Textbook *of* GYNECOLOGY

Textbook *of* GYNECOLOGY

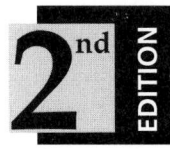

Larry J. Copeland, M.D.
Professor and Chair, Department of Obstetrics and Gynecology
The Ohio State University
College of Medicine and Public Health
The Arthur G. James Cancer Hospital and
Richard J. Solove Research Institute
Columbus, Ohio

Associate Editor

John F. Jarrell, M.D.
Professor, Department of Obstetrics and Gynecology
University of Calgary
Chief Medical Officer
Calgary Regional Health Authority
Calgary, Alberta, Canada

Illustrator: *Rebekah Dodson*

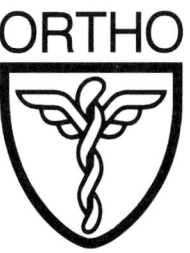

W.B. SAUNDERS COMPANY
A Harcourt Health Sciences Company

Philadelphia • London • New York • St. Louis • Sydney • Toronto

W.B. SAUNDERS COMPANY

A Harcourt Health Sciences Company

The Curtis Center
Independence Square West
Philadelphia, Pennsylvania 19106

Library of Congress Cataloging-in-Publication Data

Textbook of gynecology / [edited by] Larry J. Copeland ; associate
   editor, John F. Jarrell ; illustrator, Rebekah Dodson. — 2nd ed.
      p.   cm.
   Includes bibliographical references and index.
   ISBN 0-7216-5552-1
   1. Gynecology.   I. Copeland, Larry J.   II. Jarrell, John F.
   [DNLM: 1. Genital Diseases, Female.   WP 140 T3551 2000]
RG101.C744   2000
618.1—dc21
DNLM/DLC   99-26169

TEXTBOOK OF GYNECOLOGY   ISBN 0–7216–5552–1

Printed in the United States of America

Last digit is the print number: 9   8   7   6   5   4   3   2   1

To My Family:
My wife and life partner, Lisa, for her love and support,
My daughters, Laura Lee, Nicole, and Kelly,
for the joy and love they have brought to my life,
My parents, Alex and Fran Copeland,
for their nurturing and encouragement to pursue excellence.

and

In memory of
Felix N. Rutledge, M.D.
(November 20, 1917–June 21, 1997)
master surgeon, educator, researcher, mentor, friend, and
a role model for a generation of gynecologic oncologists

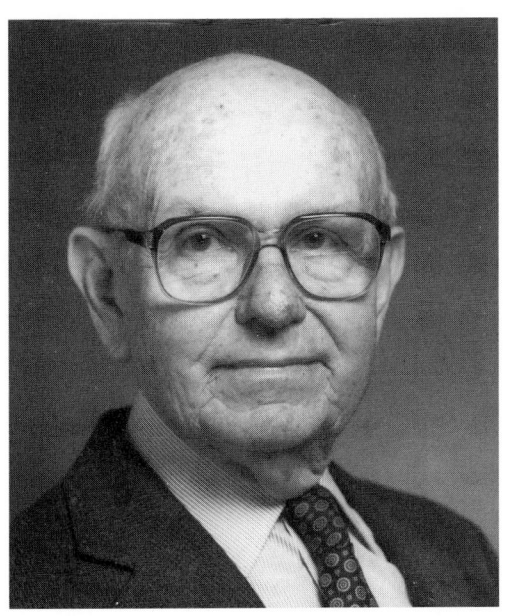

Contributors

Fredrick R. Abrams, M.D.
Retired Associate Clinical Professor of OB/GYN, University of Colorado Health Sciences Center; Professor of Public Affairs, University of Colorado Graduate School of Public Affairs Center; Visiting Professor, ILIFF School of Theology, Executive Director, Center for Health Ethics and Policy, Denver University/Colorado University Consortium, Denver, Colorado
Ethical Issues in Gynecology

Katherine L. Adelson, R.N.C., M.S., N.P.
OB-GYN Nurse Practitioner, Syracuse, New York
Miscellaneous Benign Disorders of the Upper Genital Tract: Cervix, Uterus, Ovary, Fallopian Tube, Peritoneum, Retroperitoneum, Para-adnexa

Mark D. Adelson, M.D.
Clinical Professor, Department of Obstetrics and Gynecology, State University of New York Health Science Center at Syracuse, Syracuse, New York
Miscellaneous Benign Disorders of the Upper Genital Tract: Cervix, Uterus, Ovary, Fallopian Tube, Peritoneum, Retroperitoneum, Para-adnexa

Barbara L. Anderson, Ph.D.
Professor, Departments of Psychology and Obstetrics and Gynecology, The Ohio State University, Columbus, Ohio
Psychological Adjustment for the Gynecologic Cancer Patient

Vicki V. Baker, M.D.
G.W. Morley Professor of Obstetrics and Gynecology, University of Michigan, Ann Arbor, Michigan
Molecular Biology and Applications to Gynecology

Deborah Bartholomew, M.D.
Associate Professor, Department of Obstetrics and Gynecology, The Ohio State University, Columbus, Ohio
Gynecologic Pathology: Challenges to Accurate Diagnosis

J. Thomas Benson, M.D., F.A.C.S., F.A.C.O.G.
Director, Urogynecology and Reconstructive Pelvic Surgery; Clinical Professor, Obstetrics and Gynecology, Indiana University School of Medicine; Attending Physician, Methodist Hospital, Indianapolis, Indiana
Urinary Incontinence

Jonathan S. Berek, M.D.
Professor and Vice-Chair, Chief of Gynecology, Director, Gynecologic Oncology, Department of Obstetrics and Gynecology, University of California Los Angeles School of Medicine, Los Angeles, Jonsson Comprehensive Cancer Center. Chief of Gynecology, Rhonda Fleming Women's Clinic, University Medical Center, Los Angeles, California
Immunology and Immunotherapy in Gynecologic Oncology

Matthew P. Boente, M.D.
Chief, Division of Gynecologic Oncology, Department of Surgical Oncology, Fox Chase Cancer Center, Philadelphia, Pennsylvania
Preoperative Evaluation and Preparation for Gynecologic Surgery

Diana C. Bodurka-Bevers, M.D.
Assistant Professor of Gynecologic Oncology, University of Texas, M.D. Anderson Cancer Center, Houston, Texas
Cervical Cancer

Linda Brubaker, M.D., F.A.C.S., F.A.C.O.G.
Associate Professor, Department of Obstetrics and
Gynecology, Rush Medical College; Director,
Section of Urogynecology and Reconstructive
Pelvic Surgery, Rush Presbyterian St. Luke's
Medical Center, Chicago, Illinois
Abnormalities of Pelvic Support

Thomas W. Burke, M.D.
Professor of Gynecologic Oncology, University of
Texas M.D. Anderson Cancer Center, Houston,
Texas
Adenocarcinoma of the Endometrium

Demetra L. Burrs, M.D.
Physician Instructor, Santa Clara Valley Medical
Center, San Jose, California
*Lesbian Health: Therapeutic Perspectives for
Sexual Minorities*

Joanna M. Cain, M.D.
University Professor, The Pennsylvania State
University Chair of OB/GYN, PSU/College of
Medicine, Hershey, Pennsylvania; Director, OB/
GYN/WH, Penn State Geisinger Health System,
Harrisburg, Pennsylvania
Palliative Care and End-of-Life Care in Gynecology

Brian M. Casey, M.D.
University of Texas Southwestern Medical Center
at Dallas, Assistant Professor, Obstetrics and
Gynecology, Dallas, Texas
Lower Genital Tract Infections

David A. Clark, M.D., Ph.D.
Professor, Departments of Medicine, Molecular
Medicine, Pathology, Obstetrics and Gynecology,
McMaster University; Staff Physician, Hamilton
Health Sciences Corporation, Hamilton,
Ontario, Canada
Reproductive Immunology for the Nonimmunologist

Daniel L. Clarke-Pearson, M.D.
James M. Ingram Professor of Gynecology
Oncology, Duke University School of Medicine;
Director of Gynecologic Oncology, Duke Medical
Center, Durham, North Carolina
*Preoperative Evaluation and Preparation for
Gynecologic Surgery*

David E. Cohn, M.D.
Instructor, Department of Obstetrics and
Gynecology, Fellow, Division of Gynecologic
Oncology, Washington University School of
Medicine, St. Louis, Missouri
*Gastrointestinal Complications: Prevention
and Management*

John A. Collins, M.D.
Professor, Department of Obstetrics and
Gynecology and Clinical Epidemiology and
Biostatistics, McMaster University; Active Staff,
Hamilton Health Sciences Corporation, Hamilton,
Ontario, Canada
Design and Methodology of Clinical Studies

José M. Colón, M.D.
Associate Professor, UMD-New Jersey Medical
School, Newark, New Jersey; Assistant Attending,
Director, IVF Program, Center for Reproductive
Medicine, Hackensack University Medical Center,
Hackensack, New Jersey
Assisted Reproductive Technologies

Larry J. Copeland, M.D.
Professor and Chair, Obstetrics and Gynecology,
The Ohio State University; Professor of Obstetrics
and Gynecology, The Arthur G. James Cancer
Hospital and Richard J. Solove Research Institute,
The Ohio State University, Columbus, Ohio
*Clinical Anatomy of the Pelvis; Urinary Tract Injury
and Fistula; Uterine Sarcomas; Papillary Serous
Carcinoma of the Peritoneum; Germ Cell, Stromal,
and Miscellaneous Ovarian Neoplasms; Gestational
Trophoblastic Neoplasia*

Bernard Corenblum, M.D., F.R.C.P.(C)
Professor, Department of Medicine, University of
Calgary; Consulting Endocrinologist, Foothills
Provincial General Hospital, Calgary, Alberta,
Canada
Disorders of Prolactin Secretion

Susan M. Cox, M.D.
Associate Professor of Obstetrics and Gynecology,
University of Texas Southwestern Medical Center;
Assistant Dean for Professional Education,
Dallas, Texas
Lower Genital Tract Infections

M. Yusoff Dawood, M.D., Ch.B., M.Med., M.D.
The Berel Held Professor of Obstetrics, Gynecology
and Reproductive Sciences; Director, Division of
Reproductive Endocrinology, Department of OB/
GYN/Reproductive Sciences, University of Texas
Medical School at Houston, Houston, Texas
Menopause

Salim Daya, M.B., Ch.B., M.Sc., F.R.C.S.(C)
Professor, Department of Obstetrics and
Gynecology, and Clinical Epidemiology and
Biostatistics, McMaster University, Staff Physician,
Hamilton Health Sciences Corporation, Hamilton,
Ontario, Canada
*Reproductive Immunology for the Nonimmunologist;
Habitual Abortion*

Mark G. Doherty, M.D.
Texas Oncology, San Antonio, Texas
Clinical Anatomy of the Pelvis

Oliver Dorigo, M.D.
Fellow, Department of Obstetrics and Gynecology,
University of California School of Medicine,
Los Angeles, California
*Immunology and Immunotherapy in
Gynecologic Oncology*

Maxine Dorin, M.D.
Associate Professor, Department of Obstetrics and
Gynecology, University of New Mexico School of
Medicine; Residency Program Director,
Albuquerque, New Mexico
Biopsychosocial Topics in Women's Sexual Health

Stephen S. Falkenberry, M.D.
Assistant Professor, Department of Obstetrics and
Gynecology, Brown University School of Medicine;
Director of Education and Training, Breast Health
Center, Women and Infants Hospital, Providence,
Rhode Island
Breast Cancer

Arthur C. Fleischer, M.D.
Professor of Radiology, Professor of Obstetrics and
Gynecology, Chief, Diagnostic Sonography,
Vanderbilt University Medical Center, Nashville,
Tennessee
Diagnostic Imaging

Jeffrey M. Fowler, M.D.
Associate Professor and Director of Gynecologic
Oncology, The Arthur G. James Cancer Hospital
and Richard J. Solove Research Institute, The Ohio
State University, Columbus, Ohio
Urinary Tract Injury and Fistula

Lisa M. Fromm, Ph.D.
Assistant Professor, Department of Obstetrics and
Gynecology and Psychiatry, University of New
Mexico School of Medicine, Albuquerque, New
Mexico
Biopsychosocial Topics in Women's Sexual Health

David M. Gershenson, M.D.
Professor and Deputy Chairman, Department of
Gynecology, The University of Texas M.D.
Anderson Cancer Center, Houston, Texas
Epithelial Ovarian Cancer

Alan N. Gordon, M.D.
Clinical Associate Professor, University of Texas
Southwestern Medical Center, Dallas, Texas;
Clinical Associate Professor, Texas Tech University
School of Medicine, Lubbock, Texas; Director of
Gynecologic Research, US Oncology, Sammons
Cancer Center, Baylor University Medical Center,
Dallas, Texas
Vulvar Neoplasms

Keith Gordon, Ph.D.
Clinical Research Scientist, Organon Inc, West
Orange, New Jersey
Reproductive Physiology

Calvin A. Greene, M.D.
Clinical Associate Professor, University of Calgary;
Division Chief of Reproductive Endocrinology and
Infertility, Director of the Regional Fertility
Programme, Department of Obstetrics and
Gynecology, University of Calgary, Calgary,
Alberta, Canada
Investigation of the Infertile Couple

Benjamin E. Greer, M.D.
Professor, Department of Obstetrics and
Gynecology; Director, Division of Gynecologic
Oncology, University of Washington Medical
Center, Seattle, Washington
*Gastrointestinal Complications: Prevention and
Management*

Michael M. Guarnaccia, M.D.
Fertility Center of New England, Reading,
Massachusetts
Endometriosis and Adenomyosis

Deborah J. Harrington, M.D.*
Assistant Professor of Psychiatry, University of
New Mexico School of Medicine. Assistant Director,
Psychiatry Consultation-Liaison Service, University
of New Mexico Hospital, Albuquerque,
New Mexico
Biopsychosocial Topics in Women's Sexual Health

Kenneth D. Hatch, M.D.
Professor and Head, Department of Obstetrics and
Gynecology, University of Arizona, Tucson, Arizona
Urinary Tract Injury and Fistula

David L. Hemsell, M.D.
Director, Division of Gynecology, and Professor,
Obstetrics and Gynecology, University of Texas
Southwestern Medical Center at Dallas. Attending
Physician, Parkland Memorial Hospital, Dallas,
Texas
Antibiotic Use in Gynecology

Michael P. Hopkins, M.D.
Professor, Department of Obstetrics and
Gynecology, Northeast Ohio University College of
Medicine, Rootstown, Ohio; Chairman, Department
of Obstetrics and Gynecology, Akron General
Medical Center, Akron, Ohio
Vaginal Neoplasms

*Deceased

James R. Hutchison, M.D.
Clinical Associate Professor, Department of Obstetrics and Gynecology, University of New Mexico School of Medicine; Vice President, Medical Staff Affairs, Presbyterian Healthcare Services, Albuquerque, New Mexico
Liability in Gynecology

John F. Jarrell, M.D.
Professor, Department of Obstetrics and Gynecology, University of Calgary; Chief Medical Officer, Calgary Regional Health Authority, Calgary, Alberta, Canada
Reproductive Toxicology

Sangita K. Jindal, Ph.D.
Assistant Professor, UMD New Jersey Medical School, Department of Obstetrics and Gynecology and Women's Health, Newark, New Jersey; Laboratory Supervisor, Center for Reproductive Medicare, Hackensack University Medical Center, Hasbrouck Heights, New Jersey
Assisted Reproductive Technologies

Henry M. Keys, M.D.
Professor and Chairman, Department of Radiation Oncology; Professor, Department of Obstetrics and Gynecology, Albany Medical College, Albany, New York
Basic Principles of Radiation Therapy

Edward D. Kim, M.D.
Assistant Professor of Urology, Scott Department of Urology, Baylor College of Medicine, Houston, Texas
Male Infertility

Moon H. Kim, M.D.
Professor, Department of Obstetrics and Gynecology; Director, Division of Reproductive Endocrinology, University of California Irvine Medical School, Irvine, California
Dysfunctional Uterine Bleeding

Vernon J. King, M.D.
Assistant Professor, Department of Radiation Oncology, Albany Medical College; Clinical Service Lead Physician, Department of Radiation Oncology, Albany Stratton VA Medical Center, Albany, New York
Basic Principles of Radiation Therapy

Hans-B. Krebs, M.D.
Clinical Professor, George Washington School of Medicine, Washington, D.C.; Director of Gynecologic Oncology, The Inova Fairfax Hospital, Falls Church, Virginia
Premalignant Lesions of the Cervix

Robert J. Kurman, M.D.
Richard W. Telinde Professor of Gynecologic Pathology, Johns Hopkins University School of Medicine. Director, Gynecologic Pathology, The Johns Hopkins Hospital, Baltimore, Maryland
Endometrial Hyperplasia

George S. Lewandowski, M.D.
Clinical Assistant Professor, Department of Obstetrics and Gynecology, The Ohio State University, James Cancer Hospital and Solove Research Institute, Columbus, Ohio
Management of Common Genitourinary and Gastrointestinal Conditions

Kenneth J. Lipetz, Ph.D., H.C.L.D.
Department of Obstetrics and Gynecology, UMD New Jersey Medical School, Newark, New Jersey
Assisted Reproductive Technologies

Gary H. Lipscomb, M.D.
Associate Professor and Director, Division of Gynecology, Department of Obstetrics and Gynecology, University of Tennessee, Memphis, Tennessee
Ectopic Pregnancy

Larry I. Lipshultz, M.D.
Professor of Urology, Scott Department of Urology, Baylor College of Medicine, Houston, Texas
Male Infertility

Jacquelyn S. Loughlin, M.D.
Associate Professor, Department of Obstetrics, Gynecology, and Women's Health, UMDNJ-New Jersey Medical School, Newark, New Jersey
Assisted Reproductive Technologies

Douglas J. Marchant, M.D.
Emeritus Professor of Surgery and Obstetrics and Gynecology, Tufts University School of Medicine, Boston, Massachusetts; Adjunct Professor, Brown University; Director Emeritus, Breast Health Center, Women and Infants Hospital, Providence, Rhode Island
Breast Cancer

Maurie Markman, M.D.
Director, Cleveland Clinic Taussig Cancer Center; Chairman, Department of Hematology and Medical Oncology, The Lee and Jerome Burkons Research Chair in Oncology, The Cleveland Clinic Foundation, Cleveland, Ohio
Chemotherapy

David A. Martin, M.D.
Baptist Regional Cancer Center, Knoxville, Tennessee
Postoperative Infections in Gynecology and Infectious Complications in Gynecologic Oncology

Otoniel Martínez-Maza, Ph.D.
Professor, Obstetrics and Gynecology and
Microbiology and Immunology, University of
California School of Medicine, Los Angeles,
California
*Immunology and Immunotherapy in
Gynecologic Oncology*

L. Stewart Massad, M.D.
Associate Professor, Rush Medical College;
Chairman, Division of Gynecologic Oncology, Cook
County Hospital, Chicago, Illinois
Fallopian Tube Neoplasms

Wayne S. Maxson, M.D.
Co-Director, Northwest Center for Infertility and
Reproductive Endocrinology and IVF Florida,
Margate, Florida
*Dysmenorrhea, Premenstrual Syndrome, and Other
Menstrual Disorders*

Teresita McCarty, M.D.
Associate Professor, Department of Psychiatry,
University of New Mexico School of Medicine.
Chief, Consultation Psychiatry, University of New
Mexico Hospital, Albuquerque, New Mexico
Biopsychosocial Topics in Women's Sexual Health

John S. McDonald, M.D.
Professor of Anesthesiology, Professor of Obstetrics
and Gynecology, The Ohio State University,
Columbus, Ohio
Chronic Pelvic Pain

Thomas W. McDonald, M.D.
Clinical Associate Professor, University of
Tennessee Medical Center; Consultant for
Gynecologic Oncology, Department of Obstetrics
and Gynecology, St. Mary's Medical Center,
Knoxville, Tennessee
Hysterectomy: Indications, Types, and Alternatives

Peter G. McGovern, M.D.
Assistant Professor, UMD New Jersey Medical
School, Department of Obstetrics and Gynecology
and Women's Health, Newark, New Jersey;
Associate Director, Center for Reproductive
Medicine, Hackensack, New Jersey
Assisted Reproductive Technologies

Mitchell Morris, M.D.
Professor of Gynecologic Oncology, Vice President
for Information Services and Healthcare Systems,
The University of Texas M.D. Anderson Cancer
Center, Houston, Texas
Cervical Cancer; Adenocarcinoma of the Endometrium

Robert A. Munsick, M.D., Ph.D.
Emeritus Professor of Obstetrics and Gynecology,
Indiana University School of Medicine,
Indianapolis, Indiana
Pregnancy Termination

David Muram, M.D.
Professor of Obstetrics and Gynecology, State
University of New York Health Sciences Center at
Brooklyn, New York
Developmental Abnormalities

David G. Mutch, M.D.
Associate Professor, Director, Division of
Gynecologic Oncology, Washington University
School of Medicine. Staff Physician, Barnes-Jewish
Hospital, St. Louis, Missouri
Fallopian Tube Neoplasms

James L. Nicklin, M.B.B.S., F.R.A.C.O.G., C.G.O.
Senior Lecturer, University of Queensland;
Gynecologic Oncologist, Royal Womens Hospital
and The Wesley Hospital, Brisbane, Queensland,
Australia
Uterine Sarcomas

Theodore H. Niemann, M.D.
Assistant Professor, Department of Pathology, The
Ohio State University College of Medicine,
Columbus, Ohio
Papillary Serous Carcinoma of the Peritoneum

Sergio Oehninger, M.D.
Associate Professor, Department of Obstetrics and
Gynecology, Eastern Virginia Medical School,
Norfolk, Virginia
Reproductive Physiology

Katherine A. O'Hanlan, M.D.
Attending Physician, Stanford Medical Center,
Palo Alto, California
*Gynecologic Pathology: Challenges to Accurate
Diagnosis; Lesbian Health: Therapeutic Perspectives
for Sexual Minorities*

Joseph A. O'Keane, B.M., F.R.C.S.(C)
Clinical Associate Professor, University of Calgary,
Calgary, Alberta, Canada
Investigation of the Infertile Couple

David L. Olive, M.D.
Professor and Chief, Division of Reproductive
Endocrinology and Infertility, Department of
Obstetrics and Gynecology, Yale University School
of Medicine, New Haven, Connecticut
Endometriosis and Adenomyosis

George Olt, M.D.
Associate Professor, Department of Obstetrics and
Gynecology, Division of Gynecologic Oncology,
Penn State University College of Medicine,
Hershey, Pennsylvania
*Preoperative Evaluation and Preparation for
Gynecologic Surgery*

James W. Orr, Jr., M.D.
Clinical Professor, Department of Obstetrics and Gynecology, University of South Florida, Tampa, Florida; Director, Gynecologic Oncology and Gynecologic Oncology Research, Lee Cancer Center, Ft. Myers, Florida
Intraoperative Technique; Postoperative Care

Pamela F. Orr, R.N., O.C.N.
Clinical Research Nurse, Lee Cancer Center, Ft. Myers, Florida
Postoperative Care

T. V. N. Persaud, M.D., Ph.D., D.Sc., F.R.C.Path.(Lond.), F.F.Path.(R.C.P.I.)
Former Professor and Head, Department of Anatomy; Professor of Pediatrics and Child Health; Associate Professor of Obstetrics, Gynecology, and Reproductive Sciences, University of Manitoba, Faculties of Medicine and Dentistry. Consultant in Pathology and Clinical Genetics, Health Sciences Centre, Winnipeg, Manitoba, Canada
Embryology of the Female Genital Tract and Gonads

Matthew A. Powell, M.D.
Fellow, Gynecologic Oncology, Department of Obstetrics and Gynecology, Washington University School of Medicine, St. Louis, Missouri
Clinical Anatomy of the Pelvis

Susan M. Ramin, M,D.
Associate Professor, University of Texas at Houston; Director, Division of Maternal-Fetal Medicine, University of Texas at Houston, Houston, Texas
Lower Genital Tract Infections

David F. Reid, M.D.
Professor of Diagnostic Imaging, Department of Radiology, University of Calgary, Foothills Hospital, Calgary, Alberta, Canada
Diagnostic Imaging

Robert L. Reid, M.D.
Professor, Department of Obstetrics and Gynecology; Head, Division of Reproductive Endocrinology and Infertility, Queen's University; Deputy Head, Department of Obstetrics and Gynecology, Kingston General Hospital, Kingston, Ontario, Canada
Amenorrhea

Roger S. Rittmaster, M.D.
Principal Clinical Research Physician, Metabolic Diseases, Urology and Dermatology Clinical Development, Glaxo Wellcome Research and Development, Research Triangle Park, North Carolina
Hyperandrogenism

Laura Weiss Roberts, M.D.
Associate Professor of Psychiatry, University of New Mexico School of Medicine; Director, Psychiatric Empirical Ethics Group, Albuquerque, New Mexico
Biopsychosocial Topics in Women's Sexual Health

Gustavo Rodriquez, M.D.
Associate Professor of Gynecologic Oncology, Duke University School of Medicine, Durham, North Carolina
Preoperative Evaluation and Preparation for Gynecologic Surgery

Brigitte M. Ronnett, M.D.
Assistant Professor, The Johns Hopkins University School of Medicine; Assistant Professor, Department of Pathology, The Johns Hopkins University School of Medicine and Hospital, Baltimore, Maryland
Endometrial Hyperplasia

Zev Rosenwaks, M.D.
Professor, Department of Obstetrics and Gynecology, Center for Reproductive Medicine, Cornell University, New York, New York
Dysmenorrhea, Premenstrual Syndrome, and Other Menstrual Disorders

Carolyn D. Runowicz, M.D.
Professor, Albert Einstein College of Medicine; Director, Division of Gynecologic Oncology, Department of Obstetrics, Gynecology and Women's Health, The Jack D. Weiler Hospital of the Albert Einstein College of Medicine and Montefiore Medical Center, Bronx, New York
Benign Breast Disease and Screening for Malignant Tumors

Joseph S. Sanfilippo, M.D.
Professor, Obstetrics and Gynecology, MCP Hahnemann School of Medicine, Philadelphia, Pennsylvania; Chairman, Department of Obstetrics and Gynecology, Allegheny General Hospital, Pittsburgh, Pennsylvania
Pediatric and Adolescent Gynecology

Nanette F. Santoro, M.D.
Associate Professor and Director, Division of Reproductive Endocrinology, Albert Einstein College of Medicine, Bronx, New York
Assisted Reproductive Technologies

Alberto E. Selman, M.D.
Assistant Professor, Division of Gynecologic Oncology, Department of Obstetrics and Gynecology, Clinical Hospital, Universidad de Chile, Santiago, Chile
Papillary Serous Carincoma of the Peritoneum

Margaret Sevcik, M.Sc.
Research Analyst, Calgary Regional Health
Authority, Calgary, Alberta, Canada
Reproductive Toxicology

Kaylen M. Silverberg, M.D.
Texas Fertility Center, Austin, Texas; Clinical
Assistant Professor, Division of Reproductive
Endocrinology/Infertility, The University of Texas
Health Center at San Antonio, Texas
Endometriosis and Adenomyosis

David E. Soper, M.D.
Professor and Director, Division of Benign
Gynecology, Department of Obstetrics and
Gynecology, Medical University of South Carolina,
Charleston, South Carolina
Upper Genital Tract Infections

I. Keith Stone, M.D.
Professor and Chairman, Department of Obstetrics
and Gynecology, University of Florida College of
Medicine, Gainesville, Florida
*Benign and Preinvasive Lesions of the Vulva and
Vagina*

Pamela Stratton, M.D.
Special Assistant in Gynecology and Clinical
Research; Developmental Endocrinology Branch,
National Institute for Child Health and Human
Development, National Institute of Health,
Bethesda, Maryland
*Human Immunodeficiency Virus in Nonpregnant
Women*

Gavin C.E. Stuart, M.D.
Professor and Chairman, Department of Oncology;
Director, Tom Baker Cancer Center, Calgary,
Alberta, Canada
Diagnostic Imaging

Phillip G. Stubblefield, M.D.
Professor and Chairman, Department of Obstetrics
and Gynecology, Boston University School of
Medicine; Director of Obstetrics and Gynecology,
Boston Medical Center, Boston, Massachusetts
Contraception

Togas Tulandi, M.D., F.R.C.S.(C)
Professor, Department of Obstetrics and
Gynecology; Director, Division of Reproductive
Endocrinology and Infertility, McGill University,
Montreal, Quebec, Canada
Reproductive Surgery

Derek van Amerongen, M.D.
National Medical Director, Anthem Blue Cross and
Blue Shield, Cincinnati, Ohio
Managed Care and Health Policy

Henry Wagner, Jr., M.D.
Associate Professor, Department of Radiation
Oncology, University of South Florida; H. Lee
Moffett Cancer Center, Tampa, Florida
Basic Principles of Radiation Therapy

Cheryl K. Walker, M.D.
Assistant Professor, Department of Gynecology and
Obstetrics, Stanford University, Stanford, California
*Reproductive Tract Infections: Sexually Transmitted
Diseases; Human Immunodeficiency Virus in
Nonpregnant Women*

John J. Ward, M.D.
Tri-State Gastroenterology Associate, Edgewood,
Kentucky
*Management of Common Genitourinary and
Gastrointestinal Conditions*

Edward J. Wilkinson, M.D.
Professor and Vice Chairman, Department of
Pathology; Immunology and Laboratory Medicine;
Adjunct Professor, Department of Obstetrics and
Gynecology; Chief, Division of Anatomic
Pathology, University of Florida College of
Medicine, Gainesville, Florida
*Benign and Preinvasive Lesions of the Vulva and
Vagina*

Basil Ho Yuen, M.B., Ch.B., F.R.C.S.C.
Professor, Department of Obstetrics and
Gynecology; Head, Division of Reproductive
Endocrinology and Infertility, Faculty of Medicine,
University of British Columbia; Member, Active
Staff, Vancouver Hospital and Health Sciences
Centre, Vancouver, British Columbia, Canada
Medical Management of Infertility

Preface

While the objects and goals of producing this work have not changed from the first edition, there have been a number of developments in many areas of gynecology. Those who read the first edition, will find this edition more comprehensive with new chapters in managed care, lesbian health, chronic pelvic pain, peritoneal carcinomas, and terminal care for the oncology patient. In addition all chapters have been either rewritten with new contributors or updated. The most noticeable recent developments include new information in the field of genetics and molecular biology, current therapies for acquired immunodeficiency syndrome, updating of newer antibiotic therapies, indications and complications of minimally invasive surgery, and updates in the management of malignant diseases of the female genital tract. This work was again written with the intent of representing an authoritative and contemporary state-of-the-art resource, and any information that appears dated is more the responsibility of my tardiness with meeting production delays rather than the contributors. Constructive criticisms from the readers are also invited.

Larry J. Copeland

Preface to First Edition

Gynecology is currently reaping the benefits of a rapid growth in basic and clinical information developed over the past 15 to 20 years. Much of this recent progress is secondary to the development of the gynecologic subspecialties, in particular oncology and reproductive endocrinology. Advances in patient care include the dramatic improvement in the treatment of germ cell tumors of the ovary. Also, in vitro fertilization, an idea only a few years ago, is now available in many centers throughout the world. While these success stories are significant, there lie ahead even greater challenges—the prevention, arrest, and treatment of acquired immunodeficiency syndrome and the puzzles of molecular biology.

The *Textbook of Gynecology* has been written to serve as a current learning resource sufficiently brief and focal for students, yet with adequate depth and referencing for residents, fellows, and practicing clinicians. Sixty-six chapters cover the spectrum of clinical gynecology, including the basic sciences (anatomy and physiology), developmental problems, reproductive problems, menstrual abnormalities, endocrinopathies, infectious diseases, age-related problems, operative gynecology, psychosocial aspects, breast diseases, common benign gynecologic disorders, premalignant neoplasias, oncology, pathology, molecular biology, ethics, and medical-legal aspects. Alterations in normal anatomy and physiology are reviewed in describing clinical disorders, but the emphasis is on diagnosis, treatment, and future developments. In addition to early diagnosis and appropriate intervention, preventive aspects of patient care are emphasized. Although the inevitable writing and production delays may have dated some of the presented material, the *Textbook of Gynecology* has been written with the intent of representing a contemporary state-of-the-art resource.

The editing of this work has been a personal learning experience, and readers are invited to send me constructive comments.

Larry J. Copeland

Acknowledgments

Whoever said the second edition of a text is always easier than the first has a critic in this Editor. The magnitude of the project becomes more clear when all but the final chapter has been completed. Nevertheless, the Editor sincerely appreciates the commitment to excellence exhibited by all of the contributors. The Editor also gratefully acknowledges William R. Schmitt, Editorial Manager, at W.B. Saunders, whose continuous support and encouragement were critical in completing the work. Additional special thanks is extended to Joan Sinclair and Sunny Kim who were instrumental in finalizing the production process. Also, the administrative support provided by my secretary, Sally Bourne, is sincerely acknowledged and appreciated.

Contents

I

Scientific Foundation of Gynecology

Embryology of the Female Genital Tract and Gonads

T. V. N. Persaud

SEX DETERMINATION AND DIFFERENTIATION

The chromosomal and genetic sex of the embryo is established at the time of fertilization, when the male pronucleus of the spermatozoon fuses with the female pronucleus of the oocyte to form the zygote. The chromosomal complement of the zygote is 44 autosomes and two sex chromosomes, half derived from each of the parents. The chromosomal and genetic sex of the offspring depends on whether the X-bearing female pronucleus is fertilized by an X- or Y-bearing male pronucleus. If fertilization occurs between a spermatozoon with 22 + Y chromosomes and an oocyte with 22 + X chromosomes, the offspring will be a male. A female child will result when a spermatozoon with 22 + X chromosomes enters an oocyte (Moore and Persaud, 1998).

Many genes are involved in sex differentiation, but it is the testis-determining factor (TDF) gene in the short arm (sex-determining region) of the Y chromosome that directly influences gonadal sex differentiation. Two X chromosomes are required for the development of the female phenotype. A number of genes and regions of the X chromosome have special roles in sex determination.

The male determinant (TDF) regulates gonadal sex by directing the formation of seminiferous tubules from the primary sex cords. For the development of the ovary, no such organizing influence is required because it is the absence of the H-Y antigen that leads to ovarian development (Wachtel et al, 1975, 1984). Thus, in embryos with the XX chromosome constitution, the gonads become ovaries.

The gonads of male and female embryos are morphologically indistinguishable until the seventh week of development. Nevertheless, the type of gonads present in the embryo determines sexual differentiation of the genital ducts and external genitalia (Fanghänel and Wendler, 1989). In contrast to male sexual differentiation, which depends on testicular hormones and their metabolites, female sexual differentiation occurs even in the absence of the ovaries and apparently is not under hormonal influence (Reyes et al, 1973).

OVARIAN DEVELOPMENT

Genital or gonadal ridges appear as thickenings of the celomic epithelium medial to the developing mesonephric kidneys. The primordial germ cells migrate from the yolk sac to the region of the gonadal ridges. These primordial germ cells give rise to the germinal cells in the ovary. The mesothelium covering the gonadal ridges forms the germinal epithelium from which cords of cells proliferate and grow into the underlying mesoderm (Fig. 1–1) (Van Wagenen and Simpson, 1965; Jirásek, 1977).

Primordial Germ Cells

More than a century ago, Weissmann (1885) had postulated that the germ cells are segregated quite early during cleavage, and Hertig et al (1956) reported observing a primordial germ cell among eight inner cell mass cells of a $4^1/_2$-day-old unimplanted human blastocyst. In any case, the primordial germ cells represent a highly specialized ontogenetic cellular line (Fanghänel and Wendler, 1989). They can be observed in presomite embryos (17 to 20 days) among the endodermal cells of the allantois and adjacent parts of the yolk sac, in the region of the hindgut (Eddy et al, 1981). The primordial germ cells are relatively large and round cells (15 to 20 μ), with round nuclei and pale cytoplasm. These cells contain much glycogen, and alkaline phosphatase activity has been demonstrated in both the cell membrane and nucleus (Jirásek, 1977).

The primordial germ cells migrate from the yolk sac by ameboid movement along the dorsal mesentery close to the hindgut and then laterally to the gonadal ridges (Fig. 1–1) (Witschi, 1948; Jirásek,

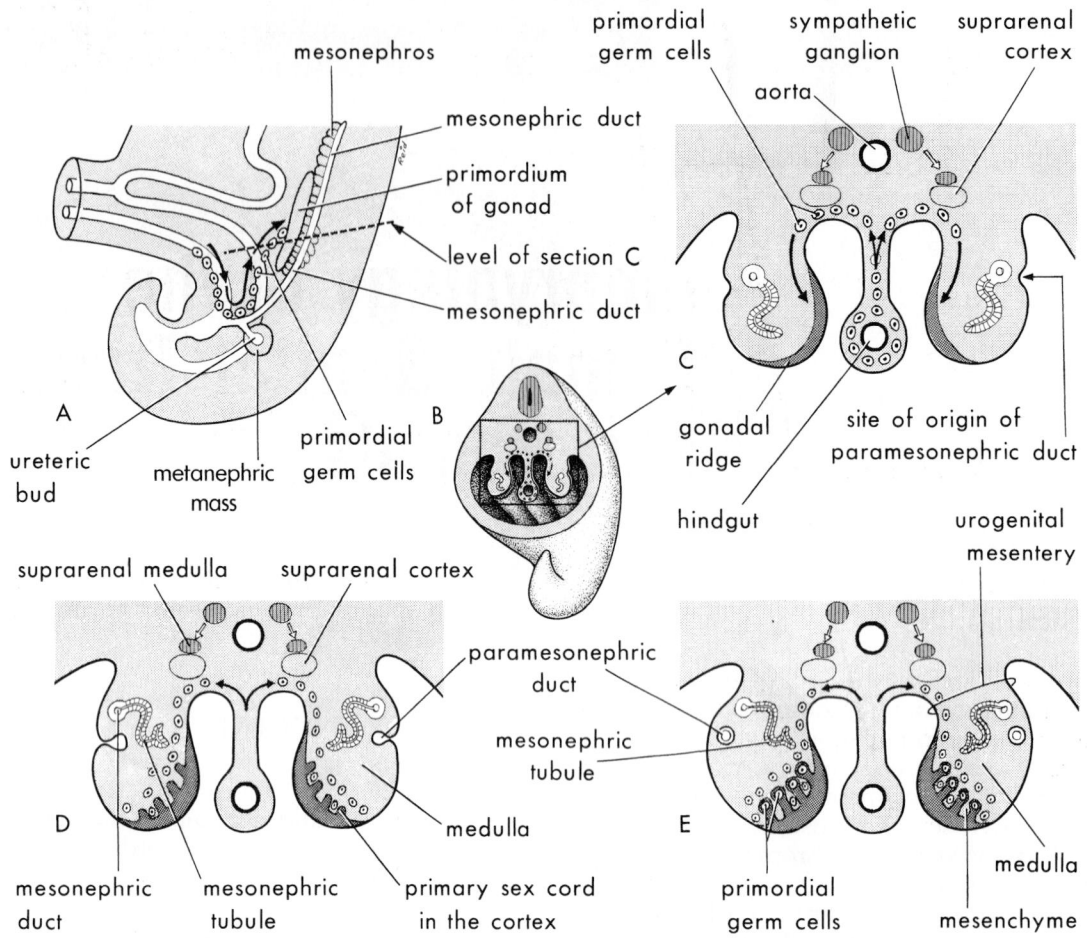

Figure 1–1

A, Sketch of a 5-week embryo, illustrating the migration of primordial germ cells from the yolk sac. *B*, Three-dimensional sketch of the caudal region of a 5-week embryo, showing the location and extent of the gonadal ridges on the medial aspect of the urogenital ridges. *C*, Transverse section showing the primordium of the suprarenal glands (adrenal glands), the gonadal ridges, and the migration of primordial germ cells into the developing gonads. *D*, Transverse section through a 6-week embryo, showing the primary sex cords and the developing paramesonephric ducts. *E*, Similar section at later stage showing the indifferent gonads and the mesonephric and paramesonephric ducts. (Adapted from Moore KL, Persaud TVN: The Developing Human. 6th ed. Philadelphia: WB Saunders Company, 1998, with permission.)

1977). The mechanisms maintaining the primordial germ cells during their migration and the factors controlling their proliferation and guidance are largely unknown (Eddy et al, 1981; Wylie et al, 1985; Makabe and Motto, 1989). Experimental studies on mouse primordial germ cells in vitro indicate that the genital ridges exert long-range effects on the migratory population of primordial germ cells and that chemotropic factors released from the genital ridges guide their migration into the genital ridge (Godin et al, 1990).

Even though Jost (1958) maintained that germ cells do not persist outside the genital ridge, delayed migration of primordial germ cells has been observed from the yolk sac to the gonadal ridge. This could cause the hindgut mesothelium to proliferate, result-ing in the formation of supernumerary ovarian tissue (Cruikshank and Van Drie, 1982).

The primordial germ cells, which are called oogonia in the female, enter the gonadal ridges by the sixth week of development. Jirásek (1977) detected primordial germ cells in somite embryos (stages XII to XVII, 26 to 44 days). He was able to do so because, during differentiation, alkaline phosphatase activity and glycogen disappear from the endodermal cells of the allantois and of the gut but are still present in the primordial germ cells (Fig. 1–2). No differences were found in the number, morphology, or migratory pattern of the primordial germ cells in genetic male and female embryos (Fig. 1–3). For the development of the gonads, the inductive influence of the primordial germ cells is essential.

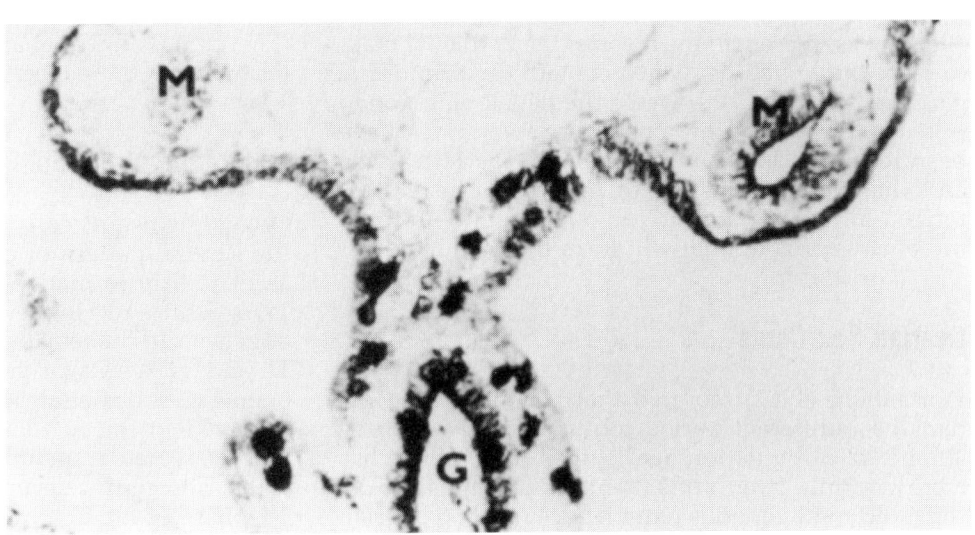

Figure 1–2
Migrating germ cells (dark) in a 3.5-mm-long human embryo (28 days, Streeter stage XII). G, gut; M, mesonephric vesicle. (Alkaline phosphatase, × 37.) (From Jirásek JE: Morphogenesis of the genital system in the human. In Blandau RJ, Bergsma D [eds]: Morphogenesis and Malformation of the Genital System. New York: Alan R Liss, Inc, for the National Foundation–March of Dimes, 1977:13, with permission.)

Gonadal Anlage

As the primordial germ cells colonize the genital ridges, the coelomic epithelium proliferates markedly and penetrates the underlying mesenchymal stroma to form the anlage of the gonads (Fanghänel and Wendler, 1989). Irregularly arranged columns of epithelial cords, called the *primitive sex cords*, are formed. The primitive sex cords are connected to the surface epithelium, and it is not possible to distinguish between male and female embryos. This stage of gonadal development is referred to as the "indifferent" stage (Minh et al, 1989c; Moore and Persaud, 1998).

The morphologic features of the gonadal anlage of a 7.4-mm embryo are as follows: (1) a thickened mesoblastic (primitive coelomic) epithelium, or cortex; (2) primitive sex cords connected to the surface epithelium; (3) loose mesenchymal cells; and (4) the colonizing primordial germ cells. There is some discussion as to the origin of the gonadal anlage, except for the primordial germ cells. Because the tissue of the gonadal anlage is relatively undifferentiated, Jirásek (1977) suggested that it cannot be classified as either epithelial or mesenchymal in origin.

Histologic studies of the developing human ovary suggest that both the coelomic mesothelium and the primary mesenchyme contribute to the gonadal ridge (Minh et al, 1989c). These investigators found that up to the sixth week, following migration of the primordial germ cells, the anlage of the ovary is established by the mesothelium. Between the 6th and

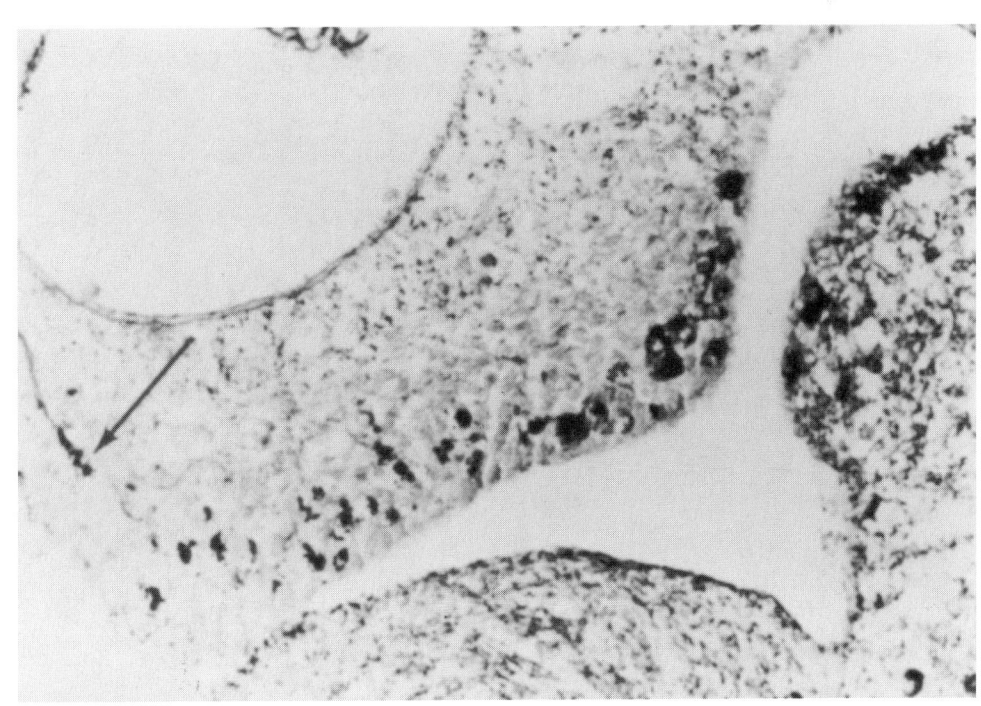

Figure 1–3
Formation of the genital ridge in a 10-mm embryo (Streeter stage XVI). Note the glycogen-rich primordial germ cells (dark). The basement membrane of the mesodermal epithelium ends laterally (*arrow*) to the gonadal primordium. (PAS stain, × 100.) (From Jirásek JE: Morphogenesis of the genital system in the human. In Blandau RJ, Bergsma D [eds]: Morphogenesis and Malformation of the Genital System. New York: Alan R Liss, Inc, for the National Foundation–March of Dimes, 1977:13, with permission.)

10th weeks, mesenchyme invades the epithelial mass to form the sex cords, which contain the primordial germ cells. By the 10th week, the developing gonad is distinct from the mesonephros. Two zones have been recognized in the fetal ovary by the 12th week: an outer zone consisting of epithelial clusters arranged in rosettes around the oocytes, and an inner mesenchymal zone that will form the medulla.

Ovarian Sex Cords

Wartenberg (1982) reported that "in the female gonad the indifferent period terminates between day 40 and 42 of ovulation age," when the embryo has a crown-rump length of 23 mm. From days 40 to 50, the indifferent gonad is remodeled so that an ovarian cortex differentiates from the medullary cords (Fig. 1–4). The human ovary develops a cortex after sexual differentiation, and this appears to depend on the mesonephros.

Transformation of the indifferent gonads of genetically female embryos into ovaries occurs during the eighth week (45- to 55-day-old embryos, 18 to 25 mm long) (Jirásek, 1977). In contrast to the testicular cords, the ovarian sex cords regress in female embryos. They are broken up into cell clusters, which are located in the medulla and contain groups of primitive germ cells. The surface coelomic epithelium continues to proliferate, giving rise to a second generation of sex cords, which are mainly located in the cortex of the gonad. The epithelium of the cortical cords penetrates the underlying mesenchyme but eventually breaks up into clusters of cells, each surrounding one or more primordial germ cells. The surrounding epithelial cells give rise to the follicular cells, and the primordial germ cells become oogonia

(Fig. 1–5) (Fanghänel and Wendler, 1989; Moore and Persaud, 1998; Spencer et al., 1996).

Maturation of the Follicles

Oogenesis begins early in human development, and the general pattern of oocyte differentiation, as well as of follicle formation, is known (Baker and Sum, 1976; Scott and Hodgen, 1990). The time of onset of oogenesis in the fetal ovary was found to be between 11 and 12 weeks of gestational age, when meiosis begins (Gondos et al, 1986). Cyclic AMP is probably involved in the regulation of oocyte maturation in the preovulatory mammalian follicle (Tsafriri et al, 1996). The germ cells enter the diplotene stage of the prophase of the first meiotic division during the formation of the primary oocytes. The primary oocytes remain dormant at this stage until puberty, when ovulation occurs. Shortly before ovulation, the first meiotic division of the primary oocyte is completed to form the secondary oocyte and the first polar body. This is followed by the second meiotic division to form the mature oocyte (ovum) and the second polar body, but only after a sperm has penetrated the secondary oocyte.

Whereas the early fetal ovary is characterized by the presence of meiotic oocytes and by the absence of isolated primary follicles, the late fetal ovary is characterized by the abundance of primary follicles and by the absence of growing follicles with many layers of granulosa cells. Minh et al (1989c) reported that at 16 weeks the fetal ovary contained several million primordial follicles, each an oocyte surrounded by a layer of granulosa cells originating from the coelomic epithelium. Mesenchymal cells of the cortical stroma separated the follicles. By the

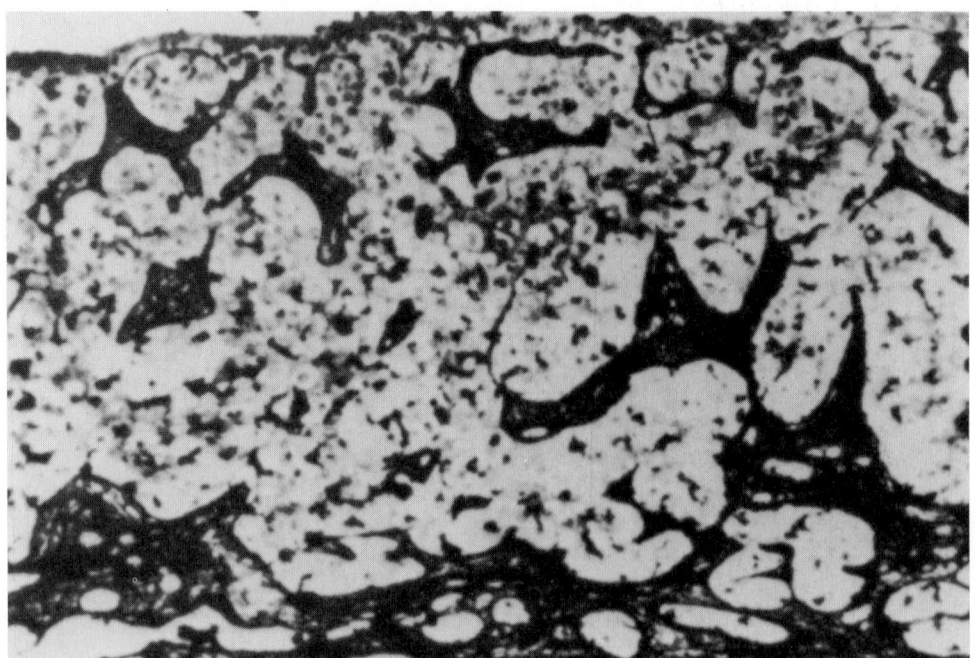

Figure 1–4
Epithelial cortical and medullary groups of an embryonal ovary are separated from the interstitial connective tissue (45-mm fetus). (Gomori's impregnation, × 50.) (From Jirásek JE: Morphogenesis of the genital system in the human. In Blandau RJ, Bergsma D [eds]: Morphogenesis and Malformation of the Genital System. New York: Alan R Liss, Inc, for the National Foundation—March of Dimes, 1977:13, with permission.)

DEVELOPING OVARIES

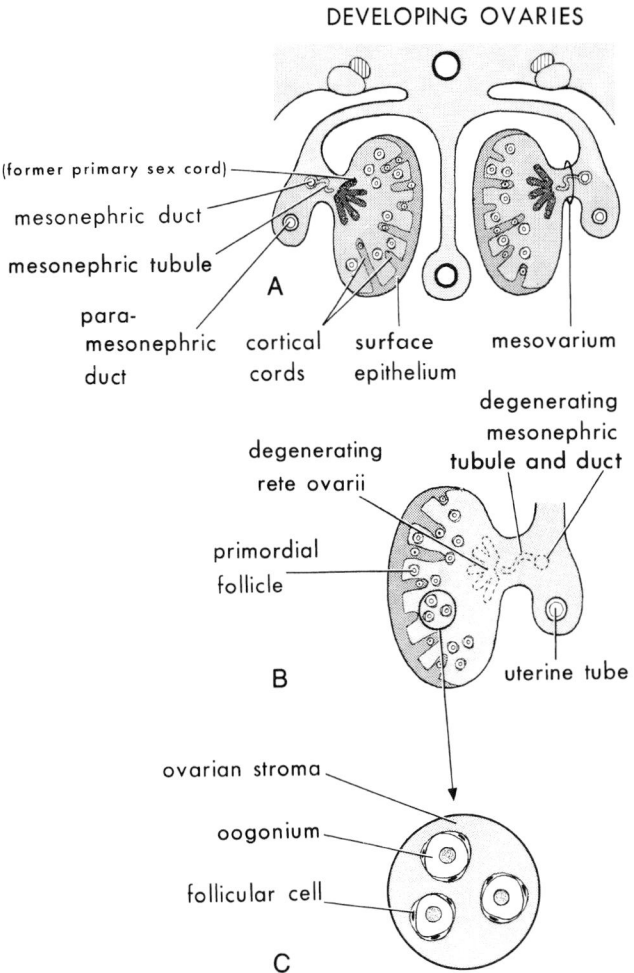

Figure 1–5
Schematic sections illustrating differentiation of the ovaries. *A,* At 12 weeks, ovaries begin to develop in the absence of a Y chromosome. Cortical cords have extended from the surface epithelium, displacing the primary sex cords centrally into the mesovarium, where they form the rudimentary rete ovarii. *B,* At 20 weeks, ovary shows the primordial follicles formed from the cortical cords. *C,* Section from the ovarian cortex of a 20-week fetus, showing three primordial follicles containing oogonia. (Adapted from Moore KL, Persaud TVN: The Developing Human. 6th ed. Philadelphia: WB Saunders Company, 1998, with permission.)

perinatal period, the ovary has growing follicles with multilayered granulosa cells (Jirásek, 1977). The human fetal ovary is considered to be functionally quiescent (Reyes et al, 1973).

The role of the interstitial cells that are present in the human fetal ovary at midgestation remains unclear. These cells are different from theca cells but are similar to the primary interstitial cells, which occupy much of the ovary in other mammalian species. Ultrastructural studies of these cells in 12 fetuses between 12 and 40 weeks of gestation revealed features particularly associated with steroid production. Because these cells are more abundant at 18 weeks of gestation around the sex cords in the medulla of the ovary, it has been suggested that they may influence the development of the sex cords or primordial follicles (Konishi et al, 1986).

At 15 to 20 weeks of age, there are as many as 7 million germ cells in each ovary. Because of degeneration, the number decreases to 2 million primary oocytes in the ovaries of a newborn. By the time of puberty, there are about 40,000 primary oocytes remaining in the ovaries. Only about 400 of these will become secondary oocytes and are extruded at ovulation, once every month, during the reproductive cycle (Moore and Persaud, 1998). For information on the development of the vascular supply of the follicle, see Gordon et al (1995).

THE GENITAL TRACT

Paramesonephric (Müllerian) Ducts

The genital tract differentiates later than do the gonads. During the indifferent period of gonadal differentiation, the urinary system of the embryo consists of a functional mesonephros and remnants of the pronephros. The paired mesonephric (wolffian) ducts run craniocaudally to the hindgut region and open into the primitive cloaca of embryos that are 26 to 32 days old (4 to 5 mm long, stages XII to XIII). By the end of the fourth week, an epithelial invagination appears in the mesodermal lining on the anterolateral side of each urogenital ridge. These epithelial invaginations, located lateral to the mesonephric ducts, eventually give rise to paired paramesonephric or müllerian ducts (Fanghänel and Wendler, 1989; Moore and Persaud, 1998).

By the 35th day, the primordium of the paramesonephric duct appears as a solid cord of epithelial cells that extends retroperitoneally in the direction of the cloaca. According to Jirásek (1977), this cellular cord, which will give rise to the paramesonephric duct, contacts the mesonephric duct and gradually becomes canalized as it grows along its epithelium. The paramesonephric ducts cross the mesonephric ducts ventrally to meet the column of cells from the opposite side. The paramesonephric ducts then run medial to the mesonephric ducts and close to the dorsal wall of the urogenital sinus (Figs. 1–6 and 1–7).

In contrast to the mesonephric ducts, which open into the urogenital sinus, the tips of the paramesonephric ducts make contact only with its dorsal wall. At this area of contact, the endodermal epithelium of the urogenital sinus proliferates and gives rise to the müllerian tubercle (Fig. 1–8). By the 65th day, the parallel-running lower part of the paramesonephric ducts begins to fuse with degeneration of the medial walls. The result is that a single midline uterovaginal canal is formed (Fig. 1–9).

As a result of the paramesonephric duct crossing the mesonephric duct ventrally, to meet its counterpart of the other side in the midline, a broad trans-

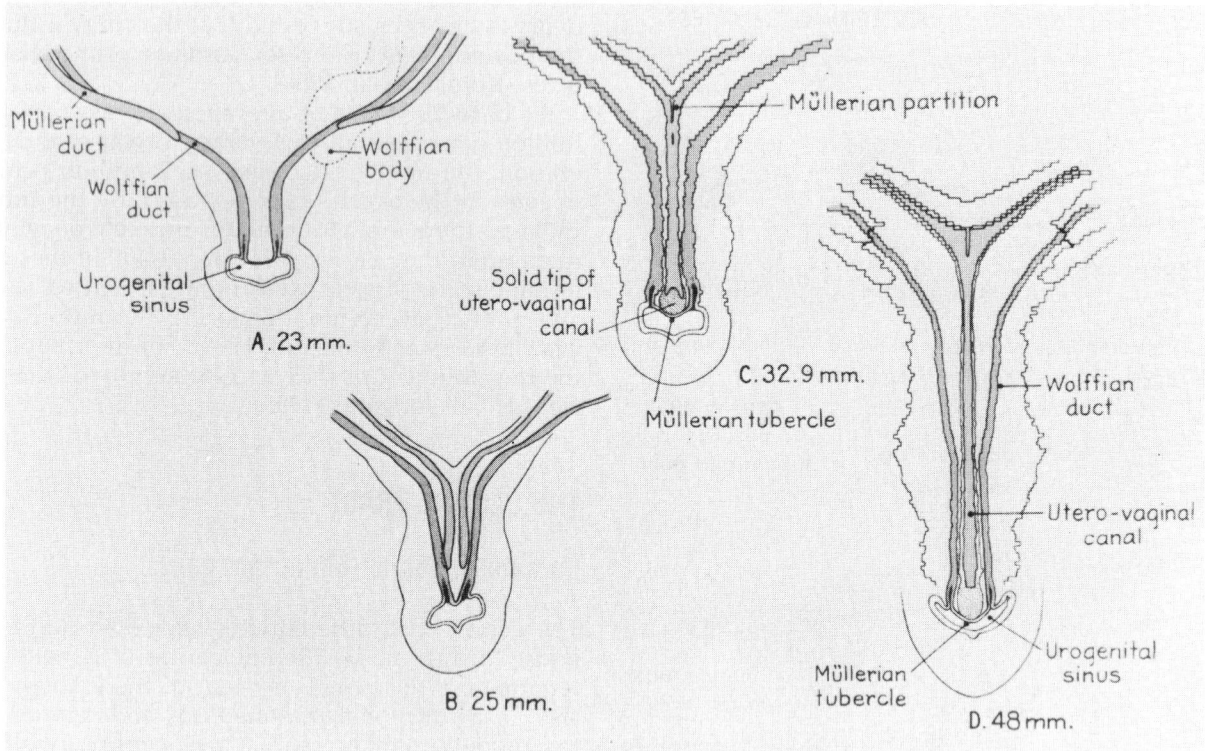

Figure 1-6

Development of the human uterus and vagina at different stages. *A*, Paramesonephric (müllerian) ducts lie lateral to the mesonephric (wolffian) ducts. The paramesonephric ducts are not yet in contact with the urogenital sinus. *B*, The paramesonephric ducts have crossed the mesonephric ducts anteriorly, are parallel to each other in the midline, and have grown caudally to almost reach the posterior wall of the urogenital sinus. The paramesonephric duct are fusing, and a müllerian tubercle is evident. *C*, The müllerian ducts have fused to form the uterovaginal primordium. *D*, The caudal tip of the fused lower ends of the paramesonephric ducts is solid, forming the sinovaginal bulbs. Fusion of the paramesonephric ducts is completed to form a uterovaginal canal. (From Koff A: Development of the vagina in the human fetus. Contrib Embryol Carnegie Inst Wash 1933;24:59, with permission.)

verse peritoneal fold is established on each side. These mesenchymal folds will form the broad ligament when the ducts fuse. The broad ligament of the uterus then extends from the lateral sides of the fused paramesonephric ducts (uterovaginal primordium) to the pelvic wall, anterior to the rectum and behind the primitive bladder (Fig. 1–10) (Moore and Persaud, 1998).

The cranial end of the epithelial invagination in the region of the mesonephros becomes the ostium of the uterine tube, at which fimbriae are formed. The caudal end of the uterovaginal canal comes in contact with the dorsal wall of the urogenital sinus. At this site of contact, as mentioned earlier, the epithelium of the endodermal sinus proliferates to form the paramesonephric or müllerian tubercle. Between the müllerian tubercle and the urogenital sinus, a solid cord of cells, known as the vaginal plate, appears. Because of cellular proliferation, the vaginal plate thickens and elongates, with the consequence that the distance between the urogenital sinus and the müllerian tubercle gradually increases.

The Uterine Tubes and the Uterus

Each paramesonephric duct can be divided into three parts: a cranial vertical part, a middle horizontal part, and a caudal vertical part, the tip of which makes contact with the urogenital sinus. The cranial vertical and the middle horizontal regions of the paramesonephric duct give rise to the uterine tube on each side. From the fused caudal vertical parts of the paramesonephric ducts, the uterus is derived (Fig. 1–11).

The epithelium of the uterus and uterine tubes is derived from the paramesonephric duct, and the surrounding mesenchyme gives rise to the connective tissue and muscle (Witschi, 1970; Jirásek, 1977; O'Rahilly, 1977; Konishi et al, 1986; Minh et al, 1989a).

According to Minh et al (1989a), the uterus has a "dual embryology." Histologic and immunohistochemical studies of embryos and fetuses of different gestational ages revealed that the endometrium, its stroma, and the transitional area between the endo-

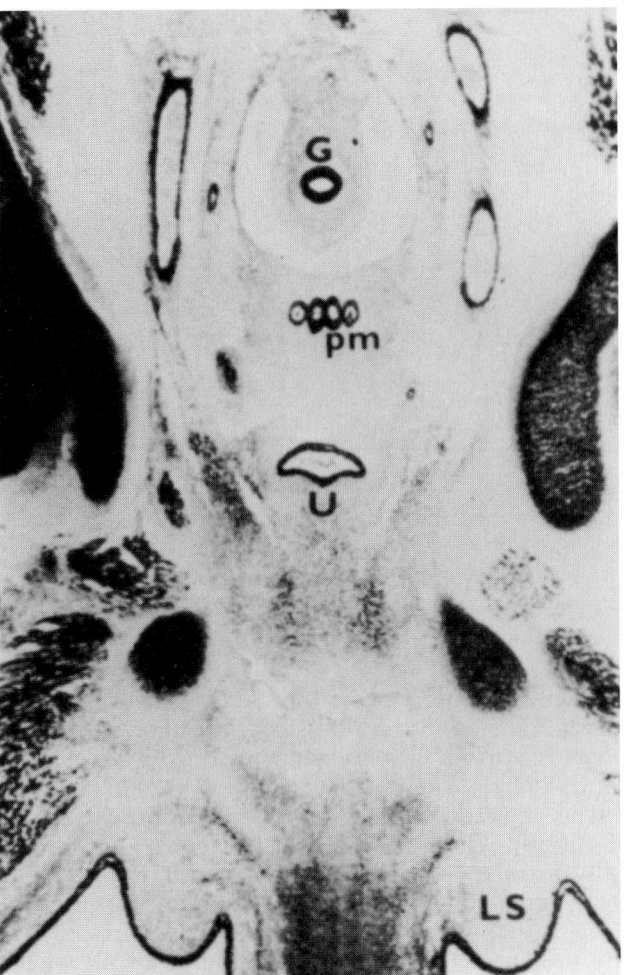

Figure 1–7
Parallel mesonephric (m) and paramesonephric (p) ducts in a 26-mm embryo (Streeter stage XX). U, urogenital sinus; G, gut; LS, labioscrotal swelling. (PAS, Alcian blue, × 32.) (From Jirásek JE: Morphogenesis of the genital system in the human. In Blandau RJ, Bergsma D [eds]: Morphogenesis and Malformation of the Genital System. New York: Alan R Liss, Inc, for the National Foundation–March of Dimes, 1977:13, with permission.)

metrium and myometrium are of coelomic origin. In agreement with earlier observations, the myometrium and the connective tissue are attributed to primary mesenchyme. This viewpoint is further supported by ultrastructural investigation of smooth muscle development in the human fetal uterus. Konishi et al (1986) found that uterine smooth muscle cells originate from undifferentiated mesenchymal cells. Smooth muscle differentiation begins in the human fetal uterus at 19 weeks of gestation, and the myometrium is formed in the outer layer of the wall of the uterus by 31 weeks. The outer layer of the wall of the uterus can be distinguished from the inner layer, which corresponds to the endometrial stroma. Moreover, a differentiation of the mesenchyme to form the smooth muscle and endometrial stroma of the fetal uterus appears to be under the influence of estrogen and progesterone during pregnancy.

VAGINA

Whereas there is general consensus as to the embryologic origin of the uterine tubes and uterus, the development of the vagina remains controversial. Several theories have been proposed for its formation (for reviews, see Hunter, 1930; Koff, 1933; Bulmer, 1957; Matéjka, 1959; Prins et al, 1976; Jirásek, 1977; O'Rahilly, 1977; Robboy et al, 1982; Gasser, 1985; Minh et al, 1989b). Two main theories should be mentioned. Hunter (1930) had suggested that the entire vagina is formed from the lower end of the fused paramesonephric ducts. He described a solid epithelial cord of cells, "the vaginal cord as it may be termed," the central part of which degenerates to form "a continuous lumen, the vagina." In contrast, Koff (1933) concluded from his studies that only "the upper part of the vagina develops from the paramesonephric ducts, while the lower portion, about one fifth, is formed from the sinovaginal bulbs, which arise from the epithelium of the urogenital sinus." This "dual origin" concept for the formation of the vagina has survived over the years and is still a debated issue (O'Rahilly, 1977; Gasser, 1985). The problem often relates to the extent of contribution from the uterovaginal primordium, one third or a fifth, to the vaginal epithelium. The account that follows is an attempt to consolidate these different structural and functional concepts.

Prerequisite for vaginal development to occur is that one or both ends of the paramesonephric ducts should come in contact with the endodermal epithelium of the urogenital sinus. In addition, the caudal part of the uterovaginal primordium should not regress prior to the induction of the vaginal plate (Jirásek, 1977).

The basement membrane of the epithelial cells in the müllerian sinus tubercle disappears by the eighth week, and, as a result of rapid cellular proliferation, paired sinovaginal bulbs are formed on each side of the fused paramesonephric ducts. The proliferative zone is replaced by a multilayered solid epithelial cord, the vaginal plate, between the 12th and 15th weeks. The vaginal plate separates the tips of the fused paramesonephric ducts, cranially, from the urogenital sinus (Fig. 1–12).

The origin of the cells forming the bilateral sinovaginal bulbs has been a contentious issue. Koff (1933) considered the sinovaginal bulbs to be derived from the urogenital sinus, a view shared also by Bulmer (1957) and Fluhmann (1960). Forsberg (1965, 1973) suggested that the vaginal plate epithelium is derived from the mesonephric duct, and, according to Witschi (1970), the lateral wings of the mesonephric duct blastema and the solid tips of the paramesonephric ducts contribute to the formation of the sinovaginal bulbs. Another theory proposed that the sinovaginal bulbs are derived from two sources, the paramesonephric ducts and the urogenital sinus (Wells, 1959).

Much of the controversy revolving around the origin of the sinovaginal bulbs, the vaginal plate, and

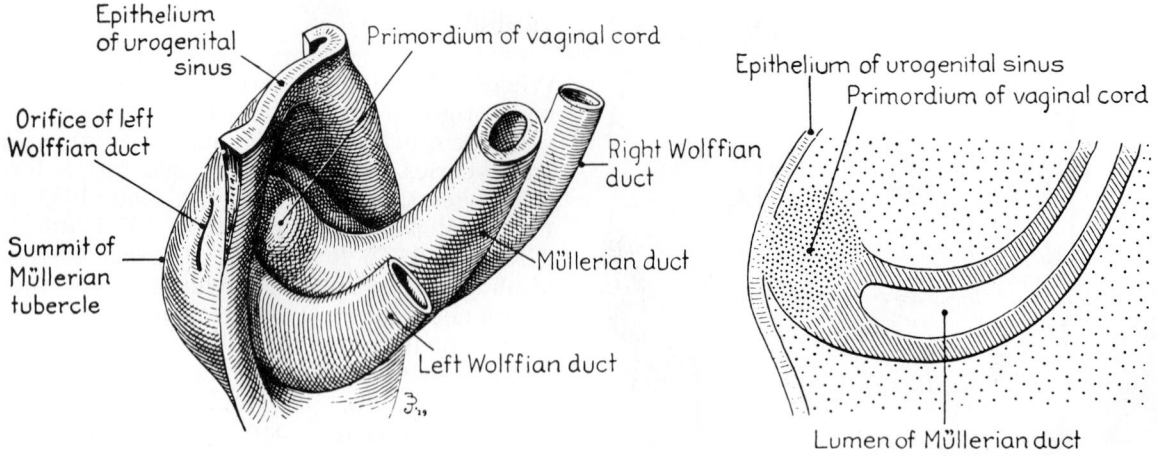

Figure 1–8
The müllerian tubercle of a 48-mm embryo. *Left*, Wax-plate reconstruction of the epithelial derivatives (×115). *Right*, schematic sagittal section of the same specimen. (From Hunter RH: Observations on the development of the human female genital tract. Contrib Embryol Carnegie Inst Wash, 1930;22:91, with permission.)

the vagina is largely due to species differences, insufficient closely staged specimens for studies, and the lack of accurate reconstructions (O'Rahilly, 1977; Gasser, 1985). Minh et al (1989b) reported on a series of 12 embryos between 4 and 8 weeks of age and 21 fetuses between 9 and 25 weeks of gestation. These investigators maintained that the vaginal plate is derived solely from the urogenital sinus and, furthermore, that the entire vagina is derived from the vaginal plate. The present consensus is that the vaginal

epithelium is derived from the endoderm of the urogenital sinus and that the surrounding mesenchyme gives rise to its fibromuscular wall (Moore and Persaud, 1998).

The vaginal plate can be seen in embryos that are about 60 to 70 mm long, and by about 140 mm it is fully formed. At 16 weeks, the cells in the center of the vaginal plate desquamate, thereby forming the lumen of the vagina (Koff, 1933). The formation of the lumen of the vagina is completed by 18 weeks,

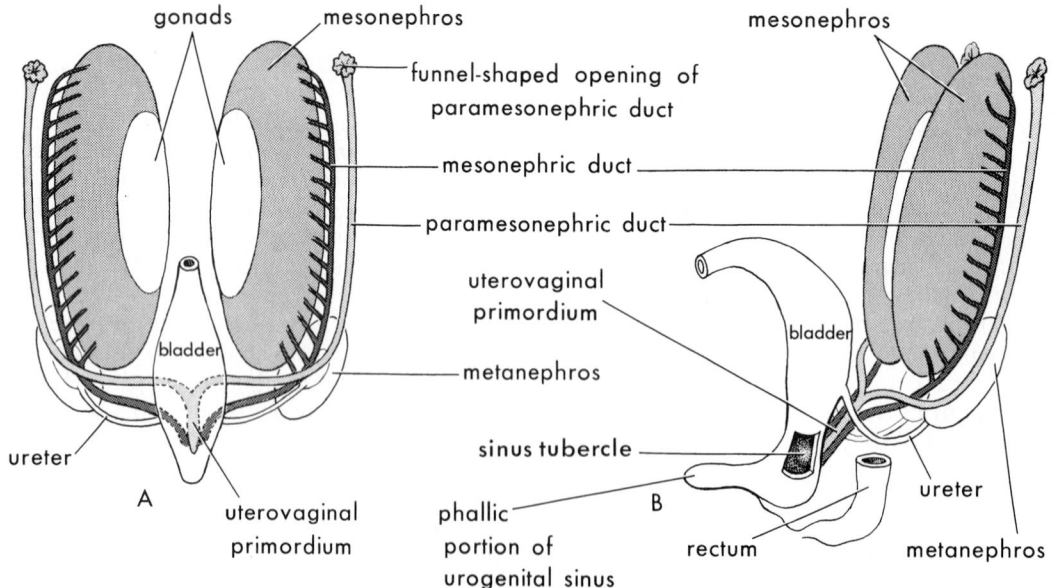

Figure 1–9
A, Sketch of a frontal view of the posterior abdominal wall of a 7-week embryo, showing the two pairs of genital ducts present during the indifferent stage. *B*, Lateral view of a 9-week fetus showing the sinus tubercle (formerly called the müllerian tubercle) on the posterior wall of the urogenital sinus. It becomes the hymen in females and the seminal colliculus in males. (Adapted from Moore KL, Persaud TVN: The Developing Human. 6th ed. Philadelphia: WB Saunders Company, 1998:287, with permission.)

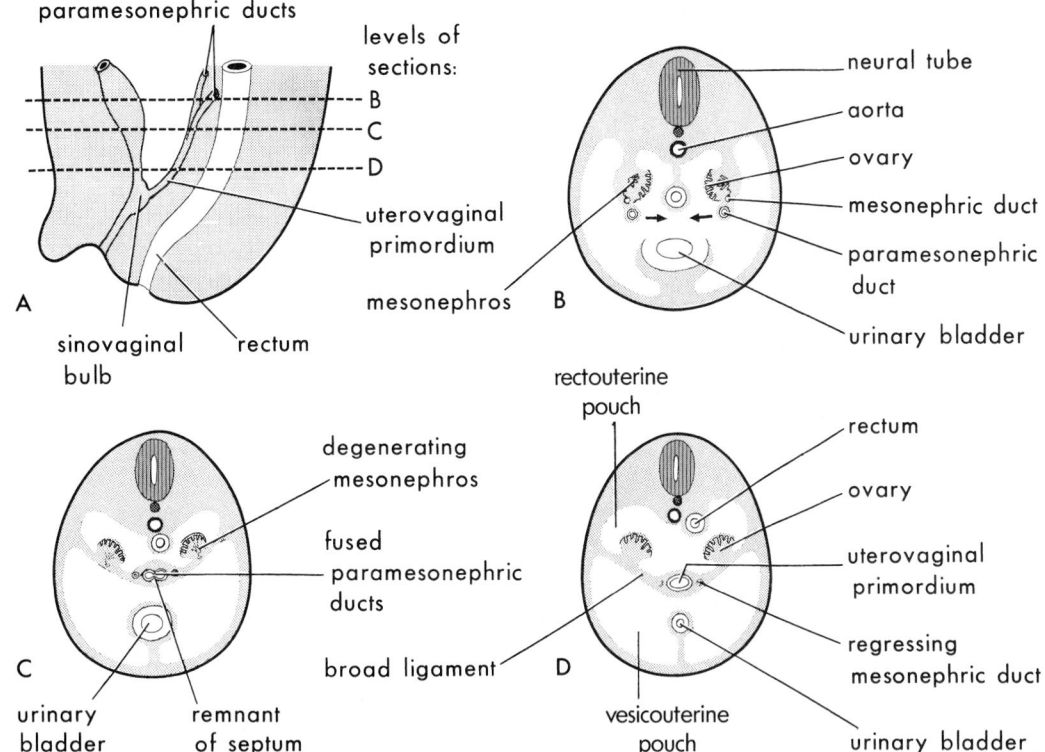

Figure 1–10

A, Schematic drawing of a sagittal section of the caudal region of an 8-week female fetus. *B*, Transverse section showing the paramesonephric ducts approaching each other. *C*, Similar section of a more caudal level, illustrating fusion of the paramesonephric ducts. A remnant of the septum that initially separates them is shown. *D*, Similar section showing the uterovaginal primordium, broad ligament, and pouches in the pelvic cavity. Note that the mesonephric ducts have regressed. Remnants of these ducts may persist as vestigial ducts of Gartner or give rise to cysts. (Adapted from Moore KL, Persaud TVN: The Developing Human. 6th ed. Philadelphia: WB Saunders Company, 1998, with permission.)

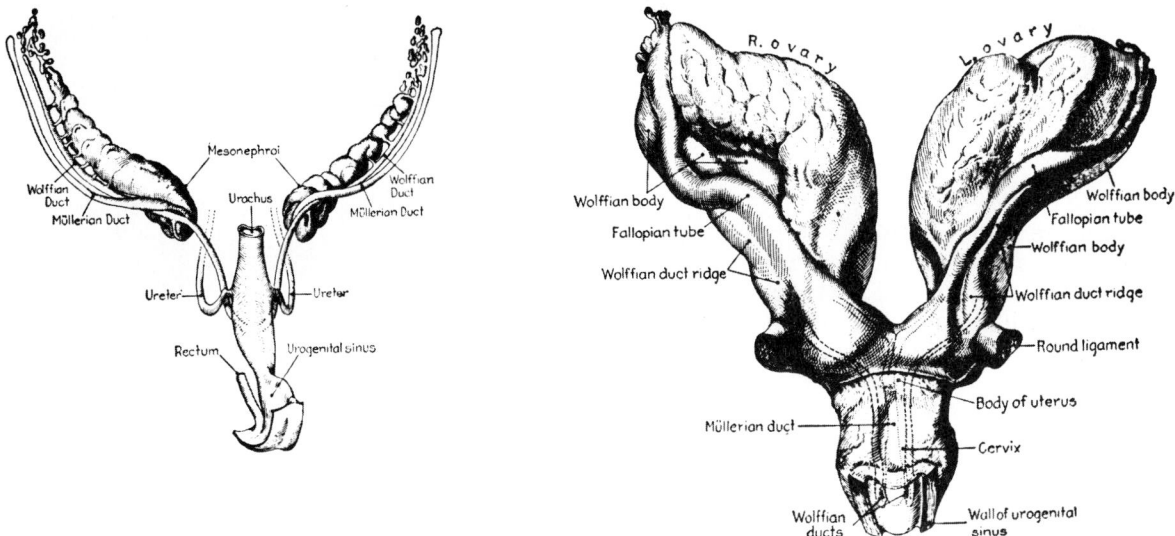

Figure 1–11

Reconstruction of the developing female genital tract of two embryos: 23 mm crown-rump (CR) length (*left*) and 36 mm CR length (*right*). In the latter, the paramesonephric (müllerian) ducts are fused to form a uterovaginal primordium. The junction between the body and cervix of the developing uterus is constricted. The uterine (fallopian) tubes are formed from the unfused parts of the paramesonephric ducts. (From Hunter RH: Observations on the development of the human female genital tract. Contrib Embryol Carnegie Inst Wash 1930;22:91, with permission.)

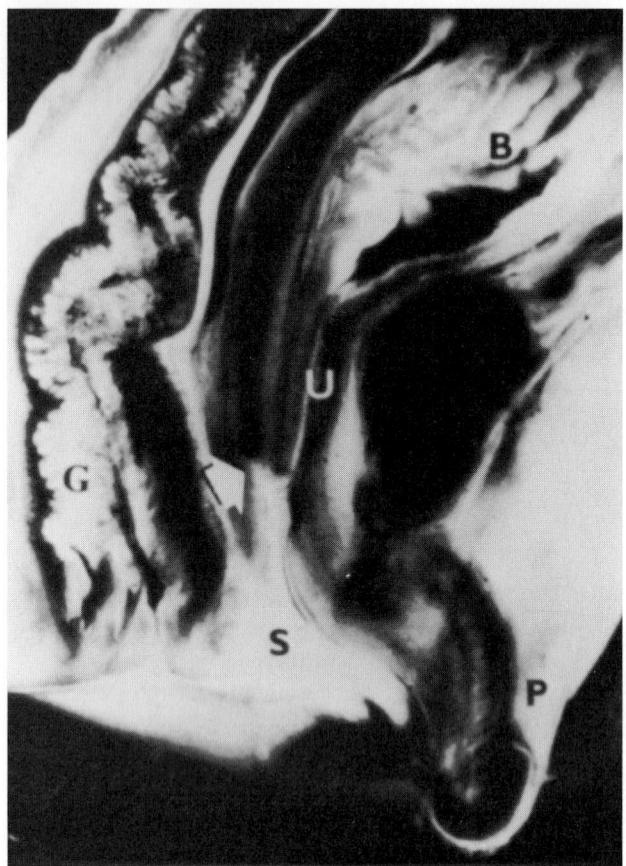

Figure 1–12
Sagittal section through the pelvis of a 150-mm-long female fetus. The urinary bladder (B), urethra (U), urogenital sinus (S), phallus (P), and gut (G) can be distinguished. The section was incubated for alkaline phosphatase activity. The border between the entodermal part of the vagina and the uterovaginal canal (*arrow*) is distinct (× 40). (From Jirásek JE: Morphogenesis of the genital system in the human. In Blandau RJ, Bergsma D [eds]: Morphogenesis and Malformation of the Genital System. New York: Alan R Liss, Inc, for the National Foundation–March of Dimes, 1977:13, with permission.)

ies on a series of embryos and fetuses that the entire vagina is derived from the vaginal plate.

The lumen of the vagina is separated from the urogenital sinus at its lower end by a thin membrane called the *hymen*. Several theories have also been proposed for the formation of the hymen (Hunter, 1930; O'Rahilly, 1977). It is usually considered to be the junction between the sinovaginal plate and the urogenital sinus. Histologic studies of the hymen led to the suggestion that it is formed passively by invagination of the posterior wall of the urogenital sinus, resulting from expansion of the caudal end of the vagina. The cells covering both surfaces of the hymen are therefore endodermal in origin because they are derived from both the vaginal primordium and the urogenital sinus (Mahran and Saleh, 1964).

CERVIX

Bulmer (1957) described a fusiform swelling (Koff, 1933) at the junction of the two types of paramesonephric epithelium, columnar and stratified "polygonal," in the 94-mm fetus as the site of the future cervix. In normal development of the uterus and vagina, the original columnar epithelium of the vagina and cervix (Koff, 1933; Bulmer, 1957) is converted

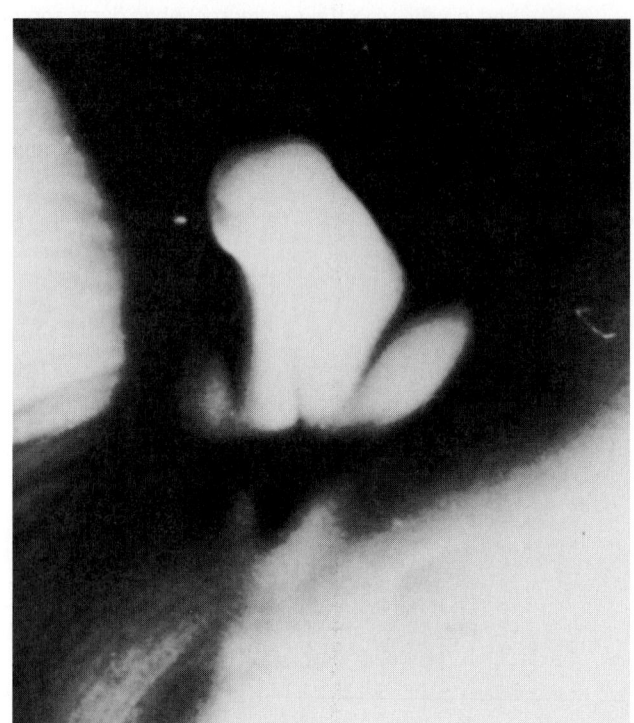

Figure 1–13
Indifferent external genitalia with labioscrotal swellings laterally from the phallus (30-mm embryo) (Streeter stage XXIII). (From Jirásek JE: Morphogenesis of the genital system in the human. In Blandau RJ, Bergsma D [eds]: Morphogenesis and Malformation of the Genital System. New York: Alan R Liss, Inc, for the National Foundation–March of Dimes, 1977:13, with permission.)

and, according to Witschi (1970), the growth of the vagina proceeds caudally from the cranial end of the vaginal plate. The anterior and posterior fornices appear as solid ring-like epithelial expansions around the lower end of the uterine canal. O'Rahilly (1977) described cavitation in the vaginal plate at 151 mm and the formation of a complete vaginal lumen, except for the solid fornices at its cephalic end, by 162 mm. At about 180 mm, the fornices are hollow and well established. With the enlargement and canalization of the vagina throughout its entire length, the genital canal now communicates with the exterior (Bulmer, 1957). According to Bulmer (1957), the upgrowth from the urogenital sinus "extends throughout the entire region of the vagina by the 140-mm stage, and forms the whole of its epithelial lining." This concept is supported by the findings of Minh et al (1989b), who concluded from their histologic stud-

into a stratified squamous epithelium. The epithelial junction at the site of the external os of the cervix with the vagina is squamocolumnar. The findings of Koff (1933) and others (Forsberg, 1965; Witschi, 1970) indicate that the cervix is of paramesonephric origin, but it seems likely that the urogenital sinus gives rise to its mucous membrane (Fluhmann, 1960). To what extent the paramesonephric ducts and urogenital sinus each contribute to the formation of the cervix remains debatable (Gasser, 1985).

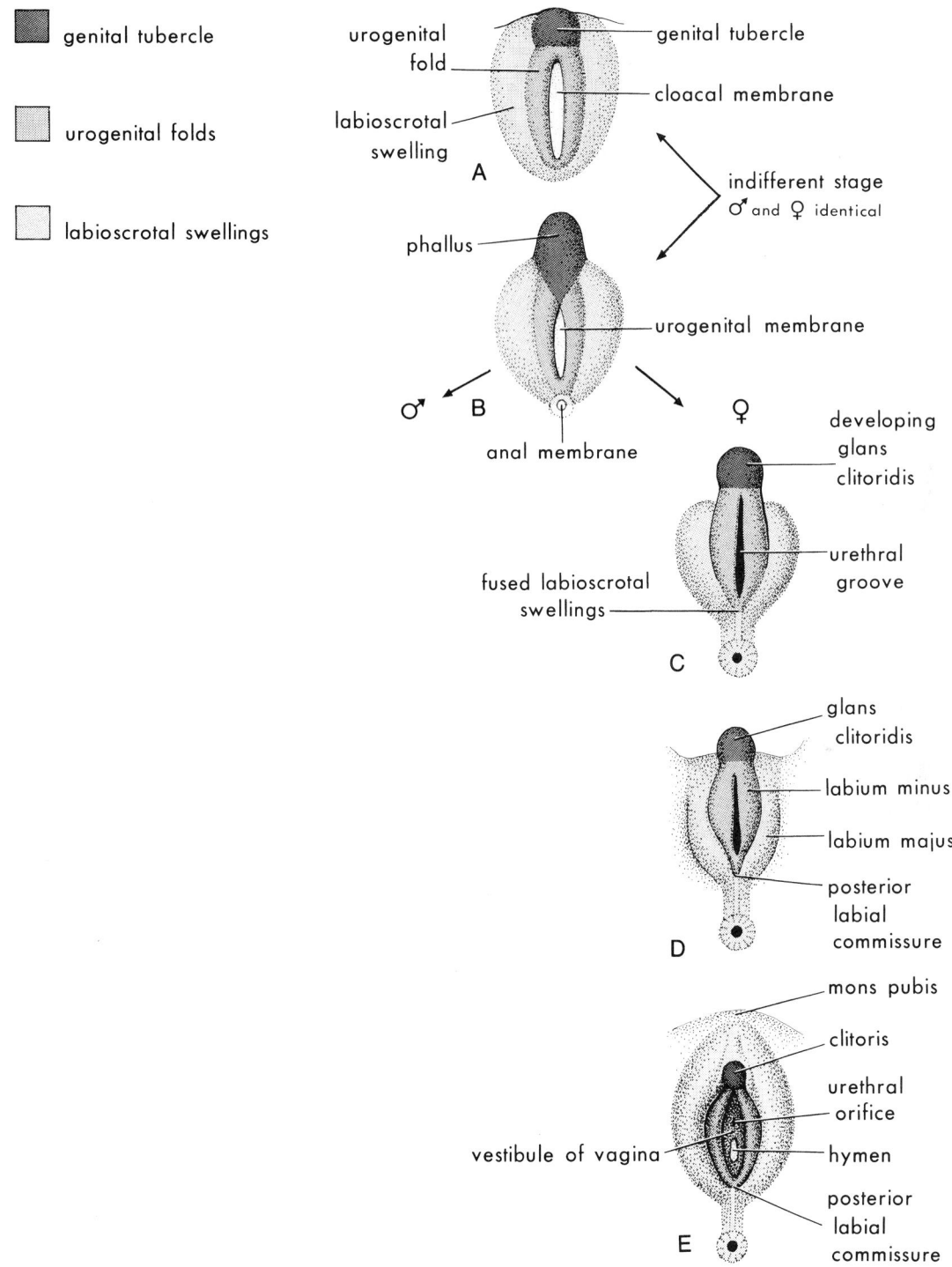

Figure 1-14
A and B, Diagrams illustrating development of the external genitalia during the indifferent stage (fourth to seventh weeks). C–E, Stages in the development of female external genitalia at 9, 11, and 12 weeks, respectively. (Adapted from Moore KL, Persaud TVN: The Developing Human. 6th ed. Philadelphia: WB Saunders Company, 1998, with permission.)

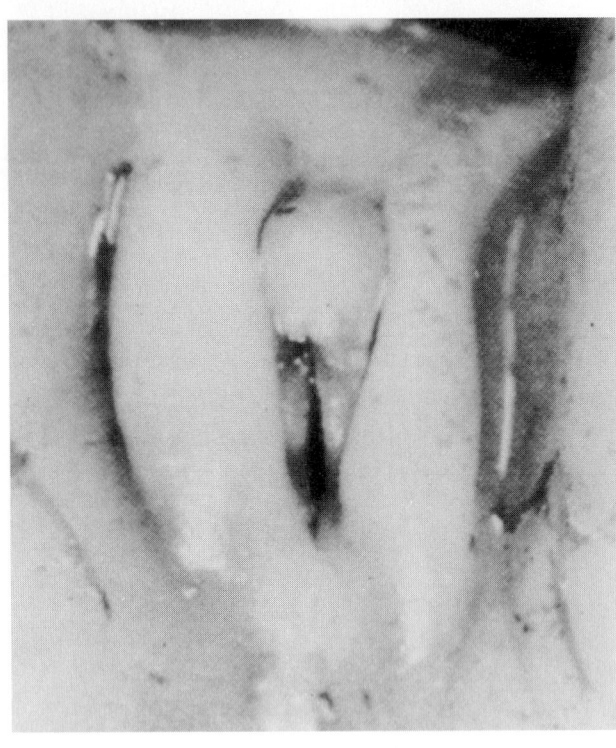

Figure 1–15
Female external genitalia in a 120-mm fetus. Labia majora, clitoris, and labia minora are easily distinguished. (From Jirásek JE: Morphogenesis of the genital system in the human. In Blandau RJ, Bergsma D [eds]: Morphogenesis and Malformation of the Genital System. New York: Alan R Liss, Inc, for the National Foundation–March of Dimes, 1977:13, with permission.)

Table 1–1. ADULT DERIVATIVES AND VESTIGIAL REMAINS OF EMBRYONIC UROGENITAL STRUCTURES*

MALE	EMBRYONIC STRUCTURE	FEMALE
Testis	**Indifferent Gonad**	*Ovary*
Seminiferous tubules	**Cortex**	*Ovarian follicles*
Rete testis	**Medulla**	Rete ovarii
Gubernaculum testis	**Gubernaculum**	*Ovarian ligament*
		Round ligament of uterus
Ductuli efferentes	**Mesonephric Tubules**	Epoophoron
Paradidymis		Paroophoron
Appendix of epididymis	**Mesonephric Duct**	Appendix vesiculosa
Duct of epididymis		Duct of epoophoron
Ductus deferens		Duct of Gartner
Ureter, pelvis, calyces, and collecting tubules		*Ureter, pelvis, calyces, and collecting tubules*
Ejaculatory duct and seminal vesicle		
Appendix of testis	**Paramesonephric Duct**	Hydatid (of Morgagni)
		Uterine tube
		Uterus
Urinary bladder	**Urogenital Sinus**	*Urinary bladder*
Urethra (except *navicular fossa*)		*Urethra*
Prostatic utricle		*Vagina*
Prostate gland		*Urethral and paraurethral glands*
Bulbourethral glands		*Greater vestibular glands*
Seminal colliculus	**Sinus Tubercle**	Hymen
Penis	**Phallus**	*Clitoris*
Glans penis		*Glans clitoridis*
Corpora cavernosa penis		*Corpora cavernosa clitoridis*
Corpus spongiosum penis		*Bulb of the vestibule*
Ventral aspect of penis	**Urogenital Folds**	*Labia minora*
Scrotum	**Labioscrotal Swellings**	*Labia majora*

*Functional derivatives are in italics.
From Moore KL, Persaud TVN: The Developing Human. 6th ed. Philadelphia: WB Saunders Company, 1998:333, with permission.

The junction between the body of the uterus and the cervix appears as a slight constriction in the fused part of the paramesonephric ducts at 16 weeks of gestation. The vagina becomes canalized and increases in size, but the surrounding mesenchymal tissue differentiates into a firm, confining mass around the endocervical region of the fused müllerian ducts between 8 and 10 weeks. In late gestation and at term, the stroma of the cervix contains only loose and cellular connective tissue, with numerous blood vessels, and is devoid of any muscle fibers (Gasser, 1985).

EXTERNAL GENITALIA

The appearance of the external genitalia in both sexes is similar between the sixth and eighth weeks of development. During this indifferent stage of external genitalia development, mesoderm from the caudal end of the primitive streak migrates toward to cloacal membrane (5- to 10-mm embryos, 30 to 35 days old), which is located between the primitive umbilical cord and the tailbud. A midline elevation, the genital tubercle, appears in front of the cloacal membrane at 6 weeks (Figs. 1–13 and 1–14).

The cloacal membrane becomes subdivided by the urorectal septum into an anterior urogenital membrane and the posterior anal membrane, and at the same time the cloacal folds give rise to urogenital folds and anal folds. Between the urogenital folds lies a common vestibule into which both the urethra and the vagina will open after the urogenital membrane disappears. Lateral to the urogenital folds, a second pair of swellings, known as the *labial swellings* in the female, appear (Fig. 1–14).

By the seventh week of embryonic development, the urogenital folds and the labial swellings are fully developed and, with further differentiation and growth, will give rise to the labia minora and the labia majora, respectively (Moore and Persaud, 1998). Feminization of the external genitalia, which begins in 40- to 50-mm fetuses and is completed in 250- to 300-mm fetuses (Fig. 1–15), results from the absence of androgens or from androgen insensitivity (Jirásek, 1977).

The indifferent stage of the external genitalia extends until the 9th week of development, and, by the end of the 12th week, the external genitalia have acquired characteristics different from those of the male (Moore and Persaud, 1998). Thus transformation of the paramesonephric ducts into the uterine tubes and uterus as well as the feminization of the external genitalia occurs because of the lack of androgens. There is no reason to believe that the fetal ovaries have any morphogenetic role (Reyes et al, 1973; Jirásek, 1977; Wachtel, 1984).

The genital tubercle enlarges to form a phallus that develops into the clitoris. The labial swellings enlarge considerably. They extend anterior to the clitoris, forming the mons pubis, and posteriorly to form the posterior labial commissure (see Fig. 1–14) (Clara, 1966; Moore and Persaud, 1998).

Table 1–1 provides a summary of the adult functional derivatives, as well as vestigial remnants, of embryonic urogenital structures.

REFERENCES

Baker TG, Sum OW: Development of the ovary and oogenesis. Clin Obstet Gynecol 1976;3:3.

Bulmer D: The development of the human vagina. J Anat 1957; 91:490.

Clara M: Entwicklungsgeschichte des Menschen. Leipzig: VEB Georg Thieme, 1966.

Cruikshank SH, Van Drie DM: Supernumerary ovaries: update and review. Obstet Gynecol 1982;60:126.

Eddy EM, Clark JM, Gong D, Fenderson BA: Origin and migration of primordial germ cells in mammals. Gamete Res 1981;4: 333.

Fanghänel J, Wendler D: Zur Entwicklung und Differenzierung der inneren weiblichen Geschlechtsorgane. Z Klin Med 1989; 44:1429.

Fluhmann CF: The developmental anatomy of the cervix uteri. Obstet Gynecol 1960;15:62.

Forsberg J-G: Origin of vaginal epithelium. Obstet Gynecol 1965; 25:787.

Forsberg J-G: Cervicovaginal epithelium: its origin and development. Am J Obstet Gynecol 1973;115:1025.

Gasser RF: The prenatal development of the cervix vagina and vulva. The Colposcopist 1985;17:1.

Godin I, Wylie C, Heasman J: Genital ridges exert long-range effects on mouse primordial germ cell numbers and direction of migration in culture. Development 1990;108:357.

Gondos B, Westergaard L, Byskov AG: Initiation of oogenesis in the human fetal ovary: ultrastructural and squash preparation study. Am J Obstet Gynecol 1986;155:189.

Gordon JD, Shifren JL, Foulk RA, et al: Angiogenesis in the human female reproductive tract. Obstet Gynecol Surv 1995;50: 688.

Hertig AT, Rock J, Adams EC: A description of 34 human ova within the first 17 days of development. Am J Anat 1956;98: 435.

Hunter RH: Observations on the development of the human female genital tract. Contrib Embryol Carnegie Inst Wash 1930; 22:91.

Jirásek JE: Morphogenesis of the genital system in the human. In Blandau RJ, Bergsma D (eds): Morphogenesis and Malformation of the Genital System. New York: Alan R Liss, Inc, for the National Foundation–March of Dimes, 1977:13.

Jost A: Embryonic sexual differentiation (morphology, physiology, abnormalities). In Jones HW Jr, Scott WW (eds): Hermaphroditism, Genital Anomalies and Related Endocrine Disorders. Baltimore: Williams & Wilkins, 1958:15.

Koff AK: Development of the vagina in the human fetus. Contrib Embryol Carnegie Inst Wash 1933;24:59.

Konishi I, Fujii S, Okamura H, et al: Development of interstitial cells and ovigerous cords in the human fetal ovary: an ultrastructural study. J Anat 1986;148:121.

Mahran M, Saleh AM: The microscopic anatomy of the hymen. Anat Rec 1964;149:313.

Makabe S, Motta PM: Migration of human germ cells and their relationship with the developing ovary: ultrastructural aspects. Prog Clin Biol Res 1989;296:41.

Matéjka M: Die Morphogenese der menschlichen Vagina und ihre Gesetzmässigkeiten. Anat Anz 1959;106:20.

Minh HN, Smadja A, Hervé de Sigalony JP, Orcel L: Étude histologique de la gonade a différenciation ovarienne au cours de l'organogenèse. Arch Anat Cytol Pathol 1989c;37:201.

Minh HN, Hervé de Sigalony JP, Smadja A, Orcel L: Nouvelles acquisitions sur l'embryogénèse de l'utérus. Rev Fr Gynecol Obstet 1989a;84:713.

Minh HN, Hervé de Sigalony JP, Smadja A, Orcel L: Nouvelles acquisitions sur l'embryogénèse du vagin. J Gynecol Obstet Biol Reprod 1989b;18:589.

Moore KL, Persaud TVN: The developing human. 6th ed. Philadelphia: WB Saunders Company, 1998.

O'Rahilly R: The development of the vagina in the human. In Blandau RJ, Bergsma D (eds): Morphogenesis and Malformation of the Genital System. New York: Alan R Liss, Inc, for the National Foundation–March of Dimes, 1977:123.

Prins RP, Morrow P, Townsend DE, Disaia PJ: Vaginal embryogenesis estrogens and adenosis. Obstet Gynecol 1976;48:246.

Reyes FI, Winter JSD, Faiman C: Studies on human sexual development. I. Fetal gonadal and adrenal sex steroids. J Clin Endocrinol Metab 1973;37:74.

Robboy SJ, Taguchi O, Cunha GR: Normal development of the human female reproductive tract and alterations resulting from experimental exposure to diethylstilbestrol. Hum Pathol 1982;13:190.

Scott RT Jr, Hodgen GD: The ovarian follicle: life cycle of a pelvic clock. Clin Obstet Gynecol 1990;33:551.

Spencer SJ, Cataldo NA, Jaffe RB: Apoptosis in the human female reproductive tract. Obstet Gynecol Surv 1996;51:314.

Tsafriri A, Sang-Young C, Zhang R, et al: Oocyte maturation involves compartmentalization and opposing changes of cAMP levels in follicular somatic and germ cells: studies using selective phosphodiesterase inhibitors. Dev Biol 1996;178:393.

Van Wagenen G, Simpson ME: Embryology of the Ovary and Testis. *Homo sapiens* and *Macaca mulatta*. New Haven, CT: Yale University Press, 1965.

Wachtel GM, Ohno S, Koo GC, Boyse EA: Possible role for H-Y antigen in the primary determination of sex. Nature 1975;257:235.

Wachtel SS: Human sexual development. J Endocrinol Invest 1984;7:663.

Wartenberg H: Development of the early human ovary and role of the mesonephros in the differentiation of the cortex. Anat Embryol 1982;165:253.

Weissmann A: Die Kontinuität des Keimplasmas als Grundlage einer Theorie der Vererbung, 1985. (Cited by Baker and Sum, 1976).

Wells LJ: Embryology and anatomy of the vagina. Ann NY Acad Sci 1959;83:80.

Witschi E: Migrations of the germ cells of human embryos from the yolk-sac to the primitive gonadal folds. Contrib Embryol Carnegie Inst Wash 1948;32:67.

Witschi E: Development and differentiation of the uterus. In Mack HC (ed): Prenatal Life. Detroit: Wayne State University Press, 1970:11.

Wylie CC, Stott D, Donovan PJ: Primordial germ cell migration. In Browder LW (ed): Developmental Biology. Vol 2. New York: Plenum Publishing Co, 1985:433.

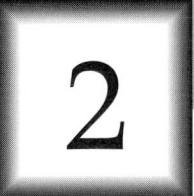

Mark G. Doherty
Larry J. Copeland
Matthew A. Powell

Clinical Anatomy of the Pelvis

Nothing is more essential to the success of an operation and the avoidance of surgical morbidity than a complete understanding of relevant anatomy. The reintroduction of surgical innovations such as the paravaginal suspension of vagina (Richardson et al. 1981) and the sacrospinous vaginal suspension (Randall and Nichols, 1971; Nichols and Randall, 1989) makes more obvious the need for thorough understanding of pelvic anatomy. Mere knowledge of uterine anatomy no longer suffices to allow a broad and deep surgical repertoire in the care of the female patient. Familiarity with normal structure and function is essential for comprehension of normal physiologic changes and pelvic pathology; it aids effective surgical planning, reduces frequency of avoidable surgical complications, and allows the successful and rapid resolution of those that are unavoidable.

This chapter concentrates on adult anatomy and its clinical relevance. Normal anatomic variants and the physiologic changes of pregnancy and aging are beyond the scope of this chapter. For the sake of easier conceptualization and understanding, the traditional division of pelvic anatomy into internal versus external anatomy is expanded. Immediately apparent to the clinician is surface and external anatomy; this is discussed first. The bones, ligaments, and musculature of the parietal pelvis are the framework on which the viscera rest; these are next to be presented. Genital, urinary, and gastrointestinal viscera and their ligaments are presented next. Because of the clinical and anatomic proximity of the appendix to the right adnexa and the frequency with which gynecologists encounter pathology from it and operate on it, pertinent aspects of its anatomy and relationships are also included.

The chapter covers the following topics: surface and external anatomy, parietal pelvis, pelvic viscera and ligaments, and appendix. Clinical and surgical correlative examples are given to enhance understanding of the relevance of anatomy to the practice of gynecology.

SURFACE AND EXTERNAL ANATOMY

Confusion and inconsistency exist in day-to-day clinical conversation, in clinical texts, and in the clinical literature regarding a correct definition of "perineum." Some gynecologic clinicians commonly refer to the perineum as all nonvulvar tissue below the pelvic diaphragm. Other clinicians use the term *perineum* when referring to the more specific *perineal body*. Anatomists commonly attribute *all* tissues below the pelvic diaphragm as belonging to the perineum. The perineum can be divided into the *urogenital triangle* (bounded by the ischial tuberosities and pubic symphysis) and the *anal triangle* (bounded by the ischial tuberosities and coccyx) with the perineal body in the margin of both (Fig. 2–1). For the sake of ease of understanding, we conform to common anatomic terminology rather than redefine the confusing clinical terms.

Urogenital Triangle

Vulva

The vulva is the most superficial of the tissues of the urogenital triangle. The vulvar external genitalia consist of the mons veneris, the labia majora, the labia minora, the clitoris, the urethral meatus, the vestibule and its glands, and the hymen. The boundaries of the vulva are the genitocrural folds laterally and the perineal body posteriorly. Cranially, there is no definite boundary to the vulva; the surface of the mons veneris is contiguous with that of the lower abdomen. The pubic tubercles, however, have often been described as the anterosuperior border of the external genitalia.

Vulvar tissues serve as sensory and erectile tissue for sexual intercourse, to direct the urinary stream during micturition, and to prevent passive retrograde entry of foreign material into the genital tract. The *mons veneris* (mons pubis) is a mound of fibrofatty tissue overlying the superior pubic rami, and

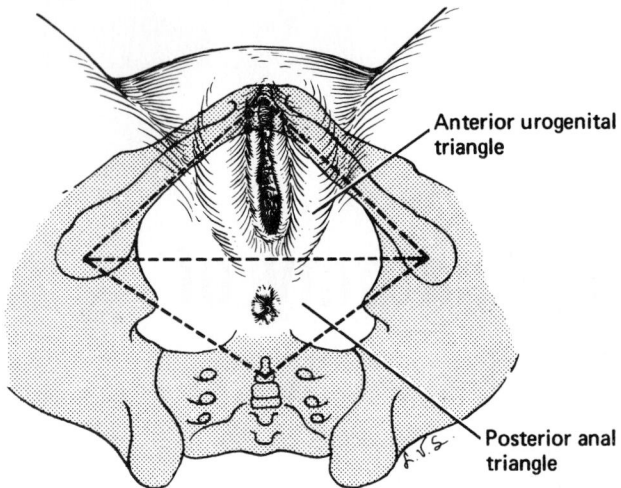

Figure 2–1
Urogenital and anal triangles. (Modified from Krantz KE: Anatomy of the female reproductive system. In Pernoll ML [ed]: Current Obstetric & Gynecologic Diagnosis & Treatment. 7th ed. Norwalk, CT: Appleton & Lange, 1991:31, with permission.)

the pubic symphysis and pubic tubercles (Fig. 2–2). It is covered with hair- and eccrine gland–bearing, keratinized squamous epithelium. Subcutaneous fibrous strands that suspend the mons course superiorly and medially from the anterior labia majora and mons, and radiate through the fatty *Camper's fascia* to insert centrally on the anterior inferior abdominal wall (conjoint tendon and linea alba). The round uterine ligament passes through the lateral mons after exiting the external inguinal ring, ramifies, then inserts in the subcutaneous tissues of the anterior labium majus.

Blood is supplied to the mons through two branches of the femoral artery, the external pudendal and the superficial epigastric vessels. Sensation in the mons is primarily a function of cutaneous branches of nerve roots T12 and L1 (iliohypogastric and ilioinguinal nerves in the anterior abdominal wall). The lateral mons is also innervated by small branches of the ilioinguinal and genitofemoral nerves. Lymphatics converge with those draining the labia and clitoris and drain into the superior and medial groups of inguinal lymph nodes (Plentl and Friedman, 1971).

The *labia majora*, paired prominent folds of lateral vulvar skin, course inferiorly, posteriorly, and laterally from the mons veneris, around the central vulvar structures; taper as they pass posteriorly; and join together posteriorly and medially at the *posterior fourchette* and at a midline raphe superficially overlying the perineal body. They are approximately 8.0 cm in length and 2.5 cm in width; this is highly variable depending on the degree of obesity. Entirely covered with sweat gland– and sebaceous gland–bearing, keratinized squamous epithelium, the exposed thick lateral and inferior surfaces are hair-bearing and are often pigmented. The medial surface

is thinner, has no hair follicles, is usually nonpigmented, and has a higher concentration of sebaceous gland opening. The subcutaneous tissue is richly vascularized areolar connective tissue and lobular fat, contiguous with Camper's fascia.

Blood is supplied to the anterior labium majus primarily through the external pudendal artery and end branches of the artery of the round ligament. The mid to posterior labium majus is supplied by posterior labial branches of the internal pudendal artery. Likewise, the sensory innervation is from more than one source. Anteriorly, the labium majus is supplied by the ilioinguinal nerve and the genital branch of the genitofemoral nerve. Most innervation of the mid to posterior labium majus is from the posterior labial branch of the pudendal nerve; however, a significant amount of sensation of this portion of the labium majus is from labial branches of the posterior and medial femoral cutaneous nerves of the thigh (Fig. 2–3).

A rich network of lymphatics courses through the rete pegs parallel to the skin surface (superficial vulvar lymphatics). A communicating parallel layer immediately overlies the deep fascia, musculature, and periosteum of the perineum (deep vulvar lymphatics). These coalesce with lymphatics from the mons and central vulvar structures and drain into the medial and superior ipsilateral inguinal lymph node groups.

The labia majora are analogous to the scrotum. Muscular remnants analogous to the male dartos can be seen histologically in the most superficial tissues of the labium majus.

CLINICAL CORRELATES

The rich innervation of the labium majus from multiple sources in addition to the pudendal nerve—in particular the

- ilioinguinal and genitofemoral nerves and the posterior femoral cutaneous nerve of the thigh— accounts for the frequent inadequacy of labial analgesia after a pudendal nerve local anesthetic block
- The high concentration of glands and hair follicles in a moist, relatively anoxic environment with skin surfaces frequently apposed and in motion lends itself to frequent development of folliculitis, especially in the obese or diabetic patient. If not promptly recognized or improperly treated, this can progress to necrotizing fasciitis. Chronic, recurrent folliculitis (hidradenitis suppurativa) of the mons and labia is a well-described entity that results from a complex interaction of genetics, bacterial organisms, and abnormally increased androgens.
- Benign proliferations of eccrine tissues (such as hidradenoma) or other indigenous tissues (e.g., lipoma, fibroma, etc.) can be mistaken for malignant tumors of the vulva.
- Numerous dermal infectious and inflammatory conditions affect the mons and labia majora. Because of the relative moistness of the area and the differing

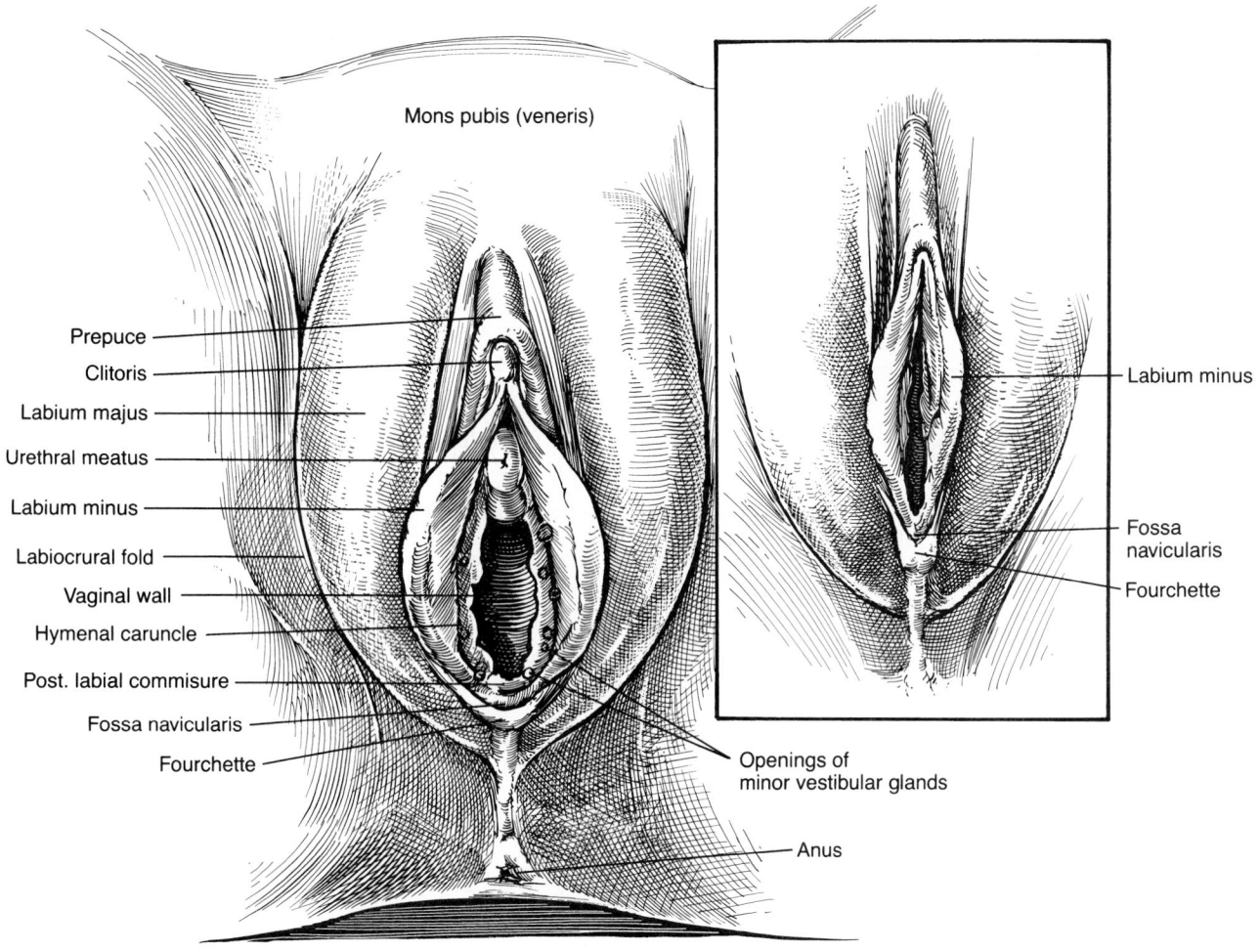

Mons pubis (veneris)

Prepuce
Clitoris
Labium majus
Urethral meatus
Labium minus
Labiocrural fold
Vaginal wall
Hymenal caruncle
Post. labial commisure
Fossa navicularis
Fourchette

Labium minus

Fossa navicularis
Fourchette

Openings of minor vestibular glands

Anus

Figure 2–2
External structures of the female perineum. Labia minora are spread to show detail of vestibule. The introitus (*inset*) is usually closed in most females.

microbial flora, they are more common than at most other external locations.

- Epithelial inclusion cysts (keratin/sebaceous material–filled cysts) have a predilection for the labium majus and only require treatment if symptomatic.
- The comprehensive management of many vulvar malignancies requires treatment of the inguinal lymph nodes, the primary lymphatic drainage of the vulva.
- The posterior anal triangle lacks a subcutaneous tissue plane. The superficial anal sphincter attaches directly to the perianal skin, thus limiting ease of dissection.
- Vulvar hematomas result from laceration of vessels in the superficial fascia by any type of trauma and are most commonly seen secondary to vaginal delivery. Blood loss is usually limited by Colles' fascia and the urogenital diaphragm. Fascial boundaries cause the expanding hematoma to extend to the skin, and visible ecchymosis will result. ∎

The anatomy of the *labium minus* is more dependent on age, parity, and vulvar disease than that of the labium majus—the size, location, and promi-

nence to external examination vary greatly among individuals. Paired, they are composed of dense connective and richly vascular erectile tissues covered by keratinizing squamous epithelium. Adipose tissue is rarely found in the labium minus. The epithelium contains no hair follicles or sweat glands; the sebaceous glands are more sparse than in the labium majus and are more numerous on the medial surface. Approximating 5 cm by 0.75 cm, the labia minora are thinner and shorter than the labia majora. Thicker anteriorly, they arise from fusion of skin overlying the clitoral prepuce (*anterior labial commissure*) with that of the clitoral frenulum. They taper and course posteriorly and laterally around the urethral meatus and vestibule, then join in the midline to form the posterior labial commissure. The infolded area separating the *posterior labial commissure* from the posterior fourchette is termed the *fossa navicularis*, which becomes more attenuated as parity and age increase.

Blood is supplied to the anterior labium minus by clitoral branches of the internal pudendal artery. The

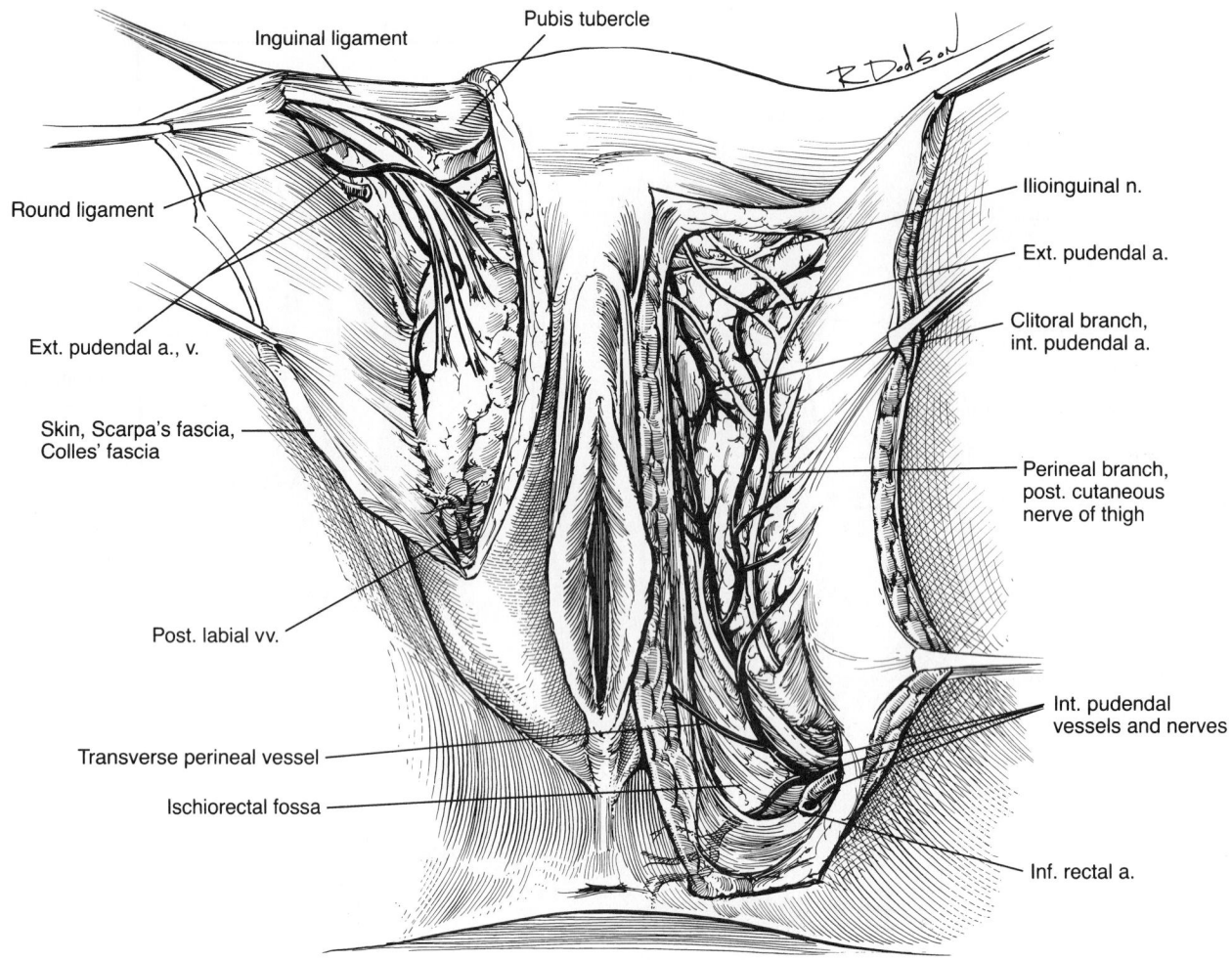

Figure 2–3
Arterial and neural supply of the perineum. Insertion of round uterine ligament.

mid to posterior labium is supplied directly by labial branches of the internal pudendal artery. Innervation is parallel to that of the blood supply; the anterior labium minus is supplied by branches of the clitoral nerve, and the remainder of the labium is served by labial branches of the pudendal nerve. Lymphatics are arranged similarly to those of the labium majus and drain into ipsilateral inguinal lymph nodes. The labia minora are analogous to penile urethra and portions of ventral penile skin.

CLINICAL CORRELATES

- At birth, labial tissues are occasionally fused (synechiae). This usually requires the application of topical estrogens to dissolve the synechiae; only rarely should mechanical separation be used.
- With chronic hypoestronism or chronic vulvar conditions, the labium minus itself can resorb into or fuse with adjacent vestibular or labium majus tissues, usually progressive from posterior to anterior, and can cause vulvovaginal stenosis (kraurosis vulvae).
- Labial edema can occur in situations of increased abdominal fluid (postoperatively, ascites) in the 10%

to 20% of women with patency of the canal of Nuck.

The *clitoris* is located at the anteriormost extent of the labia minora, midway between the anterior labia majora. It is a highly innervated erectile body consisting of two crura, a shaft, and a glans. The shaft and glans are together approximately 2 cm in length and less than 1 cm in diameter. Each of the two *crura* is composed of a bundle of cylindrical elastic and vascular erectile tissue (*corpora cavernosa*) that is subcutaneous and adherent to periosteum of the inferior pubic ramus (Fig. 2–4). Each crus courses medially and superiorly along the medial aspect of the inferior pubic ramus, uniting with its opposite counterpart at the midline (at approximately two thirds of the length) to form the shaft. At their juncture to form the shaft of the clitoris, the crura are adherent superiorly to the perichondrium of the pubic symphysis and are suspended from pubic bones by a suspensory ligament. They compose approximately one half the length of the clitoris and are encased on three sides by the ischiocavernosus muscle.

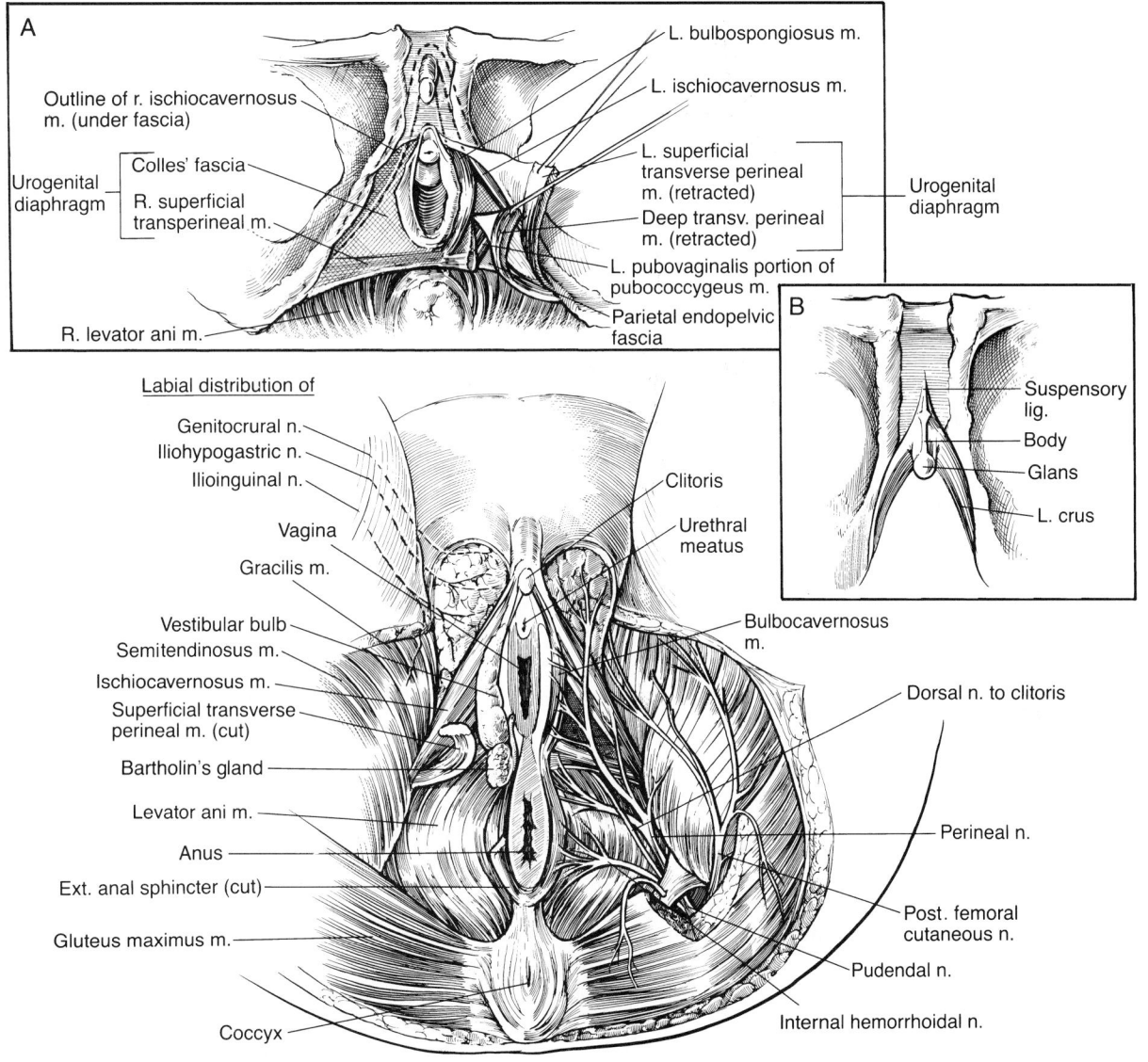

Figure 2–4
Deep structures of the perineum. *A*, Inset details the urogenital diaphragm. *B*, Inset details clitoral structure and position.

The *shaft*, or *body*, of the clitoris is formed by fusion of the two corpora cavernosa after they angulate anteriorly and inferiorly. The shaft constitutes approximately one fourth of the length of the clitoris. The distal one fourth of the clitoris, the *glans*, is composed of erectile and sensory nerve tissues and is partially hidden by skin folds, the *prepuce* anteriorly and the *frenulum* posteriorly. The glans and a portion of the shaft are covered with thin keratinizing squamous epithelium without sweat glands or hair follicles, although there are a few sebaceous glands. The glans is the most highly innervated portion of the clitoris.

The vascular supply of the clitoris is entirely from the internal pudendal artery, the shaft and glans being supplied by the dorsal clitoral artery, the terminal branch of the internal pudendal artery. The vessels of the crura and the ischiocavernosus muscle freely communicate with those of the vestibular bulb. Innervation of the clitoris is entirely from the terminal branch of the pudendal nerve, the dorsal clitoral nerve, supplying the shaft and glans.

Direct lymphatic communications between clitoris and deep pelvic lymph nodes have been demonstrated by anatomic study. Additionally, channels to contralateral lymph node groups from lateral vulvar structures have been demonstrated (Plentl and Friedman, 1971). In general, however, these communications are not clinically or functionally important. The clinically important lymphatic drainage of the clitoris is to *bilateral* superficial inguinal lymph nodes. The clitoris is homologous to the penis but contains no urethral tissue. The prepuce is analogous to the male foreskin.

CLINICAL CORRELATES

- Carcinoma of the vulva involving the clitoris can metastasize to both superficial and deep inguinal lymph node groups. Surgical or radiotherapeutic management of this disorder must take this into account.
- Although sometimes constitutional or familial, congenital or acquired clitoral hypertrophy is usually defined by a clitoral width greater than 1 cm. Hormonal (e.g., adrenal hyperplasia, virilizing ovarian tumors) causes are potentially life-threatening and must be ruled out. Because the hypertrophy is not reversible, clitoral revision or amputation may become necessary to preserve gender identity and sexuality.
- Clitoral agenesis is very rare. Clitoral splitting or duplication is caused by a failure of the corpora to fuse in the midline. This is often associated with bladder exstrophy, epispadias (urethral opening cephalad to the clitoris), and complete or partial absence of the pubic symphysis. ∎

The *vestibule* can be thought of as a broad, short, cylindrical area separating internal from external genitalia. Its external boundaries are the clitoris anteriorly, the medial labia minora laterally, and the fourchette posteriorly. The internal boundary includes the hymenal ring. The vestibule is perforated by the urethra and the vaginal orifice. The overlying skin is thin and composed of thinly keratinized squamous epithelium with essentially no epidermal adnexal structures. Blood supply to the vestibule and its structures is from direct branches of the internal pudendal artery. Sensory innervation is supplied by branches of the pudendal nerve. Lymphatic drainage is similar to that of the labia.

The *hymenal ring* widely differs from individual to individual because of the wide variations in initial conformation and subsequent sexual activity and parity. In most adult females, what remains is usually a series of epithelialized fibrous remnants, circumferential and just distal to the vaginal orifice. These remnants, termed *hymenal caruncles*, demarcate vulva from vagina. The midline *urethral meatus* is situated 2 to 3 cm directly posterior to the clitoris and equally distant from the vaginal opening.

The *bulbs of the vestibule* are paired structures that lie adjacent to the lateral "wall" of the vestibule bilaterally and deep to the subcutaneous tissues of the labia (Fig. 2–4). They are composed of erectile tissue, an intertwining network of capillaries and venous sinusoids separated by septa of areolar connective tissue. Similar to tissues of the clitoris, they become engorged during sexual arousal.

The *major vestibular (Bartholin's) glands* are paired structures, each located just deep to the posterior one third of the vestibular and labial structures, and are embedded in and adherent to the posterior vestibular bulb. They are round, lobulated glands, approximately 1 cm in diameter, consisting of cuboidal mucinous cells. Each usually has a single 0.2-cm-

diameter, 1- to 2-cm-long duct lined by transitional epithelium that courses anteromedially to empty into the posterolateral vestibule at the juncture of the hymen and labium minus. A few drops of mucoid material are secreted by them during sexual arousal. The male counterparts are the bulbourethral (Cowper's) glands.

The *minor vestibular glands* are simple tubular glands of columnar mucin-secreting cells approximately 0.5 cm in depth and up to 0.1 cm in diameter. They are arranged in a U-shaped distribution around the vestibule laterally and posteriorly (see Fig. 2–2). The ducts empty into the groove between the labia minora and the external surface of the hymen (Friedrich, 1983). Their function is unknown.

CLINICAL CORRELATES

- The thin mucosal fold of the hymen can be imperforate in some individuals. If unrecognized and untreated prior to menarche, this condition can lead to hematocolpos, hematometra, and even hemoperitoneum or endometriosis.
- Urethral caruncle—exstrophy and shortening of the urethra—occurs secondary to hypoestrogenic changes in the vagina with resultant traction upon the urethral meatus. It is occasionally symptomatic enough (bleeding, dysuria, discharge) to require surgical therapy.
- The vulva can be a site of severe pain and discomfort for patients and yet examination of the vulva will often appear anatomically normal. Vulvodynia (vulvar pain) was systematically defined by the International Society for the Study of Vulvar Diseases (ISSVD) Committee on vulvodynia in 1991. The five defined categories are vulvar vestibulitis (most common), essential (dysthetic) vulvodynia, cyclic vulvovaginitis, vulvar dermatoses (lichen sclerosis, lichen planus, etc.), and vulvar papillomatosis (McKay et al, 1991).
- Vulvar vestibulitis (chronic vestibulitis) has received a great deal of attention in both the medical and lay press. The etiology of the disorder is currently unknown. Human papillomavirus, herpes simplex virus, and disorders of oxalate excretion have been studied and do not appear to be the cause, but can be contributing factors. Treatment should be conservative, with surgical management used only as a last resort.
- Occlusion of the vestibular gland duct can predispose to acute infection of the gland. Ductal occlusion is commonly associated with gonorrheal or chlamydial infections. In the case of the major vestibular gland, this infection is commonly termed *Bartholin*'s adenitis, which can progress to abscess, cellulitis, and fasciitis. In many patients, this is a recurring entity requiring surgical management. Occlusion of the major vestibular gland duct *without* infection can lead to a pseudocystic accumulation of mucin, commonly known as *Bartholin's cyst*.
- Chronic inflammation of the minor vestibular glands is less common but, when evident, usually manifests as

vulvar pain or vaginal outlet dyspareunia. Foci of tender erythema at the gland ostia (Woodruff and Parmley, 1983) are seen. Symptoms can be severe or persistent enough to require surgical management. A similar condition of the major vestibular gland ducts has been described (Peckham et al, 1986). Adenomas of the minor vestibular glands occur (Axe et al, 1986).

- The major vestibular gland is the site of origin of the majority of vulvar adenocarcinomas. Transitional cell, squamous, and adenoid cystic carcinomas also originate in this organ (Copeland et al, 1986). These neoplasms are frequently initially misdiagnosed as adenitis or abscess—beware of the diagnosis of "Bartholin gland adenitis or abscess" in the older patient.
- The high degree of vascularity of the bulb of the vestibule results in susceptibility to trauma. Disruption of vessels at this site can occur with physical trauma (athletic or motor vehicle injuries, sexual assault, obstetric injury) or with severe coagulopathy and is the usual source of the "vulvar" or "labial" hematoma. ∎

Perineal Muscles and Urogenital Diaphragm

Deep to the cutaneous and subcutaneous tissues of the perineum lie the perineal musculature and the urogenital diaphragm (see Figs. 2–4 and 2–17).

The superficialmost layer of these tissues is a thin membranous layer of fascia, called *Colles' fascia*, contiguous with Scarpa's abdominal fascia. Directly deep to this layer lie the three paired superficial perineal muscles: the ischiocavernosus, bulbocavernosus, and superficial transverse perineal muscles. As previously described, the *ischiocavernosus* surrounds the crus of the clitoris, is densely adherent to the medial surface of the inferior pubic ramus, and is approximately semicircular in cross section. The *bulbocavernosus* overlies and surrounds the bulb of the vestibule. The tapered narrow anterior end inserts on periosteum at the pubis, behind the clitoris. Circular in cross section, it broadens as it courses posteriorly, then medially, and the posterior margin inserts into the central perineal tendon. In concert with its contralateral partner, it effectively surrounds the distal vagina and vestibule. The *superficial transverse perineal muscle* is a flat, narrow, strap-like muscle coursing transversely and medially from its origin on the ischial ramus to insert on the central perineal tendon. These three muscles are vascularized and innervated by the terminal perineal branches of the pudendal vessels and nerve. They are drained by the inguinal lymph nodes. Each has a male homolog.

Deep to these tissues lies the *urogenital diaphragm* (see Fig. 2–4). This tough triangular conglomeration of fascia and paired muscles extends from the ischial tuberosities to the pubic symphysis along the inferior pubic ramus. It is perforated by the urethra and vagina. Its major function seems to be support of the urethra and maintenance of normal urethrovesical position. Its degree of strength and integrity is highly variable with age, parity, trauma, sexual activity, and hormonal status.

The major constituent of the urogenital diaphragm is the *deep transverse perineal muscle*. Slightly broader and flatter than its superficial counterpart, it courses medially from its origin on the inferior ischial and pubic rami. Anteriorly at the midline, it forms a raphe with its opposite partner. This raphe is perforated by the urethra and vagina. Posteriorly at the midline, the muscle inserts into the central pelvic tendon. The posterior free edge of the diaphragm is bolstered by the parallel posterior free edge of the superficial transverse perineal muscle. The superficial surface of the muscle is invested with a fascial layer, the *inferior*, or *superficial*, *urogenital fascia*. Likewise, the deep surface of the muscle is invested with the *superior*, or *deep*, *urogenital fascia*.

Although the major constituent of the urogenital diaphragm is the deep transverse perineal muscle, its tough fascial envelope also contains the pudendal vessels and nerves and their clitoral branches. The site of perforation of urogenital diaphragm by the urethra is the *external urethral sphincter*.

The *central perineal tendon* lies posterior to the vestibule and vagina and anterior to the anus and rectum. Also called the *perineal body*, it too is highly variable in size and consistency, being influenced mostly by parity and trauma. The overlying skin has comparatively little fat. It is composed of the tendinous insertions of the following muscles (from superficial to deep): the bulbocavernosus, external anal sphincter, superficial transverse perineal, deep transverse perineal, and puborectalis muscles, and a portion of the pubococcygeus muscle.

Directly deep to the urogenital diaphragm and the ischiorectal fossa is the *pelvic diaphragm*.

CLINICAL CORRELATES

- Kegel's exercises, used to aid patients with stress urinary incontinence and with excessive perineal laxity, are designed to strengthen the perineal and urogenital diaphragm muscles, which in turn increase urethral resting pressure and partially restore the normal urethrovesical angle.
- The bulbocavernosus and transverse perineal muscles are thought to be those most responsible for vaginismus.
- Stretching of and trauma to the urogenital diaphragm can interfere with normal urethrovesical position and support of the bladder, predisposing to cystocele or stress urinary incontinence.
- The superficial transverse perineal and the bulbocavernosus are the two muscles often cited as being the muscles incised in a midline episiotomy. In fact, the central perineal tendon is the major structure incised, which includes tendinous insertions from many muscles. Widely debated to this day, the episiotomy is believed by many to decrease the

prevalence of excessive perineal body attenuation and to decrease trauma to urogenital and pelvic diaphragms. The use of the "prophylactic episiotomy" is often touted but is unproven (Goodlin, 1983; Wilcox et al, 1989).

- The central peroneal tendon can be disrupted by trauma, inflammatory disease, infection, or surgery, which can lead to formation of a fistulous tract with the vagina or vestibule.
- Attenuation of the perineal body, along with diastasis of the puborectalis and pubococcygeal portions of the levator ani muscle (usually secondary to obstetric trauma), allows the formation of rectocele. Meticulous perineoplasty (or perineorrhaphy), the reconstruction of the perineal body, an adjunct to posterior colporrhaphy, is used to increase the likelihood of successful rectocele repair.
- Rotational pedicled flaps of bulbocavernosus muscle, its overlying fat pad (the "Martius flap"), or both (McCall and Bolten, 1956) can be used for repair of difficult vaginal fistulas. ∎

Anal Triangle

The skin overlying the anal triangle is gland- and hair-bearing, keratinized, stratified squamous epithelium. The *anus* is the terminal opening of the intestinal tract (Fig. 2–5). It is covered by stratified squamous epithelium loosely attached to an underlying vascular plexus and connective tissue, giving it a stellate external appearance. Internally, at a distance of 2 to 4 cm, the anus adjoins the rectum, and squamous epithelium changes to columnar epithelial cells. This irregular transverse line of metaplastic demarcation is termed the *pectenate*, or *dentate*, *line*. Longitudinal vein-containing *anal columns* pass from this line distally for another few centimeters before merging with the anal wall. Small out-pouchings of mucosa between columns along the pectinate line are termed *anal valves*.

The *external anal sphincter*, a superficial ring of skeletal muscle, round to elliptical in cross section, surrounds the distal anus. It is surrounded by a fibrofascial capsule and may be divided into superficial and deep components. This capsule is densely adherent anteriorly to the central perineal tendon and posteriorly to the anococcygeal body. Its function is to aid in fecal continence. A circular arrangement of smooth muscle at the lowermost extent of large bowel is termed the *internal anal sphincter*.

Posterior to the anus lies the *anococcygeal body*, a conglomeration of fibrous tissue securing the external anal sphincter to the coccyx (see Figs. 2–16 and 2–17). It is formed by the fibrotendinous insertions of the pubococcygeus and iliococcygeus portions of the levator ani. Posterior to the central perineal tendon and urogenital diaphragm and lateral to the anus are the *ischiorectal fossae*. These paired triangular areas are bounded posterolaterally by the gluteal muscles and medially by the anus, anal sphincter,

and puborectalis. Although mostly filled with adipose tissue, the termination of the posterior perineal and para-anal branches of the pudendal and inferior rectal arteries and nerves pass through here. The lymphatic drainage of these areas is to inguinal, pararectal, and inferior rectal lymph node groups.

Directly deep to the ischiorectal fossa is the *pelvic diaphragm*. The posterior portion of the levator ani muscle encircles the anorectal junction just deep to the external sphincter before inserting into the anococcygeal body. Its sling-like action angulates the rectum anteriorly, aiding in maintenance of fecal continence.

Blood is supplied and drained in the anal triangle by the inferior rectal vessels, terminal branches of the internal pudendal vessels. Likewise, innervation is supplied by the inferior rectal nerve, a terminal branch of the internal pudendal nerve. Lymphatic drainage of this area is to superficial inguinal lymph nodes.

CLINICAL CORRELATES

- Because of coexistence in a similar "environment" and its physical contiguity with the vulva, the skin of the anal triangle is subject to many of the same dermal disorders, such as infection with *Candida*, herpesvirus, and human papillomavirus; dystrophic disorders; and the like.
- Premalignant conditions such as squamous intraepithelial neoplasia and Paget's disease frequently coexist or independently affect the skin of the anal triangle.
- Hemorrhoids—redundancies of the venous components of the anal columns—may expand to quite large proportions and prolapse from the anus. Predisposing factors include pregnancy, chronic constipation, portal venous hypertension, or any disorder that results in increased intra-abdominal pressure. They may become thrombosed or infected.
- Anal fissure, a mucosal tear at the site of the anal valve, is usually caused by constipation. This condition may progress to abscess and fistula.
- Pararectal abscess may lead to development of a rectovaginal or rectoperineal fistula.
- Inflammatory bowel disease affecting the anus, particularly Crohn's disease, may secondarily involve the perineum and form ulcers or fistulas.
- Because of proximity to the anus and the major vestibular glands and the increased propensity for overlying skin to develop folliculitis, the ischiorectal fossae are frequent sites of abscess.
- Because the inferior rectal vessels pass through the ischiorectal fossae, this area is a common site of traumatic or obstetric hematoma, especially with mediolateral episiotomy or laceration.
- Rectovaginal fistulas below the levator ani may be successfully repaired either transvaginally or transanally.
- Stretching of the pudendal nerve, such as seen with traumatic childbirth, chronic constipation, or other

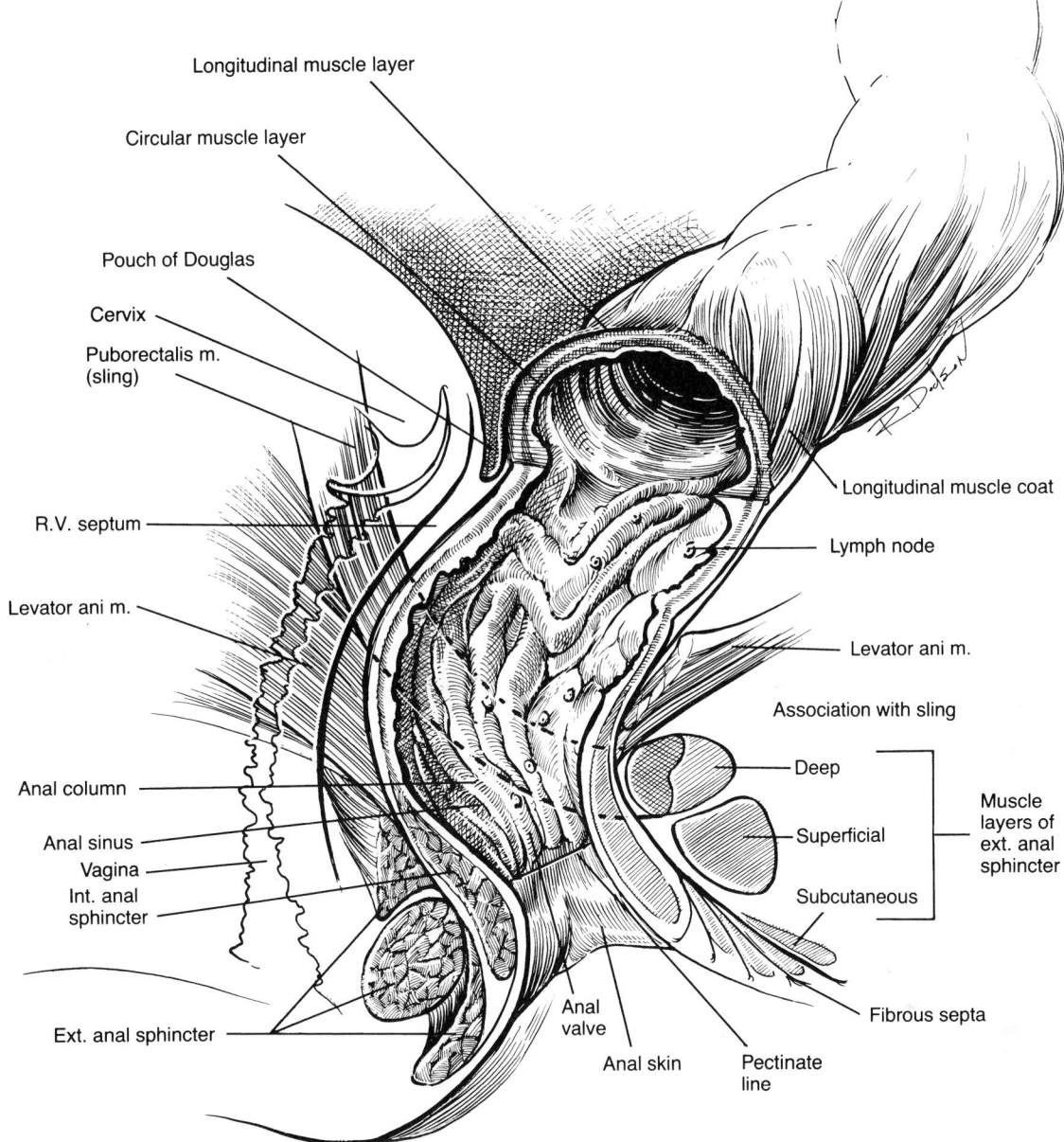

Longitudinal muscle layer

Circular muscle layer

Pouch of Douglas

Cervix

Puborectalis m.
(sling)

R.V. septum

Levator ani m.

Anal column

Anal sinus

Vagina

Int. anal
sphincter

Ext. anal sphincter

Longitudinal muscle coat

Lymph node

Levator ani m.

Association with sling

Deep

Superficial

Subcutaneous

Muscle
layers of
ext. anal
sphincter

Fibrous septa

Anal
valve

Anal skin

Pectinate
line

Figure 2–5
Details of rectum, anus, and supporting structures, showing relationships to the vagina and cervix.

defects of pelvic support, can lead to pudendal nerve damage and immediate or delayed anorectal incontinence. Primary neurologic disease can cause identical symptoms. Fecal continence can be maintained despite extensive physical disruption of the sphincter as long as the controlling neural pathways remain undamaged. Fecal incontinence in nursing homes and long-term care facilities has been reported in 33% to 47% of patients. (Borrie, 1992). There have been technological advances in the evaluation of anal incontinence. Anal manometry, pelvic floor electromyography, anal sonography, and defecography can provide objective evidence of defects. Careful history taking and physical examination remain essential. ∎

Inguinal Region

The importance of the inguinal region to the gynecologist is that it harbors lymphatic structures that may be affected by the infectious or neoplastic conditions of the vulva, distal vagina, perineum, anus, distal rectum, buttocks, and lower extremities (Fig. 2–6. Additionally, because portions of the inguinal region are innervated by branches of the ilioinguinal, genitofemoral, and obturator nerves, gynecologic conditions may initially present with inguinal pain.

The superficial tissues of the inguinal region are supplied by a variety of *cutaneous nerves*. The medialmost inguinal region is supplied proximally by the ilioinguinal nerve and the genital branch of the gen-

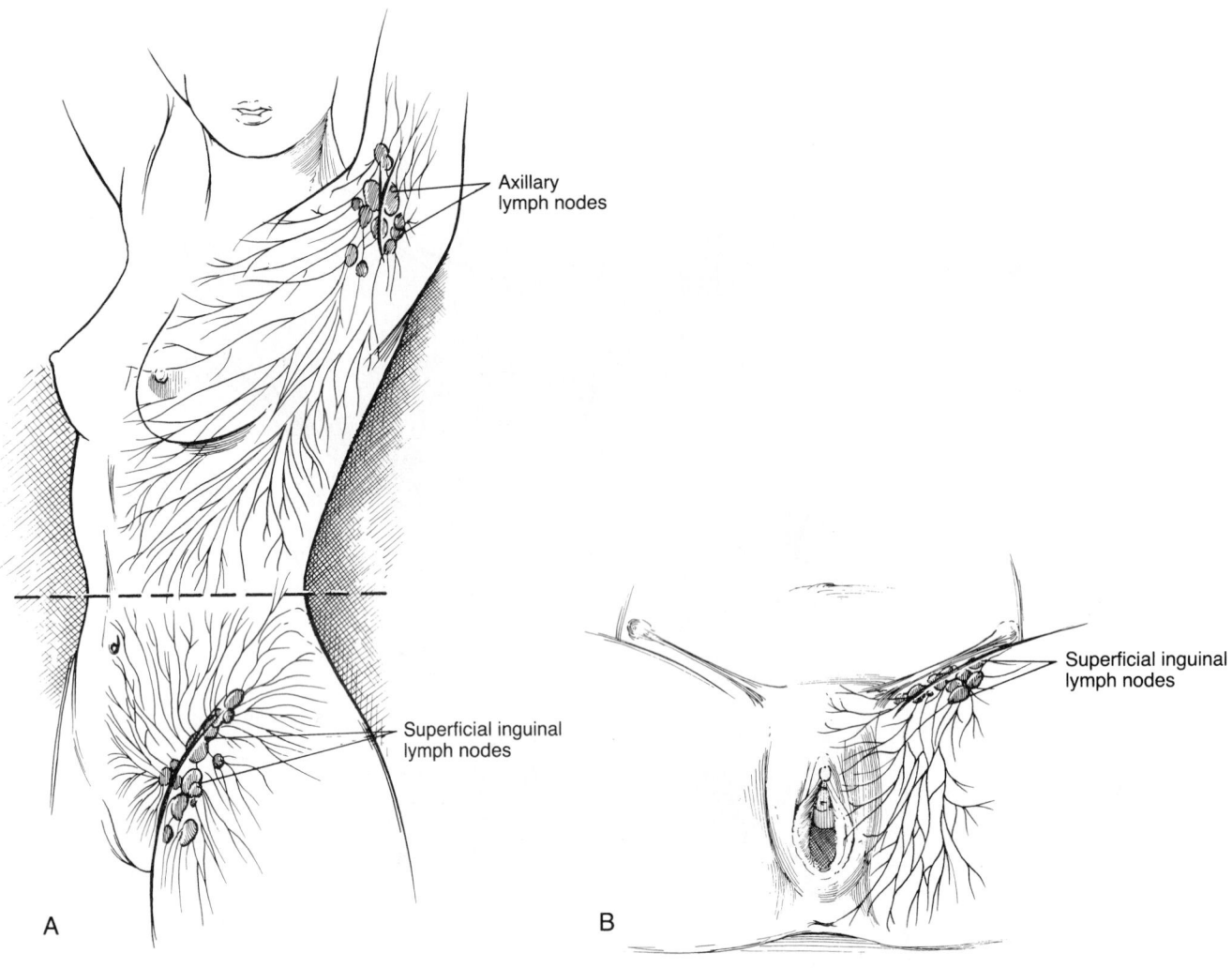

Figure 2–6
A, Lymphatic drainage of the abdominal wall. *B*, Lymphatic drainage to the inguinal region.

itofemoral nerve. Distally, sensation is supplied by a cutaneous branch of the obturator nerve. The mid-inguinal region is supplied proximally by femoral branches of the genitofemoral nerve and distally by branches of the intermediate femoral cutaneous nerve. The lateral inguinal region is almost exclusively innervated by branches of the lateral femoral cutaneous nerve.

The traditional borders of the *inguinal triangle* are the inguinal ligament superiorly and medially, the sartorius muscle laterally, and the adductor longus muscle medially (Fig. 2–7). The anterior border of the triangle is thought to be the membranous layer of superficial fascia (contiguous with Scarpa's fascia of the lower abdomen) immediately deep to the sub-cutaneous fat (Camper's fascia).

The floor of the inguinal triangle is formed by the pectineus, psoas, and iliacus muscles (mnemonic, PePsI), from medial to lateral. As the deep fascia of the thigh (fascia lata) passes medially over the in-guinal triangle, it is perforated by many small lym-phatics and is called the *cribriform fascia*. It separates

the inguinal region into superficial and deep com-partments. Additionally, there exists a 1.5- to 3.0-cm window in the fascia lata over the proximity of the femoral vessels as they approach the inguinal liga-ment, which is called the saphenous opening (also known as the fossa ovale), through which several superficial arteries and veins communicate with the femoral vessels.

The major contents of both compartments of the inguinal triangle are vascular and lymphatic. In the superficial compartment, the *saphenous and accessory saphenous veins* course superiorly in subcutaneous fat before passing through the saphenous opening di-rectly into the femoral vein. Also passing through the saphenous opening are three sets of paired ves-sels originating from and draining into the femoral vessels: the *superficial epigastric vessels* that course su-periorly in the subcutaneous tissues of the abdomi-nal wall, the *superficial circumflex iliac vessels* that course laterally and superiorly toward the superior gluteal and inferolateral lumbar region, and the *su-perficial (or external) pudendal vessels* that supply the

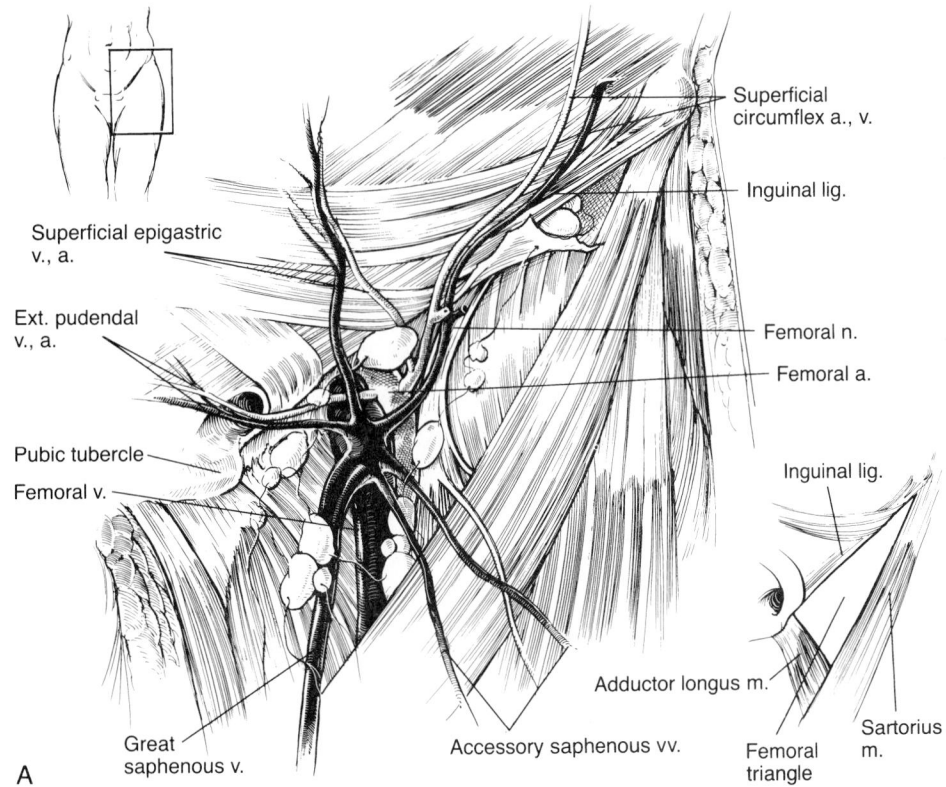

Figure 2-7
Contents and borders of the inguinal triangle. *A,* Inset details inguinal triangle borders. *Illustration continued on following page*

anterior labia after coursing medially and then inferiorly. The remaining vessels that originate from the femoral vessels in the inguinal triangle are usually not directly relevant to the gynecologic surgeon.

Structural lymphatic anatomy has been well outlined (Plentl and Friedman, 1971). *Functional* inguinal anatomy has been described, based upon investigation of vulvar cancer treatment with conservative surgery (DiSaia et al, 1979). The lymph nodes of the superficial compartment (*superficial inguinal lymph nodes*) receive lymphatics from many areas. Afferent lymphatics from abdominal wall, vulva, anus, and buttocks are generally arranged in a pattern parallel and inferior to the inguinal ligament (the "horizontal group") located cephalad to the saphenous opening. Inferior to the saphenous opening, they are arranged along the saphenous vein and drain the superficial thigh and leg. These so-called vertical groups communicate directly with the deep inguinal lymph node group by lymphatics that pass directly through the cribriform fascia. There is a trend in the current clinical literature to call the lymph nodes in the superficial compartment superficial inguinal lymph nodes and to refer to the deeper nodes as femoral nodes.

The major contents of the deep compartment of the inguinal triangle are, from lateral to medial, femoral nerve, femoral artery, femoral vein, and femoral canal. The femoral vessels together are circumferentially invested by a continuation of iliacus and trans-

versus abdominis muscle fasciae (the *femoral sheath*) that protrudes into the thigh along the vessels for a distance of 2 to 3 cm inferior to the inguinal ligament (Fig. 2-8). The space it encompasses is termed the *femoral canal*. The femoral canal is compartmentalized: the lateral compartment contains the femoral artery, the intermediate compartment accomodates the femoral vein, and the medial compartment is traditionally described as containing one to several lymph nodes and all efferent lymph vessels from the deep inguinal lymph nodes. The proximal opening of the medial compartment of the femoral canal is termed the *femoral ring*. A useful mnemonic for the contents of the femoral sheath is NAVEL (*nerve, artery, vein, empty, lymphatic*), which names these structures laterally to medially (Fig. 2-8).

The *deep inguinal lymph nodes* are found in the deep inguinal compartment. They are generally arranged in a vertical fashion, surround the femoral vessels, condense medially to pass through the femoral sheath and under the inguinal ligament, and course along the external iliac vessels. Their afferents are of two types, those that course upward from the deep thigh and leg along the limb vasculature, and the perforating lymphatics from the superficial inguinal node group.

The *femoral artery and vein* supply blood to and drain the hip, thigh, leg, and foot. The *femoral nerve* arises from the lumbar plexus, passes through the

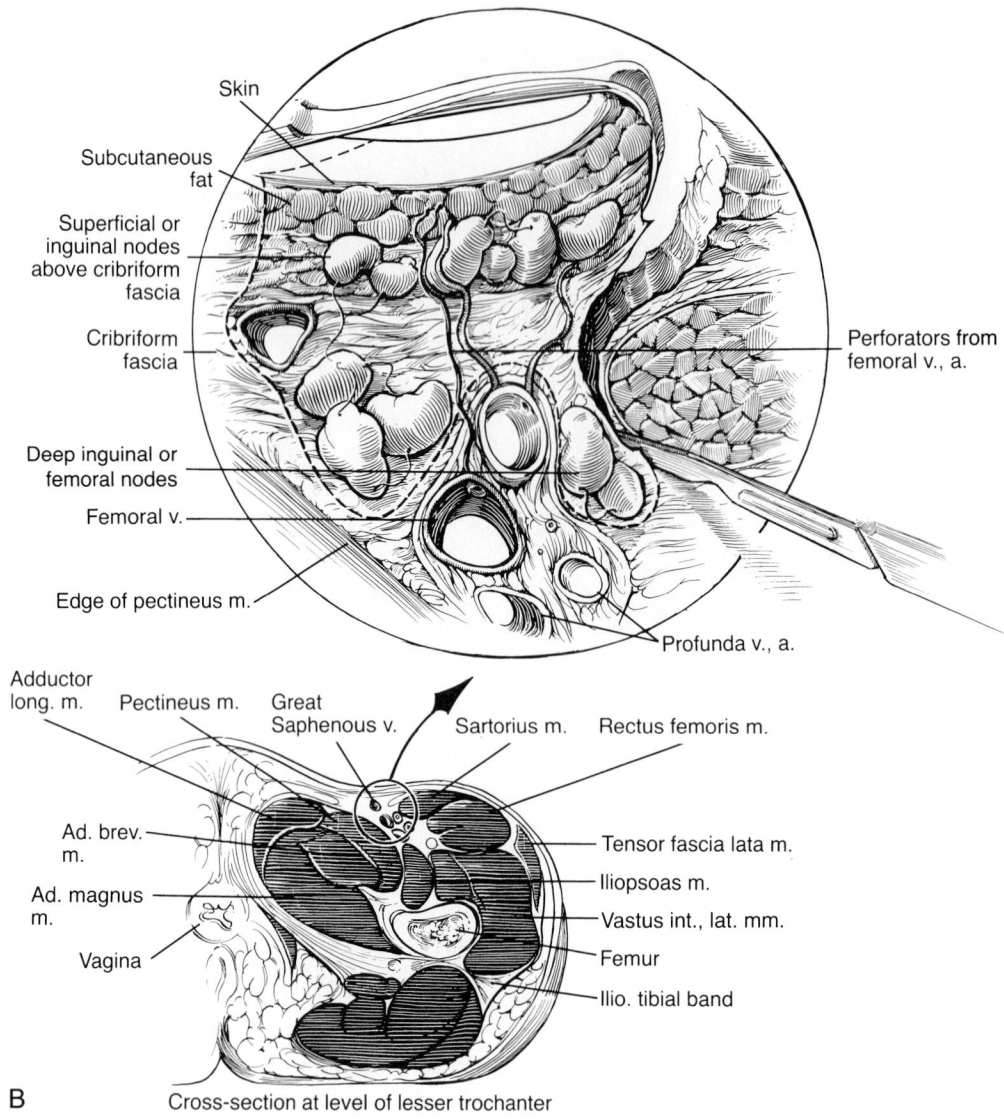

Skin

Subcutaneous fat

Superficial or inguinal nodes above cribriform fascia

Cribriform fascia

Deep inguinal or femoral nodes

Femoral v.

Edge of pectineus m.

Perforators from femoral v., a.

Profunda v., a.

Adductor long. m.
Pectineus m.
Great Saphenous v.
Sartorius m.
Rectus femoris m.

Ad. brev. m.

Ad. magnus m.

Vagina

Tensor fascia lata m.
Iliopsoas m.
Vastus int., lat. mm.
Femur
Ilio. tibial band

B

Cross-section at level of lesser trochanter

Figure 2–7
Continued B, Cross-sectional anatomy of the inguinal triangle.

psoas muscle, then parallels the muscle as it passes underneath the inguinal ligament, innervating muscles of the anterior compartment of the thigh. Additionally, skin of the thigh is innervated anteriorly and medially by its intermediate and medial femoral cutaneous branches. The femoral nerve also gives rise to the saphenous nerve, which supplies sensation to the anteromedial skin of the leg and foot.

CLINICAL CORRELATES

- The femoral ring (the proximal opening of the medial compartment of the fascial sheath) is the site of origin of femoral hernia. Females are more predisposed to this hernia than are males because of their wider pelvis and wider femoral sheath.
- Lymphadenopathy in the inguinal region can occur from any subclinical or clinical exposure to infectious

agents or malignancy. It is often symptomatic or noticeable enough to the patient to be of great concern. One must keep in mind that these lymph nodes drain abdominal, anorectal, buttock, and lower extremity areas in addition to vulvar and perineal structures. Each of these areas must be carefully examined when inguinal lymphadenopathy is present.

- Knowledge of the sequential and generally orderly fashion with which squamous carcinoma of the vulva involves the draining inguinal lymph nodes is responsible for the high success rate of its treatment. Intricate knowledge of the lymphatic anatomy and behavior of this cancer has led to the validation of less morbid conservative surgical procedures with success equal to that of traditional radical procedures (Berman et al, 1989).
- The inguinal region is a frequent site of referred ureteral pain.

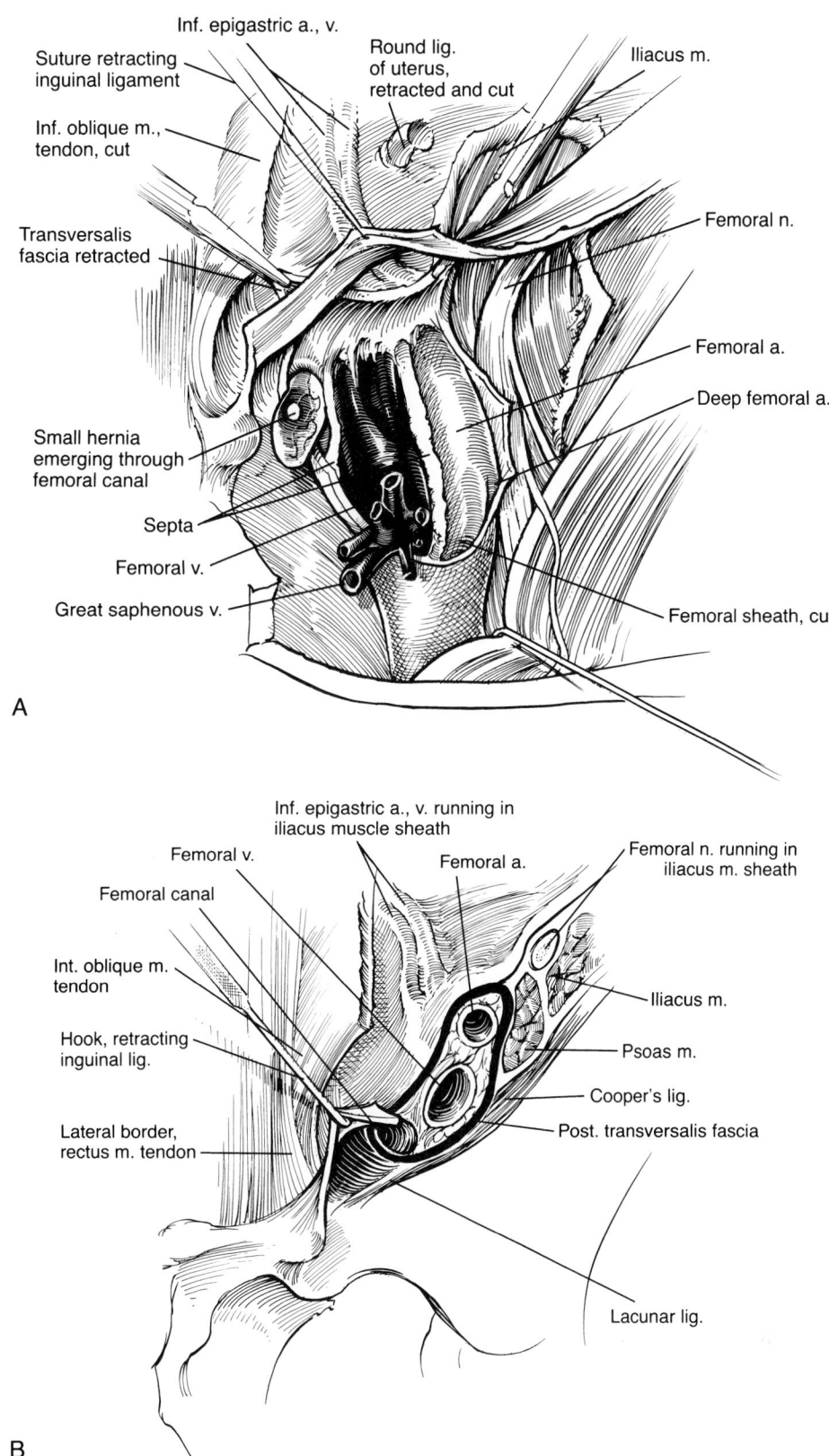

Inf. epigastric a., v.

Suture retracting
inguinal ligament

Round lig.
of uterus,
retracted and cut

Iliacus m.

Inf. oblique m.,
tendon, cut

Transversalis
fascia retracted

Femoral n.

Femoral a.

Deep femoral a.

Small hernia
emerging through
femoral canal

Septa

Femoral v.

Great saphenous v.

Femoral sheath, cut

A

Inf. epigastric a., v. running in
iliacus muscle sheath

Femoral v.

Femoral a.

Femoral n. running in
iliacus m. sheath

Femoral canal

Int. oblique m.
tendon

Hook, retracting
inguinal lig.

Lateral border,
rectus m. tendon

Iliacus m.

Psoas m.

Cooper's lig.

Post. transversalis fascia

Lacunar lig.

B

Figure 2–8
Details of the femoral sheath, canal, and ring.

- The femoral nerve can be injured by exaggerated positioning of the surgical patient, as with the lithotomy position; by the use of self-retaining retractors (especially with transverse lower abdominal incisions); or with radical vulvoinguinal surgery. The resulting sensory changes include cutaneous anesthesia or dysesthesia of the anterior and medial thigh and the anteromedial leg and foot. Motor losses seen are limitation of leg extension (loss of quadriceps femoris function) and reduction of thigh flexion (loss of sartorius and pectineus function).
- "Sentinel" node biopsy in the management of breast cancer has received a great deal of excitement. A "sentinel" node is a lymph node that, when sampled and negative for tumor, should indicate that additional nodes more distal on the lymph chain (further away from the tumor) are also negative. The use of "sentinel" node biopsy in the management of vulvar cancer has been studied. Some authorities believe that the decision to perform a pelvic node dissection in addition to groin sampling with vulvar cancer staging/treatment could be based on the status of one of two "sentinel" nodes called Cloquet's node and Jackson's node. The node of Cloquet (also known as the node of Rosenmuller or upper deep femoral node) is the most superior deep inguinal node, located medial to the femoral vein beneath the cribriform fascia. Cloquet's node is absent in over 50% of cases (Borgno et al, 1990). Jackson's node is the distalmost external iliac node accessed via the groin, located anatomically cephalad to Cloquet's node. The reliability of the "sentinel" nodes remains to be proven. Anatomically, neither node can actually be considered "sentinel." Both nodes can be bypassed by lymphatic flow, and Cloquet's nodes are frequently unobtainable. For these reasons, coupled with the fact that pelvic nodes are often treated with radiation if the groin nodes (two or more) are positive, emphasis on sentinel node analysis in management of vulvar cancer is mostly of historical significance. (Homesly et al, 1986). ∎

Abdominal Wall

A thorough understanding of the anatomy of the abdominal wall, especially that of the lower abdomen, is indispensible for avoidance of incisional complications. Additionally, because the pelvis is contiguous with the abdominal cavity, pelvic genital pathology frequently manifests with abdominal wall symptoms.

The abdomen's external surfaces are commonly divided into quadrants, delineated by horizontal and vertical lines through the umbilicus. Additionally, clinicians commonly refer to suprapubic, periumbilical, hypogastric (suprapubic), and epigastric areas as locations of abdominopelvic symptoms and findings.

The blood supply to the abdominal wall is multicentric and rich in anastomoses (Fig. 2–9). Superficial and inferior structures close to the midline are supplied by the *superficial epigastric vessels*. The deeper midline fascial and subfascial structures in the area of the rectus sheath are supplied by the inferior and superior epigastric arteries. The *inferior epigastric artery* arises from the external iliac artery and courses cephalad directly underneath the rectus muscle and anterior to the posterior rectus sheath and peritoneum. At the level of the umbilicus, it anastomoses with the *superior epigastric vessels*, which also course cephalad to anastomose with the internal thoracic vessels.

The upper quadrants are supplied by continuations of the *intercostal vessels* originating from the thoracic aorta. The lateral abdominal wall is supplied with branches of the *lumbar vessels*, direct branches of the abdominal aorta. Lower quadrants are supplied by *superficial* and *deep circumflex iliac vessels*, originating respectively from the inguinal and external iliac vessels. The lumbar and intercostal branches freely anastomose with branches of the phrenic and axillary vessels. All abdominal wall vessels richly anastomose with each other, assuring adequate blood supply to muscle and fascia when one or more vessels are absent or interrupted.

Somatic innervation of the abdominal wall is supplied by *thoracic nerve roots T7 through T12* and by *lumbar nerve root L1* branches, which terminate in the iliohypogastric and ilioinguinal nerves. A simple way to remember this is that two nerve roots separate each landmark; the epigastrium is served by T7, the umbilicus by T10, and the suprapubic and lower quadrant regions by L1. These nerves have both sensory and motor functions. The major sensorimotor nerves are the inferiormost six thoracic nerve roots (which pierce and innervate the rectus sheath contents, then pass anteriorly to innervate skin) and the L1 nerve root (which does not pierce the rectus sheath, but passes medially and inferiorly as *iliohypogastric* and *ilioinguinal nerves* to innervate skin of lower quadrants). These nerves also innervate the adjacent parietal peritoneum.

The lymphatic drainage of the abdominal wall is simply conceptualized. Tissues superficial to the rectus sheath, at and below the umbilicus, drain to the superficial inguinal lymph nodes. Those superficial tissues superior to the umbilicus drain to the axillary lymph nodes. Those areas within and deep to the rectus sheath follow their adjacent blood vessels and drain into internal thoracic, para-aortic, and external iliac lymph nodes.

Understanding of the abdominal wall layers, muscles, and tendons is not as easily accomplished. The superficial fascia of the abdominal wall is composed of two layers: the fatty superficial layer (*Camper's fascia*) and the deeper membranous layer (*Scarpa's fascia*). Camper's fascia is contiguous with the subcutaneous fatty tissues of mons, thigh, back, and thorax and greatly varies in thickness between individuals. Scarpa's fascia attenuates and disappears over the anterior thorax superiorly. Inferiorly, it passes over the inguinal ligament, where a portion fuses to the

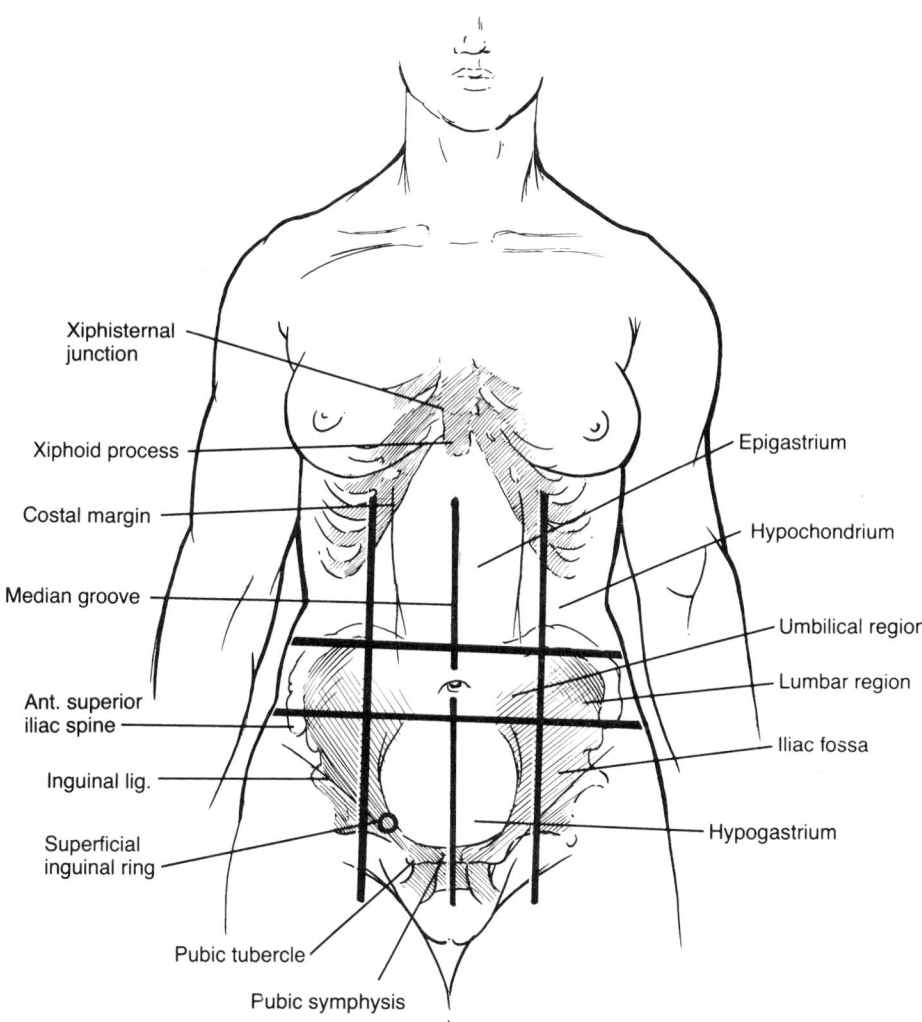

Figure 2–9
Abdominal wall superficial anatomy and regions.

Labels (top to bottom, left side):
Xiphisternal junction
Xiphoid process
Costal margin
Median groove
Ant. superior iliac spine
Inguinal lig.
Superficial inguinal ring
Pubic tubercle
Pubic symphysis

Labels (right side):
Epigastrium
Hypochondrium
Umbilical region
Lumbar region
Iliac fossa
Hypogastrium

fascia lata just below the inguinal ligament and a portion passes more inferiorly to attenuate and disappear in the mid-thigh. It is contiguous with Colles' fascia of the vulva and perineum.

The deeper musculotendinous structures are next encountered. A thick central linear aponeurosis of longitudinal tendinous structures, termed the *linea alba*, is perforated by the umbilicus. Narrower and parallel inferior to the umbilicus, it thins and broadens as it passes caphalad, and inserts upon the sternum and adjacent tissues. It is relatively avascular and without significant innervation.

The longitudinal *rectus muscle* (Fig. 2–10) is encased by a tough aponeurotic tendinous sheath (frequently misnamed the "fascial sheath") for most of its length. Anchored transversely to the *rectus sheath* at several sites by tendinous inscriptions, its function, in addition to support and protection of abdominal viscera, is to assist in flexion and stability of the thoracolumbar spine. The muscle arises from the xiphoid process and costal cartilages, courses caudally, and inserts horizontally on the superior and posterior surfaces of the pubis. A small accessory muscle, the *pyramidalis*, is frequently present. It arises

from the pubis but immediately courses superiorly and medially to insert on the linea alba. The lateral border of the rectus, frequently palpable, is called the *semilunar line*. From the level of the anterior superior iliac spine caudally, the posterior "fascia" of the rectus sheath is absent. This abrupt termination of the posterior wall of tendinous sheath forms a horizontal line called the *arcuate line* (also called the *semicircular line of Douglas*). Peritoneum and *transversalis fascia* are immediately posterior to rectus muscle below the arcuate line. Blood is supplied to these muscles and their adjacent fascia by the inferior and superior epigastric vessels.

The lateral abdominal wall is formed by three broad, flat, thin muscles and their tendons:

1. The *external oblique muscle* arises from the ribs and costal and intercostal structures and courses medially and inferiorly. The muscle body inserts on the anterior iliac crest. Medially, the tendon fuses with those of the other two muscles to form the *conjoint tendon*, which inserts into the linea alba. The inferior margins of the tendons of each muscle coalesce to form the inguinal ligament.

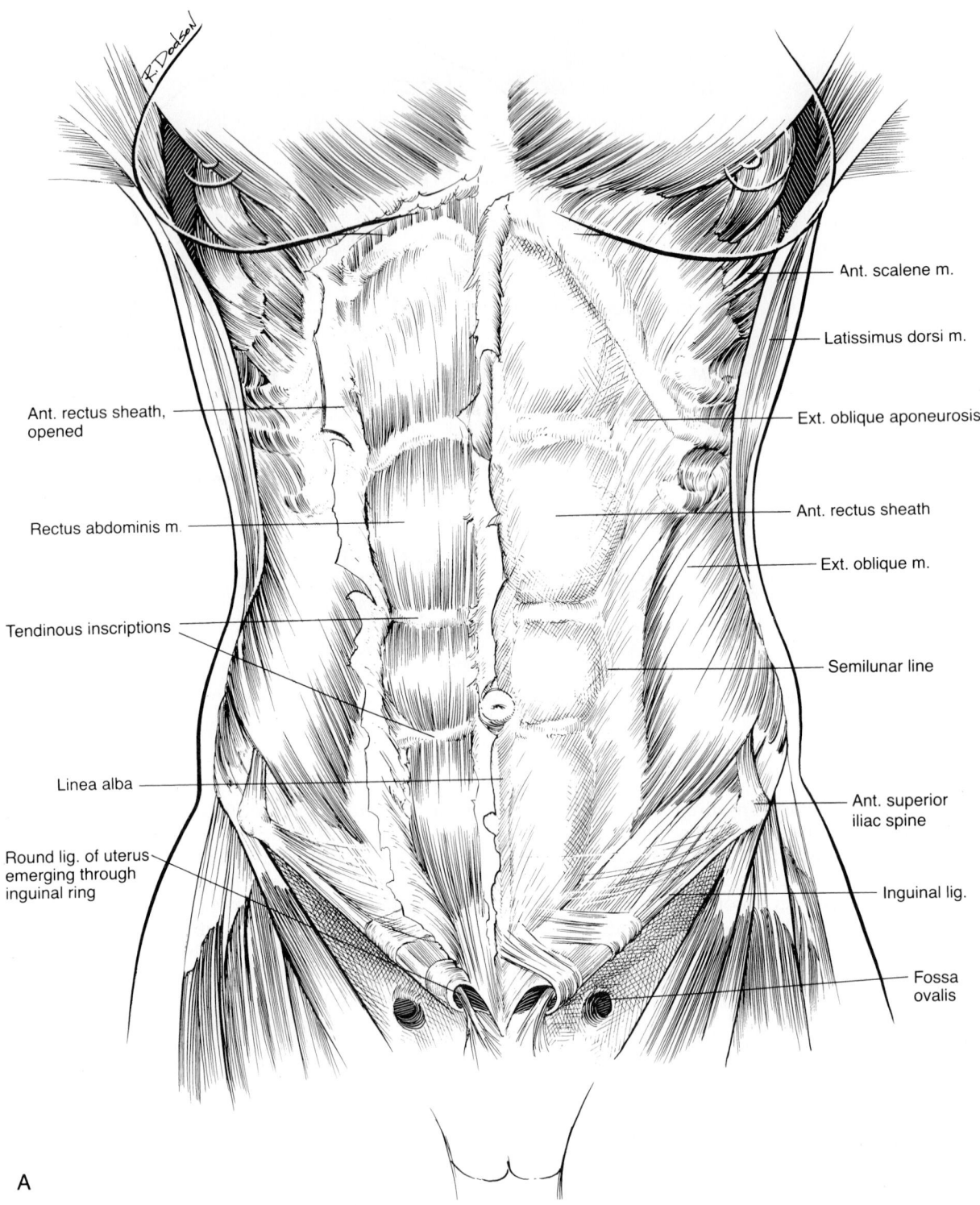

Ant. scalene m.

Latissimus dorsi m.

Ant. rectus sheath, opened

Ext. oblique aponeurosis

Rectus abdominis m.

Ant. rectus sheath

Ext. oblique m.

Tendinous inscriptions

Semilunar line

Linea alba

Ant. superior iliac spine

Round lig. of uterus emerging through inguinal ring

Inguinal lig.

Fossa ovalis

A

Figure 2–10
A and *B*, Muscles and tendons of the abdominal wall. *Illustration continued on opposite page*

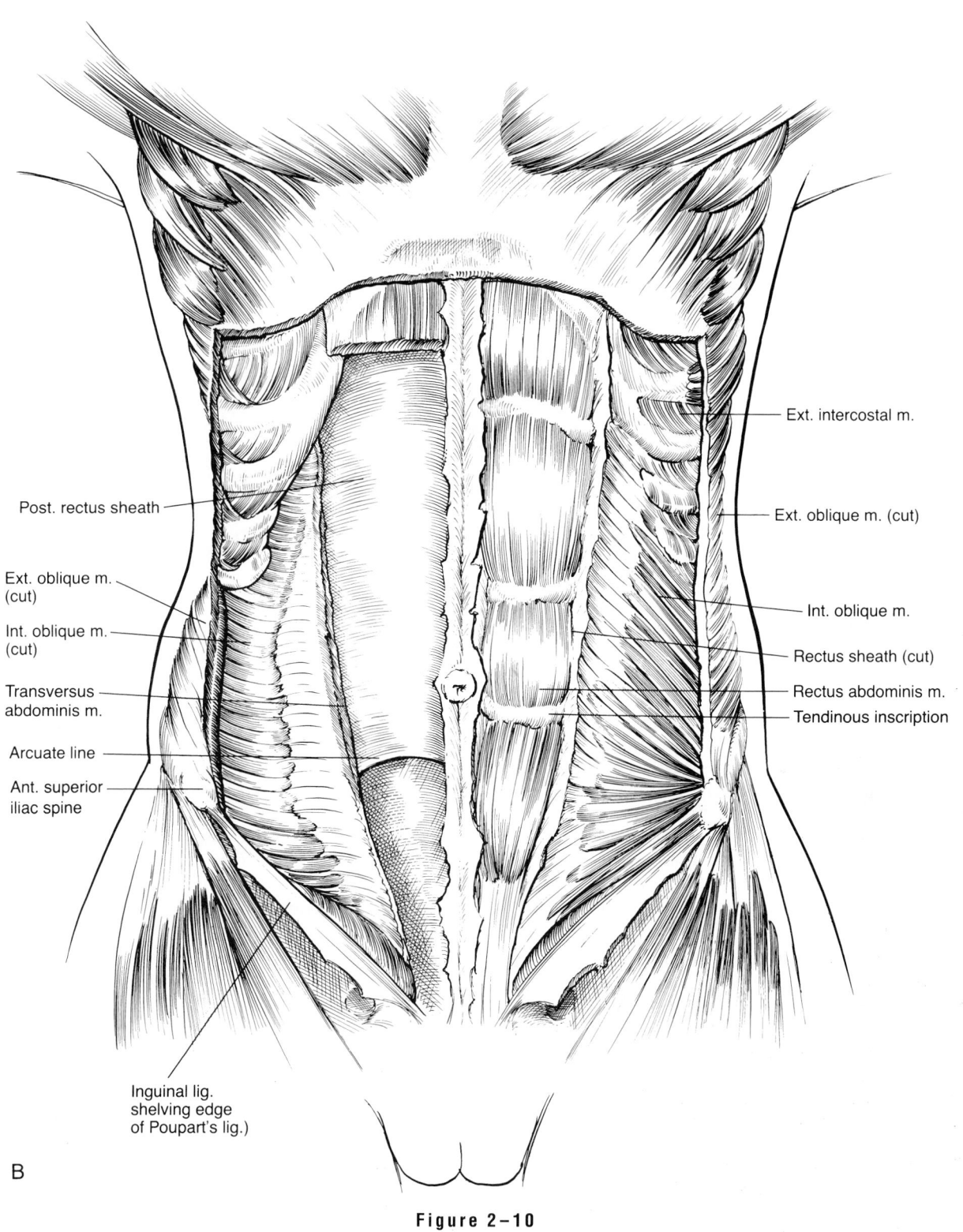

Ext. intercostal m.

Post. rectus sheath

Ext. oblique m. (cut)

Ext. oblique m. (cut)

Int. oblique m.

Int. oblique m. (cut)

Rectus sheath (cut)

Transversus abdominis m.

Rectus abdominis m.

Tendinous inscription

Arcuate line

Ant. superior iliac spine

Inguinal lig. shelving edge of Poupart's lig.)

B

Figure 2–10
Continued

Illustration continued on following page

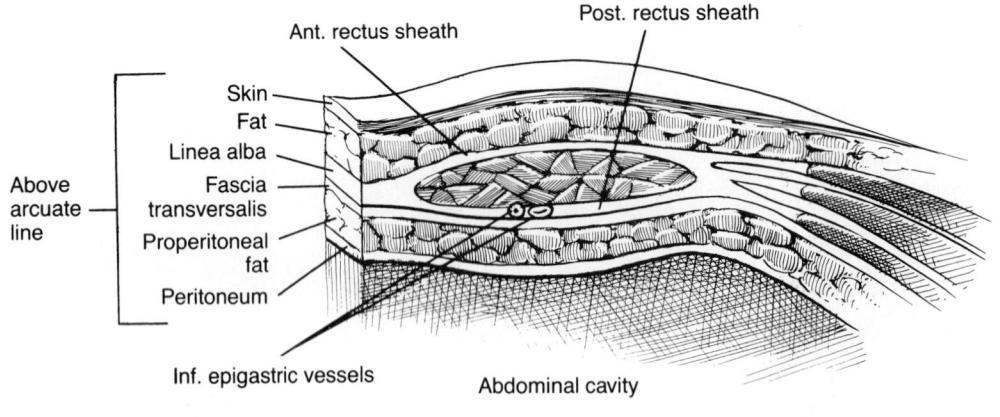

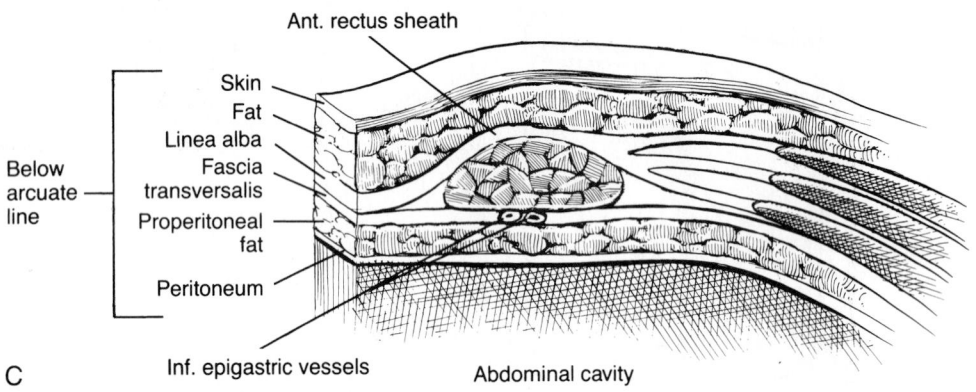

Figure 2-10

Continued C, Cross sections of abdominal wall above and below the arcuate line.

2. The *internal oblique muscle*, just deep to the external oblique, originates from the lumbar fascia and anterior iliac crest, courses cephalad and medially, and inserts superiorly on the ribs and costal margin and medially with the linea alba.
3. The *transversus abdominis muscle*, the deepest of the three, originates from the anterior iliac crest, lumbar fascia, and costal and intercostal structures. It courses directly medially to insert upon the linea alba.

In addition to protection of abdominal viscera, these three muscles contribute to latral flexion and lateral rotational stability of the thoracolumbar spine. The tendinous insertions of these muscles form the rectus tendinous sheath as they course medially. Above the arcuate line, their arrangement is similar to that seen in Figure 2–10. Below the arcuate line, the posterior rectus sheath is usually "absent."

The *inguinal canal* is also formed by these three muscles and their tendons (Fig. 2–11). The canal is approximately 4 cm in length; its inferior wall is the inguinal ligament and its reflections on pelvic bone. It extends from the internal to the external inguinal ring. The *internal inguinal ring* is a hiatus approximately 1 cm in diameter in the transversus abdominis muscle, which is approximately halfway along the inguinal ligament. The midportion of the canal is formed by a similarly sized hiatus in the internal oblique muscle. The *external inguinal ring* is a 1-cm hiatus in the conjoint tendon just lateral to the pubic tubercles. The only barrier of abdominal contents to the internal inguinal ring is the peritoneum and its overlying *transversalis fascia*, a thin membranous structure posterior to rectus muscle that also constitutes the posterior wall of the inguinal canal. The inguinal canal therefore passes obliquely through the anterior abdominal wall, medially and inferiorly, and parallel to its inferior wall, the inguinal ligament. The superior and anterior walls of the canal are the inferior portions of the three muscles and their tendons.

Contents within the inguinal canal are the round uterine ligament as it passes on its way to insert into the labium majus and the *ilioinguinal nerve*, a branch of the nerve roots T12 and L1. This nerve supplies motor innervation to the inferior portions of the three lateral abdominal wall muscles and sensory innervation to the inferiomedial abdominal wall and anterior external genitalia. Also within the canal are fused vestigial remnants of a peritoneal diverticulum, the *processus vaginalis* (also known as the *canal of Nuck*), which may extend into the labium majus.

The *umbilicus* is a hiatus through the midline abdominal wall tendinous structures through which fetal vessels communicate with the placenta. This hi-

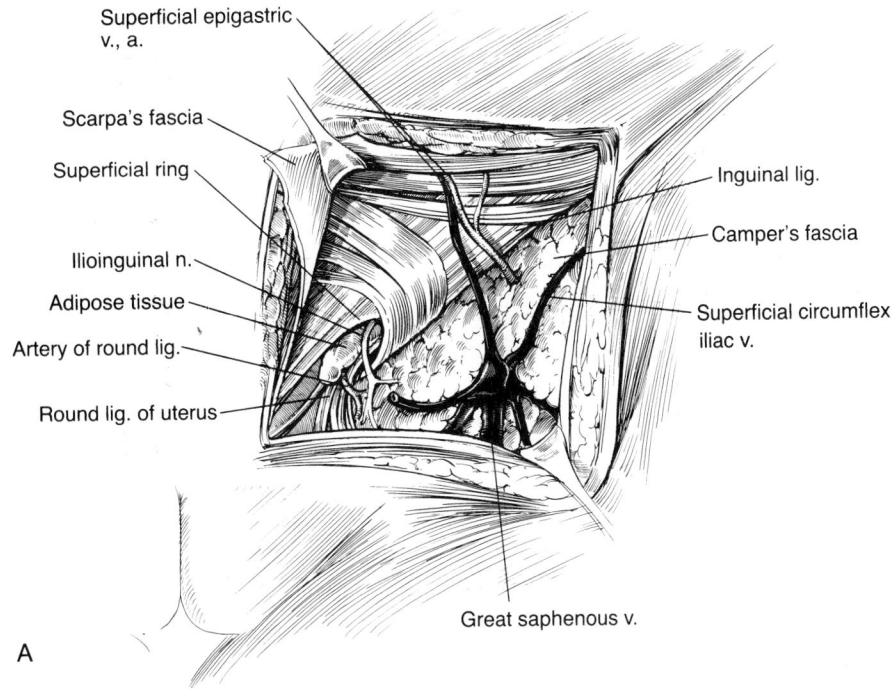

Superficial epigastric
v., a.

Scarpa's fascia

Superficial ring

Ilioinguinal n.

Adipose tissue

Artery of round lig.

Round lig. of uterus

Inguinal lig.

Camper's fascia

Superficial circumflex
iliac v.

Great saphenous v.

A

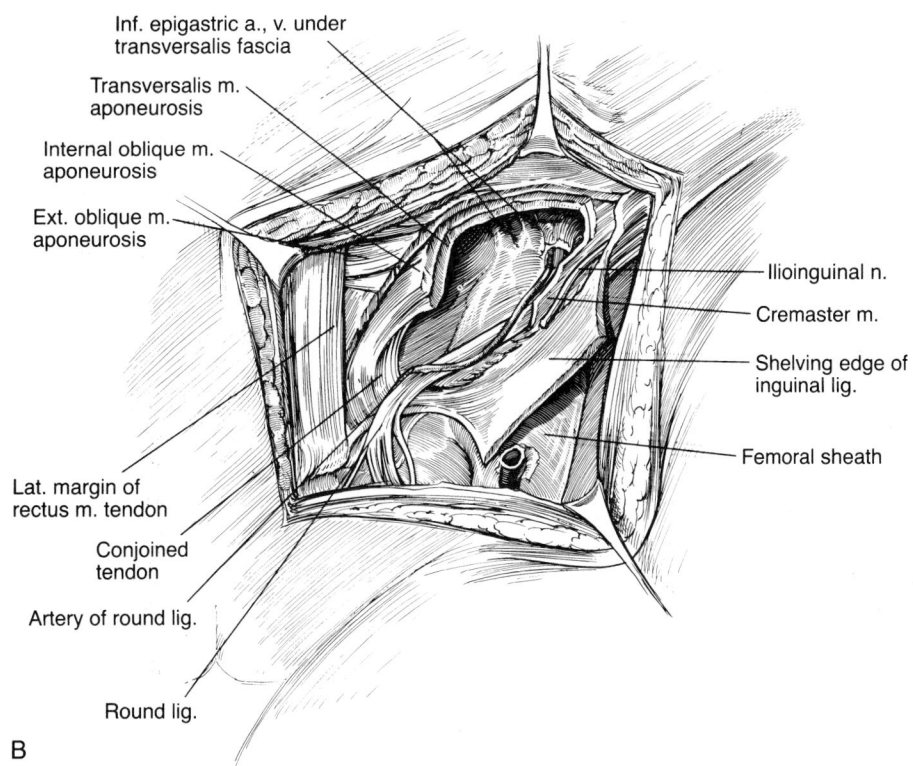

Inf. epigastric a., v. under
transversalis fascia

Transversalis m.
aponeurosis

Internal oblique m.
aponeurosis

Ext. oblique m.
aponeurosis

Lat. margin of
rectus m. tendon

Conjoined
tendon

Artery of round lig.

Round lig.

Ilioinguinal n.

Cremaster m.

Shelving edge of
inguinal lig.

Femoral sheath

B

Figure 2–11
Details of the inguinal canal.

atus is of widely varying dimensions, but in most adults it is completely fused. Camper's and Scarpa's fascias are absent at this site, and the abdominal skin is indented.

Between the musculotendinous layers of the abdominal wall and the parietal peritoneum lies a varying amount of preperitoneal adipose tissue. Through these extraperitoneal tissues course several vestigial structures. Caphalad to the umbilicus courses the obliterated umbilical vein, the *round hepatic ligament*. It extends directly from the umbilicus to the falciform ligament. Caudal to the umbilicus, the termination of each internal iliac artery, the *obliterated umbilical arteries*, course upward and medially along the abdominal wall from the lateral border of the bladder to the umbilicus and are termed the *lateral umbilical ligaments*. As they converge upon the umbilicus, they approximate the vertical midline subumbilical *median umbilical ligament*. This single fibrous structure extends directly from the anterior midline bladder to the umbilicus. A fibrotic remnant of the fetal allantois, it is also termed the *urachus*; in most individuals, the lumen has been obliterated.

The *parietal peritoneum* is a highly innervated membranous layer of tissue less than 1 mm in thickness that lines the entire abdominal cavity. It is contiguous with the parietal peritoneum of the pelvic cavity, with the exterior (through the fallopian tubes, uterine cavity, and vagina), and with the abdominal and pelvic visceral peritoneum. It is composed of an inner layer of cuboidal or flattened mesothelium with several underlying layers of collagen and fibroblasts. Like the rest of the peritoneum, it is highly innervated. Its blood supply and innervation derive from vessels and nerves of adjacent muscles, tendons, and bones. Lymphatic drainage is to the lymph node groups closest to the involved area in the horizontal plane. A large proportion of the ureteral blood supply is through peritoneal vessels, both within the pelvis and outside of it.

CLINICAL CORRELATES

- The superficial epigastric vessels are the usual source of postoperative *prefascial (subcutaneous) hematomas* from transverse incisions used to gain access to the lower abdomen and pelvis. During laparoscopic procedures, avoidance of the superficial epigastric vessels during placement of secondary trocars is usually possible in thin patients. Transillumination of the abdomen with the laparoscopic light source can allow for external visualization and avoidance of these vessels.
- The majority of postoperative *subfascial hematomas* are from disrupted branches of the inferior epigastric vessels and can occur regardless of the type of lower abdominal incision. The epigastric vessels may be the cause of incisional hematomas with either muscle- or tendon-splitting incisions. Injuries to the inferior epigastric vessels during placement of secondary trocars in laparoscopic procedures are reduced by the surgeon's understanding of internal abdominal anatomic landmarks. The inferior epigastric vessels can be followed as they depart from the space bordered medially by the medial umbilical ligament and laterally by the exit of the round ligament into the inguinal canal. Occasionally, in obese patients, identification is difficult, and simply placing the trocar lateral to the rectus sheath (6 to 7 cm lateral to the midline) should avoid injury to the vessels.
- The Pfannenstiel incision is a popular incision used by gynecologic surgeons. *Pfannenstiel syndrome* is due to entrapment or injury to the iliohypogastric or ilioinguinal nerves. Knowledge of the anatomic locations of these nerves is vital to avoiding injury and recognizing this as a potential cause of severe abdominal wall pain (Sippo et al, 1987). The nerves travel between the internal and external oblique aponeuroses, penetrating the external oblique aponeurosis just medial to the anterior superior iliac spine, then travel inferiorly along the inguinal ligament. Injury may result by extending the incision beyond the lateral aspect of the rectus muscle into the internal oblique muscle and transecting the nerve. Also, incorporating the nerves in the suture closure or scar formation involving one of the nerves can lead to pain. Diagnosis is made by injecting a local anesthestic to obtain a nerve block. If this is successful, repeat injection or surgical interruption or possible release of the nerve is indicated.
- The avascular nature of the linea alba, in combination with its inherent strength, accounts for the popularity of the vertical midline lower abdominal incision. (However, its avascular nature contributes to its susceptibility to necrosis with subsequent disruption if it is not reapproximated using proper surgical technique.)
- *Indirect* inguinal hernia, the most common form of inguinal hernia, is the herniation of abdominal contents and peritoneum through the internal inguinal ring and into the inguinal canal. In most individuals, it is prevented by several anatomic factors: the transversalis fascia, the oblique nature of the canal through the abdominal wall, the virtual closure of the canal with muscle contraction, the weakest areas of the abdominal wall (the inguinal rings) being separated by some distance, and protection of the region by the flexed thigh. Patency of the processus vaginalis and conditions that increase intra-abdominal pressure or decrease fascial integrity predispose to this condition.
- *Direct* inguinal hernia is the herniation of peritoneum and abdominal contents through the posterior wall of the inguinal canal, medial to the inferior epigastric vessels, lateral to rectus muscle, and superior to the inguinal ligament (Hesselbach's triangle).
- The remnants of the patent processus vaginalis can enlarge, forming cysts of the canal of Nuck that are often confused with inguinal hernias. These may occur anywhere within the inguinal canal or anterior labium majus.
- Spigelian or lateral ventral hernias tend to occur along the line of Spigelius (semilunar line located at the lateral edge of the rectus muscles), often at the level of the arcuate line (semicircular line of Douglas). The herniation typically passes through the transversus abdominis and internal oblique muscles but not the external oblique aponeurosis. The pain caused by this rare hernia can often be confused with pelvic pathology.
- The attenuation of the tendinous layers of the abdominal wall at the umbilicus (or failure of fusion during early childhood) and the lack of inherent strength of the peritoneal layer predispose this area of

the abdominal wall to herniation. Acquired umbilical hernias most commonly occur in women and the obese. Likewise, attenuation of the linea alba (from multiple childbirths, abdominopelvic mass, malnutrition, chronic ascites) may cause rectus diastasis and midline lower abdominal hernias.

- Portal venous hypertension may cause recanalization of the umbilical vein, which then anastomoses with other abdominal wall vessels. The resulting pattern of engorged veins radiating from the umbilicus is the so-called caput medusae.
- Persistent patency of all umbilical blood vessels, which can complicate any umbilical or paraumbiliucal incision, has been described.
- Persistent patency of the urachus can lead to vesicocutaneous fistula after surgical interruption or after urethral obstruction. Patency of portions of the urachus can lead to cystic dilation (the "urachal cyst").
- Irritation of the parietal peritoneum, such as with peritonitis or incision, predisposes to a reflex autonomic dysfunction of bowel, the adynamic ileus. The highly innervated nature of the peritoneum accounts for the increased pain and comparatively prolonged postoperative ileus experienced by patients undergoing laparotomy rather than laparoscopic or vaginal operation. Additionally, rich innervation of the parietal and visceral peritoneum accounts for most of the pain experienced with culdocentesis and paracentesis.
- Because a significant proportion of ureteral blood supply is through peritoneal vessels, care should be taken with pelvic operation to avoid extensive separation of the ureter from peritoneum. ∎

THE PARIETAL PELVIS

The parietal pelvis consists of the bones, muscles, and ligaments that are the framework on which the pelvic viscera rest; it confines the abdominal contents inferiorly and provides support for the spine.

The bony pelvis is formed by four bones: the two hip (innominate) bones, the sacrum, and the coccyx. These bones form the borders of the *true pelvis*. The inferior margin of the true pelvis is the pelvic diaphragm; the iliopectineal line defines the superior limit of the true pelvis. The *false pelvis*, that area contained by the iliac fossae, lumbar vertebrae, and lower abdominal wall, is contiguous with both the true pelvic and the abdominal cavities. Because the false pelvis is of little gynecologic significance, further mention of *pelvis* refers to the true pelvis.

The *innominate bones* are each composed of the pubis, the ilium, and the ischium, which articulate at the acetabulum (Figs. 2–12 and 2–13). The *acetabulum* is a saucer-like depression on the lateral surface of the innominate bone that articulates with the femoral head. Each thin *ilium* articulates with the superior sacral ala, or wing, at the sacroiliac joint and curves laterally, then anteriorly, to the acetabulum. Externally palpable landmarks include the *posterior* and *anterior superior iliac spines*. The *pubis* forms the anterior border of the true pelvis. Its body is separated from its opposite counterpart by a vertically oriented discoid cartilaginous joint, the *pubic symphysis*. As it extends laterally from the midline, the pubis divides into a superior and an inferior ramus,

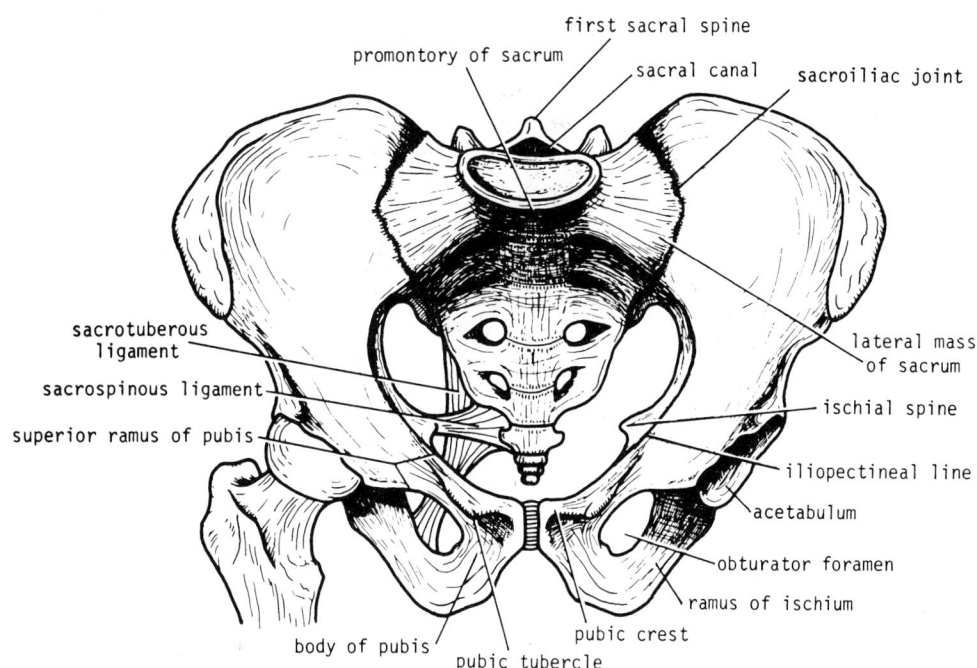

Figure 2-12
Bony pelvis, anterior view. (Modified from Snell RS: The Pelvis: Part I. The pelvic walls. In: Clinical Anatomy for Medical Students. Boston: Little, Brown & Co, 1973:267, with permission.)

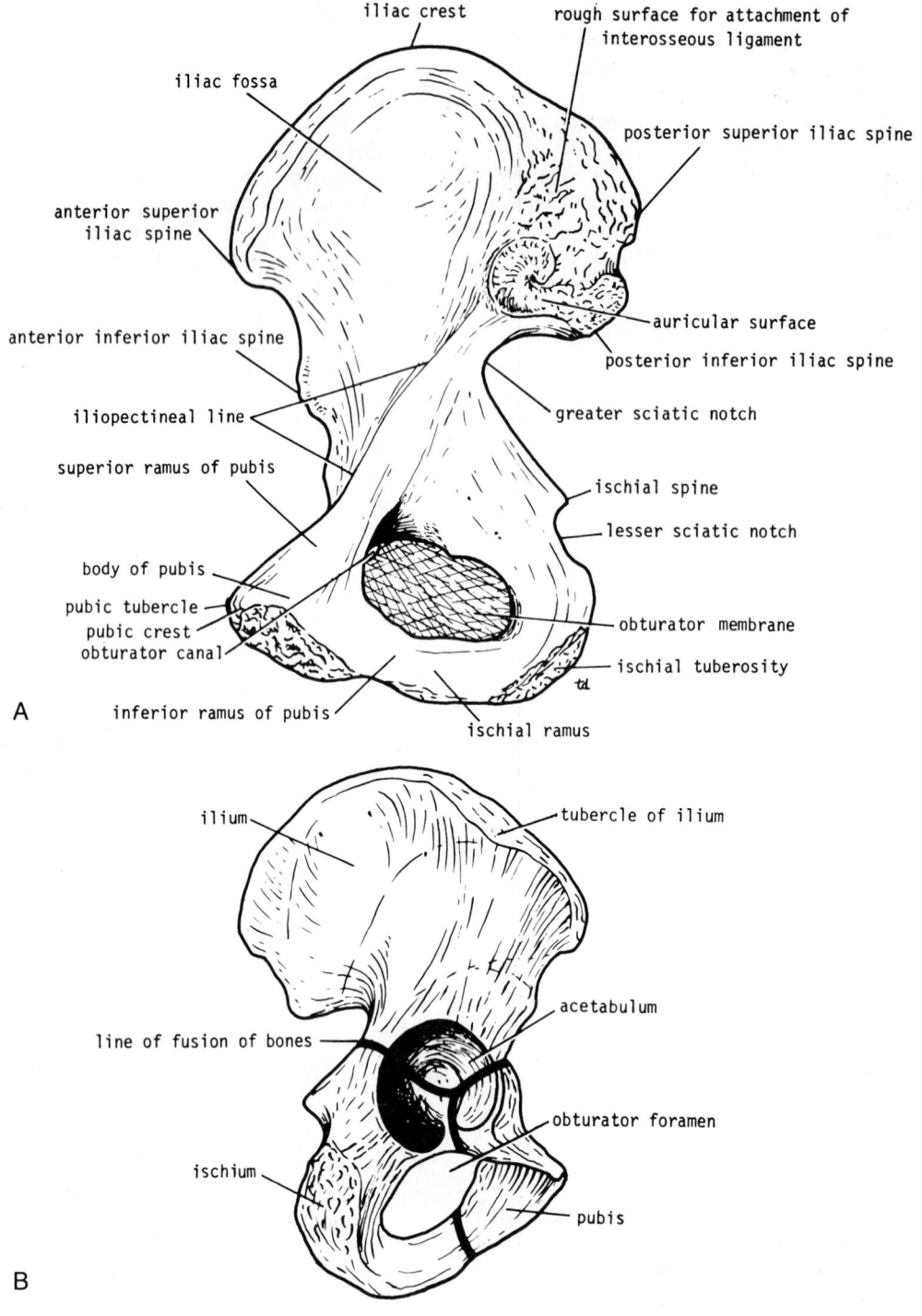

Figure 2-13
Bony pelvis. *A*, Medial view. *B*, Lateral view. (Modified from Snell RS: The pelvis: Part I. The pelvic walls. In: Clinical Anatomy for Medical Students. Boston: Little, Brown & Co, 1973:273, with permission.)

each of which adjoins an ischial ramus. The pubis forms the medial half of the obturator foramen. Externally palpable landmarks include the *pubic tubercle*, the attachment point of the inguinal ligament to the pubic bone. The *ischium* arises at the acetabulum, courses inferiorly, then curves medially, branching into two rami, which in turn fuse with the corre-

sponding ramus of the pubis. The ischium forms the lateral half of the obturator foramen. Externally palpable landmarks include the *ischial tuberosity*. The posteromedial border of the ischium gives rise to a protrusion, the *ischial spine*, palpable in most patients through the lateral vagina. The ischial spine divides the posterior border of the ischium into the greater sciatic notch, which is superior to the spine, and the lesser sciatic notch, which is inferior to it.

The posterior border of the pelvis is demarcated by the sacrum and coccyx. The *sacrum* consists of five vertebrae fused to form a single pyramid-shaped bone; the base of this inverted pyramid articulates with the fifth lumbar vertebra. The apex of the pyramid articulates inferiorly with the coccys. The sacrum and coccyx curve together anteriorly. Superiorly, one pelvic border is found at the *sacral promontory*, an anterior prominence of the superior portion of the first sacral vertebra. Laterally, the first and second sacral vertebrae articulate with the ala of the ilium to form the sacroiliac joint. The *sacral foramina* harbor vessels and lymphatic tissue. Anterior sacral nerve roots also exit from the foramina here, course laterally, and form the *sacral nerve plexus* (nerve roots S1 through S4) and the *pudendal nerve*. The sacral nerve plexus adjoins the lumbosacral trunk to become the sciatic nerve and provides major sensorimotor input to the sciatic nerve. The *coccyx*, composed of four fused rudimentary vertebrae also arranged in an inverted pyramid inferior to the sacrum, is the insertion point for the coccygeus muscle from the ilium, for the sacrospinous ligament, and for the anococcygeal body.

Situated immediately anterior to the sacrum lies the *median sacral artery*, a direct branch of the aorta. Its complementary vein drains into the left common iliac vein. Within the same retroperitoneal space lie the pelvic portion of the *sympathetic trunk* laterally and the more anterior *presacral nerves* and *pelvic (parasympathetic) splanchnic nerves*. On the posterior surfaces of the sacral vertebrae, the *sacral canal* contains neural and related structures terminating the spinal column, and terminates in the caudal *sacral hiatus*, which is often palpable.

Communications through the walls of the pelvis include the obturator foramen, the greater sciatic foramen, and the lesser sciatic foramen. The *obturator foramen* is occluded inferiorly by the broad flat *obturator internus muscle*, which arises from the rami of the pubis and ischium, passes posteriorly, converges to form a tendon, leaves the pelvis by the *lesser sciatic foramen*, and inserts upon the greater trochanter of the femur. Its function is lateral rotation of the thigh. There is a small defect in the obturator internus muscle and its underlying membrane, the *obturator canal*, through which the obturator nerve and vessels leave the pelvis. The *obturator nerve* arises from the lumbar plexus (nerve roots L2 through L4) and provides sensory and motor innervation to the medial compartment of the thigh.

The paired *sacrospinous ligaments* arise from the lateral border of the fourth and fifth sacral vertebrae and coccyx, course laterally and anteriorly, and converge to insert on the ischial spines. They are essentially inseparable from the paired triangular *coccygeus muscles*, which abut the levator ani complex (Figs. 2–14 and 2–15). The *sacrotuberous ligament*, broader than the sacrospinous ligament and slightly

exterior to it, arises on each side from the lower half of the lateral sacrum, and passes inferiorly and medially to insert on the ischial tuberosity. These three structures divide the lateral plane of the pelvis into the two sciatic foramina. The *piriformis muscle* bilaterally arises from the anterior sacrum and the posterior ilium, passes through the *greater sciatic foramen* with the sciatic nerve to the exterior, converges to form a tendon, and inserts on the greater trochanter of the femur. Like the obturator internus muscle, it also acts as a lateral rotator of the thigh. The *sciatic nerve* exits the pelvis and provides sensory innervation to the posterior and lateral thigh and anterior, lateral, and posterior leg and foot. It supplies motor innervation to the muscles of the posterior compartment of the thigh and all leg and foot muscles.

Other structures that exit from the pelvis at the greater sciatic foramen are the gluteal vessels and the internal pudendal artery. The internal pudendal artery enters the ischiorectal fossa with the pudendal nerve through the lesser sciatic foramen and travels within a fascial sheath (the *pudendal*, or *Alcock's, canal*) along the lower margin of the obturator internus muscle to later branch into inferior rectal, perineal, and clitoral branches within the urogenital diaphragm.

The floor of the pelvis, the *pelvic diaphragm*, is composed of the muscular *levator ani* complex, a paired saucer-like sling of muscle that attaches to the posterior, lateral, and anterior pelvis (Figs 2–16 and 2–17). It is perforated by two foramina. The vagina and urethra pass through the anterior hiatus, and the rectum passes through the posterior one. Although composed of multiple muscular components, the levator muscle acts as a unit to aid in control of micturition, to aid in fecal continence, and to prevent herniation of abdominopelvic viscera. There are three components of the levator ani. Anterior and most medial is the *puborectalis muscle*, which arises from the pubis, courses posteriorly, encircles the vagina, forms a raphe with its opposite counterpart between the vagina and rectum, and then continues posteriorly to encircle the rectum, decussating into the midline anococcygeal body. The posteriormost component of the levator ani is the *iliococcygeus muscle*, which arises from a tendinous condensation on the inner border of the obturator internus muscle (the *arcuate line*, also called the *arcus tendineus fascia pelvis*, or *white or White's line*), courses centrally and inferiorly, inserts into the anococcygeal body, and is contiguous with the anterior border of the coccygeus muscle. The intermediate component, the *pubococcygeus muscle*, likewise arises from the pelvic arcuate line and pubis, courses centrally and inferiorly, and inserts into the anococcygeal body. There is little, if any, space separating these muscles in the normal patient, and the pelvic arcuate line appears as a single tendinous condensation on the lateral pelvic wall. The importance of the levator plate (not the pelvic visceral ligaments) as the prime support of the pelvic viscera was first substantiated by levator myography (Berglas and Rubin, 1953).

The fusiform *psoas muscle* passes inferiorly and laterally through the false pelvis, attenuating as it passes underneath the mid-inguinal ligament to insert upon the lesser trochanter of the femur. Its anteromedial surface is a border of the false pelvis. The triangular *iliacus muscle* arises from the iliac crest and partially fills the iliac fossa as it courses inferiorly, parallel and lateral to the psoas. It attenuates as it passes under the inguinal ligament and inserts into the psoas tendon. It also is one of the borders of the false pelvis. Both muscles are responsible for thigh flexion at the hip and for internal rotation of the thigh.

The course and origin of *pelvic blood vessels* (see Fig. 2–14) are highly variable from individual to individual. Even within the same individual, the blood supply is bilaterally identical in only 50% of instances, usually because of variation in parietal branching patterns of the internal iliac artery (Braithwaite, 1952). The *aorta* bifurcates at the level of the fourth lumbar vertebra in most people. The resultant common iliac vessels course inferiorly and laterally approximately 5 cm, along the medial surface of the psoas muscle through the false pelvis. Each common iliac artery then branches at approximately the upper third of a line from anterior superior iliac spine to

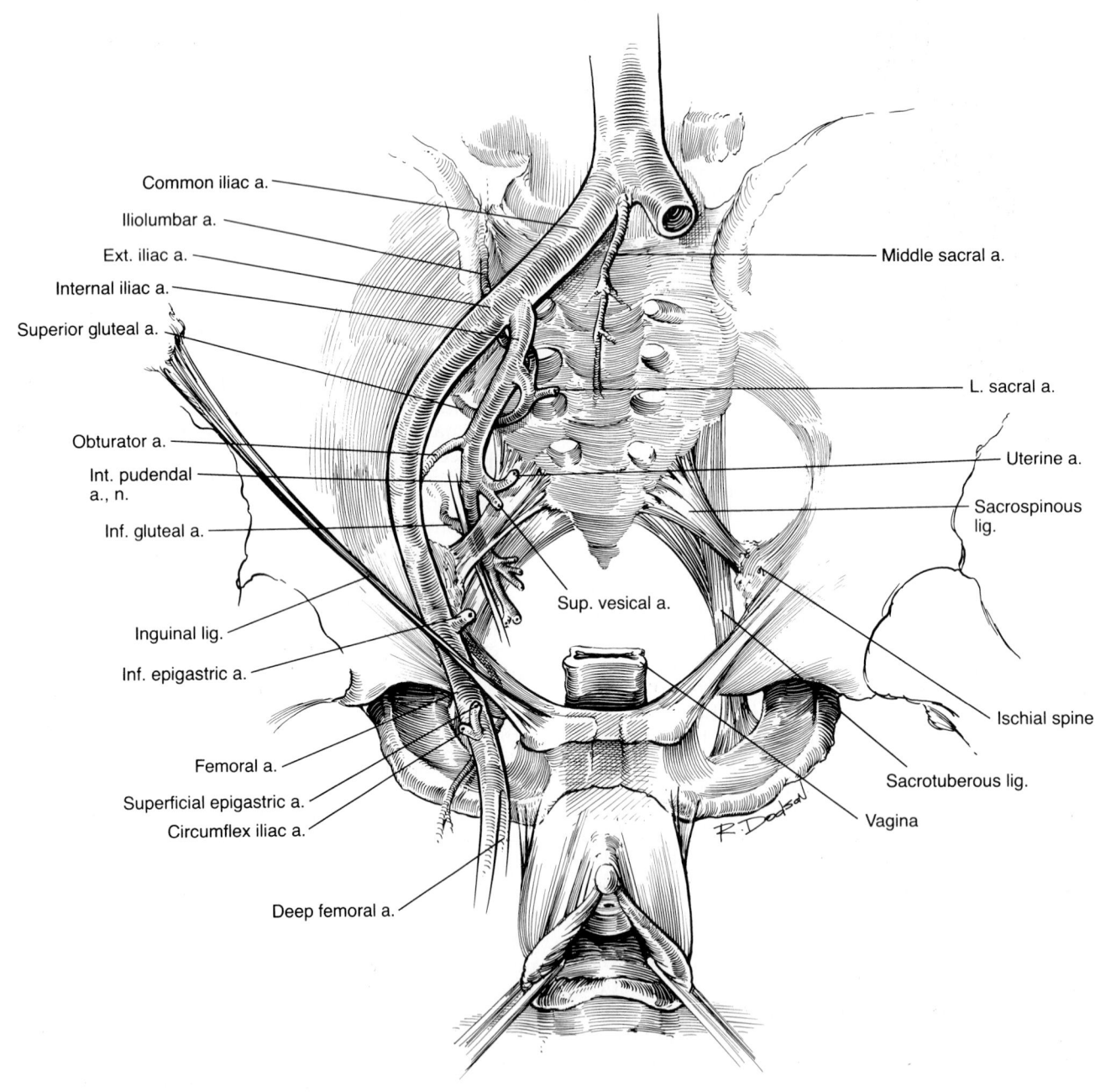

Figure 2–14
Pelvis with detail of internal iliac artery and branches.

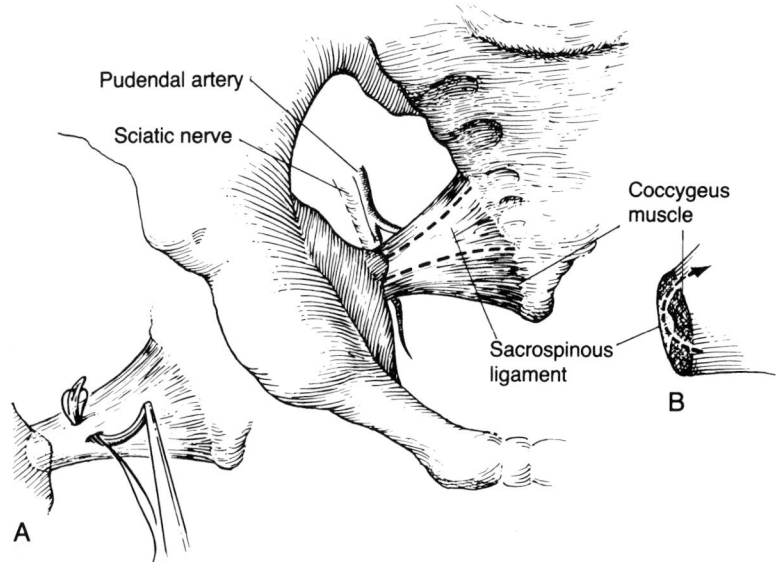

Figure 2–15
Coccygeus muscle, sacrospinous ligament, and adjacent structures. (Modified from Nichols DH, Randall CL: Massive eversion of the vagina. In: Vaginal Surgery. 3rd ed. Baltimore: Williams & Wilkins, 1989:339, with permission.)

pubic tubercle into its external iliac and internal iliac branches. The *external iliac artery* continues in the same direction as the common, gives origin to the inferior epigastric artery, and then passes underneath the inguinal ligament to become the femoral artery. The *internal iliac artery* courses inferiorly, medially, and posteriorly from its origin to supply the parietal pelvis, pelvic viscera, and buttocks. Its length is an average of 4 cm, and it divides into anterior and posterior divisions or trunks. Although four different branching patterns are described (Roberts and Krishingner, 1967), the following branches are identifiable in most females:

1. Anterior division
   • Parietal branches
     – Obturator artery
     – Internal pudendal artery
     – Inferior gluteal artery
   • Visceral branches
     – Obliterated umbilical artery
     – Superior vesical artery
     – Middle rectal artery
     – Uterine artery
     – Vaginal (inferior vesical) arteries
2. Posterior division
   • Parietal branches
     – Iliolumbar artery
     – Lateral sacral artery
     – Superior gluteal artery

Each arterial branch has a venous counterpart with a similar course and branching pattern. Although it is nearly impossible to identify pelvic vessels other than the iliacs by their point of origin, they can be readily identified by caliber, course, and the end-organ or structure served. These characteristics are much more constant from side to side and from individual to individual.

The ureter generally lies medial to and in close proximity to the internal iliac artery along the entire length of the artery.

The sensory *genitofemoral nerve* closely approximates the psoas muscle and the external iliac artery until it bifurcates approximately at the inguinal ligament. The genital branch passes through the inguinal canal to innervate the vulva; the femoral branch continues under the inguinal ligament to provide sensation to the mid-inguinal region.

The *parietal pelvic fascia* covers the internal surfaces of the pelvic muscles and bones and pelvic diaphragm. It is membranous and provides no structural support except at the point the levator ani inserts on it at the pelvic arcuate line. It reflects on and becomes contiguous with the visceral endopelvic fascia. The *parietal peritoneum* lines the pelvic walls, is contiguous with the peritoneum of the false pelvis and abdomen, and is reflected toward the mid-pelvis on the pelvic viscera.

CLINICAL CORRELATES

• Pathology within nearby articulating joints (lumbar intervertebral, sacroiliac, hip, and pubic symphysis), especially in the aged patient, frequently leads the gynecologic practitioner to search for visceral pathology as a cause of pelvic symptoms.
• Retropubic surgery, particularly the Marshall-Marchetti-Krantz retropubic urethropexy, may cause chronic inflammation and pain in the pubic symphysis (pubic symphysitis).
• Another site of female hernia is the obturator foramen. The hernial sac dissects along the obturator vessels and nerve through the obturator canal. This type of hernia occurs most frequently in females and in the elderly and malnourished.
• Inflammatory or malignant pelvic disease can involve the psoas muscle so that a patient has pain with

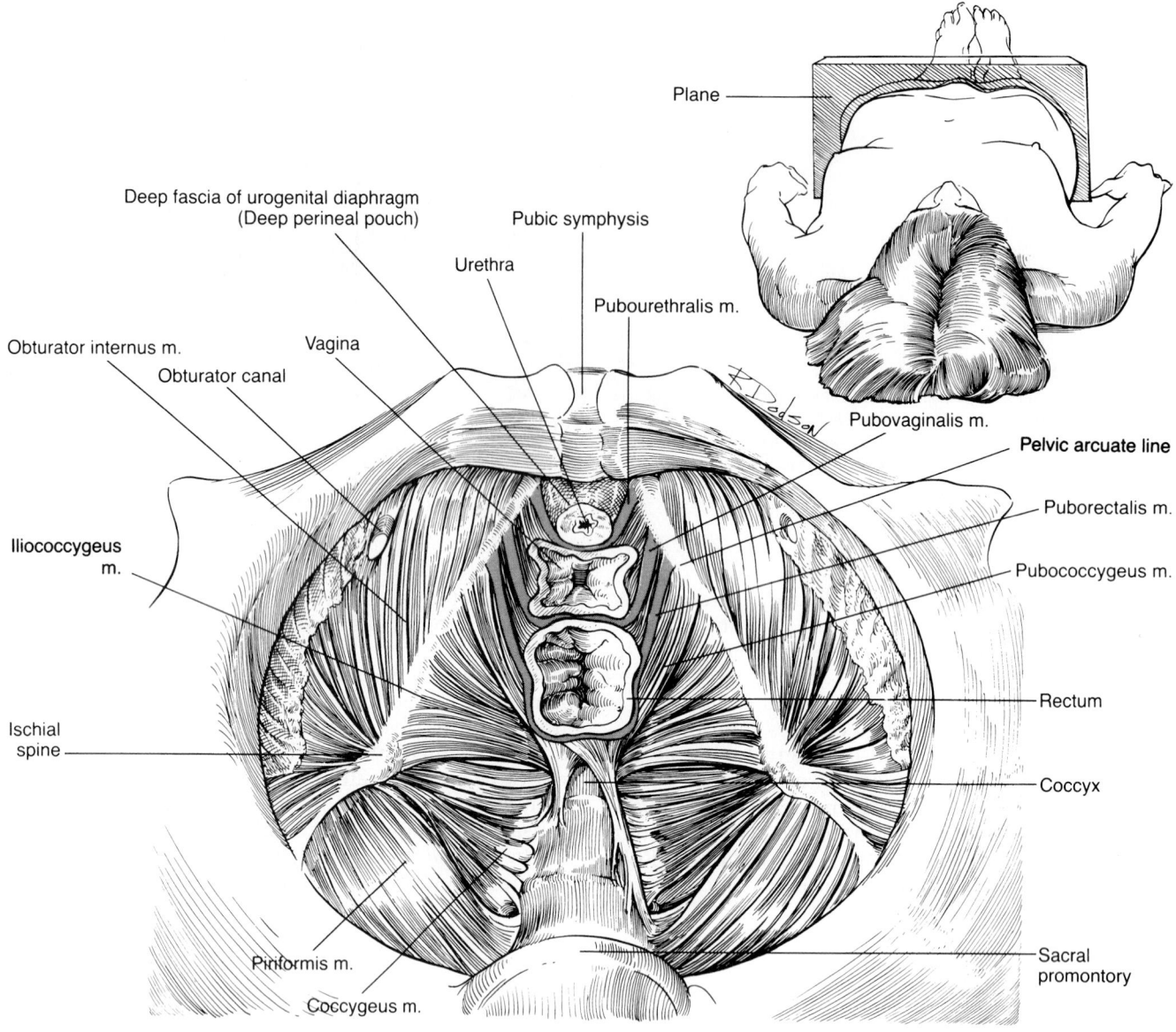

Figure 2–16
Pelvic floor from above.

thigh flexion or has excessive psoas rigidity (positive psoas sign). Likewise, in the presence of a similar disorder affecting the obturator internus muscle, lower quadrant pain will be elicited by rotation of the flexed thigh (positive obturator sign).

- Attenuation or diastasis of the levator ani or its raphes predisposes to rectocele and cystocele formation. Successful repair of a rectocele cannot occur without restoration of the original position of the levator muscle.
- Some patients with cystocele are believed to have bladder herniation secondary to rupture of the normal fascial attachment between lateral vagina and the pelvic arcuate line (also called the white line, White's line, or arcus tendineus fascia pelvis; named after George White, who in 1909 described the first paravaginal repair). Surgical restoration of this

relationship (the paravaginal suspension) (Richardson et al, 1981) corrects the cystocele and may also correct stress urinary incontinence.
- The vaginal apex can be sutured to coccygeus muscle and sacrospinous ligament in cases of vaginal eversion (Nichols, 1982). The proximity of pudendal vessels and nerves, and of the sciatic nerve, predisposes to their damage with improperly placed sutures (see Fig. 2–15).
- Because of the close proximity of the median and lateral sacral vessels to pelvic visceral nerves, profound hemorrhage may result from presacral neurectomy. The sacral vessels are also often encountered in such procedures as abdominal sacral colpopexy and pelvic exenteration. These vessels are frequently difficult to visualize because they are embedded in the dense presacral connective tissue. This dense tissue prevents

Symphysis pubis

Pubococcygeus m.

Rectum

Puborectalis m.

Urethra

Vagina

Iliococcygeus m.

Anococcygeal body

Coccyx

Ischiococcygeus m.

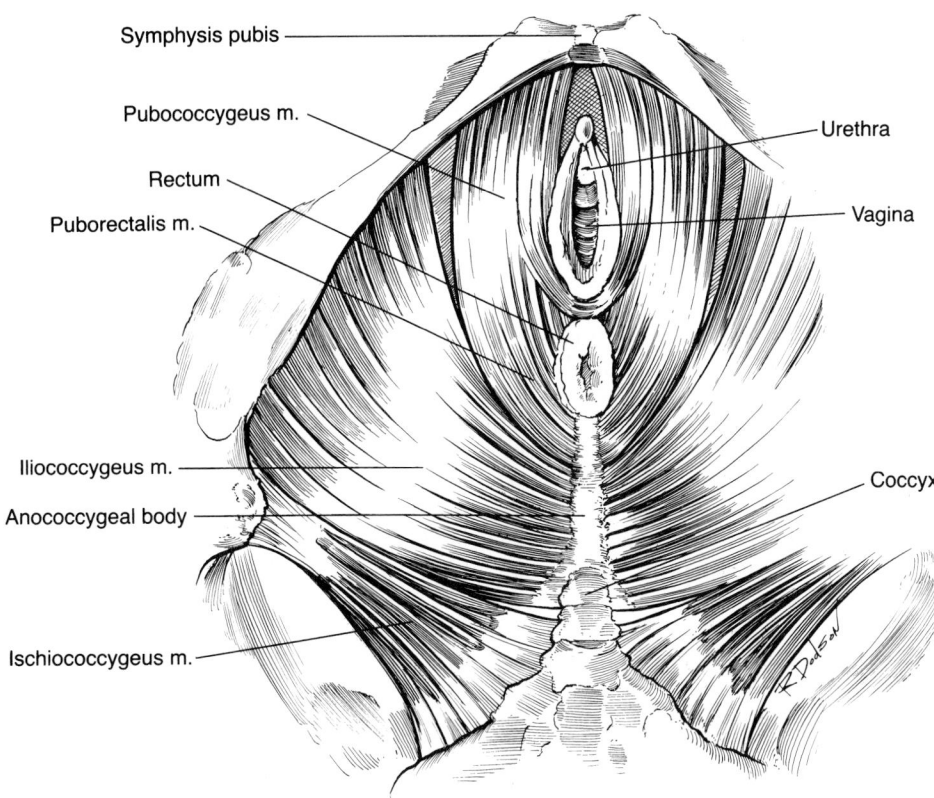

Figure 2–17
Pelvic floor from below.

clamping, clipping, or suture ligature of the vessel. A "thumb tack" to compress the vessel against to sacrum has been used successfully to control bleeding.

- Internal iliac artery (hypogastric artery) ligation has been used for the control of pelvic hemorrhage. Specifically, the anterior division of the internal iliac artery should be ligated, thereby sparing the posterior branch that gives rise to the iliolumbar, lateral sacral, and superior gluteal arteries. If one is not able to isolate the anterior division, the artery can be ligated proximal to the bifurcation. The posterior division of the internal iliac artery is usually identified 3 to 4 cm distal to the bifurcation of the common iliac artery; it initially tends to run posteromedially, then turns lateral, and when ligated can lead to gluteal claudication. Ligation of the anterior division of the internal iliac artery does not halt blood flow: it merely reduces pulse pressure (by as much as 85%), allowing hemostasis to occur more readily. Because of at least three critical arterial anastomoses (lumbar to iliolumbar, median sacral to lateral sacral, and superior rectal to middle rectal), flow within the artery is maintained, although reversed (Burchell and Olson, 1966), thereby maintaining blood flow to pelvic viscera, buttocks, and vulva. Pregnancy can occur after ligation (Mengert et al, 1969). Because of the proximity of this artery to pelvic veins and ureter, complications do occur: this has led to more focal hemorrhage control, such as with uterine artery ligation or arteriography and arterial embolization. These critical anastomoses also maintain blood flow

to the lower extremity from the pelvic viscera in cases of chronic occlusion of the external iliac or femoral artery.

- Extensive anastomoses exist between pelvic veins and presacral and epidural veins. In this valveless system, pelvic processes (malignancy, infection, thrombophlebitis, etc.) may directly extend to the central nervous system.
- Obturator nerve injury, occasionally seen with pelvic lymphadenectomy or exenteration, leads to sensory deficits over the medial thigh and motor deficits of the muscles of the medial fascial compartment of the thigh. This is manifested by weak thigh adduction. Unlike injury to other major motor nerves that traverse the pelvis, injury to this nerve is often not noted by the patient or is easily compensated.
- Sciatic nerve injury can occur from exaggerated positioning of the patient, as with the dorsal lithotomy and the modified lithotomy ("jack-knife" or "ski") positions, currently popular for laparoscopy, urologic surgery, or exenteration. In this position, stretching of the sciatic nerve between the greater sciatic notch and the fibular head can result in damage, usually to its lateral portion (the peroneal trunk). The resultant dysfunction of the peroneal nerve leads to sensory dysfunction of the posterior and lateral leg and foot. Motor dysfunction leads to calf muscle dysfunction and inability to dorsiflex the foot (footdrop).
- The genitofemoral nerve is frequently interrupted during pelvic lymphadenectomy, temporarily interfering with sensation to inguinal and vulvar areas.

• Pelvic malignancy can secondarily involve any of the pelvic nerves, leading to a wide array of sensory and motor disorders. ∎

PELVIC VISCERA

Ligaments

All pelvic ligaments are normally paired, and many form the boundaries of potential pelvic spaces. These ligaments serve mostly to stabilize pelvic viscera in the sagittal and coronal planes; they do little to provide axial or longitudinal support. They may be divided into two groups: those that do not demarcate potential pelvic spaces and those that do. The former group consists of round uterine, round ovarian, broad, and ovarian suspensory ligaments. They can stretch extensively with uterine or adnexal enlargement.

The *round uterine ligament* is the first ligament seen when inspecting the anterior pelvis (Fig. 2–18; see also Fig. 2–21). Composed mostly of fibrous tissue with a small admixture of smooth muscle, it arises from the anterior uterine cornu, courses anteriorly and laterally, enters the inguinal canal and travels through it, ramifies, and inserts in the labium majus. It provides no structural support to the uterus except to limit movement of the uterine fundus. Its blood supply is from a branch of the uterine artery proximally (Sampson's artery) and of the inferior epigastric artery distally. The male homolog is the lower portion of the testicular gubernaculum.

The *broad ligament* (Fig. 2–18) is really no more than a reflection of peritoneum from the serosa of the uterus laterally to the parietal peritoneum of the lateral pelvic wall and upward from the pelvic floor. It is composed of an anterior and a posterior leaf containing uterine vessels, nerves, and lymphatics, the fallopian tube in the upper border, the round ligaments of uterus and ovary, a portion of the ureter, and the epoöphoron and paroöphoron. The leaves become contiguous superiorly where they surround the diameter of the fallopian tube and form the free upper edge. The posterior leaf becomes contiguous with the medial surface of the ovarian suspensory ligament. Inferiorly, the layers separate as they descend to cover the pelvic floor and join the parietal peritoneum. This ligament does little more than prevent lateral motion of the uterine fundus during locomotion. The ovary is attached to its posterior leaf by the mesovarium.

Extending from the posterior uterine cornu to the medial pole of the ovary is the *round ovarian ligament* (also called the utero-ovarian ligament). Its 2.5-cm length is adherent anteriorly to the posterior leaf of the broad ligament. Its counterpart in the male is the upper portion of the testicular gubernaculum. The *mesovarium* is a peritoneal fold attaching anterior ovary to posterior leaf of broad ligament. It conducts the vessels, nerves, and lymphatics to and from the ovarian hilum. The *epoöphoron and paroöphoron* are vestigial remnants of the mesonephric duct within the broad ligament and mesovarium. The *suspensory ligament of the ovary*, like the broad ligament, is also merely a peritoneal reflection and has no fascial component. Termed the *infundibulopelvic ligament* by many clinicians, it contains the ovarian vessels, nerves, and lymphatics. Arising at the posterolateral pelvic brim near the sacroiliac joint, it courses infer-

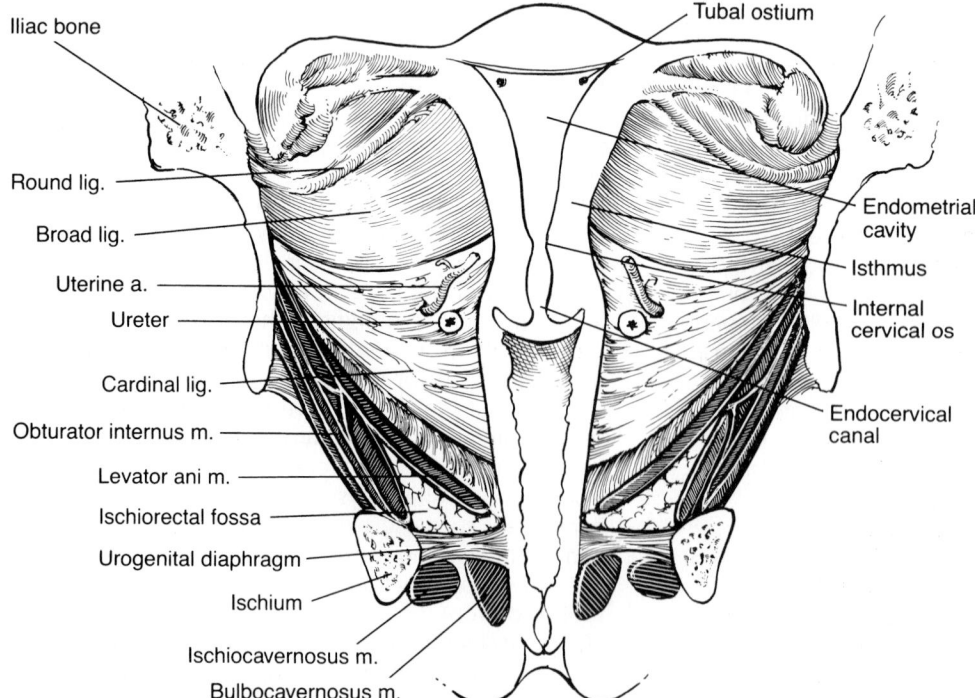

Iliac bone

Tubal ostium

Round lig.

Broad lig.

Uterine a.

Ureter

Cardinal lig.

Obturator internus m.

Levator ani m.

Ischiorectal fossa

Urogenital diaphragm

Ischium

Ischiocavernosus m.

Bulbocavernosus m.

Endometrial cavity

Isthmus

Internal cervical os

Endocervical canal

Figure 2–18
Coronal section of pelvis.

iorly and medially. Its lateral leaf becomes contiguous with parietal peritoneum of the lateral pelvic wall. The medial leaf becomes contiguous with the posterior leaf of the broad ligament medially and the uterosacral ligament and rectouterine pouch inferiorly. It aids in limitation of adnexal motion during locomotion.

The remaining major pelvic visceral ligaments are condensations of the endopelvic fascia, are paired, and demarcate the peripheral potential pelvic spaces. They have more significant structural and functional roles and are not generally stretched to a great degree with uterine or adnexal enlargement.

The *endopelvic fascia* is connective tissue that covers and supports the pelvic viscera. It is contiguous with the thin, membranous parietal pelvic fascia that overlies inner surfaces of the pelvic muscles and periosteum. Its condensation in the region of the uterus is termed *parametrium* by clinicians. These fascial condensations form the two more important structural uterine ligaments—the cardinal and the uterosacral—and the structurally important vesical ligament—the pubocervical ligament. The parametrium contains lymphatic channels from the central pelvic viscera to the internal iliac and obturator lymph nodes. A few parauterine lymph nodes may exist in the parametrium. The broad ligament, along with its con-

tents, is also referred to by some as being a parametrial structure.

The *cardinal ligament*, also known as the transverse cervical, or Mackenrodt's, ligament, lies within the base of the broad ligament. It is a condensation of fascia and smooth muscle, just lateral to the cervix and upper third of the vagina, which courses posteriolaterally to attach to the membranous fascia of the lateral wall of the pelvic diaphragm. At the cervix, it is contiguous with the uterosacral ligament, but as they leave the cervix they separate, the uterosacral passing almost directly posteriorly. The cardinal ligament contains blood vessels from the internal iliac complex and lymphatics and is perforated by the ureter (through "Wertheim's tunnel") as the ureter courses anteriorly and medially around the cervix into the bladder (Figs. 2–18 and 2–19). It conducts important nerves from the pelvic autonomic plexus to the uterus and bladder.

The *uterosacral ligament* lies just medial and inferior to the suspensory ovarian ligament, forming the lateral walls of the rectouterine pouch. An excellent analogy is that the uterosacral ligament's configuration is similar to a fan: it is thick and almost round in cross section at its attachment to the posterolateral cervix, vaginal fornix, and cardinal ligament; as it passes posteriorly, it quickly attenuates, widens, and

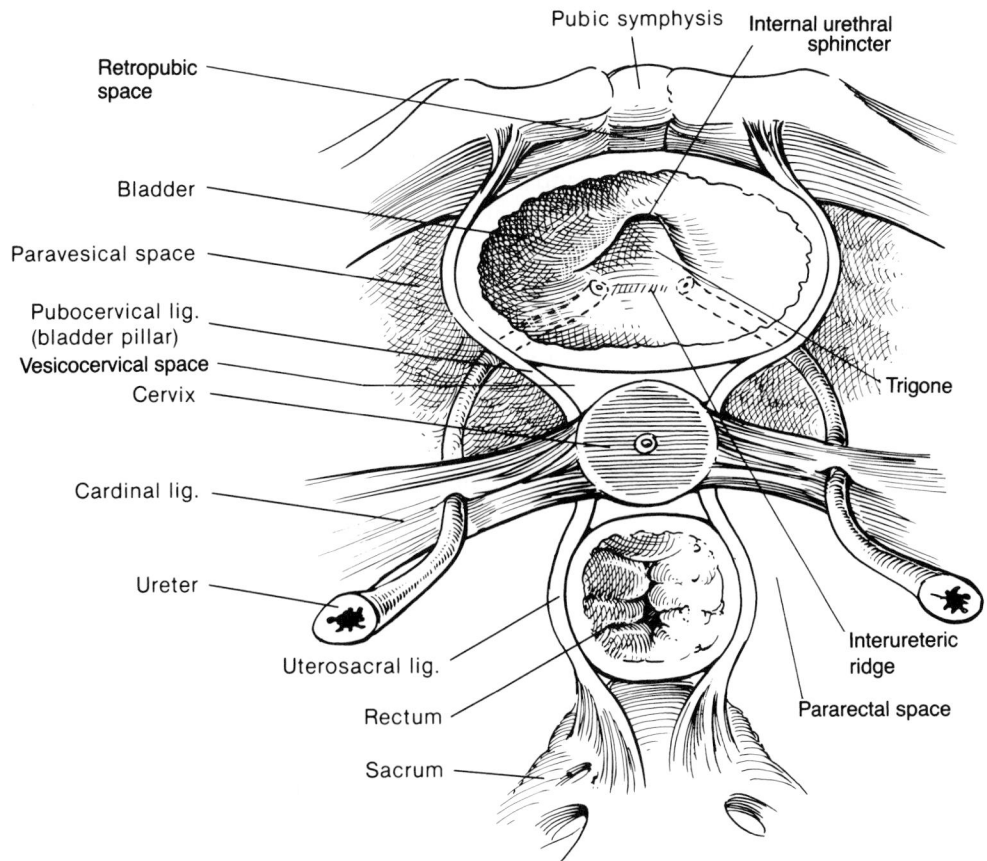

Figure 2–19
Visceral pelvic ligaments and pelvic retroperitoneal spaces.

broadens. The distal ureter is adherent to its lateral surface and runs along its length for a short distance. More posteriorly, the ligament passes lateral to the rectum; it and its pararectal fat are adherent medially. The ligament is perforated lateral to the rectum by the middle rectal artery, which passes medially from the internal iliac artery. After it passes lateral to the rectum, the ligament curves medially to form the "rectal pillars" of the posterolateral rectum and inserts on the lateral sacral periosteum (see Fig. 2–19). Like the cardinal ligament, it also conducts autonomic nerve branches to the rectum, uterus, and bladder. It contains a few lymphatic vessels to presacral lymph nodes that are not clinically important.

Traditionally, it was thought that these two ligaments played an active role in axial support of uterus and cervix. More recently, those who have extensively studied the functional anatomy of the pelvic floor have determined that the urogenital and pelvic diaphragms, not the ligaments, are the structures that prevent visceral prolapse (Berglas and Rubin, 1953; Nichols and Randall, 1989; Zacharin, 1989). The ligaments merely function to position the viscera at the point at which they are most efficiently supported by these diaphragms.

The thin *pubocervical ligament* arises vertically from the posterior periosteum of the medial pubic bone, just lateral to the symphysis, in the retropubic space. Its most superior component (*pubovesicocervical ligament*) passes directly posteriorly, just lateral to the bladder, and invests on the cervix (Fig. 2–19). The thick condensation of this component between bladder base and anterior cervix lateral to the midline is called by many the "bladder pillars." The inferior and contiguous component of the pubocervical ligament, the shorter *pubourethral ligament*, extends from the anterior and posterior medial pubis inferiorly to surround the urethra in a sling-like conformation. The male homolog of the pubocervical ligament is the puboprostatic ligament. Illustration of the structure and function of these ligaments has been elegantly provided by Zacharin (1963) and by Milley and Nichols (1971).

CLINICAL CORRELATES

- Enlargement of the uterus with traction upon the round uterine ligament may result in inguinal or labial pain. It is often seen in pregnancy, is associated with ambulation, and is frequently worse on the right side because of dextrorotation of the uterus. This pain often has to be differentiated from the pain of labor.
- The round uterine ligaments are important surgical landmarks. Division of this ligament and the adjacent peritoneum allows access to the retroperitoneal portion of the broad ligament (uterine vessels) and the suspensory ovarian ligament (ovarian vessels and ureter).
- When the uterine position was formerly believed to be pathologically abnormal, plication or transposition of the round uterine ligaments (the "uterine

suspension" operation) was used to "restore" the uterus to its "normal" position, in the process unnaturally angulating the vagina superiorly from its usual horizontal position. This widening of the rectouterine pouch predisposes to enterocele.
- The epoöphoron and the paroöphoron may cystically enlarge and cause a "paraovarian" and broad ligament cyst. These vestigial structures are remnants of the mesonephric kidney in the embryo. They are homologous to the efferent ductules of the testis.
- Parametrial thickening is best detected during rectovaginal examination, without which a pelvic examination is never complete. Parametrial thickening or nodularity (generally within the cardinal and uterosacral ligaments) may signify malignancy, "pelvic inflammatory disease," endometriosis, prior pelvic radiotherapy, or inflammation from gastrointestinal disease.
- Surgical interruption of the cardinal and uterosacral ligaments proximal to their cervical insertions, such as with radical pelvic surgery, also interrupts significant autonomic nerves. A substantial number of these patients will have subsequent bladder atony, rectal atony, or both.
- Failure to properly secure the stump of the cardinal or uterosacral ligament to the vagina during hysterectomy may predispose to later vaginal eversion.
- The McCall culdeplasty, the plication of uterosacral ligaments to each other and to the vaginal cuff and wall, is commonly performed at vaginal hysterectomy to prevent and treat enterocele (McCall, 1957). Other techniques for culdeplasty at the time of abdominal hysterectomy include the Halban and Moschcowitz procedures. Both procedures obliterate the posterior cul-de-sac in an effort to prevent and treat enterocele. ■

Potential Spaces

In the pelvis, there are several potential spaces bounded by ligaments that are relatively avascular. The existence of these spaces allows the independent movement or enlargement of one organ system without affecting the others. Their avascular nature and proximity to critical pelvic structures explain their inclusion by every accomplished pelvic surgeon in the critical knowledge base.

Four potential spaces are of greatest utility to the gynecologist. The retropubic space (of Retzius) and paravesical spaces are both regularly developed and utilized by the surgeon treating incontinence (Fig. 2–19). The pararectal spaces allow access to the internal iliac and uterine arteries and identification of the position and course of ureter. The vesicocervical space must be developed to perform total hysterectomy. The remaining two spaces, the rectovaginal and retrorectal spaces, are not regularly utilized except by the general or radical pelvic surgeon.

Knowledge of the boundaries and the usual site of access to these potential spaces is critical to help avoid damage to vital structures and develop the spaces in an avascular manner. The *retropubic space* (of Retzius) is usually entered just inferior to the pubic symphysis, superior to the parietal peritoneum. It is bounded anteriorly by the transversalis fascia and laterally by the medial umbilical ligaments. The inferior border is the pubic symphysis and the adjacent superior pubic rami with Cooper's ligament. The floor of the *retropubic space* is formed by the urethra, paraurethral ligaments, and bladder. The *paravesical spaces* (paired) are usually entered through the parietal peritoneum in the space between the medial umbilical ligament (obliterated umbilical artery) and the external iliac vein. The boundaries of the paired spaces are anteriorly the pubic symphysis, posteriorly the cardinal ligament, medially the obliterated umbilical artery, and laterally the obturator internus muscle on the pelvic sidewall. The *pararectal spaces* (paired) are usually entered through the peritoneum in the space between the ureter and internal iliac artery. The boundaries of the paired spaces are anteriorly the cardinal ligament, posteriorly the sacrum, medially the rectum, and laterally the internal iliac artery. The *vesicocervical space* is located between the bladder and cervix. It is bounded superiorly by the vesicouterine peritoneal reflection, which is its usual site of entry. The inferior and lateral borders are the vesicocervical ligament and vesicouterine ligaments (bladder pillars), respectively. The *rectovaginal space* is a potential space, as the name implies, between the rectum (posterior) and vagina (anterior). The lateral boundaries are the rectal pillars, which are continuous with the uterosacral ligaments. The inferior aspect of the space is the perineal body. The space is usually entered abdominally through the reflection of the peritoneum from the vagina onto the rectum in the pouch of Douglas or via the perineal route. Finally, the *retrorectal* (presacral) space is bounded anteriorly by the rectum and posteriorly by the sacrum. The lateral borders are the pararectal spaces. The space is usually entered via the pararectal spaces or perineally by transecting the anococcygeal ligament.

CLINICAL CORRELATES

- Identification and development of the peripheral pelvic spaces is requisite for performance of radical hysterectomy or pelvic exenteration. Paravesical, pararectal, vesicocervical, and rectovaginal spaces must be developed for radical hysterectomy. For exenteration, the rectorectal space is dissected in substitution for the rectovaginal space, in addition to those necessary for radical hysterectomy. It may be necessary to develop these spaces with difficult oöphorectomy or hysterectomy to prevent damage to adjacent ureter, vessels, or rectum.
- Development of the retropubic and paravesical spaces may be necessary for surgical correction of urinary

incontinence. The retropubic urethropexy procedure includes development of the retropubic space, placement of sutures in paraurethral fascia, and anchoring them to retropubic tissues. ∎

Viscera

The *uterus*, a thick-walled, hollow, muscular organ in the configuration of an inverted pear, is positioned centrally in the pelvis (Figs. 2–20 through 2–22). It is broader transversely and is covered on its anterior, superior, and posterior surfaces by a medial continuation of the broad ligament peritoneum. This layer is also contiguous with that of the bladder (vesicouterine pouch) and the pelvic sidewalls and rectum (rectouterine pouch). Only the anterior cervix is not covered with peritoneum. Although size varies considerably, dimensions approximate 8 × 5 × 3 cm in the nulliparous patient and weight approximates 90 g.

Longitudinally, the uterus is divided into the apex, or *fundus*, the intermediate body, or *corpus*, and the lower *cervix*. The lateralmost extent of the fundus is termed the *cornu*. The corpus' triangular lumen (in Fig. 2–18) is contiguous with that of the fallopian tubes proximally and the cervix distally. The corpus is separated from the cervix by a circumferential constriction termed the *isthmus*. The fundus and body are almost entirely composed of smooth muscle.

Upon section, the uterus is seen to be organized into three layers (Figs. 2–20 and 2–21). The 0.25- to 0.75-cm-thick luminal lining of the fundus and corpus is columnar epithelium arranged in crypts and glands with surrounding stroma, the *endometrium*. The middle and thickest layer of the uterus is the *muscular layer*, composed of interdigitating bundles of smooth muscle. It varies from 1 to 2 cm in thickness. The outer layer, the *serosa*, is the layer of visceral peritoneum, a single layer of cuboidal or flattened mesothelium.

The portion of the cervix that protrudes into the vaginal lumen and generally rests against the posterior wall of the vagina is termed the *portio vaginalis*. The superficial tissue of the portio vaginalis, which is readily viewed on speculum examination, is termed the *ectocervix*. The lumen of the *external cervical os*, usually 0.5 to 0.75 cm in diameter in the nullipara, opens into the wider *endocervical canal*, narrows again at the isthmus to form the *internal cervical os*, and then adjoins the endometrial cavity (Fig. 2–18). The amount of muscular tissue in the cervix is markedly less than that in the fundus and corpus, the cervix being mostly fibrous and composed mainly of collagen with a small proportion of smooth muscle and elastin. The endocervical epithelium is composed of mucosecretory columnar epithelium in longitudinal ridges.

The uterus is generally positioned at right angles to the axis of the almost horizontal upper vagina (anteversion). The fundus is often bent forward on the

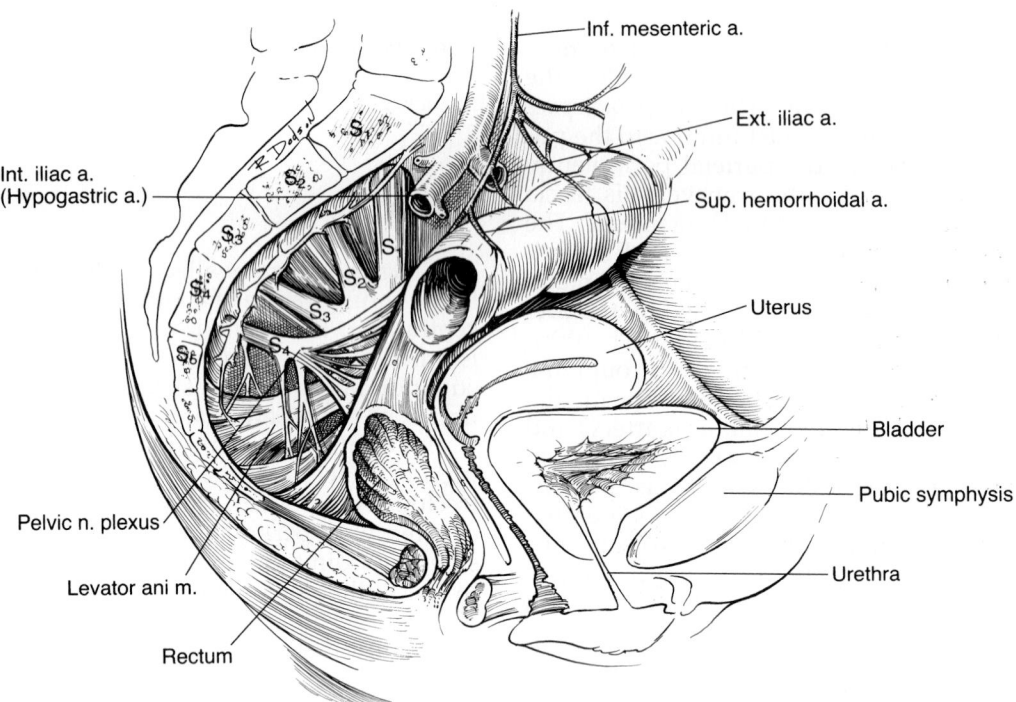

Figure 2–20
Pelvic viscera, sagittal section.

cervix (anteflexion). Retroflexion, retroversion, and neutral positioning are variants of normal, unless acquired.

Anterior to the uterine fundus lies the superior surface of the bladder and vesicouterine pouch with its contents. The cervix is adjacent to the posterior bladder dome and trigone. The rectouterine pouch and its contents lie posteriorly. The fallopian tube enters the uterus at the superior cornual region. The round ligaments of ovary and uterus attach laterally, just below this level. Lateral to the uterine body and fundus lie the broad ligament and uterine vessels. The ureter passes anteriorly, then medially, lateral to the cervix through the cardinal ligament (Figs. 2–19 and 2–22).

The uterine arterial supply is from the *uterine artery*, a branch of the internal iliac artery, which passes superiorly and medially from its origin, through the broad ligament, adjoins the cervix at the level of the internal cervical os, and passes upward along the lateral margin of the corpus and fundus within the broad ligament, anastomosing with tubal branches of the ovarian artery. It is closely approximate to the ureter, crossing over it at right angles, 1.0 to 1.5 cm lateral to the cervix. A descending branch supplies the cervix and anastomoses with the blood supply of the vagina. The uterine vein drains into the internal iliac vein; a portion of fundal venous drainage is into the ovarian veins. Most of the lymphatic drainage of the uterus is through the cardinal ligament to the internal iliac and obturator

lymph nodes. Portions of the fundus, however, drain to para-aortic nodes through the tubal and ovarian lymphatics and to superficial inguinal lymph nodes through the round uterine ligament. Nerves are supplied from the pelvic autonomic plexus through the cardinal and uterosacral ligaments.

CLINICAL CORRELATES

- The cervical transformation zone, that area of the ectocervix that undergoes metaplasia of epithelium from glandular to squamous—extending from original to current squamocolumnar junction—is the area at greatest risk for the development of premalignant and malignant squamous lesions. Cervical conization and a variety of ablative procedures address this disease by removing the epithelium at risk.
- Sutures are often placed in the lateral cervix to encircle the cervical branch of the uterine artery and reduce blood loss from cervical surgery.
- Epithelial (Nabothian) inclusion cysts of the cervix result from traumatic invagination of the surface epithelium. These cysts are lined by nonkeratinizing squamous epithelium, and generally no therapy is required.
- The endocervix is lined with abundant parasympathetic nerve endings. Transcervical manipulation of the cervix, as with an endocervical curettage or endometrial biopsy, can stimulate these nerves and lead to a vasovagal reaction. A vasovagal reaction is characterized by hypotension with

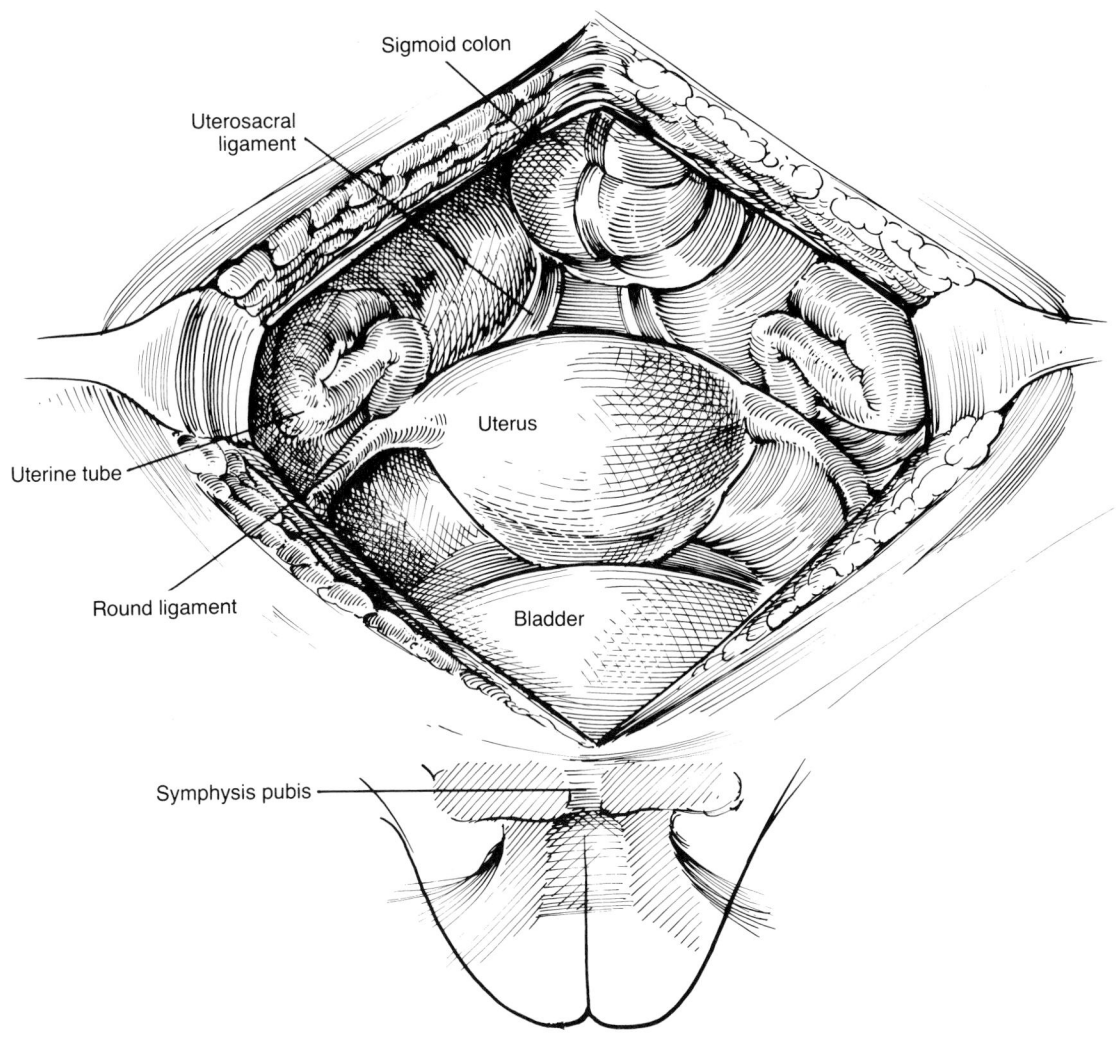

Figure 2–21
Pelvic viscera, view from above.

concurrent bradycardia. Management is usually only supportive care and reassurance; on rare occasions, measures such as atropine or smelling salts may be necessary to resuscitate the patient.

- Acquired uterine retroversion may signify malignant or inflammatory disease posterior to the uterus. Uterine retroposition may also predispose to pelvic entrapment if the uterus enlarges (e.g., as in leiomyomata or pregnancy).
- Ablation of sensory nerves from the uterus and adnexae that intermingle with the autonomic pelvic nerves (the presacral neurectomy) has been reported to provide symptom relief. Because of proximity of the hypogastric nerves to sacral vessels, hemorrhage may result from their interruption.
- *L*aparoscopic *u*terosacral *n*erve *a*blation (the LUNA procedure) has likewise been reported to provide relief of chronic pain (Lichten and Bombard, 1987). Because of its adherence to the lateral surface of the uterosacral ligament, the ureter is prone to injury here (Grainger et al, 1990). Great care must be taken to

avoid damage to the ureter during this procedure; ablation should involve only the medialmost portion of the ligament.
- Hemisection of the uterus in the sagittal plane (morcellation) is performed to aid difficult vaginal hysterectomy. The midsagittal plane is used most frequently, to minimize hemorrhage from the uterine artery on the lateral margin of the uterus.
- Perforation of the uterine corpus in the midline at the time of dilatation and curettage may lead to peritonitis but rarely to hemorrhage. Perforation of the lateral corpus or cervix may produce broad ligament hematoma, secondary to damage of the laterally positioned uterine vessels. Perforation of the anterior cervix may penetrate the bladder, especially when the bladder is full. Avoidance of vesical damage is one of the reasons that bladder drainage should usually precede pelvic operation. Posterior cervical perforation may penetrate the relatively fixed rectum.
- In gynecology, descriptive anatomic names for pelvic organs are derived from the Latin root. The surgical

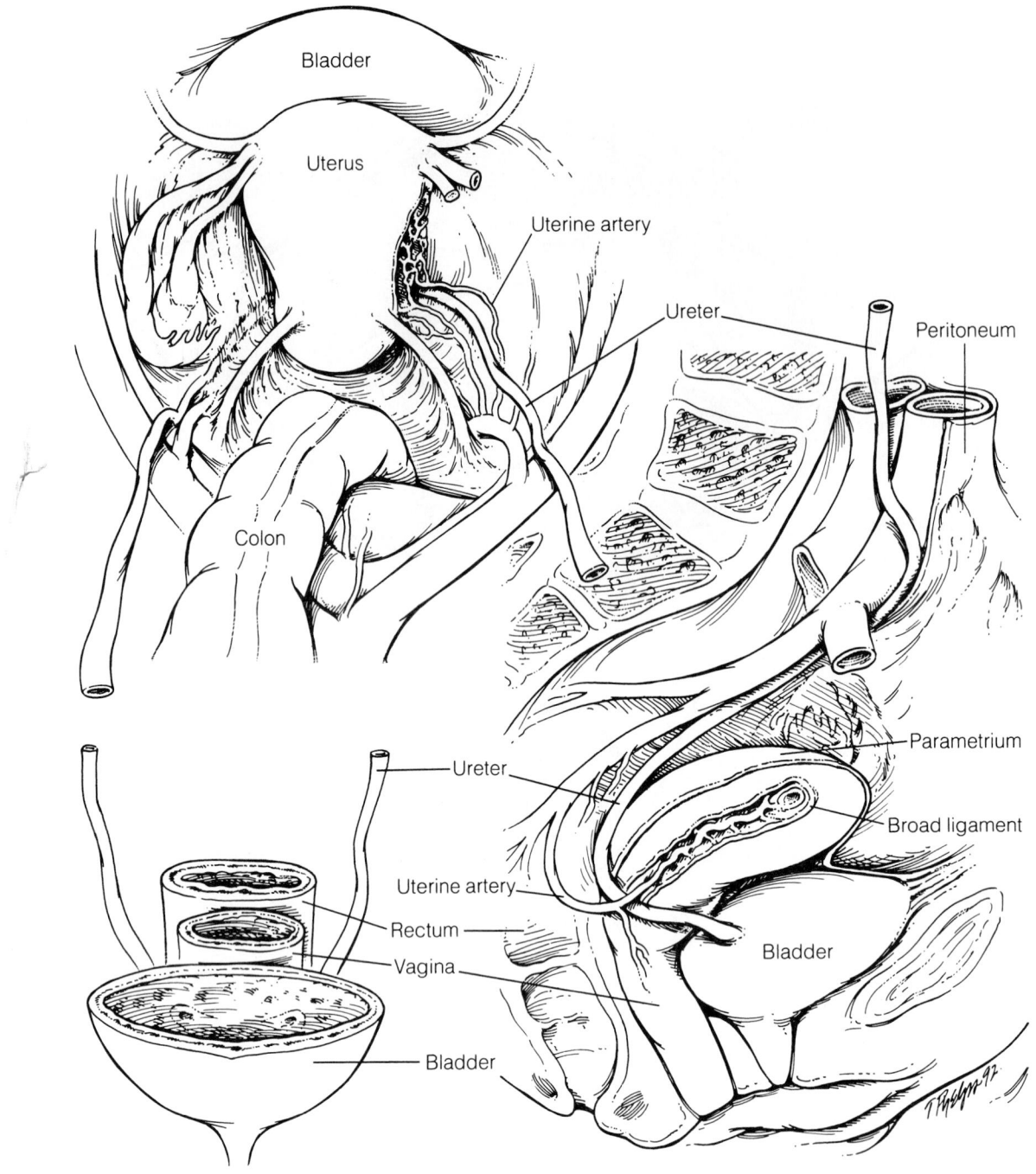

Figure 2–22
Relation of ureter to pelvic structures. (Modified from Tarkington MA, Gilbert RN, Bresette JF: Minimizing danger of iatrogenic ureteral injuries. Contemp Ob/Gyn 1992;37:99. Reprinted with permission of the artist, T. Phelps.)

procedures undertaken on a given organ are named for the Greek root. Examples with the Latin/Greek meanings:

Vagina (sheath)/*Kolpos* (fold), as in colpectomy, colposcopy, and so forth

Cervix (neck)/*Trachelos* (neck), as in trachelectomy

Uterus (womb)/*Hystera* (womb), as in hysterectomy, hysteroscopy, and so forth ■

The *vagina* is a musculoepithelial tubular organ connecting the cervix to the exterior. The lining of rugate, nonkeratinized, non–hair-bearing squamous epithelium allows for expansion without rupture and restoration to original conformation. There is an outer thin layer of contractile smooth muscle.

The vagina is not cylindrical; it is sigmoid in sagittal section (see Figs. 2–5 and 2–20) and H-shaped in cross section (see Fig. 2–16). The diameter of the upper two thirds is greater than that of the lower third. It is also larger in diameter than the portio vaginalis of the cervix; the resultant circular groove of attachment is termed the *vaginal fornix*. The posterior vaginal wall is 10 to 12 cm in length, 2 to 3 cm longer than the anterior wall. The vagina rests on the rectum, which in turn is supported by the levator plate, and is fairly horizontal for the proximal two thirds of its length. Progressing distally, the vagina then passes at a 45- to 55-degree angle through the pelvic and urogenital diaphragms to empty into the vulvar vestibule (see Fig. 2–20).

Anatomic relations include the cervix superiorly; the bladder base, bladder trigone, and urethra anteriorly; the ureter anterolaterally to the anterior fornix; the cardinal ligament laterally; the rectum and anus inferiorly, then posteriorly; and the rectouterine pouch posteriorly.

The arterial supply to the upper vagina is from the descending cervical branch of the uterine artery and the superior vesical branch of the internal iliac artery. The midvagina is supplied mostly from vaginal (inferior vesical) and middle rectal branches of the internal iliac artery. The distal vagina is supplied by pudendal and inferior rectal branches of the internal pudendal artery. The rich anastomotic network thus formed is termed by some the vaginal *azygous artery*. A venous plexus coalesces laterally to drain into internal iliac veins. Lymphatic drainage of the upper two thirds of the vagina is to internal iliac and obturator lymph nodes; the lower third drains to these *and also* to the superficial inguinal lymph nodes. Nerve supply to the vagina is from the pelvic autonomic plexus; distally, it is also from the perineal branches of the internal pudendal nerve.

CLINICAL CORRELATES

- Persistence of portions of the mesonephric duct is sometimes evident along lateral walls as Gartner's duct cysts. Rarely, an ectopic ureter may open into the cyst, leading to incontinence.
- Removal of the vagina (colpectomy), or fixation of the anterior to the posterior wall (colpocleisis), can be performed to treat complicated forms of genital prolapse in patients no longer considering coitus.
- A transverse vaginal septum is a rare condition (1 in 80,000 women) wherein a septum is located two thirds of the way up the vagina. This can lead to primary amenorrhea with the development of hematocolpos, hematometra, and even endometriosis.
- Contrary to popular belief, the vaginal epithelium is stratified, nonkeratinizing squamous epithelium *without* glands. Vaginal lubrication occurs from transudation of fluid from a rich vascular plexus that surrounds the vagina. The vascular plexus also allows many drugs (estrogens, progesterones) to be readily absorbed vaginally. ■

The *ovary* is suspended from the posterior leaf of the broad ligament by a peritoneal fold, the *mesovar-*

ium, through which its blood supply and nerves course. The ovary itself is a cribriform, almond-shaped organ of approximately $4 \times 2 \times 2$ cm. The position of the ovary in the pelvis varies considerably; it may be suspended vertically from the broad ligament in the lateral pelvis, or it may be adherent to the pelvic sidewall. If the broad ligament has been stretched or the uterus retroverted, it may lie in the rectouterine pouch just posterior to the cervix. Except for the mesovarial surface (the ovarian *hilum*), the ovary is almost entirely covered with visceral peritoneum, which is a single layer of cuboidal or flattened mesothelial cells. The more medial pole is attached to the uterine cornu by the round ovarian ligament. The more lateral pole is adjacent to the fimbriated end of fallopian tube. When sectioned, the ovary may be divided into the outer *cortex*, which contains most of the ovarian follicles, their support structures, and their remnants; and the inner *medulla* which is composed of vessels and a hormonally functional stroma. The follicles of the cortex greatly vary in size. After ovulation, a *corpus luteum* is formed in the cortex, which is usually grossly seen as a 0.5- to 1.5-cm yellow subcapsular nodule; usually only one is grossly visible without section. Follicles and corpora lutea may enlarge the ovary to a diameter of 6 cm without being thought to be pathologically distended. The corpora lutea further degenerate to white *corpora albicantia*, usually not seen without ovarian section.

Blood is supplied by the *ovarian artery*, a direct branch of the aorta. Frequently, it branches into two to five smaller arteries after originating from the aorta before supplying the ovary. It descends over the anterior psoas muscle, enters the ovarian suspensory ligament at the pelvic brim, courses medially and inferiorly to the ovary, then supplies the ovary through the broad ligament and its mesovarium. The artery then passes on to supply the mesosalpinx and fallopian tube and anastomoses with ascending branches of the uterine artery. The venous drainage consists of several ovarian veins that follow the course of the arteries. On the right, the *ovarian veins* unite into one dominant vein, which drain into the vena cava. On the left, the ovarian venous plexus coalesces and drains into the left renal vein. The ovarian vessels are the major structures within the ovarian suspensory ligament. Innervation of the ovary is from the aortic autonomic plexus and travels along the vessels. The lymphatic vessels follow the course of the blood vessels and drain into paraaortic and paracaval lymph nodes.

CLINICAL CORRELATES

- Because of a rich anastomotic network with branches from the internal iliac artery, ligation of the ovarian arteries seems not to lead to ischemic ovarian necrosis and not to prevent ovulation or pregnancy (Mengert et al, 1969). It may, however, lead to cystic degeneration of the ovary.

- Although ovarian vessel diameters are small, their origin is directly from the aorta or directly into the vena cava, causing relatively high-pressure systems. The arteries often split into two to five branches before reaching the ovary. The ovarian veins run as a rich plexus of multiple veins called the *pampiniform plexus* of veins. This leads to many small vessels loosely connected in the ovarian vascular pedicle, all subject to retraction upon transection. For these reasons, ovarian vascular pedicles are frequent sites of gynecologic postoperative pelvic hematoma, the others being the divided uterine artery and the unsecured lateral vaginal angle. Many advocate double suture ligature of the ovarian suspensory ligament to help avoid hematoma formation.
- Because of proximity to the ureters, ligation of the ovarian vessels may result in ureteral damage
- The ovary is suspended in the pelvis by three attachments: the round ovarian ligament (utero-ovarian), the suspensory ligament of the ovary (infundibulopelvic ligament), and the mesovarium. The ovary is suspended and not fixed in the pelvis, allowing torsion (twisting of the ovary on its blood supply) to occur. The most common etiology of torsion is an ovarian mass (50% to 60% of the time), and usually the fallopian tube is also involved. There is a predilection for the right ovary to torse (50% more commonly). This is likely due to the sigmoid colon's location on the left side of the pelvis, decreasing mobility of the left ovary.
- Before puberty, the surface of the ovary is smooth. Ovulation causes the ovary to become progressively scarred and distorted with release of the ovum and formation of the corpus luteum. ∎

The *fallopian tube*, 10 to 15 cm long, lies at the upper border of the broad and ovarian suspensory ligaments, except for the infundibulum, which is relatively free on its mesosalpinx (Fig. 2–23). Because of attachments to the broad and ovarian suspensory ligaments, the tube courses laterally and posteriorly from its origin on the uterine cornu. Its attachment to these ligaments, the *mesosalpinx*, transmits vessels, lymphatics, and nerves to and from the tube. The tube is divided into the narrow *interstitial portion* (which passes through the muscular wall of the uterus), 1 to 2 cm in length. The *isthmus* is the narrowest but most muscular region, 4 cm in length, immediately adjacent to the uterine fundus. The *ampulla*, the broader continuation of the tube 4 to 6 cm in length, is where fertilization occurs. At the funnel-like *infundibulum*, the fallopian tube abruptly widens to 1.0 to 1.25 cm, and from it arise 20 to 25 motile extensions, the *fimbriae*, which surround the tubal *ostium*. The tube averages about 0.75 cm in diameter before broadening at the infundibulum. The tubal lumen is lined by ciliated columnar epithelium. As the tubal ostium is approached from the cornual insertion, the epithelium displays more extensive folds (plicae), so that at the ampulla it has an almost papillary appearance in cross section (Fig. 2–23). The muscular wall of the tube is composed of an inner circular and an outer longitudinal layer of smooth muscle. The outer serosal layer is typical visceral peritoneum.

Blood is supplied by tubal branches of the ovarian artery and its anastomosis with the uterine artery. Nerves are from the pelvic autonomic plexus. Lymphatic drainage is similar to that of the ovary.

CLINICAL CORRELATES

- Because of the intimate relationship of ovary to fallopian tube, tubal masses are usually misdiagnosed

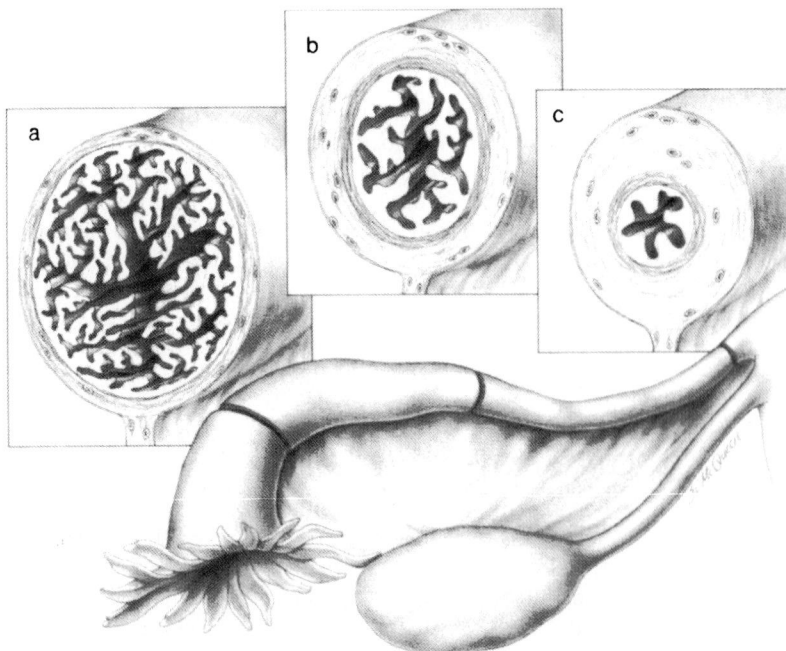

Figure 2–23
Fallopian tube cross-sections, *a*, Infundibulum. *b*, Ampulla. *c*, Isthmus. (From Droegemueller W: Anatomy. In Herbst AL, Mishell DR Jr, Stenchever MA, Droegemueller W, [eds]: Comprehensive Gynecology. 2nd ed. St. Louis: Mosby–Year Book, 1992:55, with permission.)

as ovarian neoplasms in the patient who is not acutely ill. They usually *are* the site of genital pathology (tubal pregnancy, "pelvic inflammatory disease") in the acutely ill patient.

- The fallopian tube is unusually susceptible to pain from adhesive disease when compared with other abdominal muscle-walled organs. Adhesive disease may also predispose to infertility or ectopic pregnancy.
- Mesonephric duct remnants of varying size—hydatid cysts of Morgagni—are frequently found adherent to the distal tube.
- Hysterosalpingography (initially described by Rindflesch in 1910) can be used to evaluate the patency of the fallopian tubes. Occlusion at the most proximal segment has been observed presumably secondary to muscle spasm and is not necessarily indicative of tubal pathology. Anatomic dissection has failed to identify a defined sphincter apparatus. Attempts at relieving the spasm with local anesthetics, systemic sedatives, and intravenous glucagon have been used. ∎

The *ureter* enters the pelvis at the common iliac artery bifurcation and is retroperitoneal for its entire course. It follows the course of the internal iliac artery for a short distance (slightly anterior and medial to it) until it passes near the ischial spine. Here, the ureter changes direction, coursing anteriorly along the lateral surface of the uterosacral ligament, passes into the base of the broad ligament, enters the cardinal ligament "tunnel" (of Wertheim) directly under the uterine artery, just lateral to the cervix, passes lateral to anterior vaginal fornix, exits from the cardinal ligament "tunnel," and then curves medially around the anterior fornix to enter the bladder obliquely near the trigone. The ureters adjoin the bladder approximately 5 cm apart and course obliquely to enter the trigone, where the internal orifices are approximately 2.5 cm apart. The ureters continually taper as they approach the bladder; diameter at the pelvic brim may approach 1 cm, whereas that at the bladder is 0.5 cm (see Figs. 2–19 and 2–22).

The majority of ureteral blood supply in the pelvis is from peritoneal vessels branching indirectly from the iliac vessels. There is also usually a direct vascular branch from the uterine vessels lateral to the cervix, and from the superior vesical vessels adjacent to the bladder. These vessels feed those of the ureteral adventitia, which has an extensive anastomotic network.

CLINICAL CORRELATES

- The ureter may be damaged during gynecologic surgery as a result of its proximity to surgically critical portions of the female genital organs. There are three common sites of surgical interruption in the pelvis. The first is at the pelvic brim, where it lies near the ovarian vessels and may be interrupted during oöphorectomy. The second is within the cardinal ligament adjacent to the uterine artery, where it may be interrupted during ligation of the uterine vessels, by cardinal ligament division, or by attempts to achieve hemostasis at the lateral vaginal angle. The third is near the ureterovesical junction, where it may be damaged during dissection of the bladder from the cervix and upper vagina, during placement of hemostatic suture for cervical surgery, or during vesical plication for cystocele repair (see Fig. 2–22).
- In some patients with distorted anatomy, the peristaltic action of the ureter may be the only criterion that assists the pelvic surgeon in distinguishing it from vessels or ligaments. Peristalsis alone does not imply a patent ureter. Identification of Auerbach's plexus of vessels surrounding the ureter can also aid in its identification.
- Because of its extensive vascular supply from the peritoneum, devascularization of the ureter may occur with extensive dissection of the ureter from its adjacent peritoneum, causing a subsequent ischemic fibrosis, obstruction, or fistula. During resection of adherent pelvic masses, radical hysterectomy, exenteration, and urologic procedures such as urinary diversion, attempts should be made to keep as much ureter attached to its adjacent peritoneum as possible. Because of the anastomoses within the ureteral adventitia, devascularization does not occur with interruption of small segments of ureteral blood supply unless the adventitia itself is damaged.
- Duplication of the urinary collecting system (double or bifid ureter) can occur in 1% to 4% of women and is often associated with müllerian anomalies. ∎

The *urinary bladder* is a hollow organ composed of interdigitated layers of smooth muscle (see Figs. 2–20 and 2–21). Its shape varies with degree of urinary distention: the unfilled bladder resembles a three-sided pyramid, lying on its side. The *apex* of the bladder is closely associated with the posterior pubic symphysis, and gives rise to the median umbilical ligament (obliterated urachus of the anterior abdominal wall). The *base* of the bladder is the portion that is separated from the cervix and upper vagina only by the avascular vesicocervical space. The superior wall of the bladder is the only surface covered externally with visceral peritoneum; this forms the floor of the *vesicouterine pouch*. The superior wall of the bladder distends to a greater degree than the other walls when the bladder is filled with urine. The two inferolateral walls of the bladder lie adjacent and parallel to the levator plate and obturator internus muscle. The *neck* of the bladder is that funnel-shaped portion adjacent to the urethral origin, also termed the internal urethral sphincter. It is not a true sphincter, only a thickening of interdigitating detrusor muscle prior to its passing distally to become muscle of the urethra. The *trigone*, the most nonexpansile portion of bladder wall, is covered internally by a smooth layer of transitional epithelium. The ureteral orifices, the interureteric ridge, and the internal urethral orifice demarcate the borders of the trigone.

The internal portion of bladder is covered with a redundant layer of stratified transitional cell epithelium. The redundancy of this mucosal layer accounts for the great capacity of the bladder to distend without mucosal rupture and for its wrinkled appearance outside the trigone in the undistended state. The outer portion of bladder is encased by endopelvic fascia.

The bladder is related superiorly by loops of ileum or pelvic colon in the vesicouterine pouch and by the fundus of the anteverted uterus posteriorly to the cervix and upper vagina, laterally to the paravesical space and pelvic sidewall, and anteriorly to the pubic symphysis.

The blood supply to the bladder is mostly through the *superior vesical artery*; the vaginal (inferior vesical) branches of the internal iliac artery also contribute. Between the endopelvic fascia and the outer layer of bladder is a venous plexus that drains into the internal iliac veins. Lymphatics drain to the internal and external iliac and obturator lymph nodes. The nerve supply is from the pelvic autonomic plexus via the uterosacral and cardinal ligaments.

CLINICAL CORRELATES

- Loss of vesical support by damage to the urogenital diaphragm or its endopelvic fascia can predispose to herniation of the bladder into the vaginal lumen—cystocele. Cystocele can also be caused by prolapse of pelvic viscera secondary to loss of levator plate support.
- Damage to the bladder near the vaginal apex at the time of hysterectomy may lead to vesicovaginal fistula.   ∎

The *urethra* gradually tapers along its length and conducts urine from the bladder lumen to the vulvar vestibule (see Figs. 2–20 and 2–24). This musculoepithelial tube is from 3 to 5 cm in length and 1.00 to 1.75 cm in diameter, extending downward and forward under the pubic symphysis to the external meatus. It is closely approximated posteriorly by the anterior vaginal wall and anteriorly by the pubic symphysis. It is suspended from the pubis by the pubourethral ligaments. The upper third of the urethra is composed of interdigitating bundles of smooth muscle, and the middle third by an inner circular layer of smooth muscle (the internal [involuntary] urethral sphincter) and an outer layer of longitudinal muscle. The lower third of urethra, at the level of the urogenital diaphragm, is composed of both smooth and skeletal muscle and is lined with squamous epithelium. Muscular fibers from the urogenital diaphragm and the ischiocavernosus and bulbocavernosus muscles interdigitate with the urethra here to form the external (voluntary) urethral

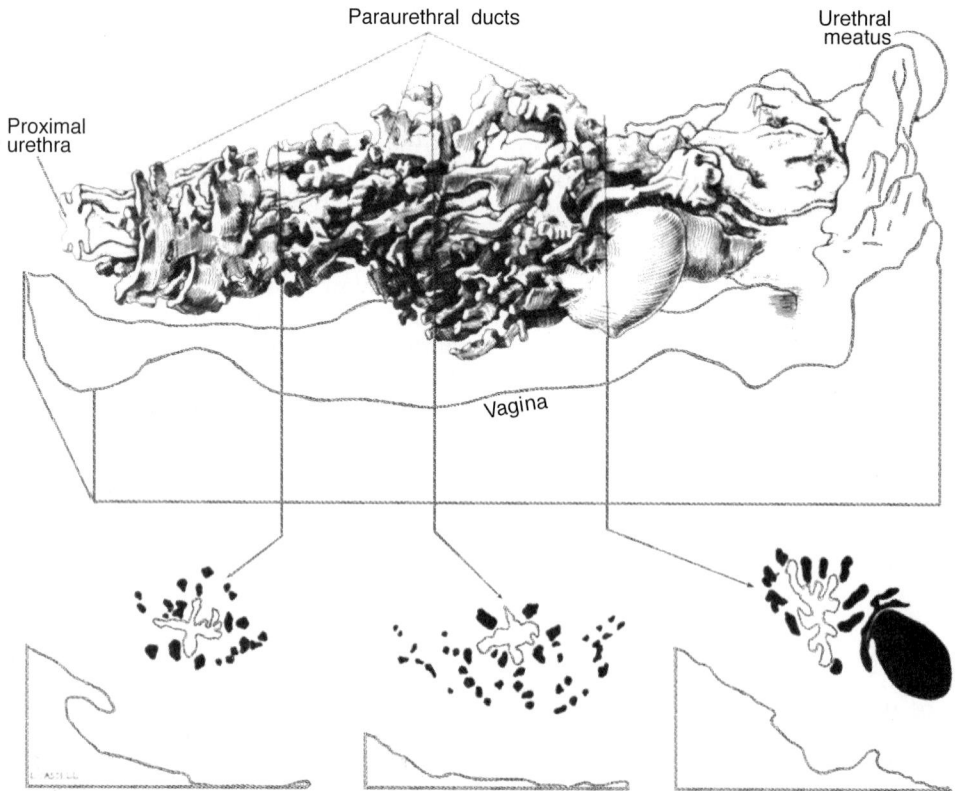

Figure 2–24
Paraurethral glands. (Modified from Huffman JW: The detailed anatomy of paraurethral ducts in the adult human female. Am J Obstet Gynecol 1948;55:86, with permission.)

sphincter. Stratified transitional epithelium lines the upper two thirds of urethra. There is a rich submucosal vascular plexus. The posterolateral wall of the distal urethra is perforated by a lumen (duct) of the paired *paraurethral (Skene's) glands*, branched tubular glands that run parallel to the distal 1 cm of urethra before emptying into its lumen (Fig. 2–24). In some, the gland ostia are external to the urethra.

The blood supply of the upper two thirds of the urethra is anastomotic from that of the anterior vagina. Blood to the lower third is from the clitoral and labial branches of the internal pudendal artery. Lymphatics of the upper two thirds follow the adjacent vessels; the lower third drains to the superficial inguinal nodes. Innervation is a continuation of that of the bladder from the pelvic autonomic plexus.

CLINICAL CORRELATES

- Urethral diverticulum, an outpouching of urethral mucosa toward the vaginal wall or even into the vaginal lumen, should be suspected in all cases of anterior vaginal wall mass or with chronic recurrent cystitis or urethritis.
- The urethral mucosa and submucosa is estrogen-responsive, as is the epithelium of the bladder trigone. In the hypoestrogenic state, the urethral mucosa and submucosa atrophy, increasing the luminal diameter of the urethra, decreasing the urethral pressure, and predisposing to urinary incontinence.
- Paraurethral glands may be sites of gonococcal or chlamydial infection and may actually form a paraurethral abscess. ■

A continuation of the sigmoid colon 12 to 15 cm in length, the *rectum* is composed of a complete outer longitudinal layer of smooth muscle and an inner circular one. The mucous membrane and inner muscular layer form three transverse folds (valves), two on the left and one on the right. Its epithelial lining is that of mucus-secreting columnar epithelium arranged in crypts. The lateral and anterior surfaces of the upper third of the rectum are covered by a visceral peritoneal reflection from the parietal peritoneum of the pelvic sidewalls, and the middle third (anteriorly only) is covered by an upward reflection from the rectouterine pouch, whereas the lower third has no serosal peritoneal covering. The rectum begins where the sigmoid colon loses its mesentery, adjacent to the upper sacral vertebrae, and it has no appendices epiploicae. The proximal rectum closely follows the contour of the sacrum and coccyx directly posterior to it. The distal rectum is closely approximate to the posterior vagina along most of the vagina's length. Because of the extensive nature of the junction of anterior rectum and posterior vagina, only the most proximal portion of the posterior vagina is immediately adjacent to the peritoneal cavity. The distal rectum closely parallels the course of the vagina through the pelvic diaphragm, being angu-

lated anteriorly by the puborectalis portion of the levator ani.

The *rectouterine pouch* (the cul-de-sac, or pouch of Douglas)—the most dependent portion of the peritoneal cavity—is formed by the reflection of the pelvic sidewall parietal peritoneum over the anterior rectum and posterior vagina, and may contain ileum or sigmoid colon. The *rectovaginal septum* is composed of peritoneal layers fused before birth, which undergo subsequent fibrosis and replacement by collagen and elastic fibers—the so-called layer of Denonvilliers' fascia. It extends from the rectouterine pouch distally to the central perineal tendon and forms the anterior border of rectovaginal space (Milley and Nichols, 1969).

The vascular supply to the rectum is from the superior rectal vessels (the terminal branch of the inferior mesenteric vessels); proximally, the midportion is supplied by the middle rectal vessels, and the portion outside the pelvic diaphragm is supplied by the inferior rectal branch of the pudendal vessels. Innervation is from the pelvic autonomic plexus. A few pararectal lymph nodes exist just external to the rectal wall. The lymphatic drainage from these nodes then follows the respective vessels to drain into internal iliac and inferior mesenteric lymph nodes. The short segment of rectum that is below the pelvic diaphragm also drains to the superficial inguinal lymph nodes.

CLINICAL CORRELATES

- Damage to rectum at the time of hysterectomy may lead to rectovaginal fistula.
- The rectum, because of intimate proximity to the vagina, rectovaginal septum, levators, and central perineal tendon, is prone to damage during posterior colporrhaphy.
- The rectouterine pouch can be entered through the posterior vaginal fornix with a needle as a diagnostic test for intraperitoneal hemorrhage or ascites (culdocentesis). Incision here (posterior colpotomy) can allow access to the pelvis to drain a pelvic abscess or to perform fallopian tubal ligation.
- Rectocele—herniation of the anterior rectum into the vaginal lumen—occurs because of defects in the central perineal tendon or rectovaginal septum. Levator diastasis may be a contributing factor. Proper rectocele repair includes repair of levator diastasis, reapproximation of septal remnants, and reconstruction of the central perineal tendon.
- Diverticulitis, an inflammatory disorder from infection surrounding mucosal outpouchings through the circular muscular layer of the large intestine, does not occur in the rectum; however, it can occur in other portions of pelvic colon, simulating disease of the genital tract.
- Enterocele—herniation of peritoneum and small bowel through the pelvic floor—usually occurs through the rectouterine pouch. It may be due to failure of fusion of the fetal rectovaginal septum

(congenital), or it may be acquired. After retropubic urethropexy, a predisposition to enterocele has been noted. Inadequate suspension of the vagina to cardinal and uterosacral ligaments after hysterectomy may also lead to vaginal eversion and enterocele. Successful repair usually includes removal of the peritoneal sac and reduction of the rectouterine pouch.

- The abdominal enterocele repair adapted from Moschowitz's repair of rectal prolapse obliterates the rectouterine pouch by successive concentric purse-string suture plications of its peritoneum. The proximity of the ureters to the lateral peritoneum of the rectouterine pouch predisposes to their damage during this operation.
- The rectouterine pouch may become secondarily obliterated by malignant or inflammatory pelvic disease, predisposing to rectal damage during gynecologic surgery.
- The rectouterine pouch is easily palpated during rectovaginal examination. Tumor implantation, endometriosis, and adnexal enlargement, which otherwise might not be palpable with bimanual pelvic examination, are often palpable here.
- The juncture between superior rectal and middle rectal veins is an important systemic-portal anastomosis and is prone to the development of extensive varices (hemorrhoids) with portal venous hypertension ∎

THE APPENDIX

The *vermiform appendix* is a hollow musculoepithelial continuation of the cecal portion of the colon, varying in length from 7.5 to 15 cm. Its width is usually 0.75 cm. On the medial side of the cecum, the three colonic taeniae converge to form a complete outer longitudinal layer of muscle, encasing the inner circular layer and epithelial layer. The appendiceal lumen is formed by a layer of mucus-secreting columnar epithelium arranged in crypts, and is narrower at the appendiceal-cecal junction. This configuration of the lumen may lead to retention of fecal material and inspissation—formation of an appendicolith. The appendiceal wall contains a relative abundance of lymphoid tissue compared with other intestinal structures. Except for its mesenteric attachment, the *mesoappendix*, the appendix is entirely covered by the visceral peritoneum. The mesoappendix, a continuation of the cecal mesentery, contains the appendiceal vessels, nerves, and lymphatics. A varying amount of mesoappendix is attached to the appendix; as much as one third of the appendix may not have an adjacent mesenteric structure.

Although the appendix is generally located in the right iliac fossa, its actual position is highly variable. The two most common positions are (1) coiled behind or medial to the cecum, anterior to the psoas (almost two thirds of cases), and (2) hanging downward into the pelvis along the right pelvic wall (al-

most one third of cases) (Wakeley, 1933). It is actually fixed retrocecally in 15% of individuals and freely mobile in the rest.

The *appendiceal artery* is a terminal branch of the ileocolic branch of the superior mesenteric artery, which passes posterior to the ileum through the mesoappendix. The appendiceal veins drain into the superior mesenteric network. The appendix is one of few intestinal areas without extensive vascular anastomoses, accounting for the propensity for ischemia to develop at this site after focal vascular insult. Appendiceal nerve supply is from sympathetic and vagal branches to the aortic autonomic plexus. A few small lymph nodes may exist in the mesoappendix; from there the lymphatic drainage is to superior mesenteric lymph nodes.

CLINICAL CORRELATES

- In 70% of patients, appendicitis is caused by luminal occlusion of the appendix, leading sequentially to bacterial overgrowth, greater than normal intraluminal pressure, vascular thrombosis, ischemia, gangrene, and localized peritonitis. Secondary perforation, generalized peritonitis, abscess formation, and death may follow if the condition is not promptly recognized or appropriately treated. In the younger population, luminal occlusion can be brought about by lymphatic hypertrophy secondary to what would otherwise be a minor viral infection. In this group, maximal incidence of appendicitis follows a seasonal variation, with peak prevalence in spring and fall. In the adult patient, the occlusion is usually caused by an appendicolith, is independent of seasonal variation, and may be associated with a low-bulk diet.
- The initial pain of appendicitis is generally visceral, dull, vague, and located in the periumbilical region. As the disease progresses and localized peritonitis develops, the pain shifts to the right lower quadrant and becomes sharp and precise. If the peritonitis becomes generalized, the pain again becomes nonlocalized. These symptoms and signs may be quite variable or less specific with the retrocecal appendix. A positive right psoas or obturator sign may be evident. Hyperesthesia over areas supplied by the femoral nerve or the lateral femoral cutaneous nerve may be present as a result of the proximity of these structures to the retrocecal appendix.
- Because of its proximity to the right ureter, inflammation of the ureter by appendicitis with a resultant "pyuria" may lead the clinician to inappropriately diagnose pyelonephritis.
- Likewise, the proximity of the appendix to the right adnexa may lead to the incorrect diagnosis of salpingitis or tubo-ovarian abscess. Pelvic ultrasound and barium enema are frequently performed, but are of value only when there are positive findings. Because this is rarely the case, they are not helpful adjuncts in confirming a diagnosis of appendicitis. Diagnostic laparoscopy should be freely used if the diagnosis of an acute pelvic or right lower quadrant

disorder is in doubt. Patients with an acute abdomen should generally undergo laparotomy.

- A secondary salpingitis may result from appendicitis and should lead to either aggressive antibiotic therapy (especially in those of low age and parity) or concomitant salpingectomy (if childbearing has been completed).
- In patients having disease processes that distort anatomy, the base of the appendix may be found by searching for the confluence of the three taeniae coli on the cecum. ■

REFERENCES

Axe S, Parmley T, Woodruff JD, Hlopak B: Adenomas in minor vestibular glands. Obstet Gynecol 1986;68:16.

Berglas B, Rubin IC: Study of the supportive structures of the uterus by levator myography. Surg Gynecol Obstet 1953;97:677.

Berman ML, Soper JT, Creasman WT, et al: Conservative surgical management of superficially invasive vulvar carcinoma. Gynecol Oncol 1989;35:352.

Borgno G, Micheletti L, Barbero M, et al: Topographic distribution of groin lymph: a study of 50 female cadavers. J Reprod Med 1990;35:1127.

Borrie MJ: Incontinence in institutions: costs and contributing factors. Can Med Assoc J 1992;147:322.

Braithwaite JL: Variations in origin of the parietal branches of the internal iliac artery. J Anat 1952;86:423.

Burchell RC, Olson G: Internal artery ligation: aortograms. Am J Obstet Gynecol 1966;94:117.

Copeland LJ, Sneige N, Gershenson DM, et al: Bartholin gland carcinoma. Obstet Gynecol 1986;67:794.

DiSaia PJ, Creasman WT, Rich WM: An alternate approach to early cancer of the vulva. Am J Obstet Gynecol 1979;133:825.

Friedrich EG Jr: The vulvar vestibule. J Reprod Med 1983;28:773.

Goodlin RC: On protection of the maternal perineum during birth. Obstet Gynecol 1983;62:393.

Grainger DA, Soderstrom RM, Schiff SF, et al: Ureteral injuries at laparoscopy: insights into diagnosis, management, and prevention. Obstet Gynecol 1990;75:839.

Homesley HD, Bundy BN, Sedlis A, Adcock L: Radiation therapy versus pelvic node resection for carcinoma for the vulva and distal vaginal malignancy. Obstet Gynecol 1986;68:733.

Lichten EM, Bombard J: Surgical treatment of primary dysmenorrhea with laparoscopic uterine nerve ablation. J Reprod Med 1987;32:37.

McCall ML: Posterior culdeplasty: surgical correction of enterocele during vaginal hysterectomy. Obstet Gynecol 1957;10:595.

McCall ML, Bolten KA: Martius' Gynecological Operations. Boston: Little, Brown & Co, 1956;327.

McKay M, Frankman O, Horowitz BJ, et al: Vulvar vestibulitis and vestibular papillomatosis: report of the ISSVD Committee on Vulvodynia. J Reprod Med 1991;36:413.

Mengert WF, Burchell RC, Blumstein RW, Daskal JL: Pregnancy after bilateral ligation of internal iliac and ovarian arteries. Obstet Gynecol 1969;34:664.

Milley PS, Nichols DH: A correlative investigation of the human rectovaginal septum. Anat Rec 1969;163:443.

Milley PS, Nichols DH: The relationship between the pubourethral ligaments and the urogenital diaphragm in the human female. Anat Rec 1971;170:281.

Nichols DH: Sacrospinous fixation for massive eversion of the vagina. Am J Obstet Gynecol 1982;142:901.

Nichols DH, Randall CL: Vaginal Surgery. 3rd ed. Baltimore: Williams & Wilkins, 1989.

Peckham BM, Maki DG, Patterson JJ, Hafez GR: Focal vulvitis: a characteristic syndrome and cause of dyspareunia. Am J Obstet Gynecol 1986;154:855.

Plentl AA, Friedman EA: Lymphatic System of the Female Genitalia. Philadelphia: WB Saunders, 1971.

Randall CL, Nichols DH: Surgical treatment of vaginal inversion. Obstet Gynecol 1971;38:327.

Richardson AC, Edmonds PB, Williams NL: Treatment of stress urinary incontinence due to paravaginal fascial defect. Obstet Gynecol 1981;57:357.

Roberts WH, Krishingner GL: Comparative study of human internal iliac artery based on Adachi classification. Anat Rec 1967;158:191.

Sippo WC, Burghardt A, Gomec AC: Nerve entrapment after Pfannensteil incision. Am J Obstet Gynecol 1987;157:420.

Wakeley CPG: The position of the vermiform appendix as ascertained by the analysis of 10,000 cases. J Anat 1933;67:277.

Wilcox LS, Strobino DM, Banft G, Dellinger WS: Episiotomy and its role in the incidence of perineal lacerations in a maternity center and a tertiary hospital obstetric service. Am J Obstet Gynecol 1989;160:1047.

Woodruff JD, Parmley TH: Infection of the minor vestibular gland. Obstet Gynecol 1983;62:609.

Zacharin RF: The suspensory mechanism of the female urethra. J Anat 1963;91:423.

Zacharin RF: Functional anatomy of the pelvic floor. Contemp Ob/Gyn Suppl 1989;34:111.

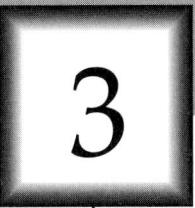

3

Keith Gordon
Sergio Oehninger

Reproductive Physiology

The previous version of this chapter, which appeared in the first edition of the *Textbook of Gynecology*, was entitled "Hypothalamic-Pituitary-Ovarian-Uterine Axis." The current title is more general and, accordingly, a slightly broader approach to the content has been taken, while still covering the same fundamentals. As always, a chapter of this kind is selective in the information portrayed and the interpretation of the data. Furthermore, it is necessarily incomplete in the treatment of many topics. No single chapter of this length can do justice to the tremendous wealth of information generated on the topic of reproductive physiology.

Our understanding of reproductive physiology is built on the foundations established by previous generations of basic and clinical researchers. In this review chapter, we rely heavily on data derived from nonhuman primates because they constitute the best animal model for human reproductive physiology. Data from subprimate species are used where there is a lack of appropriate primate data. In this decade, molecular biology has become the technique of choice for many studies, just as radioimmunoassay was some 20 years ago. Techniques come and go and are continually being improved upon at such a rate that they are almost out of date as soon as one becomes comfortable with them. Nonetheless, even though the tools of the trade have changed, the questions to which they are applied are still surprisingly unchanged. It is humbling to go back and read some of the early classical papers from 50 years ago (Markee, 1940; Green and Harris, 1947; Harris, 1948), or even earlier (Hartman, 1929).

Before we leave the preamble and get down to business, there is one final point that we wish to emphasize. What is now commonly referred to as the "normal" cycle with respect to the human female reproductive axis is in fact *abnormal* in its frequency of occurrence, when considered in evolutionary terms. The number of "normal" cycles experienced by a woman today differs greatly from the number of reproductive cycles experienced by women during most of human existence. From a genetic and physiologic standpoint we remain nearly identical to our ancestors of 10,000 years ago, yet our reproductive habits have changed dramatically. There can be little doubt that some of the common gynecologic problems encountered today are at least partially a consequence of this change in the character of the female reproductive experience (Eaton et al, 1994) (Table 3–1).

Before we get into specifics concerning how the reproductive axis operates, it is important to introduce the components of the system (the hardware). Then we will discuss the regulation of each component before finally putting all the components together and trying to deal with the full complexities of reproductive physiology.

COMPONENTS OF THE FEMALE REPRODUCTIVE SYSTEM

The Hypothalamus

The hypothalamus can be considered as the central processing unit of the reproductive system. It integrates the inputs from many sources and sends out the signal that drives the whole reproductive axis, namely gonadotropin-releasing hormone (GnRH).

Hypothalamic control of pituitary function is achieved via two mechanisms. The hormones (vasopressin, oxytocin, etc.) of the hypothalamic-neurohypophyseal system (posterior pituitary), produced in the magnocellular hypothalamic neurons, are released into the systemic circulation by axon terminals. The hormones of the anterior pituitary are under the influence of the hypothalamic releasing and inhibiting hormones, which reach the anterior pituitary via the specialized hypothalamic-pituitary portal system (see Fig. 3–1).

The hypothalamus is located at the base of the brain above the pituitary gland. Its anatomic boundaries are imprecise and do not necessarily equate with its functional activity. Further complication is introduced by the lack of clear boundaries between the cellular nuclei, which are often referred to in articles concerning hypothalamic function (Riskind and Martin, 1995).

Table 3-1. REPRODUCTIVE EXPERIENCE AND RISK OF WOMEN'S CANCERS

	REPRODUCTIVE CONTRASTS		SIGNIFICANCE FOR CANCER RISK		
	Hunter-Gatherers	Americans	Breast	Endometrium	Ovary
Age at menarche	16.1	12.5	+	+	
Age at first birth	19.5	24.0 (all)	+		
		26.5 (educated*)			
Menarche to first birth: time elapsed (years)	3.4	11.5 (all)	+		
		14.0 (educated*)			
Duration of lactation per birth	2.9 yrs	3.0 months	+		+
Completed family size†	5.9	1.8	+	+	+
Age at menopause	47	50.5	+	+	
Total number of ovulations	160	450‡			+

*Women with at least some education beyond high school.
†Mean number of live births in women who survive to age 50.
‡For women who have not used oral contraceptives.
From Eaton SB, Pike MC, Short RV, et al: Women's reproductive cancers in evolutionary context. Q Rev Biol 1994;69:353, with permission.

The median eminence is a specialized region of the floor of the third ventricle from which protrudes the pituitary stalk. Together with the upper stalk, this area forms the contact zone between terminals of the tuberoinfundibular neurons and the capillaries of the hypophyseal portal veins. The median eminence is classically thought to be part of the hypothalamus. However, Page (1996) put forth the view that the median eminence should be considered as part of the neurohypophysis. In his schema the pituitary gland is composed of a neurohypophysis (median eminence, infundibular stem, and neural lobe) and an adenohypophysis (pars tuberalis, pars intermedia, and pars distalis; Fig. 3–2). As we will see in later sections, thinking of the median eminence in this new anatomic schema may help explain some of the

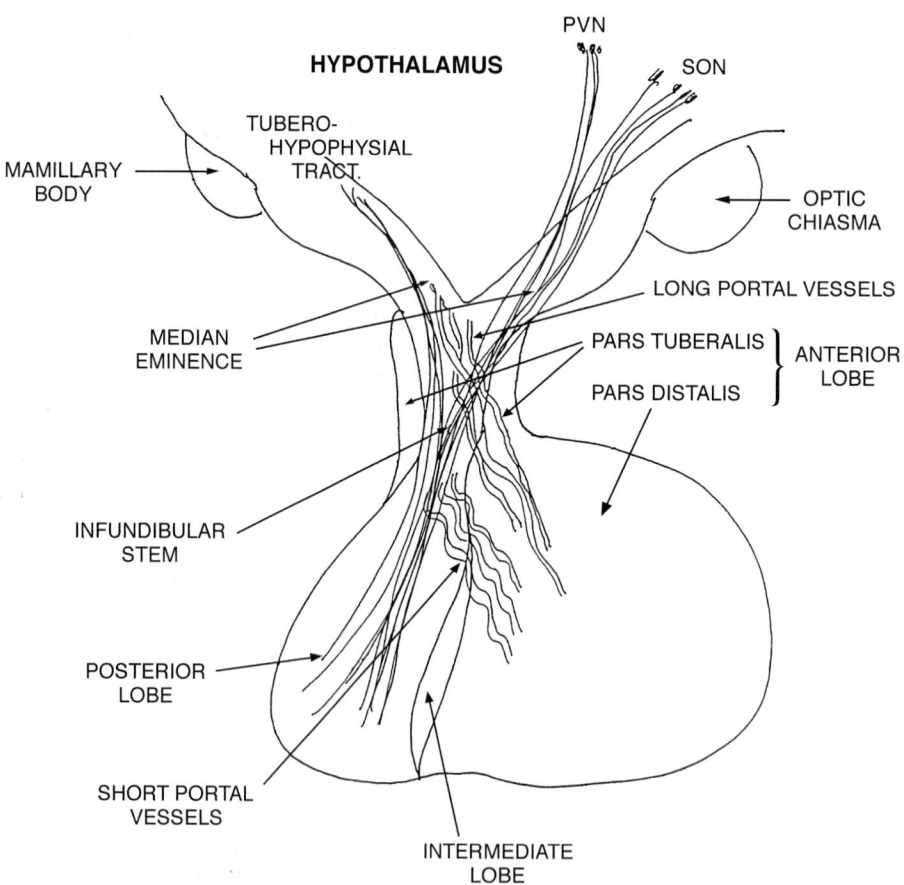

Figure 3-1
The hypothalamic-pituitary portal system. PVN, paraventricular nucleus; SON, supraoptic nucleus.

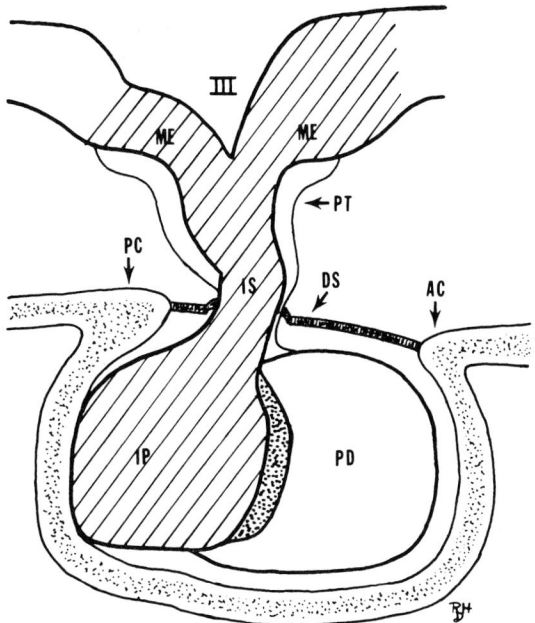

Figure 3–2
Midsagittal section of the human pituitary gland. The neurohypophysis (*hatching*) consists of the median eminence (ME), infundibular stem (IS), and infundibular process (IP; also called the neural lobe). The adenohypophysis consists of the pars tuberalis (PT), which is applied to the ME and IS and lies in the subarachnoid space above the diaphragma sellae (DS), and the pars distalis (PD), which is within the sella turcica beneath the DS. The region of aggregated melanotropes corresponding to the pars intermedia of lower forms is indicated by the *stippled area* between the PD and the IP. AC, anterior clinoid; PC, posterior clinoid; III, third ventricle. (From Page RB: Sellar and parasellar tumors: anatomy and physiology of the adenohypophysis. In Wilkins RH, Rengachary SS [eds]: Neurosurgery. 2nd ed, Vol 1. New York: McGraw-Hill, 1996: 1221, with permission.)

anomalies in the data obtained in earlier studies of the neuroendocrine regulation of the gonadal axis.

The hypothalamic regulating hormones produced in the cell bodies of various parts of the brain and hypothalamus flow down along nerve fibers to the infundibulum, the structure that forms the floor of the third ventricle of the brain and extends down to connect the hypothalamus with the pituitary. The perigomitolar capillary network is the site where these hormones enter the circulation. Larger parallel capillaries, formed from these capillaries, constitute the long portal vessels that run down the pituitary stalk and terminate in the capillaries of the anterior lobe. There are also short portal vessels that originate in the distal part of the pituitary stalk and the posterior lobe. These short portal vessels also enter the anterior lobe and terminate in capillary beds (Fig. 3–1). A common misconception is that the hypothalamus is protected by the blood-brain barrier, whereas it is actually readily permeable to the systemic circulation.

The Pituitary

The pituitary gland consists of two major components, the neurohypophysis (posterior lobe) and the adenohypophysis (anterior lobe). The pars intermedia (intermediate lobe) is sometimes considered as part of the anterior pituitary and is usually all but ignored in reference to the human pituitary because of its poorly developed nature and apparent lack of function. The neurohypophysis can be further divided into the median eminence, the infundibular stem, and the neural lobe. The anterior pituitary can similarly be divided into the pars tuberalis (which together with the infundibular stem forms the pituitary stalk) and the pars distalis (anterior lobe). The anterior pituitary gland has the highest blood flow of any organ in the body (0.8 ml/g/minute) but receives its blood supply indirectly, via the hypophyseal portal system (Riskind and Martin, 1995). Despite its close proximity to the brain, the anterior pituitary virtually lacks innervation except for a small number of nerves located in close proximity to the blood vessels. The anterior pituitary is composed of numerous cell types, including the classical somatotrophs (growth hormone), lactotrophs (prolactin), thyrotrophs (thyroid-stimulating hormone [TSH], gonadotrophs (luteinizing hormone [LH] and follicle-stimulating hormone [FSH] and corticotrophs (adrenocorticotropic hormone, melanocyte-stimulating hormone, and β-endorphin). The somatotrophs, which constitute approximately 50% of the cell population, are primarily found in the lateral wings of the anterior pituitary. The lactotrophs constitute 10% to 30% of the cell population, are scattered throughout the anterior pituitary and can often be found juxtaposed with gonadotrophs. Lactotrophs are subject to hyperplasia during pregnancy (Cinti et al, 1985) and some may be recruited from the bihormonal population of somatomammotrophs. Corticotrophs constitute approximately 20% of the anterior pituitary cell population, thyrotrophs constitute only 5% of the cell population, and gonadotrophs make up the other 15% or so. Current thinking is that gonadotrophs secrete both LH and FSH (Horvath and Kovacs, 1995).

The Ovaries

It is puzzling, that, in articles in the professional literature, one often sees the ovaries referred to in the singular (e.g., Adashi, 1994) when they are almost always found as a pair in mammals. The ovaries are ever-changing multicompartmental structures. In the adult ovary, gametogenic and endocrine functions are coordinated to produce the cyclical process of follicular development, ovulation, corpus luteum (CL) formation, and, if pregnancy does not occur, CL regression. The coordinated events in the ovaries of higher primates are directed toward the cyclic release of a single mature oocyte into an endocrine milieu that will foster implantation and embryonic development.

The Uterine Endometrium

The uterus is a very dynamic organ specialized to nurture the developing conceptus. In primates the uterus is unicornuate. Anatomically the uterus lies in the pelvis between the bladder and the rectum, and can be divided into three parts: the fundus (the top), the corpus (the body), and the isthmus (the neck), which leads into the cervix. The lining of the uterus is composed of the endometrium and a surrounding muscular myometrium. The endometrium undergoes dramatic monthly cyclic changes in morphology and biochemical characteristics. The endometrial cycle is characterized by proliferation, secretory differentiation of estrogen-primed endometrium and, in the absence of conception, degeneration (culminating in menses) and regeneration. The cyclic changes in the endometrium are largely under the control of ovarian estrogen and progesterone via their respective receptors. However, it is becoming increasingly clear that numerous growth factors, peptides, and enzymes act as intermediaries between the steroids and the endometrial tissue.

The Mammary Glands

Lactation is a part of reproduction (a fact that is often overlooked, especially in today's hectic clinical settings). In fact, the ability to lactate is a fundamental feature of all female mammals. Accordingly, the mammary glands must also be included in the list of components of the reproductive system. The primary role of the breasts is to provide nutrition for newborn infants up through the stage when they can digest and thrive on other food sources. However, in addition to providing an ideal source of nutrition, the breast also plays an important immunologic role (Wagner, 1996) and acts as a transducer in the complex pathway involved in ensuring that birth intervals are sufficiently long to enable the successful rearing of the current cohort of young before the birth of subsequent offspring (Gordon et al, 1993).

The Big Picture

The ultimate goal of reproduction is to produce viable offspring that will themselves be capable of living a full life and reproducing themselves. Many different reproductive strategies have evolved. Choosing how, when, and where to reproduce represents the key strategy for the survival of a species and represents the integration of the relative risks and benefits of each component of the reproductive process. In order to achieve this goal, all of the anatomic hardware described previously has to func-

tion in a highly coordinated manner. This marvelous degree of coordination is achieved through the close interplay of the nervous and endocrine systems.

HYPOTHALAMIC-PITUITARY-OVARIAN INTERACTIONS

Menstrual cyclicity and timely ovulation are the result of the precise integration of a series of events occurring within the different components of the reproductive system. The integrity of three of these processes is essential to the phenomenon of cyclicity: (1) the activity of the GnRH pulse generator; (2) the pituitary secretion of gonadotropins; and (3) the estradiol (E_2)-positive feedback for the preovulatory LH surge, oocyte maturation, and CL formation.

The GnRH Pulse Generator

In its unmodulated state (removed from the influence of higher centers and of the ovarian steroids), the GnRH pulse generator has a frequency of approximately one discharge per hour, which results in the release of a bolus of GnRH into the pituitary portal circulation (Hotchkiss and Knobil, 1994). The pituitary gonadotropes respond to each GnRH stimulus by discharging a pulse of LH and FSH into the peripheral circulation. During the follicular phase of the cycle, the GnRH pulse generator operates at the same frequency as in its unmodulated state, causing the release of circhoral packets of GnRH. In response to this relatively unvarying gonadotropic stimulus, the graafian follicle develops and matures, secreting increasing quantities of E_2, which rises in the peripheral circulation. When, in the course of follicular maturation, plasma E_2 levels exceed a threshold level (~250 pg/ml for >36 hours), the inhibitory (negative feedback) effect of the steroid is suddenly reversed and the pituitary discharges the preovulatory surge of LH and FSH (positive feedback). A change in GnRH pulse frequency or amplitude is not required for the normal time course of the preovulatory gonadotropin surge. The ovary responds to the gonadotropin surge by increasing the production of E_2 and progesterone. This results in a sharp rise of estrogen in the circulation associated with a small increase in progesterone secretion, which precedes ovulation by a few hours. This preovulatory increase in progesterone may play a role in the full development of the gonadotropin surge in humans.

Under the influence of LH, the ruptured follicle luteinizes and the rapidly developing CL secretes increasing quantities of progesterone. Although progesterone reduces the frequency of the hypothalamic GnRH pulse generator, the amplitude of the resulting LH pulses are proportionally increased and the mean LH levels in the circulation differ little from those found during the follicular phase. The CL and its production of progesterone have an absolute requirement for LH. During the luteal phase and in the presence of progesterone, follicular development does not occur. If pregnancy does not ensue, the CL involutes about 14 days after its formation, progesterone levels decline to follicular-phase levels, and menstruation occurs. This is followed by the return of the GnRH pulse generator to the circhoral frequency of the follicular phase, removal of the progestational block to follicular recruitment, and the beginning of a new ovarian cycle.

This basic form of operation of the neuroendocrine control system that governs the ovarian cycle of higher primates is subjected to modulation by a host of inputs from the central nervous system and from the surrounding environment, which impinge on the GnRH pulse generator and the other components of the hypothalamic-pituitary-ovarian system.

Gonadotropin-Releasing Hormone

Initially it was thought that the secretion of each anterior pituitary hormone was controlled by the actions of both releasing and inhibiting substances produced by the hypothalamus (Schally et al, 1973) acting in concert to regulate pituitary secretions. Thus it was assumed that there would be two gonadotropin-releasing hormones: FSH-releasing hormone (FSH-RH) and LH-releasing hormone (LH-RH) (Schally and Kastin, 1971; Schally et al., 1971a). In 1971, two laboratories independently reported the isolation of a putative luteinizing hormone–releasing factor (Amoss et al, 1971; Schally et al, 1971b, 1971c). Subsequent determination of its structure from porcine (Baba et al, 1971; Matsuo et al, 1971b) and ovine (Burgus et al, 1972) sources and its chemical synthesis (Matsuo et al, 1971a) and characterization led to the term *gonadotropin-releasing hormone* because it affected both FSH and LH synthesis and release (Schally et al, 1971a). However, the controversy over whether there are two separate gonadotropin-releasing hormones corresponding to the two gonadotropins continues (Schally and McCann, 1995). The terms *LH-RH* and *GnRH* are used synonymously in the scientific literature (with the latter term prevailing) and, because we still lack any definitive proof of a separate FSH-RH, we use the term GnRH in this chapter.

GnRH Neuronal System

The classical neurosecretory hypothesis (Green and Harris, 1947; Harris, 1948) holds that hypothalamic neurons release their signals into the hypothalamic-pituitary portal blood system, which then passes down the pituitary stalk into the anterior pituitary gland. GnRH is the key hypothalamic hormone for the regulation of reproductive function. Yet the GnRH neurosecretory system is very diffuse, with individual neurons located in many different regions of the brain. Furthermore, it has been estimated that there are only 1200 to 1600 GnRH-immunoreactive neurons in the rat (Ronnekleiv et al, 1989; Malik et al, 1991) and, in the rhesus monkey, the largest number of GnRH-immunoreactive neurons was found to be 2000 in a 3-day-old male (Silverman et al, 1982). In mice it has been clearly shown that GnRH neurons differentiate from the olfactory placode at around midgestation. These neurons migrate through the nasal septum and enter the ventral forebrain with the central roots of the nervus terminalis and vomeronasal nerves (Schwanzel-Fukuda and Pfaff, 1989; Wray et al, 1989a, 1989b). Subsequent studies with other species, including rhesus monkeys (Ronnekleiv and Resko, 1990), indicate that the olfactory origin and migratory pathway are general characteristics of mammals. The clinical relevance of this is seen in Kallmann's syndrome, in which a failure of this migratory system is believed to be causal for the hyposmia and hypogonadotropism commonly seen in patients with this syndrome (Schwanzel-Fukuda et al, 1989). GnRH neurons are typically oval or fusiform in shape, with simple, unbranched dendritic processes from one or both poles of the cell. Axons emerge either directly from the cell body or from a dendrite, and the dendrite may assume a beaded appearance and become axonal. GnRH neurons have a large, centrally placed nucleus and a thin rim of cytoplasm. The cytoplasm typically contains many stacks of rough endoplasmic reticulum, one or more Golgi bodies, and neurosecretory granules (Silvermann et al, 1994). In a study of thick, unembedded sections obtained from rhesus and pigtailed macaques, Silverman et al (1982) reported GnRH-immunoreactive cell bodies in the preoptic area, the periventricular hypothalamic zone from the level of the anterior hypothalamus to the premammillary nuclei, the infundibular nucleus, the supraoptic nucleus, several septal nuclei, the nervus terminalis, and the amygdala. GnRH-immunoreactive axons were observed to innervate the portal vessels in the median eminence, the organum vasculosum of the lamina terminalis, the medial mammillary nuclei, the epithalamus, and the amygdala.

The Hypothalamic Pulse Generator

The hypothalamus of mammals contains an oscillator, or pulse generator, that in the unmodulated state (disconnected from the influence of higher centers and the ovarian steroids) exhibits a periodicity of approximately 1 hour in monkeys and humans. It is the activity of this pulse generator that drives the events downstream at the pituitary, ovarian, and uterine levels via the actions of GnRH on the gonadotropins (LH and FSH), which in turn regulate the production of the gonadal steroids (E_2 and progesterone). A lack of activity of the pulse generator or derangement in the pulse frequency has adverse consequences for the reproductive process. The term *pulse generator* is often used synonymously with

GnRH pulse generator and implies that the GnRH cell bodies and/or neurons are the source of the pulses.

Studies of the relationship between GnRH and LH/FSH pulses have been complicated by the inaccessibility of the vascular system connecting the hypothalamus with the pituitary. Peripheral levels of GnRH have been reported to change with the menstrual cycle in women (Elkind Hirsch et al, 1982); however, the episodic nature of the secretion cannot be studied with peripheral sampling. Various techniques have been developed to circumvent this problem, including push-pull perfusion, microdialysis, cerebrospinal fluid sampling, and hypothalamic-pituitary portal blood sampling (Table 3–2). It is this latter technique that has allowed the most detailed evaluations to be made and, when combined with microdialysis of specific hypothalamic nuclei, provides a powerful tool to dissect the interactions of the various neuropeptides and other factors in the regulation of hypothalamic-pituitary function.

Extensive experimental studies in a variety of animal species have shown a high degree of correspondence between hypothalamic GnRH release and the episodic release of LH and, to a lesser extent, FSH. This relationship has been best characterized in sheep, in which a reliable method for collecting blood directly from the hypothalamic-pituitary portal system, originally developed by Clarke and Cummins (1982), has been modified by Alain Caraty and the group of Fred Karsch and utilized to perform extensive characterizations of the nature of GnRH secretion during the estrous cycle of the ewe (Karsch et al, 1997).

Based on the close correlation between GnRH and pulses of LH in the above studies (Fig. 3–3), extrapolation is made in many studies that the detection of peripheral pulses of LH equates with the activity of the GnRH neuronal output. There is overwhelming evidence that each LH pulse is the result of a GnRH pulse. However, whether all GnRH pulses result in LH pulses is not so clear. Small pulses of GnRH have been observed in the portal blood of sheep without concomitant LH pulses being seen in peripheral blood (Clarke, 1983).

In the rhesus monkey, it appears that the GnRH pulse generator is located within the mediobasal hypothalamus and probably within the region of the arcuate nucleus. This conclusion is based on studies in which the medial basal hypothalamus was isolated from all other areas via the use of a Halasz knife (Krey et al, 1975). These studies demonstrated that, even when the medial basal hypothalamus was completely deafferented, pulsatile LH continued. Furthermore, lesions within these islets had no effect on pulsatile LH secretion unless they obliterated the arcuate nucleus (Plant et al, 1978) (Fig. 3–4).

Using this hypophysiotropic clamp monkey model, Knobil (1980) showed that changing the mode of GnRH administration from pulsatile to continuous led to a refractoriness of the pituitary gland to GnRH stimulation. This desensitization of the adenohypophyseal gonadotropes by the continuous exposure to GnRH (or its long-acting analogs) has been studied extensively, but the cellular mechanisms underlying the phenomenon remain to be completely clarified (Fig. 3–5) (Belchetz et al, 1978; Hodgen, 1990).

Additional support for the view that the GnRH pulse generator is an intrinsic property of the mediobasal hypothalamus come from the demonstration of rhythmic, pulsatile release of GnRH at an appropriate frequency from superfused rat (Bourguignon and Franchimont, 1989), guinea pig (McKibbon and Belchetz, 1986), human (Rasmussen et al, 1989) and monkey (K. Gordon, unpublished observation) hypothalamic fragments in vitro (Fig. 3–6). Furthermore, recent studies with the immortalized GnRH neuronal cell line GT-1 have shown that

Table 3–2. TECHNIQUES USED TO EVALUATE HYPOTHALAMIC INFLUENCE ON THE PITUITARY

TECHNIQUE	SPECIES USED ON	REFERENCES
Push-pull perfusion	Rats	Ramirez et al (1991)
	Monkeys	Spies et al (1997)
	Rabbits	Ramirez et al (1991)
		Spies et al (1997)
	Sheep	Levine et al (1982)
Microdialysis	Rats	Levine and Powell (1989)
	Rabbits	Spies et al (1997)
	Sheep	Robinson (1995)
Cerebrospinal fluid sampling	Monkeys	Xia et al (1992)
Hypothalamic-pituitary portal blood sampling	Sheep	Clarke and Cummins (1982)
		Karsch et al (1997)
Pituitary venous effluent sampling	Horses	Irvine and Alexander (1987)
In vitro perifusion	Guinea pigs	McKibbon and Belchetz (1986)
	Rats	Gallardo and Ramirez (1977)
	Monkeys	Levine et al (1985)
	Humans	Rasmussen et al (1989)

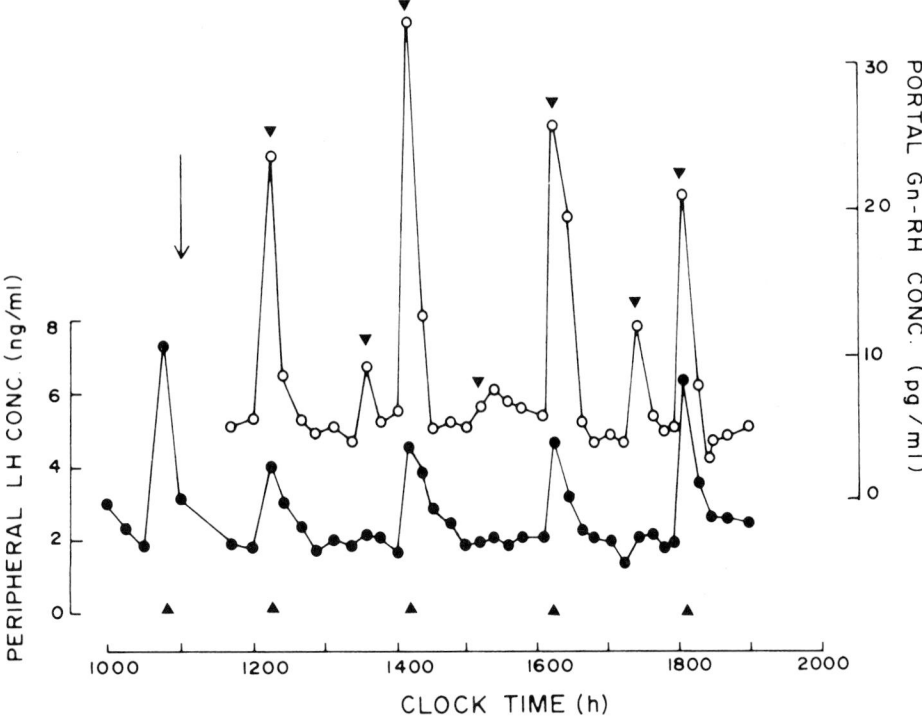

Figure 3–3
Concentrations of gonadotropin-releasing hormone (GnRH) in the hypothalamic-hypophyseal portal plasma and luteinizing hormone (LH) in the jugular venous (peripheral) plasma of an ovariectomized ewe. *Arrow* indicates the time at which the portal vessels were cut. Pulsatile secretory episodes (•• for LH and ∘∘ for GnRH) were defined as having occurred when the value in a given sample exceeded that of the previous sample by three times the standard deviation of the previous sample. (From Clarke IJ, Cummins JT: The temporal relationship between GnRH and LH secretion in ovariectomized ewes. Endocrinology 1982;11:1737, with permission. © The Endocrine Society.)

these cells themselves have an endogenous rhythm and release GnRH in pulses (Martinez de la Escalera et al, 1992).

Striking increases in multiunit activity that are always synchronous with the initiation of LH pulses measured in the peripheral circulation have been recorded from a number of species, including rhesus monkeys (Fig. 3–7). The relationship between these volleys of electrical activity and the initiation of LH pulses is absolute in that increases in electrical activity are always associated with an LH pulse (Wilson et al, 1984). This one-to-one relationship is maintained when the frequency of these events is decreased by barbiturate anesthesia, morphine administration, and other pharmacologic manipulations (Hotchkiss and Knobil, 1994). The activity of this presumptive GnRH pulse generator is markedly suppressed by α-adrenergic blockers and antidopaminergic agents, but not by β-adrenergic blockers (Hotchkiss and Knobil, 1994). A single IV injection of morphine to ovariectomized rhesus monkeys can bring about an immediate cessation of pulse generator activity. Furthermore, the endogenous opiate β-endorphin, injected into the third ventricle of such primates, also causes the arrest of pulsatile LH secretion (Ferin et al, 1984). Because opioids decrease GnRH pulse frequency, it follows that their action must be exerted at the level of the hypothalamus rather than at the level of the pituitary gland.

Although the GnRH pulse generator has been localized to the arcuate region of the mediobasal hypothalamus by the classical neuroendocrinologic techniques already described, the cellular origins of those signals remain uncertain. Clearly, each pulse of

GnRH released into the portal circulation must represent the synchronous discharge of a number of GnRH neurons that are sparse and widely distributed. What integrates the activity of these GnRH neurons remains a challenging enigma. Could the GnRH pulse generator be a single pacemaker cell or group of cells? In any event, the secretion of a pulse by this group of neurosecretory neurons can almost be equated to a digital signal within the context of the nervous system (Lincoln et al, 1985). The pulse is probably generated by an explosive increase in the spike activity of such a group of neurons linked synaptically, whereas synchrony and duration of activation are probably controlled via local circuit interconnections (Lincoln et al, 1985). Pulse frequency and amplitude are thus major modulatory mechanisms for control within this neuroendocrine transduction system.

As has already been alluded to, the hourly administration of GnRH to monkeys with intact ovaries (but bearing mediobasal hypothalamuc lesions that have abolished endogenous GnRH secretion) restores normal ovulatory menstrual cycles (Knobil, 1980). It follows from these observations and similar ones in women with hypothalamic amenorrhea (Crowley and McArthur, 1980; Santoro et al, 1986) that changes in the circhoral frequency or amplitude of the GnRH stimulus are not required for normal follicular development, the initiation and induction of the preovulatory gonadotropin surge, ovulation, CL formation, progesterone secretion, or luteolysis (Hotchkiss and Knobil, 1994). The fact remains, however, that during the luteal phase of the ovarian-menstrual cycle, a marked reduction in the fre-

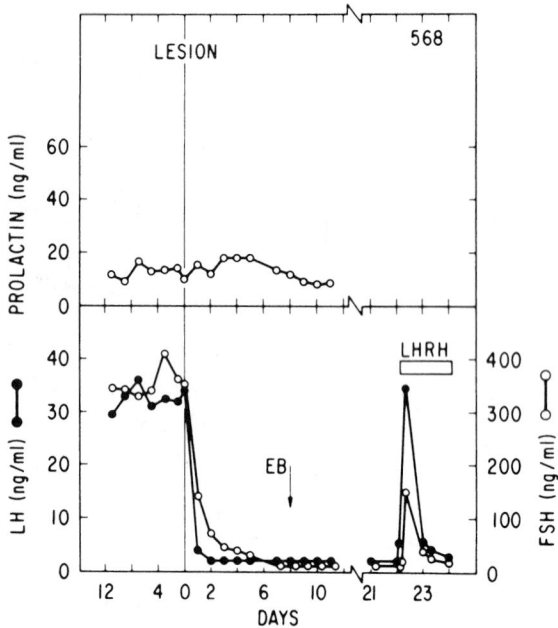

Figure 3-4

Reduction in serum luteinizing hormone (LH) and follicle-stimulating hormone (FSH) concentrations and abolition of the positive feedback action of estradiol in an ovariectomized rhesus monkey following placement of a radiofrequency lesion (on day 0) in the arcuate region and the dorsal aspect of the posterior median eminence. The injection of estradiol benzoate (EB), 42 μg/kg on day 8, is indicated by an *arrow*. The continuous intravenous infusion of gonadotropin-releasing hormone (LHRH, *horizontal bar*) at a dose of 6.8 μg/hour resulted in only a transient discharge of gonadotropic hormones. (From Plant TM, Krey LC, Moossy J, et al: The arcuate nucleus and the control of gonadotropin and prolactin secretion in the female rhesus monkey [*Macaca mulatta*]. Endocrinology 1978;102:52, with permission. © The Endocrine Society.)

quency of the GnRH pulse generator does indeed occur (Yen et al, 1972; Filicori et al, 1984; Healy et al, 1984). The consequences of this modulation in pulse generator frequency in the control of the menstrual cycle are not clear at present; however, they surely do not have a major physiologic importance because repetitive ovulatory menstrual cycles occur when driven by pulsatile GnRH administration at an unchanging follicular phase frequency (Knobil, 1980).

Conversely, the reduction in frequency of GnRH administration to mediobasal hypothalamus–lesioned (but otherwise normal) monkeys has a profound influence on follicular development and ovulation in the rhesus monkey (Pohl et al, 1983). Thus the pattern of GnRH production is as important as the quantity of the decapeptide released into the portal circulation. Deviation from the physiologic frequency can lead to changes in the concentration of LH and FSH in the circulation as well as in the ratio of one to the other (Wildt et al, 1981). The active menstrual cycle can evolve in response to unvarying pulsatile GnRH stimulation, implying that the role of GnRH in the control of gonadotropin secretion, including the induction of the preovulatory surge

(Marut et al, 1981), while essential and obligatory, is nonetheless a permissive one (Knobil, 1980; Hotchkiss and Knobil, 1994). Other observations have provided compelling support for this hypothesis that the ovary is the principal *zeitgeber* ("pelvic clock") of the rhesus monkey menstrual cycle, controlling the duration of the ovarian-menstrual cycle through its feedback mechanisms (Knobil, 1980; Hodgen, 1982; Ferin et al, 1984; Knobil and Hotchkiss, 1988).

Important therapeutic implications are derived from these observations:

1. To stimulate gonadotropin secretion in GnRH-deficient patients, treatment requires intermittent (pulsatile) administration of the decapeptide. This approach has been successful in the induction of ovulation and of puberty (Knobil, 1980) as well as spermatogenesis and fertility (Santoro et al, 1986).
2. To suppress gonadotropin secretion, treatment necessitates continuous infusion of the decapeptide. Similar effects are observed with GnRH agonists, which, after internal amino acid substitutions, are more resistant to enzymatic degradation and therefore exert a longer lasting effect (Hodgen, 1989; Gordon and Hodgen, 1992c). GnRH agonists are used extensively for the treatment of certain kinds of precocious puberty (Comite et al, 1981) and when medical castration or "medical hypophysectomy" (Hodgen, 1990) is desired for control of endometriosis, or, in conjunction with ovulation induction protocols, for assisted reproduction (Gordon and Hodgen, 1992b).
3. Because of the indirect evidence supporting the increased opioid activity in patients with hypothalamic amenorrhea (Quigley et al, 1980), specific opiate antagonists might be useful adjuncts to restore gonadotropin secretion and ovarian function in such women (Wildt and Leyendecker, 1987).

Pituitary Gonadotropes: GnRH Action and Secretion of FSH and LH

GnRH Action

The mechanism of action of GnRH on gonadotropin secretion includes binding of the decapeptide to specific receptors in the pituitary gonadotropes, followed by stimulation of intracellular responses leading to increased synthesis and secretion of LH and FSH into the circulation. The relative contributions of cyclic adenosine monophosphate (cAMP) and calcium to the cellular actions of GnRH have been controversial, but current evidence favors the importance of calcium-dependent processes in the acute mobilization and release of gonadotropins from storage granules in the gonadotropes (Catt et al, 1994). The actions of calcium- and phospholipid-dependent factors (Hirota et al, 1985) and possibly those of cyclic nucleotides in the long-term effects of GnRH are believed to be mediated through activation of protein kinases and phosphorylation of regulatory substrates in the target cell. It is likely that both calcium-

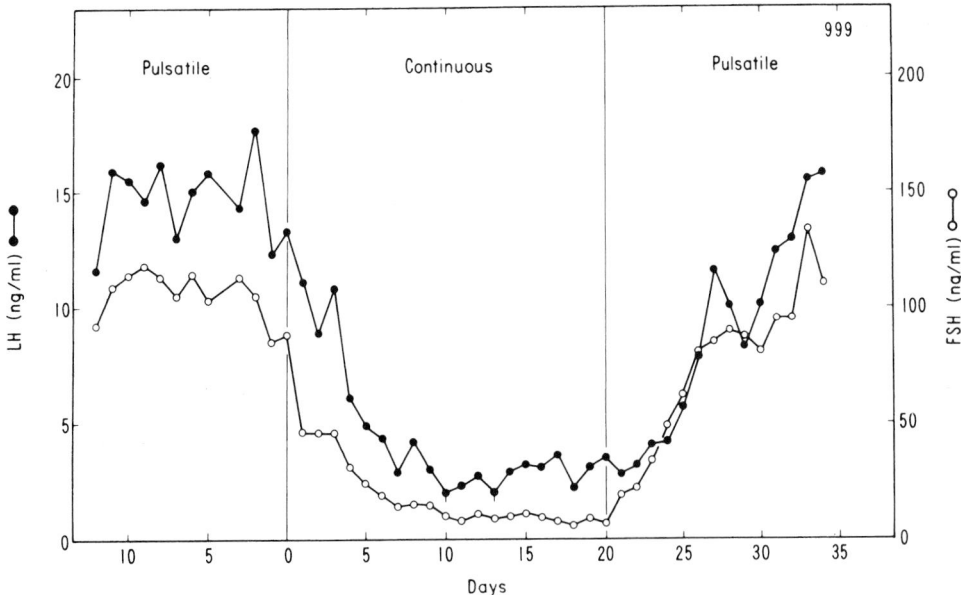

999

Figure 3–5
Inhibition of gonadotropin secretion in a rhesus monkey with a hypothalamic lesion when an intermittent gonadotropin-releasing hormone (GnRH) replacement regimen (1 μg/minute for 6 minutes every hour) was replaced by a continuous infusion of the decapeptide beginning on day 0. This inhibition was gradually reversed when the pulsatile mode of GnRH administration was reinstituted on day 20. The small vertical lines below some data points indicate levels below the sensitivity of the assay. (From Belchetz P, Plant TM, Nakai Y, et al: Hypophysial responses to continuous and intermittent delivery of hypothalamic GnRH. Science 1978;202:631, with permission. Copyright 1978 by the AAAS.)

calmodulin– and calcium-phospholipid–dependent protein kinases are regulators in the stimulation of LH release by GnRH and that arachidonic acid metabolites of the lipoxygenase pathway are also involved in the process (Fig. 3–8) (Conn, 1994; Marshall, 1995). The mechanism by which protein phosphorylation leads to increased synthesis and release of gonadotropins has yet to be clarified, but probably involves ribosomal phosphorylation and

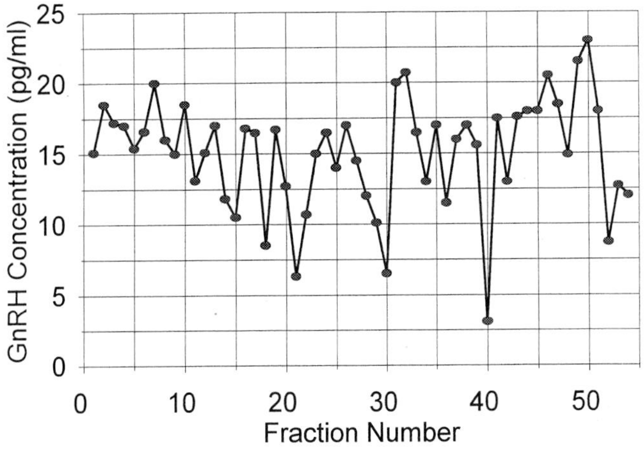

Figure 3–6
Pulsatile release of GnRH from cynomolgus monkey hypothalamus in vitro. Monkey hypothalamus superfused with M199 for 8 hours; 10-minute fractions collected and analyzed for GnRH.

modulation of translational systems within the gonadotrope. The activation of a protein element in the contractile cytoskeleton-vesicle complex within the gonadotrope also has been proposed to occur after phosphorylation, leading to extrusion of the hormone-containing granules (Kraicer, 1975).

Binding of GnRH to the gonadotropes is followed rapidly by capping or aggregation of the receptor-bound peptide and by the development of blebs into which gonadotropins become concentrated before their release (secretion) from the cell. This regional sequestration of secretory granules can be so marked as to deplete the remainder of the cell of gonadotropin, suggesting that much of the stored hormone within individual gonadotropes can be released during the secretory response to GnRH. In addition to the release of preformed gonadotropins from secretion granules, there is evidence for increased synthesis of α and β subunits during states of enhanced gonadotropin secretion. The amounts of both α and β messenger ribonucleic acids (mRNAs) are regulated by gonadal steroids, and the pituitary content of the α subunit mRNA is increased fourfold to eightfold during the preovulatory LH surge in the normal estrous cycle of sheep (Landefeld and Kepa, 1984). The stimulatory effect of E_2 on gonadotropin synthesis is complemented by the ability of pulsatile GnRH stimulation to enhance the rate of formation of LHα and LHβ subunits in the gonadotrope, a combined action that is maximally effective around the time of the preovulatory LH surge. Research (Kaiser et al, 1995) has shown that, at least in rats,

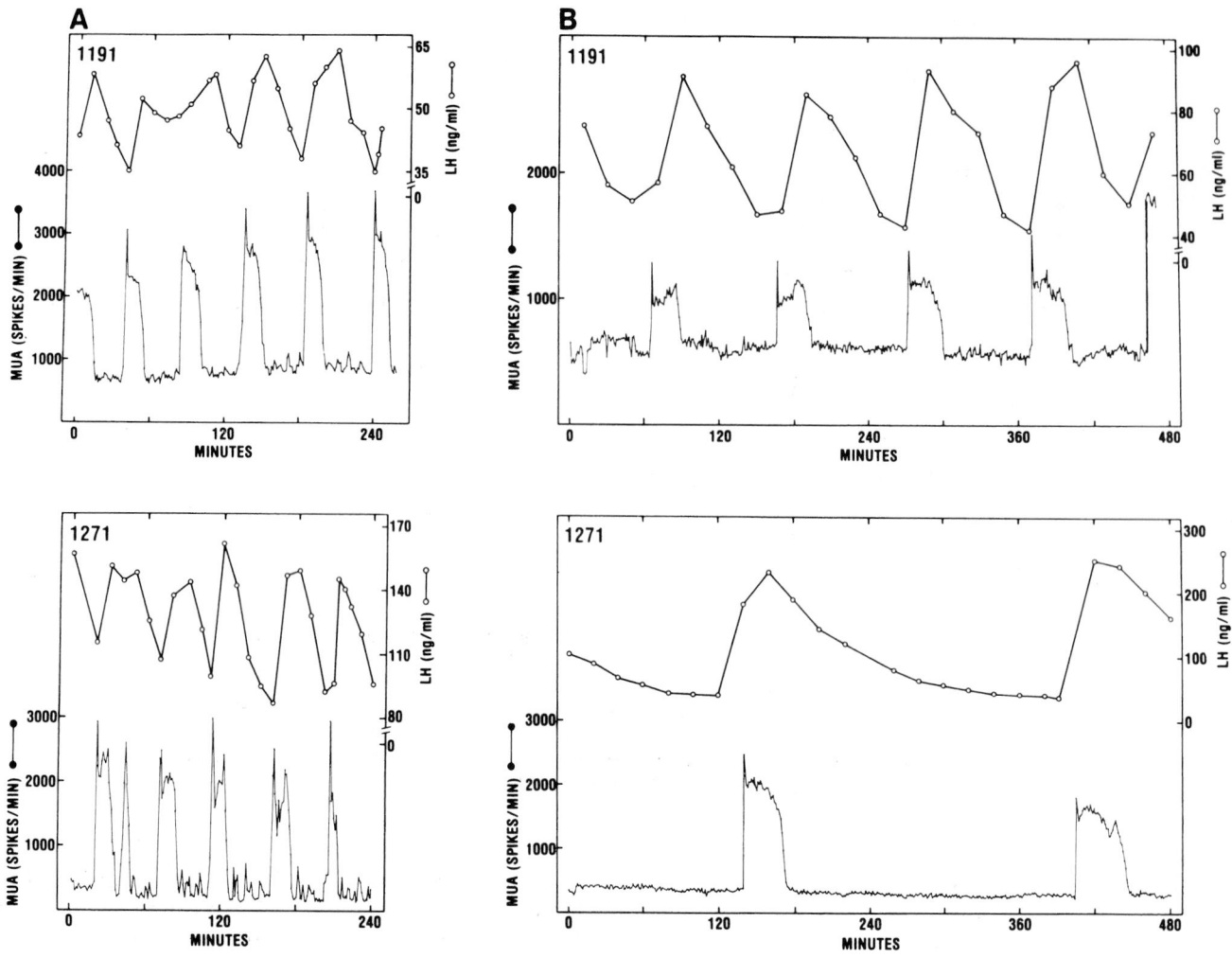

Figure 3–7
The relationship between hypothalamic pulse generator activity (multiunit activity [MUA]) and luteinizing hormone (LH) pulses in the peripheral circulation of ovariectomized rhesus monkeys bearing electrodes chronically implanted in the mediobasal hypothalamus. The coincidence of MUA volleys and LH pulses is absolute. In conscious restrained animals (A), MUA volleys and LH pulses occur at approximately hourly intervals. Each MUA volley characteristically begins abruptly, rising 100% to 600% over baseline within 1 minute, and, after a brief (1 to 2 minutes) overshoot, plateaus at a markedly increased level of variable duration, then terminates suddenly. Circulating LH levels rise within 5 minutes' start of the MUA volley. Thiopental anesthesia (B) causes a prolongation of each individual MUA and LH secretory episode as well as a reduction in the frequency of both events. (From Wilson RC, Kesner JS, Kaufman JM, et al: Central electrophysiologic correlates of pulsatile LH secretion in the rhesus monkey. Neuroendocrinology 1984;39: 256, with permission. Courtesy of Karger, Basel.)

the expression of the common α subunit and LHβ subunit genes are optimally stimulated when cell surface density of GnRH receptors is relatively high, whereas FSHβ subunit gene expression is optimally stimulated when the density of GnRH receptors is low.

Follicle-Stimulating Hormone

Follicle-stimulating hormone is a heterodimeric glycoprotein composed of two dissimilar, noncovalently linked α- and β-chains (Reichert and Ward, 1974). The α-subunit is composed of 92 amino acids and is common to FSH, LH, TSH, and human chorionic gonadotropin (hCG). Five disulfide bonds contribute to

its tertiary structure. The β subunit is composed of 115 amino acids that are specific for FSH. Six disulfide bonds contribute to its tertiary structure. The α and β subunits are held together by an unusual loop formed by a portion of the β subunit, termed the "seat belt," that wraps around the α subunit (Moyle and Campbell, 1995).

The primary function of FSH in the female is to stimulate the aromatization process by which androgens are converted to estrogen (Dorrington et al, 1975; Armstrong and Papkoff, 1976). FSH also stimulates FSH receptors, LH receptors, inhibin, activin, and insulin-like growth factor-I (Bley et al, 1992) and may stimulate granulosa cell division (Yong et al, 1992). Various types of FSH exist and are distin-

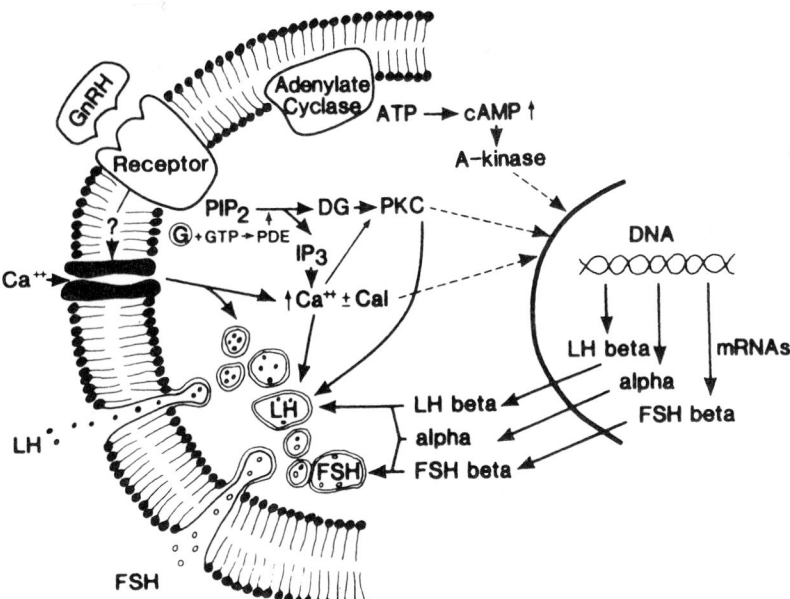

Figure 3-8
Mechanisms involved in GnRH action on the gonadotroph. *Dashed lines* indicate pathways where the mechanisms are unknown. cal, calmodulin; DG, diacylglycerol; G, G protein; IP$_3$, inositol triphosphate; PDE, phosphodiesterase (phospholipase C); PIP$_2$, phosphatidylinositol-(4,5)-phosphate; PKG, protein kinase C. (From Marshall JC: Regulation of gonadotropin secretion. In deGroot LJ [ed]: Endocrinology. 3rd ed. Philadelphia: WB Saunders, 1995:1993, with permission.)

guished by their sialic acid content. High estrogen levels induce the secretion of less sialylated molecules with higher receptor affinity and an increased clearance rate (Ben-Rafael et al, 1995).

Luteinizing Hormone

Luteinizing hormone is also a heterodimeric glycoprotein composed of two dissimilar, noncovalently linked α- and β-chains (Pierce and Parsons, 1981). The α subunit is composed of 92 amino acids and is common to FSH, LH, TSH, and hCG. As with FSH, the β subunit of LH is 115 amino acids long and wraps around the α subunit.

The primary function of LH is to stimulate the theca to produce the androgens (mainly androstenedione), which then diffuse across the cell membrane into the granulosa cells, where they are aromatized into E$_2$ in the presence of FSH (Mills, 1977; Piquette et al, 1991).

Regulation of LH and FSH Secretion

The problem of establishing the cellular origin of LH and FSH in the anterior pituitary has been a subject of controversy for many years. A separate cellular origin for these two hormones was formulated long ago on the basis of nonparallel correlations (Farquhar et al, 1975). However, immunocytochemical studies have confirmed that FSH and LH are present in the same cells, although the concentration of these hormones seems to vary from cell to cell (Tougard and Tixier-Vidal, 1994).

LH and FSH are glycoprotein hormones consisting of two different noncovalently linked α and β subunits. Both gonadotropins have the same α subunit in combination with a hormone-specific β subunit. These subunits are synthesized as precursors that undergo post-translational maturation. Glycosylation occurs on both the α and β subunits. Immuno-

cytochemical studies have delineated the secretory pathway of these hormones in a given cell (Bousfield et al, 1994).

Studies have shown that the anterior pituitary gland contains a family of FSH isohormones with different molecular weights, isoelectric properties, bioactivities, and circulatory half-lives; microheterogeneity of carbohydrate moieties is believed to be responsible for these isoforms (Dahl et al, 1988). Deglycosylation of purified pituitary glucoprotein hormones by chemical or enzymatic means generates antagonists that bind to receptors but block the action of native hormones and steroidogenesis (Sairam, 1980). Further studies have demonstrated the existence of a naturally occurring antihormone (FSH antagonist) in women treated with a GnRH analog (Dahl et al, 1988).

Subtle changes in the properties of pituitary and circulating forms of LH and FSH have also been observed in animals after changes in the gonadal steroid–pituitary feedback mechanism (Yen, 1991). In the rat, androgen treatment increases the biologic activity of pituitary FSH relative to its immunoreactivity and reduces the rate of clearance of FSH from the circulation (Bogdanove et al, 1974). In the rhesus monkey, ovariectomy is followed by changes in the properties of LH and FSH, which show a slight increase in molecular size and are cleared less rapidly from the circulation (Peckham and Knobil 1976). It is likely that these changes in pituitary gonadotropins depend on alterations in the carbohydrate composition of the hormone molecules and, specifically, on their degree of sialylation (Dufau et al, 1977).

Ovarian Feedback Mechanisms

The negative feedback control of pituitary function is one of the central concepts in endocrinology (Hotchkiss and Knobil, 1994); it was first suggested by Moore and Price (1932). Estrogen exerts an exquisitely sensitive negative feedback effect on the release of pituitary FSH. In contrast, the influence of estrogen on LH release varies with concentration and duration of exposure. Similar to its action on FSH, estrogen first commands a negative feedback relationship with LH. At high levels, however, estrogen is also capable of exerting a positive feedback effect on LH and FSH release—a response dependent on the strength and duration of the estrogen stimulus (Knobil, 1980; Marut et al, 1981). The site(s) of action of these feedback loops may be either directly on the gonadotrope, to alter responsiveness to GnRH, or indirectly at a suprapituitary level to modulate the frequency and/or amplitude of the GnRH pulses.

The mechanism(s) by which GnRH release is modulated by E_2 remain unclear for a number of reasons. First, the overwhelming majority of GnRH neurons lack estrogen receptors (Shivers et al, 1983; Watson et al, 1992; Lehman and Karsch, 1993). Second, GnRH neurons are few in number and widely dispersed throughout the brain, making them difficult to study with conventional techniques. Third, because estrogen receptors are found on so many different cells in the brain and are so widely distributed, identification of the potential interneurons with functional significance is challenging.

The secretion of gonadotropins, particularly FSH, is also under control of inhibin, a nonsteroidal inhibitor present in follicular fluid. Inhibin is a peptide moiety synthesized by the granulosa cells and secreted into the follicular fluid and ovarian venous effluent. It is capable of exerting a suppressive action on FSH secretion from the pituitary gland and may participate in the control of ovarian follicular development (Channing et al, 1980). In the rhesus monkey, porcine follicular fluid extracts inhibit FSH secretion when given during the follicular phase of the cycle, thereby interrupting follicular development and ovulation (Stillman et al, 1983). The role of inhibin in the control of gonadotropin secretion in the physiologic context, however, remains to be elucidated (Burger et al, 1995). Interestingly, inhibin belongs to a family of peptides some of which have structural similarities, including inhibins A and B, activins, and follistatins (Ying, 1988). Dimers of the β subunits of inhibin (activin) stimulate FSH secretion, whereas α,β-inihibin shows the characteristic inhibitory effect (Ling et al, 1986; MacLachlan et al, 1986).

OVARIAN PHYSIOLOGY: THE NATURAL OVARIAN-MENSTRUAL CYCLE

Follicular Development

Whereas many follicles may begin their developmental course at each ovarian-menstrual cycle, typically only a single follicle sustains its inherent gametogenic potential; all others succumb to atresia, finally having forfeited their latency (Goodman and Hodgen, 1983). Thus the vast majority of ovarian follicles are destined to undergo atresia, which is now thought to involve apoptotic cell death of the follicle cells (Hughes and Gorospe, 1991; Tilly et al, 1991; Hsueh et al, 1994). The provision of more gonadotropins during stimulated or induced cycles (clomiphene citrate or human menopausal gonadotropins [hMGs]) will violate the normal mono-ovular quota. On a controlled basis, this is a desirable effect to recover multiple eggs and facilitate in vitro fertilization (IVF). However, the alternate risk is to have impaired (qualitatively) the normality of the growing follicle and the sequelae of the ovarian-menstrual cycle, both of which are requisite for the establishment of a viable pregnancy (Hodgen, 1986).

At birth, there are approximately 200,000 to 400,000 healthy nongrowing follicles in human ovaries, each containing one oocyte. However, by the time reproductive age is reached, the number has probably fallen to less than 100,000 and continues to decline thereafter at a fairly steady rate until the fourth decade of life. At that time, there is a marked acceleration of the rate of depletion. Depletion of this nongrowing pool is the result of follicles becoming atretic or initiating follicular growth. The initiation of follicular growth occurs continuously and is thought to be at least partially gonadotropin independent. However, in the absence of appropriate gonadotropic support, follicles do not develop beyond the early antral stage, and atresia occurs. The time required for early growing follicles to attain the preantral stage is unknown but is probably at least on the order of several months (Gougeon, 1996).

In primates, early antral follicles can be seen in ovaries without regard to the stage of the cycle and even before puberty. The ability of gonadotropins to modulate follicular development depends not only on the circulating levels of gonadotropins but also on the expression of appropriate receptors by the potential target cells in the ovaries. Because early antral follicles are FSH responsive and are present throughout the menstrual cycle as a consequence of the continual supply of preantral follicles from the primordial pool, it is generally acknowledged that there is a constant source of maturing follicles for final maturation to the preovulatory stage under the influence of appropriate hormonal stimulation.

Normally, within the first half of the follicular phase of the menstrual cycle, many follicles begin to develop from either the primary to the secondary stage or all the way from primordial to secondary follicles. This process is known as "recruitment" (Fig. 3–9) (diZerega and Hodgen, 1981a). Thus a cohort of resting follicles begins a well-characterized pattern of growth and development, ultimately providing the species' characteristic ovulatory quota of eggs. This pattern of growth has been termed the "trajectory of follicle growth," with gonadotropins providing the "thrust" and ovarian factors the "guidance" along the trajectory (Fig. 3–10) (Goodman and Hodgen, 1983).

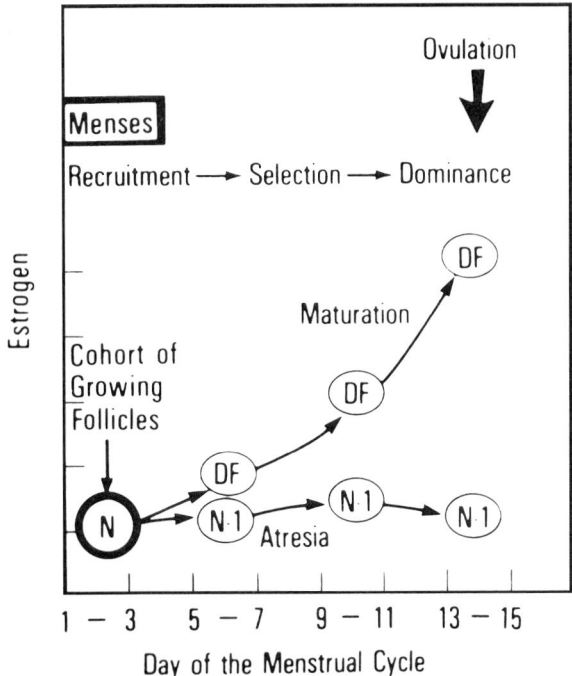

Figure 3–9
Time course for recruitment, selection, and ovulation of the dominant ovarian follicle (DF) with onset of atresia among other follicles of the cohort. (From Hodgen GD: Physiology of follicular maturation. In Jones HW Jr, Jones GS, Hodgen GD, Rosenwaks Z [eds]: In Vitro Fertilization, Norfolk. Baltimore: Williams & Wilkins, 1986:8, with permission.)

Recruitment of primordial follicles is not wholly dependent on gonadotropins and may be only enhanced by these hormones (Fauser and Van Heusden, 1997). During a typical menstrual cycle, several morphologically indistinct follicular-ovarian structures grow through cycle day 5 to 6; loss of any of these follicles does not delay timely ovulation. In contrast, after about cycle day 7, this multipotentiality is lost; typically, only one follicle will be capable of proceeding to timely ovulation. This one follicle, destined to ovulate and form the CL, is termed the *dominant follicle*. Destruction of the dominant follicle, such as by selective cautery, results in a frameshift delay of approximately one follicular phase until the next ovulation (Goodman and Hodgen, 1978; diZerega and Hodgen, 1981a). This period, during which all the recruited follicles become qualitatively equal in potential, is the time of "selection" (Fig. 3–9). That the process of selection is predetermined by some intrinsic aspect of a particular follicle seems unlikely, but, once dominance is acquired, it is certainly not transferable. No other follicle can immediately take the place of the dominant follicle. After selection of the single dominant follicle, all others become destined for atresia (Kenigsberg and Hodgen, 1987). Whereas these concepts were developed in the monkey model (Hodgen, 1982), Baird (1983) has confirmed these findings in women.

It is accepted that selection is begun and completed only during the cycle in which ovulation occurs (diZerega and Hodgen, 1981a). In contrast, the time of recruitment and thus the total length (duration) of the trajectory are unknown. Based on present evidence, the duration of the trajectory in macaques and women appears to be not less than about 2 weeks. It has been hypothesized that, in the physiologic setting of the ovarian menstrual cycle, the folliculogenic actions of gonadotropins (principally FSH) are permissive at tonic levels and the steroidogenic actions of gonadotropin (principally LH) are graded. If FSH at tonic levels is actually permissive to folliculogenesis (Goodman and Hodgen, 1983), graded effects observed may be attributable to supraphysiologic (supratonic) levels. Graded actions of gonadotropins on steroidogenesis (and perhaps on inhibin secretion) are necessary for ovarian mechanisms to control circulatory gonadotropins near the tonic setpoint so that the mechanisms of follicle selection are effective (Hodgen, 1986).

Beginning 5 to 6 days before the onset of menstruation, there is a concordant decline in plasma levels of estradiol, progesterone, and inhibin as a result of the gradual demise of the CL, which is associated with a reciprocal elevation in plasma FSH levels (the so-called intermenstrual FSH rise) (Roseff et al, 1989). It has been hypothesized that this rise in FSH is responsible for the recruitment of the cohort of follicles for the subsequent cycle, from which the single dominant follicle will ultimately be selected.

Induction of FSH receptor expression is of paramount importance in the mechanism whereby primary committed follicles become responsive to FSH. Presumptive FSH receptors are reported to first appear in rat primary follicles when the granulosa cells change shape from flattened squamous to cuboidal (Mulheron et al, 1989).

In primate ovaries, autoradiographic localization of FSH receptors is evident in the granulosa cells of some preantral follicles and in virtually all antral follicles, including the dominant follicle (Zeleznik et al, 1981). LH receptors are confined largely to the outer boundary, presumably the thecal layer, of nearly all antral follicles, with the dominant follicle also showing binding over the granulosa cells. These findings have been confirmed and extended in more recent studies in rats. Camp et al (1991) utilized a quantitative reverse transcription–polymerase chain reaction amplification scheme to measure the relative levels of FSH and LH receptor mRNAs and in situ hybridization to localize the FSH and LH receptor transcripts. FSH receptor mRNA was confined to the granulosa cells of healthy developing follicles, whereas LH receptor mRNA was localized predominantly in the theca cells of small follicles on estrous morning, with their appearance in the granulosa cells of growing follicles by diestrous morning. LH receptor mRNA was also found in the interstitial tissues and CLs throughout much of the estrous cycle.

The control of this acquisition of FSH responsiveness has been under investigation for over 50 years

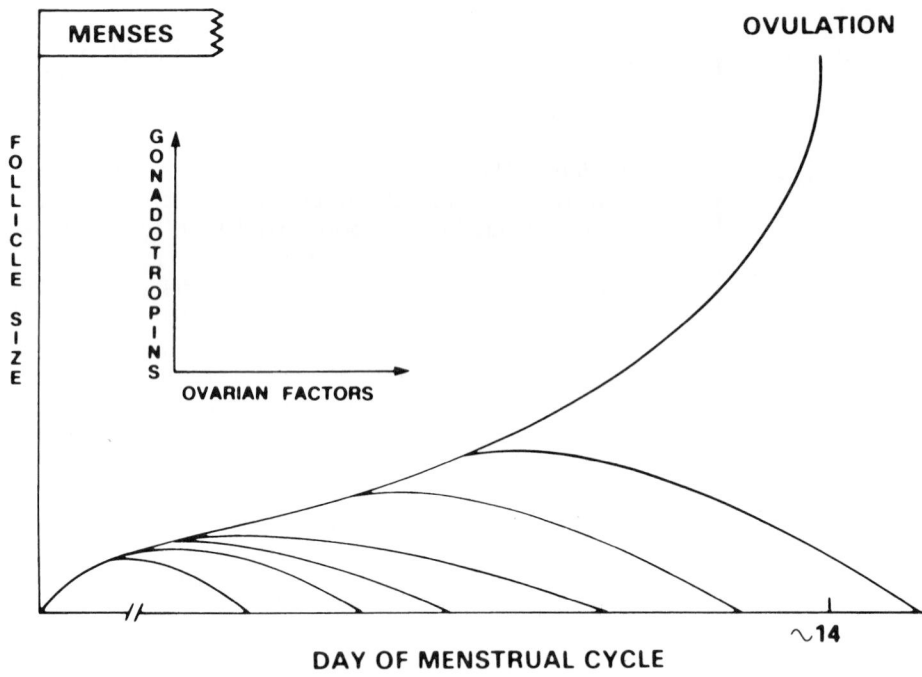

Figure 3–10
Proposed relationship between gonadotropins and ovarian factors in regulating maturation or atresia along the so-called trajectory of follicle growth. (From Hodgen GD: Physiology of follicular maturation. In Jones HW Jr, Jones GS, Hodgen GD, Rosenwaks Z [eds]: In Vitro Fertilization, Norfolk. Baltimore: Williams & Wilkins, 1986:8, with permission.)

(Hisaw, 1947) yet remains ill-defined. Research has suggested that activin may be one of the factors that stimulates granulosa cells to express FSH receptors (Hasegawa et al, 1988; Fig. 3–11). Furthermore, activin may influence the steroidogenic activity of the granulosa cells through the induction of follistatin (Findlay, 1993).

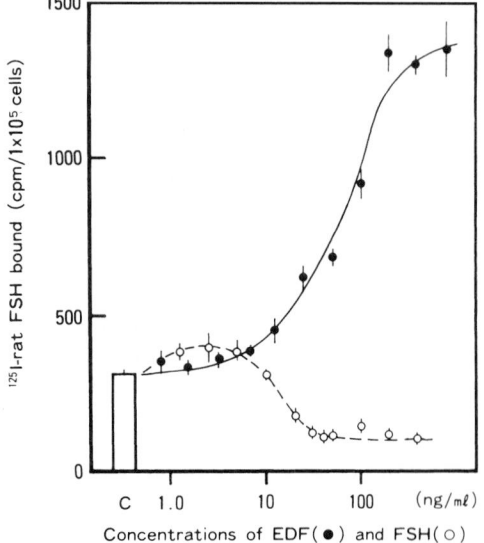

Figure 3–11
Effects of FSH (○) and erythroid differentiation factor (EDF; activin A) (●) on the number of FSH binding sites in granulosa cells. (From Hasegawa Y, Miyamoto K, Abe Y, et al: Induction of follicle stimulating hormone receptor by erythroid differentiation factor on rat granulosa cell. Biochem Biophys Res Commun 1988;156:668, with permission.)

In monkeys (Zeleznik et al, 1981) morphometric analysis of ovaries collected during the late follicular phase indicates that the percentage of the theca layer occupied by blood vessels in the dominant follicle is almost twice that of the other small follicles in the ipsilateral or contralateral ovary. This observation, plus the preferential uptake of intravenously administered hCG (diZerega and Hodgen, 1980; Zeleznik et al, 1981) by the dominant follicle, suggests that blood flow to individual follicles may be instrumental in the selective maturation of the dominant preovulatory follicle in primates.

It is well known that the developing dominant follicle is the primary source of the rising tide of E_2 seen in the peripheral circulation toward the end of the follicular phase. This E_2 has been hypothesized to serve many purposes: (1) preparation of the endometrium for implantation, (2) initiation of the preovulatory gonadotropin surge, and (3) selection of the dominant follicle.

A working hypothesis has been put forward as to how E_2 controls follicular selection (Zeleznik, 1993). There are certain assumptions. Because preantral folliculogenesis is inherently asynchronous, owing to the continued exit of follicles from the primordial pool, there will always be a maturationally distinct distribution of early antral follicles within the ovaries available for continued maturation under the influence of FSH. As FSH levels rise consonant with the demise of the CL, these follicles are stimulated to grow and, when aromatase induction is sufficient to cause peripheral estrogen levels to increase, FSH secretion is inhibited by the negative feedback actions of E_2 at the hypothalamic-pituitary level (probably mostly at the pituitary level), thus depriving the other follicles of their gonadotropic support. If this model is accurate, then certain predictions can be made.

First, administration of E_2 during the early follicular phase, before a leading follicle emerges, would cause a premature fall in FSH levels that would, in turn, interrupt timely follicular development. Studies conducted in rhesus monkeys showed that a premature elevation in systemic estrogen concentrations from 50 to 80 pg/ml on days 3 to 6 of the follicular phase produced a modest decline in FSH levels and interrupted folliculogenesis until the exogenous estrogen was removed and FSH levels rose again, whereupon folliculogenesis was resumed and ovulation occured 12 to 14 days later (Zeleznik, 1981).

Second, interference with the negative feedback actions of E_2 on pituitary FSH secretion should result in the selection and support of multiple follicles. This prediction has been shown to be true in many reports of studies in which passive immunization of monkeys to E_2 was undertaken (Zeleznik et al, 1985), or in which administration of estrogen antagonists such as clomiphene citrate have been used to induce multiple ovulations (Adashi, 1995).

In 1978, Brown demonstrated that there was a threshold level of FSH necessary for the development of a single follicle. This theory was directly tested in rhesus monkeys by Zeleznik and Kubik (1986). Rhesus monkeys had their endogenous gonadotropins suppressed with daily administrations of a GnRH antagonist. Four such monkeys were given human FSH and human LH intravenously in a pulsatile manner (one 3-minute pulse/hour). The amount of FSH per pulse (initially 24.5 ng/kg/pulse) was increased on day 5 (to 49 ng/kg/pulse) and again on day 8 (to 98 ng/kg/pulse) before serum E_2 levels rose above baseline. Upon detection of the rise in E_2 levels, the amount of FSH per pulse was decreased by 12.5%/day. The amount of LH per pulse (200 ng/kg/pulse) was held constant throughout. Despite the progressive decline in FSH as a result of the 12.5% decrease per day, serum levels of E_2 continued to rise in a manner indistinguishable from that seen during spontaneous follicular phases (see Fig. 3–12). The authors found that a threshold level of FSH (15 to 20 mIU/ml) had to be achieved to initiate follicular development as measured by E_2 production. Given the vagaries of the assay systems used to make the comparison, the authors concluded that this is comparable to that seen during the early follicular phase in these monkeys. They also concluded that the plasma level of FSH needed to maintain preovulatory follicular maturation is less than that necessary to initiate preovulatory growth.

However, not everyone is in agreement with the above hypothesis. Gougeon and Testart (1990) raised the objection that, if the "passive inhibition" theory were correct, then it should be possible to correct this effect by exogenous gonadotropins. They were un-

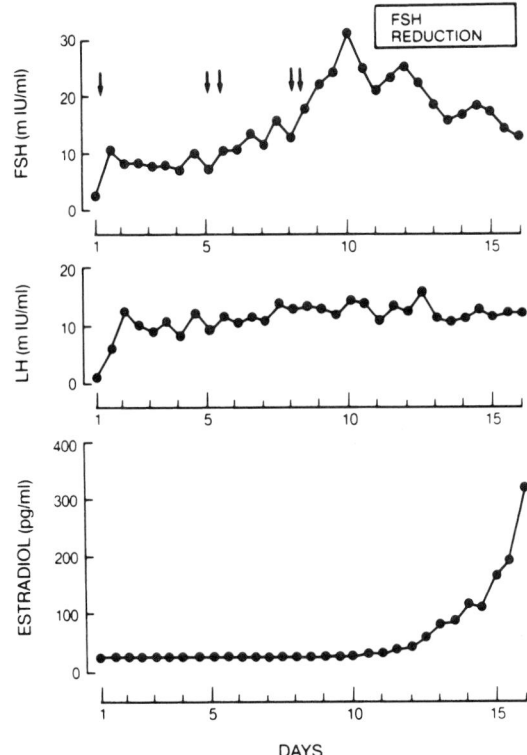

Figure 3-12
Plasma gonadotropin and estradiol concentrations in a cynomolgus monkey infused with hFSH and hLH at a frequency of one pulse per hour. The *first arrow* indicates the initiation of hFSH and hLH infusion. The subsequent *double arrows* indicate a doubling of the amount of hFSH given per pulse. As indicated at the top of the figure, the amount of FSH delivered per pulse was reduced by 12.5%/day after the initial rise in serum estradiol concentrations. (From Zeleznik AJ, Kubik CJ: Ovarian responses in macaques to pulsatile infusion of follicle-stimulating hormone (FSH) and luteinizing hormone: increased sensitivity of the maturing follicle to FSH. Endocrinology 1986;119:2027. Copyright The Endocrine Society, with permission.)

able to demonstrate such an effect when 225 IU of hMG was administered to women during different phases of the menstrual cycle.

The dominant follicle and its successor, the CL, make up the "dominant structures" of the ovarian cycle, having remarkable authority over both intraovarian (bilateral) and systemic events regulating folliculogenesis (Goodman and Hodgen, 1983). In the natural cycle, although either ovary may provide the dominant follicle in any given cycle, once the dominant follicle has been selected, the two ovaries are partitioned into that which is gametogenically active and that which is gametogenically inactive. Necessarily, ovarian function is then asymmetric. However, after corpus luteum demise, the follicular apparatus of both ovaries become symmetric; at that time, probably local ovarian factors in conjunction with gonadotropin actions initiate a typical follicle trajectory (diZerega and Hodgen, 1981a; Goodman and Hodgen, 1983).

Ovulation

The most prominent physiologic marker of impending ovulation is the midcycle LH surge. Within the microenvironment of the dominant follicle, three major events occur at this time:

1. *Resumption of meiosis I.* At this time, the oocyte resumes nuclear maturation, as evidenced by germinal vesicle breakdown, transition from prophase I to metaphase I stage, and extrusion of the first polar body (metaphase II stage). Nuclear maturation occurs, probably in synchrony with cytoplasmic and zona pellucida maturation in preparation for fertilization (Oehninger et al, 1991). The intracellular processes that account for these maturational changes are not fully understood but may involve oocyte factors as well as follicular paracrine factors (growth agents, inhibin, and so on), steroids, and gonadotropins.
2. *Luteinization.* Although there is some increased progesterone secretion before the onset of the LH surge, the exposure of the follicle to the midcycle high LH levels magnifies the extent and degree of transformation of the follicular stromal cells from an estrogen- and protein-secreting apparatus to predominantly steroid secretion (mainly progesterone, E_2, and androstenedione). The fact that late follicular phase progesterone secretion starts either before or immediately after the first perceptible changes in the endogenous LH pulse amplitude or frequency may implicate an independent intraovarian mechanism that begins to shift ovarian steroidogenesis and/or secretion toward progesterone even before initiation of the LH surge (Marut et al, 1981; Hoff et al, 1983; Collins et al, 1984).
3. *Ovulation.* The exact mechanism by which follicle rupture occurs and the oocyte, surrounded by the cumulus oophorus, is released is not completely understood. Gonadotropins (especially LH) stimulate prostaglandin secretion, plasminogen activator release, and mucification of the cumulus; enzymatic digestion of the follicular wall seems to be one of the principal mechanisms leading to ovulation.

Because the peak of the midcycle LH surge cannot be accurately defined (although it is frequently used as a reference point), the onset of the LH surge should be used to monitor menstrual cycles because it permits a relatively precise reference for timing hormonal and intrafollicular dynamics at midcycle (Hoff et al, 1983; Schenken and Hodgen, 1983). During the last 2 to 3 days before the onset of the midcycle surge, the incremental rate of circulatory E_2 (doubling time 61.3 hours) parallels that of progesterone and 17α-hydroxyprogesterone (17α-OHP) (Marut et al, 1981). This concomitant rise of progestins and E_2 may reflect the acquisition of LH receptors on the granulosa cells of the dominant follicle and the resulting ability to initiate biosynthesis of

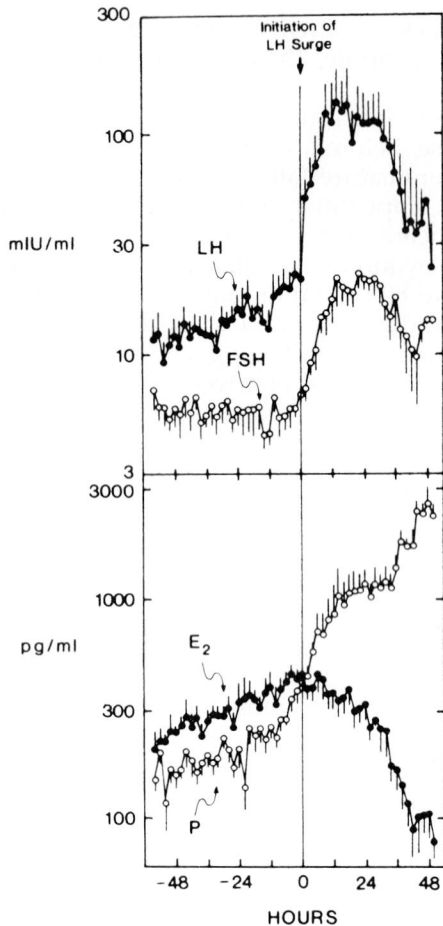

Figure 3–13

Mean (± SE) luteinizing hormone (LH), follicle-stimulating hormone (FSH), estradiol (E_2), and progesterone (P) levels measured every 2 hours for 5 days at midcycle in seven studies. Data were centered at the initiation of the gonadotropin surge. Note that the data were plotted on a logarithmic scale. (From Hoff JD, Quigley ME, Yen SSC: Hormonal dynamics at midcycle: a reevaluation. J Clin Endocrinol Metab 1983;57:792, with permission. © by the Endocrine Society.)

17α-OHP and progesterone (Fig. 3–13) (McNatty et al, 1979; Hoff et al, 1983).

Prediction of ovulation can be achieved by the correlation of clinical parameters (biologic shift of estrogen in end-target organs), follicular development and growth by ultrasonography, and E_2, progesterone, and LH determinations in blood. In IVF cycles monitored as described (nonstimulated, natural cycle), Garcia et al (1981) found that a 28-hour interval from the ascending limb of the LH surge seems to be the "ideal time" for collection of mature preovulatory oocytes (Figs. 3–14 through 3–16) (Veeck, 1986). The precise time interval between the onset of the LH surge and ovulation in women remains uncertain, but available data suggest that ovulation occurs 1 to 2 hours before the final phase of progesterone rise, or 34 to 35 hours after the onset of the LH surge (Hoff et al, 1983).

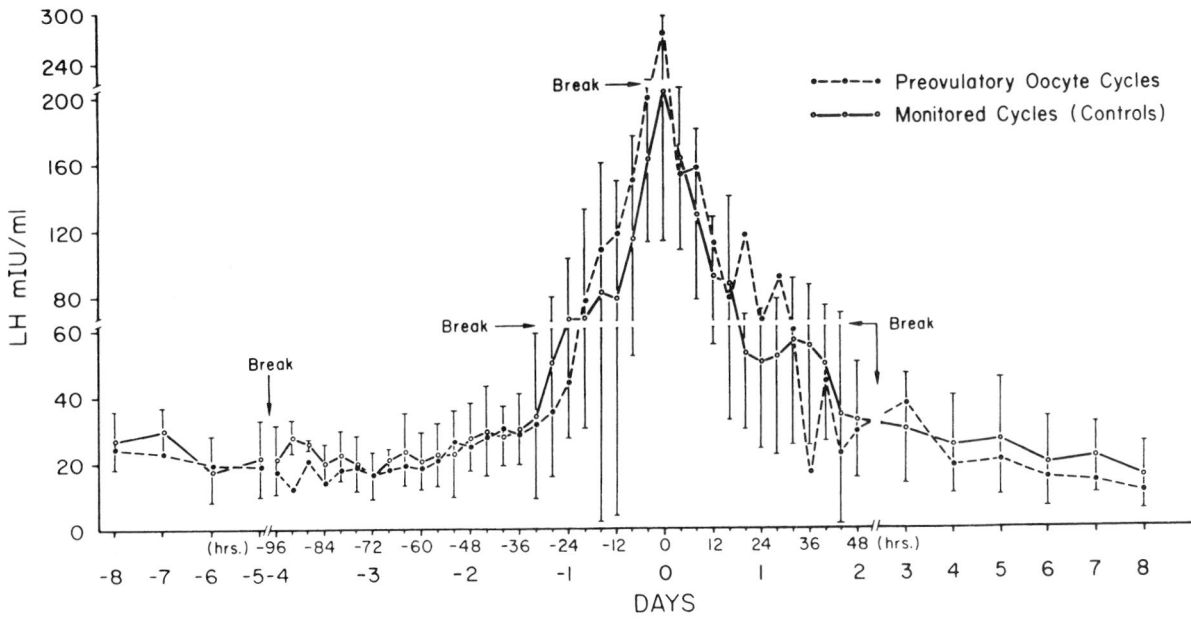

Figure 3–14
Daily and every-4-hours serum luteinizing hormone (LH) levels from day −8 to day +8 in 50 menstrual cycles normalized to the day of the LH peak. *Solid bar*, controls (mean ± SE); *broken line*, preovulatory oocyte group. (From Garcia J, Jones GS, Wright GL: Prediction of the time of ovulation. Fertil Steril 1981; 36:308, with permission of The American Fertility Soceity.)

The processes of ovulation (follicular rupture) and oocyte maturation are closely synchronized and coordinated in the ovarian follicle by appropriate gonadotropin stimuli. Extensive studies of the mechanism of ovulation demonstrate that gonadotropins stimulate ovarian steroids, enzymes, chemical inflammatory mediators, and smooth muscle contrac-

tions interacting locally within the somatic elements of the follicle. Experimental approaches using the in vitro perfused rabbit ovary provided important information regarding synchronization of follicle rupture and oocyte maturation (Yoshimura and Wallach, 1987). In this system, prostaglandins, norepinephrine, histamine, or streptokinase can induce follicle

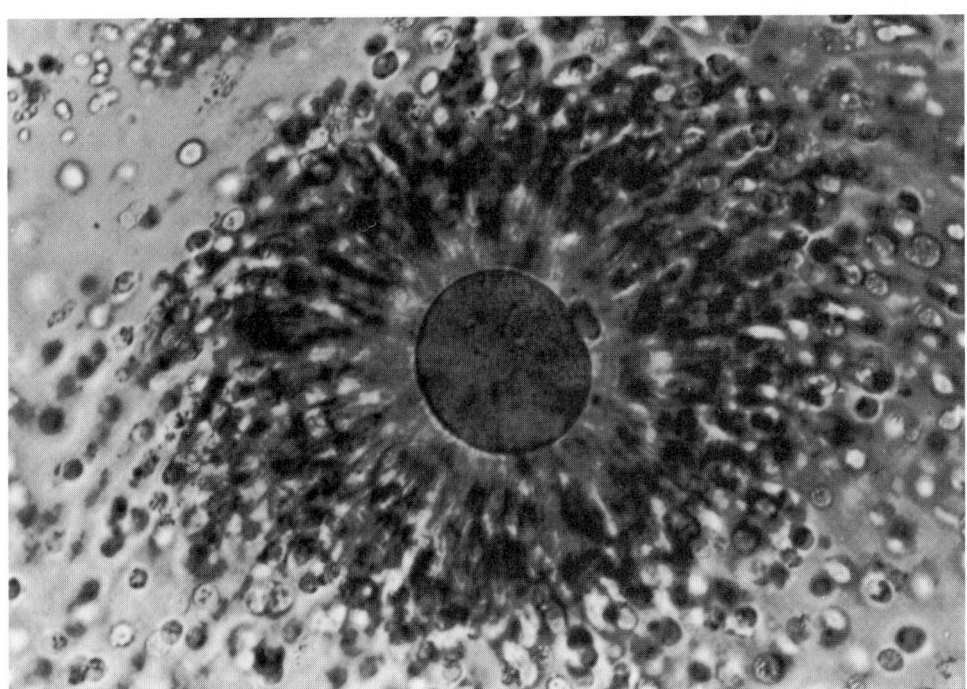

Figure 3–15
Typical mature or preovulatory human oocyte. (From Veeck LL: Morphological estimation of mature oocytes and their preparation for insemination. In Jones HW Jr, Jones GS, Hodgen GD, Rosenwaks Z [eds]: In Vitro Fertilization, Norfolk. Baltimore: Williams & Wilkins, 1986:81, with permission.)

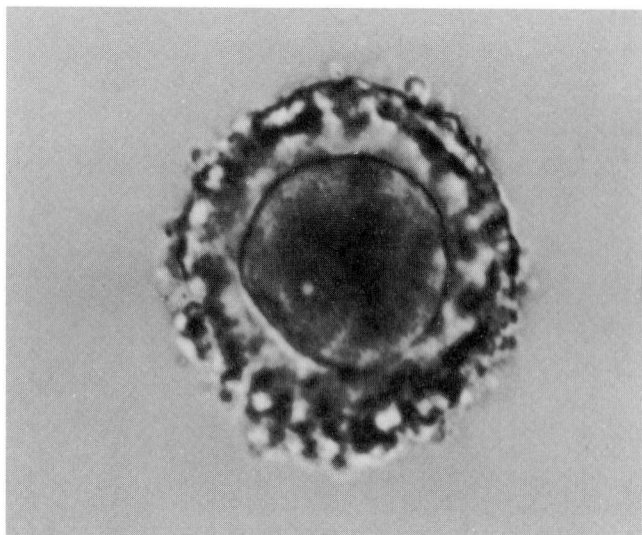

Figure 3–16
Typical germinal vesicle–bearing immature human oocyte.
(From Veeck LL: Morphological estimation of mature oocytes
and their preparation for insemination. In Jones HW Jr, Jones
GS, Hodgen GD, Rosenwaks Z [eds]: In Vitro Fertilization,
Norfolk. Baltimore: Williams & Wilkins, 1986:81, with
permission.)

rupture but not oocyte maturation. These compounds presumably alter the apical region of the follicle wall through vascular, enzymatic, or inflammatory influences that facilitate follicle disruption
and mature ovum discharge.

It has been appreciated for many years that biochemical parameters of mammalian ovulation could
exist in the absence of ovarian follicle rupture (Kerin
et al, 1983). It has been reported that the incidence
of recurrent luteinized unruptured follicle (LUF) syndrome may be high in women with infertility and
also in patients with endometriosis (Brosens et al,
1978; Schenken et al, 1984). Whatever the real incidence of the LUF syndrome is in these patients, it is
tempting to speculate that lesions or dysfunctions in
any one of the specific processes of proteolysis, mucification, smooth muscle contraction, or angiogenesis might be identified in this condition (Kenigsberg and Hodgen, 1987).

Ovarian Hormonogenesis

FSH is the prime inducer of ovarian maturation and
is responsible for the development of granulosa cell
responsiveness to several other hormones. The action of the granulosa cell products ensures optimal
folliculogenesis and oocyte maturation conducive to
the release of a fertilizable oocyte. Because FSH receptors are present exclusively in the granulosa cells,
various effects of FSH are believed to be mediated
through granulosa cells (Table 3–3) (Hsueh et al,
1984).

According to the two-cell, two-gonadotropin hypothesis for ovarian estrogen biosynthesis, LH stimulates the synthesis of androgens from cholesterol in
the theca interna (Falck, 1959; Short, 1962). Androgens diffuse across the lamina basalis (basement
membrane) and are converted to estrogens by the
aromatase enzyme present in the granulosa cells
(Fig. 3–17). This hypothesis provides a useful model
for understanding follicular estrogen biosynthesis in
many species. Notwithstanding, Kenigsberg and
Hodgen (1987) have shown that, in primates, "pure"
FSH of urinary origin is capable of stimulating ovarian E_2 secretion at a level not dissimilar from that
obtained by the same dose of urinary hMG containing an equal ratio of FSH to LH. Furthermore, un-
diminished E_2 production was observed when pure
FSH was administered in the presence of a GnRH
antagonist that maintained a relatively hypogonadotropic state with regard to endogenous gonadotropin secretion (Fig. 3–18). This finding does not necessarily negate the two-cell theory of ovarian
steroidogenesis. It does, however, open to question
the previous assumptions about the relative importance of FSH and LH. In the primate ovarian cycle,
it seems that FSH is of far greater importance, such
that a very modest presence of LH is sufficient,
whereas the quantity of FSH is crucial to ovarian
stimulus response.

Multiple studies have demonstrated the complexity of function and regulation of the granulosa cells
(Fortune and Armstrong, 1978; McNatty et al, 1979).
Hsueh and co-workers (1984) visualized the granulosa cell as a model hormonal target cell under endocrine control (classical gonadotropin hormone
control), neuromodulatory control (by neurotransmitters released by the ovarian neuronal innervation), paracrine control (i.e., androgens), and autocrine modulation (ultrashort loop regulation of
granulosa cell function by estrogens). To correlate
follicular and oocyte maturation, numerous studies
have focused on follicular fluid constituents. Table
3–4 presents those substances found in follicular
fluid, ranging from steroids and pituitary hormones
to mucopolysaccharides and nonsteroidal factors
(ovarian peptides). The follicular concentrations of
all of these substances vary depending on the follicular maturational stage; therefore, attempts have
been made to assess their potential role as markers
of oocyte maturation (Fritz and Speroff, 1982; Pellicer
et al, 1987). Several factors present in the follicular
fluid and egg vestments may have a significant impact on sperm function. It has been established that
progesterone, which is present in the follicular milieu at high concentrations, stimulates a rapid and
potent calcium influx into sperm. Calcium is a well-
known regulator of sperm functions crucial to fertilization, like the acrosome reaction and hyperactivated motility. Together with zona pellucida
components, progesterone and other local female
components are probably essential in the regulation
of sperm functions in the vicinity of the ovulated
egg.

Table 3-3. FSH–STIMULATED FUNCTION PARAMETERS IN CULTURED GRANULOSA CELLS

1. Enhancement of steroidogenesis
   a. Estrogen biosynthesis: induction of aromatases
   b. Progesterone and 20α-hydroxyprogesterone biosynthesis
      Induction of cholesterol side-chain cleavage enzymes and mitochondrial cytochrome P_{450} activity
      Induction of 3β-hydroxysteroid dehydrogenase
      Induction of 20α-hydroxysteroid dehydrogenase
2. Induction of specific plasma membrane receptors
   a. LH receptor formation
   b. Prolactin receptor formation
   c. β₂-Adrenergic receptor formation (coupling)
   d. Lipoprotein receptor formation
   e. FSH receptor formation
   f. EGF receptor formation
3. Secretion of nonsteroidal cell products
   a. Inhibin
   b. Plasminogen activator
   c. Prostaglandins
   d. Proteoglycans (mucopolysaccharides)
4. Stimulation of general cell functions
   a. DNA synthesis
   b. Protein synthesis
   c. Glucose uptake and lactate formation
   d. Cell round-up and aggregation
   e. Gap junction formation
   f. Microvilli formation
5. Plasma membrane–related processes
   a. Adenyl cyclase activation and cAMP formation
   b. Formation of cAMP binding protein
   c. Phosphodiesterase activation
   d. Increases in plasma membrane microviscosity

Abbreviations: cAMP, cyclic adenosine monophosphate; EGF, epidermal growth factor; LH, luteinizing hormone.
From Hsueh AJW, Adashi EY, Jones PB, Welsh TH: Hormonal regulation of the differentiation of cultured ovarian granulosa cells. Endocr Rev 1984;5:76, with permission. © By the Endocrine Society.

PHYSIOLOGY OF THE CORPUS LUTEUM

The midcycle gonadotropin surge serves three purposes: (1) it induces the final maturation of the oocyte, (2) it triggers the cascade of events that leads to ovulation of the oocyte, and (3) it provides the primary stimulus for the conversion of the follicle into a CL. There are two major processes that occur during the differentiation of the CL from the follicle: (1) conversion of granulosa cells into luteal cells, and (2) the disruption of the basement membrane between the granulosa and thecal layers of the follicle such that an influx of vascular elements can develop into the luteinizing granulosa layer.

It is now recognized that the CL is composed of dynamic populations of luteal and nonluteal cells, with the numbers and characteristics of cell populations changing during the luteal life span. In recent studies, three distinct size groups of luteal cells have been isolated from nonhuman primate CLs—small (15 μm), medium (16 to 20 μm) and large (>20 μm)—along with several nonluteal cell types, including vascular endothelial cells, immune system cells, and fibrocytes (Stouffer, 1996).

The CL secretes as much as 40 mg of progesterone per day during the midluteal phase of the ovarian cycle. The precursor for progesterone is cholesterol, and studies suggest a major role for low-density lipoprotein (LDL) cholesterol as a factor regulating progesterone biosynthesis (Carr et al, 1982; Brannian and Stouffer, 1993). The vascularization of the CL allows for a mechanism by which LDL cholesterol gains access to the luteinizied granulosa cells (Fig. 3–19).

Luteal cells contain specific LH-CG receptors that bind gonadotropin and activate adenylate cyclase, leading to an acute cAMP-mediated increase in progesterone production. The luteinized theca cells continue to respond to the LH pulses with both E₂ and progesterone synthesis and secretion. They continue to multiply and divide and, if pregnancy ensues, these cells respond to hCG stimulation from the conceptus and constitute the CL of pregnancy. Studies in monkeys (Healy et al, 1984) and women (Filicori et al, 1984) have demonstrated that progesterone from the CL is secreted in a pulsatile manner. As the luteal phase progresses, the LH pulse frequency falls dramatically from a high of one pulse every 90 minutes during the early follicular phase to a low of one pulse every 7 to 8 hours during the late luteal phase (Ellinwood et al, 1984), with a concomitant increase in pulse amplitude.

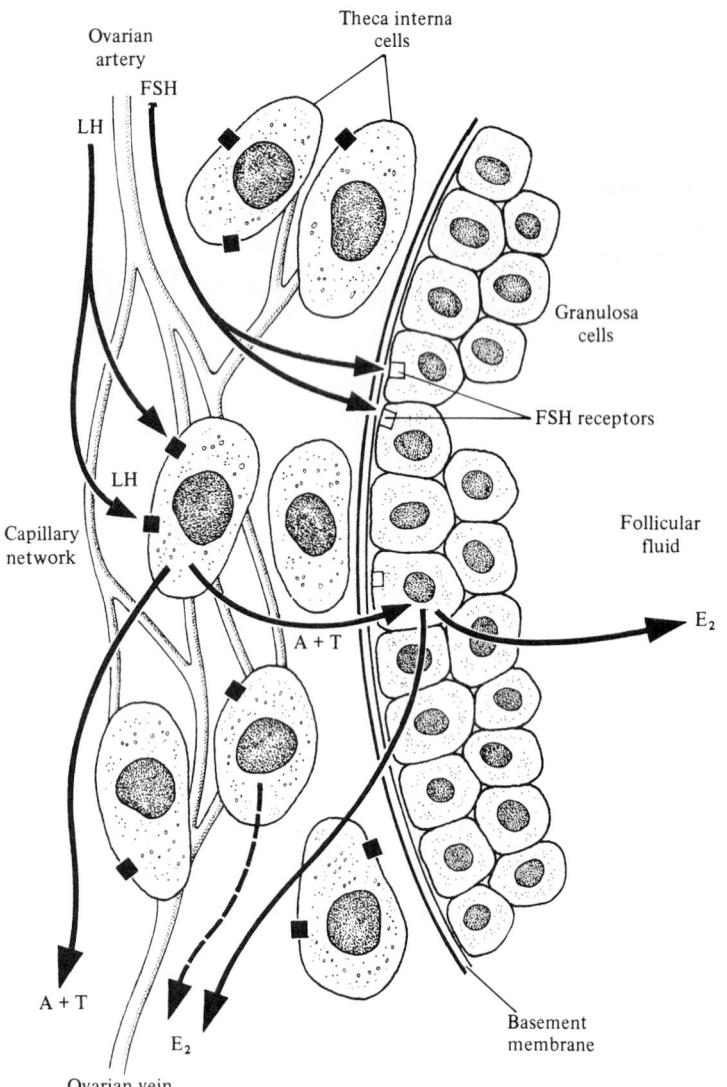

Figure 3-17
Diagram of action of gonadotrophins on the follicle and the synthesis of estrogens. Luteinizing hormone (LH) interacts with receptors on the theca cells (■) to stimulate production of androgens and small amounts of estradiol (E_2). Follicle-stimulating hormone (FSH) activates the aromatase enzyme system in the granulosa cells by interacting with receptors (□). A, androstenedione; T, testosterone. (From Baird DT: The ovary. In Austin CR, Short RV [eds]: Hormonal Control of Reproduction. Vol 3. Cambridge: Cambridge University Press, 1984:101, with permission.)

The capacity of luteal tissue for progesterone synthesis can be extended by chorionic gonadotropin (hCG in women, mCG in monkeys) as a result of either implantation or administration of exogenous hCG. In many respects, the events of the luteal phase of the ovarian cycle are consequences of preceding follicular phase activities (diZerega and Hodgen, 1981b). Indeed, the process of luteiniziation begins even before the time of ovulation. The same specialized gonadal stromal cells that support recruitment, selection, and maintenance of the dominant follicle transform from producers of estrogens and follicular regulatory proteins to producers of progesterone, inhibin, and other luteal products. A series of studies by Zelinski-Wooten, Aladin Chandrasekher, and colleagues (Aladin Chandrasekher et al, 1991, 1994; Zelinski-Wooten et al, 1991, 1992) have defined how the duration of the midcycle LH surge has an impact on subsequent ovarian events. Clearly, different exposure times are needed for various different events, with at least 18 hours being required for oocyte mat-

uration and more than 48 hours required for full luteal phase function and duration (Table 3–5).

Despite significant advances in the past decades, the factor(s) responsible for the regression of the CL at the end of the menstrual cycle remain enigmatic. Clearly the uterus is not the source of the luteolytic signal in primates because hysterectomy does not extend the life of the CL (Neill et al, 1969). Prostaglandin $F_{2\alpha}$ ($PGF_{2\alpha}$) is the apparent luteolytic agent in many nonprimate species, and $PGF_{2\alpha}$ can induce luteolysis in primates. However, administration of prostaglandin inhibitors does not extend the life span of the CL in primates. Thus, a physiologic role for endogenous $PGF_{2\alpha}$ in the initiation of luteolysis in primates remains unsubstantiated. The declining frequency of LH pulses during the luteal phase, already alluded to above, led researchers to speculate that this was causally related to luteolysis. However, studies have unequivocally shown that luteolysis cannot be solely the result of declining LH support, because artificially maintaining the frequency of LH

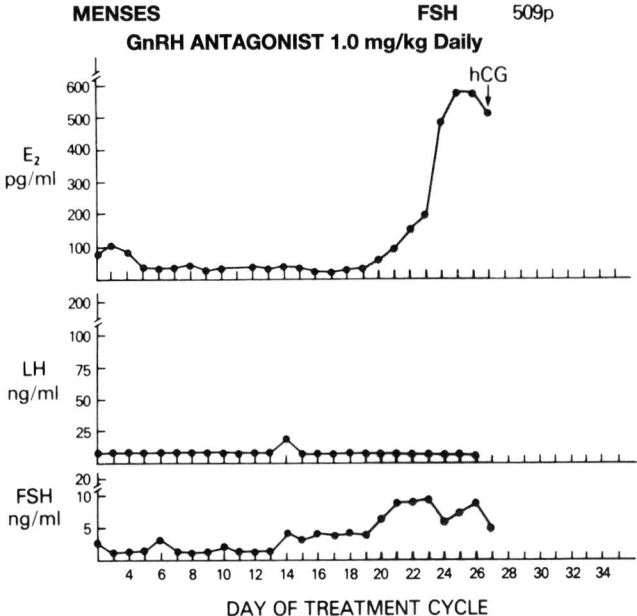

Figure 3-18

GnRH-antagonist (Ac-pClPhe[1], PClDhe[2], DTryp[3], DArg[6], DAla[10])-GnRH-HCl administration, followed by follicle-stimulating hormone (FSH) therapy, in intact cycling monkeys. Note suppression of endogenous gonadotropin secretion and ovarian responsiveness to FSH treatments, as indicated by elevations of estradiol (E_2) in serum. (From Hodgen GD: Physiology of follicular maturation. In Jones HW Jr, Jones GS, Hodgen GD, Rosenwaks Z [eds]: In Vitro Fertilization, Norfolk. Baltimore: Williams & Wilkins, 1986:8, with permission.)

Table 3-4. SUBSTANCES FOUND IN FOLLICULAR FLUID

Plasma proteins
Steroid-binding protein
Enzymes
   Steroid biosynthesis enzymes
   Aromatase
   Plasminogen
Mucopolysaccharides (proteoglycans)
   Hyaluronic acid
   Chondroitin sulfate
   Heparin sulfate
Steroids
   Estrogens
   Androgens
   Progestins
Pituitary hormones
   Follicle-stimulating hormone
   Luteinizing hormone
   Prolactin
   Oxytocin
   Vasopressin
Nonsteroidal ovarian factors
   Inhibin
   Oocyte maturation factor
   Follicle regulatory protein
   Luteinizing inhibitor
   Luteinizing stimulator
   Gonadotropin surge inhibiting factor (attenuin)

pulses (via exogenous pulsatile GnRH administration) does not extend the life span of the CL (Zeleznik and Hutchison, 1987).

According to Zeleznik and Hillier (1996), the most plausible explanation for luteal regression is that the CL regresses as a result of its ever-decreasing ability to respond to plasma levels of LH that prevail throughout the luteal phase. Recall that extended function of the CL beyond the 2 weeks of the non-fertile cycle is critical to the establishment of pregnancy. This is achieved via the actions of CG secreted by the blastocyst and syncytiotrophoblast. However, the mechanism(s) whereby CG extends the life span of the CL remain unclear. Perhaps CG provides a more "intense" stimulus to the luteal cells, thereby rescuing the CL.

PHYSIOLOGY OF THE ENDOMETRIUM

During the reproductive years, most women tend to have menstrual cycles of a relatively consistent length, which is considered to be normal at 28 ± 7 days. The luteal-secretory phase is more consistent at approximately 14 days, whereas the follicular-proliferative phase accounts for most of the variability in cycle length. For each woman, there is a tendency for longer cycles at the extremes of the reproductive years: perimenarche and perimenopause (Fig. 3-20) (Treolar et al, 1967). Both intervals are characterized by disordered follicular development and less frequent ovulation than in midreproductive life, and are accompanied by a higher incidence of dysfunctional uterine bleeding.

The primate endometrium is a complex tissue composed of various cell types (luminal and glandular epithelia, stromal fibroblasts, vascular smooth muscle cells, etc.) that are all targets for gonadal sex steroid action. Furthermore, these cellular components possess an endogenous endocrine activity producing prolactin, prostaglandins, and several other substances (Kenigsberg and Hodgen, 1987; Giudice and Ferenczy, 1996). Factors related to embryo implantation are locally produced and play an important role in the establishment of pregnancy (Dey, 1996). Recent studies have greatly increased the amount of knowledge on the preimplantation embryo and the molecular biology of the uterus. The initial, mutual recognition of the developing embryo and the endometrium probably involves a tight physical contact, perhaps mediated by the pinopodal extensions of the superficial luminal epithelium. Multiple endocrine (estrogen and progesterone) and local (adhesion molecules such as integrins, leukemia inhbitory factor, and other cytokines) factors are probably operational to ensure timely implantation. The expression of immunosuppressive factors, such as glycodelin-A and others, is also regulated in a spatial and temporal manner in order to abolish rejection of the embryo at early stages of implantation.

The endometrium is composed of two distinct tissue compartments: the upper transient functionalis,

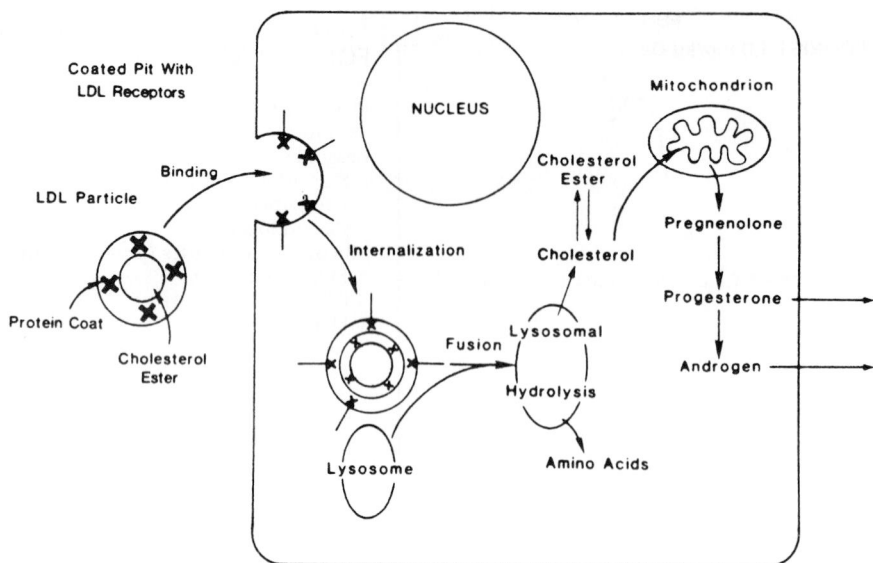

Figure 3–19

Source of ovary cellular cholesterol. Circulating low-density lipoprotein (LDL) particles, containing a cholesterol ester core surrounded by a protein coat, bind to specific cell membrane receptors. The LDL receptor complex is internalized and fuses to lysosomes. The cholesterol ester is hydrolyzed to cholesterol and the protein coat to amino acids. The free cholesterol is either stored as re-esterified cholesterol or transferred to mitochondria, where the side chain cleavage enzymes convert it to pregnenolone. (From Adashi EY: The ovarian life cycle. In Yen SSC, Jaffe RB [eds]: Reproductive Endocrinology. 3rd ed. Philadelphia: WB Saunders Company, 1991:204, with permission.)

which is formed and shed during each cycle, and the deep germinal basalis, which persists from cycle to cycle (Fig. 3–21). The primate endometrium has a distinctive arterial supply that arrives via the radial arteries, which arise from the arcuate arteries within the myometrium. After passing through the myometrial-endometrial junction, the radial arteries divide to form smaller basal arteries, which supply the basal portion of the endometrium, and the spiral arterioles, which continue upward to supply the functionalis (Fig. 3–21). The changes in the histologic appearance of the endometrium during the ovarian-menstrual cycle were well characterized almost 50 years ago (Fig. 3–22) (Noyes et al, 1950). A normal menstrual period lasts 4 ± 1 days, with most of the menstrual effluvient being expelled in the first 24

Table 3–5. EFFECTS OF GONADOTROPIN SURGES OF DIFFERENT DURATIONS ON SUBSEQUENT PERIOVULATORY EVENTS IN RHESUS MONKEYS DURING ARTIFICIAL IVF CYCLES

OVULATORY STIMULUS*	SURGE DURATION (HOURS)	OOCYTE MATURATION[†] (0/+)	GRANULOSA CELLS[‡] PR Expression (0/+)	GRANULOSA CELLS[‡] Progesterone Production In Vitro	LUTEAL PHASE[§] (DAYS)
None	0	0	0	×	0
GnRH × 1	4–6	0	0	2×	0
GnRH × 3	8–10	0	0	3×	0
GnRHag × 2	>14	0	0	5×	0
hLH × 1	18–24	+	0/+	15×	1–6
hLH × 2	36–48	+	+	15×	8–18
hCG × 1	>48	+	+	20×	11–13

Abbreviations: GnRH, gonadotropin-releasing hormone; GnRHag, GnRH agonist; hCG, human chorionic gonadotropin; hLH, human luteinizing hormone; PR, progesterone receptors.
*On day 10 of artificial cycles, monkeys (*n* = 3 to 6 per group) received various treatments to produce surge levels (100 ng/ml) of bioactive gonadotropin.
[†]Resumption of meiosis as judged from collection of oocytes at metaphase I or II, 27 hours after the ovulatory stimulus.
[‡]Cells were stained immunocytochemically for PR and incubated in vitro for 24 hours to assess progesterone production.
[§]Interval of more than 1 ng/ml progesterone in serum from the ovulatory stimulus to menses.
From Stouffer RL: Corpus luteum formation and demise. In Adashi EY, Rock JA, Rosenwaks Z (eds): Reproductive Endocrinology, Surgery, and Technology. Philadelphia: Lippincott-Raven, 1996:254, with permission.

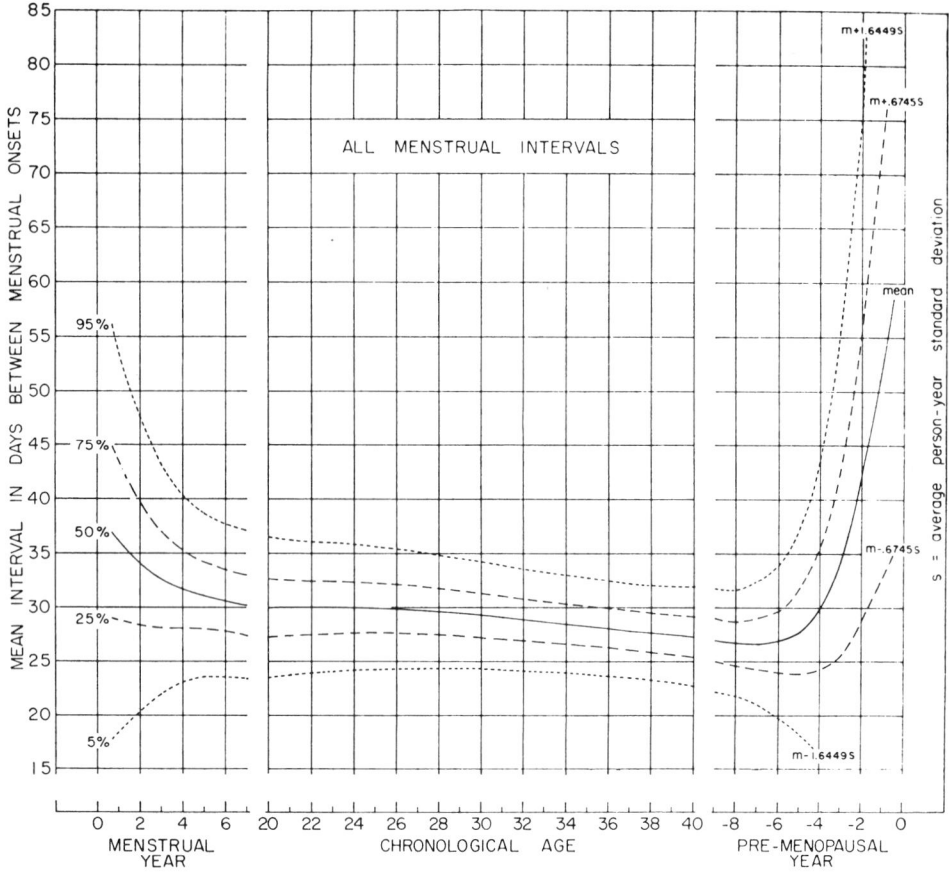

Figure 3-20
Mean menstrual cycle lengths in a large population of women. (From Treolar AE, Boynton RD, Benn BG, Brown BW: Variation of human menstrual cycle through reproductive life. Int J Fertil 1967;12:77, with permission.)

hours. Subsequent to this interval of sloughing, the proliferative phase begins with growth and proliferation of glands and stroma from an initial endometrial height of 0.5 to 5.0 mm, the maximal endometrial height that is achieved in the periovulatory interval. These events are predominantly estrogen dependent. The glands are straight and tubular and the cells lining the glands are in a pseudostratified configuration. Neither intracellular vacuoles nor luminal secretion are evident at this stage. The stroma in the proliferative phase is tightly packed and uniform. Although impressions can be made about whether endometrium is in an early, mid, or late proliferative phase, dating of this phase of the cycle is generally of little clinical utility (Kenigsberg and Hodgen, 1987).

The secretory phase of the endometrium has been extensively studied, and precise evaluation of the changes throughout the luteal-secretory phase is of considerable clinical relevance. With the appearance of progesterone in the periovulatory interval, the glands of the endometrium begin to show secretory activity. The first sign of this activity is the appearance of glycogen-rich secretory vacuoles within the cytoplasm of the glandular cells. These vacuoles are always seen in a subnuclear position on day 18 of the idealized 28-day cycle. After this, increasingly abundant luminal secretion is evident throughout the secretory phase, with peak secretory activity occurring on day 20. Both E_2 and progesterone levels are high coincident with these events. The stromal reaction to these high ambient hormone levels is edema, which, in the setting of no new accumulation in endometrial height, results in a coiling and compaction of endometrial glands and blood vessels. After the stage of maximal stromal edema on day 22, the perivascular stromal cells begin to accumulate eosinophilic cytoplasm and a characteristic decidualized appearance on day 23 of the cycle known as perivascular or periarteriolar "cuffing." This decidual response is next detected in the periluminal subcapsular region on day 25, and the two areas are connected by sheets of decidua on day 26. At this stage, a certain diagnosis of pregnancy might be fortuitously made by finding an implantation site on biopsy, but the absence of such an area does not exclude an early gestation (Kenigsberg and Hodgen, 1987). From this point on, the presence or absence of pregnancy determines the fate of the endometrium. E_2 and progesterone withdrawal will result in

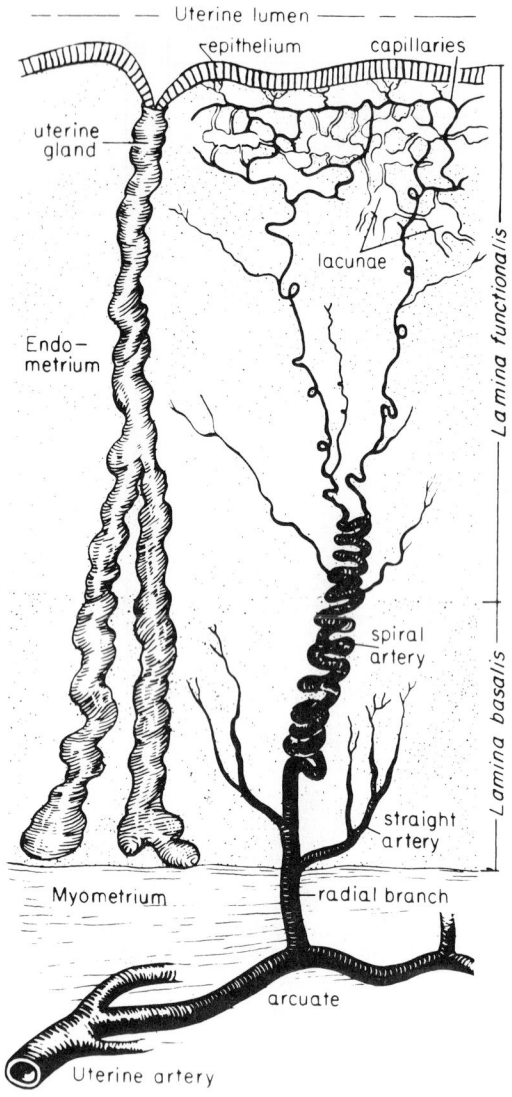

Uterine lumen
epithelium capillaries
uterine gland
lacunae
Endo-metrium
Lamina functionalis
spiral artery
straight artery
Lamina basalis
Myometrium
radial branch
arcuate
Uterine artery

Figure 3–21
Diagrammatic representation of the glands and vasculature of the human endometrium. (From Blandau RJ: The female reproductive system. In Weiss L [ed]: Histology, Cell and Tissue Biology. 5th ed. New York: Elsevier Biomedical, 1983:932, with permission.)

stromal fragmentation, interstitial hemorrhage, and tissue sloughing down to the basal layer. CL rescue by CG with continuous high levels of progesterone results in the diffuse decidualization of pregnancy.

Figure 3–23 shows progesterone and hCG levels in a patient undergoing in vitro fertilization/embryo transfer (IVF/ET) after hMG/hCG stimulation. Exogenous hCG is detectable on day 10. After day 10, the hCG reflects the endogenous production that has rescued the CL function (Jones, 1986). Serum β-hCG values in pregnant and nonpregnant patients after IVF/ET are shown in Figure 3–24 (Muasher and Garcia, 1986). Notice that a viable pregnancy and one that will end in a clinical miscarriage show the same trend in the first weeks after conception. However, preclinical abortions are characterized by an

early decrease in β-hCG levels, occurring even before the expected menses. Preclinical abortions occur also after natural conception, and their significance after IVF/ET cycles has been discussed by Acosta et al (1990).

The effects of estrogen and progesterone on the endometrium depend on the presence of hormone receptors in the target tissue. Estrogen and progesterone act on the endometrial cells by altering their structure and function through a general effect on RNA transcription and protein synthesis. These effects are mediated by specific high-affinity receptor sites that exhibit a remarkable cyclic change during the menstrual cycle. Both estrogen receptors (ER) and progesterone receptors (PR) are localized in the nuclei of epithelial and stromal cells in the functionalis and basalis layers of the endometrium. ER content is highest in the late proliferative endometrium and decreases gradually throughout the postovulatory phase of the cycle in the epithelium, and even more rapidly in the stroma (Bergeron et al, 1988a). PR content in the functionalis layer increases from early to late proliferative phase and remains high in the early secretory phase (Bergeron et al, 1988b). PR content of glandular epithelium decreases during the secretory phase, while the stroma and myometrium maintain significant PR content (Lessey et al, 1988). These results suggest that the notion that PR are up-regulated by estradiol and down-regulated by progesterone is probably an oversimplification.

Toward the end of the nonfertile cycle, steroid hormone levels decline, initiating the onset of menses. The results of several studies indicate that the endometrial production of prostaglandins, which may act as vasoconstrictors, increases at this time. This can also explain the increased uterine contractions at the time of uterine menses. In addition, fibrinolytic activity reaches maximum levels at the time of menstruation in the shed endometrium (Todd, 1964). The noncoagulability of menstrual blood probably is the result of such increased activity.

PUBERTY

Puberty is not an event. It is a process through which a complex series of interrelated physiologic changes occur leading to the development of a reproductively mature adult. Human puberty combines two processes: adrenarche (increased secretion of androgen precursors from the adrenal gland) and gonadarche (activation of hormonogenesis and gametogenesis by the gonads). Adrenarche usually begins several years before gonadarche. However, adrenarche can occur without gonadarche and vice versa, so these developmental processes should be viewed as independent, albeit temporally overlapping, phenomena.

The mechanism(s) regulating the onset of puberty remain unclear. The hypothalamic-pituitary-gonadal (H-P-G) axis becomes functional during early fetal development. By day 50 to 55 of gestation, the GnRH

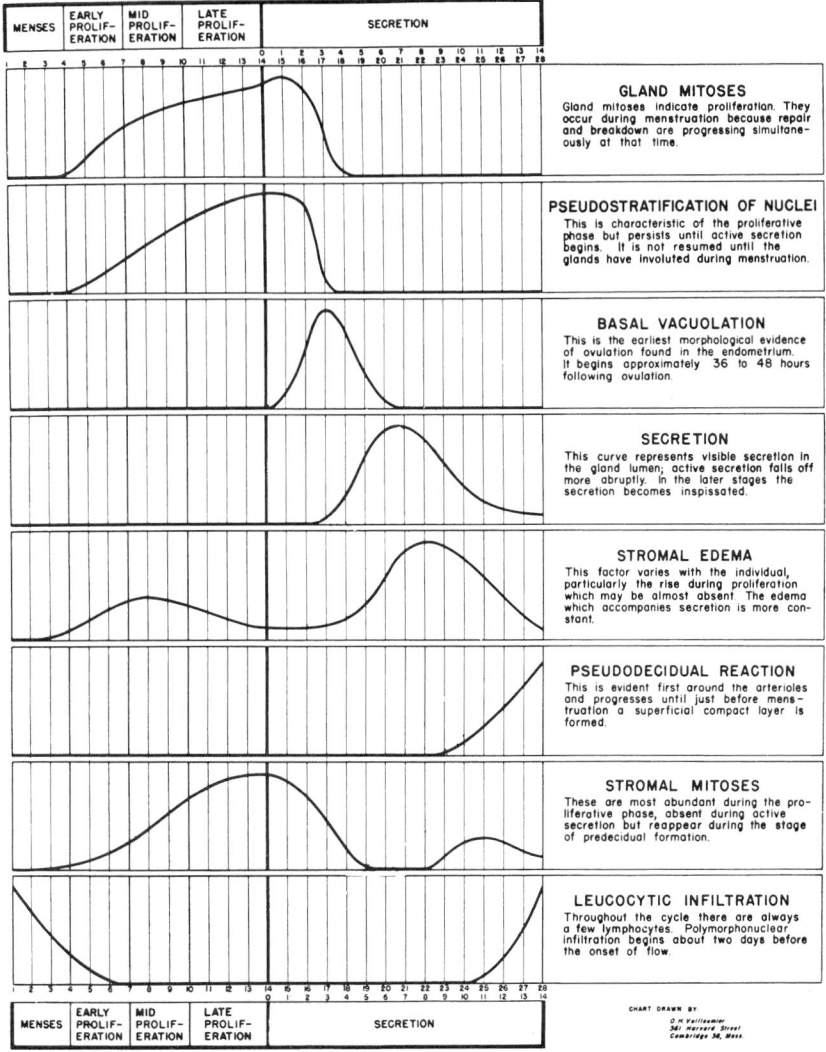

DATING THE ENDOMETRIUM
APPROXIMATE RELATIONSHIP OF USEFUL MORPHOLOGICAL FACTORS

Figure 3–22
Characteristic histologic changes in the endometrium throughout the menstrual cycle. (From Noyes RW, Hertig AT, Rock J: Dating of the endometrium biopsy. Fertil Steril 1950;1:3, with permission of The American Fertility Society.)

neuronal system is sufficiently developed in both male and female rhesus monkeys to control gonadotropin secretion (Ronnekleiv and Resko, 1990).

Clearly, appropriate pulsatile delivery of GnRH is key to the whole process. This is drammatically illustrated by the fact that ovulatory menstrual cycles can be initiated in juvenile female monkeys when pulsatile GnRH is administered (Wildt et al, 1980). Furthermore, the juvenile GnRH neurons themselves can be driven to secrete sufficient GnRH to support normal puberty by intermittent administration of N-methyl-D-aspartic acid (Gay and Plant, 1988).

Recall that in both boys and girls the H-P-G axis remains active during the first year or so of life, is inhibited during childhood, and reactivates during the pubertal interval, typically with the appearance

of sleep-induced LH increments. Thus the first essential question regarding the regulation of puberty should be how the GnRH neuronal system is turned off, rather than how it is turned on.

Whether this hiatus in activity of the GnRH pulse generator is due to active inhibition, or lack of needed excitatory input, or possibly a combination of both, remains unclear. In the neural inhibitory schema, there is direct (or indirect via interneuronal contacts) inhibition of the GnRH neurons. In prepubertal children, the H-P-G axis is very sensitive to the negative feedback effects of gonadal steroids. Furthermore, the sensitivity of the H-P-G axis is known to change as development toward puberty progresses. This became known as the "gonadostat" theory of puberty (Grumbach et al, 1974). However,

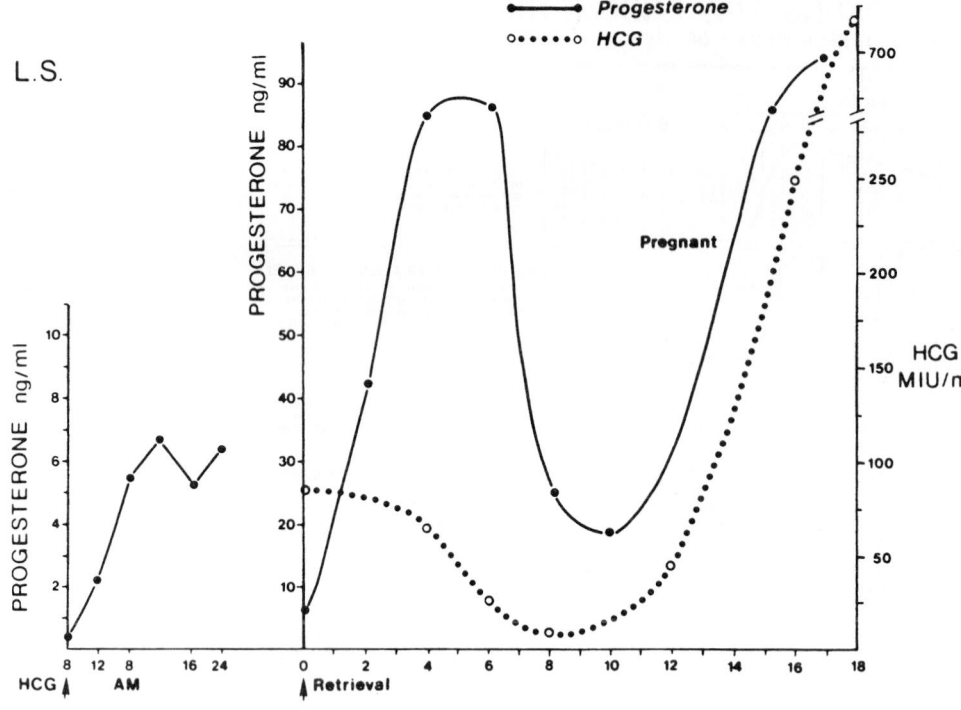

Figure 3–23
Serum progesterone and β-hCG levels in a patient undergoing in vitro fertilization/embryo transfer (hMG/hCG cycle) who was delivered of a term pregnancy. (From Jones GS: Luteal phase in a program for in vitro fertilization. In Jones HW Jr, Jones GS, Hodgen GD, Rosenwaks Z [eds]: In Vitro Fertilization, Norfolk. Baltimore: Williams & Wilkins, 1986:221, with permission.)

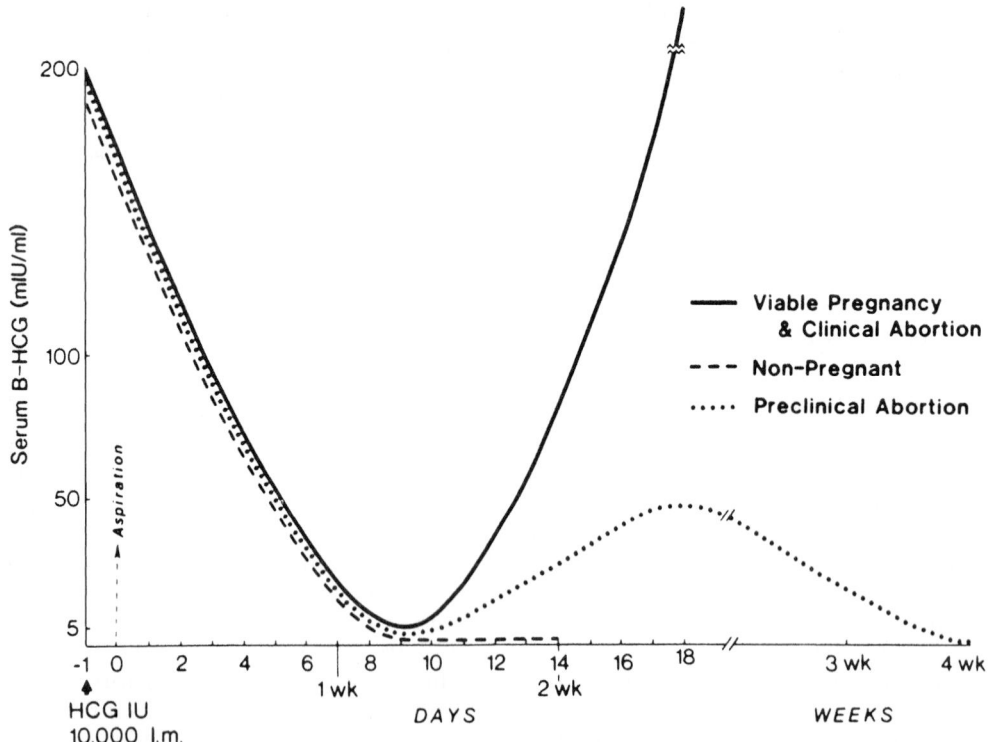

Figure 3–24
Serum β-hCG levels in pregnant and nonpregnant women following in vitro fertilization/embryo transfer. (From Muasher SJ, Garcia JE: Pregnancy and its outcome. In Jones HW Jr, Jones GS, Hodgen GD, Rosenwaks Z [eds]: In Vitro Fertilization, Norfolk. Baltimore: Williams & Wilkins, 1986:30, with permission.)

there is no compelling evidence to support the notion that the initiation of puberty in primates is triggered solely by a decrease in gonadostat sensitivity. In fact, it has now been clearly demonstrated that the presence or absence of the monkey or human gonad has little impact on the timing of pubertal onset (Conte et al, 1975; Ross et al, 1983; Plant, 1994). Work from Terasawa's lab (Mitsushima et al, 1994) strongly suggests that the GnRH neuronal system is restrained by inhibitory inputs from GABAergic neurons during this inhibitory phase.

In the neural stimulation schema, the activity of the juvenile GnRH neurons, while sufficient to maintain biosynthetic potential and minimal release of gonadotropins, lacks the requisite stimuli or capacity for full function. It has long been argued that the onset of puberty is linked to some growth-tracking device or to the degree of adiposity of the individual. Preliminary support for the latter concept was provided by Chehab et al (1997), who demonstrated that normal prepubertal female mice treated with leptin (a recently characterized hormone secreted from adipose tissue) reproduce up to 9 days earlier than controls. From these results, the authors speculated that leptin may act as a signal triggering puberty.

USE OF GONADOTROPINS FOR STIMULATION OF OVULATION

The normal process of selection of the single dominant follicle leading to ovulation and luteal phase function in the natural cycle can be overridden by supraphysiologic gonadotropin stimulation of the ovary. Typically, exogenous gonadotropin therapy allows several recruited follicles to avert atresia. Although their development is not perfectly synchronous, a few follicles are likely to mature enough for ovulation, fertilization, and implantation to ensue (Hodgen, 1982, 1986; Kenigsberg and Hodgen, 1987). This supraphysiologic stimulation is desirable for enhanced oocyte recovery for IVF/ET programs (Hodgen, 1981; Rosenwaks and Muasher, 1986). Luteal steroidogenesis in the stimulated cycle cannot be assessed by a comparison with luteal steroidogenesis in the natural cycle. The ratio of estrogen to progesterone is an important determinant of the endometrial response pattern. Thus the adequate support of the luteal function in pregnancy with exogenous progesterone may overcome a possible excessive E_2 stimulation that can occur with supraphysiologic gonadotropin levels and may ensure that the endometrial pattern is adequate and conducive to normal implantation (Jones, 1985).

Different gonadotropin preparations are available today for the treatment of ovulation disorders. These preparations include a combination of FSH and LH, purified FSH, and the more recently developed recombinant FSH and LH. Recombinant gonadotropins produced by genetic engineering technology will undoubtedly represent an important treatment modality in various fertility disturbances.

The induction of ovulation is a vital part of therapy for infertility. An understanding of the processes involved in the rescue of the single follicle in the natural cycle should provide the clinician with a better understanding of what might be the most appropriate approach to ovulation induction in various clinical conditions. Rather than using one protocol for all conditions of ovulation induction, the choice of protocol should be based upon the specific clinical problem. A few examples follow.

Ovulation Induction in Amenorrhea

Normogonadotropic Amenorrhea

Here, the goal is to recruit only one, or possibly two, follicles and to avoid multiple pregnancies. In normogonadotropic amenorrhea, the patient may have a normal baseline level of endogenous FSH, but FSH does not rise above threshold levels. Exogenous FSH is therefore required, and a low to moderate dose of FSH (one or two ampules of hMG) will bring the plasma FSH level above threshold in 2 or 3 days. Sometimes, because of the variability of sensitivity, one might need to increase the dosage (a step-up approach) during therapy (Taymor, 1996). Ovulation is routinely triggered by hCG administration when the lead follicle(s) reach the appropriate size.

Severe Hypopituitary Amenorrhea

In this situation, a deficiency of both FSH and LH exists. When there is almost complete absence of LH, hMG has been shown to be superior to purified FSH of either pituitary or urinary origin (Taymor, 1996). In this case, as opposed to the normogonadotropic amenorrhea, both FSH and LH are needed for adequate follicular growth.

Polycystic Ovarian Disease

In this condition, plasma levels of LH are usually high, with normal FSH levels. Adrenal and ovarian androgens are usually elevated. Small doses of human urinary or recombinant FSH administered daily over a 2- to 3-week period can result in ovulation that usually follows hCG triggering. Because of the multifollicular ovarian condition, these patients need to be monitored very closely to avoid the risk of hyperstimulation and multiple pregnancy. Many of these patients can be initially treated with clomiphene citrate, which will increase the levels of FSH and LH in the early follicular phase. Clomiphene citrate, an antiestrogen, exerts its effect at the hypothalamic-pituitary level, thereby indirectly stimulating ovarian function (Adashi, 1984) (Fig. 3–25). However, on occasion, the antiestrogenic effect of clomiphene may have a detrimental action at the level of the cervical mucus and/or endometrium.

CLOMIPHENE THERAPY
(CONVENTIONAL)

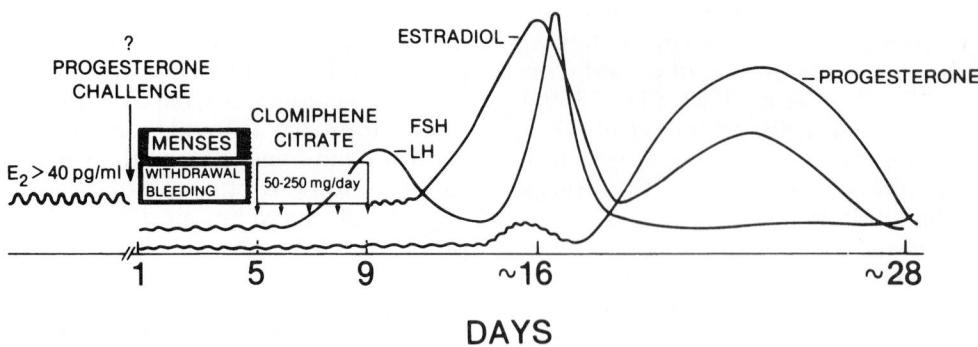

Figure 3–25

Conceptual illustration of a conventional regimen of clomiphene citrate for induction of ovulation. Note that circulating estradiol (E$_2$) levels (best results at or above 40 pg/ml) must be high enough to augment the transient elevation of serum follicle-stimulating hormone (FSH) and luteinizing hormone (LH) derived from clomiphene treatment. Spontaneous menses or progesterone withdrawal bleeding indicates sufficient estrogen for endometrial proliferation and ovulation induction. (From Kenigsberg D, Hodgen GD: Physiology of the menstrual cycle and ovarian function: clinical correlates and implications. In Rosenwaks Z, Benjamin F [eds]: Gynecology: Principles and Practice. New York: Macmillan, 1987:11, with permission.)

Controlled Ovarian Hyperstimulation

The goal in controlled ovarian hyperstimulation is the recruitment of a large number of follicles containing a fertilizable oocyte for retrieval and further embryo transfer. The Norfolk IVF program has primarily used various gonadotropin regimens for ovarian stimulation in assisted reproduction. The goal of recruitment and development of multiple follicles can be readily accomplished with the use of hMG alone, with hMG in combination with pure FSH, or with pure FSH alone (Fig. 3–26). The approach should mimic the physiologic conditions during the natural ovarian-menstrual cycle when, in the early follicular phase, relatively high levels of FSH recruit follicles from the gonadotropin-sensitive pool (diZerega and Hodgen, 1981a; Garcia et al, 1981) (Fig. 3–27). It has been shown in the primate model that a "step-down" dose regimen leads to more synchronized follicular maturation than a "step-up" dose regimen, resulting respectively in a narrower versus wider ovulatory window (Abassi et al, 1987) (Fig. 3–28). For IVF, patients should be assessed in regard to their ovarian reserve through an evaluation of day 3 serum levels of FSH, LH, and E$_2$ in a basal cycle (Muasher et al, 1988; Scott et al, 1989, 1990). Using this simple diagnostic test, three categories of patients can be individualized (Fig. 3–29):

1. *Normal or intermediate responders*—These patients have a normal FSH/LH ratio and are usually stimulated with either a combination of FSH and LH or FSH alone beginning with four ampules daily and proceeding in a step-down fashion until hCG is administered.
2. *High responders*—These patients have polycystic ovarian (PCO) disease syndrome or PCO-like dis-

ease, characterized by a higher LH/FSH ratio. These patients, as mentioned earlier, have a greater risk for hyperstimulation and therefore their treatment should be initiated with a lower dose of FSH (two ampules daily), proceeding in a "step-down" fashion until hCG is administered.
3. *Low or poor responders*—This group of patients has remained a major challenge because of the poor pregnancy results achieved in these cases. These women have a "perimenopausal" ovarian function that is diagnosed by the presence of high FSH levels on cycle day 3 or a high E$_2$ level at the beginning of a cycle. Typically, these patients are stimulated with higher doses of FSH (six or eight ampules daily), but the low number and poorer quality of oocytes retrieved usually lead to low pregnancy rates.

The evolution of the ovarian stimulation approaches in the Norfolk program is based on the recognition that individualization of gonadotropin therapy appropriate to the patients, pretreatment characteristics, and therapeutic response are the keys to good management with gonadotropins. One should keep in mind that the administration of a high dosage of hMG or FSH may induce the development of many follicles, but that, if stimulation is excessive, too short, or too prolonged, immature or postmature eggs may be obtained, with subsequent failed or abnormal fertilization and cleavage and, ultimately, reduced embryo quality. Furthermore, such treatment may significantly decrease the incidence of the sometimes dramatic, severe ovarian hyperstimulation syndrome.

A crucial factor in obtaining the optimum number of mature oocytes is the timing of hCG administration. The administration of hCG serves as a trigger

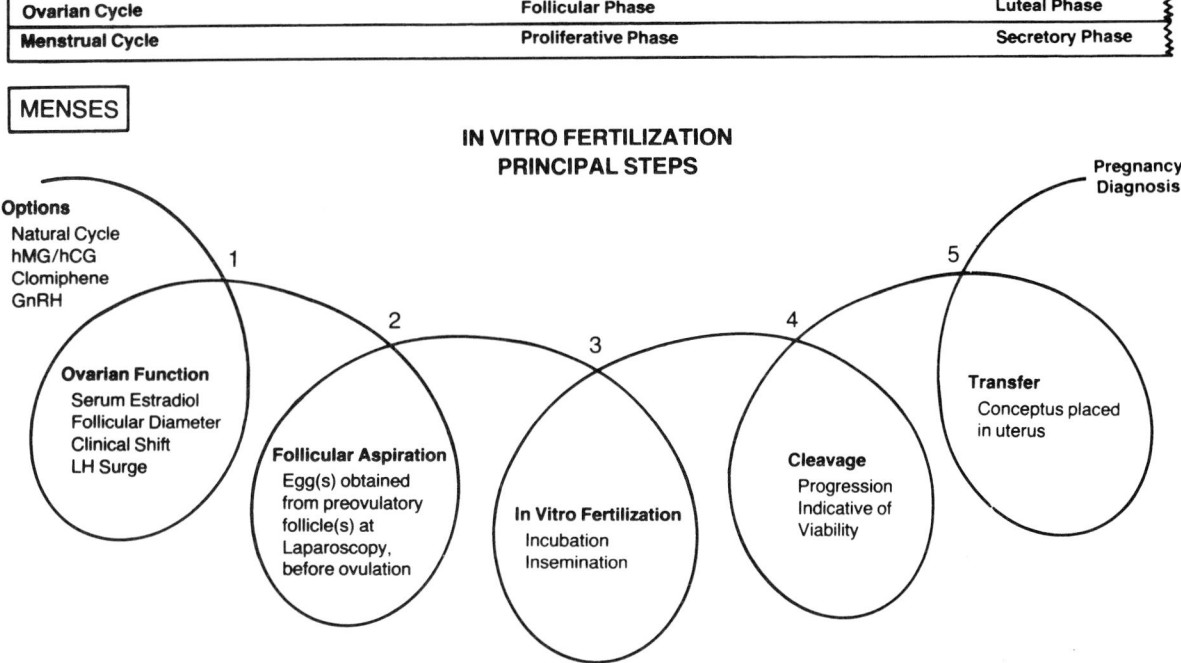

Ovarian Cycle	Follicular Phase	Luteal Phase
Menstrual Cycle	Proliferative Phase	Secretory Phase

MENSES

IN VITRO FERTILIZATION PRINCIPAL STEPS

Pregnancy Diagnosis

Options
Natural Cycle
hMG/hCG
Clomiphene
GnRH

1

2

3

4

5

Ovarian Function
Serum Estradiol
Follicular Diameter
Clinical Shift
LH Surge

Follicular Aspiration
Egg(s) obtained
from preovulatory
follicle(s) at
Laparoscopy,
before ovulation

In Vitro Fertilization
Incubation
Insemination

Cleavage
Progression
Indicative of
Viability

Transfer
Conceptus placed
in uterus

Figure 3–26
The five principal steps in in vitro fertilization/embryo transfer (IVF/ET) therapy. Hormonal stimulation of the ovarian cycle is of crucial importance for collection of several oocytes of high quality. The success of the first and second steps greatly influences the pregnancy rate after one or more pre-embryos are transferred to the uterus. (From Hodgen GD: Physiology of follicular maturation. In Jones HW Jr, Jones GS, Hodgen GD, Rosenwaks Z [eds]: In Vitro Fertilization, Norfolk. Baltimore: Williams & Wilkins, 1986:8, with permission.)

for final egg maturation and commences luteinization of the granulosa cells, which is essential for estrogen and progesterone production during the luteal phase (Hodgen, 1982; Oehninger et al, 1989). It has been shown that the production of progesterone may be inadequate after gonadotropin stimulation and, therefore, routine IVF patients are supplemented with progesterone (25 to 50 mg daily) during the luteal phase of the cycle. The classical studies of Csapo et al (1972) examining pregnancy maintenance after luteectomy or oophorectomy in women showed that the luteal-placental shift occurs approximately 8 weeks after the last menstrual period. Therefore, we routinely continue progesterone supplementation a few weeks beyond luteal-placental shift in IVF cycles.

GnRH ANALOGS

Physiologic Basis for Clinical Application of GnRH Agonists and Antagonists

The physiologic and therapeutic potency of GnRH prompted efforts to synthesize long-acting and potent agonistic and antagonistic analogs. In the past 20 years, hundreds of GnRH analogs have been synthesized (Rivier et al, 1996), representing the effort of many research laboratories and pharmaceutical companies.

The principal goals behind the development of GnRH agonists were to increase the affinity for GnRH receptors and to increase resistance to enzymatic degradation and thereby extend the plasma half-life of the analog (Karten and Rivier, 1986). This was achieved by making selective substitutions of D-amino acids for glycine at position 6 and replacement of the carboxyl-terminal glycine-amide residue by an ethylamide group (Karten and Rivier, 1986). Most of the GnRH agonists currently commercially available share these features. The GnRH agonists derive their therapeutic impact by way of pituitary intolerance to continuous stimulation. Initially, the GnRH agonist induces increased LH/FSH secretion, which is part of the so-called flare effect. Depending on the dose regimen and mode of delivery of the GnRH agonist, the flare effect typically subsides within about 7 to 10 days and is followed by down-regulation. Thereafter, the GnRH agonist achieves and sustains a reversible hypogonadotropic state reminiscent of prepubertal conditions, which can be maintained as long as adequate GnRH agonist treatment is continued. When treatment is stopped, pituitary gonadotropin secretion usually resumes within 2 weeks, with full restoration of gonadal function in about 6 weeks.

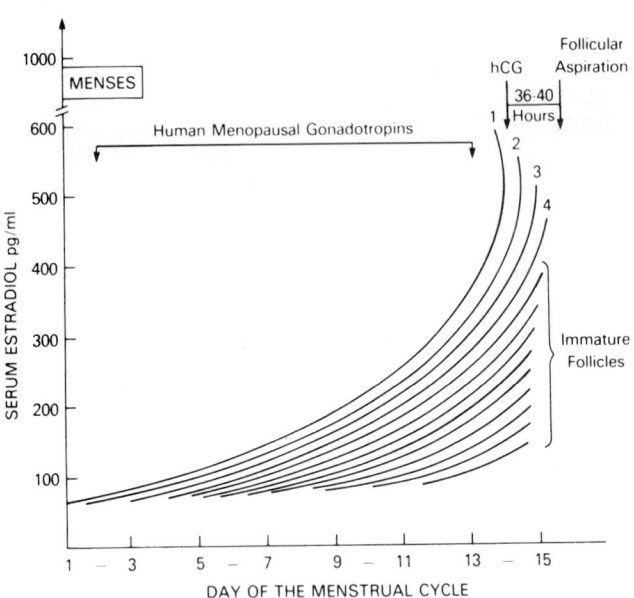

Figure 3-27
Human menopausal gonadotropin (hMG)–stimulated follicular
maturation overrides selection of a single follicle in the natural
cycle. Note that only a few follicles can be regarded
quasisynchronously. If human chorionic gonadotropin (hCG) is
given too late, advanced follicles may yield postmature eggs of
low viable potential. (From Hodgen GD: Physiology of follicular
maturation. In Jones HW JR, Jones GS, Hodgen GD,
Rosenwaks Z [eds]: In Vitro Fertilization, Norfolk. Baltimore:
Williams & Wilkins, 1986:8, with permission.)

Initially, the rationale behind the development of
early GnRH antagonists was similar to that behind
the GnRH agonists but with additional efforts directed toward substitution of the amino acids important for biologic response (His[2] or Trp[3]). These
early (first-generation) GnRH antagonists were effective in vitro and at high doses in in vivo antiovulatory assays (Coy et al, 1982), but there were problems
with histamine release side effects both locally and
systemically (Schmidt et al, 1984; Morgan et al, 1986;
Sundaram et al, 1988). In some instances this was
later determined to be due to the combination of D-
Arg at position 6 with a cluster of hydrophobic aromatic amino acids in the amino-terminal region.
Together these structural features conferred
unacceptably high allergic effects to these compounds (Karten and Rivier, 1986). As a consequence
of these early findings, the focus of attention shifted
to concentrate on the simultaneous enhancement of
potency and reduction of the histamine-release effects. A number of second-generation GnRH antagonists were soon synthesized. One of these compounds, known as *Nal-Glu*, showed particularly
promising potency both in vitro and in vivo. In addition, the median effective dose for in vitro histamine release was 1.6 µg/ml which, although far below that for native GnRH (328 µg/ml), was about a
10-fold improvement over earlier compounds (Rivier
et al, 1986). Nevertheless, local reactions in the form
of transient erythema and induration continued to
be a problem for human volunteers, but no systemic
effects were noted (Jockenhovel et al, 1988; Pavlou et

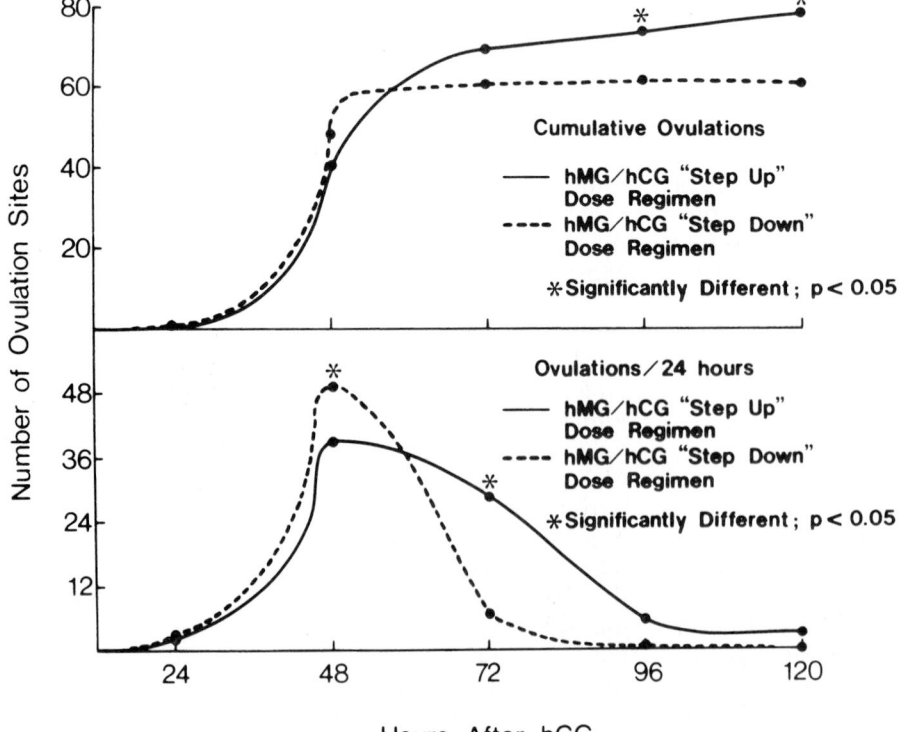

Figure 3-28
Top, Cumulative ovulations from 24
to 120 hours after human chorionic
gonadotropin (hCG) in a "step-up"
(n = 8) versus "step-down" (n = 8)
dose regimen. *Bottom,* Ovulations
per 24 hours after hMG/hCG. The
ovulatory pattern is skewed toward
72 to 96 hours when the "step-up"
hMG protocol was used. Conversely,
the "step-down" regimen for hMG
may allow greater synchronization of
ovulation. hMG, human menopausal
gonadotropin. (From Abassi R,
Kenigsberg D, Danforth D, et al:
Cumulative ovulation rate in human
menopausal/human chorionic
gonadotropin–treated monkeys:
"step-up" versus "step-down" dose
regimens. Fertil Steril 1987;47:1019,
with permission of The American
Fertility Society.)

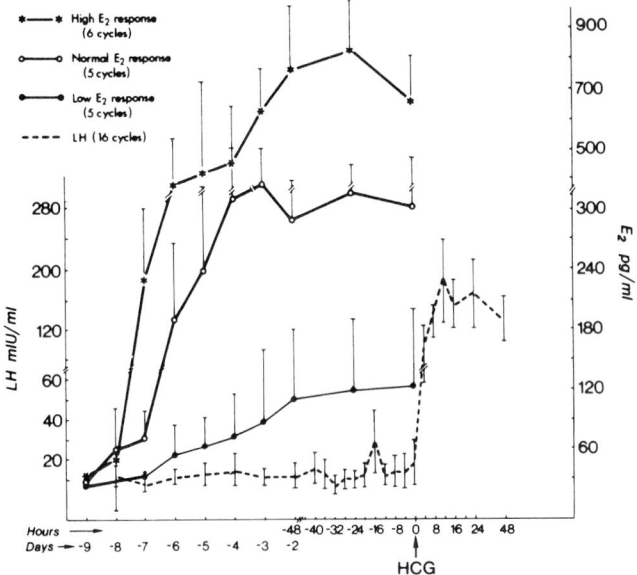

Figure 3-29
Estradiol response patterns to the 2hMG (2 ampules of hMG) protocol. *Note:* The endogenous luteinizing hormone (LH) surge is suppressed in all patients despite estradiol levels, which exceed the usual midcycle levels. (From Ferrareti AP, Garcia JE, Acosta AA, Jones GS: Serum luteinizing hormone during ovulation induction with human menopausal gonadotropin for in vitro fertilization in normally menstruating women. Fertil Steril 1983;40:742, with permission of The American Fertility Society.)

al, 1989; Bremner et al, 1991). This process of enhancing potency while reducing histamine-release effects continued and has now brought forth a third generation of GnRH antagonists. This new generation of GnRH compounds (e.g., Antide), is finally approaching the desired combination of higher potency with lower impact (Leal et al, 1991). They too, however, have come with their own problems. Some compounds are difficult to dissolve in water owing to their inherent hydrophobicity (e.g., Antide); others are expensive to synthesize. Progress continues with more soluble versions of Antide (A75998) and other compounds.

Differential Effects of GnRH Antagonists Versus Agonists

The first step in the action of GnRH, like other peptide hormones, is to bind to its specific receptor on the plasma membrane of its target cells, in this case the gonadotropes (Clayton and Catt, 1981). These receptors have at least two functions: (1) to recognize and bind to the hormone, and (2) to transmit a signal to regions of the cell where its response will be initiated. The immediate effect of GnRH binding to its receptor is to cause release of presynthesized (stored) LH/FSH into the circulation. The binding of GnRH, however, also affects the synthesis and storage of LH

and FSH over a matter of hours and may induce long-term changes in morphology of the pituitary gonadotrope (Clayton, 1988). The initial rapid release of LH depends on the mobilization of intracellular calcium, whereas the sustained release depends on the entry of extracellular calcium through the opening of receptor-activated channels (Chang et al, 1986; Huckle et al, 1988).

GnRH binds to these specific pituitary receptors; these then aggregate, cap, and become internalized. The binding causes a cascade of intracellular signal transduction events that culminate in the release of LH and FSH (Naor, 1990). GnRH agonists mimic the effects of a constant infusion of GnRH, whereby the GnRH receptors become occupied and internalized and undergo down-regulation. The pituitary desensitization accompanying GnRH agonist therapy may in part involve postreceptor mechanisms, whereby increased levels of immunoreactive but biologically inactive FSH and LH are secreted (Meldrum et al, 1984; Dahl et al, 1986).

Although GnRH antagonists also bind specifically to GnRH receptors, they do not cause the release of LH/FSH from the gonadotrope (Chillik et al, 1987; Gordon and Hodgen, 1993). Blum and Conn (1982) and Conn et al (1982) have described a process of receptor dimerization, which they suggest may be essential for GnRH analog–induced gonadotropin release. GnRH antagonists do not normally induce receptor dimerization; however, when artificially induced to do so, they behave like agonists and induce LH/FSH release. In other words, the formation of receptor microaggregation is sufficient to stimulate a transmembrane signal and produce a stimulatory effect.

GnRH Analogs in Controlled Ovarian Stimulation

To date, the majority of IVF programs use a combination of GnRH agonists and gonadotropins for the recruitment of multiple fertilizable oocytes (Palermo et al, 1988; Droesch et al, 1989; Meldrum et al, 1989). The most favored protocol involves the so-called long-term suppression protocol or luteal suppression, in which the GnRH agonist is started in the midluteal phase of the preceding cycle. In this case, desensitization of the pituitary occurs following the agonistic effect, and, after endometrial shedding occurs as a result of estrogen deprivation, stimulation is begun with gonadotropins. Typically, the GnRH agonist is continued, together with gonadotropin stimulation, until hCG administration. This combined protocol has provided numerous benefits, including improved oocyte quality, recruitment of more mature oocytes, and a decrease in cycle cancellation, all of which have translated into more and better embryos to be transferred and/or cryopreserved for future use. Clearly, there is a major consensus for the clinical use of GnRH agonists as adjunct therapy in assisted reproduction. Other regimens (i.e. flare-up, ultra-short, or ultra-long protocols), are also used with more or less similar efficiency. The GnRH agonists are being used in an effort to overcome inappropriate or untimely interference from the pituitary ovarian dynamics (Knobil, 1980). The results in normal and high-responder patients have been extremely successful. However, efforts toward improving the outcome in low-responder patients through the design of newer and more efficient strategies are warranted.

Although the approach of using GnRH agonist desensitization for controlled ovarian stimulation is widely used clinically, its full potential has not been realized with respect to its use as a key to understanding the normal process of follicular development. This is because the agonists lack precision as scientific tools in suppressing LH and FSH secretion. We are now on the verge of improvement in the way pituitary ovarian function can be precisely controlled in humans, and of further advances in our understanding of the requirements for follicular growth and luteal function. These advances should be brought about by the introduction of the new GnRH antagonists into clinical practice (Gordon and Hodgen, 1992a, 1992b, 1992c) and the availability of FSH preparations produced by means of recombinant DNA technology that have half-lives similar to that of FSH produced by the pituitary (Bouchard et al, 1994).

Initial pilot studies using a new generation of GnRH antagonists have confirmed the potential applications of these drugs in controlled ovarian superovulation for IVF (Felderbaum et al, 1995; Olivennes et al, 1995; Reissmann et al, 1995). Their use would probably lead to simplified methods of stimulation whereby gonadotropin stimulation is followed by the use of the GnRH antagonist in the late follicular phase to avoid an untimely LH surge. In addition, it may allow the triggering of ovulation with a GnRH agonist or GnRH itself, if hyperstimulation is feared (Olivennes et al, 1996). If the initial results using GnRH antagonists are confirmed by larger randomized studies, the good tolerance and efficacy that have been observed suggest a bright future for these products in assisted reproductive technologies (Gordon et al, 1992).

Other Uses of GnRH Analogs

Because of their potency in producing a medical hypophysectomy, the GnRH agonists are presently being used to treat many conditions, including endometriosis, leiomyomas, precocious puberty, and prostate cancer (Comite et al, 1981; Hodgen, 1989; Oehninger et al, 1989; Gordon and Hodgen, 1992b, 1992c; Benegiano et al, 1993). Many studies have confirmed that various GnRH agonists are potent therapeutic agents for the management of endometriosis and bring about not only the suppression of

endometrial lesions, but also relief of symptoms (Moghissi, 1993). These results are comparable to those using danazol and progestational agents. A novel aspect of treatment with GnRH agonists in patients with endometriosis is the addition of estrogen and/or progesterone to alleviate hypoestrogenic symptoms and to prevent the loss of bone mineral content (Benegiano et al, 1993).

Leaving aside endometriosis, the pharmacologic treatment of uterine leiomyomata, either as an adjunct or as a substitute to surgical management, still represents the most important gynecologic application of GnRH analogs (Benegiano et al, 1993). In these cases, the use of GnRH agonists can be advocated in at least five different situations:

1. As an adjunct before laparotomic hysterectomy
2. As an adjunct before laparotomic myomectomy
3. As an adjunct before laparoscopic myomectomy
4. As an adjunct to hysteroscopic myomectomy
5. As an alternative to surgery

In all cases, the adequate clinical management of patients with leiomyomata using GnRH agonists will depend upon a clear understanding of benefits and risks in an individualized fashion.

OVARIAN FAILURE: APPLICATION OF OOCYTE DONATION PROGRAMS

At 16 to 18 weeks of fetal life, the first signs of ovarian differentiation are expressed by the onset of rapid mitotic multiplication of gonial endowment, reaching 6 to 7 million germ cells by 20 weeks. This represents the maximum gonial content of the gonad. From this point, germ cell content irretrievably decreases until, some 50 years later, the stored-up germ cells are finally exhausted. The menopause is usually preceded by a 2- to 10-year period when regular menstrual cycles become progressively more irregular, with a shortening of the follicular phase (Sherman and Korneman, 1975). During this transitional period, ovulation occurs erratically and FSH and LH reach high "menopausal" levels, even in the presence of plasma estrogen levels within the menstrual range.

Follicles are virtually absent in the postmenopausal ovaries. Data support the view that decline of the follicular reserve with accelerated loss and ultimate exhaustion is the immediate cause of the menopausal transition. Therefore, the regulation of follicular depletion may change during the final phase of reproductive life.

Besides the physiologic menopause, there are other causes for premature oocyte loss (Hoek et al, 1997). These can be divided into three main groups (De Moraes-Ruehsen and Jones, 1967):

1. Decreased number of germ cells (failure of germ cell migration during fetal life)

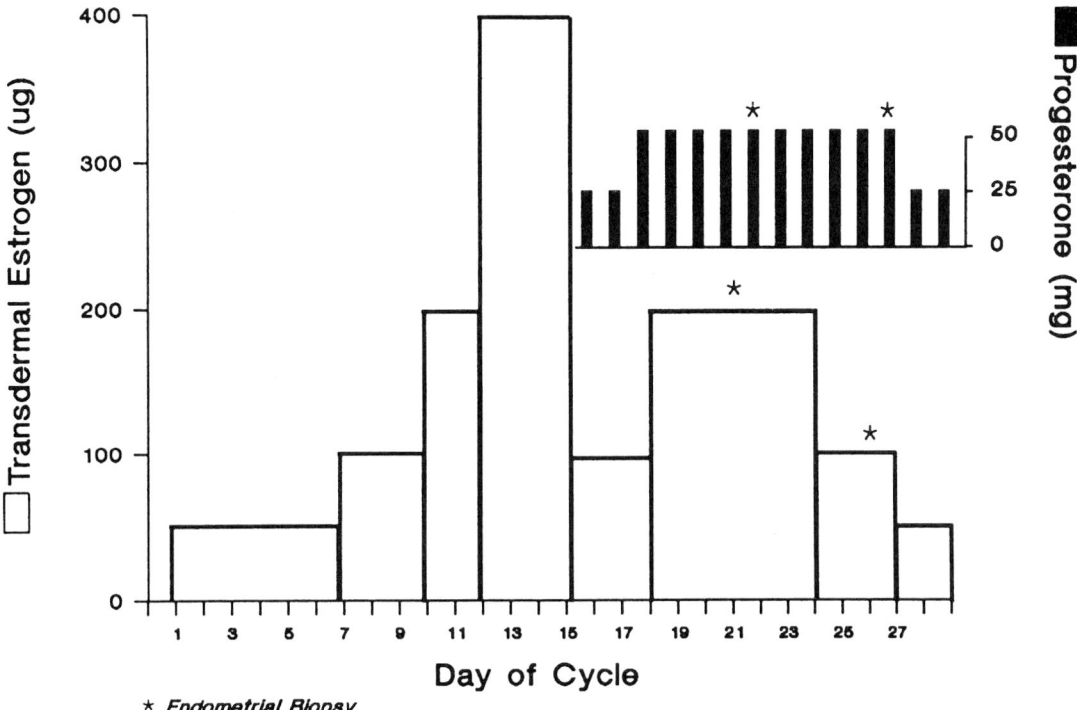

Figure 3–30

Twenty-eight–day replacement protocol used in donor egg program consisting of transdermal estrogen (estradiol) and progesterone sequential administration. (From Droesch K, Navot D, Scott R, et al: Transdermal estrogen replacement in ovarian failure for ovum donation. Fertil Steril 1988;50:931, with permission of The American Fertility Society.)

2. Accelerated atresia (gonadal dysgenesis), the prototype of which is Turner's syndrome, with a karyotype of 45,XO, and others
3. Acquired or postnatal germ cell destruction (through immune, infectious, or iatrogenic cause, such as after chemotherapy or radiotherapy)

Recently, the successful transfer of donor oocytes, fertilized in vitro, to recipient endometria has extended the use of IVF technology for conditions in which the female gametes are absent or not readily accessible for harvest, or gamete abnormality results in IVF failure.

Oocyte donation is offered to patients with premature oocyte loss (premature ovarian failure) and also to prior poor responders to IVF therapy. The process requires the synchronization of the ovulatory phase in the donor with endometrial maturation in the recipient. The temporal window of endometrial receptivity and, indeed, the window of transfer in humans have not been conclusively established, but current protocols aim to transfer the conceptus into a defined endometrial bed, characterized histologically as day 17 to day 19 endometrium (Trounson et al, 1983; Rosenwaks, 1987).

Hodgen (1983) reported a high pregnancy rate in oophorectomized recipient (surrogate) monkeys whose hormones were replaced with subcutaneous E_2 and progesterone capsules, with a tolerance of 3 days of asynchrony between embryo and endome-trium. The following year, Lutjen et al (1984) had similar success with a woman presenting with ovarian failure. Several steroid replacement protocols are being used in recipient women devoid of ovarian function or with poor ovarian function (Droesch et al, 1988) (Fig. 3–30). Typically, oocyte donors are selected based upon young age and usually prior fertility; these volunteers may provide a large number of mature, fertilizable oocytes that are thereafter inseminated with the recipient's husband's sperm and transferred to the uterus of the recipient. The recipient is therefore subjected to a very simple therapeutic regimen of estrogen and progesterone supplementation that she has to continue until the placenta establishes its endocrine functions. Because of the fertile status of the donors and the adequate endometrial preparation of the recipients, pregnancy rates in the oocyte donor program have been outstanding.

REFERENCES

Abassi R, Kenigsberg D, Danforth D, et al: Cumulative ovulation rate in human menopausal/human chorionic gonadotropin-treated monkeys: "step-up" versus "step-down" dose regimens. Fertil Steril 1987;47:1019.

Acosta AA, Oehninger S, Hammer J, et al: Preclinical abortions: incidence and significance in the Norfolk in vitro fertilization program. Fertil Steril 1990;53:673.

Adashi EY: Clomiphene citrate: mechanism(s) and site(s) of action—a hypothesis revised. Fertil Steril 1984;42:331.

Adashi EY: Endocrinology of the ovary. Hum Reprod 1994;9:815.

Adashi EY: Ovulation induction: clomiphene citrate. In Adashi EY, Rock JA, Rosenwaks Z (eds): Reproductive Endocrinology, Surgery, and Technology. Philadelphia: Lippincott-Raven, 1995: 1181.

Aladin Chandrasekher Y, Brenner RM, Molskness TA, et al: Titrating luteinizing hormone surge requirements for ovulatory changes in primate follicles. II. Progesterone receptor expression in luteinizing granulosa cells. J Clin Endocrinol Metab 1991;73:584.

Aladin Chandrasekher Y, Hutchison JS, Zelinski-Wooten MB, et al: Initiation of periovulatory events in primate follicles using recombinant and native human luteinizing hormone to mimic the midcycle gonadotropin surge. J Clin Endocrinol Metab 1994;79:986

Amoss M, Burgus R, Blackwell R, et al: Purification, amino acid composition and N-terminus of the hypothalamic luteinizing hormone releasing factor (LRF) of ovine origin. Biochem Biophys Res Commun 1971;44:205.

Armstrong DT, Papkoff H: Stimulation of aromatization of exogenous and endogenous androgens in ovaries of hypophysectomized rats in vivo by follicle-stimulating hormone. Endocrinology 1976;99:1144.

Baba Y, Matsuo H, Schally AV: Structure of the porcine LH- and FSH-releasing hormone. II. Confirmation of the proposed structure by conventional sequential analyses. Biochem Biophys Res Commun 1971;44:459.

Baird DT: Factors regulating the growth of the preovulatory follicle in the sheep and human. J Reprod Fertil 1983;69:343.

Belchetz PE, Plant TM, Nakai Y, et al: Hypophysial responses to continuous and intermittent delivery of hypothalamic gonadotropin-releasing hormone. Science 1978;202:631.

Benegiano G, Primiero FM, Villani C: GnRH analogues in the management of uterine leiomyomas and other benign gynecological situations. In Lunenfeld B, Insler V (eds): GnRH Analogs: The State of the Art, 1993. Pearl River, New York: Parthenon Publishing Group, 1993:55.

Ben-Rafael Z, Levy T, Schoemaker J: Pharmacokinetics of follicle-stimulating hormone: clinical significance. Fertil Steril 1995;63: 689.

Bergeron C, Ferenczy A, Shyamala G: Distribution of estrogen receptors in various cell types of normal, hyperplastic, and neoplastic human endometrial tissues. Lab Invest 1988a;58:338.

Bergeron C, Ferenczy A, Toft DO, et al: Immunocytochemical study of progesterone receptors in the human endometrium during the menstrual cycle. Lab Invest 1988b;59:862.

Bley MA, Simon JC, Estevez AG, et al: Effect of follicle-stimulating hormone on insulin-like growth factor-I-stimulated rat granulosa cell deoxyribonucleic acid synthesis. Endocrinology 1992;131:1223.

Blum JJ, Conn PM: Gonadotropin-releasing hormone stimulation of luteinizing hormone release: a ligand-receptor-effector model. Proc Natl Acad Sci U S A 1982;79:7307.

Bogdanove EM, Campbell GT, Blair ED, et al: Gonad-pituitary feedback involves qualitative change: androgens alter the type of FSH secreted by the rat pituitary. Endocrinology 1974;95:219.

Bouchard P, Charbonnel B, Caraty A, et al: The role of GnRH during the periovulatory period: a basis for the use of GnRH antagonists in ovulation induction. In Filicori M, Flamigni C (eds): Ovulation Induction: Basic Science and Clinical Advances. Amsterdam: Excerpta Medica, 1994:291.

Bourguignon J-P, Franchimont P: Puberty-related increase in episodic LHRH release from rat hypothalamus in vitro. Endocrinology 1989;114:1941.

Bousfield GR, Parry WM, Ward DN: Gonadotropins: chemistry and biosynthesis. In Knobil E, Neill JD, (eds): The Physiology of Reproduction. 2nd ed. New York: Raven Press, 1994:1749.

Brannian JD, Stouffer RL: Native and modified (acetylated) low density lipoprotein-supported steroidogenesis by macaque granulosa cells collected before and after the ovulatory stimulus: correlation with fluorescent lipoprotein uptake. Endocrinology 1993;132:591.

Bremner WJ, Bagatell CA, Steiner RA: Gonadotropin-releasing hormone antagonist plus testosterone: a potential male contraceptive. J Clin Endocrinol Metab 1991;73:465.

Brosens IA, Koninckx PR, Corveleyn PA: A study of plasma progesterone, oestradiol 17β, prolactin and LH levels, and of the luteal phase appearance of the ovaries in patients with endometriosis and infertility. Br J Obstet Gynecol 1978;85:246.

Brown JB: Pituitary control of ovarian function—concepts derived from gonadotropin therapy. Aust N Z J Obstet Gynecol 1978;18:46.

Burger HG, Farnworth PG, Findlay JK, et al: Aspects of current and future inhibin research. Reprod Fertil Dev 1995;7:997.

Burgus R, Butcher M, Amoss M, et al: Primary structure of the ovine hypothalamic luteinizing hormone-releasing factor (LRF). Proc Natl Acad Sci U S A 1972;69:278.

Camp TA, Rahal JO, Mayo KE: Cellular localization and hormonal regulation of follicle-stimulating hormone and luteinizing hormone receptor messenger RNAs in the rat ovary. Mol Endocrinol 1991;5:1405.

Carr BR, MacDonald PC, Simpson ER: The role of lipoproteins in the regulation of progesterone secretion by the human corpus luteum. Fertil Steril 1982;38:303.

Catt KJ, Reinhart J, Mertz LM, et al: The GnRH receptor: molecular structure and calcium signalling mechanisms. In Bouchard P, Caraty A, Coelingh Bennink HJT, Pavlou SN (eds): GnRH, GnRH Analogs, Gonadotropins and, Gonadal Peptides. New York: Parthenon Publishing, 1994:95.

Chang JP, McCoy EE, Graeter J, et al: Participation of voltage-dependent calcium channels in the action of gonadotropin-releasing hormone. J Biol Chem 1986;261:9105.

Channing CP, Schaerf FW, Anderson LD, Tsafriri A: Ovarian follicular and luteal physiology. In Greep RO (ed): International Review of Physiology, Vol 1: Reproductive Physiology III. Baltimore: University Park Press, 1980:117.

Chehab FF, Mounzih K, Lu R, Lim ME: Early onset of reproductive function in normal female mice treated with leptin. Science 1997;275:88.

Chillik CF, Itskovitz J, Hahn DW, et al: Characterizing pituitary response to a gonadotropin-releasing hormone antagonist in monkeys: tonic follicle-stimulating hormone/luteinizing hormone secretion versus acute GnRH challenge tests before, during, and after treatment. Fertil Steril 1987;48:480.

Cinti S, Sbarbati A, Marelli M, Osculati F: An ultrastructural morphometric analysis of the adenohypophysis of lactating rats. Anat Rec 1985;212:381.

Clarke IJ: Variable patterns of gonadotropin-releasing hormone secretion during the estrogen-induced luteinizing hormone surge in ovariectomized ewes. Endocrinology 1983;133:1624.

Clarke IJ, Cummins JT: The temporal relationship between gonadotropin releasing hormone (GnRH) and luteinizing hormone (LH) secretion in ovariectomized ewes. Endocrinology 1982;111:1737.

Clayton RN: Mechanism of GnRH action in gonadotrophs. Hum Reprod 1988;3:479.

Clayton RN, Catt KJ: Gonadotropin-releasing hormone receptors: characterization, physiological regulation, and relationship to reproductive function. Endocr Rev 1981;2:186.

Collins RL, Williams RF, Hodgen GD: Endocrine consequences of prolonged ovarian hyperstimulation: hyperprolactinemia, follicular atresia, and premature luteinization. Fertil Steril 1984; 42:436.

Comite F, Cutler GB, Rivier J, et al: Short-term treatment of idiopathic precocious puberty with a long-acting analogue of luteinizing hormone-releasing hormone: a preliminary report. N Engl J Med 1981;305:1546.

Conn PM: The molecular mechanism of gonadotropin-releasing hormone action in the pituitary. In Knobil E, Neill JD (eds): The Physiology of Reproduction. 2nd ed. New York: Raven Press, 1994:1815.

Conn PM, Rogers DC, Stewart JM, et al: Conversion of a gonadotropin-releasing hormone antagonist to an agonist. Nature 1982;296:653.

Conte FA, Grumbach MM, Kaplan SL: A diphasic pattern of gonadotropin secretion in patients with the syndrome of gonadal dysgenesis. J Clin Endocrinol Metab 1975;40:670.

Coy DH, Horvath A, Nekola MV, et al: Peptide antagonists of LH-RH: large increases in antiovulatory activities produced by basic D-amino acids in the sixth position. Endocrinology 1982; 110:1445.

Crowley WF Jr, McArthur JW: Simulation of the normal menstrual cycle in Kallman's syndrome by pulsatile administration of luteinizing hormone-releasing hormone (LHRH). J Clin Endocrinol Metab 1980;51:173.

Csapo AL, Pulkkinen MO, Ruttner B, et al: The significance of human corpus luteum in pregnancy maintenance: I. Preliminary studies. Am J Obstet Gynecol 1972;112:1061.

Dahl KD, Bicsak TA, Hsueh AJW: Naturally occurring antihormones: secretion of FSH antagonists by women treated with a GnRH analog. Science 1988;239:72.

Dahl KD, Pavlou SN, Kovacs WJ, Hsueh AJW: The changing ratio of bioactive to immunoreactive follicle-stimulating hormone in normal men following treatment with a potent gonadotropin releasing hormone antagonist. J Clin Endocrinol Metab 1986; 63:792.

De Moraes-Ruehsen M, Jones GS: Premature ovarian failure. Fertil Steril 1967;18:440.

Dey SK: Implantation. In Adashi EY, Rock JA, Rozenwaks Z (eds): Reproductive Endocrinology, Surgery, and Technology. Philadelphia: Lippincott-Raven, 1996:421.

diZerega GS, Hodgen GD: Fluorescence localization of luteinizing hormone/human chorionic gonadotropin uptake in the primate ovary. II. Changing distribution during selection of the dominant follicle. J Clin Endocrinol Metab 1980;51:903.

diZerega GS, Hodgen GD: Folliculogenesis in the primate ovarian cycle. Endocr Rev 1981a;2:27.

diZerega GS, Hodgen GD: Luteal phase dysfunction infertility: a sequel to aberrant folliculogenesis. Fertil Steril 1981b;35:489.

Dorrington JH, Moon YS, Armstrong DT: Estradiol-17β biosynthesis in cultured granulosa cells from hypophysectomized immature rats: stimulation by follicle-stimulating hormone. Endocrinology 1975;97:1328.

Droesch K, Muasher SJ, Brzyski R, et al: Value of suppression with a gonadotropin-releasing hormone agonist prior to gonadotropin stimulation for in vitro fertilization. Fertil Steril 1989;51:292.

Droesch K, Navot D, Scott R, et al: Transdermal estrogen replacement in ovarian failure for ovum donation. Fertil Steril 1988; 50:931.

Dufau ML, Hodgen GD, Goodman AL, Catt KJ: Bioassay of circulating LH in the rhesus monkey: comparison with radioimmunoassay during physiological changes. Endocrinology 1977; 100:1557.

Eaton SB, Pike MC, Short RV, et al: Women's reproductive cancers in evolutionary context. Q Rev Biol 1994;69:353.

Elkind-Hirsch K, Ravnikar V, Schiff I, et al: Determinations of endogenous immunoreactive luteinizing hormone-releasing hormone in human plasma. J Clin Endocrinol Metab 1982;54: 602.

Ellinwood WE, Norman RL, Spies HG: Changing frequency of pulsatile luteinizing hormone and progesterone secretion during the luteal phase of the menstrual cycle of rhesus monkeys. Biol Reprod 1984;31:714.

Falck B: Site of production of estrogen in rat ovary: a study in microtransplants. Acta Physiol Scand 1959;163(Suppl 47):1.

Farquhar MG, Skutelsky EH, Hopkins CR: Structure and function of the anterior pituitary and dispersed pituitary cells: in vitro studies. In Farquhar MG, Tixier-Vidal A (eds): The Anterior Pituitary. New York: Academic Press, 1975:83.

Fauser BCJM, Van Heusden AM: Manipulation of human ovarian function: physiological concepts and clinical consequences. Endocr Rev 1997;18:71.

Felderbaum RE, Reissmann T, Kupker W, et al: Preserved pituitary response under ovarian stimulation with hMG and GnRH antagonist (Cetrorelix) in women with tubal infertility. Eur J Obstet Gynecol 1995;61:151.

Ferin M, Van Vugt D, Wardlaw S: The hypothalamic control of the menstrual cycle and the role of endogenous opioid peptides. Recent Prog Horm Res 1984;40:441.

Filicori M, Butler JP, Crowley WE Jr: Neuroendocrine regulation of the corpus luteum in the human: evidence for pulsatile progesterone secretion. J Clin Invest 1984;73:1638.

Findlay JK: An update on the roles of inhibin, activin, and follistatin as local regulators of folliculogenesis. Biol Reprod 1993; 48:15.

Fortune JE, Armstrong DT: Hormonal control of 17β-estradiol biosynthesis in proestrous rat follicles: estradiol production by isolated theca versus granulosa. Endocrinology 1978;102:227.

Fritz MA, Speroff L: The endocrinology of the menstrual cycle: the interaction of folliculogenesis and neuroendocrine mechanisms. Fertil Steril 1982;38:509.

Gallardo E, Ramirez VD: A method for the superfusion of rat hypothalami: secretion of luteinizing hormone-releasing hormone (LH-RH). Proc Soc Exp Biol Med 1977;155:79.

Garcia J, Jones GS, Wright GL: Prediction of the time of ovulation. Fertil Steril 1981;36:308.

Gay VL, Plant TM: Sustained intermittent release of gonadotropin-releasing hormone in the prepubertal male rhesus monkey induced by N-methyl-DL-aspartic acid. Neuroendocrinology 1988;48:147.

Giudice LC, Ferenczy A: The endometrial cycle. In Adashi EY, Rock JA, Rozenwaks Z (eds): Reproductive Endocrinology, Surgery, and Technology. Philadelphia: Lippincott-Raven, 1996: 271.

Goodman AL, Hodgen GD: Between ovary interaction in the regulation of follicular growth, corpus luteum function, and gonadotropin secretion in the primate ovarian cycle: I. Effects of follicle cautery and hemiovariectomy during the follicular phase in cynomolgus monkeys. Endocrinology 1978;104:1304.

Goodman AL, Hodgen GD: The ovarian triad of the primate menstrual cycle. Recent Prog Horm Res 1983;39:1.

Gordon K, Danforth DR, Williams RF, Hodgen GD: New trends in combined use of gonadotropin-releasing hormone antagonists with gonadotropins or pulsatile gonadotropin-releasing hormone in ovulation induction and assisted reproductive technologies. Curr Opin Obstet Gynecol 1992;4:690.

Gordon K, Hodgen GD: Evolving role of gonadotropin-releasing hormone antagonists. Trens Endocrinol Metab 1992a;3:17.

Gordon K, Hodgen GD: GnRH agonists and antagonists in assisted reproduction. Baillieres Clin Obstet Gynecol 1992b;6:247.

Gordon K, Hodgen GD: Will GnRH antagonists be worth the wait? Reprod Med Rev 1992c;1:189.

Gordon K, Hodgen GD: Basis for differential therapeutic roles of GnRH agonists versus antagonists in clinical practice. Infertil Reprod Med Clin North Am 1993;4:201.

Gordon K, Kaufmann RA, Williams RF: Physiologic and psychologic adaptations in the puerperium. In Moore TR, Reiter RC, Rebar RW, Baker VV (eds): Gynecology & Obstetrics: A Longitudinal Approach. New York: Churchill Livingstone, 1993:625.

Gougeon A: Regulation of ovarian follicular development in primates: facts and hypotheses. Endocr Rev 1996;17:121.

Gougeon A, Testart J: Influence of human menopausal gonadotropin on the recruitment of human ovarian follicles. Fertil Steril 1990;54:848.

Green JD, Harris GW: The neurovascular link between the neurohypophysis and adenohypophysis. J Endocrinol 1947;5:136.

Grumbach MM, Roth JC, Kaplan SL, Kelch RP: Hypothalamic-pituitary regulation of puberty: evidence and concepts derived from clinical research. In Grumbach MM, Grave GD, Mayer FE (eds): The Control of Onset of Puberty. New York: Wiley, 1974: 115.

Harris GW: Neural control of the pituitary gland. Physiol Rev 1948;28:139.

Hartman CG: The homology of menstruation. JAMA 1929;92: 1992.

Hasegawa Y, Miyamoto K, Abe Y, et al: Induction of follicle stimulating hormone receptor by erythroid differentiation factor on rat granulosa cell. Biochem Biophys Res Commun 1988;156: 668.

Healy DL, Schenken RS, Lynch A, et al: Pulsatile progesterone secretion: its relevance to clinical evaluation of corpus luteum function. Fertil Steril 1984;41:114.

Hirota H, Hirota T, Aguikera G, Catt KJ: Hormone-induced redistribution of calcium-activated phospholipid-dependent protein kinase in pituitary gonadotrophs. J Biol Chem 1985;260: 3243.

Hisaw FL: Development of the graafian follicle and ovulation. Physiol Rev 1947;27:95.

Hodgen GD: In vitro fertilization and alternatives. JAMA 1981; 246:590.

Hodgen GD: The dominant ovarian follicle. Fertil Steril 1982;38: 281.

Hodgen GD: Surrogate embryo transfer continued with estrogen-progesterone therapy in monkeys: implantation, gestation and delivery without ovaries. JAMA 1983;250:2167.

Hodgen GD: Physiology of follicular maturation. In Jones HW Jr, Jones GS, Hodgen GD, Rosenwaks Z (eds): In Vitro Fertilization, Norfolk. Baltimore: Williams & Wilkins, 1986:8.

Hodgen GD: General applications of GnRH agonists in gynecology: past, present, and future. Obstet Gynecol Surv 1989;44: 293.

Hodgen GD: Uses of GnRH analogs in IVF/GIFT. Contemp Obstet Gynecol 1990;35:10.

Hoek A, Schoemaker J, Drexhage HA: Premature ovarian failure and ovarian autoimmunity. Endocr Rev 1997;18:107.

Hoff JD, Quigley ME, Yen SSC: Hormonal dynamics at midcycle: a reevaluation. J Clin Endocrinol Metab 1983;57:792.

Horvath E, Kovacs K: Anatomy and histology of the normal and abnormal pituitary gland. In DeGroot LJ (eds): Endocrinology. 3rd ed. Philadelphia: WB Saunders Company, 1995:160.

Hotchkiss J, Knobil E: The menstrual cycle and its neuroendocrine control. In Knobil E, Neill JD, et al (eds): The Physiology of Reproduction. 2nd ed. New York: Raven Press, 1994:711.

Hsueh AJW, Adashi EY, Jones PBC, Welsh TH: Hormonal regulation of the differentiation of cultured ovarian granulosa cells. Endocr Rev 1984;5:76.

Hsueh AJW, Billig H, Tsafriri A: Ovarian follicle atresia: a hormonally controlled apoptotic process. Endocr Rev 1994;15:707.

Huckle WR, McArdle CA, Conn PM: Differential sensitivity of agonist- and antagonist-occupied gonadotropin-releasing hormone receptors to protein kinase C activators: a marker for receptor activation. J Biol Chem 1988;263:3296.

Hughes FM, Gorospe WC: Biochemical identification of apoptosis (programmed cell death) in granulosa cell: evidence for a potential mechanism underlying follicular atresia. Endocrinology 1991;129:2415.

Irvine CHG, Alexander SL: A novel technique for measuring hypothalamic and pituitary hormone secretion rates from collection of pituitary venous effluent in the normal horse. J Endocrinol 1987;113:183.

Jockenhovel F, Bhasin S, Steiner BS, et al: Hormonal effects of single gonadotropin-releasing hormone antagonist doses in men. J Clin Endocrinol Metab 1988;66:1065.

Jones GS: Use of purified gonadotropins for ovarian stimulation in IVF. Clin Obstet Gynecol 1985;12:775.

Jones GS: Luteal phase in a program for in vitro fertilization. In Jones HW Jr, Jones GS, Hodgen GD, Rosenwaks Z (eds): In Vitro Fertilization, Norfolk. Baltimore: Williams & Wilkins, 1986:221.

Kaiser UB, Sabbagh E, Katzenellenbogen RA, et al: A mechanism for the differential regulation of gonadotropin subunit gene expression by gonadotropin-releasing hormone. Proc Natl Acad Sci U S A 1995;92:12280.

Karsch FJ, Bowen JM, Caraty A, et al: Gonadotropin-releasing hormone requirements for ovulation. Biol Reprod 1997;56:303.

Karten MJ, Rivier JE: Gonadotropin-releasing hormone analog design. Structure function studies toward the development of agonists and antagonists: rationale and perspective. Endocr Rev 1986;7:44.

Kenigsberg D, Hodgen GD: Physiology of the menstrual cycle and ovarian function: clinical correlates and implications. In Rosenwaks Z, Benjamin F, Stone ML (eds): Gynecology: Principles and Practice. New York: Macmillan, 1987:11.

Kerin JF, Kirby C, Morris D, et al: Incidence of the luteinized unruptured follicle phenomenon in cycling women. Fertil Steril 1983;40:620.

Knobil E: The neuroendocrine control of the menstrual cycle. Recent Prog Horm Res 1980;36:53.

Knobil E, Hotchkiss J: The menstrual cycle and its neuroendocrine control. In Knobil E, Neill JD, et al (eds): The Physiology of Reproduction. 1st ed. New York: Raven Press, 1988:1971.

Kraicer J: Mechanisms involved in the release of adenohypophyseal hormones. In Tixier-Vidal A, Farquhar MG (eds): Ultrastructure of Biological Systems, Vol 7: The Anterior Pituitary. New York: Academic Press, 1975:21.

Krey LC, Butler WR, Knobil E: Surgical disconnection of the medial basal hypothalamus and pituitary function in the rhesus monkey. I. Gonadotropin secretion. Endocrinology 1975;96: 1073.

Landefeld TD, Kepa J: Pituitary α-subunit mRNA amounts during the sheep estrous cycle. J Biol Chem 1984;259:12817.

Leal JA, Gordon K, Danforth DR, et al: Antide: a "third generation" GnRH antagonist with minimal histamine release. Drugs of the Future 1991;16:529.

Lehman MN, Karsch FJ: Do gonadotropin-releasing hormone, tyrosine hydroxylase-, and β-endorphin-immunoreactive neurons contain estrogen receptors? A double-label immunocytochemical study in the Suffolk ewe. Endocrinology 1993;133:887.

Lessey BA, Killam AP, Metzger DA, et al: Immunohistochemical analysis of human uterine estrogen and progesterone receptors throughout the menstrual cycle. J Clin Endocrinol Metab 1988; 67:334.

Levine JE, Bethea CL, Spies HG: In vitro gonadotropin-releasing hormone release from hypothalamic tissues of ovariectomized estrogen-treated cynomolgus monkeys. Endocrinology 1985; 116:431.

Levine JE, Pau K-YF, Ramirez VD, Jackson GL: Simultaneous measurement of luteinizing hormone-releasing hormone and luteinizing hormone release in unanesthetized, ovariectomized sheep. Endocrinology 1982;111:1449.

Levine JE, Powell KD: Microdialysis for measurement of neuroendocrine peptides. Methods Enzymol 1989;168:166.

Lincoln DW, Fraser HM, Lincoln GA, et al: Hypothalamic pulse generators. Recent Prog Horm Res 1985;41:369.

Ling N, Ying SY, Ueno N, et al: Pituitary FSH is released by a heterodimer of the β-subunits from the two forms of inhibin. Nature 1986;321:779.

Lutjen P, Trounson A, Leeton J, et al: The establishment and maintenance of pregnancy using in vitro fertilization and embryo donation in a patient with primary ovarian failure. Nature 1984;307:174.

MacLachlan RI, Robertson DM, Burger HG, de Kretser DM: The radioimmunoassay of bovine and human follicular fluid and serum inhibin. Mol Cell Endocrinol 1986;46:175.

Malik KF, Silverman A-J, Morrell JI: Gonadotropin releasing hormone mRNA in the rat: distribution and neuronal content over the estrous cycle and after castration in males. Anat Rec 1991; 231:457.

Markee JE: Menstruation in intraocular endometrial transplants in the rhesus monkey. Contrib Embryol Carnegie Inst Wash 1940;28:219.

Marshall JC: Regulation of gonadotropin secretion. In deGroot LJ (ed): Endocrinology. 3rd ed. Philadelphia, WB Saunders Company, 1995:1993.

Martinez de la Escalera G, Choi ALH, Weiner RI: Generation and synchronization of gonadotropin-releasing hormone (GnRH) pulses: intrinsic properties of the GT1-1 GnRH neuronal cell line. Proc Natl Acad Sci U S A 1992;89:1852.

Marut EL, Williams RF, Cowan BD, et al: Pulsatile pituitary gonadotropin secretion during maturation of the dominant follicle in monkeys: estrogen positive feedback enhances the biological activity of LH. Endocrinology 1981;109:2270.

Matsuo H, Arimura A, Nair RMG, Schally AV: Synthesis of the porcine LH- and FSH-releasing hormone by the solid-phase method. Biochem Biophys Res Commun 1971a;45:822.

Matsuo H, Baba Y, Nair RMG, et al: Structure of the porcine LH- and FSH-releasing hormone. I. The proposed amino acid sequence. Biochem Biophys Res Commun 1971b;43:1334.

McKibbin PE, Belchetz PE: Prolonged pulsatile release of gonadotropin-releasing hormone from the guinea pig hypothalamus in vitro. Life Sci 1986;38:2145.

McNatty KP, Makris A, DeGrazia C, et al: The production of progesterone, androgens, and estrogens by granulosa cells, thecal tissue and stromal tissue from human ovaries in vitro. J Clin Endocrinol Metab 1979;49:687.

Meldrum DR, Tsao Z, Monroe SE, et al: Stimulation of LH fragments with reduced bioactivity following GnRH agonist administration in women. J Clin Endocrinol Metab 1984;58:755.

Meldrum DR, Wisot A, Hamilton F, et al: Routine pituitary suppression with leuprolide before ovarian stimulation for oocyte retrieval. Fertil Steril 1989;51:455.

Mills TM: Effect of luteinizing hormone and cyclic adenosine 3′,5′- monophosphate on steroidogenesis in the ovarian follicle of the rabbit. Endocrinology 1977;96:440.

Mitsushima D, Hei DL, Terasawa E: γ-Aminobutyric acid is an inhibitory neurotransmitter restricting the release of luteinizing hormone-releasing hormone before the onset of puberty. Proc Natl Acad Sci U S A 1994;91:395.

Moghissi KS: GnRH agonists in the management of endometriosis. In Lunenfeld B, Insler V (eds): GnRH Analogs: The State of the Art, 1993. Pearl River, New York: Parthenon Publishing Group, 1993:49.

Moore GR, Price D: Gonad hormone functions, and the reciprocal influence between gonads and hypophysis with its bearing on the problem of sex hormone antagonism. Am J Anat 1932;50: 13.

Morgan JE, O'Neil CE, Coy DH, et al: Antagonistic analogs of luteinizing hormone-releasing hormone are mast cell secretagogues. Int Arch Allergy Appl Immunol 1986;80:70.

Moyle WR, Campbell RK: Gonadotropins. In Adashi EY, Rock JA, Rozenwaks Z (eds): Reproductive Endocrinology, Surgery, and Technology. Philadelphia: Lippincott-Raven, 1996:683.

Muasher SJ, Garcia JE: Pregnancy and its outcome. In Jones HW Jr, Jones GS, Hodgen GD, Rosenwaks Z (eds): In Vitro Fertilization, Norfolk. Baltimore: Williams & Wilkins, 1986:238.

Muasher SJ, Oehninger S, Simonetti S, et al: The value of basal and/or stimulated serum gonadotropin levels in prediction of stimulation respose and in vitro fertilization outcome. Fertil Steril 1988;50:298.

Mulheron GW, Quattropani SL, Nolin JM: The ontogeny of immunoreactive endogenous FSH and LH in the rat ovary during early folliculogenesis. Proc Soc Exp Biol Med 1989;190:91.

Naor Z: Signal transduction mechanisms of Ca^{2+} mobilizing hormones: the case of gonadotropin-releasing hormone. Endocr Rev 1990;11:326.

Neill JD, Johansson EDB, Knobil E: Failure of hysterectomy to influence the normal pattern of cyclic progesterone secretion in the rhesus monkey. Endocrinol 1969;84:464.

Noyes RW, Hertig AT, Rock J: Dating the endometrium biopsy. Fertil Steril 1950;1:3.

Oehninger S, Brzyski RG, Muasher SJ, et al: In-vitro fertilization and embryo transfer in patients with endometriosis: impact of a gonadotropin releasing hormone agonist. Hum Reprod 1989; 4:541.

Oehninger S, Veeck L, Franken D, et al: Human preovulatory oocytes have a higher sperm-binding ability than immature oocytes under hemizona assay conditions: evidence supporting the concept of "zona maturation." Fertil Steril 1991;55:1165.

Olivennes F, Fanchin R, Bouchard P, et al: Scheduled administration of a gonadotropin-releasing hormone antagonist (Cetrorelix) on day 8 of in-vitro fertilization cycles: a pilot study. Hum Reprod 1995;10:1382.

Olivennes F, Fanchin R, Bouchard P, et al: Triggering of ovulation by a gonadotropin-releasing hormone (GnRH) agonist in patients pretreated with a GnRH antagonist. Fertil Steril 1996;66: 151.

Page RB: Anatomy and physiology of the adenohypophysis. In Wilkins RH, Rengachary SS (eds): Neurosurgery. 2nd ed, Vol 1. New York: McGraw-Hill, 1996:1221.

Palermo R, Amodeo G, Navot D, et al: Concomitant gonadotropin-releasing hormone agonist and gonadotropin treatment for the synchronized induction of multiple follicles. Fertil Steril 1988;49:290.

Pavlou SN, Wakefield G, Schlechter NL, et al: Mode of suppression of pituitary and gonadal function after acute or prolonged administration of a luteinizing hormone-releasing hormone antagonist in normal men. J Clin Endocrinol Metab 1989;68:446.

Peckham WD, Knobil E: The effects of ovariectomy, estrogen replacement and neuraminidase treatment on the properties of the adenohypophysial glycoprotein hormones of the rhesus monkey. Endocrinology 1976;98:1054.

Pellicer A, Diamond MP, De Cherney AH, Naftolin F: Intraovarian markers of follicular and oocyte maturation. J In Vitro Fertil Embryo Transfer 1987;4:205.

Pierce JG, Parsons TF: Glycoprotein hormones: structure and function. Annu Rev Biochem 1981;50:465.

Piquette GN, LaPolt PS, Oikawa M, Hsueh AJW: Regulation of luteinizing hormone receptor messenger ribonucleic acid levels by gonadotropins, growth factors, and gonadotropin-releasing hormone in cultured rat granulosa cells. Endocrinology 1991; 128:2449.

Plant TM: Puberty in primates. In Knobil E, Neill JD (eds): The Physiology of Reproduction. 2nd ed. New York: Raven Press, 1994:453.

Plant TM, Krey LC, Moossy J, et al: The arcuate nucleus and the control of gonadotropin and prolactin secretion in the female rhesus monkey (Macaca mulatta). Endocrinology 1978;102:52.

Pohl CR, Richardson DW, Hutchison JS, et al: Hypophysiotropic signal frequency and the functioning of the pituitary-ovarian system in the rhesus monkey. Endocrinology 1983;112:2076.

Quigley ME, Sheehan KL, Casper RF, Yen SSC: Evidence for increased dopaminergic and opioid activity in patients with hypothalamic hypogonadotropic amenorrhea. J Clin Endocrinol Metab 1980;50:949.

Ramirez VD, Pickle RL, Lin WW: In vivo models for the study of gonadotropin and LHRH secretion. J Steroid Biochem Mol Biol 1991;40:143.

Rasmussen DD, Gambacciani M, Swartz W, et al: Pulsatile gonadotropin-releasing hormone release from the human mediobasal hypothalamus in vitro: opiate receptor-mediated suppression. Neuroendocrinology 1989;49:150.

Reichert LE, Ward DN: On the isolation and characterization of the alpha and beta subunits of human pituitary follicle-stimulating hormone. Endocrinology 1974;94:655.

Reissmann T, Felderbaum R, Diedrich K, et al: Development and applications of luteinizing hormone-releasing hormone antagonists in the treatment of infertility: an overview. Hum Reprod 1995;10:1974.

Riskind PN, Martin JB: Functional anatomy of the hypothalamic-anterior pituitary complex. In: DeGroot LJ (ed): Endocrinology. 3rd ed. Philadelphia: WB Saunders Company, 1995:151.

Rivier JE, Jiang G-C, Koerber SC, et al: GnRH antagonists: design, synthesis and side effects. In Filicori M, Flamigni C (eds): Treatment with GnRH Analogs: Controversies and Perspectives. London: Parthenon Publishing Group, 1996:13.

Rivier JE, Porter J, Rivier CL, et al: New effective gonadotropin releasing hormone antagonists with minimal potency for histamine release in vitro. J Med Chem 1986;29:1846.

Robinson JE: Microdialysis: a novel tool for research in the reproductive system. Biol Reprod 1995;52:237.

Ronnekleiv OK, Naylor BR, Bond CT, Adelman JP: Combined immunohistochemistry for gonadotropin-releasing hormone (GnRH) and pro-GnRH, and in situ hybridization for GnRH messenger RNA in rat brain. Mol Endocrinol 1989;3:363.

Ronnekleiv OK, Resko JA: Ontogeny of gonadotropin-releasing hormone-containing neurons in early fetal development of rhesus macaques. Endocrinology 1990;126;498.

Roseff SJ, Bangah ML, Kettel LM, et al: Dynamic changes in circulating inhibin levels during the luteal-follicular transition of the human menstrual cycle. J Clin Endocrinol Metab 1989;69: 1033.

Rosenwaks Z: Donor eggs: their application in modern reproductive technologies. Fertil Steril 1987;47:895.

Rosenwaks Z, Muasher SJ: Recruitment of fertilizable eggs. In Jones HW Jr, Jones GS, Hodgen GD, Rosenwaks Z (eds): In Vitro Fertilization, Norfolk. Baltimore: Williams & Wilkins, 1986:30.

Ross JL, Loriaux DL, Cutler GB Jr: Developmental changes in neuroendocrine regulation of gonadotropin secretion in gonadal dysgenesis. J Clin Endocrinol Metab 1983;57:288.

Sairam MR: Deglycosylation of ovine pituitary lutropin subunits: effects on subunit interaction and hormone activity. Arch Biochem Biophys 1980;204:199.

Santoro N, Filicori M, Crowley WF Jr: Hypogonadotropic disorders in men and women: diagnosis and therapy with pulsatile gonadotropin releasing hormone. Endocr Rev 1986;7:11.

Schally AV, Arimura A, Baba Y, et al: Isolation and properties of the FSH and LH-releasing hormone. Biochem Biophys Res Commun 1971a;43:393.

Schally AV, Arimura A, Kastin AJ: Hypothalamic regulatory hormones. Science 1973;179:341.

Schally AV, Arimura A, Kastin AJ, et al: Gonadotropin-releasing hormone: one polypeptide regulates secretion of luteinizing and follicle-stimulating hormones. Science 1971b;173:1036.

Schally AV, Baba Y, Arimura A, et al: Evidence for peptide nature of LH and FSH-releasing hormones. Biochem Biophys Res Commun 1971c;42:50.

Schally AV, Kastin AJ: Stimulation and inhibition of fertility through hypothalamic agents. Drug Therapy 1971;1:29.

Schally AV, McCann SM: The privileges of a Nobel Laureate. Fertil Steril 1995;64:452.

Schenken RS, Asch RH, Williams RF, Hodgen GD: Eitiology of infertility in monkeys with endometriosis: luteinized unruptured follicles, luteal phase defects, pelvic adhesions, and spontaneous abortions. Fertil Steril 1984;41:122.

Schenken RS, Hodgen GD: Follicle-stimulating hormone induced ovarian hyperstimulation in monkeys: blockade of the luteinizing hormone surge. J Clin Endocrinol Metab 1983;57:50.

Schmidt F, Sundaram K, Thau RB, Bardin CW: [Ac-D-Nal(2)^1, 4FD-Phe^2, D-Trp^3, D-Arg^6]-LHRH, a potent antagonist of LHRH, produces transient edema and behavioral changes in rats. Contraception 1984;29:283.

Schwanzel-Fukuda M, Bick D, Pfaff DW: Luteinizing hormone-releasing hormone (LHRH)-expressing cells do not migrate normally in an inherited hypogonadal (Kallmann) syndrome. Mol Brain Res 1989;6:311.

Schwanzel-Fukuda M, Pfaff DW: Origin of luteinizing hormone-releasing hormone neurons. Nature 1989;338:161.

Scott RT, Hofmann GE, Oehninger S, Muasher SJ: Intercycle variability of day 3 follicle-stimulating hormone levels and its effect on stimulation quality in in vitro fertilization. Fertil Steril 1990;54:297.

Scott RT, Toner JP, Muasher SJ, et al: Follice-stimulating hormone levels on cycle day 3 are predictive of in vitro fertilization outcome. Fertil Steril 1989;51:651.

Sherman BM, Korneman SG: Hormonal characteristics of the human menstrual cycle throughout reproductive life. J Clin Invest 1975;55:699.

Shivers BD, Harlan RE, Morrell JI, Pfaff DW: Absence of oestradiol concentration in cell nuclei of LHRH-immunoreactive neurones. Nature 1983;304:345.

Short RV: Steroid in the follicular fluid and the corpus luteum of the mare: a "two-cell type" theory of ovarian steroid synthesis. J Endocrinol 1962;24:59.

Silverman AJ, Antunes JL, Abrams GM, et al: The luteinizing hormone-releasing hormone pathways in rhesus (Macaca mulatta) and pigtailed (Macaca nemestrina) monkeys: new observations on thick, unembedded sections. J Comp Neurol 1982:211;309.

Silverman A-J, Livne I, Witkin JW: The gonadotropin-releasing hormone (GnRH), neuronal systems: immunocytochemistry and in situ hybridization. In Knobil E, Neil JD, et al (eds): The Physiology of Reproduction. 2nd ed. New York: Raven Press, 1994:1683.

Spies HG, Pau K-YF, Yang S-P: Coital and estrogen signals: a contrast in the preovulatory neuroendocrine networks of rabbits and rhesus monkeys. Biol Reprod 1997;56:310.

Stillman RJ, Williams RF, Lynch A, Hodgen GD: Selective inhibition of follicle-stimulating hormone by porcine follicular fluid extracts in the monkey: effects on midcycle surges and pulsatile secretion. Fertil Steril 1983;40:823.

Stouffer RL: Corpus luteum formation and demise. In Adashi EY, Rock JA, Rozenwaks Z (eds): Reproductive Endocrinology, Surgery, and Technology. Philadelphia: Lippincott-Raven, 1996:251.

Sundaram K, Didolkar A, Thau R, et al: Antagonists of luteinizing hormone releasing hormone bind to mast cells and induce histamine release. Agents Actions 1988;25:307.

Taymor ML: The regulation of follicle growth: some clinical implications in reproductive endocrinology. Fertil Steril 1996;65:235.

Tilly JL, Kowalski KI, Johnson AL, Hsueh AJW: Involvement of apoptosis in ovarian follicular atresia and postovulatory regression. Endocrinology 1991;129:2799.

Todd AS: Localization of fibrinolytic activity in tissues. Br Med Bull 1964;20:210.

Tougard C, Tixier-Vidal A: Lactotropes and gonadotropes. In Knobil E, Neill JD (eds): The Physiology of Reproduction. 2nd ed. New York: Raven Press, 1994:1711.

Treolar AE, Boynton RD, Benn BG, Brown BW: Variation of human menstrual cycle through reproductive life. Int J Fertil 1967;12:77.

Trounson A, Leeton J, Besanko M, et al: Pregnancy established in an infertile patient after transfer of a donated embryo fertilised in vitro. Br Med J 1983;286:835.

Veeck LL: Morphological estimation of mature oocytes and their preparation for insemination. In Jones HW Jr, Jones GS, Hodgen GD, Rosenwaks Z (eds): In Vitro Fertilization, Norfolk. Baltimore: Williams & Wilkins, 1986:81.

Wagner CL, Anderson DM, Pittard WB: Special properties of human milk. Clin Pediatr 1996;35:283.

Watson RE, Langub MC, Landis JW: Further evidence that most luteinizing hormone-releasing hormone neurons are not directly estrogen responsive—simultaneous localization of luteinizing hormone-releasing hormone and estrogen receptor immunoreactivity in the guinea pig brain. J Neuroendocrinol 1992;4:311.

Wildt L, Hausler A, Marshall G, et al: Frequency and amplitude of GnRH stimulation and gonadotropin secretion in the rhesus monkey. Endocrinology 1981;109:376.

Wildt L, Leyendecker G: Induction of ovulation by the chronic administration of naltrexone in hypothalamic amenorrhea. J Clin Endocrinol Metab 1987;64:1334.

Wildt L, Marshall G, Knobil E: Experimental induction of puberty in the infantile female rhesus monkey. Science 1980;207:1373.

Wilson RC, Kesner JS, Kaufman J-M, et al: Central electrophysiological correlates of pulsatile luteinizing hormone secretion in the rhesus monkey. Neuroendocrinology 1984;39:256.

Wray S, Grant P, Gainer H: Evidence that cells expressing luteinizing hormone-releasing hormone mRNA in the mouse are derived from progenitor cells in the olfactory placode. Proc Natl Acad Sci U S A 1989a;86:8132.

Wray S, Nieburgs A, Elkabes S: Spatiotemporal cell expression of luteinizing hormone-releasing hormone in the prenatal mouse: evidence for an embryonic origin in the olfactory placode. Dev Brain Res 1989b;46:309.

Xia L, Van Vugt D, Alston EJ, et al: A surge of gonadotropin-releasing hormone accompanies the estradiol-induced gonadotropin surge in the rhesus monkey. Endocrinology 1992;131:2812.

Yen SSC: The human menstrual cycle: neuroendocrine regulation. In Yen SSC, Jaffe RB (eds): Reproductive Endocrinology. 3rd ed. Philadelphia: WB Saunders Company, 1991:273.

Yen SSC, Tsai CC, Naftolin F, et al: Pulsatile patterns of gonadotropin release in subjects with and without ovarian function. J Clin Endocrinol Metab 1972;34:671.

Ying SY: Inhibins, activins and follistatins: gonadal proteins modulating the secretion of follicle-stimulating hormone. Endocr Rev 1988;9:267.

Yong EL, Baird DT, Yates R, et al: Hormonal regulation of the growth and steroidogenic function of human granulosa cells. J Clin Endocrinol Metab 1992;74:842.

Yoshimura Y, Wallach EE: Studies of the mechanism(s) of mammalian ovulation. Fertil Steril 1987;47:22.

Zeleznik AJ: Premature elevation of systemic estradiol reduces serum levels of follicle-stimulating hormone and lengthens the follicular phase of the menstrual cycle in rhesus monkeys. Endocrinology 1981;109:352.

Zeleznik AJ: Dynamics of primate follicular growth: a physiological perspective. In Adashi EY, Leung PCK (eds): The Ovary. New York: Raven Press, 1993:41.

Zeleznik AJ, Hillier SG: The ovary: endocrine function. In Hillier SG, Kitchner HC, Neilson JP (eds): Scientific Essentials of Reproductive Medicine. Philadelphia: WB Saunders Company, 1996:133.

Zeleznik AJ, Hutchison J: Luteotropic actions of LH on the macaque corpus luteum. In Stouffer RL (ed): The Primate Ovary. New York: Plenum Press, 1987:163.

Zeleznik AJ, Hutchison JS, Schuler HM: Interference with the gonadotropin-suppressing actions of estradiol in macaques overrides the selection of a single preovulatory follicle. Endocrinology 1985;117:991.

Zeleznik AJ, Kubik CJ: Ovarian responses in macaques to pulsatile infusion of follicle-stimulating hormone (FSH) and luteinizing hormone: increased sensitivity of the maturing follicle to FSH. Endocrinology 1986;119:2025.

Zeleznik AJ, Schuler HM, Reichert LE: Gonadotropin-binding sites in the rhesus monkey ovary: role of the vasculature in the selective distribution of human chorionic gonadotropin in the preovulatory follicle. Endocrinology 1981;109:356.

Zelinski-Wooten MB, Hutchison JS, Aladin Chandrasekher Y, et al: Administration of human luteinizing hormone (hLH) to macaques after follicular development: further titration of LH surge requirements for ovulatory changes in primate follicles. J Clin Endocrinol Metab 1992;75:502.

Zelinski-Wooten MB, Lanzendorf SE, Wolf DP, et al: Titrating luteinizing hormone surge requirements for ovulatory changes in primate follicles. I. Oocyte maturation and corpus luteum function. J Clin Endocrinol Metab 1991;73:577.

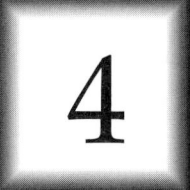

4

Reproductive Immunology for the Nonimmunologist

David A. Clark
Salim Daya

The concept of immunity dates from ancient times. The Romans noticed that a soldier contracting smallpox from the enemy and surviving the disease did not contract it a second time; such men were placed in the front line of the battle phalanx nearest to the infectious enemy, where presumably they did not live long enough for their acquired resistance to wear off. Similarly, the Greek historian Thucydites recorded that Athenians who had survived the plague could be sent to tend the sick without fear of contracting the illness again. In an outbred population, of which humans are a good example, reproduction also creates a confrontation. The conflict is between genetically foreign material from one person and the immune system of the other. For example, the female genital tract is repeatedly exposed to male ejaculate composed of spermatazoa, seminal plasma, and small numbers of lymphocytic cells, all of which may elicit an immune response in the female (Beer and Billingham, 1976). With conception and implantation, the cells of the fetoplacental unit express antigens (usually proteins) coded by the father's genes (paternal antigens) to which the mother may react. After parturition, the breast-fed infant is exposed to maternal lymphocytes that may recognize alien paternal antigens on cells lining the intestine and pass beyond to interact with cells within the fetus (Beer and Billingham, 1976). On this basis, the immune system of the mother might be expected to block essential reproductive processes; a woman would have to conceive on her first exposure to ejaculate, and one pregnancy would cure her of the "disease" forever (unless she found a new partner with antigens different from her previous male); and breast-feeding would be prohibited to protect the neonate.

The immunologist interested in determining the mechanisms permitting successful reproduction, as well as the role of failure of such mechanisms in reproductive pathology, and in harnessing and controlling mechanisms relevant to determining the success or failure of reproduction may be deemed a reproductive immunologist. The scope of reproductive immunology is expanded beyond this focus by studies on the role of immunology in ovarian and testicular failure, in endometriosis, and in reproductive tract cancers (particularly those in which the antigens of an oncogenic virus may be present), and studies on the role of lymphomyeloid cells and their products, which may play a role in uterine bleeding, resistance to sexually transmitted diseases, preeclampsia, intrauterine growth restriction, and premature parturition. Of course, immunologic techniques and assays are widely used to study reproductive tract pathology and in hormone immunoassays, but that does not define reproductive immunology. Table 4–1 summarizes the current scope of the discipline.

In this chapter, we review the structure and function of the immune system and comment briefly on the role of host resistance (immunity) in some of the problems described above. It will not be possible to discuss in detail all of the topics outlined in Table 4–1; that would require an entire textbook on its own. More detail on some of the areas in Table 4–1 may be found in chapters dealing with specific diseases.

THE HOST RESISTANCE/IMMUNE SYSTEM

The type of immunity noted in ancient times was "acquired" resistance, specific for the particular disease-causing agent and commonly induced nowadays, where necessary, by a deliberate vaccination with antigen (usually the foreign protein of the pathogen). Protection is induced by the activation of thymus- and bone marrow–derived (T and B) lymphocytes with receptors specific for the antigen (Janeway and Travers, 1996; Roitt et al, 1996). In fact, antigens usually bear multiple different sites where the arrangement of amino acids or sugars allows recognition; the unit that is recognized is called an epitope, and antigens with multiple epitopes are called

Table 4-1. SCOPE OF THE DISCIPLINE OF REPRODUCTIVE IMMUNOLOGY

AREA OF INQUIRY	CLINICAL RELEVANCE
1. Gamete immunology	Infertility caused by immune responses to gametes
	Contraceptive vaccines—gamete antigens
2. Autoimmunity	Ovarian/testicular failure/infertility
	Anti-phospholipid antibodies
	Endometriosis
3. Pregnancy immunology	Contraceptive vaccine—β-hCG as immunogen
	Implantation failure
	Spontaneous abortions—mechanism & treatment
	Pre-eclampsia/IUGR
	Premature parturition
	Transplacental traffic into fetus:
	• anti-blood group and autoantibodies
	• maternal cells—tolerance and chimerism/GVH and immunodeficiency
	• antigen—prenatal immunization of fetus via maternal immunization
	Transplacental traffic into mother—isolation of fetal cells for genetic testing
	Pregnancy-induced remission of arthritis
	Pregnancy-induced alteration in response to infections
4. Menstrual cycle and maternal cells	Role in bleeding and repair: IUD and Norplant
5. Antibodies, cells, cytokines in breast milk	?Effect on neonate
6. Immune defenses in reproductive tract	Sexually transmitted diseases/HIV
7. Immunodiagnosis	The entire spectrum of normal and abnormal

Abbreviations: GVH, graft-versus-host disease; β-hCG, β-human chorionic gonadotropin; HIV, human immunodeficiency virus; IUD, intrauterine device; IUGR, intrauterine growth retardation.

multivalent. The antigen-activated T and B cells develop into effector T cells and plasma cells producing antibody, respectively.

Phagocytic Cells

Some individuals exposed for the first time to a pathogen may not contract any disease, and are said to have natural resistance. We now know that the immune system has evolved (apologies to any creation science devotees) in a series of "layers." The most primitive layer derived from the ability of eukaryotic cells to distinguish themselves from other cell types; such self/not-self discrimination is based on complementary surface receptors. In a higher vertebrate, similar processes may explain how a homogenate of dissociated cells from different organs gather together when allowed to settle out onto a culture dish and grow; liver cells gather into one area, heart cells in another, and so forth. Refusal to bond or collaborate with a foreign invader can provide a potent mechanism of defense. Indeed, in our intestines, a bacterium wishing to pass through the mucosal epithelial lining (or even remain in the intestine when contents are flowing fast) must first bind to specific molecules on the epithelial cell processes (pili). In terms of active host resistance, the most primitive defender is the phagocytic cell. Modeled on the ameba, which can tell a live ameba (same as self) from a dead ameba from a paramecium, and so on, the macrophage recognizes foreign microorganisms and cells and tries to engulf them. The engulfee within a phagocytic vacuole in the cytoplasm of the macrophage is then bombarded with the discharge of the contents of lysosomes of the engulfor, with the objective of reducing the engulfee to amino acids, fatty acids, simple carbohydrates, and the like that can be excreted or recycled by the organism. Polymorphonuclear leukocytes represent a variation on this theme, and act more rapidly than macrophages. The importance of phagocytic cells, particularly neutrophils, is obvious from the outcome when the granulocyte count is reduced to zero by radiation or cytotoxic cancer chemotherapy drugs; the bugs take over, and the patient dies no matter how much specific acquired immunity exists. These phagocytic processes are part of inflammation and repair.

Phagocytosis may be enhanced by a series of soluble enzymes called complement (C) (Janeway and Travers, 1996; Roitt et al, 1996). Bacterial lipopolysaccharides together with factor B and properdin present in the blood can cleave (activate) the third component of complement (C3). Activated C3 binds to the bacterium and binds to C3 receptor of the membrane of phagocytic cells. Activated C3 activates C5, which can similarly bind to the bacterium and to receptors of the phagocyte membrane. Eventually, C9 may be activated, resulting in formation of pores in the cell membrane, and this leads to osmotic lysis. It is unclear if host defense ever requires activation of complement components beyond C3. C5-deficient mice thrive and survive free of fatal infection in the real world.

Natural Killer Cells

If phagocytic cells were sufficient to protect the integrity of a distinct multicellular organism, Mother Nature (the gender balancer for politically correct creationists) would have gone no further. But as the technology of warfare has become more and more sophisticated over the course of history, so it has been with host resistance mechanisms. The next layer of the system to develop involved cellular mechanisms for destroying antigen-bearing nucleated cells without having to phagocytose them. Indeed, this principle was already developing at the level of the phagocyte. Polymorphonuclear leukocytes could release their granules externally (exocytosis) and the enzymes would digest the invader (along with some of the self); if the invader was in your arm, you sacrificed your arm. Eosinophils, a variant of the polymorphonuclear leukocyte, discharged granules containing a 12-kDa molecule called major basic protein, which is very toxic to large multicellular organisms (e.g., parasites such as worms) (Janeway and Travers, 1996; Roitt et al, 1996). Macrophages secreted nitric oxide and free radicals, which, in turn, generated toxic peroxides. In the next layer of development, the release of effector molecules became much more focused and was restricted to the foreign cell with which the effector (killer) cell of the host made contact. The prototype was the natural killer (NK) cell. (The reason these were called "natural" will be explained later on.) NK cells recognize primitive embryonic cells (as do macrophages), viral and chemically altered self cells, and tumor cells. The NK cell delivers the molecule perforin to its nucleated cell target at the point of cell-cell contact, and the membrane of the target develops holes. This can be detected in a test tube if the cytoplasm of the target has been labeled with the isotope ^{51}Cr; the isotope leaks from the cells within 30 minutes of damage (Clark, 1977). By such a process, NK cells can kill bacteria (Garcia-Penarrubia et al, 1989a, 1989b). There are three other pathways of killing. Perforin (stored in granules in the cytoplasm of the NK cell) is dispensed to the target along with another enzyme, granzyme, which causes the DNA of the target cell to fragment; hence, granzyme is called fragmentin (Jans et al, 1996). Two other mechanisms lead to a similar fragmentation. One involves the cytokine tumor necrosis factor-α (TNF-α), which can be delivered to the target either in soluble secreted form or by direct contact with the cell membrane of the NK cell, with which TNF-α may be associated (Peck et al, 1989; Berke, 1997). A similar phenomenon is triggered by the membrane-associated FAS ligand (Berke, 1997). When the NK cell membrane contacts the target cell membrane, FAS ligand on the NK cell binds to FAS, the receptor on the target, and this leads to scissoring of the DNA into fragments. The consequence of fragmenting the DNA is that the cells undergo apoptosis (where they implode or crinkle up) rather than exploding outwardly from osmotic effects (lysis), as seen when their membrane is damaged by perforin. The DNA scissoring can be detected in a test tube if the target has had its DNA labeled with ^{3}H-thymidine or a similar nucleotide. There may also be delayed release of a ^{51}Cr label.

There are other NK-related effector cells. Natural cytotoxic (NC) cells can be distinguished from the NK cells of laboratory mice by surface markers and by the different range of targets they can kill, including target cells resistant to NK cell–derived perforin (Clarke et al, 1994). TNF-α in the membranes of the NC cells may explain their cytotoxicity. In the uterine endometrium and in the decidua that develops during pregnancy, there are NK-lineage cells that lack the surface crystallizable fragment (Fc) receptor (CD16) for immunoglobulin (Ig)G; CD16 is present on NK cells in the blood (Clark et al, 1994b). In the pregnant mouse, the NK-lineage cells develop into large (>20 μ diameter) cells with cytoplasmic granules containing TNF-α. These cells are like NC cells, and appear able to kill fetal trophoblasts, unlike conventional NK cells, but they do not readily kill targets lysed by conventional NK cells from other sites (Clarke et al, 1994). In the human uterus, the NK-lineage cells are also granulated, do not become so large, are inefficient killers of the targets of blood NK cells, are unable to lyse fetal trophoblast (unless modified as described below), and may produce a variety of interleukins and growth factors. NK cells in blood or uterine lining can secrete the cytokine γ-interferon, which activates macrophages (Ferry et al, 1991; Clark et al, 1994b; Parr et al, 1995; King et al, 1996; Lachapelle et al, 1996). Macrophages in turn produce TNF-α, which further activates NK cells; macrophages also produce the cytokine interleukin (IL)-12, which, like IL-2, can turn a conventional NK cell into a cytokine-activated killer with much greater potential to inflict damage on an otherwise resistant target cell (i.e., a tumor cell) (Nishimura et al, 1995; Salvucci et al, 1996). While fetal trophoblast cells that have been cultured in vitro may be lysed by such cells, it is unclear that freshly isolated trophoblast or trophoblast in situ can be killed (Ferry et al, 1991; King et al, 1996). Macrophages activated by γ-interferon become better able to deal with intracellular pathogens they have phagocytosed and that prove resistant to the normal concentration of digestive enzymes. Cytokines also activate vascular endothelium, leading to adhesion of lymphomyeloid cells from blood, clotting, and bleeding (Clark, 1992). Such a process may be regularly seen in normal menstruation, where the outer two thirds of the uterine lining is shed. This shedding has been called the "parturition of failed fertility" (Casey and MacDonald, 1990). As will be seen, similar processes may cause pregnancy failure.

T Cells

NK cells and macrophages are part of the innate resistance system. This system has a low-level basal state of activation such that it is always ready to react to an invader. Activity can be increased by the pathways described above, but, when danger has passed, activity returns to normal. The response to a second challenge is no different than on the first exposure. Thus one cannot acquire an immunity that deals with an invader more effectively so as to prevent disease at the time of a second encounter. The next layer of defense that developed solved this problem. Lymphocytic cells, like NK cells, developed surface receptors allowing specific recognition of distinct antigens. The recognition system of NK cells and macrophages did not confer specificity in the same way. Indeed, NK cells do have receptors for self antigens (Lanier et al, 1997). The self antigen recognized is now called a major histocompatibility complex (MHC) antigen. MHC antigens may be divided into class I and class II. Class I antigens in humans include classical human lymphocte antigens (HLAs) A, B, and C, which express the allodeterminants of each individual; these allodeterminants are frequently the target of specific immune responses. HLA-G and HLA-E are truncated (shorter) class I MHC molecules that lack allodeterminants but are important in human pregnancy, as will be discussed. Class II MHC antigens are called HLA-D. Class I determinants are usually present on all nucleated somatic cells, whereas class II antigens are restricted to macrophages and certain lymphocytes with antigen-specific receptors. Class I MHC antigens are recognized by a receptor called KIR (killer inhibitory receptor) that is present on NK cells. This reaction inhibits the NK cell. When self MHC antigen is *missing* on a target, the NK cell becomes active and kills; it is thus said that NK cells recognize "missing self."

The new development was an NK-like cell with a receptor for foreign peptide bound to the groove in MHC class I or class II self molecules. These cells have been called T cells (or thymus-derived cells) because most of these types of cells present in blood, spleen, and lymph node differentiate within the thymus during intrauterine development of the fetus, where their receptors for self MHC antigen are altered/mutated; most of the T cells die in the thymus, and T cells capable to reacting with "self" are largely eliminated (Janeway and Travers, 1996; Roitt et al, 1996). Each of the T cells that successfully "graduates" and leaves the thymus bears a receptor for a peptide of just one structure; that is, its receptor fits best to a particular peptide, and less well with others. The result of binding is activation, proliferation, and differentiation into a *clone* of activated effector cells all with the same receptor and specificity; when these cells revert to a quiescent, nonactivated state, they may persist as memory cells.

T cells, unlike NK cells, recirculate. Of course, NK cells in arterial blood may pass via capillaries back into venous blood and again be pumped via the heart to the arterial side of the circulation (Springer, 1995; Janeway and Travers, 1996; Roitt et al, 1996). The type of recirculation we are speaking about here is very different. Naive T cells, sometimes called "virgin" T cells because they have never been stimulated by antigen outside the thymus, may leave the blood when passing through blood vessels perfusing

lymph nodes or spleen. To simplify this presentation, we will confine our comments to lymph nodes. The naive T cells exit from the blood via high endothelial venules (which have a thickened endothelium) into the paracortical and medullary region in the center of the lymph node. Here there are abundant antigen-presenting cells that have picked up antigen drained to the node from peripheral tissues via afferent lymphatics. The concentration of naive T cell traffic increases the likelihood that a T cell able to recognize and react with a foreign antigen will do so. Antigen-activated T cells leave the lymph node and enter the bloodstream via efferent lymphatics; once the "activated" T cell has become quiescent, it becomes a memory cell. Memory cells maintain an increased surface concentration of adhesion molecules (present on activated T cells), which allows the cell to react more vigorously to the same antigen on a second encounter (Springer, 1995; Janeway and Travers, 1996; Roitt et al, 1996). Both activated T cells and memory cells have a diminished number of the molecules that allow them to behave as naive virgin T cells but gain molecules that facilitate their emigration into peripheral tissues, particularly at sites of inflammation. In addition to lymphocyte function antigen-1 (LFA-1) expression, there is/are very late antigen(s) (VLAs). Inflammation activates vascular endothelial cell surface expression of co-ligands such as intercellular adhesion molecule-1 (ICAM-1), which binds to T-cell surface LFA-1 molecules, and other co-ligands for VLA(s) that facilitate emigration from blood into tissue (Springer, 1995; Janeway and Travers, 1996; Roitt et al, 1996).

Antigen-primed T cells can remain at a site of inflammation or antigen challenge and create/enhance a local immune response, or, as with memory cells, enter an afferent lymphatic channel and, like antigen, travel to the regional lymph node. Indeed, T cells primed in a lymph node can effectively transfer the reaction in its entirety to the tissue level where the response may become independent of the original reaction in the node (Orsosz et al, 1986). Even when there is no foreign antigen or inflammation, activated and memory T cells preferentially exit the bloodstream into tissues, possibly as a result of increased surface receptors for low-level ICAM-1 expression on the endothelium. Furthermore, the vascular endothelial cells from different organs express organ-specific molecules (addressins) that enable lymphocytes primed locally to return to the same organ/tissue. Addressins also enable certain populations of naive T cells to localize in specific organs, in skin or mucosal surfaces. This is of particular importance for immune responses generated at mucosal surfaces; selected subsets of naive T cells are stimulated and the primed T cells depart the regional nodes and return to the mucosal surface. Indeed, immunity generated at one mucosal surface (e.g., the intestine) may be expressed at several mucosal surfaces (e.g., the gut, lung, eye, reproductive tract). Figure 4–1 illustrates some of the pathways that govern lymphocyte traffic.

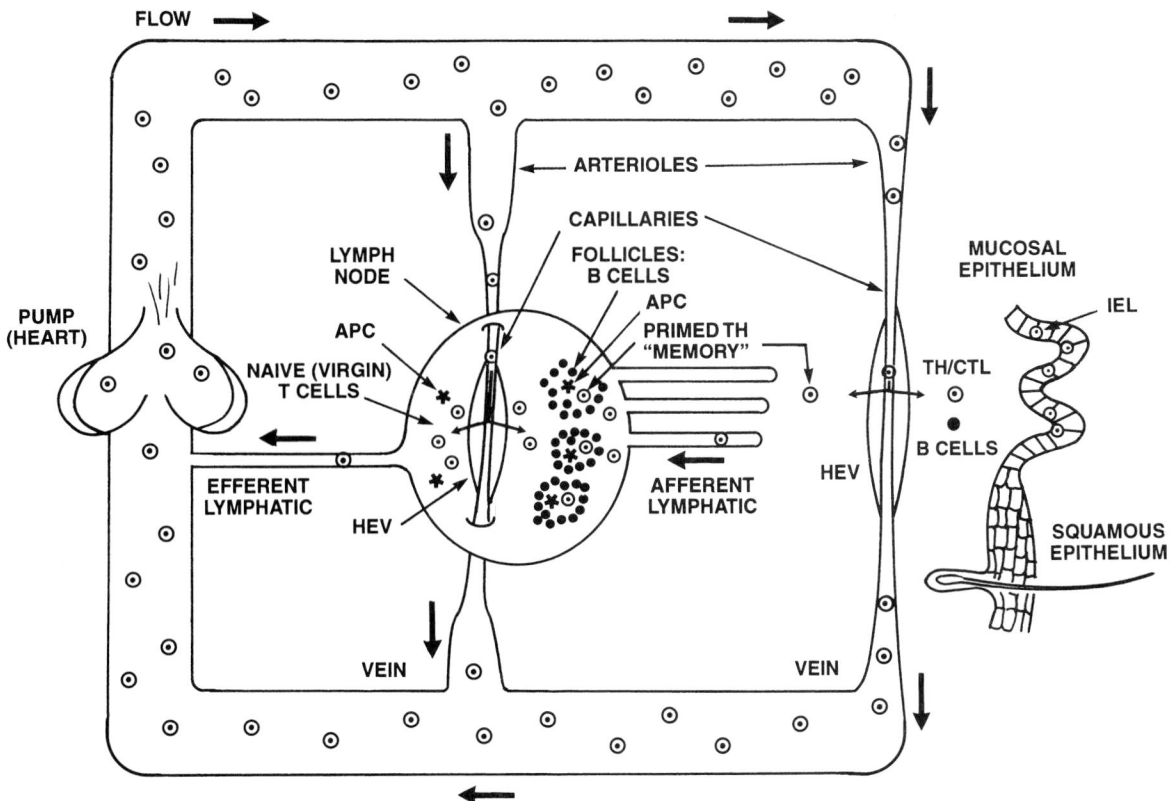

Figure 4-1
Circulation and recirculation of naive immunocompetent and antigen-activated/memory T cells in vivo. APC, antigen-presenting cell—a macrophage-related cell, usually with a dendritic shape; HEV, high endothelial venule(s); IEL, intraepithelial lymphocyte.

There are two distinct functional types of effector T cell, the cytotoxic T cell (CTL) and the cytokine-producing T cell (Janeway and Travers, 1996; Roitt et al, 1996). Cytotoxic T cells lyse nucleated cells bearing the antigen. The other type of T cell produces cytokines. Studies of cloned cytokine-producing T cells indicate there may be different types of these cells depending on the types of cytokines produced (Janeway and Travers, 1996; Roitt et al, 1996). For example, helper T cells of the T_H1 type produce IL-2, γ-interferon, granulocyte-macrophage colony-stimulating factor (GM-CSF), TNF-α, and tumor necrosis factor-β (TNF-β). These cytokines activate and attract macrophages and NK cells, and stimulate generation of CTLs. The cytokine-producing T cells have the ability to mediate cellular immunity and delayed-type hypersensitivity, and to provide "help" for certain immune responses. Classically, CTLs have been $CD8^+$ and cytokine-producing cells $CD4^+$, but this is far from an absolute restriction, and whether CD8 or CD4 is present depends on whether the antigen is presented with a class I MHC antigen (to which $CD8^+$ cells bind) or a class II MHC antigen (to which $CD4^+$ cells bind). T_H2-type T cells secrete IL-3, IL-4, IL-5, GM-CSF, and IL-10. IL-3 stimulates mast cell growth and IL-5 stimulates eosinophils, which are important in allergy and in defense

against parasites. T_H0 cells produce some cytokines of the T_H1 and T_H2 subsets and may be viewed as having not made a decision about which to become. The full implication of these T_H2-type cytokines requires a discussion of the next step in evolution of antigen-specific immune defenses.

B Cells

A late evolutionary development following the invention of T cells was the bone marrow–derived lymphocyte or B cell. These cells have a different type of surface receptor for antigen that is not dependent upon MHC, and they differentiate into a clone of plasma cells that secrete soluble antibody (Janeway and Travers, 1996; Roitt et al, 1996). The receptor on the B cell is a form of membrane-bound antibody of the IgM type, and the plasma cell may secrete an IgM that polymerizes five receptor-type molecules into a pentamer that is so large it stays within the vascular system, or the cells may change the non–antigen reactive end of the two heavy chains (in the Fc of antibody digests) to make an IgG, IgA, or IgE (Janeway and Travers, 1996; Roitt et al, 1996). The particular Fc dictates function. IgM agglutinates and activates complement via binding C1;

subsequently, via C4 and C2, there is activation of C3 that can bind to the antigen. IgG can also activate complement and facilitates phagocytosis via receptors on phagocyte membranes. IgA is selectively produced by B cells that home to epithelial surfaces, particularly in the bronchus and intestinal tract (facilitated by addressins as with T cells); two IgA molecules become linked by a J piece and are transported through the epithelium to the surface, where the IgA remains stuck to the mucus layer (Janeway and Travers, 1996; Roitt et al, 1996). Such an antibody binds antigen before it can pass through the epithelium; this is called antigen exclusion. IgE fixes to receptors on tissue mast cells and activates their release of vasoactive products should antigen appear (Janeway and Travers, 1996; Roitt et al, 1996). TNF-α may be released by mast cells, among other products that cause fluid and mucus secretion, smooth muscle spasm, and capillary leakiness. The local manifestation of this immediate hypersensitivity is the wheal and flare in the skin, bronchospasm in the lung, and diarrhea in the gut; the systemic manifestation of circulating mast cell products is anaphylaxis. IgG or IgA complexed with antigen can be deposited in tissues as immune complexes and cause inflammation.

Immune responses by B cells usually require "help" from T_H2-type T cells. T_H1 cells inhibit T_H2 cells and vice versa. These interactions facilitate switching from cellular to humoral immunity. T help to B cells occurs when the T cell recognizes antigen on the B-cell surface in association with B-cell membrane class II MHC antigen; the T_H2 cell cytokines IL-4 and IL-10 act as B-cell growth factors, and IL-5 may facilitate maturation along the IgE pathway (Janeway and Travers, 1996; Roitt et al, 1996). T-cell activation also requires "help." Antigen binding to the T-cell receptor (TCR) is not sufficient. For cells destined to become CTLs, T_H1 cell–derived cytokines may suffice, but what helps the helper cell? Macrophage-derived IL-1 was once thought to be sufficient, but we now know that a second signal (besides signal 1 from the TCR) is provided by either B7 molecules on the macrophage or by CD40 molecules (which are particular types of adhesion molecules). B7.1 derived T_H1-type differentiation and B7.2, T_H2-type cells (Janeway and Travers, 1996; Larsen et al, 1996; Roitt et al, 1996). Blocking these second signaling pathways leads to tolerance of allografts (Larsen et al, 1996). Hence, the second signal is very important. Figure 4–2 illustrates some of the details of signaling.

γδ T Cells

A recent discovery has been the γδ T cell (Janeway and Travers, 1996; Kaufmann, 1996; Roitt et al, 1996). Unlike T cells with αβ-type TCRs, γδ TCRs can recognize antigen without the requirement for MHC antigens. γδ T cells may develop without a sojourn in

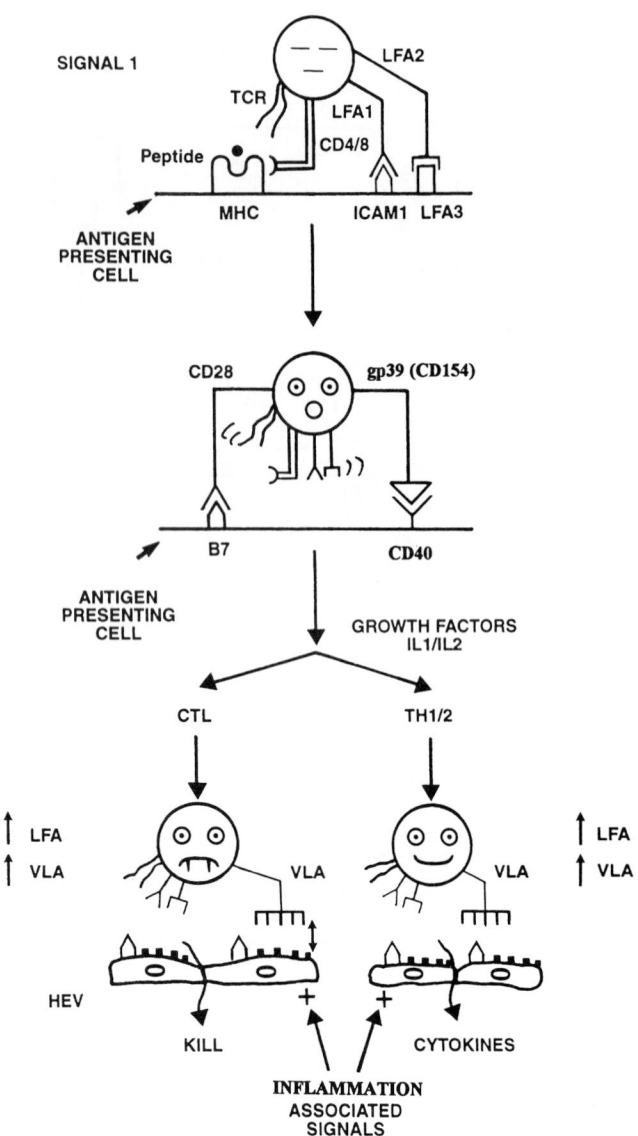

Figure 4–2

An illustration of cell surface molecules involved in activation of immunocompetent T cells. TCR, T-cell receptor that specifically recognizes foreign peptide in the groove in the MHC molecule; LFA-1 (CD11a), lymphocyte function antigen-1, which interacts with ICAM-1; LFA-2 (CD2), the receptor binding sheep red blood cells, which interacts with LFA-3; LFA-3, interacts with LFA-2 on other lymphocytes; CD28, reacts with B7.1/7.2; CD40, reacts with CP39.

the thymus, may lack CD4 and CD8, tend not to recirculate, and accumulate at mucosal surfaces and in skin (Janeway and Travers, 1996; Kaufmann, 1996; Roitt et al, 1996). In mucosa, they may be present *within* the epithelium as intraepithelial lymphocytes (IELs), although not all IELs are of the γδ phenotype. γδ T cells tend to have cytoplasmic granules, similar to NK cells, can be cytotoxic to targets *resistant* to killing by conventional NK cells and CTLs, and can produce T_H1- and T_H2-type cytokines. It is unclear whether second signals are required for activation of γδ T cells or what they might be; some γδ T cells respond to antigen without the requirement that MHC antigen be present, and γδ T cells may respond to heat shock proteins expressed on injured epithelial cells, and by certain microorganisms (e.g., *Chlamydia*) (Dieterle and Wollenhaupt, 1996). It is quite possible that γδ T-cell development in evolution preceded the "invention" of αβ T cells. The αβ T cells develop in a gut-related outpouching that creates the thymus, and γδ T cells may develop in gut epithelium that becomes their "home," so one may envisage γδ T cells as those cells that decided, after their education and maturation, to stay put, and αβ cells as T cells educated in gut-associated tissue that leave it and recirculate. Mature αβ T cells that encounter antigen and develop into effector cells may also tend to remain localized and remain at the site of confrontation with antigen. Some γδ T cells recirculate, however.

Helper and Suppressor Cells

T_H cells activated at the site of antigen in tissues are believed to percolate down afferent lymphatics to lymph nodes, where in the outer cortex they can serve to help antigen-primed B cells develop; these B cells form follicles (Fig. 4–1). In birds, B cells develop from precursors into immunocompetent cells capable of responding to antigen in a gut-related organ, the bursa of Fabricius, associated with the cloaca (rectal end of the gastrointestinal tract) (Janeway and Travers, 1996; Roitt et al, 1996). Birds have been closely related to the dinosaurs, and, in the more evolutionarily advanced mammalian species, the role of the bursa is carried out by cells in bone marrow.

But what happens if foreign material cannot be eliminated? Would continuous proliferation and activation of effector cells not cause the organism to swell up and explode? Indeed, regulators are required. Just as there are helper cells, there are suppressor cells. NK cells and macrophages can have suppressive effects, as can B cells, but the suppressor cells of greatest interest are of the T lineage. Both TCR αβ and γδ T cells can have suppressive effects that go beyond the phenomenon of a T_H1-type T_H, producing cytokines that block T_H2 and vice versa. Suppression at mucosal surfaces is particularly important, because it is that site that we encounter antigen that we cannot or do not want to mount an immune response against—food! Oral tolerance is mediated by TGF-β–producing T_H3 cells (Chen et al, 1994). Similar T cells (with TCR γδ) are described later with respect to the uterus during pregnancy.

REPRODUCTIVE TRACT IMMUNOLOGY

Now that we have our immune system, let us look specifically at the reproductive tract. The reproductive tracts of both males and females are mucosal organs that interface with the outside world.

Male Reproductive Tract

The male testis possesses afferent lymphatics, and there are T and B cells in the circulation that can recognize and react with testicular antigens (Head and Billingham, 1985). If effector cells and antibody are produced, the individual may have orchitis and problems with spermatogenesis (Tung, 1995). A vasectomy can cause reflux of sperm antigens into the host such that antibody is elicited. Locally produced IgG and IgA that gains access to the lumen can agglutinate and immobilize sperm, leading to infertility, and peritubular antigen-antibody reactions can cause inflammation. A reverse vasectomy or repeat reverse vasectomy may fail to restore fertility and may boost antisperm antibody levels locally. At one time there was a concern that systemic antigen-antibody complexes might form and accelerate development of atherosclerosis, as shown using primates, but epidemiologic evidence suggests this is not applicable to man (Kovacs and Frances, 1983).

What prevents spontaneous immune responses from arising and destroying the testes in a man (or ovaries in a woman)? There is good evidence that suppressor T cells specific for gonad antigens prevent such responses (Tung, 1995). In addition, an allograft placed within the testis has some protection against rejection (Head and Billingham, 1985). This phenomenon also occurs with allografts to the anterior chamber of the eye and brain, which are said to be "immunologically privileged sites." A primary immune response leading to rejection is not triggered, but, if the animal is immunized systemically, the graft is rejected. The immune privilege in the testis is thought to be largely due to cells that suppress immune reactivity—possibly the testosterone-producing Leydig cells (Head and Billingham, 1985).

The testis is drained by a series of tubules that form the epididimus, vas deferens, and seminal vesicles, which empty into the urethra via the prostate gland. These tubes are lined by epithelium with IELs. IgA may also be locally produced and secreted, particularly at the level of the prostate. Indeed, much of the sperm antibody in ejaculate may enter the pre-ejaculate at the level of the prostate and seminal vesicle.

The immune defenses of the male genital tract are relevant to various pathogens that may ascend the urethra, such as the gonococcus. Human immunodeficiency virus (HIV) is also present in significant quantity in ejaculate and must derive from a local source. Understanding local defense mechanisms within the male reproductive tract and their integration with systemic immunity is a subject of active research (Anderson, 1996).

Female Reproductive Tract

The female reproductive tract and its immune defenses is better understood than that of the male, in part because is easier to access the relevant sites and to obtain tissues, as every obstetrician-gynecologist will realize. The female reproductive tract is also the site at which immunologic confrontations occur. On one hand, the genetically undesirable organisms must be suppressed/eliminated; on the other, the genetically desirable (e.g., male spermatozoa and the fetus) must be tolerated even if the mother must compromise her defenses. There may be limits inherent in such compromises that are relevant to "disease."

HOST EFFECTOR SYSTEMS IN REPRODUCTIVE DISORDERS

Problems with Ins and Outs

The vagina is the closest female reproductive tract interface to the outside world, is colonized by microbial flora, is subject to invasion by bacteria and fungi from the adjacent rectal effluent, and is exposed to antigen-containing ejaculate. A low pH maintained on the stratified squamous epithelium of the vagina helps to suppress potential bacterial invaders and inactivates spermatozoa. At the time of ovulation, the environment becomes more hospitable to spermatozoa, the mucus plugging the cervical os that guards entry into the uterus becomes more penetrable, and both sperm and attached bacteria can ascend (Sanchez et al, 1989). It is thought bacteria may also ascend at the time of menstruation, but, surprisingly, endometritis is quite rare. When spermatozoa are deposited in the vagina, there is a polymorphonuclear efflux from the vaginal wall, and the invader is disposed of. There may be sufficient systemic absorption to produce an immune response, but except for an anaphylactic response to seminal plasma antigen, sensitization to sperm is detectable with only very sensitive techniques (Clark, 1991). Some women may develop antisperm antibodies. These are usually IgG and IgA in class, and are released by plasma cells in the cervix. Exactly how they are induced (i.e., what is the site of sensitization) is unknown. Orally ingested sperm can induce a mucosal IgA response that leads to antibodies in the genital tract (Clark et al, 1987). In a rat model, infertility was induced, and in mice, abortions (Clark et al, 1987). Antisperm antibodies are not specific for the sperm of one male but react with sperm from all males. It is difficult to predict the functional effect an antibody will have (some antibodies decrease sperm motility and others may stimulate it!). Sperm bear CD46, which prevents complement action; if there were complement in the vagina or cervical canal together with IgG (which can fix complement), no damage would be expected, but fortunately complement levels are very low and CD46 appears to have another function, adherence of sperm to the ovulated oocyte (Taylor et al, 1994).

There has been considerable interest in immunosuppressive factors in seminal plasma acting to prevent maternal immune responses to foreign antigens of the male, and to passengers such as bacteria and viruses (e.g., HIV). Much of the suppression of lymphocyte responses shown in vitro can be explained by an artifact. The serum used in the in vitro assay contains monoamine oxidase, which converts spermine and spermidine in seminal plasma into toxic (and hence suppressive) products (Lea et al, 1991). Seminal plasma contains high concentrations of prostaglandin E, which can be immunosuppressive. Such activity if present is not essential for pregnancy because washed sperm introduced directly into the uterus generate successful pregnancies. However, seminal plasma may contain factors, such as TGF-β, that can be absorbed and increase the implantation rate by stimulating GM-CSF production (Coulam, 1994; Robertson et al, 1997). The actual mechanism is unknown.

There is an internal interface of the reproductive tract with the peritoneal cavity. During normal menstruation, some of the endometrium may be transported retrograde via the fallopian tubes into the peritoneal cavity and elicit an immune response (Evers, 1994; Koninck, 1994; Daya, 1996). The basis for the immune response is unknown, but a reaction to heat shock protein by γδ T cells would be one possible mechanism. In most women, retrograde menstruation seems to have no adverse effect; in others, there appears to be activation of cells of the immune system to produce cytokines such as IL-1, TNF-α, and γ-interferon (Evers, 1994; Koninck, 1994; Daya, 1996). Some, but not all, of these women may show visible features of early endometriosis. With advanced endometriosis and scarring, cytokine levels are lower. The cytokines can interfere with oocyte fertilization and blastocyst implantation so as to cause infertility. There may also be effects after implantation that lead to abortion, as discussed later (Daya, 1996). Endometriosis regresses with a pregnancy. This is likely hormonal because regression can be induced independently of a pregnancy so as to reduce cytokine levels and enhance reproductive success (Taketani et al, 1992; Daya, 1996).

The Problem of Pregnancy Success and Failure

Although globally the problem of pregnancy is too many (and, hence, overpopulation), in industrialized nations, unwanted pregnancies and inability to have a successful pregnancy are the major medical concerns. Talwar et al (1997) have developed a vaccine that reversibly immunizes women to human chorionic gonadotropin to produce safe, long-term contraception. Because the objective is to reduce population fertility, a small failure rate is acceptable. Unwanted pregnancies, whether intrauterine or ectopic, have surgical and medical solutions that are not immunologic, and infertility is currently dealt with by surgical methods such as in vitro fertilization/embryo transfer rather than by immunologic methods. A possible exception may be the use of seminal plasma suppositories or intravenous gamma globulin (IVIg) to enhance implantation rates (Coulam, 1994; Clark et al, 1997). The mechanism of such effects is uncertain and will not be discussed further. That leaves the problem of recurrent miscarriages as a basis for reproductive failure, and this area has attracted a great deal of immunologic interest.

Human reproduction is surprisingly inefficient. Of 100 fertilized oocytes, 50 fail before or at the time of implantation, probably as a result of anatomic/structural/chromosomal defects, 15 to 20 implant and fail as chemical pregnancies, 5 to 10 become spontaneous abortions of clinically recognized pregnancies, and 25 reach term (Lea and Clark, 1991). With clinical spontaneous abortions, one may see several patterns. There may be a single loss associated with several live births (sporadic spontaneous abortion), a series of consecutive losses, or a mixture of successful pregnancies and losses. Five percent to 15% of pregnancies may end in a sporadic loss, and 2% to 4% in recurrent sequential losses. There is a high frequency of chromosomal anomalies in abortus tissue derived from chromosomally normal parents, and, among the recurrent loss group, there appears to be a subset of women who have a high rate of recurrent chromosome problems (Coulam et al, 1996). However, a significant proportion of losses are karyotypically normal, and, although anatomic, infectious, endocrine, and parental chromosome abnormality mechanisms are commonly sought, there is good reason to suspect *most* abnormalities are incidental to the problem (Clark and Coulam, 1995; Clark et al, 1996b; Coulam et al, 1997). This is not to deny that, on occasion, such mechanisms may lead to abortion, but, currently, immunologic/immunologically modifiable mechanisms have taken center stage. These may be summarized as follows:

1. *Endometriosis and/or unexplained infertility*: High levels of cytokines are thought to lead to embryo damage that later presents as a pregnancy failure (Muzikova and Clark, 1995; Daya, 1996).
2. *Anti-phospholipid antibodies*: These may bind to trophoblast to prevent fusion of the cytotrophoblast into a syncytium, and may promote thrombosis with ischemic death of the embryo (Rote et al, 1994).
3. *Higher than normal blood and endometrial NK cell activity plus an impaired maternal immune response to antigens on the implanted embryo* (Clark and Coulam, 1995; Coulam et al, 1995; Lachapelle et al, 1996; Clark et al, 1997): This immune recognition is thought to act to suppress NK activity (Szekeres-Bartho, 1993; Clark et al, 1994a, 1996a; Aoki et al, 1995; Jalali et al, 1996; Kwak et al, 1996; Arck et al, 1997).

Such a classification is not without controversy, because it is new. For many years, *endometriosis* was dismissed as a cause of miscarriages because the miscarriage rate was not higher in women with endometriosis than in women with a similar degree of infertility and no endometriosis. However, endometriosis is what you see. What causes the abortions is what you do *not* see (i.e., the cytokines), and both groups of women have abnormally elevated levels (Daya, 1996). Hormone suppression using a gonadotropin-releasing hormone agonist suppresses cytokine levels, but it is uncertain if that alone will reduce the abortion rate in accordance with prediction (Taketani et al, 1992; Daya, 1996). On the basis of chance alone, some women with endometriosis or unexplained infertility will belong to group 3, which is discussed below. *Anti-phospholipid antibodies* are a recognized cause of second trimester losses, and a convincing case can be made where antibody titers are high and placental infarcts are found. A role for these antibodies in the more common problem of *first*-trimester losses is controversial because we do not know how to identify which antibodies are pathogenic (Coulam et al, 1997).

The *NK cell* hypothesis has arisen out of consideration of the embryo as a graft bearing paternal antigens foreign to the mother (Clark et al, 1996a). Initially, it was thought abortion might represent antigen-specific immune rejection mediated by killer T cells, as occurs in allografts of kidney, heart, and skin. Successful pregnancy was explained by local active suppression by trophoblast cell–activated maternal suppressor cells in the uterus (Clark et al, 1996a). However, studies of animal models of abortion conclusively demonstrated that abortion occurred if T cells were eliminated, that the trophoblast was resistant to these rejection mechanisms, and that immunization against paternal antigens, even if transplantation immunity was stimulated, was more likely to prevent than to cause abortion (Coulam and Clark, 1994; Clark et al, 1996a). In humans, any sensitized killer T cells that could on occasion be found followed rather than preceded abortions (Sargent et al, 1988). It was subsequently suggested that T cells recognized trophoblasts and produced cytokines that caused growth of trophoblasts—the immunotrophism hypothesis. An essential premise was that the trophoblast was immunogenic and served as a barrier between the tissues of the fetus (which were rejectable by maternal T cells) and the mother's immune system (Chaouat et al, 1983; Clark et al, 1996a). Animal and human studies suggested that the trophoblasts do not stimulate conventional T cells, that there is no impervious barrier because maternal and fetal cells cross in both directions, and that much of the intrauterine cytokine production is from epithelium, trophoblast, and other nonimmunological cells (Clark et al, 1996a). It was also shown that activated NK cells could not kill freshly isolated trophoblast in vitro, but that in vivo injection of activated NK cells caused abortion (Ferry et al, 1991; Clark et al, 1996a). The latter effect is therefore most likely related to production of abortion-causing cytokines such as IL-1, TNF-α, and γ-interferon (Clark et al, 1996a). It is possible that NK cell–derived cytokines act through or in synergy with macrophages, which become a major source of TNF-α in response to the γ-interferon produced by NK cells (Clark et al, 1996a). As mentioned above, there are data implicating NK cells in abortion of embryos of normal karyotype, and immunization of both animals and humans with allogeneic (paternal) leukocytes reduces NK activity, as does infusion of IVIg (Aoki et al, 1995; Kwak et al, 1996). Both types of treatments may reduce the risk of a subsequent abortion (Clark et al, 1997). However, the NK cell hypothesis is controversial because

1. NK activity fluctuates in normal individuals, often increasing with a minor viral infection (but head colds do not cause abortions!); careful standardization is needed for reliable and reproducible quantitation if functional activity is used (Pross and Maroun, 1984). One laboratory has standardized NK cells by dividing the percentage of $CD56^+$ cells by the total number of blood lymphocytes (Coulam et al, 1995; Kwak et al, 1996).
2. Psychological stress is proposed to be important in abortions (and has been shown to be preventable by immunotherapy in mice) (Clark et al, 1996a, 1997). However, stress is known to reduce NK activity.
3. NK cells, even if preactivated with cytokines such as IL-2, do not kill *fresh human* trophoblasts that have not been first cultured in vitro (Ferry et al, 1991; King et al, 1996). Human syncytiotrophoblasts (but not cytotrophoblasts) bear an 80-kDa paternal alloantigenic molecule to which the woman makes an IgG antibody during pregnancy, and it has been argued that this antibody may block killing by NK cells and elutes when trophoblasts are incubated in vitro (Jalali et al, 1996). There is no good evidence, however, that this antibody is present on cytotrophoblast cells that are exposed to NK cells in the decidua, and no good evidence the antibody is present in the first trimester, when most spontaneous abortions need to be prevented.

The solution to such puzzling issues has been made more difficult by contradictory results of trials of immunotherapy of abortion and claims that psychotherapy (TLC) is as effective (Clark et al, 1997). Invariably, such trials are small, the patients are heterogeneous, chromosome abnormalities in fetal trophoblast have not been excluded, and there is no information about NK cell levels/activity or effect of treatment on this parameter. Nevertheless, current data indicate there may be a subset of patients who may benefit from immunization with paternal mononuclear leukocytes or *possibly* from repeated IV infusions of pooled human gamma globulin (Clark and Coulam, 1995; Clark et al, 1996b, 1997). The latter issue is currently under review pending analysis of the raw patient data from completed randomized

trials. For injection of allogeneic leukocytes, blood bank precautions to prevent transmission of infectious agents and graft-versus-host disease are required (Coulam and Clark, 1994). Gamma globulin is considered to be reasonably safe, and a low-IgA preparation is available for use in patients lacking IgA (who may have anaphylaxis with the usual preparations), but there is no standard of potency (and different preparations are known to vary in their properties) (Clark et al, 1997). At present, it would seem advisable to karyotype failing first-trimester trophoblasts and to have patients investigated and treated in a center specializing in the investigation of recurrent miscarriages. As previously mentioned, it is not known if those patients with elevated NK levels are the same or different from those with elevated levels of cytokines in peritoneal fluid ($\pm$ endometriosis), and what may be the effect of immunologic treatments on the latter. The data supporting the use of IVIg to treat recurrent miscarriage patients are much weaker that the data supporting the use of paternal blood mononuclear leukocytes because the number of patients in randomized controlled trials in the former is much smaller than in the latter. In patients with an autoimmune contraindication to the use of paternal leukocytes, IVIg *may* be a reasonable consideration.

Hypertension/Pre-eclampsia in Pregnancy

Pregnancy in a women with prior hypertension can aggravate the problem, and pre-existing renal disease also predisposes to hypertension. The development of hypertension in a previously normal individual, a more common scenario, represents the most common complication of pregnancy (Clark, 1994). There is a familial predisposition, and the first pregnancy with the current partner and multiple pregnancies pose the highest risk. The underlying problem is inadequate perfusion of the trophoblast by maternal blood, usually because extravillous trophoblast fails to sufficiently invade and alter the muscular walls of the maternal spiral arteries (Clark, 1994). "Sufficiently" means that the invasion affects the entire decidual portion and inner one third of the myometrial portion of the artery. "Alter" means the vessels become flaccid, high-capacitance conduits able to supply sufficient blood for fetal growth. In a normal singleton pregnancy, the problem arises in the third trimester. The fetoplacental unit then send out signals that increase maternal blood pressure so as to improve perfusion. If the maternal blood pressure does not increase sufficiently, the fetus may be growth restricted (Clark, 1994). Various mechanisms for the pressor effect have been postulated, but release of the potent vasoconstrictor endothelin seems most likely (Clark et al, 1992; Mastrogiannis et al, 1992; Schiff et al, 1992). Systemic vascular and renal damage by deportation of trophoblast membrane vesicles into the circulation seems to lead to proteinuria and vasospasm (Clark, 1994).

It has been postulated that immunologic factors may contribute to the causation of pregnancy-induced hypertension. The evidence has been weak with one exception. Patients with significant levels of anti-phospholipid antibodies may be at greater risk of developing hypertension/pre-eclampsia (Allen et al, 1996). By contrast, it is proposed that a maternal immune response to the antigens of her mate, in particular antigens in semen, may prevent pre-eclampsia (Clark, 1994). Is this due to immune stimulation that activates mechanisms that block NK cell retardation of trophoblast invasion in the decidua? Or may there be an immunotrophic stimulation of trophoblast growth and invasion? Reproductive immunologists hope to determine the precise stimulus needed and the mechanism of action of immunity in preventing hypertension/pre-eclampsia. Natural immunization, where deemed desirable, may be achieved by ensuring 6 to 12 months of exposure to the partner's semen prior to conception (Clark, 1994). A randomized interventional trial would be required to validate such a suggestion but is unlikely to prove feasible in a typical North American population.

While we are still on the topic of immunotherapy using IVIg, we should mention that IVIg may be a credible alternative to heparin plus acetylsalicylic acid for therapy of pathogenic anti-phospholipid antibodies, and it can prevent pathogenic antibodies (such as anti-Rh and autoantibodies) from crossing the placenta into the fetus (Clark et al, 1997).

Premature Parturition

The sequelae of prematurity, the most common cause of low birth weight, represent a major long-term health burden. Most prematurity is unexplained and is thought to have a psychosocial basis. Intervention trials have shown little impact on prematurity (Graham et al, 1992). There has been considerable interest in the cellular and molecular mechanisms of parturition and in development of tocolytic drugs to suppress premature activation of such mechanisms. Stimuli that activate cytokines that cause abortion seem also to stimulate parturition (Chaouat, 1994; Steinborn et al, 1996). Abortions can be prevented by immunotherapy but there is no evidence immunotherapy can affect premature labor (in the laboratory mouse [Chaouat, 1994]). Intravenous injection of the cytokine TGF-β2 has been able to prevent premature parturition in cytokine-treated rabbits (Bry and Hallman, 1993). In humans, TGF-β2 can be nephrotoxic. Immunologically activating endogenous TGF-β2–producing cells to prevent premature parturition would be potentially more physiologic (Clark et al, 1996a) but remains to be tested.

REFERENCES

Allen JY, Tapia-Santiago C, Kutteh WH: Antiphospholipid antibodies in patients with preeclampsia. Am J Reprod Immunol 1996;36:81.

Anderson DJ: The importance of mucosal immunology to problems in human reproduction. J Reprod Immunol 1996;31:3.

Aoki K, Higuchi K, Yagami Y: Suppression of natural killer cell activity by monocytes following immunotherapy for habitual aborters. Am J Reprod Immunol 1995;33:465.

Arck PC, Ferrick DA, Steele-Norwood D, et al: Murine T cell determination of pregnancy outcome. I. Effects of strain, αβ T cell receptor, γδ T cell receptor, and γδ T cell subsets. Am J Reprod Immunol 1997:492.

Beer AE, Billingham RE: The Immunobiology of Mammalian Reproduction. Englewood Cliffs, NJ: Prentice-Hall, 1976.

Berke G: Killing mechanisms of cytotoxic lymphocytes. Curr Opin Hematol 1997;4:32.

Bry K, Hallman M: Transforming growth factor-β2 prevents preterm delivery induced by interleukin 1α and tumor necrosis factor-α in the rabbit. Am J Obstet Gynecol 1993;168:1318.

Casey ML, MacDonald PC: Biomolecular mechanisms in human parturition: activation of uterine decidua. In d'Arcangues C, Fraser IS, Newton JR, Olind V (eds): Contraception and Mechanisms of Uterine Bleeding. Cambridge: Cambridge University Press, 1990:304.

Chaouat G: Synergy of lipopolysaccharide and inflammatory cytokines in murine pregnancy: alloimmunization prevents abortion but does not affect the induction of preterm delivery. Cell Immunol 1994;157:328.

Chaouat G, Kolb JP, Wegmann TG: The murine placenta as an immunological barrier between mother and fetus. Immunol Rev 1983;75:31.

Chen Y, Kuchroo VK, Inobe J, et al: Regulatory T cell clones induced by oral tolerance: suppression of autoimmune encephalomyelitis. Science 1994;265:1237.

Clark BA, Halvorson L, Sachs B, Epstein FH: Plasma endothelin levels in preeclampsia: elevation and correlation with uric acid levels and renal impairment. Am J Obstet Gynecol 1992;166:962.

Clark DA: Regulation of cytotoxic T lymphocytes. PhD. thesis, University of Toronto, 1977.

Clark DA: Controversies in reproductive immunology. Crit Rev Immunol 1991;11:215.

Clark DA: Cytokines in uterine bleeding. In Alexander NJ, d'Arcangues C (eds): Steroid Hormones and Uterine Bleeding. Washington, DC: AAAS Press, 1992:263.

Clark DA: Does immunological intercourse prevent pre-eclampsia? Lancet 1994;344:969.

Clark DA, Arck PC, Jalali R, et al: Psycho-neuro-cytokine/endocrine pathways in immunoregulation during pregnancy. Am J Reprod Immunol 1996a;35:330.

Clark DA, Chaouat G, Mogil R, Wegmann TG: Prevention of spontaneous abortion in DBA/2-mated CBA/J mice by GM-CSF involves CD8+ T-cell-dependent suppression of natural effector cell cytotoxicity against trophoblast target cells. Cell Immunol 1994a;154:143.

Clark DA, Chaput A, Slapsys RM, et al: Suppressor cells in the uterus. In Gill TJ III, Wegmann TG (eds): Immunoregulation and Fetal Survival. New York: Oxford University Press, 1987:63.

Clark DA, Coulam CB: Is there an immunological cause of repeated pregnancy wastage? Adv Obstet Gynecol 1995;3:321.

Clark DA, Daya S, Coulam CB, Gunby J, and the Recurrent Miscarriage Immunotherapy Trialists Group: Implications of abnormal human trophoblast karyotype for the evidence-based approach to the understanding, investigation, and treatment of recurrent spontaneous abortion. Am J Reprod Immunol 1996b;35:495.

Clark DA, Gunby J, Daya S: The use of allogeneic leukocytes or IV IgG for the treatment of patients with recurrent spontaneous abortions. Transfus Med Rev 1997;11:85.

Clark DA, Vince G, Flanders KC, et al: CD56+ lymphoid cells in human first trimester pregnancy decidua as a source of novel TGF-β2-related immunosuppressive factors. Hum Reprod 1994b;9:2270.

Clarke GR, Roberts TK, Smart YC: Natural killer and natural cytotoxic cells are present at the maternal-fetal interface during murine pregnancy. Immunol Cell Biol 1994;72:153.

Coulam CB: Immunotherapy for spontaneous abortion. In Hunt JS (ed): Immunobiology of Reproduction (Serono Symposia USA). New York: Springer-Verlag, 1994:303.

Coulam C, Clark DA: Immunotherapy for recurrent miscarriage. Am J Reprod Immunol 1994;32:257.

Coulam CB, Clark DA, Beer AE, et al: Current clinical options for diagnosis and treatment of recurrent spontaneous abortion. Am J Reprod Immunol 1997;38:57.

Coulam CB, Goodman C, Roussev RG, et al: Systemic CD56$^+$ cells can predict pregnancy outcome. Am J Reprod Immunol 1995; 33:40.

Coulam CB, Stephenson M, Stern JJ, Clark DA: Immunotherapy for recurrent pregnancy loss: analysis of results from clinical trials. Am J Reprod Immunol 1996;35:352.

Daya S: Endometriosis and spontaneous abortion. Infertil Reprod Med Clin North Am 1996;7:759.

Dieterle S, Wollenhaupt J: Humoral immune response to the chlamydial heat shock proteins hsp60 and hsp70 in Chlamydia-associated chronic salpingitis with tubal occlusion. Hum Reprod 1996;11:1352.

Evers JLH: Endometriosis does not exist; all women have endometriosis. Hum Reprod 1994;9:2206.

Ferry BL, Sargent IL, Starkey PM, Redman CW: Cytotoxic activity against trophoblast and choriocarcinoma cells of large granular lymphocytes from early pregnancy decidua. Cell Immunol 1991;132:140.

Garcia-Penarrubia P, Bankhurst AD, Koster FT: Experimental and theoretical kinetics study of antibacterial killing mediated by human natural killer cells. J Immunol 1989a;142:1310.

Garcia-Penarrubia P, Koster FT, Kelley RO, et al: Antibacterial activity of human natural killer cells. J Exp Med 1989b;169:99.

Graham AV, Frank SJ, Zyzanski SJ, et al: A clinical trial to reduce the rate of low birth weight in an inner-city black population. Fam Med 1992;24:439.

Head JR, Billingham RE: Immune privilege in the testis. II. Evaluation of potential local factors. Transplantation 1985;40:269.

Jalali GR, Arck PC, Chaouat G, et al: Immunosuppressive properties of monoclonal antibodies and human polyclonal alloantibodies to the R80K protein of trophoblast. Am J Reprod Immunol 1996;36:129.

Janeway CA Jr, Travers P: Immunobiology. 2nd ed. New York: Current Biology Ltd/Garland Publishing Inc, 1996.

Jans DA, Jans P, Briggs LJ, et al: Nuclear transport of granzyme B (fragmentin-2): dependence on perforin in vivo and cytosolic factors in vitro. J Biol Chem 1996;271:30781.

Kaufmann SH: γδ and other unconventional T lymphocytes: what do they see and what do they do? Proc Natl Acad Sci U S A 1996;93:2272.

King A, Jokhi PP, Burrows TD, et al: Functions of human decidual NK cells. Am J Reprod Immunol 1996;35:258.

Koninck P: Is mild endometriosis a condition occurring intermittently in all women? Hum Reprod 1994;9:2202.

Kovacs GT, Frances M: Vasectomy: what are the long term risks? Med J Aust 1983;2:564.

Kwak FM-Y, Kwak JYH, Ainbinder SW, et al: Elevated peripheral blood natural killer cells are effectively suppressed by immunoglobulin G infusions in women with recurrent spontaneous abortions. Am J Reprod Immunol 1996;35:2250.

Lachapelle MH, Miron P, Hemmings R, Roy DC: Endometrial T, B and NK cells in patients with recurrent spontaneous abortion. J Immunol 1996;156:4027.

Lanier LL, Corliss B, Phillips JH: Arousal and inhibition of human NK cells. Immunol Rev 1997;155:145.

Larsen CP, Elwood ET, Alexander DZ, et al: Long-term acceptance of skin and cardiac allografts after blocking CD40 and CD28 pathways. Nature 1996;381:434.

Lea RG, Clark DA: Macrophages and other migratory cells in endometrium relevant to implantation. Balmieres Clin Obstet Gynecol 1991;5:25.

Lea RG, Harper J, Banwatt D, et al: The detection of spermine and spermidine in human IVF supernatants and their relation to early embryo-associated suppressor activity. Fertil Steril 1991;56:771.

Mastrogiannis DS, Kalter CS, O'Brien WF, et al: Effect of magnesium sulfate on plasma endothelin-1 levels in normal and preeclamptic pregnancies. Am J Obstet Gynecol 1992;167:1554.

Muzikova E, Clark DA: Is spontaneous resorption in the DBA/2-mated CBA/J mouse due to a defect in "seed" or in "soil"? Am J Reprod Immunol 1995;33:81.

Nishimura T, Watanabe K, Lee U, et al: Phenotypic and functional characteristics of in vivo-induced interleukin-12-activated killer cells. Immunol Lett 1995;48:167.

Orsosz CG, Zinn NE, Sirinek LP, Ferguson RM: In vivo mechanisms of alloreactivity: II. Allospecificity of cytotoxic T lymphocytes in sponge matrix allografts as determined by limiting dilution analysis. Transplantation 1986;41:84.

Parr EL, Chen HL, Parr MB, Hunt JS: Synthesis and granular localization of tumor necrosis factor-alpha in activated NK cells in the pregnant uterus. J Reprod Immunol 1995;28:31.

Peck R, Brockhaus M, Frey JR: Cell surface tumor necrosis factor (TNF) accounts for monocyte- and lymphocyte-mediated killing of TNF-resistant target cells. Cell Immunol 1989;122:1.

Pross HF, Maroun JA: The standardization of NK cell assays for use in the study of biological response modifiers. J Immunol Methods 1984;68:235.

Robertson SA, Mau VJ, Hudson SN, Tremellen KP: Cytokine-leukocyte networks in the establishment of pregnancy. Am J Reprod Immunol 1997;37:438.

Roitt I, Brostoff J, Male D: Immunology. 4th ed. London: Mosby (Times Miror) Ltd, 1996.

Rote NS, Lyden TW, Vogt E, Ng AK: Antiphospholipid antibodies and placental development. In Hunt JS (ed): Immunobiology of Reproduction (Serono Symposia USA). New York: Springer-Verlag, 1994:285.

Salvucci O, Mami-Chouaib F, Moreau JL, Theze J: Differential regulation of interleukin-12- and interleukin-15-induced natural killer cell activation by interleukin-4. Eur J Immunol 1996;26:2736.

Sanchez R, Villagran E, Concha M, Cornejo R: Ultrastructural analysis of the attachment of human spermatozoon after in vitro migration through estrogenic cervical mucus. In J Fertil 1989;34:363.

Sargent IL, Wilkins T, Redman CWG: Maternal immune responses to the fetus in early pregnancy and recurrent miscarriage. Lancet 1988;2:1099.

Schiff E, Ben-Baruch G, Peleg E, et al: Immunoreactive circulating endothelin-1 in normal and hypertensive pregnancies. Am J Obstet Gynecol 1992;166:624.

Springer TA: Traffic signals on endothelium for lymphocyte recirculation and lymphocyte emigration. Annu Rev Physiol 1995;57:827.

Steinborn A, Kuhnert M, Halberstadt E: Immunomodulating cytokines induce term and preterm parturition. J Perinat Med 1996;24:381.

Szekeres-Bartho J: Endocrine regulation of the immune system during pregnancy. In Chaouat G (ed): Immunology of Pregnancy. Boca Raton, FL: CRC Press, 1993:151.

Taketani Y, Kuo TM, Mizuno M: Comparison of cytokine levels and embryo toxicity in peritoneal fluid in infertile women with untreated or treated endometriosis. Am J Obstet Gynecol 1992; 167:265.

Talwar GP, Singh OM, Gupta SK, et al: The HSD-hCG vaccine prevents pregnancy in women: feasibility study of a reversible safe contraceptive vaccine. Am J Reprod Immunol 1997;37:153.

Taylor CT, Bijan MM, Kingsland CR, Johnson PM: Inhibition of human spermatozoon-oocyte interaction in vitro by monoclonal antibodies to CD46 (membrane cofactor protein). Hum Reprod 1994;9:907.

Tung KS: Elucidation of autoimmune disease mechanism based on testicular and ovarian autoimmune disease models. Horm Metab Res 1995;27:539.

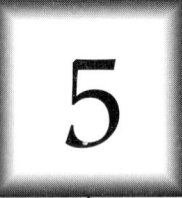

Arthur C. Fleischer
Gavin C. E. Stuart
David F. Reid

Diagnostic Imaging

As a result of significant technological developments in imaging modalities, the diagnosis of gynecologic disease processes has undergone dramatic advances. In particular, the application of intracavitary forms of ultrasonography, computerized tomography (CT), and the introduction of magnetic resonance imaging (MRI) have revolutionized the assessment of both congenital and acquired abnormalities.

Images are produced through the interaction of different forms of energy on the tissues under investigation. Specifically, the principal types of electromagnetic radiation used are x-rays in plain radiography and CT, gamma rays in nuclear medicine, and radio and magnetic waves in MRI, with high-frequency sound waves being employed in ultrasonography (Table 5–1). Both gamma rays and x-rays produce ionizing radiation, whereas radio waves and ultrasound do not.

All the energy forms discussed, including high-frequency sound waves, can cause physiologic changes. These effects vary form simple tissue heat to the production of free radical molecules, bubble formation, and cataracts, depending on the modality employed. However, *no* significant tissue effects have been demonstrated in vivo at the energy levels employed in diagnostic imaging (Budinger, 1981; American Institute of Ultrasound in Medicine, 1988; Bushong, 1988; Merritt, 1989; Shellock, 1989; Prasad et al, 1990).

The detail and sharpness of the images relate to two variables:

1. *Spatial resolution* is defined with respect to line pairs or, simply put, how many lines can be separated within a millimeter. The higher the spatial resolution, the smaller the detail that can be seen. For example, the visualization of microcalcifications on mammographic film is a result of high spatial resolution.
2. *Contrast resolution* allows the separation of tissues with similar soft tissue characteristics. Examples include the separation of white matter and gray matter in the brain and the defining of distinct muscle planes in the pelvis with MRI and CT.

Table 5–2 characterizes the difference in spatial and contrast resolution between the imaging modalities. Plain radiography offers the highest spatial definition, but CT and MRI provide far superior contrast resolution.

Contrast agents enhance the visualization of specific organs within the body. CT and MRI also employ contrast enhancement to augment nonenhanced studies. CT protocols include barium or water-soluble contrast to opacify the bowel, tampons to delineate the vagina, and intravenous ionic or non-ionic contrast agents to enhance the vascular properties of the organs investigated. Gadolinium-diethylenetriaminepenta-acetic acid (Gd-DTPA) has been approved as a contrast agent for MRI, with several other paramagnetic materials being investigated for this application (Engelstad and Wolf, 1988; Wolf, 1989).

PLAIN RADIOGRAPHS

Plain films of the pelvis and abdomen are indicated as initial screening studies in patients presenting with symptoms that may be related to gynecologic disease. Cholecystitis, renal or ureteric calculi, pancreatitis, bowel obstruction, bowel perforation, organomegaly, inflammatory bowel disease, metastatic processes, and abscesses may be confirmed or suggested on radiographs. Specific gynecologic disease processes can be diagnosed with plain radiographs. Pelvic masses, ascites, calcified leiomyomas, and teeth or fat within dermoid cysts may be demonstrated (Fig. 5–1). Intravenous pyelography and barium or water-soluble contrast gastrointestinal tract examinations are often indicated as further studies in the investigation of pelvic diseases.

GYNECOLOGIC SONOGRAPHY

Gynecologic sonography has become the diagnostic modality of choice for evaluation of women with a variety of pelvic complaints. This technique is widely utilized in both imaging departments and gy-

Table 5-1. ELECTROMAGNETIC SPECTRUM IN DIAGNOSTIC IMAGING

MODALITY	ENERGY (electron volts)	FREQUENCY (Hertz)	WAVELENGTH (meters)	
	10^{10}	10^{24}	10^{-16}	
	10^9	10^{23}	10^{-15}	
	10^8	10^{22}	10^{-14}	
	10^7	10^{21}	10^{-13}	Gamma rays
	10^6 (1 MeV)	10^{20}	10^{-12}	X-rays
X-ray imaging	10^5	10^{19}	10^{-11}	
	10^4	10^{18}	10^{-10}	
Gamma ray imaging	10^3 (1 keV)	10^{17}	10^{-9}	
Radionuclide imaging	10^2	10^{16}	10^{-8}	
Visual imaging	10^1	10^{15}	10^{-7}	Ultraviolet
	10^0	10^{14}	10^{-6}	
	10^{-1}	10^{13}	10^{-5}	Visible light
	10^{-2}	10^{12}	10^{-4}	(1 micron)
	10^{-3}	10^{11}	10^{-3}	
	10^{-4}	10^{10}	10^{-2} (1 cm)	Infrared
	10^{-5}	10^9	10^{-1}	
	10^{-6}	10^8	10^0	
Magnetic resonance imaging	10^{-7}	10^7	10^1	Microwaves
	10^{-8}	10^6	10^2	
	10^{-9}	10^5 (MHz)	10^3 (1 km)	
	10^{-10}	10^4	10^4	
	10^{-11}	10^3 (kHz)	10^5	Radiowaves
	10^{-12}	10^2	10^6	

necologists' offices and has high patient acceptance. Occasionally, additional tests such as MRI or CT are needed for either confirmation or further evaluation of patients who undergo diagnostic sonography. This overview of diagnostic sonography followed by sections that describe evaluation of common gynecologic problems. The reader is referred to several excellent texts on this topic for more detailed information (Hricak, 1996; Fleischer et al, 1997a; Smelka et al, 1997; Thurman et al, 1997).

Instrumentation and Technique

Diagnostic sonography can be performed using the transabdominal approach, wherein the uterus and adnexa are imaged through a distended urinary bladder; the transvaginal approach, wherein the probe proximity to the uterus and ovaries affords detailed pelvic evaluation; and the transvaginal color Doppler approach, which allows assessment of blood flow within the pelvic organs.

Transabdominal sonography affords a global depiction of the uterus and adnexal regions as well as the lower abdomen. It is performed utilizing a distended urinary bladder that acts to displace bowel out of the pelvis (Fig. 5–2). This technique may be limited by subcutaneous and/or pelvic fat, which acts as a scatterer of ultrasound. Transabdominal sonography includes images obtained in the sagittal and transverse planes.

Transvaginal sonography provides more detail for evaluation of the uterus and the adnexal regions (Fleischer et al, 1995a). There are a variety of probes available for, this including curvilinear probes, electronically steered transducers, mechanical sector transducers, and rotating multitransducer probes (Fig. 5–3). The transvaginal probe is first covered by a condom prior to its insertion. Gel can be added to optimize contact with the vaginal wall. Some probes have a footprint that provides a smaller scanning space and therefore are easier to use on postmenopausal women. In general, the curvilinear electronically steered probes are best suited for transvaginal sonography because of their high line density.

The technique for transvaginal sonography begins with images of the uterus as a pelvic landmark followed by images of both adnexal regions. The op-

Table 5-2. SPATIAL AND CONTRAST RESOLUTION CHARACTERISTICS

IMAGING MODALITY	SPATIAL RESOLUTION (mm)	CONTRAST RESOLUTION (mm at 0.5%)
Radiography	0.1	10
Computed tomography	0.5	4
Nuclear medicine	0.5	2
Ultrasonography (axial)	1.5 at 1 MHz	10
	0.2 at 10 MHz	10

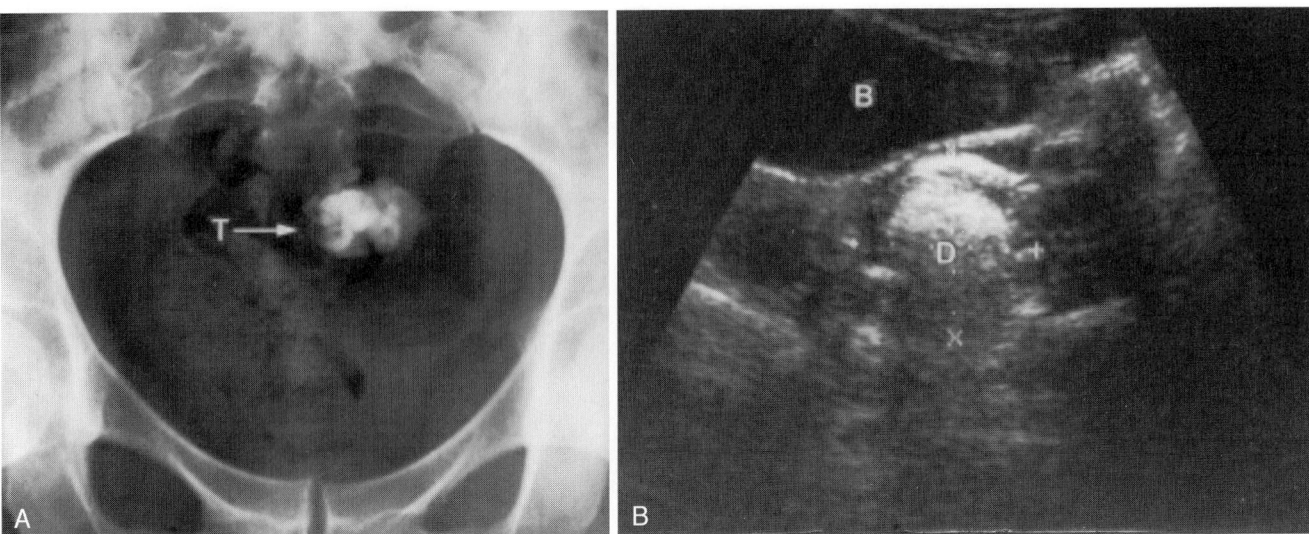

Figure 5–1
A, Radiograph of pelvis. Calcified teeth (T) within an ovarian dermoid tumor. B, Transverse ultrasonogram of dermoid tumor. B, bladder; D, dermoid.

erator may use the hand not holding the probe to provide gentle abdominal pressure to bring the adnexal structures nearer the probe for better visualization. By using the probe as a means to apply gentle pressure against the uterus and ovaries, one can obtain information as to the presence or absence of adhesions. If the uterus and ovaries move smoothly after pressure is applied, adhesions are unlikely. However, if the adnexa are adhesed to the uterus or cul-de-sac, pressure with the probe will not show this displacement.

Transvaginal color Doppler sonography involves evaluation of blood flow to and surrounding the ovaries and the uterus. Once a particular area shows a color signal, the range gate on the pulsed Doppler can be employed to obtain a specific waveform. The waveform can be characterized by the relative impedance using either the resistive index ([maximum systolic velocity − minimum diastolic velocity]/maximum systolic velocity) or the pulsatillity index ([maximum systolic velocity − minimum diastolic velocity]/mean velocity). Transvaginal color Doppler sonography is highly operator dependent but provides data on relative flow to the uterus and ovaries. Amplitude color Doppler sonography is more sensitive to blood flow than frequency-based color Doppler, which is dependent on frequency shifts. However, amplitude color Doppler sonography is degraded by motion.

Uterine Bleeding

Transvaginal sonography has a vital role in the evaluation of the patient presenting with uterine bleeding (Granberg et al, 1996). In the premenopausal woman, bleeding is commonly due to anovulation, whereas in the postmenopausal woman, bleeding can be due to endometrial atrophy, submucosal fi-

broid, or endometrial pathology such as hyperplasia or cancer.

It is important to consider patients presenting with bleeding in the perimenopausal period as different from those in the postmenopausal period. It is also important to realize that women with normal cycles can have endometrial thicknesses up to 12 mm, as opposed to the postmenopausal patient, in whom the normal bilayer endometrial thickness is between 5 and 8 mm (Fig. 5–4).

Transvaginal sonography has an important role in evaluating patients who are bleeding on hormone replacement therapy or tamoxifen. These patients represent a particular problem for the gynecologist in differentiating scheduled or expected bleeding from abnormal bleeding patterns. In general, patients who have an endometrial thickness of less than 5 mm and are postmenopausal typically have endometrial atrophy, whereas, at endometrial thicknesses above this, several types of abnormal endometrial histologies may be present (Goldstein et al, 1990). At thicknesses over 8 mm, endometrial abnormalities include hyperplasia and cancer. These entities may be missed on endometrial biopsy but still present on transvaginal sonography.

If the endometrium appears abnormally thickened and/or irregularly textured, sonohysterography provides a secondary test for delineation of polyps, submucosal fibroids, and synechiae (Fig. 5–5), (Parsons and Lense, 1993). Sonohysterography, which utilizes instillation of saline within the uterine lumen, is of particular help in evaluating patients for polyps or submucosal fibroids. Polyps are typically echogenic and invaginate between the endometrial layers. When color Doppler sonography is used, the vascular pedicle can be demonstrated. Submucosal fibroids, in contrast, are typically hypoechoic and may extend into the uterine lumen. The amount of myo-

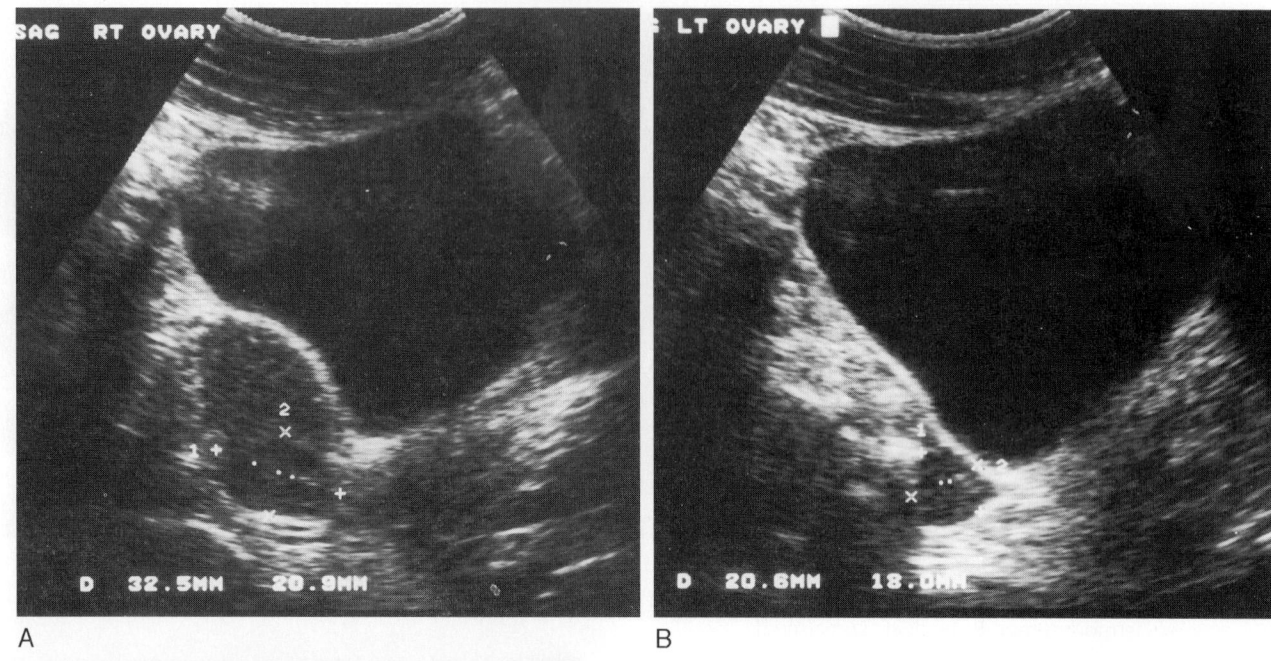

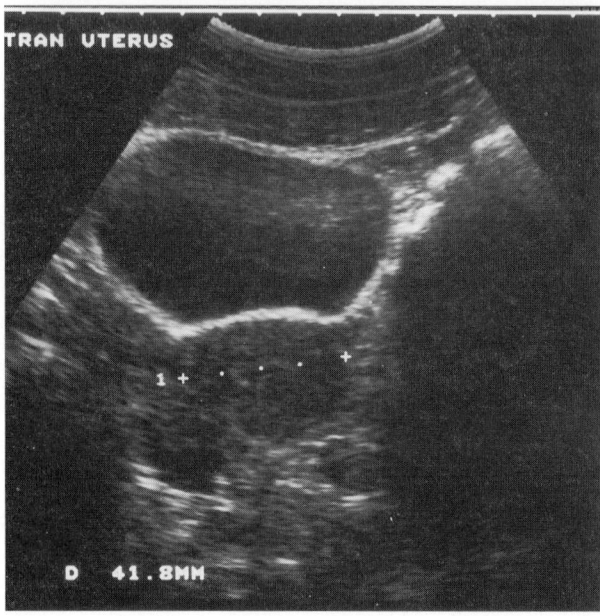

Figure 5–2
Transabdominal sonography (TAS). *A*, TAS in the sagittal plane showing the right ovary (between cursors). *B*, Sagittal TAS showing left ovary (*between cursors*). *C*, Transverse TAS showing uterus (*between cursors*) and ovaries.

metrial involvement in fibroids is important to assess because, if a fibroid is confined to the submucosal and intramural areas, it may be removed by wire loop resection. Synechiae appear as hypoechoic or echogenic thin interfaces that course between the two endometrial layers. Their extent can be outlined by sonohysterography (Fleischer et al, 1997b).

Endometrial cancer typically appears as endometrial thickening and irregular texture (over 9 to 10 mm). One may assess the possibility of invasion by complete delineation of the hypoechoic interface representing the inner myometrium. Invasive tumors will distort this layer of inner myometrium (Fleischer et al, 1987).

Pelvic Mass

In patients presenting with a pelvic mass, transvaginal sonography affords the delineation of the internal consistency and location of the mass, as well as associated disorders involved (Fig. 5–6). Larger pelvic masses are best delineated using the transabdominal approach. Color Doppler sonography of pelvic masses provides additional information as to the presence or absence of possible torsion and, in some cases, whether a mass is probably benign or malignant (Fig. 5–7).

Physiologic cysts typically demonstrate a smooth wall and no internal echoes. Their origin from the

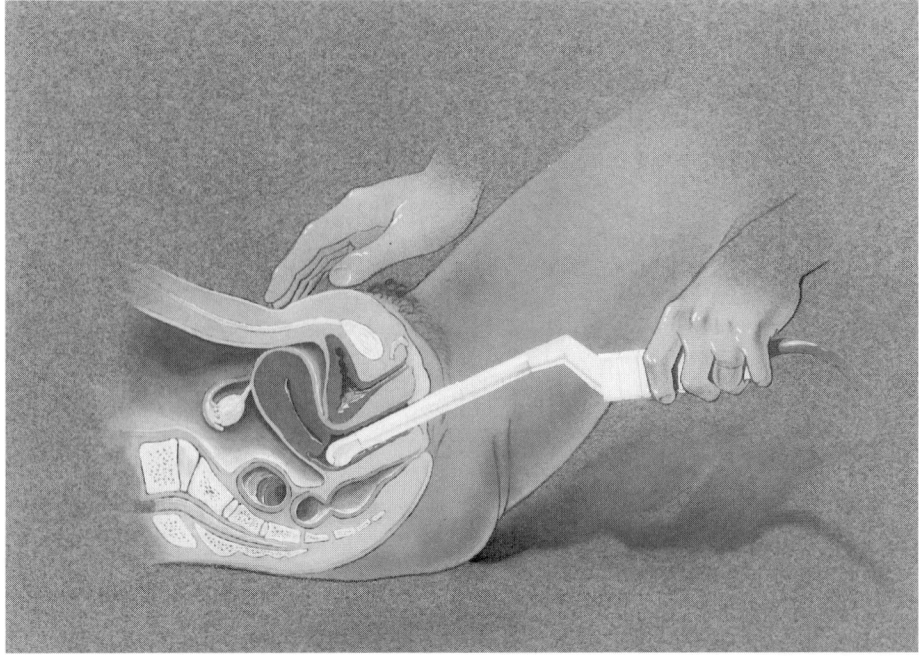

A

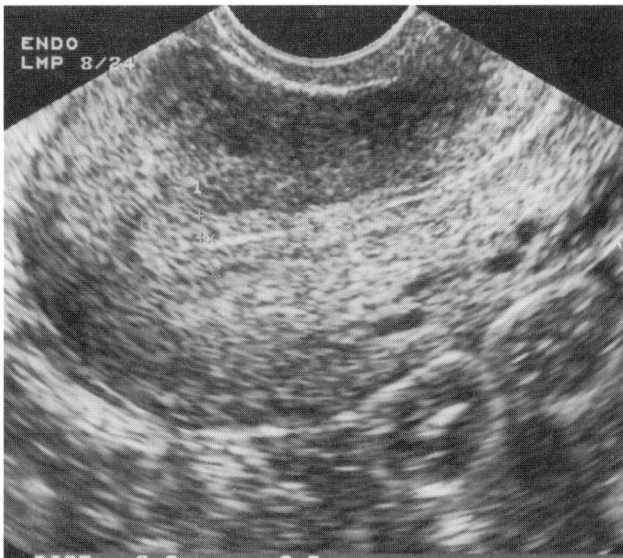

B

Figure 5–3
Transvaginal sonography (TVS). *A,* Diagram showing technique used in transvaginal sonography. The operator's free hand can palpate the adnexa in an attempt to bring it closer to the transducer for more detailed evaluation. (Drawing by Paul Gross, MS.) *B,* Typical TVS image of anteflexed uterus showing bilayer endometrial thickness of 5.8 mm (*between cursors*). Also depicted are arcuate vessels in the outer myometrium and the inner, middle, and outer layers of myometrium. *Illustration continued on following page*

ovary can usually be documented by transvaginal sonography. It has now been reported that up to 15% of postmenopausal asymptomatic women have adnexal cysts, and the complete evaluation of these cysts by transvaginal sonography is required to document the probability of regression (Wolf et al, 1991). The physiologic cysts may spontaneously regress, whereas cystic ovarian tumors may continue to enlarge over several cycles. Hemorrhagic cysts can be identified by the thin fibrin strands within the mostly cystic mass, whereas masses with irregular papillary excrescences and thickened internal septations must be considered suspicious for ovarian tumors.

There are certain findings that are specific for a particular type of pelvic mass. One of these is the "ground glass" appearance of endometriomas; the other is the echogenic focus typically found within dermoid cysts that represents hair or calcified components (see Fig. 5–6).

Transvaginal color Doppler sonography provides an indication as to whether or not a mass is benign or potentially malignant (Fleischer et al, 1996a, 1996b). Typically, malignancies have abnormal tumor vessels that demonstrate low-impedance and high-velocity flow. Although the actual cutoff point for the impedance values distinguishing benign from malignant masses remains unsettled, it is clear that

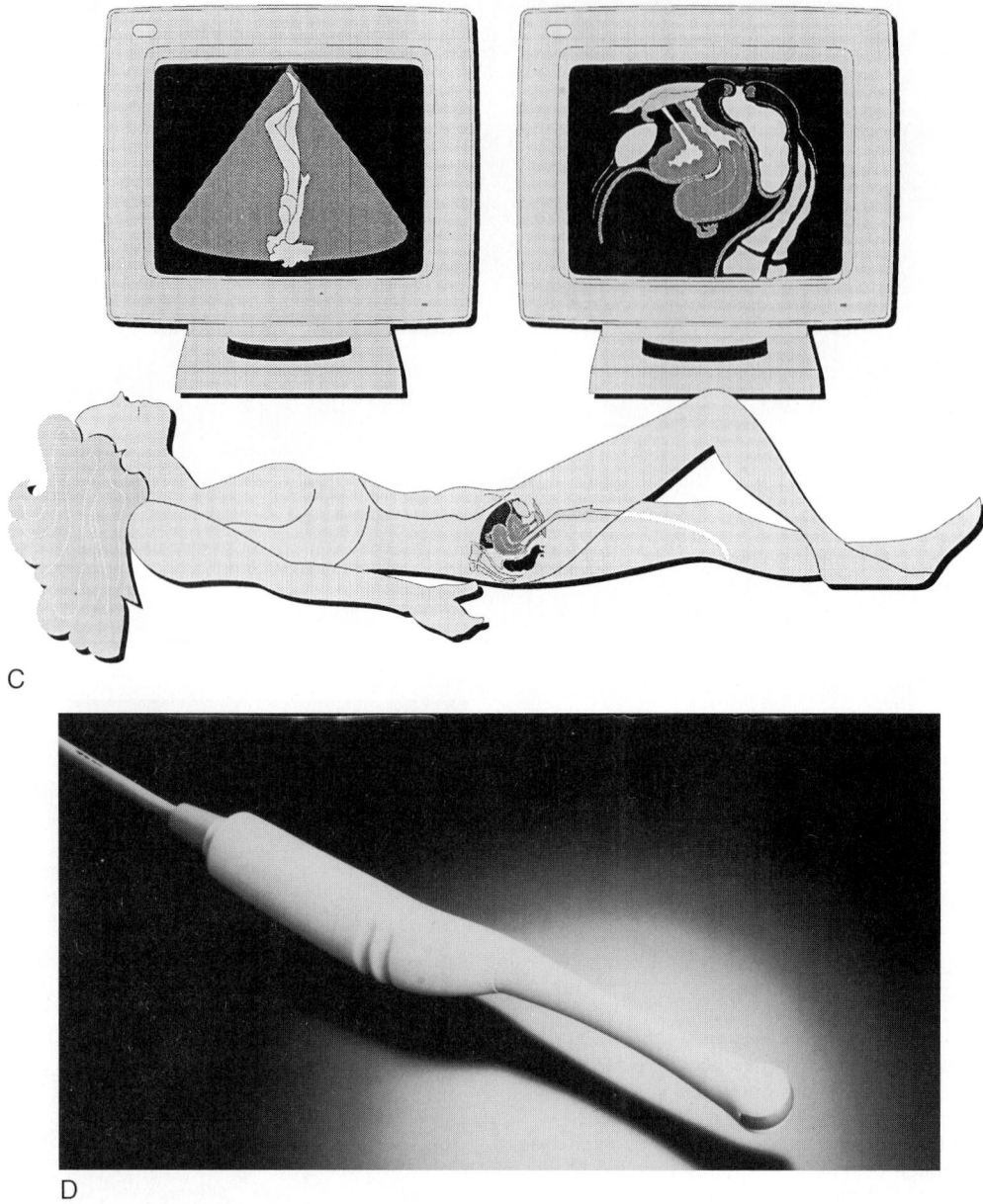

Figure 5–3

Continued C, Orientation of image on TVS. The image is shown as if the patient was oriented with her head to the floor. The top of the image represents the most posterior aspect on a sagittal image. Thus the anatomy is tilted 90 degrees from the true plane of imaging. (Courtesy of P. Jeanty, M.D., Ph.D.) *D,* Typical transvaginal probe with convex linear array. This probe has high line density and has selectable frequencies for scanning. *Illustration continued on opposite page*

this test provides a means for early detection of ovarian cancer as well as a means to determine which patient should be subjected to surgery and what type of surgery is appropriate (see Fig. 5–7).

Pelvic Pain

Transvaginal sonography has an important role in evaluating the patient with pelvic pain (Fig. 5–8). In particular, color Doppler sonography reveals the presence or absence of ovarian torsion by demonstration of lack of flow within the ovary itself (Fleischer et al, 1995b). Typically, the torsed ovary is enlarged and has small hypoechoic follicles along its periphery with increased echogenicity centrally. Documentation of the presence of intraovarian venous flow is a good sign in the exclusion of torsion, but the completeness and chronicity of the disorder makes its diagnosis difficult at times. Tubal torsion can also occur in patients who had typical bilateral tubal ligation. In this disorder, a fusiform cystic

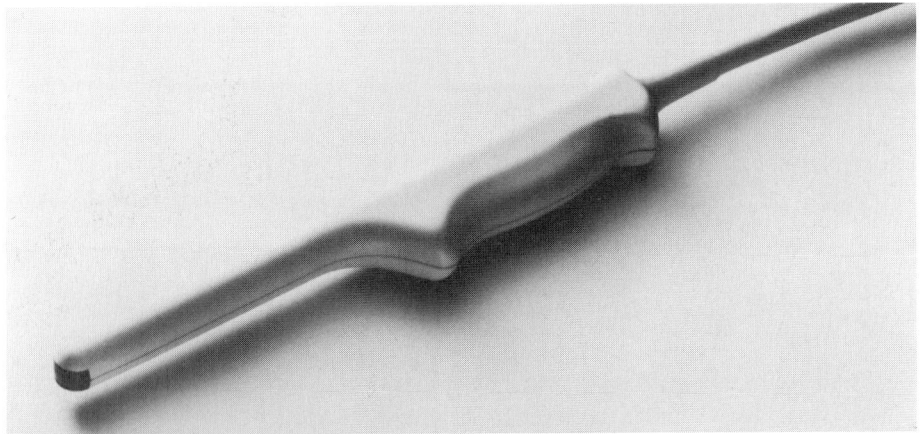

E

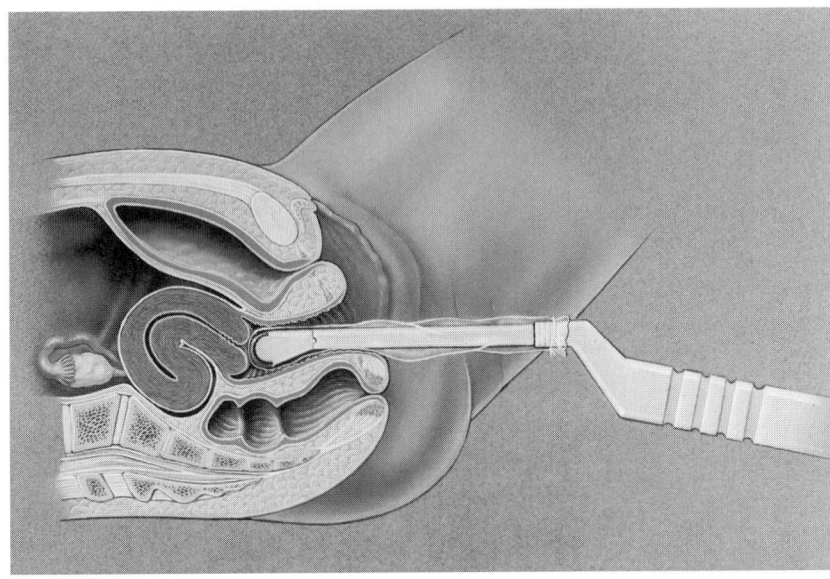

F

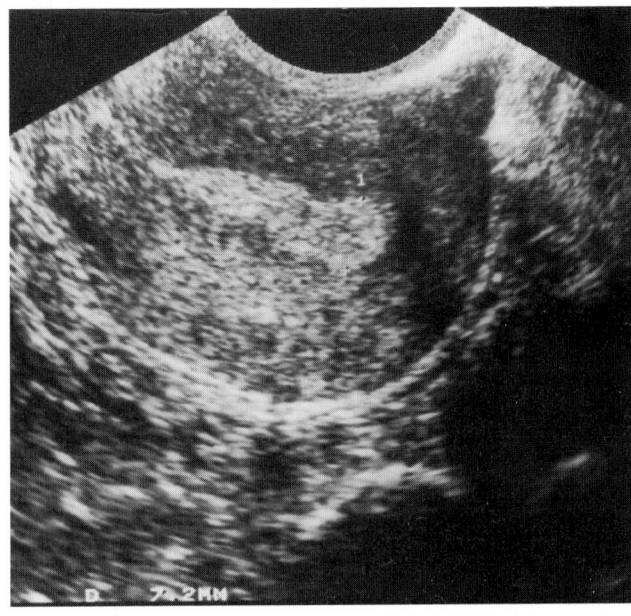

F

Figure 5-3

Continued *E*, Another transvaginal probe with even tighter curved array best utilized for older women with relatively small and atrophic vaginas. *F*, Diagram (*left*) and image (*right*) of retroflexed uterus seen in sagittal plane on TVS. The uterine fundus is displayed to the right of the image because it is retroflexed. The endometrium (between cursors) is echogenic and relatively thick, consistent with secretory phase development. (Drawing by Paul Gross, MS.) *Illustration continued on following page*

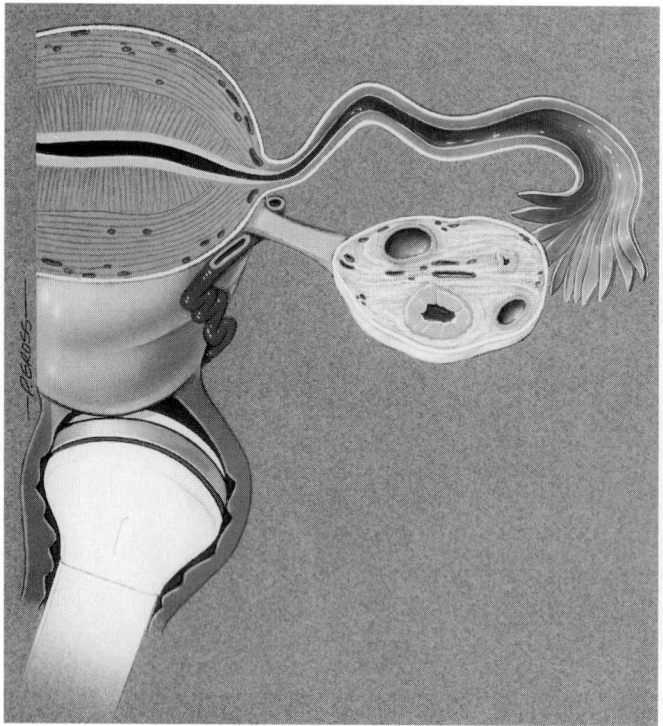
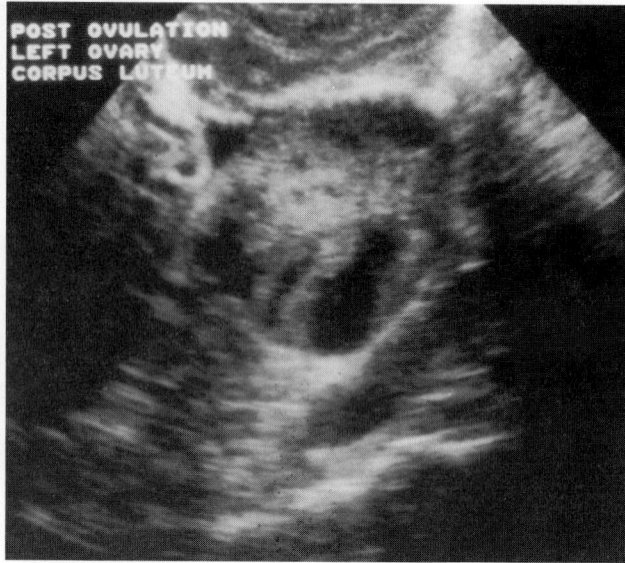

G

Figure 5-3

Continued G, Diagram (*left*) and image (*right*) of adnexal structures obtained on TVS. The left ovary is seen as well as a corpus luteum with a thick and irregular wall within the left ovary. (Drawing by Paul Gross, MS.)

structure is seen with absent or reversed diastolic flow in the wall of the tube.

Another cause of chronic pain is endometriosis and adenomyosis. Typically, endometriomas demonstrate the hemorrhagic component as the "ground glass" sonographic appearance. The small endometriotic implants typical of this disease, however, cannot be detected in most cases. Adenomyosis, which involves endometriotic implants within the myometrium, can be identified on transvaginal sonography as areas of increased echogenicity that distort the inner layer of myometrium (Fig. 5–8E) (Rheinhold et al, 1996). In some cases, color Doppler sonography can be utilized for distinguishing areas of adenomyosis from uterine fibroids, which typically have a more defined peripheral type of blood flow configuration.

Other causes of pelvic pain that can be detected by sonography include appendicitis and renal calculi (Fig. 5–8I). In appendicitis, a fusiform structure is seen in the right lower quadrant with a total outer-to-outer dimension greater than 6 mm. When evaluating for appendicitis, a linear array transducer is recommended, applied with gentle continued pressure on the abdomen. In some cases, an appendicalith can be seen in an abnormal appendix as an echogenic focus. Renal calculi may be identified in the ureteropelvic junction or in the ureterovesicular

junction as echogenic foci with shadowing (Laing et al, 1994). Color Doppler sonography can establish the exact location of the ureteral orifices, and these may be useful to identify the distal ureter and any calculi that may be lodged in this region.

Ultrasound-Guided Procedures

Transvaginal sonography can be utilized for aspiration of cystic masses as well as for follicular aspiration (Fig. 5–9). For this purpose, a needle guide is attached to the shaft of the probe that makes the needle course in a prescribed path to the area of interest. Follicular aspiration is used in in vitro fertilization, and similar principles can be used for aspiration of cystic masses. Some patients that have chronic pain with a cystic mass; aspiration may be a helpful means to assess whether the presence of the mass is associated with pelvic pain. Peritoneal cysts and tubo-ovarian abscesses may be drained using a similar approach.

Transrectal sonography (Fig. 5–9E, F) can be utilized for guided dilatation and curettage in those patients in whom the cervix cannot be identified on visual examination or when lacrimal duct dilitation of a stenotic cervix is not successful. For this procedure, the transrectal probe with the linearly arranged

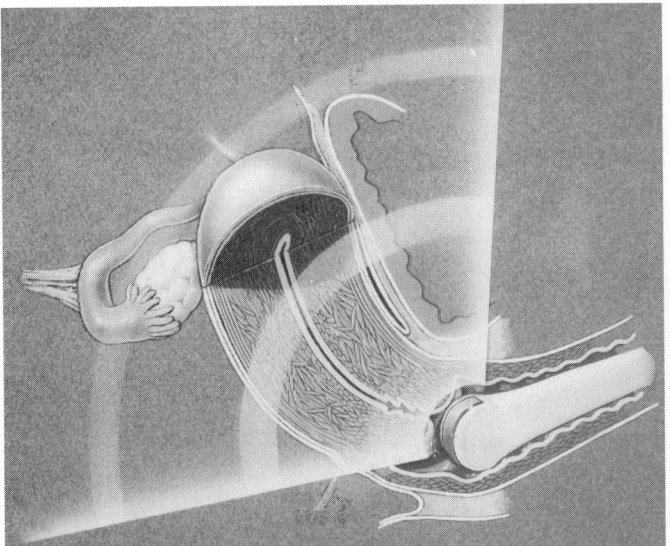

A

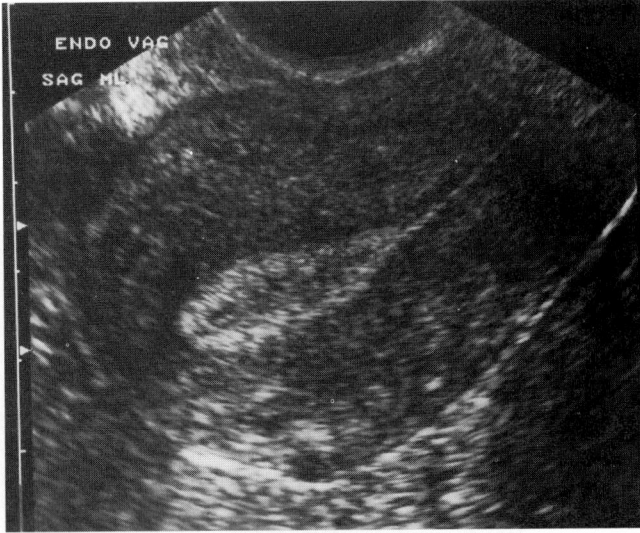

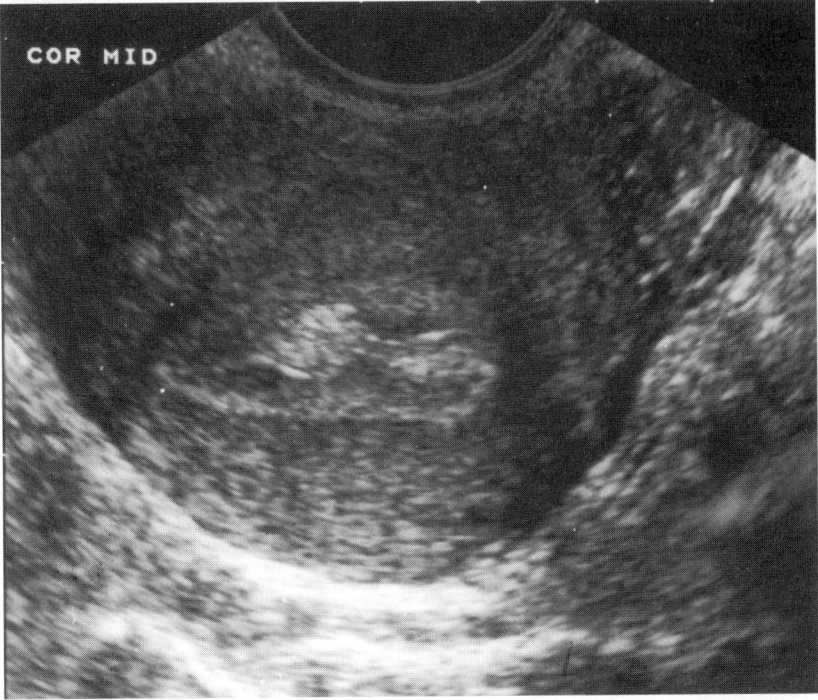

B

Figure 5–4

Endometrial evaluation. *A*, Diagram (*left*) and image (*right*) of typical secretory-phase endometrium appearing as an echogenic interface within the central portion of the uterus. *B*, Coronal image showing an echogenic mass insinuated between the endometrium indicative of polyp. *Illustration continued on following page*

transducer helps identify the position of the dilator relative to the external cervical loss. Once through the os, the dilator can be seen relative to the lesion and the surrounding myometrium, thereby decreasing the possibility of uterine perforation. Transabdominal sonography through a distended urinary bladder may also be used to guide intrauterine operative procedures.

Infertility

Transvaginal sonography provides vital information in the assessment of follicular maturation. The mature follicle averages approximately 20 mm in dimension, and in some cases a clump of tissue along the wall representing the cumulus can be seen (Fig. 5–10).

Text continued on page 126

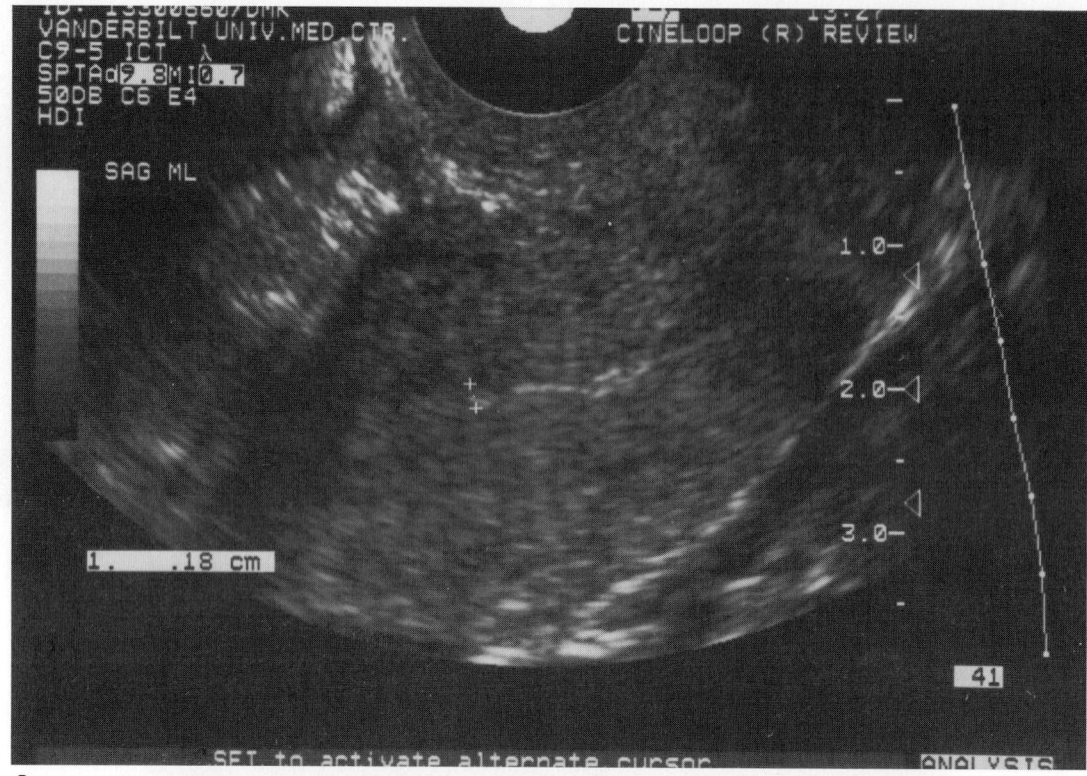

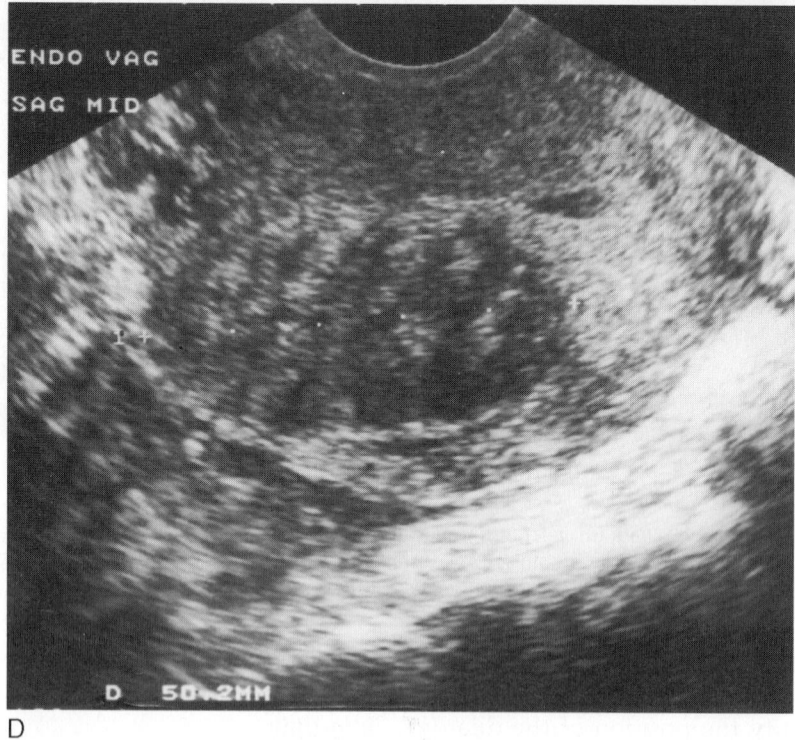

Figure 5–4

Continued *C,* Very thin (<2-mm) endometrium in patient with atrophic endometritis presenting with uterine bleeding. *D,* Endometrium displaced by large submucosal and intramural fibroid in a patient presenting with bleeding. The displacement of the endometrium by the fibroid and its extension within the middle layer of myometrium can be discerned. *Illustration continued on opposite page*

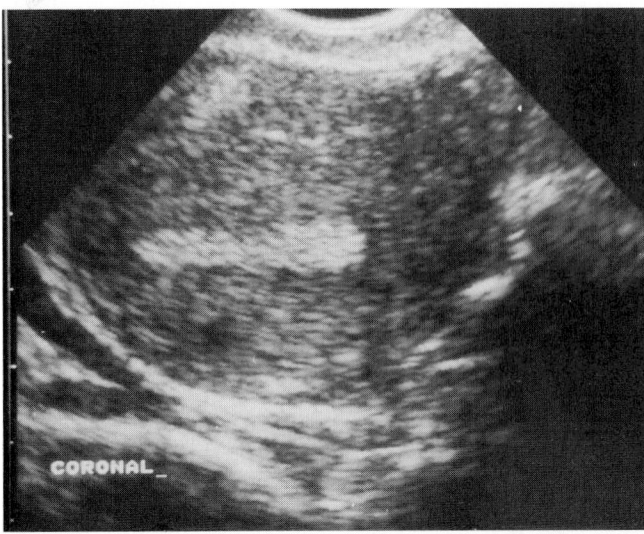

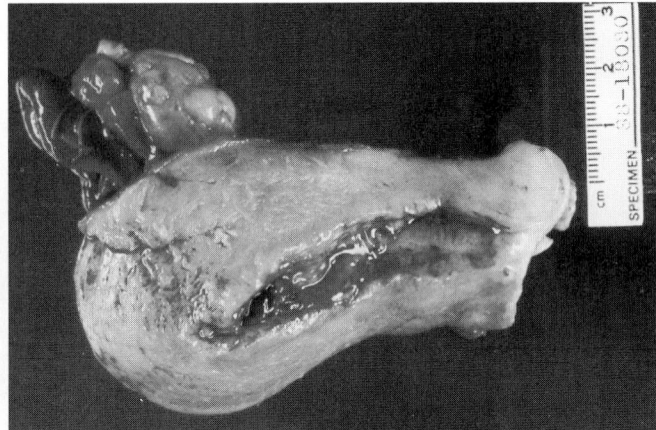

E

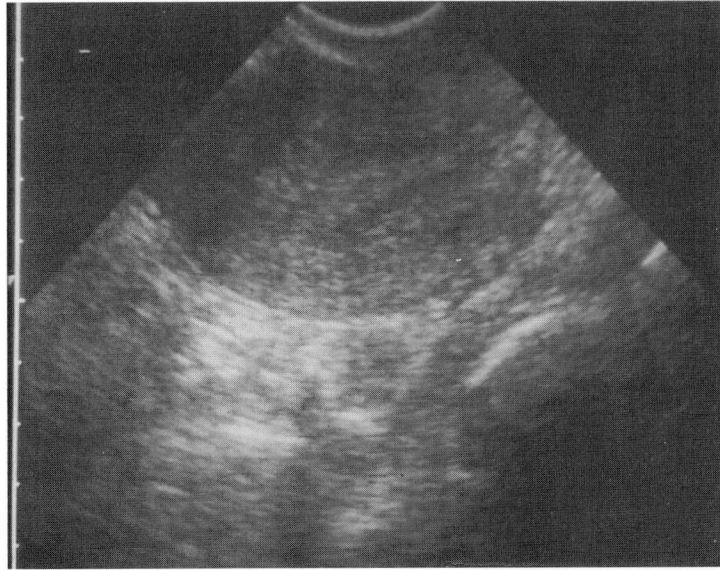

F

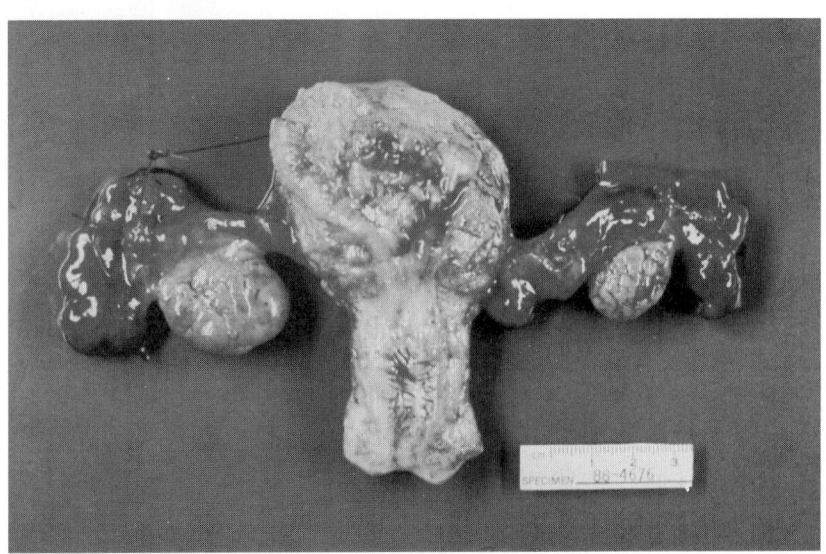

Figure 5–4

Continued *E*, TVS (*left*) and specimen (*right*) of noninvasive endometrial cancer. The echogenic interface arising from the endometrium is distinct, indicating lack of myometrial extension. *F*, TVS (*left*) and specimen (*right*) of invasive endometrial cancer as evidenced by loss of hypoechoic line near the fundus, representing invasion into the inner layer of myometrium.

F

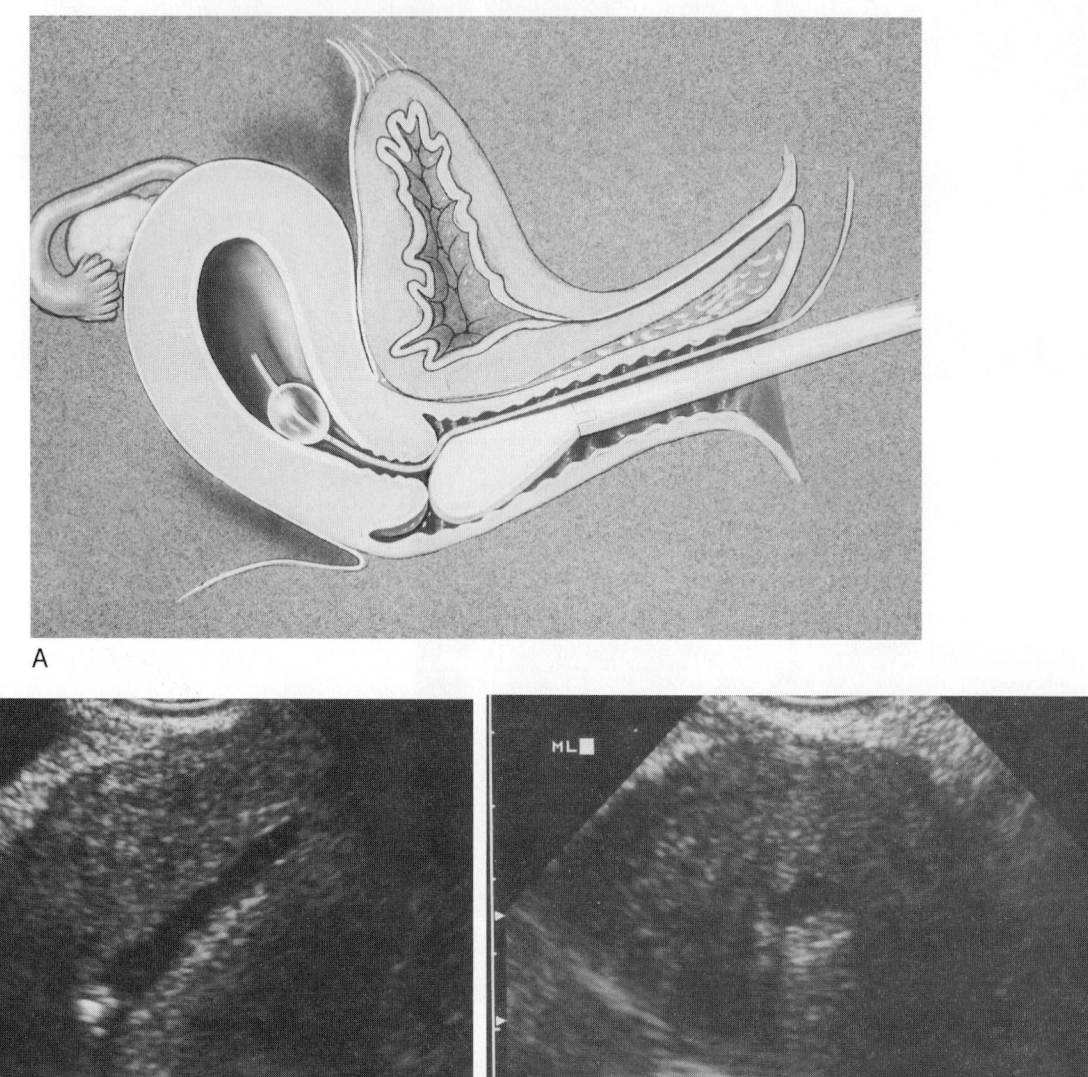

A

B

Figure 5–5

Sonohysterography. *A,* Sonohysterography can be performed using either a modified insemination catheter or a balloon-tipped catheter. If only the endometrium is to be evaluated, a thin, flexible catheter can be used. However, a balloon-tipped catheter is preferred if evaluation of the tubes is required. (Drawing by Paul Gross, MS.) *B,* Normal endometrium after instillation of saline in long (*left*) and short (*right*) axis. *Illustration continued on opposite page*

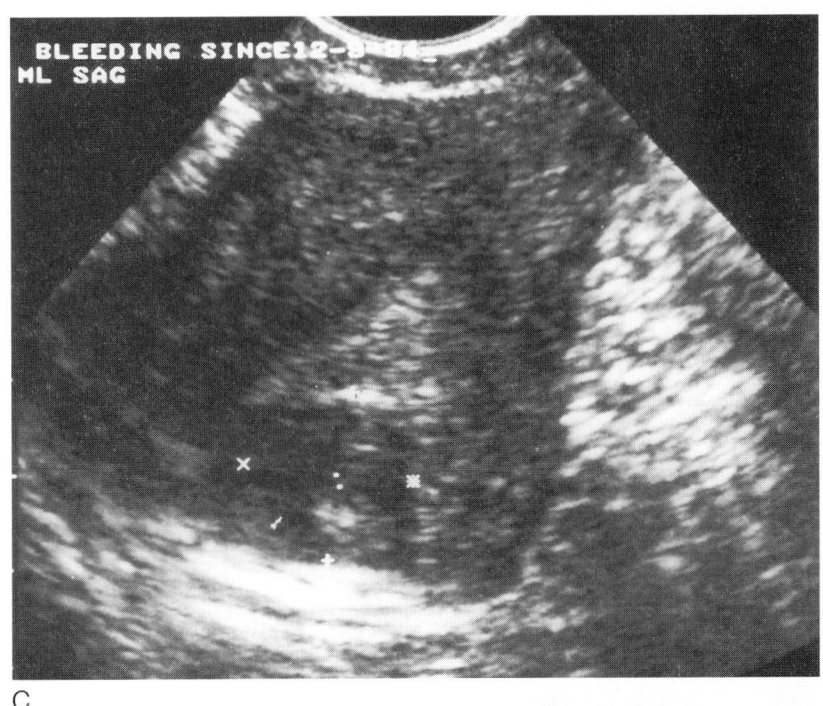

C

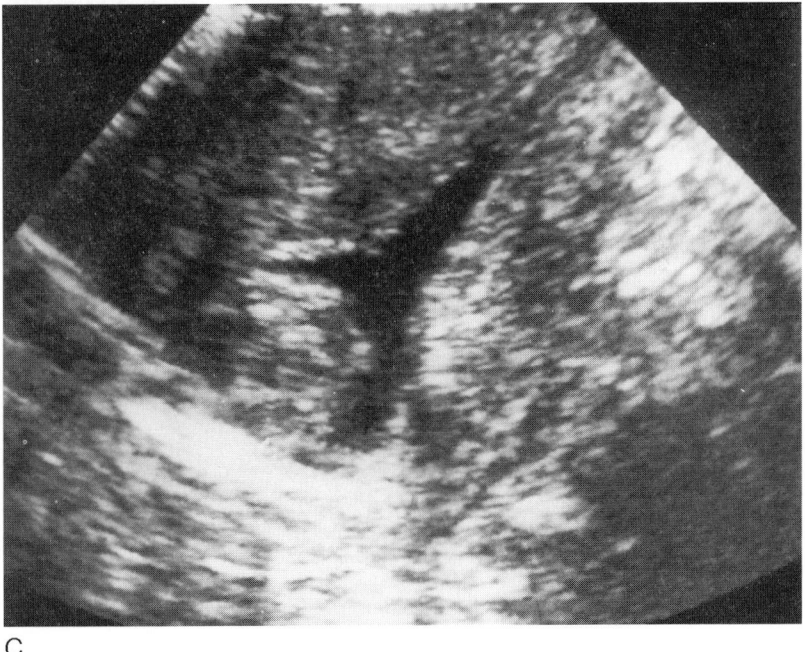

C

Figure 5–5

Continued *C*, Submucosal fibroid (*between cursors*) clearly shown on sonohysterogram to protrude into the uterine lumen. *Left*, before saline instillation; *right*, after. *Illustration continued on following page*

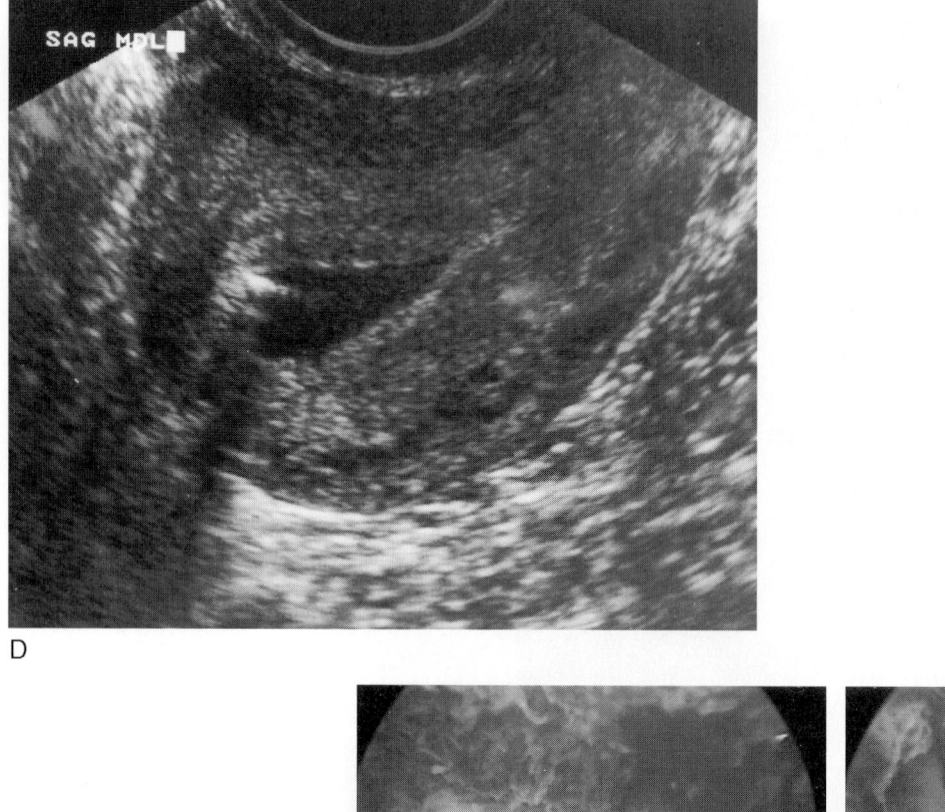

D

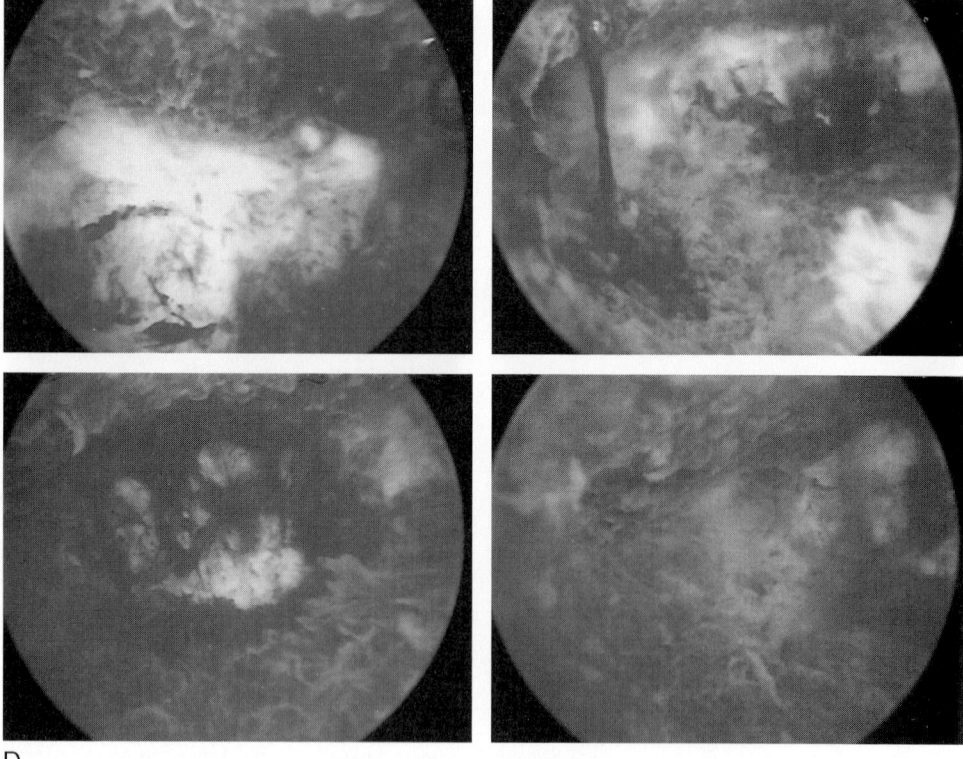

D

Figure 5–5

Continued D, Sonohysterogram (*left*) before saline instillation and hysteroscopic findings (*right*) in a patient with uterine synechiae appearing as echogenic linear interface near the fundus. (Courtesy of E. Eisenberg, MD)

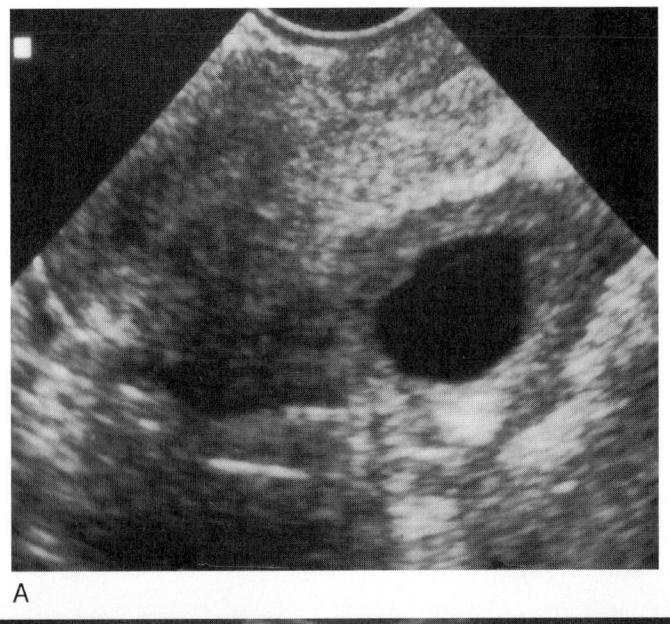

A

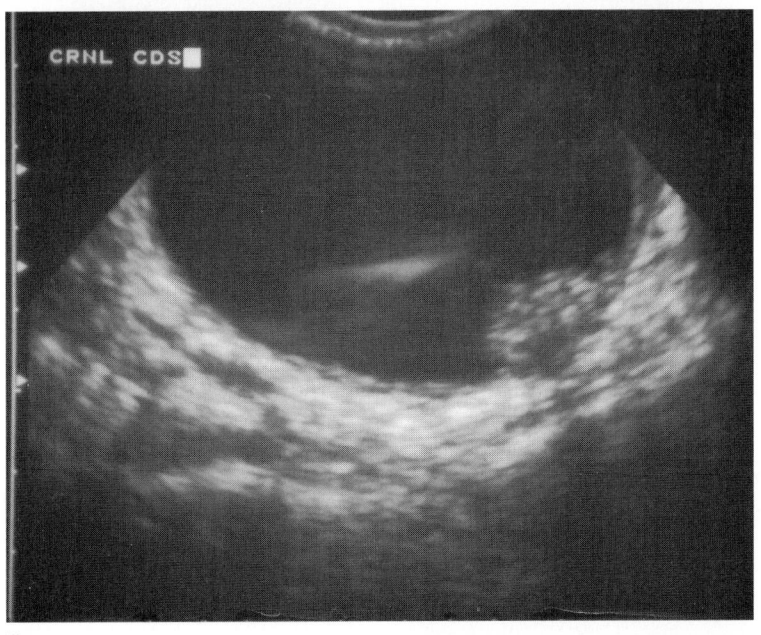

B

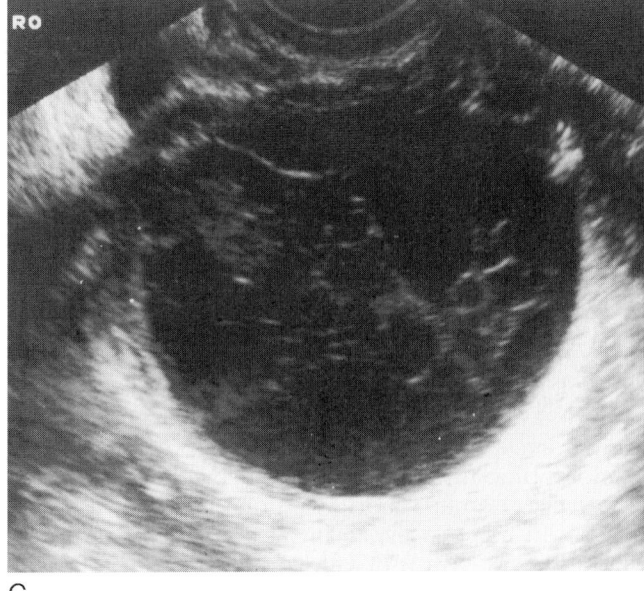

C

Figure 5–6

Pelvic masses. *A,* TVS of a mostly cystic left adnexal mass that had a thick and irregular wall. This was found to be a stage I ovarian cancer. *B,* TVS showing papillary excrescence arising from wall of an ovarian tumor. This finding is highly indicative of tumor. *C,* TVS of cystadenoma showing thin septations within a predominately cystic mass. *Illustration continued on following page*

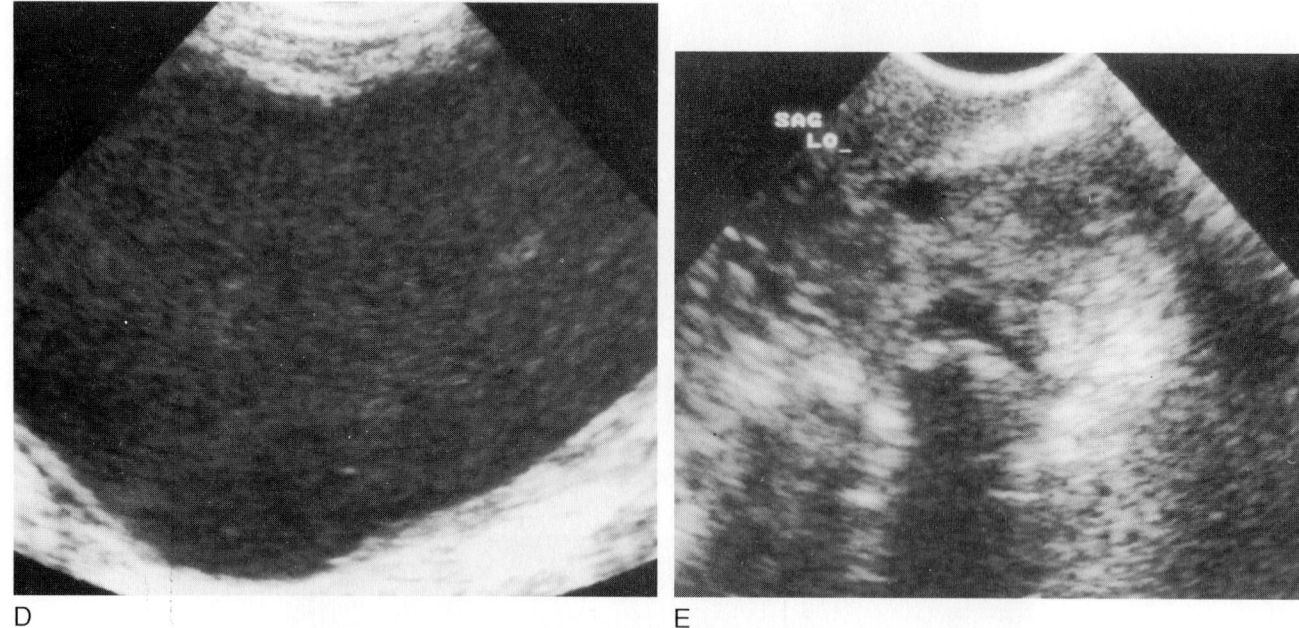

D   E

Figure 5–6
Continued   D, "Ground glass" appearance of a typical endometrioma. *E*, Echogenic focus with shadowing within dermoid containing teeth.

The endometrium should be assessed as well in infertility patients because abnormal response to ovulation induction may produce an inappropriately thickened and overly mature endometrium or, conversely, a relatively thin and atrophic-appearing endometrium. The optimal endometrial thickness in the periovulatory period is between 7 and 11 mm, with a multilayered appearance (Fleischer et al, 1990a). The multilayered appearance is typical of peri-ovulatory development with adequate estrogen exposure.

Ectopic Pregnancy

Transvaginal sonography has an important role in the detection and evaluation of patients with possible ectopic pregnancy (Fleischer et al, 1990b). First, it can confirm an intrauterine pregnancy by the presence of a gestational sac at 5 to 6 weeks. If an intrauterine pregnancy is not detected, transvaginal sonography can find the adnexal mass created by the ectopic pregnancy itself. These masses tend to have a ring that is echogenic with a central hypoechoic area. These masses are separate from the ovary and on color Doppler can be shown to be hyper-, hypo-, or isovascular to the surrounding corpus luteum (Emerson et al, 1992) (Fig. 5–11). The transvaginal sonographic findings should be correlated to quantitative β-human chorionic gonadotropin (β-hCG) levels. In most cases, an intrauterine gestational sac should be seen at β-hCG levels of between 1500 and 3000 mIU/ml (International Reference Preparation)

in an intrauterine pregnancy. β-hCG values may double normally (2 days) in the early stages of development but typically plateau or decrease as pregnancy progresses.

HYSTEROSALPINGOGRAPHY

As stated earlier, the introduction of contrast media to enhance the evaluation of pelvic structures is well established. Hysterosalpingography (HSG) was first described in 1910 by Rindflesch, who used bismuth as the contrast agent.

Presently, HSG is performed for evaluation of uterine and tubal abnormalities in infertility disorders. Specifically, these indications include (Aunet and Ellem, 1967; Schwartz et al, 1975; Kasby, 1980; Holst et al, 1983):

1. Demonstration of tubal anatomy and patency (Figs. 5–12 and 5–13)
2. Visualization of uterine myomata, polyps, or synechiae (Fig. 5–14)
3. Localization of intrauterine contraceptive devices (IUCDs)
4. Demonstration of cervical incompetence
5. Assessment of the uterine cavity prior to radiotherapy protocols

Neither HSG nor sonography necessarily precludes the need for laparoscopic or hysteroscopic assessment.

Currently, HSG is performed during the follicular phase of the menstrual cycle, after menstruation but

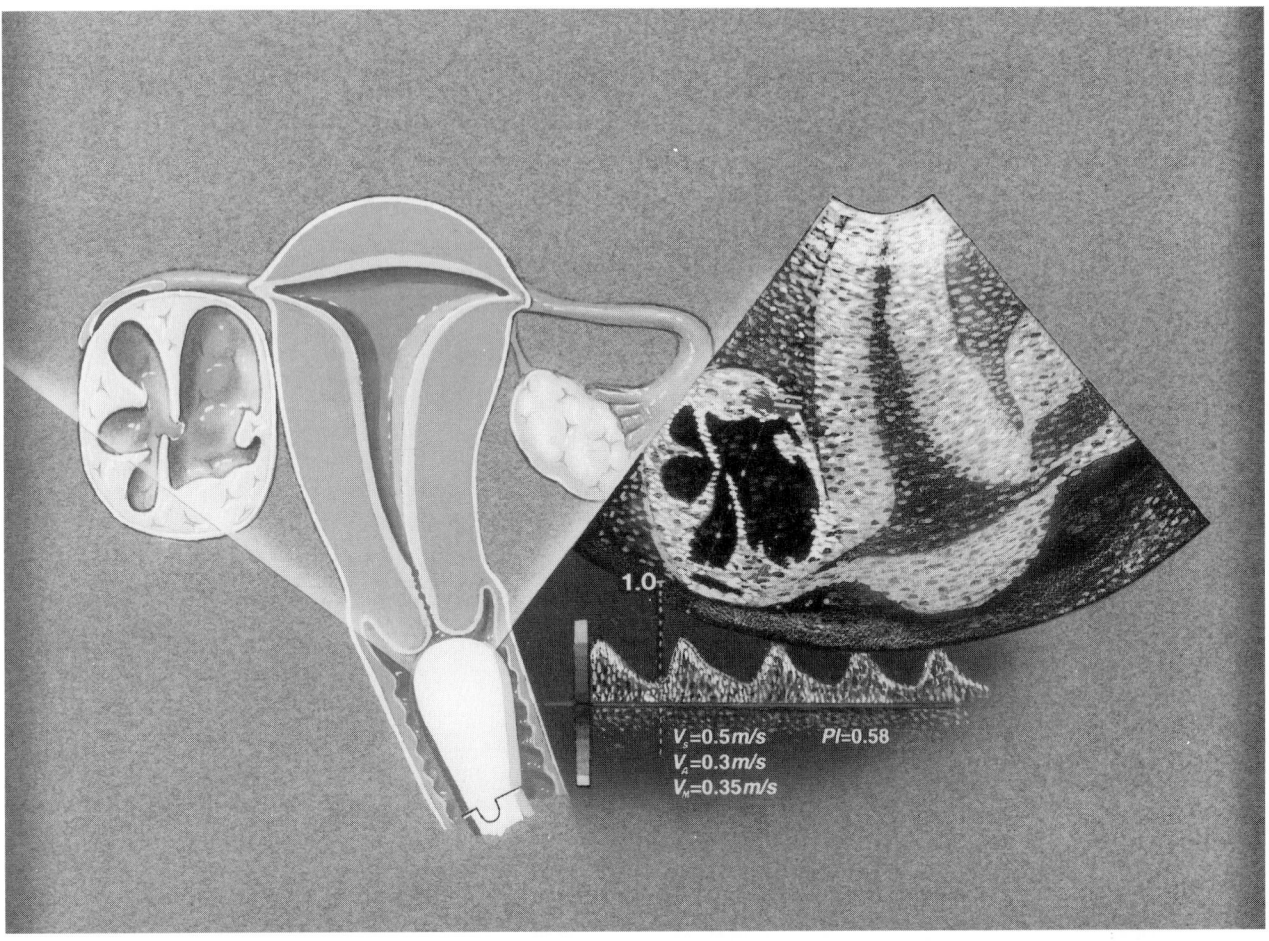

1.0

$V_s=0.5\,m/s$ $PI=0.58$
$V_d=0.3\,m/s$
$V_m=0.35\,m/s$

A

Figure 5–7
Transvaginal color Doppler sonography (TV-CDS) of pelvic mass. *A,* Diagram showing TV-CDS of right ovary. The Doppler line of sight can be manipulated to obtain signals from within the ovarian mass. The flow can be quantitated by either resistive index or pulsatility index. (Drawing by Paul Gross, MS.)
Illustration continued on following page

before ovulation. This timing prevents the possibility of the formation of endometriosis, pelvic infection, or ectopic pregnancy or the irradiation of a fertilized oocyte. The oocyte is in a more radiation-resistant stage in the luteal phase (Amendola, 1989).

Contraindications to HSG include

1. Acute pelvic inflammatory disease
2. Recent dilatation and curettage
3. Acute hemorrhage
4. Allergic hypersensitivity to iodinated contrast media

The complications are rare and include uterine or tubal rupture, hemorrhage or shock, and lymphatic or venous extravasation (Fig. 5–15). Oil embolization accounts for several of the few deaths reported. Post-procedural infections are reported in between 0.5% and 6% of patients but are less frequent with the use of prophylactic antibiotic coverage. Irradiation of a fertilized oocyte has occurred despite precautions. Several studies have failed to demonstrate any ad-

verse effects on the fetus or pregnancy. However, every effort should be made to prevent accidental exposure of a developing fetus to x-rays.

The contrast materials currently employed are either oil-soluble or water-soluble iodine-containing agents. Proponents of the oil-based agents maintain that there is less pain after peritoneal spill, a superior image quality, and an enhanced pregnancy rate in females with unexplained infertility following salpingography (29% to 78% with oil-based versus 10% to 13% after water-based studies). Despite these factors, a trend has developed toward the use of water-soluble agents (Soules and Spadoni, 1982). This has been partly the result of concern for the potential for foreign body granulomatous reactions and the risk of embolization following venous or lymphatic intravasation.

The most common oil-based contrast is ethiodol. In the water-soluble group of agents, diatrizoate (Sinografin, Hypaque 60, Renografin 60) or iothalamate (Conray 60) is the principal compound used.

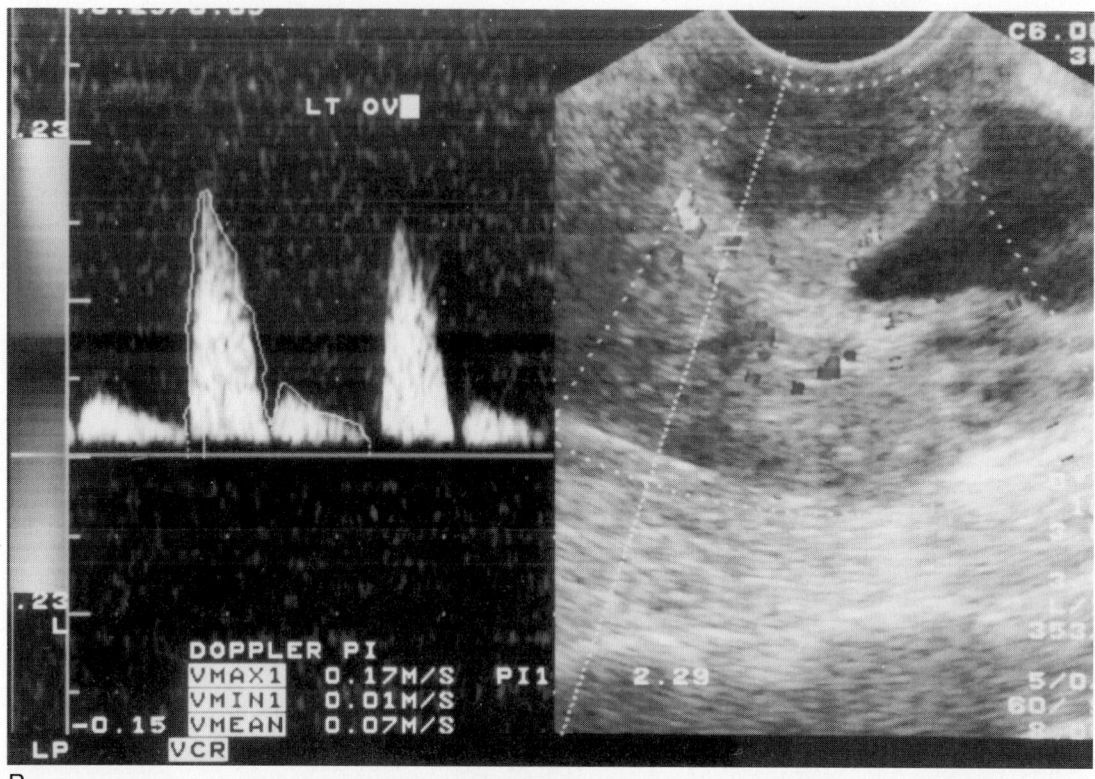

B

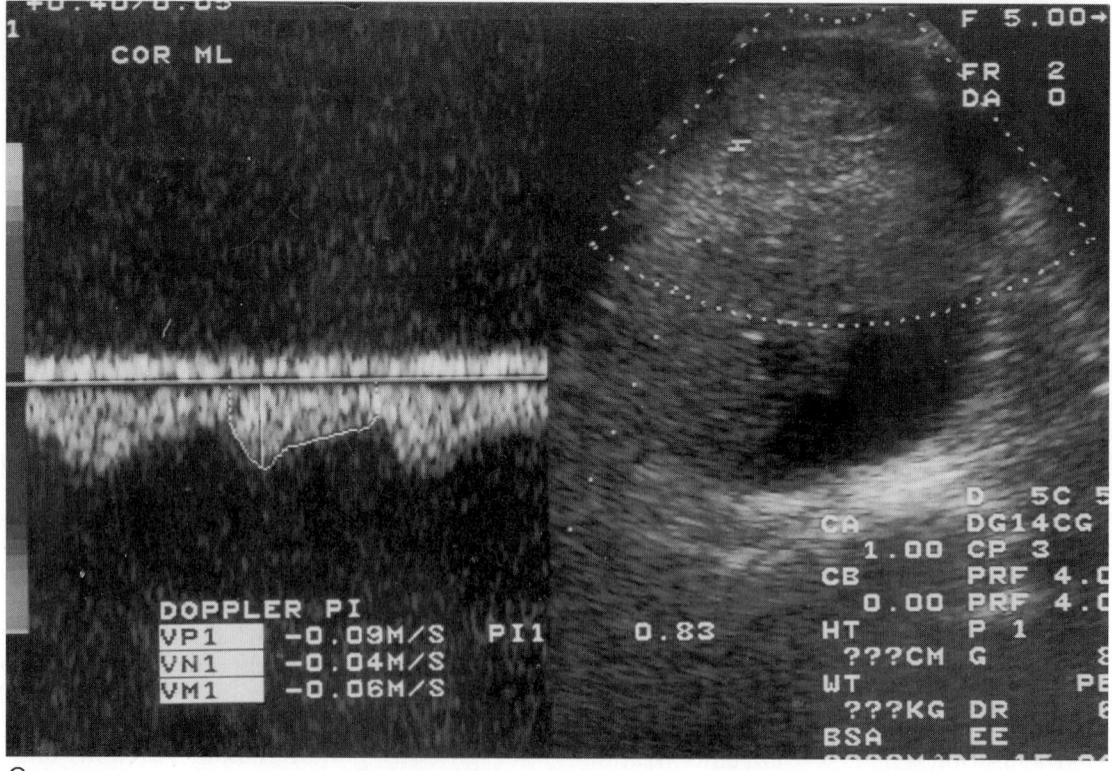

C

Figure 5–7

Continued B, Even though this mass demonstrated irregular cystic areas, the flow within it showed high impedance indicative of benign pathology. This was found to be a hemorrhagic corpus luteum cyst. C, As opposed to the mass shown in B, this mostly solid mass with cystic areas had low impedance within it, highly indicative of ovarian cancer. *Illustration continued on opposite page*

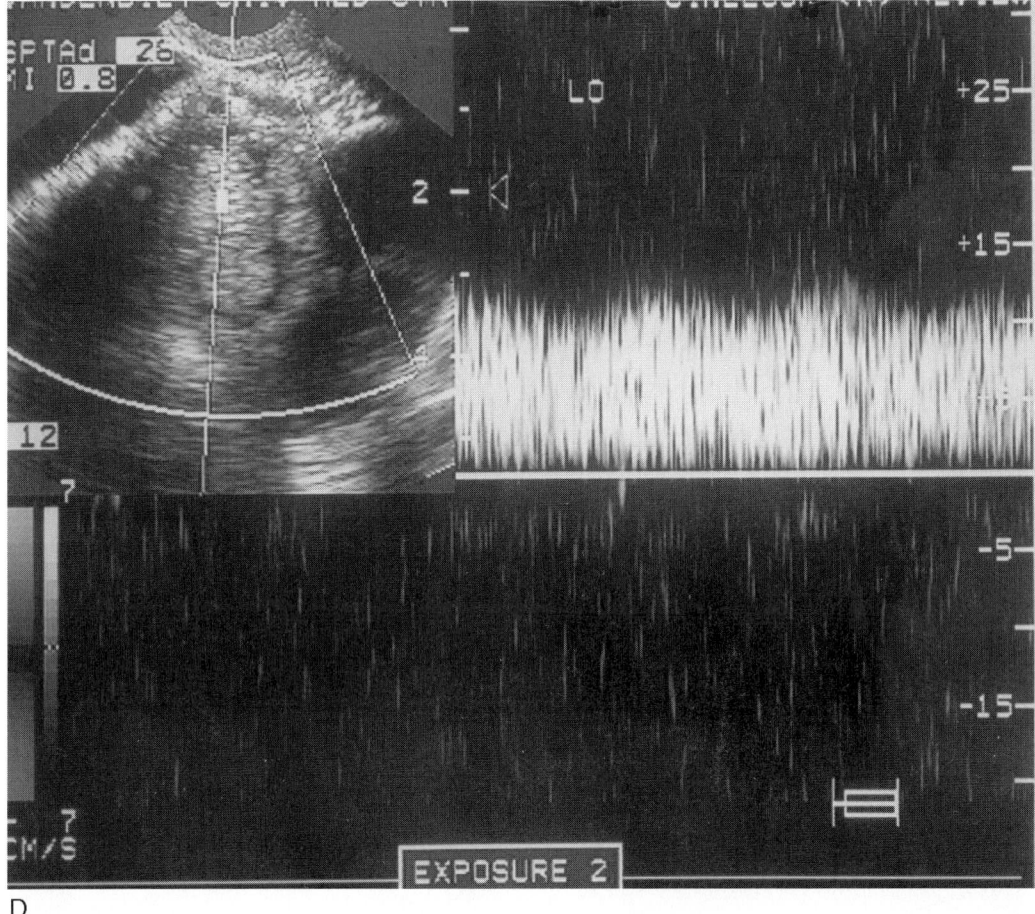

D

Figure 5–7

Continued D, Within this ovary, which contained two mature follicles, there was a papillary excrescence containing a vessel that had very low-impedance flow. This was an ovarian cancer adjacent to two mature follicles in an infertility patient undergoing ovulation induction.

Winfield and colleagues (1982) believe that there is more postprocedural discomfort with Sinografin than with the other agents. The new non-ionic materials are more expensive than the above-mentioned ionic agents but, presumably, reduce the rate of systemic discomfort and the incidence of significant allergic reactions associated with the other agents. This fact has yet to be established with HSG. The advent of other methods to investigate the uterine cavity and fallopian tubes, including MRI, may alleviate the need to perform HSG in patients at risk.

Repeated pregnancy loss raises concern for a uterine anomaly. Distinguishing a bicornuate uterus from a septate uterus can be difficult (Fig. 5–16). (Reuter et al, 1989). The HSG only visualizes the uterine cavity and provides no information regarding the total morphology. The HSG findings of a partial septate uterus are subtle and include a very acute angle between the uterine cavities. An arcuate uterus is the most common anomaly but is of no clinical significance. Uterine hypoplasia is best evaluated with HSG. HSG is also of value in assessing the diethylstilbestrol (DES)-exposed female. A T-shaped

uterine cavity is identified in 16% of daughters of DES-exposed women. Other features include constricting bands affecting the corpus, a widened lower two thirds of the uterine body, or a small endometrial cavity with an irregular or lumpy inner surface. The main uterine cavity volume in DES-exposed women is 49 ml versus 90 ml in normal subjects (Fig. 5–17). The incidence of associated vaginal clear cell adenocarcinoma in the DES daughters is approximately 0.14% to 1.4% per 1000 exposed (Herbst et al, 1975).

COMPUTED TOMOGRAPHY

The anatomy of the pelvis is well demonstrated on CT. The presence of extraperitoneal fat and the relative absence of motion artifacts enable excellent resolution to be obtained.

Opacification of the gastrointestinal tract is necessary to prevent the misinterpretation of nonopacified bowel as a pathologic mass and to evaluate the spread of disease beyond these structures (Marks

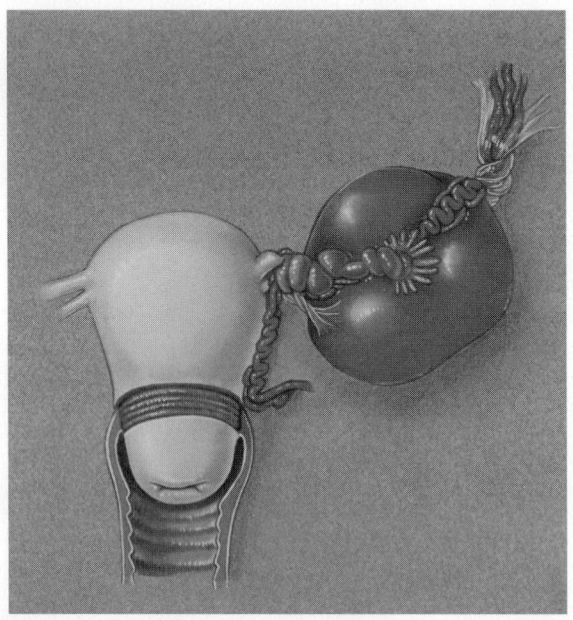

A

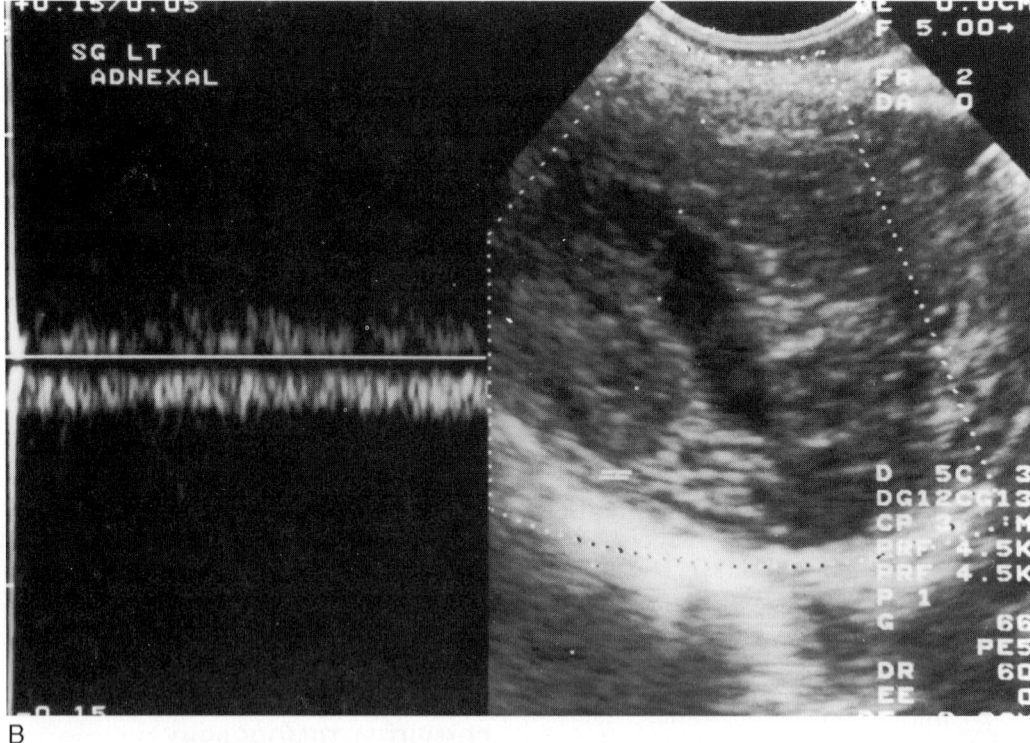

B

Figure 5–8

Pelvic pain. *A*, Diagram showing torsed hemorrhagic ovary. The dual blood supply to the ovary is twisted at both the infindibulopelvic and ovarian ligaments. (Drawing by Paul Gross, MS.) *B*, TV-CDS of patient with left ovarian mass that demonstrated arterial and venous flow in the periphery. This hemorrhagic mass was aspirated and the ovary salvaged. Partial torsion was present at time of surgery. *Illustration continued on opposite page*

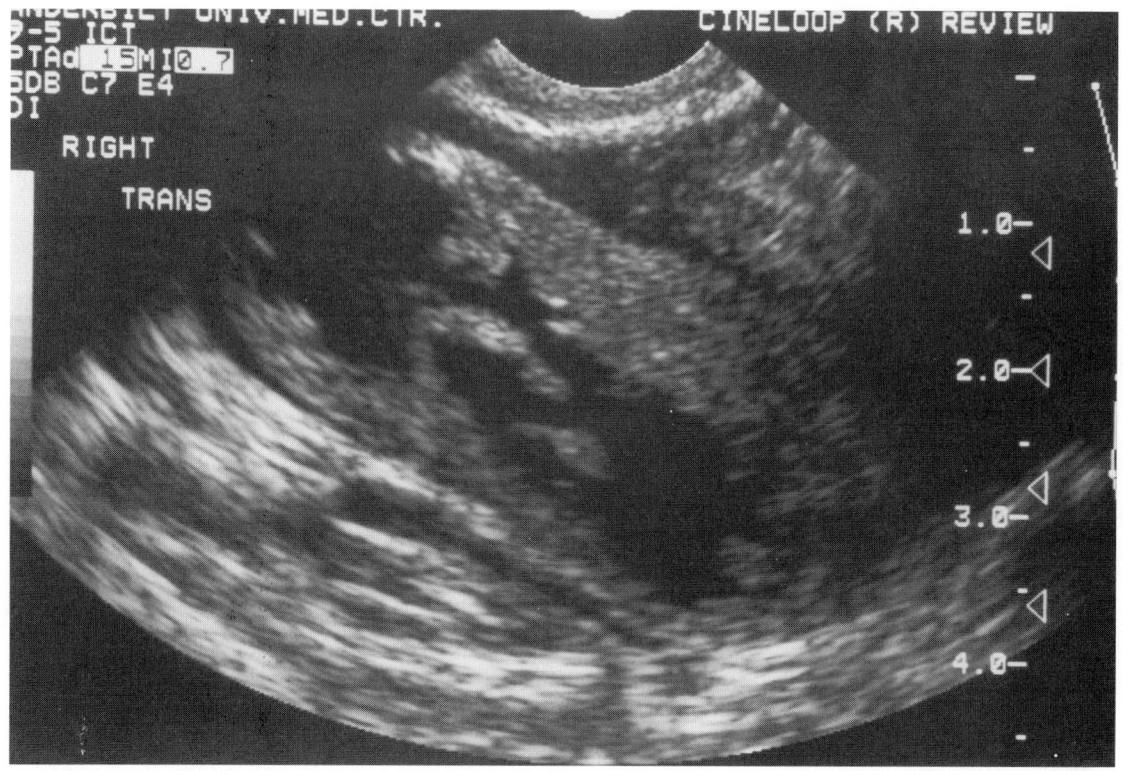

C

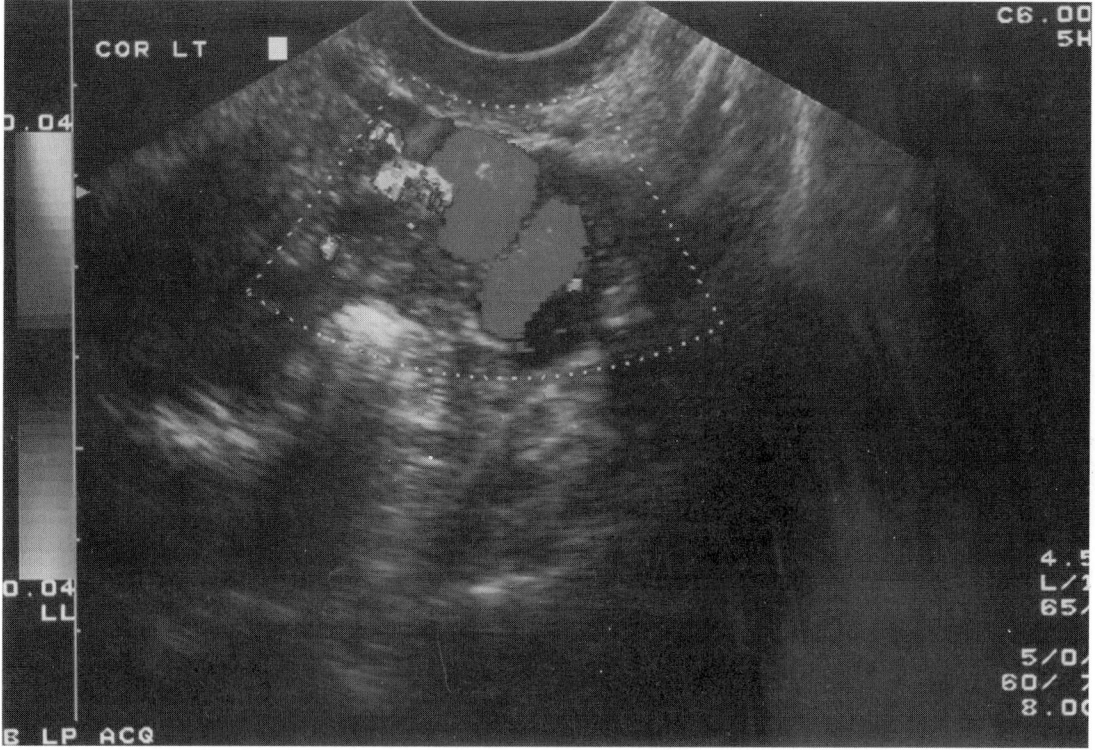

D

Figure 5-8

Continued C, Enlarged and thickened tube secondary to tubal torsion. This condition is associated with tubal ligation and subsequent agglutination of the tubal fimbria and accumulation of fluid within the tube. *D*, Color Doppler sonography showing distended ovarian veins in patient with pelvic congestion syndrome. *Illustration continued on following page*

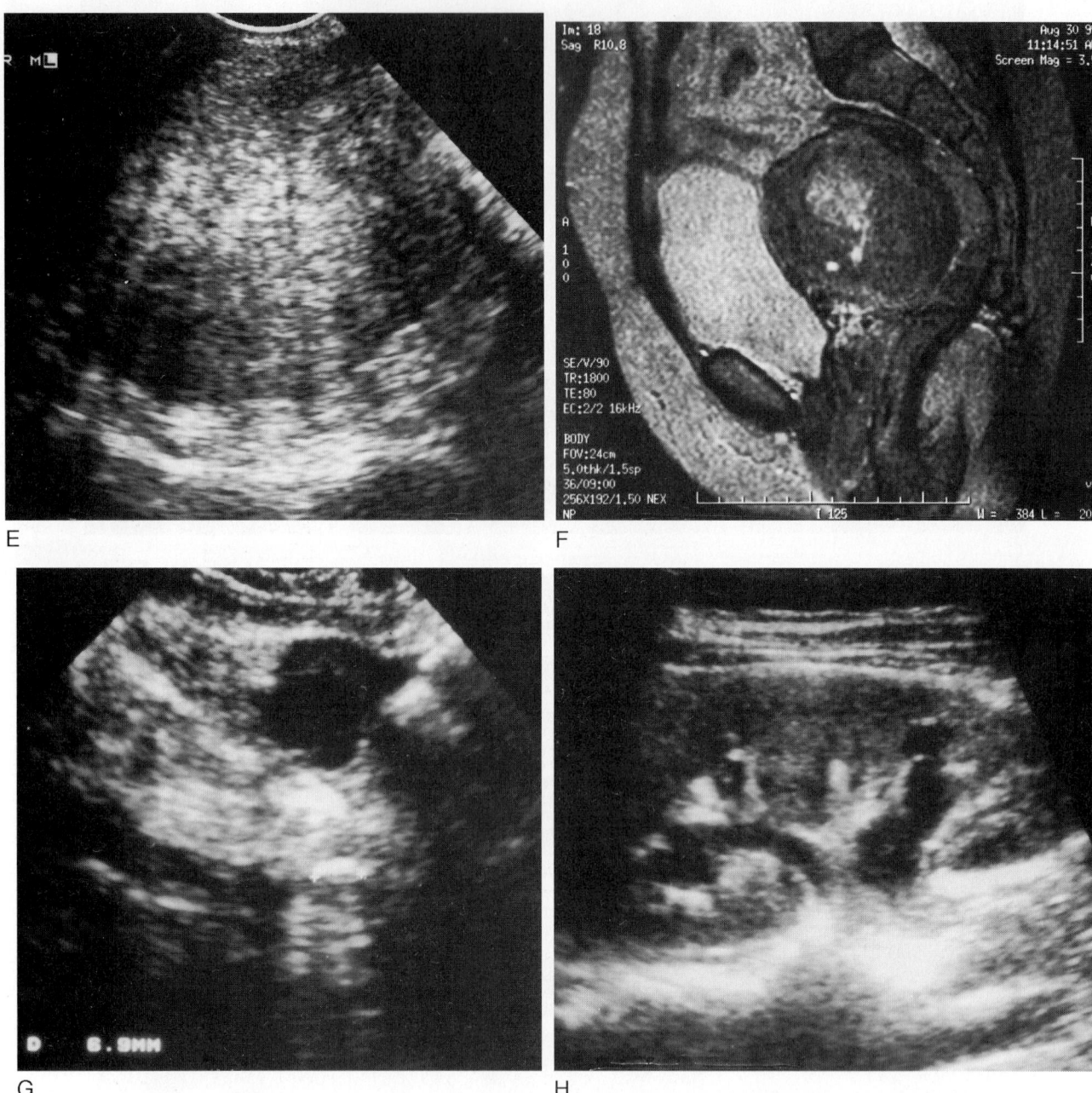

Figure 5–8

Continued *E*, TVS showing asymmetric enlargement and irregular echogenicity at the myometrium suggestive of adenomyosis. *F*, MRI of patient in *E* showing high signal areas on this T$_2$-weighted image indicative of hemorrhagic foci within the myometrium diagnostic of adenomyosis. *G*, TVS showing echogenic focus with shadow at the distal ureter (*between cursors*). This represented a renal calculus at the ureterovesicular junction. *H*, Same patient as in *G* showing mild hydronephrosis of the right kidney. *Illustration continued on opposite page*

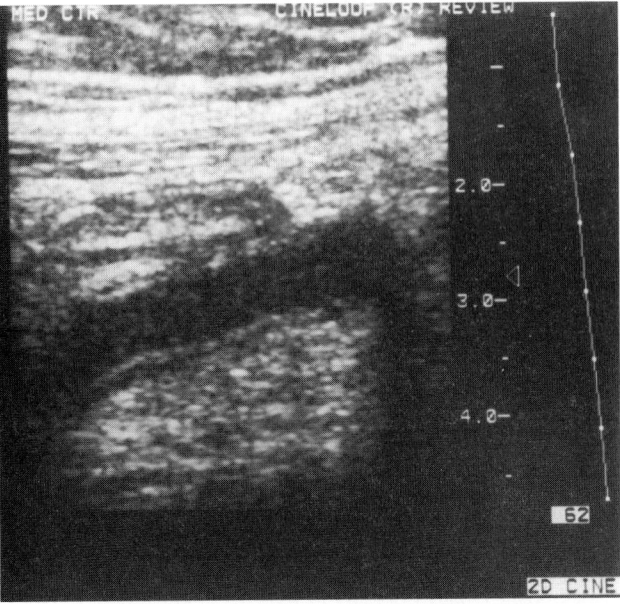

Figure 5-8
Continued *I*, Thickened appendix in a patient with pelvic pain. This patient had appendicitis at surgery.

et al, 1980). A dilute solution of barium or water-soluble contrast is ingested several hours prior to the study, with additional contrast administered immediately before the examination. A dilute contrast enema may also be given. A tampon is inserted to de-fine the vagina from the parametrial structures (Amman and Walsh, 1985). Intravenous contrast is also given to opacify the bladder and blood vessels. The contrast further enhances the vascular properties of organs such as the myometrium of the uterus. Bladder wall assessment may necessitate cystoscopy.

CT protocols typically involve 10-mm-thick slices with 10-mm interval shifts. The scan usually begins at the level of the iliac crest and proceeds to the symphysis or inferior ischial tuberosities. Slices 5 mm thick or smaller may be obtained if desired. Although patients are usually scanned in the supine position, decubitus (on the side) or prone positioning can permit evaluation of tumor fixation by demonstrating rigidity of pelvic structures (Amman and Walsh, 1985).

Axial scanning is usually satisfactory, although reformatting of the images into sagittal or coronal planes may provide further information. However, the quality of the reformatted images available with CT cannot match the flexibility or detail obtained by MRI.

CT is currently indicated for (Levitt et al, 1978; Korobkin et al, 1979; Lee and Mark, 1989)

1. Evaluation of masses located along the pelvic side walls and presacral space or within the false pelvis
2. Staging of pelvic cancer
3. Detection of tumor recurrence
4. CT-guided biopsy
5. Assessment and drainage of pelvic abscesses

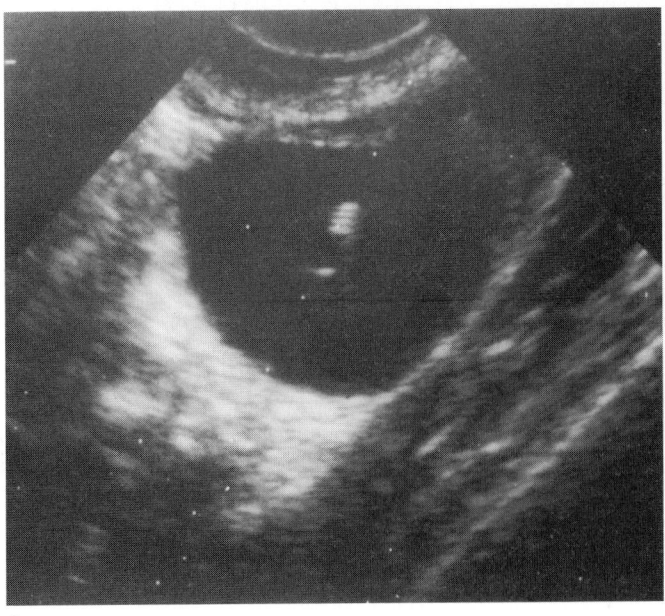
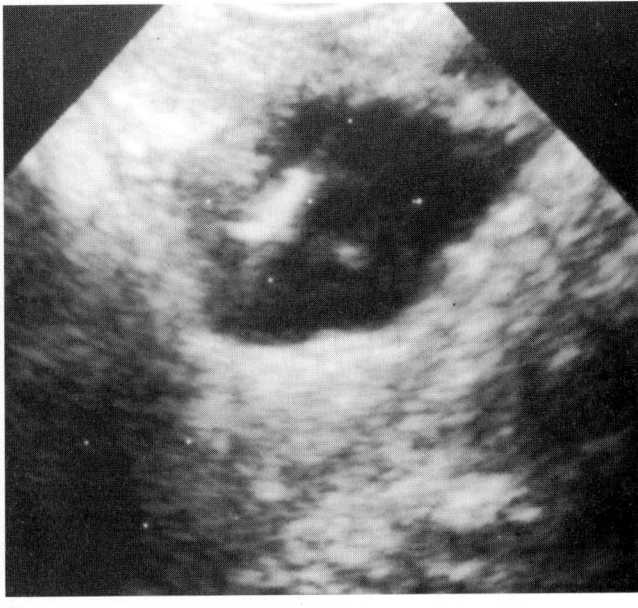

A B

Figure 5-9
Sonographically guided procedures. *A*, Aspiration of smooth-walled cyst in patient undergoing ovulation induction. The tip of the needle appears as parallel echogenic interfaces that are within the cyst. *B*, Guided aspiration of peritoneal cyst in patient with chronic pelvic pain. The tip of the needle is very well seen within the mostly cystic mass. *Illustration continued on following page*

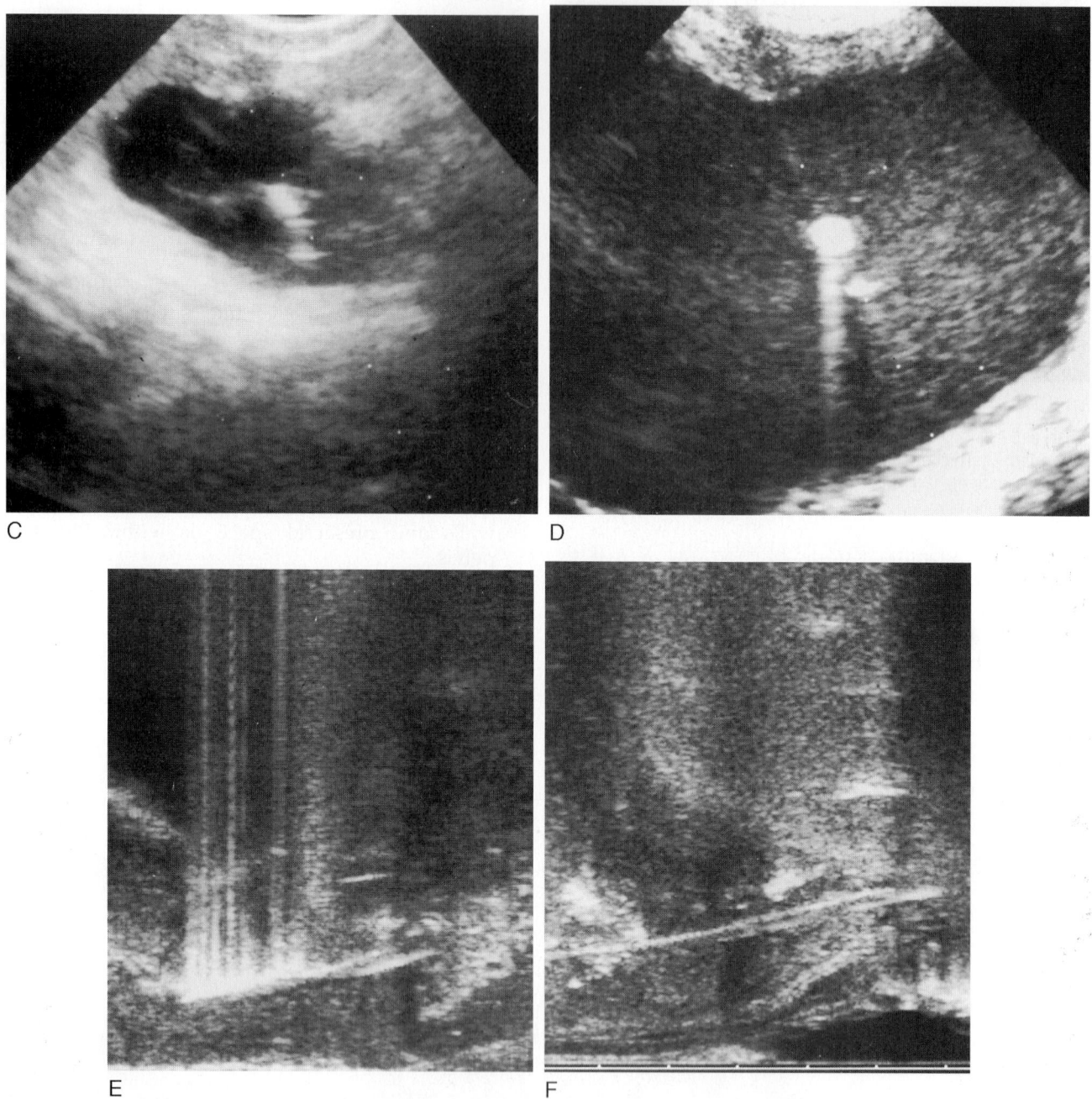

C

D

E

F

Figure 5–9

Continued *C,* Guided aspiration of tubo-ovarian abscess that contributed to defervescence of fever. *D,* Guided aspiration of endometrioma. Much of the material was organized clot and could not be aspirated. *E,* Transrectal sonography–guided dilatation and curettage in patient with cervical stenosis. Initial sonogram showing dilator adjacent and through the internal cervical os. *F,* Same as *E* documenting good position within the uterine lumen after sonography was used to place dilator past the cervix.

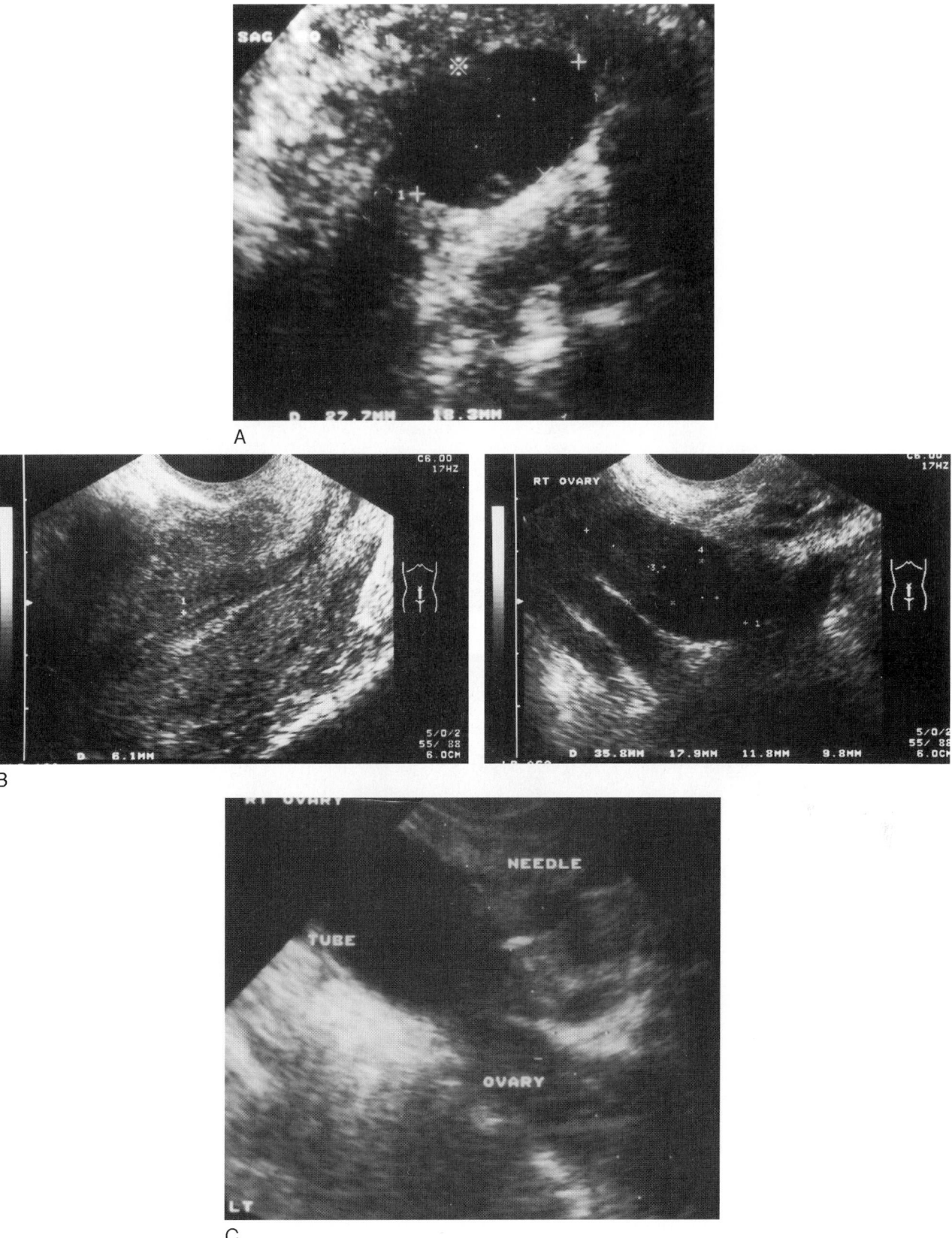

Figure 5–10

Infertility. *A*, Transvaginal sonogram of right ovary containing mature follicle (*between cursors*). The cumulus oophorus can also be delineated. *B*, Midcycle endometrial findings associated with mature follicle indicative of concordant development of follicle and endometrium. The multilayered appearance of the endometrium is seen in the periovulatory phase. *C*, Image taken during guided follicular aspiration. The needle path is adjusted to exclude the adjacent hydrosalpinx.

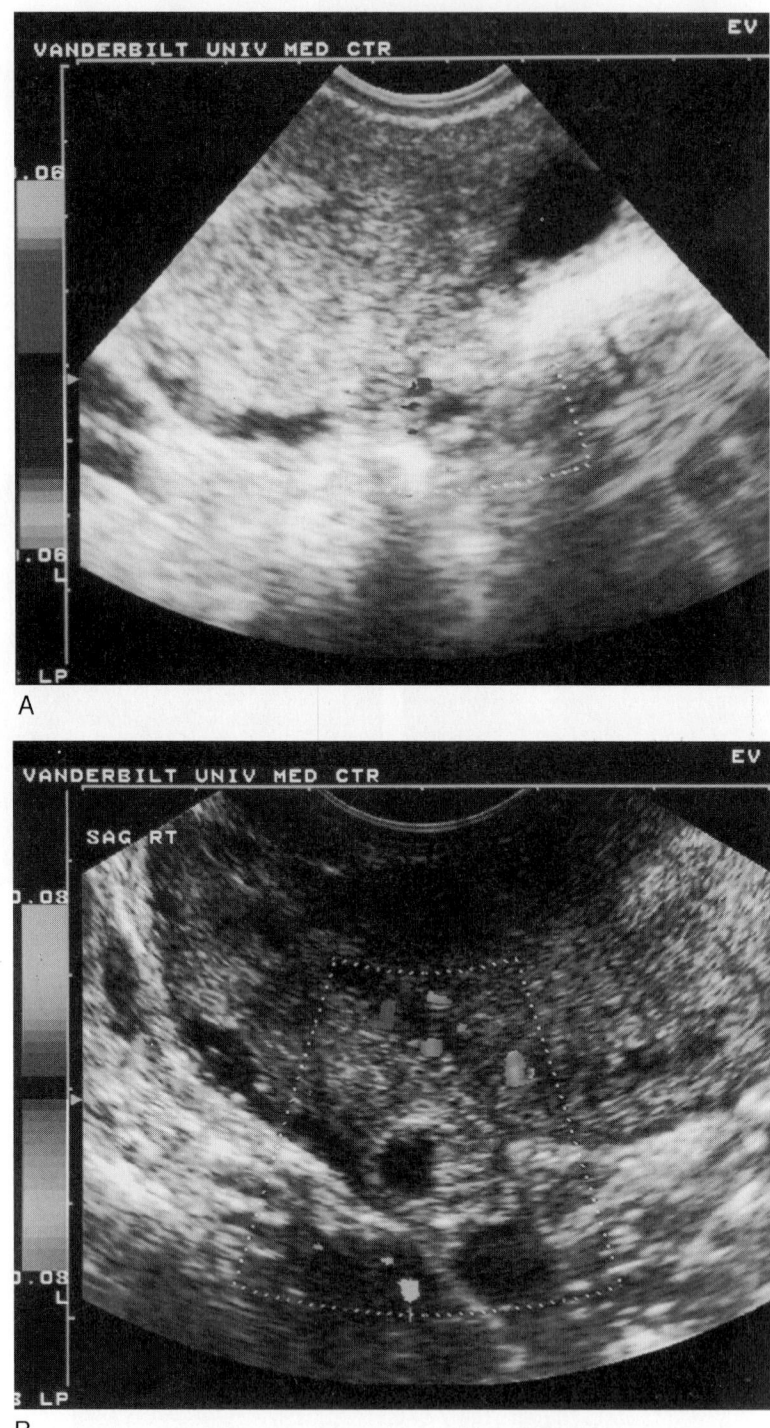

Figure 5–11
Ectopic pregnancy. *A*, TV-CDS of a hypovascular ectopic pregnancy separate from the ovary. *B*, TV-CDS of an ectopic pregnancy surrounded by intratubal hemorrhage.

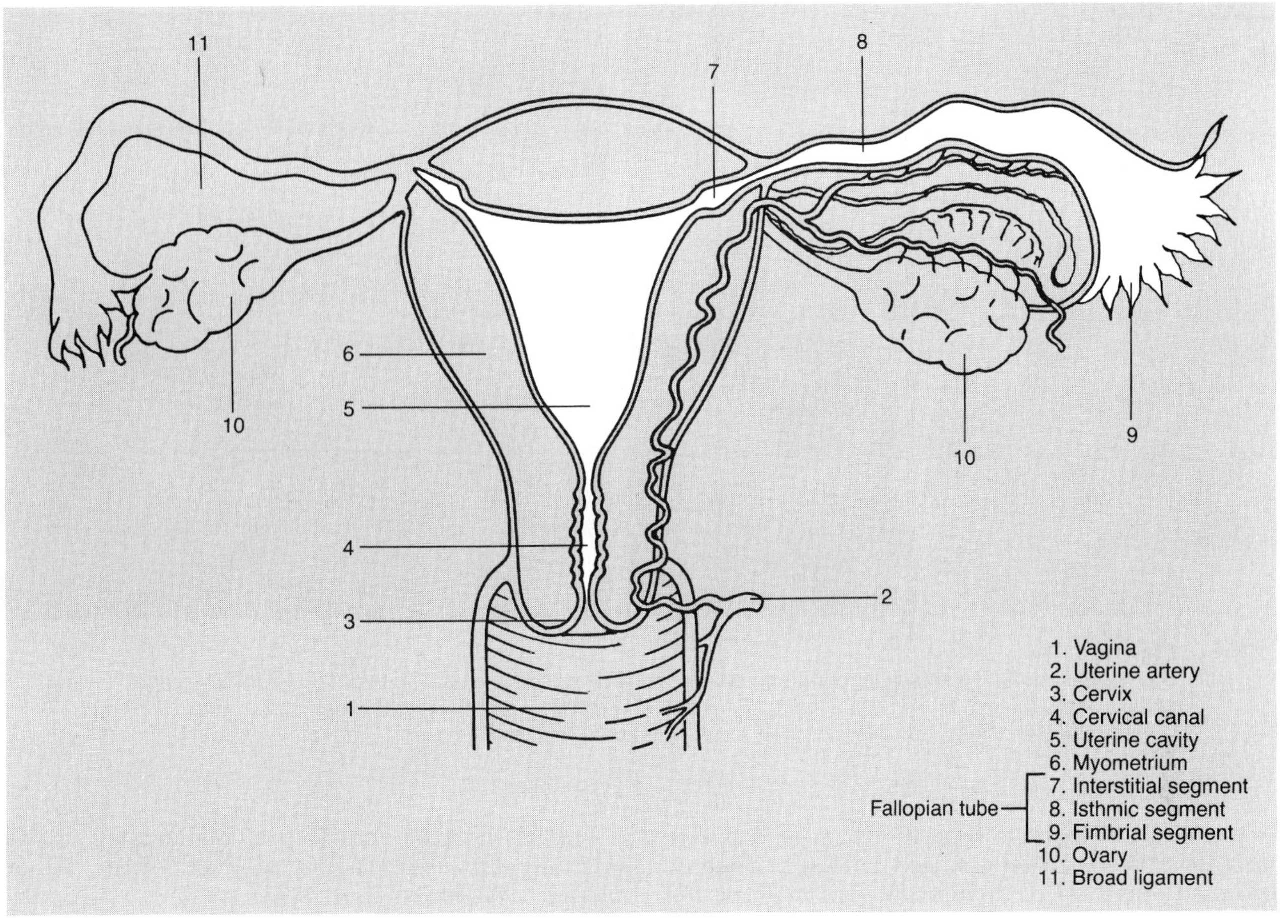

Figure 5-12
Uterus and adnexa.

1. Vagina
2. Uterine artery
3. Cervix
4. Cervical canal
5. Uterine cavity
6. Myometrium
Fallopian tube — 7. Interstitial segment
8. Isthmic segment
9. Fimbrial segment
10. Ovary
11. Broad ligament

Uterus

Uterine evaluation is optimally performed with intravenous infusion. The normal myometrium demonstrates enhancement. The uterine contour is smooth (Gross et al, 1983).

Uterine enlargement is commonly a result of leiomyoma. The appearance includes

1. A lobulated contour
2. An intramural mass distorting or obliterating the uterine cavity
3. An irregular, low-density mass

Approximately 3% of fibroids demonstrate dense calcification (Fig. 5–18) (Friedman et al, 1982; Togashi et al, 1984). The homogeneity is variable, depending on the presence or absence of hyaline, fatty, or cystic degeneration. Leiomyomas, particularly tumors in subserosal, submucosal, and intraligamentous locations, cannot be consistently distinguished from uterine or ovarian malignancies by the CT appearance alone (Korobkin et al, 1979; Lee and Marx, 1989).

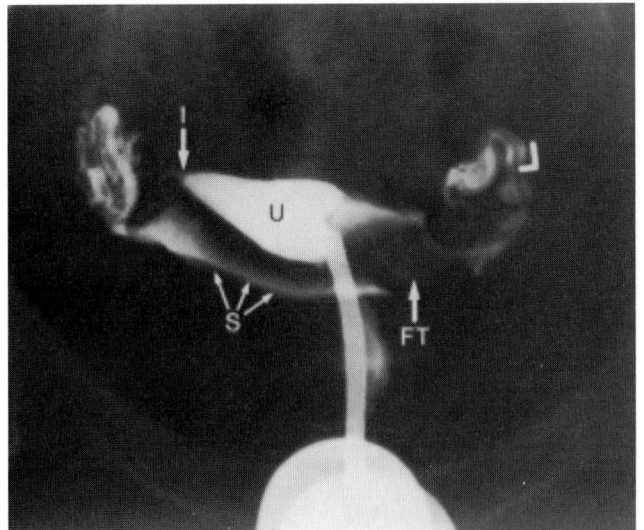

Figure 5-13
Normal hysterosalpingogram. Slightly retroflexed uterine cavity with smooth contour, normal fallopian tubes, and bilateral free spill into the peritoneal cavity. FT, fallopian tube; I, isthmus; S, free spill; U, uterine cavity.

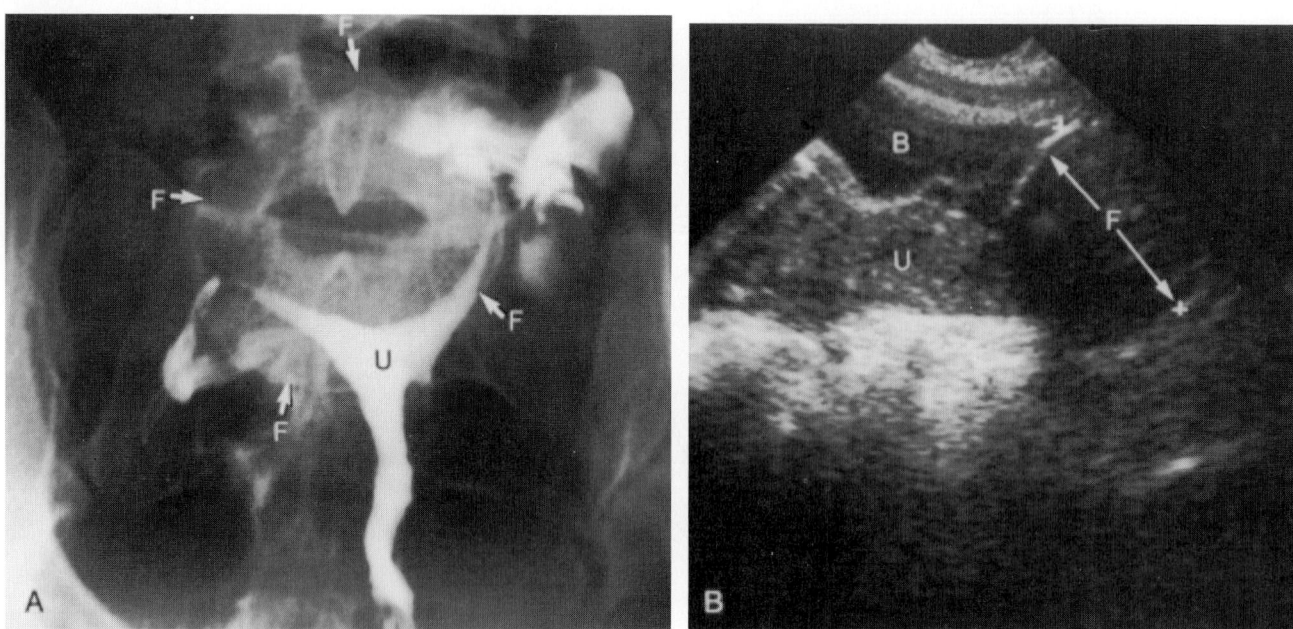

Figure 5–14
Uterine fibroid. *A*, Hysterosalpingogram demonstrates large calcified mass (leiomyoma) distorting uterine cavity. F, fibroid (*arrows*); U, uterine cavity. *B*, Ultrasound scan in same patient. A large hypoechoic mass in the fundus of the uterus is shown. B, bladder; F, fibroid; U, uterus.

Myometrial invasion and peritoneal spread of endometrial cancer can be assessed with CT. Usually more than one third of the uterine wall must be involved to be detected. CT does not generally play a significant role in the management of early stage I or II disease (tumor confined to the uterus).

The features of endometrial malignancy include (Hamlin et al, 1981; Scott et al, 1981; Walsh and Goplerad, 1982; Balke et al, 1983)

1. A low-density mass within the uterine cavity or parenchyma

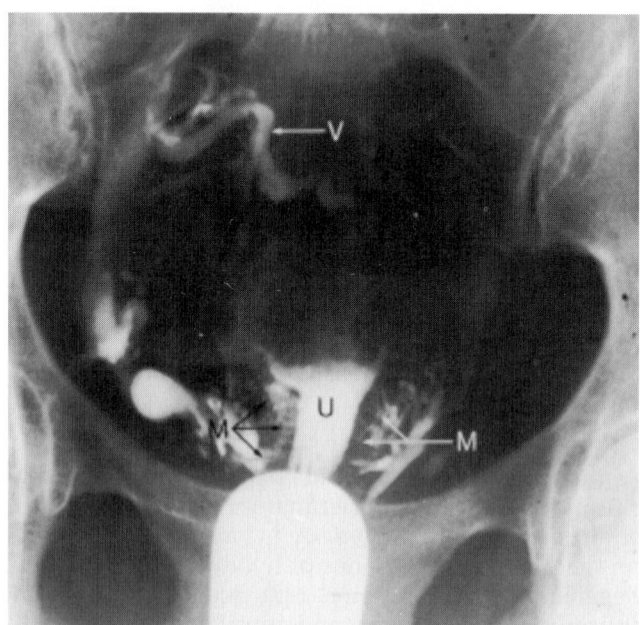

Figure 5–15
Extravasation. Hysterosalpingogram shows extravasation of contrast into myometrium (*arrows*) and into ovarian vein. M, myometrium; U, uterine cavity; V, ovarian vein.

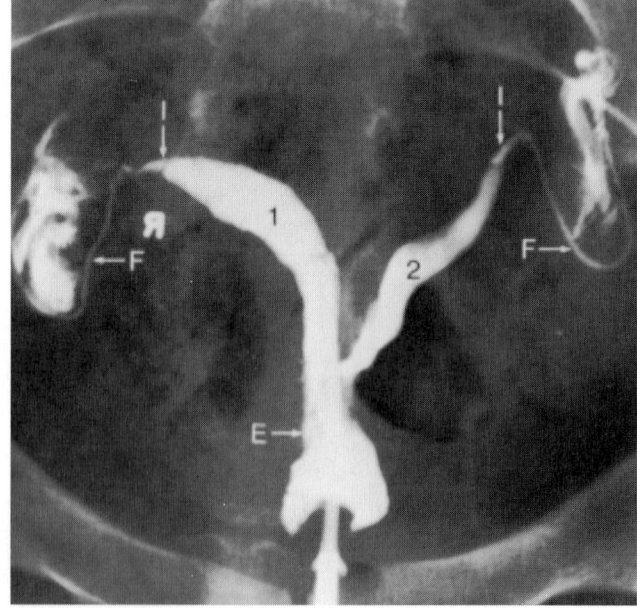

Figure 5–16
Bicornuate uterus. Hysterosalpingogram demonstrates two paired lumens with one cervix. 1 and 2, uterine cavity; E, endocervical canal; F, fallopian tube; I, isthmus.

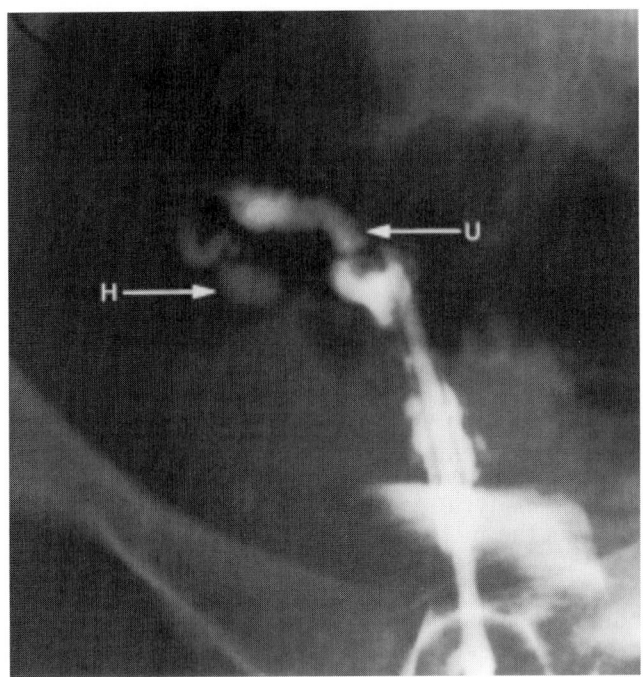

Figure 5−17
DES-exposed uterus. Hysterosalpingogram shows small irregular uterine cavity, and a hydrosalpinx. Note the associated unicornuate anomaly. H, hydrosalpinx; U, uterine cavity, unicornuate.

2. A mass obstructing the endometrial canal with resultant fluid-filled uterine cavity
3. Focally enhancing regions within a hypodense lesion

In demonstrating tumor confined to the uterus, CT has an accuracy between 83% and 92%; in docu-

menting extrauterine extension, it has an accuracy of approximately 95%. Accuracy increases with the higher stages and has the greatest clinical significance in upgrading stage III disease (pelvic sidewalls or nodes) to stage IVA (bladder or rectal involvement) or stage IVB disease (intra-abdominal or hepatic metastases) (Walsh and Goplerad, 1982; Balke et al, 1983; Sawyer and Walsh, 1988).

Lymph node involvement can be evaluated by CT. However, because the architecture of the nodes cannot be assessed accurately, the only criterion of pathology is size. Tumor within nodes of normal size is not detected. Also, enlarged nodes resulting from reactive hyperplasia or other cause of inflammation appear identical to nodes enlarged by malignancy (Lee et al, 1978; Walsh et al, 1980). Lymphangiography, therefore, provides the only evaluation of nodal architecture. CT criteria for abnormal nodes vary with site. Retroperitoneal nodes should be smaller than 1 cm in diameter. Pelvic nodes should measure less than 1.5 cm, with nodes larger than 2.0 cm considered to be pathologically enlarged. CT has an accuracy between 70% and 90% in detecting lymph node metastases (Gore, 1989). CT also is able to evaluate the iliac and obturator lymph nodes, which are not visualized with lymphangiography.

Other uterine malignancies include sarcomas with a typically nonspecific, bulky uterus (Sawyer and Walsh, 1988); trophoblastic gestational neoplasms with inhomogeneous uterine enlargement (Davis et al, 1984); and metastatic disease with homogeneous masses often indistinguishable from primary lesions.

CT is of value in planning radiation therapy and for post-treatment assessment (Walsh and Goplerad, 1981). A baseline study following treatment may enable differentiation of pelvic adhesions and radiation

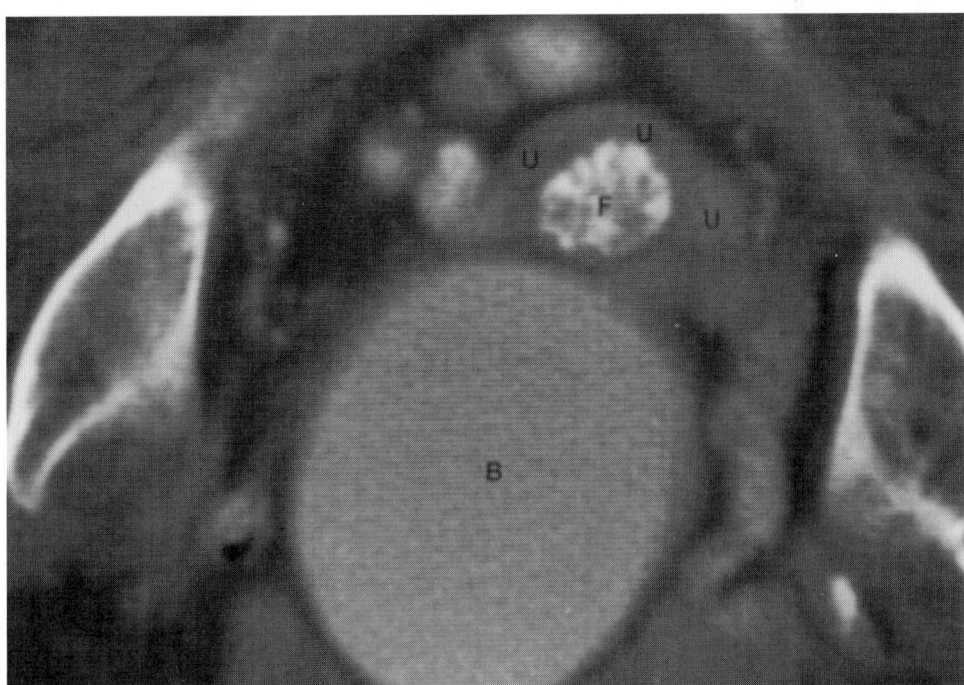

Figure 5−18
Calcified leiomyoma (fibroid). CT scan demonstrates calcification within mass demonstrated in 3% of fibroids. B, bladder; F, fibroid; U, uterus.

fibrosis from tumor recurrence (Gore, 1989). False-negative studies can result from underestimating small metastases. Peritoneal involvement is often manifested with ascites.

Cervix

Carcinoma of the cervix is staged according to criteria of the International Federation of Gynecology and Obstetrics (FIGO) Classification (Sawyer and Walsh, 1988). With respect to CT, the criteria are adapted as shown in Table 5–3.

Stage IA and stage IIIA disease are best determined by clinical examination (Walsh and Goplerad, 1991). The primary role of CT in cervical cancer is to determine whether spread is beyond the cervix and involves the parametrium (Vick et al, 1984a, 1984b).

The classical appearance of tumor is that of a solid mass with areas of decreased attenuation and decreased contrast enhancement compared with the normal cervix. The features of localized tumor without extension include (Sawyer and Walsh, 1988)

1. Smooth borders of the tumor mass
2. Absence of soft tissue lesions or stranding within the parametrial fat
3. Absence of spread into the surrounding ureteric fat planes

CT staging accuracy increases with advanced disease. CT is very limited in staging disease confined to the cervix (stage I) or beyond the cervix but without parametrial involvement (stage IIA). CT overstages parametrial extension in 40% to 70% of patients and is less accurate than physical examination for detecting vaginal invasion (Whitley et al, 1982). CT underestimates pelvic side wall extension and lymph node metastases in 10% to 20% of patients. Microscopic invasion is not detected.

In summary, CT is indicated in determining parametrial extension but tends to overstage stage IB disease and understage stage IIB and IIIB tumors.

Table 5–3. STAGING OF CARCINOMA OF THE CERVIX

STAGE	FEATURE
I	Confined to the cervix
II	Beyond the cervix
IIA	No parametrial involvement
IIB	Parametrial involvement but not to pelvic wall
III	Extension to pelvic sidewall or lower third of vagina; all cases of hydronephrosis
IIIA	No extension to pelvic wall
IIIB	Pelvic sidewall extension or hydronephrosis
IV	beyond true pelvis or to urinary bladder or rectum
IVA	Bladder or rectal involvement
IVB	Para-aortic or inguinal lymph node enlargement (>1.5–2.0 cm.) or intraperitoneal metastases

From Sawyer RW, Walsh JW: CT in gynecologic pelvic diseases. Semin Ultrasound CT MR 1988;9:122, with permission.

The overall accuracy of staging is between 58% and 88%. Recurrent disease may be difficult to distinguish from fibrosis. Post-treatment baseline examinations are of value. Fifty per cent of recurrences involve distant metastases (Walsh et al, 1981). CT of the chest, abdomen, and pelvis should be performed in 1 to 2 years for follow-up.

Ovaries

Normal ovaries are not routinely identified on CT. The majority of ovarian masses are benign cysts with a homogeneous appearance, smooth walls, and attenuation between 0 and 10 Hounsfield units (i.e., water density) (Gross et al, 1983). Sonography still remains the modality of choice. Serous and mucinous cystadenomas make up approximately 20% of benign tumors and demonstrate septations frequently (Sawyer et al, 1985). Cystic teratomas can be diagnosed if fat-fluid levels are demonstrated. Other features include water or fat density mass with globular or rim calcification (Friedman et al, 1982; Skaane and Huebeses, 1983; Williams et al, 1983). The diagnosis of malignant peritoneal implants relies principally on the site of spread and the presence of adjacent ascites rather than on actual size of the tumor mass (Fig. 5–19) (Hulnick et al, 1984).

Adnexa

The differential diagnosis of solid adnexal masses on CT is extensive and nonspecific. Abscesses may be demonstrated in the dependent cul-de-sac, but inflammatory disease and endometriosis generally have nondiagnostic features (Fishman et al, 1983).

Malignant neoplasms are disseminated, often by surface implantation and intraperitoneal spread. The site of origin is frequently indeterminate. Mesenteric spread may appear as ill-defined soft tissue masses surrounded by fat or bowel. Psammomatous calcification may be present in up to one third of serous cystadenocarcinomas and can be identified by CT (Mitchell et al, 1986). Krukenberg tumors, representing metastases from the gastrointestinal tract, are mistaken in more than 30% of cases for a primary ovarian tumor (Fig. 5–20) (Cho and Gold, 1985).

Summary

CT remains an important modality in assessing local tumor extent and in detecting metastases. CT is accurate in postoperative abscess detection. Drainage is easily performed in many cases. Similarly, the application of CT in percutaneous biopsy for tissue diagnosis is well established (Welch et al, 1989).

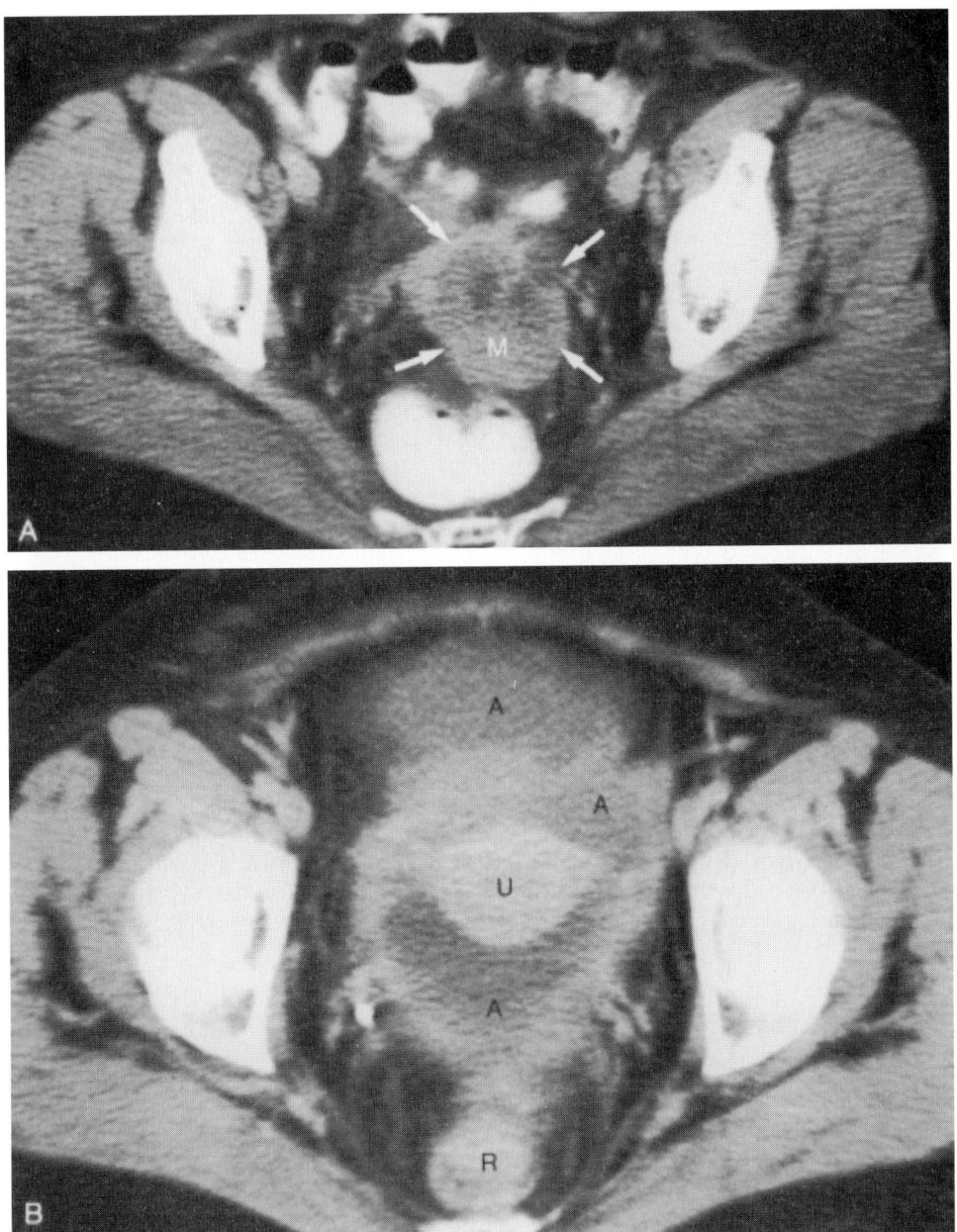

Figure 5 – 19

A, CT image demonstrates a large mass with mixed attenuation (*arrows*), representing ovarian carcinoma (M). *B*, CT scan shows malignant ascites (A) from ovarian carcinoma. R, rectum; U, uterus. *Illustration continued on following page*

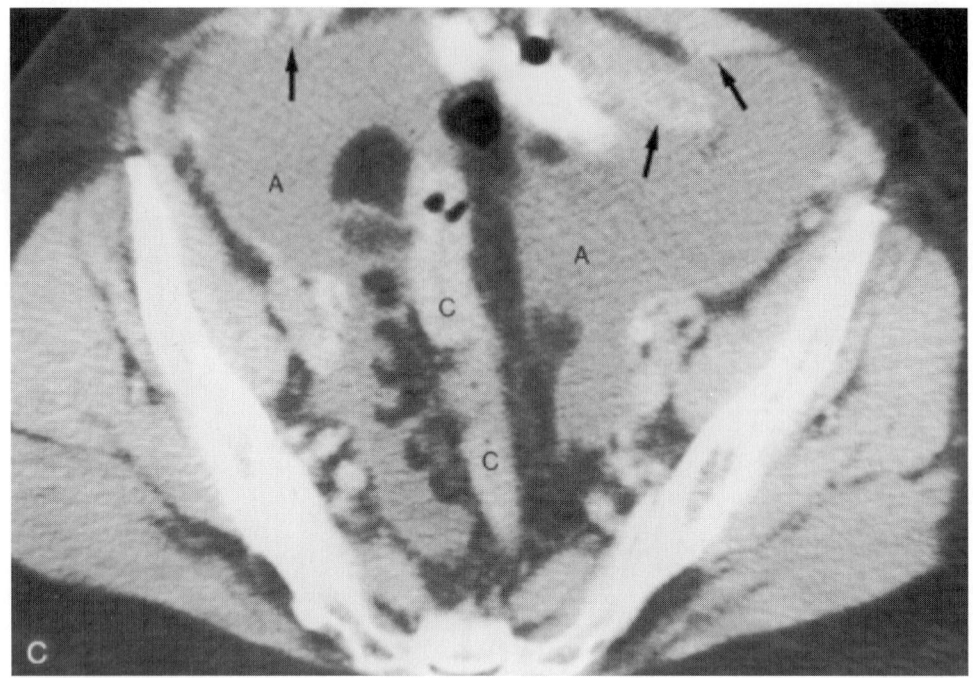

Figure 5-19
Continued   C, CT scan of a patient with stage IV ovarian cancer. Scan at the level of the iliac crests demonstrates omental tumor cake (*arrows*) with ascites (A) and fixed sigmoid colon (C).

MAGNETIC RESONANCE IMAGING

The development of MRI has resulted in significant advances in the evaluation of pelvic structures. As a result of rapid technological advances, the applications stated in printed form are frequently outdated.

The principal advantages of magnetic resonance (MR) scanning are as follows (Pykett et al, 1982; Axel, 1984; Bies et al, 1984; Lupetin, 1988; Loeffler and Laub, 1990):

1. There is no ionizing radiation (radio waves and magnetic fields are the energy sources).
2. Multiplanar imaging permits superior spatial resolution in oblique, sagittal, or other anatomic planes.
3. Soft tissue contrast resolution, superior to that in sonography and CT, is obtained. A wide range of different contrast parameters can be evaluated
4. Vascular structures can be imaged without contrast. Recent fast-scan techniques permit "MRI an-

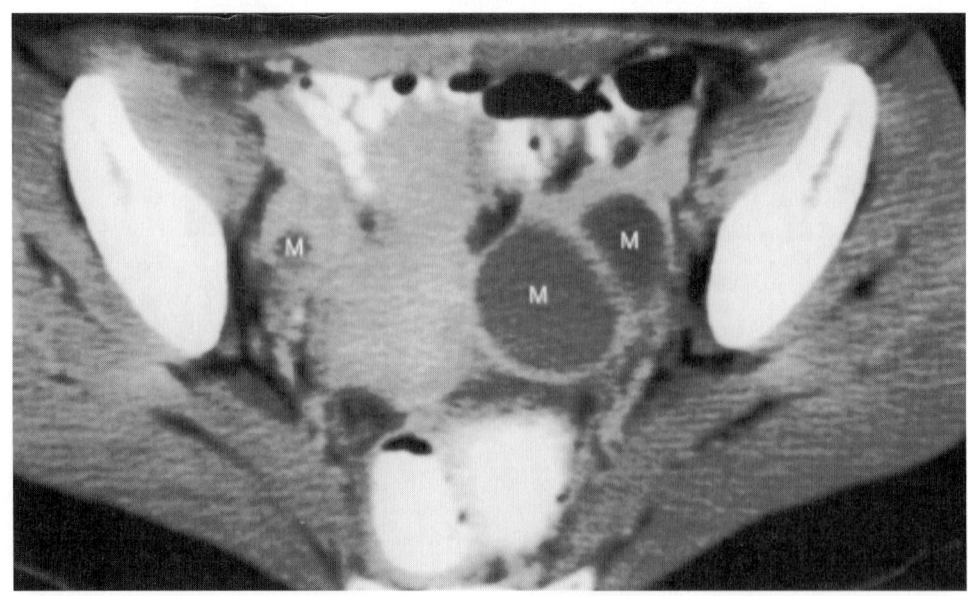

Figure 5-20
CT scan of Krukenberg tumor. Nonspecific masses within the right and left ovaries represent metastases (M) from a gastric neoplasm.

giography" (Edelman et al, 1990), although degradation of the image results.

5. Degradation of the image by cortical bone hardening artifact does not occur as with CT.
6. The potential with spectroscopy for in vivo (in body) tissue characterization with respect to tumor involvement, response to therapy, or staging exists.

Organic chemists are required to interpret spectroscopy. At present, this application is not a clinical reality (Aisen and Chenevert, 1989; Bottomley, 1989).

The amount of information available with MRI is both an advantage and a disadvantage. To obtain the maximum information, complex protocols have been developed for each organ system.

The limitations of MRI include the following (New et al, 1983; Dunn et al, 1985; Laakman et al, 1985; Powers et al, 1989):

1. Patients with pacemakers, intracranial aneurysm clips, certain heart valves, metallic foreign bodies around the orbits, and cochlear implants cannot be imaged.
2. Patients on ventilators and other life support equipment cannot be easily scanned. Nonferrous monitors are available but are not yet widely used.
3. The length of time to acquire an image is greater than with CT or ultrasonography. Continual advances decrease this factor. Newer fast-scan techniques with acronyms such as "FLASH" and "GRASS" permit dynamic imaging with very short acquisition times.
4. Interventional procedures, including abscess drainage and biopsy, cannot be performed with MRI.
5. Cost of installation is higher than with CT. Shielding from the effects of the strong magnetic fields and against external radio signals adds to the cost for the patient.
6. Claustrophobic patients are harder to scan than with CT. Certain scanner configurations minimize this effect.
7. Artifacts resulting from motion, the presence of ferromagnetic materials, patient positioning, rapid blood flow, and other imaging factors, such as field size, chemical shift, or eddy currents, are becoming more and more recognized.
8. There is an absence of signal from calcium and cortical bone. Characteristic features, such as teeth within a dermoid, cannot be imaged.

A detailed discussion of the physics of MRI (Bushong, 1988) is beyond the scope of this chapter. However, simply put, MRI permits the localization of different nuclei within the tissues of interest. Although there are several nuclei of medical interest, the hydrogen proton is the principal nucleus utilized for imaging. This application is the result of two factors:

1. Hydrogen constitutes approximately 80% of all nuclei in the human body.

2. Hydrogen nuclei are strongly magnetic.

In order to produce an image, energy must be transferred to the hydrogen nucleus, which in turn releases this energy in a manner related to certain tissue characteristics. The energy frequency introduced by a radio wave must match exactly the rate at which the nucleus wobbles in the magnetic field (a property referred to as resonance—hence the term *magnetic resonance*).

With hydrogen in a 1-tesla field (the tesla is the unit of magnetic strength), this frequency is 42.6 MHz. If an oxygen nucleus is used, the radio frequency would be 5.8 MHz. Note is made that the frequency modulation (FM) radio band is between 88 and 100 MHz; as a result, the installations must be shielded against external radio waves. By employing complex pulse sequences, an image can be developed. In reality, the image represents the distribution of hydrogen in water molecules and fat molecules and the interaction of water with macromolecules, such as proteins.

The MR image is not as tissue specific as was originally hoped, and overlap of the signal intensity or brightness of different tissues occurs (Sugimura et al, 1990). The appearance of tumor may be identical to that in normal tissues and may even overlap with the signal from hemorrhage and abscesses. MRI, however, may have application in distinguishing fibrosis from the recurrence of malignancy.

The image produced is the result of different intrinsic characteristics of the tissues. The properties include

1. *Spin density* (SD), a measure of the number of mobile hydrogen nuclei available to produce a signal (with cortical bone, the hydrogen is so tightly bound that no signal results).
2. *Spin lattice relaxation time* (T_1) relates to the time required to give up the energy acquired by the radio pulse. T_1-weighted images tend to demonstrate excellent anatomic detail.
3. *Spin-spin relaxation time* (T_2) involves the time for molecules to return to a baseline energy as a result of nuclei interacting with other nuclei. T_2-weighted images accentuate the differences between normal and abnormal structures but tend to show poorer spatial resolution than do T_1-weighted images. T_2 has been described as similar to comparing the time required to fall down between skaters who are shackled together and skaters who are free to move independently.

The radio pulse is given in specific complex sequences that are described by such terms as *partial saturation*, *spin echo*, and *inversion recovery*. The differences between these sequences predominantly involve the time between succeeding pulses or repetition time (TR), the time between echo signals (TE), or a feature referred to as inversion delay time (TI). These parameters affect the contrast between tissues and bias the image toward a greater or lesser T_1, T_2, or SD contribution.

Signal intensity refers to the brightness or whiteness of the image. Simply put, tissue with short T_1 characteristics appears bright on T_1-weighted studies. Molecules with long T_2 times have a bright image on T_2-weighted examinations. T_1 and T_2 are independent of each other.

Although motion artifact is usually not a factor in the pelvis, many protocols advocate patient fasting or glucagon, 1 mg intravenously, to minimize intestinal motion (Weinreb et al, 1984). Some authors recommend ferric ammonium citrate or solutions of Gd-DTPA to opacify the bowel (Wesbey et al, 1983; Winkler and Hricak, 1986; Laniado et al, 1988).

A tampon is usually not required as with CT to define the vagina, unless rectal tumor involvement is of concern. A Foley catheter may be used to define the urethral course. Urine appears as a low-intensity or dark region on T_1-weighted studies and high-intensity or white region on T_2-weighted examinations.

MR magnets have field strengths varying between 0.15 and 1.5 tesla. A strength of 2 tesla is an imposed regulatory limitation, although field strengths exceeding 11 tesla have been produced in laboratories. For spectroscopy, high magnetic fields are required.

The analysis of the internal female pelvic organs has undergone significant advancement with the application of MR scanning.

Uterus

T_2-weighted studies provide superior anatomic detail of the corpus, isthmus, and cervix (Fig. 5–21) (Hricak, 1986; Hricak et al, 1988; Kim et al, 1990).

The appearance of the uterus is dependent on the hormonal stimulation, varying with the phase of the menstrual cycle or exogenous estrogens (Demas et al, 1986). In the later secretory phase, the myometrium becomes brighter as the glands accumulate water. Oral contraceptives also affect the myometrial and endometrial appearance, with the separation between the layers becoming indistinct (McCarthy et al, 1986). A dark line or low-intensity signal defines the inner third of the myometrium as with ultrasound and most likely represents decreased water content (McCarthy et al, 1989).

MRI permits excellent delineation of congenital abnormalities (Fig. 5–22) (Mintz et al, 1988). The morphologic pattern of the bicornuate uterus has been well demonstrated with visualization of two bright or high-intensity regions surrounded by a dark junctional zone. Differentiation from a septate uterus can be accomplished with recognition of the low-intensity or dark fibrous septum between the cavities. Distinguishing between the two entities may not be possible. Unicornuate uteri, DES-

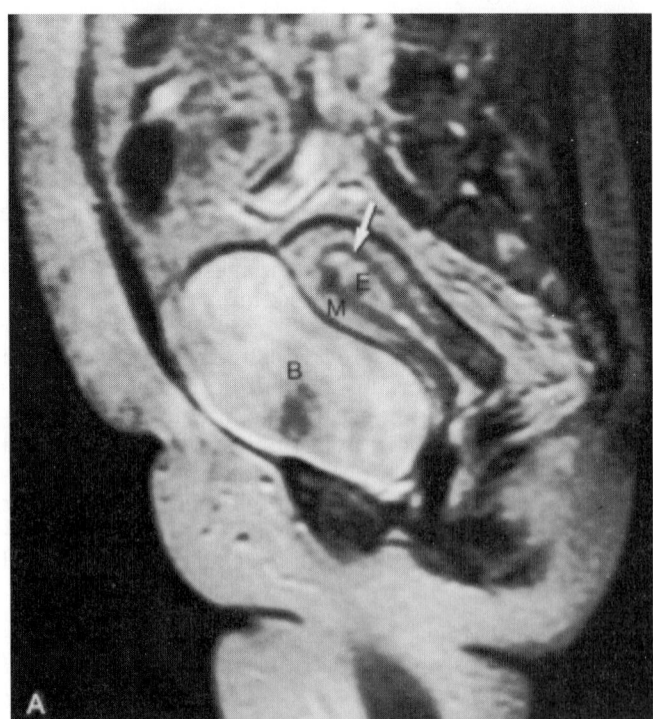

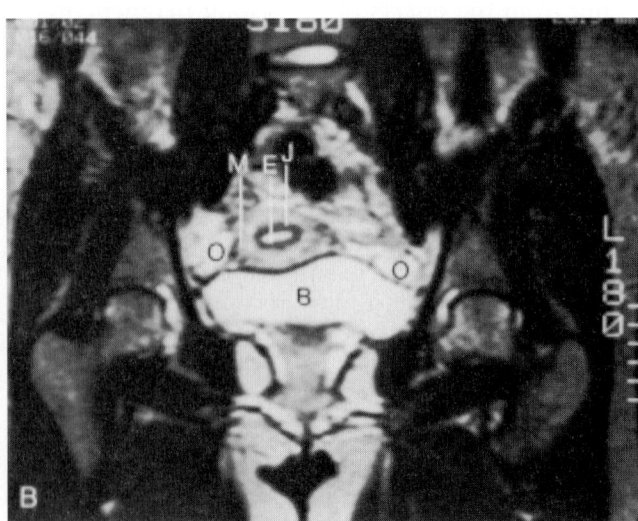

Figure 5–21

A, Sagittal MRI demonstrates a normal uterus (TR/TE = 2500/80, 1.5 T). The low-intensity junctional zone (*arrows*) can be distinguished from the high-intensity endometrium (E) and the medium-intensity myometrium (M). B, urinary bladder. *B*, Coronal MRI demonstrates intrauterine zonal anatomy in a normal pelvis on a predominately T_2-weighted image (TR/TE = 2000/80, 1.5 T). B, urinary bladder; E, endometrium; J, junctional zone; M, myometrium; O, ovary.

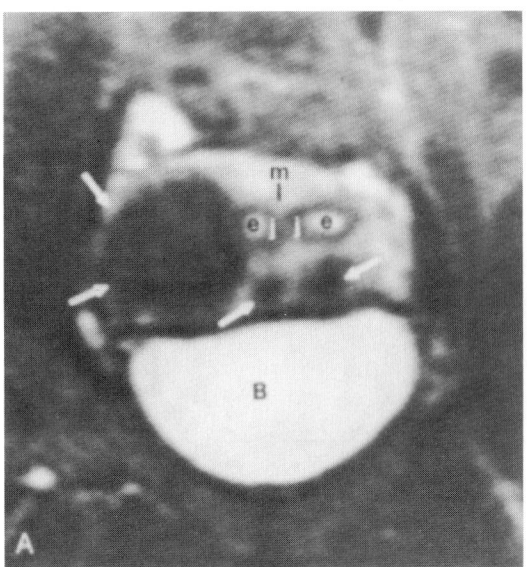
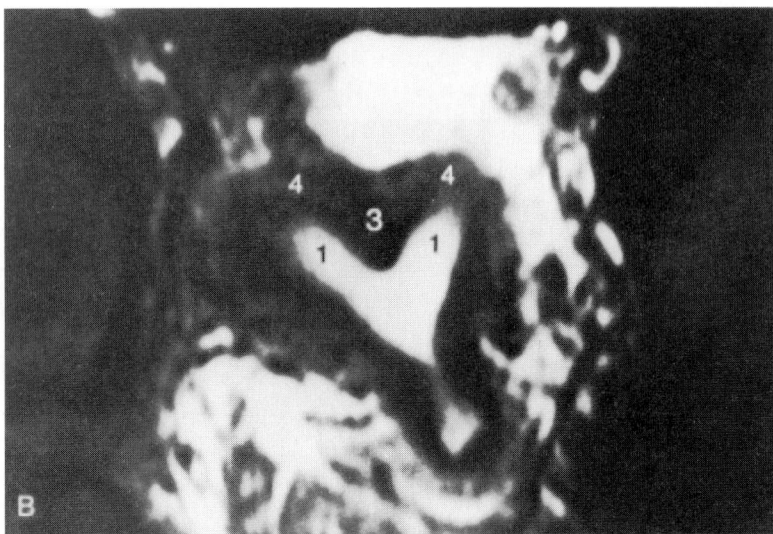

Figure 5–22

A, Coronal scan of a bicornuate uterus (TR/TE = 2500/80, 1.5 T). Fibroids (*arrows*) are shown within the myometrium. Two separate endometrial cavities are visualized. b, urinary bladder; e, endometrium; j, junctional zone; m, myometrium. (From Mintz MC, Thickman DI, Gussman D, Kressel HY: MR evaluation of uterine abnormalities. AJR 1987;148:287, with permission. © by The American Roentgen Ray Society.)
B, Axial MRI demonstrates a septate uterus with the septum (3) separating the endometrial cavities (1). 4, myometrium. (TR/TE = 2000/80, 1.5 T.) (From Mintz MC, Grumbach K: Imaging of congenital uterine anomalies. Semin Ultrasound CT MR 1988;9:167, with permission.)

exposed uteri, and uterine hypoplasia have been studied with MRI (van Gils et al, 1989).

MRI has proved to be an excellent diagnostic modality for pathology involving the myometrium (Weinreb et al, 1989). Leiomyomas can be separated from normal myometrium (Fig. 5–23). MRI can detect small lesions missed by ultrasonography and provides superior assessment of their number, size,

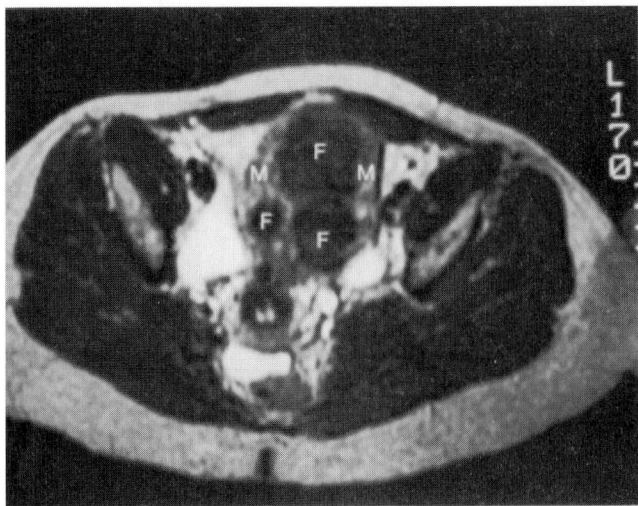

Figure 5–23

Coronal MRI demonstrates multiple low-intensity uterine fibroids (F) within medium-intensity myometrium (M) on a T_2-weighted study (TR/TE = 2500/80, 1.5 T).

and location. The appearance again varies, depending on the degree of degeneration of the fibroid.

The pattern for adenomyosis on MRI is that of a diffusely enlarged uterus with a wide, low-intensity or dark band surrounding the endometrium (Togashi et al, 1989b). This appearance does not depend on stage of menstrual cycle. Focal areas may mimic leiomyomas (Mark et al, 1987).

The Lippes loop and copper-7 IUCDs can be imaged without producing artifacts (Mark and Hricak, 1987).

Gestational trophoblastic disease produces a characteristic appearance with regions of signal void. This lack of signal is due to hypervascularity and disruption of the normal zonal anatomy between the myometrium and the endometrium. Post-treatment studies have shown a return to the normal dark junction band and uterine volume (Hricak et al, 1986a).

Endometrial carcinoma presents as widening of the endometrial cavity in the postmenopausal patient, with disruption of the low-intensity junction zone between the myometrium and the endometrium (Worthington et al, 1986; Fishman-Javitt et al, 1987). However, in some normal postmenopausal women, the junctional zone may not be demonstrated (Posniak et al, 1990). Also, adenomatous hyperplasia can appear identical to endometrial carcinoma. The overall accuracy of MRI in staging endometrial carcinoma has been reported to be as high as 92% (Hricak et al, 1987).

Metastases cannot accurately be distinguished from either benign or malignant uterine neoplasms

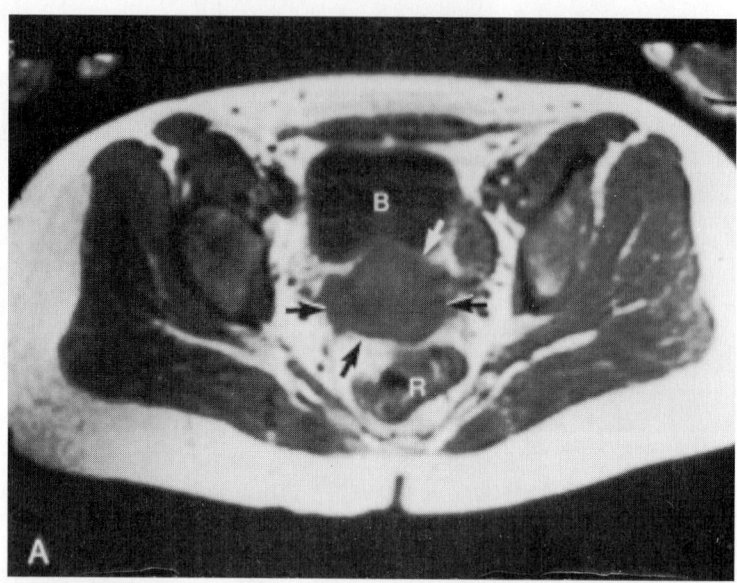

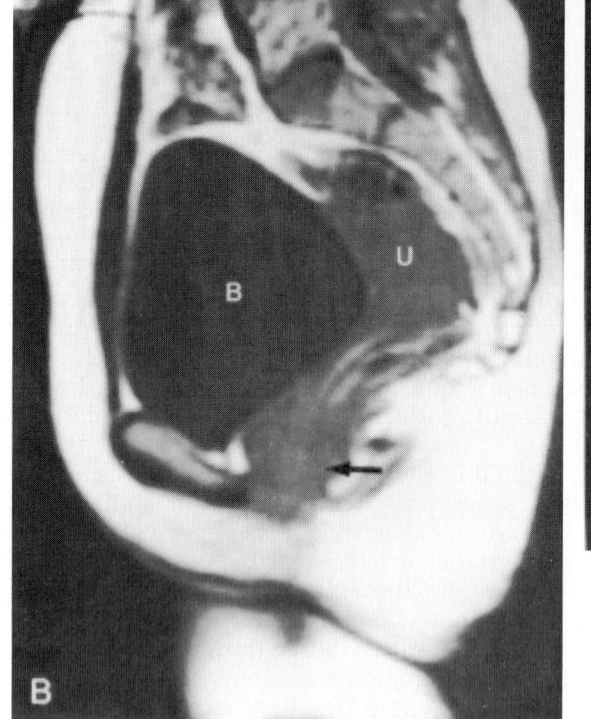

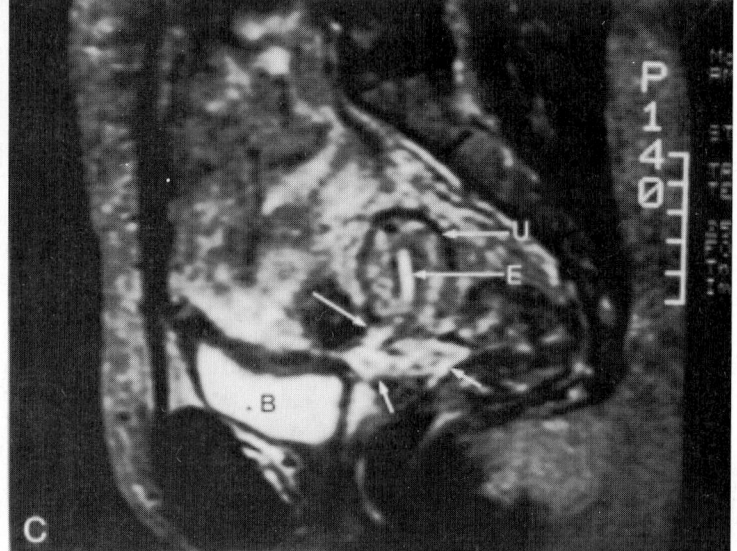

Figure 5-24

A, Coronal MRI demonstrates enlarged cervix proven to represent stage I squamous carcinoma of the cervix (*arrow*) (TR/TE = 400/17, 1.5 T). B, urinary bladder; R, rectum. *B,* Sagittal MRI of same patient as in *A* shows an enlarged cervix (*arrows*) and a normal uterine body (TR/TE = 2000/80, 1.5 T). B, urinary bladder; U, uterine body. *C,* Sagittal MRI of a different patient with treated cervical cancer (TR/TE = 2000/80, 1.5 T). Cervix shows increased intensity with stranding in the surrounding tissue planes (*arrows*). The uterine body is normal. B, bladder; E, endometrial stripe; U, uterus.

(Hricak et al, 1985). The appearance of sarcomas is also nonspecific on MRI (Shapeero and Hricak, 1989).

Cervix

Cervical carcinoma and parametrial extent have been accurately assessed with MRI (Fig. 5–24) (Togashi et al, 1986; Chang and Hricak, 1988). Typically, carcinoma demonstrates a brighter image than the normal low-intensity fibrous stroma. Tumors were more consistently identified by MRI in contrast to CT (80% versus 67%) (Kim et al, 1990). Tumors not visualized were stage IB of small size or lower. Studies have shown superior tumor staging with overall accuracy rates of 83% for MRI versus 63% for CT and 76% for clinical staging (Togashi et al, 1989). MRI has an accuracy of 77% in assessment of the thickness of stromal invasion and can provide an estimate of tumor volume (Waggenspack et al, 1988).

Lymphangitic spread is based on lymph node size. Ovaries and bowel loops can mimic lymph nodes on MRI as with CT.

Adnexa

Sonography still remains the method of choice for evaluating ovarian masses. In more than 80% of menstruating women, the ovaries have been demonstrated with MRI (Dooms et al, 1986).

Most teratomas characteristically demonstrate a signal similar to fat with regions of wall thickening (Togashi et al, 1987; Mitchell, 1988). Hemorrhagic cysts reveal bright-intensity signals on both T_1- and T_2-weighted sequences similar to fat (Dooms et al, 1986). The appearance of blood depends on the age of the hemorrhage. Follicular cysts have a bright appearance on T_2-weighted studies, and polycystic ovaries are clearly depicted. Proteinaceous material restricts the movement of water molecules, resulting in a bright appearance on T_1-weighted images (Brown et al, 1985).

As with ultrasound and CT, MRI is limited in detecting small endometrial implants (Arrive et al, 1989; Zawin et al, 1989). MRI remains nonspecific in distinguishing benign from malignant foci.

MR scanning has been applied in detecting ovarian vein thrombosis (Mintz et al, 1987), for placental localization, and for assessing cervical incompetence (McCarthy et al, 1985).

Summary

The application of MRI in pelvic imaging continues to be evaluated and defined. MRI enables superior staging of tumor in contrast to CT as a result of its greater soft tissue contrast and multiplanar capabilities.

NUCLEAR MEDICINE

Diagnostic imaging in nuclear medicine is based on the intravenous administration of a radiopharmaceutical tracer attached to a carrier molecule. The carrier molecule either is part of a physiologic pathway (such as phosphate complexes, which are taken up during bone metabolism) or is a form of macromolecule such as antibodies, colloid particles, and red blood cells. The patient is scanned with a gamma camera to detect the gamma rays emitted by the tracer. This scanning is performed anytime from minutes up to many hours after the injection. New technical advances, including the single-photon emission computed tomography (SPECT) camera, which allows tomographic-like studies, have improved the resolution of this modality.

Positron emission tomography (PET) has proved to be a sophisticated tool for in vivo noninvasive biochemical studies in patients. However, PET scanning requires expensive cyclotron technology. Short-lived positron emitters, such as oxygen-15, nitrogen-13, and carbon-11, permit physiologic metabolic pathways to be studied in disease states (McAfee et al, 1990).

Bone scintigraphy is sensitive for the detection of early bone turnover. The underlying mechanism of increased tracer uptake is nonspecific and can indicate recent trauma, infection, or neoplastic processes. Osseous metastases are detected in more than 98% of cases. Most metastases show increased uptake of the tracer, although approximately 1% can appear as cold (absent uptake) lesions.

Pelvic infection can be examined with gallium-labeled citrate or indium-labeled leukocyte imaging. Gallium may be taken up in normal physiologic healing or may be excreted with bowel activity. Indium-labeled studies do not have the disadvantage of bowel uptake and appear to be superior for pelvic imaging of infectious processes.

Recent developments in nuclear medicine have centered on tumor imaging agents, that is, the labeling of specific monoclonal antibodies (MoAbs), which are incorporated into tumors (McAfee et al, 1990). Extensive resources are being applied to MoAb labeling for tumor localization and treatment. At present, the procedures are primarily experimental and have only limited application (Epenetos et al, 1986a, 1986b). In one study with radiolabeled antibodies to ovarian carcinoma, the tumor level was only 0.015% of the injected dose per gram (Epenetos et al, 1986b). Many tumors are polyclonal, which complicates the technique. The potential for significant advancement in tumor detection and treatment within the next few years is still thought to be high.

REFERENCES

Aisen AM, Chenevert TL: MR spectroscopy: clinic perspective. Radiology 1989;173:593.

Amendola MA: Conventional radiographic contrast procedures. In Fischer MR, Kricun ME (eds). Imaging of the Pelvis. Queenstown, MD: Aspen Publishers, 1989.

American Institute of Ultrasound in Medicine: Bioeffects considerations for the safety of diagnostic ultrasound. J Ultrasound Med 1988; (Suppl):S4.

Amman AM, Walsh JW: Normal anatomy and technique of examination. In Walsh MA (ed): Computed Tomography of the Pelvis. New York: Churchill Livingstone, 1985:1.

Arrive L, Hricak H, Martin MN: Pelvic endometriosis: MR imaging. Radiology 1989;171:687.

Aunet WL, Ellem N: Hysterosalpinography. Radiol Clin North Am 1967;5:105.

Axel L: Blood flow effects in magnetic resonance imaging. AJR 1984;143:1157.

Balke DM, Van Dyke J, Lee JKT, et al: Computed tomography in malignant endometrial neoplasms. J Comput Assist Tomogr 1983;7:677.

Bies JR, Ellis JH, Kopecky KK, et al: Assessment of primary gynecologic malignancies: comparison of 0.15 T resistive MRI with CT. AJR 1984;143:1249.

Bottomley PA: Human in vivo NMR spectroscopy in diagnostic medicine: clinical tool or research probe? Radiology 1989;170:1.

Brown JJ, van Sonnenberg E, Gerber KH, et al: Magnetic resonance relaxation times of percutaneously obtained normal and abnormal body fluids. Radiology 1985;154:727.

Budinger TF: Nuclear magnetic resonance (NMR) in vivo studies known thresholds for health effects. J Comput Assist Tomogr 1981;5:800.

Bushong SC: Biological Effects of MRI in Magnetic Resonance Imaging. St. Louis: CV Mosby, 1988:326.

Chang VC, Hricak H, Thurnher S, et al: Vagina: evaluation with MR imaging: Part II. Neoplasms. Radiology 1988;169:175.

Cho KC, Gold BM: Computed tomography of Krukenberg tumours. AJR 1985;145:285.

Davis WK, McCarthy S, Moss AA, et al: Computed tomography of gestational trophoblastic disease. J Comput Assist Tomogr 1984;8:1136.

Demas BE, Hricak H, Jaffe RH, et al: Uterine MR imaging: effects of hormonal stimulation. Radiology 1986;159:123.

Dooms GC, Hricak H, Ischolakoff D: Adnexal structures: MR imaging. Radiology 1986;158:639.

Dunn V, Coffman CE, McGowan JE, et al: Mechanical ventilation during magnetic resonance imaging. Magn Reson Imaging 1985;3:169.

Edelman RR, Mattle HP, Atkinson DJ, et al: MR angiography. AJR 1990;154:937.

Emerson DS, Cartier MS, Altieri LA, et al: Diagnostic efficacy of endovaginal color Doppler flow imaging in an ectopic pregnancy screening program. Radiology 1992;183:413.

Engelstad BL, Wolf GL: Contrast agents. In Stark DD, Bradley WG (eds): Magnetic Resonance Imaging. St. Louis: CV Mosby, 1988:161.

Epenetos AA, Hooker G, Krausz T, et al: Antibody guided irradiation of malignant ascites in ovarian vein cancer: a new therapeutic method possessing specificity against cancer cells. J Obstet Gynecol 1986a;68:71.

Epenetos AA, Snook D, Durbin, et al: Limitations of radiolabelled monoclonal antibodies for localization of human neoplasms. Cancer Res 1986b;46:3183.

Fishman EK, Scatarige JC, Saksouk FA, et al: Computed tomography of endometriosis. J Comput Assist Tomogr 1983;7:257.

Fishman-Javitt MC, Stein HL, Lovecchio HL: MRI in staging of endometrial and cervical carcinoma. Magn Reson Imaging 1987;5:83.

Fleischer A, Cullinan J, Peery C, Jones H: Early detection of ovarian carcinoma with transvaginal color Doppler ultrasonography. Am J Obstet Gynecol 1996a;174:101.

Fleischer A, Dudley B, Entman S, et al: Myometrial invasion: sonographic assessment. Radiology 1987;162:307.

Fleischer A, Javitt M, Jeffery B: Clinical Gynecology. Philadelphia: Lippincott-Raven, 1997a.

Fleischer A, Johnson J, Tait D: Amplitude and frequency based transvaginal color Doppler sonography of ovarian masses: correlation with microvascularity. Ultrasound Int 1996b;3:118.

Fleischer A, Kepple D: Transvaginal Sonography: A Text Atlas. Philadelphia: Lippincott-Raven, 1995a.

Fleischer A, Stein S, Cullinan J, Warner M: Color Doppler sonography of adnexal torsion. J Ultrasound Med, 1995b;14:523.

Fleischer AC, Herbert CN, Hill GA, et al: Transvaginal sonography: applications in infertility. Semin Ultrasound CT MR 1990a;11:71.

Fleischer AC, Pennell RG, McKee NS, et al: Ectopic pregnancy: features of transvaginal sonography. Radiology 1990b;174:375.

Fleischer AC, Vasquez JM, Cullinan JA, Eisenberg E: Sonohysterography combined with sonosalpingography: correlation with endoscopic findings in infertility patients. J Ultrasound Med 1997b;16:381.

Friedman AC, Pyatt RS, Hartman DS, et al: CT of benign cystic teratomas. AJR 1982;138:659.

Goldstein SR, Nachtigall M, Snyder JR, et al: Endometrial assessment by vaginal ultrasonography before endometrial sampling in patients with postmenopausal bleeding. Am J Obstet Gynecol 1990;163:119.

Gore RM: Computed tomography. In Fischer MR, Kricun ME (eds): Imaging of the Pelvis. Queenstown, MD: Aspen Publications, 1989:247.

Granberg G, Karlsson B, Wikland M, Grill B: Transvaginal sonography of uterine and endometrial disorders. In Fleischer A (ed): Sonography in Ob/Gyn: Principles and Practice. Stamford, CT: Appleton & Lange, 1996:851.

Gross BH, Moss AA, Mihara K, et al: Computed tomography of gynecologic disease. AJR 1983;141:765.

Hamlin DJ, Burgenen FA, Beecham JB: CT of intramural endometrial carcinoma: contrast enhancement is essential. AJR 1981;137:551.

Herbst AL, Poskanzer DC, Robboy SJ, et al: Premature exposure to stilbestrol: a prospective comparison of exposed female offspring with unexposed controls. N Engl J Med 1975;292:334.

Holst N, Abyholm T, Borgersen A: Hysterosalpingography in the evaluation of fertility. Acta Radiol Diagn 1983;24:253.

Hricak H: MRI of the female pelvis: a review. AJR 1986;146:1115.

Hricak H: MRI of Pelvis. London: Martin Dunitz Publisher, 1996.

Hricak H, Chong YC, Thurnher S: Vagina: evaluation with MR imaging. Radiology 1988;169:169.

Hricak H, Demas B, Braga C, et al: Gestational trophoblastic neoplasm of the uterus: MR assessment. Radiology 1986a;161:11.

Hricak H, Schriock E, Lacey C, et al: Gynecologic masses: value of MRI. Am J Obstet Gynecol 1985;153:31.

Hricak H, Stern JL, Fisher MR, et al: Endometrial carcinoma staging by MR imaging. Radiology 1987;162:297.

Hricak H, Tscholakoff D, Heinrich LW, et al: Uterine leiomyomas: correlation of MR, histopathologic findings and symptoms. Radiology 1986b;158:385.

Hulnick DH, Negibow AJ, Balthazar IJ, et al: Computed tomography in the evaluation of diverticulitis. Radiology 1984;152:491.

Kasby CB: Hysterosalpingography: An appraisal of current indications. Br J Radiol 1980;53:279.

Kim SH, Cho BI, Lee HP, et al: Uterine cervical carcinoma: comparison of CT and MR findings. Radiology 1990;175:45.

Korobkin M, Callen PW, Fisch AE: CT of the pelvis and retroperitoneum. Radiol Clin North Am 1979;17:301.

Laakman RW, Kaufman B, Hans JS, et al: MR imaging in patients with metallic implants. Radiology 1985;157:711.

Laing F, Benson C, DiSalvo D: Distal ureteral calculus detection with vaginal US. Radiology 1994;192:545.

Laniado M, Kornmesser W, Hamm B, et al: MR imaging of the gastrointestinal tract: value of Gd-DTPA. AJR 1988;150:817.

Lee JKT, Marx MV: Pelvis. In Lee JKT, Sagel SS, Stanley RJ (eds): Computed Body Tomography with MRI correlation. 2nd ed. New York: Raven Press, 1989:851.

Lee JKT, Stanley RJ, Sagel SS, et al: Accuracy of CT in detecting intra-abdominal and pelvic lymph node metastases from pelvic cancers. AJR 1978;131:675.

Levitt RG, Sagel SS, Stanley RJ, et al: Computed tomography of the pelvis. Semin Roentgenol 1978;13:193.

Loeffler W, Laub G: Magnetic resonance angiography. J Can Assoc Radiol 1990;41:19.

Lupetin AR: Female pelvis. In Stark DD, Braley WG Jr (eds): Magnetic resonance imaging. St. Louis: CV Mosby, 1988:1265.

Mark AS, Hricak H: Intrauterine contraceptive devices: MR imaging. Radiology 1987:162:311.

Mark AS, Hricak H, Heinrich LW, et al: Adenomyosis and leiomyoma: differential diagnosis with MR imaging. Radiology 1987;163:527.

Marks WM, Goldberg HI, Moss AA, et al: Intestinal pseudotumors: a problem in computed tomography solved by directed techniques. Gastrointest Radiol 1980;5:155.

McAfee JG, Kopecky RT, Frynoyer PA: Nuclear medicine comes of age: its present and future roles in diagnosis. Radiology 1990;174:609.

McCarthy S, Scott G, Majundar S, et al: Uterine junctional zone: MR study of water content and relaxation properties. Radiology 1989;171:241.

McCarthy S, Tauber C, Gore J: Female pelvic anatomy: MR assessment of variations during the menstrual cycle and with use of oral contraceptives. Radiology 1986;160:119.

McCarthy SM, Stark DD, Filley RA, et al: Obstetrical magnetic resonance imaging: maternal anatomy. Radiology 1985;154:421.

Merritt CR: Ultrasound safety: what are the issues? Radiology 1989;173:304.

Mintz MC, Levy DW, Axel L: Puerperal ovarian vein thrombosis: MR diagnosis. AJR 1987;149:1273.

Mintz MC, Thickman DI, Gussman D, et al: MR evaluation of uterine anomalies. Semin Ultrasound CT MR 1988;9:167.

Mitchell DG: MRI of the adnexae. Semin Ultrasound CT MR 1988; 9:143.

Mitchell DG, Hill NC, Hill H, et al: Serous carcinoma of the ovary: CT identification of metastatic calcified implants. Radiology 1986;158:649.

New PF, Rosen BR, Brady TJ, et al: Potential hazards and artifacts of ferromagnetic and nonferromagnetic surgical and dental materials and devices in nuclear magnetic resonance imaging. Radiology 1983;147:139.

Parsons A, Lense J: Sonohysterography for endometrial abnormalities: preliminary results. J Clin Ultrasound 1993;21:87.

Posniak HV, Olson NC, Dudiak CM, et al: MR imaging of uterine carcinoma: correlation with clinical and pathological findings. RadioGraphics 1990;10:15.

Powers T, Lum A, Patton JA: Abdominal MRI artifacts. Semin Ultrasound CT MR 1989;10:2.

Prasad N, Wright DA, Ford JJ, et al: Safety of 4-T MR imaging: study of effects on developing frog embryos. Radiology 1990; 174:251.

Pykett IL, Newhouse JH, Buoana FS, et al: Principles of nuclear magnetic resonance imaging. Radiology 1982;143:157.

Reuter KL, Daly DC, Cohen SM: Septate versus bicornate uteri: errors in imaging diagnosis. Radiology 1989;172:749.

Rheinhold C, McCarthy S, Bret P, et al: Diffuse adenomyosis: comparison of endovaginal US and MR imaging with histopathologic correlation. Radiology 1996;199:151.

Sawyer RW, Vick CW, Walsh JW, et al: CT of benign ovarian masses. J Comput Assist Tomogr 1985;9:784.

Sawyer RW, Walsh JW: CT in gynecologic pelvic diseases. Semin Ultrasound CT MR 1988;9:122.

Schwartz PE, Kohorn El, Knowlton AN, et al: Routine use of hysterography in endometrial carcinoma and postmenopausal bleeding. Obstet Gynecol 1975;45:378.

Scott WW Jr, Rosenstein NB, Seigelman SS, et al: The obstructed uterus. Radiology 1981;141:767.

Shapeero LG, Hricak H: Mixed müllerian sarcoma of the uterus: MR imaging findings. AJR 1989;153:317.

Shellock FG: Biological effects and safety aspects of magnetic resonance imaging. Magn Reson Q 1989;5:243.

Skaane P, Huebeses KH: Computed tomography of cystic ovarian teratomas with gravity-dependent layering. J Comput Assist Tomogr 1983;7:837.

Smelka R, Reinhold C, Ascher S: MRI of Abdomen and Pelvis. New York: John Wiley & Sons, 1997.

Soules MR, Spadoni CR: Oil versus aqueous media for hysterosalpingography: a continuing debate based on many opinions and few facts. Fertil Steril 1982;38:1.

Sugimura K, Carrington BM, Quivey JM, et al: Postirradiation changes in the pelvis: assessment with MR imaging. Radiology 1990; 175:805.

Thurman A, Jones M, Cohen D: Gynecologic Imaging. Baltimore: Williams & Wilkins, 1997.

Togashi K, Nishimura K, Itoh K, et al: Uterine cervical cancer: assessment with high-field MR imaging. Radiology 1986;160: 431.

Togashi K, Nishimura K, Itoh K, et al: Ovarian cystic teratomas: MR imaging. Radiology 1987;162:669.

Togashi K, Nishimura K, Nakono Y, et al: Cystic pedunculated leiomyomas of the uterus with unusual CT manifestations. J Comput Assist Tomogr 1984;10:642.

Togashi K, Nishimura K, Sagoh T, et al: Carcinoma of the cervix: staging with MR imaging. Radiology 1989a;171:245.

Togashi K, Ozasa H, Konishi I, et al: Enlarged uterus: differentiation between adenomyosis and leiomyomata with MR imaging. Radiology 1989b;171:531.

van Gils AP, Thum RT, Falke TH, et al: Abnormalities of the uterus and cervix after diethylstilbestrol exposure: correlation of findings on MR and hysterosalpingography. AJR 1989;153: 1235.

Vick CW, Walsh JW, Wheelock JB, et al: CT of the normal and abnormal parametria in cervical cancer. AJR 1984a;143:597.

Vick CW, Whitley NO, Walsh JW, et al: Computed tomographic evaluation of parametrial extension from cervical cancer. RadioGraphics 1984b;4:787.

Waggenspack GA, Amparo EG, Hannigan EV, et al: MRI of cervical carcinoma. Semin Ultrasound CT MR 1988;9:158.

Walsh JW, Amendola MA, Hall DJ, et al: Recurrent carcinoma of the cervix: CT diagnosis. AJR 1981;136:117.

Walsh JW, Amendola MA, Konerding KF, et al: Computed tomography detection of pelvic and inguinal lymph node metastases from primary and recurrent pelvic malignant diseases. Radiology 1980;137:157.

Walsh JW, Goplerad DR: Prospective comparison between clinical CT staging in primary cervical carcinoma. AJR 1981;137:997.

Walsh JW, Goplerad DR: Computed tomography of primary, persistent and recurrent endometrial malignancy. AJR 1982;139: 1149.

Weinreb JC, Barkoff ND, Megibow A, Demopoulos R: The value of MR imaging in distinguishing leiomyomas from other solid pelvic masses when sonography is indeterminate. AJR 1990; 154:295.

Weinreb JC, Maravilla KR, Redman HC, Nunnally R: Improved MR imaging of the upper abdomen with glucagon and gas. J Comput Assist Tomogr 1984;8:835.

Welch JJ, Sheedy PF, Johnson CD, et al: CT guided biopsy: prospective analysis of 1,000 procedures. Radiology 1989;171:493.

Wesbey SE, Brasch RC, Engelstad BL, et al: Nuclear magnetic resonance contrast enhancement study of gastrointestinal tract of rats and a human volunteer using nontoxic oral iron solutions. Radiology 1983;149:175.

Whitley NO, Brenner DE, Francis A, et al: Computed tomographic evaluation of carcinoma of the cervix. Radiology 1982; 142:439.

Williams AG, Nettler FA, Wick JD: Cystic and solid ovarian neoplasms. Semin Ultrasound 1983;4:166.

Winfield AC, Henderson-Slayden R, Wentz AC, et al: Hysterosalpingography: comparison of Conray 60 and Sinografin. AJR 1982;138:599.

Winkler ML, Hricak H: Pelvic imaging with MR: techniques for improvement. Radiology 1986;158:848.

Wolf GL: Current status of MR imaging agents: special report. Radiology 1989;172:709.

Wolf SI, Gosink BB, Feldesman MR, et al: Prevalence of simple adnexal cysts in postmenopausal women. Radiology 1991;180: 65.

Worthington JL, Balfe DM, Lee JKT, et al: Uterine neoplasms: MR imaging. Radiology 1986;159:725.

Zawin M, McCarthy S, Scoutt L, et al: Endometriosis: appearance and detection at MR imaging. Radiology 1989;171:693.

6

Design and Methodology of Clinical Studies

John A. Collins

Clinical studies are designed to help physicians make clinical judgments and decisions. Typically physicians' decisions initially concern the choice of diagnostic tests; having arrived at a diagnosis, the clinician then forecasts a likely prognosis. Of course, there will be decisions about treatment, which depend on the balance between benefits and risks; and the discussions may involve judgments about etiology, that is, the cause of the condition, and the likelihood of side effects from the treatment.

Evidence from randomized clinical trials is the most appropriate type of evidence needed to address treatment effectiveness in reproductive endocrinology and infertility. Although randomized clinical trials are needed to avoid bias in estimating treatment effects, diagnostic questions are adequately addressed by well-designed cohort studies, prognosis studies generally comprise follow-up case series, and questions of causation or harm usually are addressed by means of case-control studies. Knowledge of study methodology is thus important to help physicians to assess the relative merits of results that are the product of different design architectures. This chapter discusses the study designs that are most likely to be of clinical value, making use of examples from the field of reproductive endocrinology and infertility. The focus is on the design of studies that relate most clearly to clinical decisions: (1) case series, from which one can learn about prognosis, or the clinical course of a given disease; (2) diagnostic test evaluations (cohort studies); (3) comparative evaluations of the effectiveness of treatment (cohort studies and randomized clinical trials); and (4) overview analysis, a set of quantitative methods that summarize published studies. Space does not allow complete coverage of epidemiologic methods, and therefore the topics of etiology and economic analysis, which also bear on clinical practice, are not covered here. The viewpoint adopted is that of the clinical reader; although guidelines for readers reflect the rules that must be followed by those who are

designing clinical studies, the methodologic detail required for that purpose should be sought from other sources (Petrie, 1982; Friedman et al, 1985; Kelsey et al, 1986). Before discussing study design, a preliminary section draws attention to the increasing importance of published material in clinical decision making. A second introductory section on relevance indicates how to select the studies that are most relevant to the patients in one's practice. Clinical practice is more beneficial for patients and more satisfying for physicians when it is effective. It is the purpose of this chapter to help the reader develop an understanding of clinical study design so that evidence obtained directly from the published original literature can be applied to make clinical decision making more effective.

WHY SHOULD CLINICIANS LEARN STUDY DESIGN?

Knowing the elements of study design enables clinicians to select only the best evidence and thus save time in their busy schedules. Medical practice evolves rapidly and, in fast-developing fields such as reproductive endocrinology and infertility, new information can overwhelm the orderly revision of protocols and management practices. Each year there are more journals and more published studies. Each new development raises questions about whether to adopt new methods and modify old protocols. The answer to questions about changes in clinical practice should depend on the quality of the study design; how trustworthy is each claim about the effectiveness of new methodology? The judicious clinician will incorporate only the best of the new research evidence into his or her practice.

Obviously, published evidence is just one of many factors that influence clinical decisions. The experience, views, and preferences of the patient and the physician may affect or even dominate the action that is finally taken. The question of how research evidence is incorporated into medical practice has been the subject of three general fields of study. The first field is decision analysis, which attempts to assemble all of the published evidence that is related to a single decision pathway. More formally, decision analysis comprises the study of evidence for the utility of diagnostic and treatment decisions to determine the value of practice protocols. Decision analysis is an extension of the algorithm for clinical care, and it makes use of clinical outcomes to quantify the effect of a decision at each node in the decision tree (Richardson and Detsky, 1995a, 1995b). A second field of study deals with how patient and physician preferences influence clinical decision making. One theoretical model that has been applied within the general area of reproductive medical care postulates that decisions to prescribe are based in part on preformed attitudes and perceptions of social pressures from both patients and peers (Ajzen and Fishbein, 1980). Much of the support for such models comes from studies of behavior, and there is very little systematized research to indicate to what extent such formally tested models or the results of decision analysis are generalizable in medical practice. A third area of study evaluates the means by which innovative ideas and technology diffuse among medical professionals. This research takes into account how changes in practice occur at the local level, and relies on qualitative research evidence obtained during interviews of physicians (Greer, 1988). More study is needed because the acknowledged elements of physician learning (age, type of practice, sources of drug information, and number of professional journals read) explain only a small portion of the observed variance in prescribing patterns (Eraker and Politser, 1988).

The informal scheme shown in Figure 6–1 incorporates elements from studies on clinical decision making. It shows how published research evidence may be integrated with personal experience, the views of respected authorities, and the wishes of patients to implement clinical decisions, including those in the field of reproductive endocrinology and infertility.

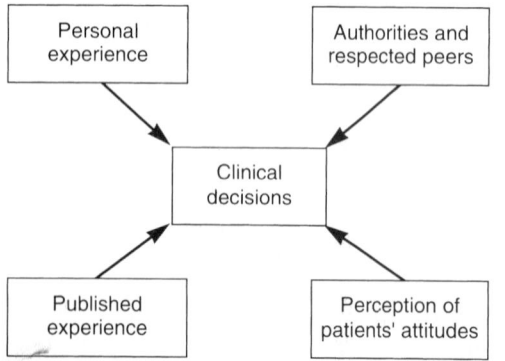

Figure 6–1
Elements of decision making in medical practice.

Personal experience can have a powerful influence on decision making. Years after randomized clinical trials showed that bromocriptine therapy was an ineffective treatment for unexplained infertility, the unproven therapy continues to be prescribed in some practices, presumably on the basis of lower quality evidence: conceptions appear to have followed its use (Wright et al, 1979). Also, personal experience with rare side effects can have an unwarranted inhibiting effect on future practices. The physician whose patient has experienced a quadruplet pregnancy after clomiphene therapy is likely to be extremely cautious about prescribing that drug in future.

The perception of patient's attitudes is a further important component of the clinical decision-making process. Women with reproductive problems and couples with infertility in the 1990s are better equipped than ever before to participate in decision making, a fact that is in part a benefit of the greater public interest in health during the 1980s. This means that, to a greater extent than ever before, clinical decisions can be tailored to the needs of the individual.

Authorities and respected peers also influence individual management decisions. Information is available from external sources in the form of published textbooks, review articles, continuing medical education meetings, annual meetings of clinical societies, hospital rounds and curbside consultations. In an important and valid way, each of these sources makes a contribution to the development of practice protocols, and to clinical decisions.

The main purpose of this chapter is to address the remaining component of the model in Figure 6–1—that is, the published research evidence. Evidence from well-designed clinical studies can reach both the physician and the patient and contribute powerfully to effective clinical practice. The astounding growth in physicians' use of personal computers to access data bases such as Medline indicates that patient problems are increasingly likely to be resolved with the aid of recently published material. The shift in emphasis toward published research evidence may, however, be impeded by two very practical hurdles: clinicians frequently find that the literature is inconsistent, and no one has the time to read all of the papers that might be relevant to a single clinical question. The usefulness of the published research evidence is directly related, however, to the quality of the individual papers, and methodologic quality depends in turn on the authors' attention to study design. As knowledge of study design improves, it is becoming increasingly recognized that, if one selects only the studies with the highest methodologic quality, there is a greater probability that the results will be more consistent (Oxman et al, 1993). Thus focusing on methodologic quality allows the physician to be ruthless in selecting only the papers that are of the highest quality so that the priceless hours that are available for clinical reading can be more productive. For the individual reader, the relevance of a given study to the patients in one's practice is the most important and overriding consideration. Relevance and the issues that determine whether a given paper is applicable to the reader's practice are discussed in the next section.

DETERMINING WHETHER PUBLISHED MATERIAL IS APPLICABLE IN CLINICAL PRACTICE

Physicians are highly motivated to provide better health care, and many do so in part by reading a broad range of literature in order to keep up with new mechanisms of disease and developments in other specialties. Without diminishing the importance of novel concepts, which abound in the challenging clinical and biologic literature, the more appropriate reading for clinicians is that which will have value for patients, leading to more effective therapy, better efficiency, or fewer side effects. To be applicable in practice, then, published material should be relevant to the problems and solutions that occur in practice, encompass representative subjects who are similar to our patients, arise from a persuasive study design, and have not only statistical but also clinical significance.

Relevance (Fig. 6–2)

No one can judge better than the individual specialist whether the new information encountered every day is relevant to his or her patients and their problems. Thus it becomes important to evaluate the clinical sampling frame in the published studies. Do all of the subjects included in the study have the clinical problem as it presents in ordinary practice? If not, the results of the study may not facilitate the decisions that are made from day to day. Second, is the particular prognostic characteristic, diagnostic test, or treatment important in everyday clinical work? Expensive, elaborate, and time-consuming methodology may be interesting but impractical, and it does not make sense to apply valuable reading time in this way.

Representativeness (Fig. 6–2)

A related issue in determining whether a study is worth reading has to do with whether the demography of the study subjects represents the patients in one's practice. For example, are the subjects similar to those in one's practice with respect to age range, education, and pregnancy history? In the case of disorders such as endometriosis, is the reported range of severity typical of the stages seen in one's practice? In studies of infertility, the duration of infertility is an important prognostic characteristic; academic

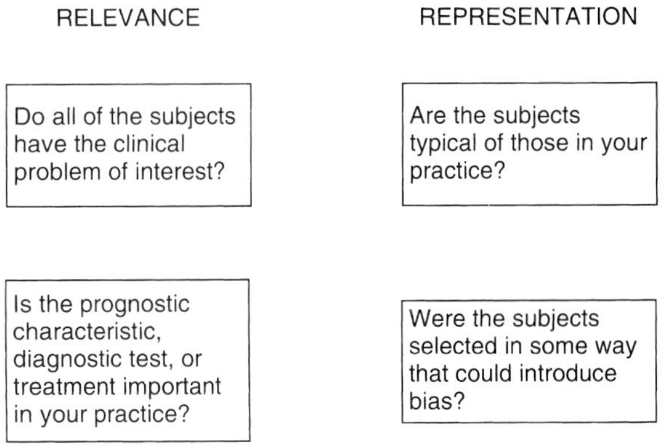

Figure 6–2
Relevance and representation issues in the interpretation of clinical literature.

clinics generally have long waiting lists and longer mean duration of infertility. Thus reported pregnancy rates may be much lower than those observed in practice, and the effect of interventions may be different than in patients with short durations of infertility.

Quality of Study Design

When there is a choice, clinicians should read only the highest quality of evidence that is available; Table 6–1 summarizes the categories of study designs in order of decreasing methodologic quality (Chalmers, 1989). For a number of reasons, the results of *randomized clinical trials* yield the most reliable information with respect to the value of therapy in clinical practice. For the evaluation of both causation and therapy, the randomized clinical trial is the most powerful design because it minimizes bias; also, statistical theory is based on the fundamental importance of chance, which can exist only after randomization. *Cohort studies* are in a second class of quality,

Table 6–1. CLASSIFICATION OF STUDY DESIGNS FOR CLINICAL RESEARCH

I. Experimental Studies
 A. Randomized clinical trials: efficacy trials, management trials, diagnostic trials
 B. "*n* of one" studies: suitable for measurable outcomes but not for terminal events such as pregnancy
II. Observational Studies
 A. Comparative studies
  1. Cohort analytic studies: cases are identified by exposure to an agent or by the inherent characteristics of the individuals (prospective or retrospective)
  2. Case-control studies: cases are identified by the occurrence of a disease or outcome (retrospective)
 B. Descriptive studies: surveys, case series, case reports

Table 6–2. METHODS OF MEASUREMENT IN CLINICAL RESEARCH STUDIES

1. Laboratory Measurements
   a. Research methodology: polymerase chain reaction, blot methodology, growth factors
   b. Clinical methodology: radioreceptor assays, radioimmunoassays, monoclonal antibody methods
2. Clinical Measurements
   a. Physical: blood pressure, weight
   b. Imaging: bone density, endometrial thickness
3. Scores: body mass index, socioeconomic class
4. Counts: hot flushes, number of births, number of deaths, number of oocytes
5. Surveys: categorical and continuous responses to questionnaires

and within this class better designs will be those that also minimize bias. *Case-control studies* represent a third class of persuasiveness, but there are few circumstances in which case-control methodology can be adopted for the evaluation of therapy. Case-control studies find a much more important and widespread application in the study of causation, a subject that is not covered in this chapter (Schlesselman, 1982). Finally, *descriptive studies* can yield important prognostic information, but for understanding the relative value of therapies these noncomparative designs are not helpful.

It is important to recognize that this ordering of study quality is not materially influenced by the type of measurement chosen for a given study. Although advanced laboratory methodology may lend scientific credibility to the accuracy of the results from an individual study, accurate methodology needs to be applied in a randomized design if it is to have an influence on changing clinical practice (Table 6–2). With a randomized design, the simple counting of events may be just as convincing as an elaborate and precise assay method.

Clinical and Statistical Significance

The final point in determining the relevance of published material to our practice is the significance of the study result. The concept of *statistical significance* is in common usage and requires little explanation in this context. It has come to be accepted that a probability (p) of less than 0.05 represents a result that is considered statistically significant, regardless of the test statistic on which the result is based. Conventionally, then, when the probability is less than 1 in 20 that the observed result might have arisen by chance, we are prepared to accept that an effect exists. Having said so, it is important to take into consideration the effect of chance on the performance of multiple comparison tests. The greater the number of comparison tests that are carried out, the greater is the chance that any single one of them may be associated with a p value less than 0.05. For the practicing clinician, a simple (and conservative) approx-

imation to account for the effects of multiple analyses consists of dividing the conventional value (0.05) by the number of statistical comparisons performed; one then uses the new figure as a guide to statistical significance (Lachin, 1982). For example, a trial of an in vitro fertilization (IVF) protocol modification might report five comparisons between cycle results with the new and the standard protocol: number of oocytes, fertilization rates, implantation rates, clinical pregnancy rates, and ongoing pregnancy rates. The appropriate p value would be 0.01—that is, 0.05 divided by 5, the number of comparison statistical tests performed.

Also of importance is *clinical significance*. For example, if a clinical IVF study found that in protocol A one retrieved 8.6 oocytes, while in protocol B one retrieved 8.9 oocytes, the difference might be highly significant if the comparison was made in a large number of cycles. Notwithstanding this statistical significance, the observed difference would be of no importance to the individual patient, and of only marginal importance to protocol designers. Thus, in the interpretation of clinical results, both statistical and clinical significance should be taken into account. These concepts of significance, together with an awareness of the quality of a given study design, the clinician's intrinsic knowledge of the practicability of published interventions, and the comparability of the research subjects with one's patients, all combine to aid in selecting only the worthwhile published research evidence.

CASE SERIES: THE ROLE OF CLINICAL OBSERVATIONS

The majority of published clinical reports fall into the general class of descriptive studies, consisting of case series, case reports, and other studies that are noncomparative in nature. Their usefulness lies in providing information on the prognosis and course of a clinical disorder. Such designs are not useful to evaluate treatment efficacy, but, in relation to follow-up after treatment, these studies provide important information on side effects and complications of therapy. Meticulous study methodology can make the results of follow-up studies more valuable to our understanding of clinical events. A good example is the demonstration that bone density is diminished among young athletes with amenorrhea (Drinkwater et al, 1990). Given that this bone loss may be reversed by changing activity or therapy, the observation has important clinical relevance. A hypothetical example can serve to illustrate study design for prognostic studies; other investigators interested in the bone density results have decided to design a study in which bone density and other conditions and events would be followed over time among similar athletic subjects. Careful attention to detail in the design of such studies can reduce bias of various kinds and improve the effectiveness of the findings

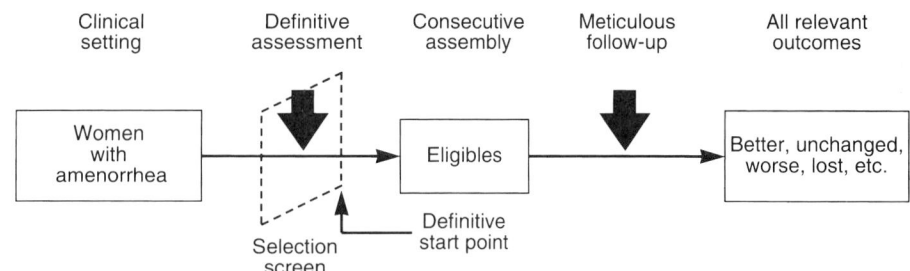

Figure 6-3
An overview of clinical methodology for case series and studies of prognosis.

when applied in clinical practice. The important design issues fall naturally under the headings of recruitment, follow-up, and analysis (Fig. 6–3).

Recruitment

Recruitment is a critical process because detailed care in sample specification sets the stage for all that follows. Although a case series can be assembled retrospectively, these studies have more value when inclusion and exclusion criteria are established prior to recruitment. In the example shown in Figure 6–3, women with amenorrhea would be the general focus of study, but the *inclusion criteria* properly should specify more detail: women with secondary amenorrhea of more than 6 months' duration, referred to a specific clinical setting, within a specified age range, all of whom were subjected to a specified complete and definitive assessment. This assessment should rule out similar but ineligible conditions, and provide information at the starting point with regard to demographic and clinical data and details such as exercise activity that are necessary to initiate the subsequent observations. As the subjects pass through this selection screen, *exclusion criteria* would also be applied; for example, women who are over age 40 years or those who have a history of cancer chemotherapy might be excluded. In order to reduce bias, it is mandatory to recruit subjects in a consecutive manner. If omissions of some subjects are inevitable, then a record should be maintained describing the characteristics of those who refused or were otherwise unable to participate in the study so that readers can evaluate whether the remaining subjects are typical. Institutional review board approval and consent of the subjects are usually required for such studies, even if the clinical procedures are those that would normally be indicated, because the data on study subjects may be reviewed by nonclinical personnel, creating a potential invasion of privacy. Many of the decisions at the point of enrollment require trade-offs between credibility and generalizability. Ensuring that the group under study is as homogeneous as possible (by the use of extensive and strict inclusion and exclusion criteria) means the results of a given study will be more credible. However, if many of the eligible subjects are eliminated by selection screens and refusal to participate, the remaining subjects will not be typical, and the study

results may not be generalizable to other clinics or practices.

Follow-up

Careful follow-up always begins with a definitive starting point. In the example shown in Figure 6–3, the starting point would be selected from among several options: the date of the last menstrual period at the start of the period of amenorrhea, the date of presentation to the specified clinical settings, or the date of the baseline assessment, if a physical measurement such as bone density was the key feature of follow-up. If the case series is one in which observations are made during and after the treatment of the subjects, then the start date may coincide with the first date of the specified treatment. The decision depends upon the specific question, but the starting point must be uniform for all subjects. During the period of follow-up, reasonable contact should be maintained with all subjects. Widely spaced intervals of contact tend to lead to increased loss to follow-up, whereas overly frequent follow-up visits can lead to noncompliance. Because the frequency of interurban mobility in the reproductive age group in North America is high, follow-up at 3-month intervals is often indicated to ensure that contact is maintained with the maximum number of subjects.

Outcome Assessment

A revealing measure of the quality of a given case series is the completeness of the outcome assessment. In the example in Figure 6–3, the outcomes might include return of menses, initiation of cyclic medication, or the induction of ovulation, among other possibilities. Other clinically relevant events that might occur during such a follow-up would include pregnancy and loss to follow-up. In the given example, a set of measured outcomes such as bone density and endometrial thickness might also be available for the observed subjects.

All of the clinically relevant outcomes should be reported in sufficient detail to understand what happened to each subject. In many clinical studies the outcome is dichotomous; an event does or does not occur. For example, in studies of infertility, the outcome of interest is pregnancy, and each subject experiences either a successful event (conception) or no event (failure to conceive). That dichotomy is useful for statistical purposes and is the basis of survival or life table analysis. For a more complete understanding of the outcome of such a study, however, one would want to know, for those subjects who conceived, the rate of live births, perinatal deaths, abortions, and ectopic pregnancies and, for those who did not conceive, the rate of loss to follow-up, the frequency of adoption, and the rate with which couples resolved or discontinued their interest in infertility management.

Where the follow-up is reasonably short, a simple statement of the proportion of subjects who experience each relevant outcome, together with confidence limits, would provide the important clinical information. This statement might be amplified to include a comparison combined with appropriate statistics, if the case series is one that naturally divides the subjects into two or more groups on the basis of age or some other inherent characteristic. In many follow-up studies, because events occur over time, a more precise estimate of the clinical importance of such events can be gained with the use of survival analysis.

Survival Analysis

Survival analysis is a class of statistical procedures for estimating an event rate over time. Such events are usually referred to as failures, although the event may in fact be a success, such as pregnancy. Because these procedures were first introduced in clinical practice for the study of cancer, the term *survival analysis* is now applied whenever an analysis makes use of time to an event or life table procedures. Life table procedures or product limit estimates of cumulative event rates, together with appropriate statistical methods, can evaluate the significance of an event over time in a univariate or multivariate analysis (Cox and Oakes, 1984). In every case, the time-table of clinical events occurring among subjects must be restated for purposes of life table analysis (Fig. 6–4). In this new example, women with amenorrhea received treatment for infertility and their experience was recorded. Subject 1 was in the study for approximately 9.5 months before conceiving, and subject 2 was in the study for approximately 18 months. If our analysis is to be restricted to 2 years of entry and follow-up, then subject 2 would not be considered to have experienced an event even if she conceived in month 25. Subject 3 became lost to follow-up after approximately 9 months because the casebook was not closed when she moved away without notice. Subject 4 is considered not eligible because registration occurred after assembly was completed.

Although in designing any case series it is important to take note of all clinically relevant outcomes, for the purposes of survival analysis only one outcome can be considered in an individual analysis. In the original example shown in Figure 6–3, one analysis could evaluate time to menses, or time to a request for treatment, but not both. Also, the investigation can evaluate loss to follow-up as an event, by making use of that element of the data collection. Survival analysis also allows for comparisons between groups. For a case series that consists of a single group under study, some natural division in the subjects might be worthy of study. For the subjects in Figure 6–3, does the return to menses occur earlier

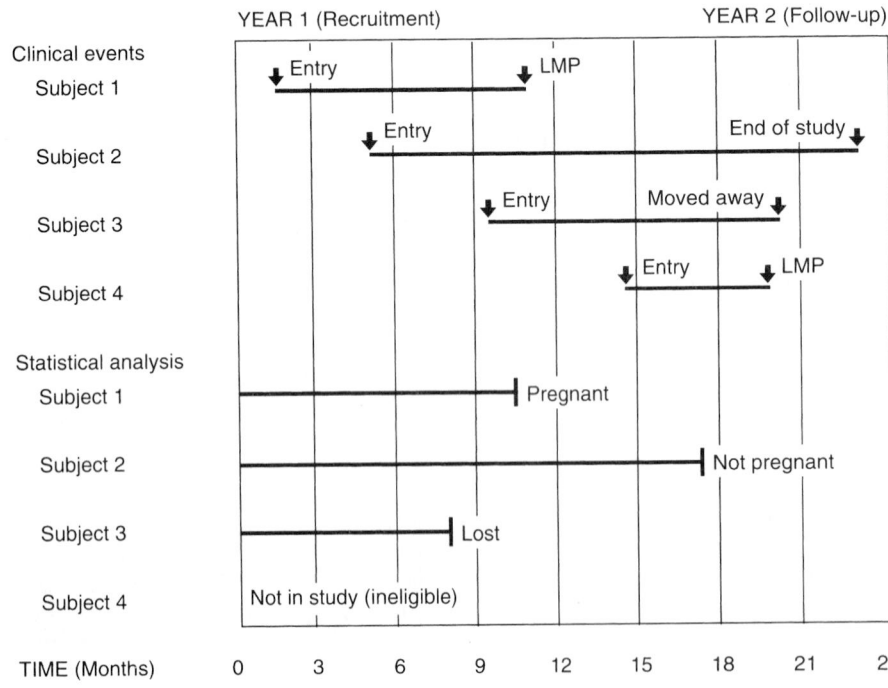

Figure 6–4
The conversion of clinical events to time under observation for statistical analysis. LMP, Last menstrual period.

among younger subjects than among those older than, say, age 30? For such purposes, one can use either the confidence limits of the estimates of cumulative events, or statistical tests based on the *chi-square statistic* (Table 6–3). The latter method is preferable because it compares data from all of the intervals of observation (Peto et al, 1977). It is possible that one or more baseline characteristics might predict an outcome such as the return of menses among women with amenorrhea. The investigator may wish to know whether the influence of age is most important, or does the presence of other characteristics in different proportions within the two age groups lead to a better clinical outcome in the younger women? Most computer programs offer a choice of statistics for the comparison of cumulative event rates stratified by one or two predictor variables. In order to evaluate more than one or two predictor variables, it is preferable to make use of a multivariate type of survival analysis.

Multivariate forms of survival analysis can be used for making inferences about the effects of treatments, prognostic factors, exposures, and other covariates on the survival function, or event rate. The *proportional hazards model* is used most frequently in clinical studies (Cox, 1972). Unlike other methods, the proportional hazards model is nonparametric and adapts to the data as distributed; therefore, its use does not assume a normal or other discrete distribution and the transformation of data is not required. With proportional hazards analysis, one can evaluate the occurrence of an event such as the return of menses over a period of time, while adjusting for the effect of prognostic factors (such as age, previous menstrual history, body mass index, etc.). The analysis also allows for events that may arise in the course of follow-up, such as treatment (or weight loss during follow-up in the Fig. 6–3 example), through the use of "time-dependent" covariates. The analyst must ensure that the hazard or event rate is proportional in each stratum of subjects, a condition that is not often limiting. When one wishes to compare two groups, the analysis yields a *relative risk* or relative probability of the outcome in one group (e.g., the older women with amenorrhea) compared with a reference group (the younger women). This relative risk is adjusted because it takes into account the baseline differences between the groups, events

during observation, and time to return of menses or completion of study. The expression of relative risks with their confidence limits can be directly applied in clinical decisions, and the inferences can also be useful in understanding the biologic implications of clinical observations. It must be noted, however, that although the issues may be compelling questions, and the statistical analysis may be sophisticated, even the most powerful statistical analysis cannot compensate for the bias that arises from post-hoc analyses, such as those that are possible within uncontrolled studies.

Although the design has limitations, case series may have an important role in the development of the clinical understanding of prognosis, and in stimulating further studies through the generation of hypotheses that can be evaluated in more powerful designs.

STUDY DESIGN FOR THE EVALUATION OF DIAGNOSTIC TESTS

The diagnostic process in clinical medicine consists of the application of tests that have been selected on the basis of information from the history and physical examination, to confirm or rule out the presence of disease. In practice, the number of diagnostic tests ordered in response to a given set of clinical conditions varies widely from clinician to clinician. An awareness of the principles of study design for the evaluation of diagnostic tests can serve two purposes in clinical practice: first, that knowledge can be used to increase the efficiency and economy of diagnostic protocols in current use; second, that knowledge can be used to evaluate the clinical literature. Space does not permit a thorough discussion of the use of diagnostic tests for other purposes, such as the monitoring of therapy, or as screening tests. Just as more effective therapy can be beneficial for patients and more satisfying for clinicians, a more accurate and better directed diagnostic process also leads to superior practice.

Basic Elements of Diagnosis

The clinical use of a diagnostic test is for prediction; a given test result predicts the likelihood of disease

Table 6–3. HYPOTHETICAL FOLLOW-UP STUDY AMONG EUGONADOTROPHIC UNMARRIED WOMEN AGES 18 TO 44 YEARS WITH SECONDARY AMENORRHEA

AGE GROUP	NUMBER OF SUBJECTS	TIME (MONTHS) TO RETURN TO REGULAR MENSES Mean	SD	CUMULATIVE PROPORTION "CURED" AT 12 MONTHS (% ± 95% CL)	CHI-SQUARE 1 df	p Value
18–30 years	25	8	6	64 ± 11%		
31–44 years	32	11	7	43 ± 8%	4.3	0.04

Abbreviations: CI, confidence interval; df, degree of freedom.

Table 6-4. DEFINITION OF POSITIVE AND NEGATIVE PREDICTIVE VALUES

PARAMETER	CALCULATION	DEFINITION
Positive predictive value (PPV)	$a/(a + b)$	Probability of true disease given an abnormal test result
Negative predictive value (NPV)	$d/(c + d)$	Probability of no disease given a normal test result
Prevalence	$(a + c)/n$	Frequency of true disease among all those tested

in the individual patient. The aggregate of the test results in all patients can show which tests are better at discriminating between disease and nondisease states. The practical value of the diagnostic test result is expressed by the predictive values: the *positive predictive value*, or proportion of diseased individuals among those with an abnormal test result; and the *negative predictive value*, or the proportion of individuals without disease among those with a normal result (Table 6-4). Discrimination is usually expressed in terms of *sensitivity*, the likelihood that an abnormal test result will occur among diseased people, and *specificity*, the likelihood that a normal test result will occur among normal people.

Two-by-Two Table

Reduced to its fundamental purpose, the diagnostic test predicts the presence or absence of disease, and thus the outcome is usually dichotomous. If a perfect test existed, its results also would be clearly divided into two distinct categories. Thus the basic element for the evaluation of diagnostic tests is the two-by-two table, illustrated in Figure 6-5. In such tables, the accepted diagnostic criterion for the outcome, that is, the gold standard, is the basis for the assessment of the diagnostic test result. Sensitivity and specificity can be defined from the cells of the table:

$$\text{Sensitivity} = a \div (a + c)$$

$$\text{Specificity} = d \div (b + d)$$

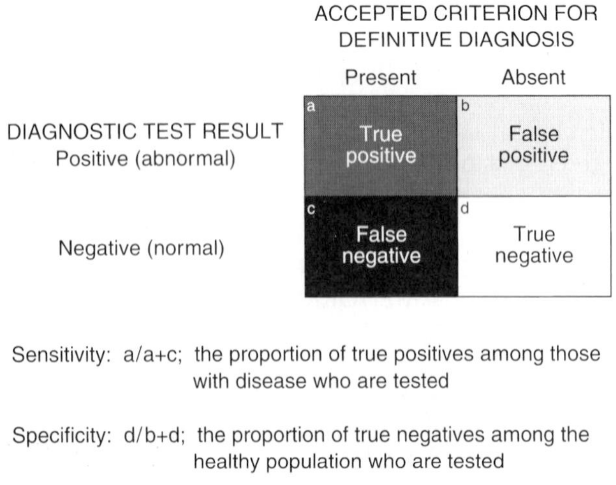

Sensitivity: a/a+c; the proportion of true positives among those with disease who are tested

Specificity: d/b+d; the proportion of true negatives among the healthy population who are tested

Figure 6-5
The conventional two-by-two table for the assessment of a diagnostic test.

The total of true positives and true negatives $(a + d)$ as a proportion of all subjects is the expression of the overall accuracy of the diagnostic test. The predictive values also can be defined according to the cells of the two-by-two table (Table 6-4).

Gold Standard

Central to the understanding of studies that evaluate diagnostic tests is the selection of a criterion or reference standard. The ultimate standard in the case of infertility, for example, is a live-born child, because that is the outcome of interest to the infertile couple. It follows that the disease state is continuing infertility and the normal state is the occurrence of live birth. Not all diagnostic studies in the field of infertility are based on so definite an outcome, however, because one must often make use of substitute standards such as clinical pregnancy or successful fertilization during IVF cycles. Although the use of substitute standards can help to clarify the relationships between fertility factors and improve our understanding of reproductive processes, the gold standard is the most definitive approximation of the outcome of interest that is available for study. The use of such a high standard is not without problems, because other factors may intervene between the test result and the measurement of the standard.

Effect of Prevalence

A further consideration in the understanding of study designs for the evaluation of diagnostic tests is the effect of the prevalence of disease on diagnostic test results. Often the subjects collected in a diagnostic study are not representative of those seen in clinical practice. The study patients are selected (some have probably dropped out after completing only a part of the screening protocol); and the study subjects usually come from the more severe end of the spectrum of disease (only those who could not be managed in a community hospital would be referred to a tertiary center where such studies are done). Thus the prevalence of disease, or of severe disease, is often higher in reported subjects than among those seen in day-to-day practice. Also, the results of the test under study might determine whether the reference test is performed. In the literature on the relative accuracy of hysterosalpingography and laparoscopy in the diagnosis of tubal patency, the prevalence of bilateral tubal obstruction in 18 reports in the aggregate data is 33%, compared

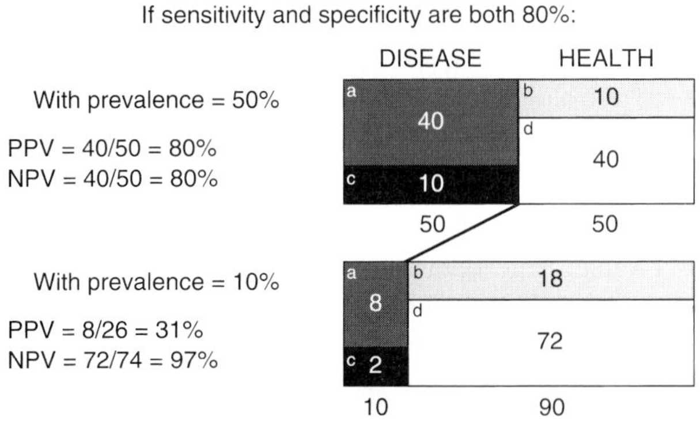

If sensitivity and specificity are both 80%:

DISEASE   HEALTH

With prevalence = 50%

PPV = 40/50 = 80%
NPV = 40/50 = 80%

	DISEASE	HEALTH
a	40	b 10
c	10	d 40
	50	50

With prevalence = 10%

PPV = 8/26 = 31%
NPV = 72/74 = 97%

	DISEASE	HEALTH
a	8	b 18
c	2	d 72
	10	90

Figure 6 – 6

The effect of changes in prevalence on negative predictive value (NPV) and positive predictive value (PPV) of a diagnostic test.

with 10% or less in the average infertility practice (Collins, 1988). The prevalence is high in the reported studies because a normal hysterosalpingogram may not lead to a laparoscopy, and these normal results are thus excluded from the study sample. Such large discrepancies in prevalence have an effect on the predictive values, as shown in Figure 6–6. If a diagnostic test with 80% sensitivity and 80% specificity is applied in a group of 100 individuals where the prevalence of disease is 50%, both the positive and the negative predictive values will be 80%. If the same diagnostic test is applied among 100 individuals where the prevalence is 10%, however, the positive predictive value falls to 31% and the negative predictive value rises to 97%. Depending on whether the positive or the negative predictive value is more useful, a reasonably discriminating test (good sensitivity and specificity) may turn out to be more or less valuable when it is applied in clinical practice. Thus diagnostic tests may be less useful when the results are in subjects with a typical spectrum of disease, even though the test appears to be valuable among highly selected patients in a given published report. With the impact of these principles of diagnostic testing in mind, one can be better prepared to examine studies designed to evaluate diagnostic tests (Sackett et al, 1985).

Sample Specification

Once again, recruitment is the key to a successful study; the clinical setting in which subjects are identified and the predetermined inclusion and exclusion criteria should be specified in advance and followed meticulously (Fig. 6–7). It is essential to define a uniform start point for the observations if there is a time interval between the test and the determination of the reference standard. In studies to evaluate diagnostic tests, as in studies of prognosis, consecutive assembly is important to avoid bias in the recruitment of subjects.

Diagnostic Test Result

In a diagnostic assessment, the test result divides the sample into two groups (normal result vs. abnormal result) in a reasonably unbiased manner. Thus random allocation is not strictly necessary provided that the outcome assessment is not conditioned by the test result.

Because the study in question is based on a diagnostic test, some information is needed on how the test result is expressed, and supporting data should indicate the accuracy of and reproducibility of the test methodology. Given the nature of biologic data, the results of diagnostic tests are often distributed in ways that are not clearly dichotomous. Thus it becomes necessary to choose a cut point in the range of diagnostic test results, in order to define normal and abnormal. Although sensitivity and specificity can be considered to be stable properties of a diagnostic test, because they do not change when different proportions of diseased and well patients are tested, these properties do fluctuate mutually when different cutoff values are chosen (Griner et al, 1981). Thus the choice of a cut point reflects a trade-off between better sensitivity and better specificity. Several methods exist for choosing a cut point when a diagnostic test is under evaluation. The highest value of the mean of sensitivity and specificity may be used to select the optimum cut point. Also, when sensitivity is plotted against specificity in a receiver operating characteristics curve, an ideal diagnostic

Figure 6 – 7

An overview of methodology for clinical studies to evaluate diagnostic tests.

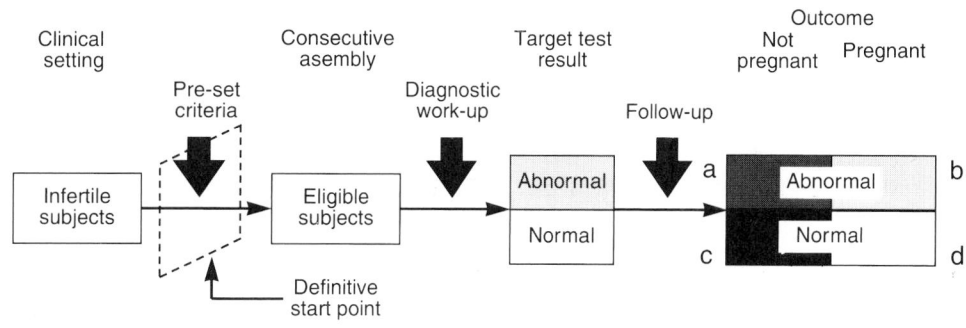

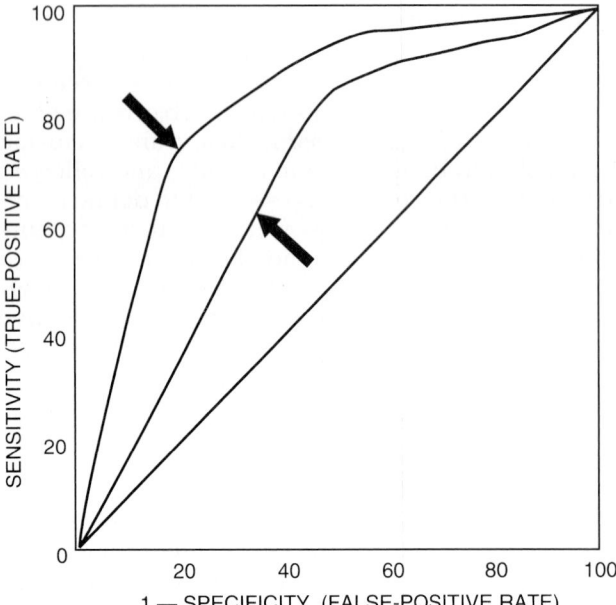

Figure 6–8
Receiver operating characteristics curve to aid in the selection of an optimum cut point for a diagnostic test.

test cut point would fall on that point of the curve that lies closest to the upper left-hand corner of the plot (Fig. 6–8) (Jaeschke et al, 1994a, 1994b).

Which Diagnostic Test Properties Should Be Evaluated?

If the study design has satisfactory selection criteria, and the consecutive assembly of a representative set of subjects, there remains the choice of which diagnostic test property should be the focus of the diagnostic test evaluation. Although sensitivity and specificity are often used to determine the overall quality of one diagnostic test compared with other similar tests, these properties are less useful to the

clinician because they express only the likelihood that an abnormal test result will occur among diseased people (sensitivity), and the likelihood of a normal test result among normal people (specificity). For clinical purposes the predictive values are most useful, provided one takes into account the shift in these values that occurs in response to changes in prevalence. Also useful are the *likelihood ratios* (LRs), which describe in numerical terms the relative worth of each type of test result; based on sensitivity and specificity, LRs show virtually no response to variability in prevalence. Finally, an estimate of agreement such as the kappa statistic can be useful as a global indicator of the value of a given diagnostic test (Eden et al, 1989). Although LRs and kappa are infrequently used to evaluate diagnostic tests, the potential clinical value of these expressions merits further consideration.

Because of the above-noted limitations of predictive values, in some situations the LRs may be preferable estimators of test quality. LRs separately quantify the performance of abnormal and normal test results and, because they are derived from sensitivity and specificity, do not fluctuate with prevalence (Schecter and Scheps, 1985). The likelihood ratio for a normal test (LR−) expresses the likelihood of disease over the likelihood of nondisease with normal test results. The likelihood ratio of an abnormal test (LR+) expresses the likelihood of disease over the likelihood of nondisease given abnormal test results. The quality of the diagnostic test is expressed by increasing distance from unity (LR+) or decreasing distance from unity (LR−) (Fig. 6–9). With some diagnostic tests, negative predictive values and normal test results are less useful because of the extremely low prevalence of disease, or because other untested conditions caused the diseased state (e.g., normal test results in a diagnostic assessment of male infertility do not necessarily predict a fertile state). The use of LRs permits an assessment of the abnormal test in isolation; if the abnormal test result performs extremely well, a dysfunctional normal test result may be more acceptable.

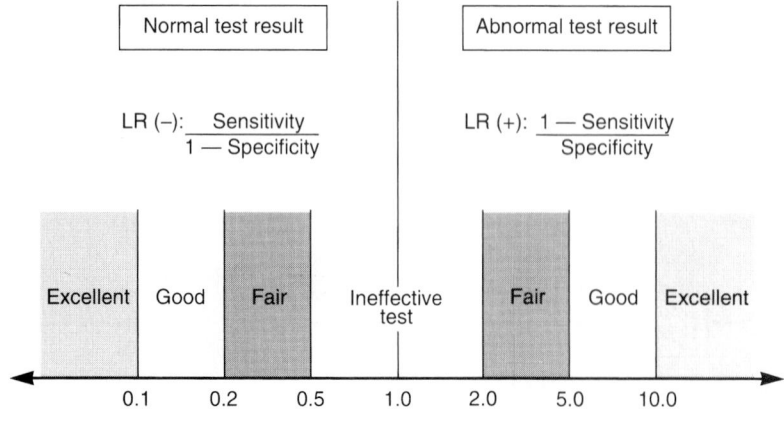

Figure 6–9
The definition and distribution of the likelihood ratios (LRs) to estimate the quality of a diagnostic test.

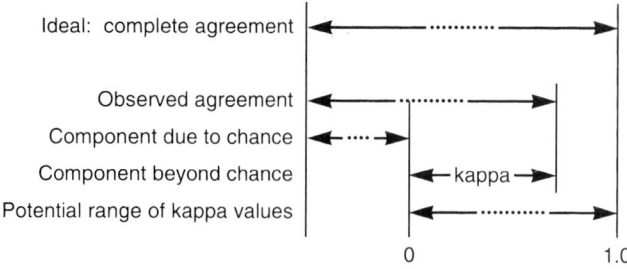

Figure 6–10
Definition and illustration of kappa as estimate of agreement between independent ratings of an observation.

When one is evaluating several diagnostic tests, another choice is the *kappa statistic*, which is an estimate of the agreement beyond chance (Fleiss, 1981). If one considers the diagnostic test and the gold standard to be two independent ratings of disease or nondisease, then a portion of the observed agreement is due to chance (Fig. 6–10). Kappa is the ratio of the observed excess beyond chance over the maximum possible excess beyond chance, and it usually varies from 0 to 1. Kappa values less than 0.4 represent poor agreement, and values greater than 0.75 reflect excellent agreement.

Studies that evaluate diagnostic tests, if carefully planned, can reduce bias and also achieve representativeness. As with the development of therapy, where explanatory trials may be necessary before one can plan management trials, two stages may be required in the development of a diagnostic test. In the first stage, the test should be evaluated in a relatively pure and homogeneous selected clinical group to determine whether the test makes an isolated and independent contribution to the diagnostic evaluation. To evaluate its effectiveness in practice, however, the test should be evaluated in a typical sample of subjects who have a broad spectrum of disorders similar to the clinical problem of interest.

STUDY DESIGNS FOR THE EVALUATION OF TREATMENT: COHORT STUDIES

In traditional epidemiology, cohort studies take note of what happens to exposed and nonexposed subjects during a period of time to estimate the relative risk of a given outcome. The exposure in question may be some inherent or external noxious influence that is postulated to have an effect on the outcome event (Kelsey et al, 1986). This conventional use of cohort studies can be modified to evaluate treatment; in such cases the exposure is defined as the treatment under study. In cohort studies adapted for this purpose, a treated group is compared with an untreated group, or a new treatment is compared with a standard treatment. Cohort study designs are less powerful than studies based on random allocation because the allocation to one group or the other in cohort studies arises as a result of physician or patient choice, which can lead to important baseline differences between the groups. Any apparent difference between the results might then be due to baseline differences in prognostic variables rather than to the treatment in one group. Cohort studies may be carried out in a prospective manner, when the investigators set out the sample specification in advance and begin to recruit patients according to an explicit protocol. In retrospective cohort studies, the investigators go back in time to document events in patient records, where the groups to be compared are defined by the exposure (treated, not treated).

Sample Specification

In the hypothetical example in Figure 6–11, the investigators are interested in the effects of a drug on facial hirsutism. They would then gather together patients who exceeded a specified threshold of hairiness, subject them to a definitive assessment, and select those who are eligible according to preset criteria. In this design, as in previous study types, consecutive assembly of the eligible subjects is essential in order to avoid the bias that arises from the informal exclusion of certain patients. A complete clinical description of the subjects is also essential, because it is very likely (as we shall see in a moment) that the treatment groups will differ in some fundamental ways. An estimate of the required sample size should be calculated, based on reasonable predictions of the expected differences between the groups, as evaluated by conventional significance and power

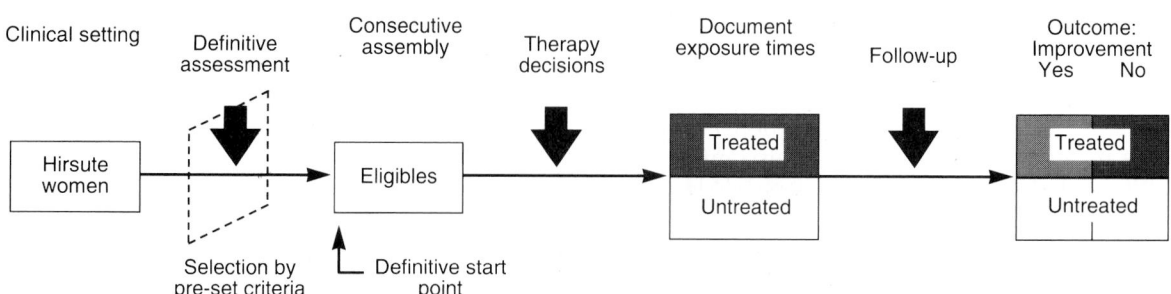

Figure 6–11
Methodology for a cohort analytic comparative study.

considerations. (Sample size considerations are discussed further in the section on randomized trials.)

Document the Exposure

Because cohort studies take place in clinical practice settings, therapy decisions will be based on practice algorithms and patient need. To be useful, however, studies should report more detail than would ordinarily be needed in patient management. Details of dosage, starting and finishing dates, compliance, and concurrent medications are an essential part of the record. In the given example of women with facial hirsutism, decisions to prescribe treatment will occur much more commonly where the hirsutism is severe, thus leading to an obvious difference between the treated and untreated groups. In this case a detailed description of the baseline extent of excess hair is essential, and the scoring system should preferably be one that has been independently validated.

Follow-up to Outcome

The results of cohort analytic comparative studies are more convincing when the outcome is clear cut and well defined. Examples of such clear outcomes include pregnancy and the return of menses. Where the outcome is based on an objective assessment by an independent observer, as would occur when a radiologist reports on the number of ovarian follicles in response to a cycle of superovulation, reasonably convincing results are also possible. In the case of the example here or any other subjective assessment, and particularly if the assessment of response is being graded by the same individual who prescribed the treatment, a range of biases are introduced that seriously undermine the credibility of the results.

Methods of expressing the treatment effect in cohort comparative studies are shown in Table 6–5. *Odds ratios* are usually reported from case-control studies, and relative risks from cohort studies. When *b* and *d* are large numbers relative to *a* and *c*, however, the odds ratio is a near approximation of the relative risk. It would be unusual to find, after a cohort analytic comparative study had been completed, that the comparison groups were equal in all important respects. Even in that rare instance there might be differences in unknown determinants of outcome. Thus it is unlikely that the unadjusted relative risk could serve to represent the true treatment effect. Far more likely is the condition where baseline differences in the comparison groups also influence the likelihood of a successful outcome. Thus, although simple assessments of outcome such as the relative risk or the odds ratio are preferable, a multivariate analysis that adjusts for these baseline differences is usually required. This is not the place to consider which of numerous methods is appropriate, or the relative merits of each type of methodology.

Table 6–5. METHODS OF ANALYSIS FOR COHORT COMPARISON STUDIES

Relative risk	$[a/(a + b)]/[c/(c + d)]$
Odds ratio	ad/bc
Adjusted odds ratio	Logistic regression
Adjusted relative risk	Proportional hazards analysis

Both logistic regression and proportional hazards analysis are reasonably accessible, comprehensible, and practicable for clinical investigators.

Table 6–6 summarizes the strengths and weaknesses of cohort analytic studies when applied to the assessment of treatment. The most important strength of these studies is that the observations are made in the course of ordinary practice because the subjects are not selected on the basis of protocols and consent to randomization. Despite these strengths, the bias that arises from baseline differences and other sources created a serious problem in the interpretation of the results, and thus in their application in clinical practice.

STUDY DESIGN FOR THE EVALUATION OF THERAPY: RANDOMIZED CLINICAL TRIALS

The role of chance is a fundamental assumption in the application of statistical theory, and random allocation to treatment groups is the means by which the play of chance is ensured in clinical studies. Thus randomization is the key element of a comparative study design, and the absence of randomization detracts from the credibility of a given study. The introduction of randomization is not by itself sufficient to reduce bias, however, and clinical investigators must pay careful attention to issues in the assembly of groups, in the maneuver, and in the definition of the outcome and its analysis (Friedman et al, 1985). The assembly, the maneuver and the outcome assessment are the key elements in the development

Table 6–6. STRENGTHS AND WEAKNESSES OF COHORT ANALYTIC STUDIES WHEN USED FOR THE EVALUATION OF THERAPY

STRENGTHS

The subjects are representative of clinical practice
The selection is unbiased by trial protocols
More than one treatment group can be simultaneously evaluated
All reasonable outcomes may be assessed

WEAKNESSES

Crucial baseline differences are common
The bias of both doctor and patient determine the treatment group
There may be competing interventions in a single subject
The analysis is complicated by different treatment and observation times

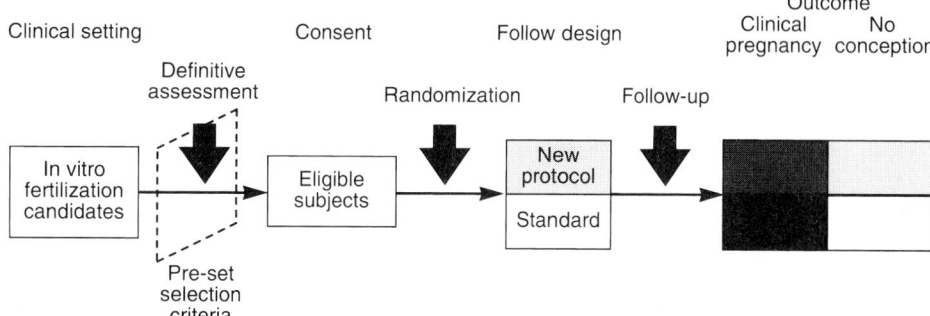

Figure 6–12
Methodology for a randomized clinical trial.

of the question, which is the essential first step in the design of a randomized clinical trial (Fig. 6–12).

Sample Specification

Having defined the target population in a clear and specific way, eligibility rules need to be established so that one can achieve a balance between homogeneity and heterogeneity. One would achieve a homogeneous sample by selecting similar subjects who are highly selected after careful screening. This is a good strategy for explanatory trials, which are designed to evaluate the efficacy of a single treatment in isolation from other influences. Use of heterogeneous samples, in which one accepts typical clinical subjects, is a good strategy for management trials. In management trials one wants to include subjects who will be typical of those with disease in the population in order to evaluate how effective the treatment might be in the average health care setting. Thus the inclusion and exclusion criteria should be carefully developed in the light of the purpose of the trial. The criteria should be based on knowledge of demographic data within the target population so that one can be reasonably sure that the sample size requirements can be met from among the eligible group. When the question covers subjects who might come from two prognosis groups (as in an IVF trial where some candidates might have a degree of seminal deficiency), the investigators should consider stratifying the subjects so that equal numbers within each prognosis group are randomly allocated to each treatment group.

The required sample size is dependent upon both statistical and clinical considerations. The clinical considerations require investigators to take into account the success associated with standard therapy, and the improvement with the new therapy that would be important enough to make a difference in clinical management. That difference is usually referred to as the clinical difference, or δ. The statistical considerations begin with conventional estimates of *type I error* (α), which allows for the possibility that the results with the new therapy might be better than the standard therapy purely by chance; in statistical terms we accept this possibility in 1 of 20 trials ($\alpha = 0.05$). Usually the new treatment could be better or worse than the standard treatment, so that one would consider a two-tailed α (α_2). When $\alpha_2 = 0.05$, or 5%, it represents the sum of the extreme 2.5% of each side of the normal distribution. Less frequently, the new protocol can only be better than the standard protocol, and one would make use of only one half of the probability curve and consider a one-tailed α ($\alpha_1 = 0.05$); there is a corresponding reduction in sample size. Investigators also need to allow for *type II error* (β), that is, the error of not discovering a true difference when it exists. Conventional levels of β are usually set in the range of 0.1 to 0.2, so that the trial would have 90% or 80% power, respectively, to detect a true difference. The way in which the interplay among these statistical and clinical considerations may affect sample size is shown in Figure 6–13. In general, the sample size requirement is increased by reductions in α, β, or δ. The process of arriving at an appropriate sample size thus involves both statistical input and clinical judgment (Lachin, 1982).

The Maneuver

A number of issues need to be sorted out with respect to randomization. First, randomization should be as free of bias as is practically possible. A random number generator should be used, and ideally the allocation should be determined by telephone, or by some process that is removed from the clinical care setting. All other attempts to allow chance to determine allocation are open to systematic bias, so that the use of hospital numbers, alternate days, and so on are not acceptable methodology.

The intervention itself should be exactly specified, and numerous methodologic details need to be worked out in the administration of the alternate treatments, in order to ensure that blinding is not only possible but carried out. Double blinding is always preferable, but, in the case of a clear and well-defined outcome, practical considerations may take precedence. Investigators who are designing studies of treatment in normal clinical settings must take pains to reduce the extent of co-intervention (the administration of other treatments) and contamination (the cross-contamination of one treatment arm by the administration of the other treatment). Compliance

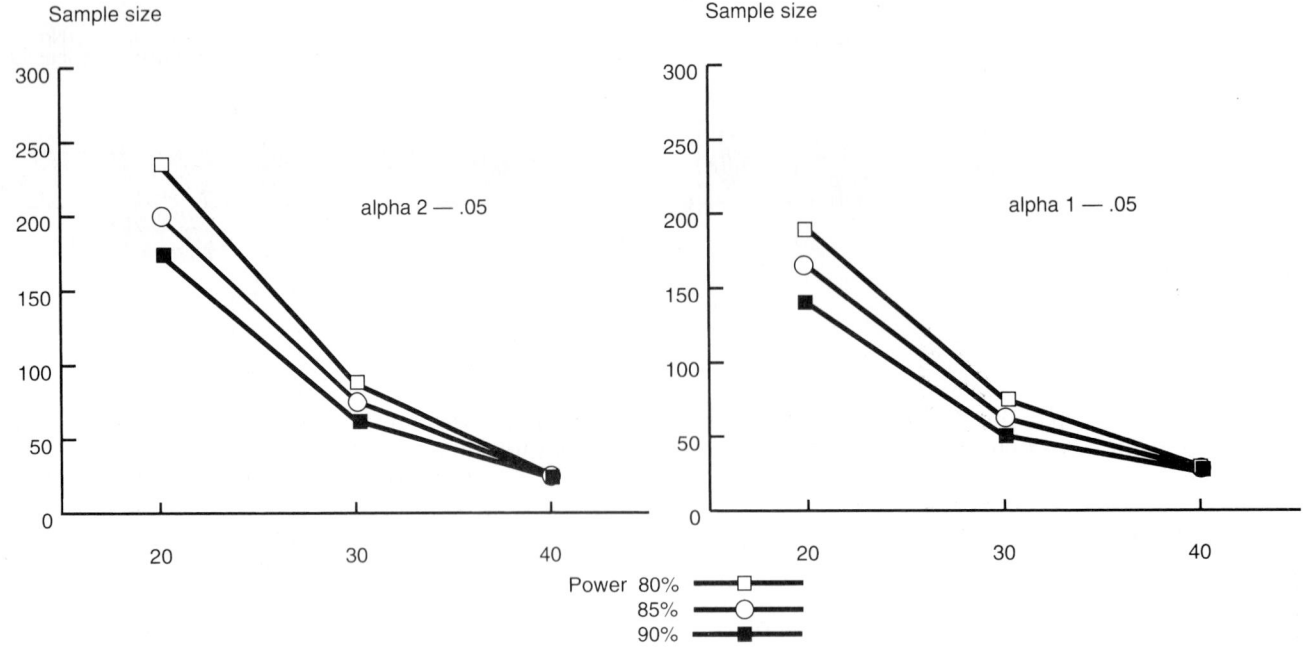

Figure 6–13

The interplay among α (type I error), β (type II error), and δ (the clinical difference) in the estimation of sample size for clinical trials: expected outcome with new treatment (20%, 30%, 40%) versus standard therapy (10%).

and loss to follow-up are other issues that should be taken into account in developing the final sample size requirements.

The phrase "randomized, controlled, double-blind, crossover trial" has come to be recognized as the gold standard of therapy trials. The appropriateness of a crossover design must be reviewed, however, in studies associated with treatments in the field of reproductive endocrinology and infertility. Crossover designs were developed so that each patient receives both the experimental and the control treatments. They are most applicable where there is considerable variability between patients and less variability from time to time in the same patient. The crossover design is appropriate only when there are short-term changes resulting from therapy and when these changes are rapidly reversed (Petrie, 1982). Such a design is useful in chronic disease states, where it is very likely that the baseline state of the disorder will not change during the entire period of the trial before and after the crossover. Crossover designs have been used effectively, for example, in the assessment of estrogen therapy for menopausal hot flushes. However, crossover designs are not appropriate in studies with an endpoint such as pregnancy, because the endpoint is final and the baseline state of the disorder is unalterably changed. Individuals who conceive during the first period are not available for study during the second period, thus introducing imbalance. Trials in which treatment is randomly allocated in the first cycle and then alternated are open to the same criticism. If treatment is randomly allocated in each cycle, the random se-

quence should be stratified by cycle, in order to take into account the lower prognosis in subsequent cycles. There are now a sufficient number of randomized clinical trials in reproductive medicine to test whether the crossover design has an influence on the magnitude of the reported treatment effect. The empirical evidence indicates that the crossover design overestimates the treatment effect by about 75%, after adjusting for differences among the reported trials (ESHRE Capri Workshop, 1996).

The Outcome and Analysis

In defining the question at the beginning of the design process, the investigator must determine which specific outcome among the range of choices that usually exists will be defined as the primary outcome. In the example given in Figure 6–12, a range of outcomes are recorded in IVF protocols. One might consider, for example, the number of oocytes retrieved, the number of embryos transferred to the uterus, the proportion of pregnancies including chemical pregnancies, the proportion of clinical pregnancies, or live birth. In making such a choice, the investigator should lean very heavily toward live birth, the clinical outcome that is of primary interest to the subject, and therefore of primary interest from the health care evaluation standpoint. Other outcomes are important, and may be considered in secondary analyses, but for the purpose of communicating the results of the trial, a specific and clearly defined primary outcome is essential. In any publication describing such a trial, one would expect to find evidence that this primary outcome also was the basis for the planning of sample size.

In the analysis, the question is finally put to the test. In a specified target population, those subjects who were exposed to alternate interventions are found to have different outcomes. Did these differences arise by chance, were they due to unintended maldistributions in the groups, or is it possible to infer that there was a true difference in the two interventions? The investigators first should compare the treatment groups with respect to important clinical prognostic variables, to demonstrate that the expected balance was achieved through randomization. Given that such balance was achieved, a univariate comparison of the two groups can determine whether the difference in the outcome is statistically significant. When there is imbalance between the groups despite the random allocation, the primary outcome must be assessed while accounting for these differences with the use of a multivariate statistical method.

By comparison with case series and cohort studies, randomized clinical trials represent an elaborate and expensive method of evaluating therapy. Nevertheless, because randomization reduces bias, justifies the use of statistical methodology, and allows for concealment or blinding, clinical readers increasingly will remain unconvinced about studies to evaluate therapy unless those studies are based on meticulously worked out randomized designs.

USE OF OVERVIEW ANALYSIS IN CLINICAL PRACTICE

It is frequently the case that the literature does not readily yield the answer to a clinical question because of discrepant results in the various publications that address the question. Variability among published studies can arise from numerous factors, the most important of which is chance; in 10 clinical studies of a given treatment that in truth has no effect, the results would be distributed around, but not necessarily at, zero. Differences from one study to

another also may arise from differences in the selection of subjects and in their baseline characteristics. More importantly, studies may differ on the basis of their methodologic quality (Oxman et al, 1994; Schulz et al, 1995). Treatment effects are most impressive in studies without internal controls, intermediate in cohort analytic studies, and least impressive in well-designed randomized trials (Sackett et al, 1985). Thus, if one accepts only the studies with superior methodologic quality, disparities in the reported results may be diminished.

Regardless of the reasons for the variability in the published data, clinicians must somehow or other synthesize the information so that it can be applied to the management of patients. In the past, the narrative review was commonly used to address the variability in the literature. With narrative reviews the clinical audience depends upon the subjective judgments of an informed and authoritative reviewer. For many years the literature review has been a routine step along the way to evaluating a new therapy, and thus such reviews have been an important and traditional component of the scientific evaluation of clinical issues.

More recently the science of reviewing research has been improved by the use of objective criteria for identifying studies and a quantitative approach to the assessment of the published studies (Light and Pillemer, 1984). In this approach, which is variously called *meta-analysis* or *overview analysis*, the steps in the review are in a general way similar to those required for the design of an individual study. The first and most important step is the formulation of a precise question. The second step is to set up rules for the inclusion of an appropriate set of studies, the rules being based on relevance to the question and the methodologic quality of the studies. Next the investigator aggregates the data, making use of techniques that evaluate whether the combined results are statistically acceptable. Finally, the results require interpretation to determine if they are applicable and useful (Fig. 6–14). Thus, overview analysis can allow an objective evaluation of controversial issues by restricting the evidence to the highest quality studies, and combining the results of those studies.

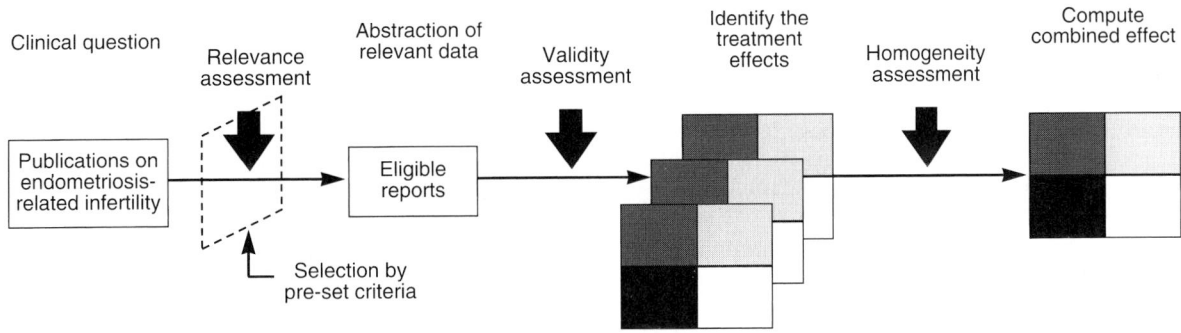

Figure 6–14
An outline of methodology for meta-analysis or overview analysis.

Refining the Question

In many cases, the definition of the question begins with the outcome of interest. It is important for the reviewers to define that outcome in a way that will be generally acceptable, and thus available in the largest number of studies in the literature. Second, there should be a careful and explicit definition of the treatment or exposure of interest. This exposure also needs to be refined in a very specific way. If one is considering long-term effects of hormone replacement therapy among postmenopausal women, for example, is the exposure of interest considered to be estrogen alone, or estrogen in some combination with progesterone? Both exposures are important, but they are parts of two separate questions. Investigators planning an overview analysis should clearly define such issues at the outset. The final point in the refinement of the question addresses the target population in which the treatment or exposure has been used. Specification here is also essential, because some treatments of interest to the investigator may have been applied in populations of which only a fraction comprise the target population of interest to the investigator. An example is the frequent occurrence in reports on hormone replacement therapy of a mixture of premenopausal and post-menopausal subjects.

Inclusion Criteria

The next step in the conduct of an overview analysis is to set up inclusion criteria that will determine which papers in the published literature are relevant to the specified question, and whether the relevant papers have sufficient validity to be included. The relevance criteria follow directly from the question, and validity criteria usually consist of one or two key methodologic characteristics. A stringent methodologic criterion would allow one to include only randomized studies; depending on the available literature, less stringent criteria might be necessary. In the case of long-term effects, as, for example, in the assessment of breast cancer risk among users of estrogen replacement therapy, randomized studies are rare; in this case, an acceptable methodologic criterion would be a requirement that the controls in cohort and case-control studies should be internal controls. In this context, internal controls would imply that the investigators had equal access to the control group, and were not relying solely on population statistics for their estimates of breast cancer rates in unexposed individuals.

Once these relevance and validity criteria for inclusion have been established, a systematic search of the published and unpublished literature is carried out. Such a search is initially easy because of the availability of several electronic data bases, but the effort to be complete may require hand searching of some journals and the review of the bibliographies of retrieved citations.

Assessment of Eligible Studies

At this stage, data from the relevant studies are abstracted and the methodologic details of each study are further reviewed, so that the studies can be stratified in order of methodologic criteria. In observational studies, the methodologic criteria could include, for example, the extent to which exposure was ascertained, the equivalence of the outcome ascertainment in the exposed and unexposed groups, the proportion of nonparticipation, and the range of potential covariates. In a well-designed overview analysis, these issues of relevance and methodologic quality would be assessed independently by the investigators, and a measure of inter-rater agreement such as kappa would be reported to support the findings (Fleiss, 1979). Because it is possible that some studies might be excluded during this state of evaluation, on the basis of relevance or methodologic criteria, it is important that such decisions be made according to preset criteria, in order to minimize selection bias.

Aggregating the Results

The most common method for aggregating the results of reported trials in the clinical literature is based on the summation of two-by-two tables, a method that estimates the common odds ratio with its 95% confidence limits (Mantel and Haenszel, 1959). Several other methods might be adopted for statistically combining the results of the different studies. The tally approach simply adds up the votes (number of studies) in favor of a therapy effect and those against. Multiple regression methods also can be applied (Greenland, 1987). Regardless of the method adopted for combining the results of studies, before one draws inferences from the combined data, it is important to estimate variability among the studies, and for this purpose a test of statistical homogeneity is applied (Breslow and Day, 1980).

Given that reasonable homogeneity has been demonstrated, and that there are reasonable clinical grounds for combining the relevant studies, the studies can be ordered according to the estimate of study methodologic quality and displayed as in Figure 6–15. When the 95% confidence limit of the common odds ratio and the weight of the evidence from individual studies is clearly above 1, the given treatment is definitively effective. More often, however, although the odds ratio is in the beneficial range, the confidence limits overlap unity and the treatment is considered to be promising but not proven, and thus in need of further study. In the analysis of observational studies, heterogeneity is often unavoidable; attempts should be made through the use of graphical

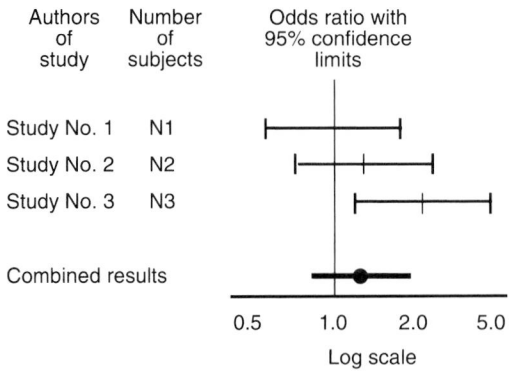

Authors of study	Number of subjects	Odds ratio with 95% confidence limits
Study No. 1	N1	
Study No. 2	N2	
Study No. 3	N3	
Combined results		

0.5   1.0   2.0   5.0

Log scale

Figure 6–15
Expression of the results of overview analysis.

displays or regression analysis to identify the source or sources of the heterogeneity (Greenland, 1987). While the methodology is still developing, the application of appropriate guidelines for the quantitative review of the literature allows more definitive conclusions to be reached, and may tend toward reducing clinical disagreement on important questions in reproductive endocrinology and infertility. The published literature is increasing in volume and improving in methodologic quality. Because it is also much more accessible to clinicians, published data will have a growing impact on how we conduct clinical work. Knowledge of the design and methodology of clinical studies is a key component in the selection of better quality information to aid in the continuing refinement of practice protocols.

REFERENCES

Ajzen, I, Fishbein M: Understanding Attitudes and Predicting Social Behavior. Englewood Cliffs, NJ: Prentice-Hall, 1980.

Breslow NE, Day NE: The Analysis of Case-Control Studies. In Davis W (ed). Statistical Methods in Cancer Research. Volume 1. Lyon: International Agency for Research on Cancer, 1980:136.

Chalmers I: Evaluating the effects of care during pregnancy and childbirth. In Chalmers I, Enkin E, Keirse MJNC (eds): Effective Care in Pregnancy and Childbirth. Oxford: Oxford University Press, 1989:3.

Collins JA: Diagnostic assessment of the infertile female partner. Curr Probl Obstet Gynecol Fertil 1988;9:1.

Cox DR: Regression models and life tables. J R Statis Soc Soc B 1972;34:187.

Cox DR, Oakes D: Analysis of Survival Data. New York: Chapman and Hall, 1984.

Drinkwater BL, Bruemner B, Chesnut CH: Menstrual history as a determinant of current bond density in young athletes. JAMA 1990;263:545.

Eden JA, Place J, Carter GD, et al: The diagnosis of polycystic ovaries in subfertile women. Br J Obstet Gynaecol 1989;96:809.

Eraker SA, Politser P: How decisions are reached: Physician and patient. In Dowie J, Elstein A (eds): Professional Judgment: A Reader in Clinical Decision Making. New York: Cambridge University Press, 1988:379.

ESHRE Capri Workshop: Guidelines to the prevalence, diagnosis, treatment and management of infertility, 1996. Hum Reprod 1996;11:101.

Fleiss JL: Confidence intervals for the odds ratio in case-control studies: the state of the art. J Chron Dis 1979;32:69.

Fleiss JL: Statistical Methods for Rates and Proportions. 2nd ed. Toronto: John Wiley and Sons, 1981.

Friedman LM, Furberg CD, DeMets DL: Fundamentals of Clinical Trials. 2nd ed. Littleton, MA: PSG Publishing Company, 1985.

Greenland S: Quantitative methods in the review of epidemiologic literature. Epidemiol Rev 1987;9:1.

Greer AL: The state of the art versus the state of the science. Int J Technol Assess Health Care 1988;4:5.

Griner P, Mayewski R, Mushlin A: Selection and interpretation of diagnostic tests and procedures: principle and applications. Ann Intern Med 1981;94:557.

Jaeschke R, Guyatt G, Sackett DL: Users' guides to the medical literature. III. How to use an article about a diagnostic test. Are the results of the study valid? JAMA 1994a;271:389.

Jaeschke R, Guyatt GH, Sackett DL: Users' guides to the medical literature. III. How to use an article about a diagnostic test. B. What are the results and will they help me in caring for my patients? JAMA 1994b;271:703.

Kelsey JF, Thompson WD, Evans AS: Methods in Observational Epidemiology. New York: Oxford University Press, 1986:366.

Lachin JM: Statistical elements of the randomized clinical trials. In Tygstrup N, Lachin JM, Juhl E (eds): The Randomized Clinical Trial and Therapeutic Decisions. New York: Marcel Dekker, 1982:77.

Light RJ, Pillemer DB: Summing Up: The Science of Reviewing Research. Boston: Harvard University Press, 1984.

Mantel N, Haenszel W: Statistical aspects of the analysis of data from retrospective studies of disease. J Natl Cancer Inst 1959; 22:719.

Oxman AD, Cook DJ, Guyatt GH: Users' guides to the medical literature. VI. How to use an overview. JAMA 1994;272:1367.

Oxman AD, Sackett DL, Guyatt GH: Users' guide to the medical literature. 1. How to get started. JAMA 1993;270:2093.

Peto R, Pike MC, Armitage P, et al: Design and analysis of randomized clinical trials requiring prolonged observation of each patient: II. Analysis and examples. Br J Cancer 1977;35:1.

Petrie A: The crossover design. In Tygstrup N, Lachin JM, Juhl E (eds). The Randomized Clinical Trial and Therapeutic Decisions. New York: Marcel Dekker, 1982:199.

Richardson WS, Detsky AS: Users' guides to the medical literature. VII. How to use a clinical decision analysis. A. Are the results of the study valid? JAMA 1995a;273:1292.

Richardson WS, Detsky AS: Users' guides to the medical literature. VII. How to use a clinical decision analysis. B. What are the results and will they help me in caring for my patients? JAMA 1995b;273:1610.

Sackett DL, Haynes RB, Tugwell P: Clinical Epidemiology: A Basic Science for Clinical Medicine. Boston: Little, Brown and Company, 1985.

Schechter MT, Scheps SB: Diagnostic testing revisited: pathways through uncertainty. Can Med Assoc J 1985;132:755.

Schlesselman JJ: Case-Control Studies: Design, Conduct, Analysis. New York: Oxford University Press, 1982.

Schulz KF, Chalmers I, Hayes RJ, Altman DG: Empirical evidence of bias: dimensions of methodological quality associated with estimates of treatment effects in controlled trials. JAMA 1995; 273:408.

Wright CS, Steele SJ, Jacobs HS: Value of bromocriptine in unexplained primary infertility: a double-blind controlled trial. Br Med J 1979;1:1037.

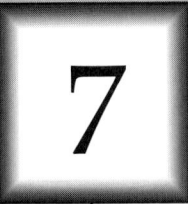

Gynecologic Pathology
Challenges to Accurate Diagnosis

Deborah Bartholomew
Katherine A. O'Hanlan

In few fields of medicine is a working knowledge of anatomic pathology more essential to clinical practice than in gynecology. An appreciation of how the study of morphology lends insight into the pathogenesis of disease and ultimately influences treatment decision is critical for effective communication between clinicians and pathologists. Limitations on time, changing resident training requirements, and an increased emphasis on primary care have caused many training programs to eliminate a rotation in pathology. Managed care has resulted in increased utilization of larger, regional laboratories that may be located a considerable distance away from the clinical setting; hence, direct communication with the pathologist may be difficult or even impossible. Burgeoning technology and the development of adjunctive tests such as immunohistochemical studies and diagnostic molecular techniques to facilitate diagnosis have resulted in subspecialization in pathology. The constant challenge to the general pathologist to maintain expertise in all areas of pathology is enormous. Despite these obstacles, teamwork and communication between clinicians and pathologists is critical for optimal patient care. Clinical correlation is as essential to the practice of pathology as accurate microscopic diagnosis is to the selection of appropriate therapy. This chapter highlights several diagnostic problem areas in gynecologic pathology with the hope of promoting improved understanding and communication and more realistic expectations between pathologists and clinicians.

VULVA

Specimen Procurement

Pertinent historical information should be included on the pathology requisition form, noting any medical problems, history of skin disease or atopy, and medication use and any potential exposure to irritants. This information may be important because primary skin disease and secondary reactions, although rarely limited to the vulva, can initially present as vulvar disease. Specific symptoms and duration of lesions and any treatments tried, whether self-medicated or prescribed, should be included in the history.

A detailed description of the appearance of the lesion is essential. A basic knowledge of dermatology and the appropriate vocabulary is valuable in describing and evaluating vulvar findings to determine if biopsy is needed. Shave biopsies, although common in dermatology, are rarely useful in gynecology. An adequate specimen obtained with a Keye's punch, which includes the underlying dermis, is necessary for proper evaluation of vulvar lesions. If the lesion is ulcerated, then the biopsy should be taken from the edge of the ulcer. Condyloma accuminata are usually easily diagnosed by simple inspection, but, if clinical suspicion for a verrucoid carcinoma exists, a deep biopsy is needed. Diagnosis is aided by finding the characteristic bulbous pushing interface of the neoplasm with the underlying dermis. A superficial biopsy may result in a false diagnosis of condyloma accuminata even though verrucous carcinomas lack koilocytosis (Fig. 7–1). Condyloma in children often lack classical verrucoid features and may appear as small, fleshy, single or coalescent papules (Frasier, 1994). Biopsy is essential for diagnosis. Koilocytosis may be minimal, and further evaluation for human papillomavirus (HPV) by molecular diagnostic techniques may be needed. Seborrheic keratosis may mimic vulvar intraepithelial neoplasia (VIN) and basal cell carcinomas. VIN is variable in appearance and has little relation of appearance to grade. Multiple biopsies should be taken to exclude underlying invasion, especially in solitary, thick hyperkeratotic lesions.

Pathology Evaluation

White lesions of the vulva have an extensive differential, including lichen sclerosus, squamous hyperplasia, lichen simplex chronicus, lichen planus, psoriasis, VIN, and carcinoma. Biopsy is usually diagnostic. Lichen sclerosus can usually be distinguished by its clinical appearance but may be associated with areas of squamous hyperplasia, thus

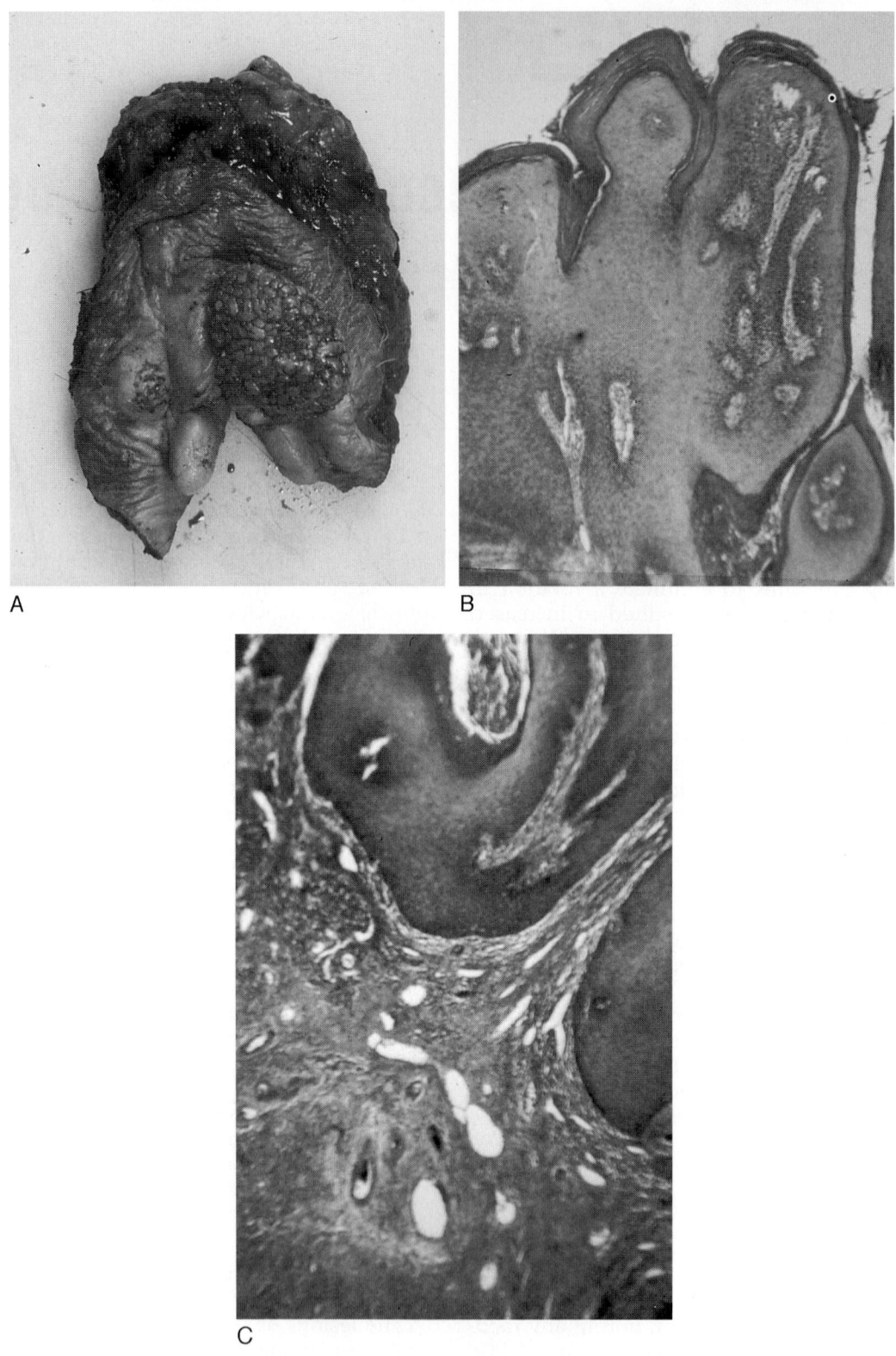

Figure 7–1

A, Warty appearance of verrucous carcinoma. *B,* Superficial biopsy resembling condylomata. *C,* Diagnostic pushing border of verrucous carcinoma.

complicating the classical presentation. Biopsy is remarkable for loss of the rete ridges, subepithelial edema, and homogenization of the dermis. Lichen planus is distinguished from lichen sclerosus by the band-like infiltrate of lymphocytes beneath the epidermis, lack of the acellular subepithelial zone, and preservation of the rete. Clinical changes of the vulvar skin are often the end result of a prolonged "itch-scratch" cycle. The lesion may appear white and thickened with accentuated skin markings as a result of hyperkeratosis and epithelial hyperplasia. The inciting agent may not be apparent, even with microscopy. Obesity or incontinence with resultant chafing and maceration may explain the symptoms and findings. The microscopic finding of edema and eosinophils suggests contact dermatitis. If not immediately apparent, methenamine silver stains can be done to evaluate for fungi. Squamous hyperplasia is distinguished by hyperplasia and widening of the rete ridges, termed *acanthosis*, and by variable degrees of hyperkeratosis. If a more specific diagnosis can be made, then the diagnosis of squamous hyperplasia should not be used. Lichen simplex chronicus is often the end result of chronic irritation and is characterized by prominent acanthosis, hyperkeratosis, and an associated superficial chronic inflammatory infiltrate. Psoriasis may involve the vulva and is characterized by even-length acanthosis and collections of polymorphonuclear cells in the superficial epidermis, called Munroe abscesses. Cytonuclear atypia characterizes VIN. Bowenoid papulosis is a clinical term and should not be used as a pathology diagnosis.

Superficially invasive squamous cell carcinoma, as defined by the International Society for the Study of Vulvar Disease, is a diagnosis of exclusion and is only made if all diagnostic criteria are met (Kneale, 1984). The pathology report should mention the gross diameter of the lesion, which must be less than 2 cm. The depth of invasion is measured from the site of invasion to the tip of the highest neighboring dermal papillae (Fig. 7-2). Invasion must be measured with the aide of an ocular micrometer and cannot exceed 1 mm (Wilkinson, 1991). Tumor thickness and vascular space involvement should be mentioned, but do not influence the diagnosis of superficially invasive squamous cell carcinoma. Gynecologists should perform only punch biopsies of clinically suspicious vulvar lesions, deferring excisional biopsies for therapeutic resection until the diagnosis is known and the appropriate excision can be planned, thus avoiding repeat excisions by gynecologic oncologists. If a wide local excision is done, margins must be addressed in the surgical pathology report, including the deep stromal margin. Frozen sections for evaluation of surgical margins are limited by potential sampling error.

Benign Conditions That Mimic Malignancy

Papillary hidradenoma, a benign neoplasm of sweat gland origin that may ulcerate through the overlying skin, has been misdiagnosed as vulvar adenocarcinoma. The exceedingly rare primary vulvar adenocarcinoma can be excluded by the noninfiltrative growth pattern and lack of a stromal response. Hidradenomas are also characterized by an epithelial cell layer surrounded by myoepithelial cells (Fig. 7-3). Minute biopsy specimens can be difficult to diagnose with certainty, unless the double cell layer is found. VIN may extend down skin appendages for a depth of 2.7 mm in hair-bearing areas (Shatz et al, 1989). Tangential cutting may give the appearance of invasion into the dermis. Multiple step sections may reveal continuity with a hair follicle. Keys to the diagnosis of true invasion are loss of polarity, eosinophilia, premature keratinization of the neoplastic cells, and a reactive stromal response. Treatment of condyloma with podophyllin results in marked

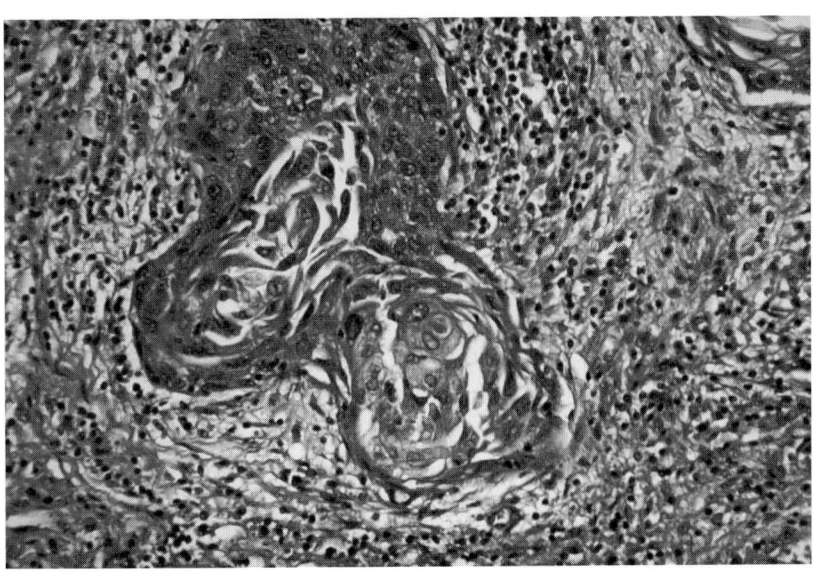

Figure 7-2
Superficial invasion arising from a skin appendage involved with VIN III.

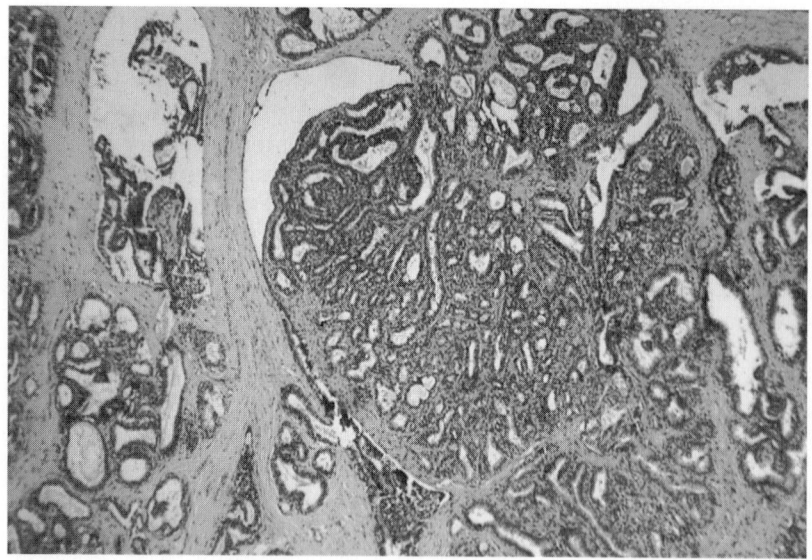

A

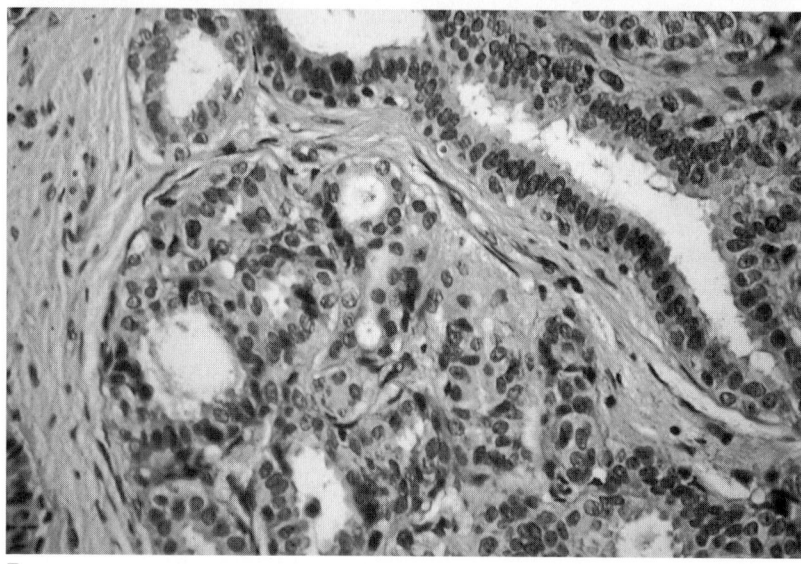

B

Figure 7–3

A, Hidradenoma of the vulva. Low-power view is suggestive of adenocarcinoma. *B*, Diagnostic double cell layer with surrounding myoepithelial cell layer.

atypia that can suggest malignancy. Communication with the pathologist is usually all that is needed to resolve the question. Keratoacanthomas may be confused with squamous cell carcinoma. Clues to the correct diagnosis include the symmetry of the lesion and the lack of irregular infiltration into the dermis (Rhatigan and Nuss, 1985). Pseudoepitheliomatous hyperplasia may overlie dermal lesions such as a granular cell tumors. A superficial biopsy may suggest a primary squamous neoplasm and mask the primary lesion (Wolber, 1991).

Diagnostic Difficulties

Distinction between superficial spreading melanoma, VIN, and noninvasive Paget's disease can be difficult on microscopic exam. Fortunately, most pathologists are well aware of this diagnostic pitfall

(Fig. 7–4). Paget cells may contain intracytoplasmic melanin, as can VIN; thus simple stains for melanin are not diagnostic. Immunohistochemical studies with a panel of antibodies will establish the diagnosis and are also extremely helpful in distinguishing invasive Paget's disease from a melanoma or poorly differentiated squamous cell carcinoma (Table 7–1). Paget's disease may extend beyond the clinically recognized lesions, and wide margins are needed for complete excision. Immunohistochemical stains have not been found to have an advantage over standard microscopic evaluation in assessing surgical margins (Ganjei et al, 1990). A careful search for an associated adenocarcinoma must be undertaken if the diagnosis of noninvasive Paget's disease is made.

A specific subtype of squamous cell carcinoma is termed warty carcinoma and must be distinguished from condyloma accuminata. Both contain koilocytes

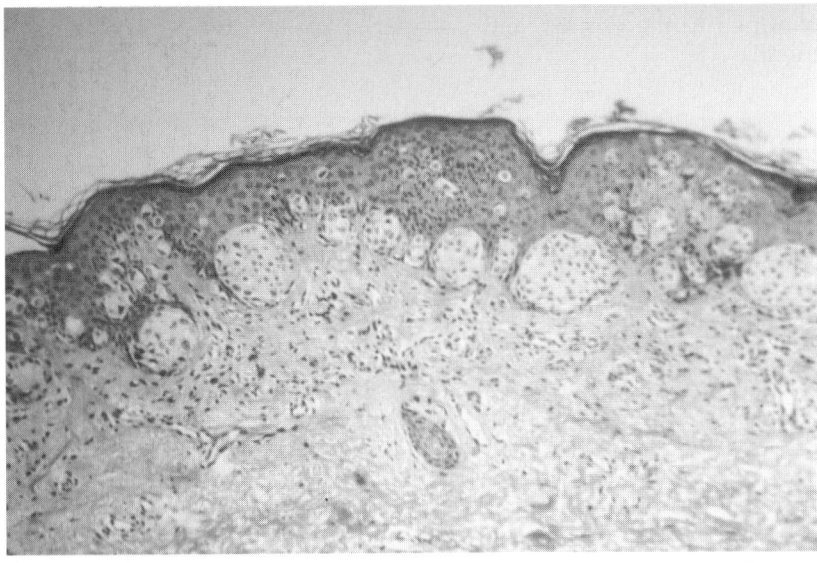

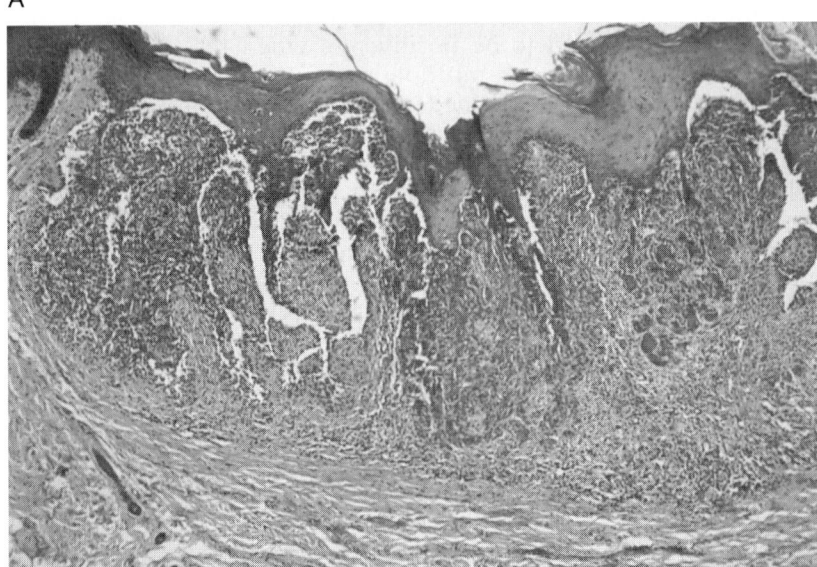

Figure 7–4
A, Paget's disease of the vulva. *B*, Superficial spreading melanoma of the vulva.

and marked atypia. Differentiation is made possible with a deep biopsy, which reveals the irregular infiltrative pattern of stromal invasion present in warty carcinomas. The diagnosis of verrucous carcinoma also requires a deep biopsy, which will reveal the characteristic bulbous, pushing margin of squamous cells. True koilocytosis with the requisite nuclear atypia is not seen in verrucous carcinoma, nor are fibrovascular cores.

Primary adenocarcinoma of the vulva is quite rare and usually arises from the Bartholin's glands (Copeland et al, 1986). Usually the neoplasm has overgrown any remaining glandular elements by the time diagnosis is made. Clues as to the site of origin include location at the site of the Bartholin gland, remnants of the gland, or a direct transition and exclusion of metastatic disease. Ectopic breast tissue, sweat glands, and vulvar endometriosis may also

give rise to vulvar adenocarcinomas (Wick et al, 1985).

Metastatic disease to the vulva is certainly not uncommon and must always be considered as a distinct possibility (Dehner, 1973). Direct extension from a primary vaginal or cervical tumor is usually easily diagnosed. Metastatic adenocarcinoma may arise from primary endometrial, ovarian, and breast carcinoma. Distinction between metastatic breast carcinoma and carcinoma arising from ectopic breast tissue can be difficult. Metastatic breast carcinoma will not be associated with in situ changes or normal breast tissue (Curtin and Murthy, 1997). Choriocarcinoma can metastasize to the vulva, although the more frequent site is the vagina. Clues to metastatic disease include normal, uninvolved overlying vulvar epithelium, absence of a preneoplastic lesion, multifocal and multinodular nests of tumor primarily confined to the dermis, and vascular space involvement.

CERVIX

Specimen Procurement

All clinically relevant information, including previous cytology or biopsy results, colposcopic findings, and a current diagnostic impression, must be included on the pathology requisition form. This information will allow the pathologist to correlate all diagnostic studies and to search for an explanation for any discrepancies. If margins are important, all cervical excisional specimens, whether they are obtained with a scalpel, electrocautery, or laser, must be oriented. Specimens that are fragmented or removed piecemeal without proper designation are difficult to interpret. If margins are not important or are clinically expected to be positive, as when the specimen is removed with multiple passes, this information should be mentioned on the requisition form. If it is essential to know the exact cervical location of disease, open the specimen at 3:00 and pin it to a tongue blade. This can easily be done by the operating surgeon in the operative suite and facilitates orientation, fixation, and cutting of the specimen. If multiple passes are needed to remove the entire lesion or if the tissue is fragmented, then the appropriate exocervical or endocervical specimen margins may be inked and so designated on the tissue requisition form. Multicolored permanent ink is now available and can be useful if several different margins need to be designated on one specimen. Many clinicians keep India ink in their office colposcopy suite. It is often helpful to the pathologist for the surgeon to draw the lesion, explain the technique used to remove the specimen, label each individual piece of tissue and areas of specific interest, and submit each separately.

Pathology Evaluation

The surgical pathology report should state the prefixation dimensions, including the length of excision of the endocervical canal, and the cervical stromal depth. Sections should be made every 1 to 2 mm, and the number of sections taken and blocks submitted stated on the report. Clinicians should read the surgical pathology report to ensure that enough sections were taken, especially if disease is not confirmed. The pathology report should list the most clinically significant diagnosis first and clearly state which margins are involved and the degree of involvement. Three margins are clinically significant: the exocervical, endocervical, and the deep stromal margins (Fig. 7–5). Cervical intraepithelial neoplasia (CIN) may extend down endocervical clefts for up to 5.2 mm of cervical stromal depth, and surgical

Table 7–1. IMMUNOHISTOCHEMICAL STAINS IN VULVAR LESIONS

ANTIGEN	MELANOMA	PAGET'S DISEASE	VIN/SCC
CEA	–	+	–
S100	+	–	+/–
HMB-45	+	–	–
GCDFP-15	–	+	–
HMW Keratin	–	–	+
B72.3	–	+	–

Abbreviations: CEA, carcinoembryonic antigen; GCDFP, gross cystic disease fluid protein; HMW, high molecular weight; SCC, squamous cell carcinoma; VIN, vulvar intraepithelial neoplasia.
Data from Mazoujian et al (1984), Shah et al (1987), and Helm et al (1992).

"cut through" of a neoplastic endocervical cleft is a significant finding and should be conveyed in the report (Anderson and Hartley, 1980) (Fig. 7–6). In a significant number of electrocautery excisions, evaluation of the margins may be difficult because of coagulation artifact, and all limitations should be stated. Coagulation artifact can limit the pathologist's ability to assess margins, especially the endocervical margin (Krebs et al, 1993). For this reason, loop electrocautery excisions should not be done by inexperienced surgeons to address endocervical glandular atypia on biopsy or endocervical curettage (Kennedy et al, 1995). If microinvasive disease is diagnosed, the depth of invasion as measured with a micrometer, the site from which the measurement was taken, the presence or absence of vascular space involvement or confluency of tumor nests, and the width of the lesion should be clearly stated in the report. A prior biopsy induces repair, inflammation, and reactive stromal change. If entrapped neoplastic cells are present, the biopsy site may be confused with a focus of invasion. Artifactual clefts surround-

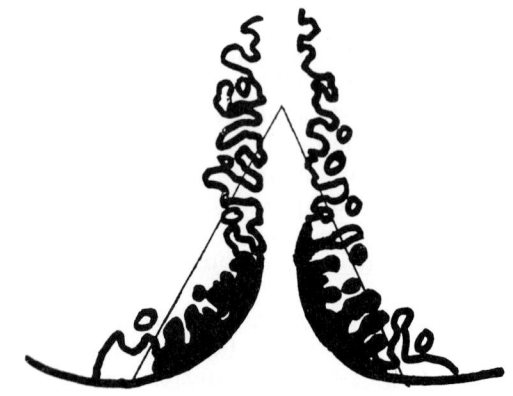

Figure 7–5
Large ectocervical lesion with extension up the canal and down endocervical clefts. Cone biopsy margins would reveal negative ectocervical and endocervical margins, but a positive deep stromal margin that "cuts through" disease residing in endocervical clefts.

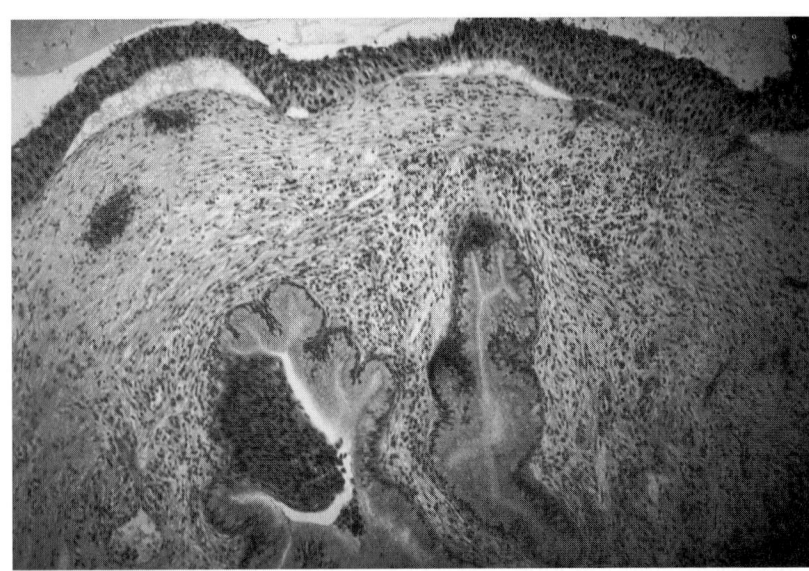

Figure 7–6
Cervical intraepithelial neoplasia extending down endocervical clefts.

ing neoplastic cells may give the appearance of vascular space involvement. If in doubt, endothelial cells may be confirmed by immunohistochemical staining for factor VIII antigen. There are very few indications for frozen section evaluation of a cone biopsy. Sampling will be limited, and loss of cytonuclear detail may inhibit the ability to diagnose microinvasion. A frozen section may be useful to diagnose obvious frank invasion. When a hysterectomy is performed for residual or persistent cervical neoplasia, the entire cervix should be processed like a cone biopsy.

Cytology Specimen Procurement

The Papanicolaou (Pap) smear can be credited with a significant decline in cervical cancer mortality. However, the diagnostic accuracy of the Pap smear has been questioned because of falsely negative smears. On analysis, the majority of the false-negative smears are due to sampling error and the rest, screening or interpretive error (Koss, 1989). Studies have shown that optimum sampling with specific inclusion of the endocervical component is achieved with a combination of spatula and brush (Schumann et al, 1992). Other studies have shown that the device used may trap cells within the fibers and contribute to sampling error (Rubio, 1977). Technological advances are now available to address these limitations. Automated Thin Prep monolayer preparations can address sampling limitations. Rinsing the collecting device in a fluid medium may decrease trapping of cells by the sampling device. Smear quality is optimized by presenting the collected cells as a homogeneous sample without obscuring inflammation or blood (Hutchinson et al, 1994). A simple clinical technique that samples the ectocervix first with the spatula, followed by brush endocervical sampling, will decrease blood contamination of the smear. The endocervix is often friable and bleeds after brush sampling. False-negative results caused by screening error can be reduced by computerized rescreening of negative smears with PapNet (Koss et al, 1994). Small cells with high-grade dysplasia that are few in number may be missed entirely during manual screening or misinterpreted as atypical metaplastic cells (Hatem and Wilbur, 1995). Computerized screening excels in finding these rare small cells.

Cytology Evaluation

The Bethesda System has simplified communication by standardizing terminology. Specific criteria for diagnosis are now available for each diagnostic category (Kurman and Solomon, 1994). The adequacy statement gives important feedback to clinicians, but should not be misused. A major survey of laboratories gave median rates of unsatisfactory and limited smears of 0.5% to 0.9%, but with a range of 0% to 20% (Davey et al, 1992). Recommendations to improve the quality of the smear, such as the use of estrogen to resolve the atypia associated with severe atrophy, may provide very useful feedback to the clinician.

It is important for clinicians to know the rate of abnormalities reported by their cytology laboratory. Clearly, the vast majority of smears are normal, and rates of atypical squamous cells of undetermined significance (ASCUS) far in excess of 5% are unacceptable in any patient population (Davey et al, 1994). In general, the rate of ASCUS should not exceed three times the total rate of squamous intraepithelial lesions found in the population. When ASCUS is diagnosed, an attempt should be made to distinguish potentially neoplastic from reactive changes and further qualify the diagnosis in the report. Strict criteria should be utilized in assigning cases to the ASCUS category. Benign cellular changes should not be included. Hyperkeratosis and parakeratosis are rarely associated with neoplasia, which, if present, is usually of low grade (Cecchini et al, 1990). These findings may be included in the benign cellular changes or ASCUS category, depending on the lab.

Atypical glandular cells of undetermined significance (AGUS) may be associated with high-grade squamous intraepithelial lesions three times as often as with ASCUS (Taylor et al, 1993). As in the squamous category, considerable difficulty is encountered in distinguishing true neoplasia from benign reactive and reparative processes. Benign processes that can simulate neoplasia include tubal or ciliated metaplasia, endometriosis, microglandular hyperplasia, endocervical polyps, the Arias-Stella reaction during pregnancy, and cervicitis. The intrauterine contraceptive device (IUD) can induce atypia in both endocervical and endometrial cells resembling the atypia seen in carcinoma (Gupta et al, 1978). Even normal lower uterine segment endometrium dragged down by the sampling brush has been confused with glandular neoplasia. High-grade CIN extending into endocervical clefts can take on glandular features on cytologic examination and be diagnosed as AGUS. Distinction between atypical endocervical and endometrial cells is usually possible, but the predictive ability of the qualifier that states whether neoplasia or a reactive process is favored is not as well tested as with atypical squamous cells (Goff et al, 1992). Tubal or ciliated metaplasia is probably the most frequent cause of diagnostic difficulty and may occur after a cone biopsy in more than 30% of cases (Jonasson et al, 1992). Endometriosis may occur after cone biopsy and is not an infrequent cause of AGUS (Symonds et al, 1997). Regenerative atypia of the endocervical epithelium after treatment may cause confusion during cytologic follow-up, and has even been confused with carcinoma (Geirsson et al, 1977).

Both clinicians and pathologists would agree that koilocytosis is frequently overcalled on cervical smears and biopsies. Pseudokoilocytosis may occur with *Trichomonas* infection and with atrophy. Strict attention to the requirement for nuclear enlargement and atypia will establish a higher threshold for the diagnosis of koilocytes. Correlation of cytology, colposcopic findings, and subsequent biopsies can be an educational exercise that benefits both the pathologist and the clinician. Some laboratories have found in situ hybridization tests for HPV DNA useful for educational and quality assurance purposes (Richart and Nuovo, 1990). The clinical utility of these studies has yet to be established with certainty.

Benign Conditions That Mimic Malignancy

Awareness of the possibility of benign and hyperplastic conditions of the cervix that may simulate carcinoma will help the pathologist avoid diagnostic errors. Atypical forms of microglandular hyperplasia have been mistaken for adenocarcinoma (Fig. 7–7). A careful search will usually disclose areas of more typical microglandular hyperplasia with squamous metaplasia. The biopsy will also lack mitotic figures and significant atypia (Young and Hart, 1989). Endocervical tunnel clusters can be distinguished from minimal deviation adenocarcinoma by the characteristic lobular arrangement and lack of an infiltrative pattern. Mesonephric hyperplasia must be distinguished from well-differentiated endocervical adenocarcinoma, clear cell carcinoma, and mesonephric carcinoma. The lack of stromal infiltration is key to the distinction. Occasional mitotic figures and mild atypia may be present in mesonephric hyperplasia, which adds to the diagnostic difficulty (Ferry and Scully, 1990).

Arias-Stella reaction involving the endocervical epithelium during pregnancy may be misinterpreted

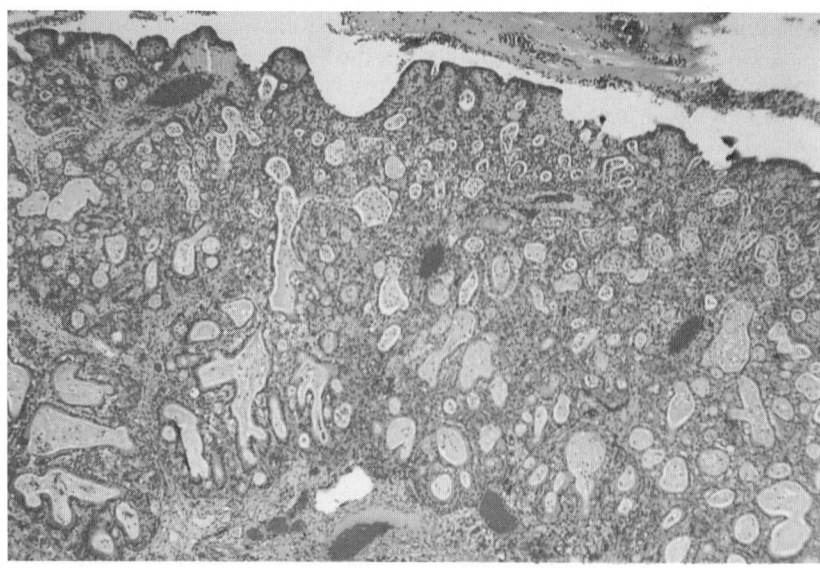

Figure 7–7
Florid microglandular hyperplasia of the cervix.

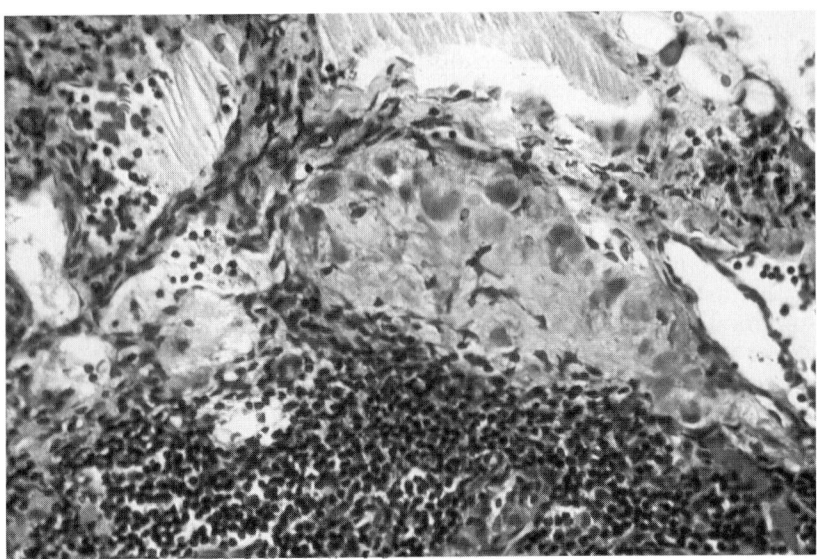

Figure 7–8
Decidual change in pelvic lymph nodes during pregnancy.

as a clear cell carcinoma; however, the former lacks a stromal response and the characteristic variation in architectural patterns present in clear cell carcinoma. Decidual change may occur in lymph nodes during pregnancy and be confused with metastatic squamous cell carcinoma of the cervix. Informing the pathologist that the patient is pregnant is usually all that is needed to resolve the question, but, if needed, immunohistochemical studies for keratins will make the distinction (Covell et al, 1977) (Fig. 7–8). *Actinomyces israelii*, a filamentous gram-positive bacteria with characteristic "sulfur granules," can be diagnosed on Pap smear (Keebler et al, 1983). Often present in women with IUDs, special silver stains can be confirmatory but are usually not necessary. Some cases of pelvic actinomycosis can mimic advanced cervical carcinoma, with a dense fibrotic reaction, fistulas, and hydroureter formation. This emphasizes the need for a recent Pap smear prior to any surgery, as well as the need to include the history of an IUD,

even if remote, on the cytology request form. When clinically essential, a preoperative smear can be processed and interpreted in a few hours.

Diagnostic Difficulties

Minimal deviation adenocarcinoma (MDA) is extremely difficult to diagnose by biopsy, and usually a cone biopsy is required (Kaminski and Norris, 1983). The bland cytonuclear characteristics have led even the most experienced pathologist to an incorrect diagnosis (Fig. 7–9). The key to diagnosis is the finding of infiltrative glands deep within the cervical stroma far removed from the expected gland field. The stroma may be innocuous or reactive. Staining for carcinoembryonic antigen (CEA) may be helpful, if positive, and can help to differentiate MDA from benign lesions (Michael et al, 1984). Difficulty may be encountered in distinguishing a stage II endo-

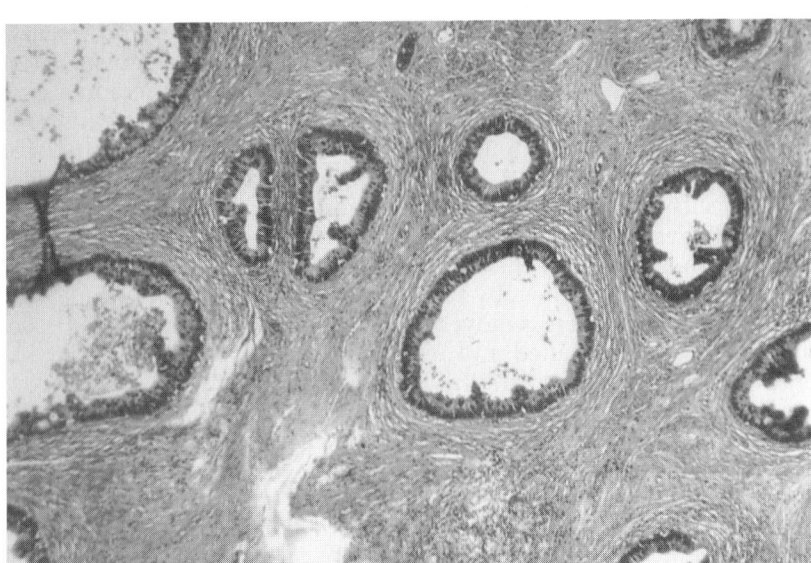

Figure 7–9
Minimal deviation adenocarcinoma of the cervix mimics normal glandular epithelium.

metrial adenocarcinoma from a primary endocervical adenocarcinoma, especially the endometrioid subtype. Although considerable overlap exists, immunoperoxidase studies may be helpful. Endometrial carcinomas usually lack CEA and stain positive for vimentin, whereas endocervical carcinomas will usually stain positive for CEA and negative for vimentin (Dabbs et al, 1986). Small cell carcinoma of the cervix may be difficult to discern from primary or metastatic lymphoma or poorly differentiated squamous carcinoma. The distinction is important for prognosis and treatment. Adjunctive tests with immunohistochemical staining and electron microscopy may be needed (Gersell et al, 1988). Lymphomas are distinguished by the presence of leukocyte common antigen (LCA) and small cell carcinomas by positive staining for neuron-specific enolase and chromogranin. Electron microscopy will reveal the diagnostic neurosecretory granules of small cell cervical carcinoma.

UTERUS

Specimen Procurement

Office sampling devices, when used properly, have been shown to be as accurate as operative dilatation and curettage (Stovall et al, 1989). Sampling inadequacy frequently occurs as a result of patient bleeding and in the setting of an atrophic endometrium. Cornual lesions, polyps, and leiomyomata may be underdiagnosed regardless of sampling technique. Whenever cancer is a possibility, assurance that the specimen obtained is representative of the entire uterine cavity is essential. Many clinicians use a thin plastic cannula attached to a syringe. The endometrium is aspirated down to the basalis while rotating the cannula 360 degrees. Such thorough sampling needs to be noted on the pathology requisition form to convey to the pathologist that the specimen is indeed representative of the entire endometrial cavity. This enables the pathologist to render a confident diagnosis even with a scanty specimen and limits concern for potential sampling error.

Aggressive uterine compression during examination under anesthesia should be avoided if peritoneal fluid will be obtained for cytology examination. Tumor cells may be forced through the fallopian tubes and result in a false-positive peritoneal wash. Prior to handing off the specimen, the surgeon should always determine, by visual inspection, if the entire cervix has been removed. The uterus should then be properly opened and examined by the operating surgeon prior to closing the peritoneum. Using large scissors, the uterus is opened bilaterally from the external cervical os at the 3 and 9 o'clock positions and extended to each cornua. The bivalved uterus allows inspection of the entire endometrial cavity and also facilitates fixation (Fig. 7–10). The endometrium is prone to rapid autolysis if the uterus

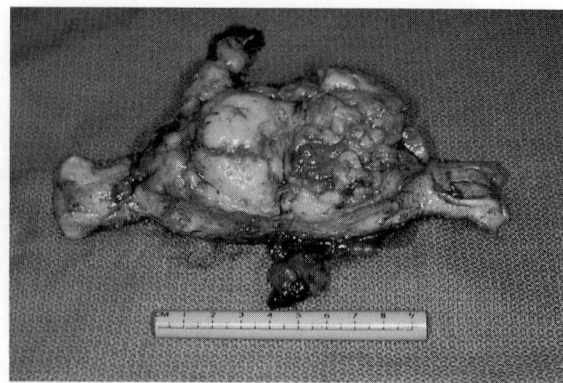

Figure 7–10
Bivalved uterus with exophytic endometrial cancer.

is not opened prior to placement in a fixative. If a pathologist is not available and inspection of the uterine cavity is suspicious for malignancy, the endometrium and myometrium can be serially sectioned to grossly assess for myometrial invasion (Fig. 7–11). This simple technique has excellent correlation with the final microscopic determination of depth of invasion and allows the surgeon to determine if lymph node sampling is needed (Doering et al, 1989).

Pathology Evaluation

When a pathologist is available, the surgeon may ask for a frozen section to determine the depth of myometrial invasion, if any, and to assess for cervical involvement. It is useful to reassess the grade of the tumor because the tumor grading at the initial endometrial sampling may not be accurate (Heller et al, 1994). Frozen section evaluation is particularly useful to determine if lymph node sampling is indicated. The pathologist should take multiple longitudinal parallel sections through the cervical canal and lower uterine segment. It is important to distinguish between downgrowth of an endometrial carcinoma confined to endocervical clefts and direct infiltration into cervical stroma. Similar detailed microscopic analysis should be undertaken to distinguish true myometrial invasion from extension down adenomyosis (Fig. 7–12). Such detailed analysis may not be possible on frozen section because of sampling limitations and less than ideal preservation of detail, but should be the standard on permanent section microscopy.

Large leiomyomas should be sectioned and inspected for areas of hemorrhage or necrosis, especially if solitary. Examination of the interface between the leiomyoma and the underlying myometrium can be informative. Typical leiomyomata have a pseudocapsule of compressed smooth muscle and will bulge away from the underlying myometrium when sectioned. A leiomyosarcoma may show

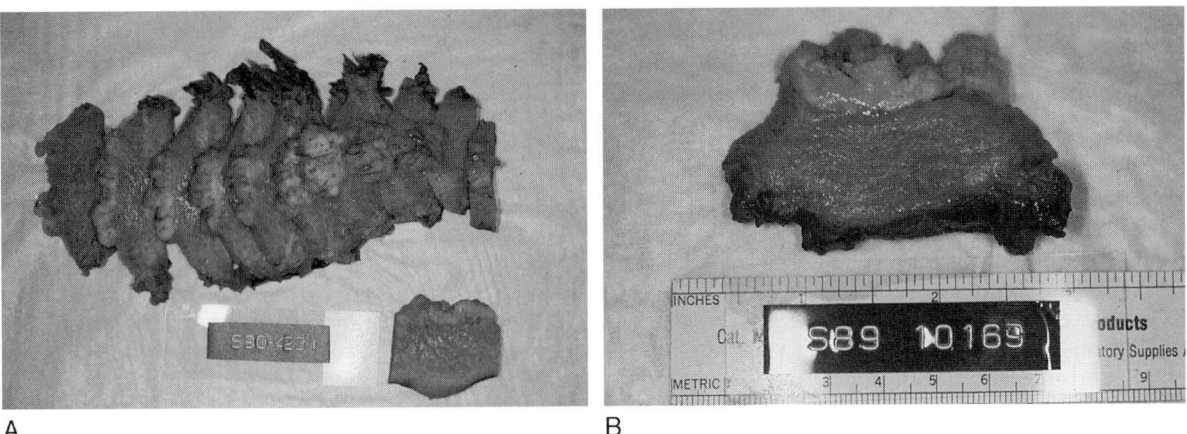

Figure 7–11
A, Serial sections of the uterus. B, Gross inspection of the myometrium for invasion. There is none.

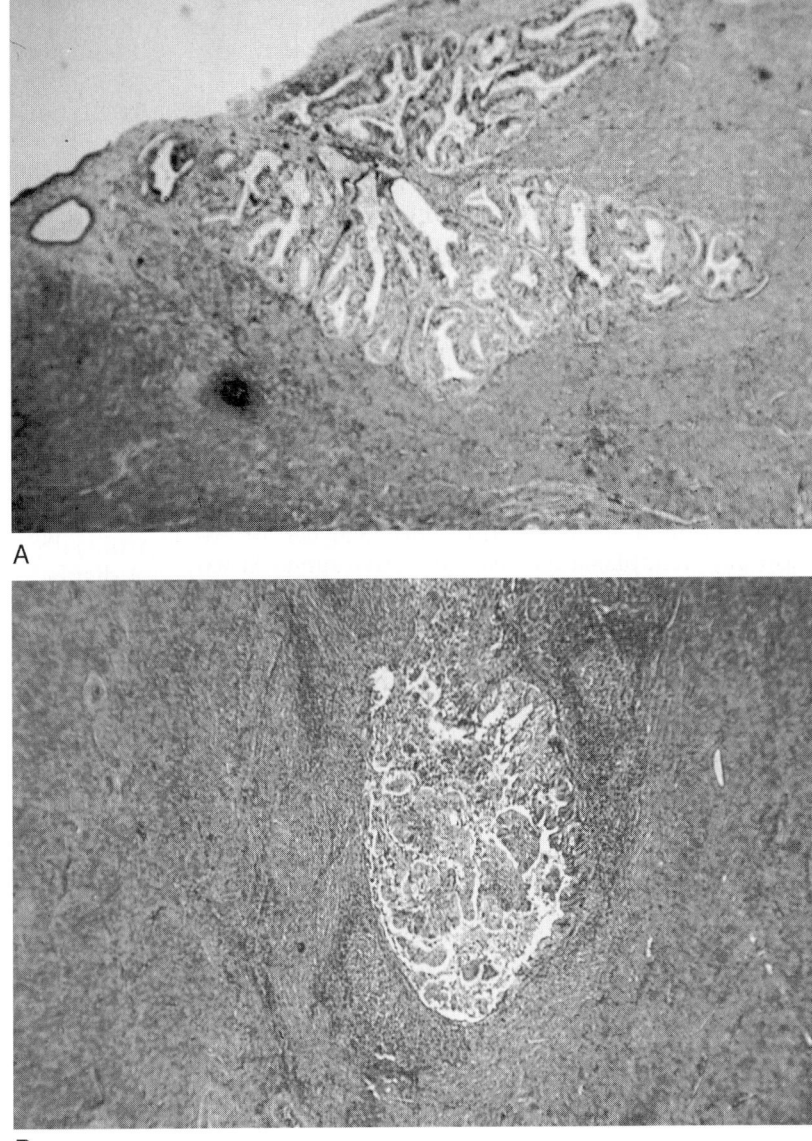

Figure 7–12
A, Superficial myometrial invasion. B, Extension of endometrial adenocarcinoma down adenomyosis.

gross multifocal infiltration into the underlying myometrium as well as hemorrhage and necrosis. A cellular leiomyoma is often solitary, large, and soft to palpation, and may even appear to infiltrate into the interfacing myometrium (Oliva et al, 1995). The examining pathologist should generously sample any grossly atypical leiomyoma. One section per centimeter of diameter is usually sufficient. Distinction between the various subtypes of smooth muscle neoplasia is based on mitotic figure counts and the presence or absence of cytonuclear atypia and necrosis. Frozen sections cannot be relied on to exclude malignancy based on mitotic figure counts. Reliable mitotic figure counts are obtained with thin permanent sections, adequate staining, and standardized magnification with 10× wide-field oculars and a 40× high-dry objective (Kempson and Hendrickson, 1988). Considerable variation may exist within a neoplasm, and all areas of high cellularity and atypia should be counted. Benign stromal nodules cannot be distinguished from a low-grade endometrial stromal sarcoma on endometrial curettage, because it is essential to evaluate the stromal-myometrial interface; therefore, a hysterectomy is often required.

Benign Conditions That Mimic Malignancy

Endometrium, whether benign or neoplastic, may be associated with different types of metaplasia involving either the glandular epithelium or stroma. An awareness of the types and significance of metaplastic epithelium is important to avoid confusion with carcinoma and unnecessary hysterectomy (Hendrickson and Kempson, 1980). Metaplasias do not require treatment provided that the entire uterine cavity has been adequately sampled to exclude any associated hyperplasia or carcinoma. Papillary metaplasia may be misinterpreted as papillary serous carcinoma of the endometrium and clear cell or eosinophilic metaplasia as clear cell carcinoma. Arias-Stella change of the endometrial epithelium during pregnancy has been confused with clear cell carcinoma (Arias-Stella, 1972) (Fig. 7–13). Objective criteria are available to establish the diagnosis of endometrial carcinoma and should be utilized especially when exuberant metaplasia suggests carcinoma (Kurman and Norris, 1982). A useful microscopic finding to diagnose endometrial carcinoma is the reactive fibrous change of the endometrial stroma called desmoplasia (Fig. 7–14). Hyperplastic glands present within an endometrial polyp may be falsely interpreted as carcinoma because of fibrous stroma present within polyps, especially if the specimen is fragmented during curettage or biopsy. Atypical polypoid adenomyoma, a benign proliferation of endometrial epithelium intimately associated with smooth muscle, has been misdiagnosed on curettage as endometrial carcinoma invading into muscle or as a malignant müllerian mixed tumor (Young et al, 1986). Atypical polypoid adenomyomas

generally occur in premenopausal women and have less cytologic atypia than carcinoma. Menstrual endometrium has been misdiagnosed as primary endometrial carcinoma as a result of the breakdown and necrosis with artifactual crowding of the glandular epithelium. Clumping of predecidual stromal cells during menstrual sloughing of the endometrium has resulted in a mistaken diagnosis of metastatic poorly differentiated carcinoma to the endometrium. Needless to say, the suspected "primary" was never found and subsequent immunohistochemical staining of the cells for keratins was negative. Stromal reaction to adenomyosis may simulate a low-grade endometrial stromal sarcoma if adjacent endometrial glands are not readily apparent. Further sections will clarify the diagnosis.

The rare diagnosis of benign metastasizing leiomyoma after hysterectomy always raises concern as to the adequacy of prior pathologic evaluation of the uterus. The specimen has often been discarded and only a few sections were taken of a "fibroid." Deportation of smooth muscle to the lung from intravenous leiomyomatosis or leiomyomata must be distinguished, if possible, from well-differentiated metastases of a leiomyosarcoma. Disseminated leiomyomatosis peritonei consisting of multiple intra-abdominal nodules of smooth muscle can also be mistaken for metastatic leiomyosarcoma. Leiomyosarcomas are usually obvious, with easily recognized numerous mitotic figures, florid atypia, and associated necrosis. Atypical or symplastic leiomyomata have significant atypia but few mitotic figures, whereas mitotically active leiomyomas have frequent mitotic figures but lack atypia (O'Connor and Norris, 1990). Pregnancy and high-dose progestational agents have been found to be associated with increased mitotic figure counts in leiomyomata (Tiltman, 1985). In these cases, extensive sampling and mitotic figure counts will be required to exclude a leiomyosarcoma. Myxoid leiomyosarcomas have artificially lowered mitotic figure counts as a result of displacement of smooth muscle cells by the myxoid ground substance and relative hyocellularity (King et al, 1982). Epithelioid smooth leiomyomas should be considered sarcomas with only five to nine mitotic figures per 10 high-power fields examined (Kurman and Norris, 1976b). An intermediate category of smooth muscle tumors exists in which malignant potential is uncertain (Table 7–2).

Diagnostic Difficulties

The basalis endometrium should be recognized by the pathologist and not used for diagnosis because the irregularity and crowding of the glands may result in overdiagnosis of hyperplasia or carcinoma. Sampling techniques may result in "telescoping" of the glands and artifactual crowding. Metastatic disease to the endometrium does occur, most notably from ovary, breast, and gastrointestinal carcinomas,

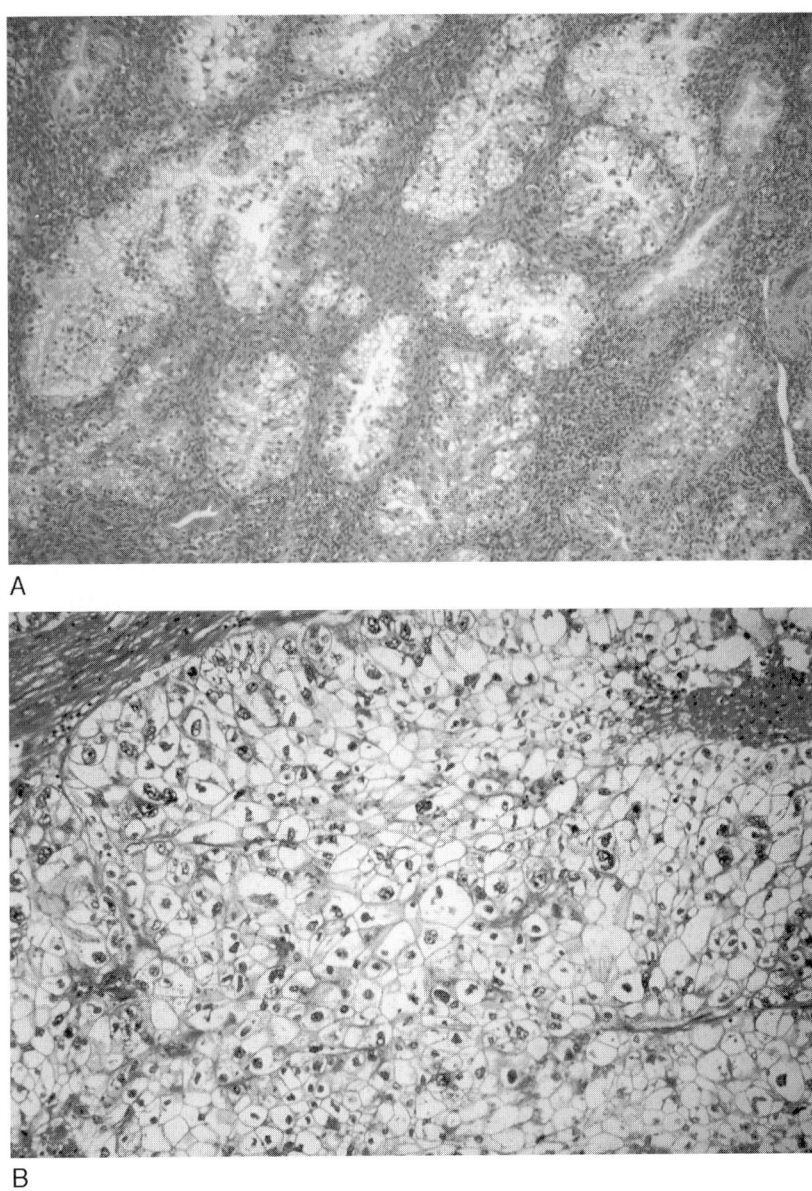

Figure 7–13
A, Arias-Stella reaction of the endometrium during pregnancy. *B*, Clear cell carcinoma of the endometrium.

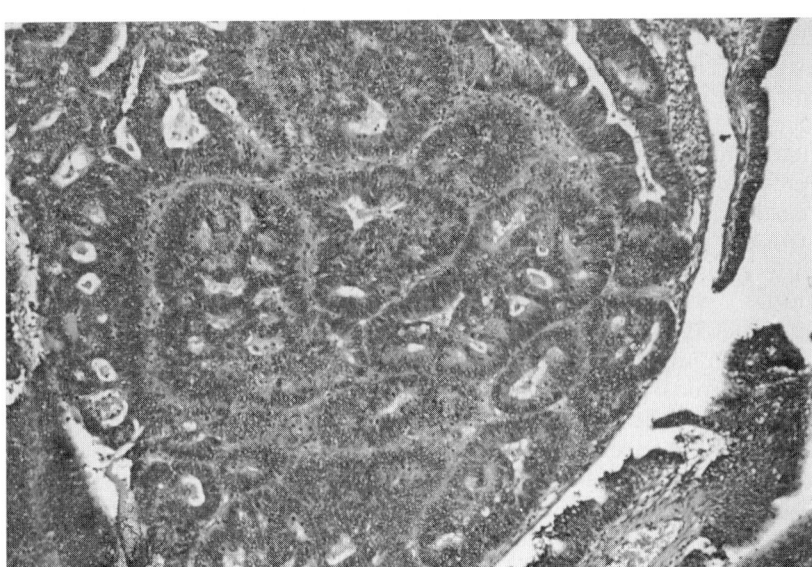

Figure 7–14
Well-differentiated adenocarcinoma of the endometrium with reactive desmoplastic stroma.

Table 7–2. SMOOTH MUSCLE NEOPLASMS OF UNCERTAIN MALIGNANT POTENTIAL

Leiomyoma with atypia with 2–5 MF/10 HPF

Leiomyoma with necrosis with abnormal MF, no atypia

Epithelioid leiomyoma with 2–5 MF/10 HPF

Symplastic leiomyoma with <10 MF/10 HPF, diffuse moderate atypia

Symplastic leiomyoma with <10 MF/10 HPF, focal moderate atypia

Intravascular smooth muscle tumor, gross or microscopic, with 2–5 MF/10 HPF

Parasitic leiomyoma with 2–5 MF/10 HPF

Cellular leiomyoma with 5–10 MF/10 HPF, minimal atypia

Infiltrating leiomyoma with 2–5 MF/10 HPF

Disseminated peritoneal leiomyomatosis with 5–9 MF/10 HPF

Myxoid leiomyoma with MF

Abbreviations: HPF, high-power fields; MF, mitotic figures.
Data from Kempson and Hendrickson (1988) and Bell et al (1994).

and should always be considered in the differential (Kumar and Hart, 1982). A high-grade primary mucinous carcinoma of the endometrium should be viewed with suspicion because most primary endometrial mucinous tumors are very well differentiated. Consideration should be given to the more common possibility of a metastatic gastrointestinal tumor. Papillary or villoglandular endometrial carcinoma should be distinguished from both typical endometrioid and papillary serous tumors, because there are distinct differences in prognosis and treatment (O'Hanlan et al, 1990). Distinction is based mainly on the absence of significant cytonuclear atypia in a villoglandular carcinoma, whereas papillary serous carcinomas are high-grade neoplasms. Another useful clarifying feature is the thin, delicate stromal stalks of the villoglandular tumor, whereas the papillary serous tumor has thick vascular stalks (Fig. 7–15). Endometrial stromal nodules may be difficult to distinguish from cellular leiomyomata (Oliva et al, 1995). Reticulin staining will show a fine, regular reticulin framework surrounding individual stromal cells in an endometrial stromal nodule. The differential of an endometrial stromal sarcoma includes poorly differentiated or undifferentiated endometrial carcinoma and metastatic disease, including lymphoma and breast carcinoma. Immunohistochemical studies for LCA and keratins can help to establish the diagnosis (Kempson and Hendrickson, 1988). A rare variant of endometrial stromal sarcomas shows sex cord differentiation and results in confusion with malignant mixed mesodermal tumors, adenosarcomas, and endometrial carcinomas (Clement and Scully, 1976).

OVARY

Specimen Procurement

All clinicians should be skilled in the gross evaluation of an adnexal mass to assess the likelihood of malignancy. This skill is absolutely essential if conservative laparoscopic removal of the adnexal mass is to be attempted. The cortical surface of the ovary and the peritoneal surfaces should be inspected for papillary excrescences, adhesions, or implants. Any pelvic fluid should be aspirated and sent for cytologic examination. A gentle pelvic wash can then be done with normal saline and the fluid aspirated. Forceful irrigation may detach aggregates of mesothelial cells, which appear papillary on microscopy. Heparin is not necessary, but the fluid should be transported to the cytology laboratory without delay. If the fluid must be shipped, then a commercial preservative or absolute alcohol should be added in equal volumes. The adnexal mass should be removed intact, without rupture of the cortical surface, because it has been shown that intraoperative rupture of stage I ovarian cancer may worsen the prognosis (Sainz de la Cuesta et al, 1994). Even benign characteristics, such as a single unilocular cyst less than 8 cm in size, do not preclude malignancy (Maiman et al, 1991). Laparoscopy and biopsy of grossly suspicious ovarian tumors has been associated with trocar site tumor implantation and should be performed only when definitive thorough debulking and staging can be accomplished at the same operation (Hsiu et al, 1986). When the decision is made to proceed with laparoscopic adnexal mass removal, it is imperative that surgeons understand that, on reexploration, gynecologic oncologists upstage approximately 30% of putative stage I ovarian neoplasms (Snider et al, 1991). Aspiration cytology of cysts is controversial and difficult to interpret, may be associated with tumor spillage, and can even result in a false diagnosis of cancer (Stanley et al, 1991).

Pathology Evaluation

Gross evaluation and frozen section of the intact adnexal mass can be performed by a pathologist. If a pathologist is not available, gross evaluation, including inspection of the interior of the cyst, can be accomplished by the surgeon away from the operative field. A specific note should be made in the operative report as to whether the cortical surface of the ovary was intact to visual inspection, because the pathologist will not be able to assure surface integrity if the mass was opened by the surgeon. Once removed, the ovary can be opened and the internal surface inspected for any solid areas, excrescences, or papillations (Fig. 7–16). Endometriomas usually have a thick cyst wall and contain blood, and benign cystic teratomas contain sebum and hair (Fig. 7–17). Both are easily diagnosed by gross inspection. Cystade-

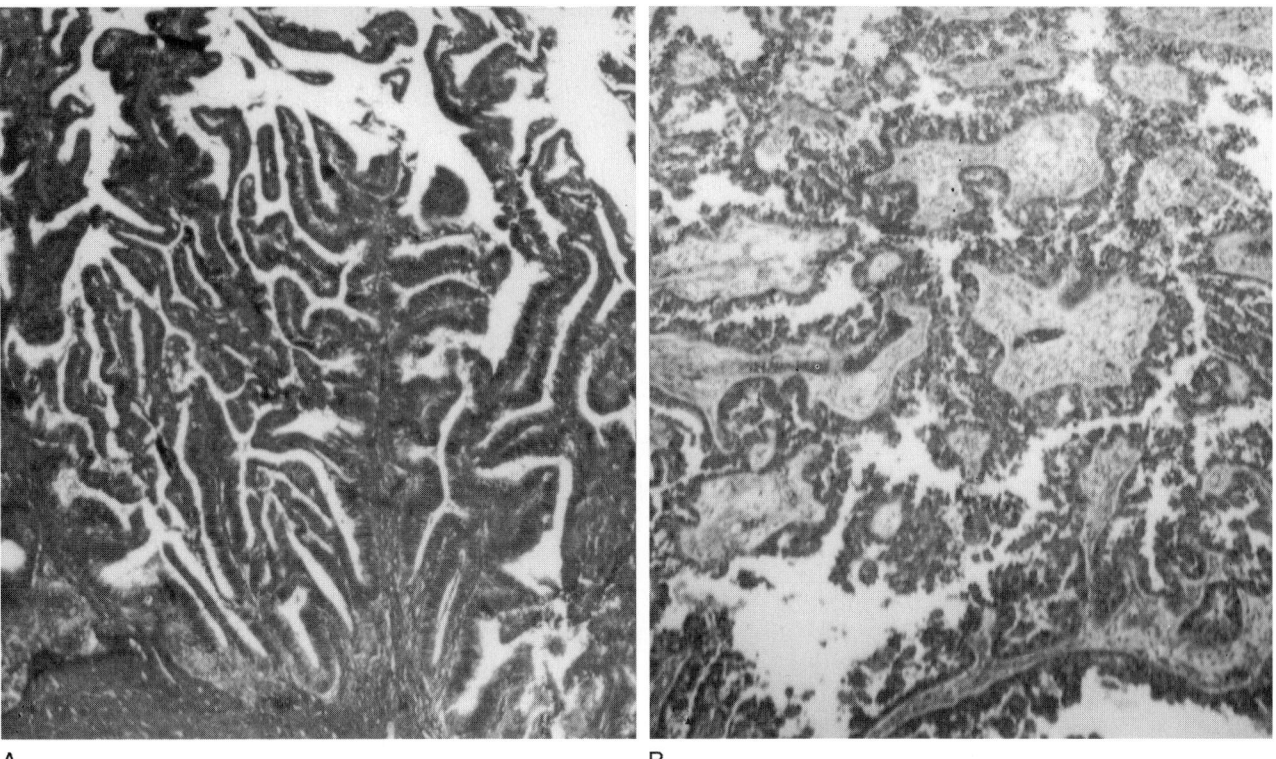

A   B

Figure 7–15
A, Papillary endometrial adenocarcinoma (villoglandular). B, Papillary serous carcinoma of the endometrium. (From O'Hanlan KA, Levine PA, Harbatkin D, et al: Virulence of papillary endometrial carcinoma. Gynecol Oncol 1990;37:112, with permission.)

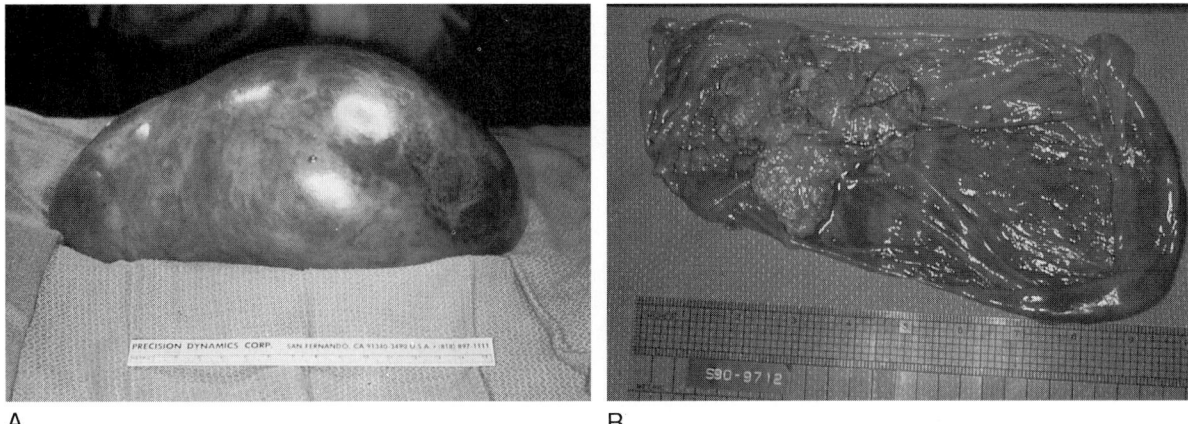

A   B

Figure 7–16
A, Large cyst with an intact, smooth cortical surface. B, Opened cyst with a solid orange growth confirmed to be a germ cell tumor.

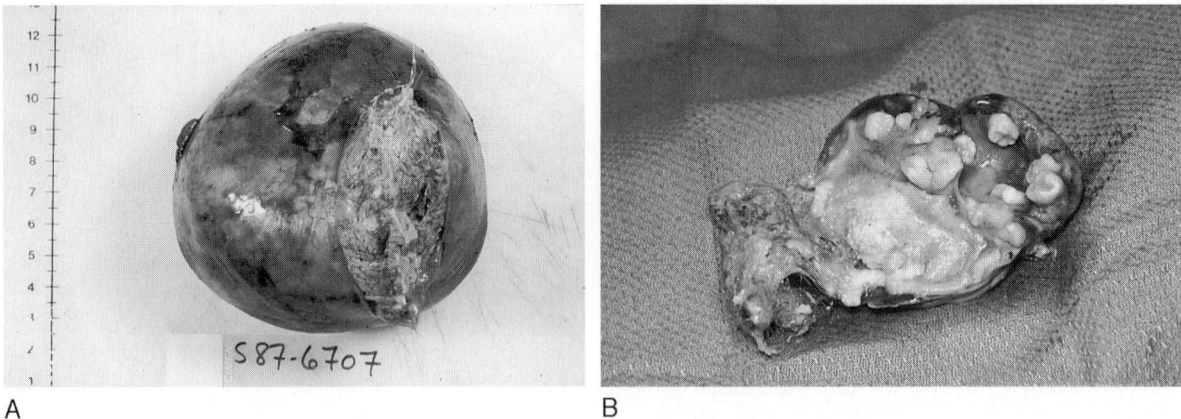

A   B

Figure 7–17
A, Ovarian cyst with a nonintact cortical surface extruding hair and sebum. *B*, Interior of the cyst with teeth and hair compatible with a benign cystic teratoma.

nofibromas contain small, firm papillations on the interior lining of the cyst, whereas borderline tumors show a more exuberant, friable growth. Any solid areas should be regarded as highly suspicious for malignancy. Protocols for the pathologic examination of adnexal masses are now available (Scully et al, 1995). Appropriate decisions as to the need for further surgery, staging, or referral can be made based on the gross evaluation and, if available, the frozen section result. A diagnosis of a borderline tumor cannot be made on frozen section evaluation because this is a diagnosis of exclusion and requires multiple sections, especially in the case of a mucinous tumor (Menzin et al, 1995) (Fig. 7–18). Regardless, any suspicion of malignancy on frozen section, whether the final diagnosis is a borderline tumor or a carcinoma, warrants complete surgical staging. An ability to assess the likelihood of malignancy based on gross inspection can be an invaluable tool to optimize patient care with appropriate staging or to facilitate prompt referral.

Gynecologic oncologists will attempt to debulk all metastases of ovarian carcinoma to leave only minimal, if any, residual disease. Small and large intestinal resections are common. Metastases to the bowel wall have been found to invade deeply, accessing the intestinal lymphatic channels and spreading both transversely to the mesenteric nodes and longitudinally along the subserosal myenteric lymphatics (O'Hanlan et al, 1995). Hence, a wide resection of involved bowel, obtaining 5-cm margins longitudinally, that includes a sizeable wedge of mesentery should be obtained. Pathologists should evaluate the submitted mesenteric nodes for metastatic disease. The depth of invasion through the bowel wall, presence or absence of lymphatic space, and surgical margin involvement should be specifically noted on the report.

Benign Conditions That Mimic Malignancy

A few interesting, rare disease processes may mimic ovarian cancer with diffuse abdominal spread or

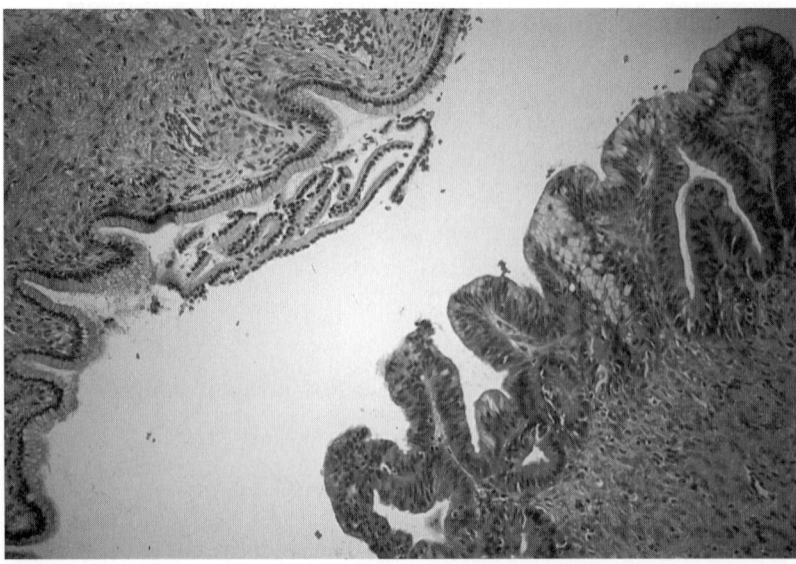

Figure 7–18
Focus of mucinous carcinoma of low malignant potential (*bottom right*) in an otherwise benign mucinous cystadenoma (*top left*).

"carcinomatosis" on visual inspection of the pelvis. Pelvic tuberculosis and schistosomiasis may simulate metastatic ovarian cancer, as can a diffuse peritoneal foreign body reaction resulting from keratin leakage from a benign cystic teratoma. Teratomas, both mature and immature, may be associated with multiple peritoneal implants of mature neural tissue, or "gliomatosis" (Robboy and Scully, 1970). A florid decidual reaction during pregnancy has been mistaken for metastatic disease (Bersch et al, 1973). Diffuse peritoneal leiomyomatosis can result in peritoneal nodularity suspicious for malignancy. Any mesothelial proliferation incited by peritoneal irritation can be associated with psammoma bodies and, although reactive in nature, may be confusing on microscopy.

Diagnostic Difficulties

Epithelial Cell Tumors

Florid mesothelial hyperplasia secondary to effusions or peritoneal inflammation may be mistaken for epithelial implants of ovarian cancer with errors made in surgical staging and in interpretation of the pelvic wash (Clement and Young, 1993). Peritoneal and omental involvement with endosalpingiosis may be misinterpreted as intra-abdominal dissemination of a borderline tumor, especially if atypia or psammoma bodies are present (Zinsser and Wheeler, 1982; McCaughey et al, 1984; Bell and Scully, 1990). A minimum of one section per centimeter of omentum is required if grossly negative for disease. A complete and detailed evaluation of implants associated with borderline tumors is necessary because distinction between benign endosalpingiosis, noninvasive desmoplastic, and invasive implants is important for prognosis and treatment (Bell et al, 1988; Copeland et al, 1988). Hyperplastic mesothelial cells and benign glandular inclusions of endosalpingosis may occur in lymph nodes and be confused with metastatic disease (Ehrmann et al, 1980; Clement et al, 1996). Although rare in occurrence, a peritoneal malignant mesothelioma must be distinguished from an advanced-stage primary ovarian papillary serous adenocarcinoma (Daya and McCaughey, 1990). Immunohistochemical studies can be helpful in distinguishing a primary mesothelial process from a carcinoma, particularly in the interpretation of

peritoneal fluid cytology (Table 7–3). On occasion, it may be necessary to perform electron microscopy to clarify the diagnosis. Extraovarian serous neoplasia has been diagnosed after bilateral oophorectomy, and consideration must be given to the possibility of a residual remnant of ovarian tissue, especially if the surgery was technically difficult (Pettit and Lee, 1988). Primary peritoneal carcinomas have occurred in carriers of a BRCA1 gene mutation after prophylactic oophorectomy. Considerable difficulty may be encountered in distinguishing a primary papillary peritoneal neoplasm with secondary ovarian surface involvement from a serous surface papillary ovarian carcinoma of the ovary with peritoneal metastatic spread. Often the distinction is based on the primary location of the majority of the tumor volume. Diffuse peritoneal disease associated with ovarian cortical surface implants that have a "stuck on" appearance is compatible with a peritoneal primary (Bell and Scully, 1990).

Distinction of epithelial subtypes may require extensive sampling, mucin stains, and, occasionally, immunohistochemical studies. A poorly differentiated endometrioid carcinoma is difficult to distinguish from a serous carcinoma unless sampling discloses foci of better differentiation or areas of squamous or clear cell metaplasia. Mucin stains may help to distinguish poorly differentiated mucinous adenocarcinomas. Although not specific, the presence of specific tumor-associated antigens, cancer antigen 125 (CA-125), CEA, and cancer antigen 19-9 (CA-19-9) on immunohistochemical staining may support a tentative diagnosis. CA-125 is predominantly seen in serous carcinomas, but is also frequently expressed by endometrioid carcinomas. CEA and CA-19-9 are primarily expressed by mucinous tumors but can also be detected in endometrioid carcinomas and a rare serous carcinoma (Neunteufel and Breitenecker, 1989). Overlap is considerable, but strong staining of a particular tumor-associated antigen along with supporting morphologic features may help establish the diagnosis.

In contrast to the other epithelial subtypes, mucinous neoplasms show extensive histologic variation within a single specimen. Extensive sampling is required because foci of invasion or borderline features may exist within an otherwise benign-appearing tumor. It is recommended that one block be taken for every 1 to 2 cm of tumor (Hart and Norris, 1973). It is essential that the appendix be removed when a

Table 7–3. IMMUNOHISTOCHEMICAL STAINS TO DISTINGUISH MESOTHELIAL FROM EPITHELIAL CELLS

ANTIGEN*	MESOTHELIOMA	CARCINOMA
CEA	Negative (10–20% positive)	Positive
TAG-72	Negative (5% positive)	Positive (poorly differentiated negative)
Leu-M1	Negative (focal positive)	Positive

*CEA, carcinoembryonic antigen; Leu-M1, myelomonocytic marker; TAG-72 tumor-associated glycoprotein, B72.3 antibody.
Data from Battifora and Kopinski (1989), Bollinger et al (1989), and Wick et al (1989).

mucinous tumor of the ovary is suspected, especially if pseudomyxoma peritonei is present. Mucinous tumors of the appendix may be found on histologic examination and may represent the primary lesion with secondary metastatic disease to the ovary (Young et al, 1991) (Fig. 7–19).

Endometrioid carcinomas may mimic Sertoli cell tumors. The surrounding ovarian stroma may be vacuolated and resemble lutein cells, resulting in confusion with Sertoli-Leydig cell tumors (Roth et al, 1982). The endometrioid pattern of yolk sac tumors may look like an endometrioid carcinoma of the ovary, but occurs in younger patients (Clement et al, 1987). Further sections and diligent examination will disclose more characteristic features of the neoplasm.

Clear cell carcinomas of the ovary are pleiomorphic, composed of multiple patterns including the diffuse, tubulocystic, and papillary morphologies. A metastatic renal cell carcinoma to the ovary will lack this variation in pattern (Young and Hart, 1992). Dysgerminoma of the ovary can be distinguished from a clear cell carcinoma by the characteristic lymphocytic infiltrate surrounding nests of tumor cells. Yolk sac tumors lack the hobnail cells characteristic of clear cell carcinomas and, on further analysis, will be found to contain classic Schiller-Duval bodies and patterns specific to germ cell tumors (Fig. 7–20). Immunostaining with antibodies for α-fetoprotein (AFP) and Leu-M1–related antigen will distinguish yolk sac tumors from clear cell carcinomas (Zirker et al, 1989). Clear cell carcinomas of the ovary are also frequently associated with endometriosis (Shevchuk et al, 1981).

Although malignant mixed mesodermal tumors generally occur in older women, they have been confused with immature teratomas. Besides the disparity in age at presentation, mixed mesodermal tumors lack any ectodermal or endodermal derivatives. Immature teratomas characteristically contain immature neural elements.

Sex Cord–Stromal Tumors

Sex cord–stromal tumors may be a source of diagnostic confusion. Granulosa cell tumors of the diffuse pattern have been misdiagnosed as small cell carcinomas, lymphomas, and metastatic melanoma, but most commonly as poorly differentiated or undifferentiated carcinomas (Young and Scully, 1982) (Fig. 7–21). Further sectioning of the tumor will usually disclose the other characteristic patterns of granulosa cell tumors (Fig. 7–22). Very few tumors have the grooved "coffee bean" nuclei typical of a granulosa cell tumor. A feature common in granulosa cell tumors is how the cells line up, or "palisade," when interfacing with another tissue type (Fig. 7–23). Granulosa cell tumors lack the prominent intranuclear inclusions of melanoma (Young and Scully, 1991a). Small cell carcinomas contain follicle-like spaces similar to granulosa cell tumors, hence the similarity and diagnostic difficulty (Dickerson et al,

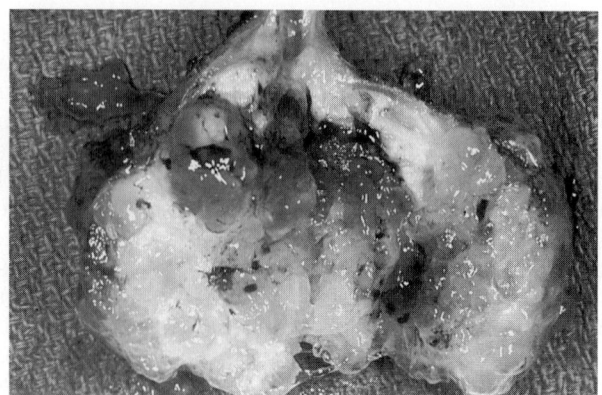

Figure 7–19
Primary mucinous neoplasm of the appendix. This was associated with pseudomyxoma peritonei and secondary ovarian involvement.

1982). Cystic, unilocular granulosa cell tumors have been mistaken for follicular cysts (Young and Clement, 1995). Juvenile granulosa cell tumors can be distinguished from yolk sac tumors by the lack of staining for AFP (Young et al, 1984). The retiform pattern of Sertoli-Leydig cell tumors may focally stain for AFP, thus exacerbating the confusion with yolk sac tumors (Talerman, 1987; Gagnon et al, 1989). An abundant mucinous epithelium or cartilage present in a heterologous Sertoli-Leydig cell tumor evokes diagnostic consideration of a mucinous carcinoma or a malignant mixed mesodermal tumor (Young and Scully, 1985).

Germ Cell Tumors

When evaluating an adnexal mass in a child, it is prudent to consider the possibility of an ovarian germ cell tumor arising in dysgenetic gonads. Preoperative karyotyping and molecular analysis for the testicular determining factor region (SRY) of the Y chromosome is helpful, because castration would be necessary for dysgenetic gonads. This may not be feasible if the child presents with an acute abdomen secondary to torsion of the mass. Germ cell tumors are not an uncommon diagnosis in pregnancy and are also frequently complicated by torsion (Krepart et al, 1978). Calcifications in association with a germ cell tumor may be the only remaining remnants of a burnt-out gonadoblastoma (Scully, 1970). Gonadoblastomas can be very small and may not be apparent on inspection of the ovary. Because an attempt is always made to perform conservative surgery and to remove only the diseased adnexa, it will spare the child a second surgery if dysgenetic gonads are diagnosed preoperatively. Germ cell tumors are frequently mixed, and a diligent search should be made to diagnose all the types present (Kurman and Norris, 1976a). An embryonal carcinoma may be difficult to discern from dysgerminoma if the characteristic clefts and spaces are not readily apparent (Fig. 7–24). If needed, immunohistochemical studies for in-

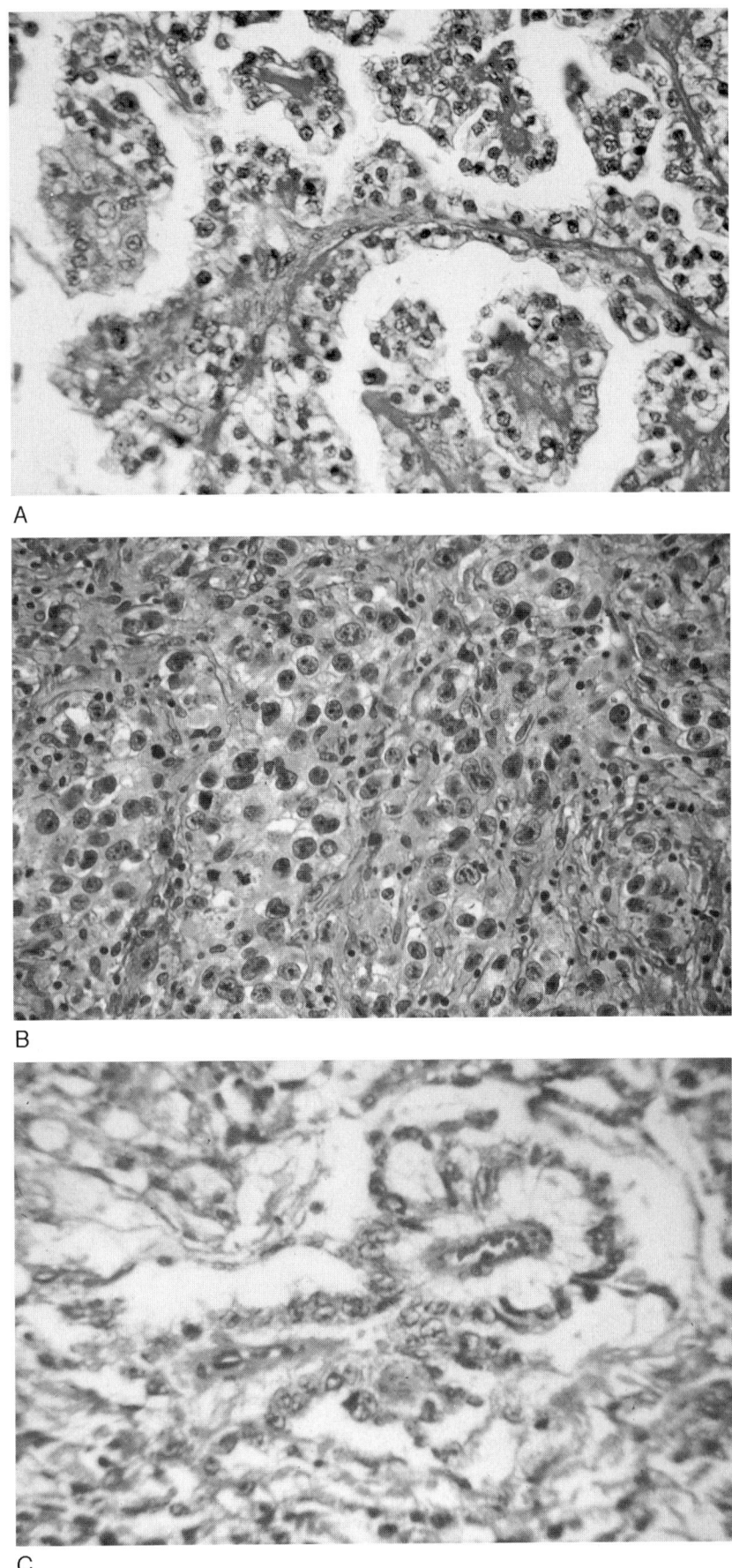

A

B

C

Figure 7-20
A, Clear cell carcinoma of the ovary. *B,*
Dysgerminoma of the ovary. *C,* Endodermal
sinus tumor with a Schiller-Duval body.

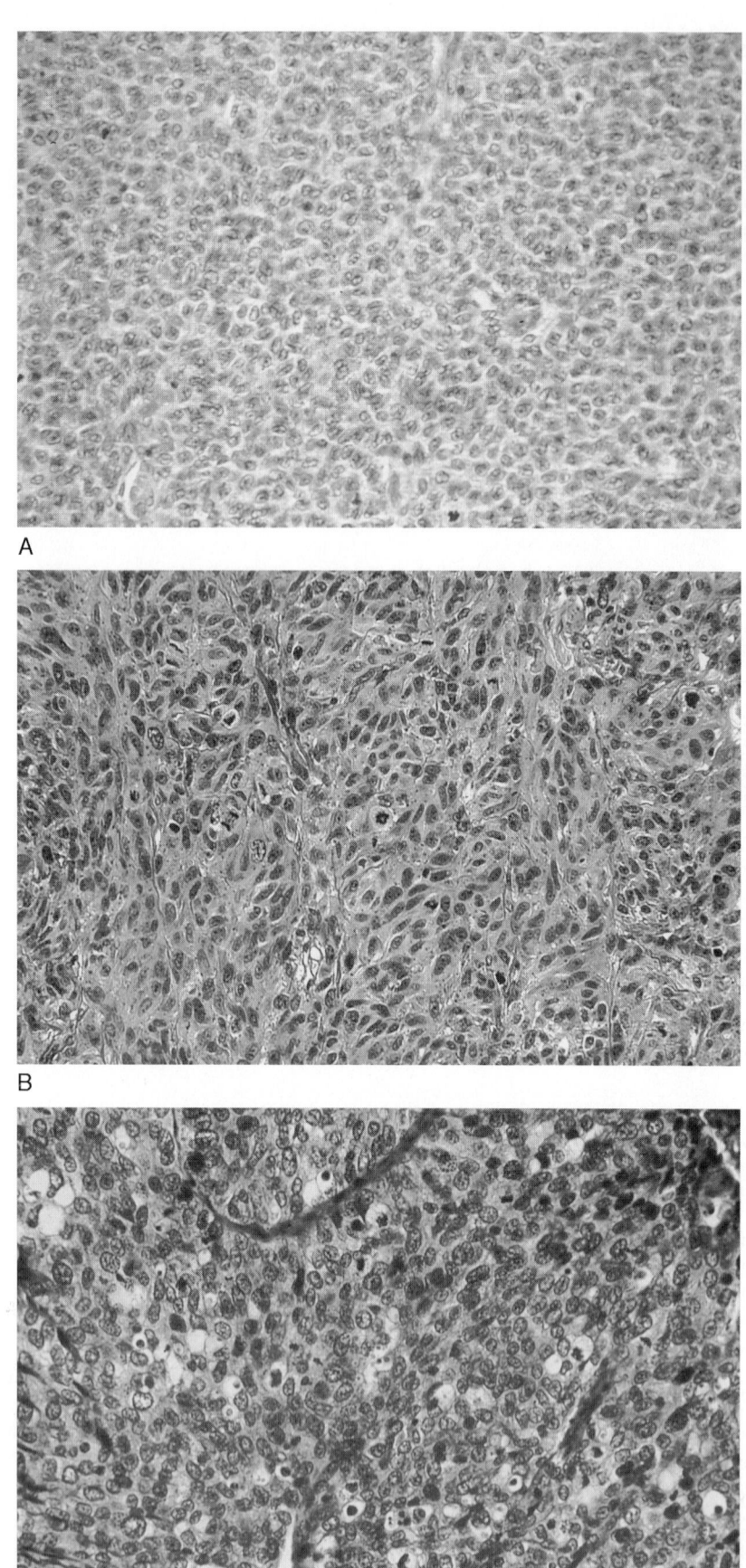

Figure 7–21
A, Granulosa cell tumor of the diffuse pattern (note "coffee bean" nuclei). B, Melanoma metastatic to the ovary. C, Undifferentiated ovarian carcinoma.

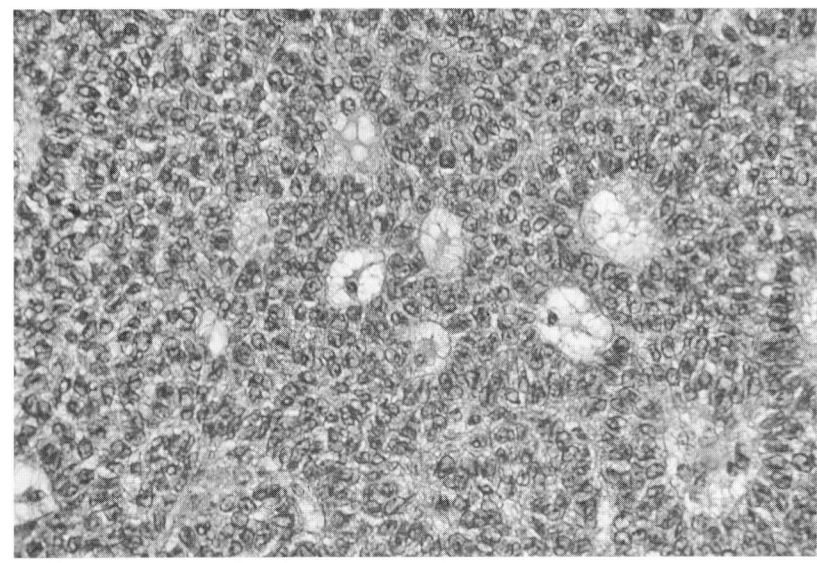

Figure 7-22
Granulosa cell tumor with Call-Exner bodies.

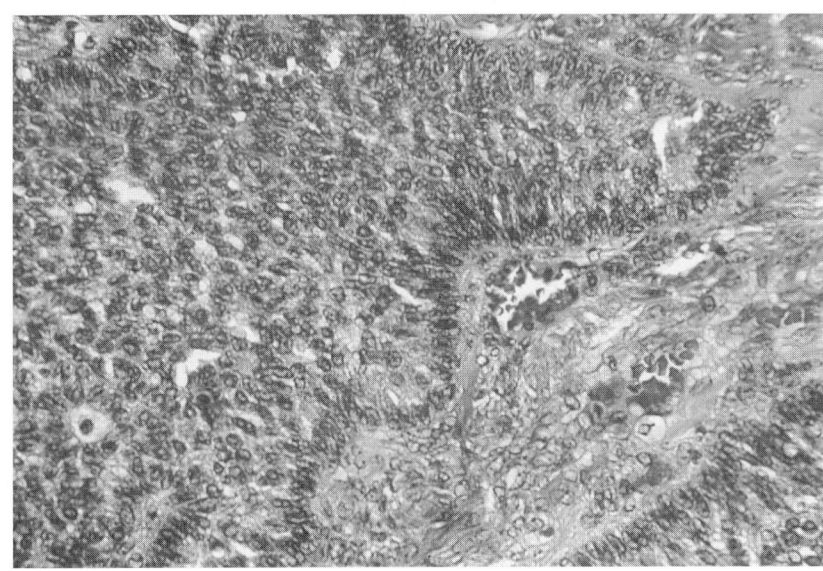

Figure 7-23
Granulosa cell tumor with characteristic orderly lining up of the cells, or "palisading."

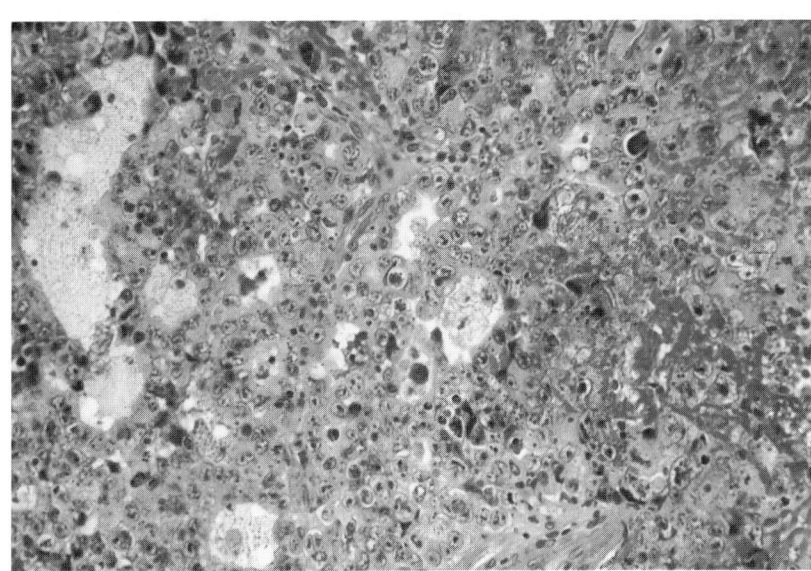

Figure 7-24
Embryonal cell carcinoma with clefts and spaces.

termediate filaments can be done. Dysgerminomas are negative for cytokeratin, whereas the other germ cell tumors that are morphologically similar, such as yolk sac tumors and embryonal carcinomas, stain positive (Miettinen et al, 1985). Embryonal carcinomas may stain positive for both AFP and human chorionic gonadotropin (hCG), whereas yolk sac tumors stain only for AFP (Kurman and Norris, 1976a). Small foci of syncytiotrophoblast may be found in dysgerminoma and will stain for hCG, but can be distinguished from a component of choriocarcinoma in a mixed germ cell tumor by the lack of cytotrophoblast, hemorrhage, or necrosis (Zaloudek et al, 1981). It is extremely rare for choriocarcinoma to exist in a pure form; it is almost invariably part of a mixed germ cell tumor, and therefore can be distinguished from a gestational choriocarcinoma. As previously discussed, yolk sac tumors must be distinguished from clear cell carcinoma. A rare pattern of a yolk sac tumor that may exist in a pure form is the hepatoid pattern, which may be similar in appearance to steroid cell tumors or metastatic hepatocellular carcinoma (Prat et al, 1982).

Metastases to the Ovary

Metastatic disease to the ovary must always be considered in the differential of a pelvic mass, both preoperatively and at microscopic evaluation. The probability of finding metastatic disease at the time of surgery for a pelvic mass has been estimated to be 7%, with primary colon cancer the most frequently misdiagnosed as primary ovarian cancer (Ulbright et al, 1984). Contiguous spread from adjacent tumors, lymphatic and hematogenous spread, and implantation can all result in secondary ovarian involvement. Breast cancer and a multitude of other primary cancers can metastasize to the ovaries and present initially as a pelvic mass. A thorough preoperative evaluation, including assessment of the gastrointestinal tract and a mammogram, will diagnose most, but not all, nongenital primary cancers. Clues to metastatic disease on gross and microscopic evaluation are presented in Table 7–4.

Table 7–4. CLUES TO METASTATIC DISEASE TO THE OVARY

GROSS EVALUATION	MICROSCOPIC EVALUATION
Bilateral ovarian involvement	Hilar location of tumor
Hemorrhage and necrosis	Multinodular pattern
Surface implants on the ovary	Vascular space involvement
Disseminated disease	Tumor necrosis

From Young RH, Scully RE: Metastatic tumors in the ovary: a problem oriented approach and review of the recent literature. Semin Diagn Pathol 1991;8:250, with permission.

Metastatic colon cancer is misdiagnosed as primary mucinous or endometrioid carcinoma of the ovary in as many as half of the cases (Lash and Hart, 1987) (Fig. 7–25). When diffuse intra-abdominal disease is apparent, it is unlikely to be a primary endometrioid carcinoma of the ovary, which usually is confined to the ovary at presentation. Ovarian mucinous carcinoma is rarely bilateral, which is common with metastatic disease. Microscopic findings specific for metastatic colon cancer have been extensively described in the literature and include "dirty" segmental necrosis of glands with a peripheral garland formation of tumor cells (Lash and Hart, 1987; Daya et al, 1992). Endometrioid carcinomas of the ovary are often associated with foci of squamous or clear cell metaplasia, and further sectioning of the tumor may help to clarify the diagnosis. Immunohistochemical staining for CEA is helpful, if supportive (Sheahan et al, 1993). The pattern of CEA staining, diffuse versus focal, may help differentiate a primary ovarian carcinoma from metastatic colon carcinoma (Fleuren and Nap, 1988). A high index of suspicion and consistent clinicopathologic correlation are often all that is needed to facilitate the diagnosis.

Delay in the initial diagnosis or recurrence of breast cancer may result in patient presentation with a pelvic mass and even with diffuse ascites and abdominal carcinomatosis (Young et al, 1981). Often characteristic patterns such as the classic "Indian filing" can be seen, but in other cases confusion may exist with primary ovarian endometrioid adenocarcinomas, granulosa cell tumors, or poorly differentiated carcinomas (Gagnon and Tetu, 1989) (Fig. 7–26). Immunohistochemical studies for gross cystic disease fluid protein-15 (GCDFP-15) may be helpful, because one study found that 71% of metastatic breast cancers stained positive (Monteagudo et al, 1991). Such diagnostic dilemmas emphasize the necessity of preoperative mammography and colon cancer screening, but even preoperative evaluation does not always exclude all nongynecologic cancers as the source of the pelvic mass.

Pancreatic cancer metastatic to the ovary can be mistaken for a primary ovarian mucinous carcinoma and may be associated with diffuse abdominal spread. Discriminating features include bilaterality, advanced disease, and tumor in vascular spaces (Young and Scully, 1989). The gastric primary in a Krukenberg tumor may be small and elude diagnosis, yet result in disseminated disease. Krukenberg tumors have been difficult to diagnose on microscopic examination when the presentation is that of a few vacuolated cells in a cellular ovarian stroma. The appearance is not unlike stromal hyperthecosis or a thecoma. Mucin staining will highlight the small signet-ring cells filled with mucin (Holtz and Hart, 1982) (Fig. 7–27). A renal cell carcinoma metastatic to the ovaries can be very similar in appearance to a primary ovarian clear cell carcinoma and may precede diagnosis of the primary neoplasm (Young and

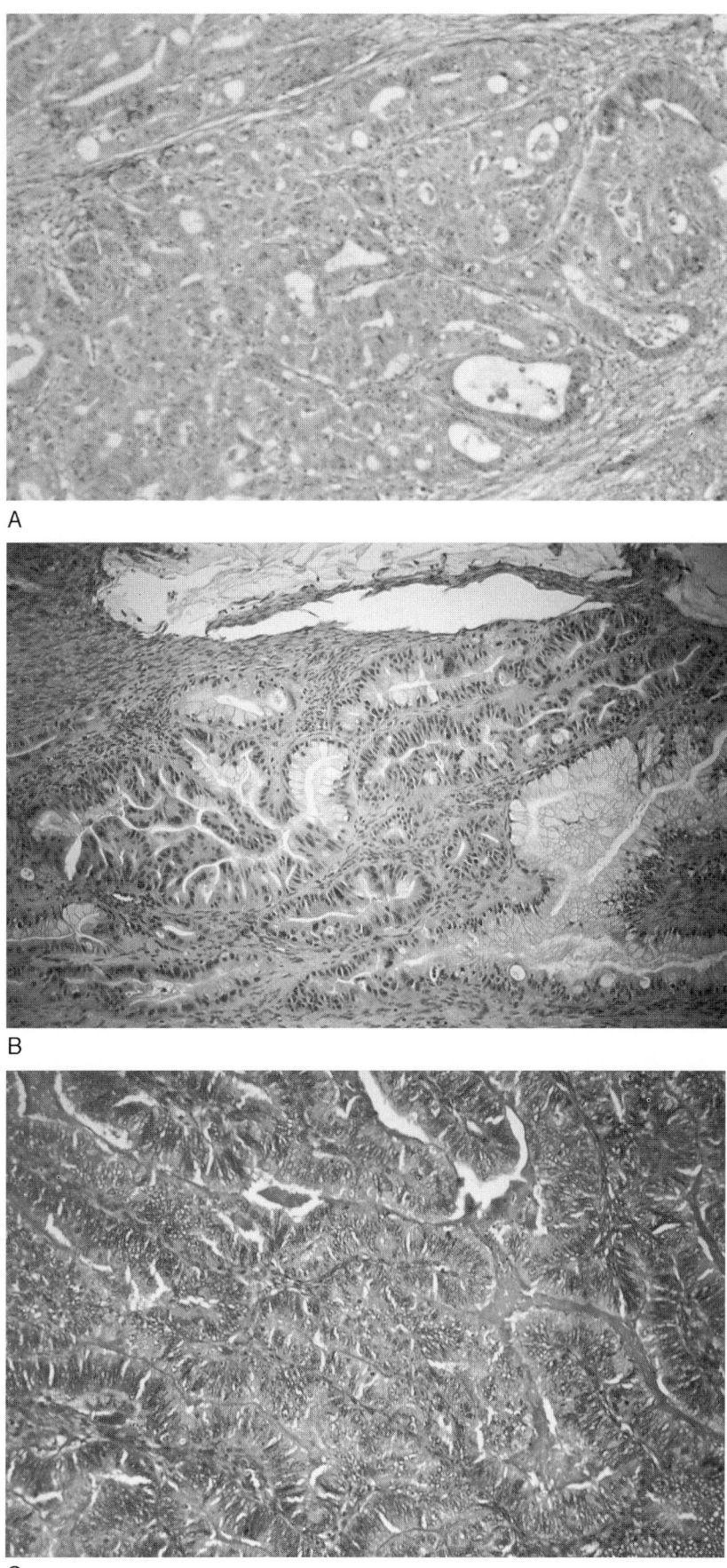

Figure 7–25
A, Metastatic colon cancer to the ovary. *B,* Primary ovarian mucinous carcinoma. *C,* Primary endometrial adenocarcinoma.

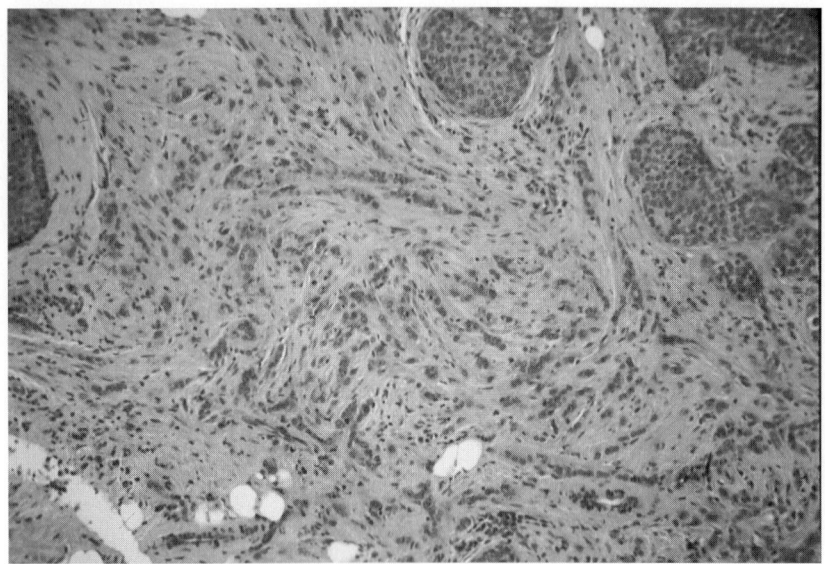

Figure 7–26
Metastatic breast carcinoma to the ovary with "Indian filing" of the cells.

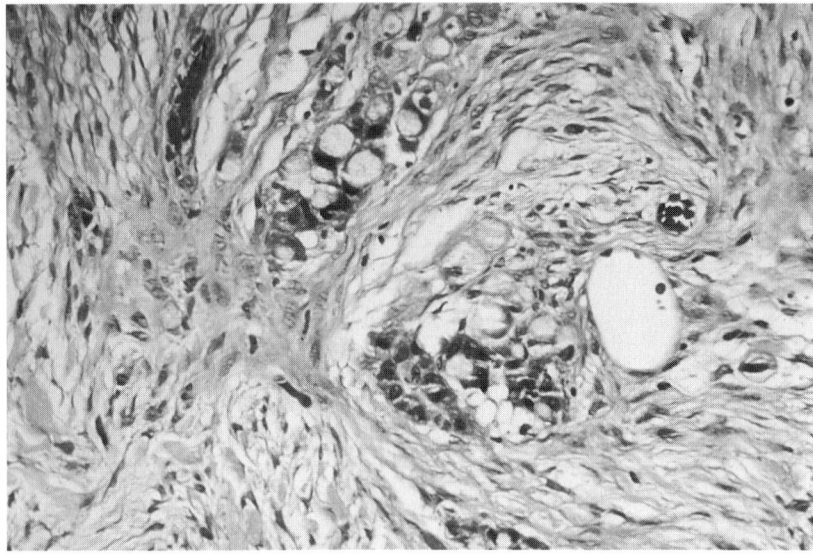

A

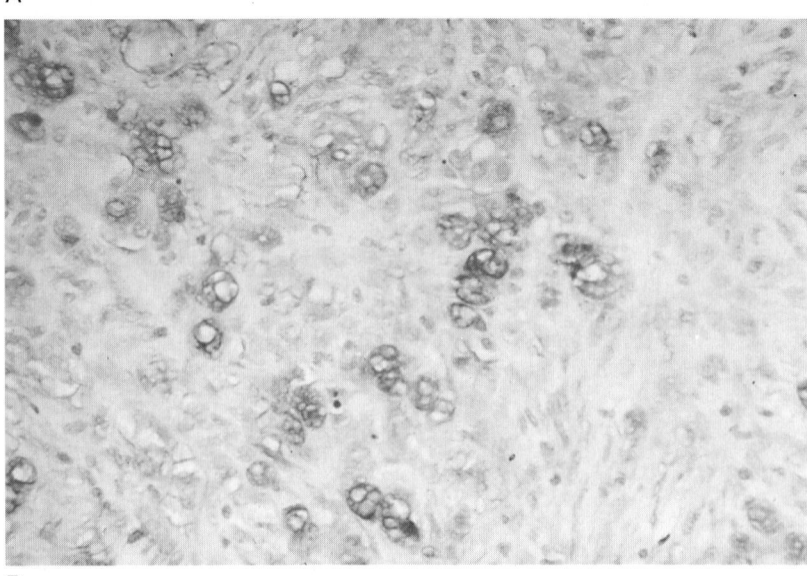

B

Figure 7–27
A, Metastatic Krukenberg tumor with signet-ring cells. *B*, Mucicarmine staining highlights the metastatic cells.

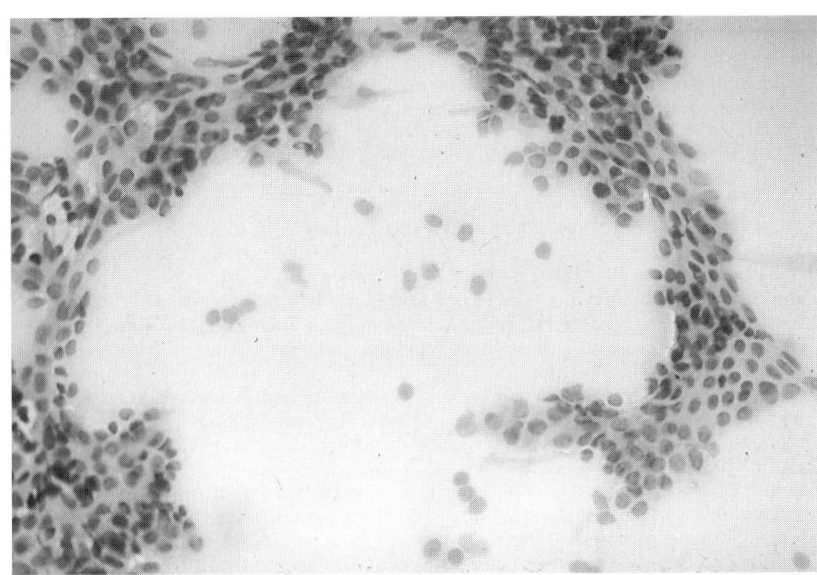

Figure 7–28
Fine-needle aspiration of the breast diagnostic for fibroadenoma.

Hart, 1992). A careful microscopic search will reveal the multiple patterns of an ovarian clear cell carcinoma, including the papillary and tubulocystic morphologies. Amelanotic metastatic melanoma can create considerable diagnostic confusion. Epithelioid cells surrounding follicle-like spaces can mimic a primary small cell carcinoma of the ovary or a juvenile granulosa cell tumor. All can occur in younger patients. Immunohistochemical studies positive for melanocytic markers such as HMB-45 and S100 protein can be invaluable in establishing the diagnosis as melanoma (Young and Scully, 1991a).

Synchronous tumors of the female genital tract do occur, and the classical example is that of an endometrioid carcinoma of the ovary with an endometrial carcinoma of the uterus (Eifel et al, 1982). The question arises: Is the ovarian disease a second primary or metastatic disease from the endometrial neoplasm? Resolution is not always easy and is often based on extensive sampling and clinical probability. It would be unlikely for a well-differentiated endometrial carcinoma with superficial myometrial invasion to be associated with ovarian metastases. Extensive sampling may reveal foci of squamous and clear cell metaplasia in the ovarian tumor, no vascular space involvement, and association with endometriosis, all of which would support a second primary in the ovary. Advances in molecular biology techniques, such as DNA loss of heterozygosity studies, or "fingerprinting" and ploidy analysis, have allowed comparison of tumor samples but are rarely necessary (Prat et al, 1991; Chuaqui et al, 1996).

BREAST

Fine-needle aspiration cytology is a valuable tool to quickly diagnose palpable breast masses. It is important to remember that the study will only be accurate if the needle enters the mass. Cytologic diagnosis may be definitive for the diagnosis of carcinoma or fibroadenoma (Fig. 7–28). Fine-needle aspiration cytology of the breast must include ductal epithelial cells for an accurate reading. An aspirate that lacks these cells or with scant cellularity cannot reliably exclude malignancy, and further diagnostic procedures, such as a biopsy, are indicated. The clinician must understand the terminology of the report and know when the sample is of inadequate cellularity; likewise, the report should state without ambiguity whether the specimen is satisfactory for evaluation. Cytology of breast discharge is of no diagnostic utility and should be discouraged.

PLACENTA

Placental site nodules have been found in the cervix and have been confused with a decidual reaction and CIN (Young et al, 1990). Normal implantation is associated with infiltration of the endometrium, myometrium, and blood vessels with intermediate trophoblast, and may be difficult to distinguish from gestational trophoblastic disease, especially on curettage. Placental-site trophoblastic tumor (PSTT) consists of intermediate trophoblast and can be difficult to distinguish from a poorly differentiated carcinoma. Foci of PSTT have been found in a postmenopausal woman mimicking a poorly differentiated carcinoma (McLellan et al, 1991). Lung metastases of malignant PSTT can simulate primary lung carcinoma. This diagnostic possibility must always be considered, especially in reproductive-age women. Fortunately, immunoperoxidase stains are diagnostic when positive for human placental lactogen and hCG (Kurman et al, 1984).

REFERENCES

Anderson MC, Hartley RB: Cervical crypt involvement by intraepithelial neoplasia. Obstet Gynecol 1980;55:546.

Arias-Stella J: Atypical endometrial changes produced by chorionic tissue. Hum Pathol 1972:450.

Battifora H, Kopinski MI: Distinction of mesothelioma from adenocarcinoma: an immunohistochemical approach. Cancer 1985;55:1679.

Bell DA, Scully RE: Serous borderline tumors of the peritoneum. Am J Surg Pathol 1990;14:230.

Bell DA, Weinstock MA, Scully RE: Peritoneal implants of serous borderline tumors: histologic features and prognosis. Cancer 1988;62:2212.

Bell SW, Kempson RL, Hendrickson MR: Problematic uterine smooth muscle neoplasms. Am J Surg Pathol 1994;18:535.

Bersch W, Alexy E, Heuser HP, et al: Ectopic decidua formation in the ovary (so-called deciduoma). Virchows Arch A Pathol Anat 1973;360:173.

Bollinger DJ, Wick MR, Dehner LP, et al: Peritoneal malignant mesothelioma versus serous papillary adenocarcinoma: a histochemical and immunohistochemical comparison. Am J Surg Pathol 1989;13:659.

Cecchini S, Iossa A, Ciatto S, et al: Colposcopic survey of Papanicolaou test—negative cases with hyperkeratosis or parakeratosis. Obstet Gynecol 1990;76:857.

Chuaqui RF, Zhuang Z, Emmert-Buck MR, et al: Genetic analysis of synchronous tumors of ovary and appendix. Hum Pathol 1996;27:165.

Clement PB, Scully RE: Uterine tumors resembling ovarian sex cord tumors: a clinicopathologic analysis of 14 cases. Am J Clin Pathol 1976;66:512.

Clement PB, Young RH: Florid mesothelial hyperplasia associated with ovarian tumors: a possible source of error in tumor diagnosis and staging. Int J Gynecol Pathol 1993;12:51.

Clement PB, Young RH, Oliva E, et al: Hyperplastic mesothelial cells within abdominal lymph nodes: mimic of metastatic ovarian carcinoma and serous borderline tumor—a report of two cases associated with ovarian neoplasms. Mod Pathol 1996;9:879.

Clement PB, Young RH, Scully RE: Endometrioid-like variant of yolk sac tumor: a clinicopathological analysis of eight cases. Am J Surg Pathol 1987;11:767.

Copeland LJ, Silva EG, Gershenson DM, et al: The significance of mullerian inclusions found at second-look laparotomy in patients with epithelial ovarian neoplasms. Obstet Gynecol 1988;71:763.

Copeland LJ, Sneige N, Gershenson DM, et al: Bartholin gland carcinoma. Obstet Gynecol 1986;67:794.

Covell LM, Disciullo AJ, Knapp RC: Decidual change in pelvic lymph nodes in the presence of cervical squamous cell carcinoma during pregnancy. Am J Obstet Gynecol 1977;127:674.

Curtin WM, Murthy B: Vulvar metastasis of breast carcinoma: a case report. J Reprod Med 1997;42:61.

Dabbs DJ, Geisinger KR, Norris HT: Intermediate filaments in endometrial and endocervical carcinomas: the diagnostic utility of vimentin patterns. Am J Surg Pathol 1986;10:568.

Davey DD, Naryshkin S, Nielsen ML: Atypical squamous cells of undetermined significance: interlaboratory comparison and quality assurance monitors. Diagn Cytopathol 1994;11:390.

Davey DD, Nielsen ML, Rosenstock W, et al: Terminology and specimen adequacy in cervicovaginal cytology: the College of American Pathologists interlaboratory comparison program experience. Arch Pathol Lab Med 1992;116:903.

Daya D, McCaughey WTE: Well differentiated papillary mesothelioma of the peritoneum: a clinicopathologic study of 22 cases. Cancer 1990;65:292.

Daya D, Nazerali L, Frank GL: Metastatic ovarian carcinoma of large intestinal origin simulating primary ovarian carcinoma: a clinicopathologic study of 25 cases. Am J Clin Pathol 1992;97:751.

Dehner LP: Metastatic and secondary tumors of the vulva. Obstet Gynecol 1973;42:47.

Dickersin GR, Kline IW, Scully RE: Small cell carcinoma of the ovary with hypercalcemia: a report of eleven cases. Cancer 1982;49:188.

Doering DL, Barnhill DR, Weiser EB, et al: Intraoperative evaluation of depth of myometrial invasion in stage I endometrial adenocarcinoma. Obstet Gynecol 1989;74:930.

Ehrmann RL, Federschneider JM, Knapp RC: Distinguishing lymph node metastases from benign glandular inclusions in low-grade ovarian carcinoma. Am J Obstet Gynecol 1980;136:737.

Eifel P, Hendrickson M, Ross J, et al: Simultaneous presentation of carcinoma involving the ovary and the uterine corpus. Cancer 1982;50:163.

Ferry JA, Scully RE: Mesonephric remnants, hyperplasia and neoplasia in the uterine cervix: a study of 49 cases. Am J Surg Pathol 1990;14:1100.

Fleuren GJ, Nap M: Carcinoembryonic antigen in primary and metastatic ovarian tumors. Gynecol Oncol 1988;30:407.

Frasier LD: Human papillomavirus infections in children. Pediatr Annals 1994;23:354.

Gagnon S, Tetu B, Silva EG, et al: Frequency of α-fetoprotein production by Sertoli-Leydig cell tumors of the ovary: an immunohistochemical study of eight cases. Mod Pathol 1989;2:63.

Gagnon Y, Tetu B: Ovarian metastases of breast carcinoma: a clinicopathologic study of 59 cases. Cancer 1989;64:892.

Ganjei P, Giraldo KA, Lampe B, et al: Vulvar Paget's disease: is immunocytochemistry helpful in assessing the surgical margins? J Reprod Med 1990;35:1002.

Geirsson G, Woodworth FE, Patten RF, et al: Epithelial repair and regeneration in the uterine cervix. I. An analysis of the cells. Acta Cytol 1977;21:371.

Gersell DJ, Mazoujian G, Mutch DG, et al: Small cell undifferentiated carcinoma of the cervix: a clinicopathologic, ultrastructural and immunocytochemical study of 15 cases. Am J Surg Pathol 1988;12:684.

Goff BA, Atanasoff P, Brown E, et al: Endocervical glandular atypia in Papanicolaou smears. Obstet Gynecol 1992;79:101.

Gupta PK, Burroughs F, Luff RD, et al: Epithelial atypias associated with intrauterine contraceptive device (IUD). Acta Cytol 1978;22:286.

Hart WR, Norris HJ: Borderline and malignant mucinous tumors of the ovary: histologic criteria and clinical behavior. Cancer 1973;31:1031.

Hatem F, Wilbur DC: High grade squamous cervical lesions following negative Papanicolaou smears: false-negative cervical cytology or rapid progression? Diagn Cytopathol 1995;12:135.

Heller D, Drosinos S, Westhoff C: Accuracy of tumor grade assigned at initial endometrial sampling. Int J Gynecol Obstet 1994;47:301.

Helm KF, Goellner JR, Peters MS: Immunohistochemical stains in extramammary Paget's disease. Am J Dermatopathol 1992;14:402.

Hendrickson MR, Kempson RL: Endometrial epithelial metaplasias: proliferations frequently misdiagnosed as adenocarcinoma. Report of 89 cases and proposed classification. Am J Surg Pathol 1980;4:525.

Holtz F, Hart WR: Krukenberg tumors of the ovary: a clinicopathologic analysis of 27 cases. Cancer 1982;50:2438.

Hsiu JG, Given Jr FT, Kemp GM: Tumor implantation after diagnostic laparoscopic biopsy of serous ovarian tumors of low malignant potential. Obstet Gynecol 1986;68:90S.

Hutchinson ML, Isenstein LM, Goodman A, et al: Homogeneous sampling accounts for the increased diagnostic accuracy using the Thin Prep® processor. Am J Clin Pathol 1994;101:215.

Jonasson JH, Wang HH, Antonioli DA, et al: Tubal metaplasia of the uterine cervix: a prevalence study in patients with gynecologic pathologic findings. Int J Gynecol Pathol 1992;11:89.

Kaminski PF, Norris HJ: Minimal deviation carcinoma (adenoma malignum) of the cervix. Int J Gynecol Pathol 1983;2:141.

Keebler C, Chatwani A, Schwartz R: Actinomycosis infection associated with intrauterine contraceptive devices. Am J Obstet Gynecol 1983;145:596.

Kempson RL, Hendrickson MR: Pure mesenchymal neoplasms of the uterine corpus: selected problems. Semin Diagn Pathol 1988;5(2):172.

Kennedy AW, Eltabbakh GH, Biscotti CV, et al: Invasive adenocarcinoma of the cervix following LLETZ (large loop excision of the transformation zone) for adenocarcinoma in situ. Gynecol Oncol 1995;58:274.

King ME, Dickerson GR, Scully RE: Myxoid leiomyosarcoma of the uterus: a report of six cases. Am J Surg Pathol 1982;6:589.

Kneale BL: Microinvasive cancer of the vulva: report of the International Society for the Study of Vulvar Disease Task Force (Proceedings of the 7th World Congress of the ISSVD). J Reprod Med 1984;29:454.

Koss LG: The Papanicolaou test for cervical cancer detection: a triumph and a tragedy. JAMA 1989;261:737.

Koss LG, Lin E, Schreiber K, et al: Evaluation of the PapNet cytologic screening system for quality control of cervical smears. Am J Clin Pathol 1994;101:220.

Krebs HB, Pastore L, Helmkamp BF: Loop electrosurgical excision procedures for cervical dysplasia: experience in a community hospital. Am J Obstet Gynecol 1993;169:289.

Krepart G, Smith JP, Rutledge F, et al: The treatment for dysgerminoma of the ovary. Cancer 1978;41:986.

Kumar NB, Hart WR: Metastases to the uterine corpus from extragenital cancers: a clinicopathologic study of 63 cases. Cancer 1982;50:2163.

Kurman RJ, Norris HJ: Malignant mixed germ cell tumors of the ovary: a clinical and pathological analysis of 30 cases. Obstet Gynecol 1976a;48:579.

Kurman RJ, Norris HJ: Mesenchymal tumors of the uterus: VI. Epithelioid smooth muscle tumors including leiomyoblastoma and clear-cell leiomyoma: a clinical and pathologic analysis of 26 cases. Cancer 1976b;37:1853.

Kurman RJ, Norris HJ: Evaluation of criteria for distinguishing atypical endometrial hyperplasia from well differentiated carcinoma. Cancer 1982;49:2547.

Kurman RJ, Solomon D: The Bethesda System for Reporting Cervical/Vaginal Cytologic Diagnoses. New York: Springer-Verlag, 1994.

Kurman RJ, Young RH, Norris HJ, et al: Immunohistochemical localization of placental lactogen and chorionic gonadotropin in the normal placenta and trophoblastic tumors, with emphasis on intermediate trophoblast and the placental site trophoblastic tumor. Int J Gynecol Pathol 1984;3:101.

Lash RH, Hart WR: Intestinal adenocarcinomas metastatic to the ovaries: a clinicopathicological evaluation of 22 cases. Am J Surg Pathol 1987;11:114.

Maiman M, Seltzer V, Boyce J: Laparoscopic excision of ovarian neoplasms subsequently found to be malignant. Obstet Gynecol 1991;77:563.

Mazoujian G, Pinkus GS, Haagensen DE Jr: Extramammary Paget's disease—evidence for an apocrine origin: an immunoperoxidase study of gross cystic disease fluid protein-15, carcinoembryonic antigen, and keratin proteins. Am J Surg Pathol 1884;8:43.

McCaughey WTE, Kirk ME, Lester W, et al: Peritoneal epithelial lesions associated with proliferative serous tumours of ovary. Histopathology 1984;8:195.

McLellan R, Buscema J, Currie JL, et al: Placental site trophoblastic tumor in a postmenopausal woman. Am J Clin Pathol 1991;95:670.

Menzin AW, Rubin SC, Nuomoff JS, et al: The accuracy of a frozen section diagnosis of borderline ovarian malignancy. Gynecol Oncol 1995;59:183.

Michael H, Grawe L, Kraus FT: Minimal deviation endocervical adenocarcinoma: clinical and histologic features, immunohistochemical staining for carcinoembryonic staining and differentiation from confusing benign lesions. Int J Gynecol Pathol 1984;3:261.

Miettinen M, Talerman A, Wahlstrom T, et al: Cellular differentiation in ovarian sex cord-stromal and germ-cell tumors studied with antibodies to intermediate-filament proteins. Am J Surg Pathol 1985;9:640.

Monteagudo C, Merino MJ, Laporte N, et al: Value of gross cystic disease fluid protein-15 in distinguishing metastatic breast carcinomas among poorly differentiated neoplasms involving the ovary. Hum Pathol 1991;22:368.

Neunteufel W, Breitenecker G: Tissue expression of CA 125 in benign and malignant lesions of ovary and fallopian tube: a comparison with CA 19-9 and CEA. Gynecol Oncol 1989;32:297.

O'Connor DM, Norris HJ: Mitotically active leiomyomas of the uterus. Hum Pathol 1990;21:223.

O'Hanlan KA, Kargas S, Schreiber M, et al: Ovarian carcinoma metastases to gastrointestinal tract appear to spread like colon carcinoma: implications for surgical resection. Gynecol Oncol 1995;59:200.

O'Hanlan KA, Levine PA, Harbatkin D, et al: Virulence of papillary endometrial carcinoma. Gynecol Oncol 1990;37:112.

Oliva E, Young RH, Clement PB, et al: Cellular benign mesenchymal tumors of the uterus: a comparative morphologic and immunohistochemical analysis of 33 highly cellular leiomyomas and six endometrial stromal nodules, two frequently confused tumors. Am J Surg Pathol 1995;19:757.

Pettit PD, Lee RA: Ovarian remnant syndrome: diagnostic dilemma and surgical challenge. Obstet Gynecol 1988;71:580.

Prat J, Bhan AK, Dickersin RG, et al: Hepatoid yolk sac tumor of the ovary (endodermal sinus tumor with hepatoid differentiation): a light microscopic ultrastructural and immunohistochemical study of seven cases. Cancer 1982;50:2355.

Prat J, Matias-Guiu X, Barreto J: Simultaneous carcinoma involving the endometrium and the ovary: a clinicopathologic, immunohistochemical and DNA flow cytometric study of 18 cases. Cancer 1991;68:2455.

Rhatigan RM, Nuss RC: Keratoacanthoma of the vulva. Gynecol Oncol 1985;21:118.

Richart RM, Nuovo GJ: Human papillomavirus DNA in situ hybridization may be used for the quality control of genital tract biopsies. Obstet Gynecol 1990;75:223.

Robboy SJ, Scully RE: Ovarian teratoma with glial implants on the peritoneum: an analysis of 12 cases. Hum Pathol 1970;1:643.

Roth LM, Liban E, Czernobilsky B: Ovarian endometrioid tumors mimicking Sertoli and Sertoli-Leydig cell tumors: sertoliform variant of endometrioid carcinoma. Cancer 1982;50:1322.

Rubio CA: The false negative smear II: the trapping effect of collecting instruments. Obstet Gynecol 1977;49:576.

Sainz de la Cuesta R, Goff BA, Fuller AF: Prognostic importance of intraoperative rupture of malignant ovarian epithelial neoplasms. Obstet Gynecol 1994;84:1.

Schumann JL, O'Connor DM, Covell JL, et al: Pap smear collection devices: technical, clinical diagnostic and legal considerations associated with their use. Diagn Cytopathol 1992;8:492.

Scully RE: Gonadoblastoma. Cancer 1970;25:1340.

Scully RE, Henson, DE, Nielsen ML, et al: Practice protocol for the examination of specimens removed from patients with ovarian tumors: a basis for checklists. Arch Pathol Lab Med 1995;119:1012.

Shah KD, Tabizzadeh SS, Gerber MA: Immunohistochemical distinction of Paget's disease from Bowen's disease and superficial spreading melanoma with the use of monoclonal cytokeratin antibodies. Am J Clin Pathol 1987;88:689.

Shatz P, Bergeron C, Wilkinson EJ, et al: Vulvar intraepithelial neoplasia and skin appendage involvement. Obstet Gynecol 1989;74:769.

Sheahan K, O'Keane JC, Abramowitz A, et al: Metastatic adenocarcinoma of an unknown primary site: a comparison of the relative contributions of morphology, minimal essential clinical data and CEA immunostaining status. Am J Clin Pathol 1993;99:729.

Shevchuk MM, Winkler-Monsanto B, Fenoglio CM, et al: Clear cell carcinoma of the ovary: a clinicopathologic study with review of the literature. Cancer 1981;47:1344.

Snider DD, Stuart GCE, Nation JG, et al: Evaluation of surgical staging in stage I low malignant potential ovarian tumors. Gynecol Oncol 1991;40:129.

Stanley MW, Horwitz CA, Frable WJ: Cellular follicular cyst of the ovary: fluid cytology mimicking malignancy. Diagn Cytopathol 1991;7:48.

Stovall TG, Solomon SK, Ling FW: Endometrial sampling prior to hysterectomy. Obstet Gynecol 1989;73:405.

Symonds DA, Reed TP, Didolkar SM, et al: AGUS in cervical endometriosis. J Reprod Med 1997;42:39.

Talerman A: Ovarian Sertoli-Leydig cell tumor (androblastoma) with retiform pattern: a clinicopathologic study. Cancer 1987;60:3056.

Taylor RR, Guerrieri JP, Nash JD, et al: Atypical cervical cytology: colposcopic follow-up using the Bethesda System. J Reprod Med 1993;38:443.

Tiltman AJ: The effect of progestins on the mitotic activity of uterine fibromyomas. Int J Gynecol Pathol 1985;4:89.

Ulbright TM, Roth LM, Stehman FB: Secondary ovarian neoplasia: a clinicopathologic study of 35 cases. Cancer 1984;53:1164.

Wick MR, Goellner JR, Wolfe JT 3rd, et al: Vulvar sweat gland carcinomas. Arch Pathol Lab Med 1985;109:43.

Wick MR, Mills SE, Dehner LP, et al: Serous papillary carcinomas arising from the peritoneum and ovaries: a clinicopathologic and immunohistochemical comparison. Int J Gynecol Pathol 1989;8:179.

Wilkinson EJ: Superficial invasive carcinoma of the vulva. Clin Obstet Gynecol 1991;34:651.

Wolber RA, Talerman A, Wilkinson EJ, et al: Vulvar granular cell tumors with pseudocarcinomatous hyperplasia: a comparative analysis with well-differentiated squamous carcinoma. Int J Gynecol Pathol 1991;10:59.

Young RH, Carey RW, Robboy SJ: Breast carcinoma masquerading as a primary ovarian neoplasm. Cancer 1981;48:210.

Young RH, Clement PB: Malignant lesions of the female genital tract and peritoneum that may be underdiagnosed. Semin Diagn Pathol 1995;12(1):14.

Young RH, Dickerson GR, Scully RE: Juvenile granulosa cell tumor of the ovary: a clinicopathological analysis of 125 cases. Am J Surg Pathol 1984;8:575.

Young RH, Gilks CB, Scully RE: Mucinous tumors of the appendix associated with mucinous tumors of the ovary and pseudomyxoma peritonei: a clinicopathological analysis of 22 cases supporting an origin in the appendix. Am J Surg Pathol 1991;15:415.

Young RH, Hart WR: Metastases from carcinomas of the pancreas simulating primary mucinous tumors of the ovary: a report of seven cases. Am J Surg Pathol 1989;13:748.

Young RH, Hart WR: Renal cell carcinoma metastatic to the ovary: a report of three cases emphasizing possible confusion with ovarian clear cell carcinoma. Int J Gynecol Pathol 1992;11:96.

Young RH, Kurman RJ, Scully RE: Placental site nodules and plaques: a clinicopathologic analysis of 20 cases. Am J Surg Pathol 1990;14:1001.

Young RH, Scully RE: Ovarian sex cord-stromal tumors: recent progress. Int J Gynecol Pathol 1982;1:101.

Young RH, Scully RE: Ovarian Sertoli-Leydig cell tumors: a clinicopathological analysis of 207 cases. Am J Surg Pathol 1985;9:543.

Young RH, Scully RE: Atypical forms of microglandular hyperplasia of the cervix simulating carcinoma: a report of 5 cases and review of the literature. Am J Surg Pathol 1989;13:50.

Young RH, Scully RE: Malignant melanoma metastatic to the ovary: a clinicopathologic analysis of 20 cases. Am J Surg Pathol 1991a;15:849.

Young RH, Scully RE: Metastatic tumors in the ovary: a problem oriented approach and review of the recent literature. Semin Diagn Pathol 1991b;8:250.

Young RH, Treger T, Scully RE: Atypical polypoid adenomyoma of the uterus: a report of 27 cases. Am J Clin Pathol 1986;86:139.

Zaloudek C, Tavassoli FA, Norris HJ: Dysgerminoma with syncytiotrophoblastic giant cells: a histologically and clinically distinctive subtype of dysgerminoma. Am J Surg Pathol 1981;5:361.

Zinsser KR, Wheeler JE: Endosalpingiosis in the omentum: a study of autopsy and surgical material. Am J Surg Pathol 1982;6:109.

Zirker TA, Silva EG, Morris M, et al: Immunohistochemical differentiation of clear-cell carcinoma of the female genital tract and endodermal sinus tumor with the use of alpha-fetoprotein and Leu-M1. Am J Clin Pathol 1989;91:511.

II

Reproduction

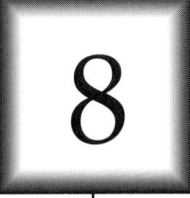

8

Developmental Abnormalities

David Muram

A nomalies of the genitalia may be divided into two major categories: those that suggest sexual ambiguity (intersex problems), and those that do not. This chapter describes the various congenital abnormalities that affect the external and internal female genital tract. The chapter also includes a brief description of the appearance and management of ambiguous genitalia.

ANOMALIES OF THE VULVA AND LABIA

As in any other part of the body, minor differences in the contour or size of vulvar structures are not unusual. Often there is considerable variation in the distance between the posterior fourchette and the anus, or between the urethra and the clitoris, giving the vulva different appearances (Huffman et al, 1981). In muscular girls the perineal body may be exceptionally thick and wide, and the vulva situated deeply between the bulging sides of the perineum, forming a "vulva retrousse." Some patients may exhibit vulvar cysts that may represent remnants of the wolffian or müllerian duct systems (Newland and Fusaro, 1991). Rare anomalies of the vulva include a caudal appendage that resembles a tail and variations in the insertion of the bulbocavernosus muscle that may alter the appearance of the labia majora and, at times, obliterate the fossa navicularis (Huffman et al, 1981; Muram and Rau, 1991). Duplication of the vulva is an extremely rare anomaly that may be associated with duplication of the urinary and intestinal tracts (Lister, 1953).

There is commonly considerable variation in the size and shape of the labia minora. One labium may be considerably larger than the other, or both labia may be unusually large (Fig. 8–1). Labial enlargement and asymmetry have been wrongly assumed by some to be the result of masturbation. The patient expects to be assured that these differences are simple minor variations that usually require no treatment. If the asymmetry is significant, or the labia are pulled into the vagina during intercourse, the hypertrophied labia may be trimmed surgically (Huffman et al, 1981).

AMBIGUOUS GENITALIA

In the absence of the Y chromosome and the *TDY* gene, the gonadal anlagen develops into an ovary, establishing female gonadal and phenotypic sex. Growth and differentiation up to 9 weeks' gestation is identical for both sexes. After this there is rapid growth and differentiation in males, but in females subsequent growth until 20 weeks' gestation is restricted to growth of the labia majora. At this stage, the urethral and vaginal orifices can be seen at the surface of the perineum. This process of feminization of the external genitalia is completed by the 26th week of gestation. These changes correspond to the development of the ovary. There is little change in the histologic appearance of the ovaries until 18 to 20 weeks of gestation, at which time follicular growth starts. Feminization of the urogenital sinus is seen shortly thereafter. So, from the temporal profile of events, it appears that development of the female external genitalia may be initiated by fetal ovarian steroids (Ammini et al, 1994).

In the presence of the Y chromosome and the *TDY* gene, the gonadal anlagen develops into a testis, establishing male gonadal and phenotypic sex. Two testicular secretions are responsible for masculinization of the fetus: müllerian inhibiting substance (MIS) and testosterone. MIS causes regression of the müllerian ducts during male embryogenesis. In addition, a number of extra-müllerian functions have been proposed for MIS, including induction of the abdominal phase of testicular descent, control of germ cell maturation, gonadal morphogenesis, and suppression of lung maturation (Lee and Donahoe, 1993). Secretion of MIS is a constitutive feature of the immature Sertoli cell, and its expression is altered only by mutations of the MIS gene (Rey et al, 1996).

Fetal Leydig cells produce an androgen, probably testosterone, that stabilizes wolffian ducts and permits differentiation of the vas deferens, epididymis, and seminal vesicles. Testosterone is converted by 5α-reductase to dihydrotestosterone, which virilizes the external genitalia. In the absence of testosterone and dihydrotestosterone, the external genitalia develop along female lines (Jost, 1947).

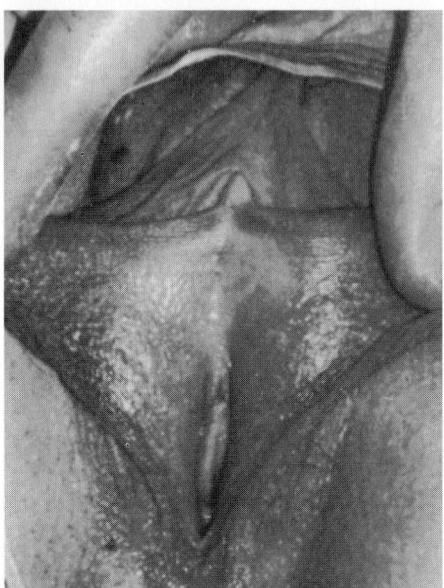

Figure 8 – 1
Bilateral labial hypertrophy in a 15-year-old girl. (From Huffman JW, Dewhurst CJ, Capraro VJ: The Gynecology of Childhood and Adolescence. 2nd ed. Philadelphia: WB Saunders Company, 1981, with permission.)

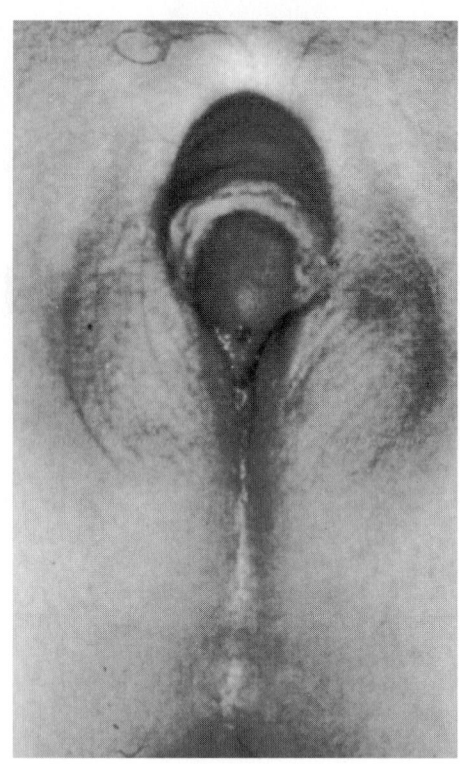

Figure 8 – 2
Genitalia of a female child with congenital adrenocortical hyperplasia. (From Huffman JW, Dewhurst CJ, Capraro VJ: The Gynecology of Childhood and Adolescence. 2nd ed. Philadelphia: WB Saunders Company, 1981, with permission.)

Ambiguous genitalia denotes partial or incomplete virilization of the external genitalia. Ambiguous genitalia may be seen, therefore, in genetic females who were virilized in utero, in undervirilized males, or in true hermaphrodites. The extent of virilization of the external genitalia depends upon the timing, length of exposure, and levels of androgens. In general, exposure to androgens after 12 weeks of gestation leads only to clitoral hypertrophy. Examination of the genitalia shows an enlarged clitoris but a normal vestibule, urethra, and vagina. The labia majora are altered by redundancy, wrinkling, and skin pigmentation (Grumbach and Conte, 1985).

Exposure at progressively earlier stages of embryologic development also leads to clitoral hypertrophy but, in addition, leads to retention of the urogenital sinus and fusion of the labioscrotal folds. In these severely virilized individuals, the labia are fused in the midline to form a median raphe (Fig. 8–2). The area of fusion may be partial or extend the entire distance from the perineum to the phallus. When extensive, the fused labia form a wrinkled, pouch-like structure that resembles the scrotum in a cryptorchid male. The vaginal opening is absent. Instead, a single opening is present that extends to a common passage connecting the urethra and vagina. If exposure occurs sufficiently early and to adequate levels of androgens, the labia will fuse to form a penile urethra (Fig. 8–3). Müllerian and gonadal development remain unaffected because neither is androgen dependent (Grumbach and Conte, 1985).

When significant ambiguity of the external genitalia is present, the true gender cannot be immediately determined. Although any anomaly in a newborn creates anxiety, abnormalities that affect the genitalia or cast doubt on the sex of the child may cause panic as the alarmed parents conjure up visions of a hopeless, lonely existence for their child. When genital ambiguity is observed, it is therefore best to explain to the parents that the sexual development of the infant is incomplete, and a few studies are required to determine whether the baby is a boy or a girl (Reindollar et al, 1987). The medical evaluation of ambiguous genitalia is discussed elsewhere in this book (see Chapter 26).

The surgical correction of genital ambiguity should be done only after the completion of the medical evaluation, which permits proper gender assignment to the neonate. Once an appropriate sex assignment has been made, surgical reconstruction of the genitalia may be required to conform the appearance of the genitalia to that of the assigned gender. The optimal time for the reconstructive procedure remains controversial. Some authors believe that a one-stage reconstructive procedure can be done early in infancy. It alleviates the need for a second procedure and, with the exteriorization of the vagina, the external genitalia appear normal (Donahoe and Gustafson, 1994).

Other surgeons believe that reconstruction of the female external genitalia is best accomplished in two stages. The first, done prior to the infant's discharge from the hospital, consists of clitoral reduction. The

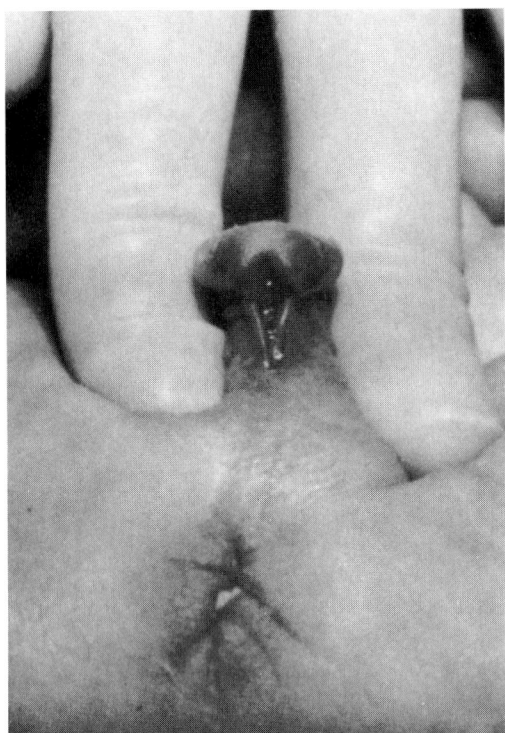

Figure 8–3
Marked masculinization resulting from congenital adrenocortical hyperplasia. The urogenital sinus has been prolonged almost to the tip of the phallus. (From Huffman JW, Dewhurst CJ, Capraro VJ: The Gynecology of Childhood and Adolescence. 2nd ed. Philadelphia: WB Saunders Company, 1981, with permission.)

surgeon should attempt to preserve the neurovascular connections to the glans. In this manner, a functional clitoris of normal size can be created. Removal of the entire clitoris is rarely indicated (Reindollar et al, 1987). The second stage, reconstruction of the vagina, should be delayed until after pubertal development. The type of surgical correction depends on the degree of virilization. If only labial fusion is present, division of the labia is all that is required. Minor degrees of narrowing of the vaginal introitus can be easily corrected using, for example, the Fenton procedure. In this procedure, a flap of vulvar skin is developed, the hymen and perineum are incised vertically, and the flap is then used to cover the perineal defect. As a result, the introital diameter is increased (8–4). When a significant narrowing is present, enlargement of the introitus may require the use of more than one flap, or even the use of a split-thickness skin graft (Monaghan, 1986).

Two-stage surgical reconstruction requires two separate procedures but has significant advantages. The appearance of the genitalia of the newborn at discharge is female-like and affirms for the parents the assigned gender, thereby helping to stabilize gender identity. Furthermore, vaginal reconstruction at a very young age may require surgical revision after puberty. Bailez et al reported their long-term follow-

up of 28 patients with salt-wasting congenital adrenal hyperplasia who underwent reconstruction of the external genitalia at an early age. Of these children, 22 (78.5%) required further vaginal reconstructive procedures to achieve a normal vaginal outlet (Bailez et al, 1992).

ANOMALIES OF THE CLITORIS

Clitoral Hypertrophy

Clitoral enlargement almost invariably suggests that the infant had been exposed in utero to elevated levels of androgens. Such enlargement of the clitoris is often associated with fusion of the labioscrotal folds, and is discussed under the section "Abnormal Sexual Differentiation." Enlargement of the clitoris caused by a benign neoplasm has been observed in a few infants. Von Recklinghausen's neurofibromatosis, lymphangiomas, and fibromas may involve the clitoris and cause enlargement (Kaneti et al, 1988). Progressive idiopathic clitoral enlargement also has been described. When an isolated neoplasm causes enlargement of the clitoris, therapy consists of excision of the neoplasm and thereby reduction of the clitoris to normal size.

Clitoral Agenesis or Duplication

Clitoral agenesis is a very rare condition (Falk and Hyman, 1971). Splitting or duplication of the clitoris represents longitudinal splitting of the clitoris, caused by failure of the corpora to fuse in the midline. Bifid clitoris usually occurs in conjunction with bladder exstrophy, epispadias, and absence or cleavage of the symphysis pubis (Fig. 8–5). The labia majora are widely separated, and the labia minora are separated anteriorly but can be traced posteriorly around the vaginal orifice. The uterus often shows a fusion deformity and the vaginal orifice is narrow (Fig. 8–6). The vagina is shortened and rotated anteriorly (Dewhurst, 1978b). The pelvic floor is incomplete, and uterine prolapse is often observed in these patients (Fig. 8–7). Other congenital anomalies may be present (e.g., spina bifida). At puberty, pubic hair growth is absent over the midline.

EPISPADIAS AND BLADDER EXSTROPHY

Failure of normal fusion of the anterior wall of the urogenital sinus results in a urethra that opens cephalad to a bifid clitoris under the symphysis pubis. Occasionally the defect is more extensive, involving the bladder and anterior abdominal wall, creating exstrophy of the bladder. Both conditions may be associated with defects involving the anterior pelvic girdle, resulting in diminished pelvic support. As previously mentioned, uterine prolapse and anterior

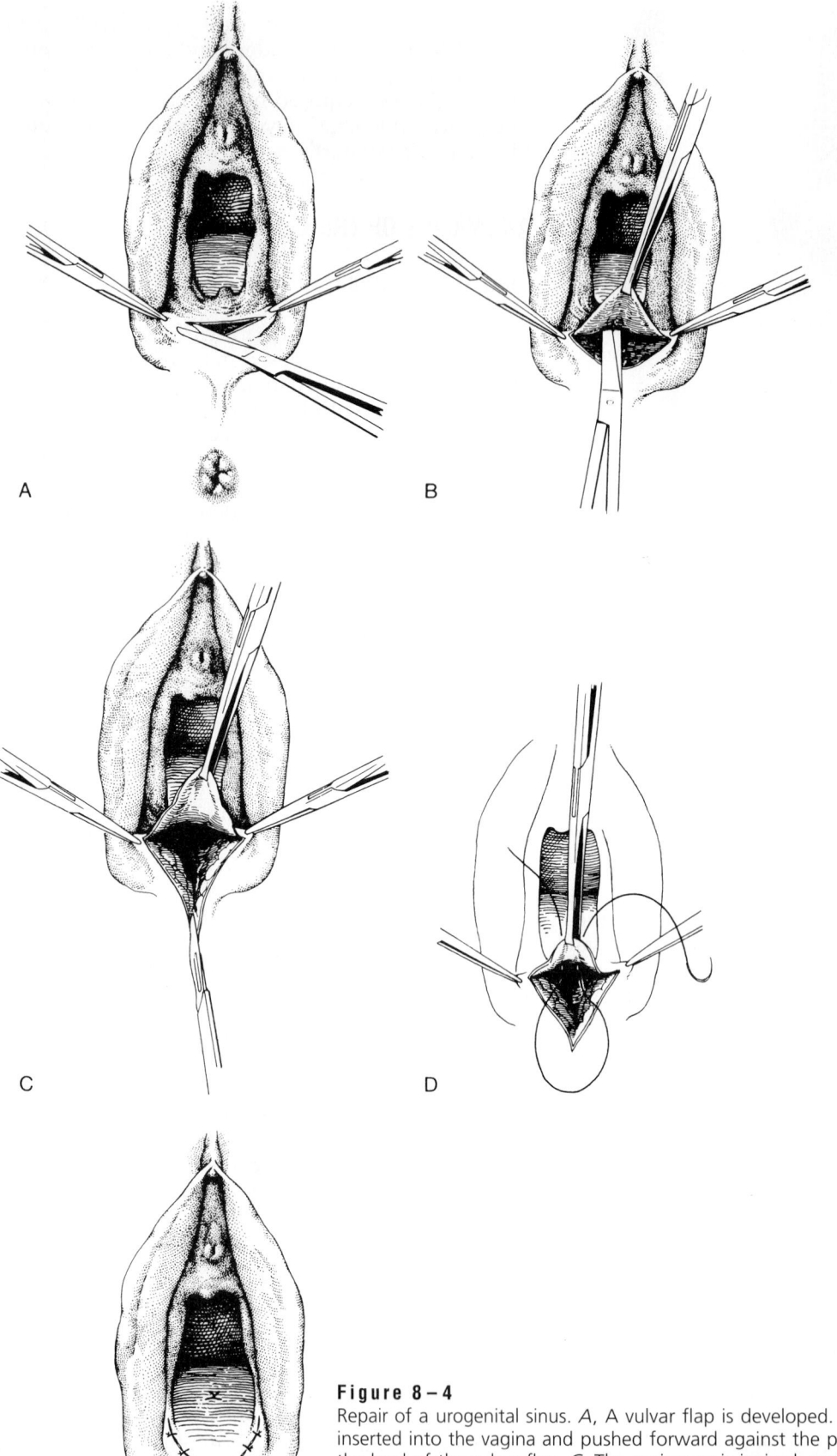

A

B

C

D

Figure 8–4

Repair of a urogenital sinus. *A*, A vulvar flap is developed. *B*, Curved Kelly forceps are inserted into the vagina and pushed forward against the perineum. The tips should be at the level of the vulvar flap. *C*, The perineum is incised, and the vaginal opening is now located at the flap. *D*, The vaginal mucosa is mobilized and sutured to the vulvar flap. In this way, the vulvar flap is used to fill the defect created by the division of the introitus. *E*, The skin incisions are closed to complete the repair. (Modified from Monaghan JM: Bonney's Gynaecological Surgery. London: Bailliere Tindall, 1986:130, with permission.)

E

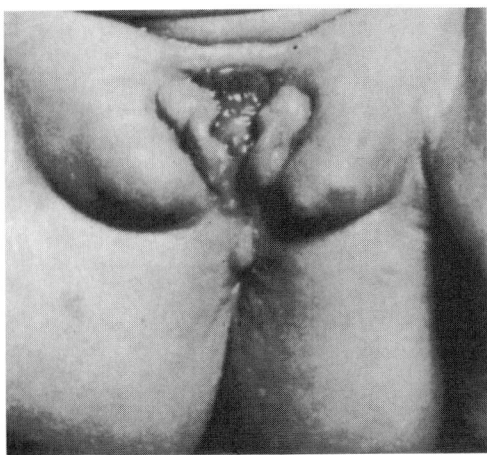

Figure 8-5
Epispadias in a newborn child. (From Huffman JW, Dewhurst CJ, Capraro VJ: The Gynecology of Childhood and Adolescence. 2nd ed. Philadelphia: WB Saunders Company, 1981, with permission.)

displacement of the vagina are commonly found in association with bladder exstrophy. Major urologic reconstruction is required immediately, but the gynecologic defects can be repaired later during the adolescent years (Dewhurst, 1978b).

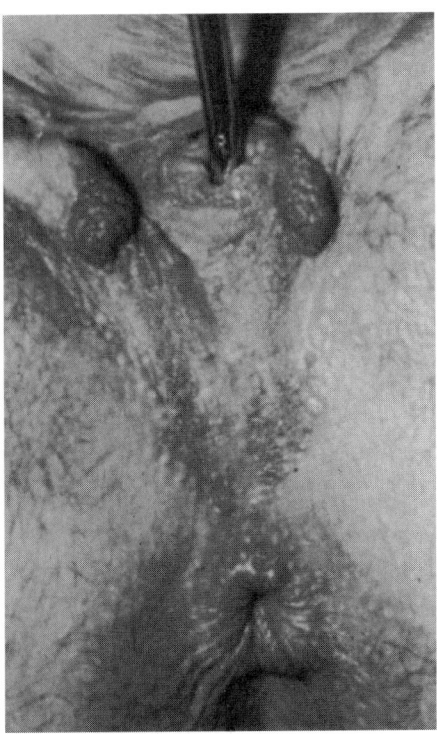

Figure 8-6
Marked constriction of the vaginal introitus in a girl with bladder exstrophy previously treated in early childhood by implantation of the ureters into the bowel and excision of the bladder mass. (From Huffman JW, Dewhurst CJ, Capraro VJ: The Gynecology of Childhood and Adolescence. 2nd ed. Philadelphia: WB Saunders Company, 1981, with permission.)

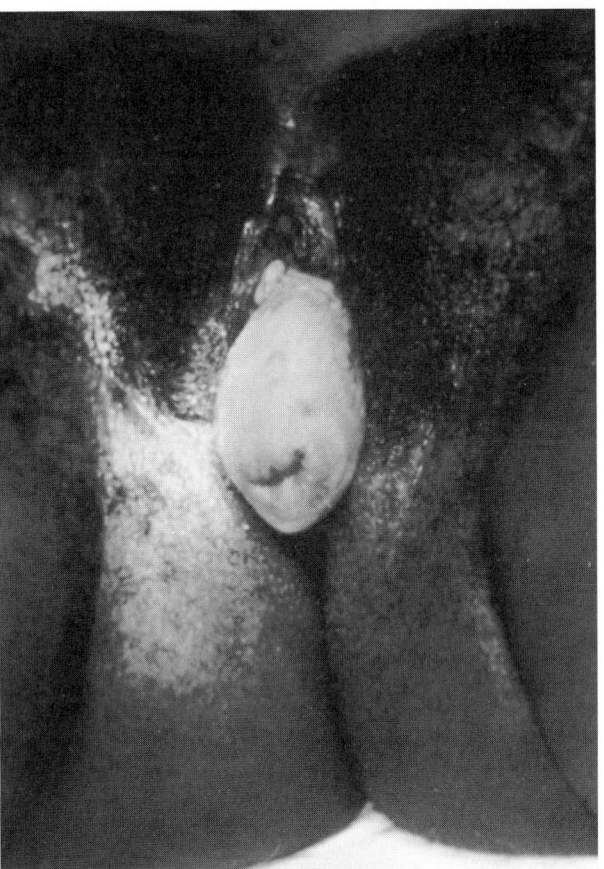

Figure 8-7
Complete uterine prolapse in a 21-year-old woman who was born with bladder exstrophy.

ANOMALIES OF THE ANUS

Failure of a newborn infant to pass meconium demands a careful evaluation because the infant may have an imperforate anus. Passage of feces through the vagina suggests a fistulous communication between the rectum and the vagina (Fig. 8-8). In general, anal and rectal anomalies are divided into two major groups: those that form a complete obstruction of the intestinal tract and those that are associated with some type of abnormal opening or fistula. A useful clinical classification has been described by Ladd and Gross (1934) (Table 8-1).

Only broad generalization can be offered regarding the management of complex cloacal anomalies, because the abnormalities are seldom alike. The principals of surgical management are as follows:

1. Obstruction of the intestinal tract must be corrected.
2. Obstruction of the urinary tract must be relieved (this may require an initial ureterostomy or cystostomy).
3. If the urogenital sinus cannot be later used as a urethra, a permanent diversion (i.e., ileal conduit) must be created.
4. If fecal contamination of the urinary tract is present, it is essential that it be corrected, usually by performing a temporary colostomy.

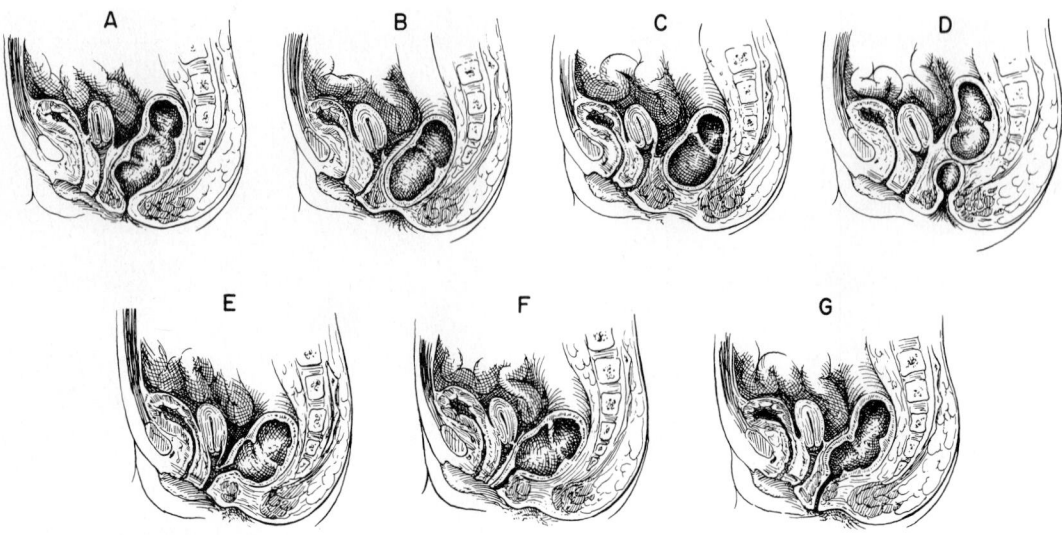

Figure 8–8
Anomalies of the rectum. *A,* Stenosis. *B,* Imperforate anus. *C,* Agenesis of anorectal canal. *D,* Atresia of large bowel at the rectosigmoid juncture. *E,* Congenital rectovaginal fistula with anorectal agenesis. *F,* Vulvorectal fistula with anorectal agenesis. *G,* Perineal-rectal fistula with anorectal agenesis. (From Huffman JW, Dewhurst CJ, Capraro VJ: The Gynecology of Childhood and Adolescence. 2nd ed. Philadelphia: WB Saunders Company, 1981, with permission.)

ANOMALIES OF THE HYMEN

Variations in the appearance of the hymen are extremely common. The orifice may vary in diameter from very small to very large (Pokorny, 1987). There may be one or more small orifices (Fig. 8–9). A thick median ridge separating two lateral hymenal orifices may suggest a septate vagina (Fig. 8–10). The hymenal diaphragm may be a thin membrane or a thickened and fibrous one, forming a firm partition. Occasionally, what initially appears to be an imperforate hymen is found to have one or more tiny openings and is called a microperforate hymen. Although most of these variants are of no clinical significance, hymenal anomalies require surgical correction if they block the escape of vaginal secretions or menstrual fluid, interfere with intercourse, or prevent an indicated vaginoscopy and treatment of a vaginal disorder (Huffman et al, 1981).

An imperforate hymen occurs when the hymen forms a solid membrane without an aperture (Fig. 8–11). It is assumed that an imperforate hymen represents a persistent portion of the urogenital membrane and occurs when the mesoderm of the primitive streak abnormally invades the urogenital portion of the cloacal membrane. When the vagina is obstructed, accumulation of vaginal secretions may distend the vagina, a condition called mucocolpos or hydrocolpos. When this occurs, the thin hymenal membrane is stretched out and forms a bulging, shiny, thin protuberance. Demonstration of vaginal patency should be part of the examination of the genitalia of the newborn, and therefore imperforate hymen should be diagnosed at birth. Unless a mucocolpos is diagnosed and the fluid

drained, the distended vagina forms a large mass that may interfere with urination, and at times may be mistaken for an abdominal tumor (Huffman et al, 1981).

In some patients, imperforate hymen and hydrocolpos can be diagnosed as early as the second trimester by antenatal sonographic evaluation. The examiner may observe a thin protruding membrane representing an imperforate hymen. Other anomalies may be present as well (Winderl and Silverman, 1995).

When the amount of vaginal fluid is small, or the obstructing membrane is thick and fibrous, an imperforate hymen forms a smooth surface between the labia minora that is similar in appearance to an absent vagina. Sonographic evaluation of the pelvis can identify the uterus, cervix, and vagina and thus distinguish between these two conditions. If the diagnosis of an imperforate hymen is not established during childhood, the condition is suspected when an adolescent girl presents with primary amenorrhea and recurrent lower abdominal pain. Menstrual flow fills the vagina (hematocolpos) and then the uterus (hematometra), and may spill through the tubes into the peritoneal cavity. The first symptom may be urinary retention caused by pressure of a large hematocolpos on the bladder and urethra. Inspection of the vulva generally reveals a dome-shaped, purplish red hymenal membrane bulging outward in response to the collection of blood above it. On rectal examination the distended vagina is palpable as a large cystic mass (Dewhurst, 1978a).

An imperforate hymen must be partially excised. If the hymen is only incised, the edges tend to coalesce and may agglutinate to reform an obstructing

Table 8–1. MALFORMATIONS OF THE ANUS
AND RECTUM

I. Anal Stenosis
II. Imperforate Anal Membrane
III. Anal and Rectal Agenesis
   A. Anal agenesis
     Female
     1. With fistula
       a. Anoperineal
         (1) Ectopic perineal anus
         (2) Anovulvar
     2. Without fistula
     Male
     1. With fistula
       a. Anoperineal
         (1) Ectopic perineal anus
         (2) Anocutaneous (covered anus)
       b. Anourethral (bulbar or membranous)
     2. Without fistula
   B. Rectal Agenesis
     Female
     1. With fistula
       a. Rectovestibular
       b. Rectovaginal
       c. Rectocloacal (urogenital sinus)
     2. Without fistula
     Male
     1. With fistula
       a. Rectourethral
       b. Rectovesical
IV. Rectal Atresia

Modified from Ladd WE, Gross RE: Congenital malformations of the
anus and rectum: report of 162 cases. Am J Surg 1934;23:167, with
permission.

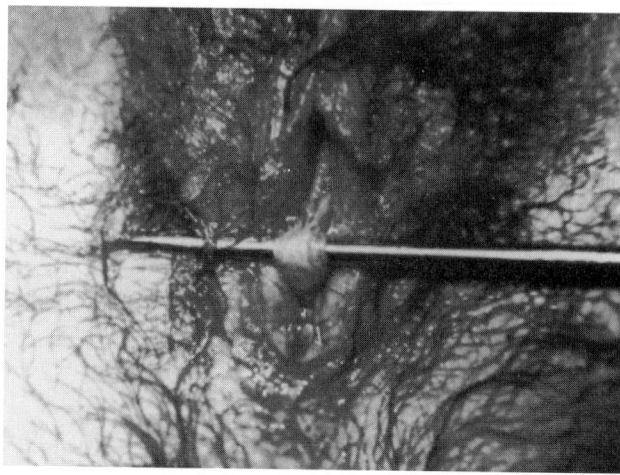

Figure 8–10
Hymen with an isolated thick median septum in an adolescent
girl.

membrane. After the initial incision, the central portion of the membrane is excised to provide a larger
aperture (Fig. 8–12). Sutures are not necessary. In
postmenarcheal girls, follow-up evaluation of the vagina and pelvis should be deferred for 4 to 6 weeks

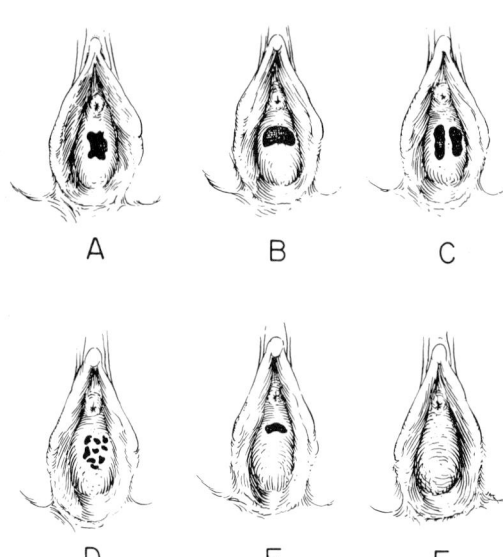

Figure 8–9
Anomalies of the hymen. *A*, Normal. *B*, Anteriorly placed
hymen. *C*, Hymenal septum. *D*, Cribriform hymen. *E*,
Microperforate hymen. *F*, Imperforate hymen. (From Huffman
JW, Dewhurst CJ, Capraro VJ: The Gynecology of Childhood
and Adolescence. 2nd ed. Philadelphia: WB Saunders
Company, 1981, with permission.)

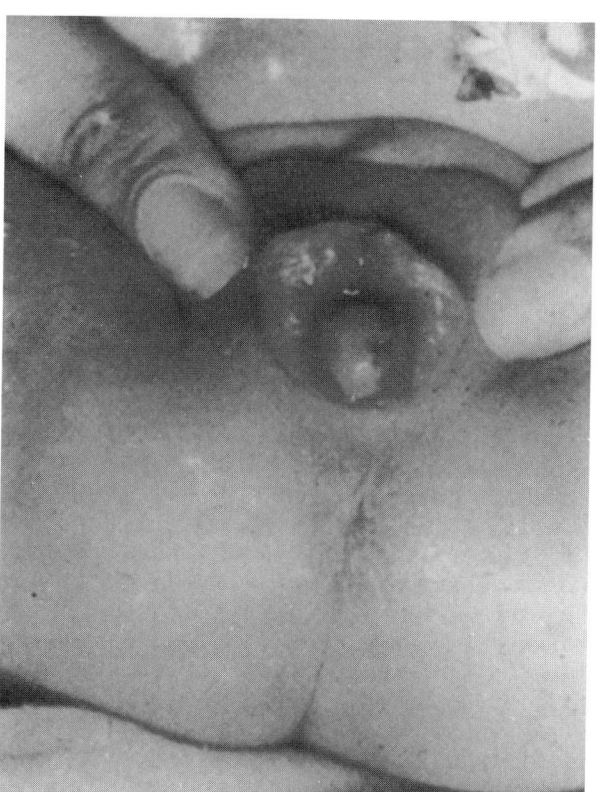

Figure 8–11
Mucocolpos in a newborn infant. (Courtesy of S. Korones.)
(From Muram D: Pediatric and adolescent gynecology. In
Pernol ML, Benson RC (eds): Current Gynecologic and
Obstetric Diagnosis and Treatment. East Norwalk, CT: Appleton
and Lange, 1987:569, with permission.)

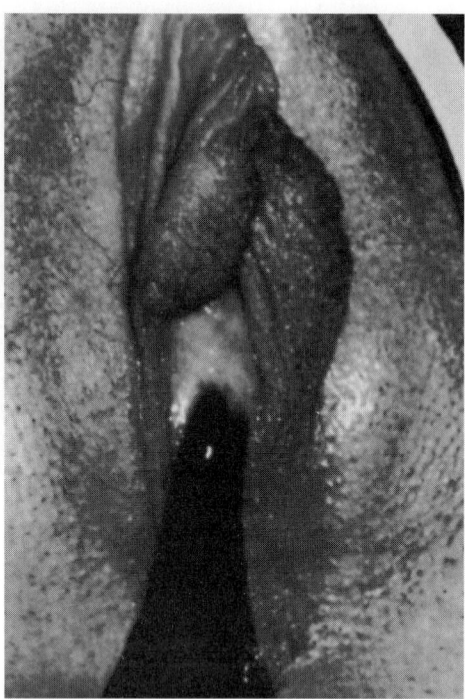

Figure 8–12
Hematocolpos. The center of the imperforate membrane has been incised, and dark blood is pouring out. Much of the redundant portion of the membrane can be snipped away with scissors to permit free drainage. (From Huffman JW, Dewhurst CJ, Capraro VJ: The Gynecology of Childhood and Adolescence. 2nd ed. Philadelphia: WB Saunders Company, 1981, with permission.)

to reduce the risk of introducing infection. Endometriosis and vaginal adenosis are known but not inevitable complications in such patients.

ANOMALIES OF THE VAGINA

Failure of Vertical Fusion

Transverse vaginal septa are the result of faulty canalization of the embryonic vagina. These septa may be without an opening (complete or obstructive) or may have a small central aperture (incomplete or nonobstructive). They are usually found in the midvagina but may occur at any level (Dewhurst, 1978a). When the septum is located in the upper vagina, it is more likely to be patent (incomplete), whereas those located in the lower part of the vagina are often complete (Fig. 8–13).

An incomplete septum is usually asymptomatic, and therefore does not require correction during childhood or early adolescence. The central aperture allows for vaginal secretions and menstrual flow to egress from the vagina. However, a complete septum will result in signs and symptoms similar to those of an imperforate hymen (Dewhurst, 1978a; Huffman et al, 1981; Jones and Rock, 1983; Rock and Azziz, 1987). Unfortunately, the diagnosis of a transverse

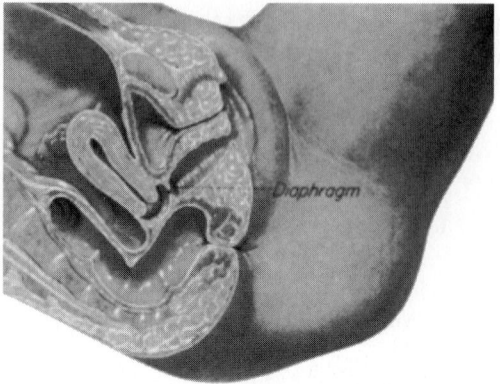

Figure 8–13
A transverse vaginal septum, as illustrated, creates a diaphragm-like fold across the vaginal canal. (From Huffman JW, Dewhurst CJ, Capraro VJ: The Gynecology of Childhood and Adolescence. 2nd ed. Philadelphia: WB Saunders Company, 1981, with permission.)

vaginal septum is often delayed until after menarche, when menstrual blood is trapped behind an obstructing membrane. If the diagnosis of a complete septum is established prior to menarche, it should be incised, creating an aperture to allow discharge. Incision of a complete septum should be done only when the upper vagina is distended and the membrane is bulging. The distention confirms the presence of an upper vaginal segment, facilitates the procedure, and reduces the risk of injury to adjacent structures (Huffman et al, 1981; Jones and Rock, 1983; Rock and Azziz, 1987).

Occasionally, there is some narrowing of the vaginal canal at the site of the septum. Because of the technical difficulties in performing intravaginal surgery on immature structures, it is best to limit the procedure only to the establishment of vaginal drainage. Surgical correction of vaginal narrowing should be performed only when the patient is contemplating initiation of sexual activity. Then the membrane should be excised along with the ring of dense subepithelial connective tissue surrounding the vagina at the level of partition. The mucosa of the upper vagina should then be sutured to the mucosa of the lower vagina (Huffman et al, 1981; Jones and Rock, 1983; Rock and Azziz, 1987). In instances where the length of the obstructing membrane is such that reanastomosis is not possible, the surgeon may leave an indwelling Lucite form in the vagina. The form allows for egress of menstrual flow and maintains vaginal patency and width. With time, re-epithelialization occurs, and the form may be removed in 4 to 6 months.

Failure of Longitudinal Fusion

Duplication of the vagina is an extremely rare condition often associated with duplication of the vulva, bladder, and uterus. Each part of the vagina is en-

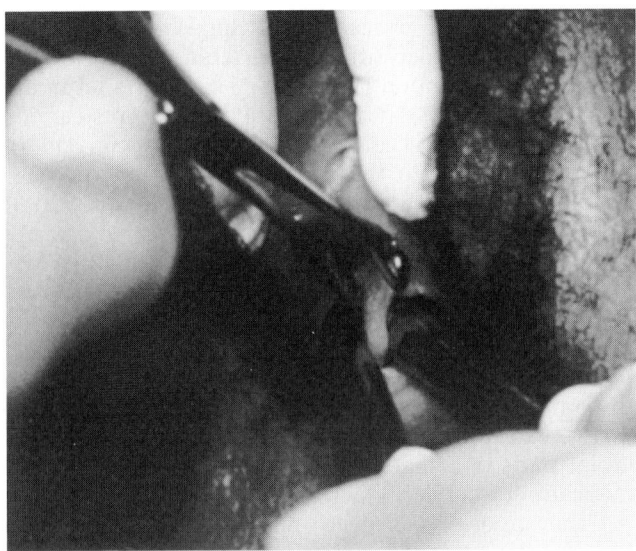

Figure 8-14
Longitudinal septum dividing the vagina. (From Muram D: Pediatric and adolescent gynecology. In Pernol ML, Benson RC (eds): Current Gynecologic and Obstetric Diagnosis and Treatment. East Norwalk, CT: Appleton and Lange, 1987:569, with permission.)

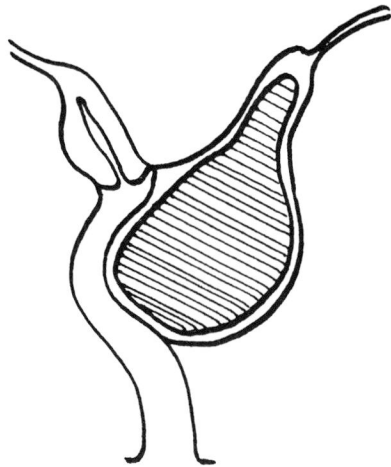

Figure 8-15
Diagram illustrating retention of blood in one half of an imperforate vagina. (From Huffman JW, Dewhurst CJ, Capraro VJ: The Gynecology of Childhood and Adolescence. 2nd ed. Philadelphia: WB Saunders Company, 1981, with permission.)

circled with a separate muscular layer (Huffman et al, 1981). The more common anomaly is one in which the vagina is encircled by one muscular layer but the cavity is divided by a longitudinal septum (Fig. 8–14). These longitudinal septa occur when the distal ends of the müllerian ducts fail to fuse properly. Failure of fusion may be limited to the vagina only or may affect the uterus as well, forming a bicornuate uterus or uterus didelphis. If asymptomatic, longitudinal septa require no treatment. Division of the septum is indicated when dyspareunia is present, when obstruction of drainage from one half of the vagina is noted, or when the physician suspects that a septum would interfere with a vaginal delivery (Jones and Rock, 1983; Rock and Azziz, 1987).

The Obstructed Hemivagina

A unicornuate or double uterus is occasionally accompanied by an anomaly of the opposite paramesonephric duct, creating a lateral vaginal wall cyst with an endometrial lining. As a result, the cyst fills with blood at menarche and produces a vaginal mass (Fig. 8–15). Excision of a small segment of the common wall between the cyst and the vagina often provides adequate drainage. Attempts to remove the cyst may involve extensive dissection with potential damage to the urethra, bladder, or ureter. The disorder is almost always associated with ipsilateral renal agenesis (Huffman et al, 1981; Jones and Rock, 1983; Rock and Azziz, 1987). Evaluation of the urinary collective system may identify a patient with ectopic ureter draining into the obstructed hemivagina (Shibata et al, 1995).

Vaginal Agenesis

Individuals with the Rokitansky syndrome are genetic females. They develop normally in adolescence and have all of the usual feminine attributes, but, because the müllerian ducts fail to develop, the uterus and vagina do not develop. However, the external genitalia are normal. A ruffled ridge of tissue represents the hymen, inside which there is an indentation marking the spot where the introitus would normally be found.

In many patients other developmental defects are present as well, affecting the urinary tract (45% to 50%), the spine (10%), and less frequently the middle ear and other mesodermal structures (Griffin et al, 1976). More recent studies have documented a much higher prevalence (up to 25%) of hearing loss among patients with Rokitansky's syndrome (Strubbe et al, 1994; Cremers et al, 1995). Therefore, any child with vaginal agenesis should undergo an evaluation of the urinary tract, spine, and hearing at some time during childhood. In addition, a chromosome analysis or serum testosterone level should be obtained in all patients with vaginal agenesis to identify the rare instances in which vaginal agenesis represents the effects of testicular activity. Neither exploratory laparotomy nor laparoscopy are indicated in patients with Rokitansky's syndrome, and the absence of the uterus can be confirmed by a pelvic sonogram.

Creation of a satisfactory vagina is the objective in treatment of vaginal agenesis, and this should be deferred until the girl is contemplating an active sexual life. Several techniques have been utilized. The nonoperative creation of a vagina using graduated vaginal dilators has been described by Frank (1938) and later by Ingram (1981). It is relatively risk free but requires motivation and patient cooperation. The area the vagina should occupy is a potential space filled with comparatively loose connective tissue that is capable of considerable indentation. The patient is given a series of dilators of graduated sizes and lengths and is taught how to place them against the vaginal dimple and apply constant pressure. This maneuver is repeated daily for 20 to 30 minutes using wider and longer dilators. The procedure takes a few months to complete and requires persistence and patience.

If gradual vaginal dilation fails, the vaginal space can be developed surgically between the urethra and bladder anteriorly and the perineal body and rectum posteriorly (Fig. 8–16). This cavity is then lined by a split-thickness skin graft overlying a plastic or soft silicone mold (McIndoe procedure) (McIndoe and Banister, 1938). Many surgeons have reported good results with this technique because of its simplicity, low morbidity, and high success rate (Alessandrescu et al, 1996). Although the use of an amnion may prevent pain and scarring at the site from which the skin graft was taken, recent fears regarding acquired immunodeficiency syndrome have rendered this method unsafe. To overcome this problem, some surgeons are experimenting with artificial membranes that can be used to line the newly created cavity. Oxidized regenerated cellulose, for example, was shown to be effective in achieving a complete and quick epithelization of the cavity (Sauer-Ramirez et al, 1995).

An alternative procedure is the Williams vulvovaginoplasty, which utilizes the labia majora to construct a coital pouch (Williams, 1964). The labia are placed under tension. A U-shaped incision is carried from the level of the urethra along the margins of the labia majora to the midpoint between the posterior fourchette and the anus. The vulvar skin is dissected from the subcutaneous fat to allow approximation without tension. Closure is in three layers. First-layer closure of the incision begins posteriorly and proceeds anteriorly, approximating the inner layer of skin. Interrupted sutures are then used to approximate the subcutaneous tissues, and then the outer layer of skin is closed over the midline (Fig. 8–17). Modifications for this procedure, using either labial pads or tissue expanders, have been reported (Muram et al, 1992; Flack et al, 1993).

Other operative procedures have been described for the correction of vaginal agenesis. Davydov and Zhvitiashivili used the peritoneum to line the newly created vaginal space. Other surgeons used cutaneous flaps to form the neovagina (Edmonds, 1994; Giraldo et al, 1996).

The use of bowel as a substitute for the absent vagina is still done in patients when there is only limited space between the bladder and the rectum or if the vascular bed is compromised. In these procedures, a loop of bowel is dissected free with its blood supply and rotated to lie in apposition to a

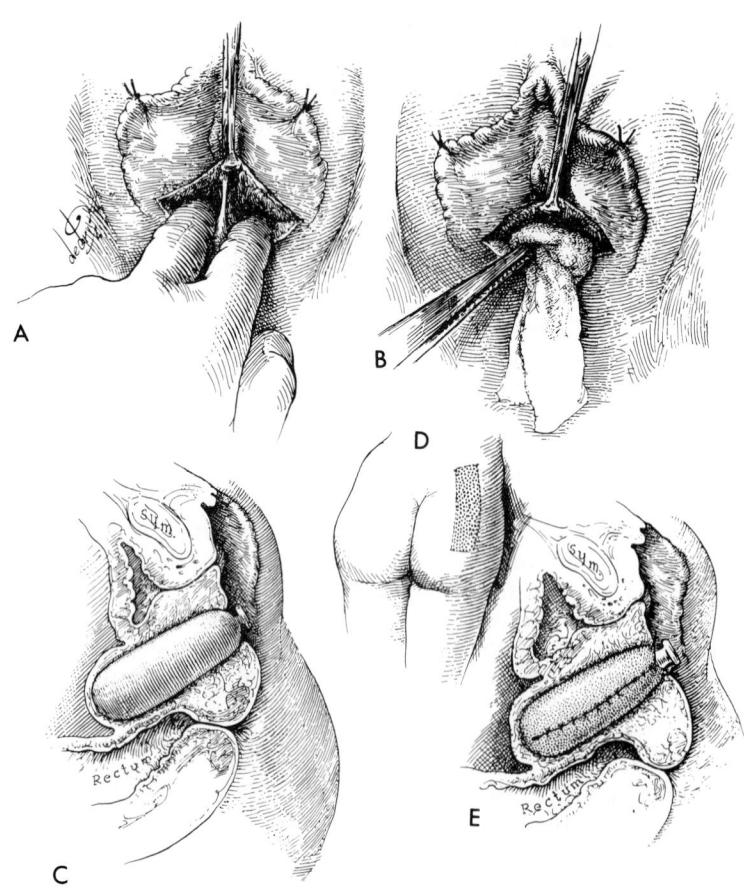

Figure 8–16

Wharton technique and McIndoe-Banister technique for the creation of a vagina. In both techniques, a channel is developed between the urethra and bladder and the rectum.

A, Dissection is more easily performed on both sides of the midline raphe in loose adventitia-like tissue by blunt finger dissection. The denser fibrous midline tissue that forms a median raphe is then cut with scissors.

B, Repeated packing of the cavity with wet gauze aids in enlarging the cavity and in controlling fine capillary bleeding.

C, Insertion of vaginal mold completes the Wharton operation; the mold keeps the canal patent while epithelialization slowly occurs.

D and *E,* Completion of the McIndoe-Banister operation. *D,* Donor site for a split-thickness skin graft. *E,* The mold, covered with the graft, is placed in the new vagina, where epithelialization promptly takes place.

(From Capraro V: Surgical correction of genital anomalies. In: Davis' Gynecology and Obstetrics. Vol II. New York: Hoeber Medical Division, Harper & Row, 1968, with permission.)

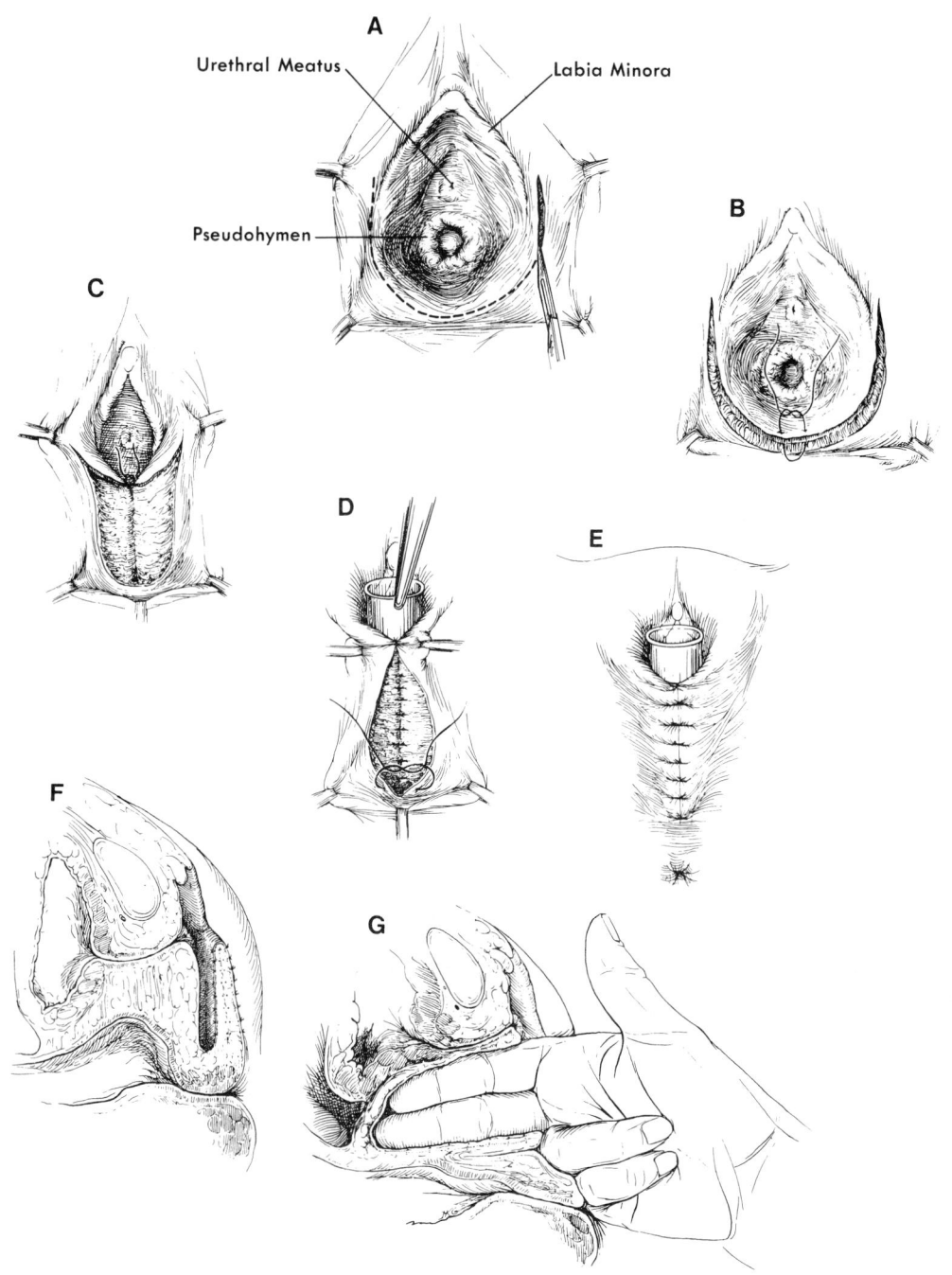

Figure 8–17

Williams' operation for the creation of a vagina.

A, The vulvar tissues are put under tension by four properly placed Allis clamps. A U-shaped incision in the skin of the medial aspects of the labia majora begins at or slightly above the level of the urethral meatus.

B and *C*, First-layer closure of the skin begins posteriorly and proceeds anteriorly. Interrupted sutures of 3-0 chromic catgut on an atraumatic needle are tied so that the knots are placed in the new vaginal cavity rather than buried in the tissue.

D, A glass tube or mold within the cavity assures its adequate diameter. A second layer of 3-0 catgut sutures brings the subcutaneous tissue together in midline.

E, A third layer of interrupted 3-0 chromic catgut sutures approximates the outer layer of skin and its subcutaneous tissue.

F, Sagittal view showing cavity of new vaginal pouch at the end of the operation.

G, Sagittal view of new vaginal canal after use of graded dilators and after coitus.

(Modified from Capraro V, Capraro E: Creation of a neovagina. Obstet Gynecol 1972;39:545, with permission from the American College of Obstetricians and Gynecologists.)

new vaginal opening. The upper edge of the loop is sutured closed. Although some patients complain of excessive mucus secretion, the results are quite satisfactory. Rare cases of bowel prolapse have been reported (Freundt et al, 1994).

Finally, a surgical modification for Frank's method, the Vecchietti procedure, had been used quite successfully in Europe. The technique uses a sphere connected to two metal wires that are guided through the potential neovaginal space to exit onto the anterior abdominal wall. The wires are then attached to an apparatus that winds and shortens the wires. The sphere is thus being pulled upward, and stretches the blind vaginal pouch. The procedure can be done using endoscopic equipment, which further simplifies the technique (Fedele et al, 1994).

Most women report satisfactory results after the surgical correction, and lead a healthy sexual life with an unimpaired emotional and sexual responsiveness. However, the surgeon should not neglect the patient's need for psychological help and guidance. This must also cover the subject of infertility, a cause of particular anguish for most women (Mobus et al, 1993). The technology of in vitro fertilization and embryo transfer now enables a woman without a uterus to have her own genetic children using a surrogate mother. This raises a host of difficult medical and legal issues for the physician who is involved in facilitating such pregnancies (Batzer et al, 1992).

Partial Vaginal Agenesis

Vaginal agenesis may be limited to only a segment of the vagina. In absence of the lower vagina, the lower vagina is not canalized and is replaced by a soft mass of tissue. Absence of the distal vagina only is identified when the upper vagina, cervix, and uterus are seen on pelvic sonogram. If the uterus has developed normally, the upper part of the vagina will fill with blood when menstruation begins (Fig. 8–18). The symptoms are similar to those associated with a transverse vaginal septum. While vulvar inspection reveals findings identical with those of vaginal agenesis, the rectoabdominal palpation reveals a large, boggy pelvic mass. Sonographic evaluation confirms the diagnosis. In these patients, the obstruction to menstrual flow must be removed. In some, drainage of the uterus can be achieved through a reconstructed vagina. In others, particularly when the uterus is rudimentary, consideration may be given to performing a hysterectomy (Huffman et al, 1981; Jones and Rock, 1983; Rock and Azziz, 1987).

UTERINE ANOMALIES

Most uterine anomalies are asymptomatic and therefore are not detected during childhood or early adolescence; often they are detected when they inter-

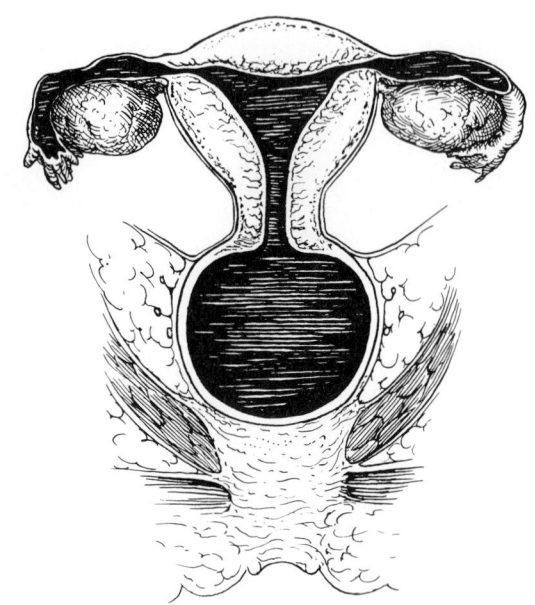

Figure 8–18
Menstrual blood collecting above an obstruction created by agenesis of the distal vagina distends the uterus and upper vagina, making a large pelvic mass. (From Huffman JW, Dewhurst CJ, Capraro VJ: The Gynecology of Childhood and Adolescence. 2nd ed. Philadelphia: WB Saunders Company, 1981, with permission.)

fere with reproduction. In comparison, obstructive anomalies that cause retention of menstrual flow cause symptoms soon after menarche.

Failure of lateral fusion of the müllerian duct may result in two separate uterine bodies. Duplication may be limited to the uterine body, the uterine body and cervix, or both the uterus and the vagina. In nonobstructed duplication, there are no symptoms related to menstruation; however, vaginal duplication may reduce the caliber of each hemivagina, resulting in dyspareunia. The longitudinal vaginal septum then requires resection. Reproduction seems to be somewhat compromised in patients with didelphic uteri. Infertility, increased rate of pregnancy wastage, and premature labor have been reported in these patients. Although some physicians attempt to prevent premature labor using cervical cerclage, Leibovitz et al (1992) have shown that the outcome of pregnancies in patients with uterine malformations was not improved by the procedure when the indication for cerclage was the malformation itself. Bicornuate or septate uteri may also interfere with reproduction. Although there is often no problem in becoming pregnant, these patients are prone to have miscarriages, malpresentation, or premature labor. A uterine septum should be removed through a hysteroscope, whereas a bicornuate uterus can be unified without the loss of myometrial tissue (e.g., Tompkin's procedure). Various surgical techniques to repair bicornuate or septate uteri have been described, but the description of those is beyond the scope of this chapter. There is no indication, how-

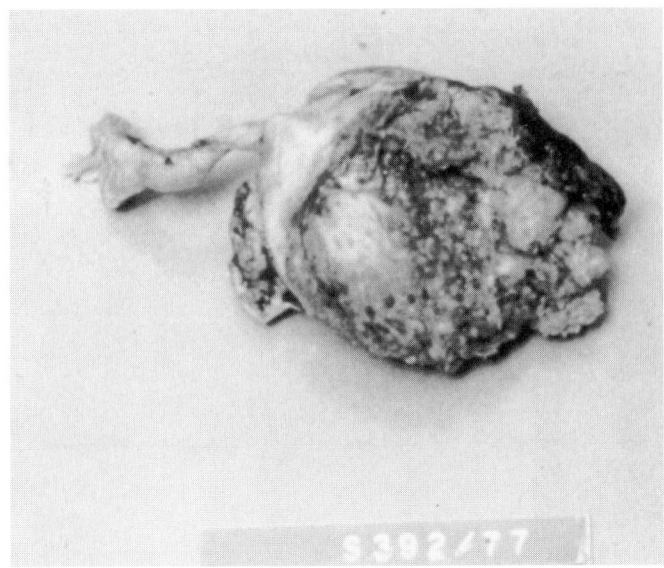

Figure 8-19
Pregnancy in a noncommunicating rudimentary uterine horn that has resulted in rupture. (From Muram D: Pediatric and adolescent gynecology. In Pernol ML, Benson RC (eds): Current Gynecologic and Obstetric Diagnosis and Treatment. East Norwalk, CT: Appleton and Lange, 1987, with permission.)

ever, for surgical intervention in patients with didelphic uteri, except for the possible removal of a vaginal septum (Jones and Rock, 1983).

Failure of lateral fusion may be associated with maldevelopment of one of the müllerian ducts, thus creating unicornuate uterus, or a unicornuate uterus with a small rudimentary uterine horn attached to it. Unicornuate uterus is usually asymptomatic. Reproduction is somewhat compromised, with increased rates of infertility, fetal wastage, and preterm labor. The rudimentary horn, however, may cause surgical emergencies, usually when it does not communicate with the other uterine cavity or the vagina. When menstruation occurs, blood is trapped within the rudimentary cavity, causing severe dysmenorrhea, hematometra, or pyometra. If pregnancy occurs in a rudimentary horn, the horn may rupture, causing a potentially fatal complication for both mother and fetus (Fig. 8–19) (Muram and Spence, 1983). Ideally, a rudimentary horn should be resected prior to conception. The tube on the affected side should be removed, but the ovary can be preserved as long as its blood supply is not impaired. If the endometrial cavity of the remaining horn is entered during the operation, cesarean section is a reasonable mode of delivery in subsequent pregnancies.

OVARIAN ANOMALIES

Supernumerary and Accessory Ovaries

At about the fifth week of gestation, the midportion of the urogenital ridge, close to the mesonephric

duct, thickens to form the gonadal ridge. Located along the urogenital ridge, an additional supernumerary ovary is infrequently found, separated from the normal ovaries. Similarly, excess ovarian tissue may be observed near a normally placed ovary and connected to it—a condition called accessory ovary (Huffman et al, 1981).

If the ovary contains testicular elements, it may be drawn by the round ligament into the inguinal canal or into the labium majus, and associated with an inguinal hernia. At the time of hernia repair, the gonad should be inspected and biopsied when indicated. If it proves to be an ovary, it should be returned to the peritoneal cavity. If testicular tissue is identified, the gonad should be removed. The ovary may be located above the pelvic brim, attached to the uterus by an elongated tube or an ovarian ligament. The ovary may be situated as cephalad as the kidney or the spleen. Ovarian malposition is more commonly observed in association with müllerian tract anomalies (Muram and Pilgrim, 1988; Meneses and Ostrowski, 1989).

Rudimentary Ovary Syndrome and Unilateral Streak Ovary Syndrome

The rudimentary ovary syndrome and the unilateral streak ovary syndrome are poorly defined entities of unknown etiology, traditionally said to be characterized by ovaries containing decreased numbers of follicles, or a unilateral streak gonad. Many cases have been associated with sex chromosomal abnormalities, particularly 45,X/46,XX mosaicism. The disorders may represent variants of gonadal dysgenesis.

Gonadal Dysgenesis

Gonadal dysgenesis denotes streak gonads in any individual, regardless of other associated somatic anomalies. In most adults with gonadal dysgenesis, the normal gonad is replaced by a white fibrous streak, 2 to 3 cm long and about 0.5 cm wide, located in the gonadal ridge. Histologically, the streak gonad is characterized by interlacing waves of dense fibrous stroma, indistinguishable from normal ovarian stroma (Fig. 8–20). Whereas oocytes are present in children and sometimes in adolescents, they are usually absent in 45,X adults. Lack of oocytes is caused by increased atresia and failure of germ cell formation (Jirasek, 1976).

The above comments notwithstanding, most patients with gonadal dysgenesis present during adolescence with delayed puberty and primary amenorrhea. If untreated, estrogen and androgen levels are decreased and follicle-stimulating hormone (FSH) and luteinizing hormone (LH) levels are increased. Estrogen-dependent organs show the predictable effects of hormonal deficiency. Breasts con-

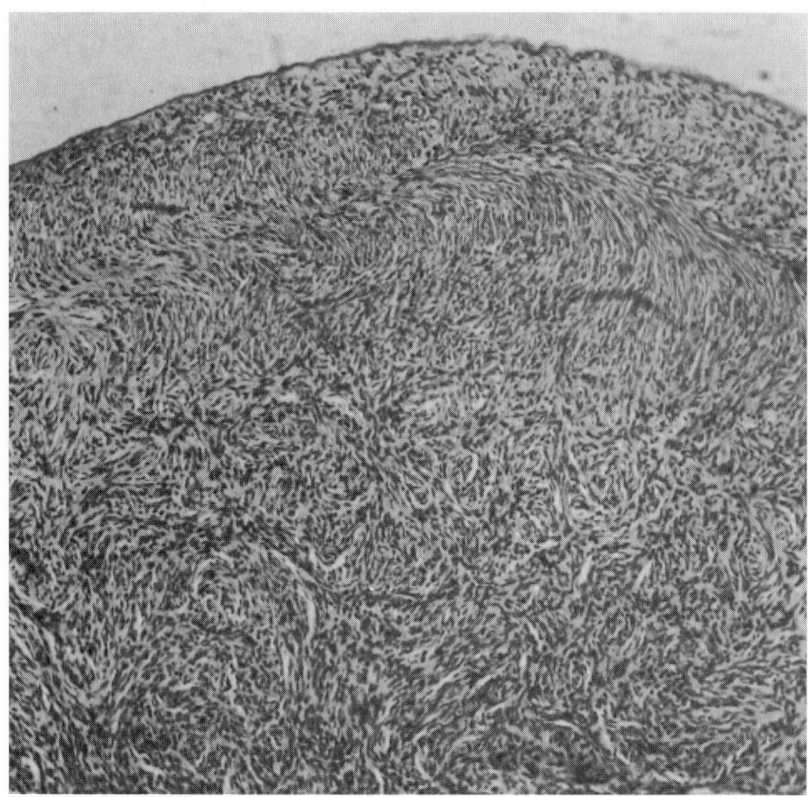

Figure 8–20
Gonadal ridge from a 15-year-old patient with gonadal dysgenesis. Medullary and cortical elements are both absent. (From Huffman JW, Dewhurst CJ, Capraro VJ: The Gynecology of Childhood and Adolescence. 2nd ed. Philadelphia: WB Saunders Company, 1981, with permission.)

tain little parenchymal tissue, and the areolar tissue is only slightly darker than the surrounding skin; the well-differentiated external genitalia, vagina, and müllerian derivatives remain small. Pubic and axillary hair fails to develop in normal quantity (Simpson, 1976; Dewhurst, 1984).

However, normal pubertal development, menstruation, and even pregnancies have been reported in adults with gonadal dysgenesis. It is possible that a few of these individuals maintain some germ cells to adulthood. Spontaneous development is more commonly observed in patients with mosaicism with a 46,XX line. The rare offspring of these women are probably not at an increased risk for chromosomal abnormalities. Patients with gonadal dysgenesis adjust quite well and function normally as adults. Furthermore, this adjustment is related not to physical stigmata, but rather to their intellectual ability and degree of achievement motivation (Aran et al, 1992). Pregnancy is possible in patients with gonadal failure using ovum donation and in vitro fertilization and embryo transfer (Bianco et al, 1992).

Many different chromosomal complements, including normal complements (XX and XY), have been associated with gonadal dysgenesis. This section includes only the most common complements.

45,X

Individuals with a 45,X karyotype have decreased height velocity before puberty, generally in the 10th to 15th percentile range. The mean adult height of 45,X females is 141 to 146 cm (Simpson, 1979, 1987b). It is assumed that the diminished height is caused by the loss of height-determining genes present on the X chromosome (Fig. 8–21). In addition, the epiphyses in patients with a 45,X complement are structurally abnormal. Cabrol et al (1996) collected growth and bone maturation data from 160 patients with Turner's syndrome. X monosomy was found in half of these patients; mosaicism or X abnormality was present in the other half. In their series, 45% of patients were small for age. When gonadal dysgenesis occurred, height velocity decreased from 2 years of age and decreased faster during adolescence, while excessive weight appeared after the age of 5 years. The final height correlated with birth weight, maternal height, and midparental height, and was not altered by spontaneous puberty (Cabrol et al, 1996).

The final height of girls with Turner's syndrome correlates well with the chromosomal abnormality. The mean heights of girls with deletion of Xq and girls with pure 46,XX gonadal dysgenesis are significantly higher than those of girls with other chromosomal abnormalities. Girls with a deletion of the entire Xp segment [46,X,i(Xq)] have the shortest stature (Cohen et al, 1995). The mean adult height of patients with XY gonadal dysgenesis is greater than that of patients with XX gonadal dysgenesis. It has been suggested that there are Y-specific growth gene(s) that promote statural growth independently

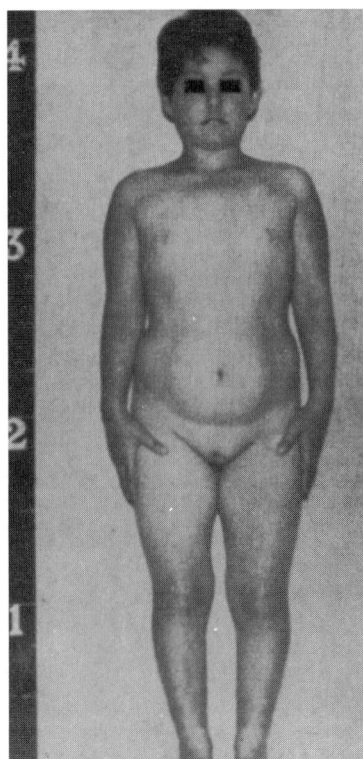

Figure 8–21
Short stature and absent secondary sexual development in a patient with 45,X gonadal dysgenesis and no other somatic features of the condition. (From Huffman JW, Dewhurst CJ, Capraro VJ: The Gynecology of Childhood and Adolescence. 2nd ed. Philadelphia: WB Saunders Company, 1981, with permission.)

Table 8–2. THE COMMON SOMATIC FEATURES OF TURNER'S SYNDROME (45,X)

Growth	Decreased birth weight
	Decreased adult height (141–146 cm)
Intellectual Function	Verbal IQ > performance IQ
	Cognitive deficits (space-form blindness)
	Immature personality, probably secondary to short stature
Craniofacial	Premature fusion of sphenoccipital and other sutures, producing brachycephaly
	Abnormal pinnae
	Retruded mandible
	Epicanthal folds (25%)
	High-arched palate (36%)
	Abnormal dentition
	Visual anomalies, usually strabismus (22%)
	Auditory deficits; sensorineural or secondary to middle ear infections
Neck	Pterygium coli (46%)
	Short broad neck (74%)
	Low nuchal hairline (71%)
Chest	Rectangular contour (shield chest) (53%)
	Apparent widely spaced nipples
	Tapered lateral ends of clavicle
Cardiovascular	Coarctation of aorta or ventricular septal defect (10% to 16%)
Renal (38%)	Horseshoe kidneys
	Unilateral renal aplasia
	Duplication ureters
Gastrointestinal	Telangiectasias
Skin and lymphatics	Pigmented nevi (63%)
	Lymphadema (38%) caused by hypoplasia of superficial vessels
Nails	Hypoplasia and malformation (66%)
Skeletal	Cubitus valgus (54%)
	Radial tilt of articular surface of trochlear
	Clinodactyly V
	Short metacarpals, usually IV (48%)
	Decreased carpal arch (mean angle 117 degrees)
	Deformities of medial tibial condyle
Dermatoglyphics	Increased total digital ridge count
	Increased distance between palmar triradii a and b
	Distal axial triradius in position t'

Modified from Simpson JL: Disorders of Sexual Differentiation: Etiology and Clinical Delineation. New York: Academic Press, 1976, with permission.

of the effects of gonadal sex steroids (Ogata and Matsuo, 1992).

Various treatments for short stature have been explored, including growth hormone, anabolic steroids, and low-dose estrogen. The effect of therapy on ultimate height is still uncertain, but the consensus is that final height is increased by 6 to 8 cm (Hintz, 1989).

Other somatic abnormalities are found in 45,X individuals. Some of the more common features are listed in Table 8–2. Assessment of renal, vertebral, cardiac, and auditory function is therefore obligatory. Although none of these features is pathognomonic, in aggregate they form a characteristic spectrum that is likely to occur in individuals with a 45,X complement. Most 45,X patients have normal intelligence. However, a 45,X patient has a slightly higher probability of being retarded, with performance IQ being lower than verbal IQ (Simpson, 1976). More recently, Ross et al (1995) have shown that girls with Turner's syndrome resemble normal subjects in terms of verbal and language abilities. However, they often show evidence of multifocal or diffuse right cerebral dysfunction and deficits generally involving nonverbal skills.

Although normal pubertal development, menstruation, and even pregnancies have been reported in adults with Turner's syndrome, only about 5% of these patients show some pubertal development, and only 3% menstruate spontaneously. While it is possible that a few 45,X individuals maintain some germ cells to adulthood, the presence of 46,XX cells should be suspected in menstruating 45,X patients. The rare offspring of 45,X women are probably not at increased risk for chromosomal abnormalities, despite some authors holding the opposite opinion (Dewhurst, 1978c).

Other X Chromosome Abnormalities

Mosaicism, the presence of two or more cell lines, is caused by nondisjunction or anaphase lag in the zygote or embryo. The final complement depends upon the stage at which the cell division occurs and upon the types of daughter cells that survive following the abnormal division. The most common form of mosaicism associated with gonadal dysgenesis is 45,X/46,XX. These individuals demonstrate fewer anomalies than do 45,X individuals. Spontaneous pubertal development occurs in 18% of patients, and menstruation in 12%. Somatic anomalies are less likely to occur and mean adult height is greater than in 45,X individuals. 45,X/47,XXX complement is less common, but, phenotypically, these individuals are similar to 45,X/46,XX individuals (Simpson, 1976).

Deletion of the X short arm often results in gonadal dysgenesis, short stature, and other of the Turner stigmata (Simpson, 1987b). The phenotypic expression depends upon the location of the break and thus the amount of X chromosome lost. In general, the more material lost, the more these individuals resemble 45,X individuals. Functioning ovarian tissue persists more often in individuals with more distal deletions (Simpson, 1987b). Patients with nonmosaic *deletions of the X long arm* usually present with premature ovarian failure (Simpson, 1987a).

Division of the centromere in the transverse rather than in the longitudinal plane results in an *isochromosome*, a metacentric chromosome consisting of isologous arms. Both arms are structurally identical and contain the same genes. An isochromosome for the X long arm is the most common X-structural abnormality, but coexisting 45,X lines (mosaicism) are common. Almost all these individuals show streak gonads. Short stature and Turner stigmata are common as well (Simpson, 1976).

45,X/46,XY

These individuals have both a 45,X cell line and at least one cell line containing a Y chromosome. The Y chromosome may be structurally abnormal. Various degrees of testicular differentiation are possible, depending on the tissue distribution of the Y cell line. As a result, a variety of phenotypes have been described, ranging from almost normal males with hypospadias to females indistinguishable from those with the 45,X Turner's syndrome (Simpson, 1976; McDonough and Tho, 1983).

When testicular differentiation fails, the external genitalia develop to be those of a normal female. Most of these individuals are normal in stature and show no somatic anomalies. However, a few may have the Turner stigmata and thus be clinically indistinguishable from 45,X individuals. At puberty, the external genitalia, vagina, and müllerian derivatives remain unstimulated (Fig. 8–22). Some pubic and axillary hair development is present, stimulated by androgens of adrenal origin. Usually, breasts fail to develop. Occasionally, an estrogen-secreting tu-

mor (e.g., gonadoblastoma, dysgerminoma) may stimulate breast growth, (Verp and Simpson, 1987), and virilization has been described as a result of gonadotropin stimulation of streak gonads (Bosze et al, 1986).

The term *asymmetric* or *mixed gonadal dysgenesis* is applied to individuals with one streak gonad and one dysgenetic testis. Such individuals usually have ambiguous external genitalia and a 45,X/46,XY complement, although occasionally only 45,X or only 46,XY cells are demonstrable. Many 45,X/46,XY individuals have normal müllerian derivatives (e.g., a uterus). Occasionally the uterus is rudimentary, or a fallopian tube may fail to develop ipsilateral to a testis. In comparison, the uterus is absent in almost all genetic forms of male pseudohermaphroditism.

Histologically, the streak gonads of 45,X/46,XY individuals are indistinguishable from the streak gonads of individuals with 45,X gonadal dysgenesis. Yet gonadoblastomas or dysgerminomas develop in about 15% to 20% of 45,X/46,XY individuals, and may develop as early as the first or second of life. Thus it is recommended that all gonadal tissue be removed as soon as the diagnosis has been established. The uterus should be preserved for menstrual function and the potential of pregnancy through donor oocytes or donor embryos. Other complements (e.g., 45,X/47,XXY; 45,X/46,XY/47,XYY) are relatively rare. Clinically, these individuals are indistinguishable from 45,X/46,XY individuals (Simpson, 1976). After puberty, patients with mixed gonadal dysgenesis exhibit variable degrees of virilization. FSH levels are high, and testicular response to human chorionic gonadotropin (hCG) in terms of testosterone secretion is also variable, ranging from minimal to almost a normal response (Mendez et al, 1993).

47,XXX

The 47,XXX syndrome is relatively common, occurring in about 0.1% of liveborn females. As a group, these women appear to be physically normal females but are more likely to be mentally retarded or mentally ill than are 46,XX women. The IQ of 47,XXX women is 16 points below that of their sibs (Robinson et al, 1979). Somatic anomalies are usually not present in 47,XXX individuals, although some 47,XXX individuals have craniofacial anomalies. Ovarian dysfunction of unknown etiology has been described among 47,XXX individuals. They may experience delayed menarche or premature ovarian failure. Reported pregnancies have shown that most offspring have been chromosomally normal; however, it is prudent to offer these women antenatal chromosome testing.

48,XXXX AND 49,XXXX

Almost all patients with 48,XXXX and 49,XXXX have subnormal intelligence or mental retardation. In ad-

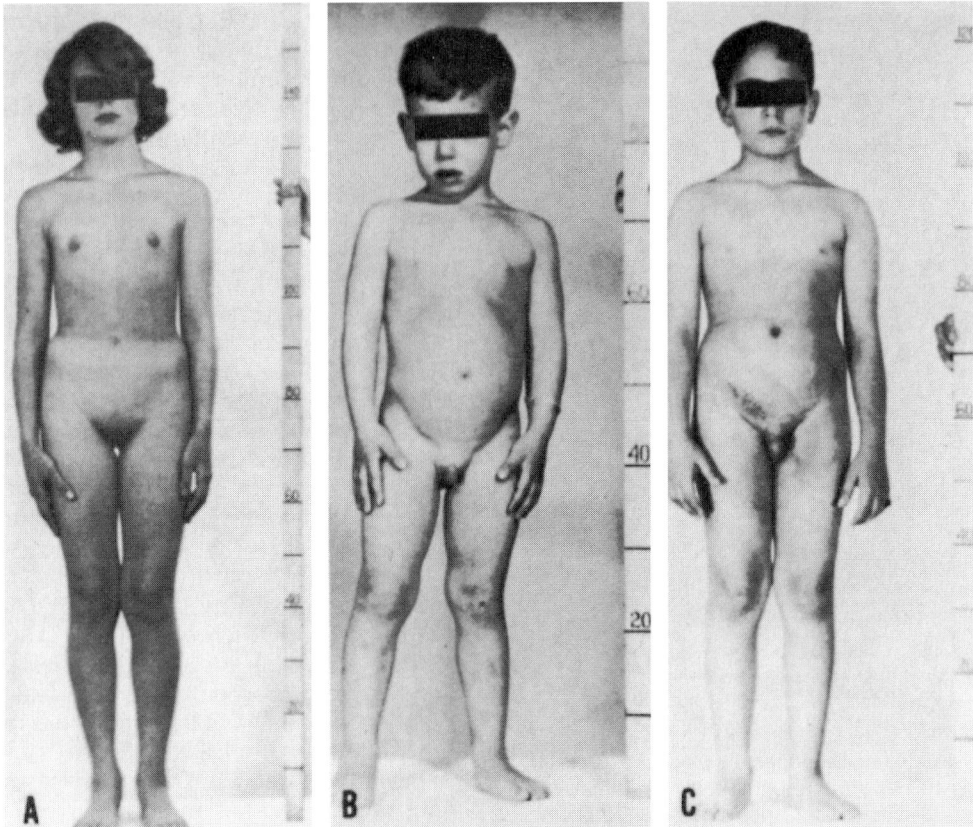

Figure 8–22

Three patients with 45,X/46,XY sex chromosome mosaicism who illustrate highly varied phenotype in this variant of gonadal dysgenesis.

A, Patient 1, a phenotypic female, was 15 years, 4 months of age, She had shortness of stature (−3.1 SD), increased number of pigmented nevi, puffiness over dorsum of fingers, and broad and short hands; she was also sexually infantile (breast development seen in photograph followed estrogen therapy), except for sparse pubic and axillary hair. Titer of urinary gonadotropin was >80 mU/day.

B, Patient 2, a 3½-year-old child, had ambiguous external genitalia, perineal hypospadias, and undescended gonads. He was of average height and had a broad chest and a duplication of left kidney.

C, Patient 3, an 8½-year-old phenotypic male with penile urethra and unilateral undescended gonad, was of average height and had cubitus valgus, short fourth metacarpals, and puffiness of dorsum of fingers. By 15 years of age, male secondary sexual characteristics were well advanced and scrotal testis, which was normal in histologic appearance, measured 4.0 × 2.4 cm.

(From Wilson JD, Foster DW: Williams Textbook of Endocrinology. 7th ed. Philadelphia: WB Saunders Company, 1985:352, with permission.)

dition, many have craniofacial abnormalities reminiscent of Down's syndrome (e.g., hypertelorism, slanting palpebral fissures, a broad nasal bridge).

XX Gonadal Dysgenesis

Gonadal dysgenesis has been observed in 46,XX individuals (Simpson, 1976; Dewhurst, 1984). Most of these individuals are normal in stature, and the somatic features of Turner's syndrome are usually absent (Simpson, 1976, 1979). However, the streak gonads of affected individuals are indistinguishable from those of individuals who have gonadal dysgenesis as a result of an abnormal chromosomal complement. Likewise, the patient presents during adolescence with absent pubertal development and gonadal failure.

Gonadal dysgenesis in 46,XX individuals may result from nongenetic causes that adversely affect gonadal tissue (e.g., infarction, mumps, neoplasia). However, the disorder has been documented in families and is inherited in an autosomal recessive fashion (Fig. 8–23). It may occur alone or coexist with other somatic anomalies (e.g., neurosensory deafness) (Christakos et al, 1969). Mendonca et al (1994) described two agonadic sisters, one with a 46,XY and the other with a 46,XX karyotype, both with normal female external genitalia and hypoplastic müllerian derivatives. They found that the XY patient had no mutations in the conserved sequence of the *SRY* gene, whereas her XX-affected sister was *SRY* negative. Using these siblings, they have concluded that an autosomal locus adversely affected gonadal development in both sexes (Mendonca et al, 1994). A

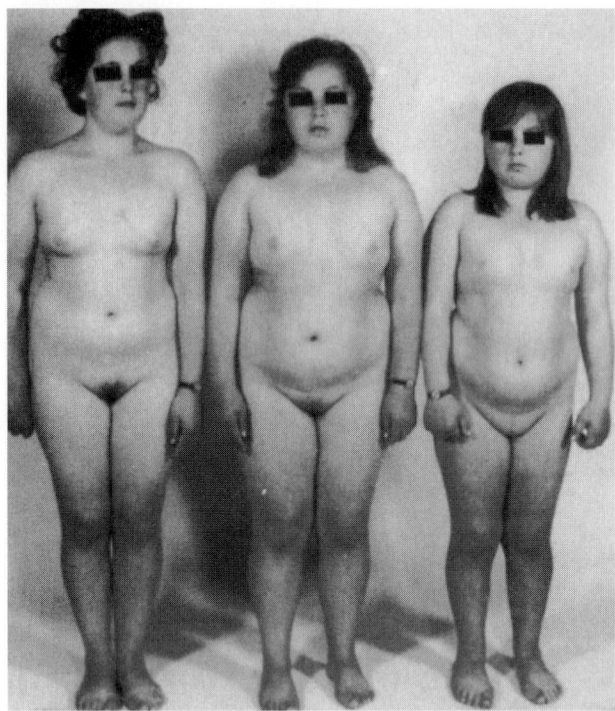

Figure 8–23
Three sisters with 46,XX familial gonadal dysgenesis. Breast growth of the eldest (*left*) is the result of estrogen therapy. (From Huffman JW, Dewhurst CJ, Capraro VJ: The Gynecology of Childhood and Adolescence. 2nd ed. Philadelphia: WB Saunders Company, 1981, with permission.)

nationwide population-based study of women born in Finland between 1950 and 1976 identified 75 patients with XX gonadal dysgenesis. The relatively large number of affected individuals identified (incidence of 1 in 8300 live-born girls) suggests a high gene frequency in the Finnish population. Most affected families originated in the north-central part of the country (Aittomaki, 1994).

XY Gonadal Dysgenesis

Gonadal dysgenesis may occur in individuals with apparently normal 46,XY chromosomal complements. The loss of testicular tissue before 7 to 8 weeks of embryogenesis would produce a female phenotype (Jost, 1947). These individuals show female external genitalia, a uterus, and fallopian tubes. Loss of gonadal tissue after MIS was produced may result in an individual with female external genitalia but a rudimentary or absent uterus. The loss of testicular tissue after 7 to 8 weeks of embryogenesis would produce an individual without a uterus, with varying degrees of virilization and genital ambiguity. The later the loss of testicular tissue occurs, the less the individual will resemble the female phenotype. It has been suggested that streak gonads in 46,XY pure gonadal dysgenesis arise from fetal ovaries and that dysgenetic testes in the partial form in 46,XY partial gonadal dysgenesis develop from ovotestis

(Berkovitz et al, 1991). Height is normal and somatic anomalies usually are absent. At puberty, secondary sexual development fails to occur. Genetic heterogeneity exists with respect to the mode of inheritance of XY gonadal dysgenesis. However, in one group of patients with 46,XY gonadal dysgenesis the disorder is transmitted in an X-linked recessive mode (Muram and Dewhurst, 1984).

Like other patients with gonadal dysgenesis who have a Y chromosome, 20% to 30% of patients develop a dysgerminoma or gonadoblastoma, often in the first or second decades of life (Simpson and Photopulos, 1976). In one series, gonadal tumors developed in 9 of 21 patients (44%). Those at greatest risk for tumor were patients with mixed gonadal dysgenesis and 46,XY pure gonadal dysgenesis. The high prevalence of gonadal tumors in these children warrants consideration of early, bilateral, prophylactic gonadectomy once the diagnosis is established with certainty (Gourlay et al, 1994). The gonads can be safely removed by laparoscopy (Arici et al, 1993; Yu et al, 1995; Ulrich et al, 1996). The uterus should be preserved because pregnancies through donor oocytes or donor embryos are feasible. However, dysgerminomas have been reported in patients without Y-chromosomal DNA. Such cases challenge the theory that Y-related DNA is necessary for the development of dysgerminoma in dysgenetic gonads (Letterie and Page, 1995).

ABNORMAL SEXUAL DIFFERENTIATION

Female Pseudohermaphroditism

Female pseudohermaphrodites are 46,XX individuals whose external genitalia fail to develop as expected for normal females. Although abnormalities of embryonic hindgut, cloacal membrane, or urogenital membrane may coexist, the anomalies are usually limited to the external genitalia.

Congenital adrenal hyperplasia (CAH) represents the most common cause of genital ambiguity in genetic females. CAH is discussed in detail elsewhere in this textbook (Chapter 28). Briefly, deficiency of one of the various enzymes required for steroid biosynthesis causes decreased production of adrenal cortisol, elevated adrenocorticotropic hormone levels, and increased quantities of steroid precursors. Excessive production of adrenal androgens during embryogenesis virilizes the external genitalia. The extent of virilization of the external genitalia depends upon the timing, length of exposure, and plasma levels of androgens. In general, exposure to androgens after 12 weeks of gestation leads only to clitoral hypertrophy. Exposure at progressively earlier stages of embryologic development leads to clitoral hypertrophy, retention of the urogenital sinus, and fusion of the labioscrotal folds. If exposure occurs sufficiently early and to adequate levels of androgens, the labia will fuse to form a penile urethra.

Müllerian and gonadal development remain unaffected because neither is androgen dependent (Cutler and Laue, 1990).

Although the syndromes of CAH account for the majority of female patients with ambiguous genitalia, some patients with genital ambiguity and normal adrenal function have been described (Park et al, 1972). Although multiple somatic abnormalities were present in these individuals, müllerian derivatives and ovaries were normal. Marked clitoral enlargement of unexplained origin sometimes results from hemangiomas, neurofibromas, or tumors.

Virilization by Maternal Androgens

Virilization of the external genitalia has been observed in newborns whose mothers received progestational agents or testosterone during the first trimester of pregnancy. The external genitalia of these infants show an enlarged phallus and fusion of the labioscrotal folds. If these drugs were taken after 12 weeks of gestation, clitoral enlargement was noted but the labia developed normally (Wilkens, 1960). Müllerian duct development and ovarian differentiation remain unaffected (Grumbach and Ducharme, 1960). It is recommended that progestational agents, often used to induce menstrual withdrawal in amenorrheic patients, not be prescribed without performing a pregnancy test. Yet, even when maternal ingestion of progestational agents occurs, not all female infants are affected. It is estimated that some degree of virilization occurs in only 2.75% of female infants whose mothers received progestogens during pregnancy (Grumbach and Conte, 1985). Furthermore, because this exposure is limited, even if virilization did occur, surgical correction is often easy, allowing for normal future reproductive function.

Of special note is the use of stilbestrol derivatives (e.g., diethylstilbestrol [DES]) during pregnancy. In addition to the potential virilizing effect on the female infant, these girls are at increased risk to develop clear cell carcinoma of the vagina as well as other müllerian tract abnormalities. Consequences of in utero exposure to DES are discussed elsewhere in this chapter.

The treatment of infants who show signs of virilization caused by placental transfer of maternal androgens consists of surgical correction of the external genitalia. Because the female infant does not produce androgens, no further virilization is anticipated, and, thus, no additional therapy is required.

Androgen-Secreting Neoplasms

Rarely, a female fetus may virilize when the pregnant mother has a virilizing adrenal or ovarian neoplasm, or when the mother suffers from a virilizing form of CAH. Under these circumstances, maternal androgens may cross the placenta and virilize the female fetus. Luteoma of pregnancy and theca-lutein cysts have been reported to cause fetal virilization

(Grumbach and Conte, 1985). Production of androgens by these lesions probably began after the pregnancy was established. Thus it is not surprising that the majority of affected infants had clitoral hypertrophy, whereas labioscrotal fusion rarely occurred. The absence of virilization in the mother does not exclude a maternal source, because the levels required to virilize the fetal external genitalia may be lower than those required to cause virilization of an adult female. Once the infant is born, therapy consists of surgical correction of the external genitalia.

Male Pseudohermaphroditism

Cytogenetic Forms

Male pseudohermaphrodites are individuals with a Y chromosome whose external genitalia fail to develop as expected for normal males. Cytogenetic forms of male pseudohermaphroditism, 46,XY gonadal dysgenesis, and variants are discussed in the section "Gonadal dysgenesis."

Central Nervous System Defects

Central nervous system defects may alter testosterone production in some individuals. However, the sex of rearing is never in doubt, and these individuals are raised as males. In these disorders inadequate stimulation of the testes is caused by the deficiency of LH and FSH. These disorders include Kallman's syndrome, isolated FSH deficiency, isolated LH deficiency, and hypopituitary dwarfism. In all of these disorders, deficiency of gonadotropins (FSH and/or LH) results in reduced production of testicular androgens. Affected males present with a small penis, small testes, and scanty beard growth. At puberty they fail to undergo normal secondary sexual development (Dewhurst, 1984; Bourguignon et al, 1985).

Deficiencies in Testosterone Biosynthesis

A variety of enzymes are required for the conversion of cholesterol to testosterone. An enzyme deficiency should be suspected if the plasma levels of testosterone are decreased while the levels of any of its precursors are increased. Detection may be difficult during infancy or in early childhood, when testosterone levels are normally low. Provocative tests (e.g., hCG, gonadotropin-releasing hormone) are usually recommended to facilitate the diagnosis (Grant et al, 1976). Inheritance is presumed to be autosomal recessive in most of these disorders. In general, the incompletely developed external genitalia consist of a small phallus, urethral opening proximal on the penis, and incomplete labioscrotal fusion (Fig. 8–24). The testes and wolffian ducts differentiate normally. Depending upon the affected enzyme, other abnormalities may coexist. Severe salt wasting and adrenals filled with foamy-appearing cells are

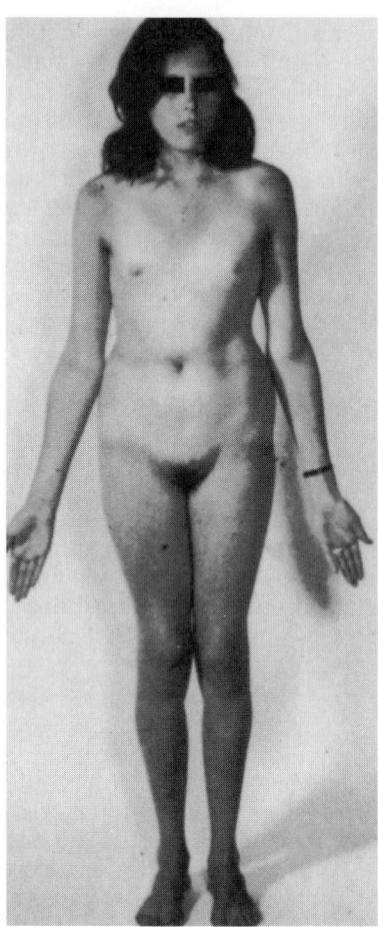

Figure 8-24
Patient with enzymatic testicular failure. The testes appear grossly normal, but plasma testosterone values are very low. (From Huffman JW, Dewhurst CJ, Capraro VJ: The Gynecology of Childhood and Adolescence. 2nd ed. Philadelphia: WB Saunders Company, 1981, with permission.)

present in patients with defects interfering with the conversion of cholesterol to pregnenolone (Kirkland et al, 1973).

In general, the degree of virilization at birth and the size of the phallus will determine the sex of rearing. If the phallus is so small as be considered inadequate for function, a serious consideration should be given to a change in the sex of rearing. Adults who were raised as boys may have to rely upon a penile prosthesis.

Agonadism (Testicular Regression Syndrome)

In individuals with agonadism, the gonads and the internal ductal system are absent, except for rudimentary derivatives of the müllerian or wolffian ducts. The external genitalia consist of a small phallus and nearly complete fusion of the labioscrotal folds. A persistent urogenital sinus is often present. Somatic anomalies (e.g., craniofacial) may coexist

(Sarto and Opitz, 1973). The etiology of the disorder is unknown. It is plausible that fetal testes formed and functioned long enough to inhibit müllerian development, yet not sufficiently long to complete the male differentiation. A study by Marcantonio et al (1994) described nine patients with this condition who showed variable degrees of virilization. Based upon this heterogeneous phenotypic expression, the authors concluded that testicular regression syndrome represents a part of the clinical spectrum of 46,XY gonadal dysgenesis. Alternatively, absence of the gonads and the ductal system may represent an abnormality caused by either defective anlage, defective connective tissue, or teratogenic action. The disorder is transmitted in an autosomal recessive fashion, but X-linked recessive inheritance cannot be excluded (de Grouchy et al, 1985).

Complete Androgen Insensitivity

Individuals with complete androgen insensitivity have bilateral testes, female external genitalia, a short blind vagina, and no müllerian derivatives. The karyotype is 46,XY. At birth, affected individuals have normal-appearing female genitalia. Some individuals show clitoral enlargement and labioscrotal fusion, and the term *incomplete (partial) androgen insensitivity* is applied to these patients. The two disorders are genetically distinct, and heterogeneity exists for each.

At puberty, individuals with complete androgen insensitivity show adequate breast development, but, although the breasts contain normal ductal and glandular tissue, the areolae are often pale and underdeveloped. Pubic and axillary hair is usually sparse or even absent (Fig. 8–25). The vagina is short and ends blindly; occasionally it is represented merely by a dimple. The müllerian derivatives are ordinarily absent, but occasionally rudimentary tubes may be present (Ulloa-Aguirre et al, 1990). Absence of the müllerian derivatives is easily understood. The anti-Müllerian hormone (AMH) secreted by the fetal Sertoli cells is not an androgen, and, thus, müllerian regression occurs in individuals with androgen sensitivity just as in normal males. Height is appropriate for males, and therefore is slightly increased compared to normal women. The testes are usually normal in size but may be located anywhere along the path of embryonic testicular descent—in the abdomen, inguinal canal, or labia majora. If located in the inguinal canal, the testes may be associated with inguinal hernias. In fact, although inguinal hernias are relatively rare in females, they may be found in about one half of all individuals with androgen insensitivity. It is therefore recommended to determine the cytogenetic status of prepubertal girls who present with inguinal hernias, especially if a gonad can be palpated within the inguinal canal.

Complete androgen insensitivity involves end-organ insensitivity to androgens. Baseline plasma

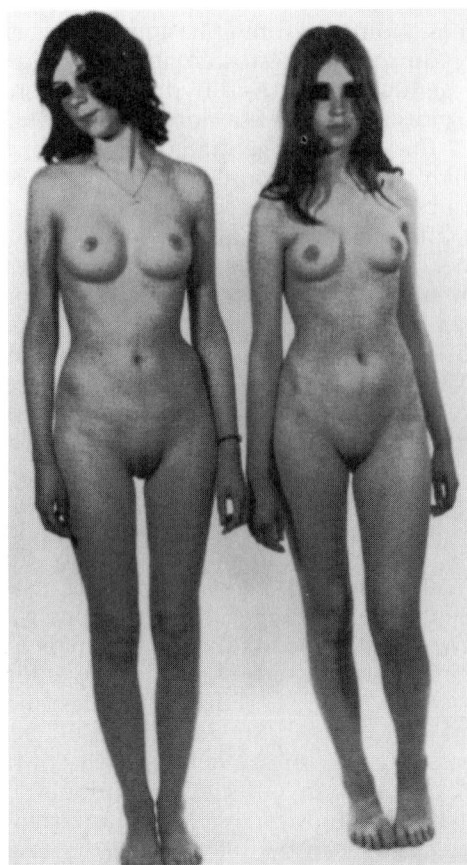

Figure 8–25
46,XY "sisters" with androgen insensitivity. (From Huffman JW, Dewhurst CJ, Capraro VJ: The Gynecology of Childhood and Adolescence. 2nd ed. Philadelphia: WB Saunders Company, 1981, with permission.)

testosterone levels are within the normal male range, yet the patients fail to virilize. In addition, hyperplastic Leydig cells and elevated LH levels suggest an abnormal response of the gonadal-hypothalamic axis. These high LH concentrations in late puberty are comparable to values found during early puberty in castrated individuals and children with gonadal dysgenesis. The sudden increase of LH in late puberty is most probably caused by defective testosterone receptors in the pituitary or hypothalamus. In contrast, FSH concentrations continuously show levels in the normal male or female range with no rise during adolescence (Schmitt et al, 1994). Tissue studies have shown that, in 60% to 70% of patients, androgen receptors are completely absent. Tissues obtained from the mothers of these individuals show the presence of just about half the concentration of receptors. In the remaining 30% to 40% of individuals, receptors are present, and it is assumed that a defect exists at a more distal step in androgen action (Pinsky and Kaufman, 1987).

The frequency of gonadal neoplasia is increased but probably no greater than 5% (Simpson and Photopulos, 1976; Verp and Simpson, 1987). The risk of malignant transformation is certainly low before 25

to 30 years of age, so it is acceptable to leave the testes in situ until after pubertal development. However, if herniorrhaphies are performed prior to puberty, the testes in the inguinal canal should be removed at that time. Otherwise, a second operative procedure (gonadectomy) will be necessary following puberty. Finally, a vaginal reconstruction should be planned, similar to the one required for patients with Rokitansky's syndrome.

Incomplete (Partial) Androgen Sensitivity

Some 46,XY individuals who were reared as females virilize during puberty, whereas other 46,XY individuals who were born with various degrees of virilization actually demonstrate pubertal breast development. Such individuals are said to have incomplete or partial androgen insensitivity. The disorder is transmitted as an X-linked recessive condition. These individuals have bilateral testes, plasma testosterone levels in the normal male range, failure to respond to androgens, absence of müllerian derivatives, and pubertal breast development in some patients and pubertal virilization in others (Fig. 8–26). (Pinsky and Kaufman, 1987; Pinsky et al, 1987). It has been postulated that partial androgen insensitivity is caused by qualitative defects of androgen receptors. With more precise genetic techniques, investigators were able to document various mutations in the *AR* gene, thereby accounting for the heterogeneity in the syndrome of incomplete androgen insensitivity (De-Bellis et al, 1994).

Although orchiectomy and vaginal reconstruction should be performed as in patients with complete androgen sensitivity, pubertal virilization may ne-

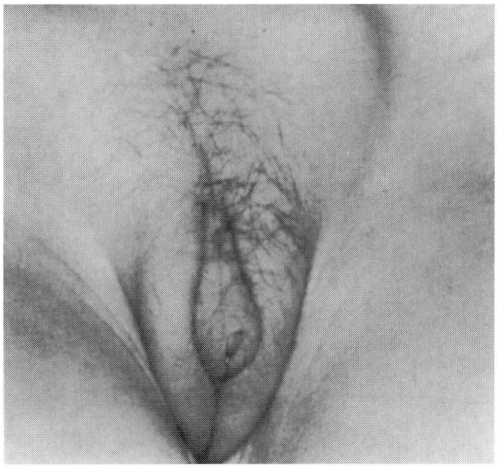

Figure 8–26
Incomplete androgen insensitivity. Note clitoral enlargement and the development of pubic hair. Both testes can be seen in the region of the external inguinal ring. (From Huffman JW, Dewhurst CJ, Capraro VJ: The Gynecology of Childhood and Adolescence. 2nd ed. Philadelphia: WB Saunders Company, 1981, with permission.)

cessitate earlier intervention. In patients who show signs of virilization early in pubertal development, as well as in those who were born with ambiguous genitalia, it is preferable to excise the gonads prior to puberty and to provide early hormone replacement therapy to induce normal female pubertal development.

5α-Reductase Deficiency

Some genetic males show ambiguous or female external genitalia at birth, yet at puberty virilize like normal males. The external genitalia consist of a small phallus, a perineal urethral orifice, and a separate blindly ending perineal orifice that resembles a vagina (Dewhurst et al, 1983). The testes are normal in size and secrete testosterone in normal amounts (Fig. 8–27). The condition is caused by a deficiency of the enzyme 5α-reductase, which converts testosterone to dihydrotestosterone (Imperato-McGinley et al, 1974).

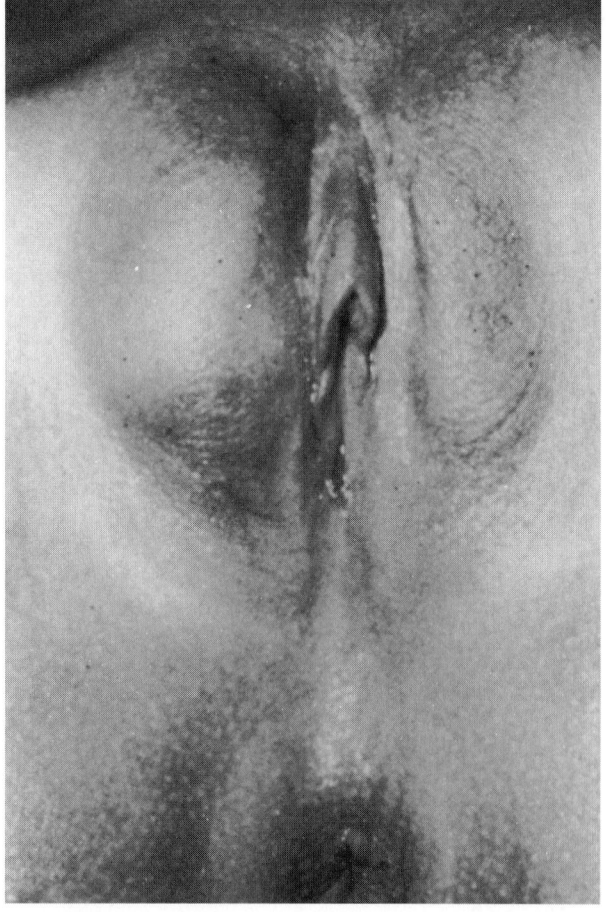

Figure 8–27
External genitalia of a child with 5α-reductase deficiency. Both testes are clearly visible. (From Dewhurst CJ, Chapman M, Muram D, Donnison B: 5-Alpha reductase deficiency in 46,XY sisters. Pediatr Adolesc Gynecol 1983;1:85, with permission. Courtesy of Springer-Verlag, Heidelberg.)

Whereas wolffian differentiation during embryogenesis requires only testosterone, virilization of the external genitalia requires dihydrotestosterone. Thus affected individuals have a normal male ductal system, but the external genitalia are predominantly female-like. In comparison, virilization during puberty can be accomplished by testosterone alone. As a result, affected individuals fail to develop breasts and, instead, show phallic enlargement, increased facial hair, muscular hypertrophy, and deepening of the voice.

The disorder is inherited in an autosomal recessive fashion. In recent years, it has become apparent that there are two genes that encode for 5α-reductase. Initially, investigators were able to clone the responsible gene (later labeled as 5α-reductase-1), but then found individuals with pseudohermaphroditism who had a normal 5α-reductase-1 gene. In these individuals, the investigators were able to identify a mutation in a second gene, now being called 5α-reductase-2. A deletion in this second gene was present in two related individuals with male pseudohermaphroditism caused by 5α-reductase deficiency (Andersson et al, 1991). Further studies showed a variety of mutations in the 5α-reductase-2 gene that may be responsible for the heterogeneity of the clinical syndrome in many affected individuals (Thigpen et al, 1992). Although carrier status in partial androgen insensitivity can be determined, the severity of the genital abnormalities in affected offspring cannot be reliably predicted. The phenotypic variation in families affected by partial androgen insensitivity is dependent on factors other than abnormalities of the androgen receptor gene alone (Batch et al, 1993).

In adults, the diagnosis is established on the basis of an elevated testosterone-to-dehydrotestosterone ratio after the administration of hCG or testosterone propionate (Greene et al, 1987). In infants, baseline levels of testosterone and dihydrotestosterone are so low that distinguishing normal from affected individuals may be difficult. An elevated urinary tetrahydrocortisol-to–5α-tetrahydrocortisol ratio may be a useful diagnostic tool in some affected infants (Imperato-McGinley et al, 1986). Early diagnosis permits proper gender assignment. If the child is to be reared as a female, removal of the gonads prior to puberty and reconstructive surgery will permit the girl to grow up to become an adult woman. If the infant is to be reared as a male, topical treatment with dihydrotestosterone cream to the external genitalia may promote phallic growth. Otherwise, corrective surgery is required to repair the genital abnormality (Odame et al, 1992).

True Hermaphrodites

True hermaphrodites display both ovarian and testicular tissue, either as a separate ovary and a separate testis or, more often, one or more ovotestes. Most true hermaphrodites (60%) have a 46,XX chromosomal complement; however, others have 46,XX/ 46,XY, 46,XY, or other complements (Simpson, 1978). The chromosomal complement varies with the geographical distribution. Of the 96 cases described in Africa, 96.9% had a 46,XX karyotype. The 46,XY karyotype was extremely rare (7%) and equally distributed throughout Asia, Europe, and North America. Chromosomal mosaicism was found in 40.5% of cases in Europe and in 21.0% of the patients in North America (Krob et al, 1994). About one third of true hermaphrodites are raised as females. Breast development usually occurs at puberty even when the external genitalia are frankly ambiguous or predominantly male (Fig. 8–28). A uterus is usually present, albeit sometimes bicornuate or unicornuate. Absence of a uterine horn usually indicates an ipsilateral testis or ovotestis (Van Niekerk, 1974; Van Niekerk and Retief, 1981). Menstruation is common, often manifested as cyclic hematuria (Raspa et al, 1986). Gonadal tissue may be located in the ovarian, inguinal, or labioscrotal regions. Ovotestis is the most common gonad found in patients with true hermaphroditism (Krob et al, 1994). A testis or an ovotestis is more likely to be present on the right than the left, whereas pure ovarian tissue is more common on the left. The greater the proportion of testicular tissue in an ovotestis, the greater the likelihood of gonadal descent.

Although oocytes are often seen, even in ovotestes, spermatozoa are rarely present (Aaronson, 1985). Pregnancies have been reported in 46,XX true hermaphrodites, usually after the removal of testicular tissue (Minowada et al, 1984). In comparison, only one true hermaphrodite apparently has fathered a child (Krob et al, 1994).

The most obvious cause of true hermaphroditism is 46,XX/46,XY chimerism. 46,XX/47,XXY cases may result from either chimerism or mitotic nondisjunction. Some authors believe that most 46,XY cases represent unrecognized forms of chimerism or mosaicism (Simpson, 1978). Some authors have suggested that the mechanism for chimerism could be fertilization of (1) the secondary oocyte and first polar body, (2) the ovum and first polar body, or (3) the ovum and second polar body, or (4) fusion of two embryos (Verp et al, 1992). However, the presence of testicular tissue in 46,XX individuals may also be caused by translocation of the testis-determining factor from a Y to an X chromosome, or to an autosome (Abbas et al, 1993; Tar et al, 1995). The presence of autosomal sex-reversal genes should be considered as well. Sibships with XX true hermaphroditism have been reported (Fraccaro et al, 1979). Familial true hermaphroditism is more likely to be characterized by bilateral ovotestes and uterine absence than are nonfamilial cases (Simpson, 1978).

The diagnosis is made after an investigation of ambiguous genitalia excludes male and female pseudohermaphroditism, and gonadal biopsy shows both testicular and ovarian elements. If the child is to be raised as a female, selective gonadal extirpation is indicated. When the child has a separate ovary and a separate testis, the testis should be removed and the ovary sampled to exclude the presence of testicular tissue. If the individual has one or more ovotestes, it is necessary to remove the testicular tissue and preserve the ovarian tissue. In 80% of ovotestes, testicular and ovarian components are juxtaposed end to end (Van Niekerk, 1974; Van Niekerk and Retief, 1981). The surgeon can easily identify and remove the testicular tissue, which is softer and darker than the ovarian tissue. The margin should be submitted for frozen section to confirm that all testicular tissue has been removed. When testicular tissue is mixed with the ovarian tissue, preservation of ovarian tissue on that side may not be possible, and the ovotestis should be excised. Rearing the infant as a male is possible depending upon the size of the phallus. Genital reconstruction, removal of müllerian structures, and selective gonadal extirpation should be performed prior to puberty.

DEVELOPMENTAL ABNORMALITIES FOLLOWING IN UTERO EXPOSURE TO DES

DES is a synthetic nonsteroidal estrogen first produced by Sir Charles Dodd in 1937. The drug was frequently prescribed to pregnant women until the early 1970s, with the intention of preventing miscarriages and other pregnancy complications. It is estimated that as many as 10 million Americans (mothers, daughters, and sons) may have been exposed to DES, either directly or in utero. The potentially devastating effects of in utero exposure to DES were first described by Herbst et al in 1971 (Herbst et al, 1971; 1974). They reported observing a rare form of vaginal cancer, clear cell adenocarcinoma, in young women ages 14 to 22 years. Cancers of this site and cell type had previously been almost unknown in women of that age group, and the occurrence of this cancer was linked to intrauterine exposure to DES. Since the mid-1970s, several follow-up studies of various DES-exposed groups have been conducted. The most notable of these in the United States have been the National Cancer Institute–initiated DES adenosis (DESAD) follow-up of 3980 DES-exposed daughters; a follow-up of 3033 DES-exposed mothers conducted by Boston University; long-term monitoring by the University of Chicago of 693 DES-exposed women and 668 placebo-exposed women who participated in a randomized trial of DES use in pregnancy, as well as offspring of both groups; and a study comparing 1706 mothers exposed to DES with an unexposed population of 1405 mothers. Much of what is known about DES exposure and its consequences has come from these studies.

The most common abnormality seen in these young women is adenosis, which denotes the presence of glandular tissue in the vagina. Adenosis is replaced by squamous metaplasia, which occurs naturally and is rarely seen in DES daughters over 30

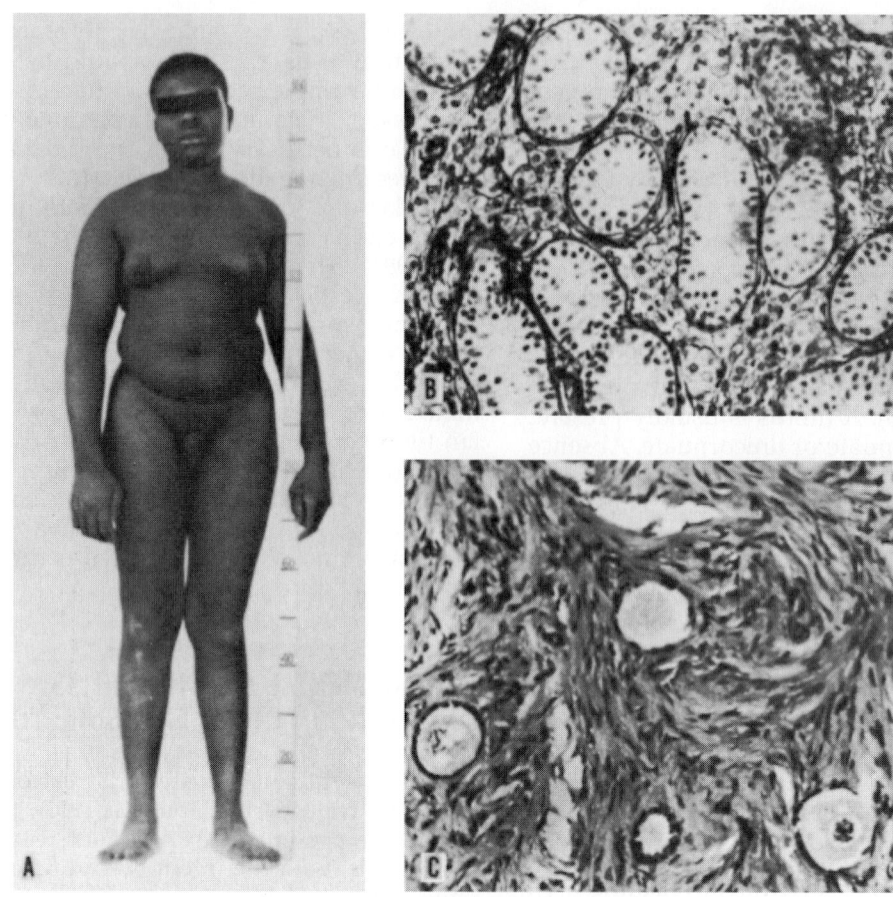

Figure 8–28

A, A 17-year-old true hermaphrodite with bilateral scrotal ovotestes and an XX sex chromosome constitution in cultures of peripheral blood and skin, a perineal hypospadias (partially repaired in photograph), moderate bilateral gynecomastia and pubic hair (recently shaved in picture), sparse axillary hair, a high-pitched voice, and absent facial hair. Height 66 inches. Urinary 17-ketosteroid 1.3 mg/day; urinary gonadotropin >10 mU, <80 mU/day. At operation a male type of urethra, bilateral scrotal fallopian tubes and ovotestes, and rudimentary bicornuate uterus and vagina attached to the posterior urethra were present.

B and *C*, Photomicrographs showing histopathology of demarcated ovarian and testicular portion of one ovotestis. *B*, Immature seminiferous tubules lined with Sertoli cells and spermatogonia and Leydig cells. *C*, Ova and follicles.

(From Grumbach MM, Barr ML: Cytologic tests of chromosomal sex in relation to sexual anomalies in man. Recent Prog Horm Res 1958;14:255, with permission.)

years old. Because adenosis is glandular and produces mucus, some affected women may have a discharge that is often mistaken for infection. This discharge does not need treatment and will lessen as the adenosis recedes.

Some DES-exposed women have demonstrable structural changes of the genital tract. Most of these changes are benign and of no clinical significance. In some DES daughters, the vagina and cervix exhibit structural changes such as a cervical "collar" or "hood" or "cocks comb." This "hood" is an extra ridge of cervical tissue that many DES daughters have. It is benign and may disappear over time. Sometimes a woman with a cervical hood may find it difficult to use a diaphragm.

Whether DES exposure in utero increases the risk of cervical or vaginal dysplasia, which may develop into squamous cell cancer, is controversial. Although initial data seemed to show no relationship between DES exposure and dysplasia, a 1984 study from the DESAD project indicated that DES exposure doubles the risk of dysplasia and of carcinoma in situ of the cervix or vagina (Robboy et al, 1984). At this time, however, it is unclear whether DES-exposed women are at an increased risk for the development of squamous cell carcinoma of the vagina and cervix. The theoretical risk of a large metaplastic T-zone requires a careful follow-up, consisting of visual inspection, digital palpation, cytology, and, when necessary, iodine staining and colposcopic evaluation. The examining physician should biopsy all atypical areas.

Clear cell adenocarcinomas are rare and occur most often in patients less than 30 years of age who have a history of in utero exposure to DES. The risk of vaginal adenocarcinoma in DES-exposed daughters increases rapidly from the onset of puberty until the early 20s. Subsequently, the risk drops dramatically, although a few cases occur in women in their 30s and 40s. It is estimated that from 1 in 1000 to 1 in 10,000 DES-exposed women will develop clear cell adenocarcinoma of the vagina and/or cervix attributable to their exposure. While some DES daughters have had both adenosis and clear cell adenocarcinoma, a progression from adenosis to cancer has not generally been seen. Boyd et al (1996) have postulated that DES exposure induces genomic instability that may later lead to the development of cancer. They have demonstrated microsatellite instability in all DES-associated tumors examined.

Researchers have documented developmental abnormalities of the upper genital tract in both male and female offspring. Congenital malformations of the genitalia have been reported three times as often by DES-exposed men as by nonexposed individuals. Nonetheless, these men were as fertile as other men. Furthermore, DES-exposed men reported no impairment of sexual function (Wilcox et al, 1995a). In females, the most common uterine abnormality is a malformed or "T"-shaped uterus, which is diagnosed by hysterosalpingogram, usually as part of an infertility evaluation.

Follow-up studies have found an increased incidence of infertility in DES-exposed daughters. DES-exposed women may also be at an increased risk for ectopic pregnancy. Estimates derived from the follow-up cohort studies suggest that ectopic pregnancy occurs in about 5.6% of pregnancies in DES-exposed women (Barnes et al, 1980). Fertility and pregnancy outcome may be adversely affected by the presence of uterine structural abnormalities. Fertility rates are lower for patients with structural abnormalities when compared with DES-exposed women with a normal hysterosalpingogram (4% and 44%, respectively) (Berger and Alper, 1986). In vitro fertilization data indicate that implantation rates are lower in women with structural abnormalities (Karande et al, 1990).

In DES-exposed women without gross genital tract abnormalities, rates of early pregnancy loss, premature labor, and premature rupture of membranes are similar to those in the general population. However, the overall risk of preterm delivery is two to three times greater in DES-exposed women with structural uterine abnormalities. Preterm labor monitoring is indicated for all DES-exposed women. Prophylactic cerclage should be considered in patients with cervical incompetence, patients who had a large cone biopsy, or patients with a grossly abnormal cervix. However, in one study, cervical incompetence was an infrequent cause of pregnancy loss even in patients with uterine abnormalities (Levine and Berkowitz, 1993).

The risk of breast cancer in women exposed to DES has also been controversial, but the weight of evidence favors an increased risk that appears 20 or more years after exposure and slowly rises to around two times normal. One study found the relative risk of breast cancer associated with DES exposure, after adjustment for demographic and reproductive variables, to be 1.35 (95% confidence interval, 1.05 to 1.74). For 30 years or more following exposure, the relative risk was not appreciably higher (1.33; 95% confidence interval, 0.95 to 1.87) than that in earlier periods (Colton et al, 1993).

Animal experiments have suggested that in utero exposure to DES may induce changes in the immune system, but these possible effects have not been well studied in humans, and their clinical significance, if any, is not known. A more recent study found that DES-exposed men and women reported rates of allergy, infection, and autoimmune diseases similar to those of unexposed individuals (Baird et al, 1996). Some investigators found a higher incidence of left-handedness among DES-exposed subjects than among controls. They concluded that intrauterine exposure to DES may have disturbed the normal process of cerebral lateralization (Scheirs and Vingerhoets, 1995). Although some studies reported an increased prevalence of abnormal uterine bleeding among DES-exposed women, the age at menarche and age at menopause were unaffected by the woman's prenatal DES exposure (Hornsby et al, 1995; Wilcox et al, 1995b). In a prospective cohort study of 198 DES-exposed women and 162 unexposed controls, Hornsby et al (1994) found that DES exposure was associated with a statistically significantly decreased duration of menstrual bleeding of approximately one-half day and a lower average daily bleeding score (self-reported). Cycle length, variability of cycle length, and symptoms of dysmenorrhea were unaffected. The authors postulated that the decreased duration and amount of menstrual bleeding among DES-exposed women was due to uterine structural changes rather than alterations in the endocrine function (Hornsby et al, 1994).

Most DES-exposed daughters are now in their early 40s. They are thus just now entering the at-risk age range for most of the hormone-related tumors (breast, ovary, endometrium). It is also unclear whether the risk of vaginal clear cell adenocarcinoma will again increase as exposed daughters approach the age at which this cancer has been most common in the unexposed population. DeMars et al (1995) reported two cases of non–clear cell mucinous adenocarcinoma in older women having a history of in utero DES exposure. In addition, the risk of cervical disease remains an open question, until new long-term follow-up data become available.

REFERENCES

Aaronson IA: True hermaphroditism: a review of 41 cases with observations on testicular histology and function. Br J Urol 1985;57:775.

Abbas N, NcElreavey K, Leconiat M, et al: Familial case of 46,XX male and 46,XX true hermaphrodite associated with a paternal-derived SRY-bearing X chromosome. C R Acad Sci III 1993;316:375.

Aittomaki K: The genetics of XX gonadal dysgenesis. Am J Hum Genet 1994;54:844.

Alessandrescu D, Peltecu GC, Buhimschi CS, Buhimschi IA: Neocolpopoiesis with split-thickness skin graft as a surgical treatment of vaginal agenesis: retrospective review of 201 cases. Am J Obstet Gynecol 1996;175:131.

Ammini AC, Pandey J, Vijyaraghavan M, Sabherwal U: Human female phenotypic development: role of fetal ovaries. J Clin Endocrinol Metab 1994;79:604.

Andersson S, Berman DM, Jenkins EP, Russell DW: Deletion of steroid 5 alpha-reductase 2 gene in male. Nature 1991;354:159.

Aran O, Galatzer A, Kauli R, et al: Social, educational and vocational status of 48 young adult females with gonadal dysgenesis. Clin Endocrinol 1992;36:405.

Arici A, Kutteh WH, Chantilis SJ, et al: Laparoscopic removal of gonads in women with abnormal karyotypes. J Reprod Med 1993;38:521.

Bailez MM, Gearhart JP, Migeon C, Rock J: Vaginal reconstruction after initial construction of the external genitalia in girls with salt-wasting adrenal hyperplasia. J Urol 1992;148(2 Pt 2):680.

Baird DD, Wilcox AJ, Herbst AL: Self-reported allergy, infection, and autoimmune diseases among men and women exposed in utero to diethylstilbestrol. J Clin Epidemiol 1996;49:263.

Barnes AB, Colton T, Gundersen J, et al: Fertility and outcome of pregnancy in women exposed in utero to diethylstilbestrol. N Engl J Med 1980;302:609.

Batch AJ, Davies HR, Evans BA, et al: Phenotypic variation and detection of carrier status in the partial androgen insensitivity syndrome. Arch Dis Child 1993;68:453.

Batzer FR, Corson SL, Gocial B, et al: Genetic offspring in patients with vaginal agenesis: specific medical and legal issues. Am J Obstet Gynecol 1992;167:1288.

Berger M, Alper M: Intractable primary infertility in women exposed to diethylstilbestrol in utero. J Reprod Med 1986;31:231.

Berkovitz GD, Fechner PY, Zacur HW, et al: Clinical and pathologic spectrum of 46,XY gonadal dysgenesis: its relevance to the understanding of sex differentiation. Medicine (Baltimore) 1991;70:375.

Bianco S, Agrifoglio V, Mannino F, et al: Successful pregnancy in a pure gonadal dysgenesis with karyotype 46,XY patient (Swyer's syndrome) following oocyte donation and hormonal treatment. Acta Eur Fertil 1992;23:37.

Bosze P, Szamel I, Molnar F, Laszlo J: Nonneoplastic gonadal testosterone secretion as a cause of vaginal cell maturation in streak gonad syndrome. Gynecol Obstet Invest 1986;22:153.

Bourguignon JP, Franchimont P, Ernould C, Geubelle F: Delayed puberty: from pathophysiology to therapy. In Venturoli S, Flanigni G, Givens JR (eds): Adolescence in Females. Chicago: Year Book Medical Publishers, 1985:389.

Boyd J, Takahashi H, Waggoner SE, et al: Molecular genetic analysis of clear cell adenocarcinomas of the vagina and cervix associated and unassociated with diethylstilbestrol exposure in utero. Cancer 1996;77:507.

Cabrol S, Saab C, Gourmelen M, et al: Turner syndrome: spontaneous growth of stature, weight increase and accelerated bone maturation. Arch Pediatr 1996;3:313.

Christakos AC, Simpson JL, Younger JB, Christian CD: Gonadal dysgenesis as an autosomal recessive condition. Am J Obstet Gynecol 1969;104:1027.

Cohen A, Kauli R, Pertzelan A, et al: Final height of girls with Turner's syndrome: correlation with karyotype and parental height. Acta Paediatr 1995;84:550.

Colton T, Greenberg ER, Noller K, et al: Breast cancer in mothers prescribed diethylstilbestrol in pregnancy: further follow-up. JAMA 1993;269:2096.

Cremers CW, Strubbe EH, Willemsen WN: Stapedial ankylosis in the Mayer-Rokitansky-Kuster-Hauser syndrome. Arch Otolaryngol Head Neck Surg 1995;121:800.

Cutler GB Jr, Laue L: Congenital adrenal hyperplasia due to 21-hydroxylase deficiency. N Engl J Med 1990;323:1806.

de Grouchy J, Gompel A, Salmon-Bernard Y: Embryonic testicular regression syndrome and severe mental retardation in sibs. Ann Genet 1985;28:154.

De-Bellis A, Quigley CA, Marschke KB, et al: Characterization of mutant androgen receptors causing partial androgen insensitivity syndrome. J Clin Endocrinol Metab 1994;78:513.

DeMars LR, Van-Le L, Huang I, Fowler WC: Primary non-clear-cell adenocarcinomas of the vagina in older DES-exposed women. Gynecol Oncol 1995;58:389.

Dewhurst CJ: Congenital malformations of the lower genital tract. Clin Obstet Gynecol 1978a;5:250.

Dewhurst CJ: Congenital malformations of the lower urinary tract. Clin Obstet Gynecol 1978b;5:520.

Dewhurst CJ, Chapman M, Muram D, Donnison B: 5 Alpha reductase deficiency in 46 XY sisters. Pediatr Adolesc Gynecol 1983;1:85.

Dewhurst Sir J: Fertility in 47,XXX and 45,X patients. J Med Genet 1978c;15:132.

Dewhurst Sir J: Female Puberty and Its Abnormalities. Edinburgh: Churchill Livingston, 1984.

Donahoe PK, Gustafson ML: Early one-stage surgical reconstruction of the extremely high vagina in patients with congenital adrenal hyperplasia. J Pediatr Surg 1994;29:352.

Edmonds KD: Sexual development anomalies and their reconstruction: upper and lower tracts. In Sanfilippo J, Muram D, Lee P, Dewhurst JC (eds): Pediatric and Adolescent Gynecology. Philadelphia: WB Saunders Company, 1994:535.

Falk HC, Hyman AB: Congenital absence of the clitoris: a case report. Obstet Gynecol 1971;38:269.

Fedele L, Busacca M, Candiani M, Vignali M: Laparoscopic creation of a neovagina in Mayer-Rokitansky-Kuster-Hauser syndrome by modification of Vecchietti's operation. Am J Obstet Gynecol 1994;171:268.

Flack CE, Barraza MA, Stevens PS: Vaginoplasty: combination therapy using labia minora flaps and Lucite dilators—preliminary report. J Urol 1993;150(2 Pt 2):654.

Fraccaro M, Tiepolo L, Zuffardio-Chiumello G, et al: Familial XX true hermaphroditism and H-Y antigen. Hum Genet 1979;48:45.

Frank R: Formation of artificial vagina without operation. Am J Obstet Gynecol 1938;35:1053.

Freundt I, Toolenaar TA, Jeekel H, et al: Prolapse of the sigmoid neovagina: report of three cases. Obstet Gynecol 1994;83(5 Pt 2):876.

Giraldo F, Solano A, Mora MJ, et al: The Malaga flap for vaginoplasty in the Mayer-Rokitansky-Kuster-Hauser syndrome: experience and early-term results. Plast Reconstr Surg 1996;98:305.

Gourlay WA, Johnson HW, Pantzar JT, et al: Gonadal tumors in disorders of sexual differentiation. Urology 1994;43:537.

Grant DB, Laurance BM, Atherden SL, et al: hCG stimulation test in children with abnormal sexual development. Arch Dis Child 1976;51:596.

Greene S, Zachmann M, Manella B, et al: Comparison of two tests to recognize or exclude 5 alpha-reductase deficiency in prepubertal children. Acta Endocrinol (Copenhagen) 1987;114:113.

Griffin JE, Edwards C, Madden JD, et al: Congenital absence of the vagina: the Mayer-Rokitansky-Kuster-Hauser syndrome. Ann Intern Med 1976;85:224.

Grumbach MM, Conte FA: Disorders of sexual differentiation. In Wilson JD, Foster DW (eds): Williams Textbook of Endocrinology. 7th ed. Philadelphia: WB Saunders Company, 1985:312.

Grumbach MM, Ducharme JR: The effects of androgens on fetal sexual development: androgen-induced female pseudohermaphroditism. Fertil Steril 1960;11:157.

Herbst AL, Kurman RJ, Scully RE: Vaginal and cervical abnormalities after exposure to stilbestrol in utero. Obstet Gynecol 1972;40:287.

Herbst AL, Robboy SJ, Scully RE, et al: Clear cell adenocarcinoma of the vagina and cervix in girls: analysis of 170 registry cases. Am J Obstet Gynecol 1974;119:713.

Herbst AL, Ulfelder H, Poscanzer DC: Adenocarcinoma of the vagina: association of maternal stilbestrol therapy with tumor appearance in young women. N Engl J Med 1971;284:878.

Hintz RL: New approaches to growth failure to Turner syndrome. Adolesc Pediatr Gynecol 1989;2:172.

Hornsby PP, Wilcox AJ, Herbst AL: Onset of menopause in women exposed to diethylstilbestrol in utero. Am J Obstet Gynecol 1995;172:92.

Hornsby PP, Wilcox AJ, Weinberg CR, Herbst AL: Effects on the menstrual cycle of in utero exposure to diethylstilbestrol. Am J Obstet Gynecol 1994;170:709.

Huffman JW, Dewhurst CJ, Capraro VJ: The Gynecology of Childhood and Adolescence. 2nd ed. Philadelphia: WB Saunders Company, 1981.

Imperato-McGinley J, Gautier T, Pichardo M, Shackleton C: The diagnosis of 5 alpha-reductase deficiency in infancy. J Clin Endocrinol Metab 1986;63:1313.

Imperato-McGinley J, Guerrero L, Gauiter T, Peterson RE: Steroid 5a-reductase deficiency: an inherited form of male pseudohermaphroditism. Science 1974;186:1213.

Ingram JM: The bicycle seat stool in the treatment of vaginal agenesis and stenosis: a preliminary report. Am J Obstet Gynecol 1981;140:867.

Jirasek J: Principles of reproductive embryology. In Simpson JL (ed): Disorders of Sexual Differentiation. New York: Academic Press, 1976:51.

Jones HW Jr, Rock JA: Reparative and Constructive Surgery of the Female Genital Tract. Baltimore: Williams & Wilkins, 1983.

Jost A: Recherches sur la differenciation sexuelle de l'embryon de lapin II. Action des androgenes de synthese sur l'histogenese genitale. Arch Anat Microsc Morphol Exp 1947;36:242.

Kaneti J, Lieberman E, Moshe P, Carmie R: A case of ambiguous genitalia owing to neurofibromatosis—review of the literature. J Urol 1988;140:584.

Karande VC, Lester RG, Masher SJ, et al: Are implantation and pregnancy outcome impaired in diethylstilbestrol exposed women after in vitro fertilization and embryo transfer? Fertil Steril 1990;54:287.

Kirkland RT, Kirkland JL, Johnson CM, et al: Congenital lipoid adrenal hyperplasia in an eight-year-old phenotypic female. J Clin Endocrinol Metab 1973;56:488.

Krob G, Braun A, Kuhnle U: True hermaphroditism: geographical distribution, clinical findings, chromosomes and gonadal histology. Eur J Pediatr 1994;153:2.

Ladd WE, Gross RE: Congenital malformations of the anus and rectum: report of 162 cases. Am J Surg 1934;23:167.

Lee MM, Donahoe PK: Mullerian inhibiting substance: a gonadal hormone with multiple functions. Endocr Rev 1993;14:152.

Leibovitz Z, Levitan Z, Aharoni A, Sharf M: Cervical cerclage in uterine malformations. Int J Fertil 1992;37:214.

Letterie GS, Page DC: Dysgerminoma and gonadal dysgenesis in a 46,XX female with no evidence of Y chromosomal DNA. Gynecol Oncol 1995;57:423.

Levine RU, Berkowitz KM: Conservative management and pregnancy outcome in diethylstilbestrol-exposed women with and without gross genital tract abnormalities. Am J Obstet Gynecol 1993;169:1125.

Lister U: Double vulva. J Obstet Gynecol Br Emp 1953;60:552.

Marcantonio SM, Fechner PY, Migeon CJ, et al: Embryonic testicular regression sequence: a part of the clinical spectrum of 46,XY gonadal dysgenesis. Am J Med Genet 1994;49:1.

McDonough PG, Tho PT: The spectrum of 45,X/46,XY gonadal dysgenesis and its implications (a study of 19 patients). Pediatr Adolesc Gynecol 1983;1:1.

McIndoe AH, Banister JB: An operation for the cure of congenital absence of the vagina. J Obstet Gynaecol Br Emp 1938;45:490.

Mendez JP, Ulloa-Aguirre A, Kofman-Alfaro S, et al: Mixed gonadal dysgenesis: clinical cytogenetic, endocrinological, and histopathological findings in 16 patients. Am J Med Genet 1993;46:263.

Mendonca BB, Barbosa AS, Arnhold IJ, et al: Gonadal agenesis in XX and XY sisters: evidence for the involvement of an autosomal gene. Am J Med Genet 1994;52:39.

Meneses MF, Ostrowski ML: Female splenic-gonadal fusion of the discontinuous type. Human Pathol 1989;20:486.

Minowada S, Fukutani K, Hara M, et al: Childbirth in a true hermaphrodite. Eur Urol 1984;10:414.

Mobus V, Sachweh K, Knapstein PG, Kreienberg R: Women after surgically corrected vaginal aplasia: a follow-up of psychosexual rehabilitation. Geburtshilfe Frauenheilkd 1993;53:125.

Monaghan JM: Bonney's Gynecological Surgery. 9th ed. London: Bailliere Tindall, 1986:129.

Muram D, Dewhurst Sir J: The inheritance of intersexuality. Can Med Assoc J 1984;130:121.

Muram D, Pilgrim P: An association of uterine and gonadal anomalies. Adolesc Pediatr Gynecol 1988;1:51.

Muram D, Rau F: Anatomic variations of the bulbocavernosus muscle. Adolesc Pediatr Gynecol 1991;4:85.

Muram D, Rau FJ, Shell DH III: Modified Williams vulvovaginoplasty: the role of tissue expanders. Adolesc Pediatr Gynecol 1992;5:81.

Muram D, Spence JEH: Rupture of a rudimentary uterine horn in an adolescent girl, followed by a successful pregnancy. Pediatr Adolesc Gynecol 1983;1:53.

Newland RJ, Fusaro RM: Mucinous cysts of the vulva. Nebr Med J 1991;76:307.

Odame I, Donaldson MD, Wallace AM, et al: Early diagnosis and management of 5 alpha-reductase deficiency. Arch Dis Child 1992;67:720.

Ogata T, Matsuo N: Comparison of adult height between patients with XX and XY gonadal dysgenesis: support for a Y specific growth gene(s). J Med Genet 1992;29:539.

Park IJ, Jones HW Jr, Melham RE: Non-adrenal familial female pseudohermaphroditism. Am J Obstet Gynecol 1972;122:930.

Pinsky L, Kaufman M: Genetics of steroid receptors and their disorders. Adv Hum Genet 1987;16:299.

Pinsky L, Kaufman M, Levitsky LL: Partial androgen resistance due to a distinctive qualitative defect of the androgen receptor. Am J Med Genet 1987;27:459.

Pokorny S: Anatomic detail of the prepubertal hymen. Am J Obstet Gynecol 1987;157:950.

Raspa RW, Subramaniam AP, Romas NA: True hermaphroditism presents as intermittent hemituria and groin pain. Urology 1986;28:133.

Reindollar RH, Tho SPT, McFonough PG: Abnormalities of sexual differentiation. Clin Obstet Gynecol 1987;30:697.

Rey R, al-Attar L, Louis F, et al: Testicular dysgenesis does not affect expression of anti-mullerian hormone by Sertoli cells in premeiotic seminiferous tubules. Am J Pathol 1996;148:1689.

Robboy SJ, Noller KL, O'Brien P, et al: Increased incidence of cervical and vaginal dysplasia in 3,980 diethylstilbestrol-exposed young women: experience of the National Collaborative Diethylstilbestrol Adenosis Project. JAMA 1984;252:2979.

Robinson A, Lubs HA, Bergsma D (eds): Sex chromosome aneuploidy: prospective studies on children. Birth Defects 1979;15:1.

Rock JA, Azziz R: Genital anomalies in childhood. Clin Obstet Gynecol 1987;30:682.

Ross JL, Stefanatos G, Roeltgen D, et al: Ullrich-Turner syndrome: neurodevelopmental changes from childhood through adolescence. Am J Med Genet 1995;58:74.

Sarto GE, Opitz JM: The XY gonadal agenesis syndrome. J Med Genet 1973;10:288.

Sauer-Ramirez R, Carranza-Lira S, Romo-Aguirre C, et al: Modification of the Abbe-Wharton-McIndoe technique using regenerated oxidized cellulose instead of a skin graft. Ginecol Obstet Mex 1995;63:112.

Scheirs JG, Vingerhoets AJ: Handedness and other laterality indices in women prenatally exposed to DES. J Clin Exp Neuropsychol 1995;17:725.

Schmitt S, Knorr D, Schwarz HP, Kuhnle U: Gonadotropin regulation during puberty in complete androgen insensitivity syndrome with testicles in situ. Horm Res 1994;42:253.

Shibata T, Nonomura K, Kakizaki H, et al: A case of unique communication between blind-ending ectopic ureter and ipsilateral hemi-hematocolpometra in uterus didelphys. J Urol 1995;153:1208.

Simpson JL: Disorders of Sexual Differentiation: Etiology and Clinical Delineation. New York: Academic Press, 1976.

Simpson JL: True hermaphroditism: etiology and phenotypic considerations. Birth Defects 1978;14:(6C)9.

Simpson JL: Gonadal dysgenesis and sex chromosome abnormalities: phenotypic/karyotypic correlations. In Vallet HL, Porter IH (eds): Genetic Mechanisms of Sexual Development. New York: Academic Press, 1979:365.

Simpson JL: Genetic control of sexual development. In Ratnam SS, Teoh ES (eds): Proceedings of the 12th World Congress on Fertility and Sterility (Singapore, 1986). Lancaster, UK: Parthenon Press, 1987a:165.

Simpson JL: Phenotypic-karyotypic correlations of gonadal determinants: current status and relationship to molecular studies. In Sperling K, Vogel F (eds): Proceedings of the 7th International Congress on Human Genetics (Berlin, 1986). Heidelberg: Springer-Verlag, 1987b:224.

Simpson JL, Photopulos G: The relationship of neoplasia to disorders of abnormal sexual differentiation. Birth Defects 1976; 12(1):15.

Strubbe EH, Cremers CW, Dikkers FG, Willemsen WN: Hearing loss and the Mayer-Rokitansky-Kuster-Hauser syndrome. Am J Otol 1994;15:431.

Tar A, Solyom J, Gyorvari B, et al: Testicular development in an SRY-negative 46,XX individual harboring a distal Xp deletion. Hum Genet 1995;96:464.

Thigpen AE, Davis DL, Milatovich A, et al: Molecular genetics of steroid 5 alpha-reductase 2 deficiency. J Clin Invest 1992;90:799.

Ulloa-Aguirre A, Carranza-Lira S, Mendez JP, et al: Incomplete regression of Müllerian ducts in androgen insensitivity syndrome. Fertil Steril 1990;53:1024.

Ulrich U, Keckstein J, Buck G: Removal of gonads in Y-chromosome-bearing gonadal dysgenesis and in androgen insensitivity syndrome by laparoscopic surgery. Surg Endosc 1996;10:422.

Van Niekerk WA: True Hermaphroditism. New York: Harper and Row, 1974.

Van Niekerk WA, Retief AE: The gonads of human true hermaphrodites. Hum Genet 1981;58:117.

Verp MS, Harrison HH, Ober C, et al: Chimerism as the etiology of a 46,XX/46,XY fertile true hermaphrodite. Fertil Steril 1992; 57:346.

Verp MS, Simpson JL: Abnormal sexual differentiation and neoplasia. Cancer Genet Cytogenet 1987;25:191.

Wilcox AJ, Baird DD, Weinberg CR, et al: Fertility in men exposed prenatally to diethylstilbestrol. N Engl J Med 1995a;332:1411.

Wilcox AJ, Umbach DM, Hornsby PP, Herbst AL: Age at menarche among diethylstilbestrol granddaughters. Am J Obstet Gynecol 1995b;173:835.

Wilkens L: Masculinization of female fetus due to use of orally given progestins. JAMA 1960;172:1028.

Williams EA: Congenital absence of the vagina: a simple operation for its relief. J Obstet Gynaecol Br Commonw 1964;71:511.

Winderl LM, Silverman RK: Prenatal diagnosis of congenital imperforate hymen. Obstet Gynecol 1995;85(5 Pt 2):857.

Yu TJ, Shu K, Kung FT, et al: Use of laparoscopy in intersex patients. J Urol 1995;154:1193.

9

Habitual Abortion

Salim Daya

DEFINITION AND EPIDEMIOLOGY

The term *abortion* is used to describe a pregnancy that terminates with death and expulsion of an embryo or fetus. The generally accepted definition used by the World Health Organization (1977) is the expulsion or extraction from its mother of a fetus or embryo weighing 500 g or less. This stage of fetal development is attained at approximately 20 weeks' gestation. Consequently, in North America a spontaneous abortion describes a pregnancy loss occurring up to 20 weeks' gestation.

INCIDENCE OF SPONTANEOUS ABORTION

The frequency of clinically recognized spontaneous abortion in the general population has been estimated to range between 10% and 15%, making it the most frequent complication of pregnancy (Warburton and Strobino, 1987) (Table 9–1). The actual rate may be higher because women may undergo complete abortion at home and not require further treatment. Consequently, epidemiologic studies involving hospital populations are likely to underestimate the incidence owing to the likelihood of underrepresentation of early abortions.

Studies attempting to determine the incidence of spontaneous abortion should not focus only on hospital patients but should include a representative sample of the population. Also, they should be prospective in design so that women can be identified early, preferably before they conceive. In one study, in which women contemplating pregnancy were recruited by radio and poster appeal and monitored during the pregnance, the overall spontaneous abortion rate among 407 pregnancies was 12.3% (Regan et al, 1989). Higher rates were observed in two older studies with larger sample sizes. In the carefully conducted field study on the island of Kauai, where over 3000 pregnancies were monitored from as early as possible (half of them before 12 weeks' gestation) until the end of the pregnancy, the overall rate of fetal loss between 4 and 20 weeks' gestation was 23.6% (French and Bierman, 1962). Similarly, using data from a well-defined segment of the population of New York City, the loss rate in pregnancies less than 20 weeks' gestation was found to be 21.6% (Shapiro et al, 1971).

In addition to the high loss rate for clinical pregnancies, it has been estimated, by using sensitive human chorionic gonadotropin (hCG) assays, that significant early fetal loss occurs soon after implantation and therefore may be unrecognized (i.e., occult abortion) (Miller et al, 1980; Edmonds et al, 1982). Edmonds et al (1982) measured hCG in alternate-day urine samples provided during the second half of the luteal phase and found that 61.9% of all aborted conceptuses were lost before 12 weeks' gestation. Furthermore, 91.7% of these losses occurred subclinically. Similarly, Wilcox et al (1988), using a more sensitive assay and more stringent criteria for defining the presence of pregnancy, reported a spontaneous abortion rate of 31%, with 69.3% of the losses occurring subclinically.

RECURRENCE RISKS OF SPONTANEOUS ABORTION

There have been several attempts to calculate the likelihood of a pregnancy proceeding to term when preceding pregnancies have terminated in spontaneous abortion. The initial estimates have been based on the assumption that the overall abortion rate consists of the sum of two independent rates, one resulting from a random factor and the other from a recurrent factor in abortion sequences. Using this assumption, Malpas (1938) calculated spontaneous abortion rates for subsequent pregnancies based on the number of previous abortions. The figures obtained were 22% after one abortion, 38% after two abortions, and 73% after three abortions. Eastman (1946) assumed that 10% of pregnancies abort sporadically and the recurrent factor causes 0.4% to abort repeatedly. Thus, following 100,000 hypothetical women through successful pregnancies, he obtained spontaneous abortion rate estimates of 13%, 37%, and 84% for one, two, and three previous spontaneous abortions, respectively. Assuming the validity of these two sets of calculations, the chance of a fourth pregnancy going to term is considerably less than that of a third pregnancy. This assumption formed the basis of the definition of *habitual abortion* to represent three consecutive spontaneous abor-

Table 9-1. PROBABILITY OF SPONTANEOUS ABORTION IN RELATION TO NUMBER OF PREVIOUS ABORTIONS*

STUDY	NUMBER OF PREVIOUS SPONTANEOUS ABORTIONS			
	0	1	2	3+
Retrospective Studies				
Stevenson et al (1959)	8.1	14.0		
Warburton and Fraser (1964)	12.3	26.2	32.2	30.2
Leridon (1976)	15.2	22.0	35.3	
Poland et al (1977)		19.0	35.0	47.0
Naylor and Warburton (1979)	13.5	23.7	25.2	40.4
Cohort Studies				
Shapiro et al (1971)	10.9	18.8		
Awan (1974)	10.4	22.1	27.4	
Prospective Studies				
Boue et al (1975a)		14.0		23.8
Lauritsen (1976)		14.2		32.5
Harger et al (1983)			16.7	30.0
Fitzsimmons et al (1983)			31.3	45.7
Regan (1988)	5.6	11.5	29.4	36.4

*Probability figures are expressed as percentages.

tions. This concept was further reinforced by a New York study of women with abortion in which women experiencing habitual abortion could be distinguished from those who experienced a single, sporadic abortion, supporting the view that habitual abortion is a valid clinical entity (Strobino et al, 1980). Women with this disorder are more likely to have chromosomally normal abortuses, have a tendency to abort later in gestation than sporadic aborters, are more likely to have previous preterm deliveries, and tend to take a longer time to become pregnant. Thus women with habitual abortion experience a well-defined clinical entity that is different from sporadic abortion.

For many years, the mathematical estimates of abortion rate were used as control rates against which the efficacy of various therapeutic regimens introduced to prevent spontaneous abortion in women threatening to abort were assessed. The reliability of these rates was challenged after evidence from a number of clinical studies suggested that the spontaneous abortion rate after three successive abortions was substantially lower than had been predicted by the earlier models (Schoeneck, 1953; Speert, 1954; Goldzieher and Benigno, 1958; Warburton and Fraser, 1959). Subsequently, data on recurrence risks for spontaneous abortion were obtained from studies ranging from retrospectively collected reproductive histories ascertained through a live-born child to prospectively collected histories ascertained through a first-trimester spontaneous abortion that had undergone karyotypic analysis (Warburton and Fraser, 1964; Boue et al, 1975b; Lauritsen, 1976). Naylor and Warburton (1979) used data from more than 14,000 reproductive histories, taking into consideration both the number of previous abortions and the sequences of abortions and live births,

in obtaining their figures for the risk of abortion (Tables 9–1 and 9–2). However, retrospective studies are often biased because they rely on factual recall by subjects whose responses may inaccurately represent the true facts. Several prospective studies have been carried out (Table 9–1) but have not included primigravidae, or women enrolled before conception. In contrast, the study by Regan (1988) was designed as a prognosis study to establish the risks of recurrent spontaneous abortion in women recruited before conception. In this report, information was available on 223 intrauterine pregnancies out of a total of 456 women enrolled into the study. Although the sample size for this report is relatively small, there were several interesting observations. In keeping with the findings of others, women with previous abortions were at greater risk of abortion in the current pregnancy (18.2%) than were primigravidae (5.6%). Also, in women who previously had only experienced abortions, there was a cumulatively higher chance that the current pregnancy would end in abortion when their past history recorded one (11.5%), two (29.4%), or three abortions (36.4%) (Table 9–1).

Despite the varied methods of ascertainment, the results of all these studies are remarkably consistent in finding an increasing risk of abortion as the number of previous abortions increases. Overall, women with habitual abortion have an approximately 40% risk of having a subsequent abortion.

INCIDENCE OF HABITUAL ABORTION

Accurate information on the incidence of habitual abortion is not yet available because population studies using random samples have not been carried

Table 9-2. SPONTANEOUS ABORTION
RISK IN RELATION TO PREVIOUS
PREGNANCY HISTORY

PREVIOUS HISTORY*	SPONTANEOUS ABORTION RISK (%)
O	12.7
OO	14.5
OOO	14.5
OOOO	13.1
X	22.8
XX	28.6
XXX	33.3
XXXX	33.3
XO	19.1
OX	27.5
XOO	20.2
OXO	23.0
OOX	29.1
XXO	35.6
XOX	18.4
OXX	27.4
XOOO	19.0
OXOO	18.5
OOXO	25.5
OOOX	34.0
XXOO	20.0
XOXO	26.3
XOOX	21.7
OXXO	22.2
OXOX	15.2
OOXX	40.8
XXXO	33.3
XXOX	33.3
XOXX	50.0
OXXX	66.7

*O, live births; X, spontaneous abortion.
Modifed from Naylor AF, Warburton D: Sequential analysis of spontaneous abortion. II. Collaborative study data show that gravidity determines a very substantial rise in risk. Fertil Steril 1979;31:282, with permission.

out. Most of the figures presently available have been derived from studies of patients attending antenatal clinics, in which the incidence of habitual abortion varied from 0.1% to 0.5% (Bishop, 1937; Javert, 1948). Assuming that each pregnancy has a 15% risk of spontaneous abortion, then one can calculate the probability of abortion in three successive pregnancies to be 0.34%, a figure that is similar to that observed in the antenatal clinics. However, based on more recent data, these figures appear to be underestimates. Data from the U.S. Department of Health and Human Services using national statistics reported that 3% of couples in the United States experience three spontaneous abortions (National Center for Health Statistics, 1982). Similarly, in the prospective follow-up study of Regan et al (1989), 4.6% of women enrolled were classified as having habitual abortion. Collectively, these observations provide an estimate for the incidence of habitual abortions as affecting 3% to 5% of couples in the reproductive age.

EFFECT OF GRAVIDITY AND AGE

Abortion-prone women have more pregnancies than successful reproducers and have their pregnancies at a later age (James, 1963). Thus the apparent relationship between gravidity and abortion may be the result of reproductive compensation. However, data from questionnaires administered to 2917 female doctors show a low incidence of abortion in the first two pregnancies and, thereafter, a steadily rising rate with increasing pregnancy order (Roman et al, 1980). Therefore, factors other than reproductive compensation may be operative. Because gravidity is closely related to age, it is possible that the increased risk of spontaneous abortion with gravidity, in part, can be ascribed to the effect of maternal age, particularly in view of the fact that chromosomal anomalies and other complications are associated with advancing maternal age. Thus the association of spontaneous abortion with maternal age may be explained by two separate and independent causes. It is well established that the risk of spontaneous abortion resulting from trisomic conceptuses increases with maternal age, especially after age 35. However, even with euploid conceptuses, the risk of abortion increases dramatically after age 35, thereby implicating an adverse maternal environment in the etiology of the abortion (Stein et al, 1980) (Fig. 9-1). Thus age and gravidity are related to abortion in a complex way.

The quality of previous pregnancies, rather than the quantity, also appears to influence the abortion risk. Gravidity includes widely differing obstetric outcomes ranging from only normal term pregnancies to only abortions. It is clear from epidemiologic studies that the risk of abortion does not change with gravidity only after live births, but the abortion risk is significantly increased if the previous pregnancy ended in abortion (Table 9-2). In the prospective study by Regan et al (1989), women whose last pregnancy had ended in abortion had a 19% chance of undergoing abortion in the study pregnancy, a significantly higher risk than in primigravidae (5%), in women whose pregnancies had all been successful (4%), and in women whose last pregnancy had been successful (5%) (Table 9-3). The greatest risk of abortion (24%) occurred in women whose obstetric histories contained only abortions.

CONCEPTION DELAY AND RECURRENT ABORTION

Women with recurrent abortion are significantly more likely than those with sporadic abortion to have a longer interpregnancy conception interval (i.e., length of time taken for conception to occur in women attempting pregnancy) (Strobino et al, 1980; Fitzsimmons et al, 1983). Approximately 51% of women with habitual abortion had unprotected intercourse for over a year before conceiving, compared with 35.6% of women with sporadic abortion

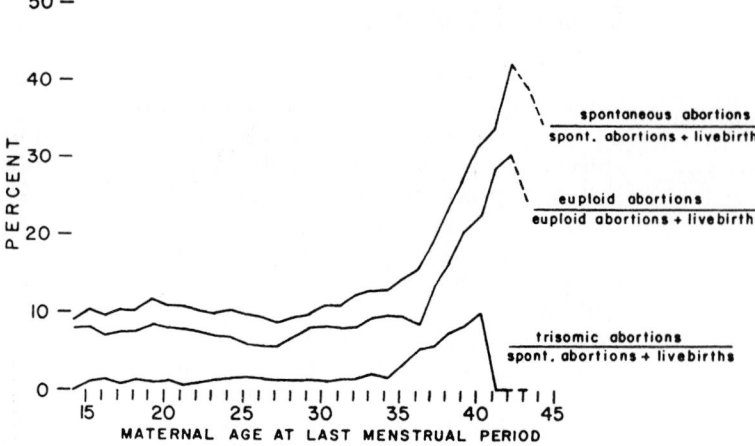

*Curves were smoothed by estimating rates at each maternal age using the number of events observed at each age and the two adjacent ages
– – – – = Denominator less than 25

Figure 9-1
Estimated rates (%) of spontaneous abortion, euploid abortion, and trisomic abortion by maternal age for private and public patients combined. (From Stein A, Kline J, Susser E, et al: Maternal age and spontaneous abortion. In Porter IH, Hook EB [eds]: Human Embryonic and Fetal Death. New York: Academic Press, 1980:107, with permission.)

(Strobino et al, 1980). The pathologic mechanism for this observation is not clear, although several hypotheses can be offered. One possibility is that women are afraid that their subsequent pregnancies will also be unsuccessful and the resulting stress may adversely influence the hypothalamus, resulting in subtle ovulatory disturbances.

ETIOLOGY OF HABITUAL ABORTION

Many factors have been suggested to have a role in the etiology of habitual abortion. Some of these are well established, whereas others are supported only by anecdotal evidence.

Genetic Factors

Successful chromosomal analysis of abortus material was first reported by Penrose and Delhanty in 1961,

Table 9-3. EFFECT OF PREVIOUS REPRODUCTIVE HISTORY ON RISK OF SPONTANEOUS ABORTION IN STUDY PREGNANCY

HISTORY	% RISK OF ABORTION
Last pregnancy aborted	19
Only abortions in the past	24
Only pregnancy aborted	20
Last pregnancy successful	5
All pregnancies successful	4
Only pregnancy successful	5
Previous termination of pregnancy	6
Primigravidae	5

Modified from Regan L, Braude PR, Tembath PL: Influence of past reproductive performance on risk of spontaneous abortion. BMJ 1989;299:541, with permission.

demonstrating triploid cells in two abortions. Thereafter, the results of cytogenetic analyses in patients with a history of two or more spontaneous abortions were reported (Schmid, 1962). This was followed by numerous studies, including a survey that established that chromosomal anomalies are a major cause of spontaneous abortion (Carr, 1967). The development of banding techniques using differential staining of chromosomes permitted a much more detailed identification of these anomalies. However, despite these developments, studies of abortus material are difficult to carry out because fetal or embryonic parts may have been expelled before a dilatation and curettage (D&C) procedure was performed, leaving only decidua for examination. Frequently, the material is unsuitable for cytogenetic preparation or may inadvertently have been fixed in preservative for histologic examination, making culture and karyotyping impossible. Also, fetal cells may not grow in culture or may be contaminated by maternal cells, thereby making evaluation difficult. Finally, because spontaneous abortions occurring early in pregnancy are less likely to require medical attention, later abortions will be overrepresented, especially in those cases where chromosome analysis is possible.

Prevalence of Chromosomal Anomalies

Early studies that demonstrated that only 20% of spontaneous abortions were the result of chromosomal anomalies were later challenged by larger studies in which anomalies were found in up to 61% of karyotyped products of conception (Boue et al, 1975b). The average proportion of anomalies calculated from a pooled data set of more than 6000 karyotyped abortuses from nine large surveys, each studying more than 200 abortuses, was 43%, with a range of 22% to 61% (Table 9-4). The principal factor influencing the proportion of chromosomal abnormalities is the gestational age distribution of the abortuses studied (Table 9-5). Apart from the lower

Table 9-4. PREVALENCE OF CHROMOSOME ANOMALIES IN SPONTANEOUS ABORTIONS

STUDY	LOCATION	NO. KARYOTYPED	NO. ABNORMAL (%)
Carr (1967)	London, Canada	227	50 (22)
Dhadial et al (1970)	London, UK	547	128 (23)
Boue et al (1975b)	Paris	1498	921 (61)
Creasy et al (1976)	London, UK	986	289 (29)
Takahara et al (1977)	Hiroshima	505	237 (47)
Therkelsen et al (1973)	Åarhus, Denmark	254	139 (54)
Hassold et al (1980)	Honolulu	1000	463 (46)
Warburton et al (1980)	New York	967	312 (32)
Kajii et al (1980)	Geneva	402	215 (54)
TOTAL		6386	2754 (43)

Modified from Creasy R: The cytogenetics of spontaneous abortion in humans. In Beard RW, Sharp F (eds): Early Pregnancy Loss: Mechanisms and Treatment. London: Royal College of Obstetricians and Gynaecologists, 1988;293, with permission.

prevalence in very early pregnancy (probably a result of the small numbers sampled), the highest prevalence of anomalies is in the 8- to 15-week gestational age range and then decreases with increasing gestation. Hence the different distribution of gestational ages represented in each survey may account for the wide range in the proportion of abortuses with an abnormal karyotype observed in Table 9-4.

Based on such information, it is now generally accepted that the cause in the majority of early spontaneous abortions is a chromosomal abnormality in the conceptus. However, the figures quoted above must be viewed with caution because they represent only those products of conception that were successfully grown in culture, thereby enabling karyotypic analysis. A summary of large surveys revealed that only 37% of 4752 specimens received were successfully cultured; the majority of cultures failed because of absence, contamination, or autolysis of fetal tissue. After the introduction in 1985 of the chorion villus biopsy for prenatal diagnosis, the problem of low diagnostic yield was circumvented. Using this technique, well-preserved villus material could be obtained from women with fetal demise that had been

confirmed by ultrasonography prior to clinical evidence of pregnancy failure (Guerneri et al, 1987). When compared with the method of culturing abortus material, direct study of chorion villus biopsy samples demonstrated a much higher prevalence of chromosomal anomalies in first-trimester abortions (67.5% vs. 55.2%) (Geraedts, 1996). Interestingly, chorion villus biopsy assessment identified an additional abnormality (usually a mosaicism) in 7% of cases studied. In several studies, a lower prevalence of chromosomal anomalies was observed in abortuses from women with habitual abortion. When the previous reproductive histories were related to the karyotype of the index abortion, no difference in the rates of spontaneous abortion among women aborting chromosomally normal and abnormal conceptions was observed (Carr, 1967; Alberman et al, 1975). However, after controlling for the fact that mothers of chromosomally normal abortions tended to be much younger than the mothers of chromosomally abnormal abortions, it became evident that the previous abortion rate was higher when the index karyotype was normal (Alberman et al, 1975). Similarly, in two prospective studies (Warburton and Fraser, 1964; Boue et al, 1975a), a higher rate of subsequent abortion was observed in women with an abortion with a normal karyotype (Table 9-6), confirming the prediction that abortions with normal karyotypes are associated with a higher recurrence risk compared with abortions with an abnormal karyotype.

Recurrent Aneuploidy

The issue of whether the karyotype of one spontaneous abortion is predictive of the karyotype of a subsequent pregnancy loss was examined using a large data base of unselected material from New York City and Honolulu (Warburton et al, 1987). The study comprised 273 women who had had at least two abortions with karyotype analysis. The authors concluded that, after accounting for the effect of ma-

Table 9-5. CHROMOSOMAL ANOMALIES AND GESTATIONAL AGE AT SPONTANEOUS ABORTION

GESTATIONAL AGE (weeks)	NO. KARYOTYPED	NO. ABNORMAL (%)
≤7	217	60 (28)
8–11	1523	790 (52)
12–15	1838	886 (48)
16–19	694	218 (31)
20–23	453	72 (16)

Modified from Kline J, Stein Z: Epidemiology of chromosomal anomalies in spontaneous abortion: prevalence, manifestation and determinants. In Bennet MJ, Edmonds DK (eds): Spontaneous and Recurrent Abortion. Oxford: Blackwell Scientific, 1987;29, with permission.

Table 9–6. RECURRENCE RISK OF ABORTION AFTER A NORMAL OR ABNORMAL KARYOTYPE IN THE INDEX ABORTUS

| STUDY | CHROMOSOMAL STATUS OF INDEX ABORTION | |
	Normal (%)	Abnormal (%)
Boue et al (1975a)	20.8	12.9
Lauritsen (1976)	26.5	13.2

Table 9–7. DISTRIBUTION OF TYPES OF CHROMOSOMAL ANOMALIES IN ABORTUSES

ANOMALY	NUMBER	%
Autosomal trisomy	1209	51
Polyploidy	516	22
Monosomy (45,X)	453	19
Structural rearrangements	97	4
Others	83	4
TOTAL	2358	100

Modified from Huisjes HJ: Spontaneous abortion. Curr Rev Obstet Gynecol 1984;8:34, with permission.

ternal age, the risk of trisomy is not increased in a second abortion following a previous abortion with trisomy, or with any other abnormal karyotype. This finding is contrary to the previously held belief that, when the first abortion studied was trisomic, there is a 71% chance that the abortion in the next pregnancy would also be trisomic (Lippman-Hand, 1980). In contrast, the risk of a nontrisomic abnormal karyotype was increased after a previous abortion with a similar karyotype. Similarly, the risk of having a chromosomally normal abortion is significantly increased if the previous abortion also had a normal karotype.

The possibility that some couples with recurrent abortion may have a tendency for aneuploid conceptions was evaluated by genetic testing (Drugan et al, 1990). Genetic counseling and amniocentesis or chorion villus sampling were offered to 305 couples with a history of two or more pregnancy losses, normal parental karyotypes, and no known risk factor for aneuploidy. The rate of aneuploid conception was significantly higher in this low-risk group compared to controls. The risk observed was 1.6%, which is similar to the risk for a 40-year-old pregnant woman.

Types of Chromosomal Abnormality in Abortus Material

Numerical errors are the most frequent abnormality in abortuses, whereas structural rearrangements are relatively rare. In a review of eight publications from 1975 to 1980, the distribution of chromosome errors was noted to be similar; after combining the data, autosomal trisomy was found to be the most common abnormality, accounting for 51% of the total group (Table 9–7). Interestingly, autosomal monosomy is a very infrequent finding. The second most frequent abnormality was polyploidy (22%), of which 16% were the result of triploidy and approximately 6% were due to tetraploidy. The third most common abnormality was monosomy X(45,X), which was present in 19% of the total group. Structural rearrangement was observed in 4%, making it the smallest subgroup of abnormalities.

The percentage of abnormal karyotypes decreases after week 12 of gestation (Table 9–5). The data for gestational ages less than 8 weeks are conflicting, in that some studies show a very low prevalence of abnormal karyotypes and others show a very high prevalence. This discrepancy may be accounted for by the fact that the number of cases studied in very early pregnancy is small, mainly because many of these patients either do not require medical intervention or the amount of tissue obtained is insufficient for successful culture. Thus these figures must be viewed with caution. However, it is entirely possible that the cause of the spontaneous abortion in very early pregnancy is nongenetic, such as maternal immune rejection. This point is discussed later in this chapter.

Comparing the gestational age distributions for chromosomally abnormal abortions, it is evident that both monosomic and trisomic abortion show modal distributions: 69% of monosomy X abortions occur between 11 and 14 weeks' gestation, and 64% of trisomy abortions occur between 11 and 13 weeks' gestation (Kline and Stein, 1987). Triploid abortions show a more uniform distribution throughout the gestational age range of 7 to 18 weeks.

AUTOSOMAL TRISOMY

The most frequent trisomy is that of chromosome 16, which is found in almost one third of all trisomies (Table 9–8). Extra chromosomes 2, 7, 13, 14, 15, 21, and 22 each account for between 5% and 10% of trisomies, while extra chromosomes 5, 6, 11, 12, 17, and 19 each comprise less than 1% of all such abnormalities (Creasy, 1988). Some autosomal trisomies are more lethal to the conceptus, resulting in early developmental arrest and unrecognizable abortion (e.g. chromosomes 1, 5, 9, and 11) (Creasy et al, 1976). Other trisomies are less lethal in early pregnancy and may be seen in fetuses surviving to a later stage of pregnancy (e.g., chromosomes 13, 18, and 22).

Although paternal nondisjunction may be a causal mechanism (Huisjes, 1984), most trisomies occur as a result of nondisjunction of the chromosomes in the occyte during meiosis or mitosis. In meiosis, homologous chromosomes do not pass into separate cells during the first meiotic division, whereas in mitosis, homologous chromatids fail to pass into separate daughter cells.

Table 9-8. RELATIVE FREQUENCY OF AUTOSOMAL TRISOMY IDENTIFIED BY BANDING TECHNIQUES—SURVEY OF NINE STUDIES

CHROMOSOME	%	CHROMOSOME	%	CHROMOSOME	%
16	30.0	2	4.6	12	0.9
9	22.8	7	4.5	17	0.6
22	10.8	8	3.7	6	0.5
21	9.2	4	2.9	11	0.2
15	7.1	20	2.5	5	0.2
13	5.5	10	2.0	19	0.1
18	4.7	X	1.3	1	0
14	4.6	3	1.2	Y	0

Modified from Creasy R: The cytogenetics of spontaneous abortion in humans. In Beard RW, Sharp F (eds): Early Pregnancy Loss: Mechanisms and Treatment. London: Royal College of Obstetricians and Gynaecologists, 1988:293, with permission.

In trisomic abortuses, the placenta generally displays hypoplastic, avascular villi with large cytotrophoblastic stromal cells (Boue et al, 1976).

MONOSOMY

Among the monosomies, the most commonly encountered is monosomy X. In contrast, monosomy Y is believed to be lethal because it has never been found (Huisjes, 1984). Monosomy X is thought to be the consequence of nondisjunction during maternal meiosis, or the result of a loss of one paternal sex chromosome during early cleavage (Chandley, 1981). Autosomal monosomies are rarely found in abortuses because they probably lead to early developmental arrest.

POLYPLOIDY

This term refers to the presence in the cell nucleus of three or more multiples of a haploid number of chromosomes. Polyploid conceptuses rarely, if ever, survive. Among the different types of polyploidy, triploidy is more commonly seen than tetraploidy. Triploidy is the result of fertilization by one diploid sperm (diandry) or two different spermatozoa (dispermy). Also, it may be seen when the first or second polar body is not extruded by the oocyte (digyny). In the majority of cases, however, the cause is likely to be dispermy (Uchida and Freeman, 1985). The villi in early triploid abortions often show hydropic changes, but, in contrast to hydatidiform moles, the trophoblast is hypoplastic and the stroma is avascular and hypocellular. Tetraploidy, in contrast, is the result of failed embryo cleavage during the first mitotic division following fertilization (Kajii and Niikawa, 1977).

STRUCTURAL REARRANGEMENTS

Structural chromosomal rearrangements, such as translocation, deletion, inversion, and ring formation, may occur de novo during gametogenesis or may be inherited from a parent carrying a balanced translocation, which can be of the reciprocal or rob-

ertsonian types. Both modes of origin seem to occur with similar frequencies (Huisjes, 1984).

OTHER ABNORMALITIES

In a minority of abortuses, the chromosomal abnormalities found are mosaic, double trisomy, sex trisomy, or other rare abnormalities (Huisjes, 1984). Sex chromosome polysomy is relatively rare in abortuses but can result in successful pregnancy (e.g., Klinefelter's syndrome [47,XXY], phenotypically normal male [47,XYY], or phenotypically normal female [47,XXX]).

Types of Paternal Chromosomal Abnormality

Early case reports, together with information from animal studies, indicated that chromosomal translocation was causally related to spontaneous abortion. Subsequently, studies were conducted to estimate the prevalence of the disorder among couples who had experienced at least two spontaneous abortions. Sample sizes and ascertainment criteria for the studies varied considerably, as did the incidence (range 0% to 21.4%) of major chromosomal abnormalities detected in the couples (Tharapel et al, 1985).

A computerized data base, generated from 200 publications on cytogenetic studies, has been set up at the University of Quebec, Canada, in which information has been recorded from 22,199 couples (44,398 individuals) ascertained through repeated spontaneous abortions, with or without other pregnancy losses (e.g., stillbirth and malformed live births) (DeBraekeleer and Dao, 1990). The distribution of the major chromosomal abnormalities, which included robertsonian translocation, reciprocal translocation, inversion, sex chromosome aneuploidy, and supernumerary chromosomes, is shown in Table 9-9. The distribution of chromosomal abnormality according to the number of spontaneous abortions (one, two, and three or more) showed a significant increase in the incidence of robertsonian and reciprocal translocations as the number of abortions increased (Table 9-10). No such correlation was ob-

Table 9–9. DISTRIBUTION OF CHROMOSOMAL ANOMALIES IN COUPLES WITH REPRODUCTIVE WASTAGE

CHROMOSOMAL ANOMALY	PREVALENCE (%)	DISTRIBUTION (%)	
		Male	*Female*
Reciprocal translocation	1.3	36	64
Robertsonian translocation	0.6	30	70
Inversion	0.2	42	58
Sex chromosome aneuploidy	0.1	27	73
Supernumerary chromosome	0.03	18	82

Modified from DeBraekeleer M, Dao T-N: Cytogenetic studies in couples experiencing repeated pregnancy losses. Hum Reprod 1990;5:519, with permission.

served with the other three major chromosomal anomalies (DeBraekeleer and Dao, 1990). Women appear more likely to be the carrier of the chromosomal abnormality (Table 9–9). A similar predominance of females to males was reported previously (Tharapel et al, 1985). One explanation is that, in humans, chromosome structural abnormalities that are compatible with fertility in females may be associated with sterility in males (DeBraekeleer and Dao, 1990).

Balanced reciprocal translocation represented the largest group of chromosomal abnormalities in couples ascertained for multiple pregnancy losses. They were observed in 1.3% of the individuals studied (i.e., 2.6% of couples had at least one partner as the carrier). This figure is 15 times higher than that observed in cytogenetic analysis of consecutive newborns. Statistical analysis of the distribution of the chromosome arms involved in these translocations using computer simulations showed that, although all chromosome arms were implicated in the exchanges, some were preferentially involved, namely, 2p, 5p, 7p, 7q, 12q, 13q, 17q, 18p and 22q (DeBraekeleer and Dao, 1990).

Balanced robertsonian translocation represented the second most common category and was seen in 0.59% of the individuals studied. The most frequently found translocation was t(13q/14q) (64.3%),

followed by t(14q;21q) (7.7%). Robertsonian translocations were six times more frequently seen in couples in whom analysis was ascertained for repeated pregnancy loss than in consecutive newborn cytogenetic analysis.

Inversions, excluding inversions of the Y chromosomes, were found in 0.19% of individuals studied. This figure is 16 times higher than reported in newborn studies. Although, in most situations, the chromosomes were found to be involved in pericentric inversions (except for chromosomes 18, 21, and 22), statistical analysis showed that only chromosomes 2, 5, 7, and 10 were not involved more often than expected. The role of pericentric inversion of chromosome 9, inv(9), in repeated pregnancy loss is still controversial.

Few cases (21 so far) of paracentric inversion have been described in couples with repeated pregnancy loss. The inversion involved chromosome arms 1p, 3q, 5q, 7p, 7q, 11q, 13q, and 14q (DeBraekeleer and Dao, 1990).

Sex chromosome aneuploidy is rarely seen in couples referred for repeated spontaneous abortion, Variation in the length of the Y chromosome is usually due to variation in the length of the distal part of the long arm. In some studies, long Y chromosome (Yq+) has been associated with an increased risk of fetal loss, although there have been other studies that did not show any relationship between the size of the Y chromosome and the risk of abortion (DeBraekeleer and Dao, 1990). These observations suggest that not all Yq+ chromosomes are identical and some may affect the viability of the fetus.

Retrospective Studies on Archived Material

The lack of chromosomal studies on previous abortions makes it difficult to attribute with confidence the causes of recurrent abortion. However, it is now possible to study sections from paraffin-embedded tissue blocks or frozen specimens stored in the pathology laboratory (Van Lijnschoten et al, 1994). Using in situ hybridization methods combined with cytochemical staining, retrospective karyotypic analysis can be undertaken. The information obtained

Table 9–10. DISTRIBUTION OF CHROMOSOMAL ANOMALIES ACCORDING TO NUMBER OF SPONTANEOUS ABORTIONS

CHROMOSOMAL ANOMALY	NUMBER OF SPONTANEOUS ABORTIONS*		
	1	*2*	*≥3*
Reciprocal translocation	0.50	1.38	1.51
Robertsonian translocation	0.36	0.62	0.66
Inversion	0.14	0.20	0.21
Sex chromosome aneuploidy	0.07	0.06	0.14
Supernumerary chromosome	0.09	0.03	0.02

*Figures expressed as percentages.
Modified from DeBraekeleer M, Dao T-N: Cytogenetic studies in couples experiencing repeated pregnancy losses. Hum Reprod 1990;5:519, with permission.

from such studies is useful in counseling patients and in estimating their prognosis for a successful outcome in subsequent pregnancies.

Assessment and Treatment

Genetic testing is essential in the management of couples who have had recurrent spontaneous abortions. In addition, they may require genetic counseling. Because it is unlikely that karyotype information would be available from the abortuses of the previous abortions, couples with normal karyotype should be allowed to attempt another pregnancy, provided that no other cause for recurrent abortion has been identified. If a trisomy had been detected in a previous abortion, genetic counseling should be recommended.

The couple with a chromosomal translocation or inversion should be counseled regarding their risk of spontaneous abortion in a subsequent pregnancy and should be encourage to under prenatal diagnosis (amniocentesis or chorionic villus biopsy) in subsequent pregnancies. Other options include the use of donor gametes and embryo biopsy. The former involves artificial insemination with donor sperm if the translocation is in the male and in vitro fertilization of donor oocytes if the translocation is in the female. In the future, embryo biopsy technology will enable preimplantation diagnosis of genetic abnormalities in embryos at the four- to eight-bastomere stage, so that normal embryos can be selected for transfer into the uterus after in vitro fertilization. The family members of affected individuals should be informed that they are also possibly at risk of being a carrier of a similar chromosomal anomaly, so that further investigation can be undertaken if they are found to be carriers, and they should be offered genetic testing in all future pregnancies.

Uterine Factors

There are four major categories of uterine abnormality that may be associated with recurrent spontaneous abortion: congenital uterine anomalies, cervical incompetence, intrauterine adhesions, and uterine fibroids.

Congenital Uterine Anomalies

Congenital uterine anomalies are frequently associated with recurrent spontaneous abortion, although a causal relationship has yet not been established. The exact incidence of such anomalies is not known, resulting in a wide range of estimates in the literature. Lack of agreement over nomenclature and diagnostic strategies have made it difficult to establish meaningful incidence figures. It was previously believed that the prevalence of uterine anomalies was 0.1% to 0.2% (Wallach, 1979; Pisnsonneault and Goldstein, 1985; Rock and Schlaff, 1985), but postnatal examinations showed a prevalence of up to 2% to 3% (Sanfilippo et al, 1986). Similarly, in asymptomatic control groups using hysterosalpingography (HSG) or hysteroscopy, the prevalence was observed to be 2% and 6%, respectively (Cooper et al, 1983; Portuondo et al, 1986).

The major evidence supporting the role of congenital uterine anomalies in recurrent abortion is the higher prevalence observed in these women. In six different reports, uterine anomalies were observed in 12% of women with recurrent abortion (Table 9–11). The rate in each study was very similar (range 10% to 23%), indicating that approximately one in every eight women with recurrent spontaneous abortion can be expected to have a congenital uterine anomaly.

MECHANISMS OF FETAL WASTAGE RESULTING FROM UTERINE ANOMALIES

Several theories have been advanced to explain the association between congenital uterine anomalies and fetal wastage (Buttram and Reiter, 1985). First, the intraluminal volume in the abnormal uterus is reduced and, when the expansile limit of the uterus is surpassed, no further growth can occur to accommodate the advancing pregnancy, which terminates in spontaneous abortion or premature labor (Strassmann, 1966). Second, inadequate vascularity may compromise a placenta implanted on the septum or medial aspect of a uterine horn (Hunt and Wallach, 1974). This theory is supported by the observation that the amount of bleeding encountered when the uterine septum is being incised is minimal. Third,

Table 9–11. PREVALENCE OF CONGENITAL UTERINE ANOMALY IN WOMEN WITH RECURRENT ABORTION

STUDY	NO. OF RECURRENT ABORTERS STUDIED	NO. WITH CONGENITAL UTERINE ANOMALY (%)
Byrd et al (1977)	59	7 (12)
Sandler (1977)	654	81 (12)
Tho et al (1979)	100	10 (10)
Harger et al (1983)	112	17 (15)
Stray-Pedersen and Stray-Pedersen (1984)	195	19 (10)
Portuondo et al (1986)	65	15 (23)
TOTAL	1185	149 (12)

increased uterine irritability and contractibility, possibly associated with alterations in serum cystine aminopeptidase activity, may cause either premature cervical thinning and dilation or placental insufficiency and/or separation, which may precipitate spontaneous abortion or premature labor (Blum, 1978). Finally, because congenital cervical incompetence is associated with congenital uterine abnormalities in approximately 30% of cases (Craig, 1973; Bennet, 1987), late abortions may occur as a result of rupture of amniotic membranes that have prolapsed through the cervix and come into contact with the relatively hostile vaginal environment (with its acid pH and bacteria). Although these theories are unsubstantiated at present, each mechanism may contribute to fetal wastage.

ETIOLOGY OF CONGENITAL UTERINE ANOMALIES

Apart from anomalies associated with in utero exposure to diethylstilbestrol (DES), the cause of congenital uterine anomalies is not known. Each of the two paramesonephric (müllerian) ducts appears 5 to 6 weeks after conception as an invagination of the coelomic epithelium lateral to the cranial extremity of the corresponding mesonephric duct. The opening of the duct persists as the abdominal ostium and the caudal tip forms a solid bud that grows in a caudal direction. Canalization of the solid core of cells then follows. The two buds fuse in the midline at about 8 to 9 weeks and eventually come into contact with the urogenital sinus. Canalization is completed shortly thereafter, by 10 to 11 weeks. Resorption of the medial septum between the two fused ducts is completed by the 19th to 20th week to form a normal uterine cavity. Thus congenital uterine anomalies can result from complete or partial failure of descent of either or both of the müllerian ducts, failure of fusion, failure of canalization, and failure of resorption of the septum.

Several familial aggregates of incomplete müllerian fusion have been reported, including multiple affected siblings and affected mother and daughter (Sarto and Simpson, 1978; Verp et al, 1983). However, the relatively infrequent recurrence among family members suggests a polygenic or multifactorial origin of the anomaly (Elias et al, 1984).

If the anomalies are related to environmental exposure, they must occur in the 8th- to 19th-week period, when fusion and canalization are occurring. To date, no specific teratogen, such as radiation, fever, drugs, or infection, has been linked to any specific anomaly (Hammond, 1989).

CLASSIFICATION OF UTERINE ANOMALIES

A variety of classification schemes have been proposed over the years. However, because it was recognized that both internal and external assessments of the uterus are necessary to evaluate the anomaly, most of these schemes have been discarded. A new and more comprehensive classification scheme based on the degree of failure of normal development of the female genital tract was proposed in 1979 by Buttram and Gibbons and was modified in 1988 by a committee of the American Fertility Society (now known as the American Society for Reproductive Medicine) (Fig. 9–2). Class I is incompatible with pregnancy. The suggestion that there may be a normal uterus and vagina with bilaterally absent fallopian tubes (class 1d) is questionable because it is embryologically impossible. Nevertheless, this classification scheme will ensure consistency and uniformity in reporting so that meaningful compilation and comparison data can be carried out, thereby overcoming a major criticism of previous classification schemes, some of which were too simple and others too complex to allow widespread acceptance and utilization.

DIAGNOSIS

The HSG is a very specific and sensitive test for the diagnosis of uterine anomalies, but it is limited to the delineation of cavities that communicate externally. Thus the presence of a noncommunicating uterine horn would not be demonstrated by this technique. All women with recurrent spontaneous abortion should undergo an HSG examination. In addition, women with a history of unexplained preterm delivery, abnormal fetal lie, or retained placenta should have an HSG performed to rule out the possibility of a uterine anomaly. It is important that the HSG be performed with appropriate traction applied on the cervix to position the longitudinal axis of the uterus in the same plane as the x-ray film so that tangential views, which provide inadequate evaluation of the uterine fundus, are not taken. However, excessive traction can create an artifact that appears as an indentation of the fundus into the uterine cavity.

Laparoscopy increases the diagnostic accuracy of the HSG and is essential for distinguishing between a bicornuate and septate uterus. These two abnormalities have a similar appearance on HSG, even though it has been suggested that a wider separation between the uterine horns is more likely in a bicornuate than a septate uterus (Hunt and Siegler, 1990). This feature is not a reliable discriminator of the two uterine anomalies. In fact, in a series of 144 patients, 38 of 39 with HSG diagnosis of bicornuate uterus were found at surgery to have a septate uterus (Buttram and Gibbons, 1979). Laparoscopy is also helpful in diagnosing the presence or absence of noncommunicating uterine horns and associated pelvic pathology, such as pelvic adhesions and endometriosis, which are often seen with uterine anomalies.

The value of hysteroscopy in the diagnosis of uterine anomalies is still being assessed. However, it is possible to resect a uterine septum through the hys-

THE AMERICAN FERTILITY SOCIETY CLASSIFICATION OF MULLERIAN ANOMALIES

Patient's Name _____ Date _____ Chart # _____

Age ____ G ____ P ____ Sp Ab ____ VTP ____ Ectopic ____ Infertile Yes ____ No ____

Other Significant History (i.e. surgery, infection, etc.) _____

HSG _____ Sonography _____ Photography _____ Laparoscopy _____ Laparotomy _____

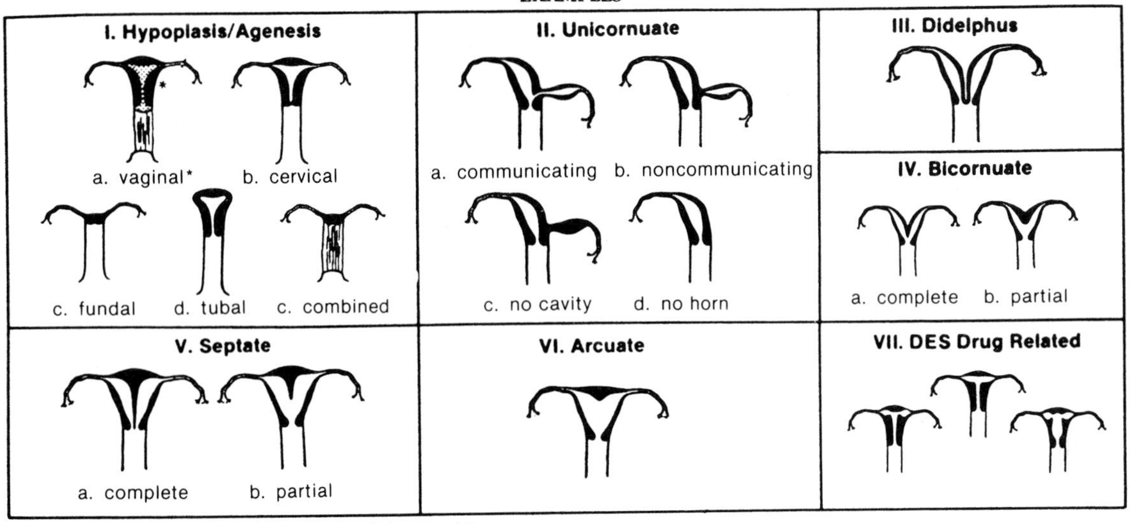

* Uterus may be normal or take a variety of abnormal forms.
** May have two distinct cervices

Type of Anomaly

Class I _____ Class V _____
Class II _____ Class VI _____
Class III _____ Class VII _____
Class IV _____

Treatment (Surgical Procedures): _____

Prognosis for Conception & Subsequent Viable Infant*

_____ Excellent (> 75%)
_____ Good (50-75%)
_____ Fair (25%-50%)
_____ Poor (< 25%)
* Based upon physician's judgment.

Recommended Followup Treatment: _____

Property of
The American Fertility Society

Additional Findings: _____

Vagina: _____
Cervix: _____
Tubes: Right _____ Left _____
Kidneys: Right _____ Left _____

DRAWING
L   R

Figure 9-2
The American Fertility Society Classification of Müllerian Anomalies. (Reproduced with permission of The American Fertility Society.)

teroscope, and this mode of management is now established.

In recent years, there has been an increase in the use of ultrasound imaging, especially with transvaginal transducers, to detect uterine anomalies in both the nongravid and pregnant uterus. The use of high-resolution, real-time, mechanical sector scanners has improved the diagnostic accuracy, and ultrasonography is now being proposed as a method for screening patients for uterine anomalies (Jurkovic and Kurjak, 1989; Daya, 1994a), but the diagnosis still requires confirmation by HSG. Clear visualization of the endometrium is necessary for a proper evaluation of the uterine cavity. Consequently, the examination should be performed during the luteal phase of the cycle because the endometrium is strongly echogenic at this time and provides a nice contrast against the relatively hypoechoic myometrium (Jurkovic and Kurjak, 1989). Scanning in a transverse uterine plane starting from the level of the cervix and progressing toward the fundus in a slow, continuous movement will clearly identify splitting of the endometrial echo in the upper portions of the uterus in the presence of a septate or bicornuate anomaly. The identification of two separate cervical canals or a division of the endometrial echo along the entire length of the uterine cavity is diagnostic of uterus didelphys.

Three-dimensional ultrasonography has the potential of significantly improving the evaluation of the uterus and is gradually being introduced into the clinical field as experience with this new method increases.

An added advantage of using ultrasonography is that an evaluation can be made of the kidneys. Urinary tract anomalies occur frequently in association with all types of uterine anomalies except class VII (DES-related) abnormality. Intravenous pyelography performed in 42 women with uterine anomalies showed abnormalities in 13 (31%), the most common of which was congenital absence of a kidney (Buttram and Gibbons, 1979). There appears to be a more frequent occurrence of urinary tract malformation in association with class I and II uterine anomalies than with those of classes III, IV, or V, (Buttram and Reiter, 1985).

The most recent technique for detecting congenital uterine anomalies is that of nuclear magnetic resonance imaging (Hamlin, 1986). Although this method is expansive, the images provided are extremely useful in distinguishing the different anomalies and in identifying noncommunicating uterine horns (Patel et al, 1997).

Physical examination is of limited value in the diagnosis of congenital uterine anomalies unless a vaginal septum or duplicate cervix is noted. Sometimes, a bimanual examination may detect the presence of two completely separate cornua, indicating the possibility of a bicornuate uterus, or the presence of a very wide fundus, which suggests that a septate uterus is a possibility.

MANAGEMENT

The management strategy depends on the type of anomaly and includes cervical cerclage, no surgical repair, and surgical correction.

Cervical Cerclage. The association of congenital uterine anomalies with cervical incompetence has led to the recommendation that a cervical cerclage procedure be performed to improve obstetric outcome (Heinonen et al, 1983; Rock and Schlaff, 1985). In fact, some clinicians advocate the insertion of a cervical suture in all cases of anomaly associated with a history of premature labor and/or recurrent abortion, or in situations in which a dilated cervical canal has been noted on HSG (Golan et al, 1989). Only if the cerclage does not improve the obstetric outcome should surgical correction of the anomaly be considered. (Abramovici et al, 1983). Although this viewpoint has its supporters, it is not the currently accepted standard of care for the management of uterine anomalies, particularly because appropriate studies have not been carried out and most of the information in the literature is based on case series.

No-Surgical-Repair Approach. Some congenital anomalies are not amenable to surgical correction and should be left alone. The following anomalies fall into this category.

Unicornuate Uterus (Class II). This malformation is the result of defective development of one of the two müllerian ducts and is frequently associated with a contralateral rudimentary uterine horn (Acién, 1992). It may also be caused by complete agenesis of all the organs derived from one urogenital ridge, resulting in unicornuate uterus and, on the contralateral side, no uterine horn or ovaries and renal agenesis or hypoplasia (Acién, 1992).

The unicornuate uterus represents 1% to 2% of congenital uterine anomalies and is associated with high rates of spontaneous abortion and premature delivery (Table 9–12). Otherwise, patients with unicornuate uterus are usually asymptomatic. Surgical correction of this anomaly is not possible because no surgical procedure will enlarge the uterus.

However, patients with a noncommunicating functional horn are at increased risk of morbidity secondary to the development of hematometrium, hematosalpinx, endometriosis, and rudimentary horn gestation and should have the horn excised. Pregnancy in a noncommunicating horn or or its fallopian tube can occur by transperitoneal migration of either sperm or ova from the contralateral side (O'Leary and O'Leary, 1963; Daya, 1986). Uterine rupture occurred by the end of the second trimester in 89% of such cases, and only 1% of the pregnancies resulted in a live birth.

Although no efficacy studies have been carried out, cervical cerclage has been suggested as a therapeutic option, especially if there is a history consis-

Table 9–12. REPRODUCTIVE OUTCOME ASSOCIATED WITH CONGENITAL UTERINE ANOMALY

TYPE OF UTERINE ANOMALY	NO. OF PATIENTS	NO. OF PREGNANCIES	SPONTANEOUS ABORTION		OUTCOME OF PREGNANCIES					
					Ectopic Pregnancy		Premature Labor		Live Birth	
			No.	(%)	No.	(%)	No.	(%)	No.	(%)
II Unicornuate	31	60	29	(48)	2	(3)	5	(17)	24	(40)
III Didelphys	54	124	53	(43)	0	(0)	23	(45)	68	(55)
IV Bicornuate	110	313	110	(35)	0	(0)	47	(23)	178	(57)
VI Septate	72	208	140	(67)	0	(0)	20	(33)	59	(28)
VI Arcuate	14	29	0	(0)	0	(0)	0	(0)	10	(34)
VII DES related	499	579	154	(27)	31	(5.4)	109	(28)	364	(63)

Data extracted from Buttram and Reiter (1985:149–199) and Bennet (1987).

tent with the presence of an incompetent cervix (Gros et al, 1974; Heinonen et al, 1983).

Uterus Didelphys (Class III). This anomaly results from complete failure of fusion of the müllerian ducts, with normal differentiation of each duct to form a cervix and hemiuterus. In 75% of cases, the vagina has a longitudinal septum as well (Sarto and Simpson, 1978). Most patients with this abnormality are asymptomatic, although some may have dyspareunia resulting from the vaginal septum. Despite the fact that premature labor is frequently associated with this anomaly and a high spontaneous abortion rate may be observed, reasonable fetal survival rates can be expected (Table 9–12).

Surgical correction is difficult, and few successes have been reported. Therefore, surgical therapy is not recommended. Cervical cerclage has been advocated and may be a reasonable strategy in patients with a history consistent with the presence of an incompetent cervix (Gros et al, 1974).

Arcuate Uterus (Class VI). This anomaly was previously classified with the septate group (Class V) (Buttram and Gibbons, 1979), but is now listed separately in the American Fertility Society (1988) classification (Fig. 9–2). Very little is known about the reproductive consequences of this type of anomaly. Incompetent cervix may be an associated finding and has been observed in 36% of patients with this anomaly (Craig, 1973). No surgical repair is recommended because the anomaly may represent a variation of normal. The management in pregnancy should include periodic assessment of the cervix to detect shortening and/or effacement, in which case cervical cerclage is indicated.

DES-Related Anomaly (Class VII). The typical upper genital tract anomalies associated with in utero exposure to DES were first reported by Kaufman et al in 1971. Several different anomalies have been described, including a T-shaped uterine cavity, abnormally small cavity, uterine constrictions, and bulbous dilation of the lower cervical segment (Buttram and Reiter, 1985). Sixty-nine per cent of exposed women had such anomalies (Kaufman et al, 1980).

Although the role of this anomaly in infertility is controversial, the available data support the observation of an increased rate of fetal wastage, with a spontaneous abortion rate of 24% and a preterm delivery rate of 15%. Overall, the rate of adverse outcomes (i.e., spontaneous abortion, ectopic pregnancy, and perinatal death), taken together, ranged from 25% to 58% in nine published studies (Kaufman and Irwin, 1987). In addition, several studies have documented not only a high first-trimester abortion rate but also a high second-trimester abortion rate (Buttram and Reiter, 1985). The latter is suggestive, but not diagnostic, of an association with incompetent cervix (Table 9–12). Previously, it was believed that patients with transverse cervicovaginal ridges were more likely to experience fetal loss, but at present there does not appear to be good evidence for such an association (Herbst et al, 1989).

In contrast to class I through VI anomalies, class VII anomalies are thought to have occurred because DES adversely affected development of the uterine muscle and thus caused areas of muscular hypertrophy and maldevelopment (Buttram and Reiter, 1985).

Currently, there is no surgical procedure that can repair class VII anomalies, although there has been a preliminary report of hysteroscopic metroplasty (Naegel and Malo, 1987). Goldstein (1978) noted that cervical incompetence was a possible complicating factor, requiring cervical cerclage, in 8 (31%) of 26 patients who delivered viable infants. Several others have reported improved fetal outcome following cervical cerclage. In contrast, others warned that prophylactic cerclage is unwarranted and recommended close observation, including weekly cervical assessment and cerclage only when there was clear evidence of incompetence (Barnes et al, 1980; Herbst et al, 1980; Sandberg et al, 1981). A prospective study, however, indicates that there is an advantage to the liberal use of cerclage (Ludmir et al, 1987). Sixty-three women were managed with weekly or biweekly cervical examinations and limited physical activity. Patients with a normal cervix and no prior loss were followed expectantly. Elective cerclage at 12 to 14 weeks' gestation was used in those with a short cervix (<1 cm in length) or in those with prior second-trimester losses. Emergency cerclages were performed for obstetric indications. Prophylactic cerclage was performed in 26 patients. In these women, the mean gestational age at delivery was 37.7 weeks and no perinatal deaths were observed. In 16 of 37 women in whom emergency cerclage was required, the mean gestational age at delivery was 36.1 weeks, with no perinatal deaths. Of the remaining 21 pregnancies with no prior second-trimester loss, no cervical changes were detected on weekly examination and the cervical length remained normal. In these women, five pregnancies ended in premature delivery at a mean gestational age of 24.4 weeks, with perinatal deaths in all of them. The remaining patients delivered at term. Until the results from controlled trials become available, the evidence from this study suggests that prophylactic cerclage in patients with class VII anomalies may have a beneficial role, even though this recommendation is not universally accepted. Nevertheless, frequent examination of the cervix in the second trimester is warranted to detect dilation and/or effacement. Ultrasound surveillance may be more useful in detecting the early cervical changes (Michaels et al, 1989; Daya, 1994b). If clinical or sonographic changes in the cervix are present, or if there is a history of repetitive second-trimester loss, then cervical cerclage is probably a wise recommendation.

Surgical Correction

Bicornuate Uterus (Class IV). This anomaly, unlike the didelphys uterus, results from failure of fusion of the müllerian ducts at the level of the fundus but complete fusion lower down in the uterus. Consequently, the uterus has a single cervix, but externally the fundus has a sagittal groove, the depth of which varies depending on the extent of the fusion defect (Fig. 9–2). In the past, both bicornuate and septate uteri were classified in the "double uterus" category, but laparoscopic findings have confirmed that the majority of uterine anomalies appearing bicornuate on HSG, in fact, are septate.

The pregnancy outcome among women with a bicornuate uterus has been difficult to quantify owing to inconsistency in classification. However, more recent data indicate that there are relatively high rates of spontaneous abortion and premature labor (Table 9–12). The abortion rate appears to be much lower than that observed with septate uteri, perhaps reflecting better blood supply in the midline indentation of the bicornuate uterus than in a uterine septum (Buttram and Reiter, 1985).

The surgical procedure of choice remains the operative procedure described by Strassmann in 1908 and popularized by his son (Strassmann, 1966) (Fig. 9–3). However, very few reports on the outcome of this surgical corrective treatment have appeared in the literature. In three papers published since 1968, in which bicornuate uteri were distinguished from septate uteri, live births were achieved in 10 of 11

(91%) pregnancies after surgical repair (Buttram and Reiter, 1985).

Septate Uterus (Class V). This anomaly results from complete or partial failure of resorption of the midline wall that is present between the two müllerian ducts after fusion and canalization have occurred. The resulting septum extends for a variable distance from the fundus down toward the cervix. The septum is always broadest at the fundus. Occasionally, the septum extends all the way down to, and including, the cervix, which appears "double" (very much like that of the didelphys uterus, but the external appearance of the uterus is normal) (Daya, 1989a).

Among the uterine anomalies, the septate uterus is the one most commonly associated with recurrent spontaneous abortion. An abortion rate of 67% was reported in an overview of 208 pregnancies in this group of uterine anomalies (Table 9–12). The abortion rate seems to be related to the depth of the septum. In 33 patients with a partial septum (class VB), the abortion rate was 70% in 69 pregnancies, whereas in five patients with a complete septum (class VA), the abortion rate was 89% in 9 pregnancies (Buttram and Reiter, 1985). As discussed previously, the high abortion rate may be explained by a variety of factors, including a decreased functional volume in the uterine cavity, inadequate blood supply to the septum where implantation may occur, or a rigid cavity caused by the stiff septum preventing appropriate growth of the gestational sac, which ultimately collapses after the membranes rupture.

Premature labor is also a relatively frequent complication associated with the septate uterus.

Abdominal Metroplasty. Surgical repair is indicated in women with a septate uterus and a history of fetal wastage. Jones and Jones (1953) described a technique in which the uterine septum was excised by means of a wedge-shaped incision and sagittal closure of the uterus. In addition to the septum, a portion of the fundus was removed, resulting in significant blood loss and a marked reduction in the amount of intrauterine space. For these reasons, this technique has found little favor outside its institution of origin, where it had been performed on 47 patients over a period of 44 years (Rock, 1981; Bennet, 1987).

The more popular abdominal procedure was described by Tompkins in 1962, and involves a sagittal incision that is made in the fundus and carried downward in an anteroposterior direction through the center of the septum until the uterine cavity is reached (Fig. 9–4). Even though the incision is relatively bloodless, vasopressor agents, such as vasopressin (Pitressin), are very useful to control bleeding by creating a relatively bloodless field.

No efficacy studies on abdominal metroplasty have been carried out to date. Nevertheless, the chance of a successful pregnancy is much higher after metroplasty. A post-treatment live birth rate of 88% and spontaneous abortion rate of 5% were ob-

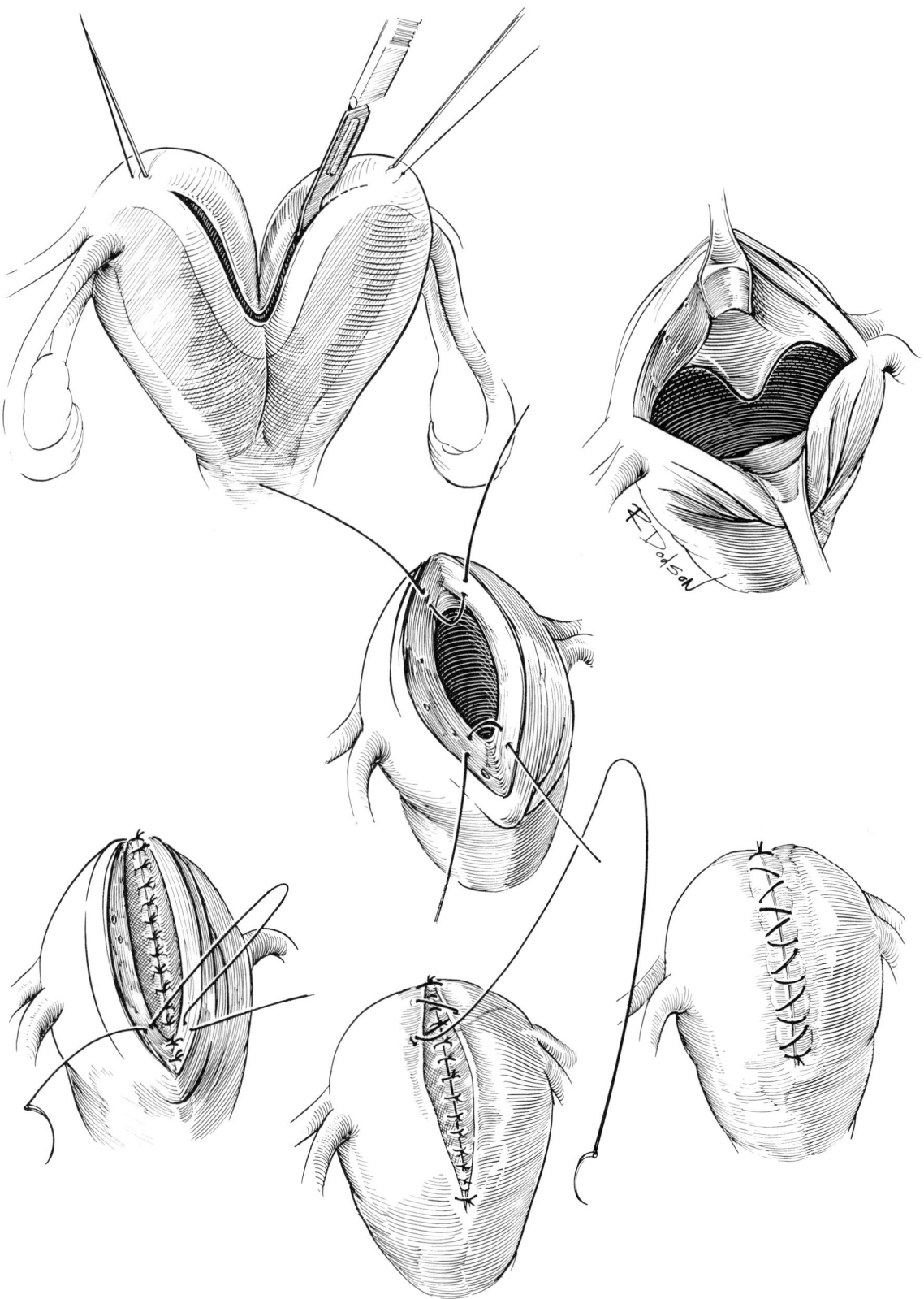

Figure 9-3
Strassmann metroplasty for bicornuate uterus.

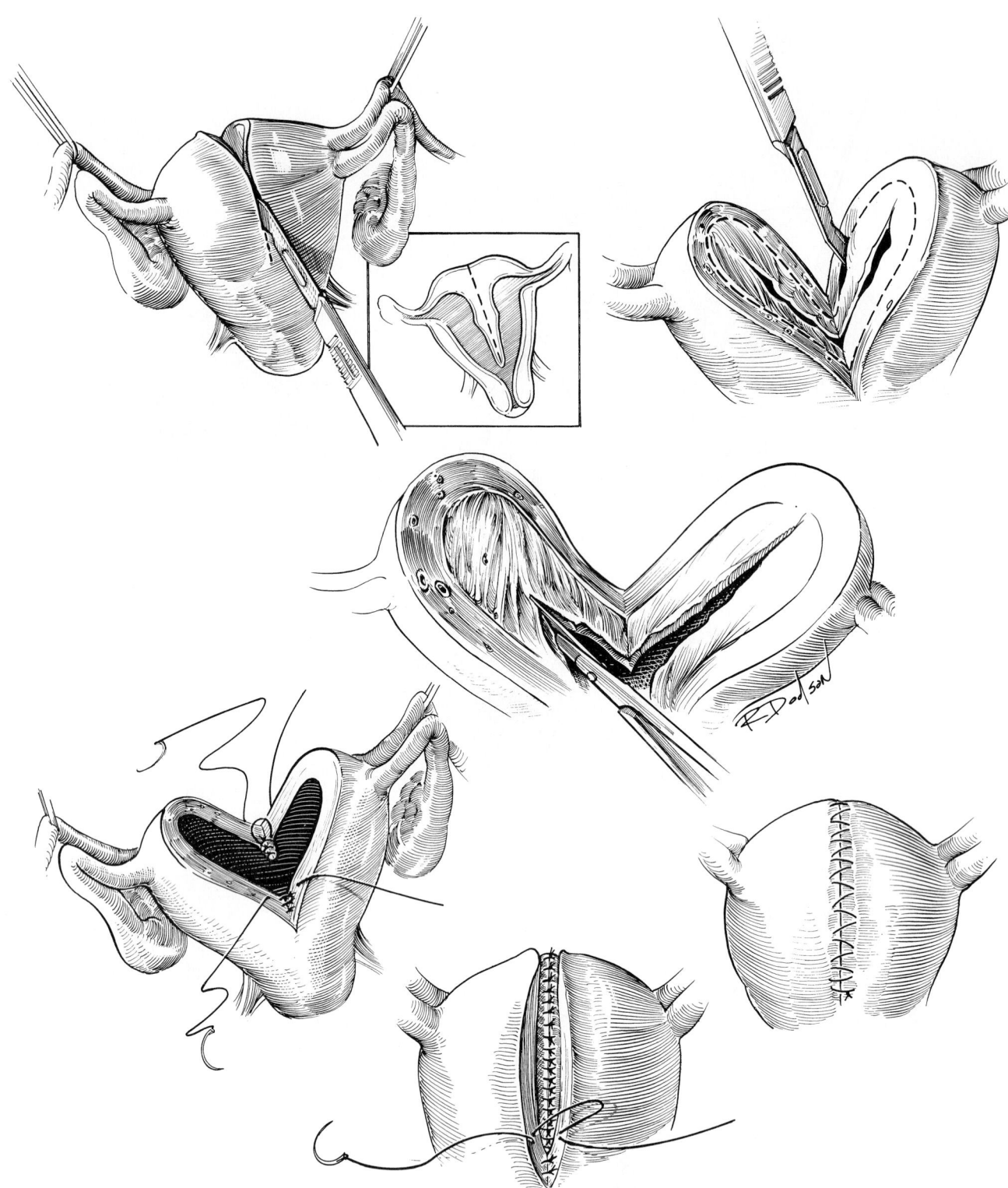

Figure 9–4
Modified Tompkins procedure. Incision of septum and reapproximation of myometrium.

served when the data from three separate reports were combined (Buttram and Reiter, 1985).

In an effort to prevent adhesions that may result from abdominal metroplasty, careful microsurgical technique with meticulous attention to hemostasis is recommended, together with the use of adjuvants or adhesion barriers and plication of the round ligaments. Cesarean section should be performed at term to avoid the risk of uterine rupture, which may occur during labor.

Hysteroscopic Repair. This method involves division of the septum through the hysteroscope. The procedure is often performed with laparoscopic guidance so that the risk of uterine perforation can be minimized.

Using the principles of the Tompkins metroplasty, the septum is incised from its apex to its base using hysteroscopic scissors. This results in retraction of the septum and a uterine cavity indistinguishable on HSG from that seen using the Tompkins method. For optimal results, the procedure should be performed in the early follicular phase of the menstrual cycle when the endometrium is still quite thin. Operating time is usually less than 1 hour and, because the septum is avascular, bleeding is minimal. Postoperatively, the use of conjugated estrogens (Premarin), 2.5 mg twice daily for 1 to 2 months, followed by medroxyprogesterone acetate (Provera), 5 mg twice daily for 10 days, has been suggested to promote healing (Hammond, 1989). A post-treatment HSG is recommended to ensure that the uterine cavity has been restored to normal. A repeat procedure is sometimes necessary if division of the septum is incomplete.

Outcome data from six series involving a total of 251 patients, of whom 81% had conceived, indicate support for this procedure, with an ongoing pregnancy rate of 90% and an abortion rate of 9%, resulting in a live birth rate of 81% (Table 9–13) (Daly et al, 1983; DeCherney et al, 1986; Fayez, 1986; Valle and Sciarra, 1986; March and Israel, 1987; Perino et al, 1987).

Resection of the septum by means of a resectoscope is sometimes used, but is applicable only if the base of the septum is narrow (<1 cm thick) (De-Cherney and Polan, 1983).

The technique of metroplasty via hysteroscopy is now a well-established and accepted first-line treatment option. The main advantages are that major abdominal surgery is avoided, the procedure is performed in an outpatient setting, immediate operative morbidity is minimized, postoperative pelvic adhesions and consequent infertility are avoided, and subsequent pregnancies do not require cesarean section for delivery.

Cervical Incompetence

Simply defined, cervical incompetence is the inability of the cervix to maintain an intrauterine pregnancy until term. Its incidence is difficult to quantify because there are no generally agreed-upon criteria for diagnosis. Consequently, figures vary from 1 in 2000 deliveries to 1 in 32 deliveries (Shortle and Jewelewicz, 1989). Its incidence among women with habitual abortion is also difficult to determine, with reports ranging from 8% to 15% (Shortle and Jewelewicz, 1989).

ETIOLOGY

The structure of the cervix has been extensively studied by Danforth (1947, 1954, 1959), who showed that it is primarily composed of collagen with approximately 10% to 15% contribution from smooth muscle. Further histologic studies have demonstrated that the smooth muscle is distributed disproportionately such that there is 29% in the upper third, 18% in the midportion, and 6.4% in the lower third of the cervix (Rorie and Newton, 1967). The relatively more muscular portion represents the internal os, which normally retains the pregnancy in utero. The cervix, which is rigid and fibrous in the nonpregnant state gradually softens during pregnancy, reaching its zenith at parturition (Editorial, 1983; McDonald, 1987). In early pregnancy, the compliance of the cervix is very low and the cervix offers some resistance to surgical dilatation, which, if forced, can easily injure the internal os mechanism or produce laceration of the cervix (McDonald, 1987). Resistance is greatest in young nulliparous women, in whom considerable damage can occur as a result of forceful dilatation.

Cervical incompetence results from a weakness in this sphincter mechanism of the internal os. Consequently the increasing pressure from the advancing pregnancy can cause amniotic membranes containing amniotic fluid to protrude through the weakened os, which may dilate painlessly and result in expulsion of the pregnancy. Rupture of membranes may also occur from the combined effect of hydrostatic pressure and the adverse vaginal environment from

Table 9–13. REPRODUCTIVE OUTCOME AFTER HYSTEROSCOPIC METROPLASTY

STUDY	NO. PATIENTS	NO. PREGNANCIES	OUTCOME OF PREGNANCY		
			Spontaneous Abortion	*Ongoing*	*Live Birth*
Daley et al (1983)	17	8	1	—	7
Valle and Sciarra (1986)	12	10	2	—	8
DeCherney et al (1986)	72	67	4	5	58
Fayez (1986)	19	16	2	—	14
March and Israel (1987)	79	63	8	7	48
Perino et al (1987)	52	39	2	7	30
TOTAL	251	203	19 (9%)	19 (9%)	165 (81%)

its relatively acidic pH and organisms. A weakened cervical state is usually the result of acquired causes, but rarely may occur from a congenital defect in the cervix.

Congenital Cervical Incompetence. In a minority (approximately 2%) of patients, no etiologic factor can be ascertained. In these women, it is presumed that an inherent weakness of the fibromusculature region at the upper end of the cervix and internal os is present (Danforth, 1959). The documentation of cervical incompetence in four pairs of sisters suggests that a familial tendency may be a factor in some women (Jennings, 1972).

As previously discussed, cervical incompetence is also associated with anomalies of the müllerian duct system. It is unclear why such an association exists, especially because detailed histologic evaluation of the uterus and cervix has not been undertaken in such anomalies. Cervical incompetence is more likely in women exposed to DES in utero (Mangan et al, 1982). It has been postulated that the fibromuscular junction in such DES-exposed women may have been displaced downward into the cervical canal, thereby affecting the structural integrity and sphincteric functioning of the internal os (Singer, 1978).

Acquired Cervical Incompetence. In a review of 329 cases, it was observed that more than 95% of patients were parous, suggesting that the most important predisposing factor for cervical incompetence is childbirth (Table 9–14) (McDonald, 19887). The majority also had a history of one or more mid-trimester abortions, and about two thirds had a D&C procedure. Trauma to the cervix resulting from such procedures, from lacerations sustained at birth (e.g., precipitous delivery, operative delivery), or following second-trimester terminations predisposes the patient to developing cervical incompetence as a consequence. Similarly, having had an induced abortion was found to be a risk factor associated with an increased incidence of subsequent mid-trimester losses among 2019 nulliparous women studied (Harlap et al, 1979). The relative risk also increased with the number of previous induced abortions. Interestingly,

the relative risk decreased after 1973, when laminaria tents were introduced for use prior to induced abortions and the technique of more gentle cervical dilatation began to be employed (Mitchell-Leef, 1989). Dilatation of the cervix to a diameter than 12 mm diameter was found to significantly increase the rate of prematurity from cervical incompetence, the safe limit being 10 mm (Johnstone et al, 1974). The maximum resistance to dilatation is believed to be encountered at 9 mm diameter, with dilatation beyond this limit possibly representing tearing of the internal os rather than true dilatation (Hulka et al, 1974).

Conization of the cervix is another important cause of cervical incompetence. Several studies have shown significantly higher rates of late spontaneous abortion and prematurity after cone biopsy. Nulliparous women in the 21 to 25 year-old age group are at highest risk, presumably because too much tissue is removed from the relatively smaller cervix, resulting in a large defect that produces cervical incompetence (Larsson et al, 1982; Moinian and Andersch, 1982). Furthermore, the risks of premature delivery and late spontaneous abortion increase in proportion with the size of the cone. In women with cone volumes greater than 4 ml, the prematurity rate was 31.7% and the second-trimester spontaneous abortion rate was 18.2%, compared with 3.2% and 6.5%, respectively, when the volume was less than 4 ml (Leiman et al, 1980). Similarly, the second-trimester abortion rate was 21.7% when the cone height was greater than 2 cm, compared with 12.3% when the height was less than 2 cm (Leiman et al, 1980). In contrast, no adverse effect on subsequent pregnancy outcome was observed when cervical dysplasia was treated with cryosurgery (Hemmingsson, 1982).

Physiologic Cervical Incompetence. There have been many case reports of cervical incompetence appearing for the first time in women with multiple gestation, with successful outcome resulting from cervical cerclage (Shortle and Jewelewicz, 1989). In a multiple pregnancy, the dilated internal os may be the consequence of rapid and excessive enlargement of the uterus and significantly higher pressure on the internal os.

DIAGNOSIS

A major difficulty in the evaluation and management of the problem of cervical incompetence is that there are no universally accepted criteria for its diagnosis. Consequently, having a high index of suspicion on the basis of the clinical history is of great importance. The classical presentation of repetitive, acute, painless second-trimester pregnancy loss without associated bleeding or uterine contractions is not commonly seen. Many patients have some bleeding and abdominal cramps as the fetus is being expelled. Often there is a history of premature rupture of membranes before the onset of contractions, or there may have been evidence of membranes bulging into the vagina. The fetus usually appears normally devel-

Table 9–14. PREDISPOSING FACTORS IN PATIENTS WITH INCOMPETENT CERVIX

PREDISPOSING FACTOR	NO. PATIENTS*	%
Parous	315	96
Midtrimester abortion	307	93
Dilatation and curettage	227	69
Cervical conization	28	9
Amputation of cervix	8	2
None	8	2

*Total number of patients studied = 329.
Modified from McDonald IA: Cervical incompetence as a cause of spontaneous abortion. In Bennet MJ, Edmonds DK (eds): Spontaneous and Recurrent Abortion. Oxford: Blackwell Scientific, 1987;168, with permission.

oped and may be alive at birth. The history of expulsion of a dead or macerated fetus generally argues against the diagnosis of cervical incompetence. Mid-trimester abortions occurring around the same gestational age in successive pregnancies is also indicative of cervical incompetence. In primigravidae patients, a history of having undergone gynecologic procedures such as D&C, cone biopsy, and so on should raise one's level of suspicion. Cervical incompetence should also be looked for in women with uterine anomalies.

The Nonpregnant Patient. Inspection of the cervix may reveal congenital anomalies or evidence of previous cervical laceration. The integrity of the cervix can be checked with a dilator. If a No. 8 Hegar dilator or a No. 15 or 17 Pratt dilator can be passed easily through the internal os, the cervix is incompetent. This test should not be performed at midcycle or during menses because a false-positive diagnosis may be made. Other tests that have been described include the intracervical balloon (Yosowitz et al, 1972), the Foley catheter traction test (Bergman and Svennerund, 1957), and the olive-tipped sound test (Durfee, 1958).

Hysterosalpingography is useful in evaluating the cervical canal. However, to properly assess the cervix with this technique, it is important to either remove the vaginal speculum or rotate it clockwise 90 degrees so that the cervical canal containing contrast material can be visualized properly and not be obscured by the radiopaque blades of the speculum. Several investigators have attempted to define cervical incompetence by measuring the width of the internal os. In one study, the internal os of the cervix in women with habitual abortion was significantly wider than in normal parous women (6.09 ± 0.98 mm vs. 2.63 ± 0.27 mm) (Ayers et al, 1982). Similarly, the isthmus was much wider in women with habitual abortion (mean 3.58 mm) than in nulliparous and parous women (Ayers et al, 1982). This finding is consistent with previous observations that indicated that cervical incompetence was associated with a diameter of the cervical isthmus of 6 mm or greater (Mann et al, 1961).

Another method of evaluating the resistance of the cervix utilizes the pressure decay curve (van Duyl et al, 1984). The initial diameter of the internal os is first determined by the size of the Hegar dilator that can be introduced into the cervix without resistance. A deflated balloon is then inserted into the cervical canal up to the level of the isthmus and filled with saline until a pressure of 250 mm Hg is achieved. Keeping the balloon volume constant, a pressure decay curve is recorded until an asymptotic value is reached, which is attributed to the relaxation point of cervical tissue at the level of the internal os. Using this technique, the resistance to dilation was found to be significantly lower in women with cervical incompetence compared with controls (van Duyl et al, 1984).

The Pregnant Patient. A patient who is pregnant and has a history of cervical incompetence or uterine anomaly should undergo periodic examinations of her cervix, beginning at 10 to 12 weeks' gestation. Effacement and/or dilation of the cervix is an indication for cervical cerclage. Also, patients should be instructed to report symptoms such as lower abdominal pressure, a "bearing-down" sensation, pressure or sensation of fullness in the vagina, and a watery or mucous discharge, because any of these symptoms may be a feature of progressive dilation of the cervix.

On routine vaginal examination, only about half of the true anatomic cervical length is accessible to the palpating finger. Consequently, the interpretation of cervical shortening is very subjective. In a double-blind study, digital measurements of cervical length did not correlate very well with measurements obtained using ultrasonography as the gold standard (Sonek et al, 1990). Thus making the diagnosis of cervical incompetence by vaginal examination in pregnancy may not be possible until the process of dilation has progressed quite far. As a result, therapy may be ineffective because it is provided too late.

Ultrasonography now enables physicians to overcome this limitation. Besides providing an objective measurement of the length of the cervix, abdominal sonography can detect dilation of the cervical canal at the level of the internal os. The cervical length in a normal second-trimester pregnancy is 2.5 to 6 cm (Zemlyn, 1981; Michaels et al, 1986; Varma et al, 1987); a length less than 2.5 cm signifies incompetence, especially if confirmed on serial assessments (Bernaschek et al, 1990). The process of cervical dilation begins at the internal os and progresses downward, culminating in prolapse of amniotic membranes into the vagina.

The advent of vaginal ultrasonography eliminated many of the problems encountered with abdominal scanning. Optimal delineation of the cervical canal along its entire length is readily possible owing to the close proximity of the vaginal probe to the cervix and the clarity of the images that are obtained (Daya, 1994b). Thus accurate measurement of the distance between the internal and external os is possible (Bernaschek et al, 1990). Also, a distended bladder is not required for transvaginal scanning as it is for abdominal scanning. Besides causing discomfort to the patient and altering the topographic relationships, a full bladder may exert too much pressure on the lower uterine segment and obscure any dilation of the internal os that may be present. Whereas the normal Y-shaped appearance of the lower uterine segment on longitudinal scans remains largely unaffected, V-shaped or U-shaped dilations of the cervical canal may go undetected with abdominal scanning (Bernaschek et al, 1990). In contrast, transvaginal scanning avoids these errors. Furthermore, the major advantage is its ability to more accurately demonstrate proximal dilation of the cervical canal, a finding that would not be obvious to the palpating finger on vaginal examination and thereby would remain undetected. A study comparing transabdominal and transvaginal sonography for evaluating the cervix demonstrated the superiority of the latter method because the lower uterine segment was easily seen in a larger percentage of patients (Brown et al, 1986).

Transvaginal scanning is also much better for evaluating "dynamic cervical incompetence," a condition in which the degree of dilation varies and may even change during the ultrasound examination (Parulekar and Kiwi, 1988). Thus the competence of the internal os can be observed on transvaginal sonography as the examiner simultaneously presses gently on the abdominal wall with a free hand. Any weakness of the internal os would be exaggerated with this method, leading to the observation of an increase in the diameter of the cervical canal (Daya, 1994b).

MANAGEMENT

Although therapeutic strategies such as bed rest, mechanical methods (e.g., Bakelite ring, Smith-Hodge pessary, Baylor balloon), and hormones (e.g., progesterone and 17α-hydroxyprogesterone caproate) have been suggested, it is generally accepted that surgical treatment is the method of choice. Cervical cerclage still remains inadequately evaluated because larger randomized studies have not been conducted. The data from 1850 cases entered into five randomized controlled trials provide a less than adequate basis for clinical decisions about the use of cervical cerclage (Grant, 1989). Prophylactic cerclage looks most promising when based on a past history of second-trimester abortion or preterm delivery.

The operations used for correction of cervical incompetence are many and varied, and there is no agreement about which technique is the most appropriate to use. However, despite the variability, all methods share the same principle of reinforcing the region of the internal os by inserting a ligature around the cervix at this level. In this manner adequate occlusion of the cervical canal is obtained and the pregnancy can be carried to a gestational age that enhances fetal survival. An ultrasound examination should be performed just prior to the cerclage to document the presence of a live intrauterine pregnancy and to rule out any obvious gross fetal anomaly. Cervical cerclage, performed as an elective procedure, is usually carried out between 13 and 15 weeks' gestation. Immediately after surgery, tocolysis with β-sympathomimetic drugs has been used to counteract uterine irritability even though no controlled studies on its efficacy have been performed. Bed rest for 24 hours is usually recommended, with full ambulation and discharge on the second to third postoperative day. Periodic ultrasonographic monitoring of the cervix is recommended to ensure effectiveness of the procedure is maintained (Daya, 1994b). A second cer-

clage occasionally may be necessary if suture displacement or erosion through the cervix is evident.

Contraindications to cervical cerclage include uterine bleeding, spontaneous rupture of membranes, uterine contractions, chorioamnionitis, and cervical dilation greater than 4 cm.

Shirodkar Cerclage. In the method described by Shirodkar (1955), a transverse anterior incision is made at the cervicovaginal junction and the bladder is pushed upward to the level of the internal os. A vertical incision is then made posteriorly at the cervicovaginal junction. A 5-mm Merseline band is drawn through these incisions to encircle the cervix and the knot is tied posteriorly, thereby avoiding the risk of subsequent erosion into the bladder by the knot. The vaginal incisions are closed with absorbable sutures. The suture can be removed at 37 to 38 weeks' gestation to allow vaginal delivery but is usually left in situ and caesarean section is recommended, especially in women desirous of more children. The original operation used a fascial band, which Shirodkar later rejected because the material is technically difficult to obtain; is slippery, resulting in knot loosening; and may undergo myxomatous degeneration from sepsis. Also the donor site leaves a scar.

McDonald Cerclage. The method described by McDonald (1957) is simple and much easier to perform than the Shirodkar cerclage. It is a closed procedure (as opposed to the open method of Shirodkar) and involves the placement of a continuous suture at the junction of the vaginal mucosa and the cervix in a purse-string fashion. A suture is drawn in and out of the stroma in four to five sites around the cervix using nonabsorbable material, such as Merseline, and the knot is tied anteriorly. The lateral blood vessels are avoided using this method, thereby eliminating the risk of ischemia of the cervix. Care must be taken to firmly anchor the suture along the posterior aspect of the cervix, because this is the area where displacement may occur. The suture is removed at 37 weeks' gestation to allow vaginal delivery.

Daya Cerclage. I have modified the method described by McDonald by using two sutures instead of one and have observed excellent results. The method requires analgesia with a regional block, usually a spinal anesthetic. The McDonald method is employed, whereby a 5-mm wide Mersilene tape is inserted at the level of the reflection of the bladder on the cervix. The knot is tied anteriorly. A second cerclage is then placed 0.5 to 1 cm below the first one. In this manner, the pressure from the advancing pregnancy is distributed over a wider area because the cervical tissue between the two sutures is held securely, thereby enhancing the effectiveness of the cerclage. I have used this method successfully for several years, with no adverse effects or complications and with a success rate of over 95% in the last 150 procedures that have been performed. The sutures are easily removed, as an office procedure, at 37 to 38 weeks' gestation.

I believe that this method eliminates the risk of the suture "cutting through" the cervix as pregnancy advances, thereby improving the effectiveness of the cerclage, which has a higher risk of failure if only one suture is inserted.

Transabdominal Cerclage. Cerclage using the transabdominal approach (Benson and Durfee, 1965; Mahran, 1978) is useful for women in whom the vaginal approach is not feasible because the cervix is short as a result of cervical amputation, cervical hypoplasia, or previous attempts at cervical cerclage that have failed. It may be performed before pregnancy is attempted because this is technically easier. However, in pregnancy, it is usually carried out late in the first trimester (i.e., around 11 weeks' gestation) after a live pregnancy has been confirmed. Several modifications of the original method have been described. Essentially, a suture is placed at the level of the internal os after the peritoneum has been opened and the bladder resected downward. The suture is placed medial to the uterine vessels. A fenestrum between the upper border of the cardinal ligament, the medial upward turn of the uterine vessels, and the terminal ureter laterally can be entered using a tonsillectomy forcep, which also allows the suture to be grasped (McDonald, 1987). The suture may be passed through or around the cardinal and uterosacral ligaments and the knot is tied anteriorly. Mersilene or nylon tape or polyvinyl ligature can be used. The peritoneum is repaired and the abdomen closed in layers. The ligature is left in situ indefinitely, and all subsequent pregnancies are delivered by cesarean section.

COMPLICATIONS

Complications from cervical cerclage include postoperative infection, immediate onset of labor, suture displacement, cervical laceration, postoperative bleeding, rupture of the membranes, fistula formation, placental abscesses, bladder injury, uterine rupture, cervical dystocia, and even material death (Mitchell-Leef, 1989). More recent studies have reported lower complication rates. Leukorrhea, which may produce an offensive odor, is commonly seen after McDonald cerclage. Reassurance is all that is necessary for the patient in whom the discharge is bothersome.

Intrauterine Adhesions

The uterine cavity may be partially obliterated by intrauterine adhesions. Occasionally, total occlusion may occur, resulting in amenorrhea. This condition is referred to as Asherman's syndrome in recognition of the person who first characterized the disorder (Asherman, 1948, 1950). Symptoms vary according to the extent of the disease but include menstrual disorders, such as hypomenorrhea, amenorrhea, and

infertility, which includes sterility and recurrent abortion. The latter was observed in 14% of 2151 patients with intrauterine adhesions (Schenker and Margalioth, 1982).

Although the incidence of intrauterine adhesions is difficult to quantify, it is encountered not infrequently (Eriksen and Kaestel, 1960). The more liberal use of HSG and hysteroscopy, coupled with greater physician awareness of the condition, are probably responsible for the increased frequency of diagnosis, but the prevalence has remained unchanged (Buttram and Reiter, 1985).

ETIOLOGY

Intrauterine trauma resulting from endometrial curettage is a common feature that leads to the development of these adhesions. The pregnant uterus is especially susceptible to this type of injury; more than 90% of the 1856 cases collected in a comprehensive review of the literature were associated with pregnancy (67% following postabortal curettage and 22% after postpartum curettage) (Schenker and Margalioth, 1982). It is more difficult to judge and control the depth of curettage in the pregnant uterus because it is so much softer. Consequently, the traumatizing effect of the procedure may result in denudation of the basalis layer of the endometrium, thereby preventing the normal regenerative process and permitting adherence of the uterine walls, which are kept apposed by postpregnancy uterine contractions. The frequency of the adhesions also depends upon the time during the puerperium when curettage was performed; the uterus is especially vulnerable during the 2nd through 4th weeks following delivery, the first 48 hours being a time of relative resistance to adhesion formation (Polishuk and Sadovsky, 1975). The hypoestrogenic state associated with postpartum lactation may act synergistically with the injury to promote adhesion formation because the stimulus to endometrial regeneration is suppressed.

Other less frequently reported causes of intrauterine adhesions include genital tuberculosis, myomectomy, diagnostic curettage, cervical manipulation (biopsy, polypectomy, etc.), curettage for menometrorrhagia, and after insertion of an intrauterine contraceptive device (IUCD) (Schenker and Margalioth, 1982). The role of infection as a predisposing factor in adhesion formation is controversial, especially because there does not appear to be a direct connection between clinical infection (fever, leukocytosis, foul discharge) and intrauterine adhesions (Schenker and Margalioth, 1982).

A relatively high percentage of cases with intrauterine adhesion was seen following curettage for missed abortion (Schenker and Margalioth, 1982). The mechanism of adhesion formation in such cases may involve placental remnants that promote fibroblastic activity and collagen formation before endometrial regeneration can take place (Carmichael, 1970). Another possibility is intravascular coagulation owing to changes in blood coagulability that causes thrombosis within the arterial vessels of the uterus, leading to fibrosis of that part of the uterus (Bernaschek et al, 1990).

CLASSIFICATION

A classification scheme based on extent of uterine cavity obliteration, as judged by hysteroscopic examination, has been proposed by March et al (1978). The minimal category was defined as involvement of less than one fourth of the uterine cavity by thin or filmy adhesions, with little or no involvement of the ostia and upper fundal area. The moderate category was associated with involvement of one fourth to three fourths of the cavity, without agglutination of the uterine walls and with only partial occlusion of the ostia and upper fundal portions of the cavity. The severe category was seen when more than three fourths of the cavity was involved, with agglutination of the wall or thick bands of adhesions and involvement of the ostia and fundal portions of the cavity.

A simpler classification, based on localization, is more practical and describes three groups (Schenker and Margalioth, 1978):

Total atresia – This very rare and severe form is defined as complete obliteration of the uterine cavity and cervical canal, with no identifiable endometrial tissue.

Corporal adhesions – These are seen in the majority of cases and vary in degree, ranging from small single adhesions that are asymptomatic to extensive adhesions that totally distort the uterine cavity.

Cervicoisthmic adhesions – These are usually identified by blockage or stenosis of the cervical canal.

The latter two groups were seen in 56% and 20%, respectively, of 1789 cases reviewed in the literature, with the remainder being made up of a combination of the two, including total atresia (Schenker and Margalioth, 1982).

DIAGNOSIS

Intrauterine adhesions should be suspected when a patient develops amenorrhea, hypomenorrhea, recurrent abortion, or infertility following curettage in pregnancy or the puerperium. If the patient has amenorrhea but has symptoms suggestive of ovulation, such as cyclic lower abdominal pain and molimina, a biphasic basal body temperature (BBT) graph, or an elevated serum progesterone level, then diagnosis is almost certain. In general, however, the patient is usually asymptomatic and the diagnosis is made with HSG or hysteroscopy.

Hysterosalpingography is performed using a cannula that is attached to the cervix with vacuum suction or is gently screwed into the cervical canal. The presence of intrauterine adhesions is demonstrated

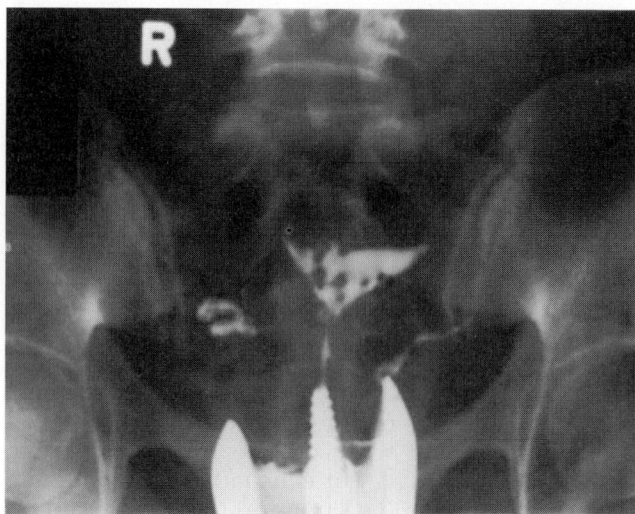

Figure 9–5
Hysterosalpingogram showing filling defects from intrauterine adhesions.

by a single or multiple lacuna-shaped filling defects of variable size within the uterine cavity. These filling defects are characterized by their irregularity, angulated form, very sharp contours, homogeneous opacity, and persistent appearance on several exposures taken at various intervals (Schenker and Margalioth, 1982). The extent will vary depending on the severity of the adhesions (Fig. 9–5). In very extensive adhesions, intravascular and intralymphatic extravasation may be seen. In cases of very minimal disease, the fine adhesions may be disrupted during the procedure by the pressure from the flow of contrast material into the uterus.

Hysteroscopy is used to confirm the HSG finding and is the only way of making a definitive diagnosis of intrauterine adhesions.

TREATMENT

The treatment regimen has four main goals: lysis of adhesions, prevention of readherence, promotion of endometrial proliferation, and verification of normal cavity restoration.

Lysis of Adhesions. Earlier attempts at surgical treatment were disappointing and led to postponement of treatment. Among eight reports of 292 women not subjected to lysis of adhesions, pregnancies occurred in 13 (45.5%) (Schenker and Margalioth, 1982). These women had a total of 165 pregnancies, of which only 50 (30%) ended in a term delivery, 38 (23%) in preterm labor, and 66 (40%) in spontaneous abortion. Thus women who do not undergo treatment for intrauterine adhesions are predisposed to reduced fertility and poor pregnancy outcome.

Lysis of adhesions by abdominal hysterotomy is rarely, if ever, indicated. In a review of the results of this treatment, 16 of 31 women conceived but, of these, only 8 delivered a healthy infant (4 requiring a cesarean hysterectomy for placenta accreta) (Schenker and Margalioth, 1982).

Transcervical lysis of adhesions is presently the treatment of choice, although there is still controversy as to whether it should be performed by blunt dissection, as is done in D&C, or by sharp disection during hysteroscopy. The former method (without additional intracavitary adjuvant therapy) was used to treat 22 women among whom 16 (73%) conceived, but 5 (31%) pregnancies ended in abortion (Michaels et al, 1986). The disadvantage of this method is not knowing whether all the adhesions have been lysed.

The advantage of the hysteroscopic approach is that adhesions can be divided under direct vision using scissors, resectoscope, or laser. The advantage of the latter two methods is immediate hemostatis, but adhesions are usually avascular and therefore are amenable to lysis using hysteroscopic scissors. Because there is no risk of significant hemorrhage, no efficacy studies comparing these different methods have been performed to enable one to draw any conclusions regarding the preferred method.

Prevention of Adherence. A major improvement in pregnancy outcome after lysis of adhesions has been achieved with the addition of adjunctive therapy to prevent adherence of the uterine walls. Methods that have worked well include placement of an IUCD or Foley catheter balloon in the uterine cavity. The mechanical device is intended to remain in place for several days to 2 weeks, although the catheter is often expelled sooner. Although no beneficial effect on subsequent pregnancy rates was observed when an IUCD or Foley catheter was used (221 of 405 [51%] and 78 of 167 [47%], respectively), the major benefit is in the probability of the pregnancy reaching term (61% and 70%, respectively) (Schenker and Margalioth, 1982). The ideal IUCD that should be used has not been identified, but one with a broad surface area, such as an Ypsilon, is preferable to a Lippes loop. A disadvantage of using an IUCD is the possibility of adhesions developing around it, making removal very difficult. For this reason, the catheter is preferred.

Promotion of Endometrial Proliferation. The administration of conjugated estrogens assists in regeneration of the endometrium and promotes healing. Despite the fact that no efficacy studies of this treatment have been carried out, there seems to be generalized agreement that estrogen therapy should be used as an adjunct to lysis of uterine adhesions. Interestingly, the repeat abortion rate after lysis of adhesions and estrogen therapy was only 5%, compared with 46% when estrogen was not used (Diamond, 1988). The doses employed varied from 1.25 to 2.5 mg/day for 1 to 2 months, often in combination with a progestational agent to induce withdrawal bleeding.

Verification of Normal Cavity Restoration. It is important to reassess the uterine cavity to verify that it is normal after treatment before permitting the patient to attempt a pregnancy. Poor reproductive outcome associated with earlier treatment regimens may have been the result of incomplete lysis of adhesions. Although HSG is easier and more practical than hysteroscopy, it is not as accurate and does not allow lysis of residual adhesions.

Pregnancies occurring after treatment for intrauterine adhesions are at higher risk for premature labor, spontaneous abortion, and placenta accreta and should be regarded as being of high risk (Schenker and Margalioth, 1982).

Uterine Fibroids

Uterine fibroids are common tumors occurring in 20% to 25% of women over the age of 30 years (Vollenhoven et al, 1990). Fibroids may be single or multiple and may be of various sizes. Each fibroid originates from smooth muscle, most probably from one cell (Vollenhoven et al, 1990). The factors responsible for the initial neoplastic transformation are not known, but at least three hormones (estrogen, growth hormone, and progesterone) are thought to influence the rate of growth of fibroids (Buttram and Reiter, 1985). Fibroids are first seen in the reproductive years and increase in size until the menopause occurs, after which regression is likely. Continuous estradiol secretion is thought to be a main underlying risk factor, although why these tumors occur in some women and not in others is unknown. Fibroids contain more high-affinity estrogen receptors than neighboring normal uterine muscle and usually depend on estrogen for growth (Editorial, 1986).

Uterine fibroids are more commonly seen than cervical fibroids and are classified as subserous (55%), intramural (40%), and submucous (5%) depending upon whether they occur just beneath the serosa, within the myometrium, or subjacent to the endometrial mucosa (Buttram and Reiter, 1985).

Premature labor, spontaneous abortion, and infertility are reproductive consequences of these tumors. Fibroids are an infrequent cause of infertility; in a review of patients undergoing myomectomy, no other cause for infertility could be found in only 2% (Buttram and Reiter, 1981). Fibroids have been associated with a higher rate of spontaneous abortion, particularly if implantation occurs in relation to a submucous fibroid. The fibroid may cause distortion and partial obliteration of the uterine cavity and may affect the vascular supply to the developing fetus. Also, the endometrium may be poorly vascularized for implantation. Other mechanisms include pressure on the gestational sac from enlarging fibroids in pregnancy and red degeneration, which may result in uterine irritability. The likelihood of disrupting the pregnancy is probably related to the number, location, and size of the fibroids (Diamond and Polan, 1989). For example, a pedunculated serous fibroid is unlikely to cause difficulty, unless uterine irritability occurs secondary to red degeneration, whereas a submucous fibroid is more likely to affect pregnancy initiation and maintenance (Diamond and Polan, 1989).

DIAGNOSIS

Approximately 30% of women with fibroids have menstrual abnormalities, most often menorrhagia (Buttram and Reiter, 1981). Chronic dull backache may be present, especially with large fibroids, and dysmenorrhea may also occur. Clinically, the diagnosis is made by palpating an irregularly or symmetrically enlarged uterus. The fibroids usually feel firm. A HSG may show an oval or round filling defect with smooth borders. The cavity may also be enlarged with irregular borders. Ultrasonography is very useful in determining the size, number, and location of fibroids and whether calcific or other degenerative changes have occurred. It is also useful in objectively evaluating growth of the fibroids over time. Laparoscopy and hysteroscopy provide useful additional information on the extent and location of the fibroids.

MANAGEMENT

Abdominal Myomectomy. Myomectomy is the most appropriate treatment for a woman with recurrent abortion who has large uterine fibroids. The high morbidity from this procedure is related to the risk of blood loss and postoperative adhesions. Various techniques have been used to minimize blood loss, including injection of vasopressin or neosynephrine around the tumor at the time of surgery and the use of clamps or tourniquets to occlude the uterine and ovarian vessels (Buttram and Reiter, 1985). Gonadotropin-releasing hormone analogs (GnRHa) have been found useful in this regard (Friedman et al, 1989). Postoperative adhesions can be minimized by ensuring adequate hemostasis, using microsurgical techniques, and avoiding multiple uterine incisions whenever possible. A single vertical midline incision is preferable. The use of adhesion-preventing barriers may further reduce adhesion formation.

Although valid studies have not been carried out, the beneficial effect of myomectomy is suggested from a review of the literature in which the abortion rate among 1941 women with fibroids was reduced from 41% preoperatively to 19% after myomectomy (Buttram and Reiter, 1985). Clearly, efficacy studies are required to confirm this finding. Until then, the recommendation for myomectomy in women with recurrent abortion should be made on an individual basis, taking into account the patient's history and clinical findings.

Hysteroscopic Resection. The use of the resectoscope for hysteroscopic treatment of submucosal uterine fibroids has been reported (Neuwirth, 1978, 1983). The resectoscope is used to shave the fibroid down to its base. Only fibroids of limited size can be resected from uterine cavities that are not too large (i.e., sounded to 10 cm or less) (Neuwirth, 1978). Strict monitoring of fluid balance is essential because the large volume of fluid that is instilled into the uterine cavity as a distending medium can be absorbed through vascular spaces that are opened by the procedure (Vollenhoven et al, 1990). Among five women who conceived after fibroid resection, none had a spontaneous abortion. This technique has the advantage of being an outpatient procedure that is relatively free from complications, but needs further evaluation as a possible alternative to myomectomy in women with recurrent abortion.

Laser Myomectomy. Endoscopic myomectomy can be performed using a CO_2 laser. The potential advantages of this approach over conventional surgery include decreased adhesion formation, better hemostasis, direct vaporization of smaller fibroids, increased precision in destroying abnormal tissue, decreased tissue injury, and improved reproductive performance (McLaughlin, 1985; Starks, 1988). The use of argon and neodymium–yttrium-aluminum-garnet (Nd-YAG) in lasers in fibroid surgery is still in its infancy. Hysteroscopic myomectomy using the Nd-YAG laser was reported in one study of five patients (Starks, 1988).

GnRH Analog Treatment. Continuous, as opposed to pulsatile, administration of GnRHa causes suppression of gonadotropin secretion by down-regulation of the gonadotropin-producing cells in the pituitary gland, thereby leading to decreased estrogen production by the ovary. The estrogen dependence of fibroids suggests that the induction of a hypoestrogenic state in patients with fibroids by using GnRHa might lead to shrinkage of these tumors. Early reports were promising, with a decrease in size of fibroids by 62% to 100% of their original volume by the end of 2 to 6 months of continuous therapy (Filicori et al, 1983; Healy et al, 1984; Maheuz et al, 1984). More recent studies have also shown similar results, with a 50% reduction in fibroid volume (Vollenhoven, 1990). The greatest reduction in uterine volume is achieved within the first 12 weeks of treatment, although not all fibroids respond in this manner. The reduction in volume appears to be dependent on the level of estrogen suppression. In women with no response, it is believed that the fibroid may be dependent on growth factors other than estrogen (Vollenhoven et al, 1990). Invariably, after therapy is discontinued, there is regrowth of the fibroids within 2 to 6 months, to pretreatment dimensions or beyond, in 40% of patients (Editorial, 1986; Vollenhoven et al, 1990). In a longer follow-up period of over 12 months, regrowth of fibroids was observed in all patients and recurrence of their pretreatment symptoms was documented in 80% (Matta et al, 1989). Thus the beneficial effect of GnRHa therapy is short lived, making it unlikely that myomectomy can be avoided in the long run. Nevertheless, it may have a role in the preoperative management of these patients. The reduction in size of the tumor may make surgical removal technically easier, especially with endoscopic methods. Also, blood loss at myomectomy after pretreatment with GnRHa is significantly lower in patients who have large fibroids (Friedman et al, 1989), presumably because the reduction in size is associated with reduced vascularity of the tumor.

Endocrine Factors

Various types of endocrine dysfunction have been reported to be associated with recurrent abortion. The most common endocrine abnormality is luteal phase deficiency (LPD) whereas diabetes mellitus, thyroid disease, and adrenal disease are observed less frequently.

Luteal Phase Deficiency

The main function of the corpus luteum is to secrete progesterone, which promotes secretory transformation of the endometrium and provides the necessary support for implantation and early pregnancy before the placenta can assume this function. This luteoplacental shift is believed to occur approximately 36 days after the luteinizing hormone (LH) surge (Lenton, 1988). Removal of the corpus luteum before 8 weeks of pregnancy is followed by abortion in 4 to 7 days. (Csapo et al, 1976). A fall in plasma progesterone precedes the abortion, which can be prevented by parenteral treatment with progesterone. Suboptimal corpus luteum function results in inadequate development of the secretory endometrium and produces the clinical entity known as luteal phase deficiency. This disorder appears to be common in women with habitual abortion, in whom prevalence figures have ranged from 25% to 60% (Balasch and Vanrell, 1987). In contrast, LPD is seen infrequently in women with infertility, suggesting that progesterone deficiency affects continuation of the pregnancy after implantation rather than affecting conception itself.

The corpus luteum is a transient endocrine gland that develops immediately after ovulation as a result of morphologic and biochemical changes in the follicle (Daya, 1990). Its life span in humans is 14 days, with a 95% confidence interval (CI) of 11.3 to 17.0 days (Lenton et al, 1984a). Arrest of falling serum progesterone levels and "rescue" of the corpus luteum by hCG secreted by the implanting blastocyst may be seen as early as 9 days after the midcycle LH surge. Induction and development of LH receptors on granulosa cells is a necessary prerequisite to luteinization and progesterone synthesis in response to LH or hCG, both of which can activate these receptors (Hanson et al, 1971).

LPD cycles are characterized by low follicle-stimulating hormone (FSH) levels in the follicular phase, low luteal phase progesterone levels, and, in some women, decreased luteal phase length (Strott

et al, 1970; Cook et al, 1983). Progesterone secretion by the corpus luteum is distributed along a parabolic curve, with maximum production occurring in the midluteal phase (Fig. 9–6) (Daya et al, 1988). Although progesterone production in LPD cycles follows a similar curve, the total output of progesterone (as measured by the area under the curve) is significantly lower than in normal cycles (Daya et al, 1988). In fact, in LPD cycles peak production occurred at day 21 (of a standardized 28-day cycle), whereas in normal cycles, this level was reached just before day 19 and was maintained until day 26 (Daya et al, 1988). The lower progesterone production in LPD results in reduced stimulation of the endometrium, thereby causing slower maturation and an inappropriate environment for blastocyst implantation and further development.

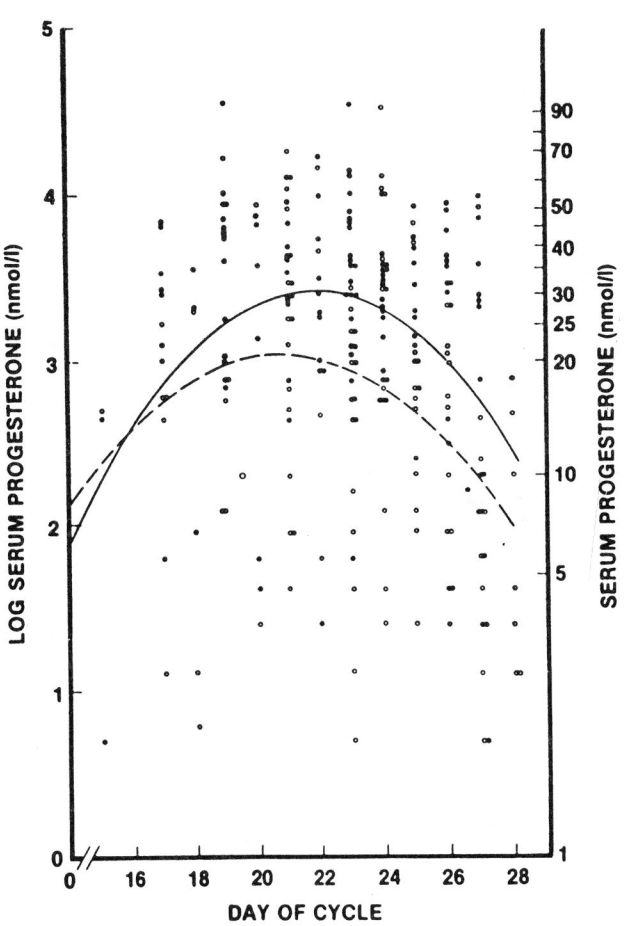

Figure 9–6
Scattered plot of serum progesterone values in the luteal phase of the menstrual cycle, from normal (●) and luteal phase–deficient (○) cycles. The best-fitting regression curves for the two types of cycle are shown: normal curve (*solid line*) and luteal phase–deficient (*broken line*). The two curves are significantly different from each other (*p* < .001). (From Daya S, Ward S, Burrows E: Progesterone profiles in luteal phase defect cycles and outcome of progesterone treatment in patients with recurrent spontaneous abortion. Am J Obstet Gynecol 1988;158:225, with permission.)

CLASSIFICATION OF LPD

Two main types of LPD have been identified: short luteal phase and inadequate luteal phase.

Short Luteal Phase. A short luteal phase is relatively uncommon (5.2%) (Lenton et al, 1984a) and is characterized by a reduced interval between ovulation and the onset of menses. The luteal phase in this condition was originally described as being 8 or fewer days from the LH peak (Strott et al, 1970) but now includes all cycles with a luteal phase of 10 days or less (Jones, 1976; DiZerega and Hodgen, 1981). Estradiol and progesterone levels in the luteal phase may be reduced because of defective follicular maturation or a defect in FSH production (Sherman and Korenman, 1974). The mean FSH levels and the FSH/LH ratio in the follicular phase have been shown to be low (Strott et al, 1970). Also, the peak progesterone level is lower and occurs earlier than in a normal cycle. Interestingly, the endometrium does not show any abnormalities with maturation. Also, there does not appear to be any effect on fertility (Smith et al, 1984), even though delayed follicular development and irregular shape and reduced size of the dominant follicle have been observed in ultrasound studies (Geisthovel et al, 1983).

Inadequate Luteal Phase. This type of luteal phase deficiency is more commonly seen. The length of the luteal phase is normal (in contrast to the short luteal phase), but the endometrium shows secretory changes that are 3 days or more behind those expected (Daya et al, 1988). The diagnosis is based on endometrial biopsy taken late in the luteal phase. Because the interobserver variability of this diagnostic test is quite wide, at least two menstrual cycles should be examined to reduce the probability of misclassification by chance. Unfortunately, the diagnosis is often accepted when there is a 2-day lag in development of the endometrium (Balasch et al, 1986). Such inconsistency in diagnostic criteria complicates any attempts to properly evaluate the role of LPD in recurrent abortion.

DIAGNOSIS OF LPD

A wide variety of diagnostic techniques has been used to characterize LPD, but as yet no universally accepted gold standard has been established.

Luteal Phase Duration. The average length of the luteal phase is relatively more consistent than that of the follicular phase, which has been observed to decrease with age. Assessment of luteal phase length with methods such as the thermal shift on BBT graphs (mean 11.8 days) (Vollman, 1977) tends to underestimate the duration when compared with measurements taken from the day of the LH peak (mean 14.1 days) (Lenton et al, 1984a). Because the length of the luteal phase in most cases of LPD is normal, the evaluation of the duration of the luteal phase using the LH peak method is only useful for the de-

tection of the short luteal phase or entity, which is not very commonly encountered. Nevertheless, a luteal phase length of 10 days or less is abnormal.

BBT Graphs. The interpretation of the BBT chart may be useful because it reflects the progesterone-mediated shift in basal temperature from ovulation to menses. Attempts to quantify this temperature rise have focused on the magnitude, rate of rise, and duration of temperature elevation (McNeely and Soules, 1988).

Although women with histologically demonstrable LPD were found to have a significantly shorter (11.8 days) luteal phase on BBT charts compared to those with normal cycles (13.4 days), there was much overlap between the two groups (Downs and Gibson, 1983). Furthermore, up to 18% of apparently normal women may have a luteal temperature elevation lasting less than 11 days (Marshall, 1963). Finally, the rate of rise in temperature does not correlate well with endometrial biopsy assessment. Therefore, the BBT chart is not a sensitive test for the diagnosis of LPD, but may give some indication of the quality of the luteal phase, especially if the duration of temperature elevation is short.

Serum Progesterone Measurement. The observation that total progesterone production in LPD cycles is lower than in normal cycles suggests that serum progesterone concentration estimation should be a reasonable test for assessing luteal function. However, because the distribution of progesterone production in the luteal phase follows a parabolic curve, daily sampling would be required to estimate total progesterone production (Fig. 9–6). Clearly, this is not a practical solution in a clinical setting. Therefore, investigators have attempted to address this problem by relying on single or multiple sampling. Several studies have assessed the value of midluteal progesterone estimation because peak levels are attained at this time. Discriminatory values for normal cycles have ranged from 9.4 to 12.5 mg/ml (approximately 30 to 40 nmol/L) (Hull et al, 1982; Abdulla et al, 1983). Unfortunately, in both studies, normal values were taken from the 10th (Hull et al, 1982) or 20th (Abdulla et al, 1983) percentile of the range in progesterone concentration observed in cycles of conception known to have higher progesterone levels. This cutoff level was too high, and was verified in a study of regularly cycling volunteers, 26% of whom did not have a single value above 12 ng/ml (39 nmol/L), which was the 10th percentile of values in conception cycles (Abdulla et al, 1983). In another study of normally cycling volunteers, the discriminatory level selected was much lower, at 6.3 ng/ml (20 nmol/L), and was estimated from the 20th percentile of values in ovulatory cycles (Wattren et al, 1984).

The variability in daily progesterone levels is quite wide and can reduce the diagnostic accuracy of this test (Daya et al, 1988). To reduce such variability, multiple estimations in the luteal phase have been

Table 9–15. MORPHOLOGIC FACTORS IN LUTEAL PHASE USED FOR DATING ENDOMETRIUM

MORPHOLOGIC FACTOR	MENSTRUAL CYCLE DAY WHEN CHANGE IS MOST APPARENT
Glandular features	
Gland mitoses	15
Pseudostratification of nuclei	14–15
Basal vacuolation	17
Secretion	20–21
Stromal features	
Stromal edema	22
Pseudodecidual reaction	28
Stromal mitoses	25
Leukocytic infiltration	28

Modified from Noyes RW, Hertig AT, Rock J: Dating the endometrial biopsy. Fertil Steril 1950;1:3, with permission.

suggested as a practical solution. In one study, the sum of three progesterone levels taken in the midluteal phase of an apparently normal cycle was found always to be higher than 15 ng/ml (48 nmol/L) (Abraham et al, 1974). This led to the recommendation of using a sum of three progesterone levels obtained every other day in the midluteal phase as a determinant of corpus luteum function. These studies were all designed to identify ovulatory cycles rather than trying to distinguish between normal and LPD cycles. Consequently, midcycle estimation of progesterone may be appropriate for the detection of ovulation. However, because endometrial maturation reflects total progesterone production, a better correlation might be found with late luteal phase progesterone estimations.

Using endometrial histology to define LPD, 91 cycle-day intervals were evaluated with receiver operator characteristic curve analysis. The optimal time in the menstrual cycle when serum progesterone levels were of value in identifying LPD was day 25 to 26 of a standardized 28-day cycle (Vollman, 1977). The discriminatory level of progesterone at this time was 21 nmol/L (sensitivity 81%, specificity 73%).

In contrast, sampling in the midluteal phase produced inferior diagnostic test properties, with the worst time interval being days 17 to 24 (Daya, 1989c), suggesting that during this period a higher discriminatory level is necessary to distinguish LPD from normal cycles. Thus the late luteal phase offers the best time for serum progesterone estimation so that the assessment of luteal phase adequacy can be undertaken with more accuracy.

Endometrial Biopsy. The endometrium undergoes a predictable sequence of changes in each menstrual cycle. After examining more than 8000 endometrial biopsies, a set of histologic criteria were established for an ideal 28-day cycle (Noyes et al, 1950). These criteria depend largely on changes in the endometrial stroma during the last week of the luteal phase (Table 9–15) and (Fig. 9–7) (Collins, 1990).

Although endometrial maturation is reasonably uniform in all areas of the uterus, some variability may be encountered. Therefore, to ensure consistency in the diagnostic test, the biopsy should be obtained from the uterine fundal area, where the endometrium is more consistently developed and is the farthest advanced. Histologic dating should be based on the most advanced area in the endometrium.

Endometrial biopsy is best performed in the late luteal phase, as close to expected menses as possible, so that the endometrial response to virtually the entire progesterone output of the corpus luteum can be examined. Specimens obtained before cycle day 25 are more difficult to date with accuracy and may re-

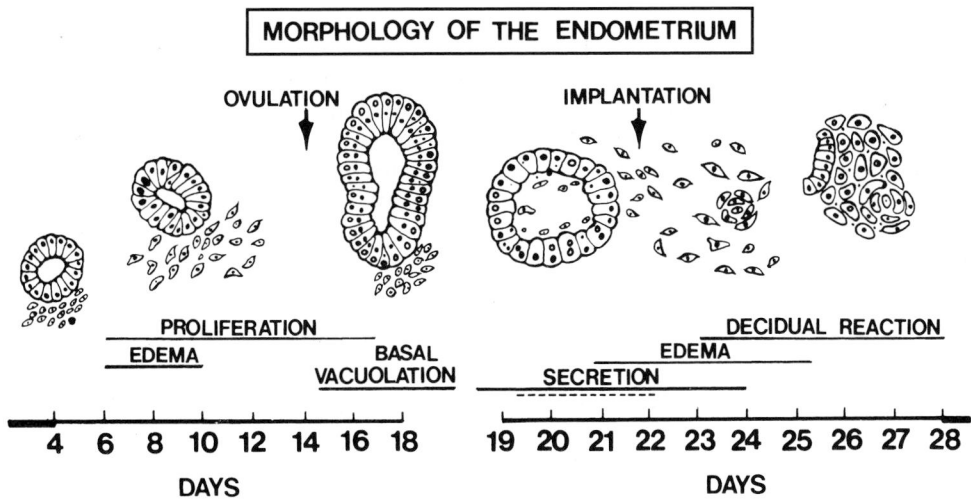

Figure 9–7
Schematic representation of the major morphologic changes that occur in the glandular epithelium and stroma of the superficial endometrium (functionalis) during an ideal 28-day cycle. (Redrawn from Maslar IA: The progestational endometrium. Semin Reprod Endocrinol 1988;6:115, with permission.)

sult in errors in the diagnosis of LPD (Kusuda et al, 1983; Cumming et al, 1985). Thus late luteal timing is preferred to reduce variability.

The definition of LPD is a 3-day or greater discrepancy between the histologic date and the chronologic date as determined by the day of onset of the menstrual period following the biopsy. At least two cycles should be examined to make this diagnosis, and, if one biopsy shows LPD and the other is normal, then a biopsy should be performed in a third cycle to resolve this discrepancy. Unfortunately, there are several studies (reviewed by Collins [1988]) that have used a 2-day lag to confirm the presence of LPD. Such lack of agreement makes it difficult to evaluate the role of LPD in reproduction.

Another source of variability may be the use of the next menstrual period to determine the chronologic date. The length of the luteal phase is relatively more constant (Lenton et al, 1984a) than that of the follicular phase (Lenton et al, 1984b). The assumption that menses occur 14 days after ovulation, therefore, is used to determine retrospectively when ovulation would have occurred so that the number of days after ovulation when the biopsy was performed can be determined. The correlation between histologic dating and chronologic dating is better and more precise when the LH peak (Li et al, 1987) or ultrasound documentation of follicle collapse (Shoupe et al, 1989) is used as a reference point for ovulation. The histologic dating assessed independently by two pathologists was within 2 days of the postovulatory day in 25 of 26 biopsies (96%) taken in 13 cycling parous women when the day of ovulation was determined by ultrasound, but in only 17 of 26 biopsies (65%) when ovulation was determined by the onset of the next menstrual period (Shoupe et al, 1989).

Intraobserver variability was studied among 63 endometrial biopsies examined on two separate occasions by the same observer, and disagreement of more than 2 days occurred in 10% (Li et al, 1989). Exact agreement was more likely in the first half of the luteal phase (32%) than in the second half (9%) (Collins, 1990).

Interobserver variability was studied among five pathologists examining 62 biopsy specimens (Scott et al, 1988). The mean interobserver variability or dating the specimens was 0.96 days (standard error 0.08), and this variability was not affected by endometrial maturity or by the presence of maturation delay (Collins, 1990).

Studies on LPD using endometrial biopsies are often biased because women with a normal result on the first biopsy are less likely to have a second biopsy (Collins, 1990). This bias may lead to erroneous estimates of the prevalence of LPD. Nevertheless, the prevalence of LPD in women with recurrent abortion is much higher than in those with infertility. LPD was found in 40% of women with recurrent spontaneous abortion when the luteal phase was evaluated with at least two endometrial biopsies (Daya et al, 1988). The probability of an abnormal second biopsy appears to be higher when the first biopsy result reveals a LPD (Collins, 1990). It has been estimated that, by chance alone, LPD can be observed in 20% of biopsies in a single cycle and in 4% of biopsies if two cycles are studied (Collins, 1988). Therefore, the diagnosis of LPD requires a maturational delay to be documented in at least two cycles.

Promising New Diagnostic Techniques

Daily Salivary Progesterone Measurements. The total progesterone output, as measured by the area under the progesterone profile curve, is significantly lower in LPD cycles than in normal cycles. Daily serum progesterone sampling is impractical, inconvenient, invasive, and costly, leading to problems with patient compliance. In contrast, analysis of saliva samples provided on a daily basis is feasible because the assay is now relatively simple and inexpensive, and the patient finds it convenient and stress-free. Levels of progesterone concentrations associated with normal luteal function have now been established (Finn et al, 1988) and may be useful to assess suboptimal progesterone production associated with LPD.

Progestagen-Associated Endometrial Protein. The level of progestagen-associated endometrial protein in serum increases during the luteal phase. In women with LPD, the levels were outside the normal CI in 83%, compared with only 16% in women with normal cycles (Joshi et al, 1986). Measurement of this protein holds promise for the diagnosis of LPD, but further study is required to determine its accuracy as a diagnostic test.

Morphometric Analysis of Endometrium. The technique of morphometric analysis has been applied to histologic dating of luteal phase endometrium using the LH peak as an indicator of ovulation (Li et al, 1988). Among 17 measurements studied, 5 were considered to be important, 4 of which pertained to glands (i.e., number of mitoses per 1000 gland cells, amount of secretion in the gland lumen, volume fraction of gland occupied by gland cell, and amount of pseudostratification of gland cells) and 1 to stroma (i.e., amount of predecidual reaction). A major drawback of this method is that it is time consuming. However, with advances in computer technology, and the use of image analysis, this may become less of a problem.

Ultrastructure of Endometrial Glandular Epithelium. Electron microscopy has been used to study the glandular epithelium of the endometrium on biopsy samples taken in the luteal phase as determined from the LH surge (Dockerty et al, 1988). The ultrastructural sequence of changes observed has been documented. Even though considerable variability in structure exists from one gland to another within a single biopsy, this technique holds promise for the diagnosis of LPD in the future.

TREATMENT

Progesterone Supplementation. The suboptimal production of progesterone in LPD suggests that the logical treatment for this condition is to provide progesterone supplementation. Whether the underlying cause is inadequate follicular development or is related to inadequate postovulatory events, supplemental progesterone should promote normal secretory transformation of the endometrium.

Although other routes of administration of progesterone include oral and intramuscular, the use of vaginal suppositories is relatively common. The patient should be instructed to monitor her cycle with a BBT graph to document ovulation and avoid premature administration, which can inhibit ovulation and, at the same time, induce a thermal shift on the BBT, giving misleading indication of a postovulatory state. Therefore, treatment should begin on the third day of persistent temperature elevation, when it can be confirmed that the shift in temperature is not a transient phenomenon. Furthermore, progesterone treatment should not be commenced before cycle day 14. The initial dose is 50 mg/day in two divided doses, an amount that is comparable to that observed during the peak of progesterone production by a normally functioning corpus luteum. Serum progesterone levels during treatment are similar to those found during a normal cycle, and the luteal phase is not prolonged by more than 2 days (Nillius and Johansson, 1971; Daya et al, 1983). An endometrial biopsy should be performed during the treatment cycle to confirm that correction of the LPD has occurred. If LPD persists, the dose may be doubled until an in-phase endometrial biopsy result has been achieved. Progesterone supplementation at this effective dose is continued until 10 to 12 weeks' gestation, by which time the placenta would have taken over the role of progesterone production from the corpus luteum. Alternatively, once pregnancy has been confirmed, a change to treatment with 17α-hydroxyprogesterone caproate, 125 mg twice weekly or 250 mg weekly, has been recommended (Wentz, 1979). Initiation of progesterone supplementation after pregnancy has been confirmed may not be effective because the endometrium has not been adequately prepared to allow postimplantation development of the fetoplacental unit.

The dose of progesterone administered intramuscularly is 12.5 mg daily. Oral administration (Maxson and Hargrove, 1985) using a micronized preparation or nasal administration (Steege et al, 1986) has been described but, to date, therapeutic efficacy studies using these preparations have not been performed in women with habitual abortion.

Synthetic progestational agents should not be used to treat LPD because they may have a lytic effect on the corpus luteum and can produce glandular stromal disparity, thereby making the situation worse (Johansson, 1971; Dallenbach-Hellwig, 1988). Also, their use in early pregnancy is contraindicated because of their teratogenic potential; the 19-nor-progestins are derivatives of testosterone and can cause masculinization of a female fetus in addition to possible cardiovascular and limb reduction defects (Wentz, 1988).

To date there have been no prospective, randomized, double-blind, placebo-controlled studies to evaluate the efficacy of treatment for LPD among women with habitual abortion. Consequently, outcome data are limited to descriptive studies in which successful pregnancies with treatment have been reported in 81% to 92% of patients (Table 9–16) (Jones and Delfs, 1951; Tho et al, 1979; Daya et al, 1988).

A meta-analysis of controlled trials of progesterone or progestational agents used in early pregnancy in women with a history of habitual abortion demonstrated a significant improvement in pregnancy outcome compared to placebo (odds ratio 3.09, 95% CI 1.28 to 7.42) (Daya, 1989b). It is important to emphasize that, in patients with habitual abortion, early pregnancy failure despite treatment may occur because of a chromosomal anomaly occurring de novo. Thus, before one concludes that treatment has failed, it is important to perform karyotypic analysis on the products of conception.

The safety of progestational treatment during early pregnancy has been studied at length. In the United States, the Food and Drug Administration (FDA) issued a warning against the use of both synthetic progestins and progesterone during pregnancy. There is no disagreement regarding synthetic progestational agents not being used because of their potential teratogenic risks. However, the issue regarding the possible teratogenic risks of progesterone use in pregnancy remains unresolved. The concern that treating patients to prevent abortion may allow more abnormal fetuses to survive to term has also been addressed. At a symposium sponsored by the American Society for Reproductive Medicine (formerly known as the American Fertility Society), Jones (1978) was unable to find any difference in the congenital anomaly rates between 155 treated and 293 untreated patients (Andrews, 1979). Similarly, Janerich and Slone (1978) indicated that no causal relationship could be demonstrated between progesterone or 17α-hydroxyprogesterone and fetal anomalies (Andrews, 1979). Neither Resseguie et al (1985), who studied 988 cases from a review of 24,000

Table 9–16. OUTCOME OF PROGESTERONE TREATMENT FOR LPD IN WOMEN WITH RECURRENT ABORTION

STUDY	NO. PREGNANCIES	SUCCESSFUL OUTCOME (%)
Jones and Delfs (1951)	34	31 (92)
Tho et al (1979)	23	21 (91)
Daya et al (1988)	16	13 (81)
TOTAL	73	65 (89)

women, nor Michales et al (1983), who reported the experience of treating women with recurrent miscarriage, found any evidence that progesterone or 17α-hydroxyprogesterone caproate was associated with congenital malformations. In a longer term study by Katz et al (1985), the outcomes in a cohort of 2754 infants born to mothers who were treated with progestational agents because of bleeding in the first trimester were assessed. 17α-Hydroxyprogesterone acetate was the most common drug to which these infants were exposed, and over half of them were exposed prior to 10 weeks' gestation. The study failed to demonstrate an incidence of fetal malformations that was higher than that expected in women with threatened abortion (Worcester et al, 1950). In all these studies, progestational agents were administered after the women had missed their expected menses. To avoid the possibility of bias in the outcomes from treatment commenced after implantation, a study was carried out to investigate the potential for teratogenesis with progesterone given during the early developmental stages of the fetus. Treatment was begun 3 to 4 days after ovulation and was continued until approximately 14 weeks' gestation (Check et al, 1986). The congenital anomaly rate was reported to be 1.3%, a rate no different from that expected by chance.

With respect to safety, no apparent toxicity has been documented with progesterone administration, even with very high doses. For example, 17α-hydroxyprogesterone caproate at doses 20 to 40 times higher than those employed in pregnancy has been used in the treatment of endometrial carcinoma without side effects other than local discomfort at the injection site (Andrews, 1979; Michaelis et al, 1983).

In November 1981, the Fertility and Maternal Health Drugs Advisory Committee to the FDA held hearings regarding the safety and efficacy of progesterone. After hearing testimony, the committee again unanimously recommended to the FDA that, on the basis of safety, progesterone and 17α-hydroxyprogesterone be excluded from the concerns regarding synthetic progestins (Wentz, 1982). Similarly, in Canada, progesterone treatment is not yet approved for use in pregnancy, but it is hoped that this view can be changed by obtaining evidence of its efficacy from randomized, controlled trials. There is no reliable evidence that indicates progesterone and 17α-hydroxyprogesterone to be teratogenic, nor is there any reason to expect them to be, because they are physiologic and used in physiologic doses (Andrews, 1979). From the evidence available, the benefits of properly prescribed progesterone therapy for LPD appear to outweigh the risks, but, before patients are offered treatment, the issues pertaining to treatment must be discussed to allow appropriate informed consent to therapy.

Clomiphene Citrate. Experimental evidence has shown that FSH deficiency during follicular growth is associated with defective corpus luteum function (DiZerega and Hodgen, 1981). The rationale for using clomiphene citrate to treat LPD is that it enhances the levels of FSH in the follicular phase (Kase, 1973). It acts by binding to the estrogen receptor in the hypothalamus, thereby inhibiting the replenishment of the receptor and interfering with the negative feedback effect of endogenous estrogens on gonadotropin secretion, possibly by altering the pattern of hypothalamic GnRH release (Kerin et al, 1985). Clomiphene is taken orally in a daily dose of 50 mg from days 5 to 9 of the menstrual cycle and may be increased to 100 or 150 mg/day, and rarely to 200 to 250 mg/day, to obtain the appropriate response. Several reports (reviewed by Daya [1990]) have shown it to be effective in treating LPD and raising progesterone levels in the luteal phase. It appears to be highly successful when used to treat LPD of the short luteal phase variety; seven of eight such women (88%) ultimately conceived in one series (Kerin et al, 1985). This observation is not unexpected because a short luteal phase is associated with FSH deficiency in the follicular phase (DiZerega and Hodgen, 1981). However, because in most cases LPD occurs in association with a luteal phase of normal duration, there is controversy regarding this treatment, especially because a large discrepancy exists between the rate of ovulation and the number of pregnancies (Garcia et al, 1977). Adding to this controversy is the paradoxical observation that clomiphene can *induce* LPD (Daya, 1990; Cook et al, 1984). Furthermore, in a significant proportion of patients with LPD, the defect remains uncorrected despite treatment. In a review of 108 patients with LPD, persistence of the defect was reported in 52% (range 41% to 78%) (Daya, 1990).

Several possibilities may account for these conflicting observations. First, estradiol is necessary to induce estrogen and progesterone receptors in the endometrium and, because clomiphene binds to estrogen receptors, it may compete with estradiol at the receptor level, producing failure of endometrial maturation as a result of inadequate receptor activation (Marut and Hodgen, 1982). In fact, inadequate numbers of estrogen and progesterone receptor sites have been observed in the endometrium of women with LPD (Levy et al, 1980). The adverse effect of clomiphene on endometrial development was also observed ultrasonographically. Women randomly assigned to treatment with human menopausal gonadotropin (hMG) had a significantly thicker endometrium than those treated with clomiphene and hMG, even though the serum concentrations of estradiol did not differ in the two groups (Gonen and Casper, 1990). Second, interference with the action of estrogen within the ovary may attenuate the response of the follicle to the increase in FSH induced by clomiphene (Marut and Hodgen, 1982). A third possibility is that clomiphene is not effective in treating a type of LPD in which the endometrium is out of phase but demonstrates synchronous development of both endometrial glands and stroma, as opposed to a second type in which asynchronous development occurs (Witten and Martin, 1985). In the former group, progesterone secretion is probably defective or inadequate, suggesting that progesterone therapy would be associated with high pregnancy rates, whereas, in the latter group, clomiphene is expected to produce better pregnancy rates (Witten and Martin, 1985).

Thus it is clear that, although clomiphene is not the first choice of treatment for habitual abortion caused by LPD, it requires careful titration when administered so that the dose that will produce the desired effect on the endometrium can be established.

Human Chorionic Gonadotropin. Human chorionic gonadotropin is an effective luteotrophic agent that has been used to treat LPD by stimulating the corpus luteum to produce progesterone. It should be effective in stimulating corpus luteum function because it can combine with LH receptors, except in those instances in which the reduced hormone production by the gland is the result of inadequate LH receptor expression. The recommended dose and frequency of hCG administration are empirically derived and vary from center to center. It has been suggested that hCG be given at the approximate time of ovulation at a dose of 5000 to 10,000 IU intramuscularly to ensure more complete luteinization (Fritz, 1988). Thereafter, hCG is given every 2 to 5 days at a dose of 1500 to 5000 IU. Treatment is discontinued after the 12th postovulatory day to avoid a high incidence of pseudopregnancy. Once pregnancy has been achieved, exogenous hCG should no longer be necessary. However, some investigators have recommended its administration be continued until the beginning of the second trimester (March, 1987). Patients must be informed that, in the absence of pregnancy, this therapy may delay the onset of menses. Also, because of the long half-life (about 12 hours) of hCG, pregnancy testing should be avoided for at least 7 days after the last hCG injection to avoid false-positive results.

There have been no controlled studies of hCG for LPD treatment, and no consensus exists on the appropriate regimen. Evidence from monkey studies indicates that premature hCG administration promotes atresia rather than luteinization (Williams and Hodgen, 1980). Furthermore, the steroid response varies with the age of the corpus luteum (Wilks and Noble, 1983; Ottobre and Stouffer, 1984). When administered immediately after the LH surge, an increase in estradiol and progesterone secretion fails to occur, whereas treatment begun on day 5 of the luteal phase is associated with a marked and sustained steroid hormone response (Ottobre and Stouffer, 1984). Treatment begun in the midluteal phase is associated with circulating levels of progesterone similar to those observed in early pregnancy, but the levels decline despite continued treatment. Finally, treatment begun in the late luteal phase is associated with a brief and attenuated progesterone response, with levels falling steadily during treatment (Wilks and Noble, 1983; Ottobre and Stouffer, 1984).

For a variety of reasons, hCG is not the drug of first choice in treating women with habitual abortion resulting from LPD. The uncertain response to treatment, the expense and logistical difficulties encountered with parenteral therapy, and problems associated with the induction of pseudopregnancy make hCG treatment relatively unattractive (Fritz, 1988). Furthermore, if the corpus luteum is hyporesponsive to endogenous hCG produced during pregnancy, then exogenous treatment is not likely to be helpful.

Gonadotropins. The evidence that the low estradiol levels in the follicular phase resulting from FSH deficiency result in LPD has led several investigators to administer FSH and hMG therapeutically (Daya, 1990). Some patients may benefit from such treatment, even though this option is time consuming, inconvenient, and expensive.

Gonadotropin-Releasing Hormone. Pulsatile GnRH treatment begun early in the cycle appears to be able to correct LPD, presumably by inducing normal folliculogenesis (Daya, 1990). Further studies have to be undertaken to evaluate this option of therapy.

Diabetes Mellitus

An association between spontaneous abortion and diabetes has been observed, but, in the absence of control groups, this inference may be questioned. Other confounding factors complicating the evaluation of a possible causal link are the lack of classification according to severity of disease and the inclusion of congenital anomalies and induced abortions in the estimation of spontaneous abortion rates. In one summary of published data, the frequency of spontaneous abortion ranged from 3.8% to 28%, with a mean for the entire sample of 1707 pregnancies of 12.3%, a rate not significantly different from that of nondiabetic women (Gellis and Hsia, 1959). In a more recent review of the literature from 1950 to 1986, 807 spontaneous abortions (10.0%) were reported among 8041 diabetic pregnancies examined (Kalter, 1987). There was no correlation between the severity of diabetes (classified according to White) and the rate of spontaneous abortion. Similarly, no increased frequency of abortion was seen in pregnancies complicated by gestational diabetes. In contrast, Miodovnik et al (1984) reported that, among insulin-dependent diabetic women, the spontaneous abortion rate was 29.5%, suggesting the existence of a causal relationship. Also, Dicker et al (1988) observed that, among 59 women attending a preconceptional clinic for intensified insulin therapy and glucose monitoring, 5 (8.5%) had spontaneous abortion, compared with 10 of 35 women (28.6%) without such strict control. It has been suggested that these adverse outcomes may be the result of abnormal magnesium metabolism. Insulin-dependent diabetic pregnant women appear to be at increased risk of magnesium deficiency owing to increased loss of magnesium in the urine; the glycosylated hemoglobin level was significantly higher and the magnesium level significantly lower in 21 pregnancies with adverse fetal outcome (17 spontaneous abortions) compared to 75 successful pregnancies (Mimouni et al, 1987).

Few studies have examined the role of maternal diabetes in recurrent spontaneous abortion. In a study of 154 diabetic patients, the frequency of two or more abortions was similar among gestational diabetics and matched controls (10.6% vs. 9.1%) and insulin-dependent diabetics and matched controls (14.6% vs. 16.7%) (Crane and Wahl, 1981).

Thus, from the available data, there is no evidence to support an association between gestational insulin-dependent diabetes that is under good control, and spontaneous or recurrent abortion. In contrast, poor glycemic control may result in an increased likelihood of abortion.

Thyroid Disease

Thyroid disease is relatively common among young women and can have adverse effects on pregnancy. In the past, thyroid disease was thought to be frequently associated with pregnancy wastage. However, the correlation was usually based on clinical and/or physical findings on laboratory tests done with older laboratory techniques (Zbella, 1989). Reports acknowledge that there is an association between thyroid disease and spontaneous or recurrent abortion, but the frequency is very small.

HYPOTHYROIDISM

Despite the fact that hypothyroidism is associated with an inability to conceive, it is found in 0.6% of pregnancies and appears to have an adverse effect on the outcome of the pregnancy. In a prospective study of hypothyroid women, higher incidences of abortion, stillbirth, congenital malformation, and prematurity were observed (Jones and Man, 1969).

In women with habitual abortion, 3 of 195 had moderate hypothyroidism and, in 2 of these women, normal pregnancies were achieved with thyroid replacement therapy (Stray-Pedersen and Stray-Pedersen, 1984).

HYPERTHYROIDISM

Very little information is available on the reproductive outcome of pregnant women with untreated hyperthyroidism because most women with this disorder have infertility or are already on treatment when they conceive. An increased rate of spontaneous abortion has been reported in women with hyperthyroidism (Kaplan, 1985). Also, in women with habitual abortion, hyperthyroidism may be detected infrequently (1 of 195 women in the study by Stray-Pedersen and Stray-Pedersen [1984]).

Endometriosis

A high prevalence of first-trimester spontaneous abortion has been reported in women with endometriosis, which, when surgically treated, is associated with a marked reduction in the abortion rate (Daya, 1996). Abortion rates prior to the diagnosis of endometriosis ranged from 22% to 63%, with an average of 33% (Damewood, 1989). Furthermore, pregnancy outcome appears to be related to the time interval before diagnosis; a significantly high abortion rate occurring within 1 to 2 years of diagnosis (Damewood, 1989). Also, it has been suggested that endometriosis is associated with recurrent pregnancy loss.

Several theories have been proposed to explain the pathogenesis of spontaneous abortion in endometriosis. One suggested mechanism is an alteration in prostaglandin secretion and metabolism (Muse and Wilson, 1982). Increased amounts of prostaglandin have been demonstrated in the endometrium (Willman et al, 1976) and peritoneal cavity (Drake et al, 1980) in patients with endometriosis. A second mechanism is corpus luteum dysfunction. In a study of luteal function in women with endometriosis, 45% had LPD, with mean progesterone levels lower than in women not having the disease (Grant, 1966). Similarly, in two other studies, high incidences of LPD (67% and 62%, respectively) were observed in patients with endometriosis (Cheesman et al, 1983; Gross, 1984). A third mechanism involves autoimmune dysfunction. Peritoneal irritation from endometriotic tissue may activate an immune response, resulting in increased numbers of peritoneal macrophages that could interfere with the implantation process (Muse and Wilson, 1982). Also, circulating antibodies to endometrium have been documented in patients with endometriosis (Williamson et al, 1982).

Despite these theories, there is much confusion and controversy in the literature regarding the association of endometriosis with reproductive wastage. Two major problems have been a lack of control patients to compare the data and selection bias. Women with recurrent abortion and who ultimately develop infertility may be found to have endometriosis. Also, women who have endometriosis and have spontaneous abortions are more likely to present for evaluation than those who have term pregnancies, in whom the endometriosis remains undetected.

The use of controls is important in any study to avoid erroneous conclusions resulting from bias. In a prospective study of 186 women with secondary infertility undergoing diagnostic laparoscopy, endometriosis was found in 52 women (Fitzsimmons et al, 1987). When this group was compared with a similar group without endometriosis, a slight but nonsignificant excess of spontaneous abortions was observed in the former group (45.3% vs. 34.4%). Similarly, in another study of secondary infertility, the spontaneous abortion rate in patients with untreated endometriosis was similar to that in the group without endometriosis (Metzger et al, 1986). Finally, in a randomized study of surgical ablation of minimal or mild endometriosis, the subsequent spontaneous abortion rates in the treated and untreated groups were similar (Marcoux et al, 1997).

Another factor that confuses the picture is the observation of an inverse relationship between severity of disease and abortion rate: 49% in patients with mild endometriosis, 25% with moderate disease, and 24% with severe disease (Wheeler et al, 1983).

Collectively, these facts argue that, if a causal relationship between endometriosis and spontaneous abortion exists, it is weak, and emphasize the fact that selection bias is a likely reason for the apparent association reported in the literature. It has been stated that roughly one third (10% to 15%) of the observed abortion rate may be attributed to the same factors that are operative in the general population, a further one third would be the result of selection bias, and the remaining third would be directly associated with endometriosis (Pittaway, 1988).

Infection

Reproductive tract infection is frequently cited as a cause of recurrent abortion, although it has been difficult to estimate the extent of its involvement. Sporadic spontaneous abortions have been attributed to a variety of organisms, including bacteria (e.g., *Listeria monocytogenes*, *Campylobacter* species, *Salmonella typhi*, *Brucella* species, *Chlamydia trachomatis*, and *Treponema pallidum*); viruses (e.g., cytomegalovirus, rubella, herpes simplex, human immunodeficiency virus, and variola); mycoplasmas (e.g., *Ureaplasma urealyticum* and *Mycoplasma hominis*); and parasites (e.g., *Toxoplasma gondii and Plasmodium*). The role of infection in recurrent abortion remains controversial because in many studies adequate control groups have not been used. Nevertheless, several microorganisms have been implicated in causing recurrent abortion; two of these are discussed below.

It is possible that ascending infection into the upper genital tract can occur early in the first trimester, before the chorioamniotic membranes fuse with the decidua, and obliterate the endometrial cavity. However, this is not a common occurrence, probably because there are several protective factors in pregnancy that prevent fetal infection. The chorioamniotic membranes act as a barrier to microorganisms. Also, amniotic fluid has bacterial inhibitory substances that provide additional protection (Watts and Eschenbach, 1988). This antibacterial activity increases as pregnancy advances (Evaldson and Nord, 1981). The placental floor behaves in the same way as the blood-brain barrier, but it is not a perfect barrier because some microorganisms can pass from the maternal bloodstream through the placenta into the fetus. The presence of immunoglobulin A (IgA) in cervical mucus may protect against ascending infec-

tion. In addition, maternal immunoglobulin (IgG) is readily transported across the placenta to the fetus and provides protection for the fetus. Finally, small amounts of immunoglobulin M (IgM) are produced in utero by the fetus, which also has the ability to activate cell-mediated immune responses.

Genital Mycoplasmas

Mycoplasmas are unique microorganisms that are neither bacteria nor viruses, but fall somewhere between these two groups. They differ from bacteria in that they have no cell wall, but instead are surrounded by a nonrigid triple-layered membrane. They differ from viruses because they contain both DNA and RNA and, therefore, are capable of self-replication. They are common inhabitants of the oropharyngeal and genital mucous membranes. *Mycoplasma hominis* and *U. urealyticum* (also called T-mycoplasma, T-strains, or ureaplasmas) can be isolated frequently from the genital tract of both men and women. Colonization appears to be directly related to sexual activity. Postpubertal women with no history of sexual activity have low rates of colonization, similar to those seen in children. Among sexually active women, colonization increases in proportion with the number of sexual partners. *Ureaplasma urealyticum* was recovered from 6% of women with no history of sexual contact, whereas, with one, two, and three or more sexual partners, the colonization rates were 38%, 55%, and 75%, respectively (McCormack et al, 1972, 1973). *Mycoplasma hominis* showed a similar pattern, occurring in 1% of women with no sexual contact and rising to 17% among those with a history of three or more partners. A similar pattern was observed among men, but the rate was lower, suggesting that women are more susceptible to colonization by genital mycoplasmas.

The role of genital mycoplasmas in recurrent spontaneous abortion is still controversial. Chromosome breaks and tetraploidy have been observed more frequently in cultures of peripheral blood lymphocytes infected with *U. urealyticum* compared to uninfected cultures (Kundsin et al, 1971). Although this finding suggests a mechanism for spontaneous abortion, similar in vivo effects on embryonic tissue have not been observed. *Mycoplasma* was also recovered significantly more frequently in tissue from spontaneous abortions in both the first and second trimesters of pregnancy compared to tissue from induced abortions (Sompolinsky et al, 1975). Also, febrile patients had a higher rate of *Mycoplasma* isolation than afebrile patients undergoing spontaneous abortion. Cervical colonization rates were similar among patients with habitual abortion and those with infertility compared to control patients, but endometrial isolates were significantly more frequent among women who had a history of spontaneous abortion (28%) or infertility (50%) than among control patients (7%) (Stray-Pedersen et al, 1978). Although suggestive of an ascending infection by mycoplasmas, specifically *U. urealyticum*, it is difficult to exclude the possibility that the necrotic products of conception became infected after demise of the fetus rather than the loss being caused by the infection. Also, studies of mycoplasmas and recurrent abortion suffer from lack of power owing to small sample sizes, because control groups also have a high frequency of colonization of the lower genital tract. Thus the size of the clinically important difference that can be detected between the control and experimental groups is small. Also prospective studies have not documented an increased rate of spontaneous abortion among women with a positive genital culture before conception (Gump et al, 1984) or at the first prenatal visit (DiMusto et al, 1973).

Efficacy studies of antibiotic treatment in couples with recurrent pregnancy wastage have not produced convincing results. Although patients with positive cervical and/or endometrial cultures treated with doxycycline had a high rate (16 of 19) of term deliveries in the next pregnancy (Stray-Pedersen et al, 1978), the lack of a control group makes it difficult to evaluate the efficacy of treatment. In another study, oral doxycycline, 200 mg initially followed by 100 mg daily for 30 days, was administered to couples with pregnancy losses (Quinn et al, 1983). Persistent colonization after treatment was treated with a similar dose for a second course, and a third course of 200 mg daily for 10 days was given when necessary. The pregnancy loss rate decreased from 96% to 48%. Unfortunately, the study was flawed by the use of historical controls, which are not appropriate for the assessment of efficacy of treatment. A subsequent controlled trial from the same institution failed to show any difference in live birth rate in women treated with erythromycin or placebo for the duration of the pregnancy (Quinn et al, 1989). Unfortunately, the sample size (30 patients) was too small for the study to have sufficient power to detect a significant improvement with treatment.

The evidence linking genital mycoplasma infection as a cause of recurrent spontaneous abortion remains inconclusive. In view of the data that are currently available and the observation that pregnancies associated with mycoplasma isolation from the genital tract appear to be at risk for poor outcome, it seems reasonable to recommend antibiotic treatment to couples with mycoplasma and a history of recurrent abortion. Prior to pregnancy, both partners can be treated with doxycycline at an initial dose of 200 mg followed by 100 mg daily for 2 weeks; cultures should then be repeated. In 5% to 10% of patients, the organism persists despite repeated treatment. Such patients could be offered erythromycin treatment during pregnancy. In addition, in women with negative cultures following treatment, genital cultures should be repeated in early pregnancy to detect and treat those patients in whom colonization recurs. It must be remembered that this recommendation is based on information derived from studies with methodologic flaws and must be interpreted with caution until well-designed controlled studies can shed more light on this controversial issue.

Listeria monocytogenes

This microorganism is a motile, microaerophilic gram-positive rod of low pathogenicity. Although infections occur in patients with reduced immunity, about half of the recognized infections with *Listeria* occur in pregnant women (Watts and Eschenbach, 1988). Rectal carriage is more common than vaginal carriage, and a major source is ingestion of contaminated foods, especially dairy products. The fetus can acquire the organism during maternal bacteremia or, rarely, as a result of ascending genital infection. Associations between listeriosis and repeated pregnancy loss usually have been based on a positive culture in the index pregnancy, with information on pregnancy loss derived from a retrospective history rather than prospective studies of further listeriosis (Ochlschlager, 1960). *Listeria monocytogenes* was recovered from 25 of 34 women with recurrent abortion compared to none of 87 controls (Rappaport and Rabinovitz, 1960). With treatment, all eight pregnant women who had positive cultures and received penicillin therapy carried their pregnancies to term. Unfortunately, no controls were included in this series, and the issue of listerosis as a cause of recurrent abortion awaits further study.

Immunologic Factors

There is increasing evidence to support immunologic mechanisms for recurrent abortion. There are two main categories of immunologically mediated pregnancy loss: autoimmune and alloimmune dysfunction.

Autoimmune Dysfunction

It has long been recognized that autoimmune conditions, such as systemic lupus erythematosus (SLE), are associated with pregnancy loss. More recently, attention has focused on the association between the presence of anti-phospholipid antibodies (aPL) and fetal loss. The anti-phospholipid antibody syndrome (APS) is now accepted as a condition associated with fetal loss, aPL, and previous thrombosis (Harris, 1986; Hughes et al, 1986). In the absence of thrombosis, the condition is referred to as subclinical autoimmunity. There is much debate about what constitutes a clinically significant elevation of aPL. In some studies, investigators have established the cut-off level at three standard deviations above the mean in a control population. A lack of consistency in the definition of an abnormal result makes it difficult to adequately review the evidence in the literature.

SYSTEMIC LUPUS ERYTHEMATOSUS

Pregnancy loss is more common among women with SLE than among normal women. The median rate of pregnancy loss among nine studies was 31% (range 10% to 46%) (Branch and Silver, 1996). Unfortunately, none of these studies included appropriately matched, prospectively acquired controls. The median rate of spontaneous abortion was 10%, a figure comparable to that of the normal population. However, the median rate of loss in the second or third trimester was 8%, a figure considerably higher than the rate of 1% to 3% seen in the normal population.

Other negative prognostic factors associated with pregnancy loss in SLE include presence of disease before conception, onset of disease during pregnancy, and presence of underlying renal disease.

Treatment. During pregnancy, treatment with low-dose aspirin and calcium supplementation is recommended to reduce the likelihood of pre-eclampsia (Branch and Silver, 1996). Women with active SLE should be advised to delay attempts to conceive until the disease is in remission. Those with moderate renal insufficiency should be counseled about the increased probability of pregnancy loss in women with severe renal disease, and should be advised against pregnancy.

ANTIPHOSPHOLIPID ANTIBODY SYNDROME

This condition is characterized by the production of moderate to high levels of aPL and at least one clinical feature, such as pregnancy loss, thrombosis, and autoimmune thrombocytopenia (Table 9–17). Laboratory tests should be positive on at least two occasions more than 8 weeks apart. Women with APS should have at least one clinical and one laboratory feature at some time in the course of their disease.

Well-established assays are available for three aPLs: (1) biologic false-positive test for syphilis (BF-STS), which is the least specific test for APS and is not evaluated routinely; (2) lupus anticoagulant (LA); and (3) anti-cardiolipin antibody (aCL). These assays all evaluate the binding of aPL moieties on negatively charged phospholipids or moieties formed by the interaction of negatively charged phospholipids with other lipids, phospholipids, or proteins (Branch and Silver, 1996). The immunoassay for aCL is calibrated against standards and measured in GPL (for IgG aCL) or MPL (for IgM aCL) units. The results are interpreted semiquantitatively as negative, low-positive, medium-positive, or high-positive (Harris, 1990). Low-positive results are of questionable clinical significance and may be found in 3% to 5% of normal individuals (Silver et al, 1996). The role of IgA aCL requires further study.

The initial reports of case series describing a relationship between aPL and pregnancy loss led to numerous publications, some in support of and others refuting the causal link. However, on the basis of several sources of evidence, an independent association between aPL and pregnancy loss seems to have been established.

1. aPL is persistently positive in a small, but clinically important, proportion of women with recurrent pregnancy loss. Although the definition of recurrent pregnancy loss (RPL) used in the literature varies from two or more losses to three or more losses, the median rates of loss in RPL versus controls are, respectively, 7% versus 0% for LA, 8% versus 2% for aCL, and 11% versus 2.5% for all aPL (Branch and Silver, 1996).
2. In prospective studies screening for aPL in early pregnancy, an increased rate of pregnancy loss has been observed among women positive for aPL (Lockwood et al, 1989; Pattison et al, 1993).
3. A significant proportion (24% to 32%) of women with aPL, followed prospectively through another pregnancy, had pregnancy losses despite treatment with glucocorticoids, heparin, low-dose aspirin, or a combination of these medications (Branch and Silver, 1996).
4. Injection of either aPL IgG fractions from women with APS or monoclonal aCL antibodies into mice in the first half of pregnancy caused fetal death (Branch et al, 1990; Blank et al, 1991).

Despite these observations, it should be noted that substantial levels of aPL may be found, albeit infrequently, among otherwise normal women. It is also clear that early pregnancy loss is infrequently caused by aPL; the pregnancy loss most specific to APS is fetal death. In a review of aPL-related pregnancy losses, a significant proportion were found to be second-trimester or early third-trimester fetal deaths (Branch et al, 1987; Oshiro et al, 1996). The high rate of fetal death among women with APS contrasts sharply with the low rate of fetal death in women with recurrent pregnancy loss. Consequently, a history of two or more early first-trimester losses without fetal death had a specificity of only 6% for the

Table 9–17. SUGGESTED CRITERIA FOR ANTIPHOSPHOLIPID ANTIBODY SYNDROME*

CLINICAL FEATURES	LABORATORY FEATURES
Pregnancy loss	Lupus anticoagulant
Recurrent pregnancy loss	Anti-cardiolipin antibody
Fetal death	IgG, medium- or high-positive
Thrombosis	Anti-phospholipid antibody
Arterial, including stroke	IgM, medium- or high-positive and lupus anticoagulant
Venous	
Autoimmune thrombocytopenia	
Other	
Coombs'-positive hemolytic anemia	
Livedo reticularis	

*Laboratory tests should be positive on at least two occasions more than 8 weeks apart. Women with APS should have at least one clinical and one laboratory feature at some time in the course of their disease.

presence of aPL (Branch and Silver, 1996). The importance of identifying aPL, therefore, lies not in its prevalence, but in its implication for the patient and the fact that it is a potentially treatable cause of pregnancy loss (Branch and Silver, 1996).

The death of the fetus is typically preceded by ultrasonographic evidence of fetal growth restriction, oligohydramnios, and fetal heart rate abnormalities, indicating hypoxemia (Branch and Silver, 1996). These effects are the consequence of placental insufficiency and reduced blood flow to the intervillons space resulting from placental vasculopathy (De Wolf et al, 1987; Erlendsson et al, 1993). Unfortunately, histologic examination of the placenta in cases of fetal death associated with APS has not always demonstrated such vasculopathy (Out et al, 1991).

Treatment. Treatment for women with aPL has included antiplatelet agents, immunosuppressive medication, and anticoagulants. Although initial reports recommended prednisone and low-dose aspirin, a placebo-controlled randomized trial demonstrated no benefit with this approach (Laskin et al, 1997). In fact, women on treatment had a higher rate of adverse effects, including hypertension, gestational diabetes, cataracts, and preterm delivery. Consequently, the current recommendation is to avoid prednisone in the treatment of recurrent pregnancy loss associated with the presence of aPL.

Heparin administration during pregnancy was introduced as treatment in the early to mid-1980s. Successful pregnancies have been reported in 75% to 93% of patients with mean daily doses ranging from 17,500 to 24,700 units (Rosove et al, 1990; Branch et al, 1992; Cowchock et al, 1992). However, in the absence of adequate controls, the efficacy of this approach awaits confirmation.

The use of heparin and aspirin, when compared with aspirin alone, was found to be efficacious in a randomized study (Rai et al, 1997). However, there have been no placebo-controlled studies with adequate power to test the efficacy of aspirin alone. Small studies have shown no beneficial effect with aspirin (Edelman et al, 1986).

Reports of case series claiming benefit from intravenous immune globulin (IVIG) have generated interest in the use of this treatment option. However, no efficacy studies have been conducted.

To date, there have been no placebo-controlled trials with sufficient power to evaluate the efficacy of any of the treatment options that have been described. Consequently, recommendations on which treatment is appropriate cannot be made at this time.

ANTINUCLEAR ANTIBODIES

Antinuclear antibodies (ANAs) have been detected in some women with recurrent pregnancy loss, the rates ranging from 5% to 29% (Cowchock et al, 1986; Edelman et al, 1986; Maier and Parke, 1989; Kwak et al, 1992; Bahar et al, 1993). However, when compared with controls, these rates were not statistically significantly different. In a much larger study, a similar proportion (16%) of women with recurrent pregnancy loss had ANAs, compared with normal nonpregnant or pregnant women (Harger et al, 1989). Although the proportion of women with recurrent pregnancy loss who had ANA titers at 1:80 or greater was higher than among controls, the outcome of a subsequent pregnancy with treatment in patients with recurrent pregnancy loss was similar in the ANA-positive and ANA-negative groups (52% vs. 67% live birth rates) (Harger et al, 1989).

Collectively, these observations suggest that routine testing for ANA is not warranted in women with recurrent pregnancy loss.

ANTITHYROID ANTIBODIES

Antithyroid antibodies, and possibly subclinical thyroid disease, have been suggested to have a causal role in recurrent pregnancy loss. Screening for antithyroid antibodies among 552 women during their first prenatal visit identified either antithyroglobulin or antimicrosomal antibodies in 20% of the women (Stagnaro-Green et al. 1990). The rate of pregnancy loss was significantly higher among those with antibodies compared to those without (17% vs. 8.4%, respectively). Similar findings have been reported by others, including observations among women achieving conception through assisted reproductive techniques (Glinoer et al, 1991; Lejuene et al, 1993; Branch and Silver, 1996).

In contrast, the findings of a more recent study raise questions about the association between antithyroid antibodies and recurrent pregnancy loss (Pratt et al, 1993). In this study, the prevalence of antithyroid antibodies among women with recurrent pregnancy loss was not significantly different from that among female blood bank controls (31% vs. 20%). It has been suggested that the discrepancy, in part, can be explained by the fact that the test has optimal predictive value only if blood samples are taken within the first few months of pregnancy (Stagnaro-Green et al, 1990).

It is clear that further study is required to evaluate the role, if any, of antithyroid antibodies in recurrent pregnancy loss so that treatment options can be identified.

Alloimmune Dysfunction

Women having spontaneous abortions of karyotypically normal pregnancies have been found to have elevated levels of natural killer (NK) cells in the blood (Clark and Coulamb, 1995). Increased levels of NK cells in normal nonpregnant women seem to be associated with a higher probability of spontaneous abortion in a subsequent pregnancy (Aoki et al, 1995). Although trophoblast at the the maternal-fetal interface is resistant to lysis by cytotoxic T cells and antibody-dependent cytotoxic cells, it is readily damaged by NK cells that have been activated by cytokines, such as interleukin-2, to become lymphokine-activated killer cells (Clark, 1991). The interaction between macrophages and NK cells may also have a role in reproductive failure by facilitating the interaction between these cells, thereby enhancing the abortion process through the release of γ-interferon (γ-IFN) and tumor necrosis factor-α (Clark, 1990; Chaouat 35 al, 1990).

Susceptibility to the effects of NK cells can be determined by local and systemic factors. The NK cells of the conventional CD 56^+16^+ type in the circulation may be found in high concentration in the uterus in women who have abortions (Lachapelle et al, 1995; Vassiliadou and Bulmer, 1995), suggesting that the cytotoxic action is at the implantation site. Furthermore, abortion does not occur when immunosuppressive activity can be detected at the implantation site.

MECHANISMS FOR ALLOIMMUNE SUPPRESSION

There are several mechanisms interacting at the maternal-fetal interface that result in pregnancy success (Daya, 1997).

Immunologic Effect of Progesterone. Pregnancy results in the activation of progesterone receptors on the surface of CD8$^+$ T cells (Szekeres-Bartho et al, 1989). These T cells are stimulated by progesterone to secrete a 34-kDa factor that suppresses cytolytic activity of NK cells. Thus a deficiency in progesterone production may lead to inadequate suppression of the cytolytic activity of NK cells and result in pregnancy failure.

Immunotrophism. Immunotrophism is a process whereby T cells become activated by placental trophoblast to produce cytokines that stimulate better growth of trophoblast (Wegmann, 1988). In this way, a robust barrier of cells is produced to more effectively resist lysis by the immune effector cells of the mother.

T Helper Cells. Primed T cells may develop along one of two pathways. The Th1 pathway results in the activation of T cells to produce abortogenic cytokines such as interleukin-1 and γ-IFN, whereas Th2 cells produce interleukin-3, -4 and -10, which promote antibody formation that blocks inflammation and NK cell activation (Wegmann et al, 1993). In normal pregnancy, there is a shift in the pattern of T-cell activation along the Th2 pathway whereby the abortogenic activity of NK cells is blocked. Trophoblast and placental cells from women with recurrent abortion have been reported to stimulate the Th1-type pattern of cytokine response (Hill et al, 1992).

Natural Suppressor Cells. In the decidua, a population of small lymphocytic cells that are believed to be neither T nor B cells can be stimulated by trophoblast to produce immunosuppressor factors (Clark et al, 1994). The activity of these cells, which release immunosuppressor molecules that are closely related to transforming growth factor-β (TGF-β) type 2, is high in successful pregnancy (Clark et al, 1988), whereas the abortion rate is increased in response to anti–TGF-β antibody administration (Clark et al, 1992). A deficiency of natural suppressor cells in the decidua is observed in approximately half of the women experiencing another abortion.

TJ6. TJ6, a novel suppressor protein produced by the decidua and thymus, may have an important role in preventing pregnancy failure (Ribbing et al, 1988; Lee et al, 1990). Although both TJ6 and TGF-β_2–like suppressor factor are produced in the decidua, these two molecules seem to be different (Merali et al, 1996). It has been suggested that, because the TGF-β_2–like suppressor molecule is detectable only after implantation, whereas TJ6 protein is present earlier, the two factors may have different but complimentary roles in ensuring pregnancy success (Merali et al, 1996). Thus TJ6 may be important in early pregnancy to facilitate early placentation by preventing cytolysis by NK cells. Ongoing viability and resistance to damage by NK cells is then provided by the release of TGF-β_2–like suppressor factor from the decidual natural suppressor cells.

TREATMENT

Failure in the normal alloimmune recognition process is believed to result in repeat abortion that is partner-specific and may be immunologically modifiable by exposing the female to her partner's antigens via a nonuterine route. Alternatively, passive immunization with IVIG may be possible because it is processed from a large pool of donors and, theoretically, should contain preformed antibodies of similar specificity.

Intravenous Immune Globulin. Although the exact mechanism of action of IVIG is not completely understood, it most likely involves immunosuppressive properties. Infusion of IVIG resulted in successful pregnancy and was associated with significant suppression of the numbers of peripheral CD56$^+$ and CD56$^+$/16$^+$ NK cells 7 days after treatment (Kwak et al, 1996), and a significant reduction in the cytotoxic activity of the NK cells (Ruiz et al, 1996).

The first pilot study of IVIG showed promise, with an 86% success rate in women who had had two or more previous abortions, and who underwent treatment in pregnancy. Since then, there have been several randomized studies, each with a small sample size, that have produced contradictory results (Daya et al, 1998). Several factors may have accounted for these findings, including lack of statistical power. A meta-analysis of the published trials suggested that there was a small beneficial effect with IVIG (Daya et al, 1998). However, a more detailed meta-analysis, using individual data from patients enrolled in randomized trials, rather than using data from the literature, was not able to demonstrate efficacy of IVIG in women with primary recurrent abortion (Daya et al, 1999). In women with secondary recurrent abortion there appears to be benefit, but further trials are required before such a conclusion can be verified. Also, issues such as dose of IVIG, duration of administration, and whether treatment should be commenced before conception or after implantation need to be addressed by conducting appropriate trials. Until then, the role of IVIG in recurrent abortion remains doubtful despite evidence of a plausible mechanism of its action in preventing abortion.

Leukocyte Immunization. Efficacy of leukocyte immunization was first demonstrated by Mowbray et al in 1985, but since then several trials have been published challenging the value of this treatment option (Cauchi et al, 1991; Ho et al, 1991; Gatenby et al, 1993). These conflicting observations have been explained, in part, on the basis of inadequate sample size, heterogeneity of study samples among trials, and the effect of co-intervention (Clark and Daya, 1991). To address this issue, a detailed meta-analysis of data from patients enrolled in randomized trials was undertaken under the auspices of the Ethics Committee of the American Society of Reproductive Immunology. A statistically significant treatment effect in favor of immunization was observed, although the magnitude of the effect was small—8% and 10% in two independent analyses (Recurrent Miscarriage Immunotherapy Trialists Group, 1994). This analysis included couples with both primary and secondary recurrent abortion and also those in which the female partner had positive autoimmune tests.

Consequently, a subgroup evaluation was undertaken after restricting the analysis to data from women with unexplained primary recurrent abortion in whom there was no evidence of anti-paternal antibody or autoimmunity (Daya et al, 1994). The likelihood of successful pregnancy was significantly higher with immunotherapy (relative risk = 1.46, 95% CI 1.19 to 1.69) (Daya et al, 1994).

Further restriction of the data to those from double-blind trials was imposed in order to reduce bias that could be introduced from a lack of blinding. The overall odds ratio was 2.42 (95% CI 1.31 to 4.47) in favor of immunotherapy (Daya, 1997). The absolute treatment effect was 21% (95% CI 6.3% to 34.9%) indicating that, for every five women treated with leukocyte immunization compared to no treatment, one additional successful pregnancy could be obtained. The effect of prior pregnancy losses was observed to be a negative prognostic factor, as shown in Figure 9–8. Furthermore, the effect of treatment appeared to be higher in women with a higher number of losses, demonstrating that immunotherapy may be even more efficacious in this more severe category of patients.

The challenge that awaits is to develop better diagnostic tests to identify women with alloimmune

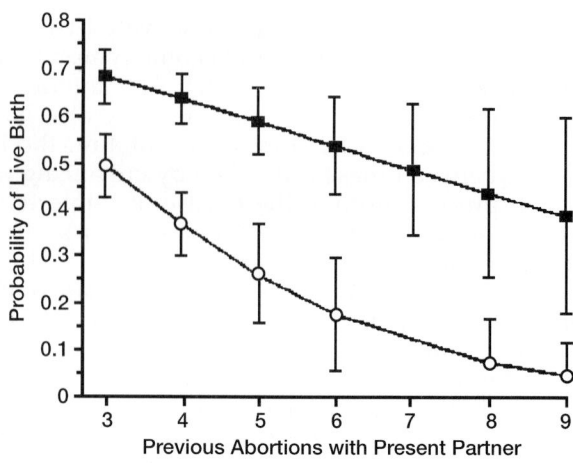

Figure 9–8
Probability of live birth with and without leukocyte immunization in unexplained primary recurrent spontaneous abortion. The probability of live birth and their standard errors are shown using the final model that predicts a successful outcome with immunization (■) and no treatment (○). (From Daya S: Immunotherapy for unexplained recurrent spontaneous abortion. Infertil Reprod Clin North Am 1997;8: 65, with permission.)

recognition failure in whom therapy can provide the best chance of success. Also, long-term follow-up studies are needed to identify whether treatment has any complications in the recipients or their offspring.

Laboratory tests should be positive on at least two occasions more than 8 weeks apart. Women with APS should have at least one clinical and one laboratory feature at some time in the course of their disease.

Environmental Factors

The possible contribution of environmental factors in causing recurrent spontaneous abortion is difficult to quantify. In couples in whom no specific cause can be identified, there is much speculation about possible environmental factors, especially because some have been associated with spontaneous abortion. Potential environmental risk factors should be reduced when possible, although one should be cautious not to ascribe a particular loss to an environmental factor unless there is strong evidence to support the finding.

A positive association between maternal cigarette smoking and spontaneous abortion has been found in many studies, including more recent studies with in vitro fertilization treatment. In one study, the odds ratio for smoking and spontaneous abortion was 1.8 (95% CI 1.3 to 2.5) (Verp, 1989). Also, among smokers there are more losses of euploid rather than aneuploid conceptuses (Alberman et al, 1976; Kline et al, 1980). Possible mechanisms by which cigarette smoking could lead to pregnancy loss include increased carboxyhemoglobin, interference with enzymes involved in oxygen transfer, decreased placental blood flow, or placental abruption, any of which might cause oxygen deprivation, deficient fetal growth, and spontaneous abortion (Harlap, 1987).

Many chemicals have been implicated in reproductive loss. Occupational exposure to anaesthetic gases may increase the risk of spontaneous abortion among exposed female personnel, but not among wives of exposed males (Verp, 1989). However, the level of exposure in the operating room today is much lower because of the use of new anaesthetic gases and effective scavenging equipment. Lead and methyl mercury are deleterious at certain levels. Wives of men exposed to vinyl chloride, chloroprene, and dibromochloropropane have suffered increased numbers of spontaneous abortions (Verp, 1989).

Considerable controversy has surrounded the potential effects of video display terminals (VDTs), the use of which has become very widespread, creating much anxiety about possible harmful effects in pregnancy. The anxiety is enhanced by the published reports of clusters of reproductive failures associated with users of VDTs, the development and sale of protective garments, and demands by trade unions for alteration of working conditions and for compensation (Blackwell and Chang, 1988). However, epidemiologic evidence has not demonstrated a statistically significant association between pregnancy failure and the use of VDTs (Blackwell and Chang, 1988). If there is an effect, it is certainly very much smaller than suggested by those who extrapolate to all users from the levels occurring in reported clusters. Surveys have shown that radiation levels from the VDT are seldom measurable above background levels with the exception of the extremely low-frequency magnetic field and static electricity (Blackwell and Chang, 1988). Levels to which operators are exposed lie comfortably below government standards for safety and are usually no greater than background forms of radiation in offices and other workplaces where VDTs are used. The Health Protection Branch of Health and Welfare Canada has measured 300 VDTs comprising 150 models, and in none of them was there measurable x-radiation above background levels (Liston, 1985). Also, no radiation was detected when some VDTs were tested in a low-level counting facility capable of measuring x-rays of low energy down to a rate of 10^{-9} rad/hr (or 10^{-7} mGy/hr)—a level 5×10^5 times less than the maximum emission rate (0.5 mrad/hr or 5 μGy/hr) allowed for television receivers and VDTs. Studies on the biologic effects of the magnetic field show equivocal results. Similarly, no adverse effect has been observed in animal studies using frequencies or levels of induced current density that pertain to VDTs.

Non-ionizing radiation emission was also examined. Microwave radiation above background has never been detected—this is to be expected because the electronic circuitry of VDTs cannot produce microwaves. Radiofrequency radiation (very low frequency) has been detected very close to the surface of some VDTs. However, the levels fall off rapidly with distance so that, at the operator position, they are either nondetectable or significantly lower than the most restrictive standard in the world. Electromagnetic fields at the power line frequency (60 Hz) have been detected. This is not surprising because such fields are associated with practically all electrical and electronic devices.

Thus, at present, it does not appear that pregnancies in women using VDTs are at risk, and the use of shielding, lead aprons, or any other protective device by VDT operators is unnecessary (Liston, 1985).

REFERENCES

Abdulla U, Diver MJ, Hipkin LJ, Davis JC: Plasma progesterone levels as an index of ovulation. Br J Obstet Gynaecol 1983;90: 543.

Abraham GE, Maroulis GB, Marshall JR: Evaluation of ovulation and corpus luteum function using measurements of plasma progesterone. Obstet Gynecol 1974;44:522.

Abramovici H, Faktor JH, Pascal B: Congenital uterine malformations as indication for cervical suture (cerclage) in habitual abortion and premature delivery. Int J Fertil 1983;28:161.

Acién P: Embryological observations on the female genital tract. Hum Reprod 1992;7:437.

Alberman E, Creasy M, Elliot M: Maternal factors associated with fetal chromosomal anomalies in spontaneous abortions. Br J Obstet Gynaecol 1976;83:621.

Alberman E, Elliott M, Creasy M, Dhadial R: Previous reproductive history in mothers presenting with spontaneous abortions. Br J Obstet Gynaecol 1975;82:366.

American Fertility Society: The American Fertility Society classification of adnexal adhesions, distal tubal occlusion, tubal occlusion secondary to tubal ligation, tubal pregnancies, müllerian anomalies and intrauterine adhesions. Fertil Steril 1988;49: 944.

Andrews WC: Luteal phase defect. Fertil Steril 1979;32:501.

Aoki K, Kajura S, Matsumoto Y, et al: Preconceptual natural killer cell activity as a predictor of miscarriage. Lancet 1995;345:1340.

Asherman JG: Amenorrhoea traumatica (atretica). J Obstet Gynaecol Br Emp 1948;55:23.

Asherman JG: Traumatic intra-uterine adhesions. J Obstet Gynaecol Br Emp 1950;57:892.

Awan AK: Some biologic correlates of pregnancy wastage. Am J Obstet Gynecol 1974;199:525.

Ayers JW, Peterson EP, Ansbacher R: Early therapy for the incompetent cervix in patients with habitual abortion. Fertil Steril 1982;38:177.

Bahar AM, Kwak JYH, Beer AE, et al: Antibodies to phospholipids and nuclear antigens in non-pregnant women with unexplained spontaneous abortions. J Reprod Immunol 1993;24:213.

Balasch J, Creus M, Marquez M, et al: The significance of luteal phase deficiency on fertility: a diagnostic and therapeutic approach. Hum Reprod 1986;1:145.

Balasch J, Vanrell JA: Corpus luteum insufficiency and fertility: a matter of controversy. Hum Reprod 1987;2:557.

Barnes AB, Colton T, Gundersen J, et al: Fertility and outcome of pregnancy in women exposed in utero to diethylstilbestrol. N Engl J Med 1980;302:609.

Bennet MJ: Congenital abnormalities of the fundus. In Bennet MJ, Edmonds DK (eds): Spontaneous and Recurrent Abortion. Oxford: Blackwell Scientific, 1987:109.

Benson RC, Durfee RB: Transabdominal cervico uterine cerclage during pregnancy for the treatment of cervical incompetency. Obstet Gynecol 1965;25:145.

Bergman P, Svennerud S: Traction test for demonstrating incompetence of the internal os of the cervix. Int J Fertil 1957;2:163.

Bernaschek G, Deutinger J, Kratochwil A: Endosonography in Obstetrics and Gynecology. Berlin: Springer-Verlag, 1990:66.

Bishop PMF: Habitual abortion: its incidence and treatment with progesterone or vitamin E. Guy's Hosp Rep 1937;87:362.

Blackwell R, Chang A: Video display terminals and pregnancy: a review. Br J Obstet Gynaecol 1988;95:446.

Blank M, Cohen J, Toder V, et al: Induction of antiphospholipid syndrome in naive mice with mouse lupus monoclonal and human polyclonal anticardolipin antibodies. Proc Natl Acad Sci USA 1991;88:3069.

Blum M: Comparative study of serum CAP activity during pregnancy in malformed and normal uterus. J Perinat Med 1978;6:165.

Boue J, Boue A, Lazar P: Retrospective and prospective epidemiological studies of 1500 karyotyped spontaneous abortions. Teratology 1975a;12:11.

Boue J, Boue A, Lazar P: The epidemiology of human spontaneous abortions with chromosomal anomalies. In Blandu RJ (ed): Aging Gametes. Basel: Karger, 1975b:330.

Boue J, Phillippe E, Giroud A, Boue A: Phenotypic expression of lethal chromosomal anomalies in human abortuses. Teratology 1976;14:3.

Branch DW, Dudley DJ, Mitchell MD, et al: Immunoglobulin G fractions from patients with antiphospholipid antibodies cause fetal death in Balb/c mice: a model for autoimmune fetal loss. Am J Obstet Gynecol 1990;163:210.

Branch DW, Rote NS, Dostal DA, et al: Association of lupus anticoagulant with antibody against phosphatidylserine. Clin Immunol Immunopathol 1987;42:63.

Branch DW, Silver RM: Autoimmunity and pregnancy loss. Infertil Reprod Med Clin North Am 1996;7:775.

Branch DW, Silver RM, Blackwell JL, et al: Outcome of treated pregnancies in women with antiphospholipid syndrome: an update of the Utah experience. Obstet Gynecol 1992;4:614.

Brown JE, Thieme GA, Shah DM, et al: Transabdominal and transvaginal endosonography: evaluation of the cervix and lower uterine segment in pregnancy. Am J Obstet Gynecol 1986;155:721.

Buttram VC, Gibbons WE: Müllerian anomalies: a proposed classification (an analysis of 144 cases). Fertil Steril 1979;32:40.

Buttram VC, Reiter RC: Uterine leiomyomata: etiology, symptomatology and management. Fertil Steril 1981;36:433.

Buttram VC, Reiter RC: Surgical Treatment of the Infertile Female. Baltimore: Williams & Wilkins, 1985:149.

Byrd JR, Askew DE, McDonough PG: Cytogenetic findings in fifty-five couples with recurrent fetal wastage. Fertil Steril 1977;28:246.

Carmichael DE: Asherman's syndrome. Obstet Gynecol 1970;36:922.

Carr DH: Chromosome anomalies as a cause of spontaneous abortion. Am J Obstet Gynecol 1967;97:283.

Cauchi MN, Lim D, Young DE, et al: Treatment of recurrent aborters by immunization with paternal cells—controlled trial. Am J Reprod Immunol 1991;25:16.

Chandley AC: The origin of chromosomal aberrations in man and their potential for survival and reproduction in the adult human population. Ann Genet (Paris) 1981;24:5.

Chaouat G, Menu F, Clark DA, et al: Control of fetal survival in CBA × DBA/2 mice by lymphokine therapy. J Reprod Fertil 1990;89:447.

Check JH, Rankin A, Teichman M: The risk of fetal anomalies as a result of progesterone therapy during pregnancy. Fertil Steril 1986;45:575.

Cheesman KL, Cheesman SD, Chatterton RT, Cohen MR: Alterations in progesterone metabolism and luteal function in infertile women with endometriosis. Fertil Steril 1983;40:590.

Clark DA: Controversies in reproductive immunology. Crit Rev Immunol 1991;11:214.

Clark DA, Coulam CB: Is there an immunological cause of repeated pregnancy wastage? Adv Obstet Gynecol 1995;3:321.

Clark DA, Daya S: Trials and tribulations in the treatment of recurrent spontaneous abortion. Am J Reprod Immunol 1991;25:18.

Clark DA, Falbo M, Rowley RD, et al: Active suppression of host-versus-graft reaction in pregnant mice. IX. Soluble suppressor activity obtained from allopregnant mouse decidua that blocks the response to interleukin 2 is related to TGF-β. J Immunol 1988;41:3833.

Clark DA, Lea RG, Flanders KC, et al: Role of a unique species of TGF-β in preventing rejection of the conceptus during pregnancy. Prog Immunol 1992;8:841.

Clark DA, Vince G, Flanders KC, et al: CD56+ lymphoid cells in human first trimester decidua as a source of novel TGFβ2 related immunosuppressive factors. Hum Reprod 1994;9:2270.

Collins JA: Diagnostic assessment of the infertile female partner. Curr Prob Obstet Gynecol Fertil 1988;11:1.

Collins JA: Diagnostic assessment of the ovulatory process. Semin Reprod Endocrinol 1990;8:145.

Cook CL, Rao CV, Yussman MA: Plasma gonadotropin and sex steroid hormone levels during early, mid-follicular and mid-luteal phases of women with luteal phase defects. Fertil Steril 1983;40:45.

Cook CL, Schroeder JA, Yussman MA, Sanfilippo JS: Induction of luteal phase defect with clomiphene citrate. Am J Obstet Gynecol 1984;149:613.

Cooper JM, Houck RM, Rigberg HS: The incidence of intrauterine abnormalities found at hysteroscopy in patients undergoing elective hysteroscopic sterilization. J Reprod Med 1983;28:659.

Cowchock FS, Reece EA, Balaban D, et al: Repeated fetal losses associated with antiphospholipid antibodies: a collaborative randomized trial comparing prednisone to low-dose heparin treatment. Am J Obstet Gynecol 1992,166:1318.

Cowchock FS, Smith JB, Gocial B: Antibodies to phospholipids and nuclear antigens in patients with repeated abortions. Am J Obstet Gynecol 1986;155:1002.

Craig CJT: Congenital abnormalities of the uterus and foetal wastage. S Afr Med J 1973;47:2000.

Crane JP, Wahl N: The role of maternal diabetes in repetitive spontaneous abortion. Fertil Steril 1981;36:477.

Creasy MR, Crolla JA, Alberman ED: A cytogenetic study of human spontaneous abortions using banding techniques. Hum Genet 1976;31:177.

Creasy R: The cytogenetics of spontaneous abortion in humans. In Beard RW, Sharp F (eds): Early Pregnancy Loss: Mechanisms and Treatment. London: Royal College of Obstetricians and Gynaecologists, 1988:293.

Csapo AI, Pulkkinen MO, Wiest WG: Effects of lutectomy and progesterone replacement therapy in early pregnant patients. Am J Obstet Gynecol 1976;115:759.

Cumming DC, Honore LH, Scott JZ, Williams KP: The late luteal phase in infertile women: comparison of simultaneous endometrial biopsy and progesterone levels. Fertil Steril 1985;43:715.

Dallenbach-Hellwig G: The endometrium in natural and artificial luteal phases. Hum Reprod 1988;3:165.

Daly DC, Walters CA, Soto-Albors CE, Riddich DH: Hysteroscopic metroplasty: surgical technique and obstetrical outcome. Fertil Steril 1983;39:623.

Damewood MD: The association of endometriosis and repetitive (early) spontaneous abortions. Semin Reprod Endocrinol 1989;7:155.

Danforth DN: The fibrous nature of the human cervix and its relation to the isthmic segment in gravid and nongravidae uteri. Am J Obstet Gynecol 1947;53:541.

Danforth DN: The distribution and functional activity of the cervical musculature. Am J Obstet Gynecol 1954;68:1261.

Danforth DN: Cervical incompetency as a cause of spontaneous abortion. Clin Obstet Gynecol 1959;2:45.

Daya S: Ectopic pregnancy resulting from transperitoneal migration of spermatozoa. Int J Gynaecol Obstet 1986;24:471.

Daya S: Classificaton of uterine anomalies. Fertil Steril 1989a;51:551.

Daya S: Efficacy of progesterone support for pregnancy in women with recurrent miscarriage: a meta-analysis of controlled trials. Br J Obstet Gynaecol 1989b;96:275.

Daya S: Optimal time in the menstrual cycle for serum progesterone measurement to diagnose luteal phase defects. Am J Obstet Gynecol 1989c;161:1009.

Daya S: Ovulation induction for corpus luteum deficiency. Semin Reprod Endocrinol 1990;8:156.

Daya S: Sonographic evaluation of uterine anomalies. In Jaffe R, Pierson R, Abramowicz JS (eds): Diagnostic Imaging in Infertility and Reproductive Endocrinology. Philadelphia: JB Lippincott Company, 1994a:63.

Daya S: The role of ultrasonography in the diagnosis and management of cervical incompetence. In Jaffe R, Pierson RA, Abramowicz JS (eds): Diagnostic Imaging in Infertility and Reproductive Endocrinology. Philadelphia: JB Lippincott Company, 1994b:93.

Daya S: Endometriosis and spontaneous abortion. Infertil Reprod Med Clin North Am 1996;7:759.

Daya S: Immunotherapy for unexplained recurrent spontaneous abortion. Infertil Reprod Clin North Am 1997;8:65.

Daya S, Gunby J, Clark DA: Intravenous immunoglobulin therapy for recurrent spontaneous abortion: a meta-analysis. Am J Reprod Immunol 1998;39:69.

Daya S, Gunby J, for the Recurrent Miscarriage Immunotherapy Trialists Group: The effectiveness of allogeneic leukocyte immunization in unexplained primary recurrent spontaneous abortion. Am J Reprod Immunol 1994;32:294.

Daya S, Gunby J, Porter F, et al: Critical analysis of intravenous immunoglobulin therapy for recurrent miscarriage. Hum Reprod Update 1999; 5 (in press).

Daya S, Ward S, Burrows E: Progesterone profiles in luteal phase defect cycles and outcome of progesterone treatment in patients with recurrent spontaneous abortion. Am J Obstet Gynecol 1988;158:225.

DeBraekeleer M, Dao T-N: Cytogenetic studies in couples experiencing repeated pregnancy losses. Hum Reprod 1990;5:519.

DeCherney AH, Polan MC: Hysteroscopic management of intrauterine lesions and intractable uterine bleeding. Obstet Gynecol 1983;61:392.

DeCherney AH, Russell JB, Graebe RA, Polan ML: Resectoscopic management of müllerian fusion defects. Fertil Steril 1986;45:726.

DeWolf F, Brosens I, Renaer M: Fetal growth retardation and the maternal arterial supply of the human placenta in the absence of sustained hypertension. Br J Obstet Gynaecol 1987;87:678.

Dhadial RK, Machin AM, Tait SM: Chromosomal anomalies in spontaneously aborted human fetuses. Lancet 1970;2:21.

Diamond MP: Surgical aspects of infertility. In Sciarra JJ (ed): Gynecology and Obstetrics. New York: Harper & Row, 1988:1.

Diamond MP, Polan ML: Intrauterine synechiae and leiomyomas in the evaluation and treatment of repetitive spontaneous abortions. Semin Reprod Endocrinol 1989;7:111.

Dicker D, Feldberg D, Samuel N: Spontaneous abortion in patients with insulin dependent diabetes mellitus: the effect of preconceptional diabetic control. Am J Obstet Gynecol 1988;158:1161.

DiMusto JC, Bohjalian O, Millar M: *Mycoplasma hominis* type I infection and pregnancy. Obstet Gynecol 1973;41:33.

DiZerega GS, Hodgen GD: Luteal phase dysfunction infertility: a sequel to aberrant folliculogenesis. Fertil Steril 1981;35:489.

Dockerty P, Li T-C, Rogers AW, et al: The ultrastructure of the glandular epithelium in the timed endometrial biopsy. Hum Reprod 1988;3:826.

Downs KA, Gibson M: Basal body temperature graph and the luteal phase defect. Fertil Steril 1983;40:466.

Drake TS, Metz SA, Grunert GM, O'Brien WF: Peritoneal fluid volume in endometriosis. Fertil Steril 1980;34:280.

Drugan A, Koppitch FC, Williams JC, et al: Prenatal genetic diagnosis following recurrent early pregnancy loss. Obstet Gynecol 1990;75:381.

Durfee RB: Surgical treatment of the incompetent cervix during pregnancy. Obstet Gynecol 1958;12:91.

Eastman NJ: Habitual abortion. Prog Gynecol 1946;1:262.

Edelman P, Rouquette AM, Verdy E, et al: Autoimmunity, fetal losses, lupus anticoagulant: beginning of systemic lupus erythematosus or new autoimmune entity with gynaecol-obstetrical expression? Hum Reprod 1986;1:295.

Editorial: Avoiding damage to the cervix. Lancet 1983;2:552.

Editorial: Uterine fibroids: medical treatment or surgery? Lancet 1986;2:1197.

Edmonds DK, Lindsay KS, Miller JF, et al: Early embryonic mortality in women. Fertil Steril 1982;38:447.

Elias S, Simpson JL, Carson SA, et al: Genetic studies in incomplete müllerian fusion. Obstet Gynecol 1984;63:276.

Eriksen J, Kaestel C: The incidence of uterine atresia after postpartum curettage: a follow-up examination of 141 patients. Dan Med Bull 1960;7:50.

Erlendsson K, Steinsson K, Johannsson JH, et al: Relation of antiphospholipid antibody and placental bed inflammatory vascular changes to the outcome of pregnancy in successive pregnancies of two women with systemic lupus erythematosus. J Rheumatol 1993;20:1779.

Evaldson G, Nord CE: Amniotic fluid activity against *Bacteroides fragilis* and group B streptococci. Microbiol Immunol 1981;170:11.

Fayez JA: Comparison between abdominal and hysteroscopic metroplasty. Obstet Gynecol 1986;68:399.

Filicori M, Hall DA, Loughlin JS, et al: A conservative approach to the management of uterine leiomyoma: pituitary desensitization by a luteinizing hormone releasing hormone analogue. Am J Obstet Gynecol 1983;147:726.

Finn MM, Gosling JP, Tallon DF, et al: Normal salivary progesterone levels throughout the ovarian cycles as determined by a direct enzyme immunoassay. Fertil Steril 1988;50:882.

Fitzsimmons J, Jackson D, Wapner R, Jackson L: Subsequent reproductive outcome in couples with repeated pregnancy loss. Am J Med Genet 1983;16:583.

Fitzsimmons J, Stahl R, Gocial B, Shapiro SS: Spontaneous abortion and endometriosis. Fertil Steril 1987;47:696.

French FE, Bierman JM: Probabilities of fetal mortality. Public Health Rep 1962;77:835.

Friedman AJ, Rein MS, Harrison-Atlas D, et al: A randomized, placebo-controlled, double-blind study evaluating luprolide acetate depot treatment before myomectomy. Fertil Steril 1989;52:728.

Fritz MA: Inadequate luteal function and recurrent abortion: diagnosis and treatment of luteal phase deficiency. Semin Reprod Endocrinol 1988;6:129.

Garcia J, Jones GS, Wentz AC: The use of clomiphene citrate. Fertil Steril 1977;28:707.

Gatenby PA, Cameron K, Simes RJ, et al: Treatment of recurrent spontaneous abortion by immunization with paternal lymphocytes: results of a controlled trial. Am J Reprod Immunol 1993;29:88.

Geisthovel F, Skubsch V, Zabel G: Ultrasonographic and hormonal studies in physiologic and insufficient menstrual cycles. Fertil Steril 1983;39:277.

Gellis SS, Hsia DY: The infant of the diabetic mother. Am J Dis Child 1959;97:1.

Geraedts JPM: Chromosomal anomalies and recurrent miscarriage. Infertil Reprod Med Clin North Am 1996;7:677.

Glinoer D, Soto MF, Bourdoux P, et al: Pregnancy in patients with mild thyroid abnormalities: maternal and neonatal repercussions. J Clin Endocrinol Metab 1991;73:421.

Golan A, Langer R, Bukovsky I, Caspi E: Congenital anomalies of the müllerian system. Fertil Steril 1989;51:747.

Goldstein DP: Incompetent cervix in offspring exposed to diethylstilbestrol in utero. Obstet Gynecol 1978;52:735.

Goldzieher JW, Benigno BB: The treatment of threatened and recurrent abortion: a critical review. Am J Obstet Gynecol 1958;75:1202.

Gonen Y, Casper RF: Sonographic determination of an adverse effect of clomiphene citrate on endometrial growth. In: Abstracts of the VIIth World Congress on Human Reproduction, Helsinki, 1990:Abstract 355.

Grant A: Additional sterility factors in endometriosis. Fertil Steril 1966;17:514.

Grant A: Cervical cerclage to prolong pregnancy. In Chalmers I, Enkin M, Keirse MJNC (eds): Effective Care in Pregnancy and Childbirth. Oxford: Oxford University Press, 1989:633.

Groll M: Endometriosis and spontaneous abortion. Fertil Steril 1984;41:933.

Gros A, David A, Serr DM: Management of congenital malformations of the uterus: fetal salvage. Acta Eur Fertil 1974;5:301.

Guerneri S, Bettio D, Simoni G, et al: Prevalence and distribution of chromosome abnormalities in a sample of first trimester abortions. Human Reprod 1987;2:735.

Gump DW, Gibson M, Ashikaga T: Lack of association between genital mycoplasmas and infertility. N Engl J Med 1984;310:937.

Hamlin DJ: Magnetic resonance imaging of bicornuate uterus with unilateral haemotometrosalpinx and ipsilateral renal agenesis. Urol Radiol 1986;8:52.

Hammond MG: Müllerian defects associated with repetitive spontaneous abortions. Semin Reprod Endocrinol 1989;7:103.

Hanson FW, Powell JE, Stevens VC: Effects of hCG and human pituitary LH on steroid secretion and functional life of the human corpus luteum. J Clin Endocrinol Metab 1971;24:606.

Harger JH, Archer DF, Marchese SG, et al: Etiology of recurrent pregnancy losses and outcome of subsequent pregnancies. Obstet Gynecol 1983;62:574.

Harger JH, Rabin BS, Marchese SG: A prognostic value of antinuclear antibodies in women with recurrent pregnancy losses: a prospective controlled study. Obstet Gynecol 1989;73:419.

Harlap S: Smoking and spontaneous abortion. In Rosenberg MJ (ed): Smoking and Reproductive Health. Littleton, MA: PSG Publishing Co Inc, 1987:75.

Harlap S, Shiono PH, Ramcharan S: A prospective study of spontaneous fetal losses after induced abortion. N Engl J Med 1979;301:677.

Harris EN: Syndrome of the black swan. Br J Rheumatol 1986;26:324.

Harris EN: The second international anticardiolipin standardization workshop: The Kingston antiphospholipid antibody study (KAPS) group. Am J Clin Pathol 1990;94:476.

Hassold T, Chen N, Funkhouser J, et al: A cytogenetic study of 1000 spontaneous abortions. Ann Hum Genet 1980;44:151.

Healy DL, Fraser HM, Lawson SL: Shrinkage of a uterine fibroid after subcutaneous infusion of a LHRH agonist. Br Med J 1984;289:1267.

Heinonen PK, Saarikoski S, Pystynen P: Reproductive performance of women with uterine anomalies. Acta Obstet Gynecol Scand 1983;61:157.

Hemmingsson E: Outcome of third trimester pregnancies after cryotherapy of the uterine cervix. Br J Obstet Gynaecol 1982;89:675.

Herbst AL, Hubby MM, Blough RR, Azizi F: A comparison of pregnancy experience in DES-exposed and DES-unexposed daughters. J Reprod Med 1980;24:62.

Herbst AL, Senekjian EK, Frey KW: Abortion and pregnancy loss among diethylstilbestrol-exposed women. Semin Reprod Endocrinol 1989;7:124.

Hill JA, Polgar K, Harlow BL, et al: Evidence of embryo- and trophoblast-toxic cellular immune response(s) in women with recurrent spontaneous abortion. Am J Obstet Gynecol 1992;166:1044.

Ho HN, Gill TJ, Hsieh HJ, et al: Immunotherapy for recurrent spontaneous abortions in a Chinese population. Am J Reprod Immunol 1991;25:10.

Hughes GRV, Harris EN, Gharavi AE: The anticardiolipin syndrome. J Rheumatol 1986;13:486.

Huisjes HJ: Spontaneous abortion. Curr Rev Obstet Gynecol 1984;8:34.

Hulka JF, Lefler HT Jr, Lachenbruch PA: A new electronic force monitor to measure factors influencing cervical dilation for vacuum curettage. Am J Obstet Gynecol 1974;120:166.

Hull MGR, Savage PE, Bromham DR, et al: The value of a single serum progesterone measurement in the midluteal phase as a criterion of a potentially fertile cycle ("ovulation") derived from treated and untreated conception cycles. Fertil Steril 1982;37:355.

Hunt JE, Wallach EE: Uterine factors in infertility—an overview. Clin Obstet Gynecol 1974;17:44.

Hunt RB, Siegler AM: Hysterosalpingography: Techniques and Interpretation. Chicago: Year Book Medical Publishers, 1990:48.

James WH: Notes towards an epidemiology of spontaneous abortion. Am J Hum Genet 1963;15:223.

Janerich, Slone: In: Transactions of the Symposium "Progesterone, Progestins, and Fetal Development, Washington, DC, 1978.

Javert CT: Habitual abortion. N Y State J Med 1948;48:2595.

Jennings CL: Temporary submucosal cerclage for cervical incompetence: report of forty-eight cases. Am J Obstet Gynecol 1972;113:1097.

Johansson EDB: Depression of progesterone levels in women treated with synthetic gestagens after ovulation. Acta Endocrinol (Kbh) 1971;68:779.

Johnstone FD, Boyd IE, McCarthy TG: The diameter of the uterine isthmus during the menstrual cycle, pregnancy and the puerperium. J Obstet Gynaecol Br Commonw 1974;81:558.

Jones: In: Transactions of the Symposium "Progesterone, Progestins, and Fetal Development," Washington, DC, 1978.

Jones GS: The luteal phase defect. Fertil Steril 1976;27:351.

Jones GS, Delfs E: Endocrine patterns in term pregnancies following abortions. JAMA 1951;146:1212.

Jones HW, Jones GES: Double uterus as an etiological factor of repeated abortion: indication for surgical repair. Am J Obstet Gynecol 1953:65:325.

Jones W, Man E: Thyroid function in human pregnancy. VI. Premature deliveries and reproductive failure of pregnant women with low butanol extractable iodines. Am J Obstet Gynecol 1969;104:909.

Joshi SG, Rao R, Henriques EE, et al: Luteal phase concentrations of a progestagen-associated endometrial protein (PEP) in the serum of cycling women with adequate or inadequate endometrium. J Clin Endocrinol Metab 1986;63:1247.

Jurkovic D, Kurjak A: Normal anatomy of the female pelvis and sonographic demonstration of pelvic abnormalities. In Kurjak A (ed): Ultrasound and Infertility. Boca Raton, FL: CRC Press, 1989:55.

Kajii T, Ferrier A, Niikawa N, et al: Anatomic and chromosomal anomalies in 639 spontaneous abortuses. Hum Genet 1980;55:87.

Kajii T, Niikawa N: Origin of triploidy and tetraploidy in man: 11 cases with chromosome markers. Cytogenet Cell Genet 1977;18:109.

Kalter H: Diabetes and spontaneous abortion: a historical review. Am J Obstet Gynecol 1987;156:1243.

Kaplan MM: Thyroid diseases in pregnancy. In Gleicher N (ed): Principles of Medical Therapy in Pregnancy. New York: Pleunum Medical, 1985;192.

Kase NG: Induction of ovulation with clomiphene citrate. Clin Obstet Gynecol 1973;16:192.

Katz Z, Lancet M, Skornik J, et al: Teratogenicity of progesterone given during the first trimester of pregnancy. Obstet Gynecol 1985;65:775.

Kaufman RH, Adam E, Binder GL, Gerthoffer E: Upper genital tract changes and pregnancy outcome in offspring exposed in utero to diethylstilbesterol. Am J Obstet Gynecol 1980;13:299.

Kaufman RH, Binder GL, Gray MT, Adam E: Upper genital tract changes associated with exposure in utero to diethyl-stilbestrol. Am J Obstet Gynecol 1977;137:299.

Kaufman RH, Irwin JF: Diethylstilboestrol exposure and reproductive performance. In Bennet MJ, Edmonds DK (eds): Spontaneous and Recurrent Abortion. Oxford: Blackwell Scientific, 1987:130.

Kerin JF, Liu JH, Phillipou G: Evidence for a hypothalamic site of action of clomiphene citrate in women. J Clin Endocrinol Metab 1985;61:265.

Kline J, Stein Z: Epidemiology of chromosomal anomalies in spontaneous abortion: prevalence, manifestation and determinants. In Bennet MJ, Edmonds DK (eds): Spontaneous and Recurrent Abortion. Oxford: Blackwell Scientific, 1987:29.

Kline J, Stein Z, Susser M, Warburton D: Environmental influences on early reproductive loss in a current New York City study. In Porter IH, Hook EB (eds): Human Embryonic and Fetal Death. New York: Academic Press, 1980:225.

Kundsin RB, Ampola M, Streeter S, Neurath P: Chromosomal aberrations induced by T-strain mycoplasmas. J Med Genet 1971;8:181.

Kusuda M, Nakamura G, Matsukuma K, Kurano A: Corpus luteum insufficiency as a cause of midatory failure. Acta Obstet Gynecol Scand 1983;62:199.

Kwak JYH, Gilman-Sachs A, Beaman KD, et al: Reproductive outcome in women with recurrent spontaneous abortions of alloimmune and autoimmune causes: preconception versus postconception treatment. Am J Obstet Gynecol 1992;166:1787.

Kwak JYH, Kwak FMY, Ainbinder SW, et al: Elevated peripheral blood natural killer cells are effectively down regulated by immunoglobulin G infusion in women with recurrent spontaneous abortions. Am J Reprod Immunol 1996;35:363.

Lachapelle H, Miron P, Hemmings R, et al: Endometrial T, B, and NK cells in patients with recurrent spontaneous abortion: altered profile and pregnancy outcome. J Immunol 1996;156:4027.

Larsson G, Grundsell H, Gullberg B: Outcome of pregnancy after conization. Acta Obstet Gynecol Scand 1982;61:461.

Laskin C, Bombardier C, Hannah ME, et al: Prednisone and aspirin in women with autoantibodies and unexplained recurrent fetal loss. N Engl J Med 1997;337:148.

Lauritsen JG: Aetiology of spontaneous abortion: a cytogenetic and epidemiological study of 288 abortuses and their parents. Acta Obstet Gynecol Scand Suppl 1976;52:1.

Lee C, Ghoshal K, Beaman KD: Cloning of a cDNA for a T-cell produced molecule with a putative immune regulatory role. Mol Immunol 1990;27:1137.

Leiman G, Harrison NA, Rubin A: Pregnancy following conization of the cervix: complications related to cone size. Am J Obstet Gynecol 1980;136:14.

Lejeune B, Grun JP, de Nayer P, et al: Antithyroid antibodies underlying thyroid abnormalities and miscarriage or pregnancy induced hypertension. Br J Obstet Gynaecol 1993;100:669.

Lenton EA: Pituitary and ovarian hormones in implantation and early pregnancy. In Chapman N, Gzudzinskas G, Chard T (eds): Implantation: Biological and Clinical Aspects. London: Springer-Verlag, 1988:17.

Lenton EA, Landgren BM, Sexton L: Normal variation in the length of the luteal phase of the menstrual cycle: identification of the short luteal phase. Br J Obstet Gynaecol 1984a;91:685.

Lenton EA, Landgren BM, Sexton L, Harper R: Normal variation in the length of the follicular phase of the menstrual cycles: effect of chronological age. Br J Obstet Gynaecol 1984b;91:681.

Leridon H: Facts and artifacts in the study of intra-uterine mortality: a reconsideration from pregnancy histories. Popul Stud 1976;30:319.

Levy C, Robel P, Gautray JP: Estradiol and progesterone receptors in human endometrium: normal and abnormal menstrual cycles and early pregnancy. Am J Obstet Gynecol 1980;136:646.

Li T-C, Dockerty P, Rogers AW, Cooke ID: How precise is histologic dating of endometrium using the standard dating criteria? Fertil Steril 1989;51:759.

Li T-C, Rogers AW, Dockerty P, et al: A new method of histologic dating of human endometrium in the luteal phase. Fertil Steril 1988;50:52.

Li T-C, Rogers AW, Lenton EA, et al: A comparison between two methods of chronological dating of human endometrial biopsies during the luteal phase, and their correlation with histologic dating. Fertil Steril 1987;48:928.

Lippman-Hand A: Genetic counseling and human reproductive loss. In Porter IH, Hook EB (eds): Embryonic and Fetal Death. New York: Academic Press, 1980:299.

Liston AJ: Video display terminals (Information letter DD-34). Ottawa: Health Protection Branch, Health and Welfare Canada, 1985.

Lockwood CJ, Romero R, Ferburg RF, et al: The prevalence and biologic significance of lupus anticoagulant and anticardiolipin antibodies in a general obstetric population. Am J Obstet Gynecol 1989;161:369.

Ludmir J, Dandon MB, Gabbe SG: Management of the diethylstilbestrol exposed pregnant patient: a prospective study. Am J Obstet Gynecol 1987;157:655.

Maheuz R, Guilloteau C, Lemay A, et al: Regression of leiomyomata uteri following hypoestrogenism induced by repetitive luteinizing hormone-releasing hormone agonist treatment: preliminary report. Fertil Steril 1984;42:644.

Mahran M: Transabdominal cervical cerclage during pregnancy: a modified technique. Obstet Gynecol 1978;52:502.

Maier DB, Parke A: Subclinical autoimmunity in recurrent aborters. Fertil Steril 1989;51:280.

Malpas P: A study of abortion sequences. J Obstet Gynaecol Br Emp 1938;45:932.

Mangan CE, Borow L, Burtnett-Rubin MM: Pregnancy outcome in 98 women exposed to diethylstilbestrol in utero, their mothers and unexposed siblings. Obstet Gynecol 1982;59:315.

Mann ED, McLarn WD, Hayt DB: The physiology and clinical significance of the uterine isthmus. Am J Obstet Gynecol 1961; 81:209.

March CM: Update: luteal phase defects. Endocr Infertil Forum 1987;10:3.

March CM, Israel R: Hysteroscopic management of recurrent abortion caused by septate uterus. Am J Obstet Gynecol 1987; 156:834.

March CM, Israel R, March AD: Hysteroscopic management of intrauterine adhesions. Am J Obstet Gynecol 1978;130:653.

Marcoux S, Maheux R, Bérubés, and the Canadian Collaborative Group on Endometriosis: Laparoscopic surgery in infertile women with minimal or mild endometriosis. N Engl J Med 1997;337:217.

Marshall J: Thermal changes in the normal menstrual cycle. Br Med J 1963;1:102.

Marut EL, Hodgen GD: Antiestrogenic action of high-dose clomiphene in primates: pituitary augmentation but with ovarian attenuation. Fertil Steril 1982;38:100.

Matta WHM, Shaw RW, Nye M: Long-term follow-up of patients with uterine fibroids after treatment with the LHRH agonist buserelin. Br J Obstet Gynaecol 1989;96:200.

Maxson WS, Hargrove JT: Bioavailability of oral micronized progesterone. Fertil Steril 1985;44:622.

McCormack WM, Almeida PC, Bailey PE: Sexual activity and vaginal colonization with genital mycoplasmas. JAMA 1972; 221:1375.

McCormack WM, Lee Y-H, Zinner SH: Sexual experience and urethral colonization with genital mycoplasmas: a study in normal men. Ann Intern Med 1973;78:696.

McDonald IA: Suture of the cervix for unsuitable miscarriage. J Obstet Gynaecol Br Emp 1957;64:346.

McDonald IA: Cervical incompetence as a cause of spontaneous abortion. In Bennet MJ, Edmonds DK (eds): Spontaneous and Recurrent Abortion. Oxford: Blackwell Scientific, 1987:168.

McLaughlin DS: Metroplasty and myomectomy with the CO_2 laser for maximising the preservation of normal tissue and minimizing blood loss. J Reprod Med 1985;30:1.

McNeely MJ, Soules MR: The diagnosis of luteal phase deficiency: a critical review. Fertil Steril 1988;50:1.

Merali FS, Arck PC, Beaman K, et al: Transforming growth factor β2-related decidual supprssor factor is not related to TJ6 protein. Am J Reprod Immunol 1996;35:342.

Metzger DA, Olive DL, Stohs GF, Franklin RR: Association of endometriosis and spontaneous abortion: effect of control group selection. Fertil Steril 1986;45:18.

Michaelis J, Michaelis H, Gluck E, Koller S: Prospective study of suspected associations between certain drugs administered during early pregnancy and congenital malformations. Teratology 1983;27:57.

Michaels WH, Montgomery C, Karo J, et al: Ultrasound differentiation of the competent from the incompetent cervix: prevention of preterm delivery. Am J Obstet Gynecol 1986;154:537.

Michaels WH, Thompson HO, Schreiber FR: Ultrasound surveillance of the cervix during pregnancy in diethylstilbestrol-exposed offspring. Obstet Gynecol 1989;73:230.

Miller JF, Williamson E, Glue J, et al: Fetal loss after implantation. Lancet 1980;2:554.

Mimouni F, Miodovnik M, Tsand R: Decreased maternal serum magnesium concentration and adverse fetal outcome in insulin dependent diabetic women. Obstet Gynecol 1987;70:85.

Miodovnik M, Lavin JP, Knowles HC, et al: Spontaneous abortion among insulin-dependent diabetic women. Am J Obstet Gynecol 1984;150:372.

Mitchell-Leef DE: Diagnosis and management of the incompetent cervical os. Semin Reprod Endocrinol 1989;7:115.

Moinian M, Andersch B: Does cervix conization increase the risk of complications in subsequent pregnancies? Acta Obstet Gynecol Scand 1982;61:101.

Mowbray JF, Liddel H, Underwood JL, et al: Controlled trial of treatment of recurrent spontaneous abortion by immunization with paternal cells. Lancet 1985;1:941.

Muse KN, Wilson EA: How does mild endometriosis cause infertility? Fertil Steril 1982;38:145.

Naegel TC, Malo JW: Hysteroscopic metroplasty in the diethyl-stilbestrol exposed pregnant patient: a prospective study. Am J Obstet Gynecol 1987;157:655.

National Center for Health Statistics: Reproductive impairment among married couples. Vital Health Stat 23 1982;11:5.

Naylor AF, Warburton D: Sequential analysis of spontaneous abortion. II. Collaborative study data show that gravidity determines a very substantial rise in risk. Fertil Steril 1979;31:282.

Neuwirth RS: A new technique for and additional experience with hysteroscopic resection of submucous fibroids. Am J Obstet Gynecol 1978;131:91.

Neuwirth RS: Hysteroscopic management of symptomatic submucous fibroids. Obstet Gynecol 1983;62:509.

Nillius SJ, Johansson EDB: Plasma levels of progesterone after vaginal, rectal or intramuscular administration of progesterone. Am J Obstet Gynecol 1971;110:470.

Noyes RW, Hertig AT, Rock J: Dating the endometrial biopsy. Fertil Steril 1950;1:3.

Ochlschlager FK: Listerosis as a possible cause of abortion: report of a case. Obstet Gynecol 1960;10:595.

O'Leary JL, O'Leary JA: Rudimentary horn pregnancy. Obstet Gynecol 1963;22:371.

Oshiro BT, Silver RM, Scott JR, et al: Antiphospholipid antibodies and fetal death. Obstet Gynecol 1996;87:489.

Ottobre JS, Stouffer RL: Persistent vs. transient stimulation of the macque corpus luteum during prolonged exposure to hCG: a function of age of the menstrual cycle. Endocrinology 1984;114:2175.

Out HJ, Kooijman CD, Bruinse HW: Histopathological findings in placentae from patients with intrauterine fetal death and antiphospholipid antibodies. Eur J Obstet Gynaecol Reprod Biol 1991;41:179.

Parulekar SG, Kiwi R: Dynamic incompetent cervix uteri. J Ultrasound Med 1988;7:481.

Patel VH, Somers S, Daya S, Markus J: The role of magnetic resonance imaging in the evaluation of congenital uterine anomalies: a comprehensive review. J Soc Obstet Gynaecol Can 1997;19:235.

Pattison NS, Chamley LW, McKay EJ, et al: Antiphospholipid antibodies in pregnancy: prevalence and clinical associations. Br J Obstet Gynaecol 1993;100:909.

Penrose LS, Delhanty JDA: Triploid cell cultures from a macerated foetus. Lancet 1961;1:1261.

Perino A, Mencaglia C, Hamou J, Cittadini E: Hysteroscopy for metroplasty of uterine septa: report of 24 cases. Fertil Steril 1987;48:321.

Pinsonneault O, Goldstein DP: Obstructing malformations of the uterus and vagina. Fertil Steril 1985;44:241.

Pittaway D: Endometriosis and spontaneous abortion. Semin Reprod Endocrinol 1988;6:257.

Poland BJ, Miller JR, Jones DC, Trimble BK: Reproductive counseling in patients who have had a spontaneous abortion. Am J Obstet Gynecol 1977;127:685.

Polishuk WZ, Sadovsky E: A syndrome of recurrent intrauterine adhesions. Am J Obstet Gynecol 1975;123:51.

Portuondo JA, Camara MM, Echanojauregui AD, Calonge J: Müllerian abnormalities in fertile women and recurrent aborters. J Reprod Med 1986;31:616.

Pratt D, Novotny M, Kaberlein G, et al: Antithyroid antibodies and the association with non-organ-specific antibodies in recurrent pregnancy loss. Am J Obstet Gynecol 1993;168:837.

Quinn PA, Barkin M, Derzko C, et al: Efficacy trial of erythromycin in the prevention of pregnancy loss. In: Abstracts of the 45th annual meeting of the Society of Obstetricians and Gynaecologists of Canada, Quebec City, 1989:Abstract 35.

Quinn PA, Shewchuck AB, Shuber J: Efficacy of antibiotic therapy in preventing spontaneous pregnancy loss among couples colonized with genital mycoplasmas. Am J Obstet Gynecol 1983;145:239.

Rai R, Cohen H, Dave M, Regan L: Randomized controlled trial of aspirin and aspirin plus heparin in pregnant women with recurrent miscarriage associated with phospholipid antibodies (or antiphospholipid antibodies). BMJ 1997;314:253.

Rappaport F, Rabinovitz M: Genital listeriosis as a cause of repeated abortion. Lancet 1960;1:1273.

Recurrent Miscarriage Immunotherapy Trialists Group: Worldwide collaborative observational study and meta-analysis on allogeneic leukocyte immunotherapy for recurrent spontaneous abortion. Am J Reprod Immunol 1994;32:55.

Regan L: Spontaneous and recurrent abortion: epidemiological and immunological considerations. In Chapman M, Grudzinskas G, Chard T (eds): Implantation: Biological and Clinical Aspects. London: Springer-Verlag, 1988:183.

Regan L, Braude PR, Tembath PL: Influence of past reproductive performance on risk of spontaneous abortion. BMJ 1989;299:541.

Resseguie LJ, Hick JF, Bruen JA, et al: Congenital malformations among offspring exposed in utero to progestins, Olmsted County, Minnesota, 1936–1974. Fertil Steril 1985;43:514.

Ribbing SL, Hoversland RC, Beaman KD: T-cell suppressor factors play an integral role in preventing fetal rejection. J Reprod Immunol 1988;14:83.

Rock JA: Diagnosing and repairing uterine anomalies. Contemp Obstet Gynecol 1981;17:43.

Rock JA, Schlaff WD: The obstetric consequences of uterovaginal anomalies. Fertil Steril 1985;43:681.

Roman EA, Alberman E, Pharoah POD: Pregnancy order and reproductive loss. Br Med J 1980;1:715.

Rorie DK, Newton M: Histological and chemical studies of the smooth muscle in the human cervix and uterus. Am J Obstet Gynecol 1967;99:466.

Rosove MH, Tabsh K, Wassersturm N, et al: Heparin therapy for pregnant women with lupus anticoagulant or anticardiolipin antibodies. Obstet Gynecol 1990;75:630.

Ruiz JE, Kwak JYH, Baum L, et al: Intravenous immunoglobulin inhibits natural killer cell activity in vivo in women with recurrent spontaneous abortion. Am J Reprod Immunol 1996;35:370.

Sandberg EC, Riffle NL, Higdon JV, Getman CE: Pregnancy outcome in women exposed to diethylstilbestrol in utero. Am J Obstet Gynecol 1981;140:194.

Sandler SW: Spontaneous abortion in perspective. S Afr Med J 1977;52:115.

Sanfilippo JS, Wakim NG, Schikler KN, Yussman MA: Endometriosis in association with uterine anomaly. Am J Obstet Gynecol 1986;154:39.

Sarto GE, Simpson JL: Abnormalities of the müllerian and wolffian duct systems. Birth Defects 1978;14:37.

Schenker JG, Margalioth EJ: Intrauterine adhesions: an updated appraisal. Fertil Steril 1982;37:593.

Schmid W: A familial chromosome abnormality associated with repeated abortions. Cytogenetics 1962;1:199.

Schoeneck F: Pregnancy patterns and fetal salvage. Obstet Gynecol 1953;1:160.

Scott RT, Snyder RR, Strickland DM, et al: The effect of interobserver variation in dating endometrial histology on the diagnosis of luteal phase defects. Fertil Steril 1988;50:888.

Shapiro S, Levine HS, Abramowicz M: Factors associated with early and late fetal loss. Adv Planned Parenthood 1971;6:45.

Sherman BM, Korenman SA: Measurement of plasma LH, FSH, estradiol and progesterone in disorders of the human menstrual cycle: the short luteal phase. J Clin Endocrinol Metab 1974;38:89.

Shirodkar VN: A method of operative treatment for habitual abortion in the second trimester of pregnancy. Antiseptic 1955;52:299.

Shortle BE, Jewelewicz R: Clinical Aspects of Cervical Incompetence. Chicago: Year Book Medical Publishers, 1989:1, 5.

Shoupe D, Mishell Jr DR, Lacarra M, et al: Correlation of endometrial maturation with four methods of estimating day of ovulation. Obstet Gynecol 1989;73:88.

Silver RM, Porter TF, van Leeuwen I, et al: Anticardiolipin antibodies: clinical consequences of "low titres." Obstet Gynecol 1996;87:475.

Singer MS, Hochman M: Incompetent cervix in a hormone exposed off-spring. Obstet Gynecol 1978;51:625.

Smith SK, Lenton EA, Landgren BM, Cooke ID: The short luteal phase and infertility. Br J Obstet Gynaecol 1984;91:1120.

Sompolinsky D, Solomin F, Elkia L: Infections with mycoplasma and bacteria in induced midtrimester abortion and fetal loss. Am J Obstet Gynecol 1975;121:610.

Sonek JD, Iams JD, Blumenfeld M, et al: Measurement of cervical length in pregnancy: Comparison between vaginal ultrasonography and digital examination. Obstet Gynecol 1990;76:172.

Speert H: Pregnancy prognosis following repeated abortion. Am J Obstet Gynecol 1954;68:665.

Stagnaro-Green A, Roman SH, Cobin RH, et al: Detection of at-risk pregnancy by means of highly sensitive assays for thyroid antibodies. JAMA 1990;264:1422.

Starks GC: CO_2 laser myomectomy in an infertile population. J Reprod Med 1988;33:184.

Steege JF, Rupp SL, Stout AL: Bioavailability of nasally administered progesterone. Fertil Steril 1986;46:727.

Stein Z, Kline J, Susser E, et al: Maternal age and spontaneous abortion. In Porter IH, Hook EB (eds): Human Embryonic and Fetal Death. New York: Academic Press, 1980:107.

Stevenson AC, Dudgeon MY, McClure H: I. Observations on the results of pregnancies in women resident in Belfast. II. Abortions, hydatidiform moles and ectopic pregnancies. Ann Hum Genet 1959;23:395.

Strassmann EO: Fertility and unification of double uterus. Fertil Steril 1966;17:165.

Stray-Pedersen B, Eng J, Reikvam TM: Uterine T-mycoplasma colonization in reproductive failure. Am J Obstet Gynecol 1978;130:307.

Stray-Pedersen B, Stray-Pedersen S: Etiologic factors and subsequent reproductive performance in 195 couples with a prior history of habitual abortion. Am J Obstet Gynecol 1984;148:140.

Strobino BR, Kline J, Shrout P, et al: Recurrent spontaneous abortion: definition of a syndrome. In Porter IH, Hook EB (eds): Human Embryonic and Fetal Death. New York: Academic Press, 1980:315.

Strott CA, Cargille CM, Ross GT, Lipsett MB: The short luteal phase. J Clin Endocrinol Metab 1970;30:246.

Szekeres-Bartho J, Reznikoff-Etievant MF, Varga P, et al: Lymphocytic progesterone receptors in normal and pathological human pregnancy. J Reprod Immunol 1989;16:239.

Takahara H, Ohama K, Fujiwara A: Cytogenetic study in early spontaneous abortion. Hiroshima J Med Sci 1977;26:291.

Tharapel AT, Tharapel SA, Bannerman RM: Recurrent pregnancy losses and parental chromosome abnormalities: a review. Br J Obstet Gynaecol 1985;92:899.

Therkelsen AJ, Grunnet N, Hjort T, et al: Studies on spontaneous abortion. In Boue A, Thibault C (eds): Chromosomal Errors in Relation to Reproductive Failure. Paris: INSERM, 1973:81.

Tho SPT, Byrd JR, McDonough PG: Etiologies and subsequent reproductive performance of 100 couples with recurrent abortion. Fertil Steril 1979;32:389.

Tompkins P: Comments on the bicornuate uterus and twinning. Surg Clin North Am 1962;42:1049.

Uchida IA, Freeman VCP: Triploidy and chromosomes. Am J Obstet Gynecol 1985;151:65.

Valle RF, Sciarra JJ: Hysteroscopic treatment of the septate uterus. Obstet Gynecol 1986;67:253.

van Duyl WA, van der Zon AT, Drogendijk AC: Stress relaxation of the human cervix: a new tool for diagnosis of cervical incompetence. Clin Phys Physiol Meas 1984;5:207.

Van Lijnschoten G, Albrechts J, Valling M, et al: Fluorescence in situ hybridization on paraffin embedded abortion material as a means of retrospective chromosome analysis. Hum Genet 1994;94:518.

Varma TR, Patel RH, Pillai U: Ultrasonic assessment of cervix in "at risk" patients. Int J Gynaecol Obstet 1987;25:25.

Vassiliadou N, Bulmer JN: Human decidual leukocytes in first trimester pregnancy pathology [abstract]. Am J Reprod Immunol 1995;33:449.

Verp MS: Environmental causes of repetitive spontaneous abortion. Semin Reprod Endocrinol 1989;7:188.

Verp MS, Simpson JL, Elias S, et al: Heritable aspects of uterine anomalies. I. Three familial aggregate with müllerian fusion anomalies. Fertil Steril 1983;40:80.

Vollenhoven BJ, Lawrence AS, Healy DL: Uterine fibroids: a clinical review. Br J Obstet Gynaecol 1990;97:285.

Vollman RF: Major Problems in Obstetrics and Gynaecology. Vol. 7. The Menstrual Cycle. Eastbourne: WB Saunders, 1977.

Wallach EE: Evaluation and management of uterine causes of infertility. Clin Obstet Gynecol 1979;22:43.

Warburton D, Fraser FC: Genetic aspects of abortion. Clin Obstet Gynecol 1959;2:22.

Warburton D, Fraser FC: Spontaneous abortion risks in man: data from reproductive histories collected in a medical genetics unit. Am J Hum Genet 1964;16:1.

Warburton D, Kline J, Stein Z, et al: Does the karyotype of a spontaneous abortion predict the karyotype of a subsequent abortion? Evidence from 273 women with two karyotyped spontaneous abortions. Am J Hum Genet 1987;41:465.

Warburton D, Stein Z, Kline J, Susser M: Chromosome abnormalities in spontaneous abortions: data from the New York Study. In Porter IH, Hook EB (eds): Human Embryonic and Fetal Death. New York: Academic Press, 1980:261.

Warburton D, Strobino B: Recurrent spontaneous abortion. In Bennet MJ, Edmonds DK (eds): Spontaneous and Recurrent Abortion. Oxford: Blackwell Scientific, 1987:193.

Wattren N, Perry L, Lilford R, Chard T: Interpretation of single progesterone measurement in diagnosis of an ovulation and defective luteal phase: observations in analysis of the normal range. Br Med J 1984;288:7.

Watts DH, Eschenbach DA: Reproductive tract infections as a cause of abortion and preterm birth. Semin Reprod Endocrinol 1988;6:203.

Wegmann TG: Maternal T-cells promote placental growth and prevent spontaneous abortion. Immunol Lett 1988;17:297.

Wegmann TG, Lin H, Guilbert L, et al: Bidirectional cytokine interactions in the maternal-fetal relationship: is successful pregnancy a Th2 phenomenon? Immunol Today 1993;14:353.

Wentz AC: Physiologic and clinical considerations in luteal phase defects. Clin Obstet Gynecol 1979;22:169.

Wentz AC: Progesterone therapy of the inadequate luteal phase. Curr Prob Obstet Gynecol 1982;6:5.

Wentz AC: Luteal phase inadequacy. In Behrman SJ, Kistner RW, Patton GW Jr (eds): Progress in Infertility. Boston: Little, Brown and Company, 1988:405.

Wheeler JM, Johnston BM, Malinak LR: The relationship of endometriosis to spontaneous abortion. Fertil Steril 1983;39:656.

Wilcox AJ, Weinberg CR, O'Connor JF, et al: Incidence of early loss of pregnancy. N Engl J Med 1988;319:189.

Wilks JW, Noble AS: Steroidogenic responsiveness of the monkey corpus luteum to exogenous chorionic gonadotropin. Endocrinology 1983;112:1256.

Williams RF, Hodgen GD: Disparate effects of human chorionic gonadotropin during the late follicular phase in monkeys: normal ovulation, follicular atresia, ovarian acyclicity and hypersecretion of follicle-stimulating hormone. Fertil Steril 1980;33:64.

Williamson HO, Youmans CD, Mancy SA: Autoimmunity to endometrium and ovary in endometriosis. Clin Exp Immunol 1982;50:259.

Willman EA, Collins WP, Clayton SG: Studies in the involvement of prostaglandins in uterine symptomatology and pathology. Br J Obstet Gynaecol 1976;83:337.

Witten BI, Martin SA: The endometrial biopsy as a guide to the management of luteal phase defect. Fertil Steril 1985;44:460.

Worcester J, Stevenson SS, Rice RG: Congenitally malformed infants and associated gestational characteristics. Paediatrics 1950;6:208.

World Health Organization: Recommended definitions, terminology and format for statistical tables related to the perinatal period. Acta Obstet Gynaecol Scand 1977;56:247.

Yosowitz EE, Hanfrect F, Kaufman RH, Goyette RE: Silicone-plastic cuff for the treatment of the incompetent cervix in pregnancy. Am J Obstet Gynecol 1972;113:233.

Zbella EA: Diabetes mellitus, thyroid disease, and adrenal disease and their contribution to spontaneous and repetitive pregnancy loss. Semin Reprod Endocrinol 1989;7:130.

Zemlyn S: The length of the uterine cervix and its significance. J Clin Ultrasound 1981;9:267.

10

Gary H. Lipscomb | Ectopic Pregnancy

An ectopic pregnancy is defined as any pregnancy in which implantation occurs at a location other than the endometrial lining. Since 1970, the first year for which statistics were compiled by the Centers for Disease Control and Prevention (CDC), the incidence of ectopic pregnancy in the United States has steadily increased from a rate of 4.5 per 1000 pregnancies to 19.7 per 1000 pregnancies (CDC, 1995). In 1992, the last year for which statistics are available from the CDC, there were an estimated 108,800 cases of ectopic pregnancy. Considering the cost in both dollars and human suffering, ectopic pregnancy has become a health problem of immense proportions. Fortunately, improved methods of diagnosis and treatment now available for ectopic pregnancy have the potential of significantly decreasing the morbidity and mortality associated with this increasing common disease.

PATHOPHYSIOLOGY

As previously noted, ectopic pregnancy occurs when the blastocyst implants in a location other than the endometrial lining of the uterus. These pregnancies are generally the result of factors that delay or prevent passage of the fertilized egg into the uterine cavity or factors inherent in the embryo that result in premature implantation. Over 98% of ectopic pregnancies occur in the fallopian tube itself. Sites for ectopic pregnancy other than the fallopian tube include the cervix (0.1%), ovary (0.5%), and abdominal cavity (0.03%). Of those ectopic pregnancies confined to the fallopian tube, approximately 93% occur in the ampullary portion, 4% in the isthmic portion, and 2.5% in the interstitial or cornual portion of the tube (Maheux, 1987). Figure 10–1 illustrates these relationships.

The exact manner in which tubal ectopic pregnancies develop within the fallopian tube remains controversial. In 1980, Budowick et al concluded that, if an ectopic pregnancy implanted in the ampullary portion of the fallopian tube, the trophoblastic tissue rapidly eroded through the epithelium of the endosalpinx and developed between the tubal lumen and serosa. However, if implantation occurred in the isthmic portion of the tube, they believed the dense muscularis of this tubal segment prevented migra-

tion of the blastocyst outside the tubal lumen. Thus a nonruptured isthmic ectopic pregnancy would always remain within the tubal lumen. Based on this theory, surgical evacuation of an isthmic ectopic pregnancy by linear salpingostomy would require entry into the tubal lumen, whereas evacuation of an ampullary ectopic pregnancy would leave the lumen undamaged. Proponents of this theory believe it is these anatomic differences in the two types of ectopic pregnancy that explain the differences in tubal patency rates following salpingostomy for ampullary and isthmic ectopic pregnancies (Decherney and Boyers, 1985). Because greater scarring and tubal blockage would be expected if the fallopian tube lumen was entered, conservative surgical procedures for ectopic pregnancy would naturally be more successful in ampullary than isthmic ectopic pregnancies.

Other authors, however, believe that the histopathologic sections appearing to show the extraluminal ectopic development of ampullary ectopic pregnancies are artifacts resulting from the cross-sectioning of two adjacent segments of the same convoluted tube. Stock (1985), in a retrospective review of 128 cases where tissue blocks were available for multiple serial sectioning, was unable to find a single case of trophoblastic invasion of the tubal muscularis by an ampullary ectopic pregnancy. Those who do not believe in the extraluminal development of ectopic pregnancies argue that the smaller lumen of the isthmic segment of the fallopian tube is inherently more prone to obstruction from scarring than the wider ampullary lumen, thus explaining the differences in tubal patency rates following conservative surgical procedures for ectopic pregnancies.

ETIOLOGY

Numerous risk factors for the development of an ectopic pregnancy have been proposed. The more commonly cited risks include prior pelvic inflammatory disease (PID), previous tubal surgery, intrauterine contraceptive device (IUCD) use, previous ectopic pregnancy, in vitro fertilization, progestin-containing contraceptives, smoking, previous abdominal surgery, and induced abortion. Two well-conducted studies have re-evaluated these classical risk factors.

273

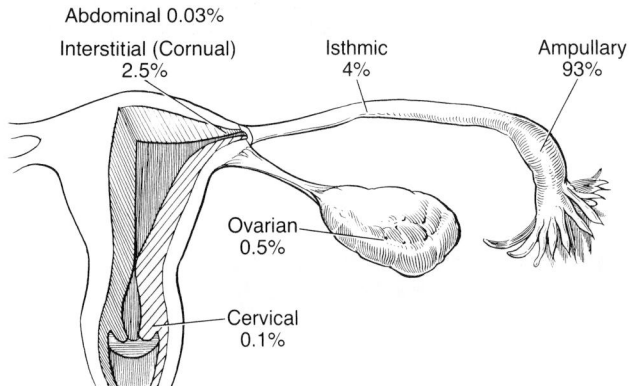

Figure 10–1
Sites of implantation in ectopic pregnancy.

In 1988, Marchbanks et al evaluated the association between ectopic pregnancy and 22 potential risk factors using a population-based case-control study. Nine variables associated with a significantly increased relative risk of ectopic pregnancy were initially identified. After conditional logistic regression, four variables remained as strong and independent risk factors: (1) current IUCD use, (2) past history of infertility, (3) prior PID, and (4) prior tubal surgery (tubal sterilization, tuboplasty, or salpingectomy). After simultaneously adjusting for the above factors, an increased risk for four other factors (previous abdominal/pelvic surgery, prior appendicitis, induced abortion, and in utero diethylstilbestrol [DES] exposure) remained. However, this increased risk did not reach statistically significant levels.

In 1996, Ankrum reported a meta-analysis of all case-control and cohort studies published in the English literature between 1978 and 1994. Previous ectopic pregnancy, previous tubal surgery, documented tubal pathology, and in utero DES exposure were found to be strongly associated with the occurrence of ectopic pregnancy. Previous genital infection (PID, gonorrhea, and *Chlamydia* infection), infertility, and more than one lifetime sexual partner were associated with a mildly increased risk.

Both of these studies confirm older previous studies showing the risk for development of an ectopic pregnancy is increased by any agent that in some way slows or prevents the fertilized embryo from reaching the uterus. Patients with histories of such risk factors—particularly those strongly associated with ectopic pregnancy, such as prior ectopic pregnancy or tubal surgery—should be screened early in pregnancy using the diagnostic modalities described later in this chapter.

PRESENTATION

Classically, the most common presenting symptoms seen with an ectopic pregnancy were pain, vaginal bleeding, and amenorrhea (Weinstein, 1985). Abdominal pain has been reported to occur in 90% to

Table 10–1. CLASSICAL SYMPTOMS OF ECTOPIC PREGNANCY

SYMPTOM	% ECTOPIC WITH SYMPTOM
Abdominal pain	90–100
Amenorrhea	75–95
Vaginal bleeding	50–80
Dizziness	20–35
Pregnancy symptoms	10–25
Passage of tissue	5–10

Adapted from Weinstein LN: Current perspective on ectopic pregnancy. Obstet Gynecol Surv 1985;40:259, with permission.

100% of ectopic pregnancies and frequently begins far in advance of tubal rupture. Other classical symptoms reported in association with ectopic pregnancy were dizziness, pregnancy symptoms, and vaginal passage of tissue. These classical symptoms are presented in Table 10–1.

The most common classical finding on physical examination is adnexal tenderness. This finding has been reported to occur in 75% to 90% of symptomatic patients (Weinstein, 1985). The presence of an adnexal mass has also been described in approximately 50% of patients with an ectopic pregnancy. However, 20% of such masses are on the side opposite the ectopic pregnancy and probably represent a corpus luteum cyst. Other classical signs associated with ectopic pregnancy were abdominal tenderness, uterine enlargement, and orthostatic changes. These classical signs are summarized in Table 10–2.

Although these classical signs and symptoms still serve as useful indicators of possible ectopic pregnancy, it must be remembered that, prior to the development of reliable and accurate techniques for evaluating patients with risk factors or minimal symptoms of ectopic pregnancy, most ectopic pregnancies were not diagnosed prior to tubal rupture. Thus many of these classical signs and symptoms are associated with advanced or ruptured ectopic pregnancies that are frequently not amenable to conservative surgical or medical treatment. Ideally, pregnant patients with risk factors or minimal symptoms suggestive of possible ectopic pregnancy should be identified and screened for this diagnosis prior to development of classical findings.

Table 10–2. CLASSICAL FINDINGS IN ECTOPIC PREGNANCY

FINDING	% ECTOPIC WITH FINDING
Adnexal tenderness	75–90
Abdominal tenderness	80–95
Adnexal mass	50
Uterine enlargement	20–30
Orthostatic changes	10–15
Fever	5–10

Adapted from Weinstein LN: Current perspective on ectopic pregnancy. Obstet Gynecol Surv 1985;40:259, with permission.

OPTIONS FOR DIAGNOSIS OF ECTOPIC PREGNANCY

Although the death rate associated with ectopic pregnancy declined almost 10-fold between 1970 and 1992, ectopic pregnancy remains the leading cause of pregnancy-related death during the first trimester and accounts for 9% of all pregnancy-related deaths (CDC, 1995). This declining death rate despite the increasing incidence of ectopic pregnancy is almost certainly the result of earlier diagnosis of the unruptured ectopic pregnancy. Diagnosis prior to tubal rupture has also allowed alternative treatment modalities to traditional salpingectomy. This earlier diagnosis has been made possible by the development of more sensitive and specific radioimmunoassays for progesterone and human chorionic gonadotropin (hCG), high-resolution transvaginal sonography, and the widespread availability of laparoscopy.

Diagnostic algorithms using these tests have been developed to simplify the management of suspected ectopic pregnancies. Initially, these algorithms relied on quantitative hCG titers and transabdominal ultrasound followed by diagnostic laparoscopy to confirm the diagnosis of ectopic pregnancy. As the sensitivity and specificity of the diagnostic tests increased, the need for laparoscopy to confirm the diagnosis decreased. Subsequently, an algorithm developed by Stovall and others (1990b) to diagnose ectopic pregnancy without the use of laparoscopy proved 100% accurate in a randomized clinical trial. This algorithm was an extension of the ectopic screening algorithm then in use at the University of Tennessee, Memphis. The current version of this nonlaparoscopic algorithm now in use at this institution is presented in Figure 10–2. The use of each of the diagnostic modalities contained in this algorithm is discussed in detail in this section. I also discuss several other classical diagnostic tests not used in this algorithm along with the rationale for their exclusion.

Serum Progesterone

Historically, use of the serum progesterone level has been proposed both as a screening tool to identify patients with potential ectopic pregnancies and to determine candidates for dilatation and curettage (D&C) to rule out ectopic pregnancy. Because progesterone concentrations associated with ectopic pregnancy are generally lower than those associated with intrauterine pregnancies, serum progesterone would appear a logical diagnostic tool for ectopic pregnancies. Unfortunately, whereas preliminary studies suggested that all ectopic pregnancies were associated with serum progesterone levels below certain threshold levels, later studies have shown considerable overlap in progesterone values for viable intrauterine pregnancies, failed intrauterine pregnancies, and ectopic pregnancies (Stovall et al, 1989b,

1990a, 1992). Although these data invalidated serum progesterone levels for the definitive diagnosis of an ectopic pregnancy, the authors of these studies suggested certain threshold levels for serum progesterone that could be used as part of a screening program for ectopic pregnancies.

Because only 1% to 2% of abnormal pregnancies (abortions or ectopic pregnancies) in the previously mentioned studies were associated with a progesterone level of 25 ng/ml or greater, patients with these levels generally do not require further evaluation for ectopic pregnancy. Exceptions would be patients at extremely high risk for ectopic pregnancy, such as those with a previous ectopic pregnancy or prior tubal ligation. Serum progesterone levels of 25 ng/ml or greater associated with an ectopic pregnancy generally indicated an ongoing and viable pregnancy that frequently exhibited cardiac activity on transvaginal ultrasound.

In these studies, a serum progesterone level less than 6.5 ng/ml was always associated with a nonviable pregnancy. However, a low serum progesterone level did not indicate whether the failed pregnancy was intrauterine or ectopic. Because this progesterone level was considered indicative of a failed pregnancy, D&C to document a failed intrauterine pregnancy could then be performed without fear of interrupting a viable pregnancy. This threshold level for pregnancy viability was subsequently lowered to 5 ng/ml and recently two viable pregnancies with serum progesterone levels of 3.9 ng/ml have been reported from the same data base (McCord et al, 1996). Thus, although a serum progesterone level of 5 ng/ml or less is highly suggestive of an abnormal pregnancy, be it intra- or extrauterine, it can no longer be considered definitive and should not be used as the sole criterion to determine candidates for D&C.

Although serum progesterone levels have not proved as valuable a diagnostic tool as previously thought, they still remain a useful screening tool for the diagnosis of ectopic pregnancies if readily available. Currently, the use of serum progesterone levels as a screening tool for ectopic pregnancy is limited by the lack of universal availability of the test itself. Many smaller laboratories do not perform the assay, and even large laboratories often perform progesterone levels only a few times a week. In these circumstances, other screening and diagnostic tools must be used to diagnose the early unruptured ectopic pregnancy.

Human Chorionic Gonadotropin

hCG levels are standardized against one of three reference preparations that are not completely interchangeable. Unfortunately, the exact reference preparation used for standardization is frequently not stated even in journal articles. The First International Standard was introduced by the World Health Or-

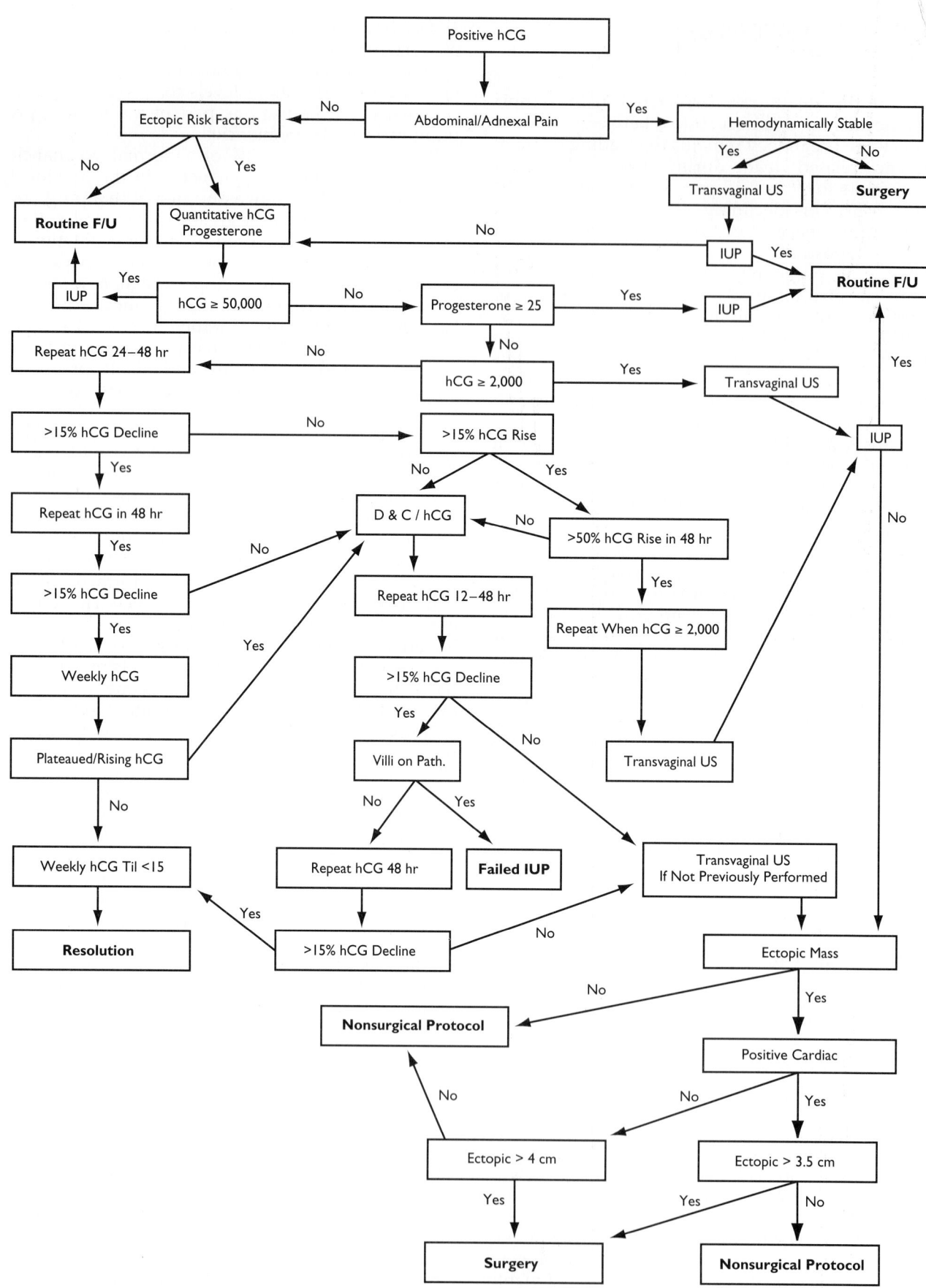

Figure 10–2
Diagnostic and treatment algorithm for ectopic pregnancy. D&C, dilatation and curettage; F/U, follow-up; IUP, intrauterine pregnancy; Path., pathology; US, ultrasound.

ganization in the 1930s. It is no longer used and is of historical interest only. The Second International Standard (2nd IS) was adopted in 1964 and is still used in some laboratories to report hCG levels. The material used to standardize the 2nd IS was relatively impure and contained large amounts of both the α and β subunits of hCG in addition to the intact hormone. Because many of the various immunoassays developed shortly after the adoption of the 2nd IS also had varying sensitivities to the α and β subunits, considerable differences in hCG titers were obtained on the same specimen by the different assays. This made correlation between the different assays difficult.

The First International Reference Preparation (1st IRP) was subsequently developed using a highly purified form of intact hCG. The 1st IRP, also known as the Third International Standard, was authorized in 1975 and should be used when reporting hCG levels. One nanogram of purified hCG is equivalent to 5.0 mIU of the 2nd IS or 9.3 mIU of the 1st IRP (Storring et al, 1980). Thus an hCG concentration referenced to the 1st IRP is roughly twice that of the same concentration referenced to the 2nd IS. All hCG levels in this chapter are referenced to the 1st IRP unless otherwise stated.

In the past, the sensitivity of available pregnancy tests was such that only a positive test was useful. Biologic and immunologic tests available in the mid-1970s frequently were not readily available, could require 24 hours or more to perform, and could detect hCG only at levels of 1500 mIU/ml or greater. Using these tests, only 50% of ectopic pregnancies had a positive pregnancy test (Hallat, 1975).

The development of rapid, extremely sensitive enzyme-linked immunosorbent assay (ELISA) pregnancy tests has simplified the diagnosis of ectopic pregnancy. Currently available quantitative assays can be performed in minutes and will detect hCG at levels of 20 to 50 mIU/ml. Using these ELISA tests, hCG can be detected in first-voided maternal urine by day 21 of the menstrual cycle (Lipscomb et al, 1993). Prior to the development of ELISA pregnancy tests, the low sensitivity of available urine pregnancy test made them unreliable with dilute urine specimens. However, the increased sensitivity of the ELISA urine pregnancy test should detect all but the earliest pregnancy without the need for a first-voided concentrated urine specimen. Likewise, these tests can be used as an initial screening test for pregnancy in patients presenting with symptoms consistent with ectopic pregnancy because all symptomatic ectopic pregnancies should have sufficiently high hCG levels to produce a positive urine test.

Serum levels of hCG can be quantified down to 2 mIU/ml using radioimmunioassay methods. The use of monoclonal antibodies to the entire hCG molecule also markedly reduces cross-reactivity to luteinizing hormone (LH), follicle-stimulating hormone, and thyroid-stimulating hormone. Using these assays, hCG can be detected in maternal serum as early as 8 days after the LH surge. Quantitative

hCG levels play a pivotal role in diagnosing the suspected ectopic pregnancy and allow for proper interpretation of the other diagnostic modalities. In intrauterine pregnancies, hCG levels rise in a curvilinear fashion until they plateau at approximately 100,000 mIU. However, the rise in hCG titers is essentially linear prior to 41 days' gestation (Daya, 1987). Because of this linearity, the rate of hCG doubling can be used to assess viability of a pregnancy.

The mean doubling time for serum hCG in a normal intrauterine pregnancy has been reported to be 1.4 to 2.1 days (Kadar et al, 1980, 1981a, 1982; Pitaway et al, 1985). However, in patients with an ectopic pregnancy, the hCG level will typically rise at a much slower rate. Based on studies of doubling times, serum hCG level will rise by at least 66% in 48 hours in 85% of normal pregnancies (one standard deviation from the mean) (Kadar et al, 1980, 1981a; Pitaway et al, 1985). Thus serum hCG levels in 15% of normal intrauterine pregnancies will rise less than this in 48 hours. However, a rise of less than 50% is more than three standard deviations from the mean and would be associated with an abnormal pregnancy 99.9% of the time. Because the interassay variability of hCG is 10% to 15%, a change of less than this amount is considered to be a plateau. Plateaued levels are the most predictive of ectopic pregnancy.

These doubling times apply only to early intrauterine pregnancies. Research by Daya (1987) has identified three gestational age ranges within which the hCG rise is linear (0 to 41 days, 41 to 57 days, and 57 to 65 days). Although the rise in hCG remains linear within each group, the rate of rise is less for each successive group, with normal 48-hour rises in hCG being 103%, 33%, and 5%, respectively, for each group. Fortunately, all normal intrauterine pregnancies should reach the discriminatory zone for both transvaginal and transabdominal ultrasound prior to 41 days' gestation.

hCG levels of 50,000 mIU/ml or greater are rarely (<0.1%) associated with an ectopic pregnancy. At hCG levels of 2000 mIU/ml or greater, transvaginal ultrasound should visualize an intrauterine sac in all normal intrauterine pregnancies (Brenaschek et al, 1988). Patients with an abnormal rise in hCG (<50% in 48 hours) or plateaued levels (±15%) may undergo D&C without fear of interrupting an ongoing viable intrauterine pregnancy. A plateaued or rising level after D&C indicates the presence of persistent trophoblastic tissue, usually an ectopic pregnancy.

Vaginal Ultrasound

The sonographic identification of an intrauterine gestational sac essentially excludes an ectopic pregnancy. The earliest sonographic finding of an intrauterine pregnancy is a gestational sac. However, intrauterine fluid accumulations may produce a pseudosac, which may be falsely interpreted as a true gestational sac. Failing intrauterine pregnancies may also appear sonographically as a pseudosac. Prior to development of a yolk sac, the double decidual sac sign (two concentric echogenic rings separated by a hypoechoic space) is the best method to differentiate a true intrauterine sac from a pseudosac.

Vaginal ultrasound permits visualization of a gestational sac at much lower hCG titers than with transabdominal scanning. Although an intrauterine pregnancy will be apparent at hCG levels of 6000 to 6500 mIU/ml with transabdominal ultrasound scanning, an experienced transvaginal sonographer should always visualize a viable intrauterine pregnancy at an hCG titer of 2000 mIU/ml (Kadar et al, 1981b; Brenaschek et al, 1988). However, the minimal hCG titer at which an intrauterine gestational sac should always be seen is not known, and thus each institution must develop its own lower limits for transvaginal detection of an intrauterine pregnancy.

The addition of color Doppler transvaginal sonography can help differentiate among a completed abortion, an incomplete abortion, and an early intrauterine pregnancy before visualization of a gestational sac. Vaginal ultrasound can also accurately image oviducts and ovaries such that ectopic pregnancies and their dimensions can be defined.

An ectopic pregnancy greater than 4 cm in greatest dimension, or the presence of adnexal cardiac activity in ectopic pregnancies larger than 3.5 cm, is a relative contraindication to methotrexate therapy. When determining candidates for methotrexate therapy, only the gestational mass or sac size is considered, and not the overall size of the hematosalpinx or hematoma. If the gestational mass cannot be distinguished from the surrounding hematoma, then the size of the entire mass must be used. Because ectopic pregnancies are generally associated with lower hCG levels than intrauterine pregnancies of similar gestation age, they can often be visualized by transvaginal ultrasound at far lower hCG levels than an intrauterine pregnancy. However, the finding of an adnexal mass in a patient with a presumed ectopic pregnancy and hCG levels less than 2000 mIU/ml should not automatically be assumed to be an ectopic pregnancy without the presence of a yolk sac, fetal pole, or cardiac activity. Frequently such masses are, in reality, corpus luteum cysts associated with an early intrauterine pregnancy.

Culdocentesis

Culdocentesis has been widely used to diagnose ectopic pregnancy. Approximately 70% to 83% of ectopic pregnancies will have nonclotting blood (positive test) on culdocentesis, but 50% to 62% of these patients will not have a ruptured fallopian tube (Cartwright et al, 1984; Romero et al, 1985; Vermesh et al, 1990). In addition, 10% to 20% of ectopic pregnancies will have either serous fluid (negative test) or no fluid/clotting blood (nondiagnostic test) at cul-

docentesis. False-positive tests will occur in 2% to 3% of culdocenteses. Historically, culdocentesis was used to decide whether to perform a laparotomy for treatment of an ectopic pregnancy or other source of bleeding (i.e., blood was found), or to proceed with diagnostic laparoscopy to obtain a definitive diagnosis. With new instrumentation, laparoscopy is now a viable treatment option even in the presence of hematoperitoneum. As a result, culdocentesis offers little clinical utility when considering diagnostic and therapeutic options for ectopic pregnancy.

Dilation and Curettage

Traditionally, D&C has played an important role in the diagnosis of ectopic pregnancy. Now, technical advances, particularly in ultrasound, frequently allow the differentiation of an ectopic or failed intrauterine pregnancy increasingly earlier in gestation and often eliminate the need for D&C. Nevertheless, D&C still plays an important role in the diagnosis of ectopic pregnancies with hCG levels below the ultrasound discriminatory zone. Except in the rare case of heterotopic pregnancy, the identification of chorionic villi in uterine contents obtained by curettage or from spontaneous passage essentially eliminates the diagnosis of ectopic pregnancy. The use of D&C also eliminates giving methotrexate unnecessarily to a patient with a failed intrauterine pregnancy.

D&C is particularly important in those patients with hCG titers below the discriminatory zone of ultrasound. In these patients, the appropriate use of hCG doubling times and serum progesterone levels is necessary to avoid the possibility of interrupting a viable intrauterine pregnancy. Patients with plateauing hCG titers (less than 15% change) or a hCG rise of less than 50% in 48 hours should undergo D&C to differentiate between a failed intrauterine pregnancy and an ectopic pregnancy. Because the diagnosis of an ectopic pregnancy can be delayed by several days after D&C while awaiting final histologic pathology, hCG titers are followed postoperatively. As noted in the ectopic pregnancy algorithm (Fig. 10–2), a serum hCG level drawn at the time of D&C is followed by a repeat level in 12 to 24 hours. Rising or inappropriately falling levels after D&C are considered diagnostic of an ectopic pregnancy.

In patients with appropriately falling hCG titers, D&C, along with its potential surgical morbidity and cost, can usually be avoided. Falling hCG titers will represent a resolving failed intrauterine pregnancy in most patients, although a small number will represent a spontaneously resolving ectopic pregnancy. Because our treatment protocol is essentially the same for spontaneously resolving ectopic pregnancies as for resolving failed intrauterine pregnancies, D&C serves little purpose in these patients. However, because the actual success rate for expectant management is less certain than with other treatment options, many clinicians still prefer to perform a

D&C to verify a failed intrauterine pregnancy in these situations. Unfortunately, villi will be absent on final histology in up to 50% of these cases (Lindahl and Ahlgen, 1986). Because only the presence of villi is diagnostic, those cases without villi require monitoring with serial hCG titers.

Laparoscopy

Laparoscopy remains the gold standard for the diagnosis of ectopic pregnancy. However, with the recent development of diagnostic algorithms that do not require the use of laparoscopy, we are rapidly moving toward a point where laparoscopy is a surgical modality rather than a diagnostic tool. As laparoscopy is eliminated, the risks, costs, and morbidity associated with diagnosis and treatment of the ectopic pregnancy are decreased.

TREATMENT OF ECTOPIC PREGNANCY

Prior to the development of surgical treatment options, mortality for presumed ectopic pregnancy was reported to be 67% (Parry, 1876). In 1884, Tait reported a series of five patients treated with salpingectomy and subsequently reported a mortality of only 5%. Laparotomy with salpingectomy soon became standard treatment for tubal ectopic pregnancy. Even today salpingectomy remains the most commonly performed procedure for ectopic pregnancies in many areas of the United States. In 1887, the first case report of a tubal pregnancy removed by opening the tube, removing the trophoblastic tissue, and suturing the tubal incision was published by Martin in the German literature. However, salpingectomy remained the treatment of choice for almost a century after this report. In fact, it was not until 1953 that a similar procedure was reported in the English literature by Stromme.

In the early 1970s laparoscopy replaced exploratory laparotomy as the preferred definitive tool for the diagnosis of ectopic pregnancies. Initially, the laparoscope was used only to diagnose a patient with an ectopic pregnancy before committing to a laparotomy, but, in 1973, Shapiro and Adler reported the first laparoscopic salpingectomy for the treatment of an ectopic pregnancy. In the 1980s, Bruhat and Decherney, along with their associates, published their experiences with the performance of laparoscopic salpingostomies as treatment for ectopic pregnancy (Bruhat et al, 1980; Decherney et al, 1981).

The most recent development in the treatment of ectopic pregnancy is the use of medical management with drugs such as methotrexate to avoid the need for surgical intervention. Although initial protocols required prolonged hospitalization and multiple doses of methotrexate and were associated with significant side effects, current protocols are performed on an outpatient basis, frequently require only one dose of methotrexate and are associated with minimal side effects.

Other options for medical treatment include the use of agents such as potassium chloride, hyperosmolar glucose, actinomycin D, prostaglandins, and RU 486. These agents may be given by direct injection into the ectopic sac or, in the case of actinomycin, prostaglandins, and RU 486, given systemically by oral, intramuscular, or intravenous administration. However, because of the limited experience with these agents, their use cannot be recommended until further data are available.

The various treatment options for ectopic pregnancy are all effective, and the most appropriate option for any particular patient depends upon the clinical circumstances, the experience of the physician, and the wishes of the patient. Each of the treatment options is discussed in detail below.

Surgical Treatment

Techniques for surgical treatment of ectopic pregnancy include salpingectomy, linear salpingostomy, linear salpingotomy, partial salpingectomy, and fimbrial expression.

Salpingectomy

Salpingectomy generally remains the surgical treatment of choice in patients who do wish to preserve future fertility. This procedure may also be appropriate in patients with a previous ectopic pregnancy in the same tube or an extensively damaged tube. Salpingectomy at the time of laparotomy is performed by cross-clamping the tubal mesosalpinx and removing the fallopian tube. In the past, cornual resection of a portion of the interstitial segment of the tube was recommended. Some surgeons further recommend suturing the round ligament to the posterior surface of the uterus (modified Coffey suspension) to cover the peritoneal defect produced by cornual resection. However, data to document a significant number of pregnancies in the remaining stump are lacking, and deep resection may predispose to uterine rupture with subsequent intrauterine pregnancy. As a result, cornual resection is not routinely performed by most gynecologists.

Salpingectomy may also be performed with the use of a laparoscope. The advantages of laparoscopic treatment include avoidance of laparotomy, decreased pain, shorter convalescence, and lower cost (Brumstead et al, 1988). Laparoscopic salpingectomy may be performed using electrocoagulation, pretied sutures, mechanical stapling devices, or combinations thereof. One technique for laparoscopic salpingectomy is illustrated in Fig. 10–3.

In the past, the performance of a "paradoxical" oophorectomy was recommended at the same time as a salpingectomy for the treatment of a tubal pregnancy (Jeffcoate, 1955). This was to ensure that ovu-

LAPAROSCOPIC SALPINGECTOMY

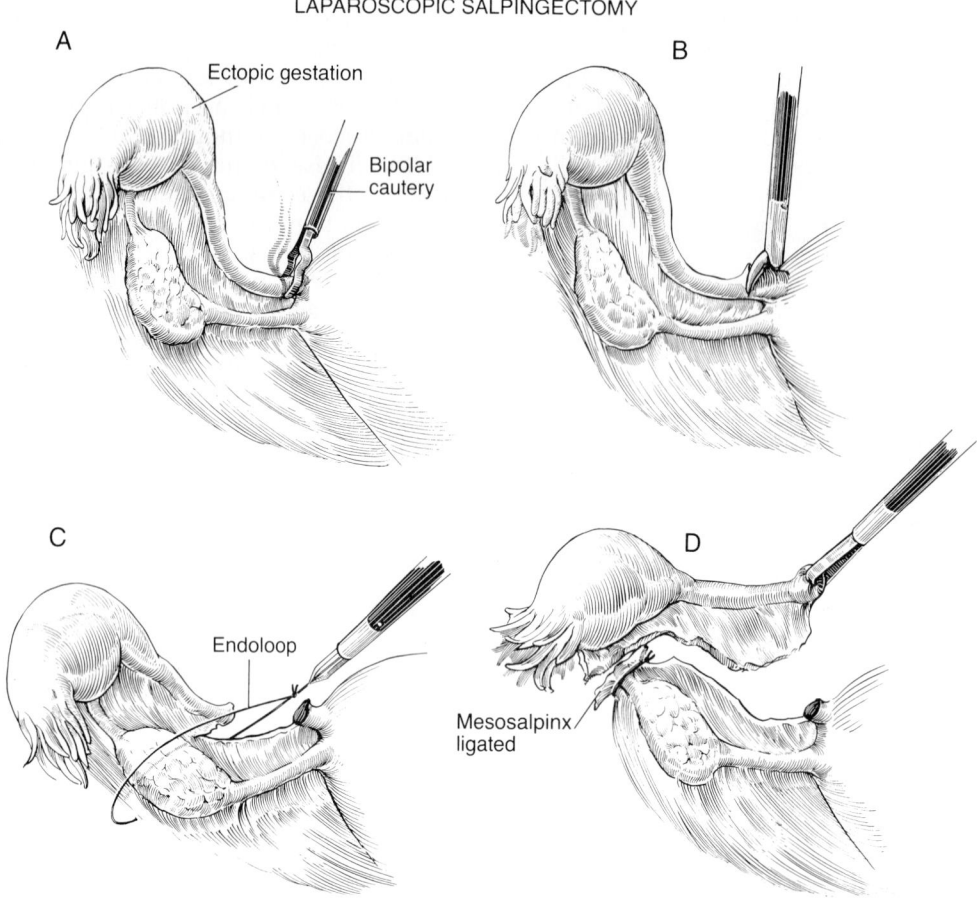

Figure 10 – 3
Technique of laparoscopic salpingectomy. *A*, Bipolar cautery utilized in the proximal portion of the fallopian tube. *B*, Transection of the fallopian tube with scissors. *C*, Placement of a pretied suture (Endoloop) around the remaining mesosalpinx. *D*, Excision of the pedicle to remove the fallopian tube.

lation occurred each month on the side with an intact fallopian tube rather than allow an ovary to function on a side where there was not a fallopian tube in close proximity. Although theoretically appealing, conception rates appear to be identical for patients treated with salpingectomy versus salpingo-oophorectomy (Franklin et al, 1973). Arguments against this practice include the possibility of future loss of the one remaining ovary to other disease processes as well as the conservation of both ovaries to serve as sources of oocytes if in vitro fertilization techniques are required for future pregnancy. Thus few authorities currently recommend paradoxical oophorectomy at the time of salpingectomy for ectopic pregnancy.

Partial Salpingectomy

Removal of only the damaged portion of the fallopian tube may be performed when future fertility is desired and more conservative procedures are not possible because of extensive damage or continued bleeding after salpingostomy. A partial salpingectomy should not be performed unless reanastomosis

is planned either immediately or as a second procedure at a later date, because repeat ectopic pregnancy in the blind distal tubal segment is possible unless the patient uses some form of contraception (Cartwright and Entman, 1984). Although minimal data exist to support either immediate or delayed repair, most surgeons prefer the delayed repair, believing repair is technically easier and more successful after resolution of the edema and inflammation accompanying an ectopic pregnancy.

Because of the low tubal patency rate following linear salpingostomy for isthmic ectopic pregnancies, some authors have advocated partial salpingectomy as the most appropriate procedure for all isthmic ectopic pregnancies (Decherney and Boyers, 1985). However, other authors believe the tubal patency rate following isthmic linear salpingostomy is acceptable (Smith et al, 1987). Given the need for a second surgery for reanastomosis as well as the inability of many patients to afford a surgery that is generally not covered by health insurance in the United States, many surgeons are reluctant to perform a partial salpingectomy unless less conservative measures are not possible.

Salpingostomy

The most common conservative surgical therapy for management of an ectopic pregnancy is linear salpingostomy. This procedure can be performed laparoscopically or with laparotomy. Although the surgical technique is similar for both the laparoscopic and the open approach, laparoscopic salpingostomy requires a much greater degree of skill and dexterity than does the same procedure performed at laparotomy. The laparoscopic technique is illustrated in Fig. 10–4.

The basics of linear salpingostomy involve the use of a scalpel, needlepoint electrode, or laser to incise the antimesenteric border of the fallopian tube over the ectopic pregnancy. The products of conception are then gently removed with graspers or thumb forceps. Vigorous removal is not recommended because this may lead to increased bleeding and damage to the tubal epithelium. The use of pressurized irrigation fluid has been suggested by some surgeons as a method of flushing additional trophoblastic tissue from the tube without increasing the risk of bleeding.

The injection of vasopressin (10 units in 20 to 50 ml of saline) prior to the linear salpingostomy can be used to markedly decrease bleeding. Injections can be made in the antimesenteric portion of tube over the ectopic pregnancy, in the mesosalpinx beneath the ectopic pregnancy, and/or in the region of the fimbria ovarica, where branches of the ovarian blood vessels enter the mesosalpinx to supply the tube. These injections can be performed laparoscopically with special laparoscopic instruments or by using standard spinal needles passed transcutaneously.

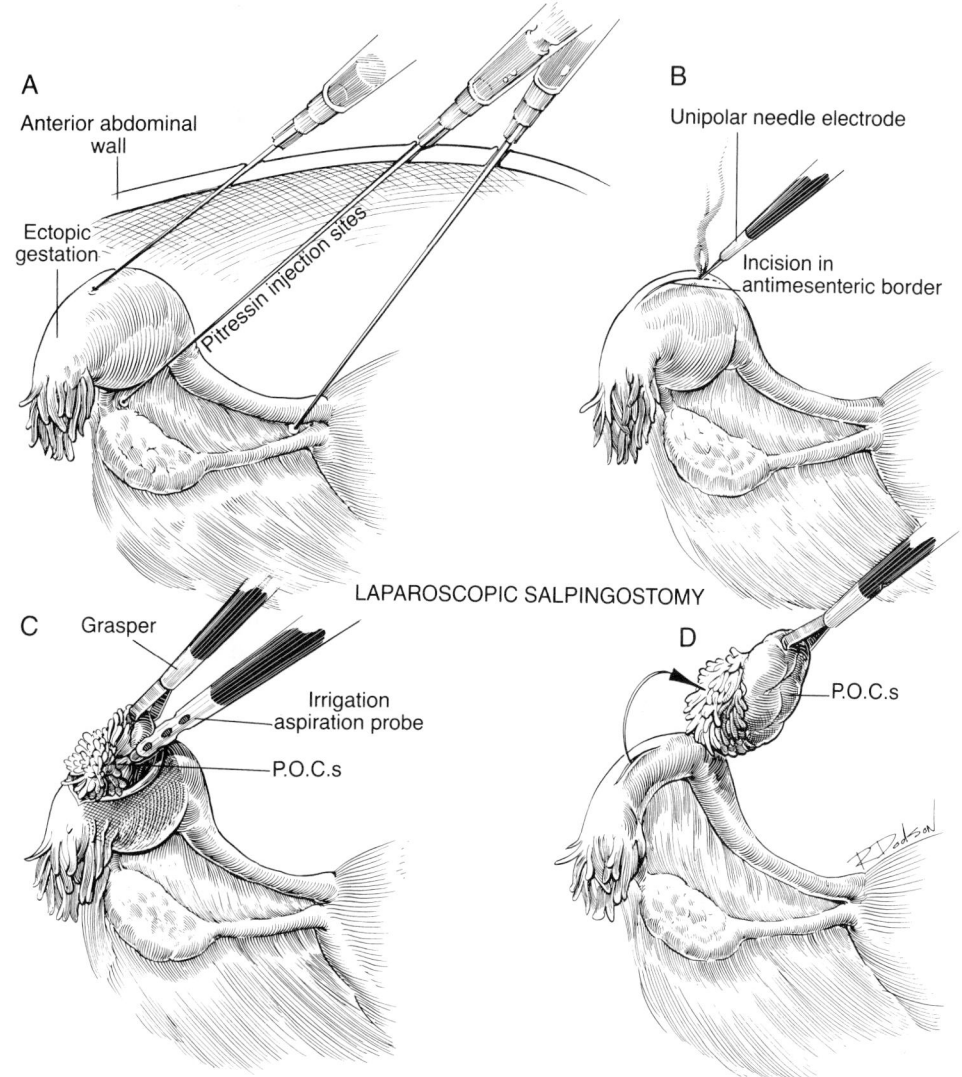

Figure 10–4
Technique of laparoscopic salpingostomy. *A*, Pitressin injection sites. *B*, Use of the unipolar needle electrode for performing the salpingostomy. *C*, Removal of the products of conception. *D*, Completion of the procedure. P.O.C.s, products of conception.

A 25-gauge spinal needle inserted using a shorter 20-gauge needle as an introducer will maintain optimum maneuverability, yet easily penetrate the tubal wall without the use of excessive countertension on the tube.

The tubal incision may be closed with fine-caliber suture (salpingotomy) or allowed to heal by secondary intention (salpingostomy). Intrauterine pregnancies have been shown to occur earlier after salpingostomy than with salpingotomy (Tulandi and Guaralnick, 1980). In addition, the presence of sutures may also favor adhesion formation. Therefore, it is generally recommended that the tubal incision be left open.

Fimbrial Expression

The use of digital pressure to extrude a fimbrial ectopic pregnancy is probably the easiest of all the conservative surgical treatments to perform. However, if the growth of ampullary ectopic pregnancies is truly extraluminal, as previously discussed, fimbrial expression would potentially be more traumatic than a surgical incision. This factor could explain the high rate of both persistent trophoblastic disease and recurrent ectopic pregnancy associated with fimbrial expression (Kooi and Kock, 1993). If this technique is to be performed, it probably should be limited to fimbrial pregnancies already in the process of being spontaneously extruded from the tube.

Methotrexate

Methotrexate is a folic acid analog that has been used extensively in medicine for the treatment of certain neoplastic diseases, severe psoriasis, and adult rheumatoid arthritis. Methotrexate inhibits dihydrofolic acid reductase, an enzyme that converts dihydrofolate to tetrahydrofolate. Tetrahydrofolates serve as carriers of one-carbon groups during the synthesis of purine nucleotides and thymidylate. Therefore, methotrexate interferes with DNA synthesis, repair, and cellular replication. Actively proliferating cells such as malignant cells, bone marrow cells, and fetal cells, as well as mucosal cells of the mouth, intestine, and urinary bladder, are generally the most sensitive to the effects of methotrexate. Methotrexate is rapidly cleared from the body by the kidneys, with 90% of an intravenous dose excreted unchanged within 24 hours of injection (Bleyer, 1978).

Until recently, methotrexate was used in gynecology only for the treatment of gestational trophoblastic disease. The first reported use of methotrexate for treatment of an ectopic pregnancy was published by Tanaka et al in 1982. In this report, an interstitial ectopic pregnancy was treated with a 15-day course of intramuscular methotrexate. Since that time, multiple reports describing the use of methotrexate for treatment of ectopic pregnancy have been published.

The initial series using methotrexate for the medical treatment of ectopic pregnancy used multiple doses of methotrexate alternating with citrovorum rescue factor. The protocols required prolonged hospital stays, lengthy courses of treatment, and higher than acceptable toxicity rates. Side effects in previous studies included changes in liver functions, bone marrow suppression, nausea, and stomatitis. Considering these side effects as well as patient costs, this form of treatment was neither attractive nor cost-effective.

Subsequently, Stovall and co-workers (1989a, 1991) at the University of Tennessee, Memphis, demonstrated that medical management of ectopic pregnancies could be performed on an outpatient basis. In this protocol, intramuscular methotrexate at dosages of 1 mg/kg of body weight was given on alternating days. Citrovorum rescue factor at dosages of 0.1 mg/kg of body weight was given on the days following methotrexate injections. Methotrexate was given only until there was a 15% decline in two consecutive daily hCG titers. A second course of methotrexate/citrovorum was given if previously falling levels plateaued or rose on two consecutive hCG titers. Using this multidose regimen, a success rate of 96% with 100 patients was obtained. Treatment was also successful in four of five patients (80%) with ectopic cardiac activity. Of the 96 successfully treated patients, 17 patients (17.7%) required only one methotrexate injection, 38 (39.6%) required two doses, 22 (22.9%) required three doses, and 19 (19.8%) received four doses. No major side effects were reported. Minor side effects included three cases of transiently elevated liver functions and two cases of stomatitis.

Single-Dose Methotrexate Protocol

A protocol using only single-dose methotrexate without the use of citrovorum rescue factor was subsequently developed at the University of Tennessee, Memphis (Stovall et al, 1991) (Table 10–3). Compared to multidose methotrexate, single-dose methotrexate is less expensive, has fewer side effects, requires less intensive patient monitoring, and has greater patient acceptance. Over 400 patients to date have been treated with this protocol with a success

Table 10–3. SINGLE-DOSE METHOTREXATE PROTOCOL

DAY	THERAPY
0	hCG ± D&C
1	hCG, AST, blood urea nitrogen, complete blood count, creatinine, Rh; methotrexate
4	hCG
7	hCG*

*With less than 15% decline in hCG level between days 4 and 7, repeat methotrexate; with more than 15% decline in hCG level between days 4 and 7, follow weekly until hCG level is less than 15 mIU/ml.

rate of approximately 94%. This success rate is similar to that obtained when a multidose protocol was followed. This success rate is particularly noteworthy because the previous limit on the size of an ectopic gestation that could be treated has been liberalized several times. Currently, the upper limit of ectopic size for medical therapy is 4 cm if cardiac activity is not present and 3.5 cm with cardiac activity.

Before treatment with methotrexate, patients must be counseled extensively about the risks and benefits of treatment, the expected course and duration of treatment, and the importance of follow-up. All patients are screened with a baseline hCG, Rh factor, complete blood count, and aspartate aminotransferase (AST), creatinine, and blood urea nitrogen levels. White blood cell counts less than $1500/mm^3$ abnormal renal function, or elevation in the liver function values more than twice the upper limit of normal are contraindications to methotrexate.

The presence of blood in the pelvis is not considered a contraindication to medical therapy. As noted previously, 50% to 60% of unruptured ectopic pregnancies will have blood in the pelvis on pelvic ultrasound, and this alone is not considered in our protocol as a reason for surgical intervention. This blood may also produce mild peritioneal signs (i.e., rebound) on abdominal examination. Although there are no data to indicate the amount of blood in the pelvis above which it is unsafe to treat medically, we empirically consider blood in the upper abdomen a strong relative contraindication to medical therapy. Stable patients with smaller amount of bloods confined to the pelvis are routinely treated medically at our institution. If there is concern that this blood is the result of active bleeding, hospitalization with observation and serial hematocrits is indicated.

Methotrexate is given intramuscularly in a dose of 50 mg/m^2 based on actual body weight. The day methotrexate is given is considered day 1. A repeat hCG is performed on days 4 and 7. If the hCG level declines less than 15 between days 4 and 7, a second dose of methotrexate is given and the protocol restarted at a new day 1. A repeat blood count and AST level are obtained before redosing. If the hCG level declines 15% or more, hCG titers are then followed weekly until less than 15 mIU/ml. If the hCG level declines less than 15% in any week, repeat methotrexate dosing is performed and the protocol restarted at a new day 1. The mean time to resolution in successfully treated patients is approximately 35 days (Stovall and Ling, 1993). However, resolution may take as long as 109 days. Tubal rupture also may be delayed, with the longest time from initial treatment to rupture in our data base occurring at 31 days.

For patients with cardiac activity, ultrasound is repeated weekly until absence of cardiac activity is demonstrated. Patients with persistent cardiac activity on day 7 are redosed. No data exist on the number of doses of methotrexate that can be safely given.

In patients with gestational trophoblastic disease, one common protocol uses a similar dose of methotrexate weekly until hCG levels are negative. Minimal side effects have been observed during this type of treatment. Nevertheless, our institution has traditionally restricted ectopic pregnancy treatments to a maximum of three injections.

During treatment, patients are required to avoid sexual intercourse, alcohol, folate-containing vitamins, and pelvic exams. Patients are also requested to avoid cabbage, onions, leeks, and other potential gas-producing foods to avoid the gastrointestinal distress from excess intestinal gas production that seems to be common following methotrexate treatment. Patients are instructed to use over-the-counter simethicone-containing antigas agents as needed for this problem.

Complications of Methotrexate Therapy

SEPARATION PAIN

Approximately 75% of patients will experience an episode of increased abdominal pain during treatment. Although the etiology of this pain is unknown, the most logical explanation is that the pain results from either tubal abortion or tubal stretching as a result of hematoma formation. Patients are advised to take ibuprofen 800 mg by mouth and lie down. If significant relief does not occur within 1 hour, patients are asked to return for re-evaluation. Hemodynamically stable patients with severe pain are admitted and observed with serial hematocrits. An ultrasound can also be obtained to document the absence of massive intra-abdominal bleeding. As noted previously, the mere presence of presumed blood in the pelvis is not an indication for surgical intervention. We believe early surgical intervention in patients experiencing separation pain may be one reason for the lower success rate reported with single-dose methotrexate therapy by other institutions.

HEMATOMA FORMATION

Following treatment with methotrexate, 56% of ectopic masses will increase in size if followed by ultrasound (Brown et al, 1991). We have observed hematomas 7 to 8 cm in size develop. Most of these patients are asymptomatic. These masses will frequently persist after the disappearance of hCG, with the longest documented time to resolution being 180 days (Brown et al, 1991).

SIDE EFFECTS

The most common side effect observed with the single-dose methotrexate protocol is excessive flatulence and bloating caused by intestinal gas formation. This problem is usually self-limiting and handled as previously described. Transient mild elevation of liver function values can occur but rarely exceeds twice the upper limits of normal. These values invariably return to normal within 2 weeks. Stomatitis generally only occurs in patients receiving more than one methotrexate injection. Viscous lidocaine can be used as needed for symptomatic relief in patients with stomatitis. Although other major side effects can occur with methotrexate, they rarely occur with the amounts and dosing intervals used with the single-dose methotrexate protocol for ectopic pregnancy.

Observation Without Intervention

The natural history of ectopic pregnancy is highly variable. At one extreme there is acute pain, hemorrhage, shock, and even death. At the other, in an asymptomatic patient, the implantation may undergo resorption or tubal abortion. When hCG titers are falling and there is no evidence of tubal rupture, nonintervention offers the freedom from chemotherapy toxicity or surgical morbidity. Success rates have been reported to be from 70% to 100% (Stoval and Ling, 1991). At our institution, all tubal ectopic pregnancy patients without cardiac activity have at least two hCG levels before treatment with methotrexate. Patients with falling levels are followed conservatively as long as hCG levels fall appropriately. However, because falling hCG levels are no guarantee against rupture, many physicians prefer to treat all diagnosed ectopic pregnancies with methotrexate regardless of the status of the hCG levels.

REPRODUCTIVE FUNCTION AFTER ECTOPIC PREGNANCY

After treatment for ectopic pregnancy, future reproductive function is of concern to the majority of patients. In a series of 527 conservative surgical procedures for ectopic pregnancy, Vermesh (1990) reported an intrauterine pregnancy rate of 54% with a recurrent ectopic pregnancy rate of 13%. However, smaller series have reported pregnancy rates as high as 82% (Langer et al, 1990). Women with normal-appearing contralateral tubes appear to have higher intrauterine and lower ectopic pregnancy rates than women with either absent or affected contralateral tubes.

In the largest single reported series of ectopic pregnancies treated with single-dose methotrexate, Stovall et al (1993) reported tubal patency in the ipsilateral tube in 51 of 62 patients (82.3%) available for hysterosalpingogram. Of the 49 patients attempting pregnancy, 79.6% became pregnant. In those patients achieving pregnancy, 87.2% had an intrauterine pregnancy and 11.8% had a recurrent ectopic pregnancy.

HETEROTOPIC PREGNANCY

Heterotopic pregnancy is the simultaneous occurrence of intrauterine and ectopic pregnancies. Classically, the incidence of naturally occurring heterotopic pregnancy has been reported as 1 in 30,000 pregnancies (De Voe and Pratt, 1948). This figure was arrived at by multiplying the ectopic rate (0.37% in 1948) by the dizygotic twinning rate of 0.8%. With the ectopic pregnancy rate now at 1.9%, the heterotopic rate for today would be 1 in 6579 pregnancies by the above formula. Any increase in the ectopic rate or multiple pregnancy rate would be expected to similarly increase the heterotopic pregnancy rate. Patients treated with clomophene citrate have been reported to have a heterotopic rate of 1 in 120 to 1 in 3000 (Tal et al, 1996). The use of menotropins for ovulation induction and in vitro fertilization techniques further increase the heterotopic rate, with estimates as high as 1 in 100 (Tal et al, 1996). Because of the differing rates of hCG and progesterone produced by heterotopic pregnancies, the algorithms for the diagnosis of ectopic pregnancy described previously in this chapter cannot be reliably used in this situation.

PERSISTENT TROPHOBLASTIC DISEASE

The continued growth of trophoblastic tissue following its apparent surgical removal is referred to as persistent trophoblastic tissue or persistent ectopic pregnancy. This condition generally occurs after incomplete removal of an ectopic pregnancy during a conservative surgical procedure. Rarely, implantation of extruded trophoblastic tissue on peritoneal or visceral surfaces can also result in persistent trophoblastic disease. Untreated, persistent trophoblastic tissue may lead to life-threatening intra-abdominal hemorrhage.

The incidence of persistent trophoblastic disease after salpingostomy ranges from 3% to 20% (Seifer et al, 1991). Seifer et al found that patients with amenorrhea less than 7 weeks or an ectopic size less than 2 cm were at increased risk for development of persistent trophoblastic disease. hCG and progesterone levels prior to surgery can also be used to identify those patients at increased risk. Lundorff and associates (1991) observed that 7 of 31 (23%) patients with a preoperative hCG level greater than 3000 mIU/ml developed persistent disease, compared to 1 of 67 (1.5%) with an hCG level below 3000 mIU/ml. Likewise, women with progesterone levels greater than 35 ng/ml or with rising hCG levels (>100 mIU/ml in 24 hours) are at increased risk to develop persistent trophoblastic disease (Hagstrome et al, 1994). The risk for persistent disease also appears to be slightly increased if the procedure is performed by laparoscopy rather than laparotomy. In a review of 157 salpingostomies for ampullary ectopic pregnancy, Seifer et al (1993) reported persistent disease in 16 of 103 patients (16%) after laparoscopic salpingostomy, and in only 1 of 54 patients (2%) following salpingostomy by laparotomy.

All patients treated for ectopic pregnancy with a conservative surgical procedure should be followed with serial hCG levels to detect persistent trophoblastic disease. An initial hCG level should be obtained in the immediate postoperative period and repeated at least weekly until it is less than 15 mIU/ml. A decline of less than 15% on consecutive hCG titers indicates persistent trophoblastic activity.

Treatment for persistent ectopic pregnancy can be surgical or medical. Surgical therapy consists of repeat salpingostomy or, more commonly, salpingectomy. Methotrexate therapy may be preferable to surgical therapy in hemodynamically stable patients. The fallopian tube is preserved and any trophoblastic tissue not confined to the tube is also treated. The single-dose methotrexate protocol described previously for ectopic pregnancy is used for treatment of persistent trophoblastic disease.

The use of prophylactic methotrexate after salpingostomy to reduce the incidence of persistent trophoblastic disease has been reported (Graczykowski and Mishell, 1997). Although prophylactic methotrexate reduced the incidence of persistent trophoblastic disease from 14.5% to 1.9%, one patient in each group still required repeat surgery. Such a treatment protocol would require treatment of 100 patients with methotrexate to prevent treating 12 patients. Furthermore, the time for the hCG levels to reach 15 mIU was only 2 days shorter (12 vs. 14 days) in the treated group. This difference was not statistically significant. Based on these data, prophylactic methotrexate cannot be advocated for routine use. However, the prophylactic use of methotrexate after conservative surgery for ectopic pregnancy may be appropriate for those patients unavailable for follow-up or at high risk for noncompliance.

SUMMARY

The incidence of ectopic pregnancy has reached epidemic proportions in the United States. Nevertheless, the mortality associated with this disease has steadily declined. This decline is primarily due to earlier diagnosis that has allowed treatment prior to rupture of the ectopic pregnancy. This earlier diagnosis is the result of improved assays for progesterone and hCG, transvaginal ultrasound, and the use of diagnostic algorithms that do not require the use of laparoscopy. Once ectopic pregnancy is diagnosed, numerous treatment options are available, including the option of medical therapy. Future developments will hopefully provide for even early diagnosis as well as data on the optimum candidates for each form of treatment.

REFERENCES

Ankum WM, Mol BWJ, Van der Veen F, Bossuyt PMM: Risk factors for ectopic pregnancy meta-analysis. Fertil Steril 1996;65:1093.
Bleyer WA: The clinical pharmacology of methotrexate: new applications for an old drug. Cancer 1978;41:36.
Brenaschek G, Rudelstorfer R, Csaicsich P: Vaginal sonography versus serum human chorionic gonadotropin in early detection of pregnancy. Am J Obstet Gynecol 1988;158:608.
Brown DL, Felker RE, Stovall TG, et al: Serial endovaginal sonography of ectopic pregnancies treated with methotrexate. Obstet Gynecol 1991;77:406.
Bruhat MA, Mahnes H, Mage G: Treatment of ectopic pregnancy by means of laparoscopy. Fertil Steril 1980;33:411.
Brumstead J, Kessler C, Gibson C, et al: A comparison of laparoscopy and laparotomy for the treatment of ectopic pregnancy. Obstet Gynecol 1988;71:889.
Budowick M, Johnson TRB, Genadry R, et al: The histopathology of the developing tubal ectopic pregnancy. Fertil Steril 1980;34:169.
Cartwright PS, Entman SE: Repeat ipsilateral tubal pregnancy following partial salpingectomy: a case report. Fertil Steril 1984;42:647.
Cartwright PS, Vaughn B, Tuttle D: Culdocentesis and ectopic pregnancy. J Reprod Med 1984;29:88.
Centers for Disease Control and Prevention: Ectopic pregnancy—United States, 1990–1992. Morbid Mortal Wkly Rep 1995;43:46.
Daya S: Human chorionic gonadotropin increase in normal early pregnancy. Am J Obstet Gynecol 1987;159:286.
Decherney AH, Boyers SP: Isthmic ectopic pregnancy: segmental resection as the treatment of choice. Fertil Steril 1985;44:307.
DeCherney AH, Romero R, Naftolin F: Surgical management of unruptured ectopic pregnancy. Fertil Steril 1981;35:21.
DeVoe RW, Pratt JH: Simultaneous intrauterine and extrauterine pregnancy. Am J Obstet Gynecol 1948;56:1119.
Franklin EW, Zeiderman AM, Laemmle P: Tubal ectopic pregnancy: etiology and obstetric and gynecologic sequelae. Am J Obstet Gynecol 1973;117:220.
Graczykowski JW, Mishell DR: Methotrexate prophylaxis for persistent ectopic pregnancy after conservative treatment by salpingostomy. Obstet Gynecol 1997;89:118.
Hagstrome HG, Hahlin M, Bennegrad-Eden B, et al: Prediction of persistent ectopic pregnancy after laparoscopic salpingostomy. Obstet Gynecol 1994;84:798.
Hallatt JG: Repeat ectopic pregnancy: a study of 123 consecutive cases. Am J Obstet Gynecol 1975;122:520.
Jeffcoate TNA: Salpingectomy or salpingo-ophorectomy? J Obstet Gynaecol Br Emp 1955;62:214.
Kadar N, Caldwell BV, Romero R: A method of screening for ectopic pregnancy and its indications. Obstet Gynecol 1981a;58:162.
Kadar N, DeCherney AH, Romero R: Receiver operating characteristics (ROC) curve analysis of the relative efficacy of single and serial chorionic gonadotropin determination in the early diagnosis of ectopic pregnancy. Fertil Steril 1982;37:542.
Kadar N, Devore G, Romero R: The discriminatory hCG zone: its use in the sonographic evaluation for ectopic pregnancy. Obstet Gynecol 1981b;58:156.
Kadar N, Freedman M, Zacher M: Further observation on the doubling time of human chorionic gonadotropin in early asymptomatic pregnancy. Fertil Steril 1980;54:783.
Kooi S, Kock HCLV. Surgical treatment for tubal pregnancies. Surg Obstet Gynecol 1993;176:519.
Langer R, Raziel A, Ron-El R, et al: Reproductive outcome after conservative surgery for unruptured tubal pregnancy: a 15 year experience. Fertil Steril 1990;53:227.
Lindahl B, Ahlgen M: Identification of chorionic villi in abortion specimens. Obstet Gynecol 1986;67:79.
Lipscomb GH, Spellman JR, Ling FW: The effect of same-day pregnancy testing on luteal phase pregnancy. Obstet Gynecol 1993;82:411.
Lundorff P, Hahlin M, Sjorblom P, Lindblom B: Persistent trophoblast after conservative treatment of tubal pregnancy: prediction and detection. Obstet Gynecol 1991;77:129.

Maheux R: Ectopic pregnancy. In Decherney AH, Polan ML (eds): Reproductive Surgery. Chicago: Year Book Medical Publishers, 1987:243.

Marchbank PA, Annegers JF, Coulam CB, et al: Risk factors for ectopic pregnancy: a population-based study. JAMA 1988;259: 1823.

Martin A: Zur Kenntniss der tubarschwangerschaft. Monatsschr Gerburtshilfer Gynakol 1887;5:244.

McCord ML, Muram D, Buster JE, et al: Single serum progesterone as a screen for ectopic pregnancy: exchanging specificity and sensitivity to obtain optimal test performance. Fertil Steril 1996;66:513.

Parry JS: Extrauterine Pregnancy: Its Causes, Species, Pathologic Anatomy, Clinical History, Diagnosis, Prognosis, and Treatment. Philadelphia, Lea & Febiger, 1876.

Pitaway DE, Reish RL, Wentz AC: Doubling times of human chorionic gonadotropin increase in early viable intrauterine pregnancies. Am J Obstet Gynecol 1985;152:299.

Romero R, Copel JA, Kadar N, et al: Value of culdocentesis in the diagnosis of ectopic pregnancy. Obstet Gynecol 1985;65:519.

Seifer DB, Diamond MP, DeCherney AH: Persistent ectopic pregnancy. Obstet Gynecol Clin North Am 1991;18:153.

Seifer DB, Gutmann JN, Grant WD, et al: Comparison of persistent ectopic pregnancy after laparoscopic salpingostomy versus salpingostomy at laparotomy for ectopic pregnancy. Obstet Gynecol 1993;81:378.

Shapiro H, Adler D: Excision of an ectopic pregnancy through the laparoscope. Am J Obstet Gynecol 1973;117:290.

Smith HO, Toledo AA, Thompson JD: Conservative surgical management of isthmic ectopic pregnancy. Am J Obstet Gynecol 1987;157:604.

Stock RJ: Histopathologic changes in tubal pregnancy. J Reprod Med 1985;30:923.

Storring PL, Gaine-Das RE, Bangham DR: International Reference Preparation of human chorionic gonadotropin for immunoassay: potency estimates in various bioassay and protein binding assay; and International Reference Preparations of the alpha and beta subunits of human chorionic gonadotropin for immunoassay. J Endocrinol 1980;84:295.

Stovall TS, Anderson RE, Ling FW, Buster JE: Improved sensitivity and specificity of a single measurement of serum progesterone over serial quantitative beta-human chorionic gonadotropin in screening for ectopic pregnancy. Hum Reprod 1992; 7:723.

Stovall TS, Kellerman AL, Ling FW, Buster JE: Emergency department diagnosis of ectopic pregnancy. Ann Emerg Med 1990a;19:1089.

Stovall TG, Ling FW: Expectant management of ectopic pregnancy. Obstet Gynecol Clin North Am 1991;18:135.

Stovall TS, Ling FW: Single-dose methotrexate: an expanded clinical trial. Am J Obstet Gynecol 1993;168:1759.

Stovall TS, Ling FW, Buster JE: Outpatient chemotherapy of unruptured ectopic pregnancy. Fertil Steril 1989a;51:435.

Stovall TS, Ling FW, Buster JE: Nonsurgical diagnosis and treatment of tubal pregnancy. Fertil Steril 1990b;54:537.

Stovall TS, Ling FW, Cope BJ, Buster JE: Preventing ruptured ectopic pregnancy with a single serum progesterone. Am J Obstet Gynecol 1989b;160:1425.

Stovall TS, Ling FW, Gray LA: Single-dose methotrexate for treatment of ectopic pregnancy. Obstet Gynecol 1991;77:749.

Stromme WB: Salpingotomy for tubal pregnancy: report of a successful case. Obstet Gynecol 1953;1:472.

Tait RL: Five cases of extrauterine pregnancy operated upon at the time of rupture. Br Med J 1884;1:1250.

Tal J, Haddad S, Gordon N, Timor-Tritsch I: Heterotopic pregnancy after ovulation induction and assisted reproductive technologies: a literature review from 1971 to 1993. Fertil Steril 1996;66:1.

Tanaka T, Hayashi H, Kutsuzawa T, et al: Treatment of interstitial ectopic pregnancy with methotrexate: report of a successful case. Fertil Steril 1982;37:851.

Tulandi T, Guaralnick M: Treatment of tubal ectopic pregnancy by salpingotomy with or without tubal suturing and salpingectomy. Fertil Steril 1980;45:292.

Vermesh M. Conservative management of ectopic gestation. Fertil Steril 1990;53:382.

Vermesh M, Graczykowski JW, Sauer MV: Reevaluation of the role of culdocentesis in the management of ectopic pregnancy. Am J Obstet Gynecol 1990;162:411.

Weinstein LN: Current perspective on ectopic pregnancy. Obstet Gynecol Surv 1985;40:259.

11

Phillip G. Stubblefield | **Contraception**

Contraception is as old as humanity. The Kahun Papyrus (Egypt, 1850 BC) describes the use of vaginal pessaries made from crocodile dung, and the Ebers Papyrus (1550 BC) details tampons made from lint soaked in fermented acacia juice to prevent pregnancy. Soranos, a Greek physician living in Rome in the second century AD, described use of vaginal plugs of wool soaked in sour oil, honey, cedar gum, pomegranate, and fig pulp to prevent conception (Himes, 1963). A number of reasonably effective means for contraception have been known for a long time: the condom since the 16th century, the cervical cap since the 1820s, the diaphragm and vaginal spermicides since the late 19th century, and intrauterine contraceptive devices (IUCDs) since early in the present century. Truly new methods are female sex steroids to prevent pregnancy, subdermal implants releasing hormones, modern methods of sterilization, and effective medicines to terminate early pregnancy.

CONTRACEPTIVE CHOICES IN THE UNITED STATES

Contraceptive choices made by U.S. couples as of 1995, as determined by a national survey carried out annually by the Ortho Pharmaceutical Corporation (Anonymous, 1995), are displayed in Figure 11–1. Oral contraception was the most common method, with voluntary contraceptive sterilization a close second. Perhaps surprisingly, the condom was the next most widely used method, and withdrawal, or coitus interruptus, was the fourth most common. A considerable portion of our population use methods of moderate or low contraceptive efficacy: condoms, withdrawal, and rhythm. Some very effective methods—progestin injection, the progestin implants, and the IUCD—are used by only a few percent. These choices are one of the reasons why 60% of U.S. pregnancies were unwanted at the time of conception, and 1.5 million legal abortions are needed each year (Mosher and Pratt, 1990). A substantial portion of our public still thinks our most effective contraceptives carry serious risk. As discussed below, these concerns are largely misplaced. For most women, unwanted pregnancy poses a far greater risk than any current contraceptive method.

Effectiveness

Theoretically, four factors should determine the effectiveness of a contraceptive method: the user's fecundability, frequency of intercourse with a fertile partner, the care with which the method is used, and the actual biologic effectiveness of the method (Steiner et al, 1996). Unfortunately, these factors cannot usually be measured directly. Fecundability, the probability of pregnancy when no contraception is used, is strongly influenced by age. Girls are relatively less fecundable immediately after menarche because of the frequent occurrence of anovulatory cycles. Fecundability improves to reach a peak in the late teens and early 20s and then declines steadily thereafter. The more frequently a couple has intercourse, the greater the probability of conception. Proper use of the contraceptive method is critical, and is also strongly influenced by personal factors such as age, race, education, socioeconomic status, and religion, and by experience with a particular contraceptive method. Thus it is not surprising that the group most often using legal abortion in the United States is 18 to 25 years old. A multivariate analysis of a large U.S. data set, the 1973 and 1976 National Surveys of Family Growth, found that four demographic factors accounted for most of the difference in contraceptive failure between different subgroups of our population: contraceptive method, intent (to delay a later desired pregnancy or to prevent pregnancy altogether), age of the user, and family income (Schirm et al, 1982). Family income is undoubtedly an indication of educational level and attitudes about many things. The biologic effectiveness of a method cannot be measured independently of these other factors, but can be estimated from large prospective studies with close medical supervision to ensure that the couples are really using the method. However, these are "best results" estimates and typically fail to include study subjects who were lost to follow-up, and cannot be applied to larger populations of people who may fail to use a method consistently for whatever reason.

Failure rates in the general U.S. population are measured every few years in national fertility surveys and form the basis for estimating "typical results." Even though pregnancy rates measured in

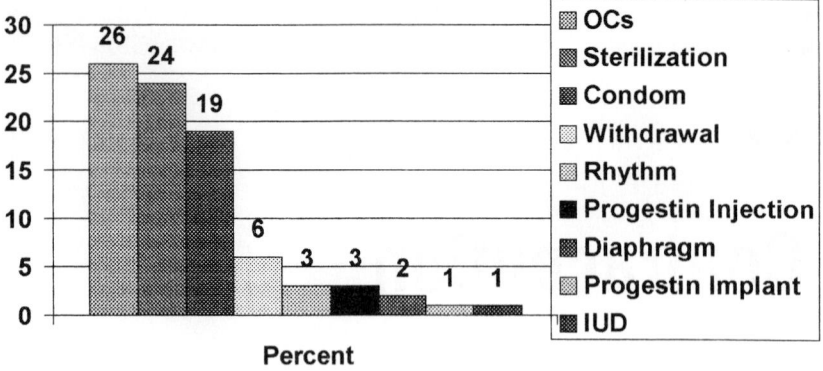

1%: Douche, Foam, Cream/Jelly alone, Sponge, Vaginal Suppository
Less than 1%, Cervical cap and Female condom

Figure 11–1
Contraceptive methods used by U.S. women, ages 15 to 50, in 1995. (From Anonymous: 1995 Annual Birth Control Study. Raritan, NJ: Ortho Pharmaceutical Corp, 1995, with permission.)

these surveys are far higher than those from prospective studies, these are also underestimates because of selective forgetting of failures that led to induced abortion. Table 11–1 represents scientific estimates from a group of experts after review of multiple published studies. The differences between "perfect use" and "typical use" result from failure to use the method consistently. Differences between the two pregnancy rates are greater for methods that require care at the time of intercourse than for the IUCD, injections, or implants, which require much less of the user. Many investigators have found that women often incorrectly understand the complexities of correct contraceptive use. Potter (1991) described a pattern seen with new oral contraceptive (OC) users: Patients skip pills because of the associated nausea, then experience breakthrough bleeding because of the missed pills and discontinue use. Continuation with a contraceptive method is less likely with methods that require constant motivation, such as the pill. Compliance and continuation are less of a problem with the IUCD, the Silastic implants, or injectable hormones. Which pregnancy rates should be quoted in advising a patient, rates for perfect use or for typical use? Both rates should be given, as an indication of the care required of the user.

Cost

Cost calculations of different contraceptive methods are complex. Some methods have a cost each time they are used (OCs, injectable progestins, condoms, and spermicide). Others have a one-time cost and provide years of benefit (Norplant, IUCDs, and sterilization). One group's attempt to compare the costs of contraceptive methods is presented in Table 11–2 (Ashraf et al, 1994).

Safety

The alternatives to sexual abstinence are contraception and pregnancy. Estimates of the risk in using a

contraceptive method must therefore include two components: health risk from complications of the contraceptive and the health risk from pregnancy should the contraceptive fail. To this equation must be added some consideration of the considerable noncontraceptive health benefits of several contraceptive methods. Age is a most important factor. Younger people have more contraceptive failures but are less likely to die from complications of contraception or from pregnancy. Computer simulation of risks of death associated with different choices for fertility control, first performed by Tietze et al (1976) and updated by Ory (1983) estimate that, for women younger than 35 years, any contraceptive method is safer than no method. At any age, Ory estimated the safest method to be diaphragm or condom backed by early, legal abortion should the method fail. This is because there is no method-related risk of death from the condom or diaphragm, and the risk of death from early abortion in the United States is very low, only 1 per 100,000 abortions. Most of our estimates of risk from contraception are based on information that is now outdated. Many cases of severe pelvic inflammatory disease (PID) and of death from septic abortion occurred with the introduction of one specific IUCD, the Dalkon Shield, which was withdrawn from the market in 1974. The older, high-dose OCs were associated with significant risk for venous thrombosis, which is markedly reduced with present low-estrogen pills. Myocardial infarction (MI) was also associated, but it is now appreciated that the risk is largely limited to older women who have other risk factors for vascular disease, most importantly cigarette smoking. With current prescribing practices and modern, low-dose OCs, a small but statistically significant risk for venous thrombosis still exists (Lidegaard, 1993), but for healthy women there is very little risk of MI (Sidney et al, 1996) or stroke (Petitti et al, 1996). Providing good contraception for women with serious illness for whom estrogen-containing OCs are contraindicated remains an important issue.

Health benefits in addition to contraception are associated with all methods. OCs reduce risk of ovarian and endometrial cancer and ectopic pregnancy.

Table 11–1. PERCENTAGE OF WOMEN EXPERIENCING CONTRACEPTIVE FAILURE DURING FIRST YEAR OF USE AND PERCENTAGE CONTINUING USE AT END OF FIRST YEAR, UNITED STATES

METHOD	% OF WOMEN EXPERIENCING ACCIDENTAL PREGNANCY WITHIN FIRST YEAR OF USE		% OF WOMEN CONTINUING USE AT 1 YEAR
	Typical Use	*Perfect Use*	
Chance	85	85	
Spermicides	21	6	43
Periodic abstinence	20		67
Calendar		9	
Ovulation method		3	
Symptothermal		2	
Postovulation		1	
Withdrawal	19	4	
Cap			
Parous women	36	26	45
Nulliparous women	18	9	58
Sponge			
Parous women	36	20	45
Nulliparous women	18	9	58
Diaphragm	18	6	58
Condom			
Female (Reality)	21	5	56
Male	12	3	63
Pill	3		72
Progestin only		0.5	
Combined		0.1	
IUCD			
Progesterone T	2.0	1.5	81
Copper T380A	0.8	0.6	78
Levonorgestrel T20	0.1	0.1	81
Depoprovera	0.3	0.3	70
Norplant*	0.3	0.3	85
Female sterilization	0.4	0.4	100
Male sterilization	0.15	0.10	100

From Hatcher RA, Trussell J, Stewart F, et al: Contraceptive Technology. 16th rev ed. New York: Irvington Publishers, 1994:113, with permission.
*Cumulative 5-year pregnancy rate for pliable tubing, divided by 5.

Barrier methods reduce risk for sexually transmitted disease, including cervical cancer. A computer simulation of risk and benefit compared five approaches to fertility control—tubal ligation, vasectomy, IUCD, condom, and combination OCs—for a population of U.S. women over age 30 (Kwachi et al, 1994). The authors used age-specific probabilities for contraceptive failure, fecundability, risk from pregnancy (delivery, spontaneous or induced abortion, ectopic), life table mortality, and mortality from specific cancers or cardiovascular disease. Between the ages of 30 and 50, use of any method of fertility control produced a net benefit of deaths prevented. This study projected increasing deaths for older men after vasectomy because the authors accepted the hypothesis that vasectomy increases risk for prostate cancer, which current studies suggest may not be real (see "Male Sterilization").

Many couples should use two contraceptive methods: hormonal contraception for excellent protection against pregnancy, and barrier contraception for protection from sexually transmitted diseases and their consequences. An increasing number of women each year do use condoms in addition to OCs (Anonymous, 1995).

Choosing a Contraceptive Method

Figure 11–2 presents an approach to helping a couple decide about contraception and demonstrates the complex interaction of patient' wishes, medical history, current physical status, goals for contraception, and need for protection against sexually transmitted disease, as well as the medical realities of specific methods.

Table 11-2. COST PER PATIENT PER YEAR OF CONTRACEPTIVE METHODS

METHOD	COST ($)	COST MULTIPLE ($)*
Vasectomy	55	Referent
Tubal ligation	118	2.14
IUCD	150	2.71
Norplant	202	3.66
DMPA	396	7.19
Oral contraceptives	456	8.27
Condoms	776	14.08
Diaphragms	1147	20.81

From Ashraf T, Arnold SB, Maxfield M: Cost effectiveness of levonorgestrel subdermal implants: comparison with other contraceptive methods available in the United States. J Reprod Med 1994;39:791, with permission.
*For every $1.00 spent on vasectomy, the amount shown would be spent on the method indicated.

COITUS INTERRUPTUS (WITHDRAWAL)

The Bible and the Koran refer to coitus interruptus (Potts, 1985). In the book of Genesis, Onan is cursed for "spilling his seed." Coitus interruptus was widely advocated in England and the United States in the 18th century and is thought, along with induced abortion and late marriage, to have accounted for most of the decline in fertility of preindustrial Europe. The most rapid decline in fertility in Europe occurred before the widespread availability of modern contraceptive methods (Potts, 1985). Coitus interruptus remains a very important means of fertility control worldwide. It is immediate availability and costs nothing. In coitus interruptus, the penis is withdrawn from the vagina just prior to ejaculation. The Oxford Study reported a failure rate of 6.7 per 100 woman-years for this method, a surprisingly low rate (Vessey et al, 1982).

There are potential problems with coitus interruptus. Neither the woman nor the man knows for sure that he will be able to withdraw in time. Another concern is that the pre-ejaculatory excretion of urethral fluids with sexual excitement may occasionally deliver live sperm that could produce conception even without vaginal ejaculation. Potts (1985) described a 1931 microscopic study of preorgasmic urethral secretions in 24 specimens from 18 individuals. Two samples contained many spermatozoa, two contained a few, and one showed occasional sperm. A more recent suggestion is that living sperm from a previous ejaculation may remain in the urethra and that urination prior to intercourse and washing after would remove this risk (Hatcher et al, 1994:344). The penis must be completely withdrawn both from the vagina and from the external genitalia as well, because pregnancy has occurred from ejaculation on the female external genitalia without penetration.

Other alterations of sexual behavior to prevent conception are oral-genital lovemaking and anal intercourse. Anal intercourse is common in some parts of the world as a means of preserving technical virginity as well as avoiding pregnancy.

LACTATION AMENORRHEA

Ovulation is suppressed for a variable period of time in women who are nursing their infants. Prolactin levels surge with each episode of suckling and reduce gonadotropin release, inhibiting ovulation (McCann et al, 1981). The duration of the antiovulatory effect is variable but is very strongly influenced by the frequency and duration of nursing, and probably by nutritional status. Women who do not nurse will have a menstruation from 1 to 3 months after birth, but women who nurse for 18 months experience amenorrhea until 8 to 13 months. Ovulation and menstruation eventually return even among women who continue to lactate. The onset of ovulation in an individual woman cannot be predicted but is unlikely prior to 6 months if no supplemental foods are given (Short et al, 1991). Pregnancy risk in the first 6 months for totally lactating women was found to be only 0.5% in one study (Hatcher et al, 1994:436). An additional method of contraception should begin at 6 months, and sooner if other foods are started to supplement lactation, because the infant will nurse less and ovulation may occur (McNeilly, 1988). Nursing may reduce breast cancer risk, but whether this is a benefit of early pregnancy or of lactation alone is unclear.

PERIODIC ABSTINENCE (RHYTHM METHOD, "NATURAL FAMILY PLANNING")

The rhythm method—pregnancy prevention by avoiding intercourse during the fertile period—has been renamed "natural family planning." Until the modern era the fertile period was thought to be close to menstruation. Soranus (AD 98–138) advised avoiding intercourse directly before and after menstruation (Himes, 1963:90), and the same advice was given by Knowlton in 1833! Three versions of natural family planning are presently taught: the calendar method, the cervical mucus method, and the sympto-thermal method. With the *calendar method*, the first day of the fertile period is estimating by subtracting 18 from the length of the shortest cycle noted during 6 to 12 months of observation. The last day of the fertile period is estimated by subtracting 11 days from the length of the longest cycle observed. The calendar method is the least effective variation. Labbock and Queenan (1989) quoted a Phillipine survey with a pregnancy rate of 40 per 100 woman-years. With the *cervical mucus method*, also known as the ovulation method or the Billings method, the woman attempts to predict the fertile period by observing the cervical mucus by feeling at the vaginal opening with her fingers. Many women can note the production of clear, watery mucus in the days immediately

General Circumstances

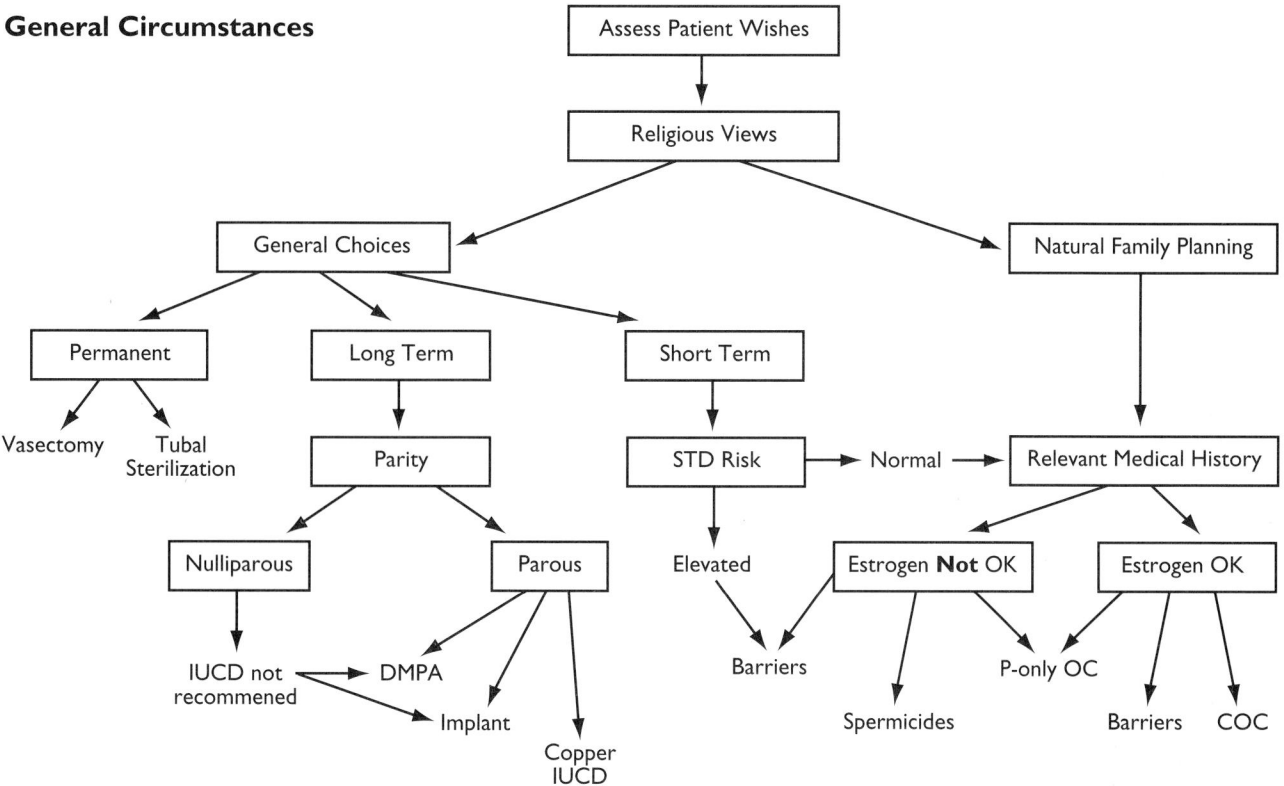

Special Circumstances

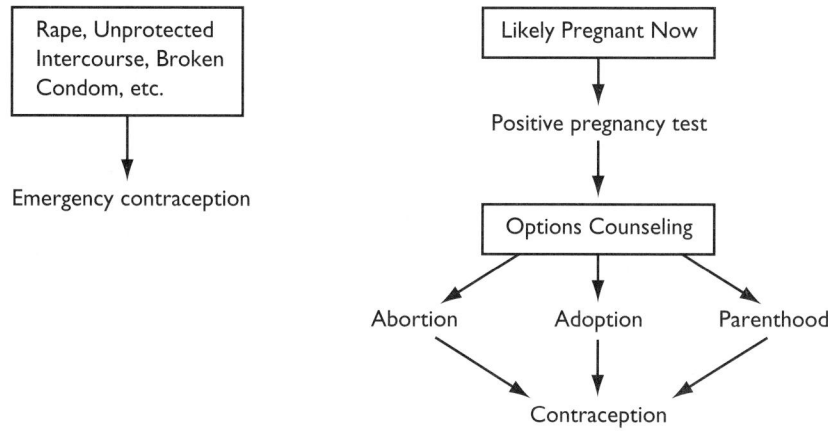

Figure 11–2
Helping couples select a contraceptive method. COC, combination estrogen-progestin oral contraceptive; DMPA, depot medroxyprogesterone acetate; P-only OC, progestin-only oral contraceptive; STD, sexually transmitted disease.

before ovulation. Under estrogen influence, the mucus increases in quantity and becomes progressively more slippery and elastic until a peak day is reached. Thereafter the mucus becomes scant and dry under the influence of progesterone until onset of the next menses. Intercourse may be allowed during the "dry days" immediately after menses until mucus is detected. Thereafter, the couple must abstain until the fourth day after the "peak" day. In the *symptothermal*

method, the first day of abstinence is predicted either from the calendar, by subtracting 21 from the length of the shortest menstrual cycle in the preceding 6 months, or by the first day mucus is detected, whichever comes first. The end of the fertile period is predicted by use of basal body temperature. The woman takes her temperature every morning and resumes intercourse 3 days after the thermal shift, the rise in body temperature that signals that the corpus luteum is producing progesterone, and hence that ovulation has occurred.

The ovulation method was studied by the World Health Organization (WHO) in a five-country study. Women who successfully completed three monthly cycles of teaching were then enrolled in a 13-cycle efficacy study. The reported pregnancy rates as calculated by the Pearl formula were 2.8 per 100 woman-years for those who always used the method (method failure) and 18.9 for those who admitted some errors in use (user failure). A critical reanalysis of the WHO study by Trussell and Grummer-Strawn (1990) calculated revised efficacy data: 3.1% probability of pregnancy in 1 year for perfect use and 86.4% probability of pregnancy during imperfect use. Even a week's abstinence around the time of actual ovulation is no insurance, because sperm may survive several days in the female genital tract. Pregnancies have been observed to occur after a single coitus 7 days prior to apparent ovulation as indicated by basal body temperature. Vaginal infections increase vaginal discharge, complicating use of the method.

Accurate advance prediction of the time of ovulation would greatly facilitate both use and efficacy of periodic abstinence. The preovulatory surge of luteotrophic hormone can be detected in the urine by daily home testing, but the tests cost $40 or more per cycle. Home monitoring of estrogen levels is also possible as a way of predicting ovulation from the preovulatory estrogen surge (Brown et al, 1991). Microcrystals in saliva are reported to indicate ovulation and form the basis for another predictive test (Rotta et al, 1992). Devices that combine an electronic thermometer with small computers are being explored in an effort to improve the accuracy of basal body temperature as a predictor of the fertile phase. Another approach is the CUE device, which measures vaginal and salivary electrical resistance. Salivary electrical resistance peaks before ovulation and can be used to predict the beginning of the fertile phase, whereas vaginal electrical resistance drops on the day of the luteinizing hormone (LH) surge and rises 1 to 2 days after ovulation, and can thus predict the end of the fertile period (Flynn, 1989). Further development of these approaches or others like them may prove useful for women in developed countries but are likely to be too expensive for the third world, where the greatest need exists.

Risks of Natural Family Planning

Avoidance of intercourse at midcycle means that, when conception does occur, it is likely to involve old gametes. Guerrero and Rojas (1975) showed that such conceptions more often lead to spontaneous abortion than do conceptions from midcycle intercourse. That failure of this method could increase birth defects has been proposed but not substantiated.

CONDOMS

The development of the condom is attributed to the 16th century Italian anatomist Fallopius, who described a linen sheath for the penis. The first serviceable condoms were made from animal intestine. The name is attributed to a Dr. Condom, a courtier of Charles II (1661–1685), who may have been the royal procurer but of whom no contemporary record exists. Casanova (1725–1798), in his "Memoirs," indicated he used condoms to prevent both venereal disease and pregnancy and wrote of "preservatives the English have invented to put the fair sex under shelter from all fear" (Himes, 1963). Condoms were used extensively in the brothels of the 18th century. Some condoms of that period discovered in a locked box in an English country home were described in the 1960s. Made around 1790 of animal intestine, they were of excellent quality (Peel, 1963). Condoms have been made in large quantities since vulcanization of rubber was developed in the 1840s. Present condoms are usually made of latex rubber, although condoms made from animal intestine are still sold and are preferred by some as better transmitting sensation. Condoms made from synthetic polymers have also been introduced (Trussell et al, 1992). The condom captures and holds the seminal fluid, thus preventing its deposition in the vagina. Condoms in the United States used to be thicker than necessary in order to prevent breakage, and this reduced sensation. A wall thickness of 0.065 to 0.085 mm was standard, but now latex condoms of only 0.010 to 0.020 mm thickness are available (Hatcher et al, 1988). Condoms prelubricated with the spermicide nonoxynol-9 have been sold for several years.

The only trial of spermicide-lubricated condoms appears to be that of Potts and McDevitt (1975), who reported a pregnancy rate of 0.83 per 100 woman-years, but the users were older, married couples who would be expected to have relatively low failure rates with all methods. The risk of condom breakage has been studied. Questionnaires given to contraception clinic patients in the United States revealed one break in 115 to 477 acts of intercourse, and that breaking usually occurred before ejaculation and seemed related to friction (Hatcher et al, 1994). Care is required if lubricants are used during intercourse. Petroleum-based products such as mineral oil markedly reduce the strength of condoms with only brief exposure. Water-based lubricants do not cause weakening of latex condoms (Voeller et al, 1989).

Benefits of Condoms

Condoms and other barriers reduce risk for sexually transmitted diseases. Several studies have demonstrated a reduction in gonorrhea and *Ureaplasma* transmission (Stone et al, 1986), and reduction of PID has also been proven (Kelaghan et al, 1982). Because tubal infertility is a sequela of PID, reduced risk of

PID should extend some protection from infertility. Indeed, a comparison of infertile women to postpartum women showed a 40% reduction in infertility with past use of condoms or the diaphragm. The greatest benefit was for methods that combined a barrier with a spermicide (Cramer et al, 1987). Condoms also offer some protection from cervical neoplasia (Kelaghan et al, 1982). In one study the relative risk of severe dysplasia among users of condoms or diaphragms was 0.4 at 5 to 9 years of use and only 0.2 when the barriers had been used for 10 years or more, a 60% to 80% reduction (Harris et al, 1980). Similar results were obtained in a North Carolina study: Ever using barrier contraception, either condoms or diaphragm, produced a 50% reduction in risk, and use for more than 2.5 years produced a 70% reduction in risk (Coker et al, 1992). Another study compared women with invasive cervical cancer to controls. The risk ratio of invasive cervical cancer was 0.4, and only 0.2 when ever-users of condoms or diaphragms were compared to never-users (Parazzini et al, 1989).

With the worldwide epidemic of acquired immunodeficiency disease, there is intense interest in the ability of condoms to prevent transmission of the human immunodeficiency virus (HIV). When tested in vitro, *Chlamydia trachomatis*, herpesvirus type 2, HIV virus, and hepatitis B were not able to penetrate latex condoms but did cross through condoms made from animal intestine (Judson et al, 1989). Additional protection is provided by the addition of the spermicide nonoxynol-9 (Judson et al, 1989; Jones et al, 1994). Follow-up of sexual partners of HIV-infected people have shown considerable protection when condoms are used (Fischl et al, 1987). In a study from Cameroon, 273 HIV-negative women at high risk because of multiple partners were given latex condoms and nonoxynol-9 suppositories and instruction in their use. Those who used the condoms and spermicide consistently had about one third the rate of seroconversion to HIV-positive status (Zenkeng et al, 1993). In a similar study in Rwanda, women whose partners received HIV testing and counseling and who were given latex condoms and spermicide had a reduction in HIV seroconversion rates from 4.1 to 1.8 per 100 person-years, and the prevalence of gonorrhea was reduced from 16% to 4% (Allen et al, 1992). Protection by condoms is not perfect. Genital contact prior to putting on the condom and breakage may explain this, but simple failure to use the condom is the more likely explanation.

Hazards of Condoms

Skin irritation of either partner from condom use has long been recognized but now is appreciated to be allergy to latex. Latex allergy can lead to life-threatening anaphylaxis and could be triggered in either partner by use of a latex condom. Use of nonoxynol-9 spermicide with latex condoms may increase risk for latex sensitization by leaching out a natural rubber protein from the latex (Blank, 1996). New barriers have been developed that can be used by couples with latex sensitivity: the female condom, which is made of polyurethane (see "Vaginal Barriers"), and the Tactylon synthetic condom soon to be available, (Trussell et al, 1992).

VAGINAL SPERMICIDES

In his 1833 pamphlet "Fruits of Philosophy," the American physician Knowlton proposed that women syringe the vagina with a solution of zinc sulfate immediately after intercourse. Suppositories made of quinine in cocoa butter were made and sold in England in the last century and continued in use until recently. The active ingredients of modern preparations are nonoxynol-9 or octoxynol, detergents that immobilize sperm. Vaginal spermicides combine the spermicidal chemical with a base of cream, jelly, aerosol foam, foaming tablet, film, or suppository. No other contraceptive method, except for periodic abstinence, has as broad a range of effectiveness. Johnson and Masters (1962) studied intercourse under laboratory conditions with a variety of preparations. The aerosol foam and one of the cream preparations provided rapid dispersal throughout the vagina. The jellies and melting suppositories provided poor distribution and would have required prolonged intercourse prior to ejaculation in order to provide significant protection from pregnancy. Aerosol-based spermicides are recommended for this reason. In widespread use in the United States, spermicides alone appear considerably less effective than condoms, diaphragm with spermicide, or the rhythm method (see Table 11–1).

Benefits of Spermicides

Nonoxynol-9 reduces risk for bacterial vaginosis (Jones et al, 1994) and sexually transmitted diseases, including HIV, and, if used with a condom or diaphragm barrier, increases the protection (Zenkeng et al, 1993). However, as noted above, nonoxynol-9 may increase latex allergy when used with latex condoms or diaphragms.

Hazards of Spermicides

One study suggested that spermicides could increase the occurrence of birth defects in babies born after contraceptive failure (Jick et al, 1981). However, it has since been shown that nonoxynol-9 is not absorbed from the human vagina (Malyk, 1983), and several studies have found no such hazard (Shapiro et al, 1982; Linn et al, 1983). A study of 30,000 women found no greater risk for miscarriage, birth defects, or low birth weight for spermicide users than for other women (Harlap et al, 1985).

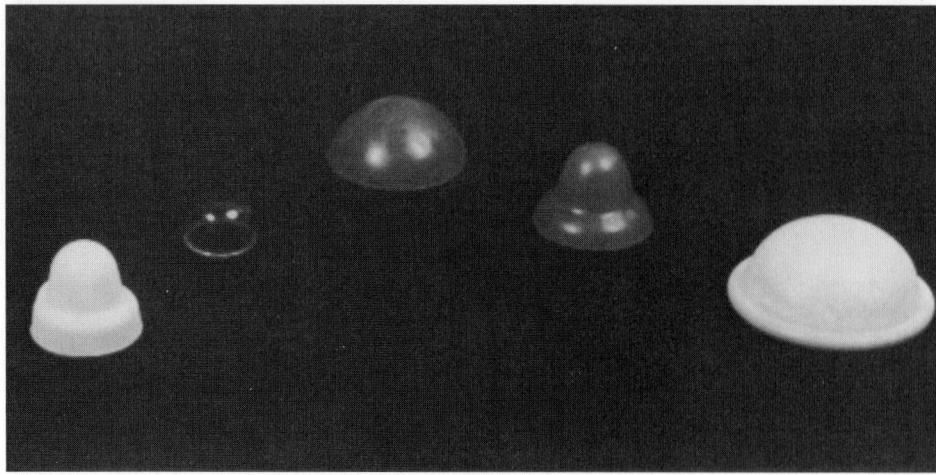

Figure 11–3
Vaginal barriers. *Left to right*, Prentiff cavity rim cervical cap, plastic cap, vault cap, vimule, and vaginal diaphragm.

VAGINAL BARRIERS

Hasse, a German physician, is given credit for invention of the rubber diaphragm. Writing under the pseudonym W. P. J. Mensinga, Hasse describe the device in an 1882 monograph. The cervical cap is even older. In 1838, another German physician, Wilde, described a rubber pessary made from a wax impression of the cervix (Bodemer, 1976). At the beginning of the 20th century, four types of vaginal barrier devices existed: vaginal diaphragm, cervical cap, vault cap, and vimule (Fig. 11–3). All are still made and sold in England. Both cervical caps and vaginal diaphragms were used in the United States until the 1950s, but only the diaphragm continued in production, probably because it was easier to fit, insert, and remove. The cervical cap was rediscovered by American women who went to England and has been reintroduced into the United States, largely through the efforts of feminist women's health centers. The vaginal barriers deserve serious attention. When used consistently they can be reasonably effective. They are safe, and they share the noncontraceptive benefits of relative protection from sexually transmitted diseases, tubal infertility, and cervical neoplasia as described for condoms.

Diaphragms

The diaphragm consists of a circular metal spring covered with fine latex rubber. There are several types as determined by the spring rim: coil, flat, or arcing. Coil-spring and flat-spring diaphragms become a flat oval when compressed for insertion. Arcing diaphragms form an arc, or half-moon, when compressed, and in my experience are the easiest to insert correctly. One manufacturer offers a diaphragm with an inner flange of soft latex (Wide Seal Diaphragm; Milex) that markedly increases the surface area of contact between the rim and the vagina and may add to the efficacy, although whether or not this is true has not been tested (Fig. 11–4). Indeed,

there appear to be no published comparative trials of the different types of diaphragms.

Diaphragms are made in diameters that increase by 5-mm increments from 50 to 90 mm. Most women can be fitted with one in the midrange, from 65 to 75 mm. Too large a diaphragm will produce discomfort and even vaginal ulcerations; however, the actual effect of diaphragm size or type upon pregnancy rates is unknown. Studies of simulated and actual intercourse under laboratory conditions by Johnson and Masters (1962) revealed the elevation of the uterus and expansion of the vaginal barrel with normal sexual excitement, which can allow slippage of the diaphragm. They noted the female-superior position and multiple mountings just prior to orgasm as likely to result in the penis being reinserted in front of the diaphragm, which would cause failure of contraception. The practitioner must not only fit the diaphragm for the patient, but must instruct her in its insertion, and verify by examination that she can insert it correctly to cover the cervix and upper vagina.

In present times, the diaphragm is always used in combination with a spermicide; however, the contri-

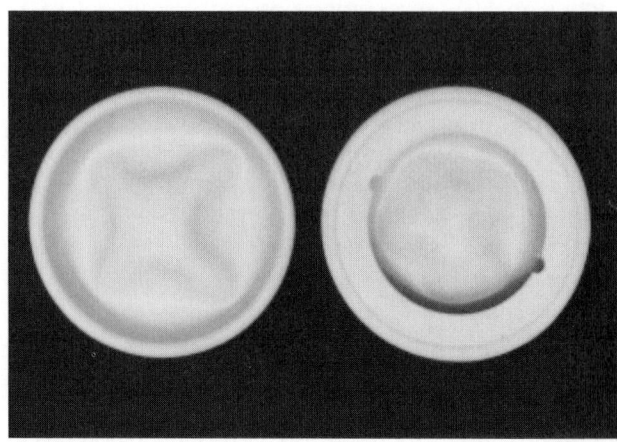

Figure 11–4
Wide Seal diaphragm (*right*) and Allflex diaphragm (*left*).

bution of the spermicide to pregnancy prevention is only now being examined. In one trial, women who used only the diaphragm only had a 12-month failure rate of 19.3 per 100 women, while those who used the diaphragm with spermicide had a pregnancy rate of 12.3 per 100 women, a difference not statistically significant in this small sample but suggesting spermicides should not be abandoned without further study (Bounds et al, 1995).

Fitting Diaphragms

The practitioner performs a vaginal examination and, with the first and second fingertips in the posterior fornix, uses the thumb of the examining hand placed against the first finger to mark where the first finger touches the pubic bone (Hatcher et al, 1994: 211). The distance from tip of the middle finger to the tip of the thumb is the diameter of the diaphragm to try first. A fitting set of diaphragms of various sizes is used. The test diaphragm is inserted and then checked by palpation. The diaphragm should open easily in the vagina and fill the fornices without pressure. The largest diaphragm that fits comfortably should be selected; too large a diaphragm will result in vaginal ulcerations. A size 65 or 70 diaphragm will fit most women. The patient is then instructed to examine herself, note the rim of the diaphragm and where it sits under the urethra and laterally, and feel for the cervix under the rubber dome. She then should remove the diaphragm and insert it herself for checking by the practitioner. If the leading edge of the diaphragm is placed into the posterior fornix, the diaphragm will open easily in the correct location. Diaphragms that do not assume an arc configuration when compressed may be accidentally inserted into the anterior fornix and, hence, fail to cover the cervix. Self-exam by the patient should reveal this malposition and lead to correction, if the patient has been properly instructed.

For contraceptive use, a teaspoon or so of water-soluble spermicidal jelly or cream is placed in the cavity of the dome and the diaphragm is inserted dome downward so that the cervix will sit in a pool of the spermicide. The diaphragm can be inserted several hours prior to intercourse. If intercourse will be repeated, additional spermicidal jelly should be inserted into the vagina without removing the diaphragm. The diaphragm is left in place at least 6 hours after intercourse to allow for immobilization of sperm. It is then removed, washed with soap and water, allowed to dry, and stored away from heat. It should not be dusted with talc because talc contains contaminating asbestos fibers, and genital dusting with talc has been linked to ovarian cancer.

Benefits of the Diaphragm

As noted in our discussion of condoms, diaphragms and other barriers provide substantial protection against sexually transmitted disease and cervical neoplasia.

Hazards of the Diaphragm

Diaphragm use appears to increase the risk for bladder infections, probably because it rests under the urethra and may hinder clearing of the bacteriuria that inevitably results from vaginal intercourse. Prolonged wearing of the diaphragm to allow for multiple acts of intercourse may be especially likely to produce cystitis. Use of a diaphragm and spermicide in a university group was associated with a relative risk for cystitis of 1.42, 2.83, and 5.68 when used 1, 3, or 5 days in the previous week (Hooton et al, 1996). When recurrent cystitis is a problem and the patient wishes to continue with a vaginal barrier, a smaller sized wide seal diaphragm or a cervical cap can be used to reduce urethral pressure. Toxic shock has been linked to diaphragm use, but the association was probably only accidental because a formal epidemiologic study comparing toxic shock cases with controls found no increased risk from diaphragm use (Davis et al, 1980).

The Cervical Cap

The cap is much smaller than the diaphragm, is also made of latex rubber but contains no metal spring in the rim, and covers only the cervix. Although it is harder to fit the cap and instruction in its use takes more time, women who have already learned to use the vaginal diaphragm readily learn to use the cap. The advantage of the cap over the diaphragm is that it can be left in place several days and hence is more convenient. Formerly, a variety of rigid caps were sold in the United States and were left in place for the entire interval between the menses. Caps are used with spermicide but, again, the contribution of the spermicide to the efficacy is not known. Modern studies of the efficacy of cervical caps have revealed a range of results. One of the better results for the Prentif Cap was a pregnancy rate of 8 per 100 woman-years with the cap left in place for as long as 5 days at a time (Koch, 1982). A randomized trial of the Prentif Cap compared to the diaphragm found equal efficacy (Berstein, 1986). A large multicenter study of 3433 women found a first year pregnancy rate of 11.3 per 100 women. Women whose pattern of use was described as "near perfect," who did not report unprotected intercourse, wore the cap for a maximum of 72 hours, and always used spermicide, had a first year pregnancy rate of 6.1 per 100, half of the overall rate (Richwald et al, 1989). A multivariate analysis of patient factors among this large group revealed that pregnancy rate increased when the cap was worn for more than 72 hours at a time. Dislodgment of the cap during intercourse or at other times was reported by 27.5% of the users at 3 months, and this along with accidental pregnancy were the main reasons women discontinued cap use. Forty-nine per cent discontinued use or were lost to follow-up by 1 year. A new version of the cervical cap, called the Femcap and made of silicone rubber, is in trials (Shihata and Gollub, 1992).

Fitting Cervical Caps

The Prentif cavity rim cervical cap is approved and available in the United States in sizes 22, 25, 28, and 31, (the size is the internal diameter of the rim in millimeters). The practitioner estimates the cervical size by inspection and palpation. In my experience, nulliparous women usually require a size 22, whereas parous women generally are fitted with a size 25. The cap is inserted by compressing it between finger and thumb and placing it through the introitus, dome outward. It is then pushed gently up to seat over the cervix. The dome is indented with the examiner's finger to create suction against the cervix. The dome should remain compressed for several seconds, indicating a good fit, and gentle lateral pressure on the rim should not dislodge the cap. Prentif caps were designed for multiparous women. The smallest size, 22 mm, is not small enough for the cervix of many nulliparous women and a good fit may not be obtained. Prior to use, the cap is one-third filled with contraceptive cream. The cap can be left is place up to 72 hours. The patient is instructed to check for dislodgment of the cap after intercourse, and an additional method such as the condom is advised until it is clear that the cap will not be dislodged.

The vimule and Dumas vault cap are not sold in the United States, although they can be obtained from the manufacturer in England.* The vimule has a thin edge, and in U.S. trials trauma to the vaginal skin was occasionally observed. There are no modern efficacy studies for either of these barriers.

Hazards of the Cervical Cap

The cap has the same theoretical risk for toxic shock as the diaphragm—perhaps more because it may be left in place longer. However, no cases were reported among the 3433 users in the large study described earlier (Richwald et al, 1989). Progression of initially negative cervical cytology to dysplasia occurred in 4% of cap wearers and less than 2% of diaphragm wearers in the National Institutes of Health–funded comparative trial (Centers for Disease Control [CDC], 1984b). In contrast, Koch (1982) found cap wearers to be protected from developing dysplasia by comparison to controls using other methods, and in other large studies development of significant cervical lesions during follow-up has been very uncommon (Richwald et al, 1989). Although it may be worn for several days at a time, the cervical cap does not

compress the urethra and has not been associated with cystitis (Koch, 1982; Richwald et al, 1989). Latex allergy is possible with the cap, as with the diaphragm and condoms.

The Female Condom

Vaginal pouches of polyurethane are available as a "female condom." The trials submitted for U.S. approval reported a pregnancy rate of 15% in 6 months. There is as yet no randomized trial comparing this device to other barriers; however, the pregnancy rate with perfect use was only 2.6%, comparable to the diaphragm and cervical cap (Trussell et al, 1994).

Sponge and Spermicide

Sea sponge appears to have been used as a barrier contraceptive since ancient times. A synthetic version of soft medical-grade polyurethane sponge permeated with 1 g of the spermicide nonoxynol-9 was sold for several years in the United States but has been withdrawn by the manufacturer. The pregnancy rate was somewhat higher than that of the diaphragm, and there was risk for toxic shock if the device fragmented during removal and part of it remained in the vagina (CDC, 1984a).

INTRAUTERINE CONTRACEPTIVE DEVICES

The German physician Richter described intrauterine insertion of silkworm gut to prevent pregnancy in the early 1900s. Graefenberg further developed the idea, first tying silver wire around strands of silkworm gut to strengthen it so it would remain in the uterus, and then moving on to pliable rings of spiral twisted silver or gold wire. His 1931 paper presented at a Planned Parenthood symposium described a large number of patients, reporting that only 1.6% of patients treated with silver rings became pregnant. Ota (1931) described a different version of intrauterine silver rings at about the same time in Japan. Lippes and Margulies carried IUCDs to the next state of development, flexible plastic devices that could be pulled into a tube for insertion without dilatation of the cervix and would then resume their original shape when released into the uterine cavity. Subsequent developments in IUCD technology included the Dalkon Shield, a plastic device with a unique multifilament tail; the progesterone-releasing IUCD (Progestasert); and the first of the copper-releasing IUCDs, the Copper T200 and the Copper 7. The Dalkon Shield was associated with a high rate of infection, and almost ended IUCD use in the United States. A third generation of improved IUCDs are in use, the high-dose copper devices such as the Copper T380A (ParaGard) and the levonorgestrel-releasing device (LevoT), which is available in Europe.

---

*Lamberts Ltd., 200 Queensbridge Rd., Dalston, London E8, England.

Mechanism of Action

IUCDs are thought to provoke a low-grade inflammatory response from the endometrium resulting in formation of a "biologic foam" containing strands of fibrin, phagocytic cells, and proteolytic enzymes released from these cells into the uterine cavity. Copper IUCDs continuously release a small amount of the metal, producing a still greater inflammatory response. All IUCDs stimulate the formation of prostaglandins within the uterus, consistent with both smooth muscle contraction and inflammation. Scanning electron microscope studies of the endometrium in IUCD-wearing women show alterations in the surface morphology of cells, especially of the microvilli of ciliated cells (El Badrawi et al, 1981). There are major alterations in the composition of proteins within the uterine cavity, and new proteins and proteinase inhibitors are found in washings from the uterus (Umapathysivam and Jones, 1980). IUCDs prevent the passage of sperm through the uterus and, hence, prevent implantation. The altered intrauterine environment also interferes with implantation of the fertilized ova, and copper devices can be used after coitus as emergency contraception. A laparoscopy study was successful about half the time in obtaining sperm in washings from the fallopian tubes of control women at midcycle, whereas among women who were wearing IUCDs there were no sperm in the tubal washings (Habashi et al, 1980). Ova flushed from the tubes at the time of tubal sterilization showed no evidence of fertilization in IUCD-wearing women (Alvarez et al, 1989). Segal and colleagues (1985) measured serum levels of the pregnancy hormone β-human chorionic gonadotropin (β-hCG) in 496 samples from 26 IUCD-wearing women. Four women were positive, but only at midcycle, a cross-reaction of the assay with the surge of luteotrophic hormone that precedes ovulation. None continued to test positive into the luteal phase of the cycle. Thus current evidence is that the IUCD is not an abortifacient, but rather that its primary mechanism of action is to prevent fertilization. The progesterone-releasing IUCD (Progestasert) contains natural progesterone in its stem, inside a polymer capsule that allows sustained slow release of the hormone over a year or more. This produces an atrophic endometrial lining. The new LevoT IUCD has additional mechanisms of action. It releases levonorgestrel, a progestin so much more potent than natural progesterone that the amount released from the IUCD is sufficient to block ovulation in many women. Blood levels of levonorgestrel are about half of those seen with the subdermal implant Norplant (Sivin and Stern, 1994).

Much of what we know of IUCDs in clinical use came from a large multicenter study carried out by Tietze and Lewit (1970). Larger versions of the same IUCD (Lippes C or D) have lower pregnancy rates and lower rates of expulsion, but more removals for pain and bleeding, than do smaller versions of the same devices (Lippes Loop A or B). Excessive menstrual bleeding and pain are the most frequent problems experienced by IUCD wearers, not infection or pregnancy. Rates of removal for pain and bleeding range from 5 to 20 per 100 woman-years. Smaller devices are better tolerated by the patient. The rediscovery by Zipper of Graefenberg's finding that certain metal wires inhibit fertility when placed inside the uterus led to the development of the small IUCD wrapped with copper wire, the Copper T200 and Copper 7 (Tatum, 1982). Another approach to improving the efficacy of a small IUCD was the development of the progesterone-releasing "T," the Progestasert. Both of these medicated, second-generation IUCDs had lower pregnancy rates than the unmedicated "T" devices, but were not consistently superior to the older Lippes Loop C or D. Third-generation IUCDs, the Copper T380A and the LevoT, are far superior. The Copper T380A (ParaGard) has bands of copper on the cross arms of the "T" in addition to the copper wire around the stem, providing a total surface area of 380 mm of copper, almost double the surface area of copper of the T200 and the Copper 7 (Fig. 11–5) The increased dose of copper clearly improves contraceptive effect and

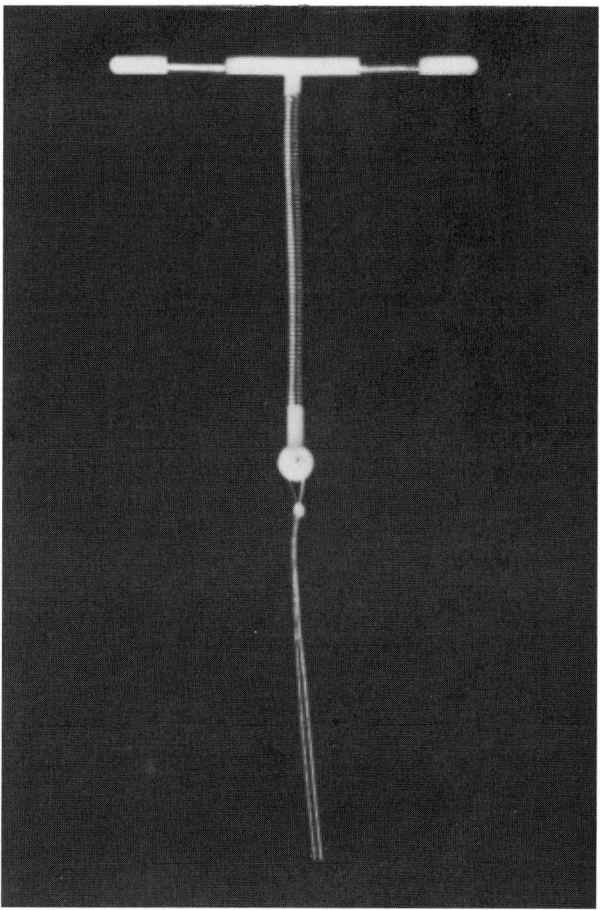

Figure 11–5
The Copper T380A (ParaGard) IUCD. (Courtesy of GynoPharma, Inc.)

Table 11–3. PREGNANCY AND ECTOPIC PREGNANCY RATES PER 1000 WOMAN-YEARS IN THE FIRST 2 YEARS OF RANDOMIZED, NON-POSTPARTUM TRIALS OF COPPER IUCDs BY DOSE

COPPER IUCDs BY COPPER SURFACE AREA	PREGNANCY RATE	ECTOPIC PREGNANCY RATE
380 mm^2		
TCu 380A	3.4 ± 0.6	0.2 ± 0.1
220–300 mm^2		
TCu 220	9.0 ± 0.8	0.3 ± 0.1
200 mm^2		
TCu 200	24.9 ± 1.7	0.6 ± 0.3
Cu7 200	25.8 ± 2.3	1.0 ± 0.4

From Sivin I: Dose and age dependent ectopic pregnancy risks with intrauterine contraception. Obstet Gynecol 1991;78:291, with permission.

markedly reduces risk for ectopic pregnancy (Table 11–3) (Sivin, 1991). This device and the LevoT had pregnancy rates of less than 0.2 per 100 woman-years and a total cumulative rate over a 7-year period of only 1.1 per 100 for the Copper T380 and 1.4 for the LevoT (Sivin and Stern, 1994). The T380A is approved for 10 years of continuous use.

IUCDs and Infection

Serious infection was very rare with modern IUCDs prior to the 1970s (Tietze and Lewit, 1970). Then two things happened: the accelerating cultural change in the Western world placed many more women at risk for sexually transmitted diseases, and a new type of IUCD was introduced. In 1974 several deaths from sepsis were reported in women wearing one particular IUCD, the Dalkon Shield (Christian, 1974). The Dalkon differed from other devices in having a multifilament tail inside a sheath, which under laboratory conditions could act as a wick, pulling bacteria from the vagina up into the uterus (Tatum et al, 1975). The other devices had tails of monofilament nylon. The Dalkon Shield was eventually withdrawn from the market. More recently, good epidemiologic studies of PID have established the precise relation between different types of IUCDs and PID. The large U.S. Women's Health study found the Dalkon Shield device to increase risk for PID by eightfold when women admitted to the hospital for PID were compared to hospitalized control women with other illnesses. In contrast, risk from the other IUCDs was markedly less: relative risk of PID was 2.2 for the Progestasert, 1.9 for the Copper 7, 1.3 for the Saf-T-Coil, and 1.2 for the Lippes Loop (Burkeman for the Women's Health Study, 1981). Increased risk was only detectable within 4 months of insertion of the IUCD, confirming a previous finding that, although bacteria are introduced into the uterine cavity with insertion, the uterus soon sterilizes itself (Mishell et al, 1966). Exposure to sexually transmitted pathogens is the more important determinant of PID than is the wearing of an IUCD. In the Women's Health

Study, women who were currently married or cohabiting and who said they had only one sexual partner in the last 6 months had no increase in PID. In contrast, previously married or single women did have marginal increase in risk, even though they had had only one partner in the previous 6 months (Lee et al, 1988). Similar findings came from a WHO study of modern copper IUCDs: PID was increased only during the first 20 days after insertion, then fell to a rate of only 1.6 per 1000 women per year, not different from the general population (Farley et al, 1992). Risk of PID was highest in the youngest women and in women with no previous pregnancy. Whether this truly a risk of the IUCD or reflects risk for PID independent of IUCD use is not clear. In U.S. practice at present, IUCDs are generally not prescribed for nulliparous women.

The only pelvic infection that has been unequivocally related to IUCDs is actinomycosis (Spence, 1978). This fungus-like bacterium is regularly found in the oral cavity, and inhabits the vagina in a small percentage of women. PID with actinomycosis appears only to have been reported in IUCD-wearing women. Rates of colonization increase with duration of use for plastic devices but appear to be much less for copper-releasing IUD's.

Ectopic Pregnancy

In considering risk of pregnancy at any site, all IUCDs are not equal. Compared with women using no contraception, IUCD-wearing women were found to have a 60% reduction in risk for ectopic pregnancy, the same reduction as was seen for users of barrier methods. Women using oral contraceptives had a 90% reduction of risk (Ory for the Women's Health Study, 1981). In a subsequent study using data from 1981 through 1986, Rossing and colleagues (1993a) found that IUCD wearers had an 80% reduction in risk (relative risk of 0.2) of ectopic pregnancy compared to women not using contraception, but, when IUCD wearers were compared to women using OCs or barriers, they experienced three times the risk of ectopic pregnancy, showing that IUCDs were not as protective as OCs and barriers. The risk for ectopic pregnancy among wearers of the Progestasert IUCD is increased (Snowden, 1977), but the LevoT and the Copper T380A confer almost complete protection (see Table 11–3) Reported rates of ectopic pregnancy with both devices are only 2 per 10,000 woman-years (Sivin, 1991; Luukkainen and Toivonen, 1995). Should pregnancy occur with an IUCD in place, it will be ectopic in 5% of cases. This is because the fallopian tubes are less well protected against pregnancy than is the uterus.

There is controversy as to whether women who have used the IUCD in the past have subsequent increased risk for ectopic pregnancy that may reflect previous tubal injury. Rossing and colleagues (1993b) found that past users of IUCDs had double the risk of ectopic pregnancy when compared to women who had never worn an IUCD. Women in this study wore first- and second-generation IUCDs, including the Dalkon Shield, but a risk from previous IUCD use was found even when the analysis was limited to women wearing then-available copper devices. Their study did not include the present higher dose copper device, the Copper T380A. Whether past use of the Copper T380A will have any effect on later risk of ectopic pregnancy is not yet known.

IUCDs and Fertility

In the Oxford Study, women gave birth just as promptly after IUCD removal as they did after discontinuing use of the diaphragm (Vessey et al, 1974). However, studies from the 1980s of women referred for infertility evaluation compared to fertile women have found history of IUCD use associated with a twofold increased risk for tubal infertility (Cramer et al. 1985). Copper devices appeared less likely to be associated with infertility, and the risk was not increased among women who reported only one sexual partner (Daling et al, 1985). Possible explanations of these conflicting results are that women in the Oxford Study were married and in their mid-20s or older at enrollment and probably at low risk for sexually transmitted infections. These studies need to be updated for modern IUCDs, and current protocols developed for IUCD placement where women are screened as described below prior to insertion.

Clinical Management of IUCDs

In general, the IUCD is better suited for older women who have had some pregnancies than for younger women who have not. Younger women have higher pregnancy rates, more expulsions, and more removals for medical reasons and are more likely to develop PID. Contraindications to IUCD use include pregnancy, history of PID or ectopic pregnancy, undiagnosed genital bleeding, uterine anomalies, and fibroid tumors of more than small size. Chronic immune suppression should be considered a contraindication. Women with such conditions are considered to be at greater risk for PID, but, in addition, the effectiveness of the IUCD may be compromised. A number of pregnancies have occurred in renal transplant patients soon after IUCD insertion. Copper allergy or Wilson's disease contraindicate copper IUCDs. IUCDs are usually inserted just after menstruation in order to be sure the patient is not pregnant. Ideally the patient should have an initial visit for a medical history, physical exam, cervical culture for gonorrhea, and immunofluorescent test for *Chlamydia*, along with detailed counseling as to risks and alternatives, and is then scheduled for insertion soon after her next menses.

IUCD Insertion

A β-hCG–specific urine pregnancy test is performed just prior to insertion. Premedication with oral prostaglandin inhibitors such as ibuprofen is strongly advised to reduce pain. Consideration could be given to antibiotic prophylaxis with a tetracycline, although this has not been demonstrated to reduce risk of PID (Walsh et al, 1994). Insertion is preceded by a pelvic exam to determine uterine size and position. The uterine cavity should be measured with a uterine sound. Depth of the cavity should measure at least 6 cm from the external os. A smaller uterus is not likely to tolerate current IUCDs (Burnhill, 1985). I routinely offer a paracervical block with 10 ml of 1% lidocaine mixed with atropine 0.5 mg to avoid vasovagal syncope and minimize discomfort. Serious cardiac arrhythmia can be seen with cervical stimulation is some women, and can be avoided by these measures. Use of a tenaculum with insertion is mandatory to prevent perforation. The cervix is exposed with a speculum, grasped with a tenaculum, and gently pulled downward to straighten the angle between cervical canal and uterine cavity; then the IUCD, previously loaded into its inserter, is gently introduced through the cervical canal. With the "T" type of devices such as the ParaGard and the Progestasert, the outer sheath of the insert is next withdrawn a short distance to release the arms of the "T," and is then gently pushed inward again to elevate the now opened "T" up against the fundus (Burnhill, 1985). Next the outer sheath and then the inner stylet of the inserter are withdrawn, and the strings are cut to project about 2 cm from the external cervical os.

As of this writing only two IUCDs are sold in the United States: the Copper T380A (ParaGard) and the Progestasert. The advantage of the Progestasert is reduced menstrual bleeding, but it must be replaced after 1 year and has a higher pregnancy rate and greater risk for ectopic pregnancy. For most women who want intrauterine contraception, the ParaGard is a better choice. IUCDs can be inserted after uncomplicated induced abortion (Rosenfield and Castadot, 1974). Insertion soon after childbirth is especially desired in third-world countries, but expulsion of present devices is frequent after postpartum insertion. The least desirable time for IUCD insertions is probably the conventional 6 weeks or so after childbirth. By this time the cervical canal has closed down but the uterus is still soft, and risk of perforation is increased.

Perforation of IUCDs through the uterine wall generally only occurs at insertion, although it may not be recognized until pregnancy occurs, infection develops, or the IUCD string disappears as the partially perforated IUCD is pulled upward through the uterine wall by uterine contractions. An exception to this is the downward migration of "T" or "7"-shaped devices, which have at times eroded through the posterior wall of the cervix into the vagina.

"Lost" IUCD

Whenever the IUCD strings cannot be found on examination, the endocervical canal is probed with the small brush used for endocervical cytology (Cytobrush) (Ben-Rafael and Bider, 1996). Gentle rotation of the brush in the cervical canal will likely retrieve the strings. If this maneuver is not successful, ultrasound is performed to visualize the IUCD inside the uterus. If it cannot be seen with ultrasound, then an abdominal radiograph is needed to search for a perforated device in the abdominal cavity. If the device is intrauterine, it can be left in place or removed under ultrasound guidance. An IUCD in the abdominal cavity should be removed, preferably by laparoscopic surgery, to prevent adhesion formation and possible bowel obstruction.

Management of PID

When PID is suspected in IUCD-wearing women, the IUCD should be immediately removed, appropriate cultures taken, and high-dose antibiotic therapy begun with drugs effective for gonorrhea, *Chlamydia*, *Bacteroides* and other anaerobes as well as the gram-negative aerobes. Pelvic abscess should be suspected and ruled out by ultrasound examination. *Actinomyces* must be considered as a possible cause, especially if the IUCD has been in place many years.

Management of IUCDs in Pregnancy

If the IUCD strings are visible, the IUCD should be removed as soon as pregnancy is diagnosed. There is a twofold increased risk of spontaneous abortion following removal, but the prospect for later septic abortion, premature rupture of the membranes, and premature birth is much greater if the device is left in than when it is removed or expelled (Tatum et al, 1976). Where the strings are not visible, an ultra-

sound exam should localize the IUCD and determine whether an unnoticed expulsion has occurred. If the IUCD is present, there are three options for management: therapeutic abortion, ultrasound-guided intrauterine removal of the IUCD, and continuation of the pregnancy with the device left in place. An informed decision should be made by the patient, with an awareness of the risks of all options. She must be aware of the risks of septic abortion, including death, should the pregnancy continue with the device in place. If the patient elects to continue the pregnancy without intervention, she must be closely observed. She should be advised to report all abnormal symptoms, such as flu-like syndrome, fever, abdominal cramping, and pain or bleeding, because symptoms may be insidious. Death has been known to occur within 72 hours of onset of symptoms. At the earliest sign of sepsis, high-dose antibiotic therapy effective against aerobic and anaerobic organisms should be started and the uterus promptly evacuated.

We have successfully removed IUCDs during pregnancy with ultrasound guidance in four cases using a small alligator forceps (Stubblefield et al, 1988). Others have reported similar success (Sachs et al, 1992). A German paper suggests removal is more likely to be successful when the IUCD is in the lower portion of the uterus or lateral to the pregnancy. If the IUCD is rostral (i.e., the gestational sac is between the cervical os and the IUCD), removal may be more likely to result in loss of the pregnancy (Wagner et al, 1980). Because 5% of pregnancies in IUCD-wearing women will be ectopic, pelvic pain, irregular vaginal bleeding, or delayed menses should be evaluated with a β-hCG−specific pregnancy test.

Duration of Use

Annual rates of pregnancy, expulsions, and medical removals *decrease* with each year of IUCD use (ParaGard Prescribing Information, 1995), and most of the risk of PID is in the first few months after insertion. Hence a woman who has had no problem with her IUCD by year 5, for example, is very unlikely to experience problems in the subsequent year. The ParaGard is approved for 10 years. Theoretically it contains enough copper for 25 years. The life span of plastic devices such as the Lippes Loop is not known. Many women have worn them for a decade or longer. Ten-year data have been reported: The 10-year cumulative pregnancy rate was only 5 per 100, and 32% of the original group were still wearing their IUCDs after 10 years (Lippes and Zielenzny, 1975). As noted, the Progestasert should be replaced after 1 year.

Actinomyces can be detected by cervical cytology. I therefore advise annual cytology for IUCD-wearing women and ask the laboratory to look for *Actinomyces*. Should *Actinomyces*-like particles be reported, I advise removal of the IUCD and treatment with oral penicillin. Patients who are still wearing inert plastic devices other than the Dalkon Shield, who still want intrauterine contraception, may continue until the menopause if they have no pelvic pain or excessive bleeding, a negative pelvic exam, and no *Actinomyces* on cervical cytology. IUCDs should be removed when menopause occurs because the uterus shrinks thereafter, making removal difficult. Women still wearing Dalkon Shield IUCDs should have them removed immediately.

IUCDs for Women with Chronic Illness

Contraception is a special problem for women with valvular heart disease because pregnancy may be a major hazard and OCs have often been considered contraindicated. The IUCD has been suggested as appropriate for these women (Anonymous, 1994), although others have expressed concern about subacute bacterial endocarditis. A long-acting IUCD such as the Copper T380A is appropriate, after thorough consideration of specific risks of pregnancy for the patient and the suitability of sterilization for her or her spouse, and, of course, with written informed consent. The American Heart Association does not recommend antibiotic prophylaxis for IUCD insertion or removal in the absence of infection, except in certain high-risk patients: those with prosthetic heart valves or a previous history of endocarditis (Dajani et al, 1990).

IUCDs are of interest for women with diabetes mellitus for whom excellent contraception is especially important but where many are concerned about estrogen-containing OCs. Kimmerle and colleagues (1993) followed 59 women with type I diabetes after insertion of a European copper IUCD (CU Safe 300) and compared them to 1150 nondiabetic women of similar age and parity. There was no difference in IUCD-related events of pregnancy, removal for pain and bleeding, or expulsion through 3 years, and the only case of PID occurred in the nondiabetic group. In another study, 160 women with type II non–insulin dependent diabetes were followed for up to 5 years after insertion of a Copper T380A device (ParaGard). None developed PID in 3066 months of observation. Event rates were as would be expected in a nondiabetic population, and 70% continued with the IUCD at 3 years (Kjos et al, 1994).

HORMONAL CONTRACEPTION

In 1940, Sturgis and Albright reported that injections of estrogen blocked ovulation in women; however, the implications of this discovery for contraception awaited the synthesis of the orally active progestins in the 1950s (Rock et al, 1956). The progestins (progesterone-like hormones) first used contained trace amounts of estrogen as a by-product of synthesis. These compounds were highly effective in producing amenorrhea and preventing conception. The pure progestins developed subsequently also prevented conception, but produced a less acceptable bleeding pattern with irregular spotting and staining. Estrogen was added back intentionally and the modern combination OC resulted. Still, these compounds would have remained as curiosities in search of medical uses, had it not been for the determined efforts of the family planning pioneer Margaret Sanger, who recognized the enormous potential of hormonal contraception to free women from slavery to reproduction. She convinced scientists to proceed with large-scale human trials and raised the funds to support the trials from private charity.

Hormonal contraceptives are female sex steroids, combinations of a synthetic estrogen and a synthetic progesterone (progestin) or a progestin only. The most widely used hormonal contraceptive is the combination OC. Progestin-only OCs are also available and are useful for specific indications—for example, in women who are breast-feeding, or who have a contraindication to estrogen. Combination OCs can be *monophasic*, with the same dose of estrogen and progestin each day, or *multiphasic*, with different doses of the steroids used through a 21-day pill cycle. Typically they are administered for 21 days beginning on the Sunday after a menstrual period, then discontinued for 7 days to allow for withdrawal bleeding that mimics the normal menstrual cycle. Both 21- and 28-day versions are available. The 28-day versions provide placebo tablets for the last 7 days so that the user simply takes one pill a day and starts a new pack as soon as the first is completed. Progestin-only OCs are taken every day without interruption. OCs currently available in the United States are listed in Table 11–4. Other forms of hormonal contraception include long-acting injectable hormones and subdermal implants that release progestins. Vaginal rings that release sex hormones are under investigation.

Steroid Hormone Action

Sex steroids were originally defined by their biologic activity. Androgens allow development of male reproductive organs in castrate male animals. Estrogens allow growth of female reproductive organs in castrate females. Progesterone maintains pregnancy after removal of the corpus luteum in subprimate species in which pregnancy is corpus luteum dependent. Receptor proteins exist in the nucleus of cells in steroid-sensitive tissues. The receptors are specific for a particular steroid hormone. The hormone diffuses out of the bloodstream and into the nucleus of the cell, where it binds to the receptor. When bound to its hormone, the receptor protein undergoes a change in its shape that allows the hormone-receptor complex to bind to specific sites on the chromatin. Binding to chromatin alters gene transcription and

Table 11-4. COMPOSITION OF ORAL CONTRACEPTIVES IN CURRENT USE IN THE UNITED STATES, 1997

TRADE NAME*	PROGESTIN† (mg)	ESTROGEN† (mg)
Progestin only		
Micronor (Nor-Q D)	NE 0.35	None
Ovrette	*d,l*-NG 0.075	None
Combination—monophasic		
Norlestrin	NEA 2.5	EE 0.050
Norlestrin-1	NEA 1.0	EE 0.050
Loestrin 1.5/30	NEA 1.5	EE 0.030
Loestrin 1/20	NEA 1.0	EE 0.020
Ovral	*d,l*-NG 0.5	EE 0.050
Lo/Ovral	*d,l*-NG 0.3	EE 0.030
Nordette (Levlen)	levoNG 0.15	EE 0.030
Ortho-Novum 1/50 (Norinyl 1 + 50)	NE 1.0	ME 0.050
Ovcon 50	NE 1.0	EE 0.050
Ortho-Novum 1/35 (Norinyl 1 + 35)	NE 1.0	EE 0.035
Modicon (Brevicon)	NE 0.5	EE 0.035
Ovcom 35	NE 0.4	EE 0.035
Demulen 1/50	ED 1.0	EE 0.050
Demulen 1/35	ED 1.0	EE 0.035
Desogen (Ortho-Cept)	Deso 0.15	EE 0.030
Ortho-Cyclen	Norg 0.25	EE 0.035
Combination—multiphasic		
Ortho-Novum 10/11		
First 10 days	NE 0.5	EE 0.035
Next 11 days	NE 1.0	EE 0.035
Ortho-Novum 7/7/7		
First 7 days	NE 0.5	EE 0.035
Next 7 days	NE 0.75	EE 0.035
Last 7 days	NE 1.0	EE 0.035
Triphasil (Tri-Levlen)		
First 6 days	levoNG 0.050	EE 0.030
Next 5 days	levoNG 0.075	EE 0.040
Last 10 days	levoNG 0.125	EE 0.030
Tri-Norinyl		
First 7 days	NE 0.5	EE 0.035
Next 9 days	NE 1.0	EE 0.035
Next 5 days	NE 0.5	EE 0.035
Ortho Tri-Cyclen		
First 7 days	Norg 0.18	EE 0.035
Next 7 days	Norg 0.215	EE 0.035
Next 7 days	Norg 0.250	EE 0.035

*Trade names are used for ease of identification. A second, identical formulation by a different manufacturer is identified in parentheses. Most formulations are available either as a 21-day or 28-day package. The 28-day package has seven placebo tablets.
†Deso, desogestrel; *d,l*-NG, *d,l*-norgestrel; ED, ethynodiol diacetate; EE, ethinyl estradiol; levoNG, levonorgestrel; ME, mestranol; NE, norethindrone; NEA, norethindrone acetate; Norg, norgestimate.

within minutes, produces changes in levels of messenger RNA, and protein synthesis begins (Spelsberg et al, 1989). Sex steroids are characterized by their affinity for specific estrogen, progesterone, or androgen receptors, as well as by their biologic effects in different systems. The synthetic estrogen ethinyl estradiol (EE) has strong affinity for estrogen receptors, equivalent to natural 17β-estradiol. The progestins have binding affinities very little greater than zero, 0.002 to 0.003 of the relative affinity of 17β-estradiol or EE (Phillips, 1990). Hence they can have no estrogen effect of any consequence except at enormous doses. Older literature suggests that some progestins may be metabolized to estrogenic compounds. Whether or not this is true seems not to have been

examined with modern techniques, but any clinical effect would be completely overwhelmed by the presence of estrogen taken with them in combination OCs.

The naturally occurring sex steroids are rapidly absorbed by the gut but go directly into the liver via the portal circulation. Here they are rapidly metabolized and inactivated; therefore, large doses are required for oral activity. The addition of the ethinyl group to carbon 17 of the steroid molecule confers oral activity by hindering degradation by the liver enzyme 17-hydroxysteroid dehydrogenase. At first sex steroids could be obtained only by isolation from biologic sources; hence only small quantities were available. Partial synthesis from plant sources and the structural alteration of adding the 17-ethinyl group made possible oral administration in doses sufficient for biologic effect at low cost.

Oral Contraceptives

Estrogens Used in OCs

OCs sold in the United States contain either of two estrogens: mestranol or EE. Mestranol is EE with an extra methyl group. It is not directly active and requires bioactivation in the liver, where the methyl group is cleaved, releasing the active agent, EE. OCs with 35 µg of EE provide the same blood levels as do OCs containing 50 µg of mestranol (Brody et al, 1989).

Progestins Used in OCs

The term *progestin* describes a large number of synthetic compounds that mimic the effect of natural progesterone but differ from it structurally (Fig. 11 –6). Progestins are divided into three classes based on their structure: *estranes* and *gonanes*, which are 19-norprogestins, structurally similar to testosterone but lacking a carbon at position 19; and *pregnanes*, which are 17-acetoxysteroids and are structurally most similar to natural progesterone. Estrane and gonane compounds are used in OCs in the United States. Medroxyprogesterone acetate (Provera), one of the pregnane compounds, is the major injectable proges-

tin. The progestins differ from each other in their affinities for estrogen, androgen, and progesterone receptors as well as their ability to inhibit ovulation, substitute for progesterone, and antagonize estrogen. Some progestins are bound directly to progesterone receptors (e.g., levonorgestrel, norethindrone, norgestimate). Others require bioactivation (Rozenbaum, 1982); for example, desogestrel is converted in the liver to the active metabolite 3-ketodesogestrel. The pharmacology of the progestins is complex. Norgestimate, for example, is directly active on the progesterone receptor (Phillips, 1990) but is also metabolized to several compounds that are also active, among them levonorgestrel. Norgestrel exists as two stereoisomers. Only levonorgestrel is biologically active. The first norgestrel OCs were mixtures of the dextro and levo forms, whereas the newer preparations contain only levonorgestrel. Three newer progestins, norgestimate, desogestrel, and gestodene, are available in Europe. Only norgestimate and desogrestrel are sold in the United States. Norgestimate, desogestrel, and gestodene are viewed as more "selective" than the other 19-norprogestins in that they have less androgenic potency by comparison with their potencies in inhibiting ovulation (Phillips, 1990). Gestodene is the most potent of the progestins in current OCs; that is, very little of it is required for antifertility effects.

Generations of OCs

Over the years since their introduction, OCs have evolved. The estrogen dose has diminished, and new

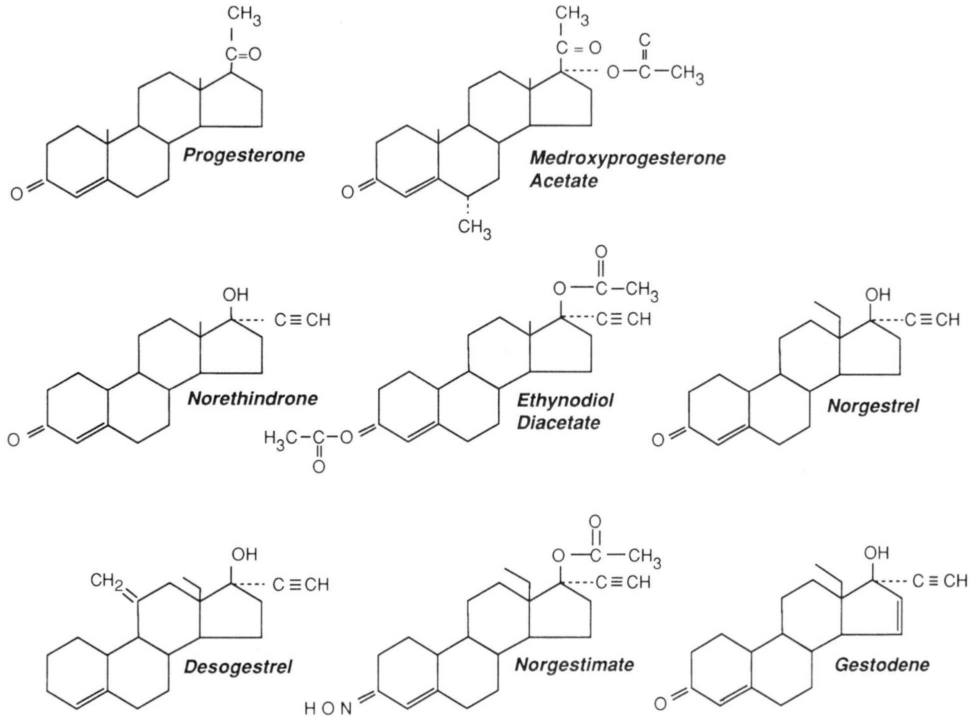

Figure 11–6
Progestins used in hormonal contraceptives.

progestins have been introduced in an effort to reduce side effects and improve safety. Three generations of OCs are recognized. One classification, as used by WHO studies of coagulation with the new progestins, is as follows (Lewis et al, 1996a). First-generation OCs are all of those containing 50 µg of EE, regardless of the progestin and its dose. Second-generation OCs are those containing 35 µg or less of EE, and a progestin other than desogestrel or gestodene. Third-generation OCs contain 30 µg or less of EE and one of the new progestins, desogestrel or gestodene. To the list of third-generation products should be added those containing 35 µg of EE and norgestimate, a new progestin widely used in the United States but less used in Europe.

Subdermal Implants

The first of the subdermal implant systems (Norplant) became available in the United States in 1991. Subdermal implants are a major advance in hormonal contraception because the constant slow release of the steroid across the wall of the Silastic rubber capsule results in constant low blood levels, in contrast to fluctuating blood levels of contraceptive steroids taken by the oral route or by injection (Fig. 11–7). OCs result in rapid rise of hormone levels followed by a rapid fall; hence, to provide enough to prevent pregnancy, much higher levels are needed for part of each day. Theoretically, contraception with the subdermal implant should be safer than OCs because much lower blood levels are needed, and, in the case of Norplant, no estrogen is given at all. Six small rods of Silastic rubber implanted under the skin provide a constant slow release of the progestin levonorgestrel for 5 or more years. Blood levels stabilize at about 0.4 ng/ml after a few months of insertion, a level considerably below

that seen with similar OCs (Shoupe and Mishell, 1989).

Vaginal Rings

Silastic rings worn in the vagina release steroid hormones that are absorbed at a constant rate, allowing contraception with blood levels of the steroids well below the peak levels that are seen with OCs. Rings containing levonorgestrel or combinations of levonorgestrel and estrogens have been studied. A large WHO trial with a ring releasing levonorgestrel at 20 µg/day produced a pregnancy rate of 3.6 per 100 woman-years (WHO Task Force on Long-Acting Systemic Agents for Fertility Regulation, 1990).

Antifertility Effects of Hormonal Contraception

Combination OCs

Ovulation can be inhibited by oral estrogen or by oral progestin alone, but large doses are required. Pharmacologic synergism is exhibited when the two hormones are combined, and ovulation is suppressed at a much lower dose of each agent. Combination OCs suppress basal follicle-stimulating hormone (FSH) and LH. OCs diminish the ability of the pituitary gland to synthesize gonadotrophins when stimulated by the hypothalamic releaser hormone gonadotropin-releasing hormone (Dericks-Tan et al, 1983). Ovarian follicles do not mature, little estradiol is produced, and there is no midcycle LH surge. Ovulation does not occur, the corpus luteum does not form, and progesterone is not produced (Ling et al, 1985). The blockade of ovulation is dose related: Low-dose OCs do not provide as dense a block and allow somewhat higher baseline FSH and LH

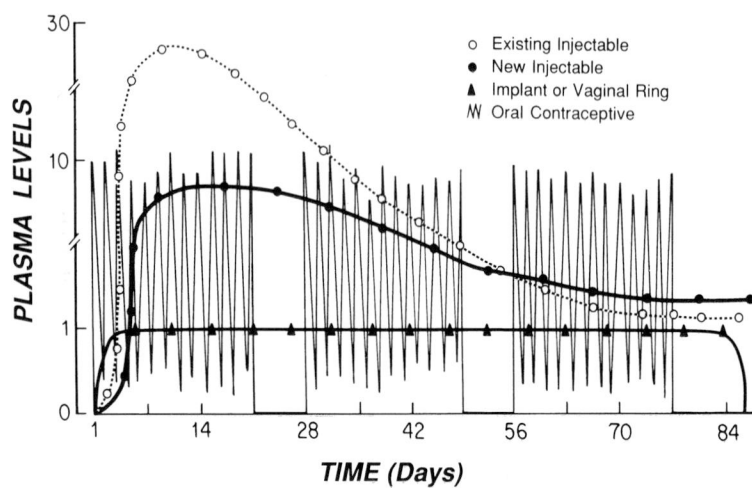

Figure 11–7
Schematic representation of the expected pharmacokinetic profiles of progestogens administered in different formulations. (Modified from Landgren BM: Mechanism of action of gestagens. Int J Gynecol Obstet 1990;32:96, with permission.)

levels than higher dose formulations (Gaspard et al. 1984). This makes ovulation more likely to occur should pills be missed, or should the patient take another medication that interferes with OC action.

Progestin-Only Preparations

The mode of action of progestin-only contraceptives depends very much on the dose of the compound (Lahteenmaki and Lahteenmaki, 1985). At low blood levels of progestin, ovulation will occur part of the time. A study of women taking the 0.3-mg norethindrone pill (Micronor) found that 40% of cycles were ovulatory and normal, 25% had inadequate luteal function, 18% showed follicular maturation but without ovulation, and in 18% follicle development was completely suppressed (Landgren, 1990). At moderate blood levels of the progestin, as with depot medroxyprogesterone acetate (DMPA), normal basal levels of FSH and LH are seen and some follicle maturation occurs. There is estradiol production and the surge of estradiol that would normally trigger pituitary release of LH occurs, but there is no answering LH surge, and hence no ovulation. At higher blood levels of progestin, basal FSH is reduced and there is less follicular activity, less estradiol production, and no LH surge, a hormonal pattern closer to that seen with combination estrogen and progestin preparations.

With Norplant there is some follicular maturation and estrogen production, but LH peak levels are low and ovulation is often inhibited (Darney, 1994). In the first year of use, ovulation is thought to occur in about 20% of cycles. The proportion of ovulatory cycles increases with time, probably as a result of the decline in hormone release, and by the fourth year 41% of cycles are ovulatory. The mechanisms of contraception with low-dose progestins are thought to include effects on cervical mucus, endometrium, and tubal motility. Progestins decrease nuclear estrogen receptor levels, decrease progesterone receptors as well, and induce activity of the enzyme 17-hydroxysteroid dehydrogenase, which metabolizes natural 17β-estradiol (Landgren, 1990). Implants offer an important advance in hormonal contraception. The sustained release allows for highly effective contraception at relatively low blood levels of the steroid. Figure 11–7 depicts expected steroid blood levels with implants, injectables, and OCs. As noted earlier, the new levonorgestrel-releasing IUCD actually functions much as does the levonorgestrel implant, providing a reservoir for sustained release and capable of inhibiting ovulation.

An additional mechanism for contraception has been discovered with the antiprogesterone mifepristone (RU 486). In the normal cycle, there is a small amount of progesterone production from the follicle just before ovulation. This progesterone appears essential to ovulation because, if the antiprogesterone is given prior to ovulation, ovulation can be delayed

for several days in women, and weekly injections of mifepristone produce complete blockade of the ovulatory cycle and amenorrhea in monkeys (Luukkainen et al, 1988; Van Uem et al, 1989).

Efficacy of Hormonal Contraception

Oral Contraceptives

If used correctly, combination OCs offer pregnancy rates as low as 2 to 3 per 1000 woman-years, but in widespread use more typical pregnancy rates are around 3 per 100, reflecting inconsistency in use (see Table 11–1). The progestin-only OCs are measurably less effective: overall, 2 to 5 pregnancies occur per 100 woman-years in the first 1 or 2 years (Vessey et al, 1982), although with perfect use much lower rates are attainable (see Table 11–1). The effectiveness of the progestin-only OCs increases with time, and the pregnancy rate is less for women who were initially on combination OCs and then switched to the progestin-only pill.

Injectable Progestins and Implants

DMPA given as a 150-mg injection every 3 months, and the levonorgestrel implant system, produce pregnancy rates lower than combination OCs, probably because they are much less subject to user error. Reported pregnancy rates with DMPA are 0.3 to 0.4 per 100 woman-years (Kaunitz, 1994). Pregnancy rates with the levonorgestrel implant system are 0.3 to 0.6 per 100 women in the first year of use, and the cumulative rate over the entire 5 years is 1.5 (Shoupe and Mishell, 1989). These methods are as effective as tubal sterilization.

Metabolic Effects of Hormonal Contraception

Blood Pressure

With older OCs the average blood pressure of most women increases very slightly during treatment. A small subset of women will have a clinically important increase that may not be evident until the patient has taken OCs for a few months, and as many as 5% of patients could be expected to develop blood pressure of greater than 140/90 mm hg. The mechanism is thought to be an estrogen-induced increase in renin substrate in susceptible individuals. Current low-dose pills have minimal blood pressure effects, but surveillance of blood pressure is still advised to detect the occasional idiosyncratic response.

Glucose Metabolism

Oral estrogen given alone has no adverse effect on glucose metabolism (Spellacy et al, 1972), but progestins appear to exhibit insulin antagonism. Older

OC formulations with higher doses of the progestins produced abnormal glucose tolerance tests in the average subject, with elevated insulin levels. The effect on glucose metabolism, like the effect on lipids, is related to androgenic potency of the progestin (Crook et al, 1988). The best information currently available comes from the very large English study of Godsland and colleagues (1990), in which 1060 women 18 to 45 years old taking different OCs and 418 women not using OCs participated in a cross-sectional study with measurement of lipids and glucose metabolism. Two levonorgestrel-EE monophasic combinations and a triphasic were compared to two norethindrone-EE monophasics and a triphasic, a desogestrel-EE monophasic combination, and three low-dose progestin-only products. Desogestrel is one of the new progestins and, like norgestimate and gestodene, has little androgenic effect. Effects on low-density (LDL) and high-density lipoprotein (HDL) and incremental areas under the curve for insulin are shown in Fig. 11–8 and incremental areas for C-peptide are shown in Fig. 11–9. Glucose metabolism was affected by all of the combinations in proportion to dose and potency of the progestin. The incremental areas under the curves for glucose, insulin, and C-peptide were increased, with levonorgestrel combinations having greater effect than norethindrone or desogestrel. Norethindrone-only preparations had no effect and levonorgestrel-only formulations increased the incremental area for glucose somewhat (Fig. 11–9).

Lipids

The higher dose OCs could have significant adverse effects on lipids (Lipson et al, 1986). Androgens and estrogens have competing effects on hepatic lipase, a liver enzyme critical to lipid metabolism. Estrogens depress LDL cholesterol and elevate HDL cholesterol, changes that can be expected to reduce risk of atherosclerosis (Knopp, 1988). Androgens and androgenic progestins can antagonize these beneficial changes, reducing HDL and elevating LDL. Estrogens elevate triglyceride. A randomized study of three OCs containing the same estrogen, 50 μg of EE, and three different progestins demonstrated more adverse lipid change with the norgestrel-containing OC than with OCs containing norethindrone or ethynodiol diacetate (Lipson et al, 1986). Such differences become more difficult to demonstrate as the dose of progestin is reduced. A multicenter study compared three triphasic OC preparations currently sold in the United States (Patsch et al, 1989). All OC groups showed small but statistically significant increases from baseline in plasma triglycerides, very-low-density lipoprotein cholesterol, and plasma apolipoprotein B (the protein component of LDL), and decreased concentrations of HDL cholesterol subfraction 2 (HDL-2). HDL subfraction 3 (HDL-3) levels increased in all three OC groups. HDL-2 is most strongly associated with protection from atheroscle-

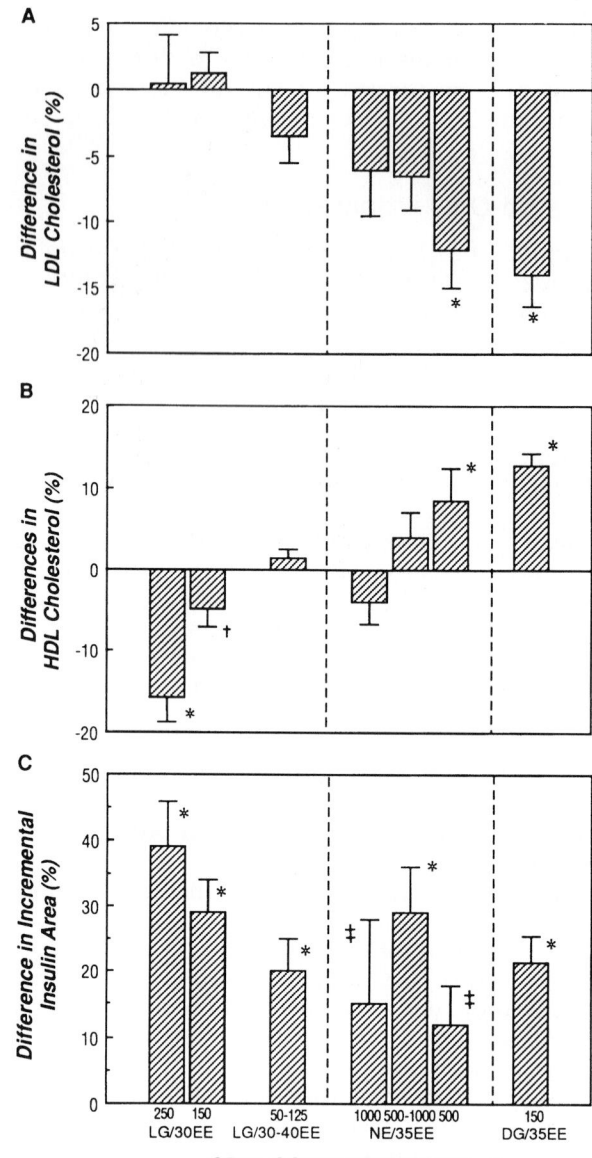

Figure 11–8

Percent differences in HDL and LDL cholesterol levels and in the incremental area for insulin in response to the oral glucose tolerance test between women taking one of seven combination oral contraceptives and those not taking oral contraceptives. The T bars indicate 1 standard deviation. The asterisk (*p* <. 001), dagger (*p* < .01), and double dagger (*p* < .05) indicate significant differences between users and nonusers in the mean values for the principal metabolic variables. DG, desogestrel; EE, ethinyl estradiol; LG, levonorgestrel; NE, norethindrone. (From Godsland IF, Crook D, Simpson R, et al: The effects of different formulations of oral contraceptive agents on lipid and carbohydrate metabolism. N Engl J Med 1990;323:1379, with permission.)

rosis; the relation of HDL-3 is not clear. The changes observed in lipids were minor but in a direction that is not desirable (Patsch et al, 1989). Whereas average lipid values of a large group show only small lipid changes with current OCs, occasional patients can have exaggerated effects. Women whose lipid levels

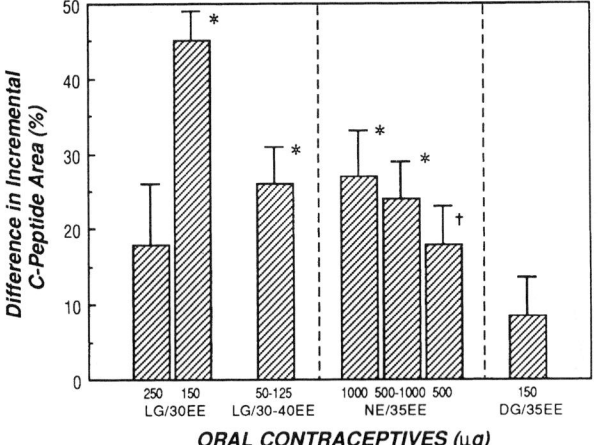

Figure 11-9
Percent differences in the incremental area for C-peptide in response to the oral glucose tolerance test between women taking one of seven combination oral contraceptives and those not taking oral contraceptives. The T bars indicate 1 standard deviation. The asterisk (*p* < .001) and the dagger (*p* < .05) indicate significant differences between users and nonusers. DG, desogestrel; EE, ethinyl estradiol; LG, levonorgestrel; NE, norethindrone. (From Godsland IF, Crook D, Simpson R, et al: The effects of different formulations of oral contraceptive agents on lipid and carbohydrate metabolism. N Engl J Med 1990;323:1379, with permission.)

are further from the mean before treatment are more likely to become abnormal during OC use. The lowest dose formulation produces less change toward abnormal HDL levels (Burkeman et al, 1989).

Third-generation OCs, containing desogestrel, gestodene, or norgestimate, have a beneficial effect on lipids (Godsland et al, 1990). As shown in Fig. 11–8, the monophasic desogestrel and low-dose norethindrone-EE combinations lowered LDL levels significantly, an effect that should be beneficial. The higher dose norethindrone-EE combinations and the triphasics containing norethindrone or levonorgestrel did not significantly alter LDL levels. Total HDL was depressed by the norgestrel monophasics and elevated by the low-dose norethindrone monophasic and the desogestrel combination. HDL-2 is most strongly related to protection from arterial disease, and was the component most affected by the OCs. Both levonorgestrel monophasics lowered HDL-2. The higher dose norethindrone monophasic lowered HDL-2, but the lower dose norethindrone combination did not affect it. Triphasic levonorgestrel lowered HDL-2 by 15%, while the triphasic norethindrone OC lowered this fraction by 8%. HDL-2 was not affected by the desogestrel combination. All combination OCs elevated HDL-3, an effect of uncertain significance (Godsland et al, 1990). Of the progestin-only formulations, the levonorgestrel product did not affect HDL-2, whereas the norethindrone product lowered it slightly. A combination OC with 30 μg of EE and norgestimate, another of the new progestins, has been compared to the low-dose levonorges-

trel combination in a large U.S. trial. The norgestimate combination had apparently beneficial effects on lipids, as did desogestrel in the study described above, whereas the levonorgestrel combination lowered HDL levels significantly (Chapdelaine et al, 1989).

Other Metabolic Effects

OCs can produce changes in a broad variety of proteins synthesized by the liver. The estrogen in OCs increases circulating thyroid-binding globulin, and thereby affects tests of thyroid function that are based on binding, increasing total thyroxine and decreasing triiodothyronine resin uptake. However, actual thyroid function as measured by free thyroxine and radioiodine tests is normal (Mishell et al, 1969).

Health Risks of OCs

Combination OCs and Vascular Disease

COAGULATION

Estrogen-containing combination OCs have a variety of effects on the coagulation system that are dose related: depression of the natural anticoagulant antithrombin III (ATIII); a mild increase in levels of prothrombin, factor VII, factor IX, and factor X; an increase in the platelet count; and effects on the interaction between platelets and the vessel walls so as to increase platelet aggregation. Normally the coagulation system maintains a dynamic balance of procoagulant and anticoagulant systems in the blood, and OCs affect both: they have both procoagulant and anticoagulant effects. For most women, fibrinolysis (anticoagulation) is increased as much as coagulation, so that the dynamic balance is maintained and abnormal thrombosis does not occur (Winkler et al, 1991).

VENOUS THROMBOSIS AND THROMBOEMBOLISM

Epidemiologic studies of the 1970s linked OC use to venous thrombosis and embolism, cerebral vascular accidents, and heart attack (Stadel, 1981a, 1981b; Royal College of General Practitioners' Oral Contraception Study, 1983). Critical rereading of the older literature on venous thrombosis reveals that absolute risk was strongly determined by other very obvious predisposing causes. For example, Maguire and colleagues (1979) investigated the role of six groups of clinical factors on risk of thrombosis with OCs: history of thrombosis or embolism, history of vascular disease, history of central vascular disorders (rheumatic heart disease, myocardiopathy, coronary artery disease, etc.), history of blood abnormalities (polycythemia, sickle cell disease or trait, leukemia, etc.), history of metabolic disease (diabetes, cancer, hypothyroidism, pelvic inflammatory disease, etc.), and surgery or trauma. Of the cases investigated, 357 were classed as predisposed; only 104 had none of the six risk factors present. In current practice women with these conditions are not given OCs. More recent studies have found much less risk (Porter et al, 1985; Farmer and Preston, 1995). Current OCs with less then 50 μg of estrogen have less measurable effect on the coagulation system, and clot-inhibiting factors seem to increase as much as procoagulant factors (Notelovitz et al, 1981, 1985). Coagulation is a very complex process, and we are hampered by the fact that our laboratory studies are much better at predicting who will bleed rather than who will clot. Smokers taking low-dose OCs demonstrate more marked activation of the coagulation system—shortening of the prothrombin time, increased fibrinogen levels, and decreased ATIII—but also have increased fibrinolysis as measured by plasminogen activity increased beyond the normal range (Notelovitz et al, 1985).

Risk of thrombosis diminishes with decreasing estrogen dose, from greater than 50 μg to 50 μg to less than 50 μg (Gerstman et al, 1991). With current OCs containing 30 to 35 μg of EE, the absolute risk of venous thrombosis is about 3 per 10,000 women per year, compared with one per 10,000 for reproductive-age women not using OCs and 6 per 10,000 for risk of thrombosis with pregnancy (Farmer and Preston, 1995). Increased risk of thrombosis is apparent by 4 months after starting combination OCs, does not increase with continued use, and disappears by 3 months after stopping OC use (WHO Collaborative Study of Cardiovascular Disease and Steroid Hormone Contraception, 1995).

Laboratory studies of large groups of women on OCs concluded that OC use was not associated with a detectable hypercoagulable state, but that individual patient factors such as family history of thrombosis, obesity, and hypertension were important (Farag et al, 1988). A concept is evolving that venous thrombosis is not a risk at all for most women on low-estrogen OCs, but rather that small subgroups are genetically predisposed. A report on individuals who experienced deep venous thrombosis prior to age 40 found that 5% to 10% had protein S deficiency, 7% had protein C deficiency, 2% to 3% had ATIII deficiency, and 3% had other identifiable abnormalities such as plasminogen deficiency or an abnormal level of fibrinogen (Gladson et al, 1988). Women with deficiencies of ATIII, protein C, or protein S are recognized to be at very high risk for thrombosis with pregnancy or estrogen therapy, but they make up a very small proportion of potential OC users (Gladson et al, 1988; Trauscht-Van Horn et al, 1992). A much more common predisposition is factor V Leiden. This recently identified mutation in the gene for coagulation factor V is found in 3% to 5% of the population. Factor V Leiden resists cleavage by activated protein C (APC), an essential limiting step in the normal process of coagulation and balancing fibrinolysis, producing the syndrome of "activated protein C resistance" (Bertina et al, 1994). In a study by Vandenbroucke and colleagues (1994), risk of a first thromboembolic episode among women using OCs who do not have the factor V mutation was estimated to be 2.2 per 10,000 woman-years. For women homozygous or heterozygous for the mutation who do not use OCs, risk was 4.9 per 10,000 woman-years. For women with the mutation who also take OCs, risk was 27.7 per 10,000 woman-years. Effect of estrogen dose was not examined. Cigarette smoking did not affect risk of thrombosis. Another study found APC resistance in 14% to 42% of women with a history of thrombosis (Bokarewa et al, 1995). Of women under age 40 who experience deep vein thrombosis, more than half have either APC resistance, protein S deficiency, protein C deficiency, or ATIII deficiency (Stubblefield, 1993). Pregnancy is even more likely to lead to thrombosis for women with inherited defects of fibrinolysis than is OC use (Trauscht-Van Horn et al, 1992).

Third-Generation OCs and Risk of Venous Thrombosis. Several studies have focused on possible differences in risk for venous thrombosis between third-generation OCs containing any of the new progestins and older OCs. All have found a small, but generally statistically significant, greater risk of thrombosis with the new OCs, even though the estrogen and its dose is the same. The large Transnational Study found an odds ratio of 1.5 for venous thrombosis risk of third-generation OCs compared to second-generation pills (Lewis et al, 1996a). A 1993 review by Stubblefield found minimal changes in the coagulation and fibrinolytic systems with OCs containing desogestrel, one of the new progestins (Stubblefield, 1993). Bias may explain the apparent increased risk for thrombosis with the new progestin combinations. Lewis et al (1996a) concluded that adverse selection accounted for the apparent increase in thrombosis. One of these types of bias is "attrition of susceptibles." First-time users of OCs include women with an unidentified increased risk for thrombosis. Because cases of venous thrombosis attributable to OCs occur during the initial months of use (WHO Collaborative Study of Cardiovascular Disease and Steroid Hormone Contraception, 1995), comparing new users to other women who have been taking one of the older OCs for some time will demonstrate an apparent increase in thrombosis with the new product that is not real. Another type of adverse selection is based on physician presumption that the new third-generation OCs are safer, and therefore new users or women with risk factors may be selectively prescribed the newer pill. The Transnational Study shows this effect very strongly. Apparent risk of thrombosis was least for the first low-dose pills introduced and greatest for those most recently introduced, even though the newest pill had the lowest estrogen dose, 20 μg rather than 30 to 35 μg of EE (Lewis et al, 1996a) (Fig. 11–10). Its apparent association with thrombosis is biologically not plausible.

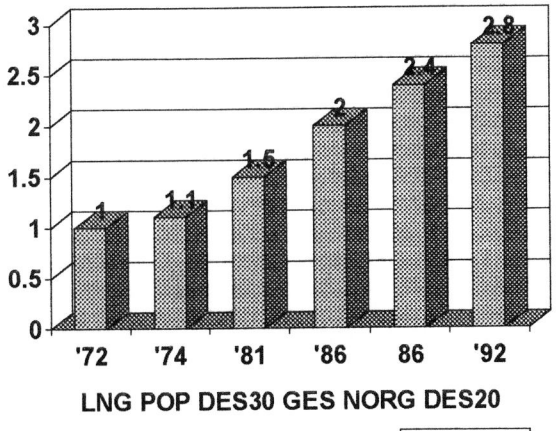

Figure 11–10
Bias in epidemiologic studies: The rate of thrombosis reported with oral contraceptive preparations for women ages 25 to 44 by year of introduction to the market in the Transnational Study. Oral contraceptives (*left to right*): LNG, levonorgestrel with 30 μg ethinyl estradiol; POP, progestin only; DES30, desogrestrel with 30 μg ethinyl estradiol; GES, gestodene with 30 μg ethinyl estradiol; NORG, norgestimate with 35 μg of ethinyl estradiol; DES20, desogestrel with 20 μg of ethinyl estradiol. (From Lewis MA, Heinemann LAJ, MacRae KD, et al: The increased risk of venous thromboembolism and the use of third generation progestagens: role of bias in observational research. Contraception 1996;54:5, with permission.)

For properly selected nonobese, normotensive, healthy women, the probability of venous thrombosis or thromboembolism occurring during treatment with present low-dose pills is low but not zero. At this time, routine screening of all women before starting OCs is unlikely to be cost effective but should be considered if there is a family history of thrombosis. Women with a personal history of thrombosis should not be given estrogen-containing OCs, but could be given the progestin-only contraceptives. Women who sustain venous thrombosis while on OCs should be evaluated with assays for ATIII, protein C, protein S, and APC resistance. It should not just be assumed that the OC was the only cause.

ISCHEMIC HEART DISEASE

Ischemic heart disease is less clearly related to OC use but was the major cause, along with stroke, of deaths attributed to OCs in the past. The principal determinants of risk are advanced age and cigarette smoking (Mant et al, 1987). A large British study found no women with MIs who were taking OCs with less than 50 μg of estrogen, although use of the lower dose preparations was comparatively infrequent at that time (Mant et al, 1987). With the OCs in use in the 1980s, smoking had a profound effect on risk. Women smoking 25 or more cigarettes per day had a 30-fold increased risk of MI (Rosenberg

et al, 1985). A large U.S. study confirms the safety of low-dose OCs as currently prescribed, where women with known risk factors are usually excluded (Sidney et al, 1996). A total of 187 women ages 15 to 44 years with confirmed MI were identified during 3.6 million woman-years of observation in the Kaiser Permanente Medical Care Program in California between 1991 and 1994, a rate of 3.2 per 100,000 woman-years. These women were compared to three controls, matched for age and location of medical care. Nearly all current users took OCs with less than 50 μg of ethinyl estradiol. Important patients factors that influenced risk of MI are summarized in Table 11–5. After adjustment for age, illness, smoking, ethnicity, and body mass index, risk of MI in current OC users was not increased (odds ratio [OR] 1.14; 95% confidence interval [CI] 0.27 to 4.72). Sixty-one per cent of heart attack victims were smokers; only 7.7% were current OC users. Of the controls currently on OCs, only 13.8% were smokers. Past users of OCs actually had less risk, although this was not statistically stable (OR 0.60, CI 0.25 to 1.44). The safety of past use of OCs was previously demonstrated by the Nurses' Health Study (Stampfer et al, 1988). With 484,096 woman-years of observation of non–OC users and 415,488 woman-years of observation of past OC users, there was no increased risk of heart attack among past users of OCs.

Third-Generation OCs and MI. The Transnational Study of third-generation OCs and venous thrombosis also addressed MI. Risk of MI was reduced by comparison with second-generation OCs, and users of third-generation OCs had no increased risk of MI when compared to nonusers of OCs (Lewis et al, 1996b) (Table 11–6). This finding is biologically quite believable because of the beneficial effect on lipids of the new progestins (Spitzer et al, 1996). Selection bias would work against this finding of benefit; hence it is likely to be real. Venous thrombosis is

Table 11–5. LOW-DOSE ORAL CONTRACEPTIVES AND RISK OF MYOCARDIAL INFARCTION: EFFECT OF SELECTED VARIABLES

VARIABLE	UNADJUSTED ODDS RATIO (95% CI)
Cigarette smoking, current	8.31 (4.74–14.57)
Treated for hypertension	4.72 (2.51–8.90)
Treated for diabetes mellitus	17.45 (5.17–58.86)
Treated for high cholesterol	3.03 (1.76–5.23)
Body mass index (quartile)	
1 (lowest)	1.00 (referent)
2	1.69 (0.85–3.73)
3	2.39 (1.22–4.68)
4 (highest)	5.60 (2.93–10.73)
Current use of oral contraceptives	0.87 (0.37–2.05)

From Sidney S, Petitti DB, Quesenberry CP, et al: Myocardial infarction in users of low dose oral contraceptives. Obstet Gynecol 1996; 88:939, with permission.

Table 11-6. RISK OF MYOCARDIAL INFARCTION FOR CURRENT USE OF DIFFERENT TYPES OF ORAL CONTRACEPTIVES

COMPARISON	ODDS RATIO (95% CI)	p VALUE	NO. EXPOSED CASES; NO. EXPOSED CONTROLS
All cases (N = 153)			
All controls (N = 498)			
Third generation v. second generation	0.36 (0.1–1.2)	0.1	6; 34
Third generation v. no current use	1.1 (0.4–3.4)	0.9	6; 34
Second generation v. no current use	3.1 (1.5–6.3)	0.003	23; 45

From Lewis MA, Spitzer WO, Heinemann LAJ, et al: Third-generation oral contraceptives and the risk of myocardial infarction: an international case control study. BMJ 1996;312:89, with permission.

rarely fatal in young women, whereas MI, although rare in the reproductive years, is frequently fatal. Hence, even if the apparent increase in venous thrombosis is real and not just the result of bias, the net effect would be reduction in deaths if the new OCs were substituted for older ones.

STROKE

OC use appeared to be linked to risk for hemorrhagic and thrombotic stroke in the 1970s (Collaborative Group for the Study of Stroke in Young Women, 1975; Vessey et al, 1984), but thereafter studies have been inconsistent. Initial studies failed to adequately deal with pre-existing risk. Modern studies have clarified this (Lidegaard, 1995; Petitti et al, 1996; WHO Collaborative Study of Cardiovascular Disease and Steroid Hormone Contraception, 1996a, 1996b). Angiographic studies of women who sustained cerebrovascular attacks while using the previous generation of OCs frequently demonstrated one of a variety of arterial lesions (e.g., stenosis, mural irregularities, beaded arteries), suggesting predisposition (Godon-Hardy et al, 1985). A rare form of cerebrovascular insufficiency, moyamoya disease, has been linked to OC use (Bruno et al, 1988).

Important new information is provided by two large studies. Petitti and colleagues (1996) identified all Kaiser Permanente Medical Care Program patients ages 15 to 44 years who sustained a fatal or nonfatal stroke in 1991–1994 in California. Three controls were randomly selected from health plan members matched for age and location of health care. A total of 408 confirmed strokes were identified during 3.6 million woman-years of observation, an incidence of 11.3 per 100,000 woman-years. Ninety-six per cent of the OC users were on pills containing less than 50 µg of estrogen. Selected risk factors for ischemic or hemorrhagic stroke are given in Table 11-7. Hypertension, diabetes, obesity, current cigarette smoking, and black race were strongly associated with stroke risk but OC use was not. Neither was OC use associated in the analysis adjusted for hypertension, diabetes, smoking status, ethnic group, and body mass index. The OR for ischemic stroke with current OC use was 0.65, a reduction in risk that was not statistically significant (CI 0.25 to 1.7). Hemorrhagic stroke was unrelated to OC use (OR 1.02, CI 0.37 to 2.83) (Petitti et al, 1996). Thirty-four per cent of women sustaining either an ischemic infarction or hemorrhagic stroke were current cigarette smokers, while only 12% and 14.2%, respectively, used OCs. There was no association between past OC use and stroke in this study, as already reported by the Nurses' Health Study (Stampfer et al, 1988).

A WHO study of cases from 1989 through 1993 in 17 countries of Europe and the developing world

Table 11-7. RISK OF STROKE IN CURRENT USERS OF LOW-DOSE ORAL CONTRACEPTIVES: EFFECT OF SELECTED VARIABLES

VARIABLE	ISCHEMIC INFARCTION*	HEMORRHAGE INFARCTION*
Cigarette smoking, current	2.66 (1.65–4.30)	2.70 (1.71–4.27)
Treated for hypertension	7.79 (3.51–17.31)	4.64 (2.14–10.06)
Treated for diabetes mellitus	7.15 (3.17–16.13)	2.50 (0.62–10.08)
Body mass index (quartile)		
1 (lowest)	1.0	1.00
2	1.60 (0.81–3.16)	0.56 (0.31–1.00)
3	2.07 (1.10–3.92)	0.82 (0.47–1.44)
4 (highest)	4.87 (2.59–9.14)	0.99 (0.57–1.71)
Current use of oral contraceptives	0.96 (0.49–1.90)	1.18 (0.65–2.16)

From Petitti D, Sidney S, Bernstein A, et al: Stroke in users of low dose oral contraceptives. N Engl J Med 1996;335:12, with permission.
*Unadjusted odds ratio (95% CI).

Table 11–8. EFFECT OF PREDISPOSING CONDITIONS AND DOSE OF ORAL CONTRACEPTIVES UPON RISK OF THROMBOTIC CEREBROVASCULAR EVENT

PREDISPOSING CONDITION*	ADJUSTED ODDS RATIO (p)
Pregnancy	1.3 (p = Nonsignificant)
Diabetes	5.4 ($p < 0.001$)
Hypertension (treated)	3.1 ($p < 0.001$)
Migraine (>once/month)	2.8 ($p < 0.01$)
Earlier thrombotic disease	5.3 ($p < 0.001$)
Other disease	8.3 ($p < 0.001$)

USE OF ORAL CONTRACEPTIVES†	ADJUSTED ODDS RATIO (95% CI)
50-µg estrogen pills	2.9 (1.6–5.4)
30- to 40-µg estrogen pills	1.8 (1.1–2.9)
Progestin-only pills	0.9 (0.4–2.4)

*From Lidegaard O: Oral contraceptives, pregnancy and the risk of cerebral thromboembolism: the influence of diabetes, hypertension, migraine and previous thromboembolic disease. Br J Obstet Gynaecol 1995;102:153, with permission.
†From Lidegaard O: Oral contraceptives and risk of a cerebral thromboembolic attack: results of a case-control study. BMJ 1993;306:956, with permission.

found some overall risk of ischemic and hemorrhagic stroke for OC users, but, unlike the Petitti et al study, included women on higher dose as well as low-dose OCs. In the WHO Collaborative Study of Cardiovascular Disease and Steroid Hormone Contraception (1996a, 1996b), the stroke risk for European women was limited to women using higher dose OCs. Those European women using low-dose OCs had no increased risk for either type of stroke. In developing countries the ORs for ischemic stroke (2.9; 95% CI 2.1 to 4) and for hemorrhagic stroke (1.8; 95% CI 1.3 to 2.3) were elevated, but this was stated to be at least partially attributable to undetected preexisting cardiovascular risk.

Current evidence supports the safety from MI or stroke for women who have no predisposing risk factors. Women with risk factors clearly are at increased risk for cardiovascular disease whether or not they use OCs, and this risk increases markedly with age. There are limited data as to risk with current low-dose OCs for women with predisposing factors. Hypertensive or diabetic women in the Nurses' Health Study who took OCs had fewer vascular events than hypertensive or diabetic women who did not, but this may well have reflected good patient selection, to limit OC use by women with more severe conditions, rather that true protection (Stampfer et al, 1988). In the case of cigarette smoking, risk is clearly additive; that is, smokers who take even low-dose combination OCs have greater risk of arterial events than smokers who do not take OCs (Lidegaard, 1993). The current practice of limiting use of combination OCs by women over 35 to nonsmokers is prudent. The effect of pregnancy, diabetes, hypertension, previous noncerebral thrombosis, and OC use on risk of thrombotic stroke among women of reproductive age in Denmark was reported by Lidegaard (1995) (Table 11–8). Risk of

stroke from OC use alone was small and dose related. Predisposed women who used combination OCs were estimated to be at greater risk, although this was based on very small numbers of cases and the data were not limited to low-estrogen OCs. Lidegaard (1995) estimated that risk of stroke for diabetic women who use low-dose OCs was increased from 5-fold for diabetes alone to 10-fold if the diabetic woman used OCs.

The effect of use or nonuse of OCs on women who smoked or had hypertension was explored in the much larger WHO Collaborative Study on Cardiovascular Disease and Steroid Hormone Contraception (1996b). Smokers on OCs had seven times the risk of ischemic (thrombotic) stroke as nonsmokers who did not use OCs, and hypertensive women had a 10-fold increased risk if they took OCs but 5-fold if they did not (Table 11–9). These data appear to be the best information available to date and still strongly suggest that risk, although strongly determined by the predisposing condition, is further magnified by OC use, even when the OCs are low dose.

Table 11–9. ODDS RATIOS (95% CI) FOR ISCHEMIC STROKE BY USE OF ORAL CONTRACEPTIVES AND PRE-EXISTING RISK FACTORS AMONG EUROPEAN WOMEN

FACTOR	NONUSER OF OCs	OC USER
Nonsmoker	1.00	2.09 (1.03–4.5)
Smoker	1.24 (0.72–2.13)	7.20 (3.23–16.1)
No hypertension	1.00	2.71 (1.47–4.99)
Hypertension	4.59 (2.39–8.82)	10.7 (2.04–56.6)

From World Health Organization Collaborative Study of Cardiovascular Disease and Steroid Hormone Contraception: Ischaemic stroke and combined oral contraceptives: results of an international, multicenter, case control study. Lancet 1996;348:498, with permission.

OCs and Neoplasia

ENDOMETRIAL CANCER

Combination OCs reduce risk for subsequent endometrial cancer. In the CDC Cancer and Steroid Hormone Study (1983b), 2 years of OC use reduced risk of subsequent endometrial cancer by 40% and 4 or more years' use reduced risk by 60%. Protection lasted until 19 years from last use, then declined when the interval from last use exceeded 20 years.

OVARIAN CANCER

Many studies have demonstrated prevention of ovarian cancer from previous use of OCs. In the large CDC Cancer and Steroid Hormone Study (1983c), a 50% reduction in ovarian cancer risk was observed for women who took OCs for 3 to 4 years, and there was some apparent benefit from as little as 3 to 11 months of past use. The benefit continued for at least 15 years after last use and did not decrease, even at 15 years.

A more recent case-control study found no protection when OCs were used for less than 3 years, but, at 3 to 4 years of use, risk of subsequent epithelial ovarian cancer was reduced by 50% (Rosenberg et al, 1994a). Longer duration of use did not increase protection. Although data were sparse for OCs with less than 50 μg of estrogen, benefit did not decrease for the low-dose formulations. National vital statistics data from England support these observations. Ovarian cancer mortality is declining in England and Wales for women under 55, and this decline has been attributed to OC use (Villard-Mackintosh et al, 1989).

CERVICAL CANCER

Cervical cancer is increased among long-term OC users. Compared to women not using OCs, typical findings in case-control studies are relative risks of 2 (Zondervan et al, 1996). A comparison of IUCD wearers to OC users found that preneoplastic lesions of the cervix progressed more rapidly among OC users (Vessey et al, 1983). It is difficult to separate out the roles of early sexual intercourse and sexual exposure to human papillomavirus (HPV) in causation (Swann and Petitti, 1982). Women who have used OCs typically started sexual relations at younger ages and, in some studies, reported more partners. Alternative choices for contraception make it harder to resolve the question because barrier contraceptives reduce risk for cervical cancer by 50% (Vessey et al, 1983). The essential risk factor is HPV. For example, presence of HPV type 16 or 18 is associated with a 50-fold increase in having a preneoplastic lesion of the cervix (Schiffman et al, 1993). Among women who have already acquired HPV, there is no further increase in risk from being on OCs (Schiffman et al, 1993), but, among women who are HPV negative, OC use doubled the risk of having such a lesion. The same increase is seen from having multiple sexual partners among those who were HPV negative. This apparent OC effect could be explained if women who used OCs were not as likely to use a barrier contraceptive as the comparison group.

Most cervical cancers are of squamous cell type. Adenocarcinomas are rare but are not as well detected by screening cytology, and may be increasing. Women who used OCs had twice the risk for adenocarcinoma of the cervix in a study by Ursin et al (1994). Risk increased with duration of OC use, reaching a relative risk (RR) of 4.4 (95% CI 1.8 to 10.8) when OC use exceeded 12 years. This study adjusted for history of genital warts, number of sexual partners, and age at first intercourse. Because adenocarcinoma is rare, absolute risk is low, with a cumulative risk to age 55 of about 1 in 1000 patients (CDC Cancer and Steroid Hormone Study, 1983a). OC use is at most a minor factor in causation of cervical cancer; however, women who have used OCs should have annual cervical cytology with use of the Cytobrush or similar technique to improve sampling of the endocervix, as should any sexually active woman.

BREAST CANCER

There is a large literature on the effects of OCs on breast cancer. For the most part the findings have been reassuring, indicating that there is no overall increase in breast cancer (CDC Cancer and Steroid Hormone Study, 1983a; Romieu et al, 1989) but that risk could be increased for small groups: women who used OCs before their first term pregnancy or who used OCs for many years (U.K. National Case-Control Study Group, 1989), nulligravid women, women who are young at time of diagnosis, and women who continue using OCs in their 40s (Caygill and Hill, 1989). A large British study found a small but statistically stable increase in breast cancer diagnosed before age 36 among OC users, but that risk was less for OCs with less than 50 μg of estrogen. Progestin-only OCs appeared to have a protective effect. Significantly, OC users who developed breast cancers had tumors of lower stage and were less likely to have positive lymph nodes than controls (Caygill and Hill, 1989). Women with a family history of breast cancer are not at increased risk with OC use compared to other women (Murray et al, 1989).

Some of the findings are difficult to interpret; for example, risk does not increase with prolonged exposure, not all what would be expected if OCs are truly causal (Schlesselman, 1989). The best information to date comes from a meta-analysis of 54 studies of breast cancer and hormonal contraceptives. The Collaborative Group on Hormonal Factors in Breast Cancer (1996) reanalyzed data on 53,297 women with breast cancer and 100,239 controls from 25 countries, representing about 90% of the epidemiologic data available worldwide. This study concluded that women have a 24% increased risk for breast cancer while taking OCs (RR 1.24, 95% CI 1.15 to 1.33). The risk falls rapidly after discontinuation, to 16% 1 to 4 years after stopping and to 7% at 5 to 9 years after stopping. Risk disappears 10 years after cessation (RR 1.01, 95% CI 0.96 to 1.05). Breast cancers diagnosed in women on OCs were less advanced clinically than those in women who had never used OCs. Results did not differ in any important way by ethnic group or reproductive or family history. There was greater risk for women who started OCs prior to age 20 relative to women who started OCs later, but, because breast cancer is so rare prior to age 20, there was no increase in actual numbers of breast cancer cases among the women who started young. A full-term pregnancy also causes a short-term increase in breast cancer risk, thought to be from the growth-enhancing effects of estrogen, but there is long-term reduction in risk, perhaps the result of induced terminal differentiation of breast cells (Melbye et al, 1997). The effects of OC use may be the same and may promote growth of existing cancers, leading to their presentation and diagnosis at an earlier age, rather than actually causing cancers to form. Most breast cancers are seen after age 50, and only now are large numbers of women with pill exposure entering this group. Some epidemiologic studies have found protection in the older age groups, although the numbers of subjects studied have been insufficient to be certain (Stadel et al, 1989). For the present, the best we can say is that risk, if it is increased, is small and goes away by 10 years after cessation of OCs.

LIVER TUMORS

OCs have been implicated in the causation of benign hepatocellular adenomas. These hormonally responsive tumors can cause fatal hemorrhage; they usually regress when OCs are discontinued. Risk is related to prolonged use (Rooks et al, 1979). The relation between OC use and hepatocellular adenoma is strong, but fortunately the tumors are rare; about 30 cases per 1 million users per year are predicted with older formulations. Presumably newer lower dose products are safer. More recently a link to hepatic carcinoma has been proposed, with small case-control studies finding risk elevated as much as 20-fold with OC use of 8 years or more (Forman et al, 1986). However, the incidence of liver cancer has increased only slightly in England, and not at all in the United States, in spite of many years of widespread OC use by a major proportion of reproductive age women (Forman et al, 1983).

Health Benefits of Hormonal Contraceptives

OCs have important health benefits (Stubblefield, 1994). The strong protective effect against endometrial and ovarian cancer was described earlier. A 50%

reduction in rates of hospitalization for pelvic infection has been reported. Chlamydial colonization of the cervix appears more likely in OC users than nonusers, but, in spite of this, there is a 40% to 50% reduction in risk for chlamydial PID (Wolner-Hanssen et al, 1990). Combined OCs confer marked reduction in risk for ectopic pregnancy, although the progestin-only OCs appear to increase risk. Other documented benefits include a significant reduction in need for breast biopsies for benign disease, reduction in dysmenorrhea, and reduction in anemia from menstrual blood loss (Vessey et al, 1974). All combination OCs offer protection from functional ovarian cysts, but protection decreases as the estrogen dose is reduced and is least with the triphasic products (Lanes et al, 1992). Women who have had symptomatic ovarian cysts should probably be treated with the slightly higher dose monophasic preparations. If progestin-only OCs are truly protective against breast cancer, then the levonorgestrel implants could be expected to confer this same very important benefit.

Fertility After OC Use

Initially there were concerns that some women might never resume spontaneous menstruation and hence be infertile after OC use. Although there is a delay of a few months in return to ovulatory cycles after discontinuing the pill, there is no permanent sterility. Women with amenorrhea for more than 6 months after stopping the pill deserve a full evaluation, because a substantial proportion of this group will eventually be diagnosed as having prolactin-producing pituitary tumors. Women who had regular cycles prior to pill use and used the pill only for contraception have very low rates for developing such tumors. It is the women who were placed on OCs because of menstrual irregularity who more often develop pituitary tumors subsequently, and presumably the slow-growing tumor was already present and producing menstrual irregularity before the OCs were started (Shy et al, 1983).

Sexuality and OCs

Occasionally women taking OCs will complain of reduced sexual interest. The effect of OCs on sexuality has been difficult to determine. However, a sensitive study by Adams and colleagues (1978) recorded all episodes of female-initiated sexual behavior throughout the menstrual cycle and noted an increase at the time of ovulation that was abolished in women who were taking OCs.

Teratogenicity of Hormonal Contraceptives

Oral contraceptives are unrelated to birth defects. A meta-analysis of 12 prospective studies with a total of 6102 women exposed to OCs compared to 85,167 unexposed women found malformations overall were not increased by OC exposure, and neither were congenital heart defects or limb reduction defects (Bracken, 1990). Progestins are still used to prevent miscarriage. A large study compared women treated with progestins (primarily medroxyprogesterone acetate) to women with the same complaint of threatened abortion who were not treated. The rate of malformation was the same among the 1146 exposed infants as among the 1608 infants born to unexposed women (Katz et al, 1985). However, estrogens taken in high doses in pregnancy can induce vaginal cancer in female offspring exposed in utero.

Interactions of OCs With Other Drugs

Some drugs reduce the effectiveness of OCs, and, conversely, OCs can augment or reduce the effectiveness of other drugs. The first type of interaction is seen with phenytoin and phenobarbital. These antiseizure drugs induce synthesis of cytochrome P_{450} enzymes in the liver and reduce plasma levels of EE in women on OCs, resulting in pregnancy (Back and Orme, 1990). There are also many case reports of OC failure in women treated with the antituberculosis drug rifampin. This drug is also a potent inducer of cytochrome P_{450} enzymes and reduces blood levels of both EE and norethindrone. Ampicillin and tetracycline have been the subjects of numerous case reports of OC failure. They kill gut bacteria (primarily clostridia) responsible for hydrolysis of steroid glucuronides in the intestine that allow reabsorption of the steroid via the enterohepatic circulation. Thus there is a theoretical basis for concern. However, in human studies to date it has not been possible to demonstrate reduced plasma levels of EE. It remains possible that the enterohepatic circulation may be much more important in rare individuals. Increased spotting and bleeding is thought to suggest interference with OC effect and probably should suggest the need for additional contraception. These same drug interactions are thought to apply with the levonorgestrel implant, where circulating levels of the contraceptive steroid are low and their further reduction can be expected to result in unwanted pregnancy. In contrast, DMPA levels are considerably higher than needed for contraception, and efficacy is thought not to be reduced by the antiepileptic drugs or rifampin.

Certain drugs actually appear to increase plasma levels of contraceptive steroids. Ascorbic acid (vitamin C) competes with EE for sulfation in the intestinal mucosa, and plasma levels of the steroid are increased when women on OCs add ascorbic acid. Similarly, parecetamol (acetaminophen) is metabolized by conjugation with glucuronide and sulfate, and women on OCs who are then treated with parecetamol can be shown to have an increase in plasma EE.

An example of the second type of interaction, OCs affecting metabolism of other drugs, is seen with diazepam and related compounds. OCs reduce the metabolic clearance and increase the half-life of those benzodiazepines that are metabolized primarily by oxidation: chlordiazepoxide, alprazolam, diazepam, and nitrazepam. Caffeine and theophylline are metabolized in the liver by two of the P_{450} isozymes and their clearance is also reduced in OC users. Cyclosporin is hydroxylated by another of the P_{450} isozymes, and its plasma concentrations are increased by OCs. Plasma levels of some analgesic drugs are decreased in OC users. Salicyclic acid and morphine clearance is enhanced by OC use; hence higher doses could be needed for adequate therapeutic effect. Clearance of ethanol may be reduced in OC users.

Clinical Chemistry Alteration With Oral Contraceptives

Because the steroids in OCs can affect liver function and the production by the liver of a number of binding proteins, OCs have the potential of altering a number of clinical laboratory tests, making the distinction between normal and abnormal more difficult in women on OCs. This concern appears to have been exaggerated, because a large study comparing OC users to pregnant and nonpregnant controls found minimal changes (Knopp et al, 1985). Hormone users were on a variety of OCs containing 50 to 100 μg of estrogen, higher doses than are used routinely today. Compared to nonpregnant women who were not using OCs, the OC users had an increase in thyroxine that is explained by increased circulating thyroid-binding protein, no change in creatinine, a slight reduction in mean fasting glucose values, a reduction in total bilirubin, a modest reduction in aspartate aminotransferase, a decrease in alkaline phosphatase, and no change in globulin.

Clinical Management of Women on OCs

Patient Selection

Food and Drug Administration (FDA)-listed contraindications to the use of OCs are present or past thrombophlebitis or thromboembolic disorders, cerebral vascular or coronary artery disease, breast cancer, estrogen-dependent neoplasm, undiagnosed genital bleeding, pregnancy, and benign or malignant liver tumors. In general, young women are good candidates for combination OCs. Most of the risk appears to be found among older women; younger women are more fertile and have the greatest need for highly effective contraception, and will benefit from the reduction in dysmenorrhea, protection from ectopic pregnancy, and reduced risk for PID and subsequent ovarian cancer. Patients who have other significant risks for thrombosis should usually not be given estrogen-containing OCs: women with prolonged immobilization after surgery or trauma, women with lupus erythematosus and the antiphospholipid syndrome, and, of course, women with a personal history of venous thrombosis, myocardial ischemia, or stroke. The most common significant risk factor is cigarette smoking. Young women should be given strong encouragement to stop smoking, whether or not they will take OCs. Women over 35 who smoke should be encouraged to use other contraceptive methods, but few physicians would presently prescribe OCs for smokers over age 40. Age 40 has been used as a mandatory cutoff for OC use in the past, but recent recommendations are that women over 40 can be considered for low-dose OCs provided they are non-obese, nonsmoking, normoglycemic, and normotensive with no family history of premature vascular disease (Mishell, 1989). There is renewed interest in 20-μg EE products for women in the older reproductive years.

The WHO (1996) has proposed a four-group classification of specific circumstances and appropriateness of contraceptive method. Group 1 includes conditions for which there is no restriction for use of the method. Group 2 are conditions where the advantages of the method generally outweigh the theoretical or proven risks. Group 3 are conditions wherein the theoretical or proven risks usually outweigh the advantages. Group 4 are conditions that represent an unacceptable health risk. Examples of each group are given in Table 11–10.

History of *migraine headache* is associated with stroke risk, and the older OCs appeared to increase this risk (Collaborative Group for the Study of Stroke in Young Women, 1975). Whether present OCs are safe for these women is unknown and is difficult to sort out, because women with migraine are frequently advised against using OCs (Lidegaard, 1995). I encourage individual consideration, and would allow a trial of low-dose OCs in such women, under close supervision after thorough neurologic evaluation. Women whose headaches become more frequent and more severe are of great concern. OC use should be terminated and other contraception substituted. After the headaches resolve, a lower dose preparation could be cautiously tried under close supervision; if headaches recur, I would consider OCs permanently contraindicated. Women who have both mitral valve prolapse and migraine should probably avoid estrogen-containing OCs.

Management of women with *hyperlipidemias* is also controversial. Older OCs were likely to make their abnormal lipid pattern worse. The low-dose norethindrone monophasic and the desogestrel and norgestimate products have beneficial effects on lipids in normal women (Godsland et al, 1990), but there are as yet no studies of their use in hyperlipidemic women. The disproportionate number of hyperlipidemic women among those who had MI on OCs signals caution (Mann et al, 1975). Women with *congen-*

ital heart disease require individual consideration based upon the pathophysiology of their particular condition, clinical status, desires for future reproduction, risk to them of a pregnancy, and contraceptive alternatives. There is published experience with the progestin-only OCs for women with cardiac disease that suggests this to be an acceptable method (Taurelle et al, 1979). There are no recent data as to the safety of low-dose combination OCs for these women. Women who will be chronically anticoagulated for their heart disease may be given oral contraceptives, and some will need them for prevention of ovulation-induced corpus luteum hemorrhages and excessive menstrual blood loss.

Epilepsy need not be considered a contraindication because OCs do not make seizure more likely (Mattson et al, 1986). With the exception of valproic acid, anticonvulsants will reduce blood levels of the contraceptive steroids; therefore, a 50-μg estrogen preparation would be recommended, and barrier contraception advised as well until it is clear that the woman will not experience breakthrough bleeding on the OCs as an indication of low steroid levels.

Women with insulin-dependent *diabetes* are at marked increased risk of heart attack and stroke compared to other women of reproductive age. Older literature suggests their risk is increased by OC use. Use of low-dose OCs in women after gestational diabetes is acceptable (Kjos et al, 1990). Common practice is to individually assess these patients, and to allow OCs for younger diabetic women who have not had vascular complications and have normal blood pressure. Some evidence that this approach works is provided by the Nurses' Health Study, which found less risk of MI or stroke among diabetics who were past users of OCs (Stampfer et al, 1988). Renal and retinal complications were not increased by OC use in young diabetic women who had used them for an average of 3.4 years (Garg et al, 1994).

Sickle cell disease has been considered a contraindication to OCs. However, androgens may be beneficial to women with sickle cell disease, and two small groups of sickle cell patients treated with OCs did not experience adverse effects (Lutcher et al, 1981; Paul Freie, 1983). There is great need for studies of women with chronic illness given OCs and followed closely.

Therapeutic Uses of OCs

OCs are prescribed for important therapeutic indications in addition to contraception. The pill that is the first choice for contraception may not be ideal for some of these other indications. Women with *recurring ovarian cysts* will require increased activity of either the estrogen or the progestin in order to be sure of suppressing gonadotropin and, hence, preventing further formation of functional ovarian cysts. The minimum dose needed is not known, but current multiphasic preparations are not sufficient.

Table 11-10. WORLD HEALTH ORGANIZATION CRITERIA FOR INITIATING AND CONTINUING USE OF COMBINED ORAL CONTRACEPTIVES CONTAINING ≤35 μg OF ETHINYL ESTRADIOL

1: CONDITION FOR WHICH THERE IS NO RESTRICTION FOR THE USE OF THE CONTRACEPTIVE METHOD
Postpartum >21 days
Post first- or second-trimester abortion
Menarche to age 40
History of pre-eclampsia
History of gestational diabetes
Major surgery without immobilization
Varicose veins
Headaches, mild
Irregular vaginal bleeding
Benign breast disease
Family history of breast cancer
Pelvic inflammatory disease and PID risk
HIV/acquired immunodeficiency syndrome
Uterine fibroids
Past ectopic pregnancy
Hypothyroid, hyperthyroid, goiter
Epilepsy
Dysmenorrhea
Endometriosis
Benign ovarian tumors

2: CONDITION WHERE THE ADVANTAGES OF USING THE METHOD GENERALLY OUTWEIGH THE THEORETICAL OR PROVEN RISKS
Age >40 years
Smoker, <age 35 years
Blood pressure 140–159/90–99 with monitoring
Diabetes, insulin dependent, no vascular disease
Superficial venous thrombosis
Known hyperlipidemias
Valvular heart disease, uncomplicated
Headaches, severe, recurrent, including migraine, but without focal neurologic symptoms
Breast mass, undiagnosed
Cervical intraepithelial neoplasia, or cervix cancer while awaiting treatment
Thalassemia
Sickle cell disease

3: CONDITION WHERE THE THEORETICAL OR PROVEN RISKS USUALLY OUTWEIGH THE ADVANTAGES OF USING THE METHOD
Lactating, 6 weeks to 6 months postpartum
Less than 21 days postpartum
Smoker, ≥35 years, light smoking (<20 cigarettes/day)
Breast cancer, past, no disease after 5 years
Biliary tract disease, current
Cirrhosis, mild

4: CONDITION THAT REPRESENTS AN UNACCEPTABLE HEALTH RISK IF THE CONTRACEPTIVE METHOD IS USED
Pregnancy
Lactating, less than 6 weeks postpartum
Smoker, over 35, >20 cigarettes/day
Blood pressure 160–179/100–109, if monitoring not available (category 3 if monitoring available)
Blood pressure 180/110 or more
High blood pressure with vascular disease
Diabetes with nephropathy, retinopathy, other vascular disease, or of >20 years' duration—category 3 or 4 depending on severity
Current or history of deep vein thrombosis/pulmonary embolism
Current or history of ischemic heart disease
Major surgery with prolonged immobilization
Valvular heart disease with complications (pulmonary hypertension, atrial fibrillation, history of subacute bacterial endocarditis)
Severe headaches with focal neurologic symptoms
Current breast cancer
Viral hepatitis, active
Cirrhosis, decompensated
Liver tumors, benign or malignant

Adapted from World Health Organization Family and Reproductive Health: Improving Access to Quality Care in Family Planning. Geneva: World Health Organization, 1996:13, with permission.

When OCs are used to produce resolution of an already existing functional ovarian cyst, the goal is short term. Higher dose formulations are needed in order to be sure of maximal effect, and surgery will be elected if the cyst does not resolve after a month or two. Typically, a preparation with 50 μg of EE is needed for maximal suppression of gonadotropins.

For the woman with *endometriosis*, the risk-benefit equation changes. Her options are continuous OCs, taken without interruption, danazol, gonadotropin-releasing hormone analog, or surgery. Therapy is generally limited in time, to 6 to 9 months. Typically higher dose OCs have been used, and 50 μg EE with norgestrel is frequently prescribed. The strongly androgenic progestin probably adds to the effectiveness. Lipids will be adversely affected, but not nearly as much as they would be by danazol. After the initial 6 to 9 months, when the patient is in remission, she could be changed down to one of the 30- to 35-μg estrogen monophasic OCs taken continuously for maintenance therapy, with presumably lower risk.

Similarly, when OCs are used to treat *uterine hemorrhage*, a higher dose of a strongly progestin-dominant pill is needed for rapid hemostasis and the production of endometrial atrophy. A 50-μg EE product with either 0.5 mg of norgestrel or 2.5 mg of norethindrone acetate would be good choices. An effective regimen is one tablet twice a day for 10 days. If it is desirable to continue the patient on OC therapy, then one of the first-line 35-μg estrogen pills would be substituted following withdrawal bleeding induced by the higher dose pill.

Women with *primary dysmenorrhea* may respond well to a first-line low-dose pill, but some will have significant persistent pain and will need a higher dose pill, and will need it over the long term. There are few comparative data, but a 30- to 35-μg estrogen monophasic may be a better first choice than a multiphasic for dysmenorrhea. *Acne* is a common reason for prescribing OCs. Although all combination OCs have been used for this purpose, a norgestimate-containing OC is specifically approved by the FDA for this indication.

Choice of OCs

As the first choice for contraceptive purposes for the average patient, I advise the 30- to 35-μg estrogen combination OCs. Breakthrough bleeding and spotting are common at first and generally improve with time. If the problem persists, one can change from a multiphasic to a monophasic version at the same estrogen level. If bleeding is still a problem, a temporary increase in estrogen proposed by Speroff (1981) should be tried: 20 μg of EE daily for 7 days while continuing the OC. The side effects of breast tenderness, mood changes, and weight gain are less common with current formulations and usually resolve after the first few cycles. If symptoms persist, the lowest dose highly effective formulation could be tried: EE 35 μg with norethindrone 0.5 mg. Nausea

is an estrogen side effect, and if persistent could be managed by changing to the 20-μg EE product. The patient with persistent breast tenderness could be switched to a pill with more progestin activity, such as 30-μg EE with 250 μg of levonorgestrel. High-progestin-potency pills produce fewer breast symptoms (Kay, 1980). The woman with worsening acne should be switched to an OC with relatively more estrogen and a less androgenic progestin. The norgestimate or desogestrel products are best for this purpose. Women who have had persistent nausea or headache on the 20-μg estrogen combination and who still desire hormonal contraception could be considered for the progestin-only minipill, but must be cautioned about the higher pregnancy rate and increased cycle irregularity. Because the progestin-only minipills do not suppress lactation and contain very small amounts of hormone, they can be used in lactating women, for whom combination pills are relatively contraindicated. All of the potentially serious complications of hormonal contraception are attributable to the estrogen component, and, in management of specific patients, the alternatives of progestin-only hormonal contraception should be remembered: progestin-only pills, injectable DMPA, and the levonorgestrel implant.

Injectable Progestin Contraceptives

The most widely used injectable is DMPA (Depo-Provera) (Kaunitz, 1994). Another injectable, norethindrone enanthate, available outside the United States, is shorter acting and must be given as 200 mg every 2 months to achieve efficacy comparable to DMPA. Once-a-month injectable combinations of estrogens and progestins are available in many countries.

DMPA, a suspension of microcrystals of the synthetic progestin, was finally approved for contraception in 1992 but had been used for more than 20 years for other indications. A single 150-mg IM dose will suppress ovulation in most women for 14 weeks or longer (Kaunitz, 1994). Contraceptive blood levels are reached within 24 hours and peak concentrations of 15 to 25 μg/ml are reached within 20 days (Kaunitz, 1994). The regimen of 150 mg every 3 months is as effective as tubal sterilization, producing pregnancy rates of approximately 0.3 per 100 women per year. Probably because of the high blood levels of the progestin, efficacy appears not to be reduced by administration of other drugs and is not dependent on the patient's weight. Women treated with DMPA experience disruption of the menstrual cycle and have initial spotting and bleeding at irregular intervals, but eventually most develop total amenorrhea, 50% by 1 year and 80% by 3 years of continued administration (Kaunitz, 1994) (Fig. 11–11). DMPA persists in the body for several months in women who have used it for long-term contraception, and return to fertility may be delayed; however, in a large study,

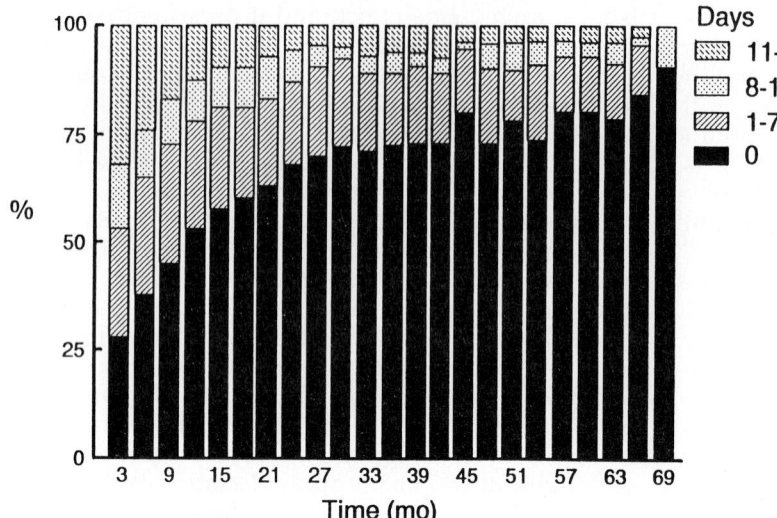

Figure 11-11
Bleeding pattern and duration of use of DMPA: percentage of women who have bleeding, spotting, or amenorrhea while taking DMPA 150 mg every 3 months. (From: Schwallie PC, Assenzo JR: Contraceptive use-efficacy study utilizing medroxyprogesterone acetate administered as an intramuscular injection once every 90 days. Fertil Steril 1973;24:331, with permission.)

70% of former users desiring pregnancy had conceived within 12 months, and 90% within 24 months (Pardthaisong, 1984).

Risks of DMPA

Loss of bone density in users of DMPA was found in one cross-sectional study (Cundy et al, 1991), but not found in another using plain radiographs of trabecular bone, which matched users and nonusers by age, body mass index, and body weight (Virutamasen et al, 1994). The sensitivity of plain radiographs for detecting osteopenia is limited. A better study used sensitive measurements of bone density in adolescent girls followed prospectively, and did find a 1.5% decrease in density per year, compared with a 1.5% increase for girls on OCs and a 2.5% increase for girls who had Norplant or did not use hormonal contraception (Cromer et al, 1996). DMPA may have reduced mean estrogen levels enough to impair the normal gain in bone density of late adolescence. More work is needed to determine the effect of longer use and the reversibility of this change.

The effect on plasma lipids of DMPA has been inconsistent, but in general DMPA users appear to have reduced total cholesterol and triglycerides, slight reduction in HDL cholesterol, and no change or slight increase in LDL cholesterol, all consistent with a modest reduction in circulating estrogen levels. In some studies the decrease in HDL and increase in LDL is statistically significant, although the values remain within the normal ranges (Fahmy et al, 1991). DMPA has not been associated with heart attack. A small elevation of glucose is seen on glucose tolerance tests in DMPA users. There are no changes in hemostatic parameters except that ATIII is sometime found to be reduced in chronic therapy (Fahmy et al, 1991). DMPA has not been linked to thrombotic episodes in reproductive-age women. However, thrombotic episodes have occurred in elderly women with advanced cancer treated with a variety of agents, including DMPA and tamoxifen (Isihizaki et al, 1992; Okada et al, 1992). Such patients are at high risk for thrombosis without treatment. Whether or not DMPA was accidentally associated or in some way causal in these cases is not known.

Women on DMPA experienced weight gain of 2 to 3 pounds more than nonusers over several years in initial studies. A study of DMPA users compared to OC and Norplant users found no significant weight change over 1 years of observation (Moore et al, 1995). Another small study had similar findings (Mainwaring et al, 1995). However, a review of studies over the last 20 years concluded that weight gain is common (Westoff, 1996). DMPA has not been associated with affective disorders and mood changes, but information is limited (Westoff et al, 1995; Westoff, 1996). Teratogenesis has not been reported with DMPA. It is safe for use by lactating women and, like other progestin-only hormonal methods, appears to increase milk production.

Benefits of DMPA

DMPA appears to have many of the noncontraceptive benefits of combination OCs: reduced anemia, reduced PID, reduced ectopic pregnancy, and reduced endometrial cancer. Several studies of DMPA and cervical cancer have found no association (La Vecchia, 1994). Adenocarcinoma risk is not increased (Thomas and Ray, 1995). Ovarian cancer has been found unrelated to DMPA use (WHO, 1991). The failure to find prevention of ovarian cancer may be because the studies were done in third-world countries with multiparous women. Reduction in ovarian cancer risk seen with OCs is greatest for women of low parity (CDC Cancer and Steroid Hormone Study, 1983c). Risk of breast cancer diagnosis during the first 4 years of DMPA use appeared slightly increased, but there was no increase in risk with long-term use and no overall increase in breast cancer risk; hence a causal relation between DMPA and breast cancer is unlikely (Chilvers, 1994).

Clinical Management of DMPA

DMPA has proven increasingly popular since its approval for contraceptive use. It offers remarkable protection from pregnancy, the convenience of a once-every-3-months injection, and freedom from estrogen-related risks. Hence it may be chosen by women who have experienced difficulties in compliance with OCs or have contraindications to their use. Ordinarily DMPA is started on the fifth day of the menstrual cycle, ensuring the absence of a pregnancy and providing immediate protection to prevent ovulation in the current cycle. It is given as a 1-ml IM injection in either the upper arm or buttocks. The 400-mg/ml preparation is not advised for contraception because bioavailability is said to be less (Kaunitz, 1994). Patients must be thoroughly educated as to the effect on menstruation: initial irregular bleeding and staining followed by complete amenorrhea by 1 to 3 years of continuous use. They must also understand that 6 to 9 months or longer will elapse after cessation of therapy before return of fertility. Persistent irregular bleeding is the most frequent complaint of women on DMPA. This can be treated by adding low-dose estrogen temporarily, as, for example, 1.25 mg of conjugated estrogens or 2 mg/day micronized estradiol for 10 to 21 days at a time. The common practice of treating bleeding problems by giving the next injection of DMPA sooner than 3 months is not effective and increases weight gain (Harel et al, 1995). Other causes of bleeding should be considered: *Chlamydia* endometritis and submucosal leiomyomata. Hence, if bothersome bleeding persists, an immunologic test for cervical *Chlamydia* and transvaginal ultrasound examination of the uterus are indicated.

Injectable Estrogen-Progestin Contraceptives

Two once-a-month injectable combinations of long-acting estrogens and progestins have been developed by the WHO: the combination of 25 mg medroxyprogesterone acetate and 5 mg estradiol cyprionate (Cyclofem) and the combination of 50 mg norethindrone enanthate plus 5 mg estradiol valerate (Mesigyna). Given once a month, both produce excellent contraceptive effect. Monthly withdrawal bleeding is like a normal menses, leading to high continuation rates (Guo-wei, 1994). A WHO study, as yet unpublished, compared coagulation parameters in women receiving either of the two monthly injectables or a combination OC containing 35 µg of EE and 1 mg of norethindrone (WHO Task Force on Long-Acting Systemic Agents for Fertility Regulation, 1993). The OC produced the expected increases in fibrinogen, factor VII, factor X, and plasminogen and a decrease in tissue plasminogen activator in-

hibitor, suggesting a compensatory increase in fibrinolysis. The injectable combinations did not induce these changes, suggesting less or possibly no effect on coagulation. This may be because the injectable estrogen is present in the subject's body for only a few days at a time, as opposed to 21 days with conventional OCs. The effect of the injectable estrogen-progestin combinations on women with factor V Leiden or other deficiencies of anticoagulation is unknown. Cyclofem, renamed "Cyclo-Provera," is undergoing U.S. trials presently.

Subdermal Implants

The levonorgestrel implant (Norplant) consists of six rods, each measuring 34 mm in length and 2.4 mm in outside diameter and containing 36 mg of the progestin levonorgestrel (Darney, 1994). Approximately 80 µg/day is released during the first 6 to 12 months after insertion. The release rate then gradually declines to 30 to 35 µg/day. Blood levels of the steroid are about 0.35 ng/ml at 6 months and remain above 0.25 ng/ml until 5 years. Plasma levels less than 0.20 ng/ml result in higher pregnancy rates. This low level of progestin produces very effective contraception, with a total number of pregnancies over 5 years of only 1.5 in 100 women (Darney, 1994). The progestin blocks the LH surge necessary for ovulation, so that over 5 years only about one-third of cycles are ovulatory. In response to the progestin, the cervical mucus becomes scant and thick and does not allow sperm penetration. U.S. trials included an older, denser walled version of Norplant, and contraceptive efficacy was less for women weighing 70 kg or more. Current Norplant devices have a less dense pliable wall and the release rate of levonorgestrel is 15% greater, so that weight is less of a problem (Darney, 1994). Some advise that heavy women should have the implants replaced after 3 years in order to maintain a very high level of pregnancy protection. Medications that increase the rate of steroid metabolism (rifampin, phenytoin, carbamazepine, phenobarbital) would be expected to reduce the efficacy of Norplant and contraindicate its use. Because of the very low blood levels of the steroid, Norplant can be used by nursing mothers (Darney, 1994). Levonorgestrel levels fall immediately with removal of the implants, and return to fertility is prompt.

Bleeding Pattern

Norplant produces endometrial atrophy. The normal menstrual cycle is disrupted, resulting in a range of possible bleeding patterns from reasonable regular monthly bleeding to frequents spotting and almost daily bleeding to complete amenorrhea. Bleeding pattern changes over time and tends to become more like a normal menstrual pattern. Women who have monthly bleeding are more likely to be ovulating and, if they become amenorrheic, must be evaluated for pregnancy. Irregular bleeding and spotting can be treated with low-dose oral estrogen, low-dose oral levonorgestrel, or ibuprofen (Hatcher et al, 1994: 306–318).

Metabolic Effects

Glucose metabolism is not altered with the use of implants. There are minimal lipid changes, with a reduction in total cholesterol and triglyceride, and either no change or minimal decrease in HDL, but maintenance of the same ratio of total cholesterol to HDL; hence, it is very unlikely that Norplant will promote development of atherosclerosis (Darney, 1994).

Adverse Events, Side Effects, and Safety

Irregular bleeding and headache are the main reasons given for discontinuation of Norplant. Side effects that are occasionally reported include acne, weight gain or loss, mastalgia, mood change, depression, hyperpigmentation over the implants, hirsutism, and galactorrhea. Symptomatic functional cysts occasionally occur. These usually resolve spontaneously over a few weeks without surgery. Should pregnancy occur, the probability of an ectopic pregnancy is increased compared to conceptions in other women; however, because pregnancy is so rare with Norplant, the total rate of ectopic pregnancies, 0.28 per 1000 woman-years, is well below that seen in the U.S. population (Darney, 1994).

The FDA has compiled all serious adverse events reported from 1991 to 1993 (Wysowski and Green, 1995). These included 24 women hospitalized for infection at the implant site, 14 hospitalized or disabled because of difficulties removing the capsules, and 14 hospitalized for stroke, 3 for thrombotic thrombocytopenic purpura, 6 for thrombocytopenia, and 29 for pseudotumor cerebri. Except for the hospitalizations related to infection and removal of the implants, the rate of occurrence of the rare illnesses did not exceed that expected in women in the reproductive years, and no causal connection was implied. More study is needed to determine whether thrombotic thrombocytopenic purpurea, thrombocytopenia, and pseudotumor cerebri are related to Norplant use. Physicians who use Norplant must learn to insert and remove the capsules properly. It is not difficult (Hatcher et al, 1994:305–306).

Seven cases of major depression, obsessive-compulsive disorder, or panic disorder have been reported in Norplant users (Wagner, 1996). Depression typically began within 1 to 3 months of insertion and resolved in 1 to 2 months after removal of the implants. It is not possible to say at present whether this is causal or accidental association.

Insertion and Removal

Norplant is inserted just beneath the skin of the inner surface of the upper arm using a 10-gauge trocar as an inserter. This is readily accomplished in a few minutes with local anesthesia. Removal of Norplant can be time consuming, but the difficulty has been overemphasized. Speroff and Darney (1992) advised use of the fingers to manipulate the end of the rod into a small skin incision, using a scalpel to nick the fibrous sheath that forms around the rod and then pushing it out with finger pressure. With the Emory technique, a some what longer incision (10 mm) is used and a hemostat forceps is used to disrupt the fibrous capsule around the ends of all of the implants before instrument removal (Hatcher et al, 1994:305–306).

Progestin-Only Contraception and Adverse Selection

Because progestin-only methods may be prescribed for women with chronic illness for whom estrogen-containing OCs are considered contraindicated, there is a real risk that these contraceptive methods will be blamed for events that would have occurred anyway because of the patient's underlying illness. In the medicolegal climate of the United States, the practitioner should document a careful discussion of risk when prescribing hormonal contraceptives for women with chronic illness.

Hormonal Contraception for Men

The same negative feedback of sex steroids that can block ovulation in women will also suppress spermatogenesis in men, but will produce lost of libido and potentially extinguish sexual performance. Replacement testosterone therapy restores libido and performance without restoring spermatogenesis. The principle was first demonstrated by Briggs and Briggs in 1974 using oral estrogen and methyltestosterone. Testosterone alone will suppress pituitary release of LH and FSH to very low levels and depress or abolish spermatogenesis, while the testosterone in the systemic circulation maintains normal sexual behavior and body habitus. Weekly doses of 200 mg achieve azoospermia in only 40% to 70% of Caucasian men; the rest become oligospermic (Knuth et al, 1989; Wallace et al, 1993). Unfortunately, pregnancy has occurred in partners of androgen-treated oligospermic men with sperm counts as low as 3 million/ ml (Wallace et al, 1992). Asian men may be more effectively treated: 100 mg weekly produced azoospermia in seven of seven Indonesian men studied (Arsyad, 1993). Combinations of DMPA plus androgen have been widely studied but also fail to achieve 100% sperm suppression in Caucasians (Swerdloff et al, 1992). Current interest is in using gonadotropin-releasing hormone analogs to suppress spermatogenesis, with long-acting androgens for replacement. One of these regimens will likely prove clinically useful, but at present costs are high and long-term safety remains to be established. Adverse lipid changes have been noted with DMPA-androgen combinations, raising the concern about vascular disease with prolonged use (Wallace et al, 1990). However, a DMPA-androgen combination reduced levels of the highly atherogenic lipoprotein A by about one third, a potential benefit (Anderson et al, 1995). Liver cancer is a concern with long-term androgen therapy (Murad and Haynes, 1980).

EMERGENCY CONTRACEPTION

Implantation of the fertilized ovum is thought to occur on the sixth day after fertilization. This interval provides an opportunity to prevent pregnancy even after fertilization. Estrogen, estrogen-progestin combinations, and copper IUCDs have been used for this purpose for many years, but many physicians have been reluctant to prescribe them, lacking an FDA indication, and many women who could have benefited have not. More than half of U.S. pregnancies were unintended at the time of conception (Brown and Eisenberg, 1995). In recent years health professionals have made a concerted effort to make postcoital contraception, renamed emergency contraception, widely available. In 1997, an FDA panel recommended use of combination OCs for this purpose (Food and Drug Administration [FDA], 1997).

Estrogens

In 1973, Morris and Van Waaganen proved first in monkeys and then in women that high-dose estrogen taken after coitus prevented pregnancy (Morris and Van Waaganen, 1973). Diethylstilbestrol, 25 mg twice a day for 5 days, was used initially. More recently, other estrogens have been substituted. EE 5 mg/day for 5 days in a study of 3000 women resulted in a pregnancy rate of only 0.15% (Haspells, 1994). Proposed mechanisms of action include altered tubal motility, interference with corpus luteum function, and alteration of the endometrium.

Estrogen-Progestin Combinations

The combination of EE 200 μg and *d,l* norgestrel 2 mg (two Ovral tablets followed by two more 12 hours later) first described by Yuspe and Smith (1982) is convenient and effective. Although the average pregnancy rate with this method is 1.8%, a study from New Zealand reported an overall failure rate of 2.3% (Kane and Sparrow, 1989). Those who took the first dose within 12 hours of intercourse experienced only 1.2% failures, whereas, of those starting more than 48 hours after intercourse, 4.5% conceived. High-dose estrogen thus appears to be more effective than the estrogen-progestin combination; however, a randomized trial found them of equal efficacy (Haspells, 1994).

Prescribing Emergency Contraception

The Yuspe method is the most widely used means for emergency contraception in the United States. Most studies of this method have used two Ovral tablets, repeated in 12 hours, started within 72 hours of intercourse. Equivalent doses of other norgestrel-containing products would be four tablets of Lo/Ovral, Nordette, Levlen, Triphasil, or Tri-Levlen rather than two tablets. Although usually started by 72 hours, there is limited information that the method may be equally effective if started within 120 hours of intercourse (Grou and Rodrigues, 1994). Nausea occurs in 30% to 66% of patients and vomiting in 12% to 22%, and prophylactic antiemetics 1 hour prior to each dose are advised (American College of Obstetricians and Gynecologists, 1996). There are no known contraindications other than an already existing pregnancy. On average, menstruation occurs within 7 to 9 days of treatment, and within 21 days in 98% of women (Yuspe et al, 1982). Nonetheless, if menses are delayed more than a few days, it is prudent to offer a sensitive pregnancy test. Because OCs have not proved to be teratogenic, presumably the Yuspe method would not be either.

Postcoital Copper IUCD

Postcoital insertion of a copper IUCD is the most effective emergency contraceptive option (Lippes et al, 1976). In a series of 879 patients treated in this fashion, only one pregnancy occurred (Fasoli et al, 1989). Haspells (1994) reported insertion of copper IUCDs as long as 7 days after coitus and had no pregnancies within 5 months of insertion. Copper is toxic to the embryo.

Danazol

Another approach is treatment with the androgen danazol. The pregnancy rate was 2% among 998 women reported (Haspells, 1994).

Postcoital Mifepristone

The antiprogesterone mifepristone (RU 486) is a highly effective postcoital contraceptive, with no apparent side effects. A three-way trial of the Yuspe method using EE-norgestrel, danazol 600 mg repeated after 12 hours, and mifepristone 600 mg as a single dose produced pregnancy rates of 2.62, 4.66, and 0%, respectively (Webb et al, 1992). Mifepristone was highly effective in inducing menstruation when taken on day 27 of the cycle, well beyond the window of 72 hours after intercourse usually recommended (Haspells, 1994). There was only one conception in 62 women treated on this protocol. As of this writing, mifepristone has received preliminary approval by the FDA for early abortion but is not yet available.

STERILIZATION

The great popularity of surgical sterilization in the United States has to do with the strong desire of individuals to control their own fertility, their concern about the safety and effectiveness of present contraceptive methods, and, most importantly, the availability of safe and reasonably easy surgical techniques. At age 30, the typical age at sterilization, most married couples have had all the children they want and face 15 or more years of continued need for contraception (Mosher, 1988). For some couples, the decision to seek sterilization will prove to be premature. Age less than 30 when sterilized, or divorce and remarriage, is a strong predictor of sterilization regret that may lead to a request for sterilization reversal (Marcil-Gratton, 1988). The availability of low-dose OCs, DMPA, the copper T380A, and the Silastic implants are providing couples with new options to avoid premature sterilization. In selecting among alternative techniques for sterilization, the physician must consider the likelihood that the patient may eventually seek reversal.

Female Sterilization

Techniques for Female Sterilization

Hysterectomy no longer is considered primarily for sterilization because the risk of morbidity and mortality from hysterectomy considerably exceeds that from tubal sterilization. Four procedures are common in U.S. practice currently (Hulka, 1993):

1. Tubal sterilization at the time of laparotomy for a cesarean section or other abdominal operation
2. Postpartum minilaparotomy soon after vaginal delivery
3. Interval minilaparotomy
4. Laparoscopy

TUBAL STERILIZATION

With the development of laparoscopy, vaginal tubal sterilization, which was associated with occasional pelvic abscess, has virtually disappeared in this country. Tubal sterilization at the time of cesarean section adds no risk of itself, other than a slight prolongation of operating time; however, cesarean has more risk than vaginal birth, and planned sterilization should not influence the decision to perform a cesarean. If there is serious concern as to the welfare of the infant, sterilization should not be done. Formerly it was taught that sterilization failure was more common if done with a cesarean section, but this has been clearly disproven (Shepard, 1974).

The tubal lesion usually elected is the Pomeroy or modified Pomeroy technique. In the classical *Pomeroy procedure*, a loop of tube is excised after ligating the base of the loop with single absorbable suture. A modification, probably most often used, is excision of the midportion of the tube after ligation of the segment with two separate absorbable sutures. This modified procedure has several names: partial salpingectomy, Parkland Hospital technique, separate sutures technique (Rimdusit, 1984), and *modified Pomeroy*. Another alternative, now abandoned because of a high rate of subsequent pregnancy, is described to prevent its reintroduction. This is the *Madlener technique* in which a loop of tube is crushed by cross-clamping its base, ligating with permanent suture, and then excising the loop. Pomeroy and partial salpingectomy procedures have failure rates of 1 to 4 per 1000 cases in the first year (Shepard, 1974). In contrast, pregnancy is almost unheard of after tubal sterilization by the Irving (1924) or Uchida (1975) method. In the *Irving method*, the midportion of the tube is excised after ligating each end of the segment with absorbable suture as for a modified Pomeroy. The proximal stump of each tube is turned back and led into a small stab wound in the wall of the uterus and sutured in place, creating a blind loop. With *Uchida's method*, a saline-epinephrine solution (1:1000) is injected beneath the mucosa of the midportion of the tube, separating the mucosa off of the underlying tube. The mucosa is incised along the antimesenteric border of the tube, and a tubal segment is excised under traction so that the ligated proximal stump will retract beneath the mucosa when released. The mucosa is then closed with sutures, burying the proximal stump and separating it from the distal stump. Uchida (1975) reported use of his technique in a personal series of over 20,000 cases with no pregnancies.

POSTPARTUM MINILAPAROTOMY

Postpartum minilaparotomy was the most common method of sterilization in the period immediately before introduction of laparoscopy, and remains a commonly used method. In the immediate postpartum state, the uterus is enlarged and the fallopian tubes lie in the midabdomen. Access to the tubes is gained through a small (3 to 4-cm) subumbilical incision. Any of the tubal sterilization methods described above is then utilized. Ideally postpartum sterilization is accomplished with the same anesthetic as used for delivery, usually a spinal or epidural block.

INTERVAL MINILAPAROTOMY

Interval minilaparotomy was probably first described by Uchida, but was rediscovered and popularized in the early 1970s with the need for large numbers of sterilizations as an alternative to the more complex and demanding laparoscopy techniques. In the nongravid state, the uterus and fallopian tubes lie deep in the pelvis. The development that allowed interval sterilization was a simple device, the uterine elevator placed on the cervix through the vagina (Osathanondh, 1974). This allows use of a short transverse suprapubic incision; the uterus and tubes are elevated upward just beneath the incision by use of the uterine elevator probe. With the tubes accessible through the small incision, a Pomeroy-type tubal ligation is usually performed, although any of the laparoscopy tubal lesion techniques described below can be substituted. Mini-laparotomy is frequently done as an outpatient procedure or with just overnight hospitalization and is readily accomplished under local anesthesia.

LAPAROSCOPY

The development of fiberoptics made possible the easy illumination of the abdominal cavity. Laparoscopy was perfected in Germany during the 1960s and began to be widely available in the United States in the early 1970s. With standard laparoscopy technique, the abdomen is inflated with a gas (carbon dioxide or nitrous oxide) via a special needle inserted at the lower margin of the umbilicus. Then a hollow sheath containing a pointed trocar is pushed through the abdominal wall at the same location, the trocar is removed, and the laparoscope is inserted into the abdominal cavity through the sheath to visualize the pelvic organs. A second, smaller trocar is inserted in the suprapubic region to allow insertion of special grasping forceps. Alternatively, an operating laparoscope can be used that has a channel for the insertion of instruments to accomplish sterilization without the need for a second puncture of the abdominal wall (Hulka, 1985; Khandwala, 1988). Laparoscopy sterilization is usually performed in the hospital under general anesthesia, but can be done under local anesthesia with intravenous sedation. Overnight hospitalization is needed only for patients with complicating pre-existing conditions.

Open Laparoscopy. Standard laparoscopy carries with it a small but definite risk of injury to major blood vessels with insertion of the sharp trocar. With the alternative technique called open laparoscopy, developed by Hasson, neither needle nor sharp trocar is used; rather, the peritoneal cavity is opened directly through an incision at the lower edge of the umbilicus. A special funnel-shaped sleeve, the Hasson cannula, is then inserted and the laparoscope introduced through it (Hasson, 1982).

Tubal Lesions for Laparoscopy. Sterilization is accomplished by any of three techniques: bipolar electrical coagulation, application of a small Silastic rubber band (Falope ring) (Yoon et al, 1977), or application of a plastic and metal clip (Hulka clip) across each tube (Hulka et al, 1973; Hulka, 1993). The Filshie clip, a simpler mechanical device for occluding the tube, has recently become available in the United States. In the bipolar electrocoagulation tech-

nique, the midisthmic portion of the tube and adjacent mesosalpinx are grasped with a special bipolar forceps and radiofrequency electrical current is applied to three adjacent areas, coagulating 3 cm of tube (Fig. 11–12). The tube alone is then recoagulated in the same places. The radiofrequency generator must deliver at least 25 watts into a 100-ohm resistance at the probe tips in order to be sure of coagulating the complete thickness of the fallopian tube and not just the outer layer; otherwise the sterilization will fail (Soderstrom et al, 1989). To apply the Falope ring, the midisthmic portion of the tube is grasped with tongs advanced through a cylindrical probe that has the ring stretched around it. A loop of tube is pulled back into the probe and the outer cylinder advanced, releasing the Silastic ring around the base of the loop of tube, producing ischemic necrosis (Fig. 11–13). If the tube cannot be easily pulled into the applicator, the operator should stop and change to electrical coagulation rather than persist and risk lacerating the tube with the Falope ring applicator. The banded tube must be inspected at close range through the laparoscope to demonstrate that the full thickness of the tube has been pulled through the Falope ring. The Hulka clip is also placed across the midisthmus, taking care that the applicator is at right angles to the tube and that the tube is completely contained within the clip before the clip is closed.

The electric and band or clip techniques each have advantages and disadvantages. Bipolar coagulation can be used with any fallopian tube. The ring and the clip cannot be applied if the tube is thickened from previous salpingitis. There is more pain during the first several hours after ring application and more analgesia will be required. The pain can be re-

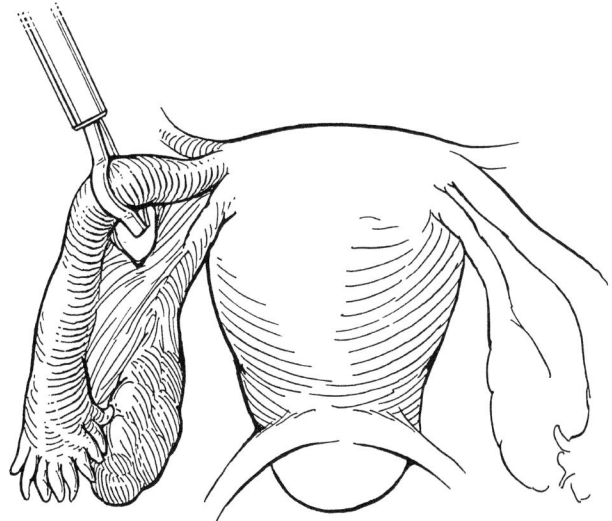

Figure 11–12
Technique for bipolar electrocoagulation tubal sterilization. (Redrawn from Novaks' Gynecology. Berek JS, Adashi EY, Hillard PA [eds]. Baltimore: Williams & Wilkins, 1996:259, with permission.)

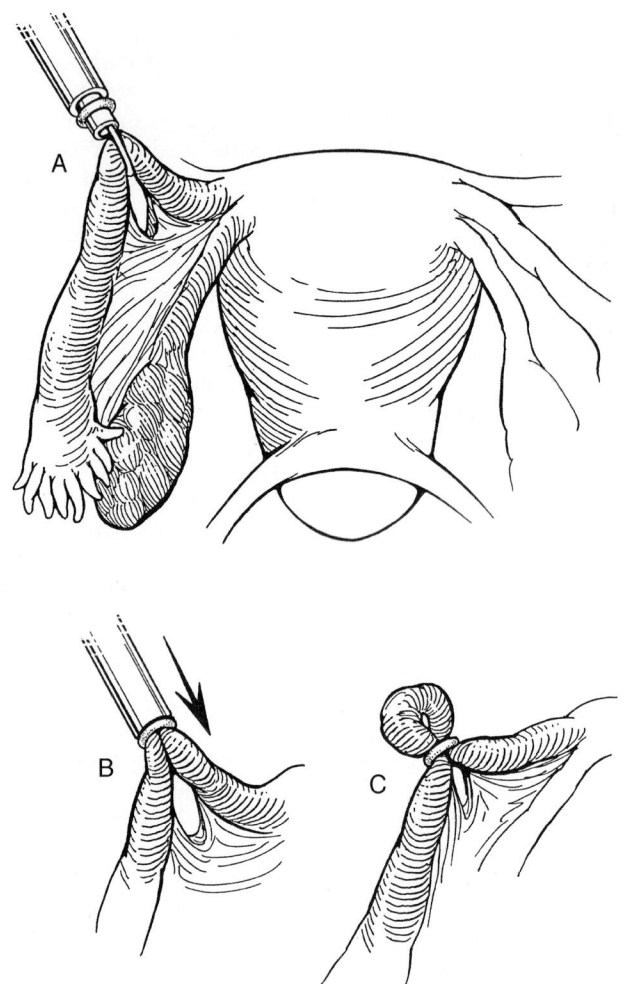

Figure 11–13
Placement of the Falope ring for tubal sterilization. (Redrawn from Novaks' Gynecology. Berek JS, Adashi EY, Hillard PA [eds]. Baltimore: Williams & Wilkins, 1996:259, with permission.)

duced by applying 2% lidocaine to the surface of the fallopian tubes before applying the Falope ring. Failures of the Falope ring or Hulka clip have to do with misapplication generally, and pregnancy, if it results, is usually intrauterine. Pregnancy after bipolar sterilization may occur from tuboperitoneal fistula and is ectopic in more than 50% of cases. If inadequate electrical energy is used, a thin band of fallopian tube remains, containing the intact lumen and allowing intrauterine pregnancy to occur. Thermocoagulation, the use of heat probes rather than electrical current, is used extensively in Germany for tubal sterilization at laparoscopy but has had little use in the United States.

Benefits of Tubal Sterilization

Tubal sterilization provides excellent, generally lifelong protection from the risks of pregnancy from a single event, the surgical procedure. Because pregnancy mortality rises steeply with age, this long-lasting protection is of great benefit. In addition, tubal sterilization reduces risk of subsequent ovarian cancer by about half. The mechanism is unknown, but it may be that of blocking access to the peritoneal cavity of oncogenic substances transported from the vagina (Weiss et al, 1991). Another advantage, little talked about, has to do with guilt. If contraception is viewed as sinful, then each pill that is taken or each condom that is used represents an act to feel guilty about. Sterilization, in this view, could constitute one sinful act for which forgiveness could be sought.

Risks of Tubal Sterilization

In the period from 1977 through 1981 there were 4 deaths per 100,000 tubal sterilization procedures in the United States. Almost half of U.S. sterilization deaths at that time were complications of general anesthesia, usually related to the use of mask ventilation for laparoscopy (Peterson et al, 1983). If general anesthesia is used for laparoscopy, endotracheal intubation is mandatory because the pneumoperitoneum increases the risk of aspiration of gastric contents. The most recent U.S. national data on mortality with tubal sterilization cover the period from 1979 to 1980 (Escobedo et al, 1989). The total case fatality rate was estimated to be 9 per 100,000 sterilizations, but only 1 to 2 per 100,000 could be attributed to the sterilization operation alone. A similar safety record has been accomplished in 50 countries worldwide: 4.7 deaths per 100,000 female sterilizations and 0.5 per 100,000 vasectomies, markedly less than the risk of death from a single pregnancy in those countries (Khairulleh et al, 1992). The rate of complications in a large series from several institutions was 1.7 per 100 sterilizations in 1983. In this multivariate analysis DeStefano et al (1983a) found that complications were increased by use of general anesthesia, previous pelvic or abdominal surgery, history of PID, obesity, and diabetes mellitus. The most common complication was unintended laparotomy made necessary to accomplish sterilization after intra-abdominal adhesions were found, and should not be considered a true complication. Initial laparoscopy methods that used unipolar electrocoagulation could produce unrecognized coagulation injuries of the bowel that could be fatal. This type of injury virtually disappeared with introduction of bipolar coagulation and the nonelectrical Falope ring and Hulka-Semens clip methods. Safety records of individual surgeons or small groups have been much better. Poindexter and colleagues (1990) performed 2827 laparoscopic sterilizations under local anesthesia and intravenous sedation using the Silastic band. Only four cases could not be completed, a technical failure rate of 0.14%, and laparotomy was never needed. Rarely, salpingitis can occur as a complication of the surgery. This occurs more often after electrical coagulation than after the nonelectrical techniques.

When tubal sterilization fails, ectopic pregnancy is likely (Kjer, 1989). The risk of ectopic pregnancy depends on the type of tubal sterilization. Hulka (1983) reported that the risk of ectopic pregnancy with sterilization failure was 16% with the Hulka-Semens clip, 38% with the Silastic ring, 44% with the Pomeroy partial salpingectomy, 59% with bipolar electrosurgical fulguration, and 73% with unipolar electrosurgery. Failures with the Falope ring or Hulka clip are often the result of misapplication of the device on the ampulla rather than the thinner isthmic portion of the tube, so that the tubal lumen is not completely occluded. This may explain the lower rate of ectopic pregnancy when failure of one of these methods occurs, in contrast to electrosurgical fulguration of the tube.

Late Sequelae of Tubal Sterilization

Increased menstrual irregularity and pain have been linked to tubal sterilization for more than 40 years. The problem is that many women develop these symptoms even though they have not had tubal surgery. Neil and colleagues (1975) studied three groups of women: those sterilized by laparoscopy with unipolar coagulation and resection of a tubal segment, those sterilized by open laparotomy with Pomeroy ligation, and those whose husbands had had vasectomies. They found the most menstrual symptoms in the first group, fewer in the second group, and the least among the wives of vascectomized men. A larger study found no menstrual function changes provided women discontinuing OCs and IUCDs were excluded (Kwak et al, 1980). Important information is provided by the Collaborative Review of Sterilization (CREST) of the CDC (DeStefano et al, 1983b). Interviews were conducted of 2546 women before tubal sterilization and then 2 years later. On average, cycle length decreased by a very small amount, 0.03 days. Fewer women reported irregular cycles after sterilization than before. The reported amount of menstrual bleeding did not increase. Women having bipolar electrocoagulation or Silastic band sterilization more often reported decreased menstrual pain at the 2-year interview, but women who had unipolar sterilization, the technique reported in the Neil et al (1975) paper, had increased pain subsequently. A 5-year follow-up of the same cohort found that reporting of menstrual pain and heavy bleeding increased over the years, but, because there was no control group of women without sterilization, this may have been the consequence of aging of the women unrelated to tubal sterilization (Wilcox et al, 1992). This issue remains unresolved. In a report by Sumiala et al (1995), uterine blood flow as measured with ultrasound was found to be altered by application of Filshie clips for tubal sterilization. Whether this alteration is permanent, and whether it would lead to symptoms, are not known.

Sterilization Failure

Most studies of pregnancy after tubal sterilization have included only 1 to 2 years of observation, and hence underestimate the cumulative failure rate over time. An important exception is the Collaborative Review of Sterilization, performed by the CDC (Peterson et al, 1996). In this study, from the time of voluntary surgical sterilization in 1978 through 1986 at one of 16 U.S. centers, a group of 10,685 women were followed with annual telephone contact for 8 to 14 years after sterilization. Pregnancies that occurred during the luteal phase of the cycle in which the sterilization was performed were excluded and true failures were measured using a life table method. Of these true failures, 33% were ectopic. Surprisingly, failures were not limited to the first year or two, but continued to appear at each year during follow-up. After 10 years, the most effective methods were unipolar coagulation at laparoscopy and postpartum partial salpingectomy, generally a modified Pomeroy procedure. Least effective were bipolar tubal coagulation and the Hulka-Clemens clip (Table 11–11). Younger women had higher risk for failure, as might be expected because of their greater fecundability. Women sterilized by the bipolar technique between ages 18 and 27 years had a pregnancy rate of 5.4% over 10 years, whereas women ages 28 through 33 had only 2% risk of pregnancy and women ages 34 through 44 at sterilization had a 0.6% pregnancy rate with the same method. This paper did not report the details of the bipolar sterilization procedure or whether the three-burn technique with adequate electrical energy was used. Unfortunately this study did not included women undergoing sterilization by the Irving or Uchida methods, which are believed to have virtually no failures.

To reduce luteal-phase pregnancy, women are advised to continue contraception until the day of surgery, and sensitive pregnancy tests are used routinely as part of preoperative testing. However, because implantation does not occur until 6 days af-

Table 11–11. TEN-YEAR LIFE TABLE CUMULATIVE PROBABILITY OF PREGNANCY PER 1000 PROCEDURES WITH DIFFERENT METHODS OF TUBAL STERILIZATION PERFORMED IN UNITED STATES, 1978–1986

METHOD	
Unipolar coagulation	7.5
Postpartum partial salpingectomy	7.5
Silastic band (Falope or Yoon)	17.7
Interval partial salpingectomy	20.1
Bipolar coagulation	24.8
Hulka-Clemens clip	36.5
Total all methods	18.5

From Peterson HB, Xia Z, Hughes JM, et al: The risk of pregnancy after tubal sterilization: findings from the U.S. Collaborative Review of Sterilization. Am J Obstet Gynecol 1996;174:1164, with permission.

ter conception, a woman could conceive just before her surgery and there would be no way to detect it. Scheduling sterilization early in the menstrual cycle obviates this problem but adds to the logistic difficulty. Another cause of failure is the finding of anatomic abnormalities, usually adhesions surrounding and obscuring one or both tubes. An experienced laparoscopic surgeon with proper instruments can usually lyse the adhesions, restore normal anatomic relations, and make a positive identification of the tube. However, in some circumstances successful sterilization will not be possible by laparoscopy, and the surgeon needs to know prior to surgery whether the patient is prepared to undergo laparotomy to accomplish sterilization in such instances. As noted, use of the nonelectrical bands and clips requires normal anatomy and tubes of normal thickness. If these conditions do not obtain but the tube can be positively identified, then electrocoagulation can usually be accomplished.

Initial electrosurgery techniques used unipolar current with coagulation of a major portion of the tube, which was then excised. This provided visual confirmation of adequate coagulation but allowed for the formation of tuboperitoneal fistulas and, eventually, ectopic pregnancy. With the development of bipolar techniques, it is no longer considered necessary to cut the tube. Attention must be paid to details of electrosurgery because there is no visual confirmation of full-thickness coagulation. Proper technique for bipolar tubal sterilization requires coagulation of three adjacent segments of tube and adjacent mesosalpinx over a length of 3 cm, followed by recoagulation of the tube alone in the same three places. Soderstrom et al (1989) has studied the effect of waveform, power output, and type of bipolar forceps and generator. Cutting current should be selected with a power output of 22 to 25 watts into a 100-ohm resistance. This will consistently produce a full-thickness tubal lesion. The circuit should include an ammeter. When the ammeter indicates zero, current flow has ceased because complete desiccation of the tissue increases electrical resistance. Use of lower power settings and coagulation current may result in coagulation of outer layers of tissue, which stops further current flow before the area around the lumen is completely coagulated, and pregnancy may result. In these cases, repeat laparoscopy will reveal only a narrow band of tissue connecting the normal tubal segments, but this narrow band contains an intact tubal lumen.

Reversal of Tubal Sterilization

Reversal of sterilization is more successful after mechanical occlusion than after electrocoagulation, because the latter method destroys much more of the tube, leaving less for the reconstructive surgeon to work with. With modern microsurgical techniques and an isthmus-to-isthmus anastomosis, pregnancy is accomplished in 75% or so of cases (Corson, 1985).

Male Sterilization

Vasectomy, excision of a portion of the vas deferens, provides permanent sterilization for men much more easily than any of the female techniques. Vasectomy is readily accomplished with local anesthesia in an office setting. The vas is palpated through the scrotum and grasped with fingers or an atraumatic forceps. A small incision is made in the skin and a loop of the vas is pulled through the incision. A small segment is then removed and a needle electrode is used to coagulate the lumen of both ends. In the "no-scalpel vasectomy," the pointed end of a forceps is used to puncture the skin over the vas, reducing bleeding from the skin edges and avoiding the need to suture the incision. Another variation is the "open-ended vasectomy," in which only the abdominal end of the vas is coagulated and the testicular end is left open. This is said to reduce congestive epididymitis after the operation (Hatcher et al, 1994: 395). Although men frequently worry that vasectomy will decrease their sexual performance, this concern has been proven groundless (Liskin et al, 1983).

Safety of Vasectomy

Vasectomized monkeys develop atherosclerosis more rapidly than controls, raising the specter that vasectomized men might suffer from increased heart attacks. Fortunately, several large-scale human studies have found no connection between vasectomy and vascular disease (Clarkson and Alexander, 1980; Goldacre et al, 1982). Several studies have linked vasectomy to later prostate cancer (Mettlin et al, 1990; Rosenberg et al, 1990, 1994b). Prostate cancer risk is largely a disease of the western world, and is strongly linked to dietary animal fat, family history, and race (Key, 1995). In the west it is more common in men of African-American ancestry and rare in men of Oriental descent. Fortunately, more recent studies report no association between vasectomy and prostate cancer. A large multiethnic case-control study from the United States and Canada compared 1642 men with prostate cancer to 1636 controls and found no overall association (OR 1.1, 95% CI 0.83 to 1.3) (John et al, 1995). There was no effect of age at vasectomy or years since the vasectomy. The OR for vasectomy was slightly increased among Japanese-Americans but was not statistically significant. Previous reports of risk may reflect undetected bias in the studies, possibly an association between higher status men, with diets higher in animal fat, being more likely than lower status men to choose vasectomy for contraception.

Reversibility of Vasectomy

Vasectomy must be regarded as a permanent means of sterilization; however, in about half of cases, modern techniques of microsurgery will reverse the procedure and allow subsequent fertility. The longer the interval since vasectomy, the poorer the results of reversal.

MEDICAL MEANS FOR PREGNANCY TERMINATION

Mifepristone (RU 486) and Prostaglandin Analogs

Termination of pregnancy by surgical means is described in Chapter 12. Safe medical means for pregnancy termination now exist and are summarized here. Mifepristone (RU 486), an analog of the progestin norethindrone, has strong affinity for the progesterone receptor but acts as an antagonist, blocking the effect of natural progesterone. Women with amenorrhea of less than 50 days and pregnancy confirmed by serum β-hCG or ultrasonography receive an oral dose of 600 mg of mifepristone on day 1. On day 3 the patient returns for administration of a prostaglandin (Ulmann et al, 1992). If treatment fails or if the patient bleeds excessively, vacuum curettage is performed. In a series of almost 17,000 cases, 600 mg of mifepristone orally followed in 36 to 48 hours by either of two prostaglandins, sulprostone or gemeprost, produced complete abortion in 95% of cases (Ulmann et al, 1992). The only significant complication to date has been three MIs with one death. All three were in women over 35 who were heavy smokers. The event occurred not from the mifepristone but at the time of administration of sulprostone, a prostaglandin E_2 analog. No MIs have occurred with the prostaglandin E_1 analog gemeprost (Anonymous, 1991). Misoprostol, another E_1 analog, seems to have fewer side effects and a greater margin of safety than sulprostone. It is very effective when combined with mifepristone and is the prostaglandin used in the U.S. trials (Peyron et al, 1993).

Methotrexate and Misoprostol

The antifolate methotrexate provides another medical approach to pregnancy termination. Widely used to treat ectopic pregnancies without surgery (Stovall and Ling, 1993), it can also be used with intrauterine gestations. In initial studies, methotrexate 50 mg/m² IM followed by misoprostol 800 μg given vaginally produced abortion in six pregnancies up to 56 days from the last menstrual period (Creinin and Darney, 1993a). Methotrexate alone without the misoprostol is also successful, although bleeding does not begin until an average of 24 days after treatment (Creinin and Darney, 1993b). Larger studies of the methotrexate-misoprostol regimen have now been published (Hausknecht, 1995). Three hundred women at 56 days or less of gestation were treated at three sites in a study by Creinin et al (1996b). All received methotrexate 50 mg/m² IM on day 1, and were given vaginal misoprostol 800 μg on day 7. Those who did not abort within 24 hours were given a second dose of misoprostol on day 8. Sixty-five percent aborted within the first 24 hours of receiving misoprostol. Abortion was delayed in the remaining patients. By 14, 28, and 35 days, 69.7%, 87.7%, and 91.7% had passed the pregnancy. Gestational age greater than 49 days or serum β-hCG greater than 40,000 IU/L were associated with reduced probability of successful abortion. The methotrexate-misoprostol method appears to be slightly less effective than mifepristone-misoprostol, takes longer to produce abortion, and results in a longer interval of vaginal bleeding after abortion, but methotrexate and misoprostol are very inexpensive drugs and are already marketed in the United States, where they are FDA approved for other indications. Drugs once approved for any indication may be used for other indications provided supporting medical literature exists (Rayburn, 1993). Mifepristone, as of this writing, has been given preliminary approval by the FDA but is still not available, and is likely to be considerably more expensive than methotrexate-misoprostol.

THE FUTURE OF CONTRACEPTION

A variety of hysteroscopic techniques for female sterilization have been evacuated and abandoned (Thatcher, 1988). Intrauterine quinacrine is of great current interest. A pellet containing this drug is inserted through the cervix into the uterine cavity during the proliferative phase of the menstrual cycle, and then repeated in the next cycle. The pregnancy rate among 9461 women who received two doses was 2.63 per 100 woman-years, and the rate of ectopic pregnancy was 0.89 per 1000 woman-years (Hieu et al, 1993). Long-term results are unknown. Improved male sterilization methods are being developed. Chinese workers have developed a method for percutaneous occlusion of the vas that has been used in more than 100,000 men, is effective, and appears to be reversible as well. Polyurethane elastomer is injected into the vas, where it solidifies and forms a plug, providing an effective block to sperm. Removal of the plugs is accomplished under local anesthesia and has resulted in return to fertility in most cases, after as long as 4 years with the plugs in situ (Zhao, 1990).

Subdermal implants are of great importance because of their convenience, remarkable efficacy, and freedom from serious side effects. A two-rod version of Norplant, Norplant II, has undergone extensive testing and has been found to be as effective as and easier to insert and remove than the six-rod system currently sold (Gao et al, 1990). Single-rod systems containing a new progestin, 3-ketodesogestrel (Implanon) are in the final phase of U.S. trials. In preliminary studies Implanon appears to be even more effective than Norplant and very easy to insert and remove (Makarainen et al, 1994). In addition, levonorgestrel in a biodegradable rod of caprolactone is in

U.S. trials (Darney et al, 1989). Unlike Norplant, the caprolactone rod does not need to be removed.

Immunologic methods for contraception have been pursued for years. Workers in India coupled the β fraction of hCG to tetanus toxoid as an adjuvant and produced anti-hCG antibody in monkeys and in humans. The vaccine is effective, and no side effects have been reported. Repeated dosing is needed to develop antibody levels in the therapeutic range; hence the method could be reversible (Talwar et al, 1993). The possibility of vaccinating men or women against certain sperm antigens is also being pursued. Perhaps one of the most promising new approaches is the use of the antiprogesterone mifepristone as a daily or once-a-month contraceptive in addition to its already proven efficacy as a safe abortifacient in early pregnancy.

Spermicidal compounds that are more effective than nonoxynol-9 and have strong antiretroviral properties are being developed. At very low concentrations, the compound 4'-acetamidophenyl 4-guanidinobenzoate inhibits the sperm enzyme acrosin, which is essential for fertilization. At the same concentrations it inhibits replication of HIV virus in vitro (Bourinbaiar and Lee-Huang, 1995). Other compounds that are both spermicidal and inhibit HIV replications—gramicidin and dextran sulfate—are in clinical trials. Widespread use of such compounds in spermicides and with condoms or diaphragms could be of enormous health benefit.

REFERENCES

Adams DB, Gold AR, Burt AD: Rise in female initiated sexual activity at ovulation and its suppression by oral contraceptives. N Engl J Med 1978;299:1145.

Allen S, Serufilira A, Bogaerts J, et al: Confidential HIV testing and condom promotion in Africa: impact on HIV and gonorrhea rates. JAMA 1992;268:3338.

Alvarez F, Guiloff E, Brache V, et al: New insights on the mode of action of intrauterine devices in women. Fertil Steril 1989;49:768.

American College of Obstetricians and Gynecologists: Emergency oral contraception. ACOG Pract Patterns 1996;2:1.

Anonymous: A death associated with mifepristone/sulprostone. Lancet 1991; 337:969.

Anonymous: Clinical challenges in contraception: a program on women with special medical conditions. In: Association of Reproductive Health Professionals Clinical Proceedings. Washington, DC: Association of Reproductive Health Professionals, 1994.

Anonymous: 1995 Annual Birth Control Study. Raritan, NJ: Ortho Pharmaceutical Corp, 1995.

Anderson RA, Wallace EM, Wu FCW: Effect of testosterone enanthate on serum lipoproteins in man. Contraception 1995;52:115.

Arsyad KM: Sperm function in Indonesian men treated with testosterone enanthate. Int J Androl 1993;10:355.

Ashraf T, Arnold SB, Maxfield M: Cost effectiveness of levonorgestrel subdermal implants: comparison with other contraceptive methods available in the United States. J Reprod Med 1994:39:791.

Back DJ, Orme ML'E: Pharmacokinetic drug interactions with oral contraceptives. Clin Pharmacokinet 1990;18:472.

Ben-Rafael Z, Bider D: A new procedure for removal of a "lost" intrauterine device. Obstet Gynecol 1996;87:785.

Berstein G: Use Effectiveness Study of Cervical Caps: Final Report (Contract No. N01-HD-1-2804). Washington, DC: National Institute of Child Health and Development, 1986.

Bertina RM, Koeleman RPC, Koster T, et al: Mutation in blood coagulation factor V associated with resistance to activated protein C. Nature 1994;369:64.

Blank A: Latex Condoms Lubricated with Nonoxynol-9 May Increase Release of Latex Protein That May Trigger Latex Hypersensitivity (Research Reports). Bethesda, MD, National Institute of Child Health and Human Development, 1996.

Bodemer CW: Concepts of reproduction and its regulation in the history of western civilization. Contraception 1976;13:427.

Bokarewa MI, Falk G, Sten-Linder M, et al: Thrombotic risk factors and oral contraception. J Lab Clin Med 1995;126:294.

Bounds W, Guillebaud J, Dominik R, Dalberth BT: The diaphragm with and without spermicide: a randomized comparative trial. J Reprod Med 1995;40:764.

Bourinbaiar AS, Lee-Huang S: Acrosin inhibitor, 4'-acetamidophenyl 4-guanidinobenzoate, an experimental vaginal contraceptive with anti-HIV activity. Contraception 1995;51:319.

Bracken MP: Oral contraception and congenital malformations in offspring: a review and meta-analysis of the prospective studies. Obstet Gynecol 1990;76:552.

Briggs MH, Briggs M: Oral contraceptives for men. Nature 1974;252:585.

Brody SA, Turkes A, Goldzieher JW: Pharmacokinetics of three bioequivalent norethindrone/mestranol-50 mcg and three norethindrone/ethinyl estradiol-35 mcg formulations: are low dose pills really lower? Contraception 1989;40:269.

Brown JB, Holmes J, Barker G: Use of the Home Ovarian Monitor in pregnancy avoidance. Am J Obstet Gynecol 1991;165(6 Pt 2):2008.

Brown SS, Eisenberg L (eds): The Best Intentions: Unintended Pregnancy and the Well Being of Children and Families. Washington, DC: National Academy Press, 1995.

Bruno A, Adams HP, Biller J, et al: Cerebral infarction due to moyamoya disease in young adults. Stroke 1988;19:826.

Burkeman RT, for the Womens' Health Study: Association between intrauterine devices and pelvic inflammatory disease. Obstet Gynecol 1981;57:269.

Burkeman RT, Zacur HA, Kimball AW, et al: Oral contraceptives and lipids and lipoproteins: Part II—relationship to plasma steroid levels and outlier status. Contraception 1989;40:675.

Burnhill MS: Intrauterine contraception. In Corson SL, Derman RJ, Tyrer LB (eds): Fertility Control. Boston: Little, Brown, and Co, 1985:272.

Caygill CP, Hill MJ: Oral contraceptives and breast cancer. Lancet 1989;1:1258.

Centers for Disease Control: Toxic shock and the vaginal contraceptive sponge. MMWR Morbid Mortal Wkly Rep 1984a;33:43.

Centers for Disease Control: Toxic shock and the vaginal contraceptive sponge. MMWR Morbid Mortal Wkly Rep 1984b;33:43 (cited in JAMA 1984b;251:1015).

Centers for Disease Control Cancer and Steroid Hormone Study: Long term oral contraceptive use and the risk of breast cancer. JAMA 1983a;249:1591.

Centers for Disease Control Cancer and Steroid Hormone Study: Oral contraceptive use and the risk of endometrial cancer. JAMA 1983b;249:1600.

Centers for Disease Control Cancer and Steroid Hormone Study: Oral contraceptive use and the risk of ovarian cancer. JAMA 1983c;249:1596.

Chapdelaine A, Desmarais JL, Derman RJ: Clinical evidence of the minimal androgenic activity of norgestimate. Int J Fertil 1989;34:347.

Chilvers C: Oral contraceptives and cancer. Lancet 1994;344:1378.

Christian CD: Maternal deaths associated with an intrauterine device. Am J Obstet Gynecol 1974;119:441.

Clarkson TB, Alexander NJ: Longterm vasectomy: effect on the occurrence and extent of atherosclerosis in rhesus monkeys. J Clin Invest 1980;65:15.

Coker AL, Hulka BS, McCann MF, Walton LA: Barrier methods of contraception and cervical intraepithelial neoplasia. Contraception 1992;45:1.

Collaborative Group for the Study of Stroke in Young Women: Oral contraceptives and stroke in young women. JAMA 1975; 231:718.

Collaborative Group on Hormonal Factors in Breast Cancer: Breast cancer and hormonal contraceptives: collaborative re-analysis of individual data on 53,297 women with breast cancer and 100,239 women without breast cancer from 54 epidemiological studies. Lancet 1996;347:1713.

Corson SL: Female sterilization reversal. In Corson SL, Derman RJ, Tyrer LB (eds): Fertility Control. Boston: Little, Brown, and Co, 1985:107.

Cramer DW, Goldman MR, Schiff I, et al: The relationship of tubal infertility to barrier method and oral contraceptive use. JAMA 1987;257:2246.

Cramer DW, Schiff I, Schoenbaum SC: Tubal infertility and the intrauterine device. N Engl J Med 1985;312:941.

Creinin MD, Darney PD: Methotrexate and misoprostol for early abortion. Contraception 1993a;48:339.

Creinin MD, Darney PD: Methotrexate for abortion at ≤42 days gestation. Contraception 1993b;48:339.

Creinin MD, Vittinghoff E, Keder L, et al: Methotrexate and misoprostol for early abortion: a multicenter trial. I. Safety and efficacy. Contraception 1996;53:321.

Cromer BA, Blair JM, Mechan JD, et al: A prospective comparison of bone density in adolescent girls receiving depot medroxy progesterone acetate (Depo Provera), levonorgestrel and oral contraceptives. J Pediatr 1996;129:671.

Crook D, Godsland IF, Wynn V: Oral contraceptives and coronary heart disease: modulation of glucose tolerance and plasma lipid risk factors by progestins. Am J Obstet Gynecol 1988;158:1612.

Cundy T, Reid OR, Roberts H: Bone density in women receiving depot medroxyprogesterone acetate for contraception. BMJ 1991;303:13.

Dajani AS, Bisno AL, Chung KJ, et al: Prevention of bacterial endocarditis: recommendations by the American Heart Association. JAMA 1990;264:2919.

Daling JR, Weiss N, Metch BJ: Primary tubal infertility in relation to the use of an intrauterine device. N Engl J Med 1985;312:937.

Darney PD: Hormonal implants: contraception for a new century. Am J Obstet Gynecol 1994;170:1536.

Darney PD, Monroe SE, Klaisle CM, et al: Clinical evaluation of the Capronor contraceptive implant: preliminary report. Am J Obstet Gynecol 1989;160:1292.

Davis JP, Chesney J, Wand PJ, Laventure M: Toxic shock syndrome: epidemiologic features, recurrence, risk factors and prevention. N Engl J Med 1980;303:1429.

Dericks-Tan JSE, Kock P, Taubert HD: Synthesis and release of gonadotropins: effect of an oral contraceptive. Obstet Gynecol 1983;62:687.

DeStefano F, Greenspan JR, Dicker RC, et al: Complications of interval laparoscopic tubal sterilization. Obstet Gynecol 1983a;61:153.

DeStefano F, Huezo C, Peterson HB, et al: Menstrual changes after tubal sterilization. Obstet Gynecol 1983b;62:673.

El Badrawi HH, Hafez ES, Barnhart MI, et al: Ultrastructural changes in human endometrium with copper and nonmedicated IUD's in utero. Fertil Steril 1981;36:41.

Escobedo LG, Peterson HB, Grubb GS, Franks AL: Case fatality rate for tubal sterilization in U.S. hospitals 1979–1980. Am J Obstet Gynecol 1989;160:147.

Fahmy K, Khairy M, Allam G, et al: Effect of depo-medroxyprogesterone acetate on coagulation factors and serum lipids in Egyptian women. Contraception 1991;44:431.

Farag A, Bottoms SF, Mammen EF, et al: Oral contraceptives and the hemostatic system. Obstet Gynecol 1988;71:584.

Farley TMM, Rosenberg MJ, Rowe PJ, et al: Intrauterine devices and pelvic inflammatory disease: an international perspective. Lancet 1992;339:785.

Farmer RDT, Preston TD: The risk of venous thromboembolism associated with low oestrogen oral contraceptives. J Obstet Gynecol 1995;15:195.

Fasoli M, Parazzini F, Cecchettie G, La Vecchia C: Post-coital contraception: an overview of published studies. Contraception 1989;39:459.

Fischl MA, Dickinson GM, Scott GB, et al: Evaluation of heterosexual partners, children, and household contacts of adults with AIDS. JAMA 1987;257:640.

Flynn AM: Natural family planning and the new technologies. Int J Gynaecol Obstet 1989;Suppl 1:123.

Food and Drug Administration (FDA): Prescription drug products; Certain combined oral contraceptives for use as postcoital emergency contraception. Notice. Federal Register 62: 8610–8612, Feb 25, 1997.

Forman D, Doll R, Peto R: Trends in mortality from carcinoma of the liver and the use of oral contraceptives. Br J Cancer 1983; 48:349.

Forman D, Vincent TJ, Doll R: Cancer of the liver and the use of oral contraceptives. Br Med J 1986;292:1357.

Gao J, Wang SL, Wu SC, et al: Comparison of the clinical performance, contraceptive efficacy and acceptability of levonorgestrel releasing IUD, and Norplant 2 implants in China. Contraception 1990;41:485.

Garg SK, Chase HP, Marshall G, et al: Oral contraceptives and renal and retinal complications in young women with insulin dependent diabetes mellitus. JAMA 1994;271:1029.

Gaspard UJ, Dubois M, Gillain D, et al: Ovarian function is effectively inhibited by a low dose triphasic oral contraceptive containing ethinyl estradiol and levonorgestrel. Contraception 1984;29:305.

Gerstman BB, Piper JM, Tomita DK, et al: Oral contraceptive dose and the risk of deep venous thromboembolic disease. Am J Epidemiol 1991;133:32.

Gladson CL, Scharr I, Hach V, et al: The frequency of type I heterozygous protein S and protein C deficiency in 141 unrelated young patients with venous thrombosis. Thromb Haemost 1988;59:18.

Godon-Hardy S, Meder JF, Dilouya A, et al: Ischemic strokes and oral contraception. Neuroradiology 1985;27:588.

Godsland IF, Crook D, Simpson R, et al: The effects of different formulations of oral contraceptive agents on lipids and carbohydrate metabolism. N Engl J Med 1990;323:1375.

Goldacre MJ, Holford TR, Vessey MP: Cardiovascular disease and vasectomy. N Engl J Med 1982;308:805.

Graefenberg E: An intrauterine contraceptive method. In: Proceedings of the Seventh International Birth Control Conference: The Practice of Contraception, 1931. (Reprinted in Langley LL [ed]: Contraception. Stroudsburg, PA: Dowden, Hutchinson, Ross, Inc, 1973:339.

Grou F, Rodrigues I: The morning after pill—how long after? Am J Obstet Gynecol 1994;171:1529.

Guerrero R, Rojas OI: Spontaneous abortion and aging of human ova and spermatozoa. N Engl J Med 1975;293:573.

Guo-wei S: Pharmacodynamic effects of once a month combined injectable contraceptives. Contraception 1994;49:361.

Habashi M, Sahwi S, Gawish S, Osman M: Effect of Lippes Loop on sperm recovery from human fallopian tubes. Contraception 1980;22:549.

Harlap S, Shiono PH, Ramcharon S, et al: Chromosomal abnormalities in the Kaiser-Permanente birth defects study, with special reference to contraceptive use around the time of conception. Teratology 1985;31:381.

Harel Z, Biro FM, Kollar LM: Depo-Provera in adolescents: effects of early second injection or prior oral contraceptives. J Adolesc Health 1995;16:379.

Harris RWC, Brinton LA, Cowdell RH, et al: Characteristics of women with dysplasia or carcinoma in situ of the cervix uteri. Br J Cancer 1980;42:359.

Haspells AA: Emergency contraception: a review. Contraception 1994;50:101.

Hasson HM: Open laparoscopy. In Zatuchni GI, Daly MJ, Sciarra JJ (eds): Gynecology and Obstetrics. Vol 6. New York: Harper & Row, 1982:1.

Hatcher RA, Guest F, Stewart GK, et al: Contraceptive Technology, 1988–1989. 14th ed. New York: Irvington Publishers, Inc, 1988:341.

Hatcher RA, Trussell J, Stewart F, et al: Contraceptive Technology. 16th rev ed. New York: Irvington Publishers, 1994.

Hausknecht RU: Methotrexate and misoprostol to terminate early pregnancy. N Engl J Med 1995;333:537.

Hieu DT, Tan TT, Tan DN, et al: 33,781 cases of non-surgical female sterilization with quinacrine pellets in Vietnam. Lancet 1993;342:213.

Himes NE: Medical History of Contraception. New York: Gamut Press, 1963.

Hooton TM, Scholes D, Huges JP, et al: A prospective study of risk factors for symptomatic urinary tract infection in young women. N Engl J Med 1996;335:468.

Hulka JF: The spring clip: current clinical experience. In Phillips JM (ed): Endoscopic Female Sterilization. Downey, CA: American Association of Gynecologic Laparoscopists, 1983.

Hulka JF: Sterilization technique. In Hulka JF (ed): Textbook of Laparoscopy. New York: Grune & Stratton, 1985:84.

Hulka JF: Methods of female sterilization. In Nichols DH (ed): Gynecologic and Obstetric Surgery. St. Louis: CV Mosby, 1993: 640.

Hulka JF, Fishbourne JI, Mercer JP: Laparoscopic sterilization with a spring clip. Am J Obstet Gynecol 1973;116:715.

Irving FC: A new method of insuring sterility following cesarean section. Am J Obstet Gynecol 1924;8:335.

Isihizaki T, Itoh R, Yasuda J, et al: Effect of high dose medroxyprogesterone acetate on coagulative and fibrinolytic factors in patients with gynecological cancers. Gen To Kagaku Ryoho 1992;19:837.

Jick H, Walker AM, Rothman KJ, et al: Vaginal spermicides and congenital disorders. JAMA 1981;245:1329.

John EM, Whittemore AS, Wu AH, et al: Vasectomy and prostate cancer: results from a multiethnic case-control study. J Natl Cancer Inst 1995;87:662.

Johnson V, Masters WH: Intravaginal contraceptive study. Phase 1: Anatomy. West J Surg Obstet Gynecol 1962;70:202.

Jones BM, Eley A, Hicks DA, et al: Comparison of the influence of spermicidal and non-spermicidal contraception on bacterial vaginosis, candidal infection and inflammation of the vagina—a preliminary study. Int J STD AIDS 1994;5:362.

Judson FN, Ehret JM, Bodin GF, et al: In vitro evaluations of condoms with and without nonoxynol 9 as physical and chemical barrier against Chlamydia trachomatis, herpes simplex virus type 2 and human immunodeficiency virus. Sex Transm Dis 1989;16:251.

Kane LA, Sparrow MJ: Postcoital contraception: a family planning study. New Zealand Med J 1989;102:151.

Katz Z, Lancet M, Skornik J, et al: Teratogenicity of progestogens given during the first trimester of pregnancy. Obstet Gynecol 1985;65:775.

Kaunitz AM: Long acting injectable contraception with depot medroxyprogesterone acetate. Am J Obstet Gynecol 1994;170: 1543.

Kay CR: The happiness pill. J R Coll Gen Pract 1980;30:8.

Key T: Risk factors for prostate cancer. Cancer Surv 1995;23:63.

Khairulleh Z, Huber DH, Gonzales B: Declining mortality in international sterilization services. Int J Gynaecol Obstet 1992;39: 41.

Khandwala SD: Laparoscopic sterilization: a comparison of current techniques. J Reprod Med 1988;33:463.

Kelaghan J, Rubin GL, Ory HW, et al: Barrier-method contraceptives and pelvic inflammatory disease. JAMA 1982;248:184.

Kimmerle R, Weiss R, Berger M, Kurz KH: Effectiveness, safety and acceptability of a copper intrauterine device (CU Safe 300) in type I diabetic women. Diabetes Care 1993;16:1227.

Kjer JJ: Ectopic pregnancy subsequent to laparoscopic sterilization. Am J Obstet Gynecol 1989;160:1202.

Kjos SL, Ballagh SA, La Cour M, et al: The copper T380A intrauterine device in women with type II diabetes mellitus. Obstet Gynecol 1994;84:1006.

Kjos SL, Shoupe D, Douyan S, et al: Effect of low dose oral contraceptives on carbohydrate and lipid metabolism in women with recent gestational diabetes: results of a controlled, randomized, prospective study. Am J Obstet Gynecol 1990;163: 1822.

Knopp RH: Cardiovascular effects of endogenous and exogenous sex hormones over a woman's lifetime. Am J Obstet Gynecol 1988;158:1630.

Knopp RH, Bergelin RO, Wahl PW, et al: Clinical chemistry alterations in pregnancy and with oral contraceptive use. Obstet Gynecol 1985;66:682.

Knowlton C: Fruits of Philosophy: A Treatise on the Population Question. London: J. Watson, 1833. (Cited in Langley LL [ed]: Contraception. Stroudsburg, PA: Dowden, Hutchinson, Ross, Inc, 1973:134.

Knuth UA, Yeung CH, Nieschlag E: Combinations of 19 nortestosterone hexyloxyphenylpropionate (Anadur) and depot medroxyprogesterone acetate (Clinovir) for male contraception. Fertil Steril 1989;51:1011.

Koch JP: The Prentif contraceptive cervical cap: a contemporary study of its clinical safety and effectiveness. Contraception 1982;25:135.

Kwachi I, Colditz GA, Hankinson S: Long-term benefits and risks of alternative methods of fertility control in the United States. Contraception 1994;50:1.

Kwak HM, Chi IC, Gardner SD, et al: Menstrual pattern changes in laparoscopic sterilization patients whose last pregnancy was terminated by therapeutic abortion. J Reprod Med 1980;25:67.

La Vecchia C: Depot-medroxyprogesterone acetate, other injectable contraceptives, and cervical cancer. Contraception 1994;49: 223.

Labbok MH, Queenan JT: The use of periodic abstinence for family planning. Clin Obstet Gynecol 1989;32:387.

Lahteenmaki PL, Lahteenmaki P: Concentration dependent mechanisms of ovulation inhibition by the progestin ST-1435. Fertil Steril 1985;44:20.

Landgren BM: Mechanism of action of gestagens. Int J Gynaecol Obstet 1990;32:95.

Lanes SF, Birman BA, Walker AM, et al: Oral contraceptive type and functional ovarian cysts. Am J Obstet Gynecol 1992;166: 956.

Lee NC, Rubin GL, Borucki R: The intrauterine device and pelvic inflammatory disease revisited: new results from the Women's Health Study. Obstet Gynecol 1988;72:721.

Lewis MA, Heinemann LAJ, MacRae KD, et al: The increased risk of venous throboembolism and the use of third generation progestagens: role of bias in observational research. Contraception 1996a;54:5.

Lewis MA, Spitzer WO, Heinemann LAJ, et al: Third generation oral contraceptives and the risk of myocardial infarction: an international case control study. BMJ 1996b;312:88.

Lidegaard O: Oral contraceptives and risk of a cerebral thromboembolic attack: results of a case-control study. BMJ 1993;306: 956.

Lidegaard O: Oral contraceptives, pregnancy and the risk of cerebral thromboembolism: the influence of diabetes, hypertension, migraine and previous thromboembolic disease. Br J Obstet Gynaecol 1995;102:153.

Ling WY, Johnston DW, Lea RH, et al: Serum gonadotropin and ovarian steroid levels in women during administration of a norethindrone-ethinyl estradiol triphasic oral contraceptive. Contraception 1985;32:367.

Linn S, Schoenbaum SC, Monson RR, et al: Lack of association between contraceptive usage and congenital malformation in offspring. Am J Obstet Gynecol 1983;147:923.

Lippes J, Malik T, Tatum HJ: The postcoital copper-T. Adv Plann Parent 1976;11: 24.

Lippes J, Zielezny M: The loop decade. Mount Sinai Med J 1975; 4:353.

Lipson A, Stoy DB, La Rosa JC, et al: Progestins and oral contraceptive-induced lipoprotein changes: a prospective study. Contraception 1986;34:121.

Liskin LS, Pile JM, Quillin WF: Vasectomy—safe and simple. Popul Rep D 1983;11(5):62.

Lutcher CL, Harris P, Henderson PA, et al: Lack of morbidity from oral contraception in women with sickle cell anemia. [abstract]. Clin Res 1981;29:863A.

Luukkainen T, Heikinheimo O, Haukkamaa M, Lahteenmaki P: Inhibition of folliculogenesis and ovulation by the antiprogesterone RU 486. Fertil Steril 1988;49:961.

Luukkainen T, Toivonen J: Levonorgestrel releasing IUD as a method of contraception with therapeutic properties. Contraception 1995;52:269.

Maguire MG, Tonascia J, Sartwell PE, et al: Increased risk of thrombosis due to oral contraceptives: a further report. Am J Epidemiol 1979;110:188.

Mainwaring R, Hales HA, Stevenson K, et al: Metabolic parameters, bleeding, and weight changes in U.S. women using progestin only contraceptives. Contraception 1995;51:149.

Makarainen L, Tuomivaara L, Alapiessa U, Van Beek A: Contraception with 3 keto desogestrel implant. In: Abstracts of the 14th meeting of the International Federation of Gynecology and Obstetrics, Montreal, 1994, abstract FC059.2.

Malyk B: Nonoxynol-9: Evaluation of Vaginal Absorption in Humans. Raritan, NJ: Ortho Pharmaceutical Corp, 1983.

Mann JI, Vessey MP, Thorogood M, et al: Myocardial infarction in young women with special reference to oral contraceptive practice. Br Med J 1975;2:241.

Mant D, Villard-Mackintosh L, Vessey MP, et al: Myocardial infarction and angina pectoris in young women. J Epidemiol Community Health 1987;41:215.

Marcil-Gratton N: Sterilization regret among women in metropolitan Montreal. Fam Plan Perspect 1988;20:222.

Mattson RH, Cramer JA, Darney PD, et al: Use of oral contraceptives by women with epilepsy. JAMA 1986;256:238.

McCann MR, Liskin LS, Piotrow PT, et al: Breast feeding, fertility and family planning. Population Reports Series J, No. 24. Population Information. Baltimore: John Hopkins University, November–December 1981.

McNeilly AS: Suckling and the control of gonadotropin secretion. In Knobil E, Neil JD, Ewing LI, et al (eds): The Physiology of Reproduction. New York: Raven Press, 1988:2323.

Melbye M, Wohlfahrt J, Olsen JH, et al: Induced abortion and the risk of breast cancer. N Engl J Med 1997;336:81.

Mettlin C, Natarajan N, Huben R: Vasectomy and prostate cancer risk. Am J Epidemiol 1990;132:1056.

Mishell D: Correcting misconceptions about oral contraceptives. Am J Obstet Gynecol 1989;161:1385.

Mishell DR Jr, Bell JH, Good RG, Moyer DL: The intrauterine device: a bacteriologic study of the endometrial cavity. Am J Obstet Gynecol 1966;96:119.

Mishell DR Jr, Colodyn SZ, Swanson LA: The effect of an oral contraceptive on tests of thyroid function. Fertil Steril 1969;20:339.

Moore LL, Valuck R, McDougall C, Fink W: A comparative study of one year weight gain among users of medroxyprogesterone acetate, levonorgestrel implants and oral contraceptives. Contraception 1995;52:215.

Morris JM, Van Waaganen G: Interception: the use of post ovulatory estrogens to prevent implantation. Am J Obstet Gynecol 1973;115:101.

Mosher WD: Fertility and family planning in the United States: insights from the National Survey of Family Growth. Fam Plann Perspect 1988;20:207.

Mosher WD, Pratt WF: Contraceptive Use in the United States (Advance Data. No. 182). Washington, DC: National Center for Health Statistics, 1990.

Murad F, Haynes RC: Androgens and anabolic steroids. In Gilman AG, Goodman LS, Gilman A (eds): Goodman and Gilman's The Pharmacological Basis of Therapeutics. 6th ed. New York: Macmillan, 1980;1448.

Murray PM, Stadel BV, Schlesselman JJ: Oral contraceptive use in women with a family history of breast cancer. Obstet Gynecol 1989;73:977.

Neil JR, Hammond GT, Nobel AD, et al: Late complications of sterilization by laparoscopy and tubal ligation: a controlled study. Lancet 1975;2:669.

Notelovitz M, Kitchens CS, Coone L, et al: Low dose oral contraceptive usage and coagulation. Am J Obstet Gynecol 1981;141:71.

Notelovitz M, Levenson I, McKenzie L, et al: The effects of low dose oral contraceptives on coagulation and fibrinolysis in two high risk populations: young female smokers and older premenopausal women. Am J Obstet Gynecol 1985;152:995.

Okada Y, Horikawa K: A case of phlebothrombosis of lower extremity and pulmonary embolism due to progesterone. Kokyu To Junkan 1992;40:819.

Ory HW: Mortality associated with fertility and fertility control: 1983. Fam Plann Perspect 1983;15:57.

Ory HW, for the Women's Health Study: Ectopic pregnancy and intrauterine contraceptive devices: new perspectives. Obstet Gynecol 1981;57:137.

Osathanondh V: Suprapubic mini-laparotomy, uterine elevation technique: simple, inexpensive and out-patient procedure for interval female sterilization. Contraception 1974;10:251.

Ota T: A new method of temporary contraception. Kinki Fujinka Gakkai Zashi 1931;18:147.

Paragard Prescribing Information. Raritan, NJ: Ortho Pharmaceutical Corp, 1995.

Parazzini F, Negri E, La Vecchia C, et al: Barrier methods of contraception and the risk of cervical neoplasia. Contraception 1989;40:519.

Pardthaisong T: Return of fertility after use of the injectable contraceptive Depo-Provera: updated analysis. J Biosoc Sci 1984;16:23.

Patsch W, Brown SA, Gotto AM, et al: The effect of triphasic oral contraceptives on plasma lipids and lipoproteins. Am J Obstet Gynecol 1989;161:1396.

Paul Freie HM: Sickle cell diseases and hormonal contraception. Acta Obstet Gynecol Scand 1983;62:211.

Peel J: Manufacture and retailing of contraceptives in England. Popul Studies 1963;17:113.

Peterson HB, DeStefano F, Rubin GL, et al: Deaths attributable to tubal sterilization in the United States, 1977–1981. Am J Obstet Gynecol 1983;146:131.

Peterson HB, Xia Z, Hughes JM, et al: The risk of pregnancy after tubal sterilization: findings from the U.S. Collaborative Review of Sterilization. Am J Obstet Gynecol 1996;174:1161.

Petitti DB, Sidney S, Bernstein A, et al: Stroke in users of low dose oral contraceptives. N Engl J Med 1996;335:8.

Peyron R, Aubery E, Targosz V, et al: Early termination of pregnancy with mifepristone (RU486) and the orally active prostaglandin misoprostal. N Engl J Med 1993;328:1509.

Phillips A: The selectivity of a new progestin. Acta Obstet Gynecol Scand Suppl 1990;152:21.

Poindexter AN, Abdul-Malak M, Fast JE: Laparoscopic tubal sterilization under local anesthesia. Obstet Gynecol 1990;75:5.

Porter JB, Hunter JR, Jick H, et al: Oral contraceptives and nonfatal vascular disease. Obstet Gynecol 1985;66:1.

Potter L: Oral contraceptive compliance and its role in the effectiveness of the method. In Cramer J, Spilker B (eds): Medical Compliance in Patient Care and Clinical Trials. New York: Raven Press, 1991.

Potts M: Coitus interruptus. In Corson SL, Derman RJ, Tyrer L (eds): Fertility Control. Boston: Little, Brown and Co, 1985:299.

Potts M, McDevitt J: A use-effectiveness trial of spermicidally lubricated condoms. Contraception 1975;11:701.

Rayburn WF: A physician's prerogative to prescribe drugs for off-label uses during pregnancy. Obstet Gynecol 1993;81:1052.

Richwald MA, Greenland S, Gerber MM, et al: Effectiveness of the cavity rim cervical cap: results of a large clinical study. Obstet Gynecol 1989;74:143.

Rimdusit P: Separate stitches tubal sterilization, a modified Pomeroy's technique: an analysis of the procedure, complications and failure rate. J Med Assoc Thailand 1984;67:602.

Rock J, Pincus G, Garcia CR: Effects of certain 19-nor steroids on the normal human menstrual cycle. Science 1956;124:891.

Romieu I, Willett WC, Colditz GA, et al: Prospective study of oral contraceptive use and risk of breast cancer in women. J Natl Cancer Inst 1989;81:1313.

Rooks JB, Ory HW, Ishak KG, et al: Epidemiology of hepatocellular adenoma: the role of oral contraceptive use. JAMA 1979;262:644.

Rosenberg L, Kaufman DW, Helmrich SP, et al: Myocardial infarction and cigarette smoking in women younger than 50 years of age. JAMA 1985;253:2965.

Rosenberg L, Palmer JR, Zauber AG, et al: Vasectomy and the risk of prostate cancer. Am J Epidemiol 1990;132;1051.

Rosenberg L, Palmer JR, Zauber AG, et al: A case-control study of oral contraceptive use and invasive ovarian cancer. Am J Epidemiol 1994a;139:654.

Rosenberg L, Palmer JR, Zauber AG, et al: The relationship of vasectomy to the risk of cancer. Am J Epidemiol 1994b;140:431.

Rosenfield AJ, Castadot RG: Early postpartum and immediate postabortion IUD insertion. Am J Obstet Gynecol 1974;118:1104.

Rossing MA, Daling JR, Voigt LF, et al: Current use of an intra-uterine device and the risk of tubal pregnancy. Epidemiology 1993a;4:252.

Rossing MA, Daling JR, Weiss NS, et al: Past use of an intrauter-ine device and risk of tubal pregnancy. Epidemiology 1993b;4:245.

Rotta L, Matechova E, Cerny M, Pelak Z: [Determination of the fertile period during the menstrual cycle in women by moni-toring changes in crystallization of saliva with the PC2000 IMP-CON minimicroscope]. Cesk Gyneckol 1992;57:340.

Royal College of General Practicioners' Oral Contraception Study: Incidence of arterial disease among oral contraceptive users. J R Coll Gen Pract 1983;33:75.

Rozenbaum H: Relationships between chemical structure and bi-ological properties of progestogens. Am J Obstet Gynecol 1982;142:719.

Sachs BP, Gregory K, McArdle C, Pinshaw A: Removal of retained intrauterine contraceptive devices in pregnancy. Am J Perinatol 1992;9:139.

Schiffman MH, Bauer HM, Hoover RN, et al: Epidemiologic ev-idence showing that human papilloma virus infection causes most cervical intraepithelial neoplasia. J Natl Cancer Inst 1993;85:958.

Schirm AL, Trussell J, Menken J, Grady WR: Contraceptive failure in the United States: the impact of social, economic and dem-ographic factors. Fam Plann Perspect 1982;14:68.

Schlesselman JJ: Cancer of the breast and reproductive tract in relation to use of oral contraceptives. Contraception 1989;40:1.

Segal S, Alvarez-Sanchez F, Adejeuwon CA, et al: Absence of cho-rionic gonadotropin in sera of women who use intrauterine devices. Fertil Steril 1985;44:214.

Shapiro S, Slone D, Heinonen O, et al: Birth defects and vaginal spermicides. JAMA 1982;247:2381.

Shepard MK: Female contraceptive sterilization. Obstet Gynecol Surv 1974;29:739.

Shihata AA, Gollub E: Acceptability of a new intravaginal barrier contraceptive device (Femcap). Contraception 1992;46:511.

Shoupe D, Mishell DR: Norplant: subdermal implant system for long term contraception. Am J Obstet Gynecol 1989;160:1286.

Short RV, Lewis PR, Renfree MB, Shaw G: Contraceptive effects of extended lactational amenorrhoea: beyond the Bellagio Con-sensus. Lancet 1991;337:715.

Shy KK, McTiernan AM, Daling JR, Weiss NS: Oral contraceptive use and the occurrence of pituitary prolactinoma. JAMA 1983;249:2204.

Sidney S, Petitti DB, Quesenberry CP, et al: Myocardial infarction in users of low dose oral contraceptives. Obstet Gynecol 1996;88:939.

Sivin I: Dose and age dependent ectopic pregnancy risks with intrauterine contraception. Obstet Gynecol 1991;78:291.

Sivin I, Stern J: Health during prolonged use of levonorgestrel 20 micrograms/d and the copper TCu 380A intrauterine contra-ceptive devices: a multicenter study. Fertil Steril 1994;61:70.

Snowden R: The progestasert and ectopic pregnancy. Br Med J 1977;1:1600.

Soderstrom RM, Levy BS, Engel T: Reducing bipolar sterilization failures. Obstet Gynecol 1989;74:60.

Spellacy WN, Buhi WC, Birk SA: The effect of estrogens on car-bohydrate metabolism: glucose, insulin, and growth hormone studies on 171 women ingesting Premarin, mestranol and eth-inyl estradiol for six months. Am J Obstet Gynecol 1972;114:378.

Spelsberg TC, Rories C, Rejman JJ: Steroid action on gene ex-pression: possible roles of regulatory genes and nuclear accep-tor sites. Biol Reprod 1989;40:54.

Spence MR: Cytologic detection and clinical significance of Ac-tinomyces israeli in women using intrauterine contraceptive devices. Am J Obstet Gynecol 1978;131:295.

Speroff L: A brief for low-dose pills. Contemp Ob/Gyn 1981;17:27.

Speroff L, Darney PD: A Clinical Guide for Contraception. Bal-timore: Williams & Wilkins, 1992:117.

Spitzer WO, Lewis MA, Heinemann LAJ, et al: Third generation oral contraceptives and risk of venous thromboembolic disor-der: an international case-control study. BMJ 1996;312:83.

Stadel BV: Oral contraceptives and cardiovascular disease. I. N Engl J Med 1981a;305:612.

Stadel BV: Oral contraceptives and cardiovascular disease. II. N Engl J Med 1981b;305:672.

Stadel BV, Schlesselman JJ, Murray PA: Oral contraceptives and breast cancer. Lancet 1989;1:1257.

Stampfer MJ, Willett WC, Colditz GA, et al: A prospective study of past use of oral contraceptive agents and risk of cardiovas-cular diseases. N Engl J Med 1988;319:1313.

Steiner M, Dominik R, Trussell J, Hertz-Picciotto I: Measuring con-traceptive effectiveness: a conceptual framework. Obstet Gy-necol 1996;88:24S.

Stone KM, Grimes DA, Magder LS: Personal protection against sexually transmitted diseases. Am J Obset Gynecol 1986;155:180.

Stovall TG, Ling FW: Single dose methotrexate: an expanded clin-ical trial. Am J Obstet Gynecol 1993;168:1759.

Stubblefield PG: The effects on hemostasis of oral contraceptives containing desogestrel. Am J Obstet Gynecol 1993;168:1047.

Stubblefield PG: Health benefits beyond contraception. Int J Fertil 1994;39(Suppl 3):132.

Stubblefield PG, Fuller AF, Foster SG: Ultrasound guided intra-uterine removal of intrauterine contraceptive device in preg-nancy. Obstet Gynecol 1988;72:961.

Sturgis SH, Albright F: The mechanism of estrin therapy in the relief of dysmenorrhea. Endocrinology 1940;26:68.

Sumiala S, Pirhonen J, Tuominen J, et al: Increased uterine and vascular resistance following Filshie clip sterilization: prelimi-nary findings obtained with color Doppler ultrasonography. Clin Ultrasound 1995;23:511.

Swann SH, Petitti DB: A review of problems of bias and con-founding in epidemiologic studies of cervical neoplasia and oral contraceptive use. Am J Epidemiol 1982;115:10.

Swerdloff RS, Wang C, Bhasin S: Developments in the control of testicular function. Baillieres Clin Endocrinol Metab 1992;6:451.

Talwar GP, Singh D, Pal R, et al: A birth control vaccine is on the horizon for family planning. Ann Med 1993;25:207.

Tatum HJ: Medicated intrauterine devices. In Sciarra JJ, Zatuchni GI, Daly MJ (eds): Gynecology and Obstetrics, Vol 6: Fertility Regulation, Psychosomatic Problems, and Human Sexuality. Philadelphia: Harper & Row, 1982:Chap 29.

Tatum HJ, Schmidt FH, Jain AK: Management and outcome of pregnancies associated with copper-T intrauterine contracep-tive device. Am J Obstet Gynecol 1976;126:869.

Tatum HJ, Schmidt FH, Phillips D, et al: The Dalkon Shield con-troversy: structural and bacteriological studies of IUD tails. JAMA 1975;231:711.

Taurelle R, Ruet C, Jaupart F, et al: Contraception using a pro-gestogen only minipill in cardiac patients. Arch Mal Coeur 1979;72:98.

Thatcher SS: Hysteroscopic sterilization. Obstet Gynecol Clin North Am 1988;15:51.

Thomas DB, Ray RM: Depot medroxyprogesterone acetate (DMPA) and risk of invasive adenocarcinoma and adenosqua-mous cardinomas of the uterine cervix. WHO Collaborative Study of Neoplasia and Steroid Contraceptives. Contraception 1995;52:307.

Tietze C, Lewit S: Evaluation of intrauterine devices: ninth progress report of the Cooperative Statistical Program. Stud Fam Plan 1970;1:1.

Tietze C, Bongaarts J, Schearer B: Mortality associated with the control of fertility. Fam Plann Perspect 1976;8:6.

Trausht-Van Horn JJ, Capeless EL, Easterling TR, Bovil EG: Preg-nancy loss and thrombosis with protein C deficiency. Am J Ob-stet Gynecol 1992;167:968.

Trussell, J, Grummer-Strawn L: Contraceptive failure of the ovu-lation method of periodic abstinence. Fam Plann Perspect 1990;22:65.

Trussell, J, Sturgen K, Strickler J, Dominik R: Comparative con-traceptive efficacy of the female condom and other barrier methods. Fam Plann Perspect 1994;26:66.

Trussell J, Warner DL, Hatcher R: Condom performance during vaginal intercourse: comparison of Trojan-enz and Tactylon condoms. Contraception 1992;45:11.

Uchida H: Uchida tubal sterilization. Am J Obstet Gynecol 1975; 121:153.

U.K. National Case-Control Study Group: Oral contraceptive use and breast cancer risk in young women. Lancet 1989;1:973.

Ulmann A, Silvestre L, Chemama L, et al: Medical termination of early pregnancy with mifepristone (RU486) followed by a prostaglandin analogue: study in 16,639 women. Acta Obstet Scand 1992;71:278.

Umapathysivam K, Jones WR: Effects of contraceptive agents on the biochemical and protein composition of human endometrium. Contraception 1980;22:425.

Ursin G, Peters RK, Henderson BE, et al: Oral contraceptive use and adenocarcinoma of cervix. Lancet 1994;344:1390.

Van Uem JFHM, Hsiu JG, Chillik CF, et al: Contraceptive potential of RU 486 by ovulation inhibition: I. Pituitary versus ovarian action with blockade of estrogen-induced endometrial proliferation. Contraception 1989;40:171.

Vandenbroucke JP, Koster T, Briet E, Reitsma PH: Increased risk of venous thrombosis in oral contraceptive users who are carriers of factor V Leiden mutation. Lancet 1994;344:1453.

Vessey M, Doll R, Peto R, et al: A long term follow up study of women using different methods of contraception—an interim report. J Biosoc Sci 1974;8:373.

Vessey M, Lawless M, Yeates D: Efficacy of different contraceptive methods. Lancet 1982;1:841.

Vessey MP, Lawless M, Yeates D: Oral contraceptives and stroke: findings in a large prospective study. Br Med J 1984;289:530.

Vessey M, McPherson K, Lawless M, Yeates D: Neoplasia of the cervix uteri and contraception: a possible adverse effect of the pill. Lancet 1983;2:930.

Villard-Mackintosh L, Vessey MP, Jones L: The effects of oral contraceptives and parity on ovarian cancer trends in women under 55 years of age. Br J Obstet Gynaecol 1989;96:783.

Virutamasen P, Wangsuphachart S, Reinprayoon D, et al: Trabecular bone in long term depot-medroxyprogesterone acetate users. Asia Oceania J Obstet Gynaecol 1994;20:269.

Voeller B, Coulson AH, Bernstein GS, et al: Mineral oil lubricant causes rapid deteriorization of latex condoms. Contraception 1989;39:95.

Wagner H, Schweppe KW, Kronholz HL, et al: Moglichkeiten der extraktion von intrauterinpessaren bei eingetretener schwangerschaft. Geburtzh Gynakol Praxis 1980;31:1317.

Wagner KD: Major depression and anxiety disorders associated with Norplant. J Clin Psychiatry 1996;57:152.

Walker AM, Jick H, Hunter JR, et al: Vasectomy and non-fatal myocardial infarction. Lancet 1981;1:13.

Wallace EM, Aitken RJ, Wu FC: Residual sperm function in oligozoospermia induced by testosterone enanthate administered as a potential steroid male contraceptive. Int J Androl 1992;15:416.

Wallace EM, Gow SM, Wu FC: Comparison between testosterone enanthate-induced azoospermia and oligozoospermia in a male contraceptive study. I: Plasma luteinizing hormone, follicle stimulating hormone, testosterone, estradiol, and inhibin concentrations. J Clin Endocrinol Metab 1993;77:290.

Wallace EM, Wu FCW: Effect of depot medroxyprogesterone acetate and testosterone oenanthate on serum lipoproteins in man. Contraception 1990;41:63.

Walsh TL, Bernstein GS, Grimes DA, et al: Effect of prophylactic antibiotics on morbidity associated with IUD insertion: results of a pilot randomized controlled trial. Contraception 1994;50:319.

Webb AMC, Russell J, Elstein M: Comparison of Yuszpe regimen, Danazol and Mifepristone (RU486) in oral postcoital contraception. Br Med J 1992;305:927.

Weiss NS, Lee NC, Peterson HB: Tubal sterilization, hysterectomy, and the subsequent occurrence of epithelial ovarian cancer. Am J Epidemiol 1991;134:362.

Westoff C: Depot medroxyprogesterone acetate contraception: metabolic parameters and mood changes. J Reprod Med 1996; 41:401.

Westoff C, Wieland D, Tiezzi L: Depression in users of depo-medroxyprogesterone acetate. Contraception 1995;51:351.

Wilcox LS, Martinez-Schnell A, Peterson HB, et al: Menstrual function after tubal sterilization. Am J Epidemiol 1992;135:1368.

Winkler UH, Buhler K, Schindler AE: The dynamic balance of hemostasis: implication for the risk of oral contraceptive use. In Runnebaum B, Rabe T, Kissel L (eds): Female contraception and male fertility regulation. Advances in Gynecological and Obstetric Research Series. Confort, England: Parthenon Publishing Group, 1991:85.

Wolner-Hanssen P, Echenbach DA, Paavonen J, et al: Decreased risk of symptomatic chlamydial pelvic inflammatory disease associated with oral contraceptives. JAMA 1990;263:54.

World Health Organization: Depot medroxyprogesterone acetate (DMPA) and the risk of epithelial ovarian cancer: The WHO Collaborative Study of Neoplasia and Steroid Contraceptives. Int J Cancer 1991;49:191.

World Health Organization: Improving Access to Quality Care in Family Planning: Medical Eligibility Criteria for Contraceptive Use. Geneva: World Health Organization, 1996:13.

World Health Organization Collaborative Study of Cardiovascular Disease and Steroid Hormone Contraception: Venous thromboembolic disease and combined oral contraceptives: results of international multicenter case-control study. Lancet 1995;346:1575.

World Health Organization Collaborative Study of Cardiovascular Disease and Steroid Hormone Contraception: Hemorrhagic stroke, overall stroke risk, and combined oral contraceptives: results of an international, multicenter, case-control study. Lancet 1996a;348:505.

World Health Organization Collaborative Study of Cardiovascular Disease and Steroid Hormone Contraception: Ischaemic stroke and combined oral contraceptives: results of an international multicenter, case control study. Lancet 1996b;348:498.

World Health Organization Task Force on Long-Acting Systemic Agents for Fertility Regulation: Microdose intravaginal levonorgestrel contraception: a multicentre clinical trial. Contraception 1990;41:105.

World Health Organization Task Force on Long-Acting Systemic Agents for Fertility Regulation, Special Programme of Research, Development and Research Training in Human Reproduction: Study 87907: Comparative Study of Effects of Two Once-Monthly Injectable Contraceptives (Cyclofem and Mesigyna) and One Combined Oral Contraceptive on Coagulation and Fibrinolysis (Draft Report of Final Analysis). WHO, Geneva, April 1993.

Wysowski DW, Green L: Serious adverse events in Norplant users reported to the Food and Drug Administration's MedWatch Spontaneous Reporting System. Obstet Gynecol 1995;86:154.

Yoon IB, King TM, Parmley TH: A two-year experience with the Falope ring sterilization procedure. Am J Obstet Gynecol 1977; 127:109.

Yuzpe AA, Smith R: Use of hormonal steroids for pregnancy interception. In Sciarra JJ, Zatuchni GI, Daly MJ (eds): Gynecology and Obstetrics. Vol 6: Fertility Regulation, Psychosomatic Problems, and Human Sexuality. New York: Harper & Row, 1982:Chap 26.

Yuzpe AA, Smith RP, Rademaker AW: A multicenter clinical investigation employing ethinyl estradiol combined with dl-norgestrel as a postcoital contraceptive agent. Fertil Steril 1982; 37:510.

Zenkeng L, Feldblum PJ, Oliver RM, Kaptue L: Barrier contraceptive use and HIV infection among high risk women in Cameroon. AIDS 1993;7:725.

Zhao SC: Vas deferens occlusion by percutaneous injection of polythane elastomer plugs: clinical experience and reversibility. Contraception 1990;41:453.

Zondervan KT, Carpenter LM, Painter R, Vessey MP: Oral contraceptives and cervical cancer—further findings from the Oxford Family Planning Association Contraceptive Study. Br J Cancer 1996;73:1291.

12

Robert A. Munsick | **Pregnancy Termination**

This chapter acquaints the reader with many safe, useful methods to terminate unhealthy, unsafe, and unwanted pregnancies. Also, some of these techniques diminish the risks that attend management of inevitable, incomplete, and missed abortions. Treatment of all these conditions has improved tremendously because of the demand in the 1960s for legalization of abortion. Thus most modern abortion methods are no more than 35 years old, yet have so improved as to make abortion one of the safest operations in modern gynecology.

This chapter contains many personal observations. It concentrates on surgical abortion, the most frequently used method, which is divided artificially into three procedures, menstrual aspiration (MA), dilatation and suction (D&S), and laminaria and evacuation (L&E). Medical methods of terminating pregnancies are described for the second trimester; interception and very early medical abortions are described in Chapter 11. Hern's book (1990) details many aspects of the practice of abortion that are not addressed here.

In the 19th century, largely because abortions were so dangerous, state laws were enacted that forbade abortion except to save lives or the health of women. In the 1960s several states liberalized their abortion laws, and, on January 22, 1973, the U.S. Supreme Court made abortion a woman's constitutional right with its *Roe v Wade* decision.

EPIDEMIOLOGY OF ABORTION IN THE UNITED STATES

Most of the following data concern abortion in the United States. They originate from the Centers for Disease Control and Prevention (CDC) of the U.S. Public Health Service (Lawson et al, 1994; Koonin et al, 1996) and from the Alan Guttmacher Institute (AGI) in New York City (Henshaw and Van Vort, 1994). Detailed annual data for the United States have been maintained since 1972, but mortality data are not yet available for the past few years.

According to CDC data, the annual number of abortions performed increased rapidly immediately before and with the 1973 *Roe v Wade* decision (about 600,000 in 1972), reached about 1,300,000 in the mid-1980s, peaked at about 1,400,000 in 1990, and fell

slightly since then, reaching 1,359,145 in 1992. According to Henshaw and Van Vort (1994), who reported AGI abortion statistics, there were 1,590,000 abortions in 1992, the lowest number recorded by the AGI since 1979 (AGI numbers of abortions always exceed those of the CDC). Although the annual decrease in cases is relatively small, it is significant.

The *abortion rate* is the number of abortions performed per 1000 women of reproductive age (15 to 44 years). It reflects the total number of abortions performed. Abortion rates increased from 13/1000 in 1972 to 25/1000 in 1980 and fell slightly in 1992 to 23/1000. Another statistic, the *abortion ratio*, may reflect more accurately the prevalence of unwanted pregnancies, for it compares the number of legal abortions performed per 1000 live births in the population studied. Abortion ratios were 180 in 1972, about 360 throughout most of the 1980s, and 335 in 1992. Abortion ratios are highest for the youngest ($\leq$ age 15) and oldest ($\geq$ age 40) groups of women, about 450/1000 live births in 1992. Lowest abortion ratios are seen in women ages 30 to 34, 183/1000 live births in 1992. For abortion rates, the highest group is 20 to 24 years old and the lowest groups are at the extremes of age.

As demand for abortions expanded, so did services. The number of women who obtained out-of-state abortions plummeted in the 1970s and has remained low for all but a few states.

Henshaw and Van Vort (1994) noted that abortion facilities decreased from 2582 in 1988 to 2380 in 1992. Although facilities have decreased at 65 per year, most of the decrease has been in hospitals where abortions are performed, not in clinics. In the United States, 69% of abortions are performed in clinics and less than 1% in hospitals (Henshaw and Van Vort, 1994). The cadre of trained abortion providers is also diminishing. Reparatory measures are being planned to correct this problem (Grimes, 1993).

The ratio of white to black women who underwent abortions decreased from 3.34 in 1972 to 1.94 in 1987; for 1992 the ratio of white to "black plus other" women who underwent abortions was 1.64 (Koonin et al, 1996). These data appear to indicate greater acceptance, availability, and affordability of abortions for minority and disadvantaged groups.

There has been a remarkable increase in the proportion of suction and evacuation procedures, whereas sharp curettage, instillation, and hysterotomy-hysterectomy abortions have diminished from about one third in 1972 to less than 1% of all abortions in 1992. This shift can largely be attributed to the proportion of abortions performed at or before 8 weeks, which has swelled in the same time frame from 34% to greater than 50% of abortions. The more dangerous terminations, performed from 16 weeks upward, have decreased from about 9% to about 5% of all abortions. Teenagers are most likely to have late abortions.

Abortion mortality has steadily dwindled since the legalization of abortion, even though the number of procedures has spiraled. Legal abortion case-fatality rates (legal, induced, abortion-related deaths per 100,000 legal abortions) plunged after the early years (4.1 in 1972 and 1973 and 3.4 in 1974 and 1975) to less than 1.0 in all but one year since 1979. For 1990, the case-fatality rate had fallen to 0.3 (Koonin et al, 1996). Reasons for the decline in mortality are many but are principally related to the greater proportion of aspiration procedures.

The CDC has shown clearly that decreasing abortion mortality rates are associated with two variables that confound one another: performance at earlier gestational ages and use of aspiration. Between 1972 and 1987 the case-fatality rates by method were: 0.5 for suction curettage, 3.7 for evacuation, 7.1 for instillation, and 51.6 for hysterotomy-hysterectomy (Lawson et al, 1994). Other noteworthy mortality risk factors, and their relative risks (RRs) were race (black, 2.3; white, 1.0), parity (≥ 3, 2.5), advanced reproductive age (25 to 29, 1.2; ≥ 40, 3.1), advanced gestational age (≤ 8 weeks, 0.4; ≥ 21 weeks, 12.0), and abortion procedure used (aspiration, 1.0; evacuation, 6.8; instillations, 13.0; hysterectomy-hysterotomy, 95.0).

The later in pregnancy that abortions are performed, the more dangerous they are, but the mortality rate does not meet that of carrying a pregnancy to term (5 to 10 maternal deaths/100,000 live births) until abortions are done after about 16 to 18 weeks. L&E appears to be safer than instillation or prostaglandin (PG)-induced abortions until about 18 weeks (Lawson et al, 1994), after which there are inadequate data to choose between the case-fatality rates for L&E, PG, or instillation. The combined methods of Hern and colleagues (1993) may be found to be significantly safer than others for late second- and for third-trimester procedures.

LOCATION OF ABORTION SERVICES

When abortion was legalized, the medical profession was unprepared for the massive changes in methodology and attitudes that swept the country. Most gynecologists hospitalized their patients and performed infrequent abortions in an operating room under general anesthesia, using Hegar dilators and sharp curettage as in diagnostic dilatation and curettage (D&C) operations. Such operations were quickly found to be dangerous and were limited to early pregnancies. For pregnancies exceeding 10 to 12 weeks but less than about 16 weeks, a "hands off" policy was wisely adopted; terminations were deferred until 16 or more weeks, when they were performed by instillation or by hysterotomy or hysterectomy. Thus the locus for most abortion procedures was the hospital, and hospitalizations for purposes of abortion provoked myriad intractable social, political, and personnel problems. Where hospitals allowed abortions, there often were inadequate beds, operating rooms, and anesthesiologists. Many midtrimester procedures were performed on labor and delivery units, where patients often had to progress through 24 to 48 hours of abortive labor before delivering the fetus, often in bed and unattended. Nurses and paramedical personnel who staffed these units were usually prejudiced toward childbirth and against abortion, and often dealt rudely with aborting patients. Women desiring abortions came to deplore hospitals, where they found that their identities were sometimes divulged from medical records, hospital personnel, and laboratory reports.

Patients, nurses, physicians, and hospitals became acutely aware that better locations were sorely needed for the administration and conduct of abortions services. Kaltreider and co-workers (1979) presented arguments against hospitalization and for outpatient abortion care, especially with midtrimester cases. Free-standing clinics were born, devoting themselves to abortion services, principally in the first trimester.

Problems have persisted, however. Many women find it embarrassing and sometimes threatening to identify themselves for abortion care, sometimes having to brave throngs of chanting, screaming, insulting antiabortion demonstrators who surround clinic sites. An at-home, nonsurgical mode of abortion is sought that requires no hospital or clinic exposure, no divulgence of identity, and reasonable safety. For early pregnancies, such a method appears to be imminent in drugs such as mifepristone and misoprostol (see Chapter 11).

ABORTION COUNSELING

When abortion is sought, empathic, honest, educated, thorough counseling is vital to

1. Recognize ignorance, ambivalence, or coercion
2. Provide detailed explanations of the risks and benefits of the procedure
3. Discuss the two major alternatives to abortion (carrying to term and raising the infant or placing it for adoption)
4. Acknowledge that the fetus is killed
5. Obtain knowledgeable informed consent
6. Warn of possible postoperative complications and their symptoms

7. Help the woman wisely plan her future reproductive preferences, including her best future method of birth control
8. Allow more time, if necessary, for her to cogitate, based upon the information she has just been given.

Most counselors for these important tasks are nurses, social workers, or other health professionals with special training. When ambivalence or serious psychological problems are recognized, most such cases should be deferred and referred for expert psychological or psychiatric consultation. Although it is not necessary for counselors to be females, it is often easier for patients to relate to knowledgeable, sympathetic women. In addition to the above tasks, it is often very helpful for the patient to have this same person accompany her during the operation.

HISTORY AND PHYSICAL EXAMINATION

Menstrual dates are often inaccurate, especially when patients may prevaricate to reduce fees. Even when dates are seemingly solid, accurate abdominal and pelvic assessments of gestational age are vitally important to choose properly the best methods of cervical dilation and termination, and for discovering abnormalities of the pelvis and uterine position. Little has been published on the accuracy of abdominal or bimanual vaginal estimates of gestational age. Because these estimates are so important, a brief account of my studies is presented.

Without knowing the date of the last menstrual period or having an ultrasound estimate of gestational age, I examined more than 1000 successive patients prior to abortion, first abdominally and then bimanually, and estimates of gestational age for each method were recorded based on uterine size, softening, Dickinson's sign, palpation of fetal parts, and audibility of fetal heart tones by stethoscope. Vernier calipers were used to measure fetal foot, leg, and arm lengths, and fetal ages were determined by averaging formula-derived weeks from each of these mensurations (Munsick, 1987). There was a tendency to underestimate gestational age by a mean of 0.5 to 1.0 week before 12 weeks and to overestimate by about 1.5 weeks after 18 weeks. It was unusual to be able to diagnose pregnancy, much less estimate its duration, before 8 weeks. Mean bimanual estimates were in almost perfect accord with mean actual weeks from 10 to 18 weeks. Variability was slightly greater for abdominal (standard deviation [SD] 1.7 weeks) than vaginal (SD 1.55 weeks) estimates.

The uterus was palpable abdominally earlier than is usually described. According to many textbooks, the uterus first becomes palpable at 12 weeks, yet, as Table 12–1 shows, I was able to feel it in 75% of 253 gravidas at 10 to 11 gestational weeks and in 39% of 31 gravidas at 6 to 7 weeks. Marked obesity and uterine retrodisplacement diminished the prevalence of abdominal uterine palpability until the 15th

Table 12–1. PREVALENCE OF ABDOMINALLY PALPABLE UTERI ACCORDING TO WEEKS OF GESTATION

WEEKS OF GESTATION	SUBJECTS	PALPABLE ABDOMINALLY Palpable	Percent
6–7	31	12	39
8–9	123	72	59
10–11	253	190	75
12–13	208	184	88
14–15	166	161	97
16–17	157	157	100
18–23	86	86	100

week. Beginning at 12 weeks, if the uterus could be felt, obesity caused bimanual estimates to be greater than actual. Retrodisplacement did not materially influence estimates because, although it is difficult to appreciate the entire uterus when it is retroverted, I usually compensated upward for my estimates. Among nine twin pregnancies there was no tendency to overestimate gestational age until 15 or more weeks. Thus abdominal estimates of gestational age are quite reasonable at and beyond 10 gestational weeks but are improved by careful bimanual palpation.

In many clinics, largely to establish fees, ultrasound assessment of gestational age precedes a physician's examination. This approach often saves clinic and patient time but should *never* supplant the physical examination (see "Ultrasound" below).

LABORATORY STUDIES

In the interests of cost, efficiency, and reality, not every desirable test can be performed. An Rh type and, when Rh(D) negative, an indirect Coombs' test are mandatory. I used to obtain rubella titers and gonorrhea cultures, but their value was judged inadequate to continue them. A complete blood count, Papanicolaou smear, and *Chlamydia* and human immunodeficiency virus tests, may be worthwhile, depending on the population being treated.

ULTRASOUND

Sonography has added materially to the safety of abortion, but it need not be depended upon for all patients. For uteri difficult or impossible to assess because of obesity, leiomyomata, or uterine retrodisplacement, it can be invaluable to estimate gestational age. Its desirability also depends on the surgeon's ability to compensate safely for underdiagnoses of gestational ages. Other than establishing fees, need for ultrasound should be based on historical and physical data and the physician's skills, but not on routine.

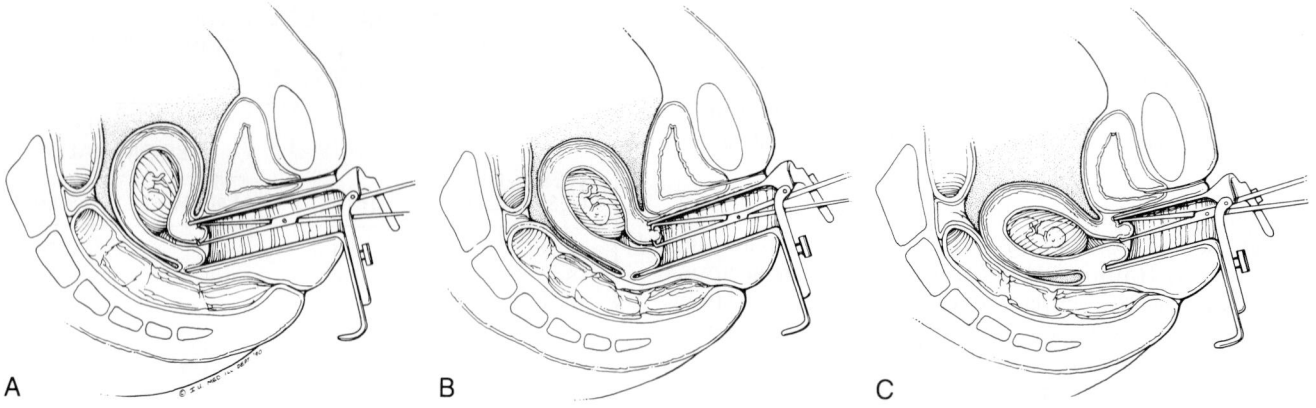

Figure 12-1
Large (A), medium (B), and small (C) Graves specula. The longer specula tend to trap the cervix high, whereas short ones allow the cervix to descend and the uterus to straighten, helping to prevent perforations at the angulated cervicouterine junction. Cervical descent also allows instruments better access high in the uterine cavity and allows them to be opened wider.

During difficult extraction operations, ultrasound equipment should be immediately available to the surgeon, and vaginal probe sonography is desirable to assess the intrauterine presence of very early pregnancies, especially with uterine retrodisplacement.

PHYSICIAN COMPORTMENT

Often, the physician will never have met the patient, whose only clinic acquaintance may be her counselor. To set her at ease and make her experience less stressful, her first impression of her doctor is extraordinarily important. Professional attire, a pleasant smile, a warm introduction, and a handshake work wonders. A conspicuous initial hand-washing provides the patient with both psychological solace and microbiologic prophylaxis.

SURGICAL ABORTION

Three general methods of surgical abortion are discussed: menstrual aspiration, dilatation and suction, and laminaria and evacuation. Hysterotomy and hysterectomy are rarely needed to treat concomitant gynecologic problems or for lifesaving emergencies, but these dangerous operations are no longer considered part of abortion practice and are mentioned no further.

Cervical Exposure

Once the patient had been assessed and the duration of pregnancy determined, the cervix must be exposed, either to commence the procedure or to insert laminaria tents. An organoiodine antiseptic solution is usually used to prepare the vulva, perineum, and vestibule, but a history of sensitivity to it or to iodine should be sought, because anaphylaxis from topical exposure to povidone-iodine has been reported (Waran and Munsick, 1995).

A Graves speculum is usually chosen to expose the cervix. Figure 12-1 shows the cervical effects of using different sizes of specula. The larger the uterus, the greater the need for a *short* speculum to draw the cervix down and allow the uterus to become less angulated. Specula recommended to visualize the cervix during abortion procedures are listed in Table 12-2. The Moore-Graves is basically a medium Graves speculum that has been foreshortened, and whose anterior and posterior blades have a significantly wider proximal circumference. This allows instruments more maneuverability within the speculum and permits easier egress of specimens. For small and medium Graves specula, the handle should usually be widely opened to allow easier access and motion through the proximal blades. When using a Moore-Graves speculum, the handle may not need to be separated at all.

Difficulties with cervical exposure accompany four physical characteristics:

Table 12-2. RECOMMENDED SPECULA FOR CERVICAL EXPOSURE DURING D&S AND L&E OPERATIONS PERFORMED UNDER LOCAL ANESTHESIA

SPECULUM TYPE	WEEKS OF GESTATION	
	4–12	*12–20*
Small Graves	Excellent	Excellent*
Moore-Graves	Excellent	Excellent
Medium Graves	Second choice	Second choice to risky
Large Graves	Risky	Risky
Weighted	Do not use	Do not use

*For L&E operations at and beyond about 18 weeks, a small Graves speculum may provide inadequate space for the products of conception and some instruments.

1. Uterine retroflexion, with its anterior, sometimes retropubic cervix
2. Underdeveloped gluteal musculature or marked lack of steatopygia, both of which place the entire pelvis low and at a difficult angle from which to visualize the cervix
3. Relaxed vaginal sidewalls that collapse and hide the cervix
4. Extreme obesity, especially of the medial thighs

With the first two problems, cervical exposure can usually be achieved by tilting the foot of the table up or by elevating the patient's buttocks with pillows. For the third problem most practitioners use a large Graves speculum, but, for abortions, sometimes a perforated condom stretched over a medium or Moore-Graves speculum works well, with the condom resisting inward encroachment by the vaginal walls. In the fourth case, severe obesity of the thighs, buttocks, and perineum, standard lithotomy position sometimes provides nothing but the view shown in Figure 12–2A. The medial thighs abut each other and obscure the perianal, perineal, and vulvar regions. Probably because of the greater depth created by vulvar and paravaginal fat, the cervix may be unreachable with a speculum even if the vulva is visualized by retracting the medial thighs. An unreported expedient, the supine knee–chest position, is shown in Figure 12–2B. It provides nearly perfect results for visualizing the cervix, vulva, and perianal regions in such women. Most patients can hold their own thighs up and maintain them there for several minutes. Thigh adduction is unnecessary. The pudendum, perineum, and perianal areas come into view immediately (Fig. 12–2C), and cervical exposure becomes easy. When the cervix has been exposed and a tenaculum has secured it, the feet can be placed back in stirrups, usually without losing sight of the cervix. I have used this maneuver 14 times when I could not find the cervix in obese patients wanting abortions. In every case it has worked an apparent miracle, not only allowing cervical visualization but, in all but two cases, also allowing easy visualization with the shorter Moore-Graves or small Graves speculum. The supine knee–chest position has several advantages over the Sims position: (1) it is rapidly attained, (2) it usually allows a quick return to lithotomy position, (3) it provides surgeons the comfort of working seated, and (4) it retains the familiar anatomic relationships of the lithotomy position. This technique has not been as successful for women with very high, retropubic cervices or extremely redundant vaginal sidewalls.

Analgesia and Anesthesia

Cumulative data from the CDC and elsewhere have documented that general anesthesia is an important cause of abortion deaths (Lawson et al, 1994). The risks are not so strong as to interdict general anesthetics, especially for women who must have addi-

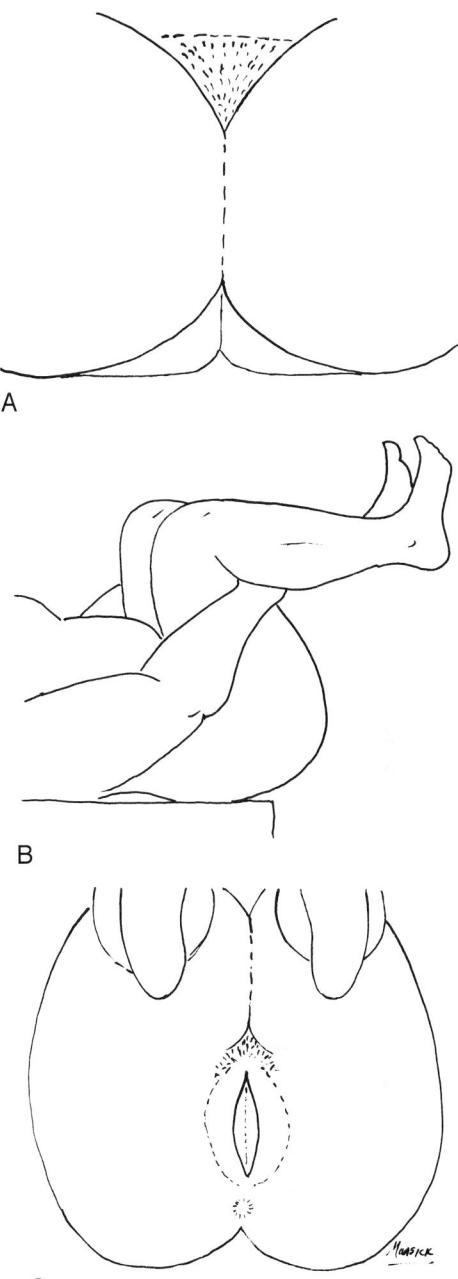

Figure 12–2
A, While in standard examining position, the patient's thighs obscure the entire pudendum. *B,* The supine knee–chest position permits cervical visualization and generous pudendal exposure (shown in *C*).

tional indicated procedures or who cannot tolerate the procedure while awake.

In the interests of safety and economy, pregnancies are usually terminated while using a form of analgesia, a local anesthetic, or both. Wiebe and Rawling (1995) showed that a nonsteroidal anti-inflammatory analgesic drug given 30 minutes before D&S significantly diminished discomfort before and after abortions. They advised buffering lidocaine solutions to obviate burning, found that slow injections hurt less than rapid ones, and that delaying dilation for several minutes after injections was unnecessary. Miller and colleagues (1996) emphasized the need for anesthetic safety, even in using local anesthetics, and found that buffered isotonic saline injections may be as effective as 1% lidocaine for paracervical anesthesia in D&S operations. These studies require confirmation. Minimal cervical dilation was used, additional analgesic or tranquilizing drugs were sometimes used without randomization, and the statistically significant results appeared possibly to lack clinical importance.

Using laminaria tents, local anesthetic drugs are usually given for aspirations and evacuations but are likely unnecessary, because there is seldom need for cervical dilation. In patients who dread or forbid needles or who have experienced local anesthetic drug reactions, I proceed with no drugs and find little difference in discomfort, provided the procedure is an MA, where no dilation is performed, or one in which laminaria tents were used for cervical dilatation.

For injections I prefer 0.5% lidocaine. It is usually injected with a plastic syringe through a 23-gauge disposable spinal needle. A 3- to 6-ml dose is infiltrated into the anterior cervical lip outside of the cervical canal, and the swollen area is vertically grasped with a single-toothed tenaculum (see Fig. 12–3). Analgesia is instantaneous and almost always complete. Paracervical anesthesia can be administered in small, multiple, intrastromal doses bilaterally, or by uterosacral injection at the cervicoforniceal junctions with about 8 ml of 0.5% lidocaine bilaterally at the 4 and 8 o'clock positions, just under the epithelium, intentionally producing large, pale blebs and relying on drug diffusion. These injections are facilitated by using the tenaculum to *push* the cervix cephalad and contralateral to the intended injection site (Fig. 12–3). Oxytocin, 10 IU or more, can be given in the local anesthetic injection of the paracervical block. It causes uterine hypertonus in this dose but results in spasm of the lower uterine segment such that evacuation may be difficult. For this reason, I have totally abandoned use of prophylactic uterotonic drugs.

I do not buffer the 0.5% lidocaine: some women feel momentary, slight burning during the anterior cervical injection, almost none feel the tenaculum, and few feel the paracervical injection at all. Avoiding deep infiltrations and achieving superficial blebs at the cervicovaginal junctions diminishes the risk of rapid lidocaine absorption and resultant systemic reactions, which are usually manifested by transient tinnitus, numbness of the tongue and lips, and lightheadedness. Symptoms are evanescent and not serious unless excessive, toxic doses have been used.

Cervical Manipulation and Traction

The most common injurious consequence of abortion is cervical laceration (Schulz et al, 1983). This was

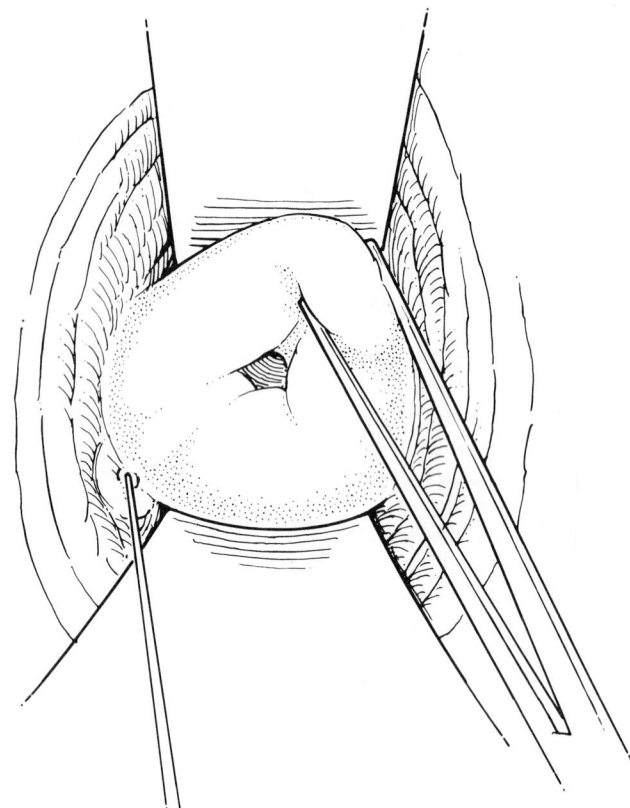

Figure 12–3
The cervix is grasped vertically with a tenaculum through its infiltrated, locally anesthetized anterior lip and is pushed upward and laterally to expose each cervicovaginal fornix for paracervical block.

particularly so in the 1970s, before laminaria tents were widely used and Hegar dilators were in vogue. Injuries may be caused by forcible dilation per se but are often a consequence of firm traction on the tenaculum. Tenaculum tears can cause significant hemorrhage and may be very difficult to repair under local anesthesia.

For abortions beyond 7 weeks, the cervix should be grasped vertically, not horizontally (Fig. 12–3). A generous bite significantly reduces but does not guarantee against lacerations. Use of preoperative laminaria tents in lieu of force is the only near-guarantee against cervical lacerations.

Uterine Sounding

In pregnancy, the uterus is soft and can be easily penetrated by any firm device, but especially by thin, sharp uterine sounds. Although *uterine* sounding is generally proscribed, endocervical exploration with a sound is not infrequently desirable and occasionally used to (1) determine the direction of the canal, (2) provide slight dilation for tent insertions, or (3) help select the size of flexible cannula to use (see "Menstrual Aspiration" below).

Cervical Dilation

Of all the steps involved in surgical abortion, cervical dilation is by far the most important. With inadequate dilation, cervical and uterine trauma are common and incomplete uterine emptying can occur, inviting hemorrhage and infection.

Forcible Dilation

In most clinic settings, abortions are performed between 7 and 10 gestational weeks and cervical dilation is accomplished quickly, using graduated rigid metallic or plastic dilators to 9 mm or less. However, underestimation of gestational age can occur and may require dilating the cervix to diameters of 11, 12, 13, or even 14 mm. Molin (1993) showed that dilating the cervix to 9 mm was accompanied by a phenomenon of sudden "giving in" of cervical resistance 12.5% of the time. This occurred in 66.7% of experiments when dilation was taken to 11 mm and suggests that the cervical stroma is disrupted. It occurred in nulliparous and multiparous women. Forced dilation may cause lacerations of the upper endocervix or lower uterus and may also result in unapparent but permanent cervical incompetence and future obstetric morbidity from recurrent midtrimester abortions and premature labors (Harlap et al, 1979). The latter possibility requires a large, randomized clinical trial to document whether cervical incompetence is caused by forced dilation, and, if so, whether or not using laminaria tents can prevent it.

It has been repeatedly shown that the Hegar dilator, still used in most operating rooms for diagnostic D&C operations, has no place in abortion practice. It is too blunt and requires excessive force for dilation. Instead, Pratt, Hawkins-Ambler, or Denniston dilators, which have much greater tapers, should be used (Hulka et al, 1974). Profiles of Hegar and Pratt dilators with approximately equal diameters are contrasted in Figure 12–4. Hegar size (diameter in millimeters) can be converted to French (or Pratt) size (circumference in millimeters), by multiplying by pi (3.14159), or, roughly, by 3. Thus an 11-mm Hegar dilator or vacuum cannula converts to 11 × 3.14159 = 34.5575, or 35 Pratt size (see also Table 12–4 below). Such conversions are often required when dilating or checking tent-provoked dilation with Pratt dilators while using vacuum cannulae that are customarily sized in diameters. Even with Pratt dilators, there is risk of traumatizing the cervix, so three more admonitions are offered:

1. Use a generous, vertical tenaculum bite on the cervix.
2. Dilate gradually, using the least possible increments in dilator size.
3. Dilate only as far as necessary for the instruments needed. Forcible dilation beyond a 31 to 35 Pratt size is likely excessive.

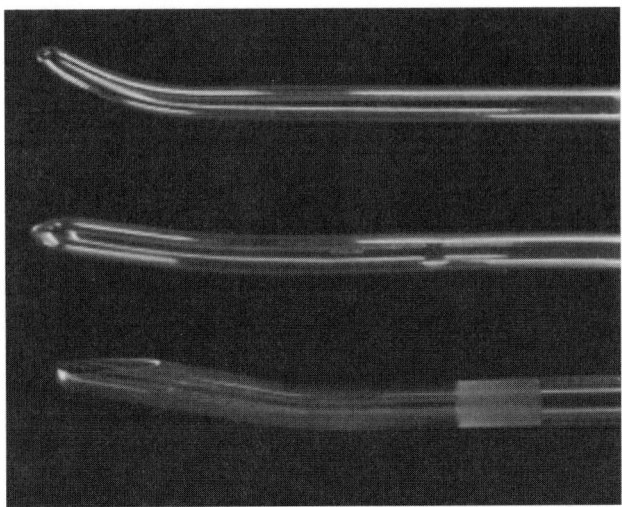

Figure 12–4
Number 35 Pratt dilator (*top*), 11-mm Hegar dilator (*middle*), and an 11-mm vacuum cannula (*bottom*), showing the greater taper of the preferred Pratt-type dilator.

Laminaria Tents

Laminaria tents are *Laminaria japonicum* seaweed stems (stipes) that are allowed to absorb water from the cervical stroma and mucus, thus dilating the cervix by dehydrating its stroma, by expanding, and possibly by releasing PGs. They are sterilized with ethylene oxide and desiccated. *Laminaria japonicum* comes from the northern sea waters of Japan, where it is a food staple and, when fermented, was the original, turn-of-the-20th-century source of the flavoring agent monosodium glutamate. Other biologic products that swell, such as the "slippery elm," came from the earth, and so frequently contained gas gangrene and tetanus *Clostridium* spores that they were discontinued. Hale and Pion (1972) thoroughly reviewed the use of these valuable adjuncts to abortion practice, and most of their observations still hold.

Although manufacturers warn that spores may persist even after sterilization, these are likely only seaweed spores. There has not been a reported increase in infections after their intracervical use. Indeed, Bryman et al (1988) conducted a randomized, nonblinded study of first-trimester abortions, comparing the infectious postabortal complications of 130 patients who underwent forcible cervical dilation with those of 115 patients who were dilated with laminaria tents. Gestational weeks were almost identical. In the two groups there were, respectively, 3/130 versus 0/115 perforations ($p = 0.3$), 10/130 versus 0/115 cases of endometritis ($p = 0.003$), and 17/130 versus 2/115 ($p = 0.001$) patients returned to the hospital because of pain. The authors concluded that forcible dilation probably is more destructive to tissues than the gentle dilation from laminaria tents, and that forcibly injured tissue likely acted as a nidus for infection.

Prepared tents look like smooth sticks. They are commonly 60 mm long and are sold in as many as

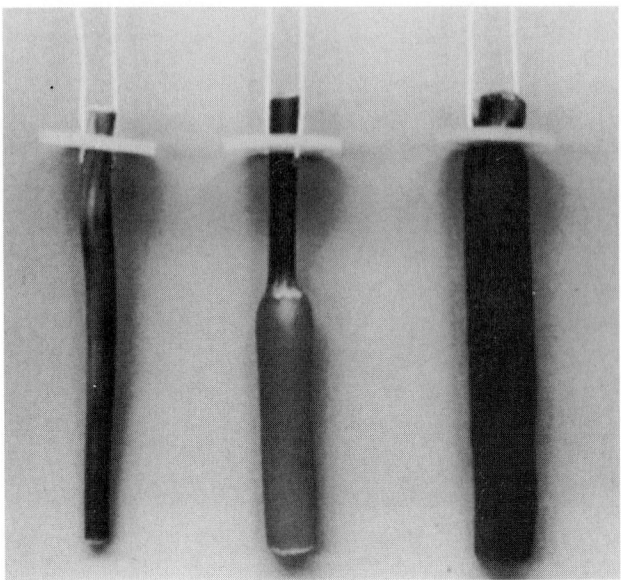

Figure 12–5
Laminaria tents. *Left*, Untreated tent. *Middle*, Tent has been dipped overnight in water only on its lower half. *Right*, Tent has been totally submerged overnight. Note the plastic collars that prevent uterine migration and strings that allow easy removal.

and swelling is time dependent, as seen in an in vitro experiment illustrated in Figure 12–6. Accurate data regarding in vivo cervical dilation rates are unavailable, but it seems reasonable to use laminaria sticks for about 4 to 6 hours for a doubling of size, and for 16 or more hours nearly to treble their diameters.

Insertion is accomplished after antiseptically preparing the cervix and stabilizing it with a tenaculum placed on the anterior cervical lip. A tent is grasped with a ring forceps at its collared end (because the collars must be removed when multiple tents are inserted, I no longer use collared ones), allowing it to swivel and follow the endocervical canal. The tent may be dipped in sterile lubricant to facilitate penetration, especially when multiple tents are placed. Firm downward traction on the cervix aids insertion by straightening the cervicouterine angle. When the canal resists insertion, it is occasionally helpful to sound it. The tent is introduced until its tip is just visible at the os or, if a collar is present, until the plastic is flush with the portio. During insertion, the tent's string can catch on a speculum knurl nut. To prevent this annoyance, begin by twirling the string around the shank of the forceps. To prevent later extrusion, use ring forceps to tamp a dry tampon made of wool or cotton sponges against the cervix as the speculum is withdrawn.

Vasovagal reactions to insertions are rare and seldom severe. They usually follow excessively tight packing with multiple tents. Cramps usually respond to a few minutes of rest. Moderate menstrual-like cramps are common, especially in the first hour and again after several more hours. Seldom do cramps cause insomnia.

Infrequently, the tampon, with or without the tents, may fall out during the night or the next day. This is far more commonly seen with retroverted uteri. Extrusion of the tents occasionally requires in-

six sizes, based on their widths: jumbo, extra thick, thick, medium thick, thin, and extra thin. Even within these groups diameters vary somewhat. For dry, medium-thick tents, diameters are usually 3 to 4 mm. Figure 12–5 shows them before and after being submerged in water overnight. The one that was only half submerged illustrates that there is very little vertical permeability to water, so it is senseless to moisten the exposed cervical end hoping to accelerate or magnify swelling. Their absorption of water

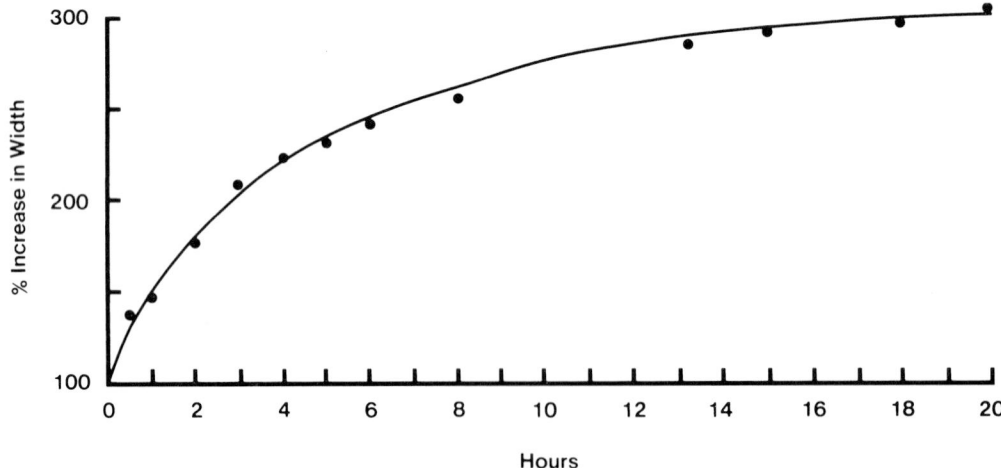

Figure 12–6
Three medium-thick laminaria tents were simultaneously submerged in water, and their diameters were measured with calipers 1.0 cm from their tips at the elapsed hours shown on the abscissa. Although doubling of width occurs in about 3 hours, tripling requires about 20 hours. All points are averaged measurements.

sertion of more tents or forced dilation, but cervical dilatation is usually adequate.

Worrisome management decisions arise when patients fail to return or change their minds about having the procedure done and want the tents removed. Two reports have addressed this problem. In one, two gravidas, both at 22 weeks' gestation, changed their minds after 2 and 3 days with multiple laminaria tents in place. Their pregnancies continued to term without complications (Van Le and Darney, 1987). The second report was from Israel, where 17 patients continued their pregnancies after their tents were removed. Fourteen proceeded to term, two had premature deliveries, and one aborted 2 weeks later; none, including three with positive *Chlamydia trachomatis* cultures, evidenced infection (Schneider et al, 1991). I have reviewed my experience with 11 similar patients. All were given prophylactic antibiotics, none developed a uterine infection, and eight carried their pregnancies to viability, with each neonate surviving. Thus emphasis should continue to be placed on patients being certain of the decision to abort before inserting laminaria tents, but, for those women who change their minds, the tents can be removed and the pregnancy continued. Prophylactic antibiotic coverage for a week with a safe drug such as erythromycin, amoxicillin, ampicillin, or a cephalothin is recommended, along with careful follow-up.

When the procedure is to be done, the tampon is removed, often with the strings of the tent if they are long enough to have been ensnarled with the tampon. Otherwise, tent removal requires digital extrication or direct speculum identification and extraction. On rare occasions, there is such "hour-glassing" and lack of dilation at the level of the internal os that a significant pull is required. On rare occasions there may be need to add more tents to provide greater removal room or to resort to their morcellation and piecemeal removal. Demurring from overtight packing should nearly obviate this rare problem.

I studied cervical dilation from single laminaria tents used for 20 to 24 hours, comparing results from thin, medium-thick, and thick sizes. Dilation was ascertained with Pratt dilators, beginning large and progressing incrementally downward until one fit without resistance. This size was defined as the achieved cervical dilation. Several variables were analyzed for their potential effects on achieved dilation—parity, prior cesarean section, and weeks of gestation, as determined by fetal extremity lengths (Munsick, 1987). Neither parity nor prior cesarean sections influenced dilation at all—identical dilations were obtained for nulliparous and multiparous women at similar weeks of pregnancy, but increasing gestational age positively influenced dilation. This salutary, statistically significant, linear relationship is shown in Figures 12–7 and 12–8. Parallel slopes but significantly different regression lines were found for different sizes of laminaria tents (Fig. 12–8). I have long preferred medium-thick tents because they (1) provide almost as much dilation as thicker ones, (2) can be used incrementally much easier than thick ones, and (3) appear less likely to perforate than do thin ones. The data shown in Figures 12–7 and 12–8 should not be taken to mean that these are the limits of dilation at any specific week. Use of tents usually *softens the cervix*, making further dilation easy. This was documented quantitatively by Atienza et al (1980a) with a force-sensing instrument that disclosed that less force was necessary for cervical dilation after use of laminaria tents.

With multiple laminaria tents, tenaculum stabilization is almost always desirable. Each tent is inserted next to a prior one until adequate numbers have been reached or more than moderate force is necessary for insertion. The number of tents should depend mostly on gestational duration, but also on

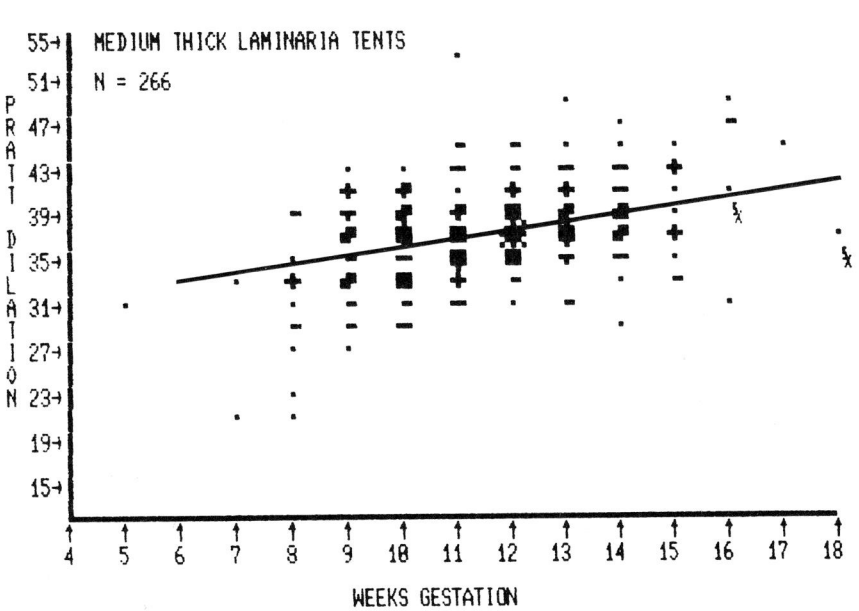

Figure 12–7
Cervical dilation (French size) versus weeks of gestation (*abscissa*) for single medium-thick laminaria tents used 20 to 24 hours in 266 subjects of mixed parities.

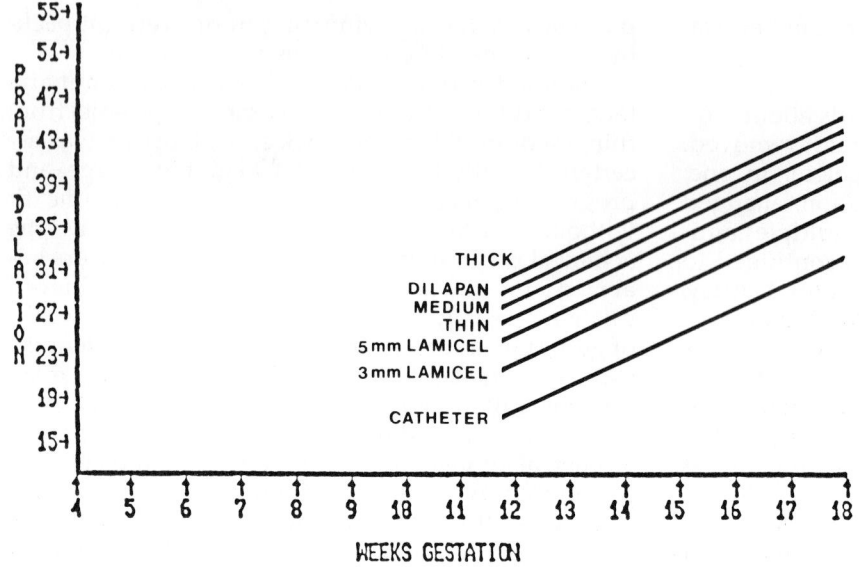

Figure 12–8
Cervical dilation after 20 to 24 hours from thick, medium-thick, and thin laminaria tents; 4-mm Dilapan; 3-mm and 5-mm Lamicel osmotic dilators; and a No. 10 French red rubber Nélaton catheter.

operator experience and instrument preferences, accuracy of gestational age estimates, type of tent used, and the duration of their placement (Table 12–3, Fig. 12–9) (Munsick and Fineberg, 1996). The cervical dilatation one can expect from one to nine medium-thick tents used for 16 to 26 hours is shown in Figure 12–9, based on the following multiple linear regression formula, (Munsick and Fineberg, 1996):

$$\text{Pratt dilation} = 12.36 + (2.35 \times$$

$$\text{medium-thick tents}) + (1.79 \times \text{weeks gestation})$$

More than nine tents can sometimes be inserted at a single application, but inadequate data were available to formulate their effects.

If cervical dilatation is inadequate after removing the tents, further forcible dilation may be performed, or, often safest, multiple new tents may be inserted and dilatation rechecked several hours to a day later.

Allowing 2 or even 3 days will almost always provide adequate dilation without injuring the cervix or risking infection. Often, after about 18 to 20 weeks' gestation, more than one application of multiple tents is advisable (Munsick and Fineberg, 1996; Hern

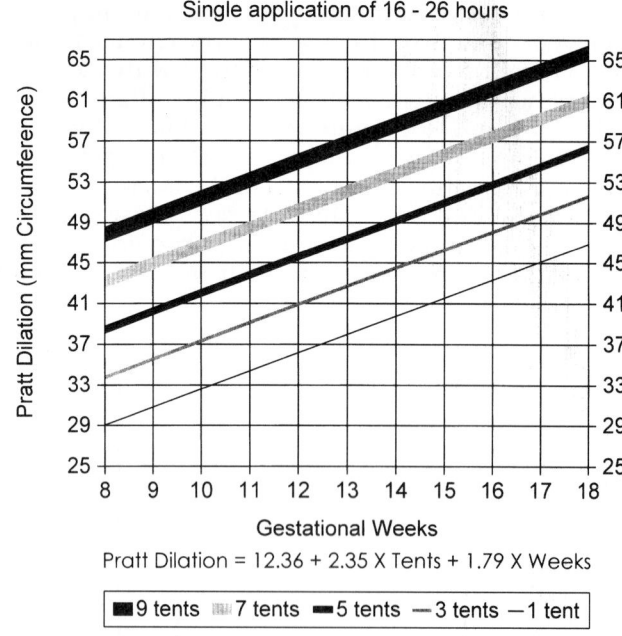

Single application of 16 - 26 hours

Pratt Dilation = 12.36 + 2.35 X Tents + 1.79 X Weeks

■ 9 tents ▨ 7 tents ▬ 5 tents —— 3 tents — 1 tent

Figure 12–9
Multiple linear regression formulas provided these parallel lines comparing achieved Pratt dilation against weeks of gestation with 1, 3, 5, 7, and 9 medium-thick laminaria tents left in situ for 16 to 26 hours. For 2, 4, 6, and 8 tents, the reader may interpolate between the lines, solve the formula shown, or use Figure 1 of Munsick and Fineberg (1996), which shows all nine lines. (Modified from Munsick RA, Fineberg NI: Cervical dilatation from multiple laminaria tents used for abortion. Obstet Gynecol 1996;87:726, with permission from the American College of Obstetricians and Gynecologists.)

Table 12–3. RECOMMENDED NUMBER OF MEDIUM-THICK LAMINARIA TENTS USED 16 TO 26 HOURS FOR ASPIRATION (L&S) AND EVACUATION (L&E) OPERATIONS

ESTIMATED WEEKS OF GESTATION	NUMBER OF TENTS
5–7	None; MA is recommended
8–11	One
12–14	Three (two will do)
15–17	Five or more (four will do for 15–16 weeks)
18–20	More than six; plural insertions may be required
>20	Plural insertions of multiple tents for 2 or more days are often advisable

Modified from Munsick RA, Fineberg NI: Cervical dilatation from multiple laminaria tents used for abortion. Obstet Gynecol 1996;87:726, with permission from the American College of Obstetricians and Gynecologists.

et al, 1993) (Table 12–3). Under such circumstances, patients should be alerted to the possibility of their needing to return more than once.

Osmotic Dilators

Although Nélaton's catheters have been advocated to dilate the cervix for abortion (Manabe and Manabe, 1981), my results showed that they could not compare with laminaria tents (Fig. 12–8). Dilation was also studied for synthetic osmotic dilators: 3-mm- and 5-mm wide Lamicels (Cabot Medical Corporation) made from compressed polyvinyl alcohol impregnated with anhydrous magnesium sulfate (Nicolaides et al, 1983; Wheeler and Schneider, 1983); and Dilapans (Brenner and Zuspan, 1982), osmotic dilators composed of very hygroscopic Hypan, a polyacrylate hydrogel, used for a manufacturer's *unrecommended* 20 to 24 hours. Their resultant dilations, by weeks of gestation, are also shown in Figure 12–8. It should be emphasized that these two types of synthetic osmotic dilators are recommended for brief use—6 hours or even less—and not day-long as used by me. The following conclusions seem fair when comparing them with laminaria tents. Dilapans have the advantage of swelling extremely rapidly, allowing terminations to be performed within only a few hours of insertion. Disadvantages, especially if they are left in for more than a few hours, include fragility and fragmentation in the cervix, the string pulling off from the dilator, and foreshortening during dilation such that neither cervical os dilates. These factors resulted in frequent inadequate overall dilation and in trapping of Dilapans within the cervix. Lamicels have the advantages over laminaria tents of causing virtually no cramping while in situ, easy removal, and swelling relatively rapidly (Nicolaides et al, 1983; Wheeler and Schneider, 1983; Grimes et al, 1987). Disadvantages I found with 20- to 24-hour use included less dilation than with laminaria tents and the frequent occurrence of the postabortal syndrome (see "Immediate Complications" below). Both osmotic types can be used plurally.

Short-term use of tents has been studied rather widely with favorable results when dilation is required for 10 or less gestational weeks. Only the study of Kline and co-workers (1995) noted the positive slope of regression of dilatation against the weeks of gestation. In that study, dilation from thick laminaria tents was compared with 3-mm Lamicels and 3-mm Dilapans after 6 hours. Dilatation was significantly less with Lamicels and there were problems removing Dilapans. These factors favor laminaria tents, which, even singly, are effective enough at 6 hours to achieve adequate dilation even for 12- to 14-week pregnancy aspirations. Dilapans are now unavailable in the United States.

Menstrual Aspiration

"Menstrual aspiration" and "menstrual regulation" are euphemisms for very early abortion, usually done between 4 and 7 weeks, using aspiration without cervical dilatation (Brenner and Edelman, 1977; Munsick, 1982). Rather, a flexible plastic cannula with diameter of 4, 5, 6, or 7 mm is introduced through the cervical canal into the uterine cavity. Suction is applied using a special syringe whose barrel is braked to prevent its unplanned, rapid, jolting descent after withdrawal. Thus there is almost no risk of the barrel's slipping and forcing its attached cannula through the uterus. The vacuum obtained is actually greater than most commercial vacuum aspirators can accomplish. The cannula and syringe used for MA are shown in Figure 12–10.

The technique is simple. Before beginning, the barrel of the syringe should be pushed forward until no air remains in it. Some kits contain a stiff, removable, plastic obturator within the cannula, which I do not use unless such stiffness is necessary. Sounding is not advised by most operators, but it can help to determine cervical direction, the resistance of the canal, and its patency. The cannula diameter in millimeters should usually match the weeks of gestation. The chosen cannula is inserted just to the uterine

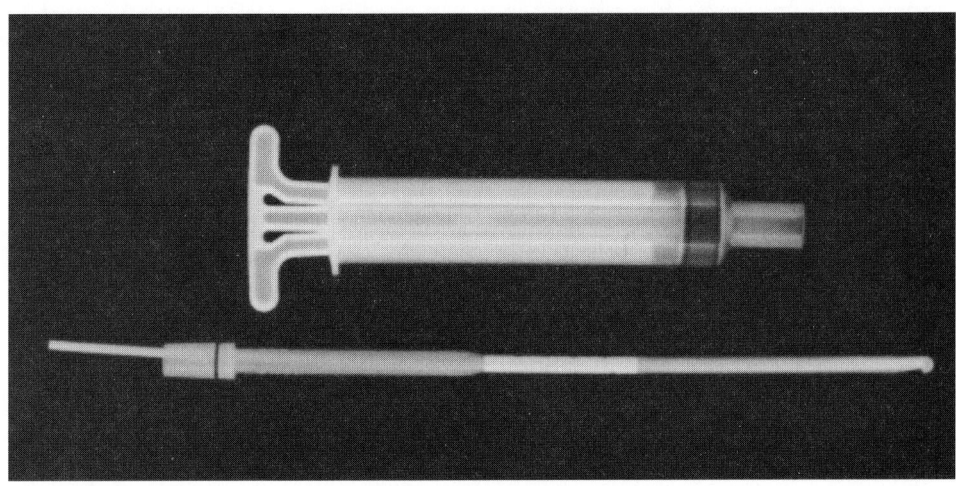

Figure 12–10
Cannula (5-mm) with its enclosed, stiff plastic obturator and O-ringed juncture, and the syringe used for menstrual aspiration.

fundus and withdrawn a centimeter, and the syringe attached securely to it, being certain that the sealing "O-ring" engages into the syringe orifice. To apply requisite traction on the syringe's barrel and avoid its sudden release, the syringe is grasped with one hand and the ipsolateral elbow firmly anchored into the operator's hip or rib cage. The other hand is used to apply traction on the barrel. The barrel is withdrawn fully and its brake secured. For pregnancies greater than 6 weeks, the syringe may fill with blood and require emptying once or twice before POC are obtained.

For 5- to 6-week pregnancies, a 5-mm cannula usually suffices, whereas at 6 to 7 weeks 6-mm cannulas are preferable. For 7- to 8-week procedures, 7-mm cannulae are often best if they will pass the cervical canal and if operators wish to proceed this far with MAs instead of using D&S. Although MA can be successfully performed beyond 7 weeks, the rate of incomplete abortion increases, so I limit them to 4 to 7 weeks. I am usually successful in estimating actual gestational age from the size of the aspirated placenta, but in the last 5 years I have missed pregnancies, some progressing normally, in 5/885 (0.56%) procedures. Of these, three eventuated in incomplete abortions and in two (0.23%), despite having aspirated pathologically documented placentas, the pregnancies continued, apparently normally, until they were aborted later by L&E. Incomplete abortions result from MA in about 2% to 3% of cases, the same as for D&S.

Aspiration (Suction) Abortion (D&S)

With the liberalization of abortion laws that occurred in the mid-20th century, first in Japan, then in Eastern Europe and mainland China, radical improvement in methodology was sought. One of the most important advancements was the introduction and rapid improvement of uterine aspiration equipment and methods. Dorothea Kerslake did much to popularize aspiration in England and the United States and, although many of the features described in her review are now passé, her account is worth reading (Kerslake and Casey, 1967).

For pregnancies of 8 to 14 weeks, aspiration is by far the safest and easiest method. One should use a commercial vacuum machine that rapidly evacuates the dead space and provides negative pressure of about 500 to 700 mm Hg. The greater the negative pressure the better. Suction is rather ineffective if less than 600 mm Hg vacuum is applied, and the lower the atmospheric pressure, the less will be the vacuum.

For two reasons, the vacuum apparatus should be checked before beginning each procedure: first, the hidden hoses within the machine could have been reversed, causing pressure and potential air embolism rather than suction; and, second, hoses or the cannula may be kinked, obstructed, or insecure, resulting in insufficient vacuum. Negative pressure can be checked as follows:

1. Cover the end of the tubing with a finger to be certain there is suction, not pressure.
2. Note the vacuum on the gauge, being certain it is satisfactory.
3. When the vacuum is broken by sliding the occluding ring of the vacuum cannula back, ensure that suction is also broken within the trap bottle, as indicated by a drop to 0 mm Hg on the gauge. In many systems, bottles contain plastic folds that can plug a vacuum port, so the vacuum does not break when the cannula is vented.

From about 8 to 14 gestational weeks, a cannula should be chosen that has the same or a slightly greater outer diameter than the estimated weeks of gestation. If dilatation is inadequate, the POC may often be minced and aspirated with persistent use of a less than sufficiently wide cannula. Suction is highly appropriate for pregnancies of 13 to 14 gestational weeks, provided that laminaria tents are used to dilate and soften the cervix. Cannulas larger than 14 mm are manufactured; however, most are metallic and lose three advantages of plastic ones: (1) lightness for easy manipulation, (2) transparency to see what is being aspirated, and (3) no need to modify the bottle or suction port so as to fit the larger tubing. The experiences of Stubblefield et al (1978) with 12- and 15.9-mm cannulas are compared with mine, using 14-mm cannulas, in Table 12–4. For

Table 12–4. ASPIRATION SUCCESS RATES USING 12-, 14-, AND 15.9-mm VACUUM CANNULAE

GESTATIONAL WEEKS	12-mm CANNULA*			15.9-mm CANNULA*			14-mm CANNULA[†]		
	Yes	No	%	Yes	No	%	Yes	No	%
13	9	2	82	10	0	100	9	0	100
14	4	7	36	7	3	70	12	2	86
15–16	0	9	0	6	5	55	2	25	7
17–18	0	3	0	0	9	0	0	11	0

*Data from Stubblefield PG, Albrecht BH, Koos B, et al: A randomized study of 12-mm and 15.9-mm cannulas in midtrimester abortion by laminaria and vacuum curettage. Fertil Steril 1978;29:512.
[†]Munsick (unpublished data).

pregnancies greater than 12 to 13 weeks, both larger sizes have indubitable advantages over the 12-mm cannula.

For MA and D&S operations, cannula techniques are nearly identical. Some surgeons use an in-and-out piston motion, rotating the cannula only when no further tissue is obtained. I recommend insertion to the fundus, backing away at least 1 cm, and beginning suction without moving the cannula at all, observing what happens. If minimal blood or tissue is obtained, I begin slow rotation, pausing when tissue is obtained. A piston motion is used only to free placenta where it is seen. In subjects with a very high cervix and uterus, as with prior cesarean section or great obesity, longer vacuum cannulae are available and are occasionally very helpful.

The procedure is concluded when all POC have been removed. This is indicated by (1) final aspiration of bubbly blood or nothing, and (2) a dramatic increase in the adherence of the cannula to the uterine wall such that it is difficult to move. If the location of the cannula cannot be determined, suction should be broken to determine its position or it should be withdrawn and reinserted; strong-arming the cannula against vacuum resistance may perforate the uterus. While the operator is suctioning during an MA or D&S, the cannula may feel unusually free, indication that its orifice or base is obstructed by placenta or a fetal part. It is then necessary to break suction, remove the cannula, and clear it. With aspiration completed, a ring forceps and sharp curette are used to check the cavity for residual POC and for abnormal architecture. Finally, freed decidua and POC are reaspirated.

One other caveat is necessary concerning vacuum aspiration. When evacuating hydatidiform moles, whoever controls the vacuum machine's on–off switch should be alert to turn it off immediately upon command, because the first bottle can fill extraordinarily rapidly, spill over into and beyond the second catch-trap, and befoul the machine, requiring that it be repaired or replaced.

Uterine Instrumentation

Additional instruments are required for L&E and are sometimes desirable for D&S and for placental delivery after instillation and uterotonic methods. For MA operations, a 5- or 6-mm cannula that will pass through the cervix is usually the only instrument used. Some surgeons use a No. 0 sharp curette when a 6- or 7-mm cannula has passed.

Following aspiration in most D&S operations, ring or Sopher forceps are used to explore and empty the cavity, following which large, sharp curettage is performed. Finally, repeat aspiration is used to remove loose decidua and placental fragments.

For L&E operations, both the fetus and the placenta are usually removed with the same forceps. Ring forceps may be useful, however, especially with

Table 12–5. PRATT DILATION REQUIRED FOR D&S AND L&E INSTRUMENTS*

INSTRUMENT	PRATT DILATION (mm)
No. 0 sharp curette	19–21
No. 6 sharp curette	33
Vacuum cannula	Diameter (mm) × pi
Ring (sponge) forceps	35
Sopher forceps	35–37
Bierer forceps	45

*All values vary somewhat, depending on cervical compliance.

poor cervical dilation or when the uterine cavity has shrunken dramatically following removal of most products of conception (POC). However, for most evacuation operations the size of the fetus and placenta will require forceps with greater length, width, grasp, and compressing power than a simple sponge forceps. The instrument I use most commonly is the Bierer forceps. Smaller than the Bierer forceps and useful when the cervix is less well dilated is the Sopher forceps. For very high uteri that compel a very long forceps reach, Hern's forceps are very useful. Table 12–5 shows the approximate dilation needed to introduce several of the instruments used in D&S and L&E operations.

Laminaria Tent Dilatation and Evacuation (L&E)

Surgical abortions beyond 12 to 14 weeks were once considered anathema, and almost all second-trimester terminations were conducted by instillation or by hysterotomy or hysterectomy. Cates et al (1982) exploded this taboo. At and beyond 17 gestational weeks in the Meadowbrook Clinic in Minneapolis, MN, serious complications occurred in 1/227 (0.44%) cases with D&E, 20/884 (2.26%) cases with hypertonic saline instillations, and 8/623 (1.28%) cases with $PGF_{2\alpha}$ instillations. Respective RRs were 1.0, 5.14, and 2.91. Largely as a result of this publication and the finding that D&E carried a lower mortality rate than instillation (Lawson et al, 1994), L&E has become the most common procedure used in the United States to terminate midtrimester pregnancies.

Instillation or PG continued to be used when fetal anomalies and genetic abnormalities indicated abortion and unmacerated specimens were desired for pathologic, cytogenetic, and biochemical studies. Even this indication has now given way to L&E, which has been found to provide the same information with greater safety and patient convenience (Shulman et al, 1990).

Placenta previa, usually diagnosed by ultrasound or by grasping the placenta at the internal os during an L&E operation, is extremely worrisome to surgeons inserting laminaria tents or performing L&E operations. Thomas et al (1994) compared blood loss during L&E procedures on 23 patients with ultrasound-diagnosed placenta previas versus 108 L&E controls without previas. Means and SDs of blood loss were 77 ± 58 ml and 56 ± 25 ml, respectively (p = 0.009), but the difference in blood loss had dubious clinical significance and the only clinical hemorrhage was seen in a control subject. Of approximately 3000 L&E operations my colleagues and I performed in the past 20 years, no patient, including those with placenta previas, has required a blood transfusion or laparotomy.

Many reports have recently documented the safety of L&E. Jacot et al (1993), with an 89% follow-up, found complications among 5.1% of 2908 D&S patients versus 2.9% of 447 D&E subjects. None of the complications was life-threatening. Schneider et al (1996), with 88% follow-up, assessed the complications and later reproductive performances of women after 171 L&E operations performed between 18 and 22 weeks. There was one case of atony and one later D&C for retained POC. Intraoperative ultrasound was used in nine cases. There were no life-threatening complications nor was there evidence of cervical injury in the 50 women who conceived and delivered, only two prematurely and without apparent cervical incompetence.

When L&E is planned for pregnancies beyond 15 weeks, some operators use a 12- or 14-mm vacuum cannula to aspirate much of the amniotic fluid before beginning evacuation. However, membranes usually rupture when ovum forceps are introduced, and there is usually no need to waste a cannula and tubing. That amniotomy can lead to amniotic fluid embolism from transcervical entry to the maternal circulation during L&E has not been documented.

Regardless of one's choice of forceps, they should be inserted into the uterine cavity and opened wide enough to secure large POC. Resident physicians learning to perform L&E operations are consistently too trepidant to open the forceps wide enough. Two hands may be necessary to obtain an adequate forceps grip. If no tissue is grasped, time should not be wasted removing the forceps they should be opened wider to try again until tissue is encountered. When POC are secured, the forceps is forcibly closed to compress the part. The placenta often delivers whole but may be fragmented. The fetus usually macerates and, to be certain that all parts are removed, should be studied for completeness during extraction. Resistance is often felt as tissue is brought down into the lower uterine segment and cervix. Continued traction should be applied firmly but slowly and the forceps and specimen rotated and even corkscrewed to aid its delivery. With compression of the cranium, white cerebral matter usually oozes from the cervix. Often this indicates that the skull is compressed enough to pass.

When sizable fetal parts are retained, the most common one is the head. When it cannot be found,

the fetus should not be assumed to be anencephalic. One or more of the following strategies can be used:

1. Reach it in the cornua.
2. Grasp posteriorly just above the endocervix (the forceps may be passing anterior to it).
3. Apply vacuum with a 12- or 14-mm cannula, hoping to adhere to the retained part, and apply traction while maintaining suction, delivering it or at least causing its descent (this is the only case where suction is not broken when removing the vacuum cannula from the cervix).
4. If these maneuvers fail to identify and secure it, use ultrasound to locate it and guide the forceps to it.

If these repeated strategies fail, it may be necessary to begin oxytocin or a PG to augment uterine contractions and cause its expulsion.

Curettage

After D&S or L&E, sharp curettage is usually desirable to palpate large residual POC, free adherent placental fragments, and feel that the uterine walls are uniformly gritty. Perfect smoothness often indicates that the curette is against POC. If the curette is held loosely with the thumb on top of the handle and fingers below it, gentle palpation and scraping can be performed without unnecessarily denuding decidua or invading myometrium. The largest possible sharp curette should be used, usually a No. 6 for L&E operations.

Examination of the POC

To be certain that all POC are present, it is mandatory that the operator examine the specimen from each MA, D&S, or L&E operation. With L&E this is usually easy, because the POC are large and are inspected as the procedure transpires.

With D&S, the vacuum trap bag should be removed, inverted, emptied, and inspected to be sure of the procedure's completion. The suction trap bag is usually *not* sterile, so the operator must not contaminate gloves or instruments with it. A quick glance will usually determine that the POC are or are not complete; gloved, digital palpation often helps to localize firm, hidden fetal parts. When done, the POC should again be carefully inspected in bright light away from the patient. At 10 weeks, almost all pregnancies except those with blighted ova contain an obvious fetus. At 9 weeks, more than half do, but at 8 weeks it usually cannot be found without a protracted search. I make it a practice to perform foot, leg, and arm length measurements and to record the averaged formula-derived weeks of gestation from these (Munsick, 1987).

With MA, one is usually even less certain of having obtained the placenta. A careful search may be required to identify it or to conclude that reaspiration is needed. A rapid, easy, and dependable method of identifying early placenta is as follows. The D&S specimen is placed or the MA syringe material injected into a clear plastic or glass bowl containing 100 to 200 ml of tap water and the container repeatedly decanted and refilled with water until tissue is clearly seen. The placenta is usually a pale ball of fluffy tissue and is best identified when the container is held over a dark surface while lighting it strongly from the side or back. If the placenta is not seen, it should be sought out within extruded clots. If it is not there either, suggestive small tissue fragments can be observed under a low-power or dissecting microscope, compressing them on a slide in water under a coverslip. The microscope condenser should be racked down with the iris diaphragm nearly closed. Typical villous placenta and the ragged appearance of decidua are shown in Figure 12–11. The gross and microscopic tests for placenta are extraordinarily specific and sensitive (Munsick, 1982).

For medicolegal reasons, most clinics send specimens to pathologists. Unless they are abnormal, it seems wasteful to perform microscopic sections on those with a fetus.

Postoperative Observation, Medications, and Activity

Most women recover rapidly from their cramps, which are usually gone within 30 minutes. If they persist longer than this they should be abating (see discussion of postabortion syndrome under "Immediate Complications" below). It is well to observe patients for about an hour.

For women who are Rh(D) negative and unsensitized to Rh(D), human anti-Rh(D) immunoglobulin should be injected as follows: 50 µg for gestations of 12 weeks or less, or a standard 300-µg dose if greater than 12 weeks. This is another good reason to measure fetal extremity lengths as a gold standard of gestational age.

The effectiveness of prophylactic antibiotics for preventing postabortal endomyometritis has been repeatedly studied. Sawaya et al (1996) used meta-analysis of 12 such reports published since 1966 and concluded that prophylactic antibiotics reduced infections by 42%. RRs with 95% confidence intervals (CIs) in the antibiotic-treated versus control groups were overall, 0.58 (0.47 to 0.71); with prior pelvic inflammatory disease (PID), 0.56 (0.37 to 0.84); and with a positive *Chlamydia* culture, 0.38 (0.15 to 0.92). The authors advised prophylactic antibiotics for all patients, both at low and high risk. No specific antibiotic was recommended, but tetracyclines or imidazoles were identified for their safety, tolerance, cost, relative lack of hypersensitivity reactions, and infrequent bacterial resistance.

How long physical and coital activity should be delayed or avoided, if at all, has never been adequately studied. It is probably best that patients avoid strenuous activity for a day or two and refrain from coitus until bleeding has ceased.

A dependable method of birth control should be begun very shortly after the termination. With conception of the aborted pregnancy, many women have used undependable contraceptive methods or no method at all. This is an excellent opportunity to

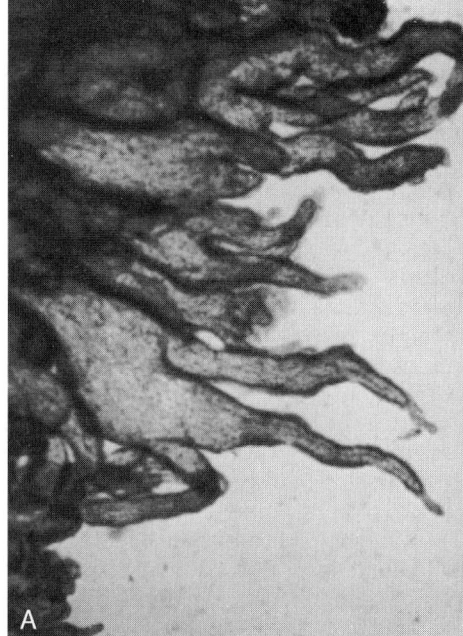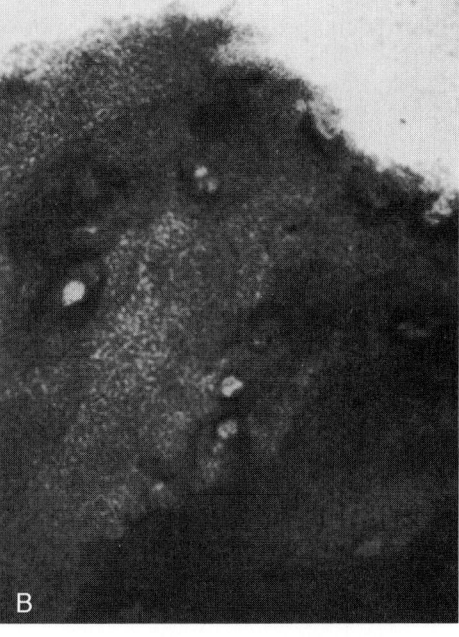

Figure 12–11
A, A fragment of 5½ weeks placenta in water under a coverslip, seen by low-power microscope. Note the villi and presence of surface cytotrophoblast. *B,* Decidua is thick, has ragged edges and tortuous glands, and often has prominent arterioles (*not shown*).

counsel women and to ensure adoption of dependable methods that are acceptable to them. Because ovulation can occur as early as 10 days after early terminations, oral contraceptive drugs should be begun within only a few days of the procedure.

Postabortally, ergot alkaloids have been routinely prescribed by some clinics, but they are dangerous. They have caused coronary arteriospasm and myocardial infarctions in two reported postabortal Japanese women (Fujiwara et al, 1993). The first subject was 38, a smoker who was treated with 0.75 mg methylergonovine daily for 10 days when she had a myocardial infarction. Angiography later showed normal coronary vessels but documented coronary angiospasm from a small challenge dose of ergot. The second subject was 42, also a smoker, and was given 0.25 mg of methylergonovine immediately after her abortion. Symptoms of myocardial infarction occurred 4 hours later. One month later, coronary angiography was normal but vasospasm occurred when the catheter touched a coronary artery ostium. No ergot challenge was given. The authors mentioned having heard of two other such cases and warned against prescribing ergot for women older than 30 to 35 years, especially if they smoke.

Immediate Complications

Cervical lacerations, uterine perforations, hemorrhage, and anesthetic complications are the usual immediate complicating features of these surgical procedures.

As previously mentioned, a generous vertical cervical tenaculum grasp and use of laminaria tents almost obviate *cervical lacerations*. If laceration results from pulling vigorously on a large fetal part through an inadequately dilated internal cervical os, the tear usually lies near the insertions of the uterosacral ligaments and uterine vessels and may be difficult to repair even abdominally. Hysterectomy is sometimes required. The same is true of lateral and anterolateral uterine lacerations, because hemorrhage may be rapid and entirely hidden intra-abdominally or retroperitoneally.

Grimes et al (1984) reported *uterine perforations* were decreased when laminaria tents were used for dilation instead of forced dilation. In a series of 145 uterine perforations during 84,850 abortions performed between 1982 and 1992, Lindell and Flam (1995) found that perforations were almost exclusively a D&S complication. About one half of these patients had exploratory operations; 18 were hemorrhaging but none had bowel injuries. Sixty-nine perforations occurred during vacuum aspirations (probably from the cannula), 30 resulted from use of Hegar dilators, and 45 were thought to be from sharp curettes or forceps. Lindell and Flam's recommendation was to observe patients following a recognized perforation, performing laparotomy, not laparoscopy, only if abdominal pain increases or signs of hemorrhage appear.

Perforations through the fundus are usually less serious. If the procedure has been completed when the perforation is discovered, observation for several hours is required, as recommended by Lindell and Flam (1995). When the procedure has not been completed, the best course will depend on surgical judgment: for anterior or posterior lacerations from a dilator or closed forceps, discontinuing the procedure and observing for hemorrhage are appropriate. A repeat procedure may be performed days later, preferably with generous use of laminaria tents and chariness when approaching the probable area of perforation. If there is any doubt about the wisdom of observation or of blindly repeating the procedure later, perform it in the operating room under laparoscopic or minilaparotomy guidance. When sharp instruments have perforated and there is concern regarding bowel damage, formal laparotomy with thorough bowel exploration should be favored over laparoscopy.

Hemorrhage may also result from uterine atony, a bleeding diathesis, or general anesthesia. Management should address the cause. With general anesthesia, blood loss is increased using all general anesthetic drugs but is especially risky when halogenated agents are employed. These should be avoided for abortion operations and, if used, immediately discontinued in the event of hemorrhage. Uterine atony, especially after terminations occurring at greater than 12 weeks, may be recognizable both from the hemorrhage itself and the soft, flabby uterine "feel" during final sharp curettage. Atony usually responds to curettage itself, but bimanual massage may be required and is effective. An ergot alkaloid such as ergonovine maleate or methylergonovine maleate can also be effective.

A distinct syndrome, known as the *postabortion syndrome* (PAS), occurred in about 22/2493 (0.8%) of their D&S operations before Sands and colleagues (1974) began routine administration of 0.05 mg ergot. After its use the rate dropped to 1/1829 (0.05%). My own rate of PAS is about 0.7% without use of uterotonic drugs. Whether or not 0.05 mg of an ergot alkaloid could cause coronary angiospasm is unknown, but I agree with the counsel of Fujiwara et al (1993) and prefer not to use such medications unless atony dictates their administration. With PAS there is usually scant vaginal bleeding in the first 30 minutes, and cramps increase rather than dissipate. As the pain increases, such patients become more "vagal"—the heart rate slows, there is profuse diaphoresis, clamminess, and often some faintness. Blood pressure is not greatly altered. The uterus may have enlarged to a size equal to or greater than its size before the operation and it and the entire lower abdomen are tender, while the upper abdomen is not. Clots usually are not expressible. Ergot alkaloids can be administered but usually cause more pain and fail to correct the problem—retained intrauterine clots obstructing egress of liquid and clotted blood. A dramatic cure follows re-emptying of the uterus with sponge forceps and a large sharp curette. Anesthesia is unnecessary. Seldom are retained secundines found, and recurrence is rare but can occur in the ensuing hour, so observation is advisable for at least that long. Ergot treatment may be advisable for the subsequent 24 hours unless the patient is a smoker and is older than 30 years (see above).

Amniotic fluid embolism is an extremely rare complication of abortion, but because of its lethality it accounted for 12% of CDC-reported legal abortion deaths during one 6-year period (Guidotti et al, 1981). In that series of 12 presumed and 3 autopsy-proved cases, estimated RRs by procedure were D&S, 0; instillation, 1; and hysterotomy-hysterectomy, 1.5. By weeks of gestation, RRs were $\leq$ 12 gestational weeks, 0.0; 13 to 15 weeks, 1.0; 16 to 20 weeks, 9.0; and $\geq$ 21 weeks, 24.0. These authors suggested that amniocentesis sites may have allowed passage of amniotic fluid into the maternal circulation. Greatly forced cervical dilation for evacuation, without autopsy-disclosed lacerations, may have contributed to fatal coagulopathy, possibly from amniotic fluid embolism, in one case (Osathanondh et al, 1981). In a similar autopsy-diagnosed case of coagulopathy, amniotic fluid embolism was confirmed after forced cervical dilation to 49 Pratt during a D&S operation (Cates et al, 1981). In the report by Osathanondh et al (1981), two additional fatal cases of coagulopathy followed use of laminaria tents for evacuation, but the adequacy of dilation was not stated.

Delayed Complications

Most delayed complications are infectious, hemorrhagic, psychological, or related to infertility.

As already noted, prophylactic antibiotics prevent *infections*. Several of my patients with severe *Trichomonas vaginalis* infections rapidly developed severe acute endomyometritis following abortions. Without proof of its causing the pelvic infection, I usually treat trichomoniasis for several days before performing terminations. In a double-blind, randomized study, Larsson et al (1992) studied the association of bacterial vaginosis (BV) with the postabortal prevalence of pelvic infections. BV was diagnosed in 174 pregnant women seeking abortions. They were randomized to placebo and metronidazole groups (500 mg three times daily for 10 days, beginning the week before abortion). PID occurred in 3.8% of the metronidazole and 12.2% of the placebo-treated ($p <$ 0.05) groups. When endomyometritis occurs postabortion, patients should be vigorously treated with antibiotics in accordance with standard regimens.

Sometimes, especially after very early terminations by MA or D&S, extremely *heavy bleeding* occurs 3 to 6 days later. It usually abates with several hours of bed rest. In my experience, repeat curettage has always failed to disclose POC and is usually unnecessary. Other than in the above time frame, heavy or persistent bleeding calls for repeat aspiration or for sharp curettage, especially if the uterus is boggy or enlarged. With incomplete abortions, the cervix is usually patulous, so a 7-mm MA cannula passes easily and aspiration under local anesthesia typically solves the problem.

Clearly, salpingitis can extend directly or by lymphatics from the endomyometritis that complicates abortion. Some such infections must cause tubal occlusion and *infertility*. Nevertheless, these cases are infrequent and difficult to demonstrate, even in large statistical studies. Frank et al (1993) were unable to find a significantly decreased fertility rate ratio following 433 abortions versus 1035 deliveries studied anterospectively, or in 9299 abortion patients studied retrospectively. If studies compared subsequent fertility rates among women with postabortal infections against those without infections, diminished fertility might be found. Asherman's syndrome, scarring and adhesions of the uterine cavity, can complicate abortions but usually only following severe infections of retained secundines after illegal, incomplete, and missed abortions.

Occurrence of *failed abortion* with MA and D&S is reason enough to emphasize the importance of a follow-up examination in 3 to 4 weeks, and sooner should symptoms of pregnancy persist for more than a few days. β-Human chorionic gonadotropin (β-hCG) is assayed by many physicians and clinics at the follow-up visit. This is a logical step, provided that the patient is at least 3 weeks postabortion and the assay is not so sensitive as to detect a level of less than about 100 IU/ml. It has been shown that serum hCG becomes undetectable at a mean of 30 days postabortion. The disappearance time depends upon its level at the time of the abortion (Aral et al, 1996).

Investigators have repeatedly sought to find severe *psychological consequences* accruing from induced abortions. Individual cases of depression, suicide, and other manifestations of mental disorder have been reported, but careful statistical analyses have not confirmed a significantly larger number of such cases than would have been expected by chance alone (Gilchrist et al, 1995). In a different vein, Zeanah et al (1993) found, among 23 women who had pregnancies terminated because of anomalous fetuses, that 17% had major postabortal depressions and 23% sought later psychiatric assistance. They concluded that such women are at approximately the same significant risk of psychological morbidity as women with perinatal losses.

Several studies have shown a slight increase in the *risk of breast carcinoma* among women who have had induced abortions. Daling et al (1996) found that, among white women ages 45 or less who had been pregnant and aborted at least once, the odds ratio for breast cancer was 1.2 with 95% CI of 1.0 to 1.5. The risk was limited to previously aborted nulliparas. This possible 20% increased rate is disturbing but is still subject to statistical sampling errors and bias. Even larger studies will undoubtedly be forthcoming.

NONSURGICAL SECOND- AND LATE FIRST-TRIMESTER ABORTION

Instillation

Several substances have been found to induce abortion when injected into the amniotic cavity.

Formalin

Initial instillation abortions were accomplished with this toxic chemical. It never achieved popularity and is no longer used.

Hypertonic Glucose

Because of its inefficiency and a propensity to cause serious infections, this method was also abandoned.

Hypertonic Saline

Instillation of hypertonic saline was the most popular method of accomplishing midtrimester abortions from the mid-1960s to the mid-1980s, and remains the most commonly employed instillation method. Transabdominal amniocentesis is used to remove 50 to 200 ml of fluid, which is replaced with about 200 ml of 23% aqueous sodium chloride solution. Labor ensues within about 24 hours and usually requires another 12 to 24 hours for expulsion to occur. Placental extraction is often necessary. Coagulopathy is a regularly detectible laboratory phenomenon that is usually not serious but can be fatal. Uterotonic drugs are often used to hasten uterine contractions and may add to the risk of coagulopathy. Oxytocin, whether given in intravenous megadosage alone or as an adjunct to hypertonic saline, has caused fatalities from water intoxication, possibly increased the risk of amniotic fluid embolism, and, by causing persistent, powerful uterine contractions, has caused extrusion of the fetus through the lower uterine segment into the posterior vaginal fornix, forming cervicovaginal or uterovaginal fistulae. Severe hypernatremia and hypertension are other complications of hypertonic saline use.

Herabutya and Prasertsawat (1994) provided a useful comparison of hypertonic saline with PGE_2 gel for midtrimester abortions. For 125 hypertonic saline abortions, the mean ($\pm$ SD) induction time was 31.7 ± 9.2 hours, whereas for 24 PGE_2 cases, induction took an extremely variable 28.4 ± 27.7 hours. Placentae were retained in 63% of the hypertonic saline and 25% of the PGE_2 groups.

Hypertonic Urea

A hypertonic solution containing 80 g of urea and 5 to 10 mg of $PGF_{2\alpha}$ decreased the latency period and labor time to 16 hours for this instillation technique, a significant improvement in induction time, and probably in safety, over using hypertonic saline (Burkman et al, 1976).

Uterotonic Induction of Abortion

Oxytocin in massive amounts infused intravenously had been used occasionally since the 1950s to induce missed abortions. Because of frequent failures, long induction times, and occasional cases of water intoxication, it never became popular. Meanwhile, newer PGs and their analogs were developed and used clinically. Some of these could be given intramuscularly, intravenously, vaginally, intracervically, and even orally. The greatest disadvantages of most PGs are their high cost, instability (some require refrigeration or fresh suppository preparation), short half-lives, and frequent side effects of asthmatic attacks, hyperpyrexia, vomiting, and diarrhea. Also, whereas hypertonic instillations usually cause fetal death, the PGs often do not; this can lead to neonatal resuscitative quandaries and pediatric dilemmas managing living abortuses.

Another potentially serious complication of uterotonic midtrimester abortion is uterine rupture. Atienza et al (1980b) first warned of the potential for uterine scar dehiscences with midtrimester abortions. Their case entailed uterine rupture through a prior cesarean section scar during a hypertonic urea instillation abortion. Among 75 women aborted with hypertonic urea who had had prior cesarean sections, they also described a longer abortion induction time and more frequently retained placentas. Their experience also included six uterine ruptures that were unassociated with prior uterine operations. Chapman et al (1996) have added their experience with midtrimester uterine ruptures with and without prior cesarean section scars. They retrospectively studied the uterotonically induced abortions of 606 women, 79 (13%) of whom had cesarean scars. All abortions were performed for fetal indications between 11 and 28 gestational weeks. Patients with cesarean scars did not require curettage more frequently than those without them, but they did require more blood transfusions (11.4% vs. 5.3%, $p = 0.04$) and their uterine ruptures significantly outnumbered controls (3.8% vs. 0.2%, odds ratio 20.8 to 1.0 and $p = 0.008$).

For the reasons described above, prior cesarean section should be considered a relative contraindication to nonsurgical midtrimester abortions. For L&E operations done on patients with prior cesarean scars, a report by Schneider et al (1994) found no serious complications among 70 subjects successfully terminated between 14 and 22 weeks. Patients with uterine scars who want midtrimester abortions might best be referred for L&E operations, provided that competent operators are available.

Most recent research with uterotonically induced midtrimester abortions has been centered on newer prostaglandins and analogs of the PGE group: dinoprostone (PGE_2), sulprostone (PGE_2), gemeprost (PGE_1), and misoprostol (a PGE_1 analog). Of these, the most exciting abortifacient prospect is misoprostol, because it is widely available, economical, and stable and can be administered safely and effectively by mouth or per vaginam.

Jain and Mishell (1994) studied 55 subjects who were at 12 to 22 weeks gestation and had fetal demises, fetal anomalies, or medical indications for abortion. Their 24 hour success rates were 81%(22/27) for PGE_2 (20 mg vaginally every 3 hours) and 89%(25/28) for misoprostol (200 µg vaginally every 12 hours). Side effects of PGE_2 versus misoprostol were fever, 63%/4%; severe pain, 63%/57%; vomiting, 33%/4%; and diarrhea, 30%/4%. The results with misoprostol were significantly better for pyrexia, vomiting, and diarrhea. The same investigators found that laminaria tents did not improve the abortifacient speed or efficiency of misoprostol (Jain and Mishell, 1996).

Bygdeman and Swahn (1985) first showed that uterine activity was increased from PGs after administration of the progesterone antagonist mifepristone (RU 486). Their conclusions were based on only a few in vitro observations but appear to have been confirmed by studies that have shown a more rapid and effective abortifacient response to mifepristone when a PG was administered for early first-trimester abortions. In the second trimester, too, mifepristone may improve the efficacy of PGs. Ho and Ma (1993) completed a trial with 13 second-trimester women randomized to receive either 600 mg of mifepristone or a placebo 36 hours before 0.5 mg sulprostone was given intramuscularly every 6 hours. With mifepristone the median induction time was 4.6 hours, and with placebo 20 hours. The amount of PG given was significantly less in the mifepristone group. Despite very few observations, they found that both differences were statistically significant and concluded that mifepristone is helpful in PG-induced cases. Webster and co-workers (1996) compared 36- to 48-hour pretreatments with 200 versus 600 mg of mifepristone for 70 women undergoing midtrimester abortions with misoprostol. Induction intervals were both 6.9 hours and the median dose of misoprostol was 1600 µg (three doses) in each group. Intervention was needed to deliver the placenta in about 11.4%. They concluded that the dose of mifepristone could be dropped to 200 mg. It would be satisfying to see if the abortifacient action of misoprostol in the second trimester is truly much improved by mifepristone.

SELECTIVE ABORTION

The abortion of one fetus, hoping to retain or protect one or more others in a multifetal pregnancy, is known as selective abortion or selective reduction of pregnancies. This has usually been done under careful ultrasonic guidance while a transabdominal needle is introduced into or near the heart of the targeted fetus and potassium chloride or a digitalis drug is injected to cause fetal asystole.

For triplets reduced to twins, Macones et al (1993) achieved a mean 35.6 weeks' gestational age for postreduction twins versus 31.2 weeks for triplets (p = 0.002) and perinatal mortality rates of 30/1000 versus 210/1000 (p < 0.001). These reductions were done between 9 and 12 weeks by transabdominal, transamniotic, transthoracic intracardiac potassium chloride injections. Lipitz et al (1994) compared outcomes of 106 triplet pregnancies managed expectantly against 34 in which reductions to twins were performed. Loss of the entire pregnancy occurred before 25 gestational weeks in 20.7% of triplets managed expectantly and in 8.7% of the reduced group. Successful pregnancy, defined by the discharge home of at least one infant, occurred in 88.2% of reduced pregnancies and in 74.5% of triplets managed expectantly. Reduction significantly lowered prematurity rates (p < 0.001), low birth weights (p < 0.001), and very low birth weights (p < 0.001).

Depp et al (1996) studied 236 multifetal (three or more) pregnancies successfully reduced to twins and compared their birth sizes and gestational ages with those of natural twins. Growth retardation was found in 19.4% of natural twins, 36.3% of twins reduced from triplets, 41.6% of sets reduced from quadruplets and 50% of those reduced from even greater numbers. They concluded that perinatal survival is improved by reduction and that the incidence of growth retardation is also decreased, but not to that of natural twins.

METHODOLOGIC OVERVIEW

For very early terminations (i.e., less than 8 weeks' gestation), MA is safe and effective, but there is much to be said for the use of mifepristone and misoprostol. Anonymity is nearly guaranteed; there may be no need to travel to an office, clinic, or hospital; costs should become minimal; success is greater than 90%; few medical personnel are required; blood loss is about the same as for MA; and only a minority of patients require curettage for bleeding or retained POC.

Later in the first trimester, dependable nonsurgical methods have not yet been developed that are quick, have a low incidence of retained placenta, and promise minimal blood loss. Uterine aspiration done in an outpatient setting still appears best.

For the second trimester, and possibly the third, L&E must be favored over instillation and uterotonic methods, provided that there are trained personnel to do it. L&E is safer, is quicker, and does not require hospitalization. The last reason is itself persuasive (Rooks and Cates, 1977).

REFERENCES

Aral K, Gurkan Zorlu C, Gokmen O: Plasma human chorionic gonadotrophin levels after induced abortion. Adv Contracept 1996;12:11.

Atienza MF, Burkman RT, King TM: Forces associated with cervical dilatation at suction abortion: qualitative and quantitative data in studies completed with a force-sensing instrument. In Naftolin F, Stubblefield PG (eds): Dilatation of the Uterine Cervix. New York: Raven Press, 1980a:343.

Atienza M, Burkman RT, King TM: Midtrimester abortion induced by hyperosmolar urea and prostaglandin $F_{2\alpha}$ with previous cesarean section: clinical course and potential for uterine rupture. Am J Obstet Gynecol 1980b;138:55.

Brenner WE, Edelman DA: Menstrual regulation: risks and "abuses." Int J Gynaecol Obstet 1977;15:177.

Brenner WE, Zuspan K: Synthetic laminaria for cervical dilation prior to vacuum aspiration in midtrimester pregnancy. Am J Obstet Gynecol 1982;143:475.

Bryman I, Granberg S, Norström A: Reduced incidence of postoperative endometritis by the use of laminaria tents in connection with first trimester abortion. Acta Obstet Gynecol Scand 1988;67:323.

Burkman RT, Atienza MF, King TM, et al: Intra-amniotic urea and prostaglandin F2a for midtrimester abortion: a modified regimen. Am J Obstet Gynecol 1976;126:328.

Bygdeman M, Swahn M-L: Progesterone receptor blockage: effect on uterine contractility and early pregnancy. Contraception 1985;32:45.

Cates W Jr, Boyd C, Halvorson-Boyd G, et al: Death from amniotic fluid embolism and disseminated intravascular coagulation after a curettage abortion. Am J Obstet Gynecol 1981;141:346.

Cates W Jr, Schulz KF, Grimes DA, et al: Dilatation and evacuation procedures and second-trimester abortions. JAMA 1982;248:559.

Chapman SJ, Crispens M, Owen J, et al: Complications of midtrimester pregnancy termination: the effect of prior cesarean section. Am J Obstet Gynecol 1996;175:889.

Daling JR, Brinton LA, Voigt LF, et al: Risk of breast cancer among white women following induced abortion. Am J Epidemiol 1996;144:373.

Depp R, Macones GA, Rosenn MF, et al: Multifetal pregnancy reduction: evaluation of fetal growth in the remaining twins. Am J Obstet Gynecol 1996;174:1233.

Frank P, McNamee R, Hannaford PC, et al: The effect of induced abortion on subsequent fertility. Br J Obstet Gynaecol 1993;100:575.

Fujiwara Y, Yamanaka O, Nakamura T, et al: Acute myocardial infarction induced by ergonovine administration for artificially induced abortion. Jpn Heart J 1993;34:803.

Gilchrist AC, Hannaford PC, Frank P, et al: Termination of pregnancy and psychiatric morbidity. Br J Psychiatry 1995;7:243.

Grimes DA: Clinicians who provide abortions: the thinning ranks. Obstet Gynecol 1992;80:719; discussion, Obstet Gynecol 1993;81:318.

Grimes DA, Ray IG, Middleton CJ: Lamicel versus laminaria for cervical dilation before early second-trimester abortion: a randomized clinical trial. Obstet Gynecol 1987;69:887.

Grimes DA, Shulz KF, Cates WJ Jr: Prevention of uterine perforation during curettage abortion. JAMA 1984;51:2108.

Guidotti RJ, Grimes DA, Cates W Jr: Fatal amniotic fluid embolism during legally induced abortion, United States, 1972–1978. Am J Obstet Gynecol 1981;141:257.

Hale RW, Pion RJ: Laminaria: an underutilized clinical adjunct. Clin Obstet Gynecol 1972;15:829.

Harlap S, Shiono PH, Ramcharan SA, et al: A prospective study of spontaneous fetal losses after induced abortion. N Engl J Med 1979;301:677.

Henshaw SK, Van Vort J: Abortion services in the United States, 1991 and 1992. Fam Plann Perspect 1994;26:100.

Herabutya Y, Prasertsawat P: Midtrimester abortion using hypertonic saline or prostaglandin EZ gel: an analysis of efficacy and complications. J Med Thai 1994;77:148.

Hern WM: Abortion Practice. Boulder, CO: Alpengio Graphics, Inc, 1990.

Hern WM, Zen C, Ferguson KA, et al: Outpatient abortion for fetal anomaly and fetal death from 15-34 menstrual weeks' gestation: techniques and clinical management. Obstet Gynecol 1993;81:301.

Ho PC, Ma HK: Termination of second trimester pregnancy with sulprostone and mifepristone: a randomized double-blind placebo-controlled trial. Contraception 1993;47:123.

Hulka JF, Lefler HT, Anglone A, et al: A new electronic force monitor to measure factors influencing cervical dilation for vacuum curettage. Am J Obstet Gynecol 1974;120:166.

Jacot FRM, Poulin C, Bilodeau AP, et al: A five-year experience with second-trimester induced abortion: no increase in complication rate as compared to the first trimester. Am J Obstet Gynecol 1993;168:633.

Jain JK, Mishell DR Jr: A comparison of intravaginal misoprostol with prostaglandin E2 for termination of second-trimester pregnancy. N Engl J Med 1994;331:290.

Jain JK, Mishell DR Jr: A comparison of misoprostol with and without laminaria tents for induction of second-trimester abortion. Am J Obstet Gynecol 1996;175:173.

Kaltreider NB, Goldsmith S, Margolis AJ: The impact of midtrimester abortion techniques on patients and staff. Am J Obstet Gynecol 1979;135:235.

Kerslake D, Casey D: Abortion induced by means of the uterine aspirator. Obstet Gynecol 1967;30:35.

Kline SB, Meng H, Munsick RA: Cervical dilation from laminaria tents and synthetic osmotic dilators used for 6 hours before abortion. Obstet Gynecol 1995;86:931.

Koonin LM, Smith JC, Ramick M, et al: Abortion surveillance—United States, 1992. MMWR Abortion Surveill Summary 1996;45:1.

Larsson PG, Platz-Christensen JJ, Thejls H, et al: Incidence of pelvic inflammatory disease after first-trimester legal abortion in women with bacterial vaginosis after treatment with metronidazole: a double-blind, randomized study. Am J Obstet Gynecol 1992;166:100.

Lawson HW, Frye A, Atrash HK, et al. Abortion mortality, United States, 1972 through 1987. Am J Obstet Gynecol 1994;171:1365.

Lindell G, Flam F: Management of uterine perforations in connection with legal abortions. Acta Obstet Gynecol Scand 1995;74:373.

Lipitz S, Reichman B, Uval J, et al: A prospective comparison of the outcome of triplet pregnancies managed expectantly or by multifetal reduction to twins. Am J Obstet Gynecol 1994;170:874.

Macones GA, Schneider G, Pritts E, et al: Multifetal reduction of triplets to twins improves perinatal outcome. Am J Obstet Gynecol 1993;169:982.

Manabe Y, Manabe A: Nelaton catheter for gradual and safe cervical dilatation: an ideal substitute for laminaria. Am J Obstet Gynecol 1981;140:465.

Miller L, Jensen MP, Stenchever MA: A double-blind randomized comparison of lidocaine and saline for cervical anesthesia. Obstet Gynecol 1996;87:600.

Molin A: Risk of damage to the cervix by dilatation for first-trimester-induced abortion by suction aspiration. Gynecol Obstet Invest 1993;35:152.

Munsick RA: Clinical test for placenta in 300 consecutive menstrual aspirations. Obstet Gynecol 1982;60:738.

Munsick RA: Similarities of Negro and Caucasian fetal extremity lengths in the interval from 9 to 20 weeks of pregnancy. Am J Obstet Gynecol 1987;156:183.

Munsick RA, Fineberg NI: Cervical dilation from multiple laminaria tents used for abortion. Obstet Gynecol 1996;87:726.

Nicolaides KH, Welch CC, MacPherson MBA, et al: Lamicel: a new technique for cervical dilation before first trimester abortion. Br J Obstet Gynaecol 1983;90:475.

Osathanondh R, Stubblefield PG, Golub JR, et al: Coagulopathy associated with midtrimester dilatation and evacuation. Adv Plan Parent 1981;16:30.

Rooks BR, Cates W Jr: Emotional impact of D&E vs. instillation. Fam Plann Perspect 1977;9:276.

Sands RX, Burnhill MS, Hakim-Elahi E: Postabortal uterine atony. Obstet Gynecol 1974;43:595.

Sawaya GF, Grady D, Kerlikowske K, et al: Antibiotics at the time of induced abortion: the case for universal prophylaxis based on a meta-analysis. Obstet Gynecol 1996;87:884.

Schneider D, Golan A, Langer R, et al: Outcome of continued pregnancies after first- and second-trimester cervical dilation by laminaria tents. Obstet Gynecol 1991;78:1121.

Schneider D, Bukovsky I, Caspi E: Safety of midtrimester pregnancy termination by laminaria and evacuation in patients with previous cesarean section. Am J Obstet Gynecol 1994;171:554.

Schneider D, Halperin R, Langer R, et al: Abortion at 18-22 weeks by laminaria dilation and evacuation. Obstet Gynecol 1996;88:412.

Schulz KF, Grimes DA, Cates W Jr: Measures to prevent cervical injury during suction curettage abortion. Lancet 1983;1:1182.

Shulman LP, Ling FW, Meyers CM, et al: Dilatation and evacuation for second-trimester genetic pregnancy termination. Obstet Gynecol 1990;75:1037.

Stubblefield PG, Albrecht BH, Koos B, et al: A randomized study of 12-mm and 15.9-mm cannulas in midtrimester abortion by laminaria and vacuum curettage. Fertil Steril 1978;29:512.

Thomas AG, Alvarez M, Friedman F Jr, et al: The effect of placenta previa on blood loss in second-trimester pregnancy termination. Obstet Gynecol 1994;84:58.

Van Le L, Darney PD: Successful pregnancy outcome after cervical dilation with multiple laminaria tents in preparation for second-trimester elective abortion. A report of two cases. Am J Obstet Gynecol 1987;156:612.

Waran KD, Munsick RA: Anaphylaxis from povidone-iodine. Lancet 1995;345:1506.

Webster D, Penney GC, Templeton A: A comparison of 600 and 200 mg mifepristone prior to second trimester abortion with the prostaglandin misoprostol. Br J Obstet Gynaecol 1996;103:706.

Wheeler RG, Schneider K: Properties and safety of cervical dilators. Am J Obstet Gynecol 1983;146:597.

Wiebe ER, Rawling M: Pain control in abortion. Int J Gynaecol Obstet 1995;50:41.

Zeanah CH, Dailey JV, Rosenblatt MJ, et al: Do women grieve after terminating pregnancies because of fetal anomalies? A controlled investigation. Obstet Gynecol 1993;82:270.

13

Investigation of the Infertile Couple

Calvin A. Greene
Joseph A. O'Keane

T he likelihood of pregnancy in an ovulatory cycle in a healthy young couple, or fecundability, is 20%. After 3 months 57%, 6 months 72%, 12 months 85%, and 24 months 93% of couples having unprotected intercourse will have achieved a pregnancy (Guttmacher, 1956). Infertility is usually defined as 1 year of unprotected intercourse without achieving a pregnancy. The prevalence of infertility is variously reported depending on the population being studied. However, overall it is believed to affect 10% to 15% of reproductive-age couples and increases with age (Mosher and Pratt, 1991). Infertility will affect one in seven couples when the woman is 30 to 34 years of age, one in five at age 35 to 39 years, and one in four when the female is between 40 and 44 years (Speroff et al, 1989). Approximately 30% of couples in the United States seek assistance from physicians to aid their chances of increasing fertility.

DEMOGRAPHICS

It appears that, although the prevalence of infertility is stable at present, the demand for infertility diagnosis and treatment has grown rapidly in the last decade (Gray, 1990). Many factors have contributed to increased infertility consultations. The most important reason is that the "baby boomers" are now entering their late reproductive years and are contributing to a large demographic cohort presenting with infertility. This has resulted from deferral of childbearing due to late marriage and career and other lifestyle choices. French data from studies of the pregnancy rate in women with azoospermic partners undergoing therapeutic donor insemination have demonstrated a profound decline in pregnancy rates with advancing reproductive age. Over 12 cycles of insemination, pregnancy rates were 74% in women less than 31 years, 62% in those between 31 and 35 years, and 54% in women who were older than 35 years (Federation CECOS, 1992). There is also a significant increase in spontaneous abortion rates with increasing age, from 10% between ages 25 and 29 years to 18% between ages 30 and 35 years and 34% in women over the age of 40 (Munnes et

al, 1995). Because of changing social attitudes, it is now more socially acceptable to seek out treatment than was previously the case. With infertility treatments being more publicized, readily available, and successful, more couples find them an acceptable option. Finally, there is a relative sparsity of babies available for adoption, forcing couples to seek infertility treatment to establish a family. All of these influences have significantly increased the number of couples presenting with infertility.

CAUSES OF INFERTILITY

Relative frequencies of etiologic factors associated with infertility are listed in Table 13–1. The ranges reflect the difficulty in precisely identifying the cause of a couple's infertility. Except in cases of azoospermia, anovulation, or bilaterally occluded fallopian tubes, it cannot be stated with certainty that the finding of an abnormal fertility test is necessarily the definitive cause of the disorder. Furthermore, reduced fertility in many couples may be the result of a combination of factors in both members of the relationship that together cumulatively result in subfertility or infertility.

INFERTILITY HISTORY

Infertility is a couple problem, and assessment of male and female factors should be undertaken simultaneously. It is helpful for each member of the relationship to fill out a gender-oriented detailed fertility questionnaire (Tables 13–2 and 13–3) and for the male partner to complete a semen analysis prior to the initial consultation. After reviewing the questionnaire responses, further inquiry is undertaken as indicated. The historical review will identify all past and present health problems and may provide clues to the possible cause of the couple's infertility. In addition, it should identify and assess the concerns and expectations of each of the partners.

Table 13–1. DIAGNOSIS ASSOCIATED WITH INFERTILITY

	% OF INFERTILE COUPLES
Tubal and peritoneal factors	25–35
Male factor	20–35
Ovulation disorders	15–25
Unexplained	10–20
Cervical	3–5
Other	1–5

Female History

In the assessment of the female partner, a careful menstrual history will usually allow discrimination between ovulatory and anovulatory women (see "Ovulation Detection"). A history of weight gain, progressive hirsutism, galactorrhea, and medication use may elucidate the etiology of an ovulation disorder. Heavy, prolonged, or intermenstrual bleeding may suggest abnormalities of the uterus such as pol-

Table 13–2. FEMALE INFERTILITY QUESTIONNAIRE

Demographic information
  Name
  Age
Fertility history
  Length of infertility
  Reproductive history
  Menstrual history
    Menarche
    Cycle length
    Duration of menses
    Dysmenorrhea
    Premenstrual molimina
Sexual history
  Coital history
  Timing and frequency of intercourse
  Use of lubricants
Marital history
Occupational and recreational activities
  Toxic factors
    Alcohol
  Smoking
    Tobacco
    Marijuana
  Drug abuse
    Cocaine
Previous investigations for the assessment of infertility
  Endocrine tests
  Laparoscopy
  Hysterosalpingography
  Rubella titer
  Progesterone and other endocrine tests
  Pap test results
Past medical illnesses
  Pelvic and abdominal surgery
  Genital tract infections
  Other significant medical or surgical illnesses
General inquiry
  Family history
  Allergies
  Medications

Table 13–3. MALE INFERTILITY QUESTIONNAIRE

Demographic information
  Name
  Age
Fertility history
  Length of infertility
  Reproductive history
Sexual history
  Coital history
  Timing, technique, and frequency of intercourse
  Use of lubricants
Marital history
Occupational and recreational activities
  Thermal factors
  Toxic factors
  Alcohol
  Smoking
    Tobacco
    Marijuana
  Drug abuse
    Cocaine
Previous investigations for the assessment of infertility
  Endocrine tests
  Results of urologic consultations
  Semen analysis
Past medical illnesses
  Pelvic and abdominal surgery
  Testicular trauma or surgery
  Genital tract infections
  Other significant medical or surgical illnesses
General inquiry
  Family history
  Allergies
  Medications

yps or fibroids, or lesions of the cervix. When menstrual flow is decreased, particularly after surgery within the uterine cavity, uterine synechiae may be present. Deep dyspareunia or significant dysmenorrhea may indicate pelvic pathology such as adhesions or endometriosis. Prior abdominal or pelvic surgery, use of an intrauterine contraceptive device, a history of sexually transmitted disease, and particularly a history of ectopic pregnancy suggest tubal factor infertility (Stock, 1990).

Review of the sexual history may reveal improper timing of intercourse or the use of a spermicidal vaginal lubricant. Intercourse frequency in most couples is two to three times per week. Less frequent sexual activity may interfere with timely conception. A history of diethylstilbestrol (DES) exposure in utero may suggest uterine cavity or cervical abnormalities (Burke et al, 1981). Women should be informed of the negative influence of cigarette smoking on fertility and encouraged and helped to stop (Howe et al, 1985). Confirmation of rubella immunity is sought and, if the patient is not immune, she should be vaccinated. A 3-month interval after vaccination is required before attempting pregnancy. Recent cervical cytology should be reviewed to ensure it is benign. All women should receive 0.4 to 1.0 mg of folic acid supplementation daily for at least 6 weeks prior to attempting conception to reduce the risk of neural tube defects (Medical Research Council Vitamin Study Research Group, 1991).

Male History

Review of the male partner's history is essential. Childhood surgery for correction of hernias, testicular torsion, trauma, cryptorchidism, postpubertal mumps orchitis, or other testicular or epididymal infections suggest male factor infertility. Prenatal exposure to DES may be associated with genital tract abnormalities and low sperm counts (Stillman, 1982) Delayed sexual maturity, decreased libido, and poor beard growth may be indicative of a chromosomal abnormality or an endocrinopathy. A history of impotence may be suggestive of a psychological problem or an organic lesion such as a prolactinoma. Heavy marijuana, alcohol, and cocaine use may reduce sperm counts. Cigarette smoking depresses sperm density and may also decrease motility (Stillman et al, 1986). Anabolic steroids, environmental toxins, radiation, nitrofurantoin, sulfasalazine, tetracyclines, erythromycins, spironolactone, and antineoplastic drugs can adversely affect sperm quality and quantity. Diabetic neuropathy and α-blockers, such as methyldopa, guanethidine, and reserpine, can cause retrograde ejaculation and ejaculatory dysfunction, respectively. A reduced semen volume and poor sperm counts may also be seen in males who have undergone prostate or bladder neck surgery. Elevated scrotal temperatures have a negative impact on sperm motility and can be caused by febrile illnesses, high environmental temperatures, and varicoceles.

Psychological Aspect

Fertility is a shared problem, and both partners should always be seen, if at all possible together. All investigations and treatment should be carried out with full cognizance of the deep psychological implications of infertility in a couple's life, particularly with regard to emotional and sexual well-being. Couples will require answers to such questions as "Why can't we have a child?" or "What are my chances of conceiving with this treatment?" The suffering of infertility can be compounded by intrusive investigations, and it is of paramount importance to investigate and treat an infertile couple expeditiously and efficiently and to avoid unnecessary repetitive testing. It is also important to proceed at a rate that the couple themselves dictate with respect to investigations and treatments.

PHYSICAL EXAMINATION

Female Examination

After completion of the history, a physical examination of the female partner is undertaken. Evidence of thyroid dysfunction is sought and the size and consistency of the gland assessed. Signs of androgen excess, including balding, acne, hirsutism, and clitoromegaly, are evaluated. Evidence of galactorrhea is sought at the time of the breast examination. The abdomen is examined for scars, tenderness, and masses. The external genitalia, vagina, and cervix are inspected and bimanaual and rectovaginal examinations are performed to assess the size and mobility of the reproductive organs and to palpate for endometriotic nodules. Appropriate microbiologic specimens are collected if a genital tract infection is suspected or if the patient is at high risk for a sexually transmitted disease.

Male Examination

Examination of the male partner who has normal libido and a satisfactory semen analysis will likely not contribute to finding the cause for a couple's infertility (Dunphy, 1989). Abnormal body habitus and eunuchoidal proportions are noted when present and may indicate a chromosomal abnormality such as Klinefelter's syndrome (XXY). Decreased body hair, gynecomastia, hypogonadism, and the lack of smell (Kallman's syndrome) suggest an endocrinopathy. Genital examination is performed standing, and the patient is asked to perform a Valsalva maneuver to check for the presence of a varicocele. Assessment of the urinary meatus is important to detect hypospadias and epispadias, both of which may interfere with sperm deposition in the vagina vault. Testicular volume is measured with an orchidometer and should be at least 20 cm^3 (Prader, 1966). The testicle is carefully checked for masses and consistency. Epididymal induration or dilation may indicate previous infection and obstruction. The vas is identified and followed to exclude congenital absence. A rectal examination is performed to assess the prostate gland and the seminal vesicles.

INFERTILITY WORK-UP (Fig. 13–1)

The three main components that are necessary to achieve a pregnancy are satisfactory production and insemination of sperm by the male, and ovulation and tubal patency in the female. Other lesser factors include adequacy of the luteal phase, cervical and uterine factors, and the absence of anti-sperm antibodies. Many components of human reproduction, such as observation of successful fertilization and embryo development, are not amenable to investigation unless the couple undergo in vitro fertilization (IVF). Although the diagnosis of sterility may be relatively straightforward, the diagnosis of subfertility can be fraught with difficulties (Hargrove and Elton, 1986). Whereas absolute bilateral tubal blockage, azoospermia, and anovulation are undoubtedly associated with infertility, many less absolute factors

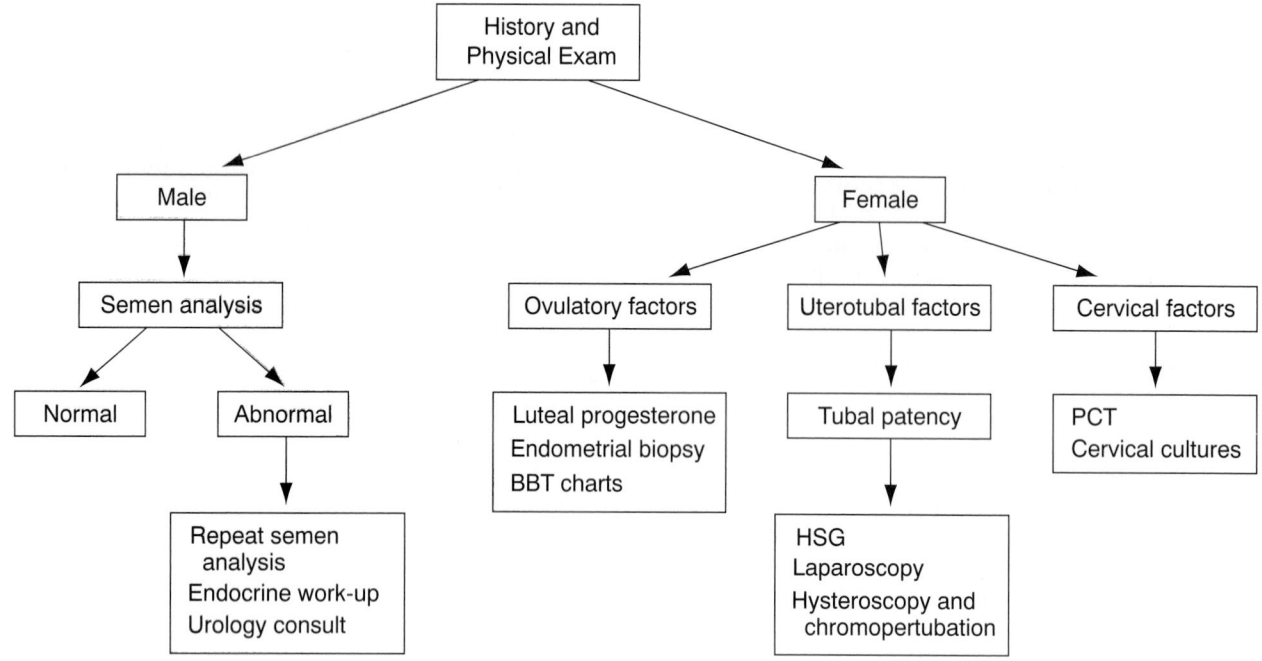

Figure 13 – 1
Basic work-up of the infertile couple. BBT, basal body temperature; PCT, postcoital test.

have different impacts in couples. For example, oligospermic males may achieve a pregnancy with a very fertile female and, vice versa, subfertile females may achieve a pregnancy with a very fertile male. Thus the results of investigations must be placed in a clinical paradigm of the couple and interpreted therein.

After reviewing the infertile couple's history and completing relevant physical examinations, the information is collated and the appropriate work-up is undertaken. The need for syphilis, human immunodeficiency virus, and hepatitis B testing is determined by the geographical prevalence of the diseases and the degree to which the patients may be at risk for those conditions. Women with a history of menorrhagia require a complete blood count. If signs and symptoms of thyroid dysfunction are present, a thyroid-stimulating hormone (TSH) determination is ordered. The semen analysis is confirmed to be normal and then tests are performed to confirm ovulation, establish fallopian tube patency, and exclude negative cervical factors. In some clinics an endometrial biopsy is still performed to rule out luteal-phase deficiency. A second semen analysis is usually requested within 1 or 2 months, particularly if abnormalities are seen in the first specimen.

INVESTIGATION OF THE FEMALE FACTOR

Ovulation Detection

Serum Progesterone Determinations

Women with regular 25- to 35-day menstrual cycles with premenstrual moliminal symptoms are ovula-

tory at least 95% of the time (Rosenfeld and Garcia, 1976). Ovulation can be documented by an elevated luteal-phase progesterone level, a biphasic basal body temperature chart, luteinizing hormone (LH) surge detection, secretory endometrial biopsy results, or serial follicular monitoring (Queenan et al, 1988). Generally a midluteal serum progesterone assay is ordered because it is easy, inexpensive, and reliable. A serum progesterone level greater than 15 nmol/L (5 ng/ml) performed on day 21 of an idealized 28-day cycle provides biochemical confirmation of ovulation. The probability of ovulation drops between 60% and 90% in the presence of oligomenorrhea, depending on the extent of the irregularity, and will thus reduce the likelihood of pregnancy over a given time interval. Correction of ovulatory abnormalities is highly rewarding, and, if no other causes of infertility are present, the prognosis is excellent, with pregnancy usually occurring within a few months of initiation of treatment. An appropriate endocrine assessment is indicated in women with oligomenorrhea or amenorrhea that includes TSH, LH, follicle-stimulating hormone (FSH), prolactin, and total testosterone. The most common endocrinopathy associated with ovulatory abnormalities is the polycystic ovarian syndrome. It is not helpful to complete an endocrine profile in regularly cycling women.

Basal Body Temperature Charting

Ovulation is triggered by a LH surge in response to high serum estradiol levels produced by granulosa cells of the preovulatory follicles. At the time of the LH surge, a temperature nadir is reached that results

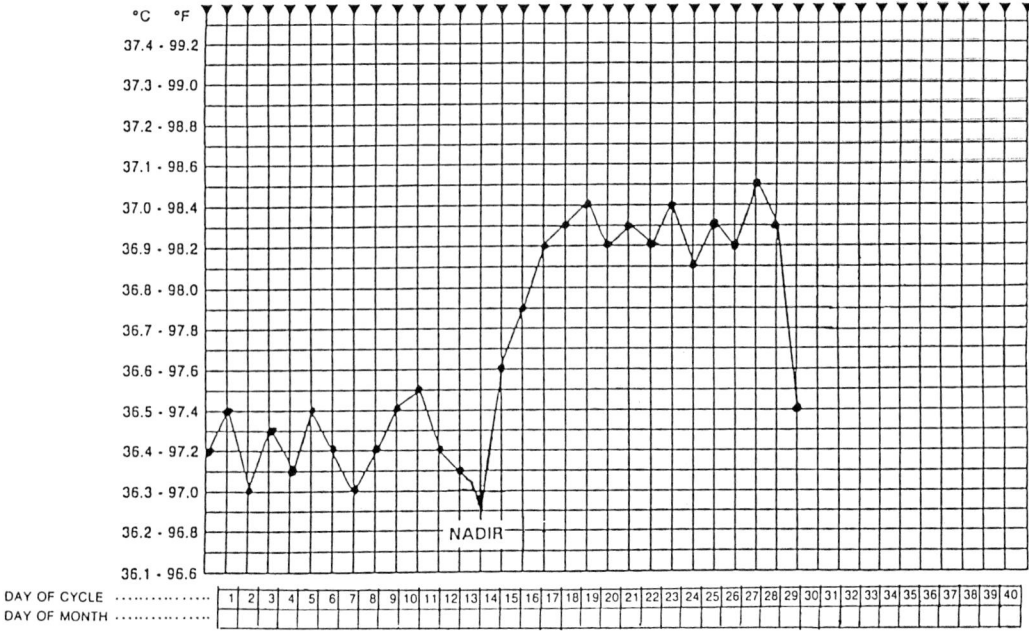

Figure 13–2
Basal body temperature chart.

from high serum estradiol levels. Following ovulation, because of the thermogenic effect of progesterone, basal body temperature rises by approximately 0.5° to 1.0°F (0.3° to 0.6°C) above baseline and is sustained, on average 14 days, unless pregnancy occurs (Fig. 13–2). Basal body temperature charting, when it shows a consistent and typical biphasic pattern, can be used to confirm ovulation and even time intercourse. Some couples who use this method may become obsessed with determination of basal body temperatures and feel they must adhere to a rigid schedule of intercourse. This obsession should be discouraged because it can adversely affect their sexual relationship. Sperm can survive in the female reproductive tract for at least 48 hours in the periovulatory period. Therefore, couples having an intercourse frequency of two to three times per week will likely have living sperm in the upper reproductive tract most of the time. Scheduling intercourse is therefore unnecessary. Couples who engage in infrequent sexual relations and who wish to rely on basal body temperature determinations to detect the fertile time should schedule intercourse every second day between 4 days prior to and 2 days after anticipated ovulation. Despite the above limitations and possible disadvantages, basal body temperature charting may be useful, particularly in the initial infertility assessment, but should be discontinued after a few months.

Day 3 FSH and Estradiol Levels

A day 3 FSH value is a marker of ovarian reserve, indicating "biologic" rather than "chronologic" age. It may be more predictive than chronologic age of the potential success of assisted reproductive technology (ART) procedures (Toner et al, 1991). The FSH level has also been shown to be predictive of cancellation rates of ART cycles (Scott et al, 1989). The FSH elevation is a result of reduced gonadal inhibin production. If the FSH level is elevated in one cycle and normal in the subsequent cycle, it is still prognostically significant for suboptimal ovulatory function. In one study of 28 women who were found to have one elevated and one subsequent normal FSH level in ART cycles, it was noted that all patients behaved as low responders in both cycles (Scott et al, 1989). A level of over 15 IU (Second International Standard) is generally predictive of a poor prognosis. In addition to elevated day 3 FSH, an elevation of estradiol (over 80 pg/ml or 294 pmol/L) on the same cycle day independently predicts a higher IVF cycle cancellation rate and a lower pregnancy rate. In one IVF study no pregnancies were achieved, and there was a 33% cancellation rate when the estradiol level was more than 100 pg/ml on day 3. The worst prognostic group was that with combined elevated FSH and estradiol (Smotrica et al, 1995).

Clomiphene Citrate Challenge Test

Various stimulatory test, including the clomiphene citrate challenge test (CCCT), have been used to predict success of ART procedures. FSH is measured on days 3 and 10 of a cycle in which clomiphene citrate is administered at 100 mg from days 5 to 9. If the day 3 FSH level is greater than 15 IU or the combined values greater than 26 IU, the test is regarded as abnormal. This test not only has prognostic significance for ART cycles, but also predicts chances for pregnancy in the general infertility population (Scott and Hoffman, 1995).

It is important to appreciate that FSH and estradiol values are not absolute indicators of potential fertility or ART success. However, this information can be used for counseling and individualized decision making by couples and their clinician (Wallach, 1995). The critical levels of FSH and estradiol will vary from lab to lab and must be interpreted in light of one's own center's experience.

Endometrial Biopsy (Luteal-Phase Defect)

Sequential estrogen and progesterone preparation of the endometrial lining is required for successful embryo implantation. After follicular-phase estrogen priming and ovulation, the endometrium matures under the influence of progesterone produced by the corpus luteum. An adequate luteal phase lasts approximately 11 to 14 days. The process of endometrial maturation occurs in a predictable and orderly manner, and biopsies can be pathologically dated. Retrieval of endometrial tissue from the fundus of the uterus can be accomplished without anesthesia using a Novak curette, endometrial pipelle, or other commercially available disposable instrument. The procedure is undertaken immediately before or up to 20 hours after menses commences, in a cycle during which the patient has protected herself against possible conception. The sample is placed in formalin and interpreted by a pathologist familiar with histologic endometrial dating (Noyes et al, 1950). The first day of the menstrual flow is designated as postovulatory day 14. To determine luteal adequacy, the actual cycle day of the biopsy is compared to the histologic day determined by the pathologist. A luteal-phase defect is said to be present if there is a difference of 3 or more days between the histologic and actual dates. In order to establish the diagnosis, the defect must be identified in two separate menstrual cycles. An alternate method of determining the anticipated postovulatory day, which may be more accurate, is to count forward from the day of the LH surge (Shoupe et al, 1989).

Luteal-phase defect may impair implantation and maintenance of early pregnancy. The incidence of this condition is said to be 3% to 4% of all infertile couples when the above diagnostic criteria are employed (Peters et al, 1992). It occurs as a result of recurrent postovulatory deficiency of progesterone and/or progesterone effect on the endometrium. However, progesterone levels do not correlate with the appearance of the endometrial biopsy in a reliable way and therefore cannot be used to diagnose luteal-phase defect (Soules et al, 1989). Several clinical conditions, including hyperprolactinemia, have been proposed, but have not been proven, to interfere

with the luteal phase and cause infertility. The alleged common underlying deficiency of the progesterone effect is proposed to be caused by defective folliculogenesis. Therefore, treatments for luteal-phase deficiency rely on the elimination of the underlying etiologic disorder, or improvement of folliculogenesis with clomiphene citrate, gonadotropins, or supplementation with exogenous progesterone.

Throughout the four decades since the concept of luteal-phase deficiency was introduced, the significance of this proposed cause of infertility has been debated. Evidence against the existence of this disorder is found in studies that find out-of-phase cycles frequently occurring in fertile women (Wentz et al, 1990). However, the most compelling evidence against its existence is a study that showed no difference in pregnancies in treated and untreated patients despite documenting out-of-phase biopsies in conception cycles (Balasch et al, 1992). It is doubtful whether routine assessment for luteal-phase deficiency in the work-up of infertility is useful, and this test has been abandoned for this reason by many infertility centers.

Postcoital Tests

Fertility is dependent on the sperm successfully gaining access to the upper reproductive tract through the cervix, allowing fertilization of the oocyte to occur in the fallopian tube. During most of the menstrual cycle, sperm transport is inhibited by unfavorable cervical mucus. However, under the direct influence of increasing preovulatory estradiol levels, cervical mucus becomes alkaline, thin, elastic, clear, and acellular, thus favoring the survival, storage, and transport of motile sperm to the upper tracts. After ovulation, under the influence of progesterone, the mucus once again becomes thick, tenacious, and opaque and the barrier to sperm transport is restored.

Cervical factor infertility may result from alteration in the quality or quantity of cervical mucus. Surgical procedures of the cervix, including electrocautery, loop excision, laser ablation, cryotherapy, and conization, can result in destruction of the mucus-secreting glandular tissue of the cervix. Cervical mucus quality can also be compromised by cervical infections, which may be manifested by a thick yellow or green discharge. Cervical cultures should be performed and the appropriate treatment initiated when indicated, with special attention given to successful culture for *Chlamydia* infections.

The postcoital test (PCT) was first described in 1866 by Marion Sims and further promoted by Max Huhner in 1913 (Speert, 1958). The test was further refined by developing a cervical mucus score for five characteristics of the postcoital test. These include spinnbarkheit (stretchability), ferning, viscosity, cellularity, and the number of motile sperm present (Moghissi, 1976).

A PCT is scheduled 2 to 3 days before ovulation as predicted by average cycle length calculations, basal body temperature charts, ultrasound follicular monitoring, or detection of the LH surge in serum or by commercially available urine testing kits. Couples are advised to abstain from intercourse for 48 to 72 hours before the test and to present for the procedure 2 to 12 hours following intercourse. A warmed speculum is placed to expose the cervix and mucus is collected from the endocervix by tuberculin syringe aspiration, nasal polyp forceps, or a commercially available collection system. The distribution of the sperm in the mucus is relatively uniform, and the sample may be obtained from anywhere in the endocervical canal. The volume is measured, the pH determined by pH paper, and the sample placed on a microscope slide. Spinnbarkheit is estimated by using a coverslip to draw the mucus from the slide and measuring its stretchability. The coverslip is then put in place and the specimen examined by high and low power under a light microscope.

What constitutes a satisfactory PCT is a matter of some debate and is clinic specific. The optimal pH ranges from 7.0 to 8.5. Outside of this range, excessively acidic mucus immobilizes sperm, whereas increased alkalinity may reduce sperm viability. Spinnbarkheit greater than 9 cm is considered optimal. Examination under the microscope will confirm the presence of ferning (graded 1 through 4) and excessive cellularity (> 11 cells per high-power field) (Moghissi, 1979). The World Health Organization (WHO) *Laboratory Manual* (WHO, 1992) states that 10 motile sperm seen per high-power field 2 to 3 hours after intercourse indicates a normal test. However, the actual number of motile sperm is controversial. It would seem reasonable to consider the test favorable provided a minimum of three progressively motile sperm are observed per high-power field. If no sperm are seen, coital adequacy should be questioned and an aspirate from the posterior vaginal fornix evaluated. The presence of anti-sperm antibodies in either the sperm or the cervical mucus should be considered if the sperm are seen to be immotile or shaking or otherwise fail to exhibit progressive forward motility.

As a diagnostic tool, the PCT test has limited usefulness in the investigation of the infertile couple. The test results confirm coital adequacy, the characteristics of the sperm in the cervical mucus, and the interaction between these two. If the test is normal, then it is likely that these parameters are not the cause of the couple's infertility. However, the converse of this statement is not true, and therefore the validity of the PCT is questionable. One author found no difference in pregnancy rates whether large numbers, very few, or even no sperm were seen in the test (Collins et al, 1984). It has also been demonstrated that women can have a negative PCT and still have sperm found in posterior cul-de-sac aspirates, confirming successful sperm transport (Asch, 1976). An important review of the literature concerning PCTs was published outlining the problems in the performance and interpretation of this diagnostic test (Griffith and Grimes, 1990). The test was shown to have wide ranges in sensitivity and specificity, thus calling into question its validity and therefore its ability to predict prognosis and direct treatment. Until properly designed clinical trials are completed, the utility of the PCT in the assessment and treatment of an infertile couple must be determined by each physician or clinic and individual experience.

It is the practice in many clinics not to routinely submit all patients to a PCT during the course of their fertility investigations. The most frequent cause of a poor PCT result is improper timing within the menstrual cycle. Patients can find this test distasteful and "scheduled lovemaking" stressful. When looked at critically, the results add little to the infertility assessment.

Uterine Factors

A large number of abnormalities of the uterus have been proposed to interfere with conception, but few have been proven to do so. These include the T-shaped uterine cavity resulting from in utero exposure to DES, fibroids, polyps, synechiae, and müllerian anomalies. These abnormalities of the uterus may be identified in up to 5% of infertile patients. However, there are insufficient data to implicate these conditions as causes for infertility, and successful pregnancy often occurs in the presence of these conditions. The frequent finding of abnormalities of the uterus in infertility patients does not necessarily constitute an indication for surgical intervention. These abnormalities are often demonstrated by hysterosalpingography (HSG), ultrasound, or hysteroscopy.

Hysterosalpingography

HSG (Fig. 13–3) is scheduled in the first 10 days of the menstrual cycle, 2 or 3 days after cessation of menses, to ensure the patient is not pregnant and to prevent retrograde dissemination of menstrual products. It has been reported that the incidence of iatrogenically induced pelvic infection after HSG is less than 1% in the low-risk population and as high as 3% in high-risk patients (Stumpf and March, 1980). Risk factors for postprocedure infection include a history of pelvic inflammatory disease, positive antichlamydial antibodies, dilated fallopian tubes, and cervicitis at the time of HSG. Evidence of any acute or chronic genital tract infection mandates postponement of the procedure and appropriate treatment of any infections prior to rescheduling. Prophylactic antibiotic treatment is advocated by many clinics and should be given to all high-risk patients (Pittaway et al, 1983). HSG is often uncomfortable for the patient, and an antiprostaglandin analgesic is advised 30 minutes prior to the procedure.

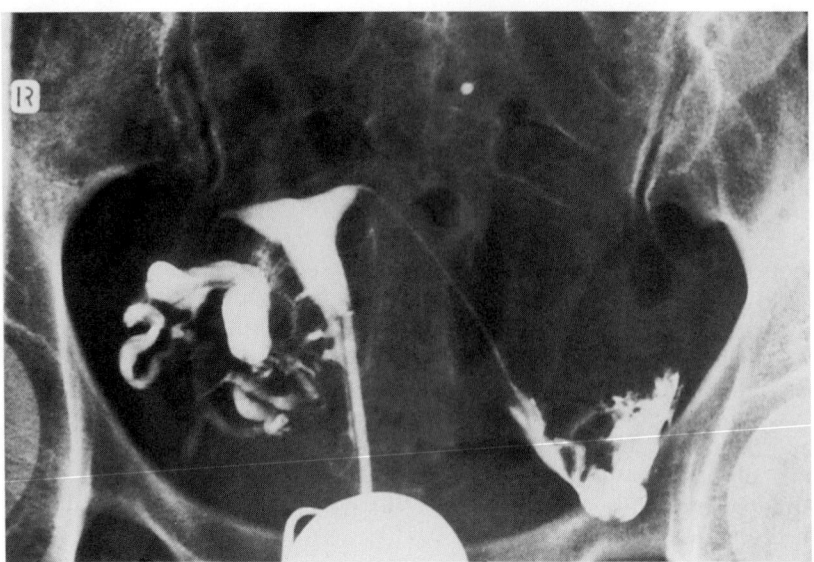

Figure 13–3
Hysterosalpingography. Bilateral hydrosalpinges are seen.

HSG is undertaken in a warm radiology room staffed with qualified personnel and equipped with a fluoroscopic image intensifier. A warmed speculum exposes the cervix, which is then carefully cleaned with a suitable antiseptic solution. A tenaculum is placed either on the anterior or posterior cervix for traction and manipulation. A suitable cannula with a sealing acorn tip, a commercially available suction device, or a No. 8 Foley or other catheter is placed so that the dye is injected above the internal cervical os. Balloon catheters are not recommended because the expanded balloon may interfere with visualization of the uterine isthmus. After placement of the injecting apparatus, a syringe with 10 ml of oil- or water-based iodinated contrast medium is attached and the speculum removed from the vagina. Fluoroscopy of the pelvis is undertaken and permanent films taken. The normal uterine cavity is in fact a potential space and can be outlined and tubal patency demonstrated usually with less than 5 ml of contrast material. The dye should be injected slowly under continuous fluoroscopic visualization to prevent excessive patient discomfort or tubal spasm and to examine the endometrial cavity for filling defects. If a questionable lesion is seen in the uterine cavity, it may be possible to aspirate the injected dye and repeat the examination with re-injection. Air bubbles can be differentiated from filling defects by rolling the patient and observing bubble displacement. Using the tenaculum for manipulation, the uterine cavity can be straightened for maximum visualization in the anteroposterior plane. Filling of the fallopian tubes and free spill of the medium usually occurs quickly and is confirmed when it is seen to outline the surrounding bowel.

Tubal obstruction is usually readily identified by HSG but must be distinguished from proximal tubal spasm. Slow injection with warm dye, intermittent injections over time, and manipulation of the uterus with the tenaculum may facilitate free spill of the dye. Aside from falloposcopy, HSG is the only method of assessing the internal architecture of the fallopian tube, and a permanent film is usually taken, as the dye traverses the fallopian tube, for later evaluation. Unilateral tubal spasm or preferential flow is suggested when one normal-appearing fallopian tube rapidly fills and spills and the other side fails to visualize, thus reflecting movement of the dye along the path of least resistance rather than a true tubal blockage. A delayed follow-up x-ray may be taken if there is a question of impaired dissipation of the dye into the peritoneal fluid. Some advise a 24-hour delayed film when oil-based contrast medium has been used and free spill has not been documented to improve the diagnostic accuracy of HSG (Bateman et al, 1987).

HSG is primarily a diagnostic procedure, although it has been suggested that it may have therapeutic benefits, particularly when oil-based contrast medium is used, with an increase in pregnancies being noted after the examination (Rasmussen et al, 1991). The potential disadvantages of using an oil-based dye compared to a water-based medium include its low absorption rate, its increased propensity to cause peritoneal granulomas, and the concern regarding oil embolization. In one study the incidence of intravasation of dye was 6.9%. In the six patients in whom embolization was documented, serious sequelae were not observed (Nunley et al, 1987). However, if vascular intravasation is noted, it is imperative that the procedure be terminated.

Ultrasound

As in other areas of obstetrics and gynecology, ultrasound screening is playing an increasingly important role in the diagnosis and treatment of infertility disorders (Table 13–4). Transabdominal scanning

Table 13-4. DIAGNOSTIC USES OF ULTRASOUND IN FEMALE INFERTILITY

Uterus
  Size
  Fibroids
    Size
  Adenomyosis
  Endometrial assessment
    Endometrial thickness and development
  Asherman's syndrome
  Polyps
  Müllerian anomalies
Ovaries
  Ovarian localization
  Polycystic ovaries
  Endometriosis
  Follicular monitoring
  Luteinized unruptured follicles
Fallopian tube
  Hydrosalpinges
  Peritubal cysts and fluid-filled adhesions
  Inflammation of the fallopian tube

through a full bladder and vaginal scanning are complementary techniques to assess the reproductive organs. Vaginal scanning (Fig. 13–4) is usually preferred because a high-frequency transducer (5 to 7.5 MHz) can be placed closer to the uterus, ovary, and fallopian tube, providing superior quality resolution of these pelvic organs.

In addition to the structural elements of the ovary that can be studied by ultrasound, folliculogenesis, ovulation, and luteogenesis can be studied in great detail. Subtle abnormalities that may interfere with fertility and their identification may direct specific treatment and in some patients provide further insight into the etiology of "unexplained infertility" (Pierson et al, 1995). Failure of the ovarian follicle to rupture and release the cumulus/oocyte complex can be identified by careful follicular monitoring. This syndrome, luteinized unruptured follicle, has been proposed as a cause of infertility in some patients (Haines, 1987).

Hysterosalpingosonography

Transcervical injection of an echo contrast suspension into the uterine cavity at the time of real-time transvaginal sonography with color Doppler is now possible. This technique will outline polyps, submucous fibroids, adhesions, intrauterine contraceptive devices, and abnormalities of the configuration of the uterine cavity. In addition, the suspension can be seen flowing through the fallopian tubes; confirmation of free spill is made with dissemination of the medium through to the peritoneal cavity. The addition of color Doppler to this technique has been reported to improve visualization (Peters and Coulam, 1991). The diagnostic accuracy of hysterosalpingosonography compared to HSG appears to be excellent in skilled hands. However, this test is not widely available (Stern et al, 1992).

The most recent developments in reproductive ultrasonography include Doppler duplex scanning and computer-generated three-dimensional ultrasound images. Transvaginal Doppler duplex scanning allows noninvasive evaluation of the profound vascular changes in the ovaries and uterus during the menstrual cycle (Campbell et al, 1993). These blood flow changes may detect abnormalities in ovulation, corpus luteum function, and uterine receptivity and aid in the diagnosis and treatment of infertility disorders. Highly detailed computer-generated three-dimensional ultrasound images will allow further delineation of follicular development in the ovary. Clinical applications of these innovative ultrasound technologies are currently being evaluated.

Hysteroscopy

Assessment of the endometrial cavity is a part of the infertility work-up to identify fibroids, müllerian anomalies, polyps, and synechiae. Hysteroscopy affords direct visualization of the endometrial cavity and is more sensitive than HSG in detecting some intrauterine abnormalities (Siegler, 1977). HSG, par-

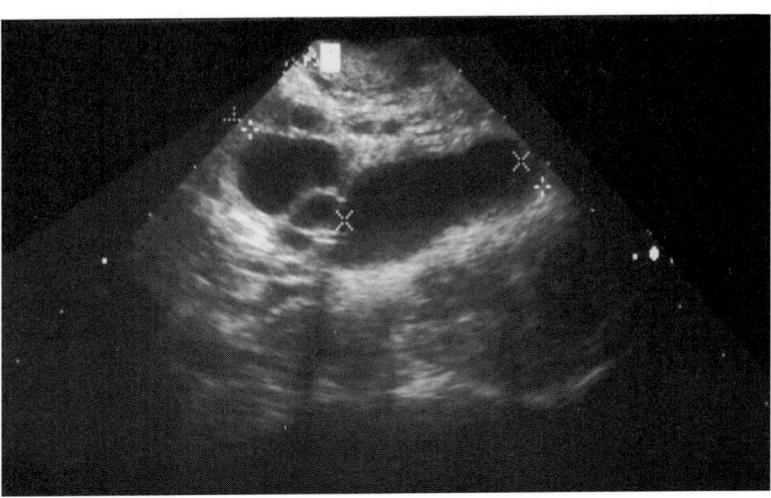

Figure 13-4
Vaginal ultrasound examination. x–x measures a hydrosalpinx. -,--x shows two cystic structures within the ovary that are follicles.

ticularly if not carefully performed by experienced personnel, can miss subtle intrauterine lesions and also result in false-positive filling defects (Taylor et al, 1986). In addition to seeing more abnormalities on hysteroscopy, lesions can be accurately characterized and, where indicated, treated by operative hysteroscopy. Müllerian anomalies can be accurately characterized by either HSG or hysteroscopy in conjunction with laparoscopy.

Hysteroscopy can be performed as an office procedure with local anesthesia or alternately at the time of laparoscopy. Minimal or no cervical dilatation is required. Small rigid panoramic hysteroscopes are usually employed for diagnostic hysteroscopy and saline or CO_2 used as the distending medium. The best view of the cavity is obtained in the proliferative phase. The procedure should not be performed during menstruation or in the presence of infection of the genital tract. Endometrial biopsy may be undertaken following hysteroscopy when indicated to sample the endometrial lining. Dilatation and curettage is not indicated in the assessment of infertility. Systematic recording of hysteroscopic findings is essential, and video recording provides excellent permanent documentation.

Laparoscopy

Patients with abnormal HSG or those who have not conceived within 6 months of normal HSG should proceed to laparoscopy. This 6-month time interval is indicated to allow spontaneous conception to occur after HSG, because this procedure has been shown to enhance fertility (Rasmussen et al, 1991). HSG and laparoscopy are complementary. It is not unusual for the fallopian tubes to appear blocked on HSG and to be found to be patent at laparoscopy (Levinson and Marlow, 1980). Laparoscopy is the only procedure that can precisely define the pelvic and abdominal anatomy, including the tubo-ovarian relationships; determine the presence and impact of adhesions on fertility; identify endometriosis; characterize ovarian cysts; and accurately assess dye transit through the fallopian tubes. Approximately 20% of patients will have abnormal laparoscopic findings in the face of apparently normal HSG (Philipsen and Hansen, 1981). In the presence of significant signs and symptoms of endometriosis, a history of intra-abdominal sepsis, an extended duration of infertility, or advanced reproductive age, some patients elect to proceed directly to laparoscopy and forgo the HSG. This allows more expedient completion of the infertility assessment so that appropriate fertility-enhancing treatments can be initiated.

Laparoscopy can be performed at any time in the menstrual cycle provided the patient is not pregnant or menstruating. Avoiding the time of menstruation will eliminate the concerns of retrograde deposition of menstrual products into the pelvic cavity and reduce the possibility of intravasation of indigo car-

mine dye at the time of chromopertubation. This outpatient procedure is usually performed under general anesthesia and endotracheal intubation with the patient in the dorsal lithotomy position. A gynecologic examination is completed and the bladder is catheterized as necessary. Diagnostic hysteroscopy may be undertaken if desired after the application of the cervical tenaculum and before placement of a uterine mobilizer. This mobilizer facilitates uterine manipulation and chromopertubation. Trocar insertion is undertaken through a small subumbilical incision with or without prior creation of a pneumoperitoneum according to the experience and training of the laparoscopist. Under direct vision, a suprapubic trocar is placed so that a blunt calibrated probe can be introduced into the cavity for manipulation. Further ports are placed as necessary if operative procedures are to be undertaken. Inspection of the abdominal and pelvic cavities should be completed systematically, taking advantage of the magnification afforded by the laparoscope. Chromopertubation with indigo carmine dye is carefully performed through the uterine manipulator to demonstrate filling and spill of dye from the fallopian tubes. Methylene blue dye is avoided because of rare methemoglobin reactions. To provide a permanent operative record that can be reviewed with the patient and/or colleagues, videotaping of the laparoscopy is recommended. Endometriosis, adnexal adhesions, tubal occlusion, and müllerian anomalies can also be classified and recorded on standard forms available through the American Society of Reproductive Medicine.

Falloposcopy

In vivo conception and early embryo development occurs within the oviductal lumen. The functions of the fallopian tube include oocyte pickup, providing a site for fertilization and early embryo development, and transportation of the embryo to the uterine cavity. In order for this to occur, the ciliated epithelial lumen must not only be patent but also able to synthesize embryotrophic factors. Falloposcopy is the only method to directly visualize the luminal architecture (Kerin et al, 1990). Falloposcopy is performed with a linear eversion catheter used in conjunction with a microendoscope and allows characterization of internal oviductal pathology. This information may be helpful in predicting future reproductive potential, including chances for pregnancy and the likelihood of having an ectopic pregnancy (Dunphy and Greene, 1995). Falloposcopy may also be useful in cases of apparent unilateral occlusive disease because it may also reveal disease in the contralateral patent fallopian tube. This can aid in predicting pregnancy prognosis and assist in choosing appropriate therapy (Scudamore et al, 1994). The linear eversion catheter has also been successfully used to open blocked fallopian tubes (Dunphy and

Greene, 1994). Falloposcopy is a new technology that is presently being evaluated on a research basis.

INVESTIGATION OF THE MALE FACTOR

Semen Analysis

The semen analysis has traditionally been the cornerstone of male infertility investigation. Although it is extensively used, it is a relatively poor predictor of fertility potential unless semen parameters are grossly abnormal (Aitken et al, 1991). To provide standardization and quality control, the WHO has published sequential editions of laboratory manuals entitled *Laboratory Manual for the Examination of Human Semen and Semen-Cervical Mucus Interaction* (WHO, 1992) (Table 13–5). The manual also provides definitions for normal and abnormal findings (Table 13–6).

Significance of the Semen Analysis

In a long-term study of over 2000 untreated couples presenting for infertility assessment with sperm counts below 5 million and motility less than 20%, it was shown that the semen analysis was a poor predictor for indicating which couples would ultimately achieve a pregnancy (Collins et al, 1993). In a retrospective analysis, the most prognostic semen parameters in predicting pregnancy were male age (reflecting the wife's age), the percentage of morphologically normal sperm, and sperm motility (Bostofte et al, 1990). Unless there is absolute azoospermia, routine semen analysis has limited prognostic significance. To date videocinematographic computer-assisted semen analysis (CASA) has not proven to be more predictive of pregnancy than routine semen analysis.

It is exceedingly important to properly interpret the semen analysis. It is surprising that men with what appears to be very deficient semen parameters can have a normal reproductive history. If there are sperm present and they are motile, then natural con-

Table 13–6. NOMENCLATURE FOR NORMAL AND PATHOLOGIC FINDINGS IN SEMEN ANALYSIS

Normal	As defined in Table 13–5
Oligozoospermia	Sperm concentration <20 million
Asthenozoospermia	<50% spermatozoa with forward progression; <25% spermatozoa with rapid progression
Teratozoospermia	<30% spermatozoa with normal morphology
Oligoasthenoteratozoospermia	Disturbance of all 3 variables (combinations of 2 prefixes may also be used)
Azoospermia	No spermatozoa in the ejaculate
Aspermia	No ejaculate

Data from World Health Organization Laboratory Manual (1992).

ception is possible. However, as the semen abnormalities increase the chances for natural conception correspondingly decrease. The lower the number of normal living motile sperm in the ejaculate and the greater the age of the female partner, the more likely the infertility specialist is to recommend treatment with ART. Depending on the results of methods to isolate sperm (swim-up techniques) from the ejaculate, treatment may include timed intrauterine insemination or even IVF with intracytoplasmic sperm insertion (ICSI). With the latter technology, men with only a few living sperm can produce a pregnancy.

Some papers have purported to show a decline in seminal parameters in the general population over the last 50 years (Carlsen et al, 1992). This study analyzed 61 papers published between 1938 and 1991, studying the semen characteristics of 14,947 males. These supposedly "normal" fertile males demonstrated a significant decline in sperm density from 113 million in 1940 to 66 million in 1990, a decline of over 40%. However, there is much doubt as to the validity of this conclusion because higher quality controlled studies using more consistent methodology and therefore fewer potential biases have not documented this decline (Fisch et al, 1996).

Collection

At least two semen samples collected on separate occasions by masturbation are recommended. Each sample is obtained after abstaining from ejaculation for a minimum of 2 days, but not longer than 3 days. The complete ejaculate should be collected in a sterile container provided by the clinic or laboratory and examined within 1 hour of collection. General semen examination includes determining the time required for the semen to become liquified, the volume, the consistency, and the pH. Microscopic evaluation of the ejaculate involves determination of the sperm density, total count, motility (percentage of moving sperm), morphology (shape), and agglutination

Table 13–5. NORMAL SEMEN VALUES

Volume	2.0 ml or more
Sperm concentration	$\geq 20 \times 10^6$ spermatozoa/ml
Total sperm count	$\geq 40 \times 10^6$ spermatozoa per ejaculate
pH	7.2–7.8
Motility	50% or more with forward progression *or* 25% or more with rapid progression 60 minutes after ejaculation
Morphology	30% or more with normal forms
Vitality	75% or more living
White cell count	<1 per 10^6/ml
Immunobead test	<20% of spermatozoa with adherent particles

Data from World Health Organization Laboratory Manual (1992).

("clumping"). The presence of elements other than sperm, such as white blood cells and bacteria, is also noted. A normal ejaculate has more than 20 million sperm/ml. More than 50% of the sperm should be forward moving, and more than 30% should have normal shapes (WHO, 1992) (Table 13–5).

Sperm Morphology

The usual criteria for assessing sperm morphology are those proposed by the World Health Organization (1992). However, various investigators have proposed more stringent markers to evaluate sperm morphology. There is some evidence that strict-criteria sperm morphology scores are more predictive of fertilization both in vivo and in vitro than is routine morphology assessment. Patients with less than 4% normal forms have a low IVF fertilization of about 8% of oocytes. Those with scores between 4 and 14% had higher fertilization rates, and patients having morphologic scores in excess of 14% had the highest fertilization rate (Grow et al, 1994). A prospective study on the predictive value of sperm morphology by computer analysis as an index for fertilization at IVF demonstrated a fertilization rate of 45% if normal morphology was 0% to 4%, and an 82% fertilization rate in the group with greater than 14% morphologically normal sperm (Kruger et al, 1996).

Tests That Assess Sperm Function

The poor predictive value of the semen analysis is understandable because of the diverse physiologic functions of sperm. Measurement of many factors important for fertilization, such as capacitation, zona pellucida recognition and binding, acrosome reaction, and fusion to the oolemma, is fraught with difficulties. A number of different tests have been developed that attempt to predict whether sperm have the ability to fertilize an oocyte. The most useful tests are the sperm penetration assay and the zona binding test.

SPERM PENETRATION ASSAY

When the zona pellucida is enzymatically removed from hamster eggs, the resulting denuded oocytes lose their species-specific barrier to fertilization and can be penetrated by any mammalian sperm. The sperm penetration assay (SPA) can provide insight into the potential for sperm to capacitate, acrosome react in the absence of the zona binding, fuse with the oocyte membrane, and decondense in the ooplasm (Zaneveld and Jeyendran, 1992). Studies have concluded that the SPA is a good predictor of IVF fertilization with a very low false-positive rate (Aitken, 1994; Wolf et al, 1996). However, with the advent of ICSI, the sperm penetration assay has essentially been abandoned by many centers because it is costly, lacks prognostic value, and is expensive (Wolf et al, 1996).

ZONA BINDING TEST

Sperm is required to bind to the zona pellucida of the oocyte before fertilization can occur. Therefore, the assessment of this parameter has potential to predict sperm fertilizing capability. The zona binding test utilizes nonliving human oocytes from surgically removed ovaries or oocytes from IVF that failed to fertilize. Usually the oocyte is bisected and the patient's sperm sample added to the hemi-oocytes. Sperm from a fertile donor is added to control hemi-oocytes for comparison. Calculations are made based on the degree of zona binding in each of the dishes and the hemizona index (HZI) derived. Franken et al (1993) demonstrated that a HZI of less than 30% predicted failed fertilization 70% of the time. When the HZI was greater than 30%, there was an 85% probability of fertilization. In one study using multiple regression analysis, it was demonstrated that the HZI results have the highest predictive power for fertilization success or failure when compared to other sperm parameters (Oehninger et al, 1992). It has been confirmed that there is high specificity and sensitivity for HZI results predicting fertilization outcome (Coddington et al, 1994). A consensus workshop in advanced andrology recommended that the HZI test be completed at the advanced stages of the andrology work-up (ESHRE Andrology Special Interest Group, 1996). However, there are many problems with the test, especially the procurement of human oocytes, the cost, and appropriate standardization of the test.

Anti-Sperm Antibodies

Sperm proteins are known to be very allergenic, and many sperm antibodies have been identified in the female serum and cervical mucus, as well as in the serum and semen of men. In both sexes these antibodies form after exposure of the sperm to the immune system in the vascular compartment. In the male, anti-sperm antibodies are formed following a breach of the blood-sperm barrier that may occur following trauma, infection, testicular torsion, or surgery (including vasectomy) on the testes or genitourinary tract.

The principal classes of antisperm immunoglobulins (Igs) are IgA, IgG, and IgM. These antibodies have been shown to bind to the whole sperm surface, and/or alternately to the tail, midpiece, or head of the sperm. Antibodies may be immobilizing or spermotoxic. The class of detected and the site of attachment of the antibodies to sperm vary in different patients, as does their potential impact on fertility. Anti-sperm antibodies identified in the serum were earlier thought to impair infertility (Menge et al, 1982). However, a more recent prospective trial failed to detect a relationship between infertility and circulating serum anti-sperm antibodies in men or women (Eggert-Kruse et al, 1989). In contrast, anti-sperm antibodies that are bound to the surface of the sperm in large numbers or found in the cervical mucus are significant.

Anti-sperm antibodies on the sperm surface are best detected by the direct immunobead test. IgG, IgA, and IgM can be screened for simultanaeously with commercially available isotype-specific immunobeads (GAM IBT) (Pattinson and Mortimer, 1987). The bead attachment to sperm is observed under a phase-contrast microscope and the location of the bound antibody observed. There is disagreement in the literature as to the immunoglobulin isotype and the binding location that have the most negative impact on fertilization and sperm motility. However, the results of in vitro studies have demonstrated a negative impact on fertilization when heavy concentrations of anti-sperm antibodies bind to the sperm head, interfering with sperm-oocyte fusion, or when they bind to the sperm tail and interfere with motility. Some infertility clinics screen all men for seminal anti-sperm antibodies, whereas others screen only those couples with an abnormal PCT or those with reduced sperm motility.

Endocrinologic Work-up of the Male

Although endocrine causes of male infertility are rare, measurements of FSH, LH, testosterone, and prolactin are indicated in males with reduced semen volume or signs of androgen deficiency to differentiate primary from secondary hypogonadism. Measurement of FSH will distinguish those patients with azoospermia, normal virilization, normal testicular size, and obstruction from those with impaired spermatogenesis secondary to seminiferous tubule failure. Men with obstructive azoospermia will have a normal FSH, whereas those with seminiferous tubule failure will have elevated FSH. A prolactin level is obtained to rule out a prolactinoma when the FSH is low because increased prolactin may interfere with gonadotropin secretion. These patients may present with galactorrhea, gynecomastia, impotence, headaches, and visual disturbances. A low FSH can be associated with Kallman's syndrome or panhypopituitarism. Although rare, endocrine causes of failed spermatogenesis can generally be treated successfully with hormone therapy.

Testicular Biopsy

Testicular biopsy is indicated in azoospermic males to determine if their condition is due to outflow tract obstruction or a spermatogenic disorder. Fine-needle aspiration or open biopsies can be obtained under either local or general anesthesia. It is desirable that sufficient resources be available at the time of open biopsy under general anesthesia to surgically correct any potentially reversible obstruction. Alternately, if an inoperable lesion or a nonobstructive process is identified, attempts can be made to recover sperm

from the epididymis or testicular tissue for cryopreservation and later use with IVF/ICSI. In men with bilateral congenital absence of the vas deferens, genetic work-up is indicated because many will be carriers of one of the cystic fibrosis genes. Ninety-five per cent of men with cystic fibrosis have congenital absence of the vas (Angulano et al, 1992).

Karyotype Analysis

Karyotypic assessment will detect genetic causes of infertility in men with azoospermia and severe oligospermia. For example, Klinefelter's syndrome (XXY) has an incidence of 1 in 650 live births and is a common cause of azoospermia. XXY-XY mosaics may also present with severe seminal abnormalities. As many as 5% of males presenting with severe seminal abnormalities have identifiable microdeletions of the long arm of the Y chromosome (Simoni et al, 1997). These microdeletions can now be detected by molecular genetic techniques and will be likey become part of the routine assessment for male infertility in the near future.

RESULTS OF INVESTIGATIONS

Couples can be triaged into various groups based on the cause of their infertility as determined by the infertility investigation.

Group 1: Normal Semen Analysis and Ovulatory Cycles, Abnormal HSG

The female partner requires further investigation with laparoscopy and/or hysteroscopy. If abnormalities are found at the time of laparoscopy, adhesiolysis or other surgical correction may be appropriate. The majority of tubal corrective surgeries can now be performed laparoscopically. The decision to proceed with surgery or refer for IVF should be determined by the severity of the pelvic/tubal pathology and the age of the female partner (Benadiva et al, 1995).

Group 2: Abnormal Semen Analysis and Ovulatory Cycles, Normal HSG

The male partner will require referral to an andrologist and further therapy may be instituted depending on the pathology found. This may include varicocele ligation if one is present. In cases of severe oligospermia or azoospermia, further investigation is required, such as measurement of FSH, testosterone, and prolactin. When complete azoospermia is found, consideration is given to performing a testicular biopsy to determine if spermatogenesis is present. A karyotypic assessment is performed in most males with severe oligospermia or azoospermia, particularly if IVF/ICSI is being considered as therapy.

Group 3: Normal Semen Analysis, Ovulatory Dysfunction

The etiology of anovulation can be elucidated by appropriate biochemical testing for FSH, LH, testosterone, prolactin, and TSH. Ovulation can often be induced with clomiphene citrate or human menopausal gonadotropins. Pulsatile gonadotropin-releasing hormone can be used in the treatment of hypothalamic amenorrhea. The prognosis for ovulation disorders is very good. Generally a test for tubal patency is performed after successful induction of ovulation after three cycles if a pregnancy has not been achieved. HSG is usually performed first and, if pregnancy has not occurred within 6 months, HSG is followed by laparoscopy.

Group 4: Unexplained Infertility

Unexplained infertility is diagnosed in a couple in whom the standard investigations have shown no overt abnormalities. In other words, the semen analysis is satisfactory, there is laboratory confirmation of ovulation, the endometrial cavity has a normal configuration by HSG or hysteroscopy, and tubal patency and the pelvic anatomy as assessed by laparoscopy are normal. It has been shown that 15% to 60% of couples with unexplained infertility will conceive within 1 year without any intervention, and 40% to 80% conceive by 3 years (Hull, 1992). The most important prognostic variable for predicting the chance of future conception is maternal age. The overall duration of infertility, whether primary or secondary, and semen count, particularly if significantly compromised, will also help to predict the overall prognosis (Collins et al, 1995). Unexplained infertility is often treated empirically with clomiphene citrate for up to six cycles. This can double the pregnancy rate (Deaton et al, 1990). Further treatment may consist of ovulation induction with menopausal gonadotropins plus intrauterine insemination or IVF if this is unsuccessful.

CONCLUSION

The number of couples presenting with infertility is increasing. Assessment of the couple should be organized and efficient and take into account their emotional needs and concerns. It is imperative that all investigations be critically evaluated and placed in the clinical paradigm of the individual couple. Treatment should be evidence based and goal oriented.

REFERENCES

Aitken RJ: On the future of the hamster oocyte penetration assay. Fertil Steril 1994;62:17.
Aitken RJ, Irvine DS, Wu FC: Prospective analysis of sperm-oocyte fusion and reactive oxygen species generation as criteria for the diagnosis of infertility. Am J Obstet Gynecol 1991;164:542.
Angulano A, Oates RD, Amos JA, et al: Congenital bilateral absence of the vas deferens: a primary genital form of cystic fibrosis. JAMA 1992;267:1794.
Asch RH: Laparoscopic recovery of sperm from peritoneal fluid in patients with negative or poor Sims-Huhner test. Fertil Steril 1976;27:1111.
Balasch J, Fabreques F, Creus M, et al: The usefulness of endometrial biopsy for luteal phase evaluation in infertility. Hum Reprod 1992;7:973.
Bateman BG, Nunley WC Jr, Kitchin JD, et al: Utility of the 24-hour delay hysterosalpingogram film. Fertil Steril 1987;47:613.
Benadiva CA, Klingman I, Davis O, Rosenwaks Z: In vitro fertilization versus tubal surgery: is pelvic reconstructive surgery obsolete? Fertil Steril 1995;64:1051.
Bostofte E, Bagger P, Michael A, et al: Fertility prognosis for infertile men: results of follow-up study of semen in infertile men from two different populations evaluated by the Cox regression model. Fertil Steril 1990;54:1100.
Burke L, Antonioli D, Friedman EA: Evolution of diethylstilbestrol-associated genital tract lesions. Obstet Gynecol 1981;57:79.
Campbell S, Bourne TH, Waterstone J, et al: Transvaginal color blood flow imaging of the periovulatory follicle. Fertil Steril 1993;60:433.
Carlsen E, Giwercman A, Keiding N, et al: Evidence for decreasing quality of semen during the past 50 years. BMJ 1992;305:609.
Coddington CC, Oehninger SC, Olive DL, et al: Hemizona index (HZI) demonstrates excellent predictability when evaluating sperm fertilizing capacity in in vitro fertilization patients. J Androl 1994;15:250.
Collins JA, Burrows EA, Willan AR: Occupation and the follow-up of infertile couples. Fertil Steril 1993;60:477.
Collins JA, Burrows EA, Willan AR: The prognosis for live birth among untreated infertile couples. Fertil Steril 1995;64:22.
Collins JA, So Y, Wilson EH, et al: The postcoital test as a predictor of pregnancy among 355 infertile couples. Fertil Steril 1984;41:703.
Deaton JL, Gibson M, Blackmer KM, et al: A randomized, controlled trial of clomiphene citrate and intrauterine insemination in couples with unexplained infertility or surgically corrected endometriosis. Fertil Steril 1990;54:1083.
Dunphy BC, Greene C: Failed reversal of sterilization: transcervical transtostial recannulation of occluded fallopian tube. Am J Obstet Gynecol 1994;171:274.
Dunphy BC, Greene CA: Falloposcopic cannulation, oviductal appearances and prediction of treatment independent intrauterine pregnancy. Hum Reprod 1995;10:3313.
Dunphy BC, Kay R, Barratt CLR, et al: Is routine examination of the male partner of any prognostic value in the routine assessment of couples who complain of involuntary infertility? Fertil Steril 1989;52:454.
Eggert-Kruse W, Gerhard I, Tilgen W, et al: Clinical significance of crossed in vitro sperm-cervical mucus penetration test in infertility investigation. Fertil Steril 1989;52:1032.
ESHRE Andrology Special Interest Group: Consensus Workshop in Advanced Diagnostic Andrology Techniques. Hum Reprod 1996;11:1463.
Federation CECOS, Schwartz D, Mayo JM: Female fecundability as a function of age: results of artificial insemination in 2193 nulliparous women with azoospermic husbands. N Engl J Med 1992;306:404.
Fisch H, Feldshuh J, Goluboff ET, et al: Semen analyses in 1,283 men from the United States over a 25-year period: no decline in quality. Fertil Steril 1996;65:1009.
Franken DR, Kruger TF, Oehninger S, et al: The ability of the hemizona assay to predict human fertilization in different and

consecutive in vitro fertilization cycles. Hum Reprod 1993;8:1240.

Gray RH: Epidemiology of infertility. Curr Opin Obstet Gynecol 1990;2:154.

Griffith CS, Grimes DA: The validity of the postcoital test. Am J Obstet Gynecol 1990;162:615.

Grow DR, Oehninger S, Seltman HJ, et al: Sperm morphology as diagnosed by strict criteria; probing the impact of teratozoospermia on fertilization rate and pregnancy outcome in a large in vitro fertilization population. Fertil Steril 1994;62:559.

Guttmacher AF: Factors affecting normal expectancy of conception. JAMA 1956;161:855.

Haines CJ: Luteinized unruptured follicle syndrome. Clin Reprod Fertil 1987;5:321.

Hargrove TB, Elton RA: Fecundability rates from the infertile male population. Br J Urol 1986;58:194.

Howe G, Westhoiff C, Vessey M, et al: Effects of age, cigarette smoking and other factors on fertility: findings in a large prospective study. Br Med J 1985;290:1697.

Hull MGR: Infertility treatment: Relative effectiveness of conventional and assisted conception methods [review]. Hum Reprod 1992;7:785.

Kerin JF, Williams DB, San Roman GA, et al: Falloposcopic classification and treatment of Fallopian tube lumen disease. Fertil Steril 1990;57:731.

Kruger TF, Ozgur K, Lacquet FA, et al: A prospective study on the predictive value of normal sperm morphology as evaluated by computer (IVOS). Fertil Steril 1996;66:285.

Levinson CJ, Marlow JL: Evaluation of patients for microsurgery. Clin Obstet Gynecol 1980;23:1195.

Medical Research Council Vitamin Study Research Group: Prevention of neural tube defects: results of the Medical Research Council Vitamin Study. Lancet 1991;338:131.

Menge AC, Medley NE, Mangione CM, et al: The incidence and influence of antisperm antibodies in infertile human couples on sperm cervical mucus interactions and subsequent fertility. Fertil Steril 1982;38:439.

Moghissi K: Postcoital test: physiologic basis, technique and interpretation. Fertil Steril 1976;27:117.

Moghissi K: The cervix in infertility. Clin Obstet Gynecol 1979;22:27.

Mosher WD, Pratt WF: Fecundity and infertility in the United States: incidence and trends. Fertil Steril 1991;56:192.

Munnes LE, Alcani M, Tompkin G, et al: Embryo morphology, developmental rights, maternal age for correlation with chromosomal abnormalities. Fertil Steril 1995;46:382.

Noyes RW, Hertig AT, Rock J: Dating the endometrial biopsy. Fertil Steril 1950;1:3.

Nunley WC, Bateman BG, Kitchin JD, et al: Intravasation during hysterosalpingography using oil-base contrast medium—a second look. Obstet Gynecol 1987;70:309.

Oehninger S, Toner JP, Muasher SJ, et al: Prediction of fertilization in vitro with human gametes: is there a litmus test? Am J Obstet Gynecol 1992;167:1760.

Pattinson HA, Mortimer D: Prevalence of sperm surface antibodies in the male partners of infertile couples as determined by Immunobead screening. Fertil Steril 1987;48:466.

Peters AJ, Coulam CB:Hysterosalpingography with color Doppler ultrasonography. Am J Obstet Gynecol 1991;164:1530.

Peters AJ, Lloyd RP, Coulam CP: Prevalence of out-of-phase endometrial biopsy specimens. Am J Obstet Gynecol 1992;166:1738.

Philipsen T, Hansen BB: Comparative study of hysterosalpingography and laparoscopy in infertile patients. Acta Obstet Gynaecol Scand 1981;60:149.

Pierson RA, Olatunbosum OA, Chizen DR: Ultrasonography and ovulation induction. JSOGC 1995;Aug:739.

Pittaway DE, Winfield AC, Maxson W, et al: Prevention of acute pelvic inflammatory disease after hysterosalpingography: efficacy of doxycycline prophylaxis. Am J Obstet Gynecol 1983;147:623.

Prader A: Testicular size: assessment and clinical importance. Triangle 1966;7:240.

Queenan JT, O'Brien GD, Bairns GD, et al: Ultrasound scanning of the ovaries to detect ovulation. Fertil Steril 1988;34:105.

Rasmussen F, Lindequist S, Larsen C, et al: Therapeutic effect of hysterosalpingography: oil versus water soluble contrast media—a randomized prospective study. Radiology 1991;179:75.

Rosenfeld DL, Garcia CR: A comparison of endometrial histology with simultaneous plasma progesterone determinations in infertile women. Fertil Steril 1976;27:1256.

Scott RT, Hoffman GE: Prognostic assessment of ovarian reserve. Fertil Steril 1995;63:1.

Scott RT, Toner JP, Muasher SJ, et al: Follicle stimulating hormone level on day 3: a predictor of in vitro fertilization outcome. Fertil Steril 1989;51:751.

Scudamore IW, Dunphy BC, Cooke ID: Falloposcopic comparison of unilateral and bilateral proximal tubal occlusive disease. Hum Reprod 1994;9:340.

Shoupe D, Mishell DR Jr, Lacarra M, et al: Correlation of endometrial maturation with four methods of estimating day of ovulation. Obstet Gynecol 1989;73:88.

Siegler AM: Hysterography and hysteroscopy in the infertile patient. J Reprod Med 1977;18:143.

Simoni M, Carani C, Gromoll J, et al: Screening for deletions of the Y chromosome involving the DAZ (Deleted in Azoospermia) gene in azoospermia and severe oligozoospermia. Fertil Steril 1997;67:542.

Smotrica DB, Widra EA, Gindoff PR, et al: Prognostic value of day 3 estradiol on in vitro fertilization outcome. Fertil Steril 1995;64:136.

Soules MR, McLachlan RI, Ek M, et al: Luteal phase deficiency: characterization of reproductive hormones over the menstrual cycle. J Clin Endocrinol Metab 1989;69:804.

Speert H: Obstetric and Gynecologic Milestones. New York: Macmillan, 1958:271.

Speroff L, Glass RH, Kase NG: Clinical Gynecologic Endocrinology and Infertility. 4th ed. Balimore: Williams & Wilkins, 1989:516.

Stern J, Peters AJ, Coulam CB: Color Doppler ultrasonography assessment of tubal patency: a comparison study with traditional techniques. Fertil Steril 1992;58:897.

Stillman RJ: In vitro exposure to diethylstilbestrol: adverse effect on the reproductive tract and reproductive performance in male and female offspring. Am J Obstet Gynecol 1982;142:905.

Stillman RJ, Rosenberg MJ, Sachs BP: Smoking and reproduction. Fertil Steril 1986;46:545.

Stock RJ: Histopathology of fallopian tubes with recurrent tubal pregnancy. Obstet Gynecol 1990;75:9.

Stumpf PG, March CM: Febrile morbidity following hysterosalpingography: identification of risk factors and recommendations for prophylaxis. Fertil Steril 1980;33:487.

Taylor PJ, Leader A, Pattison HA: Diagnostic hysteroscopy. In Hunt RB (ed): Atlas of Female Infertility Surgery. Chicago: Year Book, 1986:182.

Toner JP, Philput CP, Jones CS, et al: Basal follicle stimulation hormone levels as a better predictor of in vitro fertilization performance than age. Fertil Steril 1991;55:784.

Wallach E: Pitfalls in evaluating in ovarian reserve. Fertil Steril 1995;63:12.

Wentz AC, Kossoy L, Parker RA: The impact of luteal phase inadequacy in an infertile population. Am J Obstet Gynecol 1990;162:937.

Wolf JP, Rodrigues TL, Bulwa S, et al: Fertilizing ability of sperm with unexplained in vitro fertilization failures, as assessed by the zona-free hamster egg penetration assay: its prognostic value for sperm-oolemma interaction. Fertil Steril 1996;65:1196.

World Health Organization: WHO Laboratory Manual for the Examination of Human Semen and Semen-Cervical Mucus Interaction. Cambridge: Cambridge University Press, 1992:44.

Zaneveld LJD, Jeyendran RS: Sperm function tests. Infertil Reprod Clin North Am 1992;3:353.

14

Medical Management of Infertility

Basil Ho Yuen

Ovulation Induction

Disorders of ovulation are common causes of infertility that can be effectively treated with ovulation-inducing agents. In anovulatory women, ovulation induction therapy restores fertility to that of a normal population (Hull et al, 1982). The role of ovulation induction in the management of infertile women with anovulatory states included in World Health Organization (WHO) Groups I through III are discussed in this chapter. The three relevant groups of WHO anovulatory states are summarized as follows:

Who Group I: These women are estrogen deficient with nonelevated follicle-stimulating hormone (FSH) and prolactin levels and no space-occupying lesion in the hypothalamic-pituitary region. They have amenorrhea and do not bleed in response to progestin challenge.

Who Group II: These women are not estrogen deficient and they have nonelevated FSH and prolactin levels. They typically experience oligomenorrhea but they may have anovulatory cycles or amenorrhea with bleeding in response to a progestin challenge. Included in this group are women with polycystic ovary syndrome (PCOS).

WHO Group III: These women are estrogen deficient with elevated FSH levels but nonelevated prolactin levels. They have amenorrhea and may experience vasomotor symptoms typical of ovarian failure.

Groups I and II are common anovulatory groups. Group III women with ovarian failure are not amenable to successful stimulation (O'Herlihy et al, 1980; Surrey and Cedars, 1989) but can be treated with oocyte donation.

PRE-TREATMENT CONSIDERATIONS

Whenever possible, identifiable factors known to cause or suspected of causing anovulation should be eliminated before pharmacologic treatment. For example, underweight or overweight women should attempt to normalize their weight, nutritional problems should be corrected, and, whenever feasible, stress should be alleviated. If excess exercise is a factor, this should be corrected as well. When employing complicated ovulation protocols, such as one in which human menopausal gonadotropin (hMG) or a FSH preparation is used, treatment should be carried out in a facility equipped for undertaking such treatment protocols.

AGENTS USED IN THE INDUCTION OF OVULATION

Clomiphene Citrate

Clomiphene citrate (CC) is a triphenylethylene derivative that possesses estrogen agonist and antagonist actions. Since its introduction into clinical use in the 1960s, CC has become widely used as the first-line agent in ovulation induction therapy. CC is well absorbed from the gastrointestinal tract and slowly cleared from the circulation. The compound is supplied as a racemic mixture of chemical isomers—enclomiphene and zuclomiphene. Enclomiphene possesses the greater estrogen-antagonistic actions. Clomiphene can be detected in the circulation up to 1 month after an oral dose (Mikkelson et al, 1986). The compound is excreted in the feces (Schreiber et al, 1966) and has been shown to enter the ovarian follicular fluid (Oelsner et al, 1986). CC binds and occupies estrogen receptors for several weeks.

The mechanism by which CC stimulates follicular maturation and ovulation is not fully understood. An important site of action is at the hypothalamic-pituitary axis, where the antiestrogenic action of CC, at the level of the hypothalamus, blocks the negative feedback response to estrogen. As a result, there is an augmentation of gonadotropin release (Clark and Markaverich, 1982). The increased luteinizing hormone (LH) pulse frequency in response to CC is consistent with a hypothalamic mode of action involving increased gonadotropin-releasing hormone (GnRH) release (Kerin et al, 1985). Follicular maturation occurs in response to the enhanced gonadotropin production. Estradiol (E_2) secretion then increases within normal or supraphysiologic levels 5 to 10 days after the last tablet (Fedele et al, 1989). The midcycle LH surge resulting from the rising E_2 levels triggers ovulation and luteinization of mature follicles.

CC also exerts pharmacologic effects in the genital tract. In vitro, CC inhibits progesterone production from human granulosa cells in a dose-dependent manner, suggesting a role in the luteal defects associated with treatment (Ho Yuen et al, 1988). Antiestrogenic actions of CC have been observed in the uterus, cervix, and vagina (Clark and Markaverich, 1982). Collectively, these effects (referred to as the "antifertility" actions of CC) imply that CC may interfere with normal endometrial maturation, cervical mucus production, and luteal function.

Indications

The most useful indication for CC is in WHO Group II women, in whom high ovulation rates can be expected. In contrast, in WHO Group I women, who lack endogenous estrogen production, ovulation rates in response to CC appear lower; however, this does not preclude the use of clomiphene in this group of women. Spellacy and Cohen (1967) reported good results in this group of women, with an 80% rate of ovulation and a 35% pregnancy rate. Without a previous history of CC unresponsiveness, a course of CC could be tried in WHO Group I women before proceeding to more complicated agents such as pulsatile GnRH and exogenous gonadotropins.

Contraindications

Pregnancy, liver disease, undiagnosed genital tract and breast disease, a history of hypersensitivity or untoward side effects in response to CC, and ovarian failure are contraindications to the use of CC.

Method of Administration and Monitoring of Treatment

CC may be commenced between the second and the fifth day of a spontaneous or progestin-induced vaginal bleed without affecting the outcome of treatment (Wu and Winkel, 1989). The starting dose is 50 mg daily for 5 days, with the cycle monitored by basal body temperature (BBT) records and luteal progesterone levels. If anovulation persists, the dose may be increased by 50-mg increments to 200 mg daily over three to four treatment cycles. In patients with a tendency to developing ovarian enlargement, pain, and other side effects, treatment may be initiated at lower doses (Dodge et al, 1986). In response to CC, 80% of anovulatory women ovulate and about 40%

conceive within six ovulatory cycles on CC. Approximately 50% of pregnancies are conceived at the starting dose of 50 mg daily for 5 days, with an additional 20% of ovulating women achieving pregnancy at the 100-mg dose level. Thus 70% of women conceiving with the use of CC achieve this at daily doses of between 50 and 100 mg (Gysler et al, 1982). Few additional pregnancies will be conceived by increasing the daily dose up to 200 mg or more for 5 days. In a review of 14 publications appearing between 1964 and 1983, ovulation occurred in 74% of 8229 patients with ovulatory dysfunction treated with CC, with 31% of these women conceiving pregnancy (Gillis, 1996). Overweight women require a higher dose of CC to achieve ovulation (Shepard et al, 1979). If pregnancy is not conceived after three or four ovulatory cycles of CC, treatment should be discontinued and alternate forms of therapy considered. Pelvic examination and ultrasonography may be required if ovarian enlargement is suspected. Additional dose increases are not required in the presence of regular ovulatory cycles, biphasic BBTs, or midluteal progesterone values of 15 ng/ml (48 nmol/l) or greater (Radwanska and Swyer, 1974).

Use of Glucocorticoids

In anovulation associated with elevated androgens (the PCOS subset of WHO Group II), daily low-dose glucocorticoid therapy suppressed serum levels of LH, testosterone, androstenedione, and adrenal androgens (Ho Yuen and Mincey, 1983), with resumption of spontaneous ovulation; conception of pregnancy can follow without any other treatment. If ovulation has not occurred by 1 month after starting a glucocorticoid, CC may be added in standard doses while the glucocorticoid is continued. Higher ovulation and conception rates occurred in hyperandrogenic women when CC was given with dexamethasone (Daly et al, 1984). Dexamethasone 0.25 to 0.5 mg or prednisone 5 to 7.5 mg is commenced at night. Because glucocorticoid side effects occur at the higher doses, caution is required when such doses are used. Alternate-day as compared to daily treatment reduces side effects of glucocorticoid therapy in hyperandrogenic women (Avgerinos et al, 1987). Glucocorticoids are discontinued once pregnancy is conceived. If androgen levels remain elevated, treatment should be discontinued and further evaluation undertaken.

Failure to Respond to CC

Empirical use of human chorionic gonadotropin (hCG) 5000 to 10,000 IU given IM about 5 days after the last CC tablet may be followed by ovulation. In some women ovulation is delayed or fails to occur despite apparently adequate preovulatory E_2 levels. Documentation of follicular maturation with E_2 (300 pg/ml [1100 pmol/L] or greater) and ultrasound (leading follicle of 18 mm or greater) allows timing of the administration of hCG to coincide with the time of follicular maturation (Hammond, 1983). If androgen levels are elevated, a trial of glucocorticoid therapy could be helpful if this has not already been tried. In euprolactinemic women exhibiting CC unresponsiveness, there is no convincing evidence that bromocriptine enhances the action of CC. In addition bromocriptine may cause troublesome side effects, so its empiric use is not recommended.

Complications of Treatment

Vasomotor flushes, visual symptoms (10% or more); abdominal bloating or pain (5% or more); nausea, vomiting, irritability, fatigue, headache, and mastalgia (1% to 2%); allergic dermatitis and/or urticaria, weight gain, urinary frequency, constipation, diarrhea, and reversible hair loss (less than 1%) may occur (Gillis, 1996). Multiple pregnancies are conceived in 7.9% of women. The frequency of twins is about 7% and triplets 0.5%. Higher order multiple gestations rarely occur with clomiphene therapy (Adashi, 1986). An association between neural tube defects and ovulation-inducing agents, including CC, was suggested; however, other studies have failed to confirm such an association (Kurachi et al, 1983; Mills et al, 1990; Rosa, 1990).

Pulsatile GnRH

Indications

The most useful indication for pulsatile GnRH is in WHO Group I women in whom endogenous GnRH production is decreased (Coelingh Bennink, 1989; Carr and Reid, 1990). Administration of pulsatile GnRH in WHO Group I women results in ovulation rates of 85% to 95% per treatment cycle, with pregnancy rates of 20% to 30% per cycle, depending on the dose and route of administration. Cumulative conception rates in this group can exceed 90% after six cycles of treatment (Coelingh Bennink, 1989; Carr and Reid, 1990). In women experiencing a failure to respond to pulsatile GnRH, hMG becomes indicated.

In WHO Group II women, pulsatile GnRH is less successful in inducing ovulation. In a series of patients with PCOS, most being treated intravenously, 67% ovulated and 34% conceived (Coelingh Bennink, 1989). The spontaneous abortion rate of 36% included chemical pregnancies.

Contraindications

Significant organic lesions of the brain and/or pituitary, undiagnosed genital tract or breast disease, hypersensitivity to GnRH, ovarian failure, and pregnancy are contraindications to the use of pulsatile GnRH.

Method of Administration and Monitoring of Treatment

Pulses are administered at 60- to 120-minute intervals using a portable infusion pump. Absorption and bioavailability are better with IV therapy (Handelsman et al, 1984); however, disadvantages include local discomfort, the inconvenience of an IV, and the potential for thrombophlebitis. SC administration is more practical and simpler. SC treatment may be initiated at 5 to 10 μg/pulse and increased in increments of 10 μg every 5 days to a maximum of 40 μg/pulse (Carr and Reid, 1990).

With IV therapy, heparin 100 U/ml of diluent is added to maintain patency in the IV line. Because of the greater safety of pulsatile GnRH, the intensive monitoring usually used for exogenous gonadotropin therapy is not needed. Many patients will experience follicular maturation followed by a spontaneous LH surge and ovulation. Once ovulation has been documented, the pump can be discontinued and divided doses of hCG (1000 to 2500 IU) given every 3 to 4 days for luteal support; alternately, the pump can be continued throughout the treatment cycle (Carr and Reid, 1990).

In some women more intensive monitoring may be required. In these cases the ovarian response can be monitored by ultrasonography and rapid serum E_2 assays every few days, followed by a single injection of hCG 5000 to 10,000 IU to trigger ovulation once a dominant follicle (18-mm diameter) and preovulatory E_2 levels (about 300 pg/ml, or 1100 pmol/L) have been documented (Loucopoulous et al, 1984). On this protocol, additional luteal support is not required so the pump can be discontinued once the ovulating dose of hCG has been given.

Complications

Mild ovarian hyperstimulation occurs in about 2.5% of treatment cycles. Multiple gestations (twins and, rarely, higher order multiples) were observed in 13% of conceptions (30 of 231) (Coelingh Bennink, 1989). In response to pulsatile GnRH administration, endogenous GnRH secretion simulates the physiologic pattern, with the maintenance of normal negative feedback mechanisms promoting maturation of a single dominant follicle. Such intrinsic control mechanisms may be overridden by large IV doses or hCG given to trigger ovulation (Bogchelman et al, 1982).

There is a small risk of thrombophlebitis with IV treatment. Cellulitis and infection are rare complications of SC administration. The overall risks of these complications are less than 1% (Hopkins et al, 1989). Urticaria, anaphylaxis, and refractory responses to therapy associated with antibodies to GnRH have occurred sporadically (about 3%) (Coelingh Bennink, 1989; Carr and Reid, 1990). The risk of spontaneous abortion or congenital abnormalities in GnRH-induced pregnancies is not increased (Coelingh Bennink, 1989).

Exogenous Gonadotropins

Indications

The most useful indication for exogenous gonadotropins is failure of other techniques of inducing ovulation. The essential requirements for treatment are patients with responsive ovaries and anatomically intact genital tracts. Currently the preparations of exogenous gonadotropins available for clinical use are derived from the urine of postmenopausal women. Human menopausal gonadotropins contain 75 IU FSH and LH in a 1:1 ratio. Preparations with high FSH content, pure FSH (pFSH), are also available for clinical use. Recombinant FSH preparations will be available for clinical use in the near future. Details concerning patient selection criteria are outlined in Figure 14–1.

Contraindications

High FSH levels (ovarian failure), significant space-occupying lesions of the brain or pituitary, undiagnosed genital tract and breast pathology, hypersensi-

tivity to gonadotropin preparations, and pregnancy are contraindications to exogenous gonadotropins.

Method of Administration and Monitoring of Treatment

The individually adjusted scheme for exogenous gonadotropin administration (Brown, 1986) allows for the close monitoring of the response and the capability of making adjustments in treatment according to the response of the individual woman. The usual starting dose of hMG is between 75 and 225 IU given IM (or SC, depending on preparation), adjusted according to the serum E_2 response. As follicular maturation progresses, ultrasound findings and E_2 levels are employed to decide on further dose adjustments and when to stop hMG and induce ovulation with hCG (Fig. 14–2).

Overweight women require higher doses of hMG to induce ovulation, and they experience lower success rates. Lower pregnancy rates occur in women over 80 kg in weight (Hardiman and Ginsberg, 1996). Thus weight reduction is useful if it can be achieved before treatment is begun. In WHO Group I women,

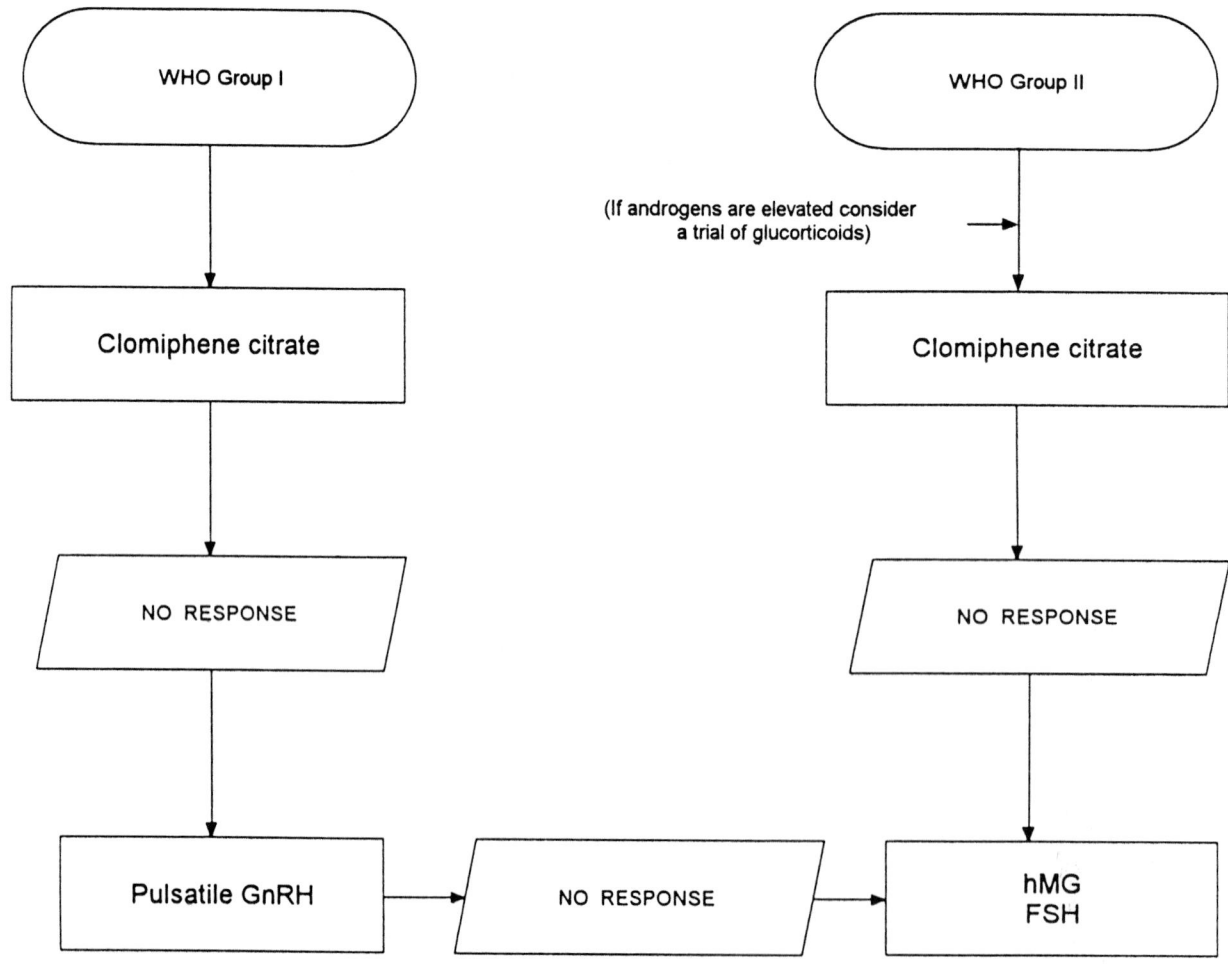

Figure 14–1
Management of WHO Group I and Group II anovulation.

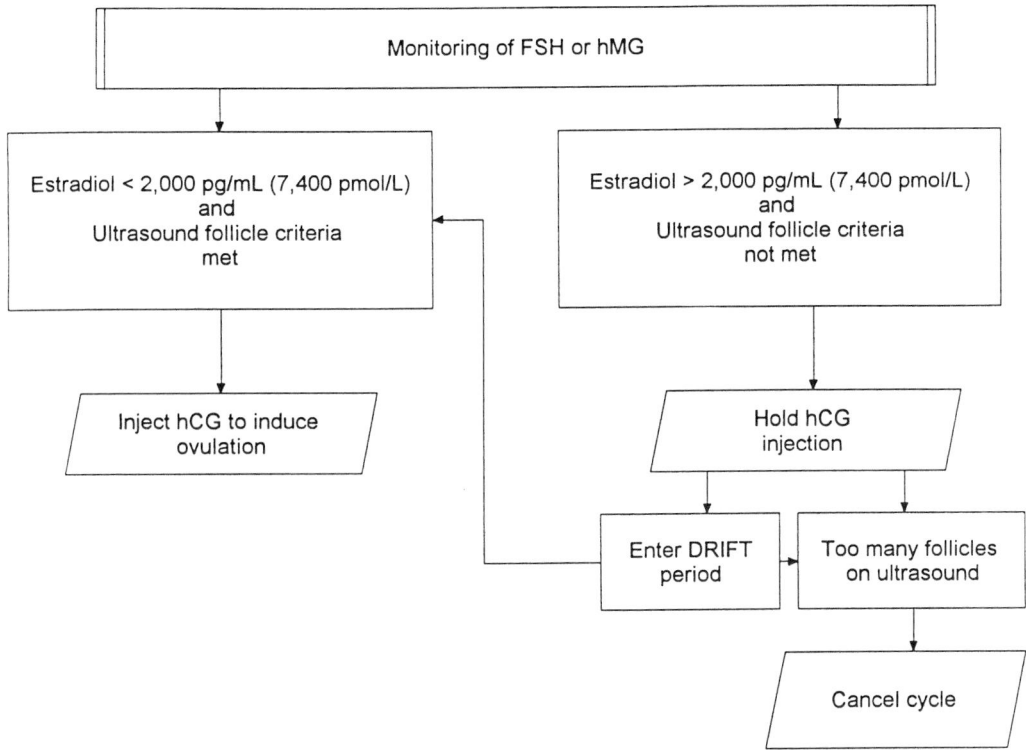

Figure 14-2
Monitoring scheme for administration of exogenous gonadotropins.

the requirements for hMG given IM appear higher, regardless of body weight (Chong et al, 1986).

The routine monitoring of the ovarian response to hMG stimulation is based on frequent serum E_2 assays and transvaginal ultrasound used in a complementary manner. Higher ovulation rates occurred when estrogen levels were stimulated above the normal range (Brown, 1986). Multiple ovarian follicular development seen on ultrasound occurred in 80% of gonadotropin-stimulated cycles as compared to 5% to 10% of natural cycles (Ritchie, 1985). There is a narrow margin of safety between the clinically effective dose of hMG that results in successful uncomplicated stimulation and doses that can cause complications, notably ovarian hyperstimulation syndrome (OHSS) and multiple pregnancy.

During the phase of active follicular growth, it is ideal to see patients daily. When E_2 reaches or exceeds 500 pg/ml (approximately 1500 to 2000 pmol/L), monitoring with ovarian ultrasound can be initiated. Stimulation is then continued to reach a level of E_2 around 1000 to 1500 pg/ml (3700 to (5500 pmol/L) (Ho Yuen et al, 1981; Ho Yuen and Pride, 1990; and Leader, 1994), with two to three leading follicles greater than 14 mm in diameter. Previous experience (summarized in Table 14-1) has shown that, with E2 levels between 1000 and 1500 pg/ml (3700 to 5500 pmol/L) at the time of giving hCG, high rates of ovulation can be expected. The likelihood of severe OHSS is reduced if the woman ovulates with hCG at E_2 levels below 1000 pg/ml (3700

pmol/L). Further details of monitoring treatment and cycle management are outlined in Figure 14-2.

If the follicular sizes on ultrasound do not meet the criteria noted, stimulation may be continued provided E_2 levels do not exceed 2000 pg/ml (7400 pmol/L). When ultrasound criteria are met at lower E_2 levels, the ovulating dose of hCG is administered. A single 10,000-IU dose of hCG is usually injected, and intercourse is advised on the day of hCG administration and for 2 to 3 days thereafter. Because multiple doses of hCG may increase the risk of OHSS, a single dose of hCG is preferred. The luteal phase is monitored with a basal temperature record and progesterone level 5 to 7 days after the ovulating

Table 14-1. RATES OF OVULATION AT VARIOUS ESTRADIOL LEVELS

CIRCULATING ESTRADIOL WHEN hCG GIVEN		CYCLES OVULATING	
pg/ml	pmol/L	Number	Per Cent
<500	<1800	5/10	50
500–1000	1800–3700	20/25	80
1000–1500	3700–5500	18/18	100
>1500	>5500	3/3	100

(Adapted from Ho Yuen B, Sy L, Cannon W: Regulation of ovarian and luteal function during treatment with exogenous gonadotropins in anovulatory infertility. Am J Obstet Gynecol 1981;140:629, with permission.)

dose of hCG. If pregnancy is conceived, an ultrasound scan is arranged 6 weeks after ovulation.

Abundant small follicles (11 or more, 5 to 8 mm in diameter) and intermediate-size follicles (9 to 15 mm in diameter) at the time of hCG correlate with a higher rate of ovarian hyperstimulation (Blankstein et al, 1987; Golan et al, 1990), and the cycle may have to be aborted, especially if the estrogen levels exceed acceptable limits. Leader (1994) recommended the cycle be cancelled, with the avoidance of intercourse, when the total number of follicles in both ovaries exceeds 30, especially when E_2 levels are high (defined as exceeding 6000 pmol/L). For further details on cycle monitoring and complications, the reader is referred to reviews by Ho Yuen and Pride (1990), Pride et al (1990), and Leader (1994).

In an attempt to avoid cancellation of biochemically overstimulated cycles (E_2 exceeding 5400 pmol/L), a series of WHO Group II patients were managed by a controlled drift period (Urman et al, 1992). This involved a schedule where further hMG injections were withheld but monitoring continued with daily assays of serum E_2 and frequent follicular ultrasound examinations. The mean E_2 level at the start of the drift, was 9249 pmol/L, dropped to safer levels (average 2945 pmol/L, a drop of 64%). After a drift period of 1 to 8 days (average 2.8 days), the ovulating dose of hCG was given. The clinical pregnancy rate per cycle was 25%, the multiple pregnancy rate was 50% (twins in all instances), and the severe OHSS rate was 2.5%. During the drift, the number of lead follicles continues to increase in size in spite of declining E_2 concentrations. Caution and experience are required when attempting the drift method.

Results of Treatment

In WHO Group I women, a cumulative pregnancy rate of 89% after six treatment cycles is contrasted with a cumulative pregnancy rate of 43% over the same duration of treatment in WHO Group II women, with a per cycle fecundity of 26% in WHO group I and 10% in WHO group II (Fluker et al, 1994). Insler (1988) tabulated pregnancy rates from a total of 2791 pregnancies. The overall per cycle fecundity was 14.3%, with a conception rate of 34.7% per patient.

The better success in response to ovulation induction in Group I women as compared to Group II women is well documented (Ho Yuen and Pride, 1990), but the reasons for this difference are not fully understood. In patients with PCOS and in superovulatory states, androgens have been associated with impaired folliculogenesis, atresia, and poor oocyte quality (McNatty et al, 1979; Coney, 1984; Moon et al, 1990). The high endogenous LH levels present in PCOS patients may also contribute to the poor outcome in this group, because excess LH induces precocious oocyte maturation and impairs oocyte quality (Howles et al, 1986; Homburg et al, 1988).

Pulsatile Administration of Gonadotropins

Pulsatile administration may be an option for women in poor prognostic categories (usually WHO Group II) who exhibit erratic responses to the IM route of administration (Ho Yuen et al, 1989). In addition, pulsatile IV administration had a significant dose-sparing action as compared to the IM route. Ovulation can also be induced by pulsatile SC administration of hMG and pFSH (Nakamura et al, 1986, 1989).

PURE FSH

Because of the elevated ratio of LH to FSH in PCOS and the potential for high endogenous LH levels in compromising oocyte quality, the low LH content in pFSH preparations provides a theoretical advantage for anovulatory PCOS patients. However, proof of the expected superiority of pFSH in terms of pregnancy rates has remained elusive. Venturoli and associates (1987) were unable to demonstrate significant advantages of pFSH over hMG in PCOS patients. When a slow protocol with pFSH was compared to a conventional protocol in women with PCOS, the slow protocol resulted in a longer duration of stimulation, development of more single as opposed to multiple follicles, and fewer cancelled cycles as a result of concerns for hyperstimulation without a significantly improved pregnancy rate (Buvat et al, 1989). In a series of PCOS patients, a low-dose regimen of pFSH (as compared to a conventional protocol) eliminated complications associated with ovarian hyperstimulation and multiple pregnancies; however, the pregnancy rates were not significantly improved (Homburg et al, 1995a). The slow pFSH protocol confer some advantages over the conventional protocol, but these protocols do not improve the pregnancy rates. In patients with PCOS, SC pulsatile pFSH had a dose-sparing action as compared to hMG given in a similar manner (Nakamura et al, 1989).

In women undergoing in vitro fertilization (IVF) treatment (Out et al, 1995), lower doses of recombinant FSH, as compared to urinary FSH, resulted in the retrieval of a larger number of oocytes. Pregnancy rates in cycles receiving fresh embryos were not significantly different. However, when data from thawed frozen embryo replacements were included, the combined (fresh plus frozen thawed) pregnancy rate for recombinant FSH was significantly higher.

hMG COMBINED WITH CC

When CC 100 mg daily for 7 days was used followed by hMG given daily using a variable dosage regimen, the rate of ovulation was increased and the dose of hMG used per cycle was decreased by about 50%, but pregnancy rates were not improved (Jarrell et al, 1981).

GnRH ANALOGS COMBINED WITH hMG

Use of GnRH analogs in WHO Group II women can effectively eliminate the premature LH surge and potentially synchronize follicular development in response to stimulation with exogenous gonadotropins. To date, in prospective controlled studies, the adjunctive use of GnRH analogs with exogenous gonadotropins in WHO Group II women have not been shown to improve pregnancy rates or complications such as OHSS (Dodson et al, 1987; Dodson, 1990). Retrospective studies suggest that GnRH analog co-treatment reduces the miscarriage rates in women with PCOS undergoing ovulation induction with hMG (Homburg et al, 1993).

GROWTH HORMONE COMBINED WITH hMG

Women with PCOS exhibit altered growth hormone (GH) kinetics. In a trial comparing the effects of GH as an adjunct to GnRH and hMG for ovulation induction in PCOS, no clinically beneficial effects of GH co-treatment could be demonstrated (Homburg et al, 1995b). Co-treatment with GH and hMG in WHO Group I patients showed that the addition of GH reduced the gonadotropin dose needed to achieve ovulation (European and Australian Multicentre Study, 1995).

Complications of Gonadotropin Treatment

Multiple Pregnancies. hMG resulted in an overall multiple pregnancy rate of 26.6%, with rates for triplets 3.5%, quadruplets 1%, and quintuplets 0.3% (Blankstein et al, 1984). A more recent series noted an overall multiple pregnancy rate of 16%, with a rate of 22% in WHO Group I women and 13% in WHO Group II women (Fluker et al, 1994). In high multiple pregnancies (triplets or higher), selective reduction of pregnancy offers an alternate to aborting the entire pregnancy (Lynch and Berkowitz, 1990).

Ectopic Pregnancy. The incidence of ectopic pregnancy conceived in women during exogenous gonadotropin therapy was reported to be 2.7% (Gemzell et al, 1982).

Spontaneous Abortion. The overall spontaneous abortion rate has been found to be about 28%. Women in WHO Group II may experience higher spontaneous loss rates as compared to those in Group I (Oelsner et al, 1978; Ben-Rafael et al, 1983; Fluker et al, 1994).

Ovarian Hyperstimulation Syndrome. Mild, moderate, and severe ovarian hyperstimulation rates vary between 8.4% and 23%, 0.5% and 7%, and 0.5%

and 6.5%, respectively (Golan et al, 1989; Pride et al, 1990).

Congenital Abnormalities. As noted earlier, ovulation-inducing agents, including exogenous gonadotropins, have not been shown to increase the rates of congenital abnormalities (Thompson and Hansen, 1970; Kurachi et al, 1983; Lunenfeld and Lunenfeld, 1989; Mills et al, 1990; Rosa, 1990).

Sex Ratio. There is no difference in the sex ratio (male to female births) in conceptions following exogenous gonadotropin therapy as compared to spontaneous conception of pregnancy (Lunenfeld and Lunenfeld, 1989; Murphy and Seagroat, 1989).

PREMATURE OVARIAN FAILURE (WHO GROUP III)

Premature ovarian failure may be defined as hypergonadotropic hypogonadism and amenorrhea occurring before age 40. Women with ovarian failure may exhibit spontaneous remissions during which ovarian function may resume, with spontaneous conception of pregnancy occurring. In a series 63 women with secondary amenorrhea (referred to as secondary ovarian failure), etiologic factors were chromosomal abnormality in 2 (3%), surgery in 16 (18%), chemotherapy in 3 (5%), idiopathic in 29 (46%), autoimmune in 11 (18%), and radiation in 1 (<1%). Of these 63 women, 7 (11%) ovulated. One woman ovulated spontaneously, with the remaining six women ovulating after receiving estrogen-progestin replacement treatment. The prognosis for ovulation was better in women whose ovarian failure was associated with surgery or chemotherapy. Three women (5%) conceived. A trial of estrogen-progestin therapy should be considered before more invasive treatment such as oocyte donation. In another 23 women with primary amenorrhea (referred to as primary ovarian failure), none of the women ovulated (Kreiner et al, 1988).

Attempts at stimulating ovulation with exogenous gonadotropins in a placebo-controlled trial of women with ovarian failure demonstrated that follicular maturation and rates of ovulation during gonadotropin treatment did not differ significantly from those seen during placebo treatment (van Kasteren et al, 1995). These results are consistent with other attempts at inducing ovulation with gonadotropins in ovarian failure patients (Surrey and Cedars, 1989).

For women with premature ovarian failure, the use of oocyte donor procedures is of benefit. Indications for oocyte donation include women with impaired or absent ovarian function from a number of causes, including premature ovarian failure, gonadal dysgenesis, previous radiation or chemotherapy, and previous ovarian surgery. The donor undergoes superovulation followed by oocyte retrieval as in conventional IVF treatment. The donor oocytes are then inseminated in vitro with sperm from the recipient's partner. The embryos are then transferred to the recipient's uterus either during a cycle that is hormonally synchronized with that of the donor, or at a later date after cryopreservation. The replacement of "fresh embryos" usually results in better pregnancy rates than do embryos subjected to cryopreservation.

The results of donor oocyte IVF/embryo transfer performed in the United States and Canada in 1992 (Assisted Reproductive Technology in the United States and Canada, 1992) revealed a higher pregnancy rate in donor oocyte cycles (37% per transfer, 625 of 1699) as compared to IVF (24% per transfer, 5279 of 21,870). The miscarriage rates were 15% for donor cycles versus 20% for IVF. Multiple pregnancy rates were 37% for donor oocytes and 33% for IVF. Further information on oocyte donor procedures can be found in the review by Moomjy et al (1995).

OVARIAN CANCER

A report in 1992 based on findings from a combined analysis of 12 U.S. case-control studies of ovarian cancer by the Collaborative Ovarian Cancer Group raised concerns about the possible increased risk of ovarian cancer associated with the use of ovulation-inducing agents. Pooled data from three studies that collected data on the previous use of fertility medications suggested increased risks for invasive epithelial tumors (odds ratio of 2.8, 95% confidence interval 1.3 to 6.1) (Whittemore et al, 1992), borderline epithelial tumors (Harris et al, 1992), and nonepithelial cancers (Horn-Ross et al, 1992) in infertile women who used fertility medications as compared to women without a diagnosis of infertility and fertility drug treatment. Using a population-based cancer registry and record linkage, Rossing et al (1994) reported a higher risk of borderline or invasive ovarian tumors in infertile women undergoing prolonged treatment with clomiphene. Clomiphene treatment in excess of 12 cycles increased this risk, whereas durations less than this interval with this agent and hMG did not increase this risk. A nationwide case-control study from Israel (Shushan et al, 1996) found that the use of hMG elevated the risk in a subgroup of women with borderline epithelial ovarian cancer. Venn et al (1995) studied Australian women undergoing IVF ovulation induction and compared them with a control group (infertile women enrolled for IVF but not receiving treatment for a number of reasons and those undergoing "natural cycle" IVF). The risk of ovarian cancer was not significantly increased in IVF patients.

These studies are limited by a number of factors that should be taken into consideration when interpreting the results. There may be recall bias (patients with infertility are more likely to report fertility drug use than controls), and information on the type of drug used, the duration of exposure, the duration of follow-up, rates of ovariectomy in groups of women compared, and the control group used for comparison are often not available. In some studies the control groups were women without a diagnosis of infertility. Because infertility is a risk factor for ovarian cancer, such studies may overestimate this risk. Potential confounding factors, such as the prevalence of oral contraceptive usage (protective effect), parity (protective effect), and other factors that could potentially influence the risk of developing ovarian cancer were not fully excluded. The number of women taking fertility medications in the published studies was small, so the attempts at estimating risks must be considered imprecise. The information available on the etiology of infertility is also limited, so effects of treatment of ovarian abnormalities that increase the cancer risk in the women to start with cannot be defined. At the present time this is a controversial and unresolved matter awaiting future definitive studies (for further details, see review by Bristow and Karlan, 1996). The practical implication for the clinician is to provide appropriate counseling for women being offered ovulation induction therapy, to carefully select women who may benefit from such treatment, to limit the overexposure of individual women to stimulation cycles, and to have a high degree of suspicion for the possibility of ovarian cancer before, during, and after ovulation induction therapy.

REFERENCES

Adashi E: Clomiphene citrate-initiated ovulation: a clinical update. Semin Reprod Endocrinol 1986;4:255.

Assisted Reproductive Technology in the United States and Canada: 1992 results generated from the American Fertility Society/Society for Assisted Reproductive Technology Registry. Fertil Steril 1994;62:1121.

Avgerinos P, Cutler G, Tsokos G, et al: Dissociation between cortisol and adrenal androgen secretion in patients receiving alternate day prednisone therapy. J Clin Endocrinol Metab 1987; 65:24.

Ben-Rafael Z, Dor J, Mashiach S, et al: Abortion rate in pregnancies following ovulation induced by human menopausal gonadotropin/human chorionic gonadotropin. Fertil Steril 1983; 39:157.

Blankstein J, Mashiach S, Lunenfeld B: Ovulation Induction and In-Vitro Fertilization. Chicago: Year Book Medical Publishers, 1984:111.

Blankstein J, Shalev J, Saadon T, et al: Ovarian hyperstimulation syndrome: prediction by number and size of preovulatory follicles. Fertil Steril 1987;47:597.

Bogchelman D, Lappohn RE, Janssens JL: Triplet pregnancy after pulsatile administration of gonadotrophin releasing hormone. Lancet 1982;2:45.

Bristow RE, Karlan BY: Ovulation induction, infertility and ovarian cancer risk. Fertil Steril 1996;66:499.

Brown JB: Gonadotropins. In Insler V, Lunenfeld B (eds): Infertility: Male and Female. New York: Churchill Livingstone, 1986: 359.

Buvat J, Buvat-Herbaut M, Marcolin G, et al: Purified follicle-stimulating hormone in polycystic ovary syndrome. Fertil Steril 1989;52:553.

Carr SJ, Reid R: Ovulation induction with gonadotropin-releasing hormone (GnRH). Semin Reprod Endocrinol 1990;8:174.

Chong AP, Rafael RW, Forte CC: Influence of weight in the induction of ovulation with menopausal gonadotropin and human chorionic gonadotropin. Fertil Steril 1986;46:599.

Clark JH, Markaverich BM: The agonist-antagonist properties of clomiphene: a review. Pharmacol Ther 1982;15:476.

Coelingh Bennink HJT: Pulsatile administration of LHRH for induction of ovulation. In Shaw RW, Marshall JC (eds): LHRH and its Analogues. Toronto: Wright, 1989:92.

Coney P: Polycystic ovarian disease: current concepts of pathophysiology and therapy. Fertil Steril 1984;46:667.

Daly DC, Walters C, Soto-Albors C, et al: A randomized study of dexamethasone in ovulation induction with clomiphene citrate. Fertil Steril 1984;41:844.

Dodge S, Strickler R, Keller D: Ovulation induction with low doses of clomiphene citrate. Obstet Gynecol 1986;67(3 Suppl):63S.

Dodson WC: Gonadotropin-releasing hormone (GnRH) analogs as adjunctive therapy in ovulation induction. Semin Reprod Endocrinol 1990;8:198.

Dodson WC, Hughes CL, Whitesides DB, Haney AF: The effect of leuprolide acetate on ovulation induction with human menopausal gonadotropins in polycystic ovary syndrome. J Clin Endocrinol Metab 1987;65:95.

European and Australian Multicentre Study: Cotreatment with growth hormone and gonadotropin for ovulation induction in hypogonadotropic patients: a prospective, randomized, placebo-controlled, dose-response study. European and Australian Multicenter Study. Fertil Steril 1995;64:917.

Fedele L, Brioschi D, Marchini M, et al: Enhanced preovulatory progesterone levels in clomiphene citrate-induced cycles. J Clin Endocrinol Metab 1989;69:681.

Fluker MR, Urman B, MacKinnon M, et al: Exogenous gonadotropin therapy in World Health Organization Groups I and II ovulatory disorders. Obstet Gynecol 1994;83:189.

Gemzell C, Guillome J, Wang CF: Ectopic pregnancy following treatment with gonadotropins. Am J Obstet Gynecol 1982;143:761.

Gillis MC (ed): Compendium of Pharmaceuticals and Specialties. Ottawa: Canadian Pharmaceutical Association, 1996:1345.

Golan A, Ron-El R, Herman A, et al: Ovarian hyperstimulation syndrome: an update review. Obstet Gynecol Surv 1989;44:430.

Gysler M, March C, Mishell D, Bailey E: A decade's experience with an individualized clomiphene treatment regimen including its effects on the postcoital test. Fertil Steril 1982;37:161.

Hammond MG, Halme JK, Talbert LM: Factors affecting the pregnancy rate in clomiphene citrate induced ovulation. Obstet Gynecol 1983;62:196.

Handelsman DJ, Jansen RPS, Boylan LM, et al: Pharmacokinetics of gonadotropin-releasing hormone: comparison of subcutaneous and intravenous routes. J Clin Endocrinol Metab 1984;59:739.

Hardiman P, Ginsberg J: Ovulation induction. In Ginsberg J (ed): Drug Therapy in Reproductive Endocrinology and Infertility. London: Arnold, 1996:86.

Harris R, Whittemore AS, Itnyre J, for the Collaborative Ovarian Cancer Group: Characteristics relating to ovarian cancer risk: collaborative analysis of 12 US case-control studies. III. Epithelial tumors of low malignant potential in white women. Am J Epidemiol 1992;136:1204.

Ho Yuen B, Mari N, Duleba A, Moon YS: Direct effects of clomiphene citrate on the steroidogenic capability of human granulosa cells. Fertil Steril 1988;49:626.

Ho Yuen B, Mincey E: Role of androgens in menstrual disorders of nonhirsute women, and the effect of glucocorticoid therapy on androgen levels in hyperandrogenic women. Am J Obstet Gynecol 1983;145:152.

Ho Yuen B, Pride SM: Induction of ovulation with exogenous gonadotropins in anovulatory infertile women. Semin Reprod Endocrinol 1990;8:186.

Ho Yuen B, Pride SM, Burch-Callegari P, et al: Clinical and endocrine response to pulsatile intravenous gonadotropins in refractory anovulation. Obstet Gynecol 1989;74:763.

Ho Yuen B, Sy L, Cannon W: Regulation of ovarian and luteal function during treatment with exogenous gonadotropins in anovulatory infertility. Am J Obstet Gynecol 1981;140:629.

Homburg R, Armar N, Eshel A, et al: Influence of serum luteinising hormone concentrations on ovulation, conception, and early pregnancy loss in polycystic ovary syndrome. Br Med J 1988;297:204.

Homburg R, Levy T, Ben-Rafael Z: A comparative prospective study of conventional regimen with chronic low-dose follicle-stimulating hormone for anovulation associated with polycystic ovary syndrome. Fertil Steril 1995a;63:729.

Homburg R, Levy T, Ben-Rafael Z: Adjuvant growth hormone for induction of ovulation with gonadotrophin-releasing hormone agonist and gonadotrophins in polycystic ovary syndrome: a randomized, double-blind, placebo controlled trial. Hum Reprod 1995b;10:2550.

Homburg R, Levy T, Berkovitz D, et al: Gonadotropin-releasing hormone agonist reduces the miscarriage rate for pregnancies achieved in women with polycystic ovarian syndrome. Fertil Steril 1993;59:527.

Hopkins CC, Hall JE, Santoro NF, et al: Closed intravenous administration of gonadotropin-releasing hormone: safety of extended peripheral intravenous catheterization. Obstet Gynecol 1989;74:267.

Horn-Ross PL, Whittemore AS, Harris R, Itnyre J, for the Collaborative Cancer Group: Characteristics relating to ovarian risk: collaborative analyis of 12 US case-control studies. VI. Nonepithelial cancers among adults. Epidemiology 1992;3:490.

Howles CM, Macnamee MC, Edwards RG, et al: Effect of high tonic levels of luteinizing hormone on outcome of in-vitro fertilization. Lancet 1986;1:521.

Hull MRG, Savage PE, Bromham DR: Anovulatory and ovulatory infertility: results with simplified management. Br Med J 1982;284:1681.

Insler V: Gonadotropin therapy: new trends and insights. Int J Fertil 1988;33:85.

Jarrell J, McInnes R, Cooke R, Arronet G: Observations on the combination of clomiphene citrate-human menopausal gonadotropin-human chorionic gonadotropin in the management of anovulation. Fertil Steril 1981;35:634.

Kerin JF, Liu JH, Phillipou G, Yen SSC: Evidence for a hypothalamic site of action of clomiphene citrate in women. J Clin Endorinol Metab 1985;61:265.

Kreiner D, Droesch K, Navot D, et al: Spontaneous and pharmacological induced remissions in patients with ovarian failure. Obstet Gynecol 1988;72:926.

Kurachi K, Aano T, Minagawa T, Miyake A: Congenital malformations of newborn infants after clomiphene induced ovulation. Fertil Steril 1983;40:187.

Leader A: Ovarian hyperstimulation syndrome. J SOGC 1994;16:1895.

Loucopoulous A, Ferin M, Vande Wiele R, et al: Pulsatile administration of gonadotropin-releasing hormone for induction of ovulation. Am J Obstet Gynecol 1984;148:895.

Lunenfeld B, Lunenfeld E: Ovulation induction: HMG. In Seibel MM (ed): A Comprehensive Text. Norwalk, CT: Appleton & Lange, 1989:311.

Lynch B, Berkowitz RL: Multiple pregnancy reduction. Semin Reprod Endocrinol 1990;8:242.

McNatty KP, Smith DM, Makris A, et al: The microenvironment of the human antral follicle: interrelationships among the steroid levels in antral fluid, the population of granulosa cells, and the status of the oocyte in vivo and in vitro. J Clin Endocrinol Metab 1979;49:851.

Mikkelson T, Kroboth P, Cameron W: Single dose pharmacokinetics of clomiphene citrate in normal volunteers. Fertil Steril 1986;42:331.

Mills JL, Simpson JL, Rhoads GG, et al: Risk of neural tube defects in relation to maternal fertility and fertility drug use. Lancet 1990;2:103.

Moomjy M, Cholst I, Davis OK, et al: Donor oocytes in assisted reproduction—an overview. Semin Reprod Endocrinol 1995;13:173.

Moon YS, Yun YW, King A: Detrimental effects of superovulation. Semin Reprod Endocrinol 1990;8:232.

Murphy M, Seagroat V: Sex ratio in singleton and multiple births. Lancet 1989;2:215.

Nakamura Y, Yoshimura Y, Tanabe K, Izuka R: Induction of ovulation with pulsatile subcutaneous administration of human menopausal gonadotropin in anovulatory infertile women. Fertil Steril 1986;46:46.

Nakamura Y, Yoshimura Y, Yamada H, et al: Clinical experience in the induction of ovulation and pregnancy with pulsatile subcutaneous administration of human menopausal gonadotropin: a low incidence of multiple pregnancy. Fertil Steril 1989;51:423.

Oelsner G, Barnea E, Mullen M, et al: Simultaneous measurements of clomiphene citrate in plasma and follicular fluid in women undergoing IVF and ET. In: Proceedings of the American Fertility Society, 1986, abstract 39.

Oelsner G, Serr G, Mashiach S, et al: The study of induction of ovulation with menotropins: analysis of 1897 treatment cycles. Fertil Steril 1978;30:538.

O'Herlihy C, Pepperell R, Evans JH: The significance of FSH elevation in young women with disorders of ovulation. Br Med J 1980;281:1447.

Out HJ, Mannaerts BMJL, Driessen SGAJ, Coelingh Bennink HJT: A prospective randomized, multicentre study comparing recombinant and urinary follicle stimulation hormone (Puregon vs Metrodin) in in-vitro fertilization. Hum Reprod 1995;10:2534.

Pride SM, James C, Ho Yuen B: The ovarian hyperstimulation syndrome. Semin Reprod Endocrinol 1990;8:247.

Radwanska E, Swyer GIM: Plasma progesterone estimation in infertile women under treatment with clomiphene citrate and chorionic gonadotropin. Br J Obstet Gynecol 1974;81:107.

Ritchie WGM: Ultrasound in the evaluation of normal and induced ovulation. Fertil Steril 1985;43:167.

Rosa F: Ovulation induction and neural tube defects. Lancet 1990;336:1327.

Rossing MA, Daling JR, Weiss NS, et al: Ovarian tumors in a cohort of infertile women. N Engl J Med 1994;331:771.

Schreiber E, Johnson J, Plotz E, Wiener M: Studies with 14C labelled clomiphene citrate. Clin Res 1966;14:287.

Shepard M, Balcameda J, Leija C: Relationship of weight to successful induction of ovulation with clomiphene citrate. Fertil Steril 1979;32:641.

Shushan A, Paltiel O, Iscovich J, et al: Human menopausal gonadotropin and the risk of epithelial ovarian cancer. Fertil Steril 1996;65:13.

Spellacy WN, Cohen WD: Clomiphene treatment of prolonged secondary amenorrhea associated with pituitary gonadotropin deficiency. Am J Obstet Gynecol 1967;97:943.

Surrey ES, Cedars MI: The effect of gonadotropin suppression on the induction of ovulation in premature ovarian failure patients. Fertil Steril 1989;52:36.

Thompson CR, Hansen LM: Pergonal (menotropins): a summary of clinical experience in the induction of ovulation. Fertil Steril 1970;21:844.

Urman B, Pride SM, Ho Yuen B: Management of overstimulated gonadotropin cycles with a controlled drift period. Hum Reprod 1992;7:213.

van Kasteren YM, Hoek A, Schoemaker J: Ovulation induction in premature ovarian failure: a placebo controlled randomized trial combining pituitary suppression with gonadotropin stimulation. Fertil Steril 1995;64:273.

Venn A, Watson L, Lumley J, et al: Breast and ovarian cancer incidence after infertility and vitro fertilization. Lancet 1995;346:995.

Venturoli S, Paradisi R, Fabbri R, et al: Induction of ovulation in polycystic ovary: human menopausal gonadotropins or human urinary follicle stimulating hormone? Int J Fertil 1987;32:66.

Whittemore AS, Harris R, Itnyre R, for the Collaborative Ovarian Cancer Group: Characteristics relating to ovarian cancer risk: collaborative analysis of 12 US case-control studies. II. Invasive epithelial ovarian cancers in white women. Am J Epidemiol 1992;136:1184.

Wu C, Winkel C: The effect of therapy initiation day on clomiphene therapy. Fertil Steril 1989;52:564.

15

Togas Tulandi | Reproductive Surgery

The surgeon's skill and experience, his or her preference of the technique and proper patient selection play a more important role. . .

Togas Tulandi (Tulandi and Bugnah, 1995)

Reproductive surgery plays an important role in the management of infertility. Indeed, infertility investigations will not be complete without a laparoscopy examination. Laparoscopy is done not only for diagnostic purposes, but also for the treatment of a variety of conditions such as endometriosis, periadnexal adhesions, and tubal occlusion. The results are similar to those with laparotomy. Laparoscopy is associated with short hospitalization time, lower incidence of ileus, less adhesion formation, and faster recovery. Operating in a closed environment prevents tissue drying, one of the causes of adhesion formation. Also, contamination with glove powder or lint is less likely to occur with laparoscopy. The pneumoperitoneum gas acts as a tamponade, reducing bleeding and allowing spontaneous coagulation of minor bleeding. Because of these advantages, most reproductive procedures should be done by laparoscopy. This chapter reviews the surgical treatment of infertility, surgical modalities, and the techniques and results.

PREOPERATIVE INVESTIGATIONS AND COUNSELING

Before a reproductive surgery is undertaken, the patient and her male partner should be fully investigated to exclude other causes of infertility. Laparoscopy should complement hysterosalpingography and not replace this important radiologic examination. Patients with hysterosalpingographic findings of tubal occlusion should be managed differently from those with patent tubes. Hysterosalpingography, especially with oil-based contrast medium, could be therapeutic (Schwabe et al, 1983).

Preoperative counseling is very important. For laparoscopy, patients should be advised about the implications of the procedure and the possibility of extending a diagnostic laparoscopy to become a therapeutic operative laparoscopy in the same set-

ting. The possibility of unexpected findings of severe pelvic disease that cannot be laparoscopically corrected should also be discussed. The side effects of laparoscopy (shoulder pain, abdominal discomfort, etc.) and the possible risks should be communicated. The alternatives of laparoscopic surgery versus reproductive surgery by laparotomy versus in vitro fertilization (IVF), the chance to conceive, and the risk of ectopic pregnancy after a particular reproductive surgery must be fully discussed. Women who request reversal of tubal sterilization generally have a more complex marital status, and in some cases psychological counseling might be required (Marcil-Gratton et al, 1988).

LAPAROSCOPY

The basic principles of reproductive surgery include gentle handling of the tissue, meticulous hemostasis, the use of magnification, the use of delicate instruments and fine inert sutures, and accurate approximation of tissues. It is important to reduce tissue drying by irrigating the peritoneal surfaces more or less continuously with Ringer's lactate solution. Advances in technology, including instrumentation and video imaging, have led to rapid progress in laparoscopic surgery. Operative laparoscopy, however, demands a higher degree of technical skills and a greater variety of equipment than does diagnostic laparoscopy or tubal sterilization. Knowledge of anatomy and pathology and the familiarity of the surgeon with the instruments are mandatory.

Laparoscopy is performed while the patient is under general anesthesia with endotracheal intubation. An intrauterine cannula is inserted into the uterus to allow manipulation of the uterus and for chromopertubation. A disposable plastic intrauterine cannula is preferable to a metal instrument. The balloon at the end of the cannula permits adequate occlusion of the cervix, preventing leakage of the chromopertubation fluid into the vagina. Under low lithotomy position, the patient is placed horizontally until insertion of the laparoscope into the abdominal cavity. Using Allen stirrups or knee braces, the thighs are placed almost parallel to the abdomen. This will facilitate manipulation of instruments. The lateral aspect of the knee should be well padded to prevent

383

peroneal nerve compression. An intravenous line is inserted through the patient's arm on the assistant's side and the arm on the side of the operating surgeon should be placed by the patient's side and protected with an ulnar pad. An extended arm will interfere with the surgeon's mobility. To ascertain that the bladder is empty throughout the procedure, an indwelling catheter is left inside the bladder and is removed at the end of the operation.

When extensive adhesion or advanced endometriosis requiring extensive dissection in the vicinity of the large bowel is suspected, a bowel prep is indicated. Shaving of the abdomen and pubic area is not required. The patient is placed in deep Trendelenburg position to allow mobilization of the intestines and good pelvic visualization. Depending upon the size of the patient, adequate pneumoperitoneum is usually obtained with 2 to 3 liters of carbon dioxide (CO_2) gas. The laparoscope is introduced using an infraumbilical entry.

Diagnostic and Therapeutic Laparoscopy

Diagnostic laparoscopy should always be done using two laparoscopic forceps. The purpose of the forceps is to manipulate the tubes and ovaries. It is not uncommon to see "normal adnexa," but, when the forceps is used to mobilize the ovary, the ovary is found to be adhered to the lateral pelvic wall with endometriotic implants underneath. Examination of the posterior cul-de-sac is also facilitated by using the forceps to retract the intestines. Tubal patency is evaluated by chromopertubation using a dilute solution of methylene blue dye.

Laparoscopy examination should be done thoroughly and described in detail. The fallopian tubes should be inspected from the origin of the tubes to the fimbriated ends. The fimbria should be carefully evaluated for evidence of fimbrial phimosis or even hydrosalpinx. It is not sufficient to note that "the tubes are patent." Patent tubes per se does not mean normal tubes. Fimbrial phimosis and open hydrosalpinx are conditions that can be misleadingly reported as "patent tubes" mainly because the chromopertubation dye is present in the cul-de-sac. The entire ovarian surface must be inspected for the presence of endometriotic implants or adhesions that immobilize the ovaries to the posterior broad ligaments. The rest of the abdominal cavity, including the diaphragm and the liver, should be carefully inspected. An incomplete or undetailed laparoscopy report might lead to a repeat laparoscopy examination. A standardized method of reporting by using the American Fertility Society (AFS) (1988) classification of adnexal adhesions, distal tubal occlusion, endometriosis, and tubal occlusion secondary to tubal ligation is recommended.

In recent years, more therapeutic procedures are done by laparoscopy. Magnification can be affected by the use of a laparoscope. Depending upon the lens and the distance between the end of the scope and the operative field, magnification of up to 8-fold can be achieved. Because of this magnification, minor bleeding looks worrisome. Accordingly, hemostasis is more absolute than at laparotomy. It must be noted that the pneumoperitoneum acts as a temporary tamponade and that bleeding may occur after the gas is evacuated from the abdominal cavity. Inspection of the operative field after instillation of approximately 500 to 1000 ml of Ringer's lactate ("examination under water") allows identification of bleeding points. In a rat model instillation of large amount of Ringer's lactate prevented adhesion formation (Pagidas and Tulandi, 1992). Operative laparoscopy is done as an extension of a diagnostic or screening laparoscopy.

Setup

The setup should ideally involve two video monitor screens. The monitors are placed on each side of an instrument table installed at the end of the operating table between the patient's legs. The surgeon stands facing one monitor on the opposite side and the assistant faces the second monitor. For a one-video-monitor setup, the monitor is placed at the end of an operating table between the patient's legs for easy viewing by both the surgeon and the assistant.

A surgical team familiar with operative laparoscopy is invaluable. These individuals are responsible for the operation of monopolar or bipolar electrosurgical generators, laser, and suction irrigator. They should be knowledgeable about all laparoscopic instruments and should know how to find backup instruments in a short notice.

Trocar Insertion

The primary trocar is inserted via a 10-mm infraumbilical incision. Direct trocar insertion without the use of Veress needle can be done using a disposable trocar. It has a retractable inner trocar and its tip is always sharp. In nonobese women, the Veress needle or primary trocar is inserted at 45 degrees from horizontal. The aortic bifurcation in nonobese women is located about 0.4 cm cranial to the umbilicus. Because in obese women the bifurcation is approximately 2.5 cm cranial to the umbilicus, the angle of insertion can be safely increased (Hurd et al, 1992). In patients who have undergone multiple laparotomies and in patients with a large pelvic mass, an open laparoscopy is recommended. After insertion of the laparoscope, the abdominal cavity should first be evaluated for possible inadvertent injury by Veress needle or trocar.

Two to three additional 5-mm trocars are usually required. These trocars are inserted just above the pubic hairline, lateral to the deep epigastric vessels or on the midline. Injury to the deep epigastric vessels is avoided by transilluminating the abdominal wall before trocar insertion and by visualization of the vessels on the peritoneal surface of the anterior abdomen by the laparoscope. The vessels, which are located lateral to the obliterated umbilical artery, should be avoided. If removal of a large specimen via the trocar is anticipated, one of the secondary trocars should be 10 or 15 mm. A morcellation can be done via this trocar. The trocars should always be inserted under direct laparoscopic control. The use of a forefinger as a guard to prevent inserting the trocar too deeply is valuable.

An incisional hernia may occur if the incision is 10 mm or more. A deep suture with 2-0 polyglycolic acid (Dexon) or polyglactin (Vicryl) to approximate the fascia is required. This is particularly necessary for a nonmidline incision.

Surgical Modalities

Dissection can be achieved by using various modalities such as scissors, electrical energy, or surgical lasers. The use of heat in laser and electrosurgery gives a combination of cutting and coagulation properties, but it is associated with a thermal effect that may impair reproductive function.

Electrosurgery

Electrosurgery is the most common coagulative method used for hemostasis. There are three types of electrical current. *Coagulating current* causes cellular dehydration, and its main effect is hemostatic. The current is characterized by intermittent periods of electrical inactivity. The *cutting current* is a continuous current that causes actual explosion of the cell membrane because of the intense heat generated within the tissue itself. A blend between cutting and coagulation current is called a *blended current*.

In the *unipolar system*, electrons flow from the electrosurgical unit to the active electrode. From the tip of the electrode, the current will flow through the air to the tissue. The current is then conducted through the body to the ground plate attached to the patient and returns to the electrosurgical unit. This electrical current may damage vital structures, including intestines. Such areas of thermal damage may not be recognized at the time of surgery. The newer generators, however, are safer than the original spark gap generators, and the use of a unipolar electrode of short duration reduces the risk of electrical injury.

In the *bipolar system*, the current from the electrosurgical unit flows to the active electrode of the bipolar forceps (the shorter paddle of the forceps), through the intervening tissue to the inactive electrode (the longer paddle), and back to the electrosurgical unit. Only tissue in the forceps is affected and no ground plate is required. Thus the effect is focused and damage to adjacent tissues is minimized.

Argon Beam Coagulator

An argon beam coagulator is not an argon laser, but a modification of a unipolar system. The difference is that electrons from a needle electrode flow through space to the tissue via argon gas; therefore, the energy is delivered to the tissue in a "nontouch" technique. Tissue effects are the same as with unipolar cautery (Daniell, 1993). The plume of argon gas that sprays around the electrode has a blast effect on the tissue. This is useful to blow away any debris or blood from the tissue. Another advantage is the lack of smoke production. However, this modality does not allow fine cutting.

One of the concerns regarding this surgical modality is an immediate increase in intra-abdominal pressure resulting from the sudden burst of argon gas during the procedure leading to air embolism.

Laser

The original and the most commonly used laser is the carbon dioxide (CO_2) laser. It is the most precise laser and leads to minimal thermal injury. Unlike other lasers, such as argon, neodymium:yttrium-aluminum-garnet (Nd:YAG), and potassium-titanyl-phosphate (KTP) lasers, the CO_2 laser has limited coagulation properties. The wavelength and the different absorption characteristics of these lasers determine their action. In short, lasers with a long wavelength are more effective for tissue vaporization but poor for coagulation. Lasers with a short wavelength, in contrast, have good coagulation but poor vaporization properties. Newer lasers that can be transmitted through a fiber include the holmium:YAG, erbium:YAG and CO lasers.

The word *laser* stands for "*l*ight *a*mplification by *s*timulated *e*mission of *r*adiation." A laser beam has special characteristics: it is coherent (all waves are in phase with each other), collimated (parallel), and monochromatic (same wavelength and energy). The original CO_2 laser delivered continuous laser energy to the tissue. To decrease the amount of thermal injury, the superpulse laser was developed. This laser pulses 100 to 900 times per second, allowing a regular cooling-off period. A longer cooling-off period is incorporated in a newer ultrapulse laser. It delivers high-power energy (up to 500 W) at 25 pulses per second over a short duty cycle; this allows rapid vaporization with less thermal damage and less charring of the tissue.

Laser energy can be delivered to the tissue as a free beam ("nontouch" or "noncontact") or by heated probe contact. In the noncontact delivery, the laser beam interacts with tissue. Delivery can be achieved through an articulated arm, through a laparoscope as a wave guide (CO_2 laser), or using fiberoptic cable (argon laser). In contact delivery, the laser energy is concentrated at the end of a sapphire, ceramic, or metallic tip or at the end of tapered fibers. The effects are then predominantly cautery effects. One of the advantages of using laser via the built-in channel of the laparoscope is that it makes one of the secondary trocars unnecessary. This trocar can then be used for an extra ancillary instrument.

Ultrasonic Vibrating Scalpel

The ultrasonic scalpel is an instrument that potentially causes minimal tissue injury with good hemostasis. Ultrasonically activated, the scalpel blade moves longitudinally at 55,000 vibrations per second while cutting the tissue. Because little heat is produced, thermal injury is minimal. The vibration of the ultrasonic scalpel is said to generate low heat at the incision site, and the combination of the vibration and the heat causes the proteins to denature. The denatured proteins form a coagulum that seals the bleeding vessels.

The ultrasonic scalpel produces less tissue injury on porcine skin than electrosurgery or CO_2 laser (Hambley et al, 1988). The tissue effects of an ultrasonic scalpel and a regular scalpel were compared (Tulandi et al, 1994). Compared to that of a regular scalpel, the use of ultrasonic scalpel is associated with very minimal bleeding. It causes tissue blanching without charring and with minimal smoke production. The two modalities subsequently produce similar acute inflammatory changes and adhesion formation.

Sharp Dissection and Hydrodissection

Sharp and hydrodissection are done without heated instruments. Therefore, the risks of thermal damage and the problem with smoke production are eliminated. After years of tissue dissection with laser and electrosurgery, my present preference is sharp dissection. This is facilitated by hydrodissection using a suction irrigator. Sharp and hydrodissection are particularly useful for the enucleation of an ovarian cyst, for the excision of deep endometriotic implants, or for dissection around important organs such as ureter, bladder, intestines, and great vessels. Hemostasis is usually achieved by bipolar electrocoagulation.

Suturing

Suture placement through the laparoscope requires considerable skill. This is done for organ reconstruction, approximation of tissue planes, and establishment of hemostasis. Two suturing methods, extracorporeal and intracorporeal knot tying, are used.

The easiest method is *extracorporeal knot tying* using a knot pusher. After the tissue is sutured, the needle is withdrawn through the trocar and the suture is tied extracorporeally. Instead of using a complicated knot, a single or double throw knot can be made. The loop is then pushed into the abdominal cavity and tightened. The procedure is repeated two to three times until the knots are secured. The best knot pusher is made of metal with a fenestration at its tip. It is important to use suture material that slips easily, such as polydioxanone suture (PDS). This technique, however is not appropriate for suturing with suture material that does not easily slip, such as polyglactin or polyglycolic acid. Also, fine suture materials smaller than 6-0 break easily when tied extracorporeally. Alternatively, *intracorporeal knot tying* can be done. This is performed using a conventional instrument tying or a "twist" technique (Toppel, 1994).

Laparoscopic suturing, especially with intracorporeal knot tying, can be tiresome and time consuming. However, with patience and experience, it can be mastered and is a valuable endoscopic skill. This will allow completion of procedures similar to those achieved by laparotomy. Some examples are eversion of the mucosal flap at terminal salpingostomy, approximation of an ovarian defect after ovarian cystectomy, and tubal anastomosis.

Clinical Results

It was initially believed that the results of laser surgery are superior to those of conventional techniques. However, there are randomized clinical studies comparing reproductive surgery using laser and electrosurgery by laparotomy in which similar results were found (Tulandi and Vilos, 1985; Tulandi, 1986). The degree of postsurgical adhesion is also comparable. Thus there is little advantage to using laser for reproductive surgery. The clinical results show that reproductive surgery is safe and effective whether using sharp dissection, electrosurgery or laser energy. The results are independent of the surgical modality used. The surgeon's skill and experience, his or her preference of technique, and proper patient selection play a more important role (Tulandi and Bugnah, 1995).

SURGICAL TREATMENT OF SPECIFIC DISORDERS

Periadnexal Adhesions

It is obvious that women with bilateral tubal occlusion will not spontaneously conceive, but spontaneous pregnancy can occur in women with periadnexal adhesions. Tulandi et al (1990) evaluated pregnancy occurrence among women with periadnexal adhesions with or without salpingo-ovariolysis. They found that the pregnancy rate in the treated group was superior to that in the untreated group (Fig. 15–1). These results suggest that salpingo-ovariolysis increases the pregnancy rate in infertile women with periadnexal adhesions. The ectopic pregnancy rate between the treated and nontreated group, was similar, however. This suggests that the intrinsic damage to the fallopian tube plays a more important role in

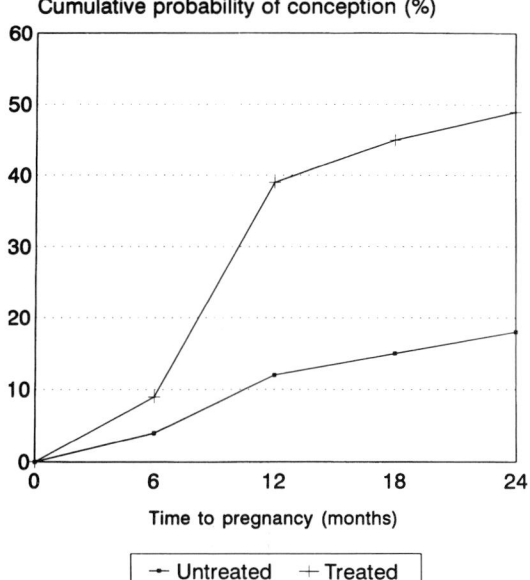

Cumulative probability of conception (%)

Time to pregnancy (months)

-*- Untreated   -+- Treated

Figure 15–1
Cumulative probability of conception among infertile women with periadnexal adhesion who were treated by lysis of adhesions and who were not treated.

the development of ectopic pregnancy than the adhesions, but the presence of adhesions decreases the chance to conceive.

Salpingo-Ovariolysis

Salpingo-ovariolysis is done by stretching the adhesions with the help of a laparoscopic forceps and an intrauterine cannula and then dividing them. Adhesions that are vascular should be first coagulated or vaporized with laser. Lysis of adhesions can be done with laparoscopic scissors, electrocautery, or laser. The results are similar. The overall pregnancy rate after laparoscopic salpingo-ovariolysis is 60% and the ectopic pregnancy rate is 5% (Tulandi and Bugnah, 1995). However, not all adhesions can be liberated by laparoscopy. Severe and dense adhesions cannot be completely liberated. In these patients, the pregnancy rate after salpingo-ovariolysis by laparotomy is poor (10% to 15%). Patients with severe and dense adhesions will gain more from IVF than from reproductive surgery.

Distal Tubal Occlusion

Terminal Salpingostomy

Laparoscopic salpingostomy is done in the same manner as salpingostomy by laparotomy (Fig. 15–2). The tubal opening is created using a laser, needle-point unipolar electrode, or laparoscopic scissors. To maintain the eversion of the neo-ostium, the mucosal flap is everted without tension using a few interrupted sutures of 6-0 polyglactin, or with laser or

electrocoagulation. Laser eversion is done by defocusing the CO_2 laser and directing the beam 0.5 cm from the margin of the flap. Retraction of the mucosal flap creates an eversion. This can also be accomplished by using a light electrocoagulation with a bipolar cautery. The same principle may be followed using other type of lasers. Because of the concerns of thermal damage and the fact that a thick hydrosalpinx does not evert with laser or electrical energy, the use of sutures is preferred. The intussusception technique is also helpful to evert the mucosal flap and to minimize the number of sutures (McComb and Paleologou, 1991).

It is important to evaluate the pregnancy rate after a reproductive surgery according to the tube with the least damage. After all, pregnancy tends to occur more from the better fallopian tube. Outcomes following laparoscopic salpingostomy are shown in Table 15–1. The small number of patients in some of the studies, the different degrees of tubal damage, the variations in length of follow-up and the different operating surgeons make it difficult to compare the results of these various techniques (Gomel, 1977; Daniell and Hebert, 1984; Dubuisson et al, 1990; Canis et al, 1991). Depending upon the degree of tubal damage, the intrauterine pregnancy rate after salpingostomy ranges between 10% and 80% (Fig. 15–3) (Schlaff et al, 1990; Canis et al, 1991). Using salpingoscopy to evaluate tubal mucosa, Marana et al (1995) reported that the term pregnancy rate in women with normal tubal mucosa was 64%. They found that salpingoscopic assessment of the tubal mucosa is of greater prognostic value than the AFS classifications for adnexal adhesions and distal tubal occlusion. In general, patients with bilateral hydrosalpinx may be expected to achieve better results following IVF than salpingostomy by laparotomy. However, laparoscopic salpingostomy is a reasonable alternative for selected patients who do not wish or cannot afford IVF, or for those who are found to have hydrosalpinx at the time of diagnostic laparoscopy.

Fimbrioplasty

Fimbrial phimosis is a partial obstruction of the distal end of a fallopian tube. On chromopertubation, the tube is dilated but patent as indicated by the passage of chromopertubation dye from a narrow tubal opening. This is due to the presence of peritoneal adhesive bands surrounding the terminal end of the tube. The longitudinal rugae of the tube are usually well preserved. The treatment of this condition is fimbrioplasty. It is done by dividing the peritoneal adhesive bands that surround the terminal end of the fallopian tube. It can also be done by inserting two graspers into the tubal lumen and spreading them apart. In some cases, several interrupted sutures of 6-0 or 8-0 polyglactin (Rx Vicryl) may be required to maintain the eversion of the fimbria.

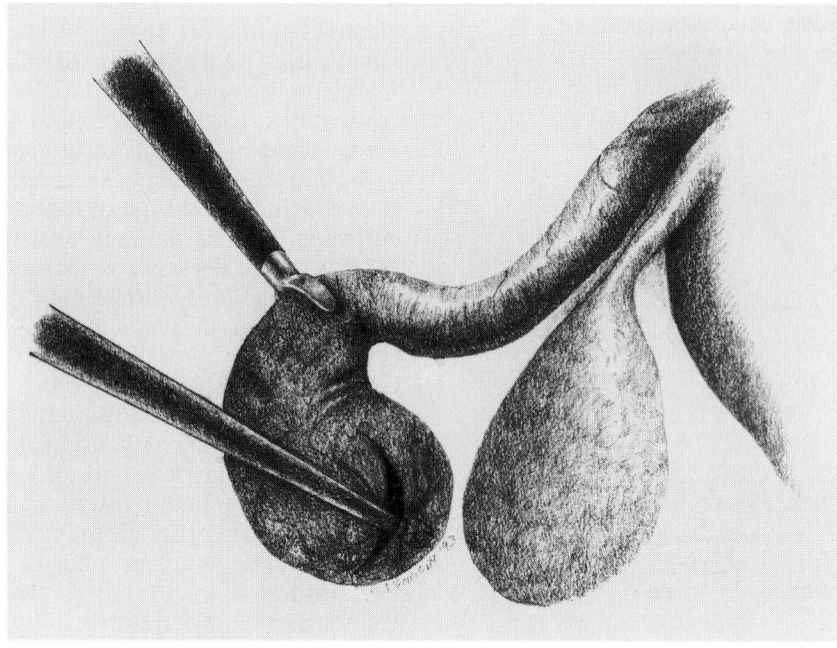

A

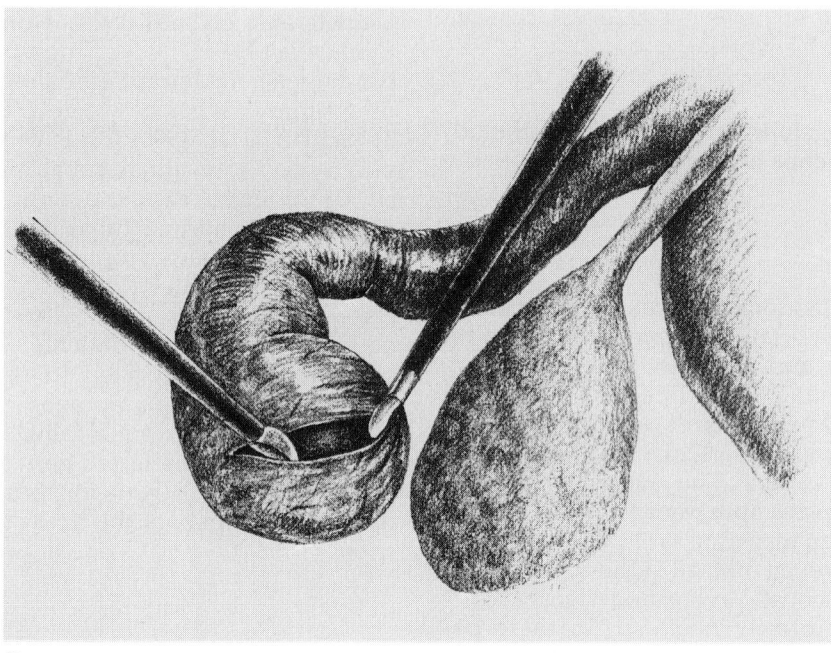

B

Figure 15–2
Laparoscopic salpingostomy. *A,* Incision at the avascular line of the hydrosalpinx. *B,* Enlargement of the neo-ostium by stretching the opening. *Illustration continued on opposite page*

Evaluation of the results of fimbrioplasty is complicated by the facts that most authors do not distinguish between salpingostomy and fimbrioplasty. The overall pregnancy rate after laparoscopic fimbrioplasty is 31% to 35% (Tulandi, 1995). These results are comparable to those obtained by laparotomy. Higher pregnancy rates (60%) have also been reported. Gomel and Erenus (1990) reported successful deliveries in 19 of 40 patients (47.5%) after laparoscopic fimbrioplasty. The ectopic pregnancy rate after this procedure is 5% to 10%.

Proximal Tubal Occlusion

The hysterosalpingographic finding of "bilateral cornual occlusion" must be followed by selective tubal catheterization for several reasons. Histopathologic

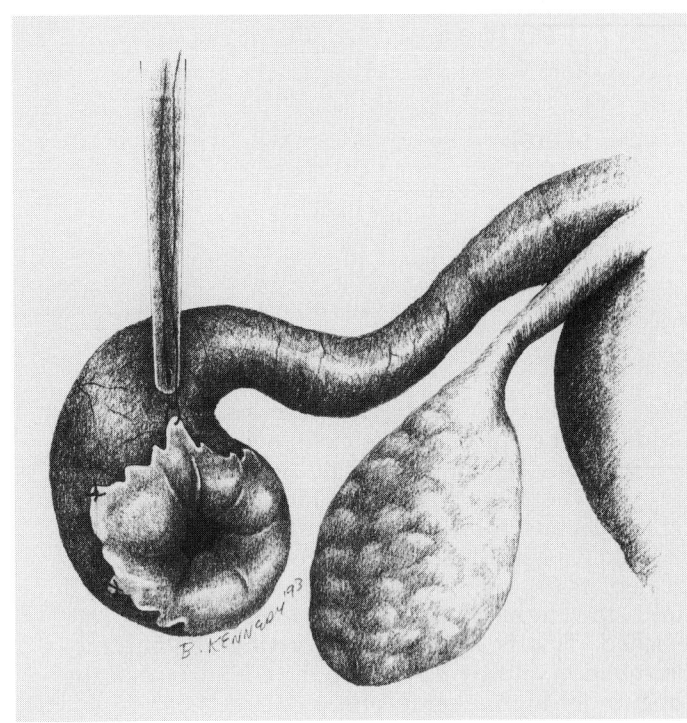

Figure 15–2
Continued   *C*, Eversion of the mucosal flap with sutures. (From Tulandi T: Atlas of Laparoscopy and Hysteroscopy Techniques for Gynecologists. London: WB Saunders Company, 1999:35, with permission.)

C

analysis of resected tubes with cornual occlusion diagnosed by hysterosalpingography and/or laparoscopy showed a variety of findings (Sulak et al, 1987), including normal (20% of the tubes), in which case the etiology was presumed tubal spasm; amorphous debris or minimal adhesions (40%); and extensive fibrosis or salpingitis isthmica nodosa (about 40%). It is also not uncommon to find a combination of proximal and distal tubal occlusion (bipolar tubal blockage). Reconstructive surgery in women with bipolar blockage is associated with a pregnancy rate of only 12% at 2.5 years' follow-up (Patton et al, 1987).

Selective Tubal Catheterization

In women with proximal tubal occlusion diagnosed by hysterosalpingography, selective tubal catheterization has become the next logical step (Daniell and Miller, 1987; Confino et al, 1988; Novy et al, 1988; Thurmond, 1995). Transcervical selective catheterization of the tube can be done by purely tactile method or under ultrasound, hysteroscopic, or fluoroscopic control, or with the aid of a falloscope. It is most practical to use this technique in conjunction with a hysterosalpingograph that shows proximal tubal occlusion. The procedure is done by inserting a 3- to 5-French catheter with a guide wire into the tubal ostium.

Selective tubal catheterization is associated with more than 90% patency rate of at least one of the tubes and 58% pregnancy rate (Thurmond and Rosch, 1990). However, in women who do not conceive by 6 months, it appears that 50% of the tubes are reoccluded. The procedure can then be repeated.

Women who failed tubal catheterization can be offered IVF or reconstructive tubal surgery. Prior to laparotomy, a laparoscopy examination should be done to ascertain that the distal tube is normal. Women with bipolar tubal disease are better treated with IVF.

Tubocornual Anastomosis

The traditional treatment of cornual occlusion is uterotubal implantation. In this procedure, the intramural portion of the tube is resected, a hole is bored into the uterine cornua, and the remaining distal part of the tube is reimplanted into the uterus. The disadvantages of this technique are excessive bleeding and the fact that the new uterotubal junction is unphysiologic, leading to a low pregnancy rate (Rock et al, 1979). Because the intramural part of the tube is almost always patent, a more successful procedure is a tubocornual anastomosis. The pregnancy rate after tubocornual anastomosis (57.7%) (McComb, 1986) is superior to that after implantation (29%) (Rock et al, 1979).

The procedure is done by laparotomy by first injecting a dilute solution of vasopressin (0.2 units/ml of physiologic saline) into the uterine cornua. Vasoconstriction will occur, and the remaining bleeding spots can later be coagulated. The occluded portion of the tube is circumferentially incised from the surrounding myometrium with a unipolar needle electrode. The tube is transected with a microscissors. The procedure is repeated 2 mm at a time until patency is reached (Fig. 15–4). This is indicated by the passage of methylene blue solution, which is injected

Table 15–1. OUTCOMES FOLLOWING LAPAROSCOPIC SALPINGOSTOMY

STUDY	NO. OF PATIENTS	FOLLOW-UP (yr)	INTRAUTERINE PREGNANCY (%)	ECTOPIC PREGNANCY (%)
Gomel (1977)	9	1	44.4	0
Daniell and Hebert (1984)	21	>1	19.0	5.0
Dubuisson et al (1990)	34	>1	29.4	2.9
Canis et al (1991)	87	>3	33.3	6.9
TOTAL	151		31.5	3.7

into the uterine cavity transcervically or transfundally. The cut surface is examined under magnification. Any remaining fibrotic tissue should be resected. Where the tube is undamaged, the normal mucosal pattern and the muscular architecture can be seen. The occluded portion of the distal tube is treated in the same manner. The tube is transected until the lumen and normal-looking tissue are reached. This is established by retrograde chromopertubation and by inspecting the cut surface of the tube under high magnification.

The two cut ends of the tubes are approximated with several interrupted sutures of 6-0 polyglactin in the mesosalpinx. Four interrupted 8-0 polyglactin sutures are then circumferentially placed in the muscularis layers under ×10 magnification. The procedure is facilitated by placing the first suture at 6 o'clock position. A second layer of 6-0 to 8-0 polyglactin is used to approximate the seromuscularis.

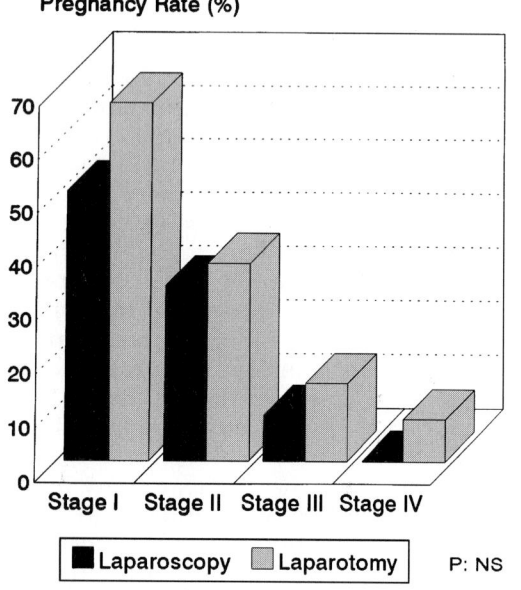

Pregnancy Rate (%)

■ Laparoscopy ▨ Laparotomy   P: NS

Figure 15–3
Pregnancy rates after salpingostomy by laparoscopy and by laparotomy. The results depend on the degree of tubal damage (stage I to IV). (Adapted from Canis M, Mage G, Pouly JL, et al: Laparoscopic distal tuboplasty: report of 87 cases and a 4-year experience. Fertil Steril, 1991;56:616, with permission.)

Midtubal Occlusion

Tubal Anastomosis

The most frequent cause of midtubal occlusion is tubal sterilization. Tubal anastomosis is repair that provides the most successful reproductive results (Gomel, 1980; Winston, 1980; Rock et al, 1987). There is an inverse relationship between the total tubal length and the surgery–conception interval. A short tube is usually due to sterilization by electrocoagulation or partial salpingectomy (Pomeroy method). The type of anastomosis in this situation is ampullary-isthmic anastomosis, which is associated with a less favorable outcome than isthmic-isthmic anastomosis. Rock et al (1987) reported that the term pregnancy rate after tubal anastomosis is 75% in women with a tubal length of 4 cm or over and 19% in women with a shorter tube. They also found that ectopic pregnancy and abortion rates are higher among women sterilized with monopolar cautery. The surgical technique is similar to that described for tubocornual anastomosis (Fig. 15–5).

Tubal anastomosis has also been done by laparoscopy (Koh, 1995). It remains to be seen whether the results are similar to those with microsurgical technique. Alternatively, a laparoscopy-assisted tubal anastomosis can be done. Here, under laparoscopic control, the occluded portions of the fallopian tube are delivered out of the abdominal cavity through a 3-cm midline minilaparotomy incision and a microsurgical tubal anastomosis is done. The procedure is done on an outpatient basis and the principles of microsurgical technique are maintained.

Transposition of the Fallopian Tube

Intrauterine pregnancies have been reported after tubal anastomosis using contralateral tubal segments (Gomel and McComb, 1985; Goldberg and Friedman, 1988; Okamura et al, 1988) in a few women with an unusual pelvic anatomy. The tubal segments are first mobilized and the distal segment is then anastomosed to the opposite proximal segment.

Endometriosis

Several studies have shown that the results of conservative surgical treatment for endometriosis by

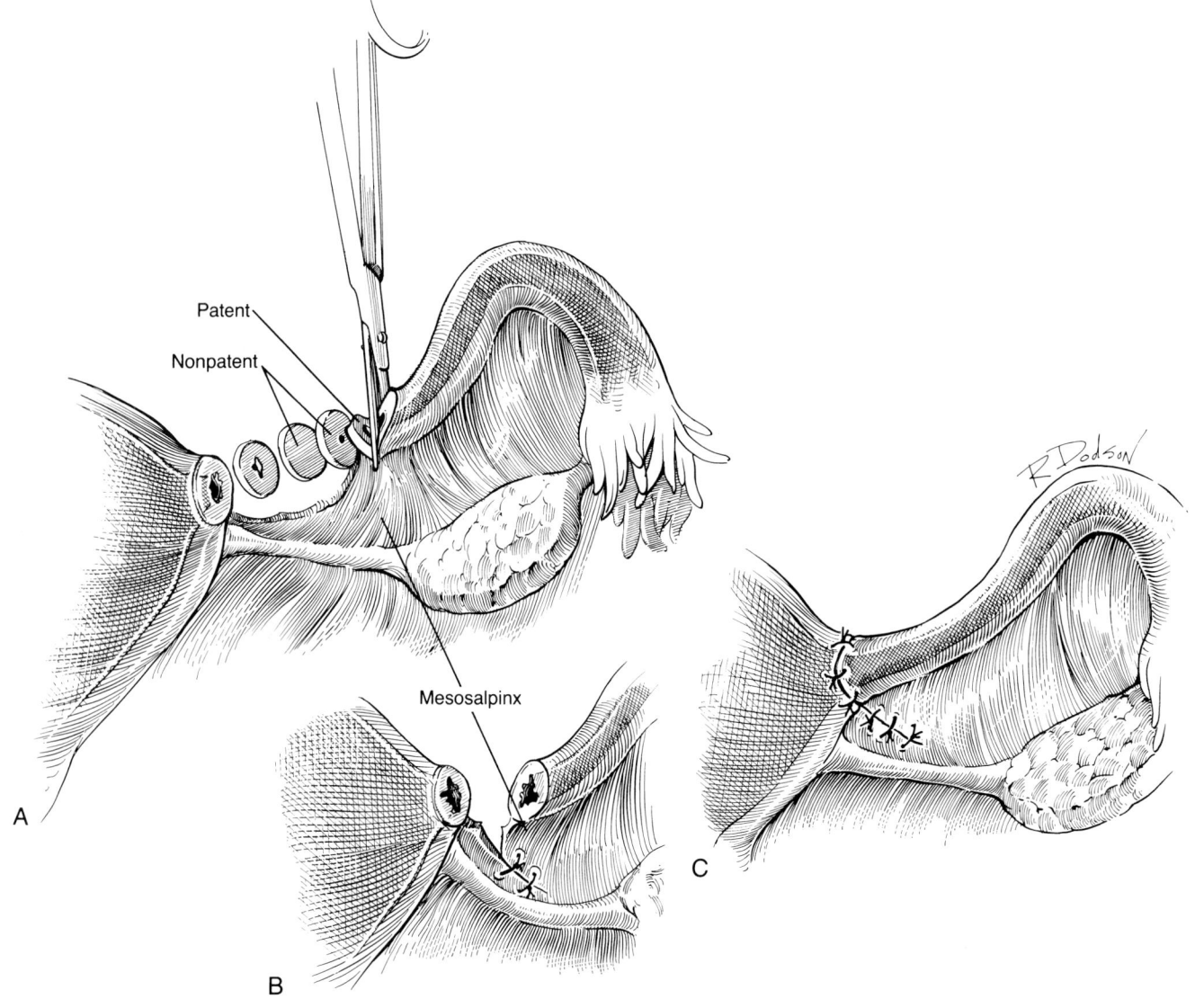

Figure 15–4
Tubocornual anastomosis. *A*, The occluded tube is resected 2 mm at a time until patency is reached. *B*, The two cut ends of the tube are approximated by several interrupted sutures of 6-0 polyglactin in the mesosalpinx. *C*, Tubocornual anastomosis has been completed.

laparoscopy are similar to or better than those by laparotomy (Cook and Rock, 1991; Nezhat et al, 1989; Adamson et al, 1993, 1994; Hughes et al, 1993). Laparoscopic treatment of endometriosis is associated with a high fecundity rate even in the presence of advanced disease, and there is a trend of increased early pregnancy rates. This is achieved by lysis of adhesions, excision of endometriotic implants, and excision of endometriomas. The incidence of pregnancy (70%) is independent of the stage of endometriosis (Olive and Martin, 1987; Nezhat et al, 1989) and of the surgical modality used, but is directly related to the duration of infertility. Adamson et al (1993) reported that laparoscopic treatment of endometriosis is superior to medical treatment. They also found that the laparoscopic approach is superior to laparotomy (Fig. 15–6). Recently, a randomized

Canadian study showed that laparoscopic treatment of minimal and mild endometriosis increased the pregnancy rate (Marcoux et al, 1997).

Excision of Endometriosis

Endometriotic implants can be coagulated electrosurgically or vaporized with the laser, but excision results in a more complete removal of the lesions (Redwine, 1994). Often a seemingly small endometriotic lesion on the peritoneum represents the tip of a deep endometriotic nodule. This will not be recognized without excision of the lesion. Excision is done by grasping the portion of the peritoneum harboring endometriosis (Fig. 15–7). A small incision is made on the peritoneum and the peritoneum is undermined, separating it from the underlying struc-

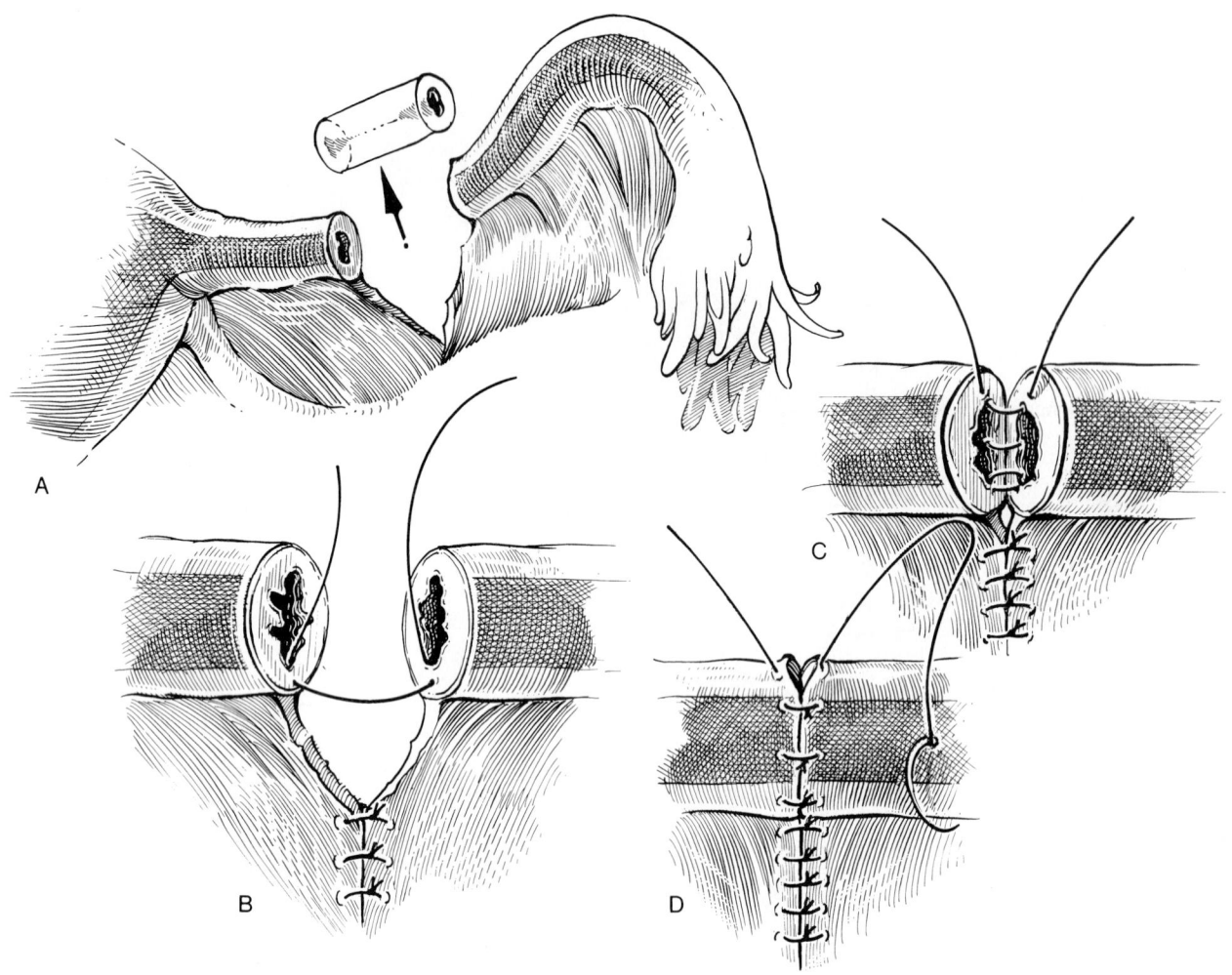

Figure 15–5
Tubal anastomosis. *A*, The occluded part of the tube has been excised until patency is reached. *B*, Approximation of the two cut ends of the tube by several interrupted sutures in the mesosalpinx. First suture of 8-0 polyglactin should be placed at 6 o'clock position (*arrow*). *C*, Four to five interrupted sutures of 8-0 polyglactin have been placed at the muscularis layer. *D*, The second layer of 6-0 to 8-0 polyglactin is used to approximate the seromuscularis.

tures. This is done by blunt dissection and hydro-dissection using a solution of Ringer's lactate or physiologic saline under pressure. The abnormal peritoneum including the endometriotic lesion, is excised. This technique is applicable for endometriosis over the ureter, over the bladder, or in the recto-vaginal septum.

Excision of Ovarian Endometrioma

The technique of removal of an endometrioma is similar to ovarian cystectomy in general. However, rarely an endometrioma can be enucleated intact. The chocolate-colored content of the cyst often escapes during the dissection. In this situation, the cyst's content should be drained and lavaged. A cleavage plane is created between the cyst wall and the ovarian capsule. Using two grasping forceps for traction and countertraction, the cyst wall is sepa-

rated from the ovarian tissue (Fig. 15–8). Bleeding form the inner surface of the ovarian defect can be electrocoagulated using a bipolar forceps.

Because ovarian endometriomas tend to be bilateral, it is important to examine the opposite ovary. Occasionally, the cyst wall is so intimately adherent to the ovarian tissue that a cleavage plane cannot be created. This is not uncommonly found in a small ovarian endometrioma. In this case the contents of the cyst are aspirated and the cyst is repeatedly irrigated. The top of the cyst, including the associated "ovarian capsule," is decapitated. Care should be taken not to remove excessive ovarian tissue. If a cleavage plane is still not found, after ascertaining that there is no suspicious lesion, the inner surface of the cyst wall is destroyed either with laser or electrocoagulation. Because of the possibility of leaving some cyst wall and of destruction of ovarian follicles, this technique should be rarely used. Usually, the

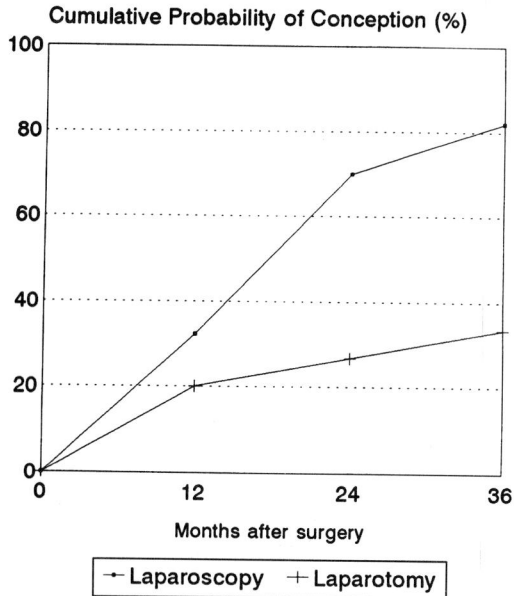

Figure 15–6
Cumulative probability of conception after treatment of moderate and severe endometriosis by laparoscopy and by laparotomy. (Adapted from Adamson GD, Hurd SJ, Pasta DJ, Rodriguez BD: Laparoscopic endometriosis treatment: is it better? Fertil Steril, 1993;59:35, with permission.)

ovarian defect collapses. If the ovary is gaping, two or three sutures of 4-0 or 5-0 polydioxanone or tissue sealant can be used to approximate the edges of the ovarian tissue. The ovarian capsule can also be inverted by coagulating the inner side of the ovarian opening approximately 1 cm from its margin. Inversion of the ovarian capsule approximates the ovarian opening.

Ectopic Pregnancy

Because of the relatively higher incidence of ectopic pregnancy (5% to 10%), patients who conceive following reproductive surgery must be followed by serial serum β-human chorionic gonadotropin (β-hCG) measurements and early transvaginal ultrasound examination. This approach allows detection of early and unruptured tubal ectopic pregnancy that can be conservatively treated by laparoscopy (DeCherney et al, 1985; Pouly et al, 1986) or medically (Stovall and Ling, 1993). The value of conservative management of tubal ectopic pregnancy has been well established. It increases the number of live births (from 30% to 50% to 50% to 80%) and the risk of recurrent ectopic pregnancy is similar to that after salpingectomy (10% to 15%). The procedure of choice is laparoscopic linear salpingostomy.

To date, surgical treatment of ectopic pregnancy remains the definitive and universal treatment, and it can be safely done by laparoscopy. The incidence of persistently elevated serum β-hCG levels is similar to that with laparotomy (5%), and it can be treated by a single-dose methotrexate injection. As more evidence has accumulated, it has become clear that tubal rupture and hemoperitoneum can still occur after expectant or medical management of ectopic pregnancy (Tulandi, 1994). These treatments should be done with utmost care and patients should be closely monitored. Surgical treatment is required when clinically indicated or when the serum β-hCG levels fail to decline and/or the dilated tube in the region of the ectopic pregnancy fails to subside. The reproductive outcome after medical treatment with methotrexate and after laparoscopic salpingostomy is depicted in Table 15–2.

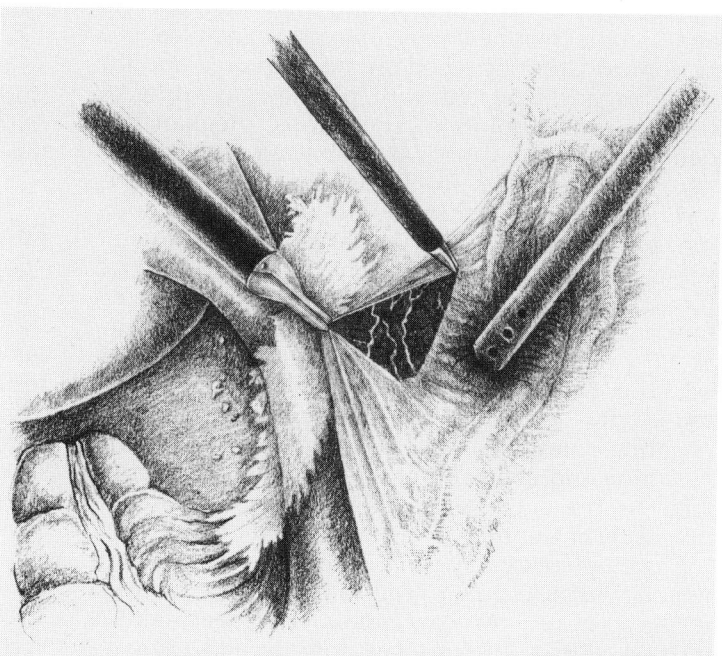

Figure 15–7
Excision of endometriosis. The peritoneum adjacent to the endometriosis on the right uterosacral ligament is grasped with a forceps and stretched medially. An incision is made on the peritoneum. The ureter is displaced laterally by the suction irrigator. (From Tulandi T: Atlas of Laparoscopy Technique for Gynecologists. London: WB Saunders Company, 1994: 27, with permission.)

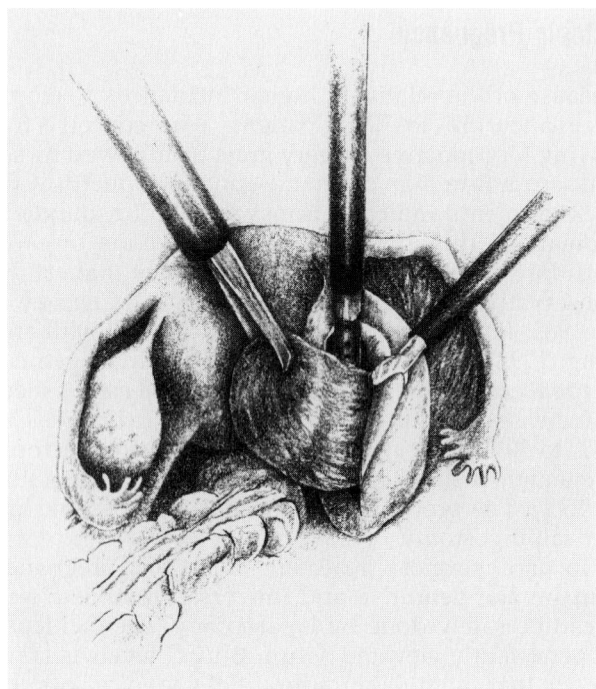

Figure 15–8
Stripping an endometriotic cyst wall using two grasping forceps for traction and countertraction. (From Tulandi T: Atlas of Laparoscopy Technique for Gynecologists. London: WB Saunders Company, 1994:49, with permission.)

In the presence of persistent bleeding or ruptured tube, a salpingectomy is an alternative. This is also the procedure for women who do not wish to preserve their fertility. If the patient is unstable, an immediate laparotomy should be done.

Linear Salpingostomy

The presence of hemoperitoneum should not prevent laparoscopic treatment of ectopic pregnancy. Using a suction irrigator, the blood can be evacuated and the pelvic organs irrigated with physiologic saline or Ringer's lactate solution. The ectopic pregnancy is identified and the tube is immobilized with a laparoscopy forceps (Fig. 15–9). Using a 22-gauge injection needle inserted through a 5-mm portal, a solution of vasopressin (0.2 units/ml of physiologic saline) is injected into the wall of the tube at the area of maximal distention. This will allow surgery with minimal bleeding. A 10- to 15-mm longitudinal incision is made on the maximally distended antemesosalpinx wall of the tube. The products of conception are flushed out of the tube with high-pressure irrigating solution. Using a combination of hydrodissection and gentle blunt dissection with a suction irrigator, the entire products of conception are removed from the tube. Evacuation of the gestational products piecemeal with a forceps is not recommended because it may lead to incomplete removal of the products of conception. The specimen is grasped with a 10-mm claw forceps and then re-moved from the abdominal cavity. A laparoscopic bag may be useful for removal of large fragments of placental tissue.

The tube is carefully irrigated and inspected "under water" for hemostasis. Bleeding points can be coagulated with bipolar coagulation. The tubal incision is left open to heal by secondary intention. Because of the risk of persistent ectopic pregnancy, one serum β-hCG measurement should be done approximately a week after salpingostomy. Persistent ectopic pregnancy can be treated with a single dose of methotrexate (50 mg/m² of body surface, or approximately 1 mg/kg body weight intramuscularly).

Salpingectomy

In salpingectomy for ectopic pregnancy, the tube is immobilized with a grasping forceps. The tubal segment to be excised is coagulated with a bipolar cautery and then cut. The procedure is repeated on the mesosalpinx of the tubal segment to be excised and on the distal portion of the tube. A recently developed "tripolar" forceps allows simultaneous bipolar coagulation and cutting. Partial salpingectomy or distal salpingectomy can be done. The tube is removed and careful hemostasis is done as described above.

Expectant and Medical Management

Expectant treatment of ectopic pregnancy should be reserved for those patients with serum β-hCG of less than 2500 mIU/ml and declining and a tubal diameter of 2 cm or less. A select group of patients with early and unruptured tubal pregnancy can be treated by systemic methotrexate injection. The treatment is especially effective in those with serum β-hCG levels of less than 5000 mIU/ml and serum progesterone levels of less than 10 ng/ml. Methotrexate has also found its place in the management of persistently elevated serum β-hCG after surgical treatment. Transvaginal administration of methotrexate precludes surgery and general anesthesia, but about one third of the patients subsequently require further treatment.

Polycystic Ovarian Syndrome

The oldest treatment for polycystic ovarian syndrome (PCOS)-related anovulation is bilateral ovarian wedge resection by laparotomy. A decrease in testosterone secretion occurs after this procedure. This frees the inhibited hypothalamic-pituitary axis and allows ovulation to occur. It also removes the local intraovarian androgen blockade that prevents normal follicular development. Another possible explanation is reduction in ovarian inhibin or stimulation of growth factor production. Ovarian wedge resection, however, is associated with a high incidence of periadnexal adhesions that may jeopardize fertility (Donesky and Adashi, 1995).

Table 15-2. REPRODUCTIVE OUTCOME AFTER MEDICAL TREATMENT OF ECTOPIC PREGNANCY
WITH METHOTREXATE AND AFTER LAPAROSCOPIC SALPINGOSTOMY*

TREATMENT	STUDY	TOTAL NO. OF PATIENTS	NO. OF PATIENTS ATTEMPTING PREGNANCY	NO. OF PREGNANCIES (%)		
				Total	Intrauterine	Ectopic
Methotrexate, single dose	Stovall and Ling (1993)	120	49	39/49 (79.6)	34/49 (69.4)	5/49 (12.8)
Salpingostomy	Pouly et al (1986)	223	118	102/118 (86.4)	76/118 (64.4)	26/76 (25.5)

*Methotrexate treatment was administered to a select group of patients with an ectopic pregnancy less than 3.5 cm in greatest diameter. Salpingostomy was done in most patients with ectopic pregnancy.

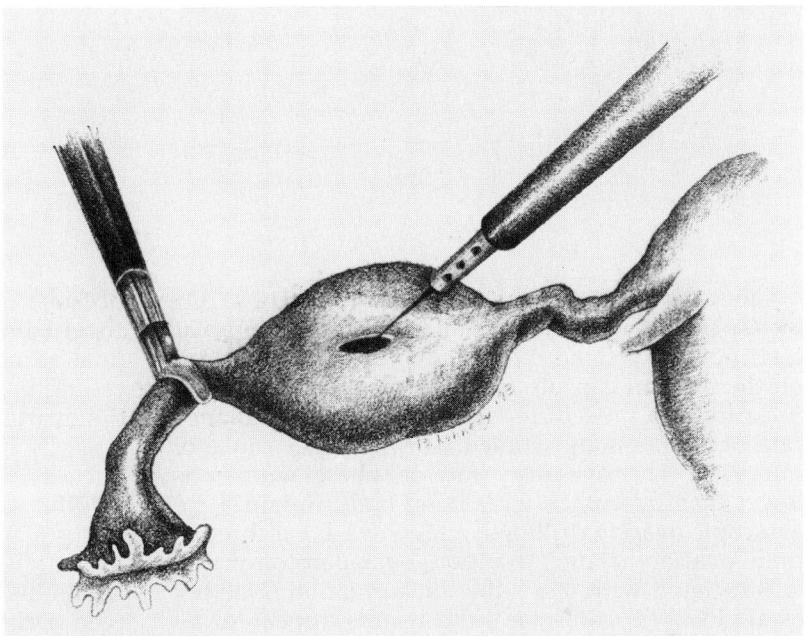

A

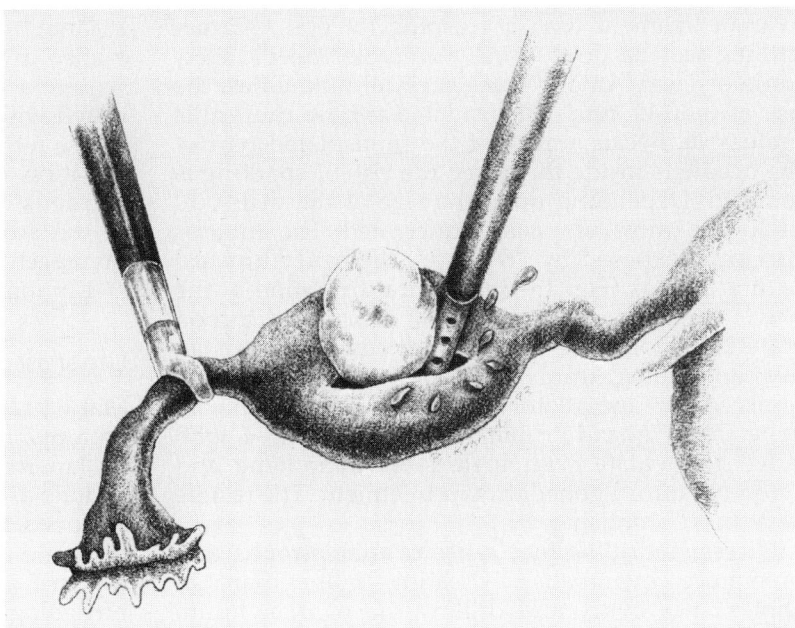

B

Figure 15-9
Linear salpingostomy for ectopic pregnancy. *A,* A longitudinal incision is made on the antemesosalpinx of the tube using a unipolar needle electrode inserted into a built-in channel of a suction irrigator. *B,* The needle electrode is removed and, by using a suction irrigator, the gestational products are flushed out of the tube. (From Tulandi T: Atlas of Laparoscopy and Hysteroscopy Techniques for Gynecologists. London: WB Saunders Company, 1999:50, with permission.)

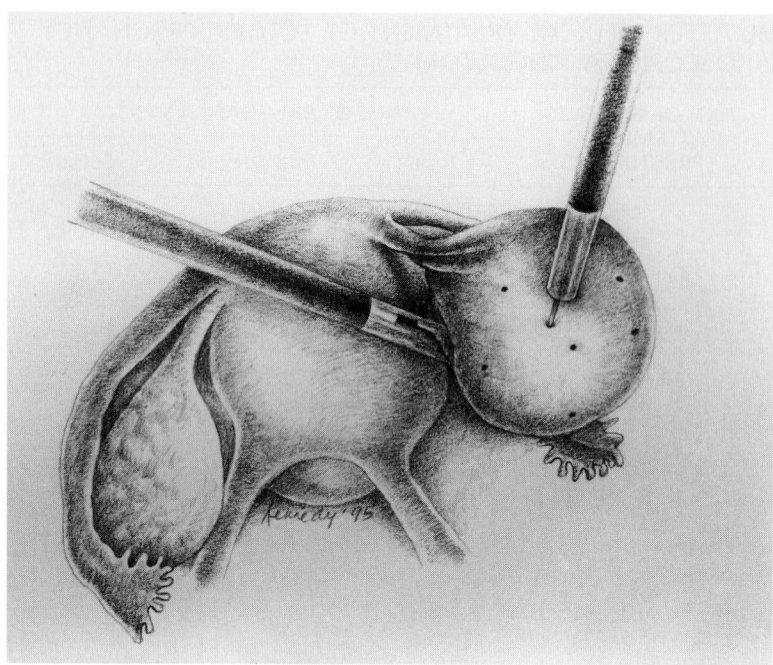

Figure 15–10
Ovarian drilling on the anterior aspect of the ovary using a unipolar needle electrode.

Gjönnaes (1994) first reported treatment of PCOS by laparoscopic ovarian drilling. Using a unipolar electrode, he created 8 to 15 craters 2 to 4 mm deep on the ovarian capsule of each ovary. The ovulatory rate after the procedure was 92%, with a pregnancy rate of 84%, among women with no other cause of infertility. The ovulatory rate in obese women is lower than in women with lower body weight. Laparoscopic ovarian drilling is a less invasive technique than ovarian wedge resection by laparotomy and is associated with less adhesion formation (Naether et al, 1993). Furthermore, the results appear to be superior.

Ovarian drilling is done by grasping the utero-ovarian ligament with a grasping forceps. Ovarian drilling can be done using a unipolar needle electrode or laser. Among these surgical modalities, the use of a 40-W unipolar insulated needle cautery is preferable. Because most of the uninsulated part of the needle is inside the ovary, the risk of sparking is reduced. Depending upon the size of the ovary, 10 to 20 punctures per ovary are created. The anterior surface is exposed by "flipping" the ovary upward with a forceps (Fig. 15–10). Liberal irrigation of the pelvic cavity to remove necrotic debris and carbon materials should be done at the completion of an ovarian drilling. In my institution, this technique is reserved for anovulatory women with PCOS who have failed gonadotropin treatment or those who failed to ovulate with high-dose clomiphene and could not afford gonadotropin treatment. The results have been promising.

Excessive drilling may cause ovarian atrophy and premature menopause. Creating more than 20 "holes" per ovary and drilling the ovarian hilum should be avoided. This may jeopardize the blood supply to the ovary and may also cause bleeding.

Because of the concern of adhesion formation, the coagulation on the ovarian surface should be as minimal as possible. After all, the purpose of the procedure is to reduce the androgen-producing cells in the ovarian stroma.

Myoma

Myoma is found in 25% of women over the age of 35. Its high prevalence suggests that not all women who harbor myoma should undergo surgery for its removal. However, those with excessive uterine bleeding, those with pressure symptoms caused by a large uterine mass, and some infertile women whose myoma is distorting the uterine cavity may require a myomectomy. Myomectomy is often associated with adhesion formation that may further decrease fertility. Adhesion can be decreased by an application of adhesion barrier on the myomectomy incisions or by a second-look laparoscopy and lysis of the adhesions. The overall pregnancy rate after myomectomy and second-look laparoscopy is 66.7% at 12 months' follow-up (Tulandi et al, 1993).

Laparoscopic Myomectomy

Many procedures that previously necessitated a laparotomy, including myomectomy, can be performed by laparoscopy. Laparoscopic excision of a myoma is done as by laparotomy. A pedunculated myoma is removed by coagulating the pedicle with a bipolar forceps and then excising the myoma. For intramural myoma, a solution of vasopressin (0.2 units/ml of physiologic saline) is first injected into the myometrium adjacent to the myoma using a laparoscopic injection needle. The myometrium over the fibroid is incised until the myoma is seen. The myoma is then enucleated using a laparoscopic scissors and blunt or hydro-dissection. Blood vessels encountered during the dissection should be coagulated. Myomas of up to 10 to 15 cm in diameter can be removed using a 15-mm serrated-edged macromorcellator. The uterine incision is closed in two layers. Larger specimens can be removed also via a posterior colpotomy opening.

Laparoscopic myomectomy, however, may lead to inadequate multilayered uterine closure. Indentations of the previous myomectomy incision and uterine fistulae have been noted (Nezhat et al, 1991, 1994). This might represent a structural defect. Uterine dehiscence in late pregnancy and uterine decapitation a few weeks after a laparoscopic myomectomy have also been reported (Harris, 1992; Dubuisson et al, 1995). It is important that the surgeon have expertise in laparoscopic suturing.

Women with diffuse myomas with >3 myomas of ≥5 cm, with a large leiomyomatous uterus (>18 weeks size after luteinizing hormone releasing hormone analog treatment), or with a myoma larger than 15 cm and those who desire a hysterectomy are not candidates for laparoscopic myomectomy.

Laparoscopy-Assisted Myomectomy

Laparoscopy-assisted myomectomy is done by enucleating the myoma partially by laparoscopy. The partially enucleated myoma is grasped with a claw forceps or held with a laparoscopic myoma screw that is inserted suprapubically via a 10-mm trocar. The incision is enlarged transversely enough to accommodate the myoma and the myoma is delivered from the abdominal cavity (Fig. 15–11). The enucleation is continued extracorporeally and the uterine defect is repaired. Closure of the myometrial cavity is done with interrupted sutures of 1-0 of polyglactin and the serosal layer is approximated with 4-0 polyglactin suture. I remove as many myomas as possible from one uterine incision. An incision is made vertically and, before incising, I infiltrate a dilute solution of vasopressin (0.2 unit/ml) into the site of the incision. The uterus is replaced into the abdominal cavity and the abdominal incision is closed. Laparoscopy is resumed and liberal irrigation of the abdominal cavity with a solution of Ringer's lactate is performed. At the completion of the procedure, I instill 500 to 1000 ml of Ringer's lactate solution into the peritoneal cavity.

The main advantage of laparosopy-assisted myomectomy is the ease of multilayered uterine closure without prolonging the duration of surgery (Tulandi and Youssef, 1997). This is especially important for women of reproductive age. Laparoscopy-assisted myomectomy is as effective as myomectomy by laparotomy, but it is associated with a smaller incision, shorter duration of hospitalization, faster recovery, and possibly less bleeding. Perhaps this is due to the "tourniquet effect" of the abdominal wall.

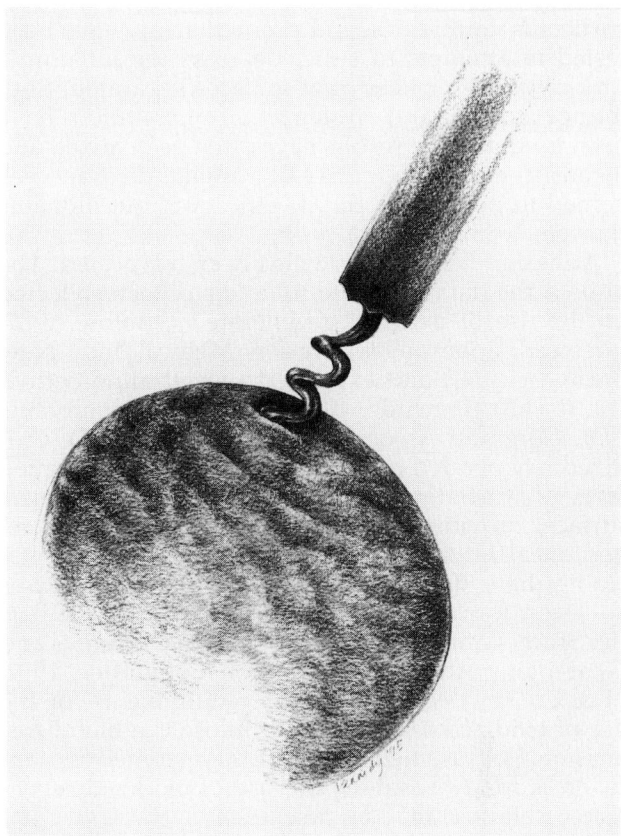

Figure 15–11
Laparoscopy-assisted myomectomy. The partially enucleated myoma is held with a myoma screw and is delivered from the abdominal cavity. The abdominal incision is large enough to accommodate the myoma.

Because abdominal packing is not used, the return of intestinal function is faster. It remains to be seen whether this technique is associated with less adhesion formation.

Laparoscopic Myoma Coagulation

Reduction of the size of a myoma can be done by coagulating its blood supply with a Nd:YAG laser or with long bipolar needle electrodes. It appears that the procedure is effective and regrowth of the myoma does not occur (Goldfarb, 1994). However, it is associated with adhesion formation that may impair future fertility. Uterine rupture following this procedure has been reported. Its long-term risks are still unknown. This technique is not recommended for women of reproductive age.

ADHESION PREVENTION

Despite the use of microsurgical principles and liberal irrigation of the peritoneal cavity, reproductive surgery is still a frequent cause of adhesion formation. A wide variety of substances, including glucocorticoids, antibiotics, and promethazine, have been tested in attempts to either decrease the inflammatory response or keep raw surfaces separated. Both intraperitoneal and systemic administration have been used, but the results have often been mixed and inconsistent. High-molecular-weight dextran has gained in popularity, but its efficacy is questionable (Jansen, 1985).

Adhesion barriers have also been advocated. The bulk of the data compiled to date has been collected on the use of oxidized regenerated cellulose (TC7, Interceed; Johnson & Johnson Medical Inc., New Brunswick, NJ) and expanded polytetrafluoroethylene (PTFE) (Preclude, GoreTex-Surgical Membrane; W.B. Gore and Associates, Inc., Flagstaff, AZ). Oxidized regenerated cellulose is a specifically designed fabric that gelatinizes and adheres to the peritoneal surface, providing a protective barrier. Natural reperitonealization is expected in 7 to 10 days. Several studies have demonstrated that this fabric decreases adhesion formation (Interceed (TC7) Adhesion Barrier Study Group, 1989; Sekiba, for the Obstetrics and Gynecology Adhesion Prevention Committee, 1992; Li & Cooke, 1994). One of the requirements for the use of oxidized regenerated cellulose is a blood-free incision. Because hemostasis at the myomectomy incision is rarely absolute, the use of oxidized regenerated cellulose may be precluded.

Expanded PTFE has been used widely in vascular grafts and orthopedics. The mechanism of action is based on the principle that surgically injured tissues heal without forming adhesions if the traumatized surfaces in apposition are mechanically separated to allow each surface to heal independently. For the purpose of adhesion prevention, PTFE is produced in thin sheets (0.1 mm) with an average pore size of less than 1 μ. This material prevents adhesion formation and reformation regardless of the type of tissue injury or whether hemostasis is achieved. It is particularly useful for prevention of postmyomectomy adhesion. In randomized studies, it was found that expanded PTFE decreases postmyomectomy adhesions (Table 15–3) and pelvic side wall adhesions (Surgical Membrane Study Group, 1992; Myomectomy Adhesion Study Group, 1995). Haney et al

(1995) found that its efficacy is superior to that of oxidized regenerated cellulose. In contrast to oxidized regenerated cellulose, PTFE is nonabsorbable and must be anchored to the tissue. It is for this reason that PTFE is not popular among gynecologists.

REPRODUCTIVE SURGERY VERSUS IVF

Advances in assisted reproductive technologies have led to improvement of their results. This has also led to the question whether reconstructive surgery should still be done (Benadiva et al, 1995). The field of reproductive surgery, especially endoscopic surgery, has also improved markedly. Furthermore, if successful, one surgery may lead to several pregnancies. Assisted reproductive technology and reproductive surgery can be complementary (Winston and Margara, 1991). Young women with tubal disease can be offered surgery, whereas older women with their rapid decline in fertility are better treated with IVF. IVF should be the first line of treatment for women with a severe degree of hydrosalpinx, those with extensive and dense adhesions, and those with bipolar tubal occlusion (proximal and distal tubal occlusion). For tubal anastomosis, however, the superior results of microsurgical procedures are well established. IVF and reproductive surgery are alternative methods of treatment for infertility caused by tubal disease.

REFERENCES

Adamson GD, Hurd SJ, Pasta DJ, Rodriguez BD: Laparoscopic endometriosis treatment: is it better? Fertil Steril 1993;59:35.

Adamson GD, Pasta DJ: Surgical treatment of endometriosis-associated infertility: meta-analysis compared with survival analysis. Am J Obstet Gynecol 1994;171:1488.

American Fertility Society: The American Fertility Society classifications of adnexal adhesions, distal tubal occlusion, tubal occlusion secondary to tubal ligation, tubal pregnancies, Mullerian anomalies and intrauterine adhesions. Fertil Steril 1988; 49:944.

Benadiva CA, Kligman I, Davis O, Rosenwaks Z: In vitro fertilization versus tubal surgery: is pelvic surgery obsolete? Fertil Steril 1995;64:1051.

Canis M, Mage G, Pouly JL, et al: Laparoscopic distal tuboplasty: report of 87 cases and a 4-year experience. Fertil Steril 1991;56: 616.

Confino E, Friberg J, Gleicher N: Preliminary experience with transcervical balloon tuboplasty. Am J Obstet Gynecol 1988;159: 370.

Cook AS, Rock JA: The role of laparoscopy in the treatment of endometriosis. Fertil Steril 1991;55:663.

Daniell JF: Laparoscopic use of the argon beam coagulator. In Sutton C, Diamond MP (eds): Endoscopic Surgery for Gynaecologists. London: WB Saunders Company, 1993:71.

Daniell JF, Herbert CM: Laparoscopic salpingostomy utilizing the CO₂ laser. Fertil Steril 1984;41:558.

Daniell JF, Miller W: Hysteroscopic correction of cornual occlusion with resultant term pregnancy. Fertil Steril 1987;48:490.

DeCherney AH, Silidker JS, Mezer HC, Tarlatsis BC: Reproductive outcome following two ectopic pregnancies. Fertil Steril 1985;43:82.

Donesky BW, Adashi EY: Surgically induced ovulation in the polycystic ovary syndrome: wedge resection revisited in the age of laparoscopy. Fertil Steril 1995;63:439.

Table 15–3. ADHESIONS ON MYOMECTOMY SITES COVERED WITH EXPANDED PTFE AND UNCOVERED (CONTROL)

	PTFE	CONTROL	p
Adhesion free	15/27 (55.6%)	2.27 (7.4%)	0.0003
Adhesion score	1.88 ± 0.46	7.55 ± 0.57	0.0001

From Myomectomy Adhesion Study Group: An expanded-polytetrafluoroethylene barrier (Gore-Tex surgical membrane) reduces postmyomectomy adhesion formation. Fertil Steril 1995;63:491, with permission of the American Society for Reproductive Medicine (The American Fertility Society).

Dubuisson JB, Cavett X, Chapron C, et al: Uterine rupture during pregnancy after laparoscopic myomectomy. Hum Reprod 1995; 10:1475.

Dubuisson JB, De Jolinière JB, Aubriot FX, et al: Terminal tuboplasties by laparoscope: 65 consecutive cases. Fertil Steril 1990; 54:401.

Gjönnaes H: Ovarian electrocautery in the treatment of women with polycystic ovary syndrome (PCOS): factors affecting the results. Acta Obstet Gynecol Scand 1994;73:407.

Goldberg JM, Friedman CI: Microsurgical fallopian tube transposition with subsequent term pregnancy. Fertil Steril 1988;50:660.

Goldfarb HA: Removing uterine fibroids laparoscopically. Contemp Obstet Gynecol 1994;39:50.

Gomel V: Salpingostomy by laparoscopy. J Reprod Med 1977;18:265.

Gomel V: Microsurgical reversal of female sterilization: a reappraisal. Fertil Steril 1980;33:587.

Gomel V, Erenus M: Prognostic value of the American Fertility Society's (AFS) Classification for distal tubal occlusion (DTO). In: American Fertility Society 46th Annual Meeting Program Supplement (P-097). Washington, DC: American Fertility Society, 1990:S-106.

Gomel V, McComb P: Microsurgical transposition of the human fallopian tube and ovary with subsequent intrauterine pregnancy. Fertil Steril 1985;43:804.

Hambley R, Hebda PA, Abell E, et al: Wound healing of skin incisions produced by ultrasonically vibrating knife, scalpel, electrosurgery, and carbon dioxide laser. J Dermatol Surg Oncol 1988;14:1213.

Haney AF, Hesla J, Hurst BS, et al: Expanded polytetrafluroethylene (Gore-Tex Surgical Membrane) is superior to oxidized regenerated cellulose (Interceed TC7) in preventing adhesions. Fertil Steril 1995;63:1021.

Harris WJ: Uterine dehiscence following laparoscopic myomectomy. Obstet Gynecol 1992;80:545.

Hurd WH, Bude RO, DeLancey JOL, Pearl ML: The relationship of the umbilicus to the aortic bifurcation: implications for laparoscopic technique. Obstet Gynecol 1992;80:48.

Interceed (TC7) Adhesion Barrier Study Group: Prevention of postsurgical adhesions by Interceed (TC7), an absorbable adhesions barrier: a prospective, randomized multicenter clinical study. Fertil Steril 1989;51:933.

Jansen RPS: Failure of intraperitoneal adjuncts to improve the outcome of pelvic surgery in young women. Am J Obstet Gynecol 1985;153:363.

Koh CH: Microsurgical laparoscopic tubal resection and anastomosis: techniques and results. In: Tuboperitoneal Infertility and Ectopic Pregnancy. Références en Gynécologie Obstétrique N° Spécial–Congrés Vichy–IFFS 1995;102.

Li TC, Cooke ID: The value of an absorbable adhesion barrier, Interceed in the prevention of adhesion reformation following microsurgical adhesiolysis. Br J Obstet Gynaecol 1994;101:281.

Marana R, Rizzi M, Muzii L, et al: Correlation between the American Fertility Society classifications of adnexal adhesions and distal tubal occlusion, salpingoscopy, and reproductive outcome in tubal surgery. Fertil Steril 1995;64:924.

Marcil-Gratton N, Duchesne C, St-Germaine-Roy S, Tulandi T: Profile of women who request reversal of tubal sterilization: comparison with a randomly selected control group. Can Med Assoc J 1988;138:711.

Marcoux Ś, Maheux R, Berube Ś, and the Canadian Collaborataive Group in Endometriosis. Laparoscopic surgery in infertile women with minimal or mild endometriosis. N Engl J Med 1997;337:217.

McComb P: Microsurgical tubocornual anastomosis for occlusive cornual disease: reproducible results without the need for tubouterine implantation. Fertil Steril 1986;46:571.

McComb P, Paleologou A: The intussusception salpingostomy technique for the therapy of distal oviductal occlusion at laparoscopy. Obstet Gynecol 1991;78:443.

Myomectomy Adhesion Study Group: An expanded-polytetrafluoroethylene barrier (Gore-Tex surgical membrane) reduces post-myomectomy adhesion formation. Fertil Steril 1995;63:491.

Naether OGJ, Fischer R, Weise HC, et al: Laparoscopic electrocoagulation of the ovarian surface in infertility patients with polycystic ovarian disease. Fertil Steril 1993;60:88.

Nezhat C, Crowgey S, Nezhat F: Videolaseroscopy for the treatment of endometriosis associated infertility. Fertil Steril 1989; 51:237.

Nezhat C, Nezhat F, Bess O, et al: Laparoscopically assisted myomectomy: a report of a new technique in 57 cases. Int J Fertil 1994;39:39.

Nezhat C, Nezhat F, Silfen SL, et al: Laparoscopic myomectomy. Int J Fertil 1991;36:275.

Novy ML, Thurmond AS, Patton P, et al: Diagnosis of cornual obstruction by transcervical fallopian tube cannulation. Fertil Steril 1988;50:434.

Okamura H, Furuki Y, Matsuura K, Honda Y: Microsurgical transposition of the human fallopian tube: report of a successful case of pregnancy. Fertil Steril 1988;50:980.

Olive DL, Martin DC: Treatment of endometriosis-associated infertility with CO_2 laser laparoscopy: the use of one- and two-parameter exponential models. Fertil Steril 1987;48:18.

Pagidas K, Tulandi T: Effects of Ringer's lactate, Interceed (TC7) and Gore-Tex surgical membrane on post surgical adhesion formation. Fertil Steril 1992;57:199.

Patton PE, Williams TJ, Coulam CB: Results of microsurgical reconstruction in patients with combined proximal and distal tubal occlusion: double obstruction. Fertil Steril 1987;48:670.

Pouly JL, Mahnes H, Mage G, et al: Conservative laparoscopic treatment of 321 ectopic pregnancies. Fertil Steril 1986;46:1093.

Redwine D: Treatment of endometriosis. In Tulandi T (ed): Atlas of Laparoscopic Technique. Philadelphia: WB Saunders Company, 1994:23.

Rock JA, Guzick DS, Katz E, et al: Tubal anastomosis: pregnancy success following reversal of Falope ring or monopolar cautery sterilization. Fertil Steril 1987;48:13.

Rock JA, Katayama KP, Martin EJ, et al: Pregnancy outcome following uterotubal implantation: a comparison of the reamer and sharp cornual wedge resection techniques. Fertil Steril 1979;31:634.

Schlaff WD, Hassiakos DK, Damewood MD, Rock J: Neosalpingostomy for distal tubal obstruction: prognostic factors and impact of surgical technique. Fertil Steril 1990;54:984.

Schwabe MG, Shapiro SS, Haning RV: Hysterosalpingography with oil contrast medium enhances fertility in patients with infertility of unknown origin. Fertil Steril 1983;40:604.

Sekiba K, for the Obstetrics and Gynecology Adhesion Prevention Committee: Use of Interceed (TC7) absorbable adhesion barrier to reduce postoperative adhesion reformation in infertility and endometriosis surgery. Obstet Gynecol 1992;79:518.

Stovall TG, Ling FW: Single dose methotrexate: an expanded clinical trial. Am J Obstet Gynecol 1993;168:1759.

Sulak PJ, Letterie G, Coddington C, et al: Histology of proximal tubal occlusion. Fertil Steril 1987;48:437.

Surgical Membrane Study Group: Prophylaxis of pelvic side wall adhesion formation with Gore-Tex Surgical Membrane: a multicenter clinical investigation. Fertil Steril 1992;57:921.

Thurmond AS: Technique and results of simple recanalization. In: Tuboperitoneal Infertility and Ectopic Pregnancy. Références en Gynécologie Obstétrique N° Spécial–Congrés Vichy–IFFS 1995;93.

Thurmond AS, Rosch J: Fallopian tubes: improved technique for catheterization. Radiology 1990;174:571.

Toppel H: Intracorporeal suturing. In Tulandi T (ed): Atlas of Laparoscopic Technique. Philadelphia: WB Saunders Company, 1994:17.

Tulandi T: Salpingo-ovariolysis: a comparison between laser surgery and electrosurgery. Fertil Steril 1986;45:489.

Tulandi T: Medical and surgical treatment of ectopic pregnancy. Curr Opin Obstet Gynecol 1994;6:149.

Tulandi T: Distal tubal obstruction: microsurgery versus operative laparoscopy. In: Tuboperitoneal infertility and ectopic pregnancy. Références en Gynécologie Obstétrique N° Spécial–Congrés Vichy–IFFS 1995;188.

Tulandi T, Bugnah M: Operative laparoscopy: surgical modalities. Fertil Steril 1995;63:237.

Tulandi T, Chan KL, Arseneau J: Histopathologic and adhesion formation study after incision using ultrasound vibrating scalpel and regular scalpel. Fertil Steril 1994;61:548.

Tulandi T, Collins JA, Burrows E, et al: Treatment-dependent and treatment-independent pregnancy among women with periadnexal adhesions. Am J Obstet Gynecol 1990;162:354.

Tulandi T, Murray C, Guralnick M: Adhesion formation and reproductive outcome after myomectomy and second-look laparoscopy. Obstet Gynecol 1993;82:123.

Tulandi T, Vilos GA: A comparison between laser surgery and electrosurgery for bilateral hydrosalpinx: a 2 year follow-up. Fertil Steril 1985;44:846.

Tulandi T, Youseff H. Laparoscopic assisted myomectomy for large uterine myomas. Gynaecol Endosc 1997;6:105.

Winston RML: Microsurgery of the fallopian tube: from fantasy to reality. Fertil Steril 1980;34:521.

Winston RML, Margara RA. Microsurgical salpingostomy is not an obsolete procedure. Br J Obstet Gynaecol 1991;98:637.

16

Male Infertility

Edward D. Kim
Larry I. Lipshultz

With recently evolved diagnostic and therapeutic techniques now available for the infertile couple, even the most severe male factor problems are now potentially treatable. Men previously considered irreversibly infertile may now initiate their own biologic pregnancies. Many of these significant changes have been provided by intracytoplasmic sperm injection (ICSI), one of the major medical milestones of the 20th century. Despite this important technical advance, proper patient evaluation remains essential because a male factor is found to be contributory in up to 50% of infertile couples. The temptation to omit or to offer a compromised male evaluation as a result of the erroneous thought that the success of ICSI bypasses the need for a proper andrologic evaluation must be avoided. Thus the emphasis of this chapter is on the essentials of a basic male factor evaluation, as well as the impact of these new reproductive technologies on decision-making strategies.

MALE REPRODUCTIVE SYSTEM

Embryology and Anatomy

In the human, the embryologic precursor to the gonad is the urogenital ridge, which forms in the fourth gestational week on the posterior abdominal wall on either side of the dorsal midline. Eventually, this mesoderm differentiates into the somatic elements of the testis or ovary. Extragonadal entoderm of the yolk sac gives rise to the germinal elements destined to become gonocytes. These gonocytes must migrate in order to reach their final resting place in the genital ridges. Differentiation into a testicle is dependent upon the proper expression of the testis-determining factor gene located on the Y chromosome. This is separate and distinct from the H-Y gene. The exact differentiation process is not well understood in the human, but eventually differentiation does occur, and there is descent of the testicles out of the abdominal cavity into their respective hemiscrota (Huckins and Hellerstein, 1991).

There are three principal cell populations within the testis: Leydig cells, Sertoli cells, and spermatogonia. These cell populations are located in two distinct intratesticular compartments. In the interstitium *between* the tubules are located the Leydig cells, which produce testosterone. *Within* the seminiferous tubules are located two specialized groups of cells. The first group are the Sertoli cells, which extend from the basement membrane to the lumen and demonstrate tight junctions between adjacent cells. These tight junctions form the blood-testis barrier. A number of proteins, including androgen-binding protein and transferrin, are produced by the Sertoli cells. Various growth factors, inhibin, and a number of other poorly understood but important secretory products are also produced by the Sertoli cells. The second cell population *within* the seminiferous tubule are the spermatogonia. Ultimately, in the adult male these undergo mitosis to form primary spermatocytes, with subsequent meiosis resulting in the formation of secondary spermatocytes. Following a second mitotic division, the formation of spermatids is complete. This maturation process lasts approximately 70 days. Transport through the epididymis and ductal elements requires another 10 to 14 days.

The testes in the adult male measure approximately 4×2 cm and have a volume of 20 cm^3 or more. One gonad is located in each hemiscrotum. The testicles are covered by the tunica albuginea. Fibroseptae divide the testicle into 200 to 300 discrete areas of packed seminiferous tubules. Common drainage channels from all of these elements eventually lead through the rete testis to the epididymis via the efferent ducts. The epididymis is located on the posterior aspect of the testis. The caput (head), corpus (body), and cauda (tail) measure a total of 6 meters in length when unwound. The epididymis secretes luminal proteins and has important sperm maturation functions related to attainment of the sperm's full maturity, motility, and functional capabilities. The epididymis eventually leads to the convoluted vas. This tightly coiled portion of the vas extends for several centimeters and becomes the straight portion of the vas. The vas deferens transports sperm from the epididymis and courses through the inguinal canal into the pelvis and retroperitoneum, where it joins with the seminal vesicles to form the ejaculatory duct complex behind the prostate. The ejaculatory ducts exit the prostate in the area of the verumontanum. The prostate is primarily a glandular structure that is hormonally sensitive to testosterone and dihydrotestosterone. It contains a significant amount of fibrostromal elements, including smooth muscle.

Sperm are transported through the urethra with excretory products from a number of other exocrine glands. These include the bulbourethral glands, the prostate, and the seminal vesicles. Only 5% of the normal ejaculate is composed of sperm. A significant portion (60%) has its origin in the seminal vesicles. Thirty per cent comes from the prostate and approximately 5% from the bulbourethral glands. Seminal vesicle fluid factors cause initial coagulation of the semen, whereas prostatic proteolytic enzymes initiate semen liquefaction.

The arterial blood supply to the testis consists primarily of the internal spermatic (gonadal) artery and is augmented by the deferential and cremasteric (external spermatic) arteries. The internal spermatic artery originates from the infrarenal portion of the aorta and courses through the inguinal canal with the spermatic cord. The main venous drainage is the internal spermatic vein, while the minor venous drainage is through the deferential and cremasteric veins. These routes of drainage communicate freely with each other. The left internal spermatic vein drains into the left renal vein, while the right internal spermatic vein empties into the vena cava.

Ejaculation and Emission

Ejaculation is the propulsion of semen through the urethra. Three events must take place:

1. The emission or deposition of fluid from the seminal vesicles and ampullae of the vasa into the posterior urethra
2. The closure of the bladder neck
3. The antegrade ejection of these intraurethral contents

The basic neurophysiology is well understood. The impulses governing this event originate in the thoracolumbar cord (T10 to L2). Preganglionic cholinergic fibers within the hypogastric nerves are used to carry the signals from the thoracolumbar cord to the ganglia within each of these accessory sex glands. From this point on, α-adrenergic neurons directly innervate the specific elements within the accessory sex organs. Bladder neck closure is a sympathetically mediated event under both α-adrenergic and cholinergic influence. Opening of the external sphincter (just prior to ejaculation) is an event mediated by the somatic nervous system (pudendal nerve). If the bladder neck fails to close, retrograde ejaculation occurs. If the T10 to L2 pathways are disrupted, there may be no emission. The normal sequence is erection, orgasm, emission, and ejaculation. However, it is possible to have an erection with orgasm but no emission. Alternatively, a man may have an erection and orgasm with emission, but retrograde ejacula-

tion; or a man with no erection may have an orgasm and antegrade ejaculation (Thomas, 1983).

EVALUATION

Because 85% of "fertile couples" conceive within 1 year of unprotected intercourse, the couple concerned about their fertility traditionally is evaluated after 12 months of unprotected intercourse that has yielded no pregnancy. However, our preference is to evaluate the male partner whenever he presents, because delays in evaluation are associated with fewer successful outcomes and may contribute unnecessarily to stress in these couples.

It is important to consider all aspects of the male in the treatment of the couple. Therefore, a full account of the past medical and surgical history is obtained (Tables 16–1 through 16–4) and routine semen analyses are performed. Numerous laboratory tests have been devised and employed, but discussion here deals only with those most widely used and clinically appropriate. Results must be interpreted in their clinical context and not considered alone. However, it is not necessary to examine all aspects of sperm function in all patients.

HISTORY

Much can be learned of the patient's problem by careful questioning. We determine the age of the patient and that of his partner, how long they have been married, and how long they have been trying to initiate pregnancy. In addition, we ask about coital timing mechanisms; specifically, whether the couple uses basal body temperatures, urine luteinizing hormone (LH) surge monitoring, or intercourse not timed to any specific day. Because sperm are viable for approximately 48 hours, and ova for 12 to 24 hours, intercourse should be planned every other day around the time of ovulation to maximize the chance of placing viable sperm in contact with the ovum in the fallopian tube during the egg's period of viability (Wilcox et al, 1995). One should also ask about the use of vaginal lubricants such as K-Y Jelly, petroleum jelly, or skin lotions, which all may have spermatotoxic effects (Tagatz et al, 1972, Schoeman and Tyler, 1983; Frishman et al, 1992).

Table 16–1. CONGENITAL ANOMALIES

Sexual ambiguities (intersex problem), chromosomal abnormalities
Receptor or gonadotropin abnormalities
Gonadotropin synthesis abnormalities
Gonadotropin action abnormalities
Müllerian ductal regression abnormalities
Cryptorchidism
Microphallus
Hypospadias

Table 16–2. PRIMARY TESTICULAR FAILURE

Klinefelter's syndrome (XXY)
XYY
Vanishing testes syndrome (in utero or early postnatal torsion)
Noonan's syndrome
Varicocele
Myotonic dystrophy
Orchitis (mumps, gonorrhea)
Cryptorchidism
Chemical exposure
Irradiation to testes
Spinal cord injury
Polyglandular failure
Idiopathic oligospermia or azoospermia
Germinal cell aplasia (Sertoli cell–only syndrome)
Idiopathic testicular failure
Testicular torsion
Testicular trauma
Diethylstilbestrol (maternal use during pregnancy resulting in in utero estrogen exposure)
Testicular tumor with subsequent irradiation therapy, chemotherapy, or surgery (retroperitoneal lymph node dissection or orchiectomy)

Table 16–4. ACQUIRED EXTRATESTICULAR CAUSES OF INFERTILITY

Obstructive
Inflammatory
Infectious
Congenital (e.g., Kartagener's syndrome, immotile cilia syndrome)
Surgical
Immunologic
Ejaculatory dysfunction
    Spinal cord injury
    Retroperitoneal lymph node dissection
    Diabetes mellitus
    Multiple sclerosis
    Transverse myelitis
    Pharmaceuticals (antihypertensives, antipsychotics)

We also seek to determine whether either partner has initiated a pregnancy in either the current or a previous relationship. Any previous evaluation and therapy are noted and recorded in detail. Frequently, the male has received medical therapy (e.g., clomiphene citrate) for a presumed male factor but with little or no monitoring. If a patient presents already on medication, we obtain serum follicle-stimulating hormone (FSH), (LH), and testosterone levels as a baseline during therapy. Later, once the patient has ceased medication for a period of 2 to 3 months, we again obtain an endocrine profile to establish his physiologic norm.

Also noted is the patient's occupation, with specific attention paid to factors in the work environment that might be deleterious to testicular function.

Table 16–3. SECONDARY TESTICULAR FAILURE

Delayed puberty
Kallmann's syndrome
Isolated gonadotropin deficiency
Prader-Labhart-Willi syndrome
Lawrence-Moon-Biedl syndrome
Central nervous system irradiation
Prepubertal panhypopituitarism
Postpubertal panhypopituitarism
Hypogonadism secondary to hyperprolactinemia
Adrenogenital syndrome
Chronic liver disease
Chronic renal failure/uremia
Hemochromatosis
Cushing's syndrome
Malnutrition
Massive obesity
Sickle cell anemia
Hyper/hypothyroidism
Anabolic steroid use

These would include exposure to chemicals, radiation, or extreme heat. Ingestion of various drugs and medications is noted; specifically, the extent to which the patient partakes of alcohol, tobacco, and recreational drugs. Not only have alcohol (Van Thiel et al, 1975), nicotine (Evans et al, 1981), marijuana (Kolodny et al, 1974) and cocaine (Berul and Harcleode, 1989) been recognized as gonadotoxins, but so have sulfasalazine (Levi et al, 1979), cimetidine (Van Thiel et al, 1979), and high-dose nitrofurantoin (Nelson and Steinberger, 1952). Additionally, anabolic steroids that act as male contraceptives are becoming more widely abused by athletes (Jarow and Lipshultz, 1990). Exposure to extreme heat should also be considered. Hot showers are potentially much less detrimental than the use of hot tubs, where heat is applied directly and continuously to the testicles.

The patient's medical history often reveals factors that could have had significant impact upon his fecundity. We note any systemic processes, including hepatitis, renal dysfunction, diabetes mellitus, nervous system disorders, and sinopulmonary diseases, and any previous infections that might have impaired testicular function or ductal patency. Prepubescent mumps usually does *not* cause orchitis, although it is seen in 19% of postpubescent males with the mumps virus. Mumps orchitis is usually unilateral (67%) rather than bilateral (33%); testicular atrophy occurs in 36% of affected men, with impaired fertility in up to 13% (Beard et al, 1977). We also make specific inquiries about tuberculosis, any sexually transmitted disease (*Chlamydia*, *Mycoplasma*, gonorrhea, syphilis, human immunodeficiency virus, condyloma, *Trichomonas*), and any trauma to the genitalia or spine. Pelvic or spinal trauma, such as that sustained in a motor vehicle accident or in a fall, is of great interest because there may have been disruption either of innervation, causing ejaculatory dysfunction, or of the ductal elements of the vas deferens, causing obstruction. A history of premature ejaculation and other sexual dysfunction is also noted.

The surgical history is important because a simple herniorrhaphy or hydrocelectomy in the past may have resulted in vasal or epididymal obstruction. Other surgical procedures of great interest are those performed on the bladder or in the bladder neck area or any transurethral procedure, such as a transurethral resection of the prostate gland or incision of the bladder neck. Any of these operations can cause complete or partial retrograde ejaculation. All testicular surgeries should be noted. An orchiectomy may have been performed for torsion, trauma, or a tumor. Fifty per cent of men with testis tumors have sperm counts below 10 to 20 million/ml at presentation (Presti et al, 1993; Foster and Donohue, 1995). Contralateral testicular function may not return to normal for 4 to 5 years after chemotherapy or radiation treatment (Meistrich et al, 1989; Oates and Lipshultz, 1989). An orchiopexy may have been performed for cryptorchidism or torsion. Previous retroperitoneal or pelvic surgery for tumors (retroperitoneal lymph node dissection in the face of a testicular tumor) may result in anejaculation or anemission as a result of interruption of sympathetic innervation (Donohue et al, 1990).

A pertinent history may also elicit information about familial infertility associated with cryptorchidism, cystic fibrosis, congenital absence of the vas deferens, or androgen receptor deficiency. However, such a history does not necessarily indicate a pathologic disease process in the patient under study.

The next task in dealing with the infertile male is a thorough review of systems. The presence of persistent headaches, changing visual fields, or anosmia would suggest the possibility of a central nervous system tumor. The complaint of frequent pneumonia, bronchial infections, or sinusitis suggests the presence of the immotile cilia syndrome (Kartagener's) or one of its variables, or Young's syndrome. The finding of galactorrhea is pathologic and requires further investigation to rule out a prolactin-secreting tumor.

PHYSICAL EXAMINATION

The importance assigned to the history should also be reflected in the physical examination, which includes measurement of height, weight, and blood pressure. A complete examination of the body, including the breasts, abdomen, and genitalia, and a digital rectal examination of the prostate should be performed. Examination of the genitalia begins with viewing all skin surfaces, including the prepuce, glans, and meatus. It is important to retract the foreskin and examine the distal penis, glans, and coronal area for any abnormalities. The meatus is examined for size, location, and patency, because hypospadias may be a contributing factor in the couple's infertility. The presence of any coronal or subcoronal lesions is noted. These would include syphilitic chancre, herpetic ulcers, carcinoma, condyloma acuminatum, erythroplasia of Queryat, and "pearly papules." The

presence of meatal or urethral discharge should be noted and a urethral culture performed if a sexually transmitted disease is suspected.

Next, the entire scrotum is examined. Careful palpation of the testicles will demonstrate any parenchymal abnormalities such as tumor, granuloma, or fibrosis. The presence and contour of the testicles, epididymides, and vasa deferens must be verified. The epididymis may be found to be enlarged, tender, indurated, or warm, all of which are signs of acute epididymitis. Alternatively, it may be somewhat nodular, firm, and granular. These are signs of chronic epididymitis with associated obstruction, such as that caused by a nonspecific inflammation or a tubercular or bacterial agent. At this point, scrotal and peritesticular abnormalities can be noted. There may be testicular atrophy, or cryptorchidism. Additionally, there may be scrotal skin lesions such as cysts and other dermatopathologies.

The patient, in the standing position, should be examined for a hydrocele or a hernia (direct, indirect, or femoral). After the patient has been standing for several minutes in a warm room, the physician should palpate the scrotum for the presence of varicoceles. This is achieved by having the patient perform a Valsalva maneuver while the physician identifies the vas deferens and other cord structures. A *large varicocele* can be seen easily without the aid of the Valsalva maneuver. It appears as a peritesticular mass or a "bag of worms" above the testicle. On palpation, the varicocele will feel like multiple, dilated yet compressible tubules. A *moderate varicocele* may be palpated without the Valsalva maneuver, and this again will feel like a compressible mass above the testicle; however, it does not distort the scrotal skin. A *small varicocele* can be felt only as an "impulse" when the Valsalva maneuver is performed. It may be necessary to repeat this maneuver several times until one is confident of the findings. Subclinical (nonpalpable) varicoceles can be diagnosed by various methods, including venography, high-resolution scrotal ultrasound, color flow Doppler ultrasound, hand-held Doppler stethoscope, radioisotope scanning, and thermography. Because deleterious effects of subclinical varicoceles on testicular function have not been consistently demonstrated, their repair is quite controversial. We currently take no action if we find these nonpalpable vascular lesions on ultrasound (Bsat and Masabni, 1988; McClure et al, 1991).

One should pay close attention to the groin and pubic area because a herniorrhaphy in the remote past may have left a small scar that is easily missed and often forgotten. Vasal injury may have occurred. Next, the patient should undergo a rectal examination for the size, consistency, and shape of the prostate as well as evaluation of the seminal vesicles. Any periprostatic or perirectal masses or intrarectal abnormalities are noted. These include atrophy or aplasia of the prostate or seminal vesicles or a large cystic midline mass (e.g., an ejaculatory duct cyst).

LABORATORY EVALUATION

With a myriad of infertility-related laboratory tests available, judicious use of laboratory resources is required. Our preliminary laboratory examination consists of two semen analyses and quantification of serum FSH, LH, and testosterone values. Prolactin levels should be obtained when clinically indicated. Because most of the patients seen at the Scott Department of Urology have already undergone preliminary evaluation and have complicated problems, evaluation also includes semen testing for the presence of anti-sperm antibodies using an immunobead assay and for leukocytospermia using a monoclonal antibody assay. Further specialized testing is dictated by clinical indications.

MacLeod's classical paper (1951) on semen quality in fertile and infertile couples offers the "gold standard" by which to measure the "limits of adequacy" of bulk semen parameters. These reflect threshold values of ejaculate volume, sperm density, viability, motility (forward progression), and morphology. Achieving a pregnancy is increasingly arduous and becomes statistically less probable when these values are not met (Table 16–5). If the first semen analysis is abnormal, then further investigation is indicated. Several semen analyses collected over a 3- to 6-week interval would be helpful in gathering further data points regarding the bulk semen parameters of volume, sperm density, motility, forward progression, morphology, viscosity, and agglutination, as well as pyospermia, the presence of bacteria, and liquefaction. There may be mild seasonal variation (Levin et al, 1990), deleterious effects of fevers or viral episodes, or subtle environmental toxins such as extreme thermal exposure contributing to abnormalities. If the bulk semen parameters have shown persistent abnormalities, then further investigations should be undertaken. Variations in the findings between laboratories may reflect differences in techniques and experience, rather than fluctuating semen quality.

Semen Analysis

A semen analysis should be collected in a standardized manner that dictates a 2- to 3-day period of sexual abstinence before the specimen is collected, precludes use of spermatocidal lubricants, and requires use of a wide-mouthed, non–sperm-toxic plastic or glass container for collection. Delivery and processing of the semen within 1 to 2 hours of its collection is mandatory. For patients who have difficulty with masturbation, we recommend a semen collection device (e.g., SCD Male-FactorPak; Hamilton-Thorn Research, Wenham, MA).

Following collection and proper labeling of the specimen, various laboratory determinations are made. Initially, the specimen resembles a coagulated, semitranslucent gel. However, in 3 to 15 minutes, liquefaction should occur. Viscosity can be assessed in a qualitative manner (i.e., the sperm should pour drop by drop). The volume should be determined to the nearest 0.1 ml using a graduated test tube. A pH meter or nitrazine strips will indicate the acidity if it is to be determined. Either a hemocytometer (Neubauer) with a 1:20 dilution (1:10 if a low number of sperm are seen on the initial count) or a Makler counting chamber (Sefi-Medical Instruments, Haifa, Israel) with no dilution is used to estimate the sperm density. Motility is measured as a percentage of moving sperm. Measurement of forward progression is a subjective assessment of the quality of sperm movement. The quality of movement is determined on a scale of 0 to 4:

0 = no movement
1 = poor, weak forward progression
2 = moderate, somewhat definite forward progression
3 = good forward progression
4 = excellent, bullet-like forward progression

In our laboratory, an undiluted aliquot of semen on a wet mount is used under a phase-contrast microscope for assessment of the percentage of sperm motility as well as morphology.

Computer-assisted semen analyses (CASA) have been introduced into the armamentaria of physicians studying male infertility. These systems, which base their analyses on video image motion analysis, include the Hamilton-Thorn Motility Analyzer (Hamilton-Thorn, Wenham, MA), and CellTrack (Motion Analysis Corporation, Santa Rosa, CA). These systems excel at measuring both rectilinear and curvilinear velocities. However, they tend to overestimate the total sperm density and to underestimate the sperm motility for a variety of reasons, among which is an inability to distinguish between a nonmotile sperm and a piece of sperm-sized debris or other cellular elements. Inadequate preparation of material, improper calibration of machines, and limitations of computer software in allowing for samples with very high and very low sperm density affect results. Operator-dependent settings influence the CASA; while their clinical efficacy remains debatable, their use in research may be important.

It is also essential to determine whether round cells are white blood cells or immature sperm. This

Table 16–5. SEMEN ANALYSIS: NORMAL VALUES

Volume	1.5–5.0 ml
Count	>20 million/ml (possibly >10)
Motility	>60%
Forward progression	>2 (scale 0–4)
Morphology	>60% oval forms

And

No significant pyospermia or hematospermia
No significant sperm agglutination
No hyperviscosity

may be determined with discriminating testing of semen using monoclonal antibodies specific for white blood cells (Wolff and Anderson, 1988), or by using specific stains. Counts are made per high-power field per 100 sperm or per ejaculate. The presence of bacteria requires further evaluation, as does hematospermia. The seminal vesicles can be assessed indirectly with qualitative fructose determinations, which, if positive, are suggestive of their presence and functional integrity.

Hormone Testing

Evaluation of couples suspected of male factor infertility should include assessment of the hypothalamic-pituitary-gonadal axis with serum determinations of FSH, LH, testosterone, and prolactin (Cunningham and Lipshultz, 1986). This axis is depicted in Figure 16–1. In general, FSH values increase as the mature germ cell population decreases. Inhibin from Sertoli cells inhibits FSH release, whereas activin from the Leydig cell stimulates FSH release. Both inhibin and activin belong to the transforming growth factor-β protein family (Lee et al, 1989). In addition to their endocrine action, it is likely that they regulate cell growth and differentiated function. Testicular dysfunction causes compensatory increases in FSH and, to a lesser extent, LH values. The prognosis is especially poor in azoospermic or oligospermic males with an FSH greater than three times normal.

Leydig cell function is reflected in values of LH and testosterone. If there is a history of delayed puberty, decreased libido, or impotence, then LH and testosterone values can be helpful. Hypogonadotropic hypogonadism in the adult male with incomplete sexual maturation is characterized by relatively low values of serum FSH and LH. Conversely, low FSH and LH values in a sexually mature individual

would suggest that there is a central, or pituitary, etiology such as a hypothalamic or pituitary tumor. By determining the prolactin level, one may identify either a microadenoma or a macroadenoma. Evaluation of the sella turcica can be best performed with magnetic resonance imaging (MRI), although computerized tomography (CT) is often adequate.

Estradiol serum values are important if there is a question of increased peripheral conversion of testosterone to estradiol, as in a very obese patient, one with gynecomastia, or one suspected of having end-organ resistance to testosterone.

Anti-sperm Antibodies

Because there is normally an intact blood-testis barrier, the presence of anti-sperm antibodies would be expected only if there had been some exposure of the patient's blood to sperm antigens. Serum anti-sperm antibodies have been detected in men having a history of vasectomy (80%; Alexander and Anderson, 1979), testicular biopsy (17%; Hjort et al, 1974), cryptorchid testes (13%; Haas, 1987), and testicular torsion or trauma (Broderick et al, 1989; Krarup, 1978). However, semen anti-sperm antibodies are thought to be of more biologic significance.

Although the presence of anti-sperm antibodies is generally thought to be pathologic, not all affected men have problems with infertility (Marshburn and Kutteh, 1994). In general, infertile men have been found to have a higher incidence of anti-sperm antibodies than their age-matched controls (Rumke and Hekman, 1977). The typical signs of anti-sperm antibody autoimmunity would include disorders of sperm movement in association with clumping or immobilization, impaired cervical mucus–sperm interaction, and impaired sperm-ovum penetration (Haas et al, 1980; Haas, 1986). Immunoglobulin G (IgG) and immunoglobulin A (IgA) anti-sperm antibodies have the greatest clinical relevance. The patient's serum, seminal plasma, and spermatozoa can be assayed for the presence of these antibodies. A number of techniques exist for detecting antibodies, including polyacrylamide beads coated with specific monoclonal antibodies (Immunobead) as well as the historically important Kibrick method (macroagglutination). We prefer the immunobead test because the location and class (IgG, IgA) of antibody binding, such as to the head, neck, or tail, can be determined.

Semen White Blood Cell Assays

Monoclonal antibody technology has been applied as a dependable method for the identification of leukocytes in semen. Round cells in the semen may represent either immature germ cells or leukocytes, and specific identification cannot be determined based on routine semen analysis or specific stains, such as peroxidase, Papanicolaou, or Giemsa (Wolff and Ander-

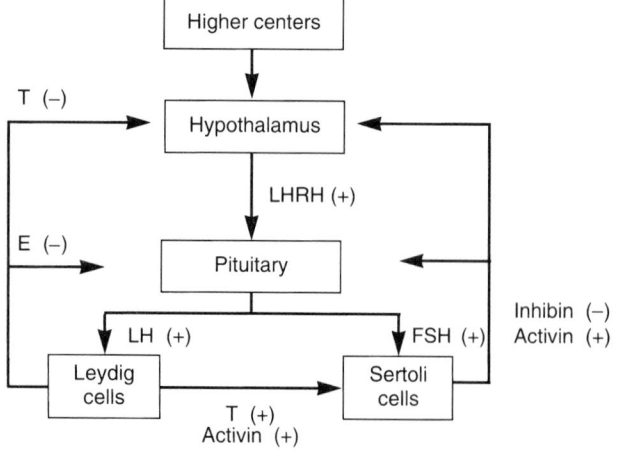

Figure 16–1
Hypothalamic-pituitary-gonadal (HPG) axis. E, estradiol; FSH, follicle-stimulating hormone; LH, luteinizing hormone; LHRH, luteinizing hormone–releasing hormone; T, testosterone.

son, 1988). However, using monoclonal antibodies against the common leukocyte antigen CD45, the detection of granulocytes, lymphocytes, and macrophages is possible. Only with proper identification of the type of "round cells" can appropriate treatment be instituted.

The significance of elevated concentrations of leukocytes within the semen is that their presence indicates infection or inflammation within the male reproductive tract (Wolff, 1995). If semen and urethral cultures are negative, then a trial of anti-inflammatory agents and antioxidant therapy may be tried. White blood cells are deleterious because of their ability to stimulate the release of reactive oxygen species. Antimicrobial therapy may be used even when cultures are negative, although results are variable (Yanushpolsky et al, 1995). Seminal leukocytes are also likely to inhibit sperm motility as a result of the release of large quantities of reactive oxygen species.

Cervical Mucus Migration Studies

The most widely utilized subjective method of evaluating interaction of sperm and cervical mucus is the postcoital test. The cervical mucus is examined 2 hours after intercourse in the periovulatory phase. The presence of 20 or more motile sperm per high-power field is considered "normal." This subjective test reflects the limitations associated with the prediction of ovulation and the timing of examination of the mucus. For these reasons, many false-negative (i.e., abnormal) results can be expected. More objective systems have been developed (Penetrak, Serono Laboratories, Inc., Norwell, MA; TruTrak, Humagen, Inc., Charlottesville, VA) that allow for a more standardized measurement of sperm-mucus interaction. These systems involve comparison of the interaction of the husband's and donor sperm with the wife's mucus and with (bovine) mucus substrate as a control.

Sperm Penetration Assay

Since it was described by Yanagimachi and coworkers in 1976, the sperm penetration assay (SPA) has been used clinically as a test of sperm function and, in the laboratory, as a means of studying the physiology of fertilization. The use of the SPA as a measure of fertility is based upon the theory that, whereas healthy sperm will penetrate most specially processed hamster ova and produce a significant amount of polyspermy (multiple sperm per egg), unhealthy sperm will penetrate a lower percentage of ova and produce a lesser degree of polyspermy. Despite general agreement as to the theory behind the SPA, the precise methodology of the assay varies significantly among laboratories. Most commonly, the scoring is based upon the percentage of ova that have been penetrated, with the lower limit of normal penetration being 10% to 30%.

Investigators at Baylor College of Medicine have found that, by optimizing each step in the SPA, they can usually achieve ova penetration of 100% of oocytes in most patients (Johnson et al, 1995). Determination of the number of sperm penetrations per ova (*sperm capacitation index*) has significantly increased the sensitivity of the assay. With a lower limit of normal being five penetrations per ovum, it has been found that couples with a normal SPA have a 95% chance of fertilizing human ova in vitro, as compared to couples with a negative SPA, who have a 50% chance of fertilizing human ova in vitro. In those couples with normal semen parameters, a positive SPA is generally predictive of success of fertilization in vitro, whereas a negative SPA may suggest that a couple has a lower chance of successful in vitro fertilization (IVF) and may do better with ICSI.

Strict Morphology

Strict morphology evaluation of sperm, in contrast to the World Health Organization's conventional morphologic assessment, defines specific "strict" criteria or measurement parameters of sperm shape related to the acrosome, head, neck, midpiece, and tail (Kruger et al, 1986). After staining a semen smear, at least 200 sperm are manually classified according to the established criteria. Newer computerized methods show promise for hastening this otherwise time-consuming process (Kruger et al, 1995). The importance of strict morphologic assessment is that results correlate with the success of IVF fertilization. In men with normal strict morphology (i.e., >14% normal forms), successful fertilization was demonstrated in 88.3% of oocytes (Kruger et al, 1988). However, in men with strict morphologies of less than 4% normal forms, normal fertilization was present in only 7.6% of oocytes. Although experiences are still somewhat limited, fertilization, implantation, and pregnancy rates using teratozoospermic samples and ICSI do not appear to be significantly affected in comparison to those results using normal strict morphology specimens (Hall et al, 1995; Svalander et al, 1996).

Other Tests

A number of other sperm function tests have been described in the literature, but few have found wide use or acceptance. These include use of a CASA system to determine the percentage of sperm in a hyperactivated motility state (suggestive of capacitation) and measuring the number of sperm that respond with a set pattern of swelling following exposure to a hypo-osmotic medium (hyper or mild swelling). In addition, tests to define the acrosome reaction have included the staining of acrosomal membranes (trypan blue, rose bengal) or the use of other acrosome-identifying techniques incorporating peanut lectins, calcium ionophore A23187 treatment, monoclonal antibodies, and chlortetracycline fluorescence. Finally, the hemizona assay has also been described but is not commonly used because of decreased availability of intact ova following more widespread application of ICSI.

DIAGNOSTIC PROCEDURES

Testicular Biopsy

Testicular biopsies and touch imprint (cytologic) preparations are used for differentiating between obstruction and testicular failure as a cause of azoospermia or severe, unexplained oligospermia. In most instances, a unilateral biopsy alone is sufficient. However, bilateral biopsies may be considered if the presence of asymmetric lesions is noted. The formal, "open" biopsy technique involves scrotal exploration and inspection of the vas deferens and epididymis following delivery of the testis when the testicular biopsy is obtained. One can readily determine the presence or absence of the vasa deferens and their relative size or identify signs of obstruction in the epididymides. A preferred, less invasive method is the "window" technique. Although this does not allow visualization of the entire ductal system, it does provide a valid biopsy. It is performed in the outpatient setting using a spinal anesthetic, a light general anesthetic, or local infiltration alone.

During the biopsy, the healthier testis is isolated and brought anteriorly with its overlying skin pulled taughtly. Following instillation of 1% lidocaine, a 1- to 2-cm incision is made down through the subcutaneous tissues to the level of the tunica vaginalis. This is incised and secured with small hemostats and a "window" is created by the use of a small eyelid retractor. The tunica albuginea is then bathed in 1% lidocaine for approximately 1 minute and a 3- to 5-mm incision is made with a No. 15 scalpel blade. When gentle pressure is applied to the testis, a small number of seminiferous tubules will protrude. These are excised with a sharp, curved scissors and, with jeweler's forceps, the excised tissue is touched lightly to a sterile glass slide that is then immediately sprayed with a fixative. The original specimen itself is placed in either Bouin's, Zenker's, or a buffered glutaraldehyde solution. Formalin is to be avoided because it may cause destruction or distortion of the delicate seminiferous tubular structures. Hemostasis is meticulously obtained with a bipolar electrocautery. The tunica albuginea, vaginalis, and scrotal skin are closed with individual layers of 4-0 chromic suture. This technique minimizes the formation of adhesions that can make future exploration very difficult.

Interpretation of the testicular touch preparation cytology is directed toward the identification of mature sperm (Kim and Lipshultz, 1996). After staining with hematoxylin-eosin or a Papanicolaou stain, all spermatogenic cells are easily seen. In some instances, late maturation arrest cannot readily be distinguished from obstruction with a routine paraffin-fixed biopsy because the sperm within the seminiferous tubules resemble spermatids in their late stages.

Specific histologic diagnoses determined from examination of the biopsy are the following:

1. *Normal*: Leydig cells, Sertoli cells, and germinal components are normal in both presence and relative number.
2. *Hypospermatogenesis*: A proportional decrease in all of the germinal elements, either mild, moderate, or severe, in some or all of the tubules is present.
3. *Maturation arrest:* Because of the lack of mature germinal elements, there are increased relative numbers of either primary or secondary spermatocytes (early arrest) or spermatids (late arrest).
4. *Sertoli cell—only*: Indicates an overall lack of germinal elements within the seminiferous tubules.
5. *End-stage fibrosis:* Severe tubular sclerosis with hyalinization and associated Leydig cell hyperplasia may also be found. This is not a pathognomonic finding for Klinefelter's disease because there are other causes of a very similar histologic pattern, including end-stage infections, inflammatory and ischemic insults, and prior radiation or chemotherapeutic exposures.

A newer technique for the assessment of the testis biopsy employs computer-assisted image analysis, which provides a quantitative method for categorizing abnormalities of intratubular cell content (Kim et al, 1997). Based on DNA content and morphology characteristics, testis biopsy image analysis avoids many of the limitations of our present purely qualitative analysis system. This technique's significant advantage over flow cytometry is the ability to distinguish between 1N cell types (i.e., the spermatozoa and spermatids). Image analysis has important implications in redefining our current purely qualitative testis biopsy interpretation, and could replace or add an additional classification to this present system.

The testis biopsy may also be used therapeutically, in combination with sperm harvesting during an ICSI/IVF cycle. The indications for testicular extraction of sperm include obstruction and testicular failure (Devroey et al, 1996). When normal spermatogenesis and an epididymal obstruction are present and sperm cannot be retrieved from the epididymis secondary to significant scarring, either an open or percutaneous testicular biopsy may be performed. The only condition in which percutaneous testicular sperm aspiration (TESA) is appropriate is in the obstructed testis. In this situation, large numbers of sperm are present for retrieval and the chances of successful recovery are high. Numerous needle passes may still be required, however, increasing the chances of injury to the testicular blood supply and resultant testicular damage.

The open testis biopsy is known as testicular sperm extraction (TESE) and is appropriate for both obstruction and testis failure. A much larger biopsy is typically required for testis failure because fewer sperm are being produced. Sperm retrieval from testicular tissue is performed using various combinations of vortexing, mincing, and separation of sperm from other cellular elements.

Vasogram

The vasogram is a radiographic study undertaken at the time of proposed microsurgical repair of an obstructed ductal system. Vasography was previously considered the traditional imaging study for the evaluation of ejaculatory duct obstruction. However, because of its moderately invasive nature with attendant risk of damage to the vas deferens, transrectal ultrasound (TRUS) with seminal vesiculography has become the preferred initial diagnostic method for ejaculatory duct obstruction. Vasography has its importance in diagnosing proximal vas deferens obstructions.

We prefer a vasography technique in which the vas deferens is microsurgically incised and the lumen identified. A complete vasal transection is not necessary and may, in fact, be counterproductive because of ultimate scarring. A sample of effluxing fluid from the testicular end of the vas deferens is examined for sperm under a standard microscope (400×). If none are found and there is a normal testicular biopsy, then there is likely an epididymal obstruction. If sperm are present in the vasal fluid, then we inject methylene blue or indigo carmine into the abdominal vas and check the urine for the presence of blue dye by catheterization. Alternatively, a radiograph can be obtained if contrast material is used (i.e., a formal vasogram). If there are sperm present and if there is patency toward the abdominal end, then the vasotomy site can be closed microsurgically with 10-0 monofilament, double-armed suture to avoid stricture or leakage. In this situation, partial obstruction of the ejaculatory ducts resulting from cyst formation should be considered. We *never* inject toward the epididymis because this can actually produce an epididymal blockage as a result of inadvertent rupture of the delicate epididymal tubules.

TRUS of the Prostate

Because of its excellent visualization of the seminal vesicles, prostate, and ejaculatory ducts, TRUS has become an important diagnostic technique in the evaluation of the infertile male (Kim et al, 1996). TRUS for infertility purposes is commonly performed with the patient in the lateral decubitus, knee-to-chest position using a high-resolution 6.5- to 7.5-MHz probe. Indications for TRUS are presented in Table 16–6.

Table 16–6. TRANSRECTAL ULTRASOUND IN MALE INFERTILITY

ABSOLUTE INDICATIONS
Low-volume azoospermia in the absence of testicular atrophy
Low-volume severe oligospermia (concentration <5 million/ml)
Abnormal digital rectal examination

RELATIVE INDICATIONS
Normal-volume azoospermia or severe oligospermia in the absence of testicular atrophy
Severe motility defects with a normal physical examination and hormonal profile
Ejaculatory abnormality
   Anejaculation
   Hematospermia
   Painful ejaculation
   Unexplained retrograde ejaculation
History suggestive of genital duct abnormality
   Unilaterally nonfunctioning or absent kidney
   History of severe hypospadias

A significant recent advance is the use of TRUS as the first-line diagnostic modality for evaluation of ejaculatory duct obstruction (Carter et al, 1989). Men with ejaculatory duct obstruction may present with primary infertility and azoospermia (no sperm present) or severe, unexplained oligoasthenospermia (severely depressed sperm density and motility). Thus absolute indications for performing TRUS include low-volume azoospermia and low-volume severe oligoasthenospermia in the absence of testicular atrophy (Hellerstein et al, 1991). Certainly, one must first be sure that retrograde ejaculation is not present. Ejaculatory duct cysts, ejaculatory duct calcification, ejaculatory duct dilation, and seminal vesicle dilation visualized on TRUS are all consistent with ejaculatory duct obstruction. Although obstruction should be suspected in patients with a transaxial seminal vesicle width of more than 1.5 cm (Jarow, 1993), seminal vesicle dilation does not occur in every patient, especially if a concurrent epididymal obstruction resulting from a "blowout" is present.

Complete obstruction of the ejaculatory ducts has been described and is characterized by low ejaculate volumes and azoospermia. *Partial obstruction* of the ejaculatory ducts can produce a wide spectrum of seminal fluid abnormalities (Ruiz Rubio et al, 1995). There may be azoospermia to normospermia in association with low-normal to very low ejaculate volumes. Motility usually is significantly diminished (<30%). Partial and complete obstruction of the ejaculatory ducts can be secondary to infection, stone, catheterization, trauma, congenital or acquired cyst formation, and other idiopathic causes.

Seminal Vesiculography

TRUS combined with seminal vesiculography has greatly reduced the need for the more invasive, open vasography, still considered by some as the "gold standard" for identifying distal ejaculatory duct obstruction but carrying a risk of vasal scarring. With a 35-cm long 21-gauge Williams needle (or a 30-cm 17-gauge oocyte retrieval needle), the seminal vesicles may be aspirated transrectally under ultrasound guidance. The presence of numerous sperm in the seminal vesicles is suggestive of obstruction at the ejaculatory duct in men with azoospermia or severe oligospermia (Jarow, 1994). This technique may be especially helpful in identifying the unilaterally obstructed ejaculatory duct or partially obstructed ejaculatory duct when sperm are present in the ejaculate but ultrasonographic findings are equivocal. Seminal vesiculography may be performed after transrectal aspiration with the injection of nonionic contrast. Fluoroscopy, combined with radiographs after instillation of 5, 10, and 20 ml of contrast, provides ideal imaging.

Transurethral resection of the ejaculatory ducts (TURED) is a relatively noninvasive procedure and is performed in an outpatient setting with little patient discomfort. TURED is the treatment of choice for men with ejaculatory duct obstruction, and may be assisted with the intraoperative use of TRUS for identifying the location of an obstructing cyst and determining the depth of resection. A series reported by Turek and colleagues (1996) demonstrated improvements in semen parameters in 65% of men and pregnancies in 20% of couples after TURED. Postoperative semen analyses can be obtained in as few as 3 weeks and can lead one rapidly into the next stage of treatment.

DIAGNOSTIC ALGORITHMS

Azoospermia and Elevated FSH (Three Times Normal)

The previous algorithm for decision making for testicular biopsy recommended that men with azoospermia, testicular atrophy, and serum FSH levels greater than three times normal had testicular failure and were hopelessly infertile. Because a diagnosis other than severe intrinsic testicular failure was highly unlikely, the couple was offered artificial insemination with donor sperm (AID) or adoption. However, with the introduction of ICSI, these men are potentially able to father their own biologic offspring because sperm may be present in 30% of their testis biopsies (Kim et al, 1997a). Using the previously discussed technique of testicular sperm extraction, ongoing pregnancy rates per transfer as high as 31% (5/16 cycles) have been reported (Devroey et al, 1996).

Abnormal Semen Analysis and FSH (Less Than Three Times Normal)

If the FSH is less than three times normal or normal, then the possibility of exposure to exogenous toxins such as heat, chemicals, or radiation should be investigated. The patient's medical history will reflect any illnesses experienced in the 3 to 6 months preceding his original visit and semen analysis. Theoretically, these events could cause transient alterations in the quality of sperm. In such an event, repetition of the semen analysis in 3 to 6 months is recommended.

Although the physical examination may reveal a varicocele, all men with varicoceles are not infertile. It is our belief that infertile men with varicoceles should have their vascular lesions repaired only in the absence of any other identifiable and correctable abnormality. In general, varicocele correction should be performed prior to any attempts at sperm manipulation and assisted reproductive technologies. Following varicocelectomy, 70% of patients have improved bulk semen parameters and 40% to 60% may establish a pregnancy (Marks et al, 1986; Magdar et al, 1995). Techniques of varicocele repair include surgical ligation (open or laparoscopic) or percutaneous embolization. If physical examination reveals no evidence of a varicocele and the index of suspicion for a subclinical varicocele is not high, then one should review the isolated abnormal bulk semen parameters as a key to possible therapy.

FSH Deficiency

If serum FSH is measured first and is below normal, then a full examination of gonadotropins LH, testosterone, and prolactin) should be undertaken. If LH, FSH, and prolactin levels are all decreased, then hypogonadotropic hypogonadism strongly suggested. If the FSH and LH levels are low and the prolactin level is elevated, there may be a pituitary anomaly. Pituitary neoplasms are evaluated with MRI or CT imaging. If a microadenoma is found (i.e., no gross distortion of the pituitary is visualized), then bromocriptine (Parlodel) can be given. Pituitary surgery (e.g., transsphenoidal approach) is reserved for larger adenomas.

SPECIFIC PARAMETER ANOMALIES

Disorders of Volume

If the volume is less than 1.5 ml, then one must make certain that there has been no collection error. A common occurrence is that the initial portion of the ejaculate is missed or not collected, or a portion of the ejaculate has been spilled from the container. Another cause of low semen volume is retrograde ejaculation, which is seen often in young diabetics and in men who have had bladder neck surgery for various lower urinary tract obstructions. If retrograde ejaculation is suspected, the patient should be instructed to ejaculate and then to urinate. More than 5 million sperm/ml in a postejaculate urine (PEU) is very good evidence that retrograde ejaculation has occurred. Treatment with sympathomimetics should be undertaken in an effort to first ascertain whether medical therapy can improve bladder neck closure. If this is not successful, then alkalinization of the urine can be instituted with oral sodium bicarbonate prior to ejaculation and the bladder specimen voided or obtained by catheterization for subsequent centrifugation and artificial insemination. Bladder washing with an alkalinized medium prior to ejaculation can also be used (Braude et al, 1987; Nijman et al, 1987). If there is no retrograde ejaculation, then one should be suspicious of ejaculatory duct blockage.

If there is a low volume on the semen analysis in the absence of any other seminal fluid findings, artificial insemination with the husband's semen (AIH) should be considered. Ultimately, two specimens might be collected on the same day if the total motile count is suboptimal.

An uncommon cause of low volume is hypoandrogenicity, which might be expected in association with low FSH and LH levels and may be seen in patients with hyperprolactinemia. Endocrine therapy should be undertaken to increase FSH and LH levels once a central nervous system lesion has been excluded.

On occasion, the volume of the ejaculate may be greater than 5.0 ml. This necessitates the evaluation of the patient for possible urination during ejaculation, especially if the volume is considerably larger and overly acidic. Split ejaculates for AIH can be obtained. The initial portion of the ejaculate generally contains the greatest concentration of sperm, while the latter portions are more likely to contain secretions from the seminal vesicles. Currently, mechanical concentration is often performed to concentrate the sperm for AIH protocols.

Disorders of Viscosity

If the viscosity of the specimen is such that there is essentially no liquification, then chemical or mechanical treatments may be attempted. These have included use of chymotrypsin, pepsin, and anti-inflammatory agents. Mechanical processing with a 22-gauge needle may be of some utility.

Disorders of Movement

Motility and forward progression are the two parameters that are perhaps the most important to measure in the evaluation of any male for fertility. If the motility and/or the forward progression are decreased, and there is no indication of a varicocele, then an etiology should be sought.

If anti-sperm antibodies are found, one can initially consider mechanical sperm washing or a swim-up technique to theoretically minimize anti-body adherence. However, these procedures have not been very successful. The use of steroids (prednisone) is somewhat controversial and should be undertaken with care (Hendry et al, 1986). We use a course of prednisone consisting of 20 mg daily for 3 weeks, followed by 10 mg daily for the last week. The patient and physician should be well informed of all potential side effects, which include acne, insomnia, gastrointestinal ulcers, and aseptic necrosis of the hip, although the latter is extremely rare. The antibody-related problems of impaired sperm-ova binding and/or penetration of the cervical mucus or zona pellucida despite medical therapy, sperm washing, and IVF appear to be bypassed with ICSI. A study by Nagy et al (1995) of 55 cycles of ICSI for men with positive anti-sperm antibodies demonstrated a normal fertilization rate of 75.7%, an embryo transfer rate of 96.4%, and fetal sac formation as detected by ultrasonography of 26.4%. Based on this study's excellent results, ICSI may become the primary treatment for this immunologic condition because fertilization and pregnancy rates are not significantly affected when high quantities of anti-sperm antibodies are present.

If there is decreased forward progression and motility but no anti-sperm antibodies are found, then the presence of a subclinical infection must be suspected. A culture of the semen or inspection of the semen using a specific white blood cell stain or monoclonal antibody will give definite information about the presence of white blood cells. If there is no infection, then semen processing or empirical medical therapy may be considered. A number of studies have reported the use of nonsteroidal anti-inflammatory drugs in the treatment of nonspecific asthenospermia. Their use was initially discussed in the 1970s and, more recently, in the 1980s when newer nonsteroidal agents were employed (Abbatiello et al, 1975; Moskovitz et al, 1988). These drugs are relatively well tolerated; however, the data for efficacy are inconclusive.

Disorders of Density

If the density is low and all other bulk parameters are normal, and there is no evidence of a varicocele, then empirical medical therapy, such as tamoxifen or clomiphene citrate, may be considered. As is well known, there have been few definitive, double-blind, randomized studies that show that any of these therapies work well. Mechanical concentration with intrauterine insemination and IVF are realistic alternatives. The reported success rate with these oligoasthenospermic patients is lower than that for IVF with normal males (Van Uem et al, 1984), hence the increased use of IVF with ICSI.

Azoospermia

If no sperm are found in repeat semen analyses, one must be certain that the laboratory centrifuged the specimen to assess for the presence of even a rare sperm, which suggests severe oligospermia rather than azoospermia. If no sperm are present, then one must examine the PEU for retrograde ejaculation. If sperm are absent in the PEU, then the physical examination is very important. The absence of palpable vasa is suggestive of congenital bilateral absence of the vasa deferens, a condition that is associated with the carrier status for cystic fibrosis mutations in approximately 55% of such patients (Schlegel et al, 1996). Because unilateral renal agenesis is seen in 13% of these individuals (Jarow et al, 1989), renal ultrasound is recommended. These patients are also at risk for abnormalities of the seminal vesicles, vasal ampullae, and epididymides.

If the physical examination, serum FSH, and TRUS are unremarkable, then one should proceed with a testicular biopsy with touch imprint cytology. A normal biopsy would be indicative of a problem in delivery (obstruction) of sperm from the testis to the urethra. These obstructive lesions would include abnormalities of structures within the testicle itself (e.g., the rete testis, efferent ductules, epididymis, and vas deferens) or occult lesions of the ampulla of the vas and the ejaculatory duct. However, these abnormalities are not always easily identified preoperatively. One method is to perform a scrotal exploration, allowing visualization of the testicle and epididymis, in conjunction with microsurgery if needed. If the epididymal tubules appear to be obstructed or enlarged and are indurated, then epididymal obstruction should be considered, possibly secondary to trauma or previous infection, and an epididymovasostomy would be appropriate. An adequate history will indicate whether there have been inguinal incisions or hydrocelectomies. Any previous surgery in the inguinal area or the scrotum may have compromised the vasal drainage. A vasogram with contrast material will demonstrate the point of obstruction. Likewise, threading a 0-Prolene suture through the abdominal vas will give the point of obstruction in centimeters when removed and measured.

For men with congenital bilateral absence of the vas or other uncorrectable obstructive lesions, epididymal sperm harvesting techniques are now available in conjunction with ICSI. Sperm may be harvested from the epididymis using an open technique known as *microepididymal sperm aspiration* (MESA) (Schlegel et al, 1995) or percutaneously with a procedure known as *percutaneous epididymal sperm aspiration* (PESA) (Craft et al, 1995). MESA involves microsurgically opening an individual tubule in the epididymis and harvesting sperm. PESA is the passage of a needle through the scrotal skin into the epididymis while aspirating for sperm. We prefer MESA because of excellent recovery and the ability to cryopreserve sperm for later IVF/ICSI cycles. PESA is limited by its blind nature and the attendant potential risk of damage to the delicate epididymal tubules, but has significantly lower associated costs.

Because of significantly better results in comparison with conventional IVF, ICSI is the treatment of choice for men with obstructive azoospermia. Pregnancy rates of approximately 50% per cycle have been obtained with ICSI, in contrast to 10% with standard IVF (Silber et al, 1994; Schlegel et al, 1995).

The treatment of severe male factor infertility has been revolutionized with the important and exciting advance provided by ICSI. Men previously considered hopelessly infertile and untreatable by prior methods are now potentially able to initiate their own biologic pregnancy because only one viable sperm is required for injection into an oocyte. Although the first success using this technique was reported by Palermo et al as recently as 1992, ICSI is now being performed by most major IVF centers in the United States.

Because this procedure has had a significant impact in the treatment of otherwise untreatable infertile males, an understanding of rational male factor indications is critical (Table 16–7). After evaluation of a couple with severe male factor infertility, provided that no reversible or correctable abnormalities exist, the decision to proceed with assisted reproductive technologies may be discussed. Although strict guidelines for patient selection have not been established, in general, at least 1 million motile sperm after sperm-washing techniques are required for intrauterine insemination (Dodson and Haney, 1991). Failed previous cycles of intrauterine insemination, female infertility factors, or severe impairments of the semen parameters will positively influence the decision to proceed with an IVF cycle. Because a thorough discussion of the decision-making pathways for pursuing assisted reproductive technologies is beyond the scope of this article, the reader is referred to reviews by Dawood (1996) and Tucker (1995).

Indications for ICSI include severe impairments of sperm density (oligospermia), motility (asthenospermia), morphology (teratospermia), and function in which therapeutic interventions to improve the abnormal parameter have failed or are unlikely to work. Obstructive azoospermia requiring sperm retrieval, as in congenital bilateral absence of the vas deferens, failed vasectomy reversal, and acquired

---

Table 16–7. MALE FACTOR INDICATIONS FOR ICSI

Severe oligospermia (decreased sperm concentration)
Severe asthenospermia (decreased sperm motility)
Abnormal sperm morphology (teratospermia)
Immunologic infertility
Obstructive azoospermia requiring microepididymal sperm
    aspiration (MESA)
  Congenital bilateral absence of the vas deferens
  Failed vasectomy reversal
  Acquired epididymal or vasal obstruction
Abnormal sperm function
  Defective acrosome reaction or capacitation
  Abnormal sperm penetration

epididymal or vasal obstruction, is also a prominent indication for ICSI. Many of these specific indications have been discussed already throughout this chapter. Because it appears that even the most severe sperm defects are treatable with ICSI, female factors such as age and oocyte quality are being examined more closely and will likely prove to be the main determinants of success (Sherins et al, 1995). Poorer results with ICSI have been observed in women over 40 years of age, likely because of the higher rate of aneuploidy and diminished oocyte retrieval after ovarian hyperstimulation in these older patients. The reader is referred to Chapter 17 for a discussion of the technical aspects of assisted reproductive technologies.

Although every man having difficulty initiating a pregnancy could have ICSI performed, clearly ICSI is not appropriate for everyone. Many men can have improvements in their semen parameters after a proper evaluation and treatment, and thus avoid ICSI. The significant costs of an IVF cycle with ICSI, as well as the potential complications to the female, must be taken into consideration before recommending this procedure as the couple's next therapeutic step.

Disorders of Ejaculation

Ejaculatory physiology was described earlier. Dysfunctions usually involve the sympathetic pathways and include multiple sclerosis, transverse myelitis, diabetes mellitus, retroperitoneal lymph node dissection (for testicular carcinoma), and, most commonly, spinal cord injury (Brindley, 1984; Eid, 1992). Electroejaculation and penile vibratory stimulation are successful in yielding semen specimens in up to 85% of these patients (Brindley, 1981; Perkash et al, 1985; Wheeler et al, 1988; Stewart and Ohl, 1989; Löchner-Ernst et al, 1996; Nehra et al, 1996), but the major problem has been poor sperm quality as manifest by motilities averaging only 11% to 22% with poor functional characteristics (Denil et al, 1992; Buch and Zorn, 1993). Using IVF, more than 50 pregnancies have been achieved in the United States alone (Moalla et al, 1987; Chung et al, 1995).

CONCLUSION

Since the first edition of this textbook was published, rapid and significant changes have evolved in the diagnosis and treatment of the infertile male. Certainly, ICSI has become a possibility for every patient with previously untreatable testicular failure. Although substantial revisions in this chapter have been made consistent with these newer diagnostic and therapeutic advances, the basics and the importance of a comprehensive male factor evaluation have remained the same. Investigation of testicular function should be pursued in patients with semen

abnormalities. Tests of sperm function and specific identification and quantification of white blood cells and anti-sperm antibodies are required if infection, immunologic causes of infertility, or other sperm function defects are suspected. If an abnormality is encountered, then further appropriate testing should be performed. Thorough investigation of the past medical history, surgical history, and use of medications is of special interest and should not be neglected. The physician can best recommend a specific therapy only after a careful evaluation of both members of the infertile couple. Despite the increased use of high technology procedures in the treatment of male infertility, a back-to-the-basics approach in evaluation is clearly in the best interest of the couple and will ultimately provide the best therapeutic results.

REFERENCES

Abbatiello ER, Kaminsky M, Weisbroth S: The effects of prostaglandins and prostaglandin inhibitors on spermatogenesis. Int J Fertil 1975;20:177.

Alexander NJ, Anderson DJ: Vasectomy: consequences of autoimmunity to sperm antigens. Fertil Steril 1979;32:253.

Beard CM, Benson RC Jr, Kelalis PP, Elveback LR: The incidence and outcome of mumps orchitis in Rochester, Minnesota, 1935–1974. Mayo Clin Proc 1977;52:3.

Berul CI, Harcleode JE: Effects of cocaine hydrochloride on the male reproductive system. Life Sci 1989;45:91.

Braude PR, Ross LD, Bolton VN, Ockenden K: Retrograde ejaculation: a systematic approach to non-invasive recovery of spermatozoa from postejaculatory urine for artificial insemination. Br J Obstet Gynaecol 1987;94:76.

Brindley GS: Electroejaculation: its technique, neurologic implications and cases. J Neurol Neurosurg Psychiatry 1981;44:9.

Brindley GS: The fertility of men with spinal cord injuries. Paraplegia 1984;22:337.

Broderick GA, Tom R, McClure RD: Immunological status of patients before and after vasovasostomy as determined by the immunobead antisperm antibody test. J Urol 1989;142:752.

Bsat F, Masabni R: Effectiveness of varicocelectomy in varicoceles diagnosed by physical examination versus Doppler studies. Fertil Steril 1988;50:321.

Buch JP, Zorn BH: Evaluation and treatment of infertility in spinal cord injured men through rectal probe electroejaculation. J Urol 1993;149(5 Pt 2):1350.

Carter SSC, Shinohara K, Lipshultz LI: Transrectal ultrasonography in disorders of the seminal vesicles and ejaculatory ducts. Urol Clin North Am 1989;16:787.

Chung PH, Yeko TR, Mayer JC, et al: Assisted fertility using electroejaculation in men with spinal cord injury—a review of literature. Fertil Steril 1995;64:1.

Craft I, Tsirigotis M, Bennett V, et al: Percutaneous epididymal sperm aspiration and intracytoplasmic sperm injection in the management of infertility due to obstructive azoospermia. Fertil Steril 1995;63:1038.

Cunningham GR, Lipshultz LI: Diseases of the testes and male sex organs. In Kohler PO (ed): Basic Clinical Endocrinology. New York: John Wiley and Sons, 1986:263.

Dawood MY: In vitro fertilization, gamete intrafallopian transfer, and superovulation with intrauterine insemination: efficacy and potential health hazards on babies delivered. Am J Obstet Gynecol 1996;174:1208.

Denil J, Ohl DA, Menge AC, et al: Functional characteristics of sperm obtained by electroejaculation. J Urol 1992;147:69.

Devroey P, Nagy P, Tournaye H, et al: Outcome of intracytoplasmic sperm injection with testicular spermatozoa in obstructive and non-obstructive azoospermia. Hum Reprod 1996;11:1015.

Dodson WC, Haney AF: Controlled ovarian hyperstimulation and intrauterine insemination for treatment of infertility. Fertil Steril 1991;55:457.

Donohue JP, Foster RS, Rowland RG, et al: Nerve-sparing retroperitoneal lymphadenectomy with preservation for ejaculation. J Urol 1990;144:287.

Eid JF: Electroejaculation. AUA Update Series 1992;XI(Lesson 10): 73.

Evans HJ, Fletcher J, Torrance M, Hargreave TB: Sperm abnormalities and cigarette smoking. Lancet 1981;1:627.

Foster RS, Donohue JP: Fertility in testicular cancer patients. AUA Update Series 1995;XIV(Lesson 19):153.

Frishman GN, Luciano AA, Maier DB: Evaluation of Astroglide, a new vaginal lubricant: effects of length of exposure and concentration on sperm motility. Fertil Steril 1992;58:630.

Haas GG: The inhibitory effect of sperm associated immunoglobulins on cervical mucus penetration. Fertil Steril 1986;46:334.

Haas GG: Antibody-mediated causes of male infertility. Urol Clin North Am 1987;14:539.

Haas GG, Sokoloski J, Wolf DP: The interfering effect of human IgG antisperm antibodies on human sperm penetration of zona-free hamster eggs. Am J Reprod Immunol 1980;1:40.

Hall J, Fishel S, Green S, et al: Intracytoplasmic sperm injection versus high insemination concentration in-vitro fertilization in cases of very severe teratozoospermia. Hum Reprod: 1995;10: 493.

Hellerstein DK, Meacham RB, Lipshultz LI: Transrectal ultrasound and partial ejaculatory duct obstruction in male infertility [abstract 279]. J Urol 1991;145:282A.

Hellstrom WJ, Tesluk H, Deitch AD, de Vere White RW: Comparison of flow cytometry to routine testicular biopsy in male infertility. Urology 1990;35:321.

Hendry WF, Treehuba K, Hughes L, et al: Cyclic prednisolone therapy for male infertility associated with autoantibodies to spermatozoa. Fertil Steril 1986;45:249.

Hjort T, Husted S, Linnet-Jepsen P: The effect of testis biopsy on autosensitization against spermatozoal antigens. Clin Exp Immunol 1974;18:201.

Huckins C, Hellerstein DK: Development of the testes and establishment of spermatogenesis. In Lipshultz LI, Howards SS (eds): Infertility in the Male. 2nd ed. St. Louis: Mosby–Year Book, 1991:3.

Jarow JP: Transrectal ultrasonography of infertile men. Fertil Steril 1993;60:1035.

Jarow JP: Seminal vesicle aspiration in the management of patients with ejaculatory duct obstruction. J Urol 1994;152:899.

Jarow JP, Espeland MA, Lipshultz LI: Evaluation of the azoospermic patient. J Urol 1989;142:62.

Jarow JP, Lipshultz LI: Anabolic steroid-induced hypogonadotropic hypogonadism. Am J Sports Med 1990;18:429.

Johnson A, Bassham B, Lipshultz LI, Lamb DJ. A quality control system for the optimized sperm penetration assay. Fertil Steril 1995;64:832.

Kim ED, Gilbaugh JH III, Patel VP, et al: Testis biopsies frequently demonstrate sperm in azoospermic men with significantly elevated follicle-stimulating hormone levels. J Urol 1997a;157: 144.

Kim ED, Greer JA, Abrams J, Lipshultz LI: Testicular touch preparation cytology. J Urol 1996;156:1412.

Kim ED, Lin WW, Abrams J, Lipshultz LI: Testis biopsy image analysis effectively quantifies spermatogenic cell types. J Urol 1997b;157:147.

Kim ED, Lipshultz LI: Role of ultrasound in the assessment of male infertility. J Clin Ultrasound 1996;24:437.

Kolodny RC, Masters WH, Kolodny RM, Toro G: Depression of plasma testosterone levels after chronic intensive marijuana use. N Engl J Med 1974;290:872.

Krarup T: The testis after torsion. Br J Urol 1978;50:43.

Kruger TF, Acosta AA, Simmons KF, et al: Predictive value of abnormal sperm morphology in in vitro fertilization. Fertil Steril 1988;49:112.

Kruger TF, Du Toit TC, Franken DR, et al: Sperm morphology: assessing the agreement between the manual method (strict criteria) and the sperm morphology analyzer IVOS. Fertil Steril 1995;62:134.

Kruger TF, Menkveld R, Stander FS, et al: Sperm morphologic features as a prognostic factor in in vitro fertilization. Fertil Steril 1986;46:1118.

Lee W, Mason AJ, Schwall R, et al: Secretion of activin by interstitial cells in the testis. Science 1989;243:396.

Levi AJ, Fisher AM, Hughes L, Henry WF: Male infertility due to sulfasalazine. Lancet 1979;2:276.

Levin RJ, Mathew RM, Chenault BC, et al: Differences in the quality of semen in outdoor workers during summer and winter. N Engl J Med 1990;323:12.

Löchner-Ernst D, Stöhrer M, Kramer G, et al: Long term results of a fertility program in spinal cord injured males. [abstract 224]. J Urol 1996;155:366A.

MacLeod J: Semen quality in one thousand men of known fertility and eight hundred cases of infertile marriages. Fertil Steril 1951;2:115.

Magdar I, Weissenberg R, Lunenfeld B, et al: Controlled trial of high spermatic vein ligation for varicocele in infertile men. Fertil Steril 1995;63:120.

Marks JL, MacMahon R, Lipshultz LI: Predictive parameters of successful varicocele repair. J Urol 1986;136:609.

Marshburn PB, Kutteh WH: The role of antisperm antibodies in infertility. Fertil Steril 1994;61:799.

McClure D, Khoo D, Jarvi K, Hricak H: Subclinical varicocele: the effectiveness of varicocelectomy. J Urol 1991;145:789.

Meistrich ML, Chawla SP, Da Cunha MF, et al: Recovery of sperm production after chemotherapy for osteosarcoma. Cancer 1989; 63:2115.

Moalla M, Bergaoui N, Cammoun M, et al: Retrograde ejaculation disclosing retroperitoneal fibrosis [letter]. Ann Med Interne (Paris) 1987;138:669.

Moskovitz B, Lin R, Nasscar S, Levin DR: Effect of diclofenac sodium (Voltaren®) on spermatogenesis of infertile oligospermic patients. Eur Urol 1988;14:395.

Nagy ZP, Verheyen G, Liu J, et al: Results of 55 intracytoplasmic sperm injection cycles in the treatment of male-immunological infertility. Hum Reprod 1995;10:1775.

Nehra A, Werner MA, Bastuba M, et al: Vibratory stimulation and rectal probe electroejaculation as therapy for patients with spinal cord injury: semen parameters and pregnancy rates. J Urol 1996;155:554.

Nelson WD, Steinberger E: The effect of turadoxyl upon the testis of the rat. Anat Rec 1952;112:367.

Nijman JM, Schraffordt-Koops H, Oldhoff J, et al: Sexual function after bilateral retroperitoneal lymph node dissection for nonseminomatous testicular cancer. Arch Androl 1987;18:255.

Oates RD, Lipshultz LI: Fertility and testicular function in patients after chemotherapy and radiotherapy. Adv Urol 1989; 2: 55.

Palermo G, Joris H, Devroey P, Van Steirteghem AC: Pregnancies after intracytoplasmic injection of single spermatozoon into an oocyte. Lancet 1992;340:17.

Perkash I, Martin DE, Warner H, et al: Reproductive biology of paraplegics: results of semen collection, testicular biopsy and serum hormone evaluation. J Urol 1985;134:284.

Presti JC, Herr HW, Carroll PR: Fertility and testis cancer. Urol Clin North Am 1993;20:173.

Ruiz Rubio JL, Fernandez Gonzales I, Quijano Barrosa P, Herrero Payo JA, et al: The value of transrectal ultrasonography in the diagnosis and treatment of partial obstruction of the seminal duct system. J Urol 1995;153:435.

Rumke P, Hekman A: Sterility: an immunologic disorder? Clin Obstet Gynecol 1977;20:691.

Schlegel PN, Palermo GD, Alikani M, et al: Micropuncture retrieval of epididymal sperm with in vitro fertilization: importance of in vitro micromanipulation techniques. Urology 1995; 46:238.

Schlegel PN, Shin D, Goldstein M: Urogenital anomalies in men with congenital absence of the vas deferens. J Urol 1996;155: 1644.

Schoeman MN, Tyler JP: Effects of surgical lubricants on semen analysis. Clin Reprod Fertil. 1983;2:275.

Sherins RJ, Thorsell LP, Dorfmann A, et al: Intracytoplasmic sperm injection facilitates fertilization even in the most severe forms of male infertility: pregnancy outcome correlates with maternal age and numbers of eggs available. Fertil Steril 1995; 64:369.

Silber SJ, Nagy ZP, Liu J, et al: Conventional in-vitro fertilization versus intracytoplasmic sperm injection for patients requiring microsurgical sperm aspiration. Hum Reprod 1994;9:1705.

Stewart DE, Ohl DA: Idiopathic anejaculation treated by electroejaculation. Int J Psychiatry Med 1989;19:263.

Svalander P, Jakobsson A-H, Forsberg A-S, et al: The outcome of intracytoplasmic sperm injection is unrelated to "strict criteria" sperm morphology. Hum Reprod 1996;11:1019.

Tagatz GE, Okagaki T, Sciarra JJ: The effect of vaginal lubricants on sperm motility and viability in vitro. Am J Obstet Gynecol 1972;113:88.

Thomas AJ: Ejaculatory dysfunction. Fertil Steril 1983;39:445.

Tucker MJ: Micromanipulative and conventional insemination strategies for assisted reproductive technology. Am J Obstet Gynecol 1995;172(2 Pt 2):773.

Turek PJ, Magana JO, Lipshultz LI: Semen parameters before and after transurethral surgery for ejaculatory duct obstruction. J Urol 1996;155:1291.

Van Thiel DH, Gavaler JS, Lester R, Goodman MD: Alcohol induced testicular atrophy. Gastroenterology 1975;69:326.

Van Thiel DH, Gavaler JS, Smith WI, Gwendolyn P: Hypothalamic-pituitary-gonadal dysfunction in men using cimetidine. N Engl J Med 1979;300:1012.

Van Uem JFHM, Acosta AA, Swanson RJ, et al: Male factor evaluation and results in the Norfolk IVF Program. Fertil Steril 1984;41:1025.

Wheeler JS, Walter JS, Culkin DJ, Canning JR: Idiopathic anejaculation treated by vibratory stimulation. Fertil Steril 1988;50: 377.

Wilcox AJ, Weinberg CR, Baird DD: Timing of sexual intercourse in relation to ovulation. N Engl J Med 1995;333:1517.

Wolff H: The biologic significance of white blood cells in semen. Fertil Steril 1995;63:1143.

Wolff H, Anderson DT: Immunohistologic characterizations and quantifications of leukocyte subpopulations in human semen. Fertil Steril 1988;49:497.

Yanagimachi R, Yanigimachi Y-H, Rogers BJ: The use of zona-free animal ova as a test system for the assessment of the fertilizing capacity of human spermatozoa. Biol Reprod 1976;15:471.

Yanushpolsky EH, Politch JA, Hill JA, Anderson DJ: Antibiotic therapy and leukocytospermia: a prospective, randomized, controlled study. Fertil Steril 1995;63:142.

17

Assisted Reproductive Technologies

José M. Colón
Peter G. McGovern
Jacquelyn S. Loughlin
Kenneth J. Lipetz
Sangita K. Jindal
Nanette F. Santoro

Conception in the human is a chance event. Sperm, an egg, and a working female reproductive tract are necessary for natural pregnancy to occur. A normal ejaculate contains as many as 300 million motile sperm (Wasserman, 1987). When deposited in the vagina at ovulation, sperm penetrate the cervical mucus, travel into the uterine cavity, and enter the fallopian tubes, where fertilization usually occurs. The attrition of sperm in human reproduction is relatively large. It has been estimated that around 500 sperm reach the vicinity of the egg at the time of fertilization (Settlage et al, 1973). At the present time there is no clear evidence of any signal from either gamete that brings them together. Given these circumstances, the fecundity rate in normal couples is around 25% per cycle. Eighty-five to 90% of couples who have intercourse around the time of ovulation, and in whom the female partner ovulates every month, achieve pregnancy within 1 year (Mosher and Pratt, 1990).

In the presence of abnormalities of the sperm, of the egg or ovulation, and/or of the female reproductive tract, the chances of conception decrease. If there are low numbers of sperm in the ejaculate, fewer sperm will reach the fallopian tube for fertilization. With fewer sperm, the chance that one will meet the egg is lower. If the egg is abnormal, or if ovulation is not regular, the chance of conception decreases. If the fallopian tubes are blocked or function improperly, the egg or the sperm may not reach the tube for fertilization to occur, the fertilized egg may reach the endometrial cavity at a suboptimal time for implantation, or it may never reach the endometrial cavity at all. Abnormalities of the endometrium itself may decrease the chance of implantation.

Assisted reproductive technologies (ART) have been designed to improve the chances of conception and pregnancy by overcoming male factor infertility and ovulatory dysfunction, as well as anatomic factors. ART have been defined as "any techniques designed to produce pregnancy which require the in-

volvement of third parties for success" (Toner and Hodgen, 1993). The general working hypothesis of ART is that increasing the relative concentration of available gametes for fertilization increases the chances of pregnancy. Conception rates will increase if there are more sperm and eggs, and/or more sperm per egg(s) for fertilization. Controlled ovarian hyperstimulation (COH) achieves the maturation of multiple eggs for fertilization. Increasing the relative concentration of sperm in the vicinity of the egg(s) increases the chance of fertilization. A number of methods have been developed to separate or "wash" sperm from seminal plasma, and use the cells to increase the concentration of sperm in the vicinity of the egg(s) in vivo or in vitro. Increasing either the number of sperm or the number of eggs should increase the chance of fertilization. Increasing both sperm and eggs should optimize success.

The birth of Louise Brown in 1978 following in vitro fertilization and embryo transfer (IVF-ET) (Steptoe and Edwards, 1978) marked the beginning of a revolution in the field of human reproduction and infertility that resulted in the development of a number of new therapies for couples who previously could not have children. Parallel with the development of new treatment modalities and techniques, research in human reproduction increased tremendously. As a result, our knowledge has expanded and previously held concepts in the field have changed radically. The revolution in our field has influenced more than our medical approach to reproduction: it has affected some of the most basic societal concepts, such as the definition of parenthood. As an example, the use of donor oocytes in human IVF has been successful since 1984 (Lutjen et al, 1984). Such developments have necessitated the ethical and moral examination of the new or changing concepts and techniques regarding human reproduction, and have required the revision and enactment of laws to protect the parties involved (Ethics Committee of the American Fertility Society, 1986; Ethics

Committee of the American Society for Reproductive Medicine, 1997). This chapter focuses on the knowledge acquired over the last 20 years that will be of clinical use to obstetrician-gynecologists involved in the care, management, and counseling of women and couples requiring ART.

SPERM PREPARATION FOR ART

Semen consists of seminal fluid with sperm and other cellular debris from the urogenital tract. The seminal fluid contains prostaglandins, enzymes, proteinase inhibitors, and other bioactive materials that protect the sperm in the vaginal environment, but that would be detrimental to the fertilization process in the fallopian tube or in vitro, in the laboratory (Äumuller and Seitz, 1990; Kanwar et al, 1979). For example, seminal fluid contains a "decapacitation" factor that prevents the sperm from undergoing capacitation. Sperm must undergo capacitation to be able to fertilize an egg. Furthermore, the seminal fluid is an irritant in the uterine cavity that, when introduced in the womb, causes strong contractions of the myometrium (Hanson and Rock, 1951). Thus sperm for ART must be separated or "washed" from the seminal fluid to achieve capacitation, and to be used inside the female reproductive tract. Sperm is processed for ART in several ways, variations of which are described below. During processing, the sperm are separated from the seminal fluid and are allowed to undergo capacitation. In the final sample, a concentrated number of motile sperm are resuspended in a small volume of protein-supplemented medium for use in ART.

The *"swim-up" method* generally gives excellent results when used to process samples with normal sperm concentration and motility. Processing by swim-up involves dividing the semen sample into 0.5-ml aliquots per centrifuge tube in order to decrease the time of centrifugation required to pellet the sperm from the seminal fluid. Diluting the semen 2:1 with protein-supplemented medium to decrease the viscosity of the fluid through which the cells must pellet further facilitates centrifugation. Centrifugation is kept to 10 minutes at speeds not exceeding $400 \times$ g to avoid excessive damage to the sperm membranes (Aitken and Clarkson, 1987; Fulgham and Alexander, 1990). The supernatants comprised of seminal fluid and medium are removed and the remaining pellets are overlaid with 0.5 ml of fresh medium. Motile sperm in the pellets are allowed to "swim up" into the medium for 60 minutes at 37°C. The swim-up supernatants are collected and pooled from all the tubes, and centrifuged at $300 \times$ g for 5 minutes. The final sperm pellet consisting of capacitated, motile sperm is resuspended in a small volume (0.5 ml) of medium and used for ART.

Semen may also be processed through a discontinuous gradient of silica particles (Isolate TM; Irvine Scientific, Santa Ana, CA), or bovine albumin (Yates et al, 1989). *Density gradient centrifugation* generally optimizes the separation of sperm from seminal fluid in samples with initial low sperm counts and/or sperm motility. Each milliliter of semen is placed undiluted on a column of 90% and 45% silica/medium in centrifuge tubes. The preparations are centrifuged for 20 minutes at approximately $400 \times$ g. Pellets of sperm are combined, washed with medium to remove the silica matrix, and resuspended in 0.5 ml of fresh medium as the final sample.

A *sperm wash* involves dividing undiluted semen into 1-ml aliquots, centrifugation for 5 minutes at 300 $\times$ g, removal of the supernatant, and resuspension of the pellet in 0.5 ml of fresh protein-supplemented medium as the final sample. This processing method is recommended for semen samples with severely low sperm counts and motility, which would not yield adequate numbers of motile sperm with more vigorous processing.

CONTROLLED OVARIAN HYPERSTIMULATION

Advances in our understanding of ovulation and of the hormonal mechanisms that control it have allowed for the development of therapies to control and enhance the ovulatory process (controlled ovarian hyperstimulation) to obtain multiple eggs for ART. Ovulation in humans depends on the coordinated activity of the hypothalamic-pituitary-ovarian axis (Knobil, 1980). Cells in the arcuate nucleus in the medial basal hypothalamus secrete pulses of gonadotropin-releasing hormone (GnRH) into the portal circulation that stimulate synthesis and secretion of the pituitary gonadotropins luteinizing hormone (LH) and follicle-stimulating hormone (FSH). Neuroendocrine input from the central nervous system and the hormonal environment in the hypothalamic-pituitary axis modulate the amplitude and frequency of the GnRH pulses necessary for normal ovulation. Responding to the GnRH pulsatile stimulus, the pituitary secretion of LH and FSH pulses results in follicular growth and oocyte maturation, ovulation, formation of a corpus luteum, and secretion of estradiol, inhibin, progesterone, and other factors by the ovary (Gougeon, 1996). The ovarian hormones feed back to modulate the pituitary secretion of gonadotropins, and prepare the endometrium for implantation and pregnancy.

COH is a deliberate manipulation of the hormones regulating ovulation in order to achieve the maturation of multiple eggs in lieu of the single, dominant egg ovulated in a natural cycle. COH followed by insemination or egg retrieval will yield more eggs for fertilization, increasing the chance of pregnancy. A number of agents and protocols have been used for COH in assisted reproduction. Human menopausal gonadotropin (hMG) preparations purified from the urine of postmenopausal women are the main agents used for COH. hMG preparations have been used alone, in combination with clomiphene citrate, or with GnRH agonists (GnRHa; see below) to achieve the maturation of multiple eggs for ART.

The first use of gonadotropins to induce ovulation was reported by Gemzell and associates (1958). These authors injected human pituitary extracts containing LH and FSH to induce follicular development. Because the supply of human pituitaries from cadavers was limited, other sources of gonadotropins were sought. Lunenfeld and associates (1962) reported the first pregnancy following the administration of human gonadotropins extracted from the urine of postmenopausal women (hMG).

Gonadotropin Preparations Used for COH

Gonadotropin preparations derived from menopausal urine include Pergonal, Metrodin, and Fertinex (Serono, Norwell, MA), and Humegon (Organon, West Orange, NJ). Urinary gonadotropin extraction by immunochromatography provides preparations with equivalent amounts of FSH and LH activity. Pergonal and Humegon contain 75 or 150 IU of FSH and LH per ampule. Because FSH is the critical gonadotropin for folliculogenesis, efforts have been directed at increasing the FSH:LH ratio in the gonadotropin preparations, and at providing preparations of pure FSH devoid of any LH activity. Metrodin is a urinary gonadotropin preparation with decreased LH content and increased FSH activity (75 IU FSH:<1 IU LH). Metrodin is the result of passage of a urinary gonadotropin preparation through an immunoactivity column prepared with an antibody to human chorioinic gonadotropin (hCG). Because of the cross-reactivity of LH with the hCG antibody, LH is retained in the column. Fertinex is a highly purified FSH preparation following immunoextraction of FSH from Metrodin using monoclonal antibodies and reverse-phase high-performance liquid chromatography. Fertinex contains less than 0.1 IU LH/1000 IU of FSH (Baird and Howles, 1994; Flamigni et al, 1994).

The next generation of gonadotropin preparations is the recombinant gonadotropins (Loumaye et al, 1995). Serono has developed Gonal F, and Organon has developed Follistim, both produced in vitro by genetically engineered Chinese hamster ovary cells. The recombinant preparations have no LH activity at all. The specific activity of these preparations is similar to that of Fertinex, in the range of 10,000 IU of FSH/mg of protein. Unlike Fertinex, the recombinant preparations are completely free of any non-FSH, urinary human protein. Available clinical studies, suggest that the recombinant gonadotropins provide equivalent stimulation and success after IVF as that obtained with hMG (Germond et al, 1992; Hornnes et al, 1993; van Dessel et al, 1994; Recombinant Human FSH Study Group, 1995; Out et al, 1997).

Injections of gonadotropins achieve supraphysiologic levels of FSH in the circulation that override the normal ovarian hormone feedback mechanisms that control the pituitary secretion of gonadotropins. The high levels of LH and FSH in the circulation result in the growth and development of multiple follicles in both ovaries, instead of the single, dominant follicle characteristic of an unstimulated cycle (Corsan and Kemmann, 1991; Ginsburg and Hardiman, 1991). COH with gonadotropins is started in the early follicular phase, around day 3 of the cycle. This procedure is believed to rescue the cohort of follicles that would have degenerated under normal conditions without hyperstimulation.

Response to COH is monitored over time with (1) serial measurements of the size of the growing follicles with ultrasound examinations, and (2) serial determinations of the concentration of estradiol in the serum, which increases proportionally with follicular maturation. The gonadotropin injections are continued until the follicles reach the appropriate size and the estradiol level confirms follicular maturation. At this point the gonadotropin therapy is stopped and the patient receives an injection of hCG, a surrogate LH surge needed for the final maturation of the eggs, and the stimulus for ovulation. COH is used to increase the number of eggs available at the time of intercourse, at the time of insemination, or for oocyte retrieval for IVF or gamete intrafollicular transfer (GIFT). Intercourse is advised every other night starting the day after the hCG injection. Inseminations and retrievals for IVF or GIFT are planned 34 to 36 hours following the surrogate LH surge. The side effects of gonadotropin therapy are described below.

Human menopausal gonadotropins have been used in combination with clomiphene citrate for COH (Kerin J et al, 1984; Qigley et al, 1984; Vargyas et al, 1984; Rogers et al, 1986). Generally the two medications are used sequentially, clomiphene citrate followed by hMG stimulation. Even though reported fertilization rates are high, pregnancy rates are not improved, and the cancellation rates are higher than those following the use of hMG combined with GnRHa.

The use of GnRHa in conjunction with gonadotropins for COH has afforded better control of the cycle, and has provided versatility to tailor specific COH protocols to specific groups of patients (Meldrum, 1989; Meldrum et al, 1989; Cedars et al, 1990; Hughes et al, 1992). GnRHa are chemically altered forms of GnRH, the hypothalamic signal that stimulates release of pituitary LH and FSH. Native GnRH is a decapeptide with a relatively short half-life of 2 to 4 minutes. GnRHa are long-acting analogs of GnRH that resist metabolism. Their relatively long half-life in the portal circulation disturbs the pulsatile nature of the GnRH stimulus necessary for the normal pituitary release of LH and FSH. The use of GnRHa paradoxically results in the shutdown of pituitary gonadotropin secretion and induces a hypogonadal state (Vickery and Nestor, 1987). The pituitary response to GnRHa administration is biphasic: an initial agonistic phase during which circulating levels of LH and FSH rise is followed by pituitary desensitization and down-regulation with shutdown of gonadotropin secretion. The short periods of hypoestrogenism from GnRHa use in COH are unlikely to have any long-term harmful effects (Quagliarello, 1993). Menopause-like symptoms such as hot flushes are common. Patient education and reassurance are usually enough to overcome these transient side effects.

The two GnRHa generally used for COH in the United States are Lupron (Tap Pharmaceuticals, Deerfield, IL) and Synarel (Searle, Chicago, IL). Lupron for COH is usually administered as 1-mg daily subcutaneous injections; Synarel is administered as an intranasal spray delivering 200 μg twice daily.

Protocols for COH

A number of protocols have been tried for COH, sometimes tailored to the response manifested by different groups of patients. Three protocols combining the use of GnRHa and gonadotropins are described here: one for patients with a normal response to COH (the standard, "long" protocol); one for "poor responders" (the GnRHa microdose "flare" protocol); and a protocol for "hyper-responders" (the "coasting" protocol).

Standard "Long" Protocol

In the standard, long protocol, GnRHa therapy is started during the midluteal phase of the cycle preceding stimulation with gonadotropins. Because the GnRHa is started after ovulation, ovarian function is little affected in the cycle in which the GnRHa is initiated. However, by the time of menses, the pituitary will be desensitized and thus "shut down," LH and FSH will be absent, and a new cycle will not be initiated as long as the GnRHa therapy is continued. The rationale for the standard long protocol is that follicular recruitment for a nonstimulated cycle begins during the late luteal phase of the preceding cycle (Gougeon, 1996). The falling levels of estrogen, progesterone, and inhibin in a nonpregnancy cycle that trigger menses also trigger a relative rise in gonadotropins that initiate follicular recruitment for the subsequent cycle. By the time of menses, the hormonal mechanisms that recruit and eventually select the dominant follicle destined to ovulate are in place. The later gonadotropins are started following menses, the more chances that some follicles from the original cohort will have been irreversibly selected out. Suppressing these selecting mechanisms with GnRHa pituitary desensitization during the intercycle period provides a larger pool of follicles for subsequent hMG stimulation. GnRHa therapy is continued through menses and through the days of

gonadotropin administration, until administration of the hCG injection, the surrogate LH surge. Because the pituitary gonadotropes are shut down, the gonadotropin injections can be started any time after the onset of menses during GnRHa suppression. COH with gonadotropins is monitored with serial ultrasound examinations and with serial measurements of serum estradiol as described for the use of gonadotropins alone. hCG is administered once follicular size and maturity is reached. Similar to what was described with the use of gonadotropins alone, intercourse, insemination, or egg retrieval for IVF or GIFT is scheduled relative to the hCG injection.

The need for luteal support following COH and oocyte retrieval has been advocated. It has been hypothesized that the use of a GnRHa with resultant pituitary gonadotrope shutdown up to the time of the artificial LH surge requires luteal support following ovulation. Smitz and associates (1987) demonstrated a dramatic fall in the serum levels of estradiol and progesterone approximately 8 days after the hCG injection. It has also been postulated that COH cycles followed by egg retrieval require luteal support because the granulosa cells that secrete progesterone in the corpus luteum are aspirated from the ovaries along with the eggs at the time of retrieval (Kreitmann et al, 1981). A number of authors have reported on the use of additional injections of hCG (e.g., 5000 IU 6 days after or 3000 IU every 3 to 4 days after the initial hCG injection) to support the corpus luteum (Casper et al, 1983; Smith et al, 1989; Belaisch-Allart et al, 1990). Alternatively, daily intramuscular or intravaginal progesterone can be administered to support the endometrium following COH for oocyte retrieval (Herman et al, 1990; Claman et al, 1992). Because additional hCG can increase the incidence of ovarian hyperstimulation syndrome (OHSS, see below (Smitz et al, 1992), progesterone supplementation may provide a safer alternative.

GnRHa Microdose "Flare" Protocol

A number of protocols have been proposed for patients who respond poorly to standard COH (Muasher, 1993; Olivennes et al, 1993; Scott, 1996). Poor responders can include, among others, older women (> 37 to 40 years old), women with elevated FSH levels, or women who have had an inadequate previous response to COH (low levels of periovulatory serum estradiol, or a small number of mature follicles at the time of hCG injection). Increasing the dose of gonadotropins alone does not improve the results of COH significantly in poor responders (Karande et al, 1990; Hoffmann et al, 1989; Land et al, 1996). The GnRHa microdose, flare protocol (Scott and Navot, 1994) takes advantage of a number of clinical observations regarding enhanced ovarian response to COH, and utilizes the physiologic, biphasic response to GnRHa administration as part of the stimulation protocol. First, following the report by Gonen and associates (1990) that pituitary suppression with oral contraceptives enhances the ovarian response to COH for IVF, patients are treated with low-dose oral contraceptives the month preceding stimulation. Second, the observation by Navot and associates (1991b) that very low doses of GnRHa every 6 hours can produce sustained ovarian hyperstimulation is used to improve the response to COH. This is in contrast to the suppression observed following higher dose GnRHa treatment. Patients on the GnRHa microdose flare protocol inject 20 µg of Lupron subcutaneously twice a day, instead of the 1 mg daily used in the standard protocol. Third, the biphasic response to GnRHa administration is used as part of the stimulation protocol. A number of flare protocols have been used that take advantage of the initial agonistic phase of the normal response to GnRHa administration. The GnRHa is started in the early follicular phase (day 2 or 3 of the cycle) instead of in the luteal phase of the cycle preceding stimulation. The induced initial elevation of endogenous circulating gonadotropins following initiation of GnRHa administration is used to initiate follicular stimulation. Gonadotropin administration started 2 to 3 days after initiating GnRHa therapy sustains follicular growth as pituitary down-regulation ensues (Garcia et al, 1990; Padilla et al, 1990, 1991, 1996; Jacobson et al, 1991). In practical terms, patients take 21 days of low-dose oral contraceptives. On the third day after discontinuing the oral contraceptives, the patients start GnRHa administration: Lupron 20 µg SC bid. On the third day of Lupron administration (6 days after stopping oral contraceptives), the patients start gonadotropin stimulation. The Lupron and gonadotropin stimulation is monitored with serial pelvic ultrasound examinations and serum estradiol determinations as in the standard protocol. hCG is administered when the follicles reach critical size, and follicular maturation is confirmed with a corresponding elevated serum estradiol level. Scott and Navot (1994) reported that the GnRHa microdose flare protocol successfully enhanced ovarian responsiveness in a group of patients who had previously experienced a poor response to COH for IVF. Schoolcraft and associates (1997) reported similar improvement in response to COH in poor responders using a variant of the GnRHa microdose, flare protocol, with the addition of growth hormone to the stimulation regimen. (In addition, pregnancy rates following IVF in poor responders may be improved by performing assisted zona hatching [AZH; see below] on the embryos prior to transfer [Schoolcraft et al, 1994].

"Coasting" Protocol

Another group of patients who require distinct management are the "hyper-responders," the patients who manifest an exaggerated sensitivity to gonadotropin stimulation, with the development of exceedingly large numbers of growing follicles and greatly elevated levels of serum estradiol concentrations (Smitz et al, 1990; Navot et al, 1992). Patients with polycystic ovarian syndrome (PCOS) oftentimes exhibit exquisite sensitivity to stimulation with gonadotropins. These patients are generally anovulatory or oligoovulatory, and may have hormonal abnormalities including an elevated LH:FSH ratio, increased androgens, and steady-state, elevated estrogen levels. COH in these patients can result in poorly controlled responses. Pituitary and ovarian suppression with GnRHa prior to stimulation does not change the sensitivity of the ovary to hMG (Dodson et al, 1989). In some instances levels of estradiol may exceed 3000 pg/ml in the serum in the absence of mature, preovulatory follicles based on size criteria. These patients are at high risk of developing severe OHSS (see below). Because of the high health risk secondary to OHSS, the cancellation rate in this group of patients is high. Because hCG promotes OHSS and pregnancy is accompanied by high levels of hCG, one option for hyper-responders who undergo egg retrieval for IVF is to freeze all embryos and to postpone the embryo transfer to a nonstimulated cycle (Frederick et al, 1995). However, pregnancy rates after the transfer of frozen-thawed embryos are lower than after the transfer of "fresh" embryos, possibly because the freeze-thawing process may damage some embryos (Levran et al, 1990). Because these patients may have elevated LH:FSH ratios, it has been suggested that gonadotropin stimulation with high FSH:LH preparations may be advantageous. The theoretical advantages of the use of purified FSH over hMG for COH in patients with PCOS have not been borne out in clinical trials (Baird and Howles, 1994). One alternative for COH has been to try small doses of gonadotropins, with increments of as little as one half of an ampule per day when necessary (Shoham et al, 1991; Homburg et al, 1995). In addition, "coasting," or withholding gonadotropin stimulation after reaching a critical level of serum estradiol (regardless of follicular size), and monitoring the serum estradiol until it falls to a "safe" level, when hCG is administered, has been shown to be effective in the management of hyperresponders (Urman et al, 1992; Ben-Nun et al, 1993; Sher et al, 1993, 1995; Benadiva et al, 1997). The cycle for an identified hyper-responder may consist of ovarian suppression with oral contraceptives for 21 days with concurrent GnRHa therapy at suppressive doses (1 mg SC daily) started during the third week. Low-dose gonadotropin stimulation (as low as 75 IU/day) is started after menses. The GnRHa therapy is continued through the low-dose gonadotropin stimulation until the hCG dose is administered. Follicular monitoring consists of serial pelvic ultrasounds and serial monitoring of the serum estradiol concentration. If the serum estradiol increases over 3000 pg/ml, the patient is "coasted": gonadotropin stimulation is discontinued while the patient continues on GnRHa suppression. The serum estradiol is monitored daily and the hCG injection is administered when the estradiol level falls below 3000 pg/ml. Not only is OHSS prevented, but also a "fresh" embryo transfer can follow on the cycle of retrieval, following COH for IVF in hyper-responders. It is, of course, still prudent to monitor these patients closely for the development of OHSS.

Complications of Ovarian Stimulation/COH

There are three potentially serious complications related to medications used for COH and for COH itself: (1) OHSS, (2) an increased incidence of multiple gestations, and (3) a reported and questionable association between medications used for ovulation induction and for COH and an increase in the risk of developing ovarian cancer (Schenker and Ezra, 1994). *OHSS* is a poorly understood, self-limiting condition characterized by a shift of fluid from the intravascular space into the abdominal cavity (Golan et al, 1989). OHSS is iatrogenic, can be life threatening, and is largely preventable. Mild cases present with ovarian enlargement to less than 5 cm, weight gain, and abdominal distention and discomfort. Moderate OHSS presents with ultrasound evidence of ascites and ovaries between 5 and 10 cm in size. Clinical ascites with hypovolemia, oliguria, hemoconcentration, electrolyte imbalance, and ovarian size greater than 10 cm characterize severe OHSS. Critical OHSS is life threatening and presents with tense ascites that may be accompanied by hydrothorax, renal failure, thromboembolic phenomena, and/or acute respiratory distress syndrome. Critical OHSS requires monitoring in an intensive care unit (Dourron and Williams, 1996). Mild OHSS may be seen in up to 25% of patients who undergo COH (Blankenstein et al, 1987). The severe and critical forms of OHSS have an incidence of 1% to 2%. OHSS is generally associated with excessively high serum estradiol levels, greater than 1500 pg/ml. Even though OHSS has been reported with relatively low estradiol levels, the severity of OHSS is generally proportional to the elevation of the serum estradiol concentration. The full-blown syndrome does not develop unless the ovulatory dose of hCG is administered. Thus it is critical to monitor patients undergoing COH closely because OHSS is potentially preventable. At the present time there is no specific therapy for OHSS other than supportive measures until the disorder resolves over time. Mild and moderate forms of OHSS can be managed on an outpatient basis with decreased activity, close monitoring, and reassurance. The severe and critical forms of OHSS require hospitalization to monitor and maintain vital functions. In critical cases, pregnancy termination may be considered.

COH for assisted reproduction results in a high rate of *multifetal pregnancies*. Multifetal gestations place both the mother and the fetus at increased health risks (Schenker and Ezra, 1994). Increased maternal risks include a higher incidence of preeclampsia, placental abruption, placenta previa, cesarean section, and postpartum hemorrhage. The fetuses have a higher risk of prematurity, early and late abortion, stillbirth, and perinatal morbidity and mortality. The economic costs associated with multifetal gestations are much higher than the costs of a singleton pregnancy (Callahan et al, 1994; Neuman et al, 1994). Limiting the number of embryos transferred into the uterus or into the tubes after IVF, and limiting the number of eggs transferred for GIFT, can reduce the incidence of multifetal gestation. Selective reduction during the early second trimester of pregnancy can reduce the number of fetuses in high-order multiple gestations to improve the chance of a favorable outcome of pregnancy (Evans et al, 1993). The risk of terminating the pregnancy as a result of fetal reduction is in the range of 10%.

A number of case reports, case-control, and cohort studies have raised the question of a possible association between the use of ovulation-inducing medications—clomiphene citrate and hMG—and an increased *risk of ovarian cancer*. In a comprehensive review and critical analysis of published studies on this topic, Bristow and Karlan (1996) concluded that, although an association between ovulation induction and ovarian cancer appears to exist, a causal effect has not been demonstrated. Confounding factors such as infertility and nulliparity in the populations reported are independent risk factors for the development of ovarian cancer. Infertile and, in many cases, nulliparous women make up the populations of women undergoing infertility treatments. These women, already at a higher risk for ovarian cancer, use ovulation-inducing medications and undergo COH. The question of the oncogenic potential of ovulation-inducing medications has not been answered but cannot be ignored. The National Institute of Child Health and Human Development and the National Cancer Institute are funding investigations that will hopefully shed more light on this issue (Bristow and Karlan, 1996). In the meantime, however, given the available information, no recommendation has been issued not to use these medications, or to use them differently than in the manner in which they are presently prescribed (Riddick, 1993; Spirtas et al, 1993). Clearly, open-ended usage of these medications or persistent COH cycling in couples with an exceedingly poor prognosis should only be undertaken after careful disclosure and informed consent.

COH–INTRAUTERINE INSEMINATION

Intrauterine insemination (IUI) is the artificial placement of washed sperm in the uterine cavity at the time of ovulation, instead of depositing the semen in the vagina or in the cervix. It is postulated that placing relatively large numbers of sperm high in the uterine cavity, close to the tubal ostia, increases the number of sperm entering the fallopian tubes, the site of fertilization. Performing an IUI following COH increases the number of sperm entering the fallopian tube from the endometrial cavity as well as the number of eggs entering the tube from the peritoneal cavity. Increasing the numbers of gametes in the fallopian tube, the site of fertilization, appears to increase appreciably the chances of pregnancy. IUI requires sperm, an ovary, and a functioning female reproductive tract, including the uterus and at least one working fallopian tube.

IUI has been used in the treatment of infertility for a variety of indications. Historically the efficiency of IUI has been difficult to establish. It has been difficult to compare results between published studies following IUI because studies have differed, among other factors, in the indications for IUI, in the extent of the infertility work-up of couples, in the method of sperm preparation used, and in the timing and number of inseminations used in a cycle of IUI (Allen et al, 1985). Dodson and associates (1987) were the first to report the use of COH and IUI to treat infertility in women with normal pelvic anatomy. The authors reported on 85 infertile couples who underwent a total of 148 cycles of COH-IUI. The overall pregnancy rate per couple in this report was 27%, which equaled or exceeded the reported results for IVF and GIFT at the time. Subsequent studies of COH-IUI reported conflicting results, likely because of differences in the COH protocols used, with different endpoints of the hyperstimulation (Dodson and Haney, 1991). Studies that utilized aggressive protocols of COH resulting in the growth and maturation of multiple follicles achieved better results than studies in which less aggressive forms of COH induced the growth of smaller numbers of follicles. Gagliardi and associates (1991) from our institution reported a 26.5% pregnancy rate per IUI following a very aggressive protocol of COH, which combined pituitary suppression with GnRHa followed by ovarian stimulation with gonadotropins. The high pregnancy rate achieved in these patients compared favorably with more expensive treatments such as IVF. The resulting multiple pregnancy rate of 36% was equivalent to the multiple pregnancy rate reported for IVF.

The clinical management of COH-IUI involves timing the IUI approximately 36 hours following the hCG injection. On the day of insemination, the sperm are washed, loaded into a sterile plastic catheter attached to a syringe, and deposited into the uterine cavity through the vagina and the cervix. COH-IUI is effective in the treatment of ovulatory dysfunction, mild to moderate male factor infertility, unexplained infertility, minimal to mild endometriosis, and other forms of infertility that exclude bilateral tubal disease. Therapy can thus be tailored to the individual patient: patients with a poor prognosis, such as older women, can receive very aggressive treatments, whereas patients with better prognoses, such as young women with ovulatory disorders, can be managed less aggressively.

The goal of COH-IUI is to achieve pregnancy without subjecting the patient to serious complications such as OHSS and multiple gestations. The main complication of IUI is endometritis following the introduction of washed sperm into the uterine cavity. Sacks and Simon (1991) reported a prevalence of infectious complications following IUI on the order of 1.83 per 1000 patients. Aseptic technique in the preparation of the sperm sample, and careful technique at the time of IUI to avoid contamination of the insemination catheter, are essential in the prevention of infections.

IN VITRO FERTILIZATION AND EMBRYO TRANSFER

IVF is extracorporeal fertilization in the laboratory, rather than in vivo fertilization in the fallopian tube. Even though IVF can follow retrieval of a dominant follicle in a natural cycle (Paulson et al, 1994), greatly improved conception rates are achieved following COH with the retrieval of multiple mature eggs (Trounson et al, 1981). Placing the eggs in close proximity to a relatively large number of sperm in the laboratory increases the chance of fertilization. Transferring more than one embryo into the uterus increases the likelihood of implantation and pregnancy (Paulson and Marrs, 1986).

The history of IVF in humans is relatively short (Perone, 1994). Rock and Menkin (1944) were the first to report the successful fertilization of human eggs in the laboratory. Eggs for these investigations were recovered at the time of laparotomy, were fertilized in the laboratory, but were never transferred into a uterus. Subsequent clinical advances such as the successful extraction of menotropins from the urine of menopausal women that are used to achieve the maturation of multiple eggs in patients increased the efficiency of the procedure. The development of endoscopic surgery using fiberoptics allowed for the laparoscopic retrieval of eggs, obviating the use of laparotomy. Steptoe and Edwards (1978) were the first to report the birth of a child, Louise Brown, following laparoscopic retrieval of eggs with IVF-ET. Elizabeth Carr, born in 1981, was the first child conceived in vitro in the United States (Jones et al, 1982). Subsequently, improvements and standardization of embryology laboratory techniques have simplified the requirements for the successful establishment of clinical IVF programs. Advances in ultrasound technology in the 1980s, such as the development of vaginal transducers for visualization of the ovaries and for the transvaginal aspiration of follicles, have transformed oocyte retrievals into procedures that can be performed without general anesthesia. In 1994, 6114 babies were born in the United States following IVF-ET (Society for Assisted Reproductive Technology and American Society for Reproductive Medicine, 1996).

The initial indication for IVF in the human was tubal disease, because IVF bypasses the fallopian tubes. IVF today is used to treat tubal infertility as well as male factor infertility, immunologic infertility, infertility secondary to endometriosis, and unexplained infertility. A cycle of IVF proceeds as follows. Following a course of COH, the female partner undergoes ultrasound-guided, transvaginal, needle aspiration of follicles under intravenous sedation or regional anesthesia. The retrieval itself can be performed in less than an hour. The patient goes home on the same day. On the day of egg retrieval, the male partner provides a semen sample from which the sperm are separated or washed for insemination of the eggs. The number of sperm used per egg depends on the quality of the semen sample. If the semen sample is normal in terms of volume, sperm count, motility, and morphology, 50,000 to 100,000 sperm/egg are used. In cases of mild to moderate male factor infertility, 500,000 sperm/egg are used (Wolf et al, 1984). Even though only one sperm fertilizes an egg, inseminating in vitro with less than 50,000 sperm/egg decreases the rate of fertilization; inseminating with more than 500,000 sperm/egg increases the rate of polyspermy, the penetration of the egg by more than one sperm. The sperm and the egg(s) are placed in an incubator under controlled conditions for fertilization to occur. The inseminated eggs are kept in the incubator and examined 16 to 18 hours later for the presence of two pronuclei, confirming fertilization. The zygotes are then returned to the incubator to allow for cleavage to occur. Forty-eight to 72 hours after the retrieval, the patient returns for embryo transfer.

The number of embryos transferred is a critical decision that influences the success of the procedure. The decision depends on several factors, such as the number and quality of available embryos, the age of the patient, and the ability to tolerate a higher risk of multiple pregnancy. Increasing the number of embryos transferred increases the pregnancy rate as well as the rate of multiple gestations. Because multiple gestations place the mother and fetuses at risk for complications of pregnancy and prematurity, the number of embryos transferred would ideally optimize the chance of pregnancy while maintaining the rate of multiple gestations as low as possible. The embryos to be transferred are loaded into a catheter that is introduced into the endometrial cavity through the vagina and cervix. The embryo transfer takes minutes to complete and does not require any anesthesia. In our program, we keep the patient supine for 30 minutes after transfer, after which she is allowed to go home. Embryos that are not transferred can be cryopreserved for uterine transfer at a later date.

The Society for Assisted Reproductive Technology (SART) of the American Society for Reproductive Medicine (ASRM) established the United States IVF Registry and publishes annual reports of ART in the United States. The last report from SART covers ART procedures for the year 1994 (Society for Assisted Reproductive Technology and American Society for Reproductive Medicine, 1996). In 1994, 249 programs reported 23,254 egg retrievals for IVF-ET resulting in 6114 clinical pregnancies (26.3% per retrieval). A clinical pregnancy is defined by the identification of a gestational sac in the uterine cavity using ultrasound imaging. A total of 4912 babies were delivered (21.1% per retrieval). Of these, 63.7% were singletons, 28.3% were twins, 5.9% were triplets, and 0.6% were higher order multiple deliveries. The spontaneous abortion rate was 19%, and the ectopic pregnancy rate was 3.9%. Of neonates delivered, 2.7% had a birth defect.

The complication rate of IVF-ET is relatively small (Schenker and Ezra, 1994). The risks and side effects of COH have already been discussed. From the retrieval, the patient is exposed to the risks of intravenous sedation or of regional anesthesia. The needle used for follicular aspiration can damage organs adjacent to the ovaries in the pelvis—the bowel, the bladder, the uterus, and vascular structures. Both the egg retrieval and the embryo transfer can result in pelvic infection. The rates of spontaneous abortion, ectopic pregnancy, and multifetal pregnancy are higher following ART than following natural conception. There is no evidence that IVF-ET increases the rate of congenital malformations (Schenker and Ezra, 1994).

Gamete Intrafallopian Transfer

GIFT is the placement of gametes—sperm and eggs—directly in the fallopian tube where fertilization takes place. COH and egg retrieval yield multiple eggs. Similar to IUI, GIFT achieves a supraphysiologic number of gametes in the fallopian tube(s), increasing the chance that sperm will meet with an egg at the natural site of fertilization. Unlike IUI, where sperm deposited in the endometrial cavity have to find their way into the fallopian tube and the egg(s) must be picked up by the tubal fimbriae, GIFT assures an extraordinary number of gametes in the fallopian tube and thus increases the chance of conception.

The first human pregnancy following GIFT was reported by Asch et al in 1984, 6 years after the first reported birth from IVF (Steptoe and Edwards, 1978). GIFT was developed as an alternative to IVF in couples in whom the female partner had at least one normal fallopian tube, or for couples for whom IVF was morally or religiously unacceptable. Initially the success from IVF was relatively poor, the cost of IVF was high, its complexity limited the availability of the procedure, and it was ethically controversial (Perone, 1991; Mastroyannis, 1993). Fertilization in vivo following GIFT provided some theoretical advantages over IVF and bypassed some of the ethical problems raised by IVF. It has been suggested that in vivo fertilization in the fallopian tube provides growth factors, hormones, and nutrients, some of which are undefined, that cannot be artificially reproduced in the IVF laboratory. The validity of these claims has yet to be established. Because fertilization occurs in the fallopian tube, the natural site where the sperm penetrates the egg, there is no need for a laboratory capable of establishing the controlled conditions necessary for fertilization, cleavage, and subsequent development of the embryo for 48 to 72 hours prior to uterine transfer. Because it is simpler to establish a GIFT program than an IVF-ET program, the general availability of ART is increased. Guidelines from the ASRM, however, emphasize the need for a laboratory with full IVF-ET capacity for those cases in which the fallopian tubes cannot be cannulated following egg retrieval, and for those cases in which eggs are recovered in excess of the number recommended for tubal transfer (American Fertility Society, 1990).

The indications for GIFT are the same as for IVF-ET, with the exception that GIFT requires the availability of at least one functioning fallopian tube (Mastroyannis, 1993). GIFT has thus been used to treat male factor infertility, unexplained infertility, immunologic infertility, and infertility secondary to endometriosis. Occasionally a patient may require GIFT because the cervix does not allow cannulation for inseminations or embryo transfer following IVF (e.g., a patient with severe cervical stenosis following surgery for neoplasia of the cervix). GIFT involves COH to induce the growth and maturation of multiple follicles and eggs. Oocyte retrieval and cannulation of the fallopian tube(s) has been performed in a variety of ways. The egg retrieval can be done transvaginally via ultrasound-guided follicular aspiration under intravenous sedation, transabdominally via laparoscopy under general anesthesia, or at the time of laparotomy under general or regional anesthesia. The GIFT can be performed at the time of laparoscopy or laparotomy. Cannulation of the fallopian tube(s) via hysteroscopy through the vagina, cervix, and uterus has been described but is not as effective as, and has not replaced, abdominal GIFT (Jansen and Anderson, 1993). Just about every combination of egg retrieval and GIFT procedure has been tried and reported. Following follicular aspiration, the retrieved eggs and a sample of washed sperm are loaded into a catheter that is cannulated into the fallopian tube(s) via laparoscopy or mini-laparotomy for GIFT. In those cases in which both tubes are available and normal, there is no advantage to performing GIFT in two fallopian tubes versus only one (Haines and O'Shea, 1991; Penzias et al, 1991). Generally a total of four eggs are used for GIFT, with 50,000 to 100,000 sperm per cannulated tube. Following GIFT, there is no need for the patient to return for embryo transfer. If a large number of eggs have been recovered, the remaining eggs undergo IVF followed by cryopreservation for embryo transfer at a subsequent time.

The main disadvantage of GIFT when compared to IVF is that GIFT requires a second procedure, a laparoscopy or a laparotomy, to cannulate the fallopian tube(s). Either a laparoscopy or a laparotomy is more invasive than an embryo transfer and involve greater risk and cost. IVF-ET bypasses the fallopian tubes entirely. Furthermore, in those cases where extra ova are not available for IVF following GIFT, fertilization cannot be confirmed if the patient does not become pregnant. Fertilization failure, although rare, can be a cause of infertility which would be discovered only using IVF, and which can be overcome with intracytoplasmic sperm injection (ICSI).

In 1994, 3692 retrievals for GIFT resulted in 1342 clinical pregnancies (36.3% per retrieval) and 1054 delivered babies (28.5% per retrieval). Of the deliveries, 63.6% were singletons, 29.2% were twins, 6.5% were triplets, and 0.6% were higher order multiple deliveries. Of the clinical pregnancies, 22.5% were lost, 3.2% were ectopic, and 1.8% of the neonates delivered had a birth defect (Society for Assisted Reproductive Technology and American Society for Reproductive Medicine, 1996). The success of GIFT over the years has consistently been higher than the success of IVF-ET. Patient selection likely accounts to a large degree for the higher success rate achieved with GIFT. Generally patients who undergo GIFT have less severe forms of infertility than those who undergo IVF-ET. For example, couples with a higher severity of female anatomic infertility, with higher degrees of male factor infertility, and with higher stages of endometriosis will be channeled toward IFV-ET rather than GIFT. Couples with relatively good sperm counts and adequate fallopian tubes are channeled toward GIFT. Large prospective, randomized, controlled studies comparing IVF-ET to GIFT in equivalent populations are lacking. Similarly unavailable are large, prospective, randomized controlled trials comparing GIFT to COH and IUI. Both of the latter treatments achieve the same end: a supraphysiologic number of gametes in the fallopian tubes, the site of fertilization. GIFT is more expensive and requires egg retrieval and surgical access to the fallopian tubes, with the respective anesthesia and surgical risks. COH combined with IUI is easier, safer, and far less expensive.

GIFT has the same risks and complications as IVF-ET regarding COH and follicular aspiration. However, with GIFT the patient must also consider the risks of anesthesia and surgery for tubal cannulation; that is, a laparoscopy under general anesthesia, or a laparotomy under general or regional anesthesia (Schenker and Ezra, 1994).

Zygote Intrafallopian Transfer/Tubal Embryo Transfer

Zygote intrafallopian transfer (ZIFT) and tubal embryo transfer (TET) are variations of GIFT where transfer into the fallopian tubes occurs following egg retrieval and IVF. With ZIFT the zygote, a fertilized egg, is transferred into the fallopian tubes at the stage prior to cleavage. ZIFT is performed 17 to 18 hours after insemination of the eggs at the pronuclear stage (Devroey et al, 1986; Matson et al, 1987; Yovich et al, 1987; Pool et al, 1990). With TET, an embryo at the two to eight-cell stage is transferred 45 to 50 hours after retrieval (Balmaceda et al, 1988, 1992). The indications for ZIFT and TET are the same as for GIFT and all require at least one functioning fallopian tube. Both assume that the fallopian tube provides a natural and superior environment for early development and transfer into the uterine cavity than the IVF laboratory and a transcervical uterine transfer. Furthermore, fertilization can be confirmed, and the products of abnormal fertilization (e.g., polyploidy) or abnormal early development (slow, asymmetrical, highly fragmented cleavage) can be identified to prevent the tubal transfer of abnormal products of conception. The SART report for 1994 includes 800 retrievals for ZIFT, of which 278 resulted in a clinical pregnancy and 233 delivered a liveborn child (34.8% and 29.1%, respectively, per retrieval); 67.5% of the deliveries were singletons, 27.7% were twins, 4.8% were triplets, and none were quadruplets. The ectopic pregnancy rate per clinical pregnancy was 3.1%, and 2.4% of neonates had a functional or structural defect (Society for Assisted Reproductive Technology and American Society for Reproductive Medicine, 1996).

The risks for ZIFT and TET are the same as for GIFT. The results of tubal transfer procedures are similar among themselves, and no advantage has been shown for ZIFT or TET over GIFT (Yovich et al, 1988; Balmaceda et al, 1992; Society for Assisted Reproductive Technology and American Society for Reproductive Medicine, 1996). As discussed for GIFT, patient selection may explain the superior results that are apparent after tubal transfer when compared to transcervical uterine transfer (Yovich et al, 1988). In fact, two prospective studies showed no advantage of tubal transfer over transcervical uterine transfer (Tanbo et al, 1990b; Balmaceda et al, 1992).

INTRACYTOPLASMIC SPERM INJECTION

ICSI is the mechanical introduction of a single sperm into the egg. It is a micromanipulation technique for assisted fertilization. A single sperm is aspirated into a glass micropipette and injected into the cytoplasm of the egg. Some of the early steps in fertilization are bypassed—sperm recognition, binding, attachment, and penetration of the zona pellucida, and fusion of the sperm-egg membranes to deliver the genetic material of the sperm into the egg. Because ICSI is a form of IVF, it can be performed in women with nonfunctioning fallopian tubes. Whereas traditional IVF requires 50,000 to 100,000 sperm for insemination of the eggs, ICSI can be performed with a minimal number of sperm—essentially one per egg.

ICSI is one of a number of techniques developed to assist fertilization in cases of fertilization failure. Unexplained fertilization failure follows the insemination of eggs with an adequate number of sperm of normal motility and morphology. Fertilization failure can occur following insemination of eggs with relatively low numbers of sperm and/or with sperm with abnormal motility and/or morphology. It is also hypothesized that fertilization failure can result from abnormalities of the zona pellucida, the egg membrane, or both. A number of micromanipulation procedures were developed to bypass the zona pellucida and the egg membrane in an effort to avoid fertilization failure. Zona drilling (Gordon et al, 1988), partial zona dissection (Cohen et al, 1989), and subzonal sperm injection (Ng et al, 1988) were early micromanipulation attempts to effectively introduce sperm to the egg. They have all been supplanted by ICSI. ICSI, the direct injection of one sperm into the cytoplasm of the egg, bypasses both the zona pellucida and the egg membrane. Palermo et al, (1992) reported the first infants born following ICSI. ICSI has been so successful in achieving fertilization and pregnancy that it has replaced all forms of assisted fertilization (Palermo et al, 1996a).

ICSI is generally performed when sperm recovery is too poor for IVF-ET (Yovich and Stanger, 1984). ICSI has been performed with sperm from severely oligospermic men (Palermo et al, 1993), with sperm recovered from the epididymis (Tournaye et al, 1994), and with sperm recovered from testicular biopsy (Schoysman et al, 1993). Tesarik and associates (1995) and Araki and associates (1997) reported pregnancies and live births following ICSI with spermatids recovered in the ejaculate and from testicular biopsy of patients with azoospermia. Even though successful pregnancy and delivery has been achieved in the mouse following ICSI of secondary spermatocytes (Kimura and Yanagimachi, 1995), similar results in the human have yet to be reported (Cha et al, 1997).

ICSI is a form of assisted fertilization in vitro. Couples undergoing ICSI require the same preparation and management as couples undergoing traditional IVF-ET. The female partner undergoes COH followed by follicular aspiration for egg retrieval. The sperm used for the procedure are separated from the seminal plasma, epididymal fluid, or testicular tissue, washed, and placed in a solution of polyvinyl pyrrolidone (PVP; ICN Biochemicals, Cleveland, OH). The viscous solution of PVP slows the sperm down and facilitates the handling of the motile cells. The PVP solution also coats the injection pipette, preventing the cells from sticking to its walls during the micromanipulation procedure. The micromanipulation procedure is performed using a microscope. Prior to aspirating the sperm into the injection micropipette, a single motile sperm is immobilized by lowering the micropipette over its tail against the bottom of the petri dish or slide. The immobilized sperm is aspirated into the micropipette tail-first for microinjection. A metaphase II egg is held with a microsuction pipette with the extruded polar body at 12 or 6 o'clock, and a single sperm is injected deep into the cytoplasm. The microinjected eggs are placed in an incubator, where fertilization is completed and the fertilized eggs proceed to cleave to the embryo stage. The embryos are replaced into the uterus 2 to 3 days later.

The success rate of ICSI for the treatment of severe male factor infertility is comparable to the success rate of IVF-ET in couples with no male factor infertility (Daya, 1996; Palermo et al, 1996a). The latest national statistics from SART do not specifically list results of ICSI procedures (Society for Assisted Reproductive Technology and American Society for Reproductive Medicine, 1996). However, review of the literature indicates that fertilization rates, implantation rates, and pregnancy rates are similar between ICSI and IVF-ET. Even though ICSI bypasses the zona pellucida and the oolema, possible filters of abnormal sperm during fertilization in vivo, there is no evidence that ICSI increases the rate of congenital malformations. Because ICSI is performed as part of an IVF cycle, patient preparation, management, and risks are equivalent to those for IVF-ET. With ICSI, however, there is an additional risk of damage to the eggs during the micromanipulation procedure in the range of 6% to 13% (Daya, 1996; Palermo et al, 1996a).

ASSISTED ZONA HATCHING

AZH is a process by which the zona pellucida is disrupted artificially following IVF, prior to embryo transfer, to presumably aid the embryo in the hatching process (Cohen, 1991; Liu et al, 1993; Dokras et al, 1994). Prior to implantation, the embryo discards the zona pellucida, or "hatches" from it, to contact the endometrial surface. It has been proposed that AZH may improve pregnancy rates in the presence of abnormalities of the zona pellucida that may prevent the natural hatching process (Cohen, 1991). It is hypothesized that the zona pellucida and its function may be altered with aging. Abnormalities of the zona pellucida could also be iatrogenic, secondary to exposure to laboratory conditions during IVF or during freeze-thawing in cases of embryo cryopreservation. Even though some clinical observations support the hypothesis that defects of the zona pellucida may be a cause of infertility, the concept remains in the realm of hypothesis.

A number of methods have been described for AZH. While holding the embryo with a suction micropipette, the zona pellucida can be disrupted mechanically with a microneedle (partial zona dissection; Cohen et al, 1990a), with a laser (Strohmer and Feichtinger, 1992), or chemically with acidic Tyrode's solution (zona drilling; Cohen et al, 1992). A defect of approximately 30 μm in diameter appears optimal to maintain the structural integrity of the embryo and to facilitate hatching. Following AZH, the embryo is transferred into the uterus. Because disruption of the zona pellucida may render the embryo(s) susceptible to attack by bacteria, leukocytes, or other immunologic agents, antibiotic coverage (tetracycline 250 mg four times daily) and low-dose immunosuppression (methylprednisolone 16 mg daily) has been recommended for patients undergoing embryo transfer after AZH. Patients take the medications for 4 days starting the night after egg retrieval (Cohen et al, 1990b).

Cohen and associates (1992) reported increased implantation and pregnancy rates after AZH of embryos with an abnormally thick zona pellucida and of embryos with poor morphology. Tucker and associates (1991) reported similar findings after performing AZH in frozen-thawed embryos prior to transfer. AZH has also been reported to be beneficial in "poor prognosis" patients: women with elevated FSH levels, older patients, and patients with a history of IVF failure (Cohen et al, 1992; Schoolcraft et al, 1994).

AZH has potential adverse effects. It is possible to damage the embryo with the microneedle, with laser energy, or with the acidic Tyrode's solution. AZH may expose the embryo to mechanical damage during the embryo transfer. AZH may result in abnormal hatching: blastomeres could be lost through the defect in the zona pellucida; the embryo may hatch too early, before the endometrium is ready for implantation; or partial extrusion of the embryo with "partial trapping" may result in an increased rate of identical twins. Available literature suggests that AZH can be performed safely, and that the complications from the procedure can be kept to an acceptable minimum, if proper technique is used and attention is paid the size of the gap created.

ARTIFICIAL INSEMINATION BY DONOR

Therapeutic or artificial insemination by donor (AID) was the most common form of treatment for severe male factor infertility before the extensive use of ICSI. The use of cryopreserved donor sperm is still indicated for azoospermic or severely oligospermic couples, for males with known genetic or hereditary disorders that place biologic offspring at high risk, for Rh-positive males whose female partners are Rh-negative and severely Rh-isoimmunized, and for single or lesbian women wishing to achieve pregnancy. In addition, cryopreserved sperm allows for storage and concentration of oligozoospermic samples for use in ART, for storage of sperm by the male partner in cases of temporary absence, and for preservation of sperm in cases in which the male must undergo medical treatments such as chemotherapy or pelvic radiation, which may impair his fertility or render him sterile (American Association of Tissue Banks, 1996).

The requirements for donor selection and screening are stringent and costly. The American Association of Tissue Banks (1996) and the ASRM (1993) have published guidelines for the screening and use of donor sperm. Donors are recruited via personal contact, lectures, or public advertisements (i.e., newspaper, radio). Currently donors are screened with personal histories (medical, family, and social/sexual), physical examination, and laboratory testing. The screening tests required for sperm donors as stated by the American Association of Tissue Banks (1996) and the ASRM (1993) are presented in Table 17–1. If all tests are negative and the semen analysis is normal, semen specimens may be collected. However, the specimens must be kept frozen in quarantine for a minimum of 6 months before patients can use them. At the end of the 6-month quarantine, the sperm donor is again tested to ensure that his health status has not changed. If the screening tests are negative, the specimens that have been under quarantine for the full 6-month period are released for clinical use. Donors who continue to provide samples for extended periods of time must therefore be rescreened every 6 months to continue to release their samples for clinical use. If there is a change in the donor's health status, all frozen specimens are discarded.

All sperm banks use donors for a finite time span. Because the retirement of a donor is dependent on the number of pregnancies produced by the donor, and on the specific cutoff of the sperm bank, sperm banks must establish mechanisms by which clinics, institutions, and private offices will provide feedback information regarding pregnancies achieved by the different donors (Verp, 1987).

Donors should be of legal age but younger than 40 years of age (Bordson and Leonardo, 1991). Donors are generally compensated for the time and expense incurred in providing the semen samples. Sperm donation has traditionally been anonymous. However, nonanonymous sperm donations have been arranged. Nonanonymous donors should be screened and managed following the same protocols used with anonymous donors. Psychological evaluation and clearance of donors and recipient couples should be pursued as necessary, and may be considered mandatory in the setting of nonanonymous sperm donation. Consent for the use of sperm donation must be signed by both parties of a couple using donor sperm to achieve pregnancy. The sperm donor should also sign consent releasing his sperm samples for clinical use. The status of anonymity should be explicit and clear in the consents signed by the donor and the recipient couple involved.

The selection of a sperm donor from an accredited sperm bank is usually left to the patients with advice from their physician. The sperm should be ordered

Table 17–1. GUIDELINES FOR SCREENING OF POTENTIAL SPERM DONORS

	INITIAL SCREENING	POSTQUARANTINE
Medical history	Yes	Yes
Family history	Yes	No
Sexual/social history	Yes	Yes
Semen analysis testing	Yes	Yes
Microbiology testing		
Gonorrhea	Yes	Yes
Mycoplasma	Yes	Yes
Chlamydia	Yes	Yes
Genital culture	Yes	Yes
Serologic testing		
HIV-1	Yes	Yes
HIV-2	Yes	Yes
CMV	Yes	Yes
HTLV-I/II	Yes	Yes
RPR	Yes	Yes
Hepatitis B antigen	Yes	Yes
Hepatitis B core antibody	Yes	Yes
Hepatitis C virus antibody	Yes	Yes
Laboratory testing		
Sickle cell anemia	Yes	No
Tay-Sachs disease	Yes	No
Blood type/Rh	Yes	No
Total protein	Yes	Yes
ALK-P	Yes	Yes
Total bilirubin	Yes	Yes
Direct bilirubin	Yes	Yes
LDH	Yes	Yes
AST	Yes	Yes
ALT	Yes	Yes

Abbreviations: ALT, alanine aminotransferase; ALK-P, alkaline phosphatase; AST, aspartate aminotransferase; CMV, cytomegalovirus; HIV-1 and -2, human immunodeficiency virus types 1 and 2; HTLV-I/II, human T-cell lymphotropic virus types I and II; RPR, rapid plasma reagin test.

and scheduled to arrive at the physician's office or to the andrology laboratory at least 1 to 2 days prior to the day of use. One or two frozen donor sperm vials will be needed depending on the procedure for which the sperm are to be used. Because all sperm banks claim a distinct, specialized freezing procedure, the sperm bank–specific thawing instructions should be followed.

OOCYTE DONATION

Oocyte donation is defined as any ART procedure in which oocytes from a third party (oocyte donor) are used to attempt to establish a pregnancy in another person (usually the infertile patient, although a surrogate carrier can be used). Trounson and associates (1983) reported the first case of oocyte donation. A single excess oocyte obtained by surgical oocyte retrieval from an infertile woman was fertilized with donor sperm and transferred into a different infertile recipient in a natural cycle. Pregnancy resulted, but unfortunately ended in a spontaneous abortion at 10 weeks. Lutjen and associates (1984) reported the first live birth after oocyte donation in a 25-year-old woman with premature ovarian failure who had artificial preparation of the endometrium with estrogen and progesterone. Navot and associates (1986) presented a series of eight patients with ovarian failure in which two conceived after oocyte donation. All patients had first undergone a preparatory cycle of estrogen-progesterone replacement, with normal endometrial biopsies on cycle days 17 and 21.

Sauer and associates (1990) first applied the technique of oocyte donation to reproductive-age women 40 years or older with premature ovarian failure and achieved a live birth rate of over 50%/cycle. Several years later, the same group (Sauer et al, 1993b) used oocyte donation to achieve pregnancy in a small group of women over 50 years of age after natural menopause. They applied a screening protocol to exclude applicants with metabolic, gynecologic, or cardiovascular disease. After the transfer of four to five embryos, 14 women undergoing 21 cycles of embryo transfer achieved a 33% ongoing pregnancy rate. Despite their screening evaluations, significant obstetric complications were seen. Five of seven women had their pregnancies complicated by preterm labor, preeclampsia, intrauterine growth retardation, or gestational diabetes mellitus. Fetal outcomes, however, were excellent despite the complicated prenatal course.

The outstanding success of oocyte donation for women with ovarian failure led to the application of this technology to different groups of patients: women with elevated FSH levels, women with a poor response to COH, women with previous failed IVF cycles, women with transmissible genetic diseases, and older reproductive-age women (≥40 years) who were still cycling normally (Serhal and Craft, 1989; Sauer et al, 1994). Oocyte donation

proved to be highly successful in all these groups and is now the treatment of choice for women with infertility caused by poor/absent ovarian function or poor oocyte quality.

Source of Donor Oocytes

Based on local regulations and availability, a number of sources of donor oocytes have been utilized. Known volunteers (usually unpaid), anonymous volunteers (paid and unpaid), and excess ova from patients themselves undergoing IVF (sometimes with the recipients assisting financially with the cycle costs) have all been reported to work well. Whatever the source, all oocyte donors should be screened with medical and family histories and laboratory testing for infectious diseases, in accordance with local guidelines (in the United States: American Society for Reproductive Medicine, 1993).

Endometrial Preparation

More has been written about hormonal preparation of the endometrium than about any other aspect of oocyte donation. Initial reports utilized varying doses of hormones, often along with GnRHa in cycling recipients, in an attempt to mimic the changing hormone levels seen in the natural cycle (Lutjen et al, 1984; Navot et al, 1986). Over time, it has become clear that constant doses of estrogen and progesterone are just as adequate for endometrial preparation (Yaron et al, 1995; Serhal and Craft, 1989). Different routes of administration have been reported: oral, transdermal, sublingual, and parenteral estrogen; and vaginal, oral, and parenteral progesterone. All seem to provide adequate endometrial preparation. Concurrent use of GnRHa for pituitary suppression appears unnecessary in cycling recipients, particularly when higher doses of estrogen are utilized (Remohi et al, 1994; Yaron et al, 1995).

Early investigators employed a preparatory cycle in which hormone replacement was given and an endometrial biopsy was performed in the luteal phase to verify that the endometrial response was in phase with the hormone replacement protocol. Because the vast majority of patients had adequate, in-phase biopsies (Sauer et al, 1993a), most groups no longer utilize endometrial biopsy to assess endometrial preparation prior to the cycle of embryo replacement.

Endometrial thickness appears to be a critical variable. Hofmann and associates (1996) found that an endometrial thickness of 7 mm or greater was 100% reliable in predicting normal endometrial biopsy results. Different groups have found the critical endometrial thickness to range from 6 to 10 mm. We have used 8 mm as the minimum acceptable endometrial thickness. The literature is inconsistent with regard to the importance of the endometrial pattern.

Opinions are divided between investigators who found the favorable "triple-line" pattern to be critical (Shapiro et al, 1993; Coulam et al, 1994; Bustillo et al, 1995) and those who did not (Hofmann et al, 1996).

The duration of estrogen administration has also been studied. Younis and associates (1992) found a critical follicular phase length of 12 to 19 days, with dramatic declines in success with either shorter or longer durations of estrogen treatment. This hypothesis has been dispelled by subsequent larger studies. In 865 oocyte donation cycles, Yaron and associates (1995) found no difference in pregnancy rates in recipients treated with estrogen alone for periods ranging from 5 to 35 days. Remohi and associates (1995) evaluated 186 cycles of oocyte donation and found stable pregnancy rates of 50% or greater in patients treated with up to 65 days of estrogen alone. Thus, above a minimum treatment duration of 5 days, the length of the artificial "follicular phase" does not seem to be important.

In contrast, the duration of progesterone replacement prior to successful embryo transfer—the window of implantation—is far more precise. Navot and associates (1991a) achieved pregnancies with embryos transferred on progesterone replacement days 1 through 6. Meldrum (1993) found lower pregnancy rates in recipients over age 40 when using daily doses of 50 mg of intramuscular progesterone. Pregnancy rates improved to match those seen in younger recipients when 100 mg of intramuscular progesterone was used daily. Similarly, Weckstein and associates (1993) added vaginal progesterone suppositories (50 mg bid) to their usual parenteral regimen of 100 mg of intramuscular progesterone daily. No difference was seen in younger patients, but recipients age 40 or older experienced significant improvements in implantation and pregnancy rates. Miles and associates (1994) compared serum and tissue levels after vaginal versus parenteral administration of progesterone. They found much lower serum levels but much higher tissue (endometrial) levels of progesterone after vaginal administration.

In successful implantations, hormonal support is usually continued through the luteal-placental shift. Most groups continue hormonal support until 8 to 14 weeks of gestation. However, there are several case reports of successful pregnancies in functionally agonadal recipients who discontinued their medications for significant periods of time during the first weeks of pregnancy (Kapetanakis and Pantos, 1990; Stassart et al, 1995).

Recipient Age and Oocyte Donation

Recipient age seems to have little or no effect on the chance of pregnancy. Although a few studies demonstrated lower pregnancy rates in older recipients (Levran et al, 1991; Borini et al, 1996), most investigators have found excellent pregnancy rates in all recipients regardless of age or diagnosis (Serhal and Craft, 1989; Pantos et al, 1993; Balmaceda et al, 1994; Sauer et al, 1994; Legro et al, 1995; Lydic et al, 1996). Successful pregnancies have been reported in recipients in the early seventh decade (Borini et al, 1995).

Spontaneous Abortion and Oocyte Donation

The use of younger, often fertile, donors has led to a much lower incidence of pregnancy loss after oocyte donation in comparison to other ART procedures. Coulam and associates (1996) compared pregnancy loss patterns after various ART procedures. The total incidence of pregnancy loss, preclinical and clinical, was much lower after oocyte donation (14%) when compared to frozen-thawed embryo transfer (32%), IVF (40%), and ICSI (47%). For comparison, pregnancy loss rates in women over 40 years of age using their own oocytes are generally found to be 50% or higher.

Risks of Oocyte Donation

The risks of oocyte donation, although small, are not negligible. With the increasing use of this technique, all the known complications of embryo transfer (ectopic implantation, heterotopic pregnancy, pelvic infection/abscess) will certainly be seen. Obstetric complications are seen more frequently in oocyte donation pregnancies. Higher than expected frequencies of placental abruption, preterm labor, cesarean delivery, intrauterine growth retardation, hypertensive disorders, and gestational diabetes mellitus have been seen in recipients 45 years or older (Antinori et al, 1995; Sauer et al, 1993b). This has occurred despite rigorous screening protocols for gynecologic, metabolic, and cardiovascular disease in the recipients. Several groups have reported as high as a 65% rejection rate for potential recipients. The psychosocial effects of oocyte donation will take more time to be fully realized. Limited evidence to date (Applegarth et al, 1995) suggests that families created through oocyte donation have no major difficulties.

Indications/Techniques

It has been recommended that prospective recipient couples undergo the following precycle evaluations:

Male

1. Testing for infectious diseases (human immunodeficiency virus [HIV], hepatitis B and C, syphilis)
2. Semen analysis with Kruger morphology, and trial sperm processing

Female

1. Testing for infectious diseases (HIV, hepatitis B and C, syphilis)

2. Testing for cervical disease (Papanicolaou smear, cultures for gonorrhea and *Chlamydia*)
3. Uterine cavity assessment (saline sonogram or hysteroscopy)
4. Uterine sounding (trial of transfer)
5. At age 45 years or older, when clinically indicated: stress electrocardiogram, diabetes screening, mammography, cholesterol level, blood urea nitrogen/creatinine level, electrolytes, thyroid-stimulating hormone level, and liver function studies

In addition, couples are seen individually and together by a mental health professional in order to ensure that they have prepared themselves to deal with the psychosocial issues involved in accepting genetic material from a third party, and in raising the resulting offspring.

Prospective oocyte donors undergo screening as outlined in the ASRM's guidelines for gamete donation (American Society for Reproductive Medicine, 1993):

1. General medical health (history and physical)
2. Low risk for sexually transmitted diseases (history and questionnaire)
3. No significant family history of transmissible disease (history, questionnaire, genetic counseling as needed)
4. Testing for infectious diseases (HIV, hepatitis A, B, and C, gonorrhea, syphilis, *Chlamydia*, Cytomegalovirus, mycoplasma)
5. Mental health evaluation
6. Selected laboratory testing for genetic carrier status based on ethnicity (Caucasian—cystic fibrosis; Ashkenazi Jewish—cystic fibrosis, Tay-Sachs disease and Gaucher's disease; African-American/Mediterranean/Asian—hemoglobin electrophoresis, complete blood count).

Cycle synchronization can be performed in cycling donors and recipients using GnRHa or low-dose oral contraceptives for varying periods of time (hormone replacement therapy alone may be manipulated as needed for noncycling recipients). We find low-dose oral contraceptives to be the simpler, inexpensive alternative for patients without any contraindications to their use. The recipient's cycle may be timed to the donor's cycle, or vice versa. If necessary, both the donor's and the recipient's cycles may be controlled. Our program performs cycle synchronization so that the recipient begins estrogen replacement in the form of 5 mg of intramuscular estradiol valerate every 3 days (Feinman et al, 1993) 1 week before the donor is expected to begin gonadotropin stimulation. This provides 3 to 4 weeks of estrogen preparation of the recipient endometrium, and allows enough time for a dosage increase in patients with an inadequate endometrial response (< 8 mm endometrial thickness). Progesterone replacement is started on the evening that the donor takes hCG, and embryo transfer is performed on the fifth day of progesterone supplementation. If pregnancy occurs, estradiol and progesterone are continued at the same doses for 8 weeks after the embryo transfer (10 weeks of gestation).

Results

Oocyte donation is becoming an increasingly popular solution for infertile patients. The 3119 cases of egg donation reported in 1994 nearly doubled the 1802 reported in 1992 (American Fertility Society and Society for Assisted Reproductive Technology, 1994; Society for Assisted Reproductive Technology and American Society for Reproductive Medicine, 1996). Oocyte donation provides exceptional success for women who otherwise have an exceedingly poor prognosis. The latest SART statistics indicate a 47% live birth rate per cycle of egg donation, which compares quite favorably with the 21%, 29%, and 29% live birth rates/cycle reported from IVF, GIFT, and ZIFT, respectively (Society for Assisted Reproductive Technology and American Society for Reproductive Medicine, 1996).

Future Developments

A major challenge under active investigation is how to improve methods of embryo assessment, so that fewer embryos with a better chance of implantation can be replaced. Advances in the area of embryo assessment will hopefully allow the continuation of excellent success rates while minimizing the unwanted complication of multiple pregnancy.

There are two other areas of investigation specific to oocyte donation that are worthy of discussion. The first is the attempt to improve embryo freezing and thawing techniques, so that the same excellent results now seen with fresh embryo transfer can be achieved with frozen, quarantined embryos. Hamer and associates (1995) reported a 21% ongoing pregnancy rate with frozen-thawed donor embryos, which were transferred after a 6-month quarantine period with repeat donor HIV screening. Most oocyte donation programs currently prefer fresh embryo transfers in order to achieve the best possible pregnancy rates. Despite extensive donor screening, tragedies such as HIV transmission from donor sperm (Stewart et al, 1985) are bound to occur eventually with the fresh transfer of donated oocytes. As Hamer and associates (1995) pointed out, "There is no logical reason for treating these donated tissues differently. . . . An increased pregnancy rate will not be of any comfort to a recipient who is inadvertently infected with HIV."

The second area of progress involves the simplification of donor stimulation. The use of gonadotropins for COH allows for the retrieval of a large number of donor oocytes but dramatically increases the cycle costs and decreases the acceptability of this technique to prospective donors. Seibel (1995) reported a 27% live birth rate per cycle after using clomiphene citrate alone for COH in oocyte donors. No cycles were cancelled, one to five oocytes per donor were retrieved, and one to four embryos were transferred into each recipient. In a subset of cycles in which the semen parameters were normal and the donors had a good response to clomiphene citrate (defined as one or more follicles with a mean diameter of 19 mm and a serum estradiol of 500 pg/ml or greater), a 50% ongoing pregnancy rate was achieved. These results compare favorably with donor stimulation using gonadotropins. Future development of this technique will certainly be of interest.

AGE AND FERTILITY

Female Age and Fertility

The dramatic influence of female age on fertility has been historically evident. Comparisons of fertility rates in noncontracepting populations over the last five centuries reveal remarkably similar findings: fertility starts to decrease at about age 30 to 32 years, with a precipitous decline after 40 years of age (Maroulis, 1991). There exists some experimental evidence in humans to help explain this phenomenon. A group of investigators counted the number of ovarian follicles in ovaries from pathology specimens or autopsy. They found a steady decline in follicle numbers until age 37 to 38 years, at which time an accelerated loss of follicles occurred (Faddy et al, 1992; Richardson et al, 1987).

The age-related decline in female fecundity is also seen in couples undergoing treatments for infertility. A large multicenter study of over 2000 nulliparous women with azoospermic husbands undergoing natural cycle-donor sperm inseminations found lower success rates starting at age 31 years, with women over 35 years having a cycle fecundity half that of younger women (Federation CECOS, 1982). Stovall and associates (1991) studied 751 donor insemination cycles and found a significant decline in monthly fecundity in women age 35 years or older; their results were unchanged when they examined the subset of their patients who had normal findings at diagnostic laparoscopy.

Similar findings are seen with more aggressive infertility treatments. Dickey and associates (1991) examined over 700 hMG-IUI cycles and noted significantly reduced fecundity in women 35 years or older (6% versus 13% in younger patients). Tan and associates (1992) reported on the outcome of over 5000 IVF cycles; women 35 years or older experienced a significantly lower chance of successful pregnancy. The live birth rate per cycle for women over 40 years was less than 5%. A study of over 5000 IVF cycles in France (FIVNAT, 1990) found a gradual decrease in success with age and noted that the pregnancy rate declined more rapidly beginning at about age 36 to 37 years. Finally, Craft and associates (1988) exam-

ined the results of 1071 GIFT procedures; they noted a gradual decline in pregnancy rates with increasing age, with a marked decrease at age 40 years. The live birth rate in women 40 years and older was further worsened by a nearly 50% incidence of miscarriage —a not uncommon finding in this age group (Feldberg et al, 1990). Thus the age-related decline in female fecundity persists, despite the use of superovulation and/or ART techniques.

Tests of Ovarian Reserve

Despite the general decline in population fecundity with increasing age, clinical experience has shown that there is considerable individual variability within patients, regardless of chronologic age. This has led researchers to investigate tests of ovarian reserve, which attempt to assess an individual woman's fecundity.

BASAL FSH

Early work by Sherman and Korenman (1975), and by Sherman and associates (1976) studied older reproductive-age women with regular cycles and established the pattern of early perimenopause: a shortened follicular phase in association with early and midfollicular FSH elevations, as compared to younger groups. Their hypothesis was that the oocyte–granulosa cell complexes of older women were deficient in the production of estradiol and inhibin, the mediators of pituitary negative feedback. In the absence of sufficient suppression by these ovarian-derived mediators, pituitary FSH secretion would remain higher than normal during the early follicular phase. Similar observations have been made by Lenton and associates (1988), Lee and associates (1988), and Reyes and associates (1977). A significant increase in FSH levels in women is detectable at age 39 years.

This information about aging of the reproductive axis was then applied to the specific case of infertile women. Cameron and associates (1988) studied the cycles of 10 women (ages 29 to 39; mean = 32 years) with regular menses who had failed an IVF treatment cycle. They identified significant FSH elevations throughout the menstrual cycle and termed this syndrome occult ovarian failure. (Since that time, diminished ovarian reserve has been the term most frequently used to describe patients with elevated basal FSH levels.)

Muasher and associates (1988) were the first to correlate basal FSH levels measured on cycle day 3 with IVF outcome. They found lower estradiol responses, lesser numbers of oocytes obtained and embryos transferred, and a lower pregnancy rate in the patients with elevated basal FSH levels. They also noted a poor correlation between basal FSH levels and patient age. A subsequent study (Toner et al, 1991) of nearly 1500 IVF cycles confirmed both the predictive value of basal FSH measurements and the

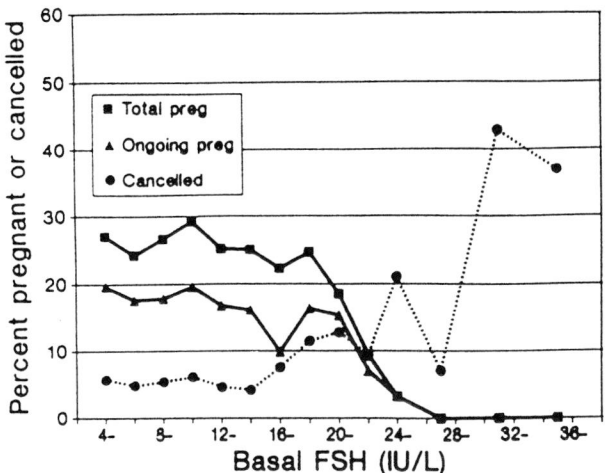

Figure 17-1
Outcome of 1478 IVF cycles as a function of basal FSH. (From Toner JP, Philput CB, Jones GS, Muasher SJ: Basal follicle-stimulating hormone level is a better predictor of in-vitro fertilization performance than age. Fertil Steril 1991;55:784. © 1991 The American Society for Reproductive Medicine [formerly the American Fertility Society], with permission.)

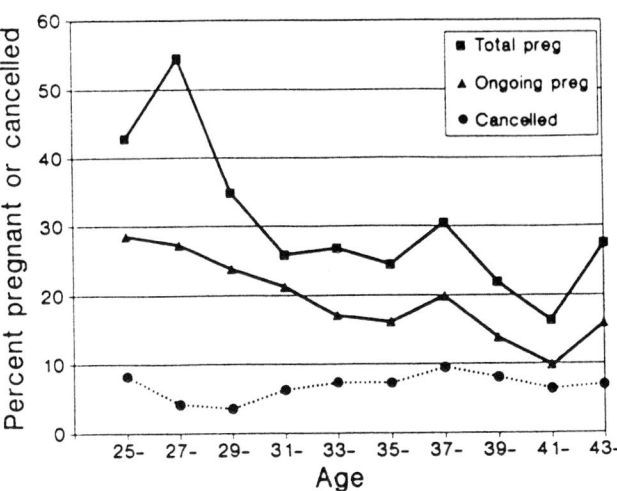

Figure 17-2
Outcome of 1478 IVF cycles as a function of patient age. (From Toner JP, Philput CB, Jones GS, Muasher SJ: Basal follicle-stimulating hormone level is a better predictor of in-vitro fertilization performance than age. Fertil Steril 1991;55: 784. © 1991 The American Society for Reproductive Medicine [formerly the American Fertility Society], with permission.)

poor correlation with patient age. Figures 17-1 and 17-2 illustrate their results. It can be clearly seen that, although success rates declined with advancing age, there was no clear age cutoff at which treatment was useless. Conversely, with increasing basal FSH levels, a very distinct value (FSH ≥25 mIU/ml) above which no successful pregnancies occurred can be seen. These initial reports have since been validated by a number of investigators (Table 17-2). The one notable drawback to this body of evidence is that, with one exception (Pearlstone et al, 1992), the prognostic value of basal FSH measurements has been examined only in populations undergoing IVF or GIFT. Pearlstone and associates found a nearly 10-fold difference in hMG-IUI cycle fecundity in patients of the same age who had varying basal FSH levels (Figure 17-3). These data argue convincingly for the independent adverse prognostic significance of advancing age and elevated basal FSH levels.

Four points deserve mention. First, treatment-independent successful pregnancies continue to occur in women with diminished ovarian reserve, albeit at a lower rate. What has been shown is that patients with diminished ovarian reserve tend to respond poorly to attempts at COH (superovulation). This may be because they are already undergoing endogenously elevated FSH stimulation.

Second, critical FSH levels are assay and laboratory dependent (Hershlag et al, 1992). It has been suggested that each institution establish its own standards for diminished ovarian reserve, but this may not always be feasible. Correlations between different assays are poor. A simple rule of thumb (which seems to agree with published data) is that patients with FSH levels within 20% above or below the upper follicular phase normal limit represent a

borderline group, while patients with basal FSH values greater than 20% above the upper limit of normal have diminished ovarian reserve and an extremely poor prognosis. (As an example, the assay currently used at our institution reports 4 to 13 mIU/ml as the normal follicular phase range; we find patients with basal FSH levels of 10.5 to 15.5 [13 ± 20%] to have a borderline success rate, while patients with higher basal FSH levels [≥16 mIU/ml] have almost no chance for successful pregnancy with infertility treatment.)

Third, longitudinal studies have demonstrated significant intercycle basal FSH variability, with increasing variation seen in patients with higher levels of FSH (Brown et al, 1995). Patients with intermittently elevated basal FSH levels had a prognosis as poor as patients with persistently elevated FSH levels. In other words, a woman's fecundity seems to be defined by her worst, not her best, FSH level (Scott et al, 1990).

Fourth, it has been reported that an abnormally elevated basal estradiol level, regardless of FSH level, is also a marker for diminished ovarian reserve and a poor prognostic indicator (Licciardi et al, 1991). A high basal estradiol level may suppress what would otherwise be an elevated basal FSH level. A basal estradiol level greater than 50 to 60 pg/ml is abnormal, and we suggest measuring basal FSH and estradiol levels 1 day earlier in a subsequent cycle.

CLOMIPHENE CITRATE CHALLENGE TEST

A patient's response to the administration of clomiphene citrate has been proposed as a dynamic test of ovarian reserve. The clomiphene citrate challenge

Table 17–2. LIVE BIRTH/ONGOING PREGNANCY RATES IN PATIENTS WITH NORMAL OR ABNORMAL BASAL FSH LEVELS*

STUDY/POPULATION	TEST CRITERIA	PREGNANCY RATE	
		Abnormal	*Normal*
Muasher et al (1988)/IVF	FSH ≥ 25 = abnormal	0% 0/5	13% 10/75
Scott et al (1989)/IVF	FSH ≥ 25 = abnormal FSH < 15 = normal	4% 2/56	17% 92/541
Toner et al (1991)/IVF	FSH ≥ 25 = abnormal FSH ≤ 10 = normal	0% 0/80	18% 104/576
Pearlstone et al (1992)/hMG-IUI, age ≥40 yr	FSH ≥ 25 = abnormal	0% 0/76	4% 14/326
Ebrahim et al (1993)/IVF or GIFT+	FSH > 11.5 = abnormal FSH < 11.5 = normal *different assay	8% 1/12	16% 16/99
Huyser et al (1995)/IVF or GIFT	FSH ≥ 11.7 = abnormal FSH < 11.7 = normal *different assay	6% 1/16	20% 23/113
TOTAL		1.6% 4/245	15.0% 259/1730

*The detection rate for the presence of diminished ovarian reserve was 12% (245/1975).

test (CCCT) involves administering clomiphene citrate 100 mg on cycle days 5 through 9, with measurement of FSH levels on cycle days 3 and 10. Navot and associates (1987) tested 51 women age 35 or older with unexplained infertility and normal basal FSH levels and found that 18 of 51 (35%) had an exaggerated FSH response to clomiphene citrate (day 10 FSH > 26 mIU/ml). Despite extensive treatment,

including superovulation and ART in most patients, this group demonstrated only a 6% clinical pregnancy rate, versus 42% in the group with a day 10 FSH less than 26 mIU/ml. This test has since been utilized in a variety of populations (Table 17–3): general infertility (Scott et al, 1993, 1995), IVF (Tanbo et al, 1989; Loumaye et al, 1990), and previous poor IVF responders (Tanbo et al, 1990a). A poor response to

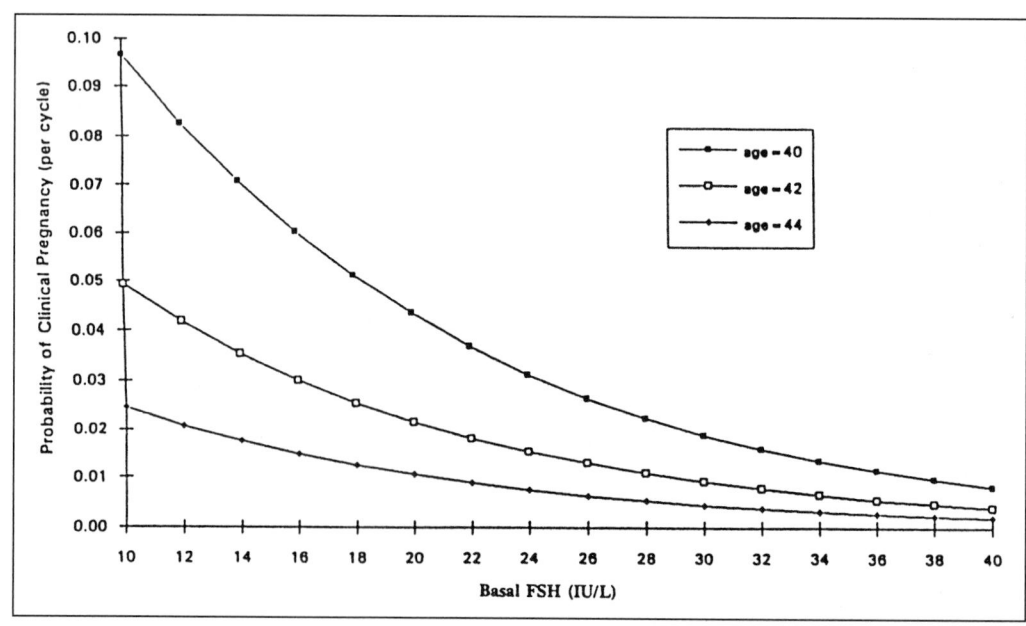

Figure 17–3
Cycle fecundity (clinical pregnancies) as a function of both basal FSH and age (women age ≥ 40, hMG/IUI). (From Pearlstone AC, Fournet N, Gambone JC, et al: Ovulation induction in women age 40 and older: the importance of basal follicle-stimulating hormone level and chronological age. Fertil Steril 1992; 58:674. © 1992 The American Society for Reproductive Medicine [formerly the American Fertility Society], with permission.)

Table 17-3. CLINICAL PREGNANCY RATES IN PATIENTS WITH NORMAL OR ABNORMAL CCCT RESULTS*

STUDY/POPULATION	TEST CRITERIA	PREGNANCY RATE	
		Abnormal	*Normal*
Navot et al (1987)/Unexplained infertility, age ≥35 yr	Day 10 FSH ≥26	6% 1/18	42% 14/33
Loumaye et al (1990)/IVF	Day 3 + day 10 FSH ≥26	0% 0/20	28% 26/94
Tanbo et al (1990a)/Previous poor IVF responders	Day 7 FSH ≥26 (CC days 3–7)	4% 1/25	22% 4/18
Scott et al (1993)/General infertility	Day 3 or day 10 FSH >10 *different assay	9% 2/23	43% 92/213
Tanbo et al (1989)/IVF	Day 7 FSH >26 (CC days 3–7)	8% 2/26	76% 63/83
Scott et al (1995)/General infertility	Day 3 or day 10 FSH >10 *different assay	5% 4/83	49% 245/505
TOTAL		5.1% 10/195	49% 444/946

*The detection rate for the presence of diminished ovarian reserve was 17% (195/1141).

the CCCT has been found in all of these studies to be highly predictive of a lower success rate with infertility treatment.

The CCCT has several advantages over basal FSH testing. The CCCT has a higher detection rate, picking up at least 50% more patients with diminished ovarian reserve compared to FSH testing alone. The currently available literature regarding these two tests of ovarian reserve is compared in Tables 17–2 and 17–3. Approximately 5% of patients with diminished ovarian reserve as defined by the CCCT achieve pregnancy.

OTHER TESTS

Other provocative tests of ovarian reserve have been proposed:

- The estradiol response to early-follicular-phase GnRHa administration, or the GnRHa stimulation test (Padilla et al, 1990; Winslow et al, 1991)
- The FSH response to early-follicular-phase GnRHa administration (Muasher et al, 1988; Fenichel et al, 1989)
- The estradiol response to a standard dose of gonadotropins (Metrodin 300 IU/day) or the exogenous FSH ovarian reserve test (Olivennes et al, 1993)

Seifer and associates (1997) reported that IVF patients with lower day 3 serum inhibin-B levels had lower clinical pregnancy rates (7%) than patients with higher levels (26%). Although they may eventually become useful screening tools, these tests have only been evaluated in limited numbers of ART patients; there is insufficient evidence at present to recommend them for general usage.

Based on current evidence, we continue to utilize basal FSH screening as the test of choice for diminished ovarian reserve. The lower yield compared to the CCCT is compensated for by the high reliability of an abnormal test (>98% accuracy in predicting therapeutic failure).

Causative Factors

There is limited evidence to date to explain why some women retain excellent fertility through the early to mid-40s, whereas others develop diminished ovarian reserve a decade or more earlier. The question naturally arises as to whether the age-related decline in fertility is due to uterine or ovarian factors. Navot and associates (1994) used the model of oocyte donation to attempt to answer this question. These authors transferred embryos from younger donors to both younger (<40 years) and older (≥40 years) recipients. They found identical pregnancy and miscarriage rates in both groups of recipients. Meldrum (1993) reviewed the available literature and concluded that the decreased uterine receptivity seen in older women could be corrected by supraphysiologic progesterone replacement. The outstanding success of oocyte donation (see above) reported by many groups—most of which employed supraphysiologic progesterone replacement—argues convincingly that ovarian factors are predominantly responsible for the age-related decline in female fecundity.

It is well known that smoking increases a woman's risk of infertility (Laurent et al, 1992). Cramer and associates (1994) studied basal FSH levels in a large group of perimenopausal women. They found that current smokers or former smokers with a 10 pack-year or longer smoking history had significantly higher basal FSH levels when compared to non-smokers. Sharara and associates (1994) screened a general infertility population and found a higher incidence of abnormal CCCT results in current smokers (12%) when compared to nonsmokers (5%). Thus there are reasonable data to support the hypothesis that smoking accelerates the development of diminished ovarian reserve.

Unilateral oophorectomy (Khalifa et al, 1992) and pelvic adhesions (Bowman et al, 1993) have also been reported as risk factors for decreased ovarian reserve.

When to Test for Diminished Ovarian Reserve

There are significant similarities between semen analysis and ovarian reserve screening. Both tests are inexpensive, noninvasive, and highly predictive of the success of both traditional and more advanced infertility treatments. These two tests are more reliable and less expensive and invasive than traditional tests employed in the evaluation of infertility: postcoital test, endometrial biopsy, hysterosalpingography, and diagnostic laparoscopy. These facts argue strongly for the performance of these tests as initial steps in the infertility evaluation, certainly before subjecting patients to costly and/or invasive procedures such as surgery or gonadotropin stimulation. Our current practice is to screen all infertile women (regardless of age) with basal FSH and estradiol levels as initial steps in their infertility evaluation. The low yield in younger patients (< 30 years) is more than adequately compensated for by the low cost, lack of complications, and excellent predictive value of an abnormal test (> 98% accuracy in predicting therapeutic failure). In view of the risks and high costs of ART today, it is imperative to attempt to identify patients who may not respond to specific therapies in order to guide them appropriately to reach their reproductive goals.

PREIMPLANTATION GENETIC DIAGNOSIS

Preimplantation genetic diagnosis (PGD) is the use of techniques of molecular biology at the time of assisted reproduction to diagnose genetic disease in the embryo, prior to transfer into the uterus. PGD can be performed early in the zygote stage (Verlinsky et al, 1990); late in the blastocyst stage, 5 to 6 days postfertilization (Muggleton-Harris et al, 1995); or at a time between, in a four- to eight-cell stage embryo (Handyside et al, 1989; Hardy et al, 1990; Tarín et al, 1992). Biopsy of the zygote involves removal of the first polar body (PB) for analysis. PB biopsy is technically more difficult than performing the biopsy at a later stage of development. Because the PB contains only maternal genetic material, detection of paternal genetic defects is not possible with this procedure. Furthermore, because the PB contains single-stranded DNA, only one copy of the gene in

question is present. PB biopsy is prone to error if abnormal cross-over at the time of PB formation results in the loss of the gene in question. Blastocyst biopsy from a 5- to 6-day embryo is technically easier than PB biopsy. The ability to extract more than one cell from a 5- to 6-day embryo enhances the accuracy of PGD by supplying multiple cells for analysis, greatly reducing the chance of misdiagnosis (Muggleton-Harris et al, 1995). However, transfer of 5- to 6-day embryos results in lower pregnancy rates than transfer of earlier embryos. Harper (1996), in a review of the procedure, reported on nearly 200 cycles in which PGD had been performed, and from which 50 pregnancies and 30 deliveries resulted.

The laboratory techniques necessary to perform PGD were developed in the late 1980s. Handyside and associates (1990) reported the first clinical case in which PGD was successfully applied. This initial work was specifically aimed at preventing the transmission of X-linked recessive genetic disorders, and resulted in the transfer of only female embryos after the elimination of embryos identified as male. PGD is currently used in research settings in which it is desirable for couples to avoid a pregnancy when the defect is known, a genetic probe is available, and the couple has already produced an affected child.

The process for obtaining a cell(s) or a blastomere(s) for PGD is simple but highly invasive (Tarín and Handyside, 1993). In a commonly used method, the embryo is held in place with the help of a suction micropipette. A small hole is made in the zona pellucida of the embryo using acidified Tyrode's solution. A second pipette is then passed through the opening in the zona pellucida and a blastomere(s) is gently pulled out of the embryo. The embryo is placed back in culture and the blastomere(s) are analyzed. To date there have been no published reports of serious abnormalities in babies born following embryo biopsy for PGD.

Following embryo biopsy, the removed cell(s) are processed for genetic analysis. Polymerase chain reaction (PCR) and fluorescent in-situ hybridization (FISH) are the two techniques in current usage. PCR is a technique used to amplify small fragments of DNA in a relatively short period of time (usually 2 to 6 hours). It is used to identify specific gene defects. The DNA is amplified exponentially to quantities large enough for electrophoretic analysis. Saiki and associates (1985) first described the technique of PCR in the diagnosis of sickle cell anemia. The sequence of base pairs flanking the DNA fragment to be amplified must be known, and is used to synthesize the "primers" used in the reaction. The primers are short, single-stranded oligonucleotides complementary to the base pairs framing the DNA fragment undergoing amplification. The primers direct DNA polymerase to synthesize new complimentary DNA in the intervening region. The primers, the DNA fragment to be amplified, and excess free single nucleotides are incubated with a specific heat-resistant DNA polymerase. The amplified DNA can be identified by agarose electrophoresis with an ethidium bromide stain. One of the more reliable and rapid methods available to examine the amplified DNA for genetic errors is through the use of heteroduplex formation. The amplified DNA is mixed with DNA from normal and affected individuals. The mixture is denatured at high temperature (92°C), cooled down to allow formation of hetero- and homoduplexes, and separated by electrophoresis. Analysis of the resultant bands allows determination of whether the amplified DNA is affected or not.

FISH analysis uses chromosome-specific, fluorochrome-labeled probes (complementary DNA sequences) to identify DNA abnormalities. It is currently useful for detection of large chromosomal errors (e.g., trisomies, monosomies, or translocations). The tissue is treated with a protease that allows the probes access to the nuclear DNA. Heating denatures the DNA and the probes are added in a hybridization buffer. The probes hybridize with the complementary DNA. After extensive washing, the tissue is examined under fluorescence microscopy for identification of the fluorochrome-labeled probes. The number and color of the probes are recorded and the diagnosis is determined (Carson and Buster, 1995).

These techniques are not free of potential problems requiring caution with the interpretation of the results. Embryo misdiagnosis has been reported (Harper and Handyside, 1994). DNA contamination at the time of PCR will lead to abnormal or no results or will produce nonspecific amplification. Other problems with PCR include amplification failure, preferential amplification of one allele, or the complete failure of one allele to amplify (Handyside, 1996). FISH can also be plagued by hybridization failure, as well as by nonspecific hybridization that results in uninterpretable findings.

PGD has been used successfully to screen for cystic fibrosis (Handyside et al, 1992) as well as to detect single gene defects in disorders such as Tay-Sachs disease, hemophilia, and sickle cell disease. The indications for PGD continue to expand as our understanding of the genetic basis of many diseases increases. PGD can also be used to improve the efficiency of ART, possibly in specific groups of patients. Chromosomal analysis using FISH for sex chromosomes and selected autosomes has revealed a high incidence of aneuploidy at conception (Munne et al, 1993). FISH and/or PGD in the older patient population, where the rate of aneuploidy may be as high as 50%, would allow for the selection of chromosomally normal embryos for transfer. This may increase the pregnancy rates following ART in this group of poor-prognosis patients (Munne et al, 1995).

APPROACH TO THE INFERTILE COUPLE

Infertility therapy is changing. Outcome information in the form of randomized, prospective clinical trials is scarce. Market influences and patient preferences, along with physician bias, often dictate which recommendations are made. The advent of high-cost ART technology has complicated decision making. Restrictions on utilization of ART technology have been forthcoming from health insurance companies in the United States, further affecting physician recommendation and patient preference. These influences have been felt in a number of ways.

The success of ART therapy has had a great bearing on enthusiasm for its utilization. Indeed, ART has now supplanted several formerly appropriate medical and surgical fertility treatments. The statistical arguments for increased ART utilization can be made in several ways.

The cost per baby born from IVF is highly dependent upon the population treated and the pregnancy rate. For example, a cost-benefit analysis performed in 1993 (Neumann et al, 1994) noted a very high cost per baby born from IVF ($66,667, with a range from $44,000 to $211,940). However, several assumptions made in this 1994 publication, which used IVF data from 1992 data bases, bear re-examination. It was assumed that an IVF cycle costs $7000 to $11,000. Current IVF cycle costs are showing evidence of decline, with some "high-volume" centers offering costs of less than half those used for the calculations by Neumann and associates (1994). It was assumed that 14% of cycles would be canceled. Current estimates of cycle cancellation in many programs are well under 10%. No cost-benefit analysis of cryopreservation and subsequent transfer of frozen embryos was applied. It was further assumed that the probability of a live birth per initiated cycle was 12%, when currently the national average of live births per retrieval is close to 20% (Society for Assisted Reproductive Technology and American Society for Reproductive Medicine, 1996) and many programs are reporting per-retrieval success in excess of 35% to 40%. The Neumann et al paper also assumed that the probability of a successful delivery with IVF declined with each failed attempt. This assumption is not borne out by actual practice, because patients undergoing IVF are often intensively prescreened and rescreened before re-entry into another cycle. Couples with a poor prognosis are steered away from this form of treatment, and many couples will not continue after a failed initial attempt. Finally, the presence of male factor infertility, formerly a major impediment to clinical success, particularly in older reproductive-age women, was taken as a very adverse prognostic factor and resulted in the highest cost per delivery in the Neumann et al data. Current practice at most infertility clinics includes a referral for ICSI for the most severe cases of male infertility, rendering the diagnosis of "male factor infertility" virtually obsolete.

Thus, although the Neumann et al (1994) analysis is entirely valid for the assumptions made, these assumptions must be challenged in the face of current clinical practice. As costs decrease, pregnancy rates

Table 17-4. COST PER DELIVERY OF TREATMENTS BASED UPON THEIR PROBABILITY OF SUCCESS AND PER CYCLE COSTS

PROCEDURE/COST	PROBABILITY OF DELIVERY	COST PER BABY BORN
Clomiphene-IUI/$1000*	0.1	$10,000
	0.2	$ 5,000
	0.3	$ 3,333
Gonadotropin-IUI/$2000†	0.1	$20,000
	0.2	$10,000
	0.3	$ 6,667
	0.4	$ 5,000
IVF/$4000‡	0.1	$40,000
	0.2	$20,000
	0.3	$13,333
	0.4	$10,000
	0.5	$ 8,000
IVF/$8000§	0.1	$80,000
	0.2	$40,000
	0.3	$26,667
	0.4	$20,000
	0.5	$16,000

*Cost of a cycle of clomiphene with IUI and follicular monitoring; reported fecundability of 16%.
†Cost of gonadotropin-IUI ovulation induction; reported fecundability ranges from 16% to 27%.
‡Low-end current costs for IVF cycle; fecundability varies per program and population treated.
§High-end current costs for IVF cycle.

increase, and ART is used more selectively, it becomes more and more "cost effective." For example, at a 30% pregnancy rate, with a per-cycle cost of $8000, the cost per baby born is $26,667 (Table 17-4). One can readily appreciate from Table 17-4 that, as IVF cycle costs decrease and pregnancy rates increase, the cost per baby born can render ART competitive with alternate forms of therapy (i.e., tubal surgery).

In fact, the converse argument to the Neumann et al data is persuasively presented by Penzias and DeCherney (1996). As the per-cycle fecundability of IVF procedures exceeds the natural population rate of approximately 20%, treatments with low monthly fecundability become less and less desirable, particularly in women of more advanced reproductive age. In such women, the odds of ever conceiving must be balanced against the detrimental effect of time. Table 17-5 gives calculated cumulative per cent pregnancies by monthly pregnancy rates. If one were to assume a constant probability of success with IVF,

even after repeated cycles (which is probably not the case), then 99.5% of all couples would conceive within 24 cycles of therapy. This is clearly an overly optimistic set of assumptions, in that most couples who pursue IVF are limited financially or emotionally to two or three attempts. However, with a monthly fecundability of 20%, three IVF attempts will result in a near-50% probability of pregnancy. It is unlikely that success per cycle drops substantially within the first three cycles. Therefore, reason would argue that alternative forms of fertility therapy ought to be able to offer a couple probabilities of pregnancy competitive with "real-life" IVF utilizations of up to three cycles or 50%. Furthermore, the 50% figure should be cumulative over a reasonable period of use (i.e., 1 to 2 years for post-tuboplasty outcome, 3 to 6 months for superovulation-insemination, etc.).

Ultimately, in response to the question "How should IVF be utilized?", an individual practitioner must take into account his or her own outcome data, the outcome data of local ART programs, and key

Table 17-5. CALCULATED CUMULATIVE PER CENT PREGNANT BY MONTHLY PREGNANCY RATE (FECUNDABILITY)

MONTH	20%	10%	5%	4%	3%	2%	1%	0.1%
1	20	10	5	4	3	2	1	0.1
3	49	27	14	12	9	6	3	0.3
6	74	47	27	22	17	11	6	0.6
	87	61	37	31	24	17	10	0.9
12	93	72	46	39	31	22	11	1.2
18	98	85	60	52	42	31	17	1.8
24	99.5	92	71	63	52	38	21	2.4

From Penzias AS, DeCherney AH: Is there ever a role for tubal surgery? Am J Obstet Gynecol 1996;174:1218, with permission.

individual features of the couple under treatment. For example, a couple in whom the female partner is 27 years old and has tubal disease, for whom a multiple pregnancy is perceived as highly undesirable and a multifetal pregnancy reduction is unacceptable, must be treated as relatively "risk-averse" for aggressive ART therapy. Such a couple might choose tubal reconstructive surgery, with its attendant risks of ectopic tubal pregnancy and low monthly fecundability (about 3% for many cases of distal tubal disease). Conversely, the same couple, if the female partner were 40 years old, would be considerably worse candidates for tubal surgery because of the additive, age-related reduction in monthly fecundability for the female partner. There are no hard-and-fast rules to guide the course of treatment for infertile couples, and physicians and patients must still negotiate and communicate in an atmosphere of trust and concern.

In the United States, the absence of mandated health insurance coverage for ART, a free-market economy, and absence of regulation has driven success rates up relative to the rest of the world. This has resulted in a significant increase in the numbers of multiple pregnancies and increased utilization of multifetal pregnancy reduction procedures (Haning et al, 1996). The costs to society of multifetal pregnancy are great, and the contribution of ART procedures to the overall multifetal pregnancy rate is believed to be substantial (Callahan et al, 1994). Aggressive use of ART is capable of changing the face of infertility therapy and shifting, perhaps increasing, the global costs of medical care for the infertile couple. This is likely the case when sophisticated technology assists older reproductive-age women, who have more complicated pregnancies but good neonatal outcomes (Bianco et al, 1996). However, appropriate usage of ART procedures has the potential to provide the most efficient attainment of pregnancy. The evolving role of ART hinges on each individual's definition of "appropriate." The policy that will provide for the greatest good is not yet known and awaits large-scale outcome studies.

It is the philosophy of the authors that, in the absence of outcome data to the contrary, ART procedures should be used judiciously, and infertility therapy should be diagnosis based. The following guidelines are based upon principles of good clinical management and the ethical principle of beneficence ("do no harm"). Absolute infertility factors are sought out aggressively and early in the work-up, and less clinical time and effort is devoted to expensive searches for mild or "relative" infertility, such as cervical mucus factors or varicoceles causing minor degrees of semen abnormalities. This is similar in attitude to an infertility managed care plan developed by Bates and Bates (1996). However, unlike that plan, our utilization of ART is more limited and medical and surgical therapy is applied more liberally. Using this philosophy in the context of a managed care health plan, the authors have attained the highest quartile of overall pregnancy rates with the lowest quartile of ART utilization for all of the plan's providers (data unpublished).

Couples with infertility (defined as 1 year of unprotected intercourse without conception, or 6 months of unprotected intercourse in women over the age of 35) undergo a standard minimum work-up at the New Jersey Medical School. Ovulation is assessed by clinical history, basal body temperature chart, or positive urinary midcycle LH surge using a home monitoring kit. Tubal patency is evaluated by hysterosalpingogram; if findings are positive, laparoscopy and/or hysteroscopy are performed as indicated. Unilateral tubal patency is not routinely taken as an indication for laparoscopy. Semen analysis is performed; if abnormal, repeat semen analysis is obtained within a subsequent sperm cycle.

Once a basic evaluation has been made, specific therapy is prescribed based upon the disorder(s) identified. Couples with unexplained infertility proceed through an empiric paradigm with superovulation (using clomiphene or gonadotropins with or without a GnRHa) plus IUI prior to consideration for IVF. Couples with severe oligoasthenospermia are candidates for IVF with ICSI.

It is no longer self-evident that medical management is superior to IVF for unexplained infertility. With reference to Table 17–4, it is apparent that, because successful pregnancies can be achieved with IVF at greater and greater percentages and lower cost, this treatment may supplant most other forms of infertility therapy. Therefore, local IVF success rates, complications such as multiple pregnancy, and patient preference will continue to govern the health care choices that are made. This is a critical principle for the referring physician to keep in mind when considering a couple ready for a subspecialist referral.

ETHICAL/LEGAL ISSUES IN ART TECHNOLOGY

Gamete Donation

ART technology has reshaped the ways in which families are created. The liberal use of donor gametes and the advent of oocyte donation have created a new generation of children who were conceived and carried in ways that were previously unimaginable. These processes have a number of consequences.

Donor insemination has been with us for years. Psychologically, when survey data are assessed, couples who have conceived and borne children via AID appear to be more than adequately well adjusted and involved in relatively strong marital relationships. These data would suggest that the rare but well-publicized disastrous outcomes are not representative of the whole experience. However, several lessons were learned from the AID experience that have informed the advent of oocyte donation and influenced its policies.

First, sperm donors should be accessed from outside the immediate health care institution. People who care for infertile couples or their spouses or relatives are inappropriate choices for sperm donors, despite their ready availability. Anonymity should be maintained scrupulously, if this is the policy that has been agreed to. Sperm donors who bring their specimen to the front of a doctor's waiting room in the early morning hours when there is only one patient waiting risk identification. Screening for sexually transmitted diseases and quarantining of donor semen are now routine, but the lesson was learned painfully and only after several documented cases of HIV transmission had occurred. Conditions in which the donor will wish to breach anonymity should be spelled out in detail in advance of the procedure. Such a policy is becoming more common, but the long-term implications are not yet known. Finally, the liberal use of psychological counseling for couples who are considering this option is strongly recommended. The insemination of one man's wife with another man's sperm, despite its context, is an excessively stressful event for the male partner, and the acute and chronic psychological risks of this procedure need to be appreciated.

Oocyte donation appears to carry fewer psychological risks to the recipient couple. Overall, the satisfaction that an infertile woman receives from the ability to conceive and carry the pregnancy is very affirming in most cases, as is the more immediate mother-child bonding that results. This is not to say that adoptive bonds are inferior, but they are by definition delayed. The ability of the recipient mother to nurse her infant also provides great satisfaction for many women. Most rewarding is the treatment of couples in whom the woman had been presumed irreversibly infertile and unable to ever carry a pregnancy, such as a young woman with Turner's syndrome. The ability to offer these women an eventual chance to conceive via gamete donation improves their self-esteem and lessens their sense that they are radically different from other young women. At the New Jersey Medical School, we have utilized known as well as anonymous oocyte donors. Follow-up studies appear favorable, and donor characteristics have been described by our group (Bartlett, 1991).

Similar to sperm donors, oocyte donors must be screened rigorously. The ASRM (1993) has published guidelines that form an excellent standard of care. When known donors are to be used, it is important to sequester the donor privately and offer her a "medical excuse" to avoid the possibility of subtle or overt coercion. In general, gamete donation techniques are relatively safe and do not often tread on frightening ethical turf.

When anonymous oocyte donors are used, the primary motivation is financial. Young women who seek to gain financially from the procedure and tolerate it well frequently request to be donors again.

How many trials of oocyte donation are safe for a young woman? Should a woman who has never been pregnant be allowed to risk possible long-term consequences of oocyte donation, despite her informed consent? Are there long-term risks of infertility? Are there long-term risks of repetitive use of gonadotropins? In the absence of answers to these questions, most practitioners limit the use of oocyte donors to two or three attempts. This provides a practical compromise between the arduous task of selecting suitable women (about 1 in every 10 who are screened by a physician are actually found to be suitable) and the potential hazards of repeat cycles. Ethical issues in anonymous oocyte donation often involve disclosure. Because this is an elective procedure, how much should the recipient couple be told about the donor? Should the donor's IQ be disclosed (as if this guaranteed high-IQ oocytes!)? Should it be disclosed to a couple if the egg donor is homosexual? How should a breach of confidentiality be handled (e.g., a curious recipient who accesses the donor's file and identifies her)? All of these situations have come up in IVF clinics. Group discussions in which these issues are brought to the forefront and articulated clearly, and involvement of hospital ethics committees when appropriate, can be useful in finding appropriate resolutions to these difficult issues.

Ethical controversies also occur when the disposition of cryopreserved embryos is not declared in advance. In the case of a couple from Kentucky who was killed in an airplane crash, the cryopreserved embryos from their IVF attempt could not be readily claimed. Similar situations arise in the event of divorce or the death of one partner. Advance directives for all the potential outcomes can avoid some of these difficulties. A further difficulty arises with the issue of very-long-term embryo storage. It is believed, but not known, that human embryos will survive indefinitely in liquid nitrogen storage. Yet prolonged storage increases the probability of human or technical error leading to an inappropriate thawing or destruction of the embryo. To avoid this level of liability, many institutions will not store embryos long term. A well-publicized government-mandated thawing of many embryos was carried out by British IVF centers. The Ethics Committee of the American Society for Reproductive Medicine (1997) published guidelines regarding the disposition of abandoned embryos. The personhood of embryos is currently unclear. Although they represent potential human beings, cryopreserved embryos have an overall low probability of implantation per embryo, and legal pundits are at a loss to characterize their "rights." This debate is unlikely to be resolved in the near future.

Surrogacy

Gestational surrogacy involves the practice of utilizing another woman, not the gamete donor, as the "gestational carrier." The gestational carrier then forfeits the offspring to the recipient couple after delivery. This procedure makes genetic motherhood possible for women with intact ovaries who cannot (because of hysterectomy) or should not (because of pre-existing medical conditions) carry a pregnancy to term.

There are many issues of ethical and legal concern involving gestational surrogacy. After the well-publicized MaryBeth Whitehead case in the 1990s, gestational surrogacy was outlawed by several states, including New Jersey. Potential harm to the "gestational" mother is the concern highlighted by the Whitehead case, and motivated this legal action. It is important to note that such a custody battle also has negative implications for the development of the child. Further concerns that frivolous, even cosmetic usage of gestational surrogacy by women who do not wish to alter their figures by pregnancy have resulted in a loss of enthusiasm for this technology. Finally, arguments that gestational surrogates can be exploited have led to doomsday scenarios of impoverished women being herded into "colonies" to support the pregnancies of well-to-do women who do not want to invest the time and effort into actually carrying a pregnancy or giving birth. Although the dialogue continues, there appears to be high potential for abuse of this technology.

Professional Abuse

Finally, abuse of these technologies by medical professionals has been documented all too frequently. The nature of ART is that it is a fast-paced, technology-driven field of endeavor. The technology of ART is not subjected to rigorous scientific testing in a controlled atmosphere because of lack of funding and patient demand. Thus technical advances that appear successful on cursory evaluation are immediately adopted and utilized to provide greater success in terms of attainment of pregnancy. The attainment of many pregnancies (whether done judiciously, cost effectively, and safely or not) is then exploited by advertisers to increase the patient flow into the ostensibly "successful" clinic, creating the potential for acquisition of enormous wealth through innovation.

There is nothing inherently wrong with such a paradigm in a capitalistic society. However, inappropriate exploitation of this model results in abuses to patients. Examples exist wherein ART centers have portrayed their statistics inappropriately, to appear to attain more pregnancies than they actually did. There are also examples of physicians who "manufacture" bogus new technical advances and advertise them heavily in order to lure patients to their clinics. Physicians have also been responsible for driving up the multiple pregnancy rates from ART by transferring excessive numbers of embryos, thereby attaining more pregnancies at the expense of much higher

multiple pregnancy rates. Most disturbingly, there have been examples of physicians engaging in completely undisclosed forms of gamete manipulation and substitution in an almost sociopathic fashion. It is doubtful that these dubious practices, which impact negatively on the entire field and are often generalized by the media, can ever be regulated from within the field. Ultimately, it is likely that external regulation will limit the numbers of embryos available for transfer or hold centers accountable for all aspects of their practice, in addition to the clinical pregnancy rate.

CURRENT CONTROVERSIES IN ART

To Freeze or Not to Freeze?

Semen cryopreservation has been in clinical use for nearly a century. Despite the technical ability to freeze and thaw male gametes successfully, individual oocytes perform poorly after cryopreservation. Only a handful of pregnancies worldwide have resulted from cryopreservation and subsequent thawing of human oocytes. Conversely, fertilized human pre-embryos respond reasonably well to freezing and thawing, and appear to retain about two thirds of their capacity to implant (Levran et al, 1990). Nonetheless, because a frozen-thawed embryo is of lesser overall viability, there is increasing enthusiasm for fresh embryo transfer. However, aggressive fresh transfer of human embryos will result in a larger percentage of multiple pregnancies, which shifts considerable cost to the maternal-fetal medicine specialist (Callahan et al, 1994). Despite the impression of patients and infertility physicians to the contrary, it is not "Buy one, get one free." Setting the appropriate number of embryos for transfer and saving embryos for freezing is an ongoing controversy that involves issues of access to IVF as well as avoidance of multiple pregnancy. For example, a couple with health insurance coverage for a single IVF attempt and little means to pay for additional attempts may desire a different disposition for their embryos than another couple with the means to pursue many attempts. From the perspective of the insured couple, the single IVF attempt may prompt the sense that they are "going for broke," and very aggressive embryo transfers may be requested. However, the health care burdens imposed by knowingly risking multiple pregnancies will not tolerate such a practice for long. Unlike European countries, in which IVF is government regulated but also government insured, the United States is motivated by a more individualistic, autonomous ethic. The eventual outcome of this controversy is unclear at the present.

The Future of the Human Species

The Darwinian concept of survival of the fittest has been applied to reproductive processes. There is reason to believe that a natural "winnowing out" of abnormal pregnancies is a manifestation of this concept, because miscarried pregnancies are frequently chromosomally abnormal, with a poor chance of neonatal survival. The ability to perform high-tech manipulations on gametes that we suspect are defective (severely abnormal, immotile sperm, aged oocytes) has led to concern that the products of these pregnancies might be abnormal or that we will create subsequent generations of individuals who are dependent upon ART technology to reproduce. Although increased chromosomal anomalies are found in oocytes of women of advanced reproductive age (Munne et al, 1993), there does not appear to be a significant increase in abnormal babies born. This suggests that the winnowing out process functions in utero effectively to protect older women against an ART-enhanced further increase in genetically abnormal offspring. With respect to apparently defective sperm that are injected into oocytes, a report by Palermo and associates (1996b) reveals no increase in adverse outcomes of 382 ICSI-produced deliveries. However, microdeletions of the Y chromosome have been reported in severely oligospermic men (Foresta et al, 1997; Pryor et al, 1997; Simoni et al, 1997), leading to the concern that transmission of reproductive defects may be facilitated by this form of ART. Screening of such men has been recommended by some. Overall, the argument that ART is "devolving" the human species does not appear sound at the present time. Clearly, as procedures become more aggressive, they need to be studied carefully to determine their risks.

Utilization of ART

Several arguments have been presented that suggest that ART is not utilized enough in the United States. Theoretically, proper use of this powerful technology should result in a greater effectiveness in attaining pregnancies in the fastest possible time frame. The problem is that "proper use" is defined differently by different people. Two scenarios currently exist: one in which ART is utilized early and repeatedly in infertility centers, after a very cursory initial workup, and a second in which ART is typically withheld as the "court of last resort" for an infertile couple in whom other treatments are inappropriate, or for whom there is no alternative (i.e., complete bilateral occlusion of the fallopian tubes). At present, neither scenario is sufficiently data based to provide adequate outcomes for policy development. The next decade should bring these important outcomes to light as physicians and patients struggle together to provide rapid, safe, and effective treatments for the painful problem of infertility.

REFERENCES

Aitken RJ, Clarkson JS: Cellular basis of defective sperm function and its association with the genesis of reactive oxygen species by human spermatozoa. J Reprod Fertil 1987;81:459.

Allen NC, Herbert CH, Maxson WS, et al: Intrauterine insemination: a critical review. Fertil Steril 1985;44:569.

American Association of Tissue Banks: Standards of semen banking. In: AATB Standards of Tissue Banks. Alexandria, VA: American Association of Tissue Banks, 1966:87.

American Fertility Society: Revised minimum standards for in vitro fertilization, gamete intrafallopian transfer, and related procedures. Fertil Steril 1990;53:225.

American Fertility Society and Society for Assisted Reproductive Technology: Assisted reproductive technology in the United States and Canada: 1992 results generated from the American Fertility Society/Society for Assisted Reproductive Technology Registry. Fertil Steril 1994;62:1121.

American Society for Reproductive Medicine: Guidelines for gamete donation:1993. Fertil Steril 1993;59(Suppl 1):1S.

Antinori S, Versaci C, Panci C, et al: Fetal and maternal morbidity and mortality in menopausal women aged 45–63 years. Hum Reprod 1995;10:464.

Applegarth L, Goldberg NC, Cholst I, et al: Families created through ovum donation: a preliminary investigation of obstetrical outcome and psychosocial adjustment. J Assist Reprod Genet 1995;12:574.

Araki Y, Motoyama M, Yoshida A, et al: Intracytoplasmic injection with late spermatids: a successful procedure in achieving childbirth for couples in which the male partner suffers from azoospermia due to deficient spermatogenesis. Fertil Steril 1997;67:559.

Asch RH, Ellsworth LR, Balmaceda JP, Wong PC: Pregnancy after translaparoscopic gamete intrafallopian transfer. Lancet 1984;2:1034.

Äumuller G, Seitz J: Protein secretion and secretory processes in male sex accessory glands. Int Rev Cytol 1990;121:127.

Baird DT, and Howles CM: Induction of ovulation with gonadotropins: hMG versus purified FSH. In Filicori M, Flamigni C (eds): Ovulation Induction: Basic Science and Clinical Advances. Amsterdam: Elsevier Science B.V, 1994:135.

Balmaceda JP, Alam V, Roszjtein D, et al: Embryo implantation rates in oocyte donation: a prospective comparison of tubal versus uterine transfers. Fertil Steril 1992;57:362.

Balmaceda JP, Bernardini L, Ciuffardi I, et al: Oocyte donation in humans: a model to study the effects of age on embryo implantation rate. Hum Reprod 1994;9:2160.

Balmaceda JP, Gastaldi C, Remohi J, et al: Tubal embryo transfer as a treatment for infertility due to male factor. Fertil Steril 1988;50:476.

Bartlett JA: Psychiatric issues in non-anonymous oocyte donation. J Psychosom Med 1991;32:433.

Bates GW, Bates SR: The economics of infertility: developing an infertility managed care plan. Am J Obstet Gynecol 1996;174:1200.

Belaisch-Allart J, De Mouzon J, Lapousterle C, Mayer M: The effect of HCG supplementation after combined GnRH agonist/HMG treatment in an IVF programme. Hum Reprod 1990;5:163.

Benadiva CA, Davis O, Kligman I, et al: Withholding gonadotropin administration is an effective alternative for the prevention of ovarian hyperstimulation syndrome. Fertil Steril 1997;67:724.

Ben-Nun I, Shulman A, Ghetler Y, et al: The significance of 17 β-estradiol levels in highly responding women during ovulation induction in IVF treatment: its impact and prognostic value with respect to oocyte maturation and treatment outcome. J Assist Reprod Genet 1993;10:213.

Bianco A, Stone J, Lynch L, et al: Pregnancy outcome at age 40 and older. Obstet Gynecol 1996;87:917.

Blankenstein J, Shalev J, Saadon T, et al: Ovarian hyperstimulation syndrome: prediction by number and size of preovulatory ovarian follicles. Fertil Steril 1987;47:597.

Bordson BL, Leonardo VS: The appropriate upper age limit for semen donors: a review of the genetic effects of paternal age. Fertil Steril 1991;56:397.

Borini A, Bafaro G, Violini F, et al: Pregnancies in postmenopausal women over 50 years old in an oocyte donation program. Fertil Steril 1995;63:258.

Borini A, Bianchi L, Violini F, et al: Oocyte donation program: pregnancy and implantation rates in women of different ages sharing oocytes from a single donor. Fertil Steril 1996;65:94.

Bowman MC, Cooke ID, Lentin EA: Investigation of impaired ovarian function as a contributing factor to infertility in women with pelvic adhesions. Hum Reprod 1993;8:1654.

Bristow RE, Karlan BY: Ovulation induction, infertility, and ovarian cancer risk. Fertil Steril 1996;66:499.

Brown JR, Liu HC, Sewitch KF, et al: Variability of day 3 follicle-stimulating hormone levels in eumenorrheic women. J Reprod Med 1995;40:620.

Bustillo M, Krysa LW, Coulam CB: Uterine receptivity in an oocyte donation programme. Hum Reprod 1995;10:442.

Callahan TL, Hall JS, Ettner SL, et al: The economic impact of multiple-gestation pregnancies and the contribution of assisted reproductive techniques to their incidence. N Engl J Med 1994; 331:244.

Cameron IT, O'Shea FC, Rolland JM, et al: Occult ovarian failure: a syndrome of infertility, regular menses, and elevated follicle-stimulating hormone concentrations. J Clin Endocrinol Metab 1988;67:1190.

Carson SA, Buster JE: Diagnosis and treatment before implantation: the ultimate prenatal medicine. Contemp OB/GYN 1995; 40:71.

Casper RF, Wilson E, Collins JA, et al: Enhancement of human implantation by exogenous chorionic gonadotropin. Lancet 1983;2:1191.

Cedars MI, Surey E, Hamilton F, et al: Leuprolide acetate lowers circulating bioactive luteinizing hormone and testosterone concentrations during ovarian stimulation for oocyte retrieval. Fertil Steril 1990;53:627.

Cha KY, Oum KB, Kim HJ: Approaches for obtaining sperm in patients with male factor infertility. Fertil Steril 1997;67:985.

Claman P, Domingo M, Leader A: Luteal phase support in invitro fertilization using gonadotrophin releasing hormone analogue before ovarian stimulation: a prospective randomized study of human chorionic gonadotrophin versus intramuscular progesterone. Hum Reprod 1992;7:487.

Cohen J: Assisted hatching of human embryos. J In Vitro Fertil Embryo Transfer 1991;8:179.

Cohen J, Alikani M, Trowbridge J, Rosenwaks Z: Implantation enhancement by selective assisted hatching using zona drilling of human embryos with poor prognosis. Hum Reprod 1992;7: 685.

Cohen J, Elsner C, Kort H, et al: Impairment of the hatching process following IVF in the human and improvement of implantation by assisted hatching using micromanipulation. Hum Reprod 1990a;5:7.

Cohen J, Malter H, Elsner C, et al: Immunosuppression supports implantation of zona pellucida dissected human embryos. Fertil Steril 1990b;53:662.

Cohen J, Malter H, Wright G, et al: Partial zona dissection of human oocytes when failure of zona pellucida penetration is anticipated. Hum Reprod 1989;4:435.

Corsan GH, Kemmann E: The role of superovulation with menotropins in ovulatory infertility: a review. Fertil Steril 1991;55: 468.

Coulam CB, Bustillo M, Soenksen DM, Britten S: Ultrasonographic predictors of implantation after assisted reproduction. Fertil Steril 1994;62:1004.

Coulam CB, Opsahl MS, Sherins RJ, et al: Comparisons of pregnancy loss patterns after intracytoplasmic sperm injection and other assisted reproductive technologies. Fertil Steril 1996;65: 1157.

Craft I, Al-Shawaf T, Lewis P, et al: Analysis of 1,071 GIFT procedures: the case for a flexible approach to treatment. Lancet 1988;1:1094.

Cramer DW, Barbieri RL, Xu H, Reichardt JKV: Determinants of basal follicle-stimulating hormone levels in premenopausal women. J Clin Endocrinol Metab 1994;79:1105.

Daya S: Overview analysis of outcomes with intracytoplasmic sperm injection. J SOGC 1996;18:645.

Devroey P, Braeckmans P, Smitz J, et al: Pregnancy after translaparoscopic zygote intra-fallopian transfer in a patient with sperm antibodies. Lancet 1986;1:1329.

Dickey RP, Olar TT, Taylor SN, et al: Relationship of follicle number, serum estradiol, and other factors to birth rate and multiparity in human menopausal gonadotropin-intrauterine insemination cycles. Fertil Steril 1991;56:89.

Dodson WC, Haney AF: Controlled ovarian hyperstimulation and intrauterine insemination for the treatment of infertility. Fertil Steril 1991;55:457.

Dodson WC, Hughes CL, Yancy SE, Haney AF: Clinical characteristics of ovulation induction with human menopausal gonadotropins with and without leuprolide acetate in polycystic ovary syndrome. Fertil Steril 1989;52:915.

Dodson WC, Whitesides DB, Hughes CL, et al: Superovulation with intrauterine insemination in the treatment of infertility: a possible alternative to gamete intrafallopian transfer and in vitro fertilization. Fertil Steril 1987;48:441.

Dokras A, Ross C, Gosden B, et al: Micromanipulation of human embryos to assist hatching. Fertil Steril 1994;61:514.

Dourron NE, Williams DB: Prevention and treatment of ovarian hyperstimulation syndrome. Semin Reprod Endocrinol 1996;14: 355.

Ebrahim A, Rienhardt G, Morris S, et al: Follicle-stimulating hormone levels on cycle day 3 predict ovulation stimulation response. J Assist Reprod Genet 1993;10:130.

Ethics Committee of the American Fertility Society: Ethical considerations of the new reproductive technologies. Fertil Steril 1986;46(3):Suppl 1.

Ethics Committee of the American Society for Reproductive Medicine: Ethical considerations of assisted reproductive technologies. Fertil Steril 1997;67(5):Suppl 1.

Evans MI, Dommergues M, Wapner RJ, et al: Efficacy of transabdominal multifetal pregnancy reduction: collaborative experience among the world's largest centers. Obstet Gynecol 1993; 82:61.

Faddy MJ, Gosden RG, Gougeon A, et al: Accelerated disappearance of ovarian follicles in mid-life: implications for forecasting menopause. Hum Reprod 1992;7:1342.

Federation CECOS, Schwartz D, Mayaux MJ: Female fecundity as a function of age: results of artificial insemination in 2,193 nulliparous women with azoospermic husbands. N Engl J Med 1982;306:404.

Feinman M, Sher G, Massaranni G, et al: High fecundity rates in donor oocyte recipients and in-vitro fertilization surrogates using parenteral oestradiol valerate. Hum Reprod 1993;8:1145.

Feldberg D, Farhi J, Dicker D, et al: The impact of embryo quality on pregnancy outcome in elderly women undergoing in-vitro fertilization-embryo transfer (IVF-ET). J In Vitro Fertil Embryo Transfer 1990;7:257.

Fenichel P, Grimaldi M, Olivero JF, et al: Predictive value of hormonal profiles before stimulation for in-vitro fertilization. Fertil Steril 1989;51:845.

FIVNAT, Piette C, deMouzon J, et al: In-vitro fertilization: influence of women's age on pregnancy rates. Hum Reprod 1990;5: 56.

Flamigni C, Venturoli S, Dal Prato L, Porcu E: Purified FSH: characteristics and applications. In Filicori M, Flamigni C (eds): Ovulation Induction: Basic Science and Clinical Advances. Amsterdam: Elsevier Science B.V, 1994:125.

Foresta C, Ferlin A, Garolla A, et al: Y-chromosome deletions in idiopathic severe testiculopathies. J Clin Endocrinol Metab 1997;82:1075.

Frederick JL, Ord T, Kettel LM, et al: Successful pregnancy outcome after cryopreservation of all fresh embryos with subsequent transfer into an unstimulated cycle. Fertil Steril 1995;64: 987.

Fulgham DL, Alexander NJ: Spermatozoa washing and concentration techniques. In: Keel BA, Webster B (eds): CRC Handbook of Laboratory Diagnosis and Treatment of Infertility. Baltimore: CRC Press, 1990:193.

Gagliardi CL, Emmi AM, Weiss G, Schmidt CL: Gonadotropin-releasing hormone agonist improves the efficiency of controlled ovarian hyperstimulation/intrauterine insemination. Fertil Steril 1991;55:939.

Garcia JE, Padilla SL, Bayati J, Baramki TA: Follicular phase gonadotropin-releasing hormone agonist and human gonadotropins: a better alternative for ovulation induction in in vitro fertilization. Fertil Steril 1990;53:302.

Gemzell CA, Diczafalusy E, Tillinger G: Clinical effect of human pituitary follicle-stimulating hormone (FSH). J Clin Endocrinol Metab. 1958;18:1333.

Germond M, Dessole S, Senn A, et al: Successful in-vitro fertilization and embryo transfer after treatment with recombinant FSH [letter]. Lancet 1992;339:1170.

Ginsburg J, Hardiman P: Ovulation induction with human menopausal gonadotropins- a changing scene. Gynecol Endocrinol 1991;5:57.

Golan A, Ron-El R, Herman A, et al: Ovarian hyperstimulation syndrome: an update review. Obstet Gynecol Surv 1989;44:430.

Gonen Y, Jacobson W, Casper RF: Gonadotropin suppression with oral contraceptives before in vitro fertilization. Fertil Steril 1990;53:282.

Gordon JW, Grunfeld L, Garrisi GJ, et al: Fertilization of human oocytes by sperm from infertile males after zona pellucida drilling. Fertil Steril 1988;50:68.

Gougeon A: Regulation of ovarian follicular development in primates: facts and hypotheses. Endocrin Rev 1996;17:121.

Haines CJ, O'Shea RT: The effect of unilateral versus bilateral tubal cannulation and the number of oocytes transferred on the outcome of gamete intrafallopian transfer. Fertil Steril 1991;55:423.

Hamer FC, Horne G, Pease EHE, et al: The quarantine of fertilized donated oocytes. Hum Reprod 1995;10:1194.

Handyside AH: Preimplantation genetic diagnosis today. Hum Reprod 1996;11(Suppl 1):139.

Handyside AH, Komtogianni EH, Hardy K, Winston RML: Pregnancies from biopsied human preimplantation embryos sexed by Y-specific DNA amplification. Nature 1990;344:768.

Handyside AH, Lesko JG, Tarín JJ, et al: Birth of a normal girl after in vitro fertilization and preimplantation diagnosis testing for cystic fibrosis. N Engl J Med 1992;327:905.

Handyside AH, Pattinson JK, Penketh RJA, et al: Biopsy of human preimplantation embryos and sexing by DNA amplification. Lancet 1989;1:347.

Haning RV, Seifer DB, Wheeler CA, et al: Effects of fetal number and multifetal reduction on length of in vitro fertilization pregnancies. Obstet Gynecol 1996;87:964.

Hanson FM, Rock J: Artificial insemination with husband's sperm. Fertil Steril 1951;2:162.

Hardy K, Martin KL, Leese HJ, et al: Human preimplantation development in vitro is not adversely affected by biopsy at the 8-cell stage. Hum Reprod 1990;5:708.

Harper JC: Preimplantation diagnosis of inherited disease by embryo biopsy: an update of world figures. J Assist Reprod Genet 1996;13:90.

Harper JC, Handyside AH: The current status of preimplantation diagnosis. Curr Obstet Gynecol 1994;4:143.

Herman A, Ron-El R, Golan A, et al: Pregnancy rate and ovarian hyperstimulation after luteal human chorionic gonadotropin in in vitro fertilization stimulated with gonadotropin-releasing hormone analog and menotropins. Fertil Steril 1990;53:92.

Hershlag A, Lesser M, Montefusco D, et al: Interinstitutional variability of follicle-stimulating hormone and estradiol levels. Fertil Steril 1992;58:1123.

Hofmann GE, Toner JP, Muasher SJ, Jones GS: High-dose follicle stimulating hormone (FSH) ovarian stimulation in low responder patients for in vitro fertilization. J In Vitro Fertil Embryo Transfer 1989;6:285.

Hofmann GE, Thie J, Scott RT Jr, Navot D: Endometrial thickness is predictive of histologic endometrial maturation in women undergoing hormone replacement for ovum donation. Fertil Steril 1996;66:380.

Homburg R, Levy T, Ben-Rafael Z: A comparative prospective study of conventional regimen with chronic low-dose administration of follicle-stimulating hormone for anovulation associated with polycystic ovary syndrome. Fertil Steril 1995;63:729.

Hornnes P, Groud D, Howles C, Loumaye E: Recombinant human follicle stimulating hormone treatment leads to normal follicular growth, estradiol secretion, and pregnancy in a World Health Organization Group I anovulatory woman. Fertil Steril 1993;60:724.

Hughes EG, Fedorkow DM, Daya S, et al: The routine use of gonadotropin releasing hormone agonists prior to in vitro fertilization and gamete intrafallopian transfer: a meta-analysis of randomized controlled trials. Fertil Steril 1992;58:888.

Huyser C, Fourie FLR, Pentz J, Hurter P: The predictive value of basal follicle-stimulating and growth hormone levels as determined by immunofluorometry during assisted reproduction. J Assist Reprod Genet 1995;12:244.

Jacobson A, Galen D, Milani H, et al: A novel superovulation regimen: three-day gonadotropin-releasing hormone agonist with overlapping gonadotropins. Fertil Steril 1991;56:1169.

Jansen RP, Anderson JC: Transvaginal versus laparoscopic gamete intrafallopian transfer: a case-controlled retrospective comparison. Fertil Steril 1993;59:836.

Jones HW, Jones GS, Andrews MC, et al: The program of in vitro fertilization at Norfolk. Fertil Steril 1982;38:14.

Kanwar KC, Yanagimachi R, Lopata A: Effects of human seminal plasma on fertilizing capacity of human spermatozoa. Fertil Steril 1979;31:321.

Kapetanakis E, Pantos KJ: Continuation of a donor oocyte pregnancy in menopause without early pregnancy support. Fertil Steril 1990;54:1171.

Karande VC, Jones GS, Veek L, Muasher SJ: High-dose FSH stimulation at the onset of the stimulation at the onset of the menstrual cycle does not suppress the IVF outcome of low-responder patients. Fertil Steril 1990;53:486.

Kerin J, Warnes G, Quinn P, et al: In vitro fertilization and embryo transfer program, Department of Obstetrics and Gynecology, University of Adelaide at the Queen Elizabeth Hospital, Woodville, South Australia. J In Vitro Fertil Embryo Transfer 1984;1:63.

Khalifa E, Toner JP, Muasher SJ, Acosta AA: Significance of basal follicle-stimulating hormone levels in women with one ovary in a program of in-vitro fertilization. Fertil Steril 1992;57:835.

Kimura Y, Yanagimachi R: Development of normal mice from oocytes injected with secondary spermatocyte nuclei. Biol Reprod 1995;53:855.

Knobil E: The neuroendocrine control of the menstrual cycle. Recent Prog Horm Res 1980;36:53.

Kreitmann O, Nixon WE, Hodgen GD: Induced corpus luteum dysfunction after aspiration of the preovulatory follicle in monkeys. Fertil Steril 1981;35:671.

Land JA, Yarmolinskaya MI, Dumoulin JCM, Evers JLH: High-dose human menopausal gonadotropin stimulation in poor responders does not improve in vitro fertilization outcome. Fertil Steril 1996;65:961.

Laurent SL, Thompson SJ, Addy C, et al: An epidemiologic study of smoking and primary infertility in women. Fertil Steril 1992;57:565.

Lee SJ, Lenton EA, Sexton L, Cooke ID: The effect of age on the cyclical patterns of plasma LH, FSH, oestradiol, and progesterone in women with regular menstrual cycles. Hum Reprod 1988;3:851.

Legro RS, Wong IL, Paulson RJ, et al: Recipient's age does not adversely affect pregnancy outcome after oocyte donation. Am J Obstet Gynecol 1995;172:96.

Lenton EA, Sexton L, Lee S, Cooke ID: Progressive changes in LH and FSH and LH:FSH ratio in women throughout reproductive life. Maturitas 1988;10:35.

Levran D, Ben-Shlomo I, Dor J, et al: Aging of endometrium and oocytes: observations on conception and abortion rates in an egg donation model. Fertil Steril 1991;56:1091.

Levran D, Dor J, Rudak E, et al: Pregnancy potential of human oocytes—the effect of cryopreservation. N Engl J Med 1990;323:1153.

Licciardi FL, Liu HL, Berkeley AS, et al: Day 3 estradiol levels as prognosticators of pregnancy outcome in in-vitro fertilization, both alone and in conjunction with day 3 FSH levels. In: Abstracts of the Thirty-eighth Annual Meeting of the Society for Gynecologic Investigation, 1991:169, abstract 141.

Liu HC, Cohen J, Alikani M, et al: Assisted hatching facilitates earlier implantation. Fertil Steril 1993;60:871.

Loumaye E, Billion JM, Mine JM, et al: Prediction of individual response to controlled ovarian hyperstimulation by means of a clomiphene citrate challenge test. Fertil Steril 1990;53:295.

Loumaye E, Campbell R, Salat-Baroux J: Human follicle-stimulating hormone produced by recombinant DNA technology: a review for clinicians. Hum Reprod Update 1995;1:188.

Lunenfeld B, Sulimovici S, Rabau E, Eshkol A: L' induction de l'ovulation dans les aménorrhées hypophysaires par un traitement combiné de gonadotrophines urinaires ménopausiques et de gonadotophines chorioniques. C R Soc Fr Ginecol 1962;5:30.

Lutjen P, Trounson A, Leeton J, et al: The establishment and maintenance of pregnancy using in-vitro fertilization and embryo donation in a patient with primary ovarian failure. Nature 1984;307:174.

Lydic ML, Liu JH, Rebar RW, et al: Success of donor oocyte in in-vitro fertilization-embryo transfer in recipients with and without premature ovarian failure. Fertil Steril 1996;65:98.

Maroulis GB: Effect of aging on fertility and pregnancy. Semin Reprod Endocrinol 1991;9:165.

Mastroyannis C: Gamete intrafallopian transfer: ethical considerations, historical development of the procedure, and comparison with other reproductive technologies. Fertil Steril 1993; 60:389.

Matson PL, Blackledge DG, Richardson PA, et al: Pregnancies after pronuclear stage transfer. Med J Aust 1987;146:60.

Meldrum D: GnRH agonists as adjuncts for in vitro fertilization. Obstet Gynecol Surv 1989;44:314.

Meldrum DR: Female reproductive aging—ovarian and uterine factors. Fertil Steril 1993;59:1.

Meldrum DR, Wisot A, Hamilton F, et al: Routine pituitary suppression with leuprolide before ovarian stimulation for oocyte retrieval. Fertil Steril 1989;51:455.

Miles RA, Paulson RJ, Lobo RA, et al: Pharmacokinetics and endometrial tissue levels of progesterone after administration by intramuscular and vaginal routes: a comparative study. Fertil Steril 1994;62:485.

Mosher W, Pratt W: Fecundity and Infertility in the United States, 1965–1988 (Advance Data from Vital and Health Statistics, No. 192). Hyattsville, MD: National Center for Health Statistics, 1990.

Muasher SJ: Treatment of low responders. J Assist Reprod Genet 1993;10:112.

Muasher SJ, Oehninger S, Simonetti S, et al: The value of basal and/or stimulated serum gonadotropin levels in prediction of stimulation response and in-vitro fertilization outcome. Fertil Steril 1988;50:298.

Muggleton-Harris AL, Glazier AM, Pickering S, Wall M: Genetic diagnosis using polymerase chain reaction and fluorescent in-situ hybridization analysis of biopsied cells from both the cleavage and blastocyst stages of individual cultured human preimplantation embryos. Hum Reprod 1995;10:183.

Munne S, Lee A, Rosenwaks Z, et al: Diagnosis of major chromosome aneuploidies in human preimplantation embryos. Hum Reprod 1993;8:2185.

Munne S, Sultan KM, Weier HU, et al: Assessment of numeric abnormalities of X, Y, 18, 16 chromosomes in preimplantation human embryos before transfer. Am J Obstet Gynecol 1995;172:1191.

Navot D, Bergh PA, Laufer N: Ovarian hyperstimulation syndrome in novel reproductive technologies: prevention and treatment. Fertil Steril 1992;58:249.

Navot D, Bergh PA, Williams M, et al: An insight into early reproductive processes through the in-vivo model of ovum donation. J Clin Endocrinol Metab 1991a;72:408.

Navot D, Drews MR, Bergh PA, et al: Age-related decline in female fertility is not due to diminished capacity of the uterus to sustain embryo implantation. Fertil Steril 1994;61:97.

Navot D, Laufer N, Kopolovic J, et al: Artificially induced endometrial cycles and establishment of pregnancies in the absence of ovaries. N Engl J Med 1986;314:806.

Navot D, Rosenwaks Z, Anderson F, Hodgen GD: Gonadotropin releasing hormone agonist-induced ovarian hyperstimulation: low dose side effects in women and monkeys. Fertil Steril 1991b;55:1069.

Navot D, Rosenwaks Z, Margalioth EJ: Prognostic assessment of female fecundity. Lancet 1987;2:645.

Neuman PJ, Gharib SD, Weinstein MC: The cost of a successful delivery with in vitro fertilization. New Engl J Med 1994;331:239.

Ng SC, Bongso A, Sathananthan AH, et al: Pregnancy after transfer of multiple sperm under the zona. Lancet 1988;2:790.

Olivennes F, Fanchin R, deZiegler D, Frydman R: "Poor responders": screening and treatment possibilities. J Assist Reprod Genet 1993;10:115.

Out HJ, Reimitz PE, Coelingh Bennink HJT: A prospective, randomized study to assess the tolerance and efficacy of intramuscular and subcutaneous administration of recombinant follicle-stimulating hormone (Puregon). Fertil Steril 1997;67:278.

Padilla SL, Bayati J, Garcia JE: Prognostic value of the early serum estradiol response to leuprolide acetate in in-vitro fertilization. Fertil Steril 1990;53:288.

Padilla SL, Dugan K, Maruwschak V, et al: Use of flare-up protocol with high dose human follicle stimulating hormone and human menopausal gonadotropins for in vitro fertilization in poor responders. Fertil Steril 1996;65:796.

Padilla SL, Smith RD, Garcia JE: The Lupron screening test: tailoring the use of leuprolide acetate in ovarian stimulation for in vitro fertilization. Fertil Steril 1991;56:79.

Palermo GD, Cohen J, Rosenwaks Z: Intracytoplasmic sperm injection: a powerful tool to overcome fertilization failure. Fertil Steril 1996a;65:899.

Palermo G, Colombero LT, Schattmen GL, et al: Evolution of pregnancies and initial follow-up of newborns delivered after intracytoplasmic sperm injection. JAMA 1996b;276:1893.

Palermo G, Joris H, Derde MP, et al: Sperm characteristics and outcome of human assisted fertilization by subzonal insemination and intracytoplasmic sperm injection. Fertil Steril 1993;59:826.

Palermo G, Joris H, Devroey P, Van Steirteghem AC: Pregnancies after intracytoplasmic injection of single spermatozoon into an oocyte. Lancet 1992;340:17.

Pantos K, Meimeti-Damianaki T, et al: Oocyte donation in menopausal women aged over 40 years. Hum Reprod 1993;8:488.

Paulson RJ, Marrs RP: Ovulation stimulation and monitoring for in vitro fertilization. Curr Probl Obstet Gynecol Fertil 1886;9:497.

Paulson RJ, Sauer MV, Francis MM, et al: Factors affecting pregnancy success in human in-vitro fertilization in unstimulated cycles. Hum Reprod 1994;9:1571.

Pearlstone AC, Fournet N, Gambone JC, et al: Ovulation induction in women age 40 and older: the importance of basal follicle-stimulating hormone level and chronological age. Fertil Steril 1992;58:674.

Penzias AL, Alper MM, Oskowitz SP, et al: Comparison of unilateral and bilateral tubal transfer in gamete intrafallopian transfer (GIFT). J In Vitro Fertil Embryo Transfer 1991;8:276.

Penzias AS, DeCherney AH: Is there ever a role for tubal surgery? Am J Obstet Gynecol 1996;174:1218.

Perone N: Gamete intrafallopian transfer: historic perspective. J In Vitro Fertil Embryo Transfer 1991;8:1.

Perone N: In vitro fertilization and embryo transfer, a historical perspective. J Reprod Med 1994;39:695.

Pool TB, Ellsworth LR, Garza JR, et al: Zygote intrafallopian transfer as a treatment for nontubal infertility: a 2-year study. Fertil Steril 1990;54:482.

Pryor JL, Kent-First M, Muallem A, et al: Microdeletions in the Y chromosome of infertile men. N Engl J Med 1997;336:534.

Quagliarello J: Safety of GnRH agonists: short-term side effects and cyst formation. Semin Reprod Endocrinol 1993;11:112.

Quigley M, Schmidt C, Beauchamp P, et al: Enhanced follicular recruitment in an in vitro fertilization program: clomiphene alone versus a clomiphene/human menopausal gonadotropin combination. Fertil Steril 1984;42:745.

Recombinant Human FSH Study Group: Clinical assessment of recombinant human follicle-stimulating hormone in stimulating ovarian follicular development before in vitro fertilization. Fertil Steril 1995;63:77.

Remohi J, Gutierrez A, Cano F, et al: Long oestradiol replacement in an oocyte donation programme. Hum Reprod 1995;10:1387.

Remohi J, Gutierrez A, Vidal A, et al: The use of gonadotrophin-releasing hormone analogues in women receiving oocyte donation does not affect implantation rates. Hum Reprod 1994;9:1761.

Reyes FI, Winter JSD, Faiman C: Pituitary-ovarian relationships preceding the menopause: a cross-sectional study of serum follicle-stimulating hormone, luteinizing hormone, prolactin, estradiol, and progesterone levels. Am J Obstet Gynecol 1997; 129:557.

Richardson SJ, Senikas V, Nelson JF: Follicular depletion during the menopausal transition: evidence for accelerated loss and ultimate exhaustion. J Clin Endocrinol Metab 1987;65:1231.

Riddick DH: AFS response to the possible association between ovulation inducing agents and ovarian cancer (memorandum sent by the American Fertility Society (AFS) to the AFS membership). Birmingham, AL: American Fertility Society, 1993.

Rock J, Menkin MF: In vitro fertilization and cleavage of human ovarian eggs. Science 1944;100:105.

Rogers P, Molloy D, Healy D, et al: Cross-over trial of superovulation protocols from two major in vitro fertilization centers. Fertil Steril 1986;46:424.

Sacks PC, Simon JA: Infectious complications of intrauterine insemination: a case report and literature review. Int J Fertil 1991; 36:331.

Saiki RK, Scharf S, Faloona F, et al: Enzymatic amplification of (β-globin genomic sequences and restriction site analysis for diagnosis of sickle cell anemia. Science 1985;230:1350.

Sauer MV, Miles RA, Dahmoush L, et al: Evaluating the effect of age on endometrial responsiveness to hormone replacement therapy: a histologic, ultrasonographic, and tissue receptor analysis. J Assist Reprod Genet 1993a;10:47.

Sauer MV, Paulson RJ, Ary BA, Lobo RA: Three hundred cycles of oocyte donation at the University of Southern California: assessing the effect of age and infertility diagnosis on pregnancy and implantation rates. J Assist Reprod Genet 1994;11: 92.

Sauer MV, Paulson RJ, Lobo RA: A preliminary report on oocyte donation extending reproductive potential to women over 40. N Engl J Med 1990;323:1157.

Sauer MV, Paulson RJ, Lobo RA: Pregnancy after age 50: application of oocyte donation to women after natural menopause. Lancet 1993b;341:321.

Schenker JG, Ezra Y: Complications of assisted reproductive techniques. Fertil Steril 1994;61:411.

Schoolcraft WB, Schlenker T, Gee M, et al: Assisted hatching in the treatment of poor prognosis in vitro fertilization candidates. Fertil Steril 1994;62:551.

Schoolcraft WB, Schlenker T, Gee M, et al: Improved controlled ovarian hyperstimulation in poor responder in vitro fertilization patients with a microdose follicle-stimulating hormone flare, growth hormone protocol. Fertil Steril 1997;67:93.

Schoysman R, Vanderzwalmen P, Nijs M, et al: Pregnancy after fertilization with human testicular spermatozoa. Lancet 1993; 342:1237.

Scott RT: Evaluation and treatment of low responders. Semin Reprod Endocrinol 1996;14:317.

Scott RT, Hofmann GE, Oehninger S, Muasher SJ: Intercycle variability of day 3 follicle-stimulating hormone levels and its effect on stimulation quality in in-vitro fertilization. Fertil Steril 1990;54:297.

Scott RT, Leonardi MR, Hofmann GE, et al: A prospective evaluation of clomiphene citrate challenge test screening of the general infertility population. Obstet Gynecol 1993;82:539.

Scott RT, Navot D: Enhancement of ovarian responsiveness with microdoses of gonadotropin-releasing hormone agonist during ovulation induction for in vitro fertilization. Fertil Steril 1994; 61:880.

Scott RT, Opsahl MS, Leonardi MR, et al: Life table analysis of pregnancy rates in a general infertility population relative to ovarian reserve and patient age. Hum Reprod 1995;10:1706.

Scott RT, Toner JP, Muasher SJ, et al: Follicle-stimulating hormone levels on cycle day 3 are predictive of in-vitro fertilization outcome. Fertil Steril 1989;51:651.

Seibel MM: Toward reducing risks and costs of egg donation: a preliminary report. Fertil Steril 1995;64:199.

Seifer DB, Lambert-Messerlian G, Hogan JW, et al: Day 3 serum inhibin-B is predictive of assisted reproductive technologies outcome. Fertil Steril 1997;67:110.

Serhal PF, Craft IL: Oocyte donation in 61 patients. Lancet 1989; 1:1185.

Settlage DS, Motoshima M, Tredway DR: Sperm transport from the external cervical os to the fallopian tubes in women: a time and quantitation study. Fertil Steril 1973;24:655.

Shapiro H, Cowell C, Casper RF: The use of vaginal ultrasound for monitoring endometrial preparation in a donor oocyte program. Fertil Steril 1993;59:1055.

Sharara FI, Beatse SN, Leonardi MR, et al: Cigarette smoking accelerates the development of diminished ovarian reserve as evidenced by the clomiphene citrate challenge test. Fertil Steril 1994;62:257.

Sher G, Salem R, Feinman M, et al: Eliminating the risk of life-endangering complications following overstimulation with menotropin fertility agents: a report on women undergoing in vitro fertilization and embryo transfer. Obstet Gynecol 1993;81: 1009.

Sher G, Zouves C, Feinman M, Maassarani G: "Prolonged coasting": an effective method for preventing severe ovarian hyperstimulation syndrome in patients undergoing in-vitro fertilization. Hum Reprod 1995;10:3107.

Sherman BM, Korenman SG: Hormonal characteristics of the human menstrual cycle throughout reproductive life. J Clin Invest 1975;55:699.

Sherman BM, West JH, Korenman SG: The menopausal transition: analysis of LH, FSH, estradiol, and progesterone concentrations during menstrual cycles of older women. J Clin Endocrinol Metab 1976;42:629.

Shoham Z, Patel A, Jacobs HS: Polycystic ovarian syndrome: safety and effectiveness of stepwise and low-dose administration of purified follicle-stimulating hormone. Fertil Steril 1991; 55:1051.

Simoni M, Gromoll J, Dworniczak B, et al: Screening for deletions of the Y chromosome involving the DAZ (Deleted in Azoospermia) gene in azoospermia and severe oligospermia. Fertil Steril 1997;67:542.

Smith EM, Anthony FW, Gadd SC, Masson GM: Trial of support treatment with human chorionic gonadotrophin in the luteal phase after treatment with buserelin and human menopausal gonadotrophin in women taking part in an in vitro fertilization programme. BMJ 1989;298:1482.

Smitz J, Camus M, Devroey P, et al: Incidence of severe ovarian hyperstimulation syndrome after gonadotrophin releasing hormone agonist/hMG superovulation for in-vitro fertilization. Hum Reprod 1990;5:933.

Smitz J, Devroey P, Braeckmans P, et al: Management of failed cycles in an IVF/GIFT programme with the combination of a GnRH analogue and HMG. Hum Reprod 1987;2:309.

Smitz J, Devroey P, Faguer B, et al: A prospective randomized comparison of intramuscular or intravaginal natural progesterone as a luteal phase and early pregnancy supplement. Hum Reprod 1992;7:168.

Society for Assisted Reproductive Technology and American Society for Reproductive Medicine: Assisted reproductive technology in the United States and Canada: 1994 results generated from the American Society for Reproductive Medicine/Society for Assisted Reproductive Technology Registry. Fertil Steril 1996;66:697.

Spirtas R, Kaufman SC, Alexander NJ: Fertility drugs and ovarian cancer: red alert or red herring? Fertil Steril 1993;59:291.

Stassart JP, Corfman RS, Ball GD: Continuation of a donor oocyte pregnancy in a functionally agonadal patient without early oestrogen support. Hum Reprod 1995;10:3061.

Steptoe PC, Edwards RG: Birth after the re-implantation of a human embryo. Lancet 1978;2:366.

Stewart GJ, Cunningham AL, Driscoll GL, et al: Transmission of human T-cell lymphotropic virus type III (HTLV-III) by artificial insemination by donor. Lancet 1985;2:581.

Stovall DW, Toma SK, Hammond MG, Talbert LM: The effect of age on female fecundity. Obstet Gynecol 1991;77:33.

Strohmer H, Feichtinger W: Successful clinical application of laser for micromanipulation in an in vitro fertilization program. Fertil Steril 1992;58:212.

Tan SL, Royston P, Campbell S, et al: Cumulative conception and livebirth rates after in-vitro fertilisation. Lancet 1992;339:1390.

Tanbo T, Abyholm T, Bjoro T, Dale PO: Ovarian stimulation in previous failures from in-vitro fertilization: distinction of two groups of poor responders. Hum Reprod 1990a;5:811.

Tanbo T, Dale PO, Abyholm T: Assisted fertilization in infertile women with patent fallopian tubes: a comparison of in vitro fertilization, gamete intrafallopian transfer and tubal embryo stage transfer. Hum Reprod 1990b;5:266.

Tanbo T, Dale PO, Abyholm T, Stokke KT: Follicle-stimulating hormone as a prognostic indicator in clomiphene citrate/human menopausal gonadotropin-stimulated cycles for in-vitro fertilization. Hum Reprod 1989;4:647.

Tarín JJ, Conaghan J, Winston RML, Handyside AH: Human embryo biopsy on the second day post insemination for preimplantation diagnosis: removal of a quarter embryo retards cleavage. Fertil Steril 1992;58:970.

Tarín JJ, Handyside AH: Embryo biopsy strategies for preimplantation diagnosis. Fertil Steril 1993;59:943.

Tesarik J, Mendoza C, Testart J: Viable embryos from injection of round spermatid into oocytes [letter]. N Engl J Med 1995;333:525.

Toner JP, Hodgen GD: The future of assisted reproductive technologies. In Marrs RP (ed): Assisted Reproductive Technologies. Boston: Blackwell Scientific Publications, 1993:218.

Toner JP, Philput CB, Jones GS, Muasher SJ: Basal follicle-stimulating hormone level is a better predictor of in-vitro fertilization performance than age. Fertil Steril 1991;55:784.

Tournaye H, Devroey P, Liu J, et al: Microsurgical epididymal sperm aspiration and intracytoplasmic sperm injection: a new effective approach to infertility as a result of congenital bilateral absence of the vas deferens. Fertil Steril 1994;61:1045.

Trounson A, Leeton J, Besanko M, et al: Pregnancy established in an infertile patient after transfer of a donated embryo fertilized in-vitro. BMJ 1983;286:835.

Trounson AO, Leeton JF, Wood C, et al: Pregnancies in humans by fertilization in vitro and embryo transfer in the controlled ovulatory cycle. Science 1981;212:681.

Tucker MJ, Cohen J, Massey JB, et al: Partial dissection of the zona pellucida of frozen-thawed human embryos may enhance blastocyst hatching, implantation, and pregnancy rates. Am J Obstet Gynecol 1991;165:341.

Urman B, Pride SM, Ho Yuen B: Management of overstimulated gonadotropin cycles with a controlled drift period. Hum Reprod 1992;7:213.

Van Dessel HJ, Doderwinkel PF, Coelingh-Bennink HJ, Fauser BC: First established pregnancy and birth after induction of ovulation with recombinant human follicle-stimulating hormone in polycystic ovary syndrome. Hum Reprod 1994;9:55.

Vargyas J, Morente C, Shangold G, Marrs R: The effect of different methods of ovarian stimulation for human in vitro fertilization and embryo replacement. Fertil Steril 1984;42:745.

Verlinsky Y, Ginberg N, Lifchez A, et al: Analysis of the first polar body: preconception genetic diagnosis. Hum Reprod 1990;5:826.

Verp MS: Genetic issues in artificial insemination by donor. Semin Reprod Endocrinol 1987;5:59.

Vickery BH, Nestor JJ: Luteinizing hormone-releasing hormone analogs: development and mechanism of action. Semin Reprod Endocrinol 1987;5:353.

Wasserman PM: Early events in mammalian fertilization. Annu Rev Cell Biol 1987;3:109.

Weckstein LN, Jacobson A, Galen D, et al: Improvement of pregnancy rates with oocyte donation in older recipients with the addition of progesterone vaginal suppositories. Fertil Steril 1993;60:573.

Winslow KL, Toner JP, Brzyski RG, et al: The gonadotropin-releasing hormone agonist stimulation test—a sensitive predictor of performance in the flare-up in-vitro fertilization cycle. Fertil Steril 1991;56:711.

Wolf DP, Byrd W, Dandekar P, Quigley MM: Sperm concentration and the fertilization of human eggs in vitro. Biol Reprod 1984;31:837.

Yaron Y, Amit A, Mani A, et al: Uterine preparation with estrogen for oocyte donation: assessing the effect of treatment duration on pregnancy rates. Fertil Steril 1995;63:1284.

Yates CA, Thomas C, Kovacs GT, de Kretser DM: Andrology, male factor infertility and IVF. In Wood C, Trounson AO (eds): Clinical In Vitro Fertilization. Berlin: Springer-Verlag, 1989:95.

Younis JS, Mordel N, Lewin A, et al: Artificial endometrial preparation for oocyte donation: the effect of estrogen stimulation on clinical outcome. J Assist Reprod Genet 1992;9:222.

Yovich JL, Blackledge DG, Richardson PA, et al: Pregnancies following pronuclear stage tubal transfer. Fertil Steril 1987;48:851.

Yovich JL, Stanger JD: The limitations of in vitro fertilization from male with severe oligospermia and abnormal sperm morphology. J In Vitro Fertil Embryo Transfer 1984;1:172.

Yovich JL, Yovich JM, Edirisinghe WR: The relative chance of pregnancy following tubal or uterine transfer procedures. Fertil Steril 1988;49:858.

18

Reproductive Toxicology

John F. Jarrell
Margaret Sevcik

There has been an enhanced awareness of the possible impact of drugs and environmental chemicals on human health in general and on reproductive function in particular (Schrader and Kanitz, 1994; Semenza et al, 1997; Cole et al, 1998; deKrester, 1998; Hansen et al, 1998). Examples stimulating this awareness of reproductive risk include the induction of sterility in men exposed to dibromochloropropane (Goldsmith, 1997), adverse effects on male fertility from occupational exposure to nitrous oxide (Buckley and Brodsky, 1988), reports of increased incidence of congenital malformations after environmental exposure to trichlorfon (Czeizel, 1996), and spontaneous abortion after occupational exposure of nurses to antineoplastic drugs (Gold and Tomich, 1994). In the case of occupational and environmental exposure, it is very difficult to establish causal relationships between a given exposure and reproductive outcome (Fishbein, 1992). A significant reduction in the sex ratio (fewer males) since 1970 has been reported in Canada and the United States; this observation requires evaluation from an environmental perspective (Allen et al, 1997; Davis et al, 1998). It is of interest that, coincident with the emergence of the environmental movement and a greater public awareness of issues, the new reproductive technologies are providing new and vital information regarding human procreation (Forti and Serio, 1993; Lee, 1994; Lipshultz, 1996). The use of in vitro fertilization (IVF) and embryo transfer technology as therapy (Hughes et al, 1990) and the hamster egg penetration test as diagnosis (Ahmadi et al, 1996) has opened the domain of the gonads and the embryo to innovative toxicologic assessment (Scialli, 1986, 1992; Winston et al, 1993; Hinch et al, 1997).

This chapter introduces the subspecialty of reproductive toxicology, which applies basic principles of toxicology to the medical specialty of obstetrics and gynecology.

GENERAL PRINCIPLES OF TOXICOLOGY

Toxicology is the qualitative and quantitative study of the injurious effects of chemical and physical agents on living systems. Injury to living systems can be loosely defined as alterations in structure or function that impair the physiology of the organism being studied. Although the changes may take place at the very basic level of cellular structure or function, toxicologists often measure outcomes that are far removed from the initial interaction of the chemical with the cells. The reason for this is that toxicologists are also interested in applying these findings to the evaluation of safety and prevention of injury to humans and to all useful forms of life (Hayes, 1989).

Toxicity can be defined by certain parameters, such as the nature of the injury (acute versus chronic; neurotoxic, carcinogenic, mutagenic, reproductive, or metabolic) and the duration of the injury (reversible or irreversible). In addition, the dose-response relationship, the spectrum of adverse effects, and the treatment and prevention of injury are critical components. The presence of a dose-response effect is the pillar of toxicology. Paracelsus as early as 1567 recognized that the only difference between a therapeutic agent and a poison was the amount administered. Simply defined, *dose-response* is the graded response of an individual to increases in the amount of an agent applied (Hayes, 1989).

Response of an individual is dependent on variables such as age, sex, and, more recently, genetic predispositions for sensitivity or resistance to different chemicals, as well as dose and route of exposure. Information about dose and exposure is rarely available for human populations, especially in cases of accidental poisoning or environmental contamination. Interindividual differences and calculating dosages received make the job of the toxicologist especially challenging to generalize results to the general population.

The difficulty of knowing the actual dose a population has received is compounded by the problem of knowing what relevent reproductive outcomes should be used to assess toxicity. Although there may be an abundance of end points well known to any clinician involved with reproductive care, reproductive toxicologists still debate valid markers of toxicity (Williams et al, 1990; Mattison, 1991; Fowle JR III and Sexton, 1992; Lasley et al, 1993; Mattison,

1993; Weinberg et al, 1993; Weinberg and Zhou, 1997; Kriek et al, 1998; Lasley and Overstreet, 1998). This is discussed in greater detail in the section "Biomarkers and Toxicity Testing for the Clinician."

MECHANISM OF TOXICITY

Just as in pharmacology, where an understanding of the drug effect is critical to the use of a particular drug, the mechanism of toxicity of reproductive toxicants is similarly important. By understanding the mechanism by which a chemical exerts an effect, one is better able to predict the possible outcomes on human health, especially when mechanisms are determined in experimental models. Mattison (1983a, 1983b) has provided an excellent template to describe the mechanism of action of reproductive toxicants. According to Mattison, one can think of toxins as being either direct-acting or non-direct-acting on reproductive systems.

Direct-Acting Toxins

Toxicants that function by means of structural similarity to an endogenous chemical signal (agonists and antagonists) or by chemical reactivity are considered direct-acting toxins. An example of this would be the exogenous steroids such as diethylstilbestrol (Golden et al, 1998; Pennie et al, 1998; Shiau et al, 1998), oral contraceptives (Pennie et al, 1998), and cimetidine (Schmidt et al, 1990). The importance of the total burden of estrogens, both naturally occurring and excreted from women taking synthetic estrogen and progesterone replacement therapy, has been stressed (Rall and McLachlan, 1980; Wide, 1980). Nonsteroidal agents that act via receptor interaction include polycyclic aromatic hydrocarbons (PAHs) (Foster et al, 1993; Wolff and Landrigan, 1994; Sonnenschein and Soto, 1998; Toppari and Skakkebaek, 1998). Direct action of toxicants can also occur via intrinsic chemical reactivity or inherent chemical activity, such as that seen with the effects of certain alkylating agents (Kumar et al, 1972) and ionizing radiation (Mandl, 1961). These agents have direct effects on information macromolecules of the cells (DNA), which are essential for cellular survival. As radiation passes through the tissues and oxidizes intracellular water, free radical species of oxygen are produced, ultimately inducing peroxidation of tissues and the destruction of cells (Dobson and Felton, 1983, Mettler and Moseley, 1985; Jarrell et al, 1987).

Metabolic activation, which controls the development of indirect toxic damage to the cells, is critical to the understanding of drug effect in the mammalian system (Sipes and Gandolfi, 1991). Most drugs or chemicals that enter the body are lipid soluble so that they readily pass through biologic membranes. In the absence of any alteration in the structure of the drug, they tend to persist in a fatty environment.

There are two major paths for the alteration of the drug's structure and facilitation of excretion. *Phase I reactions* include the processes of oxidation, reduction, and hydrolysis. The enzymes involved in these reactions include primarily the cytochrome P_{450} enzymes, but in addition amine oxidase, epoxide hydrolase, alcohol, aldehyde, and ketone oxidation and reduction processes are present. *Phase II reactions* are energy dependent because they are biosynthetic and result in covalent bonding of some form to the drug in a conjugation reaction. These processes confer aqueous solubility and ionization at physiologic pH, thereby potentiating excretion. When a xenobiotic (foreign chemical) enters the body and undergoes phase I metabolic activation, it is essential for the phase II "detoxification" enzymes to conjugate the metabolite for safe excretion. Overloading of either of these two systems results in the toxicity that a chemical exerts.

Although biotransformation can result in the elimination of certain drugs and chemicals, it is also responsible for the activation and augmentation of certain toxicants. The reactive intermediates can be toxic by virtue of the extent of production of metabolites that are capable of combining with certain cellular targets; they may deplete glutathione and they may saturate major pathways for detoxification so that minor pathways become functional. It has been suggested that the relative sensitivity of certain target tissues may be a function of their ability to activate a toxicant within an organ compartment.

Although biotransformation occurs predominantly in the liver, lesser degrees of activity are found in such varied tissues as the intestines, kidney, lung, gonads, and skin. The process of biotransformation within the gonads is a particularly interesting concept because transformation within certain compartments of the ovary may result in the delivery of an activated species to an ovarian target that would not occur if the process depended exclusively on hepatic effects (activated species are short lived and have local effects from the point of biotransformation). The recognition of the ovary as an important site of drug activation and detoxification has only begun to be appreciated by toxicologists (Bengtsson and Rydstrom, 1983; Djuric et al, 1990; Jarrell et al, 1992; Todoroff et al, 1998).

Indirect-Acting Toxins

Indirect-acting reproductive toxins are those that act by altering the metabolism of drugs via induction or inhibition of enzymes essential in these processes (Marks et al, 1982). Halogenated hydrocarbons induce cytochrome P_{450} activity which is subsequently involved in chemical activation. Exposure to these compounds produces not only a primary effect but also a secondary effect by inducing the genetic expression of other enzymes that influence future response to chemical assaults. Enzyme induction is not limited to xenobiotic-metabolizing enzymes. There is also evidence that enzymes important for steroidogenesis can be regulated in this manner. In a sense, then, indirect-acting toxins can have a direct effect on reproduction (Safe et al, 1991; Balaguer et al, 1996).

BIOMARKERS AND TOXICITY TESTING FOR THE CLINICIAN

There has been a trend to enhance the role of the obstetrician-gynecologist in the measurement of important markers of health effects resulting from priority chemicals. This has developed because of the access to such relevant tissues as placentaes, semen, granulosa cells, and oocytes with the advent of the new assisted reproductive technologies. Because the intrinsic nature of the specialty has been to study the causes and the treatments of reproductive loss, it has become a matter of combining these data with exposure data to develop circumstantial evidence for reproductive toxicants. In recent years, more rigorous attention has been paid to the methodologic assessment of these data, and the quality of evidence regarding chemical exposure and reproductive effects has improved (Schrader, 1992; Lasley et al, 1993).

One way to assess the effects of chemical exposures on human health and reproduction has been through the identification of relevant biomarkers (Mattison, 1989; Mattison, 1991; Fowle and Sexton, 1992; Mattison, 1993; Lasley and Overstreet, 1998). Biomarkers are defined as indicators signaling events in biologic systems or samples. They can be classified as those that measure exposure, effect, or susceptibility. Exposure biomarkers estimate the amount to which an organism is exposed rather than the dose that has been administered. Even when we know how much of a chemical has entered the environment (for instance, if there is a well-documented chemical spill), the dose of chemical that the indivdual may receive is often different. In this case, a credible exposure biomarker tells us not only the dose the individual receives but also the bioavailability of that chemical. Bioavailability is an important concept to regulators, who need to know how much chemical an organism can be exposed to before the levels become toxic to the organism. It also suggests how readily environmental contaminants become biologic contaminants.

A biomarker of effect predicts the probability and severity of an important health effect with a given dose or exposure. A biomarker of susceptibility classifies individuals on the basis of certain factors that are more likely to demonstrate an adverse outcome after exposure compared to a control population. These factors may include sex, age, geographic distribution, and genetic makeup. More recently, attention has been given to genetic predispositions for susceptibility because the acceptance and spread of

new molecular techniques has made this more easy to study.

From a clinical perspective, the diagnostic test assessment of an individual patient or a clinical trial is generally directed to effects or adverse health outcomes. These can be categorized as (1) mechanistic, (2) descriptive, or (3) surveillance. Any single test can be useful in more than one category. For example, the measurement of serum follicle-stimulating hormone (FSH) is used to establish that an agent has caused damage to the Sertoli cell (mechanistic); that it has interfered with the inhibin control of homeostatic levels of FSH (descriptor of pathophysiology); and that, in a large group of workers exposed to this agent, there is a high frequency of elevated FSH levels (surveillance). Virtually any test can be used in the estimation of effect, and the acceptance from a toxicity point of view depends on the specific need, cost, and utility.

The use of biomarkers for the determination of either exposure or susceptibility is a more recent trend. The availability of serum, follicular fluid, and semen from patients undergoing IVF provides important sources of tissues for the measurement of trace amounts of such priority chemicals as polychlorinated biphenyls (PCBs) and pesticides (Jarrell et al, 1993b). The availability of certain complementary DNA (cDNA) probes has allowed investigators to begin to assess genotype susceptibility; in addition, these probes can be used as exposure biomarkers (Gonzalez et al, 1991; Stegeman and Lech, 1991; Rumsby et al, 1996; Abbot et al, 1999; Mahajan and Rifkind, 1999; Walker et al, 1999).

Tables 18–1 and 18–2 highlight biomarkers for reproduction that are primarily used to measure chemical effects (effect biomarkers). There is a true need to merge the technologies of priority chemical health effects and analytic methodology to establish the markers of exposure and susceptibility.

A critical concept in biomarker acceptance relates to how reproductive end points reflect alterations in the normal physiology of the organism. The caveat of biomarkers, then, is grounded in the reality that, to know what is adverse, one needs to know what

Table 18–1. BIOMARKERS FOR MALE REPRODUCTIVE TOXICOLOGY

BIOMARKERS OF PHYSIOLOGIC DAMAGE
Hamster egg penetration with human sperm
Monoclonal antibodies to specific sperm sites
Computer-assisted semen analysis
cDNA probes in reproductive tissues
Epididymal function tests
Sertoli cell function tests
Measures of testicular stem cells
Comparative animal and human germ cell exposures

BIOMARKERS OF GENETIC DAMAGE
Chromosomal studies of spermatozoa
DNA adduct and marker studies of spermatozoa
Mechanisms of the induction of hereditable mutations in
  experimental animals

Table 18-2. BIOMARKERS FOR FEMALE REPRODUCTIVE TOXICITY

BIOMARKERS OF GERM CELL DAMAGE

The relationship of oocyte cytogenetics, follicular fluid, serum, and tissue contamination with priority chemicals

Oocyte chromosomal studies (oocytes that fail to cleave during IVF)

Measures of oocyte aneuploidy

DNA adduct and probe studies of granulosa cells and oocytes

BIOMARKERS OF DEVELOPMENT AND AGING

Specificity of sexual development

Menarche evaluation

Age-related menstrual changes

Loss of gonadal stem cells

Measures of hypothalamic and central nervous system function

BIOMARKERS OF CYCLIC OVARIAN FUNCTION

Available markers of ovulation (salivary and urinary steroids)

Measures of specific characteristics of menstrual function

Preimplantation endometrial tissue studies

Development of ovarian perfusion for toxicity assessment

BIOMARKERS OF EARLY EMBRYONIC DEVELOPMENT

Measures of tubal motility

Practical human chorionic gonadotropin assays

Preimplantation markers of embryonic health

IVF outcomes under the influence of priority exposures

Genetic assessment of the preimplantation embryo

---

is the norm. In this respect, continued efforts at understanding the reproductive physiology of humans and the model systems we use to test priority chemicals are essential to validate these markers. Several excellent resources on the assessment of reproductive effects are available, and the reader is referred to these (Mattison, 1989, 1991; Mattison et al, 1990; Lasley and Shidler, 1994; Moore et al, 1995; Williams et al, 1995a, 1995b; Weijin and Olsen, 1996).

Understanding how normal reproductive physiology is influenced by chemical perturbation is a complicated process because we now know that the ovary (for example) is not a passive player in the outcome of events. In fact, there is good evidence to suggest that the processes that regulate the normal function of the ovary are also capable of the modification of those processes that relate to toxic effects. For example, in mice, a specific female dominant lethal effect is present when the females are treated in the periovulatory period (Generoso et al, 1987; Katoh et al, 1989). This suggestion of periovulatory vulnerability is supported by the observation that there is induction of ovarian aryl hydrocarbon hydroxylase during the estrous part of the cycle in rats, and the enzyme that is capable of the activation of benzo(*a*)pyrene is further stimulated with gonadotropin (Jarrell et al, 1992; Aten et al, 1992). When we consider for a moment the known risk factors for ovarian cancer—incessant ovulation and the postmenopausal state—these observations take on added significance (Heintz et al, 1985; Alper et al, 1986).

ENVIRONMENTAL CONSIDERATIONS

There is an important parallel between the handling of chemicals in the body and in the environment. Just as these agents are subjected to the processes of exposure, uptake, bioavailability, biotransformation, storage in fat depots, and elimination in the body, these same chemicals undergo important processes in the environment (Carey et al, 1987). Human health regulators and environmental monitoring agencies are concerned with the growing evidence of widespread contamination of the environment with persistent potentially toxic chemicals (Christenson, 1998; Foster, 1998; Klotz, 1999; Sheehan et al, 1999). Perhaps another characteristic of many of these chemicals is that their reproductive effects are poorly understood if at all investigated. More recent developments in the reporting of such factors as abortion rates, congenital abnormalities, and sex ratios associated with exposure data suggest that these contaminants have adverse reproductive effects.

An example of why we should consider the toxicology of the individual and the environment in the same manner is the chlorinated organic chemical hexachlorobenzene (HCB). Although this chemical was banned in the 1970s and was responsible for an important poisoning in Turkey during the 1950s (Dogramaci, 1962; Peters et al, 1987), production of the chemical continues as a result of by-product formation during the industrial manufacturing of pentachlorophenol and other chlorinated chemicals (Courtney, 1979). Various studies have shown that serum and fat levels of HCB in humans vary according to occupational exposure and geographic distribution (Newsome et al, 1995; Liljegren et al, 1998; Schecter et al, 1998). HCB is relatively stable without substantial metabolism and is persistent in both sediments and fatty tissues owing to its lipid solubility. HCB has been isolated in various bodies of water, including the Great Lakes, as well as the birds and fish that inhabit these areas (Frank et al, 1978; Niimi, 1979; Weseloh et al, 1990; Rostad et al, 1999). Again because of the lipid solubility, HCB undergoes an important process of biomagnification. As one ascends the food chain, there is a tendency for a greater accumulation of HCB in fat deposits (Bro-Rasmussen, 1996). This is a consequence of the greater intake and life span of the larger species. HCB has been isolated by autoradiography in the ovarian tissues of a number of species, including fish and birds (Allen-Gil et al, 1997). These findings take on more significance with the observation that HCB (in addition to PCBs and dichlorophenyltrichloroethane, or DDT) is isolated with some frequency from the ovarian follicles of women undergoing IVF in Germany, Austria, and various areas in Canada (Trapp et al, 1984; Schlebusch et al, 1989; Jarrell et al, 1993c).

Although these findings indicate contamination and not necessarily toxicity, the observations of Iatropoulous et al (1976) indicate that HCB affects the health of the ovary of the rhesus monkey in a number of ways, including a reduction in the number of primordial follicles. Reports indicate that a similar effect can be identified in cynomologous monkeys, and the degree of damage appears to be consistent with the concentration of HCB in the serum and total absorbed dose (Jarrell et al, 1993a). An important consideration of this study by Jarrell et al is that ovotoxicity was demonstrated at doses that were well below those that cause characteristic HCB-induced porphyria. A 45-year follow-up of women exposed to HCB as children found a positive relationship between serum HCB levels and lifetime risk of spontaneous abortion (Jarrell et al, 1998).

In animal models the administration of HCB can be associated with damage to the structure of the ovary (Singh et al, 1990; Sims et al, 1991), relationship of the trace amounts in the follicular fluid to oocyte destruction is uncertain. These observations point to a need to explore the intraovarian compartmental relationships to a greater degree, particularly in response to the factors that regulate the distribution and biologic effects of this chemical. There is now an abundance of literature to suggest that the effects of HCB toxicity are enhanced by ovarian hormones and that toxicity is greater in the females of species studied than in the males (Pereira et al, 1982; Rizzardini and Smith, 1982; To-Figueras et al, 1991; D'Amour et al, 1992). Although the mechanisms of HCB toxicity are still to be elucidated, there is good evidence to suggest that the sex difference in toxicity to HCB might be related to iron turnover or factors that regulate glutathione, an important substrate for phase II conjugation reactions with HCB (Hershko and Eilon, 1974; Igarashi et al, 1983; Uhlig and Wendel, 1992).

The PAHs are similar to HCB as far as their environmental characteristics are concerned. They are persistent, ubiquitous contaminants of the environment that are turning up in bodily fluids and tissues of animals, avian species, and human beings with frightening regularity (Menichini, 1992; Lodovici et al, 1995; Branisteanu and Aiking, 1998). Examples of PAHs include the PCB congeners, 2,3,7,8-tetrachloro-p-dioxin (dioxin), and dioxin-like compounds. These chemicals are exogenous ligands for a critical intracellular receptor found in most cells and species, the aryl hydrocarbon hydroxylase, or Ah, receptor. The Ah receptor has been extensively studied for its role in induction of important drug-metabolizing enzymes, most notably members of the cytochrome P_{450} family, $CYP1A1$. The Ah receptor also induces phase II enzymes, so it is an important mediator in the balance of activation and detoxification of xenobiotics (Gonzalez, 1990; Nebert et al, 1993; Bock, 1994).

Studies on the Ah receptor and PAHs have also established the role of the hormonal milieu in resulting toxicity of these chemicals. Co-administration of estrogen with dioxin results in greater toxicity, suggesting that endocrine factors are important determinants of toxicity of these chemicals (Wang et al, 1998). Ah receptor activity of the ovary has been well established and, to date, the location, ontogeny, and function of the ovarian Ah receptor has remained elusive in spite of its suspected role in ovarian toxicity or mediation from PAHs (Bengtsson et al, 1987; Silbergeld and Mattison, 1987).

The corollary approach is to link adverse outcomes to certain chemicals. Evaluation of the human sex ratio could be considered an example of this approach (James, 1998, 1999; Rogan et al, 1999). The report of reductions in sex ratio in Canada and the United States since 1970 is raising the need to evaluate this biomarker from an environmental perspective (Allen et al, 1997; Davis, 1998). It is known that the sex ratio is a sensitive biomarker for effect of a chemical or adverse event (James, 1997a, 1998b; Michalek et al, 1998). There are several studies linking changes in the sex ratio to occupational or environmental chemical exposures (Whorton et al, 1994; James, 1996, 1997a, 1997b) and drug treatments, as in the case of ovulation induction drugs such as clomiphene citrate (Dickey et al, 1995; James, 1995). Hypotheses abound regarding the influence of environment on the sex ratio, and chemicals such as clomiphene citrate and dioxin (with antiestrogenic effects) could alter the hormonal milieu during critical periods in embryo sex selection (Fischer, 1990). The relationship of the environment to sex ratio is not confirmed, but ovulation induction drugs may be a model system for studying this process of sex selection in our species (Williams et al, 1995a, 1995b; Weijin and Olsen, 1996).

APPLIED REPRODUCTIVE TOXICOLOGY

To this point, reproductive toxicology has not provided a substantial basis for clinical intervention, and the emphasis has been mechanistic in approach. This is because of the uncertainties experienced when one is confronted with the most concrete applications of the principles of reproductive toxicology, that of the human subject soon to be exposed to and rendered sterile from radiation and chemotherapy. Despite several experiments in animals, there is no conclusive evidence that the gonads can be protected from these agents by any form of pharmacologic therapy, including oral contraceptives or agonists of gonadotropin-releasing hormone (Ataya et al, 1985; Jarrell et al, 1987, 1991). In the absence of a clear therapeutic maneuver, it is possible that the most effective option that individuals have at their disposal is the use of the new assisted reproductive technologies, which include the use of donor sperm, semen cryopreservation, oocyte donation, and embryo cryopreservation (Sauer and Paulson, 1984; Meldrum et al, 1989; Levran et al, 1990; Meistrich, 1993). It is evident that the availability of these treatments is still not generally appreciated. This may be a function of the severity of the primary illness, but it may also reflect the lack of discussion of options with the patient at the time of therapy in the presence of some of the most toxic compounds ever produced by humans (Ataya et al, 1989).

REFERENCES

Abbott BD, Schmid JE, Brown JG, et al: RT-PCR quantification of AHR, ARNT, GR and CYP1A1 mRNA in craniofacial tissues of embryonic mice exposed to 2,3,7,8-tetrachlorodibenzo-p-dioxin and hydrocortisone. Toxicol Sci 1999;47:76.

Ahmadi A, Bongso A, Ng SC: Intracytoplasmic injection of human sperm into the hamster oocyte (hamster ICSI assay) as a test for fertilizing capacity of the severe male-factor sperm. J Assist Reprod Genet 1996;13:647.

Allen BB, Brant R, Seidel JE, Jarrell JF: Declining sex ratios in Canada. Can Med Assoc J 1997;156:37.

Allen-Gil SM, Gubala CP, Wilson R, et al: Organochlorine pesticides and polychlorinated biphenyls (PCBs) in sediments and biota from four US Arctic lakes. Arch Environ Contam Toxicol 1997;33:378.

Alper MM, Garner PR, Seibel MM: Premature ovarian failure. J Reprod Med 1986;31:699.

Ataya KM, McKanna JA, Weintraub AM, et al: A luteinizing hormone-releasing hormone agonist for the prevention of chemotherapy-induced ovarian follicular loss in rats. Cancer Res 1985;45:3651.

Aten RF, Duarte KM, Behrman HR: Regulation of ovarian antioxidant vitamins, reduced glutathione, and lipid peroxidation by luteinizing hormone and prostaglandin $F_{2\alpha}$. Biol Reprod 1992;46:401.

Balaguer P, Joyeux A, Denison MS, et al: Assessing the estrogenic and dioxin-like activities of chemicals and complex mixtures using in vitro recombinant receptor-reporter gene assays. Can J Physiol Pharmacol 1996;74:216.

Bengtsson M, Rydstrom J: Regulation of carcinogen metabolism in the rat ovary by the estrous cycle and gonadotropin. Science 1983;219:1437.

Bengtsson M, Dong Y, Mattison DR, Rydstrom J: Mechanisms of regulation of rat ovarian 7,12-dimethylbenz[a]anthracene hydroxylase. Chem Biol Interact 1987;63:15.

Bock KW: Aryl hydrocarbon or dioxin receptor: biologic and toxic responses. Rev Physiol Biochem Pharmacol 1994;125:1.

Branisteanu R, Aiking H: Exposure to polycyclic aromatic hydrocarbons in occupational versus urban environmental air. Int Arch Occup Environ Health 1998;71:533.

Bro-Rasmussen F: Contamination by persistent chemicals in food chain and human health. Sci Total Environ 1996;188 Suppl 1:S45.

Buckley DN, Brodsky JB: Nitrous oxide and male fertility. Reprod Toxicol 1988;1:93.

Carey AE, Dixon TE, Yang HSC: Environmental exposure to hexachlorobenzene in the USA. In Morris CR, Cobral JRP (eds): Hexachlorobenzene—Proceedings of an International Symposium. Lyon: IARC Scientific Publications, No. 77, 1987:115.

Christensen FM: Pharmaceuticals in the environment—a human risk? Regul Toxicol Pharmacol 1998;28:212.

Cole DC, Eyles J, Gibson BL: Indicators of human health in ecosystems: what do we measure? Sci Total Environ 1998;224:201.

Courtney KD: Hexachlorobenzene (HCB): a review. Environ Res 1979;20:255.

Czeizel AE: Human germinal mutagenic effects in relation to intentional and accidental exposure to toxic agents. Environ Health Perspect 1996;104 Suppl 3:615.

D'Amour M, Charbonneau M: Sex-related difference in hepatic glutathione conjugation of hexachlorobenzene in the rat. Toxicol Appl Pharmacol 1992;112:229.

Davis DL, Gottlieb MB, Stampnitzky JR: Reduced ratio of male to female births in several industrial countries: a sentinel health indicator? JAMA 1998;279:1018.

DeKrester DM: Are sperm counts really falling? Reprod Fertil Dev 1998;10:93.

Dickey RP, Taylor SN, Curole DN, Rye PH: Infant sex ratio after hormonal ovulation induction. Hum Reprod 1995;10:2465.

Djuric Z, Maviya VK, Deppe G, et al: Detoxifying enzymes in human ovarian tissues: comparison of normal and tumor tissues and effects of chemotherapy. J Cancer Res Clin Oncol 1990;116:379.

Dobson RL, Felton JS: Female germ cell loss from radiation and chemical exposures. Am J Indust Med 1983;4:175.

Dogramci I: Porphyria turcica. Turk J Pediatr 1962;4:129.

Fishbein L: Exposure from occupational versus other sources. Scand J Work Environ Health 1992;18(Suppl 1):5.

Fischer K: A rapid evolution mechanism may contribute to changes in sex ratio, multiple birth incidence, frequency of auto-immune disease and frequency of birth defects in Clomid conceptions. Med Hypotheses 1990;31:59.

Forti G, Serio M: Male infertility: is its rising incidence due to better methods of detection or an increasing frequency? Hum Reprod 1993;8:1153.

Foster WG: Endocrine disruptors and development of the reproductive system in the fetus and children: is there cause for concern? Can J Public Health 1998;89 Suppl 1:S52.

Foster WG, Pentick JA, McMahon A, Lecavalier PR: Body distribution and endocrine toxicity of hexachlorobenzene (HCB) in the female rat. J Appl Toxicol 1993;13:79.

Fowle JR, Sexton K: EPA priorities for biologic makers research in environmental health. Environ Health Perspect 1992;98:235.

Frank R, Braun HE, Holdrinet M, et al: Residues of organochlorine insecticides and polychlorinated biphenyls from Lakes Saint Clair and Erie, Canada—1968–76. Pestic Monit J 1978;12:69.

Generoso WM, Rutledge JC, Cain KT, et al: Exposure of female mice to ethylene oxide within hours of mating leads to fetal malformation and death. Mutat Res 1987;176:269.

Gold EB, Tomich E: Occupational hazards to fertility and pregnancy outcome. Occup Med 1994;3:435.

Golden RJ, Noller KL, Titus-Ernstoff L, et al: Environmental endocrine modulators and human health: an assessment of the biological evidence. Crit Rev Toxicol 1998;28:109.

Goldsmith JR: Dibromochloropropane: epidemiological findings and current questions. Ann N Y Acad Sci 1997;837:300.

Gonzalez FJ: Molecular genetics of the P_{450} superfamily. Pharmacol Ther 1990;45:1.

Gonzalez FJ, Crespi CL, Gelboin HV: cDNA-expressed human cytochrome P_{450}'s: a new age of molecular toxicology and human risk assessment. Mutat Res 1991;247:113.

Hansen H, De Rosa CT, Pohl H, et al: Public health challenges posed by chemical mixtures. Environ Health Perspect 1998;106 Suppl 6:1271.

Hayes WJ: General principles. In Wayland J, Hayes JR, Laws ER Jr (eds): Handbook of Pesticide Toxicology. New York: Academic Press, 1989:1.

Heintz APM, Hacker NF, Lagasse LD: Epidemiology and etiology of ovarian cancer: an overview. Obstet Gynecol 1985;66:127.

Hershko HC, Eilon L: The effect of sex difference on iron exchange in the rat. Br J Haematol 1974;28:471.

Hinsch E, Ponce AA, Hagele W, et al: A new combined in-vitro test model for the identification of substances affecting essential sperm functions. Hum Reprod 1997;12:1673.

Hughes SF, Haney AF, Hughes CL Jr: Use of human cumulus granulosa cells for in vitro screening of reproductive toxicants. Reprod Toxicol 1990;4:11.

Iatropoulos MJ, Hobson F, Knauf V, Adams HP: Morphological effects of hexachlorobenzene toxicity in female rhesus monkeys. Toxicol Appl Pharmacol 1976;37:433.

Igarashi T, Satoh T, Ueno K, Kitagawa H: Sex-related difference in the hepatic glutathione level and related enzyme activities in rat. J Biochem 1983;93:33.

James WH: Clomiphene citrate, gonadotrophin and sex ratio of offspring. Hum Reprod 1995;10:2465.

James WH: Reproductive effects of male dioxin exposure. The use of offspring sex ratios to detect reproductive effects of male exposure to dioxins. Environ Health Perspect 1997a;105:162.

James WH: The sex ratio of offspring sired by men exposed to wood preservatives contaminated with dioxin. Scand J Work Environ Health 1996;22:267.

James WH: Paternal lead exposure, offspring birth weight, and sex ratio. Am J Ind Med 1997b;32:315.

James WH: Sex ratio of offspring of residents of a highly polluted housing site. Scand J Work Environ Health 1998b;24:74.

James WH: Re: the use of offspring sex ratios in the search for endocrine disruptors. Environ Health Perspect 1998a;106:A472.

James WH: Re: Male pesticide exposure and pregnancy outcome. Am J Epidemiol 1999;149:290.

Jarrell JF, McMahon A, Barr RD, YoungLai EV: The agonist (d-leu-6,des-gly-10)-LHRH ethylamide does not protect the fecundity of rats exposed to high dose unilateral ovarian irradiation. Reprod Toxicol 1991;5:385.

Jarrell JF, McMahon A, Villeneuve D, et al: Hexachlorobenzene toxicity in the monkey primordial germ cell without induced porphyria. Reprod Toxicol 1993a;7:41.

Jarrell JF, Sevcik M, Stuart G: Regulation of total ovarian glutathione content in the rat. Reprod Toxicol 1992;6:133.

Jarrell JF, Villeneuve D, Franklin C, et al: Contamination of human ovarian follicular fluid and serum by chlorinated organic compounds in three Canadian cities. Can Med Assoc J 1993c; 148:1321.

Jarrell JF, YoungLai EV, McMahon A, et al: Effects of ionizing radiation and pretreatment with (d-leu-6,des-gly-10) luteinizing hormone-releasing hormone ethylamide on developing rat ovarian follicles. Cancer Res 1987;47:5005.

Jarrell J, Gocmen A, Foster W, et al: Evaluation of reproductive outcomes in women inadvertently exposed to hexachlorobenzene in southeastern Turkey in the 1950's. Reprod Toxicol 1998; 12:469.

Katoh M, Cacheiro NL, Cornett CV, et al: Fetal anomalies produced subsequent to treatment of zygotes with ethylene oxide or ethyl methanesulfonate are not likely due to the usual genetic causes. Mutat Res 1989;210:337.

Klotz LH: Why is the rate of testicular cancer increasing. CMAJ 1999;160:213.

Kriek E, Rojas M, Alexandrov K, Bartsch H: Polycyclic aromatic hydrocarbon-DNA adducts in humans: relevance as biomarkers for exposure and cancer risk. Mutat Res 1998;400:215.

Kumar R, Biggart JD, McEvoy J, McGeown MG: Cyclophosphamide and reproductive function. Lancet 1972;1:1212.

Lasley BL, Gold EB, Nakajima ST, et al: Classification of adverse reproductive effects can be improved by measurements of multiple biomarkers for ovarian toxicity and early fetal loss. J Toxicol Environ Health 1993;40:423.

Lasley BL, Shidler SE: Methods for evaluating reproductive health of women. Occup Med 1994;9:3.

Lasley BL, Overstreet JW: Biomarkers for assessing human female reproductive health, an interdisciplinary approach. Environ Health Perspect 1998;106 Suppl 4:955.

Lee S: Male infertility. Lancet 1994;344:415.

Levran E, Dor J, Rudak E, et al: Pregnancy potential of human oocytes: the effect of cryopreservation. N Engl J Med 1990;323: 1153.

Liljegren G, Hardell L, Lindstrom G, et al: Case-control study on breast cancer and adipose tissue concentrations of congener specific polychlorinated biphenyls, DDE and hexachlorobenzene. Eur J Cancer Prev 1998;7:135.

Lipschultz LI: "The debate continues"—the continuing debate over the possible decline in semen quality. Fertil Steril 1996;65: 909.

Lodovici M, Dolara P, Casalini C, et al: Polycyclic aromatic hydrocarbon contamination in the Italian diet. Food Addit Contam 1995;12:703.

Mahajan SS, Rifkind AB: Transcriptional activation of avian CYP1A4 and CYP1A5 by 2,3,7,8-tetrachlorodibenzo-p-dioxin: differences in gene expression and regulation compared to mammalian CYP1A1 and CYP1A2. Toxicol Appl Pharmacol 1999;155:96.

Mandl AM: The radiosensitivity of germ cells. Biol Rev 1961;39: 288.

Marks GS, Zelt DT, Cole SP: Alterations in the heme biosynthetic pathways as an index of exposure to toxins. Can J Physiol Pharmacol 1982;60:1017.

Mattison DR: The mechanisms of action of reproductive toxins. Am J Indust Med 1983a;4:65.

Mattison DR: The mechanism of action of reproductive toxins. In Mattison DR (ed): Reproductive Toxicology. New York: Alan R. Liss, 1983b;149.

Mattison DR: Biologic Markers in Reproductive Toxicology. Washington, DC: National Academy Press, 1989:6.

Mattison DR: An overview of biological markers in reproductive and developmental toxicology: concepts, definitions and use in risk assessment. Biomed Environ Sci 1991;4:8.

Mattison DR, Plowchalk DR, Meadows MJ, et al: Reproductive toxicity: male and female reproductive systems as targets for chemical injury. Environ Med 1990;74:391.

Mattison DR: Sites of female reproductive vulnerability: implications for testing and risk assessment. Reprod Toxicol 1993;7 Suppl 1:53.

Meistrich ML: Potential genetic risks of using semen collected during chemotherapy. Hum Reprod 1993;8:8.

Meldrum DR, Wisot A, Hamilton F, et al: Artificial agonadism and hormonal replacement for oocyte donation. Fertil Steril 1989;52:509.

Menichini E: Urban air pollution by polycyclic aromatic hydrocarbons: levels and sources of variability. Sci Total Environ 1992;116:109.

Mettler FA Jr, Moseley RD Jr (eds): Medical Effects of Ionizing Radiation. Orlando, FL: Grune & Stratton, 1985.

Michalek JE, Rahe AJ, Boyle CA: Paternal dioxin and the sex of children fathered by veterans of Operation Ranch Hand. Epidemiology 1998;9:474.

Moore JA, Daston GP, Faustman E, et al: An evaluative process for assessing human reproductive and developmental toxicity of agents. Reprod Toxicol 1995;9:61.

Nebert DW, Puga A, Vasilou V: Role of the Ah receptor and the dioxin-inducible [Ah] gene battery in toxicity, cancer, and signal transduction. Ann N Y Acad Sci 1993;685:624.

Newsome WH, Davies D, Doucet J: PCB and organochlorine pesticides in Canadian human milk—1992. Chemosphere 1995;30: 2143.

Niimi AJ: Hexachlorobenzene (HCB) levels in Lake Ontario salmonids. Bull Environ Contam Toxicol 1979;23:20.

Paracelsus (Theophrastus ex Hohenheim Eremita): Von der Besucht. Dillingen: 1567.

Pennie WD, Aldridge TC, Brooks AN: Differential activation by xenoestrogens of ER alpha and ER beta when linked to different response elements. J Endocrinol 1998;158:R11.

Pereira MA, Herren SL, Britt AL, Khoury MM: Sex difference in enhancement of *GGTase*-positive foci by hexachlorobenzene and lindane in rat liver. Cancer Lett 1982;15:95.

Peters H, Cripps D, Gocmen A, et al: Turkish epidemic of hexachlorobenzene porphyria: a thirty year study. Ann N Y Acad Sci 1987;514:183.

Rall DP, McLachlan JA: Potential for exposure to estrogens in the environment. In McLachlan JA (ed): Estrogens in the Environment. New York: Elsevier/North Holland, 1980.

Rizzardini M, Smith AG: Sex difference in the metabolism of hexachlorobenzene by rats and the development of porphyria in females. Biochem Pharmacol 1982;31:3543.

Rogan WJ, Gladen BC, Guo YL, Hsu CC: Sex ratio after exposure to dioxin-like chemicals in Taiwan. Lancet 1999;353:206.

Rostad CE, Periera WE, Leiker TJ: Distribution and transport of selected anthropogenic lipophilic organic compounds associated with Mississippi River suspended sediment, 1989–1990. Arch Environ Contam Toxicol 1999;39:248.

Rumsby PC, Yardley-Jones A, Anderson D, et al: Detection of CYP1A1 mRNA levels and CYP1A1 Msp polymorphisms as possible biomarkers of exposure and susceptibility in smokers and non-smokers. Teratog Carcinog Mutagen 1996;16:65.

Safe S, Astroff B, Harris M, et al: 2,3,7,8-tetrachlorodibenzo-*p*-dioxin (TCDD) and related compounds as antioestrogens: characterization and mechanism of action. Pharmacol Toxicol 1991; 69:400.

Sauer MV, Paulson RJ: Oocyte donation to women with ovarian failure. Contemp Obstet Gynecol 1984;34:125.

Schecter A, Ryan JJ, Papke O: Decrease in levels and body burden of dioxins, dibenzofurans, PCBs, DDE and HCB in blood and milk in a mother nursing twins over a thirty-eight month period. Chemosphere 1998;37:1807.

Schlebusch H, Wagner U, van der Ven H, et al: Polychlorinated biphenyls: the occurrence of the main congeners in follicular and sperm fluids. J Clin Chem Clin Biochem 1989;27:663.

Schmidt G, Kannisto P, Owman C: Histaminergic effects on the isolated rat ovarian artery during the estrous cycle. Biol Reprod 1990;42:762.

Schrader SM: Data gaps and new methodologies in the assessment of male fecundity in occupational field studies. Scand J Work Environ Health 1992;18(Suppl 2):30.

Schrader SM, Kanitz MH: Occupational hazards to male reproduction. Occup Med 1994;9:405.

Scialli AR: The reproductive toxicity of ovulation induction. Fertil Steril 1986;45:315.

Scialli AR: Advances in reproductive toxicology. Curr Opin Obstet Gynecol 1992;4:359.

Semenza JC, Tolbert PE, Rubin CH, et al: Reproductive toxins and alligator abnormalities at Lake Apopka, Florida. Environ Health Perspect 1997;105:1030.

Sheehan DM, Willingham E, Gaylor D, et al: No threshold dose for estradiol-induced sex reversal of turtle embryos: how little is too much? Environ Health Perspect 1999;107:155.

Shiau AK, Barstad D, Lorai PM, et al: The structural basis of estrogen receptor/coactivator recognition and the antagonism of this interaction by tamoxifen. Cell 1998;95:927.

Silbergeld EK, Mattison DR: Experimental and clinical studies on the reproductive toxicology of 2,3,7,8-tetrachlorodibenzo-p-dioxin. Am J Ind Med 1987;11:131.

Sims DE, Singh A, Donald A, et al: Alterations of primate ovary surface epithelium by exposure to hexachlorobenzene: a quantitative study. Histol Histopathol 1991;6:525.

Singh A, Sims DE, Jarrell J, Villeneuve DC: Hexachlorobenzene toxicity in the monkey ovary: II. Ultrastructure induced by medium (1.0 mg/kg) dose exposure. In Michael JR, Ingram P (eds): Analysis of Environmental Toxicants. San Francisco: San Francisco Press, 1990:13

Sipes GI, Gandolfi AJ: Biotransformation of toxicants. In Klassen CD, Amdur MO, Doull J (eds): Casarett and Doull's Toxicology: The Basic Science of Poisons. New York: McGraw-Hill, 1991:88.

Sonnenschein C, Soto AM: An updated review of environmental estrogen and androgen mimics and antagonists. J Steroid Biochem Mol Biol 1998;65:143.

Stegeman JJ, Lech JJ: Cytochrome P-450 monooxygenase systems in aquatic species: carcinogen metabolism and biomarkers for carcinogen and pollutant exposure. Environ Health Perspect 1991;90:101.

To-Figueras J, Gomez-Catalan J, Rodamilans M, Corbella J: Studies on sex differences in excretion of sulphur derivatives of hexachlorobenzene and pentachloronitrobenzene by rats. Toxicol Lett 1991;56:87.

Todoroff EC, Sevcik M, Villeneuve DC, et al: The effect of photomirex on the in vitro perfused ovary of the rat. Reprod Toxicol 1998;12:305.

Toppari J, Skakkebaek NE: Sexual differentiation and environmental endocrine disruptors. Baillieres Clin Endocrinol Metab 1998;12:143.

Trapp M, Bauklough V, Bohnet HG, Heeschen W: Pollutants in human follicular fluid. Fertil Steril 1984;42:1465.

Uhlig S, Wendel A: The physiological consequences of glutathione variations. Life Sci 1992;51:1083.

Walker NJ, Portier CJ, Lax SF, et al: Characterization of the dose-response of CYP1B1, CYP1A1, and CYP1A2 in the liver of female sprague-dawley rats following chronic exposure to 2,3,7,8-tetrachlorodibenzo-p-dioxin. Toxicol Appl Pharmacol 1999;154:279.

Wang W, Smith R 3rd, Safe S: Aryl hydrocarbon receptor-mediated antiestrogenicity in MCF-7 cells: modulation of hormone-induced cell cycle enzymes. Arch Biochem Biophys 1998;356:239.

Weijin Z, Olsen J: Offspring sex ratio as an indicator of reproductive hazards. Occup Environ Med 1996;53:503.

Weinberg CR, Zhou H: Model-based approaches to studying fertility and contraceptive efficacy. Adv Contracept 1997;13:97.

Weinberg CR, Baird DD, Rowland AS: Pitfalls inherent in retrospective time-to-event studies: the example of time to pregnancy. Stat Med 1993;12:867.

Weseloh DV, Mineau P, Struger J: Geographical distribution of contaminants and productivity measures of herring gulls in the Great Lakes: Lake Erie and connecting channels 1978/79. Sci Total Environ 1990;91:141.

Whorton MD, Haas JL, Trent L, Wong O: Reproductive effects of sodium borates on male employees: birth rate assessment. Occup Environ Med 1994;51:761.

Wide M: Interference of lead with implantation in the mouse: effect of exogenous estradiol and progesterone. Teratology 1980;21:1987.

Williams J, Gladen BC, Schrader SM, et al: Semen analysis and fertility assessment in rabbits: statistical power and design considerations for toxicology studies. Fundam Appl Toxicol 1990;15:651.

Williams FLR, Lloyd OL, Ogston SA: Offspring sex ratios as an index of pollution hazard in residential environments. Occup Environ Med 1995a;52:622.

Williams FLR, Ogston SA, Lloyd OL: Sex ratios of births, mortality, and air pollution: can measuring the sex ratios of births help to identify health hazards from air pollution in industrial environments? Occup Environ Med 1995b;52:164.

Winston NJ, Braude PR, Johnson MH: Are failed-fertilized human oocytes useful? Hum Reprod 1993;8:503.

Wolff MS, Landrigan PJ: Environmental estrogens. Science 1994;266:526.

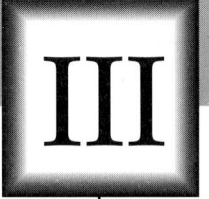

III

General Gynecology

19

Ethical Issues in Gynecology

Fredrick R. Abrams

This chapter has been written in an attempt to offer practical guidance for a gynecologist who desires to follow ethical recommendations for choices that must continually be made in the changing world of medical practice. The use of the word *recommendations* is deliberate because it acknowledges that any guidance is biased because it is written from a particular standpoint. This chapter's standpoint is that of an obstetrician-gynecologist with over 40 years of practice and 20 years a student of bioethics. A smattering of the several time-honored theories and principles that are basic for guidance in behavior and decision making is offered, but only to point to the direction for further study to discern the roots for the recommendations. Even as epitomes, they are woefully oversimplified.

ROLE OF A GYNECOLOGIST

Gynecologists are present at each of life's major passages: birth, reproduction, and death. Vicariously, they have experienced episodes of which most individuals have little or no previous experience. By acting as a guide, physicians can be of great service, helping patients through sometimes wonderful, often frightening, usually unfamiliar, terrain. The patient is a traveler. Almost all patients know where they wish to go, but their level of sophistication regarding how to get there varies widely. The doctor knows the territory, the pitfalls, the short cuts, the detours, and the questions to ask the traveler. If there are reasonable choices, which is preferred: safety or comfort, time or money? Which of these alternate routes suit the traveler's temperament? The traveler is not steered to a hotel simply because the guide owns a share in it. Nor does an ethical guide bar a suitable road because less profit lies in that direction. However, he or she might offer information or advice in the traveler's interest to persuade her to seek a different destination.

VALUES IN A PLURALISTIC COMMUNITY

Medical ethics is different from *physician ethics.* Medical ethics involves the means to search for that which is right, not wrong, and good, not evil, in solving ethical dilemmas and making difficult decisions. Equally, it is the guide for a code of individual behavior in the doctor-patient relationship. What makes a given dilemma an issue of *medical* ethics is that the dilemma arises in a medical environment. *Physician* ethics is the highly variable individual value system to which a particular physician may currently adhere.

Because of the variety of cultures, faiths, and beliefs from which patients and doctors come, the values that they hold may vary widely. A patient bringing a unique problem to several physicians may get a different response from each because there is no single ethical code to which all physicians subscribe. Doctors, nurses, and health care workers have valuable experience, but their usual professional training affords them no special expertise in discerning which of the human values at issue is the correct human value.

SEARCH FOR ETHICAL THEORIES

Scholars have searched for principles that would permit persons to live in peace with justice, decrying the use of force. Three principal modes of evaluating actions predominate in decision-making systems: An action is right if it is well motivated (deontology); an action is right if its outcome is good (utilitarianism); and an action is right if it is the action a virtuous person of good character would endorse (virtue ethics) (Graber, 1988).

Immanuel Kant (1724–1804) is regarded as the philosopher who best epitomized *deontology* (Kant, 1959) He grounded morality in what is called a categorical imperative, an unconditional duty. One version of this is to "act only according to that maxim by which you can at the same time will it to become universal law." This is one of many versions of the "golden rule." A second imperative is to "act so that you treat humanity, whether in your own person or in that of another, always as an end and never as a means only." In other words, do not exploit persons. In essence, if specified duties are honored, an act is

459

considered moral by Kantian premises regardless of (unpredictable) consequences.

John Stuart Mill (1806–1873) is generally regarded to have best formulated *utilitarianism* (Mill, 1971). His major principle was epitomized as "actions are right in proportion as they tend to promote happiness, wrong as they tend to produce the reverse of happiness." In essence, whatever produces good consequences is right. This and the related body of theories are also called "consequentialism." Most students find that each of these systems in its pure form has flaws and fuzzy boundaries, that they are not mutually exclusive, and that in fact they often lead to the same conclusion by different routes. For example, utilitarians, acting to achieve the greatest balance of value over disvalue, nevertheless often apply Kant's imperative of universalizability as a guideline. They subject their decisions to the test of whether their action could always be expected to yield the most good. Almost all deontologic systems include the principle of universalizability and the maxim that persons must never be used merely as means. Nevertheless, they use utility not as an ultimate principle, but as a guideline to help decision making.

The third theory, *virtue or character ethics*, has a venerable history as well, with extensive discussion of what comprises these traits found in the works of Plato and Aristotle. Most recent references in medical ethics concern the doctor-patient relationship. Even those who do not agree that this is a stand-alone ethical theory (because of inability to agree upon what is virtuous) concede that some virtues are necessary, but not sufficient, for regulating behavior between strangers. Edmund Pellegrino, one of the leading proponents for the primacy of virtue in practice, noted "its adherents demand more of themselves than the prevailing morality. No matter to what depths a society may fall, virtuous persons will always be the beacons that light the way back to moral sensitivity; virtuous physicians ought to be the beacons that show the way back to moral credibility for the whole profession." (Pellegrino and Thomasma, 1988:000). Further discussion of virtue theory can be found in the section "Role of the Ethical Physician."

PRINCIPLES TO GUIDE ETHICAL DECISIONS

Four principles set forth by Beauchamp and Childress (1994) are useful to screen choices. They are respect for autonomy, beneficence, nonmaleficence, and justice. These principles do not act as pathways leading to correct answers but, rather, as boundaries that, if not violated, permit at least an ethically defensible position to be attained.

Other approaches are used to flesh out or to complement principles. *Casuistry* (Jonsen and Toulmin, 1988), starting from cases that are similar, uses analogy to reach new conclusions. Working from the case to a principle when possible, it shies away from too-rigid use of rules, looking to differences in circumstances from case to case to help make decisions. (For further information, the reader is referred to the September 1995 issue of *Kennedy Institute of Ethics Journal* (Vol. 5, No. 3), which was devoted to critique and defense of "Principlism".)

Finally, no discussion of contemporary medical ethics would be complete if it failed to consider the role of *feminine-feminist ethics*. Like casuistry, this ethics also addresses context, tends away from principles, and stresses more the relationships of persons involved in dilemmas. It expands beyond its probable roots of gender oppression to decry other instances of potential abuse of power disparity, as in racism, ageism, and, of course, the doctor-patient relationship. It incorporates more communitarian ideas and the notions of care and nurturance (Wolf, 1996).

Principle of Respect for Autonomy

Respect for autonomy is respect for self-determination, self-rule. Consent and truth-telling are based on this ethical principle. How else could a patient make reasonable plans unless she were aware of her true health status and aware of the complexities of choosing a course of treatment? Respect is due any competent person's judgments, even when they conflict with her doctor's. Courts consistently uphold a patient's right to accept or reject treatment, even life-sustaining treatment; they acknowledge, with those who take respect for autonomy seriously, that regrettable and even tragic decisions will sometimes be made by competent persons. Autonomy does not mean simply doing what you want. Kant pointed out that behavior from habit or desire or other nonconsidered, nonreasoned behavior was not autonomous. Certain categories of patients may be incompetent and, therefore, not autonomous. Such patients include the organically demented, the delirious, the unconscious, the intoxicated, the depressed, and the delusional mentally ill. Underage patients are incompetent by law. Drug addicts are usually incompetent and certainly not autonomous. Prisoners or others under various types of duress are not autonomous.

Principle of Nonmaleficence

Nonmaleficence is a time-honored principle, often summarized in the Latin *primum non nocere*, or "first, do no harm." That aphorism could be the minimal basis for governing an entire society: a negatively stated golden rule. In medicine, it is sometimes an impossible injunction because potent beneficial interventions do carry harm (e.g., radiation and chemotherapy). The rule must be modified to advance a proportionate balance of burden and benefit. Treatments with known harms or risk of harm may ethically be offered to an informed patient. Although autonomy is the basis for much of the need for informed consent, nonmaleficence also contributes to its foundation. Naive patients may reasonably be expected to be unaware of all potential problems with certain medical interventions. Conversely, doctors are responsible to know, consider, and reveal the possibilities of actions in which they participate, certainly those that can, with a little thought, be foreseen. For example, in vitro fertilization and embryo transfer in which cryopreservation will be used can predictably pose a problem of disposition of excess embryos. Multiple-embryo transfer can predictably result in multiple gestation with its concomitant risks and the possible option of selective termination. Physicians who undertake the clinical interventions without settling these questions with the patients in advance are ethically remiss.

Although it is clear that gratuitous harm is eschewed by ethical practitioners, less clear but no less critical is the avoidance of harm by negligence. Gynecologists who fail to inform patients of the need and value of preventive tests, such as Papanicolaou (Pap) smears, have violated this ethical precept. Obstetricians who do not advise patients of the availability of genetic screening tests, such as those for Tay-Sachs disease, similarly are at fault.

Also, the interpretation of what constitutes harm must be clarified so that patients and physicians are speaking the same language. To a Jehovah's Witness, death is not the worst harm. Eternal damnation from being transfused with blood is a much greater harm and clearly of more concern than one's brief earthly life. A scientist must acknowledge that those things that have not been proven are not necessarily untrue. When a clearly competent adult has an earnest belief, it ought to be respected, even when it is outside of another person's belief system. This does not mean that a physician who believes a patient is making a poor decision must retreat silently. The doctor would be remiss if years of experience and professional knowledge were simply ignored. Explanation, clarification, and persuasion are tools to be used to advance the doctor's viewpoint, but coercion is *prima facie* wrong.

Principle of Beneficence

Beneficence to medical professionals is a duty because that is precisely what they profess—to do good for others. To others, charity or benevolence is praiseworthy but not obligatory. However, doing good is the very essence of a doctor's role. Once again, as in defining harm, the parallel question arises: How can good be defined? If a physician does not define good in the context of the unique clinical situation, and in consideration of the competent patient's estimation of good, conflict of values may arise. Physicians are attuned to searching for the optimal clinical intervention in terms of physical health, prolongation of life, and relief of suffering. Sometimes health and sometimes life are not paramount values for the patient. It is here that respect for autonomy and beneficence clash. The doctor's role and values may vary from those of other physicians and patients.

Society recognizes a parentalistic role in child rearing and chastises a parent for permitting a child to endanger himself or herself by acting recklessly. Similarly, some physicians take a parental role, as a "parent" to a child, arguing that the doctor knows best and that the patient will be grateful in the future for having had specific behavior coerced in the present. A different physician might intervene in a less directive manner, only long enough to ascertain that the patient is indeed competent and is clearly aware of the consequence of her choice, despite the fact that it is not one that the physician believes to be in the best interests of her health. Once satisfied that this is truly the case and having failed to persuade her otherwise, the physician might assist her. Alternatively, the physician might withdraw once other medical coverage could be found.

Principle of Justice

Justice is a principle that, when stated generally, says equals must be treated equally and unequals must be treated unequally. How to clarify the relevant equalities or inequalities is more elusive. Justice in daily activities is more readily understood as "fairness." People should get what they deserve, both burdens (like taxes) and benefits (like Medicare). Individual practice decisions may sometimes need to be made within the principle of justice. For example, gynecologists acting as triage agents for group practice or hospitals ought to make decisions on the basis of medical need, never on ability to pay. Race or ethnic origin almost never has a clinical bearing on priority of service or quality of care and, therefore, ought not to influence decisions. Refusing to care for a patient with acquired immunodeficiency syndrome (AIDS) because of personal risk imposes more of the burden on colleagues who are willing to do their fair share. Such behavior is unfair and unethical.

However, justice is a principle more usually applied at a macroallocation level in the distribution of resources. Gynecologists ought to be well aware of the problems of access to health care. As good citizens with a particular constituency to represent, they need to participate in societal efforts to improve access and to donate charitably their time and skill. There is much more to be said about the problems of ensuring a basic decent minimum of health care and to explore regarding the arguments, pro and con, of prioritization, rationing, and health care as a right. These problems need to be dealt with by society at large and are beyond the scope of this chapter.

DILEMMAS

Even when physicians conscientiously attempt to act within ethical boundaries, dilemmas arise when principles are in conflict. For example, physicians wish to use their skills to preserve health in accordance with the principle of beneficence; when a Jehovah's Witness exercises the autonomous right to refuse a blood transfusion at the risk of losing his or her life, these two principles clash. There is some evil that will occur and/or some good that will not, no matter what decision is made. That is why medical ethics is often referred to as "the logic of tragedy."

THE IDEAL ETHICAL OBSERVER

The concept of the ideal ethical observer was expressed first in a journal of philosophy by Roderick Firth (1952). Later, Norman Fost, in commenting on issues now classified as "Baby Doe" cases, brought it into the medical literature. Firth described this ideal observer as being

Omniscient: knowing all the facts and data about the clinical issue in question
Omnipercipient: knowing how all the concerned parties feel and how they would react to different action decisions
Dispassionate: not without emotion but, rather, having the ability to avoid emotional clouding of issues
Disinterested: not uncaring about the problem but, rather, having no conflict of interest that would bias decisions
Consistent: not illogically deciding contrarily when like circumstances should lead to like decisions

DECISION PROCESS

Trying to duplicate this paragon, a physician confronting a dilemma could systematically apply it to the problem at hand. This is not a linear process progressing stepwise to an answer, but one of feedback and interaction among concerned parties essential to the process of problem resolution.

1: Gather All the Medical Facts That Are Accessible

Doctors are often forced to make decisions with less than complete information. However, facts may quickly settle questions that were previously thought to be "ethical questions." For example, a person admitted to an emergency room in cardiac arrest need have no attempts at resuscitation, once you learn she has a DNR order and has been inappropriately transferred from a *home* hospice program.

2: Gather the Value Data From All Interested Parties

Often, there is more than one appropriate answer to a dilemma, arising from legitimate differences in underlying basic beliefs concerning, for example, sanctity versus quality of life, the meaning of suffering, the meaning of food, or the importance of physical and/or mental integrity. Determining who has the right to make the decision may be the only way to decide an issue. A competent, informed patient should decide for herself. When the patient is incapacitated and unable to make decisions (and has not provided for a proxy decision maker) then the closer another person is to the effects of a decision, the more weight his or her opinion should carry, provided no ethical principle will be violated.

3: Use the "Principles" to Make a First Pass at the Situation (Autonomy)

An informed, competent patient makes her own decisions. The physician may enlist help if her capacity to make choices is in doubt. A psychiatrist may be helpful, and the staff that has attended the patient probably has the best sense of her decision-making ability. One must remember that refusal of the optimal medical treatment is *not* an indicator of incompetence. Often partial capacity is sufficient. The patient need not be able to count backward from 100 to decide whether or not she wishes her leg amputated. The physician should determine quickly if there are advance directives or an appointed decision maker. Is there someone who knows what the patient desires (substituted judgment)? If not, what is in her *best interests*? Is restraining a patient to intubate her for nasogastric feeding, because she repeatedly pulls the tube out, a violation of duty (nonmaleficence)? Or would it be a more serious violation of duty to fail to nourish her (beneficence)? What are the special circumstances that have a bearing? For example, would it make a difference if she had multiple system failure from metastatic cancer? Would the use of dialysis be a reasonable use of resources under those circumstances (justice)?

4: Present the Data to Those Concerned for Discussion

Physicians may wish to enlist the help of an ethics committee, not to make decisions but to widen the scope of information and opinion for the benefit of the decision makers (usually the patient and/or the family with the help of the attending physician). The ethics committee is an area where feminine-feminist theory has truly been put into action. The committee, sensitive to the special context of a given case, serves to balance the power disparity by offering facts, information, and support in a caring manner to those responsible for difficult decisions. Ideally, with the patient and family present, committee members offer their experience and knowledge without imposing decisions.

The physician should clarify misunderstandings of the facts or unrealistic appraisals of the situation. He or she should also raise significant considerations aside from the ethical, such as economic factors and pertinent law that must be followed. The whole enterprise of decision making is a process, not a single episode. Other *medical* consultants may be helpful, but doctors steeped in the science of medicine too often forget about the clergy. They are extremely important to many patients.

Follow Up

After the consultation process, when sufficient time has elapsed, often further action is needed. Sometimes this consists of no more than emotional support for those involved after difficult decisions have been made, such as refusing chemotherapy or a proxy decision to forgo artificial feeding, or for parents who have declined surgery for a severely malformed newborn. At other times the patient or family needs more specific help—for example, from social services to connect to the proper agency or support system.

ROLE OF THE ETHICAL PHYSICIAN

In the practice of medicine, no less than in most of life's behavior, ethical considerations govern most of our actions. With society depending more on laws and regulations to govern medical practice, we will soon be in as sorry a moral state as business today finds itself. Medicine is not a business; it is a service. Profit cannot be its purpose. In the first and last analysis, medicine depends on the integrity of its practitioners and their relationship to their patients. The expansion of the theory of physician character and virtue that follows is in part empirical, but it will rarely find disagreement, even among those who do not follow the recommendations. It should be noted that ethical guidelines are for those who are seeking a basis for ethical behavior. They are not useful for those who do not wish to behave ethically.

In the most recent challenge to the integrity of the profession presented by some aspects of managed care, there are conflicts of interest setting the doctor's income against the patient's health. This and other conflicts of interest are addressed in the section "Profession-Fiduciary Relationship," which discusses the virtuous physician's reaffirmation of a commitment to practice in the patient's interest. Virtuous physicians are also guided by the Kantian imperative, "never to use a person as a means, only"—never to exploit. This imperative also applies to the "boundary issues" that deal with sexual exploitation. The aforementioned section and the section "Consent and Competence" speak also to recent ethical transgressions in artificial reproduction where embryo owners and recipients both were violated. Embryos were inserted into recipients who were unaware that other persons who had formed the embryos for their own use had not given permission for donation. What may be considered "old" virtues continue to apply to newer issues. Indeed, there are few areas where the character of the physician is not relevant to performance.

UNIVERSAL PRECEPTS

Profession-Fiduciary Relationship

Medicine is a profession. A profession has a unique body of knowledge. Competence is determined best by peers. There is a moral core that peers enforce. Society recognizes a profession, subsidizes it, and gives it privileges, often including monopoly. In turn, a profession has a fiduciary relationship with those it serves. All are aware of the disparity in knowledge, and the more knowledgeable contractor agrees to use the knowledge to benefit the person seeking aid. *First and foremost, then, a doctor practices for the benefit of the patient.* This means that a gynecologist must take care to avoid *self-deception*, because economic incentives are perverse. Depending on the means of payment, a doctor may profit by withholding treatment when patients are capitated or a portion of reimbursement is withheld until year-end costs are calculated. Conversely, overtesting and overtreating are encouraged in a pure fee-for-service situation. Referral to facilities in which a doctor has a financial interest are suspect. Any deception or misrepresentation to a patient of a physician's qualifications or incidence of favorable outcomes, with the knowledge of the likelihood of her getting less than optimal care, is unethical.

Consent and Competence

As medicine becomes less of a mystery and consumers become more educated, there has evolved an obligation to involve patients more in their care decisions by informing them of choices, alternatives, risks, and harms, as well as benefits. Consent has become such a universal ethical imperative that it has been incorporated into law. It is designed to show respect for a patient's autonomy by ensuring the patient's role in choosing alternative treatment or no treatment at all, after the patient has been made aware of the burdens and benefits of the choices. Clearly, a patient must be competent to make such a choice. She must understand the proposed treatment, must be able to consider it rationally, and must be able to consciously communicate about it. Consent is not a piece of paper with "high-tech" jargon and some signatures. Rather, it is the culmination of a process of interaction between patient and physician (President's Commission for the Study of Ethical Problems in Medicine and Medical and Behavioral Research, 1982) that is sometimes brief but, as the intervention carries more risk, often is the culmination of a series of diagnostic procedures, reports, and discussions. Consent is more evidence of the patient's involvement in her care, mutual respect, and the fiduciary relationship.

Cure and Care

A physician has a duty to continue caring even when cure is no longer possible. If death is inevitable, the "art" of medicine must advance as the "science" must retreat. Many physicians hold themselves responsible or fear that patients do so when their best efforts have failed to effect a cure. Doctors need to be made aware that their presence continues to be comforting to patients, even when the goal has changed from cure to care. A brief visit on rounds or even a telephone call buoys the spirit of patients who have little else going for them. Recognizing interventions that add nothing to living but simply prolong the dying process is extremely important. Reflexively using the potent tools of our profession simply because they are there, because we do not know what else to do, is worse than useless. Learning to use the palliative treatments correctly is ethically imperative. It is a physician's duty to help patients and their families face the reality of death and prepare for it as best as possible. Certainly, the value of advance directives ought to be raised before a crisis makes them irrelevant. More often, it is the physician's, rather than the patient's, inability to face the imminence of death that inhibits these important discussions and decisions.

Mutual Respect for Autonomy and Conscience

Respecting a patient's autonomy and helping to achieve her health goals are of great importance for an empathetic physician. However, a patient must also respect the physician's autonomy, and care must be taken to violate no one's conscientious objection to any medical intervention. Yet, if there is a conflict, a doctor must not abandon a patient but must find a way for continued care. Respect for autonomy is a two-way street. Patients and doctors must respect each other's rights to self-determination. A gynecologist has a duty to inform patients about his or her values regarding issues likely to arise in gynecologic practice. Inhibitions against abortion, sterilization, prenatal diagnosis, premarital sexual activity, or other daily occurrences in practice need to be made clear, preferably before crises arise, necessitating a

change of physician or risking the hazards of abandonment.

Professional Responsibility for Quality

A doctor cannot look away from bad practices by others. He or she must act on behalf of the patient and the integrity of the profession to protect patients from poor or inhumane treatment.

Confidentiality

Confidentiality is a time-honored ethical guide. Without the freedom to disclose all information that may be of aid in her care, a patient cannot receive the benefit of her doctor's knowledge. Sometimes this can be critical. Therefore, she must be able to rely on the privilege of confidentiality. This has met its most difficult test in recent times with the challenge of AIDS, whose virus is deadly. Nondisclosure of seropositive status by a patient to a person who has the right to expect safety in their relationship poses an enormous dilemma for the doctor who shares this knowledge.

Professional Competence

A doctor must constantly update his or her knowledge base. Patients are entitled to a physician who practices medicine according to current community standards. If his or her experience falls short of the mark, the fiduciary relationship compels consultation with a knowledgeable colleague. Practicing beyond one's competence can never be in the patient's interest and violates ethical standards.

IN CONCLUSION: A PHYSICIAN'S AFFIRMATION

In order to be worthy of self-respect, I pledge to respect others who place their trust in me as a professional in the healing arts. Therefore:

I will practice my art and my science to benefit my patients.

I will disclose to my patients that which I know of their disease and any hazards of the remedies I might suggest, that I may guide them to choose the course that suits them best.

I will offer care and comfort when they are ill, and, when death becomes inevitable, I will ease their way as best I can in keeping with their expressed plan.

I will recognize their right to self-determination and, if conflicts should arise with my own ethical constraints, make them aware, without judging wherein we differ, that they should consider seeking help elsewhere for their complaints.

I will intercede on their behalf within the scope of my authority if I perceive they are being treated without regard for their humanity.

I will hold in confidence that which is seen or heard in my role as physician.

I will ever be a student to sharpen my skills and further my knowledge that I may be a better clinician.

If I act in this way I may aspire to join the men and women who, through the ages, have approached the loftiest ideals of the healing mission, for I will have earned the faith and trust, which is the strongest tie in the bond between patient and physician.

F. R. Abrams
A Physician's Affirmation, 1976

REFERENCES

Cited References

Beauchamp TL, Childress JF: Principles of biomedical ethics. 4th ed. New York: Oxford University Press, 1994.

Firth R: Ethical absolutism and the ideal observer. J Philosophy Phenomenological Res 1952;12:317.

Graber LC: Basic theories in medical ethics. In Monagle J, Thomasma DC (eds): Medical Ethics. Rockville, MD: Aspen Publishers, 1988.

Jonsen AR, Toulmin S: The Abuse of Casuistry. Berkeley: University of California Press, 1988.

Kant I: Foundations of the Metaphysics of Morals (Whitebeck L, transl). Indianapolis, IN: Bobbs-Merrill Co, 1959.

Mill JS: In Gorovitz S (ed): Utilitarianism with Critical Essays. Indianapolis, IN: Bobbs-Merrill Co, 1971.

Pellegrino ED, Thomasma DC: For the Patient's Good. New York: Oxford University Press, 1988.

President's Commission for the Study of Ethical Problems in Medicine and Medical and Behavioral Research. Making Health Care Decisions. Vol. 1. Washington, DC: U.S. Government Printing Office, 1982

Wolf SM (ed): Feminism and Bioethics. New York: Oxford University Press, 1996.

Additional Readings

American College of Obstetricians and Gynecologists. Opinions of the ethics committee (intermittent ongoing publication). Washington, DC.

American College of Obstetricians and Gynecologists. (See also monographs and statements from the National Advisory Board for Ethics in Reproduction, the Ethics Committee of The American Society for Assisted Reproduction, and the Society for Assisted Reproduction Technology)

Engelhardt HT Jr: The Foundations of Bioethics. 2nd ed. New York: Oxford University Press, 1996.

Faden R, Beauchamp TL: A History and Theory of Informed Consent. New York: Oxford University Press, 1986.

Graber GC, Beasley AD, Eaddy JA: Ethical Analysis of Clinical Medicine. Baltimore: Urban and Schwarzenberg, 1985.

Jonsen A, Siegler M, Winslade W: Clinical Ethics. 4th ed. New York: McGraw-Hill, 1998.

Reich WT (ed): Encyclopedia of Bioethics. New York: Simon & Schuster Macmillan, 1995.

20

Managed Care and Health Policy

Derek van Amerongen

Managed care is now the dominant model for medical care delivery in the United States. Its rise to prominence during the 1990s evoked intense controversy in both the lay and medical communities. It has also caused major changes in a variety of accepted tenets of American medicine. The managed care era can be dated as beginning in earnest in 1993 with the defeat of the comprehensive health plan reform proposed by President Clinton. With the Federal government effectively removed from the forefront of reform, the private sector was left to deal with the challenge of changing decades of entrenched policy and practices. Prior to this time, it was traditional for physicians entering practice to know little if anything about the mechanics of a medical practice, or to even spend much time contemplating the larger issues of national health policy and how it affects medical care delivery. That is no longer a realistic approach for the modern physician. It is increasingly important that all participants in our medical care system understand the new landscape and have a working knowledge of the issues. One must appreciate the antecedent events that led to the creation of managed care, what one's role in this system is and can be, and what the ongoing evolution of managed care will bring forth. For gynecologists, who span the roles of both primary care providers and specialists, this is particularly necessary. The obstetrician-gynecologist often serves as the woman's first point of entry into the medical care system, and so must be prepared to navigate it efficiently in order to provide her with the optimal level of care (American College of Obstetricians and Gynecologists, 1996).

BACKGROUND: A SYNOPSIS OF THE EVOLUTION OF AMERICAN MEDICINE

To be able to put the current situation into proper context, one must be familiar with the evolution of medical practice in this country. Since World War II, medicine has been a lucrative, highly regarded profession, with unparalleled autonomy for its members. This was not part of its early tradition. Medicine in America had always been a "cottage industry," with solo practitioners functioning independently. Before 1900, and the Flexner reforms, most medical schools were proprietary, with 6-month curricula that were repeated over two years (Starr, 1982:82–91). Until organized medicine persuaded most state legislatures in the early 1900s to grant licensure exclusively to allopathic physicians, competition between homeopaths, naturopaths, allopaths, and others was intense. Prior to the 1920s, few medical doctors had or desired hospital privileges. Most treatments, births, deaths, even surgeries, occurred outside the hospital. Specialists, including obstetrician-gynecologists, were rare. Payment for medical services was made in cash or barter. Being a doctor was not a particularly prestigious or well-compensated profession. During the Depression, several "homes" were established for destitute physicians. Medicine itself was rudimentary, without antibiotics or sophisticated diagnostics and with few drugs.

This all changed radically with the emergencies imposed by World War II. With 10 million men and women under arms, the demands upon the medical system were immense. Within a span of 5 years, entire specialties were invented to meet the needs of modern warfare and public health (Starr, 1982:337–351). By the late 1940s, the growth in hospital-based medicine had become exponential, facilitated in large measure by ambitious government programs such as the Hill-Burton Act, which subsidized hospital construction. Simultaneously, new reimbursement mechanisms were devised that dramatically increased the revenue available to both physicians and hospitals. Two events were instrumental in this development: Blue Cross and Blue Shield plans that began in the 1930s but spread nationally after the war, and the institutionalization of employer-sponsored health insurance. The latter arose from wartime wage and price controls meant to control inflation. Defense industries, unable to pay workers more yet desperate to attract them, began offering health insurance as a benefit. By the 1950s, this practice had become the norm. For the next four decades, the primary route to insurance in this country would

467

be through employers (Bodenheimer and Sullivan, 1998).

Medical insurance was based on a fee-for-service model, that is, a physician or hospital would be paid according to a fee schedule for services rendered to an insured party. This permitted huge revenues to flow into a medical system that 20 years earlier had been based on barter and small cash transactions. It also enabled unprecedented autonomy on the part of the providers to perform almost any service they deemed valid, and receive full compensation. Very quickly the majority of medical costs in America were borne by a third party (Phelps, 1992).

On numerous occasions, presidents and Congresses had attempted to impose some rationality on the disjointed and decentralized medical care system, akin to the national health insurance programs in Britain, Germany, Canada, and most of the Western countries. In 1914, 1937, 1947, 1963, 1973, and 1993, such plans were proposed and ultimately defeated. Each attempt did lead to some incremental change, such as the introduction of Medicare and Medicaid in 1964 after the Kennedy-Johnson proposal was rejected. Yet not until the most recent event was the private sector both in a mood to aggressively address health care reform and given the green light by the federal government.

Preparing the way prior to 1993 was a decade of spiraling medical inflation, often in double digits, that had resulted in some employers paying as much for health insurance for an employee as in wages (Letsch, 1993). General Motors, the largest private purchaser of medical care in the world, estimated it added $1000 to the price of each new car because of health care costs for its workers. The rise in uninsured Americans also caused great consternation. Because of the high cost of insurance, millions were forced to use emergency rooms for routine care; the vast majority of these were people working for small businesses. Furthermore, despite the huge outlays for medical care, higher than any other nation on earth, the United States traditionally scored poorly on international surveys of health status indicators (Anderson, 1997). The problems of the cost of, and access to, medical care became a key issue in the 1992 presidential campaign, perhaps the first time health care had become an important election year topic. Clearly there was a medical care crisis that affected individuals, the delivery system, and those who were paying for the care but not seeing positive results.

One incremental reform that was to pave the way for the response of the private sector was the federal Health Maintenance Organization (HMO) Act of 1973 (Fox, 1996). HMOs had been around for many years, beginning as prepaid group practices and cooperative health plans, and later as health insurance plans such as the Kaiser plan on the West Coast. Yet, until the 1970s, HMOs were uncommon options for most Americans and were still somewhat experimental. The HMO Act required large employers to offer an HMO option to their employees, and set various standards for an HMO to be federally qualified. After modest growth during the 1970s and 1980s, HMOs were poised to serve as the alternative to the traditional fee-for-service system. Thus, in 1993, using the experience gained in the HMO field, particularly in California, health policy analysts were ready with an answer to the question of where to go once the government had stepped back from the reform process. The result was what we now call managed care.

THE ELEMENTS OF MANAGED CARE

In order for the practitioner to understand his or her role in the managed care framework, it is important to know what problems managed care is designed to correct. One might summarize the major deficiencies of the traditional system as follows:

- Dramatic variation in care, in terms of the types of treatments prescribed for given diagnoses, where and when the care is given, by whom, and so forth (Wennberg and Gittlesohn, 1973). For example, the rate of hysterectomy varies widely between states and between urban and rural settings (Mechcatie, 1997). In theory there should be a medical justification for a higher rate in Indiana than in Ohio, yet there is no evidence that supports a different rate between the adjacent states. The discrepancies become even more pronounced when East and West Coasts, and the United States and European countries, are compared.
- An absence of relationship between the health status (meaning the various indicators that provide a summation of one's medical condition) of a population (e.g., the people of a certain region, or the employees of a large company) and the interventions they receive or do not receive. We would expect a population that is getting more surgery, or more medications, or more hospitalizations to have different health outcomes than a matched group, yet this is not the case (Evans, 1994).
- A lack of correlation between health status and dollars spent. Again, one would intuitively expect a group that has significantly more money to spend on medical care to be healthier than a control group, but studies fail to demonstrate this (Schieiber and Poullier, 1993).
- No consistent definition of quality. Historically, there was no attempt to spell out what high-quality care consisted of or how it should be delivered. Quality was very much in the eye of the beholder, and consumers (including patients, employers, the government, and insurers) were left to fend for themselves. As a result, medical decisions were rarely based on objective data and tended to revolve around nonmedical issues (who is geographically near, who is established in the community, etc.).

As the cost of medical care approached 14% of the gross domestic product, serious questions were raised as to what benefit was being accrued to the national health. Medicare was being forced to raise premiums, state budgets were running deficits because of growing Medicaid costs, employers were dropping medical coverage, and the like. There seemed to be no attempt to deliver value for the health care service. Managed care was seen as a method to render value for the expenditures on medical services. By *value*, one means obtaining health outcomes that justify the costs. Therefore, the objective of managed care is to accomplish the following:

1. Lead consumers and providers (meaning physicians and hospitals, but also other medical professionals such as nurse midwives, and nurse practitioners) to make quality-conscious decisions in delivering medical care. The industrial quality management literature demonstrates that high-quality processes result in lower costs (Scholtes, 1994). One need only look at the phenomenal leaps in quality in the U.S. auto industry at the same time it has achieved its greatest profitability in history. Raising the quality of care will result in improved patient outcomes. This is the path to creating value in medical care.
2. To move from a *medical care* focus (i.e., treating the individual patient, which we do very well in American medicine) to a *health care* focus (i.e., improving the health of a population, which has been problematic for the U.S. medical care system).
3. To determine the wisest allocation of limited resources. Although this may appear to suggest rationing of medical care, a concept many Americans object to strenuously, it merely recognizes the obvious. There are only so many dollars that can be allotted to medical care. For example, if a new test or procedure comes on the market and many patients request it, from where does the money to cover it come? The insurance company has already collected the premium that the payer (the employer or government) has budgeted. Does the insurer go back to the payer to ask for more money (that would ultimately come from the subscriber or taxpayer)? Or does the insurer divert funds allocated to other treatments or programs? For instance, does one cut prenatal care to perform more bone densitometry studies? These are difficult questions, with no easy or correct answer.

Managed care has come to mean any medical care that involves some form of organized delivery system with the kind of quality, cost, and review oversight that will be explained below. HMOs are characterized by restrictive networks, minimal co-payments, and tight utilization rules. They have been joined by preferred provider organizations (PPOs) and point of service (POS) plans. Both PPOs and POSs are looser, more customer-friendly models devised in the wake of concern about the constraints of HMOs. However, with this loosening has also come a dilution of the quality indicators and cost savings seen in HMOs.

These goals are accomplished in the following ways. Understand that this is an evolutionary process, a work in progress. The endpoint, when these strategies are fully defined and universally implemented, is probably decades away. Nevertheless, substantial movement has already been made in this direction.

Standards for Quality Measurement

As mentioned, prior to the 1990s no organization had consistently defined, evaluated, and monitored quality of care delivered across a continuum. Managed care's focus encompasses the entire spectrum of disease as part of improving outcomes and being more relevant to the needs and experiences of patients. Hence the care that occurs in a doctor's office, as well as the inpatient hospital, is surveilled. Chart reviews of patients who may never be admitted or operated upon are reviewed as part of this process, frequently by means of office site reviews with the practitioner. The standards used have come from a variety of sources: the medical literature, guidelines produced by professional societies such as the American College of Obstetricians and Gynecologists (ACOG), benchmarking against other health plans, and others. It is hoped that, as health plans gain more experience in quality improvement, and as organizations such as the ACOG become more proactive in developing quality measures, there will be consensus on the standards used that will facilitate adherence for the practitioner. Currently the most influential quality accreditation organization for health plans is the National Committee on Quality Assurance (NCQA). Originally established by employers to bring some consistency into the field of quality assessment, many states and large companies now require NCQA certification for a health plan to participate in their programs. One newer addition is the Foundation for Accountability (FACCT), which seeks to go several steps beyond the NCQA framework by emphasizing longitudinal outcomes over time. A recurring theme of all quality activity is to attribute accountability to providers for outcomes (by assessing providers on the outcomes they generate, not just on what processes are in place) and to continually raise the bar on what is to be considered acceptable performance (Mohlenbrock, 1998).

Information Sharing

Sharing information with the stakeholders in the health care delivery process means including not just the traditional dyad of patient and physician, but also other providers, payers, and interested parties (such as consumer groups). It may be jarring for a physician to consider that data on outcomes and procedure rates may be reviewed by others. However, as long as the majority of medical costs are paid by third parties, and the issue of meeting various health status indicators remains, there will be a number of groups who are legitimately interested in this information and have an expectation to receive it. Profiling of physicians, hospitals, health plans, and so on will be a hallmark of medical practice going forward. Health plans have to be accountable as well for providing data back to employers and communicating regularly with the members on important health issues. They are also responsible for data sharing with the NCQA and various governmental organizations.

Realigning Incentives

The traditional fee-for-service paradigm is based on a piecework mentality: payment for each procedure or encounter. This is why the idea of prepaid medical care was so radical in the early days of HMOs. The fundamental problems with the cottage industry approach to medicine are that it rewards overutilization (hence variation in care, as noted above), is a disincentive to preventive care, and does little to engender the value mindset that can lead to improved outcomes. The backlash against managed care has been fostered by the reaction to the cost-cutting measures designed to change these incentives. Despite concerns among physicians and hospitals that these measures would reduce income and revenues, most recent surveys show a steady increase in both. Payers have been gratified to see substantial flattening of the medical care inflation of the 1980s. It is apparent that, as the decade ends, costs will begin to rise again as health plans loosen their restrictions and state and federal mandates, such as those requiring coverage for 48-hour postpartum hospital stays, take hold (Winslow, 1998).

Considerable innovation continues to occur in devising new formulas to reimburse providers while creating incentives for them to concentrate on appropriate utilization of resources, emphasize preventive care, monitor quality, and accept accountability for health outcomes. One term that is important to understand is *capitation*: A physician or practice accepts prepayment for services based on the number of patients (or, in insurance terms, *members*) who are assigned to that physician for care (Kongstvedt, 1996). Typically these are primary care physicians who are responsible for a set range of covered services (*benefits*, which vary depending on the specifics of the member's contract as purchased by the employer). Note that the amount paid is the same regardless of the volume or type of services delivered. The physician therefore has an incentive to keep his or her patients healthy, coordinate care, and avoid preventable adverse events. For example, a pediatrician would want to ensure that his patients are fully immunized, and a gynecologist would be sure her patients have mammograms and Pap smears. Capitated physicians tend to be primary care providers because they, unlike most specialists, are better prepared to oversee the wide range of health parameters that must be attended to in order to maintain and improve health status. There is a danger in accepting capitation: If a physician is unable to influence the care a patient receives, there will be less ability to prevent adverse health outcomes and control costs. It is also important that the managed care entity protect the primary care provider through reinsurance that absorbs costs beyond a certain level for high-cost patients. For these reasons, it is unlikely that most physicians will be asked to accept either the service or financial risk that capitation represents. Rather, other combinations involving discounts on standard fee schedules, performance guarantees, and global rates (one flat fee to cover all the services related to a given treatment; obstetricians were the pioneers in establishing global fees as the preferred mechanism of payment for routine prenatal care) are more commonly seen.

Aside from the provider, the patient is being called upon to participate more in the expenses of medical care. Cost sharing via such tools as copayments is very common. It is a way to communicate to the lay public that medical care, although usually paid for indirectly through taxes and payroll deductions, is not free but has significant costs. It encourages patients to include cost as a factor when making medical care decisions. Many critics of managed care see this as a serious detriment. Their concern is that needed care will be foregone because of the cost to an individual. Although studies have not shown this to be the case (Selby et al, 1996), bodies such as the NCQA look carefully for evidence of underutilization of needed services by a health plan's membership.

On the hospital side, diagnosis-related groups (DRGs), introduced by the Health Care Financing Administration (HCFA) in 1983 to control spiraling Medicare costs, have been quite effective in bringing costs down and reducing the length of inpatient stays, without adverse effects on medical outcomes (McIlrath, 1996). In fact, most hospitals have become very efficient because of the incentives inherent in DRGs, as evidenced by the steady increase in hospital profits over the past decade. One new incentive, designed to replace DRGs, is a per diem rate specific to a given procedure or diagnosis. By paying only a certain amount per day in the hospital, health plans seek to avoid having patients spend days in the hospital when little or no acute care is being given, usually during the last 2 or 3 days of a DRG-standard stay. As with physician reimbursement, new hospital and ancillary models of reimbursement are constantly in development.

Networking Systems of Care

Establishing systems of care organized along high-quality, cost-effective networks is a keystone of managed care delivery, tying in many of the elements discussed above. Health plans and payers identify quality providers using well-publicized standards, implement guidelines and outcomes tracking within the networks, then direct their members to them. Ideally the providers in the networks, chosen because of their demonstrated ability to produce quality results in an efficient manner, will deliver care that is better and less costly. Patients are obligated as part of their insurance contracts to use certain networks or shoulder much or all of the cost for accessing an outside provider (another example of realigning incentives). The benefit to the providers is the opportunity to tap into a stream of patients who will preferentially use their services. By designing a network with all the components necessary to deal with medical problems on a continuum, versus in a disjointed fashion, the patient will receive the most appropriate care. In gynecology, such a network would consist of primary care physicians, gynecologists, specialists such as reproductive endocrinologists, outpatient and inpatient facilities, and ancillary services such as home IV care, durable medical equipment, and visiting nurses. Such a network would be better able to address long-term medical problems such as diabetes, heart disease, and congenital defects by having services in place to deal with the different stages of chronic illness. As mentioned earlier, the classical paradigm in medicine was to focus solely on the acute episode of an illness. With so many people living longer, and the chronic disease burden a growing issue, the longitudinal course of disease must be routinely considered. For the patient, the network has significant potential benefits. By staying "in network," the patient's cost sharing is minimized; the providers are familiar with the resources available and with the particular health plan and its rules; and quality, utilization, and outcomes data are more easily collected and shared.

Increased Rational Use of Resources

Based on the needs of a population, managed care tries to allocate resources in a more appropriate manner than the disjointed fashion of the fee-for-service system. Such an approach might be to deny entry into a managed care network to a new hospital being built in an area with available capacity, given the significant oversupply of hospital beds. It is important that these efforts do not result in denial of needed care or underuse of critical services.

TRENDS FOR THE FUTURE

It is beyond the scope of this brief discussion to provide the physician with a deep understanding of where managed care is going. It is hoped that some familiarity with the context in which managed care was born, as well as some key concepts of what managed care is designed to accomplish, will make further study easier. To this end, it is worthwhile to consider what trends are occurring in medical care delivery. Being aware will permit the physician to more accurately assess how these changes will affect the practice of gynecology in the future.

A shift towards generalists is well underway, and will continue. Family physicians have been among the main beneficiaries of managed care as policy makers looked for someone to fill the gatekeeper role. Without a physician to coordinate care, the patient may quickly become lost in the medical system. Multiple specialists may be consulted with little to show for it, and medications prescribed without consideration of other medications or allergies; patients often do not know whom to talk to for objective advice on treatments. A common scenario is back pain: does the patient go to an orthopedist, a neurologist, or a neurosurgeon? Or does he or she simply need to lose weight and exercise? Such assessments may seem straightforward, but without a coordinator for these situations, the patient may spend months and thousands of dollars before an answer is obtained. The ACOG has promoted the role of primary care physician for the obstetrician-gynecologist. The challenge will then be for obstetrician-gynecologists to become comfortable filling it.

There will be continued growth in physician income and hospital revenues. Despite reductions in fee schedules and DRG payments, providers have shown surprising ingenuity in maintaining revenues (Jaklevic, 1998). This may well mean longer hours and more patients per session, but there appears to be little evidence that most providers are suffering economically.

There will increasing emphasis on adherence to best practices, guidelines, critical pathways, and the like. This will be an important indicator for the HCFA and health plans to assess the quality efforts of providers. The more a physician group can document the use of these guidelines (for example, the ACOG Criteria Sets) in daily practice, the higher it will rank and the greater the opportunity to participate in managed care networks. Of course, if one believes that guidelines do in fact improve care, these providers will also see better outcomes. In some respects this will be welcome news for academicians who have devoted their careers to identifying the optimal ways to treat disease, only to see the majority of practitioners ignore those recommendations (Rosenthal et al, 1997). The success of this trend will be reflected in the amount of improvement that can be documented in the health status indicators of a defined population.

Informations systems, also known as medical informatics, will become increasingly critical to maintaining an active medical practice. Managed care relies heavily on tracking information: details about office encounters, procedures, tests, medications, and the like. This allows the measurement of progress in health status discussed above, as well as supporting the compensation system for providers, identifying emerging medical problems, and establishing a data base for utilization and cost-of-care figures. Hence the physician who derives significant patient volume from managed care will be responsible for collecting and reporting much of this information. This will require the hardware and network connections to do so, as well as computer training and expertise on the part of the staff and the physician. For those raised on computers in the classroom, this will not be as much of a leap as for older physicians who are not as comfortable with this technology. Nevertheless, it will be a must for full participation in health plans in the next few years. This will closely parallel the rising importance of the Internet as a source of medical information and as a way to do business, such as electronic submission of claims to the insurance company and transmission of referrals to other doctors.

Despite the concerns over loss of autonomy as a result of managed care, and the inclusion of a range of stakeholders in decisions of medical policy, the influence of physicians in developing new delivery models is increasing. Prior to the 1950s, most hospital administrators were physicians. With the advent of the hospital as a large conglomerate, managers trained in medical administration and business took over. This trend is now reversing itself as more physicians, anxious to be included in the breakneck change occurring in medicine, obtain advanced business training and assume the administration roles previously reserved for nonphysicians. This is bringing a strong medically oriented point of view to the direction of many hospitals, medical corporations, health plans, and the like. It is creating an opportunity for physicians to have significant input to strategic decisions about the future directions of medical care delivery (van Amerongen, 1998).

Hospitals have been the center of medical care for almost 50 years. As more care is moved to the outpatient, ambulatory, and home settings, the hospital's role is different. It will no longer be the center of a system, but a part of a range of services available to the practitioner, to be used for a selected case depending upon the specifics involved. Coupled with this will be a continuation of the consolidation of the elements of the provider system. Hospitals will continue to merge to gain market share. Physician groups will merge with each other as well as be bought out by large hospital networks. Physician management organizations will continue to purchase practices, making many physicians either partners in a larger corporation or salaried employees. Health plans and large employers will do more direct contracting with provider groups, as long as those groups can demonstrate competence in performing managed care functions (i.e., utilization manage-

ment, data collection, etc.). As provider networks grow larger, they may be tempted to enter the insurance arena by offering managed care plans, serviced by their physician and hospital members, to major companies in their local service area. To date, however, provider-sponsored HMOs have had a poor track record because of the difficulty in managing medical costs while delivering care (Bellandi, 1998).

CHALLENGES

Just as there are opportunities for physicians as a result of the trends outlined above, there are pressing challenges as well. These must be addressed on the national, local, and individual levels. It is hoped that such organizations as the ACOG will provide the needed support to the practitioner to accomplish this.

First and foremost is actually achieving an improvement in the health of a *population* versus an *individual*. This goal requires not only the infrastructure to support it, but the philosophical support as well. Gynecologists have a unique role to play as principle physicians for women. They must understand and accept the concept of moving beyond a medical system to a health system if they are to be successful in a managed care world. As mentioned, managed care is an evolutionary process. Five or 10 years from now, the framework of the process will look very different, but it is necessary to be conversant and comfortable with the present structure in order to be prepared to move on to the next level.

Educating the public on what *quality* means is necessary. Surveys generally demonstrate an ignorance of the medical definition of quality: Lay respondents usually equate access and choice of provider with quality, not necessarily level of skill or competence or demonstrated outcomes. In order for patients to select high-quality providers, and avoid the poor performers, they must understand what is being measured, and its importance in achieving a desired result. This education is also needed if those who devote the resources to become high-quality providers wish to be appropriately recognized and rewarded as such.

Designing a satisfactory reimbursement plan will be essential to properly aligning incentives. On the one hand, it is necessary that physicians be adequately compensated. On the other, the era of being able to bill at usual and customary rates without accountability is over. The incentives that foster excess utilization of some procedures and treatments, as identified by best practices and benchmarking, must be eliminated. Incentives that encourage underutilization or withholding needed care must be avoided too. Generating value in terms of outcomes with respect to cost and resources must be the objective. This will also impact the issue of physician autonomy, which will continue to evolve with the delivery system.

The consumer and legislative backlash to managed care has resulted in literally thousands of bills being introduced to regulate and modify health plans (Weissenstein, 1998). Some have been supported by organized medicine and provider groups. Although primarily directed at health plans, this activity may have unintended consequences for the practitioner. It may preclude large medical groups from forming their own provider-sponsored health plans in the future, as an effort to put physicians in direct contact between employers and patients. Furthermore, "legislation by body part"—mandates imposed to correct real or imagined abuses by requiring certain treatments regardless of medical value—imposes significant strains on all parts of the delivery system.

SUMMARY

Managed care is an imperfect model, with serious flaws and shortcomings. Yet to date it is the only viable alternative to the outdated fee-for-service system. It was apparent that change in American medicine was inevitable, and, once a critical mass was reached in terms of cost, excess utilization, unsatisfactory outcomes, and the failure of the federal government to take the lead, a rapid transformation did occur. The current stage of this evolution is managed care, which has caused much upheaval across the board because of the fundamental restructuring it entails. Yet the new directions brought about by this way of delivering care have numerous opportunities for both physicians and patients. Managed care offers a greater role for implementing best practices and establishing a higher level of quality performance. It is remaking the standard patterns of the medical system and creating new roles for hospitals, physicians, and ancillary providers, and is bringing a new group of stakeholders into the process. With time and increasing sophistication on the part of all those involved and interested in health, managed care will likely evolve into the type of medical delivery process that will truly foster improved health. This will present physicians with important challenges that must be addressed to maintain the central role that doctors have in medical care.

REFERENCES

American College of Obstetricians and Gynecologists. Guidelines for Women's Health Care. Washington, DC: American College of Obstetricians and Gynecologists, 1996:34.

Anderson GF: In search of value: an international comparison of cost, access and outcomes. Health Affairs 1997;16(6):163.

Bellandi D: Georgia hospital-owned HMOs rack up losses. Mod Healthcare 1998;April 27:4.

Bodenheimer T, Sullivan K: How large employers are shaping the health care marketplace. N Engl J Med 1998;338:1003.

Evans RG: Why Are Some People Healthy and Others Not? New York: Aldine deGruyter Press, 1994.

Fox PD: An overview of managed care. In Kongstvedt P (ed): The Managed Care Handbook. Gaithersburg, MD: Aspen Publishers, 1996:3.

Jaklevic MC: Doc income still rising: AMA data. Mod Healthcare 1998;March 30:3.

Kongstvedt PR: Compensation of primary care physicians in open panel plans. In Kongstvedt PR (ed): The Managed Care Handbook. Gaithersburg, MD: Aspen Publishers, 1996:120.

Letsch SW: National health care spending in 1991. In Inglehart JK (ed): Debating Health Care Reform. Bethesda, MD: Project HOPE, 1993:145.

McIlrath S: DRGs for doctor pay. Am Med News 1996;October 28:27.

Mechcatie E: Vaginal hysterectomy procedures up, CDC says. OB/GYN News 1997;November 15:15.

Mohlenbrock WC: The physician imperative: define, measure and improve health care quality. Physician Executive 1998;24:47.

Phelps CE: Health Economics. New York: Harper Collins, 1992.

Rosenthal G, Harper DL, Quinn LM, Cooper GS: Severity adjusted mortality and length of stay in teaching and nonteaching hospitals. JAMA 1997;278:485.

Schieber GJ, Poullier JP, Greenwald LM: Health care spending, delivery and outcomes in OECD countries. In Inglehart JK (ed): Debating Health Care Reform. Bethesda, MD: Project HOPE, 1993:162.

Scholtes P: The Team Handbook for Educators. Madison, WI: The Joiner Associates, 1994:I-9.

Selby JV, Fireman BH, Swain BE: Effect of a copayment on use of the emergency department in a health maintenance organization. N Engl J Med 1996;334:635.

Starr P: The Social Transformation of American Medicine. New York: Basic Books, 1982.

van Amerongen D: Hospital-sponsored networks: the rush to consolidate and the future of medical practice. Physician Exec 1997;23:4.

van Amerongen D: Networks and the Future of Medical Practice. Chicago: Health Administration Press, 1998.

Weissenstein E: Managed care bills take shape. Mod Healthcare 1998;May 18:4.

Wennberg J, Gittlesohn A: Small area variation in health care delivery. Science 1973;182:1102.

Winslow R: Health care inflation revives in Minneapolis despite cost cutting. Wall Street J 1998;May 19:A-1.

SUGGESTED READING

These texts delve more deeply into managed care issues than is possible in a brief chapter, and are recommended to begin the learning process about the future for the U.S. medical care system.

Kongstvedt P (ed): The Managed Care Handbook. Gaithersburg, MD: Aspen Publishers, 1996. *A detailed text on the basics of managed care and insurance, with explanations of all the important elements and functions.*

Starr P: The Social Transformation of American Medicine. New York: Basic Books, 1982. *A Pulitzer-prize winning study of the evolution of American medicine and the political and sociological trends that have shaped it.*

van Amerongen D: Networks an the Future of Medical Practice. Chicago: Health Administration Press, 1998. *An analysis of how the delivery system is evolving as managed care attains adolescence, and what the next stages will mean to physicians.*

21

Biopsychosocial Topics in Women's Sexual Health

Teresita McCarty
Lisa M. Fromm
Laura Weiss Roberts
Maxine Dorin
Deborah J. Harrington

Women's health care has been defined as "the prevention, screening, diagnosis, and management of conditions that are unique to women, more prevalent in women, more serious among women, have different risk factors for women, and/or require different interventions in women." (ACP Committee on Women's Health, 1997). This chapter seeks to help prepare physicians to provide sound women's health care by examining four highly important but often neglected clinical topics: women's sexual response, sexual dysfunction and sexual disorders, sexual violence, and professionalism in gynecologic care.

WOMEN'S SEXUAL RESPONSE

The brain is the most important organ of human sexuality. The sexual development of the brain itself is influenced by the prenatal and postnatal hormonal environment, by genotype, and by subsequent learning and experience (Kelly, 1985). Although peripheral manifestations of human sexual responsiveness are what patients ask about, physicians must remain aware that illnesses and medications have central as well as peripheral effects upon sexual function. Because chemical treatments of sexual dysfunctions are limited, many interventions to improve sexual function are based on the brain's ability to learn. In the clinical context, this learning occurs when patients receive anticipatory guidance, education, and, when appropriate, a referral for behavioral therapy, sex therapy, and/or psychotherapy.

Phases of the Female Sexual Response Cycle

The sexual response cycle of women is characterized by four sequential phases: excitement, plateau, orgasm, and resolution. Two basic physiologic changes occur during the sexual response cycle: vasoconges-

tion and increased neuromuscular tension or myotonia. Vasocongestion occurs only in the external and internal genitalia and in the female breasts: myotonia occurs throughout the body. Table 21–1 shows the timing and integration of the phases and physiologic changes.

Excitement Phase

The excitement phase lasts a few minutes to several hours and is affected by physical as well as psychological conditions. Vasocongestion and myotonia both occur in the excitement phase. In the *breast*, the first evidence of excitement is nipple erection caused by involuntary muscle fiber contraction. The nipples do not necessarily erect simultaneously or to the same degree. They may increase in length from 0.5 to 1.0 cm, and the base diameter of the nipples may increase by 0.25 cm. During the excitement phase, increased blood flow generates an increase in the size of the breasts. The amount of increase varies among women.

In the *clitoris*, the venous engorgement causes an increase in size and consistency of the organ. The clitoris becomes hard, and in approximately 10% of women it is elongated. By stimulating the mons pubis area, which is in proximity to the clitoris, the response time can be shortened. In the *labia majora*, the response pattern for nulliparous women is different than for multiparous women. This difference can be attributed to changes in the anatomic relationship caused by birth trauma. In nulliparous women, the labia majora become thinner and flatten against the perineum. The movement of the labia in an upward and outward direction away from the vaginal opening is secondary to the venous engorgement of the labia majora and vasocongestion of the outer one third of the vagina. In multiparous women, the labia majora become rapidly congested and distended but lack the thinning seen in nulliparous women. There may be movement of the labia away from the vaginal opening but not to the same extent as seen in

Table 21–1. PERIPHERAL MANIFESTATIONS OF THE FEMALE SEXUAL RESPONSE CYCLE

	EXCITEMENT PHASE*	PLATEAU PHASE†	ORGASMIC PHASE‡	RESOLUTION PHASE§
Skin	No change	Sexual flush: inconstant; may appear on abdomen, breasts, neck, face, thighs; may resemble measles rash	No change	Flush disappears in reverse order
Breasts	Nipple erection, venous congestion, areolar enlargement	Venous pattern prominent; size may increase $1/4$ over resting state; areolae enlarge, impinge on nipples so they seem to disappear	No change	Return to normal
Clitoris	Glans: diameter increased Shaft: variable increase in diameter; elongation occurs in only 10% of subjects	Retraction: shaft withdraws deep into swollen prepuce	No change (shaft movements continue throughout if thrusting maintained)	Shaft returns to normal position in 5–10 sec; full detumescence in 5–10 min
Labia majora	Nullipara: thin down, flatten against perineum Multipara: rapid congestion and edema; increase to 2–3 times normal size	Nullipara: may swell if Phase 2 unduly prolonged Multipara: become enlarged and edematous	No change	Nullipara: increase to normal size in 1–2 min or less Multipara: decrease to normal size in 10–15 min
Labia minora	Color change: bright pink in nullipara and red in multipara Size: increase 2–3 times over normal	Color change: bright red in nullipara, burgundy red in multipara Size: enlarged labia form a funnel into vaginal orifice	Proximal areas contract with contractions of lower third	Return to resting state in 5 min
Vagina	Transudate appears 10–30 sec after onset of arousal Drops of clear fluid coalesce to form a well-lubricated vaginal barrel (aids in buffering acidity to neutral pH required by sperm)	Copious transudate can continue to form; quantity of transudate generally increased by prolonging preorgasm stimulation	No change	Some transudate collects on floor of the upper two thirds formed by its posterior wall (in the supine position)
Upper two thirds	Balloons: dilates as uterus moves up, pulling anterior vaginal wall with it; fornices lengthen; rugae flatten	Further ballooning occurs, then wall relaxes in a slow, tensionless manner	No change; fully ballooned out and motionless	Cervix descends to seminal pool in 3–4 min
Lower third	Dilation of vaginal lumen occurs; congestion of walls proceeds gradually	Maximum distention reached rapidly; contracts lumen of lower third; contraction around penis aids thrusting traction of clitoral shaft via labia and prepuce	3–15 contractions of lower third and proximal labia minora at 0.75-sec intervals	Congestion disappears in seconds; if no orgasm, congestion persists for 20–30 min
Uterus	Ascends into false pelvis in Phase 1	Contractions: strong sustained contractions begin late in Phase 2	Contractions strong throughout orgasm; strongest with pregnancy and masturbation	Slowly returns to normal position
Rectum			Inconstant rhythmic contractions	All reactions cease within a few seconds

*Duration: minutes to hours.
†Duration: 30 seconds to 3 minutes.
‡Duration: 3 to 15 seconds.
§Duration: 10 to 15 minutes; if no orgasm, 0.5 to 1 day.
From Sherfey MJ: The Nature and Evolution of Female Sexuality. New York: Random House, 1972, with permission.

nulliparous women. The *labia minora* increase two or three times in size in both nulliparous and multiparous women. As a consequence of the distention, the labia minora may protrude between the labia majora and in fact may extend the length of the vaginal vault by 1 cm. There is a color change to a bright pink hue in the nulliparous female and to a red hue in the multiparous female.

In the *vagina*, the first signal of effective sexual stimulation is the appearance of a clear vaginal secretion occurring within 10 to 20 seconds after the initiation of effective sexual stimulation. The sexual stimulation can be physical or psychological. The vaginal secretion is a transudation through the vaginal walls from the dilated venous plexus encircling the vaginal vault, and the maximal production is during the excitement phase. The appearance of droplets on the walls of the vagina is followed by coalescence of these droplets to form a well-lubricated vaginal vault that is smooth and slippery. This transudate aids in buffering the normal acidity of the vagina to a neutral pH, enhancing sperm survival. In the upper two thirds of the vagina, there is a ballooning effect with lengthening and distention. As the vagina dilates, the uterus and cervix simultaneously move upward and backward, pulling the anterior wall of the vagina with them and flattening the normal folds of the vaginal rugae. The vaginal length may increase up to 3 cm and the diameter by as much as 4 cm. The normal pink-red hue of the vaginal walls in an unstimulated vagina undergoes a change in the excitement phase to a darker purple color, which is caused by vasocongestion. The outer one third of the vagina gradually undergoes this color change as well as dilation in the excitement phase.

Plateau Phase

With adequate sexual stimulation, the sexual tension increases and the plateau phase is reached. Unlike the longer lasting excitement phase, this phase lasts only 30 seconds to 3 minutes. In the *skin and breasts*, a sexual flush is observed in 75% of females. This occasionally occurs late in the excitement phase and may be influenced by the temperature of the environment. This superficial vasocongestive flush begins at the epigastrium and spreads upward over the breasts, progressively involving the neck, face, and forehead. The flush may or may not progress over the lower abdomen, the thigh, the arms, the lower back, and even at times the buttocks. A consistent finding is that the appearance of the sexual flush in females correlates with the intensity of sexual tension. In the *breasts*, the vasocongestive phenomenon causes a further increase in size by as much as 25% over the resting state. The areolae enlarge, with a resulting illusion of a decrease in the size of the erect nipples. There is also a prominent venous pattern over the breast skin.

The *clitoris* elevates and retracts behind the clitoral hood, which does not normally interfere with the attainment of orgasm. The clitoral hood is contiguous with the labia minora, and, with the traction caused by penile or digital thrusting, there may be adequate stimulation to reach the orgasmic phase. In the *vagina*, the production of vaginal secretion continues, although not at the same rate as in the excitement phase. If the plateau phase is prolonged, the production may slow down. Continuing vasocongestion causes as much as a one-third decrease in the size of the lumen of the outer one third of the vagina established during the excitement phase. This anatomic change creates the orgasmic platform. The tenting effect, which began in the excitement phase (with the movement of the uterus and the cervix upward into the pelvis), creates an anatomic basin for seminal fluid in the posterior wall of the vagina. Maximal displacement of the uterus occurs at the end of the plateau phase. The uterus develops strong uterine contractions lasting 1 to 2 minutes late in this phase while the cervix swells and changes to a patchy purple hue.

Orgasmic Phase

The orgasmic phase is the release of vasocongestion and myotonia that developed in prior phases. It is an involuntary climax that occurs only when a threshold of maximal sexual tension is reached. This is the shortest of all the phases, lasting only a matter of seconds. This phase is sensorially focused on the pelvis, and there are *no changes observed in the skin, the breasts, the clitoris, the labia majora, and the upper two thirds of the vagina*. The *labia minora* in proximity to the vaginal opening contract with the contractions of the lower one third of the vagina or orgasmic platform. The involuntary reflexive muscle contractions of the orgasmic platform occur in 0.8-second intervals. There may be 3 to 15 contractions during orgasm. The uterine contractions initiated in the late plateau phase continue into the orgasmic phase and are found to be strongest during pregnancy and masturbation.

Resolution Phase

The final phase of the sexual response cycle is the resolution phase, which is a physiologic reversal back through the plateau and the excitement phases to the unstimulated state. The resolution phase is the most variable in its length and is dependent on the outcome of the previous phases. If orgasm is achieved, this phase can be as short as 15 minutes; when orgasm is not achieved, it may be as long as 1 day. With continued sexual stimulation, especially during the reversal through the plateau phase, multiple orgasms may be achieved.

In the *skin*, the sex flush disappears in reverse order of its appearance. There may also be a coincidental appearance of a fine sheen of perspiration, which is not indicative of the amount of physical energy expended but correlates with the intensity of the orgasm. The *breasts* decrease in size as the venous engorgement is drained and normally take 5 to 10 minutes to return to the unstimulated state. The time it takes for the breasts to return to normal depends on the size of the drainage system, so it could take longer than 10 minutes. The areolae decrease in size, with the reverse illusion of the nipples becoming erect when the erection of the nipples is actually slower to subside.

The *clitoris* returns to normal position in 5 to 10 seconds, and full return to prearousal state is achieved in 5 to 10 minutes. In the absence of orgasm, the return to prearousal state can take as long as 6 hours and often is accompanied by discomfort and irritation. The *labia majora* return rapidly to the midline position in both nulliparous and multiparous women. Divergence from the resolution pattern occurs at this stage, with the nulliparous women having an increase to normal size in 1 to 2 minutes, whereas multiparous women have a decrease in their labia majora to normal size over a longer, 10- to 15-minute period. The labia minora lose their vivid coloring over approximately 5 minutes and return to the prearousal state.

In the *vagina*, some of the transudate and semen (if present) collect in the vaginal basin on the floor of the posterior wall of the upper two thirds of the vagina in the supine position. The cervix then descends in the seminal pool over a 3- to 4-minute period and is patulous for 10 minutes. Meanwhile, the vasocongestion of the orgasmic platform disappears in seconds, and there is an increase in the lumen size of the outer one third of the vagina. The upper two thirds of the vagina returns more slowly to its collapsed prearousal state. The color of the vaginal wall requires 10 to 15 minutes to return to its normal pigment. The uterus descends with the cervix back to its normal position in the pelvis.

SEXUAL DYSFUNCTION

Assessment of Sexual Function: An Approach to the Sexual History

A woman's sexual health, her past sexual experiences, and her current sexual concerns represent clinically important data. Indeed, physicians who regularly ask sexual function questions in the course of obtaining patients histories have found that about half of their clinic patients experience problems with sex, and 91% of patients report they consider a physician asking about sexuality to be appropriate (Ende et al, 1984). Even without specific questioning, up to 10% of patients will spontaneously report having sexual difficulties (Pauly and Goldstein, 1970). Table 21–2 provides an outline for key elements of the sexual history.

Ironically, exploration of the sexual history may not occur because of the care provider's personal attitudes or discomfort with the topic—*not* because of patients' reluctance to respond to questions related to sexuality. For example, a study of senior medical students revealed that they were likely to perform inadequate sexual histories if they were shy, were unsympathetic regarding patients' psychosocial problems, believed that the sexual history was unimportant, or felt insecure and poorly trained (Merrill et al, 1990). A second study showed that medical students overall were less willing to speak with homosexual patients than with heterosexual patients (Arnow et al, 1989). A study that surveyed women college students and faculty revealed 72% were not willing to discuss sexual problems or activity because their physician seemed disinterested, rushed, or uncomfortable discussing sex, or they felt their physician was only interested in the physical aspects of gynecology (Weiss and Meadow, 1979). Such findings suggest the importance of clinician attitude and ability in caring for the sexual health of patients.

Consequently, the *first task of sexual history-taking* is overcoming obstacles to inquiring about the sexual health of patients, such as (1) having a poor knowledge base related to sexual topics; (2) feeling uncomfortable or judgmental about patients' sexual behaviors, orientation, and identities; (3) being distressed by patients' stories of sexually related violence; and (4) feeling worried that patients will misunderstand or be offended by questions connected to their sexual health. Remaining mindful and undaunted by these barriers will allow clinicians to provide better care to their patients.

Thus, despite the awkwardness that may arise, introducing the topic of sexual health is necessary in obtaining a medical history. It is helpful to forewarn a new patient about this aspect of the medical evaluation by having her complete an intake questionnaire that includes questions regarding sexual functioning. This may give the patient time to prepare for physician-directed inquiries and may increase her willingness to discuss sexual concerns. The physician can begin the interview by asking straightforward questions such as age of menarche, number of pregnancies, outcome of pregnancies, past and current use of contraception, numbers of partners, and attention to "safer sex" practices. For example, if a woman of reproductive age is not using contraception, this clinical "finding" is valuable to discuss. The answer may lead to further understanding of the patient's sexual orientation, childbearing concerns, sexual activity or abstinence, religious attitudes, and knowledge level related to sexuality. If a woman does not use "safe sex," this may allow for a discussion of risk associated with certain sexual behaviors and of the potential impact of sexually transmitted infections. *The flow of the sexual history thus moves from more concrete, factual information to more personal, psychosocially rich material along a series of related topics.* Physician-initiated questions about sexuality will

Table 21-2. SEXUAL HISTORY DOMAINS

General Information

Patient	Age, occupation, education, ethnic-cultural-religious background, gender identity, marital status

Childhood Sexuality

Family attitudes about sex	Modesty, nudity, religion, siblings
Learning about sex	Information sources; too soon, too late?
Childhood sexual beliefs	Conception, birth, body parts, gender differences
Childhood sexual activity	Genital self-stimulation, pleasure, guilt, consequences, peer sexual play, sexual abuse or exploitation by same sex or opposite sex

Physical Sexual Development

Secondary sex characteristics	Acceptance of changes, weight, size, hair distribution
Menses	Age at onset, previous awareness, reaction, social support
Pregnancies	Age, planned, number, result, breast-feeding, effect on sexual adjustment
Menopause	Age, interventions, physical and emotional adaptation

Adolescent and Adult Sexuality

Masturbation	Frequency, guilt, orgasm
Necking and petting	Age started, partners, type of activity
Body image	Body habits, gender identity, peer acceptance, self-esteem
Sex practices	Type, frequency, initiation, partners, contraception, disease protection, enjoyment, pain, orgasm
Sex in relationship	Sexual compatibility, mutual and reciprocal satisfaction, enjoyment, masturbation
Extramarital sex	Partners, attachment, frequency, emotional results, relationship effects
Sexual illnesses	Genital trauma or surgery, mastectomy, hysterectomy, sexually transmitted diseases
Sex after loss of relationship	Sex outlets, family attitudes, personal attitudes, fantasies
Sex trauma	Violence, rape, resultant fears
Sex variations	Bestiality, pedophilia, voyeurism, exhibitionism, fetishism, transexualism, transvestism

Modified from Schiff M, Fromm LM, McCarty T, et al: Sexuality (APGO Learning Objectives no 53). In Mattox JH (ed): Core Textbook of Obstetrics and Gynecology. St. Louis: CV Mosby Company, 1998:488, with permission.

make it much easier for patients to ask their own sexual questions (Table 21–3).

The specific approach to obtaining a sexual history will vary with the patient and the clinical situation. Some patients may require special sensitivity in the asking of sexual questions. This is perhaps obvious in the evaluation of a new adolescent patient. Although adolescents range from the sexually naive to the very experienced, even the sexually sophisticated teen may feel apprehensive about discussing sexual issues with an older, authoritative stranger. A physician should approach this patient with care, because alienating the adolescent may permanently color her attitude toward future health care providers. An effective approach to the adolescent can begin by instructing her about the normal stages of sexual development. Interspersing sexual questions throughout the interview with less threatening social and medical questions may help to reduce her anxiety. When rapport is established between the adolescent and the provider, more intimate questions can be introduced. Certain clinical situations, such as the case of the patient of any age who requests a human immunodeficiency virus (HIV) test, require greater attunement and awareness of the patient's physical status and psychological health. In a third

example, sexual problems may arise in established patients who have already given a full sexual history at their first visit. An alert provider will remember to ask sexual questions as conditions change for the patient. Open-ended questions regarding sexual enjoyment, effects of new medications, or effects of surgery (Table 21–4) and illness on sexual functioning can be effective in increasing communication regarding sexual issues and allow the physician the opportunity to anticipate problems before they develop. An illustration of this anticipatory approach occurs when a patient is premenopausal. Before a decrease in her natural vaginal secretions occurs, a frank discussion on the possible need for artificial lubrication can be introduced along with information on hormonal replacement. This gives the patient psychological "permission" to use lubrication, permission to continue to have sexual relationships in menopause, and permission to open up discussion regarding libido, hormones, and current sexual issues.

Like other clinical phenomena that are associated with social stigma, an area that always requires great care is the issue of childhood sexual trauma. These issues will often not be revealed in response to open-ended questions from the clinician; they may not be-

Table 21-3. SOME COMMONLY ASKED QUESTIONS ABOUT SEXUALITY

1. How does masturbation relate to physical health, psychological adjustment, and general sexual relations? Is masturbation normal or wrong?
2. Are my genitals (breasts) normal? Too small? Too large?
3. Is sex during my period safe? Can I get pregnant during my period?
4. What is normal sexual activity in frequency and pattern? Am I or my partner normal, oversexed, or undersexed?
5. Does orgasm of the woman affect conception in any way? Pregnancy? Delivery?
6. How does a woman know when she has an orgasm? Why isn't it always clear? How does my partner know?
7. Are there any contraceptives that increase or decrease libido?
8. Will contraceptives like birth control pills or foams prevent transmission of sexually transmitted diseases?
9. Are anal and oral intercourse a part of normal sexual activity?
10. Will pregnancy or childbearing affect sexuality? How?
11. Will sterilization affect sexual performance or desire?
12. Will hysterectomy affect sexual performance or desire?
13. Will menopause affect sexual performance or desire?
14. What effects on sexual activities are due to aging?
15. Is it OK not to have sex?
16. How might homosexuality affect my or my partner's being a parent?
17. Can withdrawal immediately before ejaculation or douching immediately after prevent pregnancy? Can pregnancy occur without going "all the way"?

Adapted from Diamond M: Sex and reproduction: conception and contraception. In Green R (ed): Human Sexuality. Baltimore: Williams & Wilkins, 1979; modified from Schiff M, Fromm LM, McCarty T, et al: Sexuality (APGO Learning Objectives no 53). In Mattox JH (ed): Core Textbook of Obstetrics and Gynecology. Chicago, CV Mosby Company, 1998:490, with permission.

come clarified without direct but sensitive questioning. To overcome natural barriers to discovery of childhood sexual trauma, for instance, one can ask if anything physically or sexually frightening ever happened to the patient as a child or as a young adult. The patient's response indicates whether it is

Table 21-4. POSTINTERVENTION (ILLNESS, MEDICATIONS, SURGERY) SEXUAL HISTORY

- Have you noticed a change in sexual function since . . . ?
- Has there been a change in your interest in sex, feelings of sexual desire?
- Has there been a change in your ability to become sexually aroused/turned on/excited?
- Has there been a change in your ability to reach orgasm/peak/climax?
- Has there been a change in how often you are sexually active?
- Do you feel pain or physical discomfort with sexual activity?
- Are you experiencing any emotional reactions such as embarrassment, fear, or shame since . . . ?

Adapted from Segraves RT, Schiavi RC, Wise TN: Assessing and Managing Antidepressant-Induced Sexual Dysfunction: A Physician Guide. Memphis: Physicians Postgraduate Press, Inc, 1993, with permission.

necessary to question her further on disturbing touches, molestation, and rape. Sexual traumas of childhood are such a violation of a person's sense of self that disclosure may be difficult, the reaction to the events may be confused or fragmented, and medical or psychological consequences denied. The perpetrator may threaten injury to the victim to prevent discovery, and the child frequently is made to feel she is at fault. Shame, fear, and guilt evoke the need to push or set aside the memories from everyday awareness or to continue to conceal the experience. Especially if the child reported the incident and was not believed and protected, irreparable damage to her sense of self-worth and ability to trust in caregivers is possible. If one obtains this kind of sexual history, it is important to discover if the patient has successfully resolved the issues and obtained any necessary treatment for the psychological as well as the physical consequences. If significant emotional symptoms remain, the patient should have a careful and appropriate referral for psychological treatment as well as continued medical follow-up.

In sum, obtaining a complete sexual history from a patient is not an easy task. Yet an accurate sexual history in the context of a larger medical evaluation can uncover organic causes for sexual dysfunction, prevent undesired pregnancies, interrupt the spread of sexually transmitted diseases, and help in alleviating suffering. Moreover, it may offer reassurance and helpful information about patient concerns ranging from normal development to fears of serious disease. With patience, empathy, knowledge of human sexuality, and professionalism, the sexual history may be gathered competently and a therapeutic dialogue regarding sexual health established.

Causes of Sexual Dysfunction

Sexual dysfunction may be transient, intermittent, or enduring, and it is, by its clinical definition, distressing to the individuals who experience its various manifestations. Illness, or the treatments provided for illness, are frequent triggers for sexual dysfunction. Sexual dysfunction may also be associated with mental illnesses and with situational or enduring psychological distress. Sexual dysfunction may resolve spontaneously or may require specific treatment.

Negative Sexual Effects of Illness

Many sorts of illnesses may cause sexual dysfunction among many women. The psychological and physiological effects of mental or physical illness can alter any or all phases of the female sexual response cycle. For instance, chronic and acutely ill patients alike may experience significant and wide-ranging sexual problems such as lack of desire, disinterest, malaise, or guilt related to their underlying illnesses; physical discomfort with sexual activity; or anorgasmia secondary to pain or altered neurologic function. Some diseases have a direct impact on sexual functioning because they affect the areas in the brain or in the body that regulate sexual activity. This is particularly true when the disease is neurologic, neuromuscular, or endocrinologic in nature. In these categories, the peripheral nervous system, the hypothalamic-pituitary-gonadal axis, and the end organs themselves (vulva, vagina, cervix, and uterus) may be directly affected. It is important to note that sexual dysfunction resulting from medical illnesses may persist long after resolution of the medical symptoms. Mental illnesses are also commonly complicated by sexual dysfunction. For example, depressive disorders may be characterized by diminished libido or arousal, and sometimes orgasmic dysfunction. Bipolar disorder patients may become hypersexual while manic but then suffer a loss of sexual interest and function during the depressed phase of the illness. Rituals, fears of contamination, or an obsessive need for cleanliness may preclude sexual activity in patients with obsessive compulsive disorder. Patients with post traumatic stress disorder (PTSD) or generalized anxiety may suffer many fears that prevent interest or enjoyment. Of course, substance abuse may have immediate and long-term effects on sexual performance depending on the substance used, the dosage, and the duration of use (American Psychiatric Association, 1994). Examples of illnesses associated with sexual dysfunction are listed in Table 21–5.

Negative Sexual Effects of Medications

Although there is now an emphasis on obtaining information from female research subjects, clinical reports and studies of men are the primary sources of information about the sexual side effects of medications. Although changes in sexual functioning in men may be more apparent than in women, the belief is that medications induce similar changes in both sexes. It is also assumed, but seldom verified, that a medication that causes impotence in men will impair excitement and orgasm in women. More research is necessary in order to clarify the true impact of most medications on women's sexual functioning.

Medications especially likely to cause sexual dysfunction are antihypertensive agents, histamine$_2$ receptor blockers, and psychotropic medications, including antidepressants (Abramowicz, 1987) (Table 21–6). Whereas most medications have an adverse effect on sexual function, there are some drugs (e.g., androgens) that can actually increase libido or increase the tendency to orgasm (Table 21–7). Moreover, it is reported that low dose of alcohol and marijuana may increase sexual desire, but these and other illicit drugs that are central nervous system depressants (e.g., narcotics, barbiturates), commonly will diminish sexual desire and inhibit sexual functioning.

Examples of Sexual Dysfunction

Two clinical examples of sexual dysfunction are dyspareunia and vaginismus. In *dyspareunia*, patients complain of painful intercourse. It is important to determine whether this pain is located at the introitus or deeper, and whether the pain occurs as the penis is introduced to the vagina, with deep thrusting of the penis, and/or throughout intercourse. Additionally, questions of onset, duration, and symptoms associated with the pain are important in helping to evaluate the complaint. *Pain at the onset of intercourse* has many causes. On a physical examination, it is easy to diagnose an infection, an irritative process from an external source, a congenital malformation, an injury from birth trauma, or an infection of the bladder or urethra. A very inflamed, tender vulva is a clue to look for infection, deodorants, detergents, or even the lubricants and spermicide used during sexual activity as the culprit. Dyspareunia may be due to dryness from premature penetration (inadequate time spent in the excitement phase), medications interfering with lubrication, or estrogen-deprived states such as menopause. When the pain is reproduced on palpation of the bladder and urethra, cystitis or urethritis must be considered. Pain from malformation and injuries is usually apparent or can be localized with a Q-tip. *Pain from deep thrusting* of the penis is more likely to result from pathologic pelvic anatomy; consequently, it is important to eliminate pelvic disease as a cause. Adhesions caused by surgical procedures or infection, endometriosis, pelvic inflammatory disease, ectopic pregnancy, ovarian cysts, and pelvic tumors must be considered. Finally, fear of pain associated with intercourse may aggravate dyspareunia.

Vaginismus is defined as involuntary spasms of the paravaginal and levator ani muscles and manifests itself whenever vaginal entry is attempted. In its milder form it causes dyspareunia, and in its most severe form it prevents vaginal entry. The latter is a common cause of unconsummated marriages. Because it is a conditioned reflex, it can be reproduced within insertion of the speculum during the pelvic examination. Vaginismus often has a psychological component: the stimulus for the conditioned response may be related to feelings of guilt, fear, anger, and/or loss of control. These patients may have a history of rape, sexual abuse, or other difficulties associated with sexuality. For these reasons, dyspareunia and vaginismus illustrate the importance of a biopsychosocial evaluation of sexual dysfunction.

Overview of Therapeutic Approaches to Sexual Dysfunction

Until the middle of this century, the human sexual response was viewed as a single continuous event. That is, it spanned from lust to orgasm without differentiation. Therefore, the disorders of sexual response were believed to originate from a single pro-

Table 21–5. MEDICAL CONDITIONS THAT INTERFERE WITH SEXUAL FUNCTIONING IN WOMEN

Neurologic Disorders Affecting Sex Centers in Brain
Arnold-Chiari malformation
Cardiovascular accident
Central nervous system tumors
Encephalitis
Head trauma
Hypothalamic lesions
Pituitary tumor
Temporal lobe epilepsy

Neurologic Disorders Affecting Spinal Cord and Peripheral Nerves
Alcoholic neuropathy*
Amyotropic lateral sclerosis
Diabetes mellitus*
Herniated lumbar disc
Lumbar canal stenosis
Multiple sclerosis*
Myelitis (polio)
Neoplastic spinal cord disease
Paraplegia and other spinal cord injuries
Peripheral neuropathies
Posterior urethral rupture
Radical pelvic surgery
Retroperitoneal lymphadenectomy
Surgical sympathectomy
Syringomyelia
Tabes dorsalis
Vitamin deficiencies

Cardiovascular and Pulmonary Disease
Asthma
Cardiac disease
Coronary artery disease
Hypertension*
Postcoronary syndrome
Poststroke syndrome

Endocrine Disorders
Acromegaly
Addison's disease
Cushing's disease
Diabetes mellitus*
Hypopituitarism
Pituitary tumor
Prolactin-secreting pituitary adenoma
Thyroid deficiency*
Testosterone deficiency* (natural aging, chemotherapy or surgical removal of adrenals, ovaries or pituitary)

Renal and Urologic Disorders
Chronic renal failure
Chronic interstitial cystitis*
Cystitis
Dialysis
Nephritis
Urethral prolapse
Urethritis

Gynecologic Disorders
Causes of pain on manipulation
 Labial pathology (infections, injury)*
 Clitoral problems (irritation, lesions, hypersensitivity)
Causes of pain on entry
 Hymenal irregularities
 Vulvovaginitis* (*Candida albicans, trichomonas, herpes, atrophy, chemical irritation*)*
 Bartholin's and skene glands (cyst, infection)
 Inadequate lubrication*
 Trauma (episiotomy, operative scarring)*
Causes of mid/deep vaginal pain
 Congenital shortened vagina
 Pelvic inflammatory disease
 Endometriosis*
 Fixed uterine retroversion
 Ovarian pathology
 Pelvic congestion
 Uterine contractions on orgasm (from hypoestrogenic states)
 Pelvic tumors
 Surgical adhesions

Miscellaneous
Anemia
Arthritis
Carcinoid syndrome (elevated serotonin)
Degenerative diseases
Hemochromatosis
Infections (e.g., acquired immunodeficiency syndrome)
Malnutrition
Liver disease (hepatitis, alcoholic cirrhosis, postmononucleosis hepatitis)
Lower bowel disease*
Malignancies (advanced)
Musculoskeletal disorders*
Pelvic fracture
Radiation therapy
Surgical procedures*

*Frequent cause of sexual difficulties.
From Roberts LW, Fromm LM, Bartlick BD: Sexuality of women through the life phases. In Wallis LA (ed): Textbook of Women's Health. Philadelphia: Lippincott-Raven, 1998:772, with permission.

found cause. It was not until the 1970s that Helen Kaplan introduced the contemporary perspective (Kaplan, 1969, 1974). She described the existence of a sexual desire phase that has no physiologic basis as defined by Masters and Johnson (1970). She combined the excitement phase with the plateau phase because they both involve vasocongestion, and she maintained the orgasmic phase by itself. Because there are no known disorders associated with resolution phase, she eliminated it. Her triphasic model of sexuality incorporates three phases: sexual desire, excitement, and orgasm. Disorders associated with

each of the phases are discussed below along with their treatment.

Treatment of Sexual Complaints Resulting from Illness or Medication

For treatment of sexual complaints in the context of medical or mental illness, it is helpful to note that the sexual effects of brief illnesses usually are temporary and require no therapy. Sexual dysfunction caused by more persistent health problems may be best dealt with by addressing the underlying illness

Table 21-6. MEDICATIONS AND SUBSTANCES THAT ADVERSELY AFFECT SEXUAL FUNCTIONING

Psychotropics
Tricyclic antidepressants
  Clomipramine (Anafranil)
  Amitriptyline (Elavil)
  Doxepin (Sinequan)
  Imipramine (Tofranil)
  Nortriptyline* (Aventyl)
  Desipramine* (Norpramin)
Monoamine oxidase inhibitors
  Isocarboxazid (Marplan)
  Phenelzine (Nardil)
  Tranylcypromine* (Parnate)
Serotonin uptake inhibitors[†]
  Fluoxetine (Prozac)
  Paroxetine (Paxil)
  Sertraline (Zoloft)
  Fluvoxamine (Luvox)
  Venlafaxine (Effexor)
Mood stabilizers/anticonvulsants
  Lithium carbonate*
  Valproate* (Depakote)
  Carbamazepine (Tegretol)
  Phenytoin (Dilantin)
  Phenobarbitol (Dosette)
Antipsychotics/neuroleptics
  Phenothiazines
    Chlorpromazine (Thorazine)
    Fluphenazine* (Prolixin)
    Perphanazine* (Trilafon)
    Thioridazine (Mellaril)
  Other
    Haloperidol* (Haldol)
    Thiothixine* (Navane)
    Risperidone (Risperdal)

Anxiolytics/tranquilizers[†]
Benzodiazepines

Diuretics
Thiazide type
  Chlorthalidone (Hygroton)
Loop diuretics
  Furosemide (Lasix)
Potassium sparing
  Spironolactone (Aldactone)

Antihypertensives
Reserpine (Serpasil)
Methyldopa (Aldomet)
Guanethidine (Ismelin)
β-Blockers
  Propranolol (Inderal)
  Atenolol* (Tenormin)
  Metoprolol (Lopressor)
  Bisoprolol* (Zebeta)
  Timolol (Timoptic)
  Betaxolol* (Betoptic)

α_1-Blockers*
Prazosin* (Minipress)
Doxazosin* (Cardura)

α_2-Blockers
Clonidine (Catapres)
Guanfacine (Tenex)

Angiotensin-converting enzyme inhibitors*
Captopril* (Capoten)
Enalapril* (Vasotec)

Calcium channel blockers*
Amlodipine* (Norvasc)
Verapamil* (Calan, Isoptin)
Diltiazem* (Cardizem)

Anticancer drugs
Vinblastine (Methotrexate)
5-Fluorouracil (Efudex)
Tamoxifen* (Nolvadex)

Cold/allergy medications
Chlorphenirmaine[†] (Chlor-Trimeton)
Diphenhydramine hydrochloride (Benadryl)
Pseudoephedrine[†] (Sudafed)

Antiulcer medications
Cimetidine (Tagamet)
Famotidine* (Pepcid)
Nixatidine* (Axid)

Anorectics
Phentermine (Ionamin, Fastin)
Fenfluramine (Pondamin)
Phenylpropanolamine* (Mahuang, Ephedra, Mormon tea, Dexatrim, Acutrim, Ayds)
Diethylpropion (Tenuate)
Mazindol (Sandrex)

Drugs of abuse[†]
Alcohol
Barbiturates
Cannabis
Cocaine
Opioids
Methylphenidate
Amphetamine
Nicotine

Hormones
Progesterone
Cortisol

*Thought to have fewer sexual side effects than others in class.
[†]May sometimes heighten sexual responsivity.

and/or by treating the aggravating symptoms when possible. Placing the origin of the sexual difficulty in the desire, arousal, or orgasmic phase facilitates evaluation and treatment. By informing a patient of the possible sexual effects of an illness or its treatment, sexual dysfunction in many cases may be prevented. Sometimes patients reveal a pre-existing sexual dysfunction when informed of possible sexual side effects of a new illness or therapy. However, one cannot assume that patients who seem reconciled to their chronic illness have adapted well to the associated sexual dysfunction. Delving into the patient's adjustment may uncover poor adaptations on the part of the patient and her partner.

When medication results in sexual dysfunction, alterations can sometimes be made to alleviate the problem. The dosage of the medication can be decreased until sexual functioning returns and then gradually increased to adequate therapeutic levels. If this is not an option, sexual activity can be scheduled to occur just before the next medication dose, when the blood level of the drug will be at its nadir. If neither of these choices is feasible, an attempt should be made to find an alternative medication with a different mechanism of action. Sometimes an alternative medication is not possible, so the patient must remain on the medication that causes sexual dysfunction. Fortunately, as time passes, the patient may find that the side effect of the drug diminishes (tachyphylaxis), and she may learn techniques useful in maximizing her sexual response. The health care provider should be aware of the possible side effects of the prescribed drugs and discuss them with the patient. The patient will then be less alarmed if a sexual dysfunction develops and will be more likely to seek assistance.

Sex Therapy

Sex therapy involves a combination of education, behavioral therapy, and psychodynamic therapy. The severity of the psychological dysfunction will determine which therapy is appropriate. Although sex therapy can be performed with individuals, it is best when both partners participate. Sex therapy can be used effectively as an adjunct to medical management for organically caused sexual dysfunction. It is important that the contribution of the underlying medical disease be recognized, but how much of the

Table 21-7. MEDICATION CLASSES WITH VARIABLE EFFECTS ON SEXUAL RESPONSIVENESS

DRUG	LIBIDO	EFFECT ON SEXUAL FUNCTION	
		Arousal or Erection	*Orgasm or Ejaculation*
Hormonal Agents			
Androgens	Increased	Increased (men)	Increased in men
GnRH	Decreased in men	Decreased in men	Decreased in men
Estrogens	Decreased in men; variable in women	May cause impotence in men	Delay
Thyroxin	Increased	—	—
Adrenal steroids	Decreased in high doses	—	—
Alcohol/Drugs of Abuse			
Alcohol	Initially increased	Reduced	Impaired; correlates with blood levels
Barbiturates	Reduced	Reduced	—
Narcotics	Impaired in high doses	Impaired in high doses	Impaired in high doses
Amphetamines/cocaine	Enhanced with low doses; reduced with high doses	Decreased with chronic use	Increased with low doses; diminishes with high doses
Marijuana	Variable	Decreased in chronic hashish users	—
Psychotropic Agents			
MAO-inhibiting antidepressants	May be increased	—	Impaired
Phenelzine	Reduced in 30%	—	—
Tricyclic antidepressants	May be impaired	May be impaired	May be impaired; may cause spontaneous seminal emission
Imipramine	Reduced in 20%	—	27% of women report orgasmic delay
Clomipramine	Reduced	—	96% anorgasmic
Serotonin uptake inhibitors			
Fluoxetine	—	May be impaired; vaginal anesthesia	May be impaired; 24–75% report orgasmic delay
Sertraline	Reduced/no change	—	47% report orgasmic delay
Paroxetine	Reduced	—	20–30% orgasmic delay
Venlafaxine	Reduced	—	20–30% orgasmic delay
Fluoxamine	—	—	10–12% orgasmic delay (dose related)
Lithium carbonate	Reduced; impaired	Impaired	—
Neuroleptic agents	May be decreased	Impaired (rarely priapism)	Retrograde ejaculation rarely
Antianxiety agents	Variable	Impaired with chronic use	—
Miscellaneous antidepressants			
Trazodone	None; increased	None; may cause priapism	None; may be impaired, rarely spontaneous orgasms
Nefazodone	No change	—	No effect
Bupropion	Increased	Report of clitoral priapism	7% orgasmic delay
Mirtazapine	—	Reduced nocturnal erections; no change daytime	Initial reports no effect

Abbreviations: GnRH, gonadotropin-releasing hormone; MAO, monoamine oxidase.
Data from Kaplan (1979, 1983), Rees (1983), Seagraves (1998); adapted from Cummings JL: Clinical Neuropsychiatry. Orlando, FL: Grune & Stratton, 1985:244, with permission. Copyright © 1985 by Allyn & Bacon.

dysfunction can be attributed to the disease may be difficult to delineate.

Emotional or psychological *conflicts* may cause sexual dysfunction. A patient's *immediate emotional response* to the initiation of physical intimacy has a direct impact on the outcome of the sexual experience. Distaste, ignorance, fear, anger, anxiety, and detachment can all interfere with positive sexual responsiveness. Distaste for an unclean partner; ignorance of anatomy and normal sexual function-

ing; fear of failing to satisfy; anger directed toward the partner for an unrelated event; anxiety about work, household chores, and/or bills; and spectatoring (detachment) are examples of immediate emotions that interfere with sexual response. These are usually easily treated by brief behavioral or supportive therapy.

Dysfunctions originating from the more profound or enduring conflicts may require long-term psychotherapy. These conflicts may be the result of cultural or religious teachings or the result of conditioned fears from personal experience, such as rape. These experiences have enormous power to elicit an unconscious response during any phase of sexual activity. The unconscious nature of sexual dysfunction caused by such conflicts is more difficult to treat and less likely to resolve.

DISORDERS OF SEXUAL DESIRE AND THEIR TREATMENT

A disorder of sexual desire is defined as a persistent lack of interest in sexual activity. A *primary disorder* is diagnosed when interest never existed, and a *secondary disorder* is diagnosed when interest existed at one time but is now lost. Secondary disorders are commonly caused by organic dysfunctions, situational conditions, or inhibitions. Illness, stress, and rape are examples of reasons for a secondary disorder. Treatment of a primary disorder of sexual desire involves psychotherapy and sex therapy. Treatment of a secondary disorder of sexual desire involves uncovering and treating the underlying cause.

DISORDERS OF SEXUAL EXCITEMENT AND THEIR TREATMENT

A disorder of sexual excitement occurs when vasocongestion fails to effect and preserve sufficient lubrication and engorgement during sexual activity. Commonly there is an accompanying problem with orgasm. After a thorough evaluation for organic causes, the psychological causes need to be uncovered. Disorders of sexual excitement are most often treated using a combination of behavioral and insight-oriented therapy.

Behavioral therapy for disorders of sexual excitement involves the couple. In the first step, each partner is interviewed individually, and then the couple is interviewed together to gather a complete history and to gain insight into their individual and joint difficulties. The treatment requires participation of both partners to prevent the tendency of one partner to blame the other. During this step of therapy, the couple is prohibited from engaging in any sexual activity except as prescribed by the therapist. The next step begins with relaxed, nonsexual touching and open communication. Once the couple is comfortable with this step, they progress to exploration of the erotic areas of their bodies. Next, the therapist prescribes specific sexual stimulation or masturbation. The goals of therapy are to provide accurate information, to decrease performance fears, and to increase open communication. Once reassured that they and their bodies function normally, the couple resume normal sexual activity.

Similarly, vaginismus responds successfully to sex therapy involving gradual dilation of the vagina opening with either lubricated fingers or graduated dilators. When the largest dilator or the patient's three middle fingers can be comfortably introduced into the vagina, the patient is ready for penile penetration.

INHIBITION OF ORGASM AND ITS TREATMENT

Orgasm can be achieved only if a maximal tension threshold is reached through stimulation, and involuntary reflexive contractions of the genital muscles occur. Inhibition of orgasm can range from mild to total and may occur under voluntary or unconscious control. *Primary preorgasmia* occurs when an orgasm has never been achieved by a woman either with stimulation from coitus or masturbation. This is an uncommon and serious dysfunction treated by prescribing masturbation and practicing Kegel exercises. Kegel exercises are performed by contracting the pubococcygeal muscles that are necessary to stop urination. *Secondary inhibition*, or *anorgasmia*, occurs in women who have experienced orgasm previously. This is a common complaint and can be treated successfully with sex therapy, especially if it arises from more superficial immediate emotional responses. If deeper factors exist for either primary or secondary inhibitions of orgasm, psychotherapy may be required.

Paraphilias

Sexual variations or paraphilias associated with sexual dysfunction need to be examined if the sexual practices cause patient distress. The degree of distress is often associated with the degree of acceptance and accommodation by the partner. Deeper factors leading to these less common sexual practices need not be examined when the sexual activity occurs between consenting adults. However, a physician must attempt to uncover any *illegal* sexual activity, such as child sexual activity, and report it to the appropriate authorities when necessary. Table 21–8 contains a list of paraphilias and descriptions.

SEQUELAE OF SEXUAL VIOLENCE

Interpersonal violence and the unethical use of power are often expressed via sexualized conduct. This section discusses child sexual abuse, rape, and domestic violence. These are topics that distress all involved, including the treating physicians. An effective response requires an informed physician who maintains equanimity and an attitude of compassion while responding to the patient on the foundation of the available knowledge and with specific skills. Each of the three topics is defined, statistics are provided to indicate the magnitude of the problem, and any unique features are discussed. Then the duties of the physician, including obtaining the history, performing the examination, providing treatment, and anticipating and managing possible sequelae, are described.

Table 21-8. PARAPHILIAS

PARAPHILIA	DESCRIPTION
Fetishism (nonliving object)	Sexual excitement or gratification is derived from substitution of some inanimate object, or some part of the body, for a human love object. The inanimate love object is often associated with some part of the body (i.e., underwear, stocking, shoes). This is a sexual disorder peculiar to men, although kleptomania in women, sometimes a source of sexual excitement, is also considered a fetish.
Transvestism	Sexual excitement or gratification from wearing the clothing and enacting the role of the opposite sex
Zoophilia (beastiality)	Sexual gratification through intercourse with animals
Pedophilia	Pathologic sexual interest in children of the same or opposite sex; the disorder is most commonly attributed to adult males
Exhibitionism	Exposure of the body, especially the genitalia, as a means of attracting sexual attention or achieving sexual excitement or gratification; the term is popularly used synonymously with "show-off"
Voyeurism	Sexual pleasure derived from watching others, especially those in the nude; synonymous with "peeping Tom"
Masochism	Sexual pleasure from enduring physical or psychologic pain, which may be self-inflicted or inflicted by others
Sadism	Sexual excitement or gratification from inflicting physical pain on others; also refers to excessive cruelty not necessarily associated with sexual behaviors
Pyromania	Sexual excitement and gratification from starting and watching fires; at times the pyromaniac achieves chief pleasure from witnessing the extinction of a fire; this apparently reassures him or her that underlying feelings can be controlled

Child Sexual Abuse

Definition

Child sexual abuse is sexual activity involving a child and an adult or significantly older child (Larson et al, 1994). The much older term, *incest*, is the "sexual exploitation of a child by an older person in a parental role" (Goodwin, 1989). *Legally*, incest occurs when the child and the older person are defined as "related." Because many unrelated people assume authority in a child's life, the *clinical* definition of incest is expanded to include unrelated people who act in parental roles. Using the newer terminology, child sexual abuse, allows legal and social services structures originally developed to protect children from physical abuse to intervene in cases of sexual abuse as well (Goodwin, 1989). The terms *incest* and *sexual abuse* are used interchangeably except when prevalence data specific to incest are presented.

Incidence and Prevalence

Statistics regarding child sexual abuse vary widely. The principal sources of data are federal epidemiology studies, child protection and law enforcement data, and retrospective studies of adults (Finkelhor, 1994). In a review in which 19 adult prevalence studies were factored into annual child protective agency reports, Finkelhor estimated that 500,000 children a year become child sexual abuse victims. Of those cases, 150,000 end up being reported and substantiated. In the vast majority of child sexual abuse cases, the child knows the assailant. Rimsza and Niggemann (1982) reported that only 18% of children were assaulted by strangers. In the same study, 51% of the children suffered a single assault and nearly 33% suffered repeated assaults over a period ranging from 1 week to 9 years.

The prevalence of child sexual abuse in the United States is conservatively estimated at 20% of all girls (Finkelhor, 1994). The average girl's incestuous experience lasts 4 years and includes more than 20 sexual occurrences during those years (Courtois, 1988). The extent and severity of the sexual abuse often increase with time. Incest most commonly begins between ages 7 and 13 years (Finkelhor, 1994), but at least 11% are first abused before the age of 5 years (Russell, 1986). Data from survey studies consistently underestimate the number of women who were abused at a very young age (Herman and Schatzow, 1987). Memories are stored differently in preverbal and early verbal children, and, when questioned as adults, these women may be unable to report in a coherent manner the sexual trauma they experienced as children.

Russell (1986) gathered rigorous data, and the findings indicate a fairly uniform percentage of incest victims across most ethnic groups in the United States. Ninety per cent of sexual abuse is perpetrated by men (Finkelhor, 1994) and women raised with stepfathers were more likely to have been abused than women raised with their biologic fathers. Large percentages of prostitutes, up to 65%, report childhood sexual abuse (James and Meyerding, 1977; Silbert and Pines, 1981; Steele and Alexander, 1981; Browne and Finkelhor, 1986). Adult retrospective studies find that girls in upper-income families may be sexually abused more often than those of lower socioeconomic status (SES) (Russell, 1986), although children from lower SES households are more likely to turn up on child protective case loads (Finkelhor, 1994). Lesbian women experience a significantly higher (Gundlach, 1977) rate of childhood incest:

38% (Simari and Baskin, 1982) compared with 20% of the general population. Risk factors that show up consistently "are children who are separated from their parents or children whose parents have problems that substantially compromise their ability to supervise and attend to their children." (Finkelhor, 1994:48). Finkelhor continues to warn that too much reliance on these criteria will cause many abused children to be overlooked.

Belief and Skepticism

Victims of child sexual abuse may not appear credible. We expect a logical history, with congruence of fact and emotion. When this does not happen, we begin to doubt the veracity of the patient. Sgroi et all (1982) suggested that incest is one of those clinical situations in which the reward for denial on the part of the physician may even exceed the reward for denial by the patient. When a child reports an incest experience, physicians must begin a series of reports, examinations, and referrals that may seem to be outside their role. The results are often unsatisfactory: angry parents, medical confusion, and wrenching exposure to horrible human conduct. It is much easier to decide the child's story is not credible and keep "Pandora's box" closed.

The way children tell us about events depends on their developmental stage. Very young children may act out part of the story while talking about unrelated issues. Their narrative mixes fantasy and reality. A school-age child can supply the facts but often lacks the "appropriate" emotional responses. Goodwin (1989) pointed out that teenagers commonly tell about their incest experiences at the precise moment they are least likely to be believed. For example, they choose to tell about incest with their stepfather when they become pregnant by their boyfriend. Although such a revelation is seen as a lie to distract from irresponsible behavior, it actually makes psychological sense to tell about the abuse at the time when the adolescent's sexual activity has become obvious. The topic has now been opened for discussion, as if the adolescent has been given permission to tell.

Patients sometimes revert to the emotional and cognitive age at which the abuse occurred when they first begin to talk about it. This creates cognitive dissonance for the physician and feels manipulative and irritating, so the patient's account is not believed. However, if the patient had to partition those memories out of everyday awareness, it makes psychological sense that the patient has to return to that original feeling and cognitive state to gather enough information to tell about the experience.

Physicians may also disbelieve their patients when the accounts become too horrible. Skepticism is the scientific stance; it is also the stance that allows a physician to maintain emotional equilibrium in the face of terrible realities. Historically, physicians have not been good at recognizing or reporting the physical effects of child abuse. Believing that incest does

not occur or that it occurs but does not warrant investigation in *this* patient permits the physician to maintain his or her own defenses.

RAPE

Definition

Rape is forcible carnal knowledge of a female against her will. This includes completed sexual assaults and attempts to commit sexual assault by force or threat of force (Federal Bureau of Investigation [FBI], 1989). In recent years, rape laws have been revised to include forced intercourse regardless of the victim's mental state (drugged, unconscious), sexual assault on children by family and nonfamily members, date rape, and marital rape.

Incidence and Prevalence

In one study of a community population, 44% of women reported an attempted or completed rape, and 24% reported a completed rape (Russell, 1982). There has been a striking increase in sexual assault reports over the prior two decades. There were 97,464 forcible rapes (72 of every 100,000 women in the United States) reported in 1995 (FBI, 1995), contrasted with slightly over 37,000 rapes reported in 1970 (Burgess and Holmstrom, 1974). The FBI estimated that only 10% to 20% of sexual assaults are reported to the authorities (Geist, 1988), and independent studies support the fact that rape is one of the most under-reported crimes (Binder, 1981; Russell, 1982).

Single women ages 17 through 25 years are at the highest risk of being raped. Up to 50% of college women report acquaintance or "date" rape (Rose, 1993). A non-Hispanic white woman with some college education has a 26% chance of being raped in her lifetime. Three quarters of the victims know their assailant, and over half experience harm or threat of harm (Sorensen et al, 1987). Approximately one third of all sexual assaults include oral or anal penetration in addition to vaginal penetration. Forty per cent of rape victims suffer nongenital injuries in addition to the sexual assault (Geist, 1988). At highest risk of injuries are older women and children (Hayman and Lanza, 1971). Fighting back during the sexual assault not only increases the risk of injuries requiring medical attention but also increases the victim's chances of escaping the assailant before completion of the rape (Marchbanks et al, 1990).

Misconceptions

Because physicians play a central role in gathering evidence and helping the victim cope with the aftermath of sexual assault, they must be careful to be knowledgeable and to avoid common misconceptions about rape. Patients can experience an even greater sense of violation when the treating physician holds judgmental attitudes about the causes and consequence of rape. One misconception is that rape is a crime of sexual passion and the rapist is "over-sexed" or "sexually frustrated." In fact, *rape is an act of violence* in which the rapist uses sexuality to show dominance and/or to humiliate the victim. Groth et al (1977) defined two types of rape: the power rape and the anger rape. Power rapes are most common, outnumbering anger rapes by 2 to 1. The *power rapist* wants control over another human being. His goal is to achieve submission in the victim and reassure himself that he is not inadequate or worthless. The power rapist often has the fantasy that his victim will eventually come to like the act. It is not his conscious intent to harm the victim, so it is not surprising that victims of power rapes are rarely injured physically. The *anger rapist* wants to abuse or degrade the victim. He uses sexuality to release hatred and rage. He beats the victim, sexually assaults her, and frequently forces her to perform degrading acts. A subtype of the anger rape is the anger excitation or sadistic variety. In this type of rape, violence is erotically stimulating to the rapist. The focus of violence or torture may be on sexual areas of the victim's body, and in many cases the victim does not survive (Hicks, 1988). A rapist may move from one type of rape to another, may commit multiple rapes, and often becomes more violent as he continues to rape.

Another misconception is that the victim brings an attack upon herself, and that she deserves to be raped because of her actions, intoxicated state, or manner of dress. Regardless of the circumstances, however, *no one deserves* the degrading and illegal act of sexual assault. A nonjudgmental attitude is important, especially when asking how the patient responded to the rapist. Reassurance that the patient was correct in how she handled the assault is therapeutic (Burgess and Holmstrom, 1976). The fact that the patient survived means that she handled the situation well.

Domestic Violence

Definition

Domestic violence occurs between partners in an ongoing relationship (Goldberg and Tomlanovich, 1984). A *battered woman* is defined as a woman over the age of 16 years who has been physically abused on at least one occasion at the hands of an intimate male partner (Rounsaville and Weissman, 1977-1978). The *battered wife syndrome* is a symptom complex that occurs when a woman receives deliberate, severe, and repeated (more than three times) physical abuse from her husband, with the most minimal injury being severe bruising (Parker and Shumacher, 1977). Violent acts have been classified from the least to the most severe. The range includes verbal abuse, threats of violence, throwing an object or throwing an object at someone, pushing, slapping, kicking, hit-

ting, beating up, and threatening with and without use of a weapon. Although battering is most often viewed as physical abuse, psychological battering is an integral part of the syndrome. Many definitions also include concepts of intentionality and the repetitive nature of the assaults (Richwald and McCluskey, 1985).

Incidence and Prevalence

In the United States, women are more likely to be assaulted, injured, raped, or killed by a male partner than by any other type of assailant (Browne and Williams, 1987). Approximately 40% of all American marriages will experience at least one incident of violence. Between 2 and 6 million women are battered annually (Stark et al, 1979; Straus et al, 1980), which translates to one woman being battered every 5 to 16 seconds, assuming only one act of domestic violence per couple per year. One in nine women who present to the emergency room has been found to come for care in response to domestic violence, regardless of the original chief compliant (Abbott et al, 1995). It is estimated that between one third and one half of all female homicide victims are killed by their male partners (Gelles and Cornell, 1983). As staggering as these statistics are, they do not reflect unreported crimes, and woman battering is frequently unrecognized

Relationship to Child Abuse

When a woman is battered by her partner, it is very likely that her children are also beaten. In one study, 53% of men who battered their partners also mistreated their children, and one third of the men threatened to batter their children. Of the women in the same relationship, 28% said they had abused their children, with 6% threatening to batter their children at the time of their evaluation (Walker, 1984).

Battering During Pregnancy

Physical abuse during pregnancy has been termed prenatal child abuse. Battering may intensify or begin when a woman is pregnant. In one study of 742 pregnant women, 82 (11%) of the women reported having experienced battering in the past, and 29 of these women stated that the battering was continuing during the current pregnancy. An increase of abuse during pregnancy was reported by 21%, whereas 36% noted a decrease in abuse (Hillard, 1985). Violence during pregnancy is frequently directed at the abdomen, whereas battering in the nonpregnant state generally affects the regions of the head, chest, breasts, and arms (Hilberman, 1980).

Why Women Stay in Battering Relationships

Women stay in battering relationships for a variety of reasons: low self-esteem, expecting to be abused because of a family history of violence, fear and isolation, helplessness, economic dependence, beliefs about marriage and relationships, self-blame because of societal attitudes toward battered women, and minimization when the abuse is not frequent or severe.

A woman may have *low self-esteem* before she enters an abusive relationship, but she also may acquire it as a result of the relationship. At one time, mental health professionals believed that a person's basic sense of self-worth was established during childhood and formed primarily by the influence of parental figures. We now know that, even in adult life, other adults can seriously affect how we feel about ourselves and contribute to the development of major psychiatric disorders.

Sometimes a victim stays in the relationship because of *distorted expectations* resulting from a family history of violence. She has always been battered: It is familiar, and she does not expect to be treated any other way. Therapeutically, it is important to recall that psychological development for the most part parallels physical development in that growth occurs through the taking of a series of small steps (Benjamin, 1984). A victim's first step, then, may be to choose someone who is *less* physically abusive than her parents. To a victim with a history of violence, a healthy relationship would feel unfamiliar: she would not know how to respond, and she would not have a sense of belonging. There *are* victims who choose a partner who is the exact opposite of the battering parent: those who do may have trouble tolerating any type of conflict.

Fear and isolation are also reasons that a victim stays in a battering relationship. The victim feels that the batterer knows where she is and what she is doing at all times. In fact, many batterers do physically follow their victims. The victim believes that, if she reaches out to family, friends, or health professionals, the batterer will find out and punish her, and she is *usually* right. This fear of retaliation motivates the victim to deny the abuse when asked about it. Because of the batterer's characteristic jealousy and need for control, he punishes the victim for even talking to others, which causes her to become isolated. Fear also disables the victim from acting on her own behalf, which creates a feeling of profound *helplessness*, further contributing to low self-esteem. No individual feels good about herself when she feels helpless, especially when other people feel that taking action would remedy her situation. It is hard for most people to empathize with the helplessness of the battered woman.

Battered women are often *economically dependent* on their partners, and even more so if children are involved. Although it is true that victims come from all economic levels, frequently victims have little training and few marketable skills. They are afraid they will have to go on welfare. The abuser typically controls the money and leaves the victim with no access to cash, checks, or important documents. An-

other reason women stay is because of *beliefs about marriage and relationships*. A woman may believe in the sanctity of marriage and that she would be committing a sin to leave the relationship. If the victim's families are of the same religious convictions, which they usually are, the family may also pressure the woman to remain in the relationship. *Societal attitudes* are important, and many people still view women as being in a subservient role in relation to men (so they should take what they get). Some react to the battered woman as if she is a masochist; that is, that she is sick and enjoys the battering. This is a way of *blaming the victim* and taking the responsibility away from the battering person. There is no evidence that battered women are masochistic (Hofeller, 1983).

Victims with a history of violence believe that battering is to be expected as a part of any close relationship. Many feel that *they* are failures if the relationship fails because they have been socialized to believe that a successful identity comes from a relationship with a man. Often the less frequent or severe the battering, the more likely a victim will be to minimize the importance of it and to stay in the relationship. When the frequency and severity increase and/or extend to children, a woman may be more likely to leave the relationship; conversely, she may feel less like she can leave at that point because of her even greater loss of self-esteem. Often a woman finally leaves because she is convinced that she and/or her children will be killed.

Approach to the Interview

Interviewing the Child Sexual Abuse Patient

When dealing with the child victim of a sexual assault, physicians handling the case are likely to experience strong emotions. Physicians can minimize psychological trauma to the child if they keep evidence of these feelings in check and maintain a professional posture. The child's perception of the initial evaluation will set the tone for subsequent examinations and interviews. Providing the child with a sense of safety in a warm, sensitive environment is of utmost importance. When a child victim appears in the emergency room, she should be escorted to a private room immediately, and the examination should be given high priority. The child may remain with her parents (or caregivers), but she should not be left alone with them at any time. The approach to the child victim varies with the level of maturity of the child. It is helpful to use the child's own terms for body parts and names for family members during the evaluation. The child should be interviewed without the parents present because in many instances the parent was the perpetrator or in some way assisted the perpetrator. Older children should be interviewed separately because they may not want their parents to know some secrets or about prohibited behaviors. The parents should also be interviewed without the victimized child present so that they may talk openly and provide history that they may not want the child to hear.

To obtain the history from the *very young child* (Sanders, 1986), observation is often the only source of information. Look for signs of withdrawn behavior, easy startling, developmental delay, excessive attachment to strangers, and failure to thrive. Where there is a high likelihood that sexual abuse occurred, it is often best to immediately consult with and form a team of professionals who have fairly specialized areas of expertise. Those trained and skilled in interviewing the very young, those with knowledge of pediatric normal and abnormal anal and genital anatomy, and documentation experts with equipment and the technical knowledge to obtain considerate but high-quality video and photo documentation may all be helpful (Kerns et al, 1994).

In *school-age and adolescent victims*, be aware that the child may know that she is being sexually misused but may withhold or retract reports of abuse to protect the perpetrator. Common reasons for this are fear of retaliation; awareness of the consequences on the family unit if she reports; and feelings of anger, shame, and guilt from involvement in the abuse. Again, observe for sexual behaviors or knowledge inappropriate for the level of development. The adolescent victim may seem to react as an adult but may still need more reassurance and support. In all cases, the history-taking process should not be hurried because this may be perceived as interrogation instead of gathering data. All cases of incest, rape, and molestation involving minors must be reported to the police and child protective services.

With *adults* in nonemergent situations, questions about childhood sexual experiences should be routine because the prevalence of sexual abuse is so high in the general population. Women are often grateful to finally speak freely with a professional about the experience. Knowing your patient has been sexually abused allows you to anticipate possible adverse reactions from physical examinations, diagnostic procedures, or life transitions like childbearing.

Patients who have vague, fragmented memories of childhood sexual abuse present a greater challenge to the physician. In the extreme case, these patients have a confusing constellation of physical symptoms that may make sense only in the context of the forgotten childhood sexual trauma. Symptom patterns encountered in some of these confusing cases of "forgotten" or dissociated incest include obviously sexual symptoms (anorgasmia, dyspareunia, promiscuity), nonspecific back pain, abdominal pain, chronic pelvic pain, headaches, self-mutilation, eating disorders, gastrointestinal complaints, substance abuse, breathing difficulties, musculoskeletal disorders, and sleep and memory disturbances. Patients with a large number of these physical symptoms, in the absence of physical disease, may have a somatization disorder, which is frequently seen as a consequence of childhood sexual abuse.

History from a Rape Victim

The gender of the physician is usually not an issue. A caring male physician can conduct a competent and yet therapeutic interview and a defensive female physician can be countertherapeutic. However, when a rape victim prefers to talk with a female physician and it is not possible, there are ways the male physician can reduce the victim's apprehension. The physician should focus on the nonsexual, violent aspects of the rape and attempt to identify with the victim and empathize with her emotional state. One must be cautious not to relate in a manner that could be perceived as ingratiating or patronizing.

When the victim arrives in the emergency room, she should be escorted immediately to a private room, but she should not be left alone. Prompt evaluation should be the priority. In an unhurried and supportive manner, the physician can provide much-needed reassurance to the rape victim that she is safe. When taking the history, record all the details the patient can recall and use direct quotes from the victim whenever possible. The history will guide the physical examination and will help the police investigation.

The emotional responses of the rape victim are typically described as either expressive or controlled (Burgess and Holmstrom, 1974). The rape victim with an expressive presentation may display anger, fear, anxiety, crying, tremulousness, or irritability. It is important to be tolerant and not take emotional outbursts personally. In a controlled presentation, the victim may appear calm or subdued. The lack of expression does not indicate the absence of strong emotions; in fact, it may mean exactly the opposite. A victim's emotional presentation may vary throughout the examination. Victims often become upset when describing aversive acts such as sodomy or fellatio. Remain reassuring and nonjudgmental while informing the patient that these are common practices among rapists. This approach will help minimize feelings of shame in the victim.

Domestic Violence History

Unlike the emergency physician, the physician in the office setting may not be confronted with the acute signs or symptoms pathognomonic for battering. An accurate diagnosis in either setting depends on the physician's incorporating appropriate questions into routine history taking and maintaining an index of suspicion. The patient should be asked if she has ever been physically hurt by someone close to her. This question during history taking encourages reporting of battering experiences in childhood as well as adulthood. Asking this question initially may encourage the patient to bring up the abuse at a later time even if she does not admit to it initially. The message is given that discussion of battering is appropriate in the medical setting. It is important that physicians reassure the patient that they will not intervene on her behalf unless directed to do so.

A physician might *suspect* battering if (in relating her history) the patient is shy, embarrassed, evasive, jumpy, frightened, or weepy (Billy, 1983). These affective states are more pronounced if the battering is recent or if the patient is being seen in the emergency room. Overt depression, excessive use of alcohol and other drugs or medications, and a history of suicidal ideation and/or attempts may be present. A woman who describes herself as accident prone may be camouflaging repeated incidents of battering. Particularly suspicious is a male partner who insists on staying close to the woman, who attempts to answer questions for her, or who bullies and criticizes the staff.

Somatic complaints typical of battered women include headache, insomnia, choking sensations, hyperventilation, gastrointestinal symptoms, and/or chest, pelvic, and back pain. Often there are frequent visits to the physician, and there may be noncompliance with advice and recommendations of the physician (Vilken, 1982).

Physical Examination

Examining the Sexually Abused Child

The child must be examined whether or not she or her parents agree to the examination (Sproles, 1985). Begin with a general physical examination with attention to the Tanner stage of sexual development before examination of the genitalia. Each step of the procedure should be explained as the examination progresses. A small child may accept an examination of the genitalia more readily when in the frog-leg position (feet together on the table and knees apart) or with knees pulled to the chest while sitting on a parent's lap. An older child may be examined in the position used for a lithotomy on the examination table, with the adolescent in stirrups.

The objectives of the physical examination are similar to those in the adult with a few exceptions. The hymen should be examined when appropriate and abnormalities and evidence of injury noted. If the hymen is torn or the introitus stretched, an examination using a speculum should be performed. If visualization of the vaginal mucosa is necessary, a nasal speculum or children's Pederson speculum can be used to visualize lesions. Expertise in the pediatric genital examination and familiarity with the evolving field of pediatric normal, abnormal, and post-trauma anatomy is crucial (Kerns et al, 1994). All postpubertal girls should have a pelvic examination. The physician needs to keep in mind that this may be the first gynecologic examination that the child has experienced. Efforts should be made to respect a teenager or prepubescent girl's modesty and to explain procedures at each step.

Examining Adult Rape Victims

Regardless of previous sexual activity, when the first gynecologic examination occurs in proximity to a rape, the psychological result can be devastating. The victim needs to be led through the first gynecologic examination with sensitivity and patience. The older rape victim may react strongly to the assault because of conservative attitudes about sexuality or pre-existing feelings of vulnerability that intensify following an assault. The older rape victim is more likely to have been physically injured as well. Most emergency rooms have evidence packets with instructions for the examination and gathering of physical evidence. When examining a rape victim, it is necessary to remember that one of the objectives of a rapist is to control the victim. The victim will suffer the effects of this loss of control for days, weeks, or even years. Make every effort to let the control rest with the patient because this will benefit her in the short term but may also affect the long-term outcome and the development of psychological symptoms. Ask permission at every stage of the examination, while encouraging the patient to talk and ask questions.

Nonemergent Gynecologic Examinations

Nonemergent gynecologic examinations and invasive procedures in patients who have experienced sexual violence in the past also require great sensitivity. Physicians are perceived as powerful, authoritative figures, and much of what we do is intrusive and sometimes causes discomfort and pain. An adult who was the victim of childhood sexual abuse or adult rape may not respond at her best during any kind of gynecologic procedure or examination because it can be quite similar to the original abuse. It takes active planning to make the best of a difficult situation. Orient the patient to the setting and the procedure before beginning. Ask if she has had previous pelvic examinations and how she felt during and afterward. Tell the patient how and where she will be touched before touching her. Truthfully warn her if discomfort or pain can be expected. Some patients may want to have a trusted friend present.

When a specific procedure is planned, the previously traumatized patient may experience incredible anticipatory anxiety. Such patients may need more preoperative medication than most and often do better if they are first on the operating room schedule to prevent escalating anxiety. Use medications that promote dissociation (amnesia), such as the ultra-short-acting benodiazepines (Good, 1989), with great care. They can remove the patient's usual defenses against intrusive memories so the patient feels the sexual abuse is happening in the present. These guidelines are not necessary for all patients who experienced sexual abuse in childhood, but they are a good place at which to begin building a therapeutic relationship with the patient.

Treatment

Child Sexual Abuse and Rape

These patients should have treatment for injuries, pregnancy, and sexually transmitted diseases. Treatment for obvious physical injuries is usually readily understood and accepted by the patient. The risk of pregnancy may be less apparent to the victim. The pregnancy rate from a single episode of unprotected intercourse ranges from 1% to 1.5%. The patient must be informed of the risk of pregnancy as well as the methods and risks of pregnancy prevention. Rape victims have a 1 in 30 chance of contracting gonorrhea and a 1 in 1000 chance of contracting syphilis (Hicks, 1988). The patient is also at some risk of contracting viral infections such as herpes, hepatitis, and HIV. The possibility of contracting a chronic, potentially fatal sexually transmitted disease can perpetuate the victim's sense of being in a life-threatening situation.

The issue of whether or not the victim plans to report the crime should be brought up at some point in the evaluation. Educating the victim that assailants are likely to rape again may encourage her to press charges. Although it is important to encourage reporting of the crime, the decision ultimately rests with the victim. She should never be pressured into reporting because this could be psychologically harmful. The physician's duty to maintain confidentiality does not change if the patient is a victim of a sexual assault. The patient's consent should be obtained before talking with family or police.

The disposition of the pediatric patient may be less clear-cut than that of an adult. If the home environment is not safe for the child, foster placement or admission to the hospital must be arranged immediately. If the home environment is considered safe by those involved in the case, a follow-up appointment may be arranged on an outpatient basis approximately 5 days after the assault. This visit may be used to go over results, re-examine injuries, and evaluate the emotional status of the child.

Patients who use denial, repression, or dissociative defenses when stressed may forget instructions given them by their physicians. As the caregiver, it helps to write down specific instructions to avoid unnecessary compliance problems. Those who have been recently victimized or those who were victimized frequently as children have little trust and sometimes think in rather concrete ways. These patients are likely to take statements quite literally during the regression that accompanies evaluation and illness. If a physician says "I'll be back in a minute," meaning a short time, the patient can get very anxious, feel abandoned, and become angry as the minutes tick by. Although the physician intended to convey concern and reassurance, the patient experiences the delay as one more false promise. It is better to allow plenty of time and say, "I'll be back within the hour unless there is an emergency."

Domestic Violence/Battered Women Treatment

Because the gynecologist is often a battered patient's primary care provider, it is important to establish a trusting relationship with the victim and provide a nonjudgmental and empathic environment. Furthermore, the physician can validate the importance of the problem, educate the victim, and provide appropriate referrals.

First, a nonjudgmental attitude is imperative, even though the physician may be exasperated by repeated contacts with a woman who appears to be unable to leave the battering situation. Frequently, it is harder for male than for female physicians to empathize because men are less frequently victims of physically overpowering crimes such as domestic violence and rape. Men are conditioned to have a feeling of power and believe that they can and should intervene on their own behalf if they are violated. Women are conditioned in the opposite manner.

A woman may admit to being battered in response to questions during history taking or in response to questions arising from the physician's suspicion of abuse. When she does admit to being battered, it is appropriate to ask how she feels about it and how she feels about the relationship. She is likely to say that she hates the violence, but sometimes he is nice to her and she thinks it will get better. Empathizing with the victim's response to the kind side of the batterer is helpful to the woman's self-esteem and the patient-physician relationship. A physician might say, for example, that "certainly there must be times when he is very kind, or a person like you would not have chosen him in the first place." Physicians base this statement on their knowledge of the research that there are times when batterers are in fact "wonderful" and victims are *not* masochistic. If the victim feels respected by the physician, she is more likely to ally herself with him or her and be receptive to his or her suggestions, even though she may not act on those suggestions immediately.

It is important that the physician, as a trusted authority, validate that the abuse is inappropriate, that it *must* stop, and that there is *nothing* the victim does to deserve to be beaten. This directly addresses the fact that many women think that battering is to be expected as a part of any close relationship.

Education regarding the cycle of violence is another critical intervention (Walker, 1984). Victims often recognize the pattern in the cycle of violence when it is explained to them, and the fact that the physician is knowledgeable about the pattern helps them to believe the physician when he or she describes the escalating nature of the violence.

There are three phases to the cycle: the tension-building phase, the acute battering incident, and the loving contrition phase. During the first phase, tension gradually escalates. The batterer engages in name calling, various mean and intentional behaviors, and/or physical abuse. He expresses dissatisfaction and hostility but he is not yet explosive. The woman attempts to calm and please the batterer; she does what she thinks will avoid his becoming aggravated with her and she does not respond to his hostile actions. Sometimes she is successful in calming him down, at least for a little while, and this reinforces her idea that she can control her partner's tendency to batter. After a while, however, she realizes that sometimes she can control his actions and sometimes she cannot, and so it makes her feel as if the abuse is noncontingent, that is, that the abuse will happen no matter what she does. This is the beginning of the pattern of "learned helplessness." The tension continues to escalate, and eventually the victim feels unable to stop the angry response from the batterer. "Exhausted from the constant stress, she usually withdraws from the batterer, fearing she will inadvertently set off an explosion. He begins to move more oppressively toward her as he observes her withdrawal; tension between the two becomes unbearable" (Walker, 1979).

Without intervention, the second phase, also called the acute battering incident, becomes inevitable. This phase is characterized by an uncontrollable discharge of tension that is built up during the first phase. Typically, the batterer unleashes a barrage of verbal and physical abuse that leaves the woman severely shaken and injured. Injuries, when they occur, do so during this phase. Sometimes the victim attempts to precipitate the inevitable explosion so that she can feel in control of where and when it occurs. Precipitating the explosion also allows her to take better precautions so that she can minimize her injuries and pain. Police are called during this phase, if they are called at all. When the batterer finally stops the physical and psychologic abuse, the phase is concluded. There is then a sharp reduction in tension, which is reinforcing to the batterer because he sees the battering as a way to relieve his tension.

In the third phase, the batterer apologizes profusely, offers assistance to his victim, and shows kindness and remorse. He may shower her with gifts and make promises about how he will behave in the future. In fact, the batterer himself may believe that he will never again allow himself to be violent. The woman wants to believe that the batterer will not hurt her again, and her hope is renewed in his ability to change. Even if the batterer does not try to make up for his abusive behavior or make promises to his victim, the woman feels inclined to stay in the relationship just because the battering is over with for now, the tension is less, and in a sense things are better. This third phase positively reinforces the woman in terms of her choice to stay in the relationship.

With repeated cycles, there is an increase in the first phase, the violence becomes more acute and dangerous in the second phase, and there is a decrease in the third phase. The batterer no longer puts much energy into obtaining forgiveness because he now feels in control of the victim. At this point, the

Table 21-9. EXIT PLAN FOR THE BATTERED WOMAN

1. Pack changes of clothing for yourself and your children. Pack extra toilet articles, medicine, and an extra set of keys to the house and car. Ask a friend or neighbor to store the suitcase.
2. Try to save even the smallest amount of money over time.
3. If possible, keep extra cash, your checkbook, and savings account book with a friend. You may need identification such as birth certificates, social security card, voter registration, utility bills, or driver's license to enroll your children in school or arrange financial assistance.
4. Take something special for each child, such as a toy, a book, or a blanket.
5. Take any important financial records, such as rent receipts or title to the car.
6. Know exactly where you could go, even in the middle of the night, and how you could get there.
7. Locate the nearest shelter for victims of domestic violence through the telephone book, your local social service agency, or the domestic violence hotline (1-800-333-SAFE or 1-800-873-6363 for hearing impaired).
8. Find out if your local police department has an "automatic arrest" policy and how it is enforced. An automatic arrest policy means that a police officer can arrest an alleged batterer if the officer has behavioral evidence that domestic violence has taken place. This policy takes the onus off the victim in that she does not have to be responsible for the abuser's arrest.
9. Call for help. It is important that you tell someone.
10. *Remember:* The most important consideration is to keep yourself and your children safe.

victim's self-esteem is very low and her sense of helplessness is very high.

Physicians can help the victim to see that, if the abuse has occurred once, the chances are extremely high that the abuse will happen repeatedly. They should explain to the victim that research into the cycle of violence shows that the abuse usually becomes worse over time, and all too frequently results in death. Perhaps the victim will ask what she can do to get out of the situation. The physician can offer guidelines presented in Table 21-9.

Nonmedical and Multidisciplinary Personnel

The *police* may be involved when domestic violence or sexual assault has been reported. They take statements; notify the domestic, sex, or children's crime unit of the alleged assault; and may take photographs of the victim. The police officer is also responsible for receiving and transporting the evidence gathered by the physician. *Social services workers* are very helpful, but their role may vary tremendously depending on availability, training, and institutional expectations. Often a social worker with specific training and expertise in child abuse, domestic violence, or rape will participate in the evaluation. The social worker's responsibilities may include notification of the family of the victim, notification of child protective services when applicable, evaluation of the social situation, and arrangement for alternative housing and outpatient counseling referrals. The social worker often provides important reassurance and emotional support for the victim during the examination and on follow-up visits. Various community agencies and volunteer groups may also play important roles. Patient advocates, victims assistance resources, and emergency foster parents may all interact and provide services under some circumstances.

Legal Issues

Three legal issues concern physicians: state laws, medical records, and photographs. Each of these issues relates to patient-physician confidentiality.

When there is suspicion or evidence of child abuse, physicians in all 50 states and the District of Columbia have a duty to report it. If a battered woman is making homicidal or suicidal threats, the physician should obtain a psychiatric evaluation. In most states, the physician is not required to report incidences of battering in decisionally capable adults, so the physician cannot do so without the victim's permission.

> All medical records can be subpoenaed. However, the physician has the responsibility and is not liable for recording a patient's statement or medical facts or for rendering an expert, medical opinion. As with all medical records, direct patient quotes are appropriately bracketed with the introduction "Patient stated . . . ." Medical opinions such as "suspected abuse" or "injuries suggestive of battering" do not contain legal liability. Photographs are an excellent way to document the presence of injuries. The physician is not liable if the patient signs a waiver to have the photograph taken. An identifying feature of the patient such as the hand or face should be included in the shot. The photos should be placed in a sealed envelope, which is signed and dated by the patient. The release should be affixed to the envelope (Chez, 1988).

Possible Enduring Psychological and Medical Consequences of Sexual Violence

Childhood Psychological Manifestations of Sexual Abuse

In recognizing the victim of sexual abuse, the following behavioral and psychological symptoms may indicate that such an activity has occurred: sleep disturbances, weight loss, fearfulness, bed-wetting, school phobia, deterioration in school performance, sexually provocative behavior, sexual acting out toward peers, promiscuity, depression, suicidal ideation or attempts, isolativeness, withdrawn behavior, and delinquent behavior. These symptoms may continue after the child has been placed in a safe environment, and active psychological intervention may be required.

Patients with incest histories often have specific complaints about eating and sleeping. Some patients with eating disorders describe vomiting to get a sensation out of their throat (seen in those forced to perform fellatio), wanting to vomit on someone, or wanting to be so thin (or fat) that the perpetrator of the abuse would lose interest (Goodwin et al, 1988). Sometimes the eating disorder is associated with a fear of pregnancy. These can be rather ingenious defenses in a relatively powerless child but are quite maladaptive over the course of life.

Sleep disturbances are common after an acute trauma, and they also occur as sequelae in chronic trauma. Patients describe nightmares of an intruder in their room. Many children are awakened from sleep to find the molester in action and would prefer to think of the events as dreams rather than as actual events. They may try to delay sleep as long as possible and position their bed so it faces the door to remain alert and protect themselves. These behaviors frequently persist in adults.

SOMATIZATION BEHAVIORS AND SOMATOFORM DISORDERS

Women with somatization behaviors or somatoform disorders have physical symptoms, suggesting a physical disorder, that cannot be explained by physiologic or organic findings, and there is evidence the physical symptoms may be linked to psychological factors or conflicts (American Psychiatric Association, 1994).

Somatoform disorders are a diverse group and include *conversion disorders* and the earlier *Briquet's syndrome* with chronic physical complaints in multiple systems. Conversion disorders are unexplained, abnormal physical signs with a known psychological conflict at the root and no known somatic abnormality as the etiology. A specific conversion syndrome, *pseudocyesis*, is a patient's persistent, false belief that she is pregnant. There are several case reports of adolescents with pseudocyesis who were subsequently found to be incest victims (Hardwick and Fitzpatrick, 1981; Roybal and Goodwin, 1989). How often this occurs is unknown. Briquet's syndrome includes sexual problems, conversion symptoms, depression, and anxiety. Women with somatization report high rates of childhood sexual abuse and anorgasmia (Morrison, 1989). They have many sexual and menstrual difficulties (Goodwin and Guze, 1979) along with a negative self-image (Gelinas, 1983; Bagley and Ramsey, 1986; Browne and Finkelhor, 1986), and many report amnesia (Othmer and DeSouza, 1985). These symptoms are common in incest victims in general, and women who experience somatic symptoms unexplained by organic pathologic factors also report higher rates of sexual abuse in childhood (Loewenstein, 1990).

It is important to carefully evaluate possible cases of somatization for actual or developing physical illness because overlooked illness eventually explains some 50% of apparent somatoform disorders (Stefansson et al, 1976; Ford and Folks, 1985; Goodyer, 1985). When the symptoms clearly fit a somatoform pattern, questions about abuse (sexual and physical) should be repeated. The symptoms are sometimes the only overt manifestation of the abuse.

Most physical symptoms are mediated by the brain, and we are only beginning to understand the possible pathways involved in the production of the symptoms that seem to be associated with child sexual abuse. When the abuse begins at a very young age, before the child has any vocabulary to associate with the experience, there is some evidence that memory is visual rather than verbal and information is *stored as a somatic or "body" memory* (Terr, 1988; van der Kolk, 1994). Just as phantom limb pain can appear years after a limb has been removed, the brain can "remember" sensations that have no current peripheral neural origin. Finally, a frequent psychological defense used by victims of any trauma is a kind of amnesia or dissociation (Putnam, 1985; van der Kolk, 1986). These patients frequently have patchy, disjointed memories of the abuse events, and they may not be able to associate the current symptoms with physical sensations or injuries they received as part of the violence they experienced.

CHRONIC PELVIC PAIN AND GASTROINTESTINAL SYMPTOMS

Thirty-six per cent of patients with chronic pelvic pain and normal gynecologic examinations spontaneously report a history of incest (Gross et al, 1980-1981). Because many women do not report incest unless specifically asked, it is not surprising that incest reports increase to 64% when patients are directly questioned about sexual abuse during the diagnostic interview (Walker et al, 1988). Patients with chronic pelvic pain also have more chronic abdominal discomfort, dysmenorrhea, and headaches when compared with nonabused women (Draijer, 1989). Drossman (1995) found that 44% of the female patients in a gastroenterology clinic reported prior physical or sexual abuse. The percentage rose to 53 among patients in whom no organic etiology could be found for the gastrointestinal symptoms. The abuse history was also associated with a poorer prognosis, including pain that was more severe than that of other patients.

THERAPEUTIC APPROACH

Somatization disorders are a complex group; the possibility of undiagnosed medical disorders always remains a consideration, but many cases of somatization seem strongly associated with childhood abuse. Unnecessary medical intervention does not provide symptom relief in true somatization disorder or chronic pelvic pain without a pathophysiologic basis. These patients risk iatrogenic injury and unnecessary expense for ineffective treatment as well

as continued discomfort. Continued medical care in close conjunction with psychological treatment is recommended.

When a somatization disorder or physical syndrome related to abuse is suspected, the patient should be referred for psychiatric evaluation. The findings must be presented very carefully because patients often hear "there's nothing wrong with you" or that the symptoms are "all in your head," even when that is not what the physician intended to say. Alternatively saying, "The test results have been normal, so the cause of your symptoms is still unknown, but I would like you to see a psychiatric consultant to assist you in coping with this uncertainty and to help me with thinking about your symptoms" often works much better. It establishes that the physician is committed to working with the patient, acknowledges any patient frustration, and establishes the consultant as a resource for both the patient and the physician.

Often women who experienced incest are very successful in many spheres of life. Some of these overtly successful women suffer serious constriction or chaos in their emotional relationships (Herman and Schatzow, 1987). Many of these women excel in the "care-taking" professions. They may not, however, take very good care of themselves.

Psychological Sequelae of Rape

Psychological trauma is a common consequence of rape. Nadelson et al (1982) found that, 1 to 2 1/2 years after sexual assault, 40% of the victims had sexual difficulties, restricted dating, suspiciousness, fear of being alone, and depression stemming from the rape. Burgess and Holmstrom (1979) surveyed victims 4 to 6 years after they had been raped. Thirty-seven per cent of the victims felt back to normal after a period of years, and 20% did not feel that they had fully recovered. How the rape victim reacts to the assault in the short and long term depends not only on the experience of the assault but also on the victim's life situation, social support, personality style, and previous emotional symptoms (Notman and Nadelson, 1976; Frank and Anderson, 1987; Nadelson, 1989). Very few rape victims seek help in the period immediately following the rape. The majority of women delay treatment until some time after the initial assault (Koss and Burkhart, 1989). The efficacy of crisis intervention has not been ascertained, although we know that experiences in the immediate crisis period may have positive or negative consequences on long-term adjustment (Notman and Nadelson, 1976; Calhoun et al, 1982).

RAPE TRAUMA SYNDROME

Burgess and Holmstrom (1974) first described the rape trauma syndrome. The syndrome is divided into two phases: the disorganization phase, which may last days to weeks, and the reorganization phase, which may last months to years.

The *disorganization phase* includes a variety of emotional and somatic symptoms. Emotional symptoms may be fear of injury, fear of being raped again, fear of death, anxiety, humiliation, embarrassment, guilt, anger, and thoughts of revenge. These emotions may be expressed or controlled as described previously. Somatic symptoms are general body or localized soreness; abdominal pain; nausea; vaginal, anal, or oral complaints; sleep disturbances; and appetite loss.

During the *reorganization phase*, the victim attempts to restructure her personality and her life. She may change her telephone number, change her appearance, or move to a new house or city. Burgess and Holmstrom (1974) reported that 48% of the respondents in their study changed residences in the period immediately after the rape. It is during this phase that sexual dysfunctions such as lack of desire, sexual aversion, anorgasmia, and vaginismus develop. Phobias toward men, sex, or aloneness develop as well. Symptoms such as depression, paranoia, insomnia, nightmares, and flashbacks are also likely to appear during this phase.

A chronic state of maladaptive responses may signal the development of PTSD (Nadelson, 1989). These symptoms include (1) intrusive thoughts, nightmares, or flashbacks of the event or experiencing psychological distress that symbolizes the traumatic event; (2) diminished interest in significant activities, avoidance of thoughts or situations that stimulate recollection of the trauma, isolation, diminished ability to experience emotions, and loss of hope for the future; and (3) symptoms of increased arousal, such as sleep difficulties, anger outbursts, hypervigilance, difficulty in concentrating, exaggerated startle response, and autonomic reaction to an event that symbolizes the traumatic event (American Psychiatric Association, 1994). In addition, sexual assault victims sometimes experience eating disorders, chronic anxiety, chronic depression, substance abuse, phobias, and sexual dysfunctions. Patients may describe deterioration or inability to function in work, social, or school settings. If symptoms of these disorders are noted on follow-up, a referral to a qualified mental health professional is in order.

The physician will often encounter women with these psychological and physical symptoms but without the history that the patient has been a victim of rape. Chronic somatic complaints, unexplainable pelvic pain, or persistent vaginal discharge unresponsive to treatment may result from previous sexual trauma (Walker et al, 1988; Koss et al, 1990).

Sexualized Behavior of Patients Toward Clinicians

"Sexualized" behavior by patients should be viewed as efforts to communicate clinically important information. Indeed, this phenomenon may reveal much about the patient's past sexual experiences or current conflicts surrounding sexuality. Child sexual abuse victims can appear to be very seductive, the result of an oversexualized childhood, or may exhibit an apparent defenseless naïveté. This demeanor makes the patient vulnerable to repeated victimization. The seductiveness can be very subtle, and it is not necessarily sexual. The patient may tell the physician that he or she is a wonderful doctor, and the physician may feel at his or her best when helping this particular patient. It is easy to get carried away when the patient's gratitude reinforces the aims of a concerned physician. Patients who have been the victims of previous sexual exploitation are most likely to be further victimized by sexual contact with their treating professional (Feldman-Summers and Jones, 1984). Obstetrics and gynecology is one of the specialties characterized by a high risk of improper sexual contact between patient and physician (Kardner et al, 1973; Burgess, 1986).

When clinicians repeatedly experience sexual attraction to patients, they should examine this problem carefully, monitor their behavior closely, and seek supervision to minimize their risk for professional misconduct. Several states have passed laws making sexual contact with patients a criminal offense. When defined by law, the doctor-patient relationship can continue to exist long after the last office visit. Mandatory reporting of sexual liaisons between physicians and patients is also required in some states (Bemmann and Goodwin, 1989). Physicians should be familiar with local laws. Even in states without specific legal prohibitions, it is important to understand that the patient's demeanor may be a symptom of previous abuse, and the goal of treatment is symptom reduction, not symptom exploitation.

Summary

Child sexual abuse, including incest, is prevalent. A physician must notify officials when children are sexually mistreated just as when they are physically mistreated. Sexual abuse has direct medical consequences of injury from premature sexual activity, consanguineous pregnancy, and sexual diseases. Less obvious medical consequences are overuse of medical services to treat physical symptoms without a physiologic basis, avoidance of health maintenance examinations because of unresolved fears, and further sexual victimization. Preventing possible adverse reactions to routine examinations and procedures is easily accomplished with simple steps to allay anxiety.

Rape is an intimate act of violence that can have devastating physical and psychological consequences in which physicians will be increasingly called upon to intervene. The gynecologist can minimize the initial trauma to the rape victim by approaching her with empathy and preparing her for possible physical and psychologic reactions to the assault. The physician has the additional responsibility of recognizing poor adjustment in the period immediately after the rape and making appropriate referrals. Equipped with the facts, the physician can make a positive difference in the rape victim's physical and emotional well-being.

The obstetrician and gynecologist frequently acts as a woman's primary care physician and is often best positioned to identify the battered woman and intervene on her behalf. However, a lack of understanding and frustration with why women stay in a violent relationship often affect the physician's desire to help. The solution to most physicians seems quite obvious: "She should just leave." Professional knowledge of the underlying fears, needs, and emotions together with patient education and consistent and persistent support, may eventually help the woman change her situation.

PROFESSIONALISM IN GYNECOLOGIC CARE

For clinicians to provide appropriate patient care, they must have a genuine understanding of the professional boundaries and ethical duties inherent to their work with patients. Therapeutic relationships are always founded on trust. Their aim is simply to improve the well-being of patients. Their nature is complex, and it is necessarily one of inequality because of the relative vulnerability of the patient who seeks care as a result of her need for understanding, information, and treatment. Consequently, it is the duty of the clinician to create a context of respect, safety, and clarity when exploring sexual health with patients. Moreover, it is the duty of physicians to recognize the clinical meaning of their encounters with patients. For example, if the discussion of sexual issues with the patient becomes erotically stimulating or gratifying to the caregiver, it is important to understand that this is a clinical finding that requires interpretation—it does not represent an authentic wish by the patient to become sexually involved. Professionalism in gynecologic care is grounded in respect for women. It encompasses humanistic and ethical expression in the physician-patient relationship.

REFERENCES

Abbott J, Johnson R, Koziol-McLain J, Lowenstein SR: Domestic violence against women: incidence and prevalence in an emergency department population. JAMA 1995;273:1763.
ABIM Subcommittee on Clinical Competencies in Women's Health: Core Competence in Women's Health: What Internists Need to Know. Philadelphia: Clinical Competence and Communications, 1997.
Abramowicz M (ed): Drugs that cause sexual dysfunction. Med Lett Drugs Ther 1987;29:65.
ACP Committee on Women's Health: Comprehensive women's health: the role and commitment of internal medicine. Am J Medicine 1997;103:451.

American Psychiatric Association: Diagnostic and Statistical Manual of Mental Disorders. 4th ed. Washington, DC: American Psychiatric Press, 1994.
Arnow PM, Pottenger LA, Stocking CB, et al: Orthopedic surgeons' attitudes and practices concerning treatment of patients with HIV infection. Public Health Rep 1989;104:121.
Bagley C, Ramsay R: Sexual abuse in childhood: psychosocial outcomes and implications for social work practice. Social Work Hum Sex 1986;4:33.
Bemmann KC, Goodwin J: New laws about sexual misconduct by therapists: knowledge and attitudes among Wisconsin psychiatrists. Wis Med J 1989;88:11.
Benjamin LS: Principles of prediction using the structural analysis of social behavior. In Zucker RA, Aronoff J, Rabond AJ (eds): Personality and the Prediction of Behavior. New York: Academic Press, 1984:121.
Billy BJ: Life patterns and emergency care of battered women. J Emerg Nurs 1983;9:251.
Binder RL: Why women don't report sexual assault. J Clin Psychiatry 1981;42:437.
Browne A, Finkelhor D: Impact of child sexual abuse: a review of the research. Psychol Bull 1986;99:66.
Browne A, Williams KR: Resource availability for women at risk: its relationship to rates of female-perpetrated partner homicide. Paper presented at the American Society of Criminology Annual Meeting, Montreal, Canada, November 11–14, 1987.
Burgess AW. Gynecologist-patient sexual abuse: II. An evaluation of victims. In Burgess AW, Hartman CR (ed): Sexual Exploitation of Patients by Health Professionals. New York: Praeger, 1986:74.
Burgess AW, Holmstrom LL: Rape trauma syndrome. Am J Psychiatry 1974;131:981.
Burgess AW, Holmstrom LL: Coping behavior of the rape victim. Am J Psychiatry 1976;4:413.
Burgess AW, Holmstrom LL: Rape: sexual disruption and recovery. Am J Orthopsychiatry 1979;49:648.
Calhoun KS, Resick PA, Ellis EM: Victims of rape: repeated assessment of depressive symptoms. J Consult Clin Psychol 1982;50:96.
Chez RA: Woman battering. Am J Obstet Gynecol 1988;158:1.
Courtois CA: Healing the Incest Wound: Adult Survivors in Therapy. New York: WW Norton & Co, 1988.
Draijer N: Long-term psychosomatic consequences of child sexual abuse. In van Hall EV, Everaerd W (eds): The Free Woman: Women's Health in the 1990's. Cornforth, United Kingdom Parthenon, 1989.
Drossman DA: Sexual and physical abuse and gastrointestinal illness. Scand J Gastroenterol Suppl 1995;208:90.
Ende J, Rockwell S, Glasgow M: The sexual history in general medical practice. Arch Intern Med 1984;144:558.
Federal Bureau of Investigation: Crime in the United States, 1989. Washington, DC: Federal Bureau of Investigation, 1989.
Federal Bureau of Investigation: Crime in the United States, 1995. Washington, DC: Federal Bureau of Investigation, 1995.
Feldman-Summers S, Jones G: Psychological impacts of sexual contact between therapists or other health care practitioners and their clients. J Consult Clin Psychol 1984;52:1054.
Finkelhor D: Current information on the scope and nature of child sexual abuse. Future of Children 1994;4:31.
Ford CV, Folks DG: Conversion disorders: an overview. Psychosomatics 1985;26:371.
Frank E, Anderson BP: Psychiatric disorders in rape victims: past history and current symptomology. Compr Psychiatry 1987;28:77.
Geist RF: Sexually related trauma. Emerg Med Clin North Am 1988;6:439.
Gelinas D: The persisting negative effects of incest. Psychiatry 1983;46:312.
Gelles RJ, Cornell CP (eds): International perspectives on Family Violence. Lexington, MA: DC Heath, 1983.
Goldberg WG, Tomlanovich MC: Domestic violence, victims and emergency departments: new findings. JAMA 1984;251:3259.
Good MI: Substance-induced dissociative disorders and psychiatric nosology. J Clin Psychopharmacol 1989;9:88.

Goodwin DW, Guze SB: Psychiatric Diagnosis. 2nd ed. New York: Oxford University Press, 1979.

Goodwin J: Sexual Abuse: Incest Victims and Their Families. 2nd ed. Chicago: Mosby–Year Book, 1989.

Goodwin J, Cheeves K, Connell V: Defining a syndrome of severe symptoms in survivors of severe incestuous abuse. Dissociation 1988;1:11.

Goodyer IM: Epileptic and pseudoepileptic seizures in childhood and adolescence. J Am Acad Child Psychiatry 1985;24:3.

Gross RJ, Doerr H, Caldirola D, et al: Borderline syndrome and incest in chronic pelvic pain patients. Int J Psychiatry Med 1980-1981;10:79.

Groth AN, Burgess AW, Holmstrom LL: Rape: power, anger and sexuality. Am J Psychiatry 1977;134:1239.

Gundlach RH: Sexual molestation and rape reported by homosexual and heterosexual women. J Homosex 1977;2:367.

Hardwick PJ, Fitzpatrick C: Fear, folie and phantom pregnancy: pseudocyesis in a fifteen year old girl. Br J Psychiatry 1981;139:558.

Hayman CR, Lanza C: Sexual assault on women and girls. Am J Obstet Gynecol 1971;109:480.

Herman J, Schatzow E: Recovery and verification of memories of childhood sexual trauma. Psychoanal Psychol 1987;4:1.

Hicks DJ: The patient who's been raped. Emerg Med Clin North Am 1988;20:106.

Hilberman E: Overview: The "wife beater's wife" reconsidered. Am J Psychiatry 1980;137:1336.

Hillard PJ: Physical abuse in pregnancy. Obstet Gynecol 1985;66:185.

Hofeller KH: Battered Women, Shattered Lives. Palo Alto, Calif: R&E Research Associates, Inc, 1983.

James J, Meyerding J: Early sexual experience and prostitution. Am J Psychiatry 1977;134:1381.

Kaplan HS: Disorders of Sexual Desire. New York: Brunner-Mazel, 1969.

Kaplan HS: The New Sex Therapy. Vol 1. New York: Brunner-Mazel, 1974.

Kardener SH, Fuller M, Mensh IN: A survey of physicians' attitudes and practices regarding erotic and nonerotic contact with patients. Am J Psychiatry 1973;130:1077.

Kelly DD: Sexual differentiation of the nervous system. In Kandel ER, Schwartz JH, Jessell TM (eds): Principles of Neural Science. 3rd ed. New York: Elsevier, 1991:960.

Kerns DL, Terman DL, Larson CS: The role of physicians in reporting and evaluating child sexual abuse cases. Future of Children 1994;4:119.

Koss MP, Burkhart BR: A conceptual analysis of rape victimization. Psychol Women Q 1989;13:27.

Koss MP, Woodruff WJ, Koss PG: Relation of criminal victimization to health perceptions among women medical patients. J Consult Clin Psychol 1990;58:147.

Larson CS, Terman DL, Gomby DS, et al: Sexual abuse of children: recommendations and analysis. Future of Children 1994;4:4.

Loewenstein RJ: Somatoform disorders in victims of incest and child abuse. In Kluft RP (ed): Incest-Related Syndromes of Adult Psychopathology. Washington, DC: American Psychiatric Press, 1990.

Marchbanks PA, Lui KJ, Mercy JA: Risk of injury from resisting rape. Am J Epidemiol 1990,132:540.

Masters WH, Johnson V: Human Sexual Response. Boston: Little, Brown, 1970.

Merrill JM, Laux LF, Thornby JI: Why doctors have difficulty with sex histories. South Med J 1990;83:613.

Morrison J: Childhood sexual histories in women with somatization disorder. Am J Psychiatry 1989;146:239.

Nadelson CC: Consequences of rape: clinical and treatment aspects. Psychother Psychosom 1989;51:187.

Nadelson CC, Notman MT, Zackson H, Gornick J; A follow-up study of rape victims. Am J Psychiatry 1982;139:1266.

Notman MT, Nadelson CC: The rape victim: psychodynamic considerations. Am J Psychiatry 1976;133:408.

Othmer E, DeSouza C: A screening test for somatization disorder (hysteria). Am J Psychiatry 1985;142:1146.

Parker B, Schumacher DN: The battered wife syndrome and violence in the nuclear family of origin: a controlled pilot study. Am J Public Health 1977;67:760.

Pauly IB, Goldstein SG: Prevalence of significant sexual problems in medical practice. Med Aspects Hum Sex 1970;4:48.

Putnam FW: Dissociation as a response to extreme trauma. In Kluft RP (ed): Childhood Antecedants of Multiple Personality. Washington, DC: American Psychiatric Press, 1985.

Richwald GA, McCluskey TC: Family violence during pregnancy. Adv Int Matern Child Health 1985;5:87.

Rimsze ME, Niggemann EH: Medical evaluation of sexually abused children: a review of 311 cases. Pediatrics 1982;69:8.

Rose DS: Sexual assault, domestic violence and incest. In Steward DE, Stotland NL (eds): Psychological Aspects of Women's Health. Washington, DC: American Psychiatric Press, 1993:447.

Rounsaville B, Weissman MM: Battered women: a medical problem requiring detection. Int J Psychiatry Med 1977–1978;8:191.

Roybal L, Goodwin J: The incest pregnancy. In Goodwin J (ed): Sexual Abuse: Incest Victims and Their Families. Chicago: Mosby–Year Book, 1989.

Russell DEH: The prevalence and incidence of forcible rape and attempted rape of females. Victimology 1982;7:81.

Russell DEH: The Secret Trauma: Incest in the Lives of Girls and Women. New York: Basic Books, 1986.

Sanders CG: Evaluating child abuse cases. Resident Staff Physician 1986;32:21.

Seagraves RT: Antidepressant-induced sexual dysfunction. J Clin Psychiatry 1998;59(Suppl 4):48.

Sgroi S, Porter FS, Blick LC: Validation of child sexual abuse. In Sgroi S (ed): Handbook of Clinical Intervention in Child Sexual Abuse. Lexington, MA: DC Heath, 1982:39.

Silbert MH, Pines AM: Sexual child abuse as an antecedent to prostitution. Child Abuse Negl 1981;5:407.

Simari CG, Baskin D: Incestuous experiences within homosexual populations: a preliminary study. Arch Sex Behav 1982;11:329.

Sorensen SB, Stein JA, Siegel JM, et al: The prevalence of adult sexual assault. Am J Epidemiol 1987;126:1154.

Sproles EJ: The Evaluation and Management of Rape and Sexual Abuse: A Physician's Guide (Publication No 85-1409). Washington, DC: U.S. Department of Health and Human Services, 1985.

Stark E, Fliteraft A, Frazier W: Medicine and patriarchal violence: the social construction of a "private event." Int J Health Sci 1979;9:462.

Steele BF, Alexander H: Long-term effects of sexual abuse in childhood. In Mrazek PB, Kempe CH (eds): Sexually Abused Children and Their Families. Oxford, England: Pergamon, 1981:223.

Stefansson JG, Messina JA, Meyerowitz S: Hysterical neurosis, conversion type: clinical and epidemiological considerations. Acta Psychiatr Scand 1976;53:119.

Straus MA, Gelles RJ, Steinmetz SK: Behind Closed Doors: Violence in American Families. New York: Doubleday, 1980.

Terr L: What happens to early memories of trauma? A study of twenty chldren under age five at the time of documented traumatic events. J Am Acad Child Adolesc Psychiatry 1988;27:96.

Van der Kolk B: Psychological Trauma. Washington, DC: American Psychiatric Press, 1986.

van der Kolk BA: The body keeps score: memory and the evolving psychobiology of posttraumatic stress. Harvard Rev Psychiatry 1994;1:253.

Vilken RM: Family violence: aids to recognition. Postgrad Med 1982;71:115.

Walker E, Katon W, Harrop-Griffiths J, et al: Relationship of chronic pelvic pain to psychiatric diagnoses and childhood sexual abuse. Am J Psychiatry 1988;145:75.

Walker L: The Battered Woman. New York: Harper & Row, 1979.

Walker LE: The Battered Woman Syndrome. New York: Springer, 1984.

Weiss L, Meadow R: Women's attitudes toward gynecologic practices. Obstet Gynecol 1979;54:110.

22

Lesbian Health
Therapeutic Perspectives for Sexual Minorities

Katherine A. O'Hanlan
Demetra L. Burrs

In nearly every gynecologic practice, clinicians knowingly or unknowingly provide care to sexual minorities: lesbians, bisexuals, intersexuals, and transsexuals. As more and more information about the diversity of human sexual anatomy and expression comes into peer review, access to culturally competent healthcare improves. Routine gynecologic care is important for lesbians, bisexuals, intersexuals, and transsexuals and requires an understanding of salient demographics in order to ensure compliance with standard screening guidelines. Additionally, many are creating families, seeking insemination and obstetrical services. Regardless of whether these patients have shared information about their orientation or status with the clinician, it is useful for the obstetrician-gynecologist to have some knowledge about the health demographics and special needs of the lesbian population. In October 1997 the Institute of Medicine convened a subcommittee to study lesbian health issues. The conclusions of the committee were that not enough was known about lesbian health and that more research was needed (Institute of Medicine, 1999). This chapter presents a review of the current literature.

Over 50 years of psychological and physiologic research has documented the essential normalcy of gay men and lesbians in our society; however, this information has not reached every quadrant of even the scientific community. Minimal information is presented in medical schools and residency trainings about homosexuality, except for issues pertaining to acquired immunodeficiency syndrome (AIDS). The popular media have misrepresented homosexuals as social and moral deviants, fostering disdain. This is reinforced by the government's proscription against gay men and lesbians serving in the military or contracting for civil marriage. As a result, most homosexuals have concealed their identity, effectively allowing these negative and inaccurate stereotypes to flourish. Although research has shown that familiarity with a homosexual reduces one's prejudice (Ellis and Vasseur, 1993), many gay men and lesbians, fearing loss of job, family, and friends, still prefer to hide their orientation. Others, however, have begun to "come out" and seek what are broadly perceived to be "equal rights" with heterosexuals, such as the right to pursue job and housing free from discrimination, to serve in the military, and to contract for marriage.

Epidemiologists have shown that the distinguishing characteristics of the lesbian and gay communities are based not only on sexual behavior and attraction, but also on the psychosocial impact of living in the focus of pervasive misunderstanding and disdain (Rothblum, 1994). Sources of stress among members of the gay community include the usual daily life issues such as work, finances, and health. In addition, stress also derives from anxiety, depression, and guilt from being widely viewed as immoral and deviant, an effect compounded by the presence of the human immunodeficiency virus (HIV) epidemic. Individuals who carry multiple socially marginalized statuses (e.g., race, ethnicity, and sexual orientation) are known to carry an even higher risk of depressive distress (Mays et al, 1996). These stressors can reduce an individual's ability to make decisions, employ healthful habits, and utilize available health resources.

Health surveys have revealed that lesbians perceive that their health care providers lack knowledge of the issues salient in their lives, and that many health care providers have alienated their lesbian patients. To remedy this, a demographic profile of lesbian health is described from the available literature, with additional information about the medical and psychological effects of prejudice, followed by suggestions for clinical management and research topics for obstetricians and gynecologists. Greater knowledge about who lesbians and bisexuals are, what their medical profiles are, and what the psychological effects of societal disdain are will enable practitioners to maintain the highest standard of medical care for all of their patients, including the lesbian, bisexual, transgendered, and intersexual patient.

DEFINING LESBIAN WOMEN

In the health care context, both behavior and identity are important variables of sexuality (O'Hanlan, 1995b). A lesbian defined by behavior is a woman whose sexual practices include sexual activity with other women. A bisexual is attracted to and has sex with both men and women. Behavioral investigation focuses on variables associated with sexual activity, such as sexually transmitted diseases, sexual experimentation, and functional sexuality issues. "Are you sexual with men, women, both, or neither?" is a typical question used in the research setting or medical interview in order to elucidate a woman's sexual behavior. A woman may ostensibly identify herself as heterosexual but engage in sex only with other women. Conversely, she may identify herself socially as a lesbian but engage in sexual relations with men. The importance of the strict behavioral definition is that it avoids requiring potentially uncomfortable self-labeling; however, it misses the sociocultural identity and support systems that also impact health and behavior.

A lesbian defined by identity is a woman who participates in the lesbian sociocultural network and may or may not engage in any sexual activity with other women. A lesbian identifies with the specific social group's values and perceives herself as connected to a larger social structure that provides her with a sense of community (Friedman and Downey, 1993). The stigma of this identity is the predominant cause of ego-dystonic homosexuality and confers a majority of the psychosocial effects of homophobia: isolation, shame, diminished self-concept, self-destructive behaviors or health habits, and limited utilization of health care resources (O'Hanlan, 1995b).

Identity can be investigated in both research and medical caregiving situations with the question "Do you identify as heterosexual or straight, bisexual, gay or lesbian or homosexual, transgender, or none of these?" The identity definition of lesbianism allows an individual to categorize herself based on her sociocultural self-concept and transcends the issue of sexual behavior. The identity-based research question is complicated by the fact that the various terms for female homosexuality may not be used by all lesbians and may vary over time. Typically women who came out, or began to self-identify as homosexual, in the 1960s will call themselves "gay women." The women who came out in the 1970s and early 1980s will most often self-label as "lesbians," while women who came out in the late 1980s and more recently may use the term "queer" or "dyke." These latter two terms are actually used by some members of the lesbian community who have reclaimed their use from the derogatory, denaturing the sting of disdain. These terms are not used in the clinical setting. The term *homosexual* is generally a clinical term that neither gay men nor lesbians use socially. In this discourse, and in the preponderance of literature about lesbians, any woman who self-identifies by her response to either an identity or behavioral question is included; however, she may actually engage in heterosexual, bisexual, or homosexual activity.

Thus, adapting the definition of "women's health issues" from the Office of Research on Women's Health, lesbian health issues are those issues to which lesbians are "more susceptible, may have greater prevalence, or may be unique in developing, or be affected by differently" than nonlesbian women (Office of Research on Women's Health, 1991). The health issues of bisexual women will be considered in context with lesbians.

INCIDENCE OF LESBIANISM

Surveys from Japan, Thailand, Denmark, France, the Republic of Pelau, Great Britain, Australia, and the United States reveal that 0.2% to 6.9% of women variably describe themselves as lesbians. Most surveys from the United States suggest that not more than 3.6% of the 65 million American women, or 2.3 million citizens, are lesbians. In one report, 20% of men and 18% of women in the United States reported either homosexual attraction or behavior since age 15, but only 6.2% of men and 3.6% of women had had a homosexual contact in the past 5 years (Sell et al, 1995). Awareness of any homosexual feelings was reported in adolescence by 20% and currently by 12% of adult women (McConaghy et al, 1994). In the 1990 census count, 69,000 lesbian couples identified themselves as such (Usdansky, 1993).

DIVERSITY OF ORIENTATION

How can diversity of sexual orientation be explained? This area of discussion and research is highly controversial because it can be seen to futher stigmatize a minority of individuals and pathologize all but heterosexual orientation. Culturally competent health care is better utilized by women of color, low socioeconomic status, age, and disability. Lesbians are similarly marginalized women and will benefit from provision of culturally competent care (O'Hanlan, 1995b). While children are raised in American culture with the assumption that they are heterosexual, many lesbians recollect identifying same-sex attractions before their kindergarten year. Other women come to recognize a homosexual orientation later in life, after many years of living happily as heterosexual. The evidence in the current literature supports a multifactorial determination of heterosexual and homosexual orientation with many contributions (Pattatucci and Hamer, 1995).

Biologic Theories

Homosexuality has features of a purely biologic phenomenon, similar to handedness or hair color, because patterns indicative of genetic inheritance are observed, as well molecular and anatomic evidence (Hamer et al, 1993). Some prenatal hormones have been shown to influence brain sexual differentiation and subsequent orientation (Mac Culloch and Waddington, 1981). Females with prenatal exposure to diethylstilbesterol, or who have the salt-wasting variant of congenital adrenal hyperplasia, are more likely to be lesbians than are unaffected controls (Dittmann et al, 1992). Also, genes such as the HY-antigen complex and the X chromosome have been shown to elicit secretion of various intrauterine hormones, including testosterone, within the fetal brain that are mediated by neurotransmitters. However, the balance of prenatal hormonally mediated masculinization and defeminization of the brain can explain some of human sexual behavior, as it has in other mammals (Goodman, 1983). Levels of testosterone, androstenedione, estradiol, and progesterone measured in adult lesbians, stratifying between those who were aware of their homosexuality since an early age (so-called primary lesbians) and lesbians who became aware of their true orientation later in life or ("secondary lesbians"), showed no differences in comparison to those in heterosexual women (Dancey, 1990).

Evidence of anatomic differences comes from studies comparing the sizes, volume, and cell number of various hypothalamic and anterior commissure structures in autopsy specimens (Allen and Gorski, 1992; Levay, 1991; Swaab et al, 1992). While these findings may explain some differences in cerebral lateralization and other behaviors observed between homosexual and heterosexual men, they have not been identified in women.

A component of both male and female homosexuality is likely to be heritable as suggested by studies in clinical genetics (Bailey and Bell, 1993; Whitam et al, 1993). In one large twin study, 48% of monozygotic co-twins, 16% of dizygotic co-twine, and 6% of adoptive sisters were homosexual (Bailey et al, 1993), suggesting that sharing of genetic material co-varies with orientation more than environmental factors.

Psychological Theories

Many lesbians describe living satisfactory heterosexual early lives, even having marriages with children, and coming out at midlife or in later life. This has been associated with greater personal empowerment or heightened self-examination, after which the woman begins to express herself more fully and accurately.

Parental and social enforcement of majority expectations teaches many young lesbians to repress their feelings so as to effectively participate in the majority culture (Albro and Tully, 1979; Gonsiorek, 1981). Individuals choose a behavior in response to many environmental conditions, which results in a basic, but evolving, personal psychosexual strategy. A small

degree of orientation flexibility may result from the evolution of our capacity to learn, the complexity of the human central nervous system, and behavioral plasticity in general (Kinsey et al, 1948; Seaborg, 1984). By this process, various sexual expressions of the male and female genders can change over time from purely homosexual to bisexual to purely heterosexual to celibate, as observed in ancient Athens and modern Mediterranean/Latin cultures (Dickemann, 1983).

Lesbians are not more likely than heterosexual women to have had poor or failed relationships with men or to have been mistreated, molested, or raped by men (Gundlach, 1977; Brannock and Chapman, 1990; Bradford et al, 1994). Several studies comparing heterosexual women and lesbians confirm that lesbians do not have more negative childhood sexual experiences with males, more positive childhood sexual experiences with females, more accepting parental attitudes toward sexuality and sexual experimentation, or more distant relationships with their parents (Gundlach, 1977; Shavelson et al, 1980; Peters and Cantrell, 1991). A common misperception is held by some: that lesbians hate men (Kretzschmar, 1981). They do not. Some lesbians perceive themselves as needing to overcome multiple obstacles to achieve what some men are naturally conferred by their "in-group status" in American culture (Albro and Tully, 1979). While many heterosexual women are willing to tolerate some degree of gender bias in their social interactions to maintain their attractiveness and connection to men, a lesbian derives little benefit. Discriminatory treatment in job hiring and social interactions ultimately leads to a loss of opportunities and economic deprivation without legal recourse. A lesbian may also tire of the stigma of being considered unattractive and socially outcast, and of having her relationship denied legal recognition and support (Ferguson and Finkler, 1978).

Social and Character Preference Theories

Homosexuality in modern industrial nations has risen as a result, in part, of the demographic transition to a culture with low mortality, lower fertility, and relaxed reproductive demands, which is a more permissive environment for individual expression of diversity of sexual decisions and partner gender choices (Dickemann, 1993). With greater individual independence from the family unit, many have begun to pursue fulfillment of their social needs that is more consistent with their orientation, in preference to the orientation of the family (D'Emilio, 1993).

For some individuals, sexual arousal is based on criteria that transcend categories of genital organs (Kaplan and Rogers, 1984; Ross 1984). In many studies of males and females, androgynous individuals were more attractive than the very masculine or feminine stereotypes (Kaplan and Rogers, 1984). Many lesbians recognize their orientation later in life after very successful relations with men, and some feel this to be their choice. In summary, most investigators view sexual orientation as a multifactorial derivation of both heredity and environment that is complexly determined and diversely experienced.

LESBIAN HEALTH: THE SURVEY DATA

There are five peer-reviewed obstetric and gynecologic journal articles about lesbian health (Johnson et al, 1981, 1987a, 1987b; Johnson and Palermo, 1984; O'Hanlan, 1995a). Although it is admittedly difficult to study a hidden population, there are multiple published and unpublished reports issued from surveys distributed in various lesbian communities as early as 1980 (Mays and Cochran, 1988; Bybee 1990; Warshafsky, 1992; Bradford et al, 1994). These snowball surveys (handed out at social functions, sporting events, religious meetings) have inherent sampling bias; however, it is difficult to obtain a random sample of the lesbian population. Fortunately, the Women's Health Initiative and the Harvard Nurses' Health Study have decided to stratify their data by sexual behavior and self-labeled orientation, so more information will be available in the future. Until then, data from these large surveys can be examined to generate a profile and to stimulate and focus further research.

The mean age of women in the surveys was in the early to mid-30s, with a disproportionate number of urban and caucasian or white women, despite the fact that many studies actively sought lesbians of color and members of rural communities. Although 77% to 95% of respondents identified themselves as lesbian or primarily lesbian, 78% to 80% reported having had sex with men previously, 21% to 30% in the last 5 years, confirming that orientation identity and sexual behavior are not synonymous. Between 60% and 72% of lesbian respondents reported living in primary, marriage-like relationships, similar to the U.S. Census statistic for heterosexual women who are married, nearly 62% (Usdansky, 1993).

Lesbians were disproportionately higher educated than their heterosexual counterparts (32% vs. 17% graduate work), and received lower salaries (lesbian median under $30,000 yearly, heterosexual women over $30,000) (Usdansky, 1993).

Gynecologic Disorders

Dysmenorrhea/Pelvic Pain

Severe dysmenorrhea was reported by 38% to 54% of surveyed lesbians (Johnson et al, 1987a; Mays and Cochran, 1988; Bradford et al, 1994). Although only one study of lesbians asked about a specific diagnosis of endometriosis (Johnson et al, 1987a), the rates of nulliparity, severe dysmenorrhea, and hysterectomy suggest a high rate of endometriosis or adenomyosis among lesbian respondents. Surgical

therapy for debilitating menstrual pain not responding to nonsteroidal anti-inflammatory agents should be offered to lesbians who, with certainty, have elected not to bear children.

Menstruation

Serum hormone levels of testosterone, androstenedione, estradiol, and progesterone were measured at the same time in the menstrual cycle and were found to be the same among lifelong adult lesbians, lesbians who realized their orientation as adults, and heterosexual women (Dancey, 1990), providing no evidence for differences in menstrual irregularities or menstrual prodromata. Chronic anovulation or polycystic ovarian syndrome likely occurs with similar frequency in the lesbian and heterosexual populations. Diagnosis and treatment may be delayed for lesbians who do not disclose menstrual irregularities to the health care provider or when the clinician does not ask about the frequency of menstrual cycles. Untreated chronic anovulation can lead to endometrial hyperplasia and endometrial carcinoma. Women can be successfully protected from endometrial hyperplasia with daily combined oral contraceptives or cyclic progesterone 200 mg for 14 days following 3 months of amenorrhea.

Sexually Transmitted Diseases and Vaginitis

The incidence of vaginitis and sexually transmitted diseases is low in the lesbian population; however, every category of infection has been diagnosed and reported in lesbians. Exclusive lesbian sexual activity (sexual activity with women only) is associated with the lowest rates of infection, although exclusive lesbians have been diagnosed with bacterial vaginosis (Berger et al, 1995), Trichomonas (Johnson et al, 1981), human papillomavirus (O'Hanlan and Crum, 1996), and AIDS (Marmor et al, 1986). Women who identified as bisexual were more likely than women who identified as lesbian to contract Trichomonas, yeast, herpes, and gonorrhea, with rates of infection correlating with extent of their sexual activity with men (Johnson et al, 1987a). Chlamydia, syphilis, and gonorrhea screening is not productive among all lesbians (Johnson et al, 1981; Robertson and Schachter, 1981) but should be offered to lesbians with a history of these infections, with symptoms or signs of them, or who have been recently sexual with men.

Herpes affected 7.4% of screened lesbians (Robertson and Schachter, 1981) and may be transmitted by lesbian sexual activity (Johnson et al, 1987a). Because herpesvirus can be spread by orogenital sex, lesbians with either oral or genital lesions should refrain from sexual activity during times of clinical ulceration and be informed about the risk of occult transmission during subclinical disease.

Treatment for the sexually transmitted diseases and for vaginitis is the same for lesbians as for heterosexual women. Routine treatment of an asymptomatic female sexual partner is not indicated for *Trichomonas* or any of the other infections, but inquiry about the sexual partner should be made and testing offered if symptoms are present.

HIV has been identified in menstrual blood, the white blood cells (WBCs) of vaginal effluent, and saliva. It is thus reasonable to expect that the virus is transmissible during lesbian sexual activity, and possibly more so during menses, during vaginitis (more WBCs present), or after traumatic sexual behavior. Woman-to-woman sex is believed to confer a very low risk for contracting the AIDS virus because women in general rarely transmit the virus to their male partners, and because saliva has active antibodies that make the oral route a less likely route of viral entry. There are, however, many cases of suspected sexual transmission by lesbian sex (Sabatini et al, 1983; Marmor et al, 1986; Monzon and Capellan, 1987; Perry et al, 1989) and a report of HIV transmission to an exclusive lesbian (Troncoso et al, 1995). In addition, there are other risks for HIV within the lesbian population, such as needle sharing among injection drug users and sex with men, bisexual men, or injection drug–using men or women (Chu et al, 1990; Einhorn and Polgar, 1994; Lemp et al, 1995). One survey of San Francisco lesbians in public venues revealed that the rate of HIV infection was 1.4% (Lemp et al, 1995), with unsafe sexual practices and injection drug use as primary risk factors. Until more specific investigation of the lesbian population is undertaken, it is prudent to recommend safer sex precautions to lesbians, similar to those heterosexual women must use. A latex barrier during monogamous oral sexual activity between lesbians, with condoms covering any items inserted into the vagina, should be used for the first 6 months of their relationship, and can be discontinued once a repeat HIV test is negative or continued if positive.

Obesity

In a study of college-aged women, it was found that lesbians weighed slightly but significantly more, identified a significantly heavier ideal body weight, and expressed less concern for appearance and thinness than their heterosexual peers (Herzog et al, 1992). This is because lesbian cultural standards reject the popular pressures on women to appear "sexy" (e.g., to have tiny waistlines, large breasts, and long hair). Weight issues can become problematic because high body mass index is known to increase surgical risk for complications, as well as risk for breast, colon, and endometrial cancers (Holleb et al, 1991), heart disease, diabetes, gallstone formation, and hypertension (Namnoum, 1983). Clinicians should advise lesbian patients who are obese to modify their eating habits and exercise to reduce their disease risks.

Neoplastic Diseases

Because national probability health surveys have not asked about sexual orientation or same-sex behavior until recently, there are no comparative data on which to firmly base statements about the lesbian's risk for cancer. Demographic information from multiple lesbian surveys can be compared with established population demographics and known cancer risks, so that the lesbian's risk for each of the more common cancers can be postulated. It must be emphasized that these comparisons are only theoretical and serve only to underline the need for research.

Ovary

High parity, long duration of oral contraceptive use, tubal ligation, and rural living all reduce the risk of developing ovarian carcinoma (Holleb et al, 1991; Coker et al, 1993). Lesbians seem to cluster in the cities, are unlikely to have used oral contraceptives extensively, and are frequently nulliparous, and thus, theoretically, are at higher risk of ovarian cancer. Clinicians should counsel lesbians to consider taking oral contraceptives for 5, and preferably 10 years if they have multiple risk factors for ovarian cancer, especially an extensive family history of it. As for heterosexual women, oophorectomy should be performed when fertility is complete for women with extensive family histories or documented familial ovarian carcinoma.

Endometrium

The risk factors for endometrial cancer include obesity, a high-fat diet, and low parity, all common features of the lesbian demographic profile, suggesting a higher risk for this gynecologic cancer as well (Holleb et al, 1991). Extended use of oral contraceptives exerts a protective effect, but many lesbians have never needed this. Rather, progestins should be offered on a cyclic basis to postmenopausal women, especially obese women, to ensure shedding of the endometrium and reduction of endometrial cancer risk (Gambrell, 1988).

Cervix

Two studies have shown that less than 2.7% of lesbians developed cervical dysplasia, usually nonexclusive lesbians (Johnson et al, 1981; Robertson and Schachter, 1981). Sex with men and smoking are both risk factors for contracting human papillomavirus, the initiating agent for cervical dysplasia and cancer (Holleb et al, 1991). Some national studies have suggested that *single women*, in comparison to married women, have higher rates of cigarette abuse (U.S. Department of Health and Human Services, 1991). Although it has not been clearly demonstrated that *lesbians* smoke more than heterosexual women, the rates appear *at least* as high. Because 77% to 91% of lesbians have had at least one prior sexual experience with men (Cochran and Mays, 1988; Bybee, 1990; Bradford et al, 1994), continued surveillance by routine Pap smear is indicated. Most lesbians do not know the risk factors for cervical cancer and do not perceive themselves to be at risk (Price et al, 1996).

The interval between Pap smears for lesbians was reported to be nearly three times that for heterosexual women (Robertson and Schachter, 1981). As many as 5% to 10% of lesbian respondents in two large surveys had never had a Pap smear or had one over 10 years ago (Bybee, 1990; Bradford et al, 1994). It appears prudent to stratify patients based on their clinical histories, recommending yearly Pap tests to women with *any* of the known risk factors for cervical cancer and offering triennial Pap smears to those lesbians with none of the risk factors and a history of normal Pap smears over the 3 prior years.

Breast

Risk factors for breast cancer include nulliparity or delayed parity, alcohol abuse, obesity, and high fat intake (Willett, et al, 1987; London et al, 1989; Holleb et al, 1991). Single women have lower rates of obtaining screening mammograms and clinical breast exams and of performing breast self-exams compared to married women (U.S. Department of Health and Human Services, 1991). One fourth of lesbians over age 40 in the Michigan study had never had a mammogram (Bybee, 1990). The lack of appropriate use of screening modalities, combined with an apparent concentration of risk factors, may indicate a hidden epidemic of breast cancer among lesbians.

Colon

Obesity, a high-fat diet, a history of colon polyps, smoking, and high alcohol intake have been shown to increase risk for colon polyps and colon carcinoma (Chute et al, 1991; Giovannucci et al, 1993; 1994). Stool screening guaiac cards have been shown to result in earlier diagnosis of colon cancer and subsequent higher survival rates (Fry et al, 1989). Digital rectal exam revealing polyps or a lesion may be the earliest sign of a small cancer, and is an important part of the annual exam, which may be missed by the lesbian avoiding care.

Coronary and Cerebrovascular Diseases

Smoking and obesity are two major risk factors for coronary atherosclerosis (Leaverton et al, 1987; Manson et al, 1990). Clinical assessment of the serum cholesterol level, blood pressure, weight, and exercise and dietary history is part of routine annual screening checkups, which lesbians miss if they forego annual doctor visits.

Considering all of these factors, lesbians may experience greater morbidity or mortality from multiple cancers and heart disease, especially if they defer seeing a clinician until symptoms or signs become extreme or acute (O'Hanlan, 1991; Haynes, 1992; Robertson, 1992). If reliable demographic information about lesbian health showed a higher incidence, morbidity, or mortality from various cancers or heart disease, then screening or health education programs could be instituted and targeted to the lesbian population.

Suicide

Many families are unable to provide acceptance and approval to their lesbian daughters, which may constitute the most crucial loss these young girls experience (Schneider et al, 1989; Hunter and Schaecter, 1990; American Academy of Pediatrics, Committee on Adolescence, 1993; Hammelman, 1993). At the Hetrick Martin Institute, a gay and lesbian high school in New York City, among the lesbian adolescents surveyed who reported being rejected by their families, 44% had suicidal ideation and 41% had attempted suicide (Hunter, 1989). Among adult lesbians, more than 50% of lesbian respondents had suicidal ideation at some time in their lives, and 18% had attempted suicide (Bradford et al, 1994). In a 1991 survey conducted by the Centers for Disease Control, 27% of 11,631 high school youth reported suicidal ideation and 8% had attempted suicide (Centers for Disease Control, 1991). Whether lesbian children are committing suicide at higher rates than heterosexual youth remains unclear and deserves further scientific investigation.

Substance Abuse

Epidemiologists have criticized the many older surveys about lesbian alcoholism that were circulated among bar patrons as unreliable (Clark, 1981; Paul et al, 1991). Recent data regarding lesbian alcohol abuse indicate similar rates among heterosexual and lesbian women in the Chicago and San Francisco areas (McKirnan and Peterson, 1989; Bloomfield, 1993).

Many detoxification programs show little sensitivity to how issues of sexual orientation and homophobia may relate to addictive disorders. The success of treatment for lesbian substance abusers is reduced by avoiding core issues such as self-esteem and peer relations (Fifield et al, 1975; Morales and Graves, 1983; de Monteflores, 1986; Hellman et al, 1989; Hall 1990).

Violence

A 1992 survey by the Philadelphia Lesbian and Gay Task Force revealed that half of lesbians had endured verbal abuse and over one third had experienced some form of physical violence (Gross and Aurand, 1992). Homicides against homosexuals were reported to frequently involve mutilation and torture (Bell and Vila, 1996), and go unsolved more often than the homicides of heterosexuals (Dunlap, 1994). Psychological and emotional injury, such as phobias, post-traumatic stress syndromes, chronic pain syndromes, eating disorders, and, most commonly, depression, can also occur to victims of hate violence (Bybee, 1990; LeBlanc, 1991; Barnes and Ephross, 1994).

There is growing awareness in the medical community concerning domestic violence among heterosexuals, but there is little awareness that domestic violence also occurs in lesbian relationships (Leeder, 1988; Island and Letellier, 1991; Morrow, 1994). Victims and perpetrators were more likely to experience violence in the context of alcohol use (Schilit et al, 1990), perpetuating a cycle of denial and continuing violence. The 1988 National Lesbian Health Care Survey reported that 11% of lesbians had been victims of domestic violence by their lesbian partner (Bradford et al, 1994).

Sexuality

According to various studies, about 12% of heterosexual women and 3% of lesbians are anorgasmic, with 30% of heterosexual women and most of lesbians reporting regular orgasms (Ford and Beach, 1952; Hite, 1981). Recently, it was reported that women who had ever had sex with another woman were about as likely to have low sexual desire or sexual discomfort as women who had never had sex with another women, but about half as likely to have an arousal disorder (Laumann et al, 1999). Some 10% to 23% of lesbians self-report some degree of dysfunction (Kinsey et al, 1953; Johnson et al, 1987a). A separate survey of Seattle heterosexual women revealed that 63% self-reported dysfunction (Frank et al, 1978). This apparent discrepancy may be due to the fact that the preponderance of lesbian sexual activity consists of direct manual, digital, and mostly oral stimulation of the clitoris. However, the similarity of anatomy (Hite, 1981), the less goal-oriented sexual activity, and better communication during sex (Masters and Johnson, 1979) may also confer a heightened awareness of desirable sexual stimulation.

Family Issues

Once the basic physical survival needs for food, shelter, and safety are met, then, according to Maslow's hierarchy of needs, an individual is free to fulfill higher needs such as community and social order and, after that, intimacy and procreation. Many lesbians desire marriage and children once their rela-

tionship reaches a mutual degree of satisfaction, intimacy, and commitment. There is no scientific basis to suggest social catastrophe should the right to civil contract of marriage be extended to any citizen desiring that for which the civil institution of marriage stands: a monogamous, long-term, mutually supportive, committed relationship. Denial of this right to contract with each other is deeply corrosive to the self-concept of lesbians and can preclude the fulfillment of one's natural psychosocial needs.

Parity

Between 6% and 46% of lesbians report bearing and raising children (Mays and Cochran, 1988; Bybee, 1990; Warshafsky, 1992; Bradford et al, 1994), with another 30% to 62% interested in undergoing insemination. These figures are likely understated as a result of the recent "gay-bi boom," in which lesbians and gay men alike are newly creating their families by adoption or various insemination arrangements. Some reproductive endocrinologists refuse to inseminate women who are legally "single" but in long-term, marriage-like relationships with another woman. Acquisition of semen through a licensed sperm bank offers lesbian couples their only guarantee of sole legal custody and avoidance of infectious and heritable diseases. It is currently legal to refuse to inseminate lesbians in 41 states, but it is against the nondiscrimination policy of the American Medical Association (AMA)(Council on Scientific Affairs, AMA, 1996). Such refusal relegates lesbians to obtaining sperm through unofficial means such as sex with a male or semen from a friend (Wendland et al, 1996), with the attendant risk of custody battles and disease. Although this topic has not been formally reviewed and addressed by the American College of Obstetricians and Gynecologists, it behooves individuals and departments to create equitable policies toward their lesbian patients. Lesbian patients should be asked about their desires to bear children and counseled about the safety issues of unofficial insemination.

New technology devised to provide oligospermic heterosexual couples a genetically related baby has been applied to lesbians to provide a shared maternity and assure joint custody. After superovulating one woman, the harvested ova are fertilized and cryopreserved to be used for intrauterine insemination of the other woman in the couple. She will thus carry and deliver her domestic partner's genetic baby, but she will be legally recognized as the mother as well. Although this procedure carries risk and is expensive, heterosexual and lesbian couples alike may prefer it to obtain a genetically related fetus.

Low parity confers an increased risk for breast, endometrial, and ovarian cancers. Discussion of risk reduction methods should be undertaken once a practitioner determines that a patient will not likely bear a child. However, it should not be assumed that lesbian orientation is synonymous with nulliparity.

Obstetric Care

There are no specific obstetric risk factors conferred by lesbian sexual orientation. However, clinicians should make sure that the medical power of conservatorship papers have signed by the parents-to-be in order to assure that the lesbian couple's medical intentions are understood and respected. In times of any medical crisis, clinicians can legally only recognize a blood relative or a medical conservator. The blood relative may not be as familiar with the wishes of the patient as the domestic partner, and can override her input. Additionally, hospitals can restrict visitation privileges of nonrelatives, but not medical conservators. Unfortunately only a fraction of lesbians have taken the legal steps designating their medical conservatorship. Clinicians should encourage all lesbian couples to sign these contracts, but especially prior to planned gynecologic or obstetric procedures.

Children in Lesbian Households

Over 300 children raised in gay and lesbian households, ages 5 to 17, have been exhaustively studied, with the finding that they developed no differently than children raised in heterosexual households (Patterson, 1992). They also demonstrated no significant difference in strength of self-concept (Puryear, 1983; Huggins, 1989), locus of control (Rees, 1979; Puryear, 1983), moral judgment (Rees, 1979), or intelligence (Green et al, 1986). However, 5% of children had been taunted by their peers because of their parents' sexual orientation. Additionally, two studies suggested that children fare better when they are told about their parents' orientation in early childhood rather than later (Paul, 1986; Huggins, 1989). It has also been shown to be healthier for children when the mothers are psychologically comfortable about sexual orientation issues and involved in the lesbian/feminist community (Rand et al, 1982) and when their biological fathers, if known, are not homophobic (Huggins, 1989). The incidence of homosexuality among children with lesbian parents is similar to that of children with heterosexual parents (Green, 1978; Rees, 1979; Golombok et al, 1983; Paul, 1986; Huggins, 1989).

Aging Lesbians

Senior lesbians can become invisible and frequently lost to their community when age, poverty, and health issues compound, reordering priorities to sustain basic needs in a predominantly heterosexual setting such as a nursing home or outpatient senior community (Deevey, 1990). Among older lesbians, heightened life satisfaction is reported when they remain connected to and have activity in the lesbian community (Quam and Whitford, 1992). Sex, per se, may become less important to senior lesbians, but these women stated they still preferred being with other lesbians in their generation, or to spend their days in an intergenerational lesbian retirement community (Kehoe, 1986, 1988).

Gender-Atypical and Lesbian Children

It has been shown that gender-atypical children, the "sissy" boys and the "tomboy" girls, do have a high likelihood of eventually expressing a homosexual orientation or a trandsgender identity (Whitman and Mathy, 1991). The emerging homosexual identity appears to be reflected in children's and adolescent's attractions, fantasies, and cultural affiliations, as well as behaviors. Some parents can develop strong negative attitudes in response to their children's gender atypicality (McConaghy and Zamir, 1995), which makes the child feel uncomfortable with his or her self (Savin-Williams). Gender-atypical children should not be told "this is a normal phase," because it implies that they are expected to outgrow it. If homosexuality is acceptable in its adult expression, the infantile precursors of this expression must likewise be accepted. It important to support all children in developing a strong self-esteem, and to not stigmatize them by trying to change their gender-atypical behavior.

Sexual orientation at elementary school ages is not an issue of sex, but of orientation. Children can understand in an age-appropriate fashion that some people like others who are the same gender. Although some learn about homosexuality in their families or classrooms, most report that it is negatively portrayed to them, or they are called the perjoratives "fag," "dyke," and "queer." As a result, it is often difficult to identify any adult who is supportive of them, and they are already aware of hostile attitudes within their families and schools and among their peers (Taylor and Remafedi, 1993; Telljohann and Price, 1993).

According to many surveys of gay and lesbian youth, approximately one third know they are homosexual between ages 4 and 10, and most of the rest before age 17 (Telljohann and Price, 1993). There may, however, be a significant delay in time after recognizing a homosexual orientation within oneself and telling someone else about it (coming out). During this time of insecurity, many youths may engage in both same-sex and opposite-sex sexual behaviors, often employing unsafe methods, risking infections and pregnancy. Suicide attempts may also occur during this time of nondisclosure because of perceptions of family ostracism and social rejection (D'Augelli and Hershberger, 1993).

The process of adolescent coming out usually is seen to entail four steps: recognition within the self; exploration with others; disclosure to family or friends; and accommodation, or becoming more comfortable with one's sexual orientation (Rotheram-Borus and Fernandez, 1995). Families may experience stress and require information while supporting a child's questioning of sexual orientation. Parents, Family, and Friends of Lesbians and Gays (P-FLAG) is a nationwide organization providing information and support and is invaluable to the many who have utilized its resources. Other families may benefit from a referral to supportive psychotherapy (Hammersmith, 1987; Neisen, 1987).

INTERSEXUALITY

Intersexuality refers to the presence of important male and female characteristics in a single individual. Intersexed people may be born with ambiguous genitals (microphallus, macroclitoris, or indeterminate gender), some with female external genitalia and internal testes or male external genitalia and internal ovaries. The term "hermaphroditism" is no longer used because it does not specify which of the many conditions and phenotypes possible are present. True sexual ambiguity occurs in about 1 in 2000 or 0.05% of infants, however lesser degrees of genital ambiguity are more common. Etiologies include adrenal hyperplasia, androgen resistance, gonadal dysgenesis, and errors of androgen synthesis or metabolism (Migeon et al, 1994).

Since the late 1950s it has been standard practice to regard gender as determined solely by genital appearance. The birth of a child with ambiguous genitals was treated as a "psychosocial emergency," with gender assignment made as rapidly as possible and surgical alteration performed as needed to help the genital appearance conform more to the gender assigned. Gender was usually assigned based on surgical convenience; if the phallus was considered too small, the child was assigned female without regard to genetic or gonadal sex (Dreger, 1998). In the past several years, this model has become questioned by health professionals and ethicists, as adult intersexuals came forward to discuss how early treatment had affected them (Kessler, 1998). Many have expressed dissatisfaction with either their gender assignment or the mutilating effects of early surgery.

A new model appears to be emerging, which calls for children born with ambiguous sex anatomy to be labeled with a sex, but without performing cosmetic genital surgery. Honest disclosure, peer support, and patient autonomy are emphasized, with change of sex role and cosmetic genital surgery advocated only when requested by an informed patient (Diamond and Sigmundson, 1997).

TRANSSEXUALS

Transsexuals are often confused with homosexuals but, in fact, are quite different. Transsexual individuals have a strong belief, often from childhood onward, that they were born into a body with the wrong sex. The vast majority are heterosexual to their identified gender, but a few have a homosexual orientation. A few have been reported to have had

ambiguous genitalia as children and were arbitrarily "assigned" a gender, or had their genitals surgically revised according to the obstetrician's perspective of their infantile genitalia. In retrospect, it appears safer for children with ambiguous genitals to be assigned a name appropriate to both genders and allowed to self-identify a gender as they begin to experience themselves in context (Coleman et al, 1993).

Gender identity is thought to develop as various sex hormones affect the developing fetal brain (Giordano and Giusti, 1995; Zhou et al, 1995). Many studies of the multiple sexual-dimorphic nuclei in the brain suggest that transsexuals possess the neuroanatomy appropriate to their self-perceived gender, not their phenotypic gender (Elias and Valenta, 1992; Giordano and Giusti, 1995; Zhou et al, 1995). The obstetrician-gynecologist may be called on to provide care for females who desire sex-reassignment surgery, called female-to-male (FTM) transsexuals, or for women who have had their surgery who were previously phenotypic men, called male-to-female (MTF) transsexuals. All transsexuals should be referred to by the pronouns of their identified genders. The specific needs of each are different.

FTM Transsexuals

Young heterosexual girls, lesbians, and girls who later become FTM males may all dress as tomboys to varying degrees; however, girls who later become FTM males crossdress more frequently and are more comfortable in boy's clothes. In most survey reports they describe themselves as the consummate tomboys, experiencing clear gender dysphoria and increasing discomfort with pubertal onset of thelarche and menarche (McCauley and Ehrhardt, 1977; Ehrhardt et al, 1979). Clinicians should refer these young women, at their request, for supportive counseling to a center experienced with transsexualism and help them locate a surgeon experienced in FTM sex reassignment surgery. Prior to surgery, an FTM must live ostensibly as a male for at least 1 year, employing 200-mg testosterone injections every 2 weeks to suppress menses and induce masculine secondary sex characteristics. A laparoscopic hysterectomy and vaginectomy are part of the surgery in which the gynecologist can collaborate. Because these individuals may desire to have children, cryopreservation of unstimulated ovarian cortex during oophorectomy has been discussed as a means to preserve follicles for later insemination and gestation (Newton et al, 1996). Serum cholesterol should be monitored in these individuals as usual for all men.

MTF Transsexuals

Some young boys love to dress as women, and actually may recognize themselves to have been born into the wrong body. After they have matured, they express a strong wish to be themselves, living their lives as women. Before initiating estrogen therapy to begin the transformation, cryopreservation of banked sperm should be offered to these males (Hall and Schaffer, 1997). Once they are stabilized on a dose of estrogen that suppresses gonadotropins and produces serum estradiol levels of 200 to 400 pg/ml, spermatogenesis ceases; but it will resume in a few months if estrogen is discontinued (Lubbert et al, 1992) to allow for sperm banking. The surgery, performed long after the MTF has been living as an overt female, usually involves remodeling the skin of the penile shaft into a vagina, preserving a portion of the glans penis as a clitoris, and fashioning an opening for the urethra beneath the clitoris. Sometimes a vagina is extended by adding a split-thickness skin graft, or it can be made from a segment of colon. The final result usually forms a moist vagina and a functional orgasmic sexual response, and has a good cosmetic effect.

Squamous cell carcinomas have been documented in the neovaginas of MTF transsexuals, usually occurring 10 or more years after vaginoplasty (Imrie et al, 1986). Pap smears should be performed per the usual risk profiles, and all suspicious lesions biopsied. Mammography is probably not indicated for MTF women until after 10 or more years of estrogen stimulation because the risk of breast cancer is cumulative over time. The yearly exam needs to also include an assessment of the prostate, because this is not removed in most surgeries but may be too small to identify. If any nodularity is identified, a serum prostate-specific antigen assay and sonography should be obtained, although there are no cases yet reported of prostatic carcinoma in postoperative MTFs. The gynecologist may be consulted for the occasional stenosis of the vaginal graft, and may need to surgically revise a contracted introitus to accommodate sexual activity.

INTEGRATING SOLUTIONS

It has been shown that being a lesbian or sexual minority is not inherently (genetically, biologically) hazardous, and that orientation and gender identity are the results of prenatal and life processes beyond current understanding. However, significant health risk factors are conferred through "homophobic fallout." The process of homophobia, in which heterosexuals are unwittingly socialized against homosexuals, and gays and lesbians are conditioned against themselves, must be recognized by health care providers as a legitimate, potent health hazard.

The American Medical Women's Association (AMWA) has published a policy statement urging an end to discrimination by sexual orientation. Moreover, the AMWA encouraged:

national, state, and local legislation to end discrimination based on sexual orientation in housing, employment, marriage and tax laws, child custody and adoption laws; to redefine family to encompass the full diversity of all family structures; and to ratify marriage for lesbian, gay and bisexual people . . . creation and implementation of educational programs . . . in the schools, religious institutions, medical community, and the wider community to teach respect for all humans. (AMWA, 1993)

Medical Education

It appears essential to possess some knowledge about diversity of sexual orientation in clinical practice. This information should come from organized curricula in medical school and residency training programs. The American Psychiatric Association (APA) has sponsored a curriculum for learning about homosexuality and gay men and lesbians in psychiatric residencies, which describes educational objectives, learning experiences, and implementation strategies for sound clinical practice (Stein, 1994). This can be applied to the training in obstetrics and gynecology.

Doctor-Patient Relationship

The AMA policy statement issued in December 1994 concerning gay and lesbian health recognized the alienation of gay men and lesbians from the medical system as one of the psychological effects of ubiquitous prejudice against homosexuals (Council on Scientic Affairs, AMA, 1996). The need for a trusting and supportive relationship is essential to obtain a thorough medical history. There are numerous ways obstetricians and gynecologists can make their practices more welcoming of lesbian patients:

1. During each initial encounter, routinely ask every patient about sexual behavior by neutrally inquiring whether the patient is sexual with men, women, both, or neither. Asking a patient if she is a "lesbian" or a "homosexual" relies on the patient's definition and acceptance of the labels. Many women have sex with other women but would never use these words to describe themselves.
2. Use inclusive language in conversation with lesbian patients, employing generic terms such as "partner" or "spouse."
3. Revise office registration forms and questionnaires that require patients to identify themselves only in heterosexual terms, such as single, widowed, separated, or divorced, by adding "significantly involved" or "domestic partner." Such a small change will avoid making the lesbian patient feel invisible in your practice.
4. Provide office informational brochures for patients, especially those dealing with aspects of human sexuality, which include information about lesbianism. The American College of Obstetricians and Gynecologists offers a brochure on lesbian health that can be the first message to

a young woman questioning her orientation that she is normal and welcome in your office.

5. As should be done for the heterosexual patient, if the lesbian patient is partnered, ask if she is happy in her relationship, if she feels safe and content, because domestic violence occurs in lesbian as well as heterosexual relationships. Welcome her spouse to your next office visit, and encourage the couple to obtain a medical power of attorney document, particularly prior to elective surgery or obstetric delivery.

6. Understand that many homosexuals, transsexuals, and intersexuals can be very homophobic and ashamed, and may need referral to a therapist to deal with issues about their self-esteem. Some may have lost their families or jobs as a result of societal homophobia or hatred, while others may be stressed by the prohibitions against marriage and military service; these individuals may require reassurance and emotional support. A few supportive statements can go a long way to provide comfort and establish a trusting relationship.

7. Offer parents information and reassurance to parents that their gender-atypical children are normal, enabling the parents to accept and enjoy their children, who need their support and consistent love. Although it is impossible for parents or clinicians to predict which youth are struggling with issues of orientation and gender identity, all youth benefit from nonbiased demonstrations of the doctor's and parent's positive attitude toward these issues.

8. As an educated civic leader, facilitate acculturation of gay and lesbian youth and the children of gay and lesbian parents in the schools by encouraging school libraries to include storybooks of positive gay or lesbian family role models (Goodman, 1993; Phillip, 1993). School-based family counseling programs and after-school social support programs for gay and lesbian youth will promote a more accurate image of homosexuals. There is no evidence that such policies will cause more children to become homosexual. There is evidence that these policies will facilitate the healthy adjustment of all the children who attend.

9. Support changes in government for the health of patients. The APA and the AMWA have concluded that the effective solutions to homophobia must include legislation to ban discrimination against gay men and lesbians (Bersoff and Ogden, 1991). Government-enforced discrimination delivers a message to children that homosexual adults are unfit and undeserving citizens. Denial of marriage, military discharge of gay and lesbian service members, and immigration prohibition practices perpetuate misinformation and hatred among American youth while undermining confidence and psychological health of lesbians and gay men.

10. Provide domestic partner benefits, including medical insurance, to all registered families in practice offices.

Stanford was the first university to offer its entire benefits package to all its employees and their families. The 1992 report of the Subcommittee on Domestic Partners' Benefits of the Committee for Faculty and Staff Benefits stated:

One imagines, for example, that a decision by Stanford 40 years ago to take the lead in eradicating discrimination against blacks, women or Jews in admissions, hiring, memberships in sororities and fraternities, etc., would have been politically unpopular with many alumni, as well as with the larger political community. One also imagines that had Stanford taken such a leadership role, few in the Stanford community would look back on that decision now with anything but pride. (Fried, 1992)

With such awareness, practitioners can serve as leaders and positive examples in both the medical realm and the larger community in signaling the need for reduction of societal homophobia.

Obstetricians and gynecologists have an ethical and moral obligation to treat all women equally. Clinicians must discard those old views they innocently learned but that science does not validate. All health care providers must examine their attitudes about homosexuality, recognizing which views they hold that are not consistent with facts. Practitioners have the unique opportunity to influence others to align their attitudes with objective information. By teaching all patients about diversity of orientation, providers can reduce the pervasive yet unfounded disdain for homosexuals, facilitating maintenance of lesbians' self-esteem. Legislation proscribing discrimination and providing legal recognition for the unions of lesbian and gay families would restore legal, societal, and financial equity to this marginalized population. The subsequent increased visibility of lesbians would increase their familiarity in the community and promote greater understanding.

Each of these steps will reduce oppression of lesbians and gay men from society, as well as from their learned self-oppression within. Greater access to medical care, integration into their family and society, heightened life-satisfaction, productivity, and greater health will result once we recognize homophobia as the major health hazard it poses not only to gay and lesbian individuals, but to our entire society.

REFERENCES

Albro J, Tully C: A study of lesbian lifestyles in the homosexual micro-culture and the heterosexual macro-culture. J Homosex 1979;4:331.

Allen LS, Gorski RA: Sexual orientation and the size of the anterior commissure in the human brain. Proc Natl Acad Sci U S A 1992;89:7199.

American Academy of Pediatrics, Committee of Adolescence: Homosexuality and adolescence. Pediatrics 1993;92:631.

American Medical Women's Association: Position paper on lesbian health. J Am Med Wom Assoc 1993;49:86.

Bailey JM, Bell AP: Familiality of female and male homosexuality. Behav Genet 1993;23:313.

Bailey JM, Pillard RC, Neale MC, Agyei Y: Heritable factors influence sexual orientation in women. Arch Gen Psychiatry 1993;50:217.

Barnes A, Ephross PH: The impact of hate violence on victims: emotional and behavioral responses to attacks. Soc Work 1994; 39:247.

Bell MD, Vila RI: Homicide in homosexual victims: a study of 67 cases from the Broward County, Florida, Medical Examiner's office (1982–1992), with special emphasis on "overkill." Am J Forensic Med Path 1996;17:65.

Berger BJ, Kolton S, Zenilman JM, et al: Bacterial vaginosis in lesbians: a sexually transmitted disease. Clin Infect Dis 1995; 21:1402.

Bersoff DN, Ogden DW: APA amicus curiae briefs: furthering lesbian and gay male civil rights. Am Psychol 1991;46:950.

Bloomfield K: A comparison of alcohol consumption between lesbians and heterosexual women in an urban population. Drug Alcohol Depend 1993;33:257.

Bozett F: Children of Gay Fathers. New York: Praeger, 1987.

Bradford J, Ryan C, Rothblum ED: National Lesbian Health Care Survey: implications for mental health care. J Consult Clin Psychol 1994;62:228.

Brannock JC, Chapman BE: Negative sexual experiences with men among heterosexual women and lesbians. J Homosex 1990;19:105.

Bybee D: Michigan Lesbian Survey: A Report to the Michigan Organization for Human Rights and the Michigan Department of Public Health. Detroit: Michigan Department of Health and Human Services, 1990.

Centers for Disease Control: Attempted suicide among high school students in the United States, 1990. MMWR Morb Mortal Wkly Rep 1991;40(32):1.

Chu SY, Buehler JW, Fleming PL, Berkelman RL: Epidemiology of reported cases of AIDS in lesbians, United States 1980–89. Am J Public Health 1990;80:1380.

Chute CG, Willett WC, Colditz GA, et al: A prospective study of body mass, height, and smoking on the risk of colorectal cancer in women. Cancer Causes Control 1991;2:117.

Clark W (ed): The Contemporary Tavern. New York: Plenum Press, 1981:6.

Cochran SD, Mays VM: Disclosure of sexual preference to physicians by black lesbian and bisexual women. West J Med 1988; 149:616.

Coker AL, Harlap S, Fortney JA: Oral contraceptives and reproductive cancers: weighing the risks and benefits. Fam Plann Perspect 1993;25:17.

Coleman E, Bockting WO, Gooren L: Homosexual and bisexual identity in sex-reassigned female-to-male transsexuals. Arch Sex Behav 1993;22:37.

Council on Scientific Affairs, American Medical Association: Health care needs of gay men and lesbians in the United States. JAMA 1996;275:1354.

Dancy C: Sexual orientation in women: an investigation of hormonal and personality variables. Biol Psychol 1990;30:251.

D'Augelli AR, Hershberger SL: Lesbian, gay, and bisexual youth in community settings: personal challenges and mental health problems. Am J Community Psychol 1993;21:421.

de Monteflores C: Notes on the management of difference. In Stein TS, Cohen CC (eds): Contemporary Perspectives on Psychotherapy with Lesbians and Gay Men. New York: Plenum Press, 1986:73.

Deevey S: Older lesbian women: an invisible minority. J Gerontol Nurs 1990;16:35.

D'Emilio J: Capitalism and gay identity. In Abelove H, Barale MA, Halperin DM (eds): The Lesbian and Gay Studies Reader. London: Routledge, Inc, 1993:467.

Diamond M, Sigmundson H: Management of intersexuality: guidelines for dealing with persons with ambiguous genitalis. Arch Pediatr Adolesc Med 1997;151:1046.

Dickemann M: Reproductive strategies and gender construction: an evolutionary view of homosexualities. J Homosex 1993;24: 55.

Dittmann RW, Kappes ME, Kappes MH: Sexual behavior in adolescent and adult females with congenital adrenal hyperplasia. Psychoneuroendocrinology 1992;17:153.

Dreger AD: "Ambiguous sex"—or ambivalent medicine? Ethical issues in the medical treatment of Intersexuality. Hastings Center Report 1998;28:24.

Dunlap D: Survey on slayings of homosexuals finds high violence and low arrest rate. New York Times 1994; December 21:A-10.

Ehrhardt AA, Grisanti G, McCauley EA: Female-to-male transsexuals compared to lesbians: behavioral patterns of childhood and adolescent development. Arch Sex Behav 1979;8:481.

Einhorn L, Polgar M: HIV-risk behavior among lesbians and bisexual women. AIDS Educ Prev 1994;6:514.

Elias AN, Valenta LJ: Are all males equal? Anatomic and functional basis for sexual orientation in males. Med Hypotheses 1992;39:85.

Ellis AL, Vasseur RB: Prior interpersonal contact with and attitudes towards gays and lesbians in an interviewing context. J Homosex 1993;25:31.

Fifield L, de Crescenzo T, Latham J: Alcoholism and the Gay Community: Summary of "On My Way to Nowhere: Alienated, Isolated, Drunk: An Analysis of Gay Alcohol Abuse and Evaluation of Alcoholism Rehabilitation Services for Los Angeles County. Los Angeles: Los Angeles Gay Community Services Center, 1975.

Ford CS, Beach FA: Homosexual Behavior. New York: Harper & Brothers and Paul B. Hoeber Medical Books, 1952.

Frank E, Anderson C, Rubinstein D: Frequency of sexual dysfunction in "normal" couples. N Engl J Med 1978;299:111.

Fried B: Report of the Subcommittee on Domestic Partners' Benefits. Stanford, CA: University Committee for Faculty and Staff Benefits, 1992:37.

Friedman RC, Downey J: Neurobiology and sexual orientation: current relationships. J Neuropsychiatry Clin Neurosci 1993;5: 131.

Fry RD, Fleshman JW, Kodner IJ: Cancer of the colon and rectum. Clin Symp 1989;415:29.

Giordano G, Giusti M: Hormones and psychosexual differentiation. Minerva Endocrinol 1995;20:165.

Giovannucci E, Rimm EB, Stampfer MJ, et al: A prospective study of cigarette smoking and risk of colorectal adenoma and colorectal cancer in U.S. men [see comments]. J Natl Cancer Inst 1994;86:183.

Giovannucci E, Stampfer MJ, Colditz GA, et al: Folate, methionine, and alcohol intake and risk of colorectal adenoma [see comments]. J Natl Cancer Inst 1993;85:875.

Golombok S, Spencer A, Rutter M: Children in lesbian and single-parent households: psychosexual and psychiatric appraisal. J Child Psychol Psychiatry 1983;24:551.

Gonsiorek JC: The use of diagnostic concepts in working with gay and lesbian populations. J Homosex 1981;7:9.

Goodman JM: Lesbian, gay & bisexual issues in education. Thrust for Educational Leadership 1993;April:24.

Goodman RE: Biology of sexuality: inborn determinants of human sexual response. Br J Psychiatry 1983;143:216.

Green R: Sexual identity of 37 children raised by homosexual or transsexual parents. Am J Psychiatry 1978;13:692.

Green R, Mandel JM, Hotvedt ME, et al: Lesbian mothers and their children: a comparison with solo parent heterosexual mothers and their children. Arch Sex Behav 1986;15:167.

Gross L, Aurand S: Discrimination and Violence Against Lesbian Women and Gay Men in Philadelphia and the Commonwealth of Pennsylvania: A Study by the Philadelphia Lesbian and Gay Task Force. Philadelphia: The Philadelphia Lesbian and Gay Task Force, 1992.

Gundlach RH: Sexual molestation and rape reported by homosexual and heterosexual women. J Homosex 1977;2:367.

Hall C, Schaffer J: Gamete cryopreservation prior to sex reassignment. Unpublished manuscript from the Seahorse Medical Clinic in San Jose, CA (specializing in health for transsexuals), 1997.

Hall JM: Alcoholism in lesbians: developmental, symbolic interactionist, and critical perspectives. Health Care Wom Int 1990; 11:89.

Hamer DH, Hu S, Magnuson VL, et al: A linkage between DNA markers on the X chromosome and male sexual orientation [see comments]. Science 1993;261:321.

Hammelman T: Gay and lesbian youth: contributing factors to serious attempts or considerations of suicide. J Gay Lesbian Psychiatry 1993;2:77.

Hammersmith SK: A sociological approach to counseling homosexual clients and their families. J Homosex 1987;14:173.

Haynes S: Risk of breast cancer in lesbians. Paper presented at the Annual Meeting of the National Gay and Lesbian Health Education Foundation. Los Angeles, 1992.

Hellman RE, Stanton M, Lee J, et al: Treatment of homosexual alcoholics in government-funded agencies: provider training and attitudes. Hosp Community Psychiatry 1989;40:1163.

Herzog D, Newman K, Yeh C, Warshaw M: Body image satisfaction in homosexual and heterosexual women. Int J Eating Disord 1992;11:391.

Hite S: The Hite Report. New York: Macmillan, 1981.

Holleb A, Fink D, Murphy G: American Cancer Society Textbook of Clinical Oncology. Atlanta, GA: American Cancer Society, 1991.

Huggins SL: A comparative study of self-esteem of adolescent children of divorced lesbian mothers and divorced heterosexual mothers. J Homosex 1989;18:123.

Hunter J: Violence Against Lesbian and Gay Youth: A Report From the Hetrick Martin Institute. New York: The Hetrick Martin Institute, 1989.

Hunter J, Schaecter R: Lesbian and gay youth. In Rotheram-Borus M, Bradley J, Obolensky N (eds): Planning to Live: Evaluating and Treating Suicidal Teens in Community Settings. Tulsa: University of Oklahoma Press, 1990:297.

Imrie J, Kennedy J, Holmes J, McGrouther D: Intraepithelial neoplasia arising in an artificial vagina: case report. Br J Obstet Gynaecol 1986;93:886.

Island D, Letellier P: Men Who Beat the Men Who Love them. New York: Harrington Park Press, 1991.

Johnson SR, Guenther SM, Laube DW, Keettel WC: Factors influencing lesbian gynecologic care: a preliminary study. Am J Obstet Gynecol 1981;140:20.

Johnson SR, Palermo JL: Gynecologic care for the lesbian. Clin Obstet Gynecol 1984;27:724.

Johnson SR, Smith EM, Guenther SM: Comparison of gynecologic health care problems between lesbians and bisexual women: a survey of 2,345 women. J Reprod Med 1987a;32:805.

Johnson SR, Smith EM, Guenther SM: Parenting desires among bisexual women and lesbians. J Reprod Med 1987b;32:198.

Kaplan GT, Rogers LJ: Breaking out of the dominant paradigm: a new look at sexual attraction. J Homosex 1984;10:71.

Kehoe M: Lesbians over 65: a triply invisible minority. J Homosex 1986;12(3-4):139.

Institute of Medicine: Lesbian Health: Current Assessment and Directions for the Future. Washington, DC: National Academy Press, 1999.

Kehoe M: Lesbians over 60 speak for themselves. J Homosex 1988;16:1.

Kessler S: Lessons from the Intersexed. New Brunswick, NJ: Rutgers University Press, 1998.

Kinsey A, Pomeroy W, Martin C: Sexual Behavior in the Human Male. Philadelphia: WB Saunders Company, 1948.

Kinsey A, Pomeroy W, Martin C: Sexual Behavior in the Human Female. Philadelphia, WB Saunders Company, 1953.

Laumann EO, Paik A, Rosen RC: Sexual dysfunction in the United States: Prevalence and predictors. J Amer Med Assn 1999;281:537.

Leaverton PE, Sorlie PD, Kleinman JC, et al: Representativeness of the Framingham risk model for coronary heart disease mortality: a comparison with a national cohort study. J Chronic Dis 1987;40:775.

LeBlanc S: 8 in 10: A special report of the Victim Recovery Program of the Fenway Community Health Center. Boston, MA: Fenway Community Health Center, 1991.

Leeder E: Enmeshed in pain: counseling lesbian battering couples. Wom Ther 1988;7:81.

Lemp GF, Jones M, Kellogg TA, et al: HIV seroprevalence and risk behaviors among lesbians and bisexual women in San Francisco and Berkeley, California. Am J Public Health 1995;85:1549.

Levay S: A difference in hypothalamic structures between heterosexual and homosexual men. Science 1991;253:1034.

London SJ, Colditz GA, Stampfer MJ, et al: Prospective study of relative weight, height, and risk of breast cancer [see comments]. JAMA 1989;262:2853.

Lubbert H, Leo-Roberg I, Hammerstien J: Effects of ethinyl estradiol on semen quality and various hormonal parameters in a eugonadal male. Fertil Steril 1992;58:603.

Mac Culloch MJ, Waddington JL: Neuroendocrine mechanisms and the aetiology of male and female homosexuality. Br J Psychiatry 1981;139:341.

Manson JE, Colditz GA, Stampfer MJ, et al: A prospective study of obesity and risk of coronary heart disease in women [see comments]. N Engl J Med 1990;322:882.

Marmor M, Weiss LR, Lyden M, et al: Possible female-to-female transmission of human immunodeficiency virus [letter]. Ann Intern Med 1986;105:969.

Masters W, Johnson V: Homosexuality in Perspective. Boston: Little, Brown & Company, 1979.

Mays VM, Cochran SD: The Black Women's Relationships Project: A national survey of black lesbians. In Shernoff M, Scott WA (eds): A Sourcebook of Gay/Lesbian Health Care. 2nd ed. Washington, DC: National Gay and Lesbian Health Foundation, 1988.

Mays VM, Jackson JS, Coleman LS: Race-based perceived discrimination, employment status and job stress in a national sample of black women. J Occup Health Psychol 1996;1:319.

McCauley EA, Ehrhardt AA: Role expectations and definitions: a comparison of female transsexuals and lesbians. J Homosex 1977; 3:137.

McConaghy N, Buhrich N, Silove D: Opposite sex-linked behaviors and homosexual feelings in the predominantly heterosexual male majority. Arch Sex Behav 1994;23:565.

McConaghy N, Zamir R: Sissiness, tomboyism, sex-role, sex identity and orientation. Aust N Z J Psychiatry 1995;29:278.

McKirnan D, Peterson P: Alcohol and drug use among homosexual men and women: epidemiology and population characteristics. Addict Behav 1989;14:545.

Migeon CJ, Berkowitz GD, Brown TR: Sexual differentiation and ambiguity. In Kappy M, Blizzard RM, Migeon C (eds): The Diagnosis and Treatment of Endocrine Disorders in Childhood and Adolescence. Springfield: Charles C Thomas, 1994:573.

Monzon OT, Capellan JM: Female-to-female transmission of HIV [letter]. Lancet 1987;2:40.

Morales E, Graves M: Substance Abuse: Patterns and Barriers to Treatment for Gay Men and Lesbians in San Francisco: Report to Community Substance Abuse Services. San Francisco: San Francisco Department of Public Health, 1983.

Morrow J: Identifying and treating battered lesbians. San Francisco Med 1994;April:17.

Namnoum A: Obesity: a disease worth treating. Female Patient 1993;183:33.

Neisen JH: Resources for families with a gay/lesbian member. J Homosex 1987;14(1-2):239.

Newcomb MD: The role of perceived relative parent personality in the development of heterosexuals, homosexuals, and transvestites. Arch Sex Behav 1985;14:147.

Newton H, Aubard Y, Rutherford A, et al: Low temperature storage and grafting of human ovarian tissue. Hum Reprod 1996; 11:1487.

Office of Research on Women's Health: Report of the National Institutes of Health: Opportunities for Research on Women's Health (Executive Summary 92-3457A). Bethesda, MD: National Institutes of Health, 1991.

O'Hanlan KA: Risk of cancers and heart disease in the lesbian population. Paper presented at the Annual Meeting of the Lesbian Physicians' Conference, Taos, NM, 1991.

O'Hanlan KA: Lesbian health and homophobia: perspectives for the treating obstetrician/gynecologist. Curr Prob Obstet Gynecol Fertil 1995a;18:94.

O'Hanlan KA: Recruitment and retention of lesbians in health research trials. In: Recruitment and Retention of Women in

Clinical Studies (NIH Publication No 95-3756). Bethesda, MD: National Institutes of Health, 1995b:101.

O'Hanlan KA, Crum CP: Human papillomavirus-associated cervical intraepithelial neoplasia following lesbian sex. Obstet Gynecol 1996;88(Pt 2):702.

Pattatucci AM, Hamer DH: Development and familiality of sexual orientation in females. Behav Genet 1995;25:407.

Patterson CJ: Children of lesbian and gay parents. Child Dev 1992;63:1025.

Paul J: Growing up with a gay, lesbian or bisexual parent. Unpublished doctoral dissertation, University of California at Berkeley, 1986.

Paul J, Stall R, Bloomfield K: Gay and alcoholic: epidemiologic and clinical issues. Alcohol Health Res 1991;5:151.

Perry S, Jacobsberg L, Fogel K: Orogenital transmission of human immunodeficiency virus (HIV) [letter]. Ann Intern Med 1989; 111:951.

Peters DK, Cantrell PJ: Factors distinguishing samples of lesbian and heterosexual women. J Homosex 1991;21(4):1.

Phillip M: Gay issues: out of the closet, into the classroom: racism, fear of reprisals force black gays and lesbians to keep low profile on campus. Black Issues in Higher Education 1993;20.

Price JH, Easton AN, Telljohann SK, Wallace PB: Perceptions of cervical cancer and Pap smear screening behavior by women's sexual orientation. J Community Health 1996;21:89.

Puryear D: A comparison between the children of lesbian mothers and the children of heterosexual mothers. Unpublished doctoral dissertation, California School of Professional Psychology, Berkeley, 1983.

Quam JK, Whitford GS: Adaptation and age-related expectations of older gay and lesbian adults. Gerontologist 1992;32:367.

Rand C, Graham DL, Rawlings EI: Psychological health and factors the court seeks to control in lesbian mother custody trials. J Homosex 1982;8:27.

Rees R: A comparison of children of lesbian and single heterosexual mothers on three measures of socialization. Unpublished doctoral dissertation, California School of Professional Psychology, Berkeley, 1979.

Robertson MM: Lesbians as an invisible minority in the health services arena. Health Care Wom Int 1992;13:155.

Robertson P, Schachter J: Failure to identify venereal disease in a lesbian population. Sex Transm Dis 1981;8:75.

Ross MW: Beyond the biological model: new directions in bisexual and homosexual research. J Homosex 1984;10:63.

Rothblum ED: "I only read about myself on bathroom walls": the need for research on the mental health of lesbians and gay men. J Consult Clin Psychol 1994;62:213.

Rotheram-Borus MJ, Fernandez MI: Sexual orientation and development challenges experienced by gay and lesbian youths. Suicide Life Threat Behav 1995;25:26.

Sabatini MT, Patel K, Hirschman R: Kaposi's sarcoma and T-cell lymphoma in an immunodeficient woman: a case report. AIDS Res 1983;1:135.

Savin-Williams RC: Parental influences on the self-esteem of gay and lesbian youths: a reflected appraisals model. J Homosex 1989;17:93.

Schilit R, Lie GY, Montagne M: Substance use as a correlate of violence in intimate lesbian relationships. J Homosex 1990;19:51.

Schneider SG, Farberow NL, Kruks GN: Suicidal behavior in adolescent and young adult gay men. Suicide Life Threat Behav 1989;19:381.

Seaborg DM: Sexual orientation, behavioral plasticity, and evolution. J Homosex 1984;10:153.

Sell RL, Wells JA, Wypij D: The prevalence of homosexual behavior and attraction in the United States, the United Kingdom and France: results of national population-based samples. Arch Sex Behav 1995;24:235.

Shavelson E, Biaggio MK, Cross HH, Lehman RE: Lesbian women's perceptions of their parent-child relationships. J Homosex 1980;5:205.

Stein TS: A curriculum for learning in psychiatric residencies about homosexuality, gay men and lesbians. Acad Psychiatry 1994;18:59.

Swaab DF, Gooren LJ, Hofman MA: Gender and sexual orientation in relation to hypothalamic structures. Horm Res 1992;38: 51.

Taylor BA, Remafedi G: Youth coping with sexual orientation issues. J Sch Nurs 1993;9:26.

Telljohann SK, Price JH: A qualitative examination of adolescent homosexuals' life experiences: ramifications for secondary school personnel. J Homosex 1993;26:41.

Troncoso AR, Romani A. Carranza CM, et al: [Probable HIV transmission by female homosexual contact]. Medicina (B Aires) 1995;55:334.

U.S. Department of Health and Human Services: Health: United States Prevention Profile for 1991. Washington, DC: U.S. Department of Health and Human Services, 1991.

Usdansky M: Gay couples, by the numbers: data suggest they're fewer than believed, but affluent. USA Today 1993;April 12:1a.

Warshafsky L: Lesbian Health Needs Assessment. Los Angeles: The Los Angeles Gay and Lesbian Community Services Center, 1992.

Wendlend CL, Burn F, Hill C: Donor insemination: a comparison of lesbian couples, heterosexual couples and single women. Fertil Steril 1996;65:764.

Whitam FL, Diamond M, Martin J: Homosexual orientation in twins: a report on 61 pairs and three triplet sets. Arch Sex Behav 1993;22:187.

Whitam FL, Mathy RM: Childhood cross-gender behavior of homosexual females in Brazil, Peru, the Phillippines, and the United States. Arch Sex Behav 1991;20:151.

Willett WC, Stampfer MJ, Colditz GA, et al: Moderate alcohol consumption and the risk of breast cancer. N Engl J Med 1987; 316:1174.

Zhou JN, Hofman MA, Gooren LJ, Swaab DF: A sex difference in the human brain and its relation to transsexuality [see comments]. Nature 1995;378:68.

23

Dysmenorrhea, Premenstrual Syndrome, and Other Menstrual Disorders

Wayne S. Maxson
Zev Rosenwaks

The hormonal sequences of the menstrual cycle initiate a number of repetitive physiologic events that include ovulation and menstruation. Coincident with these events are *mittelschmerz* (periovulatory ovarian pain), premenstrual molimina, bloating, breast soreness, and menstrual cramps, symptoms that are usually considered signs of a normal menstrual cycle. When these symptoms are severe, the premenstrual syndrome (PMS) and dysmenorrhea result. Once considered "psychosomatic," these conditions are now accepted as having an organic origin, although their precise etiologies remain controversial.

Accurate diagnosis of PMS and dysmenorrhea depends on a thorough understanding of their pathology. Effective treatment necessitates a knowledge of available options and their relative risks and merits.

DYSMENORRHEA

Dysmenorrhea (from the Greek, meaning difficult menstrual flow) has been classified as primary and secondary. Secondary dysmenorrhea is defined as pain that occurs during menses and that is presumed to be the sequela of an anatomic pelvic abnormality (Table 23–1). Common causes include endometriosis, uterine leiomyomatas, and intrauterine contraceptive devices.

Primary dysmenorrhea is defined as menstrual pain that is not associated with recognized pelvic pathology. Although most women have some lower abdominal cramping during menses, these mild symptoms usually subside within several days after the onset of menses and are not sufficiently severe to interfere with daily activity. In other cases, symptoms are severe enough to require medical evaluation and therapy. Primary dysmenorrhea is unusual in the absence of ovulatory cycles. The passage of

blood or tissue through the cervical canal can also elicit cramping lower abdominal pain. However, bleeding associated with estrogen breakthrough or withdrawal in the absence of ovulation is usually relatively asymptomatic. Primary dysmenorrhea generally begins with the onset of ovulatory cycles, typically 6 months to 1 year after the onset of menarche. Symptoms of primary dysmenorrhea include a colicky abdominal pain localized to the midline or lower quadrants with radiation often noted to the lower back and legs. Accompanying symptoms may include nausea, vomiting, headaches, anxiety, fatigue, diarrhea, syncope, and abdominal bloating. In some cases, the discomfort precedes menstrual flow and may persist a varying number of days after the onset of menses.

Diagnosis

Primary dysmenorrhea can be diagnosed only in the absence of an identifiable cause of pelvic pain. When menstrual cramping begins during the teenage years, a finding of secondary dysmenorrhea is unlikely. If menstrual cramps are noted after the age of 20 in the presence of a history of regular or presumably ovulatory cycles, an organic cause must be sought.

A physical examination should be carefully performed to rule out uterine irregularity, cul-de-sac tenderness, or nodularity, which may suggest endometriosis, pelvic inflammatory disease, or a pelvic mass.

There are no specific tests diagnostic for primary dysmenorrhea. A pelvic examination is indicated at the initial evaluation. Studies used for ruling out pelvic pathology include an ultrasound scan of the pelvis to evaluate for the presence of leiomyomata, ovarian cysts consistent with endometriosis, or an

Table 23–1. CAUSES OF SECONDARY DYSMENORRHEA

TISSUE OR ORGAN SYSTEM	PATHOLOGY
Peritoneum	Endometriosis
	Allen-Masters syndrome
	Pelvic congestion syndrome
Ovary	Ovarian cysts or tumors
Fallopian tubes	Pelvic inflammatory disease (acute and chronic)
Uterus	Adenomyosis
	Uterine myomas
	Uterine polyps
	Intrauterine adhesions (Asherman's syndrome)
	Congenital malformations (bicornuate and septate uterus, blind uterine horn)
	Intrauterine contraceptive device
Cervix	Stenosis or occlusion
Vagina	Imperforate hymen
	Transverse vaginal septum

unsuspected intrauterine device. A hysterosalpingogram is an effective tool in assessing the uterine cavity, especially for the detection of endometrial polyps or submucous or intraluminal leiomyomata. An endometrial biopsy may be considered if endometritis is suspected.

Incidence

Estimates of the prevalence of primary dysmenorrhea in the normal population vary widely. Multiple studies have estimated that dysmenorrhea occurs in about 45% to 50% of women (Haman, 1945; Jeffcoate, 1967; Anderson and Ulmsten, 1978; Rosenwaks et al, 1981). A survey of 113 patients in a family practice setting showed a prevalence of dysmenorrhea of 29% to 44% of women over any 2-month period of time (Sobczyk et al, 1978).

Pathology

Dysmenorrhea has been studied at least since the days of Hippocrates, who believed that stagnation of menstrual blood secondary to cervical obstruction caused painful menstrual periods (Yikorkala and Dawood, 1978). Maimonides believed that this retention of menstrual fluid resulted in "heaviness in the body, loss of appetite, shivering, and pain in the small of the neck" (Maxson and Rosenwaks, 1987). Maimonides further believed that, when menstrual flow was regular in occurrence and adequate in amount, dysmenorrhea did not occur (Rosner and Muntner, 1971).

Cervical Obstruction

The classical belief that dysmenorrhea was secondary to mechanical cervical obstruction led to clinical trials of cervical dilation. In 1832, Mackintosh reported pain relief in 24 of 27 women who received this treatment for dysmenorrhea. J. Marion Sims, in a classical paper entitled "Nulla Dysmenorrhea nisi Obstructiva," further advanced this theory (Novak, 1924).

Severe uterine flexion was also thought to contribute to trapped menstrual blood and obstructed menses. Hysterosalpingographic studies have not substantiated this theory, and it has been observed that the relief of dysmenorrhea by cervical dilatation has been inconsistent and usually temporary.

Apart from exceptional cases, the obstructive theory is now supported only by anecdote for women with cervical patency. Cyclic cramping has been observed in women with a functioning blind uterine horn, presumably because of entrapped menstrual products, and is relieved with surgical removal of the rudimentary horn. Severe cramping secondary to complete cervical obstruction in severe cases of Asherman's syndrome has also been observed. It is unclear whether this pain is secondary to retrograde menstruation or entrapped blood.

Prostaglandins

Macht and Davis (1934) demonstrated that an extract of menstrual fluids, which they called a "menstrual toxin," had a potentiating effect on the contraction of the rat vas deferens. Pickles in 1957 posited that the extractable substance from the menstruating uterus directly stimulated myometrial contractions and could be responsible for primary dysmenorrhea (Eglinton et al, 1963; Pickles et al, 1965). Typical menstrual pain was later reproduced with long-term infusion of prostaglandin $F_{2\alpha}$ ($PGF_{2\alpha}$) (Roth-Brandel et al, 1970).

Prostaglandins are specialized, unsaturated fatty acids that contain 20 carbons with a cyclopentane ring and two side chains (Fig. 23–1). Both prostaglandin E_2 (PGE_2) and $PGF_{2\alpha}$ are important in reproduction and have been isolated from menstrual blood, urine washings, plasma, and endometrial tissues. The association of subtle alterations in prostaglandins in women with dysmenorrhea has been hampered by the short half-life and rapid metabolism of these compounds. Peripheral plasma levels are not usually indicative of the in vivo rate of production of these substances (Samuelsson et al, 1975). Despite this investigative impediment, multiple studies have demonstrated elevated menstrual fluid prostaglandin levels in women with dysmenorrhea compared to controls (Lundstrom and Green, 1978; Kessel and Coppen, 1964; Pickles et al, 1965).

Prostaglandin synthesis (Figs. 23–2 and 23–3) is initiated by lysosomal enzymes that are released in the late luteal phase of the menstrual cycle. These enzymes are stimulated and released by the action

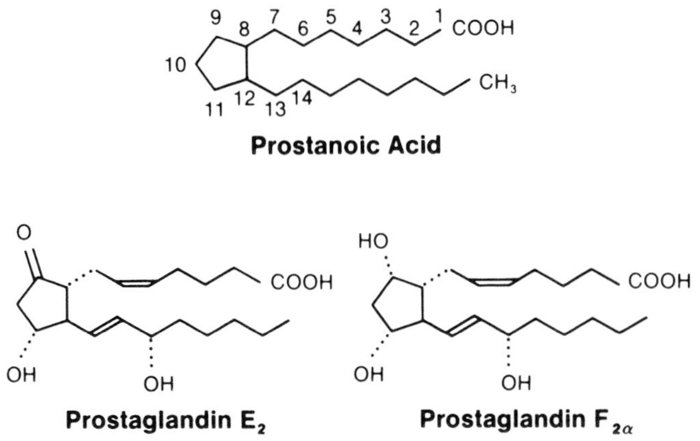

Figure 23–1
Structure of basic prostaglandins. (From Rosenwaks Z, Seegar-Jones G: Menstrual pain: its origin and pathogenesis. J Reprod Med 1980;25(4 Suppl);207, with permission.)

of gonadal steroids directly on the endometrium. Phospholipids are then released from the cell membranes and provide the precursor fatty acids that are necessary for the synthesis of prostaglandin. The first step in the conversion of arachidonic acid to prostaglandins is the formation of prostaglandin G_2 (PGG_2), a cyclic endoperoxide. This reaction is inhibited by the nonsteroidal anti-inflammatory drugs. The formation of PGE_2 and $PGF_{2\alpha}$ occurs rapidly from PGG_2.

The production of prostaglandins can be initiated by a number of factors, including peptide hormones, cyclic AMP, estrogen, progesterone, and tissue trauma. In most animal models, particularly in the hamster, rabbit, guinea pig, and ewe, it is the combination of gonadal steroids (estradiol and progesterone) that produces the highest concentration of $PGF_{2\alpha}$ in the endometrium (Green, 1979). Estradiol alone has not been found to elicit as significant an amount of $PGF_{2\alpha}$ as the combination of estrogen and progesterone (Green, 1979).

In women, concentrations of the PGE_2 and $PGF_{2\alpha}$ seem to peak in the late luteal and menstrual phases, as anticipated from the previous animal studies. As noted, serum levels of these prostaglandins are poorly reflective of these changes secondary to rapid metabolism. PGFm and PGEm, metabolites of these prostaglandins, are even more potent myometrial stimulants (Akerlund et al, 1979). PGFm levels are elevated in women with primary dysmenorrhea compared with asymptomatic controls (Ghodgaonkar et al, 1979; Rosenwaks et al, 1981).

A hypothetical schema (Fig. 23–3) has been developed to explain the interaction of endometrial prostaglandins and the succeeding events of menstrual bleeding and dysmenorrhea. With the release of lysosomal enzymes at menstruation, phospholipases are triggered, allowing the rapid release of the phospholipid precursors for prostaglandin production. Prostaglandins are synthesized rapidly and exert direct myometrial effect, causing the uterine mus-

culature to contract with resulting constriction of small endometrial blood vessels, tissue ischemia, endometrial disintegration, bleeding, and pain. The combination of increased intrauterine pressure, constriction of endometrial vessels, and the resulting tissue ischemia may be the underlying cause of primary dysmenorrhea. Prostaglandins or their metabolites may also sensitize the neuronal endings of the myometrium to other pain-producing substances, which can accentuate the symptoms.

The prostaglandin hypothesis also explains the extragenital manifestations of primary dysmenorrhea. The intravenous injection of prostaglandins can produce diarrhea, vomiting, headache, and syncope, symptoms often seen in conjunction with severe primary dysmenorrhea.

Further compelling evidence to support the prostaglandin theory is the efficacy of drugs that inhibit prostaglandin synthesis and effectively decrease pain in patients with primary dysmenorrhea (Asplund, 1952; Lundstrom et al, 1976; Chan et al, 1979; Henzl and Izu, 1979). This cause-and-effect relationship is further supported by the studies of Csapo et al (1977), which demonstrate a concomitant decrease in endometrial prostaglandins and intrauterine pressure with prostaglandin synthetase inhibitors.

Neuronal Hypothesis

The perception of pain requires transmission of impulses from the uterus to the brain. Dysmenorrhea has long been treated by surgical disruption of these pathways. Procedures such as presacral neurectomy and uterosacral ligament transection may alleviate symptoms of dysmenorrhea.

Short adrenergic neurons exist in the uterus. These neuronal fibers in the guinea pig almost completely disappear during pregnancy, and there is a decreased synthesis and turnover of neurotransmitters within the myometrium noted during and after pregnancy. Sjoberg (1979) suggested that this altered neuromuscular activity may contribute to the commonly observed decrease in menstrual pain that follows pregnancy and delivery.

Vasopressin

Vasopressin is a potent initiator of uterine myometrial contraction, and the uterus is highly sensitive to this substance during menses (Countinho and Lopes, 1968). Uterine activity can be measurably reduced when vasopressin is inhibited (Cobo et al, 1978; Fuchs et al, 1986). During menstruation, circulating vasopressin levels are increased in women; this increase is higher by fourfold in women with dysmenorrhea than in asymptomatic controls (Akerlund et al, 1979). Vasopressin can induce the contraction of the myometrium and constrict the uterine arteries without concomitant prostaglandin synthesis (Laudanski et al, 1984). Ackerlund et al (1983, 1986) demonstrated that a vasopressin antagonist can in-

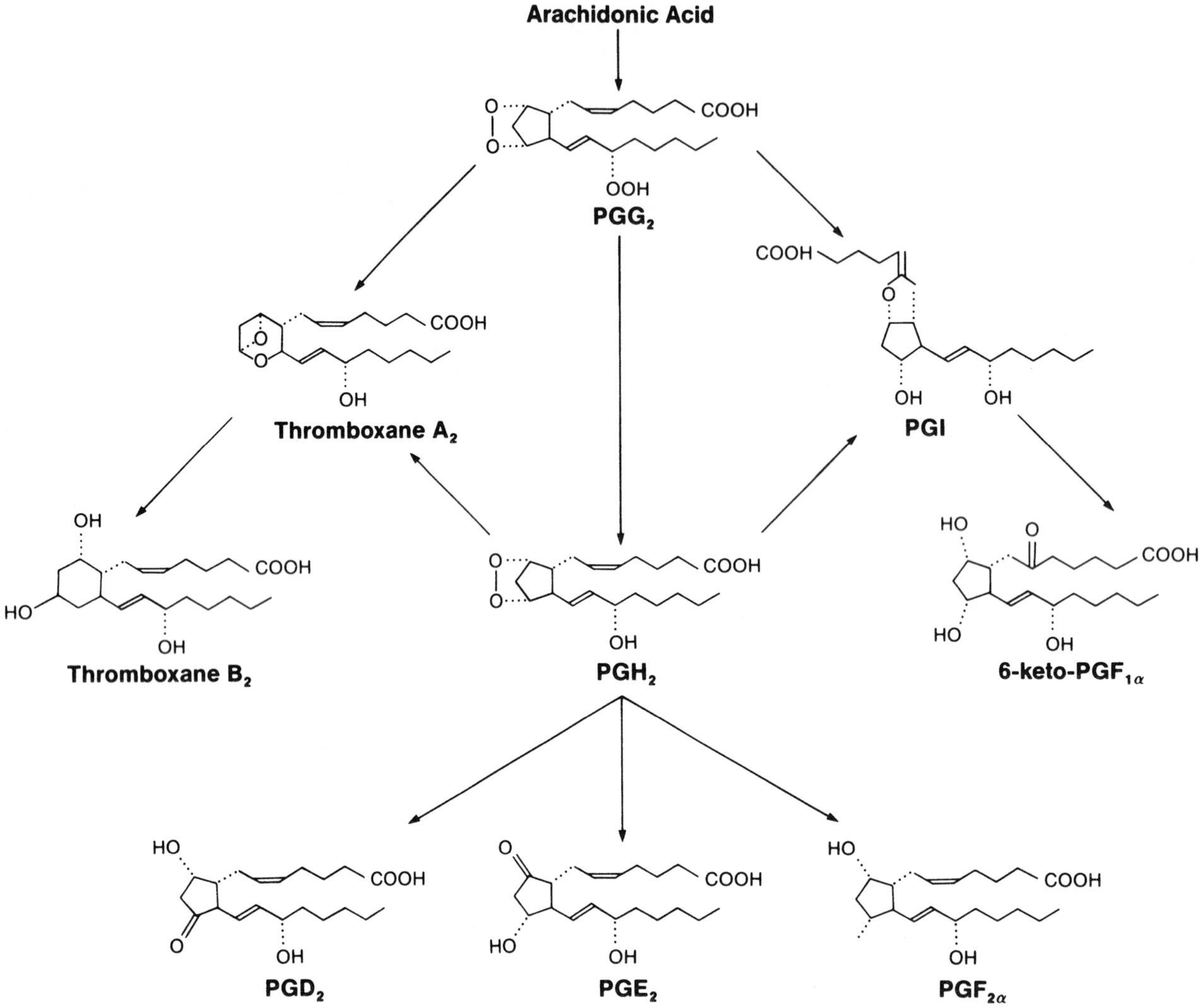

Figure 23–2
Biosynthetic pathways of prostaglandins and thromboxanes derived from arachidonic acid. PG, prostaglandin. (From Rosenwaks Z, Seegar-Jones G: Menstrual pain: its origin and pathogenesis. J Reprod Med 1980;25(4 Suppl):207, with permission.)

hibit myometrial activity in vitro, further support for vasopressin as a potential contributor to dysmenorrhea.

A placebo-controlled trial utilizing a vasopressin inhibitor showed that 50% of women with dysmenorrhea experienced alleviation of pain (Akerlund, 1987), although this treatment has not been routinely employed.

Treatment

Multiple therapies for dysmenorrhea have been proposed. Hippocrates recommended the application of heat to the external genitalia or abdomen by burning a concoction of wine, fennel, and rose oil. Other methods for applying heat have evolved, including hot compresses, heating pads, hot water bottles, and moxibustion. Moxibustion has been used by the Chinese and involves the burning of pulverized moxa rots, which are placed on ginger slices on various parts of the abdomen.

Hormonal Therapy

The association of dysmenorrhea and ovulation has been well known since its early description by Wilson and Kurzrok in 1930. Estradiol benzoate was initially demonstrated to inhibit menstruation and simultaneously relieve dysmenorrhea. Combination oral contraceptives (COCs) were then used with increasing efficacy over the succeeding decades, and it is generally accepted that first-line treatment of dysmenorrhea in young women includes consideration of COC therapy.

Oral contraceptives may decrease dysmenorrhea in several ways. Hauksson et al (1989) showed that COCs markedly decreased spontaneous uterine activity as measured by an intrauterine microtransducer. COC therapy also decreased the uterine contrac-

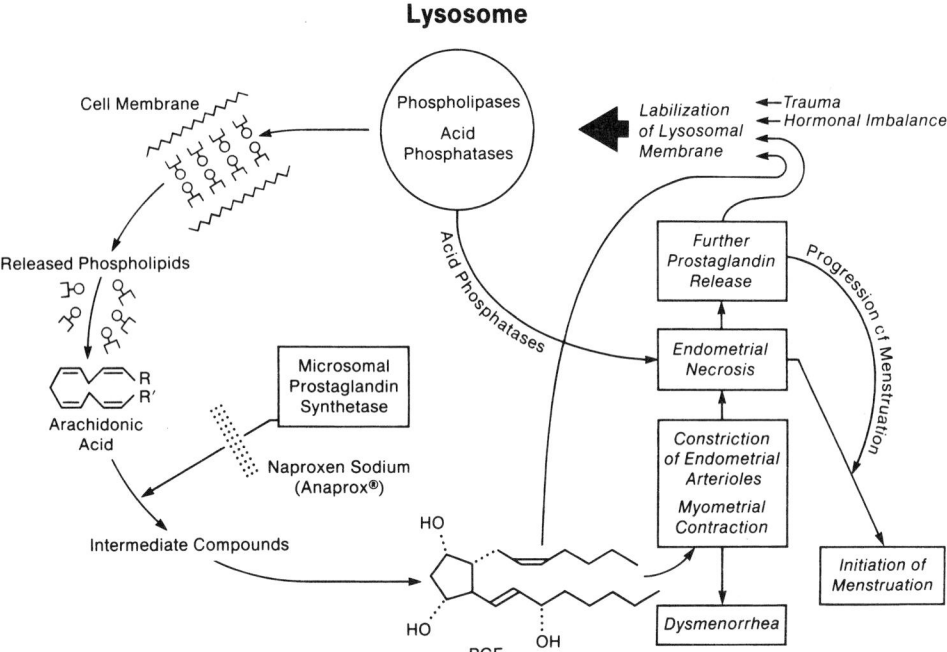

Figure 23-3
Theoretical concept of the synthesis of prostaglandins and the mechanism of naproxen sodium action. PG, prostaglandin. (From Rosenwaks Z, Seegar-Jones G: Menstrual pain: its origin and pathogenesis. J Reprod Med 1980;25(4 Suppl):207, with permission.)

tual response to both lysine vasopressin and $PGF_{2\alpha}$. This measured decrease in uterine activity correlated with a subjective decrease in the sensation of painful cramping.

Surgical Treatment

Surgical interruption of the neuronal pathways from the uterus has been used to decrease the sensation of pain with dysmenorrhea. Lee et al (1986) evaluated the presacral neurectomy in eight patients with primary dysmenorrhea. In this small study, with success defined as at least 50% pain relief by subjective recording, five patients related successful treatment and three showed no improvement. In this study, there appeared to be no difference when uterosacral transection was performed in addition to presacral neurectomy in patients with and without endometriosis or with other pelvic pathology (Lee et al, 1986).

Cervical dilatation has also been used clinically to treat dysmenorrhea. This procedure theoretically results in more efficient blood flow during menstruation, with the resultant advantage of less intrauterine accumulation of blood and prostaglandins. However, clinical experience with this modality has indicated only transient relief, and controlled studies are not available to assess its long-term efficacy.

Prostaglandin Inhibitors

Various analgesics were used empirically for treating dysmenorrhea until the publication of the prostaglandin theory for uterine contractility. In 1965, Pickles and colleagues suggested that prostaglandins may play a role in the pathogenesis of dysmenor-

rhea. Aspirin-like compounds were hypothesized to act by inhibiting prostaglandin synthesis (Vane, 1971). In 1953, Fox reported a dramatic improvement in severe dysmenorrhea with butazolidine, although the mechanism was then unknown.

The reduction in uterine symptoms from prostaglandin inhibitors is associated with documented suppression of prostaglandin production and a decrease in prostaglandin metabolites. With prostaglandin inhibitor therapy, most studies report a successful decrease in menstrual cramping in 70% to 80% of patients (Maxson and Rosenwaks, 1987).

Several possible reasons for the lack of a uniform response to prostaglandin inhibition are attractive. First, some patients may have intraperitoneal pathology such as endometriosis, uterine leiomyomata, or adenomyosis. Second, an increased activity of the alternate lipoxygenase pathway of prostaglandin metabolism may contribute to menstrual cramping. This pathway of prostaglandin production increases concentrations of leukotriene, a potent uterine muscle contractor and vasoconstrictor (Demers et al, 1975). Because the conventional prostaglandin inhibitors act primarily on the cyclo-oxygenase pathway, these agents may be ineffective in treating primary dysmenorrhea in women with increased lipoxygenase activity.

Calcium Antagonists

It is well known that calcium is necessary for the contraction of smooth muscles. Verapamil and prenylamine, antagonists of calcium transport, were shown to block spontaneous uterine activity and induced uterine contractility (Fleckenstein et al, 1971; Grün et al, 1971). The calcium blocker nifedipine decreases the amplitude of uterine contractions more than the frequency of myometrial contractions (Forman et al, 1979). Nifedipine was used in oral doses of 20 to 30 mg, with a decrease in overall uterine activity occurring within 10 to 40 minutes and lasting 3 to 5 hours (Anderson and Ulmsten, 1978; Ulmsten et al, 1978). In these patients, symptomatic improvement correlated with a measured decrease in myometrial activity.

Two small placebo-controlled trials for the treatment of dysmenorrhea showed some benefit with nifedipine (Mondero, 1983) and diltiazem 240 mg/day (Audebert et al, 1985). However, no large, long-term, controlled studies of calcium blockers are available.

Neural Stimulation

Acupuncture has also been utilized to treat dysmenorrhea. Helms (1987) compared the results using 12 needles placed in meridian points for 30 to 40 minutes with needles placed in placebo points. A trend of relief from pain with acupuncture was noted in 43 patients. However, little information appears in the English language literature to support the routine use of acupuncture for long-term treatment of dysmenorrhea.

Transcutaneous electrical nerve stimulation (TENS) is a technique for the treatment of chronic pain. TENS may work by blocking pain impulse transmission through the dorsal nerve horns and increasing local nerve cell endorphin release (Dawood et al, 1990).

Several trials using high-frequency TENS have been reported to provide relief of dysmenorrhea in approximately 30% of patients in placebo-controlled trials. There was a decrease in the need for analgesia during the first 48 hours after initiation of TENS in these patients (Lundeberg et al, 1985; Mannheimer and Whalen, 1985; Santiesteban et al, 1985; Neighbors et al, 1987).

A crossover study utilizing placebo and TENS at 100 pulses/second with 100-μsec pulses and ibuprofen, 400 mg every 4 hours, showed that 42% of patients reported excellent relief of pain with the TENS unit (Dawood et al, 1990). When the TENS unit was combined with low-dose ibuprofen, pain relief was reported in 71% of women. High-dose ibuprofen alone resulted in a decrease in pain in 74% of subjects.

A Practical Approach to Dysmenorrhea

A simple algorithm can result in effective diagnosis and treatment of women with dysmenorrhea. In patients with primary dysmenorrhea beginning during the teenage years, COCs and prostaglandin inhibitors are effective measures. For women with the progression of menstrual cramps or the onset of cramps after age 20, a careful pelvic examination, history, and possible pelvic ultrasound scan, sonohystero-

gram, or hysterosalpingogram may elucidate intrauterine or pelvic pathology. Laparoscopy is essential for women with progressive menstrual symptoms that are uncontrolled with prostaglandin inhibitors or COCs.

THE PREMENSTRUAL SYNDROMES

In 1931, Frank was credited with the first published description of the "premenstrual tension" syndrome. Despite the fact that a plethora of symptoms during the premenstruum had been described for many centuries, most clinicians up to the mid-20th century believed that the premenstrual tension syndrome was a psychosomatic condition deserving little scientific attention.

In 1953 Greene and Dalton called this condition the "premenstrual syndrome" to allow the inclusion of both somatic and psychological complaints in the symptom complex.

Clinical Presentation

Since the original description of PMS by Frank (1931), approximately 150 symptoms have been included in the list of possible premenstrual complaints (Table 23–2) (Moos, 1969). Specific clustering of symptoms has been proposed (Abraham, 1981), but studies have been unable to confirm a consistent pattern of associated complaints that can be related to a specific etiology in women with PMS.

The definition of PMS has been elusive because this condition is characterized by a wide variety of symptoms, most of which are unmeasurable by objective standards. Dalton (1985) defined PMS as the "recurrence of symptoms in the premenstruum but complete absence of symptoms in the postmenstruum." Sutherland and Stewart (1965) defined PMS as any combination of emotional or physical signs or symptoms that occur cyclically prior to menstruation and then regress or disappear during or after menstruation. The *Diagnostic and Statistical Manual of Mental Disorders, Third Edition, Revised* (American Psychiatric Association, 1987) termed PMS the "late luteal phase dysphoric disorder." The full definitions is noted in Table 23–3.

Common somatic symptoms of PMS include sensations of abdominal bloating, weight gain, breast tenderness, headache, nausea, peripheral edema, and alterations in bowel habits. Frequent behavioral changes seen with PMS include irritability, depression, difficulty with concentration, feelings of isolation and withdrawal, agitation, hostility, fatigue, craving for sugar or salt, and even suicidal ideation.

PMS is usually considered significant if the severity of symptoms interferes with a day's normal events. This general definition serves to differentiate the premenstrual molimina from the more severe symptoms characterized as PMS.

Table 23–2. COMMON SYMPTOMS ASSOCIATED WITH PREMENSTRUAL SYNDROME

AFFECTIVE
Sadness
Anxiety
Anger
Irritability
Labile mood

COGNITIVE
Decreased
  concentration
Indecision
Paranoia
"Rejection-sensitive"
Suicidal ideation

PAIN
Headaches
Breast tenderness
Joint pain
Muscle pain

NEUROVEGETATIVE
Insomnia
Hypersomnia
Anorexia
Food cravings
Fatigue
Lethargy
Agitation
Libido change

BEHAVIORAL
Decreased motivation
Poor impulse control
Decreased efficiency
Social isolation

AUTONOMIC
Nausea
Diarrhea
Palpitations
Sweating

CENTRAL NERVOUS SYSTEM
Clumsiness
Seizures
Dizziness
Vertigo
Paresthesia
Tremors

FLUID/ELECTROLYTE
Bloating
Weight gain
Oliguria
Edema

DERMATOLOGIC
Acne
Oily skin
Greasy hair
Dry hair
Hirsutism

From Rubinow D, Roy-Byrne P: Premenstrual syndromes: overview from a methodologic perspective. Am J Psychiatry 1984;141:163, with permission.

Epidemiology

Premenstrual symptoms have been described to occur in 15% to 100% of women of reproductive age (Ruble, 1977), with 5% to 10% reporting severe symptomatology at some point in their lives.

There is an intercultural variability in premenstrual complaints (Janiger et al, 1972). The prevalence of premenstrual complaints was lower among Japanese women than among American, Turkish, and Nigerian women. For African-Americans, the most frequent premenstrual complaint appeared to be headache (Abraham, 1981).

PMS symptoms may occur in adolescence. Up to 90% of adolescent females may have at least one premenstrual symptom of moderate severity, according to an evaluation of 207 teenagers by retrospective questionnaire (Fisher et al, 1989). In this study, more than 50% of adolescent women considered at least one premenstrual symptom to be severe.

Dalton et al (1987) reported a possible genetic predisposition to PMS. In monozygotic twins, 14 out of 15 sets showed PMS. This rate of sharing was significantly different from the incidence of PMS in di-

zygotic twins (7 of 16 sets) or in nontwin siblings (38 of 77). In another study, a significant correlation of PMS symptoms was found between adolescent daughters and their mothers (Widholm and Kantero, 1971).

Etiology

A single cause for PMS has not been identified. Multiple factors have been proposed, but 50 years of investigation have failed to provide a uniform hypothesis for the pathophysiology of PMS.

Behavioral, sensory, and cognitive acuity have been found to vary with the phase of the menstrual cycle. Premenstrual impairments of auditory and visual discrimination and attention span have been documented (Rausch and Janowsky, 1979). Changes in smell and taste have also been observed during the late luteal phase of the menstrual cycle, and increased reactivity to stress has been reported (Rausch and Janowsky, 1979). Furthermore, the incidence of both crimes and suicides in women have been reported to increase during the premenstruum.

Because PMS by definition depends on the occurrence of symptoms during the premenstrual cycle, a hormonal etiology has been suspected.

Hormonal Hypothesis

In a normal menstrual cycle, the interval from the initiation of menses to ovulation is termed the *follicular phase*. This phase is characterized by the rapid development of an ovarian follicle with the production of increasing levels of estradiol. The endometrium proliferates in response to this estrogen stimulation.

When sufficient estradiol is present to trigger the surge of pituitary luteinizing hormone, the *luteal phase* begins. This portion of the menstrual cycle, from ovulation to menses, is characterized by an initial drop in estradiol, followed by rising estradiol and progesterone levels that peak approximately 1 week after ovulation (1 week prior to menses). The endometrium is converted to a secretory pattern by progesterone from the corpus luteum. The end of the luteal phase is associated with progressively declining estradiol and progesterone levels, resulting in the onset of menses.

Because PMS is defined as a collection of symptoms that occur prior to menses and resolve following menstrual bleeding, PMS has been blamed on alterations in luteal estrogen and progesterone levels. Frank (1931) initially proposed that PMS was due to excessive levels of female sex hormone in the blood. Other reports, based on luteal-phase progesterone levels, endometrial biopsy specimens, and vaginal smears, suggested the possibility of inadequate corpus luteum function (Reid and Yen, 1981).

However, the attempted correlation of decreased progesterone levels with PMS symptoms has been

Table 23-3. A DIAGNOSTIC CRITERIA FOR LATE LUTEAL PHASE DYSPHORIC DISORDER

A. In most menstrual cycles during the past year, the symptoms in B occurred during the last week of the luteal phase and remitted within a few days after onset of the follicular phase. In menstruating females, these phases correspond to the week before and a few days after the onset of menses. (In nonmenstruating females who have had a hysterectomy, the timing of luteal and follicular phases may require measurement of circulating reproductive hormones.)

B. At least five of the following symptoms have been present for most of the time during each symptomatic late luteal phase, at least one of the symptoms being either (1), (2), (3), or (4):
1. Marked affective lability (e.g., feeling suddenly sad, tearful, irritable, or angry)
2. Persistent and marked anger or irritability
3. Marked anxiety, tension, feelings of being "keyed up," or "on edge"
4. Markedly depressed mood, feelings of hopelessness, or self-deprecating thoughts
5. Decreased interest in usual activities (e.g., work, friends, hobbies)
6. Easy fatigability or marked lack of energy
7. Subjective sense of difficulty in concentration
8. Marked change in appetite, overeating, or specific food cravings
9. Hypersomnia or insomnia
10. Other physical symptoms such as breast tenderness or swelling, headaches, joint or muscle pain, a sensation of "bloating," weight gain

C. The disturbance seriously interferes with work or with usual social activities or relationships with others.

Modified from American Psychiatric Association: Diagnostic and Statistical Manual of Mental Disorders. 4th ed. Washington, DC: American Psychiatric Association, 1994. Copyright 1994 American Psychiatric Association, with permission.

inconsistent. Progesterone is released in a pulsatile fashion. Therefore, even multiple progesterone samples are unreliable indices of overall corpus luteum function (Filicori et al, 1984). In fact, both decreased and increased progesterone levels in women with PMS have been reported (Backstrom and Mattsson, 1975; Reid and Yen, 1981).

In animal experiments behavior can be affected by estrogen. When female rats and cats are given estrogen implants, running and mating behaviors appear to increase (Colin and Sawyer, 1969). These effects may, at least in part, be counteracted by progesterone (Rausch and Janowsky, 1979). In contrast, in menopausal women on estrogen replacement therapy, Hammarback et al (1985) demonstrated that progesterone, not estrogen, contributed to premenstrual symptomatology.

Androgens tend to peak at midcycle and decrease before menses (Vermeulen and Verdon, 1976). Because androgens may cause an increase in sexual drive, aggression, and acne, an etiologic role for androgens in causing PMS has been investigated. No convincing association has yet been demonstrated. Prolactin levels also vary slightly during the menstrual cycle, increasing at ovulation and during the luteal phase. Women with PMS have been shown to have both normal and increased prolactin levels (Reid and Yen, 1981; Harrison et al, 1985).

A complex interaction between the monoamines serotonin, norepinephrine, and dopamine and the ovarian steroids is well known. A decrease in norepinephrine and dopamine has been associated with depression. An increase in these hormones has been linked to aggression, irritability, and even psychosis (Reid and Yen, 1981). Fluoxetine, a specific serotonin reuptake inhibitor, consistently improves the psychological symptoms of PMS when compared to placebo. However, the predictable placebo response in PMS studies, the failure of approximately 40% of PMS patients to improve with antidepressants, and

the association with PMS of somatic symptoms that are not affected by fluoxetine or alprazolam all cast shadows on the serotonin hypothesis. Although the sex steroids, directly and via conversion to catecholestrogen, have a potent effect on the monamines of the brain, the measurement of peripheral venous concentrations of these neurotransmitters and their metabolites has shown inconsistent alterations in women with PMS.

Regardless of the exact mechanism, the suppression of ovulation remains one of the most effective ways to treat PMS, presumably by reducing the cyclic fluctuation in ovarian steroids and their central nervous system sequelae (Reid and Yen, 1981; Muse et al, 1984).

Fluid Retention Theory

Because PMS is often associated with complaints of bloating and fluid retention, mineralocorticoid changes have been suspected as a potential cause of PMS symptoms. In addition, mineralocorticoids may have a central effect on mood, because one metabolite—desoxycorticosterone—has been demonstrated to bind to γ-aminobutyric acid (GABA) receptors (Majewska et al, 1986).

Serum levels of aldosterone rise before ovulation and again in the midluteal phase, to levels approximately twice those noted during the follicular phase. Aldosterone levels then drop before menstruation, suggesting an association between this hormone and the ovarian steroids. In spite of the potential theoretical connection between mineralocorticoids and PMS, studies have been unable to demonstrate any significant difference in aldosterone levels in women with PMS and controls (Munday et al, 1977; O'Brien et al, 1979).

A fluid shift without sodium or water retention has also been postulated (Oian et al, 1987). There is an increase plasma colloid osmotic pressure during the late luteal phase that could cause an increase in interstitial fluids.

Although women frequently report an increase in body weight prior to menses as one symptom of PMS, a controlled trial was unable to demonstrate any significant change in body weight from follicular to luteal phase in PMS suffers compared to women without significant PMS symptomatology (Andersch et al, 1978a).

Hypoglycemia Hypothesis

Diaphoresis, fatigue, palpitations, and headache may be caused by hypoglycemia. Although several studies initially reported an impairment in the glucose tolerance test during the second half of the menstrual cycle (Okey and Robb, 1925), subsequent studies failed to show significant differences in glucose, insulin, and glucagon levels in either the follicular or the luteal phase of the menstrual cycle in normal women and women complaining of PMS (Reid et al, 1986).

Endorphin Hypothesis

A role for an abnormality in endorphins as a potential cause of PMS is attractive because endorphins can inhibit the production of biogenic amines and can alter mood, appetite, and thirst (Reid and Yen, 1981). During the luteal phase, endogenous opioids are lower in women with PMS than in controls (Chuong et al, 1985; Facchinetti et al, 1987; Tulenheimo et al, 1987).

Vasomotor symptoms associated with PMS appear to be identical physiologically to the hot flashes of menopause (Casper et al, 1987). A link between estrogen levels and endorphins has been previously demonstrated, and it is possible that a change in endorphins induced by estrogen and central catecholamines may be associated with PMS in some patients.

Further evidence to support the endorphin hypothesis is the resemblance of some PMS symptoms to the hyperirritability and aggression associated with acute opiate withdrawal (Strickler, 1987). An opiate antagonist, naloxone, has been shown to worsen PMS and to induce PMS-like symptoms in normal volunteers (Cohen et al, 1981).

Prostaglandin Hypothesis

The association of prostaglandins and dysmenorrhea has been well demonstrated. Horrobin (1983) suggested that women with PMS have a relative decrease in PGE. Abraham (1980) suggested that this may be mediated by a deficiency in pyridoxine (vitamin B_6) and magnesium, but corroboration of this theory has been lacking.

Vitamin and Mineral Deficiencies

No clear-cut nutritional deficiencies have been consistently identified in women with PMS. Because pyridoxine acts as a co-enzyme in the final step of the biosynthesis of dopamine and serotonin, a decrease in vitamin B_6 levels in the brain could produce some symptoms of PMS. Early enthusiasm for vitamin B_6 therapy was supported by a double-blind study that showed an improvement in depression with vitamin B_6 administration in women receiving COCs (Adams et al, 1973). Although 63% of women taking vitamin B_6, 100 mg/day, during the luteal phase noted improvement in PMS (Day, 1979), another study showed no difference between women taking pyridoxine and those taking placebo (Stokes and Mendels, 1972).

Allergy Hypothesis

An allergic reaction to progesterone has been postulated as one possible cause for PMS (Shelley et al, 1965; Bierman, 1973; Korossy, 1975). Nevertheless, premenstrual urticaria is extremely rare, and a hypersensitivity to progesterone and other substances during the luteal phase has not been supported as a primary cause for PMS.

Psychological Hypothesis

The psychological symptoms are usually the most critical for women with PMS. Because many of the significant changes of PMS strongly suggest an affective disorder, an underlying psychological abnormality has been sought as the primary problem in PMS. The symptoms of tension, depression, hostility, and mood swings appear more frequent in women with severe underlying psychological problems (Keye, 1984).

Initially, PMS was thought to be a psychosomatic disorder. Benedek (1952) suggested that intense conflict over the female role was responsible for PMS symptoms. Further support for the "psychosomatic" theory was provided by a study that demonstrated that women who were premenstrual reported fewer PMS symptoms when they were deceived into thinking that the subsequent menstrual period would be delayed (Ruble, 1977).

Approximately 60% of women with a major affective disorder have been diagnosed as having a premenstrual affective syndrome (Blumenthal and Nadelson, 1988). At least 30% of women with primary recurrent depression experience their first depressive episode during a time of significant hormonal change (Kolakowska, 1975).

In a psychological review of women with PMS, between 57% and 100% of women with PMS were found to have had a prior major depressive episode at least once in their lives, in contrast to 0% to 20% of women without PMS (Halbreich and Endicott, 1985). This coincidence of major depressive disorder and PMS suggests an underlying psychological abnormality that may increase the severity of premenstrual symptoms in predisposed women.

Women with PMS reported significantly increased numbers of negative events during their daily lives compared to controls (Schmidt et al, 1990). These women also demonstrated significantly more distress associated with the occurrence of an event during the premenstrual phase than when the same event occurred during the follicular phase.

Diagnosis

Making the diagnosis of PMS has been problematic because its specific etiology is unknown and there is no objective marker that can quantitate the existence or the severity of symptomatology, or even the objective response to therapy. The diagnosis of PMS relies on a patient's self-reporting of symptoms that she feels increase significantly during the premenstruum and diminish following menses.

Retrospective symptom questionnaires were initially used in an attempt to evaluate PMS. These were adequate only as a general screen (Abplanalp et al, 1979; Magos and Studd, 1988). Retrospective tests currently in use include the Moos menstrual distress questionnaire, with 47 items in 8 symptom groups (Moos, 1969); the 19-symptom questionnaire of Abraham (1980); and the premenstrual assessment form (Halbreich et al, 1982). The best means of evaluating subjective symptoms is a prospective, daily self-assessment form that estimates relative symptom severity. Numerous menstrual calendars have been designed for the daily recording of symptoms (Reid, 1985; Magos and Studd, 1988).

Treatment Alternatives for PMS

The cornerstone of treatment for PMS remains a careful evaluation of symptoms and their chronicity. Because the placebo response rate in women with PMS is high in virtually all studies examining this condition, conservative supportive therapy may be effective in many patients.

A simplified treatment approach, emphasizing the least invasive technique first, is noted in Table 23–4. Because of the high placebo response rate, popular

Table 23–4. A PRACTICAL APPROACH TO PREMENSTRUAL SYNDROME

1. Intake history and physical examination
2. Medical evaluation
   A. Endocrine tests as indicated (thyroid-stimulating hormone, thyroxine, prolactin)
   B. Tests to rule out secondary dysmenorrhea
3. Exercise and dietary counseling
4. Psychological counseling if indicated
5. Ovulation suppression or antidepressant therapy

and inexpensive treatments have included modification of exercise, nutrition, and stress.

Exercise

Clinical studies of exercise demonstrate a reduction in anger and depression in women who exercise. It has been demonstrated that patients with mild neurotic depression did as well clinically with running as they did with psychotherapy. Exercise also can exert profound effects on the endocrine system. During exercise, levels of cortisone, testosterone, prolactin, estradiol, and growth hormones increase (Gaw et al, 1979). Exercise also increases the metabolic clearance rate of estrogen, resulting in an effective increase in circulating levels (Keizer et al, 1980). Exercise also increases β-endorphin levels (Gamberg et al, 1980; Carr et al, 1981).

Although most studies of exercise for the treatment of PMS are unconvincing, one report showed that exercise conditioning in women with PMS resulted in a decrease in somatic symptoms that correlated with increased physical conditioning (Prior et al, 1987).

Nutrition

The evidence that dietary management aids PMS symptoms remains weak, and it is unclear whether dietary changes offer a pharmacologic or a placebo effect. A study of 180 nursing students in China indicated a dose-dependent association of tea consumption with premenstrual symptoms, particularly in women drinking between four and eight cups of tea per day (Rossignol et al, 1989). Women with PMS have been described as consuming more calories, with craving for both salt and carbohydrates, during the premenstrual phase than during the follicular phase. However, a prospective study of PMS sufferers showed no alteration in dietary behavior during either phase (Wurtman et al, 1989). The improvement of PMS symptoms after a carbohydrate-enriched meal may be explained by an increase in serotonin (Wurtman et al, 1989).

Despite the absence of demonstrable nutritional deficiency in PMS and the dearth of controlled studies demonstrating efficacy, 63% of 502 physicians in the United States and Canada surveyed for the treatment of PMS in 1984 recommended dietary treatment (Lyon and Lyon, 1984). In this same study, 60% of these physicians recommended vitamins as part of their treatment for PMS, and 90% provided dietary counseling.

Pharmacologic Therapy

Some clues to the pathophysiology of PMS are suggested by the two treatment approaches most often found to be superior: ovulation suppression and selective serotonin reuptake inhibition. At least nine studies of medical or surgical oophorectomy demonstrate the clinical efficacy of ovulation suppression and implicate the cyclic fluctuation of gonadal steroids in the generation of PMS (Rubinow and Schmidt, 1995). Furthermore, the initiation of PMS-like symptoms in women receiving cyclic estrogen and progestin supports this association. However, blocking progesterone receptors with the progesterone antagonist RU-486 had no effect on PMS symptoms (Chan et al, 1994). The hormonal hypothesis of PMS is discussed above, with the link between progesterone and PMS remaining elusive. Certain metabolites of progesterone, particularly 3α-hydroxy-5α,20-one (allopregnanole) and 3α-hydroxy-5β-pregnane-30-one (pregnenolone), appear to bind to the same GABA receptors as barbiturates and benzodiazepines (Paul and Purdy, 1992). However, a deficiency of either progesterone itself or these metabolites was not identified in PMS sufferers (Schmidt et al, 1994). Furthermore, progesterone therapy has been repeatedly ineffective in most trials, even when administered by the oral route, which can increase the hypnotic metabolites of progesterone (Arafat et al, 1988; Freeman et al, 1995). Thus, neither a progesterone excess nor a deficiency of this steroid has been confirmed as a cause of PMS.

OVULATION SUPPRESSION

Because PMS symptoms by definition occur during the premenstruum in ovulatory cycles, suppression of ovulation has been an attractive approach to the therapy of PMS.

Gonadotropin-Releasing Hormone Agonists. In a double-blind, placebo-controlled study, Muse and associates (1984) demonstrated that both the physical and the behavioral manifestations of PMS could be dramatically decreased through the suppression of ovulation with gonadotropin-releasing hormone agonists (GnRHa). Called a "medical ovariectomy," the administration of GnRHa in a carefully selected group of patients with PMS resulted in low levels of estradiol and progesterone, which were maintained during the second and third months of treatment (Fig. 23–4). Cyclic symptoms of PMS were affectively attenuated in these women (Fig. 23–5).

The long-term use of GnRHa is currently impractical because of the common side effects caused by hypoestrogenism (Smith and Schiff, 1989). Daily injectable GnRHa, depot GnRHa, and nasal GnRHa are also effective in suppressing ovulation and in reducing PMS symptoms (Hammarback and Backstrom, 1988).

In a small clinical trial utilizing cyclic estrogen and progestin in addition to long-acting GnRHa, eight women with PMS showed no increase in premenstrual symptoms after the addition of the steroids (Mortola et al, 1991). This approach remains experimental because higher doses of cyclic estrogen and progesterone in women with ovarian failure or GnRHa-induced perimenopause have actually in-

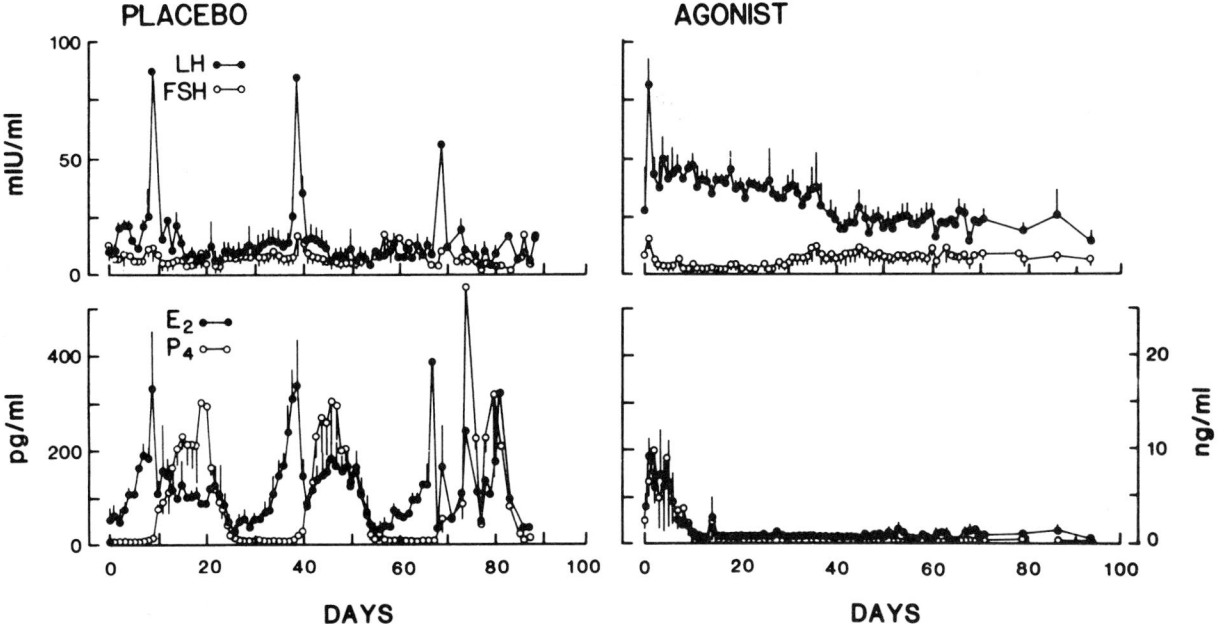

Figure 23–4
Mean concentrations (± standard error) of luteinizing hormone (LH), follicle-stimulating hormone (FSH), estradiol (E₂), and progesterone (P₄) during 90 days of placebo administration and 90 days of treatment with a gonadotropin-releasing hormone (GnRH) agonist. Data on placebo administration are standardized according to peak LH values and the onset of menses. Data on GnRH agonist treatment are normalized to the first day of administration. (From Muse KN, Getel NS, Futterman LA, Yen SSC: The premenstrual syndrome: effects of "medical ovariectomy." N Engl J Med 1984;311:1345, with permission.)

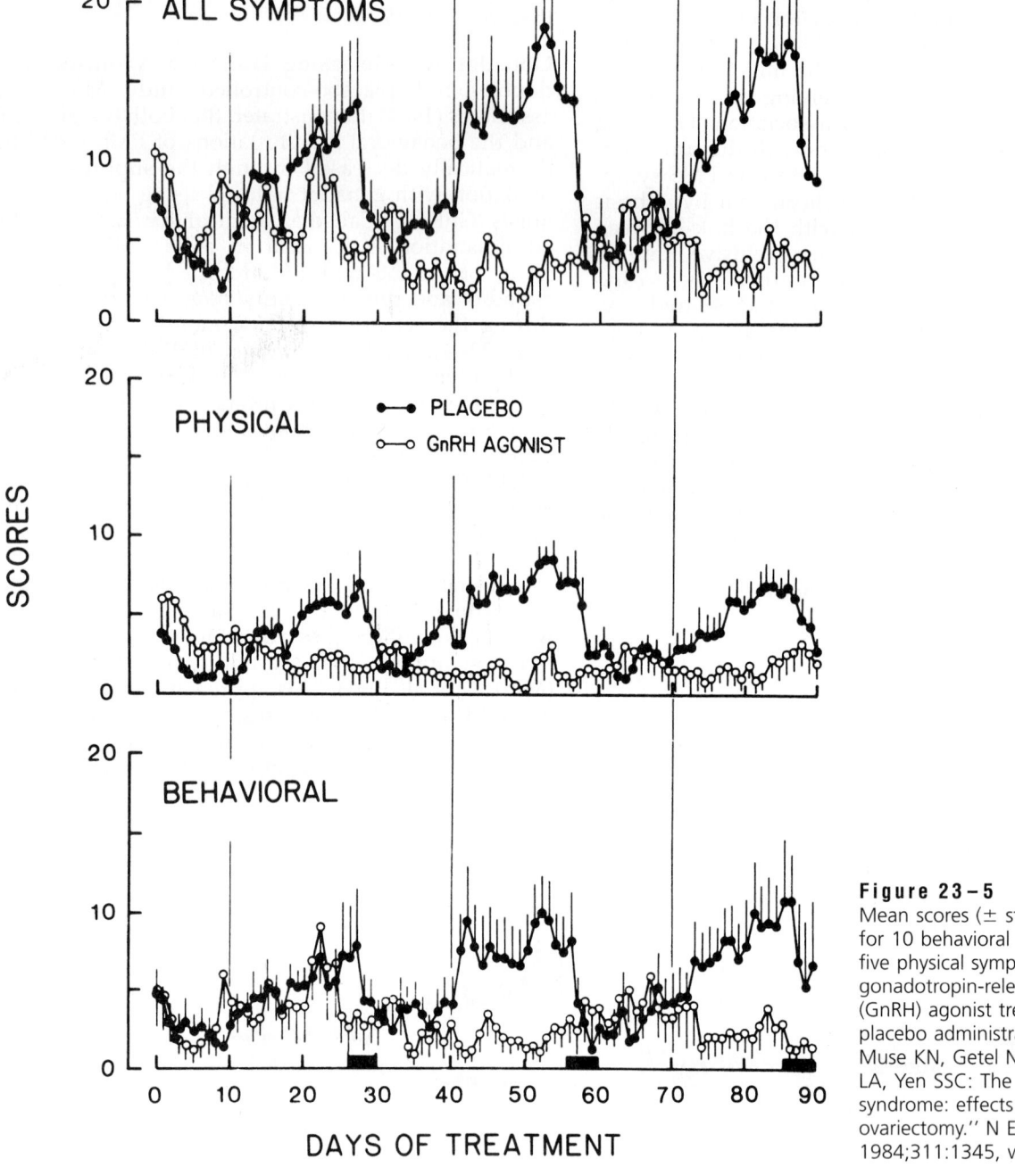

Figure 23–5
Mean scores (± standard error) for 10 behavioral symptoms and five physical symptoms during gonadotropin-releasing hormone (GnRH) agonist treatment and placebo administration. (From Muse KN, Getel NS, Futterman LA, Yen SSC: The premenstrual syndrome: effects of "medical ovariectomy." N Engl J Med 1984;311:1345, with permission.)

duced PMS-like symptoms (Hammarback et al, 1985; Magos et al, 1986a, 1986b; Hammarback et al, 1989; Muse, 1989). A subsequent 12-month trial of GnRHa with the addition of conjugated estrogen 0.625 mg daily and medroxyprogesterone acetate 10 mg daily for 10 days/month produced progressive improvement in water retention, psychological symptoms, and complaints of pain while maintaining bone density and lipid levels (Mezrow et al, 1994).

Progestins have also been effectively used to suppress cyclic hormonal fluctuations. Norethisterone enanthate, a depot progestin administered as a bimonthly injection, effectively decreased symptoms in

women who had complained of persistent PMS despite use of COCs (Gunston, 1995).

Danazol. At doses of 100 to 400 mg daily, danazol significantly improved depression, bloating, breast pain, and emotional lability in three studies (Gilmore et al, 1985; Sarno et al, 1987; Watts et al, 1987). Side effects of danazol caused dropout rates of 18% to 44%, rendering this therapy relatively impractical for long-term use. Danazol does not inhibit ovulation or change cycle length at doses of 200 mg/day (Sarno et al, 1987), mandating the use of barrier contraception. Side effects are increased further at an ovulation-suppressing dose of 400 mg or more a day (Barbieri and Hornstein, 1987).

Oral Contraceptives. The use of COCs for the treatment of PMS has been controversial. Anecdotal reports have indicated an increase in premenstrual symptomatology in PMS sufferers receiving COCs, presumably secondary to a detrimental effect of estrogen and progestin. However, in 1974 the Royal College of General Practitioners reported that the incidence of PMS in pill users was 29% lower than that in nonusers. The more progestational COCs may be associated with fewer cyclic symptoms than those with more pronounced estrogen effect (Cullberg, 1972; Kutner and Brown, 1972).

Two early placebo-controlled trials of COCs in normal women showed no change in premenstrual depression or irritability when COCs were compared with placebo (Silberfeld et al, 1971; Morris and Udry, 1972). However, the low-dose monophasic and the multiphasic COCs have not been well evaluated in this regard.

As an inexpensive and safe treatment, COCs may be tried as initial therapy for selected women with PMS. For women who continue to have symptoms during the pill-free interval, COCs can be administered on a continuous daily basis for suppression of menses and ovarian cyclicity.

Progestins. Daily progestin administration may be an effective alternative to the estrogen-containing combination COCs for ovulation suppression. Medroxyprogesterone acetate 5 to 10 mg or norethindrone acetate 5 mg daily can inhibit ovulation, suppress menses, and eliminate marked cyclic ovarian hormone production. This alternative may be preferred by women experiencing continued PMS symptomatology on estrogen-containing COCs.

Although early, uncontrolled observations of several synthetic progestins used during the luteal phase suggested efficacy for PMS treatment (Rubinow and Roy-Byrne, 1984), three controlled trials subsequently failed to show superiority over placebo (Swyer, 1955; Coppen et al, 1969; Jordheim, 1972). Synthetic progestins may be luteolytic, decreasing the production of natural progesterone by the corpus luteum. Early trials utilizing the synthetic progestin dihydrogesterone during the luteal phase suggested improvement in a variety of mood and somatic symptoms. However, a double-blind, placebo-controlled trial involving this drug demonstrated a 53% placebo response rate and a 75% drug response rate, a difference not reaching statistical significance (Haspels, 1981).

It is difficult to estimate the clinical utility during the luteal phase of treatment with either synthetic or natural progestin. In some studies, the progestins are begun during the follicular phase and may decrease PMS through the inhibition of ovulation. Varying doses and agents preclude satisfactory comparison of available studies or convincing documentation of the efficacy of any single progestational agent in treating PMS.

Progesterone. Despite extensive experience by Dalton (1985) in treating more than 30,000 women with natural progesterone, and despite the clamor of various consumer groups, only one randomized, double-blind, crossover trial has demonstrated that progesterone may be more efficacious than placebo in reducing symptoms of PMS (Dennerstein et al, 1985). This trial employed the Moos menstrual distress questionnaire as a record of daily symptoms and calculated symptom scores for the last 7 days of each cycle. The use of oral micronized progesterone 300 mg/day in 23 women was evaluated and compared with placebo. Results indicated significant improvement in anxiety, depression, stress, swelling, and hot flashes. Maximum improvement was noted during the first month of progesterone therapy.

However, numerous other prospective studies have been unable to demonstrate that progesterone is any better for the treatment of PMS than placebo (Smith, 1955; Sampson, 1979; Andersch and Hahn, 1985; Maddocks et al, 1986). Maddocks et al (1986) concluded from a 6-month study that neither progesterone nor placebo was clinically effective in improving symptomatology in women with severe PMS. Proponents of progesterone point out that the doses of progesterone were lower than 400 mg/day in these studies, which may have hampered the success of therapy.

No serious side effects of progesterone have been reported (Lauersen, 1985). Vaginal suppositories can cause moniliasis, infection, or rash. Rectal suppositories and suspension can produce flatulence, diarrhea, aggravation of colitis, abdominal cramping, and local irritation. Oral progesterone may cause dizziness and sleepiness.

ANXIOLYTICS AND ANTIDEPRESSANTS

When the psychological symptoms of PMS predominate, specific anxiolytic or antidepressive therapy is indicated when teratogenic effects are not a clinical concern.

Fluoxetine. Fluoxetine treatment for PMS is the most exciting new development in this field since the documentation of the efficacy of ovulation suppression with GnRHa. Multiple studies have demonstrated the efficacy of this serotonin reuptake inhibitor in reducing behavioral and psychological symptoms, including tension, irritability, and dysphoria (Wood et al, 1992; Pearlstein and Stone, 1994; Steiner et al, 1995). A daily dose of 20 mg was judged adequate, with fewer side effects and less menstrual irregularity (Steiner et al, 1997).

The largest collaborative study to date (Steiner et al, 1995) enrolled 405 women and ultimately evaluated 180 subjects completing the 6-month protocol. One-half of the placebo group withdrew, most because of lack of efficacy, while a similar number of women on fluoxetine 60 mg left the study, mostly secondary to side effects. One third of the women dropped out of the fluoxetine 20 mg group, with an equal number for personal reasons, protocol violations, and side effects. Overall, 52% of the women receiving fluoxetine reported at least 50% improvement during their first cycle, compared to 22% receiving placebo.

These studies utilized daily fluoxetine treatment. One case study reports on improvement in PMS symptoms with a single dose of fluoxetine during the early luteal phase (Daamen and Brown, 1992).

Lithium. Clinical trials of lithium for PMS have shown both favorable results (Sletten and Gershon, 1966; Deleon-Jones et al, 1982) and no significant difference in results between this drug and placebo (Mattson and Schoultz, 1974; Singer et al, 1974).

Alprazolam. Alprazolam is a triazolobenzodiazepine with both anxiolytic and antipanic properties. Clinical trials of alprazolam have shown mixed results when compared to placebo, with three studies indicating efficacy (Smith et al, 1987; Harrison et al, 1990; Freeman et al, 1995) and two showing no significant benefit (Dennerstein et al, 1986; Schmidt et al, 1993).

In the most recent experience of Freeman et al (1995), alprazolam 0.25 mg four times a day during the luteal phase of the cycle significantly reduced global PMS scores compared to both placebo and oral micronized progesterone. When symptom clusters were examined, alprazolam clearly improved mental function, mood, and pain scores while exerting minimal effect on physical symptoms. However, the benefits of alprazolam were far from uniform; using a clinical definition of 50% improvement in total scores, 37% of the alprazolam group improved compared to 29% of the oral progesterone group and 30% of the placebo group.

Side effects leading to cessation of therapy have been primarily drowsiness in the treatment group and lack of benefit in the placebo group.

Buspirone. This nonbenzodiazepine tranquilizer has also demonstrated favorable results in women with PMS (Rickels et al, 1989).

BROMOCRIPTINE

Bromocriptine has been shown to be effective in reducing premenstrual breast soreness. However, most clinical trials indicate that bromocriptine fails to relieve most affective and physical symptoms in PMS suffers when compared with placebo (Andersen et al, 1997; Ghose and Coppen, 1977; Kullander and Svanberg, 1979; Steiner et al, 1979). Nevertheless, clinical improvement in some affective and physical symptoms were noted in several studies (Benedek-Jaszmann and Heran-Sturtevant, 1976; Andersch et al, 1978b; Graham et al, 1978).

DIURETICS

Complaints of fluid retention and bloating have led to trials of diuretic therapy for women with somatic premenstrual complaints. Spironolactone, an aldosterone antagonist and an antiandrogen, has been studies with mixed results. O'Brien et al (1979) administered spironolactone 25 mg four times daily from days 18 to 26 of the menstrual cycle to 18 patients with PMS. Both placebo and spironolactone improved global mood assessment. Lower doses of spironolactone (25 mg daily) had no significant effect on PMS (Smith, 1955). In another study, no significant change in any symptom except bloating was noted when diuretics were compared with placebo at doses of 100 mg/day (Vellacott et al, 1987). At this time, the use of diuretics remains empirical and unproven.

PROSTAGLANDIN ANTAGONISTS AND PRECURSORS

Although prostaglandin inhibitors have been shown to be effective in the treatment of dysmenorrhea, their use for PMS during the luteal phase remains more controversial. Mefenamic acid has been evaluated in three studies with conflicting results.

In one study of 37 women with PMS, significant improvement was noted in irritability, depression, tension, abdominal pain, and headache (Wood and Jakubowicz, 1980). However, Budoff (1983) reported no significant improvement in psychological symptoms in a 7-day placebo-controlled trial. There was significant improvement in abdominal bloating, abdominal pain, edema, and premenstrual breast tenderness. In a study by Mira et al (1986), mefenamates brought about significant improvement in fatigue, headache, irritability, mood swings, and depression but no change in abdominal boating or breast pain. Significant side effects from mefanamates include gastric and esophageal irritation, diarrhea, nausea, and potential hematologic and renal changes.

Evening primrose oil, a combination of γ-linoleic acid and cis-linoleic acid, was administered with success in one study of 31 women with severe PMS (Puolakka et al, 1985). This treatment is relatively expensive, and the long-term effects remain unknown.

Surgical Therapy

In severe cases of PMS, surgical oophorectomy has been used successfully in women who no longer desire preservation of fertility (Casper and Hearn, 1990; Casson et al, 1990). Casson et al (1990) performed a total abdominal hysterectomy and bilateral oophorectomy in 14 women with severe PMS who had previously responded to danazol 200 mg twice daily for 6 to 9 months. With low-dose estrogen replacement following ovariectomy, all women demonstrated persistent improvement in PMS symptoms at 1 year follow-up.

Casper and Hearn (1990) also used danazol for ovulation suppression before considering surgical treatment. Of 14 women with severe, incapacitating PMS and a dramatic response to danazol, all noted continued complete resolution of PMS symptoms 6 months after hysterectomy and bilateral oophorectomy.

The surgical induction of menopause remains a drastic approach to PMS, requiring extensive preoperative evaluation and consultation and a clearcut, long-term trial of ovulation suppression with convincing relief.

A Practical Approach to PMS

With a condition that can result in severe debility and significant suffering, PMS patients require the same careful consideration as any other patient suspected of harboring a diagnosable medical or surgical problem. PMS is usually treatable if attention is paid to an evaluation for underlying physical and emotional factors. By definition, PMS complaints should be relieved with elimination of ovarian cyclicity. The persistence of PMS symptoms, either in women during the follicular phase or in women with obvious suppression of gonadal steroids, necessitates further medical and psychiatric investigation. Because a large number of PMS sufferers have an increased susceptibility to affective disorders, consideration of psychological or psychiatric support is important. The referral of patients for psychological evaluation is often difficult, perceived by the patient as a denial of the reality of her symptoms and as an assumption of a psychosomatic etiology. The daily symptom questionnaire and a trial of ovulation suppression are effective tools for both diagnosis and education.

Education of the patient and her family represents another cornerstone of therapy. Ongoing support from a caring health provider is important, especially in the early stages of diagnosis and therapy (Pariser et al, 1985). Ovulation suppression or antidepressant therapy have now cured most bona fide cases of PMS.

OTHER MENSTRUAL DISORDERS

Menstrual Migraine Headaches

Approximately 60% of women who suffer from migraine headaches report an increase at the time of menses, and 7% to 30% of these women experience true menstrual migraines, with headaches only occurring between 2 days prior to menses and the last day of menstrual flow (Nattero, 1982). Menstrual migraines may be more severe and less responsive to conventional therapy than noncyclic headaches.

The premenstrual dwindling of circulating estrogens and progesterone have been implicated as the principal cause for menstrual migraines. Both these hormones are known to have direct effects on the central nervous system, including the serotonergic systems. Recent evidence and the success of sumatriptan, a selective 5-hydroxytryptamine-1 (5-HT1) agonist, suggest that the pain of a migraine comes from a sterile inflammation of the dura mater mediated by release of calcitonin-gene-related peptide from the trigeminal nerve endings. Activation of the 5-HT1D presynaptic autoreceptor inhibits trigeminal neuronal firing and thus specifically prevents or ameliorates many migraine headaches. (Moskowitz and Coutrer, 1993; Goadsby and Olesen, 1996).

Menstrual migraines have been successfully treated with sumatriptan (Facchinetti et al, 1995), nonsteroidal anti-inflammatory drugs (Giacovazzo et al, 1993), estrogens (de Lignieres et al, 1986; Silberstein and Merriam, 1991; Sheftell et al, 1992), and ovulation suppression (Murray and Muse, 1997). Sumatriptan was more effective than placebo in treating menstrual migraines (73% substantial improvement within 2 hours with drug compared to 31% improvement with placebo) (Facchinetti et al, 1995). However, headaches recurred within 24 hours of initial response in 53% of patients treated with sumatriptan and 52% of women who received placebo. The nonsteroidal anti-inflammatory nimesulide significantly reduced both the severity and the duration of menstrual migraines when compared to placebo (Giacovazzo et al, 1993). Nimesulide was administered 100 mg orally three times daily for 10 days, beginning when the headache began. With treatment, headaches lasted 12 to 16 hours, compared to 57 to 69 hours with placebo.

After reviewing conflicting studies, Silberstein and Merriam (1991) concluded that COCs can generate new headaches or improve or worsen existing migraines. Because of the still-controversial fear of stroke in women who have migraine headaches while on COCs, Sheftell et al (1992) recommend the discontinuation of COCs if migraines occur or worsen during therapy. Trials of estrogen replacement during the late luteal phase have been equally disconcerting, and the clinician must resort to the imaginative medical principle of "trial and error" for long-term hormonal prophylaxis of menstrual migraines. Changing from conjugated to natural steroids, or from cyclic hormonal replacement to a continuous regimen, maybe useful in reducing the frequency or the severity of attacks (Silberstein and Merriam, 1991; Kudrow, 1975). Percutaneous estradiol (1.5 mg estradiol in 2.5 g gel) applied once daily for 7 days beginning 48 hours before the expected onset of a migraine was significantly more effective than placebo in reducing both the severity and the duration of headaches in 19 women completing both placebo and treatment arms of the study (de Lignieres et al, 1986).

The other effective method to stabilize estrogen levels premenstrually is the induction of anovulation and a hypoestrogenic state with GnRHa. Depot leuprolide acetate 3.75 mg IM monthly for 10 months significantly reduced migraine monthly scores in all months except for the first month of treatment (Murray and Muse, 1997). The addition of transdermal estradiol 0.1 mg daily and oral medroxyprogesterone acetate 2.5 mg daily increased the rate of breakthrough bleeding but did not worsen the headaches during the last 6 months of the study.

Menstrual Asthma

Although not considered a classical symptom of PMS, perimenstrual asthma represents a rare but potentially severe complication of cyclic hormonal fluctuations. A summary of five studies involving 358 patients with asthma reported that 33% to 74% of attacks occurred about the time of the menstrual flow (Settipane and Simon, 1989). Variations in reproductive hormones, with or without fluctuations in prostaglandins and their metabolism, may account for the observed increase in episodes of asthma associated with menses. One anecdotal report supported the consideration of GnRHa for the treatment of this disorder (Blumenfeld et al, 1994).

REFERENCES

Abplanalp JM, Donnelly AF, Rose RM: Psychoendocrinology of the menstrual cycle: I. Enjoyment of daily activities and mood. Psychosom Med 1979;41:587.

Abraham GE: The premenstrual tension syndrome. In McNall LK (ed): Contemporary Obstetrical and Gynecological Nursing. Vol 3. St. Louis: CV Mosby, 1980.

Abraham GE: Premenstrual tension. Curr Probl Obstet Gynecol 1981;3.

Adams PW, Rose DP, Forkard J, et al: Effect of pyriodoxine hydrochloride (vitamin B$_6$) for the depression associated with oral contraception. Lancet 1973;1:897.

Akerlund M: Can primary dysmenorrhea be alleviated by a vasopressin antagonist? Acta Obstet Gynecol Scand 1987;66:459.

Akerlund M, Haulsson A, Lundin S, et al: Vasotocin analogues which competitively inhibit vasopressin in stimulated uterine activity in healthy women. Br J Obstet Gynaecol 1986;93:22.

Akerlund M, Kostrzewska A, Laudanski T, et al: Vasopressin effects on isolated non-pregnant myometrium by deamino-ethyl-lysine-vasopressin and deamino-ethyl-oxytocin. Br J Obstet Gynaecol 1983;90:732.

Akerlund M, Stromberg P, Forsling MD: Primary dysmenorrhea and vasopressin. Br J Obstet Gynaecol 1979;86:484.

American Psychiatric Association: Diagnostic and Statistical Manual of Mental Disorders. 3rd ed, rev. Washington, DC: American Psychiatric Press, 1987;367.

Andersch B, Hahn L: Progesterone treatment of premenstrual tension—a double-blind study. J Psychosom Res 1985;29:489.

Andersch B, Hahn L, Anderson M, et al: Body water and weight in patients with premenstrual syndrome. Br J Obstet Gynecol 1978a;85:546.

Andersch B, Hahn L, Wendestam C, et al: Treatment of premenstrual tension syndrome with bromocriptine. Acta Endocrinol 1978b;88(Suppl 216):165.

Andersen RN, Steenstrup OR, Svemstrup B, Neilsen J: Effect of bromocriptine on the premenstrual syndrome: a double-blind trial. Br J Obstet Gynaecol 1977;84:370.

Anderson KE, Ulmsten U: Effect of nifedipine on myometrial activity and lower abdominal pain in women with dysmenorrhea. Br J Obstet Gynaecol 1978;85:142.

Arafat ES, Hargrove JT, Maxson WS, et al: Sedative and hypnotic effects of oral administration of micronized progesterone may be mediated through its metabolites. Am J Obstet Gynecol 1988;159:1203.

Asplund J: The uterine cervix and isthmus under normal and pathologic conditions. Acta Radiol 1952;91:1.

Audebert AJ, Colle M, Coquelin JP, Emperaire JC: Essai d'un inhibiteur calcique dans la dysmenorrhea. Press Med 1985;14:163.

Backstrom T, Mattsson B: Correlation of symptoms in premenstrual tension to estrogen and progesterone concentrations in blood plasma. Neuropsychology 1975;1:80.

Barbieri RL, Hornstein MD: Medical therapy for endometriosis. In Wilson EA (ed): Endometriosis. New York: Alan R Liss, 1987.

Benedek T: Studies in Psychomatic Medicine: Psychosexual Function in Women. New York: Roland Press, 1952.

Benedek-Jaszmann LJ, Heran-Sturtevant MD: Premenstrual tension and functional infertility: aetiology and treatment. Lancet 1976;1:1095.

Bierman SM: Autoimmune progesterone dermatitis of pregnancy. Arch Dermatol 1973;107:896.

Blumenfeld Z, Bentur L, Yoffe N, et al: Menstrual asthma: use of gonadotropin-releasing hormone analogue for the treatment of cyclic aggravation of bronchial asthma. Fertil Steril 1994;62:197.

Blumenthal SJ, Nadelson CC: Late luteal phase dysphoric disorder (premenstrual syndrome): clinical implications. J Clin Psychiatry 1988;49:469.

Budoff PW: The use of prostaglandin inhibitors for the premenstrual syndrome. J Reprod Med 1983;28:469.

Carr DB, Bullens BA, Skrinar GS, et al: Physical condition facilitates the exercise-induced secretion of beta-endorphins and beta-lipotropin in women. N Engl J Med 1981;305:560.

Casper RF, Graves GR, Reid RL: Objective measurement of hot flushes associated with the premenstrual syndrome. Fertil Steril 1987;47:341.

Casper RF, Hearn MT: The effect of hysterectomy and bilateral oophorectomy in women with severe premenstrual syndrome. Am J Obstet Gynecol 1990;1962:105.

Casson P, Hahn PM, Van Vugt DA, Reid RL: Lasting response to ovariectomy in severe intractable premenstrual syndrome. Am J Obstet Gynecol 1990;162:99.

Chan AF, Mortola JF, Wood SH, Yen SCC: Persistence of premenstrual syndrome during low-dose administration of the progesterone antagonist RU 486. Obstet Gynecol 1994;84:1001.

Chan WY, Dawood MY, Fuchs F: Relief of dysmenorrhea with the prostaglandin synthetase inhibitor ibuprofen: effect on prostaglandin levels in menstrual fluid. Am J Obstet Gynecol 1979; 135:102.

Chuong CJ, Coulam CB, Kao PC, et al: Neuropeptide levels in premenstrual syndrome. Fertil Steril 1985;44:760.

Cobo E, Cifuentes R. De Villamuzar M: Inhibition of menstrual motility during water diuresis. Am J Obstet Gynecol 1978;132: 313.

Cohen RM, Pickar D, et al: Behavior effects after high dose naloxone administration to normal volunteers. Lancet 1981;2:1110.

Colin GB, Sawyer CH: Induction of running activity by intracerebral injections of estrogen and ovariectomized rats. Neuroendocrinology 1969;4:309.

Coppen AJ, Milne HB, Outram DM, Weber JC: Dytide, norethisterone and a placebo in the premenstrual syndrome: a double-blind controlled comparison. Clin Trials J 1969;6:33.

Countinho EM, Lopes HCV: Response of the non-pregnant uterus to vasopressin as an index of ovarian function. Am J Obstet Gynecol 1968;102:479.

Csapo AL, Pulkinen MO, Henzl MR: The effect of naproxen sodium on the intrauterine pressure and menstrual pain of dysmenorrhea patients. Prostaglandins 1977;13:193.

Cullberg J: Mood changes and menstrual symptoms with different gestagen/estrogen combinations. Acta Psychiatry Scand Suppl 1972;236:1.

Daamen MJ, Brown WA: Single-dose fluoxetine in management of premenstrual syndrome. J Clin Psychiatry 1992;53:210.

Dalton K: Diagnosis and clinical features of premenstrual syndrome. In Dawood MY, McGuire GL, Demers LM (eds): Premenstrual Syndrome and Dysmenorrhea. Baltimore: Urban & Schwarzenberg, 1985:13.

Dalton K, Dalton M, Guthrie K: Incidence of the premenstrual syndrome in twins. Br Med J 1987;295:1027.

Dawood M, Yusoff MD, Ramos J: Transcutaneous electrical nerve stimulation (TENS) for the treatment of primary dysmenorrhea: a randomized crossover comparison with placebo TENS and ibuprofen. Obstet Gynecol 1990;75:656.

Day JB: Clinical trials in the premenstrual syndrome. Curr Med Res Opin 1979;6(Suppl 5):40.

de Lignieres B, Vincens M, Mauvais-Jarvis P, et al: Prevention of menstrual migraine by percutaneous oestradiol. Br Med J 1986; 293:1540.

Deleon-Jones FA, Val E, Hertz C: MHPG exertion and lithium treatment during premenstrual tension syndrome: a case report. Am J Psychiatry 1982;139:950.

Demers LM, Halbert DR, Jones DED: Prostaglandin F levels in endometrial jet wash specimens during the menstrual cycle. Prostaglandins 1975;10:1057.

Dennerstein L, Morse C, Burrows G, et al: Alprazolam in the treatment of premenstrual syndrome. In Dennerstein L, Fraser I (eds): Hormones and Behavior. New York: Elsevier Science Publishing Company, Inc, 1986:175.

Dennerstein L, Spencer-Gardner C, Gotts G, et al: Progesterone and the premenstrual syndrome: a double blind crossover trial. Br Med J 1985;290:1617.

Eglinton G, Raphael RA, Smith GN: Isolation and identification of two smooth muscle stimulants from menstrual fluid. Nature 1963;200:960.

Facchinetti F, Bonellie G, Kangasniemi P, et al: The efficacy and safety of subcutaneous sumatriptan in the acute treatment of menstrual migraine. Obstet Gynecol 1995;86:911.

Facchinetti R, Martignoni E, Petraglia F, et al: Premenstrual fall of plasma β-endorphin in patients with premenstrual syndrome. Fertil Steril 1987;47:341.

Filicori M, Butler JP, Crowley WF: Neuroendocrine regulation of the corpus luteum in the human. J Clin Invest 1984;73:1638.

Fisher M, Trieller K, Napolitano B: Premenstrual symptoms in adolescents. J Adolesc Health Care 1989;10:369.

Fleckenstein A, Grün G, Trittart H, Byon K: Uterus-Relaxation durch hochaktive Ca^{++}-antagonistische Hemmstoffe der elektromechanischen Koppelung wie Isoptin (Verapamil, Iproveratril), Substanz D 600 und Segontin (Prenylamin) (Versuche am isolierten Uterus virgineller Ratten). Klin Wochenschr 1971;49: 32.

Forman A, Andersson KE, Persson GA, Ulmsten U: Relaxant effects of nifedipine on isolated human myometrium. Acta Pharm Toxicol 1979;45:81.

Fox WM: Butazolidine. Lancet 1953;1:195.

Frank HT: The hormonal cause of premenstrual tension. Arch Neurol Psychiatry 1931;26:2053.

Freeman EW, Rickels K, Sondheimer SJ, Polansky M: A double-blind trial of oral progesterone, alprazolam, and placebo in treatment of severe premenstrual syndrome. JAMA 1995;274: 51.

Fuchs AR, Countinho EM, Xavier R, et al: Effect of ethanol on the activity of the non-pregnant uterus and its reactivity to neurohypophyseal hormones. Am J Obstet Gynecol 1986;101:997.

Gamberg SR, Garthwait TL, Hagen TC: Running increases plasma beta-endorphins in man. Clin Res 1980;28:720a.

Gaw EL: Hormonal changes with exercise. Postgrad Med J 1979; 55:373.

Ghodgaonkar RB, Dubin NH, Blake DA: 13,14-dihydro-15 keto-prostaglandin F$_{2\alpha}$ concentration in human plasma and amniotic fluid. Am J Obstet Gynecol 1979;134:265.

Ghose K, Coppen A: Bromocriptine and premenstrual syndrome: a controlled study. Br Med J 1977;1:147.

Giacovazzo M, Gallo MF, Guidi V, et al: Nimesulide in the treatment of menstrual migraine. Drugs 1993;46(Suppl 1):140.

Gilmore DH, Hawthorne RJS, Hart DM: Danazol for premenstrual syndrome: a preliminary report of placebo-controlled double-blind study. J Int Med Res 1985;13:129.

Goadsby PJ, Olesen J: Diagnosis and management of migraine. BMJ 1996;312:1279.

Graham JJ, Harding PE, Wise PH, Verriman H: Prolactin suppression in the treatment of premenstrual syndrome. Med J Aust 1978;2(Suppl 3):18.

Green K: Determination of prostaglandins in body fluids and tissues. Acta Obstet Gynecol Scand 1979;87:15.

Greene R, Dalton K: The premenstrual syndrome. Br Med J 1953; 1:1007.

Grün G, Fleckenstein A, Byon K: Hemmung der Motilität isolierter Uterus-Streifen aus gravidem und nicht-gravidem mewschlichem Myometrium durch Ca: Antagonisten und Sympathomimetica. Arnzeim Forsch 1971;21:1585.

Gunston KD: Norethisterone enantate in the treatment of premenstrual syndrome. S Afr Med J 1995;85:851.

Halbreich U, Endicott J: Relationship of dysphoric premenstrual changes to depressive disorders. Acta Psychiatr Scand 1985;71: 331.

Halbreich U, Endicott J, Schacht S, Nee J: The diversity of premenstrual changes as reflected in the premenstrual assessment form. Acta Psychiatr Scand 1982;65:46.

Haman TO: Exercises in dysmenorrhea. Am J Obstet Gynecol 1945;49:755.

Hammarback S, Backstrom T: Induced anovulation as a treatment of premenstrual tension syndrome: a double-blind cross-over study with GnRH-agonist versus placebo. Acta Obstet Gynecol Scand 1988;67:159.

Hammarback S, Backstrom T, Holst J, et al: Cyclical mood changes as in the premenstrual tension syndrome during sequential estrogen-progestagen postmenopausal replacement therapy. Acta Obstet Gynecol Scand 1985;64:393.

Hammarback S, Damber J, Backstrom T: Relationship between symptom severity and hormone changes in women with premenstrual syndrome. J Clin Endocrinol Metab 1989;86:125.

Harrison W, Sharpe P, Endicott J: Treatment of premenstrual symptoms. Gen Hosp Psychiatry 1985;7:54.

Harrison WM, Endicott J, Nee J: Treatment of premenstrual dysphoria with alprazolam. Arch Gen Psychiatry 1990;47:270.

Haspels AA: A Double-Blind Placebo-Controlled, Multicenter Study of the Efficacy of Dihydrogesterone (Duphaston) in the Premenstrual Syndrome. Lancaster, England: MTP Press, 1981.

Hauksson A, Ekstrom P, Junchnicka E, et al: The influence of a combined oral contraceptive on uterine activity and reactivity to agonists in primary dysmenorrhea. Acta Obstet Scand 1989; 68:31.

Helms JM: Acupuncture for the management of primary dysmenorrhea. Obstet Gynecol 1987;69:51.

Henzl MR, Izu A: Naproxen and naproxen sodium in dysmenorrhea: development from in vitro inhibition of prostaglandin synthesis to suppression of uterine contractions in women and demonstrations of clinical efficacy. Acta Obstet Gynecol Scand 1979;877:105.

Horrobin DF: The role of essential fatty acids and prostaglandins in the premenstrual syndrome. J Reprod Med 1983;28:465.

Janiger O, Riffenvurgh R, Kersh R: Cross cultural study of premenstrual symptoms. Psychosomatics 1972;13:226.

Jeffcoate TNA: Principles of Gynecology. 3rd ed. London: Butterworth, 1967:133.

Jordheim O: The premenstrual syndrome: clinical trials of treatment with a progestagen combined with a diuretic compared with both progestogen alone and with a placebo. Acta Obstet Gynecol 1972;51:77.

Keizer HA, Poortman J, Bunnik GJ: Influence of physical exercise on sex hormone metabolism. J Appl Physiol 1980;48:765.

Kessel N, Coppen A: The prevalence of common menstrual symptoms. Obstet Gynecol Surv 1964;19:146.

Keye W: Helping your patients cope with PMS. Clin Obstet Gynecol 1984;165:190.

Kolakowska T: The clinical cause of primary recurrent depression in pharmacologically treated female patients. Br J Psychiatry 1975;126:336.

Korossy S: Autoimmune progesterone urticaria and dermatitis. In Rajke E, Korossy A (eds): Immunological Aspects of Allergy and Allergic Diseases. Vol 3. New York: Plenum Press, 1975: 154.

Kudrow L: The relationship of headache frequency to hormonal use in migraine. Headache 1975;51(Suppl 36):1.

Kullander A, Svanberg L: Bromocriptine treatment of the premenstrual syndrome. Acta Obstet Gynecol Scand 1979;58:375.

Kutner SJ, Brown WL: Types of oral contraceptives, depression and premenstrual symptoms. J Nerv Ment Dis 1972;55:153.

Laudanski T, Kostrzewska A, Akerlund M: Interactions of vaso-pressin and prostaglandins in the non-pregnant human uterus. Prostaglandins 1984;27:441.

Lauersen NH: Recognition and treatment of premenstrual syndrome. Nurse Pract 1985;3:11.

Lee R, Stone K, Megelssen D, et al: Presacral neurectomy for chronic pelvic pain. Gynecology 1986;68:517.

Lundeberg T, Bondesson I, Lundstrom V: Relief of primary dysmenorrhea by transcutaneous electrical nerve stimulation. Acta Obstet Gynecol Scand 1985;64:491.

Lundstrom V, Green K: Endogenous levels of prostaglandin $F_{2\alpha}$ in dysmenorrheic women. Am J Obstet Gynecol 1978;130:640.

Lundstrom V, Green K, Wiqvist N: Prostaglandins, indomethacin and dysmenorrhea. Prostaglandins 1976;11:893.

Lyon KE, Lyon MA: The premenstrual syndrome: a survey of current treatment practices. J Reprod Med 1984;29:705.

Macht DI, Davis ME: Experimental studies, old and new, on menstrual toxin. J Comp Physiol Psychol 1934;18:113.

Maddocks S, Hahn P, Moller F, Reid RL: A double-blind placebo-controlled trial of progesterone vaginal suppositories in the treatment of premenstrual syndrome. Am J Obstet Gynecol 1986;154:573.

Magos AL, Brewster E, Singh R, et al: The effects of norethisterone in postmenopausal women on oestrogen replacement therapy: a model for the premenstrual syndrome. Br J Obstet Gynaecol 1986a;93:1290.

Magos AL, Brincat M, Studd JWW: Treatment of the premenstrual syndrome by subcutaneous oestradiol implants and cyclical oral norethisterone: placebo-controlled study. Br Med J 1986b; 292:1629.

Magos AL, Studd JWW: A simple method for the diagnosis of premenstrual syndrome by ultrasound of a self-assessment disk. Am J Obstet Gynecol 1988;158:1024.

Majewska MD, Harrison NL, Schwartz RD, et al: Steroid hormone metabolites are barbiturate-like modulators of the GABA receptor. Science 1986;232:1004.

Mannheimer JS, Whalen EC: The efficacy of transcutaneous electrical nerve stimulation in dysmenorrhea. Clin J Pain 1985;1:75.

Mattson B, Schoultz B: A comparison between lithium, placebo, and diuretic in premenstrual tension. Acta Psychiatr Scand 1974;225:75.

Maxson WS, Rosenwaks Z: The premenstrual syndrome and primary dysmenorrhea. In Benjamin F, Stone ML (eds): Gynecology: Principles and Practice. New York: Macmillan, 1987;81.

Mezrow G, Shoupe D, Spicer D, et al: Depot leuprolide acetate with estrogen and progestin add-back for long-term treatment of premenstrual syndrome. Fertil Steril 1994;62:932.

Mira M, McNeil D, Fraser I, et al: Mefenamic acid in the treatment of premenstrual syndrome. Obstet Gynecol 1986;68:395.

Mondero NA: Nefedipine in the treatment of dysmenorrhea. J Am Osteopath Assoc 1983;89:704.

Moos RH: The development of a menstrual distress questionnaire. Psychosom Med 1969;30:853.

Morris NM, Udry JR: Contraceptive pills and the day-to-day feelings of well-being. Am J Obstet Gynecol 1972;113:763.

Mortola JF, Flirton L, Fisher B: Successful treatment of severe premenstrual syndrome by combined use of GnRH-agonist and estrogen/progestin. J Clin Endocrinol Metab 1991;72:252a.

Moskowitz MA, Coutrer FM: Sumatriptan: a receptor-targeted treatment of migraine. Annu Rev Med 1993;44:145.

Munday M, Brush NG, Taylor RW: Progesterone and aldosterone levels in the premenstrual tension syndrome. J Endocrinol 1977;72:21.

Murray SC, Muse KN: Effective treatment of severe menstrual migraine headaches with gonadotropin-releasing hormone agonist and "add-back" therapy. Fertil Steril 1997;67:390.

Muse KN: Gonadotropin-releasing hormone agonist suppressed premenstrual syndrome (PMS): PMS symptom induction by estrogen, progestin, or both. Proceedings of the Society for Gynecologic Investigators, San Diego, CA, 1989, Abstract 75.

Muse KN, Getel NS, Futterman LA, Yen SSC: The premenstrual syndrome: effects of "medical ovariectomy." N Engl J Med 1984;311:1345.

Nattero G: Menstrual headache. Adv Neurol 1982;33:215.

Neighbors IF, Clelland J, Jackson JR, et al: Transcutaneous electrical nerve stimulation for pain relief in primary dysmenorrhea. Clin J Pain 1987;3:17.

Novak E: Dysmenorrhea in Menstruation and Its Disorders. New York: Appleton, 1924.

O'Brien PMS, Craven D, Shelby C, Symonds EM: Treatment of premenstrual syndrome by spirolactone. Br J Obstet Gynecol 1979;86:142.

Oian P, Tollan A, Fadnes HO, et al: Transcapillary fluid dynamics during the menstrual cycle. Am J Obstet Gynecol 1987;156:952.

Okey R, Robb EI: Studies of the metabolism of women: I. Variations in the fasting blood sugar level and in sugar tolerance in relation to the menstrual cycle. J Biol Chem 1925;65:165.

Pariser SF, Stern SL, Shank ML, et al: Premenstrual syndrome: concerns, controversies, and treatment. Am J Obstet Gynecol 1985;153:599.

Paul SM, Purdy RH: Neuroactive steroids. FASEB J 1992;6:2311.

Pearlstein TB, Stone AB: Long-term fluoxetine treatment of late luteal phase dysphoric disorder. J Clin Psychiatry 1994;55:332.

Pickles VR: A plain muscle stimulant in the menstruum. Nature 1957;180:1198.

Pickles VR, Hall WJ, Best FA: Prostaglandins in endometrium and menstrual fluid from normal and dysmenorrheic subjects. Br J Obstet Gynaecol 1965;72:185.

Prior JC, Vigna Y, Sciaretta D, et al: Conditioning exercise decreases premenstrual symptoms: a prospective, controlled 6-month trial. Fertil Steril 1987;47:502.

Puolakka J, Makarinen L, Vinikka L, Ylikorkala O: Biochemical and clinical effects of treating the premenstrual syndrome with prostaglandin synthesis precursors. J Reprod Med 1985;30:149.

Rausch JL, Janowsky DS: Premenstrual tension: etiology. In Freidman RC (ed): Behavior in the Menstrual Cycle. New York: Marcel Dekker, 1979;397.

Reid RL: Premenstrual syndrome. Curr Probl Obstet Gynecol Fertil 1985;8:1.

Reid RL, Greenway-Coates A, Hahn PM: Oral glucose tolerance during the menstrual cycle in normal women and women with alleged premenstrual "hypoglycemic" attacks: effects of naloxone. J Clin Endocrinol Metab 1986;62:1167.

Reid RL, Yen SSC: Premenstrual syndrome. Am J Gynecol 1981; 139:85.

Rickels K, Freeman E, Sonheimer S: Buspirone in treatment of premenstrual syndrome. Lancet 1989;1:777.

Rosenwaks Z, Jones GS, Henzl MR: Naproxen sodium, aspirin and placebo in primary dysmenorrhea: reduction of pain and blood levels for prostaglandin F alpha metabolite. Am J Obstet Gynecol 1981;140:592.

Rosner R, Muntner S: The Medical Aphorisms of Moses Maimonides. Vol 2. New York: Yeshiva University Press, 1971.

Rossignol AM, Zhang JY, Chen YZ, Xiang Z: Tea and premenstrual syndrome in the People's Republic of China. Am J Public Health 1989;79:67.

Roth-Brandel U, Bygeman M, Wiqvist N: The effect of intravenous administration on prostaglandin E_2 and $F_{2\alpha}$ on the contractility of the non-pregnant human uterus in vivo. Acta Obstet Gynecol Scand 1970;49:19.

Rubinow D, Roy-Byrne P: Premenstrual syndromes: overview from a methodologic perspective. Am J Psychiatry 1984;141:163.

Rubinow DR, Schmidt PJ: The treatment of premenstrual syndrome—forward into the past. N Engl J Med 1995;332:1574.

Ruble DN: Premenstrual symptoms: a reinterpretation. Science 1977;197:291.

Sampson GA: Premenstrual syndrome: a double-blind controlled trial of progesterone and placebo. Br J Psychiatry 1979;130:265.

Samuelsson B, Granstrom E, Green K: Prostaglandins. Annu Rev Biochem 1975;44:669.

Santiesteban AJ, Burnham TL, George KL, et al: Primary spasmodic dysmenorrhea: the use of TENS on acupuncture points. Am J Acupuncture 1985;13:35.

Sarno AP, Miller EJ, Lundblad EG: Premenstrual syndrome: beneficial effects of periodic low-dose danazol. Obstet Gynecol 1987;70:33.

Schmidt PJ, Grover GN, Hoban MC, Rubinow DR: State-dependent alterations in the perception of life events in menstrual-related mood disorders. Am J Psychiatry 1990;147:230.

Schmidt PJ, Grover GN, Rubinow DR: Alprazolam in the treatment of premenstrual syndrome. Arch Gen Psychiatry 1993;50: 467.

Schmidt PJ, Purdy RH, Moore PH, et al: Circulating levels of anxiolytic steroids in the luteal phase in women with premenstrual syndrome and in control subjects. J Clin Endocrinol Metab 1994;79:1256.

Settipane RA, Simon RA: Menstrual cycle and asthma. Ann Allergy 1989;63:373.

Sheftell FD, Silberstein SD, Rapoport AM, et al: Migraine and women: diagnosis, pathophysiology, and treatment. J Wom Health 1992;1:5.

Shelley WB, Preucel RW, Spoont SS: Autoimmune progesterone dermatitis: cure by oophorectomy. JAMA 1965;190:147.

Silberfeld S, Brast N, Noble EP: The menstrual cycle: a double-blind study of symptoms, mood, and behavior and biochemical variables using Enovid and placebo. Psychosom Med 1971;33: 411.

Silberstein SD, Merriam MD: Estrogens, progestins, and headache. Neurology 1991;41:786.

Singner K, Cheng R, Schoub M: A controlled evaluation of lithium in the premenstrual tension syndrome. Br J Psychiatry 1974;124:50.

Sjoberg N: Dysmenorrhea and uterine neurotransmitters. Acta Obstet Gynecol Scand 1979;87:57.

Sletten IW, Gershon S: The premenstrual syndrome: a discussion of its pathophysiology and treatment with lithium. Compr Psychiatry 1966;7:197.

Smith S, Rinehart JS, Ruddock VE, Schiff I: Treatment of premenstrual syndrome with alprozalam: results of a double-blind, placebo-controlled, randomized cross-over clinical trial. Obstet Gynecol 1987;70:37.

Smith S, Schiff I: The premenstrual syndrome—diagnosis and management. Fertil Steril 1989;52:527.

Smith SL: Mood and the menstrual cycle. In Sachar EJ (ed): Topics in psychoendocrinology. New York: Raven Press, 1955;19.

Sobczyk R, Braunstein ML, Solberg L: A case control survey and dysmenorrhea in a family practice population: a proposed disability index. J Fam Pract 1978;7:285.

Steiner M, Haskett R, Osmun RN, et al: Premenstrual syndrome: psychoendocrine evaluation and treatment outcome. Psychosom Med 1979;41:73.

Steiner M, Lamont J, Steinberg S, et al: Effect on fluoxetine on menstrual cycle length in women with premenstrual dysphoria. Obstet Gynecol 1997;90:590.

Steiner M, Steinberg S, Stewart D, et al: Fluoxetine in the treatment of premenstrual syndrome. N Engl J Med 1995;332:1529.

Stokes J, Mendels J: Pyridoxine and premenstrual tension. Lancet 1972;1:1177.

Strickler RC: Endocrine hypothesis for the etiology of premenstrual syndrome. Clin Endocrinol 1987;14:1.

Sutherland H, Stewart I: A critical analysis of the premenstrual syndrome. Lancet 1965;1:1180.

Swyer GIM: Treatment of premenstrual tension syndrome: value of ethisterone, mephenesin and placebo compared. Br Med J 1955;1:1410.

Tulenheimo A, Laafikainen T, Salminen K: Plasma β-endorphin immunoreactivity in premenstrual tension. Br J Obstet Gynaecol 1987;94:26.

Ulmsten U, Anderson KE, Forman A: Relaxing effects of nifedipine on the non-pregnant human uterus in vitro and in vivo. Obstet Gynecol 1978;52:436.

Vane JR: Inhibition of prostaglandin synthesis as a mechanism of action for aspirin-like drugs. Nature 1971;231.

Vellacott ID, Shroff NE, Pearce MY, et al: A double-blind placebo-controlled evaluation of spironolactone in the premenstrual syndrome. Curr Res Opinion 1987;10:450.

Vermeulen A, Verdon ZKL: Plasma androgen levels during the menstrual cycle. Am J Obstet Gynecol 1976;125:491.

Watts JF, Butt RW, Logan Edwards R: A clinical trial using danazol for the treatment of premenstrual tension. Br J Obstet Gynaecol 1987;94:30.

Widholm O, Kantero RL: A statistical analysis of the menstrual patterns of 8,000 Finnish girls and their mothers. Acta Obstet Gynecol Scand Suppl 1971;14:1.

Wood C, Jakubowicz D: The treatment of premenstrual symptoms with mefenamic acid. Br J Obstet Gynaecol 1980;87:627.

Wood SH, Mortola JF, Yuen-fai C, et al: Treatment of premenstrual syndrome with fluoxetine: a double-blind, placebo-controlled, crossover study. Obstet Gynecol 1992;80:339.

Wurtman JJ, Brzezinski A, Wurtman RJ, Laferrere B: Effect of nutrient intake in premenstrual depression. Am J Obstet Gynecol 1989;161:1228.

Yikorkala O, Dawood MY: New concepts in dysmenorrhea. Am J Obstet Gynecol 1978;130:833.

24

Dysfunctional Uterine Bleeding

Moon H. Kim

Dysfunctional uterine bleeding (DUB) is abnormal bleeding from the uterine endometrium that is unrelated to anatomic lesions of the uterus (American College of Obstetricians and Gynecologists [ACOG], 1989). It is usually associated with abnormal ovarian function and anovulation but may occur in ovulatory cycles. Prepubertal or postmenopausal uterine bleeding is a separate entity that warrants a different diagnostic and therapeutic consideration. Menstrual irregularities associated with corpus luteum defects or midcycle spotting associated with ovulation may be considered as subgroups of DUB. However, DUB is frequently a manifestation of anovulation, and the term *anovulatory uterine bleeding* might be preferred in such cases.

The diagnosis of DUB is usually made by demonstrating an anovulatory state and excluding organic causes of uterine bleeding, such as submucous fibroids, blood dyscrasias, endometrial polyps, uterine cancer, and pregnancy-related bleeding. The possibility of such lesions coexisting with anovulatory bleeding should be considered, however. The wide variations in menstrual patterns often cause difficulty in identifying abnormal bleeding. In practice, any bleeding that is excessive in duration, frequency, or amount for a particular patient should be considered abnormal and investigated accordingly.

THE NORMAL MENSTRUAL CYCLE

A normal ovulatory cycle is the consequence of endocrine interactions of the hypothalamic-pituitary-ovarian axis. In addition, the event of menstruation occurs as a result of sudden decrease in progesterone and estrogen secretion caused by the demise of the corpus luteum. In ovulatory cycles, sequential histologic changes of the uterine endometrium from proliferative phase to secretory phase reflect ovarian function, which is characterized by the cyclic pattern of estrogen and progesterone secretion. In anovulatory cycles, these predictable changes in endometrial histology and ovarian steroid hormones are missing.

The normality of menstruation is subjectively determined by the amount and duration of blood flow and by the intervals between menstrual cycles. Over the reproductive lifespan, most women experience a consistent cycle interval ranging between 25 and 34 days (Treolar et al, 1967). The secretory (luteal) phase is more consistent (14 ± 2 days) than the proliferative (follicular) phase. The duration of normal menses is 3 to 7 days. Although it cannot be accurately quantitated, blood loss in a normal menstrual period varies from 25 to 75 ml. Clinically, however, the number of pads or tampons used often gives some idea as to any changes in menstrual flow, although they are not reliable indicators of actual amount of blood loss (Chimbira et al, 1980).

DEFINITION AND CAUSE OF DUB

It is important to define clearly the meaning of the term *dysfunctional uterine bleeding*. As previously mentioned, the ACOG has defined it as abnormal bleeding from the uterine endometrium that is unrelated to anatomic lesions of the uterus. The clinical obligation is to exclude anatomic lesions of the uterus by pelvic examination and other means such as hysterosalpingogram, endometrial sampling, hysteroscopy, or ultrasonography. Virtually all variations of DUB can be related to disruption in normal ovarian function. Greater than 80% of DUB is anovulatory, and the remaining 20% is due to dysfunction of the corpus luteum or atrophic endometrium (Benjamin and Seltzer, 1987). Many anatomic lesions of the uterus, such as leiomyoma, endometrial polyps, and pregnancy-related conditions, cause uterine bleeding that must be differentiated from DUB (Table 24–1). Although no organic pathologic factors are present in the uterus, uterine bleeding secondary to such pathologic entities as blood dyscrasia, endocrinopathies, hepatic dysfunction, and other iatrogenic causes should not be considered as true DUB but rather as pseudo-DUB (Table 24–2) (Benjamin and Seltzer, 1987; ACOG, 1989).

533

Table 24-1. CAUSES OF ABNORMAL UTERINE BLEEDING

DYSFUNCTIONAL UTERINE BLEEDING
Anovulatory bleeding
Corpus luteum dysfunction (inadequate or persistent)
Atrophic endometrium

INTRAUTERINE LESIONS
Submucous leiomyoma
Endometrial polyp
Endometritis
Intrauterine contraceptive device
Endometrial carcinoma

LEIOMYOMAS OF THE UTERUS

PELVIC INFLAMMATORY DISEASE

ADENOMYOSIS

EARLY PREGNANCY COMPLICATIONS
Abortion
Ectopic pregnancy
Hydatidiform mole

Pathophysiology

A basic knowledge of normal menstrual physiology is essential to understanding the pathophysiology of DUB. Many landmark physiologic and anatomic studies of the past (Markee, 1940; Noyes et al, 1950; Bartelmez, 1957) and numerous more recent investigations (Healy and Hodgen, 1983; Wilborn and Flowers, 1984; Speroff et al, 1989) have contributed to a better understanding of the mechanisms regulating normal menstrual cycles. In ovulatory cycles,

Table 24-2. CAUSES OF PSEUDO-DUB

PELVIC DISEASES NOT DETECTED CLINICALLY
Uterine lesions (see Table 24-1)
Pelvic inflammatory disease
Endometriosis
Ovarian neoplasm (granulosa/theca cell)

VARIOUS ENDOCRINOPATHY
Hypothalamic/psychogenic
Polycystic ovary syndrome
Hyperprolactinemia
Thyroid dysfunction
Adrenal dysfunction

SYSTEMIC DISEASES
Blood dyscrasia
  Thrombocytopenic purpura
  von Willebrand's disease
  Leukemia
  Increased fibrinolysin (endometrium)
Hepatic disease
  Impaired synthesis of coagulation factors
  Impaired metabolism of sex steroids (i.e., estrogen)
  Impaired synthesis of sex hormone–binding globulin
Renal disease
  Impaired excretion of estrogens
  Obesity
Iatrogenic causes
  Anticoagulants, digitalis, oral contraceptives (breakthrough bleeding), acetylsalicylic acid

the endometrium undergoes predictable changes from proliferation as a result of estrogen stimulation in the follicular phase to the secretory pattern under progesterone effect limiting the endometrial proliferation in the luteal phase. The adequate synthesis of progesterone receptors in the endometrial epithelial cells stimulated by estrogen in the follicular phase is essential to the formation of secretory endometrium associated with characteristic alterations in the endometrial stroma (Healy and Hodgen, 1983). Exposure to progesterone alone without the estrogen priming effect will not cause endometrial bleeding when progesterone levels decline. Alternatively, estrogen will stimulate the endometrium to be proliferative. In addition, the endometrium will desquamate when estrogen levels decline sharply, resulting in uterine bleeding as in anovulatory condition.

Endometrial desquamation, or sloughing in normal menses, or DUB is limited to the so-called functional layer consisting of the stratum compactum and stratum spongiosum. The basal layer is unaffected and remains to grow and regenerate the endometrium. Although withdrawal or decline of both estrogen and progesterone results in sloughing of the functional layer of the endometrium, the progesterone withdrawal causes spasmodic vasoconstriction of the spiral arterioles followed by ischemia and desquamation of the endometrium. Studies suggest that prostaglandin may play a role in this process (Nygren and Rybo, 1983). The concentration of prostaglandins (PGs) in the endometrium of women varies at different stages of the cycle (Singh et al, 1975). The marked increase in the concentration of $PGF_{2\alpha}$ during the luteal phase probably represents an increased synthetase activity induced by the action of progesterone. $PGF_{2\alpha}$ is a potent vasoconstrictor, whereas PGE_2 and prostacyclin (PGI_2) promote vasodilation and prevent platelet aggregation. The critical ratio of $PGF_{2\alpha}$ to PGE_2 may be responsible for vasoconstriction of the spiral arterioles of the endometrium. However, the exact mechanism by which endometrial sloughing occurs is not clear.

In anovulatory uterine bleeding, the pattern of bleeding depends entirely on the duration and level of estrogen stimulation on the endometrium because progesterone influence is absent. In the absence of progesterone, the markedly reduced $PGF_{2\alpha}$-to-PGE_2 ratio may account for the uncontrolled nature of the bleeding and the absence of uterine cramps. The different patterns are shown in Table 24-3. Sometimes, despite evident ovulation, abnormal uterine bleeding may occur, although infrequently, because of a disturbance in the delicate estrogen-progesterone balance maintaining endometrial integrity: either too little progesterone (inadequate corpus luteum causing irregular ripening of the endometrium) or too much progesterone or persistent progesterone levels (persistent corpus luteum, Halban's disease causing irregular shedding of the endometrium).

There is no consistent or predictable correlation between DUB and endometrial histology. Most en-

Table 24–3. PATTERNS OF ABNORMAL UTERINE BLEEDING

Polymenorrhea	Frequent menses regularly occurring at intervals of less than 21 days
Hypermenorrhea	Excessive bleeding in amount during normal duration of regular menses
Hypomenorrhea	Decreased bleeding in amount in regular menstrual cycles
Menorrhagia	Prolonged bleeding in duration, occurring at regular intervals
Metrorrhagia	Uterine bleeding occurring at irregular intervals
Menometrorrhagia	Uterine bleeding, usually excessive and prolonged, occurring at irregular, frequent intervals

dometrial tissue in DUB shows normal proliferative endometrium (Czernobilsky, 1970). However, in the absence of progesterone interposition and prolonged exposure of the endometrium to estrogen, the endometrium in an anovulatory state may develop varying degrees of hyperplasia (cystic and adenomatous). The patients with adenomatous hyperplasia are at increased risk for atypical endometrial hyperplasia, a precursor of adenocarcimona of the endometrium.

INITIAL EVALUATION

The first step in evaluating abnormal uterine bleeding is to take a detailed history of bleeding and to establish the origin of bleeding by careful pelvic examination. Various causative factors of nonuterine bleeding should be ruled out. Inquiry about systemic diseases, general bleeding tendencies, and use of medications, such as sex hormones and anticoagulants, is important. The general physical examination requires a thorough inspection of the entire perineum to diagnose any bleeding of vulvar, urethral, and gastrointestinal origin. An examination with a speculum must be performed to confirm uterine bleeding by excluding lesions of the vagina and cervix. A bimanual examination is then performed to rule out adnexal pathologic factors and to assess uterine size, shape, and consistency.

Because DUB is a clinical diagnosis of exclusion, the next step is to rule out any pathologic condition causing uterine bleeding. It is helpful to determine whether a patient is anovulatory or ovulatory. Abnormal uterine bleeding associated with an ovulatory cycle is more likely to have an organic cause than bleeding associated with anovulation. However, the possibility of coexistence of such organic causes as submucous fibroids or endometrial polyp with anovulation should be kept in mind. Some patients may have endometrial atrophy causing uterine bleeding.

Ovulatory DUB is usually associated with premenstrual symptoms such as breast tenderness, dysmenorrhea, and weight gain and regular periodicity. It is usually caused by organic lesions, although a dysfunction of the corpus luteum may be the cause. Al-

ternatively, *anovulatory DUB* is most common in the postmenarchal and premenopausal periods. It is characteristically acyclic, unpredictable as to the onset of bleeding, and variable in the duration and amount of bleeding.

In clinical practice, a number of somewhat confusing and yet commonly accepted terms are used to describe different types of irregular uterine bleeding (Table 24–3). Anovulatory DUB often presents as metrorrhagia or menometrorrhagia. However, to avoid confusion, an accurate description of bleeding (amount, duration, and frequency) is preferred.

In most cases, the history and physical examination will greatly limit the differential diagnoses and lead to a logical and cost-effective selection of laboratory tests or diagnostic procedures to confirm the suspected etiologic factors of abnormal uterine bleeding. The history should include the patient's obstetric history and whether she plans to conceive or not. The therapeutic plan is different depending on her need for contraception, her desire to conceive, or her wish only to regulate irregular bleeding.

ETIOLOGY OF ABNORMAL UTERINE BLEEDING

Organic Causes

There are numerous conditions causing nonuterine genital bleeding that must be excluded (Table 24–4). These conditions are usually identified at a careful pelvic examination. Therefore, a complete physical examination including the pelvic area is essential. In addition, other laboratory tests, such as urinalysis for hematuria and stool examination for blood, may be performed when urinary or gastrointestinal causes are suspected.

Cervical Lesions

Bleeding resulting from cervicitis, cervical polyps, or eversion is usually of small amount, often with spotting, and intermenstrual. Most commonly, these lesions cause no bleeding. However, when easy contact bleeding or postcoital bleeding is present, further tests should be done to rule out carcinoma-

Table 24-4. ANATOMIC CAUSES OF NONUTERINE BLEEDING

CERVIX	VULVA
Neoplasia (polyps or carcinoma)	Trauma
Cervicitis	Infections/inflammations
Ectropion and eversion	Neoplasia
Ulceration	Condylomas
Condylomatous lesions	Dystrophy
Endometriosis	Varices
VAGINA	**URINARY TRACT**
Neoplasia (carcinoma, sarcoma)	Urethral caruncle
Adenosis	Urethral diverticulum
Trauma	Hematuria
Foreign body	**GASTROINTESTINAL TRACT**
Atrophic vaginitis	Hemorrhoids
Infection (vaginitis)	Anal fissure
Condylomas	Colorectal lesions

tous change. Occasionally, endometriosis of the cervix causes irregular bleeding. The most important lesion is uterine cancer, particularly of the cervix. It may present with light to heavy intermenstrual bleeding; such a history should raise suspicion and calls for thorough examination with a speculum, a cytologic smear, and a colposcopic examination when needed.

Intrauterine Lesions

Any lesion in the uterine cavity, such as submucous fibroid, endometrial polyp, or endometritis, may cause irregular bleeding. Because these lesions may not be detected clinically, the bleeding is often misdiagnosed as DUB initially. However, with a high index of suspicion and various diagnostic approaches, such cases of pseudo-DUB can be detected.

Bleeding resulting from submucous fibroids or endometrial polyps is generally cyclic at the usual intervals and menorrhagic or hypermenorrheic with premenstrual spotting. Transvaginal sonography and sonohysterography are useful in evaluating these conditions. Hysteroscopy should be considered to evaluate these conditions further. Alternatively, menometrorrhagia or intermenstrual bleeding is often associated with endometritis or intrauterine contraceptive devices.

Endometrial Hyperplasia and Cancer

Endometrial hyperplasia develops when unopposed estrogen stimulation persists, as in chronic anovulation. Bleeding occurs usually because of estrogen breakthrough. When acyclic estrogen levels are relatively low, the bleeding may be light. However, women with high levels of estrogen may have an amenorrheic period followed by acute and heavy bleeding.

Abnormal bleeding in older women must be investigated to exclude adenomatous hyperplasia with cellular atypia and adenocarcinoma of the endometrium. This is more likely seen in perimenopausal women; however, these conditions may develop in younger women with chronic anovulation during their reproductive lives.

Leiomyomas of the Uterus

Bleeding usually occurs when myomas involve the endometrial cavity because of their submucous location. Even in the absence of submucous fibroids, abnormal uterine bleeding may occur, probably because of an enlarged endometrial surface from which to bleed or venous congestion of the endometrium (Farrer-Brown et al, 1971). To assess the size and location of fibroids better, a high-resolution ultrasonogram, magnetic resonance imaging, hysterogram, or hysteroscopy may be performed (Andreyko et al, 1988).

Pelvic Inflammatory Disease

Abnormal bleeding may occur in women with pelvic inflammatory disease, probably because of its effects on ovarian function and through associated endometritis or cervicitis.

Adenomyosis

Although the diagnosis is made only after histopathologic examination of the uterus, adenomyosis is clinically suspected when a parous woman with menorrhagia and dysmenorrhea shows diffuse and often tender enlargement of the uterus. The bleeding is usually cyclic, heavy, and prolonged.

Complications of Early Pregnancy

Irregular uterine bleeding is frequently the first symptom associated with various types of abortion, ectopic pregnancy, and hydatidiform mole. A careful history, a pregnancy test (serum), and sonographic evaluation are the keys to diagnosis of these conditions. Without a high level of suspicion, it may be difficult to differentiate these conditions from DUB at times.

Endocrinologic Causes

All endocrine diseases may disturb the normal hypothalamic-pituitary-ovarian axis and cause ovulatory dysfunction by interfering with the secretion of gonadotropin-releasing hormone (GnRH), pituitary gonadotropins, and ovarian steroid hormones. Usually they are associated with anovulatory bleeding.

Hypothalamic disorders or stress-related psychogenic conditions may present with either amenorrhea or anovulatory bleeding. Most of the hypothalamic disorders are functional; however, they can be neoplasms or sequelae of inflammation. Any pituitary disorder may cause anovulation and irregular bleeding initially, which progresses eventually to amenorrhea. The most common pituitary disease during the reproductive years is hyperprolactinemia of idiopathic origin or microadenoma. Hyperprolactinemia may result in various types of menstrual disorders, including pseudo-DUB (Schlechte et al, 1980).

Thyroid disorders may cause menstrual disturbance. Although hyperthyroidism tends to cause amenorrhea, overt forms of hypothyroidism are frequently associated with menorrhagia. Menorrhagia is a complaint in as many as 45% of women with myxedema (Scott and Mussey, 1964) and in 20% of women with a subclinical form of hypothyroidism (Douglas and Greisman, 1989). Appropriate thyroid therapy usually corrects menorrhagia. Diabetes mellitus and various adrenal disorders, such as Cushing's syndrome, congenital adrenal hyperplasia, and Addison's disease, may also cause abnormal menses.

Systemic Diseases

Abnormal uterine bleeding can be one of the first signs of several serious systemic diseases. It is important for the gynecologist to keep this possibility in mind when evaluating women with irregular menstruation. The pelvic examination is normal in these cases of pseudo-DUB (see Table 24–2).

Blood dyscrasias are the most common of the systemic diseases causing irregular and usually excessive uterine bleeding. They account for about 20% of menorrhagia complaints by adolescent females (Chassens and Cowell, 1981). Several types of blood dyscrasias are more commonly associated with pseudo-DUB. Idiopathic thrombocytopenic purpura may present with menorrhagia or hypermenorrhea as the first sign even before manifesting petechiae, ecchymosis, or gastrointestinal bleeding. An accurate platelet count will lead to the diagnosis. von Willebrand's disease is a common bleeding disorder that affects both sexes and is transmitted as an autosomal dominant trait. Patients with this disease have decreased coagulation factor VIII and von Willebrand factor (vWF), a macromolecular complex with factor VIII. Other dyscrasias causing abnormal uterine bleeding include prothrombin deficiency and deficiencies of factors II, V, VII, and XI (Fraser et al, 1986). Although less common, ovulatory menorrhagia may be an early manifestation of acute leukemias with loss of clotting mechanisms. The importance of hematologic evaluation cannot be overemphasized.

Other systemic diseases causing menorrhagia are liver and renal diseases. The hepatic dysfunction results in deficient conjugation of estrogens and the decreased production of fibrinogen and clotting factors. In renal failure, the excretion of estrogen and progesterone is impaired and a disruption of the normal hypothalamic-pituitary axis results in anovulation. Menorrhagia in these disorders is usually correctable with hormone therapy.

DUB is not uncommon in the obese patient because of an increased peripheral conversion of androstenedione to estrogens in the adipose tissue, resulting in anovulation.

Various iatrogenic causes of abnormal uterine bleeding should be ruled out. These include the use of anticoagulants such as heparin, coumarin, and acetylsalicylic acid or use of digitalis or steroid oral contraceptives. Occasionally depomedroxyprogesterone acetate, GnRH analogs, and danazol are responsible for breakthrough bleeding. Needless to say, a careful history should always include a list of all current medications.

DIAGNOSTIC INVESTIGATION

The diagnosis of DUB assumes the absence of organic causes discussed already. The initial history and pelvic examination will determine a uterine source of bleeding and normal pelvic findings. Although ovulatory DUB does not occur frequently, most abnormal uterine bleeding associated with an ovulatory cycle is due to an organic cause and requires further investigation. On the basis of a good history, one must initially determine whether DUB is associated with an ovulatory or anovulatory cycle.

The history includes a detailed menstrual pattern in terms of intervals, duration, and amount of flow; a list of medications; obstetric history; sexual and contraceptive histories; and a general medical history. It should also show any recent surgical or gynecologic disorders.

The physical examination focuses on eliciting any manifestation of general medical conditions that might cause abnormal bleeding, as discussed previously (see Table 24–2). Careful examination of the thyroid, breasts, liver, and skin is essential. The presence or absence of ecchymotic lesions, obesity, and hirsutism should be noted. A pelvic examination should be completed with both inspection and bimanual palpation of the external and internal organs. The source and degree of bleeding, the size and shape of the uterus, and any adnexal abnormalities are carefully evaluated.

On the basis of the information gathered, further investigation using laboratory tests, imaging evaluations, and surgical procedures is directed at determining the patient's hemodynamic state and the causes of bleeding. A complete blood count and a Papanicolaou smear, if not performed recently, are the initial tests. A sensitive assay for β-human chorionic gonadotropin to exclude any pregnancy-related bleeding should be performed. In chronic excessive bleeding, particularly in adolescents, a coagulation study is indicated. Useful tests and procedures are listed in Table 24–5. The scope of evaluation depends on the clinical presentation of each patient and the magnitude of bleeding. For example,

Table 24–5. LABORATORY AND OTHER TESTS FOR EVALUATION OF DYSFUNCTIONAL UTERINE BLEEDING

Complete blood count, coagulation profile
Quantitative serum β-hCG
Iron concentration and binding capacity
Ovulation detection (BBT, serum progesterone)
Thyroid function tests, including TSH
Serum androgens
Serum gonadotropins and prolactin
Hepatic function tests
Endometrial biopsy
Hysterogram or hysteroscopy
Pelvic ultrasonography or magnetic resonance imaging

Abbreviations: BBT, basal body temperature; β-hCG, β-human chorionic gonadotropin; TSH, thyroid-stimulating hormone.

an endometrial biopsy is always indicated for DUB in women over 35 years of age. However, it should also be considered in younger women with increased risks for endometrial hyperplasia or cancer, such as chronically anovulatory obese women.

TREATMENT

Treatment is individualized according to the patient's age, her desire for contraception or fertility, and the severity and chronicity of the bleeding. The goals of treatment are to arrest the acute episode of bleeding, to prevent recurrences, and to induce ovulation in the patient desiring to conceive. If the pelvic examination shows a normal uterus and no systemic diseases are suspected, hormonal therapy is usually effective in managing DUB. Rarely, blood loss in DUB presents as a hemodynamically compromised state. However, patients with acute, profuse hemorrhage require aggressive treatment to stop or slow the bleeding, followed by a long-term management plan.

Acute, Profuse Bleeding

When a patient presents with acute, profuse, and uncontrollable hemorrhage, the usual steps taken for any other serious hemorrhage must be instituted immediately. Vital signs must be monitored carefully, and the hematologic evaluations should be obtained while an intravenous catheter is inserted for administration of fluids or blood as needed for stabilization. Coagulation studies and cross-matching should also be performed, and a pregnancy test is done to exclude any pregnancy-related complication. The urinary output is also recorded. A careful pelvic examination is performed to exclude organic causes of uterine bleeding, particularly malignancy and pregnancy.

In patients with acute, severe bleeding associated with unstable vital signs and a compromised hematologic finding, an operative dilatation and curettage (D&C) may be performed because this is the quickest way to stop bleeding in the absence of organic pathologic factors. However, a simpler technique of suction curettage in the office or emergency department has proven to be as effective in most cases (Hamilton and Knab, 1975). The tissue obtained will establish the histologic diagnosis. This is particularly important in women older than 35 years in whom malignancy must be ruled out. Once the acute bleeding has been controlled and the diagnosis of DUB is established, cyclic hormonal therapy using estrogen and progestin should be initiated for a few cycles.

For the acute bleeding episode that is heavy but not life threatening, medical treatment should be offered. Because most of the cases are anovulatory DUB, hormonal therapy should arrest bleeding within 24 hours. High-dose estrogen therapy, 2.5 mg of conjugated estrogen orally every 6 hours, will bring about cessation of bleeding by stimulating rapid endometrial proliferation for "healing." It has been shown to be equally effective as intravenous administration of 25 mg of conjugated estrogen every 4 hours (DeVore et al, 1982). When the bleeding stops, the treatment should be followed by either continuous administration of conjugated estrogens, 2.5 mg for 3 weeks with the addition of medroxyprogesterone acetate 10 mg daily on the last 10 days of therapy to allow for withdrawal bleeding, or the use of a combination oral contraceptive (containing 50 μg of ethinyl estradiol) for 3 weeks. An alternative approach is to try any combination oral contraceptive (i.e., Ortho-Novum 1/50 or Ovral 0.5/50), one pill two times daily for 7 days, during which the acute bleeding should be arrested, followed by one pill daily for 2 more weeks.

The mechanisms by which estrogens arrest the acute endometrial bleeding are not well understood. Among the postulated effects of high-dose estrogen therapy are an increase in coagulation factors, a direct effect on capillary vessels, and fibrin clot formation. However, these effects have been associated with the long-term use of pharmacologic doses of estrogens and not with acute administration. Intense stimulation of endometrial proliferation induced by estrogens, thus "repairing" the sloughing endometrium, may be the most important mechanism.

Because most cases of DUB involve anovulatory bleeding, the intramuscular administration of progesterone in oil (100 to 200 mg) can also arrest the bleeding. However, it will not be effective if the endometrium is completely exhausted from prolonged sloughing or under a pre-existing progesterone effect (i.e., secretory or decidual). Also, it does not work in the presence of organic causes such as submucous fibroid or pregnancy complication. Progesterone administration should be followed by 2 to 3 weeks of combination oral contraceptive pills as described previously.

Chronic, Recurrent Anovulatory Bleeding

For patients with mild to moderate recurrent bleeding or those in whom an acute episode has been resolved, there are several therapeutic options available. Treatment is based on the patient's complaint, age, and desire for fertility.

Observation only is a reasonable approach for adolescent girls with no evidence of anemia, because regular ovulatory cycles should ensue in most cases. When treatment is necessary in the adolescent who is not sexually active, cyclic administration of progestins (i.e., medroxyprogesterone acetate 10 mg orally for 10 days) for 1 to 2 months is preferred. However, if the patient is sexually active, any of the combination oral contraceptives should be offered.

For patients in the reproductive age, particularly those requiring contraception, oral contraceptives are a good choice to regulate irregular bleeding. In patients with anovulation as a manifestation of ovarian hyperandrogenism, as in the polycystic ovary syndrome, combination oral contraceptives will also help to reduce the elevated levels of circulating androgens (Givens et al, 1974). If the patient does not want or has a contraindication to the use of oral contraceptives, she may be managed with cyclic progestins (medroxyprogesterone acetate, norethindrone, etc.) to provide regular withdrawal bleeding. When fertility is desired by the patient, an induction of ovulation is indicated, with clomiphene citrate as the initial drug of choice.

In addition to conventional hormonal therapy, treatment with GnRH agonists has been tried effectively in the management of DUB (Shaw and Fraser, 1984; Fedorkow et al, 1989). Because the role of GnRH agonist therapy in DUB has not been well defined, treatment with a GnRH agonist should be considered only when the bleeding is poorly controlled with conventional hormonal treatment or in patients with contraindications for sex steroid therapy.

Abnormal Bleeding in Ovulatory Cycles

The first step in managing DUB associated with ovulatory cycles is to eliminate any organic cause if identified. In the absence of organic lesions one must consider ovulatory DUB or von Willebrand's disease.

For patients with ovulatory DUB, the cyclic administration of oral contraceptives (combination type) is often effective in stopping abnormal bleeding. Cyclic administration of progestin alone is not successful. The use of intrauterine contraceptive devices with progestin release has been reported to be effective in reducing menstrual flow (Milsom et al, 1991). Also, various nonsteroidal anti-inflammatory drugs (NSAIDs) have been shown to be effective in reducing blood loss (Chuong and Brenner, 1996). The ability of NSAIDs to block prostacyclin (PGI_2) formation explains their therapeutic effectiveness. NSAIDs are generally ineffective in treating anovulatory DUB or abnormal bleeding with organic causes. The administration of these agents starts on the day of heavy bleeding with a loading dose (i.e., ibuprofen 800 mg or mefenamic acid 1000 mg) followed by three doses (ibuprofen 400 mg or mefenamic acid 500 mg) daily for 3 days.

For those with abnormal bleeding associated with von Willebrand's disease, which affects approximately 1% of the population, desmopression acetate (1-desamino-8-D-arginine vasopressin) can be used in place of blood products. It is believed to stimulate the release of vWF. Intranasal spray or intramuscular administration is available (Chuong and Brenner, 1996).

Surgical Therapy

Although most patients with DUB can be managed by hormonal therapy, a D&C can be effective both diagnostically and therapeutically. For those older than age 35, histologic evaluation of the endometrium is essential either by an endometrial biopsy or a D&C to rule out any endometrial pathologic factors, such as hyperplasia or adenocarcinoma. The use of curettage provides only a temporary cure and should be followed by hormonal therapy in all cases.

Ablation of the endometrium by either the neodymium:yttrium-aluminum-garnet (Nd:YAG) laser or electrocoagulation through the hysteroscope has been added to the available surgical options (Baggish and Baltoyannis, 1988). Ablation is not a replacement for hysterectomy, but it is a safe alternative in those patients who are poor surgical risks or who refuse hysterectomy despite persistent menorrhagia. Preoperative treatment with danazol or a GnRH agonist for 4 to 6 weeks before hysteroscopic ablative surgery is recommended to induce endometrial atrophy, thus facilitating the surgery.

Although other therapeutic alternatives mentioned should be tried, hysterectomy is regarded as the definitive treatment of chronic DUB that does not respond to hormonal therapy or other surgical management. It is best indicated for patients who do not desire fertility or who have premalignant or significant associated pelvic pathologic factors (i.e., myoma, pelvic inflammatory disease, endometriosis). DUB per se is rarely an indication for hysterectomy.

REFERENCES

American College of Obstetricians and Gynecologists: Dysfunctional Uterine Bleeding (ACOG Technical Bulletin No 134). Washington, DC: American College of Obstetricians and Gynecologists, 1989.

Andreyko JL, Blumenfeld Z, Marshall LA, et al: Use of an agonistic analog of gonadotropin-releasing hormone (nafarelin) to treat leiomymas: assessment by magnetic resonance imaging. Am J Obstet Gynecol 1988;158:903.

Baggish MS, Baltoyannis P: New techniques for laser ablation of the endometrium in high-risk patients. Am J Obstet Gynecol 1988;159:287.

Bartelmez GW: The phases of the menstrual cycle and their interpretation in terms of the pregnant cycle. Am J Obstet Gynecol 1957;74:931.

Benjamin F, Seltzer VL: Excessive menstrual bleeding, menorrhagia, and dysfunctional uterine bleeding. In Rosenwaks Z, Benjamin F, Stone ML (eds): Principles and Practice: Gynecology. New York: Macmillan, 1987:67.

Chassens EA, Cowell CA: Acute adolescent menorrhagia. Am J Obstet Gynecol 1981;139:277.

Chimbira TH, Anderson ABM, Tunbull AC: Relation between measured menstrual blood loss and patient's subjective assessment of loss, duration of bleeding, number of sanitary towels used, uterine weight and endometrial surface area. Br J Obstet Gynaecol 1980;87:603.

Chuong CJ, Brenner PF: Management of abnormal uterine bleeding. Am J Obstet Gynecol 1996;175:787.

Czernobilsky B: Utero-ovarian pathology in dysfunctional uterine bleeding. Clin Obstet Gynecol 1970;13:416.

DeVore GR, Owens O, Kase N: Use of intravenous premarin in the treatment of dysfunctional uterine bleeding: a double-blind, randomized control study. Obstet Gynecol 1982;59:285.

Douglas LW, Greisman B: Early hypothyroidism in patients with menorrhagia. Am J Obstet Gynecol 1989;160:673.

Farrer-Brown G, Beilby JOW, Tarbit MH: Vascular patterns in myomatous uteri. J Obstet Gynaecol Br Commonw 1971;38:743.

Fedorkow DM, Corenblum B, Shaffer EA: The use of a gonadotropin-releasing hormone analog and transdermal estrogen to preserve fertility in a woman with severe menorrhagia. Fertil Steril 1989;52:3.

Fraser IS, McCarron G, Markham R, et al: Measured menstrual blood loss in women with menorrhagia associated with pelvic disease or coagulation disorder. Obstet Gynecol 1986;68:630.

Givens JR, Anderson RN, Wiser WL, Fish SA: Dynamics of suppression and recovery of plasma FSH, LH, androstenedione and testosterone in polycystic ovarian disease using an oral contraceptive. J Clin Endocrinol Metab 1974;38:727.

Hamilton JV, Knab DR: Suction curettage: the therapeutic effectiveness in dysfunctional uterine bleeding. Obstet Gynecol 1975;45:47.

Healy DL, Hodgen GD: The endocrinology of human endometrium. Obstet Gynecol Surv 1983;38:509.

Markee JE: Menstruation in intraocular endometrial implants in the rhesus monkey. Contrib Embryol 1940;28:219.

Milsom I, Anderson K, Andersch B, Rybo G: A comparison of flurbiprofen, tranexamic acid, and levonorgestrel-releasing intrauterine contraceptive device in the treatment of idiopathic menorrhagia. Am J Obstet Gynecol 1991;164:879.

Noyes RW, Hertig AW, Rock J: Dating the endometrial biopsy. Fertil Steril 1950;1:3.

Nygren KG, Rybo G: Prostaglandings and menorrhagia. Acta Obstet Gynecol Scand Suppl 1983;113:101.

Schlechte J, Sherman B, Haluci M, et al: Prolactin-secreting pituitary tumors. Endocr Rev 1980;1:295.

Scott JC Jr, Mussey E: Menstrual patterns of myxedema. Am J Obstet Gynecol 1964;90:161.

Shaw RW, Fraser HM: Use of a superactive luteinizing hormone releasing hormone (LRH) agonist in the treatment of menorrhagia. Br J Obstet Gynaecol 1984;91:913.

Singh EJ, Baccarini IM, Zuspan FP: Levels of prostaglandin $F_{2\alpha}$ and E_2 in human endometrium during menstrual cycle. Am J Obstet Gynecol 1975;121:1003.

Speroff L, Glass RH, Kase NG: Regulation of the menstrual cycle. In Clinical Gynecologic Endocrinology and Infertility. 4th ed. Baltimore: Williams & Wilkins, 1989:91.

Treolar AE, Bounton RE, Benn BG, Brown BW: Variation of human menstrual cycle through reproductive life. Int J Fertil 1967; 12:77.

Wilborn WH, Flowers CE Jr: Cellular mechanisms for endometrial conservation during menstrual bleeding. Semin Reprod Endocrinol 1984;2:307.

25

Robert L. Reid | Amenorrhea

In relation to the amount of (menstrual) discharge every woman is a law unto herself. Habits of life are apt to modify it materially. Here, again, those inured to severe labour escape more easily than their sisters petted in the lap of luxury.

G. H. Napheys (1874)

The absence of menstruation at any time between the usual ages of puberty and menopause is often a source of apprehension and uncertainty for the affected woman. Timely and accurate diagnosis rests not only on a clear understanding of the physiologic mechanisms regulating normal menstrual cyclicity but also on an awareness of a variety of embryologic, genetic, and endocrinologic aberrations that can prevent or disrupt menstrual cyclicity. This chapter provides the necessary information to allow a systematic analysis of the cause of amenorrhea. Detailed history, careful physical examination, and selective use of simple diagnostic tests will generally result in accurate diagnosis. Appropriate management of amenorrhea must respond to the patient's desires and concerns while considering the impact of the underlying disorder and its sequelae on both reproductive and nonreproductive systems.

PHYSIOLOGY OF MENSTRUATION

Under normal circumstances the female offspring has, at the time of birth, all the vital components necessary to induce menstruation. The functional responsiveness of the uterovaginal system at this time is evidenced in clinical practice by the occasional finding of withdrawal bleeding in the first week of life subsequent to priming of the endometrium of the fetal uterus by estrogens derived from the fetal-placental unit. In rare instances of precocious puberty, premature hypothalamic release of gonadotropin-releasing hormone (GnRH) activates the entire hypothalamic-pituitary-ovarian-uterine axis in the first years of life. As a rule, however, undefined central restraining mechanisms prevent pulsatile release of GnRH from the arcuate nucleus of the hypothal-amus until 8 years of age or later. This central restraint of GnRH activity cannot simply be explained on the basis of exquisite sensitivity to negative feedback from the ovary because inhibition of gonadotropin release also occurs in individuals who lack functioning gonadal tissue (e.g., Turner's syndrome) (Conte et al, 1975). Early in the pubertal transition, the pulsatile release of GnRH is maximal at night, but this pattern of GnRH secretion shifts gradually to a pattern of continuous pulsatile secretion characteristic of the adult female (Yen, 1979).

Initially, following the earliest activation of gonadotropin release, folliculogenesis is associated with anovulation in a high percentage of cases (Aoring, 1967; Durschke et al, 1974). Unopposed estrogen at this time causes gradual but progressive uterine growth and endometrial proliferation. The earliest outward manifestations of this increased estradiol secretion include breast budding, physiologic leukorrhea, and accelerated linear growth. Ovarian and adrenal androgens, acting in concert, result in the development of axillary and pubic hair.

Positive feedback responses to ovarian estradiol resulting in luteinizing hormone (LH) and follicle-stimulating hormone (FSH) surges and ovulation indicate continuing maturation of the hypothalamic-pituitary-ovarian (HPO) axis. Initially these menstrual cycles are marked by subnormal progesterone production and abbreviated intermenstrual intervals, with a gradual shift to normal corpus luteum function and fertile cycles in the first and second years (Foster, 1977; Healy and Hodgen, 1983; Reid and Van Vugt, 1987a). One of the many functions of progesterone is to increase endometrial production of prostaglandins (Eidering et al, 1990). Withdrawal of progesterone is presumed to trigger release of stored prostaglandins, evoking vasoconstriction of the spiral arterioles that supply the endometrium. This results in a synchronized and time-limited menstrual bleed as the upper two thirds of the endometrial layer is shed. Only the lower portion of the basal layer is left intact, serving as a regenerative layer for the new endometrial proliferation in the subsequent cycle. The average volume of menstrual fluid is 50 ml. Typically intermenstrual intervals ranging from 24 to 35 days (particularly when associated with premenstrual molimina) are thought to be indicative of ovulatory function (Rosenfeld and Garcia, 1976;

541

542 / Textbook of Gynecology

Table 25-1. CURRENT AGES OF PUBERTAL STAGES IN FEMALES IN NORTH AMERICA

	MEAN ± 2 SD
Breast bud (Tanner B2)	10.9 (8.9–12.9)
Presexual pubic hair (Tanner PH2)	11.2 (9.0–13.4)
Sexual pubic hair (Tanner PH3)	11.9 (9.7–14.1)
Menarche	12.7 (10.8–14.6)

From Tanner JM, Davies PWS: Pubertal data for growth velocity charts [reply]. J Pediatr 1986;109:564, with permission.

Orrell et al, 1980). Longer intermenstrual intervals are often associated with periods of anovulation, although bleeds, when they do occur, are often preceded by a brief episode of corpus luteum activity (Sherman and Korenman, 1975).

There has been a gradual but progressive fall in the mean age of menarche over the past century, largely as a result of improved nutrition and living conditions, with the mean in North America presently standing at 12.3 years (range 9 to 17 years) (Bullough 1981). Typically, menarche occurs 2 to 5 years following the first signs of breast development (Tanner and Davies, 1986) (Table 25-1).

TERMINOLOGY

Amenorrhea is the absence of menstruation. If menstruation fails to occur by age 16, it is termed *primary amenorrhea*. If there is cessation of menstruation at some time after menarche, the term *secondary amenorrhea* is applied.

From a practical point of view, the significance of amenorrhea depends not only on its timing in relation to menarche but also upon its duration and antecedent events. For example, a delay of menstruation for 1 week in a woman with otherwise regular menstrual cycles may well indicate the existence of a pregnancy, whereas a delay of 1 further week in a woman with prolonged intermenstrual intervals may represent no more than a minor variation of an underlying disorder involving menstrual cyclicity. Similarly, amenorrhea following severe head trauma is likely to elicit more anxiety than amenorrhea occurring in conjunction with a physiologic process such as postpartum lactation.

Although the designation of primary and secondary amenorrhea may make certain diagnoses more likely, and exclude other diagnoses, failure to perform a systematic evaluation exploring possible aberrations affecting the hypothalamus, pituitary, ovary, uterus, and vagina may result in misdiagnosis and inappropriate treatment.

NORMAL GENITAL DEVELOPMENT

An appreciation of normal genital development is required to understand certain forms of amenorrhea.

Testicular differentiation requires the action of testicular determinant genes located near the centromere of the short arm of the Y chromosome. Although ovarian development begins in all embryos lacking this influence, completion of ovarian development occurs only in the presence of two intact X chromosomes.

Müllerian and wolffian development begins in all embryos. Two factors produced by the fetal testes influence subsequent development. The secretion of testosterone causes local (unilateral) wolffian development resulting in the formation of the epididymis, seminal vesical, and vas deferens. Müllerian inhibiting factor (MIF), also produced by the fetal testes, causes local inhibition of development of müllerian structures. Absence of the testes results in development of normal female internal genitalia. In some circumstances the fetal testes are unable to produce testosterone (i.e., because of a defect in androgen biosynthesis), or produce testosterone that has no effect on other tissues (i.e., as a result of defective androgen receptors). This would result in a testis that produces those effects attributable to MIF but none of the differentiation normally resulting from testosterone secretion. Such individuals would have neither müllerian nor wolffian development. At other times a dysgenetic testis fails to develop both its testosterone and MIF secretory capability, hence müllerian development proceeds with formation of uterus, tubes, and upper vagina but there is no wolffian development.

External genital development proceeds along female lines except in the presence of androgens. In the normal male fetus, human chorionic gonadotropin (hCG) stimulates testosterone secretion into the systemic circulation. Testosterone is subsequently converted peripherally by the enzyme 5 α-reductase into the more potent androgen dihydrotestosterone (DHT).

In the presence of functional androgen receptors, DHT is responsible for masculinization of external genitalia in the male. Absence of testosterone secretion from a dysgenetic male gonad, inadequate testosterone secretion resulting from an androgen biosynthetic defect, or abnormal production or binding of DHT could all result in the appearance of female external genitalia and apparent primary amenorrhea at puberty.

EVALUATION OF AMENORRHEA

The differentiation between primary and secondary amenorrhea is useful only in that it may direct one's thinking toward certain disorders that are more common in these circumstances. Nevertheless, there is sufficient overlap between both categories of amenorrhea to necessitate a clear understanding of appropriate diagnostic steps in the work-up of amenorrhea. The most common causes for primary and secondary amenorrhea are listed in Tables 25-2 and

Table 25–2. MOST COMMON CAUSES OF PRIMARY AMENORRHEA

Hypothalamic/Pituitary
Deficient GnRH secretion
    Constitutional
    Systemic illness
    Extreme physical, psychological, and/or nutritional
        stress
    Isolated gonadotropin deficiency
Disturbed HPO cyclicity
    Hyperestrogenic hyperandrogenic chronic anovulation
        ("polycystic ovary syndrome")
Ovarian
Hypergonadotropic amenorrhea resulting from gonadal
    dysgenesis
Uterine/Vaginal
Agenesis (Mayer-Rokitansky-Kuster-Hauser syndrome,
    androgen insensitivity)
Obstruction
    Imperforate hymen

25–3, respectively. Awareness of these conditions and familiarity with the historical and physical clues that point to the underlying etiology will lead to correct diagnosis of the amenorrhea in the majority of circumstances.

History

A detailed history of reproductive events leading up to the occurrence of amenorrhea is essential. A history of coital exposure, contraceptive usage, and symptoms of early pregnancy may be rewarding. In the case of primary amenorrhea, a detailed history about the nature and sequence of other pubertal events is of paramount importance. A span of time in excess of 5 years since onset of puberty is suggestive of a disturbance of normal HPO relationships or outflow tract obstruction.

Questions about general health and lifestyle will expose a history of any severe systemic illness or any

Table 25–3. MOST COMMON CAUSES OF SECONDARY AMENORRHEA

Pregnancy or Breast-Feeding
Hypothalamic/Pituitary
Deficient GnRH secretion
    Extremes of physical, psychological, and nutritional
        stress
    Systemic illness
Disturbed HPO cyclicity
    Hyperestrogenic hyperandrogenic chronic anovulation
        ("polycystic ovary syndrome")
Pituitary
Hyperprolactinemia
Ovary
Hypergonadotropic amenorrhea caused by premature
    ovarian failure
Uterine
Endometrial suppression by medication (i.e., lack of
    withdrawal bleeding in an oral contraceptive user)

pattern of excessive stress (i.e., physical, psychological, or nutritional) that could impinge on normal hypothalamic function. Symptoms suggestive of hypothalamic pathology might include subtle changes in sleep, thirst, appetite, temperature regulation, and smell; in extreme cases headaches, seizures, or vomiting may be present.

Disruption of the pituitary stalk might be suggested by a history of childhood abuse, head trauma, or delayed growth or by features of panhypopituitarism with galactorrhea (Klachko et al, 1968; Miller et al, 1980). Visual field defect, headache, vomiting, and behavioral changes in children are often the earliest manifestations of craniopharyngioma (Hoff and Patterson, 1972). The predominant manifestation of a pituitary prolactinoma at an early stage is lactation, whereas tumor extension may result in retro-orbital headache or bitemporal hemianopsia. Symptoms of hypothyroidism or recent use of certain medications (phenothiazines, narcotics, metoclopramide, cimetidine, etc.) would point to other situations associated with lactotroph hyperplasia.

A history of cessation of menstrual flow followed by hot flushes or vaginal dryness suggests loss of ovarian function, which could be explained by antecedent chemotherapy, surgery, or irradiation to the pelvis. Typical menopausal-like hot flushes have been documented during the luteal phase in women with premenstrual syndrome (Casper et al, 1986); hence this symptom should only be considered as suggestive of ovarian failure until gonadal function is assessed by an FSH determination.

A history of progressive hirsutism or virilization at puberty is rare and may point toward incomplete androgen insensitivity or congenital adrenal hyperplasia (CAH). Hirsutism onsetting at a later stage is more likely to indicate polycystic ovary syndrome (PCOS) if it is gradual in onset, or an adrenal or ovarian androgen-producing lesion if progression of hirsutism is rapid and associated with virilization.

Finally, absence of bleeding following appropriate development of secondary sexual characteristics suggests either late disruption of the HPO axis or an abnormality in the outflow tract. The presence of cyclic lower abdominal pain (cryptomenorrhea) and/or urinary symptoms suggesting exogenous pressure on the bladder (sometimes interpreted as frequent urinary tract infections) point toward obstruction of the outflow tract. The absence of such pelvic symptomatology would suggest possible congenital absence of the uterus.

A history of past and present use of medication may suggest suppression of endometrial development by exogenous medications (progestin-dominant contraceptive pills, depot medroxyprogesterone acetate, luteinizing hormone–releasing hormone [LHRH] agonists, danazol). Destruction of endometrium (Asherman's syndrome) or obstruction of the uterine outflow (cervical stenosis) might be suggested by a history of postabortal dilation and curettage or cervical trauma.

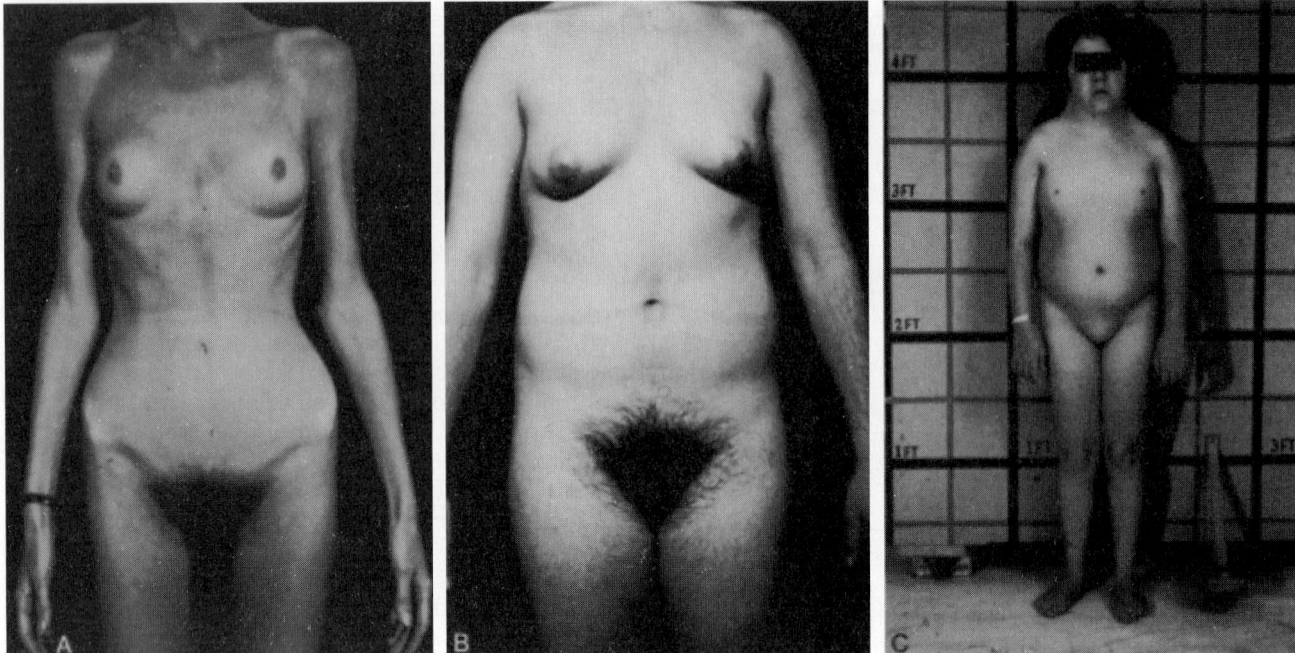

Figure 25–1
A, Typical body habitus of the undernourished individual with hypothalamic amenorrhea, *B*, Typical upper body segment obesity associated with hyperestrogenic hyperandrogenic chronic anovulation (HHCA). *C*, Typical stigmata of Turner's syndrome, including short stature, sexual infantilism, and webbed neck. Note left chest scar from surgical correction of aortic coarctation. (Photograph courtesy of R. Rebar.)

Physical Examination

A "head-to-toe" approach will ensure that the maximum amount of information is derived from physical examination.

Overall body habitus, height, weight, and arm span should be determined on the first visit. This may reveal very low body weight (decreased percentage of body fat) associated with hypothalamic amenorrhea (Fig. 25–1*A*), upper body segment obesity (a waist-to-hip girth ratio >0.85) often associated with insulin resistance and hyperandrogenism (Fig. 25–1B), or deficient linear growth suggesting an associated pituitary growth hormone deficiency or genetic cause for gonadal dysgenesis (i.e., Turner's syndrome [Fig. 25–1C]). Weight change may be of critical importance in the genesis and correction of amenorrhea and should be measured at each subsequent visit.

Stigmata of Turner's syndrome (short stature, sexual infantilism, webbing of the neck, a high-arched palate, widely spaced nipples, wide carrying angle, short fourth metacarpal) are readily apparent, although individuals with chromosomal mosaicism may show few of these features.

A rapid pulse may give a clue as to hyperthyroidism, whereas a slow pulse may be found in hypothyroidism or cases of chronic physical or nutritional stress. The eye signs of Graves' disease, such as exophthalmos, lid lag or retraction, and chemosis as well as soft moist skin, tremor, and hyperreflexia

should strengthen the impression of thyroid dysfunction and prompt appropriate blood tests to assess thyroid function. A sallow complexion of the skin with obvious orange discoloration of the palms (Fig. 25–2) (in the absence of scleral icterus) is suggestive of hypercarotinemia resulting from either excessive ingestion of low-calorie carotene-containing vegetables and fruits and/or decreased clearance of carotene. The latter may result either from hypothyroidism or functional hypothyroidism (production of biologically inactive reverse triiodothyronine) associated with starvation. In anorexia nervosa both in-

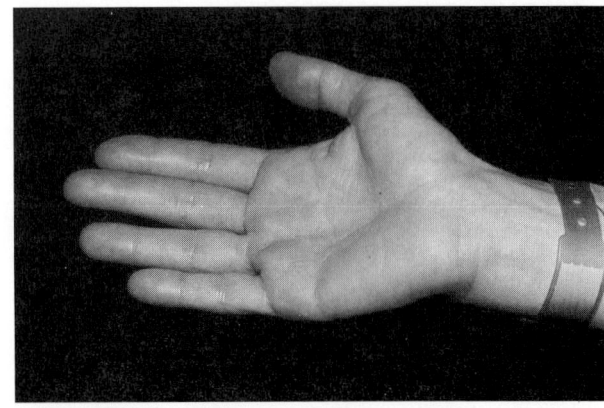

Figure 25–2
Hypercarotenemia causing orange discoloration of palm.

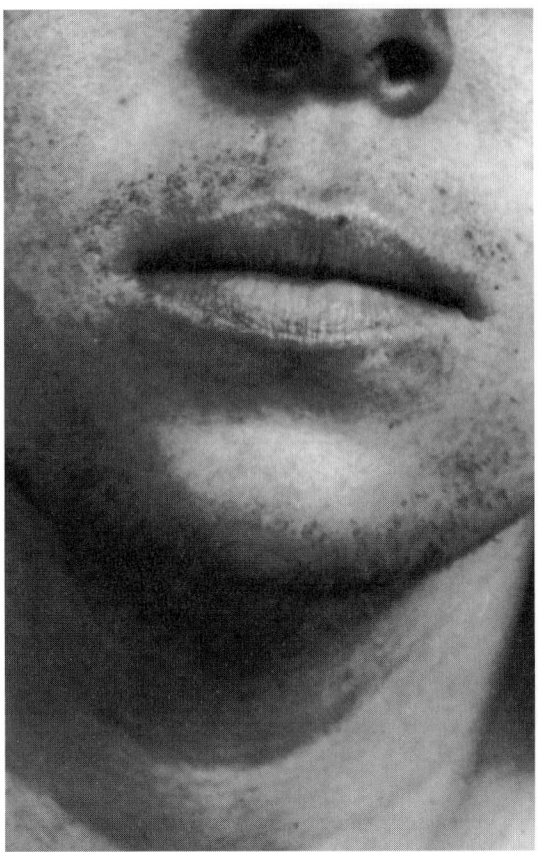

Figure 25–3
Facial hair may be overlooked in the fastidious patient. Here the patient was instructed not to shave for 48 hours to allow photographic documentation.

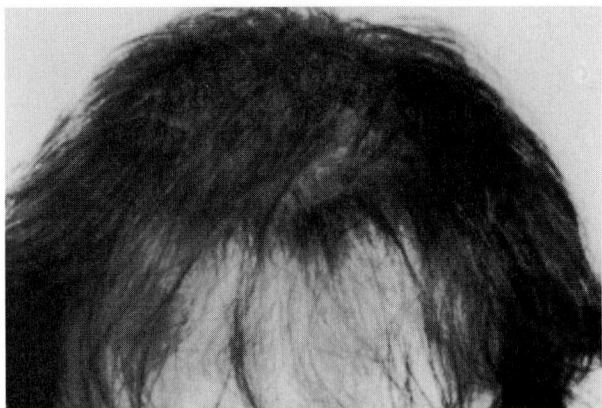

Figure 25–4
Typical frontotemporal thinning of hair with preservation of hairline in androgenetic alopecia.

creased ingestion and decreased clearance of carotene may occur.

The face should be carefully inspected for signs of hirsutism because the fastidious patient may be able to mask this sign by frequent shaving and application of makeup (Fig. 25–3). Diffuse thinning of hair in the frontotemporal region with preservation of the hairline is typical of androgenetic alopecia and is often, although not always, associated with hirsutism (Reid and Van Vugt, 1988) (Fig. 25–4). The distribution of hair on the low back, chest, abdomen, and legs should also be noted (Fig. 25–5). Evidence of marked hirsutism or virilization should raise suspicion about ovarian or adrenal neoplasm or of a severe degree of ovarian hyperthecosis associated with hyperestrogenic hyperandrogenic chronic anovulation. Rarely amenorrhea and hirsutism or virilization can result from inadvertent exposure to exogenous testosterone (Punch and Ansbacher, 1990). Hirsutism may be scored using the method of Ferriman and Gallwey (1961), in which areas of the body possessing androgen-sensitive pilosebaceous units are graded and summed. A total score of eight or more is seen in only 5% of premenopausal Caucasian women who, by definition, are said to be hirsute (Erhmann and Rosenfield, 1990).

Acanthosis nigricans is a velvety hyperpigmented skin change noted most often at the nape of the neck, in the axillae, beneath the breasts, and in the groin and upper inner thighs (Fig. 25–6). Acanthosis nigricans is usually a manifestation of severe insulin resistance and hyperandrogenism, although it can rarely signal an internal malignancy (usually adenocarcinoma of the stomach, pancreas, or colon [Barbieri et al, 1988]).

Thyroid examination may reveal a goiter (Fig. 25–7) or nodule suggesting an underlying etiology for the amenorrhea. Either hypo- or hyperthyroidism may be associated with amenorrhea (Thomas and Reid, 1987).

In addition to documenting Tanner stage of breast development, the nipples should be expressed to determine the presence or absence of galactorrhea (Fig. 25–8). Careful explanation of the rationale for this step and the presence of a female assistant during the examination should obviate potential patient concerns about sexual impropriety. Breast secretion may frequently appear clear when initially expressed and become whiter as the lipid content of secretion increases. Any secretion appearing at the nipples should be touched to a microscope slide and covered with a cover slip for subsequent examination by microscopy. Typical galactorrhea contains numerous black circles of lipid, whereas discharge from fibrocystic disease (which may be clear, brownish, or greenish) frequently shows a predominance of debris with rare fat droplets. Breast or chest wall lesions may trigger galactorrhea through a neuroendocrine reflex arc, and these should be sought (Kapcala and Lakshmanan, 1989).

Cardiac examination will rarely reveal congenital heart disease as the explanation for growth delay, or coarctation of the aorta in individuals with Turner's syndrome. Lower blood pressure in the left upper extremity, in comparison to the right, would provide additional support for the diagnosis of aortic coarctation.

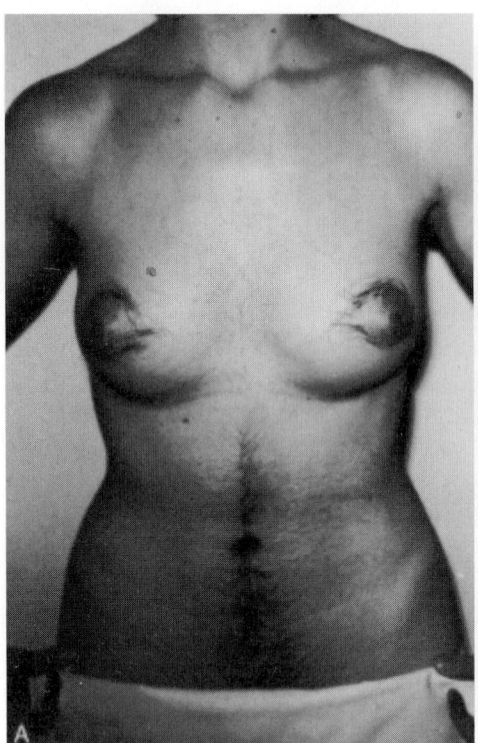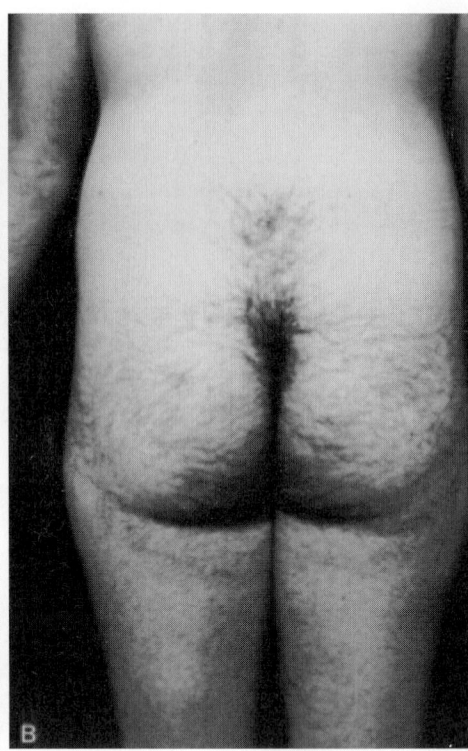

Figure 25–5
A, Abnormal hair growth on breasts, chest, and abdomen. *B*, Abnormal hair growth on back and buttocks.

Palpable adrenal masses are extremely rare but should be sought in the face of marked hirsutism. The presence of abdominal stria would point to Cushing's syndrome. A mass in the lower abdomen in association with amenorrhea most often is secondary to pregnancy but could represent hematocolpos, hematometra, or an ovarian neoplasm.

Pelvic examination forms an integral part of the evaluation of every patient with amenorrhea. In the adolescent who may never have had a pelvic examination before, the use of the educational approach (where the patient in a sitting position observes the examination in a hand mirror) usually allows visualization of the vagina and cervix (Fig. 25–9). After a brief explanation of the anatomy of the external genitalia using a lubricated cotton-tipped swab as a pointer, a decision is made as to whether or not vaginal speculum examination will be feasible based on the prior degree of maturation (estrogenization) of the vagina and the size of the hymenal ring. In those patients with no evidence of secondary sexual development, attempts to examine the genital tract even with a very small Pederson speculum are generally unrewarding. In the individual with prior estrogenization of the vagina, the use of an appropriate-sized speculum will usually allow visualization of the upper vagina and cervix without discomfort to the patient. A lubricated finger should

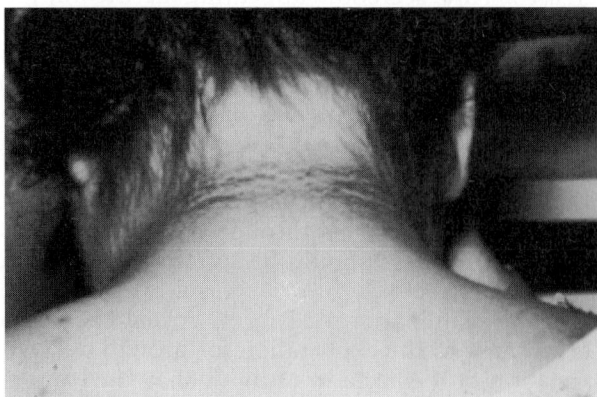

Figure 25–6
Acanthosis nigricans in a patient with obesity, insulin resistance, and hyperandrogenism.

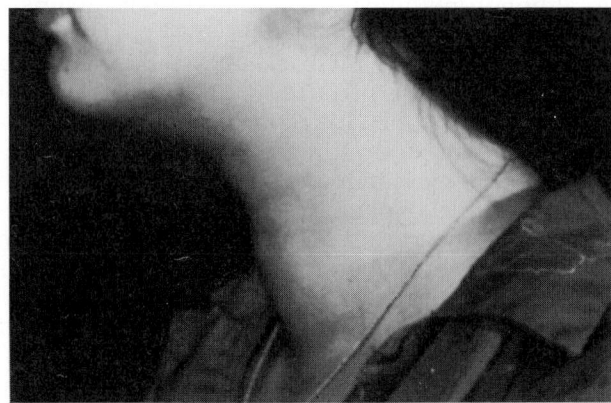

Figure 25–7
Diffuse thyroid enlargement in a hyperthyroid 19-year-old presenting with secondary amenorrhea.

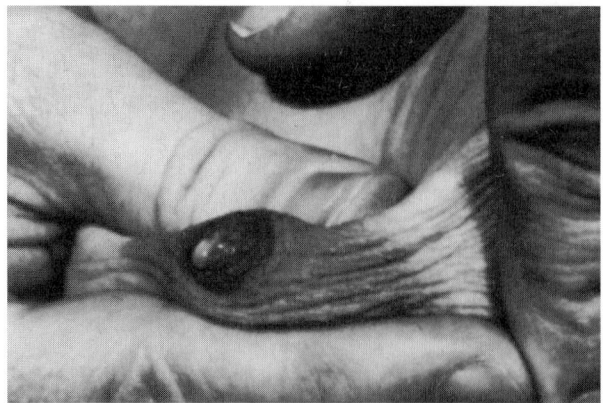

Figure 25–8
Expression of the nipple in an amenorrheic woman reveals a droplet of partially clear, partially milky fluid that can be examined microscopically for lipid droplets.

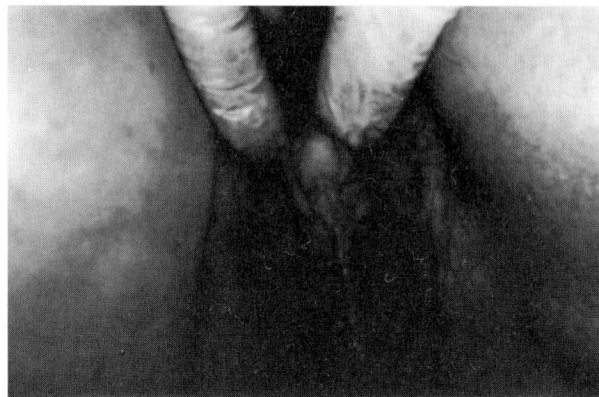

Figure 25–10
Mild clitoral hypertrophy associated with hyperandrogenism in HHCA.

always be gently inserted through the hymenal ring first to ensure adequate capacity. Initial instruction to the adolescent about how to contract and relax her vaginal sphincter muscles on the examining finger (by tightening the muscles she would use to stop urinating) better enables her to maintain the muscles in a relaxed state during the subsequent speculum examination.

Clitoral hypertrophy may be an early manifestation of virilization (Fig. 25–10). The presence of vagina and cervix rules out congenital absence of the

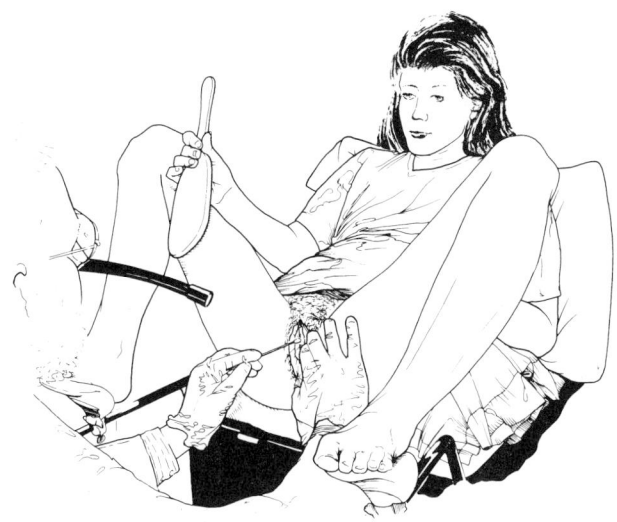

Figure 25–9
The educational pelvic examination allows a better understanding of genital anatomy and provides reassurance to the apprehensive patient. With the head and shoulders elevated, the patient uses a hand mirror to follow the perineal examination. By reflecting a flashlight beam off the hand mirror, the patient is usually able to follow the speculum examination and to visualize the vagina and cervix. (From Daicar AO: The role of the educational pelvic exam. J Soc Obstet Gynecol [Can] 1991;13:31, with permission.)

uterus and most obstructive causes of amenorrhea. The presence of cervical mucus may give further clues as to etiology. Copious watery cervical mucus is associated with the high estrogen state preceding natural ovulation or may reflect the sustained exposure to moderate estrogen levels in PCOS. The presence of tenacious cervical mucus would be more consistent with a diagnosis of recent ovulation or pregnancy. Bimanual examination may confirm enlargement of the uterus consistent with pregnancy or mild ovarian enlargement, as often seen in PCOS.

Obstruction of the vagina with a bulging, bluish membrane should suggest an imperforate hymen, whereas a thicker obstructing lesion may represent a transverse vaginal septum, the blind-ending vaginal pouch associated with androgen insensitivity or with uterovaginal agenesis (Mayer-Rokitansky-Kuster-Hauser syndrome). Rectal examination may reveal a boggy, distended hematocolpos above the site of obstruction. The depth of the vaginal canal should be determined because the adequacy of the vaginal remnant for coital function will be a consideration in individuals with androgen insensitivity or uterovaginal agenesis.

Diagnostic Investigations

In the majority of cases laboratory and other diagnostic investigations will be merely confirmatory because the diagnosis will have been established with a degree of certainty employing history and physical examination. If early pregnancy is remotely possible, this should first be ruled out with a sensitive urinary pregnancy test.

When a hypothalamic cause is suspected in the absence of obvious severe systemic disease or excessive physical, psychological, or nutritional stress, then additional neurologic evaluation is warranted to rule out tumor or infiltrative lesions. This will most often be accomplished by the use of computerized tomography (CT) scan or magnetic resonance imaging (MRI). At a minimum, patients with amenorrhea should have determinations of FSH, prolactin, and thyroid function (sensitive thyroid-stimulating hormone [TSH] and free thyroxine) (Laufer et al, 1995). Low levels of FSH and prolactin would be consistent with stress-related hypothalamic suppression, whereas an elevation of prolactin might suggest hypothalamic pathology, pituitary stalk transecction, a craniopharyngioma, or pituitary prolactinoma.

In the face of historical features or laboratory signs suggesting pituitary stalk transection, additional dynamic testing of pituitary function would be in order. Hyperprolactinemia sufficient to lead to amenorrhea in the absence of primary hypothyroidism or known use of prolactin-releasing illicit drugs or medications should elicit a search for hypothalamic or pituitary lesions employing CT scan or MRI (Blackwell, 1985).

Ovarian causes for amenorrhea will be evident with the finding of high LH and FSH levels consistent with ovarian failure. Hypergonadotropic amenorrhea should be further investigated by obtaining a karyotype in any individual under age 30. The presence of a Y chromosome would necessitate gonadectomy to avoid the risk of gonadal tumors, whereas a normal XX karyotype may indicate the need to search for coexistent autoimmune disease or endocrinopathy. Specific tests in this circumstance are outlined later.

Outflow tract obstruction will have been excluded in most circumstances by pelvic examination. With a history of recent dilation and curretage or cervical trauma, an attempt to pass a uterine sound is warranted to rule out obstructing intrauterine synechiae or cervical stenosis. A hysterosalpingogram may give more precise information about the extent of intrauterine synechiae if these are suspected (Fig. 25–11). In the event that a vaginal obstruction or anomaly is identified on physical examination, further evaluation employing pelvic ultrasound scan, vaginoscopy, hysteroscopy, laparoscopy, or MRI may be warranted. Rare cases of unilateral outflow tract obstruction may have pelvic pain and not amenorrhea as the primary presenting complaint (Goldstein et al, 1980).

Progestin Withdrawal Test

The administration of progestin has been advocated as an initial diagnostic step in the work-up of the patient with amenorrhea. Failure to have withdrawal bleeding following a course of oral progestin, such as medroxyprogesterone acetate (5 mg) or micronized progesterone (200 mg) for 7 days, would occur if prior estrogen exposure had been insufficient to cause endometrial development, if there was outflow tract agenesis or obstruction, or if the patient was pregnant. Occasionally withdrawal bleeding will not follow a 7-day course of progestin because treatment was coincidentally started in the early luteal phase.

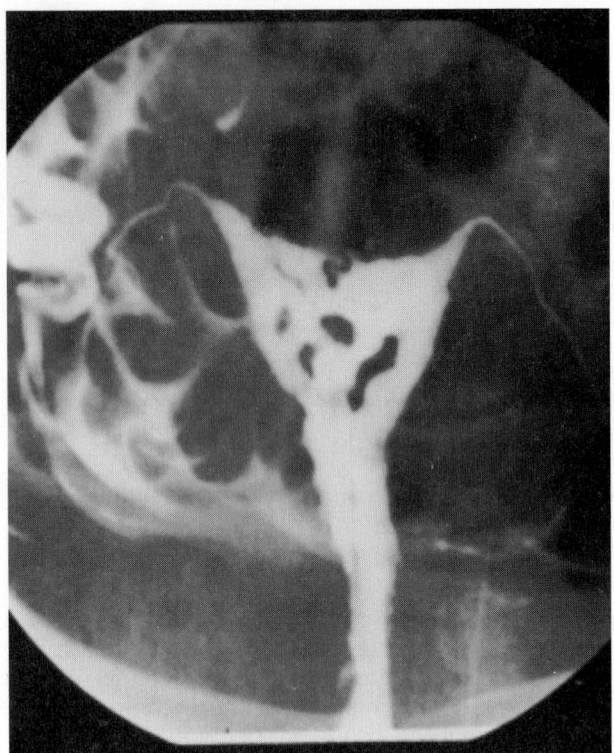

Figure 25–11
Intrauterine synechiae following postabortal dilatation and curettage as seen on hysterosalpingogram. In this case amenorrhea was not present because there was neither obliteration of the endometrial cavity nor synechiae blocking the outflow tract.

The patient's own continuing secretion of progesterone for the 14-day duration of the luteal phase would be expected to result in a delay of menstrual bleeding for up to a week following cessation of the exogenous progestin.

The routine use of the progestin withdrawal test in the evaluation of amenorrhea must be called into question. The use of exogenous progestin is no longer recommended in any circumstance where pregnancy is a possibility. If this possibility exists, a sensitive urinary pregnancy test provides rapid confirmation. The presence or absence of withdrawal bleeding after progestin has been shown to correlate poorly with serum estradiol levels (Rarick et al, 1990; Nakamura et al, 1996). This latter finding is hardly surprising because endometrial shedding following progestin is more likely to depend upon antecedent estrogen exposure than upon the present serum estradiol level. In most circumstances the diagnosis of outflow tract agenesis or obstruction should be possible through pelvic examination. Where pelvic examination is difficult, the progestin challenge test may be useful, either alone or following a short course of estrogen (Premarin 1.25 mg daily for 21 days) in order to establish that a patent and functioning uterus and vagina are present. The accuracy and simplicity of ultrasound examination, however, has largely obviated the need for this hormonal manipulation to evaluate the functional integrity of the outflow tract.

The progestin challenge test is still widely employed to gauge the estrogen status of the amenorrheic patient prior to institution of therapy. In the patient with hypothalamic amenorrhea, failure to bleed following progestin suggests that endogenous estrogen exposure is so low that an ovulatory response to the antiestrogen clomiphene citrate should not be anticipated. Withdrawal bleeding following progestin generally augurs for a favorable response to clomiphene in the infertility patient and points to the need for regularly induced endometrial shedding to avoid endometrial hyperplasia in the patient without the desire for fertility. In the patient not desiring fertility, failure to have withdrawal bleeding following progestin suggests the need for estrogen replacement to avoid sequelae of chronic hypoestrogenism (Johnston and Longcope, 1990).

Endometrial Biopsy

Although administration of exogenous progestin after a prolonged period of amenorrhea is widely believed to reduce the risk of endometrial hyperplasia by restoring the endometrium to a basal state, there has been no convincing documentation that a single withdrawal bleed will eliminate endometrial hyperplasia or exclude the possibility of coexisting endometrial carcinoma (Fig. 25–12). Where the period of amenorrhea has been prolonged in a patient with either obesity or a family history of early uterine cancer, office endometrial sampling is prudent.

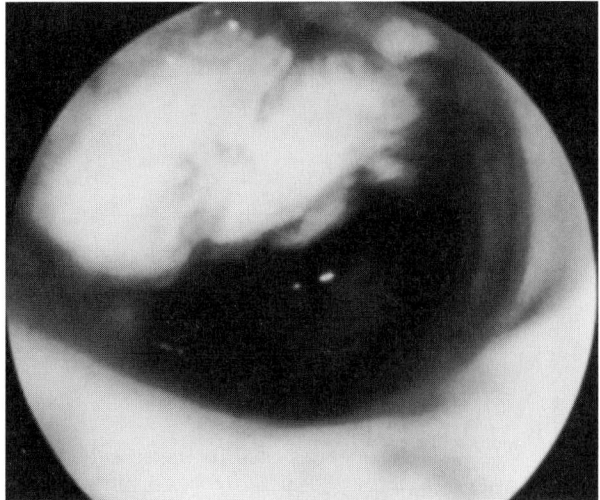

Figure 25–12
Hysteroscopic view of an endometrial cancer in an obese amenorrheic 40-year-old.

ETIOLOGIC CAUSES, SIGNIFICANCE, AND THERAPY

Hypothalamic Causes

Constitutional Delay of Puberty

In North America approximately 3% of children are delayed in developing secondary sexual characteristics (Rosenfield, 1990). The vast majority of these children will prove to have no pathology and are said to have constitutional delay in growth and development. In these circumstances the prognosis for normal stature and secondary sexual development is excellent and menarche will onset spontaneously at a later than normal stage. Typically in this disorder

1. The onset of puberty is retarded to the same extent as bone age and will begin when bone age approximates 11 years in females.
2. Prepubertal growth slows as puberty is delayed.
3. Pubertal development is not delayed past 16 years of age in females.

The condition is difficult to distinguish from isolated gonadotropin deficiency. Once puberty begins, pubertal progression and linear growth advance at normal rates. There is no underlying disorder.

It should be evident that only the eventual normal progression of puberty can definitively rule out causes other than hypogonadotropic hypogonadism. Although "watchful waiting" may appear to be the best approach to cases of apparent constitutional delay of puberty, a short course of exogenous sex hormone therapy may do much to improve self-image. For patients in whom short stature is of primary concern, a 6-month course of anabolic steroid therapy (oxandrolone 0.1 mg/kg daily) may enhance growth (Rosenfield, 1990). Subsequently, secondary sexual development is induced with a 6-month course of low-dose estrogen therapy. It is important to restrict hormone therapy in this circumstance to a 6-month course and to re-evaluate linear growth, pubertal development, bone age, and sex hormone status. A second such treatment course may be helpful if there is extreme delay. It is unusual for a child with constitutional delay of puberty to require a third course of treatment except in cases of true hypogonadotropism (Rosenfield, 1990).

Congenital GnRH Deficiency

In its most severe expression congenital deficiency of GnRH may be complete, in which case there is complete failure of development of secondary sexual characteristics. This severe variant occurs most often in association with anosmia (Kallman's syndrome [Kallman et al, 1944]) and midline craniofacial defects (Jones and Kemmann, 1976; Lieblich et al, 1982). Several different modes of inheritance of these disorders have been described, suggesting pathophysiologic heterogeneity (Ewer, 1968; Santen and Paulson, 1973; Santoro et al, 1986). At times, the GnRH deficiency may be partial or the patient may have received exogenous sex steroids, resulting in varying degrees of secondary sexual development and making the diagnosis more difficult.

Surprisingly, those individuals with anosmia may not be fully aware that their sense of smell is abnormal. Serial dilutions of a potent organic solvent such as pyridine can be used to formally determine the threshold for the sense of smell. The patient is asked to discriminate between two vials, one of which contains distilled water and the other containing the most dilute solution of pyridine. Typically individuals with Kallman's syndrome will be able to inhale 1-molar pyridine without smelling it (although they sometimes get a taste in the back of their throat). This concentration is normally enough to gag observers who are standing in the same room. Practically speaking, smell testing can be readily accomplished by asking the patient to differentiate between the smell of perfume or coffee in the clinic setting. In many circumstances, this isolated deficiency of gonadotropins, termed *isolated gonadotropin deficiency*, is not associated with anosmia or congenital facial anomaly. The diagnosis then is one of exclusion.

The initial step in evaluation is to rule out gonadal dysgenesis as an explanation for pubertal delay by confirming that concentrations of LH and FSH are low. Other causes for suppressed gonadotropins must be excluded (i.e., hyperprolactinemia; extreme physical, psychological, or nutritional stresses; central nervous system [CNS] infiltrate or tumor; pituitary stalk transection). A detailed history and selective use of ancillary tests such as the lateral skull film, CT scan, or MRI are necessary if symptoms suggest pathology. The lateral skull film will demonstrate erosion of the sella turcica or calcification in or above the sella in the majority of those patients with craniopharyngiomas (Hoff and Patterson, 1972). Its usefulness in the evaluation of prolactinomas is limited to the diagnosis of macroadenomas producing degrees of sellar disruption.

GnRH testing has been used to help establish the diagnosis in cases of delayed puberty. However, the overlap between prepubertal, hypogonadotropic, and early pubertal response is so great as to seriously limit the utility of this test (Rosenfield, 1990). Failure of development of secondary sexual characteristics by the age of 13 is an indication for intervention in such circumstances, primarily to keep the adolescent "in step" with her peers. Delayed puberty in this circumstance is seldom associated with growth delay. Most individuals with isolated gonadotropin deficiency are tall and somewhat eunuchoid in appearance at the time of presentation. Accordingly, hormone replacement therapy with estrogen only (mimicking normal puberty) in the initial 6 to 9 months of therapy, followed by therapy with cyclic estrogen and progestin for a further year before switching to a more convenient contraceptive preparation, is appropriate. Continuing follow-up is required to rule out the late development of any CNS lesion that may have been overlooked at the time of initial evaluation. Fertility can be achieved at a later date with the use of pulsatile GnRH administered either intravenously or subcutaneously by a portable pump (Fig. 25–13) (Carr and Reid, 1990; Martin et al, 1990). As with all sexually active teenagers, the use of barrier contraceptives for protection from sexually transmitted diseases should be advised in addition to the oral contraceptive.

Hypothalamic Amenorrhea

A variety of stresses (physical, psychological, or nutritional) alone or in combination may have an impact upon hypothalamic release of GnRH (Fig. 25–14) (Reid and Van Vugt, 1987b; Yamamora and Reid, 1990). Yen (1988) has postulated that the ensuing amenorrhea and reproductive quiescence evolve as an expression of endogenous hypothalamic contra-

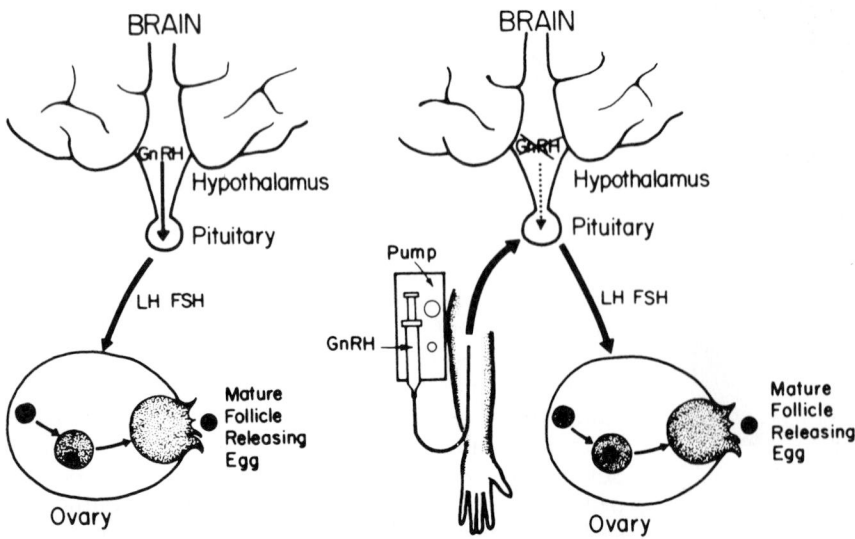

Figure 25–13
Exogenous GnRH delivered either IV or SC at 90- or 120-minute intervals will mimic endogenous hypothalamic GnRH release, triggering ovulation in 10 to 16 days in individuals with congenital or acquired deficiency of GnRH.

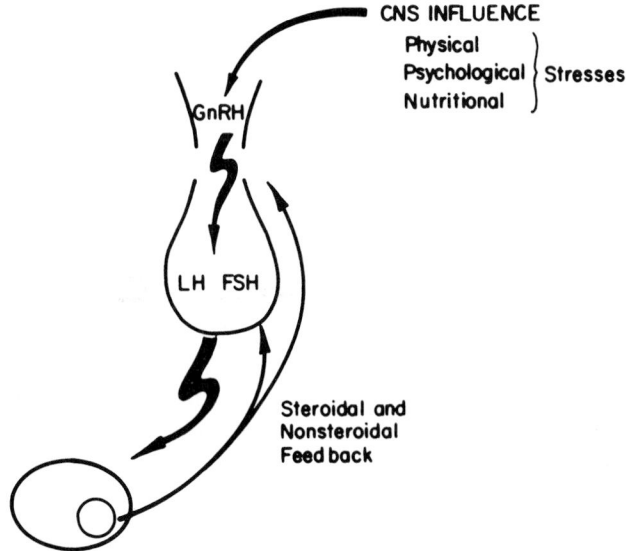

Figure 25–14
Physical, psychological, and nutritional stresses, either alone or in combination, can disrupt endogenous GnRH release. (From Reid RL, Van Vugt DA: Neuroendocrine events that regulate the menstrual cycle. Contemp Obstet Gynecol 1987;30:147, with permission.)

ception in the presence of an unfavorable environment. Although each of these components—diet, exercise, and psychological stress—may function independently, it is common for one or more of these stresses to coexist (Reid and Van Vugt, 1987b; Berga and Girton, 1989; Girton, 1989).

Widespread promotion of health and fitness has led to participation in sporting activities by unprecedented numbers of women at all competitive levels. The aspirations of parents and coaches for these young women to excel has often resulted in vigorous training programs that begin at an early age and persist throughout adolescence (Smith, 1980; Calabrese et al, 1983; Garner, 1984; Speroff, 1984). Young athletes are quick to learn about the advantages of a healthy minimum level of fatness in athletic performance and often go to great lengths to reduce body fat. This aversion to fatness is not unique to athletes: our entire society has become preoccupied with the concept that thinness and success go hand-in-hand. Weight is a function of genetics, diet, and exercise (Wilmore, 1983). Therefore, the two primary means used to achieve weight lower than that which is genetically determined are through alteration in diet or an increase in energy expenditure. Often both of these approaches are involved in the genesis of hypothalamic amenorrhea. A variety of distorted dietary patterns have been identified in both athletes and nonathletes with disturbed menstrual function (Barr, 1987; Brownell et al, 1987; Pirke et al, 1986; Highet, 1989; Nattiv et al, 1994). These range from vegetarian diets with an increased intake of fiber and decreased intake of saturated fats to eating disorders such as anorexia nervosa and bulimia (Anonymous, 1982; Mausfield and Evans, 1989; Snow et al, 1990).

It is known that most North American women, at the completion of growth around the age of 16 to 18, have 26% to 28% of their body weight as fat (Frisch and Schiff, 1986). Because this percentage of body fat is marginally above that necessary to maintain menstrual cyclicity, it is little wonder that women who diet as well as certain athletes in whom weight may fall by 10% to 15% (equating to loss of 30% of body fat) may become amenorrheic. Some, but not all, studies have found an association between the number of miles run per week and the incidence of amenorrhea (Speroff and Redwine, 1980; Sanborn et al, 1982; Shangold and Levine, 1982). The reason for discrepancies in these studies may have to do with pretraining menstrual patterns (Abraham et al, 1982; Shangold and Levine, 1982). It appears that athletes may have a higher incidence of menstrual disturbance even before they take up their athletic lifestyle. The prevalence of menstrual dysfunction in athletic women may vary with the level of athletic competition and the concomitant psychological stress. For example, as many as half of the women training for, or competing in, the Olympic Games are reported to have amenorrhea (Webb et al, 1979; Pirke et al, 1986). Oligomenorrhea was reported by 20% to 30% of long-distance runners, whereas recreational joggers have a much lower incidence of menstrual irregularity (Dale et al, 1979; Speroff and Redwine, 1980; Shangold and Levine, 1982; Garner, 1984).

The fact that variables other than weight loss may be important contributors to the ultimate determination of menstrual status is exemplified by observations of several investigators. Warren (1980) and Abraham et al (1982) found that amenorrheic ballet dancers would often reach menarche or, in the case of secondary amenorrhea, resume menstrual function without any change in weight during intervals of forced rest due to injury. They suggested that energy drain associated with intensive training might have an important modulatory effect on hypothalamic function. Amenorrhea is more likely to result when energy-demanding sports such as running are taken up by nulliparous women and those under the age of 25 (Speroff, 1984). In addition, training prior to menarche is more likely to lead to menstrual disruption than the initiation of training after menstrual function is established. Similarly, more prolonged stress occasioned by such events as separation from loved ones, incarceration, or leaving home to work or attend school, to enter religious life, or to join a military academy is reported to lead to a high incidence of amenorrhea (Drew 1961; Drew and Stifel, 1968; Anderson, 1979). That psychological stress is involved is emphasized by the observation that menses eventually resume in incarcerated women despite continued limitations on nutritional intake and in women in a military academy despite continuing physical demands (Yamamora and Reid, 1990).

In hypothalamic amenorrhea, body fat may be normal or reduced. In those women with physical or nutritional stress, obvious thinness is common together with bradycardia in an otherwise healthy individual.

Endocrine findings in hypothalamic amenorrhea include prepubertal levels of LH and FSH, low levels of estradiol, and a reduction in plasma prolactin together with loss of the nocturnal prolactin rise (Berga et al, 1989). Hypercortisolism has been demonstrated in both athletic and nonathletic women with hypothalamic amenorrhea (Loucks et al, 1989; Biller et al, 1990). Studies employing sensitive assays indicate continuing frequent low-amplitude LH pulses that are probably the result of spontaneous pituitary gonadotropin release in the absence of hypothalamic GnRH stimulation (Genazzani et al, 1990). Chronic hypoestrogenism associated with these conditions has been implicated in premature osteoporosis (Emans et al, 1990). The athletic "triad" that has become well recognized includes disordered eating, amenorrhea, and osteoporosis (Nattiv et al, 1994). Even weight-bearing exercise does not protect against osteoporosis in athletes with amenorrhea (Rockwell et al, 1990; Rencken et al, 1996).

Therapy for the individual with hypothalamic amenorrhea involves detailed counseling about the importance of lifestyle modification for the resolution of symptoms. Although patients may be admonished to gain weight, many of them are set in certain patterns of exercise and diet that they find difficult to adjust (Reid and Van Vugt, 1987b). It would be inappropriate to attempt to achieve fertility in a circumstance where the patient's nutritional status was compromised because this may ultimately have adverse effects on any offspring (Stewart et al, 1990). Many times, however, despite correction of the lifestyle stresses, ovulatory function does not return (Reid and Van Vugt, 1987b; Szmukler, 1989). Initial attempts may be made to induce ovulation employing low doses of clomiphene citrate. Theoretically, however, in the face of low endogenous estrogen production this antiestrogen therapy is not likely to be successful. The administration of GnRH using small portable pumps is a more logical and effective method for achieving ovulation and pregnancy in these patients (Carr and Reid, 1990; Martin et al, 1990). In patients who have apparent spontaneous resumption of ovulatory status, adequate corpus luteum function must be confirmed. Despite normal intermenstrual intervals, luteal-phase defects remain a significant problem in the mildly underweight and athletic woman (Prior, 1985).

The hypoestrogenism associated with hypothalamic amenorrhea may seriously impede the attainment of optimal peak bone mass during the years when calcium deposition in bone should be greatest (Ott, 1990). In the face of continuing amenorrhea, estrogen replacement and adequate calcium intake should be advised. Practically speaking, this is most easily accomplished with an oral contraceptive if inadvertent pregnancy is to be avoided or with standard forms of menopausal replacement therapy if contraception is not required (Reid and Van Vugt, 1987b). Even if ovulatory function is restored, subtle defects in corpus luteum function may be a continuing factor in bone loss (Prior et al, 1990).

Anorexia Nervosa and Bulimia Nervosa

A severe variant of hypothalamic amenorrhea is found in individuals with anorexia nervosa. Some patients may exhibit both anorexia nervosa and bulimia concurrently, while many with current bulimia nervosa (up to 50%) have a past history of anorexia nervosa (Szmukler, 1989). Specific diagnostic criteria for these two disorders are listed in Table 25–4. Garfinkle et al (1996) have questioned the need for amenorrhea as a diagnostic feature for anorexia nervosa because this feature failed to discriminate between women with anorexia nervosa and women with all features except amenorrhea across a large number of relevant variables. It is clear that psycho-

Table 25–4. CRITERIA FOR DIAGNOSIS OF ANOREXIA NERVOSA AND BULIMIA NERVOSA

ANOREXIA NERVOSA
A. Refusal to maintain over a minimal normal weight for age and height (usually 15% or more below that expected).
B. Intense fear of gaining weight or becoming fat, even though underweight.
C. Disturbance in the way in which one's body weight, size, or shape is experienced, e.g., the person claims to "feel fat" even when emaciated.
D. In females, absence of at least three consecutive menstrual cycles when otherwise expected to occur (primary or secondary amenorrhea).

BULIMIA NERVOSA
A. Recurrent episodes of binge eating (rapid consumption of a large amount of food in a discrete period of time).
B. A feeling of lack of control over eating behavior during the eating binges.
C. The person regularly engages in either self-induced vomiting, use of laxatives or diuretics, strict dieting or fasting, or vigorous exercise in order to prevent weight gain.
D. A minimum average of two binge eating episodes a week for at least three months.
E. Persistent overconcern with body shape and weight.

From Diagnostic and Statistical Manual of Mental Disorders. 4th ed. Washington, DC: American Psychiatric Association. Copyright 1994, with permission.

logical stress is often closely interrelated to the development of these disorders, because the disruption to menstrual cyclicity may occur shortly after initial weight loss or may even precede weight loss (Weiner, 1989; Yamamora and Reid, 1990).

Initial assessment of this condition must take heed of both the physical and psychological status of the patient and include a detailed account of the weight history and diet-related behaviors. Evidence of deliberate weight loss through food disposal, subterfuge, self-induced vomiting, laxative abuse, and excessive exercise together with a disordered body image, denial of thinness, and satisfaction or lack of concern at weight loss serves to differentiate this condition from other types of systemic disease resulting in wasting (Szmukler, 1989). Physical examination reveals a minimum of body fat, dry skin with lanugo hair, hypothermia, bradycardia, hypotension, cold extremities, orange discoloration of the skin associated with hypercarotenemia, and no evidence of other disease. In rare instances where laparoscopy has been indicated in such individuals for reasons other than amenorrhea, orange carotene staining of the ovaries has been noted—the so-called golden ovary syndrome.

The diagnosis of bulimia nervosa relies on the patient admitting her symptoms, which many times she is too embarrassed to do. A clue to diagnosis may come from the observation of ulcers or calluses on the skin on the dorsum of the fingers and hand resulting from regularly pushing fingers down the throat to induce vomiting. Painless enlargement of the parotid glands may also be noted, and laboratory investigation will often reveal hypokalemic alkalosis caused by repeated vomiting.

Longitudinal studies of the response to GnRH in anorexic patients during recovery have shown a shift from prepubertal gonadotropin responses to those responses typical of the mature woman (Binsbergen et al, 1990), hence this test may be useful to assess the stage of disease and predict outcome. Treatment of the patient with anorexia nervosa is best accomplished by someone experienced in techniques of behavior modification (Szmukler, 1989). Follow-up studies indicate that 50% to 75% of patients will show a favorable response to treatment in terms of weight recovery and resumption of cyclic menstruation. Psychiatric status and social adjustment remained impaired in many of these patients, with the worst prognosis for those with a long duration of illness, older age at onset, and greatest degree of pretreatment weight loss (Reid and Van Vugt, 1987b).

"Post-Pill" Amenorrhea

A number of authors have suggested that there may be a specific syndrome of secondary amenorrhea affecting some women following discontinuation of oral contraceptive (Sherman, 1966; Halbert and Christian, 1969; Larsson-Cohn, 1969). More recent publications have taken into account the fact that the incidence of secondary amenorrhea following discontinuation of the oral contraceptive is no greater than the incidence of secondary amenorrhea occurring spontaneously in the population at large (Pettersson et al, 1973). It is hardly surprising that some women, for example, lose weight while on the oral contraceptive. The development of hypothalamic amenorrhea in this circumstance would be masked by the regular withdrawal bleeding occurring while the individual continues to take the oral contraceptive but would become apparent in the months following discontinuation of oral contraceptive steroids. In one report, hypothalamic amenorrhea accounted for the so-called post-pill amenorrhea in 50% of patients evaluated (Reindollar et al, 1986). It is important, also, to recognize that a substantial percentage of women are put onto oral contraceptives because of menstrual irregularity and/or amenorrhea. In such circumstances it would not be inconsistent for the abnormal menstrual cyclicity to recur following cessation of oral contraceptives. When these factors are taken into account, no statistical correlation can be identified between the use of oral contraceptives and the subsequent occurrence of amenorrhea (Huggins and Cullins, 1990). Patients presenting with amenorrhea following use of oral contraceptives should be evaluated as any other individual with secondary amenorrhea.

Polycystic Ovarian Syndrome

Polycystic ovary syndrome—the combination of amenorrhea, obesity, and hirsutism—was first described by Stein and Leventhal in 1935. The problems in establishing a simple definition of PCOS have been identified in an excellent review by Barbieri et al (1988). Goldzier and Green (1962) documented that, among women with surgically proved PCOS, 20% had no menstrual irregularity, 59% were not obese, and 31% were not hirsute. Using histopathologic examination of ovarian tissue as the gold standard is also problematic in that ovarian tissue is available in the minority of cases and even then the supposed characteristic findings of polycystic ovaries—ovarian enlargement, a thickened ovarian capsule, absence of corpora lutea, increased number of atretic antral follicles, and stromal hyperthecosis—are not uniformly present.

The only consistent laboratory abnormalities in patients with PCOS are hyperandrogenism and insulin resistance. Insulin resistance, which is present in both lean and obese patients with PCOS, is exaggerated by obesity and is significantly higher in obese women with PCOS than in obese controls (Morales et al, 1996). The other clinical feature typical of this condition is the sustained moderate production of estrogen (from peripheral conversion of androgens to estrogen). The etiology of this syndrome remains unknown. Acronymic designations, such as Stein-Leventhal syndrome or PCOS, should be replaced by terminology that reflects the underlying biochemical abnormalities. (A simple mnemonic utilizes the vowels, *a*, *e*, *i*, *o*, and *u*: *a*ndrogen, *e*strogen, and *i*nsulin *o*versecretion of *u*nknown etiology.)

Classification of this condition as a hypothalamic cause for amenorrhea is, no doubt, an oversimplification because there is evidence pointing to abnormalities not only of the hypothalamic-pituitary unit but also involving the ovary, the periphery (including liver and skin), the adrenal gland, and the pancreas. Evidence pointing to involvement of the differing systems in the genesis of PCOS is briefly reviewed below; the reader is referred to several excellent reviews (Barbieri et al, 1988; Hutchison-Williams and Decherney, 1987; Barnes and Rosenfield, 1989; Morales et al, 1996) for additional information.

Patients with this condition have been found repeatedly to have elevated basal levels of LH together with increased pulse amplitude and pulse frequency. In contrast, FSH levels are normal or decreased. Available data suggest that elevated concentrations of estrogen may be responsible for increased sensitivity of the pituitary to GnRH stimulation of LH release and decreased pituitary secretion of FSH. The net effect of this dual gonadotropin abnormality is an increase in LH-stimulated stromal and thecal production of androstenedione and testosterone and a decrease in FSH-induced granulosa cell aromatization of androgens to estrogens, resulting in increased intraovarian androgen concentrations (Reid and Van Vogt, 1987b). Abnormal granulosa cell cytodifferentiation results in disordered folliculogenesis, oocyte degeneration, and an inability to develop a large, healthy antral follicle. In peripheral tissues, significant proportions of the testosterone and androstenedione derived from adrenal and ovarian sources are metabolized to the potent androgen 5α-DHT by the skin. This end product (DHT) increases the activity of the 5α-reductase enzyme in the skin and further enhances its own production. Hyperandrogenism also contributes to a decrease in the production of sex hormone–binding globulin, resulting in greater availability of free or biologically active testosterone, which produces in a variety of peripheral manifestations of hyperandrogenism (Fig. 25–15). Additionally, fat cells in the periphery are able to metabolize androstenedione to the weak estrogen estrone, resulting in continuing feedback augmentation of LH and suppression of FSH from the hypothalamic-pituitary unit. Adrenal androgens (primarily dehydroepiandrosterone sulfate) also contribute to the peripheral androgen pool in this condition, although studies employing GnRH agonists to ablate ovarian steroidogenesis suggest that the adrenal contributes only a small fraction (Barbieri et al, 1988).

Finally, there is evidence that hyperinsulinemia may have a direct impact upon ovarian hyperandrogenism. Clinically, the association between hyperandrogenism (HA), insulin resistance (IR), and acanthosis nigricans (AN) has been recognized and

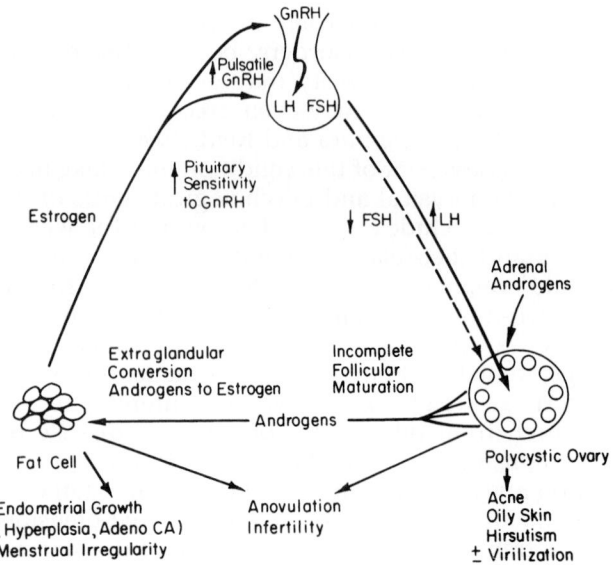

Figure 25–15

Schematic diagram depicting the clinical sequelae of aberrant gonadotropin dynamics in HHCA. (From Reid RL, Van Vugt DA: Weight related changes in reproductive function. Fertil Steril 1987;48:905, with permission of the American Fertility Society.)

described as the HAIR-AN syndrome (Barbieri and Ryan, 1983). Infusion of insulin, or glucose, which triggers release of endogenous insulin, has been shown to cause a dramatic increase in circulating androgens in hyperandrogenic women but not in non-hyperandrogenic women. It is hypothesized that insulin, through interactions with ovarian insulin-like growth factor I receptors, may stimulate androgen production (Poretsky and Kalin, 1987; Barbieri et al, 1986; Nestler et al, 1989b). It is possible that the hyperandrogenic condition is reinforced by each meal that is eaten, because the ingestion of food is followed by a compensatory increase in insulin. Indeed, studies have demonstrated that suppression of serum insulin levels with diazoxide is associated with a fall in serum testosterone and a rise in sex hormone–binding globulin in obese women with hyperandrogenism (Nestler et al, 1989b). In contrast, physiologic levels of insulin in normal women do not appear to regulate androgenic processes, as evidenced by the finding that diazoxide induces suppression of serum insulin levels in healthy nonobese women but has no impact on serum testosterone or sex hormone–binding globulin (Nestler et al, 1990).

Approximately two thirds of patients with PCOS will be obese, and most will show menstrual irregularity and features of hyperandrogenism. Menstrual cycles may occur as infrequently as once or twice per year and, in this circumstance, are generally marked by prolonged and heavy flow as endometrial tissue is sloughed. Continuous exposure to estrogen manifests itself by the production of copious amounts of watery cervical mucus, and, when the endometrium is exposed to this prolonged estrogenic stimulation, there is an increased risk of endometrial hyperplasia and carcinoma of the endometrium. Hirsutism is a gradual and progressive condition in this disorder, and virilization is only common in the most severe cases associated with stromal hyperthecosis.

Therapy for this condition depends upon the patient's needs as well as a desire to minimize the risk of future gynecologic problems such as menorrhagia leading to anemia, hirsutism, and risk of endometrial neoplasia (Reid and Van Vogt, 1987b). When fertility is desired, the primary objective is to reduce the adverse consequences of estrogen feedback on pituitary gonadotropin secretion. In the obese patient, weight loss will frequently result in correction of gonadotropin and sex steroid abnormalities, resulting sometimes in spontaneous resumption of ovulation and at other times in an attendant reduction in the required dosage of ovulation-inducing agents. The observation by Napheys, over 100 years ago, that "there are well authenticated cases of women who were stout and barren in opulence becoming thin and prolific in poverty" (Napheys, 1874) has been confirmed by studies evaluating the endocrinologic and ovulatory responses to weight loss in obese anovulatory women (Bates and Whitworth 1982; Harlass et al, 1984; Azziz, 1989; Pasquali et al, 1989). At times, hyperandrogenism is such that high local concentrations of testosterone within the ovary prevent normal folliculogenesis despite attempts at ovulation induction with agents such as clomiphene citrate. In these circumstances initial efforts must be undertaken to reduce ovarian androgen production. Although this has been tried with the use of oral contraceptives and antiandrogens such as spironolactone, the GnRH agonists have proven superior for inducing complete suppression of ovarian androgen secretion (Reid and Van Vogt, 1987b; Kelly and Jewelewicz, 1990). A similar reduction in androgen concentration is accomplished by the procedure of ovarian wedge resection and, more recently, by laparoscopic ovarian drilling (Greenblatt and Casper, 1987); however, both of these procedures carry significant risks for induction of periovarian adhesions, which may impair future fertility (Weibel and Majno, 1973).

If the patient does not desire pregnancy, then therapy is aimed at regulation of menstrual cyclicity, suppression of hyperandrogenism, and the provision of contraception where needed. The use of a combined oral contraceptive to suppress LH-induced ovarian androgen production, and to augment the production of sex hormone–binding globulin, combined with an antiandrogen such as spironolactone or cyproterone acetate, has proven effective in the management of these patients. An oral contraceptive used alone rarely will cause adequate regression in established hair growth, and spironolactone given alone creates the potential for transplacental exposure of male infants in any inadvertent pregnancies. Although spironolactone on its own may be associated with restoration of normal menstrual cyclicity, some women will develop more frequent menstrual cycles and, accordingly, the combination of this agent with an oral contraceptive combines therapy for hirsutism with optimal regulation of menstrual flow (Helfer et al, 1988; Barth et al, 1989). If the patient does not require contraception and hirsutism is not a concern, then cyclic exposure to exogenous progestin (medroxyprogesterone acetate 5 mg or micronized progesterone 200 mg orally per day for 12 to 14 days each month) will ensure regular shedding of endometrial tissue and minimize the risk of endometrial neoplasia.

Pituitary Causes

Pituitary Stalk Lesions

Damage to the pituitary stalk may result either from trauma (motor vehicle accidents, childhood abuse) or tumor (craniopharyngioma) or may be iatrogenic (following surgery for such lesions as a Rathke's pouch cyst) (Klachko et al, 1968; Hoff and Patterson, 1972; Miller et al, 1980). Typically lesions in this area result in panhypopituitarism with elevated prolactin because all trophic stimulation to the pituitary is lost along with loss of dopaminergic restraint to prolactin secretion.

The clinical presentation in such circumstances will depend on the time at which pituitary stalk disruption occurs. In childhood this condition results in growth arrest and delay or interruption of pubertal progression. After puberty is complete, the predominant features are those of amenorrhea, galactorrhea, and variable features of hypothyroidism and diabetes insipidus. Hypoadrenalism is a concern, although it may often go undetected until a time of stress. Tumors such as craniopharyngiomas often present with headache, visual field defects, and symptoms of hypothalamic dysfunction, such as somnolence and polyuria. Diagnostic testing requires the confirmation of normal pituitary responsiveness to GnRH, thyrotropin-releasing hormone, and corticotropin. Abnormalities of growth hormone secretion can be confirmed with growth hormone–releasing factor or the standard insulin-induced hypoglycemia test. Vasopressin deficiency is confirmed with a water deprivation test.

In addition to standard replacement doses of thyroxin, glucocorticoid, and mineralocorticoid (desmopressin acetate), such individuals may require growth hormone. Secondary sexual characteristics may be induced with exogenous sex steroid replacement therapy as described above. In circumstances where pubertal progression is complete, standard menopausal replacement therapy is indicated until fertility is desired. When fertility is desired, pulsatile GnRH or human menopausal gonadotropins may be used to induce ovulation and restore fertility (Carr and Reid, 1990; Leyendecker and Wildt, 1996). Subsequent to pregnancy, lifetime replacement therapy with sex steroids is indicated to reduce the risk of premature osteoporotic fractures or ischemic heart disease in addition to the control of symptomatic hypoestrogenism.

Pituitary Apoplexy

This term has been applied most often to massive infarction of the pituitary occurring in association with acute degenerative changes in pre-existing pituitary tumors (often prolactinomas). It has also been applied to the sudden infarction of nontumorous pituitary glands—most often following major obstetric hemorrhage (Reid et al, 1985). It is believed that occlusive arterial spasm of the blood supply to the anterior lobe and stalk is the initial event in postpartum pituitary necrosis. A brief period of total ischemia is followed by an attempt at re-establishment of circulation, subsequently leading to vascular congestion and thrombosis of the anterior lobe. The posterior pituitary is preserved in most circumstances because of the relative sparing of the inferior hypophyseal artery, which supplies this region.

A variety of endocrine and neurologic abnormalities may result from pituitary infarction and compression of the adjacent cavernous sinus and structures within (Fig. 25–16). Classically, postpartum pituitary necrosis (so-called Sheehan's syndrome) is often unrecognized at the time it occurs because the patient is unconscious or anesthetized during management of obstetric hemorrhage. Failure to lactate, persistent amenorrhea, and lethargy are often the earliest indicators of life-threatening anterior hypopituitarism. If the patient survives the initial insult and develops the later sequelae of pituitary infarction, dynamic tests of the hypothalamic-pituitary unit will uncover a range of pituitary deficiencies including loss of prolactin secretion (which differentiates this from pituitary stalk transection). Management involves careful evaluation of hormonal status and appropriate replacement therapy. Progression of symptoms at the time of the initial event, with loss of vision, loss of consciousness, or evidence of hypothalamic damage, indicates the need for more aggressive surgical decompression of tissues. In the long term, standard menopausal hormone replacement therapy is indicated. If and when fertility

is desired, pulsatile GnRH is ineffective and exogenous human menopausal gonadotropins are required.

Hyperprolactinemia

Hyperprolactinemia and its management is discussed elsewhere in this text (see chapter 29). In general, the higher the level of plasma prolactin, the greater the likelihood of disruption of menstrual cyclicity. Modest elevation of prolactin may merely compromise corpus luteum function, whereas higher levels often result in oligo- or amenorrhea. Amenorrhea on any occasion, and particularly in the presence of galactorrhea, should elicit a search for hyperprolactinemia (Blackwell, 1985; Howlett et al, 1989). The possibility of pregnancy should first be excluded. In the nonpregnant individual, primary hypothyroidism, drug-induced elevation of prolactin, breast or chest wall lesions in the dermatomes supplying the breast, breast feeding, and renal failure should be excluded before pursuing the diagnosis of pituitary prolactinoma (Blackwell, 1985; Thomas and Reid, 1987; Jackson, 1988; Kapcala and Lakshmanan, 1989) (Fig. 25–17). Serum prolactin does not always correlate with the size of the pituitary lesion, and most authors agree that any patient with amenorrhea or a 10 A.M. fasting serum prolactin level above 75 ng/ml warrants a baseline CT scan (or MRI).

The view that amenorrhea associated with microprolactinomas does not require treatment unless fertility is desired (Sisam et al, 1987) has been challenged based on the observations that the attendant hypoestrogenemia poses a risk of premature osteoporosis (Klibanski et al, 1980; Schlechte et al, 1983; Klibanski and Greenspan, 1986). Accordingly, failure to exhibit withdrawal bleeding following a 7-day course of oral progestin in a woman with hyperprolactinemic amenorrha is generally accepted as evidence of hypoestrogenemia sufficient to warrant treatment. Normally menstrual function and fertility are restored with the use of the long-acting dopaminergic agonist bromocriptine. Therapy may be with bromocriptine and suitable contraception or with replacement dosages of estrogen and progestin if fertility is not desired (Klibanski and Greenspan,

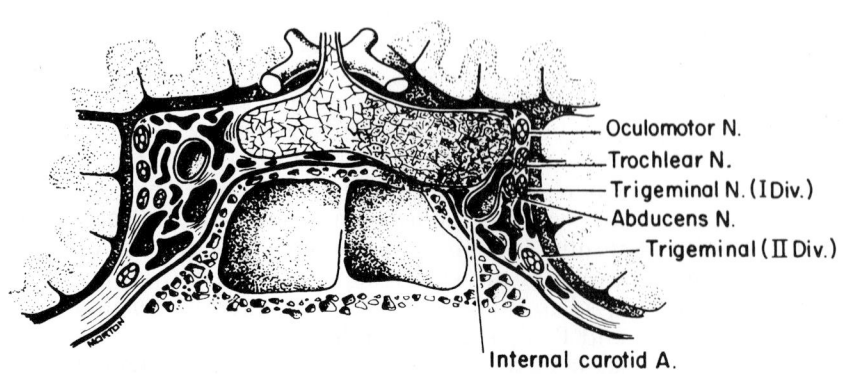

Figure 25–16

Acute pituitary infarction with secondary hemorrhage and edema may compress adjacent structures within the cavernous sinus, resulting in hypopituitarism; palsy of sympathetic nerves and/or cranial nerves III, IV, V, VI; and occlusion of the internal carotid artery with focal hemispheric dysfunction and altered consciousness. (From Reid RL, Quigley ME, Yen SSC: Pituitary apoplexy: a review. Arch Neurol 1985;42:712, with permission.)

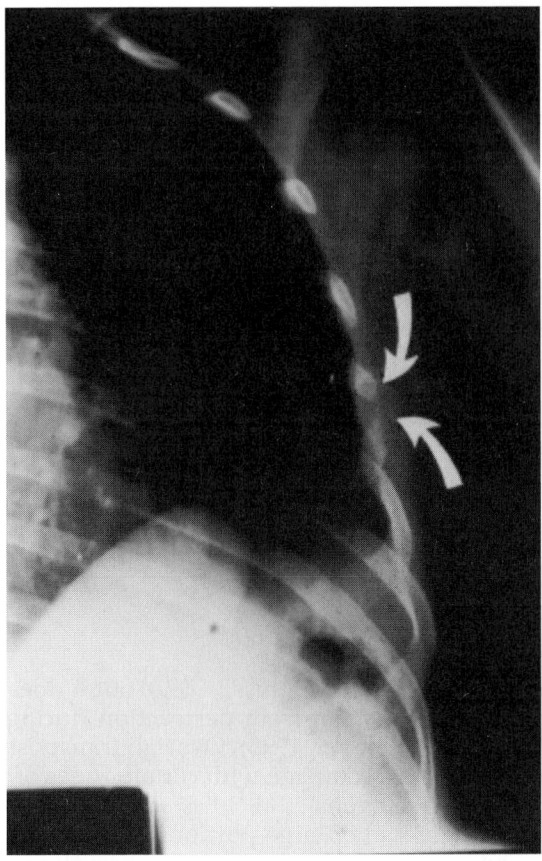

Figure 25-17
Benign osteolytic lesion (*arrows*) involving fifth rib with irritation of intercostal nerve leading to hyperprolactinemic amenorrhea. Galactorrhea and amenorrhea resolved 3 months after surgical elimination of lesion.

1986; Hartog and Hull, 1988). The theoretical risk that estrogen could adversely affect growth of prolactinomas has not been identified in practice (Frank, 1983; Frank et al, 1984).

Ovarian Causes

Hypergonadotropic Amenorrhea

Failure of gonadal tissues to respond to endogenous gonadotropins may result through a variety of different mechanisms (Table 25-5). Failure of the ovaries to develop normally is a condition termed *gonadal dysgenesis*, reported to account for up to 28% of cases of primary amenorrhea (Arman and Smentek, 1985). Premature menopause, defined as cessation of ovarian function prior to age 40, affects from 1% to 5% of North American women (Alper et al, 1986; Coulam et al, 1986). Both conditions are associated with elevated levels of the gonadotropins LH and FSH; hence the term *hypergonadotropic amenorrhea* has been used to describe this type of amenorrhea.

The marked hypoestrogenism associated with gonadal dysgenesis results in failure of secondary sex-

Table 25-5. POSSIBLE CAUSES OF HYPERGONADOTROPIC AMENORRHEA IN YOUNG WOMEN

I. Inherited characteristics
  A. Reduced germ cell number
  B. Accelerated atresia (?)
  C. Trisomy X with or without mosaicism
II. Enzymatic defects
  A. 17-alpha-hydroxylase deficiency
  B. Galactorrhea
III. Defects in gonadotropin secretion
  A. Secretion of biologically inactive forms
  B. Alpha or beta subunit defects
IV. Gonadotropin receptor and/or post-receptor defects (Resistant ovary or Savage syndrome)
V. Autoimmune disorders
  A. Associated with other endocrine disorders
  B. Isolated
VI. Congenital thymic aplasia
VII. Physical causes
  A. Irradiation
  B. Chemotherapeutic agents
  C. Viral agents
  D. Cigarette smoking
  E. Surgical extirpation
VIII. Idiopathic

From Rebar RW, Erickson GF, Coulam CB: Premature ovarian failure. In Gondos B, Riddick D (eds): Pathology of Infertility. New York: Thieme Medical Publishers Inc, 1987:123, with permission.

ual development and primary amenorrhea. In the absence of prior estrogen exposure, these individuals rarely experience typical menopausal hot flushes despite menopausal levels of estrogen. Up to 50% of patients with primary hypergonadotropic amenorrhea may have abnormal karyotypes (Portnondo et al, 1984; Reindollar et al, 1986; Rebar and Connolly, 1990). The most commonly recognized syndrome associated with hypergonadotropic amenorrhea is Turner's syndrome, which may show an XO karyotype with well-recognized clinical stigmata (short stature, webbed neck, low hairline, short fourth metacarpal) or a mosaic such as XO/XX and few somatic abnormalities (Turner, 1938) (Fig. 25-18). The ovaries from a fetus with Turner's syndrome have a normal compliment of oocytes at 18 weeks gestation but thereafter show acceleration of the normal 50-year process of oocyte loss such that the ovaries are usually oocyte depleted in the first few years of life. Often individuals with mosaicism (XO/XX) and very rarely those without evidence of mosaicism (XO) will have a period of ovulatory function resulting in pregnancy before the onset of ovarian failure (King et al, 1978). Gonadal dysgenesis in those with normal karyotypes (XX or XY) may be familial (Muram and Dewhurst, 1984).

Rarely hypergonadotropic amenorrhea can result from an enzymatic defect. In females with defective 17-hydroxylase enzyme, both adrenal and ovarian steroidogenesis are impaired, resulting in CAH (with hypertension caused by excessive mineralocorticoid production) and lack of estrogen biosynthesis at puberty. Hypertension in a patient with primary hy-

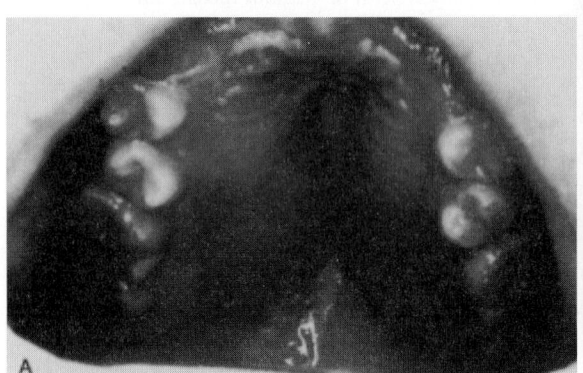
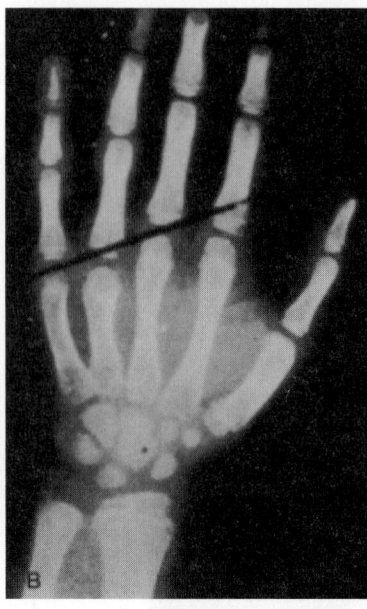

Figure 25-18
A, The high-arched palate of an individual with Turner's syndrome. B, Radiograph showing the short fourth metacarpal in Turner's syndrome. (Photographs courtesy of R. Rebar.)

pergonadotropic amenorrhea should elicit a search for this condition. Deficiency of aromatase—the enzyme responsible for conversion of C19 steroids to estrogen—has been found to be an extremely rare cause of female pseudohermaphroditism and hypergonadotropic amenorrhea (Conte et al, 1994; Bulun, 1996).

Premature ovarian failure is typically marked by increasing irregularity of menstrual cyclicity and intermittent hot flushes as ovarian function waxes and wanes leading up to complete depletion of oocytes. It occurs in association with a variety of disorders, including galactosemia (congenital deficiency of galactose-1-phosphate uridyltransferase, associated with mental retardation, hepatosplenomegaly, and renal disease), genetic abnormalities (X chromosome defects with mosaicism), autoimmune disease, and loss of ovarian function as a result of surgery or radiation or chemotherapy (Halyard et al, 1996).

Immune abnormalities may be present in up to 40% of women with this secondary hypergonadotropic amenorrhea (Damewood et al, 1986; Rebar et al, 1987; Ho et al, 1988; LeBarbera et al, 1988). Hypothyroidism caused by autoimmune thyroiditis is the most common endocrine disturbance occurring in association with premature ovarian failure. Hypoadrenalism and hypoparathyroidism, although rare, are potentially life threatening and may not be evident at the time of initial clinical presentation.

Survival of women following treatment with chemo- or radiotherapy for a variety of malignancies is becoming increasingly common (Siris et al, 1976; Schilsky et al, 1980). The dosage of irradiation together with the type of chemotherapy (single versus multiple agent) and the age at which treatment is administered will determine the likelihood that ovarian function will recover (Schilsky et al, 1980). Whether ovarian suppression with GnRH analogues will protect oocytes from chemotherapy damage is

uncertain (Ataya and Moghissi, 1989), but it does not appear to protect them from destruction during radiotherapy (Ataya et al, 1995). Ovarian transposition may avoid ovarian damage with certain types of pelvic irradiation (Covens et al, 1996).

Surgical removal of large portions of both ovaries, for conditions such as endometriosis, may also result in increased FSH levels, shorter follicular phases, and an increased incidence of twinning typical of the perimenopausal transition (Jones, 1990).

When initial investigation reveals that amenorrhea is associated with gonadotropins in the postmenopausal range, it is important to search for evidence of other autoimmune disorders or endocrinopathy (Table 25-6). A karyotype should be obtained in all

Table 25-6. REPORTED CASES OF AUTOIMMUNE DISEASE ASSOCIATED WITH PREMATURE OVARIAN FAILURE

Thyroid	26
Adrenal	8
Polyendocrinopathy (Type I)	20
Polyendocrinopathy (Type II)	19
Diabetes mellitus	1
Multiple endocrinopathy	6
Myasthenia gravis	9
Pernicious anemia	2
Idiopathic thrombocytopenia	1
Glomerulonephritis	1
Rheumatoid arthritis	1
Crohn's disease	1
Vertiligo	1
Systemic lupus erythematosus	2
Asthma	1
Ovarian lymphocytic infiltrate	3
Unspecified	15
	119/380

From LeBarbera AR, Miller MM, Ober C, et al: Autoimmune etiology in premature ovarian failure. Am J Reprod Immunol Microbiol 1988;16:115, with permission.

individuals with primary hypergonadotropic amenorrhea and on all individuals with secondary hypergonadotropic amenorrhea before the age of 30. Other blood work should include a complete blood count with differential and erythrocyte sedimentation rate, total serum protein, albumin-to-globulin ratio, rheumatoid factor, antinuclear antibody, fasting blood sugar, A.M. cortisol, serum calcium and phosphorus, serum TSH, thyroxin, antithyroglobulin, and antimicrosomal antibodies (Rebar and Connolly, 1990). If initial gonadotropin levels are merely bordering on menopausal levels, they should be repeated on at least two or three occasions at weekly intervals in conjunction with serum estradiol levels to assess the possibility of intermittent ovarian failure.

All women with premature ovarian failure should be counseled about the need for hormone replacement therapy to prevent osteoporosis (Davies et al, 1995).

Although there have been sporadic reports of ovulation induction in individuals with secondary hypergonadotropic amenorrhea employing exogenous FSH (Johnson and Peterson, 1979; Tanaka et al, 1982) or estrogen rebound (Buckler et al, 1991), pregnancies are uncommon (Hens et al, 1989). Pregnancies, when they occur, often do so while the patient is on standard menopausal replacement therapy (Surrey and Cedars, 1989; Check et al, 1990).

With the progress in in vitro fertilization and donor egg programs, it is likely that the greatest success in terms of fertility will be achieved through hormonal priming of the uterus and replacement of embryos derived from in vitro fertilization of donor eggs (Lutjen et al, 1986; Chan et al, 1987). This procedure is possible in individuals with gonadal dysgenesis despite their karyotype.

Finally, in women with premature ovarian failure, it is important to advise any offspring that they may also experience premature ovarian failure because this condition may have a hereditary tendency (Mattison et al, 1984; Krauss et al, 1987).

Male Pseudohermaphroditism Presenting as Hypergonadotropic Amenorrhea

Some individuals presenting with hypergonadotropic amenorrhea are male pseudohermaphrodites—that is, they are genetically XY with female phenotypic features. This condition results from destruction of the gonad (potential testicle) at an early stage in utero such that neither testosterone nor MIF is produced. Accordingly, development is along female lines with no secondary sexual development at puberty. Extirpation of dysgenetic gonadal tissue is necessary (Mulvihill et al, 1975; Troche and Hernandez, 1986).

Such individuals have fallopian tubes, a uterus, and a vagina and will menstruate when exogenous sex steroids are administered to complete female secondary sexual development. Such individuals, after appropriate hormonal priming, can be recipients for

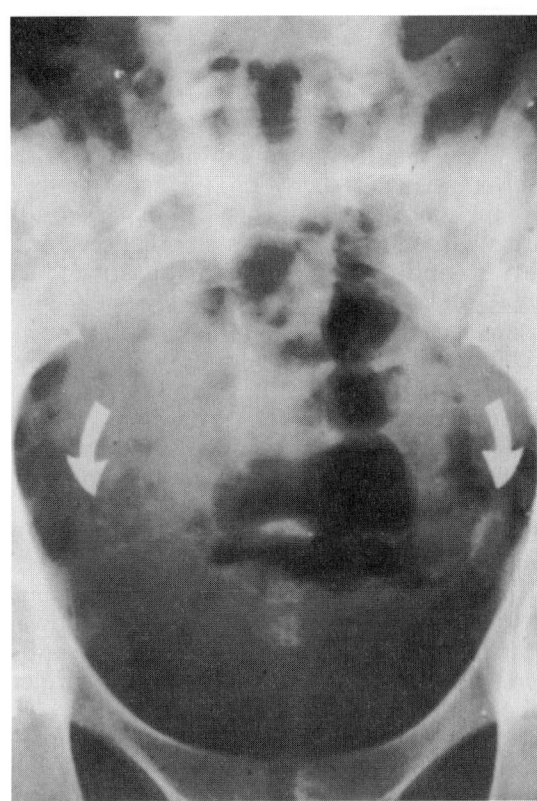

Figure 25–19
Bilateral ovoid calcifications (*arrows*) in dysgenetic gonads of an apparent female with delayed puberty at age 17. Karyotype revealed 46,XY and histopathology of gonadal tissue showed right-sided gonadoblastoma and left-sided combined gonadoblastoma and dysgerminoma.

gametes (i.e., gamete intrafallopian transfer) or embryos (after in vitro fertilization).

Patients with dysgenetic gonads and Y chromosomal material have a 15% to 25% risk of development of a gonadal neoplasm—sometimes at an early age (Mulvihill et al, 1975). Approximately 10% occur prior to the age of 10, and most neoplasms will develop under the age of 30. Although 90% of reported cases of neoplasms in dysgenetic gonads occur in individuals with a Y chromosome or Y chromosome fragments, there have been rare cases of neoplasm arising in XX individuals. Such tumors include gonadoblastomas (50%), dysgerminomas (20%), gonadoblastoma with areas of dysgerminoma (18%), and other histologic types (9%). Gonadoblastomas often contain calcium, which is identifiable on a pelvic radiograph (Fig. 25–19).

Ovarian Tumors

Approximately 5% of ovarian tumors will have some functional endocrine activity (Zhang et al, 1982; Fox, 1985). Rarely hirsutism and virilization are secondary effects resulting from the stromal reaction to an epithelial ovarian tumor; however, in most circumstances functional activity is confined to tumors of the sex cord stromal type.

The estrogen-producing granulosa tumor is the most common malignant functional tumor of the ovary. These rapidly growing tumors result in disruption of menstrual cyclicity, producing either amenorrhea or menorrhagia. Patients will experience breast enlargement and ultimately menstrual bleeding secondary to endometrial neoplasia stimulated by excessive production of estrogen. Five-year survival rates are greater than 90%, although late recurrences are common. Unilateral salpingo-oophorectomy is considered adequate treatment in the premenopausal women with a stage 1A tumor; however, total abdominal hysterectomy and bilateral salapingo-oophorectomy is usually performed when the tumor presents after the menopause.

Thecomas account for approximately 2% to 3% of ovarian neoplasms and occur most commonly in the perimenopausal woman. Estrogen production may lead to a period of amenorrhea often followed by bleeding caused by endometrial hyperplasia or carcinoma. The tumor itself is benign and surgical resection is therapeutic.

Sertoli-Leydig cell tumors (androblastomas) are characterized by marked overproduction of androgens. Initial changes noted by affected women include defeminization (amenorrhea, vaginal mucosal atrophy, and diminished breast size) followed shortly by features of hirsutism and virilization (balding, increased muscle mass, and clitoromegaly). These solid unilateral tumors grow rapidly and are often palpable. Management is conservative, with excision of the involved ovary; metastases are rare.

Lipid cell (hilus cell) tumors are small, virilizing stromal tumors occurring most commonly in postmenopausal women. Like the Sertoli-Leydig cell tumors, these cause rapid defeminization (with amenorrhea) and masculinization unless surgically removed. These tumors are rare, accounting for less than 0.1% of all ovarian tumors.

Uterine and Vaginal Causes

Despite normal hormonal changes of the menstrual cycle, menstruation may not occur if there is aplasia or obstruction of the outflow tract. Complete aplasia of the uterus, accidental or purposeful destruction of the endometrium, cervical stenosis, or vaginal obstruction may all be associated with amenorrhea. Historical factors such as the presence of cryptomenorrhea (painful monthly uterine cramps), symptoms of bladder compression, or pelvic pain typical of endometriosis suggest the possible existence of functional endometrium with obstruction to outflow. Conversely, the absence of any symptoms despite normal secondary sexual characteristics would favor a diagnosis involving lack of functional endometrial tissue. Outflow tract obstruction that has been persistent for a considerable length of time will be attended by a boggy pelvic mass (usually a hematocolpos but possibly a hematometra and/or hematosalpingies).

Uterovaginal Agenesis

The *Mayer-Rokitansky-Kuster-Hauser* syndrome involves the congenital absence of all or part of the uterus and vagina. It is frequently associated with anomalies of the urinary tract and a bony skeleton. Urinary tract malformations occur in up to 50% of patients, with vaginal agenesis and unilateral renal agenesis in 15%. Abnormalities of the vertebral column, including fusion of cervical vertebrae, have been noted in up to 25% of cases (Vasquez, 1989). Ovaries and fallopian tubes in this condition are normal, and secondary sexual development progresses in the usual fashion.

Typically patients with this condition present with primary amenorrhea. This condition is differentiated from androgen insensitivity by the presence of normal serum testosterone levels and an XX karyotype. Occasionally, rudiments of the uterus contain functional endometrium and will produce cyclic pelvic pain (cryptomenorrhea). A transverse vaginal septum may present in a similar fashion but can be excluded by further investigations, including ultrasonography (Meyer et al, 1995) and laparoscopy. Studies have shown MRI to give the most precise information about the presence or absence of intraperitoneal and retroperitoneal rudimentary müllerian structures (Fedele et al, 1990). Cavitary uterine rudiments should be removed routinely if they are large or causing cyclic pelvic pain. An intravenous pyelogram and vertebral radiographs are warranted to exclude anomalies of the renal and skeletal systems.

A functional vagina can usually be created employing a nonoperative technique with dilators (Frank, 1938; Ingram, 1981); however, surgical construction of a neovagina may be required (McIndoe, 1950; Counsellor and Flor, 1957; Rock et al, 1983). Attempts to link the vaginal pouch to a rudimentary uterus have been fraught with complications and are rarely successful (Rock et al, 1982; Pinsonneault and Goldstein, 1985).

Endometrial Suppression/Ablation

MEDICAL SUPPRESSION

At times, amenorrhea may represent nothing more than a side effect of medication given for medical ovarian suppression. The induction of amenorrhea may be the primary reason for administering such medications. Danazol, depoprovera, and, more recently, the LHRH agonists have been used to treat such pelvic conditions as endometriosis, dysmenorrhea, and menorrhagia. They may be used as preoperative preparations to shrink uterine leiomyomata or suppress endometriosis.

For some other medications amenorrhea may be an inadvertent side effect that, because it is unexpected, creates anxiety on the part of the patient. Oral contraceptives are progestin dominant and, as such, will frequently lead to gradual and progressive suppression of endometrial development. As a result, one of the established benefits of oral contraceptives is the reduction of menstrual flow and associated dysmenorrhea. Eventually some women will notice that menstrual cycles become reduced so much that the anticipated withdrawal bleed may not occur. Initially this often generates concern about possible pregnancy. On the first occasion that withdrawal bleeding fails to occur, a sensitive pregnancy test should be performed to ensure that pregnancy has not resulted from inadvertent ovulation caused by missed pills. If the affected individual takes her pills consistently and is reassured by counseling, then no intervention is required. If she wishes to have at least some withdrawal bleeding each month, it can usually be restored by simply adding supplemental estrogen (conjugated equine estrogen 1.25 mg or ethinyl estradiol 10 μg daily) during the first 10 days of the next birth control pill cycle.

Exogenous androgens applied as topical creams or ingested to promote muscle development in bodybuilding may result in amenorrhea (Punch and Ansbacher, 1990). Once the cause is identified, therapy involves removing the source of exogenous androgen.

ENDOMETRIAL ABLATION

Endometrial destruction may follow vigorous uterine curettage for postpartum hemorrhage or evacuation of an incomplete abortion (Schenker and Margolioth, 1982). Only with complete obliteration of the endometrial cavity or obstruction of uterine outflow does amenorrhea result. Hysteroscopic lysis of such dense adhesions may be problematic in that visualization and accurate entry into the endometrial cavity is made difficult by the lack of clearly defined tissue planes. Pregnancies resulting after lysis of extensive intrauterine synechiae may occasionally be complicated by abnormalities of placentation (March and Israel, 1981; Friedman et al, 1986; Townsend et al, 1990). Endometrial atrophy may inadvertently result following high doses of local irradiation.

Finally, efforts have been made to deliberately ablate the endometrium for control of menorrhagia in women whose obesity or medical conditions pose significant risks for hysterectomy (Siegler and Valle, 1988). The endometrial layer is either cauterized using the roller ball technique or actually removed with successive cuts employing the wire loop resectoscope tip (DeCherney et al, 1987; Townsend et al, 1990). Preoperative suppression of endometrial growth with an LHRH agonist facilitates this procedure and is likely to enhance success rates. In most circumstances destruction of endometrial tissue will result in amenorrhea, whereas in other cases some menstrual flow persists but menorrhagia is satisfactorily controlled (Hill and Maher, 1990; Baggish and Sze, 1996).

Cervical Stenosis or Atresia

Cervical stenosis is an uncommon cause for secondary amenorrhea. Iatrogenic causes (extensive cautery for cervical intraepithelial neoplasia) or an obstructing cervical malignancy are the most common explanations. The diagnosis can be confirmed by the sudden release of a hematometra following sounding of the cervical canal under paracervical block in the office setting. Cytology and biopsy should be performed to evaluate the possibility of malignancy if clinical features suggest this finding. Nonmalignant stenotic lesions rarely recur after sounding and/or dilatation.

Congenital cervical atresia is a rare condition often associated with other genital duct anomalies (Farber et al, 1982). Rarely is surgical correction successful, and hysterectomy therefore remains the preferred treatment.

Imperforate Hymen

Imperforate hymen occurs in approximately 1 in 1000 women. When identified in the premenarchal female it may present as a hydromucocolpos; however, it is most commonly detected as an outward-bulging bluish membrane associated with cyclic pelvic pain and primary amenorrhea. Incision and drainage should be performed under anesthesia to allow an adequate cruciate incision with resection of mucosal flaps. Adenosis, which is frequently found superior to the imperforate hymen, is gradually replaced by squamous epithelium after surgery. If imperforate hymen is not detected and treated at an early stage, the vaginal accumulation of old blood may be dramatic. Retrograde menstruation may lead to pelvic endometriosis. Failure to make an adequate incision may result in ascending infection, further compounding pelvic problems.

Transverse Vaginal Septum

Transverse vaginal septum occurs even less frequently (approximately 1 in 80,000 women). Usually these septa are located at the junction of the middle and upper third of the vagina. A boggy mass caused by accumulated blood in the vagina is palpable on rectal examination (Fig. 25–20). Resection of the septum, after careful documentation of pelvic anatomy, will restore normal vaginal function. Regrettably, this condition is most often associated with subsequent infertility if the lesion is not diagnosed and treated at an early stage, before the development of pelvic endometriosis.

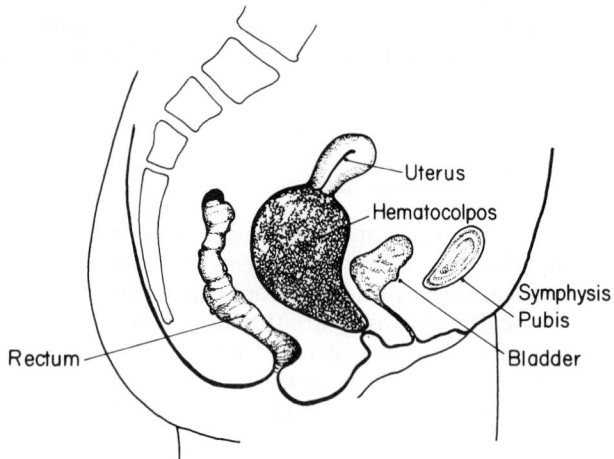

Figure 25–20
Schematic of typical findings on pelvic exam in a patient with delayed detection of transverse vaginal septum or imperforate hymen.

Male Pseudohermaphroditism Presenting as Apparent Outflow Tract Obstruction

There are a group of individuals who, despite having an XY karyotype and functioning testicular tissue, present with a female phenotype at birth, some features of normal female pubertal development, and primary amenorrhea (Kupfer et al, 1992). In this circumstance, either there is a defect of testicular androgen production or there is inadequate androgen action at target tissues (Table 25–7). In both of these forms of male pseudohermaphroditism, testosterone levels are low.

INADEQUATE ANDROGEN SECRETION

Leydig Cell Agenesis. This rare syndrome results from the absence of trophic stimulation to testicular Leydig cells caused by defective LH receptors (Ber-

Table 25–7. MALE PSEUDO-HERMAPHRODITISM PRESENTING AS UTEROVAGINAL AGENESIS

INADEQUATE ANDROGEN SECRETION
Leydig cell agenesis
Errors in androgen biosynthesis
  20,22-desmolase
  3β-ol-dehydroxygenase
  17α-hydroxylase deficiency
  17,20-desmolase
  17-ketosteroid reductase

INADEQUATE ANDROGEN ACTION AT TARGET
    TISSUES
Androgen insensitivity
  Complete testicular feminization
  Incomplete testicular feminization
  Postreceptor resistance
5α-Reductase deficiency

thezene et al, 1976; Schwartz et al, 1981). As a result, testosterone production is reduced or absent. External genitalia appear female, although occasionally they may be ambiguous. The vagina ends in a blind pouch and müllerian structures are absent because the testes continue to secrete MIF. The absence of testosterone production in utero results in failure of development of wolffian structures. Such individuals fail to respond with the expected increase in serum testosterone or 17-hydroxyprogesterone after administration of exogenous hCG. Appropriate treatment depends on the individual's gender identity and the appearance and function of external genitalia. Because intratesticular testosterone is required for spermatogenesis, these individuals are infertile (Eil, 1990).

Errors in Androgen Production. A variety of autosomal recessive disorders involving an abnormality of testosterone biosynthesis may be divided into two categories: those with defects in production of both testosterone and cortisol and those with normal cortisol production but deficient testosterone biosynthesis (Fig. 25–21). In the former category are those with defects of the enzymes 20,22-desmolase, 3-hydroxysteroid dehydrogenase, and 17α-hydroxylase. In these cases a compensatory increase in adrenocorticotropic hormone (ACTH) results in CAH. Approximately 30 cases each of 20,22-desmolase deficiency and 3-hydroxysteroid dehydrogenase deficiency have been reported. Most individuals present with severe cortisol deficiency at birth, and rarely do they survive the neonatal period. Individuals with 17α-hydroxylase deficiency are the most likely to present as females with delayed puberty. The genitalia range from ambiguous to normal female depending on the severity of the enzymatic defect. Gynecomastia may occur at puberty with little virilization. Severe glucocorticoid deficiency does not occur because of the glucocorticoid activity of corticosterone (an intermediate in the aldosterone biosynthetic pathway). Hypertension, caused by mineralocorticoid excess, a common feature in females deficient in 17α-hydroxylase, is seldom apparent in males for reasons that are uncertain. Gonadotropin and sex steroid concentrations are low. Treatment is with glucocorticoids and standard replacement with female sex steroids (Kater and Biglieri, 1994).

The second group comprises those individuals in whom the primary defect is in testosterone production alone and includes those with 17,20-desmolase and 17-ketosteroid reductase deficiencies. In these uncommon disorders, genitalia are ambiguous and virilization will occur at puberty. Unless satisfactory surgical correction for male sex-of-rearing can be anticipated, prepubertal gonadectomy and estrogen therapy are indicated.

In each of these circumstances, diagnosis of the enzymatic defect may be established by dynamic testing of adrenal function employing ACTH and hCG, with measurement of steroid intermediaries to determine the site of the enzymatic block. When

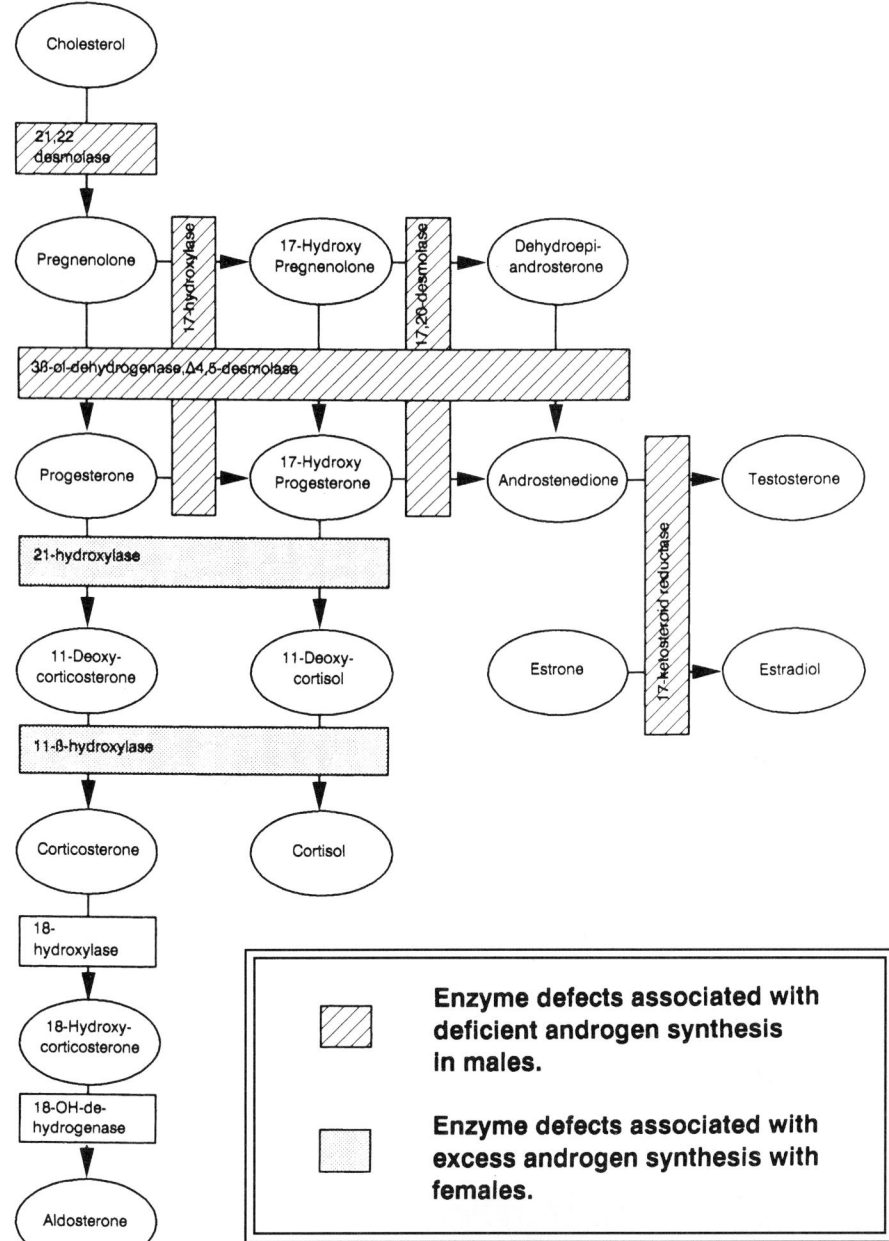

Figure 25–21
Diagram of steroid biosynthetic pathways and potential enzymatic deficiencies. In the female, 21-hydroxylase and 11-hydroxylase deficiencies can cause adrenal hyperplasia, resulting in hyperandrogenism and amenorrhea. In the male, variable degrees of pseudohermaphroditism result depending on the site and severity of the enzymatic defect in the biosynthetic pathway for androgen production.

both testosterone and cortisol pathways are involved, cortisol replacement is essential. The 21,22-desmolase and 3-hydroxysteroid dehydroxygenase deficiencies are associated with salt wasting caused by mineralocorticoid deficiency, whereas the 17α-hydroxylase deficiency may be marked by hypertension caused by mineralocorticoid excess. Sex assignment will depend upon gender identity and the potential for satisfactory virilization with exogenous testosterone. Usually only those patients with the 3-hydroxysteroid dehydroxygenase defect have any potential for male genital development. Where external genitalia show marked ambiguity or appear female, castration with subsequent estrogen replacement therapy is appropriate.

INADEQUATE ANDROGEN ACTION

Androgen Insensitivity

Complete Testicular Feminization. The most common form of male pseudohermaphroditism to account for primary amenorrhea in association with agenesis of the uterus and vagina is androgen insensitivity (Morris, 1953; Morris and Mahesh, 1963; Griffin and Wilson, 1980). Individuals with androgen insensitivity have varying degrees of target tissue androgen unresponsiveness and, accordingly, range in appearance from completely normal females without pubic or axillary hair to normal phenotypic males whose only abnormality is infertility (the mildest form). Obviously amenorrhea is a presenting complaint only in those with a severe defect in whom female gender assignment leads to the expectation of menstruation. Testes may be found either intra-abdominally, in the inguinal canals, or in the labia; these individuals may present in infancy with a diagnosis of inguinal hernia (Fig. 25–22). The majority, however, are detected at puberty when they present with primary amenorrhea.

The general appearance, breast development, and distribution of body fat are female. Axillary and pubic hair are scant or absent, although a small amount of vulvar hair is usually present. The vagina is short and ends blindly. In approximately two thirds of cases this condition is inherited as an X-linked recessive disorder (Armhein et al, 1976; Muram and Dewhurst, 1984). Diminished hypothalamic-pituitary response to the feedback effects of androgens results in elevated plasma LH levels. This further augments testosterone and estradiol secretion from the testes. The circulating concentration of estradiol is further augmented by increased peripheral aromatization of testosterone to estradiol because of the greater availability of substrate (testosterone). The elevated levels of estradiol account for the normal female secondary sexual characteristics.

Because these individuals have Y chromosomes, they are at risk for gonadal neoplasia; however, the risk appears to be considerably lower than in XY gonadal dysgenesis. Current estimates suggest that the tumor risk is less than 4% by age 30, hence gonadectomy is usually deferred until secondary sexual development is complete (Parks, 1982).

Incomplete Testicular Feminization. Incomplete testicular feminization is a relatively rare form of androgen insensitivity accounting for about 10% to 20% of cases. Clinical findings range from mild hirsutism and virilization together with primary amen-

orrhea noted at puberty in an individual with a female body habitus to the predominantly male phenotype with perineoscrotal hypospadias, peripubertal gynecomastia, normal pubic and axillary hair, cryptorchid testes, and azoospermia in the so-called Reifenstein syndrome.

Postreceptor defects. Evaluation of genital skin fibroblast androgen receptor binding has identified a distinct category of patients who would otherwise have been diagnosed as having complete testicular feminization (Eil et al, 1981). DHT binding studies reveal normal cellular androgen receptors (Collier et al, 1978). These rare patients are phenotypically female with normal female external genitalia; some have shown clitoromegaly. Breast development at puberty is varied, and some cases have shown normal pubic and axillary hair. The degree of wolffian development has not been well characterized, but müllerian structures typically are absent. Unlike testicular feminization, which typically shows an X-linked recessive pattern of inheritance, the mode of inherence of this condition has not been well established.

5α-Reductase Deficiency. The absence of the enzyme 5α-reductase results in failure of conversion of testosterone to DHT in genital tissues (Walsh et al, 1974). This condition (also known as "penis at 12 syndrome," "type II incomplete androgen resistance," and "pseudovaginal perineoscrotal hypospadias") is most prevalent in rural areas of the Dominican Republic, although other sporadic cases have been reported elsewhere throughout the world. The result is abnormal development of the external genitalia, with a hooded prepuce, a ventral urethral groove, and a urethral opening at the base of the phallus. The vaginal pouch ends blindly and forms part of a urogenital sinus. The remaining wolffian structures are well developed, and normal-appearing testes are located in the inguinal canal or labia. Other müllerian structures are absent. Masculinization at puberty may be dramatic, with deepening of the voice, phallic enlargement, and increased muscle mass, although structures such as the scrotum and prostate, which respond primarily to DHT, remain prepubertal. This disorder is inherited as an autosomal recessive condition and is expressed only in individuals with 46,XY karyotype. Plasma LH levels may be slightly elevated but other endocrine parameters are normal. DHT binding is normal in cultured fibroblasts; however, conversion of testosterone to DHT is markedly reduced.

Fertility is not achieved in patients with this condition. The primary amenorrhea in this circumstance is frequently overshadowed by the striking change in gender assignment that accompanies these changes in the rural culture of the Dominican Republic. In circumstances outside this culture, where female gender identity is well established, prepubertal gonadectomy and estrogen replacement therapy may be the preferred therapy.

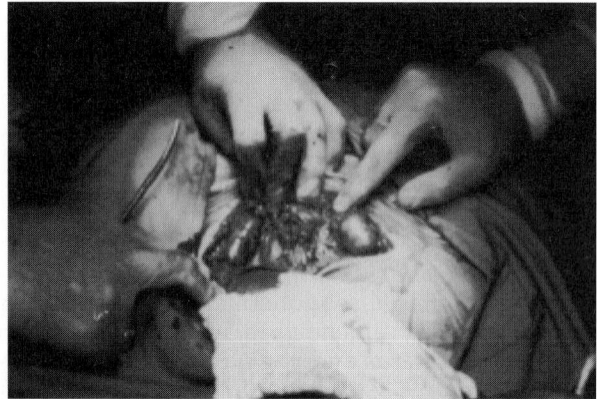

Figure 25–22
Testicles found in the inguinal canals of a 20-year-old phenotypic female with primary amenorrhea. A 46,XY karyotype, a blind vagina, elevated testosterone levels without hirsutism, and palpable inguinal masses confirm a diagnosis of complete androgen insensitivity and necessitate surgery to remove testicular tissue.

Other Endocrinopathies

Thyroid Dysfunction

HYPERTHYROIDISM

Hyperthyroidism is associated with increased production of sex hormone–binding globulin. Although the plasma concentration of total testosterone is increased, the free or active fraction of testosterone is reduced (Thomas and Reid, 1987). There is also an increased rate of conversion of androgens to estrogens in hyperthyroidism. Estrogen metabolism is altered, with preferential metabolism of estradiol to estrone by 2-hydroxylation rather than by 16α-hydroxylation. The precise effects of these changes in peripheral estrogen metabolism on hypothalamic pituitary function are unknown. Both the nutritional disturbances and the emotional upheavals associated with hyperthyroidism also may influence menstrual function (Roger, 1958). Baseline gonadotropin concentrations are frequently elevated in hyperthyroidism, and this change, together with the absence of an adequate LH surge, may be one of the causes of anovulation and menstrual dysfunction seen in this disorder (Akanade and Hockaday, 1972). Typically in hyperthyroidism menstrual function is gradually reduced and ultimately ceases. Return of normal menstrual function and fertility follows correction of the hyperthyroid state.

HYPOTHYROIDISM

Longstanding untreated primary hypothyroidism is associated with galactorrhea in 1% to 3% of cases (Kleinberg et al, 1977). Twenty-four–hour hormonal profiles show high basal levels of TSH, prolactin, and LH (Thomas and Reid, 1987). The hyperprolactinemia resulting from longstanding primary hypothyroidism has been implicated in ovulatory dysfunction ranging from inadequate corpus luteum progesterone secretion when prolactin is mildly elevated to oligomenorrhea or amenorrhea when circulating prolactin levels are high. Hypothyroidism alone without hyperprolactinemia may directly interfere with normal HPO function, resulting in menstrual disturbance. In less severe hypothyroidism, menorrhagia is common. This may result from chronic unopposed estrogenic stimulation causing acyclic shedding of the endometrium and episodes of menorrhagia (Thomas and Reid, 1987). When hypothyroidism is severe or longstanding, particularly if associated with hyperprolactinemia, amenorrhea is common. Replacement doses of thyroid hormone are therapeutic.

Adrenal Dysfunction Disease

ADRENAL HYPERPLASIA

CAH is a group of genetic disorders arising as a result of enzymatic defects in cortisol biosynthesis (White et al, 1987a, 1987b; New, 1995). Compensatory increases in ACTH production result in hyperplasia of the adrenal gland. CAH may result in amenorrhea in two ways. The most common enzymatic defect involves 21α-hydroxylase and affects approximately 1 in 5000 births. Androgen excess in the female prior to birth results in ambiguous female genitalia, and increased production of adrenal androgens thereafter results in heterosexual precocious puberty in the untreated patient. Rather than normal female pubertal development, there is primary amenorrhea associated with virilization. Reports suggest that some individuals may have late onset of CAH resulting from a mild 21-hydroxylase deficiency. Presenting features include irregular menstruation, oligo-ovulation, hirsutism, and variable degrees of virilization in the years following puberty (Lobo and Goebelsmann, 1980; Azziz et al, 1994). An elevation of serum 17-hydroxyprogesterone in the early morning hours in response to endogenous ACTH will help to make this diagnosis. Early recognition and appropriate treatment with glucocorticoid and mineralocorticoid will prevent progression of the disorder. Treatment of established hirsutism and virilization may require systemic therapy with antiandrogens and/or surgical correction of the clitoral hypertrophy.

The second form of CAH association with amenorrhea is that resulting from enzymatic blocks that prevent formation of both estrogen and androgens. This includes the 20,22-desmolase deficiency and 17α-hydroxylase deficiency as described above. In both of these disorders females will have normal genitalia at birth but will fail to develop secondary sexual characteristics at puberty because of the inability to manufacture estrogen. Few cases of the 20,22-desmolase enzymatic defect have been reported, and many of these individuals have died in the neonatal period as a result of marked glucocorticoid deficiency. Individuals with the 17α-hydroxylase deficiency may present at puberty with hypergonadotropic hypogonadism. Because of excessive production of deoxycorticosterone, these individuals have hypokalemic alkalosis and hypertension. Treatment is with replacement doses of glucocorticoid and appropriate use of exogenous estrogen to cause development of secondary sexual characteristics.

CUSHING'S DISEASE

Cushing's disease is a form of ACTH-dependent Cushing's syndrome that results from a basophilic (ACTH-producing) adenoma of the pituitary gland (Cushing, 1932). This disorder accounts for approximately 60% of cases of endogenous Cushing's syndrome. The resulting hypercortisolism and increased production of adrenal androgens produce the characteristic features of this disorder, including centripetal obesity, hypertension, proximal muscle weakness, abdominal striae, thinning of scalp hair, hirsutism, and oligo- or amenorrhea. Although not falling under the strict definition of Cushing's disease, other nonpituitary tumors may produce ectopic ACTH (or rarely corticotropin-releasing hormone), resulting in an identical symptom complex (Immura, 1980). Treatment of Cushing's disease requires elimination of the pituitary tumor, either by transsphenoidal surgery or radiation. Ectopic ACTH syndromes require treatment of the primary lesion. In circumstances where surgical elimination of excessive ACTH secretion fails or is refused, bilateral adrenalectomy may be life saving. Following successful elimination of the tumor, there is often a striking resolution of features of hirsutism, scalp hair loss, and menstrual dysfunction.

ADRENAL ADENOMA/CARCINOMA

ACTH-independent forms of endogenous Cushing's syndrome (accounting for 25% of all endogenous Cushing's syndrome) are due to adrenal adenoma (10%) and adrenal carcinoma (15%). Adrenal adenomas tend to be smaller than adrenal carcinomas at the time of diagnosis. Adrenal carcinomas are relatively inefficient synthesizers of cortisol and therefore are detected late (Hutter and Kayhoe, 1966). Production of adrenal androgens in association with these disorders may be dramatic, resulting in hirsutism, virilization, and amenorrhea. Diagnosis is confirmed using CT scan or MRI of the adrenal, with primary treatment being surgical.

REFERENCES

Abraham SF, Beumont PJV, Fraser IS, et al: Body weight, exercise and menstrual status among ballet dancers in training. Br J Obstet Gynaecol 1982;89:507.

Akanade E, Hockaday T: Plasma luteinizing hormone levels in women with thyrotoxicosis. J Endocrinol 1972;53:173.

Alper MM, Garner PR, Seibel MM: Premature ovarian failure: current concepts. J Reprod Med 1986;31:699.

Anderson JL: Women's sports and fitness programs at the U.S. Military Academy. Physician Sportsmed 1979;7:72.

Anonymous: Running, jumping and . . . amenorrhea [editorial]. Lancet 1982;2:638.

Aoring GV: The incidence of anovular cycles in women. J Reprod Fertil Suppl 1967;6:77.

Arman J, Smentek C: Premature ovarian failure. Obstet Gynecol 1985;66:9.

Armhein JA, Meyer WJ, Jones HW, et al: Androgen insensitivity in man: evidence for genetic heterogeneity. Proc Natl Acad Sci U S A 1976;73:891.

Ataya KM, Moghissi K: Chemotherapy-induced premature ovarian failure: mechanisms and prevention. Steroids 1989;54:607.

Ataya K, Pydyn E, Ramahi-Ataya A, Orton CG: Is radiation-induced ovarian failure in rhesus monkeys preventable by luteinizing hormone-releasing hormone agonists? J Clin Endocrinol Metab 1995;80:790.

Azziz R: Reproductive endocrinologic alterations in female asymptomatic obesity. Fertil Steril 1989;52:703.

Azziz R, Dewailly D, Owerbach D: Nonclassical adrenal hyperplasia: current concepts. J Clin Endocrinol Metab 1994;78:810.

Baggish MS, Sze EH: Endometrial ablation: a series of 568 patients treated over an 11 year period. Am J Obstet Gynecol 1996;174:908.

Barbieri RL, Makris A, Randall RW, et al: Insulin stimulates androgen accumulation in incubations of ovarian stroma obtained from women with hyperandrogenism. J Clin Endocrinol Metab 1986; 62:904.

Barbieri RL, Ryan KJ: Hyperandrogenism, insulin resistance, and acanthosis nigricans syndrome: a common endocrinopathy with distinct pathophysiological features. Am J Obstet Gynecol 1983;147:90.

Barbieri RL, Smith S, Ryan KJ: The role of hyperinsulinemia in the pathogenesis of ovarian hyperandrogenism. Fertil Steril 1988;50:197.

Barnes R, Rosenfield RL: The polycystic ovary syndrome: pathogenesis and treatment. Ann Intern Med 1989;110:386.

Barr SI: Women, nutrition and exercise: a review of athletes' intakes and a discussion of energy balance in active women. Prog Food Nutr Sci 1987;11:307.

Barth JG, Cherry CA, Wojnarowska F, Dawber RPR: Spironolactone is an effective and well tolerated systemic antiandrogen therapy for hirsute women. J Clin Endocrinol Metab 1989;68:966.

Bates GW, Whitworth NS: Effect of body weight reduction on plasma androgens in obese infertile women. Fertil Steril 1982;38:406.

Berga SL, Girton LG: The psychoendocrinology of functional hypothalamic amenorrhea. Psychitr Clin North Am 1989;12:105.

Berga SL, Mortola JF, Girton L, et al: Neuroendocrine aberrations in women with functional hypothalamic amenorrhea. J Clin Endocrinol Metab 1989;68:301.

Berthezene F, Forest MG, Grimand JA, et al: Leydig cell agenesis: a cause of male pseudohermaphroditism. N Engl J Med 1976;295:969.

Biller BMK, Federoff HJ, Koenig JI, Klibanski A: Abnormal cortisol secretion and responses to corticotropin-releasing hormone in women with hypothalamic amenorrhea. J Clin Endocrinol Metab 1990;70:311.

Binsbergen CJM, Coelingh Bennink HJT, Odink J, et al: A comparative and longitudinal study on endocrine changes related to ovarian function in patients with anorexia nervosa. J Clin Endocrinol Metab 1990;71:705.

Blackwell RE: Diagnosis and management of prolactinomas. Fertil Steril 1985;43:5.

Brownell KD, Steen SN, Wilmore JH: Weight regulation practices in athletes: analysis of metabolic and health effects. Med Sci Sports Exerc 1987;19:546.

Buckler HM, Evans CA, Mantora H, et al: Gonadotropin, steroid and inhibin levels in women with incipient ovarian failure during anovulatory and ovulatory rebound cycles. J Clin Endocrinol Metab 1991; 72:116.

Bullough VL: Age at menarche: a misunderstanding. Science 1981;213:365.

Bulun SE: Aromatase deficiency in women and men: would you have predicted the phenotypes? J Clin Endocrinol Metab 1996;81:867.

Calabrese LH, Kirkendall DT, Floyd M, et al: Menstrual abnormalities, nutritional patterns, and body composition in female classical ballet dancers. Physician Sportsmed 1983;1:86.

Carr SJ, Reid RL: Ovulation induction with gonadotropin-releasing hormone (GnRH). Semin Reprod Endocrinol 1990;8:174.

Casper RF, Graves G, Reid RL: Objective evidence of menopausal-like hot flushes in a woman with premenstrual syndrome. Fertil Steril 1986;47:341.

Chan CLK, Cameron IT, Findley JK, et al: Oocyte donation and in vitro fertilization for hypergonadotropic hypogonadism: clinical state of the art. Obstet Gynecol Surv 1987;42:350.

Check JH, Nowroozik K, Chase JS, et al: Ovulation induction and pregnancies in 100 consecutive women with hypergonadotropic amenorrhea. Fertil Steril 1990;53:811.

Collier ME, Griffin JE, Wilson JD: Intranuclear binding of [3H] dihydrotestosterone by cultured human fibroblasts. Endocrinology 1978;103:1499.

Conte FA, Grumbach MM, Ito Y, et al: A syndrome of female pseudohermaphroditism, hypergonadotropic hypogonadism and multicystic ovaries associated with missense mutations in the gene encoding aromatase. J Clin Endocrinol Metab 1994;78:1287.

Conte FA, Grumbach MM, Kaplan SL: A diphasic pattern of gonadotropin secretion in patients with the syndrome of gonadal dysgenesis. J Clin Endocrinol Metab 1975;40:670.

Coulam CB, Adamson SC, Annegers JF: Incidence of premature ovarian failure. Obstet Gynecol 1986;67:604.

Counsellor VS, Flor FS: Congenital absence of the vagina. Surg Clin North Am 1957;37:1107.

Covens AL, van der Putten HW, Fyles AW, et al: Laparoscopic ovarian transposition. Eur J Gynecol Oncol 1996;17:177.

Cushing H: The basophil adenomas of the pituitary body and their clinical manifestations (pituitary basophilism). Bull Johns Hopkins Hosp 1932;50:137.

Dale E, Gerlack DH, Wilhite AC: Menstrual dysfunction in distance runners. Obstet Gynecol 1979;54:47.

Damewood MD, Zacur HA, Hoffman GJ, Rock JA: Circulating antiovarian antibodies in premature ovarian failure. Obstet Gynecol 1986;68:850.

Davies MC, Guleki B, Jacobs HS: Osteoporosis in Turner's syndrome and other forms of primary amenorrhea. Clin Endocrinol 1995;43:741.

DeCherney AH, Diamond MP, Lavy G, Polan ML: Endometrial ablation for intractable uterine bleeding: hysteroscopic resection. Obstet Gynecol 1987;70:668.

Drew FL: The epidemiology of secondary amenorrhea. J Chronic Dis 1961;14:396.

Drew FL, Stifel EN: Secondary amenorrhea among young women entering religious life. Obstet Gynecol 1968;32:47.

Durschke DJ, Weiss G, Knobil E: Sexual maturation in the female rhesus monkey and the development of estrogen-induced gonadotropic hormone release. Endocrinology 1974;94:198.

Ehrmann DA, Rosenfield RL: An endocrinologic approach to the patient with hirsutism. J Clin Endocrinol Metab 1990;71:1.

Eidering JA, Nay MF, Hoberg LM, et al: Hormonal regulation of prostaglandin production by rhesus monkey endometrium. J Clin Endocrinol Metab 1990;71:596.

Eil C: Weekly clinicopathological exercises: Case 13-1990. N Engl J Med 1990;322:917.

Eil C, Loriaux DL, Schulman JD: Androgen resistance and sexual ambiguity. Contemp Obstet Gynecol 1981;17:141.

Emans SJ, Grace E, Hoffer FA, et al: Estrogen deficiency in adolescents and young adults: impact on bone mineral content and effects of estrogen replacement therapy. Obstet Gynecol 1990;76:585.

Ewer RW: Familial monotropic pituitary gonadotropin insufficiency. J Clin Endocrinol Metab 1968;28:783.

Farber M, Mitchell GW Jr, Marchant DJ: Congenital atresia of the uterine cervix: long term results. Trans Am Gynecol Obstet Soc 1982;1:113.

Fedele L, Dorta M, Brioschi D, et al: Magnetic resonance imaging in Mayer-Rokitansky-Kuster-Hauser syndrome. Obstet Gynecol 1990;76:593.

Ferriman D, Gallwey JD: Clinical measurement of body hair growth in women. J Clin Endocrinol Metab 1961;21:1440.

Foster DL: Luteinizing hormone and progesterone secretion during sexual maturation of the rhesus monkey: short luteal phases during the initial menstrual cycles. Biol Reprod 1977;17:584.

Fox H: Sex cord-stromal tumours of the ovary. J Pathol 1985;145:127.

Frank RT: The formation of an artificial vagina without operation. Am J Obstet Gynecol 1938;35:1053.

Frank S: Regulation of prolactin secretion by estrogens: physiological and pathological significance. Clin Sci 1983;65:457.

Frank S, Jacobs HS, Hull MGR: The oral contraceptive and hyperprolactinemic amenorrhea. In Cammani F, Mulles EE (eds): Pituitary Hyperfunction, Physiopathology and Clinical Aspects. New York: Raven Press, 1984:175.

Friedman A, DeFazio J, DeCherney A: Severe obstetric complications after aggressive treatment of Asherman syndrome. Obstet Gynecol 1986;67:864.

Frisch RE, Schiff I: Comparing risks in athletes and nonathletes. Contemp Obstet Gynecol 1986;28:15.

Garfinkel PE, Lin E, Goering P, et al: Should amenorrhea be necessary for the diagnosis of anorexia nervosa? Evidence from a Canadian community sample. Br J Psychiatry 1996;168:500.

Garner PR: The effect of body weight on menstrual function. Curr Probl Obstet Gynecol 1984;7:1.

Genazzani AD, Petraglia F, Fabbri G, et al: Evidence of luteinizing hormone secretion in hypothalamic amenorrhea associated with weight loss. Fertil Steril 1990;54:222.

Girton LG: The psychoendocrinology of functional hypothalamic amenorrhea. Psychiatr Clin North Am 1989;12:105.

Goldstein DP, DeCholnoky C, Emans SJ, Levanthal JM: Laparoscopy in the diagnosis and management of pelvic pain in adolescents. J Reprod Med 1980;33:25.

Goldzier JW, Green JA: The polycystic ovary. I. Clinical and histologic features. J Clin Endocrinol Metab 1962;23:325.

Greenblatt E, Casper RF: Endocrine changes following laparoscopic ovarian cautery in polycystic ovary syndrome. Am J Obstet Gynecol 1987;157:279.

Griffin JE, Wilson JD: The syndromes of androgen resistance. N Engl J Med 1980;302:198.

Halbert DR, Christian DC: Amenorrhea following oral contraceptives. Obstet Gynecol 1969;34:161.

Halyard MY, Cornella JL, Grado GL, Rizzo NR: Prolonged amenorrhea associated with total nodal irradiation for Hodgkin's disease. J Natl Med Assoc 1996;88(6):391.

Harlass FE, Plymate SR, Fariss BL, et al: Weight loss is associated with correction of gonadotropin and sex steroid abnormalities in the obese anovulatory woman. Fertil Steril 1984;42:649.

Hartog M, Hull MGR: Hyperprolactinemia: common and treatable [editorial] BMJ 1988;297:701.

Healy DL, Hodgen GD: The endocrinology of human endometrium. Obstet Gynecol Surv 1983;38:509.

Helfer EL, Miller JL, Rose LI: Side effects of spironolactone therapy in the hirsute woman. J Clin Endocrinol Metab 1988;66:208.

Hens L, Devroey P, Van Woesberghe L, et al: Chromosome studies and fertility treatment in women with ovarian failure. Clin Genet 1989;36:81.

Highet R: Athletic amenorrhea: an update on aetiology, complications and management. Sports Med 1989;7:82.

Hill D, Maher P: Treatment of menorrhagia by endometrial ablation. Med J Aust 1990;152:564.

Ho PC, Tang GWK, Ku KH, et al: Immunologic studies in patients with premature ovarian failure. Obstet Gynecol 1988;71:622.

Hoff JT, Patterson RH Jr: Craniopharyngiomas in children and adults. J Neurosurg 1972;36:299.

Howlett TA, Wass JAH, Grossman A, et al: Prolactinomas presenting as primary amenorrhea and delayed or arrested puberty: response to medical therapy. Clin Endocrinol 1989;30:131.

Huggins GR, Cullins VE: Fertility after contraception or abortion. Fertil Steril 1990; 54:559.

Hutchinson-Williams KA, Decherney AH: Pathogenesis and treatment of polycystic ovary disease. Int J Fertil 1987;32:421.

Hutter AM, Kayhoe DE: Adrenal cortical carcinoma: clinical features of 138 patients. Am J Med 1966;41:572.

Immura H: Ectopic hormone syndromes. Clin Endocrinol Metab 1980;9:235.

Ingram JM: The bicycle seat stool in the treatment of vaginal agenesis and stenosis: a preliminary report. Am J Obstet Gynecol 1981;140:867.

Jackson RL: Ecological breastfeeding and child spacing. Clin Paediatr 1988;27:373.

Johnson TR Jr, Peterson EP: Gonadotropin induced pregnancy following "premature ovarian failure." Fertil Steril 1979;31:351.

Johnston CC, Longcope C: Premenopausal bone loss—a risk factor of osteoporosis [editorial]. N Engl J Med 1990;323:1271.

Jones GS: Corpus luteum: composition and function. Fertil Steril 1990;54:21.

Jones JR, Kemmann E: Olfacto-genital dysplasia in the female. Obstet Gynecol Ann 1976;5:443.

Kallmann FJ, Schonfeld WA, Barrora SE: The genetic aspects of primary eunuchoidism. Am J Metab Defic 1944;48:203.

Kapcala LP, Lakshmanan MC: Thoracic stimulation and prolactin secretion. J Endocrinol Invest 1989;12:815.

Kater CE, Biglieri EG: Disorders of steroid 17-alphahydroxylase deficiency. Endocrinol Metab Clin North Am 1994;23:341.

Kelly AC, Jewelewicz R: Alternate regimens for ovulation induction in polycystic ovarian disease. Fertil Steril 1990;54:195.

King CR, Magenis E, Bennett S: Pregnancy and the Turner syndrome. Obstet Gynecol 1978;52:617.

Klachko DM, Winder N, Burns TW, White JE: Traumatic hypopituitarism occurring before puberty: Survival 35 years untreated. J Clin Endocrinol Metab 1968;28:1768.

Kleinberg DL, Noel G, Frantz AG: Galactorrhea: a study of 235 cases. N Engl J Med 1977;296:589.

Klibanski A, Greenspan SL: Increase in bone mass after treatment of hyperprolactinemic amenorrhea. N Engl J Med 1986;315:542.

Klibanski A, Neer R, Beitins IZ, et al: Decreased bone density in hyperprolactinemic women. N Engl J Med 1980;303:1511.

Krauss CM, Turksoy RN, Atkins L, et al: Familial premature ovarian failure due to an interstitial deletion of the long arm of the X chromosome. N Engl J Med 1987;317:125.

Kupfer SR, Quigley CA, French FS: Male pseudohermaphroditism. Semin Perinatol 1992;16:319.

Larsson-Cohn U: The length of the first three menstrual cycles after combined oral contraceptive treatment. Acta Obstet Gynecol Scand 1969;48:416.

Laufer MR, Floor AE, Parsons KE, et al: Hormone testing in women with adult onset amenorrhea. Gynecol Obstetr Invest 1995;40:200.

LeBarbera AR, Miller MM, Ober C, et al: Autoimmune etiology in premature ovarian failure. Am J Reprod Immunol Microbiol 1988;16:115.

Leyendecker G, Wildt L: From physiology to clinics . . . 20 years experience with pulsatile GnRH. Eur J Obstet Gynaecol Reprod Biol 1996;65(Suppl)S3.

Lieblich JM, Rogol AD, White BJ, et al: Syndrome of anosmia with hypogonadotropic gonadism. Am J Med 1982;73:506.

Lobo RA, Goebelsmann U: Adult manifestations of congenital adrenal hyperplasia due to incomplete 21-hydroxylase deficiency mimicking polycystic ovarian disease. Am J Obstet Gynecol 1980;138:720.

Loucks AB, Mortola JF, Girton L, et al: Alterations in the hypothalamic-pituitary-ovarian and the hypothalamic-pituitary-adrenal axis in athletic women. J Clin Endocrinol Metab 1989; 68:401.

Lutjen PJ, Findlay JK, Trounson AO, et al: Effect on plasma gonadotropins of cyclic steroid replacement in women with premature ovarian failure. J Clin Endocrinol Metab 1986;62:419.

March CM, Israel R: Gestational outcome following hysteroscopic lysis of adhesions. Fertil Steril 1981;36:455.

Martin K, Santoro N, Hall J, et al: Management of ovulatory disorders with pulsatile gonadotropin-releasing hormone. J Clin Endocrinol Metab 1990;71:1081A.

Mattison DR, Evans MI, Schwimmer WB, et al: Familial premature ovarian failure. Am J Hum Genet 1984;36:1342.

Mausfield MJ, Evans SJ: Anorexia nervosa, athletics, and amenorrhea. Pediatr Clin North Am 1989;36:533.

McIndoe A: The treatment of congenital absence and obliterative conditions of the vagina. Br J Plast Surg 1950;2:254.

Meyer WR, McCoy MC, Fritz MA: Combined abdominal-perineal sonography to assist in diagnosis of transverse vaginal septum. Obstet Gynecol 1995;85:882.

Miller WL, Kaplan SL, Grumbach MM: Child abuse as a cause of post traumatic hypopituitarism. N Engl J Med 1980;302:724.

Morales AJ, Laughlin GA, Butzow T, et al: Insulin, somatotropic, and luteinizing hormone axes in lean and obese women with polycystic ovary syndrome: common and distinct features. J Clin Endocrinol Metab 1996;81:2854.

Morris JM: The syndrome of testicular feminization in male pseudohermaphrodites. Am J Obstet Gynecol 1953;65:1192.

Morris JM, Mahesh VB: Further observations on the syndrome of "testicular feminization." Am J Obstet Gynecol 1963;87:731.

Mulvihill JJ, Wade WM, Miller RW: Gonadoblastoma in dysgenetic gonads with a Y chromosome. Lancet 1975;1:863.

Muram D, Dewhurst J: Inheritance of intersex disorders. Can Med Assoc J 1984;130:121.

Nakamura S, Douchi R, Oki T, et al: Relationship between sonographic endometrial thickness and progestin-induced withdrawal bleeding. Obstet Gynecol 1996;87:722.

Napheys GH: The Physical Life of Woman: Advice to the Maiden, Wife and Mother. Philadelphia: George MacLean, 1874:87.

Nattiv A, Agostini R, Drinkwater B, Yeager KK: The female athlete triad: the interrelationship of disordered eating, amenorrhea, and osteoporosis. Clin Sports Med 1994;13:405.

Nestler JE, Barlascini CO, Matt DW, et al: Suppression of serum insulin by diazoxide reduces serum testosterone levels in obese women with polycystic ovary syndrome. J Clin Endocrinol Metab 1989a;68:1027.

Nestler JE, Clore JN, Blackard WG: The central role of obesity (hyperinsulinemia) in the pathogenesis of polycystic ovary syndrome. Am J Obstet Gynecol 1989b;161:1095.

Nestler JE, Singh R, Matt DW, et al: Suppression of serum insulin level by diazoxide does not alter serum testosterone or sex hormone binding globulin levels in healthy non obese women. Am J Obstet Gynecol 1990;163:1243.

New MI: Steroid 21-hydroxylase deficiency (congenital adrenal hyperplasia). Am J Med 1995;98:25.

Orrell KGS, Wrixon W, Irwin AC: The clinical prediction of ovulation. Nova Scotia Med Bull 1980;59:119.

Ott SM: Attainment of peak bone mass [editorial]. J Clin Endocrinol Metab 1990;71:1082A.

Parks JS: Intersex. In Kaplan SA (ed): Clinical Pediatric and Adolescent Endocrinology. Toronto: WB Saunders Company, 1982: 339.

Pasquali R, Antenucci D, Casimirri F, et al: Clinical and hormonal characteristics of obese amenorrheic hyperandrogenic women before and after weight loss. J Clin Endocrinol Metab 1989;68: 173.

Pettersson F, Fries H, Nillius JS: Epidemiology of secondary amenorrhea. Am J Obstet Gynecol 1973;117:80.

Pinsonneault O, Goldstein DP: Obstructing malformations of the uterus and vagina. Fertil Steril 1985;44:241.

Pirke KM, Schweiger U, Laessle R, et al: Dieting influences the menstrual cycle: vegetarian versus non vegetarian diet. Fertil Steril 1986;46:1083.

Poretsky L, Kalin MF: The gonadotropic function of insulin. Endocrin Rev 1987;8:132.

Portnondo JA, Barral A, Melchos JC, et al: Chromosomal compliments in primary gonadal failure. Obstet Gynecol 1984;64: 757.

Prior JC: Luteal phase defects and anovulation: adaptive alterations occurring with conditioning exercise. Reprod Endocrinol 1985;3:27.

Prior JC, Vigna YM, Schechter MT, et al: Spinal bone loss and ovulatory disturbances. N Engl J Med 1990;323:1221.

Punch MR, Ansbacher R: Autogenic masculinization. Am J Obstet Gynecol 1990;163:114.

Rarick LD, Shangold MM, Ahmed SW: Cervical mucus and serum estradiol as predictors of response to progestin challenge. Fertil Steril 1990;54:353.

Rebar RW, Connolly HV: Clinical features of young women with hypergonadotropic amenorrhea. Fertil Steril 1990;53:804.

Rebar RW, Erickson GF, Coulam CB: Premature ovarian failure. In Riddick D, Gondos B (eds): Pathology of Infertility. New York: Thieme Medical Publishers Inc, 1987:123.

Reid RL, Quigley ME, Yen SSC: Pituitary apoplexy: a review. Arch Neurol 1985;42:712.

Reid RL, Van Vugt DA: Neuroendocrine events that regulate the menstrual cycle. Contemp Obstet Gynecol 1987a;30:147.

Reid RL, Van Vugt DA: Weight related changes in reproductive function. Fertil Steril 1987b;48:905.

Reid RL, Van Vugt DA: Hair loss in women. Obstet Gynecol Surv 1988;31:135.

Reindollar RH, Noval M, Tho SP, et al: Adult onset amenorrhea: study of 262 patients. Am J Obstet Gynecol 1986;155:531.

Rencken ML, Chestnut CH, Drinkwater BL: Bone density at multiple skeletal sites in amenorrheic athletics. JAMA 1996;276:238.

Rock JA, Reeves LA, Retto J, et al: Success following vaginal creation for mullerian agenesis. Fertil Steril 1983;39:809.

Rock JA, Zacur Hal, Dluget AM, et al: Pregnancy success following surgical correction of imperforate hymen and complete transverse vaginal septum. Obstet Gynecol 1982;59:448.

Rockwell JC, Sorensen AM, Baker S, et al: Weight training decreases vertebral bone density in premenopausal women: a prospective study. J Clin Endocrinol Metab 1990;71:988.

Roger J: Menstruation and systemic disease. N Engl J Med 1958; 259:676.

Rosenfeld DL, Garcia CR: A comparison of endometrial histology with simultaneous plasma progesterone determinations in infertile women. Fertil Steril 1976;27:1256.

Rosenfield RL: Diagnosis and management of delayed puberty. J Clin Endocrinol Metab 1990;70:559.

Sanborn CF, Martin BJ, Wagner WW: Is athletic amenorrhea specific to runners? Am J Obstet Gynecol 1982;143:859.

Santen RJ, Paulsen CA: Hypogonadotropic eunuchoidism. I: Clinical study of the mode of inheritance. J Clin Endocrinol Metab 1973;36:47.

Santoro N, Filicori M, Crowley WF: Hypogonadotropin disorders in men and women: diagnosis and therapy with pulsatile gonadotropin releasing hormone. Endocr Rev 1986;7:11.

Schenker HG, Margolioth EJ: Intrauterine adhesions: an updated appraisal. Fertil Steril 1982;37:593.

Schilsky RL, Lewis BJ, Sherins RJ, et al: Gonadal dysfunction in patients receiving chemotherapy for cancer. Ann Intern Med 1980;93:109.

Schlechte JA, Sherman B, Martin R: Bone density in amenorrheic women with and without hyperprolactinemia. J Clin Endocrinol Metab 1983;56:1120.

Schwartz M, Imperato-McGinaley J, Peterson RE, et al: Male pseudohermaphroditism secondary to an abnormality in Leydig cell differentiation. J Clin Endocrinol Metab 1981;53:123.

Shangold MM, Levine HS: The effect of marathon training upon menstrual function. JAMA 1982;143:682.

Sherman BM, Korenman SG: Hormonal characteristics of the human menstrual cycle throughout reproductive life. J Clin Invest 1975;55:699.

Sherman RP: Amenorrhea after treatment with oral contraceptives. Lancet 1966;2:1110.

Siegler AM, Valle RF: Therapeutic hysteroscopic procedures. Fertil Steril 1988;50:685.

Siris ES, Leventhal BG, Vaitukaitis JL: Effects of childhood leukemia and chemotherapy on puberty and reproductive function in girls. N Engl J Med 1976;294:1143.

Sisam DA, Sheehan JP, Sheeler LR: The natural history of untreated microprolactinomas. Fertil Steril 1987;48:67.

Smith NJ: Excessive weight loss and food aversion in athletes simulating anorexia nervosa. Pediatrics 1980;66:139.

Snow RC, Schneider JL, Barbieri RL: High dietary fiber and low saturated fat intakes among oligomenorrheic undergraduates. Fertil steril 1990;54:632.

Speroff L: The effect of exercise on the menstrual cycle. Postgrad Obstet Gynecol 1984;4:1.

Speroff L, Redwine DB: Exercise and menstrual function. Physician Sportsmed 1980;8:42.

Stein IF, Leventhal ML: Amenorrhea associated with bilateral polycystic ovaries. Am J Obstet Gynecol 1935;29:181.

Stewart DE, Robinson GE, Goldbloom DS, Wright C: Infertility and eating disorders. Am J Obstet Gynecol 1990;163:1196.

Surrey ES, Cedars MI: The effect of gonadotropin suppression on the induction of ovulation in premature ovarian failure. Fertil Steril 1989;52:36.

Szmukler GI: Treatment of eating disorders. Med J Aust 1989;151:583.

Tanaka T, Sakuragi N, Fujimoto S, et al: hMG therapy in patients with hypergonadotropic ovarian anovulation: one pregnancy case report and ovulation rate. Int J Fertil 1982;27:100.

Tanner JM, Davies PWS: Pubertal data for growth velocity charts [reply]. J Pediatr 1986;109:564.

Thomas R, Reid RL: Thyroid disease and reproductive dysfunction. Obstet Gynecol 1987;70:789.

Townsend DE, Richart RM, Paskowitz RA, Woolfork RE: "Roller ball" coagulation of the endometrium. Obstet Gynecol 1990;76:310.

Troche V, Hernandez E: Neoplasia arising in dysgenetic gonads. Obstet Gynecol Survey 1986;41:74.

Turner HH: A syndrome of infantilism, congenital webbed neck and cubitus valgus. Endocrinology 1938;22:566.

Vasquez SB: Mullerian duct agenesis and other congenital anomalies. J Adolesc Health Care 1989;2:289.

Walsh PC, Madden JD, Harrod MJ, et al: Familial incomplete male pseudohermaphroditism type 2: decreased dihydrotestosterone formation in pseudovaginal perineoscrotal hypospadias. N Engl J Med 1974;291:944.

Warren MP: The effects of exercise on pubertal progression and reproductive function in girls. J Clin Endocrinol Metab 1980;51:1150.

Webb JL, Millan DL, Stolz CJ: Gynecological survey of American female athletes competing at the Montreal Olympic Games. J Sport Med 1979;19:405.

Weibel MA, Majno G: Peritoneal adhesions and their relationship to abdominal surgery. Am J Surg 1973;126:345.

Weiner H: Psychoendocrinology of anorexia nervosa. Psychiatr Clin North Am 1989;12:187.

White PC, New MI, Dupont B: Congenital adrenal hyperplasia (1). N Engl J Med 1987a;316:1519.

White PC, New MI, Dupont B: Congenital adrenal hyperplasia (2). N Engl J Med 1987b;316:1580.

Wilmore JH: Body composition in sport and exercise: directions for future research. Med Sci Sports Exerc 1983;15:21.

Yamamora DLR, Reid RL: Psychological stress and the reproductive system. Semin Reprod Endocrinol 1990;8:65.

Yen SSC: Neuroendocrine regulation of the menstrual cycle. Hosp Pract 1979;3:83.

Yen SSC: Reproductive strategy in women. In Roland R (ed): Neuroendocrine Basis of Endogenous Contraception. Amsterdam: Excerpta Medica, 1988:231.

Zhang J, Young RH, Arseneau J, et al: Ovarian stromal tumours containing lutein or Leydig cells: a clinicopathological analysis of fifty cases. Int J Gynecol Pathol 1982;1:270.

26

Pediatric and Adolescent Gynecology

Joseph S. Sanfilippo

P ediatric and adolescent gynecology is a unique discipline that involves specific problems of the immature and maturing female reproductive system. The evaluation and management of problems in this population is age dependent and requires an understanding of developmental physiology and special examination techniques specific to each stage of pubertal development, beginning with the neonate and extending throughout childhood and into young womanhood.

PEDIATRIC AND ADOLESCENT GYNECOLOGIC EXAMINATION

The first gynecologic examination plays an important role in the reproductive health of young women. An initial positive experience of the examination as a "healthy" event may encourage these patients to acknowledge future gynecologic concerns, symptoms, and needs.

The pediatric adolescent gynecologic examination should promote the feeling of autonomy and control (Baldwin and Landa, 1995). The initial history should be taken with the patient fully clothed. Along with appropriate medical history, an assessment of the patient and her family's needs and expectations can be completed. At the same time, information can be gathered regarding the chief complaint from both the parents and the patient. Time spent talking directly to the patient will help to establish a rapport and enhance the physician's ability to complete a successful examination. Children are more likely to comply with examinations when the physician explains why the examination needs to be done and that the examination will not hurt. It is therefore important to introduce the concept and procedure of the examination before proceeding. The patient can be involved in the examination process by asking if she would like to have her accompanying adult present for the examination. Most children and teens up to age 12 to 13 prefer to be examined with a family member present, whereas older teens prefer that a nurse rather than a family member be present (Phillips et al, 1981).

Examination Techniques and Findings by Age

The hormonal milieu of different ages alters genital anatomy and reflects the reproductive physiologic state of the patient. Clinicians should recognize the various hormonal patterns, presenting complaints, and examination techniques seen in various age groups.

Birth to 8 Weeks

In the first 8 weeks of life, the vulvovaginal epithelium reflects the waning effects of residual maternal estrogen. This results in thickened, enlarged labia minora; a prominent clitoris; and thickened, prominent, estrogenized hymenal folds. Maternal estrogen exposure often stimulates a mucoid vaginal discharge and even vaginal bleeding with acute withdrawal of maternal estrogen, but these effects should wane by 2 weeks (Fig. 26–1). Persistent vaginal discharge and vaginal bleeding beyond 2 weeks of life are abnormal and require evaluation (Gidwani, 1987).

Optimal positioning will allow good visualization of vulvar structures while minimizing trauma to the patient. Appropriate positioning for newborns is either the frog-leg position (Fig. 26–2) or the supine position in the mother's lap. In the latter position, the mother holds the infant's thighs flexed against its abdomen (Fig. 26–3). In both positions, the use of labial separation or traction will assist the examiner in visualizing the vestibule (Figs. 26–4 and 26–5). With labial traction, the labia are grasped between the examiner's thumbs and index fingers and pulled slightly laterally, downward, and out toward the examiner. This maneuver places tension on the hymenal tissue by pulling the external structures away and allowing the hymen to "stand up" in the vestibule. In this age group, abnormal conditions are usually limited to vulvar presentations and invasive examinations are not usually necessary. In cases of ambiguous genitalia, a more thorough internal examination may best be completed by a rectal exam-

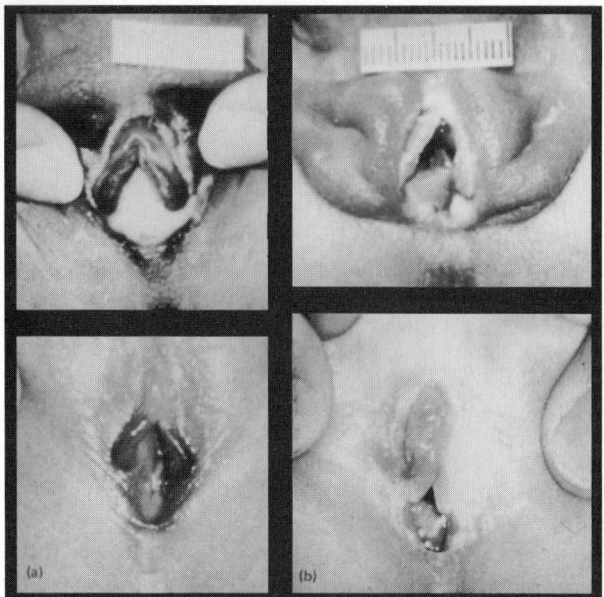

Figure 26–1
Alterations in the external genital appearances in two female infants. Each upper photograph was taken on the second day of life and the corresponding lower photograph was taken at 3 months. Note the pronounced vulvar congestion and edema in the upper photographs that have disappeared 3 months later. (From Dewhurst SJ: Patterns of childhood and adolescent gynecology. In: Practical Pediatric and Adolescent Gynecology. New York: Marcel Dekker, 1980:1, with permission.)

ination with a well-lubricated fifth digit to assess for the presence or absence of a uterus. The exposure to maternal estrogen will make the uterus prominent and palpable. Internal anatomy can be further delineated with the completion of a genitogram. These radiographic studies are completed by placing a catheter into each perineal orifice and instilling radiopaque dye, thereby outlining the urogenital sinus and rectal cavity on a lateral film.

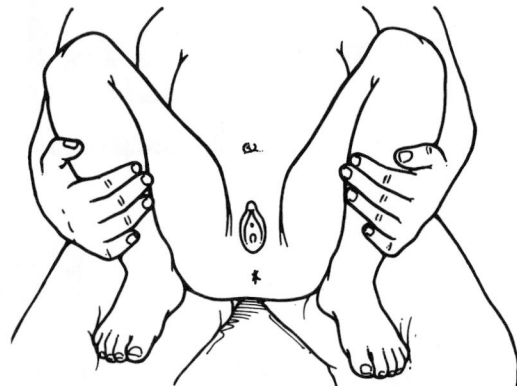

Figure 26–3
Frog-leg position in mother's lap. (From Baldwin DD, Landa HM: Common problems in pediatric gynecology. Urol Clin North Am 1995;22:161, with permission.)

Eight Weeks to Prepuberty (8 Years)

This is a unique reproductive time when the female is exposed to neither maternal nor endogenous hormones. As a result, vulvar structures and the labia majora are flat and thin, and the vaginal epithelium is atrophic, which results in little protection from infection of the vestibular mucosa. Therefore, most pediatric gynecologic presenting complaints will be about growth, development, inflammation, lesions, or reactions of the skin, the epithelium of the external genitalia, and, to a less degree, the epithelium of the vaginal canal. In addition, the cervix, uterus, and fallopian tubes are relatively hormonally inert and underdeveloped; therefore, in this population they are usually evaluated only when a neoplasm grows to a pathologically obvious size.

An examination in this age group for gynecologic complaints should begin with an overall assessment, including measurement of height and weight with

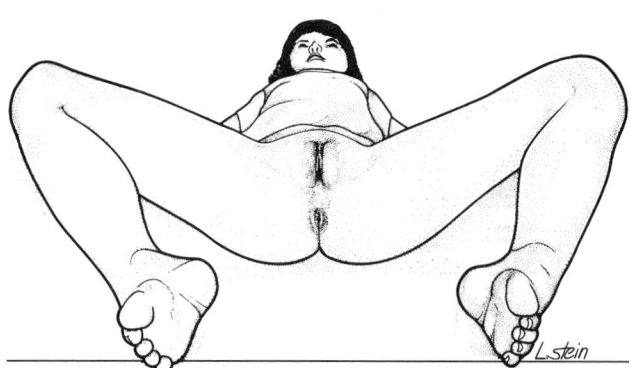

Figure 26–2
Frog-leg position. (From Giardino AP, Findel MA, Giardino ER, et al: Physical examination and laboratory specimens. In Giardino AP, Findel MA, Giardino ER, et al [eds]: A Practical Guide to the Evaluation of Sexual Abuse in the Prepubertal Child. Newbury Park, CA: Sage Publications, 1992:29, with permission.)

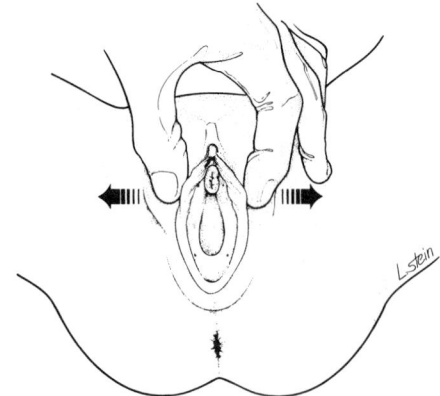

Figure 26–4
Labial separation. (From Giardino AP, Findel MA, Giardino ER, et al: Physical examination and laboratory specimens. In Giardino AP, Findel MA, Giardino ER, et al [eds]: A Practical Guide to the Evaluation of Sexual Abuse in the Prepubertal Child. Newbury Park, CA: Sage Publications, 1992:29, with permission.)

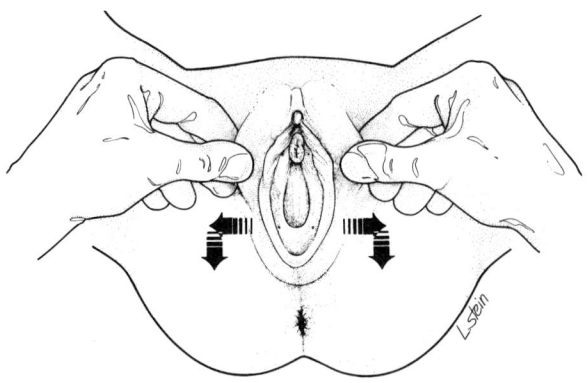

Figure 26−5
Labial traction. (From Giardino AP, Findel MA, Giardino ER, et al: Physical examination and laboratory specimens. In Giardino AP, Findel MA, Giardino ER, et al [eds]: A Practical Guide to the Evaluation of Sexual Abuse in the Prepubertal Child. Newbury Park, CA: Sage Publications, 1992:29, with permission.)

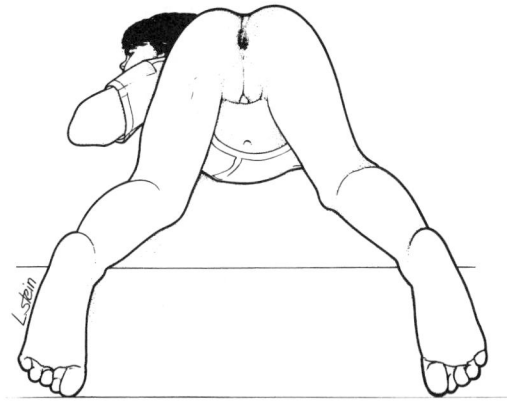

Figure 26−7
Knee−chest position. (From Giardino AP, Findel MA, Giardino ER, et al: Physical examination and laboratory specimens. In Giardino AP, Findel MA, Giardino ER, et al [eds]: A Practical Guide to the Evaluation of Sexual Abuse in the Prepubertal Child. Newbury Park, Sage Publications, 1992:29, with permission.)

appropriate plotting on growth curves. A quick "head-to-toe" assessment may aid in identifying possible endocrine abnormalities or the presence of trauma. The time spent with the patient, in addition to building further confidence and rapport, helps her to see the genital examination in the context of the entire physical examination.

These patients should be positioned for the genital examination using the frog-leg position (supine or in the parent's lap), the dorsolithotomy position with the patient's feet in stirrups or on an examiner's lap,

or with the patient sitting in the parent's lap with child's legs draped over the parent's thighs (Fig. 26−6). The knee−chest position (Fig. 26−7) may be used as an alternative way to visualize the vestibule and may provide better visualization of the hymen. In this position, the patient's face and chest rest on the examination table and the buttocks are in the air. To best visualize the vestibular structures, the examiner's thumbs should be placed at the junction of the labia majora and the buttocks and should lift upward and outward (Fig. 26−8). This will elevate the external vulvar structures and allow the hymen to "fall" into view. A hymen not easily visualized in the supine position may better be seen in the knee−chest position (Fig. 26−9). Additionally, with magnification and a relaxed patient, the lower vagina will be visualized easily in this position. The knee−

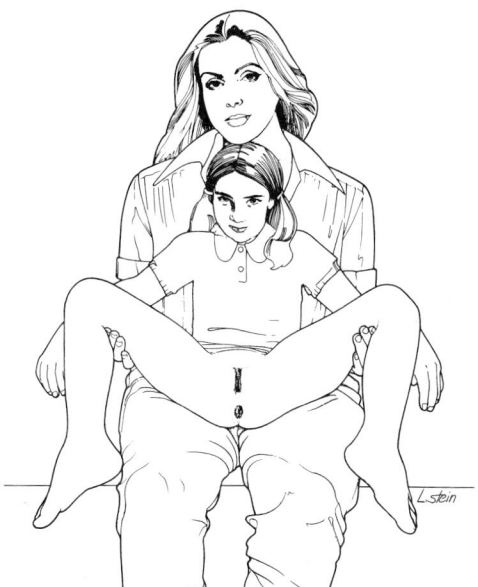

Figure 26−6
Dorsolithotomy position in parent's lap. (From Giardino AP, Findel MA, Giardino ER, et al: Physical examination and laboratory specimens. In Giardino AP, Findel MA, Giardino ER, et al [eds]: A Practical Guide to the Evaluation of Sexual Abuse in the Prepubertal Child. Newbury Park, CA: Sage Publications, 1992:29, with permission.)

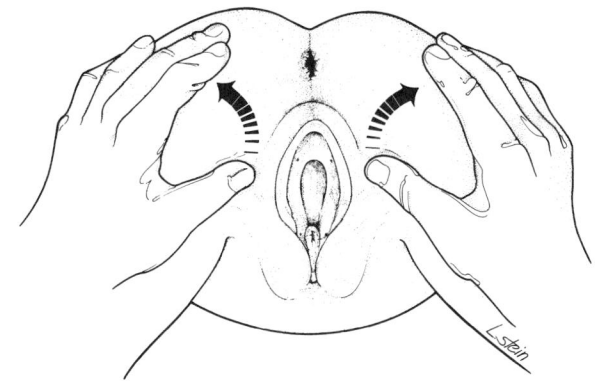

Figure 26−8
Examiner's hand placement for knee−chest evaluation. (From Giardino AP, Findel MA, Giardino ER, et al: Physical examination and laboratory specimens. In Giardino AP, Findel MA, Giardino ER, et al [eds]: A Practical Guide to the Evaluation of Sexual Abuse in the Prepubertal Child. Newbury Park, CA: Sage Publications, 1992:29, with permission.)

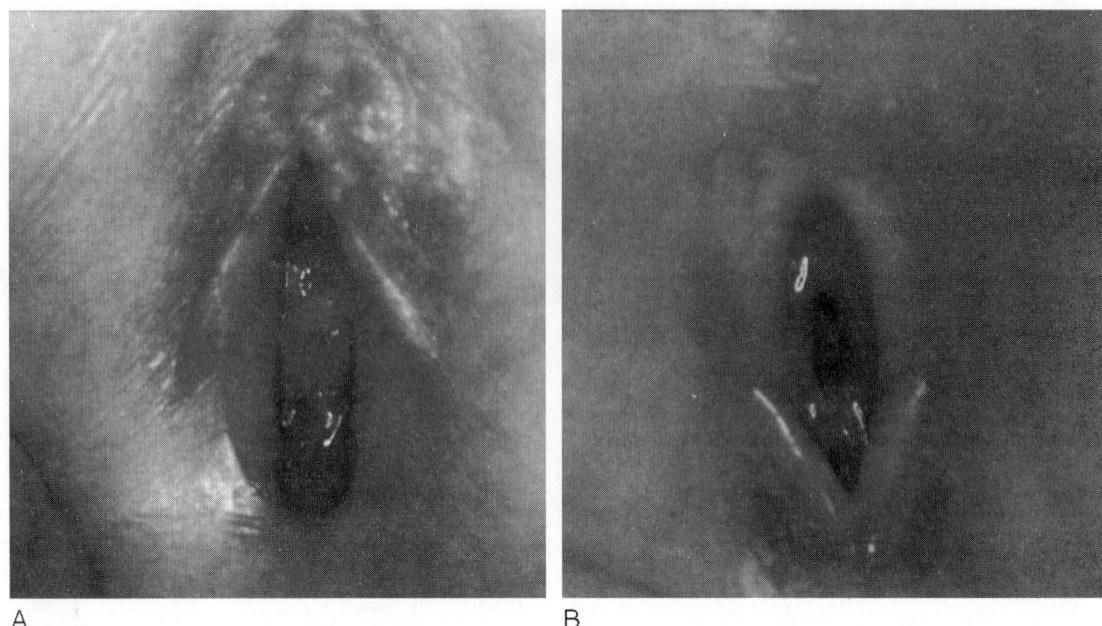

A   B

Figure 26–9
A, Hymen not well visualized in 18-month-old patient in supine position. B, Annular circumferential hymen easily seen in 18-month-old patient seen in knee–chest position. (From Chadwick DL, Berkowitz CD, Kerns DL, et al: Normal findings. In Chadwick DL, Berkowitz CD, Kerns, et al [eds]: Color Atlas of Child Sexual Abuse. Chicago, Year Book Medical Publishers, 1989:19, with permission.)

chest position can be useful in evaluating patients who may have a foreign body.

While the patient is positioned correctly, an assessment of pubic hair, external genital anatomy, clitoral size, hymenal configuration, signs of estrogenization, and perineal hygiene should be completed. The examiner will need to document the presence of each vulvar structure seen and provide some descriptive clues in the medical records from which future examining physicians can draw conclusions. It is helpful to document the location of abnormalities as on a clock face along with examination position (Fig. 26–10). An assessment of hymenal configuration is important in these young patients. A review of 1139 consecutive newborn females revealed that females are born with hymenal tissue (Jenny et al, 1987). After birth, various configurations have been noted, including crescentic, annular, or circumferential; redundant or fimbriated; and septate, microperforate or sleeve-like, or imperforate (Figs. 26–11 through 26–14). Bumps or cysts of the hymen may be seen between the 3- and 9-o'clock positions when visualized in the supine position (Figs. 26–9 and 26–15). In contrast, clefts, interruptions, or lacerations of the hymen between the 3- and 9-o'clock positions are abnormal findings and are worthy of documentation because they may indicate penetrating trauma to the vestibule area. The size of the hymenal opening is quite variable and depends on hymenal configuration, position, age of the patient, and patient relaxation. An opening greater than 1 cm in a prepubertal female combined with a posterior rim measurement of less than 2 mm may indicate penetrative trauma to the area (Fig. 26–16).

Adolescents

Adolescent girls are beginning to have anatomically and physiologically adult genitalia. Despite their similar hormonal milieu, there is a wide range of psychosocial sexual development. In this patient population, the examining physician needs appropriate interpersonal skills and sensitivity to assess the different needs of each patient based on her individual psychosocial development, maturity, and level of understanding. In preparing adolescents for their first pelvic exam, acknowledge feelings of anxiety with phrases like "Some young girls I see are worried about their first pelvic exam, that it will hurt or be embarrassing." Then explain about the examination using supplemental diagrams of external genitalia. The new computer CD-ROM "Patient Advise and Consent" (PACE) program has an introduction to the first pelvic examination with excellent graphics and explanations of pelvic anatomy. Use of such material can give the patient control and reduce fear. Encouraging the patient to participate in the examination by visualizing with a mirror or by showing her the speculum before its use may also decrease anxiety. Although in a virginal female with no problems an examination of the external genitalia is usually sufficient, a small Huffman speculum ($^1/_2$ × $4^1/_4$'') is almost always comfortable even in virginal patients if an internal examination is needed. The

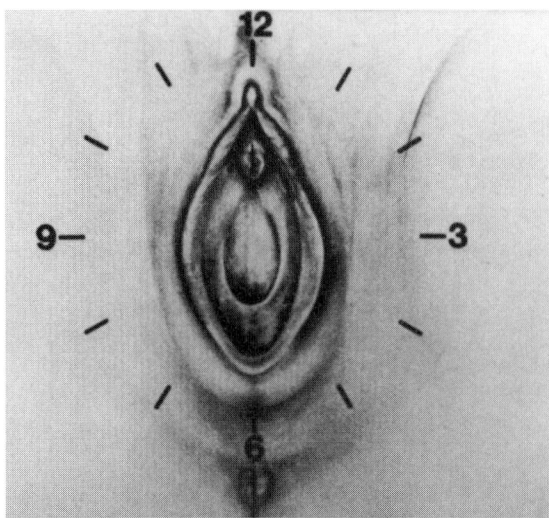

Figure 26-10
Demonstration of clock-face technique to document genital findings. (From Giardino AP, Findel MA, Giardino ER, et al: Physical examination and laboratory specimens. In Giardino AP, Findel MA, Giardino ER, et al [eds]: A Practical Guide to the Evaluation of Sexual Abuse in the Prepubertal Child. Newbury Park, CA: Sage Publications, 1992:29, with permission.)

patient will be able to see that this speculum is no wider than a tampon or her finger. Indications for a pelvic or bimanual rectoabdominal examination are listed in Table 26–1. Some pediatric gynecologists recommend an initial pelvic examination as part of well-child care in the immediate postmenarchal pa-

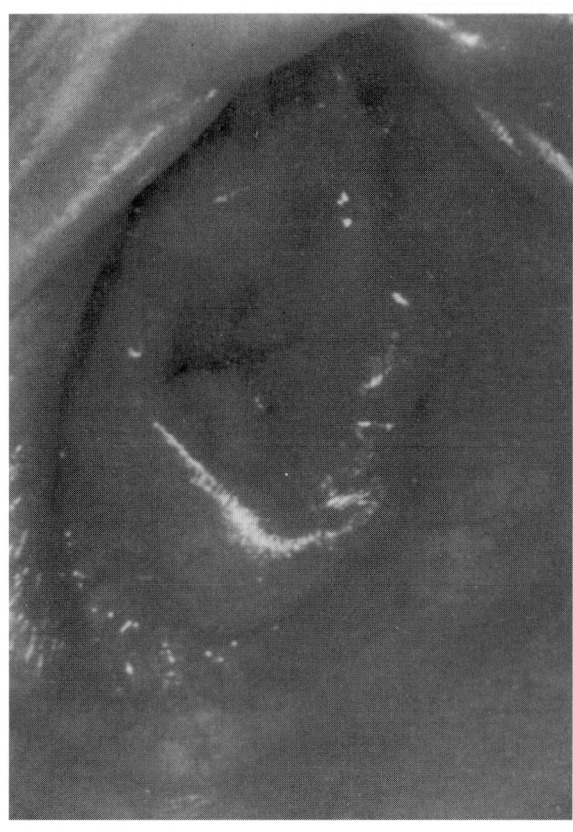

Figure 26-12
Redundant or fimbriated hymen. (From Chadwick DL, Berkowitz CD, Kerns DL, et al: Normal findings. In Chadwick DL, Berkowitz CD, Kerns DL, et al [eds]: Color Atlas of Child Sexual Abuse. Chicago, Year Book Medical Publishers, 1989: 19, with permission.)

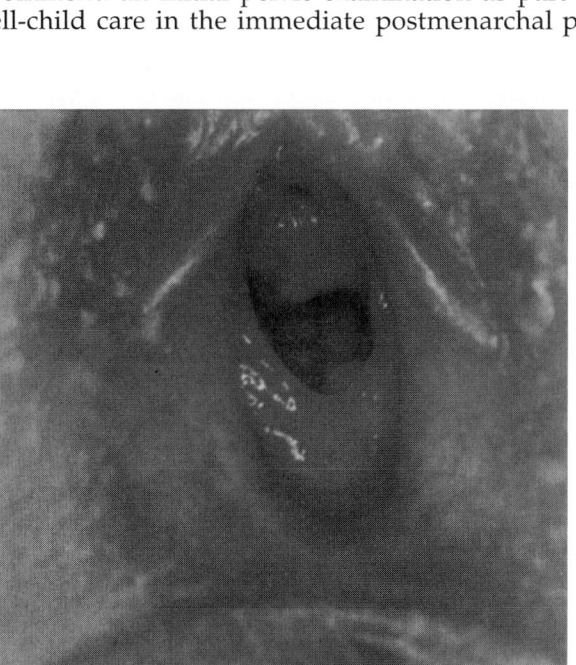

Figure 26-11
Crescentic hymen. (From Chadwick DL, Berkowitz CD, Kerns DL, et al: Normal findings. In Chadwick DL, Berkowitz CD, Kerns DL, et al [eds]: Color Atlas of Child Sexual Abuse. Chicago, Year Book Medical Publishers, 1989:19, with permission.)

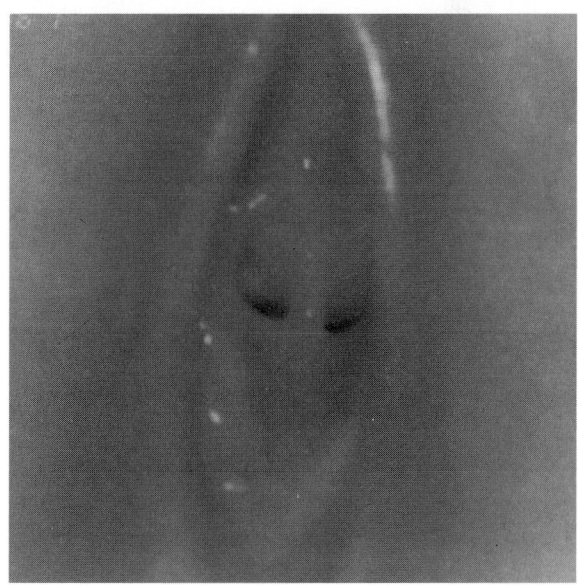

Figure 26-13
Septate hymen. (From Chadwick DL, Berkowitz CD, Kerns DL, et al: Normal findings. In Chadwick DL, Berkowitz CD, Kerns DL, et al [eds]: Color Atlas of Child Sexual Abuse. Chicago, Year Book Medical Publishers, 1989:19, with permission.)

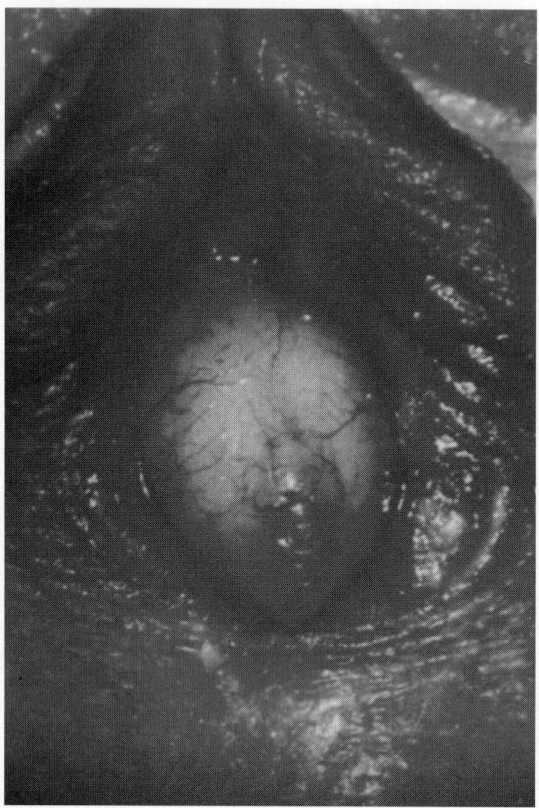

Figure 26–14
Imperforate hymen. (From Chadwick DL, Berkowitz CD, Kerns DL, et al: Normal findings. In Chadwick DL, Berkowitz CD, Kerns DL, et al [eds]: Color Atlas of Child Sexual Abuse. Chicago, Year Book Medical Publishers, 1989:19, with permission.)

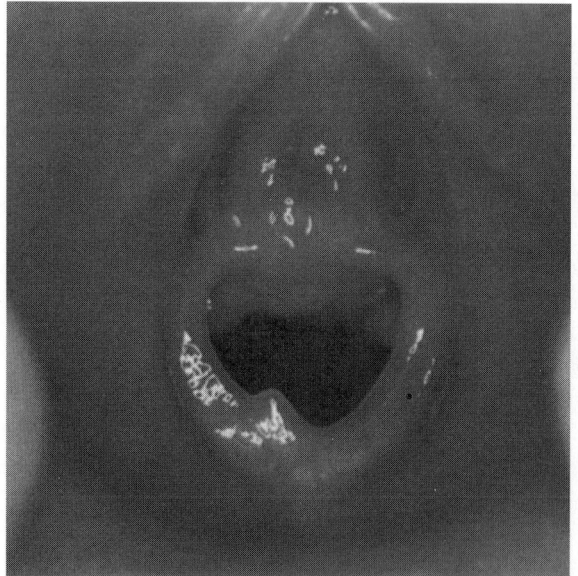

Figure 26–15
Hymenal bump (normal variant) at 7 o'clock. (From Chadwick DL, Berkowitz CD, Kerns DL, et al: Normal findings. In Chadwick DL, Berkowitz CD, Kerns DL, et al [eds]: Color Atlas of Child Sexual Abuse. Chicago, Year Book Medical Publishers, 1989:19, with permission.)

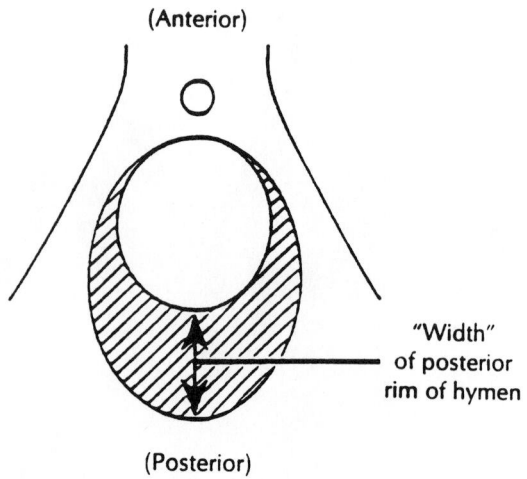

Figure 26–16
Hymenal view demonstrating posterior hymenal rim measurement. (From American Professional Society on the Abuse of Children Practice Guidelines: Descriptive terminology in child sexual abuse medical evaluations. Chicago, American Profesional Society on the Abuse of Children, 1997:1, with permission.)

tient for preventive medicine and educational purposes (Pokorny, 1996).

Placing adolescents in a semi-sitting, dorsolithotomy position with stirrups will allow better eye contact between patient and physician and further enhance a sense of control for the patient. An inspection of external genitalia with recognition of hymenal tissue and the estrogenization of the vestibule should be completed. Tanner staging assessment should be made and documented (Fig. 26–17). A vaginal-cervical examination with the use of a Huffman speculum should be completed, with a Pap smear if the patient is 18 years of age or older and/or sexually active. *Chlamydia* and gonococcal tests should be ordered if the patient is sexually active. A vaginal-abdominal bimanual exam is done to assess the uterus and adnexa.

Table 26–1. INDICATIONS FOR PELVIC EXAMINATION IN THE ADOLESCENT PATIENT

Abdominal pain
Dysmenorrhea
Vaginal discharge
Abnormal bleeding
Suspicion for STD
Pregnancy (suspected)
Amenorrhea
Sexually active—PAP smear
Suspected Müllerian anomaly

Abbreviation: STD, sexually transmitted disease.

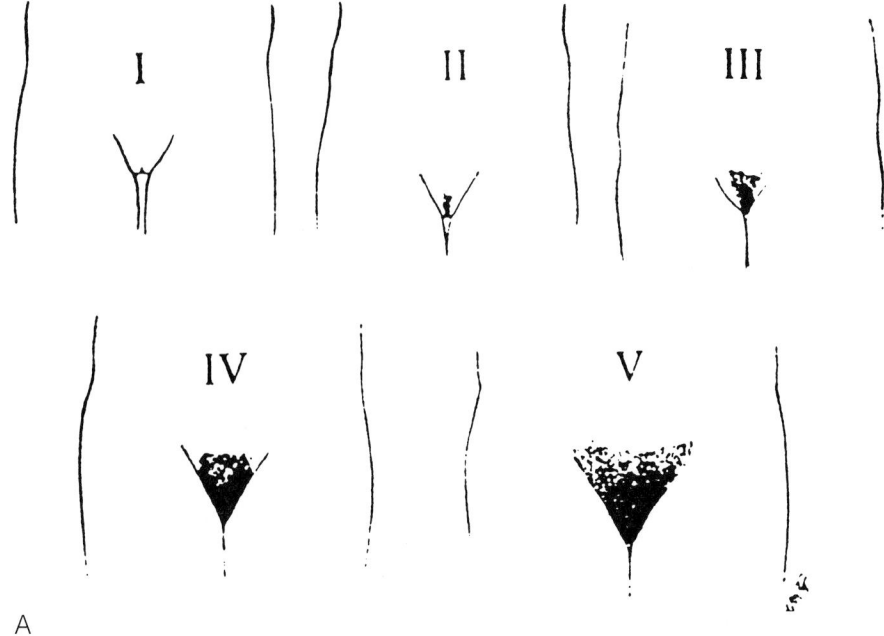

Figure 26–17
A, Tanner staging of pubic hair development. (Adapted from Marshall WA, Tanner JM: Variations in patterns of pubertal changes in girls. Arch Dis Child 1969;44:291, with permission.) *Illustration continued on following page*

Collection of Specimens

In the pediatric patient population, special care must be taken in collecting vulvovaginal specimens because of the hymen's small size, the delicate nature of the atrophic tissues, and the anxiety of the patient. A sterile Calgi swab (Hydro Med, Los Angeles, CA) moistened with sterile water or saline may be gently inserted into the vagina to obtain secretions. Regular cotton-tipped swabs are too large and may traumatize the unestrogenized epithelium, resulting in pain and possible bleeding. The use of eyedroppers has been described to first place a few milliliters of saline in the vagina and then to aspirate. The disadvantages of this technique are that this may be problematic in a moving patient and the fluid may dilute the specimen (Simmons, 1988). Pokorny and Stormer (1987) described the successful use of a double-catheter technique using butterfly-needle tubing placed inside a 12-French catheter to hold the vaginal mucosa away from the inner tubing during aspiration and thereby prevent trauma during collection (Fig. 26–18).

In most children a formal visualization of the cervix and upper vagina is not indicated. However, if the physician suspects possible internal disease, a more detailed assessment of the internal system should be completed. Fiberoptic vaginoscopy, hysteroscopy, and pediatric cystoscopy may be useful. These can be completed in the office setting in children with the use of lidocaine gel; however, physician experience and skill and cooperation of the patient are necessary for success. Without them, these

procedures should not be attempted. Many centers are performing these procedures with conscious sedation in an outpatient or emergency department setting. In uncooperative children in whom such an evaluation is needed, an examination under anesthesia is warranted.

PEDIATRIC GYNECOLOGIC CONDITIONS

Prepubertal Vulvovaginitis

Vulvovaginitis is the most common gynecologic complaint seen in the pediatric population (Grundberger and Fisch, 1982). The prepubertal vulva is predisposed to infection for many reasons. The hypoestrogenic state of the vagina, which lacks glycogen and therefore lactobacilli, creates a neutral pH that is an effective culture media for bacteria. The childhood vulva also lacks protective fatty tissue and pubic hair, which, combined with the close proximity of the vagina to the anus and poor hygiene associated with early toilet training, make infection a likely possibility (Altchek, 1995).

The differential diagnosis for pediatric vulvovaginitis is listed in Table 26–2. Most cases are due to nonspecific vulvovaginitis in which the vaginal cultures typically grow normal vaginal flora (lactobacilli, diphtheroids, *Staphylococcus epidermidis*, or α-streptococci) or gram-negative enteric organisms (Emans and Goldstein, 1990).

Respiratory, enteric, or sexually transmitted pathogens tend to be the more common specific infec-

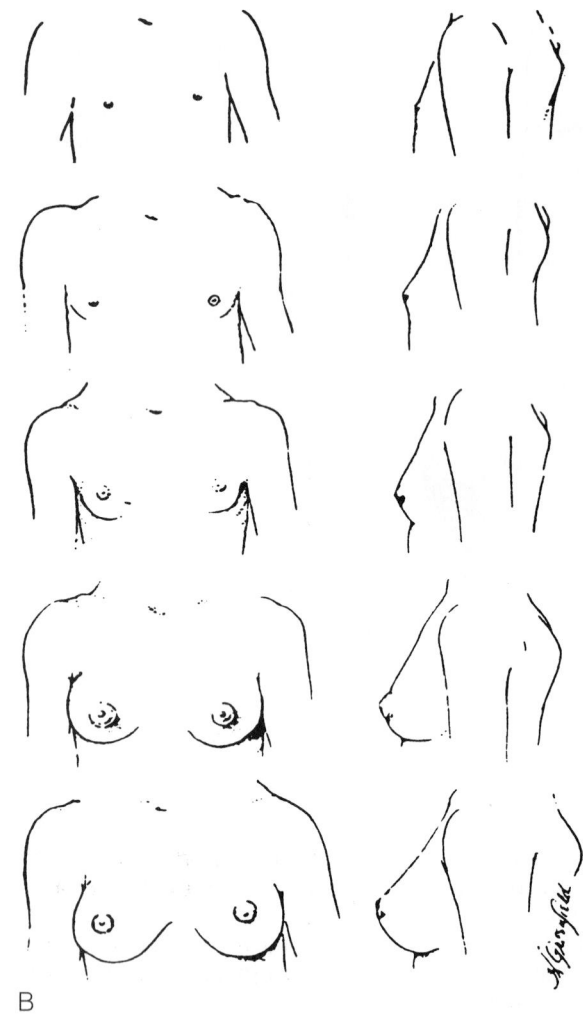

B

Figure 26-17
Continued B, Tanner staging of breast development. (From Sanfilippo JS, Pabon JE: Pediatric Endocrinology. Infertil Reprod Med Clin North Am 1995;6:1, with permission.)

tions that occur in this prepubertal age group. The common offending organisms are listed in Table 26–2. *Candida* vulvovaginitis is more commonly seen in pubertal patients unless a prepubertal patient is still in diapers and/or has recently been on antibiotics or has diabetes.

Shigella, an uncommon cause of prepubertal vulvovaginitis, deserves mention because it is commonly associated with a bloodly purulent vaginal

discharge that is recalcitrant to topical therapies. If undiagnosed, it can often lead to a work-up for precocious puberty because of the associated bleeding. The majority of the reported cases have not been associated with a recent history of diarrhea (Davis, 1975; Murphy and Nelson, 1979).

All sexually transmitted diseases (STDs) seen in adults have also been reported in children. The more commonly seen include *Neisseria gonorrhoeae* and *Chlamydia trachomatis*. Prepubertal gonococcal vaginitis is usually symptomatic with a discharge, whereas some cases of *Chlamydia* remain asymptomatic and are picked up on screening tests for sexual abuse (Siegel et al, 1995). Gonorrhea and *Chlamydia* outside the immediate neonatal period should be reported to the local Child Protective Services (CPS) authorities for investigation. The clinician should be aware that *Chlamydia* could be transmitted vertically from mother to infant and that the infant could remain colonized for up to 12 to 24 months. However, if the young patient has been treated with antibiotics for upper respiratory infections or otitis, persistent colonization is not likely (Schacter et al, 1986; Bell et al, 1987).

Important historical information regarding vulvovaginitis in children includes quantity, duration, and type of discharge; perineal hygiene; recent use of antibiotics; recent infections in the patient (upper respiratory, otitis); anal pruritus; and any behavioral changes, such as nightmares or unusual fears, that might suggest the possibility of abuse. A useful tool is to ask the patient to demonstrate her method of wiping after bowel movements. Time should be taken to ask the child questions about the possibility of anyone touching her vaginal area; this may need to be addressed both before and after the examination.

Historical information can provide clues to the etiology. Typically young girls with a short duration of symptoms (less than 1 month) more often have diagnoses of a specific nature, whereas girls with nonspecific vaginitis have symptoms of months to years before clinical presentation (Emans and Goldstein, 1980). Patients presenting with foul-smelling discharge may have a foreign body (such as toilet paper). Those with vaginal bleeding may also have a foreign body or *Shigella* or group A β-hemolytic streptococcal infections. Usually specific causes of vaginitis, such as gonorrhea or group A β-hemolytic streptococci, present with a greenish discharge,

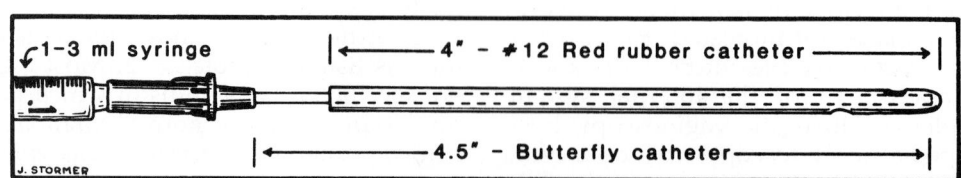

Figure 26-18
Catheter-within-a-catheter technique for specimen collection. (From Pokorny SF, Stormer J: Atraumatic removal of secretions from the prepubertal vagina. Am J Obstet Gynecol 1987;156:581, with permission.)

Table 26–2. ETIOLOGY OF PREPUBERTAL VULVOVAGINAL SYMPTOMS

NONSPECIFIC VULVOVAGINITIS

SPECIFIC VAGINAL INFECTIONS
Enteric
  Escherichia coli
  Proteus vulgaris
  Shigella
Respiratory pathogens
  Group A β-hemolytic streptococcus (*S. pyogenes*)
  Streptococcus pneumoniae
  Neisseria meningitides
  Branhamella catarrhalis
  Staphylococcus aureus
  Haemophilus influenzae
Sexually transmitted diseases
  Neisseria gonorrhea
  Chlamydia trachomatis
  Herpes simplex
  Trichomonas
  Syphilis
  Condyloma accuminatum (human papillomavirus)
Infections with other microorganisms
  Candida—vaginitis, vulvitis
Pinworm infestation
Local physical factors
  Vaginal foreign body
  Trauma
  Gynecologic: neoplasms, labial agglutination
  Urologic: urethral prolapse, ectopic ureter
  Rectal: anal fissures, pruritic
  Tight-fitting clothing
Allergic—irritant
Systemic illnesses
  Measles
  Chicken pox
  Scarlet fever
  Behçet's syndrome
  Mononucleosis
Vulvar skin disease
  Lichen sclerosis
  Psoriasis
  Seborrhea
  Atopic dermatitis
  Scabies
  Bacterial infection: impetigo
Psychosomatic vulvovaginal complaints

whereas nonspecific cases present with pruritic and vulvar erythema.

The physical examination in these cases should be tailored to the presenting complaint. Scant mucoid discharge and vestibular erythema usually are secondary to poor hygiene and should not require vaginal cultures. After a brief external examination, the physician should instruct the patient (Table 26–3) about appropriate hygiene, avoidance of irritants, and/or treatment for pinworms (Emans and Goldstein, 1990). Patients with persistent, purulent, or recurrent discharge require a general physical examination with inspection of the perineum and vaginal introitus in both the supine and knee–chest positions. Specimens should be obtained for routine vaginal culture as well as cultures for *Chlamydia* and gonorrhea. Indirect methods of testing such as immunofluorescence or antigen detection methods for

Chlamydia are inappropriate because normally occurring bacteria can cross-react and give false-positive results (Hammerschlag, 1988; Hammerschlag et al, 1988). Specimens may also be obtained for a wet mount. A rectal examination should be included as a part of this evaluation to assist in palpating for foreign bodies and detecting abnormal masses. An attempt to visualize any foreign body should be completed during the examination. Radiographs are not helpful because most foreign bodies are not radiopaque. Further evaluation for pinworms should be completed in patients with chronic complaints either with a cellophane tape test or collecting stool samples to test for ova and parasites.

Most cases of prepubertal vulvovaginitis will be of a nonspecific nature and can be treated with improved hygiene. Various therapies for nonspecific vulvovaginitis are outlined in Table 26–3. Persistent complaints of nonspecific vaginitis require that the possibility of pinworms be excluded and a trial of empirical antibiotics (i.e., amoxicillin, amoxicillin-clavulanate [Augmentin], or a cephalosporin) be given for 10 days. Patients with recurrent or persistent complaints in whom a specific etiology has been excluded may respond to a nightly dose of antibiotic for 30 to 60 days. Some patients with recurrent, transient episodes of vulvar irritation will commonly respond to tepid sitz baths and several applications of hydrocortisone cream 1%. Treatment of specific causes of prepubertal vulvovaginitis is outlined in Table 26–4.

Vaginal Bleeding

Vaginal bleeding in the pediatric patient is relatively uncommon. When it occurs, it is a cause of great anxiety to both patient and parents. Any amount of genital bleeding demands evaluation because significant causes such as a neoplasm, sexual precocity, and sexual abuse need to be excluded. Although the etiology is most often benign, a thorough work-up should be completed and more serious pathology excluded. Estrogen-withdrawal bleeding can sometimes be seen in the first few weeks of life. Beyond that time frame, the differential diagnosis includes vaginitis, foreign body, lichen sclerosus (LS), condyloma, genital neoplasms, precocious puberty, bleeding disorders, hemangiomas, polyps, and urethral prolapse. Table 26–5 provides a good summary of the differential diagnosis of vaginal bleeding in the prepubertal girl.

A complete history and physical can point one toward the diagnosis. Important findings include associated vaginal discharge; recent diarrhea; pruritis; acceleration of weight and height; other signs of bleeding disorders, such as epistaxis, petechiae, or hematomas; or history of trauma.

On physical examination, it is important to include first a general assessment prior to directing attention to the genital exam. An increased weight or height

Table 26-3. THERAPY FOR NONSPECIFIC VULVOVAGINITIS

GENERAL INSTRUCTIONS
Good hygiene with front to back wiping after bowel movements
Frequent changes of white cotton underpants to absorb discharge
Avoidance of bubble baths, harsh soaps and shampooing hair in tub
Avoid tight fitting pants and nylon tights
Sitz baths several days daily with plain warm water with gentle washing of the vulva with water or
    mild soap (Basis, unscented Dove) followed by careful drying by patting or use of blow dryer on
    cool setting
Urinate with legs spread apart and labia separated

MANAGEMENT OF ACUTE SEVERE EDEMATOUS VULVITIS
Sitz baths every 4 hours with water or colloidal oatmeal bath without use of soap
Witch hazel pads (Tucks) may be used for wiping
After acute phase, alternate sitz with painting vulva with calamine or mixture of zinc oxide (15%), talc
    (15%), and glycerin (10%) in water
In subacute phase, use topical creams on vulva like hydrocortisone 1% cream, A and D ointment
Add oral medication to decrease pruritis with hydroxyzine hydrochloride (Atarax) 2 mg/kg/day
    (divided in 4 doses) or diphenhydramine hydrochloride (Benadryl) 5 mg/kg/day (divided in 4
    doses)

MANAGEMENT OF PERSISTENT NONSPECIFIC VULVOVAGINITIS
Broad-spectrum oral antibiotics (amoxicillin, amoxicillin-clavulanate or a cephalosporin) for 10 to 14
    days; a 1- to 3-month low dose of bedtime cephalexin, amoxicillin-clavulanate, or trimethoprim/
    sulfamethoxazole in recurrent cases
Local use of antibacterial cream (Sultrin, AVC cream)
Irrigation with Betadine 1% solution
Estrogen-containing creams applied nightly to the vulva for 2 weeks then every other night for 2
    weeks
Stress hygiene

From Emans SJH, Goldstein DP: Vulvovaginal problems in the prepubertal child. In Emans SJH, Goldstein DP (eds): Pediatric and Adolescent Gynecology. 3rd ed. Boston: Little Brown & Company, 1990:67, with permission.

velocity can indicate the first sign of precocious puberty, as can early signs of breast development. Other areas of bruising or trauma can point to a traumatic injury as the etiology. Genital trauma and vulvovaginitis are often evident on inspection. The typical trauma history is that of a straddle injury, with the pattern of injury most likely involving the labia minora. A prospective review of witnessed straddle injuries in prepubertal children revealed that most straddle injuries involve the more prominent external vulvar structures, and hymenal transection in these cases is rare (Bond et al, 1995). A posterior hymenal laceration between the 3- and 9-o'clock positions is the result of a penetrative injury, and sexual abuse should be strongly considered (Muram, 1994). Helpful tips for evaluating children with active vulvar bleeding are to place 2% lidocaine jelly over the cut and then carefully irrigate with warm water

Table 26-4. TREATMENT OF SPECIFIC CAUSES OF PREPUBERTAL VULVOVAGINITIS

ETIOLOGY	TREATMENT
Group A β-hemolytic streptococcus (S. pyogenes); Streptococcus pneumoniae	Penicillin V potassium, 125–250 mg QID po × 10 days
Chlamydia trachomatis	Erythromycin 50 mg/kg/day po × 10 days
	Children >8 years of age, doxycycline 100 mg BID po × 7 days
Neisseria gonorrhoeae	Ceftriaxone 125 mg IM or Spectinomycin 40 mg/kg IM once
	Children >8 years of age should also be given doxycycline 100 mg BID po × 7 days
	Children >45 kg are treated with adult doses
Candida	Topical nystatin, miconazole, or clotrimazole cream
Shigella	Trimethoprim/sulfamethoxazole 8 mg/40 mg/kg/day po × 7 days
Staphylococcus aureus	Cephalexin (Keflex) 25–50 mg/kg/day po × 7–10 days
	Dicloxacillin 25 mg/kg/day po × 7–10 days
	Amoxicillin-clavulanate (Augmentin) 20–40 mg/kg/day of the amoxicillin po × 7–10 days
Haemophilus influenzae	Amoxicillin 20–40 mg/kg/day po × 7 days
Trichomonas	Metronidazole (Flagyl) 125 mg (15 mg/kg/day) TID × 7–10 days
Pinworms (Enterobius vermicularis)	Mebendazole (Vermox) 1 chewable 100-mg tablet, repeat in 2 weeks

From Emans SJH, Goldstein DP: Vulvovaginal problems in the prepubertal child. In Emans SJH, Goldstein DP (eds): Pediatric and Adolescent Gynecology. 3rd ed. Boston: Little Brown & Company, 1990:67, with permission.

☐ **Table 26–5.** CAUSES OF VAGINAL BLEEDING IN PREPUBERTAL GIRLS

HORMONAL
Neonatal hormonal withdrawal
Exogenous hormonal intake (birth control pills, estrogen cream)
Precocious puberty
Sex-hormone-producing tumors

INFLAMMATORY-INFECTIONS (VULVOVAGINITIS)
Inflammatory processes
Poor hygiene
Chemical irritants (soaps, cosmetics)
Infection processes
Sexually transmitted diseases (gonorrhea, *Chlamydia*)
Nonsexually transmitted diseases (*Staphylococcus aureus*, beta-hemolytic strep)
Parasitic infestations (amebiasis, *E. vermicularis*, fungal)

TRAUMA
Physical activity (bicycle riding)
Sexual abuse
Foreign bodies

UROLOGIC
Urinary tract infections (bacterial, viral, parasites)
Urethral prolapse
Hematuria

NEOPLASMS
Neoplasms
Gonadal stromal tumors (granuloma-theca cell)
Benign tumors (polyps, condyloma accuminatum)
Sarcoma botryoides

MISCELLANEOUS
Parasitic infestations of the genitorurinary tract, common in the Third World: leech
 schistosomiasis
Autoimmune diseases: lichen sclerosus, lichen simplex chronicus
Iatrogenic—exogenous hormones

From Sanfilippo JS, Wakim NA: Bleeding in the pediatric age group. Clin Obstet Gynecol 1987;30:654, with permission.

through a syringe attached to an angiocath or IV tubing. If necessary, many emergency departments now use conscious sedation to facilitate such examinations and to assist in placing sutures if needed.

Vulvovaginitis is the most common cause of vaginal bleeding in the prepubertal girl. In these patients, vulvovaginitis is most often caused by self-inoculation of bacteria, and, therefore, oropharyngeal, respiratory, and fecal bacterial organisms usually are the cause of the problem (Rau et al, 1994). Evaluation requires culture identification of the pathogen, including specific cultures for gonorrhea, *Chlamydia*, *Shigella*, and other possible pathogens. Group A β-hemolytic streptococcal infections may also on occasion be associated with vaginal bleeding. Bleeding that occurs as a result of vaginitis usually responds to local measures. Vaginitis as a result of specific organisms, such as those previously mentioned, will require oral antibiotics.

Eighteen percent of girls under the age of 13 years with vaginal bleeding with or without discharge, and 50% of those with vaginal bleeding and no discharge, can be expected to have a *foreign body*. An appropriate examination in these patients involves placing the patients in the knee–chest position to enhance visualization of the vaginal canal. The most commonly found foreign body is toilet paper, which

can usually be irrigated from the vagina with warm water by attaching a small pediatric feeding tube to a syringe filled with the irrigant and placing it intravaginally with the use of lubricant or xylocaine jelly applied to the introitus. Metallic objects may be able to be removed with forceps, but in an uncooperative patient sedation may be necessary to complete the removal.

Prepubertal girls with *urethral prolapse* usually present with painless bleeding thought to be of vaginal origin. On examination, a characteristic friable, donut-shaped, red-blue, annular mass is noted (Fig. 26–19) (Jerkins et al, 1984). This condition is more commonly seen in 5- to 8-year old black females, who may complain of dysuria, bleeding, or pain that occurs after coughing or straining or following trauma. Most cases of urethral prolapse respond to the use of a small amount of topical estrogen cream applied twice daily after a sitz bath for 1 to 4 weeks. Both the patient and the physician need to be aware that the medication is systemically absorbed and that long-term use can result in secondary sexual characteristics such as breast budding. These usually disappear after the medicine is discontinued. In patients unresponsive to medical management or in whom necrotic tissue is present, surgical therapy may be necessary.

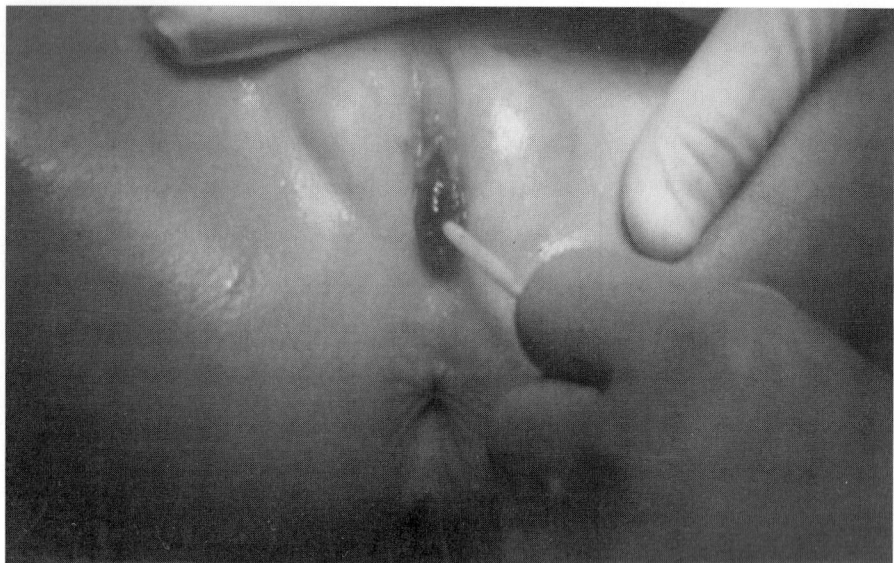

Figure 26–19
Urethral prolapse. (From Mendez MC: In Yordan EE [ed]: The PediGyn Teaching Slide Set. Philadelphia: North American Society for Pediatric and Adolescent Gynecology, 1996:slide 16, with permission.)

Rhabdomyosarcoma, the most common malignant tumor seen in the pediatric vagina, usually presents with vaginal bleeding. It characteristically arises from the anterior wall of the vagina and then expands to fill the vagina and create a visible and often palpable mass (Fig. 26–20). A review of 28 patients with rhabdomyosarcoma revealed that vaginal bleeding was the most common symptom; only 8 patients had a visible mass (Hays et al, 1988). The tumor has a bimodal age distribution with peaks at the first 2 years of life and at adolescence (LaQuaglia et al, 1994). Prognostic factors include age at diagnosis, tumor invasiveness, metastases, regional lymph node involvement, and histopathologic subtype (alveolar vs. embryonal). Embryonal subtypes are more commonly seen in the very young patient. Although in the past these patients were treated with radical pelvic exenterative surgery with only 15% survival, the combined use of intensive chemotherapy fol-lowed by limited surgical resection, preserving the bladder and rectum, and postoperative pelvic irradiation results in survival rates that are higher than 85% (Julian et al, 1995).

Lichen Sclerosus

LS, a destructive inflammatory condition of the skin with a vulvar predilection, can present in children. Most children with LS present with complaints of itching, irritation, or soreness; however, bleeding without a history of trauma or sexual abuse should prompt careful genital examination to look for the characteristic white parchment-like skin in an hourglass configuration around the introital and perianal area, with evidence of subepithelial hemorrhages, chronic ulceration, and inflammation (Fig. 26–21). There may be loss of anatomic detail, with fusion of

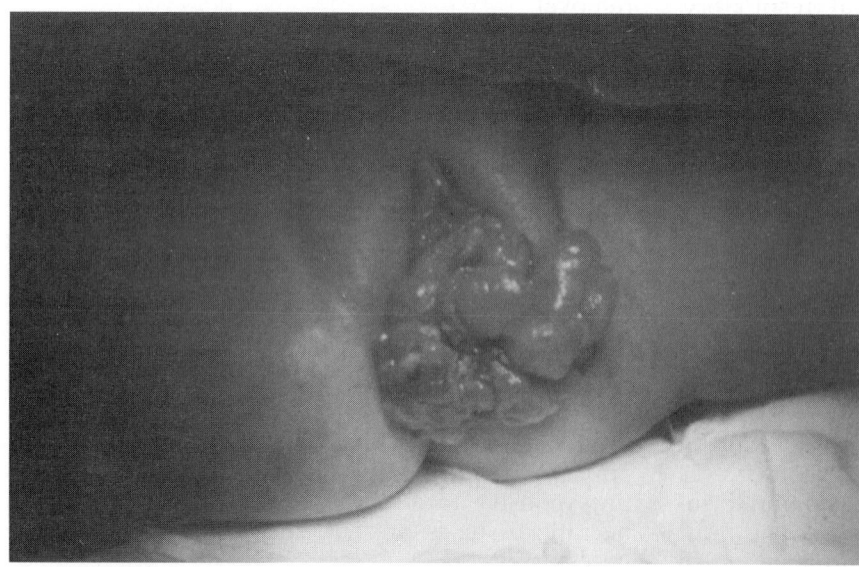

Figure 26–20
Rhabdomyosarcoma (sarcoma botryoides) protruding from the vagina of a 3-year-old girl. (From Mendez MC: In Yordan EE [ed]: The PediGyn Teaching Slide Set. Philadelphia: North American Society for Pediatric and Adolescent Gynecology, 1996:slide 124, with permission.)

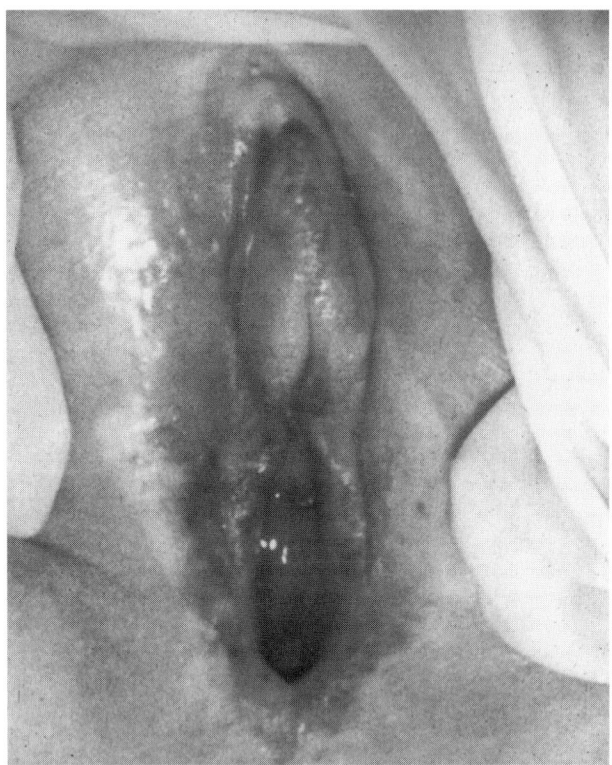

Figure 26–21
Lichen sclerosus. (From Smith SF: In Yordan EE [ed]: The PediGyn Teaching Slide Set. Philadelphia: North American Society for Pediatric and Adolescent Gynecology, 1996:slide 33, with permission.)

labia majora and minora into one structure and/or phimosis of the clitoral hood and contraction of the introitus in chronic, untreated cases. Originally LS was thought to resolve at puberty, but series with careful follow-up have revealed that many patients have symptoms or lesions into adolescence (Redmond et al, 1988). Although the true etiology of LS is unknown, there is an autoimmune association (Meyrick Thomas et al, 1988) and possibly a genetic familial component (Sahn et al, 1994).

In mild cases, symptomatic treatment is recommended, with attention to hygiene and elimination of irritants or excessive bathing with harsh soaps along with the use of protective emollients such as A and D ointment. Hydroxyzine hydrochloride (Atarax) may be given 1 hour before bedtime to decrease nocturnal itching. In unsuccessful or more severe cases, use of clobetasol propionate 0.05% applied topically several times daily for 1 to 4 weeks coupled with liberal use of emollients is successful. A randomized study comparing the use of this regimen with that of 2% testosterone propionate, 2% progesterone, and a placebo revealed that improvement in symptoms, gross aspects, and histologic features were seen only in the clobetasol-treated patients (Bracco et al, 1993). After treatment with clobetasol, regular use of emollients has been useful

(Cattaneo et al, 1996); however, because of the chronic nature of this disorder, a repeat course of steroids is sometimes necessary.

Labial Agglutination

Agglutination of the labia is a frequent occurrence in the unestrogenized child. This is an acquired condition that appears to be hormonal in origin. A 20-year study of 12,000 female patients seen with labial adhesions reported 90% of cases occurring in the first 5 months of life. The adhesions can persist from 3 months to 11 years and in rare cases into adulthood (Soifer, 1991). Most patients are asymptomatic; however, some may complain of urinary difficulties including dysuria, enuresis, deflections or interruptions of the urinary stream, and infection. These symptoms result from an obstructing membrane that covers the vagina. This causes urinary reflux into the vagina and results in urinary retention, stagnation, bacterial infection, and painful symptoms. Dysuria sometimes occurs with forceful urination that causes disruption of the agglutination and a burning sensation as urine passes over the denuded epithelial edge of the separation.

The diagnosis is made on physical examination of the external genitalia. The pathognomonic midline paper-thin bridge between the two labia is easily seen by placing gentle labial traction and shifting the labia from side to side (Fig. 26–22). Typically, the agglutination begins at the fourchette and may extend to the clitoris, often leaving only a pinpoint

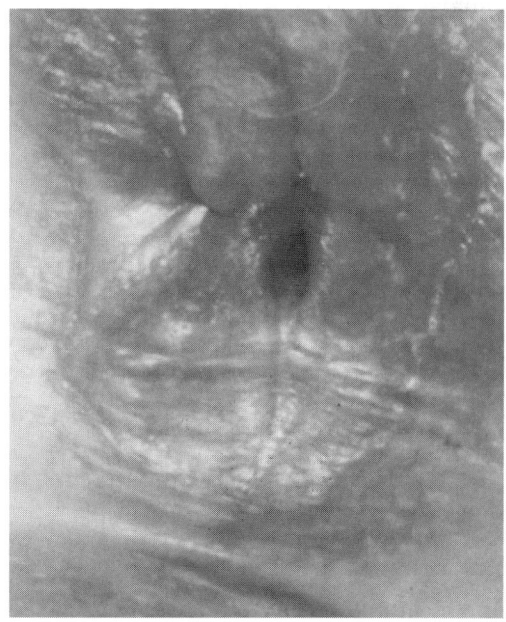

Figure 26–22
Labial agglutination. (From Yordan EE: In Yordan EE [ed]: The PediGyn Teaching Slide Set. Philadelphia: North American Society for Pediatric and Adolescent Gynecology, 1996:slide 32, with permission.)

opening and concealing the urethra, vestibule, and hymen. Therefore, this condition is sometimes confused with vaginal agenesis; however, the distinction is not difficult to make. In cases of labial agglutination, the labia are joined in the midline, whereas in cases of vaginal agenesis, the labia minora are readily seen and the hymenal ring identified.

Treatment is based on symptomatology. In those patients who have an opening large enough for adequate vaginal and urinary drainage, little treatment is necessary because the adhesions usually resolve spontaneously with the rising hormonal levels of puberty. Use of a bland ointment, such as A and D ointment, along with gentle separation of the labia may be helpful. In severe cases with complete agglutination or impaired vaginal or urinary drainage, the treatment of choice is use of topical estrogen-containing cream (Ariberg, 1975; Soifer, 1991). The cream should be applied twice daily for several weeks directly to the line of agglutination with the use of gentle labial separation or traction. A typical reason for medical treatment failure is application of the cream to the entire vulva without specific attention to the adhesion. Nightly sitz baths before application of the cream are helpful. The duration of treatment required to cause complete resolution of the membrane varies between 12 and 28 days, with an average of 14 to 28 days. Systemic signs of estrogenization can be seen with this management and may result in nipple swelling, darkening of the areola, breast enlargement, and vaginal discharge. These last up to 2 weeks after cessation of the therapy. After separation, a maintenance therapy of daily baths, good hygiene, and use of an emollient such as A and D ointment at bedtime can decrease recurrences, which are noted in 30% of cases. Recurrences are treated in the same fashion with hormonal therapy.

In some cases, the more extensive, dense adhesions fail to respond to the use of estrogen cream even with proper technique. Forceful labial separation is not recommended because it may be traumatic and/or lead to the formation of scar tissue that may not be hormonally responsive. Although forceful separation is generally contraindicated, separation of the adhesions can sometimes be accomplished in the office setting. Approximately 30 minutes after applying EMLA cream with an occlusive dressing to the vulva, the labia can be gently separated by sliding a Calgi swab along the adhesion. If this is not easily accomplished or if the patient has acute urinary retention, separation under anesthesia is recommended.

Ambiguous Genitalia

The finding of ambiguous genitalia (Fig. 26–23) in the newborn necessitates an immediate and coordinated response. The initial priority is to tell the parents that their baby is healthy but that, because the

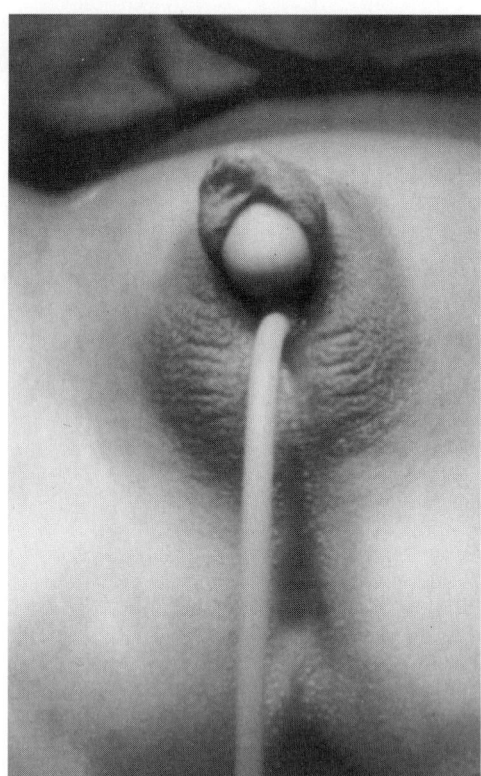

Figure 26–23
Ambiguous genitalia. (From Mendez MC: In Yordan EE [ed]: The PediGyn Teaching Slide Set. Philadelphia: North American Society for Pediatric and Adolescent Gynecology, 1996:slide 95, with permission.)

external genital development is incomplete, tests will be necessary to determine the sex of the child. The next priority is to rule out life-threatening causes of genital ambiguity such as congenital adrenal hyperplasia (CAH), which accounts for more than 90% of cases. The salt-wasting forms can lead to rapid dehydration and fluid and electrolyte abnormalities; therefore, fluid intake and output, serum electrolytes, and glucose concentration should be monitored carefully.

The differential diagnosis of a newborn with ambiguous genitalia includes three categories: female pseudohermaphroditism, male pseudohermaphroditism, and gonadal differentiation disorders (Table 26–6). *Female pseudohermaphrodites* are individuals with a 46,XX karyotype, ovaries, and masculinized or ambiguous genitalia. This category includes CAH. Those affected individuals are exposed to high levels of androgens, especially testosterone, in utero, as excess 17α-hydroxyprogesterone is converted to androstenedione and subsequently to testosterone. The entire system is driven by low cortisol levels, which produce feedback and stimulate release of adrenocorticotropic hormone (ACTH). Ninety percent of CAH cases are due to 21-hydroxylase deficiency (New, 1992; Spoudeas et al, 1993). Other forms of CAH include 11β-hydroxylase and 3β-hydroxyste-

Table 26-6. DIFFERENTIAL DIAGNOSIS OF AMBIGUOUS GENITALIA IN THE NEWBORN

FEMALE PSEUDOHERMAPHRODITISM
Congenital adrenal hyperplasia
   21-Hydroxylase deficiency
   11β-Hydroxylase deficiency
   3β-Hydroxysteroid dehydrogenase deficiency
Maternally derived androgens

MALE PSEUDOHERMAPHRODITISM
Inadequate production of testosterone
   Testosterone biosynthetic defects
      Congenital lipoid adrenal hyperplasia (Cholesterol
         side-chain cleavage enzyme deficiency)
      3β-Hydroxysteroid dehydrogenase deficiency
      17α-Hydroxylase deficiency
      17,20-Lyase deficiency
      17β-Hydroxysteroid dehydrogenase deficiency
   Leydig cell hypoplasia

PERIPHERAL UNRESPONSIVENESS TO ANDROGEN
Androgen insensitivity syndrome
5α-Reductase deficiency

GONADAL DIFFERENTIATION DISORDERS
Gonadal dysgenesis
   46,XY partial gonadal dysgenesis
   45,X/46,XY gonadal dysgenesis
True hermaphroditism

From Meyers-Seifer RH, Charest NJ: Diagnosis and management of patients with ambiguous genitalia. Semin Perinatol 1992;16:333, with permission.

roid dehydrogenase deficiencies. Steroid hormone assays can differentiate these deficiencies.

Male pseudohermaphrodites have a 46,XY karyotype, testes, and feminized or ambiguous genitalia. This may result from inadequate testosterone production or from diminished peripheral effects of testosterone as in the androgen insensitivity syndrome or 5α-reductase deficiency. In these patients, the undervirilization is the result of inadequate androgen effects, and the absence of müllerian structures is secondary to the presence of müllerian inhibiting substance produced by the testis.

Gonadal differentiation disorders include true hermaphrodites and the various types of gonadal dysgenesis (Table 26–6). True hermaphroditism may result from sex chromosome mosaicism, chimerism, translocation, or an autosomal mutant gene (Van Niekerk, 1976). The karyotypes seen in these patients are 46,XX or 46,XX/46,XY. The gonads contain varying amounts of testicular and ovarian tissue, and the various phenotypes seen are the result of the relative hormonal contribution of each gonad. Asymmetry of internal structures is often found due to variance in local effects produced by asymmetric production of androgens and müllerian inhibiting substance. Patients with gonadal dysgenesis form a heterogeneous group resulting from various chromosomal anomalies. In mixed gonadal dysgenesis, defects in the Y chromosome include translocation, deletion, and other abnormalities that involve the *SRY* region (Zah et al, 1975). The most common kar-

yotype seen is 46,XX/46,XY. The risk of neoplasia in the gonads of these individuals with gonadal dysgenesis, Y chromosomes, and undescended or abdominal testes is 30% (Scully, 1981; Verp and Simpson, 1987). As a result, these gonads and those of true hermaphrodites should be removed.

The initial evaluation of ambiguous genitalia includes a careful history, physical examination, karyotype, and serum hormonal and electrolyte assays. A thorough history of any possible hormone exposure during pregnancy as well as a detailed family history and pedigree of previous children with ambiguous genitalia must be addressed. Similarly, a history of infertility or amenorrhea in any aunts or any maternal history of CAH is also important.

The physical exam should include a detailed assessment of the external genitalia beginning with measurement of the fully stretched phallus from the tip of the glans to the pubic ramus. At term, 2.5 cm in length is 2.5 standard deviations below the mean (Feldman and Smith, 1975). The inguinal areas and labioscrotal folds must be palpated for the presence of gonads. In most cases a palpable gonad below the inguinal ligament is a testis. The perineum must be inspected for location of the urethral meatus and for the presence of a vaginal orifice. Asymmetry of the labioscrotal folds in conjunction with a unilateral palpable gonad is typically seen in cases of mixed gonadal dysgenesis or true hermaphroditism. Hyperpigmentation of the labioscrotal folds may be indicative of excess ACTH and CAH. A rectal exam should be completed to assess for the presence of a uterus or a prostate gland.

Serum must be obtained to determine the karyotype and measure the levels of 17-hydroxyprogesterone (17-OHP), 11-deoxycortisol, 17-hydroxypregneolone, dehydroepiandrosterone, testosterone, dihydrotestosterone, and electrolytes. Elevation of 17-OHP confirms the diagnosis of 21-hydroxylase deficiency. CAH is identified in over 90% of female pseudohermaphrodites. An elevation in 11-deoxycortisol is associated with 11α-hydroxylase deficiency, and elevated 17-hydroxypregneolone and dehydroepiandrosterone are indicative of 3β-hydroxysteroid dehydrogenase deficiency. Hyperkalemia and hyponatremia, which reflect hypoaldosteronism, are consistent with either 21-hydroxylase or 3β-hydroxysteroid dehydrogenase deficiencies. Hypokalemia is found with 11α-hydroxylase deficiency.

Radiologic imaging is also important in the evaluation of patients with ambiguous genitalia. A retrograde genitogram can delineate the urethra, bladder, vagina, uterus, and possible interconnecting fistulas (Fig. 26–24). A pelvic and abdominal ultrasound is useful to assess pelvic viscera as well as the kidneys and ureters. In many instances, magnetic resonance imaging (MRI) has replaced the role of ultrasonography in this capacity. An algorithm for the evaluation of newborns with ambiguous genitalia is presented in Figure 26–25.

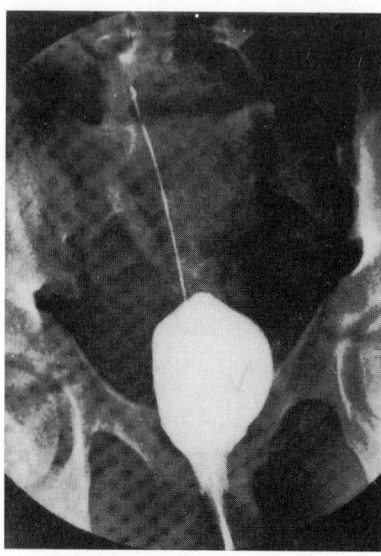
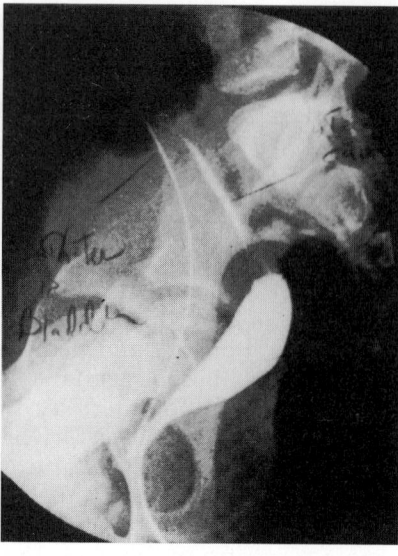

Figure 26–24
Retrograde genitogram of newborn with ambiguous genitalia. (From Sanfilippo JS, Pabon JE: Pediatric endocrinology. Infertil Reprod Med Clin North Am 1995;6:1, with permission.)

Fetal-Neonatal Ovarian Cysts

Over the past decade, the wider use of obstetric sonography has increased the detection rate of fetal and neonatal ovarian cysts, thereby presenting the gynecologist with a management dilemma. A review of the English medical literature (Kirkinen and Jouppila, 1985) regarding antenatally diagnosed cysts found them to be usually unilateral, diagnosed in the third trimester, and uncommon. The average cyst size at diagnosis is 5 × 5 cm and does not appear to change throughout the pregnancy. Most of these cysts are histologically benign, although malignancies have been reported (Ziegler, 1945; Zuspan, 1953; Pryse-Davies and Dewhurst, 1971). Polyhydramnios may be a common finding in patients with fetal cysts, but they do not seem to be associated with congenital anomalies of other organ systems. The uncommon antenatal complications result from compression of other viscera and ovarian torsion. Although larger cysts can cause compression or torsion, in utero aspiration has limited value in prenatal management. Soft tissue dystocia is rare and cesarean section is recommended only for an obstetric indication. The length of the cyst pedicle may be a better predictor of torsion than cyst size. Another review of 49 prenatally detected ovarian cysts (Muller-Leiss et al., 1992), 26 of which were treated surgically, also found torsion to be independent of cyst size. Twenty-three patients were followed sonographically, and 15 showed complete resolution in 14 months without correlation to the sonographic pattern. These authors concluded that neonatal cysts may present with a variety of sonographic patterns and need not be purely cystic. A change in the sonographic pattern from purely cystic to echogenic was typical and representative of possible hemorrhage. This was found to occur at any time, but most often during delivery.

The recommended management of ovarian cysts in this age group is conservative because disappearance is frequent and severe symptoms are rare. Spontaneous resolution of these cysts is reported to be independent of their sonographic appearance and independent of the size of the cyst. Cysts smaller than 5 cm can be safely followed with serial sonograms. Ultrasound-guided percutaneous puncture is an alternative treatment to surgery in larger space-occupying cysts that do not have a solid component (Landrum et al, 1986). Surgical intervention is thought to be indicated only when the sonographic pattern or course is atypical or in the case of an emergency.

Sexual Abuse

Sexual abuse has been defined as the involvement of children or adolescents in sexual activities that they cannot comprehend, for which they are developmentally unprepared and cannot provide informed consent, and/or that violate the social and legal taboos of society (Kempe, 1978). As stated by the American Academy of Pediatrics (AAP), these sexual activities may include all forms of oral–genital, genital, or anal contact by or to the child or nontouching abuses such as exhibitionism, voyeurism, or using the child in the production of pornography (AAP Committee on Child Abuse and Neglect, 1991).

Child sexual abuse is not uncommon. A reasonable estimate is that 20% of girls have been involved in developmentally inappropriate sexual activities during childhood for the sexual stimulation of another person (Hymel and Jenny, 1996). Children may be sexually abused in either intrafamilial or extrafamilial settings. Most perpetrators are known to the child. A review of 116 victims of sexual abuse showed 97% were abused by either a family member or a person in a position of trust and supervision of the child. None were abused by strangers (Sorenson and Snow, 1991). Children are subject to more sexual abuse by family members or caregivers, whereas ad-

1. History: family history, pregnancy (hormones, virilization inspection)
   Palpation of inguinal region and labioscrotal folds; rectal examination
   Karyotype analysis
   Initial studies: plasma 17-hydroxyprogesterone, androstenedione,
   dehydroepiandrosterone, testosterone, & dihydrotestosterone
   Serum electrolytes
   Sonogram or MRI of kidneys, ureters & pelvic contents
   Provisional Dx

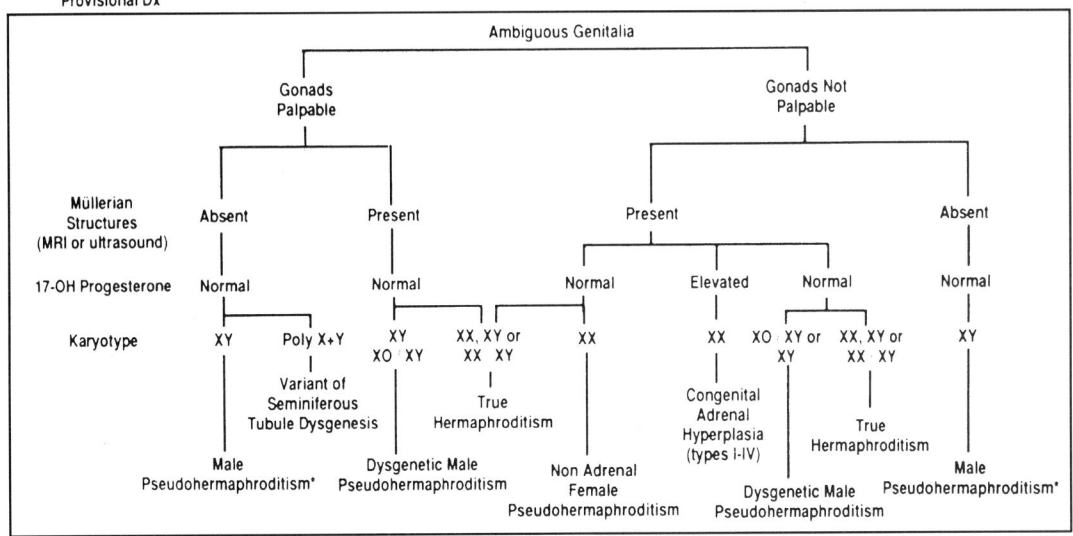

2. "Vaginogram" (urogenital sinogram): selected cases
   Endoscopy, laparotomy, gonadal biopsy: restricted to male pseudohermaphrodites, true hermaphrodites, and selected instances of nonadrenal
   female pseudohermaphroditism

   *Plasma 17-hydroxyprogesterone levels may be modestly elevated in patients with $P450_{c11}$ (Type III), 3β-hydroxysteroid dehydrogenase deficiency
   (Type IV) and are "low" in patients with $P-450_{c17}$ (Type V) and $P-450_{scc}$ deficiency (Type VI)

Figure 26–25
Steps in diagnosis of ambiguous genitalia in infancy and childhood. (From Grumbach MM, Conte FA: Disorders of sex differentiation. In Wilson JD, Fester DW [eds]: Williams' Textbook of Endocrinology. 8th ed. Philadelphia, WB Saunders Company, 1992:935, with permission.)

olescents are at higher risk of abuse by strangers. Young children are less likely to experience sexual penetration than older children. Overall, 31% of cases involve genital contact with penetration; in 45% of cases there is no penetration, and in 24% there is no direct genital contact (National Study on the Incidence of Child Abuse and Neglect, 1988). Those children living in single-parent homes, with stepparents, or in the homes of substance abusers may be at higher risk for abuse (Finkelhor, 1984). Similarly, other family risk factors associated retrospectively with child sexual abuse include poor parent–child relationships, poor relationships between parents, absence of a protective parent, and presence of a nonbiologically related male in the home.

Child victims of sexual abuse present in one of three ways: behavioral changes that are of concern, genital-rectal or medical complaints, or a specific disclosure of developmentally inappropriate sexual contact. Pregnancy in the very young adolescent should be regarded as an indication of possible sexual abuse. Genital or anal injury should raise the suspicion of abuse. In the older adolescent, eating disorders such as bulimia have been associated with a greater incidence of childhood sexual experiences (Abramson and Lucido, 1991).

History

The diagnosis of sexual abuse is established on the history obtained from the child. Physical examination is infrequently diagnostic in the absence of a history and/or specific laboratory findings (Tilleli et al, 1980). Therefore, the information from the child in cases of sexual abuse takes on a sense of legal importance because the child's out-of-court statements are sometimes the only evidence in the case. It is critical that the interview be carried out with the same attention to detail used in the collection of forensic evaluations (Myers, 1987). The initial history should be obtained from the parent or accompanying adult, followed by the child's history taken separate from and not in the presence of the accompanying adult(s). The interview should be unhurried, calm, and nonjudgmental and should include three phases. The first phase establishes rapport. The second phase of the interview will elicit details of the abuse with the use of open-ended questions. An initial question may be "Do you know why you are here today?" or "Some kids or teenagers that I see may have had someone touch them in ways that are confusing and difficult to understand by people that they know and trust. Would anything like that have ever happened to you?" These questions are followed by additional open-ended ones covering further details: who did this; what happened; where and when did it happen. It is desirable to maintain a nonjudgmental facial expression and a "tell me more" or "and then what happened" approach. Younger children may not be able to answer open-ended questions; in this circumstance, the physician may need to ask yes/no questions, remembering that consistency in the answers is important and repeat questioning may be necessary. It is important to document the interview accurately, and it might be helpful to use a hand-held tape recorder during the interview. If the child is uncomfortable with this or a tape recorder is unavailable, appropriate dictation or accurate written history listing the child's statements verbatim should be completed as soon after the interview as feasible.

Although the history is a vital portion of the sexually abused child's evaluation, those patients who present with a previous history of alleged sexual abuse in the context of divorce, custody, or visitation disputes present a complex case. Estimated frequency of false and/or unsubstantiated claims are higher in this setting. There is no single feature associated with a false allegation that can be distinguished from a true case of sexual abuse. Some clues may include a history of abuse from only the parent, a child comfortable with the discussion of her/his abuse, or a child who gives a history only with parental prompting.

Physical Examination and Collection of Evidence

Because the diagnosis of child sexual abuse is established on the basis of a child's history, the physician's diagnostic impression/conclusion should include historical and physical findings. The physical examination has been found to be normal in up to 50% of cases of sexual abuse (Rimsa and Niggemans, 1975; Adams et al, 1994). Well-designed studies concerning normal prepubertal genital anatomy are obviously difficult to obtain because the data rely on parental history to exclude the possibility of abuse. Careful studies of physical findings in children selected for nonabuse have noted findings previously described in sexually abused children, such as vestibular erythema, periurethral bands, labial adhesions, urethral dilation with labial traction, septal remnants/midline tags, and intravaginal ridges (McCann et al, 1990).

Various abnormalities of the genitalia are often confused with sexual abuse. Such conditions include LS, vaginal/vulvar hemangiomas, urethral caruncle, labial agglutination, perianal cellulitis, and vulvar trauma (Bays and Jenny, 1990). Not all genital trauma is abuse related. Some suggestive patterns of abuse include bruising, presence of pinch marks, grip marks, and scratch or burn marks on the lower trunk, genitalia, thighs, or buttocks. As compared with injuries caused by sexual abuse, straddle injuries are more often anterior and unilateral, causing external rather than internal genital damage. Anatomically, the hymen is protected from trauma with straddle injuries. In cases of penetrating sexual abuse that result in tissue damage, the injuries involve primarily the posterior commissure, fossa navicularis, and posterior hymen. As a general rule, posterior hymenal tears between the 3- and 9-o'clock positions suggest sexual abuse. Similarly, "notches" of the hymen, defined by Berenson and coworkers (1992) as concave indentations in the hymen, have not been noted between the 4- and 8-o'clock positions on the hymen in carefully accomplished studies of normal newborn infants or normal prepubertal girls (Berenson et al, 1991, 1992).

The physical examination not only provides diagnostic information by identifying residual abnormalities from the alleged actions, but also serves as a method to enforce a child's sense of normalcy. A commonly expressed fear by child victims is that someone can tell by just looking that they have been abused. This fear can be reduced by asking about this concern prior to the exam and addressing those issues during the exam.

The physical examination should be completed in a relaxed setting with the patient's mother or accompanying adult present. If a child is severely anxious, asymptomatic, and without a history of molestation within the prior 72 hours, the physician may defer the exam at the initial visit. It is important to avoid force, restraint, and "iatrogenic pain." Older, uncooperative children may function better with a supportive nurse and without the mother present. In rare circumstances, an examination under anesthesia may be necessary.

The time interval for collecting forensic medical evidence is generally considered to be within 72 hours of the alleged event. Acute cases should be evaluated immediately. A rape kit appropriately modified for child sexual assault victims should be completed, maintaining a "chain of evidence" (Table 26–7). The physical exam should begin with a general assessment, being careful to determine the presence of hematomas, edema, abrasions, bite marks, or scars. Any noted abnormalities must be recorded with either a sketch or photograph.

The genital exam should be completed using positions and techniques of labial traction as previously described, with careful inspection for bleeding, lacerations, condyloma, or secretions. It is helpful to visualize the hymen with magnification (hand lens, ophthalmoscope, or colposcope), if available. Using a moistened urethral swab (Calgi swab) to run the rim of the hymen or "floating" the hymen in a few drops of saline may allow better visualization of the hymenal edge. Instrumentation of the prepubertal child with a vaginal or nasal speculum is generally not necessary.

Hymenal diameter is a controversial subject because the dimensions have been found to vary with patient relaxation, age, and position (Heger and

Table 26-7. COLLECTING FORENSIC SPECIMENS IN SEXUAL ABUSE

1. Obtain 2–3 swabbed specimen from each body area assaulted (for sperm, acid phosphatase, P30, mouse anti–human semen-5 [MHS-5] antigen, blood group antigen determinates). Need to be air dried.
2. Mouth: swab under tongue and at buccal pouch next to upper and lower molars.
3. Vagina: Dry or moistened swab or 2-ml saline wash. Overdilution of secretions may give rise to false-negative results for acid phosphatase.
4. Rectum: insert swab at least 0.5–1 inch beyond anus.
5. Specimens should be taken from any other suspicious site in the body or clothing. Saline- or sterile water–moistened swab may be used to lift any stains suspected to be dried seminal fluid.
6. Some forensic labs request that a dry smear be made from the vaginal sample.
7. Collect a saliva specimen to determine the victim's antigen secretion status. Saliva may be collected using 3 or 4 sterile swabs on a 2 × 2″ gauze pad placed in mouth.
8. Obtain a venous blood sample from victim for antigen secretor status.
9. Save torn, bloody, or any clothing suspected to be semen stained (including tampons, pads, or diapers). These items should not be packaged in plastic bags. Sealed plastic bags will promote growth of *Candida* and other organisms that might destroy some evidence.
10. Samples of combed pubic hair or scalp hair and fingernails are sometimes taken and may be used to help identify the perpetrator.

Emans, 1990). In general, abnormal measurements in the prepubertal child are 10 to 15 mm (Emans and Goldstein, 1990). Attenuated posterior hymenal rim measurements less than 2 mm may suggest chronic penetrative injury to the hymenal and vestibular area.

Specimens for gonorrhea and *Chlamydia* should be obtained with the use of Calgi swabs. In acute assault cases, a wet-mount evaluation for trichomonads and spermatozoa and a swab slide of vaginal secretions for the forensic lab are in order.

Inspection of the perianal area should be completed in a similar fashion, and gonorrhea and *Chlamydia* cultures obtained. For suspected acute anal assault (72 hours), a swab for semen analysis for the forensic lab should be obtained. A variety of perianal findings have been considered to be the residual of anal trauma. These include perianal erythema and pigmentation, venous congestion, and anal dilation —all of which have been reported in nonabused children (McCann et al, 1988). This underscores the need to coordinate the history and physical findings. An acute anal penetrating injury requires operative evaluation with proctoscopy and possibly laparotomy, in cases in which peritoneal trauma is in question.

Included in the general assessment should be an evaluation of the mouth. Pharyngeal cultures for gonorrhea and *Chlamydia* are necessary. Forceful fellatio often results in labia frenulum tears, loose teeth, and palatal petechia. Appropriate documentation of this is required. If contact is within 24 hours, swabbing gingival surfaces for seminal products is mandatory for complete information.

The presence of semen, sperm, or acid phosphatase, or a positive gonorrhea or *Chlamydia* culture or syphilis serology, makes the diagnosis of sexual abuse a medical certainty even in the absence of a positive history (congenital forms of gonorrhea, *Chlamydia*, and syphilis excluded). Prophylaxis in not necessary in chronic or asymptomatic cases. The culture results can dictate treatment. In acute cases,

ceftriaxone (125 mg IM for patients weighing <45 kg; 250 mg IM for patients weighing >45 kg) and erythromycin (50 mg/kg/day for 7 days) should be offered. Tetanus toxoid should also be administered, as with penetrating injuries.

SPECIFICITY OF STDs FOR SEXUAL ABUSE

Most sexually abused children will not acquire an STD because the abuser may not be infectious at the time of the abuse or may not have an STD, the nature of the abuse may not be one that easily transmits a disease, and/or the prepubertal vagina is not conducive to the growth of the organism. When STDs are present, their diagnostic specificity varies. Gonorrhea or syphilis that is not acquired perinatally indicates abuse. *Chlamydia* can be vertically transmitted and may persist for months to years in vaginal and other orifices; however, it is more commonly found in sexually abused children than in non–sexually abused children. Gonorrhea is the most frequently reported STD in children who have been sexually abused (Beck-Seque and Alexander, 1987). These patients are more likely to have a vaginal discharge and be symptomatic than are those with *Chlamydia* vaginitis. As mentioned previously, it is imperative to use a culture method to diagnose the STD in prepubertal children, rather than rapid detection assessment such as radioimmunoassay and direct fluorescent antibody tests. Syphilis is not commonly detected in child victims of sexual abuse.

Condyloma acuminata are clinical manifestations of the etiologic agent human papillomavirus. Its long incubation period allows perinatal transmission to be manifested in children up to 24 months of age. The long latency period associated with this virus makes it difficult to identify the child's contact. Also, nonsexual transmission is possible, although not usual, with the same viral types as those that involve the genital tract. A single wart may express different viral subtypes at different times; therefore, viral typing may not assist in identifying all types represented. Because genital warts have been linked to sexual abuse, all cases of condyloma must be reported to CPS. Both herpesvirus types 1 and 2 are sexually transmitted and can cause both oral and genital lesions in children and adults. Perinatal transmission has been reported, and nonsexual transmission is theoretically possible. However, there are no proven cases of fomite transmission. *Trichomonas* infection in a prepubertal child outside the first week of life has a high probability of being the result of sexual abuse (Neinstein et al, 1984; Hammerschlag, 1988). Bacterial vaginosis and *Mycoplasma* have been more commonly seen in child victims of sexual abuse (Hammerschlag et al, 1985, 1987; Bump and Buesching, 1988). However, both have also been seen in normal children with genital complaints. Therefore, these organisms should not be taken as significant markers for sexual abuse.

The risk of acquisition of human immunodeficiency virus (HIV) from sexual abuse is likely to be a concern of patients and families. There have been reported cases, although it is unlikely. Currently, screening for HIV is reasonable if a child gives a history of repeated abuse by multiple perpetrators or is symptomatic or if the perpetrator is known to have acquired immunodeficiency syndrome (AIDS), is a known bisexual, or is a known intravenous drug abuser. If the screening test is initially negative, a repeat screen is indicated in 3 to 6 months after the first test. The issue of AIDS should be addressed and discussed with all victims and families.

The Centers for Disease Control and Prevention recommendations for testing for commonly encountered STDs in cases of sexual abuse of prepubertal infants and children are listed in Table 26–8.

Postdiagnosis Responsibilities

The physician's role after completion of the physical examination is first to reassure the child and the family. In most cases the examination will yield normal findings; however, the patient will be very concerned about permanent physical damage. Therefore, reassurance of the "normalcy" of the exam (if appropri-

ate) and of potentially normal reproductive capability are in order. Second, a report to CPS must be completed. All 50 states have laws requiring physicians to report suspected child abuse to the state CPS agency for further investigation. Failure to report such suspicions can result in misdemeanor or felony charges against the physician. The third responsibility involves a referral for counseling for the child and possibly family members. At a minimum, all sexually abused children, after their initial evaluation, should have a single visit with someone skilled in assessing of the emotional stress of the sexually abused child. Those patients presenting with acute assault should have a follow-up in 1 to 2 weeks. If no prophylaxis was given, repeat cultures should be obtained at this visit.

Precocious Puberty

The onset of normal puberty in 98.8% of North American girls (mean + 2.5 standard deviations) is between the ages of 8 and 13 (Zacharias et al, 1976). The first usual sign of impending puberty is increased growth rate (peak growth velocity) followed by thelarche (breast development), which occurs between the ages of 9 and 11. Pubarche, occurring at a median age of 10.5, usually follows thelarche but can occasionally precede breast development. Menarche usually occurs at 12.8 years of age and $2^1/_2$ years after thelarche. The final endocrinologic hallmark of puberty is the establishment of ovulatory menstrual cycles, which may take up to 4 years postmenarche to occur (Speroff et al, 1994).

Precocious puberty, by definition, is the onset of pubertal characteristics before the age of 8; it affects nearly 1 of every 180 normal American girls (Styne and Grumbach, 1986; Grumbach and Styne, 1992). Sexual precocity may be due to premature activation of the hypothalamic-pituitary-ovarian (HPO) axis. (Gonadotropin-releasing hormone [GnRH]-dependent, complete, or true precocity), or it may be due to autonomous sex steroid secretion (GnRH-independent, incomplete, or pseudoprecocity). Table

---

Table 26–8. RECOMMENDED TESTING FOR STDs

The U.S. Public Health Services Centers for Disease Control recommends that the following tests for STDs should be performed on all child sexual abuse victims:

1) Gonococcal (gonorrhea) cultures—pharyngeal, anal, and urethral or vaginal sites.
2) Chlamydial cultures—pharyngeal, anal, and urethral or vaginal sites. Cultures should be obtained from all sites for gonococcal and chlamydial infections since symptoms may not always be present and the infections are often found in body areas not described as contact areas during the abuse.
3) RPR or VDRL, blood tests for diagnosis of syphilis.
4) Examination for condyloma acuminata or venereal warts.
5) Herpes simplex virus cultures of any inflamed areas seen on physical examination.
6) Testing for HIV should be based on the prevalence of infection and on suspected risk.
7) In addition, for females, wet mount of urine and vaginal secretions for microscopic examination for trichomonas, and tests for bacterial vaginosis.

From Centers for Disease Control: Sexually transmitted diseases treatment guidelines. MMRW, Morbid Mortal Wkly Rep, 1989;38:40.

Table 26-9. ORIGINS OF PRECOCIOUS PUBERTY

I. Central GnRH-dependent precocious puberty
   A. Idiopathic, including familial
   B. CNS dysfunction
      1. Congenital defects
         a. Septo-optic dysplasia
      2. Destruction from tumors
         a. Craniopharyngiomas
         b. Dysgerminomas
         c. Ependymomas
         d. Ganglioneuromas
         e. Optic gliomas
      3. Destruction from other space-occupying lesions
         a. Arachnoid cysts
         b. Suprasellar cysts
      4. Excessive exposure to sex steroids
         a. Congenital adrenal hyperplasia
         b. McCune-Albright syndrome
      5. Excessive pressure
         a. Hydrocephalus
      6. Infection/inflammation
         a. Brain abscess
         b. Encephalitis
         c. Granulomas
         d. Meningitis
      7. Injury
         a. Head trauma
         b. Irradiation
      8. Redundant GnRH-secreting tissues
         a. Hypothalamic hamartomas
      9. Syndromes/phakomatoses
         a. Neurofibromatosis (with or without optic gliamas)
         b. Prader-Willi syndrome
         c. Tuberous sclerosis

II. Peripheral (GnRH-independent) precocious puberty
   A. Central
      1. Associated with severe endocrine deficiency states
         a. Chronic primary hypothyrodism
         b. Adrenal insufficiency
   B. Peripheral
      1. Ovarian tumors
         a. Granulosa cell
         b. Granulosa-theca cell
         c. Mixed germ cell
         d. Cystadenoma
         e. Gonadoblastoma
         f. Lipoid
      2. Ovarian cysts
      3. McCune-Albright syndrome
      4. Feminizing adrenal tumors
      5. Exogenous sex steroids
III. Incomplete precocious puberty
   A. Premature breast development
      1. Premature thelarche
      2. Initial presentation: precocious puberty
      3. Nonprogressive precocious puberty
      4. Exogenous sex steroids
   B. Premature pubarche
      1. Premature adrenarche
      2. Congenital adrenal hyperplasia
      3. Adrenal tumors
      4. Ovarian tumors
         a. Arrhenoblastoma (Sertoli-Leydig)
         b. Lipoid tumors
   C. Isolated vaginal bleeding
      1. Exogenous sex steroids
      2. Foreign body
      3. Hemorrhagic cystitis
      4. Hypothyroidism
      5. McCune-Albright syndrome
      6. Ovarian cyst
      7. Sexual abuse/child abuse
      8. Trauma
      9. Tumor
         a. Rhabdomyosarcoma
         b. Clear cell
         c. Endodermal carcinoma
         d. Mesonephric carcinoma
      10. Urethral prolapse
      11. Vulvovaginitis

From O'Dea LS, Siegel SF, Lee PA: Pubertal disorders: precocious and delayed puberty. In Sanfilippo JS, Muram MD, Lee PA, Dewhurst J (eds): Pediatric and Adolescent Gynecology. Philadelphia, WB Saunders Company, 1994:55, with permission.

26-9 gives an extensive list of differential diagnoses for precocious puberty.

GnRH-Dependent Sexual Precocity (True or Complete Precocious Puberty)

Idiopathic precocity is the most common cause of precocious puberty in females and results from failure of central inhibition of the GnRH pulse generator. This can be familial, in which the precocity occurs close to the age of 8 and is called constitutional. The diagnosis of idiopathic precocity is a diagnosis of exclusion and requires long-term follow-up because specific lesions may not be initially evident. Specific causes of central or GnRH-dependent sexual precocity are diverse central nervous system lesions and conditions including various tumors, trauma, encephalopathic and infectious conditions, and history of cranial irradiation (Kelch, 1991). In girls with GnRH-dependent precocity, one case with a definable central nervous system lesion is found for every 12 cases of idiopathic precocity (Grumbach and Styne, 1992).

GnRH-Independent Sexual Precocity (Pseudo- or Incomplete Precocious Puberty)

CENTRAL CAUSES

Although autonomous production of sex steroids is the most common etiology for incomplete or pseudo–precocious puberty, centrally stimulated, gonadotropin-dependent ovarian production can occur in severe glandular insufficiency syndromes such as severe hypothyroidism or adrenal insufficiency and result in sexual precocity (Wood et al, 1965; Hemady et al, 1978). The mechanism for this is not clear. In the past it was hypothesized to result from an "overlap syndrome" secondary to a condition of pituitary hyperstimulation (Van Wyck and Grumbach, 1960). In hypothyroidism, the high concentrations of thyrotropin-releasing factor were thought to cross over and stimulate the secretion of other pituitary glycoproteins, such as gonadotropins, in addition to thyroid-stimulating hormone (TSH). More recent in vitro studies have found that TSH and follicle-stimulating hormone (FSH) act through the same receptor, the FSH receptor, which may be the mechanism for the sexual precocity associated with hypothyroidism (Anasti et al, 1995). An additional associated finding in cases of precocity caused by hypothyroidism is the presence of theca-lutein ovarian cysts, which can be quite large and confuse the initial diagnostic impression (Lindsay et al, 1980; Nishi et al, 1985). Surgical resection of these cysts is not indicated unless there is adnexal or ovarian torsion. Both the precocity and the cysts will resolve with thyroid hormone replacement (Figs. 26–26 and 26–27).

PERIPHERAL CAUSES

Ovarian causes of sexual precocity are not common and account for only 3% of cases (Towne et al, 1975). They usually cause rapid pubertal changes and ovarian enlargement. In the majority of cases, the ovaries will be palpable on either rectal or abdominal examination. Solid tumors require that tumor markers be drawn preoperatively to assist in management. Conservative surgery restricted to the affected adnexa is warranted until complete pathologic diagnosis is known.

Functional ovarian cysts can cause transient estrogen production and sexual precocity. Ovarian cysts can also be associated with McCune-Albright syndrome. This is a syndrome of precocious puberty presenting with café au lait nevi with a "coast of Maine" border and polyostotic fibrous dysplasia. Because this syndrome is associated with a mutation in G protein–coupled receptors, multiple, discrete areas of autonomously functioning cells can arise in various tissues, resulting in multiple endocrinopathies (Lefkowitz, 1993). Therefore, traditional methods of treating precocious puberty are not effective. The use of testolactone, an aromatase inhibitor, to block the conversion of androgens to estrogens has been effective (Feuillan et al, 1993).

Variations of Pubertal Development

PREMATURE THELARCHE

Premature thelarche is the occurrence of isolated breast development in the absence of other clinical signs of sexual maturation in girls before age 8 years. The highest prevalence is during the first 2 years of life, and it is rare after age 4 (Grumbach and Styne, 1992). The pathophysiologic mechanism of the premature thelarche is still unknown; it has been postulated to result from increased breast sensitivity to estrogen (Ilicki et al, 1984), transient estrogen secretion by follicular cysts of the ovary (Sizonenko, 1978),

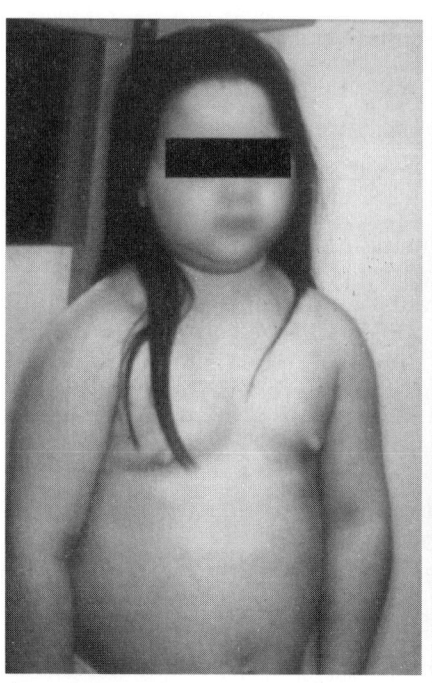
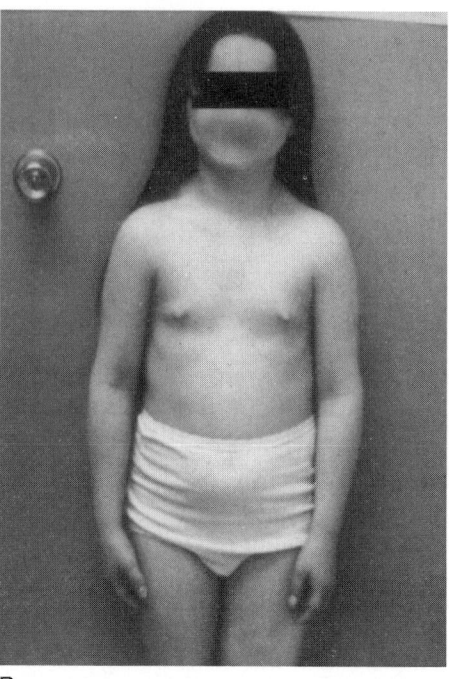

A   B

Figure 26–26
Eight-year-old girl with precocious puberty secondary to hypothyroidism. *A*, Pretreatment. *B*, Three months after thyroid replacement. (From Hertweck SP: In Yordan EE [ed]: The PediGyn Teaching Slide Set. Philadelphia: North American Society for Pediatric and Adolescent Gynecology, 1996:slide 88, with permission.)

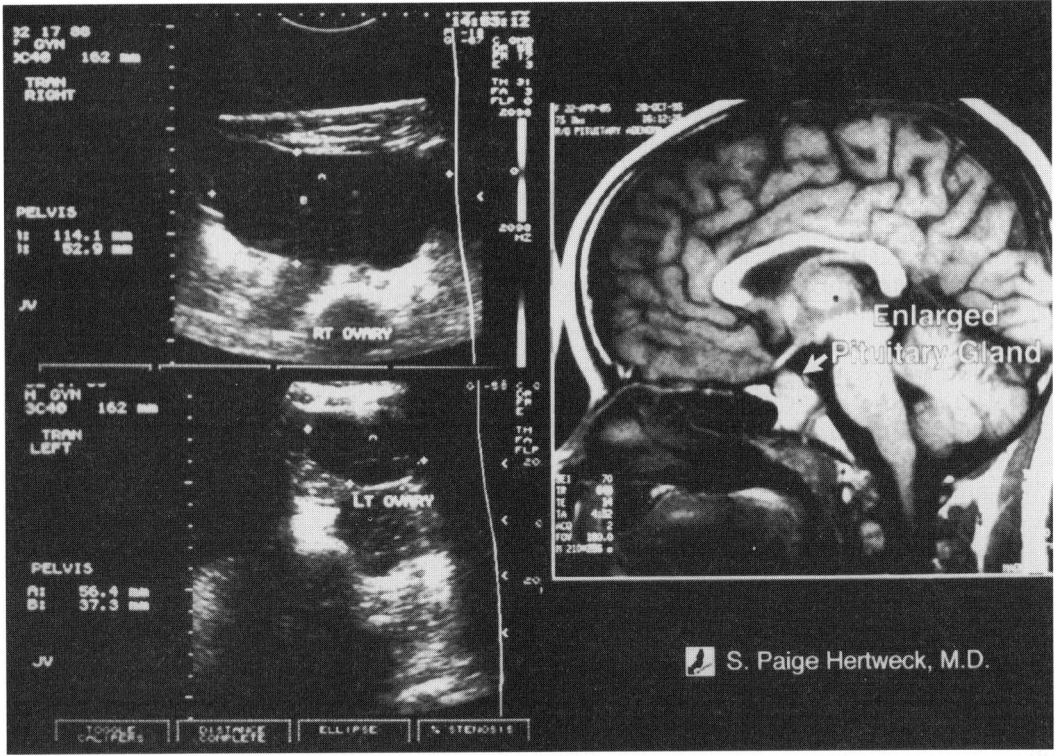

Figure 26–27
Patient in Figure 26–26*A* with theca-lutein ovarian cysts and pituitary enlargement. Both resolved after treatment. (From Hertweck SP: In Yordan EE [ed]: The PediGyn Teaching Slide Set. Philadelphia: North American Society for Pediatric and Adolescent Gynecology, 1996:slide 87, with permission.)

increased production of estrogens from precursors of adrenal origin (Dumic et al, 1982), increased dietary estrogen as a result of exogenous contamination of food (Saenz de Rodriguez et al, 1985), and transient partial activation of the hypothalamic-pituitary-gonadal axis with excessive secretion of FSH (Job et al, 1977; Reiter et al, 1975; Pasquino et al, 1980, 1985; Beck and Stubbe, 1984). These patients should be evaluated with estradiol and FSH levels, nondominant wrist radiograph for bone age, and a pelvic sonogram. In the past, premature thelarche was thought to always be a self-limited condition with no impact on the timing of puberty. However, a more recent retrospective evaluation of 100 girls originally diagnosed with premature thelarche revealed 14 progressed to precocious or early central puberty. There were no clinical or hormonal characteristics that could be established to separate the 14 children who progressed to precocity from the 86 who did not (Pasquino et al, 1995). Although the majority of cases will be self-limited, young girls presenting with premature thelarche should be monitored clinically for accelerated pubertal progression.

PREMATURE PUBARCHE

Premature pubarche (or adrenarche) is defined as the appearance of pubic hair before age 8. The causes for this condition include isolated adrenarche (increased adrenal androgen secretion or increased peripheral sensitivity to adrenal androgens), mild enzyme deficiency in adrenal steroidogenesis, and tumors. Levels of testosterone, dehyroepiandrosterone sulfate (DHEAS), and early morning 17-OHP and bone age determination can assist in the diagnosis. Follow-up data on two groups of European children with premature pubarche revealed a transient acceleration of growth and bone maturation but no negative effect on the onset of puberty, progression of puberty, or final adult height (Ibenez et al, 1992). These patients may have an increased incidence of hirsutism or polycystic ovarian disease, and therefore continued follow-up is necessary.

Evaluation and Treatment of Sexual Precocity

It is important to determine the cause of precocity, because life-threatening disease such as ovarian, central nervous system, or adrenal neoplasm must be ruled out. In addition, untreated sexual precocity results in premature epiphyseal closure with stunted final adult height. Prompt treatment prevents potential mortality and allows the patient to achieve a more normal stature.

The goal of the evaluation is to determine the source of the hormonal stimulation by beginning with a complete history and physical examination. A history of neurologic symptoms (headache, nausea, and photophobia), neurologic signs, and rapid progression of pubertal changes and abdominal complaints are indicators of a pathologic process and need for further investigation. The parents should be questioned about the access of the child to hormonal agents such as oral contraceptives (OCs) or other sex steroids.

Physical examination includes determination of height, weight, and hair distribution; thyroid gland assessment; detection of abdominal and/or pelvic masses; and skin findings such as café au lait spots seen in neurofibromatosis or McCune-Albright syndrome. A thorough neurologic and genital examination should be performed. Tanner staging is used to evaluate breast development and pubic hair distribution (Fig. 26–17).

Laboratory evaluation may include FSH, luteinizing hormone (LH), β-human chorionic gonadotropin, TSH, thyroxine, and estradiol levels. If a central mediated cause of precocious puberty is suspected, a GnRH provocation test is required (Kulin, 1987; Pescovitz et al, 1985). In cases of heterosexual precocity or precocious pubarche, 17-OHP, DHEAS, and testosterone levels are indicated. Radiologic evaluation includes wrist films for bone age, skull films, and an assessment of the central nervous system with computed tomography (CT) or MRI. Pelvic ultrasonography and/or abdominal pelvic CT imaging may be indicated in selected cases. Careful synthesis of patient age, clinical presentation, and pertinent laboratory test information can direct practical use of imaging studies.

The evaluation may point to one or more central nervous system lesions, which are usually in the vicinity of the hypothalamus. Management is complex because some lesions cannot be extirpated because of their location and may require chemotherapy and/or radiation therapy. If peripheral causes are identified, such as an ovarian or adrenal mass, the precocity is usually corrected with surgical intervention. Gonadotropin-independent, autonomous, benign ovarian cysts have been described (Lightner and Kelch, 1984). These patients do not have serum GnRH pulses, and the cysts are not suppressed with GnRH agonist therapy. The cysts may appear intermittently and present with associated vaginal bleeding. GnRH stimulation testing differentiates the autonomous cyst from that caused by true precocious puberty, which is secondary to stimulation by FSH and/or LH. If true (central) precocity is diagnosed, once a life-threatening lesion has been ruled out, the most effective therapy consists of suppression of GnRH release with GnRH agonists. This leads to a significant diminution of FSH and LH release with resultant suppression of gonadal steroid secretion. Treatment results in higher final adult height by delaying epiphyseal closure (Mansfield et al, 1983).

ADOLESCENT GYNECOLOGIC CONDITIONS

Dysfunctional Uterine Bleeding

Dysfunctional uterine bleeding (DUB) is the most frequent, urgent, gynecologic problem of the adolescent (Sanfilippo and Yussman, 1985). It is defined as excessive, prolonged, or unpatterned bleeding from the uterine endometrium that is unrelated to anatomic lesions of the uterus. Typically, these abnormal bleeding events present as minor alterations of cycle flow length, but on occasion they can be severe enough to require hospitalization. Regardless of the medical severity of the condition, the patient is very likely to be extremely concerned with her lack of normalcy. This provides the physician with a unique opportunity to assist the adolescent with her emergence into womanhood by providing appropriate education, reassurance, and treatment in the realm of confidentiality.

Anovulation or disruption of normal ovarian function accounts for more than 75% of cases of DUB. In adolescents, 95% of cases of anovulation are due to the immaturity of the HPO axis. These adolescents lack the positive feedback mechanism necessary to initiate an LH surge and subsequent ovulation despite increased follicular estrogen levels (Van Look et al, 1978; Livio et al, 1986; Neinstein, 1990). Interestingly, negative estrogen feedback is intact in these patients, because provocative testing with estrogen causes suppression of FSH and LH (Baird, 1976) and GnRH stimulation in these patients is normal, indicating a hypothalamic problem rather than a pituitary one (Livio et al, 1986; Neinstein, 1990).

Although menarche occurs at an average age of 12.8 years in the United States, the establishment of orderly ovulatory bleeding may take up to 5 years (Gidwani, 1984). McDonough and Ganett (1982) observed anovulation in 55% to 82% of the cycles from menarche to 2 years after menarche, in 30% to 55% of the cycles from 2 to 4 years, and in 0% to 20% of cycles from 4 to 5 years after menarche.

In determining whether bleeding patterns are normal or abnormal, the clinician needs to be cognizant of normal variations of the menstrual cycle. Normal menstrual cycles have been defined as a mean interval of 28 days (±7 days) with a duration of 4 days (±2 to 3 days) (Mischell, 1987). Normal menstrual flow is approximately 30 mg/cycle (Grumbach et al, 1991), with an upper limit of normal at 60 to 80 ml (Halberg et al, 1966). Therefore, bleeding occurring at an interval of 21 days or less for greater than 7 days and greater than 80 ml is considered abnormal. Definitions for various menstrual abnormalities are listed in Table 26–10.

Diagnosis

DUB is a diagnosis of exclusion (Hertweck, 1992). It is established when a patient has abnormal bleeding and when inflammatory, neoplastic, and pregnancy-

Table 26–10. DEFINITIONS OF MENSTRUAL ABERRATIONS

Polymenorrhea	Frequent irregular bleeding at less than 18-day intervals
Oligomenorrhea	Infrequent irregular bleeding at intervals of more than 45 days
Metrorrhagia	Intermenstrual bleeding between regular periods
Menorrhagia	Excessive uterine bleeding occurring regularly; synonymous with the term *hypermenorrhea*
Menometrorrhagia	Frequent, irregular, excessive, and prolonged uterine bleeding

related causes have been excluded. The causes of abnormal bleeding in the adolescent age group include anatomic lesions such as polyps, leiomyomata, vaginal adenosis, and hemangiomas; coagulation disorders such as von Willebrand's disease, idiopathic thrombocytopenic purpura, platelet defects, and thalassemia major; and pregnancy complications such as threatened, incomplete, or spontaneous abortion, ectopic pregnancy, and molar pregnancy. Patients with infections such as vaginitis, cervicitis, or pelvic inflammatory disease; trauma; foreign bodies; systemic illnesses such as adrenal, hepatic, renal, or thyroid dysfunction; or diabetes mellitus may also present with abnormal uterine bleeding. Another quite common cause of irregular uterine bleeding is medication, including complications associated with the use of hormonal contraceptive preparations (Table 26–11).

Despite the extensive possibilities, the usual diagnosis in 95% of adolescent patients with DUB remains *anovulation*. As previously stated, the most common cause of anovulation in the adolescent is

HPO axis immaturity. However, it is important to recognize that any hypothalamic dysfunction such as that associated with stress, exercise, or weight loss, as well as systemic diseases, can also affect ovulation.

The second most common cause of abnormal bleeding in the adolescent is *coagulation disorders*. Claessens and Cowell (1981), in their 9-year review, examined all admissions at a childrens' hospital for acute menorrhagia and determined that 19% were the result of primary coagulation disorders. These disorders included idiopathic thrombocytopenic purpura, von Willebrand's disease, Glanzmann's disease (a primary qualitative platelet defect), Fanconi's anemia, and thalassemia major. An underlying coagulation disorder was noted in one of four girls with severe menorrhagia and a hemoglobin of less than 10 g/100 ml and in one of two adolescents presenting at the time of menarche. Of those patients with bleeding dyscrasias, 10% present with cyclic hypermenorrhea. The most common hematologic disorder in the adolescent is thrombocytopenic purpura (Gidwani, 1984).

The initial step in evaluating abnormal bleeding involves a detailed clinical history followed by a complete physical examination. The history should be confidential, ideally obtained from the adolescent patient and not completed in the presence of the parent(s). The initial interview should focus on the current problem, including when abnormal bleeding first occurred, extent of blood loss, time of menarche, frequency of bleeding, and duration of the last menstrual period. Following this, the patients' problem can be classified into one of the categories listed in Table 26–10. The timing of bleeding is helpful in determining the cause. Abnormal bleeding that occurs cyclically at the time of normal menses or initiated with menarche is indicative of a coagulation disor-

Table 26–11. DIFFERENTIAL DIAGNOSIS OF ABNORMAL VAGINAL BLEEDING

Anovulation
Anatomic lesions
  Cervical/endometrial polyps
  Leiomyoma
  Vaginal adenosis
  Changes associated with DES exposure
  Malignancies
  Trauma
  Foreign bodies
  Hemangiomas
Coagulation disorders
  von Willebrand's disease
  Thrombocytopenic purpura
  Platelet defects
  Platelet storage pool diseases
  Thalassemia major
Pregnancy complications
  Threatened/spontaneous abortion
  Ectopic pregnancy
  Hydatidiform mole
  Retained products of conception

Infections
  Cervicitis/vaginitis
  Pelvic inflammatory disease
Systemic diseases
  Adrenal disorders
  Diabetes mellitus
  Hepatic dysfunction
  Renal dysfunction
  Thyroid dysfunction
Iatrogenic/Medications
  Tranquilizers
  Aspirin/NSAIDs
  Antineoplastic drugs
  Seizure medications
  Oral contraceptives
  Anticoagulants
Exogenous hormone

Abbreviations: DES, diethylstilbestrol; NSAIDs, nonsteroidal anti-inflammatory drugs.

der. Regular cyclic menses with intermenstrual bleeding may indicate the presence of trauma, polyp, cervical lesion, or infection. Patients with a prolonged bleeding interval with cycles greater than 21 to 40 days either have not developed negative-feedback cyclicity or have had it disrupted, or have missed one or more ovulatory cycles. This may represent an immature HPO axis, polycystic ovarian syndrome, or a central or systemic insult to the axis (i.e., stress, weight change, or adrenal-thyroid dysfunction).

A review of pubertal milestones should be evaluated to make a clinical assessment of the maturational state of the HPO axis. A sexual history should also be obtained, including sexual activity level, number of partners, number of pregnancies and outcome, contraceptive use, and proper compliance, including whether condoms are used as protection from STDs.

The medical history of patients with DUB should determine the possible presence of other medical illnesses such as diabetes mellitus or lifestyle habits (poor nutrition, excessive exercise, substance abuse, or eating disorders) that could directly or indirectly account for DUB.

The use of certain medications, such as hormonal treatments, aspirin, nonsteroidal anti-inflammatory medications, and anticoagulants, as well as radiation therapy, should be determined. If the patient is taking oral contraceptives, attention should be directed to proper compliance and concomitant use of antibiotics or seizure medications that could decrease the efficacy and may give rise to irregular bleeding. A family history of endocrine problems, malignancies, and coagulation disorders should be elicited. With respect to coagulation disorders, up to 25% of affected patients give a negative family history (Gidwani, 1984).

The physical examination should include a blood pressure and pulse assessment, which will indicate the chronicity of the condition. The general assessment will provide an estimation of body habitus, stage of secondary sexual characteristics, and stigmata of endocrine or bleeding disorders. A breast and thyroid examination should be completed with particular evaluation for galactorrhea and gland enlargement, respectively. The final portion of the examination should include an abdominal and pelvic assessment to rule out pregnancy or inflammatory and neoplastic diseases. Components of the pelvic examination include inspection of the vulvar, vaginal, and cervical areas, including a speculum examination in an effort to determine signs of pregnancy, presence of a foreign body, an infection, or an anatomic source of bleeding. A bimanual and possibly a rectovaginal examination should complete the physical examination. An adolescent who is 18 years of age should have a Pap smear, as should those teens who are younger and sexually active. *Chlamydia* and gonorrhea cultures may also be indicated for the sexually active teen who has not been screened in the recent past or since the onset of DUB.

The central laboratory tests must include a complete blood count with platelet evaluation, a blood smear, and a serum pregnancy test. This provides an index of severity, chronicity of the bleeding, and an opportunity to rule out a pregnancy. The clinical picture should influence when the following laboratory tests are ordered. For recurrent severe bleeding or onset with menarche, a coagulation profile should be completed, including liver functions, prothrombin time, activated partial thromboplastin time, and bleeding time. It is also a good idea to complete a thyroid evaluation by obtaining a TSH level. If chronic anovulation or irregular menses is present, then LH and FSH levels, thyroid studies (TSH and thyroxin), and a serum prolactin level should be considered. If hirsutism is present, total testosterone and DHEAS levels should be checked initially, with appropriate androgen evaluation if an adrenal enzyme deficiency is suspected.

Treatment

The treatment of DUB in the adolescent is based on the severity of symptomatology, with the objectives of stopping the bleeding and preventing recurrences (Table 26–12). Treatment for mild cases (defined as irregular intervals of bleeding at 20 to 60 days with a normal hemoglobin) should be supportive reassurance. Education should center around proper diet, exercise, stress management, and maintenance of a proper menstrual calendar. Usually these situations resolve after 1 to 2 years with the onset of spontaneous ovulation. Antiprostaglandin medications have been demonstrated to decrease menstrual flow and may be of benefit (Fraser et al, 1981). If contraception is needed, then an OC could be initiated. These patients need re-evaluation on a 6-month basis. In patients with severe, recurrent DUB or DUB associated with anemia, hormonal therapy is indicated. Most commonly, this is accomplished by the initiation of cyclic medroxyprogesterone acetate (Provera; the Upjohn Company, Kalamazoo, MI) or a combination OC. In the treatment of metrorrhagia or polymenorrhea, medroxyprogesterone acetate, 10 mg daily, is prescribed for 10 days/month to induce endometrial stromal stability, which is followed by withdrawal flow. This can be prescribed on calendar days 1 to 14 for 3 to 6 months. If this method is unsuccessful, beginning the medication on cycle day 14 for 10 days may be effective. After a 3- to 6-month trial, the medication may be discontinued and the condition observed for recurrence. If the adolescent needs contraception, then an OC can be used alternatively. These have the added benefit of cycle regulation in that OCs have been noted to decrease the amount of menstrual blood by at least 60% in patients with a normal uterus (Walker and Gustavson, 1983). Because the action of OCs is that of ovulation suppression, the underlying anovulatory problem is not alleviated in these patients. Therefore, the patient should be informed that the majority of individuals

Table 26–12. DUB GENERAL TREATMENT GUIDELINES

Mild DUB (menses 20- to 60-day intervals: normal Hgb)
Education (diet, exercise, stress management)
Supportive reassurance
Menstrual calendar instruction
OCs for contraceptive needs
Antiprostaglandins to decrease flow
Re-evaluate every 6 months
Severe/Recurrent DUB (± anemia)
Medroxyprogesterone acetate
10 mg qd calendar day 1–14 × 3 mo *or*
10 mg qd cycle day 14–24
or
OCs
Acute/Anovulatory Bleeding (stable patient)
50-μg estrogen-progestin OC
1 pill PO every 6 hr until bleeding stops
If no cessation—check coagulation studies
Normal coagulation—consider hysteroscopy
Cessation of menses—taper pills
1 pill PO q8h × 2 days
1 pill PO q12h × 2 days
1 pill PO twice daily × 2 days
1 pill PO qd to complete 24-cycle
Cycle on OCs c 3–6 mo
Acute/Heavy Bleeding (hypotension; HgB ≤ 7)
Hospitalize (coagulation studies)
Consider transfusion
IV Premarin 25 mg IV q6h until bleeding stops
Begin cyclic progestagen-dominant OC (Lo/Ovral; Ovral)
Begin 1 pill PO q6h × 2 days
Then 1 pill PO q8h × 2 days
Then 1 pill PO q12h × 2 days
Then 1 pill PO qd × 24
Then cycle × 2 additional mo
If no response with Premarin in 24–48 h
Re-evaluate coagulation studies
Hysteroscopy
D&C as last resort
dDAVP

Abbreviations: D&C, dilatation and curettage; dDAVP, desmopressin; Hgb, hemoglobin; OC, oral contraceptive.

will have spontaneous ovulation with maturation of the HPO axis. In a significant number, however, anovulation persists.

An acute anovulatory bleeding episode can be controlled with a 50 μg estrogen-progestin contraceptive pill. Therapy consists of one pill every 6 hours until the bleeding stops (usually within 1 to 5 days). If this does not stop the flow, causes other than anovulation must be ruled out, including the presence of myomata, polyps, or bleeding diathesis. If flow diminishes significantly or abates predictably, the OC should be tapered to one pill every day. Then the once-a-day regimen should be continued for the 21-day cycle, after which withdrawal flow will occur. The patient should be warned to anticipate a flow after therapy and may continue OCs for an additional 3 months for treatment purposes or longer if necessary for birth control. In addition to the normal therapy, these adolescents should be placed on iron therapy to compensate for decreased iron stores. Persistent oligomenorrhea, 1 to 2 years after the initial

evaluation, may necessitate further evaluation for chronic anovulation syndrome.

In cases of acute or heavy bleeding, hospitalization, with possible transfusion for hemoglobin levels of less than 7 g/dl, may be indicated. Intravenous conjugated estrogens (Premarin; Wyeth-Ayerst, Philadelphia, PA) may be administered 25 mg every 4 to 6 hours until bleeding ceases (Devore et al, 1982). Conjugated estrogen appears to have multiple, direct effects on clotting, including platelet aggregation, increased fibrinogen levels, increased factors V and IX, and decreased effectiveness of bradykinin, thereby causing hemostasis (Lindsay et al, 1986; Livio et al, 1986). After the bleeding ceases, cyclic progestagen-dominant OCs such as Ovral (Wyeth-Ayerst), Lo/Ovral (Wyeth-Ayerst), or cyclic progestins may be prescribed. The OCs should be used in a tapering fashion, one tablet four times a day for 2 days, three times a day for 2 days, twice a day for 2 days, and once a day for 24 days. The patient should then be allowed to have a withdrawal flow followed by cyclic use for an additional 3 months. A longer tapering dose may also be used in difficult cases: one tablet four times a day for 7 days, three times a day for 7 days, two times a day for 7 days, and once a day for 7 days followed by withdrawal flow and cyclic use.

In acute cases, a response to hormonal therapy is usually seen within 24 to 48 hours. If this does not occur, the patient needs re-evaluation for a coagulopathy or anatomic disorder. Curettage is the last line of attack in the adolescent and is rarely necessary. In those circumstances without response to hormonal therapy, a dilatation and curettage (D&C) and hysteroscopy is advised for diagnostic and therapeutic purposes, followed by appropriate hormonal therapy. If bleeding persists, one must suspect an anatomic abnormality not identified by the D&C. Although this unresponsiveness is rare in the adolescent, its occurrence should prompt re-evaluation. Neoplasia is also rare in the adolescent but does occur. Davis and Reindollar (1991) reported two cases of obese, anovulatory adolescents, ages 17 and 13, who had adenomatous hyperplasia, the former, with severe atypia, diagnosed by D&C and the latter by endometrial biopsy.

Another method of treating severe acute bleeding is the use of desmopressin, a synthetic analog of the neurohypothalamic nonapeptide arginine vasopressin. Classically, this has been used in the treatment of central diabetes insipidus; now it is recommended for abnormal uterine bleeding in patients with different types of hemophilia and von Willebrand's disease, as well as for patients without a coagulation abnormality (Kubrinsky and Tulloch, 1988).

Occasionally patients with longstanding use of oral contraceptives or on depot medroxyprogesterone acetate will develop irregular bleeding. Irregular bleeding in the first 10 to 14 days of the cycle may be secondary to inadequate estrogen production and result in an unstable, atrophic endometrial lining. Cyclic estrogen, in the form of conjugated estrogen

2.5 mg daily for 7 days during the first 10 to 14 days of the cycle, should control this problem.

Antiprostaglandins act on the endometrial vasculature and decrease menstrual blood loss (Anderson et al, 1976; Fraser et al, 1981). This is noted in normal women and in women with bleeding associated with chronic endometritis, as is seen with intrauterine contraceptive devices. These compounds may be prescribed in conjunction with cyclic hormonal therapy. There are numerous preparations available, none with superiority over the others. Commonly, they are initiated at the first sign of menses and continued throughout the cycle.

In rare situations in which hormonal therapy is contraindicated or bleeding is excessive and uncontrollable, the use of GnRH analogs has been recommended. Their administration suppresses gonadotropin secretion and subsequent estradiol secretion, which results in arrest of menstruation; therefore, they not only decrease menorrhagia but produce amenorrhea (McLaughlan et al, 1986). McLaughlan et al reported that, after 12 weeks of intranasal GnRH (Buserelin) treatment in four women with menorrhagia, the total menstrual blood loss decreased from 95 to 198 ml/month in the second and third treatment cycles. Limitations to long-term GnRH agonist use are osteoporosis and undesirable lipoprotein changes. Whereas these findings are reversible, the risks for this modality far outweigh the benefits for long-term treatment.

Treatments that eliminate reproductive potential, such as hysterectomy or endometrial ablation, are only rarely indicated in the adolescent patient.

Prognosis

The long-term prognosis for adolescents with irregular bleeding can be described as guarded. About 5% never ovulate, and many develop recurrent DUB and merit an endocrinologic evaluation. The importance of continued follow-up is illustrated in a 25-year prospective evaluation of adolescents with DUB (Southam and Richard, 1996). In 29 patients, 60% had continued bleeding for 2 years after initial onset. Persistent problems were noted in 50% of the patients after 4 years and in 30% after 10 years. Except in cases of blood dyscrasias, patients with normal menses before irregular bleeding had a more favorable prognosis.

Teenage Contraception and Interception

Adolescent sexuality and teenage pregnancy are major concerns of the 1990s resulting in 1 million adolescent pregnancies annually in the United States. A central problem is that, although approximately 56% of women become sexually active before their 18th birthday, most young women are sexually active long before they seek contraception. Only 40% go for medical contraceptive services within the first year after they begin intercourse (Alan Guttmacher Institute, 1988), resulting in a significant number of unwanted pregnancies.

The most important factor in providing effective contraceptive guidance to adolescents is to start counseling prior to first intercourse. It is important to recognize that most adolescents, when asked, want to talk to their physicians about contraception and STDs. Therefore, the examining physician needs to take the opportunity to introduce sexually related topics and to have some basic questions to aid in determining the adolescent's level of knowledge and cognitive development regarding sexually related issues. Questions such as the following are helpful: "What have you talked about in sex education at school?" "What would you tell a girlfriend who is going to have sex?"

It is equally important to take the opportunity to support good decision making on the part of the adolescent. Some teenagers are reluctant to admit lack of sexual activity, assuming that most peers are sexually active. The physician can use this opportunity to reinforce the wise behavior, but should remember to leave communication lines open so that future contraception needs may be provided when necessary. Spending adequate time in the first visit with an adolescent can help to establish lines of communication. In that first visit, it is important to assure confidentiality and involve the adolescent by asking open-ended questions in a nonjudgmental way.

The second most important goal in providing effective contraceptive guidance is to identify what contraceptive method the adolescent is likely to use and provide supportive counseling to help ensure continued use of the chosen method. Important factors to consider when choosing a contraceptive method for an adolescent include acceptability, effectiveness of method, frequency of intercourse, number of partners, concern about STDs, cost/access to medical care, motivation/self-discipline of the patient/partner, safety/risk factors, and personal/family religious and ethical philosophy (Slupik, 1994).

OCs may be the method of choice for the adolescent because of their ease of use, low failure rate, and multiple noncontraceptive benefits not directly related to the act of intercourse. The disadvantages include the need for daily motivation, initial cost of the physician visit, and monthly expenditure. Older adolescents in suburban residences who have experience with the use of barrier methods of contraception and have higher educational goals are much more likely to comply with OCs. Patients with multiple partners and low valuation of personal health are less likely to comply (Scher et al, 1982). Most healthy adolescents do well on any low-dose pill. Many physicians have a preference for monophasic 28-day pills for consistency.

Initial counseling should include a description of OC mechanism of action and a discussion of the need for STD protection and the risks and benefits with appropriate documentation. It may be helpful to give written and oral description and instructions. Using a 28-day pill regimen to avoid the pill-free interval confusion may also aid in adolescent compliance. It may also help to link pill taking to a daily activity (e.g., brushing teeth) and to consider a Sunday start regimen for all adolescents. Discussion of the noncontraceptive benefits may also enhance compliance.

The low cost, over-the-counter availability, and STD protection associated with condoms make them an advantageous method for teenagers. Often a partner's unwillingness to use these barriers make this choice one that is less desirable. With proper use, condom effectiveness rates approach 90% to 98%. It may be helpful to assist adolescents in being assertive about condom use by telling them how to use condoms and what to say to encourage their partner to use them, and by providing samples.

The diaphragm may be suitable for well-motivated teenagers in a stable relationship. Those teen patients who choose to use diaphragms are usually better students, are of a higher socioeconomic status, and have had fewer pregnancies than OC users (Slupick 1994). The advantages of the diaphragm for the teen are the low cost and some STD protection. Disadvantages include the necessity of physician fitting and possible disruption of foreplay.

There are multiple forms of spermicides (foams, creams, suppositories, and films). The most widely used agents are nonoxynol-9 and octoxynol-9. These methods, like the condom, have a reasonable cost, are available over the counter, have a discreet size, and do not require physician evaluation. Their use should be discussed, especially with adolescents who are relying only on barrier methods of contraception.

The female condom is a soft, loose polyurethane sheath with two flexible rings. One internal ring covers the cervix and one external ring covers the vulva. Although this is somewhat cumbersome, it has the advantage of over-the-counter availability, disposability, and female control over the use of the device. An awareness of the availability of such a device is important for adolescent protection.

Adolescents' tendencies toward multiple partners and serial monogamy, which increase the risk pelvic inflammatory disease, ectopic pregnancy, and subsequent infertility, create the basis not not recommending the use of intrauterine contraceptive devices in most adolescents. One might consider their use in an older adolescent with one or more children who has a contraindication to hormonal therapy, has failed while using OC/barrier methods and/or has no history of pelvic inflammatory disease or multiple partners.

The Food and Drug Administration approved depot medroxyprogesterone acetate (Depo-Provera) for contraceptive use in 1992. The advantage of this method for the adolescent is its use remote from the time of coitus and a pregnancy rate of less than 0.5 per 100 women annually. The associated weight gain and 20% to 30% breakthrough bleeding make counseling before use very important. Sixty percent of patients using Depo-Provera experience amenorrhea at the end of the first year of use. This can be very useful in patients in whom amenorrhea is a desired effect. The AAP has endorsed the use of Depo-Provera in mentally disabled individuals. Depo-Provera may have an adverse effect on bone mineral density, and prospective studies are under investigation. This is an important issue because bone density is reaching its peak in adolescence. With confirmation of an adverse effect on bone density, the use of Depo-Provera may require monitoring for bone loss.

Norplant subdermal implants provide highly effective and reversible contraception with a failure rate of 4.5 per 1000 users annually. Studies comparing the adolescent use of Norplant with adult use revealed an 86% to 90% satisfaction rate despite the common complaints of menstrual irregularity and weight gain (Berenson and Wiemann, 1993). Norplant has been shown to be a very effective method of birth control in the postpartum adolescent. Forty-eight postpartum Norplant users were compared with 50 postpartum OC users and evaluated 15 months later. There were no differences in the frequency of clinic visits or the incidence of STD. At 15 months, the compliance rate of Norplant users was 95% compared with only a 33% compliance rate in the OC users. In the Norplant group there was only one pregnancy; there were 19 pregnancies in the OC group. The factors associated with the choice of Norplant were multiparity and previous OC use (Polaneczy et al, 1994). Depo-Provera has been shown to be more cost-effective than Norplant unless the Norplant implant remains in place for 4 years. This reinforces the need for extensive preplacement counseling not only in adolescent users but in all women.

Adolescents need to be aware of postcoital contraception. The use of two 50 μg combination estrogen-progestin pills can be 60% to 80% effective in reducing the risk of pregnancy, if given within 72 hours of unprotected coitus and then repeated 12 hours later.

In adolescents, the best choices for contraception are hormonal methods: OCs, depot medroxyprogesterone acetate, or subdermal implants. Each patient's cognitive development needs to be assessed to determine predicted compliance with any chosen method. Frequent follow-ups are necessary to assess for compliance and weight or blood pressure changes, to answer concerns, and to screen for side effects. Because many adolescents practice serial monogamy and do not recognize this as a risk factor for acquiring STDs, reinforcing the need to use condoms in addition to contraception is necessary.

REFERENCES

Abramson EE, Lucido GM: Childhood sexual experiences and bulimia. Addictive Behav 1991;16:529.

Adams JA, Harper K, Knudson S, et al: Examination findings in legally confirmed sexual abuse: it's normal to be normal. Pediatrics 1994;94:3.

Alan Guttmacher Institute: Sex and America's Teenagers. New York: Alan Guttmacher Institute, 1988. Telephone New York City—(212) 248-1111 or 248-2203.

Altchek A: Pediatric adolescent gynecology. Comp Ther 1995; 21(5):235.

American Academy of Pediatrics Committee on Child Abuse and Neglect: Guidelines for the evaluation of sexual abuse in children. Pediatrics 1991;87:254.

Anasti JN, Flack MR, Froehlich J, et al: A potential novel mechanism for precocious puberty in juvenile hypothyroidism. J Clin Endocrinol Metab 1995;80:276.

Anderson ABM, Haynes PJ, Guillebaud J, et al: Reduction of menstrual blood loss by prostaglandin synthetase inhibitors. Lancet 1976;1:774.

Ariberg A: Topical oesrogen therapy for labial adhesions in children. Br J Obstet Gynaecol 1975;82:424.

Baird DT: Disturbance in the negative feedback loops of the pituitary ovarian axis. Clin Obstet Gynecol 1976;3:335.

Baldwin DD, Landa HM: Common problems in pediatric gynecology. Urol Clin North Am 1995;22:161.

Bays F, Jenny C: Genital and anal conditions confused with child sexual abuse trauma. Am J Dis Child 1990;144:1319.

Beck W, Stubbe P: Pulsatile secretion of luteinizing hormone and sleep-related gonadotropin rhythms in girls with premature thelarche. Eur J Pediatr 1984;141:168.

Beck-Seque C, Alexander ER: Sexually transmitted diseases in children and adolescents. Infect Dis Clin North Am 1987;1:277.

Bell TA, Stamm WE, Kuo CC, et al: Delayed appearance of *Chlamydia trachomatis* infection acquired at birth. Pediatr Infect Dis 1987;6:928.

Berenson A, Heger A, Andrew S: Appearance of the hymen in newborns. Pediatrics 1991;87:458.

Berenson AB, Heger AN, Hayes JM, et al: Appearance of the hymen in prepubertal girls. Pediatrics 1992;89:307.

Berenson AB, Wiemann CM: Patient satisfaction and side effects with levonorgestrel implants (Norplant) use in adolescents 18 years of age or younger. Pediatrics 1993;92:257.

Bond GR, Dowd MD, Landsman I, Rimsza M: Unintentional perineal injury in prepubescent girls: a multi-center, prospective report of 56 girls. Pediatrics 1995;95:628.

Bracco GL, Carli P, Sonni L, et al: Clinical and histologic effects of topical treatments of vulval lichen sclerosus: a critical evaluation. J Reprod Med 1993,38:37.

Bump RC, Buesching WJ: Bacterial vaginosis in virginal and sexually active adolescent females: evidence against exclusive sexual transmission. Am J Obstet Gynecol 1988;158:935.

Cattaneo A, Carli P, DeMarco A, et al: Testosterone maintenance therapy: effects of vulvar lichen sclerosus treated with clobetasol propionate. J Repro Med 1996;41:99.

Claessens EA, Cowell CA: Acute adolescent menorrhagia. Am J Obstet Gynecol 1981;139:277.

Davis A, Reindollar R: Adolescent endometrial hyperplasia associated with hyperinsulinemia in non-androgenized patients [abstract]. In: Proceedings of the North American Society for Pediatric and Adolescent Gynecology, Ft. Lauderdale, April 1991.

Davis TC: Chronic vulvovaginitis in children due to *Shigella flexneri*. Pediatrics 1975;56:41.

Devore GR, Owens O, Kase N: Use of intravenous Premarin in the treatment of dysfunctional uterine bleeding—double blind randomized controlled study. Obstet Gynecol 1982;59:285.

Dumic M, Tajic M, Mardesic D, et al: Premature thelarche: a possible adrenal disorder. Arch Dis Child 1982;57:200.

Emans SJH, Goldstein DP: The gynecologic examination of the prepubertal child with vulvovaginitis: use of the knee-chest position. Pediatrics 1980;65:758.

Emans SJH, Goldstein DP: Vulvovaginal problems in the prepubertal child. In Emans SJH, Goldstein DP (eds): Pediatric and Adolescent Gynecology. 3rd ed. Boston: Little, Brown & Company, 1990:67.

Feldman KW, Smith OW: Fetal phallic growth and penile standards for newborn male infants. J Pediatr 1975;86:395.

Feuillan PP, Jones J, Cutler GB: Long term testolactone therapy for precocious puberty in girls with McCune-Albright syndrome. J Clin Endocrinol Metab 1993;77:647.

Finkelhor D, et al: Sexual abuse in the National Incidence Study of Child Abuse and Neglect: an appraisal. Child Abuse Negl 1984;8:23. PMID: 6609754; UL: 84204924.

Fraser IS, Pearse C, Shearman RP, et al: Efficacy of mefenamic acid in patients with a complaint of menorrhagia. Obstet Gynecol 1981;58:543.

Gidwani GP: Vaginal bleeding in adolescents. J Reprod Med 1984; 29:417.

Gidwani GP: Approach to evaluation of premenarchal child with a gynecologic problem. Clin Obstet Gynecol 1987;30:643.

Grumbach MM, Styne DM: Puberty: ontogeny, neuro-endocrinology, physiology, and disorders. In Wilson JD, Foster DW (eds): Williams' Textbook of Endocrinology. 8th ed. Philadelphia: WB Saunders Company, 1992:1139.

Grumbach MM, Styne DM: Puberty: oncology, neuro-endocrinology, physiology disorders. In: Wilson JD, Foster DW (eds.) Williams' Textbook of Endocrinology. 8th ed. Philadelphia: WB Saunders Company, 1991.

Grundberger W, Fisch LF: Pediatric gynecological outpatient department: a report of 600 patients. Wien Klin Wochenschr 1982; 94:614.

Halberg L, Hogdahl AM, Nilsson L, et al: Menstrual blood loss —a population study: variations at different ages and attempts to define normality. Acta Obstet Gynecol Scand 1966;45:320.

Hammerschlag MR: Chlamydia and suspected sexual abuse. Pediatrics 1988;81:600.

Hammerschlag MR, Cummings M, Doraiswamy B, et al: Nonspecific vaginitis following sexual abuse in children. Pediatrics 1985;75:1028.

Hammerschlag MR, Doraiswamy B, Cox P, et al: Colonization of sexually abused children with genital mycoplasmas. Sex Transm Dis 1987;14:23.

Hammerslag MR, Rettig PJ, Shields ME: False positive result with the use of *Chlamydia* antigen detection tests in the evaluation of suspected sexual abuse in children. Pediatr Infect Dis 1988; 7:11.

Hays DM, Shimada H, Raney RB, et al: Clinical staging and treatment results in rhabdomyosarcoma of the female genital tract among children and adolescents. Cancer 1988;61:1893.

Heger A, Emans SJH: Commentary: introital diameter as criteria for sexual abuse. Pediatrics 1990;85:222.

Hemady ZS, Siler-Khoder TM, Najjar S: Precocious puberty in juvenile hypothyroidism. J Pediatr 1978;92:55.

Hertweck SP: Dysfunctional uterine bleeding. Obstet Gynecol Clin North Am 1992;19:129.

Holzgreve W, Winde B, Willital GH, et al: Prenatal diagnosis and perinatal management of a fetal ovarian cyst. Prenat Diagn 1985;5:155.

Hymel KP, Jenny C: Child sexual abuse. Pediatr Rev 1996;17:236.

Ibenez L, Virdis R, Patau N, et al: Natural history of premature pubarche: an auxologic study. J Clin Endocrinol Metab 1992;74: 254.

Ilicki A, Prager Lewin R, Kauli R, et al: Premature thelarche: natural history and sex hormone secretion in 68 girls. Acta Paediatr Scand 1984;73:756.

Jenny C, Kuyhns MLD, Arakawa F: Hymens in newborn female infants. Pediatrics 1987;80:399.

Jerkins GR, Verheeck K, Noe HN: Treatment of girls with urethral prolapse. J Urol 1984;132:732.

Job JC, Chaussain J, Garnier PE: The use of luteinizing hormone-releasing hormone in pediatric patients. Hormone Res 1977;8: 171.

Julian JC, Merguerian PA, Shortliffe LMD: Pediatric genitourinary tumors. Curr Opin Oncol 1995;7:265.

Kelch RP: Disorders of pubertal maturation. In Rudolph AM (ed): Rudolph's Pediatrics. 19th ed. Norwalk, CT: Appleton & Lange, 1991:1671.

Kempe CH: Sexual abuse: another hidden pediatric problem. The 1977 C. Anderson Aldrich Lecture. Pediatrics 1978;62:382.

Kirkinen P, Jouppila P: Perinatal aspects of pregnancy complicated by fetal ovarian cyst. J Perinat Med 1985;13:245.

Kubrinsky NL, Tulloch H: Treatment of refractory thrombocytopenic bleeding with desamino-8-D-arginine vasopressin (desmopressin). J Pediatr 1988;112:993.

Kulin HE: Precocious puberty. Clin Obstet Gynecol 1987;30:714.

Landrum B, Ogburn Pl, Feinburg S, et al: Intrauterine aspiration of a large fetal ovarian cyst. Obstet Gynecol 1986;68:11S.

LaQuaglia M, Heller G, Ghavimi F, et al: The effect of age at diagnosis in rhabdomyosarcoma. Cancer 1994;73:109.

Leftkowitz RJ: G-protein-coupled receptors: turned on to ill effect. Nature 1993;365:603.

Lightner ES, Kelch KP: Treatment of precocious pseudopuberty associated with ovarian cysts [editorial]. Am J Dis Child 1984;138:126.

Lindsay AN, Voorhess ML, MacGillivray MH: Multicystic ovaries detected by sonography. Am J Dis Child 1980;134:588.

Lindsay M, Mannucci PM, Vigano G, et al: Conjugated estrogens for the management of bleeding associated with renal failure. N Engl J Med 1986;315:731.

Livio M, et al: Conjugated estrogens for the management of bleeding associated with renal failure. N Engl J Med. 1986 Sep 18;315:731.

Mansfield MJ, Beardsworth DE, Loughlin JS, et al: Long-term treatment of central precocious puberty with a long-acting analogue of luteinizing hormone-releasing hormone: effects on somatic growth and skeletal maturation. N Engl J Med 1983;309:1286.

McCann J, Simon M, Voris J, Wells R: Perineal findings in prepubertal children selected for nonabuse: a descriptive study. Child Abuse Negl 1988;13:179.

McCann J, Wells R, Simon M, et al: Genital findings in prepubertal girls selected for nonabuse: a descriptive study. Pediatrics 1990;86:428.

McDonough PG, Ganett P: Dysfunctional bleeding in the adolescent. In Barwin BN, Belisle BS (eds): Adolescent Gynecology and Sexuality. New York: Masson Publishing, 1982:59.

McLaughlan RI, Healty DL, Burger HG: Clinical aspects of LHRH analogues in gynecology: a review. Br J Obstet Gynaecol 1986;93:431.

Meyrick Thomas RH, Ridley CM, McGibbon DH, et al: Lichen sclerosus et atrophicus and autoimmunity—a study of 350 women. Br J Dermatol 1988;108:41.

Mischell DR: Abnormal uterine bleeding. In Droegmueller W, Herbst AL, Mishell DR, et al (eds): Comprehensive Gynecology. St. Louis: CV Mosby, 1987:953.

Muller-Leisse C, Bick U, Paulussen K, et al: Ovarian cysts in the fetus and neonate—changes in sonographic pattern in the follow-up and their management. Pediatr Radiol 1992;22:395.

Muram D, Sanfilippo J, Hertweck SP: Vaginal bleeding in childhood and menstrual disorders in adolescence. In Pediatric and Adolescent Gynecology. Philadelphia: WB Saunders Company, 1994.

Murphy TV, Nelson JD: Shigella vaginitis: report of 38 patients and review of the literature. Pediatrics 1979;63:511.

Myers JEB: Role of physician in preserving verbal evidence of child abuse. J Pediatr 1987;109:409.

National Study on the Incidence of Child Abuse and Neglect. Washington, DC: U.S. Dept of Health and Human Services, 1988.

Neinstein LS: Menstrual problems in adolescents. Med Clin North Am 1990;74:1181.

Neinstein et al: Nonsexual transmission of sexually transmitted diseases: an infrequent occurrence. Pediatrics 1984;74:67.

New MI: Genetic disorders of adrenal hormone synthesis. Horm Res 1992;37(Suppl 3):22.

Nishi Y, Masuda H, Iwamori H: Primary hypothyroidism associated with pituitary enlargement, slipped capital femoral epiphysis and cystic ovaries. Eur J Pediatr 1985;143:216.

Pasquino AM, Piccolo F, Scalamandre A, et al: Hypothalamic-pituitary-gonadotropic functions in girls with premature thelarche. Arch Dis Child 1980;55:941.

Pasquino AM, Pucarelli F, Segni MS, et al: Progression of premature menarche to central precocious puberty. J Pediatr 1995;126:11.

Pasquino AM, Tebaldi L, Cioschi L, et al: Premature thelarche: a follow-up study of 40 girls. Arch Dis Child 1985;60:1180.

Pescovitz OH, Cutler GB, Loriaux DL: Management of precocious puberty. J Pediatr Endocrinol 1985;1:85.

Phillips S, Friedman SB, Seidenberg M, et al: Teenagers' preferences regarding the presence of family members, peers, and chaperones during examination of genitalia. Pediatrics 1981;68:665.

Pokorny SF: Opinions in pediatric adolescent gynecology: at what age should a virginal adolescent have her first pelvic examination? J Pediatr Adolesc Gynecol 1996;9:45.

Pokorny SF, Stormer J: Atraumatic removal of secretions from the prepubertal vagina. Am J Obstet Gynecol 1987;156:581.

Polaneczky M, Slap G, Forke C, et al: The use of levonorgestrel implants (Norplant) for contraception in adolescent mothers. N Engl J Med 1994;331:1201.

Pryse-Davies J, Dewhurst CJ: The development of ovary and uterus in the fetus, newborn, and infant: a morphological and enzyme histochemical study. J Pathol 1971;103:5.

Rau FJ, Jones CA, Muram D: Vulvovaginitis. In Sanfilippo JS, Muram D, Lee PA, Dewhurst J (eds): Pediatric and Adolescent Gynecology. Philadelphia: WB Saunders Company, 1994:187.

Redmond CA, Cowell CA, Krefchik BR: Genital lichen sclerosus in prepubertal girls. Adolesc Pediatr Gynecol 1988;1:177.

Reiter EO, Kaplan SL, Conte FA, et al: Responsivity of pituitary gonadotropins to luteinizing-hormone releasing factor in idiopathic precocious puberty, precocious thelarche, precocious adrenarche and in patients treated with medroxyprogesterone acetate. Pediatr Res 1975;9:111.

Rimsa ME, Niggeman MS: Medical evaluation of sexually abuse children: an epidemiologic study. Am J Dis Child 1975;129:689.

Saenz de Rodriguez CA, Bongiovannie AM, Conde de Borrego L: An epidemic of precocious development in Puerto Rican Children. J Pediatr 1985;107:393.

Sahn EE, Bluestein EL, Oliva S: Familial lichen sclerosus et atrophicus in childhood. Pediatr Dermatol 1994;11:160.

Sanfilippo JS, Yussman MA: Gynecologic problems of adolescence. In Lavery J, Sanfilippo JS (eds): Pediatric and Adolescent Gynecology. New York: Springer-Verlag, 1985:61.

Schacter J, Grossman M, Sweet RL, et al: Prospective study of perinatal transmission of Chlamydia trachomatis. JAMA 1986;255:3374.

Scher PW, et al: Factors associated with compliance to oral contraceptive use in an adolescent population. J Adolesc Health Care 1982;3:120.

Scully RE: Neoplasia associated with anomalous sexual development and abnormal sex chromosomes. In Josso NC (ed): The Intersex Child. Basel: Karger, 1981:203.

Siegel RM, Schubert CJ, Myers PA, Shapiro RA: The prevalence of sexually transmitted diseases in children and adolescence evaluated for sexual abuse in Cincinnati: rationale for limited sexually transmitted disease testing. Pediatrics 1995;96:1090.

Simmons PS: Office pediatric gynecology. Prim Carre 1988;15:617.

Sizonenko PC: Preadolescent and adolescent endocrinology: physiology and pathophysiology. II. Hormonal changes during abnormal pubertal development. Am J Dis Child 1978;132:797.

Slupik R: Contraception. In Sanfilippo JS, Muram MD, Lee PA, Dewhurst J (eds): Pediatric and Adolescent Gynecology. Philadelphia: WB Saunders Company, 1994:289.

Soifer H: Adhesions of the labia minora in infants and children: a 20 year study. Int Pediatr 1991;6:347.

Sorensen T, Snow B: How children tell: the process of disclosure in child sexual abuse. Child Welfare 1991;70:3.

Southam AL, Richard RM: The prognosis for adolescences with menstrual abnormalities. Am J Obstet Gynecol 1996;94:637.

Speroff L, Glass RH, Kase NG: Abnormal puberty and growth problems. In Speroff L, Glass RH, Kase NG (eds): Clinical Gynecology, Endocrinology and Infertility. 5th ed. Baltimore: Williams & Wilkins, 1994:361.

Spoudeas HA, Slater JD, Rumsby G, et al: Deoxycorticosterone, 11 beta-hydroxylase and the adrenal cortex. Clin Endocrinol 1993;39:245.

Styne DM, Grumbach MM: Puberty in the male and female. In Yen SCC, Jaffe RB (eds): Reproductive Endocrinology. 2nd ed. Philadelphia: WB Saunders Company, 1986:313.

Tilleli JA, Turek D, Jaffee AC: Sexual abuse in children. N Engl J Med 1980;302:319.

Towne BH, Mahour G, Woulley M, Issacs H: Ovarian cysts and tumors in infancy and children. J Pediatr Surg 1975;10:311.

Van Look PFA, Hunter WM, Fraser IS, et al: Impaired estrogen induced luteinizing hormonal release in young women with anovulatory dysfunctional uterine bleeding. J Clin Endocrinol Metab 1978:46:816.

Van Niekerk WA: True hermaphroditism: an analytic review with a report of 3 new cases. Am J Obstet Gynecol 1976;126:890.

Van Wyck JJ, Grumbach MM: Syndrome of precocious menstruation and galactorrhea in juvenile hypothyroidism: an example of hormonal overlap in pituitary feedback. J Pediatr 1960;57:416.

Verp MS, Simpson JL: Abnormal sexual differentiation and neoplasia. Cancer Genet Cytogenet 1987;25:191.

Walker RW, Gustavson LP: Platelet storage pool disease in women. J Adolesc Health Care 1983;3:264.

Wood LC, Olichney M, Locke H, et al: Syndrome of juvenile hypothyroidism associated with advanced sexual development: report of two cases and comment on the management of an associated ovarian mass. J Clin Endocrinol Metab 1965;25:1289.

Zacharias L, Rand WR, Wurtman RJ: A prospective study of sexual development and growth in American girls: the statistics of menarche. Obstet Gynecol Surv 1976;31:325.

Zah W, Kalderon RE, Tucci JR: Mixed gonadal dysgenesis: a case report and review of the world literature. Acta Endocrinol (Copenh) 1975;79(Suppl 197):3.

Ziegler EE: Bilateral ovarian dysgerminoma in a 30-week fetus. Arch Pathol 1945;40:279.

Zuspan F: The effect of maternal toxemia on fetal gonadal activity. Am J Obstet Gynecol 1953;66:46.

27

M. Yusoff Dawood | # Menopause

Grow old along with me!

The best is yet to be,

The last of life for which

The first was made.

    Robert Browning, "Rabbi Ben Ezra"

DEFINITIONS

Menopause refers to the final menstrual period accompanying the permanent cessation of ovarian function and menstruation. The *climacteric* refers to the transition phase from the reproductive stage of life to the nonreproductive stage in women. This transition is the period of declining ovarian function, which usually becomes clinically apparent over the 2 to 5 years around the menopause. The climacteric ultimately heralds menopause, with manifestations of progressive tissue atrophy and aging.

Perimenopause refers to the time around menopause. Although this usually refers to the 2 years before and after menopause, it is often used loosely to include an even wider time span. Because it is impossible to predict when a woman who is not quite 50 years of age might be entering menopause, the word *perimenopause* should not be loosely used unless there are objective endocrine measurements indicating clear changes in ovarian function.

An interval of 6 to 12 months of amenorrhea is usually necessary to establish the diagnosis of menopause. However, in some patients, serum follicle-stimulating hormone (FSH) and luteinizing hormone (LH) levels may be necessary to differentiate menopause from other causes of secondary amenorrhea.

AGE AT MENOPAUSE

The median age of menopause in the United States is 51.4 years, with a range of 48 to 55 years. Although it has been suggested that the age of menopause may be increasing, careful analysis indicates that it has remained unchanged for centuries. When menopause occurs at 35 years of age or younger, it is classified as *premature menopause*. Although this is a convenient classification, it should be recognized that the clinical manifestations of menopause become apparent progressively earlier as menopause occurs earlier than the usual age expected, even if it is not premature menopause by definition. Nearly 30% of American women reach menopause as a consequence of surgery (Krailo and Pike, 1983). The incidence of menopause arising from surgery increases from about the age of 22 years and plateaus at about 48 years.

Besides surgical causation, several factors affect the age at which menopause occurs, including family history of early menopause, cigarette smoking, blindness, abnormal chromosome karyotype (Turner's syndrome, gonadal dysgenesis), precocious puberty, and left-handedness, all of which produce early menopause, whereas obesity and higher socioeconomic class tend to produce late onset of menopause. Social class as a factor may be more apparent than real and is probably representative of the accompanying lifestyle, such as diet, weight, smoking, and age of menopause in the family. Several studies have shown that both a greater number of cigarettes smoked and a longer duration of smoking induced earlier menopause. The average age of menopause for left-handed women is 42.3 years; for right-handed women, 47.3 years; and for ambidextrous women, 40.7 years (Leidy, 1990). In right-handed women, menopause may occur up to as late as 56 years; in left-handed women, menopause sets in before 51 years of age.

EPIDEMIOLOGY

The number of postmenopausal women in the United States is increasing and will continue to increase as the population ages. In 1990, 52 million of 125 million women were menopausal. In 1996, the number of women beginning menopause each day was 4000. Not only is the number of postmenopausal women increasing, but from 1950 through 1991, the number of women age 65 years has tripled from 6.5 million in 1950 to 19.0 million in 1991 (Fig. 27–1) (Dawood and Tidey, 1993). From 1990 to 1994, there has been further appreciable growth in the female population of the United States who are 45 years and older, as shown in Figure 27–2. With the current life expectancy of 80 years for women projected to in-

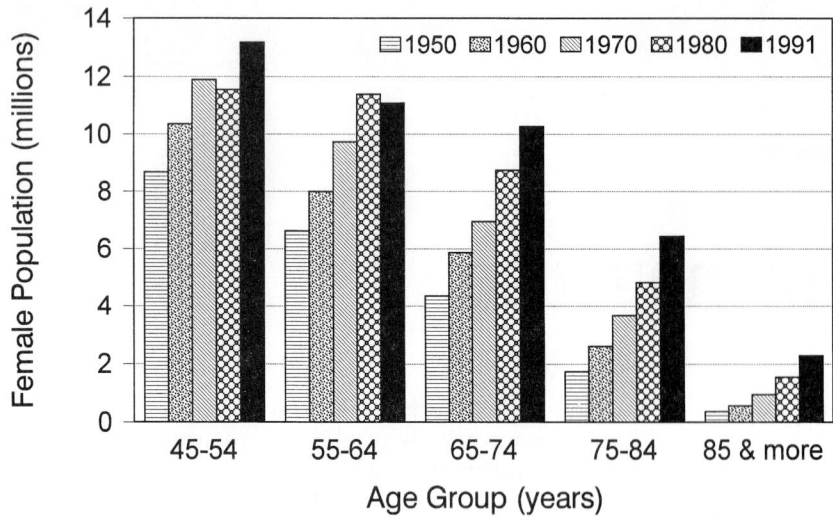

Figure 27–1
Changing trend in United States perimenopausal and postmenopausal (45 years and older) female population from 1950 to 1991. The number of women 65 years and older tripled from 1950 to 1991. (Data obtained from *Statistical Abstract of the United States 1990* [Bureau of the Census, 1992]).

crease to 81 years by 2005 (Fig. 27–3), the average woman undergoing a natural menopause will spend at least 30 years, or more than one third of her life, in the hypoestrogenic state. Thus more pronounced clinical effects secondary to long-term estrogen deprivation will appear in untreated women.

Global life expectancy, which was 55 years in 1974, will be 63 years in 2000 and almost 70 years in 2025, according to the World Health Organization. More than 20% of the world population will be older than 60 years in 2025.

ENDOCRINE CHANGES

The menopause should be looked on as a hormone-deficient state. Therefore, the metabolic sequelae and changes accompanying such a hormone-deficient state can be reversed to a large extent by correcting the hormone deficiency. The primary alteration in the reproductive endocrine system is probably in the

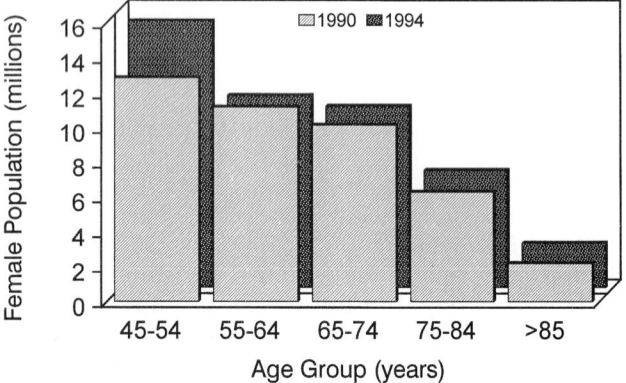

Figure 27–2
Female population in the United States of America age 45 years and older in 1994 compared with 1990. (Raw data taken from *Statistical Abstract of the United States 1995* [Bureau of the Census, 1996]).

ovary, which demonstrates decreasing responsiveness to stimulation by pituitary gonadotropins, leading to a further drop in estrogen levels.

Pituitary Hormones

For up to several years before menopause, there is a gradual increase in circulating FSH levels toward the upper limit for normal during the menstrual cycle, a concomitant decrease in serum estradiol level, no significant change in LH level, and only a slight decrease in serum progesterone. These changes are still associated with follicular maturation and corpus luteum development. After age 40, it is more common for the follicular phase to be shorter. However, serum LH levels later become elevated but still to a lesser extent than FSH levels. Ovulation is still recognized in some cases despite this increase in gonadotropins. Anovulatory cycles may be interspersed with ovulatory cycles, and consequent anovulatory bleeding may occur. Thus, clinically, there are variations and unpredictability in the amount of flow and in the duration and timing of the bleeding. Luteal-phase defects are apparently more common as menopause is approached. There can be periods of amenorrhea with elevated serum FSH and LH levels that can mimic the menopause, only to be followed a few months later by ovulatory cycles with pituitary gonadotropin levels that have returned to normal. This observation can be explained by the theory that fewer follicles are available during the episodes of high FSH and LH levels because the pituitary gland will have to secrete more gonadotropins to recruit the remaining follicles. The increasing FSH levels are probably due to the decreasing sensitivity of the follicles available for recruitment.

Finally, at the time of menopause, serum pituitary gonadotropin levels are high and estrogen levels are low. However, the levels of gonadotropin-releasing hormone (GnRH) remain unchanged. The progressive decline in ovarian follicles and the increased re-

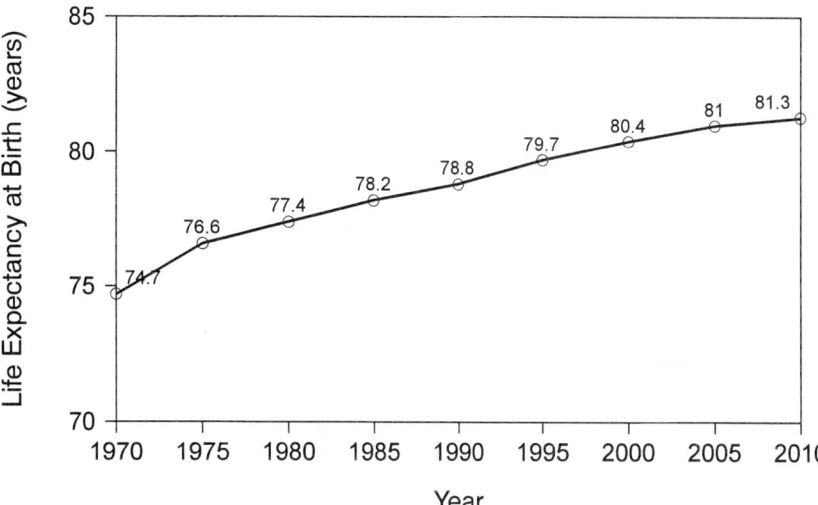

Figure 27-3
Life expectancy in females in the United States from 1970 through 2010. The life expectancies for 1995 through 2010 are projections. (From Dawood MY, Tidey GF: Menopause. Curr Probl Obstet Gynecol Fertil 1993;16;169, with permission.)

sistance to gonadotropins give rise to decreased estrogen production and also inhibin levels. The combination of decreased inhibin and estradiol levels is probably responsible for the early elevation of FSH.

Ovarian Changes

The primary basis for the progressive decrease and, ultimately, the complete cessation of the cyclic function of the female reproductive organs at the time of menopause appears to lie in the ovary itself. There is continuing progressive loss of the primordial follicles from the ovaries during intrauterine life and throughout the reproductive years until menopause. Anatomic studies, however, indicate that primordial follicles are still present during the perimenopausal and postmenopausal phases, albeit in significantly reduced numbers. The female fetus starts in utero with approximately 6 million primordial follicles, which decrease to 600,000 at birth, 300,000 at menarche, and about 10,000 or fewer near the time of menopause (Bloch, 1952). The rate of atresia of the primordial follicles is probably determined by the intrinsic genetic program of the ovary. A few immature follicles may therefore continue to undergo maturation and atresia a few years after menopause, and there are a few reports of postmenopausal ovulation.

Toward the end of the fourth decade of life, the ovaries become increasingly less responsive to stimulation by pituitary gonadotropins, and recruitment and stimulation of follicles to full maturity become increasingly difficult. As menopause approaches and as the primordial follicles decrease, ovulation becomes irregular and steadily more infrequent, finally stopping altogether. With the accompanying failure of progesterone production during the initial stages and relative lack of estrogen as follicle activity ceases completely, menstrual function stops because of insufficient estrogen to stimulate endometrial proliferation and growth. The ovary becomes smaller and

fibrotic, with atrophy of the ovarian cortex, which contains the primordial follicles. Therefore, the ovarian medulla becomes relatively more abundant with active stromal cells, which are the source of ovarian androgens. As the postmenopausal years progress, the ovaries become even more atrophic and are eventually replaced by masses of fibrotic tissue.

Extraglandular Source of Estrogen

During the premenopausal years, estradiol, the principal circulating estrogen, is made almost entirely by the maturing ovarian follicles during each cycle and is therefore primarily derived from the ovary. After the menopause, ovarian estrone production decreases markedly secondary to the failure of adequate follicular recruitment, growth, and maturation. Estradiol levels decline to 20 to 25 pg/ml or less after the menopause, and therefore estrone now becomes the principal circulating estrogen. Most of the estrogen present in the postmenopausal woman is derived from extraovarian and extraglandular production of estrone in peripheral tissues, mainly adipose tissues where androstenedione is aromatized by the enzyme aromatase to estrone. This conversion appears to be in the stroma rather than in the adipocytes. The amount of androstenedione converted to estrone in peripheral tissues is governed by the overall amount of adipose tissues. Thus slender postmenopausal women convert less of their daily production of androstenedione to estrone than obese women.

Other Hormone Changes

Serum levels of testosterone are slightly lower than in the premenopausal state. However, there is still a state of relative androgen excess compared with premenopausal levels. The levels of reproductive hormones in the postmenopausal woman compared

Table 27–1. REPRODUCTIVE HORMONE LEVELS IN POSTMENOPAUSAL WOMEN COMPARED WITH PREMENOPAUSAL WOMEN

| HORMONE | PREMENOPAUSAL | | POSTMENOPAUSAL | | |
	Plasma Level	Daily Production Rate	Plasma Level	Daily Production Rate	Tightly Bound (%)
Androstenedione	150 ng/dl	2.7 mg	90 ng/dl	16 mg	0
Testosterone	35 ng/dl	200 μg	25 ng/dl	150 μg	>90
Dehydroepiandrosterone	4–5 ng/dl		1.8 ng/ml		0
Dehydroepiandrosterone sulfate	1500 ng/ml		300 ng/ml		
Estrone	40–200 pg/ml	80–4000 μg	35 pg/ml	55 μg	0
Estradiol	40–350 pg/ml	50–500 μg	13 pg/ml	12 μg	50
Luteinizing hormone	10–40 mIU/ml		70 mIU/ml		
Follicle-stimulating hormone	10–40 mIU/ml		80 mIU/ml		
Prolactin	10 ng/ml		8 ng/ml		

From Korenman SG: Menopausal endocrinology and management. Arch Intern Med 1982; 142:1131, with permission. Copyright 1982, American Medical Association.

with the premenopausal woman are given in Table 27–1.

MENOPAUSAL SYMPTOMS AND PROBLEMS

A variety of problems or symptoms arise at or after the menopause and are summarized in Figure 27–4. Some of the problems are due exclusively to low estrogen levels or prolonged estrogen deprivation, whereas others are often aggravated or largely contributed to by the estrogen-deprived or relative estrogen-deficient status of these women.

Cardiovascular Disease

A common myth is that women are less likely to suffer from cardiovascular disease than men. Whereas only 6 of 1600 premenopausal women died of coronary heart disease in the Framingham Heart Study, the incidence rates in both men and women were similar 6 to 10 years after the menopause (U.S. Department of Health, Education and Welfare, 1974). The leading cause of death in American women of all ages is heart disease, with a rate of 287.3 per 100,000 population in 1989 (Bureau of the Census, 1992). Cancer is the next most common cause of death, with a rate of 183.0 per 100,000 population. In 1992, among 45- to 64-year-old women, malignant neoplasms accounted for 61,314 deaths, while heart disease was second with 30,700 deaths. After 65 years of age, heart disease, with 271,214 deaths, overtook the 191,204 deaths due to cancer (Bureau of the Census, 1996) (Fig. 27–5). Stroke was the third most frequent cause of death in both age groups.

Among premenopausal and postmenopausal women of the same age group, the incidence of cardiovascular disease is significantly higher in the postmenopausal women (U.S. Department of Health, Education and Welfare, 1974). In a retrospective study, Rosenberg et al (1981) estimated that the relative risk of myocardial infarction increases with decreasing age at menopause. The relative risk of myocardial infarction in women who had bilateral oophorectomy between 35 and 39 years of age rose to 2.5 and increased to 7.2 when bilateral oophorectomy was performed before the age of 35 when compared with premenopausal women. Thus the incidence of cardiovascular disease is markedly increased after the loss of ovarian function in postmenopausal women, and needs to be addressed in their management.

Several studies have focused specific attention on the effect of estrogen replacement therapy on myocardial infarction in postmenopausal women. Szklow et al (1984) found that the relative risk of myocardial infarction is reduced to 0.37 in estrogen users following surgical menopause compared with that in nonusers, indicating a protective effect of estrogen against myocardial infarction. The protective effect of estrogen against death from ischemic heart disease was further demonstrated by a reduction in the relative risk to 0.48 (Hunt et al, 1987). More recent studies using coronary arteriography have conclusively shown a significant reduction in the relative risk for coronary artery disease with estrogen use after the menopause. Selective coronary arteriography performed in 2188 postmenopausal women showed a relative risk of 0.44 for estrogen users compared with nonusers. Similarly, Gruchow et al (1988) found a significant reduction in the relative risk of developing severe coronary artery disease occlusion to 0.37 for estrogen users compared with that for nonusers. The risk for atherosclerosis in women increases significantly after the menopause. By means of radiographic examination for calcified deposits in the abdominal aorta representing intimal atherosclerosis, aortic atherosclerosis was present in 3% of premenopausal women compared with 12% of postmenopausal women (Wittemann et al, 1989). The risk for atherosclerosis is 3.4 times greater in postmeno-

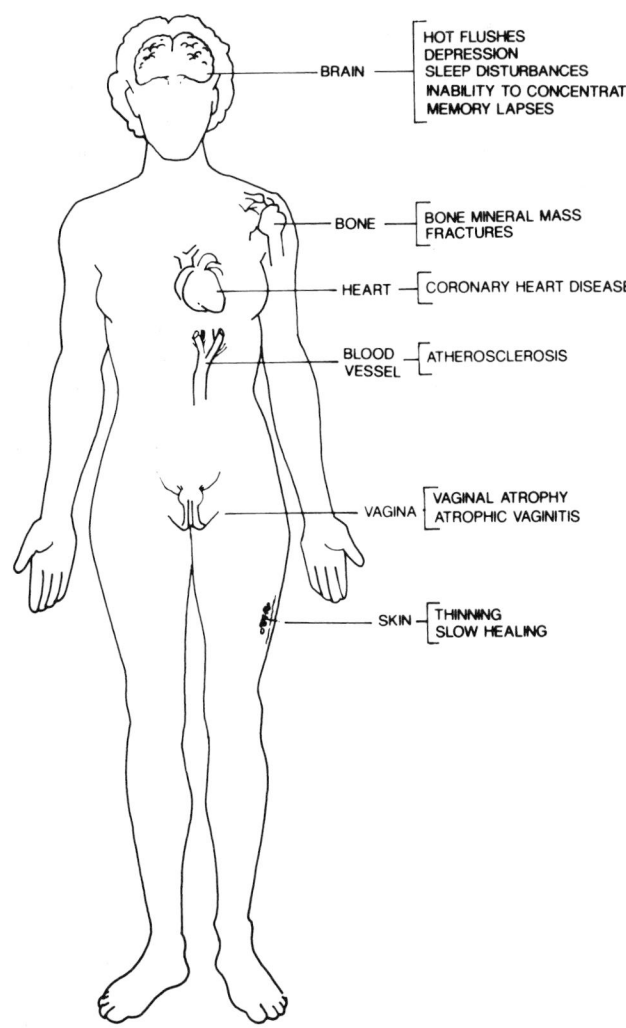

Figure 27–4
Effect of estrogen deprivation or reduced estrogen on different organ and tissue systems at or after menopause.

pausal women with natural menopause than in premenopausal women when adjusted for age and other cardiovascular risk factors. In women who underwent bilateral oophorectomy, the risk was 5.5 times greater than in premenopausal women. Parish et al (1967) found no excessive coronary atherosclerosis if women were castrated after 40 years of age but significantly more severe coronary artery disease in women castrated before age 40. An average interval of 14.4 years was required for excessive coronary atherosclerosis to become apparent in surgically castrated women.

Another way of looking at cardiovascular disease risk relates to the levels of lipids in the pathogenesis of coronary heart disease. Three lipids that have been linked to coronary heart disease and atherosclerosis are cholesterol and its two carrier proteins, the plaque-promoting low-density lipoproteins (LDL) and the plaque-sparing high-density lipoproteins (HDL) (Steinberg, 1987). Figure 27–6 illustrates the annual rate of coronary heart disease in women in relation to their serum cholesterol levels. The risk for coronary heart disease decreases by 3% for each 1% reduction in the serum cholesterol (Lipid Research Clinical Program, 1984). More recently, however, the decrease in risk is stated to be 2% for each 1% reduction in serum cholesterol level. Nevertheless, HDL and LDL are more specific indicators of coronary heart disease risk than total cholesterol (Fahraeus et al, 1982). It is claimed that, for every increase of 1 mg/dl of HDL, there is a 3% to 5% decrease in the risk of coronary heart disease, whereas for every 1% decrease in total cholesterol, there is a 2% decrease in coronary heart disease, and, for an 11% decrease in LDL, there is a decrease of only 19% in coronary heart disease. Risk factors for developing coronary heart disease based on serum cholesterol, HDL, and LDL levels are given in Table 27–2. Triglycerides have little impact on risk of cor-

Figure 27–5
Causes of deaths among females 45 years and older in the United States in 1992. (Raw data taken from *Statistical Abstract of the United States 1995* [Bureau of the Census, 1996]).

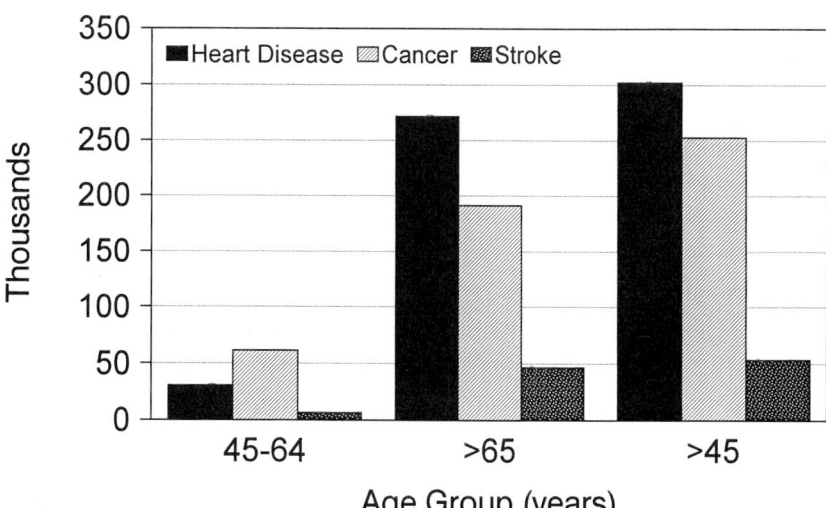

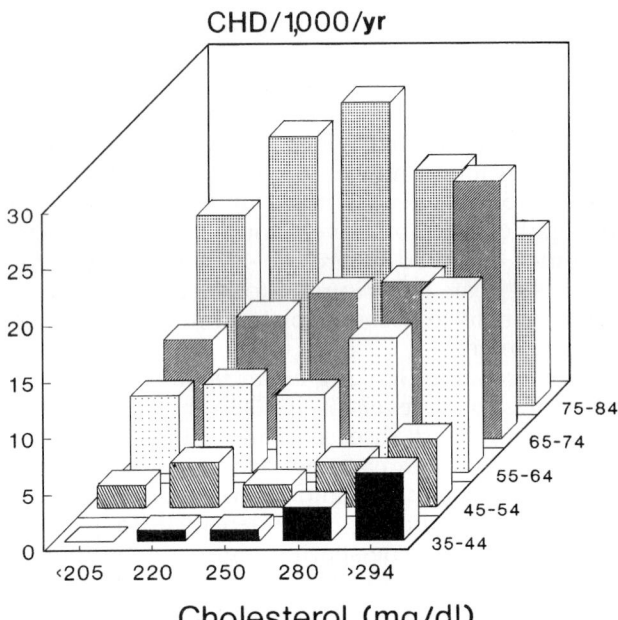

CHD/1,000/yr

Cholesterol (mg/dl)

Figure 27–6
Annual rate of coronary heart disease (CHD) in women in relation to serum cholesterol levels. (From Castelli WP: Cardiovascular disease in women. Am J Obstet Gynecol 1988; 158:1553, with permission.)

onary heart disease in women with average or high HDL but increase the risk if the HDL level is low (Fig. 27–7) (Castelli, 1986).

After the menopause, there is a considerable increase in serum cholesterol. At 35 to 44 years of age, the average cholesterol level is higher in men than in women, but by 55 to 64 years of age, women have higher cholesterol levels (Moore and Gordon, 1967; Hjortland et al, 1976). Several studies have shown that serum cholesterol increased significantly at 1 to 2 years or more after the menopause (Lindquist, 1982; Notelovitz et al, 1983). Most studies also found an increase in triglycerides, a significant increase in LDL, and a significant decrease in HDL, notably after acute estrogen withdrawal as in the case of surgical castration (Blumenfeld et al, 1983; Bonithon-Kopp et al, 1990). An endogenously low level of HDL has not been consistently found after natural menopause. More recently, lipoprotein(a) [Lp(a)], which is a cholesteryl ester–rich particle that resembles LDL cholesterol, was reported to be an indepen-

dent risk factor for myocardial infarction, stroke, and restenosis of coronary artery after bypass surgery. Serum Lp(a) levels increased significantly 3 months after oophorectomy but decreased markedly with estrogen or estrogen-progestin replacement therapy (Soma et al, 1993; Bruschi et al, 1996). Therefore, after the menopause, the lipid levels change toward a less cardioprotective pattern than before the menopause.

When postmenopausal women are placed on estrogen therapy, there is an increase in HDL, a decrease in LDL, and generally a decrease in cholesterol levels (Fahraeus et al, 1982; Wahl et al, 1983; Farish et al, 1984). The increase in HDL and the decrease in LDL, which reduce the accompanying risk for coronary artery disease, have been reported with oral conjugated estrogens, estradiol implants, intramuscular estradiol, and transdermal estradiol. There has been some contention that oral conjugated estrogens are more effective in favorably affecting the lipid pattern and levels toward cardioprotection (Wahl et al, 1983), whereas parenteral estradiol-17β does not produce the same degree of change (Farish et al, 1984). Walsh et al (1991) compared the effects of conjugated estrogen, oral estradiol, and transdermal estradiol with placebo on serum lipid levels in postmenopausal women in two randomized, double-blind, crossover studies. Conjugated estrogens (0.625 and 1.25 mg daily) and oral estradiol (2 mg daily) decreased LDL cholesterol by 15% to 19% and by 14%, respectively, through accelerated LDL catabolism, and increased HDL cholesterol by 16% to 18% and by 15%, respectively. Conjugated estrogens increased very-low-density lipoprotein (VLDL) triglyceride levels by 24% to 42%. Oral estradiol increased large VLDL apolipoprotein B by 30%. Thus the changes may protect women against atherosclerosis while minimizing the potentially adverse effects of triglyceride levels. Transdermal estradiol had no effect on serum lipoprotein levels over the 6-week period of administration.

The change in HDL and other lipoprotein levels may not necessarily be the exclusive or principal mechanism of the cardioprotective effects of estrogen. Experiments in cynomolgus monkeys indicate that the potent estrogen ethinyl estradiol, given to animals fed a highly cholesterol-rich, atherogenic diet, protected against intimal plaque formation in the vessel wall in spite of the administration of a potent progestin, levonorgestrel, and the HDL levels being low (Adams et al, 1987). Additionally, vessel

Table 27–2. LIPID PROFILE AND RISK FOR CORONARY HEART DISEASE

RISK	TOTAL CHOLESTEROL (mg/dl)	LOW-DENSITY LIPOPROTEIN (mg/dl)	HIGH-DENSITY LIPOPROTEIN (mg/dl)
Desirable	>200	<130	≥35
Borderline	200–239	130–159	
High	≥249	≥160	<35

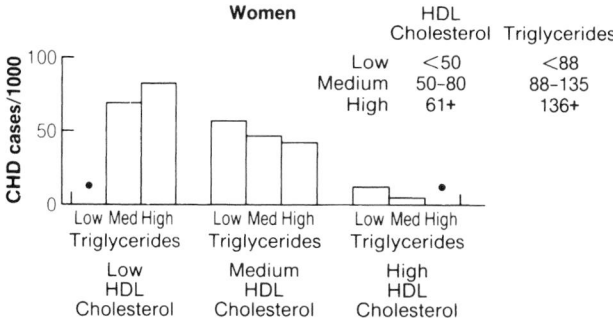

Figure 27–7
Risk for coronary heart disease (CHD) based on serum triglycerides and high-density lipoprotein (HDL) cholesterol. (From Castelli WP: The triglyceride issue: a view from Framingham. Am Heart J 1986;112:432, with permission.)

walls have estrogen receptors through which estrogens may exert a direct effect (McGill, 1989). In this regard, the uterine vessels of postmenopausal women have been found to produce significantly lower amounts of the stable prostacyclin metabolite 6-ketoprostaglandin $F_{1\alpha}$ than those of premenopausal women (Steinleitner et al, 1989). Estrogen may increase local production of prostacyclin but lower thromboxane production. Because prostacyclin is a potent vasodilator and platelet antiaggregate, whereas thromboxane is vasoconstrictive and induces platelet aggregation, there is a net balance favoring increased blood flow and reduced clotting with estrogen.

Figure 27–8 summarizes schematically the postulated mechanisms through which correction of postmenopausal estrogen deficiency may bring about cardiovascular protection against atherosclerosis. The direct action of estrogen on its receptors in the vessel walls may also play a part in the biology of the various growth factors that may be associated with the pathogenesis of vessel wall plaque formation.

One of the earliest events in atherogenesis is adherence of circulating monocytes to the arterial endothelium, followed by penetration into the intima and conversion into macrophages that ingest LDL to become foam cells and later fatty streaks. Monocytes can also promote LDL oxidation and release of lytic enzymes to contribute further to plaque formation and endothelial injury. Hormone replacement therapy reduces cellular activation of blood monocytes and platelets (Aune et al, 1995) and therefore should inhibit atherogenesis.

Tumor necrosis factor, a cytokine produced by monocytes or macrophages, stimulates these cells as well as neutrophils and vascular endothelial cells to produce and release mediators of inflammation. Detectable in human atheroma, tumor necrosis factor increases with the severity of the lesion and is a contributing factor in atheroma progression. Plasma levels of tumor necrosis factor are lower in premeno-

pausal women than in men (Balteskard et al, 1993) and are significantly suppressed with 12 months or longer of hormone replacement therapy in postmenopausal women (Aune et al, 1995).

After menopause, production of thromboxane, which is platelet proaggregatory and vasoconstrictive, is significantly increased (Balteskard et al, 1993). Hormone replacement therapy for 12 months or longer will significantly reduce plasma thromboxane levels (Aune et al, 1995).

Factor VII coagulant activity (VIIc) may be an independent predictor of coronary heart disease. Activated factor VII (VIIa) levels are positively correlated with serum cholesterol. Adjusted for age, postmenopausal women have significantly increased levels of factor VIIc and VIIa compared with premenopausal women (Scarabin et al, 1996). Administration of estrogen reverses the rise in serum levels of VIIc and VIIa.

After menopause, there is increased arterial tone and blood flow impedance in the vascular tree as reflected by an increased pulsatility index of the uterine, internal carotid, and cerebral arteries (Bourne et al, 1990; Gangar et al, 1991; Penotti et al, 1996). Administration of estrogen reduces these menopause-mediated increases in pulsatility index, improves uterine, cerebral, and cerebellar blood flow (Penotti et al, 1993; Ohkura et al, 1995); and increases aortic size (Giraud et al, 1996). Estradiol also attenuates acetylcholine-induced coronary arterial constriction in postmenopausal women with coronary artery disease through enhancement of endothelium-dependent relaxation (Collins et al, 1995).

Psychoneuroendocrine Effects

Headaches, tiredness, lethargy, irritability, anxiety, nervousness, depression, sleep difficulties, inability to concentrate, and hot flushes are symptoms for which perimenopausal and postmenopausal women frequently seek medical assistance. Many of these symptoms affect quality of life.

Hot Flush

By far the most common symptom that attracts attention is hot flushes. As many as 85% of postmenopausal women have hot flushes, with 65% having them for 1 to 5 years, 26% for 6 to 10 years, and 10% for more than 11 years (Feldman et al, 1985). Among women 60 to 62 years old, 15% reported having hot flushes. Although hot flushes usually continue for about 2 years, some women may continue to have them longer. Kronenberg (1990) found 60% of women had hot flushes for less than 7 years and 15% for more than 15 years. There is considerable variation in the frequency, intensity, and duration of hot flushes within and among individuals. Among those who are "current flushers," one third had more than

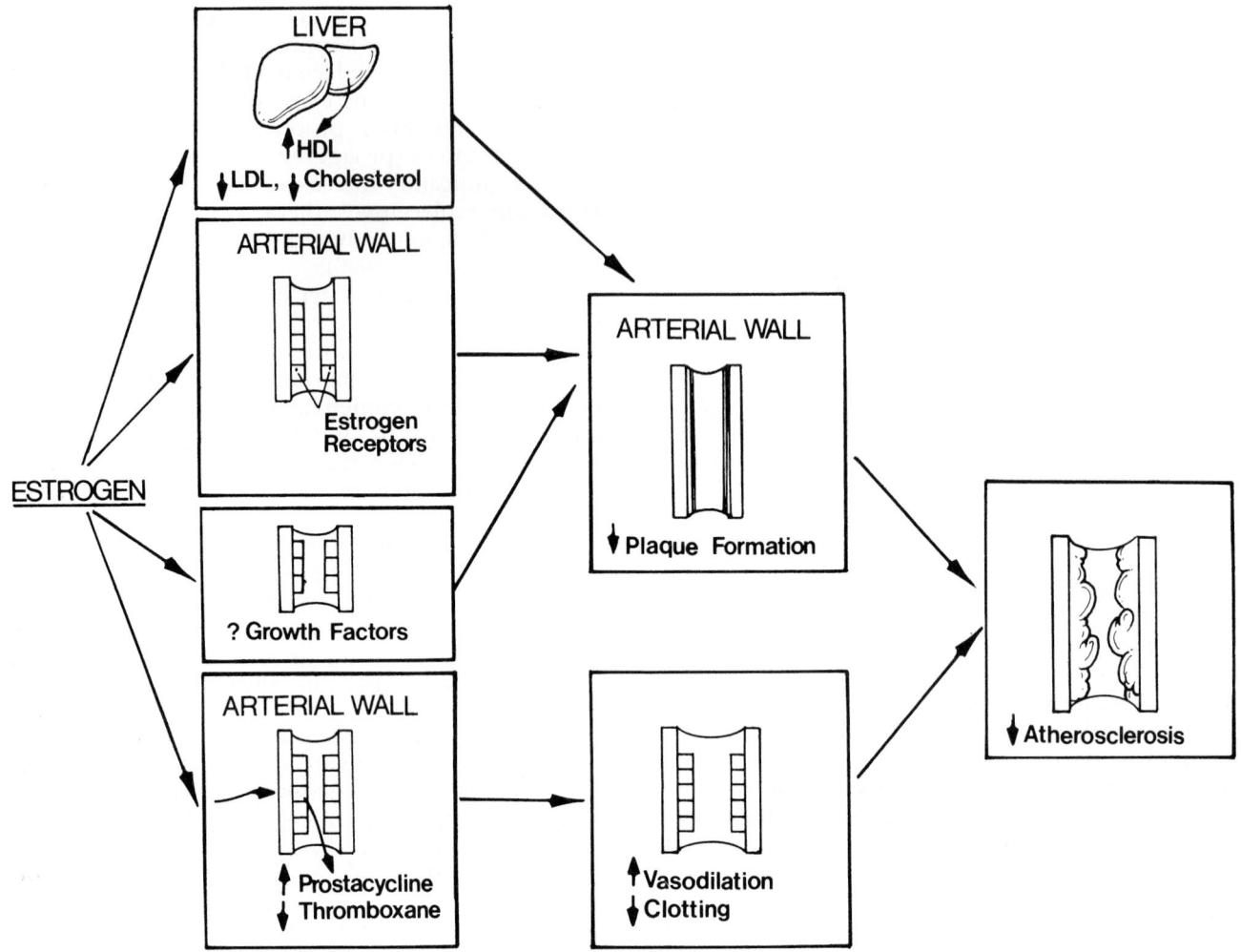

Figure 27–8
Simplified schematic representation of the postulated mechanisms through which correction of estrogen deficiency in the postmenopausal woman may confer cardiovascular protection from atherosclerosis and coronary heart disease. The effects of estrogen on growth factors and biology of the arterial vessels remain to be clarified. HDL, high-density lipoprotein; LDL, low-density lipoprotein.

10 flushes per day compared with 5 per year among "ever flushers."

Characteristically, a hot flush begins in the head and facial areas with a sensation of warmth, followed by facial flushing that may radiate down the neck and to other parts of the body. Each hot flush averages 2.7 minutes but is commonly 1 to 5 minutes long, with 17.4% of women reporting a flush of more than 1 minute and 5.7% reporting flushes of more than 6 minutes. Each flush is associated with an increase in temperature, increased pulse rate (average of 9 beats/minute and up to as many as 20 beats/minute), increased blood flow in the hand, and increased skin conductance, followed by a decline in temperature and profuse perspiration over the area of flush distribution (Fig. 27–9) (Tataryn et al, 1979). Episodes of hot flush during sleep are referred to as *night sweats*. Synchronous with the onset of each hot flush is the release of a pulse of LH.

The increase in gonadotropin release is not responsible for the mechanism of the hot flush but, rather, is an accompaniment and reflects a more central hypothalamic mechanism triggering the hot flush. Hot flushes provide a mechanism for dissipating heat through vasodilatation and perspiration in response to the thermoregulatory centers in the anterior hypothalamus around the arcuate nucleus, adjusting the core temperature of the body to a new setpoint. Thus some common stimulus of the arcuate nucleus or anterior hypothalamus appears to be directly responsible for the pulsatile increase in GnRH and therefore the LH release and the hot flush onset.

A rapid estrogen withdrawal, rather than a low estrogen level by itself, is likely to induce hot flushes. Despite high gonadotropin and low estrogen levels, women with ovarian failure resulting from gonadal dysgenesis rarely have hot flushes before exposure to normal estrogen levels; rather, hot flushes develop

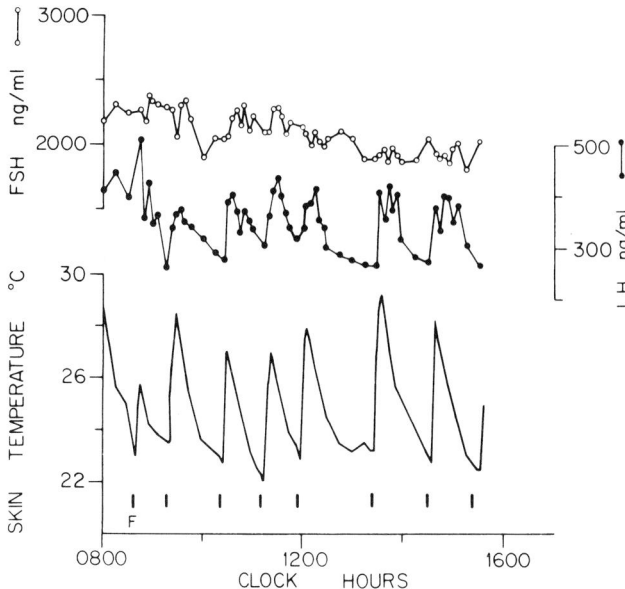

Figure 27-9
Changes in cutaneous finger temperature, serum luteinizing hormone (LH) levels, and follicle-stimulating hormone (FSH) levels in a postmenopausal woman with hot flushes. Note the close temporal relationship between the cutaneous finger temperature, serum LH (but not serum FSH) levels, and each hot flush (indicated by the vertical bars with F). (From Tataryn IV, Meldrum DR, Lu KH, et al: LH, FSH and skin temperature during the menopausal hot flush. J Clin Endocrinol Metab 1979;49:152, with permission. © by The Endocrine Society.)

upon estrogen withdrawal after such exposure. The anterior hypothalamus has estrogen and progestin receptors, and both hormones can be used effectively to treat hot flushes through binding with their respective hypothalamic receptors. Neurotransmitters that may be involved in the pathogenesis of hot flushes include norepinephrine, other noradrenergic substances, and endogenous opiate withdrawal. The central noradrenergic system in the hypothalamus triggers the hot flushes via α_2-adrenergic receptors on the noradrenergic neurons. Thus, clomidine, an α_2-adrenergic agonist, effectively alleviates hot flushes through reduction of noradrenergic release, and thereby blocks noradrenergic neuron activity associated with the rapid changes in skin temperature that occur during hot flushes and opiate withdrawal. Yohimbine, an α_2-adrenergic antagonist, induces hot flushes in postmenopausal women (Freedman et al, 1990).

Sleep

Sleep deprivation and interrupted sleep may develop in postmenopausal women. In turn, this can give rise to nonspecific complaints such as irritability, anxiety, nervousness, fatigue, forgetfulness, and inability to concentrate. Even with adequate amounts of sleep, postmenopausal women usually wake up feeling inadequately rested. Sleep-latency interval is

increased, whereas the amount of rapid eye movement (REM) sleep is decreased in postmenopausal women, probably because of the low estrogen levels. In a double-blind study, estrogen improved sleep with concomitant postslumber satiety compared with placebo treatment (Schiff et al, 1979). Although estrogen does not alter the duration of sleep significantly, the sleep-latency interval is significantly reduced and the percentage of time spent in REM sleep is significantly increased.

Mood

Hypoestrogenic levels after the menopause provide a biochemical framework for possible development of depression. Plasma free tryptophan (the fraction not bound to serum proteins) is reduced in postmenopausal women, but total plasma tryptophan levels (bound and unbound fractions) remain unchanged (Aylward, 1980). Tryptophan is an amino acid involved in the metabolism of serotonin. Alterations in serotonin levels in the brain have been implicated as a mechanism for the development of endogenous depression. Therefore, alterations in free tryptophan levels secondary to low estrogen levels in menopause can biochemically predispose the postmenopausal woman to depression. Plasma estrogen levels have been shown to be directly related to plasma free tryptophan levels. Treatment with estrogen, but not placebo, increases plasma estrogen levels, with a concomitant increase in plasma free tryptophan levels, and is accompanied by an improvement in the depression score. At the same time, changes in the environment and family circumstances of menopausal women (such as children having left the home, or the "empty nest" syndrome, and the career-oriented spouse devoting less time to the family) can be important trigger mechanisms acting on the increasingly susceptible biochemical and hormonal environment to bring about depression and mood changes.

Memory and Alzheimer's Disease

Possibly through its growth promotion of cholinergic neurons and decreased deposition of cerebral amyloid (Birge, 1996), estrogen use in postmenopausal women may lower the risk of Alzheimer's disease. Observational studies found that Alzheimer's disease developed significantly later in women taking estrogen, and the risk of developing the disease is significantly reduced with estrogen therapy (Paganini-Hill and Henderson, 1994; Tang et al, 1996).

Verbal but not spatial memory performance of postmenopausal women can be maintained with estrogen use (Kampen and Sherwin, 1994). Estrogen can probably protect from the decline in acetylcholine that normally occurs in the forebrain and frontal cortex by increasing the level of choline acetyltransferase.

Nonspecific Symptoms

Although other nonspecific menopausal complaints, such as headache, tiredness, lethargy, irritability, anxiety, and nervousness, may also be due to family, social, and personal environmental factors, double-blind studies reveal that estrogen replacement significantly reduces the symptoms compared with placebo. Thus these symptoms are also largely estrogen dependent.

Skin and Urogenital Effects

Loss of ovarian function and decreased estrogen levels after menopause reduce skin thickness secondary to a significant decrease in epidermal thickness and collagen content. Thinning of the epidermis is due to a reduced rate in epidermal cell turnover. Epidermal thickness decreases at a rate of 1.2% per year after the menopause. When estrone is given, the epidermal cell production, as reflected by tritiated thymidine uptake, is increased, leading to restoration of the epidermal thickness to the level found in premenopausal woman.

Skin collagen content in untreated postmenopausal women decreases exponentially at the rate of 2.1% per year after menopause and is significantly correlated with the number of years after menopause (Brincat et al, 1985). Estrogen replacement therapy increases skin thickness and skin collagen content, alters vascularization of the skin, and affects connective tissue by increasing the intercellular fluid content and rendering the ground substance more metachromatic and the fibroblasts more "succulent" in appearance.

As a result of postmenopausal skin thinning, the skin is clinically lax, is more transparent, has more readily visible capillaries and blood vessels, and is also more easily bruised. Healing of the skin is generally slower, but the resulting scar is less hypertrophic when union occurs.

The thickness of the vaginal epithelium is markedly reduced after menopause, and there is loss of vaginal rugae. The mechanism for this change is similar to that for the epidermis of the skin in other parts of the body, except it may be more pronounced in the vagina because of its sensitivity to estrogen. Additionally, the vaginal epithelial cells contain less glycogen, and the acidity of the vagina changes after the menopause. Thus the vagina may be small and atrophic, and secondary inflammation resulting from trauma or infection occurs much more easily. The secondary infection may therefore occur readily on top of a senile atrophic vaginitis. If a uterovaginal prolapse or descensus is present in the postmenopausal woman, decubitus ulceration occurs much more readily in a vagina that is already atrophic. Local application of estrogen cream into the vagina for 2 to 3 weeks can correct vaginal atrophy and heal atrophic vaginitis and decubitus ulceration of an atrophic vagina with gratifying results.

Coital difficulties need not arise from thinning of the vaginal epithelium as long as regular coital activity is maintained. With severe atrophy or atrophic vaginitis, however, dyspareunia may occur. Prolonged interruption of coital activity may permit significant narrowing and atrophy of the postmenopausal vagina so that resumption of coital activity after an extended abstinence may give rise to dyspareunia. Indeed, with the fear of pregnancy eliminated, improved sexual activity and response have been reported in postmenopausal women having regular coital activity.

Sexual response remains intact, but, because of age-related neuroendocrine and circulatory alterations in postmenopausal women, the timing and extent of the phases of sexual stimulation and pattern of response change. The time it takes to achieve labial and vaginal lubrication may increase from 15 to 30 seconds in the younger years to as long as 5 minutes. Excitation and elevation of clitoral tissue take longer, but the response remains intact. The number of uterine contractions with orgasm decreases, and the contractions are occasionally painful. With further aging, the duration of orgasm decreases and resolution is quicker. In addition, Masters and Johnson (1986) have also noted several changes in the physiology of the sex response after the menopause. The incidence of skin flush is decreased. Muscle tension is also decreased. The urinary meatus is distended. Increase in breast size during sexual stimulation is lacking, and secretion from the Bartholin's gland is slowed or absent. Vaginal expansion, both in length and transcervical width, as well as congestion in the outer third of the vagina (i.e., the orgasmic platform) is decreased after the menopause.

Urodynamic evaluations indicate a 30% drop in urethral closure pressure at rest and during stress in postmenopausal women because of atrophy of the urethral mucosa, which is embryologically derived from the urogenital sinus and is estrogen sensitive (Reed, 1980). Diminished support of the pelvic organs, including the bladder and urethra, can produce varying degrees of bladder and urethral prolapse and loss of the ureterovesical angle, leading to further urodynamic alterations adversely affecting the maintenance of urinary continence.

Senile urethritis or atrophic urethritis secondary to hypoestrogenism may occur in postmenopausal women. The condition is clinically characterized by urgency, frequency, dysuria, and suprapubic pain in the absence of urinary tract infection. Atrophy of the urethral mucosa and bladder trigone gives rise to the symptoms. Other urinary disturbances, such as incomplete emptying of the bladder, may be more related to neurologic dysfunction resulting from the aging process than to hypoestrogenism per se.

Estrogen replacement therapy can correct these urinary tract changes and symptoms due to postmenopausal estrogen deficit. With estrogen treatment, there is a significant decrease in trophic changes of the urinary tract and in urinary infection and a marked improvement in the cytology (Samsioe et al, 1985).

Bone Effect

Osteoporosis is one of the most significant long-term sequelae of menopause but can be readily prevented or reduced through appropriate preventive management. Among those 65 or more years of age, there are 88.0 hip fractures per 10,000 Medicare beneficiaries in women compared to 48.0 per 10,000 in men (Centers for Disease Control and Prevention, 1996). Ultradistal forearm fracture rates are five times higher in women over 65 years of age (54.0 per 10,000 Medicare beneficiaries) than in men (11.7 per 10,000). There will be twice as many women older than 65 years of age by 2000, and these numbers can be expected to double. Twenty-five per cent of women (or 5 million women) will have radiologic evidence of osteoporosis by 60 years of age. Of women living to 80 years, one in four can expect to have fractured a hip. The incidence of hip fractures in women doubles each decade after 50 years, and 85% of such fractures are in women. The true incidence of vertebral fractures in postmenopausal women is more difficult to ascertain because the fracture by itself seldom results in hospitalization. One of every three women will probably have a vertebral fracture after age 65. The estimated incidence of new vertebral fractures increases with age, reaching 29.6 per 1000 person-years in women age 85 years or older, and, with declining bone mass, the incidence increases to 42% in those with a spinal bone mineral density of 0.6 g/cm^2 (Melton et al, 1989).

In the initial period of up to 4 to 5 years after the menopause, there is accelerated loss of bone mineral mass, after which the rate of further loss is a little lower and more age related. This bone loss produces osteopenia, which is defined as decreased calcification or density of bone. Subsequently, postmenopausal osteoporosis (type I osteoporosis) occurs, usually within 15 to 20 years of the menopause. Osteoporosis is the condition in which the skeleton is sufficiently compromised by reduction in the mass per unit bone volume such that there is a significantly increased risk of skeletal failure (fracture) even in the absence of trauma. Trabecular bone is predominantly affected rather than cortical bone. Thus the three most common fractures seen in postmenopausal women are those of the vertebrae, ultradistal radius, and neck of the femur, all of which are sites of high trabecular bone composition.

White and Asian women are at greater risk for postmenopausal osteoporosis than African-American women, although the latter are twice as likely as their male counterparts to experience fractures. Whereas hypoestrogenism after menopause is a major determinant for risk of osteoporosis, other risks factors, if present, can further compound the risk as well as the severity of the osteoporosis (Aloia et al, 1985). Such risk factors are summarized in Table 27-3. Many of them are related to reduced estrogen production and/or accelerated estrogen excretion, some lifestyle factors (smoking, dietary fads), and substance abuse (alcohol, excessive caffeine). In women, peak bone mass is attained in the late 30s and is determined by genetic makeup, nutrition, exercise, and hormonal milieu. If substantial bone reserves are achieved by the late 30s, there is likelihood of greater protection against postmenopausal osteoporosis when estrogen deficiency sets in.

Several possible explanations account for accelerated bone demineralization after menopause. The frequency of new remodeling sites in bone is increased because of the accompanying estrogen deficiency, but estrogen therapy reduces loss of bone mass by reducing the frequency of remodeling sites. The presence of estrogen receptors in osteoblast or osteoblast-like cells (Eriksen et al, 1988; Komm et al, 1988) opens up the possibility of a direct action of estrogen on bone mineral deposition and resorption. The osteoblast-like cells respond physiologically to estradiol (Komm et al, 1988). Estrogens may also stimulate local production of transforming growth factor-β (TGF-β) and insulin-like growth factor-1, both of which stimulate bone formation (Ernst et al, 1988; Gray et al, 1988).

Bone balance is dependent on the equilibrium established between the bone formation activity of the osteoblasts and bone resorption activity of the osteoclasts. In estrogen-deficient states, osteoclasts grow in number and size and live longer, and as a result tend to dig deeply into the bone trabeculae. Ultimately the osteoclasts perforate the trabeculae so that not only is bone mass diminished, but the bone is also structurally weaker. Estradiol and tamoxifen exert their estrogenic effects on bone by apoptosis of the osteoclasts, and thereby reduce bone resorption (Hughes et al, 1996). The cytokine TGF-β also promotes osteoclast apoptosis. Both estrogen and tamoxifen increase the production of TGF-β by osteoblasts, and their apoptosis-promoting effect on

Table 27-3. RISK FACTORS ASSOCIATED WITH POSTMENOPAUSAL OSTEOPOROSIS

Reduced weight-for-height ratio
White or Asian ethnicity
Positive family history
Low calcium intake (lifelong)
Early menopause (or oophorectomy)
Sedentary lifestyle
Nulliparity
Alcohol abuse
High sodium intake
Cigarette smoking
High caffeine intake
High protein intake
High phosphate intake
Secondary loss (glucocorticoid therapy, hyperthyroidism, hypoparathyroidism)

osteoclasts is blocked by antibodies to TGF-β. Thus the bone-protective effect of estrogen through promotion of osteoclast apoptosis is mediated through a paracrine effect of TGF-β secreted from osteoblasts and acting on osteoclasts. Estrogens also may inhibit the production of prostaglandins, such as prostaglandin E_2, and interleukin, both of which increase bone resorption (Ernst et al, 1988; Pacifici et al, 1988).

Estrogen deficiency results in declining levels of calcitonin secreted by the thyroid. Calcitonin secreted by the thyroid opposes the effects of parathyroid hormone. Calcitonin levels are decreased by estrogen deficiency. In high-estrogen states such as pregnancy, calcitonin levels are increased, whereas in postmenopausal women undergoing oophorectomy, calcitonin levels decrease further (Whitehead et al, 1984). In postmenopausal women with osteoporosis, administration of calcitonin increases total body calcium significantly (Chestnut et al, 1981). However, it is still inconclusive whether postmenopausal estrogen replacement therapy increases calcitonin levels (Stevenson et al, 1981; Lobo et al, 1985).

Another contributory mechanism is through inadequate intestinal calcium absorption as a result of reduced intestinal conversion of vitamin D to 1,25-dihydroxyvitamin D. This conversion is estrogen dependent, and estrogen therapy increases the formation of 1,25-dihydroxyvitamin D (Gallagher et al, 1980). Reduced or inadequate calcium intake, less than the daily minimum required calcium intake of 1200 mg, may further contribute to the development of postmenopausal osteoporosis.

The principal route by which calcium is inadequately conserved in the postmenopausal woman is through urinary excretion of calcium. In postmenopausal women who are not taking estrogens, the ratio of urinary calcium to creatinine is markedly increased compared with that in premenopausal women (Frumar et al, 1980), but this is reversed with estrogen therapy. That this increased urinary calcium excretion is dependent on estrogen levels is further supported by the inverse relationship of the urinary calcium:creatinine ratio with the serum levels of estrogen as well as with the ideal body weight of the postmenopausal woman (Frumar et al, 1980). Serum calcium and alkaline phosphatase levels are not significantly altered, but urinary hydroxyproline excretion is significantly elevated in postmenopausal women. These biochemical changes indicate that urinary excretion of substances such as calcium and hydroxyproline, involved in bone mass, is increased because of estrogen deficiency in the menopause. It is suggested that estrogen promotes renal tubular reabsorption of calcium. Nordin et al (1991) have shown that the rise in urinary calcium at menopause is due to reduced tubular reabsorption of calcium secondary to the effect of estrogen deficiency on the kidney.

Estrogen replacement therapy can block the decline in bone mineral density content occurring around menopause and can also reduce fracture rates. Estrogen, but not placebo, prevents the accelerated decrease in trabecular bone mineral density content occurring over the 4- to 5-year period after menopause (Lindsay et al, 1978; Christiansen et al, 1981). In oophorectomized and naturally menopausal women who are not receiving estrogen replacement therapy, the midradius loses 15% and 18% of bone mass, the lumbar spine 23% and 25%, and the neck of the femur 25% and 28%, respectively (Richelson et al, 1984). In postmenopausal women receiving placebo, the rate of bone loss is about 1.5 mg/cm^3/year; this is reduced to 1.0 mg/cm^3/year with a daily intake of 0.3 mg of conjugated estrogens, and there is complete prevention of bone loss with 0.625 mg and 1.25 mg of conjugated estrogens daily (Lindsay et al, 1984; Genant et al, 1990). Medroxyprogesterone acetate (MPA) enhances the spinal bone density response to estrogen in postmenopausal women (Grey et al, 1996), thus providing a favorable basis for combined estrogen-progestin therapy on the bone.

Whereas bone mineral mass conservation is immediately apparent over the short term with estrogen replacement therapy, the relative risk of fractures is significantly reduced only after 4 or more years of estrogen use when sufficient amounts of bone demineralization have occurred in untreated women. Thus the relative risks of fractures of the hip and forearm are not only significantly reduced to 0.4 but also continue to be reduced even when controlled for age groups, reflecting the bone-conservation and bone-protective effects of estrogen replacement therapy (Weiss et al, 1980).

Kiel et al (1987) reported from a large cohort study that the relative risk of hip fracture in subjects who had taken estrogen at any time was 0.65 after adjustment for age and weight. The adjusted relative risk for women who had taken estrogen within the previous 2 years was further reduced to 0.34. Other studies have shown that bone loss can be partially restored, with a positive balance or gain, in women placed on estrogen therapy even if they have not been on it for many years after menopause (Christiansen and Riis, 1990; Lindsay and Hohme, 1990). Figure 27–10 summarizes schematically the mechanisms through which estrogen may mediate to bring about bone and calcium conservation.

Although postmenopausal hypoestrogenemia provides the framework for osteopenia and osteoporosis, thereby increasing susceptibility to fractures, other risk factors for falls giving rise to fractures should be considered in the overall approach to preventing fractures in postmenopausal women. In one case–control study, Grisso et al (1991) identified lower limb dysfunction, visual impairment, previous stroke or neurologic conditions, and long-acting barbiturate use as risk factors for falls associated with hip fracture. Older patients are also less likely to fall on hard surfaces but are still likely to fracture their bones. Finally, impaired balance may contribute to falls and fractures. Estrogen therapy has been shown to increase balance in postmenopausal women seek-

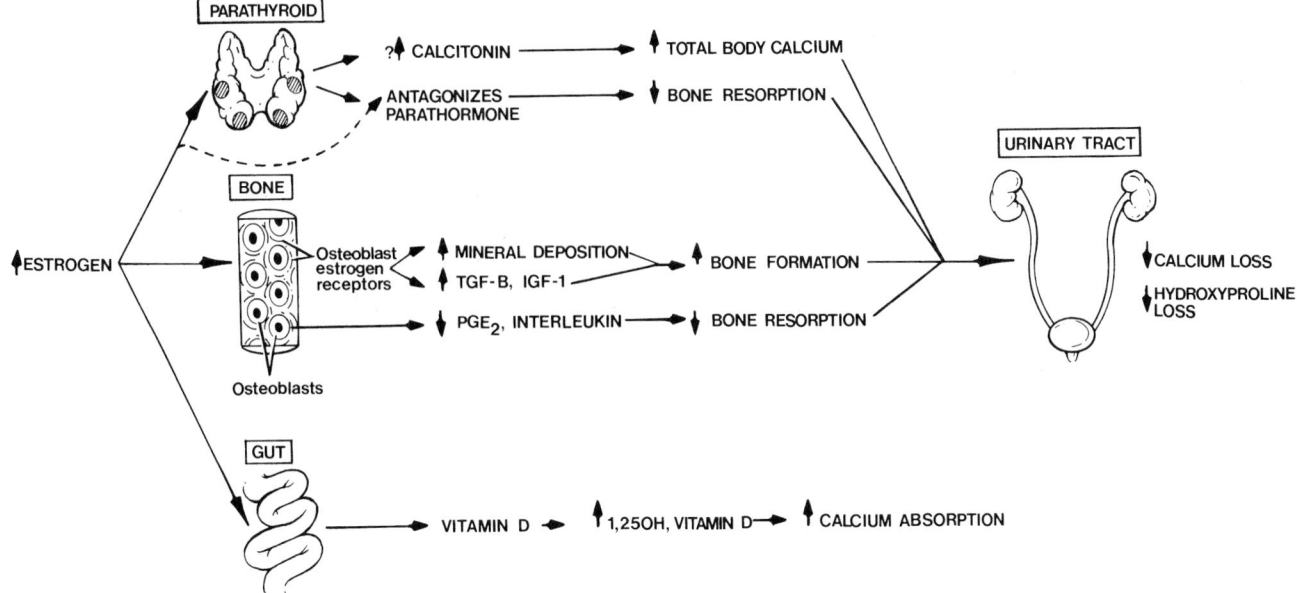

Figure 27–10
Schematic representation of the pathways of estrogen action in menopausal women to bring about bone and calcium conservation. TGF-β, transformation growth factor-β; IGF-1, insulin-like growth factor-1; PGE₂, prostaglandin E₂.

ing medical advice because of vasomotor symptoms (Hammar et al, 1996).

EVALUATION AND WORK-UP

For women who undergo natural menopause at the normal expected age, and for those who undergo hysterectomy and bilateral salpingo-oophorectomy, evaluation should include a complete history (including dietary practice) and physical examination. The work-up ought to include a Papanicolaou smear, a mammogram unless one was performed within the last year, and a lipid profile, including serum levels of cholesterol, HDL, LDL, and triglycerides.

Endometrial Evaluation

For most postmenopausal women, a baseline endometrial biopsy or curettage is neither essential nor productive. However, if the woman has irregular vaginal bleeding or abnormal findings on pelvic examination (such as abnormalities of the cervix, uterus, or adnexa) or is obese, an endometrial biopsy is advisable. A less invasive but possibly useful technique is a baseline *progestin challenge test* for identifying endometrial hyperplasia. If there is bleeding with the test, there is a high probability of endometrial hyperplasia. In 30 asymptomatic postmenopausal women, Gambrell (1986) observed that five bled after the test, and three of these had endometrial hyperplasia. In those who did not bleed, the endometrial histology was normal. Further validation of the

test indicated that, in 9 of 10 women known to have adenomatous hyperplasia, bleeding followed the test.

Vaginal sonography showing endometrial thickness of more than 5 mm has been suggested to indicate need for endometrial sampling to rule out hyperplasia (Menwissen et al, 1992), but larger definitive studies are needed to establish the reliability of this index.

Pituitary Gonadotropins and Estrogen Levels

Serum pituitary gonadotropin (FSH and LH) levels need not be routinely evaluated in the woman who has clearly begun menopause. However, if the diagnosis of menopause is not clinically clear, if there is irregular vaginal bleeding or oligomenorrhea, or if there are vasomotor symptoms without amenorrhea, measurement of serum FSH and LH levels can be helpful in making a final diagnosis. Under these circumstances, serum FSH and LH levels may be marginally elevated but not quite in the postmenopausal range. If such a result is obtained, measurement can be repeated in 6 to 8 weeks and will show further increase if the patient is menopausal.

For women in the perimenopausal phase, which is the time just before menopause, it is not uncommon to have irregular cycles with anovulatory cycles interspersed by ovulatory cycles. Therefore, periods of amenorrhea with elevated FSH and LH levels that mimic menopause can occur. In this setting, ovulatory cycles ensue a few months later and the FSH and LH levels decline to within the premenopausal range. Therefore, serum FSH and LH levels need to be repeated in such patients. These patients generally have normal or low-to-normal levels of estradiol.

Bone Mass

Because osteopenia and osteoporosis are important long-term sequelae of menopause, determination of bone mass is frequently recommended. Routine measurement of bone mass in the clinical management of postmenopausal women is questionable. Although it is informative in revealing subnormal levels of bone density, a single baseline measurement has limited predictive value as to the rate of bone loss that the individual is going to experience. Individuals starting off with a subnormal bone mass may lose bone slowly or rapidly, and likewise those with normal or above-normal bone mass may lose bone slowly or rapidly. Because bone loss after menopause is largely trabecular, measurements should use techniques for detection of this type of bone. Quantitative computed tomography (QCT) of the lumbar vertebrae and dual-energy x-ray absorptiometry (DEXA) of the same site as well as the hip (femoral neck and head) are preferable to single-photon absorptiometry, which measures largely cortical bone. DEXA is reliable and is increasingly chosen as the preferred method besides QCT. Bone density, if measured, should be tested again in 6 months or more to evaluate the rate of change.

For most patients who begin menopause without any direct evidence pointing to unusual likelihood of bone problems, bone densitometry may not be essential for management. Bone mass measurements are best reserved for research studies, for women with additional high-risk factors for osteoporosis, for those who have not received hormone replacement therapy for some time, for those who cannot be on hormone replacement therapy, for those with bone aches or backaches, and for those who may have sustained fractures.

Screening for Ovarian Cancer

Screening for ovarian cancer by a multimodal approach, including palpation of the ovaries, measurement of serum levels of ovarian antigens (such as CA-125), and ovarian ultrasonography, has been advocated. Although palpation of the ovaries is recommended as part of the routine physical examination, the value of the other screening modalities in the evaluation of menopausal women is questionable because of their sensitivity and specificity, predictive value, cost, and yield. The very few cases of ovarian cancer detected by such screening have not usually been in the early stages of the disease. These screening modalities must be evaluated further before they can be adopted as a routine.

Vaginal sonography of the ovaries and uterus is being increasingly examined as a method for early detection of ovarian cancer (Bourne et al, 1989) and endometrial cancer (Osmers et al, 1990), respectively. Vaginal sonography is an attractive, painless method (compared with endometrial biopsy) for screening such patients. It may become a routine part of the work-up of the postmenopausal patient if there is further refinement of the equipment and if clinical studies prove its reliability and predictability.

Additional Evaluation for Premature Menopause

If menopause occurs prematurely, additional evaluation should exclude abnormal sex chromosome karyotype, polyglandular autoimmune disease, and autoimmune antibodies to the ovary. Thus chromosome karyotyping and levels of circulating thyroid antibodies as well as thyroid function should be determined. Circulating levels of autoantibodies to the ovary can provide additional information on the cause of the premature menopause if the measurement is available, but this is confined more to research centers.

Other Work-up

Other appropriate work-ups should be performed when there are relevant symptoms or complaints. Such work-up may relate to urinary continence problems, psychoemotional states (depression, anxiety), and carbohydrate intolerance among those encountered in the postmenopausal age group.

MANAGEMENT

Calcium

Adequate calcium intake appears to play an important role in preventing osteoporosis and fracture (Riggs et al, 1982). The daily intake of calcium for postmenopausal women should be at least 1200 mg. Data on the American population indicate that the average daily calcium intake in adults older than 35 years is less than 800 mg. Thus supplemental calcium should further potentiate the bone mineral conservation effects of estrogen replacement therapy. However, if the daily calcium intake is more than adequate, calcium supplementation is usually not necessary. In one Dutch study, no correlations were found between habitual calcium intake of 560 to 2580 mg/day and bone mineral content of the radius, lumbar spine, and femoral neck (van Beresteijn et al, 1990). A higher body mass index had a protective effect for the appendicular skeleton but appeared to be less protective to the axial skeleton.

The contribution of calcium supplementation or increased calcium intake by itself without estrogen replacement therapy is probably small but remains to be clearly defined. Only three of seven studies demonstrated a significant reduction of bone loss when calcium intake was increased (Lindsay et al, 1987). In no study was calcium found to be as effective as estrogens. Riis et al (1987) compared the effects of calcium supplementation on bone loss in postmenopausal women in a 2-year period. Bone mineral content of the forearm, entire body, and spine decreased significantly in women receiving calcium or placebo but remained constant with estrogen treatment. Nevertheless, a high calcium intake over a lifetime appears to protect against fractures in old age by the woman having attained increased bone mass at maturity.

If calcium supplementation is needed, calcium can be given as calcium carbonate, calcium chloride, calcium lactate, calcium gluconate, bone meal, dolomite, or calcium citrate. The dose should be calculated on the basis of elemental calcium present in the preparation recommended. Calcium citrate has been advocated as being gentle to the alimentary tract and is more bioavailable than calcium carbonate. Calcium citrate inhibits calcium oxalate crystallization and should be the choice for those at risk of renal calculus formation. A simple way of administering calcium supplement is to use an antacid (Tums) which contains calcium. Certain foods or compounds promote calcium absorption, whereas others will inhibit it (Table 27–4). Therefore unbalanced or peculiar diets may have a significant impact on the bioavailability of calcium despite adequate calcium intake. Finally, calcium supplements should be given with a meal rather than during fasting or on an empty stomach, because the fraction of calcium absorbed is markedly less in the latter situations (Recker, 1985). It is best to take calcium at night so that the nocturnal release of calcium from the bone stores to meet the systemic needs can be reduced.

Patients should be counseled about balanced nutrition and the need to reduce fat and increase fiber intake if only to reduce cholesterol levels and also the risk of large-bowel neoplasia.

Exercise

Besides its positive effects on cardiovascular fitness, exercise should be advocated to retard bone loss, because prolonged immobilization results in accelerated bone demineralization. It is still inconclusive whether exercise itself increases bone mass or prevents accelerated bone demineralization at menopause (Krolner et al, 1983; Simkin et al, 1987). Krolner et al (1983) found that the bone mineral content of the spine was significantly higher in individuals who exercised regularly than in controls (Fig. 27–11). Nevertheless, exercise prevents or retards bone loss rather than producing a gain in bone mineral con-

Table 27–4. FOOD COMPOUNDS AFFECTING THE BIOAVAILABILITY OF DIETARY CALCIUM

PROMOTING ABSORPTION	INHIBITING ABSORPTION
Protein	Oxalates (leafy vegetables)
Lactose	Phytic acid (grains)
Carbohydrates	High phosphorus (meat, carbonated beverages)
Calcium-to-phosphate ratio of 1 (dairy products)	Fat
Acids (lactic, citric)	Fiber

tent. Exercise in postmenopausal women may retard osteoporosis (Oyster et al, 1984), but prolonged, excessive exercise itself may cause increased bone demineralization. Therefore, postmenopausal women should be encouraged to perform low-impact, weight-bearing exercises (such as walking, jogging, tennis, racquetball, dancing) in moderation. Compliance is likely to be better if the type of exercise chosen is part of the daily activity of the woman, consistent with her lifestyle, and easily performed without additional stress or cost.

One double-blind, placebo-controlled, randomized study compared exercise, exercise plus dietary calcium supplementation, and exercise plus estrogen-progesterone (Prince et al, 1991). In postmenopausal women with low bone density, exercise plus calcium induced significantly lower bone loss than did exercise alone. However, in women with normal bone density there was bone gain with exercise plus

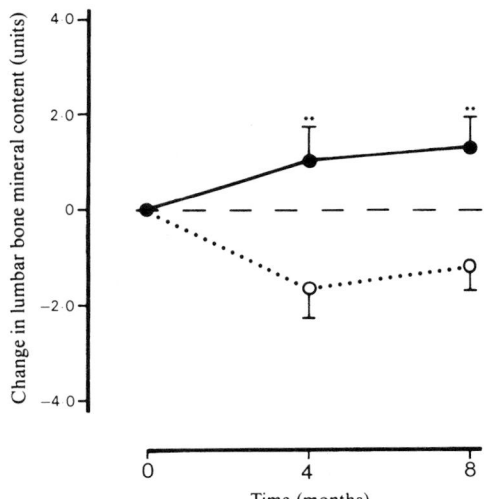

Figure 27–11
Bone mineral content of the lumbar spine in exercisers (*solid circles*) versus controls (*open circles*). (Modified from Krolner B, Toft B, Nielsen SP, Tondevold E: Physical exercise as prophylaxis against involutional vertebral bone loss: a controlled trial. Clin Sci 1983;64:541, with permission. Courtesy of The Biochemical Society and Portland Press.)

estrogen-progesterone compared with controls. Significant bone loss continued in the exercise-alone group. Exercise, therefore, is an adjunct to estrogen replacement therapy in the prevention of postmenopausal bone loss.

Estrogen Replacement Therapy

The benefits and potential risks of estrogen replacement therapy should be discussed with each patient before initiation of such treatment so that a joint decision by the patient and physician is made. From a preventive and public health standpoint, all postmenopausal women who have no contraindication to the use of estrogen should be candidates for estrogen replacement therapy because of the many therapeutic benefits that far outweigh the risk. Patients who have premature menopause, who are at high risk for osteoporosis, and who have menopausal symptoms ought to be treated with the objective of overcoming some of the problems related to estrogen deficiency. Absolute contraindications include estrogen-dependent cancers (breast cancer and melanoma), liver dysfunction, liver cirrhosis, deep vein thrombosis, pulmonary embolism, unexplained vaginal bleeding, and pregnancy. Retrospective analysis indicates that, for stages I and II endometrial cancer survivors, estrogen replacement therapy is not contraindicated because it does not decrease disease-free interval or increase the risk of recurrence (Chapman et al, 1996).

Adverse Effects

Confusion about the adverse effects of postmenopausal estrogen replacement therapy is largely due to extrapolation of the adverse effects reported from estrogen use in oral contraceptives. As the dose of estrogen used in birth control pills is brought down to as little as 30 μg of ethinyl estradiol, the incidence of life-threatening side effects is dramatically reduced. It is necessary to recognize that 0.625 mg of conjugated estrogen is approximately equivalent to 5 μg of ethinyl estradiol. Rarely is more than 1.25 mg of conjugated estrogens (equivalent to 10 μg of ethinyl estradiol) required for postmenopausal estrogen replacement therapy. Therefore, the frequency and severity of adverse estrogen effects from the birth control pill cannot necessarily be applied to potential adverse effects of postmenopausal estrogen replacement therapy. Real or potential adverse effects of postmenopausal estrogen replacement therapy may include endometrial hyperplasia and cancer, thromboembolism, stroke, hypertension, breast cancer, gallbladder dysfunction, and gallstones, as well as less life-threatening side effects such as nausea, vomiting, water retention, and breakthrough bleeding.

ENDOMETRIAL HYPERPLASIA AND NEOPLASIA

Prolonged unopposed estrogen therapy increases significantly the risk for endometrial hyperplasia and carcinoma. More than 20 case–control studies and several prospective studies have confirmed the increased risk of 3- to 25-fold. Depending on the dose and duration of estrogen therapy, the relative risk for endometrial cancer increases from threefold to fourfold with the use of postmenopausal estrogen, to sixfold with 5 or more years and 16.1 for 10 or more years of use (Cramer and Knapp, 1979; Brinton and Hoover, 1993) (Fig. 27–12). The risk for endometrial hyperplasia and carcinoma can be readily eliminated with progestin administration for 12 to 14 days each month; therefore, progestin administration is mandatory in women who still have their uterus. Progestins reduce the risk of estrogen-induced endometrial neoplasia by decreasing estrogen receptors, decreasing DNA synthesis, and increasing estrogen conversion to inactive metabolites. Estrogen and progestin therapy will also induce more complete sloughing of the endometrium or an atrophic endometrium, both of which are less likely to favor development of endometrial carcinoma. Patients who have been surgically treated for endometrial carcinoma can be given postmenopausal estrogen replacement therapy (Creasman et al, 1986; Chapman et al, 1996). It is probably best that such patients also receive progestin supplementation (Voight et al, 1991).

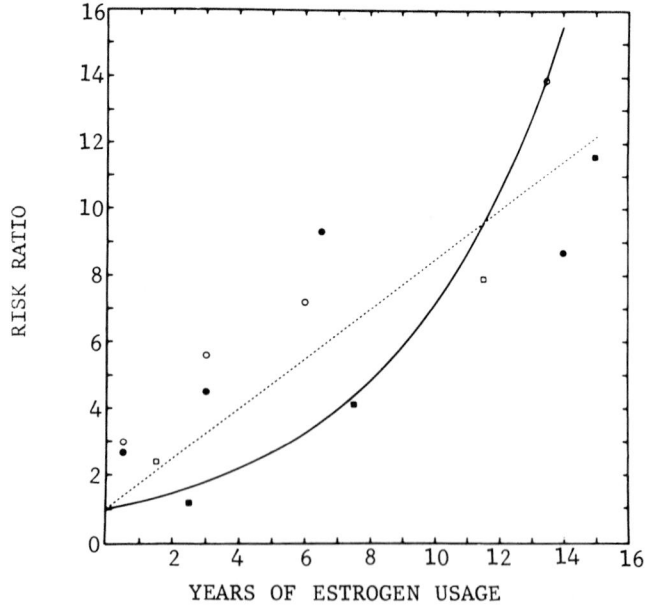

Figure 27–12
Relationship between the risk ratio for endometrial cancer and length of estrogen use based on four different studies. Each symbol (*open* and *closed circles*, *open* and *closed squares*) represents one study. (From Cramer DW, Knapp RC: Review of epidemiologic studies of endometrial cancer and exogenous estrogen. Obstet Gynecol 1979;54:521, with permission.)

The Postmenopausal Estrogen-Progestin Intervention (PEPI) trial found that women given estrogen alone were more likely to develop simple, complex, or atypical hyperplasia than those receiving placebo. Those given estrogen plus progestins continuously or by the sequential regimen had rates of hyperplasia similar to those given placebo (Writing Group for the PEPI Trial, 1996).

GALLBLADDER DISEASE

With postmenopausal estrogen replacement therapy, the incidence of gallbladder disease and gallstones is increased $2^1/_2$ times (Petitti et al, 1988). Oral estrogen, such as conjugated equine estrogens, increases biliary cholesterol by enhancing hepatic lipoprotein uptake and inhibiting bile acid synthesis (Everson et al, 1991). Therefore, the increased dietary cholesterol is diverted into bile. Formation of gallstones is due to increased cholesterol saturation in the biliary secretions. Cholecystitis and cholangitis can therefore occur secondary to the presence of the gallstones.

When different routes of estrogen administration were compared for their hepatobiliary effects, oral therapy with estradiol induced a slight, but not statistically significant, increase in cholesterol, but no change was noted with transdermal estradiol, with which the estrogen bypasses the liver (Van Erpecum et al, 1991). However, in women who had a marked increase in serum estrone after taking oral estradiol, the biliary cholesterol saturation index was increased, the relative percentage of chenodeoxycholic acid in bile was decreased, and sex hormone–binding globulin was increased. Cholesterol crystals were more likely to appear in the bile after oral therapy than with transdermal estradiol (D'Amato et al, 1989). Thus oral estrogens, especially those producing a marked increase in serum estrone, lead to an increase in the biliary lithogenic index and formation of gallstones. In women susceptible to intrahepatic cholestasis secondary to estrogens, S-adenosylmethionine can be effective in protecting against intrahepatic cholestasis when estrogen is being given (Frezza et al, 1988).

BLOOD PRESSURE

Postmenopausal estrogen replacement therapy does not appear to have any significant adverse effect on blood pressure. Three months after initiation of estrogen replacement therapy, systolic as well as diastolic blood pressures have not been found to change (Wren and Routledge, 1983). Hammond et al (1979) noted the incidence of new occurrence of hypertension to be considerably less in 301 postmenopausal estrogen users compared with 309 nonusers in a 5-year retrospective study. Mean arterial blood pressure decreased slightly with estrone replacement therapy, and blood pressure levels among mild and moderate hypertensives actually improved with postmenopausal estrogen replacement therapy (Pfeffer et al, 1979). Nonetheless, blood pressure should be documented and, if elevated, a complete work-up for hypertension should be undertaken before estrogen replacement therapy is begun. The hypertension should be treated. There is no good reason to withhold estrogen replacement therapy if the blood pressure is under control. Blood pressure should be recorded at follow-up visits for estrogen replacement therapy. There is no consensus with regard to estrogen treatment in women with sequelae of hypertension, such as thromboembolism, cerebrovascular accident, or myocardial infarction; if given estrogen, these patients require vigilant monitoring in concert with their hypertension, cardiovascular, and coagulation status.

CARDIOVASCULAR DISORDERS

There is no evidence of any significant increase in risk for stroke or myocardial infarction in normal, healthy postmenopausal women taking 0.625 to 1.25 mg of conjugated estrone, the usual dose for replacement therapy. Mortality from cardiovascular and coronary heart disease is also reduced with postmenopausal estrogen use even when controlled for age groups compared with no estrogen use (Criqui et al, 1988). Estrogen replacement therapy is also associated with a reduced mortality from myocardial infarction, with the relative risk decreased to 0.59 (Henderson et al, 1988). With one exception, all studies have consistently found a significant reduction to 0.3 to 0.7 in the relative risk for coronary heart disease, with a mean of about 0.5 in postmenopausal estrogen users. In a 10-year follow-up, the Nurses' Health Study found the overall relative risk of major coronary disease in 48,470 postmenopausal women currently taking estrogen was 0.56, irrespective of natural or surgical menopause (Stampfer et al, 1991). This protection appears to persist even at greater than 70 years of age (Sullivan et al, 1988). Although the Nurses' Health Study found no change in the risk of stroke with hormone replacement therapy, stroke mortality was noted to actually reduce to an overall risk of 0.53 with estrogen according to another report (Paganini-Hill et al, 1988).

THROMBOEMBOLISM

Earlier studies found either insufficient evidence or no association between postmenopausal estrogen use and venous thromboembolism because of lack of power in the number of subjects studied (Devor et al, 1992; RCOG Working Party Report, 1995). However, two studies have demonstrated that the relative risk of venous thromboembolism is significantly increased to 3.5 in current users of hormone replacement therapy compared to nonusers and past users (Fig. 27–13) (Daly et al, 1996; Jick et al, 1996). Depending on the dose of estrogen used, the relative risk increased from 2.1 for 0.325 mg of conjugated estrogen to 3.3 with 0.625 mg estrogen and 6.9 with

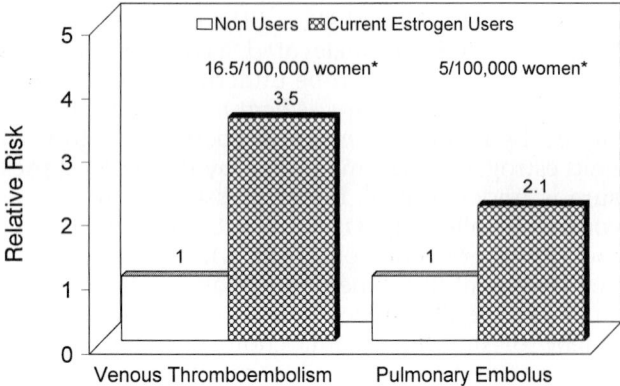

Figure 27–13
Relative risks of developing venous thromboembolism or pulmonary embolus in women using estrogen replacement therapy. *Denotes the excess or extra annual cases resulting from estrogen replacement therapy. (Data for venous thromboembolism were derived from Daly et al [1996] and Jick et al [1996] and those for pulmonary embolism from Grodstein et al [1996a].)

1.25 mg estrogen compared to nonusers (Jick et al, 1996). There is no association with past use, and the risk appears to be highest among short-term current users. The increased risk may be concentrated in new users. Therefore, current estrogen use increases the risk of venous thromboembolism 3- to 4-fold. Nevertheless, such an increased risk should be viewed against the overall low incidence of venous thromboembolism. The annual rate of idiopathic venous thromboembolism in women ages 45 to 64 years is estimated to be 27.4 per 100,000 women among hormone replacement therapy users and 10.9 per 100,000 women among nonusers, thus giving 16.5 cases per 100,000 women that may be attributed to hormone replacement therapy. Taking time into consideration, the incidence of venous thromboembolism is estimated to be 0.9×10^{-4} woman-years in nonusers compared to 3.2×10^{-4} woman-years among current estrogen users (Jick et al, 1996).

Analysis of data from the ongoing Nurses' Health Study found the risk of pulmonary embolism among current users of postmenopausal hormone replacement therapy is increased to 2.1 (confidence interval 1.2 to 3.8) when adjusted for multiple risk factors compared to nonusers (Grodstein et al, 1996a). This increased risk in pulmonary embolism among hormone replacement therapy users is similar to that noted for oral contraceptive users analyzed in the same study (Grodstein et al, 1996a). Irrespective of the cigarette smoking status, there is a consistent relationship between estrogen use and the risk of pulmonary embolism. However, it cannot be excluded that women currently using hormone replacement therapy might be undergoing more diagnostic procedures. The increased risk of pulmonary embolism notwithstanding, the additional cases that can be attributed to current postmenopausal hormone use are estimated to be only 5 cases per 100,000 woman-

years among women 50 to 59 years of age (Grodstein et al, 1996a).

BREAST CANCER

Menopause is an important event that influences the subsequent risk of breast cancer, as demonstrated by the sharp increase in incidence of breast malignancy around the time of menopause. Besides early menarche, late childbearing, and nulliparity, the age of natural menopause is associated with increased risk for breast cancer, whereas early menopause, especially involving bilateral oophorectomy, appears to reduce the risk profoundly. Increasingly, more attention is being focused on the relationship between postmenopausal estrogen replacement therapy and the risk for breast cancer.

More than 50 published studies have attempted to define the relationship between noncontraceptive estrogen use and breast cancer. The results have been conflicting, with some studies finding an increased weak, but significant, relative risk of breast cancer with estrogen replacement therapy. Given the diverse methodologies used, meta-analysis has been deployed to clarify any association between breast cancer and estrogen replacement therapy (Fig. 27–14). The weighted relative risk ranged from 1.0 to 1.07 for all women who had ever received estrogen replacement. One study reported this small increase to be significant (Sillero-Arenas et al, 1992), but all the meta-analyses (Armstrong, 1988; DuPont and Page, 1991; Steinberg et al, 1991, 1994; Sillero-Arenas et al, 1992) found significant heterogeneity, indicating that the results of the individual studies are not in close enough agreement or differ too greatly in their methodology to draw a definite conclusion.

The effects of estrogen dose, duration of exposure, family history of breast cancer, and history of benign disease were also examined. Again, there was no consistent agreement. Two of the meta-analyses (Armstrong, 1988; Dupont and Page, 1991) found a nonsignificant increase in the relative risk of developing breast cancer and receiving 1.25 mg or more of conjugated estrogen, but there was significant heterogeneity. One meta-analysis reported a significant increase in breast cancer risk after 5 years of estrogen use and a maximum increase of 30% (relative risk of 1.3) after 15 years of use (Steinberg et al, 1991), but the remaining meta-analyses found inconclusive or no effect. Again, one meta-analysis found that women with a history of benign breast disease or a family history of breast cancer had relative risks of 1.7 and 3.4, respectively, of developing breast cancer with postmenopausal estrogen use (Steinberg et al, 1991), but the other meta-analyses could not establish this. Part of the variability stems from the inclusion of European studies in which the more potent estradiol compounds were used.

The largest series to examine breast cancer risk is the Nurses' Health Study, which is an ongoing cohort of 121,700 U.S. women from 1976, when they

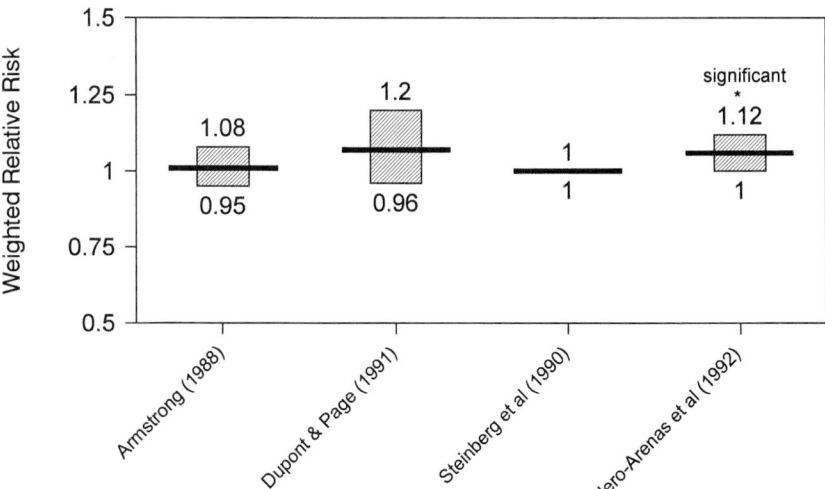

Figure 27-14
Relative risks of developing breast cancer with estrogen after menopause based on four different meta-analyses of published studies. The *vertical shaded bars* represent the 95% confidence interval, with the values given above and below the shaded bars. Two analyses found no significant effect (Armstrong, 1988; Dupont and Page, 1991), one found no effect (Steinberg et al, 1991), and one found a significant increase in risk with estrogen use (Sillero-Arenas et al, 1992).

were 30 to 55 years of age. Several analyses from this study have made the following observations. Current users of postmenopausal hormones were at 30% to 40% increased risk of breast cancer (Colditz et al, 1990). The risk increases significantly with use of more than 5 years of postmenopausal hormones (Colditz et al, 1995), such increased risk being most marked in women over 60 years. The risk of breast cancer increased with age, with a relative risk of 1.10 for current hormone users at 50 to 54 years over never-users, 1.40 for 55 to 59 years, and 1.87 for 60 to 66 years of age. It appears that the increase in risk of breast cancer for current users of postmenopausal hormone is more directly related to current age than to duration of use.

Whether addition of progestin to postmenopausal estrogen therapy alters the risk is still debatable. In nine published studies (Gambrell et al, 1983; Ewertz, 1988; Bergkvist et al, 1989; Colditz et al, 1992, 1995; Stanford et al, 1995; Kaufman et al, 1991; Yang et al, 1992; Palmer et al, 1991), one reported that addition of progestin to estrogen therapy decreased the risk (Gambrell et al, 1983), four reported increasing the risk (Ewertz, 1988; Bergkvist et al, 1989; Kaufmann et al, 1991; Yang et al, 1992), two found the risk similar to that for estrogen therapy alone (Colditz et al, 1992, 1995), and two found no association with breast cancer (Stanford et al, 1995; Palmer et al, 1991). The Nurses' Health Study found that the multivariate-adjusted relative risk of breast cancer with estrogen therapy was 1.41, and addition of progestin did not reduce this risk (Colditz et al, 1992, 1995).

In a small study, estrogen replacement therapy was positively associated with fibrocystic breast disease, the odds ratio of disease developing increasing to fivefold after menopausal estrogen use of 10 or more years (Berkowitz et al, 1985).

CARBOHYDRATE METABOLISM

The effects of estrogen on carbohydrate metabolism in normal and diabetic menopausal women have

been reported in 16 studies (Spellacy, 1987). In most of the studies, estrogen use did not affect blood glucose levels but could impair glucose tolerance. It appears that, with the more potent estrogens (mestranol, ethinyl estradiol) and with high doses, fasting blood glucose levels were lowered. In four studies in which plasma insulin levels were measured, there was no change with estrogen therapy.

In menopausal women with diabetes mellitus, estrogen treatment either did not change their carbohydrate metabolism or improved their blood glucose control, with a decreased need for exogenous insulin. Hammond et al (1979) reported a significant reduction in the frequency of diabetes mellitus in postmenopausal women taking estrogen replacement. Thus, at low doses of estrogens, no significant change in carbohydrate metabolism occurs, but changes can occur with high doses of mestranol or ethinyl estradiol. Estrogen replacement therapy may actually benefit those postmenopausal women with abnormal carbohydrate metabolism.

Nachtigall et al (1979) did not find any change in carbohydrate metabolism in both normal and diabetic postmenopausal women receiving estrogen-progestin replacement therapy. Nevertheless, diabetic postmenopausal women have a blunted response to the HDL-raising effects of estrogen and an exaggerated hypertriglyceride response that may result in attenuated cardioprotection from hormone replacement therapy (Robinson et al, 1996).

Types of Estrogen

Estrogens can be given orally, transdermally, vaginally, or as a subdermal implant. The oral and transdermal routes are the two commonly used in clinical practice in the United States.

Several estrogen preparations are available for oral administration (Table 27–5). Although conjugated estrogens (containing mainly estrone sulfate) are frequently used in the United States, ethinyl estradiol is widely used in Europe. Other oral estrogens that

Table 27–5. ORAL ESTROGENS FOR POSTMENOPAUSAL HORMONE REPLACEMENT THERAPY

PREPARATION	USUAL DAILY DOSE
Conjugated estrogens (Premarin)	0.625–1.25 mg
Ethinyl estradiol	5–10 µg
Micronized estradiol (Estrace)	1–2 mg
Estropipate (Ogen)	0.625–1.25 mg
Estradiol valerate	1–2 mg

have been and can be used for postmenopausal estrogen replacement therapy are micronized estradiol, estropipate, and estradiol valerate. The usual dose ranges for menopause therapy are listed in Table 27–5.

The choice of estrogen and its route of administration is predicated on considerations of the first-pass effect of the estrogen on the liver, acceptability of the route of administration, ease and convenience of use, patient compliance, and side effects. All of the preparations and administration routes employed are effective for relieving most menopausal symptoms, but the generic brands of estrogen have had their share of bioequivalency and bioavailability problems. The clinician should be cognizant of this and should consider this potential factor if there is reduced or no relief of symptoms. Although the use of the transdermal route reduces the need for daily dosing and avoids or reduces the first-pass effect of estrogen on the liver, the incidence of cutaneous side effects is high, and even more so in hot and humid weather. Some women prefer not to "display" their

medication needs or use, which may become apparent with the transdermal patch. With the newer matrix patch, which incorporates estradiol directly with the patch adhesive, skin irritation is less than with the earlier alcohol-based patches.

Lipoprotein levels are not altered to the same degree with parenteral estradiol-17β as with oral estrogens (Farish et al, 1984; Notelovitz et al, 1987). Colvin et al (1990) found that both estradiol-17β and estrone sulfate, when given orally, increased HDL and HDL_2 levels significantly. Although estradiol increased total cholesterol and triglycerides and did not affect LDL, estrogen sulfate decreased total cholesterol and LDL levels but did not affect triglycerides.

Estrogen Regimens

Current concepts and contemporary practice of giving oral estrogens for postmenopausal estrone replacement therapy can be simplified and narrowed to four regimens, as summarized in Figure 27–15:

1. Cyclic estrogen, given for 25 of 30 days, with progestin added on the last 12 days (days 14 to 25) and no medication for 5 days; this regimen is usually employed for a woman with her uterus intact.
2. Cyclic estrogen, given for 30 days, with progestin added during the first 12 days of the calendar month; this regimen is sometimes used for the women without a uterus who need progestin but can also be used if the uterus is in place.
3. Continuous, combined estrogen and progestin given daily and continuously throughout the month; this regimen can be adopted for the postmenopausal woman with or without a uterus.

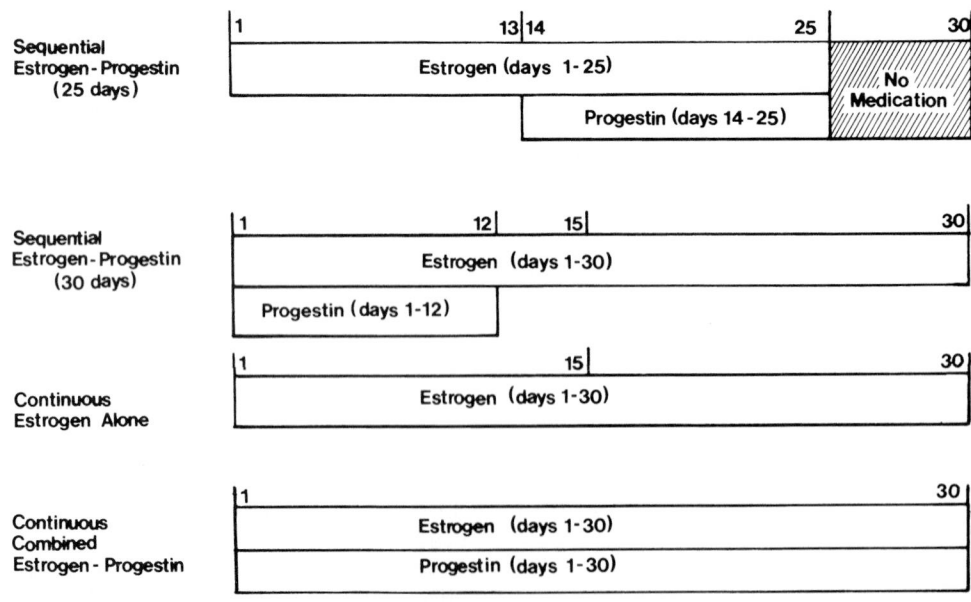

Figure 27–15
Schematic representation of the four principal regimens recommended for estrogen-progestin hormone replacement therapy in postmenopausal women.

4. Continuous estrogen given alone; this regimen is given only if the woman does not have a uterus.

CYCLIC ESTROGEN WITH PROGESTIN

Cyclic estrogen can be given either for 25 or 30 days, with progestin added for the last 12 to 14 days. Until recently, this was the regimen widely recommended and used. With the 25-day regimen, estrogen is given from days 1 through 25, with progestin added on days 14 through 25 (12 days) or days 12 through 25 (14 days); this is followed by 5 days of no medication. The basis for 5 days of no medication is unclear other than to induce a withdrawal bleeding, which may assist in preventing excessive endometrial accumulation and growth. With such a 25-day hormone replacement regimen, cyclic withdrawal bleeding is likely to occur in up to 80% of the women treated. The younger the woman, the more likely it is that bleeding will be heavy and approach that of a normal menstrual flow. Thus a woman with premature ovarian failure and premature menopause is almost certain to have a normal menstrual flow with such treatment. Also, sexual desire and arousal were significantly higher during the first 2 weeks than during the days when no hormones were taken (Sherwin, 1991). Negative moods and more psychological symptoms were reported during administration of sequential hormone with conjugated equine estrogen and medroxyprogesterone (MPA) than with estrogen alone; such symptoms, however, are attenuated by a higher estrogen-to-progestin dose ratio.

When estrogen is given for 30 days each month without a break, a progestin is added on days 19 to 30 (12 days) or days 17 to 30 (14 days). This schedule is less likely than the 25-day regimen to induce withdrawal bleeding but, nonetheless, is also complicated by bleeding. If a progestin is to be given in addition to estrogen in the postmenopausal patient without a uterus, the regimen is aligned with the calendar rather than the menstrual month. Thus estrogen and progestin are given from the first to the 12th day of the calendar month, and estrogen alone is given during the remainder of the month.

If oral conjugated estrogen is given, the usual minimum daily dose is 0.625 mg to obtain a significant antiosteopenic effect. The dose can be increased to 0.9 mg daily, but rarely is more than 1.25 mg daily needed. However, it is noteworthy that bioavailability of the estrogen is equally important as the dose because similar doses of generic preparations of conjugated estrogen have been found to have less bioavailable estrogen and have not relieved menopausal symptoms. If transdermal estradiol is given, the usual starting dose is the 0.05-mg/day patch, which gives a serum estradiol level of around 50 pg/ml. The dose can be increased to the higher dose 0.1-mg/day patch, which gives a serum estradiol level of 100 pg/ml. Most of the new matrix patches will last for 7 days, and therefore only one patch a week is required. If the woman still has her uterus, progestins should be given in a regimen similar to that for oral estrogen. A patch containing both estradiol and nonrethindrone (Combipatch) is now available for use in postmenopausal women. With such an estradiol-progestin patch, it is not necessary to give an oral progestin.

The ideal progestin for postmenopausal hormone replacement therapy should (1) protect the endometrium against hyperplasia and neoplasia, (2) have no adverse physical, psychological, or metabolic effects; and (3) not oppose the benefits of estrogen. Although several progestins have been used, MPA is often used for this purpose in the United States. In choosing a progestin for postmenopausal hormone replacement therapy, one must recognize that progestins have varying androgenic properties that can negate the favorable cardioprotective effects of estrogen on cholesterol and lipoproteins. Thus far, MPA produces fewer adverse changes in these lipids than the progestins of the 19-nor derivatives, such as norethindrone and norgestrel (Hirvonen et al, 1981; Vejtorp et al, 1986). Oral micronized progesterone is readily absorbed, can produce luteal-phase serum progesterone levels, can provoke a uterine endometrial response, and has no detrimental effect on lipoprotein profile. The usual dose is 200 or 300 mg/day as a progestin. With 300 mg, the maximum plasma concentration reached is 15 to 626 ng/ml (McAuley et al, 1996). There is considerable variation in absorption between subjects, and the extent of absorption appears to increase with age.

The progestin medrogestone (6,17α-dimethyldehydroprogesterone), a pregnane analog of 17-acetoxyprogesterone given in doses of 5 mg daily, also does not attenuate the increase in HDL induced by conjugated estrogen administration in postmenopausal women (Sonnendecker et al, 1989). Farish et al (1989) found that, when levonorgestrel was given together with estradiol in a vaginal ring, total HDL, HDL_2, and HDL_3 levels were actually reduced by 21% to 40% in postmenopausal women. Hence, it is prudent to avoid using progestins such as levonorgestrel in hormone replacement therapy.

CONTINUOUS COMBINED ESTROGEN AND PROGESTIN

Continuous combined estrogen and progestin therapy has been advocated to avoid withdrawal bleeding and thereby increase patient compliance. This regimen of hormone replacement therapy has been shown to be effective for postmenopausal hormone replacement and has had very little metabolic effect on the favorable cardioprotective lipid profile induced by estrogen alone (Upjohn Multicenter Collaborative Study, 1991a, 1991b; Archer et al, 1994; Lobo et al, 1994; Writing Group for the PEPI Trial, 1995).

With the sequential regimen of hormone replacement therapy, 75% to 80% of subjects were noted to have bleeding even 1 year after initiating treatment.

The bleeding tended to last 2 to 3 days and more with a menstrual flow type of pattern. With continuous combined therapy, bleeding occurred in only about 20% of the patients even at 1 year after beginning treatment if 2.5 mg MPA was used and in about 11% to 15% if 5 mg of MPA was used. Furthermore, the bleeding tended to be lighter, sporadic, and seldom continuous for more than a day. These observations have been made with the use of 0.625 mg conjugated estrogen. While the daily addition of MPA to estrogen in the continuous combined regimen might attenuate the overall estrogen-augmented increase in cardioprotective lipoproteins, the benefits of estrogen on lipid profile are still attained (Upjohn Multicenter Collaborative Study, 1991b; Archer et al, 1994; Lobo et al, 1994; Writing Group for the PEPI Trial, 1995). In the Nurses' Health Study analysis, addition of progestin to postmenopausal estrogen therapy was found not to attenuate the cardioprotective effects of estrogen (Grodstein et al, 1996b).

The dropout rates in the multicenter studies were not significantly different between the sequential and the continuous combined regimen, which probably reflects adequate counseling and realistic expectations of the patients by the investigators. Studies reporting surveys of patients concerning compliance with hormone replacement therapy indicate vaginal bleeding and fear of cancer as leading causes of discontinuing treatment. Nonetheless, it should be noted that continuous combined estrogen-progestin cannot be guaranteed or represented not to cause bleeding, because 15% to 26% of users will initially have bleeding and 10% to 15% will still have irregular uterine bleeding even 1 year after starting treatment; conversely, although 75% to 80% of patients may bleed with the sequential regimen, the bleeding is predictable and cyclic. These are important, practical considerations in counseling patients and in selecting regimens for hormone replacement therapy. On the basis of the currently available data base from clinical studies, either the sequential regimen of 0.625 mg of conjugated estrogen on days 1 to 25 with 5 mg of MPA on days 14 to 25 or the continuous combined regimen using 0.625 mg of conjugated estrogen and 2.5 mg of MPA daily can be used. It does not appear necessary to use 10 mg of MPA in the sequential regimen, and side effects from MPA will be less with lower doses.

The combined continuous estrogen-progestin therapy may be the preferred regimen in most cases because of the following advantages:

1. There is decreased frequency of uterine bleeding and lighter bleeding when it occurs.
2. There is higher frequency of amenorrhea 6 to 12 months after initiating treatment.
3. There is higher incidence of induced atrophic endometrium and thus a reduced risk for hyperplasia and neoplasia.
4. The progestin may have a synergistic or additive effect with estrogen to increase rather than maintain bone mass (Notelovitz et al, 1987; Christian-

sen and Riis, 1990). With the availability of the Combipatch containing estradiol and norethindrone, continuous combined estrogen-progestin therapy can also be given via the transdermal route (Ginsburg et al, 1995).

CONTINUOUS ESTROGEN ALONE

In this regimen, estrogen is given continuously without addition of any progestin. This regimen is best reserved for the woman without a uterus. Besides the absence of a need to protect the uterus against risk of unopposed estrogen, one reason for not giving a progestin is the concern that the latter hormone might attenuate the cardioprotective lipid changes induced by estrogens. However, with the doses of MPA currently used, there is no significant reversal of the cardioprotective effects of estrogen. There is no consensus as to whether a progestin should be added for women who are without a uterus. There are potential theoretical benefits for addition of progestins other than protection against endometrial hyperplasia and neoplasia (see previous discussion).

Contraindications to Estrogen Replacement Therapy

Contraindications to the use of estrogen include estrogen-dependent neoplasia, such as breast cancer, melanoma, and endometrial cancer; thromboembolism; myocardial infarction; and pregnancy. Because estrogen can stimulate proliferation of the endometrium, it should not be given to women who have active endometrial cancer. However, once the endometrial cancer has been removed by total hysterectomy and bilateral salpingo-oophorectomy, there is no contraindication to instituting estrogen replacement therapy. On the basis of concerns about the risk of thromboembolism with estrogen use, largely derived from earlier oral contraceptive studies, estrogen replacement therapy for the postmenopausal woman is discouraged if she has had thromboembolism. However, thromboembolism developing from prolonged immobilization or postoperatively should not be a contraindication to the use of estrogen replacement therapy, because this is a nonrecurring situation that has no direct relevance to estrogen. The dose of estrogen use in postmenopausal hormone replacement therapy is about three to six times lower than in currently available low-dose birth control pills (0.625 mg of conjugated estrogen is equivalent to 5 μg of ethinyl estradiol). Nevertheless, when estrogen replacement therapy is initiated in a woman who has had thromboembolism, it may be prudent to circumvent the first-pass effect of estrogen on the liver by giving her an appropriate estrogen formulation and route as well as monitoring the necessary coagulation studies.

Although myocardial infarction is often cited as a contraindication to the use of estrogen, it may be argued that a patient who has had a myocardial infarction is indeed the very patient who requires estrogen replacement therapy to lower her risk of further coronary artery disease. Nevertheless, estrogen replacement therapy should not be initiated during the acute phase of myocardial infarction but only after the patient has adequately recovered from her heart attack.

Hypertension and diabetes mellitus are not contraindications to the use of estrogen replacement therapy, but complications of these two conditions may necessitate cautious and judicious consideration of estrogen use. Hypertension itself should be evaluated and treated.

At present, it is prudent not to give estrogen replacement therapy to women who have had breast cancer and are considered to be cured (more than 10 years in remission). Withholding estrogen replacement therapy from such patients may need to be reconsidered as results of ongoing studies and trials in this population become available. Nevertheless, until definitive results document the wisdom of such a recommendation, such a treatment is best performed under a study protocol setup.

Nonestrogen Therapy to Prevent Bone Loss

For the symptomatic postmenopausal women in whom estrogen use is contraindicated, the symptoms and long-term sequelae of osteoporosis can be satisfactorily managed with alternative medication or measures. Progestins (oral Provera or intramuscular Depo-Provera) and the α-adrenergic agonist clonidine (0.2 mg to 0.4 mg daily) are effective for relief of hot flushes (Laufer et al, 1982). To a lesser extent, Bellergal, which contains a mixture of phenobarbital, ergotamine tartrate, and belladonna, is also effective for the relief of hot flushes. If estrogen is contraindicated, progestin therapy with norethindrone can prevent bone loss (Abdalla et al, 1985), and therefore postmenopausal osteoporosis. Other progestins would probably work as well. In addition, adequate calcium intake and weight-bearing exercises should further consolidate the reduction of bone loss. For those not on estrogen, a daily calcium intake of 1500 mg is recommended. Factors such as lower limb dysfunction, visual impairment, previous stroke, Parkinson's disease, neurologic conditions, and use of long-acting barbiturates that are associated with increased risk for hip fractures in women (Grisso et al, 1991) should be identified and dealt with appropriately.

Several nonestrogen medications can be used to improve or maintain bone mass (Table 27–6). Bisphosphonates can be given to treat or reduce osteoporosis and can also be added to hormone replacement therapy if there is continuing bone loss in spite of sufficient doses of estrogens. In this respect, when estradiol is given for postmenopausal hormone replacement, plasma estradiol levels of more than 300 pmol/L should be attained to prevent bone density

Table 27–6. NONESTROGEN MEDICATIONS THAT CAN IMPROVE OR MAINTAIN BONE MASS

AGENT	MECHANISM OF IMPROVING BONE BALANCE
Bisphosphonates	Inhibits bone resorption
Calcitonin	Stimulates bone formation
Fluoride	Stimulates bone formation
Vitamin D	Enhances intestinal absorption of calcium

loss in the spine and femoral neck (Studd et al, 1994). The second-generation bisphosphonates are markedly more potent than the first-generation bisphosphonates such as etidronate. The new generation of bisphosphonates includes alendronate, risedronate, and ibandronate. Alendronate has been introduced for use in postmenopausal women. It inhibits bone resorption, and the bone formed with alendronate treatment is both biochemically and histologically normal. Alendronate can be used alone or in combination with hormone replacement therapy. Alendronate significantly increases bone mass of the lumbar spine and hip compared with placebo (Chestnut et al, 1995), thereby reducing the incidence of vertebral fractures and decreasing height loss.

Vitamin D (400 to 800 IU/day) may benefit some women with osteoporosis by enhancing intestinal absorption of calcium. Subcutaneous or intranasal salmon calcitonin and subcutaneous human calcitonin are available and are effective for treating osteoporosis, but these preparations are not inexpensive. Calcitonin therapy increases vertebral bone mass; reduces the incidence of hip, vertebral, and forearm fractures; provides an analgesic effect on osteoporosis pain; and retards menopause-related loss of trabecular bone. Resistance to salmon calcitonin may develop in a third of patients treated.

Fluoride stimulates osteoblast-mediated new bone growth but may produce formation of abnormal bone and increase bone fragility. Skill is required in the dose and regimen of fluoride employed because of the narrow margin between therapeutic and toxic doses. Doses of 35 to 50 mg daily are beneficial, whereas more than 75 mg of fluoride daily may produce more fractures (Riggs et al, 1994). A slow-release, lower dose formulation of sodium fluoride is more effective in improving bone density and decreasing fracture risk (Pak et al, 1994). Prolonged treatment is usually required.

Androgens

There is increasing attention directed toward the possible need for androgen in postmenopausal hormone replacement therapy. There are few or no data available on serum testosterone levels, particularly serum free (unbound) testosterone, after menopause.

It should be noted that half the circulating serum testosterone is derived from peripheral conversion of androstenedione, while the ovaries contribute 25% and the adrenal the remaining 25% of circulating testosterone. Furthermore, with postmenopausal hypoestrogenism, the levels of sex hormone–binding globulin can be expected to decrease, therefore resulting in no change or even a net increase in serum free testosterone. Advocates of empirical use of testosterone supplement to hormone replacement therapy indicate that decrease libido in postmenopausal women is testosterone dependent and is improved, especially in post-oophorectomized menopausal women. However, there are no published data demonstrating a significant reduction in serum testosterone levels in such women. Furthermore, libido is complex and multifactorial in its etiology. Testosterone will also increase cholesterol levels, decrease HDL, and increase LDL, attenuating or negating the cardioprotective effects of estrogen or even worsening the basal postmenopausal levels of these lipids before taking estrogen. Hence, the widespread routine use of testosterone cannot be prudently recommended for hormone replacement therapy at the present time. The use of testosterone supplements should be confined to selected postmenopausal women with persistent diminished libido attributable to low androgen levels and not improved with estrogen replacement therapy. Finally, such therapy should use the lowest dose of testosterone that is effective and only for a short period of time.

Lifestyle Changes

Management of the menopausal women should include not only the prevention of clinical sequelae of chronically prolonged hypoestrogenism but also encouragement of sensible lifestyle habits to promote and maintain optimal health and quality of life. Smoking should be discouraged, and measures to discontinue smoking should be adopted. Attention should be given to reducing dietary intake of fat, increasing fiber intake, and maintaining serum cholesterol and lipoprotein levels that are cardioprotective. The patient should be advised to maintain her weight in the ideal body weight range and avoid being overweight or obese. Excessive or high intake of caffeine and indulgence in alcohol should be discouraged. Consumption of alcohol and caffeine should be in moderation.

REFERENCES

Abdalla HI, Hart DM, Lindsay R, et al: Prevention of bone mineral loss in postmenopausal women by norethisterone. Obstet Gynecol 1985;66:789.

Adams MR, Clarkson TB, Koritnik DR, Nash HA: Contraceptive steroids and coronary artery atherosclerosis in cynomolgus macaques. Fertil Steril 1987;47:1010.

Aloia JF, Cohn SH, Vaswani A, et al: Risk factors for postmenopausal osteoporosis. Am J Med 1985;78:95.

Archer DF, Pickar JH, Bottiglioni F: Bleeding patterns in postmenopausal women taking continuous combined or sequential regimens of conjugated estrogens with medroxyprogesterone acetate. Obstet Gynecol 1994;83:686.

Armstrong BK: Oestrogen therapy after the menopause—boon or bane? Med J Aust 1988;148:213.

Aune B, Oian P, Omsjo I, Osterud BI: Hormone replacement therapy reduces the reactivity of monocytes and platelets in whole blood—a beneficial effect on atherogenesis and thrombus formation? Am J Obstet Gynecol 1995;173:1816.

Aylward M: Estrogens, plasma tryptophan levels in perimenopausal patients. In Campbell S (ed): The Management of the Menopause and Post-menopausal Years. Baltimore: University Park Press, 1980:135.

Balteskard L, Brox JH, Osterud B: Thromboxane production in the blood of women increases after menopause whereas tumor necrosis factor is reduced in women compared with men. Atherosclerosis 1993;102:91.

Bergkvist L, Adami H-O, Persson I, et al: The risk of breast cancer after estrogen and estrogen-progestin replacement. N Engl J Med 1989;321:293.

Berkowitz GS, Kelsey JL, Holford TR, et al: Estrogen replacement therapy and fibrocystic breast disease in postmenopausal women. Am J Epidemiol 1985;121:238.

Birge SJ: Is there a role for estrogen replacement therapy in the prevention and treatment of dementia? J Am Geriatr Soc 1996;44:865.

Bloch E: Quantitative morphological investigations of the follicular system in women: variations at different ages. Acta Anat (Basel) 1952;14:108.

Blumenfeld Z, Aviram M, Brook GJ, Brandes JM: Changes in lipoprotein and subfractions following oophorectomy and estrogen replacement in perimenopausal women. Maturitas 1983;5:77.

Bonithon-Kopp C, Scarabin P-Y, Darne B, et al: Menopause-related changes in lipoproteins and some other cardiovascular risk factors. Int J Epidemiol 1990;19:42.

Bourne T, Campbell S, Steer C, et al: Transvaginal colour flow imaging: a possible new screening technique for ovarian cancer. BMJ 1989;299:1367.

Bourne T, Hillard TC, Whitehead MI, et al: Oestrogens, arterial status, and postmenopausal women. Lancet 1990;335:1470.

Brincat M, Moniz CF, Studd JW, et al: The long term effects of the menopause and of administration of sex hormones on collagen and skin thickness. Br J Obstet Gynaecol 1985;92:256.

Brinton LA, Hoover RN, Endometrial Cancer Collaborative Group: Estrogen replacement therapy and endometrial cancer risk: unresolved issues. Obstet Gynecol 1993;81:265.

Bruschi F, Meschia M, Soma M, et al: Lipoprotein(a) and other lipids after oophorectomy and estrogen replacement therapy. Obstet Gynecol 1996;88:950.

Bureau of the Census: Statistical Abstract of the United States 1990: The National Data Book. Washington, DC: Department of Commerce, 1992;1.

Bureau of the Census: Statistical Abstract of the United States 1995: The National Data Book. 115th ed. Washington, DC: U.S. Department of Commerce, 1996;1.

Castelli WP: The triglyceride issue: a view from Framingham. Am Heart J 1986;112:432.

Centers for Disease Control and Prevention: Incidence and costs to Medicare of fractures among Medicare beneficiaries aged > or = 65 years—United States, July 1991–June 1992. MMWR Morbid Mortal Wkly Rep 1996;45(41):877.

Chapman JA, DiSaia PJ, Osann K, et al: Estrogen replacement in surgical stage I and II endometrial cancer survivors. Am J Obstet Gynecol 1996;175:1195.

Chestnut CH III, Baylink DJ, Gruber HE, et al: Treatment of postmenopausal osteoporosis with salmon calcitonin: preliminary results. In DeLuca HF, Frost HM, Jee WSS, et al (eds): Osteoporosis: Recent Advances in Pathogenesis and Treatment. Baltimore: University Park Press, 1981:411.

Chestnut CH III, McClung MR, Ensrud KE, et al: Alendronate treatment of the postmenopausal osteoporotic woman: effect of multiple dosages on bone mass and bone remodeling. Am J Med 1995;99:144.

Christiansen C, Christensen MS, Transbol I: Bone mass in post-menopausal women after withdrawal of oestrogen/gestation replacement therapy. Lancet 1981;1:459.

Christiansen C, Riis BJ: 17β-estradiol and continuous norethisterone: a unique treatment for established osteoporosis in elderly women. J Clin Endocrinol Metab 1990;71:836.

Colditz GA, Hankinson SE, Hunter DJ, et al: The use of estrogens and progestins and the risk of breast cancer in postmenopausal women. N Engl J Med 1995;332:1589.

Colditz GA, Stampfer MJ, Willett WC, et al: Prospective study of estrogen replacement therapy and risk of breast cancer in postmenopausal women. JAMA 1990;264:2648.

Colditz GA, Stampfer MJ, Willett WC, et al: Type of postmenopausal hormone use and risk of breast cancer: 12-year follow-up from the Nurses' Health Study. Cancer Causes Control 1992;3:433.

Collins P, Rosano GM, Sarrell PM, et al: 17 Beta-estradiol attenuates acetylcholine-induced coronary arterial constriction in women but not men with coronary heart disease. Circulation 1995;92:24.

Colvin PL, Auerbach BJ, Koritnik DR, et al: Differential effects of oral versus 17β-estradiol on lipoproteins in postmenopausal women. J Clin Endocrinol 1990;70:1568.

Cramer DW, Knapp RC: Review of epidemiologic studies of endometrial cancer and exogenous estrogen. Obstet Gynecol 1979;54:521.

Creasman WT, Henderson D, Hinshaw W, Clarke-Pearson DL: Estrogen replacement therapy in the patient treated for endometrial cancer. Obstet Gynecol 1986;67:326.

Criqui MH, Suarez L, Barrett-Connor E, et al: Postmenopausal estrogen use and mortality: results from a prospective study in a defined, homogeneous community. Am J Epidemiol 1988;128:606.

Daly E, Vessey MP, Hawkins MM, et al: Risk of venous thromboembolism in users of hormone replacement therapy. Lancet 1996;348:977.

D'Amato G, Cavallini A, Messa C, et al: Serum and bile lipid levels in a postmenopausal woman after percutaneous and oral natural estrogens. Am J Obstet Gynecol 1989;160:600.

Dawood MY, Tidey GFL: Menopause. Curr Probl Obstet Gynecol Fertil 1993;16:169.

Devor M, Barrett-Connor E, Renwall M, et al: Estrogen replacement therapy and the risk of venous thrombosis. Am J Med 1992;92:275.

DuPont WD, Page DL: Menopausal estrogen replacement therapy and breast cancer. Arch Intern Med 1991;151:67.

Eriksen EF, Colvard DS, Berg NJ, et al: Evidence of estrogen receptors in normal human osteoblast-like cells. Science 1988;241:84.

Ernst M, Schmid C, Frankenfoldt C, Froesch ER: Estradiol stimulation of osteoblast proliferation in vitro: mediator roles for TGFβ, PGE₂, IGF₁ [abstract 117]. Calcif Tissue Res 1988;42(Suppl):A30.

Everson GT, McKinley C, Kern F Jr: Mechanisms of gallstone formation in women: effects of exogenous estrogen (premarin) and dietary cholesterol on hepatic lipid metabolism. J Clin Invest 1991;87:237.

Ewertz M: Influence of noncontraceptive exogenous and endogenous sex hormones on breast cancer risk in Denmark. Int J Cancer 1988;42:832.

Fahraeus L, Larsson-Cohn U, Wallentin L: Lipoproteins during oral and cutaneous administration of oestradiol-17β to menopausal women. Acta Endocrinol 1982;101:597.

Farish E, Fletcher CD, Hart DM, et al: The effects of hormone implants on serum lipoproteins and steroid hormone in bilaterally oophorectomized women. Acta Endocrinol (Kohen L) 1984:106:116.

Farish E, Hart DM, Gray CE, et al: Effects of treatment with oestradiol/levonorgestrel on bone, lipoproteins and hormone status in postmenopausal women. Clin Endocrinol 1989;31:607.

Feldman BM, Voda A, Gronseth E, et al: The prevalence of hot flash and associated variables among perimenopausal women. Res Nurs Health 1985;8:261.

Freedman RR, Woodward S, Sabharwal SC: α₂-Adrenergic mechanism in menopausal hot flushes. Obstet Gynecol 1990;76:573.

Frezza M, Tritapepe R, Pozzato G, Di Padova C: Prevention of S-adenosylmethionine of estrogen-induced hepatobiliary toxicity in susceptible women. Am J Gastroenterol 1988;83:1098.

Frumar AM, Meldrum DR, Geola F, et al: Relationship of fasting urinary calcium to circulating estrogen and body weight in postmenopausal women. J Clin Endocrinol Metab 1980;50:70.

Gallagher JC, Riggs BL, DeLuca HF: Effect of estrogen on calcium absorption and serum vitamin D metabolites in postmenopausal osteoporosis. J Clin Endocrinol Metab 1980;51:1359.

Gambrell RD Jr: Prevention of endometrial cancer with progestogens. Maturitas 1986;8:159.

Gambrell RD Jr, Maier RC, Sanders BI: Decreased incidence of breast cancer in postmenopausal estrogen-progestin users. Obstet Gynecol 1983;62:435.

Gangar KF, Vyas S, Whitehead M, et al: Pulsatility index in internal carotid artery in relation to transdermal oestradiol and time since menopause. Lancet 1991;338:839.

Genant HK, Baylink DJ, Gallagher JC, et al: Effect of estrone sulfate on postmenopausal bone loss. Obstet Gynecol 1990;76:579.

Ginsburg ES, Walsh BW, Shea BF, et al: The effects of ethanol on the clearance of estradiol in postmenopausal women. Fertil Steril 1995;63:1227.

Giraud GD, Morton MJ, Wilson RA, et al: Effects of estrogen and progestin on aortic size and compliance in postmenopausal women. Am J Obstet Gynecol 1996;174:1708.

Gray TK, Mohan S, Linkhart TA, et al: Estrogen may mediate its effects on bone cells by signalling the observation of growth factors. J Bone Min Res 1988;3:A552.

Grey A, Cundy T, Evans M, Reid I: Medroxyprogesterone acetate enhances the spinal bone density response to estrogen in late post-menopausal women. Clin Endocrinol (Oxf) 1996;44:293.

Grisso JA, Kelsey JL, Strom BL, et al: Risk factors for falls as a cause of hip fracture in women. N Engl J Med 1991;324:1326.

Grodstein F, Stampfer MJ, Goldhaber SZ, et al: Prospective study of exogenous hormones and risk of pulmonary embolism in women. Lancet 1996a;348:983.

Grodstein F, Stampfer MJ, Manson JE, et al: Postmenopausal estrogen and progestin use and the risk of cardiovascular disease. N Engl J Med 1996b;335:453.

Gruchow HW, Anderson AJ, Barboriak JJ, Sobocinski KA: Postmenopausal use of estrogen and occlusion of coronary arteries. Am Heart J 1988;115:954.

Hammar ML, Lindgren R, Berg GE, et al: Effects of hormonal replacement therapy on the postural balance among postmenopausal women. Obstet Gynecol 1996;88:955.

Hammond CB, Jelousek FR, Lee KL, et al: Effects of long term estrogen replacement therapy. Am J Obstet Gynecol 1979;133:525.

Henderson B, Paganini-Hill A, Ross RK: Estrogen replacement therapy and protection from acute myocardial infarction. Am J Obstet Gynecol 1988;159:312.

Hirvonen E, Malkonen M, Manninen V: Effects of different progestogens on lipoproteins during postmenopausal replacement therapy. N Engl J Med 1981;304:560.

Hjortland MC, McNamara PM, Kannel WB: Some atherogenic concomitants of menopause: the Framingham Study. Am J Epidemiol 1976;103:304.

Hughes DE, Dai A, Tiffee JC, et al: Estrogen promotes apoptosis of murine osteoclasts mediated by TGF-β. Nat Med 1996;2:1132.

Hunt K, Vessey M, McPherson K, Coleman M: Long-term surveillance of mortality and cancer incidence in women receiving hormone replacement therapy. Br J Obstet Gynaecol 1987;94:620.

Jick H, Derby LE, Myers MW, et al: Risk of hospital admission for idiopathic venous thromboembolism among users of postmenopausal oestrogens. Lancet 1996;348:981.

Kampen DL, Sherwin BB: Estrogen use and verbal memory in healthy postmenopausal women. Obstet Gynecol 1994;83:979.

Kaufman DW, Palmer JR, Demouzon J, et al: Estrogen replacement therapy and risk of breast cancer: results from case-control surveillance study. Am J Epidemiol 1991;134:1375.

Kiel DP, Felson DT, Anderson JJ, et al: Hip fracture and the use of estrogens in postmenopausal women: the Framingham Study. N Engl J Med 1987;317:1169.

Komm BS, Terpening CM, Benz DJ, et al: Estrogen binding, receptor mRNA and biologic response in osteoblast-like osteosarcoma cells. Science 1988;241:81.

Krailo MD, Pike MC: Estimation of the distribution of age at natural menopause from prevalence data. Am J Epidemiol 1983; 117:352.

Krolner B, Toft B, Nielsen SP, Tondevold E: Physical exercise as prophylaxis against involutional vertebral bone loss. a controlled trial. Clin Sci 1983;64:541.

Kronenberg F: Hot flushes: epidemiology and physiology. Ann N Y Acad Sci 1990;592:52.

Laufer LR, Erlik Y, Meldrum DR, Judd HL: Effect of clomidine on hot flashes in postmenopausal women. Obstet Gynecol 1982;60:583.

Leidy LE: Early age at menopause among left-handed women. Obstet Gynecol 1990;76:1111.

Lindquist O: Intraindividual changes of blood pressure, serum lipids and body weight in relation to menstrual status: results from a prospective population study of women in Goteborg, Sweden. Prev Med 1982;11:162.

Lindsay R, Fey C, Haboubi A: Dual photon absorptiometric measurements of bone mineral density increases with source life. Calcif Tissue Int 1987;41:293.

Lindsay R, Hart DM, Clark DM: The minimum effective dose of estrogen for prevention of postmenopausal bone loss. Obstet Gynecol 1984;63:759.

Lindsay R, Hart DM, Purdie P, et al: Comparative effects of oestrogen and a progestogen on bone loss in postmenopausal women. Clin Sci Mol Med 1978;54:193.

Lindsay R, Hohme JF: Estrogen treatment of patients with established postmenopausal osteoporosis. Obstet Gynecol 1990;76: 290.

Lipid Research Clinical Program: The Lipid Research Clinics coronary primary prevention trial results: II. The relationship of reduction in incidence of coronary heart disease to cholesterol lowering. JAMA 1984;251:365.

Lobo RA, Pickar JH, Wild RA, et al: Metabolic impact of adding medroxyprogesterone acetate to conjugated estrogen therapy in postmenopausal women: the Menopause Study Group. Am J Obstet Gynecol 1994;84:987.

Lobo RA, Roy S, Shoupe D, et al: Estrogen and progestin effects on urinary calcium and calciotrophic hormones in surgically-induced postmenopausal women. Horm Metab Res 1985;17: 370.

Masters WH, Johnson VE: Human Sexual Response. Boston: Little, Brown & Company, 1986.

McAuley JW, Kroboth FJ, Kroboth PD: Oral administration of micronized progesterone: a review and more experience. Pharmacotherapy 1996;16:453.

McGill HC Jr: Sex steroid hormone receptors in cardiovascular system. Postgrad Med 1989;64:8.

Melton LJ, Kan SH, Frye MA, et al: Epidemiology of vertebral fractures in women. Am J Epidemiol 1989;129:1000.

Menwissen JHJM, VenLangen H, Moret E, et al: Monitoring of oestrogen replacement therapy by vaginosonography of the endometrium. Maturitas 1992;15:33.

Moore FE, Gordon T: Serum cholesterol levels in adults. United States 1960–1962. Vital Health Stat 11 1967;22.

Nachtigall LE, Nachtigall RH, Nachtigall RD, Beckman EM: Estrogen replacement therapy: II. A prospective study in the relationship to carcinoma and cardiovascular and metabolic problems. Obstet Gynecol 1979;54:74.

National Center for Health Statistics: Health United States 1988 (DHSS Publication No [PHS]80-1232). Hyattsville, MD: National Center for Health Statistics, 1989;41.

Nordin BEC, Need AG, Morris HA, et al: Evidence for a renal calcium leak in postmenopausal women. J Clin Endocrinol Metab 1991;72:401.

Notelovitz M, Gudat JC, Ware MD, Doughtery MC: Lipids and lipoproteins in women after oophorectomy and the response to estrogen therapy. Br J Obstet Gynaecol 1983;90:171.

Notelovitz M, Johnston M, Johnston M, et al: Metabolic and hormone effects of 25-mg and 50-mg 17 beta-estradiol implants in surgically menopausal women. Obstet Gynecol 1987;70:749.

Ohkura T, Teshima HY, Isse K, et al: Estrogen increases cerebral and cerebellar blood flows in postmenopausal women. Menopause 1995;2:13.

Osmers R, Volksen M, Schauer A: Vaginosonography for early detection of endometrial carcinoma. Lancet 1990;335:1569.

Oyster N, Morton M, Linnell S: Physical activity and osteoporosis in postmenopausal women. Med Sci Sports Exerc 1984;16:44.

Pacifici R, Civitelli R, Rifas L, et al: Does interleukin-1 affect intracellular calcium in osteoblast-like cells? J Bone Miner Res 1988;3:107.

Paganini-Hill A, Henderson VW: Estrogen deficiency and risk of Alzheimers' disease in women. Am J Epidemiol 1994;140:256.

Paganini-Hill A, Ross RK, Henderson BE: Postmenopausal oestrogen treatment and stroke: a prospective study. BMJ 1988;297: 519.

Pak CYC, Sakhaee K, Piziak V: Slow-release sodium fluoride in the management of postmenopausal osteoporosis: a randomized controlled trial. Ann Intern Med 1994;120:625.

Palmer JR, Rosenberg L, Clarke EA, et al: Breast cancer risk after estrogen replacement therapy: results from the Toronto Breast Cancer Study. Am J Epidemiol 1991;134:1386.

Parish HM, Carr CA, Hall DG, King TM: Time interval from castration in premenopausal women to development of excessive coronary atherosclerosis. Am J Obstet Gynecol 1967;99:155.

Penotti M, Farina M, Sironi L, et al: Cerebral artery blood flow in relation to age and menopausal status. Obstet Gynecol 1996; 88:106.

Penotti M, Nencioni T, Gabrielli L, et al: Blood flow variations in internal carotid and middle cerebral arteries induced by postmenopausal hormone replacement therapy. Am J Obstet Gynecol 1993;169:1226.

Petitti DB, Sidney S, Perlman JA: Increased risk of cholecystectomy in users of supplemental estrogen. Gastroenterology 1988;94:91.

Pfeffer RI, Kurosaki TT, Charlton SK: Estrogen use and blood pressure in later life. Am J Epidemiol 1979;110:469.

Prince RL, Smith M, Dick IM, et al: Prevention of postmenopausal osteoporosis. N Engl J Med 1991;325:1189.

RCOG Working Party: Report of the Royal College of Obstetricians and Gynaecologists Working Party on Prophylaxis Against Thromboembolism in Gynecology and Obstetrics. London: Chameleon Press, 1995.

Recker R: Calcium absorption and achlorhydria. N Engl J Med 1985;313:70.

Reed T: Urethral pressure profile in continent women from childhood to old age. Acta Obstet Gynecol Scand 1980;58:331.

Richelson LS, Wahner HW, Meton LJ III, Riggs BL: Relative contributions to aging and estrogen deficiency to postmenopausal bone loss. N Engl J Med 1984;311:1273.

Riggs BL, O'Fallon WM, Lane A, et al: Clinical trial of fluoride therapy in postmenopausal women: extended observations and additional analysis. J Bone Miner Res 1994;9:265.

Riggs BL, Seeman E, Hodgson SF, et al: Effect of the fluoride/calcium regimen on vertebral fracture occurrence in postmenopausal osteoporosis. N Engl J Med 1982;306:446.

Riis B, Thomsen K, Christiansen C: Does calcium supplement prevent postmenopausal bone loss? N Engl J Med 1987;316:173.

Robinson JC, Folsom AR, Nabulsi AA, et al: Can postmenopausal hormone replacement improve plasma lipids in women with diabetes? The Atherosclerosis Risk in Communities Study Investigators. Diabetes Care 1996;19:480.

Rosenberg L, Hennekens CH, Rosner B, et al: Early menopause and the risk of myocardial infarction. Am J Obstet Gynecol 1981;139:47.

Samsioe G, Jansson I, Mellstrom D, Svanborg A: Occurrence, nature and treatment of urinary incontinence in a 70-year-old female population. Maturitas 1985;7:335.

Scarabin PY, Vissac AM, Kirzin JM, et al: Population correlates of coagulation factor VII: importance of age, sex, and menopausal status as determinants of activated factor VII. Arterioscler Thromb Vasc Biol 1996;16:1170.

Schiff I, Regestein Q, Tulchinsky D, Ryan KJ: Effects of estrogens on sleep and psychological state of hypogonadal women. JAMA 1979;242:2405.

Sherwin BB: The impact of different doses of estrogen and progestin on mood and sexual behaviour in postmenopausal women. J Clin Endocrinol Metab 1991;72:336.

Sillero-Arenas M, Delgado-Rodriguez M, Rodrigues-Canteras R, et al: Menopausal hormone replacement therapy and breast cancer: a meta-analysis. Obstet Gynecol 1992;79:286.

Simkin A, Ayalon J, Leichter I: Increased trabecular bone density due to bone-loading exercises in postmenopausal osteoporotic women. Calcif Tissue Int 1987;40:59.

Soma M, Osnago-Gadda I, Paoletti R, et al: The lowering of lipoprotein(a) induced by estrogen plus progesterone replacement therapy in postmenopausal women. Arch Intern Med 1993;153:1462.

Sonnendecker EWW, Polakow ES, Benade AJS, Simchowitz E: Serum lipoprotein effects of conjugated estrogen and a sequential conjugated estrogen-medrogestone regimen in hysterectomized postmenopausal women. Am J Obstet Gynecol 1989;160:1128.

Spellacy WN: Menopause, estrogen treatment, and carbohydrate metabolism. In Mishell DR Jr (ed): Menopause: Physiology and Pharmacology. Chicago: Year Book Medical Publishers, 1987:253.

Stampfer MJ, Colditz GA, Willett WC, et al: Postmenopausal estrogen therapy and cardiovascular disease. N Engl J Med 1991;325:756.

Stanford JL, Weiss NS, Voigt LF, et al: Combined estrogen and progestin hormone replacement therapy in relation to risk of breast cancer in middle-aged women. JAMA 1995;274:137.

Steinberg D: Lipoproteins and the pathogenesis of atherosclerosis. Circulation 1987;76:508.

Steinberg KK, Thacker SB, Smith SJ, et al: A meta-analysis of the effect of estrogen replacement therapy on the risk of breast cancer. JAMA 1991;265:1985.

Steinberg KK, Smith SJ, Thacker SB, Stroup DE: Breast cancer risk and duration of estrogen use: the role of study design in meta-analysis. Epidemiology 1994;5:415.

Steinleitner A, Stancyzyk FZ, Levin JH, et al: Decreased in vitro production of 6-ketoprostaglandin $F_{1\alpha}$ by uterine arteries from postmenopausal women. Am J Obstet Gynecol 1989;161:1677.

Stevenson JC, Abeyasekara G, Hillyard CJ, et al: Calcitonin and the calcium-regulating hormones in postmenopausal women: effect of estrogens. Lancet 1981;1:693.

Studd JW, Holland EF, Leather AT, Smith RN: The dose-response of percutaneous oestradiol implants on the skeletons of postmenopausal women. Br J Obstet Gynaecol 1994;101:787.

Sullivan JM, Vander Zwaag R, Lemp GF, et al: Postmenopausal estrogen use and coronary atherosclerosis. Ann Intern Med 1988;108:358.

Szklow M, Tonascia J, Gordis L, Bloom I: Additional evidence supporting a protective effect of estrogen use on myocardial infarction risk. Prev Med 1984;13:510.

Tang MX, Jacobs D, Stern Y, et al: Effect of oestrogen during the menopause on risk and age of onset of Alzheimer's disease. Lancet 1996;348:429.

Tataryn IV, Meldrum DR, Lu KH, et al: LH, FSH and skin temperature during the menopausal hot flash. J Clin Endocrinol Metab 1979;49:152.

Upjohn Multicenter Collaborative Study: Comparison of sequential versus continuous estrogen/progestin replacement therapy of serum lipid patterns. Presented at the 38th Annual Meeting of the Society for Gynecologic Investigation, San Antonio, 1991a:Abstract 491.

Upjohn Multicenter Collaborative Study: Evaluation of sequential versus continuous estrogen/progestin replacement therapy on uterine bleeding patterns and endometrial histology. Presented at the 38th Annual Meeting of the Society for Gynecologic Investigation, San Antonio, 1991b:Abstract 490.

U.S. Department of Health, Education and Welfare: Framingham Study (Publication No. 74). Washington, DC: U.S. Department of Health, Education and Welfare, 1974.

Van Beresteijn ECH, Van't Hoff MA, deWaard H, et al: Relation of axial bone mass to habitual calcium intake and to cortical bone loss in healthy early postmenopausal women. Bone 1990;11:7.

Van Erpecum KJ, Van Berge-Henegouwen GP, Verschoor L, et al: Different hepatobiliary effects of oral and transdermal estradiol in postmenopausal women. Gastroenterology 1991;100:482.

Vejtorp M, Christensen MS, Vejtorp L, Larsen JF: Serum lipoprotein changes in climacteric women induced by sequential therapy with natural estrogens and medroxyprogesterone acetate or norgestrel. Acta Obstet Gynecol Scand 1986;65:391.

Voight L, Weiss N, Chu J, et al: Progestagen supplementation of exogenous oestrogens and risk of endometrial cancer. Lancet 1991;338:274.

Wahl P, Walden C, Knopp R, et al: Effect of estrogen/progestin potency on lipid/lipoprotein cholesterol. N Engl J Med 1983;308:862.

Walsh BW, Schiff I, Rosner B, et al: Effects of postmenopausal estrogen replacement on the concentrations and metabolism of plasma lipoproteins. N Engl J Med 1991;325:1196.

Weiss NS, Ure CL, Ballard JH: Decreased risk of fractures of the hip and lower forearm with postmenopausal use of estrogens. N Engl J Med 1980;303:1195.

Whitehead MI, Lane G, Morsman J, et al: Effect of castration on calcium-regulating hormones. Maturitas 1984;6:207.

Wittemann JC, Grober DE, Kok FJ, et al: Increased risk of atherosclerosis in women after menopause. BMJ 1989;298:642.

Wren BG, Routledge AD: The effect of type and dose of oestrogen on the blood pressure of post-menopausal women. Maturitas 1983;5:135.

Writing Group for the PEPI Trial: Effects of estrogen or estrogen/progestin regimens on heart disease risk factors in postmenopausal women: the Postmenopausal Estrogen/Progestin Intervention (PEPI) Trial. JAMA 1995;273:199.

Writing Group for the PEPI Trial: Effects of hormone replacement therapy on endometrial histology in postmenopausal women: the Postmenopausal Estrogen/Progestin Intervention (PEPI) Trial. JAMA 1996;275:370.

Yang C, Daling JR, Bard PR, et al: Noncontraceptive hormone use and risk of breast cancer. Cancer Causes Control 1992;3:475.

28

Hyperandrogenism

Roger S. Rittmaster

Hyperandrogenism in women refers both to excess androgen production and to the clinical manifestations of androgen excess. These problems are not identical. On the one hand, women can have hirsutism, acne, male-pattern baldness, and anovulation with "normal" androgen levels; on the other hand, increased androgen production may or may not be associated with clinical features of androgen excess. The biochemical definition of androgen excess is also problematic. For example, the normal range for testosterone is usually based on serum levels in ovulatory women. The normal range will be lower if only nonhirsute women are included. However, hirsutism, by itself, is not abnormal. Treatment of hyperandrogenism is directed at resolving the clinical manifestations; elevated androgen levels themselves do not necessarily require therapy.

ANDROGENS

Definitions

Androgens were originally defined as compounds that could maintain male sexual behavior in castrate animals (Mainwaring, 1977). Testosterone is the major circulating androgen and is the only compound that satisfies this definition at normal plasma concentrations. However, androgens have numerous other actions, including stimulation of prostate and seminal vesicle growth in men and stimulation of androgen-dependent hair growth in men and women. Testosterone is converted to dihydrotestosterone (DHT) in the prostate, seminal vesicle, and skin by the enzyme 5α-reductase. Two isoenzymes have been cloned (Russell and Wilson, 1994). The gene for the type 1 enzyme is located on the short arm of chromosome 5. It is expressed in human liver and is the dominant isoenzyme in sebaceous glands (Luu-The et al, 1994). No individual has been identified with a deficiency of type 1 5α-reductase, and therefore its role in human physiology is unclear. However, it is important for normal partuition in female mice (Mahendroo et al, 1996). The gene for type 2 5α-reductase is located on the short arm of chromosome 2. The importance of this isoenzyme is best illustrated by men with congenital deficiency of type 2 5α-reductase (Wilson et al, 1993). Such men are

born with incomplete masculinization of the external genitalia, but, even when raised as females, they develop male sexual orientation and musculature at puberty. They do not, however, develop baldness or prostate enlargement, and they have sparse body hair, indicating that DHT is essential for androgen action in the hair follicle and the prostate. Testosterone, in contrast, appears to be the active androgen in the brain and muscle. Based on this knowledge, type 2 5α-reductase inhibitors have been developed that have been used for treatment of hirsutism, prostatic enlargement and baldness (Rittmaster, 1997a).

Testosterone and DHT are the most potent of the naturally occurring androgens. The "adrenal androgens," dehydroepiandrosterone (DHEA) and DHEA sulfate (DHEAS), and androstenedione are not androgens themselves, but exert their androgenic activity through conversion to testosterone or DHT. Thus these steroids are more properly termed *androgen precursors*. Conjugated androgens, such as androstanediol glucuronide and androsterone glucuronide, are end-products of androgen metabolism (see section on "Androgen Metabolism") and are not converted to active androgens, and therefore should properly be termed *androgen metabolites*.

Structure and Mechanism of Action

On a molecular level, androgens are steroid hormones that are capable of binding to the androgen receptor and thereby increasing the expression of androgen-sensitive genes. Antiandrogens also bind to the androgen receptor but are not themselves androgenic. Because antiandrogens compete with active androgens for the androgen receptor, they can block the action of these hormones.

The androgen receptor is part of a large family of molecules including steroid, thyroid, retinoid, and vitamin D hormone receptors (Kallio et al, 1996; Zhou et al, 1996). The androgen receptor is synthesized in the cytoplasm and, as a result of a nuclear signaling sequence in the protein structure, is rapidly transported to the nucleus. Androgens diffuse into the nucleus and then interact with the hormone-binding domain (d) of the androgen receptor (Fig. 28–1). The hormone-receptor complex then binds to a specific hormone response element on the DNA

631

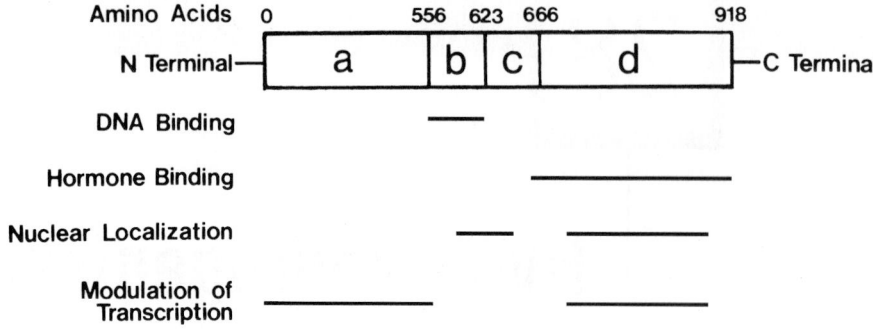

Figure 28–1

Androgen receptor. All steroid hormone receptors have similar structural features, including a hypervariable region (a), a DNA-binding domain (b), a "hinge" region (c), and a hormone-binding domain (d). The hypervariable region modulates DNA activation by the receptor. Nuclear localization sequences allow targeting of the hormone-receptor complex to the nucleus. The specificity of a steroid receptor resides in the hormone-binding domain, in the DNA-binding region, and in the region on the DNA molecule that binds the receptor (hormone response element). (Adapted from Beato M: Gene regulation by steroid hormones. Cell 1989;56:335, with permission. © Cell Press.)

through a DNA-binding domain (c) on the receptor. Androgen-dependent gene activation (domains a/b and d) results in transcription of DNA into messenger RNA, followed by translation of the mRNA into protein. Different genes are turned on by androgens in different tissues, and this regulation is controlled by tissue-specific transcription factors. These transcription factors may explain some of the variability in androgen action, such as the stimulation of hair growth on the face and the opposite effect in the scalp.

The androgen receptor is derived from a single gene, and only one form of the androgen receptor has been recognized. The differential effect of testosterone and DHT in DHT-dependent tissues can be explained by increased retention of DHT in tissues as a result of increased affinity of DHT for the androgen receptor (Grino et al, 1990) and increased potency of the DHT-receptor complex in mediating androgen action (Deslypere et al, 1992; Wright et al, 1996). The reason testosterone itself is adequate for androgen action in muscle and brain must be due to differential effects of the androgen–androgen receptor complex on gene expression, because the receptor is the same in all tissues.

Most steroid hormone receptor genes are located on autosomal chromosomes, and two defective alleles are required for phenotypic expression (autosomal recessive disorders). The androgen receptor gene, however, is located on the X chromosome, and an abnormal allele will be expressed in affected males. Many different defects in the androgen receptor have resulted in incomplete masculinization in males (see Chapter 8). No alteration of androgen receptor number or function has been found to explain hyperandrogenism in women.

Source of Androgens

Androgens originate in the adrenal glands and the ovaries, either from direct secretion or from conversion of androgen precursors to active androgens in the liver, skin, adipose tissue, and elsewhere. Average testosterone production rates from all sources are 0.2 to 0.25 mg/day in normal premenopausal women. In normal women, 30% to 50% of testosterone arises from direct secretion by the ovaries or adrenals, and the remainder comes from peripheral conversion (Fig. 28–2) (Longcope, 1986). The proportion of androgens arising directly or indirectly from the ovary and adrenals has been widely debated. In normal women, about 50% of testosterone appears to arise from each organ, although individual variability is certain to be high. In hyperandrogenic women, the variability is even greater (Moltz and Schwartz, 1986).

Early studies attempted to measure the relative contribution of the ovaries and the adrenal glands to androgen secretion by using dexamethasone to suppress adrenal function or estrogen-progestin combinations to suppress ovarian function. This approach is now known to be nonspecific because pharmacologic doses of glucocorticoids also decrease ovarian androgens, and oral contraceptives can decrease adrenal androgen production. Nevertheless, giving a 4-day course of dexamethasone (0.5 mg four times daily) causes near-maximal suppression of adrenal androgens and is unlikely to have a significant effect on ovarian androgen secretion (Ehrmann et al, 1992). Several investigators have attempted to sample steroid hormones directly in ovarian and adrenal venous effluent. For example, Kirschner and co-workers (1976) measured testosterone and androstenedione production rates in hirsute women and then used the adrenal venous concentrations of the androgens and cortisol to calculate the adrenal, and, by subtraction, ovarian contribution to the production rate of these hormones. They found that the ovary was the major site of androgen production in nearly all hirsute women. To make their calculations of adrenal steroid production, these authors assumed that adrenal androgens were secreted in parallel with cortisol. This

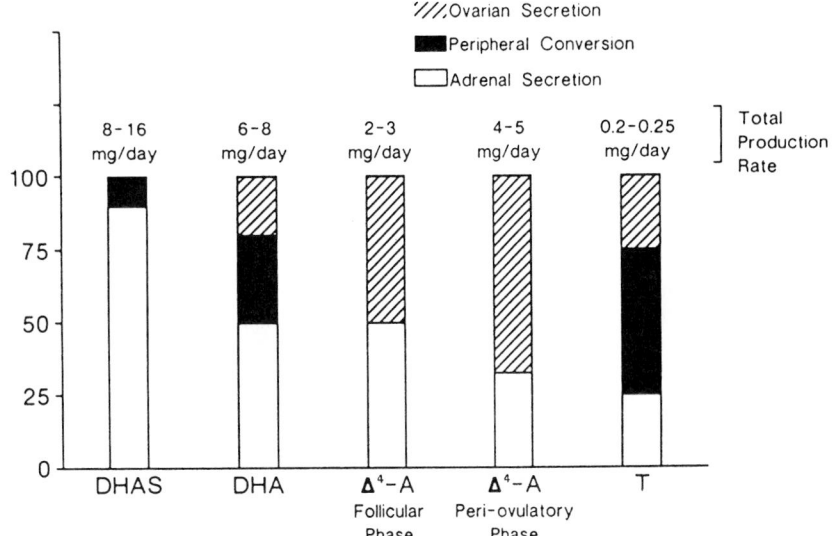

Figure 28–2
Relative contribution of adrenal secretion, ovarian secretion, and peripheral conversion of androgen precursors to androgenic steroids in normal women. DHAS, dehydroepiandrosterone sulfate; DHA, dehydroepiandrosterone; Δ⁴-A, androstenedione; T, testosterone. (From Longcope C: Adrenal and gonadal androgen secretion in normal females. Clin Endocrinol Metab 1986;15:213, with permission.)

assumption has been challenged, however, on the basis that, under the stress of catheterization, cortisol will be preferentially secreted over androgens (Rosenfield, 1976). This error would result in an underestimation of the adrenal contribution to testosterone production. Another catheterization study does, in fact, suggest that the adrenal is an important source of androgens in many hirsute women (Moltz et al, 1984).

Long-acting gonadotropin-releasing hormone (GnRH) analogs have been shown to suppress ovarian, but not adrenal, androgens in normal and hirsute women (Rittmaster, 1993b). In one study, the GnRH analog leuprolide was given to 19 severely hirsute women for 5 months, and then low doses of dexamethasone were added for an additional 4 months to suppress the remaining (presumably adrenal) androgens (Rittmaster and Thompson, 1990). In this study, women with regular menses were found to have a primarily adrenal source of serum androgens. Most women with hyperandrogenism and chronic anovulation (polycystic ovary syndrome [PCOS]) were found to have a primarily ovarian source of serum testosterone and androstenedione (Fig. 28–3), although adrenal hyperandrogenism was also present. In women with irregular menses, the higher the serum testosterone, the greater was the ovarian contribution to serum testosterone.

In summary, research to date suggests that both the adrenal glands and ovaries contribute substantially to androgen production in normal and hyperandrogenic women.

Synthesis of Androgens

Adrenal Androgen Synthesis

The pathways of adrenal steroid biosynthesis are shown in Figure 28–4. The major pathway for androstenedione synthesis from cholesterol appears to be through DHEA (Longcope, 1986). However, 17-

hydroxyprogesterone can also be an important precursor for androstenedione when the precursor is produced in excess, as in 21-hydroxylase deficiency (the most common form of congenital adrenal hyperplasia [CAH]). The two important enzymes for determining the amount of adrenal androgens produced are 3β-hydroxysteroid dehydrogenase (3β-HSD) and 17,20-lyase. The apparent activity of these enzymes varies among normal adults and may be a major determinant of the variation in adrenal androgen secretion seen in women.

At least 90% of serum DHEAS arises from the adrenal gland. DHEAS has therefore been proposed as a marker of adrenal androgen synthesis. Markedly elevated DHEAS levels are found in patients with 3β-HSD deficiency (Bongiovanni, 1984), and mildly elevated levels are also seen in the classical forms of 21-hydroxylase deficiency (New et al, 1989). However, DHEAS levels are normal in most women with late-onset 21-hydroylase deficiency (Kuttenn et al, 1985), and in some studies serum DHEAS levels have correlated poorly with adrenal testosterone and androstenedione secretion (Siegel et al, 1990). Markedly elevated serum DHEAS levels are seen in most androgen-secreting adrenal neoplasms, although pure testosterone-secreting adrenal adenomas do occur. As might be expected, some normal women have elevated DHEAS levels with no other clinical or biochemical evidence of hyperandrogenism. In summary, although serum DHEAS levels are frequently measured in hyperandrogenic women, only occasionally does measurement of this steroid provide clinically useful information.

Adrenal androgen secretion begins with adrenarche (the adrenal counterpart to gonadarche), around age 6 to 8 (Reiter and Saenger, 1997). It is characterized by an increase in serum DHEAS and, to a lesser extent, androstenedione levels. Adrenarche is adrenocorticotropic hormone (ACTH) dependent but cannot be explained by changes in ACTH or gonadotropin secretion (Parker and Odell, 1980). It occurs coincident with the development of the zona reti-

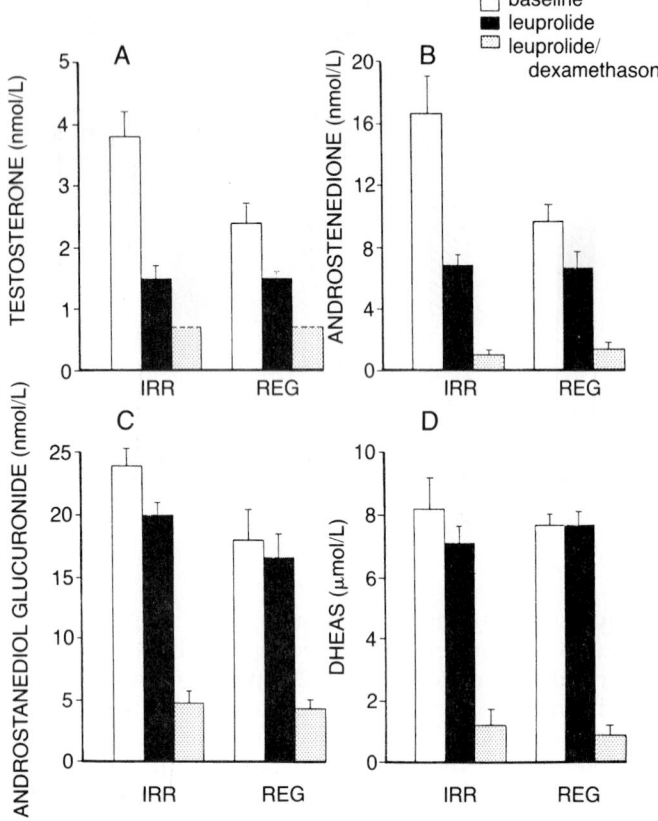

Figure 28-3

Serum testosterone (A), androstenedione (B), androstanediol glucuronide (C), and dehydroepiandrosterone sulfate (DHEAS) (D) at baseline, after ovarian suppression with leuprolide alone, and after combined ovarian and adrenal suppression with leuprolide and dexamethasone. Data are shown as a function of menstrual status. Women with irregular menses had the clinical features of polycystic ovarian syndrome. Testosterone and androstenedione arose from both ovarian and adrenal sources; DHEAS and androstanediol glucuronide arose primarily from adrenal precursors. Testosterone levels after leuprolide and dexamethasone were undetectable; the detection limit of the assay is shown. (IRR, women with irregular menses, $n = 10$; REG, regular menses, $n = 9$.) (From Rittmaster RS, Thompson DL: Effect of leuprolide and dexamethasone on hair growth and hormone levels in hirsute women: the relative importance of the ovary and the adrenal in the pathogenesis of hirsutism. J Clin Endocrinol Metab 1990;70:1096, with permission. © by The Endocrine Society.)

cularis of the adrenal cortex, supporting the hypothesis that this zone is the principle site of adrenal androgen secretion. Adrenarche is characterized by a decrease in adrenal 3β-HSD activity and an increase in 17,20-desmolase and 17-hydroxylase activity (Schiebinger et al, 1981), all of which would contribute to increased adrenal androgen precursor production. A separate pituitary-derived adrenal androgen–stimulating factor has been postulated to account for adrenarche, but convincing evidence for this is lacking. Other investigators hypothesize that the age-related increase in adrenal size causes changed in intra-adrenal steroid concentrations, which, in turn, lead to the changes in intra-adrenal enzyme activity noted above (Byrne et al, 1986). Adrenarche is independent of gonadarche, as best demonstrated by the normal adrenarche that occurs in girls with Turner's syndrome. Adrenarche can cause pubic and axillary hair growth, acne, and body odor independent of any ovarian hormone secretion. Premature adrenarche is characterized by the early development of pubic and axillary hair and should not be confused with true precocious puberty (Reiter and Saenger, 1997) (see Chapter 26).

Adult levels of adrenal androgens are reached during adolescence and then begin to decrease with age beginning in the fifth to sixth decade. The reason for this decrease is unknown, but it is not due to any changes in ACTH or cortisol secretion. There is some suggestion that an ovarian factor might be involved, because decreased adrenal androgens occur after

both natural or premature surgical menopause, even when estrogen replacement is given (Fig. 28–5) (Cumming et al, 1982).

Ovarian Androgen Synthesis

Both testosterone and androstenedione are secreted by the ovary. These steroids arise mainly from interstitial cells located in the stroma and hilus of the ovary (Longcope, 1986). Ovarian stroma is derived from the thecal cells of follicles that have undergone atresia. Thus follicular development is essential for ovarian androgen secretion. For example, the ovarian hyperandrogenism associated with severe insulin resistance only occurs during the reproductive years when atresia is an active process (Taylor et al, 1982). Because there are no known androgens or androgen metabolites that are unique to the ovary, there is no specific marker of ovarian androgen production.

Androgen secretion begins during puberty, coincident with estradiol secretion, and is dependent on luteinizing hormone (LH) stimulation. Serum androgens rise gradually during the follicular phase, peak around the time of the LH surge, and gradually fall during the luteal phase (Abraham, 1974). This temporal sequence explains why some women note an increase in acne during the luteal phase of the menstrual cycle. Ovarian androgen secretion gradually declines during the reproductive years (Mushayandebvu et al, 1996). Ovarian androgen secretion con-

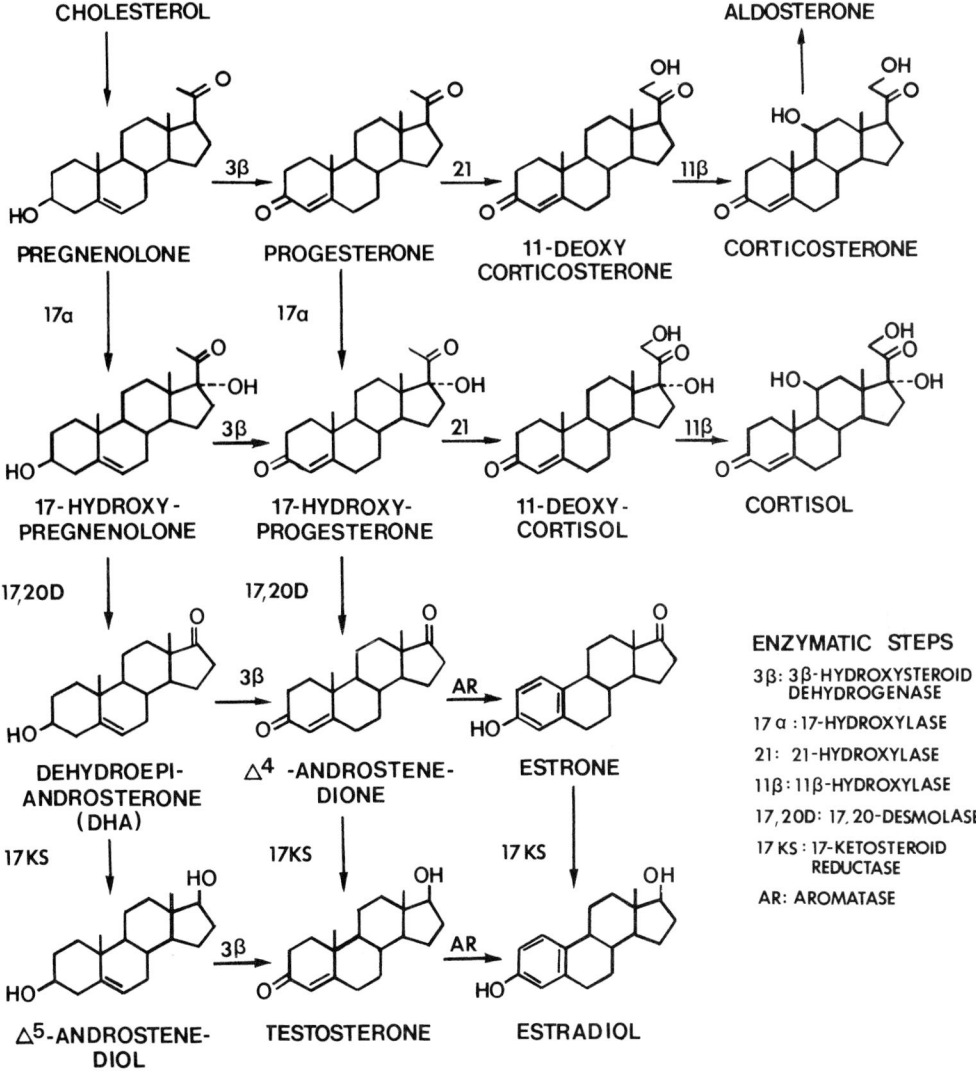

Figure 28–4
Adrenal steroidogenic pathways. Deficiencies of 3β-hydroxysteroid dehydrogenase, 21-hydroxylase, or 11β-hydroxylase lead to adrenal hyperplasia and cause shunting of cortisol precursor steroids into androgen synthesis. 11β-Hydroxylase deficiency also induces hypertension through the overproduction of the mineralocorticoid 11-deoxycorticosterone. 17α-Hydroxylase and 17,20-desmolase activity is mediated by the same enzyme, an overactivity of which has been postulated by some authors as a cause of hyperandrogenism (Rosenfield, 1990).

tinues, but does not increase, after menopause (Adashi, 1994; Sluijmer et al, 1995). Although LH levels rise, androgens do not rise further, presumably because no new follicles are being recruited and stromal development has stabilized. Because androgen secretion decreases with age (Zumoff et al, 1995), it has been argued that androgen replacement is beneficial, especially in women who have had a bilateral oophorectomy (Davis and Burger, 1996; Sands and Studd, 1995). Unfortunately, most of the studies to date have used androgen replacement that exceeds what an average premenopausal women would make. The question of whether physiologic androgen replacement is beneficial in postmenopausal women has yet to be answered in a well-designed, placebo-controlled study.

Androgen Transport in Blood

Between 1% and 2% of testosterone circulates unbound in the plasma. The remainder is bound about equally to albumin and sex hormone–binding globulin (SHBG), a glycosylated protein synthesized mainly in the liver with a molecular weight of about 90,000 (Hammond, 1990; Rosner, 1990). 17β-Hydroxysteroids, which include testosterone, DHT, and estradiol, bind with high affinity to SHBG. 17-Ketosteroids, such as androstenedione and DHEA, do not.

The "free hormone hypothesis" states that the biologic activity of a hormone is related to the proportion circulating as unbound (free) hormone (Mendel, 1989). According to this hypothesis, the higher

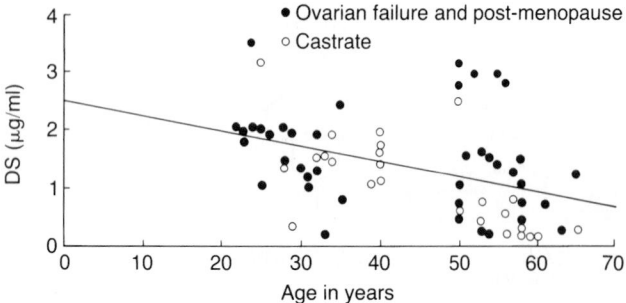

Figure 28–5

Dehydroepiandrosterone sulfate (DS) levels as a function of age in women castrated premenopausally, in women with premature ovarian failure, and in normal postmenopausal women. DS levels (mean ± standard error; μg/ml) were 2.17 ± 0.15 in normal women, 1.63 ± 0.15 in young women with premature ovarian failure, 1.29 ± 0.15 in postmenopausal women, and 0.58 ± 0.18 in postmenopausal castrated women. The lower DS levels in women with ovarian failure (regardless of estrogen replacement status) suggest the possibility that an ovarian factor may either stimulate DS production or inhibit its metabolism. (Modified from Cumming DC, Rebar RW, Hopper BR, et al: Evidence for an influence of the ovary on circulating dehydroepiandrosterone sulfate levels. J Clin Endocrinol Metab 1982;54:1069, with permission. © by The Endocrine Society.)

the free testosterone concentration, the greater will be its biologic activity. In women, testosterone does not contribute to negative feedback regulation of its own synthesis; hence, factors that tend to decrease the binding of testosterone and DHT to SHBG will tend to elevate the percentage of testosterone that is unbound and may increase its biologic activity. In addition, testosterone has a higher binding affinity to SHBG than does estradiol. Therefore, the ratio of free testosterone to estradiol decreases as the SHBG concentration increases. For example, thyroid hormone increases SHBG serum levels, and the resultant decrease in free testosterone:estradiol ratio may explain the gynecomastia seen in some men with hyperthyroidism.

Exogenous estrogens elevate serum SHBG levels by increasing hepatic production. Although oral contraceptives (OCs) decrease biologically active testosterone, this is more likely to be due to the progestin-induced suppression of ovarian testosterone production, rather than secondary to any estrogen-induced changes in SHBG. Exogenous androgens decrease serum SHBG concentrations, but the mechanism of this suppression is unknown. In vitro androgens stimulate SHBG secretion from hepatic cells (Plymate et al, 1988). SHBG levels are low in PCOS, and this association was previously thought to be related to the hyperandrogenism. However, suppression of androgen levels in PCOS with GnRH analogs does not alter SHBG levels (Nestler et al, 1991). Insulin suppresses SHBG synthesis in hepatic cells in vitro, and PCOS is associated with hyperinsulinism. Suppressing elevated insulin levels in

PCOS does lead to a rise in serum SHBG, supporting the hypothesis that insulin plays a major role in the modulation of serum SHBG levels (Nestler, 1993). The inverse relationship between serum insulin and SHBG concentrations provides an explanation for the low SHBG levels seen in obesity (Preziosi et al, 1993).

The validity of the free hormone hypothesis has been challenged. Although SHBG retards the cellular uptake of testosterone and its conversion to DHT in prostate cells (Lasnitzki and Franklin, 1972), testosterone uptake by liver and brain is greater than would be predicted from the free hormone concentration. The actual amount of bioavailable testosterone is likely to reflect a complex interaction between production and clearance rates, serum-binding proteins, endothelial transport, and capillary transit times (Mendel, 1989). SHBG may play a direct role through its cell surface receptor in modulating androgen action or uptake into cells (Nakhla et al, 1995). However, the interaction between SHBG, SHBG receptors, and androgens is complex, and the physiologic significance of cellular SHBG receptors is unknown. SHBG may also have a critically important role in development, because no individual has been discovered with an absence of SHBG, although over 1 million serum samples have been screened (Hammond, 1990).

Androgen Metabolism

Androgen metabolism in the skin is clearly an important aspect in the development of hyperandrogenism. As noted earlier, testosterone must first be converted to DHT by the enzyme 5α-reductase for the cutaneous aspects of hyperandrogenism (hirsutism, acne, male-pattern baldness) to develop. Hirsute women have increased skin 5α-reductase activity compared to nonhirsute women. Skin 5α-reductase is stimulated by androgens in vitro (Mauvais-Jarvis, 1986), and 5α-reductase activity is reduced in men with androgen resistance or deficiency.

Serum DHT has not proven to be a good marker for cutaneous hyperandrogenism, probably because it is rapidly metabolized to other compounds and inactivated by conjugation to glucuronides and sulfates (Fig. 28–6). The importance of the skin in testosterone metabolism was initially shown by Mauvais-Jarvis's group, who found that more androstanediol, a DHT metabolite, was formed from testosterone when the precursor was given percutaneously than when given orally or intravenously (Mauvais-Jarvis et al, 1970). Urinary androstanediol and serum androstanediol glucuronide levels are higher in hirsute than normal women, and many investigators have considered androstanediol glucuronide to be a marker of androgen metabolism in the skin. Much of the evidence supporting this hypothesis rests on the association between elevated serum

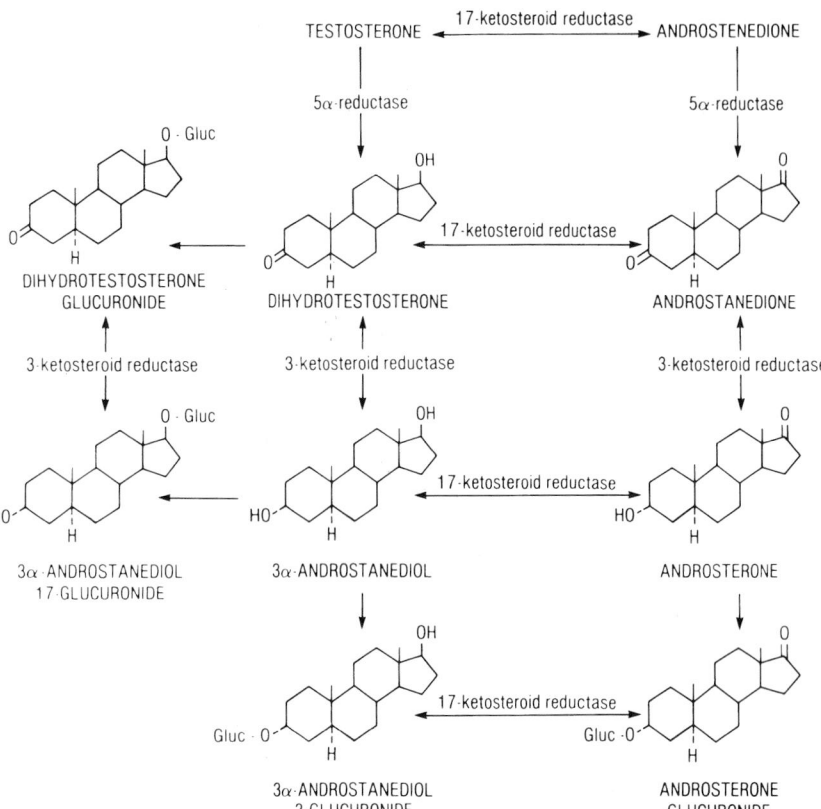

Figure 28–6
Pathways of testosterone and dihydrotestosterone metabolism. Glucuronyltransferase is the enzyme responsible for formation of glucuronide conjugates. Similarly, androgens can be conjugated to sulfates by the enzyme sulfotransferase. Androstanediol glucuronide is actually two molecules, androstanediol 17- and 3-glucuronide, with androstanediol 17-glucuronide being the predominant form in human serum. (From Rittmaster RS, Thompson DL, Listwak S, Loriaux DL: Androstanediol glucuronide isomers in normal men and women and in men infused with labeled dihydrotestosterone. J Clin Endocrinol Metab 1988;66:212, with permission. © The Endocrine Society.)

androstanediol glucuronide levels and hirsutism in both women (Horton and Lobo, 1986) and men (Lookingbill et al, 1988). In addition, Horton's group was unable to demonstrate production of androstanediol glucuronide by the liver during catheterization studies in men and concluded that this compound was formed in extrasplanchnic tissue (presumably the skin) (Morimoto et al, 1981).

In spite of the association between elevated androstanediol glucuronide levels and hirsutism, the preponderance of evidence now indicates that androstanediol glucuronide arises mainly from adrenal precursors and is an index of adrenal hyperandrogenism in hirsute women (Vermeulen and Giagulli, 1991; Rittmaster et al, 1993a). Both precursor production and 5α-reductase activity are likely to be important in determining androstanediol glucuronide levels, but the lack of correlation between androstanediol glucuronide levels and the severity of hirsutism in women or the response to medical therapy suggests that it is a poor marker of androgen action in the skin. As expected, however, androstanediol glucuronide is a marker of adrenal androgen secretion in women with CAH (Pang et al, 1991).

Serum levels of androgen sulfates have also been measured and found to circulate in concentrations up to 10 times higher than those of androgen glucuronides (Matteri et al, 1989). They also appear to arise from adrenal precursors and correlate well with DHEAS levels (Zwicker and Rittmaster, 1993).

PHYSICAL SIGNS ASSOCIATED WITH ANDROGEN EXCESS

Hirsutism, acne, muscle development, clitoral hypertrophy, male-pattern baldness, and deepening of the voice are all the result of androgen action. Acanthosis nigricans is a sign of insulin resistance, which often accompanies hyperandrogenism in women with PCOS. Taken together, these physical signs are clear evidence of androgen excess. However, androgens are present in all normal women, and their effect forms a continuum from normalcy to "virilization." Because of biologic variability in the response of the target organ, many of these clinical manifestations can be seen in some women with normal female androgen levels. Nevertheless, when they occur together, a marked elevation of serum testosterone can be expected. When recent in onset, an androgen-secreting neoplasm must be ruled out.

Hirsutism

Hirsutism is the presence of excess body hair in women (Rittmaster, 1997b). Surveys of unselected young women show that 25% to 35% have hair over the lower abdomen ("a male-pattern escutcheon"), on the chest (principally around the areolae), or on the face (mainly the upper lip) (Ferriman and Gallwey, 1961; McKnight, 1964). Furthermore, body hair growth in women increases with age (Ferriman and Gallwey, 1961). Unfortunately, these normal hair patterns are unacceptable to many women.

The pathophysiology of hirsutism is best understood in the context of the physiology of normal hair growth (Uno, 1986). The number of hair follicles is fixed before birth. Before puberty, most of the body is covered by fine, unpigmented *vellus hairs*. The coarser pigmented hair on the scalp, eyebrows, and eyelashes is called *terminal hair*. During puberty, under the influence of androgens, vellus hair is converted to terminal hair in sex hormone–dependent areas (excluding the scalp, where the opposite may occur). The transition from vellus to terminal hairs may be gradual, and hence "transitional hairs" are those hairs that have some of the features of both terminal and vellus hairs. Furthermore, the quality of terminal hair differs in different body areas. Terminal hair on the lower abdomen is not the same as terminal hair on the chin, although both are androgen dependent. The amount of terminal hair that develops depends on the amount of androgen produced, as well as the skin sensitivity to these hormones. Pubic and axillary hair follicles are sufficiently sensitive to androgens that normal female androgen levels cause terminal hair growth in these areas. Hair follicles on the face, chest, upper abdomen, and back are less sensitive and usually require increased androgen levels to form terminal hair.

Nevertheless, the range of androgen production and skin sensitivity is sufficiently large that some women have excess hair growth in all of these areas, without having a serious underlying cause of hyperandrogenism. Both androgen production and skin sensitivity to androgens are, in part, inherited features. Most women with hirsutism, therefore, have a family history of excess hair growth. The skin sensitivity to androgens is inherited as much through men as through women, and hirsutism in either parent may lead to hirsutism in their children.

Hair grows in cycles (Fig. 28–7). The active growth period is called the *anagen phase*, and its duration is the primary determinant of the length of the hair. Scalp hair has the longest anagen phase of any body hair, often up to several years; eyebrows and eyelashes have a short anagen phase. When a hair stops growing, it enters a resting, or *telogen*, phase. The duration of this phase is also variable. The number of actively growing hairs is inversely proportional to the length of telogen. Once a new hair starts to grow, the old telogen shaft is pushed out and the cycle begins again. Most investigators believe that hormonal therapy directed at hirsutism will not affect actively growing terminal hairs, and therefore treatment regimens may require a year or more to reach maximal effect.

Estrogens prolong the anagen phase in scalp hair (Lynfield, 1960) and may have a similar effect in other hair follicles. Increased circulating estrogen

Growth cycle of hair follicle

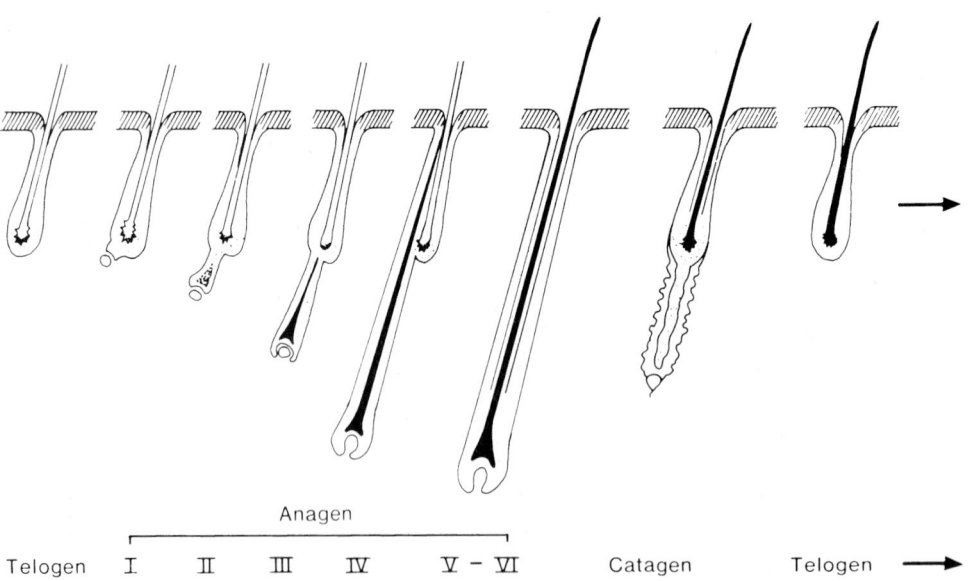

| Telogen | I | II | III | IV | V – VI | Catagen | Telogen |

Anagen: I, II, III, IV, V – VI

Figure 28–7

Hair grows in cycles. Anagen II through anagen VI are active growth phases, during which a new hair (black) replaces an old hair (white). Catagen is an involutional phase, and telogen and anagen I are resting phases. (From Rittmaster R, Uno H, Povar M, et al: The effects of N,N-diethyl-4-methyl-3-oxo-4-aza-5α-androstane-17β-carboxamide, a 5α-reductase inhibitor and antiandrogen, on the development of baldness in the stumptail macaque. J Clin Endocrinol Metab 1987;65:188, with permission. © The Endocrine Society.)

levels (i.e., OCs or pregnancy) increase the number of hair follicles in anagen, and, when the exposure to high estrogen levels ends, many hair follicles enter telogen at the same time. As the new hairs begin to grow, the telogen hairs fall out (telogen effluvium). A similar phenomenon can occur with severe illness, and affected women may need to be reassured that they are not going bald.

Several drugs have been associated with hirsutism. These include diazoxide, minoxidil, glucocorticoids, cyclosporine, and phenytoin (Tosti et al, 1994). The pattern of hair growth in drug-induced hirsutism is not restricted to androgen-dependent areas and is typically more vellus then terminal. The pathophysiology of drug-induced hirsutism is poorly understood, and the only successful treatment is to stop the offending drug.

A diffuse increase in transitional and terminal hairs is also present in women and men with familial hypertrichosis. This inherited condition has a hair growth pattern similar to drug-induced hirsutism, and includes excess hair growth over the forehead, shoulders, upper back, and flanks. It is most commonly seen in women of East Indian origin. A confusing clinical picture can arise when androgen-dependent hirsutism is superimposed on familial hypertrichosis.

Male-Pattern Baldness

Male-pattern baldness in women is common (Bergfeld, 1995). Because androgen levels are lower in women than men, the process occurs slowly and often progresses to a lesser extent. However, given enough time, or in the presence of elevated androgen levels, extensive male-pattern baldness can develop in women. Older women with male-pattern baldness often have normal androgen levels. Younger women with this condition usually have increased androgen production. A family history of alopecia is present in most women with male-pattern baldness. Increased hair follicle 5α-reductase activity is present in balding scalp in men (Dallob et al, 1994), and the same is likely true for balding women.

Beginning with puberty, in both men and women, temporal hair line recession usually occurs. This process is limited in women, and the adolescent girl with mild temporal recession can be reassured that she is not going bald. In some women, the pattern of male-pattern baldness appears different from that in men. There is prominent frontal balding, but the frontal hairline is preserved. The reason for this peculiarity is unknown. Male-pattern baldness must be distinguished from diffuse hair loss, including telogen effluvium (see previous section). Finally, diffuse, androgen-independent scalp hair thinning is common in both elderly men and women.

The treatment for male-pattern baldness in women is similar to that of hirsutism (see below). Antiandrogens are often effective at preventing further

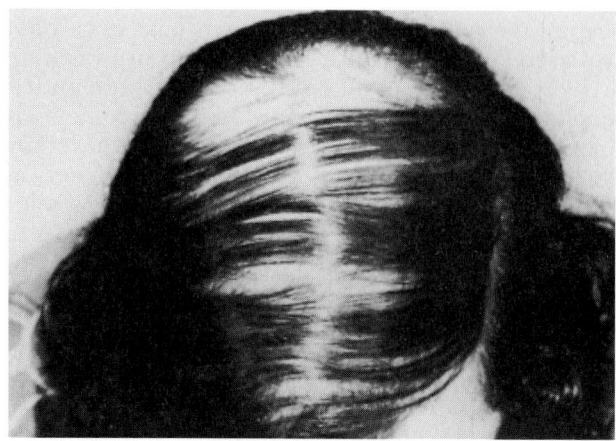
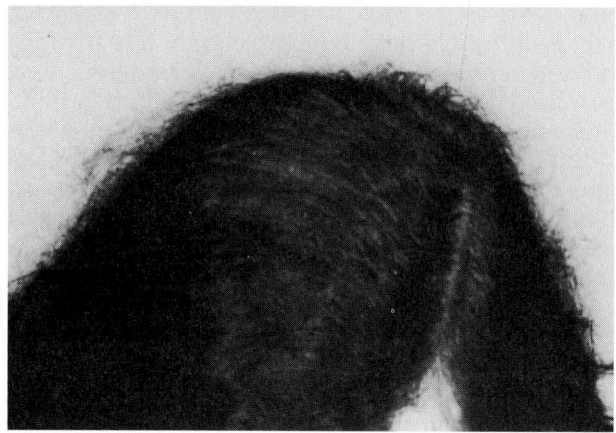

Figure 28–8
Partial reversibility of baldness in a 30-year-old woman with severe polycystic ovary syndrome treated for 2 years with the gonadotropin-releasing hormone analog leuprolide and spironolactone.

scalp hair loss, and marked improvement in balding can occur in some women (Fig. 28–8).

Acne

Androgens stimulate sebaceous glands to increase cell division and sebum production. Female androgen levels are sufficient to cause near-maximal sebum secretion, and women produce about 75% as much sebum as men (Rosenfield, 1986). Acne, which results when the outlet of the sebaceous gland becomes plugged, is dependent on the increased sebum production induced by androgens. Nevertheless, the relationship between androgens and acne is not straightforward. In spite of continuously high androgen levels, acne disappears after puberty in most men. The reason for the high incidence of acne during puberty may have more to do with rising androgen levels than with the absolute amount of circulating androgens. These fluctuating androgen levels may explain why many women note mild acne during the luteal phase of the menstrual cycle, when a modest increase in circulating androgens occurs.

Despite the fact that young women with acne have increased circulating androgens as a group (Lucky et al, 1983; Marynick et al, 1983), tonically high androgen levels in hyperandrogenic hirsute women are not usually associated with acne. Although antiandrogens can be an effective treatment for acne, the initial response is unpredictable, and some women develop transiently worse acne when antiandrogens are given. If antiandrogens are given to treat acne, they should be used in conjunction with dermatologic agents designed to prevent sebaceous gland plugging, reduce inflammation, and treat infection.

Other Signs of Androgen Excess

Increased muscle development, clitoral hypertrophy, and deepening of the voice are considered signs of marked androgen excess or "virilization." Androgen-sensitive tissues, however, exhibit a continuum of responses. These physical features are signs of virilization only because physicians are unable to distinguish mild androgenic effects in these tissues. This is best documented with clitoral enlargement. By the time most physicians recognize that clitoral enlargement has occurred, marked hyperandrogenism is usually present. However, when the cross-sectional area of the clitoris is measured (the "clitoral index"), mild to marked clitoral enlargement is found in most hirsute women (Tagatz et al, 1979). Similarly, it is reasonable to expect that mild increases in androgens in women would promote muscle development and that successful female athletes, as a group, would have higher androgen levels than nonathletic women.

Acanthosis Nigricans

Acanthosis nigricans is a dermatologic condition commonly found in obesity and PCOS, and is a sign of insulin resistance (Barbieri, 1994). It consists of thickened, hyperpigmented skin, usually developing in the skin folds of the neck and axillae (Fig. 28–9). Histologic features include papillomatosis, hyperkeratosis, and hyperpigmentation (Dunaif et al, 1991). Because of the hyperpigmentation, women may mistakenly complain of difficulty keeping the affected areas clean. The acanthosis may be missed if the neck and axillae are not examined carefully.

DIFFERENTIAL DIAGNOSIS AND PATHOPHYSIOLOGY OF HYPERANDROGENISM

Functional Hyperandrogenism

Androgen production in women is a by-product of estrogen and cortisol synthesis. Increased androgen production arises from either the adrenal glands, the

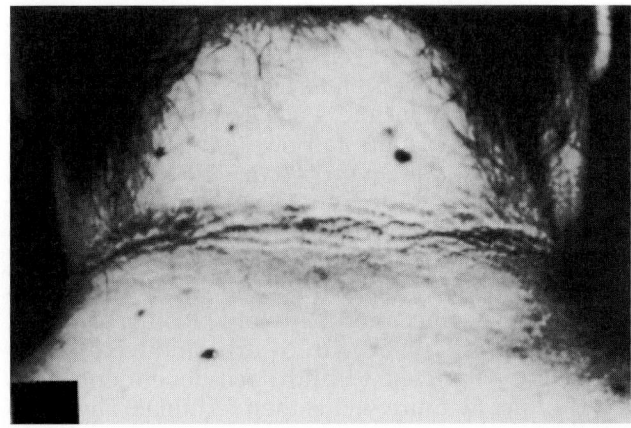

Figure 28 – 9
Acanthosis nigricans in a woman with polycystic ovary syndrome and insulin resistance. (From Barbieri RL, Smith S, Ryan KJ: The role of hyperinsulinemia in the pathogenesis of ovarian hyperandrogenism. Fertil Steril 1988;50:197. Reproduced with permission of the American Fertility Society.)

ovaries, or both (Table 28–1). Although well-defined causes of adrenal and ovarian hyperandrogenism exist, the normal range of androgen production from these organs is broad, and often no well-defined abnormality can be found. Conversely, mildly "elevated" levels of androgen precursors (DHEAS, androstenedione) and products (androgen glucuronides and sulfates) may be seen in both hirsute and nonhirsute women. The greater the androgen production (from either the ovaries or adrenals), the greater is the likelihood of hirsutism and other physical signs of hyperandrogenism. The cutaneous manifestations of androgen excess depend upon skin sensitivity to androgens. Increased skin 5α-reductase activity can result in hirsutism in some women whose androgen production is normal.

Congenital Adrenal Hyperplasia

CAH results from a deficiency of any one of the enzymes involved in cortisol biosynthesis (Fig. 28–4).

Table 28 – 1. CAUSES OF ANDROGEN-DEPENDENT HIRSUTISM

Ovarian
   Severe insulin resistance
   Virilizing ovarian tumors
Adrenal
   Congenital adrenal hyperplasia
     21-Hydroxylase deficiency
     3β-Hydroxysteroid dehydrogenase deficiency
     11-Hydroxylase deficiency
   Cushing's syndrome
   Ectopic ACTH-secreting tumors
   Virilizing adrenal tumors
Combined ovarian and adrenal
   Polycystic ovarian syndrome
   Functional hyperandrogenism

ACTH secretion is increased in response to decreased cortisol synthesis. The combination of increased ACTH stimulation of the adrenals and an enzyme deficiency results in an increase in adrenal hormone precursors before the block. In the virilizing forms of CAH (11β-hydroxylase, 21-hydroxylase, and 3β-HSD deficiencies), cortisol secretion is maintained to varying degrees (depending on the severity of the enzyme defect) at the expense of increased androgen production.

21-Hydroxylase Deficiency

All forms of CAH are inherited as autosomal recessive traits. The genetics of 21-hydroxylase deficiency, the most common form of CAH, is well described (Strachan, 1990; Miller, 1994). Two genes for 21-hydroxylase are located on the short arm of chromosome 6 within the human leukocyte antigen (HLA) locus, only one of which is functional (the other is a nearly identical pseudogene). Because of this location, 21-hydroxylase deficiency is an HLA-linked disorder. Affected individuals and carriers can be identified by HLA typing of family members. The presence of the pseudogene, with a high sequence homology to the functional gene, causes frequent mispairing during meiosis of the functional gene on one allele with the pseudogene on the other allele. If a recombination event (crossover) happens to occur within the 21-hydroxylase gene during this mispairing, at least one allele will have a nonfunctional 21-hydroxylase gene. The presence of the pseudogene explains the relatively high frequency of 21-hydroxylase deficiency.

21-Hydroxylase deficiency accounts for over 95% of individuals with adrenal enzyme defects. In the most severely affected individuals, the enzyme deficiency results in diminished cortisol and aldosterone secretion (New, 1994). This "classical" form of 21-hydroxylase deficiency presents in the neonatal period with salt wasting in both sexes and masculinization of the external genitalia of female infants (see Chapter 26). The presence of ambiguous genitalia in female neonates raises the possibility of a salt-wasting form of adrenal hyperplasia. The prognosis for affected males is worse, because the salt wasting may go unrecognized. A slightly less severe form of 21-hydroxylase deficiency may cause virilization without marked salt wasting ("simple virilizing" 21-hydroxylase deficiency). Taken together, the salt-wasting and simple virilizing forms of 21-hydroxylase deficiency occur in about 1 in 5000 to 1 in 15,000 births, depending upon the population sampled (Pang et al, 1988). Still milder enzyme defects may present in females as precocious adrenarche, PCOS, or hirsutism (Azziz et al, 1994). These "nonclassical" presentations may be indistinguishable from other causes of mild androgen excess by history or physical examination. Excess adrenal androgens during adolescence and adulthood may lead to the development of irregular menses and the

clinical features of PCOS. Nonclassical 21-hydroxylase deficiency occurs in about 1% of hirsute women and is the most common inherited metabolic disorder. An occasional individual is identified through screening programs who has the biochemical features of the disorder but no clinical manifestations of hyperandrogenism ("cryptic" 21-hydroxylase deficiency).

21-Hydroxylase deficiency is best diagnosed by measuring serum 17-hydroxyprogesterone, the substrate for the enzyme (Fig. 28–10). Studies from families with classical 21-hydroxylase deficiency indicate that heterozygous women are unaffected clinically, unless another reason for hyperandrogenism exists. In the hyperandrogenic woman, homozygous nonclassical 21-hydroxylase deficiency can be ruled out by measuring 17-hydroxyprogesterone between 7 and 9 A.M., during the follicular phase of the menstrual cycle (values may be elevated during the luteal phase). Basal 17-hydroxyprogesterone levels are usually elevated in nonclassical 21-hydroxylase deficiency, although an occasional affected woman may have normal levels in the afternoon or evening, when cortisol production is low. Values less than 6 nmol/L (200 mg/dl) rule out the diagnosis. Mildly elevated values (less than 30 nmol/L [1000 mg/dl]) may be seen in both heterozygous and homozygous nonclassical 21-hydroxylase deficiency and PCOS. To distinguish between these conditions, 17-hydroxyprogesterone should be measured basally and 30 to 60 minutes after the intravenous or intramuscular administration of 250 μg synthetic ACTH. ACTH-stimulated levels will be greater than 36 nmol/L (12000 ng/dl) in homozygous 21-hydroxylase deficiency. Lesser elevations will generally be seen with the heterozygous condition, which is not associated with hyperandrogenism (Knochenhauer et al, 1997). In PCOS, the elevated 17-hydroxyprogesterone levels usually increase minimally with ACTH stimulation, because most of the steroid is ovarian in origin (Azziz et al, 1990).

In female infants with classical 21-hydroxylase deficiency, correct gender assignment is imperative as soon after delivery as possible. Although 21-hydroxylase deficiency cannot be diagnosed on physical examination alone, it can be suspected in the infant with ambiguous genitalia, a female karyotype, and a uterus on ultrasound. If 21-hydroxylase deficiency is suspected, 17-hydroxyprogesterone and DHEAS are measured during the second day postpartum. Because these infants are genetic females with potentially normal reproductive capacity, they should be raised as females, and surgical correction of the genitalia performed at the appropriate time. Treatment includes glucocorticoid and mineralocorticoid replacement (Brook, 1990; Cutler and Laue, 1990). Initial sodium replacement in the dehydrated infant should be about 20 ml/kg 0.9% sodium chloride over the first 20 to 60 minutes, followed by fluid and electrolyte replacement according to calculated deficits and maintenance requirements. In an acute ad-

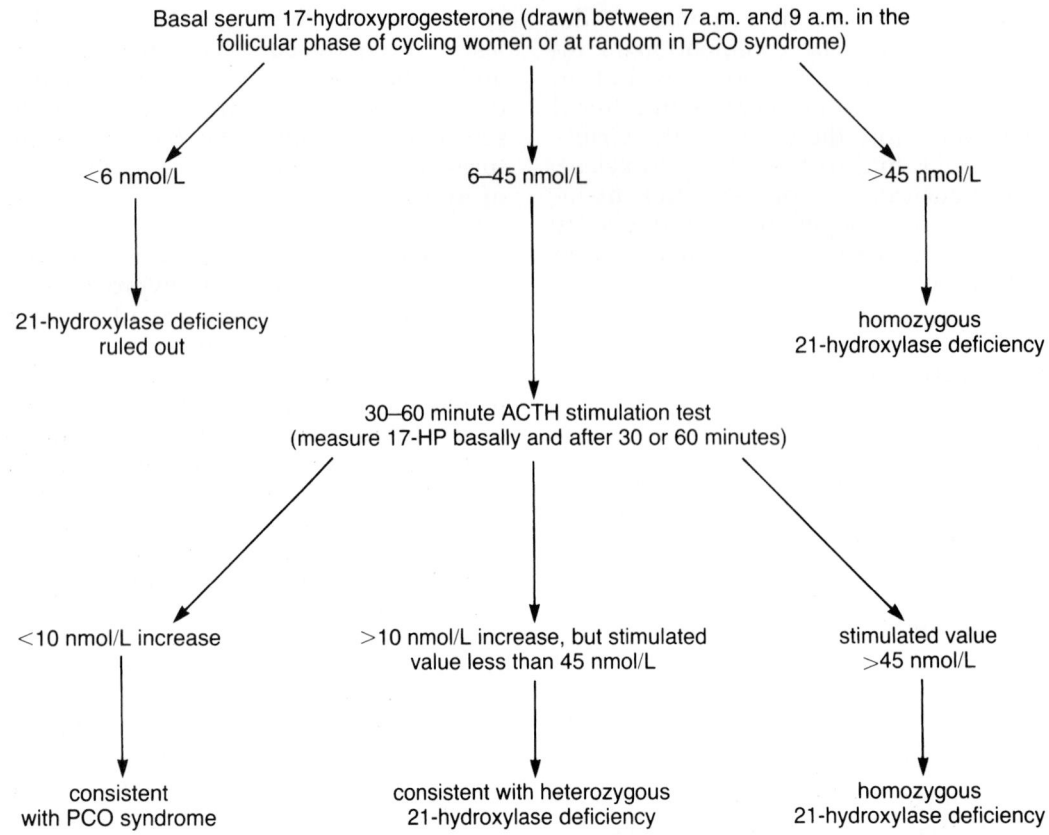

Basal serum 17-hydroxyprogesterone (drawn between 7 a.m. and 9 a.m. in the follicular phase of cycling women or at random in PCO syndrome)

<6 nmol/L

6–45 nmol/L

>45 nmol/L

21-hydroxylase deficiency ruled out

homozygous 21-hydroxylase deficiency

30–60 minute ACTH stimulation test (measure 17-HP basally and after 30 or 60 minutes)

<10 nmol/L increase

>10 nmol/L increase, but stimulated value less than 45 nmol/L

stimulated value >45 nmol/L

consistent with PCO syndrome

consistent with heterozygous 21-hydroxylase deficiency

homozygous 21-hydroxylase deficiency

Figure 28–10
Screening for 21-hydroxylase deficiency by measuring 17-hydroxyprogesterone (17-HP) in hirsute women. Other enzyme deficiencies can also cause elevated 17-HP levels; however, these are much rarer. PCO, polycystic ovary; ACTH, adrenocorticotropic hormone.

renal crisis, hydrocortisone, 25 mg IV or IM, should be given immediately as initial glucocorticoid treatment for the small infant, followed by 30 to 150 mg IV per 24 hours for the first 24 to 48 hours. Fludrocortisone (up to 300 μg/day in infants) should be given orally. If treatment is initiated before a salt-losing crisis has occurred, physiologic oral replacement of glucocorticoids and mineralocorticoids may be all that is necessary.

The best regimen for long-term glucocorticoid and mineralocorticoid replacement for classical 21-hydroxylase deficiency remains an area of ongoing debate. The goals are to optimize growth and prevent hyperandrogenism. Too much glucocorticoid will result in short stature, and too little will cause rapid advancement of height and bone age, with resulting short adult height. In order to adequately suppress adrenal steroidogenesis, superphysiologic doses of glucocorticoids are needed to prevent the hypersecretion of adrenal steroid precursors such as progesterone and 17-hydroxyprogesterone, which themselves can suppress gonadotropins and antagonize the actions of aldosterone (Helleday et al, 1993). The failure to optimally treat 21-hydroxylase deficiency is best demonstrated by the fact that, even with adequate conventional treatment, final adult height is well below expected, and that fertility problems are

common in women with this diagnosis (Premawardhana et al, 1997). Mineralocorticoid replacement is important, even in patients who have not had a salt-wasting crisis, if elevated plasma renin activity is present. Sodium depletion stimulates 17-hydroxyprogesterone and androgen production through the renin-angiotensin system. Fludrocortisone (50 to 200 μg/day) should usually be given for mineralocorticoid replacement. The dose should be adjusted to suppress plasma renin activity into the normal range. If this is not done, excessively high doses of glucocorticoid may be necessary to adequately suppress adrenal androgen production. Adequate hydrocoritsone replacement requires doses in the range of 10 to 20 mg/m²/day. In children, maintenance of a normal growth rate is essential, and growth velocity and bone age should be followed. Biochemical measurements used to assess the adequacy of hormone replacement in women include serum 17-hydroxyprogesterone, testosterone, androstenedione, and urinary 17-ketosteroids or pregnanetriol (New et al, 1989). Because suppression of serum androgens may be difficult to maintain with replacement doses of glucocorticoids, a novel proposal is to use a relatively low dose of hydrocortisone to avoid hypercortisolism and to treat any remaining hyperandrogenism with antiandrogens such as flutamide (spironolactone should be avoided because it is an aldosterone antagonist) (Van WyK et al, 1996). As with any patient with adrenal insufficiency, the dose of glucocorticoid should be doubled during periods of stress such as a viral illness. A medical alert bracelet should be worn. If precocious thelarche develops, indicating the onset of true precocious puberty, consideration should be given to treating this with GnRH analogs until the patient reaches an appropriate pubertal age (see Chapter 26).

Because of the difficulty of adequately suppressing adrenal steroidogenesis with doses of glucocorticoids that do not cause hypercortisolism, a strong case has been made for using adrenalectomy in infants with severe 21-hydroxylase deficiency (Van WyK et al, 1996). Although this approach should be considered experimental at present, there is reason to believe that it will lead to a better quality of life in affected individuals.

In families with one or more children with virilizing 21-hydroxylase deficiency, prenatal treatment of potentially affected fetuses is now becoming increasingly common in order to minimize virilization of female offspring (Migeon, 1990; Speiser et al, 1990; Mercado et al, 1995), Dexamethasone, 20 µg/kg prepregnancy weight daily in three divided doses, is given starting at the fifth to eighth week of gestation and continued until it can be determined if the fetus is an affected female. Cells from chorionic villus sampling at 8 to 11 weeks or amniotic fluid at 16 weeks are obtained for karyotyping, HLA typing, or restriction fragment length polymorphism analysis to determine the sex and the presence of the abnormal gene. Because only 25% of female offspring will be affected and half of the offspring will be male, seven of eight fetuses will not require treatment. The only significant risk to this approach is that of the diagnostic technique (about 0.3% incidence of fetal death with aminocentesis and 1% with villus sampling).

The treatment of adolescents or adults with nonclassical 21-hydroxylase deficiency is totally different. In most such subjects, cortisol and mineralocorticoid secretion are adequate and hyperandrogenism is the main concern. In such patients, anovulation is often successfully treated with small doses of glucocorticoids (e.g., 2.5 mg prednisone twice daily). Hyperandrogenism responds well to antiandrogens, such as spironolactone, and hirsutism in affected women with normal menses often responds better to antiandrogens than to glucocorticoids (Spritzer et al, 1990). Nevertheless, because of the wide range of enzyme activity and differences in end-organ sensitivity to androgens in such patients, treatment must be individualized.

3β-HSD Deficiency

3β-HSD deficiency is due to mutations in the type II 3β-HSD gene, encoding the adrenal and gonadal form of the enzyme (Simard et al, 1993; Pang, 1996).

It presents in infancy similarly to 21-hydroxylase deficiency, although ambiguous genitalia are present in both sexes (in females because of increased peripheral conversion of DHEA to testosterone and DHT via the type I enzyme, and in males because of inadequate testosterone production). The diagnosis is made by demonstrating a markedly elevated ratio of 3β-HSD precursors (Δ5 steroids) to products (Δ4 steroids)—for example, serum pregnenelone to progesterone or 17-hydroxypregnenelone to 17-hydroxyprogesterone (Fig. 28–4), or urinary pregnenetriol to pregnanetriol (the metabolic products of Δ5 and Δ4 steroids, respectively) (Bongiovanni, 1984). If only serum 17-hydroxyprogesterone or urinary pregnanetriol is measured, the mistaken diagnosis of 21-hydroxylase deficiency will be made, because these steroids will be elevated as a result of hepatic metabolism of the 3β-HSD precursors. The treatment includes both glucocorticoid and mineralocorticoid replacement as described for salt-losing 21-hydroxylase deficiency.

Rarely, a patient may have the biochemical features of 3β-HSD deficiency but present only with hyperandrogenism in adolescence (Rosenfield et al, 1980). More commonly, hyperandrogenic adolescent and adult women present with elevated Δ5 steroids and a modestly increased precursor:product ratio for 3β-HSD (greater than 2 standard deviations above the mean for normal women) (Pang et al, 1985; Siegel et al, 1990). Although these women were originally considered to represent mild forms of 3β-HSD deficiency, no evidence has been found for a 3β-HSD gene mutation in such individuals (Zerah et al, 1994; Sakkal-Alkaddour et al, 1996).

11-Hydroxylase Deficiency

11-Hydroxylase deficiency presents in female infants with virilization and with the gradual development of hypertension in both sexes (because of increased deoxycorticosterone production) (White et al, 1994). It is caused by mutations in the CYP11B1 gene, located on chromosome 22 (Geley et al, 1996). Nonclassical forms have been reported but are rare (Cathelineau et al, 1980). Although cortisol secretion is impaired, affected individuals do not present in adrenal crisis because deoxycorticosterone, mineralocorticoid, is produced in excess. The diagnosis can be made by demonstrating an increased serum 11-deoxycortisol:cortisol ratio and increased urinary deoxycorticosterone and tetrahydrodeoxycorticosterone excretion in a virilized female or hypertensive male infant. Treatment with glucocorticoids is indicated as described for 21-hydroxylase deficiency. Mineralocorticoid replacement is unnecessary.

Cushing's Syndrome

Cushing's syndrome can be divided into ACTH-dependent etiologies (pituitary tumors and ectopic

ACTH-secreting tumors) and ACTH-independent etiologies (adrenal tumors, exogenous glucocorticoids) Tsigos and Chrousos, 1996). Although any cause of glucocorticoid excess may be associated with a "drug-induced" pattern of hirsutism, only Cushing's syndrome with ACTH-secreting tumors (pituitary or ectopic) is associated with androgen-dependent hirsutism. Patients with Cushing's syndrome usually present with numerous symptoms, including truncal obesity, rounding of the face and facial plethora, striae, bruising, weakness (especially of the proximal muscles), polyuria and other symptoms of diabetes, depression, and hirsutism. Rarely is hirsutism the sole or even the primary manifestation of Cushing's syndrome. Screening for Cushing's syndrome should be done in hyperandrogenic women who present with symptoms and signs of cortisol excess (including central obesity, hypertension, and glucose intolerance), but screening does not need to be done in every obese, hirsute woman. Conversely, Cushing's syndrome must not be overlooked when it develops in a woman who already is obese or hirsute or who has PCOS.

The best screening tests for Cushing's syndrome are the overnight dexamethasone suppression test and 24-hour urinary free cortisol. For the overnight dexamethasone suppression test, 1 mg dexamethasone (two tablets) is given at 2300 hours. A serum cortisol is obtained between 700 and 900 hours the next day. Normally, serum cortisol should be suppressed to less than 5 µg/dl (140 nmol/L). False-positive tests occur in 10% to 15% of patients (Cronin et al, 1990). Reasons for false-positive tests include failure to take the dexamethasone; depression or alcoholism ("pseudo-Cushing's"); concurrent use of drugs that increase dexamethasone metabolism, such as phenobarbital, phenytoin, or coumadin; estrogen use (estrogens increase cortisol-binding globulin); and any form of moderate to serve stress, such as a concurrent illness.

A 24-hour urinary free cortisol measures the amount of unbound ("free") cortisol secreted in the urine. Most binding sites on cortisol-binding globulin are occupied at physiologic cortisol concentrations. Therefore, any increase in cortisol secretion results in a disproportionate increase in urinary cortisol. Because of the diurnal variation in cortisol secretion, a complete 24-hour collection is necessary. Normal subjects excrete less than 125 µg/day (345 nmol/day). False-positive tests occur in depressed, alcoholic, or stressed subjects, but the test is unaffected by anticonvulsants, coumadin, or estrogens. Urinary free cortisol excretion over 250 µg/day is highly suggestive of Cushing's syndrome, although any elevation requires further evaluation.

The ideal screening test is one that has no false negatives and an acceptable number of false positives. The above two tests are close to ideal, but subjects with mild Cushing's syndrome or those with episodic cortisol secretion may be difficult to diagnose. When a positive screening test is obtained, the diagnosis of Cushing's syndrome should be confirmed with a 48-hour low-dose dexamethasone suppression test. This and other tests involved in the differential diagnosis of Cushing's syndrome are best left to an endocrinologist familiar with the pitfalls in the interpretations of these tests (Tsigos and Chrousos, 1996).

Polycystic Ovarian Syndrome

Definitions and Prevalence

PCOS is a heterogeneous disorder without a simple definition. It was originally described by Stein and Leventhal (1935) as a clinical triad of hyperandrogenism, anovulation, and obesity in women with enlarged, polycystic ovaries. The pathologic features include thickening of the tunica albuginea; multiple small, atretic, subcapsular follicles; and thecal and stromal hyperplasia (Goldzieher and Green, 1962). Unfortunately, "polycystic ovarian syndrome" is a misnomer in that the morphologic changes in the ovaries appear to be secondary to the physiologic abnormalities. Any cause of hyperandrogenism can lead to anovulation and the development of polycystic ovaries, including adrenal and ovarian tumors, CAH, Cushing's syndrome, and exogenous androgens. Hence PCOS is a syndrome, not a specific disease, and the biochemical features may vary depending on the underlying etiology. Furthermore, multiple ovarian cysts may be seen with any cause of anovulation and are common in hirsute women with regular menstrual cycles (Polson et al, 1988; Clayton et al, 1992). The absence of polycystic ovaries on routine ultrasonography of the pelvis also does not rule out the diagnosis. For the purpose of this discussion, the term *polycystic ovarian syndrome* will be used to describe the clinical presentation of hyperandrogenism and oligo- or amenorrhea in women who do not have a well-defined underlying cause of their androgen excess. This definition is independent of the pathologic or ultrasonographic appearance of the ovaries. Because the severity of the clinical and biochemical abnormalities varies, at times it may be difficult to distinguish between "hypothalamic amenorrhea" in women with normal estrogen levels and "polycystic ovarian syndrome" in women with normal or near-normal androgen levels. *Hyperthecosis* is a term used to describe the pathologic findings in the ovaries of women with PCOS and severe hyperandrogenism. These women have marked stromal hyperplasia without cyst formation (Judd et al, 1973).

PCOS usually begins with puberty. Ovulatory menses may be present initially, but oligo- or amenorrhea commonly occurs soon after menarche. Mild to severe hirsutism may develop rapidly along with rising testosterone levels, raising the possibility of an androgen-secreting neoplasm. Obesity is common, and, in some women, PCOS develops after adolescence in association with weight gain. In other women, the use of OCs may delay the development of symptoms. The incidence of the clinical manifestations in PCOS depends, in part, on the type of physician to whom the patient is referred. Endocrinologists will be more likely to see obese, hirsute women. Thin women whose primary complaint is menstrual irregularity are more likely to be referred to a gynecologist.

In addition to hyperandrogenism, infertility and endometrial hyperplasia are common consequences of PCOS. Endometrial hyperplasia is due to continuous estrogen stimulation of the endometrium, unopposed by progesterone. This is a particularly worrisome problem because of the potential for progression to endometrial cancer.

Because the definitions of PCOS have varied, estimates of the prevalence of this disorder are also unclear. The clinical syndrome of hyperandrogenism with oligo- or amenorrhea is present in 1% to 4% of reproductive age women (Rosenfield, 1990). However, routine ultrasonographic screening of 257 young women not complaining of hyperandrogenism has demonstrated polycystic ovaries in 22% (Franks, 1995). All but one of the women with normal ovaries had regular menses, and 75% of the subjects with polycystic ovaries had irregular cycles (most of these women had no clinical or biochemical evidence of hyperandrogenism).

Any hypothesis concerning the fundamental defect(s) in PCOS should explain the various physical and biochemical manifestations of this syndrome (Table 28–2) (Balen et al, 1995). Hypothalamic, pituitary, ovarian, and adrenal abnormalities have all been postulated. Unquestionably, a genetic predisposition to PCOS exists, leading to one or more of the clinical features of PCOS. It is also clear that environmental factors such as weight gain can influence the expression of the disorder. These abnormalities are described individually in the following paragraphs with the goal of developing a unifying hypothesis for the pathogenesis of PCOS.

Hyperandrogenism

Women with PCOS typically have elevated levels of serum androgens (Fox et al, 1991). Free testosterone levels are elevated, in part from increased testosterone production and in part from decreased SHBG levels. Total serum testosterone is either in the upper normal range or elevated (normal <2.8 nmol/L [80 ng/dl]), and testosterone levels of 10 nmol/L or higher may be seen with severe PCOS. Similarly, serum androstenedione levels are high-normal or elevated.

Excess androgens in PCOS appear to arise from both the ovaries and adrenal glands (Rittmaster and Thompson, 1990). In general, the higher the serum level of testosterone, the greater the ovarian contribution to testosterone secretion (Rittmaster, 1996). However, adrenal hyperandrogenism is also present in many, but not all, women with PCOS, as documented by an increased adrenal androgen response to ACTH (Loughlin et al, 1986).

Several lines of evidence have contributed to our understanding of the pathophysiology of androgen excess in PCOS. GnRH analogs suppress serum testosterone, indicating that the ovarian hyperandrogenism is LH dependent (Rittmaster, 1993b). Ovulation induction also reduces serum LH and causes a rapid decrease in serum testosterone to levels seen with GnRH analogs (Blankstein et al, 1987). The enzyme primarily responsible for conversion of progesterone to androgens is the 17-hydroxylase/17,20-lyase enzyme complex (Fig. 28–4). Some investigators have postulated that increased activity of this enzyme is responsible for both the adrenal and ovarian hyperandrogenism and the development of PCOS (Ehrmann et al, 1995). If so, this is unlikely to

Table 28–2. PHYSICAL AND BIOCHEMICAL FEATURES OF PCOS*

Physical
  Obesity
  Hyperandrogenism
    Hirsutism
    Acne
    Male-pattern baldness
    Deepening of the voice
    Increased musculature
    Clitoral hypertrophy
  Oligo- or amenorrhea
  Enlarged, polycystic ovaries
  Acanthosis nigricans
Biochemical
  Elevated serum androgens (testosterone, androstenedione, DHEAS, androgen conjugates)
  Insulin resistance
  Decreased serum SHBG
  Elevated serum LH, normal serum FSH
  Low serum progesterone (anovulation)
  Normal or elevated serum estrogens
  Hyperlipidemia

*Not all features are found in all women with PCOS.

be an intrinsic enzyme defect, but rather the influence of extrinsic factors on the apparent enzyme activity. For example, the hyperinsulinemia associated with PCOS appears to increase 17-hydroxylase/17,20-desmolase enzyme activity. Lowering insulin levels with diazoxide (Nestler et al, 1991), metformin (Nestler and Jakubowicz, 1996), or troglitazone (Ehrmann et al, 1997b) is associated with a decrease in the apparent activity of this enzyme, although not all studies have found metformin to be efficacious in this regard (Ehrmann et al, 1997a). Insulin could either have a direct effect on enzyme activity or could decrease LH levels, leading to a secondary decrease in ovarian androgen production (Nestler and Jakubowicz, 1996).

The adrenal hyperandrogenism appears to be independent of ovarian androgen secretion, is not affected by ovarian suppression, and is present in hyperandrogenic women, regardless of menstrual status (Rittmaster and Thompson, 1990). Some authors have suggested that the adrenal hyperandrogenism can be explained by subtle enzyme deficiencies, similar to the more profound defects seen in CAH (Siegel et al, 1990). This hypothesis has largely been ruled out by the fact that mutations in the relevant genes have not been found in women with PCOS thought to exhibit such subtle defects in steroidogenesis. Furthermore, increased production of androgens, per se, may alter the normal ratios of precursors and products, giving the appearance of subtle enzyme defects. One study has shown that women with PCOS have an increase in the apparent activity of 11β-hydroxysteroid dehydrogenase, the enzyme responsible for metabolizing cortisol to cortisone (Rodin et al, 1994). This results in an increase in the cortisol clearance rate, leading to decreased negative feedback on ACTH secretion and a secondary increase in adrenal androgen secretion. In this study, obese women without PCOS also showed an increase in 11β-hydroxysteroid dehydrogenase activity, but not to the degree seen in weight-matched women with PCOS. It is tempting to hypothesize that hyperinsulinemia may be responsible for this increase in enzyme activity, leading to adrenal hyperandrogenism.

Hyperprolactinemia may also be a cause of adrenal hyperandrogenism in some women. Women with prolactinomas have elevated serum DHEA and DHEAS levels, and bromocryptine usually lowers the concentration of these steroids in women with marked hyperprolactinemia (Rittmaster and Loriaux, 1987). Although mild prolactin elevations (<50% increased) have been reported in up to 30% of women with PCOS (Corenblum, 1983), this hyperprolactinemia is more likely to be a result of the altered steroidal environment than a cause of it (Paoletti et al, 1995).

There has been a debate as to whether the ovarian and adrenal hyperandrogenism represents an intrinsic defect in each organ or whether the ovaries and adrenals are responding to the ambient hormonal milieu. The studies noted above provide evidence that extrinsic factors are modulating androgen production. The fact that normalization of serum LH with ovulation induction rapidly returns ovarian hormone secretion to normal argues against a primary ovarian enzyme defect (Blankstein et al, 1987). Glucocorticoid treatment can induce ovulatory cycles in some women with PCOS, suggesting that adrenal hyperandrogenism contributes to anovulation (Loughlin et al, 1986). Glucocorticoids can also enhance the ovulatory response to clomiphene in PCOS (Singh et al, 1992).

Hyperandrogenism alone can cause polycystic ovaries. This has been best demonstrated in female-to-male transsexuals given male levels of testosterone replacement (Spinder et al, 1989; Pache et al, 1991). In the study by Spinder et al, some features of polycystic ovaries developed in 25 of the 26 subjects, and 70% of the subjects met the pathologic criteria for polycystic ovaries. The analogy to PCOS is not completely appropriate, however, because the degree of testosterone elevation was much greater than is seen in PCOS.

Insulin Resistance, Obesity, Hyperlipidemia, and Hypertension

Most women with PCOS have insulin resistance when compared to weight-matched women without hyperandrogenism (Legro and Dunaif, 1996; Nestler, 1997). The insulin resistance persists even when ovarian androgens are suppressed with GnRH analogs (Dunaif et al, 1990; Lasco et al, 1995), suggesting that insulin resistance may be a cause of hyperandrogenism and not a consequence of increased androgens. The mechanism by which insulin resistance leads to the development of PCOS is probably multifactorial. Insulin stimulates androgen/steroid secretion from ovarian stroma, theca, and granulosa cells (Barbieri et al, 1986; Gilling-Smith et al, 1994; Willis et al, 1996). The results of insulin infusion studies in normal women and women with PCOS have been variable (see Legro and Dunaif, 1996, for review), probably because of the short-term duration of such studies. Suppression of insulin levels with diazoxide, metformin, or troglitazone in women with PCOS does lower serum testosterone (Nestler et al, 1989; Nestler and Jakubowicz, 1996; Ehrmann et al, 1997b), an effect that is not seen in normal women (Nestler et al, 1990). Insulin may enhance ovarian androgen secretion through a direct stimulation of the activity of steroidogenic enzymes such as the 17-hydroxylase/17,20-lyase enzyme complex (Nestler and Jakubowicz, 1996; Ehrmann et al, 1997b). Alternatively, insulin may enhance LH secretion and thereby stimulate ovarian steroidogenesis (Nestler and Jakubowicz, 1996). Adrenal androgen secretion is increased in women with PCOS, possibly as result of increased cortisol metabolism via the enzyme 11-hydroxysteroid dehydrogenase (Rodin et al, 1994), and insulin may be the factor responsible for enhanced activity of this enzyme. Hyperinsulinemia also decreases SHBG levels (Nestler, 1993). SHBG is formed in the liver, and insulin decreases SHBG secretion in hepatoma cells (Plymate et al, 1988). Although androgens themselves can lower serum SHBG concentrations, suppression of ovarian androgens in women with PCOS does not change SHBG levels (Nestler et al, 1991). However, the fall in insulin levels induced by a low-calorie diet in normal women and in women with PCOS is associated with an increase in serum SHBG levels (Kiddy et al, 1989).

Insulin resistance alone can cause PCOS. This is best demonstrated in women with the type A (decreased number and/or function of insulin receptors) or type B (insulin receptor antibodies) forms of severe insulin resistance, who develop the clinical and biochemical features of PCOS during their reproductive years (Taylor et al, 1982). In most women with PCOS, the reason for the insulin resistance is unknown. There does not appear to be any abnormality in the insulin receptor gene, and postreceptor defects have been postulated. These include abnormal phosphorylation of the insulin receptor and reduced expression of glucose transporters in adipocytes (Legro and Dunaif, 1996).

Insulin resistance in PCOS appears to result from a genetic predisposition to insulin resistance, made markedly worse by obesity. The familial predisposition to PCOS is well documented (Legro, 1995). Insulin resistance is common in relatives of PCOS women (Norman et al, 1996), and often there is a family history of non-insulin-dependent diabetes. In one twin study, although the ultrasound appearance of polycystic ovaries was often discordant among monozygotic and dizygotic twins, fasting insulin levels, body mass index, and adrenal androgen production (as assessed by androstanediol glucuronide levels) appeared to be under significant genetic regulation (Jahanfar et al, 1995). Thin women can have PCOS, but the severity of the insulin resistance and the hyperandrogenism tend to be greater in obese women with PCOS (Pasquali and Francesco, 1993). The increase in the degree of insulin resistance as a function of weight is much greater in women with PCOS than in hyperandrogenic women with regular menses or nonhirsute obese women (Rittmaster et al, 1993). Conversely, normalization of body weight in morbidly obese PCOS patients is associated with normalization of insulin sensitivity (Letiexhe et al, 1995), and weight loss alone can lead to ovulatory cycles (Bates and Whitworth, 1982; Harlass et al, 1984).

PCOS may well be the earliest manifestation of syndrome X (insulin resistance, upper body obesity, dyslipidemia, and hypertension, leading to coronary artery disease). Although the incidence of hypertension, hyperlipidemia, and diabetes is only mildly increased in young women with PCOS, retrospective studies have demonstrated that these risk factors are much more common in older women with a history of PCOS (Dahlgren et al, 1992a, 1992b). Insulin resistance may well be the cause of the increased incidence of these cardiovascular risk factors (Wild, 1995; Robinson et al, 1996), and hyperinsulinemia has also been shown to be an independent risk factor for ischemic heart disease (Despres et al, 1996).

Anovulation, Elevated Estrogens, and Abnormal Gonadotropin Secretion

Anovulation is the hallmark of PCOS, and it is inappropriate to make this diagnosis in a woman with regular, ovulatory cycles. Nevertheless, PCOS can vary in severity, and most women with PCOS will ovulate occasionally. Some women with the clinical features of PCOS will have regular menses at times, and anovulation at other times, with the periods of anovulation often coinciding with weight gain.

Anovulation in PCOS is associated with elevated estrone and free estradiol levels (Lobo et al, 1981). Because of the lack of ovarian cyclicity, the normal monthly variation in estrogen secretion is absent. In addition, increased adrenal androgen secretion may result in greater aromatization of androgens to estrogens by adipose tissue, causing elevated circulating estrogen levels. Although the total estradiol level is often normal in PCOS, the low serum SHBG concentration is associated with an elevated free estradiol level.

Anovulation and elevated LH levels are intimately linked in PCOS. About 70% of women with PCOS have an altered gonadotropin secretory pattern in which the ratio of LH to FSH is high and the midcycle gonadotropin surge is absent. Although these abnormalities in LH secretion have been offered as evidence for a primary hypothalamic defect in this condition, multiple lines of evidence suggest that the altered gonadotropin secretion is a result of the abnormal steroid milieu induced by anovulation and not the cause of it. For example, women with adrenal hyperandrogenism or an ovarian tumor may demonstrate this same gonadotropin abnormality, which is reversible when the hyperandrogenism is successfully treated (Dunaif et al, 1984). When ovulation is induced with gonadotropin administration in women with PCOS, LH levels rapidly return to normal, as does the LH response to exogenous GnRH (Blankstein et al, 1987). The abnormal gonadotropin secretory pattern resumes in these women after the subsequent cycle, if the cycle is anovulatory.

It has been postulated that the chronically elevated plasma estrogen levels seen in PCOS lead to the abnormal pattern of gonadotropin secretion and resulting anovulation. The antiestrogen clomiphene is able to induce ovulation in some women with PCOS. However, estradiol infusions suppress LH levels in both normal women and women with PCOS (Rebar et al, 1976), estrone infusions have no effect on LH secretion (Chang et al, 1982), and the aromatase inhibitor testolactone increases, rather than decreases, LH pulse amplitude and frequency (Dunaif et al, 1985). However, none of these studies addresses the concurrent problems of hyperestrogenism, hyperandrogenism, and insulin resistance, the combination of which may be required for the development of the abnormal gonadotropin secretory pattern.

The above discussion notwithstanding, some investigators postulate a primary hypothalamic defect in PCOS. Although increased LH pulse frequency has been reported by some authors in women with PCOS, a critical appraisal of this issue suggested that the elevated LH levels seen in PCOS result from increased LH pulse amplitude and not frequency (Kazer et al, 1987). A change in LH pulse frequency would suggest hypothalamic dysfunction, either primary or secondary to other factors. One widely quoted study demonstrated that four of five adolescents with PCOS had peak LH secretion during the daytime, rather than the typical nocturnal surge seen in normal adolescents (Zumoff et al, 1983). These investigators believed that these data supported a primary hypothalamic dysfunction as causing PCOS. However, this interpretation ignores the possible contribution of abnormal circulating androgen and estrogen levels to the LH secretory abnormality. Furthermore, LH pulse frequency during the early follicular phase of the adult menstrual cycle actually declines at night (Filicori et al, 1986). Normal adolescents may not be the appropriate control group for adolescent women with PCOS.

Sex steroid suppression of LH secretion involves both opioid and dopaminergic neurons (Seifer and Collins, 1990; Lanzone et al, 1995). A relative decrease in either dopaminergic or opioid tone has been postulated to cause the elevated LH levels seen in PCOS. In one study dopamine infusions suppressed serum LH (Barnes et al, 1986). In another study the dopamine agonist cabergoline decreased serum androgens and improved menstrual function in women with PCOS (Paoletti et al, 1996). Dopamine is a prolactin-inhibitory factor, and the mildly elevated prolactin levels seen in some women with PCOS suggest decreased dopaminergic tone in these women (Falaschi et al, 1986). More recent evidence, however, indicates that the elevated basal prolactin levels and the prolactin response to a dopamine antagonist are reversed by ovarian suppression, suggesting that the abnormal prolactin responses are secondary to abnormalities in ovarian function (Paoletti et al, 1995).

Opiate antagonists increase LH pulse frequency in normal women during the late follicular and luteal phases of the menstrual cycle, when endogenous estrogen and/or progesterone levels are high (Quigley and Yen, 1980). Although opiate deficiency has been postulated as a cause of increased LH secretion in PCOS, this concept has not received experimental support (Barnes and Lobo, 1985). In fact, long-term treatment with the opiate antagonist naltrexone decreased the LH response to GnRH and the insulin response to oral glucose in hyperinsulinemic patients with PCOS (Lanzone et al, 1995). However, there was no change in ovulatory status or ovarian

steroid levels in these patients, making uncertain the clinical significance of these observations.

Intraovarian Defects

Increased intraovarian androgens cause follicular atresia (Erickson et al, 1985; Daniel and Armstrong, 1986), which in turn leads to a greater mass of androgen-secreting stromal tissue. The ovaries in women with PCOS secrete more androstenedione in response to stimulation with a GnRH analog than do the ovaries of normal women (Ehrmann et al, 1992). Isolated theca cells from women with PCOS secrete more progesterone, 17-hydroxyprogesterone, and androstenedione than those from normal women, suggesting a generalized increase in steroidogenesis from the ovaries of women with PCOS (Gilling-Smith et al, 1994). Some authors have postulated intraovarian enzyme deficiencies as a cause of PCOS, and certainly 3β-HSD deficiency can affect both the ovaries and adrenal glands. However, the pattern of ovarian steroidogenesis in most women with PCOS suggests increased production of androgens without a specific enzyme *deficiency*.

17-Hydroxylase/17,20-lyase (CYP17) is the enzyme complex required specifically for the synthesis of androgens, and a "dysregulation" of this enzyme complex has been hypothesized to underlie the pathophysiology of PCOS (Ehrmann et al, 1995). Although preliminary data suggested a CYP17 polymorphism is associated with PCOS (Carey et al, 1994), more recent studies have been unable to replicate this finding (Liovic et al, 1997; Techatraisak et al, 1997). Any process that leads to an increase in ovarian or adrenal androgen secretion will give the appearance of an increase in the activity of this enzyme complex, simply because it is essential for androgen synthesis. Nevertheless, factors extrinsic to the ovary may directly or indirectly affect 17-hydroxylase/17,20-desmolase activity, leading to increased androgen production. Hyperinsulinemia is one factor that increases the apparent activity of this enzyme (Nestler and Jakubowicz, 1996). It is certainly possible that women with PCOS have a genetic defect in either the ovaries or adrenals that increases the response of these organs to extrinsic stimuli. For example, a polymorphism of the cholesterol side chain cleavage enzyme (CYP11a), which is an early step in steroid biosynthesis, has been associated with hirsutism and hyperandrogenism, although not with PCOS itself (Gharani et al, 1997). If confirmed, this finding suggests (but does not prove) that some women with PCOS are more prone to hyperandrogenism, based on a polymorphism of the CYP11a gene. Other factors, such as the severity of hyperinsulinism, must also contribute to the degree of hyperandrogenism. The fact that ovarian hyperandrogenism is rapidly reversed after ovulation indicates that ovarian hyperandrogenism is, in part, secondary to the increased LH secretion seen with hyperandrogenic anovulation, rather than a cause of it (Blankstein et al, 1987). Nevertheless, the beneficial effects of ovarian wedge resection or cauterization in some women with PCOS indicate that the ovary is not only reacting to the abnormal hormonal milieu, but also contributing in a fundamental way to the development of the syndrome.

Pathogenesis of PCOS—Summary and Hypothesis

PCOS is a heterogeneous syndrome, and multiple pathogenic mechanisms are possible. Nevertheless, the features common to most women with PCOS enable one to make predictions about the physiologic conditions leading to the development and maintenance of this disorder. These are summarized in Figure 28–11.

Most women with PCOS inherit a genetic predisposition to insulin resistance. Weight gain makes the degree of insulin resistance much worse and can lead to many of the other manifestations of this syndrome. The insulin resistance acts to magnify the androgenic milieu by suppressing SHBG and by stimulating ovarian androgen secretion. Adipose tissue itself may also directly contribute to the hyperandrogenism by converting precursors to active androgens. Most obese women are not hyperandrogenic and do not have PCOS, because they have not inherited the genetic predisposition to PCOS and are only mildly insulin resistant.

Severe hyperandrogenism alone (as in androgen-secreting neoplasms) can cause PCOS. More commonly, a combination of hyperandrogenism and insulin resistance contributes to the pathogenesis. Although the adrenal hyperandrogenism seen in PCOS may be due to a specific enzyme defect, more commonly it represents an increased secretion of adrenal androgen precursors and products, without evidence for an enzyme deficiency. It is tempting to postulate that hyperinsulinemia causes adrenal hyperandrogenism through stimulation of 11-hydroxysteroid dehydrogenase, which would lead to enhanced cortisol clearance.

The net effect of the increased androgenic milieu is to promote follicular atresia and to prevent ovulation. This resulting abnormal hormonal milieu of increased androgens, acyclic estrogen production (with elevated estrone and free estradiol levels), and low progesterone leads to increased LH and diminished follicle-stimulating hormone (FSH) secretion. These gonadotropin abnormalities further enhance stromal androgen production and decrease intraovarian aromatase, thereby increasing the intraovarian androgen:estrogen ratio and perpetuating the PCOS.

Many clinical observations can be explained by this proposed sequence of events:

1. Weight loss alone can lead to ovulation and diminished ovarian androgen secretion in some women with PCOS.
2. Adrenal suppression with glucocorticoids can induce ovulation in some women with PCOS and facilitate ovulation induction with clomiphene in others.

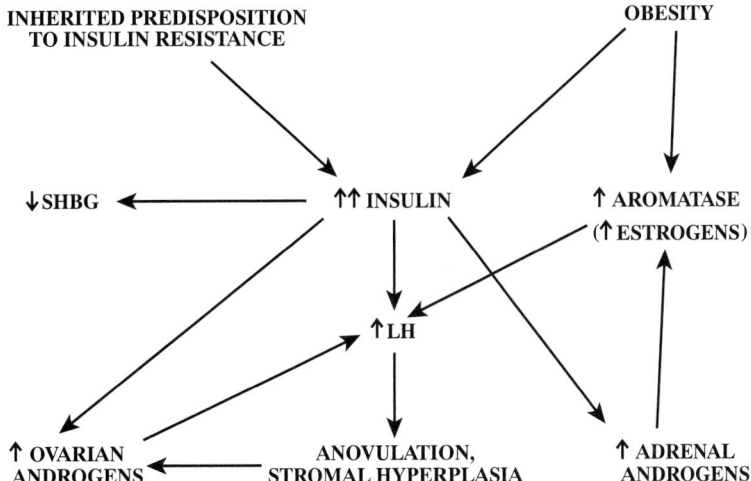

Figure 28–11

Hypothesized pathogenesis of polycystic ovarian syndrome. In this model, hyperinsulinemia is the central cause of PCOS, although increased production of androgens alone can cause the syndrome. In many patients an inherited predisposition to insulin resistance combines with obesity to cause marked insulin resistance. Hyperinsulinemia may augment androgens through at least three possible mechanisms: (1) stimulation of ovarian hyperandrogenism either through enhancing LH secretion or by stimulating 17-hydroxylase/17,20-lyase activity, (2) stimulation of adrenal hyperandrogenism through augmentation of 11-hydroxysteroid dehydrogenase activity, or (3) suppression of SHBG levels. Adipose tissue contains aromatase, the enzyme responsible for conversion of androgens to estrogens. The enhanced androgenic and estrogenic milieu leads to follicular atresia, anovulation, and tonically increased LH secretion, which further enhances ovarian androgen production.

3. GnRH analog treatment or ovulation induction will rapidly reverse the ovarian hyperandrogenism, but not the adrenal hyperandrogenism or the insulin resistance, and the ovarian hormonal abnormalities will recur once the treatment is stopped.
4. Reducing the mass of androgen-secreting ovarian tissue (wedge resection, ovarian cauterization, etc.) will permit ovulation in some women.

One group of women exists in whom the above pathogenic mechanisms are absent. An occasional anovulatory woman presents with normal to high-normal androgen levels, normal adrenal androgen responses to ACTH, normal estrogen levels, and no insulin resistance. Whether such a woman represents a variant of hypothalamic amenorrhea, very mild PCOS, a combination of the two, or a completely separate disorder is often difficult to determine.

Androgen-Secreting Neoplasms

Androgen-secreting ovarian and adrenal neoplasms are rare, accounting for much less than 1% of hyperandrogenism in women (Table 28–3). Such tumors should be ruled out in women who develop rapidly progressive signs of masculinization, although, if this begins during adolescence, PCOS is the usual cause (Friedman et al, 1985). Oligo/amenorrhea develops in reproductive-age women with androgen-secreting tumors, and postmenopausal women may present with vaginal bleeding (Surrey et al, 1988). The easiest method of screening for an androgen-secreting tumor is a serum testosterone level. Testosterone levels are usually above 5.2 nmol/L (150 ng/dl) and often are in the normal male range (>11 nmol/L) (Meldrum and Abraham, 1979). Nevertheless, lesser testosterone elevations in the appropriate clinical setting do not eliminate the diagnosis, and repeat testosterone measurements over time may be needed in questionable cases. A markedly elevated DHEAS level (>22 µmol/L [800 µg/dl]) is consistent with an adrenal neoplasm (usually a carcinoma), although pure androgen-secreting adrenal tumors do occur (Derksen et al, 1994). These tumors may be palpable on physical examination,

and can usually be seen on ovarian ultrasound or radiologically (adrenal computed tomography [CT] scan or magnetic resonance imaging [MRI]). A normal adrenal CT scan virtually rules out an adrenal tumor (Gabrilove et al, 1981); however, ovarian tumors may be too small to be visualized. Normalization of elevated testosterone levels during ovarian suppression (with OCs or GnRH analogs) or adrenal suppression (with glucocorticoids) does not rule out a neoplasm (Pascale et al, 1994). Adrenal cell rests may occur in the ovary, gonadal cells may be found in the adrenal, and ovarian tumors may aberrantly express glucocorticoid receptors. Hence, a rare ovarian tumor may be suppressible with glucocorticoids and a rare adrenal tumor may suppress with OCs. Similarly, stimulation of an adrenal cortical adenoma with human chorionic gonadotropin (hCG) was found to be due to the presence of hCG receptors in the adenoma (Leinonen et al, 1991). Selective ovarian and adrenal catheterization may localize the source of excess androgens but will not distinguish between functional disorders and neoplasms. Selective catheterization is difficult to accomplish, and, unless done by an experienced team, the results are often nondiagnostic (Surrey et al, 1988). Rarely, when the index of suspicion for an ovarian neoplasm is high, yet no tumor can be found, bilateral oophorectomy is indicated both diagnostically and therapeutically.

Androgen-Secreting Adrenal Tumors

These are adrenocortical neoplasms, of which about half are malignant. Because of the rarity of these neoplasms, large series are reported infrequently. Androgen-secreting adrenal tumors are most frequently recognized in children and young adults, although they can occur at any age (Gabrilove et al, 1981). Excess androgen secretion may occur alone or in combination with hypercortisolism or hyperaldosteronism. The pattern of steroid secretion from an adrenal neoplasm is dependent upon the enzymatic characteristics of the tumor. For example tumors deficient in 21-hydroxylase may cause virilization without glucocorticoid excess, and tumors high in aromatase may produce feminization (Freeman, 1986). Small tumors (less than 70 g) are usually benign, and larger tumors (>200 g) are more likely to be malignant (King and Lack, 1979; Richie and Gittes, 1980). Histologic features or the presence of metastases may distinguish between benign and malignant neoplasms in some individuals. In other cases, only the absence of metastases on long-term follow-up can differentiate between benign and malignant behavior.

When an adrenal tumor is suspected biochemically, an adrenal CT scan demonstrating a unilateral mass supports the diagnosis, and the absence of an adrenal mass on CT or MRI scanning essentially rules it out (tumors smaller than 1 cm may be missed, but such small tumors rarely produce enough androgen to cause virilization). The treat-

Table 28–3. ANDROGEN-SECRETING TUMORS

Adrenal
  Adrenocortical adenoma
  Adrenocortical carcinoma
Ovary
  Sex cord–stromal tumors
    Sertoli-Leydig cell tumors
      Mixed tumors
      Sertoli cell tumors (usually estrogenic)
      Leydig (hilus) cell tumors
    Granulosa-theca cell tumors (usually estrogenic)
  Luteoma of pregnancy

ment is surgical, except when extensive metastatic disease is present. However, aggressive resection of isolated metastases may permit extended survival in patients who otherwise have a poor prognosis. Cure is rare with metastatic adrenal cancer. Because adrenal carcinomas often produce hormones inefficiently, diagnosis is frequently delayed, and the cancer may be far advanced. However, virilization allows for an earlier diagnosis than is generally seen with nonsecreting adrenal carcinomas. Chemotherapy with op'DDD (mitotane) and 5-fluorouracil is helpful in less than half of these patients (Richie and Gittes, 1980; Freeman, 1986).

Androgen-Secreting Ovarian Tumors

The classification of these tumors is best understood in the context of ovarian/testicular embryology (Fox, 1985; Freeman, 1986) (Table 28–3). The primitive gonadal cells in the embryonic sex cords differentiate into granulosa cells in the ovary and Sertoli cells in the testes. Differentiation in either direction may be seen in ovarian tumors. Similarly, the stromal elements of these tumors may remain undifferentiated or develop into ovarian thecal cells or Leydig cells. Most hormone-secreting ovarian tumors are therefore broadly included under the classification of sex cord–stromal tumors, which can be subdivided into granulosa-theca cell tumors (which primarily secrete estrogens) and Sertoli-Leydig cell tumors (which primarily secrete androgens). This latter group was formerly termed arrhenoblastoma or androblastoma. Pure Sertoli or Leydig cells tumors do exist; the latter are often referred to as hilus cell tumors. A third group of sex cord–stromal tumors contain both thecal and Leydig cell elements and were formerly designated gynandroblastomas. Some hormone-secreting tumors, such as lipoid tumors, are difficult to classify histologically and may simply be poorly differentiated sex cord–stromal tumors. Finally, nonneoplastic ovarian abnormalities, including hyperthecosis and hilus cell hyperplasia (McLellan et al, 1990; Barth et al, 1997), may mimic androgen-secreting tumors. Luteomas of pregnancy, which cause recurrent hyperandrogenism during pregnancy, may or may not represent neoplasia (Shortle et al, 1987; McClamrock and Adashi, 1992).

Seventy-five to 80% of Sertoli-Leydig cell tumors are benign and are curable by surgical excision. The histologic grade may help to predict the likelihood of malignancy, although their benign nature can only be determined conclusively by the absence of metastases on long-term follow-up. Eighty per cent of these tumors are greater than 5 cm in diameter and should be detectable on pelvic exam. They are diagnosed most commonly during the reproductive years, although they can occur in any age group beyond infancy. Hyperandrogenism occurs in at least 75% of patients.

Pure Leydig (hilus) cell tumors are rare, almost always benign, and often small. Occasionally they may be undetectable even by ultrasound or diagnostic laparoscopy, their presence being suspected clinically or by selective venous catheterization and confirmed histologically after oophorectomy. They are most common in postmenopausal women. Hilus cell hyperplasia mimics hilus cell tumors and can only be differentiated pathologically, although serum androgens in women with hilus cell hyperplasia are uniformly normalized by ovarian suppression (McLellan et al, 1990).

Some women note worsening hirsutism during pregnancy. Virilization is rare, and is usually due to a luteoma of pregnancy or hyperreactio luteinalis (Shortle et al, 1987; McClamrock and Adashi, 1992). Whether these are actually different conditions is unknown. Luteomas are benign solid tumors or hyperplastic lesions consisting of luteinized ovarian cells of uncertain origin. They typically regress postpartum, only to recur with subsequent pregnancies or hCG stimulation. Most are nonsecretory and asymptomatic. Those that secrete androgens may cause virilization not only of the mother, but also of a female fetus. Elevated testosterone levels return to normal postpartum.

EVALUATION OF HYPERANDROGENISM

The evaluation of the hyperandrogenic woman includes a medical history, physical examination, and the judicious use of laboratory and other ancillary resources. The purpose of the medical evaluation is threefold: (1) to confirm and document the severity of the hyperandrogenism, (2) to rule out serious underlying disorders, and (3) to recommend appropriate treatments. Most hyperandrogenic women will not have a serious underlying disorder, but the uncommon causes of androgen excess should always be considered (Table 28–1). Rarely is an extensive evaluation necessary.

Medical History

The most important part of the medical history is determining the patient's chief complaint and how it affects her life. Although this may seem an obvious point, the physician's and patient's perception of a problem may be quite different. For example, once a serious underlying problem is ruled out, some women are unconcerned about severe hirsutism and others may be distraught over normal female patterns of body hair growth. A woman with PCOS may be pleased with lack of menses, and the risks of endometrial hyperplasia and cancer will need to be carefully explained. If a hyperandrogenic woman complains primarily of irregular menses or infertility, the extent of associated problems, such as acne, hirsutism, alopecia, deepening of the voice, and changes in libido, should be elicited. The psychological aspects of hyperandrogenism must be addressed and adequate support provided.

Beyond a routine medical history, important historical points include the onset and rate of progression of hyperandrogenism; treatment methods used to control the problem; menstrual history; drug history, including OC use; history of obesity; personal or family history of diabetes; and family history of similar hyperandrogenic problems.

Benign forms of hyperandrogenism usually begin around puberty. Nonclassical CAH may present with premature adrenarche or the early onset of menses, but more often is indistinguishable from simple hirsutism or PCOS. Although PCOS and hirsutism usually start during adolescence, the onset may occur after a period of weight gain later in life. Early OC use may delay the onset of hyperandrogenism or slow the rate of progression.

Women (and men) develop more body hair with age (Ferriman and Gallwey, 1961). Facial hair can increase indefinitely, whereas body hair usually decreases starting in the fifth decade. Thus, most hirsute women notice a gradual progression of hair growth over time. Rapidly progressive hirsutism may develop during adolescence in women with PCOS or nonclassical CAH. Rapidly progressive hirsutism or the onset of hirsutism before or after adolescence also raises the possibility of Cushing's syndrome or an androgen-secreting neoplasm. These entities can be ruled out by simple laboratory tests (see below).

Women with regular menses almost always have a benign form of hirsutism. Cushing's syndrome and androgen-secreting tumors generally cause oligo- or amenorrhea. Nevertheless, most women with hirsutism and irregular menses will have PCOS.

A complete drug history should be obtained. Occasionally physicians prescribe androgen-containing compounds for postmenopausal hormone replacement or to treat loss of libido. Female athletes using anabolic steroids may be reluctant to admit to androgen use. Although drug manuals list OCs as a cause of hirsutism, the progression of hirsutism during OC use is most likely due to inadequate ovarian suppression and/or persistence of adrenal androgen secretion.

Scalp hair loss or deepening of the voice are often considered signs of virilization. Nevertheless, women with normal testosterone levels and a family history of male-pattern baldness may report scalp hair loss. Although marked deepening of the voice (in the absence of hypothyroidism or acromegaly) suggests severe hyperandrogenism, slight changes in pitch can be seen with less severe androgen excess and will be noticed by female vocalists.

A family history of hirsutism or PCOS suggests a benign etiology. Interestingly, women with late-onset forms of CAH often have a negative family history, because these are autosomal recessive disorders and heterozygous women do not have an increased incidence of hirsutism (Knochenhauer et al, 1997). Women with PCOS often have a positive family history of diabetes, a manifestation of the familial nature of the insulin resistance.

If hirsutism is the presenting complaint, the mechanical methods used to treat the hirsutism should be carefully documented. If a woman shaves, how often? If she plucks the excess hairs or uses electrolysis, how often and for how many minutes? This type of documentation will allow the physician to assess whether improvement is occurring in response to medical therapy; it is more sensitive and may be more accurate than hirsutism scoring.

Physical Examination

The physical examination is important to assess the severity of hyperandrogenism, confirm adequate estrogenization by inspection or cytologic evaluation of the vaginal mucosa, and rule out ovarian and adrenal neoplasms. Women with PCOS may or may not have palpably enlarged ovaries, but, when present, the enlargement should be bilateral. Most ovarian tumors will present as a unilateral mass on bimanual examination. Adrenal adenomas are not palpable, but many carcinomas will be felt on careful abdominal examination. Although androgen-secreting tumors may be palpable on physical examination, the diagnosis usually depends on markedly elevated testosterone levels and the demonstration of a mass radiologically (see below).

Androgen-dependent hirsutism can be diagnosed on physical examination. If a woman develops terminal hair growth in areas where men typically become hirsute, she has androgen-dependent hirsutism. In contrast, drug-induced hirsutism (other than that caused by exogenous androgens) consists of an increased growth of long, fine hairs, that is not restricted to androgen-dependent areas of the body.

The amount and distribution of hair can be used as an index of androgen effect. The rapid onset of severe hirsutism, other than during adolescence, suggests an androgen-secreting ovarian or adrenal tumor. Although terminal hairs on the upper lip, around the areola, and over the lower abdomen are normal, hair growth over the upper back and upper abdomen suggests more severe hyperandrogenism. Nevertheless, the pattern of hair distribution is variable among hirsute women, and all degrees of hirsutism may be seen in benign forms of hyperandrogenism. Similarly, the clitoris is an androgen-responsive tissue, and varying degrees of clitoral enlargement are common in hirsute women (Tagatz et al, 1979).

The amount and distribution of hair can also be used as a semiquantitative means of assessing response to medical therapy. The most common technique used is the method of Ferriman and Gallwey (1961), which scores the amount and distribution of body hair on a scale of 1 to 4 in 11 different body areas. Unfortunately, it takes practice to be consistent with any scoring system, and interobserver variability is high.

The presence of Cushing's syndrome may be suspected by history and physical examination. Physical features suggestive of Cushing's syndrome include central obesity, increased dorsocervical and supraclavicular fat, facial plethora, hypertension, thin skin and easy bruising, striae, and proximal muscle weakness.

Laboratory Evaluation

The laboratory evaluation of hyperandrogenism is directed at ruling out serious underlying disorders and determining the cause of chronic anovulation (Table 28–4). Hormonal measurements are unnecessary to determine whether hirsutism is androgen dependent, because this can be accomplished by physical examination. Furthermore, androgen-dependent hirsutism can occur in women with normal androgen levels. Women with PCOS should have a fasting blood glucose determination to screen for diabetes and a lipid profile to screen for dyslipidemia.

In the past, physicians have expended much effort trying to determine the relative ovarian and adrenal contribution to excess androgen secretion in hirsute women. Although this approach may have been valid when the only medical therapies for hirsutism were OCs and glucocorticoids, the superiority of antiandrogens as a treatment has simplified the diagnostic approach. Because both adrenal and ovarian hyperandrogenism respond well to antiandrogens, the relative contribution of each of these organs to androgen secretion in an individual hirsute woman becomes less important.

In women with a benign history, mild to moderate hirsutism, no physical signs of Cushing's syndrome, and regular ovulatory menstrual cycles (as assessed by the presence of moliminal symptoms), a hormonal evaluation is not needed. In such a woman, the chance of a serious underlying cause of hirsutism is negligible. Although nonclassical CAH may exist

in such a woman (the approximate frequency is 1% of hirsute women), the hirsutism responds better to antiandrogens than to glucocorticoids (Spritzer et al, 1990).

In hyperandrogenic women with irregular menses, the hormonal evaluation is straightforward. In most cases serum testosterone, prolactin, 17-hydroxyprogesterone, and possibly LH and/or FSH levels are all that are necessary. A total serum *testosterone* less than 5.2 nmol/L (150 ng/dl) makes an androgen-secreting tumor unlikely. Although testosterone levels up to 12 nmol/L can be seen with PCOS or severe insulin resistance (Taylor et al, 1982), the higher the testosterone level, the more concerned the physician should be. A testosterone level should be repeated in 6 months in any woman with worsening hirsutism to ensure that it is not increasing. In PCOS, testosterone levels are either in the upper normal range or elevated ($\geq$1.8 nmol/L). Lower testosterone levels should make one reconsider the diagnosis, unless ovulation has recently occurred. Because SHBG is suppressed, free (unbound) testosterone levels are elevated in PCOS, but measurement of SHBG or free testosterone will not change the diagnosis or alter therapy.

Serum *prolactin* should be measured in women with irregular menses to rule out a prolactinoma. Mild elevations (<50% above normal) can be seen in PCOS; higher levels raise the possibility of a prolactinoma. Elevated prolactin levels do not cause hirsutism but can cause amenorrhea. Serum *17-hydroxyprogesterone* is measured to screen for 21-hydroxylase deficiency, the most common cause of CAH (Fig. 28–10).

Measurement of serum *LH and FSH* levels helps to support the diagnosis of PCOS and rule out other etiologies of amenorrhea. An elevated LH:FSH ratio is seen in many, but not all, women with PCOS. However, the pulsatile nature of LH secretion may cause an erroneous interpretation if only single values are obtained. An elevated LH:FSH ratio is ex-

Table 28–4. HORMONAL EVALUATION OF HYPERANDROGENISM*

Ovulatory menses, mild to moderate hirsutism	Routine hormonal evaluation not needed
Oligo/amenorrhea, mild to severe hirsutism	
Testosterone (nmol/L)	
<1.8	PCOS unlikely
1.8–12	Consistent with PCOS
$\geq$6	Rule out androgen-secreting tumor (adrenal CT, ovarian ultrasound)
Prolactin (μg/L; see Chapter 29)	
<30	Consistent with PCOS
>50	Suspicious for prolactinoma
LH and FSH	
↑LH, normal FSH	Consistent with PCOS
normal LH and FSH	Nondiagnostic
↑LH and FSH	Consistent with ovarian failure
low LH and FSH	Consistent with hypothalamic/pituitary dysfunction
17-Hydroxyprogesterone (see Fig. 28–10)	

*These guidelines represent a minimal evaluation for the routine hyperandrogenic woman. If the history suggests rapidly progressive hyperandrogenism, a more extensive evaluation is indicated. Unless one is willing to use glucocorticoids as a treatment, routine measurement of serum DHEAS and routine ACTH stimulation tests are unnecessary (see text).

pected with an ovulatory LH surge. Elevated FSH levels suggest ovulatory failure as a cause of amenorrhea. Low or low normal LH and FSH levels in an anovulatory woman suggest primary or hypothalamic dysfunction.

Serum *DHEAS* and *androstanediol glucuronide* are unnecessary as screening tests in hirsute women. DHEAS is not an androgen itself. An elevated level is consistent with adrenal hyperandrogenism, but, unless it is markedly elevated, it is unhelpful in the differential diagnosis of hyperandrogenism. It is usually normal in women with nonclassical 21-hydroxylase deficiency (Kuttenn et al, 1985). Elevated levels do not necessarily predict a response to glucocorticoid treatment. In women suspected of having an androgen-secreting tumor, markedly elevated DHEAS levels (>22 μmol/L [800 μg/dl]) suggest an adrenal source, although pure testosterone-secreting adrenal neoplasms do occur. Androstanediol glucuronide has been reported to be an index of androgen effect on the hair follicle (Kirschner et al, 1987; Lookingbill et al, 1988), although it is more likely to be a consequence of increased adrenal androgen secretion (see "Androgen Metabolism" section). Even as a marker of androgen action in the skin, it would add nothing to what is apparent on physical examination.

Ovarian ultrasound is also unnecessary as a screening test in hirsute women. Ovarian cysts can be seen in hirsute women with or without oligo/amenorrhea, and their presence or absence will not influence treatment.

When an androgen-secreting tumor is suspected, ovarian ultrasound and adrenal CT or MRI scanning is essential. Virtually all androgen-secreting adrenal tumors will be visualized. Although most ovarian neoplasms will be visible on transabdominal or transvaginal ultrasound, an occasional ovarian tumor will require catheterization studies to document the source of hyperandrogenism. Lack of suppression of ovarian hyperandrogenism with OCs or GnRH analogs, or lack of suppression of adrenal hyperandrogenism with dexamethasone, is consistent with a neoplasm. However, androgen suppression with these maneuvers does not rule out an androgen-secreting tumor.

TREATING THE HYPERANDROGENIC WOMAN

General Principles

Treatment of hyperandrogenism must be carefully tailored to the individual patient. For some women, the cutaneous manifestations (hirsutism, acne, or male-pattern baldness) may be the major problem. Other women may be primarily concerned with irregular menses or infertility. Associated conditions such as obesity and diabetes should be evaluated. In some obese women the hyperandrogenism and associated ovulatory dysfunction will ameliorate with weight loss. Women with PCOS and hirsutism may have psychological difficulties caused by their hyperandrogenism, and appropriate guidance should be provided. Frequently many of these concerns coexist.

Oligo/amenorrhea

All women with oligo/amenorrhea should be treated to prevent endometrial hyperplasia and cancer, if they ovulate less than about once every 2 months. In women who do not desire immediate fertility, either OCs or the cyclic administration of a progestin may be used. Because most women with PCOS do ovulate intermittently, OCs offer the advantage of both reducing ovarian hyperandrogenism and preventing conception (see following section on "Hirsutism"). Alternatively, medroxyprogesterone acetate (Provera) may be given, 5 mg daily for 12 to 14 days every 1 to 2 months.

Infertility

This topic is discussed in detail in other chapters. The treatment of choice for initial attempts at ovulation induction in PCOS is clomiphene citrate, and the majority of patients with PCOS will ovulate with this medication. Exogenous gonadotropins, or a combination of a GnRH analog followed by pulsatile GnRH administration, may be useful alternatives in clomiphene-resistance patients. Surgical options include ovarian wedge resection, which has fallen into disfavor because of the development of adhesions, and elctrocautery or laser vaporization of the ovarian capsule.

Hirsutism

Although hirsutism rarely is a manifestation of a serious underlying disorder, it can be a major cosmetic problem for women. Because hirsutism is not a disease in itself, the benefits and risks of any therapy must be carefully weighted. Nevertheless, hirsutism frequently becomes gradually worse with age, and effective treatments are available.

Mechanical Treatments

Mechanical methods of hair removal may successfully remove visible hair, although the underlying hormonal milieu is unchanged, and hair regrowth can be expected (Wagner, 1990). For mild hirsutism, bleaching and mechanical hair removal is adequate and safe. Because little scientific research has been published concerning the different methods of mechanical hair removal, misconceptions and false hopes are common.

Bleaching is most effective for increased fine (vellus) hair growth. Commercial preparations are available using hydrogen peroxide and are applied as a paste with a swab stick for periods of 15 to 30 minutes. Bleaching can be done as frequently as necessary, but skin irritation is a common problem with prolonged or excessive use. A 1% hydrocortisone cream may minimize the irritation. Bleaching of very dark hair may not totally remove the color.

Shaving is the easiest and safest method of temporarily removing visible hairs. Unfortunately, shaving of facial hair is often considered socially unacceptable for women. Shaving does not increase the rate of hair growth (Lynfield and MacWilliams, 1970), nor will it adversely affect the benefits of medical therapy. It improves the efficiency of electrolysis because the electrologist will only be removing actively growing hairs (Richards and Meharg, 1991). If the hair is sufficiently coarse, a stubble may result. Nevertheless, shaving results in an improved cosmetic appearance in virtually all hirsute women.

Plucking can effectively control mild hirsutism. Although it may also be effective for more severe hirsutism, the amount of time involved can be enormous. It is also painful. Plucking can result in folliculitis, scarring, and thickening of the skin in susceptible women. It does not slow the rate of hair growth, although there is also no evidence that it increases hirsutism.

Waxing is equivalent to mass plucking and has all of the possible side effects and complications of plucking. Nevertheless, some women find occasional waxing effective in controlling large areas of fine hair growth.

Chemical depilatory creams dissolve hairs above the skin. The result is similar to shaving, although there may be less of a stubble. The heavier the hair, the longer the cream must remain on the skin. Skin irritation is common and often necessitates discontinuation of treatment. A 1% hydrocortisone cream may lessen the irritation.

Electrolysis usually involves using shortwave thermolysis to produce locally high temperatures, which cause electrocoagulation of the hair follicle. Occasionally, a blend of shortwave and galvanic current is used to treat more resistant coarse hairs (Richards and Meharg, 1991). Electrolysis can effectively control mild to moderate hirsutism and is a useful adjunct to medical treatment in more severe cases. When combined with medical therapy, a more rapid improvement in the hirsutism can be expected. Although electrolysis is advertised as being permanent, 15% to 50% of women experience regrowth of hair after variable lengths of time (Wagner, 1990). It is unclear whether this regrowth is due to recruitment of new hair follicles or failure to destroy the hair follicles that have undergone electrolysis. Usually, electrolysis is only mildly uncomfortable, with little resulting erythema and no scarring. However, some patients are more sensitive to the discomfort and skin irritation associated with electrolysis, and ex-

cessive electrolysis can lead to skin thickening and scarring. There is no mandatory regulation or licensing of electrologists, and technical skill varies widely. As a general rule, referrals should only be directed to electrologists who have had formal training and are members of local self-regulating organizations. Electrolysis can be time-consuming and expensive.

Medical Treatments

Drug treatment is directed at suppressing ovarian or adrenal sources of androgens, or blocking androgen action in the skin (Table 28–5). Successful medical therapy results in a gradual return of terminal hair to finer, less pigmented, vellus hair. Although young women may respond best to medical treatment, a beneficial response can be expected in a majority of women regardless of age, severity of hirsutism, or serum hormone levels (Crosby and Rittmaster, 1991). Progression of hirsutism can be prevented in nearly all women, and complete resolution is possible in some patients. Complete resolution is uncommon, however, in women with severe hirsutism. Therefore, physicians should not be reluctant to institute medical therapy in young, mildly hirsute adolescents, who have a family history of moderate to severe hirsutism. Drug treatment is not a cure, and lifelong therapy may be necessary to prevent recurrence. Longstanding hair growth on the chin may be especially difficult to improve, and, at times, appears to be unresponsive to androgen blockade. In some women androgens must be suppressed to below normal or blocked with a combination of medications to cause an improvement. Generally, 6 months is needed to judge the efficacy of a given therapy. Improvement may continue indefinitely, or the hirsutism may stabilize after a period of initial improvement. The concurrent use of mechanical hair removal hastens the response to medical therapy. No drug is currently approved by regulatory agencies in the United States or Canada for treatment of hirsutism.

OVARIAN SUPPRESSION

Oral Contraceptives. OCs are designed to prevent ovulation by suppressing gonadotropin levels. Al-

Table 28–5. MEDICAL TREATMENTS OF HIRSUTISM

Ovarian suppression
 Oral contraceptives
 GnRH analogs
Adrenal suppression
 Glucocorticoids
 Ketoconazole (not recommended)
Antiandrogens
 Spironolactone
 Cyproterone acetate
 Flutamide
 5α-Reductase inhibitors (investigational)

though the original high-dose estrogen-progestin formulations caused marked gonadotropin suppression and were an effective treatment of hirsutism, the newer low-dose formulations often have only a modest effect on basal LH levels (Murphy et al, 1990). OCs also decrease adrenal androgen production, and estrogens have a direct effect on the liver to increase SHBG (Coenen et al, 1996). The result is a reduction in free testosterone levels. Progestins differ in their androgenicity (Darney, 1995) and, consequently, their effects on lipids (LaRosa, 1995). Progestins with little or no androgenicity (desogestrel, gestodine, and norgestimate) have become available in the last several years and theoretically would be better for the treatment of hirsutism. In addition, the more potent the progestational activity of an OC, the greater the suppression of LH and testosterone. On a theoretical basis, the best OC for hirsute women would be one that contains a potent antiandrogenic progestin, such as cyproterone acetate. Alternatively, OCs containing 150 μg of desogestrel combine potent progestational activity with relative lack of androgenicity.

How effective are low-dose birth control pills in treating hirsutism? No well-designed studies have been published to address this question. Uncontrolled studies have suggested that low-dose OCs are an effective treatment for hirsutism. Much controversy surrounds this issue, however, and negative studies tend not to be published. Two controlled studies with objective assessment of hirsutism found no significant improvement in hirsutism with OCs alone (Azziz et al, 1995; Heiner et al, 1995). Because hirsutism often becomes gradually worse with time, a majority of women probably achieve a modest beneficial effect on their hair growth with OCs alone. Nevertheless, results with OCs alone are frequently disappointing.

What recommendations can be given regarding the use of OCs in hirsute women? For women with PCOS and elevated testosterone levels, an OC with a potent, nonandrogenic progestin is useful to decrease circulating androgens. OCs containing 150 μg of desogestrel are the best in this regard, although there is controversy regarding a possibly increased risk of venous thrombosis with such preparations (Farmer et al, 1997). An alternative is to add cyproterone acetate to a low-progestin OC (see section on "Cyproterone Acetate"). Antiandrogens such as spironolactone can also be added to improve the efficacy of the OC.

GnRH Analogs. GnRH analogs decrease ovarian hormone secretion by suppressing LH and FSH. Because GnRH analogs all have the same mechanism of action, their effectiveness at suppressing ovarian hormone secretion depends upon the relative potency, dose, and route of administration. In sufficient dose, all should be equally effective (Rittmaster, 1995).

The use of GnRH analogs for the treatment of ovarian hyperandrogenism has been reviewed (Adashi, 1990; Rittmaster, 1993b). Because GnRH analogs have no effect on adrenal androgen secretion, their ability to suppress serum androgen levels in a given patient depends on what proportion of androgen secretion arises from the ovary. GnRH analogs work best in those hirsute women with elevated testosterone and androstenedione levels and the clinical features of PCOS (Fig. 28–12) (Rittmaster and Thompson, 1990). Women with regular menses tend to have a greater proportion of serum androgens arising from the adrenal glands and respond less well to ovarian suppression.

On a practical level, GnRH analogs are not an ideal treatment for the average hirsute woman. They are expensive, must be given parenterally, and are associated with hot flushes and other symptoms of estrogen deficiency when used alone. They also cause a loss of bone mass as a result of estrogen deficiency. However, in severely hirsute women with elevated testosterone levels and the clinical features of PCOS, they may allow a favorable response to therapy where nothing else works. However, an equally efficacious approach to androgen suppression is to add cyproterone acetate to an OC (see below). Because the goal of therapy is to suppress androgens, and not estrogens, estrogen and progesterone replacement can be added to GnRH analogs (Rittmaster and Thompson, 1990; Azziz et al, 1995; Heiner et al, 1995). Symptoms of estrogen deficiency can thus be avoided. It also makes theoretical sense

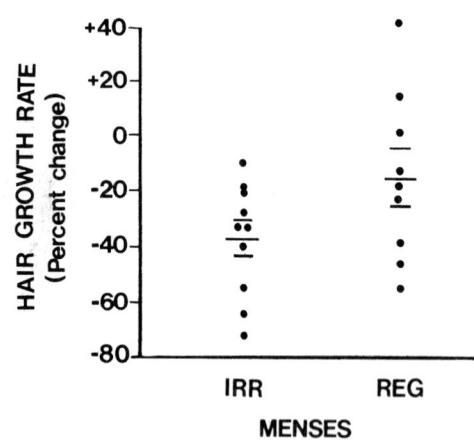

Figure 28–12

Changes in hair growth in hirsute women after 5 to 6 months of treatment with the GnRH analog leuprolide. Hair growth was measured by serially shaving an area of hirsutism and weighing the shaved hairs. Mean ± standard error is shown with bars. Women with irregular menses (IRR), who had the clinical features of polycystic ovary syndrome, responded better than women with regular menses (REG) (p = 0.07). The per cent decrease in serum androstenedione correlated best with changes in hair growth (r = .66; p = 0.002). (From Rittmaster RS, Thompson DL: Effect of leuprolide and dexamethasone on hair growth and hormone levels in hirsute women: the relative importance of the ovary and the adrenal in the pathogenesis of hirsutism. J Clin Endocrinol Metab 1990;70:1096, with permission. © by The Endocrine Society.)

to add an antiandrogen to GnRH analogs to block adrenal androgens. I have seen favorable responses by adding spironolactone to GnRH analog therapy in women who did not respond adequately to a GnRH analog alone.

The long-term effects of GnRH analogs are unknown, and this is a concern of physicians treating children with precocious puberty (Brauner et al, 1994). Normal ovulatory function occurs within 2 years of cessation of treatment in most girls treated long term with GnRH analogs for precocious puberty (Kavli et al, 1990). Over the next decade, data on the fertility potential of such women should become available. Hirsute women generally return to their pretreatment menstrual status within several months of stopping GnRH analogs. Hence, analog treatment does not appear to alter the fundamental mechanisms underlying the development of PCOS.

ADRENAL SUPPRESSION: GLUCOCORTICOIDS

Glucocorticoids were the first medical treatment for hirsutism. Their use is based on the knowledge that adrenal androgen precursors are increased in many hirsute women, whether or not an increase in ovarian androgens is also present. Although some women do achieve a reduction in hair growth with glucocorticoids, at present their use is controversial.

Glucocortocoids suppress not only adrenal androgens but also cortisol synthesis. Investigators have attempted to find a type and dose of glucocorticoid that would selectively suppress adrenal androgens. Unfortunately, clinically meaningful differences in the suppression of adrenal androgens and cortisol have not been found. This has led to a wide range of treatments, including 10 to 20 mg hydrocortisone or 2.5 to 5 mg prednisone nightly (or divided into A.M. and P.M. doses) or 0.25 to 0.5 mg dexamethasone nightly. The lower the dose, the less androgen suppression and the less chance for a beneficial response. The higher the dose, the greater is the risk of side effects of glucocorticoid excess (weight gain, nocturia, glucose intolerance, etc.). Spritzer et al (1990) compared the efficacy of hydrocortisone and cyproterone acetate (an antiandrogen) in reducing hair growth in women with nonclassical (late-onset) CAH. These are women who have a well-defined excess of adrenal androgens, and yet cyproterone acetate caused a greater reduction in hair growth than did hydrocortisone after 1 year of treatment.

Difficulties with the use of glucocorticoids to treat hirsutism are well documented. Low doses are ineffective, and higher doses are associated with weight gain, nocturia, and occasionally even more marked signs of Cushing's syndrome (Emans et al, 1988; Rittmaster and Givner, 1988; Rittmaster and Thompson, 1990). An additional problem with glucocorticoids is that about 10% to 20% of women will develop drug-induced hirsutism. Because of these problems, and the superior results with antiandro-

gens, glucocorticoids should not be used for the routine treatment of hirsutism. This is true even for women with nonclassical 21-hydroxylase deficiency, if hirsutism is the only reason for treatment.

ANTIANDROGENS

Antiandrogens competitively inhibit binding of testosterone and DHT to the androgen receptor. The three antiandrogens most widely used in North America are spironolactone, cyproterone acetate (Canada and Mexico only), and flutamide (Fig. 28–13). Their relative affinities (compared to DHT) for the human androgen receptor are: spironolactone 67%, cyproterone acetate 12.5%, and flutamide 0.08% (Eil and Edelson, 1984). However, other factors, including metabolic clearance rates, dose, and other hormonal effects, influence the efficacy of the antiandrogens. Assuming sufficient medication can be given, they all should be about equally effective. Hence, the decision as to which antiandrogen to use should be based on cost, side effects, and likelihood of compliance. Although each antiandrogen has its strong proponents, who vociferously proclaim it to be better than any other, few prospective, randomized trials with objective end points have compared antiandrogens. The published studies generally have found no significant differences in efficacy (O'Brien

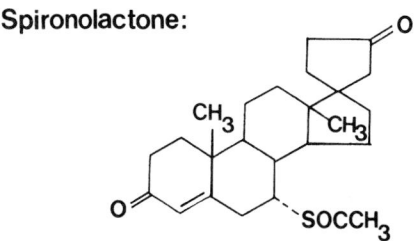

Figure 28–13
Structures of three antiandrogens used to treat hirsutism.

et al, 1991). General agreement does exist that antiandrogens are the medical treatment of choice for most hirsute women.

Spironolactone. Spironolactone is an aldosterone antagonist originally marketed for treating hypertension (Loriaux et al, 1976). After it was observed that some hirsute women taking this medication experienced decreased body hair growth, numerous studies demonstrated its efficacy in the treatment of hirsutism (Barth et al, 1989; Crosby and Rittmaster, 1991). Further research has shown that spironolactone is a potent antiandrogen, a weak progestin, and a weak inhibitor of testosterone biosynthesis. These latter two activities lead to a modest decrease in serum testosterone levels at moderate to high doses.

Although as much as 400 mg daily has been used to treat hirsutism, more commonly 25 to 100 mg twice daily is prescribed. One study suggests that efficacy is improved with higher doses, but side effects are also more frequent (Lobo et al, 1985). Some physicians prescribe spironolactone for only the first 3 weeks of the menstrual cycle, in an attempt to avoid the side effect of irregular menses. However, the incidence of irregular menses is no greater with continuous daily dosing, and the efficacy should be improved when androgens are blocked throughout the menstrual cycle.

Taking all studies together, at least a modest improvement in hirsutism can be anticipated in 70% to 80% of women who use at least 100 mg spironolactone per day for 6 months. In women with regular menses, the addition of an OC to spironolactone does not significantly increase the response rate (Crosby and Rittmaster, 1991). In women with PCOS, the combination of spironolactone and an OC is better than spironolactone alone (Fig. 28–14).

Numerous trials of topical spironolactone have been attempted. The fact that the vast majority of these studies have not been reported attests to the generally poor results with this approach. On a theoretical basis, topical applications of antiandrogens should be useful; however, finding an effective and cosmetically acceptable vehicle has proved difficult.

The most common side effect of spironolactone is increased frequency of menses. This occurs in at least 20% of women with regular menstrual cycles who are not taking an OC and often results in women having menses every 2 weeks. The pathophysiology of this side effect has not been elucidated. It usually can be treated successfully either by reducing the dose of spironolactone or by adding an OC. Nausea and fatigue can occur with high doses of spironolactone (200 to 400 mg daily). Less than 10% of women on low doses have these complaints. Although spironolactone has not been reported to cause feminization of a male fetus (Groves and Corenblum, 1995), this certainly is a theoretical possibility, and all antiandrogens should be avoided during pregnancy. As an aldosterone antagonist, spironolactone can raise serum potassium and should be avoided in women with hyperkalemia or renal insufficiency. It is pru-

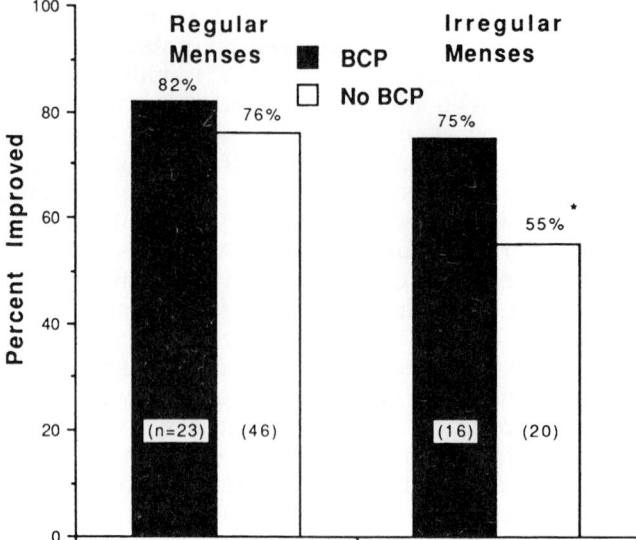

Figure 28–14
Response to spironolactone in hirsute women as a function of menstrual status and oral contraceptive use. Women with irregular menses (oligo/amenorrhea), who did not use an oral contraceptive, were less likely to respond to spironolactone treatment (*$p = 0.08$ versus the other three groups combined). BCP, birth control pill. (From Crosby PDA, Rittmaster RS: Predictors of clinical response in hirsute women treated with spironolactone. Fertil Steril 1991;55:1076. Reprinted with permission of the American Fertility Society.)

dent to monitor potassium and creatinine in patients taking spironolactone. Finally, allergic reactions to spironolactone, most commonly hives, can occur. In my experience, this is usually due to one of the incipients in the tablet, and may not recur when a different brand is used.

Cyproterone Acetate. Cyproterone acetate (CA) was initially developed as a progestin. It was discovered to be an antiandrogen when its administration to pregnant rats caused feminization of male fetuses. It is now known to be a potent progestin and antiandrogen and a weak glucocorticoid. It also induces hepatic metabolism and increases testosterone clearance. Its half-life is decreased in women receiving other hepatic enzyme inducers, such as phenobarbital. CA has a long biologic half-life, in part because it is stored in adipose tissue. Its elimination is delayed in obese women. In hirsute women, it attenuates androgen action both by competitively binding to the androgen receptor and by reducing serum testosterone levels. It is the most frequent antiandrogen used to treat hirsutism in Europe, and its efficacy has been established in numerous studies (see Miller and Jacobs, 1986, for review).

In Europe, CA (2 mg daily) is available as an OC in combination with 50 mg ethinyl estradiol (Diane) or 35 mg ethinyl estradiol (Dianette). Although such a formulation should be the birth control pill of choice in hyperandrogenic women who need contraception, higher doses of CA are generally used to treat hirsutism. In Canada and elsewhere, CA is available as a 50-mg tablet (Androcur), approved for use in prostate cancer. Originally, CA was prescribed during the first 10 to 11 days of a cyclic 21-day course of estrogen, with 7 days off both medications (Hammerstein et al, 1975). More recently, 25 to 100 mg daily has been given for the first 10 to 11 days of a birth control pill cycle, with 50 mg being the most frequent starting dose. Higher doses should be more effective, at least in theory, although side effects are also dose dependent. Because CA is a potent progestin and has a long duration of action, it is only given at the beginning of each cycle to allow sufficient time for progestin activity to fall and menses to occur. This may be one disadvantage of CA, because its antiandrogenic activity will be attenuated during the latter part of the menstrual cycle. However, CA should be better than spironolactone at suppressing the markedly elevated ovarian androgens seen in some women with PCOS. CA may also be given as a monthly intramuscular injection (Marcondes et al, 1990). However, continuous administration of CA would be expected to cause hypogonadism. The efficacy of CA in treating hirsute women is similar to that of spironolactone (Erenus et al, 1996; O'Brien et al, 1991). CA has been found to be superior to hydrocortisone in women with nonclassical CAH, suggesting that antiandrogens may be a preferable form of treatment, even in women with documented adrenal hyperandrogenism (Spritzer et al, 1990).

Side effects of CA are generally those attributable to the OC. In one study, which compared the OC Diane (2 mg CA + 5 mg ethinyl estradiol) alone with Diane plus CA (100 mg daily for 11 days each cycle), a similar incidence of many side effects was found in the two groups: menometrorrhagia (10%), acne (6%), decreased libido (10%), edema (10%), nausea (18%), headache (20%), and depression (13%) (Belisle and Love, 1986). Breast tenderness was noted in about 30% of women initially, with a decreasing incidence over time. Amenorrhea was present in 32% of women on high-dose CA after 1 month and in 15% after 9 months. Amenorrhea occurred in 0% to 4% of women on Diane alone. A mean weight gain of 1% occurred after 12 months with Diane alone and of 6% with Diane plus CA. When 50 mg CA is added daily for the first 10 days each month in women already using an OC, weight gain is uncommon. The only frequent side effect of this lower dose regimen is a 2- to 3-day delay of the onset of menses. Drug-induced hepatitis has been reported with CA, and, although this complication is rare with low doses (25 to 50 mg for 10 to 11 days monthly), it is prudent to monitor liver enzymes in patients treated with CA.

Flutamide. Flutamide is an antiandrogen that is approved for treatment of prostate cancer. It has weak affinity for the androgen receptor compared to spironolactone or CA, but, when used in adequate doses (125 to 250 mg twice daily), it is as effective as other antiandrogens. Flutamide also is a weak inhibitor of testosterone biosynthesis.

Many trials of flutamide have now been published, some claiming sensational results (Cusan et al, 1990). Although the same group has reported that flutamide is more efficacious than spironolactone, the latter was only used for 21 days each month (Cusan et al, 1994). More recent studies have found flutamide to have similar efficacy as spironolactone (Erenus et al, 1994) and cyproterone acetate (Grigoriou et al, 1996).

Flutamide has minor side effects but is well tolerated in most women. The major concern has been drug-induced hepatitis, which has a frequency of about 0.4% and can be fatal (Wysowski and Fourcroy, 1994). In North America it is five to six times as expensive as the other antiandrogens. Although it is widely used in some countries, other antiandrogens are equally effective and safer.

Other Antiandrogens. Cimetidine is a weak antiandrogen that has not proved effective for the treatment of hirsutism (Golditch and Price, 1990; Lissak et al, 1989). Ketoconazole, a potent antifungal agent, inhibits testosterone (and cortisol) synthesis and is moderately effective in hirsute women (Martikainen et al, 1988; Venturoli et al, 1990). However, the side effects and potential hepatotoxicity of ketoconazole make it a poor choice for routine use in hirsutism.

5α-Reductase Inhibitors. Finasteride (Proscar) is a 5α-reductase inhibitor approved for the treatment of benign prostatic hyperplasia (BPH). Several studies have been published on the treatment of hirsutism with 5 mg finasteride daily, and all have shown clinically significant improvement in hair growth (Moghetti et al, 1994; Ciotta et al, 1995; Wong et al, 1995; Castello et al, 1996; Tolino et al, 1996). In the only study to use an objective method of determining hair growth, finasteride and spironolactone (100 mg daily) were equally effective in reducing facial hair shaft diameter (Wong et al, 1995). No adverse side effects were reported in women taking finasteride. However, it would be expected to cause ambiguous genitalia in a male fetus exposed to this medication in the first trimester, and therefore should not be used in women who could become pregnant. Based on the fact that the 1- and 5-mg doses of finasteride demonstrated similar degrees of improvement in men with BPH (Gormley et al, 1992), and that the 1-mg dose is currently being tested for baldness, it is likely that 1 and 5 mg finasteride daily would have similar effects on body hair growth.

COMBINATION MEDICAL THERAPY

In theory, combining two medications with different mechanisms of action should lead to improved response rates in hirsute women. This hypothesis has not been rigorously tested, although many studies have been published using combinations of drugs. Before antiandrogens were available, glucocorticoids and OCs were frequently used together. At present, antiandrogens are usually used with OCs for three reasons: (1) improved efficacy (at least in women with PCOS); (2) prevention of pregnancy; and (3) prevention or treatment of irregular menses. Antiandrogens can be used with GnRH analogs in women who have both ovarian and adrenal hyperandrogenism. Combining two antiandrogens may also be possible, in an effort to avoid side effects of high doses of a single medication; however, there are few published data using this approach.

REFERENCES

Abraham GE: Ovarian and adrenal contribution to peripheral androgens during the menstrual cycle. J Clin Endocrinol Metab 1974;39:340.

Adashi EY: Potential utility of gonadotropin-releasing hormone agonists in the management of ovarian hyperandrogenism. Fertil Steril 1990;53:765.

Adashi EY: The climacteric ovary as a functional gonadotropin-driven androgen-producing gland. Fertil Steril 1994;62:20.

Azziz R, Dewailly D, Owerbach D: Nonclassic adrenal hyperplasia: current concepts. J Clin Endocrinol Metab 1994;78:810.

Azziz R, Ochoa TM, Bradley ELJ, et al: Leuprolide and estrogen versus oral contraceptive pills for the treatment of hirsutism: a prospective randomized study. J Clin Endocrinol Metab 1995; 80:3406.

Azziz R, Rafi A, Smith BR, et al: On the origin of the elevated 17-hydroxyprogesterone levels after adrenal stimulation in hyperandrogenism. J Clin Endocrinol Metab 1990;70:431.

Balen AH, Conway GS, Kaltsas G, et al: Polycystic ovary syndrome: the spectrum of the disorder in 1741 patients. Hum Reprod 1995;10:2107.

Barbieri RL: Hyperandrogenism, insulin resistance and acanthosis nigricans—10 years of progress. J Reprod Med 1994;39:327.

Barbieri RL, Makris A, Randall RW, et al: Insulin stimulates androgen accumulation in incubations of ovarian stroma obtained from women with hyperandrogenism. J Clin Endocrinol Metab 1986;62:904.

Barnes RB, Lobo RA: Central opioid activity in polycystic ovary syndrome with and without dopaminergic modulation. J Clin Endocrinol Metab 1985;61:779.

Barnes RB, Mileikowsky GN, Cha KY, et al: Effects of dopamine and metoclopramide in polycystic ovary syndrome. J Clin Endocrinol Metab 1986;63:506.

Barth JH, Cherry CA, Wojnarowska CF, et al: Spironolactone is an effective and well tolerated systemic antiandrogen therapy for hirsute women. J Clin Endocrinol Metab 1989;68:966.

Barth JH, Jenkins M, Belchetz PE: Ovarian hyperthecosis, diabetes and hirsuties in post-menopausal women. Clin Endocrinol (Oxf) 1997;46:123.

Bates GW, Whitworth NS: Effect of body weight reduction on plasma androgens in obese, infertile women. Fertil Steril 1982;38:406.

Belisle S, Love EJ: Clinical efficacy and safety of cyproterone acetate in severe hirsutism: results of multicentered Canadian study. Fertil Steril 1986;46:1015.

Bergfeld WF: Androgenetic alopecia: an autosomal dominant disorder. Am J Med 1995;98(Suppl 1A):95.

Blankstein J, Rabinovici J, Goldenberg M, et al: Changing pituitary reactivity to follicle-stimulating hormone and luteinizing hormone-releasing hormone after induced ovulatory cycles and after anovulation in patients with polycystic ovarian disease. J Clin Endocrinol Metab 1987;65:1164.

Bongiovanni AM: Congenital adrenal hyperplasia due to 3β-hydroxysteroid dehydrogenase deficiency. Pediatr Adolesc Endocrinol 1984;13:72.

Brauner R, Adan L, Malandry F, et al: Adult height in girls with idiopathic true precocious puberty. J Clin Endocrinol Metab 1994;79:415.

Brook CGD: The management of classical congenital adrenal hyperplasia due to 21-hydroxylase deficiency. Clin Endocrinol (Oxf) 1990;33:559.

Byrne GC, Perry YS, Winter JSD: Steroid inhibitory effects upon human adrenal 3β-hydroxysteroid dehydrogenase activity. J Clin Endocrinol Metab 1986;62:413.

Carey AH, Waterworth D, Patel K, et al: Polycystic ovaries and premature male pattern baldness are associated with one allele of the steroid metabolism gene CYP17. Hum Mol Genet 1994;3:1873.

Castello M, Tosi F, Perrone F, et al: Outcome of long-term treatment with the 5α-reductase inhibitor finasteride in idiopathic hirsutism: clinical and hormonal effects during a 1-year course of therapy and 1-year follow-up. Fertil Steril 1996;66:734.

Cathelineau G, Brerault JL, Fiet J, et al: Adrenocortical 11β-hydroxylation defect in adult women with postmenarchial onset of symptoms. J Clin Endocrinol Metab 1980;51:287.

Chang RJ, Mandel FP, Lu JKH, et al: Enhanced disparity of gonadotropin secretion by estrone in women with polycystic ovarian disease. J Clin Endocrinol Metab 1982;54:490.

Ciotta L, Cianci A, Calogero AE, et al: Clinical and endocrine effects of finasteride, a 5α-reductase inhibitor, in women with idiopathic hirsutism. Fertil Steril 1995;64:299.

Clayton RN, Ogden V, Hodgkinson J, et al: How common are polycystic ovaries in normal women and what is their significance for the fertility of the population? Clin Endocrinol (Oxf) 1992;37:127.

Coenen CM, Thomas CM, Borm GF, et al: Changes in androgens during treatment with four low-dose contraceptives. Contraception 1996;53:171.

Corenblum B: Hyperprolactinemic polycystic ovary syndrome. In Mahesh VB, Greenblatt RD (eds): Hirsutism and Virilism. Littleton, MA: John Wright-PSG, 1983:239.

Cronin C, Igoe D, Duffy MJ, et al: The overnight dexamethasone test is a worthwhile screening procedure. Clin Endocrinol (Oxf) 1990;33:27.

Crosby PDA, Rittmaster RS: Predictors of clinical response in hirsute women treated with spironolactone. Fertil Steril 1991;55:1076.

Cumming DC, Rebar RW, Hopper BR, et al: Evidence for an influence of the ovary on circulating dehydroepiandrosterone sulfate levels. J Clin Endocrinol Metab 1982;54:1069.

Cusan L, Dupont A, Belanger A, et al: Treatment of hirsutism with the pure antiandrogen flutamide. J Am Acad Dermatol 1990;23:462.

Cusan L, Dupont A, Gomez J-L, et al: Comparison of flutamide and spironolactone in the treatment of hirsutism: a randomized controlled trial. Fertil Steril 1994;61:281.

Cutler GB, Laue L: Congenital adrenal hyperplasia due to 21-hydroxylase deficiency. Engl J Med 1990;323:1806.

Dahlgren E, Janson PO, Johansson S, et al: Polycystic ovary syndrome and risk for myocardial infarction. Acta Obstet Gynecol Scand 1992a;71:599.

Dahlgren E, Johansson S, Lindstedt G, et al: Women with polycystic ovary syndrome wedge resected in 1956 to 1965: a long-term follow-up focusing on natural history and circulating hormones. Fertil Steril 1992b;57:505.

Dallob AL, Sadick NS, Unger W, et al: The effect of finasteride, a 5α-reductase inhibitor, on scalp skin testosterone and dihydrotestosterone concentrations in patients with male pattern baldness. J Clin Endocrinol Metab 1994;79:703.

Daniel SAJ, Armstrong DT: Androgens in the ovarian microenvironment. Semin Reprod Endocrinol 1986;4:89.

Darney PD: The androgenicity of progestins. Am J Med 1995;98(Suppl 1A):104.

Davis SR, Burger HG: Androgens and the postmenopausal woman. J Clin Endocrinol Metab 1996;81:2759.

Derksen J, Nagesser SK, Meinders AE, et al: Identification of virilizing adrenal tumors in hirsute women. N Engl J Med 1994;331:968.

Deslypere J-P, Young M, Wilson JD, et al: Testosterone and 5α-dihydrotestosterone interact differently with the androgen receptor to enhance transcription of the MMTV-CAT reporter gene. Mol Cell Endocrinol 1992;88:15.

Despres J-P, Lamarche B, Mauriege P, et al: Hyperinsulinemia as an independent risk factor for ischemic heart disease. N Engl J Med 1996;334:952.

Dunaif A, Green G, Futterweit W, et al: Suppression of hyperandrogenism does not improve peripheral or hepatic insulin resistance in the polycystic ovary syndrome. J Clin Endocrinol Metab 1990;70:699.

Dunaif A, Green K, Phelps RG, et al: Acanthosis nigricans, insulin action, and hyperandrogenism: clinical, histological and biochemical findings. J Clin Endocrinol Metab 1991;75:590.

Dunaif A, Longcope C, Canick J, et al: The effects of the aromatase inhibitor Δ^1-testolactone on gonadotropin release and steroid metabolism in polycystic ovarian disease. J Clin Endocrinol Metab 1985;60:773.

Dunaif A, Scully RE, Andersen RN, et al: The effects of continuous androgen secretion on the hypothalamic-pituitary axis in woman: evidence from a luteinized thecoma of the ovary. J Clin Endocrinol Metab 1984;59:389.

Ehrmann DA, Barnes RB, Rosenfield RL: Polycystic ovary syndrome as a form of functional ovarian hyperandrogenism due to dysregulation of androgen secretion. Endocr Rev 1995;16:322.

Ehrmann DA, Cavaghan MK, Imperial J, et al: Effects of metformin on insulin secretion, insulin action, and ovarian steroidogenesis in women with polycystic ovary syndrome. J Clin Endocrinol Metab 1997a;82:524.

Ehrmann DA, Rosenfield RL, Barnes RB, et al: Detection of functional ovarian hyperandrogenism in women with androgen excess. N Engl J Med 1992;327:157.

Ehrmann DA, Schneider DJ, Sobel BE, et al: Troglitazone improves defects in insulin action, insulin secretion, ovarian steroidogenesis, and fibrinolysis in women with polycystic ovary syndrome. J Clin Endocrinol Metab 1997b;82:2108.

Eil C, Edelson SK: The use of human skin fibroblasts to obtain potency estimates of drug binding to androgen receptors. J Clin Endocrinol Metab 1984;59:51.

Emans SJ, Grace E, Woods ER, et al: Treatment with dexamethasone of androgen excess in adolescent patients. J Pediatr 1988;112:821.

Erenus M, Gurbuz O, Durmusoglu F, et al: Comparison of the efficacy of spironolactone versus flutamide in the treatment of hirsutism. Fertil Steril 1994;61:613.

Erenus M, Yucelten D, Gurbuz O, et al: Comparison of spironolactone-oral contraceptive versus cyproterone acetate-estrogen regimens in the treatment of hirsutism. Fertil Steril 1996;66:216.

Erickson GF, Magoffin DA, Dyer CA, et al: The ovarian androgen producing cells: a review of structure/function relationships. Endocr Rev 1985;6:371.

Falaschi P, Rocco A, del Pozo E: Inhibitory effect of bromocriptine treatment on luteinizing hormone secretion in polycystic ovary syndrome. J Clin Endocrinol Metab 1986;62:348.

Farmer RD, Lawrenson RA, Thompson CR, et al: Population-based study of risk of venous thromboembolism associated with various oral contraceptives [see comments]. Lancet 1997;349:83.

Ferriman D, Gallwey JD: Clinical assessment of body hair growth in women. J Clin Endocrinol Metab 1961;21:1440.

Filicori M, Santoro N, Merriam GR, et al: Characterization of the physiological pattern of episodic gonadotropin secretion throughout the human menstrual cycle. J Clin Endocrinol Metab 1986;62:1136.

Fox H: Sex cord-stromal tumours of the ovary. J Pathol 1985;145:127.

Fox R, Corrigan E, Thomas PA, et al: The diagnosis of polycystic ovaries in women with oligo-amenorrhoea: predictive power of endocrine tests. Clin Endocrinol (Oxf) 1991;34:127.

Franks S: Polycystic ovary syndrome. N Engl J Med 1995;333:853.

Freeman DA: Steroid hormone-producing tumors in man. Endocr Rev 1986;7:204.

Friedman CI, Schmidt GE, Kim MH, et al: Serum testosterone concentrations in the evaluation of androgen-producing tumors. Am J Obstet Gynecol 1985;153:44.

Gabrilove JL, Seman AT, Sabet R, et al: Virilizing adrenal adenoma with studies on the steroid content of the adrenal venous effluent and a review of the literature. Endocr Rev 1981;2:462.

Geley S, Kapelari K, Johrer K, et al: CYP11B1 mutations causing congenital adrenal hyperplasia due to 11β-hydroxylase deficiency. J Clin Endocrinol Metab 1996;81:2896.

Gharani N, Waterworth DM, Batty S, et al: Association of the steroid synthesis gene CYP11a with polycystic ovary syndrome and hyperandrogenism. Hum Mol Genet 1997;6:397.

Gilling-Smith C, Willis DS, Beard RW, et al: Hypersecretion of androstenedione by isolated thecal cells from polycystic ovaries. J Clin Endocrinol Metab 1994;79:1158.

Golditch IM, Price VH: Treatment of hirsutism with cimetidine. Obstet Gynecol 1990;75:911.

Goldzieher JW, Green JA: The polycystic ovary. 1. Clinical and histologic features. J Clin Endocrinol Metab 1962;22:325.

Gormley GJ, Stoner E, Bruskewitz RC, et al: The effect of finasteride in men with benign prostatic hyperplasia. N Engl J Med 1992;327:1185.

Grigoriou O, Papadias C, Konidaris S, et al: Comparison of flutamide and cyproterone acetate in the treatment of hirsutism: a randomized controlled trial. Gynecol Endocrinol 1996;10:119.

Grino PB, Griffin JE, Wilson JD: Testosterone at high concentrations interacts with the human androgen receptor similarly to dihydrotestosterone. Endocrinology 1990;126:1165.

Groves TD, Corenblum B: Spironolactone therapy during human pregnancy. Am J Obstet Gynecol 1995;172:1655.

Hammerstein J, Meckies J, Leo-Rossberg I, et al: Use of cyproterone acetate in the treatment of acne, hirsutism, and virilism. J Steroid Biochem 1975;6:827.

Hammond GL: Molecular properties of corticosteroid binding globulin and the sex-steroid binding proteins. Endocr Rev 1990;11:65.

Harlass FE, Plymate SR, Fariss BL, et al: Weight loss is associated with correction of gonadotropin and sex steroid abnormalities in the obese anovulatory female. Fertil Steril 1984;42:649.

Heiner JS, Greendale GA, Kawakami AK, et al: Comparison of a GnRH agonist and a low dose oral contraceptive given alone or together in the treatment of hirsutism. J Clin Endocrinol Metab 1995;80:3412.

Helleday J, Siwers B, Ritzén EM, et al: Subnormal androgen and elevated progesterone levels in women treated for congenital virilizing 21-hydroxylase deficiency. J Clin Endocrinol Metab 1993;76:933.

Horton R, Lobo R: Peripheral androgens and the role of androstanediol glucuronide. Clin Endocrinol Metab 1986;15:293.

Jahanfar S, Eden JA, Warren P, et al: A twin study of polycystic ovary syndrome. Fertil Steril 1995;63:478.

Judd HL, Scully RE, Herbst AL, et al: Familial hyperthecosis: comparison of endocrinologic and histologic findings with polycystic ovarian disease. Am J Obstet Gynecol 1973;117:976.

Kallio PJ, Plavimo JJ, Janne OA: Genetic regulation of androgen action. Prostate 1996;Suppl 6:45.

Kavli R, Kornreich L. Laron Z: Pubertal development, growth, and final height in girls with sexual precocity after therapy with the GnRH analogue D-TRP-6-LHRH: a report on 15 girls, followed after cessation of gonadotropin suppressive therapy Horm Res 1990;33:11.

Kazer RR, Kessel B, Yen SSC: Circulating luteinizing hormone pulse frequency in women with polycystic ovary syndrome. J Clin Endocrinol Metab 1987;65:233.

Kiddy DS, Hamilton-Fairley D, Seppala M, et al: Diet-induced changes in sex hormone binding globulin and free testosterone in women with normal or polycystic ovaries: correlation with serum insulin and insulin-like growth factor-I. Clin Endocrinol (Oxf) 1989;31:757.

King DR, Lack EE: Adrenal cortical carcinoma. Cancer 1979;44:239.

Kirschner MA, Samojlik E, Szmal E: Clinical usefulness of plasma androstanediol glucuronide measurements in women with idiopathic hirsutism. J Clin Endocrinol Metab 1987;65:597.

Kirschner MA, Zucker IR, Jespersen D: Idiopathic hirsutism—an ovarian abnormality. N Engl J Med 1976;294:637.

Knochenhauer ES, Cortet-Rudelli C, Cunnigham RD, et al: Carriers of 21-hydroxylase deficiency are not at increased risk for hyperandrogenism. J Clin Endocrinol Metab 1997;82:479.

Kuttenn F, Couillin P, Girard F, et al: Late-onset adrenal hyperplasia in hirsutism. N Engl J Med 1985;313:224.

Lanzone A, Fulghesu AM, Cucinelli F, et al: Evidence of a distinct derangement of opioid tone in hyperinsulinemic patients with polycystic ovarian syndrome: relationship with insulin and luteinizing hormone secretion. J Clin Endocrinol Metab 1995;80: 3501.

LaRosa JC: Androgens and women's health: genetic and epidemiologic aspects of lipid metabolism. Am J Med 1995;98(Suppl 1A):22.

Lasco A, Cucinotta D, Gigante A, et al: No changes of peripheral insulin resistance in polycystic ovary syndrome after long-term reduction of endogenous androgens with leuprolide. Eur J Endocrinol 1995;133:718.

Lasnitzki I, Franklin HR: The influence of serum on uptake, conversion, and action of testosterone in rat prostate glands in organ culture. J Endocr 1972;54:333.

Legro RS: The genetics of polycystic ovary syndrome. Am J Med 1995;98(Suppl 1A):9.

Legro RS, Dunaif A: The role of insulin resistance in polycystic ovary syndrome. Endocrinologist 1996;6:307.

Leinonen P, Ranta T, Siegberg R, et al: Testosterone-secreting virilizing adrenal adenoma with human chorionic gonadotrophin receptors and 21-hydroxylase deficiency. Clin Endocrinol (Oxf) 1991;34:31.

Letiexhe MR, Scheen AJ, Gerard PL, et al: Postgastroplasy recovery of ideal body weight normalizes glucose and insulin metabolism in obese women. J Clin Endocrinol Metab 1995;80:364.

Liovic M, Prezelj J, Kocijancic A, et al: CYP17 gene analysis in hyperandrogenised women with and without exaggerated 17-hydroxyprogesterone response to ovarian stimulation. J Endocrinol Invest 1997;20:189.

Lissak A, Sorokin Y, Calderon I, et al: Treatment of hirsutism with cimetidine: a prospective randomized controlled trial. Fertil Steril 1989;51:247.

Lobo RA, Granger L, Goebelsmann U, et al: Elevations in unbound serum estradiol as a possible mechanism for inappropriate gonadotropin secretion in women with PCOD. J Clin Endocrinol Metab 1981;52:156.

Lobo RA, Shoupe D, Serafini P, et al: The effects of two doses of spironolactone on serum androgens and anagen hair in hirsute women. Fertil Steril 1985;43:200.

Longcope C: Adrenal and gonadal androgen secretion in normal females. Clin Endocrinol Metab 1986;15:213.

Lookingbill DP, Egan N, Santen RJ, et al: Correlation of serum 3α-androstanediol glucuronide with acne and chest hair density in men. J Clin Endocrinol Metab 1988;67:986.

Loriaux DL, Menard R, Taylor A, et al: Spironolactone and endocrine dysfunction. Ann Intern Med 1976;85:630.

Loughlin T, Cunningham S, Moore A, et al: Adrenal abnormalities in polycystic ovary syndrome. J Clin Endocrinol Metab 1986;62:142.

Lucky AW, McGuire J, Rosenfield RL, et al: Plasma androgens in women with acne vulgaris. J Invest Dermatol 1983;81:70.

Luu-The V, Sugimoto Y, Puy L, et al: Characterization, expression, and immunohistochemical localization of 5α-reductase in human skin. J Invest Dermatol 1994;102:221.

Lynfield YL: Effect of pregnancy on the human hair cycle. Invest Dermatol 1960;35:323.

Lynfield YL, MacWilliams P: Shaving and hair growth. J Invest Dermatol 1970;55:170.

Mahendroo MS, Cala KM, Russell DW: 5α-reduced androgens play a key role in murine parturition. Mol Endocrinol 1996;10: 380.

Mainwaring WIP: The Mechanisms of Action of Androgens. New York, Springer-Verlag, 1977.

Marcondes JAM, Wajchenberg BL, Aburjamra AC, et al: Monthly cyproterone acetate in the treatment of hirsute women: clinical and laboratory effects. Fertil Steril 1990;53:40.

Martikainen H, Heikkinen J, Ruokonen A, et al: Hormonal and clinical effects of ketoconazole in hirsute women. J Clin Endocrinol Metab 1988;66:987.

Marynick SP, Chakmakjian ZH, McCaffree DL, et al: Androgen excess in cystic acne. N Engl J Med 1983;803:981.

Matteri RK, Stanczyk FZ, Gentzschein EE, et al: Androgen sulfate and glucuronide conjugates in nonhirsute and hirsute women with polycystic ovarian syndrome. Am J Obstet Gynecol 1989; 161:1704.

Mauvais-Jarvis P: Regulation of androgen receptor and 5α-reductase in the skin of normal and hirsute women. Clin Endocrinol Metab 1986;15:307.

Mauvais-Jarvis P, Guillemant S, Corvol P, et al: Metabolism of radioactive 5α-androstane-3β,17β-diol. Steroids 1970;16:173.

McClamrock HD, Adashi EY: Gestational hyperandrogenism. Fertil Steril 1992;57:257.

McKnight E: The prevalence of "hirsutism" in young women. Lancet 1964;1:410.

McLellan AR, Mowat A, Cordiner J, et al: Hilus cell pathology and hirsutism. Clin Endocrinol (Oxf) 1990;32:203.

Meldrum DR, Abraham GE: Peripheral and ovarian venous concentrations of various steroid hormones in virilizing ovarian tumors. Obstet Gynecol 1970;53:36.

Mendel CM: The free hormone hypothesis: a physiologically based mathematical model. Endocr Rev 1989;10:232.

Mercado AB, Wilson RC, Cheng KC, et al: Extensive personal experience: prenatal treatment and diagnosis of congenital adrenal hyperplasia owing to steroid 21-hydroxylase deficiency. J Clin Endocrinol Metab 1995;80:2014.

Migeon CJ: Comments about the need for prenatal treatment of congenital adrenal hyperplasia due to 21-hydroxylase deficiency [editorial]. J Clin Endocrinol Metab 1990;70:836.

Miller JA, Jacobs HS: Treatment of hirsutism and acne with cyproterone acetate. Clin Endocrinol Metab 1986;15:373.

Miller W: Clinical review 54: genetics, diagnosis, and management of 21-hydroxylase deficiency. J Clin Endocrinol Metab 1994;78:241.

Moghetti P, Castello R, Magnani CM, et al: Clinical and hormonal effects of the 5α-reductase inhibitor finasteride in idiopathic hirsutism. J Clin Endocrinol Metab 1994;79:1115.

Moltz L, Schwartz U: Gonadal and adrenal androgen secretion in hirsute females. Clin Endocrinol Metab 1986;15:229.

Moltz L, Schwartz U, Sorensen R, et al: Ovarian and adrenal vein steroids in patients with nonneoplastic hyperandrogenism: selective catheterization findings. Fertil Steril 1984;42:69.

Morimoto I, Edmiston A, Hawks D, et al: Studies on the origin of androstanediol and androstanediol glucuronide in young and elderly men. J Clin Endocrinol Metab 1981;52:772.

Murphy AA, Cropp CS, Smith BS, et al: Effect of low-dose oral contraceptive on gonadotropins, androgens, and sex hormone binding globulin in nonhirsute women. Fertil Steril 1990;53:35.

Mushayandebvu T, Castracane VD, Gimpel T, et al: Evidence for diminished midcycle ovarian androgen production in older reproductive aged women. Fertil Steril 1996;65:721.

Nakhla AM, Ding VDH, Khan MS, et al: 5α-androtan-3α,17β-diol is a hormone: stimulation of cAMP accumulation in human and dog prostate. J Clin Endocrinol Metab 1995;80:2259.

Nestler JE: Sex hormone-binding globulin: a marker for hyperinsulinemia and/or insulin resistance? [editoral]. J Clin Endocrinol Metab 1993;76:273.

Nestler JE: Role of hyperinsulinemia in the pathogenesis of the polycystic ovary syndrome, and its clinical implications. Semin Reprod Endocrinol 1997;15:111.

Nestler JE, Barlascini CO, Matt DW, et al: Suppression of serum insulin by diazoxide reduces serum testosterone levels in obese women with polycystic ovary syndrome. J Clin Endocrinol Metab 1989;68:1027.

Nestler JE, Jakubowicz DJ: Decreases in ovarian cytochrome P450c17α activity and serum free testosterone after reduction of insulin secretion in polycystic ovary syndrome. N Engl J Med 1996;335:617.

Nestler JE, Powers LP, Matt DW, et al: A direct effect of hyperinsulinemia on serum sex hormone-binding globulin levels in obese women with the polycystic ovary syndrome. J Clin Endocrinol Metab 1991;72:83.

Nestler JE, Singh R, Matt DW, et al: Suppression of serum insulin by diazoxide does not alter serum testosterone or sex hormone-binding globulin levels in healthy nonobese women. Am J Obstet Gynecol 1990;163:1243.

New M, White PC, Pang S, et al: The adrenal hyperplasias. In Scriver CL, Beaudet AL, Sly WS, Valle D (eds): The Metabolic

Basis of Inherited Disease. 6th ed. New York: McGraw-Hill, 1989:1881.

New MI: 21-Hydroxylase deficiency congenital adrenal hyperplasia. J Steroid Biochem Mol Biol 1994;48:15.

Norman RJ, Masters S, Hague W: Hyperinsulinemia is common in family members of women with polycystic ovary syndrome. Fertil Steril 1996;66:942.

O'Brien RC, Cooper ME, Murray RML, et al: Comparison of sequential cyproterone acetate/estrogen versus spironolactone/oral contraceptive in the treatment of hirsutism. J Clin Endocrinol Metab 1991;72:1008.

Pache TD, Chadha S, Gooren LJ, et al: Ovarian morphology in long-term androgen-treated female to male transsexuals: a human model for the study of polycystic ovarian syndrome. Histopathology 1991;19:445.

Pang S: Genetics of 3β-hydroxysteroid dehydrogenase deficiency. Growth, Genet Horm 1996;12:6.

Pang S, Lerner AJ, Stoner E, et al: Late-onset adrenal steroid 3β-hydroxysteroid dehydrogenase deficiency. I. A cause of hirsutism in pubertal and postpubertal women. J Clin Endocrinol Metab 1985;60:428.

Pang S, MacGillivray M, Wang M, et al: 3α-Androstanediol glucuronide in virilizing congenital adrenal hyperplasia: a useful serum metabolic marker of integrated adrenal androgen secretion. J Clin Endocrinol Metab 1991;73:166.

Pang SY, Wallace MA, Hofman L, et al: Worldwide experience in newborn screening for classical congenital adrenal hyperplasia due to 21-hydroxylase deficiency. Pediatrics 1988;81:866.

Paoletti AM, Cagnacci A, Depau GF, et al: The chronic administration of cabergoline normalizes androgen secretion and improves menstrual cyclicity in women with polycystic ovary syndrome. Fertil Steril 1996;66:527.

Paoletti AM, Cagnacci A, Soldani R, et al: Evidence that an altered prolactin release is consequent to abnormal ovarian activity in polycystic ovary syndrome. Fertil Steril 1995;64:1094.

Parker LN, Odell WD: Control of adrenal androgen secretion. Endocr Rev 1980;1:392.

Pascale M-M, Pugeat M, Roberts M, et al: Androgen suppressive effect of GnRH agonist in ovarian hyperthecosis and virilizing tumours. Clin Endocrinol (Oxf) 1994;41:571.

Pasquali R, Francesco C: The impact of obesity on hyperandrogenism and polycystic ovary syndrome in premenopausal women. Clin Endocrinol (Oxf) 1993;39:1.

Plymate SR, Matej LA, Jones RE, et al: Inhibition of sex hormone-binding globulin production in the human hepatoma (Hep G2) cell line by insulin and prolactin. J Clin Endocrinol Metab 1988;67:460.

Polson DW, Adams J, Wadsworth J, et al: Polycystic ovaries—a common finding in normal women. Lancet 1988;1:870.

Premawardhana LD, Hughes IA, Read GF, et al: Longer term outcome in females with congenital adrenal hyperplasia (CAH): the Cardiff experience. Clin Endocrinol (Oxf) 1997;46:327.

Preziosi P, Barrett-Conner E, Papoz L, et al: Interrelation between plasma sex hormone-binding globulin and plasma insulin in healthy adult women: The Telecom Study. J Clin Endocrinol Metab 1993;76:283.

Quigley ME, Yen SSC: The role of endogenous opiates on LH secretion during the menstrual cycle. J Clin Endocrinol Metab 1980;51:179.

Rebar R, Judd HL, Yen SSC, et al: Characterization of the inappropriate gonadotropin secretion in polycystic ovary syndrome. J Clin Invest 1976;57:1320.

Reiter EO, Saenger P: Premature adrenarche. Endocrinologist 1997;7:85.

Richards RN, Meharg GE: Cosmetic and Medical Electrolysis and Temporary Hair Removal. Toronto, Medric Ltd, 1991.

Richie JP, Gittes RF: Carcinoma of the adrenal cortex. Cancer 1980;45:1957.

Rittmaster RS: Androgen conjugates: physiology and clinical significance. Endocr Rev 1993a;13:1.

Rittmaster RS: Use of GnRH agonists in the treatment of hyperandrogenism. Clin Obstet Gynecol 1993b;36:679.

Rittmaster RS: Gonadotropin-releasing hormone (GnRH) agonists and estrogen/progestin replacement for the treatment of hirsutism: evaluating the results. J Clin Endocrinol Metab 1995;80:3403.

Rittmaster RS: Functional hyperandrogenism. In Adashi EY, Rock A, Rosenwaks Z (eds): Reproductive Endocrinology, Surgery, and Technology. Philadelphia: Lippincott-Raven Publishers, 1996;1501.

Rittmaster RS: 5α-reductase inhibitors. J Androl 1997a;18:582.

Rittmaster RS: Hirsutism. Lancet 1997b;349:191.

Rittmaster RS, Deshwal N, Lehman L: The role of adrenal hyperandrogenism, insulin resistance and obesity in the pathogenesis of polycystic ovarian syndrome. J Clin Endocrinol 1993;76:1295.

Rittmaster RS, Givner ML: Effect of daily and alternate day low dose prednisone on serum cortisol and adrenal androgens in hirsute women. J Clin Endocrinol Metab 1988;67:400.

Rittmaster RS, Loriaux DL: Hirsutism. Ann Intern Med 1987;106:95.

Rittmaster RS, Thompson DL: Effect of leuprolide and dexamethasone on hair growth and hormone levels in hirsute women: the relative importance of the ovary and the adrenal in the pathogenesis of hirsutism. J Clin Endocrinol Metab 1990;70:1096.

Robinson S, Henderson AD, Gelding SV, et al: Dyslipidaemia is associated with insulin resistance in women with polycystic ovaries. Clin Endocrinol (Oxf) 1996;44:277.

Rodin A, Thakkar H, Taylor N, et al: Hyperandrogenism in polycystic ovary syndrome: evidence of dysregulation of 11β-hydroxysteroid dehydrogenase. N Engl J Med 1994;330:460.

Rosenfield RL: Source of androgen in hirsute women [letter]. N Engl J Med 1976;285:232.

Rosenfield RL: Pilosebaceous physiology in relation to hirsutism and acne. Clin Endocrinol Metab 1986;15:341.

Rosenfield RL: Hyperandrogenism in peripubertal girls. Pediatr Clin North Am 1990;37:1333.

Rosenfield RL, Rich BH, Wolfsdorf JI, et al: Pubertal presentation of congenital Δ⁵-3β-hydroxysteroid dehydrogenase deficiency. J Clin Endocrinol Metab 1980;51:345.

Rosner W: The functions of corticosteroid-binding globulin and sex hormone-binding globulin: recent advances. Endocr Rev 1990;11:80.

Russell DW, Wilson JD: Steroid 5α-reductase: two genes/two enzymes. Annu Rev Biochem 1994;63:25.

Sakkal-Alkaddour H, Zhang L, Yang X, et al: Studies of 3 beta-hydroxysteroid dehydrogenase genes in infants and children manifesting premature pubarche and increased adrenocorticotropin-stimulated delta 5-steroid levels. J Clin Endocrinol Metab 1996;81:3961.

Sands R, Studd J: Exogenous androgens in postmenopausal women. Am J Med 1995;98(Suppl 1A):76.

Schiebinger RJ, Albertson BD, Cassorla FG, et al: The developmental changes in plasma adrenal androgens during infancy and adrenarche are associated with changing activities of adrenal microsomal 17-hydroxylase and 17,20-desmolase, J Clin Invest 1981;67:1177.

Seifer DB, Collins RL: Current concepts of β-endorphin physiology in female reproductive dysfunction. Fertil Steril 1990;54:757.

Shortle BE, Warren MP, Tsin D: Recurrent androgenicity in pregnancy: a case report and literature review. Obstet Gynecol 1987;70:462.

Siegel SF, Finegold DN, Lanes R, et al: ACTH stimulation tests and plasma dehydroepiandrosterone sulfate levels in women with hirsutism. N Engl J Med 1990;323:849.

Simard J, Rhéaume E, Sanchez R, et al: Molecular basis of congenital adrenal hyperplasia due to 3β-hydroxysteroid dehydrogenase deficiency. Mol Endocrinol 1993;7:716.

Singh KB, Dunnihoo DR, Mahajan DK, et al: Clomiphene-dexamethasone treatment of clomiphene-resistant women with and without the polycystic ovary syndrome. J Reprod Med 1992;37:215.

Sluijmer AV, Heineman MJ, de Jong FH, et al: Endocrine activity of the postmenopausal ovary: the effects of pituitary down-regulation and oophorectomy. J Clin Endocrinol Metab 1995;80:2163.

Speiser PW, Laforgia N, Kato K, et al: First trimester prenatal treatment and molecular genetic diagnosis of congenital adrenal hyperplasia (21-hydroxylase deficiency). J Clin Endocrinol Metab 1990;70:838.

Spinder T, Spijkstra JJ, van den Tweel JG, et al: The effects of long term testosterone administration on pulsatile luteinizing hormone secretion and on ovarian histology in eugonadal female to male transsexual subjects. J Clin Endocrinol Metab 1989;69: 151.

Spritzer P, Billaud L, Thalabard JC, et al: Cyproterone acetate versus hydrocortisone treatment in late-onset adrenal hyperplasia. J Clin Endocrinol Metab 1990;70:642.

Stein IF, Leventhal ML: Amenorrhea associated with bilateral polycystic ovaries. Am J Obstet Gynecol 1935;29:181.

Strachan T: Molecular pathology of congenital adrenal hyperplasia. Clin Endocrinol (Oxf) 1990;32:373.

Surrey ES, deZiegler D, Gambone JC, et al: Preoperative localization of androgen-secreting tumors: clinical, endocrinologic, and radiologic evaluation of ten patients. Am J Obstet Gynecol 1988;158:1313.

Tagatz GE, Kopher RA, Nagel TC, et al: The clitoral index: a bioassay of androgenic stimulation. Obstet Gynecol 1979;54:562.

Taylor SI, Dons RF, Hernandez E, et al: Insulin resistance associated with androgen excess in women with autoantibodies to the insulin receptor. Ann Intern Med 1982;97:851.

Techatraisak K, Conway GS, Rumsby G: Frequency of a polymorphism in the regulatory region of the 17 alpha-hydroxylase-17,20-lyase (CYP17) gene in hyperandrogenic states [see comments]. Clin Endocrinol (Oxf) 1997;46:131.

Tolino A, Petrone A, Sarnacchiaro F, et al: Finasteride in the treatment of hirsutism: new therapeutic perspectives. Fertil Steril 1996;66:61.

Tosti A, Misciali C, Piraccini BM, et al: Drug-induced hair loss and hair growth: incidence, management and avoidance. Drug Safety 1994;10:310.

Tsigos C, Chrousos GP: Differential diagnosis and management of Cushing's syndrome. Annu Rev Med 1996;47:443.

Uno H: Biology of hair growth. Semin Reprod Endocrinol 1986; 4:131.

Van WyK JJ, Gunther DF, Ritzén EM, et al: Therapeutic controversies: the use of adrenalectomy as a treatment for congenital adrenal hyperplasia. J Clin Endocrinol Metab 1996;81:3180.

Venturoli S, Fabbri R, Dal Prato L, et al: Ketoconazole therapy for women with acne and/or hirsutism. J Clin Endocrinol Metab 1990;71:335.

Vermeulen A, Giagulli VA: Physiopathology of plasma androstanediol-glucuronide. J Steroid Biochem Mol Biol 1991;39:829.

Wagner RJ Jr: Physical methods for the management of hirsutism. Cutis 1990;45:319.

White PC, Curnow KM, Pascoe L: Disorders of steroid 11β-hydroxylase isozymes. Endocr Rev 1994;15:421.

Wild RA: Obesity, lipids, cardiovascular risk, and androgen excess. Am J Med 1995;98(Suppl 1A):27.

Willis D, Mason H, Gilling-Smith C, et al: Modulation by insulin of follicle-stimulating hormone and luteinizing hormone actions in human granulosa cells of normal and polycystic ovaries. J Clin Endocrinol Metab 1996;81:302.

Wilson JD, Griffin JE, Russell DW: Steroid 5 alpha-reductase 2 deficiency. Endocr Rev 1993;14:577.

Wong IL, Morris RS, Chang L, et al: A prospective randomized trial comparing finasteride to spironolactone in the treatment of hirsutism. J Clin Endocrinol Metab 1995;80:233.

Wright AS, Thomas LN, Douglas RC, et al: Relative potency of testosterone and dihydrotestosterone in preventing atrophy and apoptosis in the prostate of the castrated rat. J Clin Invest 1996;98:2558.

Wysowski DK, Fourcroy JL: Safety of flutamide? Fertil Steril 1994; 62:1089.

Zerah M, Rheaume E, Mani P, et al: No evidence of mutations in the genes for type I and type II 3β-hydroxysteroid dehydrogenase (3β-HSD) in nonclassical 3β-HSD deficiency. J Clin Endocrinol Metab 1994;79:1811.

Zhou Z-X, Wong C-I, Sar M, et al: The androgen receptor: an overview. Recent Prog Horm Res 1996;49:249.

Zumoff B, Freeman R, Coupey S, et al: A chronobiologic abnormality in luteinizing hormone secretion in teenage girls with polycystic-ovary syndrome. N Engl J Med 1983;309:1206.

Zumoff B, Strain GW, Miller LK, et al: Twenty-four-hour mean plasma testosterone concentration declines with age in normal premenopausal women. J Clin Endocrinol Metab 1995;80: 1429.

Zwicker H, Rittmaster RS: Androsterone sulfate: physiology and clinical significance in hirsute women. J Clin Endocrinol Metab 1993;76:112.

29

Disorders of Prolactin Secretion

Bernard Corenblum

Disordered prolactin secretion is one of the most common problems of reproductive endocrinology. In 1928, lactogenic substances were known in lower vertebrates and were extracted from the anterior pituitary by Stricker and Grueter. In lower vertebrates, prolactin is the most versatile hormone—in regard to the number and diversity of physiologic functions that it regulates. Everett, in 1954, demonstrated that disconnection of the pituitary gland from the hypothalamus resulted in enhanced prolactin secretion, showing that the major hypothalamic control is inhibitory. Meites, in 1963, confirmed the presence of a prolactin-inhibiting factor (PIF), and several investigators, especially MacLeod, in 1969 found that dopamine inhibited prolactin release from the pituitary.

Clinical descriptions of lactation disorders in humans first occurred in the Babylonian Talmud (Tractate Shabbat, page 53B). In 1855, Chiari described a syndrome of postpartum lactation associated with amenorrhea and uterine involution. Frommel further clarified this syndrome in 1882. Argonz and Del Castillo, in 1953, reported a similar syndrome that was unrelated to a preceding pregnancy. In 1954, Forbes, working with Albright, described the association of persistent lactation, amenorrhea, the presence of pituitary tumors, and low urinary follicle-stimulating hormone (FSH) levels. They hypothesized the presence of a lactogenic substance in humans. This substance was finally separated from growth hormone and was detected by bioassay in 1970 and by radioimmunossay in 1971. This resulted in an explosion of information regarding prolactin, the lactogenic substance, and its involvement in clinical disease processes. At that time, advances in neuroradiology allowed pituitary tumors to be identified, advances in neuropharmacology produced a long-acting dopamine agonist, and advances in neurosurgical techniques allowed resection of identified pituitary adenomas. Now, over two decades later, there is a general consensus on the role of prolactin secretion disorders in human disease, the natural history of such disorders, and the most appropriate therapy for these disorders.

The prolactin-secreting microadenoma is the most common primary pituitary abnormality seen in clinical practice. Hyperprolactinemia is found in 10% to 15% of nonpregnant women with secondary amenorrhea and in 1% of adult men with decreased libido and/or impotence. In one study of 119 anovulatory women, 15% had hyperprolactinemia and 7% had underlying pituitary adenomas (Greer et al, 1980). Another study of 270 women with amenorrhea described underlying hyperprolactinemia in 23% (Pepperell, 1981).

CHEMISTRY AND METABOLISM OF PROLACTIN

The most biologically active molecule of prolactin circulates in monomeric form, consisting of a 198-amino-acid polypeptide. The entire linear sequence is known. It is synthesized by the lactotrophs in the anterior pituitary gland, the placenta, other areas of the brain, and the endometrium, and occasionally by malignant tissue. The prolactin molecule is similar to the growth hormone and human chorionic somatotropin molecules, and all three may have originated from a single ancestral gene. There is continuous secretion of prolactin, superimposed with episodic secretion throughout the day, especially at night. The serum half-life is 10 minutes.

Besides its occurrence in blood, prolactin is found in amniotic fluid, milk, cerebrospinal fluid (CSF), ovarian antral fluid, and seminal fluid. Prolactin is found in the blood of the human fetus by 12 weeks and markedly increases at 25 weeks until term (Fig. 29–1). It falls to prepubertal levels by 2 months from birth. At puberty, serum prolactin levels increase in girls in association with the increase of estradiol; thus women have higher levels than men. During the menstrual cycle, the highest levels are preovulatory. During pregnancy, serum prolactin levels rise from 1 month of gestation until term, in parallel with the rise of serum estradiol and the ongoing hyperplasia of the lactotrophs of the pituitary gland (Scheithauer et al, 1990). Prolactin levels fall postpartum, returning to baseline by 3 weeks in non-nursing women but decreasing over 3 months to 1 year in

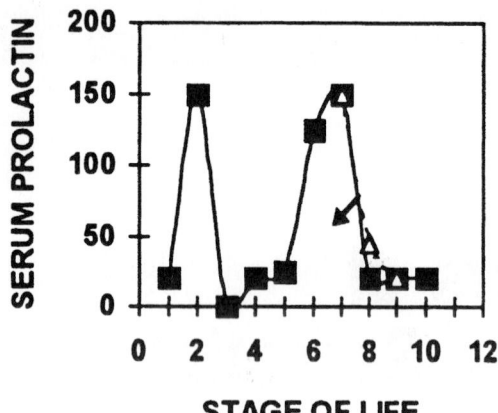

Figure 29–1
Changes of serum prolactin in a female from conception through birth, childhood, puberty, pregnancy, and adult life. 1, 10 weeks of gestation; 2, birth; 3, 3 months; 4, puberty; 5, onset of pregnancy; 6, 6 months of pregnancy; 7, delivery; 8, 1 month postpartum (*arrow* shows if the mother is lactating); 9, menstrual years; 10, menopause.

nursing women. Hyperplasia of lactotrophs disappears several months postpartum.

In humans prolactin binding occurs in the breast, ovary, testis, liver, adrenal gland, and lymphocytes. Its major role is concerned with lactation and reproduction. There are variations in circulating forms of prolactin molecules. There is heterogeneity with regard to glycosylation of prolactin.

The normal prolactin molecule consists of a single polypeptide chain with three disulfide bonds. It has a molecular mass of 23,000 daltons, whereas glycosylated prolactin has a molecular mass of 25,000 daltons but only 32% of the immunoreactivity and 50% of the bioactivity of the nonglycosylated variant (Pellegrini et al, 1988). More than one size of circulating prolactin exists, each with different biologic activities. Some are noncovalently associated aggregates. Big prolactin molecules have marked reduction in bioactivity in the Nb2 rat lymphoma bioassay and have reduced receptor binding. Circulating prolactin is readily measured by a sensitive radioimmunossay. The usual biologically active monomeric form produces excellent correlation between the radioimmunossay and bioassay. Changes in glycosylation of the monomeric form or in size (macroprolactinemia) produce poor correlation between the radioimmunoassay and bioassay. This may result in a discrepancy between clinical findings and radioimmunoassay results. A woman may have markedly elevated serum prolactin levels yet continue to have normal menses.

Variations in circulating forms and in prolactin episodic secretion throughout the day result in a range of serum prolactin levels that is skewed or polymodal in distribution in the normal population. A large minority of normal subjects do not fit a normal distribution curve. If allowance is not made for the nongaussian distribution, elevated serum prolactin lev-

els may be found in 5% to 8% of women, resulting in overdiagnosis (Jeffcoate et al, 1986). There is no general agreement on the interpretation of the prolactin assay regarding what is the absolute upper limit of normal. Discrepancies between laboratories have been due to differences not only in interpretation but also in assay methods. The same sample may produce different results in different laboratories, and they may vary in their ability to detect larger prolactin molecules. Because the prolactin values in the normal population are not normally distributed, more than the usual 2.5% of normal people may show results above the normal range. Such values may not necessarily be abnormal or indicative of a disease process. Furthermore, even in a woman with suggestive symptoms, such as those of amenorrhea or infertility, the finding of mild hyperprolactinemia may be coincidental and not necessarily causative. Thus careful interpretation of the results is necessary and must be correlated with the clinical picture. Hyperprolactinemia is only a biochemical result and requires interpretation. As in all other aspects of medicine, it is critical to treat the patient, not the laboratory test.

REGULATION OF PROLACTIN SECRETION

Synthesis and Release

Prolactin is synthesized and secreted by lactotrophs. They form up to 40% of the cells of the anterior pituitary, are especially found in the lateral wings, but are intermingled throughout the pituitary and among the other cell types, especially the gonadotrophs. Two zones of lactotrophs have been identified in the rat pituitary (Papka et al, 1986). Functional heterogeneity has been noted, because some lactotrophs secrete more prolactin than others, yet show greater responsiveness to dopaminergic inhibition (Luque et al, 1986). Not all lactotrophs demonstrate the same response to estrogen, and some secrete both growth hormone and prolactin.

Transcription of the prolactin gene results in messenger RNA (mRNA) production, and prolactin is then synthesized in the rough endoplasmic reticulum as a larger precursor peptide. The prolactin is then cleaved and stored in granules. There are both stored and newly synthesized pools of prolactin. The lactotrophs contain calcium ions. Changes in the cell membrane result in increased free ionized calcium within the cell, which then activates exocytosis, resulting in extrusion of prolactin granules. The intracellular signal may also include the lipid diacylglycerol, which with ionized calcium stimulates prolactin secretion. This mechanism may explain why deficient prolactin secretion occurs in pseudohypoparathyroidism, and enhanced prolactin release is associated with the calcium channel blocker verapamil.

Prolactin secretion is episodic, more marked during sleep and following food ingestion. The increased serum prolactin level during sleep may not fall immediately upon awakening, and thus the level of prolactin before 8 A.M. may be 20% higher than later in the day. It may be necessary to measure serum prolactin three separate times to obtain a true reading.

Control of Prolactin Secretion

Control of prolactin secretion is complex, involving both inhibitory and stimulatory factors. Classical *endocrine* systems as well as *paracrine* (locally released from one cell to act on another) and *autocrine* (acting on the cell from which it has derived) systems are involved. This complex interaction involves various neurotransmitters, peptide hormones, and steroid hormones. The endocrine control system is best understood (Fig. 29–2).

The major endocrine control is of tonic inhibition by the hypothalamus. This mostly involves the neurotransmitter dopamine. The lactotroph has high-affinity receptors specific for dopamine. Stimulation of the tuberoinfundibular dopaminergic neurons in the hypothalamus results in secretion of dopamine at the level of the median eminence. Dopamine is also derived from the tuberohypophysial dopaminergic system, whose neurons terminate in the rostral part of the pituitary gland, and the median eminence. At the lactotroph, dopamine inhibits prolactin gene transcription and thus mRNA production. Dopamine binds to D_2 receptors and decreases adenylate cyclase activity, which results in decreased intracellular cyclic AMP (cAMP) and thus decreased prolactin mRNA. Dopamine also lowers intracytoplasmic calcium levels. Nitric oxide may mediate the inhibitory action (Duvilanski et al, 1995).

Increased serum prolactin levels resulting from prolactin-secreting tumors or pharmacologic manipulation results in increased synthesis and turnover of dopamine in the median eminence, which suggests a negative feedback endocrine control for prolactin on its own secretion ("short loop" feedback).

Some PIF activity occurs other than by dopamine. γ-Aminobutyric acid (GABA) has PIF activity. Because the concentration of GABA needed to suppress prolactin seems to exceed physiologic levels, the definitive role of GABA in inhibiting prolactin secretion has not been established. Endothelin-like peptides inhibit prolactin secretion, possibly through a paracrine mechanism (Domae et al, 1992).

Prolactin synthesis and secretion are directly stimulated by estradiol. Estradiol has a direct effect on the pituitary, resulting in increased gene transcription and increased prolactin synthesis. This is best seen with pharmacologic levels of estradiol. During pregnancy, hyperplasia of the lactotrophs occurs with pituitary enlargement owing to rising serum estradiol levels. Estrogens have multiple sites of action to increase prolactin secretion, including a direct stimulatory effect on prolactin secretion, decreased hypothalamic release of dopamine into the portal system, and sensitizing the lactotroph to various stimulatory and inhibitory substances.

There is evidence for a prolactin-releasing factor (PRF) because of the response to various physiologic stimulations. These include suckling, stress, sleep, eating, pain, and hypoglycemia. All are mediated by higher brain centers. Suckling is a potent stimulus, resulting in marked increases of serum prolactin within 5 minutes. Changes in hypothalamic dopamine secretion are insufficient to mediate this response. This suggests the presence of a PRF. The PRF may include various peptides (thyrotropin-releasing hormone [TRH], vasoactive intestinal peptide [VIP], peptide histidine-isoleucine, pituitary adenylate cyclase–activating polypeptide, gonadotropin-releasing hormone [GnRH, opioids, angiotensin, cholecystokinin); steroids (estradiol); and biogenic amines (acetylcholine, serotonin, and

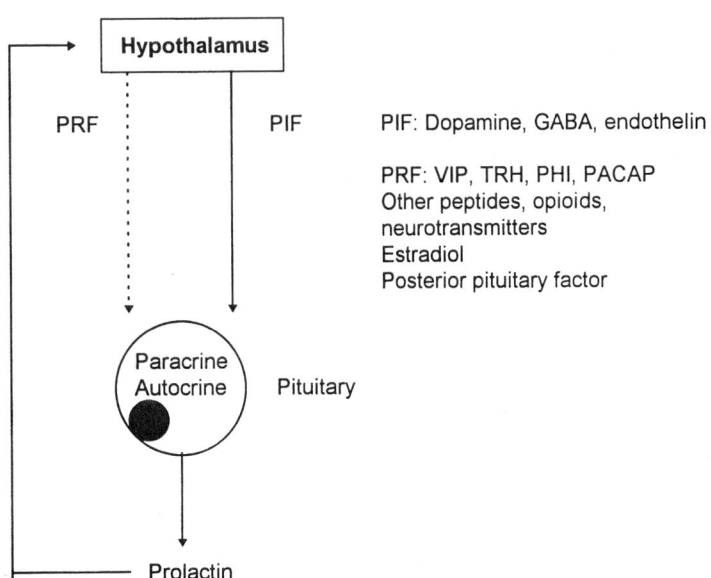

Figure 29–2

Endocrine control of prolactin secretion from the pituitary. GABA, γ-aminobutyric acid; PACAP, pituitary adenylate cyclase activating polypeptide; PHI, peptide histidine-isoleucine; PIF, prolactin-inhibitory factors; PRF, prolactin-releasing factors; TRH, thyrotropin-releasing hormone; VIP, vasoactive intestinal peptide.

histamine). The two peptides most studied as PRFs are VIP and TRH. Both are secreted into the portal blood and are stimulatory to prolactin secretion, the response of which is blunted by specific antagonists. Neither one shows marked increase during the suckling-induced increase of prolactin. Furthermore, during the suckling stimulus, there is marked increase of prolactin secretion but not of thyroid-stimulating hormone (TSH), suggesting that it is not TRH mediated.

There is evidence of a small peptide PRF from the intermediate lobe of the posterior pituitary. Removal of this area abolishes suckling-induced hyperprolactinemia (Murai and Ben-Jonathan, 1987). An animal model localized this factor to the melanotrophs (Allen et al, 1995).

Prolactin secretion remains pulsatile, despite the inhibitory presence of dopamine. These pulses originate within the pituitary gland because it persists in autotransplanted glands. This suggests the presence of paracrine or autocrine stimulation. Paracrine control of prolactin secretion may result from neighboring gonadotrophs (Denef and Andries, 1983) or folliculostellate bells (Bates et al, 1987). Under GnRH stimulation, the gonadotrophs may release angiotensin I, which then locally stimulates prolactin release from the lactotrophs. This may explain the observations that GnRH stimulates prolactin secretion (Yen et al, 1980) and the simultaneous pulsatile secretion of LH and prolactin (Casper and Yen, 1981). Folliculostellate cells inhibit the secretion of prolactin when these cells are co-cultured with lactotrophs (Bates et al, 1987), suggesting a paracrine PIF. Corticotrophs inhibit prolactin secretion by a paracrine mechanism.

VIP may have both endocrine and autocrine PRF actions. There are VIP receptors coupled to adenylate cyclase. VIP is present within lactotrophs. A VIP antagonist suppresses the spontaneous pulsatile secretion of prolactin, which occurs at basal states, suggesting an autocrine action for VIP (Nagy et al, 1988).

To summarize, both stimulatory and inhibitory control may occur from endocrine secretion of various factors (mainly from the hypothalamus), paracrine action, and autocrine secretion from the lactotroph. Autoregulation may further occur by prolactin itself, increasing dopamine turnover in the median eminence, resulting in decreased lactotroph secretion of prolactin.

Actions of Prolactin

The major role of prolactin in the adult human is lactogenic. In combination with estradiol and progesterone (and insulin, thyroxine, and cortisol), prolactin prepares the breast for lactation by stimulating lobuloacinar development; placental lactogen adds to this effect. At the breast, estradiol antagonizes prolactin-mediated milk production, so that with delivery of the placenta the elevated prolactin levels then induce milk secretion. Prolactin stimulates the formation and secretion of the milk proteins casein and lactalbumin and enhances the secretion of fatty acids, lactose, and the volume of milk secretion. The suckling stimulus sends a signal by the fourth to sixth thoracic nerves to enhance centrally mediated prolactin secretion. The reduction of prolactin secretion by dopamine agonists prevents or rapidly inhibits postpartum milk secretion. No physiologic role for prolactin secretion in the adult male has yet been established. There is no valid evidence for a direct effect on the testis.

Amniotic fluid prolactin, presumably, has a physiologic role in fetal development (Pullano et al, 1989). It may have a role in fetoplacental osmoregulation by decreasing transport of water across the amnion from the fetal side. Prolactin may contribute to maturation of the fetal lung. It may have a role in stimulating fetal growth. The prolactin production by decidual tissue is not affected by dopamine or its pharmacologic agonists.

There may be an action of prolactin on lymphocytes with a role in immunomodulation (Reber, 1993).

DISORDERS OF PROLACTIN SECRETION

Hyposecretion

The rare patient with congenital deficiency of prolactin secretion demonstrates the importance of prolactin in normal physiologic processes. Pubertal development is incomplete, and menstrual cycles are abnormal. There is no postpartum lactation, indicating that puerperal lactation is completely dependent on maternal pituitary prolactin secretion (Kauppila et al, 1987).

The classic example of decreased prolactin secretion is postpartum infarction of the pituitary gland (*Sheehan's syndrome*). The earliest clue is the absence of postpartum lactation.

The most common cause of decreased prolactin secretion is iatrogenic, by either pituitary surgery or oversuppression by dopamine agonist drugs. Hypoprolactinemia induced by overtreatment has been associated with defective progesterone synthesis in apparently normally cycling women.

Decreased prolactin secretion has been noted in the syndrome of *pseudohypoparathyroidism* as well as with destructive pituitary disorders such as hemochromatosis.

Hypersecretion

Differential Diagnosis of Hyperprolactinemia (Table 29–1)

Hyperprolactinemia is a biochemical result, not a diagnosis. It is defined as a persistently elevated serum

Table 29-1. CAUSES OF CHRONIC HYPERPROLACTINEMIA

Physiologic
Pregnancy
Lactation
Suprasellar Disorders
Infiltrate: sarcoidosis, histiocytosis X, tuberculosis
Mass: craniopharyngioma, glioma, germinoma, hamartoma, metastatic disease, abscess, aneurysm
Stalk section
Previous cranial radiation
Temporal lobe epilepsy
Pituitary Disease
Prolactinomas: microadenomas, macroadenomas
Mixed adenomas (acromegaly)
Intrasellar mass (pseudoprolactinoma)
Lymphocytic hypophysitis
Lactotroph hyperplasia
Idiopathic hyperprolactinemia
Endocrine Disease
Primary hypothyroidism
Polycystic ovary syndrome
Cushing's disease
Systemic Disease
Chronic renal failure
Cirrhosis, hepatic encephalopathy
Ectopic secretion: benign (dermoid cyst, sphenoid sinus) and malignant
Neurogenic (Chest Wall)
Burn, scar, herpes zoster, thoracotomy, nipple stimulation, esophagitis
Medications
Neuroleptics; phenothiazines, butyrophenones, tricyclic antidepressants
Antihypertensives (α-methyldopa, reserpine, calcium channel blockers)
Gastrointestinal dopamine antagonists: metoclopramide, domperidone
Narcotics
High-dose estrogen
Cocaine abuse
Macroprolactinemia

prolactin level in a nonpregnant, nonlactating woman or in a child or any male. *Transient* hyperprolactinemia may result from nonspecific stimuli, such as anaerobic exercise, nipple stimulation, coitus, emotional stress, hypoglycemia, eating, anesthesia, and surgical stress. *Chronic* hyperprolactinemia, in the absence of pregnancy or postpartum lactation, is assumed to be pathologic.

Suprasellar Disorders. At the suprasellar level, anything that interferes with dopamine delivery deinhibits prolactin secretion. Because most lesions in this area result in increased prolactin secretion, hyperprolactinemia has been referred to as the "sedimentation rate" of this part of the brain. Anatomic lesions include masses or infiltrates in the median eminence or the hypothalamus.

A syndrome of hyperprolactinemia and chronic hypogonadism, best described in males, is associated with chronic temporal lobe epilepsy. Any seizure is usually followed by a rise of prolactin, and this phenomenon has been clinically utilized to distinguish true seizures from hysterical seizures. A chronic seizure pattern originating in the temporal lobes may be less clinically obvious. Presumably, altered electrical impulses from the amygdala result in disruption of normal gonadotropin and prolactin secretion. Diagnosis is confirmed by a sleep electroencephalogram, and treatment should center on the seizure disorder (Spark et al, 1984).

Small tumors of the hypothalamus, such as craniopharyngiomas and gliomas, may be clinically and radiologically indistinguishable from pituitary tumors. Furthermore, symptoms related to hyperprolactinemia may regress with dopamine agonist therapy, adding to the confusion. Usually, galactorrhea disappears but amenorrhea persists.

Pituitary Disease. Once pregnancy and drugs have been excluded as etiologic factors in hyperprolactinemia, the most common cause is a prolactinoma. Only radiologic visualization distinguishes a prolactinoma from idiopathic hyperprolactinemia (IH), in which no tumor is visualized. Prolactinomas are discussed in greater detail later in this chapter.

Hyperprolactinemia may accompany acromegaly. This results from a mixed cell adenoma, acidophil stem cell adenoma, or mammosomatotroph cell adenoma. The features of acromegaly predominate, and treatment is directed toward resolution of the acromegaly, usually by surgery, radiotherapy, or both. Dopamine agonist therapy usually lowers levels of serum prolactin and, occasionally, growth hormone. Somatostatin analogs are more expensive but usually more effective.

Any intrasellar mass may interrupt the transport of dopamine to part of the pituitary. This relative dopamine insufficiency allows some lactotrophs to escape from inhibition, resulting in mild hyperprolactinemia. A nonsecreting mass associated with mild hyperprolactinemia is termed a *pseudoprolactinoma*. The clinical clue is that the prolactin levels seem inappropriately low for the size of the intrasellar mass. The correct diagnosis of the mass is confirmed only by pathologic examination. In one series of patients presumed to have prolactinoma, 15 of 128 masses were not prolactinomas (Bevan et al, 1987); 10 of the patients had only moderate hyperprolactinemia that was inappropriate to the size of the mass. The most common cause of pseudoprolactinoma was an intrasellar craniopharyngioma. A large mass is not likely to be a prolactinoma if the serum prolactin level is less than 100 μg/L. A patient with hyperprolactinemia resulting from a pseudoprolactinoma responds to a dopamine agonist with suppression of the hyperprolactinemia and regression of symptoms but without radiologic visualization of tumor shrinkage. The pseudoprolactinoma is important to recognize because the benign natural history of prolactinomas may not apply. The natural history of nonsecreting sellar masses is variable but is usually one of stability (Donovan and Corenblum, 1995).

Autoimmune disease may be directed toward one or more endocrine glands. In the pituitary, a lymphocytic hypophysitis is produced, with anti-pituitary antibodies directed against the lactotroph. There also may be a mass effect. There may be associated autoimmune disorders in other glands, especially the thyroid. Hyperprolactinemia is often the only manifestation, and loss of other pituitary function may not occur. Radiologic examination of the pituitary usually demonstrates an abnormal gland, but occasionally findings are normal. The patient may present with amenorrhea, galactorrhea, moderate hyperprolactinemia, and a mass on radiological study, and thus a prolactinoma may be simulated. Specific anti-pituitary or anti-lactotroph antibodies are difficult to detect in peripheral blood, so the diagnosis is confirmed only by pituitary biopsy. Thus, lymphocytic hypophysitis remains a presumptive diagnosis of moderate hyperprolactinemia in the appropriate clinical setting (Wild and Kepley, 1986).

IH is a diagnosis by exclusion of all known causes of hyperprolactinemia. For this reason, it likely consists of various disorders. Basal serum prolactin levels overlap between patients identified as having IH and those with microadenomas, and there is no dynamic test (stimulatory or suppressive) that distinguishes these two entities. Certainly, some patients diagnosed with IH have a microadenoma that is too small to be visualized but that can be detected on surgical exploration. With long-term clinical observation, about 10% of patients with IH show radiologic progression to a microadenoma, but none show progression to a macroadenoma. The natural history of IH is even better than that of microadenomas and suggests that some patients with IH form a distinct entity (Corenblum and Taylor, 1988).

Peillon et al (1991) have published a description of lactotroph hyperplasia as a cause of hyperprolactinemia.

Endocrine Disease. Hyperprolactinemia may occur in the presence of various endocrine disorders, likely by some interference with hypothalamic dopamine secretion or transport. Hyperprolactinemia may occur years before the overt presentation of Cushing's disease. A prolactinoma may be associated with the syndrome of multiple endocrine adenomatosis type I. This is associated with a tumor of the pancreatic islet cells with parathyroid hyperplasia. There may be a positive family history in first-degree relatives. A genetic test will soon be available.

Primary hypothyroidism must be considered in any patient with hyperprolactinemia or galactorrhea. It may be longstanding and borderline and may not be detected on clinical examination. For this reason, measurement of serum TSH levels is mandatory. In the presence of known pituitary disease, serum TSH should not be used to assess thyroid function. Hyperprolactinemia correlates with the duration and/or the severity of hypothyroidism. One misconception is that hyperprolactinemia in hypothyroidism results from enhanced hypothalamic secretion of TRH. There is no evidence to support such a contention. Hyperprolactinemia occurs in only 30% of

women with hypothyroidism. Furthermore, when thyroxine is administered to such hypothyroid patients, serum TSH levels decrease within days, whereas serum prolactin levels normalize within weeks or months. Hyperprolactinemia in chronic primary hypothyroidism may result from changes in hypothalamic dopamine secretion. The most likely mechanism is that hyperplasia of the thyrotrophs of the pituitary may result in an intrasellar mass effect. This would increase prolactin secretion, and it would take weeks for oral thyroxin to reverse the hyperplasia and thus the mass effect. If the cause of the primary hypothyroidism is lymphocytic (Hashimoto's) thyroiditis, concomitant lymphocytic hypophysitis may result in hyperprolactinemia.

Polycystic ovary syndrome (PCOS) is usually a clinical diagnosis. It is associated with hyperprolactinemia in 10% of cases. Patients with PCOS with hyperprolactinemia are clinically similar to those with PCOS without hyperprolactinemia. In contrast to patients with primary hyperprolactinemia, women with PCOS tend to have elevated serum luteinizing hormone (LH), testosterone, and androstenedione levels and normal withdrawal bleeding in response to progesterone challenge. It may be clinically difficult to distinguish hyperprolactinemia with PCOS from pathologic primary hyperprolactinemia because patients with the latter condition may also have oligomenorrhea. Women with PCOS have only mild intermittent hyperprolactinemia, from 25 to 40 μg/L. The pathogenesis is unknown, but it may be related to the chronic, unopposed estrogenization. This may be a direct pituitary effect of estrogen or estrogen inhibition of dopamine secretion and action. There is evidence suggestive for changes in dopamine secretion in women with PCOs (Corenblum and Taylor, 1982):

1. Elevated serum LH levels may be suppressed by an infusion of dopamine.
2. Hyperplasia of the lactotrophs is noted.
3. There is hyperresponsiveness of prolactin to an injection of TRH in women with PCOS and elevated serum LH levels.
4. A dopamine agonist may decrease serum LH and testosterone levels, restore regular menses, eliminate galactorrhea, and stabilize hirsutism. Furthermore, those who fail to respond to ovulation induction with clomiphene citrate may subsequently respond following normalization of prolactin with a dopamine agonist.

Systemic Disorders. Hyperprolactinemia may occur in the presence of several systemic disorders, which are usually obvious. The cause of hyperprolactinemia associated with chronic renal failure is unknown. Hyperprolactinemia usually does not normalize with dialysis but does so after successful renal transplantation. Even modest degrees of renal insufficiency may produce mild hyperprolactinemia. Of 59 patients with serum creatinine levels between 1.5 and 12 mg/dl, 16 had hyperprolactinemia (Hou et al, 1985). Thus, serum creatinine levels should be measured in patients with otherwise unexplained, moderate hyperprolactinemia.

Mild hyperprolactinemia occurs with progressive degrees of cirrhosis, especially alcoholic cirrhosis. Hepatic encephalopathy is associated with more moderate degrees of hyperprolactinemia. Decreased prolactin clearance by the failing liver has not been found. It has been suggested that decreased hypothalamic dopamine secretion or transport underlies the hyperprolactinemia associated with hepatic encephalopathy (Corenblum and Shaffer, 1989).

Although tissue culture studies of many malignant human cell lines have identified intracellular prolactin, systemic hypersecretion is rarely observed. Hyperprolactinemia has been associated with bronchogenic carcinoma, renal cell carcinoma, gonadoblastoma, and all stages of cervical carcinoma (Hsu et al, 1992).

A benign cause of ectopic prolactin secretion may occur with an ovarian dermoid cyst (Palmer et al, 1990). The ovarian wall contains a prolactinoma, and the hyperprolactinemia responds to oophorectomy. There may be pituitary remnants in the sphenoid sinus, and this ectopic tissue may become adenomatous.

Neurogenic Causes. Suckling is a potent physiologic stimulus for prolactin secretion. This is mediated by tactile receptors in the anterior chest wall, between T4 and T6. Any lesion that irritates this area may simulate the suckling reflex, resulting in chronic hyperprolactinemia. This has been observed with burns, rashes, irritating scars, thoracotomy, herpes zoster, or excessive nipple or breast stimulation. These causes are best identified by history and inspection of the chest wall.

Medications. Medications are the most common cause of hyperprolactinemia. Mechanisms include (1) blocking dopamine receptors (phenothiazines, neuroleptics, butyrophenones), (2) depleting dopamine (reserpine, α-methyldopa), and (3) stimulating lactotrophs (high-dose estrogens, narcotics, verapamil, cimetidine). Some neuroleptics chronically elevate prolactin, producing long-term hypogonadism and its sequelae in some patients (Zelaschi et al, 1996). This may add to the long-term morbidity of schizophrenia. Narcotics work by central endorphin pathways, either directly or by inhibiting dopamine secretion from hypothalamic nerve endings. Physiologic dosages of estrogens or the pharmacologic dosages found in 30- to 35-μg estradiol oral contraceptives do not elevate prolactin levels in a normal adult woman. High-dose estrogen replacement in a postmenopausal woman or 50-μg estradiol oral contraceptives may transiently increase serum prolactin levels but result in a return to normal within 3 months of continuous use (Josimovich et al, 1987). For this reason, a woman taking a low-estrogen oral contraceptive who is found to have hyperprolac-

tinemia should be investigated for an underlying cause.

Marked hyperprolactinemia may occur with a dopamine antagonist used for the gastrointestinal tract, such as domperidone. The antagonist also binds to dopamine receptors in the anterior pituitary gland because the pituitary lies outside the blood-brain barrier. Cocaine abuse is associated with amenorrhea, infertility, and galactorrhea in women as well as with impotence in men. Cocaine abuse also is associated with increased pulse amplitude of prolactin secretion. In a study of eight men, four had mild hyperprolactinemia, ranging from 22 to 45 μg/L (Mendelson et al, 1989).

Macroprolactinemia. Macroprolactinemia consists of increased amounts of larger prolactin molecules that are immunologically, but not biologically, active. It may consist of complexes between prolactin and immunoglobulin G (Hattori et al, 1994). Patients do not show clinical symptoms resulting from hyperprolactinemia. Massive screening of the asymptomatic population has found, that once pregnancy and drugs have been excluded, macroprolactinemia is the most common underlying cause of hyperprolactinemia (Miyai et al, 1986). Recognition of macroprolactinemia is important in order to avoid needless investigation and inappropriate therapy (Corenblum, 1990). This appears to be a benign biochemical entity, with no long-term problems yet established.

Mechanisms of Gonadal Hypofunction Resulting from Hypersecretion of Prolactin (Fig. 29–3)

Some degree of gonadal dysfunction almost always occurs in the adult of reproductive age with hyperprolactinemia. Normal ovarian function is dependent on normal pulsatile secretion of LH and FSH, and their secretion occurs in response to pulsatile GnRH release from the hypothalamus. Any abnormality in the normal secretion of GnRH may result in some degree of abnormal ovarian function. In rats, dopamine turnover in the median eminence is increased by hyperprolactinemia (short-loop feedback). In humans, dopamine infusion results in decreased frequency of LH pulses. Presumably, hyperprolactinemia acts at the hypothalamic level to increase dopamine turnover, which then inhibits GnRH/LH secretion (Ho et al, 1984). There may be a direct action of prolactin on GnRH neurons with inhibition of GnRH gene expression and release of GnRH (Milenkovic et al, 1994). Another mechanism may be an increase in opioid tone in the hypothalamus. Opioids act at the level of the median eminence to decrease GnRH secretion and thus decrease normal pulsatile release of LH and FSH, possibly by changing dopamine secretion (Grossman et al, 1981). In hyperprolactinemia, opioid receptor antagonists have been associated with return of LH and FSH secretion, presumably as a result of the return of normal pulsatile GnRH secretion (Sarkar and Yen, 1985).

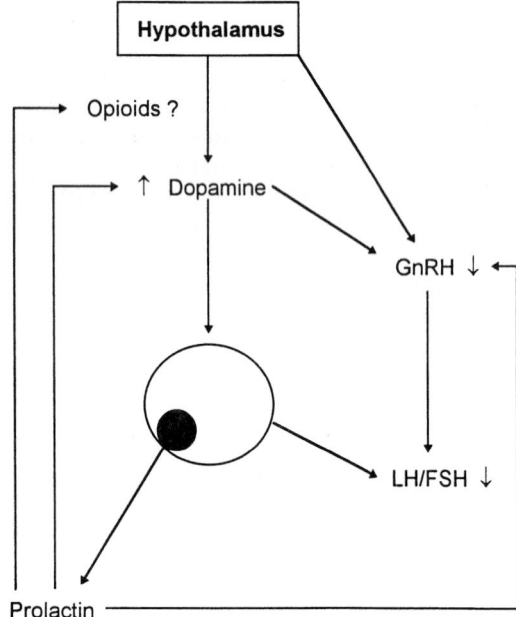

Figure 29–3
Mechanism of hypogonadism in pathologic
hyperprolactinemia. Increased prolactin secretion results in
inhibition of gonadotropin-releasing hormone (GnRH) and
secretion of luteinizing hormone/follicle-stimulating hormone
(LH/FSH).

The changes in amplitude, and especially frequency
of LH pulsation, suggest that this is mediated by
changes in secretion of GnRH. A normal serum LH
and FSH response to exogenously administered
GnRH in hyperprolactinemic women indicates normal gonadotroph function and further implies that
abnormal secretion is secondary to abnormal GnRH
release. The surgical removal of prolactin-secreting
microadenomas is associated with an increased
number of LH pulses before there is any rise of estradiol (Stevenaert et al, 1986). This suggests that the
impaired LH pulsatility is related to a central effect
of hyperprolactinemia.

Changes in LH and FSH secretion result in varying
disorders of folliculogenesis, steroidogenesis, and luteal function. Postmenopausal women with hyperprolactinemia may have low LH and FSH secretion;
however, when prolactin levels are normalized, gonadotropin levels increase to the postmenopausal
range (Scoccia et al, 1988).

Some abnormalities noted with hyperprolactinemia include loss of estrogen-induced LH secretion
(positive feedback) and loss of a normal ovulatory
response to clomiphene citrate. Suppression of normal pulsatile GnRH secretion likely results in both
of these abnormalities. The positive effect of estradiol is exerted at the pituitary under the permissive
effect of pulsatile GnRH secretion. When exogenous
pulsatile GnRH is administered, despite maintenance of hyperprolactinemia, the estradiol-induced

LH surge becomes normal as part of the midcycle
ovulatory events.

A large prolactin-secreting pituitary tumor may directly interfere with gonadotroph function. Otherwise, there is no direct effect of hyperprolactinemia
on gonadotropin secretion. Following shrinkage of
the macroadenoma by a dopamine agonist, LH and
FSH secretion usually returns to normal.

In vivo studies have shown that, if mild hyperprolactinemia is induced in normal ovulating
women throughout a menstrual cycle, follicular maturation and luteal function are abnormal (Kauppila
et al, 1982). If hyperprolactinemia is induced only
during early follicular development, abnormalities
may extend over the entire cycle. Hyperprolactinemia induced only in the luteal phase (after a normal
follicular phase) may result in abnormal luteal function, despite the pre-existing normal follicular development and ovulation (Caruso et al, 1989). The
blunted steroidogenesis of the corpus luteum is
likely due to changes in hypothalamic-pituitary secretion, because abnormal LH and progesterone secretion respond to GnRH administration. Mild hyperprolactinemia is associated with luteal-phase
insufficiency (Corenblum et al, 1976), but it is not
established whether this results from a direct luteolytic effect or from disturbed GnRH secretion; likely,
it is from the latter.

Because a normal ovulatory cycle, with normal follicular growth and release and normal corpus luteum function, may occur with exogenous pulsatile
GnRH, it appears that restoration of normal GnRH
secretion—and thus normal pituitary LH and FSH
secretion—is sufficient to overcome any direct effect
prolactin may have on the ovary. The dose of GnRH
utilized is physiologic, not different from that used
to induce a normal ovulatory cycle in women with
hypothalamic amenorrhea. This suggests that disordered secretion of GnRH is the cause of abnormal
reproductive function in hyperprolactinemic women
(Gindoff et al, 1986).

Clinical Features of Hyperprolactinemia

Symptoms of hyperprolactinemia depend on the age
and sex of the patient. In general, symptoms include
galactorrhea, oligoamenorrhea, polymenorrhea, infertility, decreased libido, and delayed pubescence in
the adolescent. Symptoms may relate to the underlying disease, such as a sellar mass, although most
prolactinomas do not produce these symptoms. In
addition, long-term sequelae of hypoestrogenization
(especially osteopenia) result in clinical problems.

WOMEN OF REPRODUCTIVE AGE

Hyperprolactinemia occurs most commonly in
women of reproductive age and is accompanied by
some form of menstrual dysfunction. In general, the
greater the degree of hyperprolactinemia, the greater
the menstrual abnormalities. Once a prolactin level

four times above normal is achieved, amenorrhea usually ensues. The greater the degree of hyperprolactinemia, the more likely there will be an underlying prolactinoma and the greater will be its size. In contrast, the degree of hyperprolactinemia has no relationship to the presence or severity of galactorrhea. The first change in the menstrual cycle would be subtle, with an inadequate luteal phase in a woman who otherwise appears to have regular ovulatory cycles, although they may be shortened. The next change may be loss of ovulation, resulting in an estrogenized anovulatory state, accompanied by infertility, polymenorrhea, or oligomenorrhea. Progressive impairment of gonadotropin secretion then results in a hypoestrogenized state, with amenorrhea, infertility, dyspareunia, and, in the long term, osteopenia. Progression through these various phases may be observed in a woman whose hyperprolactinemia was normalized with a dopamine agonist that is later withdrawn. Serum prolactin levels should be measured in all women with otherwise unexplained changes in menstrual function.

Although menstrual disorders and galactorrhea are the most common manifestations of hyperprolactinemia, there are other clinical concerns. Headaches are out of proportion to the presence of pituitary tumors. They are usually frontal and are reported as penetrating behind the eyes. The presence of headaches should suggest a search for an underlying pituitary tumor. There may be symptoms associated with a pituitary mass. Various degrees of hypopituitarism may result from compression of the stalk or of the pituitary gland, and any suprasellar extension may be associated with polyuria as a result of antidiuretic hormone insufficiency. Superior extension may produce chiasmal compression and thus peripheral visual loss, and obstructive hydrocephalus may produce papilledema. Lateral extension into the cavernous sinus may impinge on the third, fourth, or sixth cranial nerve and may produce diplopia. Superior extension to the hypothalmus may rarely result in disorders of body weight, sleeping pattern, and core body temperature. Extension to the temporal lobe may result in temporal lobe seizures. Downward extension through the sphenoid sinus may produce rhinorrhea. Gross extrasellar extension is rare, but these symptoms should be explored on initial evaluation.

Hypopituitarism becomes manifest, depending on the age and sex of the patient. A child may demonstrate loss of growth; an adolescent usually demonstrates delayed puberty and loss of growth. An adult first shows gonadal dysfunction. Symptoms and signs of hypothyroidism may occur, but the thyroid gland is small and soft on palpation. Examination of the male with hypopituitarism usually shows small testes (smaller than 4 cm in the long diameter). At a late stage, hypoadrenalism occurs with nausea, vomiting, postural lightheadedness, and loss of axillary and pubic hair. This degree of hypopituitarism is exceptionally rare among prolactinomas.

Hypoestrogenization may result in symptoms of decreased libido, dyspareunia, and vaginitis. It is usually clinically assessed by a negative withdrawal bleed in response to a progestational agent.

Longstanding hyperprolactinemia has been associated with osteoporosis resulting from various changes in bone metabolism. There may be more profound effects on trabecular bone in the spine than on cortical bone in the wrist (Schlechte et al, 1987). To date, no increase in the fracture rate has been shown. There are some reports of osteoporosis occurring in adult men with longstanding hyperprolactinemia (Taylor and Kelly, 1989). The decreased bone mineral content noted in hyperprolactinemic women is likely related to the hypoestrogenization, not the hyperprolactinemia. Hyperprolactinemic women with menses and close-to-normal serum estradiol levels have a bone mineral density similar to that in normal women. Dopamine agonist treatment of hyperprolactinemia results in some recovery of bone mineral loss (Klibanski and Greenspan, 1986).

Mild hirsutism, acne, and seborrhea have been noted in some women with hyperprolactinemia (Glickman et al, 1982). These may result from changes in androgen metabolism, but hirsutism does not occur with primary hyperprolactinemia. Some patients with hirsutism actually have PCOS with mild hyperprolactinemia.

Various psychological symptoms may occur with hyperprolactinemia. If specifically asked, many women with hyperprolactinemia report orgasmic dysfunction and decreased libido. Hyperprolactinemic women report an increased incidence of depression, hostility, and anxiety compared with amenorrheic controls (Fava et al, 1981). Normalization of prolactin levels with bromocriptine improves depression, anxiety, hostility, feelings of inadequacy, and decreased libido (Buckman and Kellner, 1985). The slow development of hyperprolactinemic symptoms may allow many young patients to adjust to both the hypoestrogenization symptoms and any psychological changes.

WOMEN OF OTHER AGE GROUPS AND MEN

The adolescent female with primary hyperprolactinemia presents with delayed or arrested puberty, such as primary amenorrhea. The elderly patient with hyperprolactinemia may present only with symptoms related to an expanding pituitary mass.

The adult male may present only with symptoms of an expanding pituitary mass. Most male patients admit to decreased libido for years and, possibly, impotence. In 1236 consecutive males presenting with impotence, only 5.3% had hyperprolactinemia (Leonard et al, 1989), and they invariably complained of decreased libido. Hyperprolactinemia does not produce gynecomastia. Adult men usually have no features of hypogonadism unless the hyperprolactinemia occurs at puberty, preventing normal development. The testes of the adult male with hyperprolactinemia are usually normal in size unless there is concomitant hypopituitarism from a mass. Oligospermia does not result from hyperprolactinemia unless more extensive hypopituitarism is present.

GALACTORRHEA

Galactorrhea is the symptom or sign suggestive of hyperprolactinemia. Nevertheless, there is no correlation between the presence or amount of galactorrhea and the degree of hyperprolactinemia. Only 30% to 80% of all women with hyperprolactinemia are found to have galactorrhea, either spontaneously or on examination. This variation in prevalence is proportional to the extent to which galactorrhea is sought and inversely proportional to the degree and duration of hypoestrogenization. The combination of galactorrhea and amenorrhea is found with a pituitary tumor in 75%. Galactorrhea is rare in prepubertal children, men, and women with primary amenorrhea. This is because the breast must first be adequately developed.

Galactorrhea may be unilateral or bilateral, continuous or intermittent, spontaneous, or expressible only with palpation. All signs have the same importance. Galactorrhea refers to any expressible milk from a nonpregnant woman who is not breastfeeding an infant. By definition, there must be the presence of fat globules, which can be confirmed by microscopic examination of an unstained drop of breast discharge or by pathologic examination with Sudan IV stain. Many breast discharges are not galactorrhea. Because the normal mature breast is a modified sweat gland, it is continually secreting fluid from the acini and possibly from the ducts. Acellular debris may be noted on microscopic examination, but fat droplets are absent.

The prevalence of galactorrhea in the adult female population is highly variable, reported to be from 0.1% to 32%. The variation depends on the population studied, how galactorrhea is defined, and to what degree it is sought. Prevalence increases with age and parity, and its occurrence may depend on the method of contraception. Hyperprolactinemia has been reported to occur in 20% to 50% of women with galactorrhea. This likely is an overestimation because galactorrhea appears to occur more frequently than has been previously recognized. Galactorrhea may be found in 5% to 10% of normal menstruating women, 90% of whom have normal serum prolactin levels. Even early studies in tertiary referral hospitals have found that, after an extensive investigation, idiopathic galactorrhea was the diagnosis, by exclusion, in over two thirds of cases (Tolis et al, 1974).

The presence of galactorrhea represents a diagnostic challenge. There must be a careful drug history, inspection of the chest wall (tactile reflex), and measurements of serum TSH and prolactin levels. If hyperprolactinemia is found, this is investigated and treated, if necessary. The presence of galactorrhea is most important when it is associated with menstrual disorders or infertility, because this systemic effect suggests the presence of hyperprolactinemia.

Galactorrhea most commonly occurs in association with regular menses and with normal serum prolactin levels as determined by radioimmunoassay. Bioassay measurements of prolactin also are normal (Johnston et al, 1985). This suggests a change in breast sensitivity for prolactin. No treatment is necessary other than reassurance. If galactorrhea is symptomatically bothersome, a dopamine agonist for 3 weeks is useful.

WHEN TO MEASURE SERUM PROLACTIN

Serum prolactin levels should be measured in the patient with galactorrhea, unexplained menstrual changes, or decreased libido, or the presence of any sellar or suprasellar mass or infiltrate (Fig. 29–4). It is important to recognize that prolactin secretion is pulsatile. Food, especially protein, may enhance prolactin secretion. Beer has long been used to support lactation and may increase serum prolactin, likely a result of the malt. The level of serum prolactin elevation is an important diagnostic tool. Values greater than 70 µg/L are usually associated with amenorrhea. Values greater than 200 µg/L are almost always due to an underlying prolactinoma, although some drugs, such as domperidone, and some suprasellar lesions, such as craniopharyngioma, may product similar elevations. Greatly elevated serum prolactin levels, despite normal regular menses, suggest the presence of macroprolactinemia. Any value less than 50 µg/L should be repeated two times. Ideally, this is done fasting, at about 9 A.M., without any sexual activity that morning. Several samples may be taken over a period of 3 hours. Because of the cost of multiple samples, the samples may be pooled for a single measurement.

It is difficult to interpret mild hyperprolactinemia as being pathologic or clinically significant in an otherwise asymptomatic patient. Symptoms may demonstrate that the biochemical measurement of hyperprolactinemia represents a true biologic entity and warrants further investigation and possible therapy.

Hyperprolactinemia may require treatment because of its effect on gonadal function and bones or because of galactorrhea. Many hyperprolactinemic patients note an improved feeling of well-being, libido, memory, and personality when hyperprolactinemia is normalized. Premature osteoporosis may be prevented or partially reversed. Thus, even when fertility or menstrual abnormalities are not clinical problems, most patients have clinical objectives that require some form of therapy for the problem of hyperprolactinemia. Specific treatment information is detailed in the section on "Prolactinomas."

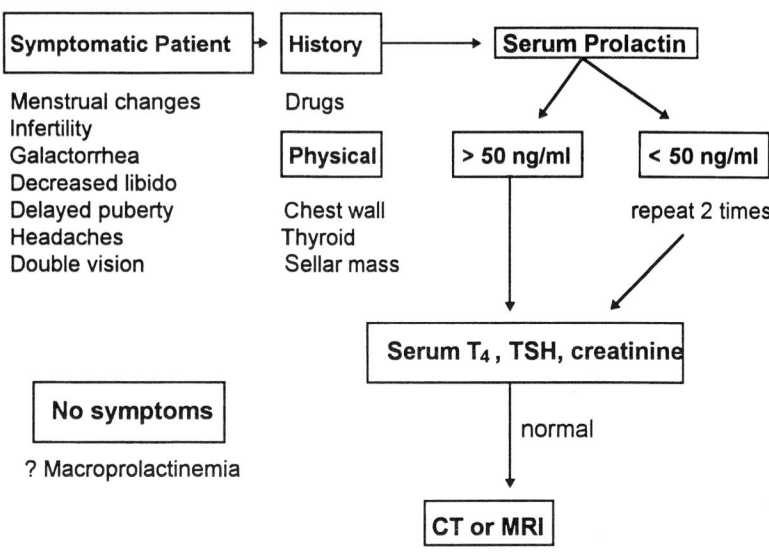

Figure 29-4
Approach to hyperprolactinemia. CT, computerized tomography; MRI, magnetic resonance imaging; T$_4$, thyroxine; TSH, thyroid-stimulating hormone.

Prolactinomas

In the asymptomatic population, mass biochemical screening for hyperprolactinemia in 10,500 adults found five subjects with prolactinomas (Miyai et al, 1986). Autopsy studies incidentally have noted pituitary tumors in 25% (Costello, 1936). When these incidental adenomas are specifically identified by immunohistochemistry, 6% to 11% of patients have prolactinomas at autopsy (Kovacs et al, 1980; Burrow et al, 1981). With incidental prolactinomas, chart reviews show no alteration in the fertility rate. The incidental prolactinoma is commonly found but is clinically insignificant.

Large prolactin tumors, *macroadenomas*, are defined as greater than 1 cm in diameter. This is an arbitrary cutoff point and is not biologically relevant. The finding of a macroadenoma at routine autopsy is a rare event; macroadenomas generally present during life as a result of clinical symptoms. The vast majority of microprolactinomas are much more common in women, whereas macroadenomas show no sex predilection. However, autopsy findings of microprolactinomas show no sex predilection.

It appears that the large, rapidly growing macroprolactinoma is a different disease entity than the small, stable microprolactinoma. It is important to recognize this difference in biology in order to select the appropriate therapy. Microprolactinomas occur more frequently in women, but this is not because symptoms are more obvious in women. In contrast, there is no sex predilection regarding macroprolac-

tinomas. Thus the majority of hyperprolactinemic women have a normal sella turcica or evidence of a microadenoma, whereas the majority of men have macroprolactinomas. When women presenting with either symptomatic microprolactinoma or macroprolactinoma are assessed in regard to mean age of presentation and duration of symptoms, there are no differences between these two groups. The macroadenoma does not result merely from passage of time; it is an entity that differs in its tumorigenesis. It shows its enhanced growth potential at the time of presentation. Finally, the response to a dopamine agonist is quantitatively different, with macroadenomas showing more marked tumor shrinkage.

Natural History

One of the unfortunate events of medical history is that, soon after the development of a radioimmunoassay for the measurement of serum prolactin (thus enabling the diagnosis of pathologic hyperprolactinemia), advances in neuroradiologic techniques allowed visualization of a pituitary mass. Once the diagnosis of prolactinomas was feasible, medical and surgical intervention was also available, with impressive results. For this reason, the natural history of the untreated prolactinoma was not initially established. Only today, after two decades, is there a better understanding of the natural history, and, with this, the therapeutic options may be better applied. It is now recognized that the vast majority of microadenomas do not progress to become macroprolactinomas. The postmortem finding of microprolactinomas in 6% to 10% of the population indicates this natural history. Clinical observations are consistent with this finding, because prolactin-secreting microadenomas are common among young women, whereas prolactin-secreting macroadenomas are rare among elderly women. Thus the transformation of microadenoma to macroadenoma is rare and the natural history of prolactin-secreting microadenomas is stable and benign. In rare instances, some prolactinomas progressively increase in size; at present, however, patients at such risk cannot be identified. In contrast, it is now evident that some women with prolactinomas will improve or even normalize without any treatment.

Various studies have defined the natural history of hyperprolactinemia. March et al (1981) reported on 43 women presumed to have prolactin-secreting microadenomas who were observed for 3 to 20 years without treatment. Progressive tumor enlargement was radiologically noted in two patients, whereas spontaneous remission of hyperprolactinemia and symptoms occurred in three. The two patients with tumors that progressed as shown on CT scan did not experience changes in symptoms, serum prolactin levels, or visual fields.

Rjosk and co-authors (1982) observed 34 hyperprolactinemic women who received no treatment over 2 to 6 years; 33 had stable or falling prolactin levels, whereas one showed increased levels and a new change in the sella suggestive of progression to a microadenoma. Of 19 patients with a microadenoma, 18 had stable serum prolactin levels and clinical course and one showed an increased serum prolactin level but without any radiologic evidence of tumor enlargement.

Koppelman and colleagues (1984) observed 25 women with hyperprolactinemia who received no treatment for an average of 11 years. Four had a macroprolactinoma, and eight had a microadenoma. Of 22 women with amenorrhea, seven developed spontaneous menses (32%). Galactorrhea was present in 19 women and resolved in 6 (32%). The mean prolactin level fell from 225 to 155 μg/L. No patient clinically worsened or demonstrated progression from a microadenoma to a macroadenoma. One subject demonstrated a slight progression of the abnormality in the skull radiograph, yet pituitary function studies and visual field examinations remained normal.

Sisam and associates (1987) reported 38 untreated women with microprolactinomas who were observed for an average of 50 months. Symptoms improved in 10 of the patients and worsened in one patient. Baseline serum prolactin levels decreased in 55% and increased in 37%. No patient showed any progression of abnormalities on CT scan.

In some reports, clinical improvement was seen in patients whose symptoms occurred after exposure to estrogen, such as from pregnancy or the birth control pill. Schlechte et al (1989) described a prospective study for 3 to 7 years of 30 untreated hyperprolactinemic women. Among 19 amenorrheic women, oligomenorrhea developed in 3 and regular menstrual periods returned in 3 others. Among 19 women with galactorrhea, 6 noted resolution. Worsening of clinical symptoms did not occur in any patient. In 4 of 14 women with initially normal radiographic studies, there was evidence of microadenomas. In contrast, four women with initial radiographic evidence of a pituitary tumor had normal radiographic findings on subsequent examination. Changes in serum prolactin concentrations did not correlate with the radiographic changes.

Not all patients studied have been untreated, but some studies have described only short-term treatment. Pepperell et al (1984) reported 98 women with mild hyperprolactinemia (prolactin levels less than four times above normal) observed for a mean of 66 months. There was spontaneous return of regular menses in 28 of 91 (31%), associated with normalization of serum prolactin levels. This finding was especially notable following bromocriptine-induced pregnancy. Radiographic evidence of tumor development was noted in nine subjects. Interestingly, four demonstrated increased basal serum prolactin levels and five noted a decrease, with some values even falling close to normal. All tumors presumably remained intrasellar and asymptomatic. Thus determination of tumor progression requires radiologic assessment, and serum prolactin levels are inadequate to screen for such a development.

One study used CT to arbitrarily separate symptomatic hyperprolactinemic women into two groups of 20 each, one group with microadenoma and the other with IH (Corenblum and Taylor, 1988). The patients were studied following discontinuation of bromocriptine after at least 1 year, and from 5 to 13 years from clinical presentation. Of the 20 women with microprolactinomas, symptoms and serum prolactin levels remained unchanged in 19, whereas 1 woman experienced complete loss of symptoms and had normal serum prolactin levels. Of the 20 women with IH, 8 had unchanged symptoms and serum prolactin levels; 9 showed improvement in symptoms, with lower basal serum prolactin levels; and 3 experienced complete loss of symptoms with normal serum prolactin levels. This study indicates that the natural history of both microprolactinoma and IH is a benign stable course, but the natural history of IH may even be better. Certainly, in the group with IH, there are various etiologic factors, with some of the patients actually harboring microadenomas; however, the better overall natural history suggests that IH may form a distinct syndrome in some women.

Initially, it had been feared that pregnancy would have an adverse effect on underlying prolactinomas. It is now clear that spontaneous pregnancy may occur in hyperprolactinemic women. Furthermore, up to one third may show normalization of serum prolactin levels without a return of symptoms following a pregnancy (Crosignani et al, 1985, 1989).

To summarize, it appears that the natural history of women with prolactin-secreting microadenomas is one of progression to a larger tumor in fewer than 5%, whereas at least 10% of the patients will spontaneously undergo remission without any treatment. Whether treatment with a dopamine agonist improves this natural history remains unknown. The natural history of women with IH is such that about 10% will show asymptomatic radiologic progression to a microadenoma, none will show progression to a macroadenoma, and about 30% will experience normalization of symptoms and serum prolactin levels with or without treatment. The natural history of untreated prolactin-secreting macroadenomas is unknown because no therapeutic intervention has not been studied. There is poor correlation of a change in the CT scan with a change in serum prolactin levels. Thus increased levels cannot be used as an indication for tumor enlargement, and serum prolactin cannot substitute for radiologic assessment.

Etiology

The etiology of prolactinomas is unknown. There have been several proposed mechanisms, which may not be mutually exclusive. They are monoclonal tumors and, thus, originate from a single cell.

ESTROGEN

Women with symptomatic prolactinomas frequently present following discontinuation of the birth control pill or after pregnancy. In retrospect, many of these women were given oral contraceptives because of menstrual irregularity. Estrogens are known to stimulate mitotic activity in the lactotrophs. In a normal pregnancy, there is hyperplasia of the lactotrophs and there may be symptomatic growth of preexisting prolactinomas. In rodents, prolactinomas may be induced by administration of high doses of estrogen. It is difficult to extrapolate these observations to humans. Autopsy-obtained pituitaries from pregnant women have found that prolactin adenomas are not more numerous or larger than those found in nonpregnant women or men (Scheithauer et al, 1990). Several careful studies, including one British prospective study of more than 200,000 woman-years of observation (Wingrave et al, 1980), have shown that there is no increased risk of prolactinoma with use of oral contraceptives. The use of oral contraceptives in women who are known to harbor prolactinomas is not associated with any deterioration in clinical status or evidence of tumor growth, nor has this occurred with physiologic estrogen replacement.

HYPOTHALAMIC DYSFUNCTION

It has been postulated that decreased hypothalamic inhibition or increased hypothalamic stimulation, or both, may induce prolactinoma formation. Prolactin secretion in response to various stimulatory and inhibitory secretagogues is almost invariably abnormal in patients harboring prolactinomas. Such abnormal prolactin secretory dynamics are likely due to changes by the tumor or hyperprolactinemia itself, as opposed to any primary underlying hypothalamic dysfunction. With successful surgical removal of prolactinomas, abnormalities in secretory function usually return to normal, but this may take months. Tumor recurrence after successful surgery may approach 50% but does not steadily increase over time. This suggests that the recurrence is due to incomplete removal, as opposed to underlying hypothalamic dysfunction giving rise to a new adenomatous state. Statements that hypothalamic dysfunction accounts for IH are unsubstantiated.

ABNORMAL VASCULAR SUPPLY

In the normal situation, the capillaries of the anterior pituitary are supplied solely by the portal venous system from the hypothalamus and do not receive any direct arterial blood. Schechter et al (1988) found arteries in 13 to 16 prolactinomas but not in control pituitary glands. It has not been established whether this is a primary event or one that is secondary to the forming adenoma. This allows one region of the anterior pituitary to receive arterial blood and thus escape from hypothalamic dopaminergic inhibition This may predispose to lactotroph hyperplasia and possibly adenoma formation. This observation may explain why patients with prolactinomas do not respond to increased hypothalamic dopamine secretion, yet suppress prolactin secretion with a dopamine agonist that is present in systemic blood. The role of arteriogenesis in the primary production of human prolactinomas remains speculative.

LOCAL PRODUCTION OF GROWTH FACTORS AND ONCOGENE TRANSFORMATION

The mechanisms of growth control within the normal pituitary gland remain to be clarified. They certainly involve extracellular messenger molecules, their receptors, and postreceptor events. Pituitary tumors secrete various growth factors, but it remains to be established whether these have any role in tumorigenesis.

Abnormal growth may reflect altered oncogene functions. Oncogenes are expressed at different stages of normal cell proliferation and differentiation and are thought to encode proteins that may control these processes. Proto-oncogene abnormalities have been found in some prolactinomas (U et al, 1988). Such changes may underlie the genetic basis for neoplastic growth, but any role remains to be established.

Pathology

Prolactinomas consist of three histologic patterns: papillary, diffuse, and ribbons of adenoma cells separated by hyalinous connective tissue. Fibrosis, especially perivascular, occurs in all forms. Prolactinomas may also contain calcification in 12%, which rarely may be sufficiently profuse to develop as a "pituitary stone." About 5% of prolactinomas are characterized by deposition of amyloid, and excessive accumulation may lead to cell necrosis.

Definitive diagnosis of a pituitary adenoma as a prolactinoma is usually achieved by immunohistochemistry, which can detect intracellular granules containing prolactin. Electron microscopy assesses ultrastructure and separates prolactinomas into two variants. The densely granulated form is relatively rare and contains many large secretory granules that occupy much of the cytoplasm. The majority of prolactinomas are sparsely granulated. Ultrastructure demonstrates an important diagnostic feature of prolactinomas: misplaced exocytosis. This is the extrusion of secretory granules at the lateral cell membrane. There are no morphologic features that can predict the biologic behavior.

Most prolactinomas are solitary lesions, but multiple tumors may occur. Local invasion into the dura and bone is common (Selman et al, 1986). There is no relationship between local invasion and size of the adenoma. Invasion is not indicative of malignancy. Features of malignancy, including cellular pleomorphism, mitotic activity, and nuclear atypia, do not apply to prolactinomas. The diagnosis of carcinoma is rare and can be made only if distant metastases are present. The invasive prolactinoma is a compressive type of lesion that is well encapsulated, although some are characterized by extensive capsular penetration and involvement of the dura, cavernous sinus, and bone.

Clinical Features

Patients with prolactinomas present with symptoms and signs that are related to prolactin hypersecretion, possibly as a result of the tumor mass if it is sufficiently large, and possibly related to deficiency in normal pituitary function. The clinical presentation for the various forms of hyperprolactinemia is shown in Table 29–2.

Diagnosis

The diagnosis of a prolactinoma is frequently obvious once the patient is assessed, serum prolactin is measured, and anatomic localization is determined by CT scan or magnetic resonance imaging (MRI). Nevertheless, caution must be exercised in diagnosis. The fact that 6% to 11% of the normal population are found to have a prolactin-secreting microadenoma at autopsy indicates that a normal serum prolactin level does not rule out the presence of a prolactinoma. Such prolactinomas are clinically silent and appear to be of no significance. Inhomogeneity, as demonstrated by a CT scan, that is compatible with a microadenoma may be seen in one third of the normal adult population and in 40% to 50% of women with hyperprolactinemia. For this reason, the CT scan must also be interpreted with discretion. MRI is also nonspecific because it demonstrates changes suggestive of a microadenoma in 10% of normal people (Hall et al, 1994). Hyperprolactinemia may be ascribed to an underlying visualized prolactinoma once a drug history has been obtained and inspection of the chest and biochemical elimination of hypothyroidism and renal failure have taken place.

The basal serum prolactin value is a useful diagnostic tool; the greater the elevation, the more likely an underlying prolactinoma exists in the symptomatic patient. A serum prolactin level of 50 μg/L indicates an underlying prolactin-secreting microadenoma in 25% of patients; 100 μg/L is associated with the diagnosis of a microadenoma in 50% of patients and greater than 200 μg/L with an underlying prolactinoma in 95% of symptomatic patients. Because prolactin is secreted episodically, a mild elevation requires multiple samples to confirm true hyperprolactinemia, and multiple samples may be

Table 29–2. CLINICAL PRESENTATION OF PRIMARY PITUITARY HYPERPROLACTINEMIA

	SERUM PROLACTIN	CT SCAN OR MRI	SYMPTOMS/SIGNS
Idiopathic hyperprolactinemia	<5 times normal	Normal	Menstrual change, galactorrhea
Microadenoma	2–10 times normal	Mass 3–10 mm	Menstrual change, galactorrhea
Macroadenoma	>10 times normal	Mass >10 mm ± extrasellar extension	Menstrual change, possibly headache, peripheral vision loss
Pseudoprolactinoma (non–prolactin secreting)	<5 times normal	Mass >10 mm ± extrasellar extension	Usually headache, possibly peripheral vision loss, galactorrhea, menstrual changes
Invasive prolactinoma	>10 times normal	Mass >20 mm with extrasellar extension	Usually headache, visual field changes, possible diplopia, some degree of hypopituitarism
Macroprolactinemia	2–10 times normal	Normal	None

required to determine that the elevation is not consistent and thus may not be important.

Various dynamic prolactin stimulation and suppression tests have been described in an attempt to identify underlying prolactinomas. To date, no single test or group of tests can practically differentiate a prolactinoma from nonadenomatous causes of hyperprolactinemia. Pituitary stimulation testing to determine the presence or absence of pituitary reserve is not sufficiently sensitive to be indicative of an underlying pituitary tumor. Such testing is not needed in patients with a normal CT/MRI scan or a microadenomatous change on CT/MRI scan. Patients harboring large prolactin-secreting pituitary tumors are at risk of hypopituitarism, and it is essential to ensure that they have adequate cortisol secretion at baseline and following stress if surgery is not being planned. This may be determined by an adrenocorticotropic hormone stimulation test of the adrenal, or insulin-induced hypoglycemia, corticotropin-releasing hormone, or metyrapone stimulation test of the hypothalamic-pituitary-adrenal axis. Postoperative pituitary stimulation testing is necessary to assess any residual hypopituitarism, especially ACTH.

Visual field examination is objectively documented using Goldmann perimetry. There must be suprasellar extension to obtain chiasmal compression. Although various visual field changes may occur, the classic abnormality is bitemporal hemianopsia. Visual field examination should be performed in all patients with macroadenomas because chiasmal compression may occur with suprasellar extension that may not be appreciated by CT scan or MRI. If an abnormality is detected, serial examinations are necessary to assess response to therapy.

An underlying anatomic problem is defined by radiologic means. Coned-down views of the sella turcica and sellar tomography yield high false-positive and false-negative rates in regard to detection of prolactinomas. The normal sella turcica has many common anatomic variants, some of which may appear as a focally thinned floor (such as a sphenoid sinus septum). One study that correlated autopsy findings of pituitary tumors with postmortem sellar tomography (Burrow et al, 1981) found that the majority of patients with microadenomas did not have associated abnormalities on sellar tomography. A normal skull film may be sufficient to rule out a large pituitary adenoma.

CT scan is the most common tool to differentiate hyperprolactinemia resulting from IH, microadenoma, macroadenoma, suprasellar lesion, and pseudoprolactinoma. Most of these categories depend on CT identification in conjunction with the basal serum prolactin value. Direct coronal CT scanning with rapid-infusion contrast enhancement is the most sensitive method of evaluating the pituitary for an underlying adenoma. Demonstration of prolactinomas is less reliable in axial sections. The CT scan is used to show a focal lesion (and thus diagnose a microad-

enoma) or a large mass, and it is used longitudinally to observe such patients or to follow the results of treatment. *Adenomas* usually appear as a hypodense lesion associated with a mass effect within the gland, such as gland enlargement, bony lesions, convex superior surface, or displacement of the infundibulum. These changes are nonspecific, so there are no absolute criteria on CT scan that are sufficient to allow a definitive diagnosis of an intrasellar adenoma, and the total findings must be interpreted together. An adenoma smaller than 5 mm may be associated with a normal sellar floor. A rounded hypodense area within the gland is associated with an adenoma but may also occur with underlying cysts, areas of necrosis, or hematomas. Thin tumoral calcifications may be identified, but these are found in only 2% of prolactinomas on CT scan.

Both the sensitivity and specificity of CT scan for identification of microadenomas has come into question. One study found that 30% of microadenomas confirmed by surgery were missed by high-resolution CT (Randall et al, 1983). Another study found underlying microadenomas on surgical exploration in only 20 of 28 patients who were shown to have focal abnormalities on CT (Teasdale et al, 1986). CT fails to identify microadenomas smaller than 3 mm in size, is about 50% accurate when adenomas are between 3 and 5 mm, and is most reliable when adenomas are larger than 6 mm. Focal, low-density abnormalities may be detected in 10% of normal subjects by CT, and upward bulging of the pituitary gland may be seen in up to 44% of normal women. This dictates cautious interpretation of a pituitary CT scan. CT is useful for indicating a large pituitary mass as well as any suprasellar disease, and the presence of calcification.

MRI is superior to CT. CT has an advantage in that it can demonstrate bony erosions and focal areas of calcification within the lesion, whereas MRI is better at defining extrasellar spread. Minimal enlargement of the pituitary gland is detected with MRI. Because of the lack of radiation, MRI may be a superior technique for serial evaluations of a known adenoma, followed with or without treatment over a prolonged course of time.

Carotid arteriography has been largely replaced by CT scan, but may still have to be performed prior to surgery to delineate the carotid arteries and to rule out a possible aneurysm.

It is impossible to diagnose a prolactinoma without visualizing the underlying lesion. A combination of an elevated serum prolactin level and an abnormal, high-resolution CT or MRI scan is highly suggestive of an underlying adenoma, but findings must agree with the clinical picture. There may be alternate causes of increased serum prolactin and of radiologic abnormalities.

Treatment

Treatment of symptomatic patients with hyperprolactinemia depends on the underlying cause. When no obvious cause is present in a symptomatic patient (IH), or if an underlying pituitary mass is visualized, treatment must consider both symptoms related to hyperprolactinemia and the mass and potential problems that may arise. In only a minority of cases is treatment not indicated, such as in a woman who menstruates at least every 2 months (spontaneously or following a progestational agent) and is otherwise asymptomatic of hyperprolactinemia or of any underlying cause. Opinions have varied regarding initial treatment between surgical removal of an adenoma or therapy with a dopamine agonist. There is now a major shift toward more conservative therapy, resulting from recognition of the benign natural history of pathologic hyperprolactinemia.

The objectives of treatment are as follows:

1. *Normalize serum prolactin.* This may not be necessary in all cases because return of estrogenization, improved libido, or loss of galactorrhea may occur in the absence of a normal serum prolactin level. The complaint of infertility usually requires a normal serum prolactin level to restore a normal menstrual cycle.
2. *Decrease tumor mass.* This is necessary in the patient with symptomatic tumor enlargement, such as visual field abnormalities. The observed natural history of untreated adenomas indicates that most prolactinoma masses do not pose immediate or long-term problems.
3. *Restore gonadal function.* This results in the return of sex steroids or can reverse infertility.
4. *Avoid any harm, such as hypopituitarism.* Any therapeutic approach must be characterized by a morbidity and mortality rate that is lower than that of the benign natural history. Therapeutic decisions for any given patient depend on the medical objectives, the presence and size of a prolactinoma, patient compliance and tolerance, and the availability of neurosurgical expertise. Most important, therapeutic decisions are influenced by the patients' personal preference, and informed consent dictates that all potential forms of therapy be explained.

NEUROSURGERY

Transsphenoidal surgery was once used aggressively to treat prolactinomas, because neither the natural history of the untreated state nor the long-term follow-up of any treatment was known. Cure is defined as normalization of serum prolactin levels and loss of symptoms related to hyperprolactinemia, usually defined as return of normal gonadal function. The surgical cure rate is inversely proportional to the size of the tumor and the preoperative serum prolactin level. Levels higher than 200 μg/L and tumors larger than 1 cm in diameter are associated with a marked decrease in cure rate and an increase in some degree of hypopituitarism (Barrow et al, 1988). The overall success rate among various reported series has ranged from 48% to 78%. This variability is due in part to the heterogeneity of surgical expertise and in part to how aggressively the adenoma and any surrounding pituitary tissue has been removed. Higher cure rates, approaching 78%, occur in regard to microadenomas; mortality is low, approximately 0.2%, with a major morbidity rate of 0.4%.

Transsphenoidal removal of a microadenoma may still be justified because of cost effectiveness and to prevent the need for prolonged treatment in some patients. Surgery certainly becomes one alternative to medical treatment in the presence of drug intolerance, resistance, or personal preference by a patient (Tyrrell et al, 1999).

With macroadenomas, the cure rate is 10% to 40%; the mortality rate, 0.9%; and the major morbidity rate, 6.5% (Vance and Thorner, 1987). Surgical treatment utilizing a craniotomy is more hazardous than the transsphenoidal approach.

Prolactin adenomas may exhibit varying degrees of fibrosis. Pretreatment with bromocriptine may increase the fibrous tissue content and negatively affect the surgical cure rate. The amount of fibrosis noted in some studies has correlated with the duration of bromocriptine therapy, but such findings have not been consistent. The increase in perivascular fibrous tissue is thought to be secondary to tumor shrinkage and to result in a denser adenoma that is more difficult to remove (Landolt and Osterwalder, 1984). Because dopamine agonist therapy usually decreases the size of a prolactinoma (which may facilitate tumor removal), many physicians pretreat prolactinomas with a dopamine agonist for 6 weeks prior to surgical removal. This gives some tumor shrinkage but is too short an interval for the induction of any fibrosis.

The initial enthusiasm for surgical removal and potential cure has been lessened by the observation of a high recurrence rate of hyperprolactinemia in patients thought to be cured. Such biochemical relapse usually occurs within 1 to 2 years after surgery but may be delayed for 5 years. The recurrence is not related to any intercurrent pregnancy. Reported recurrence rates for microadenomas have varied from 10% to 58%; for macroadenomas, the rate is up to 80% (Parl et al, 1986). Because pathologic studies have shown prolactinoma cells to be embedded within dura and bone, the recurrence is thought to be related to incomplete removal. The fact that the vast majority of patients with recurrence of hyperprolactinemia and associated symptoms are subsequently treated with long-term dopamine agonist therapy lends strong support to the use of dopamine agonists as initial treatment. If mass signs, such as visual field abnormalities, persist and if tumor shrinkage does not occur with dopamine agonist therapy, surgical resection becomes necessary.

RADIOTHERAPY

Conventional radiotherapy utilizes a linear accelerator and delivers a lesion dose of 500 to 3500 rad in 25 fractions administered over 35 days. The dose depends on the volume of the tumor. Complications are optic nerve injury, brain necrosis, and loss of pituitary trophic hormones. Long-term complications also include an increased incidence of osteogenic sarcoma and new primary brain tumors.

Heavy particle beam radiotherapy, available in a few centers, delivers 5000 to 14,000 rad in a single session without the problem of widespread scatter. It gives a greater chance of cure and is usually associated with an absence of recurrences. Complications are similar to those from conventional radiotherapy.

The major drawback of conventional radiotherapy is that it may take years for results to become manifest. Furthermore, only about one third of patients experience a return to normal prolactin levels over 3 to 13 years (Johnston et al, 1986). Also, some degree of hypopituitarism occurs in the majority of patients, increasing with each year following radiotherapy. Thus radiotherapy is seldom used as a primary treatment for prolactinomas but has an adjunctive or alternative role with macroadenomas when other forms of therapy have failed or are contraindicated.

MEDICAL THERAPY

Bromocriptine. Most drugs used to treat hyperprolactinemia are investigational (Table 29–3). The greatest clinical experience is with the dopamine agonist bromocriptine. Bromocriptine is an ergoline with a cyclic peptide side chain that is a lysergic acid derivative. It binds to dopamine receptors in both the normal and neoplastic lactotroph. After oral administration, 40% to 90% of the drug is absorbed, with a peak blood concentration occurring 2 to 3 hours later. Only 6% of the bromocriptine reaches the circulation because of the first-pass hepatic metabolism. Serum prolactin levels will be suppressed after 1 hour, will be minimal in 7 hours, and will persist for 14 hours following administration of one tablet as a result of prolonged binding to the dopamine receptor. In the circulation, 90% of bromocriptine is bound to plasma proteins. More than 95% is excreted in the feces as a result of hepatic metabolism. Studies using positron emission tomography scanning with radiolabeled bromocriptine have shown preferential uptake by pituitary adenomas. Because a single oral dose lasts for 14 hours, it is administered as two to three doses per day. Some patients show a prolonged response to once-a-day administration. Side effects are due to activation of dopamine receptors in other tissues and are dose dependent.

Bromocriptine binds to the dopamine receptor and, by acting on intracellular cAMP, decreases transcription of the prolactin gene and thus decreases synthesis and secretion of prolactin. Serum prolactin levels normalize in 95% of patients with IH, in 90% of patients with microadenomas, in 85% of patients with macroadenomas, and in 75% of patients with macroadenomas who have already failed to respond to surgical therapy. Serum LH and FSH pulsatility

Table 29–3. MEDICAL APPROACH TO PROBLEMS RELATED TO HYPERPROLACTINEMIA

Dopamine Agonists
Ergot derivatives
   Lysergic acid derivatives: bromocriptine, metergoline
   Clavine derivative: pergolide
   8-α-aminoergolines: lisuride, terguride, CU 32085, CQP 201-403, cabergoline
Nonergot derivatives (quinagolide)
Serotonin Antagonists (Metergoline)
Potentiate γ-Aminobutyric Acid (GABA) (Sodium Valproate)
Nonoral Dopamine Agonist
Intramuscular long-acting bromocriptine
Intravaginal bromocriptine, or cabergoline
Alternative Therapy to Decreasing Prolactin
Infertility
   Clomiphene citrate
   Pulsatile gonadotropin-releasing hormone (GnRH)
   Gonadotropins
Hypogonadism
   Physiologic estrogen plus progestin
   Oral contraceptive
   Testosterone for males
Protect endometrium: regular progestin-induced bleeds

returns in a few days (Fig. 29–5). Gonadal function is restored within 3 months in 90% of women and in 80% of men. Gonadal function may be restored even if the serum prolactin level does not decrease to normal, because not all measured prolactin is biologically active. Dopamine receptor–blocking drugs antagonize the action of bromocriptine.

It is worthwhile to decrease the dosage of bromocriptine to minimize both cost and side effects. The usual recommended does is 5 mg/day, but 12 of 15 patients with moderate hyperprolactinemia (less than 50 µg/L) responded to 2.5 mg/day and five of nine patients with prolactin levels between 100 and 150 µg/L responded to 2.5 mg/day (Soto-Albers et

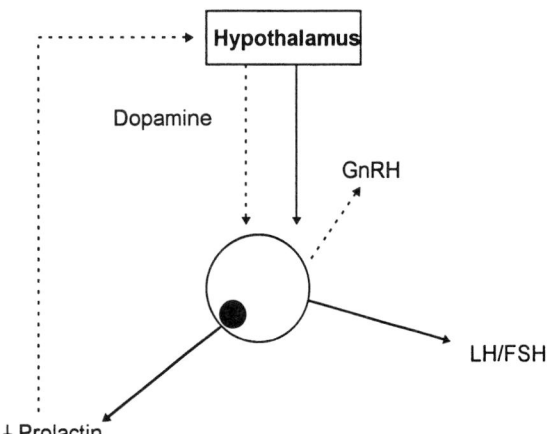

Figure 29–5

Response to dopamine agonist drug. Normalization of serum prolactin results in restoration of normal secretion of gonadotropin-releasing hormone (GnRH) and of luteinizing hormone/follicle-stimulating hormone (LH/FSH).

al, 1987). Ovulatory function was restored in 16 of 18 patients, all with serum prolactin levels greater than 100 μg/L, when 2.5 mg was taken at bedtime (DeBernal and De Villamizar, 1982). With chronic therapy, the dose of bromocriptine can usually be decreased (Liuzzi et al, 1985). This may be because the return of normal circulating levels of estradiol sensitizes the lactotroph to dopaminergic inhibition (Valcavi et al, 1985). Thus the starting and maintenance doses are often lower and the frequency of administration often less than generally recommended. In contrast, if there is no biochemical response to a dosage of 7.5 mg/day, there usually is no response to even higher doses. Chronic administration of bromocriptine for 20 years results in continued action without tachyphylaxis. There are some reports of pleuropulmonary changes associated with chronic use of high doses (Kinnunen and Viljanen, 1988). The drug has proved to be effective and safe in the pediatric age group (Blackwell and Younger, 1986).

To minimize side effects, bromocriptine is usually administered in a small dose, with food, and the dose is slowly increased to therapeutic levels. One-half tablet (1.25 mg) is initially given at bedtime with food, avoiding alcohol. After several days, a second one-half tablet may be administered in the middle of the morning meal. Gradually over the next 2 weeks 1/2 tablet a day is added each week until a full dose of 2.5 mg twice a day with food is achieved. Any initial side effects are minimized, and tachyphylaxis of these side effects usually occurs. True intolerance is uncommon. If side effects do occur, the dose should be decreased and then increased more slowly. Return of hyperprolactinemia to normal prolactin levels approaches 90%, regardless of the degree of prolactin elevation. Such results are clearly superior to those achieved by surgical treatment in all categories, but especially macroadenomas and invasive tumors.

For the treatment of infertility, prolactin should be lowered to the mid-normal range, because both mild hyperprolactinemia and hypoprolactinemia (oversuppression) may aggravate the ovulatory process. If amenorrhea persists despite normalization of serum prolactin levels and if the serum LH and FSH are not elevated, clomiphene citrate may be added to induce ovulation.

Effects of Bromocriptine Therapy. The natural history of prolactinomas following chronic bromocriptine therapy is becoming established. It appears that, when bromocriptine is discontinued, 10% to 20% of patients remain normal (Wang et al, 1987). Another 20% of women continue to maintain regular menses with only mild hyperprolactinemia, lower than the pretreatment level (Johnston et al, 1984). In one study of 75 women (52 with adenomas), bromocriptine was discontinued after 3 to 5 years. In 42 of the 75 patients, bromocriptine was restarted because of the return of symptoms. In the remaining 33 patients, there was continued normal or mild hyper-

prolactinemia without sufficient symptoms to require reinstitution of drug therapy (Rasmussen et al, 1987). Thus bromocriptine may be discontinued for 2 months every 2 years and restarted only if necessary. An intercurrent pregnancy does not adversely affect this prolonged normalization and, in fact, seems to potentiate this effect. It remains to be established whether so-called cures following bromocriptine therapy consist of patients merely following the natural history or if the "cures" represent a specific effect, such as autoinfarction.

Tumor growth is rare while patients are being treated with bromocriptine, but tumor shrinkage is a common event. The antitumor effects of ergots on prolactinomas have been noted in animals (Quadri et al, 1972) and in humans (Corenblum et al, 1975). Up to 90% of macroadenomas, even large invasive tumors, regress with bromocriptine. Conversely, a large mass that does not shrink with a dopamine agonist is not likely to be a prolactinoma, if it is associated with only moderate hyperprolactinemia. Thus tumor shrinkage and lowering of serum prolactin, in contrast to surgical results, do not depend on tumor size. Headache usually improves quickly, over 48 hours. Visual fields improve rapidly and dramatically over days, and CT scan usually shows tumor regression within 2 weeks. Usually, any hypopituitarism resolves, indicating it does not result from destruction by the pituitary tumor but, rather, from functional disconnection of the pituitary from the hypothalamus. Herniation of a tumor into the sphenoid sinus may shrink sufficiently that CSF rhinorrhea may occur.

One prospective multicenter study of 27 patients with extrasellar extension noted decreased tumor size by greater than 50% in two thirds. There was no correlation between reduction of tumor size and decrease in serum prolactin level. Visual field defects reversed in 9 of 10 patients, and menses returned in 12 of 14. Most studies indicated that tumor shrinkage occurred rapidly, but in this study tumor shrinkage in some patients was delayed for 3 to 6 months (Molitch et al, 1985). The rare tumor that increases in size despite bromocriptine is resistant because of reduced dopaminergic binding sites (Pellegrini et al, 1989).

Ultrastructural studies of prolactinomas treated with bromocriptine show regression of the rough endoplasmic reticulum and involution of the Golgi apparatus (structures involved with the translation and packaging of peptide hormones). This results in decreased volume of the cell to 60% of that of untreated adenoma cells (Saitoh et al, 1986). There is no lysozymal accumulation, cell necrosis, or endothelial cell damage. The shrinkage effects are reversible, and re-expansion of an involuted tumor may occur, sometimes rapidly. Thus caution must be exercised when bromocriptine therapy is discontinued in patients with previously large prolactinomas with extrasellar extension. With treatment of macroprolactinomas for several years, tumor regrowth is less common and of a lesser extent (van't Verlaat and Croughs, 1991).

Morphologic studies of such treated tumors show changes suggestive of cytocidal effects (Gen et al, 1984).

Tumor shrinkage is common and predictable. Thus the larger the adenoma and the greater the elevation of serum prolactin, the better the response to medical therapy as opposed to surgical therapy.

Disadvantages of Bromocriptine Therapy. Problems with dopamine agonists include cost ($0.50 to $3.00/day), side effects, and drug resistance. *Side effects* are dose related and are maximal at the onset of treatment. By starting with a low dose and increasing slowly, one may be able to minimize and often eliminate such symptoms. If side effects do occur, they usually disappear within 2 weeks. Approximately 5% of patients cannot tolerate bromocriptine in any oral form. Most dopamine agonists bind to both D_1 and D_2 dopamine receptors. The pituitary has D_2 dopamine receptors exclusively. Many of the unwanted side effects result from activation of D_1 dopamine receptors in other tissues. Side effects include

1. *Nausea* in 50% of patients and vomiting in about 5%.
2. *Orthostatic dizziness* in 20%, for 3 hours after drug administration. This rarely occurs as a severe first-dose effect. Taking the first few doses with food at bedtime is beneficial.
3. *Nasal congestion* for 2 hours after taking the medication; this can last for 6 hours. Antihistamines are not useful, but pseudoephedrine may be utilized.
4. *Miscellaneous symptoms*: headache, fatigue, abdominal cramps, constipation, somnolence, blurry vision, digital vasospasm, and nightmares.
5. With high dose, *hallucinations* and *dry mouth*.

Alcohol ingestion may initially worsen the side effects of bromocriptine. All side effects are reversible with discontinuation of the drug.

True *drug resistance* occurs in 5% of patients. This likely results from lack of functioning dopamine receptors on the adenomatous lactotroph and is unrelated to the size of the tumor or elevated serum prolactin levels. Poor compliance resulting from side effects may be presenting as drug resistance, and re-education of the patient may eliminate this problem.

Alternative Routes of Administration. Severe gastrointestinal (GI) side effects sufficient to produce noncompliance with bromocriptine may be avoided by nonoral routes of administration. Intramuscular, long-acting bromocriptine rapidly achieves therapeutic levels, maximal at 3 weeks and lasting for 6 weeks. GI side effects are minimal, yet there is a sustained decrease in prolactin and tumor size. Following a single intramuscular injection, many patients may transfer to oral bromocriptine after 1 month without recurrence of GI side effects.

Vaginally administered bromocriptine is readily absorbed and may result in prolonged therapeutic blood levels without GI side effects (Kletzky and Vermesh, 1989). A single tablet is inserted once a day either manually or with a vaginal inserter. There is no vaginal irritation or discharge. Because this technique bypasses the first-pass effect through the liver, there is a prolonged duration of action from a single tablet.

Treatment Plan. My policy is to use bromocriptine as the primary treatment for all patients with symptomatic hyperprolactinemia regardless of tumor size, if treatment is indicated. The clinical response is consistently favorable and is maintained with prolonged therapy without cumulative side effects or tumor progression (Corenblum and Taylor, 1983). Periodic discontinuation of bromocriptine is useful, considering the benign stable course of the underlying prolactinoma and the fact that some patients remain clinically normal for a long time after discontinuation of treatment. Alternate treatment is considered when compliance, intolerance, or drug resistance occurs.

Other Agents. The problems of compliance, intolerance, and resistance have led to the development of other forms of orally active agents. Most are still in the investigational stage. To date, comparative studies have demonstrated that some of the newer dopamine agonists may be more effective than bromocriptine (Webster et al, 1994). It may be clinically useful to change drugs because of patient noncompliance (with a longer acting agent) or adverse reactions. Other dopamine agonist drugs may be more potent, may have a longer duration of action (pergolide, cabergoline), or may produce fewer side effects (quinagolide [Vilar and Burke, 1994] is specific to the D_2 dopamine receptor). If the goal of therapy is to control a prolactinoma mass, therapy consists of surgery, irradiation, or both if dopamine agonists have failed. If infertility is the major complaint, ovulation induction may be attempted. Usually, administration of clomiphene citrate does not result in an ovulatory cycle when the patient is hyperprolactinemic, but it may be useful for infertility resulting from mild hyperprolactinemia and inadequate luteal phase (Corenblum et al, 1976). Women with hyperprolactinemia have various degrees of gonadal dysfunction because of a decrease in the normal pulsatile secretion of GnRH. Exogenous administration of pulsatile GnRH results in restoration of normal ovulatory cycles and normal fertility, as in women with hypothalamic amenorrhea, despite continued hyperprolactinemia. A woman with gonadotropin deficiency due to a central mass, past surgery, or irradiation responds to intramuscular gonadotropins.

A woman with estrogenized amenorrhea who does not desire a pregnancy may be treated with intermittent, progestin-induced withdrawal bleeds to protect the endometrium. If she is hypoestrogenized, restoration of estrogenization is indicated, preferably over a longer term. These women have reductions in bone mineral density that improve with return of endogenous cycles or exogenous estrogen administration. In fact, some women show resolution of hyperprolactinemia and associated symptoms when estrogen therapy has been discontinued. Thus for symptoms of hypoestrogenization and its sequelae, estrogen replacement (either physiologic or pharmacologic) is possible; it may even be preferable to bromocriptine if cost is a factor. It has been shown to be safe (Corenblum and Donovan, 1993).

Hypogonadal males may be given intramuscular testosterone, but impotence and decreased libido respond best to lowering of serum prolactin levels.

Pregnancy and Hyperprolactinemia

Symptomatic tumor growth may occur during pregnancy, but in the past this has been grossly overestimated. With normal sellas (IH) it does not occur, and with microadenomas it occurs in less than 1% of cases. Initial reports that 25% of patients with macroadenomas had symptomatic tumor growth during pregnancy resulted from pregnancies being induced with intramuscular gonadotropins. When bromocriptine is used to induce pregnancy, symptomatic tumor growth with macroadenomas is less than 5% and is most likely in patients with suprasellar extension prior to treatment (Bergh et al, 1982). A much lower incidence of symptomatic tumor growth in patients pretreated with bromocriptine may be noted because tumor shrinkage occurs, allowing room for re-expansion under the influence of rising estradiol levels. It has been suggested that treatment with either surgery or irradiation prior to inducing a pregnancy decreases symptomatic tumor growth. Because hypopituitarism may result, tumor growth may still occur, and tumor growth is relatively uncommon and easily managed, prophylactic invasive therapy is not recommended. In my experience of more than 200 pregnancies in hyperprolactinemic women, visual field abnormalities occurred twice within the same patient, headaches occurred in two other patients, and all three symptoms immediately responded to reinstitution of bromocriptine, with loss of mass symptoms (Corenblum and Taylor, 1986). For patients with pretreatment microadenomas or IH, bromocriptine is discontinued at the onset of pregnancy because the risk of tumor growth is small. Patients with macrodenomas, especially with pretreatment suprasellar extension, may either discontinue bromocriptine and be observed clinically or continue to take bromocriptine throughout pregnancy.

During pregnancy, monitoring by serial measurement of serum prolactin levels, visual field examination, or MRI is not useful. If symptomatic growth occurs, it is usually rapid. Thus it is recommended that the patient be clinically assessed every 2 months or immediately if new headaches, double vision, or loss of peripheral vision occurs. If she is clinically stable, no other monitoring is needed. If symptomatic tumor growth occurs and she is close to term, with documented fetal lung maturity, induction of labor and vaginal delivery constitute the treatment of choice. If the fetus is not mature, reinstitution of bromocriptine invariably results in regression of mass symptoms. If necessary, transsphenoidal resection of an adenoma can be performed in the second trimester. Another useful adjunct is high-dose dexamethasone.

Lactation after delivery was initially discouraged for fear that the suckling stimulus would produce tumor growth. This has been shown not to be the case, and breastfeeding may take place if desired.

Follow-up studies have demonstrated that 10% to 20% of women have regular menses and normal or mild hyperprolactinemia following delivery after a bromocriptine-induced pregnancy (Crosignani et al, 1989). Generally, a pregnancy is not detrimental to the pituitary.

Bromocriptine has not been shown to be teratogenic or associated with any problems with pregnancy, labor, or congenital abnormalities in the offspring (Turkalj et al, 1982). In one multicenter study of 64 children, psychological development was normal and the children were even precocious, with good scholastic performance (Raymond et al, 1985). Thus the overall consensus is that pregnancy is safe in women with hyperprolactinemia, even those harboring large prolactinomas. Bromocriptine is a safe drug for inducing pregnancy and, if necessary, for treating or preventing symptomatic tumor growth. New dopamine agonists have not been extensively studied in this situation.

REFERENCES

Allen DL, Low MJ, Allen RG, Ben-Jonathen N: Identification of two classes of prolactin-releasing factors in intermediate lobe tumors from transgenic mice. Endocrinology 1995;136:3093.

Argonz J, Del Castillo E: Syndrome characterized by estrogenic insufficiency, galactorrhea and decreased urinary gonadotrophin. J Clin Endocrinol Metab 1953;13:79.

Barrow DL, Mizuno J, Tindall GT: Management of prolactinomas associated with very high serum prolactin levels. J Neurosurg 1988;68:554.

Bates M, Allaerto W, Denef C: Evidence for functional communication between folliculo-stellate cells and hormone secreting cells in perifused anterior pituitary cell aggregates. Endocrinology 1987;120:685.

Bergh T, Nillius SJ, Enoksson P, et al: Bromocriptine-induced pregnancies in women with large prolactinomas. Clin Endocrinol 1982;17:625.

Bevan JS, Burke CW, Esiri MM, Adams CBT: Misinterpretation of prolactin levels leading to management errors in patients with sellar enlargement. Am J Med 1987;82:29.

Bevan JS, Davis RE: Cabergoline: an advance in dopaminergic therapy. Clin Endocrinol 1994;41:709.

Blackwell RE, Younger JB: Long-term medical therapy and follow-up of pediatric-adolescent patients with prolactin-secreting macroadenomas. Fertil Steril 1986;45:713.

Buckman MT, Kellner R: Reduction of distress in hyperprolactinemia with bromocriptine. Am J Psychiatry 1985;142:242.

Burrow GN, Wortzman G, Rewcastle NB, et al: Microadenomas of the pituitary and abnormal sellar tomograms in an unselected autopsy series. N Engl J Med 1981;304:56.

Caruso A, Lanzone A, Fulghesu AM, et al: Effect of luteal metoclopramide-induced hyperprolactinemia on pituitary and luteal responsiveness to gonadotropin-releasing hormone. Horm Res 1989;31:169.

Casper RF, Yen SSC: Simultaneous pulsatile release of prolactin and luteinizing hormone induced by luteinizing hormone releasing factor agonist. J Clin Endocrinol Metab 1981;52:934.

Chiari J, Braun C, Spaeth J: Klinik der geburtshilfe und gynakologie. Enke, Erlangen:371.

Corenblum B: Asymptomatic hyperprolactinemia resulting from macroprolactinemia. Fertil Steril 1990;53:165.

Corenblum B, Donovan L: The safety of physiological estrogen plus progestin replacement therapy and with oral contraceptive therapy in women with pathological hyperprolactinemia. Fertil Steril 1993;59:671.

Corenblum B, Patraudeau N, Shewchuk AB: Prolactin hypersecretion and short luteal phase defects. Obstet Gynecol 1976;47:486.

Corenblum B, Shaffer EA: Hyperprolactinemia in hepatic encephalopathy may result from impaired central dopaminergic neurotransmission. Horm Metab Res 1989;21:675.

Corenblum B, Taylor PJ: The hyperprolactinemic polycystic ovary syndrome may not be distinct entity. Fertil Steril 1982;38:549.

Corenblum B, Taylor PJ: Long-term follow-up of hyperprolactinemic women trated with bromocriptine. Fertil Steril 1983;38:549.

Corenblum B, Taylor PJ: Pregnancy in the hyperprolactinemic patient. Clin Reprod Fertil 1986;4:1.

Corenblum B, Taylor PJ: Idopathic hyperprolactinemia may include a distinct entity with a natural history different from that of prolactin adenomas. Fertil Steril 1988;49:544.

Corenblum B, Webster BR, Mortimer CB, Ezrin C: Possible antitumor effect of 2-bromo-ergocryptine (CB-154, Sandoz) in two patients with large prolactin secreting pituitary adenomas. Clin Res 1975;23:614A.

Costello RT: Subclinical adenoma of the pituitary gland. Am J Pathol 1936;12:205.

Crosignani PG, Mattei AM, Scarduelli C, et al: Is pregnancy the best treatment for hyperprolactinemia? Hum Reprod 1989;4:910.

Crosignani P, Scarduelli C, Brambilla G, Cavioni V: Spontaneous pregnancies in hyperprolactinemic women? Gynecol Obstet Invest 1985;19:17.

DeBernal M, De Villamizar M: Restoration of ovarian function by low nocturnal single daily doses of bromocriptine in patients with the amenorrhea-galactorrhea syndrome. Fertil Steril 1982;37:392.

Denef C, Andries M: Evidence for paracrine interaction between gonadotrophs and lactotrophs in pituitary cell aggregates. Endocrinology 1983;112:813.

Domae M, Yamada K, Hanabusa Y, Furukawa T: Inhibitory effects of endothelin-1 and endothelin-3 on prolactin release: possible involvement of endogenous endothelin isopeptide in the rat anterior pituitary. Life Sci 1992;50:715.

Donovan L, Corenblum B: The natural history of the pituitary incidentaloma. Arch Intern Med 1995;155:181.

Duvilanski BH, Zambruno C, Seilicovich A, et al: Role of nitric oxide in control of prolactin release by the adenohypophysis. Proc Natl Acad Sci U S A 1995;91:170.

Everett JW: Luteotropic function of autografts of the rat hypophysis. Endocrinology 1954;54:685.

Fava GA, Fava M, Kellner R, Mastrogiacoma G: Depression, hostility and anxiety in hyperprolactinemic amenorrhea. Psychother Psychosom 1981;36:122.

Forbes AP, Henneman PH, Griswold, et al: Syndrome characterized by galactorrhea, amenorrhea and low urinary FSH; comparison with acromegaly and normal lactation. J Clin Endocrinol Metab 1954;14:265.

Frommel R: Uber peuperale atrophie des uterus. Geburtshilfe Gynaekol 1882;7:305.

Gen M, Uozumi T, Ohta M, et al: Necrotic changes in prolactinomas after long-term administration of bromocriptine. J Clin Endocrinol Metab 1984;59:463.

Gindoff PR, Loucopoules A, Jewelwicz R: Treatment of hyperprolactinemic amenorrhea with pulsatile gonadotropin-releasing hormone therapy. Fertil Steril 1986;46:1156.

Glickman SP, Rosenfield RL, Bergenstal RM, Helke J: Multiple androgenic abnormalities, including elevated free testosterone, in hyperprolactinemic women. J Clin Endocrinol Metab 1982;55:251.

Greer ME, Moraczewski T, Rakoff JS: Prevalence of hyperprolactinemia in anovulatory women. Obstet Gynecol 1980;56:65.

Grossman A, Moult PJA, Gaillard RC, et al: The opioid control of LH and FSH release: effects of a met-enkephalin analogue and naloxone. Clin Endocrinol 1981;14:41.

Hall WA, Luciano MG, Doppman JL, et al: Pituitary magnetic resonance imaging in normal human volunteers: occult adenomas in the general population. Ann Intern Med 1994;120:817.

Hattori N, Ikekubo K, Ishihara T, et al: Effects of anti-prolactin autoantibodies on serum prolactin measurements. Eur J Endocrinol 1994;130:434.

Ho KY, Smythe GA, Lazarus L: Dopaminergic control of gonadotrophin secretion in normal women and in patients with pathological hyperprolactinemia. Clin Endocrinol 1984;20:53.

Hou SH, Grossman S, Molitch ME: Hyperprolactinemia in patients with renal insufficiency and chronic renal failure requiring hemodialysis or chronic ambulatory peritoneal dialysis. Am J Kidney Dis 1985;6:245.

Hsu CT, Yu MH, Lee CY, et al: Ectopic production of prolactin in uterine cervical carcinoma. Gynecol Oncol 1992;44:166.

Jeffcoate SL, Bacon RRA, Beastall GH, et al: Assays for prolactin: guidelines for the provision of a clinical biochemistry service. Ann Clin Biochem 1986;23:638.

Johnston DG, Haigh J, Prescott RWG, et al: Prolactin secretion and biological activity in females with galactorrhoea and normal circulating prolactin concentrations at rest. Clin Endocrinol 1985;22:661.

Johnston DG, Hall K, Kendall-Taylor P, et al: Effect of dopamine agonist withdrawal after long-term therapy in prolactinomas: studies with high-definition computerized tomography. Lancet 1984;2:187.

Johnston DG, Hall K, Kendall-Taylor P, et al: The long-term effects of megavoltage radiotherapy as sole or combined therapy for large prolactinomas: studies with high definition computerized tomography. Clin Endocrinol 1986;24:675.

Josimovich JB, Lavenhar MA, Devanesan MM, et al: Heterogeneous distribution of serum prolactin values in apparently healthy young women, and the effects of oral contraceptive medication. Fertil Steril 1987;47:785.

Kauppila A, Chatelain P, Kirkinen P, et al: Isolated prolactin deficiency in a woman with puerperal alactogenesis. J Clin Endocrinol Metab 1987;64:309.

Kauppila A, Leinonen P, Vihko R, Ylostalo P: Metoclopramide-induced hyperprolactinemia impairs ovarian follicle maturation and corpus luteum function in women. J Clin Endocrinol Metab 1982;54:955.

Kinnunen E, Viljanen A: Pleuropulmonary involvement during bromocriptine treatment. Chest 1988;94:1034.

Kletzky OA, Vermesh M: Effectiveness of vaginal bromocriptine in treating women with hyperprolactinemia. Fertil Steril 1989;51:269.

Klibansky A, Greenspan SL: Increase in bone mass after treatment of hyperprolactinemic amenorrhea. N Engl J Med 1986;315:542.

Koppelman MCS, Jaffe MJ, Rieth KG, et al: Hyperprolactinemia, amenorrhea, and galactorrhea. Ann Intern Med 1984;100:115.

Kovacs K, Ryan N, Horvath E, et al: Pituitary adenomas in old age. J Gerontol 1980;35:16.

Landolt AM, Osterwalder V: Perivascular fibrosis in prolactinomas: is it increased by bromocriptine? J Clin Endocrinol Metab 1984;58:1179.

Leonard MP, Nickel CJ, Morales A: Hyperprolactinemia and impotence: why, when, and how to investigate. J Urol 1989;142:992.

Liuzzi A, Dallabonzana D, Oppizzi G, et al: Low doses of dopamine agonists in the long-term treatment of macroprolactinomas. N Engl J Med 1985;313:656.

Luque EH, Munoz de Toro M, Smith PF, Neill JD: Subpopulations of lactotropes detected with the reverse hemolytic plaque assay. Endocrinology 1986;118:2120.

March C, Kletzky O, Dvajan V, et al: Longitudinal evaluation of patients with untreated prolactin-secreting pituitary adenomas. Am J Obstet Gynecol 1981;139:835.

MacLeod RM: Influence of norepinephrine and catecholamine-depleting agents on the synthesis and release of prolactin and growth hormone. Endocrinology 1969;85:916.

Meites J, Clemens JA: Hypothalamic control of prolactin secretion. Vitamin Horm 1972;30:165.

Mendelson JH, Mello NK, Teoh SK, et al: Cocaine effects on pulsatile seretion of anterior pituitary, gonadal, and adrenal hormones. J Clin Endocrinol Metab 1989;69:1256.

Milenkovic L, D'Angelo G, Kelly PA, Weiner RI: Inhibition of gonadotropin hormone-releasing hormone release by prolactin from GT1 neuronal cell lines through prolactin receptors. Proc Natl Acad Sci U S A 1994;91:1244.

Miyai K, Ichihara K, Kondo K, Mori S: Asymptomatic hyperprolactinemia and prolactinoma in the general population: mass screening by paired assays of serum prolactin. Clin Endocrinol 1986;25:549.

Molitch M, Elton R, Blackwell RE, et al: Bromocriptine as primary therapy for prolactin secreting macroadenomas: results of a prospective multicenter study. J Clin Endocrinol Metab 1985; 60:698.

Murai I, Ben-Jonathan N: Posterior pituitary lobectomy abolishes the suckling-induced rise in prolactin (PRL): evidence for a PRL-releasing factor in the posterior pituitary. Endocrinology 1987;121:205.

Nagy G, Mulchahey J, Neill JD: Autocrine control of prolactin secretion by vasoactive intestinal peptide. Endocrinology 1988; 122:364.

Palmer PE, Bogojavlensky S, Bhan AK, Scully RE: Prolactinoma in wall of ovarian dermoid cyst with hyperprolactinemia. Obstet Gynecol 1990;75:540.

Papka RE, Yu SM, Nikitovitch-Winer MB: Use of immunoperoxidase and immuno-gold labelling for pituitary hormones and neuropeptides. Am J Anat 1986;175:289.

Parl FF, Cruz VE, Cobb CA, et al: Late recurrence of surgically removed prolactinomas. Cancer 1986;57:2422.

Peillon F, Dupuy M, Li Uy, et al: Pituitary enlargement with suprasellar extension in functional hyperprolactinemia due to lactotroph hyperplasia: a pseudotumoral disease. J Clin Endocrinol Metab 1991;73:1008.

Pellegrini I, Gunz G, Ronin C, et al: Polymorphism of prolactin secretion by human prolactinoma cells: immunological, receptor binding, and biological properties of the glycosylated and nonglycosylated forms. Endocrinology 1988;122:2667.

Pellegrini I, Rasolonjanahary R, Gunz G, et al: Resistance to bromocriptine in prolactinomas. J Clin Endocrinol Metab 1989; 69:500.

Pepperell RJ: Prolactin and reproduction. Fertil Steril 1981;34:267.

Pepperell RJ, Martinez C, Dickinson A: The dilemma of mild hyperprolactinaemia. Aust N Z J Obstet Gynecol 1984;24:117.

Pullano JG, Cohen-Addad N, Apuzzio JJ, et al: Water and salt conservation in the human fetus and newborn: I. Evidence for a role of fetal prolactin. J Clin Endocrinol Metab 1989;69:1180.

Quadri SK, Lu KH, Meites J: Ergot-induced inhibition of pituitary tumor growth in rates. Science 1972;176:417.

Randall RV, Laws ER, Abboud CF, et al: Transsphenoidal microsurgical treatment of prolactin-producing pituitary adenomas. Mayo Clin Proc 1983;58:100.

Rasmussen C, Bergh T, Wide L: Prolactin secretion and menstrual function after long-term bromocriptine treatment. Fertil Steril 1987;48:550.

Raymond JP, Goldstein E, Konopka P, et al: Follow-up of children born of bromocriptine-treated mothers. Horm Res 1985;22:239.

Reber PM: Prolactin and immunomodulation. Am J Med 1993;95:637.

Rjosk HK, Fahlbusch R, von Werder K: Spontaneous development of hyperprolactinemia. Acta Endocrinol 1982;100:333.

Saitoh Y, Mori S, Arita N, et al: Cytosuppressive effect of bromocriptine on human prolactinomas: stereological analysis of ultra-structural alterations with special reference to secretory granules. Cancer Res 1986;46:1507.

Sarkar DK, Yen SSC: Hyperprolactinemia decreases the luteinizing hormone-releasing hormone concentration in pituitary portal plasma: a possible role for β-endorphin as a mediator. Endocrinology 1985;116:2080.

Schechter J, Goldsmith P, Wilson C, Weiner R: Morphological evidence for the presence of arteries in human prolactinomas. J Clin Endocrinol Metab 1988;67:713.

Scheithauer BW, Sano T, Kovacs KT, et al: The pituitary gland in pregnancy: a clinicopathologic and immunohistochemical study of 69 cases. Mayo Clin Proc 1990;65:461.

Schlechte J, Dolan K, Sherman B, et al: The natural history of untreated hyperprolactinemia: a prospective analysis. J Clin Endocrinol Metab 1989;68:412.

Schlechte J, Goerge E-K, Kathol M, Walkner L: Forearm and vertebral bone mineral in treated and untreated hyperprolactinemic amenorrhea. J Clin Endocrinol Metab 1987;64:1021.

Scoccia B, Schneider AB, Marut EL, Scommegna A: Pathological hyperprolactinemia suppresses hot flashes in menopausal women. J Clin Endocrinol Metab 1988;66:868.

Selman WR, Laws ER, Scheithauer BW, Carpenter SM: The occurrence of dural invasion in pituitary adenomas. J Neurosurg 1986;64:402.

Sisam DA, Sheehan JP, Sheeler LR: The natural history of untreated microprolactinomas. Fertil Steril 1987;48:67.

Soto-Albers CE, Randolph JF, Ying YK, Riddick DH: Medical management of hyperprolactinemia: a lower dose of bromocriptine may be effective. Fertil Steril 1987;48:213.

Spark RF, Wills CA, Royal H: Hypogonadism, hyperprolactinaemia, and temperal lobe epilepsy in hyposexual men. Lancet 1984;1:413.

Stevenaert A, Beckers A, Vandalem JL, Hennen G: Early normalization of luteinizing hormone pulsatility after successful transsphenoidal surgery in women with microprolactinomas. J Clin Endocrinol Metab 1986;62:1044.

Stricker P, Greuter F: Action du lobe anterieur de l'hypophse sur la montee laiteuse. C R Soc Biol 1928;99:1978.

Taylor SD, Kelly TM: Prolactinoma in a middle-aged man with an osteoporotic fracture. West J Med 1989;151:80.

Teasdale E, Teasdale G, Mohsen F, MacPherson P: High resolution computed tomography in pituitary microadenoma: is seeing believing? Clin Radiology 1986;37:227.

Tolis G, Somma M, van Campenhout J, Friesen H: Prolactin secretion in sixty-five patients with galactorrhea. Am J Obstet Gynecol 1974;118:91.

Turkalj I, Bruan P, Krupp P: Surveillance of bromocriptine in pregnancy. JAMA 1981;247:1589.

Tyrrell JB, Lamborn KR, Hannegan LT, et al: Transsphenoidal microsurgical therapy of prolactinomas: initial outcomes and long-term results. Neurosurgery 1999;44:254.

U HS, Kelley P, Lee WH: Abnormalities of the human growth hormone gene and protooncogenes in some human pituitary adenomas. Mol Endocrinol 1988;2:85.

Valcavi R, Harris PE, Foord SM, et al: The influence of oestrogens on the sensitivity of Prl, TSH and LH to the inhibitory actions of dopamine in hyperprolactinaemic patients. Clin Endocrinol 1985;23:139.

Vance ML, Thorner MO: Prolactinomas. Endocrinol Metab Clin North Am 1987;16:731.

van't Verlaat JW, Croughs RJM: Withdrawal of bromocriptine after long-term therapy for macroprolactinoma: effect on plasma prolactin and tumor size. Clin Endocrinol 1991;34:175.

Vilar L, Burke CW: Quinagolide efficacy and tolerability in hyperprolactinaemic patients who are resistant to or intolerant of bromocriptine. Clin Endocrinol 1994;41:821.

Wang C, Lam KSL, Ma JTC, et al: Long-term treatment of hyperprolactinemia with bromocriptine: effect of drug withdrawal. Clin Endocrinol 1987;27:363.

Webster J, Piscitelli G, Polli A, et al: A comparison of cabergoline and bromocriptine in the treatment of hyperprolactinemic amenorrhea. N Engl J Med 1994;331:904.

Wild RA, Kepley M: Lymphocytic hypophysitis in a patient with amenorrhea and hyperprolactinemia. J Reprod Med 1986;31:211.

Wingrave SJ, Kay CR, Vessey MP: Oral contraceptives and pituitary adenomas. Br Med J 1980;1:685.

Yan SSC, Hoff JD, Lasley BL, et al: Induction of prolactin release by LRF and LRF agonist. Life Sci 1980;26:1963.

Zelaschi NM, Delucchi GA, Rodriguez JL: High plasma prolactin levels after long-term neuroleptic treatment. Biol Psychiatry 1996;39:900.

30

Endometriosis and Adenomyosis

Michael M. Guarnaccia
Kaylen Silverberg
David L. Olive

Endometriosis and adenomyosis, conditions frequently encountered by the obstetrician-gynecologist as well as the primary care physician, continue to present difficult diagnostic and therapeutic dilemmas. Although each is frequently encountered in everyday practice, they present a contrast in terms of volume and intensity of investigative effort. Both disease entities continue to challenge the practitioner's diagnostic and clinical acumen.

Initially, endometriosis and adenomyosis were thought to be variations of the same disorder. However, we have come to understand that, despite their common feature of ectopic endometrium, they represent distinct pathophysiologic entities. Nevertheless, the two diseases continue to have many features in common. This chapter highlights both the similarities and differences of these proposed endometrium-based abnormalities, as well as differentiating fact from fiction. In so doing, we hope to give the reader a better appreciation of the limitations in current scientific understanding.

ENDOMETRIOSIS

Endometriosis is one of the most commonly encountered diseases in the reproductive-age female. However, despite its prevalence, endometriosis remains one of the most enigmatic disorders encountered by both the generalist and specialist. The wide range of signs, symptoms, and physical appearance of the lesions, combined with the apparent contradictory nature of an extensive scientific literature, has served to create confusion. This confusion has been manifested by widely divergent treatment regimens, each having a paucity of reproducible data to back it up. Indeed, it may well be that to paraphrase Sir William Osler, "he who knows endometriosis knows gynecology."

Established clinical dogma related to endometriosis is now under the close scrutiny of a large group of basic and clinical scientists. These ongoing investigations continue to challenge basic concepts related to the etiology and pathogenesis of the disease. This scrutiny has forced clinicians to rethink many long-held notions regarding diagnosis and treatment. The rapid evolution in the understanding of endometriosis makes this both a critical and an exciting time in the field. Ongoing analysis of modern advances continues to be paramount in developing a complete and accurate understanding of endometriosis.

Definition

Endometriosis is defined histologically by the presence of endometrial tissue in an ectopic location, exclusive of the myometrium. Traditionally, pathologists have required the presence of both glands and stroma with evidence of menstrual cyclicity (the presence of tissue hemorrhage or hemosiderin-laden macrophages) to firmly establish the diagnosis. The validity of each of these requirements has yet to be established. For the tissue to function as endometrium, there is evidence to indicate that glands and stroma must be present concurrently. However, pathologic function of one or the other of the tissue components (when found alone) has not been adequately assessed. For the purposes of this chapter, we will define endometriosis as the presence of either endometrial glands or stroma, or both, with or without hemosiderin-laden macrophages outside the uterine corpus. Given the fact that the vast majority of endometriosis is found in the pelvis, this is the focus of the discussion unless otherwise specified.

Pathogenesis

More than a century has passed since the original description of endometriosis (Von Rokitansky, 1860), yet we still do not know with certainty why this disease develops. Numerous theories of histiogenesis have been proposed by the leading researchers in the field, but three main theories continue to dominate current thinking (Schenken, 1989). The original theory proposed for the origin of ectopic endometriosis was *coelomic metaplasia* arising from the cells that line

687

the pelvic peritoneum. The basis of this concept derives from the observation that müllerian ducts, germinal epithelium, and pelvic peritoneum all derive from the same source—epithelium of the coelomic wall. This theory, initially advanced by the famous 19th century pathologist Robert Meyer, proposed that continuation of the process of tissue differentiation can occur selectively in certain adult tissues. However, neither he nor subsequent investigators have been able to demonstrate that these differentiated peritoneal cells can maintain a capacity for further differentiation. Several additional issues have arisen that cast doubt concerning the viability of this theory:

1. The disease is not present in males. Only a handful of case reports of endometriosis have been identified in the male; in each case, prostatic carcinoma had been treated with high-dose estrogen (Melicow and Pachter, 1967; Oliker and Harns, 1971; Pinkert et al, 1979; Schrodt et al, 1980). These few cases probably represent hyperplasia and spread from endometrial rests of the prostatic utricle, a remnant of the müllerian duct in males.
2. The implants lack uniformity within the coelomic membrane, and it is this membrane that covers both the abdominal and thoracic cavities. Although this membrane developmentally contributes to the peritoneum and pleura (Maximow, 1927; Filatow, 1933), endometriosis is seen primarily in the pelvis.
3. In all patients with endometriosis, endometrium is present. Very rarely, endometriosis may be seen in women with müllerian agenesis. However, such women invariably have a focus of endometrium present.
4. The disease occurs primarily in women of reproductive age. If the disease tissue derives from a metaplastic process, then the incidence should increase with advancing age. To explain the observed age distribution, a theory of estrogen-induced metaplasia has been invoked. However, this is not consistent with the low incidence of endometriosis in anovulatory women with chronically elevated estrogen levels.

The theory of coelomic metaplasia persisted unchallenged for many years, despite the lack of scientific evidence. It remains for proponents of this theory to validate its causal role in endometriosis.

The first major challenge to the theory of metaplasia was proposed by Sampson in 1921 when he put forth the concept of *transplantation*. This theory maintains that endometriosis originates from the uterine endometrial tissue that is transported to ectopic locations, then implants and grows. A number of routes of dissemination have been proposed, including lymphatic dissemination, vascular spread, iatrogenic transplantation, and retrograde menstruation.

The idea that "shed" endometriosis could result from lymphatic transport was first advanced by Halban in 1925 with the publication of five cases illustrating the concept. Finally, microscopic evidence of endometrial cells within lymphatics and nodes was obtained (Javert, 1949). Considerable research has established that shed endometrial cells are viable in vitro (Geist, 1933; Keettel, 1951). In addition, these cells have been viably maintained in culture for up to 2 months (Mungyer et al, 1987). Early studies done to determine the implantation capacity of such cells in vivo were initially disappointing. However, subsequent experiments involving both monkeys (TeLinde and Scott, 1950) and humans (Ridley and Edwards, 1958; Ridley, 1968) have shown that placement of endometrial tissue into ectopic locations does indeed result in endometriosis.

A second route of spread was proposed by Sampson (1925), when he introduced the concept of hematogenous transport. This was suggested by the demonstration of endometrial tissue within the pelvic veins (Javert, 1952) and reports of endometriosis at a multitude of remote sites (Ridley, 1968). However, the rarity of these cases suggests that they represent a small fraction of the cases of endometriosis.

Iatrogenic transplantation has been suggested experimentally in the subhuman primate and is further endorsed by the finding of endometrial tissue in surgical scars (Ridley, 1968). Yet most women with endometriosis have not experienced prior uterine surgery, negating this as a major cause of the disease.

The major contributing factor of retrograde menstruation in the genesis of endometriosis is now a well-established fact. Retrograde menstruation itself is a well-established phenomenon, with data available in menstruating women undergoing peritoneal dialysis (Blumenkrantz et al, 1981) or laparoscopy at the time of menses (Halme et al, 1984; Liu and Hitchcock, 1986) documenting a 76% to 90% rate of retrograde flow. In addition, it has long been known that there are viable cells within the menstrual flow, clearly demonstrated by supravital staining of endometrial cells within the menstrual discharge (Geist, 1933). Evidence also exists to support the theory that women with endometriosis have a relative hypotonia of the uterotubal junction (Ayers and Friedenstab, 1985), and endometrial tissue is refluxed into the peritoneal cavity in women with endometriosis more frequently than in controls with patent tubes but no endometriosis (Bartosik et al, 1986). Additionally, the presence of endometrial cells within the tubal lumen (Javert, 1949) and in the peritoneal fluid (Beyth et al, 1975) has been clearly established. Finally, in the baboon, intraperitoneal injection of endometrium from the proliferative or luteal phase will only occasionally result in implantation; however, the incidence is drastically higher with the injection of menstrual endometrium (D'Hooghe et al, 1994).

The anatomic distribution of endometriotic implants offers additional circumstantial evidence in support of the transplantation theory. Jenkins and colleagues (1986) assessed the anatomic distribution of endometriosis (Fig. 30–1) in a laparoscopic study

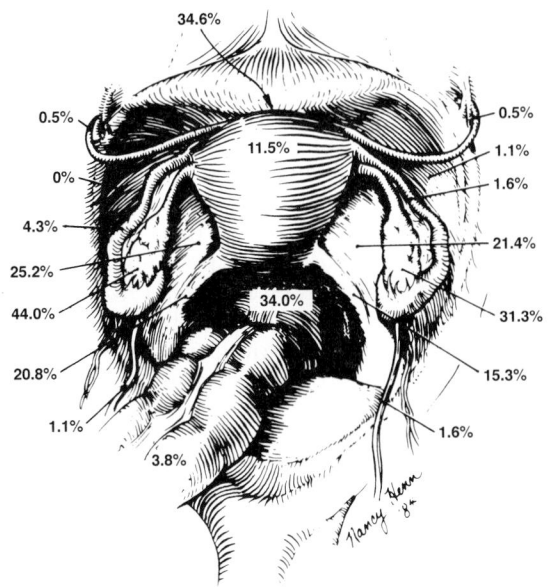

Figure 30–1
Anatomic distribution of endometriotic implants in 182 infertility patients found to have endometriosis at laparoscopy. The rates shown indicate the percentage of all with implants in a given locale. (From Jenkins S, Olive DL, Haney AF: Endometriosis: pathogenetic implications of the anatomic distribution. Obstet Gynecol 1986;67:336, with permission of the American College of Obstetricians and Gynecologists.)

of implants, adhesions, and uterine position in 182 patients. The rate of implants in dependent locations supports retrograde menstruation as a mechanism of transport. Implants and adhesions are most common in the anterior and posterior cul-de-sacs of the pelvis, as well as the paracolic gutters. Furthermore, anterior compartment endometriosis was rarely found in women with retroverted uteri, a condition in which the anterior cul-de-sac is no longer a dependent pocket. Taken together, this information confirms the importance of retrograde menstruation in the development of endometriosis. However, not all women (or even a majority of women) have endometriosis, leading one to wonder what other factors are necessary.

The *induction* theory of endometriosis is a combination of the two previously mentioned theories, coelomic metaplasia and endometrial transplantation. It states that unknown substances released from shed endometrium induce undifferentiated mesenchyme to form endometriotic tissue. Animal research in the rabbit model has attempted to validate this theory. Deposition of both fresh and denatured endometrium into the subcutaneous tissue resulted in the formation of endometrial cysts (Lavender and Normal, 1955). The demonstration of glands similar to endometrial structures adjacent to areas of subcutaneous implantation of Millipore chambers in the peritoneal cavity of rabbits supports this theory (Merrill, 1963, 1966). Of note, no endometrial stroma was induced in either of these experiments. Whether

this induction is merely the well-recognized process of stromal induction of adjacent epithelium or, instead, the induction of complete endometrium capable of growth and development is unclear.

The discrepancy between the universality of retrograde menstruation and the minority of patients with of endometriosis has led investigators to consider that the intraperitoneal environment in some women may be conducive to the development of the disease. Given this scenario, research has centered on the immune system as a likely instigator. A number of immunologic disorders are associated with the presence of endometriosis (Hill, 1992), any of which could play a role in the successful transplantation of endometrial tissue. In humans most of the research on the immunology of endometriosis is observational and involves studies on the various aspects of immune function in infertile women who have been diagnosed with the disease. A pattern of immune dysfunction can be identified from these studies: women with endometriosis appear to exhibit increased macrophage activation and decreased cell-mediated immunity.

The placement of menstrual debris into the peritoneal cavity with menses elicits a response from the body geared toward its removal, with the prime candidate being cell-mediated cytotoxicity (Dmowski et al, 1981; Steele et al, 1984). Studies have suggested that there exists a deficiency of both T-cell–mediated cytotoxicity and natural killer (NK) cell–mediated cytotoxicity in women with endometriosis. Macrophages, a key component in the function of cell-mediated cytotoxicity, are the major cell type in the peritoneal fluid, and vary throughout the menstrual cycle, being greater in the follicular phase immediately after the menses (Hill, 1988). Infertile women with endometriosis appear to possess a larger number of peritoneal macrophages compared to fertile controls. These cells have all the characteristics of tissue-differentiated mononuclear phagocytes, with the stimulus for differentiation probably being retrograde menstruation (Halme et al, 1982, 1983a, 1983b). There is evidence to suggest that peritoneal macrophages from women with endometriosis possess accentuated activation characteristics resulting in enhanced phagocytic activity and secretion of several soluble substances (e.g., proteolytic enzymes, cytokines, prostaglandins, and/or growth factors) (Halme et al, 1988). Recent investigations have documented that the increased macrophage activation in endometriosis is accompanied by their production of growth factors, including platelet-derived growth factors, epidermal growth factor, and transforming growth factor-β (Ramey and Archer, 1993). It is these growth factors that have been shown to stimulate the proliferation of endometrial stromal cells in vitro, and it has been speculated that they enhance the implantation of endometrial cells (Simms et al, 1991; Strowitzki et al, 1991; Surrey and Halme, 1991). Such data suggest that a combination of factors including the hormonal milieu and the number and secretory capacity of cells residing in the peritoneal cavity might be required to sustain the growth of ectopic endometrium, with the induction of clinical endometriosis.

Several lines of investigation have centered on interleukin-8 (IL-8) and monocyte chemotactic protein-1 (MCP-1), highly cell-specific chemoattractants in the pathogenesis of endometriosis. IL-8 is a potent angiogenic agent, chemoattractant, and activating cytokine for granulocytes, while MCP-1 is a chemoattractant and activating cytokine for monocytes and macrophages. Sources of these cytokines include endometrium (with retrograde menstrual possibly providing sufficient amounts) and peritoneal mesothelium. The concentrations of MCP-1 and IL-8 are elevated in the peritoneal fluids of women with endometriosis compared to disease-free women, and the levels correlate with the severity of the disease (Arici et al, 1995, 1996). These preliminary data serve to explain the process of endometriosis generation. Retrograde menstruation is a mandatory component, with implantation and growth requiring estrogen in conjunction with growth factors from peritoneal macrophages. In turn, these macrophages are recruited via chemoattractants such as IL-8 and MCP-1, which are produced by endometrium and/or peritoneum. Added to this may be a deficiency in the response by cytotoxic T cells and NK cells, leading to the passive promotion of endometriosis.

Epidemiology

Endometriosis has been estimated to affect between 10% and 15% of premenopausal women (Ranney, 1980). The peak incidence is in the third and fourth decades of life, but diagnosis appears to be in the range of 25 to 29 years. Approximately 4 of 1000 women ages 15 to 64 years are hospitalized annually for endometriosis (Candiani et al, 1991). The typical age at which endometriosis is diagnosed appears to be in the range of 25 to 29 years (Norwood, 1960). One report placed the mean age of symptoms at the age of 20, roughly 5 years before the mean age of diagnosis. Thus, with increased awareness and improved diagnostic capability, a decrease in the average age of diagnosis is anticipated. The latest epidemiologic data suggest that women with short cycle lengths (≤27 days) and a longer flow (≥1 week) had more than double the risk for endometriosis compared with women with longer cycle lengths and shorter duration of flow (Cramer, 1986). Cramer also found a decreased risk of endometriosis associated with smoking or exercise that was confined to women who began either habit at an early age and were heavier smokers or more strenuous exercisers.

Endometriosis is extremely rare in premenarche, having been reported in only a single autopsy examination of a stillborn (Redwine, 1989b). Its occurrence rate in adolescents is unknown, but it appears not to be rare in the teenage years. In two studies of women under age 20 with chronic pelvic pain or dysmenorrhea unresponsive to medical therapy, endometriosis was found at surgery in 47% to 65% of cases (Goldstein et al, 1980; Chatman and Ward, 1982). Simply considering the teenage years to be a single entity, however, may be misleading. A disproportionate number of cases in the early teen years are attributable to müllerian anomalies and uterine outflow obstruction (Hanton et al, 1967; Schifrin et al, 1973), whereas cases in the late teenage years tend to occur in females with otherwise normal genital tracts. Although this may represent selection bias based on when these young women undergo surgery, the fact remains that most documented instances of endometriosis in females under 17 are associated with outflow tract obstruction (Huffman, 1981).

Endometriosis is commonly believed to be rare in menopausal women. However, 2% to 4% of all women requiring laparoscopy for endometriosis are postmenopausal (Kempers et al, 1960; Punnonen et al, 1980). Although most of these women are receiving hormone replacement therapy, this is not true in all reports (Djursing et al, 1981).

Epidemiologic evaluation of the "true" prevalence of endometriosis is difficult because laparoscopy is required to make the diagnosis, but it is not possible to expose a random sample of women to the procedure. The choice of the population studied has been responsible for the large variations in observed frequency of disease. The prevalence has ranged from 2% to 48%, but these figures have been based on the populations studied. The highest rates of endometriosis are found in women undergoing laparoscopy for infertility and pelvic pain, whereas the lowest rates are in those undergoing laparoscopic tubal sterilization (Sangi-Haghpeykar and Poindexter, 1995).

The impact of selection bias is evident in a study by the Baylor Gynecologic Collaborative Group, which found a prevalence of 0.7% in women undergoing tubal anastomosis, 1.6% at laparoscopic tubal ligation, 11.3% at the time of abdominal hysterectomy, and 31% at operative laparoscopy (Wheeler, 1989). Using vaginal hysterectomy as a reference procedure by which to determine the true prevalence in the reproductive-age population, Wheeler estimated an overall prevalence of approximately 10%.

The demography of endometriosis has a highly controversial history. It was classically thought to be a disease of white middle-aged women belonging to the upper socioeconomic class, with Meigs (1949) documenting endometriosis in 28% of white women undergoing laparotomy versus only 5.8% of blacks. Numerous epidemiologic studies have disputed this myth (Chatman, 1976; Chatman and Ward, 1982; Kirshon et al, 1989), with endometriosis noted to be present in all ages, races, and socioeconomic groups. Meigs' study was limited by not controlling for confounding variables such as availability of health care, access to contraception, cultural differences regarding childbearing patterns, and attitudes toward menses and pain. Later studies demonstrated that the apparently higher endometriosis rates in whites were the result of socioeconomic factors rather than race, and controlling for such factors resulted in similar rates among the races (Scott and TeLinde, 1950; Lloyd, 1964). Investigations undertaken more recently have noted an increased rate of endometriosis among Asians in comparison to other ethnic groups (Sangi-Haghpeykar and Poindexter, 1995). They noted a higher probability of disease among Asian women (odds ratio = 8.6) compared with white women after controlling for the effect of age, number of live births, and income. When other socioeconomic factors were controlled for (i.e., marital status, income level, and education), no association with endometriosis was noted.

The possibility of a familial tendency for endometriosis was first suggested by Goodall (1943). Although initially there were few data to support this concept, Ranney (1971b) demonstrated, by retrospective analysis, what appeared to be hereditary tendencies in 53 family groups having the disease. More recently, Simpson et al (1980) and Malinak and co-workers (1980) have demonstrated a high probability of genetic influences, with the most probable mode being polygenic and multifactorial. A current search is ongoing for the endometriosis gene. The OXEGENE project has targeted sister-sister pairs with advanced, documented endometriosis as a source to identify a gene variant unique to this population. Results will be forthcoming.

Symptoms

Endometriosis, although associated with a large variety of symptoms, primarily produces pain and infertility. Despite the strong correlation with these disorders, however, the pathophysiology of the associations is not well understood. Appearance, location, depth of invasion, and other factors may all influence symptoms, as well as a number of individualized confounding variables.

When one is examining the relationship between infertility and endometriosis, two questions must be asked. First, what is the incidence of infertility in women with endometriosis? This question remains unanswered because selection bias limits the applicability of any published figures. The second question is the reverse: What is the rate of endometriosis in the infertile patient? The published range is 4.5% to 33%, with a mean of 14% (Pauerstein, 1989). One investigation demonstrated a 21% incidence of endometriosis in infertile women, whereas only 2% of fertile controls were found to have the disease (Strathy et al, 1982). Thus endometriosis is not a random finding but, rather, is well associated with infertility.

Endometriosis has been linked to aberrations in every step of the reproductive process. Moderate to severe disease can lead to marked anatomic altera-

tions and subsequent changes in the tubo-ovarian relationship. Disturbances in ovulation caused by intermittent anovulation, abnormal follicular development, and/or luteal-phase defects have been suggested as possible mechanisms (Olive and Hammond, 1985; Surrey and Halme, 1989). However, more recent studies have suggested that such abnormalities are present no more often in patients with endometriosis than in other fertile or infertile women. The role of endometriosis-associated inflammatory changes in the local peritoneal fluid environment as a cause of infertility is now an active area of investigation. Several reports have demonstrated that inflammatory cytokines within the peritoneal fluid of women with endometriosis affect sperm motility and survival, sperm-oocyte interactions, ovum pickup by the fimbria, and early embryonic development (Eisermann et al, 1988; Halme, 1989; Hill et al, 1987).

Clinical investigators also have addressed this issue. Jansen (1986) prospectively analyzed 91 women undergoing artificial insemination with donor sperm who had no apparent infertility factor. All had husbands with azospermia or severe oligospermia. Of the 91, 7 had endometriosis upon screening laparoscopy. Subsequent fertility was significantly lower in the women with endometriosis. However, the study was limited by the number of endometriosis patients, the lack of uniform criteria regarding laparoscopic diagnosis of endometriosis, and a 4% monthly conception rate among women with endometriosis (a figure far lower than that seen in most studies of endometriosis-associated infertility). A comprehensive multivariate investigation into potential pathogenic factors affecting fertility in 731 infertile women determined that endometriosis without adhesions did not alter the cumulative conception rate (Dunphy, 1989). Data on 207 couples undergoing donor insemination were analyzed by Chauhan and associates (1989); they found that recipients with no infertility problems whose partners were azospermic had the highest pregnancy rates, while rates were lowest for normal women with oligospermic partners. In addition, donor insemination recipients with treated endometriosis had higher pregnancy rates than women with other infertility factors.

Pelvic pain may well be the most common symptom of endometriosis. This particular expression of the disease may take on many forms. Dysmenorrhea is reported in 25% to 67% of women with endometriosis, with the rate clearly dependent on selection bias in the study group (Olive and Haney, 1986). Good evidence of the disease is the onset of secondary dysmenorrhea. In patients with a history of primary dysmenorrhea, increasing severity may also be a clue to the presence of endometriosis. Dyspareunia is also common, generally reported in approximately 25% in patients with documented endometriosis (Olive and Haney, 1986). The greatest incidence of dyspareunia is seen in association with uterosacral involvement. Other types of pain are also reported:

692 / Textbook of Gynecology

noncyclic lower abdominal pain in 25% to 39% and backaches in 25% to 31% (Olive and Haney, 1986).

Numerous investigators have attempted to explain the pathophysiology of endometriosis associated pain. The heterogeneity of the disease process, however, suggests that a range of pathophysiologic processes are involved. Different types of lesions cause pain via different routes. Atypical papular lesions may produce more prostaglandins than older lesions. These lesions may be responsible for functional pain symptoms, such as dysmenorrhea (Vercellini et al, 1991). Classical-appearing lesions are thought to be older or burnt out endometriosis (Koninckx et al, 1991). It is these lesions that might be more likely to provoke organic-type pain from mechanical pressure of cystic nodules and from stimulation of pain fibers by scars and stretching of areas of fibrotic infiltration, as could occur during intercourse upon deep penetration (Vercellini et al, 1991).

The depth of infiltration of endometriosis has been recognized to correlate with pelvic pain (Koninckx et al, 1991; Martin et al, 1989). Because depth cannot be easily evaluated by visual inspection alone, surgical excision is required to make an accurate evaluation. Very deep implants appear to be more active and may be found exclusively in patients with pain. Cornillie and co-workers (1990) found that nearly all women with lesions deeper than 1 cm suffer from severe pain. In this study, women with superficial (<1 mm), intermediate (2 to 4 mm), or deep (5 to 10 mm) infiltration had pain in 17%, 53%, and 37% of cases, respectively. Total lesion volume, however, has not been found to be directly related to patient symptoms. Most recently, Vercellini and co-workers (1996) found that the frequency and severity of deep dyspareunia and the frequency of dysmenorrhea were less in the patients with only ovarian endometriosis than in those with lesions at other sites. The presence of vaginal endometriosis was associated with more frequent and severe deep dyspareunia.

Adhesion formation is common in patients with endometriosis, and may be related to the degree of pain. Adhesions may cause pain by direct nerve damage, from tissue destruction and scar formation, or by devitalization and ischemia of parts of the internal pelvic organs, secondary to damage to the blood supply. Organs such as bowel or adnexa may also be adherent in abnormal areas and cause any movement to place traction on their nerve supply. Over time, scarring of the posterior uterine surface may become extensive enough to produce a fixed retroflexion possibly resulting in sacral pain caused by direct pressure. In addition, the pain may be referred to the back, lower abdomen, rectum, and thighs because of the proximity of lumbar and sacral nerves.

Dysfunctional uterine bleeding is often linked with endometriosis. Scott and TeLinde (1950) first noted the association, reporting 44% incidence of abnormal bleeding among their patients with endometriosis. However, virtually all cases were attributed to associated pathology, with few women exhibiting true dysfunctional bleeding with the disease. Similar results were later reported by Ranney (1971a). Anovulation rates in women with endometriosis are reported to be 9% to 17% (Soules et al, 1976; Radwanska et al, 1984). However, such studies lack control groups, utilize inconsistent criteria for the diagnosis of anovulation, and have not evaluated the frequency of repetitive anovulatory cycles. Thus there is not good evidence to implicate endometriosis as a cause of dysfunctional uterine bleeding.

Additionally, a diverse array of symptoms may result from implantation of endometrium on the pelvic viscera. Thus endometriosis may result in bowel-related symptoms, such as tenesmus or dyschezia, or urinary tract symptoms, such as dysuria, frequency, or urgency. Finally, endometriosis at remote sites may produce unusual site-specific complaints; examples include pleuritic pain caused by pulmonary involvement and seizures secondary to brain lesions.

Physical Findings

Physical findings associated with endometriosis are variable and dependent on the severity and location of disease as well as the character of the population under study. Common findings include nodularity or tenderness of the cul-de-sac, parametrial thickening, and adnexal masses. A retrodisplaced uterus, often fixed, has been frequently noted. Cutaneous lesions may even by present, with likely sites being the vagina, perineum, and umbilicus and within surgical scars. Rarely, significant ascites may be observed (Jenks et al, 1984).

Physical exam is of limited value in these patients because women with extensive disease often have minimal findings. Because disease manifestations often become more pronounced and areas of ectopic endometrial implantation more tender during the menses, it is often useful to examine the patient during the perimenstrual period. Deep endometriosis may be underdiagnosed clinically and, during surgery, the diagnosis can be difficult and deep endometriosis may remain undetected. Koninckx and colleagues (1996) confirmed that clinical examination during menstruation is a simple and reliable test to diagnose deep endometriosis and to decide which women should be prepared preoperatively for bowel surgery. They prospectively documented a 77% sensitivity rate for identification of deep endometriosis during menstruation, whereas there was a 36% sensitivity rate by routine clinical examination during the follicular or luteal phase.

Diagnostic Methods

Three classes of techniques have been used to diagnose and observe women with endometriosis: serum immunology, radiologic imaging, and laparoscopic examination of the peritoneal cavity. The monoclonal antibody OC-125 identifies the antigenic determinant CA-125, originally found in an ovarian epithelial tumor. This antigen has subsequently been found in the endocervix, endometrium, fallopian tube, peritoneum, pleura, and pericardium. An elevated peripheral blood concentration of CA-125 has been described in many women with endometriosis (Barbieri et al, 1986; Pittaway and Fayez, 1986). Although this discovery raised the hope of a possible blood test for endometriosis, subsequent evaluation has shown the test to be insufficiently sensitive or specific to be useful in screening (Malkasian et al, 1986; Patton et al, 1986). Furthermore, a placebo-controlled trial has questioned the value of following serum CA-125 levels to monitor treatment effect (Kauppila et al, 1988).

Development of a second-generation CA-125 assay has increased interest in its use. Hornstein and colleagues (1995) have compared the serum CA-125 concentrations in women with and without endometriosis using both the older assay and the new CA-125 assay in an effort to determine if the newer assay has improved clinical utility. They found that the sensitivity and specificity of the newer assay was slightly improved; however, they found no increase in the rate of detection of endometriosis over the old assay.

Screening for other serum proteins, such as placental protein 14 (PP-14) and antibodies to endometrial tissue, are currently being investigated. PP-14 is produced in secretory endometrium, and its concentration in the serum varies with the menstrual cycle. Active endometriosis has been shown to elevate the serum levels (Telimaa et al, 1989a). More recently, it has been shown that superficial endometriosis secreted both PP-14 and CA-125 into the peritoneal cavity and that more deeply infiltrating lesions secreted these substances into the blood (Koninckx et al, 1992). Although endometrial antibodies are detected in the serum in a high percentage of patients with endometriosis, these levels do not correlate with the severity of the disease (Wild and Shivers, 1985).

Imaging techniques have been used periodically in an attempt to diagnose endometriosis. Ultrasonography has proven to be of value in the identification of ovarian endometriomas, although the appearance of an echogenic cystic structure is not pathognomonic (Schwartz and Seifer, 1992). Guerriero and colleagues (1996) prospectively evaluated the use of transvaginal ultrasonography combined with CA-125 plasma levels to differentiate endometriomas from nonendometriotic cysts. They found that the addition of CA-125 did not improve the quality of the test. Ultrasonography is not currently useful in identifying focal implants because its sensitivity is as low as 11% (Friedman et al, 1985). In addition, Pauerstein (1989) has noted a high false-positive diagnostic rate for the identification of diffuse disease.

Magnetic resonance imaging (MRI) has now demonstrated its value in the diagnosis of endometriosis (Arrive et al, 1989; Zawin et al, 1989; Togashi et al, 1991). Some of these early studies proved disappointing, with a sensitivity of only 64%, a specificity of 60%, and predictive accuracy of 63%. When Togashi and colleagues (1991) limited their investigation to women with adnexal masses, however, the sensitivity, specificity, and predictive accuracy of the identification of endometriomas by MRI were 90%, 98%, and 96%, respectively. MRI does exhibit several limitations. The appearance of endometriosis is not pathognomonic. Although the imaging of diffuse pelvic lesions is more readily accomplished by MRI than by ultrasonography, the sensitivity remains low.

The refinement of MRI detection of diffuse endometriosis with the inclusion of both fat-suppression and fat-saturation techniques has greatly enhanced its diagnostic accuracy. Diagnosis of endometriosis by MRI using the fat-saturation technique revealed an overall sensitivity of 89%, a specificity of 71%, a positive predictive value of 95%, and a negative predictive value of 50% when compared to conventional MRI and confirmed surgically (Takahashi et al, 1994). Use of the fat-suppression technique increased the diagnostic accuracy to 77% versus 55% with conventional MRI, while overall sensitivity was increased to 61% versus 27% (Ha et al, 1994). In both studies, the detection rates were based on endometrial implants greater than 4 mm in size.

Two potential roles for MRI can be readily identified. One is the identification of endometriosis obscured by pelvic adhesions, which may prove an important screening tool prior to surgery and extensive lysis of adhesions (Zawin et al, 1989). Additionally, pelvic MRI has now been shown to be effective in the evaluation of response to medical treatment of endometriomas (Takahashi et al, 1996).

Laparoscopy remains the optimal diagnostic method for endometriosis. However, the value of this modality is directly dependent on the ability of the surgeon to recognize the lesion when visualized. Difficulty in identifying the more subtle manifestations of endometriosis may have resulted in underestimation of the prevalence of the disease among young women. Additionally, the great variety in the appearance of these lesions contributes to the potential diagnostic confusion (Table 30–1) (Jansen and Russell, 1986; Stripling et al, 1988). A recognition of

Table 30–1. MULTIPLE APPEARANCES OF ENDOMETRIOTIC IMPLANTS

Brownish, discolored peritoneum
Superficial peritoneal ecchymoses
Raised, reddish, superficial nodules
Reddish-blue invasive nodules
Fibrotic, whitish nodules
Raised, glossy, translucent blobs
Patchy, white opacified peritoneum
Reddish or bluish ovarian cysts

these "nontraditional" appearances can result in a significant increase in the frequency of diagnosis (Martin et al, 1989). The effect of this protean appearance of the disease may have resulted in a significant underestimation of endometriosis in young adults, because a pattern of evolution has been identified from more subtle-appearing lesions in the teenage years to the traditional red or black foci a decade later (Table 30–2) (Redwine, 1987). D'Hooghe et al (1996) demonstrated that endometriosis in captive baboons undergoing repeated laparoscopies is a dynamic and moderately progressive disease with periods of development, regression, and active remodeling. These fluctuations eventually led to disease progression as scored by increase in American Fertility Society (AFS) score and in both number and surface area of lesions after 9 to 13 months and after 19 to 24 months.

Given this wide variation in appearance, simple visualization cannot be relied on to rule out the disease. To this end, excision of any suspect lesions at laparoscopy, with pathologic confirmation, is essential to assess questionable aspects of the disorder (Martin and Zwaag, 1987). Still, some colorless manifestations are extremely subtle. One technique that can assist the surgeon in the identification of these subtle manifestations is the "painting" of peritoneal surfaces with bloody peritoneal fluid. By allowing the fluid to flow across the peritoneal surface, colorless endometrial lesions will be highlighted by erythrocytes as the red blood cells stream around them (Redwine, 1989a). Additionally, some have advocated the use of a "bubble test" of peritoneal surfaces utilizing bursts of saline and subsequent observation of excessive soap-like bubbling. Gleicher and colleagues (1995) demonstrated a sensitivity of 100% and a specificity of 88% for this technique, with positive and negative predictive values of 94% and 100%, respectively.

Pathology

Endometriotic implants have traditionally been described as bluish-gray "powder burns." The color is attributed to the menstrual cyclicity of the ectopic endometrium, with hemolysis and encapsulation of the debris by scarring. Frequently, the distinctive coloration is lost during surgical excision because of incision of the surrounding scar and escape of the encapsulated debris. As mentioned earlier, endometriotic implants may appear in a wide variety of presentations, including nonpigmented, clear vesicles; white plaques; and reddish petechiae or flame-like areas. These implants range from several millimeters to 2 cm in diameter. They can be superficial or invasive, with the latter often involving subperitoneal structures.

Endometriotic cysts are frequently encountered, primarily involving the ovary. At the time of menstruation, cyclic hemorrhage is retained by the surrounding cell wall, with slow reabsorption of the debris. Fresh episodes of bleeding replenish the cyst contents with each menses. Cyst fluid is often a dark, tarry, "chocolate" brown, but may also appear clear or bright red.

Fibrous adhesions often form as a response to chronic irritation of the peritoneal surfaces by the endometriotic implant and its secretory products. Foci of endometriosis are often found at the base of such adhesions.

Peritoneal pockets in the pelvis were first described in association with endometriosis by Sampson (1927). These pockets are found in roughly 18% of women with endometriosis, and two thirds of the structures have endometriotic implants either around the rim or inside the defect (Redwine, 1989b). Such pockets are thought to represent a primary developmental formation defect of the pelvic peritoneum; the ontologic relationship between these pockets and endometriosis, if any, has yet to be delineated.

Although endometriosis is often easily visualized, the disease may be missed completely by the surgeon because microscopic lesions may be present in visually normal peritoneum (Murphy et al, 1986). This phenomenon has been seen in up to 6% of women and endometriosis when biopsies were done of visually normal peritoneum and/or uterosacral ligaments (Nisolle et al, 1990b). This finding, however, has been disputed by others who claim that the original finding was secondary to "unrecognized" rather than "microscopic" disease (Redwine, 1988a).

Microscopically, endometriosis contains four major components: endometrial glands, endometrial stroma, fibrosis, and hemorrhage (Fig. 30–2). It is generally accepted that at least two of these components must be present before the lesion can be classified as endometriosis, because no individual component is itself pathognomonic.

Implants are often thought to undergo cyclic histologic changes in synchrony with normal endometrium as determined by the gonadal steroids. When carefully evaluated, however, the vast majority of implants do not demonstrate the typical cyclic histology observed within the uterus, and those that do are often asynchronous with active tissue (Metzger et al, 1988). Nisolle et al. (1994) evaluated estrogen and progesterone receptor content in both normal endometrium and peritoneal endometriotic implants; the estrogen receptor content was found to be lower in the endometriotic tissue when compared with endometrium, but the cyclic pattern was similar in both tissues. Progesterone receptor content was similar in both tissues, except during the late secretory phase in ectopic glandular epithelium, in which high persistent progesterone receptor content was observed. It is unclear whether this is due to abnormal hormonal responsiveness because of altered steroid receptor populations, an altered epithelial-stromal relationship, an aberrant blood supply, or the presence of an associated inflammatory reaction.

Table 30–2. EVOLUTION OF COLOR APPEARANCE OF ENDOMETRIOSIS WITH AGE

COLOR APPEARANCE	NO. OF PATIENTS	MEAN AGE (yr) ± SD	AGE RANGE (yr)
Clear papules only	6	21.5 ± 3.5	17–26
Clear papules plus other clear lesions	8	23.0 ± 4.0	17–28
Clear plus any others	14	23.4 ± 4.7	17–31
Red only	16	26.3 ± 5.4	16–38
Red plus any others	22	26.9 ± 5.7	17–43
All nonblack	55	27.9 ± 7.2	17–42
White plus any others	24	28.3 ± 6.9	17–43
Black plus any others	34	28.4 ± 5.8	17–43
White only	8	29.5 ± 5.9	20–39
Black only	48	31.9 ± 7.5	20–52

From Redwine DB: Age-related evolution in color appearance of endometriosis. Fertil Steril 1987;48:1063, with permission of the American Fertility Society.

The histology of the ovarian endometrioma often lacks the usual findings characteristic of the disease. The cyst wall is often nondescript, with simple cuboidal epithelium and little histologic evidence of menstrual cyclicity. Fibrous tissue often lines the cyst wall (Fig. 30–3).

Specific cycle-dependent changes in the ultrastructural appearance of normal endometrium have been described for both normal glands and stroma (Ferenczy, 1976a, 1976b). These include giant mitochondria and the appearance of nuclear channel systems coinciding with ovulation. Conversely, ectopic endometrium often fails to demonstrate these ultrastructural characteristics (Lox et al, 1984). Frequently, collagen fibrils surround the implant. Because the scarring may obliterate standard histologic features, the ultrastructural appearance may be the best means of identifying the tissue as endometriotic.

Staging Systems

A variety of classification schemes have been proposed over the years. Early attempts centered around descriptive stages derived from surgical and histopathologic findings (Table 30–3). In 1962, Riva and associates were the first to attempt a classification of endometriosis based on scalar criteria. They grouped patients based on the cumulative count of pelvic structures involved, but found their scores correlated poorly with clinical status. This attempt was the forerunner of modern classification schemes.

More recent staging systems have focused not merely on the physical manifestations but also on the prognosis (Table 30–4). Acosta and associates (1973) were the first to correlate extent of disease with pregnancy rates following conservative surgery. Their scheme was based on an anatomic description of in-

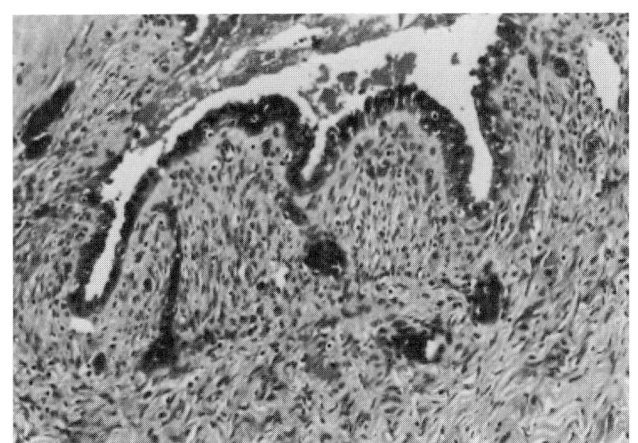

Figure 30–2
Photomicrograph of implant of endometriosis, exhibiting both glands and stroma. (Courtesy of Philip T. Valente, MD, Department of Pathology, University of Texas Health Science Center at San Antonio.)

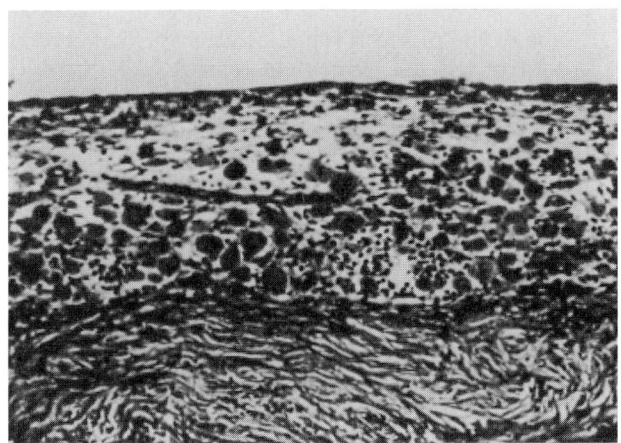

Figure 30–3
Photomicrograph of endometrioma cyst wall with numerous macrophages. (Courtesy of Philip T. Valente, MD, Department of Pathology, University of Texas Health Science Center at San Antonio.)

Table 30 – 3. EARLY ENDOMETRIOSIS CLASSIFICATION SCHEMES

Sampson (1921)	Staged by adhesions
Wicks and Larson (1949)	Histology alone
Huffman (1951)	Amount of invasion, location, pregnancy rates
Norwood (1960)	Clinical-anatomic-histologic
Riva et al (1962)	Attempted scalar criteria
Beecham (1966)	Intraoperative findings, for record keeping only
Mitchell and Farber (1974)	Similar to malignant staging

volved pelvic areas. Unfortunately, the staging was entirely arbitrary and unsupported by data; nevertheless, a rough correlation existed between severity of disease and inability to conceive. Although other related schemes were published in subsequent years, none enjoyed the widespread popularity of the "Acosta Classification."

Nevertheless, because of the lack of agreement among leading researchers in the field, the AFS convened a panel in 1978 to arrive at a consensus. The result was an innovative scheme based on the natural progression of the disease, with allowances for unilateral involvement (AFS, 1979). The stage of endometriosis was based on a cumulative score of a weighted value system related to the involvement of the peritoneum, ovaries, and fallopian tubes. In addition, an anatomic drawing was provided to depict surgical findings, including extragenital implants. In 1985, the AFS introduced a revision of this classification scheme because of numerous shortcomings that had been identified over the ensuing years. In contrast to the original scale, strong emphasis was placed upon the presence of adnexal adhesions and deep endometriotic invasion (Fig. 30–4).

The basic premise for categorization protocols is that similar stages of a disease will respond predictably to specific treatment plans, resulting in a reproducible outcome. Despite the wide range of attempts at staging the disease, all classification schemes developed to date have a number of inherent problems in fulfilling this theoretical framework:

1. None of the modern schemes attempts to correlate extent of disease with pain or risk of recurrence; only the relationship between extent of disease and fertility prognosis has been attempted.
2. All schemes are based on clinical opinion rather than any type of sophisticated statistical analysis.
3. Each classification category is arbitrarily assigned a point score that may not reflect the true relative risk of each disease locus.

4. The cutoff thresholds for each of the severity categories were chosen arbitrarily.
5. The accuracy of laparoscopic staging using these staging systems has never been assessed.

Given these shortcomings, it is of limited utility to report treatment data in terms of disease severity according to any of the published classification methods. Only more recently has scientific rigor been applied to basic and clinical investigation into endometriosis, as anecdotal reports and retrospective surveys appeared in an attempt to pass for treatment trials. The reproducibility of the revised AFS classification scheme for endometriosis has been call into question. Hornstein and colleagues (1993) found that the comparison of intraobserver and interobserver scores resulted in a change in endometriosis staging in 38% and 52% of patients, respectively. The variability was found to be high for ovarian endometriosis and cul-de-sac subscores when the revised classification was utilized.

To define adequately the relationship of various locations and extent of endometriotic lesions to the successful treatment of infertility and pelvic pain, a large, prospective study utilizing multivariate logistic regression analysis is required. Palmisano and colleagues (1993) undertook just such a study in a cohort of infertile women in whom they retrospectively evaluated the use of endometriosis staging systems to predict pregnancy rates. Pregnancy rates were analyzed using life table and cluster analyses, with combinations of endometriosis site and infertility type being evaluated with Cox's regression model. Their results showed that no anatomic site or type significantly affected prognosis, and staging systems based solely on anatomic site and the type of lesion are insufficient for predicting fertility. The relationship of pelvic pain to the stage and type of endometriotic lesions requires a different scheme, which is best illustrated by the surgical trial undertaken by Sutton and colleagues (1994). In their study

Table 30 – 4. MODERN ENDOMETRIOSIS CLASSIFICATION SCHEMES

Acosta et al (1973)	Correlates extent with pregnancy after surgery
Ingersoll (1977)	Modification of Acosta scheme
Kistner et al (1977)	Based on geographic dissemination
Buttram (1978)	Designed to select most appropriate mode of therapy
Cohen (1979)	Based on laparoscopic findings
American Fertility Society (1979)	Scalar scheme selected by committee
American Fertility Society (1985)	Revision of 1979 method

Patient's Name _____ Date_____

Stage I (Minimal) · 1-5
Stage II (Mild) · 6-15   Laparoscopy_____ Laparotomy_____ Photography_____
Stage III (Moderate) · 16-40   Recommended Treatment_____
Stage IV (Severe) · >40
Total_____   Prognosis_____ _____

PERITONEUM	**ENDOMETRIOSIS**	<1cm	1-3cm	>3cm
	Superficial	1	2	4
	Deep	2	4	6
OVARY	R Superficial	1	2	4
	Deep	4	16	20
	L Superficial	1	2	4
	Deep	4	16	20

	POSTERIOR CULDESAC OBLITERATION	Partial	Complete
		4	40

	ADHESIONS	<1/3 Enclosure	1/3-2/3 Enclosure	>2/3 Enclosure
OVARY	R Filmy	1	2	4
	Dense	4	8	16
	L Filmy	1	2	4
	Dense	4	8	16
TUBE	R Filmy	1	2	4
	Dense	4*	8*	16
	L Filmy	1	2	4
	Dense	4*	8*	16

*If the fimbriated end of the fallopian tube is completely enclosed, change the point assignment to 16.

Additional Endometriosis: _____   Associated Pathology: _____

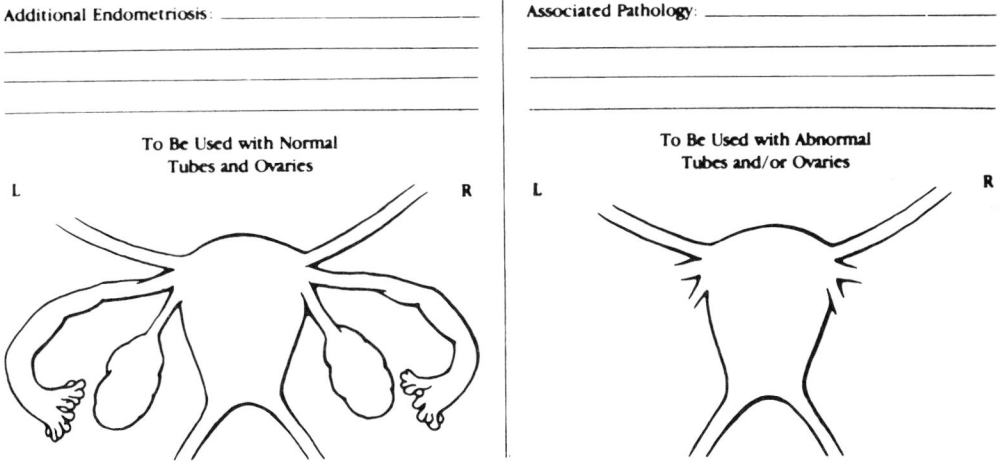

To Be Used with Normal Tubes and Ovaries   To Be Used with Abnormal Tubes and/or Ovaries

Figure 30–4
American Fertility Society revised classification, 1985. (From American Fertility Society: Research classification of endometriosis. Fertil Steril 1985;43:351, with permission of the American Fertility Society.)

assessing the efficacy of laser laparoscopic surgery in the treatment of pain associated with minimal, mild, and moderate endometriosis, they observed the poorest results in those patients with stage I disease. Conversely, patients with stage II and stage III disease experienced marked and prolonged relief of symptoms. Clearly, the standard classification of endometriosis as it relates to pelvic pain had no bearing on the severity of symptoms or surgical outcome.

Treatment

A variety of treatment options have been developed over the years in an attempt to combat endometriosis. Recommendations have included expectant management, medical therapy with a number of drugs, and surgical excision or destruction of the endometriotic lesions. It is clear that the key to developing a rational approach to the treatment of endometriosis is a thorough understanding of the pathogenesis and mechanism of adverse effects of the disease. In the absence of a general agreement on the issues, it should be no surprise that therapeutic approaches have been so diverse.

Evaluation of Treatment Options

In order to assess the relative merits of the therapeutic alternatives, it is paramount to identify outcome measures for comparison. For endometriosis, such measurable outcomes include extent of disease, pelvic pain, and infertility. Today, given the large amount of data accumulated regarding the outcomes of various treatments, rigorous adherence to a treatment regimen based solely on the scientific approach allows institution of only a few interventions of proven efficacy.

OUTCOME MEASURES

Extent of Disease. It is widely believed that endometriosis is a relentlessly progressive disease. However, longitudinal data in untreated women tend to dispute this concept. In 17 such patients observed for 6 months, 29% showed a decrease in the extent of the endometriosis (based on the revised AFS score), 24% demonstrated no change, and 47% showed a worsening of disease (Cooke and Thomas, 1989). When the patients were followed out to 12 months, progression was found in 64%, with improvement found in 27% in that time period (Mahmood and Templeton, 1990). Given the paucity of data with regard to human subjects, D'Hooghe and colleagues (1996) demonstrated that endometriosis in baboons followed with serial laparoscopies over 32 months was a dynamic and moderately progressive disease. There was a significant increase in the number of lesions and the endometriosis score, based on the revised AFS criteria. Specifically, the total number of endometriotic lesions after 24 months consisted of 69% new implants, 10% remodeled lesions, and 21% unchanged implants. However, this progression or regression must be assessed relative to a control group in order to draw useful conclusions about the natural history of endometriosis (D'Hooghe et al, 1996).

Because determination of extent of disease is by nature subjective, it can be subject to ascertainment bias on the part of the investigator. This is evidenced by one treatment trial demonstrating a decrease in adhesions as assessed by the surgeon at laparoscopy following medical therapy (Henzl et al, 1988). This effect was not present when photographic documentation was used in a similar trial (Steingold et al, 1987). Thus ascertainment bias can play a significant role in subjective study results and must be accounted for.

Pelvic Pain. Pain is a truly subjective phenomenon that is dependent on a complex interaction of pathophysiologic and psychologic factors. Pain is difficult to quantify, and it is even more difficult to evaluate the results of treatment because the types of pain are heterogeneous and an effective classification of endometriosis-related pain has yet to be established.

Two other factors are critical to evaluating pain-related treatment trials. First, relief of pain symptoms may be time dependent. Although pain relief may be substantial at the conclusion of the therapeutic intervention, once treatment is discontinued, a recurrence rate is inevitable. Evaluation of the recurrence is essential to proper evaluation of the therapeutic agent.

Second, there is generally a substantial placebo effect in the treatment of pain. Most types of pain symptoms respond to placebo, at least temporarily, at a rate of roughly 30%. However, placebo treatment of endometriosis-associated pain has shown a partial response in up to 55% of those affected (Kauppila et al, 1979). Proper evaluation of treatment of pelvic pain related to endometriosis must take the placebo response into consideration, and this can only be done by comparison to an appropriate control group.

Infertility. In regard to evaluation of the clinical response to infertility treatment, there are numerous ways to report data. Most commonly, the crude or simple pregnancy rate is used:

$$\frac{\text{Number of pregnancies}}{\text{Number of patients treated}}$$

Although simple to calculate, this figure is of little value in that pregnancy is a time-dependent phenomenon, with an increasing rate seen with longer follow-up. Two methods of correcting for this have been devised: the monthly fecundity rate (MFR) and cumulative pregnancy curve. The MFR is also simply calculated:

$$\frac{\text{Number of pregnancies}}{\text{Number of months of follow-up}}$$

Cumulative pregnancy curves are graphic constructs of the data as a function of time of follow-up and are amenable to statistical analysis by life table methodology. Both of these methods are preferable to simple pregnancy rates and should be the minimum requirement for a therapeutic trial to be considered of value. When more complex analysis is desired, a wide variety of additional statistical approaches exists. A thorough review of the advantages and disadvantages of these techniques is beyond the scope of this chapter; the reader is referred to an extensive review for further information (Olive, 1986).

Although infertility has been associated with endometriosis, except in extreme cases of extensive pelvic adhesions with tubal obstruction, the association is not absolute. In the majority of such women, there is a relative decrease in fertility reflected in a lower (but finite) rate of conception than that seen in the general population. Numerous uncontrolled trials have demonstrated pregnancy rates in untreated patients ranging from approximately 30% to 70% in early stage disease, with MRFs ranging from 5% to 11%. Similarly, women with moderate disease undergoing expectant management demonstrate an MFR of 2.9% (Olive and Lee, 1986); however, in those with severe disease, no pregnancies were noted with expectant management alone. Thus, when one is designing clinical trials to assess the efficacy of a therapeutic intervention upon fertility enhancement, the background conception rate must be considered.

STUDY DESIGN

Given the nature of the above outcome measures, it is readily apparent that uncontrolled or poorly controlled trials are of limited value. To generate meaningful information, randomized prospective trials are optimal with a controlled comparative design a minimum requirement.

A wide variety of study designs exist for treatment trials of endometriosis. Studies may be controlled or uncontrolled; if controlled, they may be controlled with historical data, concurrent nonrandomized patients, or by randomization. They may also be either retrospectively performed or carried out in a prospective manner. In endometriosis treatment trials, the vast majority of available data are derived form retrospective, uncontrolled trials. Given today's understanding of the disease, however, such studies are of little value when extent of disease, pain relief, or fertility enhancement is being evaluated. Clearly, randomized, controlled, prospective trials are required to generate significant information regarding these end points.

Additionally, the trial must be constructed and analyzed to ensure the maximal information is derived from the data generated. Objective and validated assessments of the extent of endometriosis and pain must be performed. Fertility rates must be calculated and compared in a statistically sound manner. Care must be taken to avoid the biases inherent in this type of investigation and alluded to above.

Medical Treatment

Medical therapy of endometriosis originated as a result of several distinct observations. The first was that pregnancy appeared to have a beneficial effect on the development of the disease. Although early epidemiologic data appeared to support this, it has subsequently become apparent that this effect is somewhat variable (McArthur and Ulfelder, 1965; Walton, 1977).

A second observation was the apparently hormonally dependent nature of the implants. Data in the rat and monkey conclusively demonstrated a requirement for ovarian sex steroids to maintain ectopically transplanted endometrium (DiZerega et al, 1980; Vernon et al, 1984). However, inconsistent effects of sex steroids have been noted on human endometriotic implants (Novak, 1960; Bergquist et al, 1981; Schweppe and Wynn, 1981).

Further insights have been gained by observing a number of naturally occurring states that appear to delay the onset of the disease process. Women who are at risk for endometriosis all share the common facet of altered cyclic ovulation. Thus medical strategies have been designed to create a chronic anovulatory pattern (danazol), a pseudopregnancy (continuous oral contraceptives), or a postmenopausal state (gonadotropin-releasing hormone [GnRH] analog).

Danazol

Danazol is an isoxazol derivative of 17 α-ethinyl testosterone (ethisterone). The drug is well absorbed orally and has more than 60 metabolites, many of which are hormonally active. Danazol was originally though to produce a "pseudomenopause" by lowering gonadotropins, but subsequent studies have shown this concept to be in error. In premenopausal women, danazol does not alter basal levels of gonadotropins, but rather diminishes the midcycle luteinizing hormone and follicle-stimulating hormone surge (Goebel and Rjosk, 1977; Floyd, 1980). Thus the drug creates a chronic anovulatory state to inhibit the growth and development of endometriosis.

Danazol is noted to have a number of other hormonal effects. The drug binds well to the androgen receptor (Chamness et al, 1980), less effectively to the progesterone receptor (Tamaya et al, 1978), and poorly to the estrogen receptor (Tamaya et al, 1984). These binding characteristics suggest that the capacity of the drug has a direct effect on the implants. In addition, danazol displaces testosterone and estradiol from sex hormone–binding globulin (SHBG) as well as progesterone and cortisol from corticosteroid-binding globulin; this action increases free hormone levels in the circulation, especially that of testosterone (McGinley and Casey, 1979). Finally, danazol inhibits multiple enzymes of the steroidogenic pathway (Barbieri et al, 1977).

The dosage of danazol recommended for the treatment of endometriosis has ranged from 100 to 800 mg/day and remains controversial. Originally, it was generally agreed that, to be effective, danazol must result in amenorrhea. To this end, Young and Blackmore (1977) demonstrated that 90% to 100% of women were amenorrheic at 600 to 800 mg/day, whereas 80% were amenorrheic at 400 mg/day; at 200 mg/day, only 44% ceased having menses. More recently, Vercellini and colleagues (1994) treated endometriosis patients with moderate to severe pelvic pain with very-low-dose danazol, 50 mg/day for 9 months, or depot leupron for 3 months followed by very-low-dose danazol at 50 mg/day for 6 months. They noted a significant improvement in dysmenorrhea, deep dyspareunia, and nonmenstrual pain in both treatment groups.

A number of side effects have been attributed to danazol (Table 30–5) (Buttram et al, 1982). Most result from androgenic effects of the drug, and some,

Table 30-5. SIDE EFFECTS OF DANAZOL THERAPY

SIDE EFFECTS	INCIDENCE (%)
Weight gain	85*
Muscle cramps	52
Decreased breast size	48
Flushing	42
Mood change	38
Oily skin	37
Depression	32
Sweating	32
Edema	28
Change in appetite	28
Acne	27
Fatigue	25
Hirsutism	21
Decreased libido	20
Nausea	17
Headache	17
Dizziness	10
Rash	8
Increased libido	8
Deepening of voice	7

*0-1 pound, 15%; 1-5 pounds, 22%; 6-10 pounds, 32%; 11-15 pounds, 18%; 16-20 pounds, 11%.
From Buttram VC Jr, Belue JB, Reiter RC: Interim report of a study of danazol for the treatment of endometriosis. Fertil Steril 1982;37:478, with permission of the American Fertility Society.

such as deepening of the voice, are irreversible. The occurrence of at least some side effects is a new universal phenomenon. One side effect is the adverse change in blood lipoproteins, with danazol causing a profound lowering of high-density lipoproteins (HDL) (Telimaa et al, 1989b). Although it appears that this effect is reversible shortly after discontinuation of the drug (Fahraeus et al, 1984), prolonged use of this medication may severely alter the risk of arthrosclerotic heart disease.

Good results have generally been obtained when danazol is used to treat the anatomic manifestation of endometriosis. Dmowski and Cohen (1975) demonstrated a lessening of disease in most patients and complete resolution in nearly all women with mild endometriosis. Barbieri and colleagues (1982) noted improvement in 94%. In neither of these studies was any effect noted on adhesions.

Three additional studies have attempted to assess the quantitative effect of danazol on endometriotic implants. Döberl and colleagues (1984) reduced the additive diameter of implants by 79% to 89% with the drug. Similarly, Buttram et al (1985) noted a 61% decrease in implant volume at second-look laparoscopy. Finally, Henzl and associates (1988) found danazol to produce a 43% decrease in the revised AFS classification system score.

Dickey and colleagues (1984) correlated resolution of implant to serum estradiol levels, finding that response coincided well with depth of hypoestrogenism produced. The possibility of adjusting dosages to suit individual patients based upon serum estradiol levels is intriguing and one that deserves further study.

Although each of these studies assessed the effect of danazol on implants during treatment, none looked at the rate of implant recurrence following discontinuation of the medication. One placebo-controlled trial, by Telimaa and associates (1987a), examined the effect upon implants 6 months after completion of drug therapy. In the placebo group, resolution was observed in 18%, whereas the size of the implants was estimated to be increased in 23% of patients. Conversely, 60% of those treated with danazol experienced partial or complete resolution of the endometriosis. No study has assessed the long-term effects of this drug on extent of disease.

Pain relief has been evaluated in numerous uncontrolled trials, with improvement in symptoms noted in 84% to 92% (Bayer and Seibel, 1989). A randomized, controlled study showed that danazol reduced pain significantly better than placebo throughout the treatment course and up to 6 months after discontinuation of the medication (Telimaa et al, 1987a). Few data exist on the long-term recurrence of pain, although one study suggests that symptoms recur at a rate of roughly 50% per year (Barbieri et al, 1982).

Pregnancy rates following danazol treatment vary tremendously and are confined generally to retrospective, uncontrolled reports (Bayer and Seibel, 1989). However, two randomized, prospective trials have evaluated the effects of danazol on fertility. The first consisted of 12 months of follow-up in patients either untreated or treated with danazol following the diagnosis of minimal endometriosis (Bayer et al, 1988). From life table analysis, cumulative pregnancy rates were 37.2% in the danazol-treated group and 57.4% in the untreated group (Fig. 30-5). Similar results were obtained in a second randomized comparison of danazol and placebo. In this study, consisting of patients with all stages of endometriosis, the cumulative pregnancy rate at 30 months of follow-up was 33% in the danazol group and 46% in the placebo group (Telimaa, 1988). Thus there is no evidence that danazol enhances pregnancy rates in women with endometriosis-associated infertility.

PROGESTOGENS

The use of progestational agents is gaining popularity, with a large number of options ranging from the progesterone-derived medroxyprogesterone acetate (MPA) and magestrol acetate to 19-nortestosterone derivatives, such as norethindrone and norgestrel, and retroprogesterone compounds, such as dydrogesterone. The mechanism of action of these drugs is believed to be via initial decidualization of endometrial tissue with eventual atrophy. These agents may be administered according to a variety of protocols befitting the pharmaceutical diversity of the available drugs. Today, oral administration is often preferred because of the rapid reversibility of the effect of the medication.

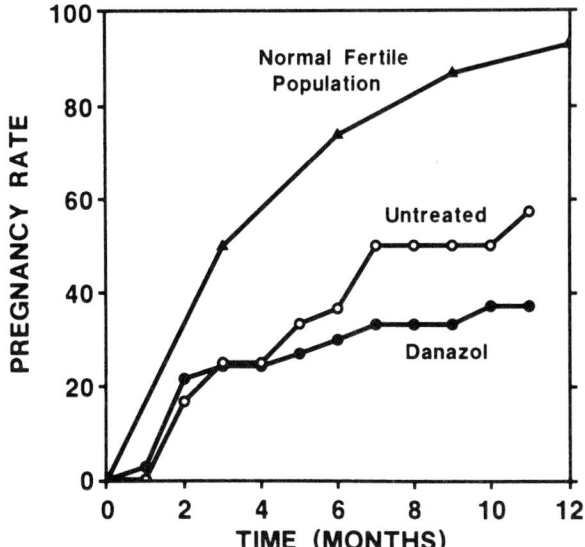

Figure 30-5
Cumulative pregnancy rates in danazol-treated and untreated patients with minimal endometriosis. The cumulative pregnancy rate in an ideal fertile population is also shown for comparison. (From Bayer SR, Seibel MM: Medical treatment: danazol. In Schenken JB [ed]: Endometriosis: Contemporary Concepts in Clinical Management. Philadelphia: JB Lippincott Company, 1989:169, with permission.) [Adapted from Cooke ID, Sulaiman RA, Lenton EA: Fertility and infertility statistics: their importance and application. Clin Obstet Gynecol 1981;8:531.])

Side effects vary greatly, depending on the specific progestogen, the dosage, the interval of treatment, and the route of administration. A common side effect is transient breakthrough bleeding, which occurs in 38% to 47% of patients (Olive, 1989b). Other side effects include nausea, breast tenderness, and fluid retention. In contradistinction to danazol, all of these adverse effects resolve upon discontinuation of the drugs. Progestogens may adversely effect serum lipoprotein levels. High-dose MPA (100 mg/day) resulted in a 26% decline in HDL cholesterol levels, a level significantly less than for placebo but only half the reduction seen with danazol (Telimaa et al, 1989b). The significance of this effect is currently unknown.

The effect of progestogens on the extent of endometriosis has been clearly defined. In a randomized, controlled, comparative trial, high-dose MPA was administered for 6 months and followed by 6 months of observation (Telimaa et al, 1987a). At the conclusion of this time, laparoscopy revealed total resolution of implants in 50% of women and partial resolution in 13%. The corresponding figures for danazol were 40% and 20%, and for placebo 12% and 6%. Thus MPA acts as effectively as danazol and significantly better than placebo in reducing disease volume, even up to 6 months after discontinuation of therapy.

Pain relief with progestational therapy also appears to be uniformly excellent. Uncontrolled trials

suggest a relief rate of roughly 90%, regardless of the progestogen used (Timonen and Johansson, 1968; Johnston, 1976; Moghissi and Boyce, 1976; Schlaff et al, 1990). In a prospective, randomized trial, high-dose MPA relieved pain symptoms to a degree comparable to danazol and significantly better than placebo (Fig. 30-6) (Telimaa et al, 1987a).

Few publications exist regarding the attempt to enhance fertility with progestogens. However, Hull and associates (1987) reported a concurrent nonrandomized, controlled, comparative trial with oral MPA, danazol, and expectant management in women with early-stage endometriosis. Cumulative pregnancy rates were no different between the three groups at 30 months of follow-up (Fig. 30-7). Telimaa (1988) reported a randomized trial between high-dose MPA, danazol, and placebo in women at all stages of disease and being followed for up to 30 months. Results demonstrated no difference in pregnancy rates among the three groups. Thus the efficacy of progestogens in treating infertility is as yet unproven.

Gestrinone. Gestrinone (ethylnorgestrienone, R2323) is an antiprogestational steroid used extensively in Europe for the treatment of endometriosis. Its effects include androgenic, antiprogestogenic, and antiestrogenic actions, although the last is not mediated by estrogen-receptor binding (Moguilewsky and Philibert, 1984). This drug is believed to enhance lysosomal degradation of the cell via a progesterone withdrawal effect Cornillie et al, 1986). This appears to be secondary to a sharp decline in estrogen and progesterone receptors as well as a substantial increase in 17 β-hydroxysteroid dehydrogenase. Additionally, there is a 50% decline in serum estradiol associated with a decrease in circulating SHBG (Robyn et al, 1984).

Gestrinone is administered orally in doses of 5 to 10 mg weekly, on a daily, twice-weekly, or three-times-weekly schedule. Side effects include androgenic and antiestrogenic sequelae (Coutinho et al, 1984). Although most side effects are mild and transient, several, such as voice changes, hirsutism, and clitoral hypertrophy, are potentially irreversible.

The effect of gestrinone on endometriotic implants has been well studied. In a randomized, placebo-controlled trial, Thomas and Cooke (1987) found improvement in the revised AFS score in 15 of 18 women (83%) taking the medication for 6 months, with 11 of 18 showing no residual disease at subsequent laparoscopic examination. Conversely, only 29% of the placebo group showed a lessening of disease. Unfortunately, no study of implant recurrence following discontinuation of treatment has been undertaken.

Relief of pelvic pain has been encouraging. In several uncontrolled trials, improvement of symptoms was noted in more than 90% of subjects while they were taking medication (Azadian-Boulanger et al, 1984; Coutinho et al, 1984). However, within 1 year

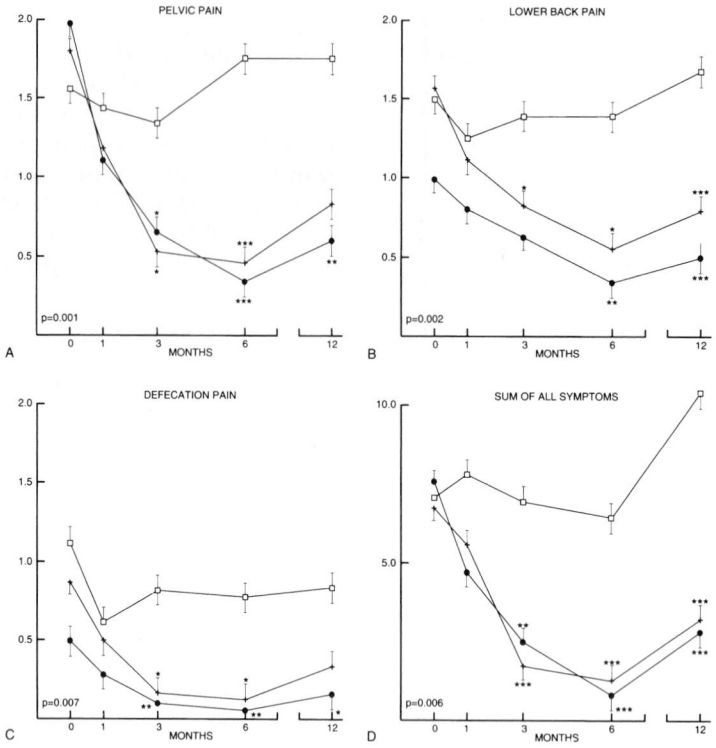

Figure 30–6

Comparison of the effects of medroxyprogesterone acetate (MPA) (+), danazol (●), and placebo (□) on (A) pelvic pain alone (p = .001 in analysis of variance), (B) lower back pain alone (p = .002), (C) defecation pain alone (p = .007), and (D) the six endometriosis-associated symptoms altogether (pelvic pain, lower back pain, defecation pain, dysuria, dyspareunia, diarrhea) (p = .006) before, during, and after the treatments. Values are given as mean ± standard error of the scores. Asterisks indicate statistical significances of differences between MPA and placebo, and danazol and placebo at different time points (Bonferroni test): *p < .05; **, p < .01; ***, p < .001. (From Telimaa S, Puolakka J, Rönnberg L, Kauppila A: Placebo-controlled comparison of danazol and high-dose medroxyprogesterone acetate in the treatment of endometriosis. Gynecol Endocrinol 1987;1:13, with permission of Parthenon Publishers.)

following discontinuation of the drug, recurrence of pain was observed in 15% to 30%.

Many researchers have investigated the effect of gestrinone upon fertility. Unfortunately, nearly all studies have been small, uncontrolled, and hetero-geneous in the cohort enrolled. An exception is a prospective trial in women with early-stage endometriosis (Thomas and Cooke, 1987). In this study, women were observed for 12 months after treatment with either gestrinone or placebo. The cumulative

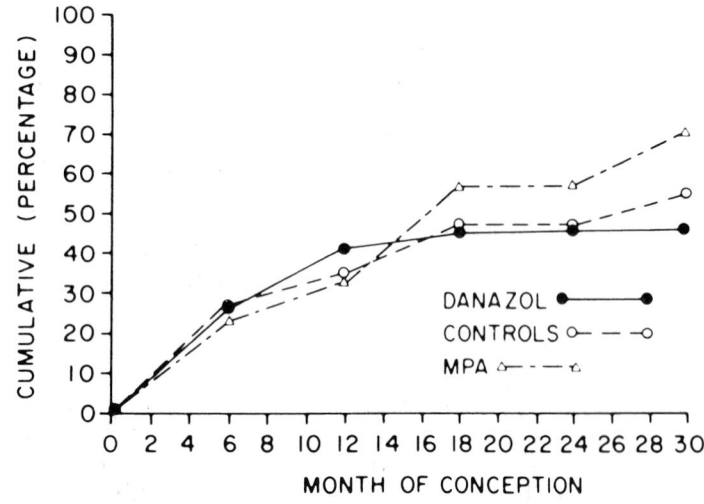

Figure 30–7

Cumulative pregnancy rates for three treatment groups with stage I and stage II endometriosis. (From Hull ME, Moghissi KS, Magyar DF, Hayes F: Comparison of different treatment modalities of endometriosis in infertile women. Fertil Steril 1987;47:42, with permission of the American Fertility Society.)

conception rate in the gestrinone-treated group (25%) did not differ significantly from those taking placebo (24%), and neither group showed differences from a concurrently studied cohort of patients with unexplained infertility (23%). Furthermore, when patients were divided by second-look laparoscopy into those with residual disease and those with total resolution, there was again no difference in conception rates. Thus there is no evidence that the treatment of endometriosis with gestrinone enhances fertility.

Mifepristone RU 486. Apart from its controversial role in pregnancy termination, mifepristone (RU 486) may well prove to be of value in a wide variety of gynecologic disorders, including endometriosis. The drug is an antiprogestational and antiglucocorticoid that can inhibit ovulation and disrupt endometrial integrity. Daily doses of the medication range from 50 to 100 mg, with side effects ranging from hot flashes to fatigue, nausea, and transient elevation in liver transaminases. No effect on lipid profiles or bone mineral density has been reported.

The ability of mifepristone to produce a regression of endometriotic lesions has been variable and apparently dependent upon duration of treatment. Trials lasting 2 months in the rodent model (Tjaden et al, 1993) and 3 months in the human (Kettel et al, 1991) failed to produce regression of disease. However, 6 months of therapy resulted in less visible disease in women (Kettel et al, 1996).

Uncontrolled trials suggest possible efficacy for endometriosis-associated pain, although numbers are small. No data have yet been collected regarding fertility enhancement.

Combination Estrogen-Progestogen. The combination of estrogen and a progestogen for treatment of endometriosis, the so-called pseudopregnancy regimen, has been utilized for 40 years. This approach, like progestational therapy alone, is believed to act via initial decidualization and growth of endometrial tissue followed by atrophy. The combination can be administered orally (with combination contraceptive pills) or parenterally. Combination oral contraceptive pills such as norethynodrel and mestranol, norethindrone acetate and ethinyl estradiol, lynestrenol and mestranol, and norgestrel plus ethinyl estradiol have all been tried. Parenteral combinations have included 17-hydroxyprogestrone or depot MPA paired with stilbestrol or conjugated estrogens.

Side effects are numerous, and include androgenic, estrogenic, and progestogenic effects. Estrogens may cause nausea, thrombophlebitis, and uterine enlargement. The 19-nortestosterone–derived progestogens may cause androgenic effects such as acne, alopecia, increased muscle mass, decreased breast size, and deepening of the voice. Noble and Letchworth (1979), in a comparative trial of norethynodrel and mestranol versus danazol, found that 41% of the pseudopregnancy group failed to complete their course of therapy because of side effects of the medication. However, dosages producing sig-

nificant side effects generally involve more estrogen than found in modern contraceptive preparations. The oral contraceptives commonly prescribed today for combination therapy are most likely to produce a progestogen-dominant picture similar to that of progestogen alone.

The efficacy of pseudopregnancy has been poorly assessed. Riva and colleagues (1962), using culdoscopy, demonstrated an 80% improvement in lesions, with an 11.8% recurrence rate at 6 months. Despite the paucity of available data, oral contraceptives remain the most commonly prescribed treatment for endometriosis symptoms.

Numerous controlled trials have evaluated pain relief, generally demonstrating improvement in 75% to 89%. A randomized clinical trial compared cyclic low-dose oral contraceptives to a GnRH agonist and found no substantial difference in the degree of relief afforded these women by the two drugs, except that the GnRH agonist provided greater relief of dysmenorrhea (Vercellini et al, 1993).

Reports of pregnancy rates in women with endometriosis-associated infertility treated with oral contraceptives are sparse and uncontrolled. None provided evidence of improvement in fertility by these medications. Adamson et al (1982), using life table analysis, was able to show that treatment with oral contraceptives had a less favorable effect on the pregnancy rate than surgical treatment or no treatment for the groups analyzed (i.e., presence or absence of adnexal lesions, anatomic structures involved, and specific types of lesions).

GnRH ANALOGS

These medications are modifications of GnRH and function to down-regulate the pituitary gland. The net effect is a decline in gonadotropins and resultant "medical oophorectomy." The clinically used analogs are listed in Table 30–6. These drugs are administered subcutaneously, intranasally, or intramuscularly, with dosage schedules varying according to the specific agonist, route of administration, and degree of pituitary suppression sought. The lowering of gonadotropin levels results in decreased ovarian stimulation and serum estradiol levels in the castrate range (Meldrum et al, 1982). The time course for this decrease is roughly 3 to 6 weeks. To the degree that endometriotic tissue is dependent on estrogen for growth, such therapy affects glandular involution and stromal atrophy of implants.

Numerous side effects have been reported, and most symptoms demonstrate an increased rate with higher dosages (Olive, 1989b). Reported side effects include transient vaginal bleeding, hot flashes, vaginal dryness, decreased libido, breast tenderness, insomnia, depression, irritability and fatigue, headache, joint stiffness, and skin changes. Comparative studies carried out with GnRH analogs and danazol have shown that GnRH agonists produce less weight gain, edema, and myalgias, whereas hot flashes, de-

Table 30-6. GONADOTROPIN-RELEASING HORMONE ANALOG EVALUATED FOR THE TREATMENT OF ENDOMETRIOSIS

STRUCTURE	TRADE NAME
[D-(but)Ser^6-des-Gly^{10}-NEt]-GnRH	Buserelin (Hoechst)
[(Imbal)-D-His^6-Pro^9-NEt]-GnRH	Histrelin (Serono)
[D-Leu^8-Pro^9-NEt]-GnRH	Leuprolide (Abbott)
[D-(2-naph)-Ala^6-GnRH	Nafarelin (Syntax)
[D-Trp^6-N-Me-Leu^7-des-Gly^{10}-Pro^9-NEt]-GnRH	Lutrelin (Wyeth)
[D-Trp^8-Pro^9-NEt]-GnRH	Lincol (Salk Institute)
[D-Ser(tBu)^6-Aza-Gly^{10}]-GnRH	Zolidez (ICI Ltd)

From Olive DL: Medical treatment: alternatives to danazol. In Schenken RS (ed): Endometriosis: Contemporary concepts in Clinical Management. Philadelphia: JB Lippincott Company, 1989:200, with permission.

creased libido, and vaginal dryness were more common (Jelley and Magill, 1986; Henzl et al, 1988).

Two major concerns are the effects of this class of drugs on the lipoprotein levels (Wheeler et al, 1993) and loss of bone mineral density (Rock et al, 1993). The latter effect is seen as early as 3 months into treatment, and may take a year or more to recover following discontinuation of therapy (Rock et al, 1993). These findings have led to alternative strategies of GnRH agonist treatment in combination with steroid hormone add-back therapy as a means of chronic administration of these drugs. Add-back is generally commenced after 3 months of unopposed agonist, and may be combination estrogen-progestogen (Friedman and Hornstein, 1993), progestogen alone (Fahraeus et al, 1986; Surrey et al, 1990), or low-dose progestogen coupled with a bisphosphonate (Surrey et al, 1993). Results have been promising, although trials have been small and duration limited to 2 years or less.

The effect of GnRH analogs on endometriotic implants is impressive in both animals (Werlin and Hodgen, 1983) and humans. Atrophic glands and stroma are the rule among biopsied implants after treatment, but Lemay and colleagues (1984) have pointed out that, although implants appear inactive, they are capable of later growth. In comparative trials, danazol or a GnRH analog produced a similar degree of regression of implants (Henzl et al, 1988; Fedele et al, 1989a; Fedele et al, 1989b).

Pelvic pain has been extensively evaluated in a variety of uncontrolled trials, with most of these studies demonstrating a diminution of symptoms in 80% or more cases during treatment. In a randomized trial of danazol and the analog nafarelin, the two drugs produced an equivalent amount of pain relief (Henzl et al, 1988). The question of recurrence, however, remains open. In this trial, most women did not note significant pain recurrence 6 months after treatment. A second study has reported a 20% recurrence of noncyclic pain but no recurrence of dyspareunia at 6 months' follow-up (Lemay et al, 1984). In yet a third trial, however, roughly half the patients noted symptomatic recurrence by 1 year (Fedele et al, 1989a). More recent data suggest that recurrence is stage dependent, with a 5-year recurrence risk of 36.9% for minimal disease but up to 74.4% for severe disease (Waller and Shaw, 1993).

Pregnancy rates following GnRH agonist therapy have been reported by numerous investigators. However, most studies suffer from small size, inconsistent staging, and variable length of follow-up. In comparative trials with danazol, no difference in the pregnancy rates has been detected at 1 year (Henzl et al, 1988; Fedele et al, 1989a). At this time, further data are required before any conclusions can be drawn concerning the efficacy of GnRH analogs with regard to enhancing pregnancy rates.

OTHER MEDICATIONS

A wide variety of additional medical therapies have been attempted in combating endometriosis. Some, such as estrogen and methyltestosterone, have been abandoned because of side effects (Karnaky, 1948; Katayama et al, 1976). Others, such as the antiestrogens tamoxifen and clomiphene, have been tested in only very small, uncontrolled trials (Haber and Behelak, 1987; Koninckx, 1987). Finally, several medications, such as pentoxifylline and verapamil, have appeared promising in the animal modal but have yet to undergo testing in human studies (Steinleitner et al, 1991).

A promising drug of the latter category is the GnRH antagonist. These medications differ from the GnRH agonist in that they produce an immediate inhibition of gonadotropin release. Thus their effect is faster and more direct than the long-acting GnRH agonist. The major problem with human use of this class of pharmaceuticals has been the annoying side effect of histamine release locally at the site of injection. This has been substantially reduced with the current group of third-generation antagonists.

ROLE OF MEDICAL THERAPY

Medical therapy directed at endometriosis appears to be of some value, depending upon the goal of treatment. If the objective is to diminish the anatomic extent of the disease (exclusive of pelvic adhesions) or to reduce pelvic pain symptoms, all of the drugs thus far evaluated are efficacious. However, few data are available regarding the long-term effectiveness of such treatments, and there is some suggestion that recurrence may be substantial in some instances.

The role of medications in the promotion of fertility is less clear-cut. To date, there is no evidence that any medical therapy alone can increase the rate of conception among infertile women with endometriosis.

Surgical Treatment

CONSERVATIVE SURGERY

Surgery is the most commonly used treatment for endometriosis. Goals are to restore normal pelvic anatomy, remove visible endometriotic lesions, and eliminate conductive pathways for pelvic pain. Such surgery is generally termed "conservative" when the ability to conceive is retained, and it may be performed either laparoscopically or via laparotomy.

In regard to conservative surgery, many potential procedures can be considered. First and foremost is the removal of all active endometrial implants utilizing an atraumatic, hemostatic method. Lysis of pelvic adhesions is also accomplished, with meticulous attention to excision of the entire fibrous tissue specimen, because endometriosis is often contained within such adhesions. Uterine suspension, ovarian suspension, and partial omentectomy may be performed to reduce postoperative adhesion formation (Olive, 1989a). To reduce pelvic pain, presacral neurectomy and/or uterosacral ligament transection have been advocated.

Sutton and colleagues (1994) assessed the efficacy of laser laparoscopic surgery in the treatment of pain associated with minimal, mild, and moderate endometriosis. They found that laser laparoscopic removal of endometriosis resulted in statistically significant pain relief compared with those patients undergoing sham laparoscopy up to 6 months after surgery. In numerous uncontrolled trials, the rates of improvement were 70% to 100% immediately after surgery (Olive, 1989a; Vancaillie et al, 1989) and 82% 1 year later (Nezhat, 1987). Longer term follow-up has shown pain reduction in 66% of patients over 5 years (Redwine, 1994). Whether such relief is due to the removal of implants and adhesions or to other adjunctive procedures remains to be clarified.

A variety of surgical instruments have been used to accomplish appropriate operative procedures. Sharp dissection is quite common, as are cautery and endocoagulation. The most common location is the peritoneal surface. Lesions on this lining can be vaporized, coagulated, or excised. Excision is the preferred method for larger lesions because of the complete removal and possession of a specimen for histologic confirmation. Endometriomas may be treated by drainage, vaporization, excision and stripping, or penetration and irrigation. Most surgeons agree that simple drainage of these structures is in-

adequate, with frequent recurrence resulting, although data to support this are limited.

Laser technology has now become a mainstay of treatment for endometriosis, including carbon dioxide, neodymium:yttrium-aluminum-garnet argon, and potassium–titanyl phosphate energy (Vancaillie and Schenken, 1989). No clear advantage has been evidenced by any one of these approaches, and it is recommended that the surgeon utilize the instruments with which he or she feels most comfortable. Although laparotomy had for many been the standard for surgical therapy, laparoscopy is increasingly important in the treatment of most, if not all, cases of endometriosis. Laparoscopy offers several advantages over laparotomy. Along with the ability to treat at the time of initial diagnosis, laparoscopy is also associated with a shortened hospital stay, reduced morbidity and recovery time, and decreased rate of adhesion formation. Additionally, for minimal and mild disease, laparoscopy and laparotomy had equivalent 3-year estimated cumulative life table pregnancy rates when meta-analysis was performed (Adamson and Pasta, 1994).

Success of surgery in ablating endometriotic implants, lysing adhesions, and restoring normal anatomy is assumed to be high. The rate of success for moderate to severe disease is proportional to adequate operative exposure and thorough, meticulous surgical technique as well as complete resection of all endometriotic tissue. However, once surgery is concluded, the patient may well be subject to the conditions responsible for initially creating the disease. The risk of recurrence of implants has scarcely been evaluated. Wheeler and Malinak (1983) noted a 40% recurrence of symptomatic disease at 9 years' follow-up (Olive, 1989a). Gordts and colleagues (1984) found recurrent disease in 28% of women after 18 months or more postoperatively. Much less success has been noted with prevention of adhesion recurrence (Adhesion Study Group, 1983; Diamond et al, 1984), but as many as 50% to 60% of those patients undergoing surgery appear to demonstrate long-term restoration of normal anatomic relationships.

Conservative surgery has been used extensively in an attempt to enhance fertility. Most studies, however, are uncontrolled. In mild endometriosis, surgical treatment has resulted in pregnancy rates ranging from 40% to 75%, with MFRs reported in the 2% to 4% range with laparotomy and up to 6.5% with laparoscopy. In women with moderate disease, pregnancy rates are nearly the same; MFRs also mirror those for mild disease. Even with severe endometriosis, success rates of 20% to 50% are reported, with MRFs approximately 1.5% with laparotomy and up to 6% with laparoscopy (Olive, 1989a).

Meta-analysis encompassing studies from 1982 through 1994 carried out by Adamson and Pasta (1994) showed that either no treatment or surgery alone is superior to medical treatment for minimal and mild endometriosis associated with infertility. They found that medical treatment merely delays the possibility of pregnancy by the duration of therapy, typically 3 to 6 months. Similarly, meta-analysis was also carried out by Hughes and associates (1993) on 25 randomized controlled trials and cohort studies. They found possible treatment benefit from laparoscopic conservative surgery, but overall they concluded that medical treatment via ovulation suppression was ineffective in the treatment of endometriosis-associated infertility. Although these medications may be considered to be an empirical intervention following the exhaustion of other treatments, the numerous side effects and the creation of the mandatory period of amenorrhea during medical treatment make the wisdom of this approach questionable.

Two retrospective, comparative trials have been reported. Guzick and Rock (1983) compared pregnancy rates in 224 women with mild or moderate endometriosis treated with either danazol or conservative surgery via laparotomy; no difference between therapies was noted in terms of subsequent success. Olive and Lee (1986) compared conservative surgery (laparotomy) to expectant management and found both modalities to be equally efficacious for mild or moderate disease. However, for severe endometriosis, surgery produced significantly better results than did no treatment. Meta-analyses have now been done (Hughes et al, 1993; Adamson and Pasta, 1994) to assess laparoscopic conservative surgery and the resultant pregnancy rates. Adamson and Pasta evaluated the pregnancy rates for surgical, medical, and no-treatment regimens, with surgical treatment involving either laparoscopy or laparotomy. Additionally, they performed meta-analysis on 25 studies previously evaluated by Hughes et al (1993). Both their results and the meta-analysis showed that either no treatment or surgery is superior to medical treatment for minimal and mild endometriosis associated with infertility. For moderate and severe disease, surgery is optimal, with laparoscopic surgery being at least as efficacious as laparotomy (Adamson and Pasta, 1994).

Clearly, conservative surgery can be efficacious in the treatment of pelvic pain and reduction of disease. However, it is not a panacea for enhancing fertility in women with endometriosis. It appears to be of value for advanced stages of the disease, as a means of correcting distorted anatomic relationships. In the absence of such anatomic distortion, the value of surgical intervention for treating infertility remains questionable.

DEFINITIVE SURGERY

When hysterectomy with salpingo-oophorectomy is performed for endometriosis, the procedure is termed *definitive surgery*. Such surgery, in conjunction with excision of existing endometriosis, is virtually certain to eliminate complaints of pain related to the disease itself. However, resulting adhesions may produce chronic pelvic pain.

When definitive surgical therapy is applied to younger women, there is increased pressure to consider preservation of one or both ovaries. The recurrence rate of pain symptomatology has ranged from 0% to 85% in published reports (Walters, 1989). More recently, patients undergoing definitive surgery with ovarian preservation were found to have a 6.1 times greater risk of developing recurrent pain and an 8.1 times greater risk of reoperation (Namnoum et al, 1995). On the basis of extensive clinical experience, Ranney (1971a) suggested four criteria by which to determine whether the ovaries should be removed:

1. Hilar areas are involved bilaterally.
2. Extensive endometriosis is present that cannot be resected.
3. A hemoperitoneum is present, necessitating emergency surgery.
4. Associated pelvic pathology is present, mandating removal.

COMBINATION MEDICAL-SURGICAL TREATMENT

Many investigators today favor combining medical and surgical approaches. Two options exist: preoperative medical treatment and postoperative hormonal intervention. Preoperative treatment has been advocated as a means of facilitating the technical aspects of surgery. Conversely, postoperative therapy has been suggested on the assumption that surgery is frequently unable to eliminate all endometriotic implants.

Unfortunately, most studies investigating these questions have serious methodologic flaws: sample sizes are small, no controlled comparisons are made, and data analysis is limited (Kaplan and Schenken, 1989). A comparison of preoperative therapy with either danazol, gestrinone, or buserelin followed by laparotomy with microsurgical excision or laparoscopy with laser excision for ovarian endometriosis was done by Nisolle and colleagues (1990a). They documented regression of endometriosis in 35% to 91% of patients depending on the preoperative medication used, but noted that hormonal treatment alone led to incomplete suppression of endometriosis. For patients with early-stage disease, Chong and associates (1990) found no differences in fertility rates after treatment with danazol, laparoscopic laser surgery, or laser surgery followed by danazol. For patients with advanced disease, a randomized study was performed comparing conservative surgery plus danazol, conservative surgery followed by MPA, and conservative surgery followed by placebo (Telimaa et al, 1987b). A confounding factor not controlled for in this study was the amount of endometriosis left behind and the ability of the surgeons to do optimal debulking. Although pregnancy rates were similar in all three groups, pain relief proved significantly better in the women undergoing combination therapy (Fig. 30–8). Thus it appears that combination therapy is the treatment of choice in order to facilitate

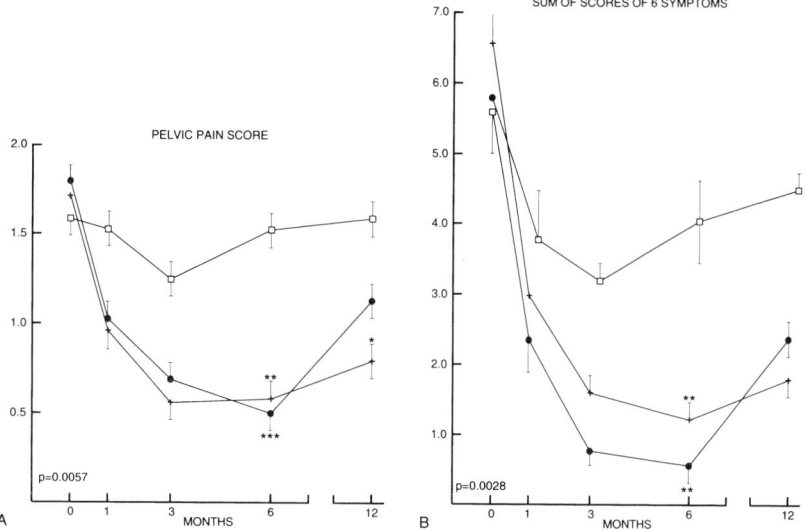

Figure 30-8

Effect of medroxyprogesterone acetate (+ — +), danazol (●—●), and placebo (■—■) on pelvic pain (A) and on six endometriosis-associated symptoms (pelvic pain, lower back pain, defecation pain, dysuria, diarrhea, and dyspareunia) (B), evaluated by symptom scores before, during, and after the treatments. Results are given as mean ± standard error of the scores. The p value indicates the statistical significance of difference between the treatment and placebo groups during the whole trial in analysis of variance. Asterisks indicate statistical significances of differences between the treatment and placebo groups at different time points in the modified Bonferroni test: *p < .05; **p < .01; ***p < .001. (From Telimaa S, Rönnberg L, Kauppila A: Placebo-controlled comparison of danazol and high-dose medroxyprogesterone acetate in the treatment of endometriosis after conservative surgery. Gynecol Endocrinol 1987;1:363, with permission of Parthenon Publishers.)

optimal surgical debulking, and to provide optimal pain relief in women with extensive disease that is not totally removed at the time of surgery.

Treatment of Symptoms

Although the majority of treatments for endometriosis are directed at eliminating the lesions themselves, some treatment regimens are designed to bypass the implants and attack the symptoms directly.

PAIN (Fig. 30-9)

One medical approach to pain relief is the use of *nonsteroidal anti-inflammatory drugs* (NSAIDs). NSAIDs act to reduce the amount of circulating prostaglandins produced by the endometriotic implants by inhibiting prostaglandin synthetase and/or antagonizing prostaglandin at its receptor. The success of these drugs has been variable with regard to endometriosis-associated pain. In a randomized, placebo-controlled study, neither aspirin, indomethacin, nor tolfenamic acid (a fenamate) decreased the premenstrual pain experienced by women with endometriosis (Kauppila et al, 1979). Tolfenamic acid resulted in a significant decrease in dysmenorrhea, whereas the two other medications failed to outperform placebo. In a second trial, naproxen sodium proved significantly better at providing relief of dysmenorrhea compared to placebo (Kauppila and

Ronnberg, 1985). These data suggest that some NSAIDs may play a role in the treatment of selected aspects of endometriosis-associated pain.

Surgical procedures for pain associated with endometriosis may involve interruption of pathways of pain conduction via uterosacral nerve ablation or presacral nerve resection. Both procedures are reserved for patients with midline pelvic pain, and may be performed by either laparoscopy or laparotomy.

The goal of *laparoscopic uterosacral nerve ablation* (LUNA) is the destruction of the uterine sensory fibers and their secondary ganglia as they exit the uterus. Accordingly, no benefit will result from a LUNA if the origin of the pain is extrauterine. Therefore, the proper selection of patients for this surgery will optimize therapeutic benefit. The procedure should be offered to those patients with central pelvic pain who have failed medical therapy. It is optimal to evaluate these women at the time of pain, with recording of the subjective evaluation of pain during examination both before and after injection of the uterosacral ligaments with a long-acting local anesthetic. During the procedure itself, approximately 1.5 to 2.0 cm of uterosacral ligaments in the region adjacent to their attachment to the cervix is excised or destroyed laparoscopically using scissors, electrosurgery, or lasers.

Studies evaluating the success rates of LUNA in the treatment of endometriosis-associated dysmen-

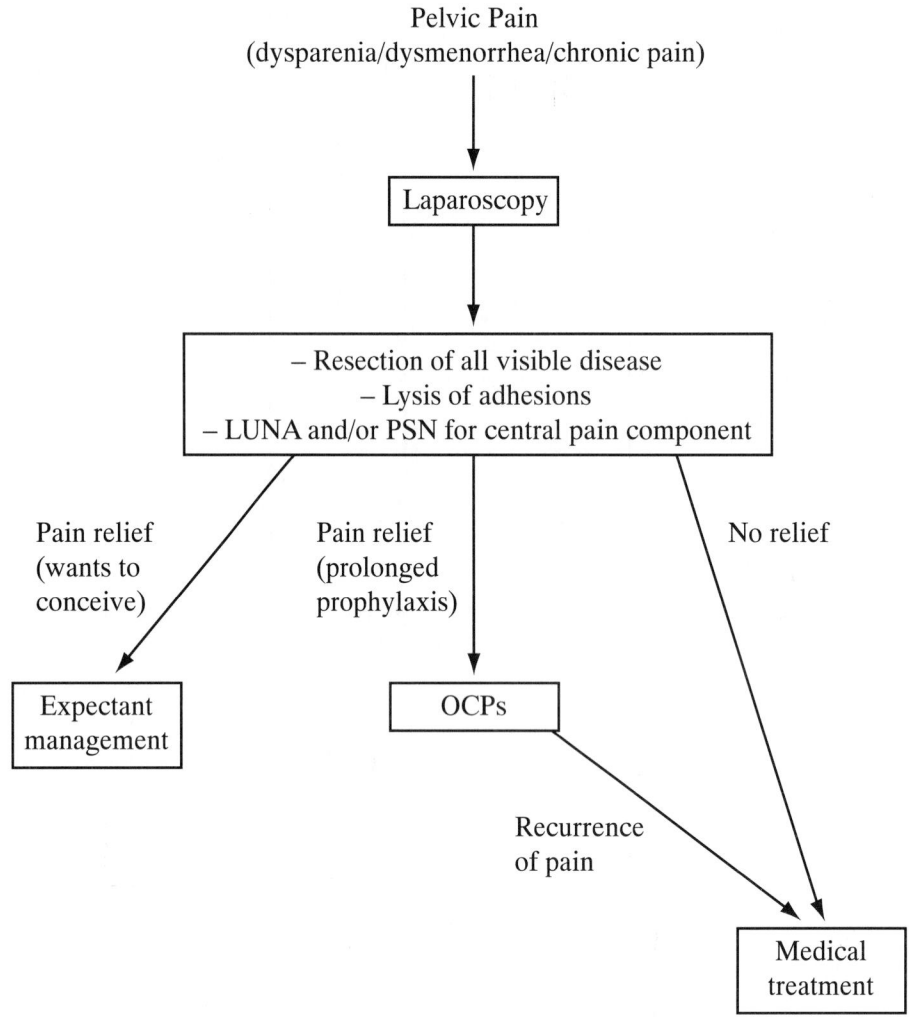

Figure 30–9
Management protocol for patients with pelvic pain caused by endometriosis. LUNA, laparoscopic uterine nerve ablation; OCPs, oral contraceptive pills; PSN, presacral neurectomy.

orrhea have shown marked improvement of dysmenorrhea ranging from 70% to 90%. When the effect of LUNA was evaluated in patients with severe incapacitating dysmenorrhea who had no pelvic pathology at laparoscopy, significant pain relief was noted in the treated group (Lichten and Bombard, 1987). Of note, though, only 44% of women had continued relief from dysmenorrhea 12 months after surgery. In another study by Sutton and colleagues (1994), women with minimal endometriosis were evaluated after either diagnostic laparoscopy followed by expectant management or LUNA with ablation of endometriosis. At 6 months after surgery, a significantly greater proportion of patients in the latter group (62%) had improvement or resolution of pain compared with the former group (23%).

Presacral neurectomy (PSN) involves interruption of the sympathetic innervation to the uterus at the level of the superior hypogastric plexus. This procedure may be performed via laparoscopy or laparotomy, but, unlike LUNA, it requires a significant degree of

surgical skill. The important anatomic landmarks are the aortic bifurcation, common iliac arteries and veins, and sacral promontory. The peritoneum over the sacral promontory is grasped and incised, and the retroperitoneal space is dissected. The retroperitoneal superior portion of the hypogastric plexus, the actual presacral nerve, is isolated below the bifurcation of the aorta, 3 or 4 cm toward the hollow of the sacrum. Once the fibers of the neural tissue have been identified, the tissue is excised for a distance of at least 2 × 2 cm over the sacral promontory. The excision is carried out medial to the ureters and common iliac vessels.

The therapeutic benefit of PSN in patients with severe endometriosis and central pelvic pain was evaluated in a prospective study by Tjaden et al (1990); they found that PSN in addition to conservative surgery was highly effective in relieving the midline component of menstrual pain. However, there was no added relief of lateral pain, back pain, or dyspareunia. Conversely, in a randomized controlled study by Candiani et al (1992), the addition of PSN to conservative surgery for moderate or severe endometriosis did not result in a greater reduction of pelvic pain than did conservative surgery alone. Thus the role of PSN in relief of endometriosis-associated pain remains controversial.

INFERTILITY (Fig. 30–10)

Infertility associated with endometriosis has been treated empirically with advanced reproductive techniques. Controlled ovarian hyperstimulation with gonadotropins results in monthly fecundity rates of 9% to 18% in women with early-stage disease; these rates are generally higher than those in women who are not treated (expectant management). A randomized comparison of three cycles of controlled ovarian hyperstimulation with 6 months of expectant management revealed a significantly higher monthly fecundity rate among the women treated with controlled ovarian hyperstimulation (15%) than among untreated women (4.5%) (Fedele

et al, 1992). The addition of intrauterine insemination also appears beneficial. In a randomized comparison of controlled ovarian hyperstimulation with and without intrauterine insemination, the combination doubled the pregnancy rate (Dodson and Haney, 1991). Experience with in vitro fertilization (IVF) for patients with endometriosis has been evaluated by Geber et al (1995), who found no difference with stimulation between patients with male factor only, tubal factor only, or unexplained infertility versus patients with endometriosis. They found that there was no difference in mean number of ampules of human menopausal gonadotropin (hMG) administered, estradiol concentration on the day of hMG administration, number of days hMG administration, mean number of oocytes retrieved and retrieval rate, fertilization rate, number of normally fertilized embryos, number of transferred embryos per cycle, or implantation rate. More importantly, the pregnancy rates were similar, as were the miscarriage rates. Additionally, they separated the endometriosis patients based on staging, according to the revised AFS clas-

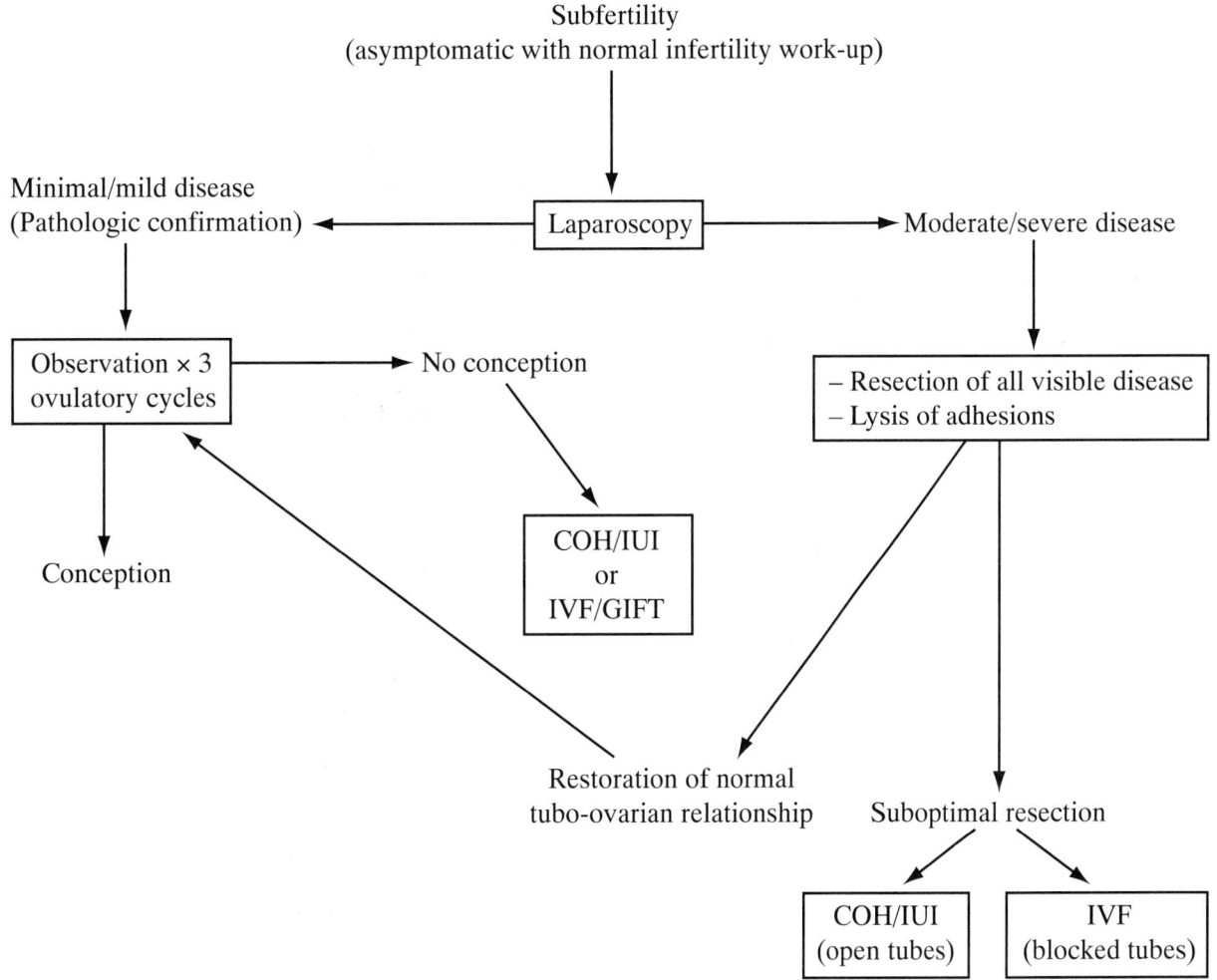

Figure 30–10

Management protocol for patients with infertility caused by endometriosis. COH/IUI, controlled ovarian hyperstimulation/intrauterine implantation; IVF/GIFT, in vitro fertilization/gamete intrafallopian transfer.

sification, and found no difference in results between stage I-II and stage III-IV disease (Geber et al, 1995). Thus, the previously held belief that endometriosis adversely affected the success rates of IVF appears to be in doubt. Additionally, the original data suggesting a difference were based on laparoscopic oocyte retrieval; therefore, a lower number of oocytes were retrieved in those patients with advanced endometriosis. The advent of transvaginal oocyte retrieval has eliminated any difference with regard to stage of disease and lower pregnancy rates.

ADENOMYOSIS

Adenomyosis was first described in 1860 by Rokitansky, who noted a condition in which endometrial glands embedded in a hyperplastic muscular stroma invaded the uterine wall. He called this condition "cystosarcoma adenoids uterinum" because the nature of the growth of these areas suggested sarcomatoid tendencies. In 1896, Cullen suggested the term "adenomyosis," and he subsequently published a review of 54 cases describing what we recognize today as adenomyosis (Cullen, 1908). Still, this entity remained somewhat obscure for many years, completely escaping mention in deQuervain's 5th edition of Clinical Surgical Diagnosis (deQuervain, 1917). In the mid-1920s, following Sampson's papers on endometriosis, Meyer (1925) aroused new interest in adenomyosis by advocating the theory of invasive endometrial hyperplasia as its etiologic mechanism. Since that time, only a handful of investigators have consistently studied adenomyosis, and investigation into its etiology and alternative diagnostic and therapeutic modalities has been especially limited.

Definition

Adenomyosis is defined as the presence of endometrial glands and stroma within the myometrium, accompanied by compensatory hypertrophy of the myometrium. Although all agree on this basic definition, the exact depth of invasion required to elicit a diagnosis of adenomyosis remains the subject of some controversy. Proposals have ranged from 1 high-powered field (1.8 mm using a 100× objective) below the endometrial surface to one third of the thickness of the uterine wall. The majority of articles written today refer to a depth of approximately 3 mm, or 1 low-powered field, below the basal layer of endometrium.

Pathogenesis

In the mid-19th century, Rokitansky (1860) described a condition in which elongated endometrial glands were found embedded in a hyperplastic endometrial stroma. He noted two variants of this condition: one in which the glands grew into the uterine musculature, and another in which they grew downward into the endometrial cavity, forming a polyp. Schatz (1883) later interpreted Rokitansky's findings to be a variant of uterine leiomyomata. He called this condition "fibroadenoma cysticus et polyposum."

Chiari (1887) subsequently described an abnormal growth of endometrial glands into the uterine musculature in the areas of the uterine cornu and proximal fallopian tube. This was the first mention of salpingitis isthmica nodosum, which he believed to be a variety of adenomyosis.

Several investigators in the 1880s and 1890s thought that adenomyosis either represented an embryonic error in müllerian cell distribution or was due to invasion of the myometrium by hyperplastic basal endometrium (Diesterweg, 1883; Ruge, 1889; Schroeder, 1892). In 1893, Hauser proposed idiopathic stromal hyperplasia as the etiology for adenomyosis. Subsequently, Von Recklinghausen (1896) proposed that adenomyosis was the result of displacement of mesonephric (wolffian) elements. He noted that these ectopic glandular elements were most commonly found on the posterior uterine wall and in the area of the uterine cornu, and he believed that these regions were more likely sites for wolffian than müllerian vestiges.

In the late 1890s and early 1900s, Meyer (1900, 1909) proposed chronic endometritis as the etiologic event that initiated invasive endometrial hyperplasia. He therefore referred to this condition as "adenomyometritis." Combining two earlier proposals, Cullen (1908) claimed that basal endometrial invasion was responsible for the majority of cases of adenomyosis, but he held out the possibility that müllerian rests could account for the encapsulated form of adenomyosis (adenomyomas). Taussig (1938) later described lymphatic transmission of endometrial components. Although this theory was used to describe pelvic endometriosis (endometriosis externa), it also offered another possible explanation for adenomyosis. Subsequently, Marcus (1961) proposed that some müllerian totipotential cells existed within the myometrium that could differentiate into endometrial cells, offering another explanation for the development of adenomyosis.

Today, we have come full circle, with most investigators believing that adenomyosis results from basal endometrial hyperplasia invading a hyperplastic myometrial stroma. Of note is the interesting observation that all organs in the human body that contain cavities also possess a submucosal region, with the exception of the uterus. It is thought that one of the main functions of this submucosa is to prevent the inward growth of glands that line these cavities.

If basal endometrial and stromal hyperplasia are, in fact, the cause of this disorder, then what etiologic event initiates this process? To date, four primary theories have been espoused: (1) heredity, (2) trauma, (3) hyperestrogenemia, and (4) viral transmission.

Heredity. Meyer (1897) initially described the finding of adenomyosis in a fetus delivered at term. Subsequently, various authors described cases of adenomyosis in young females age 4 to 14 (Emge, 1962). Because none of these young women had yet undergone menarche, hereditary transmission was suggested as the etiologic mechanism. This theory has not been evaluated further.

Trauma. Trauma has been recognized as a possible etiologic mechanism since Zaleski's elegant rabbit experiment in 1936. In that study, vigorous curettage of one pregnant rabbit uterine horn was performed while pregnancies were allowed to continue in the opposite horn. Adenomyosis was subsequently identified only in the horn that had undergone curettage. Several investigators have anecdotally described finding adenomyosis during repeat cesarean sections, and it is well known that endometrial tissue can implant after hysterotomy (Scott et al, 1954). A retrospective study of 485 cases of adenomyosis, however, failed to demonstrate any association between previous cesarean sections and the subsequent development of adenomyosis (Harris et al, 1985).

Hyperestrogenemia. In the mid-1930s, several investigators suggested that hyperestrogenemia could initiate the development of adenomyosis. Pierson (1938) treated two castrated rabbits with 0.1 mg folliculin twice a week and noted the subsequent development of adenomyosis. More recently, Huseby and Thurlow (1982) treated hybrid mice with low-dose diethylstilbestrol. These mice exhibited elevated levels of prolactin, as determined by mammary gland morphology, and they developed protrusions of endometrium into the myometrium—a phenomenon analogous to adenomyosis in humans. It was unknown in this study whether these changes were due to hyperestrogenemia or hyperprolactinemia, but Huseby and Thurlow favored hyperprolactinemia, because they could duplicate these findings by transplanting pituitary grafts into day-old mice. It should be noted that neither of these investigations definitively ruled out pre-existing adenomyosis before estrogen administration was initiated.

In a well-designed study demonstrating synergism between estrogen and prolactin, Mori et al (1984) reported an increased incidence of adenomyosis in mice that had anterior pituitary grafts. Adenomyosis did not develop initially but did so after continuous supplementation with estrogen and progesterone. Conversely, in mice that did not receive pituitary grafts but did receive continuous steroid supplementation, adenomyosis failed to develop. Therefore, it appears that in this model estrogen and/or progesterone plus prolactin maybe required for adenomyosis to develop. In addition, it appears, in similar experiments, as though bromocriptine may be able to prevent the development of adenomyosis (Mori et al, 1991).

A more recent study has suggested that estrogen is synthesized in both eutopic and ectopic endometrial tissue in women with adenomyosis, and that this estrogen may affect the growth of adenomyosis (Yamamoto et al, 1993). In this study, myometrial aromatase and estrone sulfatase activity was significantly greater in women with adenomyosis than in controls. This appears to confirm earlier work demonstrating that aromatase activity was higher in adenomyotic tissue than in normal myometrium or endometrium (Urabe et al, 1989).

Viral Transmission. Although investigators occasionally mention viral transmission as a possible etiologic mechanism, no scientific studies have evaluated this proposed process.

Histopathology

At the time of hysterectomy, the adenomyotic uterus has usually been described as globular or boggy. It is grossly enlarged in at least 60% of cases, but rarely exceeds 12 weeks' gestation in size; most weigh between 80 and 200 g (Molitor, 1971; Bird et al, 1972). In his classical article in which he found parity to be the primary determinant of uterine weight, Langlois (1970) defined the upper limits of normal uterine weight as 130 g for nulliparous women, 210 g for parity of one to three, and 250 g for parity of four or more. With these criteria, if cases with associated leiomyomata are excluded, uterine weight is not appreciably elevated by adenomyosis.

Grossly, these uteri are usually hyperemic with thickened walls (Fig. 30–11). Although most investigators have reported that the posterior wall is more frequently involved than the anterior wall, Bird et al (1972) found adenomyotic foci to be equally distrib-

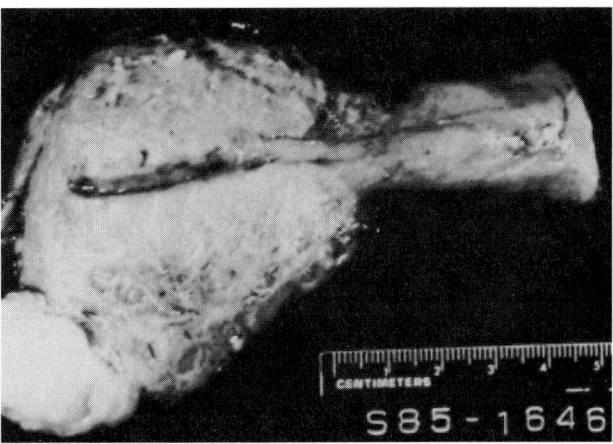

Figure 30–11
Adenomyotic uterus demonstrating asymmetric thickening of the myometrium. A leiomyoma, which frequently coexists with adenomyosis, is present at the posterior fundal aspect of the uterus. (Courtesy of Philip T. Valente, MD, Department of Pathology, University of Texas Health Science Center at San Antonio.)

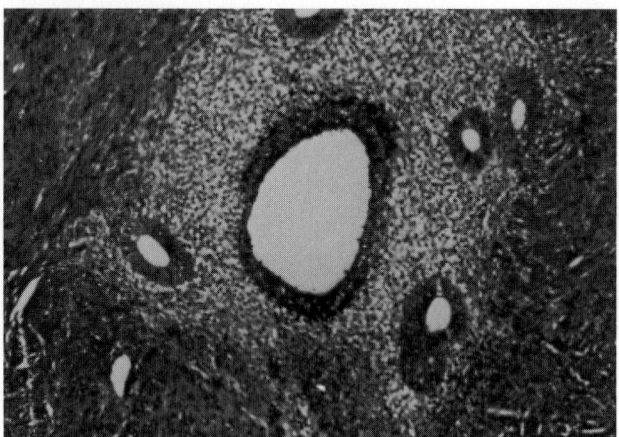

Figure 30–12
Photomicrograph depicting adenomyotic foci surrounded by hypertrophic smooth muscle cells. (Courtesy of Philip T. Valente, MD, Department of Pathology, University of Texas Health Science Center at San Antonio.)

uted when they took an additional six sections for histopathologic examination. The foci are frequently scattered diffusely throughout the myometrium but occasionally can be large and localized, forming structures called adenomyomas.

On microscopic examination, the hallmark of adenomyosis is invasion of endometrial glands and stroma into the myometrium. As noted above, the exact depth of invasion required to confirm the diagnosis remains a source of some controversy. The cells lining the adenomyotic glands resemble those of the basal endometrium. They can, however, occasionally undergo metaplasia and resemble tubal or cervical epithelium. Surrounding these glands are hypertrophic smooth muscle cells (Fig. 30–12).

Although the majority of adenomyotic glands demonstrate proliferative features, they can frequently respond to circulating hormones and can be in phase with the endometrial glands. After excluding those samples with proliferative or atrophic surface endometrium, Molitor (1971) found functional ectopic endometrium in 33% of his specimens. In addition, in his review of adenomyosis in pregnancy,

Azziz (1986) reported a 57% incidence of decidualization of adenomyotic foci.

Although it is known that adenomyotic tissue contains receptors for estrogen, progesterone, and androgens, the relative levels of these receptors are not well defined. Initially, Tamaya and associates (1979) reported finding decreased levels of estrogen and androgen receptors in 10 minced adenomyotic uteri. Progesterone receptors were absent in four of these cases and diminished in the others. These investigators also found delayed histologic dating in the adenomyotic foci and attributed this to the lower progesterone receptor levels. Subsequently, in an analysis of 319 uteri, 21 of which contained adenomyosis, estrogen receptor levels were found to be somewhat lower and progesterone receptor levels slightly higher in those uteri from patients with adenomyosis than in those from patients with no demonstrated pathology (Van der Walt et al, 1986). Obviously, more study is needed in this area.

Epidemiology

The reported incidence of adenomyosis has varied widely over the years, ranging from a low of 5.7% in 1283 uteri removed for leiomyomata to a high of 69.6% from unselected hysterectomy specimens (Table 30–7) (Cullen, 1908; Counsellor, 1938). Although some of this disparity can be explained by the use of different histologic definitions for adenomyosis, most of the variation is likely due to the degree of fervor with which pathologists pursue the diagnosis. As a result of the focal nature of this condition, the diagnosis of adenomyosis can be very difficult to make. In an excellent prospective study by Bird et al (1972), 200 consecutive hysterectomy specimens were examined histologically. When three routine sections of myometrium were examined, adenomyosis was found in 62 women. Six additional tissue blocks were then examined, three each from the anterior and posterior uterine walls, and an additional 61 cases were discovered, raising the incidence from 31% to 61.5%.

Table 30–7. INCIDENCE OF ADENOMYOSIS

STUDY	INCIDENCE (%)	COMMENTS
Cullen (1908)	5.7	1283 uteri removed for fibroids
Emge (1954)	15	1412 hysterectomy specimens
Benson and Sneeden (1958)	21.4	701 premenopausal hysterectomies
Emge (1959)	29.3	280 postmenopausal hysterectomies
Molitor (1971)	8.8	3207 hysterectomy specimens
Bird et al (1972)	31	200 consecutive hysterectomy specimens
	61.5	Same 200 cases, 6 additional histologic sections examined
Owolabi and Strickler (1977)	10	1619 hysterectomy specimens
Discepoli et al (1979)	20.6	1500 hysterectomy specimens
Thompson and Davion (1986)	15.9	702 hysterectomy specimens

Table 30-8. INCIDENCE OF ADENOMYOSIS IN HYSTERECTOMY SPECIMENS BY AGE

STUDY	NO. OF ADENOMYOTIC UTERI	PATIENT AGE					
		20-29 No. (%)	30-39 No. (%)	40-49 No. (%)	50-59 No. (%)	60-69 No. (%)	70-79 No. (%)
Emge (1962)	210	6 (2.8	48 (22.9)	99 (47.1)	48 (22.9)	8 (3.8)	1 (0.5)
Molitor (1971)	281	4 (1.4)	66 (23.5)	148 (52.7)	55 (19.6)	4 (1.4)	4 (1.4)
Bird et al (1972)	123	3 (2.4)	25 (20.4)	62 (50.4)	28 (22.7)	4 (3.3)	1 (0.8)
Thompson and Davion (1986)	112	19 (17.0)	54 (48.2)	33 (29.4)	5 (4.5)	1 (0.9)	—

A major source of difficulty in establishing the true incidence of adenomyosis lies in the fact that, although published reports may cite the number of cases of adenomyosis found in relation to patient age (Table 30-8), they uniformly fail to report the total number of hysterectomies performed in each age group. Thus the relative incidence of adenomyosis as a function of age has never been defined.

Another source of difficulty in establishing the true incidence of adenomyosis is the fact that most studies evaluate only women undergoing hysterectomies, thereby creating a selection bias. Two necropsy studies have been performed, reporting an incidence of adenomyosis in 50% and 53.7% of specimens (Lewinski, 1931; Kistner, 1964). Although these studies involve a different type of selection bias (i.e., women with hysterectomy have been excluded), they do illustrate the fact that the true incidence of adenomyosis is probably nearer the upper end of the published range.

On the surface, parity appears to correlate with adenomyosis, because up to 93% of treated patients are parous (Owolabi and Strickler, 1977; Vercillini et al, 1995). However, these figures tend to mimic those of the general population, hence their significance is called into question. If true, this would confirm an interesting paradox, because parity may be protective against endometriosis yet a risk factor for the development of adenomyosis. There does not appear to be any significant correlation between adenomyosis and race or obesity (Benson and Sneeden, 1958; Rao and Persaud, 1982). Likewise, there does not appear to be any significant predilection for adenomyosis to coexist with other specific gynecologic pathology. In a retrospective study of 134 patients undergoing hysterectomy, Vercillini et al (1995) found an essentially equal coexistence of adenomyosis with fibroids (23%), genital prolapse (26%), cervical cancer (19%), endometrial cancer (28%), ovarian cancer (28%), and ovarian cysts (21%).

Clinical Presentation

The most frequently cited profile of adenomyosis symptomatology includes the triad of abnormal uterine bleeding, secondary dysmenorrhea, and an enlarged, tender uterus. Other symptoms, such as dyspareunia and chronic pelvic pain, present less commonly (Table 30-9). Unfortunately, however, none of these symptoms (or even the triad itself) are pathognomonic for adenomyosis. Kilkku et al (1984) preoperatively assessed the symptomatology of 212 women scheduled for hysterectomy with complaints suggestive of adenomyosis or endometriosis. Because adenomyosis frequently is accompanied by other pelvic pathology, it is often difficult to attribute symptoms solely to this condition (Table 30-10). In addition, up to 35% of affected patients may be asymptomatic (Benson and Sneeden, 1958).

Abnormal uterine bleeding encompasses menorrhagia, which has been reported to affect as many as two thirds of adenomyosis patients, as well as metrorrhagia, which occurs somewhat less frequently (Emge, 1962; Molitor, 1971; Bird et al, 1972). The increased blood loss reported at the time of menstruation by these patients has been confirmed in one study (Fraser et al, 1986). Although the exact mechanisms remains unclear, the increased bleeding may result from the greater endometrial surface area found in enlarged uteri. Other postulated mecha-

Table 30-9. ADENOMYOSIS SYMPTOMATOLOGY

SYMPTOM	REPORTED INCIDENCE (%)
Menorrhagia	51-68
Metrorrhagia	11-39
Dysmenorrhea	20-46
Dyspareunia	7
Asymptomatic	3-35

Table 30-10. ASSOCIATION OF ENDOMETRIOSIS WITH OTHER GYNECOLOGIC PATHOLOGY

CONDITION	REPORTED ASSOCIATION (%)
Uterine leiomyomata	19-57
Endometrial hyperplasia	7-33
Endometriosis	0-28
Salpingitis isthmica nodosa	1-20

nisms offer a role for prostaglandins (mefenamic acid administration has been shown to reduce menstrual blood loss) or the hyperestrogenemia often noted in these patients (Fraser et al, 1986).

Dysmenorrhea is probably also related to prostaglandins, but the mechanism of dyspareunia in the absence of associated endometriosis is unknown. As with many other conditions, it appears that the severity of symptoms is associated with the extent of disease (Benson and Sneeden, 1958).

Because these symptoms are so nonspecific, it is not surprising that adenomyosis is seldom correctly diagnosed preoperatively Most investigators have reported a correct preoperative diagnosis in fewer than 10% of cases (Israel and Woutersz, 1959; Marcus, 1961; Owolabi and Stricker, 1977; Thompson and Darion, 1986). However, owing to selection bias, incomplete pathologic examination of surgical specimens, and a limited number of well-designed studies, our true ability to diagnose adenomyosis prospectively is impossible to ascertain.

Adjunctive Diagnostic Testing

Radiologic

Hysterosalpingography. Numerous investigators have explored the use of various radiologic modalities to aid in the prospective diagnosis of adenomyosis. In the largest study of hysterosalpingography (HSG) to date, Marshak and Eliasoph (1955) were able to diagnose adenomyosis correctly in only 38 of 150 patients with "proven" adenomyosis. They did not note either the total number of patients examined or the incidence of false-positive diagnosis. The most commonly described findings on HSG include endometrial diverticuli and honeycomb defects protruding into the myometrium (Siegler, 1974; Wolf and Spataro, 1988). This test is fraught with inaccuracy, however, because the myometrial spiculations frequently ascribed to adenomyosis resemble those of lymphatic or vascular dye intravasation.

Ultrasonography. Unfortunately, abdominal ultrasonography has failed to demonstrate utility as a diagnostic tool. In the late 1970s, one group proposed 5- to 7-mm irregular myometrial sonolucencies as an ultrasonographic finding characteristic of generalized adenomyosis (Walsh et al, 1979). This was subsequently disputed by Siedler et al (1987), who noted generalized uterine enlargement, normal myometrial echogenicity, and preservation of uterine contour in the majority of their patients with documented adenomyosis. Several more recent studies have failed to clarify this issue.

Transvaginal ultrasonography has only been evaluated as a diagnostic modality since the early 1990s. Fedele (1992) evaluated 43 women undergoing hysterectomy for menorrhagia with preoperative transvaginal ultrasound. He described numerous small myometrial anechoic areas with irregular hyperech-

ogenic outlines in 22 women. The sensitivity of this technique was reported to be 80% with a specificity of 74%. Other investigators have reported lower sensitivities of 48% (Ascher et al, 1994) and 53% (Wood et al, 1993). Further studies are certainly needed in this area as transvaginal ultrasonography assumes an even greater role in algorithms for gynecologic therapies.

Magnetic Resonance Imaging. MRI has been applied to pelvic pathology, and preliminary results in adenomyosis patients are encouraging (Lee et al, 1985; Mark et al, 1987). Mark et al correctly predicted adenomyosis in 8 of 20 patients studied using T_2-weighted images. Ten of the remaining 12 patients were correctly predicted not to have adenomyosis; in the other 2, radiologic diagnosis was uncertain. The investigators described a unique-appearing, wide low-signal-intensity band surrounding the normal high-signal-intensity endometrium in patients with diffuse adenomyosis. Microscopic adenomyotic foci, however, were not demonstrated. T_2-weighted imaging appears to offer significant advantages over either unenhanced or contrast-enhanced T_1-weighted imaging. MRI has also been evaluated as a technique for differentiating adenomyosis from leiomyomata (Togashi et al, 1989). Ninety-three patients were evaluated preoperatively, and the results were correlated with surgical pathology. All 16 cases of adenomyosis were correctly diagnosed preoperatively. More widespread application of this new technology, however, must await further study. In addition, cost may prohibit development of MRI as a widespread screening test.

Serum Markers

CA-125 is an antigen produced by ovarian epithelial cells. It is secreted into the blood, and its use has been advocated in a variety of gynecologic conditions. Although some have used it to predict recurrences of nonmucinous ovarian carcinomas, others have attempted to assess nonoperatively the status of recurrent endometriosis by determining serial CA-125 levels. In 1985, Takahasi et al reported elevated preoperative serum levels of CA-125 in six of seven study patients. Although elevated, these levels were significantly lower than those commonly found in patients with ovarian carcinomas. One month following hysterectomy, all patients had normal levels of CA-125. Using immunohistochemistry, these same investigators localized the CA-125 antigen to glandular epithelium present in the adenomyotic foci of eight hysterectomy specimens (Kijima et al, 1987). Another study, however, failed to reproduce these findings (Halila et al, 1987). In their report of 22 women, 11 of whom had adenomyosis, Halila and associates noted normal preoperative CA-125 levels in all adenomyosis patients. These levels did not significantly change when tests were repeated 1 and 5 weeks postoperatively. The reason for the discrepancy in these studies is not readily apparent, but it is hoped that further work will be conducted in this area.

Serum cystine aminopeptidase and leucine aminopeptidase levels have also been used as potential markers for adenomyosis. Levels of these enzymes have been reported to be elevated in several benign and malignant conditions involving the uterus and ovary (Blum and Sirote, 1977). No controlled trials have been performed to evaluate the clinical utility of these measurements.

Histopathology

As with endometriosis, histopathologic confirmation remains the gold standard in the diagnosis of adenomyosis. To this end, and in the hope of avoiding hysterectomy, two alternative tissue sampling techniques have been proposed. Popp et al (1993) described Tru-cut myometrial biopsies in 40 women performed under either laparoscopic or ultrasonographic guidance. There were no false-positive diagnosis or complications, and the sensitivity of the technique ranged from 40% to 70%, depending on the number of specimens obtained. Brosens and Barker (1995) performed myometrial needle biopsies on 40 hysterectomy specimens from 27 women with adenomyosis and 13 women without adenomyosis. They compared the histologic findings from 8 biopsies per uterus with myometrial block specimens from the same uteri, and were able to confirm adenomyosis in 12 of 27 positive specimens (sensitivity, 44%). The accuracy of the technique was dependent on the depth of glandular invasion into the myometrium, and the authors concluded that at least four biopsy specimens would have to be obtained in order to reliably diagnose adenomyosis that had invaded at least one third of the way into the myometrium. Regardless of the number of biopsy specimens obtained (up to eight), the sensitivity of diagnosing superficial adenomyosis never exceeded 9% (Brosens and Barker, 1995). Based on these findings, they concluded that this procedure should only be contemplated in a select population of prescreened patients.

McCausland (1992) described a hysteroscopic sampling technique involving removal of a 5-mm deep strip of myometrium from the posterior fundus using 70W cutting current delivered through a loop electrode. He evaluated 90 patients complaining of menorrhagia, 50 of whom had hysteroscopically normal endometrial cavities. Of those 50, 33 had significant adenomyosis, believed to be the likely etiology of their abnormal bleeding. Using a subjective scale to asses menorrhagia, McCausland concluded that the depth of invasion of the adenomyosis correlated significantly with the degree of menorrhagia.

Adenomyosis in Pregnancy

On the basis of the only large study of adenomyosis in pregnancy, an analysis of 151 uteri obtained at cesarean hysterectomy, it appears that the incidence of this condition is 17.2% (Sandberg and Cohn, 1962). Although 50 years ago it was suggested that adenomyosis in pregnancy markedly increased the risk of obstetric complications—specifically, postpartum hemorrhage, uterine atony, and uterine rupture—that has not proved to be the case (Haydon, 1942). In his excellent review of this subject, Azziz (1986) noted only 29 cases of complications in more than 80 years' worth of literature, a surprisingly low figure in light of the incidence of this entity.

Associated Gynecologic Pathology

Adenomyosis rarely occurs as an isolated finding (Table 30–10). Up to 80% of adenomyotic uteri are associated with such condition as leiomyomata, endometrial hyperplasia, peritoneal endometriosis, and uterine cancer. The fact that all of these entities, except endometriosis, are associated with prolonged estrogen exposure has been frequently cited as evidence that adenomyosis results from hyperestrogenemia. Adenomyosis occurs most frequently in association with leiomyomata (up to 57% of the time), and the similarity of symptomatology in these two conditions serves to make accurate preoperative diagnosis very difficult (Benson and Sneeden, 1958). Despite their obvious similarities, adenomyosis and pelvic endometriosis coexist in only 28% of women or less (Israel and Woutersz, 1959; Emge, 1962; Mathur et al, 1962; Moliter, 1971; Bird et al, 1972).

Salpingitis isthmica nodosum, an inflammatory process of uncertain etiology affecting the proximal fallopian tube, also occurs in association with adenomyosis. Its observed coexistent frequency was 1.4% in one study and 19.8% in another (Benson and Sneeden, 1958; Molitor, 1971). Abnormalities of the endometrial lining ranging from hyperplasia to adenocarcinoma are frequently associated with adenomyosis. The reported incidence of coexistent hyperplasia also demonstrated hyperplasia in the adenomyotic foci (Molitor, 1971). The vast majority of these cases have demonstrated simple endometrial hyperplasia (Fig. 30–13); however, atypical hyperplasia can occur. Molitor (1971) reported an incidence of 3.5% for atypical hyperplasia in an analysis of 281 adenomyotic uteri.

Adenomyosis frequently occurs in association with endometrial adenocarcinoma. In one study, 60% of 100 patients with adenocarcinoma also had adenomyosis (Marcus, 1961). Other reported incidences are much lower, at 10% to 33% (Hernandez and Woodruff, 1980). In addition to arising within the same uterus as adenomyosis, adenocarcinoma may arise from within adenomyotic foci. It appears as though the coexistence of adenomyosis does not have an impact upon the prognosis for patients with endometrial adenocarcinoma (Hall et al, 1984). Isolated reports have described other types of uterine cancer that have been reported in association with

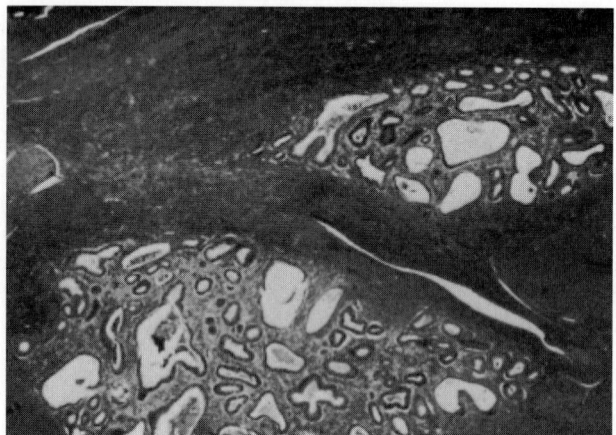

Figure 30-13
Photomicrograph of adenomyotic foci demonstrating cystic hyperplasia. (Courtesy of Philip T. Valente, MD, Department of Pathology, University of Texas Health Science Center at San Antonio.)

adenomyosis. Specifically, müllerian adenosarcoma, endometrial stromal sarcoma, and leiomyosarcoma, all of which were believed to have developed within adenomyotic foci, have been reported (Gisser and Toker, 1978; Oda et al, 1984). Although no one has specifically reported on the incidence of adenocarcinoma within adenomyotic uteri, it is thought to be relatively rare.

Treatment

The mainstay of both the diagnosis and treatment of adenomyosis remains hysterectomy. Until a safe and consistently effective method exists for directed myometrial biopsy, one will be able to diagnose adenomyosis accurately only by surgical removal of the uterus, thus effectively treating this condition simultaneously.

Concerning medical management, in the mouse model, bromocriptine has a suppressive effect upon adenomyosis (Nagasawa and Mori, 1982). Conversely, prolactin, progesterone, and possibly even growth hormone appear to accelerate the development of the disease (Nagasawa et al, 1985, 1987). RU 486, an antiprogestational agent that inhibits the effects of progesterone at uterine receptor sites, has been shown to suppress the development of adenomyosis markedly when given for up to 30 days. This finding may have some implication for future human studies (Nagasawa et al, 1989).

Anecdotal evidence exists that progesterone may exacerbate the development of adenomyosis in humans as in mice (Falk and Mullin, 1989). Danazol, an antigonadotropic derivative of 17α-ethinyl testosterone used effectively in the treatment of endometriosis, has not been extensively studied in this condition. Several small studies, however, have failed to demonstrate any benefit of treatment for 6 months

with a daily dose of either 400 or 800 mg (Lauersen et al, 1975; Ingerslev, 1977). GnRH analogs may have a potential application in treatment, but, to date, only isolated case reports have been published to evaluate this possibility.

REFERENCES

Acosta AA, Buttram VC Jr, Besch PK, et al: A proposed classification of pelvic endometriosis. Obstet Gynecol 1973;42:19.

Adamson GD, Frison L, Lamb EJ: Endometriosis: studies of a method for the design of a surgical staging system. Fertil Steril 1982;38:659.

Adamson GD, Pasta DJ: Surgical treatment of endometriosis-associated infertility: meta-analysis compared with survival analysis. Am J Obstet Gynecol 1994;171:1488.

Adhesion Study Group: Reduction in postoperative pelvic adhesions with intraperitoneal 32% dextran 70: a prospective, randomized clinical trial. Fertil Steril 1983;40:612.

American Fertility Society: Classification of endometriosis. Fertil Steril 1979;32:633.

American Fertility Society: Revised American Fertility Society classification of endometriosis: 1985. Fertil Steril 1985;43:351.

Arici A, Attar E, Tazuke S, et al: Monocyte chemotactic protein-1 (MCP-1) in human peritoneal fluid and modulation of MCP-1 expression in human mesothelial cells. In: Proceedings of the 51st Annual Meeting of the American Society of Reproductive Medicine, Seattle, 1995:S80.

Arici A, Tazuke SI, Attar E, et al: Interleukin-8 concentration in peritoneal fluid of patients with endometriosis and modulation of interleukin-8 expression in human mesothelial cells. Mol Hum Reprod 1996;2:404.

Arrive L, Hricak H, Martin MC: Pelvic endometriosis: MR imaging. Radiology 1989;171:687.

Ascher SM, Arnold LL, Patt RH, et al: Adenomyosis: prospective comparison of MR imaging and transvaginal sonography. Radiology 1994;190:803.

Ayers JWT, Friedenstab AP: Utero-tubal hypotonia associated with pelvic endometriosis. In: Abstracts of the Scientific and Poster Sessions, 41st Annual Meeting of American Fertility Society, Birmingham, 1985:131.

Azadian-Boulanger G, Secchi J, Tournemine C, Sakiz E: Hormonal activity profiles of drugs for endometriosis therapy. In Raynaud JP, Ojasco T, Martini L (eds): Medical Management of Endometriosis. New York: Raven Press, 1984:125.

Azziz R: Adenomyosis in pregnancy: a review. J Reprod Med 1986;31:224.

Barbieri RL, Canich JA, Makris A, Todd RB: Danazol inhibits steroidogenesis. Fertil Steril 1977;28:809.

Barbieri RL, Evans S, Kistner RW: Danazol in the treatment of endometriosis: analysis of 100 cases with a 4 year follow-up. Fertil Steril 1982;37:737.

Barbieri RL, Niloff JM, Bast RC Jr, et al: Elevated serum concentrations of CA-125 in patients with advanced endometriosis. Fertil Steril 1986;45:630.

Bartosik D, Jacobs S, Kelly IJ: Endometrial tissue in peritoneal fluid. Fertil Steril 1986;46:796.

Bayer SR, Seibel MM: Medical treatment: danazol. In Schenken RS (ed): Endometriosis: Contemporary Concepts in Clinical Management. Philadelphia: JB Lippincott Company, 1989:169.

Bayer SR, Seibel MM, Saffan DS, Berger MJ: The efficacy of danazol treatment for minimal endometriosis in an infertile population: a prospective, randomized study. J Reprod Med 1988;33:179.

Beecham CT: Classification of endometriosis. Obstet Gynecol 1966;28:437.

Benson RC, Sneeden VD: Adenomyosis: a reappraisal of symptomatology. Am J Obstet Gynecol 1958;76:1044.

Bergquist A, Rannevik G, Thorell J: Estrogen and progesterone cytosol receptor concentration in endometriotic tissue and intrauterine endometrium. Acta Obstet Gynecol Scand Suppl 1981;101:53.

Beyth Y, Yaffe H, Levij S, Sadovsky E: Retrograde seeding of endometrium: a sequela of tubal flushing. Fertil Steril 1975;26: 1094.

Bird CC, McElin TW, Mandalo-Estrella P: The elusive adenomyosis of the uterus—revisited. Am J Obstet Gynecol 1972; 112:583.

Blum M, Sirote P: Serum cystine aminopeptidase and leucine aminopeptidase activity in women with benign and malignant uterine and ovarian tumors. Isr J Med Sci 1977;13:875.

Blumenkrantz MJ, Gallagher N, Bashore RA, Tenckhoff H: Retrograde menstruation in women undergoing chronic peritoneal dialysis. Obstet Gynecol 1981;57:667.

Brosens J, Barker F: The role of myometrial needle biopsies in the diagnosis of adenomyosis. Fertil Steril 1995;63:1347.

Buttram VC, Belue JB, Reiter R: Interim report of a study of danazol for the treatment of endometriosis. Fertil Steril 1982;37: 478.

Buttram VC Jr: An expanded classification of endometriosis. Fertil Steril 1978;30:240.

Buttram VC Jr, Reiter RC, Ward S: Treatment of endometriosis with danazol: report of a six-year prospective study. Fertil Steril 1985;43:353.

Candiani GB, Danesino V, Gastaldi A, et al: Reproductive and menstrual factors and risk of peritoneal and ovarian endometriosis. Fertil Steril 1991;56:230.

Candiani GB, Fedele L, Vercellini P, et al: Presacral neurectomy for the treatment of pelvic pain associated with endometriosis: a controlled study. Am J Obstet Gynecol 1992;167:100.

Chamness GC, Asch RH, Pauerstein CJ: Danazol binding and translocation of steroid receptors. Am J Obstet Gynecol 1980; 136:426.

Chatman DL: Endometriosis in black women. Am J Obstet Gynecol 1976;125:987.

Chatman DL, Ward AB: Endometriosis in adolescents. J Reprod Med 1982;27:156.

Chauhan M, Barratt C, Cooke S, Cooke I: Differences in the fertility of donor insemination recipients—a study to provide prognostic guidelines as to its success and outcome. Fertil Steril 1989;51:815.

Chiari H: Zur pathologischen anatomie des eileiter-catarrhs. Ztschr Heik 1887;8:457.

Chong AP, Keene ME, Thornton NL: Comparison of three modes of treatment for infertility patients with minimal pelvic endometriosis. Fertil Steril 1990;53:407.

Cohen MR: Laparoscopy and the management of endometriosis. J Reprod Med 1979;23:81.

Cooke ID, Thomas EJ: The medical treatment of mild endometriosis. Acta Obstet Gynecol Scand Suppl 1989;150:27.

Cornillie FJ, Brosens IA, Vasquez G, Riphagen I: Histologic and ultrastructural changes in human endometriotic implants treated with the antiprogesterone steroid ethylnorgestrienone (gestrinone) during 2 months. Int J Gynecol Pathol 1986;5:95.

Cornillie FJ, Oosterlynck D, Lauweryns J, et al: Deeply infiltrating pelvic endometriosis: histology and clinical significance. Fertil Steril 1990;53:978.

Counseller VS: Endometriosis: a clinical and surgical review. Am J Obstet Gynecol 1938;36:877.

Coutinho EM, Husson JM, Azadian-Boulanger G: Treatment of endometriosis with gestrinone—five years' experience. In Raynaud J-P, Ojasoo T, Martini L (eds): Medical Management of Endometriosis. New York: Raven Press, 1984:249.

Cramer DW, Wilson E, Stillman RJ, et al: The relation of endometriosis to menstrual characteristics, smoking and exercise. JAMA 1986;255:1904.

Cullen TS: Adeno-myoma of the round ligament. Bull Johns Hopkins Hosp 1896;7:112.

Cullen TS: Adenomyoma of the Uterus. Philadelphia: WB Saunders Company, 1908.

deQuervain FJ: Clinical Surgical Diagnosis for Students and Practioners. 5th ed. New York: William Wood and Co, 1971.

D'Hooghe TM, Bambra CS, Raeymaekers BM, Koninckx PR: Serial laparoscopies over 30 months show that endometriosis in captive baboons (Papio anubis, Papio cynocephalus) is a progressive disease. Fertil Steril 1996;65:645.

D'Hooghe TM, Bambra CS, Suleman MA, et al: Development of a model of retrograde menstruation in baboons (Papio anubis). Fertil Steril 1994;62:635.

Diamond MP, Daniell JF, Martin DC, Fest J: Tubal patency and pelvic adhesions at early second-look laparoscopy following intra-abdominal use of the carbon dioxide laser: initial report of the intra-abdominal laser study group. Fertil Steril 1984;42: 709.

Dickey RP, Taylor SN, Curole DN: Serum estradiol and danazol. I. Endometriosis response, side-effects, administration interval, concurrent spironolactone and dexamethasone. Fertil Steril 1984; 42:709.

Diesterweg A: Ein Fall von Cystofibroma uteri verum. Ztschr Geburtsh Gynakol 1883;9:191.

Discepoli S, Leocata P, Giangregorio F: Adenomyosis: histological remarks about 1500 hysterectomies. Boll Soc Ital Biol Sper 1980; 56:1560.

DiZerega GS, Barber GL, Hodgen GE: Endometriosis: role of ovarian steroids in initiation, maintenance, and suppression. Fertil Steril 1980;33:649.

Djursing H, Peterson K, Weberg E: Symptomatic postmenopausal endometriosis. Acta Obstet Gynecol Scand 1981;60:529.

Dmowski WP, Cohen MR: Treatment of endometriosis with an antigonadotropin, danazol: a laparoscopic and histologic evaluation. Obstet Gynecol 1975;46:147.

Dmowski WP, Steele RW, Baker GF: Deficient cellular immunity in endometriosis. Am J Obstet Gynecol 1981;141:377.

Döberl A, Bergqvist A, Jeppsson S, Koskimies AL: Regression of endometriosis following shorter treatment with, or lower doses of, danazol. Acta Obstet Gynecol Scand 1984;123:51.

Dodson WC, Haney AF: Controlled ovarian hyperstimulation and intrauterine insemination for treatment of infertility. Fertil Steril 1991;55:457.

Dunphy BC, Kay R, Barratt CL, Cooke ID: Female age, the length of involuntary infertility prior to investigation and fertility outcome. Hum Reprod 1989;4:527.

Eisermann J, et al: Tumor necrosis factor in peritoneal fluid of women undergoing laparoscopic surgery. Fertil Steril 1988;50: 573.

Emge LA: The elusive adenomyosis of the uterus: its historical past and its present state of recognition. Am J Obstet Gynecol 1962;83:1541.

Fahraeus L, Larson-Cohn U, Ljungberg S, Wallentin L: Profound alterations of the lipoprotein metabolism during danazol treatment in premenopausal women. Fertil Steril 1984;42:52.

Fahraeus L, Sydsjo A, Wallentin L: Lipoprotein changes during treatment of pelvic endometriosis with medroxyprogesterone acetate. Fertil Steril 1986;45:503.

Falk R, Mullin B: Exacerbation of adenomyosis symptomatology by estrogen-progestin therapy: a case report and histopathological observations. Int J Fertil 1989; 34:386.

Fedele L: Transvaginal ultrasonography in the diagnosis of diffuse adenomyosis. Fertil Steril 1992;58:94.

Fedele L, Bianchi S, Arcaini L, et al: Buserelin versus danazol in the treatment of endometriosis-associated infertility. Am J Obstet Gynecol 1989a;161:871.

Fedele L, Bianchi S, Marchini M, et al: Superovulation with human menopausal gonadotropins in the treatment of infertility associated with minimal or mild endometriosis: a controlled randomized study. Fertil Steril 1992;58:28.

Fedele L, Bianchi S, Viezzoli T, et al: Gestrinone vs danazol in the treatment of endometriosis. Fertil Steril 1989b;51:781.

Ferenczy A: Studies on the cytodynamics of human endometrial regeneration. I. Scanning electron microscopy. Am J Obstet Gynecol 1976a;124:64.

Ferenczy A: Studies on the cytodynamics of human endometrial regeneration. II. Transmission electron microscopy and histochemistry. Am J Obstet Gynecol 1976b;124:582.

Filatow D: Uber die Bildung des Anfangsstadiums bei der Extremitatenetwicklung. Roux Arch EntwMech Organ 1933;127: 776.

Floyd WS: Danazol: endocrine and endometrial effects. Int J Fertil 1980;25:75.

Fraser IS, McCarron G, Markham R, et al: Measured menstrual blood loss in women with menorrhagia associated with pelvic disease or coagulation disorder. Obstet Gynecol 1986;69:630.

Friedman AJ, Hornstein MD: Gonadotropin-releasing hormone agonist plus estrogen-progesterone "add-back" therapy for endometriosis-related pelvic pain. Fertil Steril 1993;60:236.

Friedman H, Vogelzang RL, Mendelson EF, et al: Endometriosis detection by US with laparoscopic correlation. Radiology 1985; 157:217.

Geber S, Paraschos T, Atkinson G, et al: Results of IVF in patients with endometriosis: the severity of the disease does not affect outcome, or the incidence of miscarriage. Hum Reprod 1995; 10:1507.

Geist SH: The viability of fragments of menstrual endometrium. Am J Obstet Gynecol 1933;25:751.

Gisser SD, Toker C: Endometrial stromal sarcoma and leiomyosarcoma arising in adenomyosis: a possible presentation of occult extra-genital malignancy. Mt Sinai J Med 1978;45:218.

Gleicher N, Karande V, Rabin D, et al: The bubble test: a new tool to improve the diagnosis of endometriosis. Hum Reprod 1995;10:923.

Goebel R, Rjosk HK: Laboratory and clinical studies with the new antigonadotropin, danazol. Acta Endocrinol 1977;85:134.

Goldstein DP, deCholnoky C, Emans SJ, Leventhal JM: Laparoscopy in the diagnosis and management of pelvic pain in adolescents. J Reprod Med 1980;24:251.

Goodall JR: A Study of Endometriosis, Endosalpingiosis, and Peritoneo-ovarian Sclerosis: A Clinical and Pathological Study. Philadelphia: JB Lippincott Company, 1943.

Gordts S, Boeckx W, Bronsens I: Microsurgery in endometriosis in fertile patients. Fertil Steril 1984;42:520.

Guerriero S, Mais V, Ajossa S, et al: Transvaginal ultrasonography combined with CA-125 plasma levels in the diagnosis of endometrioma. Fertil Steril 1996;65:293.

Guzick DS, Rock JA: A comparison of danazol and conservative surgery for the treatment of infertility due to mild or moderate endometriosis. Fertil Steril 1983;40:580.

Ha HK, Lim YT, Kim HS, et al: Diagnosis of pelvic endometriosis: fat-suppressed T1-weighted vs conventional MR images. Am J Radiol 1994;163:127.

Haber GM, Behelak YF: Preliminary report on the use of tamoxifen in the treatment of endometriosis. Am J Obstet Gynecol 1987;156:582.

Halban J: Hysteroadenosis metastatica: die lymphogene genese der sogenannten Adenofibromatosis heterotopica. Arch Gynaekol 1925;124:457.

Halila H, Suikkari AM, Seppala M: The effect of hysterectomy on serum CA-125 levels in patients with adenomyosis and uterine fibroids. Hum Reprod 1987;2:265.

Hall JB, Young RH, Nelson JH: The prognostic significance of adenomyosis in endometrial carcinoma. Gynecol Oncol 1984; 17:32.

Halme J: Release of tumor necrosis factor by human peritoneal macrophages in vivo and in vitro. Am J Obstet Gynecol 1989; 161:1718.

Halme J, Becker S, Hammond MG, Raj S: Pelvic macrophages in normal and infertile women: the role of patent tubes. Am J Obstet Gynecol 1982;142:890.

Halme J, Becker S, Hammond M, et al: Increased activation of pelvic macrophages in infertile women with mild endometriosis. Am J Obstet Gynecol 1983a;145:333.

Halme J, Becker S, Wing R: Accentuated cyclic activation of peritoneal macrophages in patients with endometriosis. Am J Obstet Gynecol 1983b;148:85.

Halme J, Hammond MG, Hulka JF, et al: Retrograde menstruation in healthy women and in patients with endometriosis. Obstet Gynecol 1984;64:151.

Halme J, White C, Kauma S, et al: Peritoneal macrophages from patients with endometriosis release growth factor activity in vitro. J Clin Endocrinol Metab 1988;66:1044.

Hanton EM, Malkasian GD Jr, Dockerty MB, Pratt JH: Endometriosis in young women. Am J Obstet Gynecol 1967;98:116.

Harris WJ, Daniell JF, Baxter JW: Prior cesarean section: a risk factor for adenomyosis? J Reprod Med 1985;30:173.

Haydon GB: A study of 569 cases of endometriosis. Am J Obstet Gynecol 1942;43:704.

Henzl MR, Corson SL, Moghissi K, et al: Administration of nasal nafarelin as compared with oral danazol for endometriosis. N Engl J Med 1988;318:485.

Hernandez E, Woodruff JD: Endometrial adenocarcinoma arising in adenomyosis. Am J Obstet Gynecol 1980;138:827.

Hill JA, Faris HM, Schiff I, Anderson DJ: Characterization of leukocyte subpopulations in the peritoneal fluid of women with endometriosis. Fertil Steril 1988;50:216.

Hill JA: Immunologic factors in endometriosis and endometriosis-associated reproductive failure. Infertil Reprod Med Clin North Am 1992;3:583.

Hill JA, Haimovici F, Anderson DJ: Products of activated lymphocytes and macrophages inhibit mouse embryo development in vitro. J Immunol 1987;139:2250.

Hornstein MD, Gleason RE, Orav J, et al: The reproducibility of the revised American Fertility Society classification of endometriosis. Fertil Steril 1993;59:1015.

Hornstein MD, Harlow BL, Thomas PP, Check JH: Use of a new CA-125 assay in the diagnosis of endometriosis. Hum Reprod 1995;10:932.

Huffman JW: External endometriosis. Am J Obstet Gynecol 1951; 62:1243.

Huffman JW: Endometriosis in young teen-age girls. Pediatr Ann 1981;10:44.

Hughes EG, Fedorkow DM, Collins JA: A quantitative overview of controlled trials in endometriosis-associated infertility. Fertil Steril 1993;59:963.

Hull ME, Moghissi KS, Magyar DF, Hayes MF: Comparison of different treatment modalities of endometriosis in infertile women. Fertil Steril 1987;47:40.

Huseby RA, Thurlow S: Effects of prenatal exposure of mice to "low dose" diethylstilbesterol and the development of adenomyosis associated with evidence of hyperprolactinemia. Am J Obstet Gynecol 1982;144:939.

Ingerslev M: Danazol: an antigonadotrophic agent in the treatment of recurrent pelvic and intestinal endometriosis. Acta Obstet Gynecol Scand 1977;56:343.

Ingersol FM: Selection of medical or surgical treatment of endometriosis. Clin Obstet Gynecol 1977;20:849.

Israel SL, Woutersz TB: Adenomyosis: a neglected diagnosis. Obstet Gynecol 1959;14:168.

Jansen RPS: Minimal endometriosis and reduced fecundability: prospective evidence from an artificial insemination by donor program. Fertil Steril 1986;46:141.

Jansen RPS, Russell P: Nonpigmented endometriosis: clinical, laparoscopic, and pathologic definition. Am J Obstet Gynecol 1986;155:1154.

Javert CT: Pathogenesis of endometriosis based on endometrial homeoplasia, direct extension, exfoliation, and implantation, lymphatic and hematogenous metastasis. Cancer 1949;2:399.

Javert CT: The spread of benign and malignant endometrium into the lymphatic system with a note of coexisting vascular involvement. Am J Obstet Gynecol 1952;64:780.

Jelley RY, Magill PJ: The effect of LHRH agonist therapy in the treatment of endometriosis (English experience). Prog Clin Biol Res 1986;225:227.

Jenkins S, Olive DL, Haney AF: Endometriosis: pathogenetic implications of the anatomic distribution. Obstet Gynecol 1986;67: 335.

Jenks JE, Artmant LE, Haoskins WJ, Miremardi AK: Endometriosis with ascites. Obstet Gynecol 1984;63:755.

Johnston WI: Dydrogesterone and endometriosis. Br J Obstet Gynaecol 1976;83:77.

Kaplan CR, Schenken RS: Combination medical and surgical treatment. In Schenken RS (ed): Endometriosis: Contemporary Concepts in Medical Management. Philadelphia: JB Lippincott Company, 1989:279.

Karnaky KJ: The use of stilbestrol for endometriosis. South Med J 1948;41:1109.

Katayama KP, Manuel M, Jones HW Jr, Jones GS: Methyltestosterone treatment of infertility associated with pelvic endometriosis. Fertil Steril 1976;27:83.

Kauppila A, Puolakka J, Ylikorkala O: Prostaglandin biosynthesis inhibitors and endometriosis. Prostaglandins 1979;18:655.

Kauppila A, Ronnberg L: Naproxen sodium in dysmenorrhea secondary to endometriosis. Obstet Gynecol 1985;65:379.

Kauppila A, Telimaa S, Ronnberg L, Vucri J: Placebo-controlled study on serum concentrations of CA-125 before and after treatment of endometriosis with danazol or high-dose medroxyprogesterone acetate alone or after surgery. Fertil Steril 1988;49:37.

Keettel WC, Stein RJ: The viability of the cast-off menstrual endometrium. Am J Obstet Gynecol 1951;61:440.

Kempers RD, Dockerty MB, Hunt AB: Significant postmenopausal endometriosis. Surg Gynecol Obstet 1960;111:348.

Kettel LM, Murphy AA, Morales AJ, et al: Treatment of endometriosis with the antiprogesterone mifepristone (RU 486). Fertil Steril 1996;65:23.

Kettel LM, Murphy AA, Mortola JF, et al: Endocrine responses to long-term administration of the antiprogesterone RU 486 in patients with pelvic endometriosis. Fertil Steril 1991;56:402.

Kijima S, Takahashi K, Kitao M: Expression of CA-125 in adenomyosis. Gynecol Obstet Invest 1987;23:122.

Kilkku P, Erkkola R, Gronroos M: Nonspecificity of symptoms related to adenomyosis: a prospective comparative study. Acta Obstet Gynecol Scand 1984;63:229.

Kirshon B, Poindexter AN, Fast J: Endometriosis in multiparous women. J Reprod Med 1989;34:215.

Kistner RW: Principles and Practice of Gynecology. Chicago: Year Book Medical Publishers, 1964.

Kistner RW, Siegler AM, Behrman SJ: Suggested classification for endometriosis: relationship to infertility. Fertil Steril 1977;28:1008.

Koninckx PR: Pelvic endometriosis: a consequence of stress? Contrib Gynecol Obstet 1987;16:56.

Koninckx PR, Meuleman C, Demeyere S, et al: Suggestive evidence that pelvic endometriosis is a progressive disease, whereas deeply infiltrating endometriosis is associated with pelvic pain. Fertil Steril 1991;55:759.

Koninckx PR, Meuleman C, Oosterlynck D, Cornillie FJ: Diagnosis of deep endometriosis by clinical examination during menstruation and plasma CA-125 concentration. Fertil Steril 1996;65:280.

Koninckx PR, Riittinen L, Seppala M, Cornillie FJ: CA-125 and placental protein 14 concentrations in plasma and peritoneal fluid of women with deeply infiltrating pelvic endometriosis. Fertil Steril 1992;57:523.

Langlois PL: The size of the normal uterus. J Reprod Med 1970;28:1008.

Lauersen NH, Wilson KH, Birnbaum S: Danazol: an antigonadotrophic agent in the treatment of pelvic endometriosis. Am J Obstet Gynecol 1975;123:742.

Lavender G, Normal P: The pathogenesis of endometriosis: an experimental study. Acta Obstet Gynecol Scand 1955;34:366.

Lee JKT, Gersell DJ, Balfe DM, et al: The uterus in vitro MR-anatomic correlation of normal and abnormal specimens. Radiology 1985;157:175.

Lemay A, Maheux R, Faure N, Jean C: Reversible pseudomenopause induced by repetitive luteinizing hormone-releasing hormone agonist administration (Buserelin): a new approach to the treatment of endometriosis. In Raynaud J-P, Ojasoo T, Martini L (eds): Medical Management of Endometriosis. New York: Raven Press, 1984;:263.

Lewinski H: Bietrag zur Frage der Adenomyosis. Zentralbl Gynak 1931;55:2163.

Lichten EM, Bombard J: Surgical treatment of primary dysmenorrhea with laparoscopic uterine nerve ablation. J Reprod Med 1987;32:37.

Liu DTY, Hitchcock A: Endometriosis: its association with retrograde menstruation, dysmenorrhea, and tubal pathology. Br J Obstet Gynecol 1986;93:859.

Lloyd FP: Endometriosis in the Negro women. Am J Obstet Gynecol 1964;89:468.

Lox CD, Word L, Heine MW, Markwald R: Ultrastructural circulation of endometriosis. Fertil Steril 1984;41:755.

Mahmood TA, Templeton A: The impact of treatment on the natural history of endometriosis. Hum Reprod 1990;5:965.

Malinak LR, Buttram VC Jr, Elias S: Heritage aspects of endometriosis. II. Clinical characteristics of familial endometriosis. Am J Obstet Gynecol 1980;137:332.

Malkasian GD Jr, Podratz KC, Stanhope CR, et al: CA-125 in gynecologic practice. Am J Obstet Gynecol 1986;155:515.

Marcus CC: Relationship of adenomyosis uteri to endometrial hyperplasia and endometrial carcinoma. Am J Obstet Gynecol 1961;82:408.

Mark AS, Hricak IT, Heinrichs LW, et al: Adenomyosis and leiomyoma: differential diagnosis with MR imaging. Radiology 1987;163:527.

Marshak RH, Eliasoph J: The roentgen findings in adenomyosis. Radiology 1955;64:846.

Martin DC, Hubert GD, Zwaag RV, El-Aeky FA: Laparoscopic appearances of peritoneal endometriosis. Fertil Steril 1989;51:63.

Martin DC, Zwaag RV: Excisional techniques for endometriosis with the CO2 laser laparoscope. J Reprod Med 1987;32:753.

Mathur BBL, Shah BS, Bhende YM: Adenomyosis uteri: a pathologic study of 290 cases. Am J Obstet Gynecol 1962;84:1820.

Maximow A: Uber die Mesothel (Deckzellen de serosen Haut) und die Zellen der serosen Exsudate: Untersuchungen an entzundetem Gewebe und an Gewebskulturen. Arch Exp Zellforsch 1927;4:1.

McArthur JW, Ulfelder H: The effect of pregnancy upon endometriosis. Obstet Gynecol Surv 1965;20:709.

McCausland A: Hysteroscopic myometrial biopsy: its use in diagnosing adenomyosis and its clinical application. Am J Obstet Gynecol 1992;166:1619.

McGinley R, Casey JH: Analysis of progesterone in unextracted serum: a method using danazol—a blocker of steroid binding to proteins. Steroids 1979;33:127.

Meigs JV: Medical treatment of endometriosis and significance of endometriosis. Surg Gynecol Obstet 1949;89:317.

Meldrum DR, Chang RJ, Lu J, Vale W: "Medical oophorectomy" using a long acting GnRH agonist—a possible new approach to the treatment of endometriosis. J Clin Endocrinol Metab 1982;54:1081.

Melicow MM, Pachter MR: Endometrial carcinoma of the prostatic utricle (uterus masculinus). Cancer 1967;20:1715.

Merrill JA: Experimental induction of endometriosis across millipore filters. Surg Forum 1963;14:397.

Merrill JA: Endometrial induction of endometriosis across millipore filters. Am J Obstet Gynecol 1966;94:780.

Metzger DA, Olive DL, Haney AF: Limited hormonal responsiveness of ectopic endometrium: histologic correlation with intrauterine endometrium. Hum Pathol 1988;19:1417.

Meyer R: Ueber die genese der cystadenome und adenomyome des uterus, mit demonstrationene. Ztschr Geburtsch Gynakol 1897;37:327.

Meyer R: Ztschr Geburtsch Gynakol 1900;43:130.

Meyer R: Ueber entzundliche heterotope Epithelwucherungen im weiblichen Genitalgebiete und uber eine bis in die Wurzel des Mesocolon ausgedehnte benigne Wurzel des Darmepithels. Virchows Arch Pathol Anat 1909;155:487.

Meyer R: Beitrage zur lehre von der adenomyosis uteri und der adenofibrosis peritonealis. Atschr Geburtsh Gynakol 1925;89:469.

Mitchell GW, Farber M: Medical versus surgical management of endometriosis. In Reid DE, Christian CD (eds): Controversy in Obstetrics and Gynecology. Vol II. Philadelphia: WB Saunders Company, 1974:631.

Moghissi KS, Boyce CRK: Management of endometriosis with oral medroxyprogesterone acetate. Obstet Gynecol 1976;47:265.

Moguilewsky M, Philibert D: Dynamics of the receptor interactions of danazol and gestrinone in the rat: correlation with biological activities. In Raynaud J-P, Ojasoo T, Martini L (eds): Medical Management of Endometriosis. New York: Raven Press, 1984:163.

Molitor JJ: Adenomyosis: a clinical and pathologic appraisal. Am J Obstet Gynecol 1971;110:275.

Mori T, Ohta Y, Nagosawa H: Ultrastructural changes in uterine myometrium of mice with experimentally induced adenomyosis. Experientia 1984;40:1385.

Mori T, Singtripop T, Kawashima S: Animal model of uterine adenomyosis by pituitary grafting and retardation of its development by bromocriptine mesylate in Balb/C mice. In Vivo 1991;2:107.

Mungyer G, Willemsen WNP, Rolland R, et al: Cells of the mucous membrane of the female genital tract in culture: a comparative study with regard to the histogenesis of endometriosis. In Vitro Cell Dev Biol 1987;23:111.

Murphy AA, Green WR, Bobbie D, et al: Unsuspected endometriosis documented by scanning electron microscopy in visually normal peritoneum. Fertil Steril 1986;146:522.

Nagasawa H, Aoki M, Mori T, et al: Stimulation of mammary tumorigenesis and inhibition of uterine adenomyosis by suppressed progestone effects in SHN mice. Anticancer Res 1989; 9:827.

Nagasawa H, Ishida M, Mori T: Effects of treatment with prolactin or progesterone on the coincidence of mammary tumors and uterine adenomyosis in young SHN mice. Lab Anim Sci 1987;37:200.

Nagasawa H, Mori T: Stimulation of mammary tumorigenesis and suppression of uterine adenomyosis by temporary inhibition of pituitary prolactin secretion during youth in mice. Proc Soc Exp Biol Med 1982;171:164.

Nagasawa H, Noguchi Y, Mori T, et al: Suppression of normal and preneoplastic mammary growth and uterine adenomyosis with reduced growth hormone level in SHN mice given monosodium glutamate neonatally. Eur J Cancer Clin Oncol 1985;21: 1547.

Namnoum AB, Hickman TN, Goodman SB, et al: Incidence of symptom recurrence after hysterectomy for endometriosis. Fertil Steril 1995;64:898.

Nezhat C, Hood J, Winer W, et al: Videolaseroscopy and laser laparoscopy in gynaecology. Br J Hosp Med 1987;38:219.

Nisolle M, Casanas-Roux F, Wyns C, et al: Immunohistochemical analysis of estrogen and progesterone receptors in endometrium and peritoneal endometriosis: a new quantitative method. Fertil Steril 1994;62:751.

Nisolle M, Clerckx F, Casanas-Roux F, Gillerot S: Treatment of endometriosis: evaluation of preoperative therapy with danazol, gestrinone, and buserelin (nasal spray and implant). J Gynecol Obstet Biol Reprod 1990a;19:759.

Nisolle M, Paindaveine B, Bourdon A, et al: Histologic study of peritoneal endometriosis in infertile women. Fertil Steril 1990b; 53:984.

Noble AD, Letchworth AT: Medical treatment of endometriosis: a comparative trial. Postgrad Med J 1979;(Suppl 5)55:37.

Norwood GE: Sterility and fertility in women with pelvic endometriosis. Clin Obstet Gynecol 1960;3:456.

Novak ER: Pathology of endometriosis. Clin Obstet Gynecol 1960; 3:314.

Oda Y, Nakanishi I, Tateiwa T: Intramural mullerian adenosarcoma of the uterus with adenomyosis. Arch Pathol Lab Med 1987;108:798.

Oliker AJ, Harns AE: Endometriosis of the bladder in a male patient. J Urol 1971;106:858.

Olive DL: Analysis of clinical fertility trials: a methodologic review. Fertil Steril 1986;45:157.

Olive DL: Conservative surgery. In Schenken RS (ed): Endometriosis: Contemporary Concepts in Clinical Management. Philadelphia: JB Lippincott Company, 1989a:213.

Olive DL: Medical treatment: alternatives to danazol. In Schenken RS (ed): Endometriosis: Contemporary Concepts in Clinical Management. Philadelphia: JB Lippincott Company, 1989b:189.

Olive DL, Hammond CB: Endometriosis: pathogenesis and mechanisms of infertility. Postgrad Obstet Gynecol 1985;5:1.

Olive DL, Haney AF: In DeCherney AH (ed): Reproductive Failure. New York: Churchill Livingstone, 1986:153.

Olive DL, Lee KL: Analysis of sequential treatment protocols for endometriosis-associated infertility. Am J Obstet Gynecol 1986; 154:613.

Owolabi TO, Strickler RC: Adenomyosis, a neglected diagnosis. Obstet Gynecol 1977;50:424.

Palmisano GP, Adamson GD, Lamb EJ: Can staging systems for endometriosis based on anatomic location and lesion type predict pregnancy rates? Int J Fertil Menopausal Stud 1993;38:241.

Patton EP, Field CS, Harms RW, Coulam CB: CA-125 levels in endometriosis. Fertil Steril 1986;45:770.

Pauerstein C: Clinical presentation and diagnosis. In Schenken RS (ed): Endometriosis: Contemporary Concepts in Clinical Management Philadelphia, JB Lippincott Company, 1989:127.

Pierson H: Metaplastastisch entstandene knochenbildungen neben infiltrierenden epithelwucherungen im uterus des kaninchens durch follickelhormon. Ztschr Krebsforsch 1938;47:336.

Pinkert TC, Catlow CE, Straus R: Endometriosis of the urinary bladder in a man with prostatic carcinoma. Cancer 1979;43: 1562.

Pittaway DE, Fayez JA: The use of CA-125 in the diagnosis and management of endometriosis. Fertil Steril 1986;46:790.

Popp LW, Schwiederessen JP, Gaetje R: Myometrial biopsy in the diagnosis of adenomyosis uteri. Am J Obstet Gynecol 1993;69: 546.

Punnonen R, Klemi P, Nikkanen V: Postmenopausal endometriosis. Eur J Obstet Gynecol Reprod Biol 1980;11:195.

Radwanska E, Rane D, Dmowski WP: Management of infertility in women with endometriosis and ovulatory dysfunction. Fertil Steril 1984;41:775.

Ramey JW, Archer DF: Peritoneal fluid: its relevance to the development of endometriosis. Fertil Steril 1993;60:1.

Ranney B: Endometriosis: III. Complete operations: reasons, sequellae, treatment. Am J Obstet Gynecol 1971a;109:1137.

Ranney B: Endometriosis: IV. Hereditary tendencies. Obstet Gynecol 1971b;37:734.

Ranney B: Etiology, prevention, and inhibition of endometriosis. Clin Obstet Gynecol 1980;23:875.

Rao BN, Persaud V: Adenomyosis uteri. West Indian Med J 1982; 31:205.

Redwine DB: Age-related evolution in color appearance of endometriosis. Fertil Steril 1987;48:1062.

Redwine DB: Is "microscopic" peritoneal endometriosis invisible? Fertil Steril 1988a;50:665.

Redwine DB: Mülleriosis: the single best fit model of the origin of endometriosis. J Reprod Med 1988b;33:915.

Redwine DB: Peritoneal blood painting: an aid in the diagnosis of endometriosis. Am J Obstet Gynecol 1989a;161:865.

Redwine DB: Peritoneal pockets and endometriosis: confirmation of an important relationship, with further observations. J Reprod Med 1989b;34:270.

Redwine DB: Endometriosis persisting after castration: clinical characteristics and results of surgical management. Obstet Gynecol 1994;83:405.

Ridley JH: The histogenesis of endometriosis: a review of facts and fancies. Obstet Gynecol Surv 1968;23:1.

Ridley JH, Edwards IK: Experimental endometriosis in the human. Am J Obstet Gynecol 1958;76:783.

Riva HL, Kawasaki DM, Messenger AJ: Further experience with norethynodrel in the treatment of endometriosis. Obstet Gynecol 1962;19:111.

Robyn C, Delogne-Desnoeck J, Bourdoux P, Copinschi G: Endocrine effects of gestrinone. In Raynaud J-P, Ojasoo T, Martini L (eds): Medical Management of Endometriosis. New York: Raven Press, 1984:207.

Rock JA, Truglia JA, Caplan RJ, The Zoladex Endometriosis Study Group: Zoladex (Goserelin acetate implant) in the treatment of endometriosis: a randomized comparison with danazol. Obstet Gynecol 1993;82:198.

Rokitansky K: Uber uterusdrusen neubildung. Ztschr Gesellsch Aerzte Wein 1860;16:577. (Reprinted by William Wood and Co, 1917).

Ruge C: Ztschr Deburtsch Gynak 1889;16:577.

Sampson JA: Perforating hemorrhagic (chocolate) cysts of the ovary. Arch Surg 1921;3:245.

Sampson JA: Heterotopic or misplaced endometrial tissue. Am J Obstet Gynecol 1925;10:649.

Sampson JA: Peritoneal endometriosis due to menstrual dissemination of endometrial tissue into the peritoneal cavity. Am J Obstet Gynecol 1927;14:422.

Sandberg EC, Cohn F: Adenomyosis in the gravid uterus at term. Am J Obstet Gynecol 1962;84:1457.

Sangi-Haghpeykar H, Poindexter A: Epidemiology of endometriosis among parous women. Obstet Gynecol 1995;85:983.

Schatz F: Ein fall von fibroadenoma cysticum diffusum et polyposum corporis et colli uteri. Arch Gynakol 1883;22:456.

Schenken RS: Pathogenesi. In Schenken RS (ed): Endometriosis: Contemporary Concepts in Clinical Management. Philadelphia: JB Lippincott Company, 1989:1.

Schifrin BS, Erez S, Moore JG: Teenage endometriosis. Am J Obstet Gynecol 1973;116:973.

Schlaff WD, Dugoff L, Damewood MD, Rock JA: Megestrol acetate for treatment of endometriosis. Obstet Gynecol 1990;75:646.

Schrodt GR, Alcorn MD, Ibanez J: Endometriosis of the male urinary system: a case report. J Urol 1980;124:722.

Schroeder C: Handbuch der weiblichen Geschlachtsorgane. 9th ed. 1892:318.

Schwartz LB, Seifer DB: Diagnostic imaging of adnexal masses: a review. J Reprod Med 1992;37:63.

Schweppe KW, Wynn RM: Ultrastructural changes in endometriotic implants during the menstrual cycle. Obstet Gynecol 1981;58:465.

Scott RB, TeLinde RW: External endometriosis—the scourge of the private patient. Ann Surg 1950;131:697.

Scott RB, Te Linde RW, Wharton LR: Further studies in experimental endometriosis. Am J Obstet Gynecol 1954;66:1082.

Siedler D, Laing FC, Jeffrey RB, Wing VW: Uterine adenomyosis: a difficult sonographic diagnosis. J Ultrasound Med 1987;6:345.

Siegler AM: Hysterosalpingography. 2nd ed. New York: Medcom Press, 1974:112.

Simms JS, Chegini N, Williams RS, et al: Identification of epidermal growth factor, transforming growth factor-alpha, and epidermal growth factor receptor in surgically induced endometriosis in rats. Obstet Gynecol 1991;78:850.

Simpson JL, Elias S, Malinak LR, Buttram VC Jr: Heritable aspects of endometriosis. I. Genetic studies. Am J Obstet Gynecol 1980;137:327.

Soules MR, Malinak LR, Bury R, Poindexter A: Endometriosis and anovulation: a coexisting problem in the infertile female. Am J Obstet Gynecol 1976;125:412.

Steele RW, Dmowski WP, Marmer DJ: Immunologic aspects of human endometriosis. Am J Reprod Immunol 1984;6:33.

Steingold KA, Cedars M, Lu JKH, Randal D: Treatment of endometriosis with a long-acting gonadotropin-releasing hormone agonist. Obstet Gynecol 197;69:403.

Steinleitner A, Lambert J, Suarez M, et al: Immunomodulation in the treatment of endometriosis-associated subfertility: use of pentoxifylline to reverse the inhibition of fertilization by surgically induced endometriosis in a rodent model. Fertil Steril 1991;56:975.

Strathy JH, Molgaard CA, Coulam CB, Melton LJ III: Endometriosis and infertility: a laparoscopic study of endometriosis among fertile and infertile women. Fertil Steril 1982;38:667.

Stripling MC, Martin DC, Chatman DL, et al: Subtle appearance of pelvic endometriosis. Fertil Steril 1988;49:427.

Strowitzki T, Wiedemann R, Hepp H: Influence of growth factors EGF, IGF-I, and human growth hormone on human endometrial stromal cells in vitro. Ann N Y Acad Sci 1991;626:308.

Surrey E, Fournet N, Voigt B, Judd H: Effects of sodium etidronate in combination with low-dose norethindrone in patients administered a long-acting GnRH agonist. Obstet Gynecol 1993;81:581.

Surrey E, Gambone J, Lu J, Judd H: The effects of combining norethindrone with a gonadotropin-releasing hormone agonist in the treatment of symptomatic endometriosis. Fertil Steril 1990;53:620.

Surrey ES, Halme J: Endometriosis as a cause of infertility. Obstet Gynecol Clin North Am 1989;16:79.

Surrey ES, Halme J: Effect of platelet-derived growth factor on endometrial stromal cell proliferation in vitro: a model for endometriosis? Fertil Steril 1991;56:672.

Sutton CJG, Ewen SP, Whitelaw N, et al: Prospective, randomized, double-blind, controlled trial of laser laparoscopy in the treatment of pelvic pain associated with minimal, mild, and moderate endometriosis. Fertil Steril 1994;62:696.

Takahashi K, Kijima S, Yoshino K, et al: Differential diagnosis between leiomyomata uteri and adenomyosis using CA-125 as a new tumor marker of ovarian carcinoma. Nippon Sanka Fujinka Gakkai Zasshi 1985;37:591.

Takahashi K, Okada S, Okada M, et al: Magnetic resonance imaging and serum CA-125 in evaluating patients with endometriomas prior to medical therapy. Fertil Steril 1996; 65:288.

Takahashi K, Okada S, Ozaki T, et al: Diagnosis of pelvic endometriosis by magnetic resonance imaging using "fat-saturation" technique. Fertil Steril 1994;62:973.

Tamaya T, Furuta N, Motoyama T, Boku S: Mechanism of antiprogestational action of synthetic steroids. Acta Endocrinol 1978;88:190.

Tamaya T, Motoyama T, Ohono V, et al: Steroid receptor levels and histology of endometriosis and adenomyosis. Fertil Steril 1979;31:396.

Tamaya T, Wada K, Fujimoto J, Yamada T: Danazol binding to steroid receptors in human uterine endometrium. Fertil Steril 1984;41:732.

Taussig FS: A study of the lymph glands in cancer of the cervix and cancer of the vulva. Am J Obstet Gynecol 1938;36:819.

Telimaa S: Danazol and medroxyprogesterone acetate are inefficacious in the treatment of endometriosis associated with infertility. Fertil Steril 1988;50:872.

Telimaa S, Kauppila A, Rönnberg L, et al: Elevated serum levels of endometrial secretory protein PP14 in patients with advanced endometriosis. Am J Obstet Gynecol 1989a;161:866.

Telimaa S, Penttila I, Puolakka J, et al: Circulating lipid and lipoprotein concentrations during danazol and high-dose medroxyprogesterone acetate therapy of endometriosis. Fertil Steril 1989b;52:31.

Telimaa S, Puolakka J, Rönnberg L, Kaupille A: Placebo-controlled comparison of danazol and high-dose medroxyprogesterone acetate in the treatment of endometriosis. Gynecol Endocrinol 1987a;1:13.

Telimaa S, Rönnberg L, Kaupilla A: Placebo-controlled comparison of danazol and high-dose medroxyprogesterone acetate in the treatment of endometriosis after conservative surgery. Gynecol Endocrinol 1987b;1:363.

TeLinde RW, Scott RB: Experimental endometriosis. Am J Obstet Gynecol 1950;60:1147.

Thomas EJ, Cooke ID: Successful treatment of asymptomatic endometriosis: does it benefit infertile women? BMJ 1987;294:117.

Thompson JR, Davion RJ: Adenomyosis of the uterus: an enigma. J Natl Med Assoc 1986;78:305.

Timonen S, Johansson C-J: Endometriosis treated with lynestrenol. Ann Chir Gynaecol Fenn 1968;57:144.

Tjaden B, Galetto D, Woodruff JD, Rock JA: Time-related effects of RU486 treatment in experimentally induced endometriosis in the rat. Fertil Steril 1993;59:437.

Tjaden B, Schlaff WD, Kimball A, Rock JA: The efficacy of presacral neurectomy for the relief of midline dysmenorrhea. Obstet Gynecol 1990;76:89.

Togashi K, Nishimura K, Kimura I, et al: Endometrial cysts: diagnosis with MR imaging. Radiology 1991;180:73.

Togashi K, Ozasa H, Konishi I, et al: Enlarged uterus: differentiation between adenomyosis and leiomyoma with MR imaging. Radiology 1989;71:531.

Urabe M, Yamamoto T, Kitawaki J, et al: Estrogen biosynthesis in human uterine adenomyosis. Acta Endocrinol 1989;121:259.

Van der Walt LA, Sanfilippo JS, Siegel JE, Wittliff JL: Estrogen and progestin receptors in human uterus: reference ranges of clinical conditions. Clin Physiol Biochem 1986;4:217.

Vancaillie T, Schenken RS: Endoscopic surgery. In Schenken RS (ed): Endometriosis: Contemporary Concepts in Clinical Management. Philadelphia: JB Lippincott Company, 1989:249.

Vercellini P, Boxxiolone L, Vendola N, et al: Peritoneal endometriosis: morphologic appearance in women with chronic pelvic pain. J Reprod Med 1991;36:533.

Vercillini P, Parazzini F, Oldani S, et al: Adenomyosis at hysterectomy: a study on frequency distribution and patient characteristics. Hum Reprod 1995;10:1160.

Vercellini P, Trespidi L, Colombo A, et al: A gonadotropin-releasing hormone agonist versus low-dose oral contraceptive for pelvic pain associated with endometriosis. Fertil Steril 1993;60:75.

Vercellini P, Trespidi L, Panazza S, et al: Very low dose danazol for relief of endometriosis-associated pelvic pain: a pilot study. Fertil Steril 1994;62:1136.

Vercellini P, Trespidi L, De Giorgi O, Cortesi I, Parazzini F, Crosignani PG: Endometriosis and pelvic pain: relation to disease stage and localization. Fertil Steril 1996;65:299.

Vernon M, Rush M, Wilson E: Effect of pregnancy and steroids on endometrial implants in rats with surgically induced endometriosis. Fertil Steril 1984;41:105.

Von Recklinghausen D: Die Adenomyome und Cystodenome der Uterus und Tubenwandung: Ihre Abkunftvon Resten des Wolffschen Korpeus. Berlin: Hirschwald, 1896.

Von Rokitansky C: Uber Uterusdrusen-Neubildung. Ztschr Gesellsch Aerzte Wien 1860;16:577.

Waller KG, Shaw RW: Gonadotropin-releasing hormone analogues for the treatment of endometriosis: long-term follow-up. Fertil Steril 1993;59:511.

Walsh JW, Taylor KJ, Rosenfield AT: Gray scale ultrasonography in the diagnosis of endometriosis and adenomyosis. Am J Roentgenol 1979;132:87.

Walters MD: Definitive surgery. In Schenken RS (ed): Endometriosis: Contemporary Concepts in Clinical Management. Philadelphia: JB Lippincott Company, 1989:267.

Walton LA: A reexamination of endometriosis after pregnancy. J Reprod Med 1977;19:341.

Werlin LB, Hodgen GD: Gonadotropin-releasing hormone agonist suppresses ovulation, menses, and endometriosis in monkeys: an individualized, intermittent regimen. J Clin Endocrinol Metab 1983;56:844.

Wheeler JM: Epidemiology of endometriosis-associated infertility. J Reprod Med 1989;34:41.

Wheeler JM, Knittle JD, Miller JD, the Lupron Endometriosis Study Group: Depot leuprolide acetate versus danazol in the treatment of women with symptomatic endometriosis: a randomized comparison with danazol. Am J Obstet Gynecol 1993; 169:26.

Wheeler JM, Malinak LR: Recurrent endometriosis: incidence, management, and prognosis. Am J Obstet Gynecol 1983;146: 247.

Wicks MJ, Larson CP: Histologic criteria for evaluating endometriosis. Northwest Med 1949;48:611.

Wild RA, Shivers CA: Antiendometrial antibodies in patients with endometriosis. Am J Reprod Immunol Microbiol 1985;8: 84.

Wolf DM, Spataro RF: The current state of hysterosalpingography. RadioGraphics 1988;8:1041.

Wood C, Hurley VA, Leoni M: The value of vaginal ultrasound in the management of menorrhagia. Aust N Z J Obstet Gynecol 1993;33:198.

Yamamoto T, Noguchi T, Tamura T, et al: Evidence for estrogen synthesis in adenomyotic tissues. Am J Obstet Gynecol 1993; 169:734.

Young MD, Blackmore WP: The use of danazol in the management of endometriosis. J Int Med Res 1977;5:86.

Zaleski W: Adenomyosis experimentalis nach interruptio graviditatis durch curretage bei kaninchen. Zentralbl Gynako 1936; 60:1046.

Zawin M, McCarthy S, Scoutt L, Comite F: Endometriosis: appearance and detection at MR imaging. Radiology 1989;171: 693.

31

Miscellaneous Benign Disorders of the Upper Genital Tract

Mark D. Adelson
Katherine L. Adelson

Cervix, Uterus, Ovary, Fallopian Tube,

Peritoneum, Retroperitoneum,

Para-adnexa

T his chapter reviews benign conditions, excluding those associated with infection, infertility, endometriosis, pregnancy, and topics addressed in other chapters.

UTERINE CERVIX

Inflammatory Conditions

Infections of the cervix often result from sexually transmitted diseases, which account for most inflammatory problems. Inflammation of a noninfectious etiology is uncommon but can result from atrophy. This inflammation in postmenopausal women might present with symptoms of vaginal pain and burning or purulent cervical discharge unresponsive to antimicrobial and antifungal treatment. Colposcopy and endometrial biopsy should be performed to rule out malignancy. The discharge often resolves within 2 weeks after initiation of estrogen replacement therapy. The cytologic changes of inflammation noted on a Papanicolaou (Pap) smear, namely reactive atypia, hyperkeratosis, and parakeratosis, should not be confused with intraepithelial neoplasia.

Neoplasia

Neoplastic conditions of the cervix can be epithelial in nature or can originate in the stroma. At the time of clinical presentation, however, the origin of the neoplasia may not be evident.

Disorders of the Epithelium

Polyps. Cervical polyps are the most common neoplasms of the cervix, found in at least 4% of all gynecologic patients. These are often referred to as "pseudotumors," representing hyperplastic response of normal tissue. Most often presenting in perimenopausal women, postmenopausal women, and multigravidas, cervical polyps are usually found incidentally and are predominantly asymptomatic. Less commonly, polyps may be a cause of profuse bleeding or discharge. Usually several millimeters in size, these lesions may become quite large. Etiology of the polyp may be inflammatory, traumatic, pregnancy related (pseudodecidual), or unknown. The anatomic origin of the polyp is the exocervix, endocervix, or endometrium. Grossly, the polyp might be confused with an epithelial malignancy of the cervix or endometrium or with a benign or malignant stromal tumor.

Microscopically, cervical polyps are composed of endocervical epithelium (most common) or a combination of endocervical and endometrial epithelia (mixed). An endocervical polyp may arise de novo but can be seen after overvigorous eversion of the endocervix during laser conization. Fibrous tissue (probably of exocervical stromal origin) may predominate, or the polyp may be composed of vasculature. Decidualized endocervical stroma may sometimes present as a polyp during pregnancy. The pseudosarcomatous polyp is benign and represents a form of stromal cell hyperplasia.

Since the nature of the polyp is often unclear, treatment consists of excision, although carcinoma developing in a polyp is rare. If possible, the polyp is grasped with a ring forceps and twisted off at the pedicle close to its attachment. Removal of the polyp alone, when the Pap smear is abnormal, does not obviate the need for colposcopic evaluation, however. Care should be used when dealing with polyps during pregnancy because the cervix is highly vascularized during that time. Stable and benign-appearing polyps may be observed during pregnancy. In the postmenopausal patient, cervical polyps (especially if symptomatic) may be associated with endometrial polyps (57% of cases) or neoplasia. Endometrial sampling and possibly hysteroscopy with dilatation and curettage (D&C) should be considered as part of the work-up in this age group (Neri et al, 1995).

Inclusion Cysts. Epithelial (nabothian) inclusion cysts are often noted after a pregnancy. These cysts are lined by nonkeratinizing squamous epithelium and contain a dense, yellow, mucoid material. Nabothian cysts result from traumatic invagination of the surface epithelium. Epithelial inclusion cysts present a characteristic appearance, and generally no therapy is required. If the differential diagnosis is not obvious, biopsy is essential, because confusion with minimal deviation adenocarcinoma may occur (Yamashita et al, 1994). Cauterization of these cysts in cases of persistent cervicitis has been recommended. It is unclear whether these cysts act as a reservoir of infection, and the efficacy of this procedure is unknown.

Microglandular Endocervical Hyperplasia. This is a benign condition often noted in patients who are taking oral contraceptives (OCs). It has also been seen in pregnant and postpartum patients and may represent an effect of progesterone or estrogen. Although most cases are found in women of reproductive age, 6% are diagnosed in postmenopausal women. The relationship to hormonal stimulation is disputed (Greeley et al, 1995).

Typically, the lesion appears 1 to 2 cm in size, bleeds easily, and may persist even after the hormonal stimulus has been removed. Postcoital spotting may be a primary complaint. Histologically, two forms have been recognized. *Microglandular* hyperplasia, the most common form, is made up of tightly packed glandular or tubular units. *Atypical* endocervical hyperplasia is composed of benign glandular units arranged in a reticulated or solid pattern, but is sometimes mistaken for clear cell adenocarcinoma. If the diagnosis is unclear, a biopsy should be performed, although no treatment is required. It may be mistaken on Pap smear for adenocarcinoma or a high-grade squamous intraepithelial lesion. This diagnosis should be accepted with caution in the postmenopausal woman because adenocarcinoma of the endometrium and cervix may simulate microglandular hyperplasia.

Cystic Endocervical Tunnel Clusters. This benign entity may be mistaken for endocervical adenocarcinoma or hyperplasia. It can be found in 6% to 10%

of patients. Histologically, they are multifocal and small (2 to 3 mm) and consist of closely packed, dilated tubular endocervical glands. They are lined by a single layer of flattened or cuboidal cells without significant atypia, extending up to 9 mm deep.

Tubal Metaplasia. These lesions appear as normal tubal mucosa in the cervix. They may be accompanied by a variety of other benign lesions (e.g., endometriosis, microglandular or mesonephric hyperplasia). These lesions must not be confused with early endocervical glandular neoplasia.

Adenomas. Adenomas of the cervix are rare benign tumors. Depending on the predominance of fibrous or muscular tissue, these are classified as *fibroadenoma* or *adenofibroma*. A papillary variant of the adenofibroma has been recognized.

Heterologous Tissue. Heterologous tissue is rarely found in the cervix. Glia, skin (including sebaceous glands, hair, and sweat glands), and cartilage have been reported. This incidental finding must not be confused with a malignant mixed mesodermal tumor. Fourteen teratomas have been reported.

Melanosis. Melanosis of the cervix is a benign condition that must be differentiated from melanoma. Only seven cases have been reported. This darkly pigmented lesion contains a proliferation of benign melanocytes. The differential diagnosis includes endometriosis and malignant melanoma. Biopsy is mandatory. Melanosis has been reported to develop after cervical cryotherapy. Whether or not this lesion is a precursor to melanoma is unknown. Benign blue nevi have also been reported, and are similar to those seen in the dermis.

Disorders of the Stroma

Leiomyomas. Cervical leiomyomas are much less common than those occurring in the fundus, accounting for 8% of all uterine leiomyomas. These lesions are most often discovered incidentally and are generally small and asymptomatic. Rarely, prolapse from the endocervical canal occurs, resulting in bleeding or pregnancy dystocia. The histologic patterns are similar to those seen in the fundal tumors.

Mesonephric Remnants and Hyperplasia. Vestigial remnants of the distal ends of the mesonephric (Gartner's) ducts are found in 1% of cervices. These small tubules or cysts, lined by nonciliated low columnar or cuboidal epithelium, are located deep in the lateral cervical wall. They commonly form a lobular pattern, showing a distinct clustering of mesonephric tubules. The less common diffuse pattern is nonclustered. The mean size of these lesions is 14 mm. The mean age of the patient is 38 years, and rarely they present with bleeding. The pattern of florid, tubuloglandular proliferation may be confused with minimal deviation adenocarcinoma or adenocarcinoma of the endocervix (Seidman and Tavassoli, 1995).

Miscellaneous Tumors. Rare miscellaneous benign tumors include hemangiomas of the capillary or cavernous type, lymphangioma, lipoma, neurofibroma, neuroma, and ganglioneuroma.

Structural Conditions

Stenosis

Cervical stenosis is due to both congenital and acquired causes. Obstruction of the efflux of secretions from the uterus leads to pressure buildup from clear fluid (*hydrometra*), blood (*hematometra*), or infected exudate (*pyometra*). Pressure forces the intrauterine collection through the fallopian tubes and into the peritoneal cavity. When stenosis occurs in the young female, dysmenorrhea, endometriosis, or infertility may result. Stenosis in the elderly may result in painful hematometra or pyometra and may progress into peritonitis and sepsis. Stricture of the cervical canal interferes with examination of the cervix and endometrium to rule out malignancy.

Senile atrophy is an acquired cause of cervical stenosis in postmenopausal women who are not receiving estrogen replacement. This condition should be ruled out prior to initiating hormone replacement, because hematometra may result. Cervicitis may result in scarring of the endocervical canal, which produces stricture, although this is uncommon. Occasionally, trauma from childbirth results in stenosis.

Acquired cervical stenosis is most often iatrogenic. "Hot" cautery, cryocautery, and cervical conization are the most common causes (Reuter et al, 1994). The reported risk of this complication varies between 1% and 17%. A subgroup of patients at greatest risk for scarification are diethylstilbestrol-exposed women born with cervical structural abnormalities who undergo cervical surgery, notably cryosurgery. Following sharp conization, the placement of Sturmdorf or large figure-of-8 approximating sutures increases the risk of subsequent stenosis. The risk of stenosis is lowest after laser or loop electrosurgical conization of the cervix.

Treatment of acquired cervical stenosis has been largely frustrating and unproductive. In the past, progressive and repeated dilatation of the fibrotic canal was used. The procedure was either performed rapidly, with metal dilators and anesthesia, or gradually, with laminaria tents. The stenosis invariably returned. Presently, laser vaporization of fibrotic tissue around the canal with eversion of the canal results in successful elimination of the stenosis in most patients.

Anomalous Development

Anomalous development of the cervix is rare. The Mayer-Rokitansky-Kuster-Hauser syndrome, or rudimentary or absent development of the müllerian ducts, occurs once in every 5000 to 20,000 female births. Patients often have atresia of the cervix with an intact uterine fundus. Niver and colleagues (1980) reviewed the outcome of patients with cervical atresia. In 22 patients, 45 surgical procedures were performed to re-establish continuity of the uterus with the vagina and introitus. Menses was restored in eight of the patients, and pregnancy was achieved in only one. Some authors have recommended hysterectomy in these patients, whereas others have reported successful attempts to re-establish continuity (Bates and Wiser, 1985). But, the prospect for success and for restoration of fertility is ultimately poor.

UTERINE CORPUS

Inflammatory Conditions

The majority of inflammatory conditions of the uterine corpus are infectious in nature. *Pyometra* may result from any condition occluding the outflow tract (see text on cervical stenosis earlier). It may also occur without cervical stenosis, and has been reported after endometrial ablation, with an intrauterine contraceptive device (IUCD) of long duration, and in the postpartum patient. Spontaneous perforation may, especially in an elderly woman with acute abdominal pain, present as peritonitis. The morbidity and mortality are high in this situation.

Neoplasia

Disorders of the Endometrium

Polyps. Endometrial polyps are common, found in 10% of uteri examined at autopsy. They occur most commonly in women 40 to 60 years of age. The etiology is unknown. Polyps contain a variable amount of glands, stroma, and blood vessels. Endometrial polyps are generally solitary; 20% are multiple. Most originate at the fundus, usually in the cornual region. Polyps may also originate at the lower uterine segment/upper endocervix and contain mixed epithelium.

Morphologically, endometrial polyps exhibit great diversity and are classified into three main categories:

1. *Hyperplastic polyps* are derived from the basalis layer of the endometrium, are estrogen responsive, and are irregular in size and shape. These occur most frequently, resembling diffuse hyperplasia of the endometrium, but are focal and pedunculated. This type of polyp might be incorrectly diagnosed as endometrial hyperplasia or, if large, as adenosarcoma.
2. *Atrophic (or "inactive") polyps* are covered by low columnar to cuboidal glandular epithelium. The glands tend to be enlarged and cystically dilated and are typically found in postmenopausal women. These polyps result from regressive changes in a hyperplastic or functional polyp.

3. *Functional polyps* appear least often and show glandular changes resembling those of the surrounding endometrium. The surface epithelium may be "out of phase" or "dyssynchronous" compared with surrounding endometrium. This may result in a mistaken diagnosis of luteal-phase defect on endometrial biopsy. If significant amounts of muscle are identified, the polyp is referred to as "adenomyomatous."

The malignancy potential of endometrial polyps has been debated but appears to be low. Malignant transformation in a polyp is rare, but 10% to 34% of cases of endometrial cancer in postmenopausal women have been associated with polyps. In a case-control study from Sweden, the increased risk of subsequent endometrial cancer in women with endometrial polyps was estimated to be twofold (Petterson et al, 1985). They also occur two to four times more often in women taking tamoxifen.

Endometrial polyps are usually asymptomatic. The most common presenting symptom is bleeding, either intermenstrual or excessive menstrual flow (menorrhagia). In a series of 176 patients with postmenopausal bleeding, endometrial polyps were the causative factor in 45% (Cravello et al, 1998). Large polyps are more likely to be associated with bleeding.

Endometrial polyps are usually diagnosed after uterine curettage but are easily missed by the curet and the polyp forceps. Therefore, hysteroscopy is a more sensitive diagnostic test and has been advocated as the initial step in the evaluation of abnormal uterine bleeding. Hysteroscopy should be performed if D&C fails to identify the cause of bleeding or if bleeding recurs after D&C. In a study of 276 patients undergoing D&C and panoramic hysteroscopy for abnormal bleeding, hysteroscopy revealed more information than D&C in 18% of cases (Gimpelson and Rappold, 1988). Endometrial polyps accounted for 34% of the diagnoses missed by D&C.

Adenomyomas. The atypical polypoid adenomyoma grossly resembles an endometrial polyp and often involves the lower uterine segment. Microscopically, the lesion is composed of irregularly shaped, hyperplastic glands haphazardly arranged within smooth muscle. The polypoid adenomyoma, usually occurring in the reproductive years and in the perimenopausal period, is often associated with bleeding. The lesion must be differentiated from hyperplasia, carcinoma, and mixed müllerian tumors. Despite the atypical appearance, the lesion follows a benign course, although cystic degeneration has been reported. Curettage may be curative in premenopausal women who wish to preserve fertility, and in some cases pregnancy has followed. Recurrence is common, however (50%; Longacre et al, 1996). Ultimately, hysterectomy may be required to rule out malignancy.

Stromal Nodules. Endometrial stromal nodules are rare, accounting for 25% of endometrial stromal tumors (Fekete and Vellios, 1984). Grossly, the nodules are fleshy, yellow-tan, and rounded. The median size is 4 cm, ranging from 1 to 15 cm. Five per cent are multiple, and 18% are polypoid. Half of the nodules are located entirely within the myometrium in an intramural or subserosal location, with no apparent connection to the endometrium. Microscopically, the cells are identical to normal endometrial stromal cells but are surrounded by an expansile and noninfiltrative capsule, and are devoid of necrosis or cellular pleomorphism. They are cytologically indistinguishable from low-grade stromal sarcoma (which has an infiltrating growth pattern).

Clinically, 75% of endometrial stromal nodules occur in patients of reproductive age. Approximately 80% of the tumors are symptomatic, with heavy bleeding and pelvic and abdominal discomfort the most common complaints. Hysterectomy is the usual treatment, but complete excision may also be appropriate. It is important to subject the nodule, including its periphery, to complete histologic evaluation to rule out a malignancy. Endometrial stromal nodules follow a benign course and do not recur or metastasize.

Teratomas. Primary teratoma of the endometrium is also rare. To make the diagnosis, metaplasia and the presence of embryonic remnants must be ruled out. Histologically, teratoma of the endometrium resembles that seen in the ovary. These can be mature or immature (malignant).

Benign Heterologous Tissue. Benign heterologous tissue in the endometrium has been reported. This finding is accounted for by metaplastic transformation of the endometrial stromal cell or by implantation of fetal tissue after abortion and instrumentation. Heterotopic bone is most characteristically found in women with a history of repeated abortions and endometritis and probably represents implantation of fetal parts. The finding of cartilage is also associated with a history of prior abortion. This may, alternatively, develop by metaplasia, because cartilage has been found in postmenopausal women. Similarly, smooth muscle may be found in the endometrium, seen as fascicles or nodules, probably arising from metaplasia of endometrial stromal cells. Adipose tissue may represent portions of omentum (obtained by uterine perforation) or less commonly a fatty tumor. Vascular tissue may be from a low-grade stromal tumor or vascular proliferation at the surface of a polyp, rather than a hemangioma. Mature glial tissue presents in multiple foci. The etiology is probably persistent remnants from a terminated pregnancy. When glial tissue is thought to represent true neoplasia, the term *glioma* is employed. Extramedullary hematopoiesis in the endometrium has been reported in four patients.

Disorders of the Myometrium

LEIOMYOMAS

The leiomyoma is the most common neoplasm of the uterus. Found clinically in 20% to 30% of women, leiomyomas are noted in 50% of uteri at autopsy. Uterine leiomyomas are more common in black women (50%) than in white women (25%). Most leiomyomas are diagnosed in middle-aged women; they are rarely noted in females younger than 18 years of age. The youngest patient reported was a 13-year-old girl.

Otherwise known as *uterine fibroids*, leiomyomas originate in the intramural portion of the myometrium from a single clone of smooth muscle cells. With continued growth in one direction, the location may shift in relation to the myometrium. Anatomically, the lesions are categorized as *submucosal* (beneath the endometrium), *intramural* (within the myometrium but distorting neither the endometrium nor the serosa), or *subserosal* (beneath the uterine serosa). Five per cent to 10% of myomas are submucosal and are the most symptomatic. Submucosal myomas can pedunculate into the endometrial cavity or prolapse through the cervix. Subserosal myomas also become pedunculated at times. When blood supply is derived from neighboring organs, the term *parasitic myoma* is used. These myomas may be attached to omentum or intestine or may grow in a lateral direction into the broad ligament. An uncommon uterine tumor characterized by visible intravascular proliferation of benign smooth muscle is termed *intravascular (or intravenous) leiomyomatosis*. Hysterectomy is the treatment of choice. This lesion is responsive to gonadotropin-releasing hormone agonists (GnRHa), which may render debulking surgery more feasible.

Histology. Histologically, many subtypes of leiomyomas have been identified, although all appear macroscopically similar. Generally spherical and firm, the cut surfaces are white to tan with a whorled trabecular pattern. At least six histologic variants have been identified:

1. The extreme cellularity of *cellular leiomyomas* may lead to confusion with leiomyosarcoma. Cellular leiomyomas composed of small cells with scanty cytoplasm are also confused with endometrial stromal tumors.
2. *Atypical leiomyomas* contain atypical cells distributed in clusters throughout the tumor. If multinucleated giant cells are numerous, the terms *bizarre* or *symplastic* leiomyoma have been applied. These tumors are also confused with leiomyosarcomas, which have a higher mitotic count.
3. *Epithelioid leiomyomas* include leiomyoblastoma, clear cell leiomyoma, and plexiform leiomyoma. The clinical behavior of the epithelioid leiomyoma is varied. Small tumors without cytologic atypia and with circumscribed margins, extensive hyalinization, low mitotic activity, and clear cells are considered benign.
4. *Myxoid leiomyomas* contain amorphous myxoid substance, producing a soft, translucent appearance. The margins are well circumscribed and mi-

totic figures and atypia are absent. These tumors should be differentiated from leiomyosarcoma.
5. *Lipoleiomyomas* contain large areas of fat. These areas may be well circumscribed or diffuse. Pure lipoma is rare. These tumors should not be confused with mixed mesodermal sarcoma.
6. *Leiomyomas with tubules* are uncommon. Histologically, epithelium-lined tubules are noted. Mesothelial differentiation also occurs.

Many leiomyomas undergo degeneration. These secondary changes occur as the myoma outgrows its blood supply and are termed hyaline, myxomatous, calcific, cystic, fatty, carneous (red), and sarcomatous.

The mildest form is *hyaline degeneration*, found in 65% of myomas. The appearance is homogeneous, with loss of the whorled pattern and cellular detail as the smooth muscle cells are replaced by fibrous connective tissue.

Myxomatous change occurs in 15% of tumors, and *calcific degeneration* occurs in 4% to 10%, predominantly in older women. *Cystic degeneration* is found in 4% of leiomyomas and results from coalescence of hyalinized areas with liquefaction. *Fatty degeneration* occurs rarely, but may result from late-stage hyaline degeneration or necrosis.

Carneous necrosis is the most acute form of degeneration. It occurs in a rapidly growing myoma, most often in the second trimester of pregnancy, in up to 10% of pregnant patients with myomas. Acute muscular infarction causes severe pain and localized peritoneal irritation. Myomas with advanced degeneration may become secondarily infected because of the large areas of necrosis. One case of tetanus caused by *Clostridium tetani* infection has been reported.

Sarcomatous change, or malignancy developing from or occurring within a benign myoma, is very rare (2 to 3/1000).

Clinical Findings. Many patients with uterine myomas are asymptomatic, notably when the myomas are small or if slow growth allows gradual accommodation of abdominal viscera to the expanding mass. One third of patients experience pelvic pain, with acquired dysmenorrhea the most frequent complaint. Vascular compromise in the myoma, resulting in acute degeneration associated with enlargement or with torsion of the pedicle, may produce severe pain. Edematous swelling in the myoma produces a feeling of pelvic heaviness or a dull, aching sensation. Intense cramping pain may result from a prolapsing submucous myoma as the uterus tries to expel the mass.

Size and location also determine symptomatology. A very large myomatous tumor may result in increasing abdominal girth without associated pain. An anterior myoma pressing on the bladder often produces urinary frequency and urgency. A posterior myoma may produce rectal pressure, tenesmus, constipation, lower back discomfort, or sacral plexus pain. Symptoms referable to the urinary tract are more common. Bilateral ureteral obstruction can result from a large myoma filling the pelvis. Secondary polycythemia has been associated with myomas, resolving after surgical removal.

Abnormal uterine bleeding occurs in 30% of patients with leiomyomas. Menorrhagia is most common, but intermenstrual spotting and irregular periods may also result. Weakness secondary to anemia of blood loss and abnormal bleeding may result from increased endometrial surface stretched over a submucous myoma. Ulceration or atrophy of mucosa overlying the myoma might also be a cause of bleeding. In addition, distortion, dilation, and elongation of endometrial glands has been found on the wall opposite the myoma and in the endometrium along its margin. Intramural myomas may impede venous return, resulting in stasis, a change in venous drainage, and heavier flow.

Treatment. For asymptomatic leiomyomas, no treatment is required other than observation. Uterine size has been used as an indication for hysterectomy if it is greater than 12 to 14 weeks' gestation, but without scientific validation (Reiter et al, 1992). The real concern is not the absolute size of the myoma, because malignancy is rare, but the true etiology of the perceived myomatous mass. The mass must be differentiated from enlarged adnexa. The pelvic examination alone is not sufficiently sensitive to make the differential diagnosis, inasmuch as ovarian cancer is found 16% of the time after an incorrect preoperative diagnosis of leiomyoma. Pelvic sonography is the simplest and most cost-effective study to help identify the origin of the mass and locate the ovaries. If the ovaries are identified independent of the mass and appear normal on scan, a patient with a myomatous uterus is a candidate for conservative follow-up. Additionally, endometrial sampling to rule out endometrial hyperplasia and cancer should be performed in the patient with abnormal bleeding.

Indications for surgery include life-threatening uterine bleeding or a rapidly enlarging mass found in a perimenopausal or postmenopausal patient. Hysterectomy stops the bleeding and initiates the differential work-up and treatment for presumed uterine sarcoma. If the patient wishes to preserve or restore fertility, myomectomy is an alternative to hysterectomy. Before operative treatment, an attempt is made to identify and localize the myoma by scan. If a submucous myoma is diagnosed, it may be removed using the hysteroscope. Operative myomectomy via laparoscopy or laparotomy provides another conservative option. The recurrence rate after myomectomy is 15% to 45%.

Medical treatment of leiomyomas is based on the tumor response to estrogen and progesterone. For example, the rapid growth of myomas often noted during pregnancy is thought to be due to high circulating levels of estrogen. When estrogen levels decline postpartum or during menopause, leiomyomas often regress. A hypoestrogen state may be induced by the administration of a progestogen, antiestrogen (tamoxifen), danazol, or GnRHa. The efficacy of progestational agents is in question because, although some authors have demonstrated regression of the myomas, others have found no response. Ueki et al (1995) demonstrated effectiveness in reducing myoma size using danazol. A number of authors have reported tamoxifen-induced myoma growth, necessitating hysterectomy, in patients being treated for breast cancer (Kang et al, 1996). Significant regression in myoma size (50%) has been demonstrated using the antiprogesterone RU 486 (Murphy et al, 1995).

GnRHa therapy represents the most current advance in medical therapy. GnRHa produces a hypoestrogenic state by acting hypothalamically to down-regulate ovarian estrogen production. Uterine arterial blood flow is thereby decreased. A 30% to 60% reduction in myoma volume can be demonstrated by magnetic resonance imaging or sonography after treatment. Symptom reduction and elevation of hematocrit generally accompany this size decrease (Benagiano et al, 1996). Unfortunately, uterine and myoma volumes often return to baseline levels by 3 months after therapy, even with OC therapy following cessation of GnRHa. Histologically, GnRHa therapy of leiomyomata has been shown to induce an increase or decrease in cellularity, hyalinization, infarction and reduction in the number of nucleolar organizer regions and a decrease in the number of proliferating cells.

Use of GnRHa to reduce myoma size prior to surgical myomectomy potentially increases the technical ease of operation and decreases blood loss (Lumsden et al, 1994). The disadvantage of this approach is that, if pretreatment renders a myoma undetectable at the time of surgery and prevents surgical extirpation, regrowth will occur after therapy, compromising the efficacy of the entire treatment. Additionally, dissection may become more difficult because softening of the myoma results in the surrounding plane of dissection becoming less distinct. Delaying surgery 4 to 6 weeks after the last dose ameliorates this problem. Other problems with prolonged treatment include side effects such as hot flushes, decreased libido, vaginal dryness, worsening memory, osteoporosis, and inadvertent treatment of a leiomyosarcoma. Add-back therapy with estrogen and progestin or progestin alone may prevent some of these symptoms. A case of massive ascites after a single dose of GnRHa to treat fibroids has been reported.

ADENOMYOSIS

Adenomyosis is a common condition, found in 18% of hysterectomy specimens and in 53% of those from patients taking tamoxifen (Cohen et al, 1997). The term *endometriosis interna* has been applied to this disease, although this is misleading because endometriosis (externa) and adenomyosis are found together in fewer than 20% of women. In addition, these two entities are clinically different.

An association between adenomyosis and other conditions may exist, with estrogen effect the common factor suspected. Leiomyomas have been noted in 23% to 50% of cases of adenomyosis, but this percentage also represents the incidence of leiomyomas in the general population. Adenomyosis has been noted in 33% of patients with endometrial hyperplasia. In a series of 332 cases, no relationship was found between the presence of adenomyosis and other gynecologic conditions (fibroids, prolapse, ovarian cysts, and cancer) (Vercellini et al, 1995).

Adenomyosis is characterized by the finding of islands of benign endometrial glands surrounded by benign endometrial stroma. To avoid confusion with endometrium dipping into the myometrium, the location of the adenomyosis should be deeper than one half of a low-power field (2.5 mm) below the lower border of the endometrium. This lesion most commonly presents with diffuse involvement of both anterior and posterior uterine walls, resulting in a diffusely enlarged uterus. Another presentation is the encapsulated adenomyoma, described as glands and stroma surrounded entirely by muscle. On cut section, the myometrium may appear spongy and darker than unaffected myometrium.

Most women with adenomyosis are asymptomatic or minimally symptomatic. Menorrhagia or dysmenorrhea are presenting complaints, usually seen between the ages of 35 and 50 years. Most women with symptoms are multiparous. This secondary dysmenorrhea becomes increasingly severe as the disease progresses. On pelvic examination, the diffusely enlarged globular uterus is most tender immediately before and during menstruation. Ultrasonography or magnetic resonance imaging may be used for diagnosis. Treatment is generally symptomatic, with hysterectomy reserved for patients with severe symptoms. Limited surgical resection has been used in few cases. Although adenomyosis is unresponsive to hormone treatment (e.g., progestin, OCs), three cases of severe adenomyosis demonstrating regression with GnRHa, followed by conception, have been reported. Bleeding resulting in hematoperitoneum has also been reported.

ARTERIOVENOUS MALFORMATION

Arteriovenous malformation (AVM) of the uterus is a rarely diagnosed condition (Abdul-Karim et al, 1989). A tumor with extensive communication between the arterial and venous vascular systems, AVM may be congenital or acquired. Congenital lesions present with excessive uterine bleeding in the absence of any prior history of instrumentation. Acquired lesions usually appear following D&C related to abortion or gestational trophoblastic neoplasia, hysterectomy, or removal of an IUD. Endocrinologic causes of the abnormal bleeding are ruled out, and the bleeding may not respond to hormonal manipulation. Diagnosis can be made by sonography, but experience with this is minimal. Hysteroscopy may re-

veal a pulsatile mass, but the examination is often unsatisfactory if active bleeding is present. Arteriography is the definitive diagnostic procedure for AVM.

Conservative treatment includes arterial embolization, and should be offered to the patient desiring to preserve her reproductive potential. This method is not always risk free or successful, but pregnancies have been reported after such treatment. Hysterectomy is, of course, curative.

Disorders of the Serosa

The *adenomatoid mesothelioma* is diagnosed as an incidental finding in 1% of uteri. The median age of the patient is 42 years, and no associated symptoms or conditions are attributed. Grossly, these gray, round, rubbery tumors measure 0.5 to 2.0 cm and have an irregular border. Most often subserosal and found in the cornual region, the lesions may be confused with leiomyomas or adenomyomas. One half of the tumors are found in the uterus, and the remainder are generally found in the fallopian tube. Microscopically, adenomatoid mesotheliomas consist of cystic spaces lined by flat or cuboidal cells surrounded by stroma with abundant collagen, elastic tissue, and smooth muscle. Confusion with a signet-ring cell carcinoma or angioma may also occur. Simple excision of adenomatoid mesothelioma may be sufficient treatment. Because recurrence is rare, hysterectomy can be avoided (Klintorp et al, 1993).

Structural Conditions

Hematometra refers to a uterus distended with blood, and *hydrometra* indicates distention of the uterus with fluid. Both are caused by obstruction of any portion of the lower genital tract. Obstruction may be congenital, most commonly an imperforate hymen or a transverse vaginal septum. Among the most prevalent acquired lesions are senile atrophy of the endocervical canal; scarring of the isthmus by synechiae; cervical stenosis associated with surgery, radiation therapy, cryocautery, or electrocautery; malignant disease of the cervix; and cervical obstruction by tissue following suction curettage. Common signs and symptoms include an enlarged globular uterus, amenorrhea, and cramping lower abdominal pain. Secondary infection may result in pyometra. Diagnosis is suspected on history and physical examination and may be confirmed by sonography. Treatment is by D&C or by surgical correction of the obstruction.

FALLOPIAN TUBE

Neoplasia

Disorders of the Epithelium

Papillomas and Polyps. Epithelial papillomas and polyps are rare and are noted in 2% of hysterosalpingograms (Gisser, 1986). Because papillary prolif-erations may be found with salpingitis, the diagnosis of papilloma in the presence of inflammation is prob-ably unjustified. Although 20% to 60% of women with tubal polyps have associated infertility, it is not known how or why these tumors contribute to in-fertility. A case of an adenomatous polyp has been described.

Teratomas. Benign teratomas are usually located in the lumen of the tube, and fewer than 50 cases have been reported. Often cystic and small, the lesions may grow to large sizes. Most tumors have been dis-covered in women in the 31- to 40-year age group. Very rarely, a single histologic type of tissue is found. Mature thyroid tissue (two patients) and a nodule of pancreatic tissue (one patient) have been described. One occurrence with a tubal ectopic pregnancy has been reported.

Mucinous Lesions. This entity includes mucinous metaplasia, and cystadenomas. An association with adenocarcinomas in other genital tract sites and Peutz-Jeghers syndrome may exist.

Miscellaneous Tumors. Other benign tumors of mesenchymal origin are also rarely found. They in-clude hemangioma, lipoma, angiomyolipoma, gan-glioneuroma, and neurilemmoma. Cartilage has been noted in benign fibroblastic and fatty tumors.

Disorders of the Muscularis

Leiomyomas of the fallopian tube are unusual in contrast to the their uterine counterparts, with fewer than 100 reported. These benign tumors may be sin-gle or multiple and are often discovered in the in-terstitial portion of the tube. Usually coexistent with uterine leiomyomas, most tubal leiomyomas are asymptomatic. However, the tumors may undergo acute degeneration or may be associated with tubal obstruction or torsion. One occurrence in conjunction with a tubal ectopic pregnancy has been reported; perhaps the leiomyomas was the etiologic factor. The histologic features are identical to those of myomas found in the uterus.

Disorders of the Serosa

Adenomatoid Tumors. The adenomatoid tumor, or *benign mesothelioma*, is the most commonly seen be-nign tubal tumor. These tumors are found just below the serosa and are described in the section on uterine neoplasia.

Mesothelial Inclusion Cysts. Benign inclusion cysts are formed by invagination of the tubal serosa. The cysts, then, are lined by mesothelial cells. By under-going metaplasia, the cells are transformed into cells with irregular ovoid nuclei and a longitudinal nu-clear groove ("coffee bean" appearance). Benign in-clusions, or *Walthard's nests*, are common incidental findings.

Structural Conditions

Torsion

Acute torsion of the fallopian tube is a rare event, occurring in both benign and malignant tubes. Be-cause the tube and ovary share a common vascular pedicle, tubal torsion usually is accompanied by tor-sion of the ovary. The right tube is involved more often than the left. Intrinsic causes of torsion include congenital abnormalities, such as increased mobility resulting from excessive length. Pathologic pro-cesses, such as hydrosalpinx, hematosalpinx, neo-plasm, and previous surgery (notably tubal ligation), are also associated. Extrinsic causes of torsion in-clude ovarian and peritubal tumors, adhesions, trauma, and pregnancy. The usual predisposing fac-tor is unilateral enlargement of the ipsilateral ovary resulting from a benign tumor, present in 65% to 95% of patients, or a malignant tumor, present in 5% to 15%.

Torsion most often occurs in women in their re-productive years, although nine cases of torsion of a normal fallopian tube in premenarchal girls have been reported. Torsion of an accessory fallopian tube has been reported in two premenarchal girls. The most prevalent presenting complaint is acute lower abdominal and pelvic pain. This pain is usually lo-cated in the iliac fossa with radiation to the thigh and flank, with a gradual or sudden onset. Nausea and vomiting occur in two thirds of the cases. A mass is usually not palpable on examination unless there is associated torsion of the ovary. Tubal torsion has been discovered and managed laparoscopically during pregnancy and diagnosed during labor.

Preoperatively, the diagnosis of tubal torsion is made in fewer than 20% of cases. The differential diagnosis includes appendicitis, ectopic pregnancy, pelvic inflammatory disease (PID), renal colic, and rupture or torsion of an ovarian mass. Ultrasonog-raphy may reveal a thickening of the tube with in-traluminal hemorrhage. Color-flow Doppler ultra-sonography may reveal decreased adnexal blood flow. At laparoscopy, the finding of a nonviable, edematous, gangrenous, and infarcted tube prompts excision. However, with intermittent or minor de-grees of torsion, the tube may often be salvaged by untwisting and suturing it into a secure position to prevent future torsion (Gordon et al, 1994). Previous undiagnosed torsion occurring in an infant or adult may result in the finding of an absent tube (autoam-putation), as a result of resorption, or one that is calcified.

Prolapse

Tubal prolapse may occur as a complication of vag-inal hysterectomy (Hellen et al, 1993). It has been reported less frequently after posterior colpotomy and the interposition operation. Predisposing factors include pelvic infection, hematoma, intraperitoneal vaginal drains or packs, and failure to close the vaginal cuff. Clinically, this condition may present days to years after hysterectomy, with discharge or bleeding. The mass appears as a red, friable, edematous tumor at the vaginal apex. It may be acutely painful when it is manipulated or during biopsy, often differentiated from granulations, tumor, or endometriosis. The presence of herniated bowel through the vaginal incision should be ruled out prior to biopsy. A prolapsed tube can be confused with adenocarcinoma, especially when pseudogland formation is present.

Treatment includes avulsion with cautery to the base (at the vaginal mucosa) or surgical release with salpingectomy after the vaginal vault is opened. Partial salpingectomy is often performed in deference to the scarring and adhesions surrounding the tube, ovary, bladder, and bowel. Total salpingectomy has been recommended to reduce the possibility of continued pain by traction on the remaining portion of the prolapsed tube. Prolapse into a hernia sac has also been reported and may be associated with gonadal dysgenesis.

Intussusception

Intussusception of the tube has been reported. A paraovarian cyst was engulfed by the end of the tube and pulled the fimbriated end into the ampulla. Simple eversion and cystectomy permitted tubal salvage.

Congenital Anomalies

Structural congenital anomalies of the tube are infrequent. Absence of a tubal segment, tubal duplication, and accessory tubes have all been noted. Accessory tubes may be present in as many as 6% to 13% of patients and most often are bilateral. Ectopic pregnancy has been seen in the accessory tube, and a percentage of the accessory tubes have been patent. Tubes may be absent in phenotypic females in certain cases, presumably as a result of asymptomatic torsion or generalized or localized failure in development of the müllerian duct.

OVARY

Non-neoplastic Tumors

Follicle Cysts

Follicle cysts of the ovary are the most commonly occurring cystic structures found in normal ovaries. These cysts arise from temporary pathologic variation of a normal physiologic process and are not neoplastic. The tumors result from either nonrupture of the dominant mature follicle or failure of an immature follicle to undergo the normal process of atresia, with absence of follicular fluid resorption. Abnormal release of anterior pituitary gonadotropins has been postulated as an etiologic factor. Many follicle cysts lose the ability to produce estrogen; in other instances, the granulosa cells remain productive with prolonged secretion of estrogen. Solitary follicle cysts are common and may occur during all stages of growth, from fetal life to menopause. They may be found in up to 68% of premenarchal ovaries, by sonography (usually less than 10 mm in diameter). The cysts are thin walled and unilocular, usually ranging from several millimeters to 8 cm in diameter, averaging 2 cm. Follicle cysts are lined by an inner layer of granulosa cells and an outer layer of theca interna cells.

Most follicle cysts are asymptomatic, and many are discovered incidentally. The thin wall surrounding the mass predisposes them to rupture, for instance during pelvic examination. Clinically a pelvic mass may be noted on examination or the patient may present with manifestations related to increased estrogen production, such as sexual precocity, menstrual disturbances, or endometrial hyperplasia. Less commonly, both follicular and corpus luteum cysts present with signs of rupture and intraperitoneal bleeding. Although this bleeding is usually of no clinical significance, it may at times be massive and operative intervention may be necessary. This complication is more common in patients with a predisposition to bleeding, such as those on anticoagulation therapy or with bleeding diatheses.

Management of suspected follicle cysts is conservative. Most resolve within 8 to 12 weeks of observation. Treating the patient with OCs may hasten resolution of the cyst. This management strategy also applies to the young patient treated by unilateral salpingo-oophorectomy for ovarian cancer who develops unilocular ovarian cysts post-treatment (Muram et al, 1990) and in the postmenopausal patient with a simple cyst up to 5 cm in size (Auslender et al, 1996). Management of persistent or large cysts is discussed later.

Corpus Luteum Cysts

Corpus luteum cysts are less prevalent than follicular cysts. Corpora lutea are not considered to be corpus luteum cysts unless their size is at least 3 cm in diameter. The cyst results from intracystic hemorrhage, occurring as a normal part of the stage of vascularization, 2 to 4 days after ovulation. Rapid and excessive bleeding may result in rupture and hematoperitoneum. Gradual and profuse bleeding results in enlargement of the cyst, and with persistence blood is replaced by clear fluid. These cysts are normally hormonally inactive, having an average diameter of 4 cm. The yellowish orange lining consists of luteinized granulosa and theca cells. When hemorrhage occurs, it is predominantly right-sided, possibly because of higher intraluminal pressure on the right side from differences in ovarian vein architecture.

Rupture characteristically occurs during days 20 to 26 of the menstrual cycle. Most patients present with acute pain of less than 24 hours in duration, although 23% of patients present with pain for a duration of 1 to 7 days. About 17% of patients report the onset of pain during sexual intercourse. Sonography may confirm the diagnosis of the cyst and the presence of intraperitoneal fluid. A negative serum β-human chorionic gonadotropin (β-hCG) titer will usually rule out a ruptured ectopic pregnancy. Culdocentesis reveals nonclotting blood, and if the hematocrit value on the fluid is less than or equal to 15%, the patient is often successfully observed. Should the patient demonstrate significant pain, falling hematocrit level, hypotension, or tachycardia, operative intervention is necessary. Laparoscopy confirms the diagnosis, and the bleeding is controlled with cautery or laser coagulation. Laparotomy may be required in the presence of massive or vigorous bleeding. The bleeding cyst may be excised or oversewn with preservation of the ovary. Anticoagulated patients have a 31% chance for subsequent hemorrhage from a recurrent corpus luteum cyst.

Multiple Follicular Cysts

Multiple cysts of follicular origin are usually associated with elevated levels of gonadotropins. Hyperreactio luteinalis is secondary to hCG stimulation. Multiple bilateral cysts produce moderate to marked enlargement of the ovaries. The cysts are filled with clear or hemorrhagic fluid and are lined by luteinized theca interna cells and, in some cases, granulosa cells. Marked stromal edema and prominent stromal luteinization are present. This condition is found in 10% to 37% of patients with trophoblastic disease and in patients with fetal hydrops and multiple gestations. About 60% of the cases of hyperreactio luteinalis unassociated with trophoblastic disease occur with a normal singleton pregnancy (Schnorr et al, 1996). The ovarian enlargement regresses postpartum and in the first 2 to 12 weeks after evacuation of a molar pregnancy. Virilization of the patient (but not the fetus) may occur, and hemoperitoneum from cyst rupture, torsion, or ascites is an uncommon complication. This benign process may be confused with an ovarian malignancy.

Multiple Theca Lutein Cysts

Multiple theca lutein cysts, which occur iatrogenically (e.g., following ovulation induction), are referred to as "ovarian hyperstimulation syndrome." Multiple bilateral follicular cysts may also occur in up to 75% of young girls with hypothyroidism. More than 50% of these patients exhibit sexual precocity and galactorrhea. Treatment of the hypothyroidism results in regression of the cysts. Multiple cystic ovaries have been described in infants born before the 30th week of gestation. The cysts are secondary to elevated levels of follicle-stimulating hormone (FSH) and luteinizing hormone (LH). Congenital deficiency of 17-hydroxylase results in low estrogen levels and secondarily elevated levels of FSH and LH with multicystic enlarged ovaries.

Neoplastic Tumors

Surface Epithelial Tumors

SURFACE PROLIFERATIVE LESIONS

Surface proliferative lesions are found on the ovary, often incidentally. Epithelial inclusion cysts arise from invaginations of the ovarian surface epithelium that have lost connection with the surface. Although most often found in postmenopausal women, the cysts can be seen in all age groups. Most are seen microscopically, but gross cysts up to 1 cm diameter may also be noted and are usually multiple. Proliferation of mesothelial cells on the ovarian surface is generally a response to pelvic inflammation and may mimic carcinoma. Nodular and papillary stromal projections from the ovarian surface are commonly found in the late reproductive and postmenopausal age groups. These projections are composed of hyalinized stroma covered by a single layer of surface epithelium.

COMMON EPITHELIAL TUMORS

Common epithelial tumors comprise 65% of all ovarian neoplasms, and are thought to evolve from the pelvic mesothelium (coelomic epithelium) as it reflects over the surface of the ovary. Consistent with the müllerian differentiation of the epithelial surface during the transformation to neoplasia, there are five major subtypes of common epithelial tumors: serous, which are similar to fallopian tube epithelium; endometrioid, which are similar to endometrial epithelium; mucinous, which are similar to endocervical epithelium; clear cell, which are similar to endometrial epithelium during pregnancy; and transitional cell (Brenner), which are similar to urothelial epithelium. Mixed epithelial tumors contain a significant component of a second or third of these subtypes, and account for 2% of benign tumors.

Common epithelial tumors are further classified into three subtypes; two are based on architectural appearance: (1) if the glandular component is largely cystic, the prefix "cyst" is used; and (2) if the stromal component is predominant, the tumor is classified as an adenofibroma. A third subtype is based on degree of differentiation: borderline (or atypically proliferating) tumors or carcinomas, which have low malignant potential, are not discussed in this chapter. The average age of patients with benign epithelial tumors is 45 years; these tumors rarely occur before puberty.

Benign *serous tumors* make up 25% of all benign ovarian neoplasms and 60% of all ovarian serous tumors. They are bilateral in 12% of cases. The cystic form ranges in size up to 30 cm (average 10 cm) and may present in a papillary or adenofibromatous pattern. The epithelium of serous tumors varies from a flat mesotheliod to a tall columnar type, sometimes containing cilia, resembling fallopian tube epithelium. Calcified granules (psammoma bodies) representing degenerated small papillae are often found.

Benign *endometrioid tumors* have the same morphology as endometrium, consisting of epithelial and stromal elements. These occur predominantly as unilateral cystadenofibromas in older women, averaging 10 cm in diameter. The epithelium is arranged in branching tubular glands and cystic spaces. This tends to represent a proliferative or atrophic pattern. One case associated with benign omental "implants" has been reported.

Benign *mucinous tumors* constitute 20% of all benign ovarian neoplasms and 75% of all mucinous ovarian tumors. These tumors are grossly cystic, multiloculated neoplasms that may reach 50 cm in diameter and 21 kg in weight. They are bilateral in 2% of cases, and are associated with a cystic teratoma in 5% of cases. Rarely, rupture may be associated with pseudomyxoma peritonei. Microscopically, they are lined by a single layer of uniform tall columnar cells with clear homogeneous cytoplasm. About one half show an endocervical pattern, and the other half an intestinal epithelial pattern.

Benign *clear cell tumors* are lined by flattened or cuboidal polyhedral cells with clear cytoplasm. Often, hobnail cells with nuclei protruding into the glandular lumens are present. The predominant histologic pattern is that of tubules, glandular areas, papillae, and cysts scattered within varying amounts of stroma. These tumors are generally bilateral and appear lobulated. The cut surfaces display a fine honeycomb appearance with minute cysts embedded in firm rubbery stroma. Only about a dozen cases have been reported.

Benign *transitional cell (Brenner) tumors* have cellular features similar to those of Walthard's nests, which are epithelial inclusions. These inclusions can most commonly be seen beneath the serosa of the fallopian tubes, and occasionally in the hilum of the ovaries. Comprising 1% of all primary ovarian tumors, they are generally benign. Most are microscopic or are discovered incidentally. Six per cent are bilateral. Grossly the tumors appear well circumscribed, firm, and rubbery. Microscopically there are sharply demarcated epithelial nests in a fibrous stroma.

Fibroma

Ovarian fibroma comprises 3% of all benign tumors. The majority are unilateral (>90%), found in the left ovary (70%), and benign. Most patients are in the older reproductive age group. This tumor is not hormonally active, but is uncommonly associated with ascites and Gorlin's syndrome. They range in size, are hard, are white to yellow, and may contain cysts.

The cut surfaces have a whorled appearance, and microscopically appear as bundles of spindle cells with bands of hyalinized fibrous tissue. Degeneration and calcification may occur in larger tumors.

Edema

Massive edema of the ovary results in ovarian enlargement, with an average diameter of 11 cm. The ovary has a shiny, white, smooth exterior, and the cut surface is solid, tan, and gelatinous. Microscopically, foci of luteinized cells are found within the diffuse edema in 40% of cases. The average age at presentation is 21 years. Presenting symptoms include abdominal or pelvic pain, menstrual irregularities, and abdominal distention. Pain may be of sudden onset and may mimic acute appendicitis. Androgenic manifestations are present in 20% of patients, with two thirds of these virilized and the remainder exhibiting hirsutism only (Siller et al, 1995). Only one reported patient had estrogenic effects, manifested by precocious puberty. Partial or complete torsion of the ovary occurs in 50% of patients with massive edema. Three patients have been reported to have Meig's syndrome. The differential diagnosis includes fibroma, sclerosing stromal tumor, Krukenberg's tumor, polycystic ovaries, and ovarian myxoma.

Etiology of the tumor is intermittent torsion causing partial obstruction of venous and lymphatic drainage. Alternatively, the process may begin as stromal proliferation, either fibromatosis or stromal hyperthecosis, causing enlargement of the ovary and promoting torsion with subsequent edema.

Treatment generally includes oophorectomy. Wedge resection with frozen section to exclude malignancy and fixation of the ovary to prevent torsion may be successful.

Fibromatosis

Ovarian fibromatosis exhibits a similar picture and is characterized by a proliferation of collagen-producing spindle cells. In rare cases luteinized cells are seen, and foci of stromal edema and sex cord elements are found in a minority of cases. Reported patient ages range from 13 to 39 years (average 25 years). Clinical signs include menstrual abnormalities, abdominal pain, and, less commonly, virilization and hirsuitism. The endocrine manifestations disappear after oophorectomy.

Sclerosing Stromal Tumors

The sclerosing stromal tumor of the ovary is a rare neoplasm. About 90 cases have been reported. These tumors are generally diagnosed in the 20- to 30-year age group, with 75% of patients younger than 30 years old. The most common presenting symptoms are menstrual irregularities (50%) and pelvic pain (27%), although infertility, anovulation, and amenorrhea do occur. All reported cases but one are unilateral, and 65% are noted in the right ovary. The tumors range in size from 1 to 20 cm and are mostly solid. Grossly, some cystic areas may be present and the solid areas are firm, nodular, and gray-white with tan-yellow foci. Microscopically, the tumor is composed of cellular lobules or "pseudolobules" separated by edematous hypocellular zones in some areas and sclerotic bands in others. Spindle cells are admixed with epithelioid cells containing neutral lipid. These tumors share antigenic determinants and morphologic features with thecomas, from which it is postulated they may arise. Elevated levels of androgens and estrogens are produced by the tumor, and virilization may rarely occur.

Nonspecific Mesenchymal Tumors

Nonspecific mesenchymal tumors are infrequent. Only 30 cases of ovarian *leiomyoma* have been documented. Uterine leiomyomas are usually also present. Nonspecific mesenchymal tumors originate from smooth muscle in the walls of blood vessels of the cortical stroma, in the corpus luteum, and in the ovarian ligaments.

Hemangioma is considered either a hamartomatous malformation or a true neoplasm and is associated with hemangiomas in other parts of the genital tract and with hemangiomatosis. These lesions range in size from several millimeters to 11 cm. Fewer than 40 cases have been recognized. These unilateral tumors are usually found incidentally. Associated findings include abdominal distention resulting from the large mass, acute abdominal pain from torsion, ascites, and thrombocytopenia.

Lymphangioma is an even rarer tumor of vascular origin, with fewer than 10 cases reported. Ovarian *myxoma* has been reported in fewer patients yet.

Tumors of cartilage, bone, fat, and neural origin are uncommon in the ovary. *Osteoma* and *chondroma* originate from ovarian stroma, by metaplasia. Two cases of *giant cell tumor* of the ovary, indistinguishable from the tumor that originates in the bone, have been reported. Few cases of *neurofibroma*, *ganglioneuroma*, *pheochromocytoma*, and *neurilemmoma* have been found.

Adenomatoid tumors are most frequently seen in the fallopian tube or broad ligament. Only six cases of ovarian tumors have been reported.

An *ovarian tumor of probable wolffian origin* has been described. This benign tumor must be differentiated from adenocarcinoma.

Structural Conditions

Torsion

Ovarian torsion is estimated to account for 3% of gynecologic operative emergencies. Ovarian torsion and tubal torsion are concurrent in most cases. Adnexal torsion usually occurs in the reproductive age group, notably in the mid-20s. Twenty per cent of patients are pregnant at the time of diagnosis. Adnexal torsion also occurs in postmenopausal women and has been noted in 6% of ovarian tumors (Koonings and Grimes, 1989). An ovarian tumor is discovered in 50% to 60% of patients with torsion, and the tumor is most often enlarged 8 to 12 cm. Torsion of normal adnexa may also occur, usually in children. The right ovary becomes torsed more often than the left, but bilateral torsion has been reported. Torsion of a malignant tumor accounts for a minority of cases.

Patients with ovarian torsion present with acute, severe, and unilateral lower abdominal pain. The pain may relate to an abrupt change in position. Two thirds of patients have nausea and vomiting, a finding that may lead to an incorrect diagnosis, such as appendicitis or small bowel obstruction. Intermittent episodes may precede the most acute episode by days or weeks. Venous and lymphatic obstruction produce edema and a tender mass. Approximately 10% of patients have a subsequent episode involving the contralateral ovary. Color-flow Doppler sonography may be used for diagnosis and for evaluating the recovery of the affected ovary after surgical treatment.

If the patient desires to preserve fertility, treatment should be conservative. When the diagnosis is suspected, diagnostic laparoscopy should be employed. The correct preoperative diagnosis is made in only 18% to 64% of cases. If the adnexa appear viable, they are untwisted and a cystectomy is performed (Shalev et al, 1995). The adnexa should be secured to prevent future episodes of torsion. If the ovary appears nonviable or gangrenous, however, resection is advisable.

Ovarian Remnant Syndrome

Ovarian remnant syndrome is a complication of bilateral salpingo-oophorectomy. The syndrome describes postoperative remnants of ovarian cortex that become functional and cystic. Patients present with pain and a mass and may exhibit signs of hyperestrogenism or even ureteral obstruction. A similar condition, known as *residual adnexal syndrome*, describes cystic, enlarged ovaries occurring after hysterectomy with ovarian conservation. This condition probably results from compromise of the ovarian arterial or venous blood flow.

Treatment of each of these conditions is complete surgical removal of the cystic remnants, including all of the wall and surrounding adhesions. This therapy is often complicated by dense postsurgical adhesions resulting from the original surgery and by the retroperitoneal or retrocolic position of the ovarian tissue (Siddall-Allum et al, 1994).

Supernumerary Ovary

The supernumerary ovary is one of the rarest gynecologic conditions; approximately 22 cases have been reported. This condition involves a third ovary lying separate from and without direct or ligamentous attachment to the normally placed ovary. The extra ovary (often found in the omentum), is not connected to the broad, utero-ovarian, or infundibulopelvic ligament. Development of tumors in this ovary, including dermoid, mucinous cystadenoma, serous cystadenoma, endometrioma, and Brenner's tumor, have been reported.

A supernumerary ovary should be distinguished from an *accessory ovary*, which lies near the eutopic ovary and has either a direct or ligamentous attachment or is attached to the broad, utero-ovarian, or infundibulopelvic ligaments. A *lobulated ovary* is one in which the ovarian anlage has been divided into two or more lobes, separated or connected by fibrous tissue or ovarian stroma. As many as one third of patients with these ovarian anomalies have other congenital genitourinary abnormalities.

Splenic-Ovarian Fusion

Splenic-ovarian fusion is uncommon. Three cases in the newborn have been described and are of the continuous type, in which a cord-like structure connects the spleen to the left ovary. Two of these cases are associated with partially undescended ovaries as well as with other multiple congenital anomalies. An additional case involves an adult female in whom a septate uterus and a cluster of splenic nodules surrounds the otherwise normal left ovary. Another adult case was described with the continuous type. Seven cases of an accessory spleen attached to an ovary have also been documented.

Paraneoplastic Syndromes

Paraendocrine (paraneoplastic) syndromes are reported predominantly with malignant ovarian tumors and occur in 5% of all ovarian cancers. This syndrome is an endocrine disorder associated with tumor derived from nonendocrine tissue. It results from the neoplastic synthesis of hormones thought not to be made by normal gynecologic tissue. When the syndrome is caused by an excess of hormone normally produced by gynecologic tissue, such as with masculinization or feminization, the tumor is "functioning." Functioning tumors represent 10% to 20% of ovarian tumors. Virilization (or feminization, after conversion of the excess androgen to estrogen) may occur with any ovarian tumor, resulting from stromal luteinization surrounding the tumor.

Few cases of paraendocrine syndrome associated with benign ovarian tumors have been reported, most commonly with *benign cystic teratoma* (dermoid). *Dermoid cysts* are associated with masculinization, hirsutism, hypoglycemia and Cushing's disease. Sixteen cases of acquired hemolytic anemia have been reported with a dermoid, and all patients entered remission after excision of the cyst. An ad-

ditional case of hemolytic anemia resolved after excision of a degenerated *ovarian cyst*. Thrombocytopenia has been reported with *ovarian hemangioma*, with normalization of the platelet count after excision of the affected ovaries. Two cases of hypoglycemia have been noted with *ovarian fibroma*, and were resolved upon removal of the tumor. Insulin intolerance and diabetes mellitus caused by a *thecoma-fibroma* has been reported, resolving after surgical excision. Nonthrombocytopenic purpura has occurred in association with *mucinous cystadenoma*. Finally, autonomic dysreflexia was reported with a benign ovarian cyst. The paroxysmal hypertension resolved after excision of the cyst.

Hereditary Syndromes

Hereditary syndromes involving benign ovarian tumors are uncommon. *Basal cell nevus* (Gorlin's syndrome) is a rare autosomal dominant disorder with associated ovarian fibromas and basal cell carcinomas of the skin, primordial cysts of the jaw, abnormalities of bone, and soft tissue calcification. These calcified fibromas are often bilateral. Familial occurrence of *benign teratoma* has been rarely reported. *Ovarian fibromas* have been reported in four generations of a single family.

McCune-Albright syndrome is a pediatric condition characterized by polyostotic fibrous dysplasia of bones, skin pigmentation, and sexual precocity. Follicular ovarian cysts are found in these children and may play a role in the development of the precocious puberty.

Evaluation of the Unilateral Adnexal Mass in the Young Female

The unilateral adnexal mass in the young female offers a diagnostic and management challenge. Because the majority of adnexal tumors are benign and future fertility is a concern, diagnosis and treatment should be conservative. In the reproductive-age woman, most adnexal masses are likely to be of gynecologic origin. Congenital abnormalities of the uterus are uncommon, as is the pelvic kidney. These abnormalities are usually ruled out with a sonogram to visualize the pelvis and the kidneys. In addition, an intrauterine pregnancy is ruled out by sonogram and serum β-hCG determinations.

Most ovarian masses in the young patient are nonneoplastic (functional) cysts. The sonogram exhibits a simple cyst, free of internal echoes, indicating the low risk of malignancy. Color Doppler ultrasonography may help discriminate benign from malignant tumors on the basis of vascular patterns and flow (Predanic et al, 1996). Functional cysts may reach large sizes of up to 10 cm, although most are smaller than 5 cm. Simple cystic masses smaller than 8 cm are usually observed through one menstrual cycle, necessitating a subsequent sonogram. Spanos (1973) observed 286 premenopausal patients with cystic masses for 6 weeks. The patients were treated with OCs to hasten resolution of the masses. The mass resolved in 72% of the women, and the likelihood of resolution was proportional to the size of the mass. Tumors in the range of 4 to 6 cm resolved 84% of the time, those 6 to 8 cm resolved in 56% of patients, and cysts 8 to 10 cm in size disappeared in only 38% of cases. Of the 81 patients with a persistent mass who underwent laparotomy, no functional cysts were found. Endometrioma comprised 35% of the cysts, and benign teratoma accounted for 11%.

Endometriosis, tubal pregnancy, tubo-ovarian abscess, and uterine leiomyomas may present and may be accompanied by pelvic discomfort and menstrual abnormalities. These conditions usually exhibit a complex cystic or solid appearance. The CA-125 serum test may be used to evaluate the patient for ovarian cancer, but the result must be interpreted cautiously. Because ovarian cancer is uncommon in the premenopausal woman, a positive test caused by cancer is also uncommon. The proportion of false-positive tests, therefore, is increased. The most common cause of a false-positive finding is endometriosis, but the CA-125 test may also be positive from uterine leiomyomas, PID, and pregnancy. Serial serum β-hCG studies and serum progesterone levels may contribute to the diagnosis of tubal pregnancy. Any mass that is solid, persistent, or cystic and greater than 8 cm usually requires operative laparoscopy or laparotomy for proper diagnosis (Russell, 1995).

PERITONEUM, RETROPERITONEUM, AND PARA-ADNEXAL STRUCTURES

Mesothelium

Benign Cystic Mesothelioma

An uncommon condition of the peritoneum, benign cystic mesothelioma is characterized by multiple free and attached cysts lined by cytologically bland mesothelial cells (Yaegashi and Yajima, 1996). Although this condition was first described in 1928, the clinical behavior and etiology are still ill-defined. About 83% of the patients are women, with a mean age of 37 years. The most common presenting symptoms are chronic pelvic and abdominal pain. Many patients have a past history of celiotomy, 14% have had PID, and 7% have endometriosis. Cysts may range from a few millimeters up to 6 kg. Although the condition is considered benign, recurrences may be expected in 45% of patients observed for at least 1 year. Colon obstruction has been observed. Benign cystic mesothelioma must be differentiated from other reactive mesothelial lesions, cysts of lymphatic origin, and neoplasms such as adenomatoid tumor, mesothelioma, serous carcinoma of the ovary or peritoneum, and cystic lymphangioma. One case in a 2-year-old girl has been reported, preoperatively diagnosed as intra-abdominal lymphangioma. One case of calcification of the cysts in a 79-year-old women was presented, with a preoperative diagnosis of adrenal tumor or peritoneal teratoma.

Treatment consists of complete surgical excision (laparoscopy or laparotomy), with reoperation for symptomatic recurrences as needed. Response has been noted during treatment with GnRHa therapy, with regrowth noted during hormonal add-back.

Mesothelial Hyperplasia

Mesothelial hyperplasia appears as unifocal or multifocal small nodules or granulations of the peritoneum. These hyperplastic lesions may develop in response to inflammation and are found incidentally. Histologically appearing as solid, trabecular, or complex papillary or tubulopapillary patterns, these lesions display reactive atypia, mitotic activity, multinucleated cells, and limited degrees of infiltration, mimicking malignancy. Because these benign lesions may proceed to mesothelioma, patients must be followed closely. Mesothelial hyperplasia can be seen in conjunction with ovarian tumors and must be differentiated from metastatic deposits. Mucinous ascites may result.

Nonspecific Tumors

A benign melanotic complex peritoneal cyst has been described. By light and electron microscopy, the lesion imitated the pigmentation process of the skin.

Ascites

Ascites is generally associated with the presence of malignancy, most often ovarian. Ascites also occurs in association with benign ovarian tumors and with other conditions. Inflammatory conditions involving the peritoneum are uncommonly associated with ascites. Examples include lupus peritonitis, small intestinal inflammation or obstruction, PID, spontaneous bacterial peritonitis and tuberculous peritonitis, and transperitoneal migration of *Trichomonas*. Additional benign miscellaneous conditions associated with ascites include heart, liver, pancreatic, and renal disease, pre-eclampsia, ovarian hyperstimulation syndrome, intravenous leiomyomatosis, and endometriosis.

Meig's Syndrome

Meig's syndrome describes serous ascites and hydrothorax, associated with a benign ovarian fibroma or thecoma, which resolves upon removal of the tumor (Lacson et al, 1989). Ascites occurs in fewer than 1% of these tumors overall but is found in 40% of tumors larger than 10 cm in diameter. Hydrothorax is right-sided in two thirds of patients and bilateral in one quarter. *Pseudo–Meig's syndrome* refers to this condition associated with other ovarian tumors or tumors of other gynecologic origin. Included are ovarian leiomyoma, hemangioma, cystadenoma, benign cystic teratoma, struma ovarii, Brenner's tumor, broad ligament leiomyoma, and uterine leiomyoma.

Pseudomyxoma Peritonei

Pseudomyxoma peritonei refers to mucinous ascites from both benign and malignant tumors. This is to be differentiated from the serous or serosanguinous ascites noted above. The most common benign source of mucinous ascites is ovarian mucinous cystadenoma, followed by mucocele of the appendix. One case of ascites resulting from a mucinous adenoma of the fallopian tube has been reported, and two cases of endometriosis with myxoid change have resulted in mucinous ascites. We have seen one case, treated by monthly paracenteses, of a woman treated many years before for endometrial cancer who subsequently developed mesothelial hyperplasia. Because of the high viscosity of the mucus, repeated episodes of bowel obstruction may result in multiple laparotomies. Laparotomy with aggressive cytoreduction is important for controlling the reaccumulation of fluid (Sullivan and Sugarbaker, 1995). Retroperitoneal extension of the fluid presenting as a retroperitoneal cystic mass has been reported. Use of the argon beam coagulator or surgical ultrasonic aspirator may facilitate tumor removal. Intraperitoneal photodynamic therapy and radiotherapy have also been used with some success. Mixed results have occurred from the use of agents instilled into the peritoneal cavity to reduce viscosity of the ascites and to increase the efficacy of paracentesis. The solutions used include mucolytic agents (acetylcysteine), lytic enzymes (hyaluronidase, urokinase), and starches (2% to 10% dextran sulfate, 2% to 10% dextrose and water).

Leiomyomatosis Peritonealis Disseminata

Solid benign neoplasms of the peritoneum are uncommon. Leiomyomatosis peritonealis disseminata is a rare disorder characterized by multiple small nodules composed of smooth muscle and resembling carcinomatosis (Raspagliesi et al, 1996). About 60 cases have been described. Grossly, these nodules are usually gray-white, firm, and 1 to 2 cm in diameter. Excess exogenous or endogenous estrogen may be a predisposing factor, because 50% of patients have been pregnant at the time of diagnosis and one quarter of patients have a history of OC use. Five cases of malignant degeneration have been reported.

Cytoreduction of the nodules is the recommended treatment, with removal of the uterus, ovaries, and fallopian tubes if fertility is not a consideration. The nodules may regress after castration and may respond to progesterone therapy.

Splenosis

Splenosis is the autotransplantation of splenic tissue that follows traumatic rupture of the spleen and may mimic abdominal carcinomatosis. Because of the sometimes bluish appearance, the lesions may also be mistaken for endometriosis (Matonis and Luciano, 1995). These implants are most often asymptomatic and are discovered incidentally. Intraabdominal or intestinal hemorrhage occurs in a small percentage, however. Because these implants compensate in part for the asplenic state and are immunologically active, they should not be removed.

Gliomatosis

Gliomatosis is also found occasionally, characterized by multiple firm glial nodules. Although this condition is most often associated with an immature teratoma of the ovary, it has also been reported congruent with endometriosis, with mature teratoma of the ovary, and with a ventriculoperitoneal shunt. No therapy is required.

Para-adnexal Structures

Supporting Ligaments

Tumors of the supporting ligaments of the uterus are uncommon. Leiomyoma is the most commonly diagnosed benign tumor of the round ligament. Mesenchymoma, myolipoma, thecoma, and mesothelial cysts have also been reported. Leiomyoma is the prevalent benign neoplasm found in the broad ligament, but thecoma, lipoma, Brenner's tumor, and papillary cystadenoma (in association with von Hippel–Lindau disease) have also been described. Female adnexal tumor of probable wolffian origin has been reported within the broad ligament, and can present with abdominal pain. The most common tumor of the uterosacral ligament is endometriosis. Leiomyomas and mature teratoma occur rarely.

Paraovarian Tumors

Paraovarian tumors, predominantly cystic and benign, account for 10% of adnexal masses. Generally found in women of reproductive age, these tumors are usually small, asymptomatic, and incidentally discovered at laparotomy. The cysts can become quite large (up to 35 cm), however, and may cause pelvic pain, menstrual disturbances, or adnexal torsion, or present as an inguinal hernia (Azzena et al, 1994). Two thirds of the cysts arise from the mesothelium lining peritoneal inclusions, 30% from tubal epithelial (paramesonephric) origin, and 2% from mesonephric (wolffian) remnants. Identifying a separate, normal ipsilateral ovary by sonography may aid in preoperative diagnosis.

Paratubal Cysts

Paratubal cysts are found adjacent to the tube. They are generally smaller than 1 cm in diameter and are usually near the fimbriated end. Seventy-six per cent of these cysts are of paramesonephric (müllerian) origin; they are termed *hydatids of Morgagni* and represent accessory lumina. The remainder are derived from mesothelium. One case each of a leiomyoma and of a transitional cell carcinoma have been reported arising in a paratubal cyst (Thomason et al, 1995). These cysts are usually discovered incidentally and require no therapy.

Retroperitoneum

Fibrosis

Retroperitoneal fibrosis (Ormond's disease) is an uncommon condition primarily occurring between the third and sixth decades of life. Grossly appearing as a flat grayish white plaque of varying thickness, fibrosis envelops and obstructs structures of the retroperitoneal space, including the ureters, nerves, arteries, veins, and occasionally intestine. The most frequent presenting complaint is dull, colicky pain localized in the back, flank, or abdomen. Other symptoms include weight loss, gastrointestinal complaints, leg edema, and fever.

Excretory urography, computerized tomography, ultrasound, color Doppler imaging, and magnetic resonance imaging all help to establish the diagnosis. More than two thirds of patients have the idiopathic form, but 25% of cases are caused by methylsergide, a drug used for migraine headaches. A case has been reported in a patient taking a related drug, pergolide, for Parkinson's disease. Etiologic factors in the remaining patients include malignancy, surgery, radiation, trauma, retroperitoneal hemorrhage, urine extravasation, and genitourinary infection. Treatment involves surgical (laparoscopic) relief of ureteral obstruction, and suppression of the inflammatory process with immunosuppressive drugs (e.g., corticosteroids; Boeckmann et al, 1996). Successful low-dose methotrexate therapy has been reported in one patient, and tamoxifen in another. Lifelong anticoagulation should be considered for patients with vascular obstruction.

Fibromatosis

Fibromatosis (desmoid tumor) is unusual and may occur at any location in the abdominal cavity, including the pelvis (Antoniuk et al, 1993). Characterized by interlacing benign fibroblasts that are locally invasive, it is most commonly diagnosed in patients from 20 to 40 years of age, often during pregnancy. The rate of tumor growth appears to be estrogen responsive, and regression has been reported following menopause and with tamoxifen treatment. Wide radical local excision is the treatment of choice, but

recurrence is common. *Neurofibromatosis* of the genitourinary tract has rarely been reported.

Neoplasia

Retroperitoneal tumors are uncommon, and benign tumors account for only 20% of the group (Nuzzo et al, 1996). The benign neoplasms are classified as:

1. Tumors of *mesodermal* origin (lipoma, leiomyoma, fibroma, rhabdomyoma, lymphangioma, hemangioma, xanthogranuloma, mucinous cystadenoma)
2. Tumors of *neurogenous* origin (neurilemmoma, neurofibroma, ganglioneuroma, Schwannoma)
3. Tumors arising from *embryonic remnants* (mature teratoma)

Most patients present with abdominal pain and mass. Retroperitoneal cysts are much less common than solid tumors. These are classified as wolffian, chylous, dermoid, mesocolic, parasitic, or traumatic cysts. Complete excision of retroperitoneal tumors prevents recurrence. Benign neoplasms arise in retroperitoneal lymph nodes and may present as an ovarian mass. Reported benign nodal tumors include müllerian glandular inclusions, ectopic decidua, endometriosis, endosalpingiosis, nevus cell aggregates, leiomyomatosis, hemangioma, and lipoma.

Mesenteric Tumors

Tumors of the mesentery are more commonly cystic than solid (Liew et al, 1994). The classification and spectrum of solid tumors are the same as with the retroperitoneal tumors. Cystic masses are classified as

1. *Embryonic* and *developmental* (enteric, urogenital, lymphoid, dermoid, embryonic defects [i.e., chylous])
2. *Traumatic* or *acquired* (chylous)
3. *Neoplastic*
4. *Infective* or *degenerative*

Chylous and lymphatic cysts are most common. About 50% of cysts are found in the small intestine (usually ileal) mesentery and 30% in the mesocolon. The most common presenting symptom is abdominal pain, followed by nausea, vomiting, constipation and diarrhea. An abdominal mass is noted in 50% of cases. Less than 3% are malignant. Treatment includes excision or enucleation, sometimes requiring intestinal resection for complete removal. At operation, these lesions may be confused with duplication cysts of the intestine.

REFERENCES

Abdul-Karim RW, Badaway SZA, Adelson MD, et al: Uterine hemorrhage due to arteriovenous malformation in a teenage girl: diagnosis and management. Adolesc Pediatr Gynecol 1989;2:235.

Antoniuk P, Tjandra JJ, Lavery IC: Diffuse intra-abdominal fibromatosis in association with bilateral ovarian fibromatosis and oedema. Aust N Z J Surg 1993;63:315.

Auslender R, Atlas I, Lissak A, et al: Follow-up of small, postmenopausal ovarian cysts using vaginal ultrasound and CA-125 antigen. J Clin Ultrasound 1996;24:175.

Azzena A, Quintieri F, Salmaso R: A voluminous paraovarian cyst: case report. Clin Exp Obstet Gynecol 1994;21:249.

Bates GW, Wiser WL: A technique for uterine conservation in adolescents with vaginal agenesis and a function uterus. Obstet Gynecol 1985;66:290.

Benagiano G, Kivinen ST, Fadini R, et al: Zoladex (goserelin acetate) and the anemic patient: results of a multicenter fibroid study. Fertil Steril 1996;66:223.

Boeckmann W, Wolff JM, Adam G, et al: Laparoscopic bilateral ureterolysis in Ormond's disease. Urol Int 1996;56:133.

Cohen I, Beyth Y, Shapira J, et al: High frequency of adenomyosis in postmenopausal breast cancer patients treated with tamoxifen. Gynecol Obstet Invest 1997;44:200.

Cravello L, Pinelli L, Heckenroth H, et al: Contribution of hysteroscopic surgery for the treatment of postmenopausal menorrhagia. Presse Med 1998;27:1267.

Fekete PS, Vellios F: The clinical and histologic spectrum of endometrial stromal neoplasms: a report of 41 cases. Int J Gynecol Pathol 1984;3:198.

Gimpelson RJ, Rappold HO: A comparative study between panoramic hysteroscopy with directed biopsies and dilatation and curettage: a review of 276 cases. Am J Obstet Gynecol 1988;158:489.

Gisser SD: Obstructing fallopian tube papilloma. Int J Gynecol Pathol 1986;5:179.

Gordon JD, Hopkins KL, Jeffrey RB, Giudine LC: Adnexal torsion: color Doppler diagnosis and laparoscopic treatment. Fertil Steril 1994;61:383.

Greeley C, Schroeder S, Silverberg SG: Microglandular hyperplasia of the cervix: a true "pill" lesion? Int J Gynecol Pathol 1995;14:50.

Hellen EA, Coghill SB, Clark JV: Prolapsed fallopian tube after abdominal hysterectomy: a report of the cytological findings. Cytopathology 1993;4:181.

Kang J, Baxi L, Heller D: Tamoxifen-induced growth of leiomyomas: a case report. J Reprod Med 1996;41:119.

Klintorp S, Grinsted L, Franzmann MB: Adenomatoid tumor of the uterus. Eur J Obstet Gynecol Reprod Biol 1993;50:255.

Koonings PP, Grimes DA: Adnexal torsion in postmenopausal women. Obstet Gyncol 1989;73:11.

Lacson AG, Alrabeeah A, Gillis DA, et al: Secondary massive ovarian edema with Meig's syndrome. Am J Clin Pathol 1989;91:597.

Liew SC, Glenn DC, Storey DW: Mesenteric cyst. Aust N Z J Surg 1994;64:741.

Longacre TA, Chung MH, Rouse RV, Hendrickson MR: Atypical polypoid adenomyofibromas (atypical polypoid adenomyomas) of the uterus: a clinicopathologic study of 55 cases. Am J Surg Pathol 1996;20:1.

Lumsden MA, West CP, Thomas E, et al: Treatment with the gonadotrophin releasing hormone-agonist goserelin before hysterectomy for uterine fibroids. Br J Obstet Gynaecol 1994;101:438.

Matonis LM, Luciano AA: A case of splenosis masquerading as endometriosis. Am J Obstet Gynecol 1995;173:971.

Muram D, Gale CL, Thompson E: Functional ovarian cysts in patients cured of ovarian neoplasms. Obstet Gynecol 1990;75:680.

Murphy AA, Morales AJ, Kettel LM, Yen SS: Regression of uterine leiomyomata to the antiprogesterone RU486: dose-response effect. Fertil Steril 1995;64:187.

Neri A, Kaplan B, Rabinerson D, et al: Cervical polyp in the menopause and the need for fractional dilatation and curettage. Eur J Obstet Gynecol Reprod Biol 1995;26:53.

Niver DH, Borrette G, Jewelewicz R: Congenital atresia of the uterine cervix and vagina: three cases. Fertil Steril 1980;33:25.

Nuzzo G, Lemmo G, Trischitta MM, et al: Retroperitoneal cystic lymphangioma. J Surg Oncol 1996;61:234.

Petterson B, Adami H-O, Lindgren A: Endometrial polyps and hyperplasia as risk factors for endometrial carcinoma. Acta Obstet Gynecol Scand 1985;64:653.

Predanic M, Vlahos N, Pennisi JA, et al: Color and pulsed Doppler sonography, gray-scale imaging, and serum CA125 in the assessment of adnexal disease. Obstet Gynecol 1996;88:283.

Raspagliesi F, Quattrone P, Grosso G, et al: Malignant degeneration in leiomyomatosis peritonealis disseminata. Gynecol Oncol 1996;61:272.

Reiter RC, Wagner PL, Gambone JC: Routine hysterectomy for large asymptomatic uterine leiomyomata: a reappraisal. Obstet Gynecol 1992;79:481.

Reuter KL, Young SB, Daly B: Hematometra complicating conization with radiologic correlation: a case report. J Reprod Med 1994;39:408.

Russell DJ: The female pelvic mass: diagnosis and management. Med Clin North Am 1995;79:1481.

Schnorr JA, Miller H, Davis JR, et al: Hyperreactio luteinalis associated with pregnancy: a case report and review of the literature. Am J Perinatol 1996;13:95.

Seidman JD, Tavassoli FA: Mesonephric hyperplasia of the uterine cervix: a clinicopathologic study of 51 cases. Int J Gynecol Pathol 1995;14:293.

Shalev E, Bustan M, Yaron I, Peleg D: Recovery of ovarian function after laparoscopic detorsion. Hum Reprod 1995;10:2965.

Siddall-Allum J, Rae T, Rogers V, et al: Chronic pelvic pain caused by residual ovaries and ovarian remnants. Br J Obstet Gynaecol 1994;101:979.

Siller BS, Gelder MS, Alvarez RD, Partridge EE: Massive edema of the ovary associated with androgenic manifestations. South Med J 1995;88:1153.

Spanos WJ: Preoperative hormonal therapy of cystic adnexal masses. Am J Obstet Gynecol 1973;116:551.

Sullivan MH, Sugarbaker PH: Treatment of pseudomyxoma peritonei in a geriatric patient population. J Surg Oncol 1995;58:121.

Thomason RW, Rush W, Dave H: Transitional cell carcinoma arising within a paratubal cyst: report of a case. Int J Gynecol Pathol 1995;14:270.

Ueki M, Okamoto Y, Tsurunaga T, et al: Endocrinological and histological changes after treatment of uterine leiomyomas with danazol or buserelin. J Obstet Gynaecol 1995;21:1.

Vercellini P, Parazzini F, Oldani S, et al: Adenomyosis at hysterectomy: a study on frequency distribution and patient characteristics. Hum Reprod 1995;10:1160.

Yaegashi N, Yajima A: Multilocular peritoneal inclusion cysts (benign cystic mesothelioma): a case report. J Obstet Gynaecol Res 1996;22:129.

Yamashita Y, Takahashi M, Katabuchi H, et al: Adenoma malignum: MR appearances mimicking nabothian cysts. AJR Am J Roentgenol 1994;162:649.

32

Chronic Pelvic Pain

John S. McDonald

Pain in the gynecology patient is often difficult to deal with for members of the health care team at large. This diverse group of physicians includes family physicians, internists, neurologists, gynecologists, and pain practitioners. The reasons for this are varied but certainly involve the fact that pelvic pain can be expressed as either pelvic or abdominal pain, can be heavily influenced by emotional factors, and can be difficult to diagnose because of the multiple innervation pathways. Consultation for pain in strictly the pelvic area is often sought only after significant agony is endured by the patient, perhaps partly because the patient is loath to seek medical advice regarding her sexual organs unless the pain is really unbearable or not manageable with over-the-counter drugs.

This chapter offers a practical differential guide for doctors confronted with the complaint of chronic pelvic pain, outlining many of the various gynecologic and associated pelvic disorders that may be involved in the causation of the chronic pelvic pain disorders. It also covers the contribution of the chronic pain specialist to consultation and treatment of patients with chronic pelvic pain seen by specialists in many fields. Success in management of these patients must begin with a consideration of possible etiologies for pain other than those classically attributable to pelvic pain (i.e., organ pathologic processes). To accomplish this, the chapter focuses on the work-up and diagnosis of various etiologies of pelvic pain. In addition, the chapter stresses, from the outset, very important and often overlooked psychological aspects of disease processes and the problems created by them. The overall objective is to acquaint the obstetrician-gynecologist with a new, fresh, and practical approach to assisting the patient with a complaint of various gynecologic and associated pelvic disorders, so that both the physician's and patient's time will not be wasted on performing endless diagnostic and operative procedures. An appropriate time for referral to a bona fide chronic pain specialist must be recognized by the physician during his or her treatment of the patient with pelvic pain.

NEUROPATHY AS A SOURCE OF CHRONIC PELVIC PAIN

In many instances the gynecologist treating a patient with chronic pelvic pain is looking for any abnormal pathology as determined by organopathology. The reason for this orientation is that most obstetrics-gynecology training courses and clinical-pathologic conferences are centered around the concept of pelvic pain caused by organ disease processes. That concept is one of the barriers to diagnosis of pelvic pain. The primary focus of the concept is based upon organ pathology, including myoma, adenomyosis, endometrial polyps, functional cysts, and hemorrhagic ovarian cysts. This focus is so intense that physicians may be unaware of other cause of pelvic pain, such as specific point neuropathy. There have even been instances where all pelvic organs have been removed for pelvic pain without achieving effective pain relief (Baskin and Tanagho, 1992). Often the neuropathies are the primary problem in producing and generating the very intense state of pelvic pain that women have. The causes of such neuropathies can include pregnancy itself, with the stretching and growth that occurs, and the various traumas associated with pregnancy, such as the delivery of a large baby through a narrow pelvis, which could result in stretch and compression during or in the second stage of labor (Swash et al, 1985). Gynecologists in England are very much aware of this problem. For years, they have believed that pregnancy itself as well as pushing in the second stage can cause nerve stretch and resultant damage. Subsequently, women can develop neuropathies that involve the sacral outflow tracts and have malfunction and problems associated with all types of activity after delivery (Snooks et al, 1985). At Ohio State University, my colleagues and I are investigating many possible types of stretch problems of the pudendal nerve by analysis of magnetic resonance imaging (MRI) studies in an attempt to link these problems to possible etiologies, because the course of the pudendal nerve through the pelvis is so long and tortuous. In this way, we can examine what amount of stretch may occur during delivery of a baby. We may be able to show that a few millimeters of stretch can be enough to produce a stretch neuropathy.

I believe that many of the abdominal neuropathies are iatrogenic and caused during various surgical procedures (Miyazaki and Shook, 1992). One of these is the Pfannensteil incision with use of retractors. With the Pfannensteil incision, maximum pull and stretch may occur along the anatomic pathways of the ilioinguinal and the iliohypogastric nerves (Hameroff et al, 1981). Such stretching may subsequently result in pelvic pain only after several months or years (Reiter, 1990). Typically, during the development period, the pain may increase incrementally month by month until it peaks at a pain level near or at 10 on a scale from 1 to 10. Often, the patient perceives this pain to be pelvic in origin, despite the fact that it emanates from the lower lateral abdominal quadrants.

Generally speaking, there are three sensory inputs to the pelvis: (1) sympathetic, (2) parasympathetic, and (3) visceral somatic afferent (McDonald, 1996).

One of the important aspects of pelvic pain is based on what I believe is a very important neuropathy model (Sommer et al, 1995). To appreciate this model, one must understand that the nerve's vessels begin on the outside of the nerve structurally at the nerve's origin, and that they penetrate deeper and deeper along the pathway of the nerve. In a sense the vessels enshroud the nerve like a stocking. Figure 32–1 shows the rich vascularity as the vessels go deep to the nerve core, where one blood vessel is positioned in the center. All over the body these nerves penetrate into and through the middle of muscle tissue. So when there is compression from the outside, such as muscle spasm or injury, the mechanics of contraction and the effect upon the vessels result in an embarrassed vascular supply. When this occurs, the nerve transmits signals centrally that connect to the central nervous system (CNS), via first the spinal cord, then the brain. The initial stimulus may be in the form of a nerve action potential that may be interpreted centrally as the simple existence of a problem at the point of injury or the point of

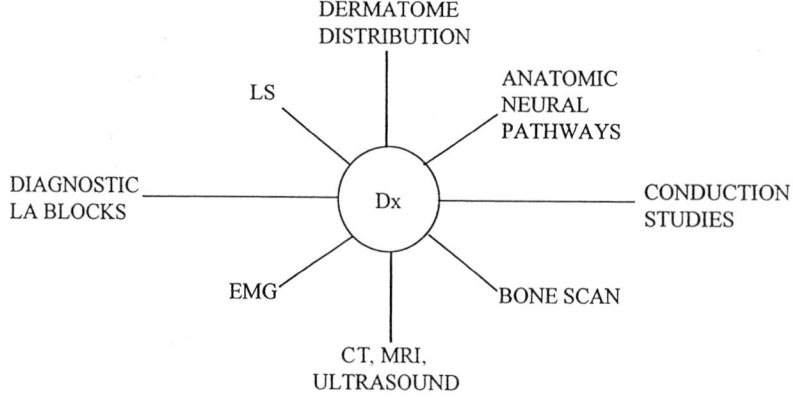

Figure 32–1
Schematic illustration of the components of the work-up for chronic pelvic pain. CT, computerized tomography, Dx, diagnostics; EMG, electromyography; LA, local anesthetic; LS, laparoscopy; MRI, magnetic resonance imaging.

input. However, eventually the DRG, which serves as the overall gate for incoming signals, may develop an intrinsic signal that may subserve the signal input from the area initially involved. After a period of time, the DRG may perpetuate such a signal even in the absence of any further painful input from the affected area (Garrison and Foreman, 1994).

The type of pain generated from a neuropathic injury is not beneficial to the patient because it may allow the development of such self-sustaining pain generators, emphasizing the negative aspects of pain signaling. One of the prime benefits of identifying such a pain generator is to eradicate the pain signal from the local area by decreasing the stimulus level enough so that the dorsal root ganglion (DRG) receives progressively weaker signaling. In doing so, it is possible to reach a balance point at which the signal is so weak that it may no longer be sensed by the spinal cord and thus is not propagated onto the brain. This technique is exactly the one used in repetitive local anesthetic nerve blockade. In the majority of patients there may be sufficient response over time such that some patients may be considered "cured" or pain free. Others may have substantial reductions in their pain states to the point that they can begin regular and normal functioning again. Pelvic pain patients are not simple cases to manage, how-ever, and some patients, even with regular improvements, may experience little pain relief because of depression and anxiety or other psychological factors.

PATIENT WORK-UP

The work-up begins on day 1 of the patient's visit with the history and physical exam, including a pelvic exam. A psychological interview is completed to assess any emotional component to the patient's pain because this can have a significant impact on treatment outcome. Finally, any necessary diagnostic studies are scheduled.

History

In the initial work up of patients with pelvic pain, a thorough history must occur first. During this time it is imperative to be a good listener. A careful discussion about location, what type of pain is present, and other specific aspects of the pain in regard to its relief and radiation must be carried out. All chronic pain patients have had their histories taken over and over again. It is frustrating for the patient to endlessly repeat these details of pain history. To avoid further repetition, the history can be recorded on a

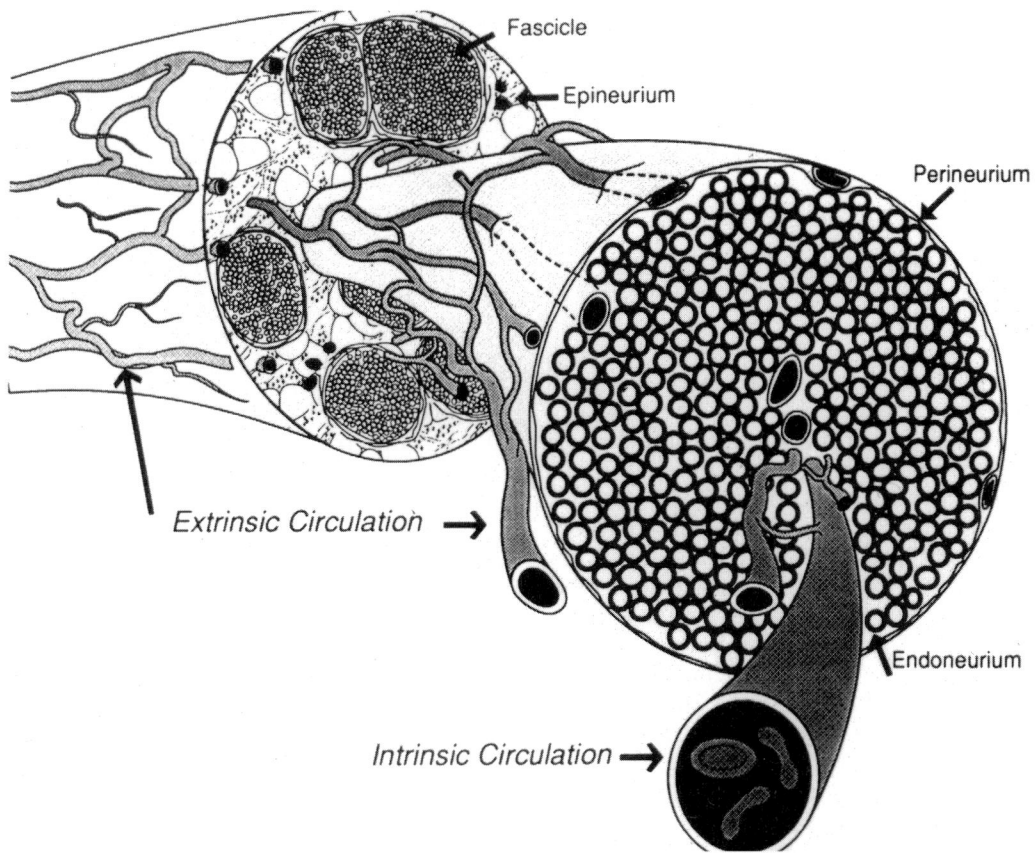

Figure 32-2
Schematic representation of the circulation in peripheral nerves. Extrinsic vessels connected to the intrinsic vasculature are vulnerable to compressive forces.

standardized form such as that shown in Figure 32–3. In addition, one of the quick reference unisex diagrams can be used to record information such as tender points (Fig. 32–4). A very quick reference to these forms can reorient the physician on return visits so that historical details do not have to be repeated.

Often pelvic pain patients have seen multiple other physicians. They may have undergone laparotomy, laparoscopy, hysterectomy, removal of tubes or ovaries or both. Some have repeated surgeries for adhesions. Some have had work-ups that include computerized tomography (CT) scans or MRIs. During the history it is important to determine, in chronologic order, the physicians who have been consulted, the diagnostic tests they instituted, the procedures they used in either diagnosis or therapy, and the medications they prescribed. Also, because the history is so focused on the pain, it is important to get some idea as to the impact the pain has had upon the function of the patient. This part of the pain history is vital because it not only illustrates the degree of difficulty the patient has had in the past but it can also be used as a reference to determine future improvement based upon the treatment regimens.

It is important to listen to the patient explain the aspects of her problem herself. A thorough history should include the salient points the patient wants to bring out; however, the physician must carefully lead the patient to make sure she stays focused on the important facts and features of her pain. Salient features include circumstances that were operative at the time the pain began, the location and migration of the pain, and the circumstances that make the pain worse or better.

Physical Exam

The initial physical exam must also be carefully carried out with strict attention to areas that may have been contributory to the pelvic pain. The examination of the abdomen, back, and lower extremities is key in ruling in or out problems that may be primary or secondary in regard to causation. The physical exam should be focused primarily upon the area of complaint that the patient has and be detailed in regard to sensorimotor function, reflexes, and obvious visual changes that are noticeable. Particular attention should be given to the pelvic organs and other tissues in respect to their anatomic relationship with nearby nerves, as well as specific innervation of pain areas during stimulation and attempts to re-create the exact pain sensations. One of the very important characteristics that differentiates the pain examination from other medical examinations. For example, if the patient has pain in her right pelvic area, the physical should begin with the abdomen and include the lower extremities. In the process of examining these areas, the physician must attempt to elicit pain by superficial and deep pressure exerted by either the examining finger or a prop such as the blunt end of a pen or pencil.

In the past, there was a tendency to encourage pain specialists to do a complete physical examination on every patient to avoid missing something that may play a role in the generation of the pain process. In cases where a patient comes to the office as a self-referral, does not have a family physician, and has not had a routine physical examination, it is of course best to complete an entire physical examination. However, when the patient is referred by her own physician, who requests a consultation for pelvic pain, then it is expensive, time consuming, and unacceptable to repeat an entire basic physical exam. In such cases, the pain medicine physical exam may be limited to the area of the pain and the areas immediately adjacent. There are some instances where restricted "area" exams may result in missed diagnoses, but this can be kept at a minimum by making sure all diagnoses include all possible contingent areas.

Pelvic Exam

The pelvic exam comprises observation of the external genitalia, Bartholin's glands, hymen, vagina, and cervix, and palpation of the cervix, uterus, vulva, ovaries, and rectovaginal septum. An important step in differentiating an abdominal versus a pelvic origin of pain is the pelvic exam. Individual maximum tender points are identified and then a comparison of the responses to abdominal versus the pelvic digital pressure can be made (Fig. 32–5). With this assessment, it becomes clear which area is the primary pain location. This pain localization can be simplified with instructions to the patient to raise her head and contract the abdominus rectus muscles. This maneuver results in maximal pain above the rectus sheath and localizes the pain to the abdomen, not pelvis.

One of the important skills in identification of pain is how to correctly use the examining hands and fingers during the physical exam. A certain level of skill must be attained in regard to discovery of these maximum tender points. Often the only examining skill medical students are taught in regard to use of their hands and fingers is in physical diagnosis, where they are taught the four basic skills of observation, percussion, palpation, and auscultation. Even then only percussion and palpation demand manual function. The use of the hands to determine painful areas in and around the area of primary pain complaint is a skill that is very important, and one that is often taught very informally and without any organized approach. Nevertheless, it is this very skill that must be learned and learned well if one is determined to work in the area of pain management. Pelvic pain diagnosis demands an extensive and experienced knowledge of the pelvic area and its anatomy and physiology. It is senseless to have general pain management specialists, who are anesthesiologists with some informal training in pain diagnosis and management, do pelvic examinations on patients when they have had no formal training in pelvic proce-

INITIAL PAIN EVALUATION   NAME:_____

DATE:_____

ROOM:_____

The Ohio State University Center for Pain Control

Columbus, Ohio

MULTIDISCIPLINARY PAIN CENTER

Initial Pain Evaluation

HISTORY:_____

_____

_____

_____

_____

_____

_____

_____

_____

_____

_____

_____

Location:_____

Quality:_____

Duration:_____

Frequency:_____

Radiation:_____

Precipitating/Relieving Factors:_____

_____

MEDICATIONS:_____

_____

_____

Figure 32–3
Ohio State University Center for Pain Control pelvic pain work-up sheet focusing on detailing the patient's pain history, including six central aspects.

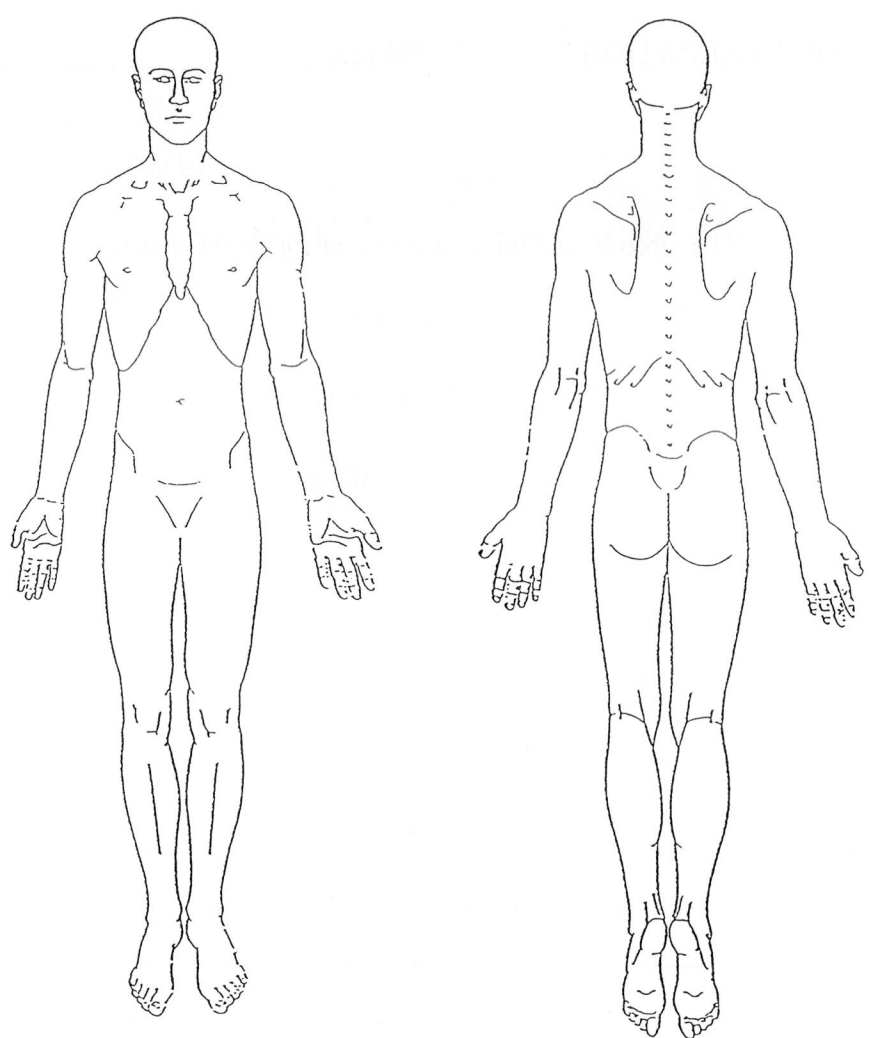

Figure 32–4
Unisex diagram used at the Center for Pain Control to record placement of maximum tender points located either by the patient or by the physician.

dures. It literally takes years to be able to learn to perform a good pelvic examination and to be able to sensitively detect subtle abnormalities that may exist in the pelvis. Furthermore, the patients who are referred with pelvic pain have already been examined repeatedly by their gynecologists. It will be quite obvious to these patients that the skills of a physician untrained in pelvic examinations are significantly different than those of their gynecologists. Finally, these are patients with long-term pelvic pain. Thus the pelvic examination itself must be modified so as to not stimulate great degrees of pain yet still enable the operator to detect abnormalities. In other words, pelvic pain is an area where pain specialists cannot expect to be effective unless they have extensive training and subsequent experience in pelvic examination.

Psychological Interview

The psychological interview is performed at the time of the first visit, often prior to the physical exami-

nation. This is important because it sets up a framework for recognition by the patient that this is a vital aspect of her health and well-being, as emphasized by its early inclusion in the work-up. Significant psychological impairment can have devastating effects upon the success of a planned program for a patient's recovery, especially in instances where it is not even suspected as being a problem. The literature is replete with articles associating childhood abuse with later sexual and psychological dysfunction, and many minor and major gynecologic pain problems have also been blamed upon such disturbances (Hameroff et al, 1981). These problems are often hidden early in physician-patient relationships because the patient is waiting for some signs of comfort and trust, or possibly because the patient has suppressed her past history to the extent that it is not available for recall without expert intervention.

The psychologist conducting the interview should work in concert with established treatment goals based on the general acceptance that there is indeed an intricate relationship between the patient's good

ABDOMINAL PELVIC EXAM:

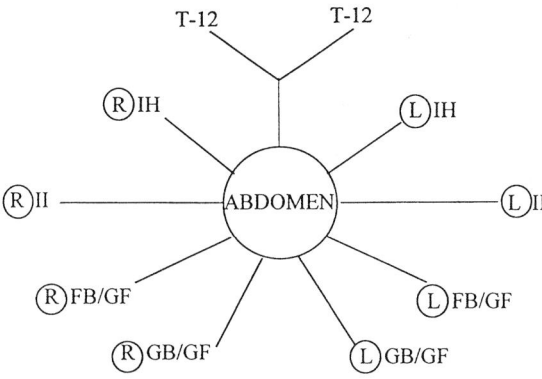

PELVIC PAIN EXAM:

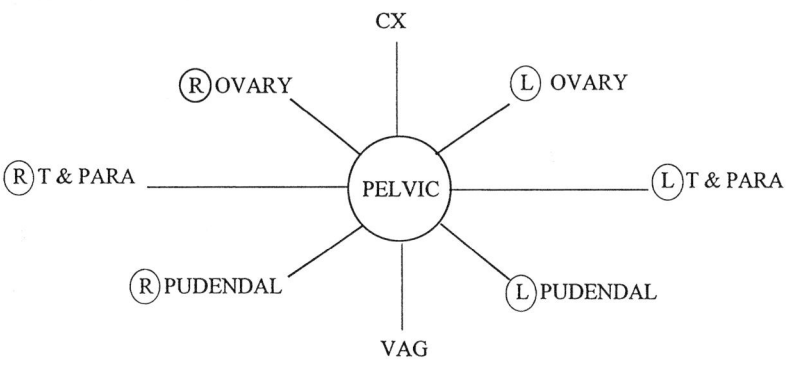

Figure 32–5
Schematic diagram used to compare abdominal and pelvic pain responses in relation to local tissues and nerves. This diagram allows the practitioner to quickly locate in a graphic way the problem that particular patient has. CX, cervix; FB/GF, femoral branch of genitofemoral nerve; GB/GF, genital branch of genitofemoral nerve; IH, iliohypogastric nerve; T-12, 12th thoracic nerve; T & PARA, fallopian tube and adnexa; VAG, vagina; II, ilioinguinal nerve.

general medical health and her psychological health. Ideally, it would be beneficial to have a psychologist schooled or experienced in the area of sexual function and the problems inherent in this very specialized care continuum. I am fortunate to work with such a psychologist, Dr. Mark Elliott, who is an expert in pelvic pain. We have developed a "dyssexualis" history that helps us to identify those patients with significant sexual dysfunction early on in the work-up (Fig. 32–6).

Functional Assessment

In pelvic pain patients it is very important to emphasize function and dysfunction just as in work-ups of regular chronic pain patients. For the most part these chronic pain patients have a significant decrease in the functional aspects of their lives. This decreased function usually has an impact on the patient from both personal and professional stand-points. From a personal standpoint, there is both a social and a psychological aspect, and from the professional standpoint, there is both an efficiency and a capability aspect. Patients often relate that function in their personal lives is as low as 20% to 30% of normal. Interestingly enough, function in their professional lives is always higher percentagewise because all patients must function in their jobs to earn money for personal survival. Thus they will endure pain during the day and remain functional, but when home at night they may become largely dysfunctional because they now must pay the price.

The initial challenge is to get to know the patient, become familiar with her history, and develop a feel for her functional status in regard to her social, psychological, and sexual interactions. The general rule of thumb in our pelvic pain clinic calls for close coordination and communication between the physician and the psychologist, who are specialists by training and by limitation in practice to pelvic pain syndromes and pain in and about the lower

Have you been treated by any other health care professionals for your pelvic pain? Yes No

  If yes, what was done:_____

_____

How would you rate the pelvic pain you are experiencing?

|----------|----------|----------|----------|----------|----------|----------|----------|----------|
1   2   3   4   5   6   7   8   9   10

  least pain ever   worst pain ever

  experienced in life   experienced in life

Over the last 2 years, about how often have you had sex with a partner?

  1+/day   3-4/week   1/week   1-2/month   <6/year

Are you comfortable with your current sexual frequency? Yes No

  If no, why are you uncomfortable?_____

Do you ever experience pain/discomfort during sexual intercourse? Yes No

  If yes, how frequently do you have pain?   always   most times   sometimes   rarely

How would you rate the intercourse pain you have most often?

|----------|----------|----------|----------|----------|----------|----------|----------|----------|
1   2   3   4   5   6   7   8   9   10

  least pain ever   worst pain ever

  experienced in life   experienced in life

What is the worst the intercourse pain has ever been?

|----------|----------|----------|----------|----------|----------|----------|----------|----------|
1   2   3   4   5   6   7   8   9   10

  least pain ever   worst pain ever

  experienced in life   experienced in life

About how long ago did the pain begin? _____

Which of the following best describes the location of your pain during intercourse?

  _____closer to the opening of the vagina

  _____deeper in the vagina

  _____both close to the opening of the vagina and deep in the vagina

  _____other (rectum, stomach, etc.), please specify _____

Is the intercourse pain worse with thrusting? Yes No

Is your pain worse with different intercourse positions (e.g., male on top, female on top, rear entry)?

  Yes   No

  If yes, what position(s) feels more painful? _____

Figure 32–6
Dyssexualis history developed by Dr. Mark Elliott for use in psychological evaluation of patients during the work-up.

abdomen. A team approach is used during the initial work-up and during the later therapy sessions by a physician board certified in both obstetrics-gynecology and anesthesiology and a psychologist who was formerly a director at the Master and Johnson Institute. Women with chronic pelvic pain are especially sensitive patients with many psychological, social, and physiologic ramifications of their pain.

Special Studies

In addition to a careful and considerate pelvic examination directly reflective of pelvic pain identification (not the usual pelvic bimanual examination), there are several procedures that must be considered basic work-up tools in practitioner's approach to pelvic pain. These include as a minimum the following studies that I believe form the basic foundation in the approach to understanding the patient with pelvic pain:

1. *Pelvic ultrasound examination.* This helps identify difficult-to-detect abnormalities that are "hidden" as a result of a patient's not allowing deep palpation because of pain.
2. *CT scan.* This is the ultimate exam for problems in the interface between the osseous and tissue planes. It may be indicated at times even in the face of anormal MRI if historical and laboratory findings point toward suspicion of abnormalities along this interface.
3. *Pelvic MRI.* This examination is the ultimate for detection of hidden tumors, masses, or even totally obscured endometriomas that may include occult neural involvement.
4. *Abdominal MRI.* This exam can rule out possible pathology in the abdomen that cannot be appreciated or cannot be detected on physical examination.
5. *Bone scan.* This is important in detecting fractures that may involve nerve distributions and cause long-term pain and disability when these fractures are not visible on plain radiographs.
6. *CA-125 values.* These may be helpful in certain situations to confirm a diagnosis that is already highly suspicious because of strong history and physical findings (e.g., endometriosis).

Ultrasound is the best imaging method currently available for early examination of the pelvis. Its advantages are its lower relative cost and the availability. The picture formed by reflection of high-frequency sound waves off of anatomic structures is the result of the various acoustic densities presented to the sound waves during penetration. Ultrasound is useful as a determinant of whether pelvic organs are normal or not and whether there is displacement resulting from other pathological entities.

The CT scan is also valuable as a diagnostic tool in determining pelvic abnormality, especially in re-lation to bony anatomy. It is performed by making a series of cross-sectional radiographs taken very close together (within 1 cm). It differs from conventional x-ray studies in that a computer is used to determine the variation in penetration of the tissues by the x-rays. Because the CT scan uses x-rays, the picture is excellent in regard to the bony relationships and thus serves as an ideal medium for evaluation of pelvic problems associated with tumor growth, tumor invasion, and distortion of pelvic anatomy.

MRI is a noninvasive diagnostic method that creates cross-sectional images of the body by use of sophisticated software and hardware. The result is a cross-sectional high-resolution image of the body. The advantage of using MRI for the evaluation of the pelvis is that the contrasting images of the tissues are sufficiently superior to the CT scan and ultrasound as to distinguish normal and abnormal tissues with a clarity not possible with these other methods.

Laparoscopy or peritoneoscopy is the spinoff of the old culdoscopy surgical technique (Slocumb, 1990; Spitzer et al, 1992). Its advantage is considerable compared to that older method, however, in that the positioning of the patient is more reasonable and both diagnostic and a considerable number of therapeutic procedures can be performed via the laparoscopic technique. It is the most widely applied diagnostic technique today in gynecology, and its application avoids many operative exploratory procedures that would have been done in the past. Its use does require significant experience and expertise, but, when used appropriately by experienced personnel, it is indeed an invaluable tool.

It is also important to record all previous such studies and to take detailed notes on dates and findings. This information can help in understanding the diagnostic and therapeutic approach taken by physicians who have previously cared for the patient. Furthermore these studies should not be repeated because of the delay in time and the added expense. A close working relationship with the doctors and staff who previously treated the patient will be necessary to utilize previous test results to best advantage.

Differential Diagnosis

The differentiation of the various operative gynecologic disease processes is very tricky, and often pelvic and low abdominal pain can be interchanged. For example, one study revealed that patients suffering from irritable bowel syndrome had over a 20% incidence of hysterectomy, revealing the confusion in regard to the origin of abdominal pain (Whitehead, 1992). One of the problems confounding the practitioner who attempts to sort out the cause of and treatment for the chronic pain patient with pelvic and abdominal pain is the fact that the etiology can be quite variable, the target organs affected quite disparate, and the intensity of the pain quite different.

This can lead to early frustrations from employing diagnostic tests that repeatedly turn up negative. It also intensifies the pressure on the physician to eventually identify an etiology and some treatment that may be beneficial. To complicate matters, some of the health care team members, such as the gynecologist, internist, or family practitioner, are not trained in the application of various diagnostic and therapeutic local anesthetic blocks, while other members of the health care team, such as the anesthesiologist, neurologist, or internist, are not versed in and have had little experience in pelvic exams. Both of these techniques, of course, are important in the work-up of such patients, and, if either is excluded a piece of the puzzle is missing that may confound the practitioner attempting to make the diagnosis.

An important aspect of the differential diagnosis is the pelvic examination, wherein various tissues and sensitive locations are carefully examined. It is at this time that maximum tender points will often be located and appreciated by the appropriately trained and experienced clinician. Among physicians not trained to understand the importance of the neuropathic aspect of pain etiology, there is a tendency to blame problems with pelvic organs that are readily apparent or adhesions that are remnants of past surgeries. The latter, however, are rarely the cause of pelvic pain and should not be just a default excuse when no other etiology for the pain is evident. At this point the clinician needs to do various diagnostic blocks to rule out different possible neuropathies that may well be the culprit. These must be done with a full understanding of and appreciation for the innervation pathways for the pelvis. This can only be achieved after many years of study of the relationships of the muscles, ligaments, bony pelvis, and neuroanatomy. Such a topic cannot be summarized in a chapter, and it is not something that can be taught in one or two or even several sessions during a "learning" visit. In instances where the initial physician has completed a work-up that reveals no obvious organic abnormalities and the patient still complains of pain, the physician in charge should consider referring the patient to a full-time pelvic pain practitioner, who will have broad-based experience in diagnosis and management of chronic pelvic pain with successful outcomes.

One of the very important associated problems in women's complaints of lower abdominal pain may be abdominal nerve entrapment. That issue was addressed by John Slocumb in 1990. This is the first of several conditions that are outlined here as a practical guide for the practitioner to consider in his or her initial work-up of the chronic pelvic pain patient.

Gynecologic Etiologies

Ilioinguinal or Iliohypogastric Neuropathy. It is possible that, during an exploratory laparotomy or laparoscopy, one may stretch, avulse, or otherwise damage either the ilioinguinal or iliohypogastric

nerve (or both in some instances). In these cases the time to neuropathy development may be protracted. The pain may begin days, weeks, or even months after the injury and gradually escalate over time from a pain of 1 to 3 on a scale of 10 to a pain of 7 to 10 eventually. Typically a burning, stabbing type of pain, it may develop to a degree that literally incapacitates the patient. Often the well-meaning doctor misses the diagnosis altogether and does not even examine this area (Fig. 32–7). The diagnosis is made by pressure applied over the area until the patient complains. This neuropathy is discussed in greater detail in the section "Example of Pelvic Pain Diagnosis and Treatment."

Genitofemoral Neuropathies. These patients come in with variable stories of low abdominal pain, or even back pain that has migrated to the front of their body and now descends into the pubic area. The pain is often incapacitating when it occurs in sharp repeated attacks. Almost all patients will have significant reductions in pain after individual nerve blocks and maximum tender point injections. It is hoped that patients will exhibit gradual reductions in pain scores over time and that they will have an increase in their function at the same time. Failure of this treatment must be viewed as an open invitation to explore further the possibility of an overlooked pathologic condition that may have been missed. For example, one patient I managed recently had been refractory to repeated therapy over time; upon surgical exploration, it was discovered that a suture had been placed around the genital branch of the genitofemoral nerve during a former hernia repair. Since the distal portion of the nerve was notably atrophic, it was resected above the area of involvement; patient follow-up has been gratifying in that the patient is now pain free.

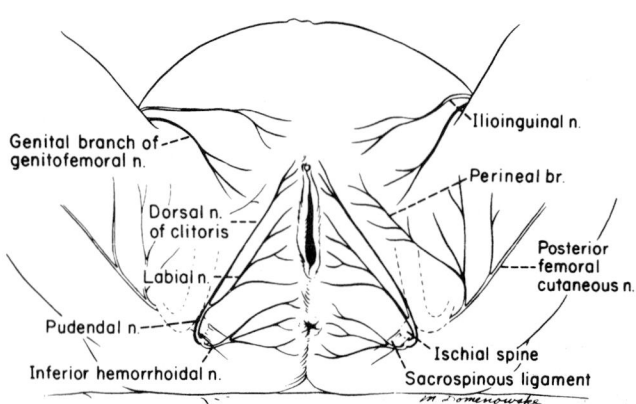

Figure 32–7
Cutaneous nerve supply of the perineum. The female perineum has multiple sources of innervation. Its primary supply is from the pudendal nerve bilaterally. Its second source of supply is from the ilioinguinal nerves bilaterally. Its third source of supply is from the genitofemoral nerve. Its fourth source is from both the S2 through S4 nerves and the anococcygeal nerve.

Bartholinitis. Infection in Bartholin's glands is the chief problem here. That often means surgical incision and drainage to reverse the effects of inflammation and sequestration of purulent matter. Complete disruption of all communicating and infected sacs should be carried out, along with placing the patient on antibiotics (Cheetham, 1985).

Skene's Urethritis. Infection in Skene's glands, a set of glands lying along the urethral orifice, is the cause of pelvic pain in this instance. Usually, heat applications and gentle pressure can empty the infected material, but rarely patients may require incision and drainage and antibiotics similar to that described for bartholinitis (Buntin, 1994).

Herpes. The chief pain problems with herpes initially include dysuria, dyspareunia, vesicular eruptions, and groin pain. These can be treated with B & O suppositories, avoidance of sex, acyclovir cream, and systemic analgesics, respectively. Long-term pain can be due to actual neuropathic changes. These are treated by identification of the involved nerve or nerves and local anesthetic blocks for pain relief trials spaced over several weeks. Some patients who are refractory to these may be considered for other methods of nerve treatment, such as cryotherapy or thermolysis. The term *focal vulvitis* should be introduced here because it is a general term that has been used in the past to describe a syndrome of general vulvar pain without evident cause (Whitehead, 1992).

Condyloma. In early stages, colposcopy helps make the diagnosis. Treatment by application of 5-fluorouracil until all wart activity appears neutralized. The skin will recover over a short period of time and develop normal texture again. In some cases, larger lesions may have to be removed by use of cryotherapy, fulgeration, or surgical excision. One of the important differentials is human papillomavirus (Ferenczy, 1995).

Vaginitis. The emphasis in cases of vaginitis is on the etiology. Possibilities include bacterial, viral, yeast, and protozoan sources. The diagnosis is made with inspection, sampling of any vaginal discharges, and examination under a microscope for identification.

Vaginismus. Causes of vaginismus may be congenital, infectious, traumatic, or psychological. Because the primary cause by far is psychological, it is important to consult a psychologist early on in the diagnosis of this malady. Some of the underlying reasons may reflect back to childhood problems that have been suppressed. The treatment regimen is complex and demands intensive therapy targeted at several positive forces that knowledgeable psychologists can institute (Reamy, 1982).

Tension Myalgia. This is an umbrella diagnosis that requires identification of the involved muscles, which could be the levator, the piriformis, or the coc- cygeus muscle groups. Tension myalgia is best treated by attempts to relieve the spasm by heat and massage or direct local anesthetic injection of the involved muscles. Follow-up with specific muscle-oriented stretching exercises will greatly help this painful condition and assist with recovery and prevention of repeated episodes.

Hymeneal Syndrome. Patients with hymeneal syndrome are a most interesting group. They are many times so distraught and histrionic that the initial practitioner may entirely miss the diagnosis due to preoccupation with the reaction the patient displays during physical and gynecologic examination. Often the patient complains so violently that a pelvic exam is not even possible (i.e., the examiner cannot get past the introitus). In other instances the examiner does get past the introitus only to find there is no evidence of pain on examination of the vagina, cervix, uterus, fallopian tubes, and ovaries. Patients usually have a history of normal, healthy sexual patterns before the onset of their vaginal pain but develop significant sexual dysfunction secondary to their disease process. This is usually manifested by symptoms of severe dyspareunia totally focused in the area of the vaginal outlet.

The past history of these patients often reveals an infection with *Candida albicans*. It would appear that repeated infections with this agent can cause irritation of the superficial nerves in an around the area of the hymeneal ring. Figure 32–8 shows the area of involvement in regard to this syndrome. Note that the perineum is richly innervated by nerves from different spinal cord segments, so that there is some overlap protection in regard to innervation. Of five patients treated by my colleagues and me, four experienced complete relief of pain and a return to normal sexual function within 8 weeks of definitive

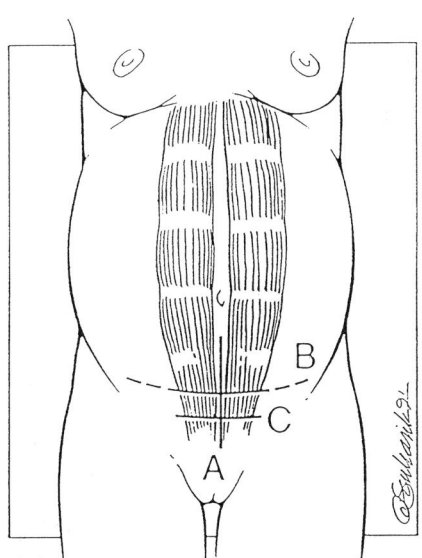

Figure 32–8
Pfannensteil incision (C); retraction of lower corners may result in neuropathy.

therapy—surgical extirpation of the hymeneal ring. In the one patient who did not have complete relief of pain there was also a significant psychological component to the problem. This patient also had had a previous hysterectomy and oophorectomy and had problems adjusting to exogenous estrogen, and thus had a thin vaginal mucosa with other associated problems.

The patient work-up must include at least three successful hymeneal blocks, which should be performed prior to consideration for surgery. In our series of patients all had repeated hymeneal local anesthetic blocks with demonstrated complete relief of symptoms. The association of the aforementioned infectious process, and specifically the offending agent, is too consistent to be coincidence. It may be that the fungus may gain deep mucous membrane penetrance, with a damaging effect upon the nerve endings, perhaps even causing a neuroma-like formation to occur (Theofrastous, 1998).

Dysmenorrhea. This problem can be so severe as to be debilitating. It necessitates the use of systemic over-the-counter analgesics, such as nonsteroidal anti-inflammatory drugs (NSAIDs), that are taken by the clock to maintain adequate analgesia. The patient also should receive a "rescue medication" for very severe crises. This may be in the form of analgesics stronger than the NSAIDs (i.e., combination drugs such as Darvocet or Fiorinal). The use of birth control pills to suppress hormonal levels may also be beneficial because they may reduce or partially eradicate the endocrine-driven aspect of the disease process. Heat or cold applications are also useful during major pain periods (Peters et al, 1991).

Ectopic Pregnancy. Although hemorrhage is the main problem in ectopic pregnancy, pain may occur as a result of peritoneal stretch or even irritation and becomes the predominant symptom from the point when actual rupture occurs. Ultrasound can now rapidly diagnose ectopic pregnancy, and laparoscopy is further diagnostic and therapeutic at the same time. In earlier days there was no concern about tubal sacrifice, but today usually tubal conservation is the concern after adequate hemostasis (Hinney et al, 1995).

Corpus Luteum Cyst. Again, a corpus luteum cyst combines a hemorrhagic event and pain when distention occurs to the point of excessive stretch of the peritoneal covering surrounding the cyst. Diagnosis is again made with ultrasound and confirmed with laparoscopy, whereby definitive surgical correction can also be carried out.

Twisted Ovarian Cyst. Some ovarian cysts can enlarge to the point that local vascular supply is embarrassed, and this can elicit pain to the degree that immediate attention is indicated. This type of pain usually develops slowly over hours or days and presents with sharp definition and radiation to the iliac fossa. Diagnosis here is also by laparoscopy, whereby definitive therapy can be accomplished with either aspiration followed by excision or total excision of the entire cyst without aspiration if there is concern about the possibility of any malignant potential.

Mesenteric Thrombosis. With thrombosis of the mesenteric artery, the pain is sudden and extremely localized, manifesting as a remarkably severe pain that is knifelike in quality. There may well be associated free blood in the abdomen on peritoneal irritation, as well as muscular rigidity. Diagnosis may be difficult, but it can be definitively made with vascular studies. Surgery is indicated as soon as possible to avoid unnecessary damage to the integrity of the nearby bowel.

Diverticulitis. Most of the involved areas in diverticulitis that cause acute or repeated chronic pain problems are the result of minute outpouchings in locally weakened intestinal wall. The diagnosis is by radiologic study, and treatment is by laparotomy and excision of the involved area if indicated. It is important to remove these damaged areas after repeated episodes because of the possibility of future rupture with resultant peritoneal leakage and inflammation (Vignati et al, 1995).

Endometriosis. Endometriosis itself is one of the major causes of pelvic pain and perhaps one of the most confounding problems because this disease can present clinically as almost anything, having the ability to mimic many other disease states. Endometrial implants may attach to many different abdominal organs and tissues. They can be in the typical form of a dark red or brown color, or they may be even colorless. The diagnosis is made on the basis of the history and definitively by laparoscopy. Currently, the most popular treatment method is medical, with suppression of both estrogen and progesterone by use of pituitary inhibitory hormones, such as the newly developed gonadotropin-releasing hormone inhibitor drugs such as Syneral. Surgical exploration via laparoscopy with laser treatment of the identified endometrial implants and sometimes surgical severance of either the uterocervical plexus (laparoscopic uterosacral nerve ablation [LUNA] procedure) or the superior hypogastric plexus (presacral neurectomy) may give permanent relief of pain (Anonymous, 1995).

Pelvic Congestion Syndrome. This is often a last thought of diagnosis. Pelvic congestion syndrome was discounted by many in the past because one could not get a clear picture of the anatomic disorder. Now, with new methods of diagnosis that utilize rapid-sequence radiographs and injection of dye into the cervical venous system, there is an acceptable means of measurement by noting the size and configuration of the venous drainage plexus on the right and left sides of the cervix. Earlier these studies were done with the patients examined when lying down;

now they are performed with the patient in the upright position (Mathis et al, 1995).

Nongynecologic Etiologies

Sympathetic Pelvic Syndrome. Many of the patients who complain of gynecologic pain have a deep pain in the pelvis not associated with physically detectable abdominal wall tenderness or myofascial disease of the abdominal musculature. This disease entity has been classified as a "sympathetic pelvis syndrome." Patients in this group present with a historical vignette that is atypical from the standpoint of identification of any single source of causation. It must be recalled that visceral disease often results in pain transmitted to cutaneous areas (referred pain), and often such pain may be interpreted as indicating primary disorders located in that specific area of the body. In other words, it is possible to have a visceral etiology of cutaneous pain in such instances. The area of innervation includes the vagina and cervix, with innervation from the pudendal nerves with derivation from S2 through S4; and the uterus, tubes, and ovaries, with innervation from the sympathetic pelvic branches of T10 through T12.

Some patients will obtain relief from repeated local anesthetic nerve blocks if the physician is patient enough and the patient detailed enough to check the progress of improvement every time and note if it is specifically the same area of pain previously identified. In the remaining patients, whose pain is relieved only during the time period determined by local anesthetic pharmacokinetics, laparoscopic surgery can be considered for one of two nerve ablation techniques, the LUNA procedure or a superior hypogastric ganglion resection. Those patients who were refractory to the local anesthetic block therapy are usually rendered pain free after the surgical resection, and these patients will have a return to normal function.

Pelvic Joint Instability. Persistent pelvic pain and pelvic joint instability in some females has been associated with precocious puberty and use of oral contraceptives prior to reproduction. Thus patients who complain of pelvic pain in which all diagnostic work-ups have been normal and who have histories of early onset of menarche associated with oral contraceptive use should be considered for possibilities of pelvic joint instability.

Pyramidal Muscle Hematoma. Hematoma of the pyramidal muscle is a rare but possible complication that may cause impingement of the sciatic, inferior gluteal, and pudendal nerves. This may result from compression of these nerves between the muscle and the iliac spine. In these cases a CT scan should help to confirm the diagnosis (Conacher, 1986).

Osteitis Pubis. Females active in competitive sports who present with pubic and adductor pain should be considered for osteitis pubis as a cause. In one study of 59 patients, recovery was slow, taking up to 7 months. There was also an associated finding of pelvic malalignment or sacroiliac dysfunction in these patients (Major, 1997).

Adductor Tendinitis. This problem is usually associated with marathon walkers or runners who suffer from acute injury to the adductor muscle of the anterior thigh, which attaches directly to the pubic ramus. It is often misdiagnosed as pelvic pain because of the complaint by the patient of diffuse ache that radiates into the involved pelvic area laterally. Diagnosis is made by running the examining finger along the medial margin of the adductor muscle up to the point of insertion on the pubic ramus. At this point the patient will suffer exquisite pain and pinpoint the pain as being located exactly at the point of insertion. A local anesthetic injection will completely eradicate the pain within minutes of injection. It may be necessary to repeat such a treatment a few times for complete eradication of the pain.

Osteoporotic Sacral Fractures. Osteoporotic sacral fractures were found to be associated with pelvic pain complaints in which other pathologic causes had been excluded (Fricker et al, 1991).

Example of Pelvic Pain Diagnosis and Treatment

Patients with ilioinguinal and iliohypogastric nerve disturbances have histories that often include surgical or other types of trauma in the area of the lower abdominal wall. The genesis of the pain is not known for sure, but suspicion falls on the retraction placed upon nerves located around an incision line that may result in overstretch and avulsion-type neural injuries. The onset of pain after the initial trauma will be variable due to the intensity of the injury and perhaps the fiber size. Many of the gynecologic patients have undergone surgery using the Pfannensteil incision, which cuts across both the ilioinguinal and iliohypogastric nerves. In addition, injury may result from retraction in the lower corners of the incision, where these nerves are located (Fig. 32-8).

Interestingly, many of the patients in this group have histories of repeated abdominal explorations of one type or another because their original physician was convinced the initial problem of intraabdominal pathology had not been solved, or perhaps that recurrent pain might be due to abdominal adhesions or other yet undefined "organ-related pathology." This is becoming less frequent as a result of the widespread use of laparoscopy, but the latter procedure in itself may cause abdominal neuropathy due to placement of the scope, obturator, or one or more ancillary sites made percutaneously. A classical example of this patient type can be seen in Figure 32-9, where the incisions can be seen and the maximal tender points are noted via the skin markers. In this case the patient initially identified eight tender points.

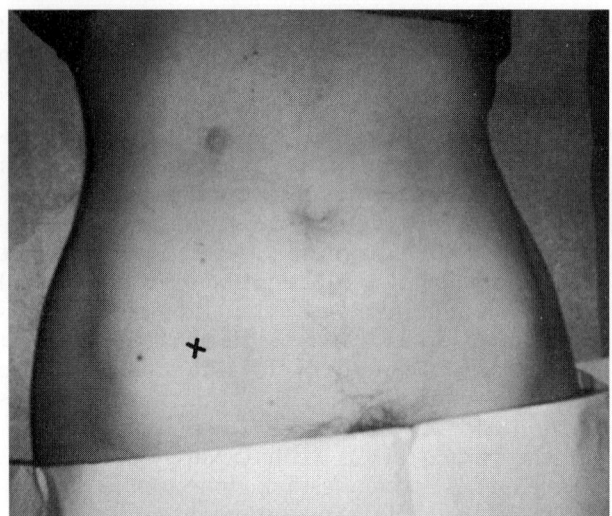

Figure 32–9
Photograph of patient abdomen showing previous incision and maximal tender points (cross marks).

These cases are managed by repeated local anesthetic nerve blocks spaced over time to take advantage of the maximal pain signal depression but not so frequently as to set up a de novo peripheral pain signal generated from mechanical stimulation alone. Most patients will fall into the responding category by 4 to 6 weeks. Those who do not can benefit from abdominal catheter placement and continuous local anesthetic irrigation of the nerves between the transversalis and oblique muscle groups (Ghia et al, 1991). Those who do not respond to that tactic can be treated with cryotherapy for destruction of those few refractory nerves still causing problems (Conacher, 1986). For ultimate failures in instances where multiple nests of neuromas may still be active and have been refractory to all the above modalities, one can consider surgical extirpation of the local nests to try to correct the problem (J. S. McDonald, unpublished results, 1996).

THERAPEUTIC PROCEDURES

In discussing therapy for pelvic pain, one must provide the patient with various options for relief, not just one. The patient needs to realize that there is just not one medium of care or one treatment method that she will be relying upon from the outset. I cannot emphasize too much how patient confidence in the physician is eroded when only one method of treatment is suggested and it begins to fail the patient once again. At such a point the patient may become demoralized and depressed because she has experienced such problems in her interaction with many previous physicians before being referred, and now even the referral physician is repeating previously unsuccessful therapy trials.

Treatment should begin with an emphasis on rapport by carefully outlining to the patient what the various problems are, what the possible etiologies may be, what the possible therapies might be, and how you and your staff will stand by the patient throughout the work-up phase and be supportive into the therapy phase. Some may not look upon this as therapy, but the concern and consideration of the physician, the eye contact, and the reaching out to touch the patient and display sincere concern are not to be underestimated in regard to their value. It is also wise to discuss with the patient how the pathology can be related to the anatomy in the area. To facilitate this, the physician may want to use anatomy book pictures to demonstrate that relationship.

Medical Therapy

It is very important to begin some therapy right away on the first visit. This can begin with administration of various systemic medications, but these should only be prescribed after careful analysis of the currently used medications and after recording the successes and failures of the medications and therapies tried in the past. This is a time-consuming process, but it is really necessary to make a breakthrough in understanding the complete medical background of the patient. At this time it is also necessary to have an in-depth conversation with the patient about her sleep habits and to consider the addition of one of the low-dose antidepressant medications such as amyltriptyline (0.25 mg taken at bedtime). The use of this regimen can aid in both decreasing the reception of pain centrally and in providing the patient with some badly needed sleep (Walker et al, 1991).

The basic foundation for treatment of non–cancer pain patients of course begins with the use of over-the-counter, readily available drugs such as salicylates and/or NSAIDs. Next comes the use of tricyclic antidepressants, believed to act by the blockage of the uptake of serotonin and norepinephrine in the CNS. Next comes the use of anticonvulsant drugs, which have also been found to be effective in certain pain syndromes such as trigeminal neuralgia. Last is the use of the opioid drugs. There are some patients and some instances when use of such opioid analgesics may have fewer side effects than the aforementioned tricyclic antidepressants and the anticonvulsant drugs. There is also a wide difference in the incidence of side effects among opioids; morphine sulfate, codeine, and pentazocine have an incidence of side effects in the range of 20%, whereas oxycodone has a side effects incidence one half of that. The adverse effects usually associated with the opioids are pruritus, drowsiness, nausea, vomiting, dizziness, headache, euphoria, dry mouth, and swelling.

Generally speaking, our clinic does not give prescriptions for opioid drugs because the clinic will eventually become a dumping ground where patients can get whatever prescriptions they ask for in regard to their previous narcotics usage pattern. Yet is it possible to have the patient continue for a short time on the opioid drugs he or she has been used to taking for pain relief by contacting the referral physician and establishing a good relationship with him or her. In doing so, we mention that we would appreciate the continuance of whatever medications the patient has been taking for the past few months, and that our aim is to gradually reduce those medications over time and substitute other drugs such as the NSAIDs. The referring physician can continue to prescribe the previous drugs for a short bridge period that we identify with him or her. This can work out nicely if there is good communication between both parties, and the referring physician realizes he or she is being helpful and supportive in the continuing management of a difficult patient.

The problem with medical therapy is that, until we try different types of pain medications on patients, we cannot say for sure which medication will have a beneficial effect and which will have no to little effect at all. Patients are becoming more and more sophisticated about pain and their rights in regard to having a decent pain relief regimen. The majority of patients should be able to get some degree of pain relief with prescription antinociceptors; if neither the planned local anesthetic nerve blocks nor the prescribed antinoceptors are effective in providing pain relief, then consideration should be given to some type of nerve destructive procedure. These methods include techniques such as cryotherapy, thermolysis, stimulation, and at times surgery.

Physical Therapy

This aspect of the treatment regimen is often overlooked, but it is vital to good recovery and adds substantially to the overall therapy regimen. The prime physical therapy methods include heat, electrical stimulation, deep ultrasound, and massage. In addition, it is important to work with professionals in the area of physical therapy so that they can devise treatment regimens for the patient that are specifically designed for her after suitable input from the physician. The professional will examine the patient, design a special mode of therapy for the patient, and follow the patient over time with feedback to the physician for follow-up purposes.

Psychological Therapy

Psychological therapy is almost always an integral part of treatment. To a great extent, successful psychological intervention is imperative for recovery and dealing with the psychological ramifications of any pain syndrome. It is based upon use of hypnosis, relaxation techniques, behavioral feedback, and group therapy. Often patients find safe harbor among other patients who have similar problems, and they have been able to work through their problems with some success.

Nerve Therapy

During the pelvic examination or shortly afterward, one may use a diagnostic blockade in the form of local anesthetic nerve block. The trial of local anesthetic nerve blocks includes the three specific sensory innervation points for the pelvis: the inferior hypogastric nerve, representing the parasympathetics; the pudendal nerve, representing the somatic afferents; and the superior hypogastric nerve plexus, representing the sympathetics. It also includes nonspecific sensory innervation points both in the pelvic area and in the abdominal area. Once the area of neuropathy is identified, a local anesthetic nerve block may or may not be effective in eradicating it. Pain relief may be immediate but may not persist over a long period of time.

Interestingly enough, many times when repeated local anesthetic nerve blocks are made to an area where there is nerve damage, an improvement may begin to develop. The exact mechanism of this improvement is still a mystery. Whether this connection is akin to an electrical link that is dissipated over time is largely conjecture. What is apparent is that, as the intensity of the input signal from the periphery lessens, there is a critical point at which the patient begins to feel significantly better. The general improvement continues over time in a step-down fashion, the reverse of the stepwise increase in pain noted in the early production of the pain process. As successful blockade occurs, these patients eventually may de-escalate from experiencing pain at a level of 8 on a scale of 10 to a 6, then to a 4, finally to a 3 or even 2. As many as 70% of patients will respond in this way. Unfortunately, there is no way to tell if a patient is in the responding group until an adequate trial period has passed.

For the 20% to 30% of patients who are nonresponders, it is important to offer alternative modes of therapy such as unique medication regimens with or without extensive physical therapy and exercise programs to aid in the healing process. The other alternative is cryotherapy or even thermolysis therapy. Both of the latter effect nerve dissolution for varying periods of time. Cryotherapy consists of freezing of portions of the involved nerve so that it undergoes cell death and in turn ceases to function. The machines available for such treatments include sophisticated circuitry to provide for identification of involved nerves by electrical stimuli and then freeze therapy to effect destruction at a chosen point immediately proximal to the involved nerve (McDowell et al, 1994).

Another type of neural therapy involves insertion of an abdominal catheter for the purpose of continuous irrigation of the involved nerves. However, this method should only be considered for use in situations where patients are refractory to the local anesthetic block therapy mentioned above. Its advantages are that it minimizes the repeated painful injections that are a necessary part of the repeat treatments, it reduces the visits necessary for repeated injections, and in some isolated cases it has given continuous pain relief instead of cyclic on-and-off pain relief (Ghia et al, 1991).

A final method of neural therapy is mentioned only for completeness and is not recommended by me for lasting pain relief. That method is surgical excision of a so-called neural bed in an area that has been repeatedly refractory to nerve block and other methods of pain relief.

Surgical Therapy

Surgical entry into the area where repeated surgical procedures as mentioned above have been ineffective is sometimes necessary because of neuroma persistence or ineffective or misdirected local anesthetic nerve blocks. It usually consists of opening of the incision and careful visualization of the incision line and wound bed to denote any obvious pathology such as suture placement around a nerve or an obvious collection of neuromas resulting from old nerve damage (Jarde et al, 1995).

Laparoscopy can be employed to treat abnormalities noted previously, such as endometriosis and adhesions. These can be either vaporized or lysed by use of the laser beam, which offers the benefit of direct focus on the exact lesion to be affected, complete destruction by the high-energy beam, and instant hemostasis at the same time. Laparotomy is used in circumstances where there is some concern about distorted anatomy from multiple adhesions, or where there is a definite diagnosis, such as by ultrasound, of a substantial mass that demands removal by laparotomy rather than by laparoscopy.

Alternative Medicine

The use of alternative medical therapy has become increasingly popular with patients who suffer from chronic pelvic pain and who have not gotten relief with traditional methods. This category of treatment options would not even have been considered 5 years ago in a discussion of pelvic pain. Today alternative medicine is promoted for good reason—it helps to make the patient feel included in her healing process and helps her to continue some of the "remedy"-oriented methods of treatment that she may have tried already. These methods include acupuncture, yoga, meditation, chiropractic, and nutritional therapy, among others.

FOLLOW-UP

In this era of longitudinal care, follow-up, and outcome orientation, it is especially important for the pain practitioner to be keyed into follow-up and outcome studies of all patients treated.

Establishing Patient Goals

The patient with chronic pelvic pain has two mutually nonexclusive goals: improved function and decreased pain. Of course, any early discussions about pain treatment results must be guarded in respect to any promises of certain definite end points. That is, it is unwise to tell a patient who presents with a pain score of 8 on a scale of 10 that, by the end of therapy, she can expect a reduction to a 2 or 1. It makes more sense to discuss the general goal over time as being to reduce the beginning pain scale from a severe category of 7 to 10 to a moderate category of 4 to 6 and then to a mild category of 1 to 3. In this way one can avoid zeroing in on a numerical score. In addition, it is very important to stress function improvement by noting the patient's function percentage from the professional and the personal standpoint. In regard to function, it is necessary to identify what the patient's level of function was at a full 100%, and then identify what it is now at the given level of pain recorded. Again, it is not wise to quote a numerical score as a goal to achieve, but to emphasize instead improved function overall. Thus the dual goal soon perceived by the patient is improved function in both the personal and professional area *and*, at the same time, reduction in her pain level.

Tracking Patient Outcome

Medical Log

The medical log consists of patient notes of medications and their effects recorded on a daily basis. This is important because patients often are given medication and very little if any feedback is noted. Thus the patient remains on the same dosage, which may either be too great or too little depending on the circumstance. Of course the goal is to reduce the level of medication the patient is on regardless of the type of medication. This can only be done if the physician notes the progress that is being made at each return visit. The individual physician may make up notebooks or use sheets of paper with standardized spaces to record on, but really any system is a workable one as long as it is something the patient is motivated to do. In other words, it is not how neat or organized it looks, it is how accurate the data input is in regard to dosage of drug, when it was taken, and the effect that is important.

Activity Log

The activity log is vital in regard to the progress that is being made. It can be kept along with the aforementioned medical log or it can be kept separately. It is best to begin the log with a notation about what the patient used to do or be capable of doing prior to the time of the pain disorder. Again, it can be merely sheets of paper on which the patient records her activity on a daily basis or it can be standardized, as for the medical log. The important point is that the patient is motivated to maintain the log. Obviously, the emphasis for the patient should be on continued activity and function regardless of the state of the pain disorder. Therefore, this instrument can be the most valuable index of the functional status of the patient and a good indicator of the progress being made with various therapeutic trials.

CONCLUSION

In the discussion of chronic pelvic pain patients presented in this chapter, I have attempted to point out the complexity of the problem these patients bring to the unwitting practitioner. On first blush there may appear to be a simple organic problem that is the primary cause of the pain. The problem is that the physical causes of chronic pelvic pain are difficult to identify and prove. Special techniques of physical examination are called for, and the physician must have a high index of suspicion for neuropathic conditions such as nerve compression and neurapraxia that result in problems such as hyperalgesia and allodynia, myofascial pain syndrome, and pressure neuropathy of the pudendal nerve, obturator nerve, and inferior hypogastric ganglion. However, in managing chronic pelvic pain, the primary question is, can a carefully constructed history, a thorough physical exam, and structured use of local anesthetic blocks over a short period of time aid in the determination of the etiology and the prediction of the success of treatment of modalities of nonsurgical therapy?

An attitude of futility develops after a period of time when trial after trial of treatment fails to alleviate the pain described by the patient. Many patients relate their frustrations in regard to multiple physician visits, laboratory studies, diagnostic studies, and surgical explorations, all without a definitive diagnosis and all without substantial reduction in pain despite changes in medication, changes in sleep patterns, changes in work habits, and extensive relaxation exercises. Most patients will confess they were at the end of their mental and physical tolerance.

After initial work-up, including operative laparoscopy, MRIs, laboratory studies, and psychological profiles, if there is no hint of a basic underlying problem, perhaps it would be prudent to consider referral of the patient to someone who specializes in management of chronic pain syndromes that involve the lower abdomen and pelvis. However, because physical causes are much more socially acceptable than psychological ones, both physician and patient continually seek to find organic pathology.

An additional frustration is that various physicians may tell patients that the pain they have may well be "in their heads." Such phrases must not be used because they rob the patient of any hope she had about getting well. This is a tragic robbery. The patient must be referred before this happens.

REFERENCES

Singh KK, Lessells AM, Adam DJ, et al: Presentation of endometriosis to general surgeons: a 10-year experience. Br J Surg 1995;82:1349.
Baskin LS, Tanagho EA: Pelvic pain without pelvic organs. J Urol 1992;147:683.
Buntin DM: The 1993 sexually transmitted disease treatment guidelines. Semin Dermatol 1994;13:269.
Cheetham DR: Bartholin's cyst: marsupialization or aspiration? Am J Obstet Gynecol 1985;152:569.
Conacher ID: Percutaneous cryotherapy for post-thoracotomy neuralgia. Pain 1986;25:227.
Drossman DA, Leserman J, Nachman G, et al: Sexual and physical abuse in women with functional or organic gastrointestinal disorders. Ann Intern Med 1990;113:828.
Ferenczy A: Epidemiology and clinical pathophysiology of condylomata acuminata. Am J Obstet Gynecol 1995;172:1331.
Fricker PA, Taunton JE, Ammann W: Osteitis pubis in athletes. Infection, inflammation, or injury? Sports Med 1991;12:266.
Garrison DW, Foreman RD: Decreased activity of spontaneous and noxiously evoked dorsal horn cells during transcutaneous electrical nerve stimulation (TENS). Pain 1994;58:309.
Ghia JN, Blank JW, McAdams CG: A new interabdominus approach to inguinal region block for the management of chronic pain. Reg Anesth 1991;16:72.
Hameroff SR, Carlson GL, Brown BR: Ilioinguinal pain syndrome. Pain 1981;10:253.
Hinney B, Bertagnoli C, Tobler-Sommer M, et al: Diagnosis of early ectopic pregnancy by measurement of the maternal serum to cul-de-sac fluid beta-hCG ratio. Ultrasound Obstet Gynecol 1995;5:260.
Jarde O, Trinquier JL, Pleyber A, et al: Treatment of Morton neuroma by neurectomy: apropos of 43 cases. Rev Chir Orthop Reparatrice Appar Mot 1995;82:142.
Major NM: Pelvic stress injuries: the relationship between osteitis pubis (symphysis pubis stress injury) and sacroiliac abnormalities in athletes. Skeletal Radiol 1997;26:711.
Mathis BV, Miller JS, Lukens ML, Paluzzi MW: Pelvic congestion syndrome: a new approach to an unusual problem. Am Surg 1995;61:1016.
McDonald JSM: Pelvic and low abdominal pain. In Lefkowitz M, Lebovits A (eds): A Practical Approach to Pain Management. Boston: Little, Brown and Company, 1996:265.
McDowell JH, McFarland EG, Nalli BJ: Use of cryotherapy for orthopaedic patients. Orthop Nurs 1994;13(5):21.
Miyazaki F, Shook G: Ilioinguinal nerve entrapment during needle suspension for stress incontinence. Obstet Gynecol 1992;80:246.
Peters AAW, van Dorst E, Jellis B, et al: A randomized clinical trial to compare two different approaches in women with chronic pelvic pain. Obstet Gynecol 1991;77:740.
Reamy K: The treatment of vaginismus by the gynecologist: an eclectic approach. Obstet Gynecol 1982;59:58.
Reiter RC: A profile of women with chronic pelvic pain. Clin Obstet Gynecol 1990;33:130.
Slocumb JC: Chronic somatic, myofascial, and neurogenic abdominal pelvic pain. Clin Obstet Gynecol 1990;33:145.
Snooks SJ, Badenoch DF, Tiptaft RC, Swash M: Perineal nerve damage in genuine stress incontinence: an electrophysiological study. Br J Urol 1985;57:422.

Sommer C, Lalonde A, Heckman HM, et al: Quantitative neuropathology of a focal nerve injury causing hyperalgesia. J Neuropathol Exp Neurol 1995;54:635.

Spitzer M, Krumholz BA: Human papillomavirus-related diseases in the female patient. Urol Clin North Am 1992;19:71.

Swash M, Henry MM, Snooks SJ: Unifying concept of pelvic floor disorders and incontinence. J R Soc Med 1985;78:906.

Theofrastous JP: The clinical evaluation of pelvic floor dysfunction. Obstet Gynecol Clin North Am 1998;25:783.

Vignati PV, Welch JP, Cohen JL: Long-term management of diverticulitis in young patients. Dis Colon Rectum 1995;38: 627.

Walker EA, Roy-Byrne PP, Katon WJ, Jemelka R: An open trial of nortriptyline in women with chronic pelvic pain. Int J Psychiatry Med 1991;21:245.

Whitehead WE: Researchers delineate scope of visceral pain syndromes. Pain Topics 1992;5:2.

33

Liability in Gynecology

James R. Hutchison

The typical physician practicing obstetrics and gynecology in 1990 was 47 years of age, had been in practice 16 years, and had been sued three times. Nearly 80% of physicians in the specialty had been sued at least once, and more than one third had been sued three or more times. The resolution time of these claims averaged almost 5 years. Slightly fewer than half of the claims involved the practice of gynecology (American College of Obstetricians and Gynecologists [ACOG], 1990). A 1996 update of this information showed the average physician to be 46 years of age, in practice for 14 years, and sued 2.3 times. A total of 73% of the physicians in the specialty had been sued at least once, and 33.7% had been sued three or more times. The time required for resolution of a claim had decreased to 4.4 years. In 1996, 38.2% of the claims were a consequence of alleged negligence in gynecologic patient care (ACOG, 1996).

Nationally, it is anticipated that more than 4000 claims of negligent care will be filed annually against physicians practicing obstetrics and gynecology. The impact of alleged negligence on gynecologic care is a major concern for the medical profession and cannot be measured by monetary value alone. Physicians practice in a litigiously oriented society that anticipates compensation for less-than-perfect outcomes. The determination of compensation falls under tort liability, and litigation is the process used to attempt a collection and disbursement of money through the legal system.

There is no question that situations of true negligent care do occur, and in these cases the injured parties should be compensated. However, it is unrealistic to assume that almost three out of every four physicians practicing obstetrics and gynecology are "bad physicians" on the basis of filed claims. This chapter examines factors associated with the crisis, identifies clinical areas of liability risk, addresses some realistic preventative measures, and reviews the process of litigation and its consequences for physicians.

WHAT IS NEGLIGENT CARE?

Distinguishing between medical "maloccurrence" and medical "malpractice" is a concept that patients and physicians often have difficulty understanding. A *medical maloccurrence* is a bad outcome that cannot be related to the quality of care rendered by the physician. Medical and surgical complications occur even when appropriate care has been given. *Malpractice* occurs when negligent care results in an adverse outcome to the patient. *Negligence*, in this instance, is defined as the failure to render the degree of care that a reasonable and ordinarily qualified physician would provide under similar circumstances.

To be successful in a lawsuit against a physician, four elements must be proven in a court of law. Those four elements are duty, breach of duty, causation, and damages. *Duty* is the physician's obligation to treat a patient after an established relationship. *Breach* of that duty occurs when the physician does not treat the patient by the accepted standards of care. This means that not performing a procedure, or performing a procedure that should not have been performed, would be a breach of duty. *Causation* refers to that element in a lawsuit that shows that the adverse outcome was a result of a deviation from the standard of practice. *Damages* are the monies awarded to the patient as relief for the health care provider's malpractice.

WHO SETS THE "STANDARDS OF CARE"?

The standard of care for gynecology is the basic care a physician must provide when compared to a reasonably competent physician, in similar circumstances, with the same training and experience. In the past, standard of care was determined by the care rendered in the local community. Now the care is judged by national standards. It is extremely difficult to establish the true standard of care. Local hospital medical staffs, third-party payers, governmental agencies, the Joint Commission for Accreditation of Healthcare Organizations, the National Committee for Quality Assurance, the American College of Obstetricians and Gynecologists, medical liability insurance companies, and the court system have all defined expected care in specific medical situations. Frequently, these organizations include disclaimers in their publications stating that the information provided should not be judged as standards of care, but only as accepted approaches to patient care. Unfortunately, the final decision as to whether these publications promote a standard of care is left to the court system. One can conclude from this information that the term *standard of care* is somewhat nebulous when it becomes a decision of the legal system.

Medical texts, specialty publications, and current medical literature can be utilized in an attempt to establish appropriate care under specific clinical situations. Unless the plaintiff can prove with a preponderance of evidence that the physician's care fell below nationally accepted treatment standards, the obligation for a patient's care has been met. Our current system uses expert witnesses to testify regarding their interpretation of the standard of care. The final decision is then made by the court or jury on the basis of testimony that may or may not have scientific validity.

PROFESSIONAL LIABILITY INSURANCE

Most practicing physicians purchase professional liability insurance. Insurance is purchased to cover the cost of the defense of claims of alleged negligent care. It is also used as the source of payment of damages for the settlement of a claim or payment of monies awarded by a court verdict within the limits of the purchased policy. The dollar amount of coverage has a specific limit per occurrence and an aggregate amount per year. The premium rate is dependent on the historical risk of the specialty, the frequency of lawsuits, and the severity of the awards.

There are two basic types of professional liability insurance. *Occurrence coverage* covers the physician for claims of alleged negligent acts that occurred during the period of time covered by the policy regardless of when the claim is filed. The second type of coverage, *claims-made coverage*, covers the physician for claims filed during the time covered by the policy. After the claims-made policy has expired, coverage ceases. For the possible filing of later claims and to protect physicians, most insurance companies provide "tail coverage" or "reporting endorsement coverage." Purchasing this additional coverage at the time of expiration of a claims-made policy enables the insured to have coverage similar to that of an occurrence coverage policy. Claims-made coverage policies are the most common type of liability insurance policies written in the United States.

A frequent but rarely successful request in medical-legal lawsuits is for punitive damages. These are damages awarded to the patient for gross negligence (willful and wanton behavior or intentional tort) and are used to punish the defendant physician as a deterrent to future occurrences. If this type of damage is awarded, it is *not* covered under most medical malpractice insurance policies and becomes the personal financial responsibility of the physician.

AREAS OF RISK IN GYNECOLOGY

For several years, the ACOG has conducted liability surveys of its membership. This has enabled the College to identify the areas of risk for practicing physicians. In 1990, approximately 42% of the total claim information involved claims of negligence for gynecologic care. By 1996, this had decreased to approximately 38% of the claims. Failure to diagnose, patient injury minor, patient injury major, abortion related, failure of sterilization, informed consent, intrauterine contraceptive device related, and patient death were the leading categories of liability. Figure 33–1 shows a comparison of these eight most frequent events by percentage that resulted in claims of medical malpractice in the 1990 and 1996 ACOG professional liability survey (ACOG, 1990, 1996).

The majority of the allegations occurred in three major areas: failure to diagnose, minor patient injuries, and major patient injuries. Under the failure to diagnose allegation, 57.2% of the cases in 1990 and 66% of the cases in 1996 involved the failure to diagnose cancer, and almost 70% of these claims were related to the failure to diagnose breast cancer. Not only was the failure to diagnose breast cancer a frequent allegation, it was also expensive—resulting in indemnity payments averaging almost $217,245 by 1996.

In 1990, the Physician Insurers Association of America (PIAA) released its *Breast Cancer Study*. This report reviewed 273 closed paid breast cancer cases that involved a delay in diagnosis. Almost 70% of the patients were under the age of 50 years, and 40% were under the age of 40 years. Mammograms were not diagnostic in 49% of the cases, and physicians often delayed biopsy despite patient self-examination concerns or physician physical examination findings, especially in younger women. In 1995, a follow-up report was released (PIAA,1995). This study of 487 closed paid cases all alleged a delay in the diagnosis of breast cancer. The average delay from time of probable discovery to actual diagnosis was 14 months. In almost 80% of these cases the mammogram results were reported as equivocal or negative. Physicians need to maintain an awareness of diagnostic protocols for breast cancer, including appropriate biopsy in patients of any age.

The 1990s have identified new potential liability risks for the gynecologist. The diagnosis of ovarian malignancy, assuming the role of primary care provider, genetic screening, medical management of ectopic pregnancy, and advanced endoscopic gynecologic surgery are worthy of mention.

The lack of evidence-based testing for the early diagnosis of *ovarian cancer* and improved outcomes has been a concern of gynecologists for many decades. Print and broadcast media have increased pa-

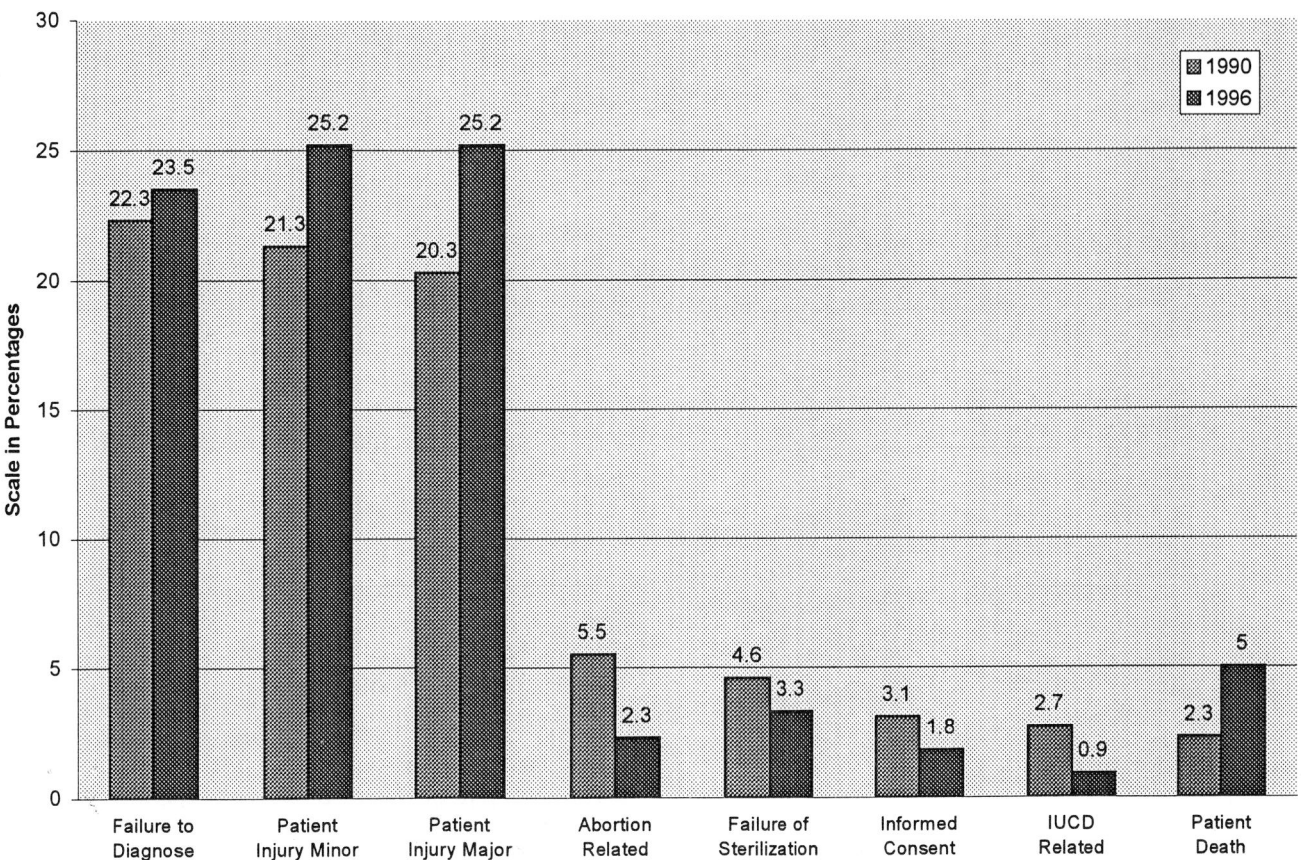

Figure 33-1
Frequency of liability risk categories, 1990 and 1995. (Data from the ACOG professional liability surveys [ACOG, 1990, 1995].)

tients' awareness that early diagnosis may be achieved with the utilization of transvaginal ultrasound examinations, genetic screening, and measurements of serum tumor marker antigens such as CA-125. In some reports, this is specifically recommended for patients with increased risk factors (i.e., first-order family history) and postmenopausal women. To date, scientific data may not substantiate the wide use of these studies for the mass screening of patients. Unfortunately, the media has proclaimed this technology as a developing standard, and physicians must counsel patients appropriately regarding current benefits and limitations of these diagnostic modalities.

Many gynecologists have assumed the role of *primary care physicians* for women. The treatment and management of diseases not involving the reproductive organs, such as asthma, hypertension, and diabetes, may become the responsibility of gynecologists with contracted health plan agreements. Gynecologists must demonstrate appropriate training and experience in the medical management of nontraditional gynecologic disease.

Genetic testing and counseling will become a major part of the practice of gynecology. Identifying the various genetic susceptibilities for many medical conditions is now a reality. Breast cancer susceptibility associated with mutations in the tumor suppressor genes BRCA1 and BRCA2 have been identified. Mutations in these genes may be associated with malfunctions of this protective function. Physicians will be confronted with the dilemma of patient selection for genetic screening, appropriate counseling of the results with the patient, costs versus benefits of this genetic information, and the associated ethical dilemmas.

Medical management of ectopic pregnancy is now an accepted therapy for this previously surgically treated condition. Proper patient selection, informed consent, and close follow-up are mandatory.

The rapid development of *advanced endoscopic gynecologic surgery* procedures has had a major impact on the specialty. The media have described laparoscopic-assisted vaginal hysterectomy as "painless hysterectomy." Patients will request this approach to their surgery, and physicians will be obliged to learn these new endoscopy techniques and offer them as options to selected patients. Most residency training programs are now teaching these techniques, and it is mandatory that, prior to performing these surgical procedures, physicians receive adequate didactic, laboratory, and preceptorship training. Failure to properly credential this approach to patient care by hospital medical staffs will place increased liability on hospitals as well as physicians.

DECREASING THE RISK OF ALLEGED NEGLIGENT CARE: RISK MANAGEMENT

The practice of gynecology, as in any medical specialty, is balanced between the science and the art of medicine. The use of both of these in the care of a patient is the obligation of the physician and is basic to the quality of that care. Ordering highly technologic tests without employing the humanistic art of medicine is fraught with danger. Conversely, ignoring the appropriate diagnostic studies and relying solely on personal attentiveness to a patient's needs is not conducive to good patient care. The following areas are important as physicians try to position themselves for the successful defense of potential litigation while providing quality care with the lowest possible patient injury.

Physician-Patient Relationship

Physicians who present themselves as hurried, noncaring practitioners set the stage for a dissatisfied patient. If an adverse outcome of care occurs, this can contribute to that patient seeking redress in the court system. The relationship established with patients not only is part of the art of medicine but also can be part of the healing process. The patient who feels that her physician is a friend as well as a professional confidant is in a better position to accept a medical maloccurrence. Knowing the patient as a person instead of a disease process improves the opportunity to help and to heal. A patient's perception of good communication with a physician and the willingness of that physician to look past the positive physical findings, laboratory/radiology reports, and procedural care develops a relationship that enhances the care plan. When a patient states that the physician "doesn't seem to care about me as a person," this is a perfect setting for alleged negligence when the outcome is less than optimal. More frequent visits to a hospitalized patient who experienced a medical maloccurrence or adverse outcome and answering the questions of both patient and family is meaningful. A physician-initiated telephone call to a patient following hospitalization or an office procedure, inquiring about her medical status, is an example of caring.

Informed Consent and Informed Refusal

Informed consent is a legal doctrine that requires a health care provider to obtain the consent of the patient for treatment rendered or surgery performed (ACOG, 1988). If documented informed consent was not obtained, a physician may be at risk when an adverse patient outcome occurs despite rendering appropriate care. Many states have specific requirements for informed consent, and physicians must be familiar with their state's legal standard.

There are two basic standards. The first is the *reasonable physician standard*, which requires the physician to supply the patient with the information customary to the rest of the medical community. The second is the *reasonable patient standard*, which requires disclosure of information a reasonable patient would want to know in the same circumstances. The process of informed consent depends on an exchange of information between the physician and the patient. Frequently, physicians rely on a patient's signature on a formal consent form as agreement to care without emphasizing the needed personal exchange of information prior to that signature. Complete informed consent probably does not exist. As a minimum, physicians should explain the diagnosis, the recommended procedure, the potential risks of the procedure, the benefits, the alternative treatments, and the expected outcome. Offering the patient another medical opinion is good practice and may provide the patient with the most comprehensive opportunity to select her appropriate care.

Informed refusal is now a recognized concept within the physician-patient relationship (ACOG, 1995). Sharing the decision making with the patient regarding a treatment or specific procedure is now the requirement of appropriate patient counseling. Patients have the right to accept or to refuse a recommendation for care. Informed refusal occurs when an informed patient rejects the physician's suggested therapy. Accurate documentation of this treatment refusal in the patient's medical record is mandatory. A signature by the patient in her record acknowledging this refusal may be beneficial.

Two exceptions to acquiring informed consent occur with true medical emergencies and in treating minors. The physician must attempt to give as much information as possible to the patient in a life-threatening situation. Documentation of that communication by the physician in the patient's record is necessary. Most states have specific statutes establishing the criteria governing the age at which a minor is permitted to give consent for medical care without parental permission. Many states provide exceptions to the law when a minor presents for diagnosis and treatment of a sexually transmitted disease, pregnancy diagnosis and care, and pregnancy termination. Knowledge of the law within the state where the physician is practicing is crucial.

In all circumstances, the treating physician must include detailed notes within the patient's record indicating that the appropriate disclosures regarding the care were communicated to the patient, including a discussion of risks versus benefits. Special informed consent forms are available and can be utilized for specific procedures. The best informed consent is establishing the patient-physician relationship, utilizing office and inpatient record documentation of the process of informed consent, and, finally, obtaining the patient's signature on a document indicating agreement to that form of therapy.

Documentation

The medical record may be used as a legal document, but our medical education may not have emphasized its importance. The legal system has alerted many physicians to the necessity of record keeping and the need for appropriate documentation of patient care. Health care providers are compensated for treating patients for a specific problem and for documenting that care. The medical record is utilized for defense during litigation, but its main function is to record a patient's history, symptoms, and physical findings; assessment of the patient; and an outline of a treatment plan. A satisfactory record should enable any qualified physician to assume the care of the patient with an understanding of the medical status and the therapy. Record keeping should encompass the following:

1. *Completeness.* Medical records must be complete. Records that do not provide documentation of all patient encounters or description of treatments are incomplete. Telephone encounters, including advice and prescribed therapies, should be promptly entered into the patient record. If a standardized form is used for obtaining a history or completing a physical exam, all blanks must be completed. If the blanks are not filled in, it is assumed that the question was not asked or the examination was not performed.
2. *Comprehensiveness.* Chart notes should be comprehensive. Progress notes in a hospital record or office notes should include the format of subjective patient complaints; objective findings, including diagnostic studies reports; assessment of the patient's status; and the plan of therapy. Including all of these in each patient encounter not only establishes the thoroughness of the care but enables other practitioners to understand the management plan.
3. *Timeliness.* Records should be completed at the time of the patient encounter. The record must be dated, and the time of the encounter and entry must be placed within the chart. In situations of critical care, the time of the entry should be recorded and, in the note, the time of the patient contact noted. Delays in the completion of an operation report for days or weeks after surgery are not acceptable. These delays may imply that the physician was overextended, was not caring, or might be recording inaccurate information.
4. *Legibility.* Records that cannot be read by the physician or other health care providers are dangerous. This suggests sloppy practice patterns and may reflect on the quality of care. Frequently physicians must defend the care of a patient many years after the event. Illegible records at that point

in time do nothing to support the standard of care rendered to the patient.
5. *Lack of alterations.* Changing or adding notes to a record out of sequence is not defensible. If a late entry is made into a patient's record, it should be labeled as a late entry and an explanation must be given within the note as to the reasons for that delay. Attempts at changing a record to promote the defense of a case are illegal and will result in embarrassment and discredit the physician's integrity.

Follow-up Documentation

Physicians must assume the responsibility of follow-up on patient treatment plans. Ordering appropriate diagnostic tests is the obligation of the physician. Following up on test reports and conveying these results to the patient also constitutes the physician's responsibility. The physician must document the follow-up conversation with the patient as well as any changes in the treatment plan. There is no defense for not responding appropriately to reports such as an abnormal mammogram or preoperative electrocardiogram.

Physician-to-Physician Communication

When a physician is going to be unavailable, conveying pertinent patient information to covering physicians and office staff is imperative. In a group practice or in a solo practice with other physicians assuming patient care, there must be documentation of the exchange of patient information to the covering physician. This coordination of patient management is expected and necessary for continuity of care. Patients must also be aware of what coverage arrangements a physician has established so they will accept the unavailability of their primary physician.

Consultation

Physicians must know their limitations. In dealing with a medical condition that would be best evaluated by another medical specialist, one should not hesitate to seek another opinion. Chart documentation of that referral and the follow-up on that referral are imperative. Documenting the offer for such a consultation demonstrates the physician's thoroughness.

THE CLAIM OF NEGLIGENT CARE

Warnings

Each day physicians deal with clinical situations that are potential sources of a claim of negligent care. The warning signs of these incidents should alert the physician to action. Anytime a complication in treatment occurs that results in an untoward outcome for a patient, the physician must record the event and advise the patient and family appropriately, with detailed documentation of that discussion. When the patient or her family expresses displeasure with the result of medical care, the physician again needs to be aware of the potential legal action. Not paying a bill or failing to return for scheduled follow-up office appointments is also a warning. A request for transfer of records to another physician, to the patient herself, or to an attorney may be the most significant indication of a potential claim of negligent care. After the physician receives the patient's authorization for record release, it is ethically and legally required that a *copy* of the patient's medical record be forwarded as requested.

The Formal Complaint

The warnings discussed above may be nothing more than warnings. If a lawsuit is filed, it will be a formal complaint of alleged negligence that will include the legal basis to support these allegations against the physician. The time period in which the patient (plaintiff) must file a lawsuit following the alleged negligence is called the *statute of limitations*; it is established by statute and may vary in each jurisdiction. After the complaint is filed with the court, the physician is served with a summons and a copy of the complaint. Each state has its own particular method for handling claims of alleged medical malpractice. Some states require review by a screening panel. If a formal complaint is received, the immediate notification of the physician's liability insurance company and attorney is indicated. At that point in time, one should never consider changing or adding to a patient's record. The physician must realize that he or she will be advised by the insurance company and attorney not to discuss the pending case with anyone except at the direction of the defense attorney.

The Process

After the filing of a formal complaint, conclusion of the process may take years. During this time, many legal activities will begin between opposing attorneys, insurance carriers, plaintiff, and defendant. The following simplification of this process is important in understanding what is expected of the physician.

Discovery

Discovery is the lengthy process performed by both the plaintiff and the defendant legal counsels and is the mechanism used to gather information about the events surrounding the case. Discovery activities may include interrogatories (lists of questions to be answered), a request for production of documents, depositions of involved parties and expert witnesses, and a request for admissions (admissions or denials in writing of a list of factual statements). Responding to these discovery procedures is a very time-consuming but extremely important obligation for the defendant physician. Unfortunately, physicians may regard this aspect of a lawsuit to be mundane and unimportant. This is the time one needs to listen to legal counsel.

One of the most important parts of discovery are *depositions*. A deposition is a question-and-answer examination under oath of the other party or potential witness named to testify at trial. Responses at deposition are evidence that can be introduced into the courtroom at the time of a trial. Preparation for a deposition is very important and is the same as preparing for a court appearance. Following the attorney's advice in this area of a lawsuit is extremely important. Remember, law is an attorney's specialty.

Trial or Settlement

After the filing of a lawsuit, facing the cost, both emotional and financial, and the risk of losing in court often motivate the parties to consider a settlement out of court. A settlement is an agreement between the parties to a financial disposition of the case without a decision on liability. A majority of cases are settled without proceeding to trial. Arbitration and mediation are frequently used in an attempt to reach a settlement. Many liability insurance companies look at the cost of litigation and frequently suggest settlement as a more financially prudent way of handling an alleged claim of malpractice. The high cost of defense and the potential of losing at trial are major concerns for insurance companies and the insured physicians. Physicians are caught in the process of negotiations and frequently feel that they need to have their "day in court" to prove that they did not commit malpractice. A prompt and early resolution of the problem without the unknown financial loss, time expenditure, and emotional trauma associated with a trial are compelling reasons to consider an out-of-court settlement. This is a very individualized decision and should be evaluated in every case on its merits after input from all concerned parties.

The Expert Witness

Much attention has been given to the testimony of the physician expert witness in the liability arena. Both parties in the process of discovery and at trial call on expert witnesses. Requirements of appropriate credentials for these expert witnesses are mandated in some states; unfortunately, however, some members of the medical profession have become "professional" experts who testify frequently and sometimes in areas where they lack expertise. These physicians are well known to the national plaintiff's bar and have gained considerable financial rewards for their expert testimony, which may or may not be substantiated in current literature or reflected in accepted standards of care. These "experts" frequently develop and state their own standards on the basis of unproven theories and often contradict themselves from testimony to testimony. After an expert witness has been identified by the plaintiff's side in the process of discovery, the deposition of that expert can be taken by the defense counsel. *It is often helpful that the defendant physician attend that deposition, not only to assist the defense attorney but also to evaluate the expert's credibility.*

If those cases go to trial, cross-examination of the professional expert witness by the defense attorney can impeach his or her credibility. Statistically, juries have excellent insight into these financially motivated testimonies. When juries are exposed to the complete information, they usually make the correct decision.

NATIONAL PRACTITIONER DATA BANK

The Health Care Quality Improvement Act of 1986 mandated the establishment of the National Practitioner Data Bank (NPDB). Expansion of this act occurred with further legislation in 1987. The act also included protection for peer review activities for hospitals and physicians. The data bank became operational in 1990. The purpose of the NPDB is to protect the public from incompetent health care providers. State licensing boards, disciplinary boards, hospitals, and other health care entities that conduct peer review on members have access to the data bank. Currently, the public does not have access to the data bank, but opening the bank to the public has been proposed.

The data bank was set up to store information on actions related to licensure status, professional competency, professional conduct, and malpractice financial settlements. For this reason, all payments in settlement or judgment for medical malpractice must be reported to the data bank and to state licensing boards. All adverse licensure actions and professional review actions in hospitals and other health care entities are reported to the data bank. Adverse actions taken against a member by professional societies that conduct formal peer review are also reported.

All hospitals must query the data bank every 2 years regarding physicians, dentists, and other health care practitioners on their staff with clinical privileges. They also must question the data bank when considering new applicants to their medical staffs. The implications of the NPDB for physicians are numerous, because the majority of gynecologists will face claims of negligent care during their lifetimes. The fact that a health care provider has been placed into this computerized bank does not necessarily imply incompetence. Because the goal of the NPDB is to improve the quality of medical care, only time will tell if the process is in fact successful.

COPING WITH THE SYSTEM

Dealing with the issue of fear of potential liability or the reaction to an actual filing of a claim of negligence creates significant emotional changes for the physician. Physicians are aware of the financial cost both to the medical profession and to society, but the enormous psychological effect on those physicians sued and their families has not been emphasized. Sara Charles, M.D., a psychiatrist from the University of Illinois College of Medicine, has written about the personal psychological implications felt by physicians as they cope with the concerns of liability (Charles et al, 1984). The decision to avoid high-risk procedures, order more laboratory and diagnostic studies, and consider early retirement is the outcome of this litigation crisis. When a physician is confronted with a claim of negligent care, it is initially met with anger, tension, frustration, and depression. Most health care providers are not willing to accept professional psychological assistance and are either too proud or embarrassed to admit their need for such help. The first correspondence a physician may receive after the filing of a lawsuit is from the liability insurance company. This correspondence commonly states that the physician should not discuss this situation with anyone except the company representative or the designated attorneys. The feeling of separation from one's professional colleagues at this time of need is then intensified. Discussing feelings without specifics regarding the case is very important. A physician's identity is threatened by this process, and support must be obtained. Many liability insurance companies and state medical societies have developed a referral system for physicians to join support groups. The families of physicians involved in litigation are also affected by the process.

Physicians need to be alerted to the signs of stress in colleagues. Sleep disorders, irritability, concentration difficulties, memory loss, and loss of self-esteem have all been reported as symptoms experienced by the sued physician. Concentrating on solutions to the financial impact on health care from this crisis without looking at the emotional effect on health care providers will do little to ease the dilemma. The emotional stress of litigation felt by health care providers, as well as the resultant effect on professional dissatisfaction, has resulted in a decreased interaction with patients and a decrease in their access to care. This is a major societal problem.

WHAT THE FUTURE HOLDS

There is little chance that a rapid solution to the litigation crisis will occur in the near future. Patients are being blocked from care, and defensive medicine has increased the cost of health care without data to support improved outcomes. The proliferation of liability claims affects the medical profession and all segments of our society. These concerns regarding the liability crisis are being addressed by both federal and state legislatures. The emphasis of legislative activity is centered on solutions to the increasing cost of health care as well as accessibility to that care. Health care providers must realize that true negligent acts do occur in the process of medical practice, and patients need to be promptly compensated for these injuries caused by an act of malpractice. We must separate true medical malpractice from medical maloccurrence. It is physicians' responsibility to assure society that they are constantly reviewing the standards for their profession and to allow only appropriately trained and qualified physicians to practice. The concept of continuous quality improvement cannot be legislated; it must be part of the practice of medicine.

Not since the turn of this century has the medical profession been confronted with such change. In the early 1890s we witnessed a change in the education of physicians from apprenticeships to scientific training. Now, almost 100 years later, we are in a modern revolution of accountability. Until recently we were accountable only to ourselves and our patients. Control of the practice of medicine and accountability is switching to the payers of health care.

The move from traditional financial reimbursement by fee for service and indemnity insurance to managed care organizations has increased liability risk for physicians. Health maintenance organizations (HMO) contract with providers and employers, and financial risk-sharing features such as capitation payments for physicians could result in physicians not furnishing medically necessary care. A physician's contract with the HMO may bar him or her from making any adverse communications about the health plan to plan beneficiaries and may bar the physician from informing patients about treatment alternatives not covered by the plan. Prior authorization for specialty referrals, adoption of practice guidelines and protocols, and confidentiality issues associated with computerized electronic records all are new potential liability risks for the physician. Mandating that physicians inform their patients of the availability of nontraditional approaches to treatment will further alienate the medical profession.

Requests by the public for access to information regarding physician liability claims history, adverse peer review activity, and adverse licensing information has prompted some states to legislate its release. Further initiatives to open the NPDB to public access continue on a federal level.

SUMMARY

This simplistic review of liability in gynecology has been an effort to focus attention on a problem that is eroding the practice of medicine. The medical profession is to blame when it supports unrealistic expectations from diagnostic procedures as well as treatment modalities. Restraint must be utilized when the purported advances of high technology are applied to health care. The benefits of this technology must be demonstrated and shown to be cost-effective. Unrealistic expectations from medical care must be addressed. The profession has a responsibility to patients to recommend cost-effective care based on outcome studies. Assuming that "more" is always "better" is no longer realistic or affordable. Following accepted standards of care, informing patients appropriately, documenting our care, performing within training experience, and honestly blending the art and science of medicine must be the ultimate goal.

REFERENCES

American College of Obstetricians and Gynecologists: Informed Consent: The Assistant. Washington, DC: American College of Obstetricians and Gynecologists, 1988.

American College of Obstetricians and Gynecologists: Professional Liability and Its Effects: Report of a 1990 Survey of ACOG's Membership. Washington, DC: American College of Obstetricians and Gynecologists, 1990.

American College of Obstetricians and Gynecologists: Informed Refusal: ACOG Committee Opinion 166. Washington, DC: American College of Obstetricians and Gynecologists, 1995.

American College of Obstetricians and Gynecologists: Professional Liability and Its Effects: Report of a 1996 Survey of ACOG's Membership. Washington, DC: American College of Obstetricians and Gynecologists, 1996.

Charles SC, Wilbert J, Kennedy EC: Physicians' self reports of reactions to malpractice litigation. Am J Psychiatry 141:563, 1984.

Physician Insurers Association of America: Breast Cancer Study. Washington, DC: Physician Insurers Association of America, 1990.

Physician Insurers Association of America: Breast Cancer Study. Washington, DC: Physician Insurers Association of America, 1995.

IV

Gynecologic Infections

34

Brian M. Casey
Susan M. Ramin
Susan M. Cox

Lower Genital Tract Infections

The most common complaint that prompts women to seek medical attention is vulvovaginitis. The symptoms include vaginal discharge, vulvar pruritis, and vaginal odor. It is not unusual for the patient with a previous history of vulvovaginitis to present with a recurrence or treatment failure of a prior infection. It is therefore of paramount importance that the physician obtain a complete history regarding prior infections and the characteristics of the current discharge, as well as a complete menstrual and sexual history. A detailed physical examination, including examination of the perineum, vulva, vagina, and cervix, should be performed. Fortunately, the etiologic agents responsible for vulvovaginitis can commonly be identified in the office or clinic by obtaining an appropriate sample of the vaginal discharge for microscopic examination. Although women complain of vaginal discharge, most of these infections involve both the vagina and cervix. In an attempt to differentiate the two, vaginitis tends to be symptomatic whereas cervicitis tends to be asymptomatic. Also, in some cases the vulva may be involved and the symptoms may be predominantly those of vulvar irritation. In this chapter, we review the clinical presentation, diagnosis, and therapy for the most common forms of vulvovaginitis (Table 34–1).

MONILIAL VAGINITIS

One of the more common benign diseases of the lower genital tract is monilial vaginitis. Monilial vaginitis is prevalent throughout the world but is seen more commonly in women living in tropical or subtropical climates. In the United States, monilial vaginitis is second only to bacterial vaginosis as a cause of symptomatic vaginitis (Fleury, 1981) and affects approximately 20% of women annually (Geiger et al, 1995). The majority of fungal vaginitis cases are caused by the genus *Candida*, with *Candida albicans* being isolated in 67% to 95% of patients (Carter et al, 1959; Dukes and Gardner, 1961; Centers for Disease Control [CDC], 1979). To date, there are over 200 strains of *C. albicans* that have been identified in

the vaginal flora, and all are equally capable of colonizing and causing vaginitis. Specifically, *Torulopsis glabrata* and *Candida* species other than *C. albicans* are pathogenic and may be responsible for fungal infection (Gardner & Dukes, 1955; Lewis et al, 1971; Oriel et al, 1972; McCormack et al, 1977). Furthermore, these organisms may account for both recurrences and treatment failures (Eschenbach, 1983; Spinillo et al, 1994).

Candida organisms, which are dimorphic, may be found in humans in different phenotypic phases. The organisms are capable of growing as a filamentous (pseudohyphae) fungus or in a yeast form. Blastospores are the phenotypic form responsible for asymptomatic colonization of the vagina as well as transmission and spread. Conversely, germinated yeast, with production of mycelia, most commonly constitute the invasive form found in the presence of symptomatic disease.

Epidemiology

Candida albicans is more frequently identified in women of childbearing age. It is unknown why *Candida* is pathogenic in some women and not in others, but commonly noted risk factors include recent use of antibiotics (especially broad-spectrum antibiotics), diabetes mellitus, immunosuppressant agents, and pregnancy (Hesseltine et al, 1934; Seelig, 1966; Oriel and Waterworth, 1975; Hopsu-Havu et al, 1980; Hurley, 1981). Importantly, *Candida* is rarely isolated from premenarchal or postmenopausal women, suggesting that there is a hormonal dependence for this infection. The growth of *Candida* is usually inhibited by the normal vaginal milieu (various lactobacilli and corynebacteria), but during pregnancy there is an increase in vaginal carriage rate as a result of an alteration in the vaginal microflora secondary to hormonal fluctuations. Also, pregnancy causes increased vaginal glycogen secondary to estrogens, vaginal thinning from progestational hormones, altered glucose metabolism, and altered sexual habits (Hopsu-Havu et al, 1980).

☐ **Table 34–1.** SIGNS, SYMPTOMS AND DIAGNOSIS OF VULVOVAGINITIS

ETIOLOGY	SYMPTOMS	CLINICAL SIGNS	DIAGNOSTIC METHOD
Monilial vaginitis	Pruritis	Thick white discharge; pH 4.0–4.7	Wet prep or KOH prep (pseudohyphae)
Trichomonas	Malodorous discharge, pruritis	Frothy, copious yellow-green discharge; pH 5.0–7.0	Wet prep (motile trichomonads)
Bacterial vaginosis	Discharge, fishy odor	Thin, gray discharge; pH 5.0–5.5	Wet prep, sniff test (clue cells)
Chlamydia	Discharge	Mucopurulent discharge, cervical erosion	Culture; MicroTrak or Chlamydiazime
Gonorrhea	Discharge	Cervical discharge	Cervical culture; Gram's stain
Genital herpes	Pain	Ulcerative, vulvar vesicles and ulcers	Virus culture, Tzank prep
Chemical	Discharge	Erythema; may be ulcerative	History and exclusion of other causes
Physiologic	Discharge	No odor or erythema	Wet prep; history, exclusion of other causes; cervical culture

Yeast may also be sexually transmitted. In women with recurrent candidiasis, *Candida* species have been identified in the ejaculates of their husbands (Gilpin, 1967). Moreover, up to 10% of men having sexual intercourse with women harboring yeast developed mycotic balanoposthitis (Oriel et al, 1972). There is, however, no direct association of yeast with other sexually transmitted diseases, nor is there a difference in yeast isolation rates between groups with and without sexually transmitted diseases.

Controversy still remains with regard to the role of oral contraceptive–induced vaginitis. An increase in yeast isolation rate without an increase in symptoms has been reported in association with oral contraceptive use (Oriel et al, 1972). In a cross-sectional survey at a large university, vulvovaginal candidiasis was associated with oral contraceptive use with a relative risk of 1.7 (95% confidence interval, 1.4 to 2.2) (Geiger et al, 1995). Additionally, women who wear tight-fitting undergarments may be at risk for yeast infection secondary to the increase in local temperature and moisture, and/or by direct irritation (Sobel, 1984). Others have also reported increased vaginal carriage rates in oral contraceptive users by way of increased adherence.

Pathogenicity

Koch's postulates have been unequivocally demonstrated for the determination of *Candida* sp. as the etiology of monilia vaginitis (Odds, 1979). The overall frequency of isolates in women with vulvovaginitis are as follows: 57% have *C. albicans*, 21% have *T. glabrata*, and 6% have *Candida tropicalis*. *Candida* virulence factors include ability to adhere to and colonize the vaginal epithelia; germination of the organism, increasing colonization and promoting tissue invasion; and ability of the original organism to switch colony types (Soll et al, 1989). Upon switching to a different colony, individual yeast cells or blastospores that vary from the original prototypic col-

ony now take on superior virulence characteristics, including an increased capacity to adhere, germinate, form mycelia, and produce proteases. It is generally believed that the ability to switch colony types contributes to the pathogenicity of *Candida*, making it capable of invading diverse body sites, altering its antigenicity, and increasing resistance to antifungal agents.

Clinical Findings

The characteristic manifestations of monilial infection are a thick, white, "cottage cheese" discharge; reddened vulvar and vaginal areas with vulvar edema; and excoriation. Raised white or yellow adherent plaques ("thrush" patches) may also be present on the epithelial surfaces (O'Brien, 1964; Odds, 1979). Intense itching is the symptom that women are likely to find troublesome and is the most frequent complaint.

Diagnosis

For accurate results, it is best to perform the pelvic examination when a woman has noted symptoms for several days and has avoided douching for at least 48 hours. Additionally, she should not have used vaginal medications for at least 5 days. The diagnosis of monilial infections is suspected on the basis of history and physical examination and can be confirmed by sampling an aliquot of the discharge and examining it under low-power light microscopy. Wet-smear microscopy of the vaginal secretion along with signs found at examination should be the first-line test in the diagnosis (Zdolsek et al, 1995). The characteristic microscopic finding is the presence of the branched and budding pseudohyphae of the candidal organisms. Other genera of yeast that are normally harbored in the vagina do not produce such pseudohyphae. To further aid the observer, a drop of 10% potassium hydroxide (KOH) may be added to the sample, which will destroy all the cells except for the fungus because the cell wall of the fungus is resistant to this concentration of alkali. The KOH preparation will detect *Candida* in approximately 80% of infected patients (McLennan et al, 1972). It may be more difficult to identify *C. albicans* on KOH preparations when present in the yeast phase. Therefore, although the saline or KOH wet preparation will usually suffice for office or clinic use, the most reliable method for identifying *Candida* species is by culture in Sabouraud's medium. Cultures on Nickerson's media are also available and have a sensitivity of 95% (Hantschke, 1981). Culture should be used when there is a clinical suspicion of vulvovaginal candidiasis but the patient has a negative microscopic exam (Zdolsek et al, 1995). In support of this, Oriel and colleagues (1972) previously observed that 50% of culture-positive women did not have pseudohyphae on wet smear.

Treatment

A thorough history regarding systemic diseases, recent use of antibiotics and other drugs, previously treated infection, and douching habits should be obtained before initiating therapy. Treatment relieves symptoms in 80% to 90% of cases, but recurrence is common. There are several therapeutic regimens (Table 34–2) available for the treatment of monilial vaginitis, including the topical use of nystatin, miconazole, clotrimazole, amphotericin B, and/or gentian violet (Teoh et al, 1977; Bentley et al, 1978; VanSlyke et al, 1981; Dennerstein and Langley, 1982; Gil-Antunanos & Palacios, 1983; Lebherz et al, 1985). These antifungal regimens have little to no vaginal absorption. Nystatin (Mycostatin), a commonly used antifungal agent, is available in vaginal suppositories, cream, or ointment. The usual dose is either one suppository (100,000 units) or one g (100,000 units/g) of the cream applied intravaginally two times a day for 7 days. A high failure rate, however, has been reported in treating pregnant women with nystatin, and recurrent infections are common (Long et al, 1956; Wallenberg and Wladimiroff, 1976; McNellis et al, 1977).

Currently, a mainstay of therapy for monilial infections is an imidazole preparation. These include miconazole (Monistat), clotrimazole (Gyne-Lotrimin or Mycelex-G), butoconazole (Femstat), tioconazole (Vagistat), and ketoconazole (Nizoral). In fact, imidazoles have been shown to be more effective in eradicating infection. Two studies comparing the cure rates of nystatin and miconazole for the treatment of monilial vulvovaginitis during pregnancy demonstrated a significantly higher cure rate with miconazole (Wallenberg and Wladimiroff, 1976; McNellis et al, 1977). Clotrimazole and miconazole have broad-spectrum activity against dimorphic fungi and yeast along with some activity against bacteria. In comparison with clotrimazole, miconazole was slightly less effective during the logarithmic growth phase of *C. albicans* but demonstrated greater fungicidal activity (Van den Bossche et al, 1975). The usual dose for both agents is one suppository or one

Table 34–2. TREATMENT REGIMENS FOR MONILIAL VULVOVAGINITIS

AGENT	DOSE
Nystatin (Mycostatin)	One vaginal tablet × 7–14 days 1 g cream bid × 7–14 days
Clotrimazole (Gyne-Lotrimin, Mycelex-G)	100-mg vaginal tablet qd × 7 days 500-mg vaginal tablet × one dose 1% cream 5 g intravaginally qd × 7–14 days
Miconazole (Monistat)	100-mg vaginal suppository qhs × 7 days 200-mg vaginal suppository qhs × 3 days 2% cream 5 g intravaginally qhs × 7 days 2% cream 5 g or lotion for topical use bid × 14 days
Tioconazole (Vagistat)	6.5% ointment (4.6 g) intravaginally × one dose
Terconazole (Terazol)	80-mg vaginal suppository qhs × 3 days 0.4% cream 5 g intravaginally qhs × 7 days 0.7% cream 5 g intravaginally qhs × 3 days
Butoconazole (Femstat)	2% cream 5 g intravaginally qhs × 3 days
Ketoconazole (Nizoral)	200-mg tablet PO qd or bid × 7–14 days
Fluconazole	150-mg tablet PO × one dose
Boric acid powder	600 mg in gelatin capsules qd × 14 days
Gentian violet	1% solution for topical use

full applicator intravaginally every night for 7 days. The cream may also be applied to the vulva to relieve the pruritis associated with monilial infection. The development of the single-dose 500-mg clotrimazole intravaginal tablet translates into a more effective and longer lasting concentration of the active agent at the infection site (Fleury et al, 1985). Some studies have shown that, 48 hours after insertion of the tablet, fungicidal quantities of drug still remain in the vaginal fluid. In a randomized study of 100 women, a 100% success rate was achieved with a single dose of this intravaginal clotrimazole tablet (Odds and MacDonald, 1981); others have reported less success (Fleury et al, 1985; Lebherz et al, 1985). The main advantage of butoconazole (vaginal cream 2%) is its 3-day regimen. This formulation has been shown in several trials to be equivalent to other topical antifungal agents. A multicenter, double-blind trial comparing butoconazole (2% cream) for 3 days with clotrimazole (200-mg vaginal tablets) for 3 days revealed microbiologic cure rates of 95% and 91%, respectively (Droegemueller et al, 1985).

Ketoconazole, an imidazole piperazine derivative, is a safe, effective, orally active preparation for the treatment of vaginal candidiasis. The usual dose is 200 mg orally twice daily for 5 days. The main advantages of ketoconazole compared to conventional therapy include convenience (oral vs. vaginal) and potential to eliminate the gastrointestinal reservoir of *Candida* (Bingham, 1984). Commonly reported side effects are abdominal pain (1.2%), pruritis (2%), and gastrointestinal upset (5%) (Talbot and Spencer, 1983). Ketoconazole therapy may lead to hepatic dysfunction from hepatocellular toxicity. This is uncommon and is usually reversible; however, one case of fatal hepatic necrosis has been reported.

The relatively new and effective triazole antifungals include terconazole and fluconazole. Terconazole has been shown to be effective therapy for *C. albicans* vulvovaginitis (Hirsch, 1989; Thomasen, 1989). The normal dosage is one applicatorful of cream intravaginally daily for 7 days or one vaginal suppository daily for 3 days. Fluconazole is a *bis*-triazole compound that is orally active and is also a safe and effective treatment of vaginal candidiasis. The usual therapy, a single dose of 150 mg, has been reported to be as effective as 7 days of intravaginal clotrimazole (van Heusden et al, 1994; Sobel et al, 1995).

A topical 1% aqueous dye, gentian violet, has been reported to be effective when applied to cervical and vaginal mucosa of women with candidiasis. The disadvantages of gentian violet include local irritation and the staining of clothing. Boric acid (one dose contains 600 mg of boric acid powder in a gelatin capsule) intravaginally has also been reported to be effective in the treatment of candidiasis. There are no serious side effects from this regimen other than a watery discharge (VanSlyke et al, 1981). Boric acid capsules should be avoided in pregnancy because of the potential of boron toxicity.

A woman with recurrent monilial vulvovaginitis, especially when lacking predisposing factors, poses a rather difficult situation for the practitioner. Some of these women may be susceptible to recurrent fungal infections because of an altered immune system. In a recent study of 151 women with a history of recurrent vulvovaginal candidiasis who were treated with either clotrimazole or ketoconazole, an extremely high recurrence rate was noted in both groups (Sobel et al, 1994). Therefore, treatment of recurrent fungal vulvovaginitis should include an initial full course of therapy followed by maintenance therapy comprised of topical therapy immediately prior to or during menstrual flow for a minimum of two cycles. If a reduction of the gastrointestinal fungal colony count is desirable, treatment of the acute episode with ketoconazole is the preferred choice. Sexual transmission may play a role in cases of recurrent fungal vaginitis, particularly in women who have a monogamous relationship. Males can be effectively treated with topical antifungal creams.

TRICHOMONAL VAGINITIS

Trichomonas vaginalis, a flagellated parasite first described by Donne in 1836, is the etiologic agent of trichomonal vaginitis. *Trichomonas vaginalis* is an anaerobic protozoan characterized by four anteriorly located flagelli and an anterior lateral undulating membrane. It is slightly larger than a leukocyte and is oval in shape (Burch et al, 1958). This organism, of which humans are the only known host, is sexually transmitted and appears to be associated with multiple sexual partners. *Trichomonas vaginalis* frequently coexists with other sexually transmitted organisms (Eschenbach, 1983). In fact, this parasite commonly exists asymptomatically in vaginal and cervical secretions in females and seminal fluid in males (McLennan et al, 1972). Although the reservoir for *T. vaginalis* may be either male or female, the male primarily functions as a vector for transmission and is more likely to be asymptomatic than the female. Approximately one in five women will develop trichomoniasis during their lifetimes. The incidence of trichomonal vaginitis is not correlated with age, day of menstrual cycle, type of contraceptive used, recent use of antibiotics, or frequency of intercourse (McLellan et al, 1982).

Clinical Findings

This organism predominantly infects the vagina, urethra, endocervix, and bladder, causing a multitude of symptoms in the reproductive woman. The primary symptom, a profuse malodorous vaginal discharge, will vary in appearance depending on the severity of inflammation and secondary infection (Foutes and Kraus, 1980). The discharge is classically described as frothy and yellow (identified in only

20% of symptomatic women), but may vary from white and watery to thick and green. The cervix can be extensively involved, and postcoital bleeding is often associated with trichomonal cervicitis. Although they are seen in less than 5% of women with active trichomoniasis, examination of the vagina and cervix may reveal the characteristic red punctate lesions (subepithelial hemorrhages) known as "strawberry patches." Additionally, vaginal and vulvar erythema, edema, and excoriation may be present when the infection is severe. The patient may complain of pruritis, burning, or dysuria, as well as dyspareunia.

Diagnosis

The diagnosis of trichomoniasis can be confirmed by microscopic examination of a wet mount. The motile flagellated trichomonads can be easily identified in 80% to 90% of infected patients (Hess, 1969; Penza and Rankin, 1970; McLennan et al, 1972). Trichomonads may also be identified on Papanicolaou-stained smears but not as reliably as with the wet-mount examination (McLennan et al, 1972). In an accuracy analysis of screening Pap smears in diagnosing trichomoniasis, 30% of patients would be treated unnecessarily. As a result, we recommend a confirmatory test prior to initiating therapy (Weinberger and Harger, 1993).

The most sensitive diagnostic technique is culture of *T. vaginalis*. Historically, however, because of the impracticality of maintaining Diamond's medium in the office setting, cultures have not been used frequently. Chintana and associates (1979) compared the sensitivities of wet-mount examinations, Papanicolaou-stained preparations, and cultures. Upon examining approximately 1200 asymptomatic female subjects, the culture method was positive in 16.5%, the wet-mount preparation in 15.5%, and the Pap smear in only 6.7%. Furthermore, one study in 600 high-risk women compared the diagnostic accuracy of two culture media against wet-mount ex-

aminations, Pap-stained smears, and a rapid immunodiagnostic method for the diagnosis of *Trichomonas* infection (Krieger et al, 1988). Of the 88 positive cultures, the Feinberg-Whittington and Diamond's culture media produced the diagnosis in 93% and 89%, respectively, while the wet prep and Pap smears were relatively insensitive, confirming the culture diagnosis in only 60% and 56%, respectively.

A newer, more sensitive test, the InPouch TV culture system (BioMed Diagnostics, San Jose, CA), has a selective fungicidal and bacteriocidal medium with a longer shelf life. This convenient culture system has been proven effective in pregnant (Draper et al, 1993) and nonpregnant (Borchardt et al, 1992) patients. Interestingly, direct immunofluorescence with monoclonal antibodies diagnosed 86% of the 88 cases and holds future promise as an adjunct to our current diagnostic methods (Krieger et al, 1988). Also, a number of polymerase chain reaction (PCR)-based tests have been developed and are highly specific for *T. vaginalis* (Riley et al, 1992; Kengne et al, 1994).

Treatment

The treatment of *T. vaginalis* is directed at eradicating this sexually transmitted organism. Acidification of the vagina or douching with a mild antiseptic or povidone-iodine are effective for symptomatic relief but are not effective for cure (Dunlop and Wisdom, 1965). The only effective treatment for *T. vaginalis* is metronidazole (Flagyl), the prototype of the 5-nitroimidazole agents (Table 34–3). It has selective activity against anaerobic bacteria and protozoa, and most isolates are exquisitely sensitive, with susceptibilities at minimum inhibitory concentrations of less than 1 μg/ml. Metronidazole is usually administered orally as a single dose of 2 g (Morton, 1972; Woodcock, 1972; Fugere et al, 1983; CDC, 1989). This method, because it is easier to administer, is less expensive and affords greater patient compliance. To minimize gastrointestinal disturbance, this dosage

Table 34–3. RECOMMENDED TREATMENT REGIMENS FOR BACTERIAL VAGINOSIS AND TRICHOMONIASIS

AGENT	DOSE
Bacterial Vaginosis	
• Metronidazole (Flagyl)	500 mg PO bid × 7 days
	250 mg PO tid × 5–7 days
• Ampicillin	250 mg PO qid × 7 days
• Clindamycin	300 mg PO bid × 7 days
• Cephalosporin	250 mg PO qid × 7 days
Trichomoniasis	
• Metronidazole (Flagyl)	2 g PO in a single dose
	250 mg PO tid × 5–7 days
	500 mg PO bid × 7 days
• Clotrimazole (Gyne-Lotrimin, Mycelex-G)*	One 100-mg vaginal tablet or applicatorful of 1% cream qd × 7 days

*Symptomatic treatment only (see text).

may be divided into two 1-g administrations, with one dose in the morning and one in the evening. An intravenous incremental dosing protocol has been proposed for women with severe symptomatic *T. vaginitis* and an allergy to metronidazole (Pearlman et al, 1996). Women with recurrent trichomoniasis may require a longer treatment period, such as 250 mg three times daily for 7 days. Both methods are more than 95% effective (Hager et al, 1980; Lossick, 1982).

Candidasis is a side effect of metronidazole, caused by the eradication of specific vaginal flora, particularly with longer treatment schedules (Aubert and Sesta, 1982). Other possible side effects include an Antabuse-like reaction if alcohol is consumed during therapy, alterations in depth perception, a metallic aftertaste, gastrointestinal intolerance, and blood dyscrasias.

Significant controversy exists concerning the possible oncogenicity, mutagenicity, and teratogenicity of metronidazole (Robinson & Mirchandani, 1965; Peterson et al, 1966; Morgan, 1978; Beard et al, 1979; Goldman, 1980; Fleury, 1981; Cantu and Garcia-Cruz, 1982; Eschenbach, 1983). Conflicting conclusions on the safety of metronidazole in pregnancy have resulted in concern about its widespread use in women with trichomoniasis. Morgan (1978) reported that metronidazole did not influence birth weight or fetal viability or increase congenital anomalies. A randomized, double-blind, placebo-controlled trial of single-dose intravaginal versus single-dose oral metronidazole therapy in culture-positive women sought to circumvent systemic use. However, a single 2-g intravaginal dose of metronidazole gel was inferior to the single oral dose regimen (Tidwell et al, 1994). Although there are no available studies supporting metronidazole as a teratogenic agent, it is commonly recommended that this drug not be prescribed during the first trimester. As an alternative, clotrimazole may be used for symptomatic relief of trichomonal infection during the first trimester. Both clotrimazole and miconazole are safe for use during pregnancy. Metronidazole may be used later in gestations for women in whom local therapy (clotrimazole) did not relieve symptoms. Additionally, it is recommended that metronidazole not be used during breast-feeding because it is excreted in breast milk (Fleury, 1981). Lactating women can be given a single dose of metronidazole, pump their breasts for 24 hours, and then resume breast-feeding.

There have been reports of *T. vaginalis* strains resistant to metronidazole (Meingassner and Thurner, 1979). However, isolation of these strains demonstrated a decreased sensitivity but not resistance to metronidazole. A recommended effective treatment option reported for resistant cases is metronidazole 2 to 4 g/day for 2 weeks. Intravenous metronidazole is usually reserved for those cases of resistant infection unresponsive to oral administration.

Controversy exists regarding the treatment of the male consort of a woman with trichomonas vulvo-vaginitis (Fleury, 1981). Some investigators believe that, because *T. vaginalis* has a short survival time in the male genital tract and with the potential Antabuse effect of metronidazole, treatment of the male consort is not warranted. However, the CDC (1989) recommends concurrent treatment of male consorts. In either case, women should be counseled to either abstain from intercourse during treatment or use a condom to prevent reinfection.

BACTERIAL VAGINOSIS

Another common cause of vaginitis is bacterial vaginosis, a term used for the entity once called nonspecific vaginitis or *Gardnerella* vaginitis. It accounts for 45% of all vulvovaginal infections in women of reproductive age (Eschenbach, 1993). This condition represents a malproportion of bacterial species in the vagina—specifically a decrease in lactobacilli and an increase in anaerobic organisms (Eschenbach et al, 1988). The salient features of this entity, which was first described by Gardner and Dukes in 1955, includes a gray, homogeneous, malodorous vaginal discharge with a pH of 5.0 to 5.5 without yeast forms or trichomonads present. The vaginal discharge is copious, and on microscopic examination stippled, granulated epithelial cells termed *clue cells* are present. Leukocytes are not prominent, and characteristic Gram's stain of the vaginal discharge reveals a predominance of *Gardnerella* and *Mobiluncus* species together with other small gram-negative rods and gram-positive cocci. The organism *Gardnerella vaginalis* (formerly *Haemophilus vaginalis* or *Corynebacterium vaginale*) is frequently isolated from the vaginal secretions (90%) (Holmes, 1981) and has been associated with this entity since its original description. Unfortunately, during the last 30 years, and particularly since the use of newer selective culture media, it is apparent that *G. vaginalis* can be detected in 40% to 50% of otherwise normal women without signs or symptoms of vaginal infection (Eschenbach et al, 1988). Also, anaerobic bacteria such as *Bacteroides* species play a major role in the pathophysiology of bacterial vaginosis (Spiegel et al, 1980). *Mobiluncus*, a small, curved, gram-negative rod, is isolated in many women with bacterial vaginosis as well; however, the role of this organism remains uncertain (Spiegel et al, 1983; Sprott et al, 1983; Roberts et al, 1984).

Bacterial vaginosis has been found in 10% to 25% of women in general obstetric and gynecologic clinics and in up to 64% of patients visiting sexually transmitted disease clinics (American College of Obstetricians and Gynecologists, 1996). Interestingly, in a 5-year survey of more than 25,000 women presenting with symptomatic vaginitis or vaginal discharge, *G. vaginalis* accounted for 33% of cases of vaginal infection, whereas *Candida* and *Trichomonas* contributed 20% and 10%, respectively (Fleury, 1981). Finally, Eschenbach and co-workers (1988) compared the use of Gram's stains with a composite of clinical criteria for the diagnosis of bacterial vaginosis in 616 randomly selected women attending a sexually transmitted disease clinic. The sensitivity, specificity, and predictive value of the Gram's stain were determined in comparison with the composite clinical criteria for this diagnosis. In summary, bacterial vaginosis was documented by clinical criteria in 33%, clue cells in 39%, and Gram's stain criteria in 47%, and *G. vaginalis* was isolated in high concentrations from 63%. Moreover, if women were divided into positive composite clinical criteria versus negative clinical criteria for bacterial vaginosis, isolation rates of *G. vaginalis* were 97% and 58%, respectively.

Special mention of bacterial vaginosis and pregnancy is warranted given the associations with several obstetric complications. Bacterial vaginosis has been associated with premature rupture of membranes, infection of the chorion and amnion, histologic chorioamnionitis, infection of amniotic fluid, and preterm delivery. In a cohort study of over 10,000 pregnant women, bacterial vaginosis was again associated with preterm delivery of low-birth-weight infants independent of other recognized risk factors (Hillier et al, 1995). Another prospective controlled trial confirmed these associations and reported a 50% reduction in bacterial vaginosis–linked preterm birth and preterm premature rupture of membranes (McGregor et al, 1995). Ultimately, then, pregnant women at risk of preterm birth or preterm premature rupture of membranes should be screened for bacterial vaginosis and treated (Hauth et al, 1995; McGregor et al, 1995).

Clinical Findings

Fifty percent of women with bacterial vaginosis are asymptomatic (Eschenbach et al, 1988). The most common complaint is nonpruritic vaginal discharge associated with a "fishy" odor, most pronounced after menses, coitus, or alkaline douche (Pheifer et al, 1978; American College of Obstetricians and Gynecologists, 1996). The discharge does not fit the classical description of discharge caused by monilial, trichomonal, or gonorrheal infections; it may be thin, gray, white, and noncharacteristic of an infection. In contrast to candidiasis or trichomoniasis, there are few if any symptoms of vulvovaginal irritation (pruritis, inflammation, or edema).

Diagnosis

The diagnosis of bacterial vaginosis is generally based upon clinical findings after excluding all other causes. The vaginal pH is usually between 5.0 and 6.0. When a small drop of KOH is added to an aliquot of the vaginal discharge, a "fishy" odor is often released (positive "sniff" or "whiff" test) (Chen et al, 1979; Fleury, 1981; Eschenbach, 1983). The alka-

Table 34-4. CLINICAL CRITERIA FOR A DIAGNOSIS OF BACTERIAL VAGINOSIS

1. pH > 4.5
2. Clue cells
3. Positive KOH
4. Homogeneous discharge

linization of the discharge by KOH, blood, or semen results in the volatilization of amines, causing the "fishy" odor. Women with trichomoniasis may have a positive whiff test, although the odor is not as pronounced (Eschenbach, 1983). Microscopic examination usually reveals a paucity of white blood cells in conjunction with clue cells. Clue cells are desquamated epithelial cells with clusters of bacteria attached to their surfaces so that the borders are obscured (Gardner and Dukes, 1955). However, up to 40% of patients with bacterial vaginosis may not have clue cells (Eschenbach, 1983).

The diagnosis can be made based on three of four clinical criteria listed in Table 34-4. Using these criteria, more than 90% of patients with bacterial vaginosis will be diagnosed correctly and the number of false-positive diagnoses will be less than 10% (American College of Obstetricians and Gynecologists, 1996).

Culture confirmation is generally not necessary unless the vaginitis is persistent after fungal and trichomonal etiologies have been eliminated. Laboratory diagnosis is confirmed by a major change in vaginal flora from a predominance of *Lactobacillus* to a mixture of anaerobic bacteria and *G. vaginalis* in the absence of lactobacilli. Gas-liquid chromatography can be used to identify the by-products of carbohydrate and protein metabolism by these anaerobic bacteria, such as the succinic acid and acetic acid produced by *Bacteroides* and *Gardnerella* species, respectively (Spiegel et al, 1983). Despite the role of anaerobes in the pathophysiology of this entity, cultures are not necessary in the diagnosis of bacterial vaginosis.

Treatment

Therapy is directed against *G. vaginalis* as well as the anaerobic bacteria. Numerous agents have been used for the treatment of bacterial vaginosis, including local agents such as sulfa creams, tetracycline vaginal tablets, 2% clindamycin cream, and metronidazole gel. Systemic agents such as tetracycline, ampicillin, cephalosporins, clindamycin, and metronidazole have also been evaluated (Table 34-3) (Smith and Dunkelberg, 1977; Pheifer et al, 1978; Fleury, 1981; Eschenbach, 1983). Ampicillin and amoxicillin are antibiotics that have activity against *G. vaginalis* in vitro; however, in vivo these organisms have been shown to possess β-lactamase activity and are not inhibited by these drugs. In addition, the other anaerobic bacteria are not sensitive to penicillins. This is apparent clinically because, 7 to 14 days after initiation of therapy with ampicillin or amoxicillin, 57% of women have persistent or recurrent bacterial vaginosis. Other less effective regimens include 250 mg of a cephalosporin four times daily for up to 7 days. Additionally, tetracyclines are contraindicated during pregnancy because of potential adverse fetal effects.

The treatment of choice and most efficacious agent for bacterial vaginosis is metronidazole (Pheifer et al, 1978; Fleury, 1981; Eschenbach, 1983). Metronidazole has excellent activity against both anaerobic bacteria and *Trichomonas*. Seven-day regimens of 500 mg twice daily and 250 mg three times a day have shown greater than 90% efficacy (American College of Obstetricians and Gynecologists, 1996). Furthermore, guidelines from the CDC list a single 2-g dose as appropriate treatment. However, this single-dose regimen is slightly less effective and results in greater gastrointestinal upset (Hager et al, 1980; CDC, 1993). Finally, oral clindamycin at a dose of 300 mg twice daily for 7 days has also been shown to be an effective regimen, but it may be more frequently associated with diarrhea (American College of Obstetricians and Gynecologists, 1996).

Two intravaginal regimens also have similar efficacy. The available agents include 0.75% metronidazole gel applied twice daily for 5 days and 2% clindamycin cream applied daily for 7 days (Hillier et al, 1990; Hillier, 1993). Also, vaginal sulfa creams are not effective against *G. vaginalis* and tetracycline vaginal tablets are contraindicated in pregnancy.

In women with persistent or recurrent bacterial vaginosis, treatment of the partner remains a controversial issue. Although bacterial vaginosis is more prevalent in sexually active women or women with other sexually transmitted diseases, there has been no evidence that concurrent treatment of partners improves the cure rate or reduces recurrence rates. However, in women with persistent bacterial vaginosis, oral treatment of their partners may be helpful. Additionally, women with recurrent or persistent bacterial vaginosis should also be screened for other sexually transmitted diseases and human immunodeficiency virus infection.

Metronidazole use should be restricted to symptomatic pregnant women after the first trimester who did not respond to initial therapy or who are penicillin allergic. Other therapies, such as sulfa cream, doxycycline, and ampicillin, have been effective in 55%, 64%, and 48% of cases, respectively (Pheifer et al, 1978; Balsdon et al, 1980). As with metronidazole, prolonged treatment with either ampicillin or a cephalosporin may be associated with candidal overgrowth.

CHLAMYDIAL CERVICITIS

Currently the most prevalent venereal disease in the United States is chlamydia. In 1985 there were an estimated 4.6 million new cases of chlamydia, with more than $1 billion (direct and indirect costs) spent on chlamydial infections annually (Gunby, 1983). However, because reporting has not been universal in the United States, the true incidence of chlamydia infection is unknown. *Chlamydia trachomatis*, an obligate intracellular parasite, is a specific human pathogen (Schachter, 1978). Fifteen serotypes of chlamydia have been identified to date and are associated with three major groups of infection; these include lymphogranuloma venereum (LGV) from serotypes L1, L2, and L3; endemic blinding trachoma from serotypes A, B, Ba, and C; and sexually transmitted diseases and perinatal infections from serotypes D through K (Grayston and Wang, 1975).

Chlamydia trachomatis depends upon the host cell for energy and nutrients because it does not contain enzyme systems able to generate ATP, and is therefore capable only of limited metabolic activity. The organism is therefore referred to as an "energy parasite." The elementary body is the particle capable of transmitting infection, and columnar epithelial cells internalize the elementary bodies by endocytosis. Within the endocytic vesicle, the elementary body changes into the reticulate or intermediate body. It is the inclusion body that is formed as a result of the multiple divisions of the intermediate body within the vesicle (Page, 1974) that can be stained with iodine, Giemsa stain, or fluorescent antibody technique.

Clinical Findings

The cervix is the site most commonly colonized with *C. trachomatis* in the female, which results in endocervicitis. The most specific clinical symptoms for chlamydial infection are purulent or mucoid discharge, postcoital bleeding and vaginitis (Ghinsberg and Nitzan, 1994). Also, asymptomatic infection may occur (Paavonen and Vesterinen, 1982). In one study of over 500 women, approximately 8% of asymptomatic controls were found to have evidence of chlamydial infection (Garozzo et al, 1993). Because *C. trachomatis* does not infect squamous cells, it is not associated with vaginitis by itself.

However, other infectious agents are frequently isolated in association with chlamydial infection. For example, multiple logistic regression analysis of a cohort of women with chlamydial endocervicitis identified four risk factors associated with isolation of *C. trachomatis*. These are *Neisseria gonorrhoeae* cervicitis, *G. vaginalis* cervicitis, purulent vaginal discharge, and age less than 25 years (Rugpao et al, 1993). Speculum examination reveals an edematous, congested cervix and possibly the presence of hypertrophy of the endocervical columnar tissue (ectropy). Mucopus is observed to be extruding from the cervical os and is characterized by 20 or more leukocytes per high-power field when examined microscopically. Chlamydia are also capable of ascending the urethra, causing nongonococcal urethritis in both men and women. Finally, *C. trachomatis* may ascend to the fallopian tubes, causing acute salpingitis and pelvic inflammatory disease (Paavonen, 1980; Mardh and Svensson, 1982; Paavonen et al, 1982).

Diagnosis

Currently, cell culture is the reference method for diagnosis of infection with *C. trachomatis*. In the past, demonstration of intracellular inclusions in genital tract scrapings were used to identify chlamydial infection. This technique has been abandoned because of poor sensitivity. In fact, Schachter and Dawson (1978) observed that cervical infections caused by chlamydia are recognized cytologically in only 20% of cases. However, if cultures or direct detection techniques are not available, cytologic examination using the Giemsa stain may prove helpful. In addition, there are serologic tests available for detection of chlamydial infections, but they are of little value except in diagnosing LGV and *C. trachomatis* pneumonitis (Woods, 1995). A complement fixation test is utilized in diagnosing LGV and a single titer of 1:64 or greater supports its presumptive diagnosis. A microimmunofluorescent test is still more sensitive for diagnosing *C. trachomatis* pneumonitis, with detection of immunoglobulin M titers of 1:32 or greater being diagnostic. However, because of the high background rates of anti-chlamydial antibodies in sexually active populations, the use of serologic tests to diagnose genital chlamydial infections is not recommended.

Newer direct methods for identification of the chlamydial organism involve the use of monoclonal or polyclonal antibodies, DNA probes, and PCR. The direct immunofluorescent antibody test was the first nonculture chlamydia detection test developed. It allows direct visualization of elementary bodies in specimens using different monoclonal antibodies available from several manufacturers. Sensitivity of this test varies greatly depending on the antibody used, prevalence of infection in the population, and the number of elementary bodies required for a positive result (Woods, 1995).

Enzyme immunoassays (EIAs) detect chlamydial lipopolysaccharides with monoclonal or polyclonal antibodies. Total processing time is 15 to 30 minutes, with sensitivities that are also variable, with a tendency to be higher in persons attending a sexually transmitted disease clinic (Woods, 1995). Also, a commercially available acridinium ester–labeled DNA probe complementary to *C. trachomatis* ribosomal RNA acid allows direct detection within 3 hours. PCR techniques are available but are limited by their expense and wide range of sensitivities. Despite variable sensitivities in all direct methods, specificities are greater than 95%.

The "gold standard" used for the diagnosis of chlamydia is isolation of the organism in tissue cul-

ture. McCoy cells, the cell line of choice, can be pretreated with either 5-iodo-2-deoxyuridine or cyclohexamate in order to enhance sensitivity. The organisms are centrifuged onto cell monolayers and incubated for 24 to 72 hours. After incubation, the monolayers can be fixed, stained, and microscopically examined for the presence of inclusion-forming units. It is important that an adequate sample of involved epithelial cells be obtained for culture because the organism cannot be isolated from the discharge alone.

Therapy

With the increasing number and improved availability of direct diagnostic tests for *C. trachomatis*, the number of documented genital chlamydial infections should increase (Lee et al, 1995). Common treatment regimens include tetracycline 500 mg orally four times daily or doxycycline 100 mg orally twice daily for 7 days. Erythromycin base is an alternative regimen at 500 mg orally four times daily for 7 days. If gastrointestinal symptoms occur, a dose of 250 mg four times daily for 14 days may be substituted. These less expensive regimens have recently given way to more costly but convenient therapies. A single dose of azithromycin (1 g) has been proven effective in treating urethral and cervical chlamydial infection (Anonymous, 1995; Weber and Johnson, 1995). Ofloxacin also offers a convenient, albeit more expensive, alternative with twice-daily dosing for 1 week.

For chlamydial infection in pregnancy, doxycycline, other tetracyclines, and ofloxacin are contraindicated. Therefore, erythromycin base is the recommended regimen. Effective alternative regimens in pregnancy include amoxicillin 500 mg three times daily for 7 days or a single 1-g dose of azithromycin. It must be remembered, however, that the safety of azithromycin in pregnancy has not been well established. Finally, it is of utmost importance that all partners of women with chlamydia be treated with one of the above regimens because it is a sexually transmitted disease.

GONOCOCCAL CERVICITIS/VAGINITIS

Gonorrhea is the most common reported communicable disease in the United States. There are an estimated 1 million new infections with *N. gonorrhoeae* in the United States each year. Specifically, it is an infection of the columnar and transitional epithelial cells of the female genital tract. Infectivity appears to be related to the presence of hair-like structures, or pili, on the bacterium that are important for the attachment of the gonococcal organism to the epithelial cell (Swanson et al, 1971). The organism, *N. gonorrhoeae*, is a gram-negative, kidney-shaped diplococcus that measures approximately 1 μ in diameter. Optimal growth of this organism occurs at 34° to 36°C, with a pH of 7.2 to 7.6 in humid aerobic conditions and 5% to 10% CO_2 (Kellogg et al, 1963).

Clinical Findings

Gonorrhea may present as cervicitis and/or vaginitis in prepubertal girls and in the early stages of disease in women of reproductive age (Schrocter and Pazin, 1970). The discharge is commonly described as profuse in volume, odorless, nonirritating, and creamy white to yellow in color. Gonococcal infection may involve the Bartholin's gland with resultant abscess formation. Furthermore, the infection may ascend to the endometrium and the fallopian tube, resulting in pelvic inflammatory disease (Rees and Annels, 1969). When the infection involves the fallopian tubes, the inflammatory exudate and the accompanying pus exude from the fimbriated ends of the fallopian tube into the peritoneal cavity, thereby involving the ovaries, the cul-de-sac, and the pelvic peritoneum. In one study of nearly 300 infertile women, those who reported previous gonococcal infection were at an increased risk of tubal infertility (Grodstein et al, 1993). Other symptomatic sequelae from this disease include arthritis, chronic endometritis, endocarditis, Fitzhugh-Curtis syndrome (gonococcal perihepatitis), and pelvic abscesses (Ackerman et al, 1965; Trimble, 1970; Holmes et al, 1971; Thompson et al, 1974; Rothbard et al, 1975).

Additionally, gonococcal infection in any trimester may have a deleterious effect on pregnancy outcome. Preterm delivery, premature rupture of membranes, chorioamnionitis, and postpartum infection are more common in women with *N. gonorrhoeae* detected at delivery (Wendel and Wendel, 1993). Also, newborns of infected mothers may develop gonococcal ophthalmia neonatorum.

Diagnosis

Culture of the urogenital tract is the reference method for diagnosis of gonococcal cervicitis/vaginitis. However, a more rapid diagnosis may be possible by direct examination of a gram-stained smear from the urogenital tract (Schmale et al, 1969; Rudolph and Printz, 1971; Woods, 1995). Microscopic examination revealing numerous white blood cells is suggestive of gonorrhea, and a Gram's stain revealing gram-negative intracellular kidney-shaped diplococci within polymorphonuclear leukocytes is more convincing.

Importantly, other *Neisseria* organisms that are normal flora of the human vagina may produce false-positive Gram's stains. Therefore, culture of the organism remains the mainstay or "gold standard" of diagnosis. Thayer-Martin selective medium is optimal for culturing these organisms. Because of the fastidious nature of *N. gonorrhoeae* and the potential toxicity of swabs to the organism, immediate plating to a culture medium at room temperature is preferred (Martin et al, 1967; Woods, 1995). The culture should be incubated immediately with a source of carbon dioxide for the critical 5% CO_2 atmosphere.

As with other sexually transmitted diseases, direct detection methods are being developed and some are commercially available. Currently an EIA for detection of *N. gonorrhoeae* is available; however, the sensitivity of endocervical specimens is less than with cervical culture. Also, an oridinium ester–labeled DNA probe allows direct detection of *N. gonorrhoeae*, and several studies indicate that its reliability is comparable to that of culture. This probe is the same probe a clinician may use for *C. trachomatis*. The advantage of this is a single probe to diagnose both infections; the disadvantage is obviously cost (Woods, 1995).

Therapy

The treatment regimens recommended by the CDC for uncomplicated gonococcal infection are listed in Table 34–5. Ceftriaxone (Rocephin), a broad-spectrum cephalosporin antibiotic, has bactericidal activity against *N. gonorrhoeae* (including penicillinase-producing strains). A single injection of 125 mg yields high bactericidal blood levels and is considered sufficient therapy. This is a reduction from the 1993 recommendation for a 250-mg injection. Cefixime, which is administered orally, has an antimicrobial spectrum similar to that of ceftriaxone but unfortunately does not reach the same bactericidal levels. Therefore, it is less efficient in cases of pharyngeal gonorrhea but is clinically efficacious in other cases of gonorrhea. Ciprofloxacin, an orally administered quinolone antibiotic, produces sustained bactericidal blood levels and is clinically effective at all anatomic sites. It is also the least expensive of all the recommended options. Ofloxacin (Floxin) is another quinolone with proven clinical efficacy. Importantly, however, quinolones should be avoided in patients less than 18 years of age and during pregnancy. Another equally effective and preferred

---

Table 34–5. TREATMENT REGIMENS FOR UNCOMPLICATED GONOCOCCAL INFECTIONS

A single dose of
- Ceftriaxone 125 mg IM, *or*
- Cefixime 400 mg orally, *or*
- Ciprofloxacin 500 mg orally, *or*
- Ofloxacin 400 mg orally

PLUS

- A regimen effective against co-infection with *C. trachomatis*, such as doxycycline 100 mg orally 2 times/ day for 7 days

alternative regimen is a single 2-g intramuscular injection of spectinomycin. This has been recommended for penicillinase-producing *N. gonorrhoeae*, which causes 2% of gonorrheal infections in the United States.

Up to 40% of persons with gonorrhea are also infected with *C. trachomatis*; therefore, follow-up therapy with an antimicrobial effective against chlamydia is recommended. It is also of paramount importance that known sexual partners of women with all forms of gonorrhea be cultured and receive appropriate antibiotic therapy. Additionally, it is recommended that cultures be repeated after antibiotic therapy to verify cure.

HERPETIC VULVOVAGINITIS/CERVICITIS

Genital herpes, a sexually transmitted disease, may be caused by herpes simplex virus type I or type II (HSV-I or HSV-II). The herpesvirus is a double-stranded DNA virus surrounded by a glycoprotein envelope (Nahamias et al, 1980). Herpes simplex virus is the most common cause of genital ulcers in the United States and other developed countries. Approximately 85% of primary genital herpes infections are due to HSV-II, whereas 15% are caused by HSV-I. Herpesvirus is endemic in the United States, with an estimated 600,000 new cases of genital herpes annually and a prevalence of more than 20 million. The incidence of symptomatic disease is 1% to 2% of the population (Corey et al, 1983), but as many as 50% to 80% of adults will have antibodies to the herpesviruses (HSV-I or HSV-II). Genital herpes appears to affect the 15- to 29-year-old age group with the highest frequency. Herpetic vulvovaginitis and cervicitis is a recurrent disease, with recurrence being three to four times more likely following infection with HSV-II compared to infection with HSV-I (Reeves et al, 1981). Interestingly, 25% of the recurrences are asymptomatic; however, asymptomatic viral excretors are known to be infective.

Clinical Findings

According to Corey and colleagues (1983), genital HSV infections occur in three distinct clinical manifestations: first-episode primary herpes, first-episode nonprimary herpes, and recurrent herpes. *First-episode primary herpes* is the initial infection in a patient without circulating antibodies to HSV-I or HSV-II. Clinically, patients suffer from severe local symptoms involving multiple painful lesions that progress from vesicles to an ulcerative stage with inguinal adenopathy. Moreover, commonly seen systemic effects include fever, malaise, myalgias, headache, and nausea. *First-episode nonprimary genital herpes* is an infection that occurs in patients with circulating antibodies to HSV-I or HSV-II. The clinical manifestations and course are comparable to those

seen in recurrent herpes, with patients having mild local symptoms lasting for a few days compared to the primary episode. The number of lesions is less and systemic manifestations of the disease are absent. Moreover, there is a shorter duration of viral shedding and the likelihood of concomitant HSV shedding from the cervix is less than with primary disease. Ultimately, the majority of cases of genital herpes will not likely present with classical lesions such as tender, grouped vesicles or ulcers. More likely, patients with herpetic infection will present with "nonspecific" genital ulcers (University of Washington School of Medicine and the CDC, 1994).

Genital HSV probably complicates pregnancy more often than appreciated. The clinical course in pregnancy has been studied in women with recently acquired recurrent genital herpes infection. Approximately 80% of these women will have symptomatic recurrences during pregnancy, with the average number of recurrent infections ranging from two to four. The risks of adverse pregnancy outcome are greatest when the initial outbreak of genital herpes is during the pregnancy. Concomitant cervical infection is common with primary genital infection, and the viral inoculum tends to be high. First-episode HSV infection early in pregnancy has been associated with an increased rate of spontaneous abortion, whereas late pregnancy primary infection is associated with an increased incidence of preterm labor (Wendel and Wendel, 1993).

Diagnosis

For patients who present with classical, painful grouped vesicles or ulcers, the diagnosis of genital herpes can be based on clinical criteria alone. Because most cases will not present in this fashion, definitive diagnosis often requires detection of the virus. Conventional cell culture remains the reference method and is the most sensitive technique for detection of HSV in clinical specimens (Corey, 1982; Corey and Holmes, 1983; Woods, 1995). Vesicles and their fluid have the highest concentration of virus particles and should be sampled if possible. The sample should be placed immediately in a viral transport medium (Hanks balanced salt solution) and refrigerated. Inoculated cell cultures are then examined for the cytopathic effect of HSV. This cytopathic effect should appear within 7 days but usually takes 3 days (Woods, 1995).

Direct detection methods have also been developed. Characteristic intranuclear inclusions may be observed in Tzanck preparations or those smears stained with Pap stain. Additionally, solid-phase and membrane EIA tests, along with enzyme-linked immunofluorescent assays, are available. In general, the sensitivity of these direct methods is less (50% to 70%) than that of cell cultures. This is especially true in nonvesicular infection (Naib et al, 1966; Brown et al, 1979; Woods, 1995).

Therapy

Treatment is directed at relieving symptoms. For cases of primary infection, acyclovir is effective at decreasing the duration of symptoms as well as the duration of viral shedding (Corey et al, 1982; Bryson et al, 1983; Anonymous, 1995). Acyclovir, a competitive inhibitor of viral DNA polymerase and DNA chain terminator, interferes with viral thymidine kinase and, therefore, viral replication. The recommended regimen for the first clinical episode of genital herpes is acyclovir 200 mg orally five times a day for 7 to 10 days or until clinically resolved (CDC, 1989). However, many clinicians consider 400 mg orally three times daily as effective and more convenient (Anonymous, 1995). Oral acyclovir is not highly effective for treatment of recurrent genital herpes, but a regimen of 200 mg twice daily may decrease or prevent recurrences of genital herpes simplex virus infection (Douglas et al, 1984; Fife et al, 1994). Topical acyclovir provides little or no benefit.

In pregnancy, the safety of acyclovir has not been firmly established; however, its use has not been associated with an increased risk of congenital anomalies. In fact, one study on acyclovir prophylaxis in pregnant women with primary herpetic infections revealed a decreased cesarean delivery rate because of a decreased presence of lesions at the time of delivery (Scott et al, 1996). Further studies on acyclovir and its prodrug esters are underway to establish their safety and efficacy in pregnancy.

CHEMICAL-INDUCED VAGINITIS

Any chemical that is placed into the vagina is a potential irritant. The list of chemical irritants is numerous and includes spermicides and the vehicles carrying the spermicides, douches and douche powders, acetic acid, and the antimicrobials used in treating other forms of vaginitis and cervicitis. Table 34–6 lists some of the known chemical irritants.

Clinical Findings

The vaginal discharge from a woman with chemical-induced vaginitis is nonspecific in nature. Micro-scopic examination of the vaginal discharge may reveal numerous white cells, without evidence of concomitant trichomonads or monilial hyphae.

Diagnosis

Chemical-induced vaginitis is suspected in a woman with a history of excessive douching or the onset of symptoms associated with use of a topical vaginal agent. Importantly, the diagnosis of chemical-induced vaginitis is a diagnosis of exclusion.

Treatment

After identification of the chemical irritant, treatment involves removal of the substance.

ENTEROBIUS VAGINITIS

The pinworm, *Enterobius vermicularis*, may cause vaginitis in the prepubescent female. *Enterobius* vaginitis occurs secondarily to the migration of the adult worm from the anus to the vaginal area. The patient will typically complain of a vaginal discharge, perineal erythema, and pruritis that is most severe at night.

Diagnosis

The diagnosis of *Enterobius* vaginitis is made by applying cellophane tape to the perianal and/or perineal area and placing the tape adhesive side down on a glass microscope slide. The characteristic double-walled *Enterobius* ova are pathognomonic for the condition.

Treatment

Treatment of *Enterobius* vaginitis involves one dose of pyrantel pamoate suspension. It is important that other family members be treated as well.

SUMMARY

Every effort should be made by the clinician to arrive at an appropriate diagnosis and institute specific therapy for lower genital tract disease. It is recommended that the clinician avoid the so-called shotgun approach because the medications employed with this approach may do more harm than good. Therapy is usually unrewarding and economically impractical in patients who are asymptomatic with their vaginal infections, except in cases of chlamydia or gonorrhea infection, which must be treated.

Table 34–6. CHEMICAL IRRITANTS OF THE VAGINA

Bubble baths	Over-the-counter drugs
Deodorant soaps	Perfumes
Deodorant sprays	Perfume-treated toilet paper
Home remedies	Spermicides
Hot tub water	Swimming pool water
Laundry detergent, especially enzyme-activated "cold water" formulas	

REFERENCES

Ackerman AB, Miller RC, Shapiro L: Gonococcemia and its cutaneous manifestations. Arch Dermatol 1965;91:227.

American College of Obstetricians and Gynecologists: Vaginitis (Technical Bulletin No 226). Washington, DC: American College of Obstetricians and Gynecologists, 1996.

Anonymous: Drugs for sexually transmitted diseases. Med Lett Drugs Ther 1995;37:117.

Aubert JM, Sesta HJ: Treatment of vaginal trichomoniasis, single 2-gram dose of metronidazole as compared with a seven-day course. J Reprod Med 1982;27:743.

Balsdon MJ, Taylor GE, Pead L, et al: Corynebacterium vaginale and vaginitis: A controlled trial of treatment. Lancet 1980;1:501.

Beard C, Noller K, O'Fallon W, et al: Lack of evidence for cancer due to use of metronidazole. N Engl J Med 1979;301:519.

Bentley S, Bournes MS, Powell A: A comparative study of miconazole nitrate pessaries and Nystan vaginal tablets in one treatment of vaginal candidiasis. Br J Clin Pract 1978;32:258.

Bingham JS: Single blind comparison of ketoconzaole 200 mg oral tablets and clotrimazole 100 mg vaginal tablets and 1% cream in treating acute vaginal candidiasis. Br J Venereal Dis 1984;60:175.

Borchardt KA, Hernandez V, Miller S, et al: A clinical evaluation of trichomoniasis in San Jose, Cost Rica using the InPouch TV test. Genitour Med 1992;68:328.

Brown ST, Jaffe HW, Zaidi A, et al: Sensitivity and specificity of diagnostic tests for genital infection with herpes virus hominis. Sex Transm Dis 1979;6:10.

Bryson YJ, Dillon M, Lovett M, et al: Treatment of first episodes of genital herpes simplex virus infection with oral acyclovir. N Engl J Med 1983;308:916.

Burch TA, Rees CW, Kayhoe DE: Laboratory and clinical studies on vaginal trichomoniasis. Am J Obstet Gynecol 1958;76:658.

Cantu JM, Garcia-Cruz D: Midline facial defects as a teratogenic effect of metronidazole. Birth Defects 1982;18:84.

Carter B, Jones CP, Creadick RN: The vaginal fungi. Ann N Y Acad Sci 1959;83:265.

Centers for Disease Control: Nonreported sexually transmitted diseases. MMWR Morbid Mortal Wkly Rep 1979;28:61.

Centers for Disease Control: 1989 Sexually transmitted diseases treatment guidelines. MMWR Morbid Mortal Wkly Rep 1989; 38(suppl):16.

Centers for Disease Control: 1993 Sexually transmitted diseases treatment guidelines. MMWR Morbid Mortal Wkly Rep 1993; 42(RR):1.

Chen KCS, Forsyth PS, Buchanan TM, et al: Amine content of vaginal fluid from the untreated and treated patients with non-specific vaginitis. J Clin Invest 1979;63:828.

Chintana J, Sucharit P, Chongsuphajaisiddhi T: A study on the diagnostic methods for Trichomonas vaginalis infection. Southeast Asian J Trop Med Public Health 1979;10:81.

Corey L: The diagnosis and treatment of genital herpes. JAMA 1982;248:1041.

Corey L, Adams HG, Brown Z, Holmes K: Genital herpes simplex virus infections: clinical manifestations, course, and complications. Ann Intern Med 1983;98:958.

Corey L, Holmes K: Genital herpes simplex virus infections: current concepts in diagnosis, therapy and prevention. Ann Intern Med 1983;98:973.

Corey L, Nahmias AJ, Guinan ME, et al: A trial of topical acyclovir in genital herpes simplex virus infections. N Engl J Med 1982;306:1313.

Dennerstein GJ, Langley R: Vulvovaginal candidiasis: treatment and recurrence. Aust N Z J Obstet Gynaecol 1982;22:231.

Donne A: Animalcules observes dans les matieres purulentes et le produit des secretions des organes genitaux de l'homme et de la femme. Acad Sci 1836;3:385.

Douglas JM, Critchlow C, Benedetti J, et al: A double-blind study of oral acyclovir for suppression of recurrences of genital herpes simplex virus infection. N Engl J Med 1984;310:1551.

Draper D, Parker R, Patterson E, et al: Detection of Trichomonas vaginalis in pregnant women with the InPouch TV culture system. J Clin Microbiol 1993;31:1016.

Droegemueller W, Adamson DG, Brown D, et al: Three-day treatment with butoconazole nitrate for vulvovaginal candidiasis. Obstet Gynecol 1985;64:530.

Dukes CD, Gardner HL: Identification of Haemophilus vaginalis. J Bacteriol 1961;81:277.

Dunlop EMC, Wisdom AR: Diagnosis and management of trichomoniasis in men and women. Br J Venereal Dis 1965;41:85.

Eschenbach DA: Vaginal infection. Clin Obstet Gynecol 1983;26:186.

Eschenbach DA: History and review of bacterial vaginosis. Am J Obstet Gynecol 1993;169:441.

Eschenbach DA, Hillier S, Critchlow C, et al: Diagnosis and clinical manifestations of bacterial vaginosis. Am J Obstet Gynecol 1988;158:819.

Fife KH, Crumpacker CS, Mertz GJ, et al: Recurrence and resistance patterns of herpes simplex virus following cessation of ≥6 years of chronic suppression with acyclovir: Acyclovir Study Group. J Infect Dis 1994;169:1338.

Fleury FJ: Adult vaginitis. Clin Obstet Gynecol 1981;24:407.

Fleury FJ, Hughes D, Floyd R: Therapeutic results obtained in vaginal mycoses after single-dose treatment with 500 mg clotrimazole vaginal tablets. Am J Obstet Gynecol 1985;152:968.

Foutes AC, Kraus SJ: Trichomonas vaginalis: reevaluation of its clinical presentation and laboratory diagnosis. J Infect Dis 1980; 141:137.

Fugere P, Verschelden G, Caron M: Single oral dose of ornidazole in women with vaginal trichomoniasis. Obstet Gynecol 1983; 62:502.

Gardner H, Dukes CD: Haemophilus vaginalis vaginitis: a newly defined specific infection previously classified as "nonspecific" vaginitis. Am J Obstet Gynecol 1955;69:962.

Garozzo G, Lomeo E, La Greca M, et al: Chlamydia trachomatis diagnosis: a correlative study of Pap smear and direct immunofluorescence. Clin Exp Obstet Gynecol 1993;20:259.

Geiger AM, Foxman B, Gillespie BW: The epidemiology of vulvovaginal candidiasis among university students. Am J Public Health 1995;85:1146.

Ghinsberg RC, Nitzan Y: Chlamydia trachomatis direct isolation, antibody prevalence and clinical symptoms in women attending outpatient clinics. New Microbiol 1994;17:231.

Gil-Antunanos S, Palacios P: Vulvovaginal candidiasis: comparative study of the therapeutic efficacy of miconazole, nystatin, econazole nitrate, clotrimazole and Amphotericin B applied topically. Revista Gine-Dips No 13, 1983.

Gilpin CA: Resistant monilial vaginitis: male aspect. Fl State Med J 1967;54:337.

Goldman P: Metronidazole: proven benefits and potential risks. Johns Hopkins Med J 1980;147:1.

Grayston JT, Wang S-P: New knowledge of chlamydiae and the diseases they cause. J Infect Dis 1975;132:87.

Grodstein F, Goldman MB, Cramer DW: Relation of tubal fertility to history of sexually transmitted diseases. Am J Epidemiol 1993;137:577.

Gunby P: Chlamydial infections probably most prevalent of STD's. Arch Intern Med 1983;143:1665.

Hager WE, Brown ST, Kraus SJ, et al: Metronidazole in vaginal trichomonas: seven day vs single dose regimens. JAMA 1980; 244:1219.

Hantschke B: Essential and possible laboratory studies in a gynecological practice of prospective vaginal candidiasis. In Illingworth HPR (ed): GynoTraveogen Monograph. Amsterdam: Excerpta Medica, 1981.

Hauth JC, Goldenberg RL, Andrews WW, et al: Reduced incidence of preterm delivery with metronidazole and erythromycin in women with bacterial vaginosis. N Engl J Med 1995; 333:1732.

Hess J: Review of current methods for the detection of trichomonas in clinical material. J Clin Pathol 1969;22:69.

Hesseltine HC, Bonts IC, Peass ED: Pathogenicity of the monilia (castellani), vaginitis, and oral thrush. Am J Obstet Gynecol 1934;27:112.

Hillier SL: Diagnostic microbiology of bacterial vaginosis. Am J Obstet Gynecol 1993;169:455.

Hillier SL, Nugent RP, Eschenbach DA, et al: Association between bacterial vaginosis and preterm delivery of a low birthweight infant: the Vaginal Infections and Prematurity Study Group. N Engl J Med 1995;333:1737.

Hillier SL, Witkin SS, Krohn MA, et al: The relationship of amniotic fluid cytokines and preterm delivery, amniotic fluid infection, histologic chorioamnionitis, and chorioamnion infection. Obstet Gynecol 1990;81:941.

Hirsch HA: Clinical evaluation of terconazole: European experience. J Reprod Med 1989;34:593.

Holmes K: Nonspecific vaginosis. Scand J Infect Dis Suppl 1981; 26:110.

Holmes K, Counts GW, Beaty HN: Disseminated gonococcal infection. Ann Intern Med 1971;74:979.

Hopsu-Havu VK, Gronroos M, Punneren R: Vaginal yeast in parturients and infestations of the newborns. Acta Obstet Gynecol Scand 1980;59:73.

Hurley R: Recurrent Candida infections. Clin Obstet Gynecol 1981;8:209.

Kellogg DS Jr, Peacock WL Jr, Deacon WE, et al: Neisseria gonorrhoeae. I. Virulence genetically linked to clonal variation. J Bacteriol 1963;85:1274.

Kengne P, Veas F, Vidal N, et al: Trichomonas vaginalis: repeated DNA target for highly sensitive and specific polymerase chain reaction diagnosis. Cell Mol Biol 1994;40:819.

Krieger JN, Tam MR, Stevens CE, et al: Diagnosis of trichomoniasis: comparison of conventional wet-mount examination with cytologic studies, cultures, and monoclonal antibody staining of direct specimens. JAMA 1988;259:1223.

Lebherz T, Guess E, Wolfson N: Efficacy of single versus multiple dose clotrimazole therapy in the management of vulvovaginal candidiasis. Am J Obstet Gynecol 1985;152:965.

Lee HH, Chernesky MA, Schachter J, et al: Diagnosis of Chlamydia trachomatis genitourinary infection in women by ligase chain reaction assay of urine. Lancet 1995;345:213.

Lewis JF, O'Brien SM, Ural UM, et al: Corynebacterium vaginale vaginitis in pregnant women. Am J Clin Pathol 1971;56:580.

Long WE, Stella JG, Benchakan V: Nystatin vaginal tablets in treatment of candidal vulvovaginitis. Obstet Gynecol 1956;8:364.

Lossick JG: Treatment of Trichomonas vaginalis infection. Rev Infect Dis 1982;4(suppl):801.

Mardh P-S, Svensson L: Chlamydial salpingitis. Scand J Infect Dis Suppl 1982;32:64.

Martin JE, Billings TW, Hackney JF, et al: Primary isolation of N. gonorrhoeae with a new commercial medium. Public Health Rep 1967;82:361.

McCormack WM, Hayes CH, Rosner B, et al: Vaginal colonization with Corynebacterium vaginale (Haemophilus vaginalis). J Infect Dis 1977;136:740.

McGregor JA, French JI, Parker R, et al: Prevention of premature birth by screening and treatment for common genital tract infections: results of a prospective controlled evaluation. Am J Obstet Gynecol 1995;173:157.

McLellan R, Spence MR, Brockman M, et al: The clinical diagnosis of trichomoniasis. Obstet Gynecol 1982;60:30.

McLennan MT, Smith JM, McLennan CE: Diagnosis of vaginal mycosis and trichomoniasis: reliability of cytologic smear, wet smear, and culture. Obstet Gynecol 1972;40:231.

McNellis D, McLeod M, Lawson J, et al: Treatment of vulvovaginal candidiasis in pregnancy: a comparative study. Obstet Gynecol 1977;50:674.

Meingassner JG, Thurner J: Strain of Trichomonas vaginalis resistant to metronidazole and other 5-nitroimidazoles. Antimicrob Agents Chemother 1979;15:254.

Morgan I: Metronidazole treatment in pregnancy. Int J Gynecol Obstet 1978;15:501.

Morton RS: Metronidazole in the single-dose treatment of trichomoniasis in men and women. Br J Venereal Dis 1972;48:525.

Nahmias A, Dowdle W, Schinazi R (eds): The Human Herpes Virus: An Interdisciplinary Perspective. (Proceedings of the International Conference on Human Herpes Virus). New York: Elsevier, 1980.

Naib ZM, Nahmias AJ, Josey WE: Cytology and histopathology of cervical herpes simplex infection. Cancer 1966;19:1026.

O'Brien JR: Nickerson's medium in the diagnosis of vaginal monilia. Can Med Assoc J 1964;90:1073.

Odds FC: Candida and Candidiasis. Baltimore: University Park Press, 1979.

Odds FC, MacDonald F: Persistence of miconazole in vaginal secretions after single applications: implications for the treatment of vaginal candidosis. Br J Veneral Dis 1981;57:400.

Oriel JD, Partridge BM, Denny MJ, et al: Genital yeast infections. Br Med J 1972;4:761.

Oriel JD, Waterworth PM: Effect of minocycline and tetracycline on the vaginal yeast flora. J Clin Pathol 1975;28:403.

Paavonen J: Chlamydia trachomatis in acute salpingitis. Am J Obstet Gynecol 1980;138:957.

Paavonen J, Vesterinen E: Chlamydia trachomatis in cervicitis and urethritis in women. Scand J Infect Dis Suppl 1982;32:45.

Paavonen J, Vesterinen E, Mardh P-A: Infertility as a sequelae of chlamydial pelvic inflammatory disease. Scand J Infect Dis Suppl 1982;32:73.

Page LA: The rickettsias. In Buchanan RE, Gibbons NE (eds): Bergey's Manual of Determinative Bacteriology. 8th ed. Baltimore: Williams & Wilkins, 1974:914.

Pearlman MD, Hashar C, Ernst S, et al: An incremental dosing protocol for women with severe vaginal trichomoniasis and adverse reaction to metronidazole. Am J Obstet Gynecol 1996; 174:934.

Penza J, Rankin JS: Infectious vaginopathies during pregnancy. Clin Obstet Gynecol 1970;13:223.

Peterson WF, Stauch JE, Ryder CD: Metronidazole in pregnancy. Am J Obstet Gynecol 1966;94:343.

Pheifer TA, Forsyth PS, Durfee MA: Nonspecific vaginitis: role of Haemophilus vaginalis and treatment with metronidazole. N Engl J Med 1978;298:1429.

Rees E, Annels EH: Gonococcal salpingitis. Br J Venereal Dis 1969; 45:205.

Reeves WC, Corey L, Adams HC, et al: Risk of recurrence after first episode of genital herpes. N Engl J Med 1981;305:315.

Riley DE, Roberts MC, Takayama T, et al: Development of a polymerase chain reaction-based diagnosis of Trichomonas vaginalis. J Clin Microbiol 1992;30:465.

Roberts MC, Hillier SL, Schoenknecht FD, et al: Nitrocellulose filter blots for species identification of Mobiluncus curtisii and M. mulieris. J Clin Microbiol 1984;20:826.

Robinson SC, Mirchandani G: Trichomonas vaginalis. V. Further observations on metronidazole (including infant follow-up). Am J Obstet Gynecol 1965;93:502.

Rothbard MJ, Gregory T, Staerns LJ: Intrapartum gonococcal amnionitis. Am J Obstet Gynecol 1975;121:565.

Rudolph AH, Printz DW: Recommendations on the diagnosis of gonorrhea. JAMA 1971;218:448.

Rugpao S, Sirirungsi W, Vannareumol P, et al: Isolation of Chlamydia trachomatis among women with symptoms of lower genital tract infection. J Med Assoc Thailand 1993;76:475.

Schachter J: Chlamydial infections. N Engl J Med 1978;298:428, 490, 540.

Schachter J, Dawson CR: Human Chlamydial Infections. Littleton, MA: PSG Publishing, 1978.

Schmale JD, Martin JE Jr, Domesick G: Observations on the culture diagnosis of gonorrhea in women. JAMA 1969;210:312.

Schrocter AL, Pazin GJ: Gonorrhea. Ann Intern Med 1970;72:553.

Scott LL, Sanchez PJ, Jackson GL, et al: Acyclovir suppression to prevent cesarean delivery after first-episode genital herpes. Obstet Gynecol 1996;87:69.

Seelig MS: The role of antibiotics in pathogenesis of Candida infections. Am J Med 1966;40:887.

Smith RF, Dunkelberg WE: Inhibition of Corynebacterium vaginale by metronidazole. Sex Transm Dis 1977;4:20.

Sobel JD: Recurrent vulvovaginal candidiasis, what we know and what we don't [editorial]. Ann Intern Med 1984;101:390.

Sobel JD, Brooker D, Stein GE, et al: Single oral dose fluconazole compared with conventional clotrimazole topical therapy of Candida vaginitis: Fluconazole Vaginitis Study Group. Am J Obstet Gynecol 1995;172:1263.

Sobel JD, Schmitt C, Stein G, et al: Initial management of recurrent vulvovaginal candidasis with oral ketoconazole and topical clotrimazole. J Reprod Med 1994;39:517.

Soll DR, Galask R, Isley S, et al: Switching of *Candida albicans* during successive episodes of recurrent vaginitis. J Clin Microbiol 1989;27:681.

Spiegel CA, Amsel R, Eschenbach D, et al: Anaerobic bacteria in nonspecific vaginitis. N Engl J Med 1980;303:601.

Spiegel CA, Eschenbach DA, Amsel R, et al: Curved anaerobic bacteria in bacterial (nonspecific) vaginosis and their response to antimicrobial therapy. J Infect Dis 1983;148:817.

Spinillo A, Nicola S, Colonna L, et al: Frequency and significance of drug resistance in vulvovaginal candidiasis. Gynecol Obstet Invest 1994;38:130.

Sprott MS, Ingham RS, Pottman RL, et al: Characteristics of motile curved rods in vaginal secretions. J Med Microbiol 1983;16:175.

Swanson J, Kraus SJ, Gotschlieh EL: Studies on gonococcus infection. I. Pili and zones of adhesion: Their relation to gonococcal growth patterns. J Exp Med 1971;134:886.

Talbot MD, Spencer RC: Oral ketoconazole in the treatment of vaginal candidosis. Curr Res Ther 1983;34:746.

Teoh SK, Asari AR, Ysof K, et al: Miconazole in the treatment of vulvovaginal candidiasis. Aust N Z J Obstet Gynaecol 1977;17:98.

Thomasen JL: Clinical evaluation of terconazole, United States experience. J Reprod Med 1989;34:597.

Thompson TR, Swanson RE, Weisner PJ: Gonococcal ophthalmia neonatorum. JAMA 1974;228:186.

Tidwell GH, Lushbaugh WB, Laughlin MD, et al: A double-blind placebo-controlled trial of single-dose intravaginal versus single-dose oral metronidazole in the treatment of trichomonal vaginitis. J Infect Dis 1994;170:242.

Trimble C: Gonococcal hepatitis simulating acute cholecystitis. Surg Gynecol Obstet 1970;130:54.

University of Washington School of Medicine and the Centers for Disease Control and Prevention: Sexually transmitted diseases treatment guidelines. Clin Courier 1994;12:1.

Van den Bossche H, Willemsens G, Van Cutsem J: The action of miconazole on the growth of *Candida albicans*. Sabourandia 1975;13:63.

van Heusden AM, Merkus HM, Euser R, et al: A randomized, comparative study of a single oral dose of fluconazole versus a single topical dose of clotrimazole in the treatment of vaginal candidosis among general practitioners and gynaecologists. Eur J Obstet Gynecol Reprod Biol 1994;55:123.

VanSlyke K, Michel VP, Rein MF: Treatment of vulvovaginal candidiasis with boric acid powder. Am J Obstet Gynecol 1981;141:145.

Wallenberg HCS, Wladimiroff JW: Recurrence of vulvovaginal candidiasis during pregnancy: comparison of miconazole versus nystatin treatment. Obstet Gynecol 1976;48:491.

Weber JT, Johnson RE: New treatments for *Chlamydia trachomatis* genital infection. Clin Infect Dis 1995;20S:866.

Weinberger MW, Harger JH: Accuracy of the Papanicolaou smear in the diagnosis of asymptomatic infection with *Trichomonas vaginalis*. Obstet Gynecol 1993;82:425.

Wendel PJ, Wendel GD Jr: Sexually transmitted diseases in pregnancy. Semin Perinatol 1993;17:443.

Woodcock KR: Treatment of *T. vaginalis* with a single oral dose of metronidazole. Br J Venereal Dis 1972;48:65.

Woods GL: Update on laboratory diagnosis of sexually transmitted diseases. Clin Lab Med 1995;15:665.

Zdolsek B, Hellberg D, Froman G, et al: Culture and wet smear microscopy in the diagnosis of low-symptomatic vulvovaginal candidosis. Eur J Obstet Gynecol Reprod Biol 1995;58:47.

35

Upper Genital Tract Infections

David E. Soper

U pper genital tract infections in women are characterized by bacterial (or rarely, viral) infection located above the internal cervical os. Their importance is underscored by their association with longstanding sequelae such as tubal factor infertility caused by pelvic inflammatory disease (PID) or life-threatening illness such as clostridial sepsis associated with septic abortion. These infections affect hundreds of thousands of women each year and are responsible for a substantial physical, emotional, and economic burden (Grimes et al, 1977; Washington et al, 1986; Washington and Katz, 1991).

ANATOMIC, IMMUNOLOGIC, AND MICROBIOLOGIC BARRIERS TO INFECTION

Nonspecific and nonimmunologic factors play an important role in providing a barrier to the penetration of bacteria across the genital mucosa, in a manner similar to the mucosa of the respiratory and intestinal tracts. These factors include antibacterial properties found in vaginal secretions, cervical mucus, endometrial secretions, and oviductal fluids. Vaginal secretions maintain the integrity of and, in conjunction with macrophage activity, offer additional protection against bacterial penetration of the vaginal mucosa. The cervical mucus, by virtue of its gel structure and cell composition, is a mechanical barrier to ascending infection. In addition, cervical mucus proteins, such as lactoferrin, possess antibacterial activity that inhibits bacterial penetration into the endometrium. The secretion of endometrial and oviductal fluids, with the help of myometrial and ciliary activity, help wash out cellular debris and possibly bacteria from the upper genital tract. Endometrial and oviductal secretions also possess lactoferrin and lysozomal enzymes with antibacterial activity (Chow et al, 1980; Ogra et al, 1981).

Like all mucosal surfaces in direct contact with the external environment, the genital tract has a common immune system that functions somewhat independently of the systemic immune system. The endocervix and uterus contain varying amounts of organized lymphoid tissue or lymphocytes scattered diffusely in subepithelial regions. These surfaces are characterized by the presence of a basement membrane or lamina propria containing immune-competent cells predominantly of the immunoglobulin A (IgA) class. Another immunologically specific factor found in genital tract secretions, in addition to immunoglobulins, is complement. These immunologic factors may contribute to a clearing of bacteria that may, in small numbers, intermittently gain entrance to the upper genital tract by physiologic mechanisms (Chow et al, 1980; Ogra et al, 1981; Kutteh et al, 1988).

The vagina and cervix are heavily colonized with a mixture of aerobic and anaerobic microorganisms. Both gonococcus and chlamydia must compete with the local microflora for adherence to mucosal epithelial cells. In addition, several bacterial species may actually inhibit the growth of these microorganisms. Although poorly understood, it appears that microbial interference plays at least some role in the protection against infection with sexually transmitted pathogens (Britigan et al, 1985).

PELVIC INFLAMMATORY DISEASE

Epidemiology

The economic consequences of PID are staggering. More than 1 million women are treated for this disease in the United States each year. Over 250,000 women are hosptialized with this diagnosis annually, and as many as 150,000 women undergo surgical procedures, many involving hysterectomy. In addition, the outpatient management of PID involves between 2 and 3 million physician visits annually. Direct costs (those associated with spending for health services) and indirect costs (output lost because of disease or premature death) are projected to approach $10 billion annually by the year 2000, with an increasing proportion covered by public payment sources.

Although there has been a decreased incidence of hospitalization for acute PID since 1983, the average annual number of women visiting private physicians

785

for this disorder has increased, suggesting a higher proportion of women with clinically mild disease associated with *Chlamydia trachomatis* (Rolfs et al, 1992). *Chlamydia trachomatis* remains the most common bacterial sexually transmitted disease (STD), in America, while rates of *Neiserria gonorrhoeae* infection have been decreasing since the 1970s.

Risk Factors

Determining a woman's risk for PID is essential for successful disease prevention and timely, effective management. Factors associated with the development of disease may be assessed in relation to the risk of exposure to the infectious agent, risk of acquiring the infection upon exposure, and risk of progression to upper genital tract infection. Risk factors may be viewed either as increasing risk or as protective (Washingon et al, 1991).

Risk factors for the development of PID primarily involve patient exposure to the sexually transmitted pathogens *N. gonorrhoeae* and *C. trachomatis* (Table 35–1). Young, sexually active women with increased numbers of sexual partners will be at the highest risk (Westron, 1980). In addition, younger age may be associated with biologic characteristics conducive to the progression of lower genital tract infections (LGTIs) to PID. These characteristics include a lower prevalence of protective antibodies, larger zone of cervical ectopy, and greater penetrability of the cervical mucus (Cates et al, 1990). Reports suggest that bacterial vaginosis (BV) may also be related to the development of PID (Eschenbach et al, 1988; Soper et al, 1994; Hillier et al, 1996). This complex alteration of vaginal flora leads to an increase in the

concentration of potentially pathogenic bacteria, particularly gram-negative anaerobic rods ("BV microorganisms") in the endocervix and/or vagina.

Race and lower socioeconomic status have traditionally been assumed to be markers for sexual behavior. It appears that these two markers are correlated with risky sexual behavior and increased risk for STDs in black men, which results in an increased risk for LGTI and subsequent PID in their female sexual partners (Washington et al, 1991).

Risk factors promoting the progression of a LGTI to PID facilitate the movement of bacteria through the cervical mucus barrier and into the endometrium and fallopian tubes. These include iatrogenic factors such as intrauterine contraceptive device (IUCD) insertion, dilatation and curettage, and hysterosalpingography that may directly transport microorganisms to the upper genital tract. Moreover, patients themselves can increase their risk for the development of PID by douching. Douche fluid can probably enter the uterine cavity, depending on the anatomy of the cervical canal, the viscosity of the cervical mucus, and the douching technique used (Wolner-Hanssen et al, 1990a).

Contraceptive practices also play a role in the development of PID. The risk of PID associated with IUCD use is primarily confined to the time of insertion. For women without risk factors for PID, IUCD use poses little risk of tubal infection (Burkman, 1996). Barrier methods of contraception (condoms or the diaphragm in conjunction with vaginal spermicides) decrease the risk for acquisition of STD and therefore protect against the development of PID. Oral contraceptives have a dichotomous role in the prevention of PID. Use of oral contraceptives increases the risk for the acquisition of lower genital tract chlamydia infection, probably as a result of a larger zone of cervical ectopy. However, using oral contraceptives decreases the risk of symptomatic PID and decreases the severity of salpingitis in patients who develop the disease (Wolner-Hanssen et al, 1990b). This decreased risk may be related to enhancement of the cervical mucus as a barrier to upper tract infection and a decrease in the menstrual blood loss, and therefore a decrease in the inoculum resulting from retrograde menstruation. An important caveat remains the fact that the risk of tubal infertility is unchanged in patients using oral contraceptives, suggesting that "silent" PID may play a role in these patients (Cramer et al, 1985).

Microbiology

The microbiology of PID has been defined by the use of lower genital tract cultures for the sexually transmitted organisms *N. gonorrhoeae* and *C. trachomatis* in patients with the clinical diagnosis of PID. In an attempt to further describe the microbiology of the upper genital tract, telescoping endometrial sampling devices and culdocentesis have been used to culture

Table 35–1. RISK FACTORS FOR PELVIC INFLAMMATORY DISEASE

Age <25 years
Correlated with sexual behavior
Lower prevalence of protective antibodies
Larger zone of cervical ectopy
Greater penetrability of cervical mucus

Microbiologic LGTI
Neisseria gonorrhoeae
Chlamydia trachomatis
Bacterial vaginosis

Behavioral risks to increase chance of LGTI
Multiple sexual partners
Sexual intercourse with high risk men
    Lower socioeconomic class
    Ethnicity

Facilitate transport to the upper genital tract
Iatrogenic procedures
    Dilatation and curettage
    IUCD insertion
    Hysterosalpingogram
Patient practices
    Douching

Abbreviations: IUCD, intrauterine contraceptive device; LGTI, lower genital tract infection.

the endometrium and purulent material from the cul-de-sac of patients with PID. Both of these techniques are associated with some contamination of the specimen with resident vaginal and/or cervical flora. Use of the laparoscope allowed investigators to sample the sites of infection without the possibility of contamination from microorganisms in the vagina or cervix (Table 35-2).

Bernoutz and Goupil in France in 1857 were the first to establish the relationship between gonococcus and PID based on autopsy studies. Since that time innumerable reports have suggested a causal relationship between *N. gonorrhoeae* and PID. Gonococci have been recovered from the cervices of 10% to 85% of women with PID (Mårdh, 1980). *Neisseria gonorrhoeae* is able to infect the endometrium and subseqently the fallopian tubes of approximately 15% to 30% of women who harbor these organisms in their lower genital tracts (Mårdh, 1980). Cultures from the cervix have confirmed the association of these organisms with laparoscopically confirmed salpingitis in between 45% and 82% of cases reported in North America (Sweet et al, 1981; Wasserheit et al, 1986; Burnham et al, 1988). Cultures from the fallopian tubes and peritoneum have confirmed the presence of *N. gonorrhoeae* in about half of those patients with lower tract infection.

Chlamydia trachomatis was first isolated from the fallopian tubes of patients with acute salpingitis by Swedish researchers (Eilard et al, 1976; and Mårdh et al, 1997). Now studies suggest that this agent may be responsible for as much as 85% of all cases of PID in Scandinavia. Isolation of *C. trachomatis* from the fallopian tubes of patients with acute salpingitis has been much more problematic in North America. Few cases of culture-proven chlamydial salpingitis have been reported by North American investigators (Sweet et al, 1981; Wasserheit et al, 1986; Fridberg et al, 1987; Burnham et al, 1988). A partial explanation of these findings includes the difficulty in culturing chlamydia, especially in the upper genital tract. The ability to isolate *C. trachomatis* from the cervix and/or upper genital tract is inversely related to the chlamydial antibody titer. Direct fluorescent antibody

stains and serologic studies suggest that the presence of this organism is responsible for as many as 65% of cases of salpingitis in some North American populations (Kiviat et al, 1986; Wasserheit et al, 1986). Geographical differences appear to exist. Moreover, chlamydial salpingitis seems to be associated with a subacute clinical presentation, which may lead patients to seek care from STD clinics or physicians' offices as opposed to reporting to an emergency room for evaluation. Differences in patient selection in these scenarios could affect the incidence of chlamydial salpingitis studied by North American investigators.

In any event, *C. trachomatis* has been cultured from the cervix, endometrium, and fallopian tubes of patients with laparoscopically confirmed salpingitis. In an experimental model, repeated inoculations of chlamydia into the fallopian tubes of the pig-tailed macaque led to distal tubal obstruction, and cervical inoculation of *C. trachomatis* serovar D was shown to induce salpingitis (Patton et al, 1987, 1990). Observations in this model document a brief (<48 hours) inflammatory reaction consisting of polymorphonuclear cell infiltration followed by progressive adhesion formation.

Haemophilus influenzae appears to be increasingly associated with acute salpingitis. This microorganism has been isolated from the cervix and fallopian tubes of patients with laparoscopically proven salpingitis (Burnham et al, 1988). In most cases these patients are severely affected, with pyosalpinx formation being the rule. Although not proven to be sexually transmitted, this microorganism is highly virulent and is capable of monoetiologic disease similar to that seen with *N. gonorrhoeae*. It appears to originate in the endocervix and ascend into the upper genital tract.

Other microorganisms not thought to be sexually transmitted have also been implicated in the pathogenesis of salpingitis. Originally culdocentesis studies suggested that as many as 80% of cases were associated with mixed infections of both aerobic and anaerobic microorganisms (Chow et al, 1975; Eschenbach et al, 1975; Cunningham et al, 1978). However, a certain amount of contamination by resident vaginal flora occurred with this procedure (Eschenbach et al, 1975; Cunningham et al, 1978; Sweet et al, 1980; Soper et al, 1991). North American laparoscopic studies confirm a polymicrobial etiology of acute salpingitis in 30% to 40% of cases (Sweet et al, 1981; Wasserheit et al, 1986; Burnham et al, 1988). These organisms are particularly found in cases associated with tubo-ovarian abscesses (TOAs). These "BV microorganisms" ascend from the vagina and/or cervix. In most cases it appears that this polymicrobial infection is the result of bacterial superinfection following the initiation of the inflammatory process by *N. gonorrhoeae* (Monif, 1980). Microorganisms of particular importance include *Escherichia coli* and gram-negative anaerobic rods such as *Prevotella* species. The *Prevotella* group of microorganisms is particu-

Table 35-2. MICROBIOLOGY OF PID*

Neisseria gonorrhoeae
Chlamydia trachomatis
Haemophilus influenzae
Polymicrobial infections
  Aerobes
    Escherichia coli
    Group B streptococcus
  Anaerobes
    Peptostreptococcus sp.
    Peptococcus sp.
    Prevotella sp.

*Commonly reported microorganisms (Sweet et al, 1981; Wasserheit et al, 1986; Burnham et al, 1988; Soper et al, 1994).

larly important because many of these isolates are penicillinase producing, making them resistant to the penicillins and the first-generation cephalosporins. In unusual cases, appendicitis or Crohn's disease can lead to a polymicrobial salpingitis by contiguous spread of microorganisms from the bowel.

The genital mycoplasmas are ubiquitous microorganisms found in the lower genital tracts of sexually active individuals that have also been isolated from the upper genital tracts of patients with salpingitis (Mårdh, 1983). Although their isolation is related to sexual activity, their role as sexually transmitted pathogens is controversial. *Mycoplasma hominis* may be an uncommon cause of acute salpingitis in North America.

Actinomyces israelii is a rare cause of severe salpingitis and TOA formation. The pathophysiology involves an ascending infection of the endometrium, fallopian tubes, ovaries, and peritoneum. In some cases, contiguous spread from the bowel associated with ruptured appendices has been noted. Clinical manifestations of this disease are protean. Patients most frequently present with longstanding abdominal pain and a palpable pelvic mass. The most significant pathogenic factors appear to be the demonstrated relationship between IUCD usage and colonization of the cervix and vagina with *Actinomyces*, and the duration of IUCD use. Diagnosis in these cases is usually made at the time of exploratory laparotomy (Schmidt et al, 1980).

Almost half of the cultures of the fallopian tubes and peritoneal surfaces are negative in patients with laparoscopic evidence of salpingitis. This may reflect a difficulty in isolating viable microorganisms when they exist in an upper genital tract rich in antibody and antibacterial secretions. However, it may also reflect failure of the investigator to culture for all potential pathogens, including viruses. Uniformly, investigators do not perform viral cultures of the endometrium and fallopian tubes. There are several case reports of herpesviruses being associated with acute salpingitis (Lehtinen et al, 1985). Cytomegalovirus has been isolated from the cervix of up to 27% of patients with acute salpingitis (Wasserheit et al, 1986). Further study is warranted in this regard to truly elucidate the role of viruses in the pathogenesis of PID.

Mycobacterium tuberculosis is the single bacterium that infects the fallopian tubes by way of hematogenous spread. Pelvic tuberculosis most commonly presents with amenorrhea and/or infertility. In addition, new-onset ascites in the reproductive-age female should elicit a work-up for tuberculous salpingitis. This agent rarely is a cause of salpingitis in western industrialized countries. However, with an increasing incidence of human immunodeficiency virus infection, pelvic tuberculosis could become more prevalent.

Pathophysiology

The majority of PID cases in the United States are caused by an ascending infection (Fig. 35–1). The prototypic model for understanding the pathophysiology of acute PID is gonococcal salpingitis; a typical scenario is presented here for explanatory purposes. A young female with multiple sexual partners develops an endocervical *N. gonorrhoeae* infection. Mucosal inflammation occurs, manifested by an influx of neutrophils attracted to the endocervical site of infection by chemotaxins. Clinical evaluation of the endocervix in such a case will reveal mucopurulent endocervicitis that will also be associated with vaginal leukorrhea. The cervical mucus barrier to ascending infection becomes altered in conjunction with either menstruation or changes in hormonal milieu, and the gonococcus gains entrance to the en-

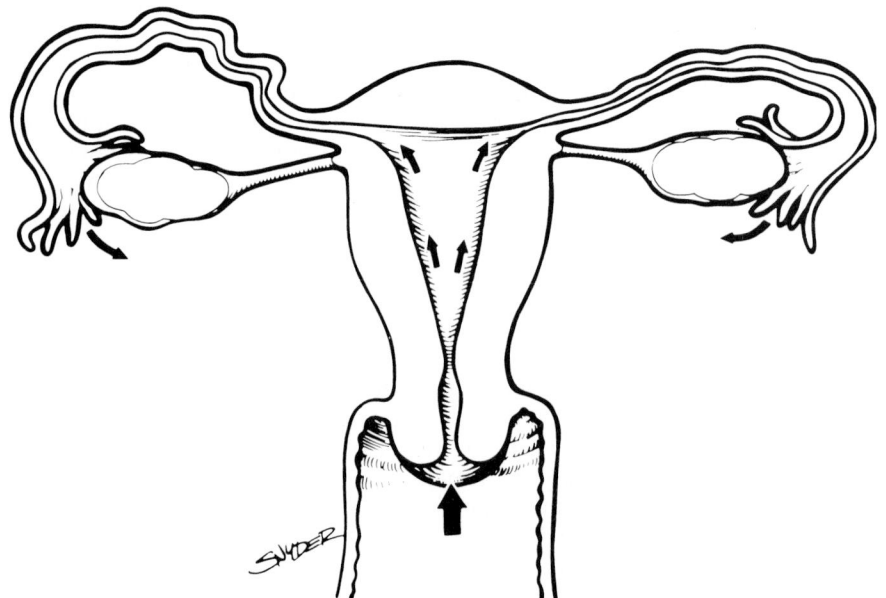

Figure 35–1
The pathophysiology of acute salpingitis involves ascending infection of pathogens found initially in the endocervix.

dometrial cavity. This ascending spread from the cervix to the endometrium may be assisted by gonococci attaching to spermatozoa and being carried up into the endometrium, or canalicular spread (capillary tube action) may occur. In the endometrium, the gonococcus stimulates an inflammatory response as manifested by neutrophilic inflammation and plasma cells secreting IgA. An endometrial biopsy will thus reveal either acute (neutrophilic) or chronic (plasma cell) endometritis or evidence of both (Kiviat et al, 1990). Metrorrhagia may occur as clinical evidence of endometritis. With continued canilicular spread, with help from a vehicle such as sperm, or by reflux of menstrual blood into the fallopian tubes, the gonococcus reaches the tubes and peritoneal surface. Gonococci then adhere to the nonciliated epithelium of the fallopian tube. Gonococcal infection of the tube promotes ciliostasis and may promote secondary infection with other bacteria that normally would have been cleared. The source of these other bacteria may be the endocervix and/or upper vagina, or they may be present as a result of a translocation phenomenon across an inflamed bowel wall. The gonococcus is able to invade the tubal mucosa and is actually transported through the tubal epithelium to be deposited in the subepithelial space. Here tissue destruction and suppuration occur and, in some cases, the microorganism gains access to the local vasculature. Suppuration leads to tubal erythema, edema, and an exudate made up of predominantly polymorphonuclear leukocytes. These changes are visually recognized as salpingitis through the laparoscope. Peritoneal inflammation is also promoted by similar mechanisms. The important concept here is that of a continuum of infection with associated signs of inflammation. PID is cervicitis-endometritis-salpingitis-peritonitis, and in some cases oophoritis with abscess formation occurs. The clinical diagnosis of PID can then be based upon the evaluation of these sites for signs of inflammation.

The role of LGTI is crucial in the development of PID. As has been outlined above, N. gonorrhoeae begins as an uncomplicated LGTI but under certain circumstances may ascend to cause acute salpingitis. An identical mechanism of infection occurs with C. trachomatis. BV is present in the majority of women with PID (Eschenbach et al, 1988; Soper et al, 1994). It appears that "BV microorganisms" also gain access to the upper genital tract from the cervix and vagina (Hillier et al, 1996). Sweet (1990) noted that isolates obtained from the endometrial cavity closely mirror those in the fallopian tube in patients with acute salpingitis. This evidence suggests that ascending infection with these potential pathogens occurs.

Diagnosis (Table 35–3)

Symptoms

Lower abdominal pain is the most frequent symptom noted in patients with PID. This reflects upper

---

Table 35–3. DIAGNOSIS OF PID

SYMPTOMS
Lower abdominal pain
Vaginal discharge
Urethritis symptoms
Proctitis symptoms
Metrorrhagia
Fever
Nausea and/or vomiting

SIGNS
Signs of a LGTI
  Leukorrhea*
    Mucopurulent endocervicitis[†]
Lower abdominal tenderness
Cervical motion tenderness
Bilateral adnexal tenderness
Palpable adnexal swelling
Temperature >38°C

LABORATORY RESULTS
Leukocytosis
Erythrocyte sedimentation rate >20 mm/hr
Elevated C-reactive protein >2 mg/dl
Endometrial biopsy = endometritis

---

*More than one white blood cell per epithelial cell on microscopy of the vaginal secretions.
[†]Green or yellow endocervical secretions on a Q-tip inserted into the endocervical canal or 30 or more white blood cells per oil immersion field on microscopy of cervical mucus.

---

genital tract inflammation involving the endometrium, fallopian tubes, and/or peritoneum. The pain is generally bilateral and is not necessarily severe. Associated symptoms generally reflect infection of other anatomic structures with N. gonorrhoeae or C. trachomatis. For example, endocervicitis may be manifested by the complaint of an abnormal vaginal discharge. Urethritis symptoms such as dysuria, urgency, and frequency may be due to concomitant infection of the urethra. Breakthrough bleeding on the birth control pill or persistent vaginal spotting following elective termination of pregnancy are other signs that may herald the onset of PID. These complaints commonly result from an endometritis that, if not treated, may progress to salpingitis. More systemic symptoms such as fever and the association of nausea with or without vomiting reflect peritoneal inflammation and severe clinical disease.

Physical Examination and Laboratory Results

Physical findings consistent with the diagnosis of PID include the presence of leukorrhea and/or cervical mucopus (Peipert et al, 1996). A saline preparation of the vaginal secretions should be microscopically examined for the presence of white blood cells. Leukorrhea can be defined as more than one polymorphonuclear leukocyte per vaginal epithelial cell. Following the cleansing of the ectocervix with a large cotton swab, a Q-tip should be placed into the endocervical canal and inspected for a green or yellow color. In addition, Gram's stain of this material after it is streaked on a slide should be examined microscopically for the presence of white blood cells. More that 30 polymorphonuclear leukocytes per oil immersion field correlates with mucopurulent cervicitis and chlamydial or gonococcal infection (Holmes, 1990). In a patient presenting with lower abdominal pain, the presence of bilateral adnexal tenderness together with signs of a LGTI (mucopus and/or leukorrhea) is associated with the laparoscopically confirmed diagnosis of acute salpingitis in 65% of cases (Westrom and Mårdh, 1984).

Additional clinical and laboratory findings supportive of infection and inflammation improve the specificity of the clinical diagnosis of PID. Elevated temperature, palpation of an adnexal complex, leukocytosis, elevated erythrocyte sedimentation rate or C-reactive protein, purulent material obtained by culdocentesis, and/or a positive test for a LGTI with N. gonorrhoeae or C. trachomatis are considered adjunctive criteria for the diagnosis of PID. The specificity of the clinical diagnosis of PID increases to greater than 90% when two or more of these criteria are associated with the findings of pain, adnexal tenderness, and leukorrhea (Table 35-4) (Westrom and Mårdh, 1984).

Endometrial biopsy is another technique used to document upper genital tract inflammation. When compared to laparoscopically confirmed salpingitis, endometritis detected with biopsy had a sensitivity of 89%, a specificity of 67%, a positive predictive value of 84%, and a false-negative rate of 22% in the diagonsis of PID (Paavonen et al, 1985). The procedure, using a Pipelle endometrial suction curette, can easily be performed in the office or in the emergency room as part of the evaluation of patients suspected to have acute salpingitis. In addition, it is indispensable in the evaluation of the endometrium of those patients undergoing diagnostic laparoscopy. Patients who fail to meet criteria for the visual diagnosis of acute salpingitis may have an acute or chronic endometritis as the sole source of their symptoms.

Laparoscopy

Use of the laparoscope has greatly enhanced our understanding of the pathophysiology of PID; however, the routine use of the laparoscope for the diagnosis of PID is not useful. The majority of patients with the clinical diagnosis of PID will respond promptly to antimicrobial therapy. Moreover, those patients without visually confirmed salpingitis still require antimicrobial therapy because of the presence of endometritis in most of these patients (Soper et al, 1994). Diagnostic laparoscopy should be considered in patients in whom the diagnosis is in question, especially if ectopic pregnancy is possible. Also, those patients failing an initial outpatient course of antibiotics are rarely visually confirmed to have salpingitis, and therefore laparoscopy should be considered for diagnosis. Many of these patients will have

Table 35-4. CRITERIA FOR CLINICAL DIAGNOSIS OF PID

CRITERIA	SPECIFICITY
Major	
Lower abdominal pain	
Signs of a LGTI	
Bilateral adnexal tenderness	61%
Minor	
Fever	
Palpable adnexal swelling	
Leukocytosis	
Elevated C-reactive protein	
Positive test for gonococcus or chlamydia	
Major + one **Minor**	78%
Major + two **Minor**	90%
Major + three **Minor**	96%

Adapted from Westrom L, Mårdh PA: Salpingitis. In Holmes KK, Mårdh PA, Sparling PF, et al (eds): Sexually Transmitted Diseases. New York: McGraw-Hill, 1984:765, with permission.

an alternative, treatable diagnosis such as endometriosis.

The minimum criteria for the visual confirmation of acute salpingitis include (1) pronounced hyperemia of the tubal surface, (2) edema of the tubal wall, and (3) a sticky exudate on the tubal surface and from the fimbriated ends when patent (Table 35-5) (Jacobson and Westrom, 1969). In some cases, erythema and edema can be overinterpreted as a result of observer bias. For this reason, Gram's stain of the peritoneal exudate to document the presence of polymorphonuclear cells is suggested. In cases of peritoneal inflammation caused by endometriosis, the peritoneal fluid will contain predominantly mononuclear cells and macrophages. Peritoneal fluid from normal patients will be lacking in cellular elements, or a few mononuclear cells or macrophages may be seen. The value of histologic evaluation of minute fimbria biopsies to pathologically confirm the visual diagnosis of salpingitis has yet to be defined.

Mild salpingitis is associated with the above minimum visual criteria. In addition, the tubes are freely mobile and the ostia appear patent. The tube may be covered with a sticky exudate. Moderate salpingitis is associated with more pronounced inflammation. Patchy fibrin deposits are on the serosal surfaces and the tubes are not freely movable. Adhesions are loose and moist, and a paraphimotic appearance may be

Table 35-5. VISUAL CRITERIA FOR THE LAPAROSCOPIC DIAGNOSIS OF SALPINGITIS

Pronounced hyperemia of the tubal surface
Edema of the tubal wall
Sticky exudate on the tubal surface or from the fimbriated ends when patent

From Jacobson L, Westrom L: Objectivized diagnosis of acute pelvic inflammatory disease: diagnostic and prognostic value of routine laparoscopy. Am J Obstet Gynecol 1969;105:1088, with permission.

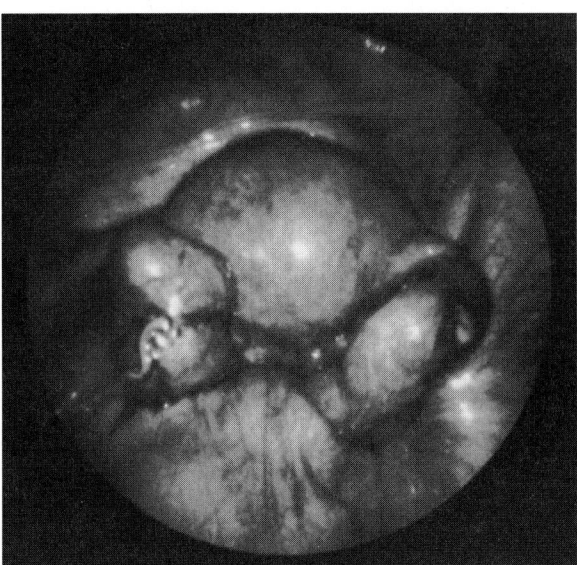

Figure 35-2
Bilateral pyosalpinges are noted. Puncture wounds from an 18-gauge spinal needle are noted to exude purulent material. (From Soper DE: Diagnosis and laparoscopic grading of acute salpingitis. Am J Obstet Gynecol 1991;164[Suppl]:1373, with permission.)

Table 35-6. LAPAROSCOPIC GRADING OF ACUTE SALPINGITIS

Mild
Tubes freely mobile
Tubal ostia open

Moderate
Inflammation more pronounced
Tubes not freely mobile
Adhesions are loose and "moist"
Paraphimosis may be present
Fimbria may be adherent

Severe
Pelvic organs adherent to one another
Pyosalpinx or tubo-ovarian complex
Omental adhesions

Data from Westrom and Mårdh (1984) and Jacobson and Westrom (1969).

present. The fimbria may appear adherent. Severe salpingitis reveals intensely congested peritoneal surfaces. Pelvic organs adhere to each other, and pyosalpinx (Fig. 35–2) or tubo-ovarian complex formation may be present (Table 35–6) (Westrom and Mårdh, 1984).

In some cases, both adnexae are not equally affected by the inflammatory process. Grading should be performed with respect to individual adnexal findings. The overall grade should reflect the most severe findings. For example, a patient with a right-sided pyosalpinx but otherwise mildly involved left tube would warrant an overall grade of severe. The severity of the grade of salpingitis is dependent for the most part on tubal mobility and patency. Therefore, an acute infectious process superimposed upon chronic adhesive changes, possibly caused by previous episode of salpingitis, will be graded as more advanced when in reality the amount of purulent exudate, side-to-side agglutination, and tubal edema and erythema may be less than an initial mild grade of gonococcal salpingitis. Despite this possibility, patients with a more severe grade of salpingitis require a longer duration of antibiotic therapy before reaching a therapeutic response (Wasserheit et al, 1986).

Atypical or "Silent Salpingitis"

More than half of women with tubal infertility have no history of PID. Antibodies to *C. trachomatis* are often present in asymptomatic women with either ectopic pregnancy or distal tubal occlusion (Moore and Cates, 1990). Moreover, morphologic changes of

the fallopian tube mucosa and physiologic alterations of ciliated epithelium were similar in patients with tubal factor infertility with and without clinically overt salpingitis (Patton et al, 1989). In addition, it is not uncommon to find endometrial infection with *C. trachomatis* in asymptomatic women with serum anti-chlamydial antibodies (Cleary and Jones, 1985; Fish et al, 1988). Women with BV may also have associated endometritis (Korn et al, 1995; Hillier et al, 1996). These data suggest the probability that patients develop tubal infection without the typical clinical signs of pelvic infection—so-called silent salpingitis. In some cases, symptoms such as metrorrhagia, abnormal vaginal discharge, or urinary tract symptoms, in the absence of pelvic pain, may represent the clinical manifestations of PID. In order to address this issue and to improve the treatment capture rate for these patients, a concept of "think PID" should be adopted. Much like the "think ectopic" concept promoted prior to the use of serum pregnancy tests, this increases awareness of subtle and often subclinical signs of upper genital tract infection, prompting evaluation and treatment.

The diagnostic criteria for silent salpingitis must therefore be less stringent and reflect the subacute or relatively asymptomatic nature of this entity (Table 35–7). Patients seen by health care workers with bilateral adnexal tenderness and signs of a LGTI or BV, even in the absence of a complaint of pelvic pain, should be treated as if they have acute salpingitis until more information is available. Obviously the specificity of the diagnosis of silent salpingitis will be lower than that of overt PID, but this is acceptable considering how much there is to be gained from the

Table 35-7. DIAGNOSTIC CRITERIA FOR "SILENT" SALPINGITIS

Signs of a lower genital tract infection
Bilateral adnexal tenderness

prompt treatment of patients with upper genital tract infection.

Treatment

Current guidelines for the treatment of PID reflect the concern that a significant number of cases will be associated with a polymicrobial infection. Recommended regimens provide empirical, broad-spectrum coverage of likely etiologic pathogens while maintaining an emphasis on coverage of both, *N. gonorrhoeae* and *C. trachomatis*. Selection of a treatment regimen must consider institutional availability, cost-control efforts, patient acceptance, and regional differences in antimicrobial susceptibility (Centers for Disease Control and Prevention, 1997). Antibiotic regimens are listed in Table 35–8.

Ambulatory management of PID utilizes a β-lactam antibiotic, administered as a single injection, followed by a 10- to 14-day course of doxycycline and metronidazole. Parenteral administration of the β-lactam antibiotic ensures compliance. Ceftriaxone and doxycycline maximize coverage against gonococcus and chlamydia, while metronidazole provides treatment for a commonly associated BV and coverage for a possible anaerobic upper genital tract infection. All patients treated in an ambulatory setting should return for repeat evaluation within 72 hours if they notice no improvement in their symptoms.

Some patients may benefit from parenteral therapy or hospitalization (Table 35–9). Generally, those patients with severe clinical disease and/or those who are unable to tolerate oral administration of antibiotics should be hospitalized. As mentioned before, patients with a questionable diagnosis should be admitted and diagnostic laparoscopy should be considered. This is especially true in cases of early pregnancy complicated by PID because ectopic pregnancy must be ruled out. Women with TOAs should receive parenteral therapy, with the decision for hospitalization relegated to the severity of their clinical disease.

Both inpatient antibiotic regimens (Table 35–8) cover *N. gonorrhoeae* and *C. trachomatis* as well as anaerobes and facultative bacteria. The combination of cefotetan or cefoxitin and doxycycline is recommended when sexually transmitted organisms are believed to play a role in the etioloy of PID. The combination of clindamycin and an aminoglycoside provides excellent coverage for mixed anaerobic and aerobic infections. Both regimens have been extensively studied and are associated with clinical cure rates in the 90% range (Peterson et al, 1991).

Parenteral antibiotics should be continued until a therapeutic response is reached (Table 35–10). This response should include total lysis of fever, normalization of the white blood cell count, total disappearance of abdominal rebound tenderness, and marked amelioration of pelvic organ tenderness. Most patients respond within 5 to 6 days; however, patients with TOA formation may take even

---

Table 35–8. CENTERS FOR DISEASE CONTROL AND PREVENTION TREATMENT GUIDELINES FOR PID

INPATIENT TREATMENT
Regimen A
    Cefotetan 2 g IV every 12 hours, or **cefoxitin*** IV 2 g every 6 hours
    PLUS
    Doxycycline 100 mg every 12 hours orally or IV
Regimen B
    Clindamycin IV 900 mg every 8 hours
    PLUS
    Gentamicin loading dose IV or IM (2 mg/kg) followed by a maintenance dose (1.5 mg/kg)
        every 8 hours
One of the above regimens is given for at least 24 hours after the patient clinically improves.
Continue therapy with:
    Doxycycline 100 mg orally 2 times a day to total of 10–14 days
    (Clindamycin 450 mg orally, 5 times daily, for 10–14 days may be considered as an alternative.)

OUTPATIENT TREATMENT
Regimen A
    Ceftriaxone 250 mg IM or equivalent cephalosporin
    PLUS
    Doxycycline 100 mg orally 2 times a day for 10–14 days
    PLUS
    Metronidazole 500 mg orally 2 times a day for 10–14 days
Regimen B
    Ofloxacin 400 mg orally 2 times a day for 10–14 days
    PLUS
    Metronidazole 500 mg orally 2 times a day for 10–14 days

*Other cephalosporins such as ceftizoxime, cefotaxime, and ceftriaxone, which provide adequate gonococcal, other facultative gram-negative aerobic, and anaerobic coverage, may be utilized in appropriate doses.
From Centers for Disease Control and Prevention: 1998 Sexually transmitted diseases treatment guidelines. MMWR Morbid Mortal Wkly Rep 1997;47:79.

Table 35–9. INDICATIONS FOR PARENTERAL THERAPY AND/OR HOSPITALIZATION OF PATIENT WITH PID

Uncertain diagnosis
  Pregnancy and PID: rule out ectopic pregnancy
  Failure to respond to outpatient therapy
Severe clinical disease
  Temperature >39°C
  Upper peritoneal signs
Suspected pelvic or tubo-ovarian abscess
Compliance with outpatient regimen questionable
Nausea/vomiting precludes oral therapy

Table 35–10. THERAPEUTIC RESPONSE

Total lysis of fever
Total disappearance of rebound tenderness
Normalization of white blood cell count
Marked amelioration of pelvic organ tenderness

longer. Patients should be continued on an oral antibiotic, usually doxycycline, to complete a 10- to 14-day course of therapy. Patients with chlamydia-associated PID can have a clinical response to antibiotics not directed at this organism and continue to be culture positive despite becoming asymptomatic (Sweet et al, 1983). This observation may be due to inhibition of the microorganism without its death. This raises the possibility of an ongoing subclinical infection causing continued tubal damage. Therefore, treatment of chlamydia-associated PID should depend not only upon a clinical response but also eradication of the microorganism as documented by a negative follow-up culture. In experimental chlamydial infections as well as in trachoma, host immune response is enhanced with subsequent infections, thus precipitating more local tissue damage.

Anaerobic microorganisms may also persist in the endometria of women having a clinical response to therapy with an antibiotic, such as ciprofloxacin, not active against these microorganisms (Crombleholme et al, 1989). Concern about their ability to cause continued upper genital tract inflammation has prompted the addition of metronidazole to the regimen A outpatient treatment recommendation (Table 35–8).

Treatment of PID involves more than just antibiotic therapy (Table 35–11). Sexual partners of patients treated for PID should be evaluated for STDs. This is true even for partners of those patients with PID who fail to test positive for *N. gonorrhoeae* or *C. trachomatis*. Approximately one third of male sexual contacts of patients with gonococcal PID will test positive for gonococcus, and many will be asymptomatic. Moreover, even sexual contacts of patients with nongonococcal PID will have a 15% incidence of culture-proven *N. gonorrhoeae* (Gilstrap et al, 1997). Chlamydia infection is also common in sexual contacts of women with PID, existing in 35% of male sexual partners (Moss and Hawkswell, 1986). Epidemiologic treatment for an uncomplicated LGTI of sexual contacts of patients with PID is in order. These contacts should receive a β-lactam antibiotic such as ceftriaxone plus 7 days of oral doxycycline. In addition, screening these individuals for sexually transmitted diseases may shed new light on the

pathogenesis of PID in the index patient as well as eliminate a reservoir for re-infection. Indeed, in many cases it is not the patient's exposure to multiple sexual partners that puts her at risk. It is the exposure to her single sexual partner who has exposed himself to many different sexual partners and is asymptomatically infected that puts her at risk.

Complications

Tubo-ovarian Abscess

TOA formation, the most severe consequence of pelvic inflammatory disease, complicates approximately 15% of cases. The pathophysiology is identical to uncomplicated salpingitis except that, presumably through an ovulation site, microorganisms gain entry to the ovarian stroma. This would lead to destruction of the ovary and formation of an abscess cavity. Alternatively, loculations of pus can occur between pelvic structures such as the tube, ovary, and uterus, and in many cases bowel becomes involved. These loculations act as abscess cavities and lead to persistent inflammation and destruction of the adjacent organs. Moreover, intraluminal pus from pyosalpinx formation is also involved.

The clinical diagnosis of TOA is based upon the previously noted criteria for the diagnosis of PID in conjunction with a palpable adnexal complex. This adnexal complex can be further characterized by sonography or computerized tomography (CT). These complexes may actually appear to be "bags of pus" or may only represent side-to-side agglutination of pelvic structures in association with tissue induration.

Treatment of TOAs should initially consist of the parenteral administration of broad-spectrum antibiotics. Hospitalization should be considered in women with severe clinical symptoms. Patients should begin showing a therapeutic response with subjective improvement of symptoms, decreasing white blood cell count, and lysis of fever within 72

Table 35–11. THERAPEUTIC APPROACH TO THE PATIENT WITH PID

Antibiotics
Follow-up
Treat sexual partners
Education regarding STDs

hours. If there is suspicion of abscess rupture or if the patient fails to respond to antibiotic therapy within 72 to 96 hours, surgical exploration should be considered. A conservative approach with unilateral adnexectomy and drainage is appropriate if future fertility or hormone production is desired (Landers and Sweet, 1985). Total abdominal hysterectomy with bilateral salpingo-oophorectomy may be reserved for those patients not desirous of future fertility or in cases in which overwhelming sepsis has developed. Laparoscopic or CT-guided drainage of TOAs is being performed with increasing frequency and is successful in selected cases.

Sequelae

Major sequelae resulting from PID include tubal factor infertility, ectopic pregnancy, chronic abdominal pain, and recurrent infection (Table 35–12). *Infertility* resulting from salpingitis is directly proportional to the severity of the inflammatory reactions of the tubes. In addition, the number of episodes of salpingitis will increase the risk for the patient of tubal factor infertility (Svensson et al, 1983). Infertility resulting from a single episode of severe salpingitis appears to occur in close to 27% of cases, falling to a low of 6% in patients with only mild disease. Patients taking oral contraceptives at the time of their diagnosis appear to have an improved prognosis. Not only are they less likely to develop salpingitis in the first place, but they generally have a less severe grade of salpingitis if they do develop upper tract disease (Burkman, 1996). Rates of tubal factor infertility also increase with subsequent episodes of PID. The patient with three or more episodes of salpingitis runs a 50% to 60% risk of tubal factor infertility (Westrom and Mårdh, 1984). Fertility prognosis does not appear to be related to the microbial etiology of acute salpingitis (Svensson et al, 1983).

There has been a fourfold increase in the number of *ectopic pregnancies* occuring in this country since 1970. This increase appears to be related to the concomitant increase in the number of cases of PID over the same period of time. Patients with a history of PID have a four- to eightfold increased risk for ectopic pregnancy (Westrom, 1975). In addition, those patients with antibody to *C. trachomatis* also have an increased risk for the development of ectopic pregnancy.

Chronic *lower abdominal pain* occurs in up to 20% of patients with a history of PID. This pain is believed to be due to pelvic adhesive disease, with over two thirds of these patients being infertile. Compounding this problem is the presence of dysparuenia in over half of these patients (Westrom, 1980).

Finally, *recurrence* of PID is common, occurring in up to 25% of patients. Distorted tubal architecture may increase the risk of subsequent infection as a result of impairment of host immune factors. Patients with PID are more likely to become re-infected with the same sexually transmitted pathogens that

Table 35–12. SEQUELAE ASSOCIATED WITH PID

Tubal factor infertility
Ectopic pregnancy
Chronic lower abdominal pain
Recurrent pelvic infection

caused their upper tract inflammation in the first place.

Fitz-Hugh–Curtis Syndrome

Fitz-Hugh–Curtis syndrome is characterized by "violin string" adhesions between the liver and anterior abdominal wall in women with gross pathologic evidence of prior tubal infection. It consists of a continuum of acute perihepatitis associated with acute salpingitis followed by the formation of perihepatic adhesions (Fig. 35–3). Both *N. gonorrhoeae* and *C. trachomatis* have been isolated from the liver capsule in patients with Fitz-Hugh–Curtis syndrome. The severity of perihepatic adhesions is associated with the severity of pelvic adhesions, suggesting that, like pelvic adhesions, the process is progressive. Occasionally chronic right upper quadrant pain necessitating laparoscopic lysis of adhesions occurs (Reichert and Valle, 1976).

Prevention of PID

The most cost-effective approach to the management of PID and its associated sequelae is prevention (Table 35–13). Because the majority of PID is caused by sexually transmitted pathogens, specifically *N. gon-*

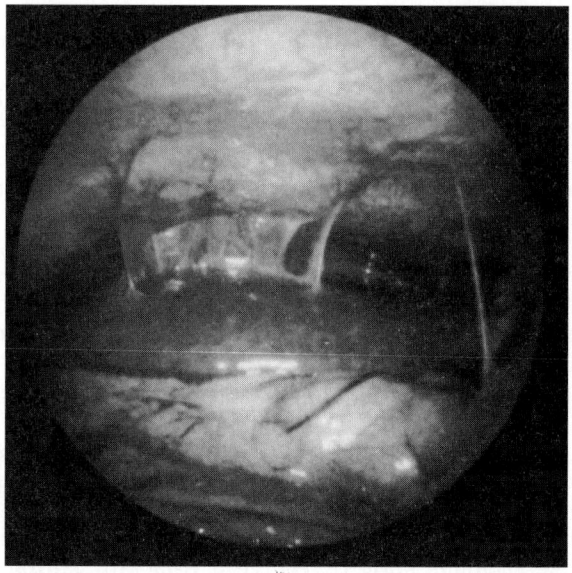

Figure 35–3
"Violin string" adhesions are visualized in this patient with Fitz-Hugh–Curtis syndrome.

Table 35–13. PREVENTION OF PID

Control of LGTIs
Liberal therapy for MPC
Increased public awareness
Stricter attitudes concerning sexual relationships
AIDS awareness
Minimize iatrogenic risk

Abbreviations: AIDS, acquired immunodeficiency syndrome; MPC, mucopurulent cervicitis.

orrhoeae and *C. trachomatis*, aggressive diagnosis and treatment of LGTIs must be undertaken. This not only includes liberal therapy for mucopurulent endocervicitis but also an increased public awareness of the dangers of lower tract infection with these pathogens (Scholes et al, 1996). In addition, patient education concerning the earliest signs of abnormality, such as an abnormal vaginal discharge, which will prompt health–care seeking behavior, in addition to education of physician providers to "think PID," will go far in decreasing the morbidity associated with overt or "silent" salpingitis. Physicians can minimize iatrogenic risks by appropriate screening and prophylaxis of those patients undergoing upper genital instrumentation, such as hystero-salpingogram.

INFECTIONS ASSOCIATED WITH ABORTION

Legal abortion is now the most frequent operation performed on American women, spontaneous abortions occur in large numbers, and illegal abortions have not been eliminated. The prevention and management of infectious complications of abortion continue to be important concerns (Grimes et al, 1981). Abortion-related infections can be categorized as those associated with retained products of conception (septic abortion) versus those occurring, after complete emptying of the uterine cavity (postabortal endometritis) (Table 35–14).

Postabortal Endometritis

Elective termination of pregnancy occurs frequently in this country, with more than 1.3 million legal abortions being performed in the United States in 1987.

Table 35–14. ABORTION-RELATED INFECTIONS

Postabortal endometritis
No retained POCs
Septic abortion
Incomplete abortion
Inevitable abortion
Threatened abortion

Abbreviation: POC, products of conception.

The risk of febrile morbidity from curettage abortion is 1 per 100 procedures, resulting in thousands of women with postabortal infections each year. Risk factors for the development of postabortal endometritis include untreated gonococcal or chlamydia cervicitis and a prior history of PID.

The pathophysiology of this infection involves bacteria, both aerobes and anaerobes, normally found in the vagina or endocervix ascending into the endometrial cavity, probably during the procedure or shortly thereafter. Women with BV have an increased risk for developing postabortal PID unless treated with metronidazole (Larsson et al, 1992). Commonly isolated microorganisms include group B streptococci, *Staphylococcus aureus*, and *Bacteroides* species. The sexually transmitted pathogens, *N. gonorrhoeae* and *C. trachomatis* are also well-known causes of postabortal endometritis. Symptoms such as fever, abdominal or uterine cramping, tissue passage, and/or foul vaginal discharge generally occur 5 or more days after the abortion procedure. Physical examination reveals uterine or parametrial tenderness with palpation. Elevated temperature may not be present (Burkman et al, 1977). Laparoscopy, if performed, does not reveal any evidence of tubal infection (Westrom et al, 1981).

Treatment consists primarily of broad-spectrum antibiotic therapy. Uterine curettage is an important adjunctive treatment for some patients, especially in cases in which retained products of conception are a possibility. Patients requiring curettage generally present with pain, vaginal bleeding, and temperature elevation. If retained products of conception are discovered, then the diagnosis of septic incomplete abortion is made.

Septic Abortion

Septic abortion most commonly refers to an infected incomplete abortion, although some patients present prior to the passage of any products of conception. Therefore any threatened, inevitable, or incomplete abortion associated with fever should be considered a septic abortion. Incomplete passage of the products of conception may follow spontaneous abortion, legal abortion, or illegal abortion. Infection of the endometrium following abortion in which the products of conception have been completely evacuated is referred to as postabortal endometritis.

The pathophysiology of septic abortion involves the ascending spread of microorganisms normally found in the upper vagina and cervix. Retained products of conception act as a nidus for the development of local infection, which can then lead to a more generalized sepsis. Bacteria migrating through the uterine wall via venous and lymphatic channels may produce cellulitis and abscesses in the broad ligaments and retroperitoneal spaces of the pelvic floor. TOAs may occur as direct extensions of intrauterine infection. In severe cases, septic pelvic thrombophlebitis may result in multiple small septic pulmonary emboli, bacteremia, and metastatic infection to other organs. Risk factors for serious infection associated with abortion include behavioral and physiologic factors. Delay in obtaining abortion, as seen in younger women for fear of involving their parents, leads to the use of instillation techniques for termination and therefore increases the risk for infection. In addition, once symptoms of infection begin, these patients take longer (mean, 7 days) to request medical attention. The use of intrauterine foreign bodies to induce abortion appears to be even more dangerous. Incomplete abortion and uterine perforation are other risk factors for the development of infection. The risk of infection following illegal termination of pregnancy is much higher than that associated with legal abortion. This is probably due to inadequate sterile technique or unsafe methods (such as intrauterine foreign body insertion) used for illegal abortion as well as a delay in seeking treatment or failure to admit to uterine instrumentation because of the patient's fear of criminal action (Grimes et al, 1981).

The use of an IUCD for contraception has greatly decreased over the past decade. However, an occasional patient will be utilizing this method for birth control. Women with an IUCD in situ should have the device removed when pregnancy is first diagnosed. Pregnant IUCD wearers have an increased risk for spontaneous abortion and an increased risk for associated febrile complications, including septic shock and death (Cates et al, 1976; Kim-Farley et al, 1978).

The most common microorganisms (Table 35–15) isolated from the blood and/or the uterine cavity in association with septic abortion are anaerobes and microaerophilic bacteria. Because these microorganisms are normally found in the upper vagina and endocervix, they may be readily introduced into the endometrial cavity during instrumentation or ascend to infect retained products of conception associated with an incomplete abortion. Bacteremia occurs in as many as 60% of patients admitted with the diagnosis. Anaerobic gram-positive cocci are the most common isolates, but *Bacteroides* species and *Clostridium* species can also play a major role in the pathogenesis of septic abortion. The most common aerobic isolates include *E. coli* and the group B streptococcus (Rotheram and Schick, 1969).

One of the most severe complications of septic abortion involves *Clostridium perfringens* bacteremia with associated shock, intravascular hemolysis, and renal failure. This distinctive syndrome is probably due to the release of α-toxin into the blood stream. The group A streptococcus (*Streptococcus pyogenes*) can also produce a fulminating illness characterized by lymphatic spread, intense pelvic cellulitis, and overwhelming septicemia. The rarity of each of these organisms in the vaginal flora, and therefore the infrequency of uterine inoculation, partially accounts for the low frequency of this complication. In addi-

Table 35–15. MICROBIOLOGY OF SEPTIC ABORTION

Anaerobes
Peptostreptococcus sp.
Peptococcus
Bacteroides bivius
*Bacteroides fragilis**
Bacteroides sp.
*Clostridium perfringens**
Clostridium sp.
Aerobes
Staphylococcus aureus
*Streptococcus pyogenes**
Streptococcus agalactiae
*Escherichia coli**
Klebsiella

*Microorganisms commonly associated with severe sepsis.
From Rotheram EB, Schick SF: Nonclostridial anaerobic bacteria in septic abortion. Am J Med 1969;46:80, with permission.

tion, variations in toxigenicity among strains, the presence or absence of uterine muscle damage, and the severity of associated septic thrombophlebitis may determine when the role of these microorganisms become dominant. The possibility of tetanus (*Clostridium tetani*) developing as a result of septic abortion should be kept in mind, especially in the setting of illegal abortion. Appropriate immunization procedures should be carried out.

Patients with septic abortion usually present with fever, chills, leukocytosis, uterine tenderness, and a foul-smelling cervicovaginal discharge. Treatment (Table 35–16) involves the use of broad-spectrum antibiotics, uterine curettage, and supportive therapy in severe cases. Antibiotic coverage (see Table 35–17) should include agents with good anaerobic activity as well as coverage for aerobic gram-negative rods. In severe cases, penicillin should be utilized to cover the possibility of infection caused by *Clostridium* species or group A streptococci, an aminoglycoside should be added to cover *E. coli*, and either clindamycin or metronidazole should be added to cover penicillinase-producing anaerobes such as *Bacteroides bivius*. Imipenem-cilistatin offers an excellent single-agent alternative with broad-spectrum coverage of all potential pathogens in this scenario.

Early evacuation of the uterus is consistent with accepted principles of débridement and drainage of infected tissues; however, its use must be tempered by sound surgical judgment. It is often best to allow the large, grossly infected uterus of an advanced pregnancy to empty spontaneously under pitocin or

Table 35–16. THERAPY FOR SEPTIC ABORTION

Antibiotics
Uterine curettage
Intensive care for severe cases

Table 35–17. ANTIBIOTIC THERAPY FOR SEPTIC ABORTION

ANTIBIOTIC	MICROORGANISM
Triple therapy	
Penicillin	All gram-positive cocci (aerobic and anaerobic), *Clostridium* sp.
Aminoglycoside (Gentamicin)	All aerobic gram-negative rods (*E. coli*)
Clindamycin or metronidazole	Anaerobic bacteria (esp. penicillinase-producing *Bacteroides*)
Single agent therapy	
Cefoxitin	Most implicated microorganisms (some aerobic gram-negative rods and *Enterococcus* will be resistant)
Imipenem/cilistatin	All implicated microorganisms

prostaglandin stimulation than to perform curettage, which may result in uterine perforation (Rotheram and Schick, 1969).

Several interventions can decrease the risk of death associated with septic abortion (Table 35–18) Availability of services for legal abortion and medical care of complications will decrease the incidence of second-trimester terminations and prompt young women with infection-related complications to seek early treatment. In addition, patient education concerning the possibility of infectious complications and the need for early return to the physician for diagnosis and treatment should be stressed. Finally, optimal therapy to include broad-spectrum antibiotic therapy and early uterine curettage will improve outcome. Despite these measures, some patients with particularly virulent infections, as seen in conjunction with group A streptococcus or *C. perfringens*, will still die.

LATE POSTPARTUM ENDOMETRITIS

Endomyometritis is the most common genital tract infection following delivery. Most endometritis presents early in the postpartum period, usually following cesarean section. These early infections are caused by a polymicrobial flora and are not further discussed. Late postpartum endometritis more commonly occurs in patients having delivered vaginally. These patients develop late postpartum endometritis

Table 35–18. PREVENTION OF DEATH ASSOCIATED WITH SEPTIC ABORTION

Minimize delays associated with abortion services
  Increase availability of abortion services
  Promote first-trimester termination over second-trimester
Minimize delays after infection has developed
  Counsel patients about signs and symptoms of infection
Optimal therapy
  Broad spectrum antibiotic therapy
  Early curettage

From Grimes DA, Cates W Jr, Selik RM: Fatal septic abortion in the United States, 1975–1977. Obstet Gynecol 1981;57:739, with permission.

between 7 and 42 days postpartum. Symptoms are usually mild and consist of fever, chills, or foul-smelling lochia. Despite the complaints of fever and/or chills, most patients are afebrile. In addition, physical examination reveals uterine tenderness. In some cases more generalized lower abdominal tenderness along with cervical motion tenderness with or without adnexal tenderness is present.

Cultures of the endometrium should be obtained for aerobic and anaerobic bacteria in these patients. In addition, cervical cultures for *N. gonorrhoeae* and *C. trachomatis* should also be performed. *Chlamydia trachomatis* is the most common microorganism associated with late postpartum endometritis. Other microorganisms associated with this clinical entity include the genital mycoplasmas and a diverse group of facultative bacteria including *Gardnerella vaginalis*. The late timing suggests that these women develop an ascending infection after delivery (Wagner et al, 1980).

Treatment should include coverage for chlamydia. Erythromycin is the drug most commonly recommended and is well tolerated in most patients treated as outpatients. Patients with more severe disease should be hosptialized and treated with an antibiotic regimen similar to those recommended for the therapy of PID (see Table 35–8). These regimens have an extended facultative and anaerobic bacterial spectrum as well as activity against *C. trachomatis*. Rarely, retained products of conception will be associated with the development of late-onset endometritis. These patients usually present with significant vaginal bleeding and will require dilatation and curettage to empty the endometrial cavity in addition to antibiotic therapy (Hoyme et al. 1986).

REFERENCES

Britigan BE, Cohen MS, Sparling PF: Gonococcal infection: a model of molecular pathogenesis. N Engl J Med 1985;312:1683.
Burkman RT: Intrauterine devices and pelvic inflammatory disease: evolving perspectives on the data. Obstet Gynecol Surv 1996;51(Suppl):S35.
Burkman RT, Atienza MF, King TM: Culture and treatment results in endometritis following elective abortion. Am J Obstet Gynecol 1977;128:556.

Burnham RC, Binns B, Guijon F, et al: Etiology and outcome of acute pelvic inflammatory disease. J Infect Dis 1988;158:510.

Cates W, Ory HW, Rochat RW, Tyler CW: The intrauterine device and deaths from spontaneous abortion. N Engl J Med 1976;295:1155.

Cates W, Rolfs RT, Aral SO: Sexually transmitted diseases, pelvic inflammatory disease, and infertility: an epidemiologic update. Epidemiol Rev 1990;12:199.

Centers for Disease Control and Prevention: 1998 Sexually transmitted diseases treatment guidelines. MMWR Morbid Mortal Wkly Rep 1997;47:79.

Chow AW, Carlson C, Sorrell TC: Host defenses in acute pelvic inflammatory disease. I. Bacterial clearance in the murine uterus and oviduct. Am J Obstet Gynecol 1980;138:1003.

Chow AW, Malkasian KL, Marshall JR, et al: Acute pelvic inflammatory disease and clinical response to parenteral doxycycline. Antimicrob Agents Chemother 1975;7:133.

Cleary RE, Jones RB: Recovery of Chlamydia trachomatis from the endometrium in infertile women with serum antichlamydial antibodies. Fertil Steril 1985; 44:233.

Cramer DW, Schiff I, Schoenbaum SC, et al: Tubal infertility and the intrauterine device. N Engl J Med 1985;312:941.

Crombleholme WR, Schachter J, Ohm-Smith M, et al: Efficacy of single-agent therapy for the treatment of acute pelvic inflammatory disease with ciprofloxacin. Am J Med 1989;87:142S.

Cunningham FG, Hauth JC, Gilstrap LC, et al: The bacterial pathogenesis of acute pelvic inflammatory disease. Obstet Gynecol 1978;52:161.

Eilard T, Brorsson J-E, Hamark B, Forssman L: Isolation of Chlamydia trachomatis in acute salpingitis. Scand J Infect Dis Suppl 1976;19(Suppl):82.

Eschenbach DA, Buchanan TM, Pollock HM, et al: Polymicrobial etiology of acute pelvic inflammatory disease. N Engl J Med 1975;293:166.

Eschenbach DA,. Hillier S, Critchlow C, et al: Diagnosis and clinical manifestations of bacterial vaginosis. Am J Obstet Gynecol 1988;158:819.

Fish ANJ, Fairweather DVI, Oriel JD, Ridgway GL: Isolation of Chlamydia trachomatis from endometriums of women with and without symptoms. Genitourin Med 1988;64:75.

Fridberg J, Confino E, Suarez M, Gleicher N: Chlamydia trachomatis attached to spermatozoa recovered from the peritoneal cavity of patients with salpingitis. J Reprod Med 1987;32:120.

Gilstrap LC, Herbert WNP, Cunningham FG, et al: Gonorrhea screening in male consorts of women with pelvic infection. JAMA 1977;238:965.

Grimes DA, Cates W Jr, Selik RM: Fatal septic abortion in the United States, 1975–1977. Obstet Gynecol 1981;57:739.

Grimes DA, Schulz KF, Cates W Jr, et al: The Joint Program for the Study of Abortion/CDC: a preliminary report. In Hern WM, Andrikopoulos B (eds): Abortion in the Seventies. New York: National Abortion Federation, 1977.

Hillier, SL, Kiviat NB, Hawes SE, et al: Role of bacterial vaginosis-associated microorganisms in endometritis. Am J Obstet Gynecol 1996;175:435.

Holmes KK, Stamm W: Lower genital tract infection in women. In Holmes KK, Mårdh PA, Sparling PF, et al (eds): Sexually Transmitted Diseases. 3rd ed. New York: McGraw-Hill, 1999:761.

Hoyme UB, Kiviat N, Eschenbach DA: Microbiology and treatment of late postpartum endometritis. Obstet Gynecol 1986;68:226.

Jacobson L, Westrom L: Objectivized diagnosis of acute pelvic inflammatory disease: diagnostic and prognostic value of routine laparoscopy. Am J Obstet Gynecol 1969;105:1088.

Kim-Farley RJ, Cates W, Ory HW, Hatcher RA: Febrile spontaneous abortion and the IUD. Contraception 1978;18:561.

Kiviat NB, Wolner-Hanssen P, Eschenbach DA, et al: Endometrial histopathology in patients with culture-proved upper genital tract infection and laparoscopically diagnosed acute salpingitis. Am J Surg Pathol 1990;14:167.

Kiviat NB, Wolner-Hanssen P, Peterson M, et al: Localization of Chlamydia trachomatis infection by direct immunofluorescence and culture in pelvic inflammatory disease. Am J Obstet Gynecol 1986;154:865.

Korn AP, Hessol N, Padian N, et al: Commonly used diagnostic criteria for pelvic inflammatory disease have poor sensitivity for plasma cell endometritis. Sex Transm Dis 1995;22:335.

Kutteh WH, Hatch KD, Blackwell RE, Mestecky J: Secretory immune system of the female reproductive tract: I. Immunoglobulin and secretory component-containing cells. Obstet Gynecol 1988;71:56.

Landers DV, Sweet RL: Current trends in the diagnosis and treatment of tuboovarian abscess. Am J Obstet Gynecol 1985;151:1098.

Larsson P, Platz-Christensen JJ, Thejls H, et al: Incidence of pelvic inflammatory disease after first trimester legal abortion in women with bacterial vaginosis after treatment with metronidazole: a double-blind, randomized study. Am J Obstet Gynecol 1992;166:100.

Lehtinen M, Rantala I, Teisala K, et al: Detection of herpes simplex virus in women with acute pelvic inflammatory disease. J Infect Dis 1985;152:78.

Mårdh Pa: An overview of infectious agents of salpingitis, their biology, and recent advances in methods of detection. Am J Obstet Gynecol 1980;138:933.

Mårdh P-A: Mycoplasmal PID: a review of natural and experimental infections. Yale J Biol Med 1983;56:529.

Mårdh P-A, Ripa T, Svensson L, Westrom L: Chlamydia trachomatis infection in patients with acute salpingitis. N Engl J Med 1977;296:1377.

Monif GRG: Significance of polymicrobial bacterial superinfection in the therapy of gonococcal endometritis-salpingitis-peritonitis. Obstet Gynecol 1980;55:154S.

Moore DE, Cates WJ Jr: Sexually transmitted diseases and infertility. In Holmes KK, Mårdh P-A, Sparling PF, Wiesner PJ (eds): Sexually Transmitted Diseases. 2nd ed. New York: McGraw-Hill, 1990.

Moss TR, Hawkswell J: Evidence of infection with Chlamydia trachomatis in patients with pelvic inflammatory disease: value of partner investigation. Fertil Steril 1986;45:429.

Ogra PL, Yamanaka T, Losonsky GA: Local immunologic defenses in the genital tract. In Barber HK (eds): Reproductive Immunology. New York: Alan R. Liss, 1981:381.

Paavonen J, Aine R, Teisala K, et al: Comparison of endometrial biopsy and peritoneal fluid cytologic testing with laparoscopy in the diagnosis of acute pelvic inflammatory disease. Am J Obstet Gynecol 1985;151:645.

Patton DL, Kuo C-C, Wang S-P, Halbert SA: Distal tubal obstruction by repeated Chlamydia trachomatis salpingeal infections in pig-tailed macaques. J Infect Dis 1987;155:1292.

Patton DL, Moore DE, Spadoni LR, et al: A comparison of the fallopian tube's response to overt and silent salpingitis. Obstet Gynecol 1989;73:622.

Patton DL, Wolner-Hanssen P, Cosgrove SJ, et al: Acute salpingitis in a pig-tailed macaque induced by cervical inoculations of Chlamydia trachomatis. Obstet Gynecol 1990;76:643.

Peipert JF, Boardman L, Hogan JW, et al: Laboratory evaluation of acute upper genital tract infection. Obstet Gynecol 1996;87:730.

Peterson HB, Walker CK, Kahn JG, et al: Pelvic inflammatory disease: key treatment and issues and options. JAMA 1991;266:2605.

Reichert JA, Valle RF: Fitz-Hugh–Curtis syndrome, a laparoscopic approach. JAMA 1976;236:266.

Rolfs RT, Galaid EI, Zaidi AA: Pelvic inflammatory disease: trends in hospitalizations and office visits, 1979 through 1988. Am J Obstet Gynecol 1992;166:983.

Rotheram EB, Schick SF: Nonclostridial anaerobic bacteria in septic abortion. Am J Med 1969;46:80.

Schmidt WA, Bedrossian CWM, Ali V, et al: Actinomycosis and intrauterine contraceptive devices: the clinicopathologic entity. Diag Gynecol Obstet 1980;2:165.

Scholes D, Stergachis A, Heidrich FE, et al: Prevention of pelvic inflammatory disease by screening for cervical chlamydia infection. N Engl J Med 1996;334:1362.

Soper DE, Brockwell NJ, Dalton HP: False positive cultures of the cul-de-sac associated with culdecentesis in patients undergoing elective laparoscopy. Obstet Gynecol 1991;164:134.

Soper DE, Brockwell NJ, Dalton HP, Johnson D: Observations concerning the microbial etiology of acute salpingitis. Am J Obstet Gynecol 1994;170:1014.

Svensson L, Mårdh PA, Westrom L: Infertility after acute salpingitis with special reference to *Chlamydia trachomatis*. Fertil Steril 1983;40:322.

Sweet RL: Pelvic inflammatory disease. In Sweet RL, Gibbs RS (eds): Infectious Disease of the Female Genital Tract. 2nd ed. Baltimore: Williams & Wilkins, 1990.

Sweet RL, Draper DL, Hadley WK: Etiology of acute salpingitis: influence of episode number and duration of symptoms. Obstet Gynecol 1981;58:62.

Sweet RL, Draper DL, Schacter J, et al: Microbiology and pathogenesis of acute salpingitis as determined by laparoscopy: what is the appropriate site to sample? Am J Obstet Gynecol 1980; 138:985.

Sweet RL, Schachter J, Robbie MO: Failure of β-lactam antibiotics to eradicate Chlamydia trachomatis in the endometrium despite apparent clinical cure of acute salpingitis. JAMA 1983;250: 2641.

Wagner GP, Martin DH, Koutsky L, et al: Puerperal infectious morbidity: relationship to route of delivery and to antepartum. *Chlamydia trachomatis* infection. Am J Obstet Gynecol 1980;138: 1028.

Washington AE, Aral SO, Grimes DA, Holmes KK: Assessing risk for pelvic inflammatory disease and its sequelae. JAMA 1991; 266:2581.

Washington AE, Arno PS, Brooks MA: The economic cost of pelvic inflammatory disease. JAMA 1986;255:1735.

Washington AE, Katz P: Cost of and payment source of pelvic inflammatory disease: trends and projections, 1983 through 2000. JAMA 1991;266:2565.

Wasserheit JN, Bell TA, Kiviat NB, et al: Microbial causes of proven pelvic inflammatory disease and efficacy of clindamycin and tobramycin. Ann Intern Med 1986;104:187.

Westrom L: Effect of acute pelvic inflammatory disease on fertility. Am J Obstet Gynecol 1975;121:707.

Westrom L: Incidence, prevalence, and trends of acute pelvic inflammatory disease and its consequences in industrialized countries. Am J Obstet Gynecol 1980;138:880.

Westrom L, Eschenbach D: Pelvic inflammatory disease. In Holmes KK, Mårdh PA, Sparling PF, et al (eds): Sexually Transmitted Diseases. New York: McGraw-Hill, 1999:783.

Westrom L, Svensson L, Wolner-Hanssen P, Mårdh P-A: A clinical double-blind study on the effect of prophylactically administered single dose tinidazole on the occurrence of endometritis after first trimester legal abortion. Scan J Infect Dis Suppl 1981; 26:104.

Wolner-Hanssen P, Eschenbach DA, Paavonen J, et al: Association between vaginal douching and acute pelvic inflammatory disease. JAMA 1990a;263:1936.

Wolner-Hanssen P, Eschenbach DA, Paavonen J, et al: Decreased risk of symptomatic chlamydial pelvic inflammatory disease associated with oral contraceptive use. JAMA 1990b;263:54.

36

Postoperative Infections in Gynecology and Infectious Complications in Gynecologic Oncology

David A. Martin

INCIDENCE AND IMPLICATIONS

Febrile morbidity and infectious complications developing during the initial postoperative course are the most common complications that occur in surgical patients. These complications increase the cost of care, require extended hospitalization, and may result in permanent morbidity.

Because of the nonspecific presentation of most infectious complications, it is often difficult for clinicians who first recognize a febrile postoperative course to be certain whether they are dealing with a patient showing atelectatic fever, a wound seroma, early signs of a necrotizing soft tissue infection, or the first evidence of a pelvic abscess that may lead to systemic sepsis. Each patient with a postoperative fever merits evaluation to determine the origin of the possible infectious process, but not all patients who have fever need antibiotics because not all are infected. Frequently, careful surveillance allows times for resolution of a noninfectious fever, and the patient thereby avoids the side effects or allergic reactions that may occur as a result of drug reactions.

Nosocomial Infection

Postoperative infections are a common type of nosocomial infection. Nosocomial infections are estimated to be related to one third of hospital deaths (Gross et al, 1980). Postoperative wound infections are responsible for approximately 24% of nosocomial infections. The other major causes of nosocomial infections are urinary tract infections (42%), pneumo-

nia (10%), and bacteremia (5%) (Haley et al, 1985b). Because hospitalized gynecologic patients frequently undergo urinary tract instrumentation or catheterization, they are at risk for nosocomial urinary tract infections. They are also predisposed to pneumonia caused by postoperative atelectasis. The mortality of a nosocomial pneumonia varies from 35% to 55% (Gross et al, 1980). It is a fundamental concern that postoperative nosocomial pneumonias are frequently due to hospital-acquired organisms that may have resistance to multiple antibiotics.

The short-term implications of postoperative infections vary with the site of infection. A postoperative incisional wound infection typically increases the length of hospitalization by 3 to 7 days, depending on whether significant cellulitis is present and on the preoperative condition that necessitated operation. For the gynecologic patient in whom prompt return of bowel function and discharge on postoperative days 2 to 7 is a typical occurrence, the wound infection that first presents on postoperative days 4 or 5 certainly impacts on the length of hospitalization.

Historically, patients with nosocomial infections complicated by bacteremia averaged an additional 30-day hospital stay. These infections are frequently due to the use of intravenous catheters or instrumentation of the urinary tract (Haley et al, 1981b). The related mortality for nosocomial bacteremia varies from 16% to 80% and is often determined by concomitant underlying illness. Approximately 70% of hospital-acquired infections are caused by gram-negative rods. Staphylococcal organisms account for most of the remainder, and, as a hospital-acquired organism, they are frequently resistant to methicillin.

Hysterectomy-Associated Infections

Gynecologic surgery patients also face special risks of soft tissue pelvic infection and of pelvic and abdominal abscess. The incidence of febrile morbidity in the patient undergoing a hysterectomy is illustrated by the report of Ledger and Child (1973) showing that 50% of patients undergoing abdominal or vaginal hysterectomy required antibiotics during the postoperative period. Hevron and Llorens (1976) reported that posthysterectomy pelvic abscesses developed in 3% of patients; the rate after vaginal hysterectomy was 4%, in contrast to 0.7% after abdominal hysterectomy.

Pelvic cellulitis is the most common major infection after vaginal hysterectomy. Serious infections occur in 25% to 50% of patients subjected to abdominal or vaginal hysterectomy when prophylactic antibiotics are not used. This high rate of infection is reduced to 5% to 15% when preoperative antibiotics are utilized. These reports also show that overall febrile morbidity, regardless of whether infection is proven, occurs much more often than do pelvic cellulitis or abscess. In contrast to the effect on true infections, the occurrence rates of febrile morbidity are not uniformly reduced with prophylactic antibiotics. Incidence rates vary on the basis of definitions used for clinical diagnosis, and they differ in some patient populations on the basis of associated risk factors. Most clinical efforts have focused on reducing these high spontaneous infection rates after gynecologic surgery and on distinguishing noninfectious fever from significant pelvic infections. To this end, much effort has been expended in identifying risk factors that increase the incidence of postoperative infection.

The remainder of the chapter discusses the evaluation of febrile postoperative patients, risk factors predisposing to infection, the use of perioperative antimicrobial prophylaxis, and the specific postoperative infections that commonly occur. Additionally, I describe separately the infectious complications of gynecologic oncology patients because they have unique risk factors for infection.

PREDISPOSING FACTORS FOR INFECTION

Defense Mechanisms

In most postoperative patients, infection does not develop. Generally, the initiation of postoperative infection is due to a breakdown of the normal host defenses in association with exposure to endogenous organisms. Surgery causes multiple defects in the host defense systems by altering the integrity of skin and mucosal epithelia and providing sanctuary sites with poor blood supply and excellent growth media for culturing the inoculum of bacteria at the surgical site. Alteration of the host defenses can occur as a result of local factors, systemic disease, or environmental effects on the systemic defenses (Table 36–1).

Table 36–1. ALTERED HOST DEFENSES: RISK FACTORS FOR POSTOPERATIVE INFECTIONS

Obesity
Chronic obstructive lung disease
Acute viral upper respiratory tract infection
Bowel obstruction
Urinary tract obstruction
Diabetes mellitus
Chronic renal failure
Malnutrition
Asplenia
General anesthesia
Immunosuppressants
    Glucocorticoids
    Azathioprine
    Cyclosporine
Radiotherapy (prior dose to operative site)

The normal defense mechanisms of the respiratory tract are the phagocytic cells, a strong cough, and mucociliary clearance. Similarly, the gastrointestinal and urinary systems maintain a defense barrier with an intact epithelial surface, phagocytic mechanisms, and, to varying degrees, high flow rates in a single direction to keep the upper gastrointestinal system and upper urinary tract sterile. The upper gastrointestinal system, in addition, has the benefit of an acid pH. In view of these normal defense mechanisms, it is easily understood how urinary or gastrointestinal obstruction promotes bacterial growth as a result of stasis. Respiratory defenses are compromised by mucociliary paralysis resulting from smoking and by secretions plugging airways in lungs that are scarred and sacculated by the changes of chronic obstructive pulmonary disease (COPD).

Systemic disease can easily affect host defense mechanisms involved in fighting bacteria. Diabetes affects leukocyte mobility and is also associated with inhibition of phagocytosis. This effect correlates clinically with the increased incidence of infection in diabetic patients. Chronic renal failure is associated with defective cell-mediated immunity.

Malnutrition is associated with decreased numbers of circulating white blood cells, decreased antibody production, and defective cell-mediated immunity. Complement levels are decreased, and the net result is decreased chemotactic ability of leukocytes and defective macrophage function.

Patients who have undergone splenectomy or who are functionally asplenic, such as adults with sickle cell disease, are at increased risk for infection. The most common postsplenectomy infections are meningitis and bacteremia caused by encapsulated organisms such as *Escherichia coli*, *Haemophilus influenzae*, *Streptococcus pneumoniae*, or *Neisseria meningitidis* (Francke and Neu, 1981). These organisms require opsonization to promote phagocytosis. Patients without a spleen have a defective complement pathway because of defective antibody production and therefore do not clear bacteria from the circulation effectively. Splenic macrophages act as the primary filter for circulating bacteria when the host is first exposed to an invading organism and prior to specific antibody production. After specific antibodies are present, phagocytes of the liver become the predominant phagocytic system.

General anesthesia compromises systemic defenses by limiting leukocyte migration. Mucociliary function is decreased by general anesthetics and, therefore, airway sterility is harder to maintain. Local anesthetics can also affect granulocyte migration. Certain narcotics, muscle relaxants, and sedatives also affect chemotaxis.

Surgical Factors

Certain surgical procedures are inherently more at risk for postoperative infection. Such procedures include bowel surgery, vaginal surgery, and surgery in infected sites. Other surgeries at high risk for infection include those with placement of a nontissue prosthesis, such as hernia repairs. The degree of wound contamination at surgery has long been known as a risk factor for infection. The greater the amount of contamination, the higher the incidence of surgical site infection. Increased tissue damage in contaminated sites compromises the defense mechanisms, as does decreased local tissue perfusion whether from local ischemia or systemic shock. Hypoxemia has the same effect.

Wound Factor: Obesity

Obese patients have a higher incidence of incisional wound infections. Incisions in areas of deep subcutaneous fat are at high risk for infection, probably because of compromised defense mechanisms related to seroma or hematoma formation, dead space in the wound, and relatively poor blood supply to adipose tissue. This topic is discussed in greater detail later in this chapter in the section "Wound infections."

PATHOGENS IN GYNECOLOGIC SURGERY SITES

Infectious complications after gynecologic surgery are caused by endogenous organisms in most cases. Those organisms are normal skin flora and normal vaginal flora. Many studies describe the bacterial species that colonize the vagina in healthy patients. These studies confirm multiple bacterial isolates from each patient, and the proportion of individual bacterial species varies with menopausal status,

menstrual cycle timing, associated medications such as antibiotics, and even the presence of neighboring malignancies. Change in vaginal flora caused by antimicrobial prophylaxis for surgery is difficult to measure with preoperative and postoperative cultures because surgery alone affects the relative numbers of vaginal organisms.

Antibiotics in current usage for prevention of postoperative infections are effective against many of the resident vaginal bacteria. Not all bacterial species present need to be sensitive to the prophylactic antibiotic used in order for that antibiotic to reduce the infection rate. Many antibiotic agents with markedly differing spectra of activity provide similar reductions in postoperative infection. Similarly, not all bacteria present in an established infection need to be sensitive to the antibiotics given in order for treatment to be effective. Treating the most virulent pathogens and those that may create a synergistic effect appears to be sufficient. When postoperative infection does occur, empiric therapy needs to be chosen with regard to the potential pathogens present. Antibiotics may assist in local containment of the infection, and host defenses then complete eradication of the organisms.

The bacterial species normally present in the vagina include gram-positive aerobic staphylococci and streptococci, particularly streptococci of groups A, B, and D (enterococci). Also present are gram-negative aerobic bacteria of the Enterobacteriaceae as well as anaerobic bacilli and anaerobic streptococci. An excellent review of the normal genital microflora and the factors affecting prevalence of various bacteria can be found in a monograph by Larsen (1985).

Rather than consider all of the possible flora, it is more reasonable to be concerned with the typical pathogens recovered from active infections. These represent a subgroup of the normal flora. The typical pathogens vary between different types of postoperative infections and between patients, depending on predisposing factors and prior antibiotic exposure or length of hospitalization. For example, the postoperative pelvic cellulitis or abscess is a polymicrobial infection of aerobic and anaerobic bacteria. In the aerobic pathogen group, *E. coli*, *Klebsiella pneumoniae*, *Proteus* species, group A and group B streptococci, and enterococci predominate. These same organisms will be recovered from urinary tract and respiratory infections as well as from incision wound infections.

The anaerobic organisms are primarily *Bacteroides* species, *Peptococcus* species, and *Peptostreptococcus* species. Particular attention has been given to *Bacteroides bivius* and *Bacteroides disiens* as aggressive pathogens. Patients who are immunosuppressed, who have previously been exposed to antibiotics, or who have been in the hospital for extended time will be colonized by less common aerobic gram-negative organisms such as *Pseudomonas* or *Enterobacter*. (See Chapter 37 for a review of antibiotic activity against specific organisms.)

EVALUATING POSTOPERATIVE FEVER

Definitions

Normal daily oral temperature fluctuations make it difficult to define fever; however, a temperature greater than 38.0°C (100.4°F) is a conventional definition of fever. Postoperative febrile morbidity is usually defined as a temperature higher than 38.3°C on two measurements at least 6 hours apart, excluding the first 24 hours after surgery (Ledger, 1980; Hemsell et al, 1983b).

Distinguishing Fever From Infection

Postoperative febrile morbidity of unknown etiology usually resolves without treatment and is generally thought to arise from inflammatory changes at the operative site as a result of tissue necrosis in surgical pedicles, resorption of hematoma and serosanguinous exudate, and atelectasis. In the gynecologic patient, fever during the first 36 postoperative hours will most often be due to a noninfectious cause, atelectasis, or urinary tract infection. Less commonly, the fever will be sustained, and then it more likely represents an incisional wound infection, operative site infection at the vaginal apex, pneumonia, or skin infections related to venous access catheters. Many patients with fever in the postoperative period do not have infection. A prospective study of general surgery patients reported by Garibaldi et al (1985) noted that 38% of the postoperative fevers were "unexplained" fever. By comparison, 26% of patients had wound infections, 21% had urinary tract infections, and 13% had respiratory infections. Unexplained fever makes up a much larger proportion (71%) of fevers if only the first 72 postoperative hours are included.

Most significant infections in the body cause fever. Any new fever or other change in clinical condition that may be associated with sepsis (even when fever is not present) should suggest occult infection. These changes in clinical condition can be subtle, and for immunosuppressed or elderly patients they may include only mental status changes, general fatigue, and lack of appetite. Infection should also be considered in patients who are hypothermic when there are other clinical signs consistent with infection. Some incisional wound infections progress rapidly, and it is crucial that these be treated promptly. Similarly, prompt recognition and proper management of pelvic cellulitis is required to avoid the life-threatening complications of pelvic abscess, septic pelvic vein thrombophlebitis, and septic shock.

Fever Triage

The initial approach to a febrile patient must include a review of the clinical events preceding the onset of fever, with particular attention to the time elapsed between surgery and the onset of fever. The patient should be queried regarding a fever preceding hospitalization, and the past history should be reviewed for any systemic disease or noninfectious causes of fever that may be reappearing during the hospitalization. Common infectious causes include chronic diverticulitis, chronic pyelonephritis, and chronic sinusitis or otitis media. Noninfectious causes include inflammatory bowel disease, thyroiditis, and drug-induced fevers. Fever may be the first symptom of a flare of alcoholic hepatitis after alcoholic indiscretion prior to admission. The more rare problems of a pre-existing febrile disease (Table 36–2) may include sarcoidosis, rheumatic fever, or collagen-vascular diseases such as giant cell arteritis, periarteritis nodosa, and systemic lupus. Tuberculosis is becoming more common once again, and the extrapulmonary sites of systemic tuberculosis in the kidney, lymph nodes, or genital system may cause fever. A hematoma may result in a low-grade fever, and this should be suspected particularly in those patients who have been given anticoagulant therapy postoperatively. This applies particularly to patients who were taking warfarin (Coumadin) prior to admission.

After the past history is reviewed, recent surgery should be considered as a source of fever. The nature of the surgery should be considered. In addition to hysterectomy-related pelvic cellulitis, other intra-abdominal surgical procedures predisposing to deep operative site infections include bowel resection with a leaking anastomosis or extended ureteral dissection with an occult urinary tract injury causing a urinoma. All incisions should be checked for a wound infection. If a patient with an infected urinary tract undergoes invasive procedures, such as manipulation of urinary stents or retrograde pyelograms, the procedure may cause acute onset of fever.

The time interval from procedure to onset of fever may help to identify the most likely cause of fever (Table 36–3). For high fevers occurring during the first 36 hours postoperatively, the clinician must consider a short list of possible infectious causes. Several of these infections are common, and the others are uncommon but dangerous.

Table 36-2. CAUSES OF FEVER UNRELATED TO SURGERY (PRE-EXISTING DISEASE)

INFECTIOUS	NONINFECTIOUS
Viral upper respiratory infection	Rheumatic fever
Chronic diverticulitis	Sarcoidosis
Chronic pyelonephritis	Collagen-vascular disease
Chronic sinusitis	Inflammatory bowel disease
Otitis media	Thyroiditis
Tuberculosis	Alcoholic hepatitis
	Addison's disease

Table 36-3. CAUSES OF POSTOPERATIVE FEVER (CATEGORIZED BY TIME TO ONSET)

EARLY FEVER (<36 hr)	LATE FEVER (>36 hr)
Unexplained fever	All of the causes of early fever
Atelectasis	Incision infection
Streptococcal cellulitis	Urinary tract infection
Incision	Pneumonia
Pelvis	Pelvic cellulitis
Peritoneal soiling by	Vaginal cuff abscess
Occult bowel injury	Pelvic abscess
Anastomotic leak	Septic thrombophlebitis
Urinoma	Deep vein thrombosis
Occult ureteral injury	Sinusitis
Ureteral obstruction	Drug fever
Clostridial cellulitis	Bacteremia
Incision site	Catheter sepsis
Pelvic operative site	Antibiotic-associated diarrhea caused by *Clostridium difficile*

Early Fever

The most common early fever is from the respiratory system. Atelectasis occurs to some degree in almost all patients who have received a general anesthetic, and this may be a noninfectious cause of fever. With atelectasis, findings may include distant breath sounds or rales, and chest films may be normal or may show volume loss or atelectatic densities at the bases. Patients with underlying lung disease may become hypoxic.

If surgery was performed on the bowel and an occult injury occurred, early intraperitoneal contamination may cause fever with development of peritonitis. Unrecognized operative injury to the ureter or bladder may do the same. Wound infections at the incision usually manifest after the fourth or fifth postoperative day. However, early-onset wound infections are generally due to highly virulent organisms and may cause significant morbidity and mortality even with prompt recognition. Examination should certainly include a survey of the incision for signs of early infection when the patient's temperature reaches 38.5°C during the first 24 hours. Group A or group B β-hemolytic streptococci may cause a rapid-onset incision infection, as may *Clostridium* species.

Delayed Fever

Postoperative fevers developing more than 36 hours after surgery may include all of the entities discussed above for early fever as well as additional infections of intra-abdominal and intrapelvic operative sites, such as pelvic cellulitis, vaginal cuff cellulitis, cuff abscess, or abdominal abscess. Nonoperative infection sites include pneumonia, urinary tract infection, or venous catheter–related sepsis. In addition, evaluation for purulent nasal drainage may identify paranasal sinusitis, which is particularly likely to occur in patients with chronic intubation by nasogastric or nasotracheal tubes. Similarly, peripheral intravenous catheters and central venous catheters may become colonized during the initial postoperative days and may cause a fever or skin site inflammation 3 to 5 days after insertion. The likelihood of development of a nosocomial urinary tract infection increases with every day of continued catheterization and increases dramatically with any opening of the closed urinary drainage system. New-onset diarrhea, particularly in the setting of recent systemic antibiotics, requires consideration of an antibiotic-associated diarrhea and checking for underlying colitis caused by *Clostridium difficile*. Postoperative pneumonia may also manifest after the initial 36 hours postoperatively and will eventually be associated with symptoms or signs of dyspnea, hypoxia, productive cough, or pleuritic chest pain. Occult venous thrombotic disease may cause a fever during this same period.

Further evaluation of these late fevers includes a bimanual pelvic examination to identify any tenderness or induration at the operative site or mass effect that may be a drainable abscess. At the incision, evidence of deep induration, tenderness, or fluctuance may appear several days after the initial fever. A common clinical course for wound infection is for a low fever to precede by several days the serous drainage and eventual spontaneous separation of an incision that appeared to be healing well for the first 3 to 5 days. Intra-abdominal infection and abscess may be associated with persistent ileus, peritoneal signs, or deep abdominal tenderness away from the area of the incision or operative site. If an intra-abdominal process is the presumed cause of fever, flat plate and upright abdominal films should be obtained to look for signs of free air, localized air-fluid levels, or a generalized ileus pattern. A chest radiograph is obtained to evaluate for subdiaphragmatic air. Lateral decubitus films may be useful in patients who cannot stand.

A suspected pelvic or intra-abdominal abscess may be confirmed and localized using computerized tomography (CT) or ultrasound studies. For evaluating an abdominal abscess, ultrasound is frequently less useful than CT scan because of the often-associated ileus and obscured imaging resulting from artifact created by small-bowel gas. Imaging studies also serve to localize the process for possible percutaneous drainage by interventional radiology. CT scan or magnetic resonance imaging (MRI) also frequently shows an occult pelvic thrombophlebitis or iliofemoral vein thrombus that has been clinically occult and may be the sole explanation for postoperative fever. If cardiac examination reveals a new murmur, an echocardiogram should be ordered to evaluate for valvular vegetations.

An adnexal abscess may present even later after surgery than a vaginal apex abscess. Tubo-ovarian abscesses may form as a complication subsequent to treatment of a vaginal apex abscess; they may also form as a primary infection of the ovary. An ovarian abscess is presumably due to bacterial invasion at sites of minimal ovarian trauma from surgery. Alternatively, a follicular cyst may become infected when ovulation occurs perioperatively.

Another late-presenting infectious complication is septic pelvic thrombophlebitis; it may be difficult to distinguish this disorder from an adnexal abscess. Both entities may present with high fevers in a delayed fashion after surgery, and septic pelvic thrombophlebitis may develop during treatment of a pelvic abscess. The examination findings may be unimpressive despite the high fever when septic thrombophlebitis is the correct diagnosis. Further examination should exclude the possibility of pharyngitis, otitis media, perianal abscess, or endocarditis. If no obvious site of infection is found, the differential diagnosis includes drug-induced fever or, for cancer patients, a tumor fever. The latter subjects are covered under the oncology topics later in this chapter.

Another iatrogenic cause of fever is transfusion-related febrile episodes from stored blood. This is usually temporally related to transfusion, does not usually cause persistent fever, and is not discussed further in this chapter.

WOUND INFECTIONS

Epidemiology

Wound Pathogens

Information gained from national multi-institutional studies has described the common organisms recovered from wound infections. A listing of the organisms by frequency of their recovery suggests to some extent the pathogenicity of the organism and reflects also the potential exposure of a given wound to that organism. Exposure to certain organisms is expected to vary by the type of procedure performed. The National Academy of Sciences (Report of Ad Hoc Committee, 1964) described the frequency of occurrence of organisms recovered from wound infections. *Staphylococcus* (coagulase-positive and coagulase-negative) was the most common isolate (61%), followed by *E. coli* (22%), *Proteus* (12%), *Pseudomonas* (13%), non-hemolytic *Streptococcus* (9.7%), and *Klebsiella* (8.7%). Similar information was reported by the National Nosocomial Infection Study from 1980 to 1982 (Hughes et al, 1983) with *Staphylococcus aureus* predominating on adult surgical services. When obstetric and gynecologic services were compared for wound pathogens, *E. coli*, enterococcus, and *Bacteroides* species were the predominant organisms.

By comparison, Moir-Bussy et al (1984) conducted a prospective study of wound infections after all types of cesarean sections in 31 hospitals. This group of patients, who underwent cesarean section with a dilated cervix, may very closely approximate gynecologic patients who undergo laparotomy and vaginal incision during the same surgical procedure; therefore, the organisms contaminating the incisions in both patient groups would be expected to be similar. That report noted the most common organisms to be enterococci (especially *Streptococcus faecalis*), *E. coli*, *Proteus* species, hemolytic non-group A streptococci, *S. aureus*, and *Staphylococcus albus*. Anaerobic organisms were found in 8% of the positive cultures. The true contribution of anaerobes to wound infections was probably not accurately reported prior to the 1980s, when good culture techniques for anaerobes became widespread.

Procedure-Related Pathogens

Perhaps a more useful method for predicting the most likely organisms in an incision wound infection is to categorize by the type of procedure performed. Type of procedure provides knowledge of organisms likely to have contaminated the tissues operated on. For example, the incision infection after a laparotomy to repair an incision hernia, when the vagina, bowel, or urinary tract has not been entered, would be expected to contain *Staphylococcus* species, *Streptococcus* species, or perhaps *E. coli*. Conversely, when abdominal hysterectomy has been performed, the vaginal organisms would then have access to the peritoneal cavity and the incision wound, and this wound may contain not only the preceding organisms but also enteric gram-negative and other anaerobic organisms, frequently in a polymicrobic infection. The same vaginal flora are causes of upper genital tract infections; in addition, whenever laparotomy is performed for complications of pelvic inflammatory disease or when a gross purulence has been encountered, these incisions are even more likely to be infected, and to be infected by the same multiple organisms found in the infections complicating hysterectomy.

Most wound infections on gynecologic services are due to multiple organisms, and it is the exception when a single organism causes the clinical infection.

Time Of Presentation

An alternative classification system is to divide the infections into *early-onset* versus *late-onset* wound infections. When early-onset infections occur, certain organisms are more likely the cause, such as *Streptococcus* and *Clostridium* species. Clinical judgment will take all of these generalizations into account and assist the clinician in the choice of empiric antibiotic coverage for those wounds that warrant antibiotic therapy.

Wound Contamination

Contamination of the surgical site predisposes to infection. A wound classification has been defined by the American College of Surgeons to take the degree of contamination into account. There are four main categories of wounds: (1) clean, (2) clean-contaminated, (3) contaminated, and (4) dirty or infected (Altemeir et al, 1976).

- *Clean-contaminated wounds* are associated with surgery wherein the vagina or respiratory tract have been entered, or where the gastrointestinal tract is entered but no gross spillage occurs. Most gynecologic surgical procedures involve this category of wounds. A typical infection rate for clean-contaminated wounds is 3% to 5%.
- *Contaminated wounds* are associated with surgery where there has been a major break in sterile technique, where there has been gross spillage of intestinal contents, or where there is infected urine and the urinary tract has been entered.
- A *dirty* or *infected wound* is one in which a collection of pus is drained or a perforated viscus or acute bacterial cellulitis is encountered.

Studies on clean wounds show that other variables can be identified as risk factors for subsequent wound infection. Even under optimal circumstances with a *clean wound*, the typical infection rate is 1% to 2%. A large prospective study has been reported by Cruse and Foord (1980) involving 63,000 surgical wounds. The authors noted a sixfold increase in infection rates in a comparison of those patients older than age 66 and those younger than age 14. Age was again confirmed to be an important variable in a later study (Mead et al, 1986), with an increased wound infection rate for patients over 50 years of age.

Cruse and Foord (1980) evaluated duration of surgical operations and reported a doubling of the infection rate for clean wounds with every additional hour of surgical time. Another finding was that incidental appendectomy would change clean wound infection rates from 1.4% to 4.5%. Type of skin preparation and various types of wound care after surgery had minimal effect. It was also noted that tissue necrosis caused by excessive use of electrocautery dramatically raised the infection rate during the initial years of use until surgeons recognized the importance of minimizing the necrotic tissue induced by cautery within a wound. During later years of their surveillance, infection rates were identical whether or not electrosurgical units were used to secure hemostasis.

Minimal skin trauma in the area of the incision predisposes to wound infection. Examples are the minimal trauma caused by shaving to remove hair in the area of the incision. Either not removing the hair or clipping the hair is preferred to shaving (Alexander et al, 1983; Olson et al, 1986). Cruse and Foord (1980) also noted that the length of preoperative in-hospital stay correlated with increased wound infections. Necrotic tissue or foreign bodies, such as suture material or implanted devices, decrease the size of the inoculum required to generate an infection. The most important factors in the etiology of incisional wound infections appear to be the degree of contamination and local factors causing a compromised host, such as necrotic tissue, foreign body sutures, or hematoma formation within the wound.

Factors that promote infection include devitalized tissue from excessive use of electrocautery, fat necrosis from retractor-induced tissue injury, foreign bodies such as suture, or use of open drains that exit through the operative incision. Any foreign body will dramatically lower the innoculum size of bacteria required to produce a wound infection. Controlled wound experiments using various sizes of innocula have shown that foreign bodies in a wound decrease innoculation size required for an infection to form by a factor of 10^3 to 10^4. For this reason, highly reactive sutures, such as silk, or the use of any suture not absolutely required in the subcutaneous and skin tissues is to be avoided. If this kind of suture is required, either a monofilament permanent suture or a relatively inert absorbable suture (e.g., polyglyconate) is preferred.

In an effort to further define a given patient's risk for a wound infection, a risk index has been reported that combines patient susceptibility factors with degree of wound contamination. The risk index was verified prospectively using patients from the SENIC Project (Study on the Efficacy of Nosocomial Infection Control) and identified high-risk and low-risk subgroups within each of the traditional wound classes as described by the degree of contamination (Haley et al, 1985a). Patients at high risk are those with multiple concomitant diagnoses, whose procedures last longer than 2 hours, who have undergone any abdominal procedure, or with contaminated or dirty/infected wounds. These risk factors are present in almost all gynecologic oncology patients undergoing abdominal surgery.

Obesity: A Wound Factor

Obesity has been repeatedly confirmed as a major risk factor for incisional wound infections and for wound separation and dehiscence even without infection. Obese patients were noted to have an eightfold higher rate of infected incisions after hysterectomy (Pitkin, 1976). An eightfold increase in wound infections was also shown for obese patients compared to normal-weight patients undergoing laparotomy (Forse et al, 1989). The risk contributed by obesity to the incisional infection rate is equal to the risk created by making an incision directly into an infected site, as reported by Barber et al (1995). Obesity is a risk for infection in many surgery sites, including laparotomy, cesarean section, sternotomy, renal transplant, and breast surgery (Forse et al, 1989; Parrott et al, 1989; Barber et al, 1995).

Placing an incision into areas of deep subcutaneous fat may be more important to the risk of incisional infections than is the patients' weight. A multivariate analysis of a prospective study on patients undergoing hysterectomy confirmed that the thickness of the subcutaneous tissue at the site of the incision was the specific risk factor for infection (Soper et al, 1995). Body weight and body mass index had a positive correlation with infection risk, but they were outweighed in importance by the depth of the subcutaneous fat at the incision site. Wound infection risk was seen to rise when the depth of the subcutaneous tissue was greater than 3 cm.

Prevention of surgical site infections in obese patients is not possible in every case, but the infection rate may be reduced by using antibiotics. Special dosing of antibiotics is required to achieve adequate blood and tissue levels in these obese patients. Forse et al (1989) noted a reduction in wound infection rates for those obese patients given prophylactic antibiotics dosed by adjusting for body weight.

Evaluation and Initial Care

Wound infections generally are evident on postoperative days 4 to 7. The preceding days are often characterized by a low-grade fever, with higher temperature spikes eventually developing. Subtle signs of infection at the wound may not be noticed until one of these higher temperature elevations is noted. The usual presentation is erythema near the incision, accompanied by edema, induration, and tenderness. If skin staples are removed, frequently the incision will spontaneously open, confirming poor healing. There may be significant drainage from deeper in the subcutaneous tissues as well.

Another common presentation of wound infections is spontaneous serous or purulent drainage from the wound accompanied by a low-grade fever. When the wound is explored, a serosanguinous discharge or hematoma can be evacuated. Occasionally, an indolent infection in an obese person features well-healed skin but eventually presents with a deep subcutaneous mass. The mass may be fluctuant and tender. When this wound is opened, purulent discharge will decompress. This presentation is often more delayed because it is not as easy to identify in the absence of significant early induration and erythema.

During inspection of wound infections, grave warning signs to note are skin crepitus caused by subcutaneous air or inappropriate skin coloration such as bruising, bronzing, or mottling. In addition, severe pain reported by the patient or skin edema spreading away from the incision even without associated erythema are signs of severe cellulitis. Associated petechiae, intermittent hypotension, or disorientation should alert the clinician to bacteremia or toxemia associated with severe infection.

Reopening Surgical Wounds

At the time an incisional wound infection is suspected, full examination of the wound is required. This usually includes removal of several skin sutures and probing of the wound with a cotton swab or aspiration with a needle and syringe to document the presence of a fluid collection and to assist with spontaneous drainage of purulent material. It is gen-

erally better to err toward opening of the incision; if any evidence of infection is found, most of the wound should be opened unless only a small hematoma is encountered. If no evidence of inflammation or purulence is identified on the initial probing of the wound, nothing has been lost because the wound will promptly re-close within several days. Conversely, if a wound infection is not managed aggressively, it may progress to a significant infection complicated by permanent morbidity.

When the wound is opened, all loculated collections should be broken up. All necrotic tissue and debris should be removed. The wound should then be packed with fine-mesh gauze and kept moist. The surface dressing should be changed frequently enough to débride the wound of any purulent material or necrotic debris that accumulates between dressing changes. Initially, changes may be required three to four times per day. As the infection improves, dressing changes will be needed less frequently.

With this method of wound cleaning, bacterial counts are frequently reduced within several days and granulation tissue will be promptly seen over the subcutaneous fat. When adequate granulation tissue is covering the surface, a decision can be made regarding allowing the wound to continue to close by secondary intention or attempting a re-closure. If the wound is allowed to heal by secondary intention, granulation tissue will continue to form and eventually the wound will contract and the skin surface will re-epithelialize. If there has been chronic distortion at the abdominal wall surface, such as may happen with obese patients or patients with previous scars in the area, the scar may be wider than if primary closure had occurred.

Re-closing Previously Infected Wounds

If it is elected to re-close the wound, this should be done when there is no further sign of inflammation or necrotic tissue and when a good granulation tissue coverage of the subcutaneous fat is present. On re-closure, there is risk for development of another wound infection. However, with proper judgment, this should be reduced to 5% to 10% of cases. Before the wound is closed, it should be sterilized with some topical disinfectant, such as povidone-iodine, followed by a saline irrigation. Skin edges can be approximated with adhesive tape bridges such as Steri-Strip. If the patient has a large amount of subcutaneous fat, the fat may not approximate throughout the incision if the surgeon simply pulls the skin edges together. In this situation, a vertical mattress suture using a large loop down to the level of the fascia may help to approximate subcutaneous tissue and avoid dead space. If sutures are required, I prefer a monofilament permanent suture, such as nylon, to reduce the incidence of infection. These sutures can be removed in 7 to 14 days. When these sutures are required, it is often useful to remove tension from the wound edges by using Montgomery straps to approximate the skin and subcutaneous tissue as a mass effect. The sutures tend to "cut" by local pressure and ischemia when there is too much tension at the skin edges.

Antibiotics

The acute management for most wounds is accomplished primarily by opening the incision. After the wound is opened, there is usually a prompt defervescence and the patient may be afebrile within 12 to 24 hours. For the majority of patients, no antibiotics are required. However, in addition to opening the wound, antibiotics are indicated when there is evidence of significant cellulitis, systemic signs suggesting bacteremia, or signs suggestive of a necrotizing infection. A strong case can also be made for adjuvant antibiotics in high-risk patients, such as diabetics, patients with uremia, patients receiving chemotherapy with decreased neutrophil counts, patients receiving systemic steroids, or patients with an incisional wound infection in a previously irradiated skin area. Moderate malnutrition or severe obesity may also be considered high-risk situations.

Early-Presenting Wound Infection

Incisional wound infections in the first 12 to 48 hours after surgery are often caused by a single pathogen. Group A or group B streptococci or clostridial species make up the majority of the early infections. These early-onset infections should be treated with antibiotics because these virulent organisms have a high potential for prompt tissue invasion. If the patient is not treated, a diffuse spreading cellulitis and systemic illness may develop. On examination, the patient will have fever and the area of the abdominal wound may show a spreading margin of cellulitis notable for erythema or other inappropriate discoloration of the skin. Infection with *Clostridium perfringens* will be associated with a watery discharge and crepitation. The skin also has a characteristic bronze appearance. The streptococcus generates a spreading infection by elaborating extracellular toxins such as hemolysin, hyaluronidase, streptokinase, streptolysin, and plasminogen-activating enzyme. The clostridial organisms elaborate collagenase, proteinase, hyaluronidase, and lecithinase.

Both the hemolytic streptococci and clostridia are highly sensitive to penicillin, and this antibiotic is recommended unless the patient is allergic to it. Of greater importance than the antibiotic is prompt débridement of all nonviable tissue. Failure to perform débridement will doom the patient to continued infection because the toxins advance ahead of the organisms and render the tissue ischemic, thereby preventing good tissue levels of antibiotic. If these infections are uncontrolled, bacteremia, necrotizing fasciitis, or myonecrosis may develop. Complications

of those severe infections include adult respiratory distress syndrome (ARDS), disseminated intravascular coagulation, or multisystem organ failure. When this type of early-onset cellulitis is noted, the infecting organism may be identified by aspirating material from the advancing margin of cellulitis and using the aspirate to perform a Gram's stain. The presence of gram-positive cocci suggests streptococci, and gram-positive rods indicate clostridia.

Therapy for streptococcal cellulitis can be initiated with aqueous penicillin in doses of 2 to 5 million units every 6 hours administered intravenously (IV). For patients who are allergic to penicillin, appropriate alternative antibiotics are vancomycin or erythromycin for streptococcal infections. For suspected clostridial infections, penicillin is the agent of choice, but additional coverage with clindamycin is recommended for other organisms usually present. For specific doses and alternative regimens, see "Necrotizing Wound Infections" later in this chapter.

Late-Presenting Wound Infections

Late-onset infections usually do not present until postoperative days 4 to 7. Fever may develop acutely, or it may have been of low grade and become a high spiking temperature later. The wound usually shows some degree of erythema and induration. Tenderness is variable and depends on the degree of associated cellulitis or pressure within the subcutaneous abscess. If the infection continues untreated, it will frequently drain spontaneously at the skin surface; however, the entire wound needs to be explored to completely evacuate all loculations.

Staphylococcus aureus is recovered from most of these incisions. Additional organisms are commonly cultured from the polymicrobial infections that are typically associated with gynecologic procedures. Most commonly, cultures of the purulent drainage will show *Staphylococcus* species, *Streptococcus* species, *E. coli*, enterococci, *Bacteroides* species, and other anaerobic bacteria. The additional organisms listed are more common when the laparotomy incision involves hysterectomy with vaginal entry, when bowel resection has contaminated the operative field, or when active pelvic inflammatory disease has been encountered in the surgical field. Wound infections in clean cases are frequently unpredictable (see "Predisposing Factors for Infection" earlier in this chapter).

Patients with late-onset infections should improve markedly within the first 12 to 24 hours after drainage. If improvement is documented, further observation and local wound care, as previously described, are all that should be required. If fever or signs of cellulitis persist, antibiotics should then be instituted.

Antibiotics

Even though there may be one predominant organism, these are frequently polymicrobial infections, and, when the vagina or gastrointestinal tract has been entered during the preceding surgery, both anaerobic and aerobic coverage should be used empirically when antibiotics are initiated. Depending on the degree of infection and nature of the preceding operation, the antibiotics chosen may consist of an aminoglycoside such as gentamicin, with ampicillin, nafcillin, or cefazolin. The preceding combination is not sufficient when anaerobic bacterial contamination is likely. For a sick patient with systemic signs of infection, triple-agent regimens of penicillin (or ampicillin) with gentamicin and either metronidazole or clindamycin is appropriate. For patients who traditionally were treated with gentamicin plus clindamycin, good alternatives include a broad-spectrum cephalosporin, such as cefoxitin, cefotaxime, or cefotetan.

Any patient initiated on cephalosporin coverage or clindamycin plus gentamicin who fails to respond to therapy should be re-evaluated for further need of local débridement or additional sites of infection, such as concomitant pelvic cellulitis or abscess. Upon failing to identify alternative explanations for failure of therapy, additional coverage for enterococcal organisms should be added to the regimen. The patient receiving clindamycin and gentamicin can be covered for enterococcus by adding penicillin to the regimen in a dose of 5 million units every 6 hours.

Necrotizing Wound Infections

Necrotizing wound infections are uncommon but of life-threatening potential; they demand prompt recognition and accurate therapy. These infections do not resolve without surgical intervention. Unfortunately, when many of these infections develop, the patient may no longer be under direct physician surveillance or the local signs may not be prominent early in the course and may be overlooked. These infections may smolder for several days prior to causing sudden onset of systemic symptoms, which then bring the patient to evaluation. Obese patients with diabetes or immunosuppressive disorders may experience a rapidly deteriorating course. These same patients are predisposed to necrotizing infections unrelated to operative incisions. Reports in the literature contain a confusing overlap of clinical syndromes, and multiple names have been given to identical processes. Some named infections do have different etiologies, but recognition and primary treatment in all cases are the same and include the need for aggressive tissue débridement.

Necrotizing infections have often been classified as *clostridial* and *nonclostridial*. This is a simplistic division from a clinical standpoint but useful for understanding etiology. Clostridial organisms are frequently present in cultures from infected wounds when they are not contributing to infection. For this reason, identification of a clostridium from an infection does not necessarily result in a diagnosis of a necrotizing clostridial infection. Furthermore, the true clostridial infections are frequently polymicrobial, with other anaerobic bacteria present.

Nonclostridial necrotizing infections are also generally polymicrobial, with the exception of several rare processes, such as streptococcal gangrene caused by *Streptococcus pyogenes* as a single organism (Giuliano et al, 1977). The clinical problem with the multiple names for the various etiologic organisms is the difficulty distinguishing the polymicrobic synergistic infections from the single-agent process using only the physical exam. The most useful concepts are related to the different tissue compartments that may be involved. The tissue involved from the onset of the infection will explain the varying presentations and associated examination findings. These are discussed next.

Clostridial Infections

CLOSTRIDIAL MYONECROSIS

The classical histotoxic clostridial infection is a clostridial myonecrosis known as "gas gangrene." This infection most commonly occurs after extremity injuries. This process is also seen after abdominal surgery or wounds contaminated by feces. *Clostridium perfringens* is a normal inhabitant of the gastrointestinal tract and frequently the vagina. It may be found in pelvic inflammatory disease and it may contaminate an abdominal incision made during treatment for this condition. The examination findings may be a sweet or "mousy" odor with a thin discharge. Bubbles may be seen in the incision or crepitus palpated in the surrounding tissue. The overlying skin becomes edematous and eventually shows erythema before undergoing color changes typical of a bruise, such as green-yellow, becoming bronze over time. The patient may appear quite ill within the first 1 to 2 days after bacterial contamination of the wound. There will be severe wound pain and malaise, and a coagulopathy will be seen in many cases. Histologically, white blood cells (WBCs) are infrequent, and there is minimal purulence (MacClennan, 1962). The skin overlying the muscle necrosis may eventually show hemorrhagic bullae; Gram's stain of this fluid may show gram-positive rods. Plain films showing gas in muscle compartments are diagnostic of anaerobic infection, whereas the presence of gas in the subcutaneous tissues may be a late finding, as are the crepitus and palpable edema.

CLOSTRIDIAL CELLULITIS

This infection is a different entity from clostridial myonecrosis. It has a slightly different presentation. The pathogenesis of a clostridial necrotizing infection is explained by the action of multiple exotoxins of clostridia. These exotoxins cause liquefaction of tissues and systemic toxicity eventuating in cardiovascular collapse. The systemic toxins explain why the patient may be in extremis before there are significant surface signs of the progressive infection present in the deep tissue. Characteristically, the infected tissue shows little inflammatory response with few WBCs, whereas gram-positive rods are present. Clostridial cellulitis generally presents within several days after a wound. A foul-smelling or sweet odor will be noted from the thin, serous discharge that may be present initially. The absence of inflammatory cells prevents the purulent discharge from forming. These wounds are characterized by severe pain. When superficial infection is primary, skin vesicles and crepitus may be seen prior to severe systemic signs. If the wound is suspicious but no crepitus is felt, soft tissue radiographs may confirm the presence of soft tissue gas.

The *Clostridium* species responsible most commonly is *C. perfringens*; however, many cases of *C. novye*, *C. histolyticum*, and *C. septicum* also occur. Other bacteria are usually also recovered by careful culture (MacClennan, 1962; Caplan and Kluge, 1976; Skiles et al, 1978).

ANTIBIOTIC CHOICES

Penicillin is the antibiotic of choice. Metronidazole, clindamycin, and chloramphenicol are also effective. For suspected clostridial infections, aqueous penicillin in doses of 5 million units every 6 hours should be used as the primary antibiotic therapy, but additional coverage should also be given for other organisms usually present as secondary pathogens. Clindamycin with gentamicin is an appropriate addition to the penicillin as long as there is no significant renal insult or myoglobinuria to complicate the aminoglycoside use. Imipenem-cilastatin alone in doses of 500 mg IV every 6 hours is also a good initial choice. Imipenem-cilastatin may be especially helpful in the patient with poor renal reserve if it can avoid the need for the aminoglycoside, but the doses may need to be adjusted. A multiagent regimen such as cefoxitin and metronidazole is also appropriate. For the patient allergic to penicillin, chloramphenicol 1 g IV, then 500 mg IV every 6 hours, is acceptable for clostridial infection.

Nonclostridial Infections (Necrotizing Fasciitis)

"Necrotizing fasciitis" is the most common term applied to nonclostridial necrotizing infections of the subcutaneous tissues. These nonclostridial infections are also life threatening and necessitate similar therapy. The term refers to the superficial fascia and subcutaneous tissue between the skin and deep muscular fascia; the latter may be secondarily involved. Other names used for this infection include "gramnegative gangrene," "nonclostridial gas gangrene," "Meleney's gangrene," "synergistic progressive bacterial gangrene," "Necrotizing erysipelas," and, when occurring on the perineum or vulva, "Fournier's gangrene." This process may also progress to involve the muscle below the deep muscular fascia. Distinguishing the multiple subcategories of necrotizing infections is of minimal importance compared to distinguishing a necrotizing from a non-necrotizing infection. The necrotizing infection must be débrided vigorously, because this is the primary treatment. By comparison, drainage may suffice for a nonnecrotizing infection.

A series of 28 cases of necrotizing fasciitis treated between 1969 and 1981 were reported by Rouse et al (1982). At the time of initial examination, all patients showed edema and "cellulitis"; however, only 12 were noted to have crepitus, 8 to have temperature above 38.3°C, 7 to have altered sensorium, and 3 to have blood pressure less than 80 mm Hg. Fifteen patients already had cutaneous gangrene at first examination, and 18 had either leukopenia or leukocytosis. In this series, nine were postoperative infections and were first noted 3 to 14 days after the initial intra-abdominal procedure. Of the 28 patients, 73% died. Eight-five per cent of the patients with diabetes and 88% of the patients with atherosclerosis died.

DIAGNOSIS

Fisher et al (1979) described the criteria for diagnosis of necrotizing fasciitis. The histologic portion of these criteria were then used by Stamenkovic and Lew (1984) for frozen section biopsy to make an early accurate diagnosis and initiate early intervention. After radical débridement, patients require another examination under anesthesia in 24 to 48 hours to confirm that all necrotic tissue has been completely removed. The large soft tissue defect created may eventually require plastic surgery reconstruction.

Necrotizing fasciitis may present with a rapid course shortly after surgery, or more commonly, several weeks after previous trauma or surgery. The nonclostridial necrotizing infections typically progress in a rapid fashion, although an occasional slowly evolving process has been reported (Wilson, 1952). Necrotizing fasciitis has many clinical similarities to the clostridial infection, such as severe pain out of proportion to local examination findings. Any discharge or exudate present will be of a thin "dishwater" type. Fever and signs of systemic toxicity may not always be present; however, if they are noted, they may be severe in the absence of significant physical findings. If only antibiotic therapy is initiated, infection will progress. Failure to respond to conventional antibiotic therapy and watery drainage from the wound are two of the earliest clues to the necrotizing process for a patient with an indolent course.

When bruising or bullae of the ischemic skin develops, the clinician will recognize the advanced infection. Figures 36–1A and 36–2 show the early skin findings of advanced necrotizing infections and the extent of débridement needed to excise all necrotic tissue. Early in its course, necrotizing fasciitis may look identical to a simple cellulitis. The skin overlying the process has an inordinate amount of edema, and associated crepitus is a common but late finding. This edema extends beyond the areas of erythema or discoloration. As the process progresses, there is a bruised appearance to the skin followed by the formation of bullae. When the skin with this appearance is incised or débrided, there will be no bleeding.

The advancing toxins and later advance of organisms in the tissue planes deep to the skin explain the innocuous appearance at the site early in the process as well as the absence of a sharp demarcation of erythema on the skin. The skin eventually loses its blood supply as a result of thrombosis of the perforating vessels that supply the dermis. The earliest signs are localized pain and edema. The rate of progression from one visible skin change to the next is variable but may be extraordinarily rapid. Large areas of skin may change from a normal appearance to a black necrotic appearance in as short a time as 6 to 8 hours. The associated changes include skin edema, erythema, bullae, ecchymoses, cyanotic or

gray color, crepitus, skin slippage between skin layers on examination, petechiae, black skin, or anesthesia on palpation (Fig. 36–1A). A high degree of suspicion and frequently repeated examinations may be required for a timely diagnosis.

Histologically, necrosis and thrombosis of arteries and veins are present. In addition, the nonclostridial necrotizing infection shows significant inflammatory infiltrate and microabscesses. The evidence of skin necrosis and crepitus should be considered advanced signs of cellulitis and require immediate operative exploration for débridement. If there is any question regarding the finding of crepitus, an x-ray film or CT scan (Rogers et al, 1984) can be more sensitive than physical examination for detecting gas. These x-ray studies may also assist with planning débridement margins because small connecting pathways of necrotic tissue may separate several larger areas from one another.

Other signs indicating the need for urgent surgical exploration of the infection site include systemic signs, such as mental status change, tachypnea, acidosis, and hyperglycemia. Local signs include cyanosis or bronze color; thin, foul drainage; blistering; extensive edema surrounding the erythematous area; and nonresistance of subcutaneous tissue to blunt probing (Fig. 36–1C), as is consistent with a liquefaction-necrosis of tissue (Ahrenholz, 1988).

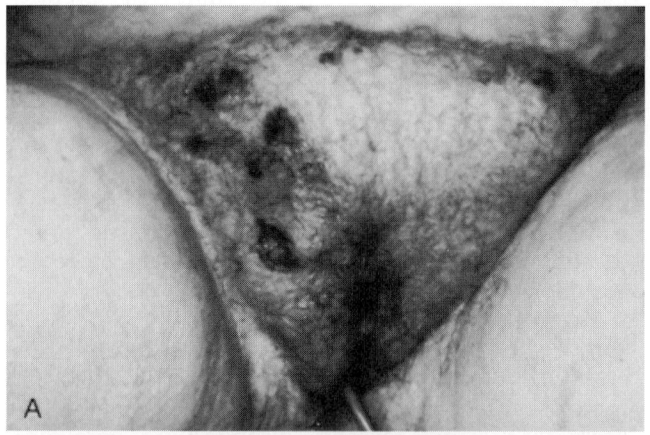
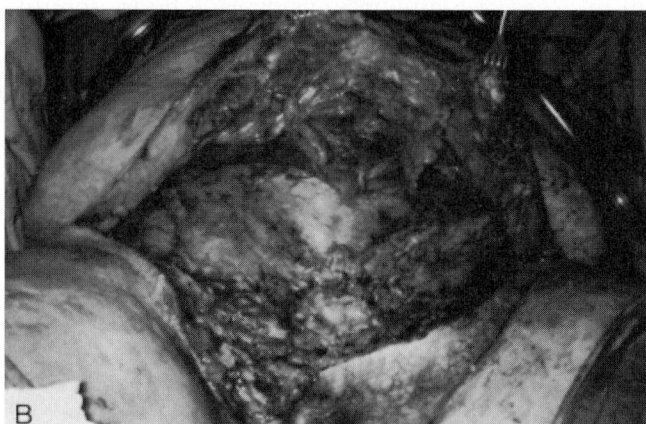
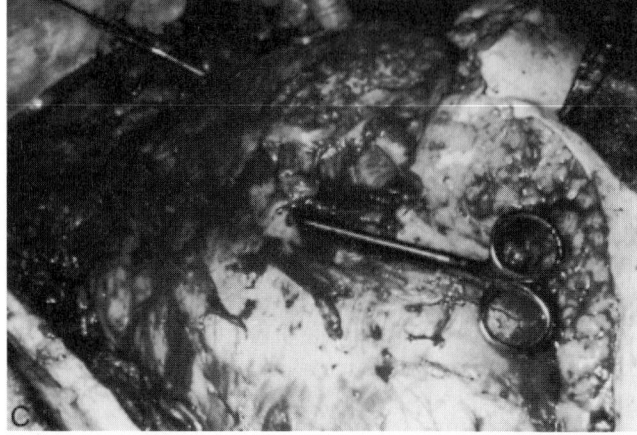

Figure 36–1
Perianal abscess in a 72-year-old obese patient. The abscess has progressed as a necrotizing fasciitis and involves the mons pubis and anterior abdominal wall. A, Note ecchymoses and bullae of the skin on the mons pubis. B, Note subcutaneous involvement at exploration, extending beyond abnormalities seen at the skin surface. Fat on the elevated pannus is discolored. C, Anterior abdominal tissue is débrided to the main abdominal fascia. Note the absence of resistance to the passage of a blunt instrument in necrotic subcutaneous tissue. (A–C, Courtesy of Dr. Richard Howard.)

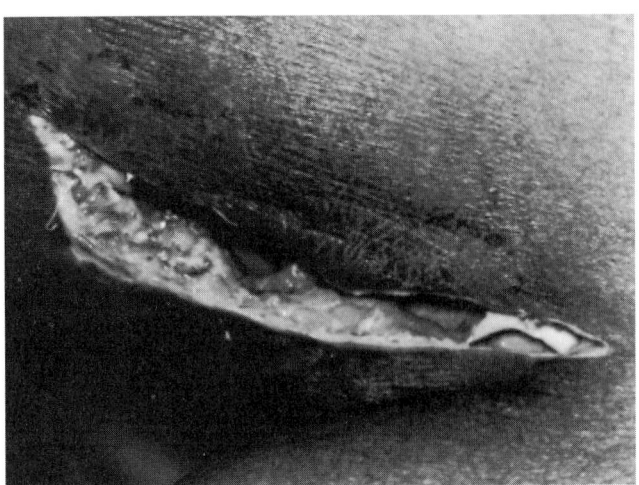

Figure 36–2
The incision shown was used for débridement in a 47-year-old black patient with diabetes. Necrotizing fasciitis of the perineum, vulva, and thigh had developed. Infection had begun as a perianal abscess. Note the skin flaps saved after extensive subcutaneous débridement in an obese thigh. Débridement was performed to the level of the deep fascia, extending to the popliteal fossa. (Courtesy of Dr. Richard Howard.)

PATHOGENS

The organisms typically recovered from nonclostridial necrotizing infections include all of the gram-negative aerobes, gram-positive aerobes, and typical anaerobes of the gastrointestinal tract. These same organisms have been listed previously in this chapter as causes of other wound infections.

Necrotizing fasciitis is a polymicrobial infection of a synergistic nature. Clostridial organisms may also be found, but a nonclostridial nature of the infection is confirmed by the histologic findings of inflammatory cells. Pathogenic organisms and several clinical presentations have been reported (Jones et al, 1979; Kaiser and Cerra, 1981; Pessa and Howard, 1985; Gozal et al, 1986). The nonclostridial gas-forming organisms include E. coli, Klebsiella, Enterobacter, Pseudomonas, anaerobic peptostreptococci, or Bacteroides. The amount of gas varies with the type of organism.

THERAPY

Prior incision wounds are completely opened, and all necrotic tissue is removed, including the superficial fascia and fat below it. Involvement of the fat or skin overlying the superficial fascia is noted grossly by green-black discoloration or histologically by intraoperative review of a biopsy specimen. All involved areas need to be removed, but, if intervention has occurred early enough to find overlying skin that is not yet involved, that skin should be allowed to remain as a flap (Baxter, 1972). The deep fascia should be opened to inspect the underlying muscle and exclude myonecrosis. Remote areas of

abnormal-appearing skin should be incised and the subcutaneous layers inspected or presented for biopsy. Wounds are left open and are packed with saline- or povidone-iodine–soaked gauze.

A caveat in the management of postoperative fasciitis is to be sure not to forget the *possibility of associated intra-abdominal sepsis.* Casali et al (1980) reported that 85% of such patients have associated intra-abdominal infection. Abdominal-pelvic CT scan may be indicated before a first débridement to assist in detecting such an occult process needing surgical attention.

Treatment of necrotizing fasciitis is predicated on early recognition, débridement, and systemic antibiotics to treat any persisting foci of infection. Extent of débridement is determined by the amount of gross necrotic tissue. The destruction of subcutaneous tissue by infection is commonly identified by the easy passage of blunt dissectors, such as cotton swabs, surgical clamps, or the operator's finger, which meets no resistance when probing the tissue. Débridement should occur until all edges bleed normally on incision, including confirmation of muscle that contracts on stimulation and bleeds when cut, if there is any suggestion of deep muscular involvement.

This infection is associated with a high mortality, which varies with the site of involvement as well as the time interval from diagnosis to initiation of therapy (Holland et al, 1975; Caplan and Kluge, 1976). Mortality associated with necrotizing fasciitis averages 39% in collected series (Ahrenholz, 1988) and has changed little over the last 50 years. Associated medical illness and delay in initiating surgical débridement appear to be the factors most predictive of poor outcome (Rouse et al, 1982). It is hoped that better systemic support will increase salvage rates. Recommendations include low-dose heparin to prevent both local tissue thrombosis and deep vein thromboembolism. Hyperalimentation is strongly recommended (Kaiser and Cerra, 1981; Majeski and Alexander, 1983).

To quickly gain control of the infection, systemic antibiotics and topical antibiotics may be useful. The topical agents, such as silver sulfadiazine (Silvadene) or mafenide acetate (Sulfamylon), may control surface infection and promote earlier granulation tissue in the area of débridement. Silver sulfadiazine should be applied every 6 hours, mafenide every 8 hours. Silver sulfadiazine should not be used for patients with sulfa allergies, and mafenide may be better at penetrating wound eschar after burns or prior to débridement.

Antibiotic Choices. The regimen administered must provide coverage of aerobic and anaerobic organisms. Patients with necrotizing fasciitis usually have a life-threatening infection, and combination regimens should therefore be used and administered intravenously. An aminoglycoside with either metronidazole or clindamycin added to either ampicillin or penicillin is recommended. For the patient with minimal systemic symptoms, a reasonable alternative is metronidazole with a broad-spectrum cephalosporin such as cefoxitin, ceftriaxone, or ceftazidime. Each of these cephlosporins provides excellent streptococcal, anaerobic, and gram-negative coverage.

If metronidazole is used, a penicillin or cephalosporin must be included to cover streptococci. Imipenem-cilastatin might be used as a single agent for the patient who is not toxic from infection and who has undergone adequate débridement. Imipenem is bactericidal and has excellent coverage of streptococcal, aerobic gram-negative, and most anaerobic organisms except rare strains of *Bacteroides fragilis*. Most clostridia are very sensitive to imipenem, with the exception of *C. difficile*. Unfortunately, *Pseudomonas aeruginosa*, coagulase-negative staphylococci, methicillin-resistant staphylococci, and *Enterococcus faecium* are resistant. Dosing for imipenem-cilastatin is 500 to 1000 mg IV every 6 hours, for the patient with normal renal function.

If an initial tissue aspirate and Gram's stain show predominantly gram-positive rods, penicillin should be included for coverage of clostridia. Other agents effective against clostridia are metronidazole, clindamycin, chloramphenicol, erythromycin, and vancomycin; these should provide excellent alternatives for a patient allergic to penicillin.

Combination antibiotic regimens that are acceptable for treating necrotizing fasciitis in the situation where the patient has a penicillin allergy include clindamycin with gentamicin (or aztreonam); chloramphenicol with either gentamicin or aztreonam; or vancomycin with metronidazole plus either gentamicin or aztreonam. Aztreonam is a monocyclic β-lactam but has a very low cross-reactive allergenicity with penicillins or cephalosporins. Vancomycin can be used despite penicillin allergy; it is bactericidal and provides excellent coverage for all staphylococci and streptococci of groups A, C, and G and most group B isolates. Enterococci are sensitive but require much higher concentration of drug. Most clostridia and microaerophilic and anaerobic streptococci are susceptible, but *Bacteroides* and gram-negative aerobes are not.

Antibiotic Dosing. Doses chosen for this discussion represent a need for high tissue levels in partially ischemic sites in a life-threatening infection. Ampicillin, 2 g IV every 4 to 6 hours, is given for a daily dose of 4 to 12 g. Aqueous penicillin G is given in high doses of 3 to 4 million units IV every 4 hours. Metronidazole should be dosed with a loading dose of 1.0 g, then 500 mg IV every 6 hours. Clindamycin, 900 mg IV, is given every 8 hours. Cefoxitin doses for this infection should be 2 g IV every 4 to 6 hours. Doses for ceftazidime should be 1 to 2 g IV every 8 hours; for ceftriaxone, the recommended dose is 2 g IV every 12 hours. Chloramphenicol is dosed at 50 mg/kg of body weight per day, given in four doses. A typical adult might receive 750 to 1000 mg IV

every 6 hours. Aztreonam, 1 to 2 g IV, is given every 6 hours.

For adults with normal renal function, vancomycin is given at 30 mg/kg/day or 2 g/day IV in two to four divided doses. Serum levels should be checked, especially when vancomycin is given with gentamicin because this situation is associated with higher incidences of nephrotoxicity. Peak serum levels should be 24 to 40 mg/L obtained 1 to 2 hours after infusion. Trough serum levels should be obtained immediately before a scheduled dose. Dose reduction is needed for patients with decreased renal function, because this is the only route of excretion.

Gentamicin is given with a loading dose of 2 mg/kg IV and maintenance doses of 1.0 to 1.7 mg/kg/day IV every 8 hours. Peak and trough serum levels are then checked at 24 to 48 hours after initial dosing, and adjustments are made as needed to avoid toxicity and ensure therapeutic levels. The peak level, obtained 30 minutes after dose infusion, should be 4 to 10 μg/ml and the trough level under 2 μg/ml.

Pharmacist assistance for pharmacokinetic calculation of optimal dosing is now commonly available; if it is not, several generalizations apply. Adjusting the dose affects mainly the peak level, and adjusting the dosing interval affects primarily the trough level. Serum creatinine levels are then monitored one to three times per week when the patient is stable, and trough levels repeated one to two times per week after initial dosing is satisfactory.

PELVIC CELLULITIS AND PELVIC ABSCESS

Cellulitis

The incidence of soft tissue pelvic infections has decreased over the years with the advent of prophylactic antibiotics; however, pelvic cellulitis remains a significant problem in gynecologic surgery. This is not unexpected, as the vagina is a field contaminated by microbes, and traumatized devitalized tissue is present following surgery. Additionally, bleeding at the operative site releases hemoglobin, and hemoglobin inhibits the ability of leukocytes to phagocytose bacteria (Sweet and Gibbs, 1990). Therefore surgical site bleeding predisposes to cellulitis or abscess.

Serious infection incidence rates following hysterectomy vary depending on the surgical method, noting differences between abdominal and vaginal hysterectomy. Pelvic abscess developed after hysterectomy in 4% of vaginal hysterectomy cases and in 0.7% of abdominal hysterectomy cases as reported by Hevron and Llorens (1976). Seventy-three per cent of these abscesses occurred at the vaginal cuff, and the remaining 27% occurred as a delayed abscess in the pelvis. Duff and Park (1980) reviewed the literature on infectious morbidity associated with vaginal hysterectomy. They reported rates of febrile morbidity ranging from 19% to 77% without prophylactic antibiotics and from 0 to 52% with antibiotic prophylaxis. Rates after β-lactam agent prophylaxis were 5% to 15%. They also estimated that pelvic cellulitis was the major infectious complication after vaginal hysterectomy and that, without prophylaxis, a soft tissue pelvic infection would develop in a total of 40% to 50% of patients.

Duff (1982) reported that, in patients undergoing abdominal hysterectomy, pelvic cellulitis developed in 19% of 91 cases during a randomized study of prophylactic antibiotics versus placebo. There were no differences in rates of cellulitis incidence between arms of the study. This rate of almost 20% in a low-risk population confirms that pelvic cellulitis is a frequent postoperative complication. Vaginal cuff abscess developed in 2 of 46 (4%) in the placebo group. Hemsell et al (1983b) reported major infections such as abscess, pelvic cellulitis, and abdominal wound infection in 32% of cases after abdominal hysterectomy in a placebo control arm not receiving prophylactic antibiotics. Febrile morbidity occurred in 40% of patients undergoing abdominal hysterectomy without antibiotic prophylaxis and in 15% of those receiving antibiotics, as reported by Ohm and Galask (1976). For gynecology patients undergoing hysterectomy, Ledger and Child (1973) reported decreases in postoperative fever from a high of 31% after abdominal hysterectomy without prophylaxis to a low of 5% with the use of prophylactic antibiotics.

From these types of studies, we could anticipate a spontaneous infection rate of 25% to 50% for vaginal hysterectomy without prophylaxis, depending on patient age, and a 4% to 8% rate of serious infections if prophylaxis is used. For patients undergoing abdominal hysterectomy, we can anticipate a spontaneous infection rate of 30% to 40% without antibiotic prophylaxis and a rate of 12% to 15% for serious infections with prophylaxis (Taylor and Hansen, 1961; Pratt and Galloway, 1965; Allen et al, 1972; Ledger et al, 1973; Ohm and Galask, 1976; Roberts and Homesley, 1978; Hemsell et al, 1983a, 1983b, 1987). As used here, "serious" infections include pelvic cellulitis , vaginal cuff abscess, pelvic abscess, and wound infections.

Pathogens

Soft tissue pelvic infections are usually caused by pathogens that arise from normal microflora of the vagina and cervix and, therefore, are usually polymicrobial. Although anaerobes are frequently the only organisms isolated, in reality these are generally mixed infections. The organisms most commonly implicated in the development of pelvic cellulitis include gram-negative as well as gram-positive aerobes and anaerobes.

The most common aerobic organisms include streptococci (groups A, B, and D), staphylococci (primarily *S. epidermidis*), *Gardnerella vaginalis*, and gram-negative enterobacteriaceae, including *E. coli*, *Klebsiella*, and *Proteus*. The important anaerobic organisms include peptococci as well as peptostreptococci and bacteroides (Sweet and Gibbs, 1990). It is the *Bacteroides* species that are currently thought to be the most important organisms with respect to the development of pelvic cellulitis and abscesses. In patients with pelvic cellulitis, it is *B. bivius* and *B. disiens* that are believed to play a key role. *Bacteroides fragilis* is occasionally isolated; however, this organism is thought to have a more important role in the development of pelvic abscesses. Additionally, clostridia and fusobacteria are occasionally isolated. Reports concerning the effects of genital malignancies and/or pelvic radiation on the normal flora of the vagina and cervix are inconsistent and contradictory.

Diagnosis

The diagnosis of pelvic cellulitis following surgery is usually straightforward. These patients typically present with fever, leukocytosis, and lower abdominal or pelvic pain. The onset of fever is usually 24 to 72 hours following surgery. Evaluation of these patients should include a careful history and physical examination as well as routine blood work, including cultures from at least two sites.

Therapy

Initiation of empirical antibiotic therapy for pelvic cellulitis is generally recommended for patients with persistent fever and leukocytosis greater than 24 hours following pelvic surgery with no identifiable source of infection. Early therapy is associated with an increased cure rate and a decreased incidence of complications, including abdominal or pelvic abscesses and septic thrombophlebitis. As previously stated, the treatment is empirical and is based on knowledge of the usual organisms involved.

Therapy should be tailored to treat gram-negative Enterobacteriaceae as well as anaerobes, particularly bacteroides. There are many accepted regimens, including combination therapy with an aminoglycoside, a third-generation cephalosporin, or aztreonam in combination with clindamycin or metronidazole. Alternatively, monotherapy is acceptable for patients who do not appear critically ill. The agents most frequently employed in the monotherapy of pelvic cellulitis include a second- or third-generation cephalosporin, such as cefoxitin, cefotetan, or cefotaxime. Additionally, any of the antipseudomonal penicillins or a carbapenem should be adequate. Therapy should be continued until patients remain afebrile for at least 48 hours with resolution of leukocytosis and pain. Failure to improve on antibiotic therapy should prompt a repeat exam and CT scan to exclude a pelvic abscess.

Abscess

True pelvic or abdominal abscesses occur in 0.5% to 4% of patients following major pelvic surgery

(Ledger et al, 1969; Hevron and Llorens, 1976). Patients often present with fever, pain, and a tender palpable mass. Abscesses following pelvic surgery may present days to months following surgery (Ledger, 1980). Typically, the mass is high in the pelvis and, therefore, not readily appreciated at the time of pelvic examination and not amenable to vaginal drainage.

The patient may look relatively well on initial presentation, with only fever and leukocytosis, or, conversely, may be in septic shock. In patients who appear critically ill, Swan-Ganz and/or arterial catheterization may be appropriate, particularly if inotropic agents are employed. Monitoring of vital signs, urine output, and mental status should be routine. If there is any alteration in mental status, hypoxemia should be ruled out and corrected with supplemental oxygen as necessary.

Diagnosis

For patients in whom a fullness is appreciated at the vaginal cuff at the time of initial examination and for patients who fail to respond to conventional therapy for presumed pelvic cellulitis, the diagnosis of a cuff abscess or infected hematoma should be entertained. Cuff abscesses or infected hematomas develop in approximately 2% of patients undergoing abdominal hysterectomy (Hevron and Llorens, 1976). The abscess or hematoma usually presents 48 to 72 hours postoperatively with fever and a fullness in the pelvis, although in many patients the fullness in the pelvis is not appreciated initially and therefore the working diagnosis is pelvic cellulitis. For patients thought to have a cuff abscess or infected hematoma, treatment includes antibiotic therapy, as outlined for patients with pelvic cellulitis, as well as drainage. Drainage is usually well tolerated, consisting of simple exploration of the vaginal cuff area. Once drainage has been facilitated, patients usually respond promptly to antibiotic therapy.

The diagnosis of an abdominal or pelvic abscess requires a high index of suspicion because palpation of a tender mass is not universal, but depends on its location. The diagnosis may be established definitively with either ultrasound or CT scan. A radionucleotide scan (gallium-67– or indium-111–labeled WBC scanning) may be employed in selected patients. This test has largely been replaced by ultrasound and/or CT scan as a result of its high false-positive rate. Ultrasound examination is fast, inexpensive, and not associated with any radiation exposure. However, it is operator dependent, and detail may be obscured by gas. Additionally, ultrasound is difficult in patients with open wounds, ileus, or an ostomy bag. Therefore, CT scan has become the diagnostic method of choice in localizing abdominal as well as pelvic abscesses, because it is the most accurate method (Moir and Robins, 1982). CT scan has an accuracy of greater than 95% in localizing intra-abdominal or pelvic abscesses. The

major drawbacks of CT are that the modality is not portable, requires a relatively cooperative patient, and is expensive.

Therapy

The treatment of intra-abdominal abscesses has become more conservative in the last few years. Initial therapy includes stabilization of the patient and initiation of broad-spectrum antibiotic therapy directed against the organisms most likely to be recovered from the abscess. These include gram-positive aerobes, facultative gram-negative aerobes, Enterobacteriaceae (E. coli, Klebsiella, Proteus, Enterobacter, and Pseudomonas), and gram-positive and gram-negative anaerobes. Combination therapy must include antibiotics effective against all of these organisms, particularly B. fragilis. Accepted combinations generally employ an aminoglycoside or a third-generation cephalosporin in combination with an antianaerobic agent. Monotherapy with such agents as cefoxitin, piperacillin, and imipenem has been reported; except for imipenem, however, results are somewhat discouraging.

After the patient is stabilized and antibiotic therapy is initiated, the mainstay of therapy is drainage of the abscess. Antibiotics serve only as an adjunct to drainage. Antibiotics are likely to be ineffective if used as the sole treatment modality because of their poor penetration into abscess cavities, inactivation in the microenvironment of the abscess, and inactivation of the drug by the high bacterial inoculum.

During the past several years, the drainage of abdominal and pelvic abscesses has changed considerably. *Percutaneous drainage* of abdominal and pelvic abscesses was initially introduced by Gerzof et al in 1979. Since then, this method has been refined significantly and is now recognized as the treatment of choice for most abdominal as well as pelvic abscesses. *Open surgical drainage* is generally reserved for patients with ruptured abscesses that are anatomically inaccessible for a safe percutaneous approach or for patients with abscesses that have not resolved after percutaneous drainage (Brolin et al, 1991). As radiologists have gained experience with percutaneous drainage, indications for its use have been greatly liberalized.

This liberalization has resulted in lower success rates and higher morbidity and mortality rates than were initially reported. In the mid-1980s, Brolin's earlier work had noted a success rate of 90% for percutaneous drainage of abdominal abscesses and a mortality of 0 in the first 24 patients treated. In a follow-up study reported in 1991, the success rate was only 76% and the mortality rate was 16%. This is in line with mortality rates reported in other series of abdominal abscesses treated by percutaneous drainage. Additionally, the 10% to 15% mortality rate associated with percutaneous drainage of abdominal as well as pelvic abscesses is similar to that reported in some series of abscesses treated by open laparotomy (Olak et al, 1986; Deveney et al, 1988). The decrease in the success rate for percutaneous drainage is largely attributed to its use in patients with multiloculated abscesses, interloop abscesses, intrahepatic abscesses, and abscesses associated with enteric fistulas. If percutaneous drainage procedures are limited to those with unilocular abscesses with no enteric communications, the success rate is 85% to 96% (Brolin et al, 1991). The complication rate associated with percutaneous drainage of abdominal as well as pelvic abscesses is approximately 15%. The major complication is sepsis, with hemorrhage occurring in fewer than 5% of patients.

Failure to demonstrate resolution of fever and leukocytosis within 4 days of percutaneous drainage generally portends a poor prognosis for percutaneous drainage (Brolin et al, 1991). Brolin and associates recommend that these patients be reassessed and perhaps be treated with open laparotomy. Criteria for removal of the catheter includes complete resolution of sepsis, minimal drainage from the catheter, and radiographic evidence of resolution of the abscess. Exploratory laparotomy is indicated in all patients in whom the diagnosis is not firm, in all patients suspected of having rupture of the abscess, and in all patients who fail to respond to percutaneous drainage.

NONOPERATIVE SITE INFECTIONS

Clostridium Difficile Colitis

Several distinct diarrhea syndromes have been recognized in association with the use of antibiotics. Multiple species of bacteria have been identified as the causative agents of antibiotic-associated diarrhea syndromes. The most common bacteria involved include S. aureus, E. coli, Salmonella, C. perfringens, and C. difficile. These bacteria achieve a large overgrowth advantage in the antibiotic setting. This overgrowth is associated with a toxin production that in turn injures colonic mucosa. The longer the exposure to antibiotics, the greater the likelihood of developing diarrhea. Approximately 20% to 30% of patients with antibiotic-associated diarrhea have a colitis caused by enterotoxic C. difficile (Bartlett et al, 1980).

Clostridium difficile is of particular importance in surgical patients because of frequent exposure to antibiotics and use of bowel preparation before surgery. Clostridium difficile infection varies in severity from mild diarrhea alone, to severe colitis with systemic symptoms but without pseudomembranes, to severe colitis with pseudomembranes that is generally associated with the most severe signs of toxicity. The most severe forms can also develop toxic megacolon and perforation with peritonitis. Severe pseudomembranous colitis is a potentially lethal disease process. Prior to availability of effective therapy, mortality rates as high as 8% were reported (Tedesco, 1977; Swartzberg et al, 1977). Mortality rises dramatically

if toxic megacolon or perforation occurs, with reported mortality rates of 35% and 50%, respectively (Morris et al, 1990).

Clostridium difficile colitis is thought to occur when antibiotics alter the normal bowel flora, leading to overgrowth of C. difficile in those patients who are carriers of this toxigenic strain. This colitis may occur after either oral or parenteral use of antibiotics and has occurred after use of all antibiotics, including metronidazole and vancomycin, which constitute the most effective therapy. The highest rate of occurrence per dose administered is seen after exposure to clindamycin; however, most cases occur with antibiotics that are more commonly used, such as ampicillin, or cefazolin.

Incidence

Clostridium difficile diarrhea occurred in 2% of the surgery patients undergoing a variety of procedures as recorded in the prospective study by McCarter et al (1996). This accounted for one third of the 6% incidence of diarrhea. These patients were admitted to vascular, trauma, and general surgery services. The diarrhea was directly responsible for extending the length of the hospital stay in 25% of the patients. The extra length of stay averaged 4 additional days. A preoperative bowel preparation was associated with an increased risk of both diarrhea and C. difficile colitis. Pseudomenbraneous colitis is more likely to occur after exposure to oral antibiotics than after parenteral antibiotics. Some cases occur without antibiotic exposure and are usually associated with cancer, intestinal obstruction, or intestinal ischemia.

The majority of hospital patients colonized with C. difficile are asymptomatic. Approximately 25% of adults recently treated with antibiotics are colonized with C. difficile. By comparison, healthy adults carry asymptomatic C. difficile in fewer than 1% of the population. Hospitalized patients are quickly colonized by C. difficile because of environmental contamination with C. difficile spores. Nosocomial outbreaks of C. difficile colitis are reported from nursing homes and hospitals. A 21% incidence of colonization with C. difficile was reported by McFarland et al (1989) in a group of hospitalized patients. Subsequent exposure to antibiotics may allow the patient to quickly become symptomatic. These epidemiologic findings constitute the basis for recommending isolation and general hygiene with infection control measures for any patient diagnosed with C. difficile colitis. The asymptomatic carrier state is not as easily eradicated with antibiotic therapy as is the infected colitis syndrome. This is apparently due to spore formation.

Pathogenesis

Clostridium difficile colitis is well described by Kelly et al (1994). Colonization by C. difficile occurs by the oral-fecal route. Spores are ingested from the environment and survive the gastric acid exposure to then return to the vegetative state in the colon. After overgrowth in the colon, the pathogenic strains of *C. difficile* produce two toxins that cause colonic mucosal injury and diarrhea: toxin A, an enterotoxin, and toxin B, a cytotoxin. A third toxin stimulates gut motility, causing diarrhea (Justus et al, 1982). The result of exposure to these toxins includes epithelial necrosis and a prominent exudate over the resulting epithelial ulcer. In the severe form with large ulcers, the overlying pseudomembrane is composed of cellular debris, leukocytes, and mucin. When pseudomembranes are present, these can be visualized with colonoscopy and give rise to the term pseudomembraneous colitis (PMC). The rectum is involved for 77% of patients who develop pseudomembranes. Pseudomembranes may be confined to the ascending colon and cecum (Tedesco et al, 1982). Actual invasion of bacteria into the bowel wall is not a typical feature of the disease, and is not likely except in neutropenic patients with severe *C. difficile* colitis. Toxin-produced damage creates the clinical syndrome.

Clinical Course

Clostridium difficile colitis typically causes watery diarrhea and a cramping type of abdominal pain. Symptoms commonly develop 4 to 7 days after beginning antibiotic therapy. A delayed onset may occur in up to one third of patients, with initial symptoms up to 8 weeks after exposure to antibiotics. Exposure to a single dose of antibiotics may be the causative event, such as is commonly used for surgical prophylaxis. In addition to diarrhea, a low-grade fever may be present and a modest leukocytosis of 15,000 to 20,000 cells/mm^3. Stool samples evaluated for leukocytes are frequently positive. Some patients may also have guaiac-positive stools. In mild cases systemic symptoms will not be found, and the physical exam may be normal or show a slight tenderness in the lower abdomen.

With severe colitis, a profuse diarrhea may develop associated with severe abdominal pain and an ileus creating abdominal distention. Concomitant systemic symptoms include fever, nausea, and evidence of dehydration. As severe colitis progresses to PMC, abdominal tenderness and diarrhea as well as systemic toxicity become even more prominent. With fulminant colitis, evidence of an acute abdomen will be found on exam and radiologic evaluation may show a toxic megacolon. Paradoxically, the diarrhea may cease and an ileus develop as the disease status worsens. In this setting, perforation and peritonitis are possible and evidence of free air within the abdomen may be found.

Clostridium difficile colitis may present as an acute abdomen. Findings may include abdominal distention resulting from dilated small bowel, colon, or both. Other findings typically include abdominal tenderness and pain, fever, and leukocytosis. The differential diagnosis includes ischemic bowel, diverticular abscess, small bowel ileus, colonic pseudo-obstruction, or volvulus. The presentation of *C. difficile* as an acute abdomen is not as rare as previously thought, occurring in a reported 7% of cases (Triadafilopoulos and Hallstone, 1991). Immediate colonoscopy was used in that study to confirm the diagnosis and decompress the colon during the procedure, thereby avoiding surgery. Two thirds of these patients had rectal sparing. The most unusual aspect of this presentation is that there is no diarrhea. These patients were successfully treated with intravenous metronidazole because of severe ileus, and several were given vancomycin through a nasogastric tube simultaneously with the intravenous metronidazole.

Diagnostic Evaluation

Finding *C. difficile* toxin in stool samples from patients with diarrhea remains the most useful and commonly performed laboratory study for the diagnosis of *C. difficile* colitis. Immunoassays detect the *C. difficile* antigens or the toxins with rapidly available results. Several enzyme immunoassays are available that can detect toxin A or toxin B with sensitivity reaching 70% to 90% and specificity as high as 75% to 100%, but the negative predictive value is 98% to 99%. A more sensitive test is a stool cytotoxin test, done as a tissue culture, but it is expensive and requires overnight testing. A latex agglutination test yields too many false-negative and false-positive results and has therefore fallen out of favor for laboratory testing. Use of stool cultures to identify *C. difficile* organisms is also not recommended because of false-positive results in 20% of samples related to identification of nontoxigenic strains. Stool cultures are only interpretable when used in combination with toxin assays. Stool culture also requires 2 or 3 days to obtain a report, and that is too slow to help most patients. Modern laboratory testing using enzyme immunoassays can provide results within several hours.

Consideration should be made for proceeding to direct inspection of the colon using sigmoidoscopy or colonoscopy in a patient with diarrhea and repeatedly negative tests for toxin in stool samples. These procedures for diagnosing *C. difficile* colitis are more likely to identify pseudomembranes when severe diarrhea syndromes are present. When stool assays are negative for toxin and patients remain seriously ill, the possibility of other causes of diarrhea should be considered, such as ulcerative colitis or diarrhea caused by other enteric pathogens. Finding the pseudomembranes can direct proper therapy for *C. difficile* in these cases, because the finding of pseudomembranes is pathognomonic for *C. difficile* colitis.

The pseudomembranes appear as yellow plaques varying from 2 to 10 mm in diameter with either normal or slightly erythematous surrounding mucosa. The majority of the disease will be found in the distal colon in the rectum and sigmoid. In a minority of cases the colitis will be confined to the proximal colon and only a full colonoscopy will identify the process (Kelly et al, 1994). It is recommended that sigmoidoscopy or colonoscopy not be performed in the presence of fulminant colitis out of fear of creating perforation. A minimal proctoscopy may be possible, and, if evidence of pseudomembranes is found in the distal colon, then the procedure can be diagnostic.

The indications for endoscopy to assist in evaluation of antibiotic-associated diarrhea are reviewed by Bartlett (1992), and include urgent need to confirm suspected PMC in the setting of an acute abdomen, or the failure of medical management.

CT scan findings can identify thick edematous colon wall areas but are nonspecific. CT scan is, however, a valuable tool for excluding other dangerous causes of the acute abdomen (Fishman et al, 1991). Air-contrast barium enema is best avoided if C. difficile colitis is suspected because it can markedly aggravate the severity of the colitis and acute symptoms. Ultrasound may be more useful for diagnosing colitis because it can show the edema in the mucosa and the specific pattern associated with the colitis can be seen if gas from the ileus does not obscure the colon. Ultrasound can be completed as a bedside study, unlike CT scanning. Ultrasound, CT scanning, and endoscopy are occasionally crucial to diagnosis because C. difficile colitis does occur in patients who test negative for C. difficile toxin by assay techniques.

Treatment

Discontinuation of the contributing antibiotic is the foundation of therapy. In many cases of mild colitis the diarrhea syndrome will resolve without any therapy beyond discontinuation of the antibiotic that initiated the syndrome. Supportive measures to treat dehydration may be needed. Any attempt to slow diarrhea should be discouraged so that elimination of toxin can be accomplished. If colitis is severe or persistent after antibiotic discontinuation, then specific therapy should be aimed at eradicating C. difficile. Antibiotic treatment directed against C. difficile is effective, with response rates of 95% to 100%. Vancomycin and metronidazole are the agents with greatest efficacy in treating C. difficile infection. Oral metronidazole in doses of 200 to 250 mg four times daily or vancomycin in doses of 125 to 500 mg orally four times daily are used. Vancomycin given IV for this condition has many recorded failures. Resolution of diarrhea usually occurs within 3 to 5 days. Ninety-five per cent of patients will be cured by a 10-day course of therapy.

Metronidazole has become the preferred first-line therapy because of an extreme price advantage when compared to oral vancomycin. Metronidazole is readily absorbed from the intestinal tract, but adequate intraluminal concentrations in the colon are maintained as a result of enterohepatic recirculation and exudation from the inflamed colonic mucosa.

For this reason intravenous metronidazole is also effective therapy.

Oral vancomycin has equal activity compared to metronidazole for treating C. difficile colitis. Vancomycin is not absorbed from the gastrointestinal tract, nor is it metabolized and excreted into the stool. For this reason oral vancomycin works well for treating C. difficile colitis, but intravenous vancomycin will not be adequate therapy.

Bacitracin is also active against C. difficile and, like vancomycin, is not well absorbed from the gastrointestinal tract. The response rate to bacitracin is similar to that of metronidazole, but the cost is similar to oral vancomycin and it tastes bad, and therefore has no real advantage.

Ten to 20% of patients initially treated for C. difficile colitis will relapse after initial therapy. Relapse occurs within 1 to 3 weeks after termination of therapy. Re-treatment even with the same antibiotic therapy will frequently be successful. It is hard to distinguish antibiotic-resistant spores from re-colonization and re-infection when identifying the etiology of apparent relapse. Development of antibiotic resistance under therapy is thought not to be the usual cause of relapse (Kelly et al, 1994). Vancomycin is not recommended as the first-line therapy for most cases of C. difficile diarrhea because of the potential for promoting the development of vancomycin-resistant E. faecium.

Symptomatic relief without antibiotic therapy can sometimes be provided with the use of cholestyramine, but recent evaluations have not shown as much benefit as did earlier reports (Ariuno et al, 1990). These medications bind the toxin but cannot be used concomitant with the specific antibiotic therapy because they bind the antibiotic as well and decrease the effectiveness of specific antibiotic therapy (Taylor and Bartlett, 1980). Cholestyramine has been advocated for use following antibiotic therapy and in patients who have had recurrent relapses of C. difficile diarrhea in hopes of binding any minimal toxin and avoiding further recurrences of colon injury that would precipitate a full-blown event (Fekety et al, 1984).

Surgical intervention is indicated if medical management has failed. Colon resection with diversion is recommended if toxic megacolon or perforation is found (Morris et al, 1990). Mortality is elevated if diversion is not performed at the time of resection.

Chemotherapy-Induced C. difficile Colitis

Chemotherapy, including several regimens used for treating ovarian cancer, has been associated with causing episodes of C. difficile diarrhea (Cudmore et al, 1982). Some patients have been treated and had relapses caused by repeat courses of chemotherapy without any re-exposure to possible offending antibiotics (Satin et al, 1989). Again, these patients may benefit from prophylactic cholestyramine or prophylactic oral metronidazole, but these are of unproven benefit. Most patients developing chemotherapy-related *C. difficile* infection have been treated with multiple chemotherapeutic agents. Methotrexate, Adriamycin, cyclophosphamide, and fluorouracil are the most commonly associated with this diarrhea. These agents are known to have significant gastrointestinal mucosal toxicity and probably disrupt the resistance barriers and the fecal bacterial balance simultaneously (Anand and Glatt, 1993). Finding blood in diarrheal stools of patients who develop diarrhea on chemotherapy should heighten the suspicion of *C. difficile* diarrhea, as reported by Kamthan et al (1992).

Neutropenic Enterocolitis

Neutropenic enterocolitis is discussed briefly because of similarities to *C. difficile* colitis in its clinical presentation and its presence in cancer patients treated with chemotherapy. A frequently associated chemotherapy agent is cytarabine. Many other chemotherapeutic agents have also caused this syndrome. This syndrome is a full-thickness necrosis of the intestine affecting primarily the right colon.

It is understood that a disruption in the bowel epithelium occurs as a result of chemotherapy. Invasion by colonic bacteria occurs secondarily and is not contained in these neutropenic patients. Presenting signs include abdominal pain, diarrhea, fever, and nausea and vomiting. Plain films of the abdomen may show loss of haustral markings in a dilated and fluid-filled cecum. Examination findings have shown rebound tenderness in 69% of patients and abdominal distention in 62% (Exelby et al, 1975). These patients may present with fever, right lower quadrant pain, and diarrhea in association with neutropenia. Pain is not present in every case; however, vomiting and bloody stools were found in approximately one third of cases.

Neutropenia has usually been present for a period of greater than 7 days prior to the onset of enterocolitis. Gram-negative bacteremia is often seen in association. Histologic studies of the bowel wall show invasion by multiple gram-negative and gram-positive bacterial species as well as yeast. The disease primarily involves the cecum, causing hemorrhage, edema, and a fibrinous exudate on the mucosa. These patients are found to be without evidence of *C. difficile* toxin, in the stool. In fulminant cases of diarrhea without *C. difficile* toxin, the possible diagnosis of neutropenic enterocolitis should be entertained and plans for surgical intervention considered, because it will usually be required. Progression to peritonitis and bowel perforation or septic shock may quickly ensue. *Clostridium septicum* is now considered to be the primary pathogen in this disease. (Scully et al, 1997). Malignant involvement of the bowel wall is not a common part of the histologic findings on resection of the colon. This disease is more commonly associated with the treatment of leukemias than it is with solid tumors; however, this may be dependent more on the agents used for treatment than the underlying type of malignancy.

Treatment of these patients requires intensive support because of the septic response. Broad-spectrum antibiotics are appropriate, and surgery must be undertaken for patients with continued intestinal bleeding or evidence of free intraperitoneal perforation. Clinical deterioration alone would also merit exploration. These issues have been reviewed by Ettinghausen (1993) and by Moir et al, (1986). Resection of the severely involved bowel has been advocated, although selective management may allow for exploration to exclude necrotic bowel or free perforation and re-closure without resection in some cases that show no perforation or necrosis at laparotomy. If signs of peritonitis develop, the patient should be explored and all necrotic bowel resected. Surgical management usually includes right hemicolectomy or total colectomy. If a subtotal colectomy is done, then diverting ileostomy rather than an anastomosis is prudent in these toxic patients. Patients without peritonitis who respond to the gastrointestinal rest often experience resolution of this process concomitant with the resolution of the neutropenia. These patients have a high mortality rate because of the underlying disease and surgical complications such as wound infection, sepsis, disseminated intravascular coagulation, and multisystem organ failure.

Neutropenic enterocolitis is uncommon compared to *C. difficile* colitis; however, it is important in the differential diagnosis of severe diarrhea syndromes associated with systemic illness and is interesting from the etiologic standpoint of being another clostridial invasive infection. As newer chemotherapeutic agents are evaluated clinically, those with associated gastrointestinal mucosal toxicity may trigger more episodes of this disease in patients with solid tumors than has historically been the case. Patients may have repeat episodes with subsequent courses of chemotherapy.

Postoperative Pneumonia

Pneumonia is the number one cause of death resulting from infection in the United States. Pneumonia is the second most common nosocomial infection. Pneumonia that develops after surgery during the postoperative hospital stay differs in many aspects from a community-acquired pneumonia. The physiologic insults causing or predisposing to the development of pneumonia in these two patient groups are different also. These differences are significant enough that nosocomial pneumonias require markedly different therapy from that required to treat community-acquired pneumonias. A single infecting organism is the causative pathogen in most cases of community-acquired pneumonia. The postoperative pneumonia is often polymicrobic, and usually does not have a specific causative organism identified.

An accurate diagnosis of an infectious pneumonia is also harder to make in the postoperative setting. The difficulty in confirming this diagnosis lies in the concomitant diseases causing noninfectious pulmonary infiltrates, or fever with respiratory symptoms. Atypical responses to drugs can also mimic a pneumonia. Nosocomial pneumonia may even be overlooked because common clinical findings may be absent. Instead of presenting with a group of signs, such as cough, a new infiltrate on chest radiograph, new fever, sputum change, and leukocytosis, the patient may exhibit only one of the above, or have all signs be very subtle or intermittent. Even when the common signs are present, they may be due to several other causes and pneumonia may not exist. Careful review of clinical experience suggests that underdiagnosis may be more common than overdiagnosis for patients not on a ventilator. Overdiagnosis may be more common for suspected ventilator-associated pneumonias.

Nosocomial pneumonia is associated with mortality rates of 28% to 37% (Wenzel, 1989). The mortality may reach 60% to 80% when there is associated bacteremia, empyema, or infection by highly virulent organisms such as *P. aeruginosa*. Pneumonia ranks third among the most common causes of nosocomial infections for surgical patients, exceeded only by wound infection and urinary tract infection. The surgeries most often complicated by pneumonia are those involving thoracic or upper abdominal incisions. Postoperative respiratory failure requiring mechanical ventilation is another predisposing factor. Elderly patients have higher rates of nosocomial pneumonia, rising from a rate of 0.5 to a rate of 1.5 cases per 100 patients under age 35 or over age 65, respectively (Haley et al, 1981a). Postoperative pneumonia continues to be a major source of morbidity and mortality on surgical services. The mortality for intensive care unit (ICU) patients who develop pneumonia is nearly 50%, in contrast to ICU patients without pneumonia, whose mortality is roughly 5%. Additionally, the mortality rate for patients with ARDS who develop an infectious pneumonia is in excess of 70%.

Risk Factors

The most common route of infection for pathogens causing a postoperative pneumonia is through aspiration of secretions from the oropharynx or nasopharynx. Any situation predisposing to aspirations of even small amounts of these pharyngeal secretions will markedly increase the risk of pneumonia. An elaborate defense mechanism normally protects the pulmonary system from infection. This defense system includes a mechanical barrier to aspiration at the glottis, a powerful mucociliary transport system to propel contaminants up the bronchial tree, secreted immunoglobulin A antibodies, and ubiquitous

Table 36–4. PULMONARY RISK FACTORS FOR POSTOPERATIVE PNEUMONIA

Chronic obstructive pulmonary disease
Asthma
Productive cough (preoperatively)
Cigarette smoking
Prolonged mechanical ventilation (postoperatively)

macrophages in the alveoli. The protective benefit of a strong cough is needed as a backup mechanism for rapid elimination of any excess mucus or trapped waste that has overwhelmed the mucociliary elevator.

Pulmonary risk factors for postoperative pneumonia are listed in Table 36–4. The underlying problem shared by patients with these risk factors is difficulty expectorating minimal aspiration events. For patients with asthma or COPD there is obstruction to air flow. Tobacco users generate increased amounts of mucus after exposure to general anesthetics, and have a depressed mucociliary function. A productive cough demonstrates an already overwhelmed primary defense system that requires forceful coughing to clear the excess waste. An endotracheal tube prevents coughing and predisposes to a constant low-grade aspiration of oral-pharyngeal bacteria.

Nonpulmonary risk factors for postoperative pneumonia are noted in Table 36–5. Histamine blockers are used to prevent gastric stress ulcers. These drugs change the gastric pH to a favorable environment for growth of pharyngeal bacteria. The normal gastric contents are free of gram-negative bacteria because of the acidic pH. Histamine$_2$ blockers predispose to developing a reservoir of bacteria in the stomach by raising the pH. Their use is associated with prompt colonization of the stomach by organisms from the oropharynx. The trachea then becomes colonized by these same organisms because of reflux and aspiration of gastric contents (duMoulin et al, 1982). A graphic demonstration of these events was reported by Torres et al (1992) in a study using a radioisotope tracer. The tracer was placed in the stomach, and then shown to rapidly be transferred to the lungs in a short (6-hour) time span for patients with endotracheal or nasogastric tubes.

There is a normal background rate of aspiration of gastric fluid in normal individuals. This aspiration

Table 36–5. NONPULMONARY RISK FACTORS FOR POSTOPERATIVE PNEUMONIA

Duration of surgery	Obesity
Location of incision	Sinusitis
Nasogastric intubation	Narcotics
Prior antibiotic use	ASA ≥ II
Enteral feeding tubes	Age over 65
CNS depression (drugs)	Malnutrition
Elevated gastric pH (H$_2$ blockers)	

Abbreviations: ASA, American Society of Anesthesiologists classification; CNS, central nervous system; H$_2$, histamine$_2$.

occurs mostly when sleeping. These small aspiration events are usually asymptomatic in healthy individuals. The presence of a nasogastric tube increases gastroesophageal reflux and aspiration of gastric contents. Incision pain contributes to pneumonia because normal respiratory tidal volumes and cough are reflexively inhibited so as to avoid pain. This predisposes to atelectasis and mucus plugging, which lead to bacterial overgrowth and pneumonia. A greater amount of diaphragmatic dysfunction, impaired cough, and pain are noted with thoracic or upper abdominal incisions, thereby increasing pneumonia risks with these incisions (Pierce and Robertson, 1977; Garibaldi et al, 1981). Malnourished patients have decreased respiratory muscle strength, stamina, and macrophage function. Pain medications and anesthetic agents depress the cough reflex and tidal volumes, thereby promoting atelectasis and prohibiting the clearance of the upper respiratory tree. For all the reasons cited, postoperative critically ill patients are three to four times more likely to develop nosocomial pneumonias than are unoperated critically ill patients.

Measures to decrease the incidence of postoperative pulmonary complications should be employed in all patients, and include incentive spirometry, early ambulation, and positioning the patient in a head-up or modified semi-Fowler position. Adequate pain control is important to the extent that it permits the patient to make deep breathing efforts and better coughs, but narcotic medications have the side effect of sedation and respiratory depression that can depress cough and large sighing breaths, and so the therapeutic window is narrow. Pain control using regional anesthesia is a good alternative if sedation is thereby avoided.

Pathogens

The oropharynx of a healthy person is predominantly colonized by anaerobes and gram-positive organisms. By contrast, ill patients quickly become colonized by gram-negative organisms on the pharyngeal mucosa. This change appears to be due to stress-induced changes of surface site binding and bacterial adherence factors that favor adherence of gram-negative bacilli. Bacteria from the hospital environment quickly colonize respiratory passages after admission. On the third to fourth day of hospitalization, healthy patients are colonized by many nosocomial pathogens. Pathogens that most commonly cause nosocomial pneumonias are the aerobic gram-negative bacilli and S. aureus. These pathogens are often resistant to many antibiotics. There is a lesser frequency of infection by those agents causing community-acquired pneumonias, such as S. pneumoniae, Legionella pneumophila, H. influenzae, and viruses. The fungal organisms are less common pathogens unless the patient is immunocompromised. Multiple organisms are commonly identified in culture or tissue studies of patients with nosocomial pneumonia, making it difficult to confirm the identify of the original pathogen. Similarly, blood cultures obtained from patients with nosocomial pneumonia are positive for more than one bacterial pathogen in 12% of patients (Bryan and Reynolds, 1984). COPD patients may represent a special subgroup at risk for nosocomial pneumonia caused by H. influenzae and Moraxella catarrhalis as a result of chronic colonization of the airways by these organisms.

Table 36–6 presents a comparison of the common pulmonary pathogens and their relative incidence in community-acquired pneumonia. A similar list is shown in Table 36–7 for nosocomial pneumonias, noting a total greater than 100% because of polymicrobial infections. The aerobic gram-negative bacilli of the Enterobacteriaceae family cause the great majority of nosocomial pneumonias. Common offending organisms include K. pneumoniae, Serratia marcescens, Enterobacter species, E. coli, P. aeruginosa, and Proteus species.

Two of the most dangerous organisms are P. aeruginosa, and the Enterobacter species. Pseudomonas aeruginosa characteristically causes a severe, rapidly progressive necrotizing pneumonia. This organism has a special affinity for respiratory epithelium, and as a frequent colonizer of the pharynx is poised to cause nosocomial pneumonia. Enterobacter species have a special advantage because they are able to quickly develop resistance to antibiotics during therapy.

Diagnosis

Criteria used to define the diagnosis of a nosocomial pneumonia are nonspecific. A working definition published by the Centers for Disease Control and Prevention (CDC) provides a reasonable framework (CDC, 1989). The CDC criteria include:

1. Onset of pneumonia greater than 72 hours after hospital admission
2. A physical examination showing rales or dullness to percussion or chest radiograph showing an infiltrate
3 At least one of the following findings:
   - Purulent sputum.

Table 36–6. COMMON PATHOGENS CAUSING COMMUNITY-ACQUIRED PNEUMONIA

Streptococcus pneumoniae	50*
Staphylococcus aureus	20%
Aerobic gram-negative bacilli	10–20%
Legionella species	
Mycoplasma pneumoniae	10–25% for all atypical pneumonia agents as a group
Moraxella catarrhalis	
Chlamydia species	
Viral	

*Percentage as incidence in cultures.

Table 36–7. COMMON PATHOGENS CAUSING NOSOCOMIAL PNEUMONIA*

COMMON ORGANISMS		UNCOMMON ORGANISMS	
S. aureus	25%[†]	S. pneumoniae	<10%
All aerobic gram-negative bacilli as a group	70%	Other enteric gram-negative bacilli	<5%
		Anaerobic mouth-flora	<2
P. aeruginosa	17%	Moraxella catarrhalis	<2
Enterobacter species	15%	Legionella species	<10
Klebsiella species	15%	Influenza A virus	<10
E. coli	15%	Aspergillus	<5
H. influenzae	15%		
Serratia marcescens	10%		
Proteus species	5%		
Candida albicans	5%		

*Total is greater than 100% because of polymicrobial pneumonias.
[†]Percentage as incidence in cultures; rates per organism vary with local ICU flora.

- Isolation of a pathogen from blood, transtracheal aspirate, biopsy specimen, or protected bronchial brushing specimen.
- Isolation of a virus in respiratory secretions.
- Diagnostic antibody titers.
- Histopathologic evidence of pneumonia.

Making an accurate diagnosis of the presence of a nosocomial pneumonia can challenge the most vigilant and experienced clinician. Overdiagnosis is common because of noninfectious causes of pulmonary infiltrates or fevers. Any patient who develops a pulmonary infiltrate during hospitalization that has lasted a week or more must be evaluated for a possible nosocomial pneumonia. The same is true for infiltrates developing after general anesthesia for surgical patients. Classical findings associated with pneumonia include fever, pulmonary infiltrate, productive cough or increase in sputum, thoracic chest pain, dyspnea, and leukocytosis in the blood cell count. Physical exam may show signs of consolidation or decreased breath sounds as a result of an effusion. The most important finding is new purulent sputum. This and other signs of pneumonia should be searched for if there is a clinical change of a pertinent type in the patient. Important changes include a changed mental status, fever, poor oxygenation, dyspnea, pleuritic pain, sputum change, or leukocytosis.

Clinically suspected pneumonia may be erroneously overdiagnosed in as many as 30% of patients with a new infiltrate, fever, or sputum increase. Noninfectious infiltrates most commonly are caused by congestive heart failure, ARDS, pulmonary emboli, or drug reactions causing pulmonary changes. Underdiagnosis of pneumonia easily occurs in hospitalized patients with other illnesses. Postoperative patients with new pneumonia may not have fever or classical signs of infiltrate or sputum, especially if elderly. More subtle signs of pneumonia may be confusion, a drop in blood oxygen saturation, or change in the respiratory rate. An increase in purulent sputum may be the most reliable finding to suggest pulmonary infection.

Elderly patients with pneumonia can be harder to diagnose early. They also have a higher mortality. Cough may be minimal and nonproductive, and sputum samples are harder to obtain. Lung consolidation may be absent. Elderly patients are less likely to have fever, leukocytosis, or increased sputum despite having a pneumonia. Elderly patients are more likely to develop confusion or lethargy as the only early sign of illness associated with a nosocomial pneumonia. Unexplained increase in respiratory rate to above 25 breaths per minute or tachycardia may precede the more typical findings of pneumonia. The differential diagnosis includes congestive heart failure, pulmonary emboli, aspiration, atelectasis, ARDS, cancer metastases, or drug responses.

Proving that infection exists and identification of the invading pathogen are both complicated by the constant polymicrobial colonization of the pharynx and upper airways. Specimens collected from the lower airways are frequently contaminated by upper airway organisms even with the most sophisticated bronchoscopic techniques. This contamination leads either to overdiagnosis when no infection exists, or to uncertainty regarding the invading pathogen. Using bronchoscopy with a protected tip technique to obtain brush cultures of the terminal airways or mini-bronchoalveolar lavage still yields false-positive and false-negative rates of 30% to 40%. These techniques may still be clinically useful when compared to the diagnostic errors when using clinical criteria alone. Patients on mechanical ventilation with fever and pulmonary infiltrates did not have pneumonia in 50% to 70% of cases (Mauldin et al, 1991). Bronchoscopic sampling techniques as well as open-lung biopsy are best reserved for patients not responding to therapy or patients on mechanical ventilation. The results need to be critically interpreted by pulmonologists experienced in the techniques.

Less invasive techniques of transtracheal aspiration are fraught with the same contamination problems as noted for bronchoscopic techniques. If the diagnosis of pneumonia is suspected, a microscopic evaluation of the sputum should be performed and Gram's stain and cultures should be done. Only Gram's stain is likely to assist in the early decisions regarding therapy. Sputum culture results are sometimes helpful for comparison to blood culture results or comparison to the antibiotic sensitivity profiles. Contamination of the lung secretions by organisms in the oropharynx limits the value of sputum analysis.

An estimate of the quality of the sputum sample can be made, looking for a predominant organism and assessing the number of squamous epithelial cells. A good specimen should have less than 10 squamous epithelial cells per low-power field, and finding more than 25 neutrophils suggests that the specimen originated from the site of active infection. Sputum samples showing predominantly gram-positive cocci or culture proven *S. aureus* are more likely to be true positives than are gram-negative bacilli and Enterobacteriaceae when evaluating postoperative patients for pneumonia. *Pseudomonas aeruginosa* is also more likely to be a true positive than are the Enterobacteriaceae. Unfortunately, the causitive organism is not present in sputum cultures in 23% of patients with bacteremia resulting from a nosocomial pneumonia (Bryan and Reynolds, 1984).

Blood cultures should be obtained prior to starting therapy for a nosocomial pneumonia. Approximately 10% of patients will be bacteremic, and this may provide the most accurate identification of the invading pathogen. Mortality rates are known to be higher for bacteremic pneumonia patients. Bacteremia may be secondary to the pneumonia, or the pneumonia may have developed secondary to bacteremia from a nonpulmonary source of sepsis. Clinical evaluation for extrapulmonary sites of infection should attempt to exclude urinary infections, sinusitis, intravascular catheter infections, and surgical

site infections. The urine should be cultured, and existing vascular access devices should be removed and the catheter cultured. Nasogastric tubes should be changed to the opposite nostril or removed, and a head CT scan obtained to evaluate for sinusitis.

A chest radiograph should be evaluated for infiltrates, effusions, or evidence of an abscess (Fig. 36–3). A decubitus film may help document an effusion. A chest CT scan should be obtained if plain films are equivocal for effusion or abscess. Any effusion present should be aspirated. Culture of the effusion may provide a pure culture of the pathogen. An empyema may require chest tube drainage. Patients with dyspnea, accelerated respiratory rate, or a changed mental status should have an arterial blood gas analysis and consideration for placement in an ICU.

Treatment

The bacterial pathogens associated with postoperative pneumonia are capable of creating a rapidly progressive pneumonia, and therefore prompt initiation of therapy may be critical to successful intervention. Left untreated, these pneumonias can evolve into lung abscesses, necrotizing pneumonia, empyema, and septic death. The treatment of postoperative pneumonia includes aggressive pulmonary toilet, maintenance of host defense mechanism with particular attention to nutrition, and antibiotic therapy. Any patient with a weak cough will benefit from vigorous pulmonary toilet. Chest physiotherapy for pulmonary toilet is initiated using vibropercussion with postural drainage. Bronchodilators and mucolytic agents may be administered in aerosolized form to further improve expectoration. Antibiotics should be started without waiting for culture results, because cultures may not accurately reflect the true

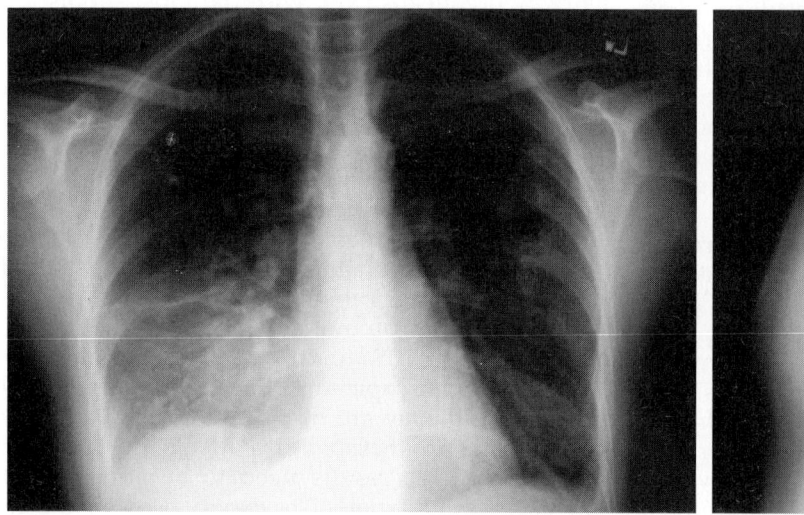
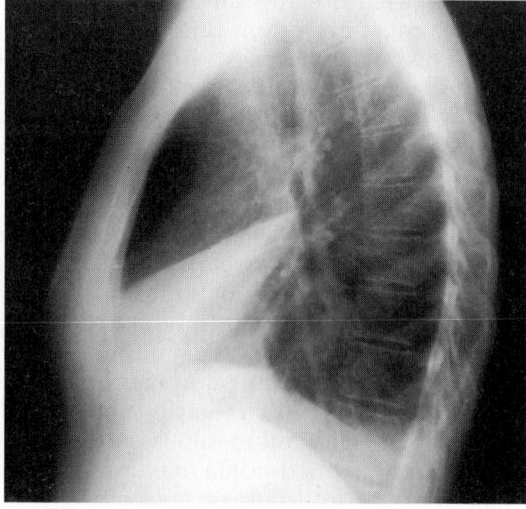

A   B

Figure 36–3
Chest radiographs of a 45-year-old patient with fever and cough 4 days after hysterectomy. *A,* Infiltrate is a right middle lobe pneumonia, with lobar consolidation seen better on lateral view. *B,* Lateral view of right middle lobe pneumonia in same patient.

pathogen, and because rapid progression of disease precludes waiting for results. An international consensus panel has endorsed empirical therapy of nosocomial pneumonia (Mandell et al, 1993). Proper therapy is crucial, as illustrated by the reported 92% mortality with inappropriate therapy compared to a 31% mortality with proper antibiotics (Celis et al, 1988).

A postoperative nosocomial pneumonia may be polymicrobial in as many as 40% of cases. The pathogens may be resistant bacteria because of recent antibiotic exposure. *Pseudomonas aeruginosa*, *Enterobacter* species, and *Acinetobacter* species are notorious for developing resistance during therapy. The preceding facts provide the basis for traditional recommendations to use combination antibiotic therapy for hospital-acquired pneumonia. Combination therapy broadens coverage, provides synergistic activity with some agents, and decreases the chance of resistance developing during therapy. Combination therapy has been proven to improve survival for pneumonia caused by *P. aeruginosa* and pneumonia complicated by bacteremia. Single-agent therapy may be of equal effectiveness compared to combination therapy for patients who do not appear ill and in whom no bacteremia or *P. aeruginosa* is involved, as has been shown in studies using imipenem, ciprofloxacin, ticarcillin–clavulanic acid, cefoperazone, ceftazidime, and aztreonam. This approach has merit because patients who are not critically ill with pneumonia do not commonly have a *P. aeruginosa* infection. Single-agent therapy avoids toxicity and expense. Nevertheless, presence or absence of bacteremia is not usually known at the time therapy is chosen.

Two common approaches to therapy are used. In the first, combination therapy is initiated and therapy is then streamlined as soon as possible if no bacteremia or *Pseudomonas* is identified. The sensitivity profile allows optimal choice of monotherapy at the time combination therapy is streamlined. The second approach is to start monotherapy and add a synergistic second agent if *P. aeruginosa* is isolated, thereby preventing emergence of resistance. The international consensus panel (Mandell et al, 1993) recommended choosing empirical therapy after assessing the severity of the illness at the time of diagnosis and the presence of patient-specific risk factors that would predict specific pathogens. Table 36–8 lists the pathogens and associated risk factors.

Single-agent therapy might be considered for a patient with only mild illness symptoms, no severe underlying disease, short antecedent hospitalization, and absence of risk factors listed in Table 36–8. The responsible organisms likely in this setting are the common nonpseudomonal gram-negative bacilli *S. aureus*, and *S. pneumoniae*, as listed for uncomplicated pneumonias in Table 36–8. Reasonable choices for single-agent antibiotic therapy aimed at these organisms are listed in Table 36–9. It should be remembered that fluoroquinolones are only modestly effective against streptococci, including *S. pneumoniae*. Therefore, these quinolones would not be the agents of choice if the sputum suggests primarily *S. pneumoniae*. They are an excellent choice if mixed gram-positive cocci and gram-negative bacilli and some *S. pneumoniae* organisms are seen on Gram's stain. Excellent serum levels after oral dosing make the fluoroquinolones a good choice for completing therapy after an initial prompt response to parenteral antibiotics. Efficacy of ciprofloxacin for empirical therapy is evidenced by the clinical response of 70% documented for ciprofloxacin during therapy for pneumonia where *S. pneumoniae* has been identified as the primary pathogen. Trimethoprim-sulfamethoxazole also provides the necessary spectrum of activity and is a useful agent for the penicillin-allergic patient. Combination antibiotic regimens should be used in all situations with risk factors predicting polymicrobial infection, resistant organisms, or possible infection by highly virulent pathogens such as underlying *P. aeruginosa*. Specific therapy may be aimed at an unusual pathogen or

Table 36–8. RISK FACTORS ASSOCIATED WITH SPECIFIC PATHOGENS CAUSING NOSOCOMIAL PNEUMONIA

RISK FACTOR	PATHOGEN
No risk factors, and not critically ill	Organisms found in pneumonias of uncomplicated hosts; *Klebsiella* species, *Enterobacter* species, *E. coli*, *Proteus* species, *S. marcescens*, *H. influenzae*, *S. pneumoniae*, *S. aureus*
Prior antibiotic use	*P. aeruginosa*, *Acinetobacter* species
Prolonged hospitalization, ICU patient, or endotracheal tube ventilation	*P. aeruginosa*
Recent abdominal or thoracic surgery: suspected aspiration	Mixed gram-negative bacilli and anaerobes
Diabetes, coma, or head injury	*S. aureus*
Corticosteroid use	*Legionella* species, *P. aeruginosa*, or *Aspergillus* species
Malignancy, neutropenia, renal failure, chemotherapy	*Legionella*, Enterobacteriaceae, or *Aspergillus* species
Severe illness	*P. aeruginosa* or other resistant Enterobacteriaceae

Table 36–9. AGENTS ACCEPTABLE FOR MONOTHERAPY OF NOSOCOMIAL PNEUMONIA FOR THE UNCOMPLICATED HOST

Cefotaxime
Ceftriaxone
Ciprofloxacin, ofloxacin, or levofloxin
Ampicillin-sulbactam
Trimethoprim-sulfamethoxazole

group of pathogens in certain clinical situations. When these situations are present, it is advisable to treat using an agent previously discussed for monotherapy plus an additional second agent that best treats the pathogen the patient is at high risk to be infected by.

Prior abdominal surgery or known aspiration both increase the risk of anaerobes. So does the presence of infiltrates confined to the dependent portions of the lungs. Ampicillin-sulbactam or ticarcillin–clavulanic acid as single agents adequately cover the aerobes of the pathogens seen in the uncomplicated-host pneumonia. Alternatively, an agent adequate for monotherapy (Table 36–9) could be used with either metronidazole or clindamycin.

Staphylococcus aureus is the second most common cause of nosocomial pneumonia, causing essentially an equivalent proportion of pneumonias as are caused by *P. aeruginosa*, at 16% and 17%, respectively. Pneumonia caused by *S. aureus* was associated with a 90% mortality prior to availability of antibiotics. A report by Watanakunakorn (1987) identified the subgroup of *S. aureus* pneumonias complicated by bacteremia as still having an 84% mortality. Bacteremia is thought to complicate 20% to 30% of *S. aureus* pneumonia cases. These patients are frequently elderly and have underlying pulmonary disease. ICU patients with staphylococcus cellulitis whose staphylococcus bacteremia originated from indwelling vascular catheters were particularly at risk to develop *S. aureus* pneumonia from hematogenous origin (Schaberg et al, 1991).

Patients with diabetes or those in a coma who develop pneumonia are at high risk for *S. aureus* in addition to the usual pathogens seen in the uncomplicated host. If methicillin-resistant staphylococci are common in the ward, ICU, or hospital, then vancomycin should be added to the agent chosen from the monotherapy agents listed in Table 36–9. Methicillin-resistant *S. aureus* is especially likely to be present if antibiotics were being administered at the time pneumonia developed. If *S. aureus* is cultured from blood, it may be either secondary to the pneumonia or the cause of the pneumonia. Empirical use of vancomycin is not recommended so as to avoid aggravating the recent problem of the emergence of vancomycin-resistant strains of *S. aureus* or of *Enterococcus*.

If *S. aureus* pneumonia is believed to have begun by oropharyngeal aspiration, then 14 to 21 days of therapy are recommended. If *S. aureus* bacteremia is identified as the hematogenous origin of the pneumonia, then 4 to 6 weeks of antistaphylococcal therapy may be necessary. This prolonged therapy is needed to adequately sterilize endovascular and other nonpulmonary sites of infection. Agents chosen for specific antistaphylococcal therapy include oxacillin, nafcillin, cefazolin, ampicillin-sulbactam, piperacillin-tazobactam, and vancomycin.

Legionella pneumonias are more likely in patients receiving corticosteroid therapy or cytotoxic chemotherapy. *Legionella* pneumonia will usually be associated with high fever, scant sputum, decreased mentation, extreme clinical toxicity, and mild liver transaminase elevations in the serum. Risk factors include immunosuppression or underlying cardiac, pulmonary, or renal disease. *Legionella* pneumonia will not respond to β-lactam antibiotic therapy. Sputum samples in these patients can be evaluated by direct immunofluorescence staining. If staining is positive, *Legionella* infection is very likely, but sensitivity is only 50% with this test. Sputum and urine can also be checked for *Legionella* antigen, but this identifies only some of the more common subtypes. Therapy for these patients consists of erythromycin, with or without rifampin, for 21 days.

Certain patients developing a nosocomial pneumonia should be considered at high risk for pneumonia caused by *P. aeruginosa*. Patients at high risk for this pathogen include those whose pneumonia develops in an intensive care unit, a prolonged hospital stay preceding pneumonia, prior antibiotic use during the hospitalization, ventilator-associated pneumonias, and severely ill patients with pneumonia. Empirical therapy for these patients should specifically cover *P. aeruginosa* in addition to the organism seen in the uncomplicated host. This group of patients is also more likely to have polymicrombial infections, and infections with organisms resistant to many antibiotics. Arbitrary definitions of severe pneumonia include high supplemental oxygen requirements (inspired O_2 concentrations above 40%), hypotension, rapid progression, or multilobar infiltrates. Proper therapy for these patients with multiple risk factors or severe illness includes coverage of the usual pathogens plus specific therapy aimed at *P. aeruginosa* (see Table 36–10 for agents with antipseudomonal efficacy).

Pseudomonas aeruginosa should be treated with dual-agent coverage to avoid development of resistance during therapy. Development of resistance during therapy is associated with treatment failures. Use of ciprofloxacin or aztreonam avoids the toxicity associated with aminoglycosides. Therapy is changed to a single oral therapy when complete defervescence has occurred. Total duration of therapy is usually 2 weeks.

Once a pneumonia is under treatment, most patients will have prompt resolution of fever and dyspnea within 2 to 3 days. Chest radiographic findings may lag behind the clinical response, but infiltrates

Table 36-10. ANTIPSEUDOMONAL ANTIBIOTICS*

Group 1: β-Lactam
   Piperacillin, azlocillin, mezlocillin, ticarcillin
   Ticarcillin–clavulanic acid, piperacillin-tazobactam
   Ceftazadime, cefoperazone, cefipime
   Imipenem-cilastatin
Group 2: Non–β-Lactam
   Ciprofloxacin
   Aminoglycosides†
   Aztreonam

*An agent from group 1 is given with an agent from group 2 for pseudomonal infections.
†Use qd dosing to ensure adequate levels are achieved in the lung tissue.

on radiograph should improve after 10 days of therapy (Fein and Feinsilver, 1993). Some authors allow up to 4 weeks for a complete resolution depending on the pathogen responsible. If the patient does not appear to be responding clinically, then initial concerns should deal with the possibility of resistant organisms requiring a change in antibiotics, or an atypical pneumonia caused by *Legionella* species or *Mycoplasma pneumoniae*. Viral pneumonia is harder to diagnose but is less likely to require a therapy. Viral pneumonia may be complicated by bacterial superinfection subsequent to the viral pneumonitis injury. This might be recognized with a change in the clinical course after initial slow resolution of pneumonia complicated by development of new infiltrates.

Recognition of an inadequate or slow response to therapy should also prompt consideration of bronchoscopy for protected specimen cultures, and consideration of high-resolution CT scan of the chest. After obtaining these specimens and repeat blood cultures, empirical addition of erythromycin or doxycycline can be done while awaiting cultural results. Other causes of pulmonary infection resistant to standard therapy are fungi such as *Aspergillus* or *Candida* species or *Pneumocystis carinii*. These organisms are more common in the immunocompromised host, such as occurs with high-dose corticosteroids, neutropenia, cancer, or human immunodeficiency virus (HIV) infection.

Ventilator-Associated Pneumonia

Persons who require prolonged mechanical ventilation are at high risk for pneumonia. Ventilator-associated pneumonia carries a high mortality compared to other hospital-acquired pneumonias. The diagnosis of pneumonia during mechanical ventilation may be difficult to make with accuracy because of other concomitant infections causing fever, or because of noninfectious causes of pulmonary infiltrates. Purulent secretions from the endotracheal tube are common after long ventilation, but pneumonia is not the cause for most. False-positive airway cultures create another diagnostic problem in this setting. New fever for a ventilated patient always raises the question of a new pneumonia, but confirmation is difficult and clinical diagnosis is incorrect 60% of the time (Meduri et al, 1994). Despite the presence of common clinical signs typical of pneumonia, a careful evaluation may show that the fever is due to atelectasis, chemical injury from aspiration, ARDS, deep vein thrombus, urinary tract infection, drug fever, sinusitis, venous catheter infection, cholecystitis, or pancreatitis.

Fagon et al (1989) reported cumulative incidences of ventilator-associated pneumonia to be 6.5% at 10 days, 19% at 20 days, and 28% at 30 days of ventilation. This report identified *S. aureus* in 33%, *P. aeruginosa* in 31%, *Acinetobacter* species in 15%, and *Proteus* species in 15% of cultures obtained by the protected-tip brush technique for retrieving pulmonary specimens. Forty per cent of specimens yielded more than one bacterial species. Seventy-five per cent of cases contained one or more gram-negative bacilli, 48% included only gram-negative bacilli, and 51% included staphylococci, streptococci, and *Corynebacterium*. Only 1% of cases were anaerobe-only isolates. Of the 49 patients with ventilator-associated pneumonia, 71% died in the hospital. This is twice the rate of the ventilated patients concomitantly studied who did not develop pneumonia. *Pseudomonas aeruginosa* and *Acinetobacter* species were associated with an 81% mortality. By comparison, other organisms identified on culture from ventilator-associated pneumonias were associated with a 55% mortality. Of the *S. aureus* cultures, 100% were methicillin resistant. This high resistance rate was deemed attributable to prior antibiotic exposure in these ICU patients. These patients can be extraordinarily difficult to manage and are usually best managed by consultation with an experienced pulmonologist.

Sepsis Syndrome and Septic Shock

Definition and Etiology

The terms *bacteremia*, *sepsis*, *sepsis syndrome*, and *septic shock* are not synonymous, but rather represent different issues in the infection process and physiologic responses to infection (Table 36–11). *Bacteremia* simply implies bacterial organisms within the bloodstream. *Sepsis* is a term historically used with many different definitions, varying from the simple state of infection to a state of septic shock, and is therefore confusing because of the nebulous meanings attached by different clinicians. *Sepsis syndrome* refers to a systemic response to the infection, and is recognized by evidence of organ dysfunction. Sepsis syndrome develops in only 25% to 30% of patients with bacteremia. The term *septic shock* is used when sepsis syndrome is associated with hypotension.

The phrase "systemic inflammatory response syndrome," or SIRS, should be used when referring to the clinical evidence of inflammation that is the body's response to some injury (Fig. 36–4). SIRS can occur as a result of infection, hemorrhagic shock,

Table 36-11. DEFINITIONS

Infection: Microbial phenomenon characterized by an inflammatory response to the presence of microorganisms or the invasion of normally sterile host tissue by those organisms

Bacteremia: The presence of viable bacteria in the blood

Systemic Inflammatory Response Syndrome: The systemic inflammatory response to a variety of severe clinical insults. The response is manifested by two or more of the following conditions:

    Temperature >38°C or <36°C

    Heart rate >90 beats/min

    Respiratory rate >20 breaths/min or $PaCO_2$ < 32 torr (<4.3 kPa)

    WBC > 12,000 cells/mm^3, <4000 cells/mm^3, or >10% immature (band) forms

Sepsis: The systemic response to infection. This systemic response is manifested by two or more of the following conditions as a result of infection:

    Temperature >38°C or <36°C

    Heart rate >90 beats/min

    Respiratory rate >20 breaths/min or $PaCO_2$ < 32 torr (<4.3 kPa)

    WBC > 12,000 cells/mm^3, <4000 cells/mm^3, or >10% immature (band) forms

Severe Sepsis: Sepsis associated with organ dysfunction, hypoperfusion, or hypotension. Hypoperfusion and perfusion abnormalities may include, but are not limited to, lactic acidosis, oliguria, or an acute alteration in mental status

Septic Shock: Sepsis with hypotension, despite adequate fluid resuscitation, along with the presence of perfusion abnormalities that may include, but are not limited to, lactic acidosis, oliguria, or an acute alteration in mental status. Patients who are on inotropic or vasopressor agents may not be hypotensive at the time that perfusion abnormalities are measured

Hypotension: A systolic BP of <90 mm Hg or a reduction of >40 mm Hg from baseline in the absence of other causes for hypotension

Multiple Organ Dysfunction Syndrome: Presence of altered organ function in an acutely ill patient such that homeostasis cannot be maintained without intervention

From ACCP/SCCM Consensus Conference Committee: Definitions for sepsis and organ failure and guidelines for the use of innovative therapies in sepsis. Crit Care Med 1992;20:866, with permission.

trauma, a burn, or other organ injury. SIRS is manifested as temperature greater than 38°C or less than 36°C, heart rate greater than 90 beats/min, respiratory rate greater than 20 breaths/min or arterial partial pressure of CO_2 less than 32 mm Hg, and WBC count greater than 12,000 cells/mm^3 or less than 4,000 cells/mm^3 or greater than 10% band forms of neutrophils. These thresholds are considered evidence only if they occur as an acute change from baseline and when no other cause exists, such as chemotherapy-induced leukopenia/neutropenia. When SIRS progresses to a severe condition, then either individual or multiple organs will fail. If cardiac or pulmonary function is inadequate, then the resulting inadequate tissue perfusion and oxygenation can lead to multiple organ dysfunction syndrome (MODS).

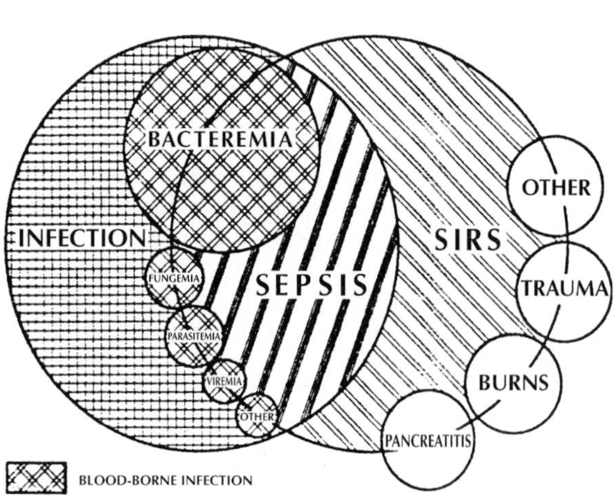

Sepsis syndrome is best defined as evidence of infection associated with a systemic response by the host, usually resulting from microbial toxins in the bloodstream. The term *sepsis* should be reserved for when a confirmed infection has caused SIRS. Some authors use the term *sepsis syndrome* to designate the clinical manifestations of sepsis. *Sepsis* and *sepsis syndrome* are interchangeable if the definitions recommended by the ACCP/SCCM Consensus Conference Committee (1992) are used, such that "sepsis is the systemic inflammatory response to infection." The severity of the septic response is recognized by whether there is evidence of organ dysfunction in addition to the infection-induced SIRS. Common signs of organ dysfunction include altered mental status, oliguria, lactic acidosis, hypotension, or other evidence of underperfusion.

Septic shock occurs as a severe form of sepsis, defined as sepsis-induced hypotension that persists after fluid resuscitation. The hypotension refractory to volume correction confirms cardiovascular dysfunction resulting from the sepsis, and the definition excludes other causes such as primary cardiogenic shock. Fortunately, only a small number of patients

Figure 36-4

Interrelationships among systemic inflammatory response syndrome (SIRS), sepsis, and infection. (From ACCP/SCCM Consensus Conference Committee: Definitions for sepsis and organ failure and guidelines for the use of innovative therapies in sepsis. Crit Care Med 1992;20:865, with permission.)

with sepsis experience septic shock. Septic shock is currently associated with a mortality of 40% (Dunn, 1994). This mortality was found to vary with the severity at diagnosis and its progression after diagnosis. Bone et al (1989) reported a mortality of 13% for sepsis syndrome without shock, 28% for sepsis syndrome presenting with shock, and 43% mortality if shock developed after the sepsis syndrome presented. The incidence of shock may be 15% to 20% for infection with coagulase-negative staphylococci (Martin et al, 1989), and 20% for gram-negative rod bacteremia (Greenman et al, 1991; Ziegler et al, 1991). Estimates suggest that sepsis results in shock in 40% of cases (Kreger et al, 1980).

Incidence

Sepsis syndrome occurs in approximately 1% of all hospitalized patients (Zimmerman and Dietrich, 1987), and is associated with a mortality rate of 30% to 40% (Marik and Varon, 1998). Sepsis and septic shock are reportedly responsible for 75,000 to 100,000 deaths per year and constitute the leading cause of death in the immediate postoperative period. Numerous risk factors have been identified, including a surgical wound, trauma, venous or urinary catheters, extremes of age, malnutrition, cancer, immunodeficiency states, immunosuppressant therapy, and chemotherapy. Certain chronic diseases such as diabetes mellitus, liver, cardiac, and renal disease also increase the risk. Other risk factors include alcohol abuse, antibiotics, invasive procedures and devices, and hypothermia.

Pathophysiology

Sepsis is caused by gram-negative bacteremia in about 50% of cases. The remaining cases are caused by gram-positive cocci, yeast, or rarely a virus. The physiologic changes underlying sepsis and septic shock are very complex; however, the primary offending agent in gram-negative sepsis appears to be endotoxin or lipopolysaccharide (LPS). LPS has three components; the O antigen, the R core antigen, and lipid A. The lipid A region of LPS is responsible for most, if not all, of the biologic activity of LPS. Directly and indirectly, LPS causes derangements of intermediary metabolism, results in the body's inability to use metabolic substrates effectively, and progresses eventually to multiple organ system dysfunction and failure. The initiating agent in sepsis syndrome and septic shock caused by gram-positive organisms is probably a toxin liberated by the organism or a part of its cell wall.

The metabolic derangement characteristic of septic shock (impaired cellular oxygen consumption) is due to a variety of factors, including hypotension, arteriovenous shunting, impaired oxyhemoglobin dissociation, direct suppression of cellular respiration, and impaired utilization of other metabolic substrates, such as glucose, free fatty acid, and protein.

Sepsis is the inflammatory response that results from a complex cascade of events mediated by a variety of cytokines and humoral factors. The primary initiator of sepsis is usually endotoxin from gram-negative bacteria, cell wall fragments or exotoxin from gram-positive cocci or yeast, or a viral antigen. When these toxins reach the circulation they cause the release of tumor necrosis factor-α (TNF-α), followed by interleukin-1, interleukin-6, interleukin-8, and platelet activating factor. These cytokines are released from endothelial cells and mononuclear phagocytes. Gram-negative LPS induces a tremendous release of TNF-α from macrophages (Luce, 1987).

Simultaneously, the complement system and coagulation cascade are activated. The cytokines of the first wave of the cascade cause arachidonic acid to be metabolized to form vasoactive leukotrienes, thromboxane A_2, and prostaglandins. Next the T cells are activated to produce interferon and interleukins. Most of the cytokines from the first and second wave are able to cause increased endothelial permeability. Complement fragments cause neutrophil activation that in turn can damage tissue by releasing free-radical oxygen species (Bone, 1991).

TNF-α and interleukin-1 cause myalgias, chills, headache, increased cardiac output, reduced systemic vascular resistance (SVR), and fever. TNF-α can depress cardiac myocyte shortening. Interleukin-2 can decrease SVR, arterial pressure, and cardiac ejection fraction. Platelet activating factor stimulates release of TNF-α, activates leukocytes, causes thrombosis from platelet aggregation, increases microvascular permeability, causes a negative inotropic effect on the heart, and may be neurotoxic and affect the brain directly. Leukotrienes increase vascular permeability, affect microcirculatory blood flow, and decrease cardiac contractility (Bone, 1991).

Sepsis is associated with large volumes of third-space losses causing hypovolemia. Several common and clinically important changes in physiology characteristically occur during sepsis, including a decrease in SVR, a maldistribution of blood flow within organs and to certain organs, and a depressed cardiac ejection fraction as a result of biventricular dysfunction that not only decreases cardiac output but fails to respond in a normal fashion when volume re-expansion is done. The best measure of cardiac dysfunction during sepsis is the stroke work index. During sepsis the decreased systolic function shows a low stroke work index. During this state, attempts at volume re-expansion yield a smaller improvement in left ventricular stroke work index than is expected for nonseptic patients (Marik and Varon, 1998). The combination of hypovolemia from third-space losses and decreased SVR plus depressed cardiac function causes hypotension leading to shock.

Diagnosis

The diagnosis of sepsis or septic shock is relatively straightforward in some instances, especially if not recognized until late in the course. The differential diagnosis of septic shock includes a wide array of disorders, although a careful history and physical examination usually can narrow the list significantly (Table 36–12). Any of the causes of shock can cause hypoperfusion and systemic hypotension.

Septic shock may present dramatically, as with gram-negative sepsis, or insidiously, as with fungemia. Fungemia usually occurs in an immunocompromised patient. Frequently, gram-positive cocci cause septic shock that develops as a slow deterioration of multiple organs, but the diagnosis is not immediately suspected because there is little or no fever for the first several days. The time into the course of septic shock is referred to as early (warm shock) or late (cold shock). Each phase is associated with characteristic hemodynamic and metabolic changes as well as with characteristic signs and symptoms (Tables 36–13 and 36–14).

The first and most important step in the recognition of sepsis and septic shock is a high index of suspicion and a knowledge of high-risk groups. The diagnosis should be suspected in any patient with hyperthermia or hypothermia, tachycardia, a change in mental status, and/or tachypnea. Those criteria noted above for SIRS are used to make a presumptive diagnosis of sepsis, pending confirmation of associated infection. In these patients, an exhaustive search should be made to identify the source of infection. The yield of blood culture specimens is highly variable, depending on the timing and number of cultures obtained as well as the growth characteristics of the particular organisms involved. Apart from a thorough history and physical examination, useful tests include blood cultures, a urine culture, a chest radiograph, a complete blood count, arterial blood gas measurements, and a metabolic profile. Tests that may be of benefit in selected patients include lumbar puncture with cerebrospinal fluid analysis, sputum Gram's stain and culture, culture of skin lesions, sinus films, an echocardiogram, a CT scan to detect an abscess, or a radiolabeled WBC study.

Table 36–12. DIFFERENTIAL DIAGNOSIS OF SEPTIC SHOCK

Anaphylaxis
Toxic shock
Drug overdose
Hyper- or hypothermia
Diabetic ketoacidosis
Pancreatitis
Addison's disease
Endocarditis/myocarditis/pericarditis
Infectious diarrhea
Myocardial infarction
Pulmonary embolus (submassive/massive)
Shock of any other etiology (hemorrhagic, etc)

From Gelder MS: Acute medical problems in the postoperative patient. In Shingleton HM, Hurt WE (eds): Postreproductive Gynecology. New York: Churchill Livingstone, 1990:543, with permission.

Table 36–13. WARM (EARLY) SHOCK

Hemodynamic changes
  Decreased peripheral vascular resistance
  Increased cardiac output
Clinical signs
  Tachycardia
  Tachypnea
  Wide pulse pressure/bounding pulses
  Hyperthermia or hypothermia
  Flushed, warm skin
  Possible subtle changes in mental status

From Gelder MS: Acute medical problems in the postoperative patient. In Shingleton HM, Hurt WG (eds): Postreproductive Gynecology. New York: Churchill Livingstone, 1990:543, with permission.

Management

Sepsis syndrome following gynecologic surgery will most frequently have its source in pulmonary infections, urinary tract infection, or operative site cellulitis and abscess. Decompression of an obstructed upper urinary tract or drainage of pelvic and abdominal abscesses are the cornerstone of management when sepsis is caused by these sources. The management of patients with bacteremia or sepsis involves identification of the source of infection and initiation of measures to eradicate the source of infection, such as incision and drainage of any abscess, débridement of necrotic tissue, chest physical therapy, or institution of appropriate antibiotic coverage. Supportive therapy includes adequate nutrition, antipyretics, and maintenance of volume status.

Empirical antibiotic therapy should be initiated when evidence of sepsis is found. Prompt initiation of antibiotics effective against the bacteria causing sepsis has been found to cut mortality of sepsis by half. The antibiotics most appropriate for empirical use are determined by the specific body site showing evidence of infection, knowledge of organisms ex-

Table 36–14. COLD (LATE) SHOCK

Hemodynamic changes
  Increased peripheral vascular resistance
  Decreased cardiac output
  Low central venous and pulmonary capillary wedge
    pressures
Clinical signs
  Tachycardia
  Tachypnea (labored/shallow)
  Hypotension
  Weak pulses
  Hyper- or hypothermia
  Cold, clammy skin
  Cyanosis
  Moderate to severe alteration in mental status
  Oliguria/anuria

From Gelder MS: Acute medical problems in the postoperative patient. In Shingelton HM, Hurt WE (eds): Postreproductive Gynecology. New York: Churchill Livingstone, 1990:543, with permission.

pected at that site, and familiarity with local antibiotic resistance patterns. Broad-spectrum antibiotics or two-agent regimens are usually recommended. Commonly used agents include third-generation cephalosporins, aminoglycosides, imipenem or meropenem, aztreonam, or extended-spectrum penicillins, including those combined with a β-lactamase inhibitor, such as ticarcillin-clavulanate, ampicillin-sulbactam, or piperacillin-tazobactam.

Patients with septic shock are frequently very difficult to manage, because attention must be directed to several organ systems simultaneously. Treatment is aimed at interrupting and reversing the pathophysiologic progression and at maintaining organ viability. Initial therapy of patients with septic shock involves hemodynamic stabilization, maintenance of adequate oxygenation, and correction of acidosis. Initiation of broad-spectrum antibiotics, and surgical procedures to débride infected tissue, drain an abscess, or relieve obstructed and infected urinary tracts or bowel are directed specifically at the cause of the sepsis.

Volume resuscitation is imperative, because this can often correct hypotension without other intervention (Marik and Varon, 1998). Sepsis is associated with large volumes of third-space losses causing hypovolemia. The combination of hypovolemia from third-space losses, with decreased SVR plus depressed cardiac function causes hypotension leading to shock. These patients may need 2 to 3 liters of fluid resuscitation at the time of diagnosis of sepsis. Another 5 to 10 liters may be needed to keep up with ongoing losses during a 24-hour period, often despite dramatic peripheral edema. Volume resuscitation to achieve adequate perfusion pressure is more important than type of volume administered. Controversy continues regarding the ideal agent to select when choosing between crystalloid, colloid, or blood products.

Hemodynamic stabilization frequently necessitates the use of a Swan-Ganz catheter because it may be impossible to determine the effects of therapeutic interventions accurately using clinical impressions alone. Poor response to volume resuscitation may be due to inadequate volume correction or to primary cardiac dysfunction. Such cardiac dysfunction may be best treated with inotropic support. Urine output may remain depressed as a result of blood flow maldistribution within the kidney even if hypotension has been corrected. Sophisticated assessment of volume status and cardiac performance relative to systemic pressure and SVR will be required in many patients to properly judge the ideal manipulation of intravascular volume, vasopressors, and inotropic agents.

The initial resuscitation from sepsis should aim to provide adequate tissue perfusion by achieving adequate systemic pressure and blood flow distribution. A goal of achieving a mean arterial pressure of 70 to 80 mm Hg and a cardiac index of 2.8 L/min/m² is recommended (Marik and Varon, 1998). The optimal

volume status is also controversial, although most authorities recommend a pulmonary capillary wedge pressure of 12 to 16 mm Hg. If hypotension is refractory to adequate volume replacement, then inotropic and pressor agent support is indicated. Hemodynamic monitoring of left and right heart pressures is needed for proper adjustment of volume and pressors over time.

It is imperative to maintain adequate oxygenation, and mechanical ventilatory support is often needed. Unfortunately, it is all too frequently impossible to maintain oxygenation, because ARDS is the most common direct cause of death. The use of steroids is very controversial; however, it is currently recommended that they be avoided (Sprung et al, 1984; Bone et al, 1987). After initial stabilization, attention is directed to identification and eradication of the source of infection.

The prognosis of patients with septic shock is clearly related to the extent of organ system failure. Evidence of failure of three or more organ systems generally portends a very poor prognosis (Dellinger, 1988). Therefore, close attention must be paid to all organ systems and immediate, aggressive measures should be implemented to reverse any abnormalities.

Transfusion-Associated Infections

The acquired immunodeficiency syndrome (AIDS) epidemic has led to a greatly increased concern regarding the risks of blood transfusion. Many transfusions are now autologous; however, when these are not available, physicians and patients alike are more likely to question the necessity of transfusion. Although HIV infection has created a new awareness of transfusion risk, blood transfusion has always been associated with risk. Acute transfusion reactions are an immediate risk, but chronic disease or death can result from acquired infection after exposure to infectious agents during transfusion. Hepatitis viruses cause acute and chronic hepatitis, and HIV infection results in AIDS. Hepatitis B virus (HBV), hepatitis C virus (HCV), and other non-A, non-B hepatitis agents occur with greater frequency than does HIV in donor blood, and are contracted as transfusion-acquired infections more often than is HIV after a transfusion. Infection by cytomegalovirus (CMV) is less common, and both malaria and trypanosomiasis are rare in the blood supply in the nited States. HCV causes 90% of cases of transfusion-associated hepatitis.

Owing to constantly improved and expanded screening techniques as well as the use of an all-volunteer donor population, the infectious risks associated with blood transfusions have continued to decrease. The development of non-A, non-B hepatitis from commercial donor blood was estimated to occur at an incidence rate of 28% per unit prior to changes in donor eligibility and advances in testing used for screening donor units. This incidence rate has fallen significantly with the use of volunteer blood (Aach and Kahn, 1980; Shorey, 1985). Additionally, the advent of more extensive screening for hepatitis-associated markers has markedly decreased the incidence of transfusion-acquired HBV as well as the incidences for HCV and the other non-A, non-B hepatitis infections.

Currently, all blood is screened for syphilis, HBV antigens, antibody to HIV, antibody to HCV, alanine aminotransferase levels, and antibody to human T-cell lymphotropic virus type I. An assay to screen for HCV infection was designed by Kuo et al in 1989 and approved in May 1990. Screening for malaria and CMV infection is not routine. Malaria is unusual except in Asian immigrants, and Asian donors should be screened for it. CMV infection associated with blood product transfusion primarily occurs with transfusion of WBCs, although it can occur with any product. The risk of transmission of a bacterial infection with blood or blood product transfusion is virtually unheard of today, except in instances of nonsterile handling of IV tubing or catheters.

Hepatitis C Virus

To gain a full understanding of the infectious risk associated with blood transfusions, one must have a knowledge of the frequency of the various transmitted diseases, and an understanding of the natural history of the disease itself once established. HCV infection may become chronic in up to 80% of cases, but clinical liver disease may occur in only 20% to 35% of cases (Schreiber et al, 1996; Sharara, 1997). Some patients who acquire hepatitis C through blood transfusion experience spontaneous resolution. Twenty-eight per cent of patients go on to have a chronic persistent hepatitis, and 13% a chronic active hepatitis; 30% to 35% develop cirrhosis at 20 years, and 23% develop fatal hepatocellular carcinoma at 30 years after infection. Approximately 1% develop fulminant hepatitis. HCV is the most common cause of cryptogenic cirrhosis, and the most common cause of liver failure requiring liver transplantation (Sharara, 1997).

Hepatitis B Virus

Among patients with transfusion-associated hepatitis B infection, 90% experience spontaneous resolution, 9% have chronic persistent hepatitis, 3% have chronic active hepatitis, 1% develop cirrhosis, 1% develop fulminant hepatitis, and 1% die from hepatocellular carcinoma several years later. The 5-year survival rate for patients with chronic persistent hepatitis is approximately 97%. For patients with chronic active hepatitis, the 5-year survival rate is approximately 86%; for patients with cirrhosis, 55%. Patients with fulminant hepatitis do very poorly; 68% to 91% of them die shortly after onset of disease. Additionally, patients with hepatocellular carcinoma

fare exceedingly poorly and die quickly after clinical diagnosis (Carson et al, 1992).

Risk of Infection with Transfusion

Hepatitis B infection causes only 5% to 10% of all cases of transfusion-associated hepatitis. The safety of transfusing patients has increased dramatically over the last 10 years. Studies during the decade of the 1980s reported that the risk for development of hepatitis B following a transfusion was approximately 1 in 200 to 300 units of blood transfused (0.063% to 0.087%) (Sugg et al, 1985; Columbo et al, 1987). Donor screening using current testing reduced the risk of transfusion-acquired HBV to 1 in 63,000 (Schreiber et al, 1996) (Table 36–15). The risk for development of transfusion-associated non-A, non-B hepatitis prior to the development of a screening test for HCV was 1% to 7% of transfused units. Because studies have shown that 44% to 85% of patients with non-A, non-B hepatitis are positive for antibody to HCV, the risk of acquiring non-A, non-B hepatitis from blood product transfusion was predicted to decrease with this better screening (Carson et al, 1992). The risk is now down to 1 in 103,000 that a patient would be transfused with a unit of blood infectious for HCV (Schreiber et al, 1996).

Mandatory screening of blood for antibody to HIV was initiated in March 1985. Prior to this, the risk for development of HIV infection was thought to be 1 in 3300 units transfused (0.03%) (Cumming et al, 1989). Currently, the risk of transfusion-associated HIV infection is estimated at 1 in 500,000 units transfused (Ward et al, 1988; Cumming et al, 1989; Schreiber et al, 1996). There is no cure for HIV infection at this time, and, once individuals have full-blown AIDS, the mortality is virtually 100%. AIDS will develop in half of transfusion-infected patients within 7 years after exposure to HIV-infected blood from transfused units (Ward et al, 1989). Almost all recipients of HIV-infected blood will become HIV positive eventually.

Unfortunately, because there is a latency period between the onset of infection and the development of antibodies to HIV infection, some donors who test negative for the antibody do, in fact, harbor the virus. The mean incubation period for transfusion-

Table 36–15. TRANSFUSION-TRANSMITTED VIRAL INFECTION: RISK OF TRANSFUSING AN INFECTED UNIT

VIRAL AGENT	RISK
HBV	1 in 63,000
HCV	1 in 103,000
HIV	1 in 493,000
HTLV	1 in 641,000
All viruses: aggregate risk	1 in 34,000

From Schreiber GB, Busch MP, Kleinman SH, et al: The risk of transfusion-transmitted viral infection. N Engl J Med 1996;334:1685, with permission.

associated AIDS is 23 months (range 10 to 43 months), and the interval to development of antibody production is approximately 2 to 3 months. New testing will soon be available to again markedly decrease this "window period" where virus is present but not recognized by current screening tests. Achieving a shorter window period will reduce the risk of transfusion-acquired AIDS even further.

Although the risk for HIV infection has directed attention to the safety of our nation's blood supply, AIDS has never been the largest contributor to overall mortality associated with transfusion. Indeed, given the exceedingly high sensitivity and specificity of the test currently employed for HIV screening and the low prevalence of HIV infection in the donor population, HIV infection accounts for a very small portion of the overall mortality risk of blood transfusion.

The major infectious risk associated with transfusion continues to be HCV. It is estimated that HCV is responsible for 97% to 98% of the mortality risk associated with blood transfusion. This should decrease considerably with the advent of the screening test for HCV.

Vascular Catheter–Related Infections

Infections that develop as complications from the use of a vascular catheter may be limited to a local process, such as insertion site cellulitis, a tunnel infection, or an abscess. The infection can also be systemic, with bacteremia or sepsis syndrome. The infection can cause a septic thrombophlebitis or a complicated endocarditis. The most common pathogen isolated from vascular catheter infections is coagulase-negative staphylococci; S. aureus is also a frequent cause of these infections, although somewhat less common than the former.

Nosocomial bacteremia prolongs hospitalization, adding significantly to the cost, and is associated with significant morbidity and mortality. The reported frequency of intravascular device–associated bacteremia varies tremendously, depending on the device used, the duration of time in use, and the clinical setting. The incidence of bacteremia is 0.2% to 0.5% for intravenous peripheral catheters, up to 7% for central venous catheters utilized for total parenteral nutrition (TPN), and anywhere from 3.8% to 12% for central venous catheters utilized for fluid and monitoring (Elliott, 1988).

The cumulative incidence of infection episodes and bacteremia events increases for each vascular device in direct correlation with length of time the device is maintained. This is true for peripheral venous catheters as well as catheters in the superior vena cava or balloon-tipped pulmonary artery catheters. The same association is true with the peripheral arterial catheters commonly used for blood pressure monitoring, but this arterial device will not be discussed further.

Bacteremia

Although the risk of sepsis related to vascular catheters is less than 1%, more than 50,000 cases of nosocomial bacteremia occur each year in the United States related to the use of intravenous devices. A case fatality rate of 10% to 20% has been associated with catheter-related bacteremia (Corona et al, 1990). The morbidity and mortality of each patient's bacteremia is largely determined by underlying illness severity and the specific type of bacteria involved. If bacteremia results in the development of acute infective endocarditis, then mortality rates vary from 10% to 15% for Haemophilus species, to 30% to 60% for S. pneumoniae, to 60% to 90% for P. aeruginosa. The most common cause of acute infective endocarditis in the United States is S. aureus, with an associated mortality rate of 40%.

Enterococcal bacteremia has become more prevalent during the last decade. Heavy use of cephalosporin antibiotics for surgical prophylaxis is one primary reason for this rising incidence. Surgical patients and, in particular, patients in the surgical ICU setting, have an unusually high proportion of enterococci causing the bacteremia events. Enterococci were the most commonly isolated blood-borne pathogen in the surgical ICU in a study by Mainous et al (1997). Of 134 bacteremic episodes, 30% involved enterococci and one fourth of these were resistant to vancomycin. In addition, 29% of these episodes were polymicrobial, with Enterococcus being only one of the organisms identified. Only 2 of the 41 episodes were associated with infected vascular catheters. An abdominal source was responsible for the majority of the enterococcal bacteremias; however, a source was not identified in 20%. The mortality associated with enterococcal bacteremia was 40%.

In this study (Mainous et al, 1997), two thirds of the cases identified Enterococcus faecalis and one third identified E. faecium on culture. One hundred per cent of the E. faecalis isolates were sensitive to vancomycin, but 72% of the E. faecium isolates were resistant. Only 1 of 28 E. faecalis isolates was resistant to ampicillin, but 12 of 14 E. faecium isolates was resistant. Of the E. faecium isolates resistant to ampicillin and vancomycin, seven were tested for susceptibility to tetracycline and all seven were susceptible and responded to therapy with doxycycline. Enterococcus faecium has been associated with a higher mortality as compared to E. faecalis (Noskin et al, 1995). The E. faecium more commonly infected debilitated patients with underlying disease such as cancer, neutropenia, renal insufficiency, or ongoing corticosteroid therapy. In this population, enterococcal bacteremia usually arose from the urinary tract or an intra-abdominal focus of infection. Only the E. faecium isolates were found to be vancomycin resistant in this study. Thirteen per cent of the enterococcal bacteremias in this study arose from central venous catheters.

The potential sources of bacterial infection associated with intravascular devices are numerous. They are usually categorized by site, such as catheter hub, insertion site, tunnel, or catheter tip. The most common point at which bacteria gain access is at the catheter insertion site. There are many risk factors for vascular device–associated infection (Henderson, 1985), including

- Extremes of age (<1 year or >60 years)
- Neutropenia
- Immunosuppressive therapy
- Loss of skin integrity secondary to burns or psoriasis, underlying illnesses, failure of personnel to perform appropriate aseptic techniques, application of contaminated creams
- Contamination of infusate or monitoring equipment
- Excessive manipulation of the system
- Formation of a fibrin sheath around the device within a vessel
- Type and composition of the catheter

Most intravascular device–related infections continue to be due to staphylococci, both *S. aureus* and *S. epidermidis*, and yeasts (Hampton and Sherertz, 1988). Staphylococci are thought to account for one half to two thirds of all cases of catheter-associated bacteremia. More unusual isolates include *Klebsiella* species, *Enterobacter*, *Serratia*, *Candida*, *Pseudomonas*, and *Citrobacter*.

Diagnosis

Catheter-associated bacteremia may be difficult to diagnose with certainty. Signs of infections, such as localized erythema or edema, are present in only about 50% of patients. Prior to the development of the semiquantitative culture technique, most laboratories used the broth culture technique on the catheter's tip. This technique proved to be very unreliable because of the high false-positive rate. The semi-quantitative culture technique, as developed by Maki et al (1977), defines a positive catheter tip culture as yielding greater than or equal to 15 colonies of bacteria per catheter tip (Maki et al, 1977). A catheter tip that is positive utilizing the semiquantitative culture technique in the absence of local or systemic infection is said to be colonized. Maki et al (1977) defined a "catheter-related infection" as a positive catheter culture associated with a clinically apparent bacteremia or signs of a local infection. A "catheter-related" bacteremia is strictly defined as the identification of the same organism in a catheter culture specimen and in either a peripheral blood culture or positive blood culture specimen obtained from the catheter.

Peripheral Vascular Catheters

Numerous risk factors for catheter-associated infections have been identified for peripheral intravenous catheters, including the type of catheter used, location of the catheter, type of placement, duration of placement, and the skill of the person placing the catheter. Steel catheters, catheters that are placed peripherally, catheters that are placed percutaneously rather than via cut-down technique, catheters in the upper extremities, catheters that are left in place less than 72 hours, and catheters that are placed by an IV team all are associated with a decreased risk of infection (Henderson, 1985). Several authors have recommended the use of antimicrobial skin ointment over the catheter insertion site; however, no studies have clearly documented the efficacy of this practice (Maki and Band, 1981).

Central Venous Catheters

The use of central venous catheters is associated with numerous potential complications, including infection, pneumothorax, thrombosis of the subclavian vein or superior vena cava, and right-sided endocarditis. The infectious complications of the central venous catheter vary, depending on whether it is a short-term catheter, as is frequently used in ICUs, or a long-term catheter, as is primarily used for repeated vascular access in chemotherapy patients or patients requiring long-term TPN.

SHORT-TERM DEVICE

Numerous risk factors have been identified that predispose to catheter infections. These include duration of catheterization, severity of the underlying illness, type of catheter used, function of the catheter, and type of dressing (Corona et al, 1990). The duration of catheterization appears to be the most important risk factor for device-associated infection (Craven et al, 1988). Triple-lumen catheters and pulmonary artery catheters have been associated with an increased risk of infection compared with single-lumen central venous catheters (Pemberton et al, 1986; Hilton et al, 1988). The use of plastic transparent dressings may increase the risk of infection compared with traditional gauze dressings (Hampton and Sherertz, 1988).

The practice of changing catheters over a guide wire is controversial. Bozzetti et al (1983) and Snyder et al (1988) suggested that there is no increased incidence of catheter-related infection or colonization. Changing a central venous catheter over a guide wire does decrease the incidence of mechanical complications associated with insertion and is more comfortable for the patient. This approach is ideally used when a fever is being evaluated but no overt signs of catheter infection are evident. Removal of the existing catheter allows the tip to be cultured to assist in diagnosis. If infection is confirmed, the recently placed catheter should usually be removed again, and a new site used the next time. Venous catheter–related infection without severe sepsis syndrome is often best treated by simply removing the catheter.

Fever will often resolve within hours of catheter removal. Antibiotics are given if severe sepsis is present, if *S. aureus* is the cause, or if fever does not resolve within hours of removing the catheter. Culture results should guide therapy.

Empirical therapy should cover staphylococci using vancomycin. Coverage for gram-negative Enterobacteriaceae or *Pseudomonas* is advisable if the patient is quite ill or immunosuppressed. Good choices for these patients include vancomycin in combination with ceftazidime, or with imipenem, or with ticarcillin-clavulanate. If sepsis syndrome or fever persist despite the preceding measures, then a survey for distant sites of infection should be completed, with cultures repeated and held long enough to evaluate if yeast are present. *Staphylococcus aureus* infection demands urgent and aggressive therapy because of the danger of endocarditis and distant seeding of the infection causing abscesses. Antibiotics are always used for *S. aureus* infections, and continued for 4 to 6 days of total therapy.

LONG-TERM DEVICES

The use of long-term central venous access devices has increased considerably in the past few decades. In 1973, Broviac and colleagues reported their initial experience with the use of a long-term indwelling right atrial catheter. The Hickman modification of the Broviac catheter provided a larger internal diameter that facilitated blood drawing (Hickman et al, 1979). More recently, a totally implantable venous access device, the Port-A-Cath, has been introduced. The complications associated with these long-term vascular access devices include those related to insertion, infection, and thrombosis. The risk of thrombotic complications is thought to be virtually the same regardless of the type of device used. The incidence of clinically apparent thrombosis associated with these devices is thought to be less than 1%; however, many cases may remain unrecognized, because a large autopsy series showed evidence of thrombosis in 17% of patients (Reed et al, 1985). The percutaneous devices are more labor-intensive because they require frequent flushing with heparin, whereas the subcutaneous ports require only monthly flushing.

The incidence of infectious complications varies tremendously, depending on the patient population and the type of device. In non-neutropenic patients, infectious complications occur in fewer than 1% of patients. Unfortunately, this number increases significantly in neutropenic patients. Additionally, the infectious complications associated with the totally implantable access device (Port-A-Cath) reportedly are significantly less than that of the Broviac or Hickman percutaneous devices (Greene et al, 1988).

Three distinct types of infections have been associated with the use of long-term percutaneous central venous catheters (Broviac or Hickman): exit site infection, tunnel infection, and catheter tip infection.

Aside from catheter-related bacteremia, other important infectious complications include suppurative thrombophlebitis and endocarditis. Hickman catheter–related infections are caused by *S. epidermidis* in 54% of cases and by *S. aureus* in 20% of cases (Press et al, 1984). A similar study showed relatively similar rates of 31% for *S. epidermidis* and 14% for *S. aureus* (Clark and Raffin, 1990).

Exit Site Infection. This infection is characterized by localized erythema, edema, and purulent discharge at the entrance site of the catheter into the skin. The most common organism isolated is *S. epidermidis*. Exit site infection for a Hickman catheter can usually be treated with intravenous antibiotics and local care without removal of the catheter. Antibiotic therapy will be successful in 85% of cases (Press et al, 1984).

Tunnel Infections. These are more difficult to treat and are usually diagnosed clinically by the presence of erythema, edema, and pain in response to palpation along the subcutaneous course of the catheter. Frequently, the catheter must be removed because only 20% to 25% of these infections can be treated with antibiotics and local care alone (Benezra et al, 1988).

Catheter Tip Infection. This infection is diagnosed when either a single blood culture specimen from the catheter is positive for an organism not usually regarded as a contaminant or when two or more culture specimens from the catheter are positive for an organism usually regarded as contaminant. Catheter tip infections can usually be treated without removal of the catheter. The antibiotic is infused through the infected port. Treatment with antibiotics is continued for at least 10 days after a negative culture specimen is obtained. If the initial infection was with *Pseudomonas*, it is usually treated for 3 to 4 weeks following a negative culture. Pseudomonal infections and other polymicrobial infections are notably difficult to eradicate. It is recommended that the catheter be removed when exit site, tunnel, or catheter tip infections are polymicrobial or are due to pseudomonal infections.

GYNECOLOGIC CANCER COMPLICATED BY INFECTION

Patients with gynecologic malignancies have long been recognized as patients at high risk for development of infection. Infection may be a direct consequence of progressive disease complicated by bowel fistulization, ureteral obstruction, or cellulitis originating in necrotic tumor. Infection also occurs as a complication of surgery or chemotherapy. These patients frequently undergo multiple hospitalizations and multiple procedures, with exposure to antibiotic-resistant pathogens.

Incidence

A retrospective survey of infectious morbidity on a gynecologic oncology service was performed on serial admissions during 1982 at the University of Minnesota. The average for these patients was three admissions each, and 11% of the patients had a serious infection diagnosed during admission. Admissions most often complicated by infection were surgical. The infectious complication rate (22%) was the highest in patients with cervical cancer undergoing operation. The postoperative infection rate for patients with uterine, ovarian, and vulvar cancer was 11% to 12% (Brooker et al, 1987).

Culture results showed that most infections were polymicrobial, and both aerobic gram-positive and gram-negative organisms and multiple anaerobes were involved. When pelvic cellulitis, peritonitis, pneumonia, pelvic abscess, or sepsis was diagnosed, organisms frequently encountered were *Pseudomonas*, *Enterobacter*, enterococci, *Candida*, *Clostridium*, and *Bacteroides*.

In 1986, a prospective study was performed at the University of Michigan on a gynecologic oncology service to assess the incidence of infection developing during hospitalization (McNeeley et al, 1990). One hundred nine infections occurred during 510 admissions, for a nosocomial infection rate of 21%. Urinary tract and wound infections were the most common. Reasons for admission included surgery, chemotherapy, and radiation treatment.

Pathogens

The most common organism isolated by culture was *E. coli*; *P. aeruginosa*, *Enterococcus*, and *S. epidermidis* were the next most frequent organisms identified. A comparison group of gynecology patients without cancer admitted to the same hospital during the same period was studied. Differences in occurrence of organisms were noted; *P. aeruginosa* caused 15% of infections for oncology patients but only 3% of the infections in gynecology patients without cancer. More importantly, the benign disease gynecology patients uniformly had gentamicin-sensitive *Pseudomonas*, whereas oncologic patients had gentamicin-resistant *Pseudomonas* in 25% of cases and another 36% had only intermediate sensitivity to gentamicin. Similarly, staphylococci were isolated from both patient groups; however, the strains of coagulase-negative staphylococci from oncologic patients were uniformly resistant to all antibiotics except vancomycin, but the strains from the benign gynecologic patients had a 20% sensitivity rate to penicillin. When only the surgical admissions were reviewed, infection developed in 28% of patients. An additional 14% were clinically diagnosed with infections, but a culture specimen was not obtainable (i.e., pelvic cellulitis), for a total infection rate of 42% being treated with antibiotics.

Risk Factors

Infection rates of this magnitude are understandable when one considers the effect of malignancy, the effect of treatment on the host, and exposure of the host to resistant pathogens during the hospital admissions. The effect of malignancy is to depress the immune response for both humoral and cytotoxic mechanisms. Treatment of malignancy with chemotherapy or radiotherapy may alter barrier defenses, predisposing to invasion by organisms. The extended surgical procedures for cancer are associated with extensive dissection and increased numbers of surgical pedicles. Each pedicle has some tissue necrosis and is easily infected if contaminated. Operative site serous effusions provide growth media for bacteria. Surgical procedures in cancer patients are frequently of extended duration when compared with benign gynecologic procedures and may involve multiple contamination sites when the urinary or gastrointestinal tract is entered.

When compared with simple extrafascial hysterectomy, postoperative infections are more common after the surgical procedures of oophorectomy with radical cytoreduction of ovary cancer, radical hysterectomy, radical vulvectomy, or pelvic exenteration. Infections that do occur may be more difficult to treat because of antibiotic-resistant organisms or because the patient is immunocompromised. Immunosuppression may be due to radiotherapy, chemotherapy, or malnutrition or may be related to medical conditions such as diabetes and renal failure. Reported incidence of severe postoperative infections, such as pelvic cellulitis or abscess, varies with the year of report. Over time, decreased infection rates reflect changes in surgical technique, the availability of improved antibiotics, and the recognition of the value of prophylactic antibiotics.

Despite these improvements, infectious complications still occur. Urinary diversion by creation of a urinary conduit can cause great infectious morbidity and mortality if a conduit anastomosis leak occurs. Delayed complications after a pelvic exenteration include pelvic abscess, sepsis, and bowel fistulization. Fistulization has historically occurred in 10% to 20% of patients.

Operative Infections in Gynecologic Oncology

Pelvic Exenteration

Tissue damage after therapeutic irradiation complicates surgery primarily because of microvascular damage. Poor healing increases the rates of fistulization and anastomotic breakdown in resected bowel or urinary system tissues treated to standard doses, and fistulization may occur after even minimal surgical manipulation of tissues that previously received high doses of radiation. As a group, gastrointestinal complications continue to be the most common complications requiring reoperation for irradiated patients who undergo exenteration.

Symmonds et al (1975) reviewed their experience with postoperative complications after pelvic exenteration. Of these patients, 31% had not received prior radiotherapy. Of 198 patients operated on between 1950 and 1971, infectious morbidity appears to have been the most frequent type of complication. Wound infection occurred in 14%, pelvic abscess in 4%, urinary infection in 11%, peritonitis or septicemia in 4%, "chest infection" in 3%, and bowel fistulization in 13%. Operative mortality was 8%, with improvement to 3% during the later portion of the series. Bowel complications of obstruction and fistula were considered the most common and most serious complications for exenteration patients. When fistulization occurs, nutrition and secondary infection are significant problems.

Morgan et al (1980) reviewed 46 exenteration patients for evidence of infectious morbidity. These patients had been treated between 1970 and 1978. None had received preoperative systemic antibiotics, but all had undergone a preoperative bowel preparation. The bowel preparation was a combined mechanical and oral antibiotic regimen. The oral antibiotics for the bowel preparation were either sulfasuxidine with neomycin, or erythromycin with neomycin. The pelvic and perineal defects were managed by leaving a pelvic pack in the open defect in 89% (41) of the patients. The pack was supposed to prevent bowel herniation and contamination in the early postoperative period. It was hoped that, by leaving the perineal wound open, the incidence of operative site abscess and cellulitis would be reduced. Of these 46 patients, 70% developed pelvic cellulitis, as diagnosed on postoperative days 2 to 30. Organisms most frequently obtained from culture of the operative site pelvic infections were *Bacteroides* species, *Peptostreptococcus, S. epidermidis, E. coli, Proteus* species, and enterococci. After patients with asymptomatic bacteriuria were excluded, 21 patients (46%) were categorized as having a major infectious morbidity. Two or more major infections in the same patient occurred in 11 of 46 patients. Specific infections in order of decreasing incidence were as follows

1. Pelvic wound infections in 67% of patients overall and "major" pelvic infections in 20% of patients
2. Abdominal wound infections in 28% and "major" abdominal wound infections in 20%, including two subfascial infections with dehiscence and one necrotizing fasciitis
3. Pyelonephritis in 15%
4. Septicemia in 15%
5. Pneumonia in 7%

Another large series of exenterations was reported by Rutledge et al (1977), covering a similar time period (1955 to 1976) and including 296 patients. During the first 90 days after surgery, sepsis was responsible for most deaths. In this series, 22% of procedures were done as primary therapy, that is, there was no preceding or concomitant radiotherapy. Additional reports have shown septicemia (21%) to be the most common postoperative complication from exenteration and usually to be due to acute urinary tract infection (Morley and Lindenauer, 1976). Postoperative mortality was 1.4%. Marked changes in technique reduced the rate of complications during the study. Significant advances included preoperative bowel preparation, preoperative antibiotic prophylaxis, use of isolated urinary conduits, creation of urinary colon conduits instead of ileal conduits, intraoperative stenting of ureteral conduit anastomoses, hyperalimentation, perioperative intensive care, and better management of the pelvic basin with peritoneal or omental coverage to avoid abscess and bowel complication. Primary closure of the perineal defect, self-suction drains, and primary reconstruction of the vagina have been further improvements in management used recently.

PROCEDURE MODIFICATIONS AND REDUCED INFECTION

Soper et al (1989) reported on the surgical morbidity of 69 pelvic exenteration patients treated between 1970 and 1987. Pelvic cellulitis was noted in 17%, pyelonephritis in 13%, wound infection or separation in 12%, and pneumonia in 3%. In the later part of this series, decreased morbidity was noted in patients for whom a transverse colon conduit was created instead of an ileal or sigmoid urinary conduit. Immediate pelvic reconstruction using gracilis myocutaneous flaps was also associated with fewer complications than when pelvic packs were left in the pelvic defect.

INTESTINAL COMPLICATIONS AND INFECTION

The Jackson Memorial Hospital/University of Miami Medical Center experience, with 92 pelvic exenterations done between 1966 and 1981, showed gastrointestinal complication rates of fistulization in 16% and obstruction in 5% (Averette et al, 1984). Fistulization uniformly was from small bowel adherent to the pelvic floor operative site. Surgical correction of a fistula was associated with a 40% mortality. Only 2 of 15 (13%) fistulas healed with conservative management, thereby avoiding reoperation. Morley and Lindenauer (1976) reported that, in 7% of cases (5 of 70), fistulas developed, and they noted the association of pelvic abscess preceding fistulization. Irradiated small bowel lying in the inflammatory exudate of the pelvic basin and in the site of pelvic cellulitis has long been the explanation for the high fistula rates associated with this procedure (Morley and Lindenauer, 1976; Rutledge et al, 1977).

As causes of fistula, even greater importance is given to anastomotic leak at points of bowel resection in these previously irradiated patients. The report from the University of Alabama (Orr et al, 1983) reviewed 125 pelvic exenterations in preirradiated patients performed from 1969 to 1981. Gastrointestinal complications accounted for 60% of all nonmalignant indications for reoperation. To create a urinary conduit, bowel resection with reanastomosis was performed in 120 patients. Conduits were constructed from distal ileum (83%), transverse colon (14%), and sigmoid colon (2.5%). Stapled anastomoses were associated with a fistula rate of 6.6% and sutured anastomoses fistulized at a rate of 10%. Postoperative fistulas developed in 18 patients; nine were rectovaginal fistulas occurring after an anterior exenteration. A small-bowel fistula developed in 10 patients (8% of exenterations). All had undergone urinary diversion by ileal conduit, for a rate of 10% (10/100) after ileal conduit. In contrast, none of 20 patients with colon conduits developed a small-bowel fistula.

Avoiding resection and reanastomosis of irradiated small bowel appears to be even more important than the method of anastomosis when one considers methods to avoid anastomotic breakdown. To minimize fistulization and all the secondary infectious complications of a fistula, it is imperative to isolate the small bowel from the denuded pelvic basin, to avoid resection and reanastomosis of irradiated bowel, and to reduce postoperative pelvic cellulitis to a minimum. Reduction of local cellulitis can best be accomplished by using preoperative bowel preparation and prophylactic antibiotics, proper drains, and primary perineal closure. Orr et al (1983) reported that using these techniques also reduced the risk of abscess or pelvic cellulitis from 33% to 19% and the rate of wound infection from 17% to 7%.

Radical Hysterectomy

For patients undergoing radical hysterectomy, Lerner et al (1980) reported a 14% rate of significant postoperative infections. No prophylactic antibiotics were routinely used. Specific infections in 108 patients were cuff cellulitis in 1%, pelvic abscess in 2%, wound infection in 3%, and urinary tract infection in 9%. Similarly, Sotto (1990) reported that, of 627 patients undergoing radical hysterectomy between 1961 and 1989, infection was the most common postoperative complication, occurring in 24%. The most common sites of infection were the urinary tract in 14%, followed by the incision site in 5.5% and the operative site in 4.7%. This infection rate occurred despite prophylactic antibiotics. The most commonly used prophylactic regimens were chloramphenicol plus gentamicin plus metronidazole *or* the combination of chloramphenicol plus metronidazole.

These rates are typical of reports from other low-risk populations who undergo radical hysterectomy; however, most published reports have been retrospective, and seldom was the purpose of the review to find infectious morbidity. The purpose of the studies was usually to identify cure rates or fistula rates, and the reviews are therefore unlikely to represent a true incidence of the more common and less complicated infections of cuff cellulitis or pelvic cellulitis.

ANTIBIOTIC PROPHYLAXIS

Incidence of postoperative pelvic cellulitis appears to vary markedly between patient populations, with some investigators reporting less than 1% without prophylaxis and others a rate of 25% to 30% in studies done to evaluate infectious morbidity. Ayhan et al (1991), reviewing 270 cases of radical hysterectomy for complications, reported the most common infection to be a urinary tract infection (6%), with wound infection in 3.5% and pelvic infection in 2.2%. Fever of unknown origin was seen in 3.5%. All patients in this report received prophylactic antibiotics consisting of either ampicillin with gentamicin or clindamycin with amikacin. These regimens were continued for 48 hours after surgery.

Sevin et al (1991) reported a randomized, double-blind, prospective comparison of cefoxitin prophylaxis in patients undergoing radical hysterectomy. Patients received either one dose preoperatively plus two doses postoperatively or three doses preoperatively plus nine doses of postoperative extended prophylaxis. Operative site infections in the pelvis or incisional wound occurred in 6% of 113 study patients, with no differences between the randomized arms. Extended prophylaxis does not seem to add additional protection beyond doses confined to the immediate perioperative time. Of note, despite prophylaxis, urinary tract infections still occurred in 32% of patients. This same group of investigators had performed a previous placebo-controlled, randomized, double-blind, prospective study using cefoxitin-extended prophylaxis before and after radical hysterectomy. That study showed a 52% surgical infection rate without prophylaxis (Sevin et al, 1984) and a significantly decreased ($p = 0.005$) rate of infection (15%) in the cefoxitin arm. The rate of pelvic cellulitis was 6 of 27 (22%) in the placebo group and none of 26 in the cefoxitin group. Infections other than surgical site infections were also decreased ($p < 0.05$).

Mann et al (1981) reported on 207 radical hysterectomy patients reviewed retrospectively for infectious morbidity. For patients who received prophylaxis, a cephalosporin was most often used. Of 172 patients receiving prophylactic antibiotics, pelvic cellulitis or abscess occurred in 7%. Of 35 patients not receiving prophylactic antibiotics, 20% developed pelvic cellulitis or abscess. Of all significant infections diagnosed, the most common were urinary tract (28%), pelvic cellulitis (23%), wound (13%), pelvic abscess (8%), and pneumonia (13%).

A more recent study by Fuchtner et al (1992) included 135 patients treated by radical hysterectomy from 1980 to 1989. Prophylactic antibiotics and pelvic self-suction drains were used. This retrospective study matched 45 patients over the age of 65 with a control group under age 65. The control group was chosen as the next two consecutive patients age younger than 65 admitted for radical hysterectomy after each elderly study patient. Overall infectious morbidity was 38% in the elderly group and 39% in the young group. Surgical site infections in the pelvis or wound occurred in 11% of the elderly group and in 10% of the young group. There were no differences noted on the basis of age.

Prospective randomized studies have not always shown a proven benefit for prophylactic antibiotics prior to radical hysterectomy. Those studies showing no benefit were usually small groups of study subjects, and limited statistically (Rosenshein et al, 1983; Marsden et al, 1985). The reported rates of significant surgical site infections after radical hysterectomy despite prophylactic antibiotics confirm that this procedure is at least as likely to cause postoperative infection as is simple abdominal hysterectomy.

Radical Vulvectomy

For patients undergoing radical vulvectomy, wound breakdown and wound infection continue to be the most frequent complications (Hacker et al, 1981). Recent progress confirms that modified radical vulvectomy procedures, and radical vulvectomy using three-incision techniques for the vulvar and groin lymphadenectomy portions of the operation, have both reduced the wound breakdown and wound infection rates. Nevertheless, infection may be a significant contributor to wound separation.

Recurrent lymphangitis and cellulitis may occur in radical vulvectomy patients who develop chronic leg edema. Prophylaxis for streptococcal skin infections of the lower extremity has been recommended. Daily oral penicillin or erythromycin is suggested.

Nonoperative Infections in Gynecologic Oncology

Infection in Neutropenic Cancer Patients

Gram-negative bacteremia in neutropenic patients was usually lethal prior to the availability of modern antibiotics. It was associated with a mortality rate of 90% in the 1950s. The mortality fell to 10% to 30% during the 1980s as a result of availability of improved broad-spectrum antibiotics coupled with the recognition that reduced mortality was dependent on empirical emergency administration of these agents (Hathorn, 1997).

DEFINITION

Neutropenia is classically defined as less than 500 to 1000 granulocytes/mm^3. Definitions for fever and neutropenia have been provided by the Infectious Diseases Society of America in the 1997 report on guidelines for care of neutropenic patients with

unexplained fever (Hughes et al, 1997). Fever is present if a single oral temperature is measured greater than 38.3°C (101°F), or persists at 38.0°C (100.4°F) or greater for at least 1 hour's duration. Neutropenia is defined as a neutrophil count less than 500/mm^3, or less than 1000/mm^3 when it can be predicted to fall to 500/mm^3 or less.

Neutropenia occurs almost entirely as an iatrogenic event resulting from cytotoxic chemotherapy. The incidence of neutropenia is increasing with the use of more aggressive chemotherapeutic regimens. Neutropenia is associated with an increased incidence of infection, which in turn leads to markedly increased morbidity and mortality if the patient is not treated appropriately. Incidence of infection during neutropenia not only increases as the absolute granulocyte count decreases but also is associated with the rapidity of the fall in the absolute granulocyte count as well as with the duration of neutropenia. Although the incidence of infection is increased with granulocyte counts below 1000/mm^3, it rises more sharply with counts below 500/mm^3 and yet even further with counts below 100/mm^3 (Bodey et al, 1966).

For all patients receiving myelosuppresive chemotherapy, blood counts should be determined at the anticipated nadir period following administration of therapy. If severe neutropenia begins, counts should be observed every few days until values rise. Patients who are neutropenic (<500 granulocytes/mm^3) should take their temperature at home every 6 to 12 hours and contact their physician immediately if body temperature is greater than 38.0°C (100.4°F). Patients should not be hospitalized because of neutropenia alone, because this does nothing but expose them to hospital-acquired pathogens that are potentially resistant to multiple antibiotics. Additionally, the patient should be instructed to avoid contact with people who are known to have contagious diseases. Not all neutropenic patients with infection have fever; therefore, other signs of sepsis should be taken seriously.

Febrile patients with neutropenia need prompt evaluation. Work-up includes a thorough history; physical examination to evaluate for a specific site of infection and for evidence of sepsis syndrome; routine laboratory evaluation, including complete blood count and platelet count; urinalysis and urine culture; chest film, and blood culture from at least two different sites. If a patient has an indwelling Hickman or Broviac catheter, at least one set of blood culture specimens is obtained from the catheter.

Evidence of sepsis may be subtle. The examining physician should be aware of increased heart rate, elevated respiratory rate, widened pulse pressure, or a change in mental status as suggested by confusion or lethargy. More obvious findings include skin lesions, abnormal lung sounds, flank tenderness over the kidneys, inflammation at intravenous catheter sites, or evidence of a perianal abscess. The oropharynx should be checked for gingival or tonsillar abscesses. A lumbar puncture would be indicated if there is evidence of mental status change or specific central nervous system signs such as headache, nuchal rigidity, or photophobia. A CT scan of the head is indicated prior to the lumbar puncture to exclude metastatic disease or evidence of elevated intracranial pressure.

Unfortunately, there is usually no readily identifiable source of infection. The clinical findings in patients with neutropenia and fever are usually very subtle because there is a blunted inflammatory response (Sickles et al, 1975). It is not unusual for the patient to have normal pulmonary exam findings yet have an infiltrate clearly demonstrated on the chest radiograph. The most common source of infection in patients with neutropenia and fever is the gastrointestinal tract. Therefore, it is not surprising that the most common isolates from blood cultures in these patients are gram-negative rods, although nationally there is an increasing incidence of infection caused by gram-positive cocci associated with indwelling catheters (Hughes et al, 1990).

In one large study from the Memorial Sloan-Kettering Cancer Center, 16% of all isolates were *E. coli*, 15% were *Klebsiella*, 8% were *Pseudomonas*, 6% were *S. aureus*, and 21% were polymicrobial (Whimbey et al, 1987). Other common organisms include coagulase-negative staphylococci, *Enterococcus* species, *S. pneumoniae*, *S. pyogenes*, and the viridans streptococcus group. Sixty to 70% of those infections documented by culture are now caused by gram-positive organisms, and many are methicillin resistant (Hughes, 1997). Only 10% to 20% of patients with fever and neutrophil counts $\leq 100/mm^3$ have positive blood cultures (Hughes et al, 1997). It is thought that the remainder of the patients probably do have some degree of bacteremia; however, the inoculum is considered to be insufficient to cultivate the organisms with our current culture techniques. Only 20% to 30% of febrile neutropenic patients will have a specific site of infection identified.

TREATMENT

Immediately following initial evaluation, empirical antibiotic therapy should be promptly initiated in all patients with neutropenia and fever (Table 36–16). Delay of therapy may allow infection to disseminate and cause increased mortality. This should be considered a medical emergency, and therapy should not be withheld pending the results of blood culture or the development of an obvious source of infection on physical examination. These patients are admitted for observation and antibiotic therapy. Current therapy for patients with neutropenia and fever usually employs two antibiotics that are active against *Pseudomonas*, but broad-spectrum coverage is required. Additional anaerobic coverage is prudent if perianal inflammation or gingivitis is found. Once antibiotic sensitivity data from cultures is available, the antibiotic therapy can then be tailored as appro-

---

Table 36–16. EMPIRICAL ANTIBIOTIC REGIMENS FOR FEBRILE NEUTROPENIA

Monotherapy
    Ceftazidime
    Imipenem-cilastatin
Dual-agent therapy
    Ceftazidime and aminoglycoside*
    Ceftazidime and vancomycin
    Ticarcillin-clavulanate and aminoglycoside
    Piperacillin-tazobactam and aminoglycoside
    Levofloxacin (or other quinolone) and aminoglycoside

*Substitute aztreonam for aminoglycoside if poor renal function or recent therapy with cisplatin.

---

priate. Antibiotics are continued until the granulocyte count has increased above 500 cells/mm^3 and the patient is afebrile and clinically stable.

Numerous effective regimens have been employed for patients with neutropenia and fever, and it is imperative that the physician know the particular sensitivity patterns of his or her locale. Patients are treated with intravenous antibiotics, including ceftazidime or imipenem-cilastatin as single-agent therapies, or dual-agent therapies using an aminoglycoside combined with either an antipseudomonal penicillin or ceftazidime. An alternative dual-agent therapy combines vancomycin with ceftazidime (Hughes et al, 1997). Aztreonam is considered in place of the aminoglycoside for any patient with impaired renal function. Aztreonam is also a good choice for patients who have recently received cisplatin because the nephrotoxicity caused by cisplatin and by aminoglycosides are synergistic. Quinolone antibiotics could be used instead of ceftazidime or a penicillin for patients with a severe β-lactam allergy, but need to be combined with an aminoglycoside.

Several reports have recommended single-agent empirical antibiotic therapy incorporating either a third-generation cephalosporin with antipseudomonal activity, such as ceftazidime, or a carbapenem, such as imipenem or meropenem. The primary argument favoring monotherapy is that monotherapy is equally effective when compared to combination therapy, but it is associated with decreased toxicity and lower cost. Unfortunately, most of the studies to date include small numbers and many are poorly designed. Additionally, in some studies patients initially treated with monotherapy were switched to combination therapy. These monotherapies do not provide coverage for coagulase-negative staphylococci, methicillin-resistant *S. aureus* (MRSA), enterococci, or viridans streptococci (Hughes et al, 1997). Therefore, most authorities recommend empirical therapy with at least two agents. A patient who is severely ill at presentation may be best treated with agents providing the best gram-positive and the best pseudomonal and gram-negative bacillary coverage at the very onset of therapy.

Imipenem-cilastatin has been compared to ceftazidime in empirical single-agent therapy for neutropenic febrile patients. Each agent had a 98% or greater success rate, and no difference was found in rate of relapse, incidence of superinfections, or need to add vancomycin or an aminoglycoside. Superinfection occurred in 22% of patients treated with either agent. Imipenem-cilastatin caused *C. difficile* colitis in 11%, where as ceftazidime caused this complication in only 4%. Imipenem is more likely to cause nausea and vomiting, more likely to cause seizures, and will need dose reduction if renal function is poor. Institutions with a long history of heavy use of ceftazidime may now have a local pattern of acquired resistance to ceftazidime. Some studies have shown febrile neutropenia patients to have a significantly higher clinical response rate to imipenem/cilastatin than to ceftazidime, but study results have not been uniform.

The primary arguments favoring combination therapy include the synergy of a β-lactam and an aminoglycoside against *Pseudomonas* and a decreased incidence of *Pseudomonas* developing resistance to a single agent during treatment (Davis, 1982). Regimens using two drugs are usually used to provide synergistic activity, prevent emergence of resistance during therapy, and ensure coverage of the full range of aerobic gram-negative organisms as well as coverage for anaerobes and gram-positive organisms. Studies show little difference in efficacy of various regimens. Dual-agent therapy most commonly uses an aminoglycoside, such as gentamicin or tobramycin, combined with an antipseudomonal penicillin or an antipseudomonal cephalosporin such as ceftazidime. The antipseudomonal penicillins include piperacillin, mezlocillin, and ticarcillin. Ticarcillin ideally is given in combination with clavulanic acid.

The recent increase in gram-positive organisms causing infection during neutropenia has generated argument for including vancomycin in the empirical first-line regimen given to these febrile neutropenic patients. Many of these gram-positive organisms can cause a rapidly lethal sepsis and many are resistant to all antibiotics except vancomycin. At institutions with a high incidence of gram-positive infections, or for patients with a high risk of gram-positive infections, such as where an indwelling vascular catheter is likely to be infected or if quinolone antibiotic prophylaxis was given, then vancomycin is justifiable as initial therapy. Neutropenic patients who receive a quinolone antibiotic as prophylaxis against infection during neutropenia have a lower incidence of gram-negative infections and a disproportionately high fraction of gram-positive infections. The empirical regimen is then streamlined as soon as culture data allow, and should be discontinued in 3 to 4 days if no evidence of infection is found. The recommended vancomycin-containing regimen for empirical therapy is vancomycin with ceftazidime (Hughes et al, 1997).

Most patients treated appropriately with empirical antibiotics for febrile neutropenia will become afe-brile in 2 to 7 days. If no organism has been identified after 7 days of treatment with the initial regimen, then antibiotics are stopped, providing that the neutrophil count has recovered to $500/mm^3$ or greater and all signs of infection have resolved. If an organism is cultured, then treatment is streamlined while maintaining coverage based on sensitivities and toxicity. However, therapy should remain broad-spectrum. It should continue for a minimum of 7 days and is stopped only with the same provisions given for those patients with negative cultures.

A group of low-risk neutropenic patients has been described. These patients are neutropenic with fever, show no signs of sepsis at admission, have no identifiable specific site of infection, are culture negative, and become afebrile within 48 hours of starting intravenous therapy. For this low-risk group, conversion to an oral regimen to complete the full course of therapy can be considered. Recommended regimens for this oral therapy include cefixime, ciprofloxacin or ofloxacin, clindamycin with ciprofloxacin, or amoxicillin–clavulanic acid plus pefloxacin (Hughes et al, 1997). Patients such as this are at low risk for complications, and could be considered for release from the hospital under careful outpatient surveillance to complete oral antibiotic therapy.

If clinical deterioration is noted during the initial several days of empirical therapy, then vancomycin is added if not currently being given, and broad-spectrum antipseudomonal gram-negative bacillary coverage is enhanced if not optimal. Serum levels of the aminoglycosides are checked to confirm adequate dosing.

Patients with neutropenia and fever who fail to respond to empirical antibiotic therapy after 72 hours should be considered for the addition of vancomycin to provide additional activity against resistant gram-positive cocci, particularly staphylococci. Patients who fail to respond should be closely monitored with serial cultures and repeat examination. New blood cultures may show emergence of resistant organisms or a new superinfection. Failing to find a new explanation for persistent fever should suggest a systemic fungal infection because up to one third of febrile neutropenic patients who fail to respond to 7 days of antibiotic therapy will have disseminated *Candida* or *Aspergillus* infections (Pizzo et al, 1982). In that setting, continuation of current antibiotics and addition of amphotericin B is considered.

Recommended practice guidelines (Hughes et al, 1997) suggest stopping antibiotics after treatment day 7 if the patient is afebrile and has a neutrophil count above $500/mm^3$. If the neutropenia persists but the patient becomes afebrile, it is reasonable to stop systemic antibiotics if the patient has been afebrile for 5 to 7 days, appears clinically well, and shows no laboratory or radiographic evidence of infection.

Patients who fail to respond to proper initial therapy within 4 to 7 days should be suspected of having a fungal infection, and antifungal therapy should be strongly considered. Fungal infection should be suspected if neutrophil counts have recovered to above 500/mm^3 but fever continues despite proper antibiotic therapy. CT scan of the abdomen may show lesions in the liver, spleen, or kidneys. If no lesions are found, antibiotics can be stopped despite fever if neutrophil counts are above 500/mm^3.

FUNGAL INFECTION

There are numerous risk factors for the development of systemic candidiasis, including prolonged duration (>7 days) of broad-spectrum antibiotic therapy, central venous catheters, recent surgery, neutropenia, immunosuppressive therapy, and central hyperalimentation (Marsh et al, 1983). The two main mechanisms involved include colonization of a central venous catheter as well as colonization and overgrowth in the gastrointestinal tract. Yeast is frequently isolated from the urine or from a throat culture in patients with neutropenia and fever. The decision then becomes whether this represents invasive disease or simply colonization. It is generally accepted that all patients with blood cultures positive for yeast have systemic candidiasis or invasive disease, and that patients in whom yeast is isolated from at least three peripheral sources (throat, urine, or wound culture) also probably have an invasive or a systemic form of candidiasis.

All patients with evidence of systemic candidiasis, as well as those patients with neutropenia and fever who have failed to respond to broad-spectrum antibiotics for 5 to 7 days, should then be treated with systemic antifungals. The treatment of choice is amphotericin B, 0.5 to 1.0 mg/kg/day. All patients should be treated to a total dose of amphotericin B of at least 15 mg/kg. Most authorities now recommend the lower daily dose (0.5 mg/kg/day) because it is thought to be just as efficacious as the higher dose but with decreased toxicity. The decision whether to continue the broad-spectrum antibiotics once antifungal therapy is initiated is a difficult one. More than 50% of patients with systemic candidiasis have a simultaneous bacteremia. Alternative therapies for fungal infections in specific circumstances include flucytosine as well as fluconazole.

GRANULOCYTE COLONY-STIMULATING FACTOR

Routine use of granulocyte colony-stimulating factor (G-CSF) is not recommended for febrile neutropenia episodes. Certain situations may warrant use of G-CSF during neutropenic fever, such as when it is possible to predict worsening or prolonged duration of neutropenia. G-CSF is indicated in the setting of neutropenia complicated by pneumonia, hypotensive sepsis, systemic fungal infection, severe cellulitis or sinusitis, multisystem failure resulting from sepsis,

or neutropenic infection failing to respond to antibiotics (Hughes et al, 1997).

Pyometra

Incidence of pyometra related to gynecologic cancers of the uterus and cervix can be estimated from several large series of patients who underwent preoperative evaluation with CT or MRI scans. Not all cases of pyometra or intrauterine fluid are related to malignancy. Carlson et al (1991) reported 20 postmenopausal patients with intrauterine fluid detected by ultrasound, and only one endometrial cancer and one cervical cancer were identified. However, three other gynecologic malignancies of the upper tract were noted. The benign cases included uterine leiomyomata and benign ovarian tumors. Small fluid accumulations within the uterus may be asymptomatic until initiation of radiotherapy, at which time active infection may occur. These intrauterine fluid collections should be recognized before initiation of treatment so as to avoid interruption of radiotherapy while infection is being treated.

Five-year survival rates have been lower in patients with cervical cancer who have pyometra than in those without pyometra. When a pyometra recurs after completion of radiotherapy or when it first develops after radiotherapy, persistent disease in the endometrial cavity has been found in 78% of cases (Yu and Yan, 1987). Of 11,284 patients treated by radiotherapy for cervix cancer, 282 pyometras were encountered, for an incidence rate of 2.5% of cervical cancers. However, this series spanned the years 1958 to 1980, and it is unlikely that all pyometras were recognized prior to the availability of accurate ultrasound and CT diagnoses.

In a similar report by Suzuki (1989), a 16% incidence of pyometra was noted among 251 cases of cervical cancer when pretreatment evaluation included imaging with CT or MRI. An unusual pyometra has been reported. It developed postoperatively after second-trimester hysterotomy performed for a patient with a stage IIb squamous carcinoma of the cervix. The pyometra developed because of the procedure prior to initiation of radiotherapy (Saunders and Landon, 1988).

When a patient with a gynecologic malignancy presents with a pyometra, the primary therapy is drainage by dilatation of the cervix and placement of a drain, such as a Malecot catheter or pediatric Foley catheter, until the patient is afebrile and drainage has ceased. In my experience, some of these patients present with signs of infection consistent with pelvic cellulitis. In this situation broad-spectrum antibiotics, as used for other pelvic infections, are indicated. It is appropriate to avoid curettage or biopsy when one is initially draining the pyometra for fear of perforation that might cause bowel injury or infectious contamination of the peritoneal cavity. After drainage and antibiotics, the patient usually can be sampled in an outpatient setting with a suction catheter at a later date if confirmation of malignancy in the endometrial cavity is required. Most pyometras related to gynecologic malignancy are associated with advanced-stage disease, such as stages II through IV cervical cancer. An occasional patient with endometrial cancer and concomitant cervical stenosis will present with a pyometra or hemato-metra and a markedly enlarged uterus. Concomitant problems frequently include ureteral obstruction, and any patient who does not promptly respond to therapy should be investigated for pyelonephritis above the urinary obstruction.

Drug-Induced Fever

Cancer patients are frequently exposed to medications that may cause fever. Fever accompanies drug reactions in up to 10% of inpatients but may be the only feature of a drug reaction in 3% to 5% of cases (Lipsky and Hirschman, 1981; Cunha, 1986). A fever is thought to be drug-induced if no other cause is evident, and if the temperature elevation is temporally associated with drug administration, or if the fever disappears within 72 hours of stopping the drug. Fever caused by a drug reaction will only rarely be associated with an elevated heart rate, unlike the tachycardia associated with fever caused by a true infection.

Drug fevers are often attributed to hypersensitivity reactions. This type of reaction is often delayed for several days into therapy and may be associated with eosinophilia. Eosinophilia occurs in 10% to 20% of cases of drug-induced fever. Another mechanism for drug-induced fever is red blood cell hemolysis caused by drugs acting as oxidants in patients with glucose-6-phosphate dehydrogenase deficiency. This inherited defect occurs most commonly in Asian and Mediterranean populations. Drugs that can cause hemolysis by this method include nitrofurantoins, sulfonamides, antimalarial agents, and antitubercular drugs.

Antibiotics are one of the most frequent drugs producing fever as a result of a hypersensitivity response (Caldwell and Cluff, 1974; Mackowiak, 1987). Penicillin and cephalosporin antibiotics are the most commonly responsible medications. Fever may also be seen with clindamycin and trimethoprim-sulfamethoxazole. New formulations of vancomycin are less likely to cause fever. Amphotericin B is also associated with fever.

Cytotoxic chemotherapy agents are also causes of drug-induced fever, and the onset is often the same day. Bleomycin predictably causes a temperature elevation after administration. Other chemotherapy agents responsible for fever include mithramycin, dacarbazine, methotrexate, vincristine, daunomycin, and cyclophosphamide. Adriamycin occasionally causes a temperature.

Cancer patients with hypercalcemia have been treated with pamidronate, and transient temperature elevations of greater than 1°C are seen in up to 25%

of patients. Occasional temperature elevations of 2° to 3°C have been seen, occurring within the first 24 to 48 hours after administration of a single dose. This fever is transient, and patients do not appear infected.

Drug-induced fever may not appear until 3 to 7 days into therapy. It usually resolves in 48 hours after the offending agent is discontinued unless excretion or metabolism is delayed. Fever may be either of low grade or as high as 43°C. The pattern is often associated with diurnal variation. Patients may have sepsis associated with rigors, leukocytosis to as high as 20,000 WBCs/mm³, and a left shift. Other findings may include myalgias, arthralgias, and headache. Helpful findings that suggest a hypersensitivity reaction include rash and hives. Patients treated with antibiotics for infection may have persistent fever after the infection has cleared. When a patient with a fever has been receiving antibiotics since very early in the postoperative course with no obvious source of infection, the diagnosis of drug-induced fever should be considered. Discontinuing antibiotics may allow resolution of the fever. Defervescence usually occurs promptly, but days may be required, as in resolution of drug-induced rashes.

Tumor-Related Fever

The diagnosis of fever resulting from tumor necrosis is one of exclusion. Tumors commonly associated with necrosis and fever include ovarian cancer, sarcomas, and choriocarcinoma. Trophoblastic disease is highly vascular, and minimal bleeding within the tumor may cause some fevers. Nonmetastatic persistent trophoblastic disease is easily infected within the uterus, and most deaths related to nonmetastatic trophoblastic disease have been due to local infection in the pelvis. For this reason, any evidence of infection beyond fever in these trophoblastic disease patients should not be attributed only to tumor fever of necrotic tissue. Aggressive therapy with drainage and antibiotics, or resection, may be needed. Similarly, progressive ovarian cancer may erode through bowel wall and may cause occult microabscesses.

The general meaning of tumor fever does not refer to true infection. It is seen in patients with pulmonary and hepatic metastases, and fever is thought to be related to the metabolic effects of the tumor or to a humoral effect in the central nervous system causing fever. After other infections are excluded, a trial of nonsteroidal anti-inflammatory medications may control the temperature.

INFECTIONS MASQUERADING AS GYNECOLOGIC CANCER

Genital Tuberculosis

Tuberculous pelvic disease may create an adnexal mass, ascites, or both, and can be difficult to distinguish from an ovarian malignancy. Genital tuberculosis may present many years after initial infection in the lungs. Seeding of various distant sites occurs, including the pelvic organs and peritoneal membranes. Peritoneal involvement may be silent or associated with ascites, and may follow a reactivation of the disease. Evidence of granulomas in the endometrium found on endometrial biopsy should create suspicion of tuberculous endometritis. However, when the peritoneal cavity is involved, fewer than 50% of patients will have endometrial involvement. Similarly, negative chest radiographic findings do not rule out the presence of genital tuberculosis. Diagnosis may not be suspected until postoperatively, when histologic evaluation of peritoneal nodules or fallopian tubes confirms the diagnosis. If the diagnosis is made without operation, antibiotic therapy may allow resolution of palpable adnexal disease. Surgery should be delayed until after treatment with antibiotics to reduce the risk of infectious complications.

Genital Actinomycosis

Urogenital actinomycosis is a rare infection of the upper genital tract and pelvis. The inflammatory changes created may fool the examiner into believing that the findings are due to advanced cervical or ovarian cancer. *Actinomyces israelii* is the most common species. This gram-positive anaerobe is a slow-growing organism and is slow to be identified at culture; however, it may be recognized by appearance on Papanicolaou smear. It may also produce a chronic endometritis with a discharge. Draining sinus tracts may form. Systemic symptoms may include weight loss and fatigue. Lymphadenopathy or hepatosplenomegaly may be seen. If the diagnosis is made by evaluation of surgical specimens, typical sulfur granules of intact colonies are seen. Fistulization may also occur as a result of ureteral or bladder invasion.

Pelvic and genital tract actinomycosis may produce signs and symptoms similar to tuberculous involvement, with an adnexal mass effect and induration. Hepatic involvement can occur from disseminated infection and cause either a solitary intrahepatic mass or multiple liver abscesses. The clinical picture is even more confusing when this hepatic involvement suggesting liver metastases is seen with pelvic findings that mimic malignancy.

When genital actinomycosis originates after gastrointestinal contamination of the peritoneal cavity, the fallopian tubes appear to be the primary site of infection and the disease may have an indolent course. If this diagnosis is made prior to operation, the adnexal mass should be allowed to respond to antibiotic therapy prior to surgery. Long-term treatment with antibiotics such as penicillin or tetracycline is needed. Penicillin in high doses may be needed to penetrate abscesses and should be given in doses of 10 to 20 million units per day IV for 2 to 6 weeks. Total therapy for 6 to 12 weeks is usually required, and oral penicillin (ampicillin, 500 mg to 1 g every 6 hours) is continued after initial response to parenteral therapy. When active infection with abscess fails to respond to antibiotics and percutaneous drainage, surgical exploration and drainage may be required.

For further information on actinomycosis, the reader is referred to reviews by Richter et al (1972) and by Schiffer et al (1975).

REFERENCES

Aach RD, Kahn RA: Post-transfusion hepatitis: current perspectives. Ann Intern Med 1980;92:539.

ACCP/SCCM Consensus Conference Committee: Definitions for sepsis and organ failure and guidelines for the use of innovative therapies in sepsis. Crit Care Med 1992;20:864.

Ahrenholz DH: Necrotizing soft-tissue infections. Surg Clin North Am 1988;68:199.

Alexander JW, Fischer JE, Boyajian M, et al: The influence of hair-removal methods on wound infections. Arch Surg 1983;118:347.

Allen JL, Rampone JF, Wheeless CR: Use of a prophylactic antibiotic in elective major gynecologic operations. Obstet Gynecol 1972;32:219.

Altemeir WA, Burke JF, Pruitt BA, et al: Manual on the Control of Infection in Surgical Patients. Philadelphia: JB Lippincott Company, 1976.

Anand A, Glatt AE: *Clostridium difficile* infection associated with antineoplastic chemotherapy: a review. Clin Infect Dis 1993;17:109.

Ariuno RE, Zhanel GG, Harding GK: The role of anion-exchange resins in the treatment of antibiotic-associated pseudomembranous colitis. Can Med Assoc J 1990;142:1049.

Averette HE, Lichtinger M, Sevin B, Girtanner RE: Pelvic exenteration: a 15-year experience in a general hospital. Am J Obstet Gynecol 1984;150:179.

Ayhan A, Tuncer ZS, Yarali H: Complications of radical hysterectomy in women with early stage cervical cancer: clinical analysis of 270 cases. Eur J Surg Oncol 1991;17:492.

Barber GR, Miransky J, Brown AE, et al: Direct observations of surgical wound infections at a comprehensive cancer center. Arch Surg 1995;130:1042.

Bartlett JG: Antibiotic-associated diarrhea. Clin Infect Dis 1992;15:573.

Bartlett JG, Taylor NS, Chang T-W, et al: Clinical and laboratory observations in clostridium difficile colitis. Am J Clin Nutr 1980;33:2521.

Baxter CR: Surgical management of soft tissue infections. Surg Clin North Am 1972;52:1483.

Benezra D, Kiehn TE, Gold JWM, et al: Prospective study of infections in indwelling central venous catheters using quantitative blood cultures. Am J Med 1988;85:495.

Bodey GP, Buckley M, Sathe YS, et al: Quantitative relationship between circulating leukocytes and infection in patients with acute leukemia. Ann Intern Med 1966;64:328.

Bone RC, Fisher CJ, Clemmer TP: Sepsis syndrome: a valid clinical entity. Crit Care Med 1989;17:389.

Bone RC, Fisher CJ, Clemmer TP, et al: A controlled clinical trial of high dose methylprednisolone in the treatment of severe sepsis and septic shock. N Engl J Med 1987;317:653.

Bone RC: The pathogenesis of sepsis. Ann Intern Med 1991;115:457.

Bozzetti F, Terno G, Bonfanti G, et al: Prevention and treatment of central venous catheter sepsis by exchange via a guidewire: a prospective controlled trial. Ann Surg 1983;198:48.

Brolin RE, Flancbaum L, Ercoli FR: Limitations of percutaneous catheter drainage of abdominal abscesses. Surg Gynecol Obstet 1991;173:203.

Brooker DC, Savage JE, Twiggs LB, et al: Infectious morbidity in gynecology cancer. Am J Obstet Gynecol 1987;156:513.

Broviac JW, Cole JJ, Scribner BH: A silicone rubber atrial catheter for prolonged parenteral alimentaton. Surg Gynecol Obstet 1973;136:602.

Bryan CS, Reynolds KL: Bacteremic nosocomial pneumonia. Am Rev Respir Dis 1984;129:668.

Caldwell JR, Cluff LE: Adverse reactions to antimicrobial agents. JAMA 1974;230:77.

Caplan ES, Kluge RM: Gas gangrene. Arch Intern Med 1976;136:788.

Carlson JA, Arger P, Thompson S, Carlson EJ: Clinical and pathologic correlation of endometrial cavity fluid detected by ultrasound in the postmenopausal patient. Obstet Gynecol 1991;77:119.

Carson JL, Russell LB, Taragin MI, et al: The risks of blood transfusion: the relative influence of acquired immunodeficiency syndrome and non-A, non-B hepatitis. Am J Med 1992;92:45.

Casali RE, Tucker WE, Petrino RA, et al: Postoperative necrotizing fasciitis of the abdominal wall. Am J Surg 1980;140:787.

Celis R, Torres A, Gatell J, et al: Nosocomial pneumonia a multivariate analysis of risk and prognosis. Chest 1988;93:318.

Centers for Disease Control: CDC definitions for nosocomial infections, 1988. Am Rev Respir Dis 1989;139:1058–1059.

Clark DE, Raffin TA: Infectious complications of indwelling long-term central venous catheters. Chest 1990;97:966.

Columbo M, Oldani S, Donato MF, et al: A multicenter, prospective study of post-transfusion hepatitis in Milan. Hepatology 1987;7:709.

Corona ML, Peters SC, Narr BJ, et al: Infection related to central venous catheters. Mayo Clin Proc 1990;65:979.

Craven DE, Kunches LM, Lichtenberg DA: Nosocomial infection and fatality in medical and surgical intensive care unit patients. Arch Intern Med 1988;148:1161.

Cruse PJ, Foord R: The epidemiology of wound infection: a 10-year prospective study of 62,939 wounds. Surg Clin North Am 1980;60:27.

Cudmore MA, Silva J, Fekety R, et al: Clostridium difficile colitis: association with cancer chemotherapy. Arch Intern Med 1982;142:333.

Cumming PD, Wallace EL, Schorr JB, et al. Exposure of patients to human immunodeficiency virus through the transfusion of blood components that test antibody-negative. N Engl J Med 1989;321:941.

Cunha BA: Drug fever. Postgrad Med 1986;80:123.

Davis BD: Bactericidal synergism between beta-lactams and aminoglycosides. Rev Infect Dis 1982;4:237.

Dellinger EP: Use of scoring systems to assess patients with surgical sepsis. Surg Clin North Am 1988;68:123.

Deveney CW, Lurie K, Deveney KE: Improved treatment of intra-abdominal abscesses. Arch Surg 1988;123:1126.

Duff P: Antibiotic prophylaxis for abdominal hysterectomy. Obstet Gynecol 1982;60:25.

Duff P, Park RC: Antibiotic prophylaxis in vaginal hysterectomy: a review. Obstet Gynecol 1980;55(Suppl):193S.

duMoulin GC, Paterson DG, Hedley-Whyte J, et al: Aspiration of gastric bacteria in antacid-treated patients: a frequent cause of postoperative colonization of the airway. Lancet 1982;1:242.

Dunn DL: Gram-negative bacterial sepsis and sepsis syndrome. Surg Clin North Am 1994;74:621.

Elliott TSJ: Intravascular-device infections. J Med Microbiol 1988;27:161.

Ettinghausen SE: Collagenous colitis, eosinophilic colitis, and neutropenic colitis. Surg Clin North Am 1993;73:993.

Exelby PR, Ghandchi A, Lansigan N, et al: Management of the acute abdomen in children with leukemia. Cancer 1975;35:826.

Fagon JY, Chastre J, Domart Y, et al: Nosocomial pneumonia in patients receiving continuous mechanical ventilation. Am Rev Respir Dis 1989;139:877.

Fein AM, Feinsilver SH: The approach to non-resolving pneumonia in the elderly. Semin Respir Infect 1993;8:59.

Fekety R, Silva J, Buggy B, Deery HG: Treatment of antibiotic-associated colitis with vancomycin. J Antimicrob Chemother 1984;14:97.

Fisher JR, Conway MJ, Takeshita RT, Sandoval MR: Necrotizing fasciitis: importance of roentgenographic studies for soft-tissue gas. JAMA 1979;241:803.

Fishman EK, Kavuru M, Jones B, et al: Pseudomembranous colitis: CT evaluation of 26 cases. Radiology 1991;180:57.

Forse RA, Karan B, MacLean LD, et al: Antibiotic prophylaxis for surgery in morbidly obese patients. Surgery 1989;106:750.

Francke EL, Neu HC: Post-splenectomy infection. Surg Clin North Am 1981;61:135.

Fuchtner C, Manetta A, Walker JL, et al: Radical hysterectomy in the elderly patient: analysis of morbidity. Am J Obstet Gynecol 1992;166:593.

Garibaldi RA, Britt MR, Coleman ML, et al: Risk factors for postoperative pneumonia. Am J Med 1981;70:677.

Garibaldi RA, Brodine S, Matsumiya S, Coleman M: Evidence for the noninfectious etiology of early postoperative fever. Infect Control 1985;6:273.

Gerzof SG, Robbins AH, Birkett DH, et al: Percutaneous catheter drainage of abdominal abscesses guided by ultrasound and computed tomography. Am J Roentgenol 1979;133:1.

Giuliano A, Lewis F, Hadley K, Blaisdell FW: Bacteriology of necrotizing fasciitis. Am J Surg 1977;134:52.

Gozal D, Ziser A, Shupak A, et al: Necrotizing fasciitis. Arch Surg 1986;121:233.

Greene FL, Moore W, Strickland G, et al: Comparison of a totally implantable access device for chemotherapy (Port-A-Cath) and long term percutaneous catheterization (Broviac). South Med J 1988;81:580.

Greenman R, Schein R, Martin M, et al: A controlled clinical trial of E5 murine monoclonal IgM antibody to endotoxin in the treatment of gram-negative sepsis: the XOMA Sepsis Study Group. JAMA 1991;266:1097.

Gross PA, Neu HC, Aswapokee P, et al: Deaths from nosocomial infections: experience in a university hospital and a community hospital. Am J Med 1980;68:219.

Hacker NF, Leuchter RS, Berek JS, et al: Radical vulvectomy and bilateral inguinal lymphadenectomy through separate groin incisions. Obstet Gynecol 1981;58:574.

Haley RW, Culver DH, Morgan WM, et al: Identifying patients at high risk of surgical wound infection: a simple multivariate index of patient susceptibility and wound contamination. Am J Epidemiol 1985a,121:206.

Haley RW, Culver DH, White JW, et al: The nationwide nosocomial infection rate: a new need for vital statistics. Am J Epidemiol 1985b;121:159.

Haley RW, Hooton TM, Culver DH, et al: Nosocomial infections in U.S. hospitals, 1975–1976. Am J Med 1981a;70:947.

Haley RW, Schaberg DR, Crossley KB, et al: Extra charges and prolongation of stay attributable to nosocomial infections: a prospective interhospital comparison. Am J Med 1981b:70:51.

Hampton AA, Sherertz RJ: Vascular-access infections in hospitalized patients. Surg Clin North Am 1988;68:57.

Hathorn JW, Lyke K: Empirical treatment of febrile neutropenia: evolution of current therapeutic approaches. Clin Infect Dis 1997;24(Suppl 2):S256.

Hemsell D, Hemsell P, Nobles B, et al: Moxalactam versus cefazolin prophylaxis for vaginal hysterectomy. Am J Obstet Gynecol 1983a;147:379.

Hemsell DL, Bawdon RE, Hemsell PG, et al: Single-dose cephalosporin for prevention of major pelvic infection after vaginal hysterectomy: cefazolin versus cefoxitin versus cefotaxime. Am J Obstet Gynecol 1987;156:1201.

Hemsell DL, Reisch J, Nobles B, Hemsell PG: Prevention of major infection after elective abdominal hysterectomy: individual determination required. Am J Obstet Gynecol 1983b;147:520.

Henderson DK: Bacteremia due to percutaneous intravascular devices. In Mandell G, Bennett JE, Dolin R, et al (eds): Principles and Practice of Infectious Diseases. 4th ed. New York: John Wiley & Sons, 1995:2589.

Hevron JE, Llorens AS: Management of postoperative abscess following gynecologic surgery. Obstet Gynecol 1976;47:553.

Hickman RO, Buckner CD, Clift RA, et al: A modified right atrial catheter for access to the venous system in marrow transplant recipients. Surg Gynecol Obstet 1979;148:871.

Hilton E, Haslett TM, Borenstein MT, et al: Central catheter infections: single versus triple-lumen catheters: influence of guidewires on infection rates when used for replacement of the catheters. Am J Med 1988;84:667.

Holland JA, Hill GB, Wolfe WG, et al: Experimental and clinical experience with hyperbaric oxygen in the treatment of clostridial myonecrosis. Surgery 1975;77:75.

Hughes JM, Culver DH, White JW: Nosocomial infections surveillance 1980–1982. MMWR Morbid Mortal Wkly Rep 1983; 32:155.

Hughes WT, Armstrong D, Bodey GP, et al: Guidelines for the use of antimicrobial agents in neutropenic patients with unexplained fever. J Infect Dis 1990;161:381.

Hughes WT, Armstrong D, Bodey GP, et al: 1997 Guidelines for the use of antimicrobial agents in neutropenic patients with unexplained fever. Clin Infect Dis 1997;25:551.

Jones RB, Hisschman JV, Brown GS, et al: Fournier's syndrome: necrotizing subcutaneous infection of the male genitalia. J Urol 1979;122:279.

Justus PG, Martin JL, Goldberg DA, et al: Myoelectric effects of Clostridium difficile: motility-altering factors distinct from its cytotoxin and enterotoxin in rabbits. Gastroenterology 1982;83: 836.

Kaiser RE, Cerra FB: Progressive necrotizing surgical infections —a unified approach. J Trauma 1981;21:349.

Kamthan AG, Bruckner HW, Hirschman SZ, et al: Clostridium difficile diarrhea induced by cancer chemotherapy. Arch Intern Med 1992;152:1715.

Kelly CP, Pothoulakis C, LaMont JT: Clostridium difficile colitis. N Engl J Med 1994;330:257.

Kreger BE, Craven DE, McCase WR: Gram-negative bacteremia IV: Re-evaluation of clinical features and treatment in 612 patients. Am J Med 1980;68:344.

Kuo G, Choo Q-L, Atler HJ, et al: An assay for circulating antibodies to a major etiologic virus of human non-A, non-B hepatitis. Science 1989;244:362.

Larsen B: Normal genital microflora. In Keith LG, Berger GS, Edelman DA (eds): Common Infections: Infections in Reproductive Health. Vol 1. Lancaster, United Kingdom: MTP Press Ltd, 1985:3.

Ledger WJ: Prevention, diagnosis, and treatment of postoperative infections. Obstet Gynecol 1980;55(Suppl):203S.

Ledger WJ, Campbell C, Taylor D, et al: Adnexal abscess as a late complication of pelvic operations. Surg Gynecol Obstet 1969; 129:973.

Ledger WJ, Child MA: The hospital care of patients undergoing hysterectomy: an analysis of 12,026 patients from the Professional Activity Study. Am J Obstet Gynecol 1973;117:423.

Ledger WJ, Sweet RL, Headington JT: Prophylactic cephaloridine in the prevention of postoperative pelvic infection in premenopausal women undergoing vaginal hysterectomy. Am J Obstet Gynecol 1973;115:766.

Lerner HM, Jones HW, Hill EC: Radical surgery for the treatment of early invasive cervical carcinoma (Stage 1B): review of 15 years experience. Obstet Gynecol 1980;56:413.

Lipsky BA, Hirschman JV: Drug fever. JAMA 1981;245:851.

Luce JM: Pathogenesis and management of septic shock. Chest 1987;91:883.

MacClennan JD. The histotoxic clostridial infections of man. Bacteriol Rev 1962;26:177.

Mackowiak PA: Southwestern Internal Medicine Conference: Drug fever: mechanisms, maxims and misconceptions. Am J Med Sci 1987;294:275.

Mainous MR, Lipsett PA, O'Brien M: Enterococcal bacteremia in the surgical intensive care unit. Arch Surg 1997;132:76.

Majeski JA, Alexander JW: Early diagnosis, nutritional support, and immediate extensive debridement improve survival in necrotizing fasciitis. Am J Surg 1983;145:784.

Maki DG, Band JD: A comparative study of polyantibiotic and iodophor ointments in prevention of vascular catheter-related infection. Am J Med 1981;70:739.

Maki DG, Weise CE, Sarafin HW: A semiquantitative culture method for identifying intravenous catheter-related infections. N Engl J Med 1977;296:1305.

Mandell LA, Marrie TJ, Niederman MS: Initial antimicrobial treatment of hospital acquired pneumonia in adults: a conference report. Can J Infect Dis 1993;4:317.

Mann WJ, Orr JW, Shingleton HM, et al: Perioperative influences on infectious morbidity in radical hysterectomy. Gynecol Oncol 1981;11:207.

Marik PE, Varon J: The hemodynamic derangements in sepsis. Chest 1998;114:854.

Marsden DE, Cavanagh D, Wisniewski BJ, et al: Factors affecting the incidence of infectious morbidity after radical hysterectomy. Am J Obstet Gynecol 1985;152:817.

Marsh PK, Tally FP, Kellum J, et al: Candida infections in surgical patients. Ann Surg 1983;198:42.

Martin MA, Pfaller MA, Wenzel RP: Coagulase-negative staphylococcal bacteremia. Ann Intern Med 1989;110:9.

Mauldin GL, Meduri GU, Wunderink RG, et al: Causes of fever and pulmonary infiltrates in mechanically ventilated patients. Am Rev Respir Dis 1991;143:A109.

McCarter MD, Abularrage C, Velasco ET, et al: Diarrhea and Clostridium difficile-associated diarrhea on a surgical service. Arch Surg 1996;131:1333.

McFarland LV, Mulligan ME, Kwok RYY, et al: Nosocomial acquisition of Clostridium difficile infection. N Engl J Med 1989; 320:204.

McNeeley SG, Hopkins MP, Ehlerova B, Roberts J: Infection on a gynecologic oncology service. Gynecol Oncol 1990;37:183.

Mead PB, Pories SE, Hall P, et al: Decreasing the incidence of surgical wound infections: validation of a surveillance-notification program. Arch Surg 1986;121:458.

Meduri GU, Mauldin GL, Wunderink RG, et al: Causes of fever and pulmonary densities in patients with clinical manifestations of ventilator-associated pneumonia. Chest 1994;106:221.

Moir C, Robins RE: Role of ultrasound, gallium scanning and computed tomography in the diagnosis of intra-abdominal abscess. Am J Surg 1982;143:582.

Moir CR, Scudamore CH, Benny WB: Typhlitis: selective surgical management. Am J Surg 1986;151:563.

Moir-Bussy BR, Hutton RM, Thompson JR: Wound infection after caesarean section. J Hosp Infect 1984;5:359.

Morgan LS, Daly JW, Monif GR. Infectious morbidity associated with pelvic exenteration. Gynecol Oncol 1980;10:318.

Morley GW, Lindenauer SM: Pelvic exenterative therapy for gynecologic malignancy: an analysis of 70 cases. Cancer 1976;38: 581.

Morris JB, Zollinger RM, Stellato TA: Role of surgery in antibiotic-induced pseudomembranous enterocolitis. Am J Surg 1990;160: 535.

Noskin GA, Peterson LR, Warren JR: Enterococcus faecium and Enterococcus faecalis bacteremia: acquisition and outcome. Clin Infect Dis 1995;20:296.

Ohm MJ, Galask RP: The effect of antibiotic prophylaxis on patients undergoing total abdominal hysterectomy. 1. Effect on morbidity. Am J Obstet Gynecol 1976;125:442.

Olak J, Christou NV, Stein LA, et al: Operations vs percutaneous drainage of intra-abdominal abscesses: comparison of morbidity and mortality. Arch Surg 1986;121:141.

Olson MM, MacCallum J, McQuarrie DG: Preoperative hair removal with clippers does not increase infection rate in clean surgical wounds. Surg Gynecol Obstet 1986;162:181.

Orr JW, Shingleton HM, Hatch KD, et al: Gastrointestinal complications associated with pelvic exenteration. Am J Obstet Gynecol 1983;145:325.

Parrott T, Evans AJ, Lowes A, et al: Infection following caesarean section. J Hosp Infect 1989;13:349.

Pemberton LB, Lyman B, Lander V, et al: Sepsis from triple- vs single-lumen catheters during total parenteral nutrition in surgical or critically ill patients. Arch Surg 1986;121:591.

Pessa ME, Howard RJ: Necrotizing fasciitis. Surg Gynecol Obstet 1985;161:357.

Pierce AK, Robertson J: Pulmonary complications of general surgery. Annu Rev Med 1977;28:211.

Pitkin RM: Abdominal hysterectomy in obese women. Surg Gynecol Obstet 1976;142:532.

Pizzo PA, Robichaud KJ, Gill FA, et al: Empiric antibiotic and antifungal therapy for cancer patients with prolonged fever and granulocytopenia. Am J Med 1982;72:101.

Pratt JH, Galloway JR: Vaginal hysterectomy in patients less than 36 or more than 60 years of age. Am J Obstet Gynecol 1965;93: 812.

Press OW, Ramsey PG, Larson EB, et al: Hickman catheter infections in patients with malignancies. Medicine 1984;63:189.

Reed W, Newman K, Tenney J, et al: Autopsy findings after prolonged catheterization of the right atrium for chemotherapy in acute leukemia. Surg Gynecol Obstet 1985;160:417.

Report of an Ad Hoc Committee of the Committee on Trauma, Division of Medical Sciences, National Academy of Sciences–National Research Council: Postoperative wound infections: the influence of ultraviolet irradiation of the operating room and of various other factors. Ann Surg 1964;160(Suppl):1.

Richter GO, Pratt JH, Nichols DR, Coulam CB: Actinomycosis of the female genital organs. Minn Med 1972;55:1003.

Roberts JM, Homesley HD: Low-dose carbenicillin prophylaxis for vaginal and abdominal hysterectomy. Obstet Gynecol 1978; 52:83.

Rogers JM, Gibson JV, Farrar WE, Schabel SI: Usefulness of computerized tomography in evaluating necrotizing fasciitis. South Med J 1984;77:782.

Rosenshein NB, Ruth JC, Villar J, et al: A prospective randomized study of doxycycline as a prophylactic antibiotic in patients undergoing radical hysterectomy. Gynecol Oncol 1983;15:201.

Rouse TM, Malangoni MA, Schulte WJ: Necrotizing fasciitis: a preventable disaster. Surgery 1982;92:765.

Rutledge FN, Smith JP, Wharton JT, O'Quinn AG: Pelvic exenteration: analysis of 296 patients. Am J Obstet Gynecol 1977;129:881.

Satin AJ, Harrison CR, Hancock KC, Zahn CM: Relapsing Clostridium difficile toxin-associated colitis in ovarian cancer patients treated with chemotherapy. Obstet Gynecol 1989;74:487.

Saunders N, Landon CR: Management problems associated with carcinoma of the cervix diagnosed in the second trimester of pregnancy. Gynecol Oncol 1988;30:120.

Schaberg DR, Culver DH, Gaynes RP: Major trends in the microbial etiology of nosocomial infection. Am J Med 1991;91(Suppl 3B):72S.

Schiffer MA, Elquezabal A, Suttana M, Allen AC: Actinomycosis infections associated with intrauterine contraceptive devices. Obstet Gynecol 1975;45:67.

Schreiber GB, Busch MP, Kleinman SH, et al: The risk of transfusion-transmitted viral infection. N Engl J Med 1996;334:1685.

Scully RE, Mark EJ, McNeely WF, et al: Presentation of case. N Engl J Med 1997;336:277.

Sevin B, Ramos R, Gerhardt RT, et al: Comparative efficacy of short-term versus long-term cefoxitin prophylaxis against postoperative infection after radical hysterectomy: a prospective study. Obstet Gynecol 1991;77:729.

Sevin B, Ramos R, Lichtinger M, et al: Antibiotic prevention of infections complicating radical abdominal hysterectomy. Obstet Gynecol 1984;64:539.

Sharara AI: Chronic hepatitis C. South Med J 1997;90:872.

Shorey J: The current status of non-A, non-B viral hepatitis. Southwestern Internal Medicine Conference. Am J Med Sci 1985;289:251.

Sickles EA, Greene WH, Wiernik PH: Clinical presentation of infection in granulocytopenic patients. Arch Intern Med 1975;119:715.

Skiles MS, Covert GK, Fletcher HS: Gas-producing clostridial and nonclostridial infections. Surg Gynecol Obstet 1978;147:65.

Snyder RH, Archer RJ, Endy T, et al: Catheter infection: a comparison of two catheter maintenance techniques. Ann Surg 1988;208:651.

Soper DE, Bump RC, Hurt WG: Wound infection after abdominal hysterectomy: effect of the depth of subcutaneous tissue. Am J Obstet Gynecol 1995;173:465.

Soper JT, Berchuck A, Creasman WT, Clarke-Pearson DL: Pelvic exenteration: factors associated with major surgical morbidity. Gynecol Oncol 1989;35:93.

Sotto LS: Radical hysterectomy with bilateral pelvic node dissection: our experience at the Philippine General Hospital. Eur J Gynaecol Oncol 1990;11:447.

Sprung CL, Caralis PV, Marcial EH, et al: The effects of high-dose corticosteroids in patients with septic shock. N Engl J Med 1984;311:1137.

Stamenkovic I, Lew PD: Early recognition of potentially fatal necrotizing fasciitis: the use of frozen-section biopsy. N Engl J Med 1984;310:1689.

Sugg U, Schneider W, Hoffmeister HE, et al: Hepatitis B immune globulin to prevent non-A, non-B post-transfusion hepatitis. Lancet 1985;1:405.

Suzuki M: Role of x-ray, CT and magnetic resonance imaging in the diagnosis of gynecological malignant tumor. Acta Obstet Gynecol Jpn 1989;41:942.

Swartzberg JE, Maresca RM, Remington JS: Clinical study of gastrointestinal complications associated with clindamycin therapy. J Infect Dis 1977;135:S99.

Sweet RL, Gibbs RS: Infectious Diseases of the Female Genital Tract. 2nd ed. Baltimore: Williams & Wilkins, 1990:75.

Symmonds RE, Pratt JH, Webb MJ: Exenterative operations: experience with 198 patients. Am J Obstet Gynecol 1975;121:907.

Taylor ES, Hansen RR: Morbidity following vaginal hysterectomy and colpoplasty. Obstet Gynecol 1961;17:346.

Taylor NS, Bartlett JG: Binding of Clostridium difficile cytotoxin and vancomycin by anion exchange resins. J Infect Dis 1980;141:92.

Tedesco FJ: Clindamycin and colitis: a review. J Infect Dis 1977;135:S95.

Tedesco FJ, Corless JK, Brownstein RE: Rectal sparing in antibiotic-associated pseudomembranous colitis: a prospective study. Gastroenterology 1982;83:1259.

Torres A, Serra-Batlles J, Ros E, et al: Pulmonary aspiration of gastric contents in patients receiving mechanical ventilation: the effect of body position. Ann Intern Med 1992;116:540.

Triadafilopolous G, Hallstone AE: Acute abdomen as the first presentation of pseudomembranous colitis. Gastroenterology 1991;101:685.

Ward JW, Bush TJ, Perkins HA, et al: The natural history of transfusion-associated infection with human immunodeficiency virus. N Engl J Med 1989;321:947.

Ward JW, Holmberg SC, Allen JR, et al: Transmission of human immunodeficiency virus (HIV) by blood transfusions screened as negative for HIV antibody. N Engl J Med 1988;318:473.

Watanakunakorn C: Bacteremic Staphylococcus aureus pneumonia. Scand J Infect Dis 1987;19:623.

Wenzel RP: Hospital-acquired pneumonia: overview of the current state of the art for prevention and control. J Clin Microbiol Infect Dis 1989;8:56.

Whimbey E, Kiehn TE, Brannon P, et al: Bacteremia and fungemia in patients with neoplastic disease. Am J Med 1987;82:723.

Wilson B: Necrotizing fasciitis. Am Surg 1952;18:416.

Yu GR, Yan YZ: Pyometra and radiotherapy of cancer of the uterine cervix—analysis of 282 patients. Chin J Oncol 1987;9:379.

Ziegler EJ, Fisher CJ, Spring CL, et al: Treatment of gram-negative bacteremia and septic shock with HA-1A human monoclonal antibody against endotoxin. N Engl J Med 1991;324:429.

Zimmerman JJ, Dietrich KA: Current perspectives on septic shock. Pediatr Clin North Am 1987;34:131.

37

Antibiotic Use in Gynecology

David L. Hemsell

Antimicrobials are among the medications most commonly prescribed by gynecologists. Administration to prevent infections in women undergoing elective surgical procedures continues to account for a large proportion of total antimicrobials administered because nosocomial infections are a major source of morbidity, prolonged hospitalization, and mortality in hospitalized surgical patients. Such application of antibiotics has prevented the development of many serious pelvic operative site infections and their sequelae. The numbers of new antibiotics and families of antibiotics that have been and are being developed since the introduction of antimicrobials into clinical medicine over 50 years ago is staggering. This occurred in attempts to overcome resistance and to expand antibacterial activity in order to increase efficacy of a single agent against a wider variety of potential pathogens. Pharmacokinetic manipulations have also resulted in agents with a prolonged half-life in serum, allowing less frequent dosing.

ANTIMICROBIAL AGENTS

β-Lactam Antibiotics

Penicillins (Bactericidal)

Penicillins effect microbial killing by blocking synthesis of bacterial cell wall mucopeptide; in subinhibitory concentrations, however, these antibiotics may be only bacteriostatic. The principal mechanism of microbial resistance to penicillins is production of β-lactamase enzymes, which hydrolyze the β-lactam ring, inactivating the antibiotic.

Activity. The principal target of the penicillins is gram-positive aerobic microorganisms, although there is limited activity against gram-negative aerobes and anaerobes. Penicillin is not particularly active against *Staphylococcus aureus*, *Bacteroides*, or *Prevotella* species. It is possible to create semisynthetic penicillins by adding various side chains to the 6-aminopenicillanic acid nucleus. This results in antibiotics that are more resistant to β-lactamases, and

very effective against bacteria such as staphylococci. Representatives are methicillin (Staphcillin) and nafcillin (Nafcil). It is possible to synthesize pencillins that are stable to gastric acid and therefore suitable for oral administration, such as penicillin-V, cloxacillin (Tegopen), ampicillin (Omnipen, Polycillin, etc.), and amoxicillin (Amoxil).

Further substitution results in parenteral penicillins with enhanced activity against both gram-positive bacteria and Enterobacteriaceae: ampicillin (Polycillin, others), carbenicillin (Geopen), and ticarcillin (Ticar). Alternate substitution results in azlocillin (Azlin), mezlocillin (Mezlin), and piperacillin (Pipracil), which are even more active against Enterobacteriaceae.

Recent research with penicillins has concentrated on enhancing antibacterial efficacy by adding a β-lactamase inhibitor, thereby theoretically negating the most important form of bacterial resistance. The three marketed enzyme inhibitors are clavulanate potassium, sulbactam, and tazobactam. Clavulanate potassium has been added to amoxicillin (Augmentin) and ticarcillin (Timentin), resulting in oral and parenteral antibiotics, respectively. Sulbactam is commercially available in combination with ampicillin (Unasyn), and piperacillin is combined with tazobactam (Zosyn) for parenteral administration.

Cephalosporins (Bactericidal)

The cephalosporin family of antibiotics has a spectrum of in vitro activity similar to that of the penicillins. In general, there is more activity against Enterobacteriaceae and less against aerobic gram-positive bacteria. The nucleus of this family of antibiotics is 7-aminocephalosporanic acid, which can be substituted at two sites rather than one. This resulted in an explosion of semisynthetic products that are classified according to appearance on the market and in vitro activity.

Activity

First Generation. First-generation parenteral cephalosporins (cephalothin [Keflin], cefazolin [Ancef, Kefzol], cephapirin [Cefadyl], and cephradine [Ve-

849

losef]) have a similar spectrum, with primary activity against gram-positive aerobic cocci (excluding enterococci and methicillin-resistant *S. aureus*) and Enterobacteriaceae such as *Escherichia coli*, *Klebsiella pneumoniae*, and *Proteus mirabilis*. This class of cephalosporins is the most active against gram-positive aerobic bacteria and least active against Enterobacteriaceae and anaerobic bacteria, although there is moderate activity against gram-positive anaerobic bacteria. An oral formulation, cephalexin (Kelfex), is available.

Second Generation. These parenteral antibiotics (cefonicid [Monocid], cefotetan [Cefotan], cefoxitin [Mefoxin], and cefuroxime [Zinacef], have expanded activity against gram-negative aerobic and anaerobic bacteria. Cefoxitin and cefotetan technically are cephamycins and not cephalosporins, and have the most activity against the gram-negative anaerobic bacteria *Prevotella* species and *Bacteroides fragilis* group. As was true for first-generation cephalosporins, there is little activity against *Enterococcus faecalis*. An oral preparation is cefaclor (Ceclor).

Third Generation. These cephalosporins are even more active against Enterobacteriaceae, including those resistant to multiple antibiotics. This is due to enhanced β-lactamase stability and high affinity for bacterial penicillin-binding proteins. The sacrifice made for enhanced gram-negative aerobic activity is decreased activity against staphylococci and anaerobes. Parenteral examples include cefmetazone (Zefazone), cefoperazone (Cefobid), cefotaxime (Claforan), ceftazidime (Fortaz), ceftizoxime (Cefizox), and ceftriaxone (Rocephin). Cefixime (Suprax) is an oral formulation.

Monobactam (Bactericidal)

The one clinically available monobactam, aztreonam (Azactam), inhibits bacterial cell wall synthesis by its high affinity for penicillin-binding protein.

Activity. Aztreonam is highly active against a wide spectrum of Enterobacteriaceae, including *Pseudomonas aeruginosa*. It has the advantage of not possessing the nephro- or ototoxic consequences of aminoglycosides. Its combination with another β-lactam antibiotic, however, may be associated with induction of high levels of β-lactamase enzyme production in some aerobic gram-negative bacteria.

Carbapenems (Bactericidal)

The first of a new class of β-lactam antibiotics released for clinical use was imipenem, which, when combined with cilastatin, a renal dehydropeptidase I inhibitor, has been marketed for clinical use as Primaxin. Meropenem (Merem) does not require combination with a renal dehydropeptidase I inhibitor, and is dosed less frequently.

Activity. This family of antibiotics has a very broad spectrum of antibacterial activity and is effective in low concentrations. It has limited activity against methicillin-resistant staphylococci and enterococci. To prevent the development of resistance, use is reserved for severe infections.

Tetracyclines (Bacteriostatic)

This family of antibiotics interferes with bacterial protein synthesis by inhibiting amino acid transfer from RNA to microsomal protein by ribosomal binding.

Activity. Tetracyclines are broad-spectrum antibiotics with in vitro activity against most aerobic gram-positive species that are sensitive to penicillin and many gram-negative species that are not sensitive to penicillin. They are well absorbed from the gastrointestinal tract and are available as both oral and intravenous formulations. They are deposited in teeth and bones during early stages of calcification, and for that reason should not be given in early childhood or to pregnant women, except for situations in which a tetracycline is the antibiotic of choice and when a short course will be indicated. Serum and tissue concentrations of doxycycline (Vibramycin) are similar after IV or oral administration, and its serum half-life is about 22 hours.

Macrolides (Bacteriostatic)

Although principally bacteriostatic, erythromycins may become bactericidal in high concentrations. They also inhibit bacterial protein synthesis by competitive inhibition of access to transfer of RNA–amino acid complexes to messenger RNA.

Activity. Erythromycins are active against pneumococci, streptococci, enterococci, and many staphylococcal and clostridial species, but they are inactive against gram-negative anaerobes. They are available in both parenteral and oral formulations, and are useful for aerobic gram-positive infections in penicillin-allergic patients.

Aminoglycosides (Bactericidal)

Aminoglycosides inhibit protein synthesis by disorganizing messenger RNA attachment to the bacterial ribosome. Bacteria may be impermeable to aminoglycosides or there may not be active transport across the cell membrane. Other forms of resistance result from a deficiency in ribosomal receptor and plasmid-mediated destruction by adenylylation, acetylation, or hydroxylation.

Activity. Gentamicin (Garamycin), tobramycin (Nebcin), amikacin (Amikin), and netilmicin (Netromycin) are active primarily against Enterobacteriaceae, including *Pseudomonas* species, although they do possess minimal activity against some gram-positive bacteria. These compounds are given only parenterally, and are oto- or nephrotoxic. Knowledge of renal function is important, and it should be monitored because dose reduction is necessary if renal function is not normal, as is true with any antibiotic that is eliminated primarily by renal excretion. Amikacin, the newest of the aminoglycosides, as a semisynthetic derivative of an early representative of this family, kanamycin. It is resistant to several of the enzymes that inactivate gentamicin, tobramycin, and netilmicin. For that reason, infectious disease specialists reserve it for the treatment of nosocomial infections caused by gram-negative pathogens in severely ill, hospitalized patients, who are frequently immunocompromised.

Sulfonamides (Bacteriostatic)

Folic acid acts as a co-enzyme in the transfer of protein fragments that are involved in the synthesis of amino acids, and hence bacterial cellular components. Bacteria sensitive to the sulfonamides are unable to utilize preformed folic acid and must synthesize it themselves.

Activity. The sulfonamides were first introduced into medicine in 1935, penicillin not becoming available until 1941. The principal use of oral sulfonamides is against Enterobacteriaceae, especially those causing urinary tract infection. The most appropriate first-line agent in uncomplicated lower urinary tract infections is sulfisoxazole (Gantrisin). Trimethoprim is also a folate antagonist; it has been combined with sulfamethoxazole (Gantanol) and is marketed as Septra for IV and oral administration. Another use for this antibiotic family is for the local application of sulfadiazine (Silvadene) cream to vulvar areas after laser vaporization or to burned areas.

Quinolones (Bactericidal)

This family of antibiotics effects bacterial killing by inhibiting DNA gyrase.

Activity. The first in this family of antibiotics available for clinical use was nalidixic acid, an oral product regarded as a urinary antiseptic. The newer and more active members of this family of antibiotics have been derived by semisynthetic synthesis. The currently marketed quinolones are norfloxacin (Noroxin), ciprofloxacin (Cipro), and levo-ofloxacin (Levoquin). It is available as an oral and parenteral agent. They are effective primarily against Enterobacteriaceae, although there is some activity against staphylococci, less activity against streptococci, and very minimal activity against anaerobic bacteria. Several newer investigational quinolones have potent antianaerobic and anti–gram-positive aerobic activity as well as potent activity against Enterobacteriaceae. Originally, quinolones were available only in an oral

formulation; many now are or soon will be available in parenteral formulations as well. The first such expanded-spectrum quinolone was trovafloxacin (Trovan), which was approved by the Food and Drug Administration (FDA) in 1998. Its spectrum of activity is comparable to that of the carbapenems, and it requires only once-daily dosing. Both parenteral and oral formulations are available. Potential liver toxicity requires careful monitoring of liver function tests.

Antifungals

Systemic fungal infections are uncommon in patients treated by the gynecologist. Amphotericin B (Fungizone) is effective for such infections but is a toxic compound. Fluconazole (Diflucan) is the most recently introduced imidazole, and is available in oral and IV formulations. It inhibits fungal cytochrome P-450 sterol demethylation with a resultant *fungistatic* effect.

Specialized Antibiotics

Lincosamides

Clindamycin (Cleocin) is used primarily in the treatment of anaerobic infections, although it does have activity against some aerobic gram-positive bacteria. Other agents such as erythromycin are potentially less toxic and more active against those species, however. Clindamycin is available in both oral and parenteral formulations. A potentially serious adverse side effect is the development of *Clostridium difficile* necrotizing enterocolitis after administration of this antibiotic. This sequela can, however, be seen after any antibiotic regimen that significantly alters colonic flora, resulting in an overgrowth of toxin producing *C. difficile*.

Chloramphenicol

This antibiotic also is bacteriostatic and is available in oral and parenteral formulation. It inhibits bacterial protein synthesis by blocking the polypeptide linkage on the messenger RNA–ribosome complex. It has a broad spectrum of antibacterial activity, including gram-negative and -positive aerobic and anaerobic bacteria. Physicians usually reserve it for patients with severe infections because of the potential for the rare development of bone marrow aplasia with resultant aplastic anemia.

Vancomycin

Vancomycin is bactericidal for most aerobic gram-positive bacteria, including staphylococci, streptococci, and enterococci, and anaerobic bacteria such as clostridia. It is primarily reserved for penicillin-allergic patients with life-threatening infections caused by gram-positive aerobic bacteria. It is not well absorbed after oral ingestion; for that reason, it can be given as treatment for antibiotic-associated pseudomembranous enterocolitis secondary to *C. difficile*. There is increasing resistance among enterococci. To prevent progression of resistance, its use should be carefully monitored.

Metronidazole

This is a 5-nitroimadazole antiprotozoal drug. It has bactericidal activity against most clinically important anaerobic bacteria. It is also the antibiotic of choice for *Trichomonas vaginalis*, intestinal amebiasis and giardiasis, and bacterial vaginosis. Serum and tissue concentrations are essentially equivalent with oral or IV administration.

MICROBIOLOGY

Interestingly, during initial research with penicillin in 1940, it was identified that certain strains of *E. coli* demonstrated in vitro resistance. In vitro testing is the ideal basis for antimicrobial selection when administration is necessary to treat established infection. With the exception of sexually transmitted disease bacterial species (see Chapters 34 and 35), the bacteria recovered from pelvic infection sites are those identified in cultures obtained from the lower reproductive tract of asymptomatic women, that is, the vaginal flora. The most commonly recovered species, presented in Table 37–1, were recovered pre-

operatively from 400 women scheduled for elective vaginal or abdominal hysterectomy for benign diagnoses.

Cultures have been obtained from the cervix and vagina prior to hysterectomy, or from the vaginal surgical margin or broad ligament areas intraoperatively, in hopes that these data might be predictive for postoperative pelvic infection (Ledger et al, 1973; Breedon and Mayo, 1974; George et al, 1975; Grossman and Adams, 1979; Mendelson et al, 1979; Hemsell et al, 1980, 1983, 1984b, 1989; Polk et al, 1980). There was no predictive value in either the preoperative or the intraoperative cultures for the development of operative site infection. There are two reports in which women who had bacterial vaginosis prior to abdominal hysterectomy had a higher incidence of operative site infection than women who did not have bacterial vaginosis (Soper et al, 1990; Larsson et al, 1991).

To be most beneficial, a culture should be obtained from infected pelvic tissues, and obtained in a manner to protect against contamination by vaginal flora. This is possible only after hysterectomy. On occasion after hysterectomy, there is an extraperitoneal collection of purulent material (abscess) or an infected hematoma above the vaginal surgical margin (cuff) that can be drained by opening the vaginal cuff. The vaginal margins appose and agglutinate soon after surgery even if they are not sutured together. Material for culture that can be obtained by aspiration most successfully avoids the potential for contamination by the bacteria that colonize the vagina. It is possible

Table 37–1. LOWER REPRODUCTIVE TRACT FLORA RECOVERED PRIOR TO ELECTIVE HYSTERECTOMY

BACTERIAL SPECIES	CATEGORY COMPOSITION (%)	TOTAL COMPOSITION (%)
Gram positive		
Aerobic bacteria		
Staphylococcus epidermidis	31	12
Enterococcus faecalis	29	11
Streptococcus species	19	7
Streptococcus agalactiae	14	5
Staphylococcus aureus	7	2
Anaerobic bacteria		
Peptostreptococcus species	96	19
Clostridium species	4	1
Gram negative		
Aerobic bacteria		
Escherichia coli	64	12
Klebsiella species	12	2
Proteus species	10	2
Enterobacter species	6	1
Other Enterobacteriaceae	8	1.5
Anaerobic bacteria		
Prevotella bivius	38	9
Prevotella species	32	8
Bacteroides fragilis group	28	7
Fusobacterium species	2	0.5

that fluid also may be collected by percutaneous transabdominal aspiration with computerized tomography (CT) guidance.

Culture results may not exactly identify *the* pathogen(s) recovered from the infection site, but will identify potential pathogens; cultures can produce from 1 to 10 different bacterial species. Researchers who are proponents for culture prior to the initiation of antimicrobial therapy believe that culture results will guide altered therapy if the initial empirical regimen fails, because one could predict which organisms were not covered by the initial regimen. Contrarily, there are those who believe that culturing at the time of failed antibiotic therapy will be more revealing because only the true pathogens should be present in that culture.

Therapy for acute pelvic infections is empirical because of the inaccessibility of uncontaminated culture material and the fact that one cannot await culture results before initiating therapy; regimen selection is based on knowledge of the variety of potential pathogens and antibacterial activity of various antibacterial agents.

INFECTIONS

Infections described in this chapter are those observed after elective pelvic surgery, primarily after vaginal or abdominal hysterectomy. One of the problems in the diagnosis of infections after hysterectomy or other pelvic operative procedures is the fact that it is common for women to develop recurrent temperature elevations, a universally accepted sign of infection. The ability to make an accurate diagnosis is confounded somewhat by the findings normally present at vaginal examination immediately following hysterectomy. As can be seen in Figure 37–1, there are usually purulent secretions in the vagina soon after hysterectomy, and the vaginal surgical margin is normally edematous, erythematous, and tender to palpation. These findings are present irre-

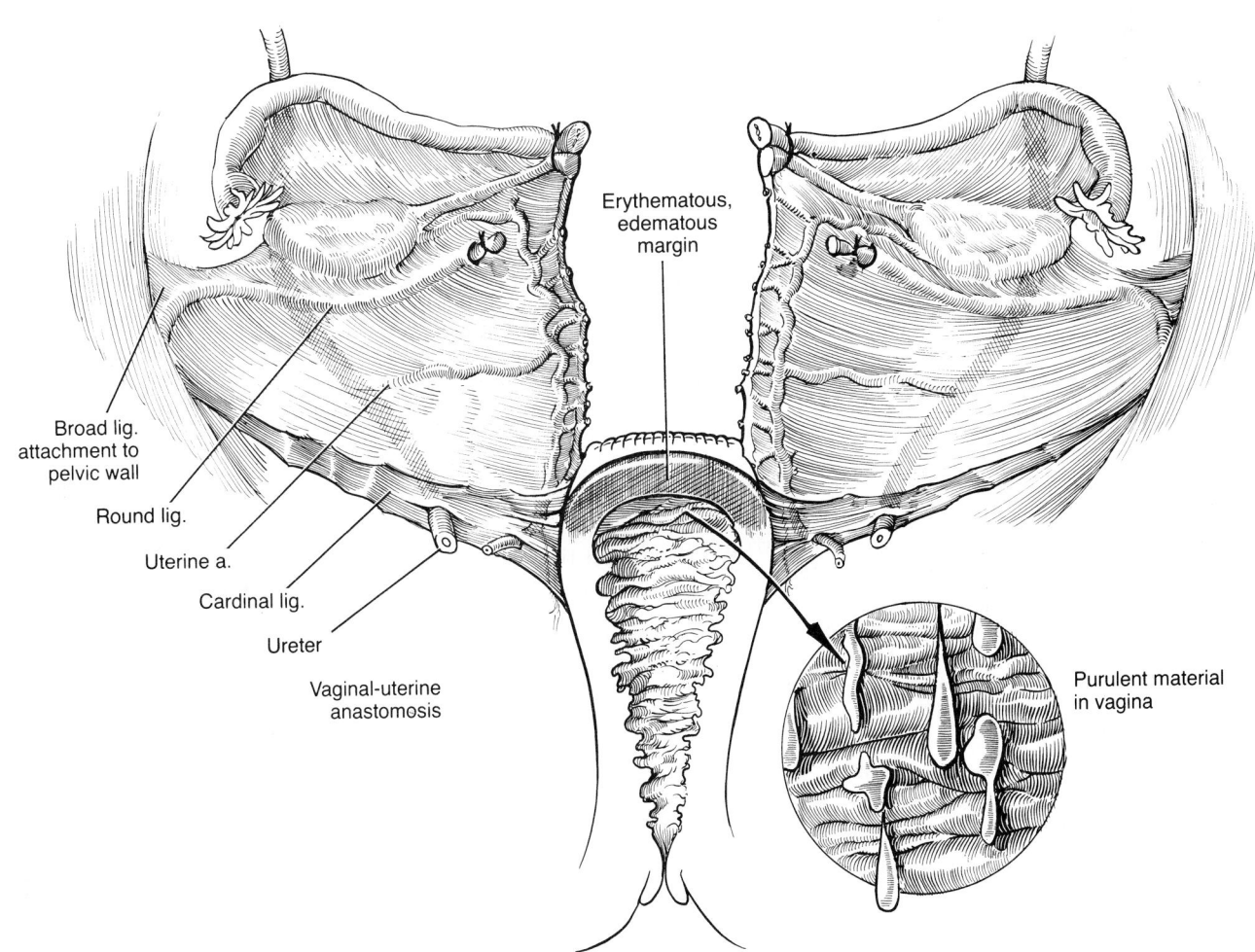

Erythematous, edematous margin

Broad lig. attachment to pelvic wall

Round lig.

Uterine a.

Cardinal lig.

Ureter

Vaginal-uterine anastomosis

Purulent material in vagina

Figure 37–1
Anterior view of the female pelvis on the second or third day following hysterectomy; the vaginal surgical margin has been closed with suture.

spective of temperature readings or patient symptoms. They should not be interpreted as an indication that infection exists or that parenteral antimicrobial therapy is necessary.

The Centers for Disease Control and Prevention (CDC) published definitions of nosocomial infections in 1988; these were revised by Horan and colleagues in 1992 to provide detail covered in the National Nosocomial Infection Surveillance (NNIS) System hospital manual. Hospital infection control teams use these definitions in their monitoring. An attending physician's or surgeon's diagnosis is an acceptable criterion for infection. Unfortately, administration of antibiotic without an infection diagnosis is not monitored, but should be.

Surgical site infection (SSI) has replaced the word *wound*, and also includes deep infection. Incisional SSI is subdivided into *superficial* (skin and subcutaneous tissue) and *deep* (fascial and muscle layers). Either must develop within 30 days of the surgical procedure, assuming that no non-human-derived implantable foreign body (fascial hernia graft) was permanently placed during the original procedure. If such occurred, a deep SSI may be diagnosed up to 1 year after surgery.

A *superficial SSI* involves only the skin and/or subcutaneous tissue and at least one of the following must be present:

1. Purulent drainage
2. Aseptically obtained organisms from fluid or tissue
3. At least one of the following signs or symptoms:
   • pain or tenderness
   • localized swelling
   • redness
   • heat

In addition, *the superficial incision is deliberately opened by the surgeon (unless the culture is negative)*. Stitch abscess and several other nongynecologic conditions are not included.

A *deep SSI* involves the incisional fascial and muscle layers if at least one of the following is present:

1. Purulent drainage from the space but not from the organ/space involved in the original surgical procedure
2. Spontaneous dehiscence or deliberate opening of the space by a surgeon when the patient has at least one of the following signs or symptoms:
   • fever (temperature >38°C)
   • localized pain
   • localized tenderness—unless the culture is negative
3. An abscess or other evidence of infection is identified:
   • on direct examination
   • during reoperation
   • by histopathologic examination
   • by radiologic examination

An *organ/space SSI* is defined as infection in any part of the anatomy other than the incision that is opened or manipulated during the surgical procedure. Twenty-three different areas of organ/space infection were listed by Horan et al (1992). Those following gynecologic surgery would include (1) vaginal cuff, (2) other . . . female reproductive tract, and possibly (3) other infection of the urinary tract, and (4) intra-abdominal, not specified elsewhere. These infections also must occur within 30 days if no implant is left (1 year if there is a implant [e.g., graft at sacral colpopexy]) and the infection appears to be related to the original procedure. At least one or more of the following must be present:

1. Purulent drainage from a drain placed through a "stab wound" into the organ space
2. Aseptically isolated organisms from fluid or tissue
3. An abscess or other evidence of infection made by
   • direct examination
   • reoperation
   • histopathology
   • radiologic examination
4. A diagnosis of infection by a surgeon or attending physician.

More than one type of SSI may be present in a given patient. The following conditions commonly diagnosed clinically are given CDC SSI assignment in parentheses where applicable.

Febrile Morbidity

The term *febrile morbidity* appeared in early literature discussing infection after hysterectomy. It was an all-encompassing term that included not only patients having infections with a specific diagnosis, but many times patients who had fever but in whom no infection source could be identified. Many such patients were given parenteral antibiotic therapy.

The literature that deals with postoperative infection in the gynecology patient includes over 30 different definitions for febrile morbidity. They range from a temperature of 37.5°C on two or more consecutive days more than 24 hours after surgery (Berkeley et al, 1988) to a temperature of 38.3°C on two occasions at least 6 hours apart more than 24 (Roy and Wilkins, 1982) or 48 (Allen et al, 1972) hours after surgery. The most frequently reported definition is 38°C on two occasions at least 6 hours apart more than 24 hours after surgery. As a descriptive term, febrile morbidity should include all women who have recurrent temperature elevations at a level specified by the operating surgeon or preferably by an infection control team. To repeat, it should not be equated with operative site infection, any infection, or the necessity for antimicrobial therapy.

Recurring temperature elevations do indicate a necessity for patient evaluation to identify the source, however. A determination of the cause of temperature elevation cannot be made without a complete physical examination; extragenital sites of infection must be excluded. Antibiotic therapy should not be initiated without a pelvic examination, or for a diagnosis of "presumed pelvic infection!"

Vaginal Cuff Cellulitis (Organ/Space SSI)

If a woman has the complaints of lower abdominal, lower back, or pelvic pain with recurrent temperature elevations, and has unexpected tenderness in the suprapubic area at depression of the abdominal wall, as well as accentuated tenderness in the area of the vaginal surgical margin but not the parametrial areas, then the diagnosis is vaginal cuff cellulitis. This is an uncommon diagnosis in the immediate postoperative period in our patients, being seen more commonly 7 to 10 days after discharge from the hospital.

Pelvic Cellulitis (Organ/Space SSI)

When host defense mechanisms and/or prophylactic antibiotics are unable to control the intraoperative bacterial inoculum to the vaginal margin, infection develops in the parametrial soft tissues of the pelvis (Fig. 37–2). This may be enhanced by the production of bacterial virulence factors such as β-lactamase enzymes (penicillinase and/or cephalosporinase), proteases, collagenases, or hydrogen peroxide; the presence of pili; or capsule formation. Patients with pelvic cellulitis have recurring temperature elevations as well as lower abdominal, pelvic, and/or low back pain, and tenderness to gentle deep depression of the lower abdominal wall over the infected area, with differential tenderness in parametrial areas at bimanual examination. This usually occurs on the second or third postoperative day.

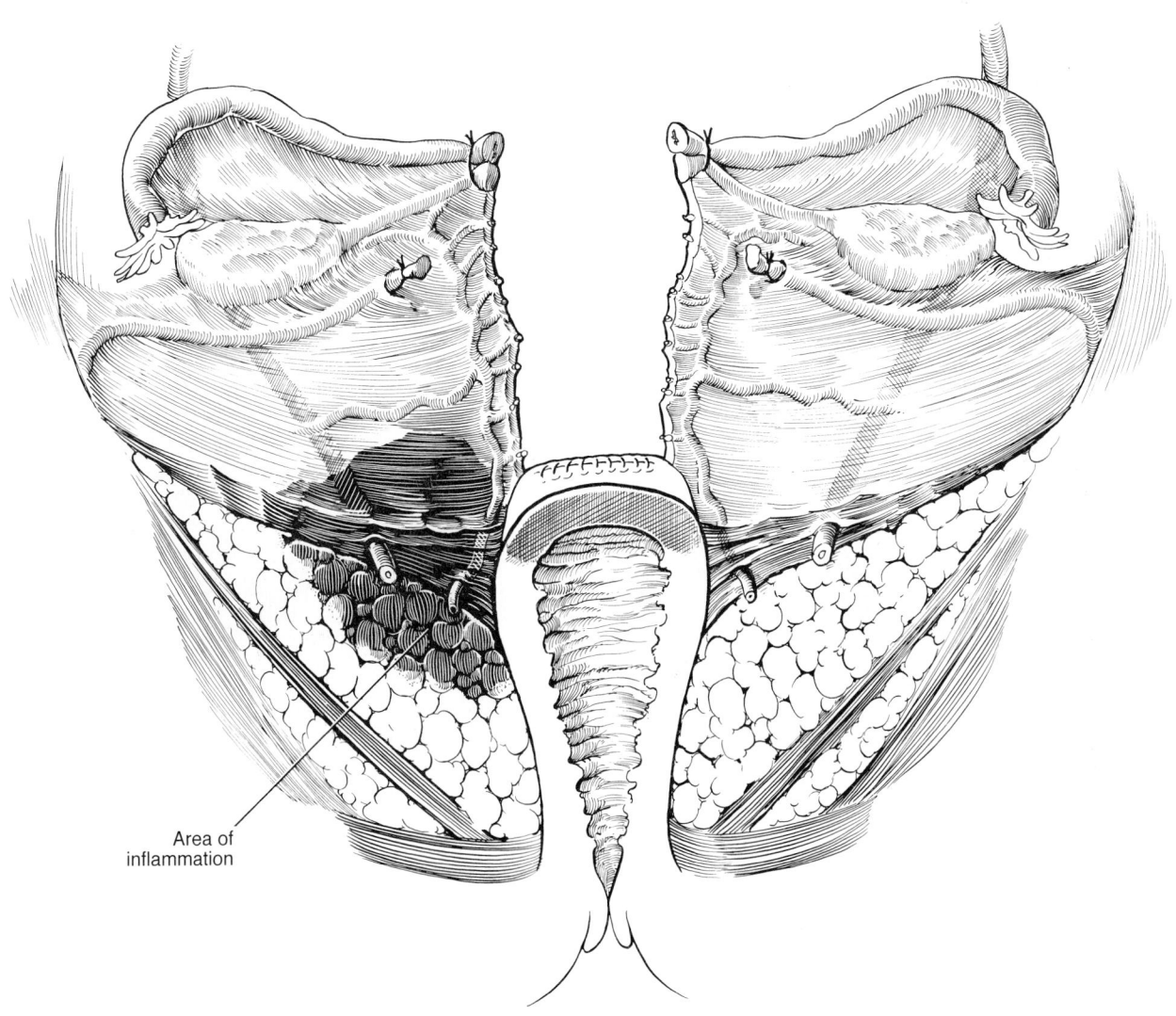

Area of
inflammation

Figure 37–2
Pelvic cellulitis. Anterior view of the female pelvis following hysterectomy with unilateral infection in the right parametrial area.

Phlegmon (Organ/Space SSI)

It is possible that an intense focal cellulitis with microabscesses may develop in a larger area of cellulitis. When this occurs, the result is referred to as phlegmon, which is usually a palpable tender mass commonly detected in the pelvis on the third or fourth postoperative day. *Ligneous cellulitis*, or woody induration, may also develop in a parametrial area. Anaerobic bacteria play a significant role in both of these infections. Pelvic cellulitis, phlegmon, or ligneous cellulitis rarely develop in parametrial areas after conization, dilatation and curettage (D&C), adnexal surgery, laparoscopy, and like procedures.

Adnexitis (Organ/Space SSI)

As can be seen in Figure 37–3, a retained adnexa may become infected after hysterectomy or other pelvic surgical procedure. The symptoms and physical findings for this infection are essentially those of pelvic cellulitis, except that the tenderness may be somewhat higher in the pelvis and the immediate paravaginal/parametrial areas are not involved. This infection can also develop after surgery for an ectopic pregnancy, tubal ligation, or other adnexal surgery, and is usually manifest on the second or third day following surgery.

Pelvic Abscess/Infected Hematoma (Organ/Space SSI)

Women with recurring temperature elevations, pain, and tenderness as above with a palpable tender pelvic mass at bimanual examination have a pelvic abscess/infected hematoma. An infected hematoma is usually not palpable early. Figures 37–4A and 37–4B depict midsagittal and coronal views of the female pelvis, respectively, in which either an infected hematoma or pelvic abscess developed following hysterectomy. The contents of the space can be drained by opening the vaginal surgical margin, usually in a treatment (examination) room on a nursing unit. One should endeavor to break up any loculations in that space. It is usually not necessary to place a drain into that space; if one is desired, closed suction drainage is superior to a passive drain. Any fluid initially collected from this space should be submitted for aerobic and anaerobic culture and sensitivity testing.

Adnexal Abscess (Organ/Space SSI)

It is possible, although rare, that an abscess or an infected hematoma may develop in a retained adnexa. This rarely occurs during the initial hospitalization, more commonly developing after discharge from the hospital. Symptoms and signs of the infec-

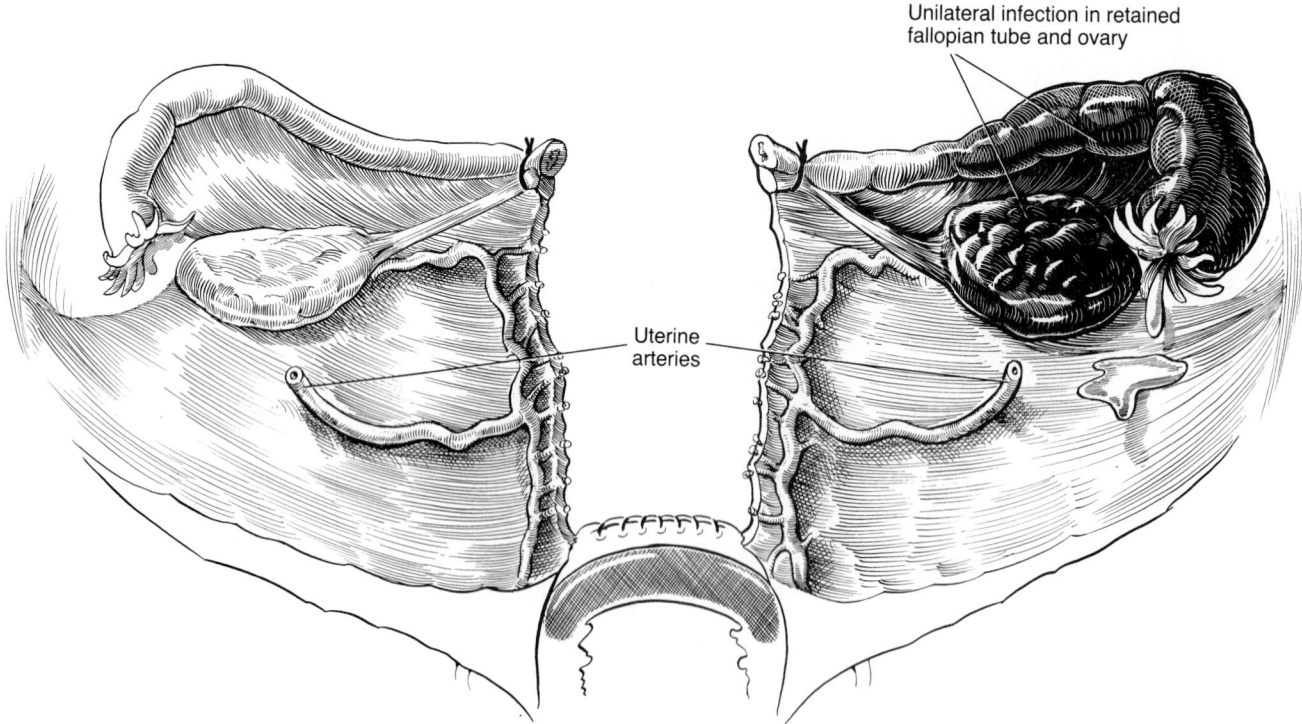

Figure 37–3
Adnexitis. Posterior view of the female pelvis after hysterectomy with cellulitis involving the right fallopian tube and ovary.

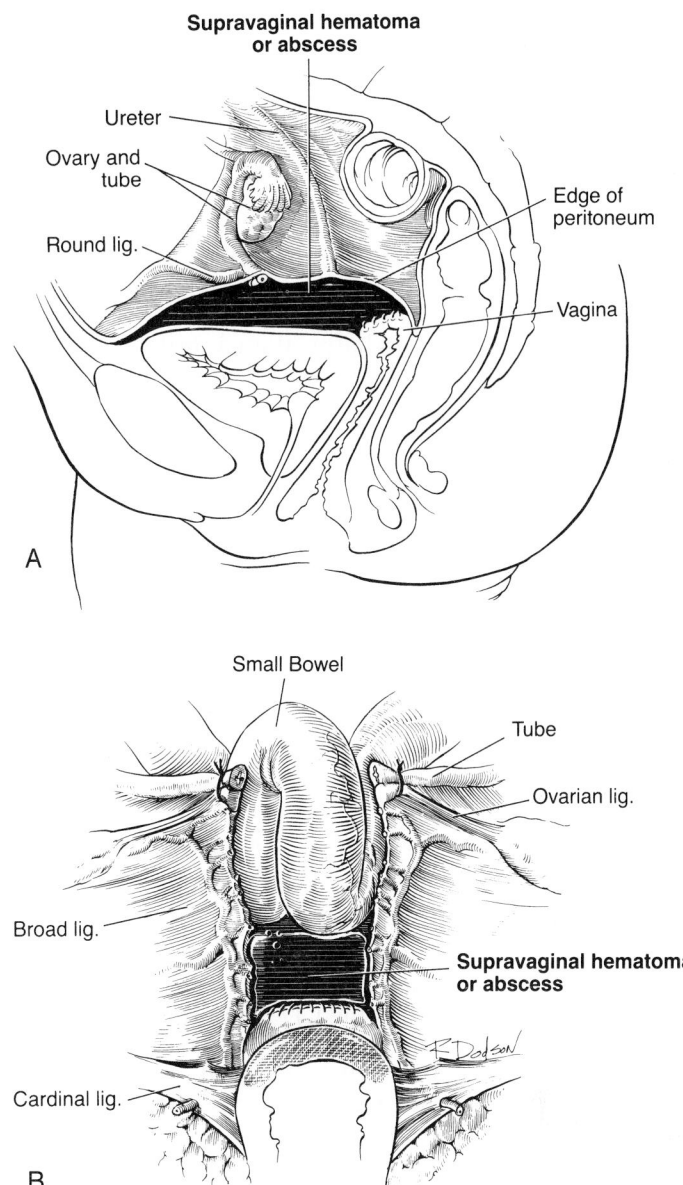

Figure 37–4
Female pelvis after hysterectomy with a supravaginal hematoma or abscess. *A*, Midsagittal view. *B*, Coronal view.

tion may be similar to those of pelvic cellulitis. The tenderness is more cephalad than that of pelvic cellulitis at bimanual examination. However, it usually causes very little in the way of symptoms until rupture 1 to 2 weeks after discharge from the hospital, causing a life-threatening condition requiring immediate surgical therapy in addition to broad-spectrum antimicrobial therapy (Ledger et al, 1969; Livengood and Addison, 1982).

Abdominal Incision Infection (Superficial and Deep SSI)

This infection is not as common as pelvic infection, and infection below the fascia occurs uncommonly enough to be classified as rare. It is seen most frequently after abdominal hysterectomy, but it may de-

velop after any transabdominal pelvic surgery. A seroma or hematoma also may develop, causing superficial dehiscence of the abdominal wall incision. If an incision opens or begins to drain, it should be evaluated, including culturing. Incision margin hyperemia is more easily diagnosed at this site than in the pelvis, and purulent drainage is diagnostic. Temperature elevations, pain, erythema, and tenderness develop usually on or after the fourth postoperative day, one day later than is observed with pelvic infection. A culture should be performed on any incision that is opened. An abscess also may develop. Infection is uncommon in the abdominal wall deep to the fascia, but evidence for such should be sought by careful examination of the fascia when superficial separation or infection develops. These infections usually are caused by the bacteria recovered from pelvic infection sites after hysterectomy, or only aerobic gram-positive bacteria if the vagina is not entered.

Epidemiology of Posthysterectomy Infections

Although most postoperative pelvic and abdominal wall infections do occur within five days following hysterectomy, many develop later. In order to identify the magnitude of the problem of postoperative infection, both early and late infections should be included. Patients must be instructed about the symptoms and signs of postoperative infection at hospital discharge because with the current prevalence of early hospital discharge, these infections will develop after the patient gets home.

It has been reported that between 20% and 70% of postoperative surgical site infections do not develop until after the patient is discharged from the hospital. This results in an under-reporting of infection rates. In a report by Gravel-Trooper et al (1995), 41.7% of the 24 infections that occurred after 469 pelvic surgical procedures developed after the patient went home. Standard surveillance detected 14 infections, 6 (25% of total) of which were detected when patients were readmitted for therapy. An additional 10 infections (41.7% of total) that developed in women who did not require admission for therapy were detected by postoperative physician surveys. Thus 66.7% of these patients developed late infections. At one time, it was thought that antibiotic prophylaxis was responsible for delayed infection, but that was not confirmed by placebo-controlled studies.

Hysterectomy is the gynecologic surgical procedure after which the highest infection rate is observed. It was 7.0% in the Gravel-Trooper et al (1995) report and just over 6% in the CDC report by Horan and co-workers (1993). That report detailed 42,509 patients undergoing a variety of surgical procedures in 95 different hospitals between January 1986 and June 1992, and who developed 52,388 infections. Of the infections that occurred in women undergoing abdominal hysterectomy, 46% were in an operative site, 22% in the abdominal incision, and 24% in the pelvis.

PREVENTING POSTOPERATIVE INFECTIONS

Ledger et al (1975) proposed guidelines for the prevention of *operative site* infection (Table 37–2). Elective pelvic surgery should not be performed in a patient who has an active urinary tract infection, upper or lower respiratory tract infection, or bacterial vaginosis.

Richards reported in 1944 that the local use of sulfonamides did not significantly reduce postoperative pelvic infection rates. Turner, however, reported in 1950 that a penicillin vaginal suppository was, in fact, superior to parenteral penicillin for the prevention of pelvic infection after vaginal hysterectomy. In 1978, Wright et al reported that vaginal antibiotic spray significantly reduced pelvic infection following gynecologic surgery. Most investigators,

Table 37–2. GUIDELINES FOR PREVENTING OPERATIVE SITE INFECTION

1. The operation should have a significant risk of operative site infection following surgery.
2. The operation should be associated with endogenous bacterial contamination.
3. The prophylactic antibiotic should have laboratory evidence of effectiveness against some of the contaminating organisms.
4. The prophylactic antibiotic should be present in the wound area, preferably prior to incision.
5. A short course of prophylactic antibiotics should be used.
6. Therapeutic agents should be reserved for therapy unless proved superior.
7. There should be clinical evidence for effectiveness of the agent selected.
8. Benefits of antibiotic prophylaxis should outweigh the risks.

however, have conducted clinical trials evaluating parenteral antibiotic, compared with either a no-antibiotic arm, a placebo, or another antibiotic regimen.

Pharmacokinetic Characteristics

An antibiotic must achieve sufficient concentration in potentially infected tissues to adequately protect the patient from clinical infection. Table 37–3 presents the many antibiotics that have been administered to clinically uninfected women for infection prevention (prophylaxis) at hysterectomy. Burke reported in 1961 that there was a 4-hour time period during which the administration of antibiotic would prevent tissue infection caused by *S. aureus* inoculated into a dermal lesion in an animal model. There are obviously no prospective human data along similar lines, but Shapiro et al (1982) reported that there was not a measurable protective effect of prophylactic antibiotic at vaginal or abdominal hysterectomy if the surgical procedure had a duration longer than 3.3 hours. Most hysterectomies and other gynecologic surgical procedures for benign diagnoses require much less time than 3.3 hours. Prolonged surgical procedure was not a risk factor for postoperative infection in 10 reported studies (Grossman et al, 1979; Roy and Wilkins, 1982; Hemsell et al, 1984b, 1985a, 1985b, 1987a, 1989; Soper and Yarwood, 1987; Wijma et al, 1987; Soper et al, 1990), but it was in four others (Fleming et al, 1954; Ledger et al, 1968; Shapiro et al, 1982; Hemsell et al, 1985c). Blood loss greater than 1000 to 1500 ml warrants a second dose.

Infection rates are usually higher after vaginal hysterectomy than after abdominal hysterectomy, which is understandable because contamination begins at the beginning of the procedure and persists throughout the procedure. Vaginal hysterectomy usually requires less operative time, however. No clinically evident benefit results from using an antibiotic agent with a prolonged half-life in serum. This has been true in both multiple- and single-dose comparative

Table 37-3. PHARMACOKINETIC VARIABLES AND COST FOR ANTIMICROBIALS GIVEN PARENTERALLY FOR PROPHYLAXIS AT HYSTERECTOMY

ANTIBIOTIC (g/dose)	NUMBER OF DOSES*	SERUM HALF-LIFE (hr)	SERUM PROTEIN BINDING (%)	AWP COST/REGIMEN[†] ($)
Cefamandole (1–2)	3	0.5–2.1	67–74	27.19–54.39
Cefazolin (1–2)	3–4	1.2–2.2	74–86	27.79–37.05
Cefmetazole (2)	1	1.2–1.3	65	14.33
Cefonicid (1)	1	3.5–5.8	>90	26.10
Cefotaxime (1)	1	0.9–1.7	13–38	10.64
Cefotetan (1)	1	2.8–4.6	76–91	11.58
Cefoxitin (2)	3	0.7–1.1	50–80	62.04[‡]
Ceftizoxime (1)	1	1.7	30	13.44[‡]
Ceftriaxone (1)	1	4–10.9	85–95	42.43[‡]
Cefuroxime (1.5)	1	1–2	33–50	15.03
Mezlocillin (4)	3	0.7–1.3	16–42	51.15[‡]
Piperacillin (2)	3	0.6–1.3	15–22	37.25

*Food and Drug Administration–approved regimen for prophylaxis at vaginal and/or abdominal hysterectomy.
†Data from Red Book Advisory Board: 1998 Drug Topics RED BOOK. Montvale, NJ: Medical Economics Company, Inc, 1998. The prices presented in Tables 37–3, 37–7, and 37–8 are for nongeneric antibiotics only. It is possible on occasion to obtain generics at a somewhat lower cost. Prices were obtained from the RED BOOK, and represent the average wholesale price (AWP).
‡AddVantage vial.

clinical prophylaxis trials. Attempts to correlate concentration of prophylactically administered antibiotic in serum and/or pelvic tissues with the subsequent development of clinical infection were unsuccessful (Hemsell et al, 1984b, 1985c).

The protein-binding capacity of an antibiotic is variably related to the half-life in serum. For example, the half-life of cephalothin in serum is 0.5 hours, with serum protein binding of 65% to 79%. Cefoxitin is similarly bound to protein in serum but has a half-life in serum that is up to 1.1 hours; that of ceforanide is 3 hours. Theoretically, if antibiotic is strongly bound to serum protein, it will not be available to produce its bactericidal or bacteriostatic effect on bacteria that are inoculated into the operative site(s). As was true for half-life in serum, there appears to be no clinically significant correlation between protein binding and postoperative surgical site infection prevention.

Antibacterial Activity

Initial prospective, randomized, placebo-controlled or no-antibiotic comparative regimens were conducted utilizing a first-generation cephalosporin, penicillin, or tetracycline. Many newer agents with an enhanced antibacterial spectrum and/or a prolonged elimination half-life also were evaluated as prophylactic agents. Few prospective data established the fact that broadening the antibacterial spectrum of an antibiotic enhanced infection prevention after gynecologic surgical procedures. Because there were small numbers of patients in the comparative arms of most studies, however, the power of the data was insufficient to detect a statistically significant difference.

If prospective, randomized, blinded studies in which there are large numbers of patients in each arm identify no difference in protection provided by older or newer agents, then older agents not commonly utilized for therapy should be administered for prophylaxis. Those agents are usually less expensive as well, as can be seen in Table 37–3. Contrarily, if it can be demonstrated that newer agents are more effective, their use would be appropriate.

Agent Administration

One prospective randomized clinical trial comparing IM with IV cefazolin at abdominal hysterectomy in 539 women identified an identical infection rate (Hemsell et al, 1990). The same comparison in 207 women undergoing vaginal hysterectomy identified a higher infection rate in women given antibiotic IM, although it was not statistically significant (Hemsell et al, 1990). Most earlier clinical trials involved IM injection of the initial and subsequent doses, whereas more recent clinical trials have evaluated IV administration. Advantages of the IV route include higher serum/tissue concentrations closer to the time the contaminating incision is performed. Disadvantages for IM injection include pain, possible nerve injury, sterile abscess or hematoma formation, and the potential necessity for another dose if an unpredicted delay occurs. Cancellation of the surgical case after dose administration makes a dose unnecessary.

Risks

If the dose is given IV in the operating room prior to the administration of anesthesia, the patient should be able to identify an allergic reaction before complete dose administration; anaphylaxis has been reported (Bloomberg, 1988). *Clostridium difficile* colitis has also been reported after even single-dose cefazolin prophylaxis (McNeeley et al, 1985). My experience is that more than one dose of antibiotic increases the likelihood for induction of resistance and pathogen selection (Hemsell et al, 1985a, 1989), another potential risk of prophylaxis. At one time it was feared that administration of an antibiotic to clinically uninfected women would result in delayed presentation of infection, resulting in a more severe infection that developed after the patient was discharged from the hospital. This has not been identified to be a problem (Ledger et al, 1973; Ohm and Galask, 1975; Hemsell et al, 1980).

PROSPECTIVE DATA

When one reviews risk factors for infection after vaginal or abdominal hysterectomy or other gynecologic surgical procedures, one finds that there is wide variation in the importance of variables contributing to infection. Undoubtedly, the most important information gained from the literature is that individual determination of these risk factors is mandatory. Ideally, an impartial group of evaluators such as an infection surveillance or infection control team would be able to accurately and impartially identify infection rates and to monitor antibiotic usage to ensure appropriate selection.

Vaginal Hysterectomy

Most prospective randomized, placebo-controlled trials, including those with as few as 14 patients in an arm (Forney et al, 1976) reported that the administration of antibiotic to clinically uninfected women significantly reduced postoperative pelvic infection. Comparative clinical trials conducted as early as that of Goosenberg and associates (1969) reported an infection rate in a no-antibiotic arm as high as 77.5%. As studies progressed from that of Allen et al in 1972 through that of Stage et al in 1982, it was observed that regimen durations gradually decreased from 5 days to only a single dose without sacrificing clinical efficacy. Infection rates in placebo groups ranged from 12% (Roberts and Homesley, 1978) to 64% (Mendelson et al, 1979). With prophylaxis, a mean infection rate of less than 6% was observed. The majority of more recent investigations involved a single dose of a variety of different antimicrobials compared to multiple doses of either the same or other agents. No single agent proved to be superior in these comparative clinical trials, perhaps because of the low power of the data.

Abdominal Hysterectomy

Infection rates in placebo-controlled, randomized studies evaluating antibiotic prophylaxis for abdominal hysterectomy ranged in early reports from 5% (Stage et al, 1982) to only 39% (Holman et al, 1978), lower than observed for vaginal hysterectomy. An equal number of trials reported no benefit from antibiotic prophylaxis as reported a significant reduction in the operative site infection rate with prophylaxis. As was true for vaginal hysterectomy, a reduction on antibiotic administration from 5 days to one dose resulted in no decrease in efficacy.

Limited power of data was responsible for lack of identification of a significant difference in many reports. When infection rate data from placebo patient groups enrolled in many prospective studies conducted in our center were combined and compared with the infection rate observed in patients in comparative arms in which women were given prophylactic antibiotic, a significant reduction was observed (Hemsell, 1991). In one meta-analysis evaluating almost 4000 women in over 20 randomized controlled trials, this difference was very significant ($p = 0.00001$) (Mittendorf et al, 1993).

Because there are no data clearly demonstrating superiority of one agent, it would be easy to recommend a dose of the least expensive agent. There is such variability in the importance of risk factors in different patient populations that it would seem more logical to combine data from reports originating in a variety of patient populations and then perform a statistical comparison. Statisticians point out that historical comparison is not valid; however, such may be an indicator for a need for further investigation.

Presented in Table 37–4 are data from prospective, randomized, placebo-controlled or blinded vaginal hysterectomy clinical trials (Lett et al, 1977; Galle et al, 1981; Hemsell et al, 1984a, 1984c, 1985c, 1987a, 1988, 1989, 1990; Maki et al, 1984; Roy and Wilkins, 1984; Soper and Yarwood, 1987; Berkeley et al, 1988; Gordon, 1988; Roy et al, 1988; Hager et al, 1989b; Multicenter Study Group, 1989; Stiver et al, 1990) comparing single-dose cefazolin, the first-generation cephalosporin for which there are the most data, to a single dose of a variety of second- or third-generation cephalosporins or extended-spectrum penicillins. These data were extracted from studies in which operative site infections were clearly defined.

An infection rate of 6.83% (28 of 410) observed with cefazolin is significantly ($p = 0.01$) higher than the infection rate of 2.98% (33 of 1108) observed in women given a single dose of extended-spectrum antibiotic at vaginal hysterectomy. The infection rate of 7.61% (41 of 539) observed after abdominal hysterectomy with single-dose cefazolin was not statistically different ($p = 0.154$) than the rate of 5.59% (39 of 698) observed in women given an expanded-spectrum antibiotic (Table 37–5) (Maki et al, 1984;

Table 37-4. SINGLE-DOSE PROPHYLAXIS AT VAGINAL HYSTERECTOMY: CEFAZOLIN VERSUS EXTENDED-SPECTRUM AGENTS

ANTIBIOTIC ADMINISTERED	STUDY	NUMBER OF PATIENTS STUDIED	PATIENTS INFECTED	INFECTION RATE (%)
Cefazolin	Lett et al (1977)	52	6	11.5
	Hemsell et al (1987a)	106	5	4.7
	Soper and Yarwood (1987)	45	4	8.9
	Hemsell et al (1990)	207	13	6.3
Cefamandole	Hemsell et al (1988)	38	1	2.6
	Multicenter Study Group (1989)	129	6	4.7
Cefonicid	Maki et al (1984)	37	0	0
	Soper and Yarwood (1987)	45	2	4.4
Cefotetan	Berkeley et al (1988)	70	1	1.4
	Gordon (1988)	18	0	0
Cefoxitin	Hemsell et al (1984a)	58	1	1.7
	Hemsell et al (1987a)	51	2	3.9
Cefotaxime	Roy and Wilkins (1984)	36	1	2.8
	Hemsell et al. (1987a)	55	3	5.5
	Hemsell et al (1988)	40	1	2.5
	Multicenter Study Group (1989)	131	5	3.8
	Hager et al (1989b)	44	1	2.3
Ceftizoxime	Roy et al (1988)	52	1	1.9
Ceftriaxone	Hemsell et al (1984c)	64	1	1.6
	Hemsell et al (1985c)	57	1	1.7
	Stiver et al (1990)	65	2	3.1
Mezlocillin	Hager et al (1989b)	41	3	7.3
Piperacillin	Hemsell et al (1989)	52	1	1.9
Carbenicillin	Galle et al (1981)	25	0	0

Roy and Wilkins, 1984; Hemsell et al, 1985a, 1985c, 1988, 1989, 1990; Eron et al, 1985; Evaldson et al, 1986; Berkeley et al, 1988; Gordon, 1988). Based on these data, the recommendations for hysterectomy prophylaxis that appear in Table 37-6 are made.

My colleagues and I learned during a subsequent prospective, randomized, blinded clinical trial that 1 g of cefotetan was statistically significantly superior to cefazolin (Hemsell et al, 1995). The infection rate was lower ($p = <0.05$), there were fewer abscesses ($p = 0.04$), and a calculated $117,000 fewer dollars were spent for the care of women given cefotetan. An additional 234 hospital days were required to treat the infections in women given cefazolin.

Abortion

Several authors (Sonne-Holm et al, 1981; Heisterberg and Peterson, 1985; Darj et al, 1987) indicate a significant reduction in postoperative infection with administration of antibiotic prophylaxis at induced abortion. The infection rate in a placebo group was as low as 3% in one study (Levallois and Rioux, 1988). Bacterial vaginosis was reported to be a risk factor for infection after this procedure, too (Larsson et al, 1992). Although a low infection rate was found, pelvic infection following elective termination might have a significant impact on future fertility. Because this is an elective surgical procedure, testing for sexually transmitted diseases can be performed and appropriate treatment given prior to surgery. There are a few data evaluating prophylaxis with spontaneous

abortion. In one prospective, randomized, double-blind clinical trial in 289 women, preoperative doxycycline did not significantly reduce the incidence of postoperative pelvic infection ($p = 0.22$) (Ramin et al, 1995). Only five women (1.7%) required antibiotic therapy.

Infertility-Related Surgery

It was reported by Pyper et al (1988) that, in 90% of women studied at laparoscopy, bacteria were carried into a previously sterile peritoneal cavity with dye injection. Unfortunately, there are no prospective randomized studies evaluating prophylaxis in this or any other type of surgery that relates to infertility. Operative-site infection is extremely low after surgery for endometriosis, ovarian wedge resection, myomectomy, or any such procedure in which the vaginal flora are not inoculated into the operative site. That may not be true for metroplasty or reconstructive tubal surgery, because the operative site may have been infected previously or because lower reproductive tract flora are inoculated into the operative site. Prospective data are lacking.

Intrauterine Contraceptive Device Insertion

Testing for sexually transmitted bacteria should be performed prior to the insertion of an intrauterine contraceptive device (IUCD). In one prospective study, there was not a significant reduction in infec-

Table 37–5. SINGLE-DOSE PROPHYLAXIS AT ABDOMINAL HYSTERECTOMY: CEFAZOLIN VERSUS EXTENDED-SPECTRUM AGENTS

ANTIBIOTIC ADMINISTERED	STUDY	NUMBER OF PATIENTS STUDIED	PATIENTS INFECTED	INFECTION RATE (%)
Cefazolin	Hemsell et al (1990)	539	41	7.6
Cefamandole	Hemsell et al (1988)	79	6	7.6
Cefonicid	Maki et al (1984)	37	0	0
Cefotetan	Berkeley et al (1988)	169	9	5.3
	Gordon (1988)	21	1	4.8
Cefoxitin	Hemsell et al (1985a)	50	2	4.0
Cefotaxime	Roy and Wilkins (1984)	55	5	9.1
	Hemsell et al (1988)	84	2	2.4
Ceftriaxone	Hemsell et al (1985c)	54	4	7.4
	Eron et al (1985)	49	2	4.1
Piperacillin	Hemsell et al (1989)	51	3	5.9
Tinidazole	Evaldson et al (1986)	49	5	10.2

tion with a 200-mg dose of doxycycline, but there was a significant reduction in unscheduled postinsertion visits (Sinei et al, 1990). Other prospective clinical trails are underway. The consequences of pelvic infection after IUCD insertion in a woman desiring future fertility are potentially such that attempts to prevent infection should be employed.

Hysterosalpingogram

The pelvic infection incidence following hysterosalpingogram is reported to occur in only up to 3.4% of cases. This is a low infection rate, and one not generally thought to be associated with the necessity for infection prevention. With the data provided by Pyper and co-workers (1988) and the potential devastating result of a pelvic infection after hysterosalpingogram, and because the basis for the test is infertility, this outpatient procedure warrants an attempt at infection prevention. As is true for IUCD insertion, testing for sexually-transmitted bacteria should be performed and treatment instituted prior

to the procedure. If a woman has a history of prior pelvic infection, and will undergo laparoscopic evaluation with chromotubation, there is no necessity for a hysterosalpingogram.

Allergic Reactions

There may be cross-allergenicity between penicillins and cephalosporins because both possess the same β-lactam ring, and many women have an undocumented history of allergic reaction to a penicillin. I have not observed an allergic reaction in a woman with such a history, or in women who have had other than a type I immediate hypersensitivity reaction who were given a cephalosporin for prophylaxis or therapy. Women who are allergic to cephalosporins as well as penicillins pose a problem. A successful regimen for that rare patient in Parkland Memorial Hospital is 100 mg oral doxycycline given at bedtime the night before surgery and again 2 hours preoperatively. The average wholesale cost of that clinically effective but unstudied regimen is

Table 37–6. RECOMMENDATION FOR SINGLE-DOSE INFECTION PREVENTION AT GYNECOLOGIC SURGERY

SURGICAL PROCEDURE	ANTIBIOTIC AGENT	DOSE (g)
Vaginal hysterectomy	Cefotetan	1 (1)
Abdominal hysterectomy	Cefazolin	1 (1)*
Elective abortion	Doxycycline	200 mg 2 hr before procedure & 100 mg 12 hr later
Infertility-related surgery		
Ovarian wedge resection	None	
Myomectomy	None	
Laser ablation of adhesions or endometriosis	None	
Reconstructive tubal surgery	Cefotetan	1 (1)
Laparoscopy with hydrotubation	Cefotetan	1 (1)
Intrauterine contraceptive device insertion	Doxycycline	200 mg 2 hr prior to insertion
Hysterosalpingogram	Doxycycline	200 mg 2 hr prior to procedure

*Cefotetan is used in Parkland Memorial Hospital because of clinical trial results (Hemsell et al, 1995).

$7.32, compared to $42.14 for a 200-mg IV dose administered over 4 hours that was ineffective in our hospital (Hemsell et al, 1985b). For a woman also allergic to tetracyclines, clindamycin 600 or 900 mg IV in the operating room would be an appropriate alternative choice.

Bacterial Endocarditis

The American Heart Association has developed revised recommendations for antibiotic administration to prevent bacterial endocarditis (Dajani et al, 1997). The most frequent cause of bacterial endocarditis after pelvic surgery is *Streptococcus faecalis*, not *S. viridans*, although both have been reported (Seaworth and Durak, 1986). For high-risk patients undergoing urethral dilatation, cystoscopy, or any surgery in which intestinal mucosa is entered, the recommendation was 2 g ampicillin plus 1.5 mg/kg gentamicin (not >120 mg) IV or IM within 30 minutes of starting the procedure, and, 6 hours later, 1 g ampicillin IM or IV or 1 g amoxicillin orally. In patients who are allergic to ampicillin, penicillin, or amoxicillin, the recommendation is 1 g vancomycin given IV over 1 to 2 hours to finish within 30 minutes of starting the procedure, and gentamicin as above. High-risk patients are those who have any type of prosthetic valve, surgically constructed pulmonary shunts or conduits, previous bacterial endocarditis, or complex cyanotic congenital heart disease (tetralogy of Fallot, great vessel transposition, etc.).

Patients who are at moderate risk are those with acquired valvular dysfunction (rheumatic heart disease), hypertrophic cardiomyopathy, mitral valve prolapse with insufficiency and/or leaflet thickening, or most other types of congenital heart disease. Their prophylaxis can be either ampicillin as above or amoxicillin 2 g orally 1 hour before the procedure. If the patient is penicillin allergic, then the recommendation is for vancomycin as above.

In special cases, prophylaxis should be given. For example, for incision and drainage of infected tissues, antistaphylococcal penicillin or a first-generation cephalosporin should be given, whereas for catheterization or urinary tract surgery in the presence of a urinary tract infection, an aminoglycoside or a third-generation cephalosporin is appropriate.

Prophylaxis is not recommended for hysterectomy, vaginal or cesarean delivery, D&C, therapeutic abortion, sterilizing procedures, laparoscopy, or urethral catheterization, but prophylaxis for vaginal hysterectomy or vaginal delivery is optional.

Bowel Preparation

If it is suspected that a surgical procedure may result in the entry into the lower gastrointestinal tract, it is wise to lower the bacterial inoculum in that location as much as possible. This can be accomplished mechanically in large part by a combination of dietary restriction (liquid intake for 1 to 2 days), a cathartic (one bottle of magnesium citrate), whole-gut lavage beginning 2 to 3 hours later, and possibly the addition of one of several different antibiotic regimens. Whole-gut lavage is usually accomplished with a volume of 4 liters of a polyethylene glycol–electrolyte (Golytely) solution given over several hours. When rectal effluent is clear, this may be stopped. Administration of a liquid such as Gatorade improves the palatability, and may be beneficial as far as electrolyte replacement is concerned.

One antibiotic regimen is the administration of 1 g of erythromycin base and 1 g of neomycin 19, 18, and 9 hours prior to the operative incision. Another regimen substitutes metronidazole for erythromycin with administration 18 and 9 hours prior to the surgical procedure. If one does not have the luxury of a controlled preparation as mentioned above, a three-dose parenteral antibiotic regimen with a second- or third-generation cephalosporin is associated with a significantly lower infection rate. Ampicillin/sulbactam has been used in that setting, but is not approved by the Food and Drug Administration (FDA) for prophylaxis.

THERAPY FOR GYNECOLOGIC INFECTIONS

Operative site pelvic and abdominal incision infections are the most common serious complications of gynecologic surgery. Fortunately, the majority of gynecologic patients who develop operative site infections are young and healthy. The primary consideration relating to empirical therapy for a woman with such an infection is clinical efficacy. If various regimens are similar in their efficacy, then regimen safety becomes the primary consideration. If regimens are similar in their efficacy and safety, then regimen costs become the important consideration. In addition to the cost of antibiotic, there are hidden costs such as the pharmacy mixing costs, the additional cost of nurse administration, and testing or monitoring that may be required, such as for aminoglycosides. These variables can add significantly to the overall cost of an antibiotic regimen.

Unfortunately, there is not a scoring system for the severity of gynecologic infection similar to that developed for trauma patients (APACHE-II) (Knaus et al, 1985). Bacteremia is an uncommon finding at initiation of therapy for gynecologic pelvic infections, and for that reason blood cultures are usually unnecessary unless suggested by the presence of extremely high temperature elevation, chills, suggestion of sepsis, and the like. Only 2% of infections after abdominal hysterectomy, as reported by Horan et al (1993), involved the bloodstream.

The most serious infections are those in which an infected hematoma or abscess developed following surgery, or in patients in whom there was evidence of generalized peritonitis associated with rupture of an abscess or perforated viscus. Immunocompromised patients or those with significant underlying diseases may also require aggressive fluid management, correction of bleeding parameters, and invasive hemodynamic monitoring in addition to intensive antimicrobial therapy and perhaps another surgical procedure.

Anaerobic bacteria are significant pathogens in intra-abdominal and soft-tissue pelvic infection. The contribution to the infection by various types of bacteria was elegantly presented in 1974 in an intra-abdominal abscess animal model by Weinstein et al. It was somewhat surprising that the combination of clindamycin (300 to 600 mg q6h to q8h) and kanamycin (0.5 g q12h) was not significantly more effective than penicillin (5 to 10 mU q6h to q8h) plus kanamycin in the treatment of women with acute pelvic infection (71.4% vs 69.6%) (Ledger et al, 1974). For patients not requiring surgery to complete infection therapy, lack of enterococcal coverage was believed to be responsible for failure of the first regimen and lack of anaerobic coverage was the presumed factor for many failures in the second regimen. Success rates reported by Ledger et al were similar to those with nonantianaerobic regimens utilized in Parkland Memorial Hospital during the 1970s (Hemsell and Cunningham, 1981).

Enterococcal isolates are recovered from many infection sites in patients who are successfully treated with a single-agent cephalosporin or a carbapenem, agents that are generally ineffective against enterococci. When that species is a pathogen in pelvic infections, or if patients have generalized peritonitis, enterococcal coverage is usually adequately provided by the addition of penicillin, ampicillin, ticarcillin, or piperacillin. Some also recommend adding gentamicin for synergism. The role of *Enterococcus* in pelvic infections is controversial. There are increasing numbers of species being isolated that produce

β-lactamase enzyme, but not enough to warrant universally adding β-lactamase enzyme inhibitor.

Monotherapy

Many different expanded-spectrum semisynthetic antibiotics have been evaluated as single-agent parenteral therapy for hospitalized women with acute gynecologic (non–pelvic inflammatory disease) infections. Obstetric infections were usually included in those evaluations, and, in many instances, it was difficult to accurately identify differential success rates of the various therapeutic regimens. Table 37–7 presents data for regimens in which these determinations could be made (Hager and McDaniel, 1963; Sweet and Ledger, 1989; Hemsell and Cunningham, 1981; Duff et al, 1982; Sweet et al, 1983, 1988; Gilstrap et al, 1984, 1986; Berkeley et al, 1985; Sweet, 1985; Giamarcellou et al, 1986; Hemsell et al, 1987b). It must be emphasized that these data may not reflect unpublished efficacy observed in many hospitals. Acute mild to moderately severe gynecologic infections usually can be successfully treated with single-agent expanded-spectrum antibiotics. There are no data establishing a superior regimen.

Combination Therapy

Women who initially respond to a single-agent regimen and then fail to respond or become more ill, and women who are immunocompromised and/or who have significant underlying disease(s), should be treated initially with combination therapy. Rivlin and Hunt (1986) reviewed the surgical management of diffuse peritonitis complicating obstetric and gynecologic infections. They reported that there was a significant decrease in mortality when antianaerobic

Table 37–7. SINGLE-AGENT PARENTERAL THERAPY FOR ACUTE GYNECOLOGIC INFECTIONS

ANTIBIOTIC	STUDY	DOSE (g)	DOSING INTERVAL	AWP COST/DAY* ($)	PATIENT/ANTIBIOTIC EFFICACY
Cefotaxime	Hemsell and Cunningham (1981)	1–2	q8h	30.84–57.09	21/21
Cefoxitin	Hager and McDaniel (1963), Sweet and Ledger (1979), Duff et al (1982), Sweet et al (1983, 1988)	2	q8h	60.70	6/8
		2	q6h	80.93	12/17
Cefotetan	Sweet et al (1988)	2	q12h	43.80	5/5
Piperacillin	Sweet et al (1988), Gilstrap et al (1984), Hemsell et al (1987b)	4	q6h	99.30	17/19
Imipenem/cilastatin	Berkeley et al (1985), Sweet (1985)	0.5	q6h	111.07	6/9
Ampicillin/sulbactam	Giamarellou et al (1986)	3	q6h	54.62	13/13
Cefoperazone	Gilstrap et al (1986)	2	q12h	65.68	12/14
Mezlocillin		4	q6h	67.08	
Trovafloxacin[†]		0.3	qd	55.63	
		0.2	qd	36.88	

*Data from Red Book Advisory Board: 1998 Drug Topics RED BOOK. Montvale, NJ: Medical Economics Company, Inc, 1998. AWP, average wholesale price.
[†]To be followed by 100 to 200 mg PO qd (when tolerating oral feedings) after the first dose; cost of 100-mg tablet is $5.94 and that of 200-mg tablet is $7.19.

antibiotics were utilized. As mentioned earlier, regimens without specific anaerobic activity had failures ranging from 30% to 50%.

The intra-abdominal abscess model of Weinstein et al (1974) established that the initial aerobic component of importance was gram-negative, namely *E. coli*. For that reason, it was common to include an aminoglycoside in combination regimens. Most facultative gram-negative aerobic pathogens of pelvic infections are very sensitive to aminoglycosides. Although dosage recommendations in general are for from 3 to 5 mg/kg/day, it is common for gynecologists to dose gentamicin, for example, at 80 mg q8h, irrespective of patient weight. This undoubtedly results in low serum peak and trough concentrations, especially following delivery in women with an increased glomerular filtration rate, but outcomes of therapy generally are successful.

Zaske et al (1981) reported that doses based on peak and trough levels ranged from 1.9 to 14 mg/kg/day, and administration was required at 6- rather than 8-hour intervals in over one half of the patients to achieve therapeutic concentrations. As depicted in Table 37–8 efficacy in regimens with gentamicin at lower doses resulted in a good clinical outcome (Ledger et al, 1974; Gall et al, 1981; Hemsell and Cunningham, 1981; Gilstrap et al, 1984, 1986; Hemsell et al, 1987b). Patients with impaired renal function require dosage reduction for β-lactam antibiotics and aminoglycosides. In patients with significantly embarrassed renal function, aztreonam should be substituted for aminoglycosides.

Over the past several years, there has been a move to once-a-day aminoglycoside dosing. If there is no pre-existing renal impairment, there is decreased risk for nephrotoxicity and no greater risk for ototoxicity with comparable efficacy with this regimen (Barza et al, 1996). Nursing, pharmacy, and cost savings are significant with this regimen. Although there are no data in women with post–gynecologic surgery pelvic infection, there are data in women with postpartum endometritis (Belliveau et al, 1995; del Priore et al, 1996) and pelvic inflammatory disease (Tulkens et al, 1988), confirming no decrease in efficacy with once-a-day dosing at 5 to 7 mg/kg.

Failure of the initial empirical regimen may indicate inadequate coverage of initial pathogens or superinfection by noncovered species. In such cases, entire regimens need not necessarily be altered, but rather selective therapy added or altered, targeted at species not predictably covered by the initial regimen. Experience with one's patient population is the best guideline to such therapy alteration. "Identical" patient populations treated in Houston and Dallas, for example, respond differently at failure of empirical single-agent cephalosporin therapy. Women failing therapy in Houston, according to Faro (personal communication), responded to the addition of ampicillin. Addition of ampicillin at similar regimen failure for patients treated in Parkland Memorial Hospital frequently resulted in no improvement, but the addition of an anaerobic-specific agent such as clindamycin, metronidazole, or chloramphenicol resulted in resolution of the symptoms and signs of infection.

There are reports of increasing resistance observed in anaerobic bacteria to clindamycin. Whether related or not, there have been an increasing number of women treated with combination antibiotic regimens containing clindamycin in our hospital who

Table 37–8. COMBINATION THERAPY FOR ACUTE PELVIC INFECTIONS

ANTIBIOTICS	STUDY	DOSE	DOSING INTERVAL	AWP COST/DOSE* ($)
Clindamycin	Ledger et al (1974), Gall et al (1981), Hemsell and Cunningham (1981), Gilstrap et al (1984, 1986), Hemsell et al (1987b)	900 mg	q8h	18.21
Gentamicin		2 mg/kg	Loading dose	4.37/80 mg
		1–1.5 mg/kg	q8h	
Metronidazole	Gall et al (1981)	15 mg/kg	Loading dose	3.79/500 mg
		7.5 mg/kg	q6h	
Gentamicin +		As above		
Ampicillin		2 g[†]	q6h	9.84
Chloramphenicol +		12.5 mg/kg	q6h	4.48/g
Penicillin		5 million units	q6h	4.80/5 million units
Substitutes/additions				
Vancomycin		1 g[†]	q12h	28.05
Tobramycin		2 mg/kg	Loading dose	3.67/80-mg vial
		1.5 mg/kg	q8h	
Amikacin		5 mg/kg	q8h	8.13/500-mg vial
Aztreonam		1 g	q8h	16.51

*Data from Red Book Advisory Board: 1998 Drug Topics RED BOOK. Montvale, NJ: Medical Economics Company, Inc, 1998. AWP, average wholesale price.
†AddVantage vial.

have not responded to the initial regimen. Substituting metronidazole for clindamycin results in resolution of the infection.

It must be remembered that infections such as pneumonia, subacute bacterial endocarditis, pyelonephritis, and septic pelvic thrombophlebitis may be responsible for "failure to respond" to an initial regimen. For that reason, other infections must be eliminated or diagnosed by careful evaluation of patients at "regimen failure." The CDC data (Horan et al, 1993) indicated that 37% of the nosocomial infections occurring after abdominal hysterectomy involved the urinary tract, and 6% were pneumonia. Drug fever must be considered. Percutaneous drainage with CT guidance usually prevents the necessity for another surgical procedure if a pelvic abscess or infected hematoma develops postoperatively and is not accessible to vaginal drainage.

It was common practice at one time to discharge all patients on oral antibiotics after successful inpatient parenteral therapy for acute postoperative infections. Several prospective studies (Gilstrap et al, 1984; Hemsell et al, 1987b; Hager et al, 1989a) have proven such practice unnecessary. However, amoxicillin–clavulanate potassium (Augmentin) provides coverage for many of the potential pathogens for acute gynecologic infections. Although expensive, it is less expensive than parenteral antibiotics. Studies are currently underway to evaluate conversion from IV to oral antibiotics in the hospital with early discharge on oral antimicrobial therapy. They may prove that this form of therapy will result in a decrease in the cost of health care without jeopardizing successful therapy in women who develop acute gynecologic infections.

REFERENCES

Allen JL, Rampone JF, Wheeless CR: Use of a prophylactic antibiotic in elective major gynecologic operations. Obstet Gynecol 1972;39:218.

Barza M, Ioannidis JPA, Cappelleri JC, Lau J: Single or multiple daily doses of aminoglycosides: a meta-analysis. BMJ 1996;312:338.

Belliveau PP, Nicolau DP, Nightingale CH, Quintiliani R: Once-daily gentamicin: experience in one hundred eighteen patients with postpartum endometritis. J Infect Dis Pharmacother 1995;1:11.

Berkeley AS, Freedman K, Hirsch J, Ledger WJ: Imipenem/cilastatin in the treatment of obstetric and gynecologic infections. Am J Med 1985;78(Suppl 6A):79.

Berkeley AS, Freedman KS, Ledger WJ, et al: Comparison of cefotetan and cefoxitin prophylaxis for abdominal and vaginal hysterectomy. Am J Obstet Gynecol 1988;158:706

Bloomberg RJ: Cefotetan-induced anaphylaxis. Am J Obstet Gynecol 1988;159:125.

Breeden JT, Mayo JE: Low dose prophylactic antibiotics in vaginal hysterectomy. Obstet Gynecol 1974;43:379.

Burke JF: The effective period of preventive antibiotic action in experimental incisions and dermal lesions. Surgery 1961;50:161.

Dajani AS, Taubert KA, Wilson W, et al: Prevention of bacterial endocarditis: recommendations by the American Heart Association. JAMA 1997;277:1794.

Darj E, Strålin E-B, Nilsson S: The prophylactic effect of doxycycline on postoperative infection rate after first-trimester abortion. Obstet Gynecol 1987;70:755.

del Priore G, Jackson-Stone M, Shim EK, et al: A comparison of once-daily and 8-hour gentamicin dosing in the treatment of postpartum endometritis. Obstet Gynecol 1996;87:994.

Duff P, Keiser JF, Strong SL: A comparative study of two antibiotic regimens for the treatment of operative site infections. Am J Obstet Gynecol 1982;142:996.

Eron LJ, Saltzman D, Sites J: Prophylaxis of infection following abdominal hysterectomy by ceftriaxone: a placebo-controlled trial. In: Program and Abstracts of the 25th Interscience Conference of Antimicrobial Agents and Chemotherapy (Abstract no 1141. Washington, DC: American Society for Microbiology, 1985:301.

Evaldson GR, Lindgren S, Malmborg AS, Nord CE: Single-dose intravenous tinidazole prophylaxis in abdominal hysterectomy. Acta Obstet Gynecol Scand 1986;65:361.

Fleming SP, Kerns PR, Locke FR: Factors influencing morbidity following vaginal hysterectomy. Obstet Gynecol 1954;4:295.

Forney JP, Morrow CP, Townsend DE, Disaia PJ: Impact of cephalosporin prophylaxis on conization-vaginal hysterectomy morbidity. Am J Obstet Gynecol 1976;125:100.

Gall SA, Kohan AP, Ayers OM, et al: Intravenous metronidazole or clindamycin with tobramycin for therapy of pelvic infections. Obstet Gynecol 1981;57:51.

Galle PC, Urban RB, Homesley HD, et al: Single dose carbenicillin versus T-tube drainage in patients undergoing vaginal hysterectomy. Surg Gynecol Obstet 1981;153:351.

George JW, Ansbacher R, Otterson WN, Rabey F: Prospective bacteriologic study of women undergoing hysterectomy. Obstet Gynecol 1975;45:60.

Giamarellou H, Trouvas G, Avlami A, et al: Efficacy of sulbactam plus ampicillin in gynecologic infections. Rev Infect Dis 1986;8(Suppl 5):S579.

Gilstrap LC III, Maier RC, Gibbs RS, et al: Piperacillin versus clindamycin plus gentamicin for pelvic infections. Obstet Gynecol 1984;64:762.

Gilstrap LC III, St. Clair PJ, Gibbs RS, Maier RC: Cefoperazone versus clindamycin plus gentamicin for obstetric and gynecologic infections. Antimicrob Agents Chemother 1986;30:808.

Goosenberg J, Emich JP Jr, Schwarz RH: Prophylactic antibiotics in vaginal hysterectomy. Am J Obstet Gynecol 1969;105:503.

Gordon SF: Results of a single-center study of cefotetan prophylaxis in abdominal or vaginal hysterectomy. Am J Obstet Gynecol 1988;158:710.

Gravel-Trooper D, Oxley C, Memish Z, Garber GE. Underestimation of surgical site infection rates in obstetrics and gynecology. Am J Infect Control 1995;23:22.

Grossman JH III, Adams RL: Vaginal flora in women undergoing hysterectomy with antibiotic prophylaxis. Obstet Gynecol 1979;53:23.

Grossman JH III, Greco TP, Minkin MJ, et al: Prophylactic antibiotics in gynecologic surgery. Obstet Gynecol 1979;53:537.

Hager WD, McDaniel PS: Treatment of serious obstetric and gynecologic infections with cefoxitin. J Reprod Med 1963;28:337.

Hager WD, Pascuzzi M, Vernon M: Efficacy of oral antibiotics following parenteral antibiotics for serious infections in obstetrics and gynecology. Obstet Gynecol 1989a;73:326.

Hager WD, Sweet RL, Charles D, Larsen B: Comparative study of mezlocillin versus cefotaxime single-dose prophylaxis in patients undergoing vaginal hysterectomy. Curr Ther Res 1989b;45:63.

Heisterberg L, Petersen K: Metronidazole prophylaxis in elective first trimester abortion. Obstet Gynecol 1985;65:371.

Hemsell DL: Prophylactic antibiotics in obstetrics and gynecology. Rev Infect Dis 1991;13(Suppl 10):S821.

Hemsell DL, Bawdon RE, Hemsell PG, et al: Single-dose cephalosporin for prevention of major pelvic infection after vaginal hysterectomy: cefazolin versus cefoxitin versus cefotaxime. Am J Obstet Gynecol 1987a;156:1201.

Hemsell DL, Cunningham FG: Combination antimicrobial therapy for serious gynecological and obstetrical infections—obsolete? Clin Ther 1981;4(Suppl A):82.

Hemsell DL, Cunningham FG, Kappus S, Nobles B: Cefoxitin for prophylaxis in premenopausal women undergoing vaginal hysterectomy. Obstet Gynecol 1980;56:629.

Hemsell DL, Heard ML, Nobles BJ, Hemsell PG: Single-dose cefoxitin prophylaxis for premenopausal women undergoing vaginal hysterectomy. Obstet Gynecol 1984a;63:285.

Hemsell DL, Hemsell PG, Heard ML, Nobles BJ: Preoperative cefoxitin prophylaxis for elective abdominal hysterectomy. Am J Obstet Gynecol 1985a;153:225.

Hemsell DL, Hemsell PG, Heard MC, Nobles BJ: Piperacillin and a combination of clindamycin and gentamicin for the treatment of hospital and community acquired acute pelvic infections including pelvic abscess. Surg Gynecol Obstet 1987b;165:223.

Hemsell D, Hemsell P, Nobles B, et al: Moxalactam versus cefazolin prophylaxis for vaginal hysterectomy. Am J Obstet Gynecol 1983;147:379.

Hemsell DL, Hemsell PG, Nobles BJ: Doxycycline and cefamandole prophylaxis for premenopausal women undergoing vaginal hysterectomy. Surg Gynecol Obstet 1985b;161:462.

Hemsell DL, Hemsell PG, Nobles BG, Heard MC: Single-dose cefamandole and cefotaxime prophylaxis at vaginal and abdominal hysterectomy. Adv Ther 1988;5:97.

Hemsell DL, Johnson ER, Bawdon RE, et al: Cefoperazone and cefoxitin prophylaxis for abdominal hysterectomy. Obstet Gynecol 1984b;63:467.

Hemsell DL, Johnson ER, Bawdon RE, et al: Ceftriaxone and cefazolin prophylaxis for hysterectomy. Surg Gynecol Obstet 1985c;161:197.

Hemsell DL, Johnson ER, Heard MC, et al: Single-dose piperacillin versus triple-dose cefoxitin prophylaxis at vaginal and abdominal hysterectomy. South Med J 1989;82:438.

Hemsell DL, Johnson ER, Hemsell PG, et al: Cefazolin for hysterectomy prophylaxis. Obstet Gynecol 1990;76:603.

Hemsell DL, Johnson ER, Hemsell PG, et al: Cefazolin inferior to cefotetan for single-dose prophylaxis in women undergoing hysterectomy. Clin Infect Dis 1995;20:677.

Hemsell DL, Menon MO, Friedman AJ: Ceftriaxone or cefazolin prophylaxis for the prevention of infection after vaginal hysterectomy. Am J Surg 1984c;148:22.

Holman JF, McGowan JE, Thompson JD: Perioperative antibiotics in major elective gynecologic surgery. South Med J 1978;71:417.

Horan TC, Culver DH, Gaynes RP, et al, for the National Nosocomial Infections Surveillance (NNIS) System: Nosocomial infections in surgical patients in the United States, January 1986–June 1992. Infect Control Hosp Epidemiol 1993;14:73.

Horan TC, Gaynes RP, Martone WJ, et al: CDC definitions of nosocomial surgical site infections, 1992: a modification of CDC definitions of surgical wound infections. Am J Infect Control 1992;20:271.

Knaus WA, Draper EA, Wagner DP, Zimmerman JE: APACHE II: a severity of disease classification system. Crit Care Med 1985;13:818.

Larsson P-G, Platz-Christensen J-J, Forsum U, Pahlson C: Clue cells in predicting infections after abdominal hysterectomy. Obstet Gynecol 1991;77:450.

Larsson PG, Platz-Christensen J-J, Thejls H, et al: Incidence of pelvic inflammatory disease after first-trimester legal abortion in women with bacterial vaginosis after treatment with metronidazole: a double-blind randomized study. Am J Obstet Gynecol 1992;166:100.

Ledger WJ, Campbell C, Taylor D, Willson JR: Adnexal abscess as a late complication of pelvic operations. Surg Gynecol Obstet 1969;129;973.

Ledger WJ, Campbell C, Willson JR: Postoperative adnexal infections. Obstet Gynecol 1968;31:83.

Ledger WJ, Gee C, Lewis WP: Guidelines for antibiotic prophylaxis in gynecology. Am J Obstet Gynecol 1975;121:1038.

Ledger WJ, Kriewall TJ, Sweet RL, Fekety RF: The use of parenteral clindamycin in the treatment of obstetric-gynecologic patients with severe infections: a comparison of clindamycin-kanamycin combination with penicillin-kanamycin. Obstet Gynecol 1974;43:488.

Ledger WJ, Sweet RL, Headington JT: Prophylactic cephaloridine in the treatment of postoperative pelvic infection in premenopausal women undergoing vaginal hysterectomy. Am J Obstet Gynecol 1973;115:766.

Lett WJ, Ansbacher R, Davison BL, Otterson W: Prophylactic antibiotics for women undergoing vaginal hysterectomy. J Reprod Med 1977;19:51.

Levallois P, Rioux J-E: Prophylactic antibiotics for suction curettage abortion: results of a clinical controlled trial. Am J Obstet Gynecol 1988;158:100.

Livengood CH III, Addison WA: Adnexal abscess as a delayed complication of vaginal hysterectomy. Am J Obstet Gynecol 1982;143:596.

Maki DG, Lammers JL, Aughey DR: Comparative studies of multiple dose cefoxitin vs. single-dose cefonicid for surgical prophylaxis in patients undergoing biliary tract operations or hysterectomy. Rev Infect Dis 1984;6(Suppl 4):S887.

McNeeley SG Jr, Anderson GD, Sibai BM: Clostridium difficile colitis associated with single-dose cefazolin prophylaxis. Obstet Gynecol 1985;66:737.

Mendelson J, Portnoy J, De Saint Victor JR, Gelfand MM: Effect of single and multi-dose cephradine prophylaxis on infectious morbidity of vaginal hysterectomy. Obstet Gynecol 1979;53:31.

Mittendorf R, Aronson MP, Berry RE, et al: Avoiding serious infections associated with abdominal hysterectomy: a meta-analysis of antibiotic prophylaxis. Am J Obstet Gynecol 1993;169:1119.

Multicenter Study Group: Single-dose prophylaxis in patients undergoing vaginal hysterectomy: cefamandole versus cefotaxime. Am J Obstet Gynecol 1989;160:1198.

Ohm MJ, Galask RP: The effect of antibiotic prophylaxis on patients undergoing vaginal operations: I. The effect on morbidity. Am J Obstet Gynecol 1975;123:590.

Polk BF, Shapiro M, Goldstein P, et al: Randomised clinical trial of perioperative cefazolin in preventing infection after hysterectomy. Lancet 1980;1:437.

Pyper RJD, Ahmet Z, Houang ET: Bacterial contamination during laparoscopy with dye injection. Br J Obstet Gynecol 1988;95:367.

Ramin KD, Ramin SM, Hemsell PG, et al: Prophylactic antibiotics for suction curettage in incomplete abortion. Infect Dis Ob/Gyn 1995;2:213.

Richards WR: An evaluation of the local use of sulfonamide drugs in certain gynecological operations. Am J Obstet Gynecol 1944;46:541.

Rivlin ME, Hunt JA: Surgical management of diffuse peritonitis complicating obstetric/gynecologic infections. Obstet Gynecol 1986;67:652.

Roberts JM, Homesley HD: Low-dose carbenicillin prophylaxis for vaginal and abdominal hysterectomy. Obstet Gynecol 1978;52:83.

Roy S, Wilkins J: Comparison of cefotaxime and cefazolin for prophylaxis of vaginal or abdominal hysterectomy. Clin Ther 1982;5(Suppl A):74.

Roy S, Wilkins J: Single-dose cefotaxime versus 3 to 5 dose cefoxitin for prophylaxis of vaginal or abdominal hysterectomy. J Antimicrob Chemother 1984;14(Suppl B):217.

Roy S, Wilkins J, Hemsell DL, et al: Efficacy and safety of single-dose ceftizoxime vs multiple-dose cefoxitin in preventing infection after vaginal hysterectomy. J Reprod Med 1988;33(Suppl):149.

Seaworth BJ, Durak DT: Infective endocarditis in obstetric and gynecologic practice. Am J Obstet Gynecol 1986;154:180.

Shapiro M, Munoz A, Tager IB, et al: Risk factors for infection in the operative site after abdominal or vaginal hysterectomy. N Engl J Med 1982;307:1661.

Sinei SKA, Schulz KF, Lamptey PR, et al: Preventing IUCD-related pelvic infection: the efficacy of prophylactic doxycycline at insertion. Br J Obstet Gynaecol 1990;97:412.

Sonne-Holm S, Heisterberg L, Hebjorn S, et al: Prophylactic antibiotics in first trimester abortions: a clinical controlled trial. Am J Obstet Gynecol 1981;139:693.

Soper DE, Bump RC, Hurt WG: Bacterial vaginosis and trichomoniasis vaginitis are risk factors for cuff cellulitis after abdominal hysterectomy. Am J Obstet Gynecol 1990;163:1016.

Soper DE, Yarwood RL: Single-dose antibiotic prophylaxis in women undergoing vaginal hysterectomy. Obstet Gynecol 1987;69:879.

Stage AH, Glover DD, Vaughan JE: Low-dose cephradine prophylaxis in obstetric and gynecologic surgery. J Reprod Med 1982;27:113.

Stiver HG, Binns BO, Brunham RC, et al: Randomized, double-blind comparison of efficacies, costs, and vaginal flora alterations with single-dose ceftriaxone and multidose cefazolin prophylaxis in vaginal hysterectomy. Antimicrob Agents Chemother 1990;34:1194.

Sweet RL: Imipenem/cilastatin in the treatment of obstetric and gynecologic infections: a review of worldwide experience. Rev Infect Dis 1985;7(Suppl 3):S522.

Sweet RL, Gall SA, Gibbs RS, et al: Multicenter clinical trials comparing cefotetan with moxalactam or cefoxitin as therapy for obstetric and gynecologic infections. Am J Surg 1988;155(5A):56.

Sweet RL, Ledger WJ: Cefoxitin: single-agent treatment of mixed aerobic-anaerobic pelvic infections. Obstet Gynecol 1979;54:193.

Sweet RL, Robbie MO, Ohm-Smith M, Hadley WK: Comparative study of piperacillin versus cefoxitin in the treatment of obstetric and gynecologic infections. Am J Obstet Gynecol 1983;145:342.

Tulkens PM, Clerckx-Braun F, Donnez J, et al: Safety and efficacy of aminoglycosides once-a-day: experimental data and randomized controlled evaluation in patients suffering from pelvic inflammatory disease. J Drug Dev 1988;1(Suppl 3):71.

Turner SJ: The effect of penicillin vaginal suppositories on morbidity in vaginal hysterectomy and on the vaginal flora. Am J Obstet Gynecol 1950;60:806.

Weinstein WM, Onderdonk AB, Bartlett JG, Gorbach SL: Experimental intra-abdominal abscess in rats: development of an experimental model. Infect Immun 1974;10:1250.

Wijma J, Kauer FM, van Saene HKF, et al: Antibiotics and suction drainage as prophylaxis in vaginal and abdominal hysterectomy. Obstet Gynecol 1987;70:384.

Wright VC, Lanning NM, Natale R: Use of a topical antibiotic spray in vaginal surgery. Can Med Assoc J 1978;118:1395.

Zaske DE, Cipolle RJ, Strate RG, Dickes WF: Increased gentamicin dosage requirements: rapid elimination in 249 gynecologic patients. Am J Obstet Gynecol 1981;139:896.

Reproductive Tract Infections: Sexually Transmitted Diseases

Cheryl K. Walker

G enital tract infections are a frequent and serious cause for morbidity in women. Aside from the acute symptoms, these infections can result in several long-term health consequences: fallopian tube scarring leading to infertility, chronic pelvic pain, and ectopic pregnancy; pregnancy loss and neonatal morbidity and mortality caused by infection of the fetus during pregnancy or delivery; genital cancers; and enhanced transmission of other sexually transmitted diseases (STDs), including the human immunodeficiency virus (HIV) (Chapter 39). Genital tract infections can be divided into STDs and infections caused by endogenous bacteria and those induced by pertubations of the vaginal ecosystem.

The United States has the highest rate of STDs in the industrialized world, with an estimated 12 million new cases annually. The cost of this epidemic is estimated to exceed $17 billion annually, including $10 billion for common STDs and their sequelae and another $6.7 billion for that proportion of HIV infections acquired through heterosexual transmission (Donovan, 1997). Teens and young adults and individuals of lower socioeconomic status living in urban areas are disproportionately at risk for acquisition of STDs.

The female genital tract is an intricate ecosystem influenced by myriad internal and external factors, including sex steroid hormone variation, menstrual bleeding, sexual activity, contraceptive and personal hygiene behaviors, antimicrobial use, presence of foreign bodies, and pregnancy and childbirth. Divided microbiologically from each other by the internal os of the cervix, the lower genital tract is colonized by a wide variety of gram-negative facultative and anaerobic bacteria that exist in harmony under normal circumstances, whereas the upper genital tract is typically sterile. Disruption of normal protective mechanisms of the lower genital tract or assault by virulent organisms may cause inflammation or infection of either compartment.

Genital tract infections, including STDs, account for the most common complaint prompting women to seek care from a health care provider. This chapter is broken down into three segments: the vaginal ecosystem, lower and upper tract infections, and prevention.

THE VAGINAL ECOSYSTEM

A complex set of interdependent mechanisms in the lower genital tract protect both it and the upper tract from disease. Endogenous components include vaginal and cervical epithelium, cervical mucus, microbial flora, vaginal fluid, and pH.

Anatomy

Histologically, the vagina is classified as noncornified, stratified squamous epithelium consisting of five layers overlying a vascular submucosa. Epithelial integrity is preserved by desmosomes between cells and occasional tight junctions. Intracellular channels facilitate movement of macromolecules, fluids, and cells to and from the vaginal surface. The vaginal surfaces of prepubertal and postmenopausal women are characterized by lack of transitional and superficial layers. Rising estradiol levels during the follicular phase in menstruating women result in epithelial thickening, which thickness is maintained through the luteal phase and sloughed during menstruation.

The histology of the cervix is separated by the transformation zone into the stratified squamous epithelium of the ectocervix and the simple columnar cells of the endocervix, both of which overlie a vascular submucosa. The ectropion is defined as the area of endocervical columnar cells visible from the lower genital tract. It comprises 50% of the cervix in most adolescents and undergoes cephalad migration during adulthood, frequently disappearing into the endocervix in menopause. Influenced to a great degree by hormonal surges, it enlarges during pregnancy and with oral contraceptive use.

Cervical Mucus

The primary source of mucus in the female genital tract is cervical goblet cells (Elstein, 1978). The amount and viscosity of cervical mucus varies widely depending on female sex steroid hormone levels. Data suggest that the high carbohydrate content of mucus may prevent adherence of pathogens to genital tract epithelial surfaces (Williams and Gibbons, 1975; Parke, 1978). Mucus also contains lactoferrin, lysozyme, defensins, antibodies, and phagocytic cells, long known to be central to primitive host defenses (Oram and Reiter, 1968; Lehrer et al, 1993; Cohen, 1994).

Microbiologic Barriers

Normal bacterial flora includes approximately 10^9 colony-forming units per gram of vaginal secretions. Bacteria commonly found in the lower tract are listed in Table 38–1. When the host is functioning appropriately, indigenous bacterial flora antagonize pathogens. For instance, *Lactobacillus* species produce a number of compounds (including lactocidin, acidolin, acidophilin, lactacin B, lactic acid, and hydrogen peroxide) that exhibit antimicrobial activity (Hughes and Hillier, 1990). When homeostasis of the vaginal ecosystem is perturbed and normal flora deranged, then pathogens are not hindered from adhering and invading mucosal surfaces.

Table 38–1. BACTERIA IN THE FEMALE GENITAL TRACT

AEROBES & FACULTATIVES	ANAEROBES
Gram-Positive Cocci	**Gram-Positive Cocci**
Streptococcus species	*Peptostreptococcus* species
S. pyogenes (Group A)	P. anaerobius
S. agalactiae (Group B)	P. asaccharolyticus
S. bovis (Group D)	P. magnus
S. canis (Groups G)	P. prevotii
viridans group	
S. pneumoniae	**Gram-Positive Rods**
Staphylococcus species	*Actinomyces* species
S. aureus	*Clostridium perfringens*
S. epidermidis	*Clostridium difficile*
S. saprophyticus	*Propionibacterium* species
Enterococcus species	*Eubacterium* species
E. faecalis (Group D)	
E. faecium (Group D)	**Gram-Negative Cocci**
	Veillonella species
Gram-Positive Rods	
Lactobacilli	**Gram-Negative Rods**
Diphtheroids	*Bacteroides* species
Gardnerella vaginalis	B. fragilis group
	B. capillosus
Gram-Negative Cocci	*Prevotella* species
Neisseria gonorrhoeae	P. bivia
	P. disiens
Gram-Negative Rods	P. melaninogenica
Escherichia coli	*Fusobacterium* species
Klebsiella pneumoniae	*Mobiluncus* species
Enterobacter species	*Porphyromonas asaccharolytica*
Proteus species	
Pseudomonas aeruginosa	

Immunologic Barriers

The lower genital tract of the female is in direct contact with the external environment and displays features of the common immune system similar to those of other mucosal surfaces (Kutteh and Mestecky, 1994). Plasma cells are abundant in the subepithelial layers of the endocervix, and to a lesser extent in the ectocervix and vagina. T-cell populations vary by site, with CD8-positive cells predominating. There are particularly high concentrations of cytotoxic T cells at the transformation zone of the cervix (Edwards and Morris, 1985). The predominant antigen-presenting cell in the endocervix and endometrium is the macrophage, and in the ectocervix and vagina, Langerhan's cells. Cervical and vaginal epithelial cells produce a wide variety of cytokines critical to host defenses, including interleukins 1α, 1β, 6, and 8; granulocyte-macrophage and macrophage colony-stimulating factors; transforming growth factor-β; macrophage inflammatory proteins 1α and 1β; and RANTES (Fichorova and Anderson, 1999).

LOWER AND UPPER TRACT INFECTIONS

Evolving resistance patterns require continuous reassessment of optimal treatments. The best resource for current data regarding diagnosis and treatment of STDs is the Centers for Disease Control and Prevention (CDC) publication entitled "STD Treatment Guidelines." Published every 2 to 4 years, it is based primarily upon a thorough review of the literature pertaining to each infection, which is then modified by expert/consensus opinion to assure that practicality. At the time of this writing, the latest version was published in 1998. Its evidence-based approach elevates it to the highest standards of quality currently available.

Chlamydia trachomatis

This obligate intracellular parasite is responsible for a wide variety of clinical syndromes, including mucopurulent cervicitis, nongonococcal urethritis, and pelvic inflammatory disease (PID). It is the leading cause of preventable infertility and ectopic pregnancy. Two problems have hampered adequate control of the spread of this infection: the fact that its signs and symptoms, if present at all, are frequently mild and nonspecific, leading to chronic infection, and that diagnostic techniques have been inadequate for widespread use as a screening or diagnostic tool.

Epidemiology

Chlamydia trachomatis is the most commonly reported infectious disease in the United States, with an estimated 4 million new cases annually at a cost of $2.4 billion (Centers for Disease Control and Prevention,

1997). Reported cases in women outnumber those in men by 6 to 1, reflecting screening programs for women. Prevalence rates in various female populations range from up to 5% in asymptomatic low-risk women to over 20% in women seen in STD clinics; by age 30, approximately 50% of sexually experienced women have serum antibodies to the organism (Stamm, 1999). Infected women are more commonly young (15 to 21 years old), nonwhite, single, users of oral contraceptives, and in a new sexual relationship or active with multiple partners (Quinn et al, 1996).

Genital tract chlamydial infections are sexually transmitted and caused most commonly by serovars D, E, F, G, H, I, J, and K; D, E, and F are the most prevalent. Although the F serotype has been isolated more commonly from women with PID (Dean et al, 1995), it has been found by some investigators to produce less inflammation and symptoms than other serovars (Batteiger et al, 1989).

Clinical Features

It appears that the most common clinical syndrome in women with genital tract chlamydial infection is one of subacute and chronic infection of mucosal surfaces in the genitourinary tract. Severity of symptoms does not reflect degree of damage in the fallopian tube or incidence of sequelae, including infertility, ectopic pregnancy, and chronic pelvic pain.

The manifestations of chlamydial infections parallel those of gonococcal infections in the genital tract. Both preferentially infect columnar cells in the urethra, endocervix, anus, and upper genital tract, and both induce extensive inflammation and scarring. Compared with gonococcal infections, chlamydial infections are more commonly asymptomatic or subclinical.

At least one third of women with endocervicitis have local signs of infection on examination (Paavonen et al, 1988). Mucopurulent discharge is identified in up to 37% of women, and hypertrophic ectopy (edema and friability) in 19%; the latter is most commonly manifested as postcoital bleeding. Two thirds of women with evidence of endocervical chlamydial infection will test positive in the urethra, and isolated urethral infection appears to be more common with increasing age (Paavonen et al, 1978). Symptoms in women with urethritis are rare, and the most common reported one is dysuria. Chlamydial infection can also occur in Bartholin's glands and throughout the upper genital tract and peritoneal cavity.

Diagnosis

Many technologies, including culture, antigen detection, DNA hybridization, nucleic acid amplification, and serology, have been employed to diagnose chlamydial infections. Ranges for sensitivity and specificity are noted in Table 38–2. As an intracellular or-

Table 38–2. ACCURACY OF CHLAMYDIAL SCREENING TESTS

TEST	SENSITIVITY (%)	SPECIFICITY (%)
PCR/LCR/TMA	85–95	99–100
Culture	70–80	100
DFA	70–75	95–99
DNA probe	65–70	95–99
EIA	50–70	95–99

Abbreviations: DFA, direct fluorescent antibody; EIA, enzyme immunoassay; PCR/LCR/TMA, polymerase chain reaction/ligase chain reaction/transcription-mediated amplification.
From Black CM: Current methods of laboratory diagnosis of chlamydia trachomatis infections. Clin Microbiol Rev 1997;10:160, with permission.

ganism, *C. trachomatis* requires a cell culture system for direct identification. Chlamydial culture systems are costly and complex, with great potential for error at each stage from specimen collection and transport through final evaluation of results. This has prompted the development of alternative technologies in the last two decades. Antigen detection products, including direct fluorescent antibody and enzyme immunoassay (EIA), detect chlamydial elementary bodies. Nucleic acid hybridization was first used in the GenProbe product to identify but not amplify chlamydial DNA; its sensitivity levels are comparable to those of antigen detection. Automated methods for detection of amplified chlamydial DNA or RNA from endocervical, urethral, and urine specimens include polymerase chain reaction (PCR), ligase chain reaction, and transcription-mediated amplification. These amplified technologies have superb sensitivity and specificity and have rapidly become the gold standard for chlamydial detection.

Given the largely subclinical and asymptomatic nature of chlamydial infection in women, a high index of suspicion and routine screening of at-risk women in populations with reasonable rates of infection are warranted. Several approaches to screening have been advocated. The CDC recommends testing (1) all women with mucopurulent cervicitis, (2) adolescents, and (3) all women 20 to 23 years of age who do not consistently use barrier contraception or who have had a new sexual partner or more than one sexual partner during the last 90 days (Centers for Disease Control and Prevention, 1997). A medical cost and outcome decision model was used to compare the CDC screening criteria with two other strategies, testing women younger than 30 and testing all women (Howell et al, 1998b). The investigators found that screening all women under 30 provided the greatest cost savings. In a separate cost-effectiveness analysis designed to determine which product should be used in screening, it was determined that amplified technologies were superior to other methods of chlamydial detection (Howell et al, 1998a). A randomized controlled trial of 2607 unmarried women between 18 and 34 years of age with epidemiologic risk factors for STD acquisition concluded that screening and treating women for chlamydial infection reduced the incidence of PID (Scholes et al, 1996).

Treatment

The most active antimicrobial agents against chlamydial infections are rifampin and the tetracyclines, followed by macrolides, sulfonamides, some fluoroquinolones, and clindamycin (Schachter et al, 1995). The CDC STD treatment guidelines for *C. trachomatis* are listed in Table 38–3. Because there has been no apparent emergence of antimicrobial resistance, once treated with doxycycline or azithromycin, test-of-cure is not recommended unless symptoms suggest reinfection.

Neisseria gonorrhoeae

Gonococcal infections are caused by the gram-negative intracellular diplococci *Neisseria gonorrhoeae*. This bacterium infects noncornified epithelium, including the endocervix, upper genital tract, urethra, rectum, and pharynx, and is transmitted sexually.

Epidemiology

Over 1 million new gonococcal infections were reported to the CDC last year. The incidence of gonococcal infection varies with age, with incidence rates from 1995 in sexually active women almost twice as high for adolescents as for women in the 20- to 24-year-old age group (Division of STD Prevention, 1995). The number of reported cases in nonwhite individuals has been consistently higher than for whites, reported as 37-fold higher in 1995. This figure could be explained only partially by the fact that nonwhites are more likely to attend publically funded clinics, which are more likely to report infections. Other risk variables for infection include low socioeconomic status, early sexual activity, and being unmarried. Gonococcal transmission has been estimated per coital act at male-to-female 50% and female-to-male 25% (Judson, 1990). In women, use of hormonal contraceptives may increase susceptibility to gonococcal infection (Louv et al, 1989).

A complex classification system has been applied to *N. gonorrhoeae*. It includes auxotyping, which categorizes according to nutritional requirements of the organism, and antigenic diversity of protein-I, the outer membrane protein present on most gonococcal isolates. These schemes are used for epidemiologic tracing purposes.

Clinical Features

Although a large proportion of women with gonococcal infection are asymptomatic, more than 75% of women with gonorrhea attending acute care facilities have symptoms (McCormack et al, 1977). Individuals with asymptomatic infection contribute disproportionately to sexual transmission because those with symptoms are more likely to seek medical care.

There is a broad range of symptoms ascribed to gonococcal infection, ranging from none to subclinical to locally symptomatic to systemically symptomatic. The endocervix is the primary site of infection in women, with concomitant urethral colonization in up to 90% of infected women (Barlow and Phillips, 1978). Infection of the urethra, rectum, Bartholin's glands, and Skene's glands is common, but rare in the absence of endocervical infection. The rectal mucosa is infected in up to 50% of women with gonococcal endocervicitis (Kinghorn and Rashid, 1979). Up to 20% of women diagnosed with gonorrhea have pharyngeal infection, but over 90% of individuals with gonococcal pharyngitis are asymptomatic.

Symptoms of endocervical infection include increased vaginal discharge, dysuria, intermenstrual bleeding, and menorrhagia, and range from minor to severe. Signs include mucopurulent cervical discharge, hypertrophic ectopy, and cervical friability. Minor symptoms deriving from rectal infection include pruritis, painless mucopurulent discharge, and rectal bleeding. Infected individuals may suffer from overt proctitis, manifested by rectal pain, tenesmus, and constipation (Kinghorn and Rashid, 1979). Anoscopy is required for adequate evaluation of the rectum, and may reveal purulent exudate associated with the anal crypts, erythema, friability, or other signs of inflammation. Pharyngeal infection may be heralded by inflammatory changes and purulent exudate.

Diagnosis

Although the specificity of Gram's staining for diagnosis of gonorrhea from endocervical specimens is high (95% to 100%), sensitivity is only 50% to 70%, making this methodology unsatisfactory for screening purposes (Wald, 1977). Diagnosis in women relies on culture using antibiotic-containing selective media, which has sensitivities of 80% to 95% (Reichart et al, 1989). The site of specimen collection influences the sensitivity, with the urethra having the highest and the rectum the lowest sensitivity because of contamination with other organisms and secretions. In the absence of site-specific symptoms (urethritis, proctitis, or pharyngitis), culturing of sites other than the endocervix is not recommended because incremental yield is small and not considered cost-effective (Judson and Werness, 1980).

Most women with lower genital tract and anorectal infections are asymptomatic, and many women with gonococcal PID are as well. For this reason, a high index of suspicion and screening of at-risk women in populations with reasonable rates of infection are warranted.

Table 38-3. SUMMARY OF 1998 TREATMENT GUIDELINES FOR CHLAMYDIA TRACHOMATIS INFECTIONS

SPECIFIC INDICATION	PRIMARY THERAPY	ALTERNATIVE THERAPY	SPECIAL NOTES
Adolescents and adults	**Azithromycin** 1 g PO single dose *or* **Doxycycline** 100 mg PO bid × 7 days	**Erythromycin** base 500 mg PO qid × 7 days *or* **Erythromycin ethylsuccinate** 800 mg PO qid × 7 days *or* **Ofloxacin** 300 mg PO bid × 7 days	Screen sexually active adolescents on annual basis. Screen women ages 20–24 years with new or multiple partners and who do not use barrier contraceptives. Sequelae from untreated infection may include PID, ectopic pregnancy, and infertility. Ofloxacin cannot be used in pregnancy and in patients ≤ 17 years old. Azithromycin 1-g sachets are less expensive than using 250-mg tablets or capsules. No test of cure indicated. HIV-positive patients receive same treatment as HIV-negative.
Pregnancy	**Erythromycin base** 500 mg PO qid × 7 days *or* **Amoxicillin** 500 mg PO tid × 7 days	**Erythromycin** base 250 mg PO qid × 14 days *or* **Erythromycin ethylsuccinate** 800 mg PO qid × 7 days *or* **Erythromycin ethylsuccinate** 400 mg PO qid × 14 days *or* **Azithromycin** 1 gram PO single dose	Erythromycin estolate is contraindicated in pregnancy. Doxycycline and ofloxacin are contraindicated during pregnancy. Insufficient data to recommend routine use of azithromycin in pregnancy. Repeat cultures 3 wk after therapy completed because of high noncompliance rates and lower efficacy of erythromycin regimens.
Ophthalmia neonatorum	**Erythromycin** 50 mg/kg/day PO divided into 4 doses for 10–14 days		Neonatal ocular prophylaxis with silver nitrate or antibiotic ointments does not prevent perinatal transmission of *Chlamydia.* Prophylactic antibiotics not indicated; treat only if symptomatic. Topical antibiotic treatment is ineffective and unnecessary if systemic antibiotics are used. Erythromycin is 80% effective; might need second course of therapy. Treat mother and partner(s).
Infant pneumonia	**Erythromycin** 50 mg/kg/day PO divided into 4 doses for 10–14 days		
Children	CHILDREN WHO WEIGH <45 KG: **Erythromycin** 50 mg/kg/day PO divided into 4 doses for 10–14 days CHILDREN WHO WEIGH ≥45 KG, BUT ARE <8 YEARS OLD: **Azithromycin** 1 PO single dose CHILDREN ≥8 YEARS OLD: **Azithromycin** 1 g PO single dose *or* **Doxycycline** 100 mg PO bid × 7 days		Consider sexual abuse in preadolescent children.

Data abstracted from Centers for Disease Control and Prevention (1998).

Treatment

In general, gonococcal isolates are sensitive to a variety of antimicrobial agents, including penicillins, cephalosporins, tetracyclines, macrolides, quinolones, rifampin, and aminoglycosides. Because resistance to several agents has developed over the last few decades through chromosomal mutations and plasmid acquisition, only single-dose antibiotics that retain greater than 95% treatment efficacy in routine sentinel surveillance for susceptibility patterns by the CDC are recommended for routine use (Centers for Disease Control and Prevention, 1998) (Table 38–4). Individuals infected with gonorrhea should also be treated for chlamydial infection because co-infection rates are high.

Vulvovaginitis

Vulvovaginitis is the most common reason for gynecologic visits, accounting for over 5 million office visits annually. This diagnosis is made in 28% of women who attend STD clinics (Kent, 1991). The term *vulvovaginitis* encompasses a broad spectrum of complaints, ranging from mild irritation to an abnormal discharge to severe pain. Characteristics that help to differentiate abnormal from normal discharge include excessive amount, yellow to green color, abnormal consistency (frothy, cottage cheesy), and abnormal odor. Etiologies can be single or multiple infectious agents or noninfectious irritants or inflammatory conditions. It is thus imperative that clinicians evaluating a woman with symptoms obtain a complete history of the current symptoms and remedies already sought, medical problems, menstruation, pregnancies, sexual behavior and practices, contraceptive practices, and vulvovaginal product use (including tampons and pads, douches, perfumes, powders, creams, lotions, and hair dyes). This should be followed by a thorough examination of the vulva, vagina, and internal organs to rule out upper genital tract infection.

Vaginal Bacteriosis (Bacterial Vaginosis)

Vaginal bacteriosis (VB), more commonly known as bacterial vaginosis, is something of a misnomer, given that the overgrowth (-osis) is of bacteria rather than the vagina itself (Huth, 1989). VB is the most common vaginal infection occurring in women of childbearing age (Berg et al, 1984). This condition may be sexually transmitted or may arise spontaneously, but is largely correlated with sexual activity (Amsel et al, 1983).

Epidemiology

Prevalence rates vary widely, depending on the population studied. A study of 13,747 pregnant women in the United States found rates ranging from 6.1%

for Asians to 8.8% for Caucasians, 15.9% for Hispanics, and 22.7% for African-Americans (Goldenberg et al, 1996). Rates are higher in STD clinic populations (24% to 37%) than in antenatal or family planning patients (Hill et al, 1983; Hallén et al, 1987; Eschenbach et al, 1988; Harms et al, 1994).

Natural History

VB develops when normal H_2O_2-producing *Lactobacillus* are replaced by high concentrations of anaerobic bacteria, such as *Gardnerella vaginalis*, anaerobes, and *Mycoplasma hominis*. It has been postulated that factors that reduce concentrations of *Lactobacillus* species below normal levels may promote overgrowth of VB-associated bacteria and thus predispose to the development of VB. Vaginal lactobacilli have been shown to inhibit *G. vaginalis*, *Mobiluncus*, and *Bacteroides* species in vitro (Skarin and Sylwan, 1986), and women with VB have been found to have lower concentrations of H_2O_2-producing strains of lactobacilli (Eschenbach et al, 1989; Hillier et al, 1992).

Clinical Features

The most consistent symptom of women diagnosed with VB is a malodorous vaginal discharge. Findings on clinical examination include presence of a thin homogeneous, white to gray, adherent vaginal discharge without signs of inflammation.

Diagnosis

Diagnosis can be made by identifying three of the following four signs: (1) adherent, homogeneous, white, noninflammatory vaginal discharge; (2) clue cells on saline wet mount; (3) elevated pH (>4.5); and (4) positive whiff test caused by release of amines when affected secretions come into contact with potassium hydroxide. Vaginal Gram's stain is an excellent diagnostic test, but culture is not (Eschenbach et al, 1988). Given the strong associations between VB and PID, endometritis, and cuff cellulitis following genital tract procedures in infected women, it is reasonable to screen for and treat VB in women about to undergo any such interventions.

Treatment

Antibiotics with broad activity against most anaerobes are highly effective in the treatment of VB. The most widely used therapy for this condition is metronidazole, in either oral or topical form, although oral and topical clindamycin preparations have been shown to have equivalent efficacy (Lugo-Miro et al, 1992; Fischbach et al, 1993; Hillier et al, 1993; Livengood et al, 1994) (Table 38–5). Treatment of sexual partners has not been shown to improve cure rates or reduce recurrences (Vejtorp et al, 1988; Mengel et al, 1989; Moi et al, 1989; Vutyavanich et al, 1993).

Table 38-4. SUMMARY OF 1998 TREATMENT GUIDELINES FOR *NEISSERIA GONORRHOEAE* INFECTIONS

SPECIFIC INDICATION	PRIMARY THERAPY	ALTERNATIVE THERAPY	SPECIAL NOTES
Uncomplicated gonococcal infections (cervicitis, urethritis, rectal)	**Cefixime** 400 mg PO single dose *or* **Ceftriaxone** 125 mg IM single dose *or* **Ciprofloxacin** 500 mg PO single dose *or* **Ofloxacin** 400 mg PO single dose **PLUS** A regimen effective against possible co-infection with *C. trachomatis*: **Azithromycin** 1 g PO single dose *or* **Doxycycline** 100 mg PO bid × 7 days	**Spectinomycin** 2 g IM × 1 dose *or* **Ceftizoxime** 500 mg IM × 1 dose *or* **Cefotaxime** 500 mg IM × 1 dose *or* **Cefotetan** 1 g IM × 1 dose *or* **Cefoxitin** 2 g IM × 1 dose with probenecid 1 go PO *or* **Lomefloxacin** 400 mg PO × 1 dose *or* **Enoxacin** 400 mg PO × 1 dose *or* **Norfloxacin** 800 mg PO × 1 dose	Azithromycin 2 g PO single dose effective but expensive and causes gastrointestinal distress; 1-g dose insufficient. **Pregnancy**—Quinolones and tetracyclines contraindicated. If cephalosporins cannot be tolerated by pregnant woman, treat with spectinomycin 2 g IM × 1 dose along with effective *Chlamydia* regimen. **Pharyngeal infections**—Recommended regimens are ceftriaxone or ciprofloxacin. Alternative therapy—A regimen effective against possible co-infection with *C. trachomatis* (see Table 38–3) **must** be included.
Gonococcal pharyngitis	**Ceftriaxone** 125 IM single dose *or* **Ciprofloxacin** 500 mg PO single dose *or* **Ofloxacin** 400 mg PO single dose **PLUS** **Azithromycin** 1 gram PO single dose *or* **Doxycycline** 100 mg PO bid × 7 day		If unable to tolerate cephalosporins or quinolones, use spectinomycin 2 g IM (only 52% effective).
Disseminated gonococcal infection (DGI) adults	**Ceftriaxone** 1 gm IM or IV q 24 h	**Cefotaxime** 1 g IV q8h *or* **Ceftizoxime** 1 g IV q8h *or* **Spectinomycin** 2 g IM q12h (if β-lactam allergic)	Hospitalization is recommended for initial therapy. Continue parenteral regimen for 24–48 hours after improvement; may then switch to one of the following to complete a full week of therapy: **cefixime**, 400 mg PO bid; **ciprofloxacin**, 500 mg PO bid; or **ofloxacin**, 400 mg PO bid. Quinolones not recommended for use in pregnant or lactating women, or in children ≤17 years old. Treat presumptively for concurrent *C. trachomatis* infection.
DGI, infants	**Ceftriaxone** 25–50 mg/kg/day IM/IV qd × 7 days, up to 10–14 days if meningitis is documented *or* **Cefotaxime** 25 mg/kg IM/IV q12h × 7 days, up to 10–14 days if meningitis is documented		
Gonococcal meningitis and endocarditis	**Ceftriaxone** 1–2 g IV q12h		Therapy for meningitis should be continued for 10–14 days and at least 4 weeks for endocarditis.

(Table continued on following page)

Table 38-4. SUMMARY OF 1998 TREATMENT GUIDELINES FOR *NEISSERIA GONORRHOEAE* INFECTIONS (*Continued*)

SPECIFIC INDICATION	PRIMARY THERAPY	ALTERNATIVE THERAPY	SPECIAL NOTES
Gonococcal conjunctivitis	**Ceftriaxone** 1 g IM × 1 dose **PLUS** Lavage of infected eye with saline solution once		
Ophthalmia neonatorum prophylaxis	**Silver nitrate (1%) aqueous solution** × 1 application *or* **Erythromycin (0.5%) ophthalmic ointment** × 1 application *or* **Tetracycline (1%) ophthalmic ointment** × 1 application		Not effective for prophylaxis of chlamydial eye disease. Prophylaxis should occur for both vaginal and cesarean deliveries. Bacitracin is not effective. Povidone-iodine has not been adequately studied.
Ophthalmia neonatorum treatment	**Ceftriaxone** 25–30 mg/kg IM/IV × 1 dose (max 125 mg)		Topical antibiotic therapy alone is inadequate and unnecessary if systemic therapy is administered. Simultaneous infection with *C. trachomatis* is possible. Use ceftriaxone cautiously in infants with elevated bilirubin levels. Treat until cultures negative at 48–72 hours.
Prophylaxis for infants	**Ceftriaxone** 25–30 mg/kg IM/IV × 1 dose (max 125 mg)		Use in infants born to untreated mothers. Simultaneous infection with *C. trachomatis* is possible. Use ceftriaxone cautiously in infants with elevated bilirubin levels. Treat mother.
Gonococcal infections in children	CHILDREN WHO WEIGH ≥45 KG: See adult regimens CHILDREN WHO WEIGH <45 KG: **Ceftriaxone** 125 mg IM × 1 dose (for uncomplicated gonococcal vulvovaginitis, cervicitis, urethritis, pharyngitis, or proctitis) *or* **Ceftriaxone** 50 mg/kg IM/IV qd (max. dose 2 g >45 kg and 1 g <45 kg) × 7 days (*for bacteremia, arthritis, or meningitis*)	CHILDREN WHO WEIGH <45 KG: **Spectinomycin** 40 mg/kg (max. 2 g) IM × 1 dose (*for uncomplicated gonococcal vulvovaginitis, cervicitis, urethritis, pharyngitis, or proctitis*)	Sexual abuse is the most common cause. For meningitis, increase duration of treatment to 10–14 days. Only parenteral cephalosporins are recommended for use among children; oral cephalosporins have not been adequately evaluated in children. Cefotaxime is only approved for gonococcal ophthalmia. Simultaneous infection with *C. trachomatis* is possible.

Data abstracted from Centers for Disease Control and Prevention (1998).

Table 38-5. SUMMARY OF 1998 TREATMENT GUIDELINES FOR VAGINAL BACTERIOSIS—CAUSATIVE ORGANISMS (*Prevotella* species, *Mobiluncus* species, *G. vaginalis*, *Mycoplasma hominis*)

SPECIFIC INDICATION	PRIMARY THERAPY	ALTERNATIVE THERAPY	SPECIAL NOTES
Nonpregnant females	**Metronidazole** 500 mg bid × 7 days (avoid alcohol during or 24 hours after) *or* **Clindamycin cream (2%)**, 1 applicator full (5 g) intravaginally qhs × 7 days *or* **Metronidazole gel (0.75%)**, 1 applicator full (5 g) intravaginally bid × 5 days	**Metronidazole** 2 g PO × 1 dose *or* **Clindamycin** 300 mg PO bid × 7 days	Only women with symptomatic disease need treatment. Treatment of male partners has *not* been shown to alter course or relapse/re-infection rate of VB. Single-dose metronidazole less effective than other regimens. Flagyl ER (metronidazole 750 mg) PO qd × 7 days also Food and Drug Administration approved for VB; no comparative data with other regimens available. Patients allergic to oral metronidazole should not be given vaginal gel. Recent meta-analysis of metronidazole does not indicate teratogenicity in humans. Intravaginal route may be preferred because of ↓ systemic side effects.
Pregnancy	FOR HIGH OR LOW RISK: **Metronidazole** 250 mg PO tid × 7 days	**Metronidazole** 2 g PO × 1 dose *or* **Clindamycin** 300 mg PO bid × 7 days *or* **Metronidazole gel (0.75%)**, one applicator full (5 g) intravaginally bid × 5 days **[low risk only]**	VB has been associated with adverse outcomes of pregnancy. Treatment of high-risk pregnant women (previous premature delivery) who are asymptomatic might reduce premature delivery. Screening and treatment suggested early in second trimester. Low-risk pregnant women who have symptomatic VB should be treated. Lower doses recommended to minimize exposure to fetus. Clindamycin vaginal gel not recommended; use associated with increase in premature deliveries.

Data abstracted from Centers for Disease Control and Prevention (1998).

In women who have a history of preterm birth or who are underweight, excellent data suggest screening and treatment of infection (Morales et al, 1994; Hauth et al, 1995). Systemic therapy seems warranted, given the fact that treatment is both for the lower genital tract infection itself and for prevention of preterm premature rupture of membranes, preterm labor, and preterm birth.

Trichomonas vaginalis

Trichomonas vaginalis is a unicellular, flagellated, motile protozoan parasite that is primarily transmitted through sexual contact. Most commonly found in vaginal secretions of pH greater than 4.5, it proliferates at the time of menstruation and is frequently associated with a large number of leukocytes.

Epidemiology

Because long-term longitudinal studies of at-risk populations have not been conducted and because many infected women are asymptomatic, accurate incidence rates are difficult to estimate. Prevalence varies significantly, depending on the population evaluated and the diagnostic method employed. In 1975 it was estimated conservatively that there were at least 3 to 4 million cases diagnosed in the United States (Rein and Muller, 1990). It is estimated that approximately one quarter of women presenting with symptoms of vaginal infection have trichomoniasis.

Clinical Features

The clinical presentation of persons infected with *T. vaginalis* is varied, with many women harboring the organism asymptomatically. Vaginal discharge may vary from minimal to copious, purulent, homogeneous, yellow-green, frothy, and irritating. Dysuria, urinary frequency, vaginal pruritis, dyspareunia, offensive genital odor, and low back pain can also be present. The "classical" frothy, yellow, copious discharge with vaginal wall erythema and "strawberry" cervix are seen in fewer than 10% of infected women. Disagreeable odor associated with a slight increase in homogeneous nonsticky, yellow-white discharge that pools in the posterior vaginal fornix is the most common presentation.

Diagnosis

The diagnosis can be made in most circumstances using microscopic evaluation of a wet mount, mixing vaginal secretions obtained from the anterior fornix with a drop or two of normal saline. The sensitivity of this method varies from 42% to 92%, depending on the reagents employed, the handling of the specimen, and the compulsiveness of the observer; sensitivity increases to approximately 80% in the hands of experienced microscopists but is about 50% for the average clinician (Fouts and Kraus, 1980; Thomason et al, 1988).

The diagnosis of trichomoniasis is made occasionally on a Papanicolaou smear. In a research setting, the sensitivity of this method varies from 52% to 67%, too low to permit its use as a screening method (Weinberger and Harger, 1993). Culture is another option for diagnosis. Special media are required that make this procedure labor intensive and costly, making this a poor choice in most clinical settings.

Treatment

Metronidazole remains the mainstay of treatment for trichomoniasis. The 2-g single-dose regimen of metronidazole is the current standard for treatment, and boasts cure rates ranging from 82% to 88% (Dykers, 1975; Fleury et al, 1977). Topical metronidazole gel has considerably lower efficacy than oral regimens for treatment of trichomoniasis because of its failure to achieve therapeutic levels in the urethra and perivaginal glands (Lohmeyer, 1974). The Food and Drug Administration (FDA) has approved a regimen of Flagyl 375 twice daily for 7 days as an alternative regimen for this infection, although there are no published clinical data to support this contention. Concurrent treatment of all sexual partners is recommended.

There was initial concern regarding the mutagenic potential of metronidazole, based on rodent data in which animals developed tumors after chronic high-dose exposure to the drug. Subsequent human studies have not substantiated these early claims. Until recently, use of metronidazole in pregnancy, particularly during the first trimester, has been discouraged strongly because of the potential for increased birth defects. No data have been presented in the English language that support this fear. The 1998 CDC Treatment Guidelines recommend that low-risk pregnant women with symptomatic trichomoniasis be treated using the 2-g single dose (Table 38–6). Studies suggest a possible relationship between *T.*

vaginalis infection and pregnancy complications such as preterm premature rupture of membranes and preterm birth. It is not clear whether routine screening and treatment of low- or high-risk pregnant women with trichomonal infection will lower these adverse outcomes.

Treatment failures occur occasionally. Reinfection by an untreated partner is the most common cause of recurrent infection, and retreatment with the standard dose is recommended. Persistence of trichomonal infection is less common. Etiologies for persistent infection include nonadherence to the treatment schedule by either the woman or her partner(s), interference with other systemic medications (especially phenytoin and phenobarbitol), and antibiotic resistance.

Vulvovaginal Candidiasis

Most commonly caused by *Candida albicans*, this infectious syndrome may also be caused by other fungi. Seventy-five per cent of women will have at least one yeast infection, nearly 50% will have more than one episode, and less than 5% will have recurrent infections (more than three per 12-month period) (Hurley and De Louvois, 1979; Geiger, 1995; Geiger and Foxman, 1996).

Epidemiology

Candidal species are rarely isolated from premenarchal or postmenopausal women, suggesting that there is a hormonal dependence for this infection. Prevalence figures are difficult to estimate, given that this is a common infection with nonspecific symptoms of vulvovaginal irritation, and use of over-the-counter medications and empirical treatment by health care practitioners has limited use of medical records to establish accurate rates of infection. Although previous work established that 80% to 92% of infections were caused by *C. albicans* (Odds, 1988), newer data suggest a mild shift toward the non-*albicans* candidal species, such as *C. glabrata* (Horowitz et al, 1992). This shift may represent the effect of widespread use of nonprescription topical azoles and suboptimal short treatment courses.

Table 38–6. SUMMARY OF 1998 TREATMENT GUIDELINES FOR *TRICHOMONAS VAGINALIS*

PRIMARY THERAPY	ALTERNATIVE THERAPY	SPECIAL NOTES
Metronidazole 2 g PO single dose	**Metronidazole** 500 mg bid × 7 days	If treatment fails, use 500 mg bid × 7 day regimen. If repeated failure, use 2 g qd × 3–5 days. **Flagyl** 375 mg PO bid × 7 days FDA approved; no clinical data available comparing its efficacy with 500 mg bid × 7 days regimen. May treat pregnant women with 2-g single dose.

Data abstracted from Centers for Disease Control and Prevention (1998).

Natural History

Although most episodes appear to be unprovoked, there are clear associations between vulvovaginal candidiasis and uncontrolled diabetes mellitus, use of antibiotics, high levels of estrogen such as may be seen in some women on oral contraceptives, and use of an intrauterine contraceptive device or vaginal sponge (Amsel et al, 1983; Foxman, 1990).

Clinical Features

Symptoms include copious vaginal discharge with vulvar and/or vaginal pruritis, and may be accompanied by burning, dyspareunia, and dysuria.

Diagnosis

Vulvovaginal candidiasis is overdiagnosed because of frequently incomplete diagnostic evaluation; at least half of women diagnosed with a yeast infection in one study had other etiologies for their symptoms (Berg et al, 1984). Diagnosis is most commonly made by identification of hyphal or spore forms of yeast on wet mount using KOH or on Gram's stain, and pH determination is usually normal ($\leq$4.5). Given the poor sensitivity of these techniques, however, the presence of appropriate symptoms and a negative microscopy should prompt use of vaginal culture (Sobel, 1997).

Treatment

Drugs from the azole and imidazole classes are considered standard of care for the treatment of vulvovaginal candidiasis. Treatment using single topical doses should be reserved for uncomplicated cases, and multiday topical and all oral regimens should be given to women with severe or complicated infections (Table 38–7). Topical drugs result in cure rates in excess of 80%, which is similar to rates of cure with oral agents. Given that oral agents pose no clear biologic advantage, patient choice should guide choice of therapeutic intervention.

Topical administration of gentian violet (1%) and intravaginal administration of boric acid capsules (600 mg of powder in a size 0 gelatin capsule) for 14 days may be used for severe or tenacious infections. Recurrent infections may require systemic treatment with fluconazole, ketaconazole, or itraconazole; long-

Table 38–7. SUMMARY OF 1998 TREATMENT GUIDELINES FOR VULVOVAGINAL CANDIDIASIS (VVC)—(*C. albicans*, other *Candida* species, *Torulopsis* species, or other yeasts)

THERAPY	SPECIAL NOTES
Butoconazole 20% cream, 5 g intravaginally × 3 days *or* **Clotrimazole** 1% cream, 5 g intravaginally × 7–14 days *or* **Clotrimazole** 100-mg vaginal tablet, × 7 days **Clotrimazole** 100-mg tablet, × 1 dose *or* **Miconazole** 2% cream, 5 g intravaginally × 7 days *or* **Miconazole** 200-mg vaginal suppository, 1 dose × 3 days *or* **Miconazole** 100-mg vaginal suppository, 1 dose × 7 days *or* **Nystatin** 100,000-unit vaginal tablet, qd intravaginally × 14 days *or* **Tioconazole** 6.5% ointment, 5 g intravaginally × 1 dose *or* **Terconazole** 0.8% cream, 5 g intravaginally × 3 days *or* **Terconazole** 80-mg suppository, 1 dose × 3 days ORAL AGENT: **Fluconazole** 150 mg PO single dose	**VVC:** Topical azole products more effective than nystatin. Self-medication with over-the-counter products advised only if diagnosed previously with VVC and same symptoms recur. Uncomplicated VVC responds to all regimens. Oral azoles, itraconazole and ketoconazole, might be as effective as topical agents, but potential toxicity and drug interactions must be considered. Complicated VVC (severe local or recurrent VVC in patient with uncontrolled diabetes or infection caused by less susceptible organism) requires 10–14 days of topical or oral therapy. Treatment of **sex partners** has not been shown to ↓ frequency of recurrences. VVC may occur more frequently in HIV+ women; treatment is the same. **Pregnancy**—Only topical azole therapies should be used. Most effective are butoconazole, clotrimazole, miconazole, and terconazole. Seven-day regimens preferred. **Recurrent vulvovaginal candidiasis (RVVC):** Defined as four or more episodes of symptomatic VVC per year. Risk factors for RVVC: uncontrolled diabetes, immunosuppression, and corticosteroid use. Optimal treatment has not been established. Initial intensive regimen of 10–14 days, followed by a maintenance regimen for 6 mo, is recommended. Ketoconazole, 100 mg PO qd for up to 6 mo, reduces frequency of episodes. Studies are evaluating a weekly fluconazole regimen. All cases of RVVC should be confirmed by culture before initiating maintenance therapy. Management of HIV+ women should be same as other women with RVVC.

Data abstracted from Centers for Disease Control and Prevention (1998).

term suppression with these agents may reduce risk of further episodes.

Treponema pallidum (Syphilis)

Syphilis is a chronic systemic sexually transmitted infection caused by the bacterium *T. pallidum*, which has been described for centuries. Endemic in Europe in the 15th century, its prevalence has declined dramatically in this century with the introduction of antimicrobial therapy and targeted disease control efforts.

Epidemiology

Prevalence of syphilis peaked during the 1940s and declined rapidly thereafter because of the development and widespread availability of penicillin. There was a resurgence of cases in the 1980s in homosexual males, injection drug users, and HIV-infected individuals that peaked in 1990 and has declined steadily since. Syphilis now appears largely concentrated in urban areas of the Southeastern United States in African-Americans (Wortley and Fleming, 1997). This has prompted many public health officials to consider policy strategies aimed at eradication of endemic syphilis in the United States (Hook, 1998).

Natural History

Although syphilis becomes a systemic process shortly following acquisition, host factors appear to affect penetration of disease. A prospective study of syphilis conducted in Oslo between 1890 and 1910 showed clearly that some individuals progressed rapidly to the late destructive stages of disease and others remained in latency for long periods of time (Bruusgaard, 1929; Gjestland, 1955). A second infamous study of the natural history of syphilis was undertaken by the U.S. Public Health Service through the Tuskegee Institute in Alabama in 1932 (Heller et al, 1946; Schuman et al, 1955; (Olansky, 1956; Rockwell et al, 1964). It was a cohort study designed to determine whether the use of arsenicals might not be more toxic than the untreated disease itself, and its study design was superior to that of the Oslo study, including autopsies in approximately two thirds of those who died during the next 20 years. However, informed consent was not obtained and study participants were not offered penicillin after it became recommended for treatment (Brandt, 1978; Jones et al, 1981). The main finding of the study was excess mortality in those with syphilis of 20% at the 12-year follow-up and 17% at the 20-year evaluation (Heller et al, 1946; Olansky, 1956).

Clinical Features

Syphilis is a systemic disease with myriad clinical presentations. Primary infection is marked by a non-tender ulcer at the site of acquisition. Secondary infection symptoms include a generalized rash (including palmar and plantar surfaces), mucocutaneous lesions, and adenopathy. A latent stage of variable duration ensues, with the early latent stage encompassing no more than 1 year of infection and the late latent stage greater than 1 year. Tertiary infection may strike the heart, nervous system, hearing, or sight, or may be manifested diffusely with gummatous changes.

Diagnosis

Although definitive diagnosis of early syphilis relies on darkfield examination of scrapings recovered from primary chancres or secondary lesions, presumptive diagnosis relies on a nontreponemal test (Venereal Disease Research Laboratory [VDRL] or rapid plasma reagin [RPR]), with confirmation by a treponemal test (fluorescent treponemal antibody, absorbed [FTA-ABS] or microhemagglutination–*T. pallidum*). Direct tests remain positive for life, whereas indirect ones revert to negative in 6 to 12 months in early syphilis and 12 to 18 months in late infection. A fourfold difference in RPR or VDRL titer designates a significant difference in disease status. In neurosyphilis, cerebrospinal fluid white blood cell levels are elevated ($>5/mm^3$) and a VDRL test is normally positive. In rare cases the VDRL test will be negative, and FTA-ABS must be used (this test has more false positives).

Treatment

Penicillin is still the treatment of choice for all stages of syphilis (Table 38–8). Parenteral penicillin G is the only therapy for neurosyphilis or any stage in pregnant women, and when infected individuals in these categories are penicillin allergic, desensitization and treatment with penicillin is warranted. The Jarisch-Herxheimer reaction manifests as an acute febrile reaction resulting from breakdown of immune complexes occurring in the first 24 hours following treatment.

Genital Herpes

Genital herpes is a chronic viral infection caused by two antigenic types of the human herpesvirus, herpes simplex virus type 1 (HSV-1) and herpes simplex virus type 2 (HSV-2). Most commonly distinguished by identification of purified type-specific proteins such as glycoproteins gG1 and gG2, HSV-1 is more commonly associated with oral-labial infection and HSV-2 is estimated to be responsible for at least 90% of genital infections. Although antibodies to HSV-1 rise through childhood, antibodies to HSV-2 are not commonly detected until puberty and seroprevalence rates rise in proportion to level of sexual activity (Johnson et al, 1989; Oliver et al, 1995), suggesting

Table 38-8. SUMMARY OF 1998 TREATMENT GUIDELINES FOR SYPHILIS—
TREPONEMA PALLIDUM

SPECIFIC INDICATION	PRIMARY THERAPY	ALTERNATIVE THERAPY	SPECIAL NOTES
Primary and secondary syphilis; early latent syphilis (<1 year)	ADULTS: **Benzathine penicillin G** 2.4 million units IM × 1 dose CHILDREN: **Benzathine penicillin G** 50,000 units/kg IM × 1 dose (up to 2.4 million units) IF PENICILLIN ALLERGIC: **Tetracycline** 500 mg PO qid × 14 days	IF PENICILLIN ALLERGIC: **Erythromycin** 500 mg PO qid × 14 days *or* **Ceftriaxone** 1 g daily (must provide 8–10 days treponemicidal levels)	If titers not ↓ 4× by 6 months after treatment for primary or secondary, **re-treat** with 3 weekly injections of benzathine penicillin G, 2.4 million units IM. Erythromycin regimen less effective than other regimens. Optimal dose and duration for ceftriaxone have not been established. **Single-dose ceftriaxone is not effective.** Test for HIV.
Late latent or latent syphilis of unknown duration; late (tertiary) syphilis (gumma and cardiovascular syphilis)	ADULTS: **Benzathine penicillin G** 2.4 million units IM/wk × 3 wk (7.2 million units total) CHILDREN: **Benzathine penicillin G** 50,000 units/kg IM (up to 2.4 million units) for 3 total doses (150,000) units/kg or 7.2 million units) IF PENICILLIN ALLERGIC: **Tetracycline** 500 mg PO qid × 4 weeks *or* **Doxycycline** 100 mg PO bid × 4 weeks		Patients are seroreactive with no other evidence of disease and should be evaluated for evidence of tertiary disease. Some recommend CSF evaluation before treatment for latent syphilis, and, if treatment fails, neurosyphilis should be considered. Pregnant women and HIV-positive patients should only receive penicillin regimens.
Neurosyphilis	**Aqueous crystalline penicillin G** 18–24 million units IV qd, administered as 2–4 million units IV q4h × 10–14 days	IF COMPLIANCE ASSURED: Procaine penicillin 2.4 million units IM qd *plus* probenecid 500 mg PO qid × 10–14 days	May occur at any stage of syphilis. Some experts add benzathine penicillin, 2.4 million units IM, following treatment in order to complete regimen for late syphilis. Follow CSF q6 months until cell count is normal. If not ↓ at 6 mo or normal in 2 yr, re-treat. If penicillin allergic, desensitize.
HIV and syphilis	PRIMARY/SECONDARY/EARLY LATENT SYPHILIS: Treat as above. Some experts recommend other supplemental antibiotics in addition to standard therapy or **benzathine penicillin G** as dosed for late syphilis. LATE LATENT SYPHILIS OR UNKNOWN DURATION: CSF exam, then treat as above for late latent or neurosyphilis based on exam results.		Neurosyphilis must be considered in differential for HIV patients with mental status changes. Evaluate at 3, 6, 9, 12, and 24 mo for treatment failure. If failure, examine CSF and re-treat as previously recommended. **Penicillin must be used;** penicillin-allergic patients must be desensitized.

(Table continued on following page)

a sexual pattern of transmission. Many use the terms *genital herpes* and *HSV-2* synonymously, although that is not strictly correct.

Epidemiology

National seroprevalence rates have been estimated based on two population-based surveys conducted by the federal government (Johnson et al, 1989; Fleming et al, 1997). The latest survey estimated the U.S. prevalence to be 21.9% in the period of study, 1988 to 1994, which represents a potential infected population of in excess of 45 million people (Fleming et al, 1997). This represented a 30% rise from the previous period of study, 1976 to 1980. Rates were higher in persons of color and in females, with cumulative lifetime incidence rates of infection reaching 80% in African-American women and 60% in African-American men, as compared with 25% in white women and 20% in white men. One of the

Table 38-8. SUMMARY OF 1998 TREATMENT GUIDELINES FOR SYPHILIS—
TREPONEMA PALLADIUM (Continued)

SPECIFIC INDICATION	PRIMARY THERAPY	ALTERNATIVE THERAPY	SPECIAL NOTES
Pregnancy and syphilis	Treat for appropriate state of syphilis. Some experts recommend a second dose of **benzathine penicillin G** 2.4 million units IM 1 wk after initial dose for women with primary, secondary, or early latent syphilis. IF PENICILLIN ALLERGIC: Desensitize patient to penicillin.	**Doxycycline** and **tetracycline** are contraindicated in pregnancy. **Erythromycin** cannot be relied upon to treat infected fetus. Insufficient data **azithromycin** or *ceftriaxone.*	Routine screening for syphilis at time of first prenatal visit. High risk should also be screened at 28 wk and at delivery. Titers should be repeated in third trimester and at delivery (monthly for high risk). Penicillin is effective in preventing transmission to and established infection in fetuses. Women treated in second half of pregnancy are at risk for premature labor and/or fetal distress. All patients who have syphilis should be offered testing for HIV.
Congenital syphilis	FOR NEWBORNS: **Aqueous crystalline penicillin G** 100,000–150,000 units/kg/day IV (50,000 units/kg IV q12h for first 7 days of life and q8h thereafter for total of 10 days) *or* **Procaine penicillin G** 50,000 units/kg IM qd (single dose) × 10 days FOR CHILDREN IDENTIFIED AT >1 MONTH: **aqueous crystalline penicillin G** 200,000–300,000 units/kg/day IV or IM (as 50,000 units/kg q4–6h) × 10 days	Insufficient data regarding use of other antibiotics	Routine screening of newborn sera or cord blood not recommended; check mother's serum. All infants born to mothers with syphilis should be evaluated with VDRL, not FTA or MHA. Treatment decisions should be based on identification of syphilis in mother, adequacy of maternal therapy, evidence of syphilis in infancy, and comparison of infant's VDRL with mother's VDRL. If more than 1 day of therapy is missed, the entire course must be restarted. Follow-up every 2–3 months until titers decline or become nonreactive in VDRL-positive infants.

Abbreviations: CSF, cerebrospinal fluid; FTA, fluorescent treponemal antibody; HIV, human immunodeficiency virus; MHA, microhemagglutination; VDRL, Venereal Disease Research Laboratory (test).
Data abstracted from Centers for Disease Control and Prevention (1998).

most important findings of the study was that less than 10% of those found to be seropositive for HSV-2 reported a history of genital herpes, suggesting a large subclinical or asymptomatic reservoir of infected individuals.

Incidence rates have been established for two small but interesting cohorts of women. In a study of 839 Swedish adolescent women, 22% acquired HSV-2 during the 15-year follow-up period (Christenson et al, 1992). A higher risk group drawn from an STD clinic in Seattle had a 3% annual incidence for HSV-2 (Wald et al, 1995).

of one person and shedding lesions or secretions from either genital or oral origin that contain viral particles from another person. Infection results in focal necrosis and balloon degeneration of cells, with production of mononucleated giant cells and intranuclear inclusions called Cowdry type A bodies. Most vesicles ultimately burst and re-epithelialize, while the virus ascends peripheral sensory nerves and enters sensory or autonomic nerve root ganglia to establish latency. Reactivation is influenced by a complex interplay of viral and host factors.

Natural History

Prior infection with HSV-1 appears to moderate clinical symptoms of infection with HSV-2 (Koutsky et al, 1992). HSV is acquired through direct contact between mucosal surfaces or small cracks in the skin

Clinical Features

There are four types of genital herpes: first-episode primary, first-episode nonprimary, recurrent, and asymptomatic. In first-episode primary infection, severity of clinical symptoms is high and the person is seronegative. First-episode nonprimary infection refers to the first recognized episode of genital herpes in individuals whose sera contain HSV antibodies; most commonly the clinical severity of these episodes is moderated by these antibodies. Recurrent infection refers to repeated episodes of genital herpes in the same individual, and is more common in those with HSV-2 infection. Finally, asymptomatic infection refers to episodes of shedding of HSV-2 from genital sites in the absence of recognizable symptoms in an individual with antibodies to the virus.

The incubation period for HSV-2 ranges from 2 to 12 days, after which symptoms typically include the development of painful, grouped, discrete vesicles. The vesicles typically evolve into pustules, which then erode into ulcers that slowly crust over, resulting in complete re-epithelialization within 15 to 20 days. In women, lesions typically occur around the introitus, the urethral meatus, or the labia. Cervical infection is extremely common, affecting up to 90% of women with first-episode genital herpes (Barton et al, 1981; Corey and Holmes, 1983). Extragenital lesions involving the buttocks, groin, thigh, hands, or eyes are more common in women than men, occurring in about 9% of those with primary infection (Benedetti et al, 1995). Anorectal infection can be seen in women, although more than 75% of these infections are asymptomatic, and there appears to be little association between anorectal HSV and recent or past anal intercourse (Koutsky et al, 1992).

Primary infection may involve a systemic response, including fever, headache, malaise, and myalgias, that can last for approximately 1 week. Local clinical symptoms include pain, itching, dysuria, vaginal or urethral discharge, and tender inguinal adenopathy that peak in severity at approximately 1 week and gradually recede over the second week of the illness. Those with serologic evidence of prior HSV-1 infection are less likely to have systemic symptoms and have a shorter course of local symptoms because of the effect of neutralizing antibodies (Notkins, 1974).

In recurrent infection, systemic symptoms are absent, and the local symptoms are milder in intensity and shorter in duration than those of first-episode infections. Approximately 90% experience a prodrome that includes mild irritation of the area where an outbreak is about to occur.

Subclinical or asymptomatic viral shedding is common. HSV has been cultured from the genital tract of individuals in the absence of identifiable lesions, and both sexual and vertical transmission of genital herpes may occur during such shedding (Brown et al, 1991; Mertz et al, 1992). Subclinical HSV shedding is highest during the first 6 months of infection, and declines thereafter. PCR genital tract swabbing has shown detectable rates of HSV-2 shedding in up to 35% of days in the 6 months following infection acquisition. In a 3-month study of 110

women with a history of genital herpes who collected daily genital swabs for evaluation by PCR, women were found to shed HSV viral particles on 55% of days when infected with HSV-2 alone and on 52% of days when co-infected with HSV-1 and HSV-2 (Wald et al, 1995).

Individuals who are unaware of their infection can frequently be taught to recognize outbreaks. Sixty-two women seropositive for HSV-2 who were not aware of their infection were shown pictures of outbreaks and taught about the mild symptomatology associated with subclinical infection; 48 of them (77%) were able to recognize their next outbreak and reported that that they had previously mistaken their symptoms (vulvar irritation and dyspareunia) for either a yeast infection or a mild reaction to a common irritant (Langenberg et al, 1989).

Diagnosis

Laboratory diagnosis of genital herpes can be accomplished by viral isolation, DNA detection, or antigen detection by EIA or fluorescent antibody from specimens obtained directly from lesions. Alternatively, serologic tests using purified type-specific proteins such as gG1 and gG2, and ICP-35 complex, can be used.

Treatment

Treatment is directed at relieving symptoms; shortening the clinical course of disease; reducing viral shedding, which thereby reduces infectiousness and potential for complications; and reducing the frequency of recurrences. The mainstays of treatment are several nucleoside analog formations, including acyclovir, famcyclovir, and valacyclovir (Table 38–9).

Human Papillomavirus

At least 35 of the over 100 documented human papillomavirus (HPV) viral types infect the genital tract (Shamanin et al, 1994). Types 6 and 11 are most commonly identified in visible genital warts, whereas types 16, 18, 31, and 45 are most commonly associated with high-grade squamous intraepithelial lesions (SILs) and squamous cancers of the genital tract.

Epidemiology

Current epidemiologic evidence using ultrasensitive detection methods for identifying HPV suggests that well over 50% of sexually active adults have been infected with one or more types of HPV. The majority of these lesions are subclinical, unrecognized, and benign (Kjaer et al, 1990; Wheeler et al, 1993; Becker et al, 1994; Heim et al, 1995). Transmission is sexual, involving close contact of genital tract skin, and ap-

Table 38-9. SUMMARY OF 1998 TREATMENT GUIDELINES FOR GENITAL HSV INFECTION (HSV-2 Usually)

SPECIFIC INDICATION	PRIMARY THERAPY	ALTERNATIVE THERAPY	SPECIAL NOTES
First clinical episode of genital herpes	**Acyclovir** 400 mg PO tid for 7–10 days or until clinically resolved *or* **Acyclovir** 200 mg PO 5×/day for 7–10 days or until clinically resolved *or* **Famciclovir** 250 mg PO tid for 7–10 days or until clinically resolved *or* **Valacyclovir** 1 g PO bid for 7–10 days or until clinically resolved		Topical acyclovir is less effective than oral; use is discouraged. First clinical episode during pregnancy may be treated with acyclovir. Safety of valacyclovir and famciclovir in **pregnancy** not established; benefits must outweigh risks.
First clinical episode of herpes proctitis or oral infection (stomatitis or pharyngitis)	**Acyclovir** 400 mg PO 5×/day for 7–10 days or until clinically resolved		Valacyclovir and famciclovir probably effective but clinical experience lacking.
Recurrent episodes	**Acyclovir** 400 mg PO tid × 5 days *or* **Acyclovir** 200 mg PO 5×/day × 5 days *or* **Acyclovir** 800 mg PO bid × 5 days *or* **Famciclovir** 125 mg PO bid × 5 days *or* **Valacyclovir** 500 mg PO bid × 5 days		Treatment must be initiated during prodrome or within 1 day of onset of lesions for patient to experience benefit from therapy
Daily suppressive therapy	**Acyclovir** 400 mg PO bid *or* **Famciclovir** 250 mg bid *or* **Valacyclovir** 250 mg bid *or* **Valacyclovir** 500 mg bid *or* **Valacyclovir** 1 g qd		Reduces frequency of HSV recurrences by at least 75% in patients with 6 or more recurrences/yr. Safety and efficacy documented with daily use of acyclovir for up to 6 yr, and with valacyclovir and famciclovir for 1 yr. After yr of suppressive therapy, discontinuation should be considered to assess rate of recurrent episodes. Valacyclovir 500 mg PO qd less effective than other valacyclovir regimens in patients with >10 episodes/yr.
Severe infection	**Acyclovir** 5–10 mg/kg body weight IV q8h for 5–7 days or until clinical resolution		
HIV+ or immunocompromised	**Acyclovir** 400 mg PO 3–5×/day until clinically resolved (if severe, see above) *or* **Famciclovir** 500 mg PO bid	If resistance suspected, **foscarnet** 40 mg/kg IV q8h until clinical resolution attained *or* topical **cidofovir 1% gel** applied to lesions qd × 5 days	All acyclovir-resistant strains are resistant to valacyclovir and most are resistant to famciclovir.
Neonatal herpes	**Acyclovir** 30–60 mg/kg/day for 10–21 days		Available data do not support routine use of acyclovir for asymptomatic infants exposed during birth process.

Data abstracted from Centers for Disease Control and Prevention (1998).

pears to be enhanced by moisture and epithelial disruption.

Natural History

Transience of HPV expression has been established in multiple cohorts (Reeves et al, 1989; Rosenfeld et al, 1992; Schneider et al, 1992; Moscicki et al, 1993; Wheeler et al, 1996). It is not clear whether this represents clearance of virus or whether the virus becomes suppressed below the level of detection; the latter appears more likely. Individuals who are immunosuppressed secondary to illnesses such as HIV, Hodgkin's disease, pregnancy, or immunosuppressive therapy may experience rapid and excessive growth of genital warts.

Clinical Features

Although most infections are asymptomatic or subclinical, there are two clinical manifestations worthy of mention: visible genital warts and SILs, particularly high-grade ones. Most visible genital warts are asymptomatic, although occasionally patients will report itching, burning, pain, or bleeding. Presence of warts at multiple sites is common, and they can assume multiple forms, including condylomata acuminata, papules, flat-topped macules, and keratotic warts. The natural history of genital warts may include spontaneous resolution, persistence, or exacerbation in size or number or both.

Diagnosis

Although there are many HPV DNA detection and typing tests available commercially, their usefulness in clinical situations remains controversial given the intermittent expression of HPV from mucosal and epidermal surfaces. Most individuals with genital warts are diagnosed clinically, based on the visible features of the lesions. The differential diagnosis for such lesions includes skin tags, vestibular papillae, nevi, and other infectious papules such as those caused by molluscum contagiosum and syphilis. Although diagnosis may be confirmed by biopsy, this is rarely needed.

Treatment

The primary goal of treating visible genital warts is the removal of symptoms. It is not clear whether removal of visible lesions reduces infectivity. Although treatment can reduce the size of warts or remove them, no known treatment has been shown to eradicate HPV from genital tract tissues. Treatment of subclinical infection has not been shown to be of benefit, and carries the risk of promotion of scarring, chronic pain, and abnormalities of skin pigmentation. Treatment should therefore be offered to those with symptomatic visible genital warts or SIL.

Choice of treatment for those with visible warts should be guided by patient preference as well as the number and size of warts. Therapies have been divided into patient-applied and provider-administered, and most require several treatment courses to effect a wart-free state (Table 38–10). Recurrences are common with all treatment modalities because it is not expected that eradication of HPV can be attained. Alternative treatments, including intralesional interferon injection and laser surgery, appear to offer no benefit when compared with the other regimens described, and both are more costly and have a higher side effect profile (Beutner and Ferenczy, 1997; Swinehart et al, 1997).

The work-up and treatment of SILs is discussed in greater detail in Chapter 52.

Pelvic Inflammatory Disease

PID is a continuum of inflammation/infection that may involve the endometrium, fallopian tubes, ovaries, perihepatic region, and intraperitoneal cavity. Despite the fact that clinical episodes are frequently subclinical or asymptomatic, serious sequelae are common, including infertility (12% to 50%), chronic pelvic pain (18%), and ectopic pregnancy (increased by 6- to 10-fold) Weström, 1985; Brunham et al, 1988; Cates et al, 1990). Infertility and ectopic pregnancy rates rise with subsequent episodes of PID, with approximately 43% of patients becoming infertile and 22% having an ectopic pregnancy, respectively, after three cases of PID (Weström et al, 1992).

Epidemiology

PID is the most common gynecologic disorder necessitating hospitalization for women of reproductive age in the United States, at a rate of 49.3 per 10,000 hospital discharges (Velebil et al, 1995). This represents only the tip of the iceberg, because the majority of women are treated for PID as outpatients (Washington and Katz, 1991), and many women with subacute or asymptomatic disease are never identified (Tjiam et al, 1985; Sellors et al, 1988). Although rare, it can occur during pregnancy and in women who have undergone tubal ligation or hysterectomy.

Natural History

The pathogenesis of PID is incompletely understood but involves some single event or set of circumstances that results in disruption of standard host immunity, which under normal circumstances protects the upper genital tract from the anaerobes and gram-negative bacteria of the vagina. How this happens remains largely speculative at this time. Damage to cervical mucous and tubal ciliated epithelium by both *N. gonorrhoeae* and *C. trachomatis* has been well documented. *Neisseria gonorrhoeae* attaches to and penetrates mucosal epithelial cells, directly causing cell destruction and irreversible damage to cili-

Table 38–10. SUMMARY OF 1998 TREATMENT GUIDELINES FOR GENITAL WARTS (Human Papillomavirus)

SPECIFIC INDICATION	PRIMARY THERAPY	ALTERNATIVE THERAPY	SPECIAL NOTES
External genital/perianal warts	PATIENT APPLIED: **Podofilox 0.5% solution or gel** (apply bid × 3 days, then off 4 days. May repeat cycle total of 4 times) *or* **Imiquimod 5% cream** (apply qhs 3 × week; wash off after 6–10 hours. May use up to 16 weeks; may clear in 8–10 weeks or sooner) PROVIDER-ADMINISTERED: Cryotherapy with liquid nitrogen or cryoprobe *or* **Podophyllin 10%–25%** in compound tincture of benzoin (wash off thoroughly in 1–4 hours after application. Repeat weekly if necessary.) *or* **Trichloroacetic acid (TCA) 80%–90%**; apply only to warts. Powder with talc or baking soda to remove unreacted acid. Repeat weekly if necessary. *or* Surgical removal	Intralesional interferon *or* Laser surgery	No therapy has been shown to eradicate or effect natural history of HPV. **Imiquimod, podifilox, and podophyllin are contraindicated in pregnancy.** Some experts advocate removal of visible warts during pregnancy. Scarring in the form of hypo- or hyperpigmentation is common with ablative therapies. If warts persist after one type of therapy, other therapies should be considered. Most experts believe combining modalities does not increase efficacy but may increase complications. Examination of sex partners is not necessary for management because of minimal risk for re-infection. Screening for subclinical genital HPV infection using DNA or RNA tests or acetic acid is not recommended. Patients with HIV may not respond as well to treatment.
Cervical warts	Dysplasia must be excluded before treatment started. Consult with expert for management.		
Vaginal warts	Cryotherapy with liquid nitrogen (cryoprobe is not recommended) *or* TCA 80%–90%: apply only to warts. Powder with talc or baking soda to remove unreacted acid. Repeat weekly if necessary. *or* Podophyllin 10%–25% in compound tincture of benzoin. Apply to treatment area, which must be dry before removing speculum. Treat ≤ 2 cm² per session. Repeat weekly.		**Podophyllin is contraindicated in pregnancy** because of systemic absorption.
Urethral meatus warts	Cryotherapy with liquid nitrogen *or* Podophyllin 10%–25% in compound tincture of benzoin. Treatment area must be dry before contact with normal mucosa. Wash off in 1–2 hours. Repeat weekly if necessary.		**Podophyllin is contraindicated in pregnancy** because of systemic absorption.
Anal warts	Cryotherapy with liquid nitrogen *or* Surgical removal *or* TCA 80%–90%; apply only to warts. Powder with talc or baking soda to remove unreacted acid. Repeat weekly if necessary.		Warts on rectal mucosa should be referred to an expert.
Oral warts	Cryotherapy with liquid nitrogen *or* Surgical removal		

Data abstracted from Centers for Disease Control and Prevention (1998).

Table 38-11. BACTERIA ISOLATED FROM THE UPPER GENITAL TRACTS OF WOMEN WITH PID

AEROBES	ANAEROBES	MYCOPLASMA BACTERIA	INTRACELLULAR
Coagulase-negative staphylococci	*Bacteroides fragilis*	*Mycoplasma hominis*	*Chlamydia trachomatis*
Group B streptococci		*Ureaplasma urealyticum*	
α-Hemolytic streptococci	*Prevotella bivius*		
Nonhemolytic streptococci	*Prevotella disiens*		
Neisseria gonorrhoeae	*Peptostreptococcus anaerobius*		
Escherichia coli	*Peptostreptococcus asaccharolyticus*		
Gardnerella vaginalis	*Peptococcus* species		

ary motility (Carney and Taylor-Robinson, 1973; McGee et al, 1981; Melly et al, 1981). In contrast, it is the host immune response to *C. trachomatis* which causes tubal scarring (Patton et al, 1983, 1987). However, little is known about the role of anaerobes in this process.

Investigators using laparoscopy have recovered a variety of microbes from the upper genital tracts of women with PID (Sweet et al, 1979; Heinonen et al, 1985; Kiviat et al, 1986; Wasserheit et al, 1986, Paavonen et al, 1987; Brunham et al, 1988; Soper et al, 1994; Arredondo et al, 1997). Pathogens include *N. gonorrhoeae*, *C. trachomatis*, anaerobes, and gram-negative organisms (Table 38-11).

Clinical Features

Whether or not a given individual develops clinically evident symptoms related to an episode of PID depends on a complex interplay between the pathogens involved and various elements of the host response. Women with minimal symptoms may report mild low abdominal pain, dyspareunia, intermenstrual or postcoital bleeding, dysuria, or an abnormal vaginal discharge. Those with a more fulminant presentation typically develop constitutional symptoms, including fever and gastrointestinal symptoms.

Between 7% and 16% of women hospitalized with PID have tubo-ovarian abscesses (Ginsburg et al, 1980). The microbiology of these abscesses is mixed, with *Bacteroides fragilis* and other *Bacteroides* and *Prevotella* species predominating.

Diagnosis

As noted above, the clinical features of PID are often enigmatic, making diagnosis difficult. Studies using laparoscopic confirmation have shown that women meeting the clinical and laboratory criteria for PID in fact do not have PID, but rather have evidence of another separate pathologic process or a normal pelvis, in up to 54% of cases (Jacobson and Weström, 1969; Chaparro et al, 1978; Heinonen et al, 1985; Kiviat et al, 1986; Wasserheit et al, 1986; Soper et al, 1994). Furthermore, there is evidence that many women with PID experience minimal or no discern-

ible symptoms (Wolner-Hanssen et al, 1990). Kahn and colleagues (1991) have demonstrated that no single historical, clinical, or laboratory finding or combination thereof had both high sensitivity and specificity for the diagnosis of PID (Table 38-12).

With these difficulties in mind, experts recommend a high index of suspicion for making the diagnosis of PID. Thus, in a woman with mild symptoms, findings of pelvic tenderness on examination is enough to make the diagnosis and prompt treatment (Table 38-13). Alternatively, a woman who presents with more severe symptoms should have one or more of the additional criteria in order to diagnose PID. Elaborate criteria may be helpful in establishing the diagnosis, but most involve diagnostic techniques either too expensive or too invasive to be used routinely.

Treatment

Treatment options for women with PID have evolved during the last three decades along with our understanding of the pathogenesis and polymicrobial nature of the infection. For the last decade, the CDC has recommended regimens with antimicrobial coverage against *C. trachomatis*, *N. gonorrhoeae*, and gram-negative and anaerobic bacteria (Table 38-14).

One question that continues to spark controversy is whether anaerobes must be eradicated in order to achieve an appropriate clinical response. Interestingly, clinical and microbiologic cure rates are excellent for several regimens that lack optimal theoretical anaerobic coverage (Crombleholme et al, 1986; Wolner-Hanssen et al, 1988; Apuzzio et al, 1989; Heinonen et al, 1989; Thadepalli et al, 1991; Wendel et al, 1991; Soper et al, 1992; Arredondo et al, 1997). A meta-analysis of antimicrobial regimen efficacy for the treatment of acute PID evaluated 21 of 34 trials published between 1966 and 1992, and found roughly equivalent short-term clinical and microbiologic cure rates for all but one of the regimens (Walker et al, 1993). This study did not include assessment of anaerobic bacterial eradication.

Table 38-15 presents an updated review of the individual and pooled clinical and microbiologic cure rates from this meta-analysis. It has been expanded

Table 38-12. ACCURACY OF DIAGNOSTIC INDICATORS FOR PID

INDICATOR	SENSITIVITY (%)	SPECIFICITY (%)
History		
Lower abdominal pain >4 days	78	54
Irregular menses	32	70
Clinical Examination		
Temperature >38°C	33	82
Palpable mass	40	76
Abnormal vaginal discharge	60	61
Laboratory Tests		
Elevated C-reactive protein	86	72
Erythrocyte sedimentation rate >15 to >25 mm/hr	72	56
Endometrial inflammation on biopsy	80	78

From Kahn JG, Walker CK, Washington AE, et al: Diagnosing pelvic inflammatory disease: a comprehensive analysis and considerations for developing a new model. JAMA 1991;266:2594, with permission.

to include data from the five clinical trials (Kosseim et al, 1991; Uri et al, 1992; Martens et al, 1993; Hemsell et al, 1994; Arredondo et al, 1997) that were published in the interim period from 1992 through 1997 and that met the original inclusion criteria for the study. It should be noted that these cure rates are roughly equivalent, with the exception of those for metronidazole plus doxycycline. Clearly, most accumulated data exist for the parenteral regimens cephalosporin/cephamycin plus doxycycline and clindamycin plus an aminoglycoside because these are the gold standards against which most newer regimens have been compared. In contrast, there are relatively few studies for the oral regimens, despite the fact that these regimens are used in approximately 75% of women with PID (Washington and Katz,

1991). Limited data exist with regard to the ability of a given antimicrobial regimen to prevent long-term sequelae. Given the dearth of data regarding the long-term effects of failure to eradicate anaerobes in women with PID, and because of the seriousness of these potential long-term sequelae, consensus opinion considers PID a polymicrobial infection and recommends broad-spectrum antimicrobial therapy.

There are at least three situations in which enhanced coverage of anaerobes in women with PID may be warranted. The first involves women in whom a tubo-ovarian abscess is identified. Tissue destruction, vascular compromise, large concentrations of anaerobes and their by-products, and local immunologic factors combine to result in an abscess milieu that is relatively impermeable to many antibiotics (Sweet, 1995). In a study that measured reduction in bacterial counts in subcutaneous abscesses, the most active antimicrobials (in order of decreasing activity) were metronidazole, clindamycin, moxalactam, and cefoxitin (Joiner et al, 1981). In the absence of comparative trials, parenteral treatment is advocated, as is the recommendation to complete the 14-day treatment course with oral metronidazole and doxycycline.

The second situation in which enhanced coverage of anaerobes in women with PID may be warranted is in women who have coexistent infection with VB. As noted above, VB is commonly associated with PID. Irrespective of the role of VB in the pathogenesis of PID or one's certainty about the need to cover anaerobes adequately to treat PID, antimicrobial treatment must be sufficient to eradicate VB when these two infections coexist. Because metronidazole is the recommended treatment for VB, a regimen including metronidazole is preferred in this situation.

HIV-infected women who develop PID are no more likely than seronegative controls to have coexistent VB (Irwin et al, 1993) or to have pathogenic bacteria, such as *N. gonorrhoeae, C. trachomatis,* or *G.*

Table 38-13. CDC CRITERIA FOR DIAGNOSIS OF PID

Minimum Criteria in Women with Mild Presentation
1. Lower abdominal tenderness
2. Cervical motion tenderness
3. Adnexal tenderness

Additional Criteria
1. Oral temperature >38.3°C
2. Abnormal cervical or vaginal discharge
3. Elevated erythrocyte sedimentation rate
4. Elevated C-reactive protein
5. Laboratory documentation of *N. gonorrhoeae* or *C. trachomatis* infection

Elaborate Criteria
1. Histopathologic evidence of endometritis on endometrial biopsy
2. Radiologic abnormalities (thickened, fluid-filled tubes with or without free pelvic fluid or tubo-ovarian complex) on transvaginal sonography or other radiologic tests
3. Laparoscopic abnormalities consistent with PID

Data from CDC, 1998. Guidelines for treatment of sexually transmitted diseases.

Table 38-14. SUMMARY OF 1998 TREATMENT GUIDELINES FOR PID—
CAUSATIVE ORGANISMS (*N. gonorrhoeae, C. trachomatis, G. vaginalis, H. influenzae,* etc.)

SPECIFIC INDICATION	PRIMARY THERAPY	ALTERNATIVE THERAPY	SPECIAL NOTES
Inpatient management	REGIMEN A **Cefoxitin** 2 g IV q6h *or* **Cefotetan** 2 g IV q12h **PLUS** **Doxycycline** 100 mg IV/PO q12h **followed by** **Doxycycline** 100 mg PO bid for 14 days total REGIMEN B **Clindamycin** 900 mg IV q8h **PLUS** **Gentamicin** 2 mg/kg IV/IM loading dose then 1.5 mg/kg maintenance dose q8h (Single daily dosing may be substituted) **followed by** **Doxycycline** 100 mg PO bid for 14 days total *or* **Clindamycin** 450 mg PO qid for 14 days total	**Ofloxacin** 400 mg IV q12h **PLUS** **Metronidazole** 500 mg IV q8h *or* **Ampicillin-Sulbactam** 3 g IV q6h **PLUS** **Doxycycline** 100 mg IV/PO q12h *or* **Ciprofloxacin** 200 mg IV q12h **PLUS** **Doxycycline** 100 mg IV/PO q12h **PLUS** **Metronidazole** 500 mg IV q8h	Parenteral therapy may be discontinued 24 hours after clinical improvement. When tubo-ovarian abscess is present, clindamycin may be preferred for continued therapy. Other generation cephalosporins may be effective but clinical data are limited. Azithromycin 500 mg IV × 2 days, followed by 500 mg PO for total of 10 days recently FDA approved. **Pregnancy**—Women should be hospitalized and treated with parenteral therapy.
Outpatient management	REGIMEN A **Ofloxacin** 400 mg PO bid × 14 days **PLUS** **Metronidazole** 500 mg PO bid × 14 days REGIMEN B **Ceftriaxone** 250 mg IM × 1 dose *or* **Cefoxitin** 2 g IM plus **Probenecid** 1 g PO × 1 dose *or* Other parenteral third-generation cephalosporin **PLUS** **Doxycycline** 100 mg PO bid × 14 days		Patients who do not respond within 72 hours to therapy should be hospitalized. Alternative oral regimens suggested include amoxicillin-clavulanic acid plus doxycycline. Insufficient data to recommend azithromycin as part of treatment regimens.

Data abstracted from Centers for Disease Control and Prevention (1998).

vaginalis, recovered from the upper genital tract (Moorman et al, 1997). In addition, although they may present with slightly more severe symptoms than HIV-uninfected controls, they respond equally well to standard antimicrobial therapy (Irwin et al, 1993; Barbosa et al, 1997).

PREVENTION

Most of what we do is secondary and tertiary prevention. Secondary prevention involves the identification, diagnosis, and treatment of those with lower genital tract infections in order to prevent spread within the community and ascension to the upper genital tract. Tertiary prevention focuses on the identification, diagnosis, and treatment of those with upper tract infection in order to prevent sequelae such as infertility and chronic pelvic pain.

This chapter deals primarily with secondary and tertiary prevention. It must not be forgotten, however, that primary prevention probably has the biggest opportunity to impact the lives of the women for whom we care. This should be our most dedicated effort. We need to learn how to talk about sex and sexual risk, and feel comfortable discussing risk reduction in explicit detail. The highest risks remain unprotected intercourse with multiple partners and

Table 38-15. SINGLE AND POOLED CURE RATES IN TREATMENT OF ACUTE PID

DRUG REGIMEN	NO. OF STUDIES	NO. OF PATIENTS	% CURED (CLINICAL/MICROBIOLOGIC)
Inpatient			
Clindamycin + aminoglycoside	11	470	91/97
Cefoxitin + doxycycline	8	427	91/98
Cefotetan + doxycycline	3	174	95/100
Ceftizoxime + tetracycline	1	18	88/100
Cefotaxime + tetracycline	1	19	94/100
Ciprofloxacin	4	90	94/96
Ofloxacin	1	36	100/97
Sulbactam-ampicillin + doxycycline	1	37	95/100
Amoxicillin–clavulanic acid	1	32	93/—
Metronidazole + doxycycline	2	36	75/71
Outpatient			
Cefoxitin + probenecid + doxycycline	3	219	89/93
Ofloxacin	2	165	95/100
Amoxicillin–clavulanic acid	1	35	100/100
Sulbactam-ampicillin	1	36	70/70
Ceftriazone + doxycycline	1	64	95/100
Ciprofloxacin + clindamycin	1	67	97/94

Adapted from Walker C, Kahn J, Washington A, et al: Pelvic inflammatory disease: metaanalysis of antimicrobial regimen efficacy. J Infect Dis 1993; 168:969, with permission. Additional data from Kosseim et al (1991), Uri et al (1992), Martens et al (1993), Hemsell et al (1994), and Arredondo et al (1997).

illicit drug use. Primary prevention efforts should be directed toward all patients, with special focus on adolescents, who have the highest incidence of STDs.

The most effective way to prevent acquisition of STDs is to avoid sexual intercourse with an infected partner. Methods to achieve this include abstinence from penetrative sexual intercourse, having both partners tested for STDs and HIV before initiating sexual intercourse, and using a new condom with each act of sexual intercourse.

When used consistently and correctly, male condoms prevent many STDs, including HIV. Cohort studies, including those of serodiscordant sexual partners, have repeatedly shown a strong protective effect for male latex condoms. However, condoms do not cover all exposed areas, allowing transmission of infections such as syphilis, HPV, and HSV. In addition, they may slip or break.

Other barrier contraceptives that may protect against the spread of STDs are female condoms, diaphragms/cervical caps, and spermicides.

Partner Notification

Patients should be advised to contact all sexual partners, even those without symptoms, and suggest they seek clinical evaluation, which should include counseling, diagnosis, treatment, and vaccination. In many states, local or state health department staff can assist.

Reporting

Reporting is a critical component of disease control efforts. Every state requires that *N. gonorrhoeae, T.* *pallidum,* and acquired immunodeficiency syndrome cases be reported to local or state officials. Most states now require *C. trachomatis,* and many require HIV reporting.

REFERENCES

Amsel R, Totten PA, Spiegel CA, et al: Nonspecific vaginitis: diagnostic criteria and microbial and epidemiologic associations. Am J Med 1983;74:14.

Apuzzio JJ, Stankiewicz R, Ganesh V, et al: Comparison of parenteral ciprofloxacin with clindamycin-gentamicin in the treatment of pelvic infection. Am J Med 1989;87:148S.

Arredondo JL, Diaz V, Gaitan H, et al: Oral clindamycin and ciprofloxacin versus intramuscular ceftriaxone and oral doxycycline in the treatment of mild-to-moderate pelvic inflammatory disease in outpatients. Clin Infect Dis 1997;24:170.

Barbosa C, Macasaet M, Brockmann S, et al: Pelvic inflammatory disease and human immunodeficiency virus infection. Obstet Gynecol 1997;89:65.

Barlow D, Phillips I: Gonorrhoea in women: diagnostic, clinical, and laboratory aspects. Lancet 1978;1:761.

Barton IG, Kinghorn GR, Walker MJ, et al: Association of HSV-1 with cervical infection [letter]. Lancet 1981;2:1108.

Batteiger BE, Lennington W, Newhall WJ, et al: Correlation of infecting serovar and local inflammation in genital chlamydial infections. J Infect Dis 1989;160:332.

Becker TM, Wheeler CM, McGough NS, et al: Sexually transmitted diseases and other risk factors for cervical dysplasia among southwestern Hispanic and non-Hispanic white women. JAMA 1994;271:1181.

Benedetti JK, Zeh J, Selke S, Corey L: Frequency and reactivation of nongenital lesions among patients with genital herpes simplex virus. Am J Med 1995;98:237.

Berg AO, Heidrich FE, Fihn SD, et al: Establishing the cause of genitourinary symptoms in women in a family practice: comparison of clinical examination and comprehensive microbiology. JAMA 1984;251:620.

Beutner KR, Ferenczy A: Therapeutic approaches to genital warts. Am J Med 1997;102:28.

Brandt AM: Racism and research: the case of the Tuskegee Syphilis Study. Hastings Center Rep 1978;8:21.

Brown ZA, Benedetti J, Ashley R, et al: Neonatal herpes simplex virus infection in relation to asymptomatic maternal infection at the time of labor [see comments]. N Engl J Med 1991;324: 1247.

Brunham RC, Binns B, Guijon F, et al: Etiology and outcome of acute pelvic inflammatory disease. J Infect Dis 1988;158:510.

Bruusgaard E: Ober das schicksal der nicht specifisch behanderlten leuktiker. Arch Dermatol Syph (Berlin) 1929;157:309.

Carney FE Jr, Taylor-Robinson D: Growth and effect of Neisseria gonorrhoeae in organ cultures. Br J Vener Dis 1973;49:435.

Cates W Jr, Rolfs RT Jr, Aral SO: Sexually transmitted diseases, pelvic inflammatory disease, and infertility: an epidemiologic update. Epidemiol Rev 1990;12:199.

Centers for Disease Control and Prevention: Chlamydia trachomatis genital infections—United States, 1995. JAMA 1997;277: 952.

Centers for Disease Control and Prevention: 1998 Guidelines for treatment of sexually transmitted diseases. MMWR Morbid Mortal Wkly Rep 1998;47:1.

Chaparro MV, Ghosh S, Nahed A, Poliak A: Laparoscopy for confirmation and prognostic evolution of pelvic inflammatory disease. Int J Gynaecol Obstet 1978;15:307.

Christenson B, Böttiger M, Svensson A, Jeansson S: A 15-year surveillance study of antibodies to herpes simplex virus types 1 and 2 in a cohort of young girls. J Infect 1992;5:147.

Cohen MS: Molecular events in the activation of human neutrophils for microbial killing. Clin Infect Dis 1994;18(Suppl 2): S170.

Corey L, Holmes KK: Genital herpes simplex virus infections: current concepts in diagnosis, therapy, and prevention. Ann Intern Med 1983;98:973.

Crombleholme W, Landers D, Ohm-Smith M, et al: Sulbactam/ ampicillin versus metronidazole/gentamicin in the treatment of severe pelvic infections. Drugs 1986;31:11.

Dean D, Oudens E, Bolan G, Padian N, Schachter J: Major outer membrane protein variants of Chlamydia trachomatis are associated with severe upper genital tract infections and histopathology in San Francisco. J Infect Dis 1995;172:1013.

Division of STD Prevention: Sexually Transmitted Diseases Surveillance, 1995. Atlanta: Centers for Disease Control and Prevention, 1995.

Donovan P: Confronting a hidden epidemic: the Institute of Medicine's report on sexually transmitted diseases. Fam Plann Perspect 1997;29:87.

Dykers JR: Single-dose metronidazole for trichomonal vaginitis: patient and consort. N Engl J Med 1975;293:23.

Edwards JN, Morris HB: Langerhans' cells and lymphocyte subsets in the female genital tract. Br J Obstet Gynaecol 1985;92: 974.

Elstein M: Functions and physical properties of mucus in the female genital tract. Br Med Bull 1978;34:83.

Eschenbach DA, Davick PR, Williams BL, et al: Prevalence of hydrogen peroxide-producing Lactobacillus species in normal women and women with bacterial vaginosis. J Clin Microbiol 1989;27:251.

Eschenbach DA, Hillier S, Critchlow C, et al: Diagnosis and clinical manifestations of bacterial vaginosis. Am J Obstet Gynecol 1988;158:819.

Fichorova RN, Anderson DJ: Differential expression of immunobiological mediators by immunized human cervical and vaginal epithelial cells. Biol Reprod 1999;60:508.

Fischbach F, Petersen EE, Weissenbacher ER, et al: Efficacy of clindamycin vaginal cream versus oral metronidazole in the treatment of bacterial vaginosis. Obstet Gynecol 1993;82:405.

Fleming DT, McQuillan GM, Johnson RE, et al: Herpes simplex virus type 2 in the United States, 1976 to 1994 [see comments]. N Engl J Med 1997;337:1105.

Fleury FJ, Van Bergen WS, Prentice RL, et al: Single dose of two grams of metronidazole for Trichomonas vaginalis infection. Am J Obstet Gynecol 1977;128:320.

Fouts AC, Kraus SJ: Trichomonas vaginalis: reevaluation of its clinical presentation and laboratory diagnosis. J Infect Dis 1980; 141:137.

Foxman B: The epidemiology of vulvovaginal candidiasis: risk factors. Am J Public Health 1990;80:329.

Geiger AM, Foxman B: Risk factors for vulvovaginal candidiasis: a case-control study among university students. Epidemiology 1996;7:182.

Geiger AM, Foxman B, Gillespie BW: The epidemiology of vulvovaginal candidiasis among university students. Am J Public Health 1995;85:1146.

Ginsburg DS, Stern JL, Hammod K, Genadry R, Spence MR: Tubo-ovarian abscess: a retrospective review. Am J Obstet Gynecol 1980;138:1055.

Gjestland T: The Oslo study of untreated syphilis: an epidemiologic investigation of the natural course of syphilitic infection based on a restudy of the Boeck-Bruusgaard material. Acta Derm Venereol 1955;35:I.

Goldenberg RL, Klebanoff MA, Nugent R, et al: Bacterial colonization of the vagina during pregnancy in four ethnic groups: Vaginal Infections and Prematurity Study Group. Am J Obstet Gynecol 1996;174:1618.

Hallén A, Påhlson C, Forsum U: Bacterial vaginosis in women attending STD clinic: diagnostic criteria and prevalence of Mobiluncus spp. Genitourin Med 1987;63:386.

Harms G, Matull R, Randrianasolo D, et al: Pattern of sexually transmitted diseases in a Malagasy population. Sex Transm Dis 1994;21:315.

Hauth JC, Goldenberg RL, Andrews WW, et al: Reduced incidence of preterm delivery with metronidazole and erythromycin in women with bacterial vaginosis [see comments]. N Engl J Med 1995;333:1732.

Heim K, Christensen ND, Hoepfl R, et al: Serum IgG, IgM, and IgA reactivity to human papillomavirus types 11 and 6 virus-like particles in different gynecologic patient groups. J Infect Dis 1995;172:395.

Heinonen PK, Teisala K, Aine R, Miettinen A: Intravenous and oral ciprofloxacin in the treatment of proven pelvic inflammatory disease: a comparison with doxycycline and metronidazole. Am J Med 1989;87:152S.

Heinonen PK, Teisala K, Punnonen R, et al: Anatomic sites of upper genital tract infection. Obstet Gynecol 1985;66:384.

Heller JR Jr, Bruyere PT: Untreated syphilis in the male Negro: II. Mortality during 12 years of observation. J Vener Dis Inform 1946;27:34.

Hemsell DL, Little BB, Faro S, et al: Comparison of three regimens recommended by the Centers for Disease Control and Prevention for the treatment of women hospitalized with acute pelvic inflammatory disease. Clin Infect Dis 1994;19:720.

Hill LH, Ruparelia H, Embil JA: Nonspecific vaginitis and other genital infections in three clinic populations. Sex Transm Dis 1983;10:114.

Hillier SL, Krohn MA, Klebanoff SJ, Eschenbach DA: The relationship of hydrogen peroxide-producing lactobacilli to bacterial vaginosis and genital microflora in pregnant women. Obstet Gynecol 1992;79:369.

Hillier SL, Lipinski C, Briselden AM, Eschenbach DA: Efficacy of intravaginal 0.75% metronidazole gel for the treatment of bacterial vaginosis. Obstet Gynecol 1993;81:963.

Hook EW 3rd: Is elimination of endemic syphilis transmission a realistic goal for the USA? Lancet 1998;351(Suppl 3):19.

Horowitz BJ, Giaquinta D, Ito S: Evolving pathogens in vulvovaginal candidiasis: implications for patient care. J Clin Pharmacol 1992;32:248.

Howell MR, Quinn TC, Brathwaite W, Gaydos CA: Screening women for chlamydia trachomatis in family planning clinics: the cost-effectiveness of DNA amplification assays. Sex Transm Dis 1998a;25:108.

Howell MR, Quinn TC, Gaydos CA: Screening for Chlamydia trachomatis in asymptomatic women attending family planning clinics: a cost-effectiveness analysis of three strategies. Ann Intern Med 1998b;128:277.

Hughes VL, Hillier SL: Microbiologic characteristics of Lactobacillus products used for colonization of the vagina. Obstet Gynecol 1990;75:244.

Hurley R, De Louvois J: Candida vaginitis. Postgrad Med J 1979; 55:645.

Huth EJ: Style notes: bacterial vaginosis or vaginal bacteriosis? [editorial; comment]. Ann Intern Med 1989;111:553.

Irwin KL, Rice RJ, O'Sullivan MJ, et al: The clinical presentation and course of pelvic inflammatory disease in HIV+ and HIV− women: preliminary results of a prospective multicenter study [abstract]. In: Abstracts of the 10th International Meeting of the International Society for STD Research, Helsinki, Finland, August 1993.

Jacobson L, Weström L: Objectivized diagnosis of acute pelvic inflammatory disease. Am J Obstet Gynecol 1969;105:1088.

Johnson RE, Nahmias AJ, Magder LS, et al: A seroepidemiologic survey of the prevalence of herpes simplex virus type 2 infection in the United States. N Engl J Med 1989;321:7.

Joiner KA, Lowe BR, Dzink JL, Bartlett JG: Antibiotic levels in infected and sterile subcutaneous abscesses in mice. J Infect Dis 1981;143:487.

Jones JH, for the Tuskegee Institute: Bad Blood: the Tuskegee Syphilis Experiment. New York: 1981:xii, 272 (8 leaves of plates).

Judson FN: Gonorrhea. Med Clin North Am 1990;74:1353.

Judson FN, Werness BA: Combining cervical and anal-canal specimens for gonorrhea on a single culture plate. J Clin Microbiol 1980;12:216.

Kahn JG, Walker CK, Washington AE, et al: Diagnosing pelvic inflammatory disease: a comprehensive analysis and considerations for developing a new model [see comments]. JAMA 1991;266:2594.

Kent HL: Epidemiology of vaginitis. Am J Obstet Gynecol 1991; 165:1168.

Kinghorn GR, Rashid S: Prevalence of rectal and pharyngeal infection in women with gonorrhoea in Sheffield. Br J Vener Dis 1979;55:408.

Kiviat NB, Wolner-Hanssen P, Peterson M, et al: Localization of Chlamydia trachomatis infection by direct immunofluorescence and culture in pelvic inflammatory disease. Am J Obstet Gynecol 1986;154:865.

Kjaer SK, Engholm G, Teisen C, et al: Risk factors for cervical human papillomavirus and herpes simplex virus infections in Greenland and Denmark: a population-based study. Am J Epidemiol 1990;131:669.

Kosseim M, Ronald A, Plummer F, D'Costa L, Brunham RC: Treatment of acute pelvic inflammatory disease in the ambulatory setting: trial of cefoxitin and doxycycline versus ampicillin-sulbactam. Antimicrob Agents Chemother 1991;35:1651.

Koutsky LA, Stevens CE, Holmes KK, et al: Underdiagnosis of genital herpes by current clinical and viral-isolation procedures [see comments]. N Engl J Med 1992;326:1533.

Kutteh WH, Mestecky J: Secretory immunity in the female reproductive tract. Am J Reprod Immunol 1994;31:40.

Langenberg A, Benedetti J, Jenkins J, et al: Development of clinically recognizable genital lesions among women prviously identified as having "asymptomatic" herpes simplex virus type 2 infection. Ann Intern Med 1989;110:882.

Lehrer RI, Lichtenstein AK, Ganz T: Defensins: antimicrobial and cytotoxic peptides of mammalian cells. Ann Rev Immunol 1993;11:105.

Livengood CH 3rd, McGregor JA, Soper DE, et al: Bacterial vaginosis: efficacy and safety of intravaginal metronidazole treatment [see comments]. Am J Obstet Gynecol 1994;170:759.

Lohmeyer H: Treatment of candidiasis and trichomoniasis of the female genital tract. Postgrad Med J 1975;50(Suppl 1):78.

Louv WC, Austin H, Perlman J, Alexander WJ: Oral contraceptive use and the risk of chlamydial and gonococcal infections [see comments]. Am J Obstet Gynecol 1989;160:396.

Lugo-Miro VI, Green M, Mazur L: Comparison of different metronidazole therapeutic regimens for bacterial vaginosis: a meta-analysis. JAMA 1992;268:92.

Martens MG, Gordon S, Yarborough DR, et al: Multicenter randomized trial of ofloxacin versus cefoxitin and doxycycline in outpatient treatment of pelvic inflammatory disease. South Med J 1993;86:604.

McCormack WM, Stumacher RJ, Johnson K, Donner A: Clinical spectrum of gonococcal infection in women. Lancet 1977;1:1182.

McGee ZA, Johnson AP, Taylor-Robinson D: Pathogenic mechanisms of Neisseria gonorrhoeae: observations on damage to human fallopian tubes in organ culture by gonococci of colony type 1. J Infect Dis 1981;143:413.

Melly MA, Gregg CR, McGee ZA: Studies of toxicity of Neisseria gonorrhoeae for human fallopian tube mucosa. J Infect Dis 1981;143:423.

Mengel MB, Berg AO, Weaver CH, et al: The effectiveness of single-dose metronidazole therapy for patients and their partners with bacterial vaginosis. J Fam Pract 1989;28:163.

Mertz GJ, Benedetti J, Ashley R, Selke SA, Corey L: Risk factors for the sexual transmission of genital herpes. Ann Intern Med 1992;116:197.

Moi H, Erkkola R, Jerve F, et al: Should male consorts of women with bacterial vaginosis be treated? Genitourin Med 1989;65:263.

Moorman A, Schwartz D, Irwin K, et al: Influence of HIV infection on the relationship of endometritis and endometrial pathogens among women with acute pelvic inflammatory disease (PID) [abstract]. In: Abstracts of the National Conference of Women with HIV, May 1997.

Morales WJ, Schorr S, Albritton J: Effect of metronidazole in patients with preterm birth in preceding pregnancy and bacterial vaginosis: a placebo-controlled, double-blind study. Am J Obstet Gynecol 1994;171:345; discussion 348.

Moscicki AB, Palefsky J, Smith G, Siboshshi S, Schoolnik G: Variability of human papillomavirus DNA testing in a longitudinal cohort of young women. Obstet Gynecol 1993;82:578.

Notkins AL: Immune mechanisms by which the spread of viral infections is stopped. Cell Immunol 1974;11:478.

Odds F: Candidosis of the genitalia. In: Candida and Candidosis: A review and Bibliography. London: Baillière Tindall, 1988: 124.

Olansky S: Untreated syphilis in the male Negro: X. Twenty years of clinical observation of untreated syphilitic and presumably nonsyphilitic groups. J Chronic Dis 1956;4:177.

Oliver L, Wald A, Kim M, et al: Seroprevalence of herpes simplex virus infections in a family medicine clinic. Arch Fam Med 1995;4:228.

Oram JD, Reiter B: Inhibition of bacteria by lactoferrin and other iron-chelating agents. Biochim Biophys Acta 1968;170:351.

Paavonen J, Saikku P, Vesterinen E, et al: Genital chlamydial infections in patients attending a gynaecological outpatient clinic. Br J Vener Dis 1978;54:257.

Paavonen J, Stevens CE, Wølner-Hanssen P, et al: Colposcopic manifestations of cervical and vaginal infections. Obstet Gynecol Surv 1988;43:373.

Paavonen J, Teisala K, Heinonen PK, et al: Microbiological and histopathological findings in acute pelvic inflammatory disease. Br J Obstet Gynaecol 1987;94:454.

Parke DV: Pharmacology of mucus. Br Med Bull 1978;34:89.

Patton DL, Halbert SA, Kuo C, Wang SP, Holmes KK: Host response to primary Chlamydia trachomatis infection of the fallopian tube in pig-tailed monkeys. Fertil Steril 1983;40:829.

Patton D, Kuo CC, Wang SP, Halbert SA: Distal tubal obstruction induced by repeated Chlamydia trachomatis salpingeal infection in pig-tailed macaques. J Infect Dis 1987;155:1292.

Quinn TC, Gaydos C, Shepherd M, et al: Epidemiologic and microbiologic correlates of Chlamydia trachomatis infection in sexual partnerships JAMA 1996;276:1737.

Reeves WC, Brinton LA, Garcia M, et al: Human papillomavirus infection and cervical cancer in Latin America. N Engl J Med 1989;320:1437.

Reichart CA, Rupkey LM, Brady WE, Hook EWD: Comparison of GC-Lect and modified Thayer-Martin media for isolation of Neisseria gonorrhoeae. J Clin Microbiol 1989;27:808.

Rein M, Chapel T: Trichomoniasis, candidiasis and the minor venereal diseases. Clin Obstet Gynecol 1975;18:73.

Rockwell DH, Yobs AR, Moore MB, Jr: The Tuskegee study of untreated syphilis: the 30th year of observation. Arch Intern Med 1964;114:792.

Rosenfeld WD, Rose E, Vermund SH, et al: Follow-up evaluation of cervicovaginal human papillomavirus infection in adolescents. J Pediatr 1992;121:307.

Schachter J, Stamm WE: Chlamydia. In Murray PR, Baron EJ, Pfaller MA, et al (eds): Manual of Medical Microbiology. Washington DC: ASM Press, 1995:669.

Schneider A, Kirchhoff T, Meinhardt G, Gissmann L: Repeated evaluation of human papillomavirus 16 status in cervical swabs of young women with a history of normal Papanicolaou smears. Obstet Gynecol 1992;79:683.

Scholes D, Stergachis A, Heidrich FE, et al: Prevention of pelvic inflammatory disease by screening for cervical chlamydial infection. N Engl J Med 1996;334:1362.

Schuman SH, et al: Untreated syphilis in the male Negro: background and current status of patients in the Tuskegee study. J Chronic Dis 1955;2:543.

Sellors J, Mahony J, Chernesky M, Rath D: Tubal factor infertility: an association with prior chlamydial infection and asymptomatic salpingitis. Fertil Steril 1988;49:451.

Shamanin V, Glover M, Rausch C, et al: Specific types of human papillomavirus found in benign proliferations and carcinomas of the skin in immunosuppressed patients. Cancer Res 1994;54:4610.

Skarin A, Sylwan J: Vaginal lactobacilli inhibiting growth of Gardnerella vaginalis, Mobiluncus and other bacterial species cultured from vaginal content of women with bacterial vaginosis. Acta Pathol Microbiol Immunol Scand B Microbiol 1986;94:399.

Sobel JD: Vaginitis [see comments]. N Engl J Med 1997;337:1896.

Soper D, Brockwell N, Dalton H: Microbial etiology of urban emergency department acute salpingitis: treatment with ofloxacin. Am J Obstet Gynecol 1992;167:653.

Soper D, Brockwell N, Dalton H, Johnson D: Observations concerning the microbial etiology of acute salpingitis. Am J Obstet Gynecol 1994;170:1008.

Stamm W: Chlamydia trachomatis infections of the adult. In: Holmes KKMP-A, Sparling PF, et al (eds): Sexually Transmitted Diseases. New York: McGraw-Hill Health Professions Division, 1999:407.

Sweet R: Mixed anaerobic-aerobic pelvic infection and pelvic abscess. In Sweet R, Gibbs R (eds): Infectious Diseases of the Female Genital Tract. Baltimore: Williams & Wilkins, 1995:189.

Sweet R, Mills J, Hadley W, et al: Use of laparoscopy to determine the microbiologic etiology of acute salpingitis. Am J Obstet Gynecol 1979;134:68.

Swinehart JM, Sperling M, Phillips S, et al: Intralesional fluorouracil/epinephrine injectable gel for treatment of condylomata acuminata: a phase 3 clinical study. Arch Dermatol 1997;133:67.

Thadepalli H, Mathai D, Scotti R, Bansel MB, Savage E: Ciprofloxacin monotherapy for acute pelvic infections: a comparison with clindamycin plus gentamicin. Obstet Gynecol 1991;78:696.

Thomason JL, Gelbart SM, Sobun JF, Schulien MB, Hamilton PR: Comparison of four methods to detect Trichomonas vaginalis. J Clin Microbiol 1988;26:1869.

Tjiam KH, Zeilmaker GH, Alberda AT, et al: Prevalence of antibodies to Chlamydia trachomatis, Neisseria gonorrhoeae, and Mycoplasma hominis in infertile women. Genitourin Med 1985;61:175.

Uri FI, Sartawi SA, Dajani YF, Masoud AA, Barakat HF: Amoxycillin/clavulanic acid (Augmentin) compared with triple drug therapy for pelvic inflammatory disease. Int J Gynaecol Obstet 1992;38:41.

Vejtorp M, Bollerup AC, Vejtorp L, et al: Bacterial vaginosis: a double-blind randomized trial of the effect of treatment of the sexual partner. Br J Obstet and Gynaecol 1988;95:920.

Velebil P, Wingo PA, Xia Z, Wilcox LS, Peterson HB: Rate of hospitalization for gynecologic disorders among reproductive-age women in the United States. Obstet Gynecol 1995;86:764.

Vutyavanich T, Pongsuthirak P, Vannareumol P, et al: A randomized double-blind trial of tinidazole treatment of the sexual partners of females with bacterial vaginosis. Obstet Gynecol 1993;82:550.

Wald A, Zeh J, Selke S, Ashley RL, Corey L: Virologic characteristics of subclinical and symptomatic genital herpes infections. N Engl J Med 1995;333:770.

Wald ER: Gonorrhea: diagnosis by Gram stain in the female adolescent. Am J Dis Child 1977;131:1094.

Walker CK, Kahn JG, Washington AE, Peterson HB, Sweet RL: Pelvic inflammatory disease: metanalysis of antimicrobial regimen efficacy. J Infect Dis 1993;168:969.

Washington AE, Katz P: Cost of and payment source for pelvic inflammatory disease: trends and projections, 1983 through 2000. JAMA 1991;266:2565.

Wasserheit JN, Bell TA, Kiviat NB, et al: Microbial causes of proven pelvic inflammatory disease and efficacy of clindamycin and tobramycin. Ann Intern Med 1986;104:187.

Weinberger MW, Harger JH: Accuracy of the Papanicolaou smear in the diagnosis of asymptomatic infection with Trichomonas vaginalis. Obstet Gynecol 1993;82:425.

Wendel GD Jr, Cox SM, Bawdon RE, et al: A randomized trial of ofloxacin versus cefoxitin and doxycycline in the outpatient treatment of acute salpinitis. Am J Obstet Gynecol 1991;164:1390.

Weström L: Influence of sexually transmitted diseases on sterility and ectopic pregnancy. Acta Eur Fertil 1985;16:21.

Weström L, Joesoef R, Reynolds G, Hagder A, Thompson SE: Pelvic inflammatory disease and fertility: a cohort study of 1,844 women with laparoscopically verified disease and 657 control women with normal laparoscopic results. Sex Transm Dis 1992;19:185.

Wheeler CM, Greer CE, Becker TM, et al: Short-term fluctuations in the detection of cervical human papillomavirus DNA. Obstet Gynecol 1996;88:261.

Wheeler CM, Parmenter CA, Hunt WC, et al: Determinants of genital human papillomavirus infection among cytologically normal women attending the University of New Mexico student health center. Sex Transm Dis 1993;20:286.

Williams RC, Gibbons RJ: Inhibition of streptococcal attachment to receptors on human buccal epithelial cells by antigenically similar salivary glycoproteins. Infect Immun 1975;11:711.

Wolner-Hanssen P, Kiviat NB, Holmes KK, et al: Atypical pelvic inflammatory disease: subacute, chronic, or subclinical upper genital tract infection in women. In Holmes KK, Mardh PA, Sparling PF, et al (eds): Sexually Transmitted Diseases, 3rd ed. New York: McGraw-Hill, 1990.

Wolner-Hanssen P, Paavonen J, Kiviat N, et al: Outpatient treatment of pelvic inflammatory disease with cefoxitin and doxycycline. Obstet Gynecol 1988;71:595.

Wortley PM, Fleming PL: AIDS in women in the United States: recent trends [see comments]. JAMA 1997;278:911.

39

Human Immunodeficiency Virus in Nonpregnant Women

Cheryl K. Walker
Pamela Stratton

Soon after human immunodeficiency virus (HIV) was identified almost two decades ago, it became one of the major causes of death worldwide (Mann et al, 1996). Fortunately, in the last 5 years, a convergence of advances in knowledge of its basic biology and improvements in diagnosis and treatment of HIV and associated diseases have transformed this infection from one of the most deadly to a chronic disease. Use of aggressive combination antiretroviral therapy has led to an unprecedented improvement in the clinical course of individuals with HIV. Advances in prevention of perinatal transmission and transfusion-acquired infections have also limited spread of the infection in several populations, thus offering hope that HIV may finally be controlled.

Before control of viral replication became the goal of treatment, a major strategy for health maintenance of HIV-infected individuals was to treat and prevent illnesses that occurred in HIV-infected persons. As acquired immunodeficiency syndrome (AIDS)–associated illnesses were delineated, some questioned whether several gynecologic conditions were more common and severe in women with HIV. In particular, immunosuppression appeared to augment infections such as human papillomavirus, pelvic inflammatory disease, vulvovaginal candidiasis, and genital herpes simplex virus. Initial data associating HIV disease with gynecologic conditions was typically observational, and few subsequent prospective studies confirmed the associations. In this chapter, we review the current state of the field of HIV medicine, and discuss gynecologic concerns specifically.

EPIDEMIOLOGY AND NATURAL HISTORY

By the end of 1997, 641,086 persons with AIDS had been reported to the Centers for Disease Control and Prevention (CDC) (Centers for Disease Control and Prevention, 1997); more than half had died. Twenty-two per cent (98,468) of adult cases were women. Epidemiologic trends mark a sustained increase in cases in blacks and Hispanics, who together account for 65% of adult cases. Geographically, the largest increases have been seen in the South and Midwest, especially in smaller cities and towns.

The epidemic is shifting from gay men and injection drug users (IDUs) to heterosexuals. Heterosexual women are the most rapidly increasing population with HIV infection. Injection drug use continues to influence the epidemic in women. Not only have 44% acquired it through injection drug use, but, of the 39% who acquired their infection through heterosexual contact, 44% had sex with an IDU; 46% were exposed by unprotected sexual intercourse and only 8% had sex with a bisexual male. The proportion of women with AIDS who have acquired HIV through coitus has increased from 19% through 1985 to 32% in 1990 and 39% in 1997.

Rates of death, opportunistic infection, and AIDS have all declined since 1995, in large part as a result of the increasing use of combination antiretroviral therapy, including protease inhibitors. Comparing data from January through September of 1996 with the same period in 1997, newly reported AIDS cases fell 14% and deaths declined by 44%; the smallest reductions were in women, blacks, and heterosexual contact cases. The number of deaths in men decreased more than in women between 1995 and 1996 (30% vs. 17%) (Centers for Disease Control and Prevention, 1997). Women may have been diagnosed later, or have had less access to care, or perhaps treatments do not work as well in women.

Rates of vertical transmission have declined precipitously since 1994, when the results of Pediatric AIDS Clinical Trials Group (PACTG) trial 076 were released and use of zidovudine in pregnancy became the standard of care. This landmark randomized controlled trial demonstrated that use of zidovudine prophylaxis during the antepartum, intrapartum, and neonatal periods reduced perinatal HIV-1 transmission by 67% (Connor et al, 1994). Adoption of

895

PACTG 076 recommendations by obstetric and pediatric care providers throughout the United States and France have resulted in dramatic declines in perinatal transmission since then (Cooper et al, 1996; Fiscus et al, 1996, 1997; Simonds et al, 1996; Mayaux et al, 1997; Thomas et al, 1997).

Without treatment or with nucleoside monotherapy, the time from initial infection to AIDS diagnosis is approximately 10 years (Enger et al, 1996). A small proportion of those with HIV maintain extremely low viral loads and stable CD4 counts over long periods of time; these "long-term nonprogressors" have some evidence of immune damage on laboratory analysis. Because there is no way to predict which people will become ill, all individuals with HIV infection are considered to be at risk for progressive disease.

Treatment advances have altered the natural history of HIV infection, contributing to an increase in the number of persons living with HIV and even AIDS. Thus AIDS surveillance is no longer able to represent characteristics of affected populations and project the need for resources for prevention and treatment. This has led 25 states to expand reporting to include those with HIV by name. Compared with AIDS data bases, persons with HIV appear more likely to be female, younger, nonwhite, and infected through heterosexual intercourse.

However, it is estimated that the prevalence of HIV is grossly underestimated. Anonymous testing, home testing, and lack of testing all contribute to underreporting. Conservative estimates suggest that there are five times as many people with HIV as those with AIDS—over 3 million with HIV, nearly 500,000 of whom are women.

PATHOGENESIS

Our understanding of the complex interplay of the HIV virus and host immunity in adults has evolved rapidly, especially since 1995. The availability of sensitive viral load assays to measure HIV levels in blood and other human tissues have allowed investigators to delineate the kinetics of HIV replication and immune system clearance within the infected host and to determine more precisely response to therapy.

Diagnosis and Screening

There are a variety of ways to test for HIV, including serologic techniques to identify antibodies to the virus or by detecting the virus with p24 antigen, nucleic acid–based tests, or peripheral blood mononuclear cell culture (Gürtler, 1996). HIV-1 is divided into clades designated "A" through "I" (collectively called "M" subtypes) and "O." Group O strains have commonly been traced to West and Central Africa.

Serology for antibody detection to HIV-1 or HIV-2 is still the most commonly used test to identify HIV infection, and an enzyme-linked immunosorbent assay (ELISA) is the preferred assay, with a Western blot for confirmation. Seroconversion takes 3 to 12 weeks after transmission of the virus, and antibodies persist for life in most individuals. Commercially available ELISA kits in the United States lack O antigens, and will thus not ascertain infection with this viral clade. Western blot assays also will not identify infection with subtype O and will detect HIV-2 inconsistently. Regulatory organizations each use slightly different criteria for the interpretation of Western blots; the CDC requires identification of two of the following bands: p24, gp41, and gp120/160.

Accuracy of HIV serology is excellent, with results reported as positive, negative, or indeterminant. Criteria for a positive test are a repeatedly positive ELISA followed by a positive Western blot. The frequency of false-positive tests in a low-prevalence population is 0.0007% (Burke et al, 1988). False-negative results range from 0.001% in a low-prevalence population (Busch et al, 1991) to 0.3% in a high-prevalence population (Farzadegan et al, 1993). The usual cause of a false-negative result is testing after infection acquisition but before seroconversion. This time period varies depending on the sensitivity of the test and ranges from 4 weeks with the newer, more sensitive tests to 6 months with traditional tests. Causes of indeterminant results include active seroconversion; late disease; cross-reacting alloantibodies from pregnancy, blood transfusions, or organ transplantation; autoantibodies with collagen-vascular diseases, autoimmune diseases, or malignancy; HIV-2; and receipt of experimental HIV-1 vaccines. People who are in the process of seroconverting should become truly positive by Western blot within 1 month.

Several other HIV tests are available for different clinical settings. HIV test kits have been developed for home use in which a fingerstick blood sample is collected and mailed to the company for analysis. Results linked to an anonymous code are available by telephone, as is counseling. Three rapid tests (SUDS by Murex, Recombigen latex agglutination assay by Cambridge Biotech, and Genie HIV-1 by Genetic Systems) are used when immediate results are important in management decisions, such as when women without prenatal care arrive in labor and wish to learn their serostatus in order to consider the use of antiretroviral drugs to reduce vertical transmission. Accuracy of the rapid tests is analogous to that of enzyme immunoassay screening tests, with negative results considered final and positive ones requiring confirmatory testing. Salivary and urine tests for immunoglobulin G (IgG) are available to health care practitioners and are both inexpensive and noninvasive. Use of these tests facilitates screening in places in which phlebotomy would be cumbersome, such as schools and correctional facilities.

Screening is recommended for women who fall into the following categories: IDUs, hemophiliacs, persons with known HIV infection, prostitutes, persons who received blood products between 1977 and 1985, sexual partners of men who have sex with men, and heterosexual persons with more than one sexual partner during the previous calendar year who have not used condoms consistently and correctly during the past 6 months (Berrios et al, 1993). Counseling and voluntary testing is recommended for all pregnant women, given the spectacular reduction in vertical transmission rates with antiretroviral prophylaxis strategies (Centers for Disease Control and Prevention, 1995). Informed consent is required by law in 41 states and recommended as a standard practice in most others.

Virology and Viral Load Tests

Measuring blood levels of the viral capsid protein p24 using an antigen capture assay has been an indirect measure of viral load. Unfortunately, p24 levels correlate poorly with viral activity and disease progression, in part because antigens may bind to circulating antibodies, creating immune complexes that escape detection by this method.

The new viral load assays are more sophisticated, precise, and sensitive than previous methods of quantifying viral activity. There are three major tests available for directly testing virus in the blood (Mulder et al, 1994; Vandamme et al, 1995). HIV RNA can be detected by target amplification (reverse transcriptase–polymerase chain reaction [Amplicor HIV-1 Monitor by Roche Molecular Systems]) for diagnostic and prognostic use. Other tests, including signal amplification with a branched-chain DNA (bDNA) (Quantiplex HIV RNA assay by Chiron) test and a nucleic acid sequence-based amplification assay (NASBA by Organon Teknika), are now available also. The first of these assays had limited sensitivity, in the range of 200 to 500 copies/ml, whereas newer tests (Roche Ultrasensitive, Chiron bDNA Version 3, and NASBA Version 2) are more sensitive, with a threshold of about 20 to 50 copies/ml.

Risk of disease progression and efficacy of antiretroviral treatment is most accurately predicted by the magnitude of viral replication, as measured by viral load tests (Jurriaans et al, 1994; Dickover et al, 1994, 1998; Coffin, 1995; Ho et al, 1995; Mellors et al, 1995; Saksela et al, 1995; Ewi et al, 1995; O'Brien et al, 1996a, 1996b, 1998; Katzenstein et al, 1996; McIntosh et al, 1996; Perelson et al, 1996; Saag et al, 1996; Kempf et al, 1998; Palumbo et al, 1998; Marschner et al, submitted). When plasma HIV RNA levels are below the level of detection, it does not mean that infection is eradicated or even quiescent; in fact, viral replication may continue in lymphatic tissues or the central nervous system (CNS) (Cavert et al, 1997; Chun et al, 1997; Perelson et al, 1997). The rapidity and magnitude of viral turnover during all stages of HIV-1 infection is greater than previously recognized, with a mean half-life of plasma virions of only 6 hours (Perelson et al, 1996).

Viral load levels obtained during the first 6 months of initial HIV infection are not accurate predictors of disease progression; levels stabilize and become more predictive at 6 to 9 months (Schacker et al, 1997). To accurately assess viral load, two baseline measurements should be obtained within 2 weeks of each other using the same test in the same lab to reduce variability. Immunizations and infections can cause transient elevations of viral load for approximately 4 weeks (Staprans et al, 1995; Brichaek et al, 1996; Stanley et al, 1996). For this reason, it is recommended that measurement of viral load be delayed at least 1 month following immunization or other infectious illness (Saag et al, 1996; Raboud et al, 1996, 1997; Deeks et al, 1997). Because different tests measure different things, it is important to utilize the same test in patient management.

Immunology

With viral replication, HIV infection progressively destroys CD4+ T lymphocytes that serve essential roles in the generation and maintenance of host immune responses (Embretson et al, 1993; Pantaleo et al, 1993; Jurriaans et al, 1994; Ho et al, 1995; Mellors et al, 1995; Saksela et al, 1995; Wei et al, 1995; O'Brien et al, 1996a, 1996b, 1998). This target preference of HIV is determined by the identity of the cell surface molecule, CD4, recognized by the HIV envelope glycoprotein (gp120) as the virus binds to and enters host cells (Weiss, 1996). Other targets include macrophages and their CNS counterparts, microglial cells, both of which may represent reservoirs of chronically infected cells. Peripheral lymphocytes comprise only about 2% of the total lymphocyte population; the rest are in other lymphoid organs. The result of systematic destruction of lymphoid organs by HIV disease is clonal deletion, sequential loss of specific types of immune responses, and loss of memory CD4+ T cells (Schnittman et al, 1990; Shearer and Clerici, 1991; Connors et al, 1997).

Progression of disease is heralded by acceleration in the rate of increases in HIV replication, decline of CD4+ T cells, and declines in host cell-mediated immune responses (Haynes et al, 1996; Koot et al, 1996). Host compensatory responses that preserve the homeostasis of total T-cell levels break down in HIV-infected persons about 18 months before development of AIDS, resulting in net loss of peripheral T cells and signaling immune collapse (Margolick et al, 1995).

Chemokines

The chemokines are a complex family of small proteins that were initially characterized through their chemotactic effects on a variety of leukocytes. They play a crucial role in recruitment and function of T lymphocytes, and T lymphocytes appear to produce a number of chemokines. The expression of two chemokine receptors, CXCR4 and CCR5, appears to be extremely important in determining sensitivity of T cells to HIV-1 infection (Ostrowski et al, 1998). HIV-1 requires interaction of the viral envelope protein with CD4 and at least one additional cell surface molecule, termed a "cofactor" or "coreceptor." Macrophage-trophic strains of HIV-1, which are largely responsible for sexual transmission, require CCR5 in addition to CD4, while the T cell–tropic viruses that emerge after infection has been established use CSCR4. Both CD4 and the appropriate chemokine receptor must be expressed on the cell surface in order for HIV-1 to enter the cell and establish an infection.

Sex steroid hormone variation in women, principally when progesterone levels are high, has long been implicated as a risk for acquisition of sexually transmitted infections (STIs) and HIV. Interestingly, CCR5 has been shown to be significantly increased ($p < 0.02$) in cervical biopsies from women with STIs and others who were progesterone predominant compared with normal controls (Patterson et al, 1998). Further in vitro studies demonstrated that progesterone increased CCR5 and CXCR4 expression in lymphocytes and monocytes/macrophages (Patterson et al, 1998). These data may provide additional biologic plausibility to the increased transmission rates for women.

PRIMARY CARE INTERVENTIONS FOR ADULT WOMEN WITH HIV

Antiretroviral Treatment

The goal of current therapeutic interventions is to maximally suppress viral replication, preserve immune function, prevent disease progression, and ultimately prolong survival. Currently, the most efficacious regimen and first line of treatment includes two nucleoside analog reverse transcriptase inhibitors combined with a potent protease inhibitor. Individual drugs in these regimens should have synergy of activity and different toxicities (Table 39–1). Also, therapeutic options should be preserved in case the regimen fails. Combination therapy drugs should be started within 2 days of one another, and should be used at therapeutic dosages.

The biggest obstacle to effective treatment is HIV's ability to develop resistance to drugs (Coffin, 1995). Development of drug resistance can be delayed and perhaps even prevented by using a combination therapy that suppresses HIV replication to undetectable levels (Montaner and Wainbert, 1996; Gulick et al, 1997; Kempf et al, 1997). Cessation of replication stops development of mutants and subsequentresistance to therapy. Patient adherence to the regimen is critical to the success of treatment. Some drug combinations should be used only if there is reason

to believe that complete suppression is likely, because HIV rapidly develops resistance to them. Examples include lamivudine and the non-nucleoside reverse transcriptase inhibitors nevirapine and delavirdine.

Because the use of combination antiretroviral therapy to maximally suppress viral load has become the standard of care in the majority of adults with HIV disease, the number of pregnancies exposed to multiple drugs has increased. This has raised questions regarding the management of antiretroviral therapy in women. Based on the best available data, the U.S. Public Health Service Task Force (1998) has developed recommendations for the use of antiretroviral agents in pregnancy for maternal health and reduction of perinatal transmission of HIV. In this document, four scenarios are presented:

- Scenario 1 describes pregnant women without prior antiretroviral therapy, and recommends use of the same parameters used in nonpregnant individuals for decisions regarding the initiation and choice of antiretroviral therapy. The PACTG 076 regimen using zidovudine should be recommended if another multiple-drug regimen is not chosen, and consideration may be given to initiation of zidovudine at the end of the first trimester.
- Scenario 2 involves women receiving antiretroviral therapy at the time pregnancy is diagnosed, and recommends continuing therapy if pregnancy is identified after the first trimester. However, if pregnancy is identified within the first trimester, counseling should involve the benefits and potential risks of these drugs, and continuation of therapy should be considered.
- In Scenario 3, women who are identified in labor and have not had prior therapy should be given the intrapartum intravenous zidovudine regimen and their infants given the neonatal regimen.
- Scenario 4 involves infants born to mothers who did not receive therapy, and recommends discussion of therapy for the woman and initiation of the neonatal regimen as soon as possible as post-exposure prophylaxis.

Immunizations and Prophylaxis

The risk of developing specific opportunistic infections is best assessed by measuring the CD4+ T-cell count (Enger et al, 1992; Stein et al, 1992; El-Sadr et al, 1994; Mellors et al, 1997). T-cell count appears to be a valid indicator of length and extent of immune damage regardless of whether or not someone is on antiretroviral therapy. CD4 counts are subject to considerable variability because of both biologicand lab methodologies (Stein et al, 1992), and can vary up to 30% in the absence of a clinically significant change in status. Trends are more important than individual values.

Table 39-1. ANTIRETROVIRAL AGENTS

NAME	ADULT DAILY DOSE*	PREGNANCY CLASS	SPECIAL CONSIDERATIONS/ SIDE EFFECTS	DRUG INTERACTIONS
Non-nucleoside Reverse Transcriptase Inhibitors (NNRTIs)				
Delavirdine mesylate (Rescriptor)	4 × 100 mg tablets tid	C	Should be taken at least 1 hour apart from didanosine and from antacids • Rash, Rx Benadryl / Atarax, hydrocortisone cream, avoid sunburn	↑ AUC of PIs **Contraindications:** Seldane, Hismanal, Xanax, Ca channel blockers, Versed, Propulsid, rifampin, ergots
Efavirenz (DMP 266) (Sustiva)	3 × 200 mg capsules qid	C	• Feeling of disengagement within 1st 2 weeks • Headaches, dizziness, N&V, insomnia—divide dose, rash—Rx Benadryl • Divide dose tid if nightmares	↓ Biaxin AUC 30% ↓ AUC of PIs **Contraindications:** Hismanal, Halcion, ergots, Propulsid
Nevirapine (Viramune)	1 × 200 mg tablet bid	C	Lead-in dosing for first 14 days of therapy; 1 × 200 mg tablet qid • Mild rash (with pruritus) continue dose q s ↑ • Severe rash—D/C drug; fever >100°F, conjunctivitis, oral lesions, Stevens-Johnson syndrome, ↑ LFTs, hives malaise, myalgia / arthralgia	Not recommended with PIs (↓ AUC)
Nucleoside Reverse Transcriptase Inhibitors (NRTIs)				
Abacavir sulfate (Ziagen)	1 × 300 mg tablet bid	C	May be taken without regard to food Nausea, vomiting, diarrhea; hypersensitivity reaction (fever, rash, GI symptoms)—do **NOT** rechallenge	Minimal
Didanosine (DDI) (Videx)	2 × 100 mg tablets bid	B	Take on an empty stomach; alcohol may exacerbate toxicity • Peripheral neuropathy—30% • Pancreatitis—15% • Elevated LFTs; diarrhea; GI upset-nausea • Photophobia—5%	Do not give cipro, dapsone, ketoconazole, TCN within 2 hours of ddI dose; avoid use of other drugs that can cause pancreatitis or peripheral neuropathy
Lamivudine (3TC) (Epivir)	1 × 150 mg tablet bid	C	• Headache, peripheral neuropathy, nausea, diarrhea, rash	Reverses AZT resistance
Lamivudine/ zidovudine (Combivir)	1 × 150 mg/ 300 mg tablet bid	C	Should not be prescribed for patients requiring dosage adjustments • Anemia; ↓ ANC, headaches, GI upset-nausea • Peripheral neuropathy, diarrhea, rash	Inhibitory with d4T
Stavudine (D4T) (Zerit)	1 × 40 mg capsule bid	C	• Peripheral neuropathy—25% • Pancreatitis—1% • Headache; elevated LFTs	Synergy with ddI. Substitute for AZT if intolerant/cytopenic.
Zalcitabine (DDC) (Hivid)	1 × 0.75 mg tablet tid	C	Should not be used concomitantly with didanosine; do not take simultaneously with magnesium/aluminum-containing antacids • Peripheral neuropathy—30% • Aphthous ulcers; transient rash; pancreatitis; urticaria	Avoid use of other drugs that can cause pancreatitis or peripheral neuropathy. Amphotericin, foscavir, and aminoglycosides may increase ddC levels.
Zidovudine (ZDV, AZT) (Retrovir)	2 × 10 mg capsules tid or 1 × 300 mg tablet bid	C	• Anemia; ↓ ANC, headaches, GI upset-nausea	Probenecid may ↑ AZT levels; AZT may alter dilantin levels; hematologic toxicity ↑ with IFN, DHPG, chemo.

Table continued on following page

Table 39 – 1. ANTIRETROVIRAL AGENTS (*Continued*)

NAME	ADULT DAILY DOSE*	PREGNANCY CLASS	SPECIAL CONSIDERATIONS/ SIDE EFFECTS	DRUG INTERACTIONS
Protease Inhibitors (PIs)				
Amprenavir (APV) (Agenerase)	8 × 150 mg capsules bid	C	Take with food • Nausea, diarrhea, rash, headache, vomiting, numbness around the mouth, abdominal pain	Each 150 mg capsule of amprenavir contains 109 IU of vitamin E. The normal adult dose of amprenavir contains 1744 IU of vitamin E. **Contraindications:** Rifampin, Hismanal, Seldane, Propulsid, Halcion, Versed, rifampin, ergots
Indinavir (Crixivan)	2 × 400 mg capsules q8h	C	Take on empty stomach 1 hour before or 2 hours after a meal; drink at least 1.5 liters of liquid daily • Kidney stones—4% • HA, insomnia, blurred vision, diarrhea, N&V, altered taste, ↑ LFTs • Weakness/fatigue/asthenia CR1 × belly • ↓ Platelets, rash, dizzy	**Contraindications:** Rifampin, Hismanal, Seldane, Propulsid, Halcion, Versed If used with ddI, take 1 hour apart on empty stomach
Nelfinavir mesylate (Viracept)	3 × 250 mg capsules tid	B	Take with a meal or light snack • Diarrhea—Imodium • N&V—Rx Pepsid • ↑ glucose/lipid	**Contraindications:** Seldane, Hismanal, Propulsid, rifampin, etc., Halcion, Versed, Nizoral 200 mg qid ↑ AUC
Ritonavir (Norvir)	6 × 100 mg capsules bid	B	Should be refrigerated; take with meals; titrated lead-in dosing; start at no less than 300 mg bid; increase by 100-mg increments bid up to 600 mg bid • Oral & UE paresthesias • Abdominal pain, diarrhea, N&V • Altered taste, weakness/ fatigue/asthenia • Labs: BUN, LFTs triglycerides, ↑ CPK, ↑ glucose/lipid	**Contraindications:** Xanax, Valium, Ambien, etc. Smoking ↓ Norvir AUC by 18% Adverse events T/T liver toxicity and altered metabolism of other drugs. Bioavailability;—Unknown
Saquinavir (Fortovase)	6 × 200 mg soft gelatin capsules tid	B	Take within 2 hours after a full meal; saquinavir taken without food may have less bioavailability • Nausea—27% • Diarrhea—4% • Rash—1% ↑ LFTs, confusion, HA ↓ Platelets, Stevens-Johnson syndrome, buccal mucosa ulcers • ↑ Glucose/lipid	**Contraindications:** Seldane, Hismanal, Propulsid, rifampin, AUC of Ca channel blockers, dapsone, dilantin Nizoral 200 mg qid ↑ AUC 5× Norvir use ↑ 20xx
Saquinavir mesylate (Invirase)	3 × 200 mg hard gelatin capsules tid	B	Take within 2 hours after a full meal; saquinavir taken without food may have less bioavailability	

*Based on manufacturer's presciding information for adults weighing ≥60 kg.
Abbreviations: AUC, adequate area under the curve; Rx, prescribe; UE, upper extremity; N&V, nausea and vomiting; BUN, blood urea nitrogen; LFTs, liver function tests; CPK, creatine phosphokinase; HA, headache; GI, gastrointestinal; D/C, discontinue; ANC, absolute neutrophil count; IFN, interferon; DHPG, dehydroxyphenylglycol.

The most commonly used opportunistic infection prophylactic regimens are listed below:

• *Pneumocystis carinii*—CD4 count less than 200/ mm^3 or prior *P. carinii* pneumonia or HIV-associated thrush or fever of unknown origin for 2 weeks: preferred, trimethoprim-sulfamethoxazole (TMP- SMX), one double-strength tablet or one single-strength tablet per day; alternatives, one double-strength tablet three times per week, TMP-SMX, dapsone, aerosolized pentamidine, atovaquone

• *Mycobacterium tuberculosis*—positive purified protein derivative (PPD) test (>5 mm induration), prior positive PPD without treatment, or contact

with an active case: isoniazid plus pyridoxine for 12 months; rifampin plus pyrazinamide
- *Toxoplasma gondii*—CD4 count less than 100/mm^3 and positive IgG serology: TMP-SMX, one double-strength tablet per day; dapsone
- *Mycobacterium avium* complex—CD4 count less than 50/mm^3: clarithromycin, 500 mg twice a day, or azithromycin, 1200 mg PO weekly; alternative, rifabutin 300 mg PO daily
- Varicella—significant exposure to chickenpox or shingles and no history of either, or negative serology: varicella zoster immune globulin, 5 vials IM, within 96 hours of exposure, best if within 48 hours; alternative, acyclovir, 800 mg PO five times per day
- *Streptococcus pneumoniae*—all patients: Pneumovax, 0.5 ml IM once; repeat once in five years
- Hepatitis B vaccines—Recombivax HB (Merck) or Engerix-B (SmithKline Beecham), are available in several formulations and dosage strengths. The vaccine is given in 3 doses, with the final booster 4 to 6 months after the primary immunization series. Immunocompromised individuals typically require higher doses to achieve immunity.
- Influenza—all patients: influenza vaccine, 0.5 ml IM, each year in October or November; alternative, amantadine, 100 mg PO twice daily, or rimantadine, 100 mg PO twice daily.

Sexual Risk Reduction: Prevention of Transmission and Pregnancy

HIV-infected persons, even those with viral loads below detectable limits, should be considered infectious and should be counseled to avoid sexual and drug-use behaviors that are associated with transmission or acquisition of HIV and other infectious pathogens. They can still transmit HIV and other STIs; also, they may acquire a multiply resistant HIV variant from another person. The only effective method to prevent sexual transmission of HIV is through the consistent and correct use of male condoms.

GYNECOLOGIC MANIFESTATIONS

Menstrual Disorders

Abnormal uterine bleeding is a frequent complaint among HIV-infected women. Controlled studies have failed to document a clinically significant direct effect of HIV or immunosuppression on menstruation (Shah et al, 1994; Ellerbrock et al, 1996). Rather, it appears that most menstrual irregularities are due to secondary factors, such as concomitant substance abuse, weight loss associated with chronic illness, cervicitis, or exogenous hormone use for contraception or appetite stimulation. Menstrual abnormalities are common in all women, and HIV-infected women

with this problem should be evaluated using the usual paradigm with special attention paid to the factors noted above.

Lower Genital Tract Neoplasia

Early in the epidemic in women, a strong association was established between detectable human papillomavirus (HPV) and HIV. This was not surprising, given that both viral infections are sexually transmitted. A dose-response effect was delineated, with expression of HPV increasing with level of immunosuppression (Centers for Disease Control, 1990; Vermund et al, 1991; Mandelblatt et al, 1992; Lipsey and Northfelt, 1993; Van Landuyt et al, 1993; Fisher and Gissmann, 1994; Northfelt, 1994; Petry et al, 1994; Stratton and Ciacco, 1994; Vernon et al, 1995). In addition, the prevalence of squamous intraepithelial lesions (SIL) was found to be two to three times higher in HIV-infected women (17% vs. 40%) (Carpenter et al, 1991; Clark et al, 1996). The association between HIV and high-grade SIL or cancer has not been substantiated by population-based studies, which have failed to identify a genital tract cancer epidemic coincident with the HIV epidemic (Coté et al, 1991; Goedert et al, 1998).

Other authors found SIL to be more extensive, with a multifocal pattern of lesions (Centers for Disease Control, 1990). Multifocal lesions were also associated with immunosuppression (Maiman et al, 1991; Clark et al, 1996). Vulvar intraepithelial neoplasia (VIN) was present in 14 of 58 HIV-infected women (24%) versus 1 of 85 uninfected controls (0.01%) in another study. Women with pigmented or raised lesions had higher rates of VIN on biopsy (Korn et al, 1996). Anal HPV/dysplasia is as common as cervical disease in HIV-infected women, making it imperative that gynecologic evaluation extend to the perianal area and suggesting a role for perianal Pap smears (Williams et al, 1994).

For HIV-infected women, the CDC and the Agency for Health Care Policy and Research recommend a baseline gynecologic evaluation, including a pelvic examination and Pap smear at baseline, in 6 months, and then annually (Kurman et al, 1994; Centers for Disease Control and Prevention, 1998). Some recommend colposcopy either at baseline evaluation or routinely to enhance identification of abnormalities in this population, who may have a higher prevalence of dysplasia and are less likely to return for follow-up. However, controlled studies have failed to determine any difference in sensitivity of Pap screening between HIV-infected and -uninfected populations (Adachi et al, 1993; Korn et al, 1994).

Once SIL has been identified, most recommend treating according to established guidelines for HIV-seronegative women. Loop excision is commonly used in clinical practice for treatment of high-grade lesions. Persistence and recurrence rates after loop excision are higher in women with HIV (18 of 30, or

60%) than in uninfected controls (10 of 80, or 13%) irrespective of size or grade of lesion (Wright et al, 1994). Women treated for preinvasive lesions of the lower genital tract should have Pap smears every 3 to 4 months for the first year and every 6 months thereafter (American College of Obstetricians and Gynecologists, 1992).

Lower Genital Tract Infections and Inflammatory Conditions

A fundamental concept to understanding the epidemiology of STIs and HIV is that of "epidemiologic synergy" (Wasserheit, 1992). The basic tenets of epidemiologic synergy are that the presence of any STI increases acquisition and transmissibility of HIV, that coexisting STIs increase HIV viral replication, and that the effects of HIV on the immune system prolong the course and therefore the infectious period of other STIs. Prevention and control of STIs is therefore crucial to HIV care (Minkoff et al. 1999). HIV-infected women should be screened for STIs on a regular basis, promptly and appropriately treated when diagnosed, and encouraged to use barrier protection during sexual intercourse.

Prevalences for specific sexually transmitted infections in HIV-positive women were established in five retrospective cohorts: trichomoniasis, 9% to 27%; *Chlamydia trachomatis*, 4% to 18%; *Neisseria gonorrhoeae*, 2% to 7%; syphilis, 3% to 22%; and genital herpes simplex virus (HSV), 4% to 18% (Carpenter et al, 1991; Clark and Kissinger, 1993). Syphilis and trichomoniasis rates were higher in IDUs after adjustment for race, age, and CD4 count, while clinically evident HPV and HSV were proportional to level of immunosuppression (Clark and Kissinger, 1993). A more recent study supports these prevalence ranges (Bersoff-Matcha et al, 1998). There is no evidence to suggest that vaginal bacteriosis, trichomoniasis, *C. trachomatis*, or *N. gonorrhoeae* have a different clinical course or manifestations in HIV-infected women.

There were concerns that chronic vulvovaginal candidiasis (VVC), defined as four or more episodes annually, was an HIV-related symptom in women. One cohort reported that the prevalence of VVC was 38%, and that VVC represented the most common presenting complaint of the women (Carpenter et al, 1991). The CDC guidelines were altered in 1991 to include VVC as a symptom of HIV. Subsequent evaluation of 66 women from the same population revealed that recurrent VVC appeared first at a median CD4 cell count of $506/mm^3$, followed by oral and esophageal candidiasis at median CD4 cell counts of $230/mm^3$ and $30/mm^3$, respectively (Imam, 1990). These findings have not been substantiated in other studies. Median CD4 cell count at diagnosis of recurrent VVC was significantly lower ($196/mm^3$) in another population (Clark and Kissinger, 1993), and the frequency of VVC appears to noticeably increase only when the CD4 cell count falls below $200/mm^3$

(Duerr et al, 1997). The correlation could be with immunodeficiency itself, or a result of the large array of therapeutic and prophylactic antimicrobial agents taken by HIV-positive women.

Pelvic Inflammatory Disease

High-risk sexual behaviors, as well as the high prevalence of coexisting genital tract infections, place many HIV-infected women at risk for pelvic inflammatory disease (PID), with the prevalence of PID in established cohorts ranging from 5% (Clark and Kissinger, 1993) to 16% (Carpenter et al, 1991). Early unblinded descriptive studies suggested that HIV-infected women with PID had lower white blood cell counts on admission and were more likely to require surgical intervention than uninfected controls (Hoegsberg et al, 1990; Korn et al, 1993). Both studies concluded that PID may be more serious in HIV-seropositive women, although many other factors, such as access to care, may have influenced the results. Unfortunately, there is no long-term follow-up in these studies.

Prospective studies have determined that HIV-infected women who develop PID are no more likely than seronegative controls to have coexistent vaginal bacteriosis (Irwin et al, 1993) or to have pathogenic bacteria, such as *N. gonorrhoeae*, *C. trachomatis*, or *Gardnerella vaginalis*, recovered from the upper genital tract (Moorman et al, 1997). In addition, although they may present with slightly more severe symptoms, including pain, fever, and pelvic masses, than HIV-uninfected controls, they respond equally well to standard antimicrobial therapy (Irwin et al, 1993; Barbosa et al, 1997).

REFERENCES

American College of Obstetricians and Gynecologists: Human Immunodeficiency Virus Infections (ACOG Technical Bulletin). Washington, DC: American College of Obstetricians and Gynecologists, No. 169. 1992:1.

Adachi A, Fleming I, Burk RD, Ho GY, Klein RS: Women with human immunodeficiency virus infection and abnormal Papanicolaou smears—a prospective study of colposcopy and clinical outcome. Obstet Gynecol 1993;81:372.

Barbosa C, Macasaet M, Brockmann S, et al: Pelvic inflammatory disease and human immunodeficiency virus infection. Obstet Gynecol 1997;89:65.

Berrios DC, Hearst N, Coates TJ, et al: HIV antibody testing among those at risk for infection. The National AIDS Behavioral Surveys. JAMA 1993;270:1576.

Bersoff-Matcha SJ, Horgan MM, Fraser VJ, Mundy LM, Stoner BP: Sexually transmitted disease acquisition among women infected with human immunodeficiency virus type 1. J Infect Dis 1998;178:1174.

Brichaek B, Swindells S, Janoff E, Pirruccello S, Stevenson M: Increased plasma human immunodeficiency virus type 1 burden following antigenic challenge with pneumococcal vaccine. J Infect Dis 1996;174:1191.

Burke DS, Brundage JF, Redfield RR, et al: Measurement of the false positive rate in a screening program for human immunodeficiency virus infections. N Engl J Med 1988;319:961.

Busch MP, Eble BE, Khayam-Bashi H, et al: Evaluation of screened blood donations for human immunodeficiency virus type 1 infection by culture and DNA amplification of pooled cells. N Engl J Med 1991;325:1.

Carpenter CC, Mayer KH, Stein MD, et al: Human immunodeficiency virus infection in North American women: experience with 200 cases and a review of the literature. Medicine 1991; 70:307.

Cavert W, Notermans DW, Staskus K, et al: Kinetics of response in lymphoid tissues to antiretroviral therapy of HIV-1 infection. Science 1997;276:960.

Centers for Disease Control: Risk for cervical disease in HIV infected women in New York City. MMWR Morbid Mortal Wkly Rep 1990;39:846.

Centers for Disease Control and Prevention: U.S. Public Health Service recommendations for human immunodeficiency virus counseling and voluntary testing for pregnant women. MMWR Morbid Mortal Wkly Rep 1995;44:1.

Centers for Disease Control and Prevention: HIV/AIDS Surveillance Report. Atlanta: Centers for Disease Control and Prevention, 1997.

Centers for Disease Control and Prevention: 1998 Guidelines for the treatment of sexually transmitted diseases. MMWR Morbid Mortal Wkly Rep 1998;47:1.

Chun TW, Carruth L, Finzi D, et al: Quantification of latent tissue reservoirs and total body viral load in HIV-1 infection. Nature 1997;387:183.

Clark R, Kissinger P, Fuller C, Abodalian SE: Squamous intraepithelial lesions among adolescent women infected with human immunodeficiency virus. J Adolesc Health 1996;19:246.

Coffin JM: HIV population dynamics in vivo: implications for genetic variation, pathogenesis, and therapy. Science 1995;267: 483.

Connor EM, Sperling R, Gelber R, et al: Reduction of maternal-infant transmission of human immunodeficiency virus type 1 zidovudine treatment. Pediatric AIDS Clinical Trials Group Protocol 076 Study Group. N Engl J Med 1994;331:1173.

Connors M, Kovacs JA, Krevat S, et al: HIV infection induces changes in CD4+ T cell phenotype and depletions within the CD4+ T-cell repertoire that are not immediately restored by antiviral or immune-based therapies. Nat Med 1997;3:533.

Cooper ER, Nugent RP, Diaz C, et al: After AIDS Clinical Trial 076: the changing pattern of zidovudine use during pregnancy, and the subsequent reduction in vertical transmission of human immunodeficiency virus in a cohort of infected women and their infants. J Infect Dis 1996;174:1207.

Coté TR, Howe HL, Anderson SS, et al: A systematic consideration of the neoplastic spectrum of AIDS: registry linkage in Illinois. AIDS 1991;5:49.

Deeks SG, Coleman RL, White R, et al: Variance of plasma human immunodeficiency virus type 1 RNA levels measured by branched DNA within and between days. J Infect Dis 1997;176: 514.

Dickover RE, Dillon M, Gillette SG, et al: Rapid increase in load of human immunodeficiency virus correlates with early disease progression and loss of CD4 cells in vertically infected infants. J Infect Dis 1994;170:1279.

Dickover RE, Dillon M, Leung KM, et al: Early prognostic indicators in primary perinatal human immunodeficiency virus type 1 infection: importance of viral RNA and the timing of transmission on long-term outcome. J Infect Dis 1998;178:375.

Duerr A, Sierra M, Feldman J, et al: Immune compromise and prevalence of Candida vulvovaginitis in human immunoeficiency virus-infected women. Obstet Gynecol 1997;90:252.

Ellerbrock T, Wright T, Bush T, et al: Characteristics of menstruation in women infected with human immunodeficiency virus. Obstet Gynecol 1996;87:1030.

El-Sadr WM, Oleske JM, Agins BD: Evaluation and Management of Early HIV Infection. Rockville, MD: Agency for Health Care Policy and Research, 1994.

Embretson J, Zupancic M, Ribas JL, et al: Massive covert infection of helper T lymphocytes and macrophages by HIV during the incubation period of AIDS. Nature 1993;362:359.

Enger C, Graham N, Peng Y, et al: Survival from early, intermediate, and late stages of HIV infection. JAMA 1996;275:1329.

Farzadegan H, Vlahov D, Solomon L, et al: Detection of human immunodeficiency virus type-1 infection by polymerase chain reaction in a cohort of seronegative intravenous drug users. J Infect Dis 1993;168:327.

Fiscus SA, Adimora AA, Schoenbach VJ: Perinatal HIV infection and the effect of zidovudine therapy on transmission in rural and urban counties. JAMA 1996;275:1483.

Fiscus SA, Adimora AA, Schoenbach VJ, et al: Importance of maternal ZDV therapy in the reduction of perinatal transmission of HIV. In: Abstracts of the 4th Conference on Retroviruses and Opportunistic Infections, Washington DC, 1997:176.

Fisher SG, Gissmann L: Convergent infections: human papillomavirus and human immunodeficiency virus. Antibiot Chemother 1994;46:134.

Goedert JJ, Coté TR, Virgo P, et al: Spectrum of AIDS-associated malignant disorders. Lancet 1998;351:1833.

Gulick RM, Mellors JW, Havlir D, et al: Treatment with indinavir, zidovudine, and lamivudine in adults with human immunodeficiency virus infection and prior antiretroviral therapy. N Engl J Med 1997;337:734.

Gürtler L: Difficulties and strategies of HIV diagnosis. Lancet 1996;348:176.

Haynes BF, Panteleo G, Fauci AA: Toward an understanding of the correlates of protective immunity to HIV infection. Science 1996;271:324.

Ho DD, Neumann AU, Perelson AS, et al: Rapid turnover of plasma virions and CD4 lymphocytes in HIV-1 infection. Nature 1995;373:123.

Hoegsberg B, Abulafia O, Sedis A, et al: Sexually transmitted diseases and human immunodeficiency virus infection among women with pelvic inflammatory disease. Am J Obstet Gynecol 1990;163:1135.

Imam N, Carpenter CC, Mayer, et al: Hierarchical pattern of mucosal candida infections in HIV-seropositive women. Am J Med 1990;89:142.

Irwin KL, Rice RJ, O'Sullivan MJ, et al: The clinical presentation and course of pelvic inflammatory disease in HIV+ and HIV− women: preliminary results of a prospective multicenter study. In: Abstracts of the 10th International Meeting of the International Society for STD Research, Helsinki, 1993.

Jurriaans S, van Gemen B, Weverling G, et al: The natural history of HIV-1 infections: virus load and virus phenotype independent determinants of clinical course? Virology 1994;204:223.

Katzenstein DA, Hammer SM, Hughes MD et al: The relation of virologic and immunologic markers to clinical outcomes after nucleoside therapy in HIV-infected adults with 200 to 500 CD4 cells per cubic millimeter. N Engl J Med 1996;335:1091.

Kempf DJ, Rode RA, Xu Y, et al: The duration of viral suppression for HIV-1 infection is predicted by plasma HIV-1 RNA at the nadir. AIDS 1998;12:F9.

Koot M, van't Wout AB, Kootstra N, et al: Relation between changes in cellular load evolution of viral phenotype, and the clonal composition of virus populations in the course of human immunodeficiency virus type 1 infection. J Infect Dis 1996;173: 349.

Korn AP, Abercrombie PD, Foster A: Vulvar intraepithelial neoplasia in women infected with human immunodeficiency virus-1. Gynecol Oncol 1996;61:384.

Korn AP, Autry M, DeRemer PA, Tan W: Sensitivity of the Papanicolaou smear in human immunodeficiency virus-infected women. Obstet Gynecol 1994;83:401.

Korn AP, Landers DV, Green JR, Sweet RL: Pelvic inflammatory disease in human immunodeficiency virus-infected women. Obstet Gynecol 1993;82:765.

Kurman RJ, Henson DE, Herbst AL, Noller KL, Schiffman MH, et al: Interim guidelines for management of abnormal cervical cytology. JAMA 1994;271:1866.

Lipsey LR, Northfelt DW: Anogenital neoplasia in patients with HIV infection. Curr Opin Oncol 1993;5:861.

Maiman M, Tarricone N, Viera J, et al: Colposcopic evaluation of HIV infected women. Obstet Gynecol 1991;78:84.

Mandelblatt JS, Fahs M, Garibaldi K, Senie RT, Peterson HB: Association between HIV infection and cervical neoplasia: implications for clinical care of women at risk for both conditions. AIDS 1992;6:173.

Mann J, Tarantola D, for the Global AIDS Policy Coalition. AIDS in the world II: global dimensions, social roots, and responses. In Mann J, Tarantola D (eds): New York: Oxford University Press; 1996:616.

Margolick JB, Munoz A, Donnenberg AD, et al: Failure of T-cell homeostasis preceding AIDS in HIV-1 infection. Nat Med 1995; 1:674.

Marschner I, Collier A, Coombs R, et al: Use of changes in plasma levels of human immunodeficiency virus type 1 RNA to assess the clinical benefit of antiretroviral therapy. J Infect Dis 1998; 177:40.

Mayaux MJ, Teglas JP, Mandelbrot L, et al: Acceptability and impact of zidovudine for prevention of mother-to-child human immunodeficiency virus-1 transmission in France. J Pediatr 1997;131:857.

McIntosh K, Shevitz A, Zaknun D, et al: Age- and time-related changes in extracellular viral load in children vertically infected by human immunodeficiency virus. Pediatr Infect Dis J 1996;15:1087.

Mellors JW, Munoz A, Giorgi JV, et al: Plasma viral load and CD4+ lymphocytes as prognostic markers of HIV-1 infection. Ann Intern Med 1997;126:946.

Mellors J, Kingsley LA, Rinaldo CR Jr, et al: Quantitation of HIV-1 RNA in plasma predicts outcome after seroconversion. Ann Intern Med 1995;112:573.

Minkoff HL, Eisenberger-Matityahu D, Feldman J, Burk R, Clarke L: Prevalence and incidence of gynecologic disorders among women infected with human immunodeficiency virus. Am J Obstet Gynecol 1999;180:824.

Montaner JS, Wainbert M: INCAS study results. In: Proceedings of a Public Meeting of the NIH Panel to Define Principles of Therapy of HIV Infection, Washington, DC, 1996.

Moorman AC, Schwartz D, Irwin K, et al: Influence of HIV infection on the relationship of endometritis and endometrial pathogens among women with acute pelvic inflammatory disease (PID). In: Abstracts of the National Conference on Women with HIV (abstract 103.6), Pasadena, CA, May 4–7, 1997.

Mulder JC, McKinney N, Christopherson C, et al: Rapid and simple PCR assay for quantitation of human immunodeficiency type 1 RNA in plasma: application to acute retroviral infection. J Clin Microbiol 1994;32:292.

Northfelt DW: Cervical and anal neoplasia and HPV infection in persons with HIV infection. Oncology 1994;8:33.

O'Brien TR, Blattner WA, Waters D, et al: Serum HIV-1 RNA levels and time to development of AIDS in the Multicenter Hemophilia Cohort Study. JAMA 1996a;276:105.

O'Brien WA, Hartigan PM, Martin D, et al: Changes in plasma HIV-1 RNA and CD4+ lymphocyte counts and the risk of progression to AIDS. N Engl J Med 1996b;334:426.

O'Brien TR, Rosenberg PS, Yellin F, Goedert JJ: Longitudinal HIV-1 RNA levels in a cohort of homosexual men. J Acquir Immune Defic Syndr Hum Retrovirol 1998;18:155.

Ostrowski MA, Justement SJ, Catanzaro A, et al: Expression of chemokine receptors CXCR4 and CCR5 in HIV-1-infected and uninfected individuals. J Immunol 1998;161:3195.

Palumbo PE, Raskino C, Fiscus S, et al: Predictive value of quantitative plasma HIV RNA and CD4+ lymphocyte count in HIV-infected infants and children. JAMA 1998;279:756.

Pantaleo G, Graziosi C, Demarest JF, et al: HIV infection is active and progressive in lymphoid tissue during the clinically latent stage of disease. Nature 1993;362:355.

Patterson BK, Landay A, Andersson J, et al: Repertoire of chemokine receptor expression in the female genital tract: implications for human immunodeficiency virus transmission. Am J Pathol 1998;153:481.

Perelson AS, Essunger P, Cao Y, et al: Decay characteristics of HIV-1-infected compartments during combination therapy. Nature 1997;387:188.

Perelson AS, Neumann A, Markowitz M, Leonard JM, Ho DD: HIV-1 dynamics in vivo: virion clearance rate, infected cell lifespan, and viral generation time. Science 1996;217:1582.

Petry KU, Scheffel D, Bode U, et al: Cellular immunodeficiency enhances the progression of human papillomavirus-associated cervical lesions. Int J Cancer 1994;57:836.

Raboud J, Montaner J, Conway B: Variation in plasma RNA levels, CD4 cell counts, and p24 antigen levels in clinically stable men with human immunodeficiency virus infection. J Infect Dis 1996;174:191.

Raboud JM, Montaner JS, Rae S, et al: Issues in the design of trials of therapies for subjects with human immunodeficiency

virus infection that use plasma RNA level as an outcome. J Infect Dis 1997;175:576.

Saag MS, Holodniy M, Kuritzkes D, et al: HIV viral load markers in clinical practice. Nat Med 1996;2:625.

Saksela K, Stevens CE, Rubinstein P, Taylor PE, Baltimore D: HIV-1 messenger RNA in peripheral blood mononuclear cells with an early marker of risk for progression to AIDS. Ann Intern Med 1995;123:641.

Schacker TW, Hughes JP, Shea T, Coombs RW, Corey L: Biological and virologic characteristics of primary HIV infection. Ann Intern Med 1998;128:613.

Schnittman SM, Lane HC, Greenhouse JJ: Preferential infection of CD4+ memory T cells by human immunodeficiency virus type 1: evidence for a role in selective T cell functional defects observed in infected individuals. Proc Natl Acad Sci USA 1990; 87:6058.

Shah PN, Smith JR, Wells C, et al: Menstrual symptoms in women infected by the human immunodeficiency virus. Obstet Gynecol 1994;83:397.

Shearer GM, Clerici M: Early T-helper cell defects in HIV infection. AIDS 1991;5:245.

Simonds RJ, Steketee R, Nesheim, et al: Impact of zidovudine use on risk and risk factors for perinatal transmission of HIV. Perinatal AIDS Collaborative Transmission Studies. AIDS 1998;12: 301.

Stanley SK, Ostrowski MA, Justement JS, et al: Effect of immunization with a common recall antigen in viral expression in patients infected with human immunodeficiency virus type 1. N Engl J Med 1996;334:1222.

Staprans SI, Hamilton BB, Follansbee SE, et al.: Activation of virus replication after vaccination of HIV-1 infected individual. J Exp Med 1995;182:1727.

Stein DS, Korvick JA, Vermund SH: CD4+ lymphocyte cell enumeration for prediction of clinical course of human immunodeficiency virus disease: a review. J Infect Dis 1992;165:352.

Stratton P, Ciacco KH: Cervical neoplasia in the patient with HIV infection. Curr Opin Obstet Gynecol 1994;6:86.

Thomas PA, Singht T, Bornschlegel K: Use of ZDV to prevent perinatal HIV in New York City (NYC). In: Abstracts of the 4th Conference on Retroviruses and Opportunistic Infections, Washington, DC, 1997:176.

U.S. Public Health Service Task Force: Use of Antiretroviral Drugs During Pregnancy for Maternal Health and Reduction of Perinatal Transmission of Human Immunodeficiency Virus Type 1 in the United States. Los Angeles: California AIDS Clearinghouse, 1998:1.

Van Landuyt H, Mougin C, Drobacheff C, et al: [Anogenital papillomavirus lesions in humans with or without HIV infection: comparison of colposcopic, histopathological and virological results]. Ann Dermatol Venereol 1993;120:281.

Vandamme AM, Van Dooren S, Kok W, et al: Detection of HIV-1 RNA in plasma and serum samples using the NASBA amplification system compared to RNA-PCR. J Virol Methods 1995; 52:121.

Vermund SH, Kelley KF, Klein RS, et al: High risk of human papillomavirus infection and cervical squamous intraepithelial lesions among women with symptomatic human immunodeficiency virus infection. Am J Obstet Gynecol 1991;165:392.

Vernon SD, Holmes KK, Reeves WC: Human papillomavirus infection and associated disease in persons infected with human immunodeficiency virus. Clin Infect Dis 1995;21:S121.

Wasserheit J: Epidemiological synergy: interrelationships between human immunodeficiency virus infection and other sexually transmitted diseases. Sex Transm Dis 1992;19:61.

Wei X, Ghosh SK, Taylor ME, et al: Viral dynamics in human immunodeficiency virus type 1 infection. Nature 1995;373:117.

Weiss RA: HIV receptors and the pathogenesis of AIDS. Science 1996;272:1885.

Williams AB, Darragh TM, Vranizan K, et al: Anal and cervical human papillomavirus infection and risk of anal and cervical epithelial abnormalities in human immunodeficiency virus-infected women. Obstet Gynecol 1994;83:205.

Wright TC Jr, Koulos J, Schnoll F, et al: Cervical intraepithelial neoplasia in women infected with the human immunodeficiency virus—outcome after loop electrosurgical excision. Gynecol Oncol 1994;55:253.

40

Management of Common Genitourinary and Gastrointestinal Conditions

George S. Lewandowski
John J. Ward

G ynecologists frequently encounter patients with symptoms referrable to the gastrointestinal and genitourinary systems. In addition, obstetricians and gynecologists are becoming increasingly involved in the initial evaluation and ongoing management of women with nongynecologic pelvic symptoms and pathology. It follows that they should possess a working understanding of these disease processes to adequately triage patients and apply contemporary screening methods to those in their practice.

This chapter begins with the development of a rational algorithm for the initial management of genitourinary and gastrointestinal conditions. In reviewing basic pathophysiology, we hope to provide sufficient background information to allow the gynecologist to understand his or her role in therapy. Finally, we review colorectal cancer screening as a model for triage and primary disease prevention.

URINARY TRACT DISEASE

The close anatomic proximity of the urethra, the vagina, and the rectum provides an important clue to the etiology of urinary tract infections (UTIs) in women. Factors that place women at greater risk than men for the development of UTIs include a comparatively shorter urethral length and the lower genital tract manipulation that may occur with sexual intercourse or gynecologic examinations and treatments.

Importantly, hypoestrogenic states are frequently encountered throughout a woman's life (pre- and postmenopause, pregnancy and lactation). Postmenopausal estrogen replacement has been incompletely adopted by patients and physicians; systemic antiestrogens are used to treat malignancies and endometriosis. Thus one may encounter atrophy of the

lower genital and urethral tissues as a result of a relative estrogen deprivation. This can clearly augment a woman's risk for lower UTI (Samsioe et al, 1985). Over one half of all women will report at least one episode of dysuria in their lives. In one half of these, a proven bacterial infection will be demonstrated. As longevity increases, a greater number of women can be expected to suffer from urinary incontinence. Complications of incontinence as well as procedures involved with its evaluation and treatment may contribute to a higher incidence of UTI.

Fortunately, lower urinary tract disorders can generally be easily diagnosed and treated, and may resolve spontaneously. In spite of this, the proper clinical management of seemingly uncomplicated UTIs requires both the appropriate choice of an antibiotic and the control of predisposing medical conditions. Contributory behavioral or hygienic influences should be vigorously pursued. A listing of some of these factors is included in Table 40-1 (Remis et al, 1987; Strom et al, 1987). Because life-threatening diseases, including pyelonephritis and sepsis, can result from persistent or recurrent infections, a failure to successfully manage the conditions listed may have serious sequelae.

Pathophysiology, Clinical Presentation, Diagnosis

Nearly all lower UTIs result from vertical transmission of rectal or vaginal flora into the urethra or bladder (Kunin, 1987; Johnson and Stamm, 1989). Urinary stasis along with factors that compromise tissue integrity allow the entry of pathogenic organisms. Bacteria commonly encountered in such infections include strains of *Escherichia coli*, *Proteus*, *Klebsiella*, and *Enterobacter*. *Staphylococcus* and *Gardnerella* species can also be involved. (Schultz et al, 1984; Ronald

Table 40-1. MEDICAL AND PSYCHOSOCIAL FACTORS THAT MAY CONTRIBUTE TO FEMALE LOWER URINARY TRACT INFECTION

MEDICAL

Diabetes mellitus
Urinary incontinence
Neurogenic bladder
Chronic catheterization
Immunosuppression
Therapy for gynecologic or other malignancy

Pregnancy
Vaginitis
Low estrogen states
Foreign body (catheter)
Renal calculi
Urethral stenosis or diverticulum

PSYCHOSOCIAL

Inadequate perineal hygiene
Urethral trauma during intercourse
Infrequent voiding

and Conway, 1988). When extraordinary factors exist, including multiple recurrent infections or profound immune suppression, infections with the yeast *Candida* may be demonstrated.

Patients with UTI ordinarily complain of painful burning upon urination, difficulty in controlling the urinary stream, or, rarely, systemic manifestations such as malaise. Initial outpatient analysis commonly starts with a "dipstick" analysis of a clean catch, midstream voided urine specimen. Urinary evidence of white blood cells, bacteria, or elevated nitrite levels (products of bacterial degradation) supports the diagnosis of UTI. Although 10,000 colony-forming units/ml urine is used as an indicator of significant bacteriuria, a symptomatic patient or one at high risk for infection would normally be treated without regard to an absolute value. Culture and antibiotic sensitivities should be obtained prior to starting treatment.

At times, empirical antibiotic therapy may be instituted at the initial visit. It would be based upon culture information, treatment success, or antibiotic exposure from prior UTI; allergy history; and a Gram's stain of the current urinary sediment. Subsequent alterations of treatment should be based upon follow-up culture and sensitivity information as well as the clinical response. Documentation of a sterile culture 1 week following the completion of therapy can be useful in decreasing the risk of recurrence attributable to persistent subclinical bacteriuria (Stamey, 1987).

Fever, chills, costovertebral tenderness, or other manifestation of systemic disease encountered during initial evaluation or therapy suggests the presence of upper urinary tract disease. Sepsis should also be considered. Management features of complicated UTIs are included in a later section.

Therapy of Uncomplicated UTIs

A range of antibiotic choices and regimens exist for use in the treatment of apparently uncomplicated UTIs. In addition to the features listed above, factors influencing antibiotic choices include an assessment of patient compliance and the cost of therapy. Excellent success has been achieved with both the 1-day and extended regimens summarized in Table 40-2 (Ronald et al, 1976; Norrby, 1990).

Features of the antibiotic itself may influence its use for a particular patient. Amoxicillin and ampicillin are frequently chosen to treat uncomplicated UTIs. Although in vitro bacterial resistence to ampicillin can exceed 25%, the high concentration of these drugs in urine often leads to a clinical cure even in the face of unfavorable sensitivites. Allergy to the penicillin derivatives is common, as are the side effects of diarrhea and rashes.

Cephalexin is but one of many cephalosporin derivatives available for the treatment of UTI. Allergic cross-reactivity to the penicillins is reported but is rarely of significance. The cephalosporins are safe, widely used, and generally well-tolerated drugs. Although newer cephalosporins may be more effective, their increased cost is an important consideration in their first-line use.

Nitrofurantoin is used almost exclusively in the early treatment of both gram-positive and gram-negative UTIs. Although generally well tolerated and effective, some GI side effects can be encountered. Pulmonary fibrosis is an unusual side effect that has been reported following the long-term use of nitrofurantoin. Because its elimination depends upon renal metabolism, nitrofurantoin should not be

Table 40-2. THERAPEUTIC REGIMENS FOR UNCOMPLICATED FEMALE URINARY TRACT INFECTION

ANTIBIOTIC	SINGLE-DOSE ORAL REGIMEN	MULTIPLE-DAY ORAL REGIMEN
Amoxicillin; ampicillin	3 g	250 mg bid
Cephalexin (Keflex)		250–500 mg qid
Ciprofloxacin (Cipro)	750 mg	250 mg bid
Floxacin (Floxin)		200–400 mg bid
Nitrofurantoin (Macrodantin)	100 mg	50–100 mg qid
Norfloxacin (Noroxin)	800 mg	400 mg bid
Sulfisoxazole (Gantrisin)	2 g	1 g qid
Trimethoprim-sulfamethoxazole (Bactrim)	160 mg/800 mg	1 double-strength tablet bid

used in patients with markedly impaired kidney function.

The sulfonamides, including sulfisoxazole and the combination of trimethoprim-sulfamethoxazole, are popular because of general effectiveness and low cost. Skin rashes and nausea are among the more common side effects.

The alteration in genital flora that may accompany any antibiotic usage can predispose to the development of yeast vaginitis. Patients should be instructed to contact the physician with symptoms; alternatively, a prescription for an appropriate antifungal compound can be provided at the start of therapy for UTI, with instructions to institute treatment should symptoms of vaginitis develop.

Phenazopyridine (Pyridium) is an oral urinary tract analgesic that may provide symptomatic relief during the initial period of therapy. A dose of 100 mg tid for 3 to 4 days will normally suffice. The patient should be cautioned that the urine will darken, taking on an orange color.

Complicated UTIs

Although the majority of UTIs will be cleared using the strategies described above, certain clinical situations may arise that require more intensive therapy and evaluation. Included among these are persistent and recurrent lower UTIs and upper UTIs (pyelonephritis).

Treatment failure for an uncomplicated UTI can be predicted by several clinical features. At times, the prescribed antibiotic regimen will not be completed, because of either bothersome side effects or the cost of therapy. Still other patients will fail to provide a follow-up culture, improperly linking improvement of their clinical symptoms with microbiologic cure (Nicolle and Ronald, 1987). The failure to identify or modify sexual or hygienic practices that lead to bacterial contamination of the urinary tract can increase the risk for recurrent infection. Specifically, suburethral or periurethral trauma from intercourse or the use of a diaphragm may predispose to recurrent UTI. In challenging cases, pericoital antimicrobial prophylaxis has been shown to be effective in decreasing recurrent UTIs (Pfau and Sacks, 1989; Stapleton et al, 1990). The importance of identifying and correcting the conditions listed in Table 40–1 cannot be overemphasized when searching for a long-term cure.

When dealing with a patient suspected of having a recurrent or persistent UTI, neither re-treatment with the failed regimen or empirical therapy with a different antibiotic is indicated. This practice may only delay the ultimate diagnosis. A second midstream voided urine or catheterized specimen should be obtained for urinalysis and culture and sensitivities, basing new treatment upon these results. A careful physical examination should be done.

The fluoroquinolones (ciprofloxacin, norfloxacin, floxacin) have recently gained widespread use in the outpatient management of complicated UTI. *Pseudomonas* coverage is an important feature of their activity. Gastrointestinal (GI) discomforts, including nausea and diarrhea, are among the side effects commonly associated with the use of these drugs. Because of their wide spectrum and greater cost, their initial use should be restricted to either the treatment of well-documented complicated infections or the management of patients with severe systemic disease.

Purulent material expressed following transvaginal urethral palpation suggests the possibility of a urethral diverticulum—a surgically correctable entity that may be present in up to 3% of women. Both clinician and patient should be alert to symptoms that suggest the presence of more serious complications, including pyelonephritis, perinephric abscess, or sepsis.

Upper UTIs can be obvious sequelae of recurrent lower UTI. The term *pyelonephritis* refers to infection within the renal pelvis involving the kidney parenchyma. Interventions including intravenous fluid, parenteral antibiotics, or a longer course of extended-spectrum oral antibiotics may be indicated (Safrin et al, 1988). Radiographic imaging may be needed to define both the cause and extent of this condition. On occasion, a renal calculus can be demonstrated on a noncontrast abdominal film. Intravenous pyelography may be needed to demonstrate hydroureter and stasis resulting from ureteral obstruction as a cause of infection. Renal ultrasound or computerized tomography may assist in identifying a perinephric abscess in a patient whose infection does not respond to intensive antibiotic therapy. In such patients, surgical drainage may be required.

Urinary tract fistulas are unusual but possible causes of chronic UTI in women. Their management is reviewed in Chapter 48.

UTI in Pregnancy

Physicians who treat women cannot ignore the possibility of pregnancy either contributing to UTI or serving as a factor to be considered in treatment planning (Samuels, 1996). Asymptomatic bacteriuria is found in 10% of pregnant women. Physiologic dilatation of the ureters has been ascribed to systemic effects of progesterone and ureteral compression resulting from the enlarging uterus. Bacterial colonization of the lower genital tract may be implicated in both preterm labor and premature rupture of the membranes. These factors underscore the value of a urine culture obtained as part of an initial prenatal assessment.

In women of reproductive age, pregnancy should be ruled out by menstrual or contraceptive history prior to the institution of any therapy. Serum pregnancy testing may be required. If bacteriuria is demonstrated on culture in a pregnant woman, antibiotic choices should be limited to the penicillins, the cephalosporins, or nitrofurantoin. The potential maternal and fetal risk from persistent or recurrent infection coupled with the pregnancy-related risk factors for urinary stasis noted above underscore the importance of demonstrating urinary sterility following therapy. When the clinical suspicion of renal calculus or other cause of ureteral obstruction is high, renal ultrasound, plain abdominal radiographs, or limited-exposure ("one-shot") pyelography should be carefully considered.

GASTROINTESTINAL DISEASES

The gynecologist plays an important role in the assessment of patients with GI disease. Gynecology patients will often present with GI complaints; more detailed history-taking may reveal gynecologic conditions with related GI manifestations. Many gynecologists currently provide primary care services; therefore they should understand the impact that the common chronic GI diseases may have upon their patients' health. Furthermore, they should be aware of and follow colorectal cancer screening guidelines.

Although many gynecologic conditions may be accompanied by GI discomfort, most are limited in both the duration and severity of associated symptoms. Evaluation should begin with a thorough history and physical. Factors including a history of travel, treatment with antibiotics, or exposure to another patient with a GI infection should be specifically addressed. Hospitalization may be required to correct dehydration and electrolyte imbalances arising from severe nausea, vomiting, and diarrhea. Minimum measures include a stool test for occult blood; a complete blood count with differential; and a stool sample for culture, ova and parasite evaluation, and a *Clostridium difficile* toxin determination. Fever, grossly bloody stools, anemia, or other systemic manifestations of disease mandates a more comprehensive evaluation.

This section provides background information on common gastroenterologic conditions, including ulcerative colitis (UC), regional enteritis (RE; Crohn's disease), diverticulitis, and the irritable bowel syndrome (IBS). These topics are followed by a brief presentation and algorithm for colorectal cancer screening. The presenting symptoms and management of gynecologic neoplasms with GI manifestations are discussed elsewhere in the text.

Inflammatory Bowel Disease

Inflammatory bowel disease (IBD) is a term that links two processes—ulcerative colitis and regional enteritis. Both diseases share a familial and racial preponderance (white > nonwhite), lead to extraintestinal manifestations that suggest a primary immunologic etiology, and have been subjects of an unsuccessful search for an infectious etiology. Medical management of UC is comparable to that of RE. In spite of these similarities, the conditions have notable clinical differences. Specifically, the role of surgical management and the risk of developing colon cancer are significantly different in UC and RE. A brief comparison of their clinical and pathophysiologic features is presented in Table 40–3.

Diagnosis and Medical Therapy

Elucidating a history of chronic diarrhea accompanied by weight loss suggests the need for evaluation with barium enema and proctoscopy (Bartram, 1977). Colonoscopy is a useful adjunct in differentiating between UC and RE, and a brief comparison of their respective endoscopic findings has been listed in Table 40–4. The results obtained from these tests should be carefully evaluated because the long-term consequences of these conditions differ significantly.

In the absence of an acute surgical emergency, medical therapy constitutes the cornerstone of management in both UC and RE. Oral sulfasalazine (3 to

Table 40–3. COMPARISONS BETWEEN ULCERATIVE COLITIS AND REGIONAL ENTERITIS

CHARACTERISTIC	ULCERATIVE COLITIS	REGIONAL ENTERITIS
Clinical		
Rectal bleeding		
Gross	Common	Rare
Occult	Rare	Common
Diarrhea	Often subtle	May be striking based upon involved bowel segment
Pace of presentation	Commonly subtle; some acutely ill	"Low-grade small bowel obstruction" or "left-sided appendicitis"
Toxic megacolon	Up to 15% of cases	Rare
Pathophysiologic		
Pathology	Diffuse, superficial involvement	Discontinuous "skip lesions," transmural
Rectal involvement	95% of cases	<50%
Extracolonic disease	Rare	Common

Table 40–4. ENDOSCOPIC FINDINGS IN INFLAMMATORY BOWEL DISEASE

ULCERATIVE COLITIS	REGIONAL ENTERITIS
Rectum often involved	Rectum ordinarily normal
Granular, friable mucosa	Rare mucosal friability
Ulcers appear in areas of mucosal inflammation	Discontinuous ulcers in normal mucosa
Diffuse erythema	"Cobblestoning"
Loss of vascular network	

Table 40–5. EXTRAINTESTINAL MANIFESTATIONS OF INFLAMMATORY BOWEL DISEASE

CONDITION	INCIDENCE AMONG PATIENTS WITH IBD
Rheumatic	10–30%
Ankylosing spondylitis	
Rheumatoid arthritis	
Reiter's syndrome	
Hepatobiliary	5–15%
Primary sclerosing cholangitis	
Cholelithiasis	
Cirrhosis	
Hepatitis	
Ocular	5–15%
Uveitis	
Episcleritis	
Neoplastic	1–5%
Cholangiocarcinoma	
Colorectal adenocarcinoma	
Small bowel adenocarcinoma	
Thrombotic	<5%
Stroke (cerebrovascular accident)	
Deep vein thrombosis	
Pulmonary embolism	
Genitourinary	<5%
Urolithiasis	
Enterovaginal fistula	
Enterovesical fistula	
Cutaneous	<5%
Erythema nodosum	
Pyoderma gangrenosum	

4 g daily) constitutes initial therapy in patients with moderate disease. A newer derivative, 5-aminosalicylate (5-ASA), is available in colon/ileum-release oral preparations as well as transrectal forms. The effects of these salicylate drugs are attributed to the inhibition of prostaglandin synthesis. Oral prednisone (20 to 40 mg daily) or a hydrocortisone enema (100 mg per rectum at bedtime) can be used to augment this therapy in refractory cases. Clinical remission can be achieved in up to 80% of patients following 2 weeks of therapy (Williams et al, 1987). The salicylates can often be reduced to maintenance levels (2 g daily) at this time. There are instances when both forms of IBD may require treatment with other immunosuppressants, including azathioprine, 6-mercaptopurine, or cyclosporine (Present et al, 1985). Patients receiving these medications require careful monitoring for serious systemic side effects, including infection and pancreatitis, and may be at greater risk for the development of malignancy. Therapy with antibiotics such as tetracycline, metronidazole, or ciprofloxacin may be used in selected cases (Davies et al, 1977). However, the risk of developing pseudomembranous colitis and toxic megacolon as a result of bacterial overgrowth by C. difficile largely precludes their use (Gilat et al, 1987). Antidiarrheal preparations, including diphenoxylate derivatives, are useful for symptomatic relief.

The gastrointestinal dysfunction common to these diseases predisposes to comparable chronic nutritional deficiencies. Weight loss is common. Low values of serum albumin, calcium, zinc, magnesium, and phosphorus reflect longstanding poor absorption through the gastrointestinal tract. Anemia is common—a result of both chronic blood loss and poor folate absorption. As a result, dietary modification and nutritional support, as well as patient and family education, are additional important components to successful therapy.

A cluster of other systemic conditions may be variably demonstrated in patients with IBD. These include musculoskeletal, dermatologic, hepatobiliary, ocular, and renal manifestations (Rankin, 1990). Details of these conditions and their relative occurrences are shown in Table 40–5. Although systemic conditions are often encountered in RE patients with colonic involvement, they are rare when the small bowel alone is affected.

Surgery in IBD

The need for surgical interventions encountered in UC and RE are surprisingly different. A significant number (10% to 15%) of patients with severe UC present with toxic megacolon. This condition requires immediate intensive medical management while preparing for prompt surgical intervention in the event of either acute decompensation (as a result of perforation or excessive hemorrhage) or a failure to improve within 1 to 2 days. Emergent colectomy is commonly used in this condition (Smith, 1989). A two-stage approach has been described (Turnbull et al, 1971) that relies upon an initial ileostomy and colostomy, followed with the curative colectomy after clinical improvement.

Surgery may also play a nonemergent role in the care of certain patients with UC. Approximately one quarter will require a colectomy with ileostomy after having failed to respond to maximum medical management. Patients with UC are at an increased risk of developing dysplastic and neoplastic changes in the colon. In one report, the risk of developing colon cancer was 23% in patients with a 20-year history of UC and 43% in patients with 35 years of active UC (Telander, 1981). Surgery for UC can also be indicated for intractable extraintestinal disease. Joint, skin, and renal manifestations are known to be associated with GI inflammation (Table 40–5); cure of these symptoms can be achieved following removal of the colon should medical management be unsuccessful (Klein et al, 1988).

Although the cost-effectiveness of screening colonoscopy has been questioned (Gyde, 1990), pancolonoscopy with directed or random biopsies is often used to survey for clinically occult colon cancer in this high-risk group. Surgery (colectomy) would be indicated if these biopsies indicated either high-grade dysplasia or cancer. When diagnosed in patients with UC, colon cancer tends to be multifocal in growth and is distributed more evenly throughout colonic segments. These neoplasms tend to be more widespread at diagnosis, attributed in part to the symptoms shared by UC and colon cancer. Some patients may elect colectomy rather than accepting yearly colonoscopy along with the increased risk of developing malignancy.

Surgery plays a notably different role in the management of RE (Shorb, 1989). The classically pan-intestinal involvement, frequent postoperative development of dense proximal adhesions, and the noncurative nature of surgery limit the role of surgery. RE is frequently complicated by small bowel obstruction, the development of fistulas, and intra-abdominal and perirectal abscesses. Over 60% of patients with RE will require at least one surgical procedure. The success of their treatment relies upon skillful surgical judgment and operative management. RE does not appear to carry the same risk as UC for the development of colon cancer. Colectomy for prophylaxis against colon cancer is clearly not indicated in RE.

In spite of the significant morbidity associated with UC and RE, survival with these diseases approaches that of the general population. Although aggressive, as noted above, colectomy is a curative procedure in UC. Death attributable to UC would ordinarily be as a result of bleeding or infection resulting from colonic perforation. Colon cancer exists as a late complication. Individuals with RE can also expect an essentially normal survival interval. Unfortunately, the lack of a medical or surgical cure emphasizes the chronic nature of this disease and subjects the patient to complications of both the disease and its treatments. The rare death directly attributable to RE will most likely result from a septic event, perhaps related to sequelae of multiple surgeries.

IBD in Pregnancy

Because IBD occurs across the spectrum of age, pregnancy and IBD will often co-exist. Male factor infertility resulting from a low sperm count is related to the use of sulfasalazine. The effect is reversed with discontinuation of therapy and is not present with other 5-ASA preparations (Chatzinoff et al, 1988; Narendranathan et al, 1989). There appears to be no effect on female fertility with UC, but increased female infertility is reported with Crohn's disease. This may represent physicians advising against pregnancy (Lindhagen et al, 1986; Mayberry and Weterman, 1986).

The outcome of pregnancies complicated by IBD mirrors that of the general population. There is a higher risk of preterm delivery in patients whose Crohn's disease is active at the time of conception or during the pregnancy (Baird et al, 1990). Vaginal delivery with episiotomy may lead to perineal involvement with Crohn's disease (Brandt et al, 1995).

IBD is treated in pregnancy essentially as in the nonpregnant state. Sulfasalazine, a combination of 5-ASA and sulfapyradine, may be absorbed after breakdown by colonic bacteria. As a result of its interference with folate metabolism, folate supplementation should exceed that normally required in pregnancy. Although sulfasalazine carries a theoretical risk for neonatal jaundice and kernicterus, its poor absorption and low protein affinity in the nonmetabolized state make these complications unlikely (Habal et al, 1993; Boulton et al, 1994).

The classes of compounds used to treat IBD in pregnancy include steroids, 5-ASA compounds, antibiotics, and immunosuppressives. Steroids have a long history of safe use in pregnancy. As newer medications, the 5-ASA drugs have a smaller base of experience but appear to be safe in pregnancy. Each of the antibiotics mentioned above for the treatment of IBD (tetracycline, metronidazole, and ciprofloxacin) has been associated with fetal malformations; their use should be avoided. Immunosuppressives such as azathiaprine, 6-mercaptopurine, methotrexate, and cyclosporine are being used more often as therapy for IBD and may be safe in pregnancy (Alstead et al, 1990), but the uncertain potential for teratogenic effects suggests that patients taking these drugs should be counseled to stop well in advance of conception.

IBD treatment can involve surgical intervention for a variety of indications, including toxic megacolon, abscesses, fistulas, or bowel obstruction. Pregnancy does not alter the indications for surgery provided that appropriate concern is directed at fetal well-being.

Diverticulitis

In Western societies, diverticular disease ranks among the more common chronic GI conditions, being demonstrated in nearly half of the population by age 80. Mucosa and submucosa pass through the circular muscle of the colon, normally at the site of penetration of a colonic arteriole, forming sac-like herniations called diverticula. The prime postulated risk factor for their development includes the adoption of a diet low in fiber, subsequently requiring a chronically increased intraluminal pressure to promote rectal evacuation. Chronic therapy is directed at relieving symptoms and includes increasing fecal bulk, thus promoting ease of evacuation.

Inflammation deep within the diverticulum may promote necrosis and perforation, leading to lower abdominal pain with or without a pelvic mass, fever, and GI bleeding. A gynecologist caring for a patient with these symptoms should include diverticulitis in the differential diagnosis and understand basic principles of its treatment. The presence of either rectovaginal or rectocystic fistulas in women who have undergone hysterectomy for benign indications should alert the clinician to the possibility of diverticulitis.

The initial therapeutic approach involves medical management, including parenteral antibiotics and bowel rest. Antimicrobial coverage is sought against *E. coli*, enterococci and anaerobes. Mild infection could conceivably be managed using ampicillin alone (500 mg every 6 hours). Broader coverage would include the addition of an aminoglycoside and clindamycin (900 mg every 8 hours) or metronidazole (500 mg every 8 to 12 hours). Alternate single-agent regimens would include cefoxitin (2 g every 6 to 8 hours) or imipenim/cilastatin (500 mg every 6 to 12 hours). Bowel rest should be achieved by dietary restriction, reserving the use of a nasogastric tube for severe nausea or vomiting. Resolution of symptoms allows for the gradual advancement of diet, focusing upon a high-residue input.

Surgery for diverticular disease should be reserved for the following indications: large bowel obstruction or perforation, hemorrhage, abscess and/or peritonitis, or the failure of medical management. Chronic diverticular disease may manifest as a colonic fistula. A skilled gynecologic surgeon can be an asset in the approach to these complex pelvic operations. Since the risk factors for diverticulosis parallel those for colon cancer, it is necessary to rule this out during the initial evaluation, or certainly after clinical stabilization has been achieved. Both endoscopy and barium enema are acceptable means to evaluate the lower GI tract. Colonoscopy offers the advantage of instantaneous biopsy evaluation of suspicious lesions.

Irritable Bowel Syndrome

IBS is an entity estimated to affect at least 10% of the general population. In Western societies, women are more than twice as likely as men to be diagnosed with IBS. In other societies, males predominate. Although the disease afflicts persons throughout life, it is most frequently diagnosed between the ages of 16 and 30. Many individuals with symptoms consistent with IBS do not seek medical attention (Drossman and Thompson, 1992).

In 1990, consistent diagnostic criteria for the diagnosis of IBS were developed by an international commission (Drossman et al, 1990). Guidelines that specified a 3-month history of either continuous or recurrent symptoms were adopted. Symptom complexes include pain relieved with defecation or pain associated with a change in frequency or consistency of stool or an irregular pattern of fecal evacuation occurring 25% of the time. This latter concept was further defined by the presence of three of the following: altered stool form or frequency; altered stool passage, including incomplete evacuation, urgency, or straining; passage of mucus per rectum; or bloating or abdominal distention. Symptoms of IBS mimic those of lactose intolerance but occur without lactose ingestion.

The pathophysiologic manifestations of IBS include altered small bowel motility and colonic motor hyperactivity associated with stress, hormonal infusion, and emotional arousal. The sigmoid muscular hypertrophy seen with diverticulosis is not seen in IBS. The etiology of the disease is unknown, although exacerbations and remissions with menstrual cycling suggest a role for hormonal influence (Camilleri and Prather, 1992).

IBS is a diagnosis of exclusion. Physical exam is usually normal but up to 75% of patients manifest excessive pain over the colon or during sigmoidoscopy. The basic evaluation would include a complete blood count and sedimentation rate. When diarrhea is a strong component of disease, testing for enteric pathogens should be obtained. Flexible sigmoidoscopy might play a role if IBD is suspected. Likewise, a colonoscopy or perhaps a barium enema should be considered if age or family history makes colon cancer is a strong consideration.

There is a significant psychosocial component to IBS. Up to 50% of patients may meet criteria for a psychiatric diagnosis—mostly depression. Cancer phobia, somatization, and the potential to overuse medical resources are not uncommon (Owens et al, 1995).

Management of IBS requires a multifactorial approach (Drossman and Thompson, 1992). Dietary interventions include increasing dietary fiber and decreasing fat. Avoidance of known precipitating situations may eliminate the stimulus for increased GI activity. Other symptomatic management would be based upon the dominant symptomatic complaint. Constipation might be improved with the use of bulk-forming agents, osmotic laxatives, and stool softeners. Cisapride 20 mg twice daily may be a useful prokinetic agent. If diarrhea is the major symptom of suspected IBS and other causes of diarrhea have been ruled out, anticholinergic antispasmodics (Dicyclomine 10 to 20 mg qid, Hyocyamine 0.125 mg every 4 hours, or Hyocyamine long-acting 0.375 mg every 12 hours) would ordinarily represent the initial therapeutic approach. Loperamide (Imodium) 2 to 4 mg every 6 to 8 hours or diphenoxylate 2.5 to 5 mg every 4 to 6 hours may be beneficial but is not preferred because dependence might result. If pain, flatulence, or bloating constitute the major symptomatology, anticholinergics and antidepressants should be considered. A prokinetic agent could also be added. The gonadotropin-releasing hormone agonist leuprolide acetate may have some effect at control-

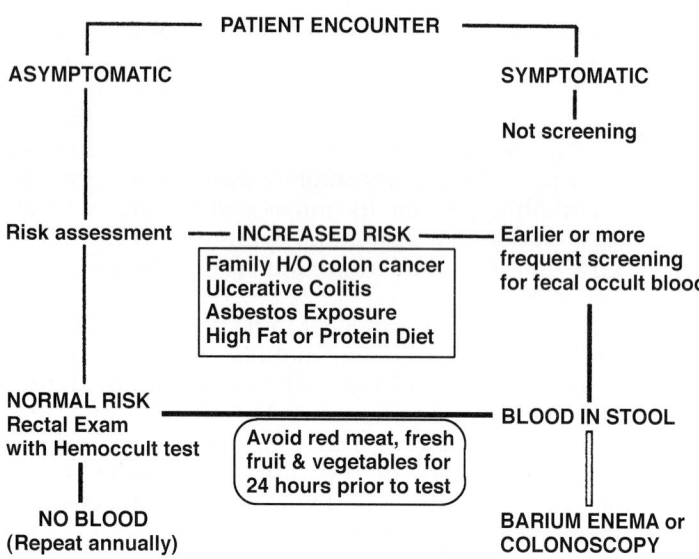

Figure 40–1
Screening algorithm for colorectal cancer. (Adapted from Mettlin C, Jones G, Averette H, et al: Defining and updating the American Cancer Society guidelines for the cancer related checkup. CA Cancer J Clin 1993;43:42, with permission.)

ling symptoms that are exacerbated by menses (Mathias et al, 1989).

Patients with IBS will require reassurance that, although their disease carries distressing symptoms, it does not represent a threat to life. It can be managed with a focus upon lessening symptoms, establishing a diet that minimizes their individual GI problems, and adopting a lifestyle that shields them from psychoemotional stimulants of IBS.

Colorectal Cancer Screening

The American Cancer Society estimated that 65,900 cases of colorectal cancer would be diagnosed in 1996 *in women*. It was also estimated that 27,500 women would die from colorectal cancer in 1996— a figure that surpasses that for all primary gynecologic malignancies *COMBINED* (Parker et al, 1996). The National Cancer Data Base has indicated that patients over age 80 are presenting with earlier stage disease. (Jessup et al, 1996). The "aging" of the U.S. population, along with the increasing involvement of gynecologists as primary care providers for women, support the inclusion of colorectal cancer screening in this chapter.

Colon cancer is found more frequently in patients with a family history of the disease, those who consume a diet high in fat and protein, persons with UC, and those exposed to asbestos. Patients with earlier stage disease at diagnosis have an improved survival and often achieve this with less morbid treatment (Fleisher et al, 1989). Much research has been directed at developing and evaluating colorectal screening modalities; details of this process lie beyond the scope of this chapter. Figure 40–1 demonstrates a proposed risk assessment–based screening algorithm that could be easily incorporated into a gynecologic practice (Mettlin et al, 1993).

SUMMARY

Gynecologists will frequently encounter patients whose symptoms may be referred to the genitourinary and GI systems. Better triage will optimize patient care. Thus an awareness of symptoms, cost-effective evaluation, and pathophysiology will allow the gynecologist to develop greater comfort in caring for women with these conditions. Cancer screening remains the responsibility of all physicians, so gynecologists should not only be aware of pertinent guidelines, but should apply them to the women for whom they care.

REFERENCES

Alstead EM, Ritchie JK, Lennard-Jones JE, et al: Safety of azathioprine in pregnancy in inflammatory bowel disease. Gastroenterology 1990;99:433.

Baird DD, Narendranathan M, Sandler RS: Increased risk of preterm birth for women with inflammatory bowel disease. Gastroenterology 1990;99:987.

Bartram C: Radiology in the current assessment of ulcerative colitis. Gastrointest Radiol 1977;1:383.

Boulton R, Hamilton M, Lewis A, et al: Fulminant ulcerative colitis in pregnancy. Am J Gastroenterol 1994;89:931.

Brandt LJ, Estabrook SG, Reinus JF: Results of a survey to evaluate whether vaginal delivery and episiotomy lead to perineal involvement in women with Crohn's disease. Am J Gastroenterol 1995;90:1918.

Camilleri M, Prather CM: The irritable bowel syndrome: mechanisms and a practical approach to management. Ann Intern Med 1992;116:1001.

Chatzinoff M, Guarino JM, Corson SL, et al: Sulfasalazine-induced abnormal sperm penetration assay reversed on changing to 5-aminosalicylic acid enemas. Dig Dis Sci 1988;33:108.

Davies PS, Rhodes J, Heatley RV, et al: Metronidazole in the treatment of chronic proctitis: a controlled trial. Gut 1977;18:680.

Drossman DA, McKee DC, Sandler RS, et al: Psychosocial factors in the irritable bowel syndrome: a multivariate study of patients and nonpatients with irritable bowel syndrome. Gastroenterology 1988;95:701.

Drossman DA, Thompson WG: The irritable bowel syndrome: review and graduated multicomponent treatment approach. Ann Intern Med 1992;116:1009.

Drossman DA, Thompson WG, Talley NJ, et al: Identification of subgroups of functional gastrointestinal disorders. Gastroenterol Int 1990;4:159.

Fleischer DE, Goldberg SB, Browning TH, et al: Detection and surveillance of colorectal cancer. JAMA 1989;261:580.

Gilat T, Suissa A, Leichtman G, et al: A comparative study of metronidazole and sulfadiazine in active, not severe, ulcerative colitis. J Clin Gastroenterol 1987;9:415.

Guthrie E, Creed F, Dawson D, et al: A controlled study of psychological treatment for irritable bowel syndrome. Gastroenterology 1991;100:450.

Gyde S: Screening for colorectal cancer in ulcerative colitis: dubious benefits and high costs. Gut 1990;31:1089.

Habal FM, Hui G, Greenberg GR: Oral 5-aminosalicylic acid for inflammatory bowel disease in pregnancy: safety and clinical course. Gastroenterology 1993;105:1057.

Jessup JM, McGinnis LS, Winchester DP, et al: Clinical highlights from the National Cancer Data Base: 1996. CA Cancer J Clin 1996;46:185.

Johnson JR, Stamm WE: Urinary tract infections in women: diagnosis and treatment. Ann Intern Med 1989;111:906.

Klein S, Mayer L, Present DH, et al: Extraintestinal manifestations in patients with diverticulitis. Ann Intern Med 1988;108:700.

Kunin CM: The concepts of significant bacteriuria. In: Detection, Prevention and Management of Urinary Tract Infections. 2nd ed. Philadelphia: Lea & Feibiger, 1987:82.

Lindhagen T, Bohe M, Ekelund G, Lalentin L: Fertility and outcome of pregnancy in patients operated on for Crohn's disease. Int J Colorectal Dis 1986;1:25.

Mathias JR, Ferguson KL, Clench MH: Debilitating "functional" bowel disease controlled by leuprolide acetate, gonadotropin releasing hormone (GnRH) analog. Dig Dis Sci 1989;34:761.

Mayberry JF, Weterman IT: European survey of fertility and pregnancy in women with Crohn's disease: a case-control study by the European collaborative group. Gut 1986;27:821.

Mettlin C, Jones G, Averette H, et al: Defining and updating the American Cancer Society guidelines for the cancer related checkup. CA Cancer J Clin 1993;43:42.

Nanda R, James R, Smith H, et al: Food intolerance and the irritable bowel syndrome. Gut 1989;30:1099.

Narendranathan M, Sandler RS, Suchindran CM, Savitz DA: Male infertility in inflammatory bowel disease. J Clin Gastroenterol 1989;11:403.

Neff DF, Blanchard EB: A multicomponent treatment for irritable bowel syndrome. Behav Ther 1987;18:70.

Nicolle LE, Ronald AR: Recurrent urinary tract infection in adult women: diagnosis and treatment. Infect Dis Clin North Am 1987;1:793.

Norrby SR: Short term treatment of uncomplicated urinary tract infections in women. Rev Infect Dis 1990;12:458.

Owens D, Nelson DK, Talley NJ: The irritable bowel syndrome:

long-term prognosis and the physician-patient interaction. Ann Intern Med 1995;122:107.

Parker SL, Tong T, Bolden S, et al: Cancer statistics. CA Cancer J Clin 1996;65:5.

Pfau A, Sacks TG: Effective prophylaxis of recurrent urinary tract infections in premenopausal women by postcoital administration of cephalexin. J Urol 1989;142:1276.

Present DH, Meltzer SJ, Wolke A, et al: Short and long term toxicity of 6-mercaptopurine in the management of inflammatory bowel disease. Gastroenterology 1985;88:1545.

Rankin GB: Extraintestinal and systemic manifestations of inflammatory bowel disease. Med Clin North Am 1990;74:39.

Remis RS, Gurwith MJ, Gurwith D, et al: Risk factors for urinary tract infection. Am J Epidemiol 1987;126:685.

Ronald AR, Boutros P, Mourtada H: Bacteriuria localization and response to single-dose therapy in women. JAMA 1976;235:1854.

Ronald AR, Conway B: An approach to urinary tract infections in ambulatory women. Curr Clin Top Infect Dis 1988;9:76.

Safrin S, Siegel D, Black D: Pyelonephritis in adult women: inpatient versus outpatient therapy. Am J Med 1988;85:793.

Samsioe G, Jansson I, Mellstrom D, Svanborg A: Occurrence, nature and treatment of urinary incontinence in a 70-year-old female population. Maturitas 1985;7:335.

Samuels P: Renal disease. In: Gabbe SG, Niebyl JR, Simpson JL (eds): Obstetrics: Normal and Problem Pregnancies. 3rd ed. New York: Churchill Livingstone, 1996:1025.

Schultz HJ, McCaffrey LA, Keys TF, et al: Acute cystitis: a prospective study of laboratory tests and duration of therapy. Mayo Clin Proc 1984;59:391.

Shorb PE Jr.: Surgical therapy for Crohn's disease. Gastroenterol Clin North Am 1989;18:111.

Smith LE: Surgical therapy in ulcerative colitis. Gastroenterol Clin North Am 1989;18:99.

Stamey TA: Recurrent urinary tract infections in female patients: an overview of management and treatment. Rev Infect Dis 1987;9(Suppl 2):S195.

Stapleton A, Latham RH, Johnson C, et al: Post-coital antimicrobial prophylaxis for recurrent urinary tract infection. JAMA 1990;264:703.

Strom BL, Collins M, West SL, et al: Sexual activity, contraceptive use and other risk factors for symptomatic and asymptomatic bacteriuria: a case-control study. Ann Intern Med 1987;107:816.

Telander RL: Surgical management of young persons with inflammatory bowel disease. Comp Ther 1981;7(5):40.

Turnbull RB Jr, Hawk WA, Wearley FL: Surgical treatment of toxic megacolon: ileostomy and colostomy to prepare patients for colectomy. Am J Surg 1971;122:325.

Williams CN, Haber G, Aquino JA: Double-blind, placebo-controlled evaluation of 5-ASA suppositories in active distal proctitis and measurement of extent using 99m-Tc-labeled 5-ASA suppositories. Dig Dis Sci 1987;32(Suppl):71S.

V

Gynecological Surgery

41

Preoperative Evaluation and Preparation for Gynecologic Surgery

Daniel L. Clarke-Pearson
George Olt
Gustavo Rodriguez
Matthew P. Boente

Successful gynecologic surgery is based on thorough evaluation and preoperative preparation of the patient and careful postoperative management. This chapter discusses approaches to the general perioperative management of patients undergoing major gynecologic surgery and specific medical problems that could complicate the surgical outcome.

MEDICAL HISTORY AND PHYSICAL EXAMINATION

Surgery that is undertaken without a thorough understanding of a patient's medical history and a complete physical examination may result in the development of otherwise preventable complications. The historical information to be obtained includes any significant medical history or medical illnesses that might be aggravated by or that might complicate anesthesia or surgical recovery. Inquiry should be made as to current medications being taken, even those discontinued within the previous months before surgery. Specific inquiries should be directed at the possibility of nonprescription drugs being taken and the use of oral contraceptives, because many patients consider these to be a routine part of their living rather than a medication. The importance of recognizing such medications is emphasized by the fact that aspirin may lead to intraoperative or postoperative bleeding. Discontinuation of aspirin several weeks prior to elective surgery is advised to avoid platelet dysfunction. Likewise, oral contraceptives should be discontinued 6 weeks before elective surgery to reduce the risk of postoperative venous thrombosis. Specific instructions must be given to the patient regarding the need to discontinue any other prescription medications before surgery as well as the recognition of those medications that should be continued (such as cardiac or antihypertensive medications). The patient should be questioned as to known allergies to medications (most commonly sulfa and penicillin) as well as other allergies to foods or environmental allergens. Because iodinated IV contrast material is used for intravenous pyelography (IVP), enhanced computerized tomography (CT) scanning, and venography or arteriography, the patient should be questioned as to her tolerance of other iodinated substances. A history of sensitivity to shellfish may be the only clue to an iodine sensitivity. A history of hypersensitivity to previous intravenously administered iodine-containing compounds should be clearly noted, and the patient should not undergo further exposure to iodine-containing compounds unless absolutely mandatory. When IV contrast must be used, corticosteroid preparation should be instituted to prevent life-threatening anaphylactic reactions.

A social history should include use of tobacco, alcohol, and illicit drugs. Smokers should be encouraged to stop smoking 6 weeks preoperatively. In these situations, nicotine patches may help the nicotine-dependent patient have improved pulmonary function. Alcohol abuse may be reflected as nutritional deficiency or bleeding disorders, which should lead to further preoperative assessment. Patients who have unusual dietary habits may also be nutritionally deficient, and further evaluation may identify those who would benefit from preoperative nutritional support. The social history should also identify the patients' support system of family, spouse, significant others, and friends who will assist in the patient's recovery from surgery.

Specific studies such as liver function tests, nutritional parameters, arterial blood gases, or pulmonary function tests should be obtained only when there is a significant history or specific risks are anticipated.

Previous surgical procedures, including such minor procedures as dilatation and curettage (D&C) or tonsillectomy, should be reviewed, including the patient's course following those surgical procedures, to identify potential complications of previous operations that might be avoided. Reaction and response to anesthetic techniques should be evaluated with

917

the anesthesiologist in charge. Inquiries should be made as to other complications, including excessive bleeding, wound infection, deep vein thrombosis (DVT), peritonitis, and bowel obstruction. Previous pelvic surgery should alert the gynecologist to the possibility of distorted surgical anatomy and possible pre-existing injury to adjacent organ systems, such as small bowel adhesions in the pelvis or ureteral stenosis from previous periureteral scarring. An IVP should be considered in such cases to establish bilateral patency of the ureters or to identify any pre-existing abnormality. Operative notes from previous pelvic operations should be obtained and reviewed to precisely determine the prior surgical procedure and surgical findings. Many times, a patient may not be entirely clear as to the extent of the procedure or the details of intraoperative findings. This is particularly important in patients who have had surgery for pelvic inflammatory disease, pelvic abscess, endometriosis, or pelvic malignancy.

Family history should be reviewed to minimize the possibility of familial traits that might complicate planned surgery. History of excessive intraoperative or postoperative bleeding, malignant hyperthermia, and other potentially inherited conditions should be sought. General review of systems should also be included in the questioning, searching for any coexisting gastrointestinal and urologic function is particularly important before undertaking pelvic surgery, and many gynecologic diseases also involve adjacent nongynecologic viscera.

A thorough physical examination must be performed preoperatively. Although many women undergoing gynecologic surgical procedures are otherwise healthy, with only pathologic factors identified on pelvic examination, other major organ systems must not be neglected in the physical examination. Identification of abnormalities such as heart murmur or pulmonary compromise should lead the surgeon to obtain additional testing and consultation to minimize intraoperative and postoperative complications.

LABORATORY EVALUATION

Preoperative laboratory studies to be obtained will depend upon the extent of the anticipated surgical procedure and the patient's general health evaluation. As a minimum for patients undergoing general anesthesia, a blood count including hematocrit, white count, and platelet count should be obtained. Serum chemistry analyses and liver function testing are rarely abnormal in the asymptomatic patient who has no significant medical history and who is not taking medications. Likewise, coagulation studies are of little value unless the patient has a significant medical history (Myers et al, 1994). In women younger than age 40, a chest film and electrocardiogram (ECG) are likewise of very low yield in identifying asymptomatic cardiopulmonary disease and

may not be necessary (Loder, 1987; Lamers et al, 1989). Conversely, women older than age 40 who are undergoing major gynecologic surgical procedures should have a chest film and ECG taken and their serum electrolytes evaluated preoperatively. Even if these studies are normal, they will serve as baseline data for comparison to other studies, that might be required in the evaluation of a postoperative complication. Specific studies such as liver function tests, nutritional parameters, arterial blood gases, or pulmonary function tests should be obtained only when there is a significant history or specific risks are anticipated. Further evaluation of adjacent organ systems should be undertaken in individual cases. For example, an IVP is helpful to delineate ureteral patency and course, especially in such cases as a pelvic mass, gynecologic cancer, or congenital müllerian anomaly. However, an IVP is not required for most patients undergoing pelvic surgery (Piscitelli et al, 1987).

A barium enema or upper gastrointestinal tract series with small bowel follow-through may be of significant value in evaluating some patients before undergoing pelvic surgery. Because of the proximity of the female genital tract to the lower gastrointestinal tract, the rectum and sigmoid colon may be involved with benign (endometriosis or pelvic inflammatory disease) or malignant gynecologic conditions. Conversely, a pelvic mass could be of gastrointestinal origin, such as a diverticular abscess or a mass of inflamed small intestines (Crohn's disease). Clearly, any patient with gastrointestinal symptoms should be further evaluated with contrast radiographs as well as a proctosigmoidoscopy, flexible sigmoidoscopy, or colonoscopy. Other imaging studies, including ultrasonograms, CT scan, or magnetic resonance imaging, are useful only in selected patients and are not considered helpful as part of the preoperative work-up of most patients.

PREOPERATIVE DISCUSSION AND INFORMED CONSENT

The rapport and trust that exist between the patient and her gynecologic surgeon begin on the initial office visit and should be built upon at each subsequent interchange. When surgery is deemed advisable, initial discussion should explain in sufficient detail to the patient the findings on examination and the results of testing, the natural history of the disease process, and the goals of the surgical procedure. This discussion should be performed in an unhurried manner and be of sufficient detail so that the patient may decide whether to go ahead with preoperative preparation. Because most gynecologic surgery is elective, the gynecologist has the opportunity to thoroughly evaluate the patient from a medical point of view, to allow the patient to develop psychological coping mechanisms, and to answer questions that may not have been initially discussed. The surgeon should make himself or herself available to discuss these questions in person or by telephone before actual hospital admission.

A few days before the anticipated surgery, another preoperative discussion should be held with the patient and key family members. These may include the spouse or other significant support person of an adult woman or the parents of a minor. Privacy should be ensured to allow thorough and frank discussion, particularly when delicate questions regarding sexuality and sexual function may be raised. Discussions in hallways or office waiting rooms are to be condemned.

The goals of this preoperative discussion should serve to allay anxiety and fears that the patient may have and to answer any questions that may have arisen in the preoperative period. The discussion should serve to further expand on many issues relative to the surgery, its expected outcome, and risks, and is the basis for obtaining the signed informed consent (Easley and Hammond, 1986). This is an educational process for the patient and her family, and explanations need to be made in understandable terms by the physician. The topics listed in Table 41–1 should be discussed, after each of which the patient and family should be invited to ask questions.

A discussion of the nature and the extent of the disease process should explain in lay terms the significance of the disease process. Is it life-threatening, or will it likely result in significant disability or dysfunction? To what extent does the disease process alter the patient's daily living? If left untreated, could the disease spontaneously resolve, or could it potentially worsen? What is the time course and natural history of the disease?

The goals of the surgery should be discussed in detail. Some gynecologic surgical procedures are performed purely for diagnostic purposes (e.g., D&C, cold knife conization, diagnostic laparoscopy, staging laparotomy), whereas most are clearly aimed at correcting an anatomic defect or a specific disease process. The extent of the surgery should be outlined, including notation of which organs will be removed. Most patients like to be informed as to the type of surgical incision and the estimated duration of anesthesia.

The expected outcome of the surgical procedure should be explained. If the procedure is being per-

formed for diagnostic purposes, the outcome will depend upon surgical or pathologic findings that are not known before surgery. When treating anatomic deformity or disease, the expected success of the operation should be discussed as well as the potential for failure. This should include a discussion of the probability of failure of tubal sterilization or the possibility that stress urinary incontinence may not be alleviated. When treating cancer, the possibility of finding more advanced disease and the potential need for adjunctive therapy (such as postoperative radiation therapy or chemotherapy) should be mentioned. Other issues of importance to the patient include discussion of loss of fertility or loss of ovarian function. These issues should be raised by the physician to make sure the patient adequately understands the pathophysiology factors that may result from the surgery and also to allow her to express her feelings regarding these emotionally charged matters.

The risks and potential complications of the surgical procedure should be discussed with the patient, including the most frequent complications of the particular surgical procedure. For most major gynecologic surgery, the risks include intraoperative and postoperative hemorrhage, postoperative infection, venous thrombosis, and injury to adjacent viscera. Because of the risks associated with blood transfusion, the patient should be clearly informed that she has the option (in elective cases) to secure autologous or donor-directed packed cells for potential transfusion. Although there is no evidence that this is cost-effective, the patient nonetheless should be given this information as part of the informed consent process.

Unanticipated findings at the time of surgery should also be mentioned. For example, if the ovaries are unexpectedly found to be diseased, it may be the best surgical judgment that they should be removed. A discussion of these unanticipated findings and the judgments that the surgeon must make intraoperatively will alleviate many instances of surprises following surgery and unhappiness on the part of the patient or her family.

The usual postoperative course should also be discussed in enough detail so that the patient understands what to expect in the days following surgery. The information as to the need for a suprapubic catheter or prolonged central venous monitoring helps the patient accept her postoperative course and avoids surprises that may be very disconcerting. The expected duration of the recovery period, both in and outside of the hospital, should be noted.

Alternative methods of therapy are also to be mentioned as part of the preoperative discussion. Other medical management or other surgical approaches should be discussed along with their potential benefits and complications. Finally, the patient should have an understanding as to the outcome of the disease should nothing be done. It should be clear to the patient following this discussion why the pro-

---

☐ **Table 41–1.** KEY ELEMENTS OF THE PREOPERATIVE DISCUSSION

1. The nature and extent of the disease process.
2. The extent of the actual operation proposed and potential modifications of this operation, depending on unexpected intraoperative findings.
3. The anticipated benefits of the operation, with a conservative estimate of successful outcome.
4. The risks and potential complications of the surgery.
5. Alternative methods of therapy, their risks, and results.
6. The likely results if the patient remains untreated.

posed surgery is the appropriate next step in her care. Witnesses to the preoperative discussion and signing of the consent form should include a family member and another member of the health care team. We believe that the preoperative informed consent discussion should be performed by the responsible surgeon and not delegated to nursing staff or house staff, who may not have full understanding of the patient's disease process, or the rapport with the patient or responsibility for her ultimate care. The informed consent discussion detailing the information given the patient should be documented in the patient's chart.

The anesthesiologist responsible for the surgical procedure should also have the opportunity to examine the patient, review her laboratory findings, and discuss the proposed anesthetic method with the patient. In many institutions, the consent to the administration of anesthetic is included in the surgical consent form, whereas in others it is a separate form that should be provided by the anesthesiologist after preoperative discussion.

GENERAL CONSIDERATIONS

Nutrition

Nutritional Status Assessment

Women having gynecologic surgery should be in an adequate nutritional state, and an accurate assessment of each patient's nutritional status should be made preoperatively. The significance of weight loss and its negative effect on surgical outcome has been recognized for decades. More recently, the Eastern Cooperative Oncology Group has reported significantly shorter median survivals in weight-losing cancer patients receiving treatment for cancer than in similar patients without histories of weight loss (DeWys et al, 1980). Clinical experience indicates that, if nutritional deficits are corrected before surgery, a quicker recovery, fewer postoperative infections, and more rapid wound healing can occur (Vogel et al, 1972; Blackburn and Bistrian, 1976). The goal preoperatively is to quantify the malnutrition and to provide appropriate preoperative nutritional supplementation.

Energy utilization varies dramatically with the fasting-feeding cycle and is influenced by every organ system as well as hypermetabolic states such as sepsis, burns, surgery, gastrointestinal disorders, and malignancy. To approximate the caloric needs, the patient's height, weight, sex, age, activity level, type of surgery required, and disease state must be taken into consideration (Table 41–2). Chronic illness such as renal, endocrine, and cardiovascular abnormalities may alter nutritional needs (Abel, 1983). Gastrointestinal problems, including short bowel syndrome, obstruction, fistula, emesis, gastric suctioning, and diarrhea (Kinney et al, 1968; Aguirre et al, 1974), and cancer-related problems, including chemotherapy,

radiation enteritis, and extensive surgery (Copeland et al, 1975; Bandy et al, 1987; Soper et al, 1989), also account for increased nutritional requirements.

Nutritional assessment of the preoperative patient is essential. The most important measurement is body weight. When recorded serially as a percentage of the ideal body weight, it is the single most influential reflection of energy and protein reserve; however, extracellular fluid or fluid overload may give a false impression that nutritional stores are unaffected.

Anthropometry is the study of the measurement of size, weight, and proportions of the human body. Tricep skinfold thickness can be used to derive a midarm fat area, which is the simplest index to measure body fat stores (Butterworth and Blackburn, 1974).

The creatinine-height index is the most sensitive indicator of protein-calorie nutrition (Nixon et al, 1980). The body's total protein reserve is estimated clinically by calculating the approximate muscle mass and visceral protein reserve. Muscle mass can be estimated from a 24-hour urine collection from which a creatinine-height index may be calculated. Visceral protein reserve is estimated by serum albumin and transferrin levels (Butterworth and Blackburn, 1974). In general, hypoalbuminemia (≤ 2.5 mg/dl) coupled with weight loss ($\geq 10\%$) is associated with excessive surgical morbidity and mortality (Baker et al, 1982; Bandy et al, 1987).

Supplemental Nutrition

Many women will require additional nutritional support in the perioperative period. The route of administration chosen to deliver the nutritional support must be decided on an individual basis. The enteral route should be considered first because it is the simplest and most economical. Contraindications include intestinal obstruction and upper gastrointestinal bleeding. Diarrhea is a relative contraindication but can almost always be managed medically. A variety of types of enteral feeding solutions exist that vary in caloric content, osmolality, fat content, protein content, lactose content, viscosity, and price. Depending on the nature of the problem, delivery may be through a nasogastric, gastrostomy, or jejunostomy tube. Vomiting and diarrhea may be alleviated by slowing the rate of the infusion, although, for the enteral route to be effective, the patient must be able to tolerate a volume of solution sufficient to deliver an adequate number of calories. Complications of enteral feeding include obstruction, aspiration, pharynx and esophageal erosions, vomiting, diarrhea, and electrolyte disturbances. Interestingly, Daley and coworkers (1992) have demonstrated significant improvements in infections and wound complications and a shorter length of hospital stay in a randomized study comparing postoperative enteral feedings supplemented with argenine, RNA, and ω-3-fatty acids as compared with a standard enteral formula.

☐ **Table 41–2.** CALORIC NEEDS IN GYNECOLOGIC SURGERY

Total Daily Calorie Requirements

Basal energy expenditure (E_b) + energy for physical activity (E_{pa}) + energy of injury of surgery (E_{surg})

1. E_b (kcal/day)
   Men = $66 + (13.7 \times W) + (5.0 \times H) - (6.8 \times A)$*
   Women = $655 + (9.6 \times W) + (1.7 \times H) - (4.7 \times A)$
   Simplified: $E_b = 22 \times W$

2. E_{pa} (kcal/kg/hr)

Activity level	Men	Women
Very light	1.5	1.3
Light	2.9	2.6
Moderate	4.3	4.1
Heavy	8.4	8.0

3. E_{surg}

	(kcal/day)
Minor surgery (e.g., appendectomy)	50–75
Cholecystectomy	100
Partial gastrectomy	150
Severe trauma	200–500
Trauma with sepsis	500–1000
Burns	% burn × 40
Fever	E_b × 0.07 × degrees of fever above 98.6°F

Net Dietary Intake = caloric intake (CI) − caloric loss (CL)

1. CI = (1) enteral
       (2) parenteral

2. CL = (1) urinary† = 100 kcal/day
       (2) fecal† = 75 kcal/day
       (3) SDA‡ = 0.6 × total kcal intake/day

Adequacy of Energy Intake

Maintenance: CI = CL
Depletion: CI < CL
Repletion: CI > CL

*W, weight (kilograms); H, height (centimeters); A, age (years).
†Values assume normal fecal and urinary losses. Values will be correspondingly higher in uncontrolled diabetes (urinary loss) or malabsorption (fecal loss). When patients are receiving parenteral feedings, stool caloric losses will be reduced.
‡SDA, specific dynamic action.
Adapted from Lubin MF, Walker HK, Smith RB: Medical Management of the Surgical Patient. 2nd ed. Reading, MA: Butterworth, 1989:9–10, with permission.

Peripheral parenteral nutrition can be delivered to supplement enteral feedings or may be given alone as a nutritional supplement. A 900-mOsm/L solution can be delivered through peripheral veins. Phlebitis, one common side effect, may be overcome by the addition of 5 mg of hydrocortisone to each liter of solution. Additional calories may be provided by peripheral intralipids. Monitoring of both parenteral nutrition and enteral alimentation by measurement of electrolytes, glucose, and transaminase should be performed approximately every 2 to 3 days for the first week and weekly thereafter to ensure normality. If the combined route of nutritional support is insufficient or intolerable, central venous nutrition should be initiated.

Total parenteral nutrition (TPN) has gained wide acceptance as a means of providing nutritional support for a variety of medical and surgical problems. The gynecologic literature has focused attention on central hyperalimentation in the setting of advanced gynecologic malignancies or in patients receiving chemotherapy. TPN is given when other routes have not or cannot meet the patient's nutritional needs. TPN must be delivered through the subclavian or internal jugular vein. Placement of this line must be performed under meticulous sterile technique, and proper daily care must be given to avoid infection. Two to 3 L/day of TPN solution will usually maintain homeostasis. Trace metals (copper, iodine, magnesium, zinc) and multivitamins are added to 1 liter each day. Folate and vitamin B_{12} must be added separately because they are incompatible with the trace metals. Essential fatty acids are supplied weekly, and iron must be given if the hyperalimentation is prolonged and bone marrow stores become depleted. In patients with cardiac, liver, or renal dysfunction, special care must be taken to adjust the sodium, potassium, and amino acid concentration to meet the patient's needs. Complications associated with TPN range from metabolic or electrolyte abnormalities to sepsis, pneumo/hemothorax, or air/catheter embolism. In experienced hands, the most frequent serious problem, catheter infection, has been reduced to around 7% (Heymsfield et al, 1980).

TPN in the preoperative setting has been reviewed by many authors, but its role remains controversial because of its risk, the cost, and the difficulty in selecting patients who might benefit from it. A predictive model of nutritional status, designed and validated by Mullen and associates (1979), exists to identify patients at risk for operative morbidity or mortality. The prognostic nutritional index (PNI) is calculated using the formula:

$$PNI = 158 - 16.6 \, [Alb] - 0.78 \, [TSF]$$
$$- 0.2 \, [TFN] - 5.8 \, [DH]$$

where ALB is serum albumin (milligrams per milliliter), TSF is triceps skinfold thickness (centimeters), TFN is serum transferrin (milligrams per milliliter), and DH is delayed skin hypersensitivity (scale of 0 to 2). Patients are classified as high risk (PNI > 50%), intermediate risk (PNI > 40%), and low risk (PNI > 40%) (Buzby, 1980).

To date, there are four prospective, randomized, controlled studies indicating a benefit for administration of preoperative TPN. Three studies have shown a decrease in the frequency of early septic events postoperatively (Heatley et al, 1979; Foschi et al, 1986; Müller et al, 1986). In these studies the patients received preoperative TPN for 7 to 20 days. Increased weight, increased tricep skinfold thickness, improved immunologic status, and improved PNI were achieved preoperatively in the fourth study (Smith and Hartemink, 1989). Improvement in survival was also shown by Mullen and colleagues (1980). However, because of the small number of patients, changing and improving surgical techniques, better antibiotics, and improvements in specific cancer and critical care treatments, all of the improvement in survival may not be due to preoperative TPN. Similarly, it has been impossible to prove or disprove the cost-effectiveness of TPN. More recently, the Veteran's Affairs Total Parenteral Nutrition Cooperative Study Group (1991) critically evaluated the role of perioperative TPN in a prospective, randomized fashion. This large study, consisting of 395 patients (60% with cancer), found an increase in infectious morbidity in patients who received TPN as compared with nontreated controls. However, severely malnourished patients who received TPN (<5% of the study group) had fewer noninfectious complications than the control patients who did not receive TPN. Finally, Brennen and colleagues (1994) completed a prospective, randomized trial that evaluated the role of TPN and the operative outcomes of 117 patients undergoing resections for pancreatic cancer. Once again, this study demonstrated no difference in mortality or length of hospital stay for the experimental (TPN) arm and, in fact, demonstrated an increase in infectious morbidity in the TPN arm.

In general, it is our opinion that, because of the expense and potential complications, perioperative TPN should be given only to those patients who are severely malnourished. In our experience, although common sense would seem to indicate that TPN would help many patients, especially in gynecologic malignancies, the available data would indicate otherwise in the vast majority of cases.

Fluid and Electrolytes

Pathophysiologic changes that occur in the perioperative period place the surgical patient at the risk of developing fluid, electrolyte, and metabolic imbalances that can lead to numerous complications both intraoperatively and postoperatively. It is not unusual for surgical patients to suffer severe preexisting fluid and electrolyte derangements as a result of inadequate oral intake, nausea and vomiting, and nasogastric suction. In addition, however, the perioperative period is associated with an increase in circulating levels of catecholamines, adrenocorticotropic hormone (ACTH), and aldosterone (Brensilver and Goldberger, 1996). Elevations in these hormones lead to both metabolic changes and fluid retention. Proper assessment and management of fluid and electrolyte status must begin preoperatively, and continues into the postoperative recovery period. Knowledge of the physiologic changes that occur perioperatively, combined with appropriate correction of deficits, is imperative for minimizing the morbidity and mortality of anesthesia and surgery.

In the average woman, total water constitutes approximately 50% to 55% of body weight. Two thirds of this water is contained in the intracellular compartment. One third is contained in the extracellular compartment, of which one fourth is contained in plasma and the remaining three quarters is in the interstitium.

Osmolarity, or tonicity, is a property derived from the number of particles in a solution. Sodium and chloride are the primary electrolytes contributing to the osmolarity in the extracellular fluid compartment. Potassium, and to a lesser extent magnesium and phosphate, are the major intracellular electrolytes. Water flows freely between the intracellular and extracellular spaces so as to maintain osmotic neutrality throughout the body. Any shifts in osmolarity in any fluid spaces within the body will be accompanied by corresponding shifts in free water from spaces of lower to higher osmolarity, thus maintaining a balance in equilibrium.

The daily fluid maintenance requirement for the average adult is approximately 30 ml/kg/day, or 2000 to 3000 ml/day (Pestana, 1989). This is offset partially by insensible losses of 1200 ml/day, which include losses from the lungs (600 ml), skin (400 ml), and gastrointestinal tract (200 ml). Urinary output from the kidney will provide the remainder of the fluid loss, and this output will vary depending on total body intake of water and sodium. Approximately 600 to 800 mOsm of solute are excreted by the kidney per day. Healthy kidneys can concentrate urine up to approximately 1200 mOsm/L, and therefore minimum output can range between 500 and 700 ml/day. The maximal urinary output capability of the kidney can be as high as 20 L/day, as seen in the patient with diabetes insipidus. In the healthy patient, the normal kidney will adjust urine output commensurate with the daily fluid intake.

The major extracellular buffer used in acid-base balance is the bicarbonate–carbonic acid system (Miller and Duke, 1983):

$$CO_2 + H_2O \rightleftharpoons H_2CO_3 \rightleftharpoons H^+ + HCO_3^-$$

Typically the body will maintain a bicarbonate–carbonic acid ratio of 20:1 in order to maintain an extracellular pH of 7.4. Both the lung and kidney play integral roles in the maintenance of normal extracellular pH, via retention or excretion of carbon dioxide and bicarbonate. Under conditions of alkalosis, minute ventilation decreases and renal excretion of bicarbonate increases such as to restore the normal bicarbonate–carbonic acid ratio. The opposite occurs with acidosis.

Ultimately, the kidney plays the most important role in fluid and electrolyte balance through excretion and retention of water and solute. Circulating antidiuretic hormone (ADH) and aldosterone help modulate the process. Hypothalamic release of ADH is sensitive to serum osmolarity and aldosterone secretion is responsive to renal perfusion. Under states of dehydration or hypovolemia, serum ADH levels increase, leading to increased resorption of water in the distal tubule of the kidney. In addition, increased aldosterone release promotes increased renal sodium and water retention. The opposite occurs in states of fluid excess. As a result, the individual with normal renal function as well as normal circulating ADH and aldosterone levels maintains normal serum osmolarity and electrolyte composition despite daily fluctuation of fluid and electrolyte intake.

Various disease states can alter the normal fluid and electrolyte homeostatic mechanisms, making perioperative fluid and electrolyte management more difficult. In patients with intrinsic renal disease, there is an inability to excrete solute and to maintain acid-base balance. In patients with the stress of chronic starvation or severe illness, there may be inappropriately high levels of circulating ADH and aldosterone, resulting in fluid and sodium retention. With severe cardiac disease, secondary renal hypoperfusion can lead to increased aldosterone synthesis and, therefore, increased sodium and water retention by the kidney. Finally, the patient with severe diabetes can have a significant osmotic diuresis as well as acid-base dysfunction secondary to circulating ketoacids. Correction and optimization of renal, cardiac, or endocrinologic disorders preoperatively is imperative, and will often rectify fluid and electrolyte abnormalities.

Fluid and electrolyte management in the preoperative and perioperative period requires a knowledge of the daily fluid and electrolyte requirements for maintenance, replacement of ongoing fluid and electrolyte losses, and correction of any existing abnormalities. Each of these three topics is considered separately.

Fluid and Electrolyte Maintenance Requirements

The normal daily fluid requirement in the average adult is 2000 to 3000 ml. The body can and does adjust to higher and lower volumes of intake via changes in plasma tonicity. Alterations in plasma tonicity induce adjustments in circulating ADH, which ultimately regulates the amount of water retained in the distal tubule of the kidney. The daily requirements for various electrolytes are shown in Table 41–3 (Magrina, 1988). In the preoperative and the early postoperative patient, it is usually only necessary to replace sodium and potassium. Chloride is automatically replaced concomitant with sodium and potassium because chloride is the usual anion used to balance sodium and potassium in electrolyte solutions. There are various commercially available solutions containing 40 mmol of sodium chloride, with smaller amounts of potassium, calcium, and magnesium, designed to meet the requirements of a patient who is receiving 3 liters of IV fluids per day. The daily requirement, however, can be met by any combination of IV fluid orders. For example, 2 liters of 5% dextrose in 0.45 N saline ($D_{5.45}NS$; 77 mEq sodium chloride each), supplemented with 20 mEq of potassium chloride, followed by 1 liter of 5% dextrose in water (D_5W) with 20 mEq of potassium chloride, would suffice.

Fluid and Electrolyte Replacement

Fluid and electrolyte losses beyond the daily average must be replaced by appropriate solutions. The choice of solutions for replacement depends on the composition of the fluids lost. Often, it is difficult to measure free water loss, particularly in patients who have high "insensible" losses from the lungs or skin or into the gastrointestinal tract. These "insensible" losses are difficult to monitor. Procurement of daily weights in these patients can be very useful. Up to 300 g of weight loss daily can be attributable to catabolism of protein and fat in the patient who is tak-

Table 41–3. DAILY FLUID AND ELECTROLYTE MAINTENANCE REQUIREMENTS

FLUID/ELECTROLYTE	REQUIREMENTS
Sodium	100–140 mEq
Potassium	40–60 mEq
Magnesium	30 mEq
Calcium	15 mEq
Carbohydrate	100–150 g
Water	1500 ml/m² body surface area

Modified from Magrina JF: Intravenous fluids and blood component therapy. Clin Obstet Gynecol 1988;31:686, with permission.

ing nothing by mouth (Pestana, 1989). Anything beyond this, however, would be due to fluid loss and should be replaced accordingly.

The patient with a high fever can have increased pulmonary and skin loss of free water, sometimes in excess of 2 to 3 L/day. These losses should be replaced with free water in the form of D_5W. Perspiration typically has one third the osmolarity of plasma, and can be replaced with D_5W or, if excessive, with 5% dextrose in 0.25 N saline.

The patient with acute blood loss needs replacement with appropriate isotonic fluid and/or blood. There are a wide range of plasma volume expanders, including albumin, dextran, and hetastarch solutions, that contain large-molecular-weight particles (>50,000 molecular weight). These particles are slow to exit the intravascular space, with about one half of the particles remaining after 24 hours. These solutions are expensive, however, and for most cases simple replacement with 0.9 N saline or lactated Ringer's solution will suffice. One third of the volume of lactated Ringer's solution or normal saline will typically remain in the intravascular space, the remainder going to the interstitium.

Appropriate replacement of gastrointestinal fluid loss is dependent upon the source of fluid loss in the gastrointestinal tract. Gastrointestinal secretions beyond the stomach, and up to the colon, are typically isotonic with plasma (Table 41–4), with similar amounts of sodium, slightly lower amounts of chloride, slightly alkaline pH, and more potassium, in the range of 5 to 10 mEq/L (Shires and Canizaro, 1991). Under normal conditions stool is hypotonic. However, under conditions of increased flow (i.e., severe diarrhea), stool contents are isotonic, with a composition similar to that of the small bowel. Gastric contents are typically hypotonic, with one third the sodium of plasma, increased amounts of hydrogen ion, and low pH.

In the patient with gastric outlet obstruction, nausea and vomiting, or nasogastric suction, appropriate replacement of gastric secretions can be provided with a solution such as $D_{5.45}NS$ with 20 mEq/L of potassium. Potassium supplementation is particularly important to prevent hypokalemia in these patients, whose kidneys attempt to conserve hydrogen ion in the distal tubule of the kidney in exchange for potassium ion.

In patients with bowel obstruction, 1 to 3 liters of fluid can be sequestered daily in the gastrointestinal tract. This fluid should be replaced with isotonic saline or lactated Ringer's solution. Patients with enterocutaneous fistulas or new ileostomies should similarly have fluid losses replaced with isotonic fluids.

Correction of Existing Fluid and Electrolyte Abnormalities

The patient who presents preoperatively with fluid and/or electrolyte abnormalities can pose a diagnostic challenge. The correct diagnosis and therapy is contingent upon a correct assessment of total body fluid and electrolyte status. The management of hyponatremia, for example, may be either fluid restriction or fluid replacement, with the treatment choice dependent upon whether there is an overall extracellular fluid excess and normal body sodium stores or decreased overall total body sodium stores and extracellular fluid. A detailed history is necessary for documentation of any underlying medical illness as well as for assessment of the amount and duration of any abnormal fluid losses or intake. Initial evaluation should include an assessment of hemodynamic, clinical, and urinary parameters in order to assess the overall level of hydration systemically as well as the fluid status of the extracellular fluid compartment. The patient who has good skin turgor, moist mucosa, stable vital signs, and good urinary output is well hydrated. Nonpitting edema is indicative of extracellular fluid excess, whereas the patient who presents with orthostasis, sunken eyes, parched mouth, and decreased skin turgor clearly has extracellular volume contraction. On a caution-

Table 41 – 4. COMPOSITION OF GASTROINTESTINAL SECRETIONS

	VOLUME (ml/24 hr)	Na (mEq/L)	K (mEq/L)	Cl (mEq/L)	HCO₃ (mEq/L)
Salivary	1500 (500–2000)	10 (2–10)	26 (20–30)	10 (8–18)	30
Stomach	1500 (100–4000)	60 (9–116)	10 (0–32)	130 (8–154)	—
Duodenum	100–2000	140	5	80	—
Ileum	3000 (100–9000)	140 (80–150)	5 (2–8)	140 (43–137)	30
Colon	—	60	30	40	—
Pancreas	100–800 (113–185)	140 (3–7)	5 (54–95)	75	115
Bile	50–800 (131–164)	145 (3–12)	5 (89–180)	100	35

From Shires GT, Canizaro PC: Fluid and electrolyte management of the surgical patient. In Sabiston DC Jr (ed): Textbook of Surgery. 14th ed. Philadelphia: WB Saunders Company, 1991:67, with permission.

ary note, a patient's overall extracellular fluid status does not always reflect the hydration status of the intravascular compartment. A patient can have increased interstitial fluid, yet be intravascularly dry, requiring replacement with isotonic fluid.

Laboratory work-up for patients who may have pre-existing fluid problems should include blood hematocrit, serum chemistries, glucose, blood urea nitrogen (BUN) and creatinine, urine osmolarity, and urine electrolytes. Serum osmolarity is mainly a function of the concentration of sodium and is given by the following equation:

$$2 \times [Na^+] \ (mEq/L) + \frac{Glucose \ (mg/dl)}{18}$$

$$+ \frac{BUN \ (mg/dl)}{2.8}$$

Normal serum osmolarity is typically 290 to 300 mOsm/kg. Blood hematocrit (Hct) can be used to estimate volume deficit according to the following equation:

$$Plasma \ deficit \ (ml) = Normal \ blood \ volume$$

$$- \left(\frac{Normal \ blood \ volume \times Normal \ Hct}{Measured \ Hct} \right)$$

Normally, the blood hematocrit will rise or fall inversely at a rate of approximately 1% per 500-ml alteration of extracellular fluid volume. The BUN-creatinine ratio is typically 10:1 but will rise to greater than 20:1 under conditions of extracellular fluid contraction. Under conditions of extracellular fluid deficit, urine osmolarity will typically be high (>400 mOsm/kg) while urine sodium concentration is low (<15 mEq/L) indicative of an attempt by the kidney to conserve sodium. Under conditions of extracellular fluid excess, or in cases of renal disease where the kidney has impaired ability to retain sodium and water, urine osmolarity will be low with urine sodium high (>30 mEq/L). Finally, changes in sodium can give insight as to the degree of extracellular fluid excess or deficit. In the average person, the serum sodium rises by 3 mmol/L for every liter of water deficit, and falls by 3 mmol/L for each liter of water excess. One must, however, be careful in making these estimates, in that the patient with prolonged water and electrolyte loss can present with low serum sodium and marked water deficit.

Specific Electrolyte Disorders

HYPONATREMIA

Because sodium is the major extracellular cation, shifts in serum sodium are usually inversely correlated with the hydration state of the extracellular fluid compartment. The pathophysiology of hyponatremia, then, is usually expansion of body fluids leading to excess total body water (Miller and Duke, 1983). The symptoms of hyponatremia are related to both the serum sodium level and the rapidity of its

fall. Acute hyponatremia will usually become symptomatic when the serum sodium falls to below 120 to 125 mEq/L, whereas, in chronic hyponatremia, symptoms may not occur until the serum sodium is below 110 mEq/L. Symptoms of hyponatremia can include anorexia, nausea, vomiting, lethargy, headaches, weakness, change in mental status, and seizures.

Hyponatremia in the state of extracellular fluid excess can be seen in patients with renal or cardiac failure as well as in conditions such as nephrotic syndrome, where total body salt and water are increased, with a relatively greater increase in the latter. Administration of hypertonic saline to correct the hyponatremia would be inappropriate in this setting. The treatment should include, in addition to correcting the underlying disease process, water restriction with diuretic therapy.

Inappropriate secretion of ADH can occur with head trauma and pulmonary or cerebral tumors and under states of stress. The abnormally elevated ADH results in excess water retention. Treatment includes water restriction and, if possible, correction of the underlying cause. Demeclocycline has been shown to be effective in this disorder via its action in the kidney.

Inappropriate replacement of body salt losses with water alone will result in hyponatremia. This will typically occur in patients who are losing large amounts of electrolytes secondary to vomiting, nasogastric suction, diarrhea, or gastrointestinal fistulas who receive fluid replacement with hypotonic solutions. Simple replacement with isotonic fluids and potassium will usually correct the abnormality. Rarely will rapid correction of the hyponatremia be necessary, in which case hypertonic saline (3%) can be administered. Hypertonic saline should be very cautiously administered in order to avoid a rapid shift in serum sodium, which will induce central nervous system (CNS) dysfunction. Common causes of hyponatremia in the preoperative patient are shown in Table 41–5.

HYPERNATREMIA

Hypernatremia is an uncommon condition that can be life threatening if severe. Symptoms usually do not develop until the serum sodium is in excess of 160 mEq/L and the serum osmolarity reaches 320 to 330 mOsm/kg. The pathophysiology is one of severe extracelluar fluid deficit. The resultant hyperosmolar state results in decreased water volume in cells in the CNS, which, if severe, can result in disorientation, seizures, intracranial bleed, and death. The causes include excessive extrarenal water loss as can be seen in patients with high fever, tracheostomy in a dry environment, extensive thermal injuries, diabetes insipidus (either central or nephrogenic), and iatrogenic salt loading. The treatment involves correction of the underlying cause (correction of fever, humidification of the tracheostomy, pitressin for con-

Table 41-5. PREOPERATIVE CAUSES OF HYPONATREMIA

Decreased total body sodium
   Diuretics
   Salt-losing nephropathy
Excess volume
   Oral or IV fluid overload
Medical
   Congestive heart failure
   Renal failure
   Cirrhosis
   Nephrotic syndrome
   Hypothyroidism
   Addison's disease
Pharmacologic
   Antidepressants
   Phenothiazines
Sulfonylureas
   Carbamazepine
Syndrome of inappropriate antidiuretic hormone secretion

trol of central diabetes insipidus) and replacement with free water either by the oral route or intravenously with D_5W. As with severe hyponatremia, marked hypernatremia should be corrected slowly.

HYPOKALEMIA

Hypokalemia may be encountered preoperatively in patients with significant gastrointestinal fluid loss (prolonged emesis, diarrhea, nasogastric suction, intestinal fistulas); in patients with marked urinary potassium loss secondary to renal tubular disorders (renal tubular acidosis, acute tubular necrosis, hyperaldosteronism, prolonged diuretic use); or as a result of prolonged administration of potassium-free parenteral fluids in patients who are taking nothing by mouth. The symptoms associated with hypokalemia include neuromuscular disturbances ranging from muscle weakness to flaccid paralysis as well as cardiovascular abnormalities, including hypotension, bradycardia, arrhythmias, and enhancement of digitalis toxicity. These symptoms rarely occur unless the serum potassium is below 3 mEq/L. The treatment is potassium replacement. Oral therapy is preferable in patients who are on an oral diet. If necessary, potassium replacement can be given intravenously in doses that should not exceed 10 mEq/hour.

HYPERKALEMIA

Hyperkalemia is encountered infrequently in preoperative patients. It is usually associated with renal impairment but can also be seen in patients with adrenal insufficiency, with the use of potassium-sparing diuretics, and with marked tissue breakdown as can be seen in patients with crush injuries, massive gastrointestinal bleeds, or hemolysis. The clinical manifestations are mainly cardiovascular. Marked hyperkalemia (potassium greater than 7

mEq/L) can result in bradycardia, ventricular fibrillation, and cardiac arrest. The treatment chosen depends upon the severity of the hyperkalemia and whether or not there are associated cardiac or ECG abnormalities. Calcium gluconate (10 ml of a 10% solution) given intravenously can offset the toxic effects of hyperkalemia on the heart. One ampule each of sodium bicarbonate and 50% dextrose with or without insulin will cause rapid shift of potassium into cells. Longer term cation exchange resins such as Kayexalate, taken either orally or by enema, will bind and decrease total body potassium. Hemodialysis is reserved for emergent conditions where other measures are not sufficient or have failed.

ACID-BASE DISORDERS

A variety of metabolic, respiratory, and electrolyte abnormalities can result in an imbalance in normal acid-base homeostasis, leading to alkalosis or acidosis. Changes in the respiratory rate will directly affect the amount of carbon dioxide that is exhaled. A respiratory acidosis will result from carbon dioxide retention in patients who have hypoventilation from CNS depression, as seen under conditions of oversedation from narcotics, particularly in the presence of concurrent severe chronic obstructive pulmonary disease (COPD). A respiratory alkalosis will result from hyperventilation either due to excitation of the CNS from drugs or pain, or iatrogenically produced from excess ventilator support. Numerous metabolic derangements can result in alkalosis or acidosis, and these are discussed further in this section. Fortunately, proper fluid and electrolyte replacement as well as maintenance of adequate tissue perfusion will help to prevent most acid-base disorders in the postoperative period.

Alkalosis. Alkalosis is a common acid-base disorder seen in surgical patients. Fortunately, mild alkalosis is usually of no clinical significance and resolves spontaneously. Several etiologic factors may include hyperventilation associated with pain; post-traumatic transient hyperaldosteronism, which results in decreased renal bicarbonate excretion; nasogastric suction, which removes hydrogen ions; infused bicarbonate during blood transfusions in the form of citrate, which is converted to bicarbonates; administration of exogenous alkali; and use of diuretics. Correction of the alkalosis can usually be easily achieved with removal of the inciting cause, as well as with correction of extracellular fluid and potassium deficits (Table 41-6). Full correction can usually be safely achieved over 1 to 2 days.

Marked alkalosis, with serum pH greater than 7.55, can result in serious cardiac arrhythmias or CNS seizures. Myocardial excitability will be particularly pronounced with concurrent hypokalemia. Under such conditions, fluid and electrolyte replacement may not be sufficient to rapidly correct the alkalosis. Acetazolamide (250 to 500 mg) orally or intravenously can be given two to four times daily to

Table 41-6. METABOLIC ALKALOSIS

DISORDER	SOURCE OF ALKALI	CAUSE OF RENAL HCO₃ RETENTION
Gastric alkalosis		
Nasogastric suction	Gastric mucosa	↓ ECF, ↓ K
Vomiting		
Renal alkalosis		
Diuretics	Renal epithelium	↓ ECF, ↓ K
Respiratory acidosis and diuretics		↓ ECF, ↓ K, ↑ Pco₂
Exogenous base	NaHCO₃, Na citrate, Na lactate	Co-existing disorder of ECF, K, Paco₂

Abbreviations: ↓ ECF, extracellular fluid depletion; ↓ K, potassium depletion; ↑ Pco₂, carbon dioxide retention.

induce renal bicarbonate diuresis. Treatment with an acidifying agent is rarely necessary and should be reserved for acutely symptomatic patients (cardiac or CNS dysfunction) or for patients with advanced renal disease. Under such conditions, HCl (5 to 10 mEq/hour of a 100-mmol/L solution) can be given via a central line. Ammonium chloride can also be given orally or intravenously but should not be given in patients with hepatic disease.

Acidosis. Metabolic acidosis can be potentially serious as a result of its effect on the cardiovascular system. Under conditions of acidosis, there are decreased myocardial contractility, a propensity for vasodilation of the peripheral vasculature leading to hypotension, and refractoriness of the fibrillating heart to defibrillation. These effects promote decompensation of the cardiovascular system and can hinder attempts at resuscitative efforts.

The primary pathophysiology of metabolic acidosis results from a decrease in serum bicarbonate level as a result of consumption and replacement of bicarbonate by circulating acids, or owing to replacement by other anions such as chloride. The proper work-up includes a measurement of the anion gap:

$$\text{Anion gap} = \text{Na}^+ - (\text{CL}^- + \text{HCO}_3^-)$$

The anion gap is normally 10 to 14 mEq/L and is composed of circulating protein, sulfate, phosphate, citrate, and lactate (Narins and Lazarus, 1984).

Patients with metabolic acidosis can be divided into two groups based on the anion gap (increased vs. normal anion gap). An increase in circulating acids will consume and replace bicarbonate ion, thus increasing the anion gap. The causes include an increase in circulating lactic acid secondary to anaerobic glycolysis, as is seen under conditions of poor tissue perfusion; increased ketoacids, as is seen in cases of severe diabetes or starvation; exogenous toxins; and renal dysfunction, which leads to increased circulating sulfates and phosphates (Demling and Wilson, 1988). The diagnosis can be established via a thorough history and measurement of serum lactate (normal < 2 mmol/L), serum glucose, and renal function parameters. Metabolic acidosis in the face of a normal anion gap is usually the result of an imbalance of the ions chloride and bicarbonate, under conditions leading to excess chloride and decreased bicarbonate. Hyperchloremic acidosis can be seen in patients who have undergone saline loading. Bicarbonate loss will be seen in patients with small bowel fistula, new ileostomies, severe diarrhea, or renal tubular acidosis. Finally, in patients with marked extracellular volume expansion, as is seen commonly postoperatively, the relative decrease in serum sodium and bicarbonate will result in a mild acidosis. A summary of the various causes of metabolic acidosis in shown in Table 41–7 (Narins and Lazarus, 1984).

The treatment of metabolic acidosis depends on the cause. In patients with lactic acidosis, restoration of tissue perfusion is imperative. This can be done through cardiovascular and pulmonary support as needed, oxygen therapy, and aggressive treatment of

Table 41-7. CAUSES OF METABOLIC ACIDOSIS

HIGH ANION GAP	NORMAL ANION GAP	
	Hyperkalemic	*Hypokalemic*
Uremia	Hyporeninism	Diarrhea
Ketoacidosis	Primary adrenal failure	Renal tubular acidosis
Lactic acidosis	NH₄Cl	Ileal and sigmoid bladders
Aspirin	Sulfur poisoning	Hyperalimentation
Paraldehyde	Early chronic renal failure	
Methanol	Obstructive uropathy	
Ethylene glycol		
Methylmalonic aciduria		

From Narins RG, Lazarus MJ: Renal system. In Vandam LD (ed): To Make the Patient Ready for Ganesthesia: Medical Care of the Surgical Patient. 2nd ed. Menlo Park, CA: Addison-Wesley, 1984:67, with permission.

systemic infection wherever appropriate. Ketosis from diabetes can be corrected gradually with insulin therapy. Ketosis resulting from chronic starvation or from lack of caloric support postoperatively can be corrected with nutrition. In patients with normal anion gap acidosis, bicarbonate losses from the gastrointestinal tract should be replaced, excess chloride administration can be curtailed, and, where necessary, a loop diuretic can be used to induce renal clearance of chloride. Dilutional acidosis can be corrected with mild fluid restriction.

Bicarbonates should not be given unless serum pH is less than 7.2, or unless there are severe cardiac complications secondary to acidosis. Furthermore, close monitoring of serum potassium is mandatory. Under states of acidosis, potassium will exit the cell and enter the circulation. The patient with a normal potassium concentration and metabolic acidosis is actually intracellularly potassium depleted. Treatment of the acidosis without potassium replacement will result in severe hypokalemia with its associated risks. A summary of the various acid-base abnormalities and associated therapies is shown in Table 41–8 (Demling and Wilson, 1988).

Antibiotic Prophylaxis

Bacteria that may contaminate the gynecologic surgical field are those that are indigenous to the vaginal tract, including both gram-positive and gram-negative aerobes and anaerobes (Table 41–9). The primary pathogenic bacteria include the coliforms, streptococci, fusobacteria, and bacteroides. Gynecologic operations that carry a significant risk of postoperative infection include vaginal hysterectomy, abdominal hysterectomy, cases involving pelvic abscess or inflammation, select cases of pregnancy termination, and radical surgery for gynecologic cancers. In these cases, organisms indigenous to the vagina may contaminate the pelvic cavity and surgical wound site. Most other gynecologic procedures are considered "clean" and have a low risk (5%) of postoperative wound infection (Flynn, 1987). Included in these are procedures confined to the abdomen, space of Retzius, perineum, and vagina.

The following are proposed guidelines for antibiotic prophylaxis in gynecologic procedures (Ledger et al, 1975):

1. The procedure should carry a significant risk of postoperative infection.
2. The surgery should involve considerable bacterial contamination.
3. The antibiotic chosen for prophylaxis should be effective against most contaminating organisms.
4. The antibiotic should be present in the tissues at the time of contamination.
5. The shortest possible course of antibiotic prophylaxis should be given.
6. The prophylactic antibiotic chosen should not be one considered for treatment should postoperative infection occur.
7. The risk of complications from the prophylactic antibiotic should be low.

The existing literature uniformly supports the use of the prophylactic antibiotics for vaginal hysterectomy; however, the use of prophylactic antibiotics for patients who undergo abdominal hysterectomy is controversial. Hirsch (1985) reviewed the placebo-controlled trials in the English and non-English literature regarding antibiotic prophylaxis in vaginal and abdominal hysterectomy. Included in the review were 48 studies encompassing 5524 patients who underwent vaginal hysterectomy, and 30 studies encompassing 3752 patients who underwent abdominal hysterectomy. In vaginal hysterectomy, prophylactic antibiotics decreased febrile morbidity from 40% in control patients to 15% in treated patients, and lowered the pelvic infection rate from 25% in control patients to 5% in treated patients. The benefits of antibiotic prophylaxis were less pronounced in the abdominal hysterectomy series; febrile morbidity was reduced in 57% of studies, whereas wound infections and pelvic infections were reduced in a minority of the studies. Overall, antibiotic prophylaxis for abdominal hysterectomy reduced febrile morbidity from 28% in control patients to 16% in treated patients, pelvic infections from 10% to 5%, and wound infections from 8% to 3%, respectively. This analysis is further complicated by a lack of series-to-series uniformity regarding criteria for fever or for diagnosis of infection requiring antibiotic therapy. Nonetheless, most investigators would agree that antibiotic prophylaxis should be used in all patients who undergo vaginal hysterectomy, as well as in selected high-risk patients who undergo abdominal hysterectomy. Factors that have been identified as placing patients at high risk for posthysterectomy infection have included low socioeconomic status, duration of surgery greater than 2 hours, presence of malignancy, and increased number of surgical procedures performed. Obesity, menopausal status, and estimated blood loss have not been shown to be risk factors for postoperative infection when evaluated by multivariate analysis (Shapiro et al, 1982; Haley et al, 1985).

The antibiotic chosen for prophylaxis for gynecologic cases should have activity against the broad range of vaginal organisms. The first- and second-generation cephalosporins are well suited given their activity against gram-positive, gram-negative, and anaerobic organisms. Most classes of antibiotics, including the penicillins, tetracyclines, sulfonamides, broad-spectrum penicillins, and cephalosporins, as well as anaerobic drugs (clindamycin/metronidazole [Flagyl]), have been shown to be effective as prophylactic antibiotics (Chodak, 1977; Davey et al, 1988; Munck and Jensen, 1989; Roy et al, 1989; Trimbos et al, 1989), although none has been demonstrated to be consistently more effective than first-generation cephalosporins.

Table 41–8. ACID-BASE DISORDERS AND THEIR TREATMENT

PRIMARY DISORDER	DEFECT	COMMON CAUSES	COMPENSATION	TREATMENT
Respiratory acidosis	Carbon dioxide retention (hypoventilation)	Central nervous system depression Airway and lung impairment	Renal excretion of acid salts Bicarbonate retention Chloride shift into red cells	Restoration of adequate ventilation Control excess carbon dioxide production
Respiratory alkalosis	Hyperventilation	Central nervous system excitation Excess ventilator support	Renal excretion of sodium, potassium, bicarbonate Absorption of hydrogen and chloride ions Lactate release from red cells	Correction of hyperventilation
Metabolic acidosis	Excess loss of base Increased nonvolatile acids	Excess chloride versus sodium Increased bicarbonate loss Lactic, ketoacidosis Uremia Dilutional acidosis	Respiratory alkalosis Renal excretion of hydrogen and chloride ions Resorption of potassium and bicarbonate	Increase sodium load Correct underlying process Waste chloride Give bicarbonate for pH <7.2 Restore buffers, protein, hemoglobin
Metabolic alkalosis	Excess loss of chloride potassium Increased bicarbonate	Gastrointestinal losses of chloride Excess intake of bicarbonate Diuretics Hypokalemia Extracellular fluid volume chloride ions	Respiratory acidosis May be hypoxia Renal excretion of bicarbonate and potassium Absorption of hydrogen and replacement	Increase chloride content Potassium replacement Acetazolamide (Diamox) to waste bicarbonate Vigorous volume Occasional 0.1 N HCl as needed

From Demling RH, Wilson RF: Fluids, electrolytes, and acid-base balance. In Decision Making in Surgical Critical Care. Philadelphia: BC Decker, 1988:114, with permission.

Table 41-9. BACTERIA INDIGENOUS TO THE LOWER GENITAL TRACT

Lactobacillus	Enterobacter cloacae
Diphtheroids	Enterobacter agglomerans
Staphylococcus aureus	Klebsiella pneumoniae
Staphylococcus epidermidis	Proteus mirabilis
Streptococcus agalactiae	Proteus vulgaris
α-Hemolytic streptococci	Morganella morganii
Group D streptococci	
Peptostreptococcus	Bacteroides species
Peptococcus	B. bivius
Clostridium	B. disiens
Gaffkya aerococcus	B. fragilis
Escherichia coli	B. melaninogenicus
Fusobacterium	

The timing of administration of the prophylactic antibiotic agent is important. Studies dating back to the work by Burke (1961) have demonstrated that antibiotics given for prophylaxis against infection are most active if present in tissues prior to contamination with an inoculum of bacteria. For patients who undergo hysterectomy, the antibiotic should be present in the tissues prior to the opening of the vaginal cuff, at which time vaginal organisms gain access to the pelvic cavity. Infusion of an antibiotic, on call to the operating room, within 30 minutes of surgery is ideal for this purpose. For long surgical procedures, particularly where there is a large blood loss or when an antibiotic agent with short half-life is used, a second antibiotic dose should be given intraoperatively.

Many prospective studies have documented that short courses of prophylactic antibiotics (24 hours or less) are as efficacious as longer ones. Several clinical trials have found that one perioperative dose of prophylactic antibiotic is sufficient (Hemsell et al, 1988, 1989; Friese et al, 1989; Munck and Jensen, 1989; Orr et al, 1990). The use of one dose of prophylactic antibiotic has many advantages, including decreased cost, decreased toxicity, and minimal alteration of host flora (selection of resistant pathogens).

Despite the advantages of using prophylactic antibiotics, the importance of good surgical technique must be emphasized. Antibiotics should not be used in lieu of correct surgical principles such as delicate handling of tissues, good hemostasis, adequate drainage, and avoidance of unnecessarily large pedicles of tissue in ligatures.

Gastrointestinal Preparation

Preparation of the lower gastrointestinal tract before elective gynecologic surgery has several goals. In most gynecologic surgery, when the gastrointestinal tract is not entered, mechanical preparation of the bowel reduces gastrointestinal contents, thus allowing more room in the abdomen and pelvis, facilitating the surgical procedure. Furthermore, even if there is a rectosigmoid colon enterotomy during surgery, the mechanical bowel preparation eliminates formed stool and reduces the bacterial contamination, thus reducing infectious complications. Mechanical bowel preparation may be accomplished by several methods (Table 41-10). The traditional use of laxatives and enemas requires at least 12 to 24 hours and generally causes moderate abdominal distention and crampy pain. In addition, nursing supervision of enema administration and the need for IV fluid replacement make this regimen relatively expensive. Randomized trials comparing traditional mechanical bowel preparation with oral gut lavage (PEG-3350 and electrolytes for oral solution, or GoLYTELY) have found that the use of approximately 4 liters of GoLYTELY (administered until the rectal effluent is clear) provides more complete, faster, and more comfortable bowel preparation (Beck et al, 1985). Furthermore, the fluid loss following gut lavage with GoLYTELY appears to be clinically insignificant. Gut lavage can usually be performed at home the day before scheduled surgery. Rarely, if the patient cannot drink the 4 liters, the GoLYTELY may be administered through a small-caliber nasogastric tube. We recommend mechanical bowel preparation to all patients who will undergo major abdominal, pelvic, or vaginal surgery.

High infection rates after colonic surgery have led to investigation of methods aimed at reducing these significant complications. Although mechanical bowel preparation is an essential part of all colonic surgery preparation regimens, it does not reduce the infection rate satisfactorily. Reduction of the number of pathogenic flora in the colon is the primary strategy to reducing infection after colonic surgery. The colon has the greatest concentration of bacteria, including both aerobes and anaerobes, in the body. Anaerobes outnumber aerobes by 1000 to 1.

After reducing the bacterial load by mechanical preparation, antibiotics should be used to further re-

Table 41-10. MECHANICAL BOWEL PREPARATION REGIMENS TO BEGIN DAY BEFORE GYNECOLOGIC SURGERY

TIME	TRADITIONAL MECHANICAL PREP	GoLYTELY
12:00 A.M.	Clear liquid diet	Clear liquid diet
12:00 P.M.	Magnesium citrate, 240 ml by mouth	GoLYTELY, 4 L by mouth over 3 hr
8:00 P.M.	Saline enemas to clear, 5% dextrose in one-half normal saline IV with 20 mg potassium chloride at 125 ml/hr	
12:00 A.M.	Nothing by mouth	Nothing by mouth

duce the bacterial count and to prevent infections following intestinal (especially colonic) surgery. Over the past decade, perioperative IV antibiotics have replaced the oral bowel preparation with neomycin and erythromycin (Fry, 1988). We routinely prescribe mechanical *and* antibiotic prophylaxis for patients who will likely undergo colorectal surgery (pelvic exenteration, ovarian cancer debulking) and for those who are at high risk for rectal injury (such as severe cases of endometriosis or pelvic inflammatory disease).

Thromboembolism Prophylaxis

Risk Factors

DVT and pulmonary embolism, although largely preventable, are significant complications occurring in postoperative patients. The magnitude of this problem is relevant to the gynecologist, because 40% of all deaths following gynecologic surgery are directly attributed to pulmonary emboli (Jeffcoate and Tindall, 1965). Pulmonary embolism is the most frequent cause of postoperative death in patients with uterine (Clarke-Pearson et al, 1983b) or cervical (Creasman and Weed, 1981) carcinoma.

The causal factors of venous thrombosis were first proposed by Virchow in 1858 and include a hypercoagulable state, venous stasis, and vessel intima injury. When the patient undergoing gynecologic surgery is specifically considered, two prospective studies have evaluated risk factors associated with the postoperative occurrence of DVT. Clayton et al (1976) studied the risk factors of 124 patients undergoing vaginal and abdominal surgery for benign gynecologic disease. Logistic regression analysis identified five factors to be associated with postoperative DVT: age, varicose veins, percentage overweight, euglobulin lysis time, and serum fibrin-related antigen. The risk factors associated with venous thromboembolic complications have also been assessed in 411 patients undergoing major abdominal and pelvic surgery (Clarke-Pearson et al, 1987). Preoperative risk factors identified in this study include age, nonwhite patients, increasing stage of malignancy, history of DVT, lower extremity edema or venous stasis changes, varicose veins, weight, and a history of radiation therapy. Intraoperative factors associated with postoperative DVT included increased anesthesia time, increased blood loss, and transfusion requirements in the operating room. The recognition of these factors, which are associated with postoperative venous thromboembolism, should allow the clinician to stratify patients into low-risk, medium-risk, and high-risk groups.

Prophylactic Methods (Table 41–11)

Over the past two decades, a number of prophylactic methods have undergone clinical trials showing significant reduction in the incidence of DVT, and a few studies have been completed that demonstrate a reduction in fatal pulmonary emboli. The ideal prophylactic method would be effective, free of significant side effects, well accepted by the patient and nursing staff, widely applicable to most patient groups, and inexpensive.

LOW-DOSE HEPARIN

The use of small doses of subcutaneously administered heparin for the prevention of DVT and pulmonary embolism is the most widely studied of all prophylactic methods. More than 25 controlled trials have demonstrated that heparin given subcutaneously 2 hours preoperatively and every 8 to 12 hours postoperatively is effective in reducing the incidence of DVT. The value of low-dose heparin in preventing fatal pulmonary emboli was established by a randomized, controlled, multicenter international trial that demonstrated a reduction in fatal postoperative pulmonary emboli in general surgery patients receiving low-dose heparin every 8 hours postoperatively (Kakkar, 1975).

Table 41–11. PROPHYLACTIC TECHNIQUES BY CATEGORY OF THROMBOEMBOLISM RISK

RISK CATEGORY	PROPHYLACTIC TECHNIQUES
Low	Graduated compression stockings (GCS)

Moderate
  Age <40 years and other risk factor(s)
  Age >40 and no other risk factors
	Intermittent pneumatic compression (IPC) (24 hr)
	Low-dose heparin (LDH) (q12h)
	Low-molecular-weight heparin (qd)
	GCS

High
  Age >60
  Cancer
	IPC (5 days)
	LDH (q8h)

Very high
  Pelvic exenteration
  Radical vulvectomy
  Prior history of DVT/pulmonary embolism
	Combination of methods (e.g., IPC and GCS or IPC and LDH)
	Inferior vena cava interruption

Trials of low-dose heparin in gynecologic surgery patients are limited, and a clear consensus as to the value of low-dose heparin in all groups of patients has not been established because of differences in patient selection and length of follow-up. Three randomized, controlled gynecologic surgery studies used the same regimen of low-dose heparin administration: 5000 units subcutaneously 2 hours preoperatively and every 12 hours for 7 days postoperatively. The trials reported by Ballard and co-workers (1973) and Taberner and associates (1978) were conducted in patients with benign gynecologic conditions (98%). All patients were older than 40 years of age, and follow-up was discontinued at the time of discharge from hospital. The American study (Clarke-Pearson et al, 1983a) evaluated a larger group of patients on a gynecologic oncology unit. Only 16% had benign gynecologic conditions, and follow-up included the first 6 weeks postoperatively.

The trial by Taberner and associates (1978) showed a 23% incidence of DVT in the control group compared with a 6% incidence of in the low-dose heparin–treated patients. This difference was statistically significant ($p < 0.05$). Unfortunately, although this was a randomized trial, the control group contained a larger number of patients with malignancy. When the cancer patients were excluded from the trial analysis, there remained no significant value to the use of low-dose heparin in patients with benign conditions. The study by Ballard and co-workers (1973) study also evaluated a group of patients who had benign gynecologic diseases. The nontreated control group had a 29% incidence of DVT, as compared with a 3.6% incidence in the low-dose heparin–treated group ($p < 0.001$). In contrast, in a randomized trial of patients undergoing major abdominal and pelvic surgery on a gynecologic oncology service (Clarke-Pearson et al, 1983a), there was no difference in the incidence of thromboembolic complications between the control group (12.4%) and the low-dose heparin–treated group (14.8%). In summary, with regard to gynecologic surgery, only the trial reported by Ballard and co-workers has found a beneficial effect of low-dose heparin in patients with benign gynecologic conditions. Taberner and associates in benign gynecology patients, and Clarke-Pearson and colleagues in gynecologic oncology patients, did not find low-dose heparin to be of benefit.

In a subsequent trial (Clarke-Pearson et al, 1990), two more intense heparin regimens were evaluated in high-risk gynecologic oncology patients. In this study, heparin was given in a regimen of either 5000 units subcutaneously 2 hours preoperatively and every 8 hours postoperatively or 5000 units subcutaneously every 8 hours preoperatively (a minimum of three preoperative doses) and every 8 hours postoperatively. Both of these prophylaxis regimens were effective in significantly reducing the incidence of postoperative DVT.

Although low-dose heparin is considered to have no effect on measurable coagulation parameters, most large series have noted an increase in the bleeding complication rate, especially a higher incidence of wound hematoma. A prolonged activated partial thromboplastin time (APTT) developed in up to 10% to 15% of otherwise healthy patients after 5000 units of heparin was given subcutaneously (Clarke-Pearson et al, 1984b). These transiently anticoagulated patients have also been noted in one carefully monitored trial of low-dose heparin in gynecology. It was these patients in whom the major bleeding complications were encountered postoperatively. Dockerty and colleagues (1983) also found that estimated blood loss increased from 246 to 401 ml in low-dose heparin–treated patients undergoing inguinal or pelvic lymphadenectomy. Retrospective studies have suggested that low-dose heparin contributed to an increased occurrence of lymphocysts (Catalona et al, 1979; Piver et al, 1983), and a prospective study demonstrated a twofold increase in retroperitoneal lymph drainage volume in patients treated with low-dose heparin (Clarke-Pearson et al, 1984b). Finally, although relatively rare, thrombocytopenia is associated with low-dose heparin use and has been found in 6% of patients after gynecologic surgery (Clarke-Pearson et al, 1984b). Although many authors believe that no monitoring of coagulation parameters is necessary for effective and safe low-dose heparin use, periodic postoperative assessment of activated thromboplastin time and platelet count seems prudent to maximize the identification of the 22% of patients who either had prolonged APTT or thrombocytopenia and who are most at risk for development of major clinical hemorrhagic complications.

LOW-MOLECULAR-WEIGHT HEPARIN

Low-molecular-weight heparins (LMWHs) are fragments of unfractionated heparin that vary in size from 4500 to 6500 molecular weight. When compared to unfractionated heparin, LMWHs have more anti–factor Xa and less antithrombin activity, leading to less effect on partial thromboplastin time. Decreased platelet inhibition and microvascular bleeding has been noted with LMWH, which may also lead to fewer complications with bleeding (Tapson and Hull, 1995). An increased half-life of 4 hours (in both IV and subcutaneous administrations) leads to increased bioavailability when compared to unfractionated heparin. This may allow once- or twice-a-day dosing. Several commercial LMWH preparations are internationally available, but only two (enoxaparin and dalteparin) have been approved by the Food and Drug Administration for DVT prophylaxis in the United States.

The investigation of perioperative LMWH prophylaxis is limited in gynecologic surgery. Four randomized controlled trials have compared LMWH to unfractionated low-dose heparin, revealing similar rates of bleeding complications (Fricker et al, 1988; Heilmann et al, 1989; Borstad et al, 1992; Kaaja et al,

1992). The rate of thromboembolism was approximately 2% in this collective group of 521 operative patients receiving LMWH prophylaxis. A recent meta-analysis of general and gynecologic surgery patients from 32 trials likewise indicated that daily LMWH administration is as effective as unfractionated low-dose heparin in DVT prophylaxis without any difference in hemorrhagic complications (Jorgensen et al, 1993). Caution should be maintained in interpretation of assimilated data involving LMWH because different anti-factor Xa activities are associated with the different preparations (Haas and Haas, 1993). In a comparison of prophylactic methods of DVT treatment, LMWH has been suggested by some investigators to be more cost-effective than low-dose heparin in general and orthopedic surgery patients, because of the convenience of once-daily dosing (Bergquist et al, 1996).

MECHANICAL METHODS

Stasis in the veins of the legs has been clearly demonstrated on the operating table and continues postoperatively for varying lengths of time. Many authors believe that the combination of stasis occurring in the capacitance veins of the calf during surgery plus the hypercoagulable state induced by surgery is the prime factor contributing to the development of acute postoperative DVT. Prospective studies of the natural history of postoperative venous thrombosis have shown that the calf veins are the predominant site of thrombi and that most thrombi develop within 24 hours of surgery (Clarke-Pearson, 1993). A growing body of literature supports the important role that the reduction of stasis by mechanical prophylactic methods plays in the prevention of postoperative DVT.

Although probably of only modest benefit, reduction of stasis by short preoperative hospital stays and early postoperative ambulation should be encouraged for all patients. Elevation of the foot of the bed 20 degrees, thus raising the calf above heart level, allows gravity to drain the calf veins and should further reduce stasis. More active forms of mechanical prophylaxis include elastic gradient compression stockings and external pneumatic leg compression.

Graded Compression Stockings. The simplicity of graded elastic stockings and the absence of significant side effects are probably the two most important reasons for their inclusion in the routine postoperative orders of many surgeons. Controlled studies of gradient elastic stockings are limited but do suggest modest benefit when carefully fitted (Scurr et al, 1977). Poorly fitted stockings may be hazardous to some patients in whom a tourniquet effect develops at the knee or midthigh (Clarke-Pearson et al, 1983b). Variations in human anatomy do not allow perfect fit of all patients to stocking sizes manufactured.

Although most postoperative DVT occurs in the first 72 hours after surgery, approximately 15% will occur 7 to 30 days postoperatively. The practice of earlier hospital discharge after major surgery raises concerns about the effectiveness of prophylaxis if it is discontinued at the time of discharge. Of the prophylactic methods available, graded compression stockings are the most logical prophylactic method to be used by the patient after hospital discharge.

External Pneumatic Compression. The largest body of literature dealing with the reduction of postoperative venous stasis deals with intermittent external compression of the leg by pneumatically inflated sleeves placed around the calf and/or leg during intraoperative and postoperative periods. Various pneumatic compression devices and leg sleeve designs are available, and the current literature has not demonstrated superiority of one system over another. In randomized, controlled trials, compression devices appear to reduce significantly the incidence of DVT on a par with low-dose heparin. In addition to increasing venous flow and pulsatile emptying of the calf veins, external pneumatic compression also appears to augment endogenous fibrinolysis, which may result in lysis of very early thrombi before they become clinically significant (Allenby et al, 1976).

The duration of postoperative external pneumatic compression has been different in various trials. Because most cases of DVT occur intraoperatively and in the first 72 hours postoperatively (Clarke-Pearson et al, 1984c), we believe that this time interval should be a minimum length for external pneumatic compression. Several investigators have found external pneumatic compression to be effective when used only in the operating room or in the operating room and for the first 24 hours postoperatively (Nicolaides et al, 1980; Salzman and Davies, 1980).

External pneumatic compression used in patients undergoing major surgery for gynecologic malignancy has been found to reduce the incidence of postoperative venous thromboembolic complications by nearly threefold (Clarke-Pearson et al, 1984c). Calf compression was applied intraoperatively and for the first 5 postoperative days. In a subsequent trial of similar patients designed to evaluate whether external pneumatic compression might achieve similar benefits when used only intraoperatively and for the first 24 hours postoperatively, there was no reduction of DVT compared with the control group (Clarke-Pearson et al, 1984a). It appears that patients with gynecologic malignancies remain at risk because of stasis and hypercoagulable states for a longer period of time than general surgical patients, and, if compression is to be effective, it must be used for at least 5 days postoperatively.

External pneumatic leg compression has no significant side effects or risks, although patient tolerance has been cited as a drawback to the use of this equipment. In our experience, less than 1% of patients request that the compression sleeves be discontinued because of discomfort. However, in order to achieve maximal effectiveness, compliance in the use of the devices is critical, and the importance of use while in bed should be stressed by nurses and physicians alike. The equipment is easily managed by the nursing staff, and, although initial capital outlay for external pneumatic compressors may seem large, Salzman and Davies (1980) calculated that the cost per patient of this prophylactic method is slightly less than that of low-dose heparin given for 7 days postoperatively.

Finally, when we compared low-dose heparin and pneumatic compression in a randomized trial, we found that both methods were equally effective in preventing DVT, although there was significantly more bleeding and transfusions given to the group who received low-dose heparin. For this reason, pneumatic compression is the cornerstone of DVT prophylaxis in our institution (Clarke-Pearson et al, 1993).

MANAGEMENT OF COMMON MEDICAL PROBLEMS

Endocrine Disease

Diabetes Mellitus

Diabetes affects approximately 6% to 7% of all women between the ages of 20 and 74 and 15% of women between the ages of 65 and 74 (Jarrett, 1986). Diabetes can cause problems that affect the cardiovascular, renal, nervous, immune, and gastrointestinal systems. Also, if serum glucose is not controlled at the time of surgery, there may be up to a twofold increase in morbidity and a threefold increase in postoperative mortality. If a patient is not known to be diabetic but exhibits hyperglycemia in the perioperative setting, a glucose tolerance test should be performed that administers a 75-g load after an overnight fast following a 3-day diet that provides 300 g of carbohydrate each day. A diagnosis of diabetes can be made if the fasting glucose is greater than 140 mg/dl or if the 2-hour test is 200 mg/dl or higher.

Cardiovascular disease in diabetic patients accounts for more than 50% of all deaths (Porte and Halter, 1981). Women with non–insulin-dependent diabetes are four times more likely to suffer from myocardial infarction than similar age-adjusted controls and may develop cardiomyopathy or congestive heart failure (CHF) in the absence of coronary artery disease (CAD). Therefore, the preoperative evaluation should include an investigation of the diabetic's cardiovascular history, especially for symptoms of CHF. The physical examination must evaluate end-organ (cardiac, renal, ocular) damage in order to assess the patient's risk for surgical complications and to prevent problems.

Approximately 50% of longstanding diabetics will have nephropathy, and 70% will be hypertensive (Porte and Halter, 1981). Relative hyperkalemia secondary to a hyporeninemic hypoaldosteronism is also seen in patients with this disease. Strict attention

to fluid and electrolytes is necessary in these patients. Diabetics also have an increased risk of acute renal failure after receiving IV iodine contrast, especially if their serum creatinine is 2.0 mg/dl or higher, other vascular disease is present, or the onset of diabetes is before age 40.

Complications of diabetes also include defects in the autonomic nervous system, which innervates the esophagus, stomach, and small intestine, that can result in decreased esophageal and intestinal motility and delayed gastric emptying. These problems increase the risk of aspiration pneumonitis. The autonomic neuropathy also causes labile changes in pulse and blood pressure, and because of this these patients are known to be at increased risk for intraoperative myocardial infarction (Page and Watkins, 1978).

Diabetes can also predispose patients to infection. There is a known predisposition to gram-negative and staphylococcal pneumonia and an increased incidence of gram-negative and group B streptococcal sepsis (Wheat, 1980). Diabetics will have a sevenfold increase in postoperative gram-negative sepsis compared with the normal population. Sepsis is most often caused by Escherichia coli from the urinary tract (Abbott, 1967). On a cellular level, diabetic patients have defects in the ability to mobilize inflammatory cells, phagocytosis function, and bacteriocidal activity in polymorphonuclear neutrophils. These defects are related to poor glucose control (Rayfield et al, 1982). Decreased amounts of collagen formation, fibroblast growth, and capillary growth also account for the increased incidence of wound dehiscence (Weringer et al, 1982; McMurry, 1985). Patients with diabetes have approximately a 10% incidence of wound infection, compared with 1.8% in the nondiabetic population (Cruse and Foord, 1973).

Surgically related stress is known to increase serum glucose levels as well as to stimulate increases in the insulin antagonists glucagon, growth hormone, cortisol, norepinephrine, and epinephrine (Goldberg et al, 1981; Nesto et al, 1988). These adverse effects, however, are not seen when diabetics receive a regional anesthetic.

Preoperative management of insulin depends on whether the disease is controlled or not at the time of surgery. Controlled patients should exhibit no glucosuria, infrequent ketoacidosis, and a hemoglobin A1c of 6% or better. Goals include avoiding ketosis, hyperglycemia, and hypoglycemia. Failure to achieve these goals places these patients at risk for fluid and electrolyte disturbances, decreased immune function, osmotic diuresis, and ketoacidosis. The management in the perioperative period is based on whether the patient's disease is diet controlled, managed with an oral hypoglycemic, or controlled with insulin. If the disease is diet controlled, then this should be continued in the perioperative setting. Approximately 50% of the calories should come from carbohydrates, 35% from fat, and 25% should come from protein.

Patients on oral hypoglycemic agents should discontinue their medication the day of surgery and may tolerate a minor operation without insulin. Oral chlorpropamide-like agents need to be stopped the day before the surgery because of their long half-lives. These patients usually require insulin in the perioperative setting. Insulin does not need to be given unless the serum glucose is above 250 mg/dl. Clearly the most important concept to remember is that patients who have never had insulin administered to them are usually very sensitive to it, and great care must be taken so that significant hypoglycemia does not occur. If these patients have major surgery, they most often require a continuous infusion of insulin in 5% dextrose with 0.1 units of regular insulin/kg/L.

For the patients who are insulin dependent, the traditional regimen of giving one third to one half of the patient's total daily requirement of insulin as intermediate-acting insulin (e.g., NPH) the morning of surgery is believed by some authors to be inadequate (Walts et al, 1981). An alternative is to admit the patient 2 days prior to surgery and begin an insulin drip at 1 to 3 units/hour. Initially, glucose levels are monitored every 1 to 2 hours. After stabilization in the 100 to 200-mg/dl range, glucose monitoring every 4 hours is adequate.

Regardless of whether the patient has mild or severe disease, intraoperative glucose control is believed to be important in the overall management of diabetes. Intravenous insulin is given intraoperatively depending on serum glucose, which is checked every hour (Meyers et al, 1986). Glucose should be maintained in the 100- to 200-mg/dl range with 5% dextrose in 0.5 N or isotonic saline. Compulsive management of diabetes in the perioperative setting will yield better postoperative and long-term results.

Diabetic ketoacidosis may be seen if the serum glucose is greater than 350 mg/dl and the concentration of ketone bodies is greater than 5 mmol/L. Serum sodium levels are not predictable and may be high or low. Serum potassium levels are normal or elevated but total body potassium is depleted. Plasma phosphate and magnesium are usually low as well, but few biochemical abnormalities are predictable. Patients are usually acidotic and the serum bicarbonate level is low. In addition, amylase levels are often elevated. Finally, the white blood cell count is usually greater than 20,000/mm^3. Treatment preoperatively involves the correction of the blood pH to 7.3 and the bicarbonate level to greater than 20 mEq/L. In nonemergent situations, these corrections should be done at least 48 hours before the surgery. Dehydration and hypovolemia must be corrected immediately, and oftentimes Swan-Ganz catheter management is necessary. Saline (0.9 N) is the fluid of choice so that extracellular fluid depletion is corrected. Intravenous insulin should be administered until the serum glucose is less than 250 mg/dl. Finally, the causes that precipitated the ketoacidosis should be addressed (e.g., infection).

Hyperthyroidism

Grave's disease is the most common cause of hyperthyroidism and affects women more than men (10:1). Also known as diffuse toxic goiter, its management depends on preoperative recognition, which is crucial to avoid a catastrophic postoperative course that usually manifests as a thyroid storm (Goldman, 1987). The typical patient is between 20 and 40 years of age and usually presents with tachycardia, diaphoresis, palpitations, flushing, and weight loss. Physical examination may reveal a diffusely enlarged thyroid gland with a smooth or lobular contour. If the patient is severely thyrotoxic, fever, exophthalmos, hyperflexia, or tremors may be seen. Bruits can be heard over the lateral thyroid lobes from increased blood flow. Circulating immunoglobulins and intrathyroidal T lymphocytes, capable of binding to the thyroidal thyroid-stimulating hormone (TSH) receptor, cause increased levels of triiodothyronine (T_3) or thyroxine (T_4). Laboratory data including total T_4, free T_3, free T_4, and TSH are useful to confirm the clinical diagnosis.

Treatment with propylthiouracil (PTU) for at least 2 weeks before surgery in doses of 100 to 200 mg every 6 hours is the best approach in most patients. PTU inhibits thyroglobulin iodination and iodotyrosine coupling. In addition, it reduces extrathyroidal conversion of T_4 to T_3. Iodine blocks hormonal synthesis and release from the thyroid gland by inhibiting iodine uptake and organification by the follicular cell. SSKI (saturation solution of potassium iodine) is given 6 to 12 drops twice daily for about 10 to 14 days prior to surgery. It is useful in hyperthyroidism secondary to Grave's disease but is not appropriate in hyperthyroidism caused by thyroiditis and may exacerbate conditions if toxic nodular goiter exists. In addition, hydrocortisone 100 mg every 8 hours decreases extrathyroidal conversion of T_4 to T_3. Sympathomimetic symptoms may be controlled with β-blockers. Propranolol 10 to 80 mg every 6 to 8 hours is the most commonly used medication for relief of palpitation, tachycardia, diaphoresis, and anxiety (Geffner and Hershman, 1992). These treatments must be implemented at least 2 weeks prior to surgery and be continued postoperatively. Normalization of laboratory values prior to 2 weeks of treatment may give the clinician a false sense of security (Goldman, 1987). In addition, a careful examination of the airway by an anesthesiologist to exclude tracheal compression or deviation secondary to goiter is necessary preoperatively. Special care should be given to the eye during surgery to avoid injury precipitated by the exophthalmos. Several other anesthesia considerations include avoiding atropine and cyclopropane, which may exacerbate tachycardia and catecholamine release.

Avoidance of methoxyflurane, which undergoes toxic biotransformation, is also advised (Roizen, 1984).

Hypothyroidism

Hypothyroidism is a common problem seen in the perioperative setting. It affects almost 1% of the population. Fifty percent of all cases are caused by previous thyroid surgery or radioactive iodine treatments. Symptoms consist of lethargy, intolerance to cold, fatigue, weight gain, constipation, dry skin, memory impairment, and apathy. Physical findings include hoarseness, periorbital edema, dry skin, goiter, brittle hair, and an increased relaxation phase of deep tendon reflexes. Preoperative studies may also reveal cardiomegaly, pleural and pericardial effusions, ascites, and peripheral edema. Severe hypothyroidism can cause a myxedematous coma, which manifests as decreased consciousness, hypothermia, hypoventilation, and CHF. Laboratory results diagnostic of these problems include an elevated TSH and normal or decreased T_4 levels.

Preoperative preparation of hypothyroid patients requires slow replacement with levothyroxine. Levels of T_3, T_4, and TSH may normalize quickly, but organ abnormalities are slower to recover. It should be recognized that T_3, if given too fast, may cause cardiovascular collapse (Murkin, 1982). A decreased incidence of postoperative CNS depression and improved wound healing have been shown to correlate with a preoperative euthyroid state. Hypothyroid patients are sensitive to drugs that require metabolic transformation for their elimination. They are also more likely to experience hypoglycemic episodes, anemia, and hypothermia. In addition, their ability to excrete free water may be impaired, making them susceptible to hyponatremia (Anderson and Hausmann, 1956). Evidence shows that hypothyroid patients have an increased incidence of intraoperative hypotension, CHF, and ileus after abdominal surgery (Siddiq and Gebhart, 1988).

Adrenal Insufficiency/Iatrogenic Steroid Use

Several conditions that the gynecologist sees will require perioperative steroid treatment. The most common is long-term steroid use. Rarely, the gynecologist is operating on a patient with adrenal insufficiency caused by Addison's disease, adrenal metastasis, or previous removal of the adrenal glands. Several questions regarding steroid use need to be answered. First, what is the duration of steroid use required to produce hypothalamic-pituitary axis suppression? Second, how long after steroid use does it take for the axis to recover well enough to tolerate the stress of surgery? Third, how does the clinician evaluate the integrity of the axis?

Abnormal cortisol responses to metyrapone or ACTH have been observed after only 3 days of ste-roid administration. Similarly, cortisol response to insulin-induced hypoglycemia is significantly reduced after 2 days of prednisone use (25 mg/day) (Stehling, 1974). It may take up to 1 year for the hypothalamic-pituitary axis to recover after large doses of corticosteroids. Therefore, a detailed history regarding any steroid use should be obtained from all patients. If the patient is unsure, a preoperative ACTH test (250 μg) may be administered and the maximum cortisol response measured. If the cortisol level is normal, it is unlikely that a patient will develop perioperative hypotension secondary to impaired cortisol secretion (Kehlet and Binder, 1973).

Women on chronic steroid suppression or with Addison's disease should receive perioperative steroids. The replacement of glucocorticoids in the perioperative period is as follows (Gann et al, 1987):

1. Hydrocortisone 100 mg IM/IV, on call to the operating room
2. Hydrocortisone 100 mg IM/IV in recovery room then every 8 hours for three doses
3. Taper to maintenance dosage by 50% per day over next 3 to 5 days until the maintenance dose is reached
4. Increase cortisol dosage to 200 to 400 mg/day if fever, hypotension, or other complications occur

Hydration and antibiotics should be given as required.

Cardiovascular Diseases

In the past, gynecologic surgeons were relatively free from concerns about cardiovascular disease in their patients undergoing surgery. Over the last 20 years, however, there has been a large increase in the postmenopausal population and a larger group of gynecologic surgery patients who have a cardiovascular risk similar to their male counterparts. Despite these factors, the incidence of perioperative cardiovascular complications has decreased markedly because of improved preoperative detection of high-risk patients, improved preoperative preparation, and improved surgical and anesthetic techniques.

Preoperative Evaluation

The goal of a preoperative cardiac evaluation is to determine the presence of heart disease, its severity, and the potential risk to the patient in the perioperative period. Patients without known symptomatic cardiac atherosclerotic disease, significant dysrhythmias, valvular disease, or CHF are at very low risk of perioperative myocardial infarction or cardiac disease. Every patient should be carefully questioned about symptoms of cardiac disease such as chest pain, dyspnea on exertion, peripheral edema, wheezing, syncope, claudication, or palpitations. Patients with a prior history of cardiac disease should be closely evaluated for worsening of symptoms, which indicates progressive or poorly controlled disease. Old records are indispensable and every effort should be made to obtain them, particularly if the patient has received treatment at other institutions. Prescriptions for antihypertensive, anticoagulant, antiarrhythmic, antilipid, or antianginal medications may be the only hint of prior cardiovascular problems. In patients without known heart disease, the presence of diabetes, hyperlipidemia, hypertension, tobacco use, or a strong family history of heart disease identifies a group of patients at higher risk for heart disease and who should be more carefully screened.

The presence of physical exam findings such as hypertension, jugular venous distention, laterally displaced point of maximal impulse, irregular pulse, third heart sound, pulmonary rales, heart murmurs, peripheral edema, or vascular bruits should prompt a more complete evaluation. Laboratory evaluation of patients with known or suspected heart disease should include a blood count and serum chemistries. Anemia is poorly tolerated by patients with heart disease, and serum sodium and potassium levels are particularly important in patients taking diuretics and digitalis. BUN and creatinine values provide information on renal function and hydration status. Blood glucose levels may detect undiagnosed diabetes. A chest radiograph and ECG are mandatory as part of the preoperative evaluation and may be particularly helpful when compared with previous studies.

Coronary Artery Disease

CAD is responsible for the major risk to cardiac patients undergoing abdominal surgery. The incidence of myocardial infarction following surgery in an adult population is approximately 0.15% (Goldman et al, 1978). However, in patients who have a prior myocardial infarction, most studies report a reinfarction rate of about 5% (Goldman et al, 1978; Steen et al, 1978; Von Knorring, 1981). The risk of reinfarction was inversely proportional to the length of time between infarction and surgery (Steen et al, 1978). At 3 months or less, the risk of reinfarction is approximately 30% and from 3 to 6 months the rate falls to 12%. Six months after myocardial infarction the risk of death as a result of a perioperative infarction is similar to that in patients who have no prior history of ischemic heart disease. Fortunately, it has been demonstrated that careful perioperative management can lower the reinfarction rate even in patients with recent infarctions (Rao et al, 1983). This is important because perioperative myocardial infarction is associated with a 50% mortality rate (Tarhan et al, 1972; Von Knorring, 1981).

Because of the high mortality and morbidity associated with perioperative myocardial infarction, much effort has been made to predict perioperative cardiac risk. Goldman and colleagues (1977) prospectively evaluated preoperative cardiac risk factors and, using a multivariate analysis, identified independent cardiac risk factors (Table 41–12). Using these factors, a cardiac risk index was created that places a patient into one of four risk classes (Table 41–13). Unstable angina, probably because it is relatively uncommon, did not appear as a risk factor, although many believe that patients with unstable angina should be considered at extremely high risk of perioperative cardiac mortality and should undergo a coronary artery angiography and revascularization procedure prior to any elective gynecologic surgery.

Subsequently, several studies have validated and modified the Goldman criteria (Zeldin, 1984; Detsky et al, 1986; Larsen et al, 1987). However, it is important to understand the limited sensitivity of these indexes. For example, most of the risk of a bad outcome in a patient undergoing pelvic exenteration lies in the risk of the procedure itself. Risk indexes may

Table 41–12. RISK FACTORS ASSOCIATED WITH PERIOPERATIVE MYOCARDIAL INFARCTION

INDEPENDENT RISK FACTORS	POINTS*
• Jugular venous distention or S_3 gallop immediately preoperatively	11
• Myocardial infarction in preceding 6 months	10
• Presence of premature atrial contractions on preoperative ECG or any rhythm other than sinus	7
• More than 5 premature ventricular contractions per minute preoperatively	7
• Evidence of significant aortic valvular stenosis	3
• Age >70	5
• Emergency operation	
• Intraperitoneal operation	3
• Poor general medical condition:	3
$\quad PO_2$ <60 or PCO_2 >50 mm Hg	
$\quad$ K <3.0 or HCO_3 <20 mEq/L	
$\quad$ BUN >50 or creatinine >3.0 mg/dl	
$\quad$ Liver disease or debilitated patient	

*Points to be added to place patient into risk class (see Table 41–13).

Table 41–13. RISK CLASS AND OCCURRENCE OF PERIOPERATIVE CARDIAC COMPLICATION

CLASS	SCORE*	TOTAL NO. OF PATIENTS	% PATIENTS WITH LIFE-THREATENING COMPLICATIONS[†] OR DEATH
I	0–5	537	5 (1%)
II	6–12	316	21 (7%)
III	13–25	130	18 (14%)
IV	≥26	18	14 (78%)

*Score derived from factors listed in Table 41–12.
[†]Life-threatening complications are documented: intraoperative or postoperative myocardial infarction, pulmonary edema, or ventricular tachycardia without progression to cardiac death.
Data from Goldman L, Caldera DL, Nussbaum SR, et al: Multifactorial index of cardiac risk in noncardiac surgical procedures. N Engl Med J 1977;297:845, with permission.

be helpful to stratify the risk of an individual within the group of exenteration patients. This explains why a high score on risk assessment in a patient undergoing an anterior colporrhaphy has a much different implication than the same score obtained on a patient undergoing exenteration.

Foster and his colleagues (1986) followed patients from the Coronary Artery Surgery Study registry who subsequently underwent major noncardiac surgical procedures. These 1600 patients had CAD and left ventricular function defined by angiography. Multivariate analysis of potential risk factors found only dyspnea on exertion and left ventricular wall motion score to be independently predictive of perioperative cardiac mortality. Contrary to Goldman et al's (1978) analysis, in this study a history of previous myocardial infarction was not an independent risk factor. The authors thought that this implied that the degree of left ventricular wall dysfunction was more critical than the less objective information provided by a history of infarction. Conversely, preoperative angiography is an invasive procedure that is less clinically feasible than clinical evaluation of risk using the criteria proposed by Goldman.

The importance of clinical predictors in preoperative assessment is underscored by the publication of the American College of Cardiology/American Heart Association task force guidelines for perioperative cardiovascular evaluation. A stepwise approach is utilized that divides patients into three groups based on major, intermediate, and minor clinical predictors (Table 41–14). Patients with major predictors present are at high risk of adverse events and require intensive evaluation. Patients with intermediate or minor clinical predictors are further evaluated by their functional status. Functional status reliably predicts adverse cardiac events (Weiner et al, 1984) and is expressed in metabolic equivalent (MET) levels. The oxygen consumption of a 40-year-old, 70-kg man at rest is 3.5 mL/kg/minute, or 1 MET. Functional capacity is classified as excellent (>7 MET), moderate (4 to 7 MET), or poor (<4 MET). The Duke Activity Status Index provides correlation between historical information and functional status (Table 41–15) (Hlatky et al, 1989).

In an effort to quantitate preoperative cardiac risk, several tests have been utilized to assess cardiovascular function. Exercise stress testing prior to surgery can identify patients who have ischemic heart disease not present at rest. These patients have been shown to be at increased risk of developing cardiac complications in the perioperative period. In a study of patients undergoing peripheral vascular surgery, Cutler and associates (1981) identified a high-risk group of patients who had ischemic ECG changes when they exercised to less than 75% of their maximal predicted heart rate. This group had a 25% incidence of perioperative myocardial infarction and an overall 18.5% cardiac mortality rate. Conversely, patients who were able to exercise to greater than

Table 41–14. CLINICAL PREDICTORS OF RISK OF PERIOPERATIVE CARDIAC EVENTS

MAJOR CLINICAL PREDICTORS	INTERMEDIATE CLINICAL PREDICTORS	MINOR CLINICAL PREDICTORS
• Unstable coronary syndromes • Decompensated CHF • Significant arrhythmias • Severe valvular disease	• Mild angina pectoris • Prior MI • Compensated or prior CHF • Diabetes mellitus	• Advanced age • Abnormal ECG • Rhythm other than sinus • Low functional capacity • History of stroke • Uncontrolled systemic hypertension

Abbreviations: CHF, congestive heart failure; ECG, electrocardiogram; MI, myocardial infarction.

Table 41–15. EVALUATION OF PREOPERATIVE FUNCTIONAL STATUS*

1 MET
   Take care of yourself
   Eat, dress, or use the toilet
   Walk indoors around the house
   Walk a block or two on level ground at 2–3 mph
     (3.2–4.8 km/hr)
   Do light work around the house like dusting or washing
     dishes
4 METs
   Climb a flight of stairs or walk up a hill
   Walk on level ground at 4 mph (6.4 km/hr)
   Run a short distance
   Do heavy work around the house like scrubbing floors
     or lifting or moving heavy furniture
   Participate in moderate recreational activities like golf,
     bowling, dancing, doubles tennis, or throwing a
     baseball or football
>10 METs
   Participate in strenuous sports like swimming, singles
     tennis, football, basketball, or skiing

*Estimated energy requirements expressed as metabolic equivalent units (METs).

75% of their maximal predicted heart rate and had no ECG evidence of ischemia had no perioperative myocardial infarctions. However, the prognostic value of stress testing was not supported in another prospective study that found that only an abnormal preoperative resting ECG was an independent risk factor (Carliner et al, 1985). However, five of six major events occurred in patients with impaired exercise tolerance, suggesting that exercise tolerance may be more important than the ECG response. The exercise stress test must be selectively applied to a high-risk population because its predictive value is dependent on the prevalence of the disease. Therefore, it is not prudent to screen all patients preoperatively; rather, it is preferable to rely on a careful history to identify a group with symptoms of cardiac disease for whom the test would be the most predictive, such as those with new chest pain or those in whom coronary disease status is unclear by history.

Exercise stress testing is limited in some patients who cannot exercise because of musculoskeletal disease, pulmonary disease, or severe cardiac disease. The dipyridamole-thallium scan may be used to overcome the limitations of exercise stress testing. This sensitive and specific study relies on the ability of dipyridamole to dilate normal coronary arteries but not stenotic vessels. Normally perfused myocardium readily takes up thallium when given intravenously. Conversely, hypoperfused myocardium does not demonstrate good uptake of thallium when scanned 5 minutes after injection. Reperfusion and uptake of thallium 3 hours after injection identifies viable but high-risk myocardium. Old infarctions are identified as areas without uptake. Several studies have shown a risk of perioperative myocardial infarction in patients with areas of reperfusion of thallium uptake ranging from 20% to 33%. However, a more recent study (Baron et al, 1994) of 457 consecutive patients indicated that preoperative dipyridamole-thallium scans did not accurately predict adverse cardiac outcomes and should therefore not be utilized for screening. The dipyridamole-thallium scan may be helpful for high-risk patients who are unable to exercise because it uses a medically induced "stress."

The resting multiple gated acquisition (MUGA) blood pool study provides another test to evaluate cardiac risk in patients who are unable to exercise. Although this test does not directly evaluate CAD, it has been shown to correlate with perioperative cardiac risk. Pasternack and co-workers (1985) studied 100 patients preoperatively with resting MUGA scans, and found the incidence of postoperative myocardial infarction was 19% if the ejection fraction was greater than 35% but increased to 75% with ejection fractions less than 35%. Another large study failed to confirm this association, and the role of preoperative MUGA scans remain unclear (Baron et al, 1994). Although left ventricular dysfunction, which can be diagnosed by echocardiography, is a predictor of perioperative cardiac morbidity, there is no evidence that resting echocardiography is helpful in predicting adverse outcomes. By utilizing dobutamine to increase heart rate, "stress" echocardiography can be performed. In a series of 300 patients, all of the 27 cardiac adverse events occurred in the 72 patients who had positive stress echocardiograms (Poldermans et al, 1995). Patients without clinical risk factors, however, rarely had positive tests (12%), thus limiting stress echocardiography as a screening test.

It is rare for patients who are less than 50 years old and who do not have diabetes, hypertension, hypercholesterolemia, or CAD to suffer a perioperative myocardial infarction. Conversely, patients with CAD are at increased risk of myocardial infarction in the postoperative period. Prevention, early recognition, and treatment are important because myocardial infarctions that occur in the postoperative period are more highly lethal than those that are not associated with surgery, with mortality rates of approximately 50%.

Nearly two thirds of postoperative myocardial infarctions occur during the first 3 postoperative days. Although the pathophysiologic factors are complex, the causes of postoperative myocardial ischemia and infarction are related to decreased myocardial oxygen supply coupled with increased myocardial oxygen requirements. Conditions commonly present in postoperative patients that decreased oxygen supply to the myocardium include tachycardia, increased preload, hypotension, anemia, and hypoxia. Those that cause increased myocardial oxygen consumption are tachycardia, increased preload, increased afterload, and increased contractility. Of all these factors, tachycardia and increased preload are the most important causes of ischemia, because both decrease oxygen supply to the myocardium while increasing myocardial oxygen demand. Tachycardia decreases the time in diastole, which is when the coronary arteries are perfused, thus decreasing the volume of oxygen available to the myocardium. Increased preload increases the pressure exerted by the myocardial wall on the arterioles within it, thus decreasing myocardial blood flow.

Other factors that have been associated with perioperative cardiac ischemia include physiologic responses to the stress of intubation, intravenous or intra-arterial line placement, emergence from anesthesia, pain, and anxiety. This stress results in catecholamine stimulation of the cardiovascular system, resulting in increased heart rate, blood pressure, and contractility, which may induce or worsen myocardial ischemia. Loss of intravascular volume because of third-spacing of fluids or postoperative hemorrhage can induce ischemia as well.

Patients with CAD may benefit from pharmacologic control of hyperadrenergic states that result from increased postoperative catecholamine production. β-Blockers decrease heart rate, myocardial contractility, and systemic blood pressure, all of which are increased by adrenergic stimulation. Perioperative β-blockade has been shown to significantly reduce arrhythmias and myocardial infarctions. Certainly, patients receiving β-blockade therapy prior to surgery should continue to receive it in the perioperative period, because abrupt withdrawal results in a rebound hyperadrenergic state.

Labetalol, a mixed α- and β-receptor blocker, may also be useful in patients with CAD who are also hypertensive, because reflex tachycardia is limited. Additionally, labetalol has been shown to have antiarrhythmic effects. In patients with asthma, which can be exacerbated by sympathomimetic β-blockers, the use of esmolol is advantageous because it is a cardioselective β-blocker without intrinsic sympathomimetic activity and thus should not cause bronchoconstriction.

Although prophylactic nitrates have been used in the perioperative period for many years, this practice remains controversial. Nitroglycerin enhances blood flow to ischemic areas, increases collateral flow, increases myocardial oxygenation, and reduces angina. The route of administration, dosage, and duration of therapy are controversial as well; thus, perioperative treatment with nitrates should be initiated in conjunction with consultation with a cardiologist (Coriat et al, 1984; Gallagher et al, 1986).

Nifedipine, a calcium channel blocker, may be given sublingually in the postoperative period. It lowers blood pressure by selectively dilating arteries and begins to decrease blood pressure in 5 minutes, with plateauing in 30 minutes (Pedersen et al, 1980). The ultimate fall in blood pressure is related to the degree of hypertension initially present because vasodilation is more profound in patients with hypertension. Care must be taken when giving this drug, because ischemia and myocardial infarction have been reported following hypotension associated with nifedipine (Lacche and Basaglia, 1983).

Congestive Heart Failure

Patients with CHF face a substantially increased risk of myocardial infarction during surgery. The postoperative development of pulmonary edema is a grave prognostic sign and results in death in a high percentage of patients. Because patients with heart failure at the time of surgery are significantly more likely to develop pulmonary edema perioperatively, every effort should be made to diagnose and treat CHF prior to operating. The signs and symptoms of CHF are listed in Table 41–16 and should be sought on preoperative history and physical exam. Patients who are able to perform usual daily activities without developing CHF are at limited risk of perioperative heart failure occurring.

To prevent severe postoperative complications, congestive heart failure must be corrected preoperatively. Treatment usually relies on aggressive diuretic therapy, although care must be taken to prevent dehydration, which may result in hypotension during the induction of anesthesia. Hypokalemia can result from diuretic therapy and is especially deleterious to patients who are also taking digitalis. In addition to diuretics and digitalis, treatment often includes the use of preload and afterload reducers. Optimal usage of these drugs and correction of CHF may be aided by the consultation of a cardiologist. In general, it is preferable to continue patients on their usual regimen of cardioactive drugs through the perioperative period. In patients with severe or intractable CHF, the perioperative measurement of left ventricular filling (wedge) pressure with a pulmonary artery catheter (Swan-Ganz) may be extremely helpful to guide perioperative fluid management (Kaplan, 1987).

Postoperative CHF results most frequently from excessive administration of intravenous fluids and blood products. Other common postoperative causes are myocardial infarction, systemic infection, pulmonary embolism, and cardiac arrhythmias. It is important to determine the cause of postoperative heart failure because successful treatment is based on simultaneous treatment of the underlying cause.

Diagnosis of postoperative CHF is often more difficult, because the signs and symptoms of CHF (listed in Table 41–16) are not specific and may result from other causes. The most reliable method of detecting CHF is by chest radiography, in which the

Table 41–16. SIGNS AND SYMPTOMS OF CONGESTIVE HEART FAILURE

- Presence of an S_3 gallop
- Jugular venous distention
- Lateral shift of the point of maximal impulse
- Lower extremity edema
- Basilar rales
- Increased voltage on ECG
- Evidence of pulmonary edema or cardiac enlargement on chest radiograph
- Tachycardia

presence of cardiomegaly or evidence of pulmonary edema is a helpful diagnostic feature.

Acute postoperative CHF frequently manifests as pulmonary edema. Treatment of pulmonary edema may include the use of intravenous furosemide, supplemental oxygen, intravenous morphine sulfate, and elevation of the head of the bed. Intravenous aminophylline may be useful if cardiogenic asthma is present. Laboratory evaluation, including an electrocardiogram, arterial blood gases, serum electrolytes, and renal function chemistries, should be expediently obtained. If the patient does not improve rapidly, she should be transferred to an intensive care unit.

Arrhythmias

Nearly all arrhythmias found in otherwise healthy patients are asymptomatic and of limited consequence. However, in patients with underlying cardiac disease, even brief episodes of arrhythmias may result in significant cardiac morbidity and mortality. Preoperative evaluation of arrhythmias by a cardiologist and anesthesiologist is important because many anesthetic agents and surgical stress contribute to the development or worsening of arrhythmias. In patients undergoing continuous cardiographic monitoring during surgery, Kuner and colleagues (1967) reported a 60% incidence of arrhythmias excluding sinus tachycardia. Although there has been some disagreement, most authors believed that patients with heart disease have an increased risk of arrhythmias. Commonly these are ventricular arrhythmias. Conversely, patients without cardiac disease are more likely to develop supraventricular arrhythmias during surgery. Those patients taking antiarrhythmic medications prior to surgery should continue on those drugs during the perioperative period. Initiation of antiarrhythmic medications is rarely indicated preoperatively, but patients in whom arrhythmias are detected prior to surgery should receive cardiology consultation.

Patients with first-degree atrioventricular (AV) block or asymptomatic Mobitz I (Wenckebach) second-degree AV block require no preoperative therapy. Conversely, those with symptomatic Mobitz II second-degree AV block or third-degree AV block should have a permanent pacemaker implanted before undergoing elective surgery. In emergency situations, a pacing pulmonary artery catheter can be used. Prior to performing surgery on patients with a permanent pacemaker, information as to the type and location of the pacemaker is important because electrocautery units may interfere with demand-type pacemakers. When performing gynecologic surgery on patients with pacemakers, it is preferable to place the electrocautery unit ground plate on the leg to minimize interference. In patients with a demand pacemaker in place, the pacemaker should be converted to the fixed-rate mode preoperatively.

Surgery is not contraindicated in patients with bundle-branch blocks or hemiblocks. Rarely do patients with conduction system disease develop complete heart block during noncardiac surgical procedures. However, the presence of left bundle-branch block may indicate the presence of aortic stenosis, which can increase surgical mortality if severe.

Valvular Heart Disease

Although there are many forms of valvular heart disease, primarily two types, aortic and mitral stenosis, are associated with significantly increased operative risk. Patients with significant aortic stenosis appear to be at greatest risk, which is further increased if atrial fibrillation, CHF, or CAD is also present. In general, patients with significant stenosis of aortic or mitral valves should have them repaired prior to undergoing elective gynecologic surgery.

Severe valvular heart disease is usually evident during physical examination. Common findings in such patients are listed in Table 41–17. The classical history presented by patients with severe aortic stenosis includes exercise dyspnea, angina, and syncope, whereas symptoms of mitral stenosis are paroxysmal and effort dyspnea, hemoptysis, and orthopnea. Most patients have a remote history of rheumatic fever. Severe stenosis of either valve is considered to be a valvular area of less than 1 cm^2, and diagnosis can be confirmed by echocardiography or cardiac catheterization.

Patients with any valvular abnormality should receive prophylactic antibiotics immediately preoperatively to prevent subacute bacterial endocarditis. Table 41–18 outlines the American Heart Association recommendations for antibiotic valvular prophylaxis.

Sinus tachycardias and other tachyarrhythmias are poorly tolerated by patients with aortic and mitral stenosis. In patients with aortic stenosis, it is important to provide sufficient digitalization to correct preoperative tachyarrhythmias, while propranolol may

---

Table 41–17. SIGNS AND SYMPTOMS OF VALVULAR HEART DISEASE

AORTIC STENOSIS
- Systolic murmur at right sternal border that radiates into carotids
- Decreased systolic blood pressure
- Apical heave
- Chest radiograph with calcified aortic ring, left ventricular enlargement
- ECG with high R waves, depressed T waves in lead I and precordial leads

MITRAL STENOSIS
- Precordial heave
- Diastolic murmur at apex
- Mitral opening snap
- Suffused face and lips
- Chest radiograph with left atrial dilation
- ECG with large P waves and right axis deviation

Table 41-18. AMERICAN HEART ASSOCIATION RECOMMENDATIONS FOR PROPHYLAXIS OF BACTERIAL ENDOCARDITIS

Standard Regimen
Ampicillin, 2 g, and gentamicin, 1.5 mg/kg IM or IV, 30 min to 1 hr before and 8 hr after procedure

Penicillin-Allergic Patients
Vancomycin, 1 g IV slowly over 1 hr, and gentamicin, 1.5 mg/kg IM or IV 1 hr before; may be repeated once in 12 hr if risk of bacteremia is prolonged

Oral Regimen for Minor Procedures in Low-Risk Patients
Amoxicillin, 3 g PO, 1 hr before and 1.5 g 6 hr later

From Katholi RE, Nolan SP, McGuire LB: The management of anticoagulation during noncardiac operations in patients with prosthetic heart valves. Am Heart J 1978;96:163, with permission.

be used to control sinus tachycardia. Patients with mitral valve stenosis often have atrial fibrillation and, if present, digitalis should be used to reduce rapid ventricular response.

Patients with mechanical heart valves usually tolerate surgery well. Management of these patients requires antibiotic prophylaxis (Table 41–18) and discontinuation of anticoagulant therapy during the perioperative period. Usually, warfarin (Coumadin) is withheld several days prior to surgery and anticoagulation is obtained by intravenous heparinization. The heparin is discontinued 6 to 8 hours prior to surgery and resumed a few days postoperatively. Ultimately the patient is returned to oral warfarin maintenance therapy. Alternatively, some authors recommend stopping the warfarin 1 to 3 days preoperatively and restarting it several days postoperatively. Both methods of management had no thromboembolic complications and had similar bleeding complication rates of approximately 15%.

In the postoperative period, patients with mitral stenosis should be carefully monitored for pulmonary edema, because they may not be able to compensate for the amount of intravenous fluid administered during surgery. Patients with mitral stenosis also frequently have pulmonary hypertension and decreased airway compliance. Therefore, they may require more pulmonary support and therapy postoperatively, including prolonged mechanical ventilation.

For patients with significant aortic stenosis, it is imperative that a sinus rhythm be maintained during the postoperative period. Even sinus tachycardia can be deleterious, because it shortens time in diastole. Bradycardia below 45 beats/minute should be treated with atropine. Supraventricular dysrhythmias may be controlled with verapamil or direct-current cardioversion. Particular attention should be provided to the maintenance of proper fluid status, digoxin levels, electrolyte levels, and blood replacement.

Hypertension

It appears that patients with a history of mild to moderate hypertension alone are at no greater perioperative risk of cardiac morbidity or mortality. However, patients with hypertension and heart disease have a 13% perioperative mortality rate. Therefore, the preoperative evaluation of patients with hypertension should emphasize diagnosis of target organ damage. Laboratory studies should include an ECG, chest radiograph, blood count, urinalysis, serum electrolytes, and creatinine. Patients with evidence of co-existent heart disease should undergo cardiac evaluation.

Patients with diastolic pressures greater than 110 mm Hg or systolic pressures greater than 180 mm Hg should have their hypertension controlled prior to surgery. During surgery, patients with chronic hypertension tend to have increased fluctuations in blood pressure. Chronically hypertensive patients are very susceptible to intraoperative hypotension because of an impaired autoregulation of blood flow to the brain, and therefore require a higher mean arterial pressure to maintain adequate perfusion. Additionally, hypertensive patients who also complain of sweating, palpitations, and headaches should be evaluated for a coexisting pheochromocytoma because this disease is associated with greatly increased perioperative mortality.

The treatment of early postoperative hypertension is usually limited to drugs that can be given parenterally, because absorption via the gastrointestinal mucosa may be diminished and transdermal absorption may be erratic in patients who are cold and are rewarming. Despite these difficulties, it is generally best to maintain antihypertensive medication postoperatively if blood pressures are elevated. Certainly, patients receiving preoperative β-blockade should be maintained on parenteral therapy to prevent rebound tachycardia, hypercontractility, and hypertension (O'Mailia et al, 1987).

Hematologic Disorders

Hematologic disorders, although infrequent in gynecology patients, can dramatically increase surgical morbidity and mortality and therefore should be routinely considered preoperatively. Preoperative evaluation should consider the following hematologic problems: (1) anemia and transfusion, (2) disorders of platelets and bleeding, (3) disorders of coagulation, and (4) disorders of white blood cells and immunity.

Anemia

The presence of moderate anemia in itself should not be a contraindication to surgery because it can be readily rectified by transfusion. However, if possible, surgery should be postponed until the cause of the anemia can be identified and the anemia corrected without resorting to the potential risks and expense of blood transfusion. Current anesthetic and surgical practice usually mandates a hemoglobin of 10 g/dl or more or a hematocrit of 30% or greater volume. Rather than strictly adhering to these levels, it is important to individualize application of these parameters for several reasons. First, more precisely, it is the circulating blood volume that provides oxygen-carrying capacity and tissue oxygenation. Although in most individuals this is accurately reflected by hemoglobin or hematocrit values, in certain situations it may not be. If there has been a recent blood loss, the hematocrit may remain normal although the blood volume is very low until the lost volume is replaced with extracellular fluid, which then results in a drop in hematocrit. Conversely, overly hydrated patients may exhibit low hematocrits or hemoglobins but may have a normal red cell mass.

Second, the patient's general physical condition determines her ability to tolerate anemia. The effects of anemia depend on the oxygen requirement of the patient, the rate at which the red cell mass decreases, the magnitude of the anemia, and the ability of compensatory physiologic mechanisms. To maintain the same cardiac output, a patient with a hemoglobin of 10 g/dl requires twice as much coronary blood flow as does a patient with a hemoglobin of 14 g/dl. Clearly, a patient with ischemic heart disease will not tolerate anemia as well as a healthy young patient. Therefore the presence of cardiac, pulmonary, or other serious illness justifies a more conservative approach to the management of anemia. Conversely, patients with longstanding anemia may have normal blood volumes and tolerate surgical procedures well. The National Institutes of Health Consensus Group (1989) has pointed out that there is no evidence that mild to moderate anemia increases perioperative morbidity or mortality.

If large perioperative blood losses are anticipated, patients with normal hematocrits are generally able to store at least three units of autologous blood preoperatively. Additionally, the use of recombinant human erythropoietin therapy may increase the amount of blood an autologous donor may store without developing anemia (Goodnough et al, 1989). Planning for intraoperative red cell recovery and reuse can also be useful in eliminating or reducing the need for homologous transfusions in selected patients.

Platelet and Coagulation Disorders

Surgical hemostasis is provided by platelet adhesion to an injured vessel, which plugs the opening as simultaneously the coagulation cascade is activated, forming a stabilizing fibrin clot. The presence of both functioning platelets and coagulation factors are thus necessary to prevent excessive surgical bleeding. Platelet disorders are more commonly encountered in the preoperative patient than are coagulation factor abnormalities.

Platelets may be deficient in both number and function. The normal peripheral blood platelet count ranges between 150,000 and 400,000/mm^3, and the normal life span of a platelet is approximately 10 days. Although there is no clear-cut correlation between the degree of thrombocytopenia and the presence or amount of bleeding, several generalizations can be made. If the platelet count is greater than 100,000/mm^3 and the platelets are functioning normally, there is little chance of bleeding during surgical procedures. Patients with a platelet count above 75,000/mm^3 almost always have normal bleeding times, and indeed a platelet count greater than 50,000/mm^3 is probably adequate. A platelet count below 20,000/mm^3 will often be associated with severe and spontaneous bleeding. Interestingly, platelet counts above 1,000,000/mm^3 are often paradoxically associated with bleeding.

If the patients platelet count is less than 100,000/mm^3, a bleeding time should be obtained. If the bleeding time is abnormal and surgery must be performed, an attempt should be made to raise the platelet count to that level by administering platelet transfusions immediately prior to surgery. In those patients with immune destruction of platelets, human leukocyte antigen donor-specific platelets may be required to prevent rapid destruction of transfused platelets. If surgery can be postponed, a hematology consultation should be obtained to identify and treat the cause of the platelet abnormality.

Abnormally low platelet counts result from either decreased production or increased consumption of platelets. Although there are numerous causes of thrombocytopenia, most are exceedingly uncommon. Decreased platelet production may be drug induced and has been most often associated with the use of thiazide diuretics or ethanol, although many other drugs have been sporadically implicated. Drugs may also cause immunologic thrombocytopenia by inducing the formation of cross-reacting antibodies that increase platelet destruction. Again, numerous drugs have been occasionally reported in this context, but certainly this mechanism has been convincingly demonstrated with quinine and sulfonamide usage. Frequently patients receiving cytotoxic chemotherapy or radiation therapy for the treatment of malignancies are thrombocytopenic.

Diseases that are characterized by decreased platelet production include vitamin B$_{12}$ and folate deficiencies, aplastic anemia, myeloproliferative disorders, renal failure, and viral infections. Inherited congenital thrombocytopenia is extremely rare. Much more commonly, thrombocytopenia results from immune destruction of platelets by diseases such as idiopathic thrombocytopenia purpura and collagen vascular disorders. Thrombocytopenia is caused by increased consumption of platelets in patients with disseminated intravascular coagulation (DIC). In a preoperative population, DIC nearly always is associated with the presence of malignancy or sepsis.

Platelet dysfunction may be inherited but it is much more likely to be acquired. Commonly prescribed drugs such as aspirin, amitriptyline, and nonsteroidal anti-inflammatory agents may cause decreased platelet function as well as numbers. Large doses of penicillin and carbenicillin have been shown to increase bleeding times. Patients who have prolonged bleeding times because of drug therapy should have those drugs withheld for 7 to 10 days before undergoing surgery. Uremia and liver disease are also common causes of poorly functioning platelets. von Willebrand's disease is the major inherited congenital disorder of platelet dysfunction. Although it is the second most common inherited coagulation disorder, it is extremely rare in a preoperative population.

Although the diagnosis of an abnormal platelet number is easily made by a blood count, the diagnosis of platelet dysfunction is most often made by a careful history and physical examination. The signs and symptoms of platelet abnormalities are easy bruisability, petechiae, bleeding from mucous membranes, or prolonged bleeding from minor cuts or wounds. A bleeding time will demonstrate clinically important platelet abnormalities. Further laboratory investigation is warranted in patients with abnormal bleeding times and should be obtained in conjunction with a hematology consultation. The preoperative evaluation must first determine the cause of the platelet abnormality so that corrective treatment can be initiated. Clearly, elective surgery should be postponed until therapy has been effected. Even in those patients in whom surgery must be performed expediently, the evaluation is helpful in predicting the magnitude of perioperative problems that may be encountered.

Disorders of coagulation factors are most often diagnosed by a thorough history and physical exam. Episodes of excessive bleeding following dental procedures, minor surgery, or childbirth, or during menses, or a family history of a bleeding diathesis may be indicators of a coagulation disorder. Inherited coagulation disorders are very uncommon, but, of these rare disorders, factor VIII deficiency (hemophilia), factor IX deficiency (Christmas disease), and von Willebrand's disease occur most frequently. There are few commonly prescribed drugs that affect coagulation factors, with the exception of warfarin and heparin. Disease states that may be associated with decreased coagulation factor levels are primarily liver disease, vitamin K deficiency (secondary to obstructive biliary disease, intestinal malabsorption, or antibiotic reduction of bowel flora), and DIC.

The use of preoperative laboratory screening for coagulation deficiencies is controversial. It appears, however, that routine screening in patients without historical evidence of a bleeding problem is not warranted. Conversely, patients who are seriously ill or who will be undergoing extensive surgical procedures should have a prothrombin time, partial thromboplastin time, fibrinogen level, and platelet count obtained preoperatively.

White Cells and Immune Function

Abnormally high or low white blood cell counts are not an absolute contraindication to surgery. However, they should be considered relative to the need for surgery. Evaluation of an elevated or decreased white blood cell count should be undertaken prior to elective surgery. Clearly patients with absolute granulocyte counts less than $1000/mm^3$ are at increased risk of severe infection and perioperative morbidity and mortality, and should only undergo surgery for life-threatening indications.

Pulmonary Disease

General Consideration

Patients undergoing abdominal surgery manifest several pulmonary physiologic changes secondary to immobilization, anesthetic irritation of the airways, and the splinting of breathing that inevitably occurs secondary to incisional pain. Pulmonary physiologic changes include a decrease in the functional residual capacity and vital capacity, an increase in ventilation-perfusion mismatching, and impaired mucociliary clearance of secretions from the tracheobronchial tree. These changes result in transient hypoxemia and atelectasis, which, if untreated, can progress to pneumonia in the postoperative period (Hotchkiss, 1988; Mohr and Jett, 1988). Postoperative pulmonary dysfunction is more pronounced in patients with advanced age, pre-existing lung disease, obesity, a significant smoking history, and upper abdominal surgery (Mohr and Jett, 1988).

The majority of postoperative pulmonary complications occur in patients who have pre-existing pulmonary disease. In these patients, the incidence of pulmonary complications is greater than 70%, as compared to the low incidence (2% to 5%) in individuals with healthy lungs. The risk of postoperative pulmonary complications is lower in patients who undergo lower abdominal as compared to upper abdominal surgery, and nonthoracic, nonabdominal surgery as compared to abdominal operation. The presence of COPD markedly increases the risk for all patients (Forthman and Shepard, 1969; Mohr and Jett, 1988).

Preoperative spirometry is of unproven value in patients undergoing abdominal surgery in whom the risk of postoperative pulmonary complications is low (Lawrence et al, 1989; Zibrak et al, 1990). In high-risk patients, preoperative spirometry should be performed with and without bronchodilators in order to identify patients who may benefit from preoperative treatment with inhaled β_2-agonists and steroids. These patients should include those with a history of chronic cough or dyspnea, evidence of pulmonary abnormalities by either physical examination or chest radiograph, and a known history of COPD, as well as those patients with a significant smoking history. In addition to the preoperative spirometric evaluation, an arterial blood gas should be performed.

Young, healthy patients rarely have abnormal chest radiographs. Therefore, chest radiographs should not be performed routinely in these patients. Most patients with abnormal chest radiographs have history or physical examination findings suggestive of pulmonary disease (Sagel et al, 1974; Loder, 1987; Lamers et al, 1989). Chest radiographs should be limited to patients over the age of 40, patients with a history of smoking, patients with a history of pulmonary disease, and patients who present with evidence of cardiopulmonary disease.

Chronic Obstructive Pulmonary Disease

COPD is the fourth leading cause of death in North America (Siafakas et al, 1995). Early diagnosis can be difficult because symptoms are usually minimal to absent until late in the course of the disease. Simple spirometry remains the easiest and most reliable method for detecting changes consistent with COPD, which is heralded by an accelerated deterioration in the forced expiratory volume in 1 second (FEV_1) as compared to baseline (Chapman, 1992).

In contrast to asthma, COPD is characterized by progressive and incompletely irreversible airflow obstruction. Cholinergic agents such as the inhaled quaternary anticholinergic drugs (ipratropium bromide) offer greater bronchodilation than that seen with β_2-agonists. In addition, less than 10% of patients will benefit from steroid therapy, in stark contrast to the majority of patients with asthma, who will benefit from the anti-inflammatory effect of steroidal therapy. Cessation of smoking decreases the accelerated rate of lung deterioration in patients with COPD. Other preventive measures include the use of pneumococcal and influenza vaccines and the initiation of bronchodilator therapy. In those patients with severe COPD, long-term oxygen therapy has been shown to significantly prolong life.

The term *COPD* has been used to encompass both chronic bronchitis and emphysema, disease entities that often occur in tandem (Flenley, 1988). Chronic bronchitis has been defined as the presence of productive cough on most days for at least 3 months per year and for at least 2 successive years (Hensley and Fencl, 1981). It is characterized by chronic airway inflammation and by excessive mucus production. The histologic changes of emphysema include destruction of the alveolar septa and distention of air spaces distal to terminal alveoli. The destruction of alveolar septa is most likely caused by serine elastase, released by neutrophils exposed to cigarette smoke (Flenley, 1988). The destruction of alveoli results in air trapping, loss of pulmonary elastic recoil, collapse of the airways in expiration, increased work of breathing, significant ventilation-perfusion mismatching, and, most importantly, ineffective cough (Blosser and Rock, 1990). The impaired ability for effective cough and clearance of secretions predis-

poses patients with COPD to atelectasis and pneumonia in the postoperative period.

Pulmonary function testing can be used to quantitate the severity of obstructive disease (Mohr and Jett, 1988). Patients with COPD will typically demonstrate impaired expiratory flow, manifested by diminished FEV_1, forced vital capacity (FVC), FEV_1/FVC, and maximal expiratory flow rate (MEFR). Arterial blood gases should be obtained preoperatively and may show varying degrees of hypoxemia and/or hypercapnia. An arterial partial pressure of oxygen (PaO_2) less than 70 mm Hg and an arterial partial pressure of carbon dioxide ($PaCO_2$) greater than 45 mm Hg are associated with a marked increase in the risk of postoperative pulmonary complications and with an increased risk of requirement for postoperative mechanical ventilation (Milledge and Nunn, 1975).

Stein and colleagues (1962) used pulmonary function testing to identify a group of surgical patients at risk for postoperative pulmonary complications. Patients at risk were selected by an abnormal single nitrogen breath test, diminished MEFR (<200 L/minute), or increased PCO_2 (>45 mm Hg). Patients with abnormal pulmonary function tests had a 70% incidence of postoperative pulmonary complications, as compared with a 3% incidence of complications in patients who had normal spirograms. In patients considered to be at high risk, the incidence of complications was highest in those undergoing abdominal surgery (92%) or thoracic surgery (78%) and lowest in those undergoing surgery outside the abdomen (26%).

In gynecologic surgical patients, the risk of postoperative pulmonary complications is confined mainly to those patients with a heavy smoking history and to patients with COPD. In these patients, prophylactic pulmonary measures should be instituted preoperatively and continued postoperatively to minimize the incidence of atelectasis and pneumonia. Several studies have suggested that preoperative pulmonary preparation of patients with preexisting lung disease can significantly decrease the incidence of postoperative pulmonary complications. In a study including 464 patients with COPD (Tarhan et al, 1973) who underwent a variety of surgical procedures, preoperative preparation, including chest physiotherapy, bronchodilators, and antibiotic therapy (for patients with positive sputum cultures), decreased the incidence of pulmonary complications from 43.1% to 23.7%. In another series of 157 patients with COPD, a 48-hour preoperative preparation including inhaled β-adrenergic agonists, oral theophylline, and chest physiotherapy resulted in improvement in measured spirometric parameters, improved PaO_2 and $PaCO_2$, and a lower postoperative pulmonary complication rate (Gracey et al, 1979). There was no correlation, however, between the degree of improvement in spirometric parameters and postoperative pulmonary outcome. In one randomized study (Stein and Cassara, 1970), poor-risk patients who stopped smoking and received bronchodilator drugs, antibiotics, inhalation of humidified gases, postural drainage, and chest physiotherapy had a significant decrease in the incidence of postoperative pulmonary complications, from 60% to 22%. In addition, the treatment group had decreased severity of complications and enjoyed a shorter length of hospital stay. Finally, the timing of administration of perioperative prophylactic pulmonary measures is important in that measures instituted preoperatively and continued postoperatively are more effective in reducing the incidence of postoperative pulmonary complications than measures instituted solely in the postoperative period (Castillo and Haas, 1985).

Our approach to the preoperative preparation of the patient at high risk for postoperative pulmonary complications includes cessation of smoking for as long as possible. Two days of smoking abstinence is sufficient for returning carboxyhemoglobin levels to normal (Anderson and Belani, 1990). However, 2 months of smoking abstinence is necessary to significantly lower the risk of postoperative pulmonary complications (Warner et al, 1989). Therefore, it is optimal to attempt cessation of smoking for as long as possible in those patients who are undergoing elective surgery. Pulmonary function should be optimized with the use of inhaler therapy preoperatively. The anticholinergic inhaled agents should form the mainstay of therapy for patients with COPD. Inhaled β-adrenergic agonists can also provide additive effects. These agents should be started at least 72 hours preoperatively, particularly in those patients who have demonstrated clinical or spirometric improvement on bronchodilators. Approximately 10% of patients with COPD will benefit from steroid therapy, and these patients can be identified with a steroid challenge (prednisone or its equivalent, 0.5 mg/kg for 2 or 3 weeks) (Chapman, 1996). In patients with a suppurative cough and positive sputum culture, a full course of antibiotic therapy can be used preoperatively whenever possible. The antibiotics used should cover the most likely etiologic organisms, *Streptococcus pneumoniae* and *Haemophilus influenzae*. Surgery should be delayed if possible in patients with acute upper respiratory infections. Finally, instruction in deep breathing maneuvers and chest physical therapy are simple to institute, and these measures can be started the evening prior to surgery (Hotchkiss, 1988).

Asthma

Approximately 5% of the U.S. population suffers from asthma (Blosser and Rock, 1990). The disease is a chronic inflammatory condition of the airways and is associated with hyperresponsiveness of the tracheobronchial tree and variable, reversible obstruction of the airways. Multiple "triggers" are known to precipitate or exacerbate asthma, including inflammatory factors (upper respiratory infections, allergens, and chemical sensitizers), and bronchospastic factors, which include exercise, cold air, emotional stress, β-adrenergic blockers, and aspirin (Hensley and Fencl, 1981; Cockroft, 1990). The management of asthma requires the use of anti-inflammatory therapy for all but those patients with the mildest asthma, in order to address the inflammatory component of the disease as well as remove inciting stimuli in those individuals in whom "triggers" can be identified. Despite the advances in the pharmacotherapeutic management of asthma over the past 10 years, morbidity and mortality from asthma have been increasing (Galant, 1990; Li, 1996).

The preoperative work-up of the asthmatic patient should direct particular attention to the pulmonary examination, chest film, arterial blood gas values, and pulmonary function testing. Pulmonary function testing should be performed with and without inhaled bronchodilators. This work-up is necessary to assess the current state of the airways as well as to reveal the presence of any underlying obstructive pulmonary disease. Although pulmonary function testing may be normal in patients who truly have mild asthma, patients with moderate to severe asthma may exhibit peak expiratory flow rates that are 60% to 80% of normal or lower (Hargreave, 1990; Li, 1996).

The pathophysiology of asthma involves a chronic inflammatory reaction in the airways; in fact, some refer to asthma as a chronic eosinophilic bronchitis (Barnes, 1989). Various mediators released in the lungs by eosinophils or macrophages induce microvascular leakage, bronchoconstriction, and epithelial damage, which blocks the distal airways. Mast cell degranulation is not involved in this inflammatory component but rather is involved with the bronchoconstriction associated with the early response to allergen. Histologic examination of the airways reveals epithelial cell injury, mucosal edema, smooth muscle hypertrophy, and hyperplasia of submucosal mucous glands.

In the past, bronchodilator therapy was the mainstay in first-line pharmacotherapy for asthma. However, the growing appreciation of asthma as a chronic inflammatory disease has led to the use of anti-inflammatory therapy as the mainstay of treatment. More recent published guidelines for the management of asthma have recommended that anti-inflammatory treatment be initiated for all but the patients with the mildest forms of asthma. The primary component of anti-inflammatory therapy is inhaled corticosteroids, and, for moderate to severe asthmatics, these agents are to be used chronically. Corticosteroids inhibit mediator release from eosinophils and macrophages, inhibit the late response to allergens, and reduce hyper-responsiveness of bronchioles (Barnes, 1989). Most asthmatics can be adequately controlled on low-dose, inhaled steroids (less than 500 μg/day). Up to 2 mg/day can be inhaled without clinically significant adrenal suppression or significant adverse systemic effects. The onset of action is slow (several hours), and up to 3 months of steroid therapy may be required for optimal improvement of bronchial hyper-responsiveness. For patients with acute exacerbations of asthma, a short course of oral steroids (40 to 60 mg of prednisone per day) may be necessary. Rarely will patients with chronic asthma require chronic oral steroid therapy. Those patients who are taking oral steroids should receive a steroid preparation perioperatively for stress coverage. A number of inhaled steroids currently are available, including beclomethasone, budesonide, and the highly potent steroid flunisolide (Wasserfallen and Baraniuk, 1996).

Until recently, β_2-adrenergic agonists were considered the first-line drugs for asthma. These drugs, inhaled four to six times daily, rapidly relax smooth muscle in the airways and are effective for up to 6 hours. Studies of β_2-agonists in chronic asthma, however, have failed to show any influence of these agents on the inflammatory component of asthma. Furthermore, some have suggested that the long-term use of this class of drugs can lead to a worsening of asthma. Thus β_2-agonists are now recommended for use for short-term relief of bronchospasm or as first-line treatment for patients with very infrequent symptoms or symptoms provoked solely by exercise.

Methylxanthines, such as theophylline, have been relegated to third-line status in the management of asthma. It is questionable whether these drugs add any additional benefit in patients who are on maximal inhaler therapy. The xanthines are limited by their narrow therapeutic window. It is necessary to achieve a serum concentration of at least 10 μg/ml, but at levels greater than 20 μg/ml significant toxicity develops, including nausea, tremor, and CNS excitation. Xanthines have a limited anti-inflammatory effect, and have no effect on bronchial hyper-responsiveness or eosinophilic degranulation. In addition, it is important to note that plasma concentrations can be altered by drugs, or environmental factors, requiring an adjustment in the theophylline dose. Smoking and phenobarbital, for example, increase clearance of theophylline by the liver, whereas clearance of theophylline is decreased with hepatic disease, cardiac failure, or the concomitant use of certain drugs, including ciprofloxacin, cimetidine, erythromycin, and troleandomycin.

Anticholinergic agents are weak bronchodilators that work via inhibition of muscarinic receptors in the smooth muscle of the airways. The quaternary derivatives such as ipratropium bromide (Atrovent) are available in an inhaled form that is not absorbed systemically. Anticholinergic drugs may provide additional benefit in conjunction with standard steroid and bronchodilator therapy but should not be used as single-agent therapy because they do not inhibit mast cell degranulation, have no effect on the late response to allergens, and do not have an anti-inflammatory effect.

Cromolyn sodium is highly active in the treatment of seasonal allergic asthma in children and young adults. It is usually not as effective in older patients or in patients in whom asthma is not allergic in character. The drug is taken by inhalation but has a relatively short duration of action (3 to 4 hours). It has a mild anti-inflammatory effect but is less effective than inhaled corticosteroids, and its role as a single agent is limited.

In asthmatics, elective surgery should be postponed whenever possible until pulmonary function and pharmacotherapeutic management are optimized. For the mild asthmatic, this may simply require the use of inhaled β-adrenergic agonists preoperatively. For the chronic asthmatic, optimization of steroid therapy will greatly decrease alveolar inflammation and bronchiolar hyper-responsiveness. Inhaled β_2-agonists should be added as needed for further control of asthma. Each drug prescribed should be used in maximal dosage before adding an additional agent. For patients undergoing emergent surgery who have significant bronchoconstriction, a multimodal approach should be instituted, including aggressive bronchodilator inhalation therapy, intravenous methylxanthines, and steroid therapy. Ideally, the steroid therapy can be instituted 3 to 6 days preoperatively. In all asthmatics, pharmacotherapeutic response can be monitored with pulmonary function testing as demonstrated by an improvement in the peak expiratory flow rate.

Renal Disease

Renal failure is defined as alterations in volume regulation and ionic composition of body fluids and inadequate excretion of body waste. Renal insufficiency (RI) is a spectrum of diseases and may be associated with a high perioperative morbidity and mortality (Pinson et al, 1986). Management of patients with RI and prevention of iatrogenically induced renal dysfunction in gynecologic surgery patients requires an understanding of the etiology of RI and the metabolic disturbances that develop secondary to RI.

The most common etiologic factors leading to end-stage renal disease include glomerulonephritis (28%), pyelonephritis (20%), hereditary factors, diabetes, and hypertensive diseases (Broyer et al, 1986).

Hematologic abnormalities, namely a chronic normocytic, normochromic anemia, are common in RI patients. As opposed to a normal patient, these women tolerate the stress of surgery well at hematocrits around 25% (Lundin et al, 1987) and routine transfusion is not necessary before surgery. Recombinant erythropoietin is successful in increasing the hematocrit when administered to anemic patients preoperatively. Up to a month may be necessary to see the desired increase (Eschbach et al, 1987).

Patients with chronic renal failure (CRF) are susceptible to strange coagulation abnormalities that are manifested as increased bleeding times. Prolonged bleeding time is thought to be due to platelet dysfunction caused by a decreased amount of factor VIII/von Willebrand antigen in serum of uremic patients. Cryoprecipitate, desmopressin, and conjugated estrogens are given to patients with CRF to improve the bleeding time (Mannucci et al, 1983; Livio et al, 1986). In addition, dialysis particularly improves these coagulation abnormalities. To date, the theoretical risk of potentiating thromboembolic phenomena with these agents has not been carefully studied. Women with chronic RI also are at increased risk for postoperative gastrointestinal bleeding and stress ulcers, and should therefore receive prophylaxis with antacids, histamine blockers, or sucralfate both pre- and postoperatively. Unless aluminum toxicity is suspected, sucralfate is a desirable choice because of its antibacterial effect on enteric flora, which reduces the incidence of nosocomial pneumonia in patients who subsequently aspirate (Driks et al, 1987).

For the uremic patient whose host defense mechanisms are depressed, broad-spectrum antibiotics are indicated preoperatively to prevent infection. Abnormalities in neutrophil and monocyte function and a depressed anergy status have all been reported in women with RI (Mullen et al, 1980; Lewis and Van Epps, 1987). Preoperative nutritional support may also help reduce these infectious complications.

Chronic RI impairs a patient's ability to excrete medications, and the metabolic derangements alter the bioavailability of many common drugs. The effect of dialysis on drug availability is also an important concept the surgeon must understand. Narcotics, barbiturates, muscle relaxants, antibiotics, and chemotherapeutic agents are medications that require renal clearance. Their metabolism may be significantly affected depending on the severity of the RI.

Fluid management is important in patients with RI. Ischemic heart disease is the most common cause of death in patients with RI, but it is not a major cause of mortality in surgical patients with impaired renal function (Broyer et al, 1986). Intravascular and extravascular fluid shifts leading to hyper- or hypotension are common and are difficult to manage because of autonomic dysfunction, acidosis, and other problems inherent to RI. Because physical examination and central venous pressure monitoring correlate poorly with left cardiac filling pressures, women with RI undergoing major abdominal and pelvic surgery may be optimally managed by invasive intraoperative monitoring with a pulmonary artery catheter. This intensive management should be continued during the first postoperative week because the reabsorption of "third-spaced" fluid will occur during this time. Prompt dialysis may avoid serious problems associated with fluid overload and hyperkalemia.

Patients on long-term maintenance dialysis are usually dialyzed 24 hours before surgery and the day after. Severe, refractory hyperkalemia may also require dialysis. If dialysis cannot be performed emergently, hyperkalemia can be treated with a 10% calcium chloride solution (5 to 10 ml). Other, less aggressive measures include $NaHCO_3$ with glucose and insulin or Kayexalate enemas. However, advances in dialysis therapy, including its availability, the timing, its metabolic consequences, its effect on hematologic abnormalities, fewer infectious complications, and improvements in pharmacology and cardiovascular management, may all improve the perioperative outcome of these patients.

Perioperative renal failure in normal patients may be divided into those cases caused by decreased renal perfusion, those caused by nephrotoxins, and those caused by both. Patients with cardiac failure, intravascular volume depletion, sepsis, or hypotension fall into the first category. Nephrotoxic medications such as aminoglycosides, IV iodinated contrast agents, some chemotherapeutic drugs, and anesthetic agents fall into the second category (Hou et al, 1983; Bullock et al, 1985; Wilkes and Mailloux, 1986). If more than one of the risk factors exist at the same time, the risk is cumulative, especially if they occur during a period of intravascular volume depletion (Meyers et al, 1986; Shusterman et al, 1987). Fluids, electrolytes, and acid-base balance need to be monitored closely in these patients, and the cause of the renal damage needs to be immediately corrected or removed.

Important measures should be taken prior to surgery in all patients with renal insufficiency or CRF. Nephrotoxic drugs should be discontinued. Most of the time, ceftazidime or aztreonam can be substituted for an aminoglycoside when a serious gram-negative infection is suspected. When this is not possible, strict attention should be paid to the pharmacokinetic characteristics of each drug. Peak and trough levels are critically important in determining the dose and timing of aminoglycoside administration (Meyer, 1986). Often after culture and sensitivity results are available, aminoglycosides can be discontinued and another less toxic antibiotic can be substituted. If renal impairment develops preoperatively as a result of nephrotoxins, surgery should be delayed until renal function returns to baseline. Diabetics should be given a limited dose of intravenous radiocontrast agents and need to be well hydrated, because they are particularly susceptible to renal injury from these materials. An adequate intravascular volume assessment should be made, and invasive monitoring may be necessary to ensure adequate left ventricular preload. Volume repletion preoperatively has been shown both in animal and clinical studies to lower the incidence of renal impairment postoperatively (Bush et al, 1981).

In conclusion, patients with RI or who develop RI in the perioperative setting pose difficult problems to the clinician. A review of the patient's renal history, including dialysis records, and an evaluation of risk factors should be part of the preoperative plan. Physical examination, serum chemistries, and invasive hemodynamic monitoring should provide information regarding the intravascular volume status and an estimate of renal perfusion. Appropriate action, including aggressive early dialysis, can then prevent hemodynamic instability and electrolyte disturbances and avert operative and postoperative complications. Patients with coagulopathies or prolonged bleeding time should be given cryoprecipitate, desmopressin, or conjugated estrogens in order to circumvent excessive intraoperative bleeding.

Liver Disease

When the liver is injured, its cells die, the reticular network breaks down, and collagen is produced to form scar tissue. This process is termed cirrhosis. The two most common forms of cirrhosis in the United States are Laennec's cirrhosis (alcohol or nutritional) and posthepatic cirrhosis. The increase in scar tissue causes a disorder in the hepatic architecture and an increase in resistance to hepatic arterial and especially portal-venous blood flow. Although a patient with mild cirrhosis may not be at any particular operative risk, most have incurred a loss of functional hepatocytes. Liver disease may cause numerous problems with nutrition, coagulation, electrolytes, encephalopathy, and sepsis both before and following surgery. The preoperative history should focus attention on questions regarding viral hepatitis, jaundice, intravenous drug use, alcohol use, previous blood product exposure, abnormal bleeding during previous surgery, or a family history of liver disease. The examination should note any jaundice, ascites, or hepatosplenomegaly. Jaundice is the result of obstruction to the outflow of bile or hepatocellular dysfunction. Clinical jaundice (serum bilirubin >3 mg/dl) indicates a significantly increased operative risk. In patients with known or suspected hepatic disease (Friedman and Maddrey, 1987), assays of serum transaminases, albumin, prothrombin time, and direct bilirubin are essential. Significant elevation of these transaminases (in the 500- to 1000-IU/L range) usually indicates hepatitis and should prompt further investigation. A prolonged prothrombin time (PT) also suggests liver dysfunction. Administration of phytomenadione (10 mg IM) for 3 days should correct the PT (Roberts and Cederbaum, 1972). However, a failure of vitamin K administration to reverse the abnormal PT indicates severe liver disease (Maze, 1986). Partial thromboplastin time, thrombin clotting time, and platelet count should also be evaluated in patients with liver disease, although their values may not correlate well with the degree of hepatic dysfunction. Increased splenic sequestration of platelets is seen in liver dysfunction, and patients with fewer than 60,000 platelets/m^3 usually require platelet transfusion preoperatively (Isaacs and Byrne, 1987). Careful evaluation of electrolytes, BUN, and creatinine are important because of the relationship between cirrhosis and the hepatorenal syndrome. Serum glucose should be monitored in patients with

liver disease because the liver controls glycogenesis, glycogenolysis, gluconeogenesis, and glycolysis.

Acute hepatocellular damage results in increased morbidity and mortality in surgical patients (Harvill and Summerskill, 1963). If after a thorough history, physical examination, and laboratory assessment the etiology of the liver disease remains unknown, a hepatologist should be consulted. After the specific diagnosis is made, the risk assessment for surgery is made using Child's classification, which has shown that morbidity and mortality are directly related to the degree of liver dysfunction (Table 41–19) (Child and Turcotte, 1964). Originally this classification was used for patients undergoing surgery for bleeding esophageal varices, but it has since been shown to be useful in patients undergoing all types of abdominal surgery and is an excellent predictor of surgical outcome in these patients (Wirthlin et al, 1974; Bloch et al, 1985).

Garrison and associates (1984) reported operative mortalities of 10%, 31%, and 76%, respectively, for each of the three Child classifications in patients having major abdominal surgery with coexistent liver disease. The Child classification was the best predictor among the 53 variables studied and correlated with other postoperative complications such as bleeding, renal failure, wound dehiscence, and sepsis. The major cause of perioperative death in this series was sepsis. These data indicate that patients with Child's Class A disease may proceed with elective surgery without excessive risk. Patient's with Child's Class B or C disease, however, should not have elective surgery until their liver disease improves or stabilizes.

Not so infrequently, the gynecologist will encounter patients with ascites. This condition is drastically different than that in patients who have ascites secondary to an ovarian malignancy. Patients with ascites resulting from cirrhosis also frequently have a hydrothorax, a pulmonary ventilation-perfusion mismatch, and decreased gastric emptying time and are at high risk of regurgitation and aspiration. If pulmonary function tests and arterial blood gases are severely compromised, a therapeutic thoracentesis or paracentesis should be considered preoperatively. Careful attention should be given to the patient's hemodynamic status because withdrawal of these transudates can result in rapid declines in blood pressure. Anesthetic considerations include administration of a histamine antagonist, a rapid sequential induction, and an awake intubation because of the high risk of regurgitation and aspiration. Intraoperative invasive hemodynamic monitoring greatly assists with fluid replacement decisions.

Additional considerations need to be made with regard to medications. Metabolism of benzodiazepines, narcotics, and muscle relaxants can be altered. Diazepam and morphine doses should be lowered and dosing intervals increased because of a prolonged effect of these agents in patients with liver impairment. Hepatic function also is greatly affected

Table 41-19. CHILD CLASSIFICATION OF SURGICAL RISK WITH LIVER DYSFUNCTION

PARAMETER	CLASS A	CLASS B	CLASS C
Bilirubin (mg/dl)	<2.0	2.0–3.0	>3.0
Albumin (g/dl)	>3.5	3.0–3.5	<3.0
Ascites	None	Easily controlled	Poorly controlled
Encephalopathy	None	Mild	Advanced
Nutritional status	Excellent	Good	Poor

From Child CG, Turcotte JG: Surgery and portal hypertension. In Child CG (ed): The Liver and Portal Hypertension. 3rd ed. Philadelphia: WB Saunders Company, 1964:50, with permission.

by the choice of anesthetic agents, because certain drugs alter the flow of blood to the liver and thus change the rate of metabolism. Isoflurane preserves blood flow at clinically effective doses and is the agent of choice in patients with liver dysfunction. Halothane's metabolites possess hepatotoxic potential, and this effect may be genetically influenced. Those at risk to develop halothane hepatitis are patients who have had previous exposure to halothane and patients who are likely to have enzyme induction secondary to barbiturates, smoking, or alcohol ingestion.

Patients with acute viral hepatitis who undergo surgery can have significant problems. These patients are hopefully identified preoperatively using serologic markers. Because of an increased risk of perioperative morbidity (12%) and mortality (9.5%), only emergency surgery is indicated during acute hepatitis. After the convalescent phase of the disease has passed and the patient is fully recovered, definitive surgery can be scheduled. In addition to these patient complications, there is also increased risk to the health care provider when viral hepatitis is encountered.

Women with chronic liver disease (chronic active hepatitis, chronic persistent hepatitis) may benefit from steroids (prednisone 20 mg/day, or azathioprine 50 mg/day and prednisone 10 mg/day) preoperatively. These modalities have been shown to result in remission in up to 80% of patients. The regimen is continued only if there is clinical, biochemical, and histologic evidence of remission. A controlled, randomized, trial of prednisone and interferon-α_{2b} has documented disappearance of the hepatitis B core antigen (HBcAg) and hepatitis B viral DNA replication in 37% of patients (Perrillo et al, 1990). Although further evaluation of this treatment is needed, it may become part of the preoperative treatment of patients with chronic hepatitis B.

Patients with encephalopathy who need to undergo surgery are at significant risk for problems. Because these women are often not able to participate in their care, they often build up secretions and are at major risk for aspiration. The condition may be provoked by constipation, sepsis, malnutrition, and dehydration. Treatment consists of catharsis and intestinal sterilization with lactulose and neomycin to decrease the number of urease-producing bacteria.

Nutritional support in the form of branched-chain amino acids should be given when severe malnourishment exists.

Patients with cirrhosis are at major risk for perioperative infection secondary to poor lymphocyte interactions and abnormal hepatic synthesis of acute phase-protein and complement. Meticulous sterile technique should be observed and appropriate broad-spectrum antibiotics should be given both preoperatively and intraoperatively. Patients with liver disease are also at significant risk for fungal infection, and prophylaxis with 30 ml of nystatin may be helpful (Brayton et al, 1970).

Patients with cirrhosis should be considered for surgery only after evaluation with the Child classification and coagulation studies have been performed. The 30% mortality rate in these patients warrants extensive preoperative preparation. Although limited information is available in the gynecologic patient, morbidity and mortality should be considered significant and infection is a major factor to contend with in these patients.

REFERENCES

Abbott TR: Anesthesia in untreated myxedema: report of 2 cases. Br J Anaesth 1967;39:510.

Abel RM: Nutritional support in the patient with acute renal failure. J Am Coll Nutr 1983;2:33.

Aguirre A, Fischer JE, Welch CE: The role of surgery and hyperalimentation in therapy of gastrointestinal-cutaneous fistulae. Ann Surg 1974;180:393.

Allenby F, Boardman L, Pflug JJ, et al: Effects of external pneumatic intermittent compression on fibrinolysis in man. Lancet 1976;2:1412.

Anderson A, Hausmann W: Triiodothyronine in myxedema coma [letter]. Lancet 1956;2:999.

Anderson ME, Belani KG: Short-term preoperative smoking abstinence. Am Fam Physician 1990;41:1191.

Baker JP, Detsky AS, Wesson DE: Nutritional assessment: a comparison of clinical judgement and objective measurements. N Engl J Med 1982;306:969.

Ballard M, Bradley-Watson PJ, Johnstone ED, et al: Low doses of subcutaneous heparin in the prevention of deep venous thrombosis after gynecologic surgery. J Obstet Gynaecol Br Commonw 1973;80:469.

Bandy LC, Chin N, Soper JT, et al: Total parenteral nutrition in poor prognosis gestational trophoblastic disease. Gynecol Oncol 1987;28:305.

Barnes PJ: A new approach to the treatment of asthma. N Engl J Med 1989;321:1517.

Baron JF, Mundler O, Bertrand M, et al: Dipyridamole–thallium scintigraphy and gated radionuclide angiography to assess car-

diac risk before abdominal aortic surgery. N Engl J Med 1994;
330:663.

Beck DE, Harford FJ, DiPalma JA: Comparison of cleansing methods in preparation for colonic surgery. Dis Colon Rectum 1985;
28:491.

Bergquist D, Lindgren B, Matzsch T: Comparison of the cost of
preventing postoperative deep vein thrombosis with either unfractionated or low-molecular-weight heparin. Br J Surg 1996;
83:1548.

Blackburn GL, Bistrian BR: Nutritional care of the injured and/
or septic patient. Surg Clin North Am 1976;56:1195.

Bloch RS, Allaben RD, Walt AJ: Cholecystectomy in patients with
cirrhosis: a surgical challenge Arch Surg 1985;120:669.

Blosser SA, Rock P: Asthma and chronic obstructive lung disease.
In Breslow MJ, Miller CJ, Rogers MC (eds): Perioperative Management. St. Louis: CV Mosby Company, 1990:259.

Borstad E, Urdal K, Handeland G, Abildgaard U: Comparison of
low-molecular-weight heparin vs. unfractionated heparin in
gynecological surgery II: Reduced dose of low-molecular-weight heparin. Acta Obstet Gynecol Scand 1992;71:471.

Brayton RE, Stokes PE, Schwartz MS, et al: Effect of alcohol and
various diseases on leukocyte mobilization, phagocytosis, and
intracellular bacterial killing. N Engl J Med 1970;282:123.

Brennan MF, Pisters PWT, Posner M, et al: A prospective randomized trial of total parenteral nutrition after major pancreatic
resection for malignancy. Ann Surg 1994;220:436.

Brensilver JM, Goldberger E: Parenteral therapy in surgical patients. In A Primer of Water, Electrolyte, and Acid-Base Syndromes. 8th ed. Philadelphia: FA Davis Company, 1996:347.

Broyer M, Brunner FP, Brynger H, et al: Demography of dialysis
and transplantation in Europe, 1984. Nephrol Dial Transplant
1986;1:1.

Bullock ML, Umen AJ, Finkelstein MS, et al: The assessment of
risk factors in 462 patients with acute renal failure. Am J Kidney Dis 1985;5:97.

Burke JF: The effective period of preventive antibiotic action in
experimental incisions and dermal lesions. Surgery 1961;50:161.

Bush HL, Huse JB, Johnson WC, et al: Prevention of renal insufficiency after abdominal aortic aneurysm resection by optimal
volume loading. Arch Surg 1981;116:1517.

Butterworth CE, Blackburn GL: Hospital malnutrition and how
to assess the nutritional status of a patient. Nutr Today 1974;9:
1.

Buzby GP, Mullen JL, Matthews DC, et al: Prognostic nutritional
index in gastrointestinal surgery. Am J Surg 1980;139:160.

Carliner NH, Fisher ML, Plotnick GD, et al: Routine preoperative
exercise testing in patients undergoing major noncardiac surgery. Am J Cardiol 1985;56:51.

Castillo R, Haas A: Chest physical therapy: comparative efficacy
of preoperative and postoperative in the elderly. Arch Phys
Med Rehabil 1985;66:376.

Catalona WJ, Kadmon D, Crane DB: Effect of mini-dose heparin
on lymphocele formation following extraperitoneal pelvic lymphadenectomy. J Urol 1979;123:890.

Chapman KR: Guidelines for the assessment and management of
chronic obstructive pulmonary disease. Can Med Assoc J 1992;
147:420.

Chapman KR: Therapeutic approaches to chronic obstructive pulmonary disease: an emerging consensus. Am J Med 1996;100:
1A-5S.

Child CG, Turcotte JG: Surgery and portal hypertension. In Child
CG (ed): The Liver and Portal Hypertension. 3rd ed. Philadelphia: WB Saunders Company, 1964:50.

Chodak GW: Use of systemic antibiotics for prophylaxis in surgery. Arch Surg 1977;112:326.

Clarke-Pearson DL: Prevention of venous thromboembolism in
gynecologic surgery patients. Curr Opin Obstet Gynecol 1993;
14:25.

Clarke-Pearson DL, Coleman RE, Synan IS, et al: Venous thromboembolism prophylaxis in gynecologic oncology: a prospective controlled trial of low-dose heparin. Am J Obstet Gynecol
1983a;145:606.

Clarke-Pearson DL, Creasman WT, Coleman RE, et al: Perioperative external pneumatic calf compression as thromboembolism prophylaxis in gynecologic oncology: report of a randomized controlled trial. Gynecol Oncol 1984a;18:226.

Clarke-Pearson DL, DeLong E, Synan IS, et al: Complications of
low-dose heparin prophylaxis in gynecologic oncology surgery.
Obstet Gynecol 1984b;64:689,

Clarke-Pearson DL, DeLong E, Synan IS, et al: A prospective
study of risk factors associated with postoperative venous
thromboembolism in gynecology. Obstet Gynecol 1987;69:146.

Clarke-Pearson DL, DeLong E, Synan IS, et al: A controlled trial
of two low-dose heparin regimens for the prevention of postoperative deep vein thrombosis. Obstet Gynecol 1990;75:684.

Clarke-Pearson DL, Jelovsek FR, Creasman WT: Thromboembolism complicating surgery for cervical and uterine malignancy:
incidence, risk factors, and prophylaxis. Obstet Gynecol 1983b;
61:87.

Clarke-Pearson DL, Synan IS, Dodge , et al: A randomized trial
of low-dose heparin and intermittent pneumatic calf compression for the prevention of deep venous thrombosis following
gynecologic oncology surgery. Am J Obstet Gynecol 1993;168:
1146.

Clarke-Pearson DL, Synan IS, Hinshaw W, et al: Prevention of
postoperative venous thromboembolism by external pneumatic
calf compression in patients with gynecologic malignancy. Obstet Gynecol 1984c;63:92.

Clarke-Pearson DL, Synan IS, Soleman RE, et al: The natural history of postoperative venous thromboembolism in gynecologic
oncology: a prospective study of 382 patients. Am J Obstet Gynecol 1984d;148:1051.

Clayton JK, Anderson JA, McNicol GP: Preoperative prediction
of postoperative deep vein thrombosis. Br Med J 1976;2:910.

Cockroft DW: Hyperresponsiveness in asthma. Hosp Pract 1990;
25:111.

Copeland EM, MacFadyen BV, Lanzotti VJ, Dudrick SJ: Intravenous hyperalimentation as an adjunct to cancer chemotherapy.
Am J Surg 1975;129:167.

Coriat P, Daloz M, Bousseau D, et al: Prevention of intraoperative
myocardial ischemia during noncardiac surgery with intravenous nitroglycerin. Anesthesiology 1984;61:193.

Creasman WT, Weed JC Jr: Radical hysterectomy. In Schaefer G,
Graber EA (eds): Complications in Obstetrics and Gynecologic
Surgery. New York: Harper & Row, 1981:389.

Cruse PJE, Foord R: A five-year prospective study of 23,649 surgical wounds. Arch Surg 1973;107:206.

Cutler BS, Wheeler HB, Paraskos JA, Cardullo PA: Applicability
and interpretation of electrocardiographic stress testing in patients with peripheral vascular disease. Am J Surg 1981;141:501.

Daley JM, Lieberman MD, Goldfine J, et al: Enteral nutrition with
supplemental argenine, RNA, and omega-3-fatty acids in patients after operation: immunologic metabolic, and clinical outcome. Surgery 1992;112:56.

Davey PG, Duncan ID, Edward D, Scott AC: Cost-benefit analysis
of cephradine and mezlocillin prophylaxis for abdominal and
vaginal hysterectomy. Br J Obstet Gynaecol 1988;95:1170.

Demling RH, Wilson RF: Fluids, electrolytes, and acid-base balance. In Eiseman B (ed): Decision Making in Surgical Critical
Care. Philadelphia: BC Decker Inc, 1988:114.

Detsky AS, Abrams HB, McLaughlin JR, et al: Predicting cardiac
complications in patients undergoing non-cardiac surgery. J
Gen Intern Med 1986;1:211.

DeWys WD, Begg C, Lavin PT, et al: Prognostic effect of weight
loss prior to chemotherapy in cancer patients. Am J Med 1980;
69:491.

Dockerty PW, Goodman JDS, Hill JG, et al: The effect of low-dose
heparin on blood loss at abdominal hysterectomy. Br J Obstet
Gynaecol 1983;90:759.

Driks MR, Craven DE, Celli BR, et al: Nosocomial pneumonia in
intubated patients given sucralfate as compared with antacids
or histamine type 2 blockers: the role of gastric colonization.
N Engl J Med 1987;317:1376.

Easley HA, Hammond CB: Informed consent in obstetrics and
gynecology. Postgrad Obstet Gynecol 1986;10:1.

Eschbach JW, Egrie JC, Downing MR, et al: Correction of the anemia of end-stage renal disease with recombinant erythropoietin: results of a combined Phase I and II clinical trial. N Engl J
Med 1987;316:73.

Flenley DC: Chronic obstructive pulmonary disease. Dis Mon 1988;34:543.

Flynn NM: Reducing the risk of infection in surgical patients. In Bolt RJ (ed): Medical Evaluation of the Surgical Patient. Mt. Kisco, NY: Futura Publishing Co, 1987:195.

Forthman HJ, Shepard A: Postoperative pulmonary complications. South Med J 1969;62:1198.

Foschi D, Gavagna G, Callioni F, et al: Hyperalimentation of jaundiced patients on percutaneous transhepatic biliary drainage. Br J Surg 1986;73:716.

Foster ED, Davis KB, Carpenter JA, et al: Risk of noncardiac operation in patients with defined coronary disease: The Coronary Artery Surgery Study (CASS) registry experience. Ann Thoracic Surg 1986;41:42.

Fricker JP, Vergnes Y, Schach R, et al: Low-dose heparin versus low-molecular-weight heparin (Kabi 2165, Fragmin) in the prophylaxis of thromboembolic complications of abdominal oncological surgery. Eur J Clin Invest 1988;18:561.

Friedman LS, Maddrey WC: Surgery in the patient with liver disease. Med Clin North Am 1987;71:453.

Friese S, Pricker JG, Willems FT, et al: Prophylaxis in gynaecological surgery: a prospective randomized comparison between single dose prophylaxis with amoxicillin/clavulanate and the combination of cefuroxime and metronidazole. J Antimicrob Chemother 1989;24:213.

Fry DE: Antibiotics in surgery: an overview. An J Surg 1988; 155(5A):11.

Galant SP: Treatment of asthma: new and time-tested strategies. Postgrad Med 1990;87:229.

Gallagher J, et al: Prophylactic nitroglycerin infusions during coronary artery bypass surgery. Anesthesiology 1986;64:785.

Gann DS, DeMaria EJ, Cambell RW: Adrenal gland. In Davis JH, Drucker WR, Forser RS, et al (eds): In Clinical Surgery. St. Louis: CV Mosby Company, 1987:2617.

Garrison RN, Cryer HM, Howard DA, et al: Clarification of risk factors for abdominal operations in patients with hepatic cirrhosis. Ann Surg 1984;199:648.

Geffner DL, Hershman JM: Beta-adrenergic blockade for treatment of hypothyroidism. Am J Med 1992;93:61.

Goldberg NJ, Wingert TD, Levin SR, et al: Insulin therapy in the diabetic surgical patient: metabolic and hormone response to low dose insulin infusion. Diabetes Care 1981;4:279.

Goldman DR: Surgery in patients with endocrine dysfunction, preoperative consultation. Med Clin North Am 1987;71:499.

Goldman L, Caldera DL, Nussbaum SR, et al: Multifactorial index of cardiac risk in noncardiac surgical procedures. N Engl J Med 1977;297:845.

Goldman L, Caldera DL, Nussbaum SR, et al: Cardiac risk factors and complications in non-cardiac surgery. Medicine 1978;57: 357.

Goodnough LT: Autologous blood donation. JAMA 1988;260:65.

Goodnough LT, Rudnick S, Price TA, et al: Increased preoperative collection of autologous blood with recombinant human erythropoietin therapy. N Engl J Med 1989;321:1163.

Gracey DR, Divertie MB, Didier EP: Preoperative pulmonary preparation of patients with chronic obstructive pulmonary disease. Chest 1979;76:123.

Haas S, Haas P: Efficacy of low-molecular-weight heparins: an overview. Semin Thromb Hemost 1993;19:101.

Haley RW, Culver DH, Morgan WM, et al: Identifying patients at high risk of surgical wound infection: a simple multivariate index of patient susceptibility and wound contamination. Am J Epidemiol 1985;121:206.

Hargreave FE, Dolovich J, Newhouse MT: The assessment and treatment of asthma: a conference report. J Allergy Clin Immunol 1990;85:109.

Harvill DD, Summerskill WH: Surgery in acute hepatitis: causes and effects. JAMA 1963;184:257.

Heatley RV, Williams RHP, Lewis MH: Preoperative intravenous feeding—a controlled trial. Postgrad Med J 1979;55:541.

Heilmann L, Kruck M, Schindler AE: Prevention of thrombosis in gynecology: double-blind comparison of LMW heparin and unfractionated heparin. Geburtshilfe Frauenheilkd 1989;49:803.

Hemsell DL, Johnson ER, Heard MC, et al: Single-dose piperacillin versus triple-dose cefoxitin prophylaxis at vaginal and abdominal hysterectomy. South Med J 1989;82:438.

Hemsell DL, Martin JN Jr, Pastorek JG II, et al: Single-dose antimicrobial prophylaxis at abdominal hysterectomy: cefamandole vs. cefotaxime. J Reprod Med 1988;33:939.

Hensley MJ, Fencl V: Lungs and respiration. In Vandam LD (ed): To Make the Patient Ready for Anesthesia: Medical Care of the Surgical Patient. Menlo Park, CA: Addison-Wesley, 1981:21.

Heymsfield SB, Horowitz J, Lawson DH: Enteral hyperalimentation. In Berk JE (ed): Developments in Digestive Diseases. Vol 3. Philadelphia: Lea & Febiger, 1980:59

Hirsch HA: Prophylactic antibiotics in obstetrics and gynecology. Am J Med 1985;78:170.

Hlatky MA, Boineau RE, Higginbotham MB, et al: A brief self-administered questionnaire to determine functional capacity (The Duke Activity Status Index). Am J Cardiol 1989;64:651.

Hotchkiss RS: Perioperative management of patient with chronic obstructive pulmonary disease. Int Anesthesiol Clin 1988;26: 134.

Hou SH, et al: Hospital-acquired renal insufficiency: a prospective study. Am J Med 1983;74:243.

Isaacs JH, Byrne MP: Pelvic Surgery: A Multidisciplinary Approach. Mt. Kisco, NY: Futura Publishing Company, 1987:14.

Jarrett RJ: Descriptive epidemiology in diabetes types 1 and 2. In: Diabetes Mellitus. Littleton, MA: PSG Publishing Company, 1986:11.

Jeffcoate TNA, Tindall VR: Venous thrombosis and embolism in obstetrics and gynecology. Aust N Z J Obstet Gynaecol 1965;5: 119.

Jorgensen LN, Willie-Jorgensen P, Hauch O: Prophylaxis of postoperative thromboembolism with low-molecular-weight heparins. Br J Surg 1993;80:689.

Kaaja R, Lehtovirta P, Venesmaa P, et al: Comparison of enoxaparin, a low-molecular-weight heparin and unfractionated heparin, with or without dihydroergotamine, in abdominal hysterectomy. Eur J Obstet Reprod Biol 1992;47:141.

Kakkar VV: Prevention of fatal postoperative pulmonary embolism by low dose heparin: an international multicenter trial. Lancet 1975;2:145.

Kaplan J: Hemodynamic monitoring. In Kaplan J (ed): Cardiac Anesthesia. New York: Grune & Stratton, 1987:179.

Kehlet H, Binder C: Value of an ACTH test in assessing hypothalamic-pituitary-adrenocortical function in glucocorticoid-treated patients. Br Med J 1973;2:147.

Kinney JM, Long CI, Gump FE, Duke JH: Tissue composition of weight loss in surgical patients. I. Elective operation. Ann Surg 1968;168:459.

Kuner J, Freseu V, Utsu F, et al: Cardiac arrythmias during anesthesia. Dis Chest 1967;52:580.

Lacche A, Basaglia P: Hypertensive emergencies: effects of therapy by nifedipine administered sublingually. Curr Ther Res 1983;34:879.

Lamers RJ, van Engelshoven JM, Pfaff A: Once again, the routine preoperative thorax photo. Ned Tijdschr Geneesk 1989;133: 2288.

Larsen SF, et al: Prediction of cardiac risk in non-cardiac surgery. Eur Heart J 1987;8:179.

Lawrence VA, Page CP, Harris GD: Preoperative spirometry before abdominal operations: a critical appraisal of its predictive value. Arch Intern Med 1989;149:280.

Ledger WJ, Gee C, Lewis WP: Guidelines for antibiotic prophylaxis in gynecology. Am J Obstet Gynecol 1975;121:1038.

Lewis SL, Van Epps DE: Neutrophil and monocyte alterations in chronic dialysis patients. Am J Kidney Dis 1987;9:381.

Li JTC: Three steps towards better management of asthma. Compr Ther 1996;22:345.

Livio M, Mannucci PM, Vigano G, et al: Conjugated estrogens for the management of bleeding associated with renal failure. N Engl J Med 1986;315:731.

Loder RE: Routine preoperative chest radiography. Anesthesiology 1987;66:195.

Lundin AP, Stein RA, Brown CD, et al: Fatigue, acid-base and electrolyte changes in exhaustive treadmill exercise in hemodialysis patients. Nephron 1987;46:57.

Magrina JF: Intravenous fluids and blood component therapy. Clin Obstet Gynecol 1988;31:686.

Mannucci PM, Remuzzi G, Pusineri F, et al: Desamino-8-D-arginine vasopressin shortens bleeding time in uremia. N Engl J Med 1983;308:8.

Maze M: Hepatic physiology. In Miller RD (ed): Anesthesia. Vol 2. New York: Churchill Livingstone, 1994;649.

McMurry JF Jr: Wound healing with diabetes mellitus. Surg Clin North Am 1985;64:35.

Meyer RD: Risk factors and comparison of clinical nephrotoxicity of aminoglycosides. Am J Med 1986;80(Suppl 6B):119.

Meyers EF, Alberts D, Gordon MD, et al: Perioperative control of blood glucose in diabetic patients: a two-step protocol. Diabetes Care 1986;9:40.

Milledge JS, Nunn JF: Criteria of fitness for anaesthesia in patients with chronic obstructive lung disease. Br Med J 1975;3:670.

Miller TA, Duke JH: Fluid and electrolyte management. In Dudrick SJ, Baue AE, Eiseman B, et al (eds): Manual of Preoperative and Postoperative Care. Philadelphia: WB Saunders Company, 1983:38.

Mohr DN, Jett JR: Clinical reviews: preoperative evaluation of pulmonary risk factors. J Gen Intern Med 1988;3:277.

Mullen JL, Buzby GP, Matthews DC, et al: Reduction of operative morbidity and mortality by combined preoperative and postoperative nutritional support. Ann Surg 1980;192:604.

Mullen JL, Buzby GP, Waldman TG, et al: Prediction of operative morbidity and mortality by preoperative nutritional assessment. Surg Forum 1979;30:80.

Müller JM, Keller HW, Brenner U, et al: Indications and effects of preoperative parenteral nutrition. World J Surg 1986;10:53.

Munck JM, Jensen HK: Preoperative clindamycin treatment and vaginal drainage in hysterectomy. Acta Obstet Gynecol Scand 1989;68:241.

Murkin JM: Anesthesia and hypothyroidism: a review of thyroxine physiology, pharmacology, and anesthetic implications. Anesth Analg 1982;61:371.

Myers ER, Clarke-Pearson DL, Olt GJ, et al: Preoperative coagulation testing on a gynecologic oncology service. Obstet Gynecol 1994;83:483.

Narins RG, Lazarus MJ: Renal system. In Vandam LD (ed): To Make the Patient Ready for Anesthesia: Medical Care of the Surgical Patient. 2nd ed. Menlo Park, CA: Addison-Wesley, 1984:67.

National Institutes of Health Consensus Group: Summary of NIH consensus development conference on perioperative red cell transfusion. Am J Hematology 1989;31:144.

Nesto RW, Phillips RT, Kett KG, et al: Angina and exertional myocardial ischemia in diabetic and non-diabetic patients: assessment by exercise thallium scintigraphy. Ann Intern Med 1988;108:170.

Nicolaides AN, Fernandes e Fernandes J, Pollock AV: Intermittent sequential pneumatic compression of the legs in the prevention of venous stasis and postoperative deep venous thrombosis. Surgery 1980;87:69.

Nixon DW, Heymsfield SB, Cohen AE, et al: Protein-calorie undernutrition in hospitalized cancer patients. Am J Med 1980;69:491.

O'Mailia J, Saunder G, Giles T: Nifedipine associated myocardial ischemia or infarction in the treatment of hypertensive emergencies. Ann Intern Med 1987;107:185.

Orr JW Jr, Sisson PF, Patsner B, et al: Single-dose antibiotic prophylaxis for patient undergoing extended pelvic surgery for gynecologic malignancy. Am J Obstet Gynecol 1990;162:718.

Page MM, Watkins PJ: Cardiorespiratory arrest and diabetic autonomic neuropathy. Lancet 1978;1(Part 1):14.

Pasternack PF, Imprato AM, Riles TS, et al: The value of the radionuclide angiogram in the prediction of postoperative myocardial infarction in patients undergoing lower extremity revascularization procedures. Circulation 1985;72(Suppl II):13.

Pedersen O, Christensen N, Ramsch K: Comparison of acute effects of nifedipine in normotensive and hypertensive man. J Cardiovasc Pharmacol 1980;2:357.

Perrillo RP, Schiffer ER, Davis GL, et al: A randomized controlled trial of interferon alpha-IIB alone and after prednisone withdrawal for the treatment of chronic hepatitis B. N Engl J Med 1990;323:295.

Pestana C: Fluids and Electrolytes in the Surgical Patient. 4th ed. Baltimore: Williams & Wilkins, 1989.

Pinson CW, Schuman ES, Gross GF, et al: Surgery in long-term dialysis patients: experience with more than 300 cases. Am J Surg 1986;151:567.

Piscitelli JT, Simel DL, Addison WA: Who should have intravenous pyelograms before hysterectomy for benign disease? Obstet Gynecol 1987;69:541.

Piver MS, Malfetano JH, Lele SB, et al: Prophylactic anticoagulation as a possible cause of inguinal lympocyst after radical vulvectomy and inguinal lymphadenectomy. Obstet Gynecol 1983;62:17.

Poldermans D, Arnese M, Fioretti PM, et al: Improved cardiac risk stratification in major vascular surgery with dobutamine-atropine stress echocardiography. J Am Coll Cardiol 1995;26:648.

Porte D, Halter JB: The endocrine pancreas and diabetes mellitus. In Williams RH (ed): Textbook of Endocrinology. Philadelphia: WB Saunders Company, 1981:715.

Rao TLK, Jacobs KH, El-Etr AN: Reinfarction following anesthesia in patients with myocardial infarction. Anesthesiology 1983;59:499.

Rayfield EG, Ault MJ, Keusch GT, et al: Infection and diabetes: the case for glucose control. Am J Med 1982;72:439.

Roberts HR, Cederbaum AI: The liver and blood coagulation: physiology and pathology. Gastroenterology 1972;63:297.

Roizen MF: Endocrine abnormalities and anesthesia: implications for the anesthesiologist. Refresher Course Anesthesiol 1984;13:161.

Roy S, Wilkins J, Galaif E, Azen C: Comparative efficacy and safety of cefmetazole or cefoxitin in the prevention of postoperative infection following vaginal and abdominal hysterectomy. J Antimicrob Chemother 1989;23:109.

Sagel SS, Evens RG, Forrest JV, Branson RT: Efficacy of routine screening and lateral chest radiographs in a hospital based population. N Engl J Med 1974;291:1001.

Salzman EW, Davies GC: Prophylaxis of venous thromboembolism: analysis of cost effectiveness. Ann Surg 1980;191:207.

Scurr JH, Ibrahim SZ, Faber RG, et al: The efficacy of graduated compression stocking in the prevention of deep vein thrombosis. Br J Surg 1977;64:371.

Shapiro M, Munoz A, Tager IB, et al: Risk factors for infection at the operative site after abdominal or vaginal hysterectomy. N Engl J Med 1982;307:1661.

Shires GT, Canizaro PC: Fluid and electrolyte management of the surgical patient. In Sabiston DC Jr (ed): Textbook of Surgery. 14th ed. Philadelphia: WB Saunders Company, 1991:57.

Shusterman N, Strom BL, Murray TG, et al: Risk factors and outcome of hospital-acquired acute renal failure. clinical epidemiologic study. Am J Med 1987;83:65.

Siafakas NM, Vermeire P, Pride NB, et al: Optimal assessment and management of chronic obstructive pulmonary disease (COPD). Eur Respir J 1995;8:1398.

Siddiq YK, Gebhart SS: Disorder of the thyroid gland. In Lubin MF (ed): Medical Management of the Surgical Patient. 2nd ed. Reading, MA: Butterworth, 1988:297.

Smith RC, Hartemink R: Improvement of nutritional measures during preoperative parenteral nutrition selected by the prognostic nutritional index. a randomized controlled trial. JPEN J Parent Enteral Nutr 1989;12:587.

Soper JT, Berchuck A, Creasman WT, Clarke-Pearson DL: Pelvic exenteration: factors associated with major surgical morbidity. Gynecol Oncol 1989;35:93.

Steen PA, Tinker JH, Tarhan S: Myocardial reinfarction after anesthesia and surgery. JAMA 1978;239:2566.

Stehling LC: Anesthetic management of the patient with hyperthyroidism. Anesthesiology 1974;41:585.

Stein M, Cassara EL: Preoperative pulmonary evaluation and therapy for surgery patients. JAMA 1970;211:787.

Stein M, Koota GM, Simon M, Frank HA: Pulmonary evaluation of surgical patients. JAMA 1962;181:765.

Taberner DA, Poller L, Burnstein RW, et al: Oral anticoagulants controlled by British comparative thromboplastin versus low dose heparin prophylaxis of deep venous thrombosis. Br Med J 1978;1:272.

Tapson VF, Hull RD: Management of venous thromboembolic disease. the impact of low-molecular-weight heparin. Chest 1995;16:231.

Tarhan S, Moffitt EA, Sessler AD, et al: Risk of anesthesia and surgery in patients with chronic bronchitis and chronic obstructive pulmonary disease. Surgery 1973;74:720.

Tarhan S, Moffitt EA, Taylor WF, Giuliani ER, Myocardial infarction after general anesthesia. JAMA 1972;220:1451.

Trimbos JB, van Lindert ACM, Heintz APM, et al: Piperacillin for prophylaxis in gynecological surgery. Eur J Obstet Gynecol Reprod Biol 1989;30:141.

Veterans Affairs Total Parenteral Nutrition Cooperative Study Group: Perioperative total parenteral nutrition in surgical patients. N Engl J Med 1991;325:525.

Vogel CM, Kingsbury RJ, Baue A: Intravenous hyperalimentation: a review of two and one-half years' experience. Arch Surg 1972; 105:414.

Von Knorring J: Postoperative myocardial infarction: a prospective study in a risk group of surgical patients. Surgery 1981;90: 55.

Walts LF, Miller J, Davidson MB, et al: Perioperative management of diabetes mellitus. Anesthesiology 1981;55:104.

Warner MA, Offord KP, Warner ME, et al: Role of preoperative cessation of smoking and other factors in postoperative pulmonary complications: a blinded prospective study of coronary artery bypass patients. Mayo Clin Proc 1989;64:609.

Wasserfallen J-B, Baraniuk JN: Clinical use of inhaled corticosteroids in asthma. J Allergy Clin Immunol 1996;97:177.

Weiner DA, Ryan TJ, McCabe CH, et al: Prognostic importance of a clinical profile and exercise test in medically treated patients with coronary artery disease. J Am Coll Cardiol 1984;3:772.

Weringer EJ, Kelso JM, Tamai IY, et al: Effects of insulin on wound healing in diabetic mice. Acta Endocrinol 1982;99:101.

Wheat LJ: Infection and diabetes mellitus. Diabetes Care 1980;3: 187.

Wilkes M, Mailloux LU: Acute renal failure: pathogenesis and prevention. Am J Med 1986;80:1129.

Wirthlin LS, Van Erk H, Malt RB, et al: Predictors of surgical mortality in patients with cirrhosis and non-variceal gastroduodenal bleeding. Surg Gynecol Obstet 1974;13:65.

Zeldin RA: Assessing cardiac risk in patients who undergo noncardiac surgical procedures. Can J Surg 1984;27:402.

Zibrak JD, O'Donnell CR, Marton K: Indications for pulmonary function testing. Ann Intern Med 1990;112:763.

42

Intraoperative Technique

James W. Orr, Jr.

Irrespective of the disease process, once an operative approach has been determined to be appropriate therapy, it is vital that the surgeon and support team constantly evaluate new techniques and continually re-evaluate all previously incorporated technical aspects of the specific procedure. This review process will assist in the elimination of unnecessary surgical steps while improving the effort to complete the chosen procedure safely and efficiently. In 1998, the economic impact of the surgical approach, as it relates to both direct and indirect costs, should be considered.

The "entire" risk of postoperative morbidity is affected by all facets of surgical planning and technique. The final surgical result can be adversely or favorably impacted by existing patient co-morbidity. To be optimally effective, surgical planning and the choice of operative technique should be decided prior to entering the operating room, recognizing that modifications and drastic changes of the planned surgical approach are frequently required pre- or intraoperatively. Although the initial surgical approach may be thoughtfully charted, inflexibility or the inability to alter the perioperative course may result in suboptimal outcome. For instance, patient factors such as glucose intolerance may be unknown or even unrecognized prior to preoperative evaluation or hospitalization. Schedule changes may be appropriate to minimize or increase surgical delay in a newly diagnosed diabetic in an attempt to improve perioperative glucose control. Older patients, particularly those who require daily medication, may not tolerate long periods of being maintained on a nothing-by-mouth order, especially if undergoing a mechanical bowel preparation. In this situation, schedule changes or hospitalization with the administration of intravenous fluids may be appropriate to maintain intravascular volume. A preoperative examination under anesthesia (EUA) may reveal important pathologic factors or dictate a change in surgical approach (i.e., abdominal, laparoscopic, or vaginal). It is important that surgeons outline these "potential" alterations of the operative algorithm during their preoperative evaluation and consultation. Although these discussions sometimes appear to "overwhelm" patients with information, extensive informed consent sets the stage and limits the risk of potential restriction on the surgical procedure. For example, a "mass" may not be apparent during an EUA. The surgeon is then faced with a dilemma: Proceed with exploration? Perform a laparoscopy? Cancel the case? The finding of cul-de-sac nodularity during EUA may suggest the benefit of a different approach or type of incision. Obviously, in these these types of situations it usually better serves the patient and the physician to alter the approach on the basis of immediate findings. Although extensive preoperative discussion may occasionally appear cumbersome, adequate preoperative information and preparation can be associated with a lessened requirement for postoperative pain medication and result in a better adaptation during recovery (Orr, 1988). This extensive type of dialogue should begin when the case is scheduled and should conclude only after complete physical and psychologic recovery.

Successful prophylaxis necessitates manipulation of existing physical, chemical, and psychologic factors. However, even in optimal situations, modification of these factors lessens risks but cannot be expected to completely eliminate perioperative complications. It is not a rare instance that one of our colleagues relates having unsuccessfully tried a method, a technique, or a drug, implying that the specific method or individual technique does not work. Although our clinical experience is important, we must realize that individuals are unable to discriminate differences in events that occur at levels of 15% or less. Additionally, surgeons tend to recall only the extremes of success or failure. To develop and maintain a successful surgical practice, it is necessary to continually review our entire personal experience and integrate these results with those of the published literature before disregarding or incorporating some potentially important new technique or methodology.

Categorization of key morbidity-related risk factors suggests that a number of fixed patient-related elements are important; however, the majority are potentially manipulated by the surgeon or surgical staff during the perioperative period (Table 42–1).

Table 42–1. FACTORS AFFECTING SURGICAL MORBIDITY

PATIENT	SURGEON
Preoperative	
Age	Preoperative stay
Immune status	Skin preparation
Co-morbid conditions	Hair removal
Obesity	Antibiotics
Nutritional status	Positioning
Urgency	Thermal control
Intraoperative	
	Surgical approach
	Experience
	Duration
	Incision
	Cautery
	Suture material
	Suture technique
	Irrigation
	Drains
	Vasoconstrictors
Postoperative	
	Wound closure
	Nutritional status
	Oxygen
	Transfusion

Table 42–2. AGE-RELATED OPERATIVE MORTALITY (EXENTERATION)

AGE (yr)	NO. OF PATIENTS	% MORTALITY
<40	24	0
41–50	36	3.3
51–60	38	7.1
61–70	23	9.9
>70	4	9.6

Modified from Orr JW Jr, Hatch KD, Shingleton HM, et al: Gastrointestinal complications associated with pelvic exenteration. Am J Obstet Gynecol 1983;145:325, with permission.

PREOPERATIVE MANAGEMENT

A number of potentially modifiable preoperative variables exist that can affect patient morbidity during gynecologic surgical procedures. Some are patient related and others can be manipulated by the surgeon.

Patient Variables

Age. Many gynecologic procedures are completed in older or elderly women. Obviously the average age, as well as the types and radicality of procedures, varies significantly among gynecologic practices. Younger women typically undergo diagnostic or therapeutic procedures for the management of pelvic pain, premalignant disease, benign masses, fertility-related problems, or refractory uterine bleeding. Older women are more likely to undergo procedures for the diagnosis and management of malignancy or pelvic relaxation. The adverse influence of advancing patient age on surgical morbidity is well known to gynecologic surgeons. Six decades ago, the age-related morbidity and mortality of an elective inguinal hernia repair in the patient older than 50 years prohibited an operative approach. Current attitudes differ as elective, emergent, and sometimes radical procedures are routinely performed in women during their seventh, eighth, and ninth decade of life. Surgically correctable problems in the elderly cannot be ignored because older women represent 12% of the U.S. population and compromise the fastest growing segment of our population. Coexisting medical problems, such as hypertension, vascular disease, and diabetes, are present in as many as 80% of the elderly (Orr, 1988; Orr and Taylor, 1994). For various reasons not just including stoic behavior and difficulties in accessing medical care, the elderly have an increased tendency for emergent medical and surgical situations. Reduced "homeostatic" reserves are the rule, with a 1% per year reduction in renal and hepatic function beginning at age 30 years and a 30% reduction of blood volume by age 75 years. With preoperative problem recognition, prompt intervention, and appropriate monitoring, the initial surgical insult is frequently well tolerated even in the eldest population; however, the alterations in physiologic reserves reduce or eliminate these patients' ability to tolerate complications. Although surgical morbidity may be increased in any gynecologic procedure, the frequency of complications associated with radical surgery (Orr et al, 1983) results in an increased risk of perioperative mortality (Table 42–2). Appropriate preoperative medical consultation should always be considered in the elderly when intervention can favorably influence outcome. Intensive postoperative surveillance and monitoring of the elderly should be the rule.

Immune Status. The direct correlation between immunocompromise and increased risk, frequency, severity, and lethality of surgical infection is an accepted fact (Orr and Shingleton, 1984). As expected, patients with advanced malignancy, particularly ovarian cancer, frequently have measurable immunologic deficits (Tunca, 1983). Unexpected immunologic alterations are also frequent in women with early-stage endometrial or cervical cancer (Orr et al, 1985). Importantly, a significant number of women with systemic disease (diabetes, rheumatism) or those taking specific medications (corticosteroids, antimitotics) may also have associated measurable or immeasurable deficits. Although individual immunologic testing may not be necessary, risk recognition and attempts at surgical risk reduction could potentially benefit this segment of the population. Regardless of the preoperative immunologic status, anesthesia, regional or general, transiently depresses host phagocytic function for 7 to 14 days (Orr and Taylor, 1994). Surgical blood loss varies dramatically with the radicality of the procedure (Table 42–3); however, transfusions are not infrequent, and the administration of blood products depresses T-lymphocyte antigen and mitogen response, mixed lymphocyte reactivity, and cell-mediated lympholysis. These deficits may persist for months or even years (Eisenkop et al, 1990). Finally, expected or unanticipated nutritional deficits are frequently present, and adversely affect both humoral and cell-mediated immunity and significantly increase the risk of infectious morbidity and poor wound healing (Orr and Shingleton, 1984).

Nutritional Status. As expected, 75% of patients with advanced ovarian cancer have nutritional deficits (Tunca, 1983); however, nutritional parameters are frequently abnormal in women with other gynecologic malignancies. Despite their clinical appearance, anthropometric measurements of triceps skinfold (body fat stores) and midarm muscle circumference (protein stores) are abnormal in as many as 50% of patients with early cervical and corpus cancer. Serum albumin levels are abnormal in 10% of patients with cervical cancer and in as many as 20% of women with corpus cancer (Orr et al, 1985). Because albumin has a relatively long half-life (20 days), these abnormalities suggest longstanding nutritional deficits. Serum iron transferrin levels, which correlate with total iron-binding capacity (serum half-life 8 days), are abnormal in more than 50% of patients with early cervical or corpus cancer (Orr et al, 1985), suggesting the presence of acute nutritional deficits in a significant number of women. Additional deficits of at least this magnitude occur in patients hospitalized for nonmalignant conditions (Orr and Shingleton, 1984). Because the potentially adverse effects of malnutrition are reversible if recognized and treated, gynecologic surgeons should become attentive to those laboratory or clinical nutritional indexes. Fortunately, even postoperative recognition and late nutritional supplementation may be beneficial (Ward et al, 1982; Mann, 1994).

Co-morbid Conditions. Coexisting medical diseases may increase the potential of operative morbidity.

These risks may be directly related to the operative procedure (i.e., risk of wound infection, bleeding) or to the disease itself (i.e., prior myocardial infarction). Unfortunately, in most situations there exists little disease-specific information to qualify risks. One report (MacKenzie and Charlson, 1988) indicated that the specific surgical risk associated with diabetes could be stratified on the basis of preoperative findings (Fig. 42–1). The risk of both cardiac and noncardiac complications was directly related to the presence of end-organ disease and not associated with the level of preoperative glucose control. In fact, diabetic patients without end-organ disease have only a 4% risk of serious noncardiac complications. In this context, it becomes imperative that preoperative surgical evaluation allow the gynecologic surgeon to identify potential concurrent illness to predict and potentially alter surgical risk with appropriate perioperative monitoring.

Surgeon Variables

Hand Washing. Maimonides first emphasized the importance of hand washing in the 11th century. The French surgeons DeChaulic in the 14th century and Paré in the 16th century recognized the importance of "surgical cleanliness." In 1857, Pasteur proposed the important effect of microorganisms in the genesis of infection. Semmelweis in 1861 indicated the importance of hand washing (with chlorinated lime) in decreasing the risk of puerperal fever. Later, Lister utilized a 1:20 solution of carbolic acid to disinfect his skin (Orr and Taylor, 1994). Unfortunately, the surgeon's hands cannot be sterilized, because 20% of the resident bacterial flora are located in nail beds or appendages beyond the reach of surgical scrubs. Therefore, the purpose of the surgical scrub is to remove transient pathogenic organisms. Although subject to debate, significant evidence exists to suggest the adequacy of a 2-minute scrub if a brush is used to scrub the skinfolds around the nails (Orr and Taylor, 1994). Friction appears necessary to remove resistant microorganisms. Although preoperative preparation is paramount, a 10- to 15-second scrub with an alcohol-containing agent after every surgical procedure will decrease the concentration of transient bacteria and inactivate the human immunodeficiency virus.

Percutaneous Injury. Glove puncture occurs in as many at 60% of all surgical procedures. Actual needle injury occurs commonly with many gynecologic procedures (Table 42–4). Regardless of technique, this risk is increased in direct proportion to the amount of surgical needle handling. However, other factors (Table 42–5) also increase these risks. Thus the surgical team's bacterial flora is frequently exposed to the incision and the patient's disease is exposed to the surgical team. It is important to decrease the risk of disease transmission through good skin preparation of both the surgeon and the patient.

Table 42–3. AVERAGE BLOOD LOSS DURING GYNECOLOGIC SURGERY

SURGICAL PROCEDURE	MEAN LOSS (ml)
Laparoscopic hysterectomy	100 ± 50
Vaginal hysterectomy	175 ± 75
Abdominal hysterectomy	250 ± 31
Radical hysterectomy/ lymphadenectomy	1126 ± 756
Abdominal hysterectomy/ lymphadenectomy	397 ± 207
Vulvectomy	250 ± 125
Ovarian debulking	1200 ± 225

Data from Orr et al (1984, 1986, 1990b) and Orr et al (unpublished data).

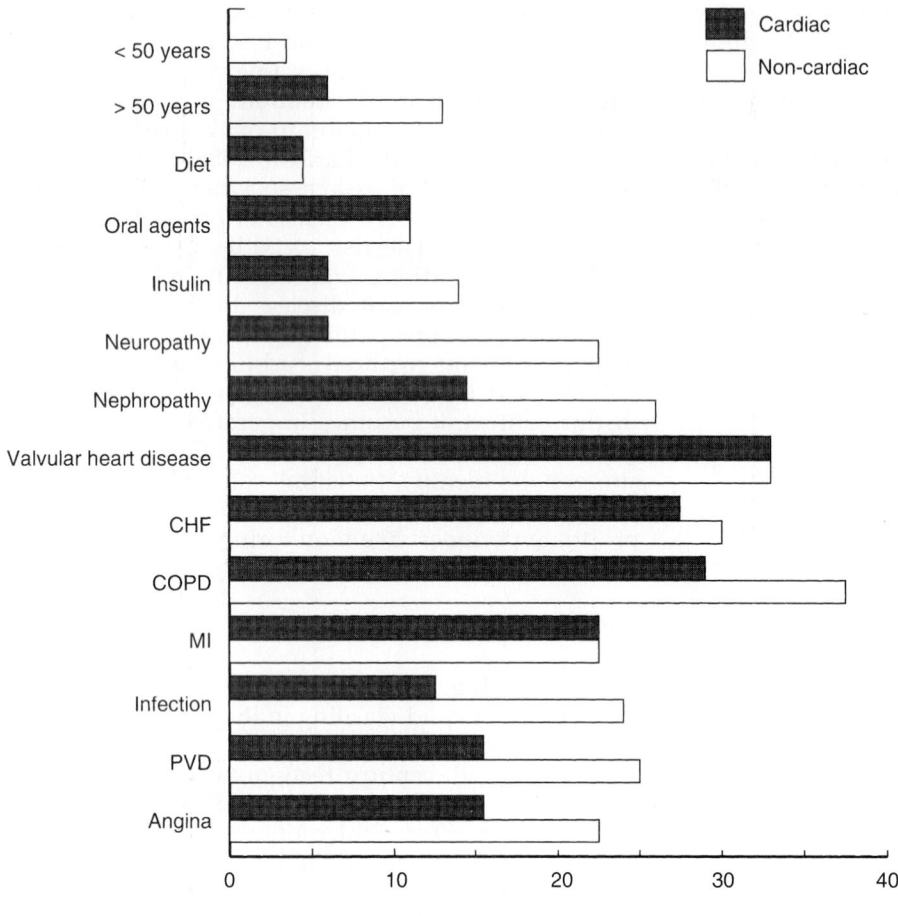

Figure 42–1
Diabetes: surgical risks. CHF, congestive heart failure; COPD, chronic obstructive pulmonary disease; MI, myocardial infarction; PVD, peripheral vascular disease. (Modified from MacKenzie CR, Charlson ME: Assessment of perioperative risk in the patient with diabetes mellitus. Surg Gynecol Obstet 1988;167:293, with permission.)

Preoperative Stay. There is reported an increased risk of surgical wound infection as the duration of preoperative hospitalization increased (Table 42–6) (Cruise and Foord, 1973). These increased risks may relate to patient variables that require a prolonged preoperative hospitalization. However, bacterial recolonization occurs within 48 hours of admission, and prolonged hospitalization potentially allows more virulent bacteria access to a "fresh" surgical wound (Orr and Taylor, 1994). Regardless, in most clinical situations it appears beneficial to maximize outpatient evaluation and minimize preoperative hospitalization.

Skin Preparation. A necessary component of every procedure involves preparation of the surgical site. The patient's skin (average area 1.8 m^2) is the largest body organ, accounting for 16% of body weight and 20% of body water (Orr and Taylor, 1994), and has a significant quantity of bacterial flora. Currently, a number of surgical preparation solutions with topical antimicrobial effects are available (Table 42–7).

Table 42–4. PERCUTANEOUS INJURIES AND RECONTACTS FOR GYNECOLOGY SERVICE AND BY SURGICAL PROCEDURE

PROCEDURE	RISK CLASS*	NO. OF PROCEDURES	NO. (%) OF PROCEDURES WITH ONE OR MORE INJURIES
Gynecology service	—	307	31 (10)
Vaginal hysterectomy	H	47	10 (21)
Abdominal hysterectomy	M	165	17 (10)
Other gynecology	L	95	4 (4)
Ovarian cystectomy	—	15	1 (7)
Salpingo-oophorectomy	—	35	1 (3)
Miscellaneous	—	45	2 (4)

*Risk class: H, high; M, medium; L, low.
Modified from Tokars JI, Bell DM, Culver DH, et al: Percutaneous injuries during surgical procedures. JAMA 1992;267:2899, with permission.

Table 42–5. FACTORS INCREASING THE RISK OF GLOVE PERFORATION

Emergency procedure
Longer operative time
Inadequate muscle relaxation
Number of sutures
Wound depth
Needle handling

Their mechanisms and rapidity of action as well as residual bactericidal effects differ (Table 42–8). Additionally, their spectrum of antibacterial or antifungal activity may vary dramatically. Not infrequently, these agents are combined to provide a more efficacious skin preparation.

Aqueous iodine alone is highly concentrated and irritating. However, iodophors (e.g., povidone-iodine [Betadine]) combine iodine with a polymer to promote slow release to overcome these effects. The most commonly used solution is 10% (1% free iodine) and may be combined with a detergent to form a scrub solution. Betadine scrub should only be used on intact skin because it is cytotoxic to fibroblasts and impedes healing of soft tissues. Chlorhexidine gluconate has broad-spectrum bactericidal activity. Solutions containing chlorhexidine gluconate, which binds to the stratum corneum (activity for 5 to 6 hours), or an iodophor are the most effective surgical scrubs with the fewest stability, contamination, or toxicity problems. Chlorhexidine gluconate, a quaternary amine, is superior in decreasing the bacterial count and is a more persistent agent (i.e., in preventing regrowth in a gloved hand) than providone-iodine. Although alcohol produces the most rapid and quantitative reduction of bacterial counts, it does have significant drying effects on the skin and is extremely volatile.

Unfortunately, few prospective studies evaluating the efficacy of specific skin preparations are available. Geelhoed and colleagues (1983) evaluated a regimen using a combination of iodine alone or with an alcohol wipe and an iodine-impregnated drape or alcohol alone with an impregnated drape. Bacterial counts at incision or closure were significantly decreased in those groups using alcohol as a part of the

Table 42–6. SURGICAL WOUND INFECTION AND DURATION OF PREOPERATIVE HOSPITALIZATION

DAYS IN HOSPITAL	CLEAN WOUND INFECTION RATE
≤1	1.1%
2–6	2.2%
7–13	2.4%
≥14	4.3%

Modified from Cruise PJE, Foord R: A 5 year prospective study of 23,649 surgical wounds. Arch Surg 1973;107:206, with permission. Copyright 1973, American Medical Association.

Table 42–7. ANTISEPSIS FOR SURGICAL DISINFECTION

| AGENT | MEAN REDUCTION IN RELEASE OF SKIN BACTERIA (%) | |
	Immediate	>3 Hr
Liquid soap	40	0
Povidone-iodine liquid soap	90	20
Chlorhexidine detergent*	75	70
Povidone-iodine aqueous solution	97	75
Isopropyl alcohol 60%	96	90
Hexachlorophene detergent	40	91
Isopropyl alcohol 70%	99.3	99.1
Isopropyl alcohol 70% plus chlorhexidine 0.5%	99.4	99.7

*The application time for chlorhexidine detergent is 3 minutes; for all other preparations it is 5 minutes.
Modified from Masterson BJ: Skin preparation. In American College of Surgeons: Care of the Surgical Patient. New York: Scientific American, 1991:22, with permission.

preoperative preparation (Fig. 42–2). More recently, other types of preparations combining alcohol, irgasan, and film formers have been studied; these preparations apparently represent rapid, safe methods of skin preparation (Gabel-Hughes et al, 1991). These particular studies suggested that the use of a specific skin preparation may decrease operating room time and cost without increasing patient risk. Although the "optimal" preoperative preparation is unknown, a simple change in technique (i.e., using alcohol) may be potentially cost-effective, particularly in short operative procedures.

Hair Removal. Despite the lack of evidence supporting its benefits, hair removal has been and remains an acceptable part of the preoperative surgical ritual. In fact, evidence to the contrary (i.e., no need for hair removal) has been present for almost two decades. Cruise and Foord (1973), in over 18,000 patients, conclusively demonstrated that clean wound infection rates were lowest when hair was not removed from the surgical field. Regardless, our surgical obsession continues, and prospective randomized studies (Alexander et al, 1983) comparing razor and clipper techniques of hair removal on the morning of surgery with removal the evening before surgery clearly demonstrate the potential benefit of clipper hair removal in the morning if deemed necessary (Table 42–9).

Thermal Control. Humans are homeotherms, having a protective core temperature with minimal organ system deviation. Until recently, thermal control has been a neglected part of the surgical procedure; however, failure to control body temperature adversely affects nearly every organ system (Table 42–10). Although each organ is potentially important, alterations in prostaglandin and arachidonic acid byproducts may result in a bleeding diathesis (Sladen, 1989). Significant bleeding increases the potential

Table 42-8. TOPICAL ANTIMICROBIALS

	ALCOHOLS	CHLORHEXIDINE	HEXACHLOROPHENE	IODINE
Mode of action	Denaturation of protein	Cell wall disruption	Cell wall disruption	Oxidation substitution by free iodine
Gram-positive bacteria	++	++	++	++
Gram-negative bacteria	++	+	−	+
Rapidity of action	++	+	±	+
Residual	−	+	+	±

Modified from Larson E: Guideline for use of topical antimicrobial agents. Am J Infect Control 1988;16:253, with permission.

need for transfusion but also potentially increases the medium for bacterial proliferation and subsequent infectious morbidity. Although anesthesia has been the monitor for these problems, surgeons can and must modify techniques in an effort to maintain temperature hemostasis. Anesthesia is associated with a decreased metabolic rate, which includes at least a 20% reduction of heat production at rest, necessitating operating room environment control. The operating room should be warm (>21°C) before draping the patient because lower temperatures encourage heat loss. Skin preparation solutions, infused fluids and blood, as well as irrigation fluids should be warmed. Thermal hot air drapes to reduce

heat losses from the head, chest, and legs should also be routine. Gastrointestinal or pleural surfaces lose fluid at rates greater than 500 ml/hour and should be exteriorized minimally or not at all to decrease losses from evaporation, conduction, radiation, and convection. The highest rate of heat loss occurs during the first hour of surgery; thus attention to detail becomes important even during shorter procedures. Although all patients are at risk, older women produce less heat, are less able to modify heat loss, and are at higher risk for hypothermia and associated problems. Importantly, high flow rates during operative laparoscopy may increase the risk of hypothermia.

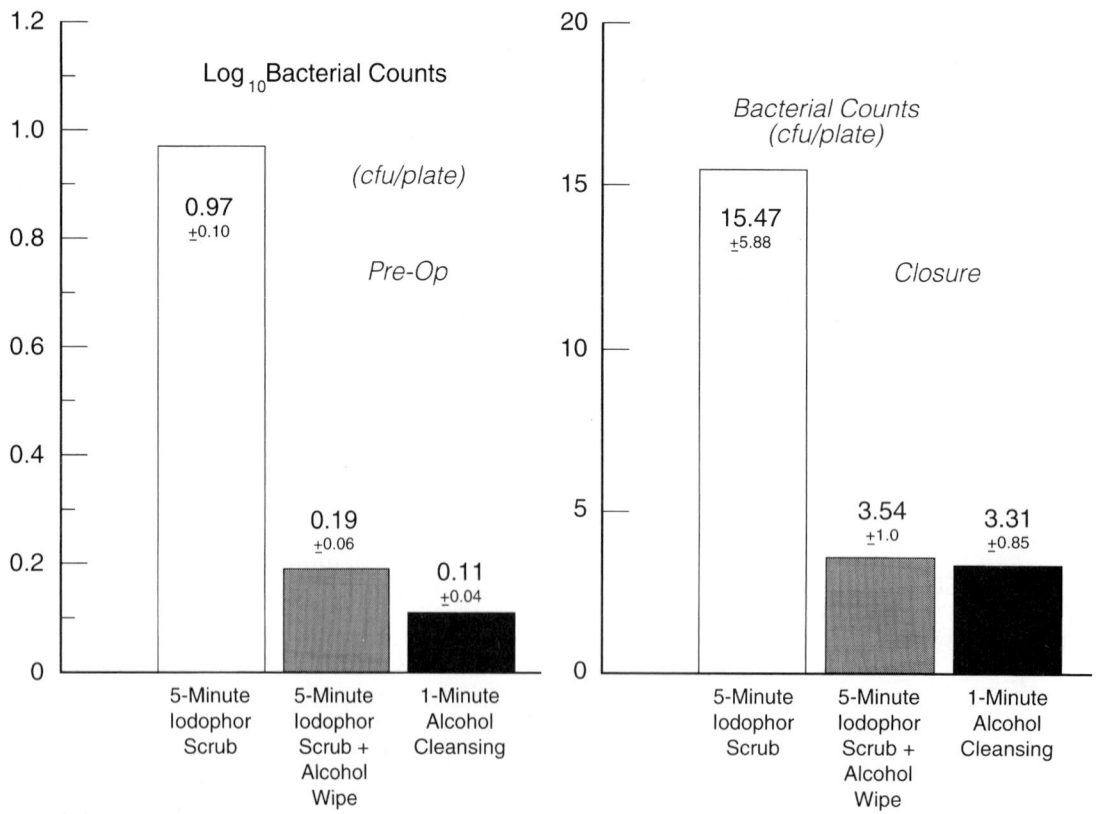

Figure 42-2
Bacterial counts with various types of skin preparation. cfu, colony-forming unit. (Modified from Geelhoed GW, Sharpe K, Simon GL: A comparison study of surgical skin preparation methods. Surg Gynecol Obstet 1983;107:265, with permission.)

Table 42-9. HAIR REMOVAL METHODS

METHOD	NO. OF PATIENTS	% INFECTION
Razor in evening	271	5.2
Razor in morning	266	6.4
Clipper in evening	250	4.0
Clipper in morning	226	1.8

Modified from Alexander JW, Fischer JE, Boyajan M, et al: The influence of hair removal methods on wound infection. Arch Surg 1983; 118:347, with permission. Copyright 1983, American Medical Association.

Table 42-10. EFFECTS OF HYPOTHERMIA

SYSTEM	ORGAN SYSTEM FUNCTIONS
Cardiovascular	Increased systemic vascular resistance
	Myocardial depression
	Arrhythmias
Respiratory	Diminished response to hypoxemia, hypercarbia
	Decreased CO_2 production
Neurologic	Delayed emergence from anesthesia, drowsiness, confusion, coma
Hematologic	Increased viscosity (ischemia)
	Thrombocytopathy
	Thrombocytopenia
	Impaired coagulation
Metabolic	Hyperglycemia
Renal	Cold diuresis (impaired sodium absorption)

Prophylactic Antibiotics. A pivotal preoperative surgeon-modified variable involves the use of prophylactic antibiotics. Gynecologic surgery for benign or malignant disease carries an inherent risk of infectious morbidity. Once present, infection alters patients' mobility, increases their exposure to additional medications, and predisposes them to additional complications. Prophylactic antibiotics decrease these risks regardless of the surgical route (laparoscopic, vaginal, or abdominal), but their protective effect varies with the duration of the procedure (Fig. 42–3). The benefit of the antibiotic prophylaxis decreases as the duration of the procedure increases. With a first-generation cephalosporin (Orr et al, 1985), this benefit is lost if the operative procedure lasts longer than 2½ hours. Although the efficacy in nonradical procedures is accepted, few studies have addressed the benefits of prophylactic antibiotics in extended hysterectomy (Orr et al, 1990b). Although factors such as operative time, blood loss, need for transfusion, and surgeon experience vary dramatically between series, the majority of published information suggests the efficacy of prophylactic antibiotics. Current information suggests that 68% of gynecologic oncologists routinely use antibiotics (Orr et al, 1990b). One fifth use them occasionally, and one sixth do not use them at all. At least two thirds of those who use antibiotics utilize a single drug; however, one in six use a multiple-drug prophylaxis regimen, with few or no data supporting this benefit. In an attempt to determine the most appropriate duration of antibiotic prophylaxis, our investigations have attempted to control important variables such as duration of preoperative hospitalization, hair clipping, or administration of antibiotic drugs and the use of small 2-0 polyglycolic acid (PGA) sutures while avoiding subcutaneous sutures and subcutaneous drains. No vasoconstrictors are used. The majority of patients receive postoperative oxygen supplementation (Knighton et al, 1984).

Over the past few years, I have reported the efficacy of single-dose prophylaxis compared with multiple-dose administration both in university practice and in a private practice (Orr, 1986, 1988b). More recently, we have evaluated single-dose prophylaxis in extended hysterectomy, including hysterectomy with lymph node resection for endometrial malignancy and radical hysterectomy for

cervical malignancy (Orr et al, 1990b). In no situation have we been able to demonstrate the clinical benefit of a multiple-dose prophylactic antibiotic regimen (Table 42–11).

Single-dose prophylaxis is apparently efficacious and certainly cost-effective. Laboratory data suggest a potential benefit (when compared with multiple doses) in wound healing (Scher et al, 1988). When comparing cefonicid, cefazolin, and controls, there was a marked decrease in wound strength as the duration of prophylaxis increased. Clinically, this related to an increase in the risk of late wound hernias. After evaluating these clinical and laboratory data, it is difficult to rationalize the use of multiple-dose antibiotic prophylaxis during any gynecologic procedure.

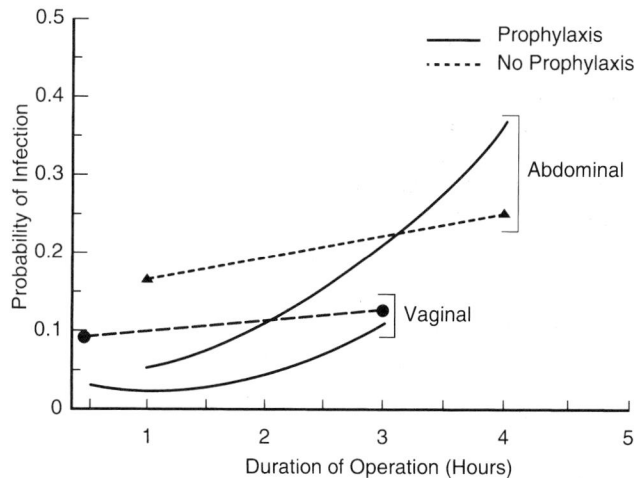

Figure 42-3
Probability of infection with and without antibiotic prophylaxis for hysterectomy. (Adapted from Shapiro M, Muñoz A, Tager IB, et al: Risk factors for infection at the operative site after abdominal or vaginal hysterectomy. N Engl J Med 1982;307: 1661, with permission.)

Table 42–11. EFFICACY OF SINGLE-DOSE ANTIBIOTIC PROPHYLAXIS

TYPE OF SURGERY	% SURGICAL SITE INFECTION	
	Single Dose	Multiple Dose
Hysterectomy*		
University	4.2	4.3
Private practice	1.7	0.0
Extended†		
Hysterectomy and nodes	2.9	6.5
Radical hysterectomy	4.2	4.5

*Data from Orr et al (1986, 1988b).
†Data from Orr et al (1990b).

Table 42–12. CEFOTETAN CONCENTRATION IN TISSUES

TISSUE (SAMPLE NO.)	MEAN TIME (min)	CONCENTRATION (μg/ml)
Plasma (51)	49 ± 25	138 ± 38
Uterus (57)	69 ± 32	46 ± 16
Parametrium (56)	68 ± 33	63 ± 24
Fat (37)	88 ± 38	17.5 ± 9
Fascia (34)	89 ± 38	44.0 ± 20

Modified from Orr JW Jr, Sisson PF, Barrett JM, et al: Pharmacokinetics and tissue kinetics of 1 gm. cefotetan prophylaxis in abdominal or vaginal hysterectomy. Am J Obstet Gynecol 1988;158:742, with permission.

Although single-dose antibiotic prophylaxis is encouraged, the exact dosage may require modification because the abdominal wall may provide an anatomic sanctuary for bacterial colonization in some clinical situations. In our report (Orr et al, 1988a), single-dose prophylaxis resulted in significantly decreased antibiotic concentrations in subcutaneous tissues compared with those in the plasma, uterus, parametrium, or fascia (Table 42–12). This effect may be exaggerated in subcutaneous tissues of obese patients or those having undergone previous pelvic radiation, in whom the blood supply may be relatively compromised. When compared with normal-weight controls, adipose levels of cefazolin in the morbidly obese are depressed when a single gram is administered intramuscularly or intravenously. However, when drug dosage is increased to 2 g and given intravenously, adipose levels equal those of normal-weight controls. Clinically, an increase in drug results in increased subcutaneous tissue drug levels and potentially decreases infection risk. In one report, 2-g intravenous dosing was associated with a significant reduction (16% vs. 5%) in wound infection in obese patients (Forse et al, 1988). Although cost-effective practice is important and single-gram dosing seems appropriate during vaginal procedures or uncomplicated abdominal procedures, consideration of higher dose administration should be given in those situations in which abdominal wall physiologic factors (obesity, previous radiation therapy) increase the risk of infection or other problems. We prefer to administer the drugs intravenously just before the operative procedure in an attempt to avoid the pain of an intramuscular injection and minimize the problems of lowered drug concentration with unexpected time delays. Concerns regarding anaphylaxis are important; however, this route does not increase risks. Administration by an anesthesiologist allows close monitoring as well as treatment should this complication occur.

A significant number of women with gynecologic cancer require intestinal surgery as part of their primary treatment, management of complications, or even palliation. In this situation, available data suggest that single-dose antimicrobial prophylaxis is as efficacious as multiple doses in the prevention of surgical site infection (Morton et al, 1989). It is apparent that mechanical bowel preparation in conjunction with parenteral prophylaxis is efficacious and should be used to prevent postoperative infection. In fact, there is little reason to omit a mechanical bowel preparation before most gynecologic procedures. If time permits, 48 hours of a clear liquid diet with cathartics is efficacious. The development of osmotic electrolyte solutions results in an adequate mechanical preparation if started the evening before surgery. Nasogastric lavage with normal saline (6 liters) can also be effectively used but results in unnecessary morbidity (i.e., insertion of nasogastric tube) and potential electrolyte and volume disturbances. The use and side effects of oral "nonabsorbable" antibiotics is no longer necessary (Bartlett and Burton, 1983).

INTRAOPERATIVE VARIABLES

The manipulation of intraoperative variables must be oriented toward a single goal: completing the procedure as efficiently and as safely as possible. The operative components affecting operative time include the incision, intraoperative techniques (particularly to increase operative exposure), use of instrumentation, and closure. Every surgeon should attempt to modify specific events to affect the outcome favorably because longer procedures are associated with an increased risk of infectious morbidity (with or without antibiotic prophylaxis), pulmonary complications, and increased blood loss (Orr, 1988).

Before addressing these components, two potential areas of intraoperative bacterial contamination require comment. Regardless of the method of measurement, bacterial recovery is consistently increased in the presence of operating room conversation (Letts and Doermer, 1983). Although this quantity of contamination may not "cause" infection, conversation frequently detracts attention from the surgical procedure and potentially adds to operative time.

The surgical "splash basin" is of unproven benefit and may provide an additional source of bacterial contamination (Baird et al, 1984). At least 75% have positive cultures and as many as 12% grow more than 100 colonies. Although bacterial contamination at relatively high levels (10^5) is required to incite surgical infection consistently (Orr et al, 1993), this level of additional contamination may tip the scale. Although using splash basins may not create risks, their lack of efficacy and their continued use demonstrate the need to examine each aspect of every procedure.

Incision

Wound healing and outcome may be related to incision placement. The selection of the abdominal incision and its placement are related to a number of factors. The actual incision placement and incision type are governed by the diagnosis, the urgency of the operation, patient habitus, the presence of a previous incision, cosmetic preferences, and the possible need for a stoma. A transverse incision has fewer adverse effects on postoperative respiratory function. In planning incisions for elective surgery, the surgeon's primary responsibility is to identify a site that allows sufficient access for successful completion of the planned operation but also allows extension of the operative field exposure if necessary. Finally, the site must allow safe closure.

The most aesthetically pleasing scar results when the long axis of the scar is in the direction of maximal skin tension. A transverse incision, although not the strongest, heals with an almost invisible scar and clinically performs very well. Clinically, transverse fascial incisions rarely suffer acute wound failure. This benefit is not related to incision strength but is likely related to less stress placed on the incision itself. In most situations, the Pfannenstiel incision is adequate for benign gynecologic procedures. If necessary, exposure can be increased by incising the rectus muscle at its insertion. The converted Cherney incision then allows increased lateral pelvic exposure as well as improved upper abdominal access. If a transverse incision is used with the preoperative anticipation of the need of additional exposure, a rectus muscle–splitting incision (Maylard) may be appropriate. If this incision is chosen, care to ligate the epigastric artery is essential.

The strongest incision is a midline incision closed with widely placed sutures incorporating nearly 1.5 cm of fascial tissue and placed at intervals of 1.5 to 2.0 cm (Orr and Taylor, 1994). Sutures placed close to the fascial edge result in tissue ischemia and a decrease in tensile strength and predispose to poor wound outcome. Although transverse incisions may not be as strong (Table 42–13), they are subjected to a different postoperative anatomic stress and perform well clinicaly (Ott et al, 1995). There appears to be no difference in the incision strength of extended

Table 42–13. CLOSURE STRENGTH OF FASCIAL INCISIONS

TYPE OF INCISION	CLOSURE STRENGTH INDEX (PARAMEDIAN WITH 7.2 = 100)
Midline incision, wide closure	318
Transverse incision	208
Transverse incision, below umbilicus	153
Midline incision, ordinary closure	150
Paramedian incision	100

Modified from Tera H, Aberg C: Tensile strengths of twelve types of knots employed in surgery, using different suture materials. Acta Chir Scand 1976;142:349, with permission.

vertical incisions through or around the umbilicus. Supraumbilical incisions may be appropriate to allow adequate pelvic exposure in the morbidly obese patient without increasing wound depth.

While incision site selection is important during primary procedures, the correct decision during repeat procedures may be more critical. Although previous scars are associated with less vascularity and an increased rate of infection, second or repeat incisions should be made at the same site if possible. If not, new parallel incisions or new incisions that transect previous scars at an acute angle should be avoided, because they compromise blood supply and predispose the site to poor healing. If the previous incision is used for reoperation, the pelvic surgeon must be cognizant of the increased risk of intraperitoneal adhesions and intestinal injury. Sharp dissection of the subcutaneous and fascial tissue above or below the incision may facilitate peritoneal entry into the peritoneum. It would appear that in many clinical situations even radical procedures can be safely performed through a transverse incision (Orr et al, 1995). Although many operative procedures can be performed through less than vertical incisions, the correct operative procedure should not be influenced by the initial incision site if less than adequate.

The surgical incision provides exposure to the intra-abdominal organs, and a single bold incision through the skin and subcutaneous tissues should be used. Multiple-stroke incisions increase the risk of infection and recoverable bacteria in a contaminated wound (Edlich et al, 1977). The technical benefit of a single incision relates to creating less surgical dead space. Unfortunately, once created, the adverse affects of surgical dead space cannot be reversed. Sutures placed to close potential dead space result in an increase in foreign body material and further increase the infection risk fourfold (Fig. 42–4). Another antiquated portion of the surgical procedure involves using multiple knives to create the abdominal incision. Multiple knives and multiple-stroke incisions only "stairstep" subcutaneous tissues and create added dead space. There is no benefit (Table

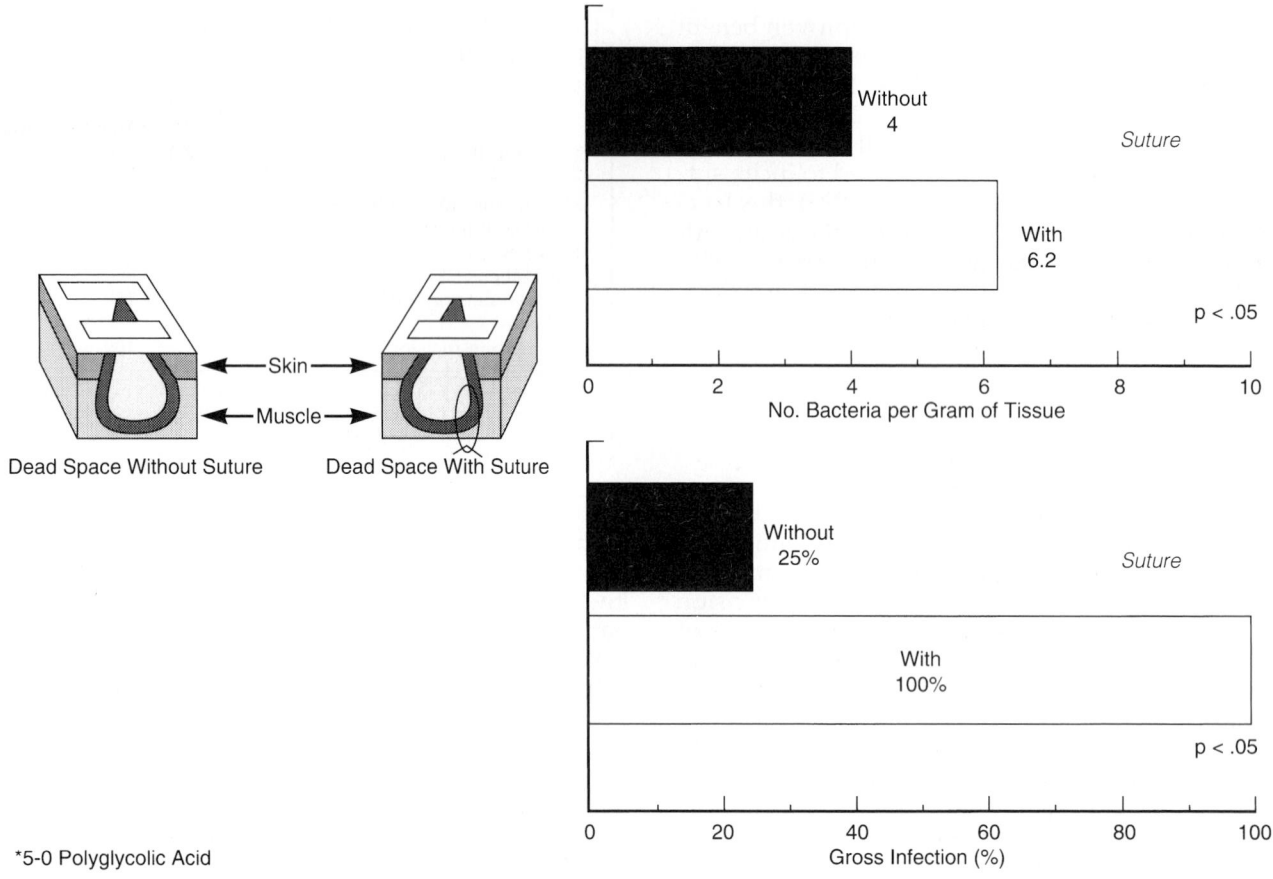

Figure 42-4
Infection results with and without suture (5-0 PGA) in dead space. Inoculum: *Staphylococcus aureus* 10⁴.

*5-0 Polyglycolic Acid

42-14) in terms of decreasing contamination or infectious risk when comparing the infection rate with one knife versus two knives in clean or clean-contaminated procedures or overall (Hasselgren et al, 1984). Additionally, charges of $5 to $12 per blade per procedure can potentially be eliminated, resulting in a favorable effect on cost control. With the exception of individual vessel control, there appears to be little benefit in incision tensile strength to using electrocautery for the skin incision (Table 42–15).

Intraoperative Techniques

Appropriate intraoperative exposure of the surgical field results in reduced operative time and potentially decreases the risk of blood loss. Our experience with a table-stabilized retractor ring has been favorable. Currently, we use the Bookwalter retractor (Codman U.S.). Positioning the ring while using multiple adjustable blades allows adequate retraction of the abdominal wall and the gastrointestinal

Table 42-14. INFECTION RATE BY NUMBER OF KNIVES USED FOR SKIN INCISION (*N* = 609 PATIENTS)

	NO. OF INFECTIONS (%)	
TYPE OPERATION	*1 Knife*	*2 Knives*
Clean	5 (3.1)	10 (5.8)
Clean-contaminated	5 (4.3)	7 (5.1)
Overall	10 (3.6)	17 (5.5)

Modified from Hasselgren P, Hagberg E, Malmer H, et al: One instead of two knives for surgical incision: does it increase the risk of postoperative wound infection? Arch Surg 1984;119:917, with permission. Copyright 1984, American Medical Association.

Table 42-15. MIDLINE FASCIAL INCISION STRENGTH BY CUTTING INSTRUMENT

INSTRUMENT	STRENGTH (g)
Scalpel	1087
Cautery cut	623
Cautery "coag"	402

From Kumagai SG, Rosales RF, Hunter GC, et al: Effects of electrocautery on midline laparotomy. Am J Surg 1991;162:620, with permission.

tract, resulting in a constant, appropriate exposure of the surgical field with minimal need for repacking or tissue trauma. The retractor can be satisfactorily used in abdominal procedures using a vertical or transverse incision (Orr et al, 1995, 1997). A vaginal retractor is also available.

Every surgical procedure results in tissue trauma and surgical debris. Irrigation with appropriate warm fluids may decrease the bacteria but, more importantly, removes potential culture media. If used, wound irrigation under pressure results in a marked reduction of recoverable bacteria as well as wound infection (Edlich et al, 1977). Any fluids used for pelvic irrigation should be completely removed so as to not interfere with postoperative macrophage function. Theoretically, hypotonic solutions (water) may potentially lyse free-floating malignant cells; however, laboratory evidence does not support its use. Isotonic irrigation (Ringer's lactate) should be used if fertility is a consideration (Fayez and Schnerder, 1989).

Vaginal surgeons frequently propose the use of vasoconstrictors to reduce blood loss and to provide a "cleaner" operative field. Unfortunately, no available information confirms this clinical impression because postoperative alterations in hematocrit and blood loss are not different. In fact, the use of vasoconstrictors decreases local blood supply, antibiotics, and local tissue oxygenation and may increase the incidence of cuff cellulitis and pelvic abscess (England et al, 1983). Additionally, systemic side effects including increased heart rate, increased ventricular irritability (50%), increased systolic pressure, hyperkalemia, and hyperglycemia are the rule (Cunningham et al, 1985). Justification for their routine use is not available.

Closure

Decisions regarding suture selection for wound edge reapproximation or vessel ligature are of vital importance to wound outcome. Lister introduced the first monofilament absorbable suture material. His use of catgut dramatically changed many techniques. In fact, today there is little role for natural suture material. It is important that the gynecologic surgeon choose the suture and method of closure in every situation based on factual information. Modifications should be made only after the surgeon's own experience has been reviewed (Orr, 1986).

The choice of appropriate surgical suture material is primarily related to the need for suture tensile strength and the duration of activity. The ideal suture loses its tensile strength over a time interval in which the injured tissue regains tensile strength. Reported information divides suture tensile strength into three categories (Orr, 1986). Steel sutures are the strongest, synthetic sutures are intermediate, and natural sutures have the lowest intrinsic initial strength. A large number of suture materials and configurations are currently available (Table 42–16). The suture's chemical composition is more important than the physical configuration in determining wound outcome.

The concepts of surgical knot tying are considered elementary to most practicing gynecologists. However, during procedures, it is not infrequent for a physician to use 6, 8, or even 10 throws in an individual suture in an effort to "secure" the pedicle. In most instances, this is only time consuming. The placement of a surgeon's square knot in chromic sutures, a surgeon's knot in PGA sutures, or a double surgeon's knot in polypropylene (Prolene) provides

Table 42–16. CHARACTERISTICS OF SUTURE MATERIALS

MATERIAL	TENSILE STRENGTH	KNOT SECURITY	REACTIVITY	DAYS TO 10% OF TENSILE STRENGTH
Permanent				
Manufactured				
Steel	4	4	1	
Polyamide (nylon)	3	3	1	
Polyesters (Dacron)	3	3	1	
Polyolefins (Prolene)	3	1	1	
Natural				
Silk	2	3	3	
Cotton	2	2	2	
Linen	2	2	2	
Absorbable				
Catgut	1	2	3	5
Chromic catgut	1	3	3	28
Polyglycolic acid	2	2	1	28
Polydioxonone sulfate	3	2	1	56
Polyglyconate	3	2	1	55

From Orr JW Jr, Taylor PT Jr: Wound healing. In Orr JW Jr, Shingleton HM (eds): Complications in Gynecologic Surgery: Prevention, Recognition, and Management. Philadelphia: JB Lippincott Company, 1994:167, with permission.

Table 42–17. KNOT STRENGTH

SUTURE	KNOT CONFIGURATION TO MAXIMUM STRENGTH (% UNKNOTTED)	
Monofilament steel	2 × 1	(92%)
Chromic	2 × 1	(72%)
Dexon	2 × 2	(74%)
Prolene	2 × 2 × 2	(98%)

Modified from Tera H, Aberg C: Tensile strengths of twelve types of knots employed in surgery, using different suture materials. Acta Chir Scand 1976;142:1, with permission.

maximal knot strength (Table 42–17) compared with an unknotted suture. Although in vivo knot slippage may occur, additional throws only increase the amount of foreign material in the surgical wound.

As previously noted, any suture material or foreign body in the surgical wound increases the risk of infection (Edlich et al, 1977). This increased rate of recoverable bacteria and risk of infection rises proportionately with the length or amount of suture material (Fig. 42–5). Clinically, this translates to attention to all aspects of suture technique, including the length of "tag" on suture material. To leave more than a 2-mm tag in a PGA suture offers little to knot security and potentially increases the risk of infection.

Even the choice of suture size has potential implications for surgical morbidity (Edlich et al, 1977). The recoverability of gram-positive or gram-negative bacteria decreases in proportion to suture size. We currently use 2-0 or smaller PGA sutures in all pelvic procedures, benign or malignant, vaginal or abdominal. Although tying these sutures may initially seem difficult, their strength, rate of absorption, and favorable effects on potential infection (McGeehan et al, 1980) and decreased pain (Rogers, 1974) suggest a patient benefit.

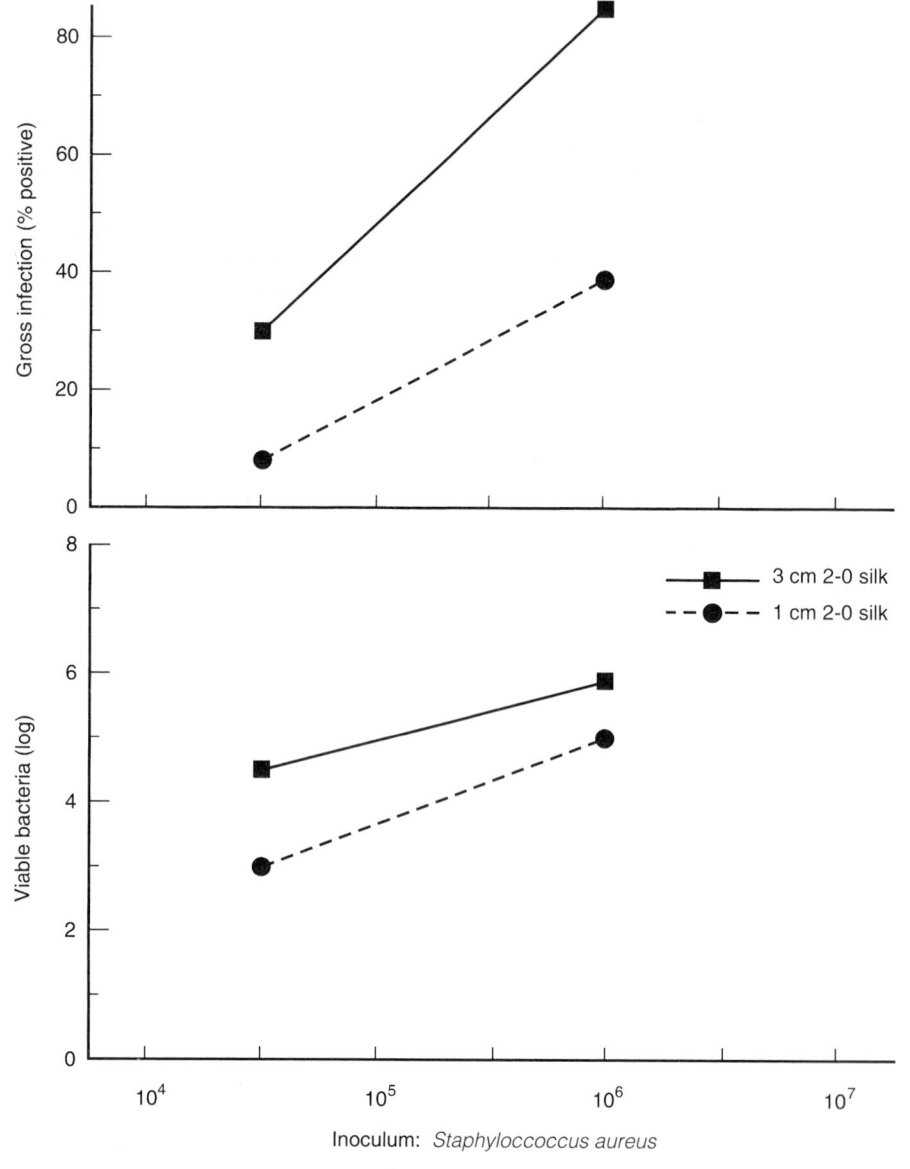

Inoculum: *Staphyloccoccus aureus*

Figure 42–5
Rate of infection risk with increased suture length. (Modified from Edlich RF, Rodehaver GI, Thacker JG, et al: Fundamentals of Wound Management in Surgery: Technical Factors in Wound Management. South Plainfield, NJ: Chirugecom, 1977, with permission.)

Table 42–18. SUTURE SIZE AND KNOT VOLUME

KNOT CONFIGURATION (THROWS)	SUTURE SIZE	KNOT VOLUME POLYGLACTIN 910
3	4-0	0.40
5	4-0	0.57
3	2-0	2.60
5	2-0	3.53

6.2   1.4

Modified from van Rijssel EJC, Brand R, Admiraal C, et al: Tissue reaction and surgical knots. Obstet Gynecol 1989;74:64, with permission from the American College of Obstetricians and Gynecologists.

When comparing the effects of suture size and knot configurations, it becomes evident that knot volume is influenced more by suture size than by the number of throws (Table 42–18). In a comparison of 4-0 and 2-0 suture material with three or five knots, increasing the number of throws increases foreign body volume by a factor of 1.4, whereas an increase in suture size increases knot volume by a factor of 6.2. The message is clear. Large sutures and multiple knots add little to the surgical procedure and are not necessarily in the patient's best interest.

Surgical hemostasis relates to a complex interaction of the coagulation cascade as well as surgical control of intermediate and large-size vessels. In an elegant, practical study by Hay et al (1989), the effects of required duration of vessel ligation and the propensity of bleeding were evaluated (Fig. 42–6). In small (1.5 to 3.5-mm) vessels, de-ligation and vessel trauma resulted in a 100% risk of bleeding at 48 hours, a 90% risk at 60 hours, a 40% risk at 72 hours, and a 30% risk at 82 hours. No bleeding occurred after 96 hours of ligation. Clinically, this suggests the adequacy of currently available synthetic (PGA) su-

ture materials and does not propose the need for a longer acting suture material (polyglyconate or polydioxanone sulfate) during pedicle tying of the pelvic portion of the operation. These data further discourage the use of silk suture, which has a significant inflammatory response and may contribute to adhesion formation (Luijendijk et al, 1996).

Broken sutures increase frustration and operative time. Tying techniques are important, but sutures are sometimes handled by instruments. Breaking strength of 5-0 monofilament is reduced by 50% when handled with a needle holder (Stamp et al, 1988). This information reiterates the fact that sutures are not designed to be manipulated by instruments. Needle carriers are intended to drive needles, not move sutures. Deviations in technique provide no benefits to the patient.

The antediluvian need to close the peritoneum can be overcome to decrease operative time without increasing potential risk. Peritoneal closure adds nothing to incisional strength and, when compared with open techniques, is not associated with an increase in wound infection, abdominal wall adhesions, or bowel obstruction (Table 42–19). If there is no benefit to close the peritoneum, only poor outcomes can result (Franchi et al, 1996). Although many methods have been unsuccessfully proposed to reduce the incidence of abdominal adhesions, data on the use of a sodium hyaluronate–based bioresorbable membrane in a randomized prospective evaluation indicate a statistical and clinical benefit for the reduction of significant intra-abdominal adhesions (Becker et al, 1996). Although further studies may be necessary, this exciting new modality may play a major role in the reduction of morbidity associated with adhesions.

Abdominal wall closure is best accomplished with sutures placed at some distance from the fascial layers. Using porometric material, Sanders et al (1977) demonstrated the benefit of widely placed, loosely

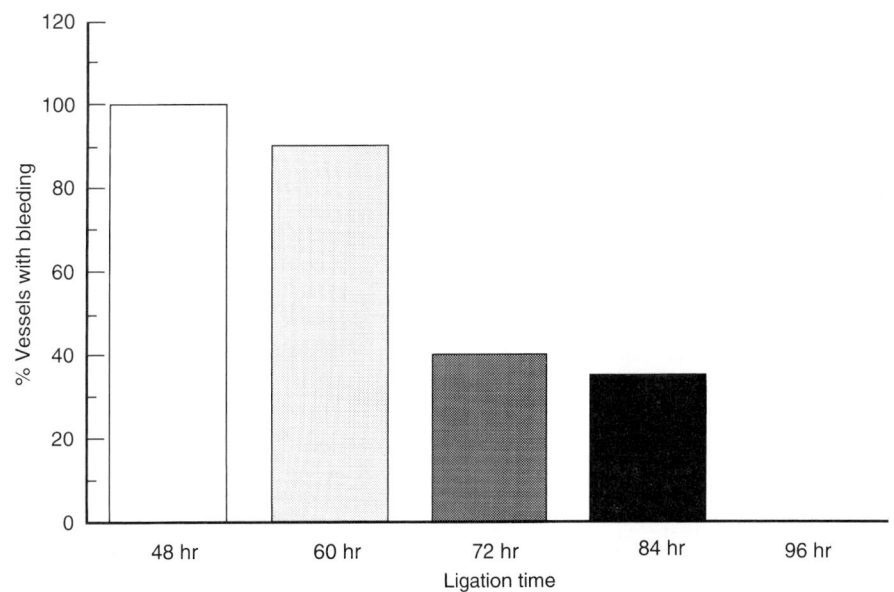

Figure 42–6
Effects of duration of vessel ligation and propensity of bleeding. (Modified from Hay DL, Von Fraunhofer JA, Masterson BJ: Hemostasis in blood vessels after ligation. Am J Obstet Gynecol 1989;160:737, with permission.)

Table 42-19. PERITONEAL CLOSURE VERSUS OPEN TECHNIQUE

	OPEN	CLOSED
Wound infection (%)	2.4	3.6
Adhesions (%)	15.8	22.2
Obstruction (%)	0	1.6

Modified from Tulandi T, Hum HS, Gelfand MM: Closure of laparotomy incisions with or without peritoneal suturing and second-look laparoscopy. Am J Obstet Gynecol 1988;158:536, with permission.

tied sutures when measuring wound-breaking pressure. The adverse effects of tightly tied fascial sutures as they relate to changes in tensile strength and wound failure energy have been documented (Fig. 42–7). There appears to be no reason or benefit to strangulate fascial tissue during fascial closure.

The obsession with closing the fascia with permanent sutures is addressed in the gynecologic literature. Absorbable sutures have different rates of tensile strength loss (Fig. 42–8), and there may be a benefit to using longer acting absorbable suture that mirrors the normal return of fascial strength. In 3 to 4 weeks, chromic or PGA sutures have little remaining tensile strength; however, the fascia has only begun its return to normalcy. Although Prolene or other permanent sutures maintain their tensile strength and theoretically offer protection against fascial dehiscence or hernia, prospective studies indicate a 10% to 20% risk of later wound pain or suture sinus problems (Orr et al, 1990a). Despite the potential problems, Prolene mesh can be safely used (even in contaminated procedures) to facilitate the closure of significant fascial defects (Brandt et al, 1995) without major risks. Full-thickness flaps may lessen the risks associated with soft tissue closure.

Prospective studies evaluating permanent suture materials for fascial closure suggest a 10% risk of chronic wound problems. Long-acting absorbable

sutures were developed in an attempt to bypass these problems. Although previous data suggested little difference, one report that evaluated PGA and polydioxanone sulfate sutures suggested that these two presumably long-acting, absorbable materials were similar in suture reactivity but markedly different in early (14 days) and late (35 days) tensile strength (Metz et al, 1990). Fortunately, both sutures performed well clinically. Although long-acting absorbable or nonabsorbable sutures are ideal for fascial repair, the surgeon must choose appropriate sutures for other portions of the operation.

In an attempt to evaluate the risk and benefits of a long-acting absorbable suture, we completed a prospective study of gynecologic incisions (Orr et al, 1990a). We attempted to stratify patients on the basis of known risk factors, and patients were randomized between an en bloc continuous closure and an en bloc interrupted far-far-near closure. Continuous closure times were decreased by one half in transverse incisions and almost 70% in vertical incisions (Fig. 42–9). Although actual times may not be important, this time difference represents a 7% decrease in a 2-hour operative procedure. No patient in this series suffered a wound dehiscence, and the risk of hernia was not altered between closure techniques (Table 42–20). These findings suggest that continuous closure using widely placed, long-acting absorbable sutures is an optimal method of fascial closure for the majority of gynecologic procedures. A prospective evaluation comparing a long-acting absorbable suture and permanent suture in a running mass closure was unable to delineate a significant difference in acute or late wound problems (Carlson and Condon, 1995).

Having mentioned the importance of the methods of closure, size of suture, and knot characteristics, the actual choice of suture material should be questioned. In the evaluation of wounds contaminated with significant *Escherichia coli* and *Bacteroides* bacteria, it becomes evident that PGA sutures are asso-

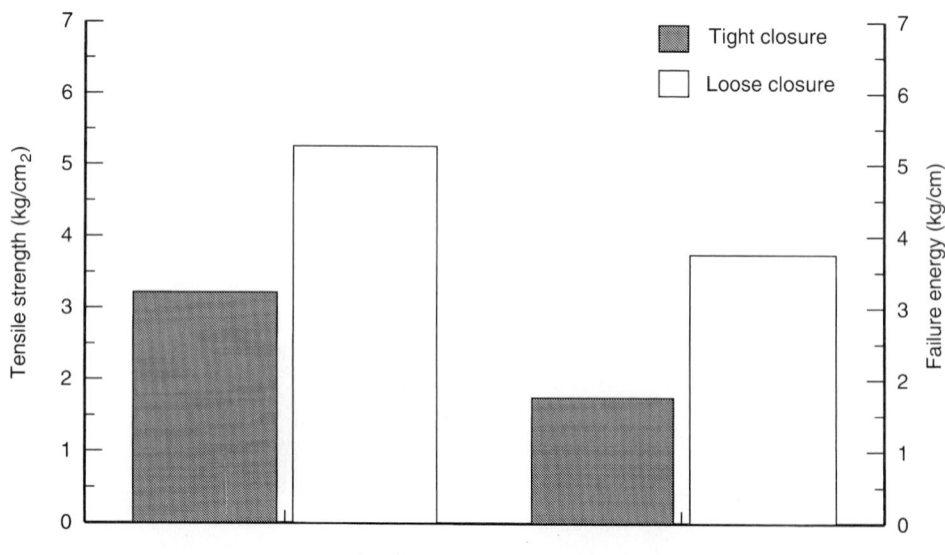

Figure 42-7
Tensile strength. (Modified from Stone KI, von Fraunhofer JA, Masterson BJ: The biomechanical effects of tight suture closure upon fascia. Surg Gynecol Obstet 1986;163:448, with permission.)

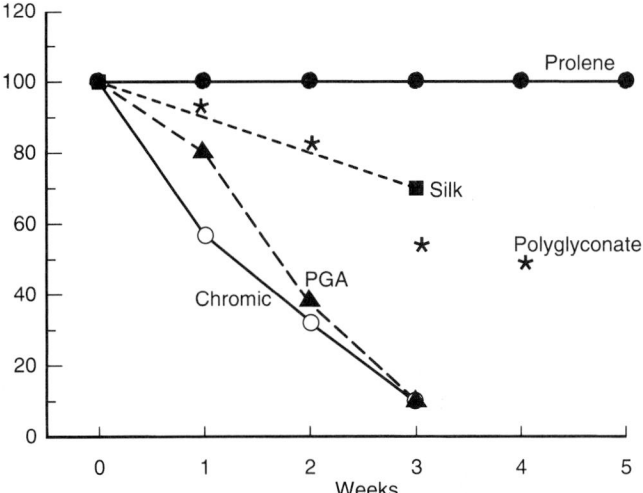

Figure 42–8
Suture tensile strength loss in vivo over time. PGA, polyglycolic acid.

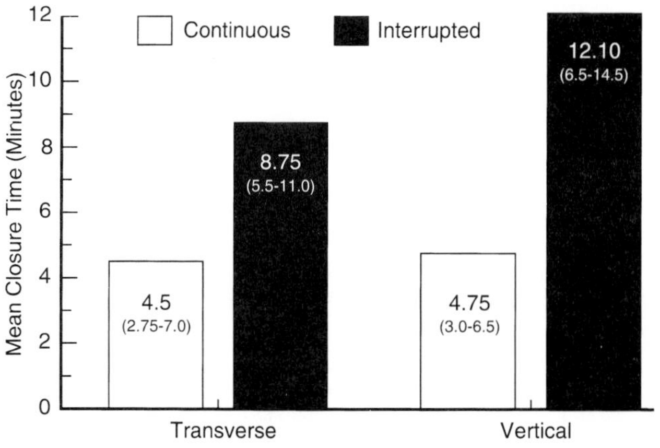

Figure 42–9
Fascial closure time by type of closure. (From Orr JW Jr, Orr PF, Barrett JM, et al: Continuous or interrupted fascial closure: a prospective evaluation of No. 1 Maxon suture in 402 gynecologic procedures. Part 1. Am J Obstet Gynecol 1990a; 163:1485, with permission.)

ciated with a reduced risk of infection (Table 42–21). In an elegant study, McGeehan et al (1980) evaluated the effect of suture material in the presence of synergistic wound sepsis in an animal model. When contaminated with a significant inoculum (6×10^5) of *E. coli* and *B. fragilis,* PGA suture material was associated with less risk of infection than catgut, nylon, silk, Prolene, or controls. This "antibacterial" effect may be related to specific suture breakdown products. PGA sutures are also associated with a decrease in incisional pain (Rogers, 1974; Orr et al, 1995), although the exact mechanism of this effect remains to be determined. We believe that using anything other than PGA sutures during the abdominal, inguinal or vulvar portion of the procedure increases the potential risk of infection and contributes to poor wound healing and poor surgical outcome.

Postoperative Wound Management

Following closure, the wound should be covered. Unfortunately, much of the information available on postoperative wound management and dressings has little scientific merit. Surgical dressings should protect the wound from contamination during epithelialization; however, their use can alter pH, cellular infiltration, moisture, or oxygen concentration. Increased moisture under occlusion facilitates epithelial migration and epithelialization. Therefore, an occlusive dressing, if not contaminated by blood or serum, should be left in place for 48 hours. Clear, semipermeable dressings allow easy wound inspection; however, collections of serum or blood should be avoided because they may accentuate poor wound healing or result in maceration. The semipermeable dressings clearly have different characteristics that can affect bacterial growth (Table 42–22). One prospective study in human volunteers suggested no clinical difference in the healing of superficial wounds. While providing a physical barrier, no dressing had the ability to stave off infection once bacteria were present.

Halstead indicated that no drainage was better than the ignorant deployment of it. There is little

Table 42–20. COMPLICATIONS WITH TYPES OF FASCIAL CLOSURE

COMPLICATION	TRANSVERSE		VERTICAL	
	Continuous	Interrupted	Continuous	Interrupted
Seroma/infection	2.6	0	5.6	3.2
Hernia				
1 Month (%)	0	0	0	0
6 Months (%)	0	0	3.9	2.4
Dehiscence (%)	0	0	0	0

Modified from Orr JW Jr, Orr PF, Barrett JM, et al: Continuous or interrupted fascial closure: a prospective evaluation of No. 1 Maxon suture in 402 gynecologic procedures. Part 1. Am J Obstet Gynecol 1990;163:1485, with permission.

Table 42–21. SUTURE MATERIAL AND SYNERGISTIC WOUND SEPSIS (*Escherichia coli/Bacteroides fragilis*, 6×10^5)

MATERIAL	% INFECTION
Control	27
Prolene	29
Silk	30
Nylon (multifilament)	48
Catgut	52
Polyglycolic acid	18

Modified from McGeehan D, Hunt D, Chaudhuri A, Rutter P: An experimental study of the relationship between synergistic wound sepsis and suture materials. Br J Surg 1980;67:636, with permission of Butterworth-Heinemann Ltd.

question that, following radical surgical procedures, a significant amount of serous fluid collects in the pelvis. As previously reported, the daily volumes are greater after a radical hysterectomy than after a total hysterectomy and pelvic lymphadenectomy and may approach 7000 ml over the initial 5 days (Orr et al, 1987). Although accumulated fluids (and their proteins) can be removed from the pelvis with drainage, there is minimal evidence that drains offer a form of risk reduction in patient care. However, their use significantly increases nursing care time.

The prophylactic use of pelvic drainage does not have a secure foundation. In fact, the use of any wound drains does not have a secure foundation. Cruise and Foord (1973) indicated that undrained incisional wounds have a much smaller risk of infection than drained wounds. We were unable to demonstrate any infection reduction benefit with pelvic drains following radical surgery (Orr et al, 1987). If drainage is necessary, it should be performed with a closed-suction apparatus. As might be expected, any drain material, latex or silicone, represents a foreign body and, when compared with no drain, increases the risk of infection and the rate of recoverable bacteria. Some proponents have suggested that there is decreased risk of lymphocyst formation with closed-suction drainage after lymphadenectomy.

We consider drains to be expensive, with the patient cost approximately $70 per drain. Drains remove significant amounts of protein and add to nursing care. We currently note a 1.0% risk of symptomatic lymphocysts in patients undergoing lymph node dissection and total hysterectomy and lymphadenectomy without the use of pelvic drains during a closed-cuff operation.

Some investigators have proposed the use of subcutaneous drains to decrease the accumulation of fluids in the abdominal wall dead space. Although proponents suggest the benefit, prospective studies have not demonstrated their efficacy. In more than 2000 patients, Farrell et al (1986) evaluated the use of subcutaneous drains with and without irrigation and found that there was no benefit in clean-contaminated procedures (Table 42–23). Although some

Table 42–22. RECOVERY OF BACTERIAL PATHOGENS FROM SEMIPERMEABLE DRESSINGS

ORGANISM/TREATMENT	PATHOGENS BY TIME (hr)*		
	25	48	72
Staphylococcus aureus			
Air exposed	7.0 ± 0.2	6.5 ± 0.6	6.8 ± 0.5
DuoDERM	7.0 ± 0.2	7.3 ± 0.2	7.0 ± 0.5
Opsite	6.4 ± 0.1	6.7 ± 0.5	6.0 ± 0.1
Vigilon	7.9 ± 0.3	7.8 ± 0.2	7.7 ± 0.1
Clostridium perfringens			
Air exposed	2.8 ± 1.0	3.0 ± 0.8	2.7 ± 0.7
DuoDERM	6.2 ± 0.7	6.7 ± 0.2	6.1 ± 0.7
Opsite	3.7 ± 0.4	3.9 ± 0.9	5.7 ± 1.6
Vigilon	5.8 ± 0.5	6.5 ± 0.4	6.2 ± 0.4
Pseudomonas aeruginosa			
Air exposed	4.3 ± 1.1	4.9 ± 0.3	5.0 ± 0.3
DuoDERM	5.9 ± 0.7	6.4 ± 0.6	6.1 ± 0.4
Opsite	6.5 ± 0.1	7.4 ± 0.3	6.9 ± 0.4
Vigilon	7.0 ± 0.4	7.3 ± 0.2	6.9 ± 0.3
Bacteroides fragilis			
Air exposed	1.3 ± 1.8	0.0 ± 0.0	0.0 ± 0.0
DuoDERM	6.4 ± 0.3	8.0 ± 0.1	8.2 ± 0.2
Opsite	1.9 ± 2.7	2.7 ± 3.8	5.0 ± 3.2
Vigilon	6.1 ± 0.7	7.6 ± 0.2	7.0 ± 0.8

*Values are given as geometric mean log colony-forming units per milliliter, ± standard deviation.
Data from Katz S, McGinley K, Leyden JJ: Semipermeable occlusive dressings: effects on growth of pathogenic bacteria and reepithelialization of superficial wounds. Arch Dermatol 1986;122:58, with permission.

Table 42–23. INFECTION RATE WITH SUBCUTANEOUS DRAINS

	% INFECTION	
CLOSURE	Clean-Contaminated	Dirty
Primary + DAB*	4.1	15.5
Catheter + DAB	3.8	9.4
Catheter + Saline	4.3	5.7
Catheter Alone	4.4	22.6

*DAB, neomycin, polymyxin, gentamicin.
Modified from Farrell MB, Worthington-Self S, Mucha P, et al: Closure of abdominal incisions with subcutaneous catheters. Arch Surg 1986;121:641, with permission.

have advocated their use in the obese (Gallop et al, 1989), until further prospective data are available, the use of subcutaneous drains cannot be advocated on a routine basis.

POSTOPERATIVE PROCEDURES

Postoperatively, several important variables can be manipulated. Delayed wound-closure techniques are applicable in many instances, especially in the presence of intra-abdominal contamination. In this situation, the timing of postoperative wound approximation becomes clinically important. Regardless of culture results, there is little need to consider secondary closure before 96 hours because the incidence of infection remains high. However, longer delays are not usually necessary because infection rates return to control values (Fig. 42–10), and local care as well as hospitalization is decreased.

The routine use of intestinal decompression has been a surgical ritual, but prospective information questions its benefit, even in intestinal surgery. In their prospective study of 513 patients, Wolff et al (1989) were unable to show a clear benefit of nasogastric compression (after gastrointestinal surgery), indicating that less than 10% of patients would require suction. It makes little sense to use prophylactic decompression in 100% of patients to potentially benefit 10% of patients. There certainly appears to be little place for routine use of the nasogastric tube if it affects only patient comfort and potential fluid losses.

Resistance to local bacterial infection remains a dynamic interplay between the number of invading organisms and host interaction. Neutrophil bacterial activity, an energy-dependent and oxygen-dependent process, is associated with a respiratory burst or increase in local oxygen utilization. Bacterial activity is extremely sensitive to local tissue oxygenation levels. When recoverable bacteria in the first postoperative day are evaluated versus recoverable bacteria in the second postoperative day, it becomes clear that oxygen supplementation may be an important method of prophylaxis. In the guinea pig model, as proposed by Burke, increased inspired oxygen concentration resulted in a lower risk of infection (Knighton et al, 1986). When combined with prophylactic antibiotics, this effect was even more pronounced (Fig. 42–11). This paper demonstrates the prophylactic efficacy of oxygen administration and questions any previous study not controlling for its use. Although routine oxygen administration may not be necessary, it should be pointed out that all patients have some relative hypoxemia postoperatively. Because granulocytes have a critical P_{O_2} for their activity, supplementation makes sense and should be considered.

Figure 42–10
Assessment of optimal time for delayed primary closure of contaminated open wounds. (Modified from Edlich RF, Rodehaver GT, Thacker JG, et al: Fundamentals of Wound Management in Surgery: Technical Factors in Wound Management. South Plainfield, NJ: Chirugecom, 1977, with permission.)

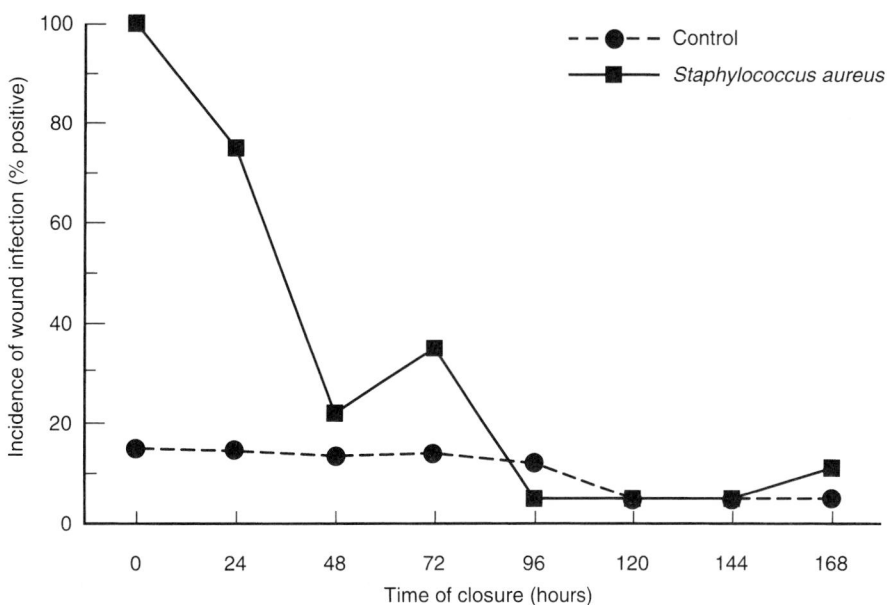

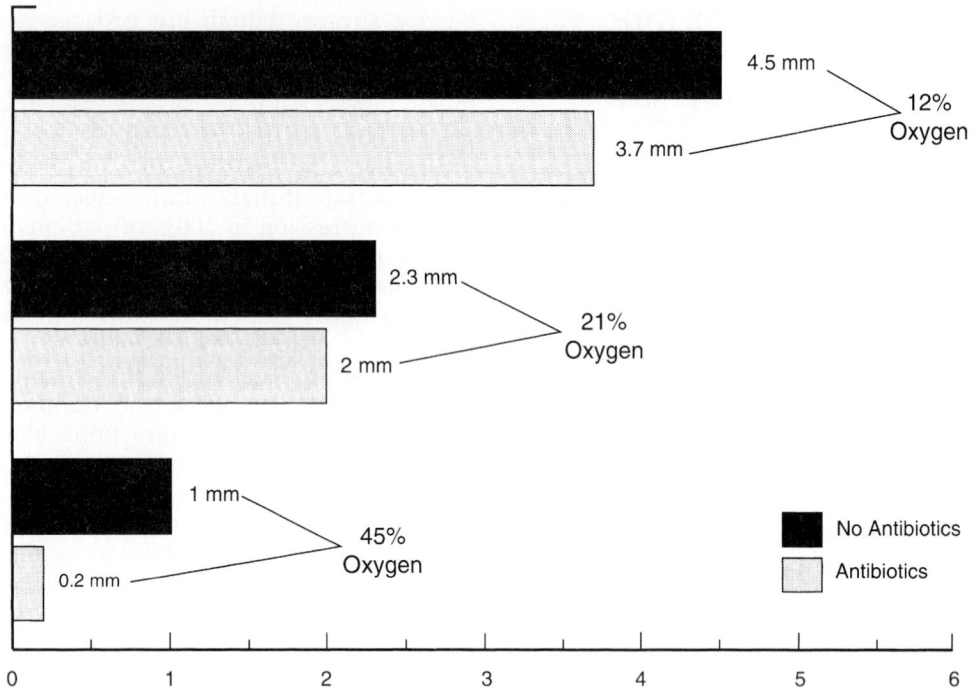

Figure 42-11
Lesion size. (Modified from Knighton DR, Halliday B, Hunt TK: Oxygen as an antibiotic: a comparison of the effects of inspired oxygen concentration and antibiotic administration on in vivo bacterial clearance. Arch Surg 1986;121:191, with permission. Copyright 1986, American Medical Association.)

REFERENCES

Alexander JW, Fischer JE, Boyajan M, et al: The influence of hair removal methods on wound infection. Arch Surg 1983;119:347.

Baird RA, Nickel FR, Thrupp LD, et al: Splash basin contamination in orthopaedic surgery. Clin Orthop 1984;187:129.

Bartlett SP, Burton RC: Effects of prophylactic antibiotics on wound infection after elective colon and rectal surgery. Am J Surg 1983;145:300.

Becker JM, Dayton MT, Fazio VW, et al: Prevention of postoperative abdominal adhesions by a sodium hyaluronate-based bioresorbable membrane: a prospective, randomized, double-blind multicenter study. J Am Coll Surg 1996;183:297.

Brandt CP, McHenry CR, Jacobs DG, et al: Polypropylene mesh closure after emergency laparotomy: morbidity and outcome. 1995;118:736.

Carlson MA, Condon RE: Polyglyconate (Maxon) versus nylon suture in midline abdominal incision closure: a prospective randomized trial. Am Surg 1995;61:980.

Cruise PJE, Foord R: A 5 year prospective study of 23,649 surgical wounds. Arch Surg 1973;107:206.

Cunningham BJ, Donnelly M, Bourke A, Murphy JF: Cardiovascular and metabolic effects of cervical epinephrine infiltration. Obstet Gynecol 1985;66:93.

Edlich RF, Rodehaver FT, Thacker JG, et al: Fundamentals of Wound Management in Surgery: Technical Factors in Wound Management. South Plainfield, NJ: Chirugecom, 1977.

Eisenkop SM, Spirtos NM, Montag TW, et al: The clinical significance of blood transfusion at the time of radical hysterectomy. Obstet Gynecol 1990;76:110.

England GT, Randall HW, Graves WL: Impairment of tissue defenses by vasoconstrictors in vaginal hysterectomy. Obstet Gynecol 1983;61:271.

Farrell MB, Worthington-Self S, Mucha P, et al: Closure of abdominal incisions with subcutaneous catheters. Arch Surg 1986;121:641.

Fayez JA, Schnerder JA: Prevention of pelvic adhesion formation by different modalities of treatment. Am J Obstet Gynecol 1989; 157:1184.

Forse RA, Karam B, Maclean LD, Christou NV: Antibiotic prophylaxis for surgery in morbidly obese patients. Surgery 1988; 106:750.

Franchi M, Donadello N, Ghezzi F, et al: A randomized study of nonclosure of the peritoneum at total abdominal hysterectomy. J Gynecol Tech 1996;2:123.

Gabel-Hughes KS, Geelhoed GW, Zalkind DL: Evaluating a new skin preparation method for invasive procedures. Complications Surg 1991;8:26.

Gallop DG, Talledo OE, King LA: Primary mass closure of midline incisions with a continuous running monofilament suture in gynecologic patients. Obstet Gynecol 1989;73:675.

Geelhoed GW, Sharpe K, Simon GL: A comparison study of surgical skin preparation methods. Surg Gynecol Obstet 1983;107: 265.

Hasselgren P, Hagberg E, Malmer H, et al: One instead of two knives for surgical incision: does it increase the risk of postoperative wound infection? Arch Surg 1984;119:917.

Hay DL, Von Fraunhofer JA, Masterson BJ: Hemostasis in blood vessels after ligation. Am J Obstet Gynecol 1989;160:737.

Knighton DR, Halliday B, Hunt TK: Oxygen as an antibiotic: the effect of inspired oxygen on infections. Arch Surg 1984;119:199.

Knighton DR, Halliday B, Hunt TK: Oxygen as an antibiotic: a comparison of the effects of inspired oxygen concentration and antibiotic administration on in vivo bacterial clearance. Arch Surg 1986;121:191.

Letts J, Doermer E: Conversation in the operating theater as a cause of airborne bacterial contamination. J Bone Joint Surg [Am] 1983;65:357.

Luijendijk RW, de Lange DCD, Wauters AP, et al: Foreign material in postoperative adhesions. Ann Surg 1996;223:242.

MacKenzie CR, Charlson ME: Assessment of perioperative risk in the patient with diabetes mellitus. Surg Gynecol Obstet 1988; 167:293.

Mann WJ Jr: Nutritional complications. In Orr JW Jr, Shingleton HM (eds): Complications in Gynecologic Surgery. Philadelphia: JB Lippincott Company, 1994:260.

McGeehan D, Hunt D, Chandhure A, et al: An experimental

study of the relationship between synergistic wound sepsis and suture materials. Br J Surg 1980;67:636.

Metz SA, Chegini N, Masterson BJ: In vivo and in vitro degradation of monofilament absorbable sutures, PDS and Maxon. Biomaterials 1990;1141.

Morton AL, Taylor EW, Lindsey G, Wells GR: A multicenter study to compare cefotetan alone with cefotetan and metronidazole as prophylaxis against infection in elective colorectal operation. Surg Gynecol Obstet 1989;169:41.

Orr JW Jr: Sutures and closures, an update. Ala J Med Sci 1986; 23:36.

Orr JW Jr: Introduction to pelvic surgery: pre- and postoperative care. In Gusberg S, Shingleton HM, Deppe G (eds): Female Genital Cancer. London: Churchill Livingstone, 1988:497.

Orr JW Jr, Barter JF, Kilgore LC, et al: Closed suction pelvic drainage following radical pelvic surgery. Am J Obstet Gynecol 1987; 155:867.

Orr JW Jr, Hatch KD, Shingleton HM, et al: Gastrointestinal complications associated with pelvic exenteration. Am J Obstet Gynecol 1983;145:325.

Orr JW Jr, Holimon JL, Orr PF: Stage I corpus cancer: is teletherapy necessary? Am J Obstet Gynecol 1997;176:777.

Orr JW Jr, Orr PF, Barrett JM, et al: Continuous or interrupted fascial closure: a prospective evaluation of No. 1 Maxon suture in 402 gynecologic procedures. Part 1. Am J Obstet Gynecol 1990a;163:1485.

Orr JW Jr, Orr PJ, Bolen DD, Holimon JL: Radical hysterectomy: does the type of incision matter? Am J Obstet Gynecol 1995; 399:406.

Orr JW Jr, Patsner B, Orr PJ: Infection in the immunocompromised women: prophylaxis, diagnosis, and treatment. In Pasorek JG III (ed): Obstetric and Gynecologic Infectious Disease. New York: Raven Press, 1993:171.

Orr JW Jr, Shingleton HM: Importance of nutritional assessment and support in surgical and cancer patients. J Reprod Med 1984;29:635.

Orr JW Jr, Sisson PF, Barrett JM, et al: Pharmacokinetics and tissue kinetics of 1 gm cefotetan prophylaxis in abdominal or vaginal hysterectomy. Am J Obstet Gynecol 1988a;158: 742.

Orr JW Jr, Sisson PF, Barrett JM, et al: Single-center study results of cefotetan and cefoxitin prophylaxis for abdominal and vaginal hysterectomy. Am J Obstet Gynecol 1988b;158(3 Part 2): 714.

Orr JW Jr, Sisson PF, Patsner B, et al: Single dose antibiotic prophylaxis for patients undergoing extended pelvic surgery for gynecologic malignancy. Am J Obstet Gynecol 1990b;162:718.

Orr JW Jr, Taylor PT Jr: Wound healing. In Orr JW jr, Shingleton HM (eds): Complications in Gynecologic Surgery. Philadelphia: JB Lippincott Company, 1994:167.

Orr JW Jr, Wilson KW, Bodiford C, et al: Pretreatment comparison of nutritional parameters in patients with cervix and corpus cancer. Trans Am Gynecol Obstet Soc 1985;111:159.

Orr JW Jr, Varner RE, Kilgore LC, et al: Cefotetan versus cefoxitin as prophylaxis in hysterectomy. Am J Obstet Gynecol 1986;154: 960.

Rogers RE: Evaluation of post-episiorrhaphy pain: polyglycolic acid vs. catgut sutures. Milit Med 1974;130:102.

Sanders RJ, Diclementi D, Ireland K: Principles of abdominal wound closure. I. Animal studies. Arch Surg 1977;112:1184.

Scher KC, Scott Conner CE, Montany PF: Effect of cephalosporins on fascial healing after celeostomy. Am J Surg 1988;155:361.

Sladen R: Inadvertent hypothermia: risks and prevention. Presented at the 40th Annual Refresher Course of the American Society of Anesthesiology, New Orleans, 1989.

Stamp CV, McGregor W, Rodeheaver GT, et al: Surgical needle holder damage to suture. Am Surg 1988;54:300.

Tunca JC: Nutritional evaluation of gynecologic cancer patients during initial diagnosis of their disease. Am J Obstet Gynecol 1983;147:893.

Ward MW, Danzi M, Lewin MR, et al: The effects of subclinical malnutrition and refeeding on the healing of experimental colonic anastomoses. Br J Surg 1982;69:308.

Wolff BG, Pembeton JH, van Heerden JA, et al: Elective colon and rectal surgery without nasogastric decompression: a prospective, randomized trial. Ann Surg 1989;209:670.

43

James W. Orr, Jr.
Pamela F. Orr

Postoperative Care

Effective perioperative risk reduction occurs when plans, methods, and technologies are instituted prior to the actual performance of a gynecologic procedure. Perioperative outcome might be considered a target, with each technique, intervention, order, or action aimed to reduce overall patient risk. The concept of developing a preoperative data base or postoperative care plan for risk reduction is predicated on the assumption that the information obtained can and will be used to modify care that ultimately results in an improved outcome. Although the skillful, successful completion of a surgical procedure remains the primary goal, final results may be unsatisfactory if a potentially life-threatening or unrecognized complication intervenes. It is accepted that, regardless of the method and extent of perioperative evaluation and surgical planning, adverse events can and will occur. A thoughtfully planned preoperative evaluation, combined with a well-executed surgical procedure and an established routine of postoperative surveillance, facilitates early recognition and timely intervention when common or unsuspected complications occur. The postoperative period is a dynamic process. With numerous hurdles (return of bowel function, ambulation, wound healing) present, the postoperative race is won with physician vigilance and awareness that significant complications require prompt recognition and appropriate management changes.

THE IMPORTANCE OF COMMUNICATION

Patient and Staff Education

Although all physicians concur in the need for an appropriate preoperative plan and good surgical technique, we believe that the sometimes seemingly less important role of patient and staff education remains a necessary, important ingredient of optimal surgical care. Apart from the actual operative procedure, direct physician-patient contact is minimal during the postoperative convalescence. In the absence of a critical care situation, even the best intentioned physician spends less than 30 minutes daily with a hospitalized patient. In contrast, nursing staff and other health care personnel spend more time (up to 70-fold) with the patient each day. A dedicated,

educated health care team composed of physicians, nurses, and other allied personnel allows individualization of care and realization of surgical goals, minimizes the adverse effects of conflicting information, and delivers a unified perioperative approach.

Although each health care provider has a designated role, continued communication between all team members during the postoperative course allows smooth transitions in treatment strategy to occur, particularly when complications arise. Additionally, knowledge as to the "whys" of postoperative care may decrease the incidence of prescribing errors or other miscommunication during the postoperative convalescence. Avoiding medication errors is particularly important, because they are reported to occur at a rate of 3.13 per 1000 written orders, or in 2.4% of admissions (Classen et al, 1997). Potential serious mistakes occur in 1.80 per 1000 orders (Lesar et al, 1990). Adverse drug events dramatically increase costs and nearly double the risk of in-hospital mortality (Bates et al, 1997; Classen et al, 1997). Almost 50% of these problems relate to the prescribing of antimicrobial, cardiovascular, or gastrointestinal drugs. A female patient receives on average 16 different drugs during postoperative convalescence (Orr, 1988), and preventing medication errors promote good care.

Although nursing notes are a method of communication, we believe that personal or open lines of communication between physician and nursing staff can improve patient care and lessens the risk of missed or miscommunication. This educational process between physicians and other members of the health care team must be updated continually, particularly when new techniques are utilized or when new personnel (physician or hospital staff) are introduced. Finally, clear, precise, timed, and dated physician's charting and orders facilitate team members' understanding of their evolving roles as well as the patient's progress.

Patient education (and informed consent) begins prior to hospitalization. Appropriate preoperative patient education is associated with a decrease in the need for postoperative analgesia, less anxiety, shorter hospital stay, and earlier postoperative ambulation (Abbott and Abbott, 1995). These ameliorating effects may affect recovery from major or minor procedures. The patient, her family, or designated support persons should be informed in understandable language as to surgical indications and possible alternatives. Initially, this may be quite simple, as in a discussion of the need for laparotomy or laparoscopy for a pelvic mass. The role and surgical steps (including important aspects such as incision placement) related to cancer staging or cytoreduction during the procedure may be straightforward. However, if benign disease is present, the actual procedure may vary in relation to additional findings, patient desires, or physician expertise. The algorithm for intraoperative decision making should be outlined to avoid misconception or unnecessary conflict during the postoperative interval. Omission of these details can only result in misunderstanding, fear, anxiety, and perhaps mistrust. These physician-patient discussions should continue during the postoperative period to allow understanding of the surgical findings as well as the possible need for additional treatment, be it hormonal replacement for estrogen deficiency or chemotherapy for an ovarian malignancy.

In general, most physicians focus on the physiologic changes that occur after surgery and, to some extent, ignore the resultant psychological alterations that might result from an operative procedure involving the reproductive tract. Although both changes are important, ignoring the latter frequently complicates postoperative recovery. Most patients are initially reluctant to discuss potential psychological or psychosexual implications of the planned procedure. However, once the physician broaches these subjects, the doors to communication usually open for free discussion. From a patient care or medicolegal standpoint, documenting the pertinent aspects of each physician-patient contact in the chart or at the time of discharge may prove helpful years after the hospitalization. Timely completion of all medical records (office and hospital) allows incorporation of even the most subtle aspects of preoperative evaluation or postoperative care and serves as a reference in the event of future problems.

Regardless of the initial patient-physician interaction, continued communication may be valuable even after the procedure is scheduled. We believe that procedure-specific, written information concerning preoperative preparation or evaluation can be given to the patient. Written instructions for physical (bowel preparation) and psychological (location of testing) aspects of perioperative care contribute to improved understanding and allay patient anxiety during this stressful waiting period. Importantly, these procedures can be safely and cost-effectively performed on an outpatient basis (Le et al, 1997). When the patient will not be seen until surgery (same-day admission), the physician or staff should communicate the results and implications of the important diagnostic studies by phone or in person before she enters the operating room. Some abnormal values or findings (e.g., the diagnosis of cancer) may

be better accepted by the patient if the physician, rather than office personnel, initiates patient contact. The importance of this continued communication is emphasized by the fact that 42% of women feel that the "diagnostic period" is their most stressful time of medical care, particularly if they are dealing with a malignant or premalignant condition (Jamison, 1978). Minimizing stress should be a goal of preoperative preparation because mental stress may increase the risk of myocardial ischemia (Gullette et al, 1997). Only with constant or appropriate communication can the physician minimize or alleviate the fear of loss of femininity or control, or even phobias of cancer that may exist.

In general, all communications should be conducted in a caring manner and, if possible, privately. An associated touch, eye contact, or even sitting on the bed can lessen the barriers to communication (Blanchard et al, 1986). Postoperatively, multiple, short discussions at the bedside in an unhurried manner can alleviate many problems and contribute to an improved physician-patient relationship. Discharge provides another important plateau. The most complete postoperative verbal instructions are likely to be forgotten by the patient during this time of happiness (going home) and anxiety (leaving the safety of the hospital). Again, we prefer to use printed postoperative instructions to reinforce discharge communications. "Generic" instructions often provide sufficient information, but more specific written instruction may be necessary in certain situation, such as care of a suprapubic catheter or open wound. The use of and communication with home health care agencies can smooth this important transition.

Physician Education

Continued physician education remains a most important element of preoperative evaluation and postoperative care. The gynecologist must devote a significant amount of attention to important patient historical factors, including previous or concurrent illness, allergies, and current medications. A thorough understanding of the entire patient should be the goal, to allow appropriate preoperative triage or consultation in an effort to lower the risk of a catastrophic postoperative event. We believe that allowing patients to delineate their problems on a preprinted checklist offers a focused insight to important coexisting medical conditions. Patient questionnaires are at least as accurate as, if not more accurate than, physician interview (Fleisher, 1996b). However, even when "questioned" on paper, the stress of the medical situation, or denial, may result in failure to mention important associated problems or intake of medications. Consequently, use of patient-volunteered information from a printed form should not abbreviate the history and physical examination. The omission of even the simplest fact, such as the use of over-the-counter drugs, may play an important role in intraoperative or postoperative management. For instance, a bleeding diathesis related to platelet dysfunction can occur for up to 10 days from ingesting a single aspirin. The importance of the physical examination and history becomes evident when one evaluates the predictability of abnormal laboratory values in patients admitted for ambulatory surgery. Well over 95% of abnormal laboratory values can be predicted by specific signs or symptoms from a history or physical examination (Johnson et al, 1988; Velanovich, 1991; Orr and Shingleton, 1994). For instance, the evaluation of exercise tolerance may be the most important determinant of cardiac risks. The likelihood of extensive coronary artery disease (CAD) is small if the patient can walk a mile without becoming short of breath (Fleisher and Eagle, 1996). Additionally, the comparative results of "specific" indicated tests (electrocardiogram [ECG], chest radiograph, nutritional studies) based on historical or physical findings are more predictive of postoperative complications than routine screening test results.

Although gynecologists undergo an intensive educational process during residency or fellowship, they must continue evaluating new concepts or methodology in an effort to improve their preoperative evaluation, intraoperative technique, or postoperative care. In specific clinical situations, the physician's expertise may be limited by experience or intention, and information must be obtained to allow appropriate patient triage. For example, a menopausal woman with a pelvic mass and an elevated CA-125 level is at significant risk for harboring an ovarian malignancy. In this situation, an optimal surgical resection is associated with an increased patient response and progression-free interval. Because as many as 20% of these women require intestinal or urinary procedures, the gynecologist may wish to obtain surgical consultation from a gynecologic oncologist or seek a referral avenue. Combined procedures, performed with "unexpected" intraoperative findings, may involve a surgical subspecialist who is reluctant to perform an extensive urinary or intestinal resection for "debulking" ovarian cancer, perhaps because of a lack of understanding of the disease process (i.e., the potential benefit of cytoreduction) or limited experience with radical debulking surgery or presumed lack of informed consent. Furthermore, the surgical consultant may prefer additional preoperative preparation (e.g., bowel preparation, parenteral nutrition) that would avoid specific procedures (colostomy) or potentially improve the likelihood of a successful postoperative recovery. Women with endometrial cancer and an elevated serum CA-125 level represent another potential subgroup who may be at increased risk to harbor extrauterine disease that requires extended surgical staging or resection. Adequate staging may further decrease patient costs (Orr et al, 1997). The patient's best interest is usually served by obtaining additional laboratory or radiologic studies or necessary

surgical assistance preoperatively. This thoughtful preoperative evaluation assists in avoiding the stress and potential adverse outcome of unnecessary intraoperative "fire drills."

In addition to the need to incorporate new techniques, suture materials, and antibiotics, most gynecologists encounter problems associated with the older population. The lack of physiologic reserve and the greater incidence of medical problems in geriatric patients may warrant a more in-depth preoperative evaluation of the cardiovascular and pulmonary systems, which may include general or subspecialty medical consultation. Unfortunately, most internists have little experience and few guidelines for consultation. Many preoperative consultations serve as a medicolegal screen, but we contend that a consultation should be considered if any existing physiologic risk factor can be favorably affected. Once involved, the consultant should take an active role in the patient's care by providing diagnostic as well as therapeutic recommendations (Golden and Lavender, 1989), which should continue throughout the entire postoperative convalescence. Although most obstetric and gynecologic training programs dedicate a significant amount of time to the fundamentals of physiology and internal medicine, constant medical advances (i.e., new antibiotics, pharmacologic cardiac stress testing) and the relative lack of postgraduate education in regard to postoperative care make it imperative that the gynecologist use consultants wisely (Houston et al, 1987). Prior to complete incorporation of new techniques or methods, local review of outcomes and results of new methodology may be prudent because experience reported from tertiary medical centers may not reflect overall practice or outcome in community settings (Warner et al, 1990).

Finally, as surgeons, we might interpret changes that promote risk reduction by less than 10% to be of little importance; however, on a national basis, prevention, even at a 1% decrease in morbidity (in more than 4 million procedures per year), should not only benefit the individual patient but also allow for effective distribution of available health care resources. In many instances, individual physicians may negate reported information in preference to their own "personal" experience. Unfortunately, few surgeons are able to discriminate between events that occur with a difference of 15% or less, thereby invalidating one's own "personal" experience unless it has been reviewed in its entirety. Few physicians scoff at the necessity of considering cost-effectiveness of specific treatments; today's cost-conscious society emphasizes the public demand that "standard of care" evolves to reflect all considerations, including efficacy and cost-effectiveness.

IMPACT OF ANESTHESIA

Once surgery has been designated as the appropriate treatment option, preparation directed toward risk reduction can be best accomplished by understanding the interaction of patient variables and the physiologic stresses of anesthesia and surgery that may adversely affect every organ system. Major pulmonary effects include impaired oxygenation and altered elimination of carbon dioxide from increased dead space ventilation. Mismatch of pulmonary ventilation and perfusion, as well as altered chest wall and diaphragm mechanics, are combined with a progressive decrease in functional residual capacity (related to shallow breathing), absent breath signs, reduced surfactant production, and microatelectasis (Orr et al, 1994). The associated premature small airway and alveolar collapse, gas trapping, and lowered vital capacity, forced expiratory volume, and functional residual volume frequently contribute to pulmonary morbidity. Anesthetic- and intubation-related epithelial desquamation, a decrease in mucus velocity, and reduced bacterial clearance predispose to pulmonary infection. These changes are more likely to be clinically apparent after an upper abdominal incision but are greatly influenced by pain, narcotics, ileus, or abdominal distention. Patients receive many (13 to 91) doses of perioperative drugs (Swartz, 1979), anesthetics, and transfusions that may reduce oxyhemoglobin affinity. Fortunately, these pulmonary effects are not usually clinically important. However, the major adverse pulmonary effects occur during the first 2 postoperative days and may persist much longer (weeks). Hypoxemia and diminished pulmonary reserve are likely well tolerated by the healthy 40-year-old but may result in catastrophic consequences for the heavy smoker, older women, or those with other associated pulmonary or cardiovascular disease. Impaired pulmonary mechanics and the presence of large anatomic shunts also predispose obese patients to the development of significant pulmonary complications.

Nearly all inhalation anesthetics are myocardial depressants, modify neural control of vascular tone, and are arrhythmogenic (Orr and Browne, 1994). Risks associated with anesthetic-induced myocardial depression are directly related to the kinetics of oxygen supply and demand. The well-vascularized myocardium is more tolerant than that with even the most minimal abnormality. Arrhythmias, occurring in as many as 27% of women during anesthesia, are common during intubation. This risk is lowest in patients with no prior history of arrhythmias (16%) and rises to approximately 26% to 34% in patients with a previous history of arrhythmias. Fortunately, fewer than 5% are clinically significant and require treatment. Additionally, hypotension (related to sympathetic block) or hypertension (related to sympathetic stimulation during induction) are not uncommon. If the former is present for 10 minutes, it is associated with a significantly increased risk (as much as eightfold) of postoperative cardiovascular complications (Charlson et al, 1990). The associated increased afterload, increased preload, expanded blood volume, and more profound anesthetic-related cardiac depression place obese patients at even greater risk for perioperative cardiovascular complications. Despite popular opinion, cardiac risks are not primarily dependent on the choice of regional versus general anesthesia or on specific agents but on the anesthesiologist's techniques, skills, methods of monitoring detection of specific problems, and appropriate intervention (Orr and Browne, 1994). The cardiac risk of regional anesthesia is not necessarily less than that of general anesthesia (Rao et al, 1983).

During anesthesia, the renal blood supply is predictably decreased by 30% to 70% of preanesthetic values (Orr, 1988). Smaller decreases occur in glomerular filtration rate (GFR); however, myocardial depression (direct or indirect) may be responsible. Intraoperative urinary osmolality is increased secondary to vasopressin release and results in lessened renal free water clearance and a decrease in renal autoregulation.

After anesthesia and surgery, literally every arm of the immune system is altered (Lennard et al, 1985). In addition to loss of normal phagocytic function and altered antibody production, abnormalities in cell-mediated immunity as well as reduced T- and B-cell levels commonly occur. Opsonic activity related to fibronectin or other glycoproteins in the reticuloendothelial system is also decreased.

Alterations in gastrointestinal function associated with anesthesia and surgery include ileus, altered hepatic function, and an increased risk of stress-related bleeding. In most clinical situations, the small intestine maintains its motility and absorptive function throughout the entire postoperative period. Gastric atony (1 to 4 days) and colon immotility (3 to 5 days) contribute to postoperative ileus (Orr and Shingleton, 1984). Duration of surgery actually has little impact on the severity of ileus, but ileus may be worsened in the presence of overt infection, excessive handling of the small bowel, retroperitoneal dissection, or bleeding. Regional anesthesia, reported to have favorable effects on colonic blood flow and healing, lowers the risk of perioperative ileus. Unfortunately, its primary use may be limited when upper abdominal exploration or manipulation is required. Regardless of the method of anesthesia, an empty gastrointestinal tract is a prerequisite to any safe anesthetic, and appropriate surgical preparation includes maintenance of the nothing-by-mouth (NPO, nil per os) status for at least 2 hours before the surgical procedure. Women with altered states of motility (e.g., pregnancy, small bowel obstruction, carcinomatosis, or ascites) may require longer periods of NPO in order to adequately empty the stomach. Regardless, most anesthetics should be performed with crash induction to protect the airway. Specific clinical conditions (i.e., proposed or possible intestinal surgery) mandate preoperative mechanical bowel preparation to decrease infectious risks. Importantly, additional oral antibiotics are not necessary and may result in nausea or intolerance to further preparation. Mechanical preparation (clear liquids for 48 hours) and cathartics can usually be completed on an outpatient basis, add little expense, and may be of significant benefit (avoiding colostomy) even with unintentional injury. For these reasons, we propose consideration of their use in the preoperative preparation of nearly every patient undergoing an abdominal procedure.

Although local metabolites, serum osmolality, partial pressure of carbon dioxide (PCO_2), partial pressure of oxygen (PO_2), systemic blood pressure, cerebral blood flow, and cerebral metabolic rate are determined by a complex interaction of perivascular hydrogen ion concentration, these values can be altered by anesthesia (Orr, 1988). Specifically, hydrocarbon inhalants increase blood flow, decrease metabolic rate, and raise intracranial pressure. This is not usually deemed a problem during gynecologic surgery, but assumes more importance in women who have problems with altered cerebral blood flow or increased intracranial pressures, particularly in older populations, women with vascular disease, or perhaps those with proven or occult metastatic disease.

Finally, muscle relaxants and anesthesia create a certain vulnerability to potential neuromuscular injury during positioning or retractor placement. The surgeon, anesthesiologist, and operating room staff must be cognizant of this potential problem. Recognition of preoperative problems (i.e., severe arthritis) as well as care during patient positioning may alleviate some of these risks. In particular instances (i.e., hip problems), patient positioning might be more safely accomplished before induction of anesthesia.

Although recognition of associated multisystem anesthetic risks is important, only 4% of surgical mortalities can be directly attributed to the anesthetic. Most surgical mortalities (79%) are related to problems stemming from the patient's coexisting medical disease; 18% occur as a direct result of the actual surgical procedure (Orr, 1988).

Intraoperative complications are likely to influence the method of postoperative care. Approximately 1 in 3000 anesthetics is associated with some significant clinical alteration of cardiac activity, including cardiac arrest. When present, the associated mortality rate approaches 50%. Serious cardiac events occur in equal frequency during anesthesia induction or maintenance. This risk is not significantly lowered by the use of regional anesthesia, which may actually lessen ventilatory control or result in hypotension. In this context, the extraordinary specifics of each preoperative patient should be discussed to allow planning of anesthesia.

Obviously, the occurrence and intraoperative management of intraoperative events impacts on the overall postoperative care plan. Hemorrhage occurs in a significant number of radical procedures, and is increased in obese women and in those receiving heparin prophylaxis. It is advisable to place large-diameter peripheral intravenous lines or, preferably, central lines shortly after induction in women "at risk" for excessive blood loss.

POSTOPERATIVE SURVEILLANCE

Although "standardized" care plans generally suffice, changes in postoperative care should be instituted according to specific findings. Obviously, these plans are influenced or modified by the degree of preoperative preparation (i.e., emergent procedure, bowel preparation) or indications (benign, malignant, palliative). At each postoperative visit, the physician should make a mental checklist and evaluate each organ system and its status during progressive recovery.

Fluid Replacement

A primary goal of postoperative care involves adequate fluid resuscitation. There is no "cookbook" approach, and requirements may differ dramatically for patients with coexisting medical disease and those with significant intraoperative or ongoing postoperative fluid losses (Shires and Canizaro, 1983; Orr, 1988; Mann, 1994). Appropriate volume replacement requires an understanding of the normal woman's physiologic makeup. Water constitutes approximately 50% ($\pm$15%) of a young woman's body weight. Aging is associated with a decrease in total percentage of body water in direct proportion to the increase in fatty tissue (fat is composed of less water per gram than muscle). Thus the latter approximates 57% of total body weight in 18-year-olds but falls to 46% in the average 60-year-old woman. Functional body fluid compartments are divided into two major components. Intracellular water makes up 30% to 40% of total body weight and extracellular water, approximately 20%. The latter is composed of intravascular volume, which represents approximately 5% of body weight; lymphatic volume, 2%; and interstitial volume, approximately 13%.

Under normal conditions, third "space" fluids, consisting of intestinal contents, ascites, and joint, intestinal, and pleural fluid are of little clinical relevance. In contrast to intravascular and extravascular volumes, third-space fluids are usually considered immobile and unresponsive to the normal physiologic mechanisms that allow free fluid flux. However, accumulation or alteration of third-space fluids may become a significant problem in patients with ascites or pleural effusions, following extensive pelvic dissection, with intra-abdominal carcinomatosis, or in conjunction with a prolonged intestinal ileus. In these situations, third-space volumes may dramatically increase, become mobile (usually at 48 to 72 hours), and have an adverse effect on hemodynamic status or require a significant alteration in the plan for fluid management. Invasive (central venous pressure, pulmonary artery pressure) monitoring of intravascular volumes may be necessary for optimal postoperative fluid replacement, particularly in women with coexisting cardiovascular problems or if initial "clinical" changes in replacement fluid or volume do not achieve their goals (Orr et al, 1986b). Importantly patients at risk for perioperative problems may benefit by preoperative saline loading (Garrison et al, 1996).

The normal chemical composition of intravascular, extravascular, and interstitial fluids differs significantly (Table 43–1). Potassium and magnesium are the primary intracellular cautions; phosphates and proteins are the principal anions. The principal cation of extracellular fluid is sodium, with chloride and carbonate being its principal anions. Extracellular fluid volume is primarily determined by total body sodium content. Under usual circumstances, the interstitial and intravascular volumes are not considered interchangeable. Clinically, this becomes an important aspect with the administration of isotonic fluids, which contribute acutely to the maintenance of intravascular volumes and blood pressure, particularly during anesthesia or during episodes of hypotension or relative hypoperfusion. These fluids later are distributed to the interstitial-to-intravascular compartments in a ratio of approximately 3:1. Thus the administration of 1 liter of isotonic fluid (after 24 hours) equilibrates and 750 ml is distributed to the interstitial space, which potentially contributes to edema of the extremities, the pulmonary parenchyma, the gastrointestinal tract, or even the central nervous system. Because dextrose solutions are equally distributed through total body water, one half of the infused free water remains in the intravenous space.

These complicated interactions, and particularly the distribution of the extracellular fluids, are determined by the balance between plasma and interstitial osmotic and hydrostatic pressures. Osmotic pressures relate to the actual number of particles present in solution of the individual fluid component. The total number of osmotic reactive particles normally varies between 200 and 310 mOsm in each compartment. The effective oncotic pressures are dependent on substances that are unable to pass through semipermeable cellular membranes. In general, dissolved proteins are the primary substances that affect osmotic pressures. Any alteration in effective oncotic pressure is associated with distribution of water. In general, hypotonicity is associated with expansion and hypertonicity with contraction of the intracel-lular fluid compartment. Hypernatremia usually results in a flux of water from the intracellular to extracellular compartment; however, clinically, most acute losses or gains in body fluid are from the extracellular compartment. Hypernatremia always implies a hypertonic state; however, hyponatremia is not necessarily equated with a hypotonic state.

In health, fluid volumes in these compartment boundaries undergo complex regulation by pressure and perfusion of the kidney modulated by antidiuretic hormone (ADH) and aldosterone (Orr, 1988). The intestinal tract has a potentially important passive role. Aldosterone influences the renal absorption of sodium and is essential to maintain a circulating volume during times of decreased intravascular volume (related to anesthesia, prolonged ileus, dehydration, or hemorrhage). Serum levels of aldosterone are regulated by adrenocorticotropic hormone and modulated by renin and input from myocardial stretch receptors. Hyperaldosteronism secondary to alterations in arterial blood volume commonly occurs during the postoperative period. Intraoperative and postoperative water retention is in large part related to the associated activity of ADH secreted from the supraoptic and paraventricular nucleus of the hypothalamus, which increases water absorption by decreasing the permeability of the renal collective ducts to water. The primary physiologic stimulus for ADH release is a rise in body fluid toxicity; however, large decreases (10% to 15%) in blood volume are associated with a dramatic increase in ADH secretion. Additional postoperative factors, including fear, pain, hemorrhage, and injury, are important potential stimulants to ADH production and secretion.

Alterations in acid-base status can have profound adverse effects on cellular function and membrane permeability. Despite the daily production of more than 20,000 mmol of carbonic acid and 80 mmol of nonvolatile acids, the normal arterial pH of 7.35 to 7.45 is tightly regulated by the kidney, the lung, and seven buffer systems. Under normal circumstances, significant alterations in pH are unusual. However, if present, persistent acidosis can result in potential catastrophic cardiac dysfunction or altered cerebral blood flow. Normally, the associated postoperative hyperaldosteronism increases renal hydrogen ion secretion, with a resultant mild postoperative meta-

Table 43–1. NORMAL FLUID COMPOSITION

CATIONS/ANIONS	PLASMA (mEq/L)	INTERSTITIAL (mEq/L)	INTRACELLULAR (mEq/L)
Na^+/Cl^-	142/103	144/114	10
K^+/HCO_3^-	4/27	4/30	150/10
$Ca^{2+}/SO_4^{2-}/PO_4^{2-}$	5/3	3/3	
$Mg^{2+}/HPO_4^{3-}/SO_4^{2-}$	3/	2/	40/150
Organic acids	5	5	
Protein	16	1	40
TOTAL	154/154	153/153	200/200

Modified from Orr JW Jr: Introduction to pelvic surgery: pre- and postoperative care. In Gusberg SB, Shingleton HM, Deppe G (eds): Female Genital Cancer. New York: Churchill Livingstone, 1988:497, with permission.

bolic alkalosis. However, postoperative events, including volume depletion (regardless of etiology) or gastric suction (acid loss), can result in significant abnormalities. Although routine monitoring of acid-base status is not usually considered necessary, specific clinical situations may necessitate obtaining this information obtained from arterial blood gases.

Given these fluid compartments, hormonal aberrations, and the potential fluid losses (Table 43–2), the "average" 70-kg woman requires a daily fluid replacement of 2000 to 2500 ml. A minimum of 800 ml (to maintain a urine osmolality of 1400 mOsm) per day of urine production is considered adequate for appropriate solute excretion. This volume of urine (0.5 ml/kg/hour) should be a minimal goal. Insensible pulmonary losses approach 800 ml/day but may be much greater in the presence of tachypnea or in women requiring mechanical ventilation. Perspiration losses (which are sodium-free) and intestinal losses equal an additional 300 ml/day. An additional 600 ml is usually required to replace other immeasurable losses, such as those related to postoperative temperature elevation, which occurs in 30% to 70% of women. During postoperative convalescence, these temperature-related losses can become important because they increase 10% for each 1°F increase in body temperature. In specific situations, other losses may require replacement. Clinically significant losses (up to 1000 ml/24 hours) may occur with closed suction pelvic drainage (Orr et al, 1986a) as well as other sources (diarrhea, vomiting). The astute clinician routinely monitors postoperative input and output and evaluates alteration in daily weights. These simple, easily obtained clinical indicators may alert the surgical team to potential problems and allow further intervention to decrease the risk of serious postoperative problems related to inadequate or excessive volume replacement.

Under optimal circumstances, the normal kidney excretes less than 10 mEq of sodium per day, whereas potassium excretion averages less than 30 mEq per day. Although these minimal requirements exist, additional electrolyte losses occur, and 75 to 100 mEq of sodium and 60 mEq of potassium should be the minimal goal of daily replacement. In general, intravenous solutions containing potassium concentration greater than 40 mEq/L are avoided in an attempt to minimize patient discomfort, venous irritation, sclerosis, or cardiac abnormalities. However, hypokalemia is a common postoperative finding. If acute replacement is necessary, safe correction can be undertaken with hourly replacement of 20 mEq of potassium chloride per 100 ml of Ringer's lactate solution via a central or peripheral route. In more than 1300 instances, the mean serum K^+ increase was 0.25 mmol/L and no life-threatening arrhythmias occurred (Kruse and Carlson, 1990). In most situations, the daily administration of 100 g of dextrose minimizes the risk of ketosis in the catabolic postoperative state. However, the clinician must be cognizant of potential nutritional defects and their adverse effects (Orr and Shingleton, 1984). Parenteral or enteral alimentation as supplementation should be considered for those patients judged preoperatively to be malnourished or for any patient in whom gastrointestinal function is not expected to return for 5 or more days postoperatively. Enteral alimentation may further lessen septic risks.

Currently, a variety of parenteral replacement or maintenance fluids are available (Table 43–3). The reliance on any routine formula or single clinical sign to determine the adequacy of volume and electrolyte replacement will be associated with more than an occasional problem. An effective postoperative plan for fluid administration must begin early and should be altered in the presence of preoperative deviation from normal fluid or electrolyte profiles or significant intraoperative or ongoing postoperative losses. Fluid requirements can be calculated on a kilogram basis, on an incremental kilogram basis, or by surface area (Mann, 1994). Regardless of the method chosen, constant monitoring of clinical variables (weight, input or output) facilitates the institution of necessary changes. Recognition of existing volume deficits that may be isotonic (loss of cellular water), hypertonic (loss of water and excess electrolytes), or hypotonic (loss of electrolytes and excess water) is important. Prediction of individual deficits should

Table 43–2. POTENTIAL POSTOPERATIVE FLUID LOSS

TYPE	MEAN VOLUME (ml/24 hr)	CATION (mEq/L)		ANION (mEq/L)	
		Na	K	Cl	HCO₃
Saliva	1500	10	26	10	30
Stomach	1500	60	10	130	
Pancreas	400	140	5	75	115
Bile	300	145	5	100	35
Small intestine	2000	140	5	104	30
Colon		60	30	40	
Lymphadenectomy drainage	300	135	4	107	

Modified from Orr JW Jr: Introduction to pelvic surgery: pre- and postoperative care. In Gusberg SB, Shingleton HM, Deppe G (eds): Female Genital Cancer. New York: Churchill Livingstone, 1988:497, with permission.

Table 43 – 3. COMPOSITION OF COMMON PARENTERAL FLUIDS

SOLUTION	CATION (mEq/L)					ANION (mEq/L)			
	Na	K	Ca	Mg	NH$_4$	Cl	HCO$_4^-$	HPO$_4^{3-}$	Protein
Plasma	142	4	5	3	0.3	103	27	3	
Intracellular fluid	10	150		40			10	150	40
Ringer's lactate*	130	4	2.7			109	28*		
0.9% sodium chloride (normal saline)	154					154			
0.45% sodium chloride (half-normal saline)	77					77			
3% sodium chloride	513					513			
5% sodium chloride	855					855			
0.9% ammonium chloride		168				168			

*Lactate in solution is converted to bicarbonate.
Modified from Orr JW Jr: Introduction to pelvic surgery: pre- and postoperative care. In Gusberg SB, Shingleton HM, Deppe G (eds): Female Genital Cancer. New York: Churchill Livingstone, 1988;497, with permission.

be made. In general, only one half of an indicated deficit is initially replaced. In symptomatic severe hyponatremia (serum Na$^+$ < 110 mEq/L), hypertonic (3%) saline and loop diuretics can be administered to increase serum sodium levels by 20 to 25 mEq/L during the initial 24 hours. More rapid repletion can result in permanent central nervous system impairment (central demyelination) (Ayus and Arieff, 1990). Parameters are then remeasured and deficits recalculated. Once deficits have been completely replaced, maintenance fluids plus ongoing losses are monitored and replaced with the appropriate parenteral fluids.

Unless the clinical situation dictates otherwise, we do not advocate routine daily monitoring of electrolytes. Certainly, women with total body potassium deficiency secondary to diuretic use, women with high-output enteric fistulas, or those with prolonged ileus require frequent electrolyte monitoring. Routine electrolyte determinations in the absence of specific indications add little benefit and increase health care costs.

Complications

Postoperative Mortality

The major causes of intraoperative and postoperative death include cardiac arrest, pneumonia, sepsis, embolic phenomena, and renal failure; however, an individual's death risk is correlated with the nature and duration of the surgical procedure. The American Society of Anesthesiologists (ASA) preoperative physical status scale developed by Dripps and the ASA (Table 43–4) allows for relative risk prediction (Table 43–5). In fact, ASA status is a strong predictor of postoperative complications and is more reliable than "routine screening" studies. The extent of underlying disease, patient age, urgency of the surgical procedure, and experience of the surgical team are additional important factors. The mortality rate per 1000 population for simple procedures, such as dilatation and curettage, is 0.1 but increases to 0.25 per

1000 for hysterectomy and to 0.3 per 1000 for oophorectomy. Radical hysterectomy and surgical staging procedures for endometrial cancer carry a mortality rate of approximately 3 per 1000, while exenterative procedures carry mortality rate of 70 to 80 per 1000 (Orr, 1988). These risks may be markedly increased for older women, those with coexisting medical disease, or those undergoing an emergent procedure.

Infectious Morbidity

As previously noted, anesthesia adversely affects white blood cell function by reducing T- and B-cell levels (by as much as 50%) as well as lymphocyte response and chemotactic activity. Both phagocytic function and levels of antibody production are abnormal after major surgical procedures. Despite these effects, there is little question that the risk of developing postoperative infection is procedure- and patient-related, and risks can be related to numerous factors (Table 43–6). Specific methods of prophylaxis are addressed elsewhere (Orr and Taylor, 1987; Orr et al, 1990). Specific individuals, including the obese, those on immunosuppressive drug therapy, the elderly, and diabetics, are at increased risk for infectious morbidity. In fact, infections account for the majority of postoperative complications and 20% of perioperative morbidity in diabetics (Roizen, 1996). Tight perioperative glucose control improves the glycemic-associated loss of granulocytic phagocytic function and restores intracellular healing activity.

Establishing the presence of postoperative infection can be difficult. Following benign gynecologic procedures, this risk is approximately 10%. The risk is no higher after radical hysterectomy but increases to 40% to 60% after exenterative surgery. The development of postoperative infection is associated with a marked increase in patient drug exposure, cost of hospitalization, and psychological morbidity. Additionally, infectious morbidity may decrease mobilization and may create other serious sequelae (embolic phenomena) or expose patients to other

Table 43–4. AMERICAN SOCIETY OF ANESTHESIOLOGISTS PHYSICAL STATUS CLASSIFICATION

STATUS	DISEASE STATE
Class I	No organic, physiologic, biochemical, or psychiatric disturbance
Class II	Mild to moderate systemic disturbance that may or may not be related to the reason for surgery
Class III	Severe systemic disturbance that may or may not be related to the reason for surgery
Class IV	Severe systemic disturbance that is life threatening with or without surgery
Class V	Moribund patient who has little chance of survival but is submitted to surgery as a last resort (resuscitative effort)
Emergency Operation (E)	Any patient in whom an emergency operation is required

Data from American Society of Anesthesiologists: New classification of physical status. Anesthesiology 1963;24: 111.

potential risks (including fistulas). Sepsis not only increases acute morbidity but also increases the risk of death for up to 5 years after the septic episode (Quartin et al, 1997). The adage "fever equals infection" should be cautiously evaluated. Careful review indicates that more than 50% of obstetric and 30% of gynecologic postoperative fevers cannot be attributed to infection (Klimek et al, 1982). When fever is present, the prudent gynecologic surgeon should first evaluate the entire patient with a careful history and physical examination, considering the clinical situation, and should avoid the "knee-jerk" reflex ordering of antibiotics.

In most patients with fever (temperature > 100.4°F, [38°C]) in the first 48 to 72 hours postoperatively, pulmonary atelectasis is thought to be a contributing cause. Frequently, incentive spirometry and ambulation suffice as interventions. Women with a smoking history or other pulmonary conditions may benefit from chest percussion and postural drainage, but incentive spirometry remains an essential component of pulmonary toilet. Chest radiographs are seldom indicated in the absence of physical symptoms or signs, unless other predisposing factors are present (i.e., immunosuppression).

The increasingly short stay associated with laparoscopic or other gynecologic surgery creates the potential problem of evaluating fever after discharge. The authors encourage examination and evaluation for those women who remain febrile for 24 hours or longer or those with markedly elevated temperature.

Fever on or after the third postoperative day is more indicative of infection, although persistent atelectasis frequently remains the culprit. The urinary tract is the most common site, and urinary infection may result from perioperative genitourinary drainage. Therefore, urinalysis and culture are appropriate for patients in whom fever develops beyond 72 hours. Empirical antibiotics should be considered for those women with an abnormal urinalysis whose culture findings are pending.

Wound infections are not uncommon, and abdominal wounds should be carefully inspected daily. Induration and erythema frequently precede tenderness and drainage by 1 to 2 days. Specimens from the purulent exudate of wounds may be obtained for

Table 43–5. MORTALITY ASSOCIATED WITH PREOPERATIVE PHYSICAL STATUS

	ASA CLASSIFICATION (%)*				
	I	*II*	*III*	*IV*	*V*
48-Hour Mortality[†]					
Elective	0.07	0.24	1.4	7.5	8.1
Emergency	0.16	0.51	3.4	8.3	9.5
6-Week Mortality[‡]					
Elective					
Low-risk	0.03	0.31	1.9	5.6	20.0
Medium-risk	0.02	1.7	7.2	17.2	31.4
High-risk	2.2	5.4	14.6	20.5	42.4

*ASA (American Society of Anesthesiologists) status: I, healthy; II, mild systemic disease; III, severe, but not incapacitating, disease; IV, incapacitating disease; V, moribund.
[†]N = 68,388.
[‡]N = 856,000.
Modified from Feigal DW, Blaisdell FW: The estimation of surgical risk. Med Clin North Am 1979;63:1131, with permission.

Table 43-6. SURGICAL FACTORS REPORTED TO AFFECT SURGICAL SITE INFECTION

Preoperative
Age
Immune status
Nutritional status
Obesity
Concurrent illness
Preoperative stay
Skin preparation
Hair clipping
Antibiotics

Intraoperative
Duration
Incision
Cautery
Suture material
Suture technique
Drains
Irrigation
Vasoconstrictors

Postoperative
Wound closure
Nutritional status
Oxygen

culture, especially in an intensive care setting, when multiple resistant organisms may be present. After a wound is opened, most patients respond to debridement and packing and do not require long-term antibiotics in the absence of significant cellulitis. The routine use of blood cultures contributes little (except cost) to the initial evaluation of postoperative fever. Again, specific circumstances, such as high fever (>103°F [39.4°C]) with shaking chills or other clinical signs or symptoms suggesting septicemia or fever in immunocompromised patients, may warrant blood cultures. In the absence of clinically or radiologically confirmed abscess, we believe that decisions based on postoperative pelvic examinations provide little useful information because pelvic induration is always present and the associated tenderness only confuses the clinical situation. However, ultrasonography may rapidly assist in the diagnosis of a cuff hematoma or hydronephrosis.

Intravenous sites may be the source of fever in the presence of thrombophlebitis. Both peripheral and central intravenous sites should be monitored daily for tenderness, erythema, or purulence, and these lines should be discontinued with the resumption of adequate oral intake of fluid. Lower extremity or pelvic deep venous thrombosis (DVT) may be associated with low-grade fever, and careful lower extremity examination may suggest the need for further evaluation and treatment.

Additional radiologic studies are rarely helpful and usually are unnecessary during the primary fever work-up. Although chest radiographs are of little benefit in the initial evaluation of the febrile, neutropenic patient, 60% of such patients evaluated for persistent or recurrent fever show findings that require

or suggest a need for a change in therapy (Orr et al, 1994b). In the absence of localizing signs or symptoms, intravenous pyelograms (IVPs) and intestinal barium studies usually contribute little. Computerized tomography (CT) adds little and is certainly not cost-effective in the early evaluation of postoperative fever, but it may have a role in evaluating patients with refractory temperature elevation because it may allow detection of unusual sites of infection (subdiaphragmatic) and localization and drainage of percutaneous abscess. Gallium scans and other radionucleotide studies (radiolabeled leukocytes) are reserved for the most refractory (and unusual) instances. In the absence of localizing evidence for infection, careful review of current medication may indicate a possible idiosyncratic drug reaction as an etiology.

When the diagnosis of infection is suspected or established, the gynecologic surgeon should use antibiotics in a logical manner based on the suspected source. Numerous antibiotics and combinations thereof are available, and, in the absence of specific microbiologic isolation, treatment should be directed toward the usual polymicrobic etiology. Each time antibiotics are ordered, four questions should be asked:

1. What is the most likely source of infection?
2. What are the most likely causative organisms?
3. What is the antibiotic or combination of antibiotics?
4. Is there a more cost-effective antibiotic or combination available?

There appears to be little justification to institute treatment with the same antibiotic used for surgical prophylaxis.

Drainage is needed for specific infections. We usually initially avoid an open surgical procedure, favoring the use of radiologically guided percutaneous drainage of an intra-abdominal or pelvic abscess if possible. Success rates with the latter are high and compare favorably with those for open drainage in terms of morbidity and cost (Fry and Clevenger, 1991). Abdominal wound infections can be easily recognized and drained. Delayed secondary closure, after at least 4 days of open wound care, can be used to safely accelerate healing and lower the costs and need for additional outpatient care (Walters et al, 1990).

Every pelvic surgeon should be familiar with the serious sequelae associated with the systemic inflammatory response syndrome (Santilli and Cerra, 1990; Bone, 1997). Although uncommon following gynecologic or obstetric procedures, its occurrence is associated with significant mortality rates. The diagnosis must be considered with the onset of multiple organ dysfunction combined with fever, leukocytosis, and a progressive deterioration in the patient's clinical status. If this syndrome is present, a diligent search for intra-abdominal or other serious infection must be undertaken. If loculated infection is present, drainage is mandatory. Surgical or percutaneous drainage requires localization for success (Shaff et al, 1988).

Pulmonary Problems

Perioperative alterations in pulmonary physiology predispose the lungs to numerous complications, particularly in high-risk groups (Table 43–7) (Jayr et al, 1988; Orr, 1988; Pett and Wernly, 1988; Orr et al, 1994a). Anesthetics, drugs, transfusions, and other intervention may adversely affect oxyhemoglobin affinity; fortunately, the tissue effect on oxygen supply is not usually clinically significant. Ventilation-perfusion abnormalities affect pulmonary closing pressures and increase the risk of postoperative atelectasis. Patients with obstructive pulmonary disease are at greater risk for pulmonary complications than are those with restrictive pulmonary disease. Even when these predisposing factors are present, diligent preoperative preparation and postoperative care can decrease the rate of pulmonary complications. Postoperative respiratory care must emphasize sustained maximum inspiration to increase alveolar inflation and maintain a near-normal functional residual capacity. Intermittent positive-pressure breathing, blow bottles, and endotracheal stimulation are only variably effective and in some situations may be harmful. Although it fails to increase diaphragmatic movement (Brooks-Brunn, 1995), incentive spirometry remains the most effective postoperative maneuver to decrease the risk of atelectasis. Once inflated, alveoli tend to remain open for at least 1 hour; consequently, any effective pulmonary maneuver should be scheduled during the patient's waking hours on a regular basis. Patient education on the importance of deep breathing exercises is most helpful when provided before the procedure and reinforced afterward.

Certain drugs (antiarrhythmics, antibiotics, diuretics) should be avoided because they potentiate neuromuscular blockade and adversely affect respiratory mechanics (Emory and Stedman, 1990).

Postoperative pulmonary infection occurs in approximately 0.4% of patients undergoing total hysterectomy for benign indications; this incidence is 2% after radical hysterectomy, 3% after exenteration, and 3% after ovarian debulking procedures (Orr and Taylor, 1987). Surgeons should be particularly cognizant of the 13% risk of significant pulmonary complications (atelectasis, pneumonia) that occur during the recovery of institutionalized patients following abdominal surgery (Cutler and Fink, 1990). These infectious risks are also increased in patients who are immunocompromised (malignancy, malnutrition) and in those undergoing long (>3 hours) operative procedures. Although pulmonary infectious risks are not affected by the administration of prophylactic antibiotics, ambulation combined with deep inspiration decreases these risks. If pneumonia occurs, unusual organisms may be responsible; broad-spectrum antibiotic coverage should be considered, particularly in the immunocompromised patient (Gleckman and de La Rosa, 1997).

In the absence of pre-existing disease or coexisting complication, respiratory insufficiency is a rare complication after nonradical surgical procedures. However, this is not true of longer procedures requiring high-volume blood replacement or ultraradical procedures, wherein postoperative respiratory compromise may complicate recovery in 25% of patients (Grant and Morton, 1988; Orr, 1988; Schuster, 1990). Spirometric preoperative risk factors have been defined (Table 43–8), and appropriate intervention (Table 43–9) can successfully alter these risks. Smoking remains an important risk factor for pulmonary complications. Acute cessation (≤24 hours) can reduce the quantity of carboxyhemoglobin and improve oxygenation. However, cessation in excess of 6 weeks is necessary to improve mucociliary clearance to baseline and lessen pulmonary risk. Specific preop-

Table 43–7. FACTORS ASSOCIATED WITH INCREASED PULMONARY RISK

History/Physical
Smoker
Chronic obstructive pulmonary disease or productive cough
Institutionalized
>60 Years
Obesity
Malnutrition
Abnormal chest radiograph

Procedure
Upper abdomen
Extensive procedure
Prolonged anesthesia (>3 hr)

Table 43–8. SPIROMETRIC PREOPERATIVE RISK FACTORS

	PULMONARY RISK*	
	Increased	*High*
FEV_1	<2.0 L: <50% predicted	<1.0 L
FVC	<50% predicted	<1.5 L
FEV_1/FVC	<50%	<35%
FEF_{25-75}	<50% predicted	
MVV		<50% predicted
$PaCO_2$		>45 mm Hg

Abbreviations: FEV, forced expiratory volume; FVC, forced vital capacity; FEF_{25-75}, forced expiratory flow at 25% versus 75% of FVC; MVV, maximal voluntary ventilation; $PaCO_2$, partial pressure of carbon dioxide.
*Pulmonary risks are also increased in the presence of an abnormal electrocardiogram or pulmonary wedge pressures greater than 30 mm Hg.
Modified from Orr JW Jr: Introduction to pelvic surgery: pre- and postoperative care. In Gusberg SB, Shingleton HM, Deppe G (eds): Female Genital Cancer. New York. Churchill Livingstone, 1988:497, with permission. Originally from Harmon E, Lillington G: Pulmonary risk factors in surgery. Med Clin North Am 1979;63:1289.

Table 43 – 9. PULMONARY PROPHYLAXIS	
Cessation of smoking (≥2 weeks)	Ambulation
Bronchodilators	Antiembolism
Chest physiotherapy	Antibiotics
Incentive spirometer	Education

erative testing can determine the likelihood of postoperative pulmonary complications and should be conducted in those patients deemed at high risk after history and physical examination.

Perioperative bronchospastic disorders are relatively rare. This complex airway response, including airway edema and increased secretions and smooth muscle contraction, is associated with or related to inflammatory changes that increase bronchial hyperresponsiveness (Bishop, 1996). Thus perioperative steroids have an increasingly important role in the management of these individuals and may be combined with the use of inhaled β-adrenergics. Theophylline adds little to this regimen during acute attacks and is of primary importance in prophylaxis, particularly nighttime bronchospasm. Its beneficial effects on mucociliary clearance and diaphragmatic contraction are likely important. Unfortunately, this drug has a low toxic/therapeutic index (Domino, 1996).

Spirometry, developed almost 150 years ago, remains the most useful test for the evaluation of lung function. This study allows identification of obstructive or restrictive disease. Intrapulmonary obstruction (asthma, chronic obstructive pulmonary disease) reduces air flow as estimated by forced expiratory volume (l second)/forced vital capacity (FEV_1/FVC). Restriction in lung volumes must be corrected for race. Measurements of functional residual capacity and derived residual volume are necessary to define true restriction because reduced vital capacity alone may reflect air trapping. Spirometry also allows measurement of maximal voluntary ventilation, an effort-dependent measurement of maximum ventilation greater than 12 to 15 seconds (standardized to liters/minute). Although it is not specific to the nature of pulmonary disease, spirometry may assist in assessing perioperative pulmonary risks. Clinical abnormalities during resting gas exchange can be evaluated by diffusion (carbon monoxide) techniques and measurement of Po_2 and Pco_2. The measurement of maximal voluntary ventilation may unmask a potential inspiratory muscle weakness. Maximal inspiratory force is the best clinical test of respiratory muscle strength (−80 cm H_2O is normal for women). Postoperative muscle dysfunction (hypoventilation) may be related to the fatigue associated with intrinsic lung disease or to other nonpulmonary causes, such as poor nutrition, electrolyte imbalance (hypokalemia or hypophosphatemia), incision placement, and sedation from narcotics. Other studies (helium-oxygen flow volume loops, closing volumes) are available, but spirometry serves as a sensitive screening tool for patients suspected of having significant lung disease (Iber, 1990). Abnormal findings should prompt either appropriate consultation or modification of the surgical plan, or both.

Specific methods of intervention (cessation of smoking for 6 weeks, treating bronchitis, optimization of bronchodilator therapy) may decrease the risk of postoperative pulmonary complications. Postoperative intervention (Table 43–10) includes deep breathing and other methods designed to increase alveolar ventilation. Continuous positive airway pressure may be of benefit for those with refractory atelectasis (Brooks-Brunn, 1995). Continuous or intermittent pulse oximetry during postoperative recovery may assist in early detection of clinical difficulties, allowing appropriate intervention (Smith, 1990). Ambroxol, a mucolytic that also promotes surfactant therapy, has been associated with a lower incidence of atelectasis and a smaller drop in Pco_2 (Brooks-Brunn, 1995).

THROMBOEMBOLISM

Postoperative DVT or pulmonary thromboembolism remains a significant problem after gynecologic surgery, occurring in as many as 50% of patients depending on the methods of detection and the risk of the population. Clinically, thrombosis above the popliteal vein is more likely to result in thromboembolus, and fibrinogen scan (nonclinical)–detected calf thromboses extend proximally in approximately 20% of patients (Farquharson and Orr, 1984). Thrombus in the proximal deep venous system is of serious clinical significance because pulmonary embolic phenomena may develop in 50% of these women.

Documentation of DVT remains an important aspect of postoperative surveillance. Contrast venography remains the accepted standard for the diagnosis of DVT in the lower extremities. Unfortunately, new thrombosis develops in 2% of patients following venography and as many as 10% of venograms are judged technically inadequate. Impedance plethysmography and compressive ultrasonography are important noninvasive preliminary studies. Compression ultrasonography is highly sensitive (>90%) for the detection of popliteal or femoral vein thrombosis (Dauzat et al, 1997). Abnormal results obtained with noninvasive methods are treated. Normal ultrasound should be followed by venograms (if there is high clinical suspicion) or by repeat ultrasonography in 1 week (low clinical suspicion). The use of a *d*-dimer may compliment a normal ultrasound. Detection is important because untreated women with pulmonary thromboembolism face a 40% chance of recurrence and at least a 20% mortality rate. The initial event may not be fatal, but 75% of patients who die as a result of pulmonary thromboembolism have evidence suggesting a recent prior embolus. Unfortunately, the diagnosis of thromboembolism had not been considered in more than 70% of patients suffering a fatal embolus (Rosenow, 1995). Although

Table 43-10. RECOMMENDED INTERVENTIONS TO PREVENT AND TREAT POSTOPERATIVE PULMONARY COMPLICATIONS

Preoperative Interventions
Modify risk factors (smoking, weight, patient education)
Optimize therapy for underlying pulmonary disease: pharmaceutical (bronchodilators, corticosteroids, antibiotics); CPT (optimize secretion management)
Educate patient regarding DBEX, positioning, early ambulation, pain management

Intraoperative Interventions
Select anesthesia
Manage airway, protect
Monitor oxygenation, acid-base status
Give periodic hyperinflations
Minimize duration of anesthesia

Postoperative Interventions
Primary management to prevent/minimize atelectasis:
    Reinforce preoperative patient education regarding DBEX, reposition frequently, ambulate early, manage pain. Give postoperative respiratory care starting in the postanesthesia care unit and continuing in surgical unit.
    Reposition and do DBEX every hour while awake with or without a device (8–10 breaths with a 3- to 5-second inspiratory hold). After education, patient may perform SMI without supervision but should be monitored regularly and coached by healthcare personnel. As patient begins ambulation, frequency of deep breathing maneuvers may be decreased.
    Assess patient for secretion management problems; implement directed cough or percussion/postural drainage as necessary. If these measures are inadequate, consider bronchoscopy. If the patient is exhibiting continued signs/symptoms of atelectasis or potential infectious problems that do not respond to the primary measures, a chest radiograph should be obtained.
Secondary interventions to treat refractory atelectasis/infections process:
    Atelectasis
      CPAP: (10–15 cm H_2O) 25–35 breaths or 5–10 min every hour while awake. PEP: similar regimen as CPAP. Both CPAP and PEP should continue a minimum of 24 hr after resolution as demonstrated by chest radiograph.
      IPPB: use only if patient has vital capacity <10 ml/kg, inspiratory capacity <1 L, or unable to voluntarily take a deep breath; prior to initiation of therapy assess for adequate trial of DBEX.
      CPT: chest percussion and postural drainage only if indicated for secretion management problems caused by acute problem or preexisting pulmonary disease.
    Infectious process
      Antibiotics
      Chest physical therapy (if needed for secretion management)

Abbreviations: CPAP, continuous positive airway pressure; CPT, chest physiotherapy; DBEX, deep breathing exercises; IPPB, intermittent positive-pressure breathing; PEP, positive end-expiratory pressure; SMI, sustained maximum inspiration.
From Brooks-Brunn JA: Postoperative atelectasis and pneumonia. Heart Lung 1995;24:94, with permission.

pulmonary emboli are common during hospitalization, as many as 50% of these occur after initial discharge, indicating the necessity of postdischarge attention to voiced complaints.

The risk of thrombogenesis is governed by Virchow's triad of altered blood flow, blood coagulation, and intimal damage (Orr, 1988). Intimal drainage commonly occurs during pelvic operations for malignancy, but overall risks are increased in the obese, smokers, and the elderly and during longer procedures. The usual intimal protection against thrombosis may be related to the effects of electrostatic repulsion, plasminogen activation, secretion of fibronectin, local production of prostacyclin, or heparinoids. Damage to endothelium that occurs during retroperitoneal or nodal dissection results in the exposure of collagen microfibrils and basement membranes, increases local coagulability, and theoretically predisposes the patient to thrombogenesis.

Vascular or venous stasis occurs with regional or general anesthesia, and 50% of postoperative DVT initially develops within 24 hours of surgery. The major risk of stasis begins at induction; therefore, to be effective, any prophylactic method should be incorporated preoperatively. Tested methods of prophylaxis include minidose heparin, dextran, venoconstrictors, and various physical techniques. Although minidose unfractionated heparin has been proclaimed as the prophylactic method of choice to decrease thrombosis, its comparative efficacy in preventing emboli following gynecologic surgery has not been documented. One study has suggested a statistical and clinical reduction in scan-detected thrombosis using an every-8-hour regimen (Clarke-Pearson et al, 1990). Subcutaneous heparin administered at 8-hour intervals decreased the risk of thrombotic (clinical or subclinical) events. However, heparin use during radical gynecologic procedures has been associated with an increased risk of bleeding and lymphocyst formation. We caution the surgeon to monitor platelet counts during subcutaneous heparin administration, because thrombocytopenia and thrombocytopenic thrombocytosis have been reported. The availability of low-molecular-weight heparin, which has a longer bioavailability and is associated with a lesser bleeding risk, should allow prophylaxis alternatives to be developed.

Pneumatic calf compression appears to be an effective method of prophylaxis. Compression stockings are intermittently inflated to 40 to 60 mm Hg, resulting in a twofold increase in venous blood velocity and an increase in systemic fibrinolytic activity. Prospective and retrospective reports indicate its benefit and suggest the need to continue use of these stockings for at least 3 postoperative days. Although cumbersome, these stockings are well tolerated, and this physical method appears to have equal or superior benefit to subcutaneous minidose heparin while subjecting the patient to little potential risk. Until information to the contrary exists, we prefer the use of a low-morbidity physical method of prophylaxis. Subcutaneous heparin is used in the rarest situation. Other prophylactic methods, such as dextran, dihydroergotamine, and warfarin therapy, remain of uncertain benefit in the gynecologic patient. Importantly, epidural anesthesia and analgesia appears to significantly reduce the hypercoagulable state associated with postoperative recovery and may reduce the risk of thromboembolic events (Carpenter, 1996). It would seem prudent to encourage some form of antiembolic prophylaxis in every woman, and mandate it in those women deemed at high risk (obesity, hypertension, cigarette smoking [Goldhaber et al, 1997]).

Most postoperative pulmonary emboli probably go unrecognized; however, clinical suspicion mandates evaluation. Systemic anticoagulation based on the clinical diagnosis of emboli is unacceptable because it may be associated with a risk of bleeding as high as 25% (Farquharson and Orr, 1984; Orr, 1988). In some situations (such as central nervous system bleeding), the mortality rate of heparin-associated bleeding approaches 50%. In fact, heparin is the leading cause of drug-related deaths in an otherwise healthy population. Although the use of low-molecular-weight heparin may lessen bleeding risks, a pulmonary evaluation should be considered prior to anticoagulation. If the ventilation-perfusion scan is normal, no additional evaluation is necessary. About 40% of patients with pulmonary embolism have high-probability scans; 40% have intermediate- and 20% have low-probability scans. However, 14%, 30%, 87%, and 18% of patients will show angiographic findings of pulmonary emboli with low-, moderate-, high-, or indeterminate-probability scans (Fiszman et al, 1998). Although ventilation-perfusion scan results serve as a guide, a minority of patients with emboli have a high-probability scan (sensitivity 41%, specificity 97%) (Orr, 1988; Hyers, 1990; Levine and Hirsch, 1990; Saltzman et al, 1990). The clinician should seek pulmonary consultation or pursue the diagnosis with angiography, if clinically indicated, because emboli may be present in a significant percentage (12% to 24%) of those patients with low-probability scans. Using scan results allows the angiographer to visualize the most suspicious area, and the angiographic study, if indicated, may require the injection of less radiographic dye. Documentation becomes most important if symptoms persist after anticoagulation, and a caval filter or interruption is required.

Once DVT or embolic phenomena are diagnosed, systemic anticoagulation is appropriate. Various nomograms related to dose, weight (Table 43–11) or dose titration (Cruickshank et al, 1991; Ginsberg, 1996) are available to assist in therapeutic anticoagulation with reduced periods of under- or over-anticoagulation (Table 43–12). Effective treatment is focused on stabilizing the venous thrombus and minimizing the risk of recurrence. Previous practice dictated heparin administration for 7 to 10 days (to stabilize the clot), with oral anticoagulants given on days 5 to 7. However, starting oral medication within 24 hours of starting heparin, with a 3- to 4-day overlap (5 days of heparin), is as effective as a longer course of heparinization (Clarke-Pearson and Rodriguez, 1994). Importantly, early adequate intravenous anticoagulation is imperative because the addition of warfarin is associated with a hypercoagulable state.

Cardiovascular Problems

Cardiovascular complications can occur following benign gynecologic procedures; however, cardiovascular disease is a common coexisting medical illness, often complicating cancer surgery (Madlon-Kay, 1987; Orr, 1988; Freeman et al, 1989; Orr and Browne, 1994). Extrapolating from demographic data, as many as 25% of patients undergoing anesthesia are at risk for or have significant cardiovascular disease (Table 43–13). Although patients with heart disease generally tolerate surgery, associated complications can be life threatening. Recognition of cardiovascular problems and alteration of the medical management or surgical plan can decrease these risks. Recent data suggest that postoperative atherosclerotic plaque rupture is a secondary phenomenon, and excess stress and catecholamine levels that cause an excess in myocardial oxygen demand are the primary cause of perioperative cardiac morbidity (Bodenheimer, 1996). The incidence of postoperative infarction peaks on days 2 and 3, following the peak occurrence of postoperative tachycardia.

Pooled data indicate the risk of perioperative myocardial infarction (MI) to be 0.15% in patients with no prior evidence of heart disease. Pre-existing cardiac disease poses an eightfold increase in the risk of postoperative MI. Temporal relationship was previously thought to be important (Table 43–14) because patients undergoing surgical procedures within 3 months of a previous MI were predicted to be at greater risk of reinfarction than those undergoing surgery after a 3- to 6-month delay. However, time interval may no longer be important in the current era of thrombolytics, angioplasty, and risk stratification after an acute MI (Orr and Browne, 1994). Unless surgery is emergent, it should be delayed after a recent MI, because mortality rates for a postoperative reinfarction approach 70%. Although mortality risks of reinfarction are higher, necessary surgery can be performed safely with intensive mon-

Table 43-11. WEIGHT-BASED HEPARIN ANTICOAGULATION NOMOGRAM

The initial dose is a bolus of 80 U/kg body weight, followed by an infusion starting at a rate of 18 U/kg/hr. The APTT is
measured every 6 hours, and the heparin dose adjusted as follows:

MEASURED VALUE	ADJUSTMENT
PTT < 35 sec (<1.2 × control value)	80 U/kg as bolus, then increase infusion rate by 4 U/kg/hr
APTT 35–45 sec (1.2–1.5 × control value)	40 U/kg as bolus, then increase infusion rate by 2 U/kg/hr
APTT 46–70 sec (>1.5–2.3 × control value)	No change
APTT 71–90 sec (>2.3–3 × control value)	Decrease infusion rate by 2 U/kg/hr
APTT >90 sec (>3 × control value)	Stop infusion for 1 hour, then decrease infusion rate by 3 U/kg/hr

5000-U BOLUS DOSE, FOLLOWED BY 1280 U/HR

APTT (sec)	BOLUS (U)	STOP INFUSION (min)	RATE OF CHANGE (ml/hr)	REPEAT APTT
>50	5000	0	+3	In 6 hr
50–59	0	0	+3	In 6 hr
60–85	0	0	0	Next morning
86–95	0	0	−2	Next morning
96–120	0	30	−2	In 6 hr
>120	0	60	−4	In 6 hr

INTRAVENOUS DOSE-TITRATION NOMOGRAM FOR APTT

The starting dose is a 5000-U bolus, followed by 40,000 U/24 hr (if the patient has a low risk of bleeding) or 30,000 U/24 hr (if
there is a high risk of bleeding).

APTT (sec)	INTRAVENOUS Rate of Change (ml/hr)	INFUSION Change in Dose (U/24 hr)	ADDITIONAL ACTION
45	+6	+5760	Repeat APTT in 4–6 hr
46–54	+3	+2880	Repeat APTT in 4–6 hr
55–85	0	0	None
86–110	−3	−2880	Stop heparin for 1 hr; repeat APTT 4–6 hr after restarting heparin treatment
>110	−6	−5760	Stop heparin for 1 hr; repeat APTT 4–6 hr after restarting heparin treatment

Modified from Ginsberg JS: Management of venous thromboembolism. N Engl J Med 1996;335:1816, with permission.

itoring. However, if possible it would seem prudent to delay surgery for 6 to 12 weeks to allow atherosclerotic plaque stabilization and myocardial healing. At least three reports have suggested that patients undergoing recent successful coronary artery bypass grafting are not at increased risk of cardiovascular complications (Orr and Browne, 1994). An America Heart Association/American College of Cardiology Task Force has recommended all patients have some form of preoperative risk stratification following an acute MI (Fleisher, 1996a).

The risk of cardiac death is 20-fold increased in women with any sign or symptom of heart disease (Madlon-Kay, 1987). Goldman (1983) determined the major cardiac risk factors associated with postoperative cardiovascular morbidity (Table 43–15). In addition, noncardiac factors, including abdominal surgery and procedures lasting longer than 3 hours, increase the risk of postoperative cardiac morbidity. Using these risk factors as an index, the risk of life-threatening or cardiac death may be predicted. Although overall cardiovascular risks can be calcu-

lated, variables not associated with postoperative cardiac complications include hyperlipidemia, smoking, diabetes, hypertension, atherosclerotic vascular disease, and mitral valve disease. In addition, ECG stress testing is not reliably predictive of cardiovascular morbidity. Finally, although "low risk" indicates a small probability, it does not exclude a patient from adverse perioperative cardiac events. The American College of Cardiology guidelines suggest that preoperative cardiac intervention is rarely necessary to lower surgical risks unless such intervention is indicated irrespective of the perioperative context (Eagle et al, 1996).

Data suggest that two thirds to three quarters of ischemic changes occur in the absence of hemodynamic change, suggesting that hemodynamic control is a necessary but not sufficient requirement to minimize the risk of cardiac ischemic (Lowenstein, 1996). Development of postoperative pulmonary edema is ominous, with mortality rates approaching 45% (Orr, 1988; Charlson et al, 1991). These risks are increased in older patients with perioperative left ventricular

Table 43-12. COMPARISON OF HEPARIN THERAPY IN NOMOGRAM AND CONTROL PATIENTS

	GROUP (Mean ± SE)		
	Nomogram	Control	P
Heparin duration (hours)	122.3 ± 6.6	118.4 ± 7.0	.69
No. of APTTs* performed	8.6 ± 0.4	6.4 ± 0.4	.005
Heparin dose (units/24 hours)	32,903 ± 1,283	28,563 ± 796	.005
No. of APTTs until first therapeutic result	2.6 ± 0.2	3.2 ± 0.3	.13
Time to first dose adjustment (hours)	8.2 ± 0.4	14.3 ± 1.0	<.0001
Time to first therapeutic result (hours)	24.3 ± 2.4	56.9 ± 6.4	<.0001

*APTT, activated partial thromboplastin time.
Modified from Cruickshank MK, Levine MN, Hirsch T, et al: A standard heparin nomogram for the management of heparin therapy. Arch Intern Med 1991;151:333, with permission.

dysfunction, an abnormal ECG, and valvular disease. A history of stable angina or β-blocker therapy does not increase these risks. Preoperative inotropic support with digoxin should be considered in those patients with a previous history of pulmonary edema, signs or symptoms of ventricular dysfunction, the presence of nocturnal angina, atrial fibrillation with a rapid ventricular response, and frequent episodes of paroxysmal atrial or junctional tachycardia. One report suggested the importance of maintaining a stable intraoperative blood pressure, because large (40-mm Hg) shifts (up or down) in mean arterial pressure (MAP) were associated with a significant increase of postoperative congestive heart failure (Charlson et al, 1991). Failure rates were highest (eightfold) in those patients receiving a small volume (<300 ml) of intravenous fluids, suggesting the importance of individualized fluid replacement. If clinical failure develops, available drugs, including ionotopes or other classes (Table 43–16), may be

needed. If the gynecologist is unfamiliar with their use in an intensive care setting, consultations should be considered.

A potentially important risk factor for those with CAD is the development of postoperative anemia. A hematocrit of 28% is the risk threshold for those undergoing vascular surgical procedures, and those with a hematocrit of less than 29% on postoperative day 2 are at increased risk for coronary events (Lowenstein, 1996). Patients with prosthetic valves, valvular disease, congenital defects, hypertrophic cardiomyopathy, and mitral valve prolapse are at increased risk for endocarditis and should be considered for antimicrobial prophylaxis (Table 43–17) (Dajani et al, 1990). Most gynecologic procedures are clean-contaminated, and antimicrobial prophylaxis consisting of ampicillin (2.0 g) plus an aminoglycoside (1.5 mg/kg, maximum dose 80 mg) should be administered perioperatively. Penicillin-allergic patients should receive vancomycin (1.0 g) and genta-

Table 43-13. PREDICTORS OF CARDIAC RISK

Historical Predictors

Age	Dysrhythmia
Previous MI	Peripheral vascular disease
Angina	Valvular heart disease
Left ventricular dysfunction	Previous CABG or PTCA
Hypertension	Risk indices
Diabetes	

Intraoperative Predictors

Classical	Dynamic
Anesthetic choice	Hypertension
Surgical site	Hypotension
Duration of surgery	Tachycardia
"Emergency" surgery	Myocardial ischemia
Hypertension	ST-T wave changes
Hypotension	TEE-demonstrated wall motion/thickening
Tachycardia	Pulmonary artery monitoring
Ventricular dysfunction	Cardiokymographic detection
Myocardial ischemia	Biochemical markers
Dysrhythmias	Ventricular dysfunction
	Arrhythmias

Abbreviations: CABG, coronary artery bypass graft; PTCA, percutaneous transluminal coronary angioplasty; TEE, transesophageal echocardiography.
From Orr JW Jr, Browne KF Jr: Cardiovascular complications. In Orr JW Jr, Shingleton HM (eds): Complications in Gynecologic Surgery: Prevention, Recognition, and Management. Philadelphia: JB Lippincott Company, 1994:1, with permission.

Table 43–14. PERIOPERATIVE MI OR MORTALITY IN PATIENTS WITH PREVIOUS MI

TIME FROM MI TO OPERATION (mo)	GOLDMAN, 1975–1976		EEROLA, 1970–1974		SCHOEPPEL, 1980		RAO, 1973–1976		RAO, 1976–1982		SHAH, 1990	
	Reinf.	Mort.	Reinf.	Mort.	Reinf.	Mort.	Reinf.	Mort.	Reinf.	Mort.	Reinf.	Mort.
0–3	4.5% (1/22)	23% (5/22)	8% (1/12)	8% (1/12)	0% (0/1)	0% (0/1)	30% (4/11)	*	5.8% (3/52)	*	4.3% (1/23)	*
4–6		5.9% (1/17)	5.9% (1/17)	0% (0/1)	0%	0% (0/8)	26% (8/31)	*	2.3% (2/36)	*	0% (0/18)	*
7–12	0% (0/13)			0% (0/1)	0% (0/8)		5% (6/127)	*	1.0% (1/104)	*	5.7% (10/174)	*
13–18		8% (1/133)			0% (0/10)	0% (0/10)	5% (6/114)	*	1.6% (4/258)	*		
19–24	3.3% (2/66)	3.3% (2/66)	4.9% (4/82)	12% (1/82)								
25–36					0% (0.26)	0% (0.26)	5% (4/81)	*	1.7% (4/235)	*		
>36 Unknown											3.3%	
Total no. of pts. with MI		8.9% (9/109)			5.7% (3/35)	3.8% (2/53)	7.7% (28/364)	4.1% (15/364)	1.9% (14/733)	0.7% (5/733)		

Abbreviations: Mort., mortality; pts., patients; Reinf., reinfarction.
*Not applicable.
From Orr JW Jr, Browne KF Jr: Cardiovascular complications. In Orr JW Jr, Shingleton HM (eds): Complications in Gynecologic Surgery: Prevention, Recognition, and Management. Philadelphia: JB Lippincott Company, 1994:1, with permission.

Table 43-15. CARDIAC RISKS AND COMPLICATIONS AFTER GYNECOLOGIC SURGERY

	CARDIAC "RISK" FACTORS	POINTS
History	Age > 70	5
	MI (<6 mo)	10
Physical	S_3, JVD	11
	Aortic stenosis	3
ECG	Arrhythmia	7
	PVC (>5/min)	7
General	PaO_2 < 60, $PaCO_2$ > 50	3
	Potassium, <3; creatinine, >3.0	
	Abnormal LFTs	
	Confined to bed	
Operation	Abdominal/thoracic	3
	Emergency	4
Total		53

CARDIAC "NON-RISK" FACTORS

Compensated CHF (Absent S_3, LVD)	MI > 6 mo prior	Hypertension
Diabetes	Peripheral vascular disease	Cardiomegaly
Bundle-branch block	Mitral disease (no failure)	Stable angina

CARDIAC RISK CATEGORIZATION

Goldman Score	Life-Threatening Complication (%)*	Mortality (%)
<5	0.7	0.2
6–12	5.0	2.0
13–25	11.0	2.0
>26	22.0	56.0

*Myocardial infarction, failure, ventricular tachycardia.
Abbreviations: CHF, congestive heart failure; ECG, electrocardiogram; LFT, liver function test; LVD, left ventricular dysfunction; JVD, jugular venous distention; MI, myocardial infarction; PVC, premature ventricular contraction; S_3, third heart sound.
Modified from Goldman L: Cardiac risks and complications of noncardiac surgery. Ann Intern Med 1983;98:504, with permission.

micin perioperatively. Patients requiring anticoagulation for prosthetic heart valves should discontinue oral anticoagulants 24 to 48 hours before surgery. Protection against thromboembolic phenomena can be accomplished with the administration of perioperative heparin and immediate reinstitution of oral anticoagulation. Only in the rarest circumstance should anticoagulation be completely reversed because the risk of cardiac death in these situations is markedly increased. Patients with peripheral vascular disease, a systemic atherosclerotic process, frequently have associated CAD, which may be silent. These patients may be best served with perioperative consultation or by undergoing noninvasive or invasive testing.

Hypertension affects 60 million Americans and is associated with CAD and congestive heart failure. Perioperative risks are increased in those with end-organ, cardiac, or renal damage. Forty percent of patients with hypertension are either untreated or inadequately treated with pharmacologic therapy (Longnecker, 1990). When compared with normals, these patients generate the highest MAP in response to laryngoscopy and intubation, and are at greatest risk for myocardial ischemia. Many (75%) require in-

traoperative or postoperative vasodilator therapy. It must be remembered that patients with hypertension may have other coexisting cardiac disease. In the absence of such disease, preoperative diastolic pressure below 110 mm Hg is not associated with increased cardiovascular risk (Orr and Browne, 1994). However, even a single preoperative dose of a β-blocker may decrease the risk of significant perioperative sequelae. In patients receiving medication, these medications should be continued (and given the morning of surgery) perioperatively to prevent rebound hypertensive effects. The combination of hypertension and diabetes may have significant risks (Grossman and Messerli, 1996). Numerous drugs are available for treatment (Laslett, 1995).

Although careful history, physical examination, and routine diagnostic studies may suffice in the typical gynecologic patient, additional studies are often necessary for those with abnormal cardiovascular findings, older women, obese women, those with an abnormal exercise capacity, or those undergoing extended or radical surgical procedures. Importantly, the stress associated with minimally invasive procedures is also associated with the same potential perioperative risks. In fact, only 17% of patients un-

Table 43-16. RECOMMENDED DOSAGES OF SPECIFIC AGENTS IN CONGESTIVE HEART FAILURE

DRUG	DOSAGE
Diuretics	
Furosemide	IV: 40 mg: maximum: 1 g/d
	PO: 40 mg/d in 1 or 2 doses, titrated to clinical response
Ethacrynic acid	IV: 50–100 mg/d
	PO: 50–400 mg/d
Bumetanide	IV: 0.5–1.0 mg; maximum: 10 mg/d
	PO: 0–10 mg/d
Metolazone	PO: 2.5–10.0 mg/d
Spironolactone	PO: 200 mg/d in divided doses
Inotropic Agents	
Digoxin	IV: For rapid digitalization, 0.75–1.0 mg; maintenance: 0.25–0.50 mg/d
	PO: Maintenance: 0.25 mg/d
Dopamine	IV: 2–5 μg/kg/min
Dobutamine	IV: 5 μg/kg/min, titrated to hemodynamic response; maximum: 20 μg/kg/min
Amrinone	IV: Bolus of 0.75 mg/kg/min, followed by infusion of 5–10 μg/kg/min
Vasodilators	
Nitroprusside	IV: 0.5–10.0 μg/kg/min, titrated to hemodynamic response
Nitroglycerin	IV: 10–15 μg/min, titrated up to 200 μg/min
Hydralazine	IV: 10–25 mg; maximum: 200 mg/d
Captopril	PO: 6.5–50.0 mg 3×/d
Enalapril	PO: 2.5–15.0 mg 2×/d
Lisinopril	PO: 5–20 mg 1×/d

From Orr JW Jr, Browne, KF Jr. Cardiovascular complications. In Orr JW Jr, Shingleton HM (eds): Complications in Gynecologic Surgery: Prevention, Recognition, and Management. Philadelphia: JB Lippincott Company, 1994:1, with permission.

Table 43-17. RECOMMENDATIONS FOR CARDIAC ANTIMICROBIAL PROPHYLAXIS*

SURGICAL PROCEDURES	CARDIAC CONDITIONS
Endocarditis Prophylaxis Recommended†	
Surgical operations that involve intestinal or respiratory mucosa	Prosthetic cardiac valves, including bioprosthetic and homograft valves
Bronchoscopy with a rigid bronchoscope	Previous bacterial endocarditis, even in the absence of heart disease
Gallbladder surgery	Most congenital cardiac malformations
Cystoscopy	Rheumatic and other acquired valvular dysfunction, even after valvular surgery
Urethral dilatation	Hypertrophic cardiomyopathy
Urethral catheterization if urinary tract infection is present‡	Mitral valve prolapse with valvular regurgitation
Urinary tract surgery if urinary tract infection is present‡	
Incision and drainage of infected tissue‡	
Vaginal hysterectomy	
Vaginal delivery in the presence of infection‡	
Endocarditis Prophylaxis Not Recommended	
Endotracheal intubation	Isolated secundum atrial septal defect
Bronchoscopy with a flexible bronchoscope, with or without biopsy	Surgical repair without residua beyond 6 months of secundum atrial septal defect, ventricular septal defect, or patent ductus arteriosus
Cardiac catheterization	Previous coronary artery bypass graft surgery
Endoscopy with or without gastrointestinal biopsy	Mitral valve prolapse without valvular regurgitation†
Cesarean section	Physiologic, functional, or innocent heart murmurs
In the absence of infection for urethral catheterization, dilatation and curettage, uncomplicated vaginal delivery, therapeutic abortion, sterilization procedures, or insertion or removal of intrauterine devices	Previous Kawasaki's disease without valvular dysfunction
	Previous rheumatic fever without valvular dysfunction
	Cardiac pacemakers and implanted defibrillators

*This table lists selected conditions and procedures but is not meant to be all-inclusive.
†In patients who have prosthetic heart valves, a previous history of endocarditis, or surgically constructed systemic-pulmonary shunts or conduits, physicians may choose to administer prophylactic antibiotics even for low-risk procedures that involve the lower respiratory, genitourinary, or gastrointestinal tracts.
‡In addition to prophylactic regimen for genitourinary procedures, antibiotic therapy should be directed against the most likely bacterial pathogen.
Modified from Dajani AS, Bisno AL, Chung KJ, et al: Prevention of bacterial endocarditis. JAMA 1990;264:2919; JAMA 1991;266:2594. Copyright 1990, 1991 American Medical Association, with permission.

dergoing radical gynecologic procedures are without associated medical problems. The 12-lead ECG has limited diagnostic capabilities. It may serve as a screen, but the resting ECG is normal in as many as 50% of patients with significant CAD. Additional noninvasive studies (echocardiography, Holter monitor, thallium scans), resting or with stress (exercise or pharmacologic), or invasive studies (angiogram) should be utilized appropriately to delineate risks. Unfortunately, even the positive predictive value of pharmacologic cardiac stress tests (dipyridamole thallium scans) is low (<70%); however, the negative predictive value is high (>98%) and a normal study is reassuring (Beller, 1991). Postoperative ECGs are important in the perioperative care for women at risk. Perioperative maintenance of normothermia significantly reduces the risk of morbid cardiac events (Frank et al, 1997), because exposure to cold may be one of the triggers that disrupt atherosclerotic plaque (Alpert and Cheitlin, 1996).

The risk of postoperative cardiac death is increased 10-fold in patients over 70 years of age, and, if reoperation is needed in the older woman, mortality rates approach 100% (Orr, 1988). Age as a risk factor is becoming increasingly important because almost 10% of the population in the United States is older than 65 years of age. In one report, using intensive preoperative evaluation, Babu et al (1980) found that only 33% of older (>68 years) patients had normal left ventricular function. Volume deficits (preload) were present in 27%, and vasodilator agents (afterload reduction) were required in 13%. Inotropic support was required in 17% of patients, and the remainder had some form of combination therapy. Importantly, 93% of patients showed improved ventricular function, and the delay (usually less than 3 days) had no apparent adverse effect on outcome. Del Guercio and Cohn (1980) evaluated 148 elderly patients who were normal by standard evaluation. Intensive invasive evaluation indicated that only 13.5% had a normal hemodynamic cardiovascular status; 22% of these were severely compromised, and the remainder (63.5%) had mild to moderate deficits. Postoperative mortality risks paralleled these deficits. Although no patient with a normal profile died, the mortality rate with mild to moderate abnormalities was 8.5%. A fatal outcome occurred in all patients who were severely compromised undergoing the original planned surgical procedures. These studies indicate the need for continuously monitoring and evaluating the cardiovascular status of older patients because their associated medical illness predisposes them to numerous postoperative complications.

At least 50% of obese patients have associated medical problems and react to anesthesia with a pronounced ventricular dysfunction (Agarwal et al, 1982; Crapo et al, 1986; Orr and Taylor, 1987). Decreased tidal capacity, lowered tidal volume, and increased work of breathing, coupled with long operative procedures and increased blood loss in these individuals, result in a marked increase in perioperative cardiovascular and pulmonary morbidity and mortality.

In patients with cardiovascular risk factors, intraoperative attention to hypotension, perfusion, and cardiovascular performance is mandatory (Estafanous, 1989; Heuser et al, 1989). Maintaining optimal myocardial kinetics in certain risk groups may necessitate invasive monitoring, including pulmonary artery catheters, or other methods of monitoring oxygen delivery. Successful treatment during the postoperative period may require continued intensive monitoring to define problems accurately and permit continuous assessment and appropriate early intervention prior to exhausting physiologic reserves. The initiation and duration of the monitoring should be in proportion to the predictability of the patient's convalescence (Orr et al, 1986b). Most patients have a short, uneventful postoperative course. Postoperative evaluation of cardiovascular status focuses on urine output, blood pressure, pulse, and hematocrit values. Occasionally, central venous pressure is measured. Unfortunately, these parameters may not predict the patient's clinical status if there is coexisting cardiovascular disease or serious illness. In fact, heart rate, MAP, hematocrit level, and central venous pressure are not early predictors of cardiovascular morbidity. These parameters become abnormal late in clinical management, making it less likely that early intervention will prove successful (Yang and Puri, 1986; Orr, 1988; Shoemaker et al, 1990; Bedford, 1991).

Even though healing is not directly influenced in critically ill patients, the hematocrit level should be stabilized at about 32% to maximize oxygen availability and ventricular function. A urine output of 0.5 ml/kg/hour should be the minimal accepted volume, because outputs approaching 2 ml/kg/hour are to be expected if postoperative cardiovascular parameters are normalized (Celoria et al, 1990).

Central venous pressures are less likely to be meaningful in patients with cardiovascular disease; in these patients insertion of a pulmonary artery catheter may therefore be required for optimal central monitoring. The catheter is not intended to obtain measurements but, rather, to facilitate manipulation of important physiologic parameters. Inadequate perfusion can be prevented or corrected early with aggressive therapy that attains supernormal circulatory values. Although routine use of pulmonary artery catheters is not advocated, those patients with serious cardiovascular disease or those who fail to respond to initial clinical management are prime candidates. In these situations, the ability to define important cardiovascular parameters clinically is only 50% to 60% (Yang and Puri, 1986; Shoemaker et al, 1990). Intraoperatively or postoperatively, patients with cardiovascular disease may require large-volume crystalloid replacement. The resultant peripheral edema can be misleading during clinical assessment. The information obtained from invasive monitoring permits evaluation and promotes directed intervention. Prior to insertion of the pulmonary artery catheter, it is important to recognize potential complications and methods to avoid them.

Finally, patients with significant cardiovascular disease might benefit from serial ECGs, because the risk for MI and other cardiovascular problems is greatest during the first 3 postoperative days. During this time, serial ECGs should be obtained in high-risk patients because at least 50% of postoperative infarctions are silent (Charlson et al, 1988). Cardiac enzymes may be necessary. Althougth creatine phosphokinase MB evaluation has been the standard, the newer evaluation of troponin, a cardiac-specific enzyme, may be more appropriate (Barash, 1996) and may allow earlier diagnosis of microinfarction (Etievent et al, 1995). Patients with a previous MI and unstable angina are at risk, but the postoperative cardiac complication rate (in noncardiac surgery) of those with prior revascularization is small. However, the operative mortality (2% to 3%) of bypass surgery and the potential complications of angioplasty should be weighed against decisions to proceed with a surgical procedure.

Although no prospective data exist (Bodenheimer, 1996), patients with New York Heart Association classification III or IV disease may benefit from coronary artery bypass surgery, and patients with significant aortic or mitral valvular heart disease may require valve replacement before abdominal surgery (Fleisher, 1996a). The interval between procedures may be quite short without adversely affecting surgical outcome. However, the risk of surgical mortality of these procedures must be evaluated prior to subjecting patients to additional surgical procedures (Table 43–18).

Hemorrhage

Intraoperative or postoperative hemorrhage is one of the most feared complications of gynecologic procedures. The risk of significant blood loss is obviously increased in procedures requiring extensive surgical dissection (i.e., endometriosis, presacral neurectomy) or after radical procedures involving cancer. However, transfusion may be necessary in as many as 8% of patients undergoing vaginal hysterectomy and 15% of women undergoing abdominal hysterectomy for benign procedures (Table 43–19). Risk reduction involves completing a careful history and examination to determine the presence of a potential bleeding diathesis. Most reports evaluating the necessity of preoperative laboratory findings suggest that careful attention to history and physical findings allows prediction of greater than 99% of inherent or acquired coagulation defects (Johnson et al, 1988; Velanovich, 1991). This information suggests little benefit of obtaining routine bleeding or coagulation studies unless blood loss is expected to be excessive, other risk factors are present (i.e., ongoing chemotherapy, obesity, previous radiation therapy),

Table 43–18. CARDIAC RISK STRATIFICATION FOR NONCARDIAC SURGICAL PROCEDURES*

High Risk (reported cardiac risk often more than 5%)
  Emergent major operations, particularly in the elderly
  Aortic and other major vascular surgery
  Peripheral vascular surgery
  Anticipated prolonged surgical procedures associated with large fluid shifts or blood loss
Intermediate Risk (reported cardiac risk generally less than 5%)
  Carotid endarterectomy
  Head and neck surgery
  Intraperitoneal and intrathoracic surgery
  Orthopedic surgery
  Prostate surgery
Low Risk (reported cardiac risk generally less than 1%)[†]
  Endoscopic procedure
  Superficial procedure
  Cataract removal
  Breast surgery

*Risk = combined incidence of cardiac death and nonfatal myocardial infarction.
†Patients in this group do not generally require further preoperative cardiac testing.
Modified from Fleisher LA, Eagle K: Screening for cardiac disease in patients having noncardiac surgery. Ann Intern Med 1996;124:767, with permission Original from American College of Cardiology/American Heart Association: 1996, with permission.

or a radical procedure is contemplated. In most instances gynecologic patients do not require the expense of a preoperative type and crossmatch because antibody screening allows rapid (<30 minutes) completion of a crossmatch. In emergency situations, type O negative blood can be given with an extremely low risk of reaction. Maximal surgical blood order schedules are available (Table 43–20) as guidelines.

Intraoperative prophylaxis against hemorrhage begins prior to incision by avoiding hypothermia, which can be associated with platelet dysfunction and a coagulopathy (Glass, 1990). Coagulation reactions are temperature dependent, and the activity of thromboxane A (a potent platelet-aggregating substance) is decreased with hypothermia. Attempts to

Table 43–19. COMPLICATION RATES IN HYSTERECTOMY

COMPLICATION	COMPLICATION RATE (%)	
	Vaginal (568)	Abdominal (1283)
Febrile morbidity*	15.3	32.3
Transfusion*	8.3	15.4
Life-threatening event	0	0.4
Rehospitalization	1.8	2.8
Death	0.2	0.1

*$p < .001$.
Modified from Dicker RC, Greenspan JR, Strauss LT, et al: Complications of abdominal and vaginal hysterectomy among women of reproductive age in the United States. Am J Obstet Gynecol 1982; 144:841, with permission.

Table 43–20. SUGGESTED MAXIMAL SURGICAL BLOOD ORDER SCHEDULE FOR ELECTIVE GYNECOLOGIC PROCEDURES

Type and Screen
Simple vaginal or abdominal hysterectomy
Oophorectomy
Ovarian wedge resection
Tuboplasty, tubal ligation
Laparoscopy
Dilatation and curettage
Elective abortion

Type and Cross	No. of Units
Complicated hysterectomy	2
Pelvic mass	2–4
Ovarian cancer	2–4
Myomectomy	2
Radical hysterectomy	4
Pelvic exenteration	6
Radical vulvectomy	2
Type and screen positive for atypical antibodies	2
Coagulopathy or bleeding disorder	2+

Modified from Clarke-Pearson DL, Rodriguez G: Hematologic complications. In Orr JW Jr, Shingleton HM (eds): Complications in Gynecologic Surgery: Prevention, Recognition, and Management. Philadelphia: JB Lippincott Company, 1994:83, with permission.

control heat loss begin with maintenance of ambient room temperature during preoperative preparation. Warming preparation and intravenous fluids should be considered, particularly if a prolonged procedure is anticipated or encountered. Finally, forced warmed air chest drapes and caps (the two major areas of heat loss) should be considered in all patients, particularly those at risk (children and the elderly), and in prolonged procedures (Orr and Shingleton, 1994). Intraoperatively, the surgeon can minimize the risk of hypothermia by avoiding prolonged exteriorization of the intestinal surfaces. All irrigation fluids should be warmed.

The single most important prophylactic method to minimize hemorrhagic risk involves a comprehensive understanding of pelvic anatomy (Kaufman et al, 1990; Fry and Clevenger, 1991) and the use of good surgical technique and adequate exposure. Dissection of safe, avascular paravesical and pararectal spaces exposes the retroperitoneum and the ureter and allows easy identification of the important pelvic vascular supply. Familiarity with this anatomy facilitates restoration of an anatomic dissection (decreasing blood loss) regardless of the intraperitoneal process and assists in exposure of all major pelvic vasculature (hypogastric artery) for ligation if intraoperative hemorrhage ensues. These methods designed to increase intraoperative exposure allow the prudent safe use of hemoclips, atraumatic vascular ligation, or other specific methods (including thumbtacks for sacral bleeding) to control blood loss even in the most difficult situation. Although hemostatic agents and pressure may help to control raw surface bleeding, we discourage their routine use and encourage the use of more direct methods (clip, suture, cautery), if necessary, to control bleeding. Vessel li-

gation, if necessary, need not be performed with permanent suture, because any suture that maintains hemostasis for greater than 96 hours protects against acute or delayed hemorrhage (Hay et al, 1989).

Continuous intraoperative surveillance of blood loss, with recognition given to the inadequacy of measured suction losses, is important. As much as 15% to 42% of intraoperative blood loss is immeasurably lost in gowns and drapes (Orr, 1988). Additionally, 38% of women may enter a radical surgical procedure with significant intravascular volume deficits and are more likely to require intraoperative and postoperative fluid resuscitation. These facts emphasize the necessity of appropriate patient monitoring and surgeon-anesthesiologist communication. A special awareness must be present concerning women with smaller blood volume or those with heart disease, for example, who may not tolerate even "insignificant" losses. Excessive blood loss should not arouse panic but should alert the anesthesiologist to institute replacement while the surgical team progresses through the procedure and attempts to maintain hemostasis. Intraoperative autotransfusion should always be considered in emergent situations (Spence et al, 1993).

In the past, many anesthesiologists in the United States had a transfusion trigger at a hemoglobin level of 9 g/dl before proceeding with elective surgery However, there is little evidence to suggest an increased surgical risk associated with compromised hemoglobin levels alone. More important is the etiology of the anemia, its effect on oxygen-carrying capacity, and coexisting myocardial kinetics. Patients with sickle cell anemia, autoimmune hemolytic anemia, thrombocytopenia, granulocytopenia, and congenital acquired coagulation defects may have specific perioperative risks and often require medical consultation. Chronic blood losses may relate to a coexisting malignancy or even metastatic disease. Importantly adaptation allows those patients with a chronic anemia (i.e., chronic renal disease) to tolerate surgery even in the presence of extremely low hemoglobin levels (unless blood loss is excessive).

Whenever an associated medical illness suggests a need for preoperative transfusion, ideally blood should be administered 24 hours preoperatively. This time span allows volume equilibration, facilitating easier fluid management as well as the improved delivery of oxygen by the repletion of red blood cell 2,3-diphosphoglycerate (DPG) levels. Normal saline is the only solution that is compatible with all blood components. Hypotonic solutions can cause hemolysis, and dextrose may result in red blood cell clumping. Ringer's solution contains calcium, which may exceed the calcium-binding capacity of citrate in the anticoagulated blood and promote clotting. Time permitting, erythropoietin administration might be considered (Spence et al, 1993).

Surveillance and recognition of postoperative bleeding is a postoperative priority. Rapid changes in hematocrit and hemoglobin levels may not occur; however, patients with blood loss usually demonstrate early clinical signs of tachycardia, followed later by hypotension. The clinician must be cognizant of the entire clinical picture because, in specific instances (high-dose β-blockers), this protective mechanism may not occur. Changes in vital signs are related to blood loss, and initial tachycardia may occur with loss of as little as a single unit, depending on the patient's total blood volume and degree of resuscitation. Smaller, thinner patients have smaller blood volumes and are potentially adversely affected by a lesser magnitude of loss. In the presence of significant blood loss, demonstrated by either alterations in vital signs or changes in hematocrit and hemoglobin levels, monitoring of central venous pressure or pulmonary artery pressures should be considered.

The initial approach to bleeding involves maintaining perfusion and oxygenation and normalizing associated coagulation defects. Establishing adequate venous access is a priority (Rudolph and Boyd, 1990). We frequently place a multilumen catheter preoperatively or intraoperatively in patients at risk for intraoperative loss or postoperative instability. Even though these lines allow volume resuscitation, eliminate the need for venipuncture, and allow central venous monitoring, they may pose an increased risk of infection when compared to single-lumen catheters. With multilumen catheters, it is imperative to minimize line interruptions, particularly if parenteral alimentation is instituted. If expectant management with transfusion of red blood cells and normalization of coagulation deficits is insufficient, invasive interventions become necessary to prevent further losses and perfusion problems. The patient who underwent a difficult surgical procedure with intraoperative hemorrhage is at highest risk for postoperative bleeding. Re-operation for hemorrhage is needed in less than 1% of gynecologic procedures and should be considered the treatment of choice with continued hemodynamic instability; however, depending on the situation, we would consider using selective arteriogram with gel foam or steel coil embolization in the management of postoperative bleeding. The interventional radiologist can rapidly identify the specific bleeding vessel and evaluate other potential bleeding sites (O'Hanlan et al, 1989). Although embolic complications can occur, this procedure avoids the risk of a repeat anesthetic and has gained widespread acceptance. It must be emphasized that good surgical judgment is mandatory to determine which patient is best suited for arteriographic embolization versus a repeat laparotomy.

Regardless of the method chosen, monitoring and continued evaluation are mandatory during temporization. In some situations, drastic maneuvers, including using the pneumatic antishock garment (MAST suit), may be necessary. Although this is rare, the surgeon should maintain a level of understanding of literally all support techniques (physical and chemical). If an open operation is necessary, adequate exposure is a prerequisite, and every potential bleeding site must be re-evaluated even if an "obvious" bleeder is recognized early. Additionally, other sites (delayed splenic bleeding following omentectomy) should be evaluated. If no specific site is recognized, we favor hypogastric ligation in the presence of documented pelvic blood loss. Technically, this procedure should be performed only after identification of the ureter and associated venous vasculature. This surgical maneuver significantly alters the vascular pulse pressure, converting the arterial supply to the pelvic viscera to a venous pressure system.

TRANSFUSION SPECIFICS AND COMPLICATIONS

If clinically indicated, component-specific blood products should be administered (Table 43–21) (Waymack, 1990). Although decisions to transfuse must be individualized, patients who are capable of doubling their cardiac output rarely have problems with losses of less than 20% of their total blood volume. Earlier replacement may be required if the preoperative hemoglobin was low or if associated medical disease (usually cardiac or pulmonary) necessitates an increased buffer in the oxygen-carrying capacity. Stored whole blood is rarely used today, and in most situations primary use of high-molecular-weight dextran hetastarch (Hespan) albumin, or other solutions allows preparation of the appropriate matched blood products. Consumptive coagulopathies infrequently occur after a single-volume transfusion because clotting elements are reduced to approximately 75% of normal levels. However, clinical bleeding does occur after a two-volume blood transfusion because clotting elements are reduced to only 10% of prebleeding levels (Orr, 1988). Although any blood product replacement has risks, massive transfusion (defined as a 10-unit transfusion or replacement of one blood volume per 24 hours) carries an even greater risk of complications.

Current blood banking techniques utilize citrate phosphate dextrose (CPD) or add adenine (CPDA-1) to permit storage at less than 6°C (42.8°F) for up to 35 days. Nearly all units are fractionated into specific components. The rapid degradation of platelets, factor V, and factor VIII is eliminated by gentle centrifugation to pack red blood cells. The serum (with 70% of platelets) is spun and separated into plasma and platelet concentrate. The plasma is rapidly frozen (−30°C [−22°F]), thawed (4°C, [39.2°F]), and centrifuged into fresh frozen plasma (FFP) and cryoprecipitate. In the absence of any serologic obstacles, ABO and Rh type testing, antibody screening, and crossmatching can be completed in less than 1 hour. Simple determination of ABO and Rh typing can be completed in less than 10 minutes. If necessary, O-negative blood can be administered with little risk of transfusion reaction or future problems with

Table 43-21. COMPONENT-SPECIFIC BLOOD PRODUCTS

RED BLOOD CELL PRODUCTS

Components	Volume	Red Cell Content	Plasma Content	Hematocrit
Whole blood	450 ml blood + 63 ml CPDA-1	200 ml	250 ml	0.40
Red blood cells	>200 ml	200 ml	60–90 ml	0.70–0.80
Leukocyte-poor red cells	Approx. 200 ml	>160 ml	40–60 ml	0.70–0.80
Washed red cells	Approx. 200 ml	180 ml	—	As desired
Frozen and deglycerolized red cells	Approx. 200 ml	180 ml	—	As desired

PLASMA AND DERIVATIVES

Components	Usual Volume	Contents
Fresh frozen plasma	>200 ml	All factors
Single-donor (stored) plasma	>200 ml	Factor VIII deficient; factor V decreased
Cryoprecipitate	10–15 ml	Factor VIII (>80 units), fibrinogen (100–350 mg)
Albumin	Varies	5% and 25%
Immunoglobulin	Varies	Varies
Coagulation factor concentrates	Lyophilized	Varies

From Clarke-Pearson DL, Rodriguez G: Hematologic complications. In Orr JW Jr, Shingleton HM (eds): Complications in Gynecologic Surgery; Prevention, Recognition, and Management. Philadelphia: JB Lippincott Company, 1994:83, with permission.

crossmatching. We prefer to minimize blood banking cost by performing a type and antibody screen without crossmatch unless more than 1000 ml of blood loss is expected.

Specific storage-related complications are related to hypothermia and biochemical changes (Rudolph and Boyd, 1990; Rutherford, 1990; Waymack, 1990). Red blood cell storage at 4°C (39.2°F) is intended to decrease cellular metabolism, maintain cellular integrity, and inhibit bacterial growth. Raising the temperature of one blood volume (10 units) to 37°C (98.6°F) requires 150 kcal and consumes 30 liters of oxygen and fuel substrate. In addition to the previously mentioned coagulopathy, hypothermia induces cardiac dysrhythmias, impairs metabolism (citrate and lactate), shifts the oxygen-hemoglobin dissociation curve to the left, increases intracellular potassium release, delays drug metabolism, increases blood viscosity, and impairs red blood cell deformability.

Other storage losses include a decrease in 2,3-DPG (85% remaining after 2 weeks, 40% after 3 weeks), hyperkalemia, decreased levels of factors V and VIII, denaturation of proteins, and red blood cell hemolysis. Although previous reports suggest the need for prophylactic calcium supplementation during massive transfusion, its use is not necessary (unless infusion rates exceed 10 ml/minute) and may be associated with ventricular dysrhythmias. Furthermore, patients with normal renal function generally do not manifest hyperkalemia, even with massive transfusions.

A newly recognized potential transfusion-related side effect is immunosuppression, which may have significant relevance in women with gynecologic cancer. A significant volume of literature is accumulating to report the adverse effects of transfusion on acute (infectious) (Wobbes et al, 1990) and long-term (failed treatment for malignancy) (Eisenkop et al, 1990) complications. In experimental models, transfusions alter the macrophage metabolism of arachidonic acid and are associated with a 150% increase in the rate of synthesis of prostaglandin E, which suppresses neutrophil and macrophage function, impairs B- and T-cell activity, and stimulates suppressor T-cell function. Additionally, levels of fibronectin (an important opsonic glycoprotein) are decreased following transfusion.

One report suggests that red blood cell transfusion adversely affects survival in patients undergoing radical hysterectomy for treatment of early-stage cervical cancer (Eisenkop et al, 1990). Others refute this finding (Soper, 1991). Methods to potentially decrease these immunosuppressive effects include the use of autologous donor blood and the use of autotransfusions in patients with nonmalignant disease. For those with malignancy, the risk of tumor cell transmission may be prohibitive; however, washed red blood cells may be used because it appears that the immunosuppression is probably related to exposure to white blood cell antigens. The use of recombinant erythropoietin, allowing preoperative donation, is an accepted methodology. Autotransfusion is contraindicated when infection is present.

The coagulopathy associated with large-volume transfusion is more severe in patients with prolonged (>1 hour) hypotension and may be in part related to the systemic effects of hypoperfusion. In the past, routine incremental prophylactic administration of FFP and platelets has been common. Today, FFP and/or platelets should be administered only if abnormal coagulation studies or clinical "oozing" is present. In the absence of severe liver disease, "clinical" component replacement for bleeding should initially incorporate platelets. Under these guidelines, it is estimated that 90% of prophylactic administration of coagulation products can be eliminated (Gravlee, 1990).

Complications that are not volume related include transfusion reaction and infection. Reactions may be hemolytic (10%), febrile (44%), or allergic (45%) (Rudolph and Boyd, 1990; Rutherford, 1990; Waymack, 1990; Spence et al, 1993). Hemolytic reactions occur in 1 of 6000 units transfused and are due to ABO incompatibility and clerical errors (which occur in 80% of reactions). A nonspecific febrile reaction can be associated with a minor determinant mismatch or with white blood cell antibodies. Leukocyte removal filters decrease this risk. Allergic reactions occur in 1% of blood transfusions. Although reactions are usually mild, anaphylaxis can occur. Recognition of any reaction should prompt immediate termination of transfusion. An often-mentioned sign of a hemolytic reaction during anesthesia is an increase in clinical "oozing." In the presence of a recognized hemolytic reaction, the focus of therapy is to preserve renal function. Therapy consists of adequate hydration and diuresis (osmotic or other) to maintain urine outputs of 1.5 ml/kg/hour. Urine alkalinization may prevent pigment sedimentation in the renal tubules.

The risk of transmission of human immunodeficiency virus is estimated to be 1 in 250,000 or 1 in 28,000 units, for the average transfusion recipient. Other important viral infections transmitted include hepatitis (3% to 5% per transfusion episode), cytomegalovirus (CMV), and Epstein-Barr virus. Approximately 80% of hepatitis infections are hepatitis C. CMV infections are transmitted via white blood cells and usually occur in immunocompromised individuals.

The overall death rate related to transfusion is approximately 0.00031% (3 per 100,000), often related to complications associated with hepatitis. Many of these deaths (>50%) can be attributed to clerical or laboratory errors.

Gastrointestinal Problems

Preoperative evaluation of coexisting gastrointestinal disease (inflammatory bowel disease, pancreatitis, liver disease) may be necessary to evaluate the risk in the proposed gynecologic procedure. For instance, women with "benign" liver disease who have significant abnormalities of serum liver function studies, abnormal coagulation studies, and ascites have an extremely high mortality rate. It behooves the physician to determine the presence of coexisting disease to optimize the medical condition and to modify the procedure and technique accordingly.

Intraoperative injury to the intestinal tract occurs in 0.2% to 0.4% of gynecologic procedures performed for benign indications, but may be increased by more than 100-fold in patients undergoing procedures for gynecologic malignancy (Alvarez, 1988). Endometriosis and pelvic inflammatory disease increase the risk of intestinal injury by as much as ninefold. The highest incidence of injury occurs during peritoneal entry and during adhesiolysis. Injury is particularly increased in the obese (2.5-fold) when properitoneal fat obscures the normal anatomy (Alvarez, 1988; Flint, 1988; Holder, 1988: Fry and Osler, 1991). Careful entry into the peritoneal cavity, adequate intraoperative exposure, and sharp dissection of intra-abdominal adhesions are important methods to minimize intestinal injury. Lacerations of the small intestine, which can occur after abdominal, vaginal, or laparoscopic surgery, are associated with low levels of bacterial contamination (Table 43–22). Regardless, appropriate parenteral antibiotics should be administered to decrease infectious risks, and copious intra-abdominal irrigation may further decrease bacterial levels. In most instances, serosal injuries can be observed; however, muscularis and mucosal injuries require layered closure. Sutures placed on an axis perpendicular to the long axis of the bowel decrease the risk of later luminal stenosis. If an enterotomy occurs, it is generally prudent to visually inspect the entire bowel surface to exclude the presence of other areas of unrecognized injury. Injury to irradiated small bowel (particularly in the terminal ileum) may require a more extensive procedure for repair, because altered blood supply and poor healing in the heavily irradiated ileum increases the risk of fistulization. In those instances, resection of the injured bowel with an ascending ileocolostomy may supplement local anastomotic blood supply and may improve the chance of primary healing.

In contrast, colonic injury, especially to the descending colon and rectosigmoid, results in significant bacterial contamination, which adversely affects healing. Simple lacerations may be repaired in a layered technique; however, as with small-intestine injury, good surgical judgment often indicates that resection and reanastamosis may be required. Intestinal stapling devices shorten the operative procedure, increase anastomotic blood supply, and result in a more consistent or reproducible repair (Orr et al, 1983a). In the absence of preoperative mechanical bowel preparation, temporary diversion of the fecal stream proximal to the repair may be required even if a primary repair is contemplated. It is our opinion that, in the absence of significant postresidency training, the gynecologist should seek additional surgical advice and assistance when faced with these clinical situations. Antibiotic irrigation of the abdominal wound should be considered, because it may decrease infectious risks in those women with intestinal intraperitoneal contamination. Endarteritis from previous radiation therapy inhibits normal intestinal healing following primary repair, and an anastomosis in heavily irradiated bowel is associated with an increased risk of stenosis, breakdown, fistula for-

Table 43-22. POTENTIAL BACTERIAL CONTAMINATION

SITE	QUANTITY	COMMENT
Vagina	10^9	90% anaerobes; 10% aerobes and facultative bacteria
Stomach	$\leq 10^4$	Gram-positive cocci and *Lactobacillus* (anaerobes rare)
Duodenum	$\leq 10^4$	Gram-positive cocci and *Enterococcus* (anaerobes rare)
Jejunum	$\leq 10^4$	Gram-positive cocci (anaerobes rare)
Ileum	$>10^4$–10^5	Aerobes plus anaerobic coliforms, *Bacteroides*, *Clostridium* (aerobic cocci rare)
Colon	10^{10}–10^{11}	90% anaerobes; 10% aerobes and facultative bacteria

Modified from Orr JW Jr: Introduction to pelvic surgery: pre- and postoperative care. In: Gusberg SB, Shingleton HM, Deppe G (eds): Female Genital Cancer. New York, Churchill Livingstone, 1988:497, with permission.

mation, and subsequent abscess formation. In these situations, anastomotic blood supply may be improved by incorporating nonirradiated bowel into the anastomosis or transposing an additional source of blood supply, such as an omental J flap. A protecting, diverting colostomy should be considered. If postoperative radiotherapy is anticipated, the potential benefit of altering the anatomy of the existing intestinal tract may be desirous. We do not recommend the routine use of synthetic mesh because it has been associated with significant complications (Patsner et al, 1990); rather, we prefer the construction of an omental J flap in the pelvis.

The prophylactic use of postoperative nasal intubation of the gastrointestinal tract after a routine gynecologic or intestinal procedure is not necessary, because fewer than 10% of patients derive any benefit from intestinal suction, whereas the remainder are subjected to the discomfort and possible electrolyte abnormalities with no favorable effects on return of bowel function (Orr, 1988). However, patients undergoing a total omentectomy may benefit from intubation during the period of gastric atony. An inflated stomach may jeopardize the integrity of vascular pedicles. Additionally, patients with preoperative ileus secondary to carcinomatosis and patients with irradiated small bowel anastomoses may benefit from nasogastric suction or intraoperative gastrostomy.

Fortunately, postoperative intestinal complications occur rarely after nonradical gynecologic surgery. However, risks increase to 8% to 10% of patients undergoing radical surgical procedures. The degree and duration of postoperative ileus are related to retroperitoneal dissection, development of retroperitoneal hematoma, or electrolyte abnormalities, and acute changes may be difficult to diagnose postoperatively. (Surgical fatigue and disbelief on the part of the physician are the biggest enemies of the judgment process.) Postoperative epidural analgesia with local anesthetics has been associated with earlier passage of flatus or bowel movements than observed with systemic patient-controlled analgesia or with epidural morphine (Carpenter, 1996).

In general, normal postoperative gastric dysfunction persists for 24 to 48 hours; however, colonic dysfunction persists for 72 to 96 hours (Orr and Shin-

gleton, 1984). Occasionally, persistent ileus becomes a significant clinical problem, creating the inability to establish the presence of intestinal obstruction. The incidence of intestinal ileus is much greater in patients with malignant disease (3% to 30%) than in those with benign disease (0.2%). Clinical small-bowel obstruction is rarely evident prior to the seventh postoperative day because the density of adhesions increases dramatically at this time. In the patient with persistent ileus, the diagnosis can usually be established by an upper gastrointestinal tract series. Ingested barium should traverse the ileocecal valve within 2 hours. Although slow transit may be associated with ileus, long delays accompanied by small bowel dilatation are usually associated with obstruction. Although some disagree, we prefer to utilize barium in these studies to improve radiologic imaging. Water-soluble contract often rapidly negotiates tight partial obstructions, making the diagnosis of small-bowel obstruction difficult to establish. In the absence of previous radiation, postoperative small-bowel obstruction can be managed successfully by intestinal suction, volume resuscitation, and nutritional support in as many as 80% of patients. Conservative or initial nonoperative therapy is less likely to be successful in the presence of previous radiation therapy or in patients with disseminated intraperitoneal disease (Alvarez, 1988; Flint, 1988; Holder, 1988).

Conservative management is not intended to promote procrastination, and must include close monitoring for associated complications (strangulation, complete obstruction). If clinical improvement occurs within 24 hours, 75% of patients progress to spontaneous resolution. If no improvement is apparent within 48 hours, only 5% will be successfully managed with nonoperative intervention (Fabri and Rosemurgi, 1991). If increasing abdominal tenderness or other symptoms suggesting peritonitis (fever, tachycardia, elevated white blood cells with left shift) develop, an immediate operation may be indicated. Mortality rates in the absence of strangulation (<1%) are dramatically increased when vascular compromise intervenes. Potential stomal sites should be determined and marked preoperatively. In the presence of previous radiation therapy, early exploratory laparotomy with lysis of adhesions and perhaps intestinal resection, reanastomosis, or intestinal bypass is advised. Although opinions differ, we prefer a bypass procedure in these situations unless clinical or intraoperative findings suggest bowel necrosis. In the latter situation, the affected bowel must be resected. If a bypass procedure is selected, the surgeon must mobilize as large a segment of proximal small intestine as possible because secondary or subsequent operative procedures are more likely to be necessary in this subgroup of patients. There is little evidence to support the routine use of long tube "stenting"; however, stents may be considered for women with irradiated bowel, extensive denuded pelvic surfaces, and especially recurrent obstructions. Fortunately, large-bowel obstruction is exceedingly rare, especially when preoperative colon function was normal.

Although routine prophylaxis for stress-related mucosal damage (SRMD) is unnecessary, it must be considered in patients at risk, those undergoing radical procedures, or those requiring intensive care. In these latter situations, SRMD can be documented in 70% to 100% of patients. Only 10% to 20% can be expected to bleed; however, SRMD becomes massive in 2% to 5% of patients and is associated with a mortality rate of 80% with or without therapy. It has become clear that prophylaxis must be directed toward the potential imbalance of aggressive gastric (bile acids, gastric acid), defensive gastric (mucosal blood flow, mucous layer prostaglandins), and mucosal factors. The primary goal of SRMD prevention or treatment relates to reversal of the underlying disease process, be it required ventilation or radical surgery. Secondary methods involve maintaining a gastric pH of 3.5 to 5.0, because pepsin is inactivated at 4.5 and gastric acid is almost completely normalized at 5.0.

Antacids, histamine$_2$, receptor antagonists, sucralfate (Carafate), and prostaglandins may all have a therapeutic role. Unfortunately, to maintain an acceptable gastric pH, antacids must be given frequently, and this subjects the patient to potential troublesome metabolic side effects. The histamine$_2$ receptor antagonists are most effectively delivered by continuous infusion; we prefer to add these to existing parenteral nutrition solutions. Sucralfate binds exposed proteins in denuded areas of the in-

testinal tract and acts as a physical barrier. It also stimulates prostaglandin E$_2$ synthesis.

Specific attention must be paid to residual drug effect (specifically sedatives and analgesics) in women with significant liver disease (Coursin, 1996). While the modified Child's classification (Table 43–23) may predict perioperative risks, the physician must be cognizant of potential drug effects or bleeding disorders associated with chronic liver disease regardless of the etiology.

The most feared postoperative intestinal complication is the development of an enterocutaneous fistula (Alvarez, 1988; Rubelowsky and Machiedo, 1991). Although more commonly associated with intra-abdominal malignancy or previous radiation therapy, the general gynecologist increases this risk with an enterostomy (either unrecognized or repaired) or devascularization of the intestinal wall during a subsequent surgical procedure. Prevention begins with careful entry into the abdominal cavity and continues with minimized bowel trauma (sharp dissection), decreasing the tension placed on intestinal segments (adhesiolysis or packing), and careful placement of abdominal wall closure sutures.

Once present, enterocutaneous fistulas present a difficult clinical situation. Management includes attempts to protect the skin, institution of total parenteral nutrition, nasogastric suction, radiographic assessment of the fistula, and development of a treatment plan. Because almost half of all enterocutaneous fistulas are associated with an intra-abdominal abscess, appropriate antibiotic coverage is indicated. In general, low-output fistulas are more likely to resolve nonoperatively than high-output ones (>500 ml/day). Fistulas in previously irradiated patients and in those with intra-abdominal carcinomatosis are unlikely to heal spontaneously. Conservative therapy using Somatostatin can be justified for at least 3 weeks; however, if healing is not apparent by 6 to 8 weeks, operative intervention will likely be necessary. Enterovaginal fistulas create a difficult problem of intestinal secretion management and often require earlier surgical intervention. Regardless, a thorough radiologic intestinal evaluation is mandatory to determine fistula complexity; that is, an apparent rectovaginal fistula may also have a small-intestine component (particularly in the pres-

Table 43–23. CHILD-PUGH CLASSIFICATION OF PREOPERATIVE RISK IN LIVER DISEASE

PARAMETER	A (Minimal risk)	B (Moderate risk)	C (Severe risk)
Serum bilirubin (mg/dL)	<2	2–3	>3
Serum albumin (g/dL)	>3.5	3–3.5	<3
PT (sec > control)	1–4	4–6	>6
CNS (coma grade)	Normal	Confused (1–2)	Coma (3–4)
Ascites	None	Easily controlled	Not easily controlled
Nutrition	Excellent	Good	Poor

From Sladen RN: Anesthetic concerns for the patient with renal or hepatic disease. ASA Annual Refresher Course Lectures 1997;271:1–7, with permission.

ence of previous radiation). In this situation, a diverting colostomy will be of little benefit. Surgical repair necessitates intestinal resection because simple isolation or oversewing the fistula site is doomed to failure.

Finally, there is little rationale supporting a routine postoperative dietary progression schedule. Patients with lesser or vaginal procedures often tolerate a regular diet during the first postoperative day, but this is usually not the case for patients undergoing radical surgery. Clinical judgment with attention to physical findings on examination during daily rounds is necessary during the reinstitution of oral feedings.

Urinary Tract Problems

The anatomic proximity of the urinary tract to the genital tract, combined with the need for intraoperative urologic evaluation, places the patient at risk for urinary postoperative complications during gynecologic procedures (Orr, 1988; Holley and Kilgore, 1994). The true incidence of urinary injury remains unknown, because many injuries are probably unrecognized and heal spontaneously. Injury to the urinary tract occurs in as many as 1.4% of patients undergoing vaginal or abdominal hysterectomy. Bladder injury is most common; however, ureteral injury is reported to occur in 0.2% of women during procedures for benign conditions. As expected, this figure is dramatically increased during surgery for gynecologic malignancy. Ureteral injury occurs in 1.7% of patients undergoing radical hysterectomy, and at least 2% of patients undergoing ovarian debulking require resection or repair of the urinary tract. Adequate exposure and sharp dissection reduce the risk of bladder injury. The risk of ureteral injury can be minimized by dissecting the retroperitoneal spaces, allowing visualization of the entire pelvic ureter as it crosses over the common iliac artery to the vaginal angle.

Following completion of the gynecologic procedure, the ureters and bladder should be routinely inspected. Recognition of urinary tract injury is extremely important because immediate repair is associated with excellent results. The bladder is a remarkable organ. In the absence of radiation, the majority of the bladder can be resected (80%) and repaired, still maintaining normal function. If bladder injury is suspected, the intravesical instillation of sterile milk assists in distinguishing the site of injury without staining the surrounding tissue. The absence of local tissue staining allows retesting after cystotomy repair. Avoiding placement of intravesical (particularly permanent or long-term absorbable) sutures during a watertight repair and institution of adequate bladder drainage (3 to 7 days) are the cornerstones of success. Care during vaginal cuff closure minimizes the risk of inadvertent injury to the bladder base. Urinary injury and a coexistent urinary tract infection mandate the use of appropriate antibiotics. Healing may be adversely affected after tolerance doses of radiation therapy that alter bladder blood supply and pliability. Cystotomy repair in this circumstance might be aided by augmentation of blood supply with an omental J-flap. Long-term (2 to 4 weeks) bladder drainage seems prudent. Management of vesicovaginal fistulas depends largely upon the extent of injury. Under no circumstance should a urinary leak be presumed to be of bladder origin; ureteral integrity must be substantiated by IVP. We favor a transvaginal repair and recommend myocutaneous pedicle grafts (bulbocavernosus flaps) in irradiated fields.

Ureteral injuries can result from devascularization, ligation, crushing, or incision (Holley and Kilgore, 1994). Devascularization injuries are rare in the absence of ureteral dissection and may not become clinically evident until the second postoperative week. If ureteral dissection is necessary, the surgeon should strive to minimize disruption of the longitudinal ureteral vascular blood supply. Ligation or crush injuries require recognition and immediate attention. Deligation or unclamping avoids unnecessary resection in 66% of patients (Orr, 1988). Where persistent ureteral blanching occurs or ureteral peristalsis does not cross the injured segment, resection (and anastomosis) or reimplantation is necessary. In general, ureteral injury in the distal one third is treated with reimplantation with bladder mobilization via a psoas hitch or Boari flap. Transureteroureterostomy may be the procedure of choice when the injury occurs proximal to the pelvic brim.

If urinary injury is unrecognized or discovered during the postoperative interval, the pelvic surgeon is faced with numerous decisions regarding the definition of the abnormality as well as management. Following diagnostic studies for localization of the ureteral leak or obstruction, placement of percutaneous nephrostomy drainage or transvesical ureteral stenting permits nonoperative diversion and salvage of the remaining renal function (Mann et al, 1983). Internalization of percutaneously placed stents can often be accomplished. In many instances, conservative management avoids the need for an open surgical procedure.

Unfortunately, information obtained from preoperative IVP has not been demonstrated to decrease the risk of ureteral injury (Piscitelli et al, 1987; Simel et al, 1988; Mushlin and Thornbury, 1989). Although unexpected findings, including upper tract abnormalities (18.3%) and congenital abnormalities (14%), are common, information obtained concerning ureteral deviation or placement cannot be translated into a lessened risk of trauma. Coexisting renal tumors are extremely rare (0.06%). Additionally, the urologic study is not without risks. At least 3% of IVPs are associated with significant adverse effects. Cost-effectiveness ratio studies indicate the need for 833 IVPs to potentially prevent a single ureteral injury. More than $3 million would have to be expended to prevent a single death. Whereas information obtained may be helpful in individual situations, contrast studies cannot be considered a substitute for good surgical technique because unusual abnormalities such as crossed ectopia may occur (Patsner and Orr, 1990).

Postoperatively the kidneys perform a vital role in maintaining body water, regulating electrolytes, maintaining acid-base balance, controlling pressure, and excreting metabolic waste and drugs. These functions are important for all patients but are especially critical for patients with pre-existing renal insufficiency. Maintenance of normal postoperative renal function becomes crucial for women who require additional therapy with potentially nephrotoxic agents (antibiotics, antifungals, chemotherapy).

In general, the degree of reduction of GFR rather than the type of renal disease is the most important factor in estimating surgical risk (Goldstein, 1983; Orr, 1988). Patients with mild (GFR >50 ml/minute) or moderate (GFR between 25 and 50 ml/minute) renal dysfunction require particular attention to electrolyte, drug, or fluid therapy. Those with severe dysfunction (GFR <10 ml/minute) often exhibit extrarenal manifestations, including anemia, hypertension, and coagulation defects. These women are at significant risk for poor wound healing and postoperative infections. In the extreme, patients on dialysis may have a surgical mortality rate approaching 4%.

Preoperative or postoperative evaluation of blood urea nitrogen level is not the most accurate index of renal function because this parameter is heavily dependent on other factors, such as protein hypercatabolism, intestinal bleeding, and urinary flow rate. The blood creatinine level, a product of creatinine phosphate metabolism, is a superior index but is closely related to body muscle mass. Complete cessation of renal function leads to daily increases in measured serum creatinine of 1 to 2 mg/dl. Lesser daily increases suggest the presence of remaining function, whereas greater rises suggest the presence of increased catabolism.

Patients requiring dialysis should undergo hemodialysis within the 24 hours preceding surgery. Dialysis may be required immediately after surgery, because these patients have an impaired ability to respond to sodium, water loads, or fluid shifts. In addition, potassium balance may be disturbed. The associated metabolic acidosis should be measured and corrected preoperatively.

Oliguria frequently occurs during the immediate postoperative period. Adequate renal function necessitates the production of at least 400 ml (17 ml/hour) of urine per day. This obligatory volume is required to excrete the daily metabolic osmotic load of 500 mOsm. Urine output is not a good index of renal function; however, if metabolic products are in constant production, a doubling of blood creatinine levels represents a 50% reduction in GFR.

Postoperative oliguria can be therapeutically and diagnostically separated into renal, prerenal, and postrenal causes (Chazan and Tilney, 1983). Prerenal failure is most common and results from inadequate renal perfusion secondary to decreased intravascular volume, decreased cardiac output, or both. Renal etiologies include secondary or primary glomerular diseases and tubulointerstitial diseases, such as acute tubular necrosis (ATN). Predisposing factors for ATN include advancing age, volume concentration, and recent MI. Drug-induced interstitial nephritis is becoming a more common cause for renal dysfunction. Postrenal etiologies include bladder outlet (catheter) obstruction and complete ureteral occlusion (unilateral or bilateral). Although postrenal etiology is unusual, the presence of anuria should arouse suspicion. In these situations, renal ultrasound can quickly determine the presence of hydronephrosis and guide the placement of percutaneous nephrostomies.

Postoperative evaluation and early recognition and treatment of oliguria is important because the development of renal failure, depending on the clinical setting, is associated with mortality rates as high as 80% (Chazan and Tilney, 1983; Goldstein, 1983). Initial physical examination may detect evidence of prerenal causes, such as cardiac dysfunction or vascular volume contraction. Urinalysis with a specific gravity greater than 1.010 suggests a prerenal etiology. Additional diagnostic studies may be necessary, and the fractional excretion of sodium is relatively specific. Importantly, these diagnostic indices are of little value if obtained during the first 24 hours following diuretic administration. The correction of postoperative prerenal volume deficits requires immediate, rapid infusion of blood or crystalloid. In specific instances (ascites, extensive dissection) third-space losses may require exceptionally large-volume replacement. In the absence of left ventricular failure, fluid challenge—not diuresis—should be the primary therapy. Prognosis of oliguria and renal insufficiency and efforts to rehydrate may be guided by monitoring vital signs or may require more invasive techniques (central venous pressure, pulmonary artery pressure). Once adequate hydration is accomplished, urinary output may be increased with furosemide, mannitol, or other diuretics.

Acute renal insufficiency requires early consultation; attention to electrolyte and acid-base balance, early dialysis (minimizing catabolic needs), and instituting adequate caloric intake become important therapeutic goals. All drugs administered should be reviewed for dosage reduction or discontinuation in an effort to minimize additional nephrotoxic effects.

Neurologic Problems

Nearly all agents used for premedication, induction, and anesthesia maintenance have subtle but lingering central nervous system effects. Short (3.5-minute) halothane anesthesia impairs psychomotor performance for 5 hours (Crosby, 1996) and natural rapid eye movement and slow wave sleep patterns are disrupted for 24 hours and may remain abnormal for days. Patients with cerebrovascular disease and transient ischemic attacks (TIAs) may require preoperative treatment that could include extracranial carotid endarterectomy, systemic anticoagulation, or medical platelet inhibition. Although no prospective studies have compared these treatment regimens, the risk of postoperative stroke after simultaneous carotid and noncarotid surgery may be as low as 2.4%, however, the risk of other thrombotic events remains high (15%). Cerebrovascular (CVA) may be increased if perioperative hypotension occurs.

Following a completed stroke, cerebral blood flow is unstable and brain metabolism is depressed. Large cerebral infarcts may take 6 to 8 weeks to resolve, and elective operations should not be undertaken during this critical recovery phase because these patients may have a 20% risk of a second CVA. An emergency procedure requires careful maintenance of adequate intravascular volume and normal or elevated blood pressure. Following a stroke, sequential cerebral computerized tomography may assist in determining the time of complete resolution of the cerebral clot and may permit optimal timing for the surgical procedure.

Patients with vertebral basilar ischemic episodes appear to have a lower stroke risk than patients who demonstrate carotid ischemia. Primary therapy for these patients includes the administration of antiplatelet drugs. The value of surgical repair of the vertebral arteries has not been tested in a controlled study.

The presence of an asymptomatic cervical bruit serves as a general index of the presence of atherosclerotic disease; however, there is no good correlation between the location or presence of an asymptomatic bruit and the risk or site of eventual brain infarction. In fact, cervical bruits have little influence on neurologic morbidity following abdominal surgical procedures. Investigation and surgical treatment of patients with an asymptomatic cervical bruit does not alter central nervous system morbidity after systemic surgery.

Peripheral neuropathies may be related to cytotoxic therapy, particularly after or during treatment with the vinca alkaloids or cisplatin. The former is more common in the elderly, and the latter is more common in the presence of hypomagnesemia. Femoral neuropathy is a clinical diagnosis of pain, initiating in the groin and radiating to the inner thigh and medial portion of the leg. This leads to secondary degrees of flexion of the hip and knee. Knee jerks are absent. Pain is increased with extension, and rotational movements of the hip are normal. Retractor injury can occur when the femoral nerve (from L-2 through L-4) is compressed between the psoas or iliacus muscle. The genital femoral nerve can be injured in a transverse incision, resulting in paresthesias over the lateral vulva and inner thigh.

Elderly patients are at particular risk for postoperative delirium. The acute mental clouding associated with delirium should not be confused with the more chronic problem of dementia (Cutler and Fink, 1990). If delirium is present, a search for organic causes (fever, sepsis, hypoxemia, hepatic insufficiency, renal failure, or MI) should be undertaken immediately. All potential drug-related etiologies should be investigated and discontinued if possible. Alcohol withdrawal may occur with a ''lower'' regular intake than expected because elderly women have less lean body mass, although an unexplained anemia, thrombocytopenia, or elevated liver function studies may suggest the diagnosis. It is important to carefully question friends or relatives. Idiopathic delirium is usually self-limiting (2 to 3 days) and is associated with sensory deprivation (Bonnet's syndrome) or sleep deprivation. It is imperative that the physician accept an idiopathic etiology as a diagnosis of exclusion. Attempts should be made by the family or health care team to continually orient the affected woman. If the postoperative patient becomes a threat to herself or others, low-dose (0.5 mg twice daily) or higher dose (1 mg every 6 to 8 hours) haloperidol may be used with special care to avoid extrapyramidal effects or hypotension.

The risk of a new focal neurologic deficit is rare (≤0.04%) and unpredictable following non-neurologic, noncardiac surgery. An asymptomatic carotid bruit is likely not a significant risk factor; however, if a documented high-grade stenosis is present, preoperative carotid endarterectomy might be considered (Crosby, 1996). Those patients with TIAs may be considered for preoperative endarterectomy prior to elective surgery. Although the perioperative period may be the time for greatest risk for reinfarction, there is little information that risks decrease with time. It would appear that perioperative hypotension is not a common cause for stroke and that most strokes are embolic or thrombotic in nature. A patent foramen ovale increases this risk.

REFERENCES

Abbott J, Abbott P: Psychological and cardiovascular predictors of anaesthesia induction, operative and post-operative complications in minor gynaecological surgery. Br J Clin Psychol 1995; 34:613.
Agarwal N, Shibutani K, Sanfilippo JA, Del Guercio LR: Hemodynamic and respiratory changes in surgery of the morbidly obese. Surgery 1982;92:226.
Alpert JS, Cheitlin MD: Update in cardiology. Ann Intern Med 1996;125:40.
Alvarez RD: Gastrointestinal complications in gynecologic surgery: a review for the general gynecologist. Obstet Gynecol 1988;72:533.
Ayus JC, Arieff AI: Symptomatic hyponatremia: correcting sodium deficits safely. J Crit Illness 1990;5:905.
Babu SC, Sharma PV, Raciti A, et al: Monitor-guided responses. Arch Surg 1980;115:1384.
Barash PG: Monitoring myocardial ischemia: a sequential clinical approach. American Society of Anesthesiologists (ASA) Refresher Course Lectures, No. 222, New Orleans, 1996.
Bates DW, Spell N, Cullen DJ, et al: The costs of adverse drug events in hospitalized patients. JAMA 1997;277:307.
Bedford RF: Central venous cannulation. Surg Rounds 1991;13:228.
Beller GA: Pharmacologic stress imaging. JAMA 1991;265:633.

Bishop MJ: Bronchospasm: successful management. America Society of Anesthesiologists (ASA) Refresher Course Lectures, No. 123. New Orleans, 1996.

Blanchard CG, Ruckdeschel JC, Fletcher VA, Blanchard EB: The impact of oncologists' behaviors on patient satisfaction with morning rounds. Cancer 1986;58:387.

Bodenheimer MM: Noncardiac surgery in the cardiac patient: what is the question? Ann Intern Med 1996;124:763.

Bone RC: Managing sepsis: what treatments can we use today? J Crit Illness 1997;12:15.

Brooks-Brunn JA: Postoperative atelectasis and pneumonia. Heart Lung 1995;24:94.Carpenter RL: Does outcome change with pain management? American Society of Anesthesiologists (ASA) Refresher Course Lectures, No. 166, New Orleans, 1996.

Celoria G, Steingrub JS, Vickers-Lahti M, et al: Clinical assessment of hemodynamic values in two surgical intensive care units. Arch Surg 1990;125:1036.

Charlson ME, MacKenzie CR, Ales K, et al: Surveillance for postoperative myocardial infarction after noncardiac operations. Surg Gynecol Obstet 1988;167:407.

Charlson ME, MacKenzie CT, Gold JP, et al: Intraoperative blood pressure: what patterns identify patients at risk for postoperative complications? Ann Surg 1990;212:567.

Charlson ME, MacKenzie CR, Gold JP, et al: Risk for postoperative congestive heart failure. Surg Gynecol Obstet 1991;172:95.

Chazan JA, Tilney NL: Oliguria in the postoperative patient. Infect Surg 1983;2:909.

Clarke-Pearson DL, DeLong E, Synan IS, et al: A controlled trial of two low-dose heparin regimens for the prevention of postoperative deep vein thrombosis. Obstet Gynecol 1990;75:864.

Clarke-Pearson DL, Rodriguez G: Hematologic complications. In Orr JW Jr, Shingleton HM (eds): Complications of Gynecologic Surgery: Prevention, Recognition and Management. Philadelphia: JB Lippincott Company, 1994:83.

Classen DC, Pestotnik SL, Evans RS, et al: Adverse drug events in hospitalized patients. Excess length of stay, extra costs and attributable mortality. JAMA 1997;277:301.

Coursin DB: Anesthetic concerns for the patient with liver disease. American Society of Anesthesiologists (ASA) Refresher Course Lectures, No. 251, New Orleans, 1996.

Crapo RO, Kelly TM, Elliott CG, Jones SB: Spirometry as a preoperative screening test in morbidly obese patients. Surgery 1986;99:763.

Crosby G: Perioperative CNS dysfunction—diagnosis and management. American Society of Anesthesiologists (ASA) Refresher Course Lectures, No. 262, New Orleans, 1996.

Cruickshank MK, Levin MN, Hirsh J, et al: A standard heparin nomogram for the management of heparin therapy. Arch Intern Med 1991;151:333.

Cutler BS, Fink MP: Postoperative complications in patients with disabling psychiatric illnesses or intellectual handicaps. Arch Surg 1990;125:1436.

Dajani AS, Bisno AL, Chung KF, et al: Prevention of bacterial endocarditis. JAMA 1990;264:2919.

Dauzat M, Laroche JP, Deklunder G, et al: Diagnosis of acute lower limb deep venous thrombosis with ultrasound: trends and controversies. J Clin Ultrasound 1997;25:343.

Del Guercio LR, Cohn JD: Monitoring operative risk in the elderly. JAMA 1980;243:1350.

Domino KB: Evaluation, preparation and management of the patient with respiratory disease. American Society of Anesthesiologists (ASA) Refresher Course Lectures, No. 152, New Orleans, 1996.

Eagle KA, Brundage BH, Ewy GA, et al: Guidelines for perioperative cardiovascular evaluation for noncardiac surgery. J Am Coll Cardiol 1996;27:910.

Eisenkop SM, Spirtos NM, Montag TW, et al: The clinical significance of blood transfusion at the time of radical hysterectomy. Obstet Gynecol 1990;76:110.

Emory WB, Stedman R: When alveolar hypoventilation occurs perioperatively: which drugs are most likely to potentiate neuromuscular blockade? J Crit Illness 1990;5:1161.

Estafanous FG: Hypertension in the surgical patient: management of blood pressure and anesthesia. Cleve Clin J Med 1989;56:385.

Etievent JP, Chocron S, Toubin G, et al: Use of cardiac troponin I as a marker of perioperative myocardial ischemia. Ann Thorac Surg 1995;59:1192.

Fabri PF, Rosemurgy A: Reoperation for small intestinal obstruction. Surg Clin North Am 1991;71:131.

Farquharson DIM, Orr JW Jr: Prophylaxis against thromboembolism in gynecologic patients. Reprod Med 1984;29:845.

Fiszman M, Haug PJ, Frederick PR: Automatic extraction of PIOPED interpretations from ventilation/perfusion lung scan reports. Proc AMIA Symp 1998:860–4.

Fleisher LA: Perioperative management of the cardiac patient undergoing noncardiac surgery. American Society of Anesthesiologists (ASA) Refresher Course Lectures, No. 223, New Orleans, 1996a.

Fleisher LA: Preoperative evaluation. Clin Anesthesiol 1996b;18:443.

Fleisher LA, Eagle K: Screening for cardiac disease in patients having noncardiac surgery. Ann Intern Med 1996;124:767.

Flint LM: Early postoperative acute abdominal complications. Surg Clin North Am 1988;68:445.

Frank SM, Fleisher LA, Breslow MJ: Perioperative maintenance of monothermia reduces the incidence of morbid cardiac events. JAMA 1997;14:1127.

Freeman WK, Gibbons RJ, Shub C: Preoperative assessment of cardiac patients undergoing noncardiac surgical procedures. Mayo Clin Proc 1989;64:1105.

Fry DE, Clevenger FW: Reoperation for intra-abdominal abscess. Surg Clin North Am 1991;71:159.

Fry DE, Osler T: Abdominal wall considerations and complications in reoperative surgery. Surg Clin North Am 1991;71:1.

Garrison RN, Wilson MA, Matheson PJ, Spain DA: Preoperative saline loading improves outcome after elective, noncardiac surgical procedures. Am Surg 1996;62:223.

Glass DD: Blood coagulation, coagulopathies and anticoagulation therapy. American Society of Anesthesiologists (ASA) Refresher Course Lectures, No. 162, Las Vegas, 1990.

Ginsberg JS: Management of venous thromboembolism. N Engl J Med 1996;335:1816.

Gleckman R, de la Rosa G: In-hospital management of pneumonia in the elderly. J Crit Illness 1997;12:163.

Golden WE, Lavender RC: Preoperative cardiac consultations in a teaching hospital. South Med J 1989;82:292.

Goldhaber SZ, Grodstein F, Stampfer JM, et al: A prospective study of risk factors for pulmonary embolism in women. JAMA 1997;277:642.

Goldman L: Cardiac risks and complications of noncardiac surgery. Ann Intern Med 1983;98:504.

Goldstein MB: Acute renal failure. Med Clin North Am 1983;67:1325.

Grant IS, Morton NS: Ventilatory support of the surgical patient. J R Coll Surg Edinb 1988;33:235.

Gravlee GP: Blood transfusion and component therapy. American Society of Anesthesiologists (ASA) Refresher Course Lectures, No. 215, Las Vegas, 1990.

Grossman E, Messerli FH: Diabetic and hypertensive heart disease. Ann Intern Med 1996;125:304.

Gullette EC, Blumenthal JA, Babyak M, et al: Effects of mental stress on myocardial ischemia during daily life. JAMA 1997;277:1521.

Hay DL, von Fraunhofer JA, Masterson BJ: Hemostasis in blood vessels after ligation. Am J Obstet Gynecol 1989;160:737.

Heuser D, Guggenberger H, Fretschner R: Acute blood pressure increase during the perioperative period. Am J Cardiol 1989;63:26c.

Holder WD Jr: Intestinal obstruction. Gastroenterol Clin North Am 1988;17:317.

Holley RL, Kilgore LC: Urologic complications. In Orr JW Jr, Shingleton HM (eds): Complications of Gynecologic Surgery: Prevention, Recognition and Management. Philadelphia: JB Lippincott Company, 1994:5:131.

Houston MC, Ratcliff DG, Hays JT, Gluck FW: Preoperative medical consultation and evaluation of surgical risk. South Med J 1987;80:1385.

Hyers TM: Efficient work-up and treatment for pulmonary thromboembolism. Contemp Intern Med 1990;April:13.

Iber C: Pulmonary function testing in clinical practice. Contemp Intern Med 1990;May:31.

Jayr C, Mollie A, Bourgain JL, et al: Postoperative pulmonary complications: general anesthesia with postoperative parenteral morphine compared with epidural analgesia. Surgery 1988;104:57.

Johnson H Jr, Knee-Ioli S, Butler TA, et al: Are routine preoperative laboratory screening tests necessary to evaluate ambulatory surgical patients? Surgery 1988;104:639.

Kaufman JL, Shah DM, Chang BB, et al: Retroperitoneal exposure technique for repair of aortic and iliac aneurysms. Surg Rounds 1990;October:62.

Klimek JJ, Afemian ER, Gracewaski J, et al: A prospective analysis of hospital-acquired fever in obstetric and gynecologic patients. JAMA 1982;247:3340.

Kruse JA, Carlson RW: Rapid correction of hypokalemia using concentrated intravenous potassium chloride infusions. Arch Intern Med 1990;150:613.

Laslett L: Hypertension preoperative assessment and perioperative management. West J Med 1995;162:215.

Le TH, Timmcke AE, Gathright JB Jr, et al: Outpatient bowel preparation for elective colon resection. South Med J 1997;90:526.

Lennard TW, Shenton BK, Borzotta A, et al: The influence of surgical operations on components of the human immune system. Br J Surg 1985;72:771.

Lesar TS, Briceland LL, Delcoure K, et al: Medication prescribing errors in a teaching hospital. JAMA 1990;263:2329.

Levine M, Hirsh J: The diagnosis and treatment of thrombosis in the cancer patient. Semin Oncol 1990;17:160.

Longnecker DR: Perioperative blood pressure control. American Society of Anesthesiologists (ASA) Refresher Course Lectures, No. 211, Las Vegas 1990.

Lowenstein E: Review of recent information on myocardial ischemia. American Society of Anesthesiologists (ASA) Refresher Course Lectures, No. 234, New Orleans, 1996.

Madlon-Kay R: Evaluation of coronary artery disease in patient having noncardiac surgery. South Med J 1987;80:1366.

Mann JW Jr: Nutritional complications. In Orr JW, Jr, Shingleton HM (eds): Complications in Gynecologic Surgery: Prevention, Recognition, and Management. Philadelphia: JB Lippincott Company, 1994:52:260.

Mann JW, Hatch KD, Taylor PT, et al: The role of percutaneous nephrostomy in gynecologic oncology. Gynecol Oncol 1983;16:393.

Mushlin AI, Thornbury JR: Intravenous pyelography: the case against its routine use. Ann Intern Med 1989;111:58.

O'Hanlan KA, Trambut J, Rodriguez LR, et al: Arterial embolization in the management of abdominal and retroperitoneal hemorrhage. Gynecol Oncol 1989;34:131.

Orr JW Jr: Introduction to pelvic surgery: pre- and postoperative care. In Gusberg SB, Shingleton HM, Deppe G (eds): Female Genital Cancer. New York: Churchill Livingstone, 1988:497.

Orr JW Jr, Barter JF, Kilgore LC, et al: Closed suction pelvic drainage following radical pelvic surgery. Am J Obstet Gynecol 1986a;155:867.

Orr JW Jr, Browne KF Jr: Cardiovascular complications. In Orr JW Jr, Shingleton HM (eds): Complications of Gynecologic Surgery: Prevention, Recognition and Management. Philadelphia: JB Lippincott Company, 1994:1.

Orr JW Jr, Hatch KD, Shingleton HM, et al: Gastrointestinal complications associated with pelvic exenteration. Am J Obstet Gynecol 1983a;145:325.

Orr JW Jr, Holimon JL, Orr, PF: Stage I corpus cancer: is teletherapy necessary? Am J Obstet Gynecol 1997;176:777.

Orr JW Jr, Holloway RW, Orr PJ: Pulmonary complications. In Orr JW Jr, Shingleton HM (eds): Complications of Gynecologic Surgery: Prevention, Recognition and Management. Philadelphia: JB Lippincott Company, 1994:52.

Orr JW Jr, Holloway RW, An PF, et al: Surgical staging of uterine cancer: an analysis of perioperative morbidity. Gynecol Oncol 1991;42:209.

Orr JW Jr, Kilgore LC, Shingleton HM: Guidelines for CV monitoring of the surgical patient. Contemp Obstet Gynecol 1986b;27:71.

Orr JW Jr, Patsner B, Orr PF: Infection in the immunocompromised woman: prophylaxis, diagnosis and treatment. In Pastorek JG (ed): Obstetric and Gynecologic Infectious Disease. New York: Raven Press, 1994b:171.

Orr JW Jr, Shingleton HM: Importance of nutritional assessment and support in the surgical and cancer patients. J Reprod Med 1984;29:635.

Orr JW Jr, Shingleton HM (eds): Complications in Gynecologic Surgery: Prevention, Recognition and Management. Philadelphia: JB Lippincott Company, 1994.

Orr JW Jr, Sisson PF, Patsner B, et al: Single dose antibiotic prophylaxis for patients undergoing extended pelvic surgery for gynecologic malignancy. Am J Obstet Gynecol 1990;162:718.

Orr JW Jr, Taylor PT: Reducing postoperative infection in the patient with gynecologic cancer. Infect Surg 1987;6:666.

Patsner B, Chalas E, Orr JW Jr: Intestinal complications associated with the use of Dexon mesh sling in gynecologic oncology. Gynecol Oncol 1990;38:146.

Patsner B, Orr JW Jr: Case report: renal agenesis with crossed ectopia diagnosed during radical hysterectomy. Gynecol Oncol 1990;37:443.

Pett SB, Wernly JA: Respiratory function in surgical patients: perioperative evaluation and management. Surg Ann 1988;20:311.

Piscitelli JT, Simel DL, Addison WA: Who should have intravenous pyelograms before hysterectomy for benign disease? Obstet Gynecol 1987;69:541.

Quartin AA, Schein RM, Dett DH, Peduzzi PN: Magnitude and duration of the effect of sepsis on survival. JAMA 1997;277:1058.

Rao TL, Jacobs KH, Ei-Etr AA: Reinfarction following anesthesia in patients with myocardial infarction. Anesthesia 1983;59:449.

Roizen MR: Perioperative management of the diabetic patient. American Society of Anesthesiologists (ASA) Refresher Course Lectures, No. 245, New Orleans, 1996.

Rosenow EC: Venous and pulmonary thromboembolism: an algorithmic approach to diagnosis and management. Mayo Clin Proc 1995;70:506.

Rubelowsky J, Machiedo GW: Reoperative versus conservative management for gastrointestinal fistulas. Surg Clin North Am 1991;71:147.

Rudolph R, Boyd CR: Massive transfusion: complications and their management. South Med J 1990;83:1065.

Rutherford C: The technique of selecting and administering blood components. J Crit Illness 1990;5:487.

Saltzman JA, Alavi A, Greenspan RH, et al: Value of the ventilation/perfusion scan in acute pulmonary embolism: results of the Prospective Investigation of Pulmonary Embolism Diagnosis (PIOPED). JAMA 1990;263:1753.

Santilli SM, Cerra FB: Understanding multiple organ failure syndrome. Hosp Physician 1990;26:52.

Schuster DP: A physiologic approach to initiating, maintaining, and withdrawing mechanical ventilatory support during acute respiratory failure. Am J Med 1990;88:268.

Shaff MI, Tarr RW, Partain CL, James AE: Computed tomography and magnetic resonance imaging of the acute abdomen. Surg Clin North Am 1988;68:233.

Shires GT, Canizaro PC: Fluid and electrolyte management of the surgical patient. In Schwartz ST (ed): Principles of Surgery. 4th ed. New York: McGraw-Hill, 1983:91.

Shoemaker WC, Kram HB, Appel PL, Flemming AW: The efficacy of central venous and pulmonary artery catheters and therapy based upon them in reducing mortality and morbidity. Arch Surg 1990;125:1332.

Simel DL, Matchar DB, Piscitelli JT: Routine intravenous pyelograms before hysterectomy in cases of benign disease: possibly effective, definitely expensive. Am J Obstet Gynecol 1988;159:1049.

Smith RP: Transcutaneous oximetry in obstetrics and gynecology. Obstet Gynecol Surv 1990;45:81.

Soper JT, et al: The clinical significance of blood transfusion at the time of radical hysterectomy. Obstet Gynecol 1991;77:165.

Spence RK, Cernaianu AC, Carson J, DelRossi AJ: Transfusion and surgery. Curr Probl Surg 1993;12:1101.

Swartz WH: Prophylaxis of minor febrile and major infectious morbidity following hysterectomy. Obstet Gynecol 1979;54:284.

Velanovich V: The value of routine preoperative laboratory testing in predicting postoperative complications: a multivariate analysis. Surgery 1991;109:236.

Walters MD, Dombroski RA, Davidson SA, et al: Reclosure of disrupted abdominal incisions. Obstet Gynecol 1990;76:597.

Warner MA, Hosking MP, Lobdell CM, et al: Effects of referral bias on surgical outcomes: a population-based study of surgical patients 90 years of age or older. Mayo Clin Proc 1990;65:1185.

Waymack JP: Sequelae of blood transfusions. Infect Surg 1990; July:41.

Wobbes T, Bemelmans BLH, Kuypers JHC, et al: Risk of postoperative septic complications after abdominal surgical treatment in relation to perioperative blood transfusion. Gynecol Obstet 1990;171:59.

Yang SC, Puri VK: Role of preoperative hemodynamic monitoring in intraoperative fluid management. Am Surg 1986;52:536.

44

Gastrointestinal Complications

David E. Cohn
Benjamin E. Greer

Prevention and Management

A gynecologist's primary role is in the management of disorders and diseases of the female reproductive tract. Given the physical proximity of the gastrointestinal system to the reproductive tract, as well as the fact that signs and symptoms of gastrointestinal pathology can mimic those of gynecologic pathology, the gynecologist may expect to be confronted with preoperative, intraoperative, and postoperative issues that relate to the gastrointestinal system. Despite this, most gynecologists are hesitant when faced with a gastrointestinal problem. This hesitancy may lie in their relatively limited experience in the operative management of gastrointestinal issues, a lack of understanding of gastrointestinal anatomy and physiology, or the acknowledgment of the potential morbidity associated with gastrointestinal complications.

Proper preoperative evaluation and management may decrease the risk of gastrointestinal complications. In the event of an intraoperative gastrointestinal complication, an understanding of the anatomy and physiology of the condition and its proper management is necessary to minimize intraoperative and postoperative complications. Likewise, gynecologic patients are at risk for postoperative gastrointestinal complications. The proper diagnosis and management of these problems is necessary for a satisfactory outcome. This chapter reviews the preoperative evaluation and management of the gastrointestinal tract, intraoperative evaluation and management of expected or unexpected gastrointestinal complications, and proper postoperative care to prevent, diagnose, and manage gastrointestinal complications associated with gynecologic surgery.

PREOPERATIVE CONSIDERATION OF THE GASTROINTESTINAL TRACT

The goal of preoperative evaluation is to identify those patients at high risk for gastrointestinal involvement by gynecologic disease prior to surgical intervention. A complete history and physical examination as it relates to the gastrointestinal tract may raise the suspicion of coexisting gastrointestinal disease associated with or related to the primary gynecologic concern.

Preoperative Investigations

A history of gastrointestinal diseases and gastrointestinal symptoms is invaluable in directing the preoperative evaluation toward the most appropriate diagnostic examinations. Ultrasonography may be used in the evaluation of symptoms of cholelithiasis. A concern for peptic ulcer disease or other upper gastrointestinal symptoms would direct an examination toward endoscopy or radiographic evaluation of the upper gastrointestinal tract and small bowel, as well as direct the postoperative management toward the early recognition of complications from peptic ulcer disease. Patients with a history of rectal bleeding, diverticulitis, or changes in stool consistency, caliber, or frequency or a strong family history for familial cancer syndromes should be further evaluated with attention to screening for coexisting lower gastrointestinal conditions with a barium enema, colonoscopy, or sigmoidoscopy (Table 44–1). These evaluations have not been shown to be beneficial or cost-effective as a screening tool in a low-risk, asymptomatic population, even in the presence of concurrent adnexal pathology. In women in the older age groups, the incidence of lower gastrointestinal pathology, including diverticulitis and carcinoma, increases, and thus preoperative screening for these diseases may be of value. Patients with Crohn's disease and ulcerative colitis should be managed in consultation with a gastrointestinal specialist.

Operative Consent

Given the potential gastrointestinal complications of gynecologic procedures, preoperative verbal and

Table 44–1. INDICATIONS FOR PREOPERATIVE BARIUM ENEMA OR FLEXIBLE SIGMOIDOSCOPY

Rectal bleeding or positive stool guaiac
History or symptoms of diverticulitis
Changes in stool caliber, consistency, or frequency
Family history suggestive of familial carcinoma syndrome

written surgical consent must reflect the need for possible gastrointestinal procedures. Consideration of indicated or incidental appendectomy, cholecystectomy, or other bowel surgery should be mentioned if not specifically indicated preoperatively in those patients in whom there is a possible need for these procedures. Specifically, patients with known or suspected endometriosis or cancer, or those in whom complicated or radical procedures are expected, are at high risk for the need for gastrointestinal procedures to be performed concurrently, and this should be reflected in their consent.

Bowel Preparation

Bowel preparation prior to abdominal exploration for gynecologic conditions is used in many conditions. Patients requiring large-bowel surgery, those undergoing laparotomy for ovarian cancer, those with possible bowel involvement by endometriosis, those undergoing multiple abdominal procedures, and those being evaluated for possible exenterative surgery should undergo preoperative bowel preparation. Wound infection rates range from 32% to 58%, and infectious complications range as high as 75% when surgery is performed on the unprepared gastrointestinal tract (Nichols et al, 1972). Colon reanastamosis should heal without leakage in 98% of patients if the bowel has been adequately prepared and the segments are well vascularized.

Preparation of the gastrointestinal tract attempts to accomplish many goals: to decrease the bulk of stool and gastrointestinal contents to increase operative space; to minimize formed stool and bacterial load; and to decrease the morbidity of intestinal surgery, including the risks of septic complications and wound infection. Therefore, bowel preparation involves the reduction of intestinal contents by a mechanical method, as well as the reduction of pathogenic intestinal flora with an antibiotic regimen.

Mechanical bowel preparation traditionally involved the use of dietary restrictions, laxatives, and enemas for greater than 24 hours, with the frequent need for intravenous volume support and correction of associated electrolyte abnormalities. Comparisons of this traditional method of bowel preparation with oral gut lavage (GoLYTELY, Braintree Laboratories, Braintree, MA) have demonstrated similar preoperative and intraoperative quantitative stool cultures, with the GoLYTELY group experiencing less weight loss, better cleansing of the colon, and less fluid and electrolyte abnormalities (Beck et al, 1985). Four liters of GoLYTELY is ingested orally the day prior to surgery, with nasogastric intubation used in those patients who cannot tolerate this regimen. The GoLYTELY method has had varied patient acceptance (Beck and Fazio, 1990).

Oral antibiotics are an important component of bowel preparation in an effort to reduce the number and concentration of pathogenic flora in the colon. Studies have demonstrated a decreased incidence of intraperitoneal and postoperative wound infection with the use of a specific regimen of oral antibiotics. The most widely utilized regimen for antibiotic bowel preparation incorporates the use of oral erythromycin base and neomycin (Table 44–2) (Clarke et al, 1977; Menaker, 1987; Fry, 1988). Substitution of metronidazole for erythromycin base has been used with similar efficacy and improved symptomatic tolerance. The timing of antibiotic administration for this regimen is based on a surgery scheduled for 8 A.M. For operations scheduled later in the day, the timing of administration should be adjusted to adhere to the 19 hours of preparation time that appears to be critical.

The use of oral antibiotics results in very little systemic antimicrobial efficacy, leading to their benefit in sterilizing the intestines. If systemic prophylaxis against infection is desired, certain criteria should be

Table 44–2. ROUTINE BOWEL PREPARATION TO REDUCE INTESTINAL CONTENT AND MICROBIAL FLORA

TIME	MECHANICAL	ANTIBIOTIC
Preoperative day 2	Clear liquid	
Preoperative day 1	Clear liquid	
Noon	Begin GoLYTELY 4 L	
1 P.M.		EM 1 g, Neo 1 g
2 P.M.		EM 1 g, Neo 1 g
8 P.M.	Enemas until clear	
	IV fluids if needed	
11 P.M.		EM 1 g, Neo 1 g
Operative day	NPO at MN	Prophylactic antibiotic

Abbreviations: EM, erythromycin base; IV, intravenous; MN, midnight; Neo, neomycin; NPO, nothing by mouth.

met to justify the use of antibiotics in this setting. The procedure should have a significant risk of infection of the operative site, the procedure should be associated with endogenous bacterial contamination, the prophylactic antibiotic to be used should be effective against the presumed contaminating organisms, and the antibiotic should be present at effective levels during the procedure. As in any therapeutic decision, the benefits of the use of prophylactic antibiotics should outweigh the risks of administration. If these criteria are met, the use of prophylactic antibiotics is appropriate. Patients should receive an intravenous dose of a first- or second-generation cephalosporin, such as cefotetan, preoperatively. Patients allergic to β-lactam antibiotics should receive a combination of metronidazole 500 mg and gentamycin 2 mg/kg intravenously preoperatively. For patients undergoing emergency colon surgery, or a procedure that is likely to include colorectal surgery, this preoperative prophylaxis may be extended to include a total of three doses (Table 44–3).

Preoperative Stoma Site Selection

Given the risks of intestinal complications in gynecologic surgery, one must consider the possible need for an abdominal stoma to be placed intraoperatively. To ensure the best result if a stoma does need to be created, evaluation and planning must take place to minimize potential complications with site selection.

Markings for stoma sites should be performed preoperatively if possible. Patients should be evaluated supine, sitting, and standing so that the surgeon can ensure a proper placement. The final selection of the stoma site should be made with the patient in the sitting position, when the natural protuberance of the abdomen is most noticeable. The most important criterion for selecting a stoma site is ensuring adequate surface area to support the stoma appliance. Application of faceplates over bony prominences, skin creases, or scars produces poor results (Fig. 44–1) (Greer and Rodriguez, 1979).

INTRAOPERATIVE MANAGEMENT OF THE GASTROINTESTINAL TRACT

Despite careful preoperative evaluation and management, there will be circumstances when the gynecologic surgeon will be faced with an expected or unexpected gastrointestinal complications. Knowledge of anatomy and physiology, as well as surgical technique should allow the clinician to properly evaluate and manage many gastrointestinal problems encountered during gynecologic surgery. Except for cases of acute abdominal emergencies, routine early exploration of the abdomen results in a consistent procedure and permits time to mobilize

Table 44–3. ANTIBIOTIC REGIMENS FOR EMERGENCY BOWEL PREPARATION
For colon surgery or clinical conditions precluding oral prophylaxis:
Cefotetan 2 g IV preoperatively, and every 12 hr for three doses
If allergic to β-lactam antibiotics, substitute:
Metronidazole 500 mg IV
or
Gentamycin 2 mg/kg preoperatively, and
Gentamycin 1.5 mg/kg every 8 hr for three doses

additional instruments and personnel if abnormalities are identified.

Exploration of the Abdomen

Abdominal exploration allows the gynecologic surgeon a unique opportunity to diagnose concurrent pathologic states that may not have been previously evaluated. A systematic method of exploration will lead to a thorough evaluation. This may be accomplished by identifying individual organ systems, or by dividing the abdomen into compartments. One system frequently used combines features of both, and incorporates both visual and proprioceptive input.

The initial examination should include the peritoneal surfaces of the diaphragm. This is especially important in cases of ovarian carcinoma, because isolated metastases have been noted in this location in early-stage ovarian cancer (Bagley et al, 1973). The left hemidiaphragm should be inspected for evidence of diaphragmatic hernia. Both lobes of the liver should be palpated for evidence of surface or intrahepatic nodularity. Small hemangiomas or cysts

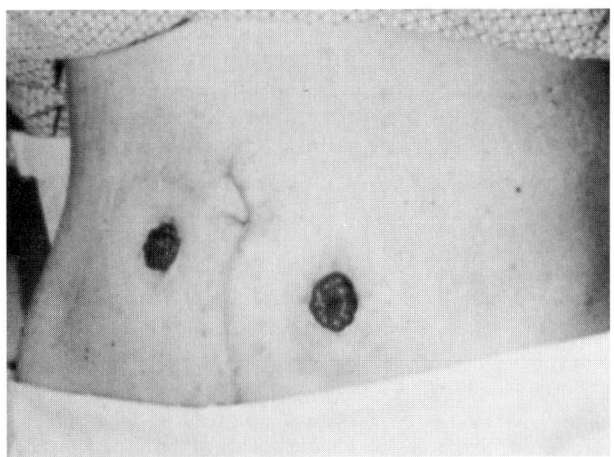

Figure 44–1
Stoma placement in a postoperative patient following a total pelvic exenteration. The stomas are well placed, with the urinary conduit higher than the colostomy. The stomas have adequate surface area for faceplate application, and the skin is without excoriation.

of the liver are common and are of no consequence. Under the right lobe of the liver lies the gallbladder, which should be palpated for abnormal wall thickening as well as for gallstones. If the gallbladder is tense and distended, it can be cupped manually and shaken gently to identify the presence of gallstones.

Directly beneath the gallbladder is the pylorus of the stomach, which is identified as a circular muscular constriction that will usually admit one finger. The first part of the duodenum can be palpated for abnormalities, including scarring from peptic ulcer disease. The lesser and greater curvatures of the stomach as well as the omentum and lymph nodes are then inspected and palpated. When palpating the stomach, one can ensure proper placement of the nasogastric tube if needed. Through the lesser sac, or through the omentum, the outline of the pancreas can be appreciated visually and with gentle palpation. Palpation of the right kidney, left kidney, and spleen completes the examination of the upper abdomen.

Attention is then turned to the lower abdomen. The cecum is identified by its taeniae coli, with three bands of outer longitudinal muscle that converge on the appendix to ease in its identification. The appendix is evaluated for abnormalities, including appendiceal fecaliths. The small bowel is then evaluated in its entirety, with inspection and palpation of serosa and mesentery. Careful attention should be paid to the location of a Meckel's diverticulum as well as to the intestinal lymph nodes. The large bowel should then be evaluated both visually and palpably. Upon the completion of a thorough exploration of the abdomen, the surgeon can direct attention to the area of initial focus, confident that no significant pathologic condition has been overlooked.

Intestinal Injury

Even in the hands of an experienced surgeon, intestinal injury is a possible complication of any gynecologic surgery. The incidence of intestinal injury is approximately 0.7% during gynecologic surgery (Table 44–4) (Dicker et al, 1982; Krebs, 1986). Of the 128 enterotomies in 17,650 patients undergoing gyneco-

logic procedures over a 10-year period, 37% occurred during entrance into the peritoneal cavity, 35% during lysis of adhesions, 10% during laparoscopy, 9% during vaginal operations, and 9% during dilatation and curettage (D&C) or dilatation and evacuation (D&E). Of these enterotomies, 25% involved the large bowel and 75% the small bowel. Gynecologic procedures identified as "uncomplicated" accounted for 72% of the cases in which enterotomy occurred. Interestingly, only 28% of patients identified as being at risk for bowel injury (adhesions, neoplasm, infection, endometriosis) were among those in whom enterotomy was discovered. Nonetheless, serosal laceration was reported to be five to nine times more common in those patients at risk for injury (Krebs, 1986). Endometriosis has been estimated to involve the bowel in 3% to 18% of cases (Weed and Ray, 1987), with the appendix being most frequently involved. Obese women and those with previous abdominal incision had a threefold higher risk of injury. This emphasizes the need for meticulous technique as well as preoperative screening to minimize morbidity and mortality.

To avoid potential bowel laceration, the peritoneum should be entered sharply with a knife and opened cephalad to a previous incision to minimize the risk to bowel adherent to the anterior abdominal wall. Tissue should be kept under tension by traction and countertraction during lysis of adhesions. An attempt should be made to dissect along anatomic planes. Bowel loop adhesions should be lysed one loop at a time, and adhesions deep in the pelvis should not be lysed until anterior loops are separated. Insertion of laparoscopic trocars outside of an old incision may reduce the risk of bowel injury. Careful dissection of tissue planes and attention to adhesions in the cul-de-sac should reduce the chances of bowel injury during vaginal surgery. Careful use and selection of instruments may reduce the chance of bowel injury during D&C and D&E.

Most significant intestinal lacerations occur during lysis of adhesions. Lacerations of the serosa and mucosa occur when the adhesion being lysed is stronger than the tissue to which it is attached. Those adhesions that have occurred following a procedure performed years prior tend to be firmer and denser than

Table 44–4. CHARACTERISTICS OF 128 INTESTINAL INJURIES RECORDED IN 17,650 PATIENTS DURING GYNECOLOGIC SURGERY

OPERATION	INJURIES (%)	% INCIDENCE
Opening peritoneum	48 (37)	0.8
Lysis of adhesions or dissection	45 (35)	0.8
Laparoscopy	13 (10)	0.4
Vaginal surgery	11 (9)	0.1
D&C/D&E	11 (9)	0.1
Totals	128 (100)	0.7

Abbreviations: D&C, dilatation and curettage; D&E, dilatation and evacuation.
Modified from Krebs HB: Intestinal injury in gynecologic surgery: a ten-year experience. Am J Obstet Gynecol 1986;155:509, with permission.

those formed following a recent procedure (Alvarez, 1988). The proper management of intestinal lacerations depends on the extent of the injury. Minor serosal defects will usually reserosalize within 72 hours. Seromuscular lacerations generally need to be repaired unless the defect is extremely shallow and without mucosal extension. These lacerations, if repaired, should be oversewn with 3-0 polyglycolic or nonabsorbable suture (i.e., silk), with the stitches being placed 0.5 cm apart. Repair of multiple adjacent seromuscular lacerations may compromise the diameter of the bowel lumen; thus a bowel resection with primary anastomosis may be the most appropriate repair technique.

Full-thickness enterotomies are important to recognize given the risk for intra-abdominal sepsis and fistula formation without adequate repair. Enterotomies should be closed in two layers after the edges are sharply trimmed, unless the bowel lumen would be compromised. Here, 3-0 delayed-absorbable suture should incorporate the full thickness of the bowel, with the knot placed on the intraluminal side of the bowel. These sutures should be placed 0.25 cm from the edge and about the same distance apart for approximation of the defect. The mucosal defect is closed over with an interrupted imbricating seromuscular layer of 3-0 silk, with stitches placed at 0.5-cm intervals. This defect should be closed perpendicular to the lumen of the bowel to minimize the risk of stenosis of the bowel lumen (Fig. 44–2). If the injury cannot be repaired without compromise of the bowel lumen or excessive tension on the wall of the bowel, resection and reanastomosis, either handsewn or stapled, should be performed. Major intestinal injuries should be repaired under the guidance of a gynecologic oncologist or general surgeon.

The principles of repair of colon injuries are as described above. For patients who sustain an injury to an unprepared large bowel, infectious complications can be minimized with the use of copious irrigation, intraoperative and postoperative intravenous antibiotics, and delayed closure of the skin. A diverting, protective loop colostomy may be the best alternative in the case of major colon injury with extensive spillage. Loop colostomies can usually be closed 3 or 4 months postoperatively without the need for laparotomy.

Gynecologic Cancer

Gynecologic cancer represents a specific situation in which the risk of gastrointestinal surgery or complications is extremely high. A series from Memorial Sloan-Kettering (Rubin et al, 1989) reported a 10.4% rate of major intestinal surgery during gynecologic oncology procedures over a 3-year period, with surgery for ovarian cancer accounting for 43% of these procedures. This is due to the fact that the majority of these cancers are densely adherent to bowel serosa, and that bowel resections are frequently nec-

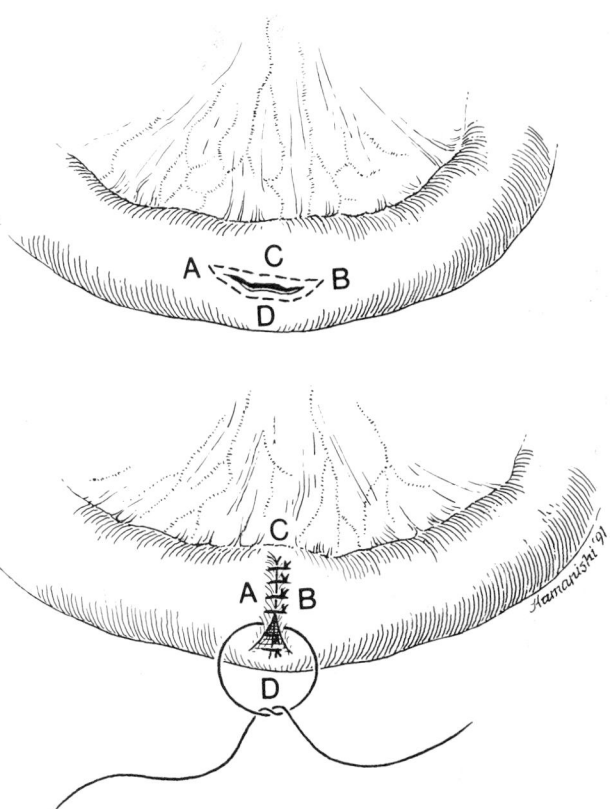

Figure 44–2
After freshening of the edges, a longitudinal intestinal laceration should be closed with a two-layer closure perpendicular to the lumen of the bowel in order to minimize the possibility of causing a stenosis to the bowel lumen.

essary for optimal cytoreduction. Fifty per cent of patients with ovarian cancer will have a bowel obstruction during their course of disease (Krebs and Goplerud, 1984). The most frequent indications for intestinal surgery were obstruction (43%) and fistula (21%). Likewise, treatments for gynecologic cancers may put patients at risk for gastrointestinal complications.

Acute radiation reactions (within the first 6 months of therapy) are usually managed medically. It is common for patients to experience watery diarrhea and cramping in the first few weeks of radiation therapy because of increased peristalsis and decreased transit time. The bowel symptoms can be treated with a low-gluten, low-lactose, and low-protein diet. Antidiarrheal and antispasmodic agents may also be beneficial. Delayed radiation enteritis (after 6 months) consists of diarrhea, possible hemorrhage, and obstruction. The incidence of significant gastrointestinal complications is between 0.5% and 5% (Smith et al, 1985). If an operative procedure is performed for a radiation-induced complication that removes the terminal ileum, supplementation with vitamin K, vitamin B$_{12}$, and bile salts is needed. Approximately 100 cm of small bowel beyond the ligament of Treitz is necessary for adequate oral nutrition.

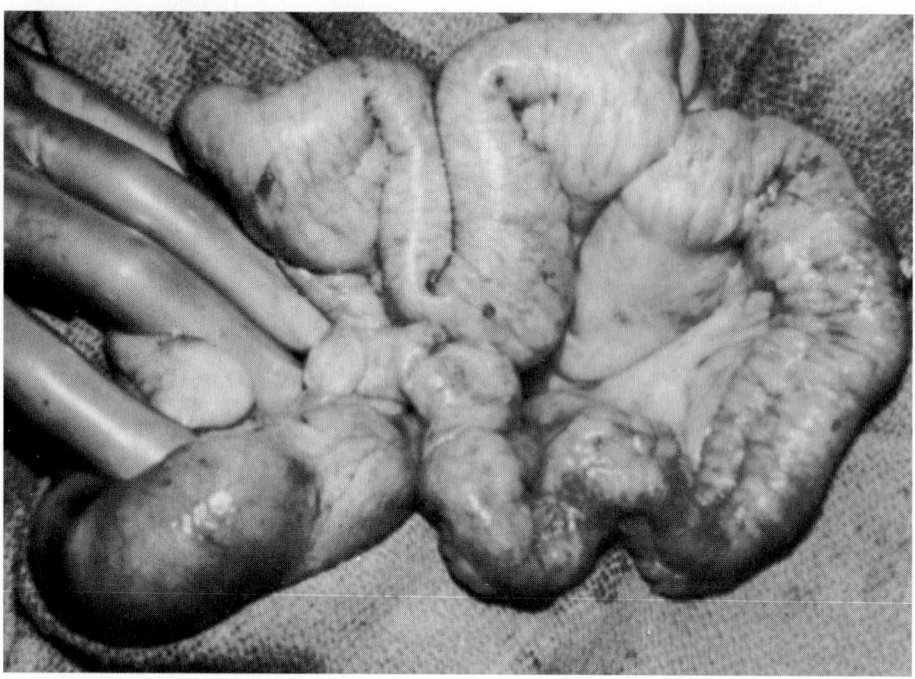

Figure 44–3
Delayed radiation fibrosis of small intestine with thickened bowel wall, stenosis of lumen, and obstruction.

Whole-abdomen radiation therapy is associated with a higher incidence of gastrointestinal complications (Cain et al, 1988). Segmental radiation fibrosis can develop, consisting of thickening of the bowel wall and stenosis of the lumen. The result is a partial or complete bowel obstruction (Fig. 44–3). Life-threatening bowel perforation can occur (Fig. 44–4). When operative intervention is necessary and feasible, the involved segment of bowel should undergo primary resection with end-to-end or end-to-side anastomosis. Although the entire bowel is sensitive to radiation therapy, the terminal ileum is the area at greatest risk. Ileocolectomy of the affected ileum and ascending colon is indicated if the section of bowel is damaged by radiation.

Appendectomy

With strict adherence to the principles of thorough abdominal exploration, the appendix should be evaluated in every operative gynecologic procedure. The incidence of interval appendectomy (1.13 per 1000) exceeds that of appendectomy for appendicitis (0.97 per 1000), with the majority of incidental appendectomies performed in women (Sugimoto and Edwards, 1987). It has previously been stated that "the appendix has been considered devoid of any useful function. The privilege of its amputation has rewarded many a fledgling physician for the pulling of retractors" (Moertel et al, 1974). Despite this thought, controversy exists concerning the practice of routine incidental appendectomy (Cooper et al, 1987).

Approximately 7% of the population will have appendicitis during their lifetime. This risk decreases throughout life, with the highest incidence occurring between the ages of 10 and 30. By the age of 75, the risk of acute appendicitis is approximately 1 in 320 (Ludbrook and Spears, 1965). Despite the decreasing incidence, the morbidity and mortality related to acute appendicitis increase with age (Peltokallio and Tykka, 1981).

Appendectomy as an incidental procedure in the younger age group has been demonstrated to be a safe surgery without an increase in morbidity or mortality over the primary surgical procedure (Westermann et al, 1986, Voitk and Lowry, 1988). Thus proper selection of patients for incidental appendectomy should decrease the incidence of acute appendicitis without incurring further risk. Guidelines for the decision to perform incidental appendectomy have been developed (Fisher and Ross, 1990). These authors recommend appendectomy in patients up to 30 years of age. In patients between 30 and 50, the decision to perform an incidental appendectomy should be left to the discretion of the surgeon. In patients older than 50 years of age, the rare occurrence of acute appendicitis combined with the increasing risk of prolonged anesthesia makes incidental appendectomy less beneficial. Along with these indications, other circumstances exist in which incidental appendectomy is recommended. In patients with appendiceal fecaliths, inflammation, appendiceal involvement of endometriosis or ovarian carcinoma, or malrotation of the gastrointestinal tract, or in whom procedures are being performed that would limit access to the appendix in the future, appendectomy is warranted. Also, patients unable to communicate symptoms of disease may benefit from appendectomy.

There exist specific situations in which the risk of performing an incidental appendectomy outweighs its benefit. Unstable patients, patients with Crohn's disease, and patients who are at risk for incomplete or delayed healing of the appendiceal stump (i.e.,

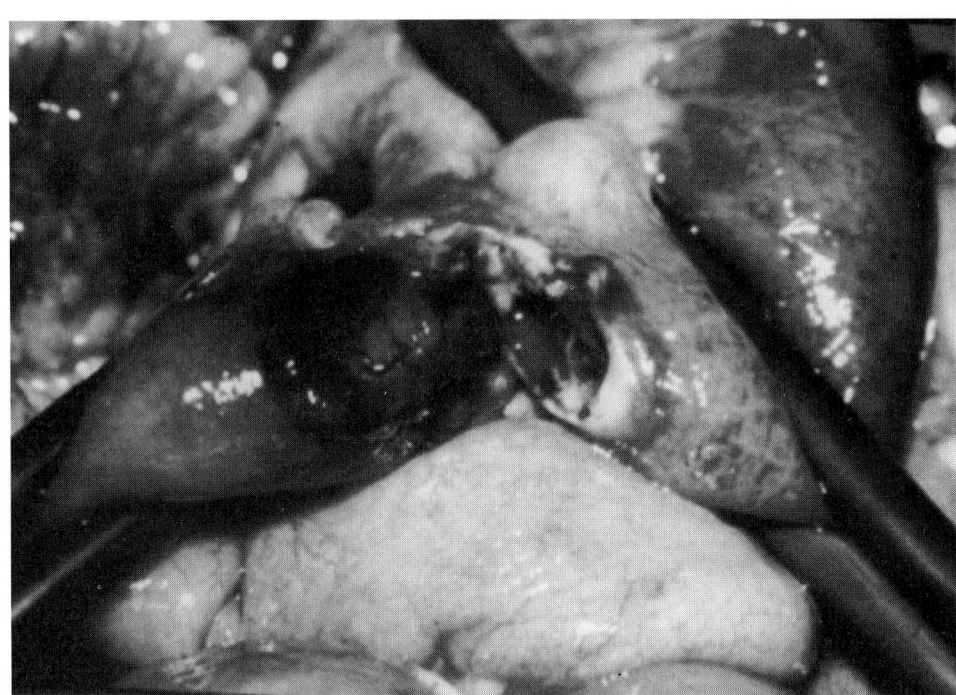

Figure 44-4
Delayed radiation reaction resulting in life-threatening small-bowel perforation.

immunocompromised patients, patients receiving radiation) should not undergo incidental appendectomy. Interest in the use of the appendix in the surgical reconstruction of the urinary system as well as in the construction of an antegrade continence enema has led some to argue against the practice of incidental appendectomy (Wheeler and Malone, 1991).

In 1983, the first laparoscopic appendectomy was reported. Since then, the feasibility and safety of the procedure have been established. Two prospective, randomized trials have compared open versus laparoscopic appendectomy, with both demonstrating a shorter hospitalization (Heinzelmann et al, 1995; Martin et al, 1995). Likewise, fewer wound infections have been reported with laparoscopic appendectomy (Attwood et al, 1992; McAnena et al, 1992). Studies have also demonstrated a decreased incidence of adhesion formation following laparoscopic appendectomy (deWilde, 1991). Whether incidental laparoscopic appendectomy will prove to be beneficial is yet to be determined, but laparoscopic appendectomy for acute appendicitis at the time of diagnostic laparoscopy for presumed gynecologic pathology may be more common as this technique becomes more popular.

Cholelithiasis

Gallstones occur in 10% of adults in the United States, with a 4:1 female-to-male ratio. The finding of previously undiagnosed cholelithiasis in the healthy patient undergoing gynecologic surgery is a common problem and poses a dilemma. Retrospectively, a majority of patients will be noted to have

had symptoms. The development of postoperative cholecystitis is well recognized (Ottinger, 1976). The triad of fasting, dehydration, and narcosis is considered to be a contributing factor. Reviews have demonstrated low morbidity when cholecystectomy is performed with hysterectomy or other major abdominal surgery for gynecologic cancer (Murray et al, 1980; Stevens et al, 1984; Patsner et al, 1989). The general surgery literature supports this concept (Saade et al, 1987). Consent of patients with known or suspected cholelithiasis should be obtained. Depending on the primary gynecologic surgery planned, incision should be made with consultation from the general surgery team. For abdominal hysterectomy, a midline incision will allow access to both the pelvis and right upper quadrant. With the decreased hospitalization time, less postoperative pain, and more rapid return to full physical activity associated with laparoscopic cholecystectomy, vaginal surgery may be performed along with a laparoscopic cholecystectomy (Reddick and Olsen, 1989; Soper et al, 1992).

Meckel's Diverticulum

Meckel's diverticulum, a remnant of the vitelline duct, occurs in approximately 2% of the population and is the most common congenital anomaly of the gastrointestinal tract. The diverticulum usually occurs in the terminal 24 to 48 inches of the ileum. When a Meckel's diverticulum is encountered at abdominal exploration, many factors must be considered in the decision to resect or observe the anomaly. Most complications from a Meckel's diverticulum occur in the pediatric age group, with the estimated lifetime risk of developing symptoms from the diverticulum being 4% (Soltero and Bill, 1976). Many complications are a result of ectopic gastric or pancreatic mucosa in the diverticulum, with resultant hemorrhage or perforation. Clinically, identification of ectopic tissue is difficult. In general, an incidental removal of a Meckel's diverticulum is recommended unless it jeopardizes the intended operation. If resection of a Meckel's diverticulum is determined to be the most appropriate surgical option, the base of the diverticulum is clamped and the pouch excised. Closure of the defect is performed with principles similar to the repair of a full-thickness intestinal laceration, with a seromuscular layer imbricated over a mucosal layer. The defect may also be repaired with a staple device. Again, care should be taken to ensure the lumen of the bowel is not compromised by the repair.

Laparoscopic Surgery

With decreased postoperative pain, shorter hospitalization, and more attractive cosmetic results, more procedures in gynecologic surgery are being performed laparoscopically. As with any surgical procedure, "minimally invasive" laparoscopic surgery carries the risk of complications. The incidence of gastrointestinal injury from laparoscopy has been reported as 1 to 2.7 per 1000 procedures (Cunanan et al, 1980; Yuzpe, 1990). It is difficult to draw conclusions from these data given that a large number of diagnostic and simple operative procedures are included in these statistics. Only one paper has reviewed the experience with operative laparoscopy (Peterson et al, 1990). Here, 155 laparotomies in approximately 37,000 operative laparoscopies were performed, corresponding to a rate of 4.2 per 1000 procedures. Of these 155 laparotomies, 96 were for hemorrhage and 59 for visceral injury. Data from the general surgery literature suggest that the incidence of penetrating bowel injury is 1.4 per 1000 laparoscopic cholecystectomies (Deziel et al, 1993).

Intestinal injury may occur as a result of either trocar insertion or thermal effects from electrocautery. Entry into the peritoneal cavity may be accomplished by insertion of a Verres needle, by direct insertion of a laparoscopy trocar, or by an open technique with a Hassan cannula (Nezhat et al, 1991). Despite a reduction in the incidence of major vascular injuries with open laparoscopy, no studies have demonstrated a decreased incidence of intestinal injury, and data suggest that open laparoscopy is associated with intestinal injury (Penfield, 1985). Insertion of trocars through a left upper quadrant site may avoid many of these intestinal complications (Reich, 1992; Childers et al, 1993). If intestinal injury is suspected during laparoscopy, management depends on the nature of the injury as well as the anatomic location of the suspected injury. Small-diameter injuries from the Verres needle may be

managed expectantly, whereas larger injuries should be repaired, either laparoscopically or by laparotomy. If a Verres needle or trocar has perforated bowel, it should be left in place to identify the site of injury that needs to be repaired. Trocar injuries to bowel must be repaired using the principles outlined previously. If technically possible, this may be done laparoscopically. If there is uncertainty as to the extent of the injury, laparotomy is prudent. Antibiotics should be used postoperatively. Colostomy may be necessary for large lacerations to unprepared bowel. Surprisingly, previous laparotomy has not been demonstrated to be a risk factor for bowel injury during laparoscopy (Chi et al, 1983). However, if a difficult laparoscopy is anticipated, preoperative bowel preparation is recommended.

Bowel injury from laser or electrocautery accounts for approximately 15% of laparoscopic intestinal injury. Many of these thermal injuries are unrecognized at the time of surgery, and thus electrical injury to the bowel accounts for much of the litigation surrounding laparoscopy (Soderstrom, 1993). Even if thermal injury is suspected during laparoscopy, it is difficult to estimate the extent of the damage by inspection, because coagulation necrosis may extend beyond the area of visual damage. The risk of bowel injury can be minimized with attention to careful technique, as well as avoiding the use of laser or electrocautery when close to bowel. If bowel injury from electrocautery or laser is suspected during laparoscopy, principles similar to those described for trocar injuries should be followed. Superficial lesions can be managed expectantly. Areas of thermal damage should be excised and reapproximated rather than oversewn to account for the lateral spread of thermal necrosis. Patients with an unrecognized thermal injury to the bowel may present 4 to 10 days later with evidence of bowel injury. This is later than the onset of symptoms from a mechanical bowel perforation, likely because of delayed bowel wall necrosis.

Vaginal Surgery

Gastrointestinal injury may also occur during vaginal surgery, including vaginal hysterectomy, colporrhaphy, episiotomy, and D&C or D&E. Likewise, a potential complication of vaginal or abdominal surgery is fistula formation. During vaginal hysterectomy, entry into the posterior cul-de-sac is performed blindly, and thus most intestinal injuries occur at this stage of the procedure. If the injured segment of bowel can be mobilized, it can be repaired vaginally. Injury to the rectosigmoid during posterior colporrhaphy should be repaired using three layers: a two-layered repair of the bowel, followed by a repair of the vaginal tissues in an effort to decrease the risk of fistulization. The bowel repair should use absorbable suture in a transverse plane, with the vaginal repair running in the opposite direction.

Bowel injury may occur during D&C or D&E following uterine perforation. In cases of simple uterine perforation, the patient may be observed in the hospital for evidence of acute bleeding or peritonitis. If symptoms develop, or if the patient becomes hemodynamically unstable, laparotomy is indicated. If intestinal injury is identified at the time of perforation, laparotomy with intestinal repair should be performed.

Knowledge of pelvic floor anatomy is crucial for repair of episiotomies. In cases of fourth-degree lacerations or episiotomy, identification and repair of the rectal mucosa, anal sphincter, and vaginal mucosa are necessary for cosmetic and functional success. Rectal mucosa can be repaired with interrupted or running 3-0 absorbable sutures with the knot tied in the lumen of the rectum. The puborectalis and capsule of the rectal sphincter is repaired with interrupted 0 delayed-absorbable suture, and the perineal defect and vaginal mucosa with either interrupted or running 3-0 absorbable suture.

Rectovaginal fistulas often result from obstetric trauma, frequently from an improperly healed fourth-degree perineal laceration. Adherence to certain principles in the surgical repair of rectovaginal fistulas is imperative for a successful result. Preoperative bowel preparation is necessary, and prophylactic intravenous antibiotics are commonly used in an effort to decrease the risk of wound infection. Fistula repair should be accomplished when infection, granulation, and edema are minimal. Data support early surgical correction of fistulas, even 2 weeks following fistula formation (Hauth et al, 1986). The repair must interrupt the continuity of the fistula, and the epithelialized tract must be excised. The rectal wall should be repaired in at least two layers to minimize tension, and there is a benefit in interposing a layer of fresh tissue between the rectum and vagina to minimize the risk of recurrence.

Abdominal Closure

Abdominal fascia provides the mechanical integrity of an abdominal closure. Likewise, it protects the abdominal cavity from contamination from a wound infection. In patients at high risk for dehiscence, especially those with intraperitoneal infection, cancer, prior or planned radiation exposure, or poor nutritional status, a stronger closure is accomplished with a modified Smead-Jones closure using a permanent or delayed-absorbable suture (Fig. 44–5). This internal retention suture provides a wide fascial anchor and avoids the suture pulling through the fascial edge. Studies in rats have demonstrated improved wound strength and decreased closure time when compared to an interrupted en bloc closure (Seid et al, 1995). Likewise, closure of the abdominal fascia can be accomplished with the use of a mass closure,

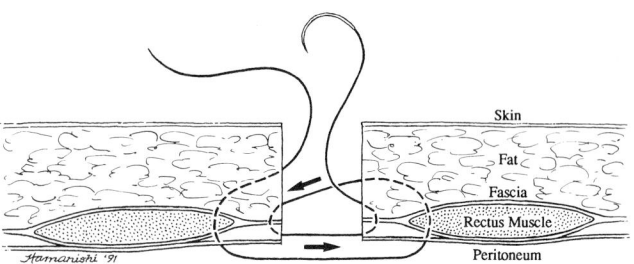

Figure 44–5
Smead-Jones internal retention suture illustrated with permanent suture, including a full stitch of the fascia and peritoneum during the first placement of the suture and only the fascia during the second placement. This placement should be in the same plane and not in a figure-of-8 configuration.

incorporating the peritoneum, rectus muscle, and rectus fascia. A delayed-absorbable, double-looped, monofilament suture (PDS or Maxon) is frequently used for this closure (DiSaia et al, 1994).

POSTOPERATIVE MANAGEMENT OF THE GASTROINTESTINAL TRACT

Postoperative management of the gynecologic patient is frequently complicated by gastrointestinal dysfunction. Management of patients depends on both preoperative factors and intraoperative findings and procedures.

Diet Management

Patients who undergo uncomplicated minor operative procedures such as laparoscopy require no specific dietary restrictions postoperatively. In many institutions, routine postoperative care of patients undergoing uncomplicated laparotomy includes restriction of oral intake until either the presence of normally active bowel sounds or the passage of flatus. The literature supports the idea of early enteral feeding after both uncomplicated and complicated (elective colorectal surgery) procedures (Reissman et al, 1995). When compared to a group of patients given an oral diet only upon resolution of their postoperative ileus, those patients given a clear liquid diet on postoperative day 1, and advanced as tolerated, had no difference in the rate of vomiting, nasogastric intubation, length of hospitalization, or overall complications. Likewise, rates of abdominal complaints and postoperative ileus were identical in patients who were fed immediately following cesarean delivery compared to those who were fed upon the return of bowel function (Kramer et al, 1996).

Nasogastric Intubation

Rarely are nasogastric tubes indicated in uncomplicated abdominal surgery. A study evaluating their routine postoperative use found that nasogastric tubes demonstrated no benefit, but led to increased patient discomfort, when compared to intraoperative orogastric tube decompression in gynecologic oncology patients who underwent extensive intraabdominal surgery (Pearl et al, 1996). Cases in which decompression of the stomach are desirable include patients in whom an omentectomy has been performed, either for staging of ovarian cancer or for use as a pedicle graft in radical surgery. If a nasogastric tube is necessary, a No. 16 French sump tube allows for suction without entrapping the gastric mucosa in the tube. Longer gastrointestinal tubes, such as Cantor or Miller-Abbott tubes, are used even less frequently, usually to stent the small bowel following resection or extensive adhesiolysis. The use of nasogastric tubes in the setting of intestinal ileus and obstruction is discussed separately.

Stress Ulcer Prophylaxis

It has been well established that the gastric mucosa is susceptible to stress. Stress ulceration of the gastric mucosa has been reported with extensive burns (Curling's ulcer), severe central nervous system injury or disease (Cushing's ulcer), shock, sepsis, and profound coagulopathy (Navab and Steingrub, 1995). Many patients who undergo gynecologic surgery remain without oral intake for many days. During this time of relative starvation, it is thought that the mucosal barrier of the stomach and duodenum may be compromised; thus many institutions recommend routine prophylaxis with histamine antagonists (H$_2$-blockers) in the postoperative setting. Studies have demonstrated that stress ulcer prophylaxis in the absence of risk factors may not be necessary (Cook et al, 1991a). Data suggest that, even in critically ill patients in the intensive care unit, the use of H$_2$-blockers does not significantly alter the incidence of stress ulceration (Zeltsman et al, 1996). The use of histamine antagonists may also increase the risk of nosocomial pneumonia by favoring gastric colonization with gram-negative bacilli (Driks et al, 1987; Tryba, 1987), although other studies have not confirmed this finding (Cook et al, 1991b). Thus the decision to use H$_2$-blockers should be individualized based on a patient's preoperative risk factors, as well as intraoperative management and expected postoperative course.

POSTOPERATIVE COMPLICATIONS OF THE GASTROINTESTINAL TRACT

Ileus

Ileus is one of the most common postoperative complications faced by a gynecologic surgeon, because most patients will experience intestinal ileus following uncomplicated or complicated abdominal or pelvic surgery. Entry into the peritoneal cavity and manipulation of the intestinal tract leads to a disorganization of intestinal motility through an unclear mechanism. Other factors causing peritoneal irritation or abnormalities of intestinal motility, such as intraperitoneal infection, unrecognized intestinal or ureteral injury, retroperitoneal hematoma, electrolyte disturbance, and narcotic use, also contribute to intestinal ileus. In most cases, the degree of ileus is minimal, and resolution is rapid and spontaneous. Following abdominal surgery, gastric emptying may be delayed 24 to 36 hours and small intestinal peristalsis and absorption may not be significantly changed. Colonic dysfunction may persist longer than gastric dysfunction, with resumption of normal function after 3 to 5 days. If signs and symptoms suggestive of intestinal dysfunction persist longer than would be expected based on preoperative evaluation and intraoperative exploration and management, further assessment is necessary to ensure that serious intestinal complications, such as intestinal obstruction, are not the cause of the prolonged course.

Clinical features of an intestinal ileus include nausea, vomiting, constipation, abdominal distention, hypoactive bowel sounds, and generalized tenderness. Physical examination should also include a pelvic examination to ensure a pelvic abscess or hematoma is not the cause of a prolonged ileus. Vital signs are usually within normal limits. Abdominal radiographs may demonstrate scattered air-fluid levels throughout loops of dilated small and large intestine. The small-bowel loops are noted transversely in a stepladder manner in the central abdomen, with shadows of valvulae traversing the complete width of the small-bowel shadow at regular intervals. Both flat (supine) and upright radiographs should be obtained. Evidence of free air under the diaphragm in an upright position is common for approximately 1 week postoperatively and is not diagnostic for a perforated viscus.

Treatment of a postoperative ileus is largely conservative, with decompression of the gastrointestinal tract and fluid and electrolyte replacement. Nasogastric suction is instituted to minimize swallowed air in the stomach and reduce gastric distention. Longer tubes, as mentioned above, are favored by some institutions. Unfortunately, the decreased intestinal motility caused by ileus makes placement of these tubes more problematic. Fluids should be replaced intravenously, and electrolytes monitored closely and replaced as needed. As the patient improves, the nasogastric tube can be clamped before it is removed, with an estimation of residual gastric fluid volumes. Diet should then be managed routinely. If patients fail to improve with conservative treatment after 2 to 3 days, other causes of prolonged intestinal dysfunction should be evaluated, including the possibility of bowel obstruction.

Small-Bowel Obstruction

Either small bowel or large bowel can become obstructed. These obstructions can be immediate or delayed, partial or complete. The approach to management of a bowel obstruction varies, depending on the clinical situation. The most common cause of small-bowel obstruction is postoperative adhesions, which account for approximately 50% of cases (Mucha, 1987). Neoplasm and herniation through an incision or mesentery account for 30% of small-bowel obstructions. The incidence of bowel obstruction with gynecologic surgery is variable. In a series reviewing a 25-year experience at a major university (Krebs and Goplerud, 1987), 83% of bowel obstructions were in patients with a history of gynecologic malignancy. Small bowel was obstructed in 77% of cases. These small-bowel obstructions were caused by extrinsic neoplasm in 62% and radiation-associated adhesions in 17% of cases. Postoperative adhesions accounted for 14% of all mechanical small-bowel obstructions.

Early small-bowel obstruction is often indistinguishable from postoperative ileus. Patients experience colicky pain, nausea, and vomiting. The volume of emesis is dependent on the location of the obstruction, with more copious emesis with a high small-bowel obstruction. Abdominal radiographs may be identical to those in patients with a postoperative ileus. In 5% of small-bowel obstructions, radiographs are normal. Thus serial radiographs may be necessary to evaluate the progression of the dysfunction. The initial treatment of obstruction is identical to that of intestinal ileus, with decompression and fluid and electrolyte resuscitation. Approximately 80% of partial small-bowel obstructions will resolve with this management scheme. A persistent small-bowel obstruction following 24 to 48 hours of conservative management is an indication for surgical exploration and management. Usually, adhesiolysis will correct the cause of the obstruction. In cases of undiagnosed intestinal laceration or extensive scarring from adhesions, a bowel resection and reanastomosis may be necessary. Patients who demonstrate clinical deterioration during conservative management warrant earlier surgical evaluation. Patients with possible large-bowel obstruction in addition to a small-bowel obstruction should have a limited barium enema to rule out a double obstruction. Operative correction should be individualized for the cause of the obstruction.

Large-Bowel Obstruction

Large-bowel obstructions are far less common than small-bowel obstructions, accounting for approximately 25% of all intestinal obstructions (Krebs and Goplerud, 1987). A 25-year review of admissions to a major university gynecology service revealed that the factors contributing to large-bowel obstruction included external compression from malignancy, strictures and adhesions from radiation therapy, intrinsic colon neoplasms, and fecal impaction. Because of its fixed position in the abdomen, the right colon is susceptible to large doses of radiation relative to the small bowel and the remainder of the colon. The effects of radiation lead to vascular compromise, ulceration, and fibrosis, leading to injury and obstructive symptoms usually 1 to 2 years following completion of the course of radiation (Kinsella and Bloomer, 1980).

Symptoms of large-bowel obstruction include colicky abdominal pain. The nausea and vomiting typical of small-bowel obstruction is less profound in a large-bowel obstruction. Patients typically experience a decrease in stool caliber and volume, and have usually been unsuccessful in alleviating their symptoms with a home bowel regimen including stool softeners, laxatives, and enemas. History and physical examination should be directed toward the underlying cause of the obstruction, including abdominal or pelvic tumors, rectal masses, or a suspicion of radiation-induced obstruction. Abdominal examination may reveal distention and tympany, with decreased bowel sounds. Abdominal radiographs demonstrate dilatation of the large bowel, noted as distended loops of bowel peripherally with irregularly spaced haustral folds that do not traverse the bowel lumen.

Large-bowel obstructions usually warrant operative intervention. The proper surgical technique should be dictated by the etiology of the obstruction, and may include decompression with a temporary loop colostomy or more complicated bowel resections and anastomoses, with or without protective colostomy. In a majority of patients, the ileocecal valve is believed to be competent. When the large bowel becomes obstructed, the ileocecal valve must be evaluated. Dilatation of the cecum more than 9 cm on abdominal radiographs requires emergent evaluation given the risk of impending perforation. Colostomy decompresses the colon and resolves this emergent situation. Conservative management of advanced colonic obstruction is not appropriate given the high mortality of perforation.

Diarrhea

It is common for patients to experience diarrhea in the postoperative period, largely as a result of the passage of intestinal secretions retained during the previous days of intestinal ileus. However, if spontaneous resolution does not occur, or if the frequency of these episodes increases, pathologic conditions should be considered. Early small-bowel obstruction may be manifested by frequent episodes of loose stool. Thus, if the clinical situation suggests obstruction, management should proceed as previously described.

Clostridium difficile colitis and associated diarrhea is a condition frequently seen following gynecologic surgery, especially following the administration of intravenous antibiotics. *Clostridium difficile*–associated colitis is caused by toxins that this organism produces. The mechanism of action of these toxins is not completely understood, but they are thought to disrupt cell membranes, microfilaments, and protein synthesis (Fekety and Shah, 1993). The critical role of antibiotic use reflects the impact of these medications on intestinal flora. The antibiotics most commonly implicated in *C. difficile* colitis and diarrhea include clindamycin, cephalosporins, and aminopenicillins, although virtually any antibiotic can be associated with this disorder (Bartlett, 1994). Diagnostic tests include a tissue culture or latex agglutination assay to detect *C. difficile* toxin. Enzyme-linked immunosorbent assay is also available, and its sensitivity has been reported to be 80 to 90%, although false-positive tests have been seen with low toxin titers.

Management of *C. difficile*–associated diarrhea includes the discontinuation of narcotics and the offending antibiotic if possible, along with treatment directed against the organism. Metronidazole 500 mg orally, three times daily, for 7 to 10 days, is effective against *C. difficile* colitis. Treatment with vancomycin is substantially more expensive and carries the added risk of selection for multiply-resistant enterococcus.

Miscellaneous

The prevention, diagnosis, and management of many gastrointestinal complications of gynecologic surgery have been reviewed. Other, less common complications deserve clinical consideration when signs or symptoms are present. Postoperative bleeding, either from an upper or lower gastrointestinal source, may occur. The most common causes of upper gastrointestinal tract bleeding include peptic ulcers, Mallory-Weiss tears, and esophageal varices. Nonsteroidal analgesics, such as ketorolac, have been reported to increase the incidence of postoperative gastrointestinal bleeding when used in high doses in older patients, and when administered for greater than 5 days (Strom et al, 1996). Most lower gastrointestinal tract bleeding originates in the colon, and less commonly in the small bowel or from an upper gastrointestinal tract source. In both cases, initial management includes medical stabilization and resuscitation. Surgical intervention is usually not necessary (Lawrence et al, 1989).

Enterocutaneous fistulas are a potential postoperative complication. Factors contributing to fistula formation include bowel injury, poor healing of an intestinal anastomosis, and bowel obstruction. Patients in whom healing is compromised, such as those with cancer, malnutrition, radiation exposure, infection, or metabolic disease, are at an increased risk for fistula formation. Initial management should include bowel rest and nutritional support. Octreotide (a long-acting somatostatin analog) decreases fistula output and may decrease the time to spontaneous closure (Martineau et al, 1996). Surgical repair should be delayed until inflammation has resolved and nutritional status has been optimized.

Pancreatitis should be considered as a postoperative complication in patients with a history of biliary lithiasis or chronic alcohol use. Careful monitoring postoperatively should lead to early diagnosis and therapy.

REFERENCES

Alvarez RD: Gastrointestinal complications in gynecologic surgery: a review for the general gynecologist. Obstet Gynecol 1988;72:533.

Attwood SE, Hill AD, Murphy P, et al: A prospective randomized trial of laparoscopic versus open appendectomy. Surgery 1992;112:497.

Bagley CM Jr, Young RC, Schein PS, et al: Ovarian carcinoma metastatic to the diaphragm—frequently undiagnosed at laparotomy: a preliminary report. Am J Obstet Gynecol 1973;116:397.

Bartlett JG: *Clostridium difficile*: history of its role as an enteric pathogen and the current state of knowledge about the organism. Clin Infect Dis 1994;18:S265.

Beck DE, Fazio VW: Current preoperative bowel cleansing methods: results of a survey. Dis Colon Rectum 1990;33:12.

Beck DE, Harford FJ, DiPalma JA: Comparison of cleansing methods in preparation for colonic surgery. Dis Colon Rectum 1985;28:491.

Cain JM, Russell AH, Greer BE, et al: Whole abdomen radiation for minimal residual epithelial ovarian carcinoma after surgical resection and maximal first-line chemotherapy. Gynecol Oncol 1988;29:168.

Chi I, Feldblum PJ, Balogh SA: Previous abdominal surgery as a risk factor in interval laparoscopic sterilization. Am J Obstet Gynecol 1983;145:841.

Childers JM, Brzechffa PR, Surwit EA: Laparoscopy using the left upper quadrant as the primary trocar site. Gynecol Oncol 1993;50:221.

Clarke JS, Condon RE, Bartlett JG, et al: Preoperative oral antibiotics reduce septic complications of colon operations: results of prospective, randomized, double-blind clinical study. Ann Surg 1977;186:251.

Cook DJ, Pearl RG, Cook RJ, et al: The incidence of clinically important bleeding in ventilated patients. J Intensive Care Med 1991a;6:167.

Cook DJ, Laine LA, Guyatt GH, Raffin TA: Nosocomial pneumonia and the role of gastric pH: a meta-analysis. Chest 1991b;100:7.

Cooper G, Taylor WS, Goldstein PJ: Incidental appendectomy: the controversy. MD Med J 1987;36:833.

Cunanan RG Jr, Courey NG, Lippes J: Complications of laparoscopic tubal sterilizations. Obstet Gynecol 1980;55:501.

deWilde RL: Goodbye to late bowel obstruction after appendicectomy. Lancet 1991;338:1012.

Deziel DJ, Millikan KW, Economou SG, et al: Complications of laparoscopic cholecystectomy: a national survey of 4292 hospitals and an analysis of 77,604 cases. Am J Surg 1993;165:9.

Dicker RC, Greenspan JR, Strauss LT, et al: Complications of abdominal and vaginal hysterectomy among women of reproductive age in the United States: the collaborative review of sterilization. Am J Obstet Gynecol 1982;144:841.

DiSaia PJ, Creasman WT, Eddy G, Montz J: Experience with a mass closure technique using continuous looped polyglyconate absorbable suture. J Am Coll Surg 1994;178:177.

Driks MR, Craven DE, Celli BR, et al: Nosocomial pneumonia in intubated patients given sucralfate as compare with antacids or histamine type 2 blockers: the role of gastric colonization. N Engl J Med 1987;317:1376.

Fekety R, Shah AB: Diagnosis and treatment of *Clostridium difficile* colitis. JAMA 1993;269:71.

Fisher KS, Ross DS: Guidelines for therapeutic decision in incidental appendectomy. Surg Gynecol Obstet 1990;171:95.

Fry DE: Antibiotics in surgery: an overview. Am J Surg 1988;155:11.

Greer BE, Rodriguez DB: Abdominal Stomas: Complications and Management. New York: Medcom, Inc, 1979.

Hauth JC, Gilstrap LC III, Ward SC, Hankins GD: Early repair of an external sphincter ani muscle and rectal mucosal dehiscence. Obstet Gynecol 1986;67:806.

Heinzelmann M, Simmen HP, Cummins AS, Largiader F: Is laparoscopic appendectomy the new "gold standard"? Arch Surg 1995;130:782.

Kinsella TJ, Bloomer WD: Tolerance of the intestine to radiation therapy. Surg Gynecol Obstet 1980;151:273.

Kramer RL, VanSomeren JK, Qualls CR, Curet LB: Postoperative management of cesarean patients: the effect of immediate feeding on the incidence of ileus. Obstet Gynecol 1996;88:29.

Krebs HB: Intestinal injury in gynecologic surgery: a ten-year experience. Am J Obstet Gynecol 1986;155:509.

Krebs HB, Goplerud DR: The role of intestinal intubation in obstruction of the small intestine due to carcinoma of the ovary. Surg Gynecol Obstet 1984;158:467.

Krebs HB, Goplerud DR: Mechanical intestinal obstruction in patients with gynecologic disease: a review of 368 patients. Am J Obstet Gynecol 1987;157:577.

Lawrence MA, Hooks VH III, Bowder TA Jr: Lower gastrointestinal bleeding. a systematic approach to classification and management. Postgrad Med 1989;85:89.

Ludbrook J, Spears GF: The risk of developing appendicitis. Br J Surg 1965;52:856.

Martin LC, Puente I, Sosa JL, et al: Open versus laparoscopic appendectomy: a prospective randomized comparison. Ann Surg 1995;222:256.

Martineau P, Shwed JA, Denis R: Is octreotide a new hope for enterocutaneous and external pancreatic fistulas closure? Am J Surg 1996;172:386.

McAnena OJ, Austin O, O'Connell PR, et al: Laparoscopic versus open appendicectomy: a prospective evaluation. Br J Surg 1992;79:818.

Menaker GJ: The use of antibiotics in surgical treatment of the colon. Surg Gynecol Obstet 1987;164:581.

Moertel CG, Nobrega FT, Elveback LR, Wentz JR: A prospective study of appendectomy and predisposition to cancer. Surg Gynecol Obstet 1974;138:549.

Mucha P Jr: Small intestinal obstruction. Surg Clin North Am 1987;67:597.

Murray JM, Gilstrap LC III, Massey FM: Cholecystectomy and abdominal hysterectomy. JAMA 1980;244:2305.

Navab F, Steingrub J: Stress ulcer: is routine prophylaxis necessary? Am J Gastroenterol 1995;90:708.

Nezhat FR, Silfen SL, Evans D, Nezhat C: Comparison of direct insertion of disposable and standard reusable laparoscopic trocars and previous pneumoperitoneum with Veress needle. Obstet Gynecol 1991;78:148.

Nichols RL, Condon RE, Gorbach SL, Nyhus LM: Efficacy of preoperative antimicrobial preparation of the bowel. Ann Surg 1972;176:227.

Ottinger LW: Acute cholecystitis as a postoperative complication. Ann Surg 1976;184:162.

Patsner B, Wann WJ Jr, Arato M, et al: Cholecystectomy accompanying major abdominal surgery for gynecologic cancer. Gynecol Oncol 1989;32:46.

Pearl ML, Valea FA, Fischer M, Chalas E: A randomized controlled trial of postoperative nasogastric tube decompression in gynecologic oncology patients undergoing intra-abdominal surgery. Obstet Gynecol 1996;88:399.

Peltokallio P, Tykka H: Evolution of the age distribution and mortality of acute appendicitis. Arch Surg 1981;116:153.

Penfield AJ: How to prevent complications of open laparoscopy. J Reprod Med 1985;30:660.

Peterson HB, Hulka JF, Phillips JM: American Association of Gynecologic Laparoscopists' 1988 membership survey on operative laparoscopy. J Reprod Med 1990;35:587.

Reich H: Laparoscopic bowel injury. Surg Laparosc Endosc 1992;2:74.

Reissman P, Teoh TA, Cohen SM, et al: Is early oral feeding safe after elective colorectal surgery? A prospective randomized trial. Ann Surg 1995;222:73.

Reddick EJ, Olsen DO: Laparoscopic laser cholecystectomy: a comparison with mini-lap cholecystectomy. Surg Endosc 1989;3:131.

Rubin SC, Benjamin I, Hoskins WJ, et al: Intestinal surgery in gynecologic oncology. Gynecol Oncol 1989;34:30.

Saade C, Bernard D, Morgan S, et al: Should cholecystectomy be done *en passant* for asymptomatic cholelithiasis? Can J Surg 1987;30:350.

Seid MH, McDaniel-Owens LM, Poole GV Jr, Meeks GR: A randomized trial of abdominal incision suture technique and wound strength in rats. Arch Surg 1995;130:394.

Smith ST, Seski JC, Copeland LJ, et al: Surgical management of irradiation-induced small bowel damage. Obstet Gynecol 1985;65:563.

Soderstrom RM: Bowel injury litigation after laparoscopy. J Am Assoc Gynecol Laparosc 1993;1:74.

Soltero MJ, Bill AH: The natural history of Meckel's diverticulum and its relation to incidental removal: a study of 202 cases of diseased Meckel's diverticulum found in King County, Washington over a 15 year period. Am J Surg 1976;132:168.

Soper NJ, Barteau JA, Clayman RV, et al: Comparison of early postoperative results for laparoscopic versus standard open cholecystectomy. Surg Gynecol Obstet 1992;174:114.

Stevens ML, Hubert BC, Wenzel FJ: Combined gynecologic surgical procedures and cholecystectomy. Am J Obstet Gynecol 1984;149:350.

Strom BL, Berlin JA, Kinman JL, et al: Parenteral ketorolac and risk of gastrointestinal and operative site bleeding: a postmarketing surveillance study. JAMA 1996;275:376.

Sugimoto T, Edwards D: Incidence and costs of incidental appendectomy as a preventative measure. Am J Public Health 1987;77:471.

Tryba M: Risk of acute stress bleeding and nosocomial pneumonia in ventilated intensive care unit patients: sucralfate versus antacids. Am J Med 1987;83:117.

Voitk AJ, Lowry JB: Is incidental appendectomy a safe practice? Can J Surg 1988;31:448.

Weed JC, Ray JE: Endometriosis of the bowel. Obstet Gynecol 1987;69:727.

Westermann C, Mann WJ, Chumas J, et al: Routine appendectomy in extensive gynecologic operations. Surg Gynecol Obstet 1986;162:307.

Wheeler RA, Malone PS: Use of the appendix in reconstructive surgery: a case against incidental appendectomy. Br J Surg 1991;78:1283.

Yuzpe AA: Pneumoperitoneum and trocar injuries in laparoscopy, a survey on possible contributing factors and prevention. J Reprod Med 1990;35:485.

Zeltsman D, Rowland M, Shanavas Z, Kerstein MD: Is the incidence of hemorrhagic stress ulceration in surgical critically ill patients affected by modern antacid prophylaxis? Am Surg 1996;62:1010.

45

Thomas W. McDonald

Hysterectomy
Indications, Types, and Alternatives

HISTORICAL PERSPECTIVE

Uterine Prolapse—An Ancient Affliction

Twenty centuries before the advent of Christianity, the Egyptians described prolapse of the uterus. The uterus, described by Aristotle as "the seat of womanhood," was considered an indispensable vital organ that somehow embodied a woman's spirit. Therefore, it is not surprising that ancient practitioners tried or suggested therapies of every imaginable type to correct prolapse before considering actual removal of the uterus (Benrubi, 1988). Ancient medical writings show that *genital prolapse* continued to plague womankind through the centuries and was the first recorded indication for hysterectomy (Emge and Durfee, 1966).

Succussion therapy and vaginal pessaries were two popular nonsurgical treatments for genital prolapse. Succussion therapy, described by Hippocrates 460–377 BC), required securing the patient to a frame by ropes and then inverting her. With the patient suspended head down, the entire frame was rapidly moved up and down so that shaking motion and gravity might return the uterus to its normal position!

Reducing the prolapsed womb to its anatomic position followed by placement of an object in the vaginal canal to prevent repeated prolapse was widely used and accepted treatment in ancient times. Soranus (AD 98–138), a Greek physician who practiced in Alexandria and Rome, said that an earlier practitioner, Diocles of Carystos (fourth century BC), had suggested using half a pomegranate soaked in vinegar for this purpose (Temkin, 1956). Over the centuries, all sorts of materials of varied shapes have been used in the vagina as a pessary for mechanical support of the prolapsed uterus.

Some remedies advocated for uterine prolapse suggest that ancient practitioners apparently believed the uterus could independently react to stimuli in its environment. This seems evident from the recommendation of Roderico de Castro (1603) to treat uterine prolapse "by attacking it with a piece of iron—red hot—as if to burn it, whereupon fright

will force the prolapsed part to recede into the vagina" (Emge and Durfee, 1966). Soranus also recorded that many of his predecessors treated uterine prolapse by applying herbs and fumigations. Pleasant odors were directed toward the woman's head and neck to coax the uterus upward while foul odors were applied to the vagina to drive the uterus back to its anatomic position. Soranus opposed these practices, stating that "the uterus does not issue forth like a wild animal from the lair, delighted by fragrant odors and fleeing bad odors" (Temkin, 1956). Soranus noted that the chronically prolapsed uterus could become gangrenous, and that the gangrenous uterus was both irreducible and a threat to life. Abandoning fumigations, Soranus recommended *surgical amputation* of the prolapsed gangrenous uterus—the earliest recorded indication for vaginal hysterectomy (Temkin, 1956).

Sporadic reports continued to document vaginal amputation of the prolapsed womb up to the beginning of the 19th century. These early cases (Alsaharavius, Arabia, 1080; Berengarius, Bologna, Italy, 1507; Andreas Cruce, Grenada, Spain, 1560; Ambrose Paré, France, 1575; Schenck, Grabenberg, Germany, 1617; Volkamer, Nuremberg, Germany, 1675) were usually performed by simple ligation of the prolapsed uterus as high as possible followed by excision with knife or cautery or by allowing the organ to slough over a period of weeks (Kennedy, 1944).

Improved Techniques and Instruments—The 19th Century

Surgeons began developing techniques and instruments around the beginning of the 19th century that gradually evolved into the vaginal hysterectomy technique used today. In 1808 Osiander of Gottingen, Germany, reported a series of eight partial vaginal hysterectomies (Cianfrani, 1960). He listed *cervical cancer* as the indication for his first operation in 1801. He described some of his instruments and techniques. When the uterus was not prolapsed, he used traction and a vaginal speculum to bring the cervix down and aid visualization. He then excised the can-

1023

cerous cervix using a scalpel and curved scissors. We know that the vaginal speculum was also used in antiquity. A bivalve speculum was found in the ruins of Pompeii, and Galen, writing in the first century AD, distinguished between a vaginal and a rectal speculum (Mathieu, 1934). However, this practical instrument seems to have been forgotten and then rediscovered for diagnostic examination and surgery by Osiander in Germany and Recamier (1816), in France (Tilt, 1881).

Cervical cancer provided the impetus for other pioneer efforts in vaginal surgery. In 1810 Wrisberg delivered a prize-winning essay to the Vienna Royal Academy of Medicine advocating vaginal hysterectomy as treatment for cervical cancer (Henrotin, 1907). In 1812, the Italian surgeon Palleta (1822) reported removing the entire uterus vaginally, although his intention was to remove only the cancerous cervix and the lower uterine segment.

Conrad Langenbeck of Gottingen, Germany, performed the *first planned vaginal hysterectomy* in 1813 and reported it in 1817 (Langenbeck, 1842). His patient was the first reported to survive this operation and in fact lived 26 years after the surgery. She was 50 years old at the time of surgery and suffered from a prolapsed womb with a hard, ulcerated cervix. We cannot conclude from existing records whether Langenbeck's indication for surgery was cervical cancer or prolapse. The success of this operation is remarkable considering that Langenbeck operated without the benefits of an assistant, anesthesia, antisepsis, hemostatic clamps, or blood transfusion. Langenbeck's colleagues were incredulous and did not believe that the entire uterus had been removed vaginally until his patient had postmortem examination 26 years after the surgery.

Blood loss and infection were the major causes of death from these early hysterectomies. By 1880 the operative mortality for vaginal hysterectomy was less than 10% compared to a 70% abdominal hysterectomy mortality rate (Morley, 1988). The concept of using the hemostatic clamp made it possible to control blood loss. Wilhelm Freund in Germany (1881) studied cadavers in his efforts to improve vaginal hysterectomy technique and recommended that "compression forceps" be applied to the broad ligaments in place of suture and ligature or only simple cautery. He left these clamps in place for several days before removing them.

Pean, a contemporary operating in France, initially worked to combine the suture and clamp technique for vaginal hysterectomy, but settled on the clamp method, which he reported in 1886. Pean extended the indications for vaginal hysterectomy beyond cervical cancer to include fibroid enlargement by developing the *morcellation technique* for vaginal removal of the uterus (Pean, 1886). His 2% mortality rate for vaginal hysterectomy was an excellent achievement for his time (Kennedy, 1944).

Surgical infection was addressed in 1867 by Joseph Lister, surgeon at Glasgow Royal Infirmary, who in-troduced antiseptic surgery when he began using carbolic acid to cleanse surgeons' hands and instruments and carbolic acid spray for airborne germs. The German surgeon and bacteriologist Robert Koch (1881) initiated aseptic surgical practice in 1876, when he suggested using steam sterilization to prevent wound infection.

Ephraim McDowell (1817) established the propriety of abdominal surgery for ovarian masses when he performed the first ovariectomy in the United States in 1809. In 1842, Heath of Manchester, England, opened the abdomen planning to perform an ovariectomy when he encountered a large fibroid uterus. He proceeded with a supracervical hysterectomy by passing ligatures through the lower uterine segment. Unfortunately, the patient died 13 hours after the surgery (Heath, 1843). Thus a large fibroid tumor became the surgical indication for the *first reported abdominal hysterectomy*, although the preoperative diagnosis was an ovarian tumor.

Walter Burnham (1854) of Lowell, Massachusetts, performed the first successful supracervical abdominal hysterectomy for fibroids in June 1853, which he also had misdiagnosed as an ovarian tumor preoperatively. Gilman Kimball (1855), also from Lowell, was the first to *correctly* diagnose uterine fibroids preoperatively and performed abdominal hysterectomy for that indication in September 1853.

First Abdominal Hysterectomy for Cervical Cancer

Cervical cancer, recognized as a condition leading to inevitable death of the patient and usually accompanied by protracted pain, foul discharge, and bleeding, was often considered to be an unsuitable indication for vaginal surgery and stimulated continued efforts to perfect the higher risk abdominal operation. Wilhelm Freund (1878) of Strasbourg reported the *first abdominal hysterectomy performed for cervical cancer*. He described many surgical principles that we apply today:

1. Antisepsis using 10% carbolic acid to scrub the patient and cleanse the vagina
2. Packing the intestines into the upper abdomen with a warm, carbolized towel
3. Successive ligation of the vessels
4. Traction on the uterus by means of a ligature through the fundus
5. Complete reperitonealization of the broad ligaments and pelvis by suture
6. Tilting the patient to elevate the pelvis (this was 12 years before Trendelenburg [1890] described this position)

Development of Radical Hysterectomy for Cervical Cancer

Other gynecologists built on Freund's work, expanding the scope of abdominal hysterectomy for cervical cancer. Mackenrodt (Germany) in 1894 described a *combined vaginal–abdominal procedure* in which the upper vagina was dissected and excised from below and then the uterus and cervix with all possible parametrial tissue were removed abdominally (Mathieu, 1934). Working independently, Emil Reis in Chicago, a former student of Freund, and John Clark, a resident of Howard Kelly's at Johns Hopkins University, both reported an *extended abdominal hysterectomy* for cervical cancer that included wide parametrial dissection, removal of the upper vagina, and a selective pelvic lymph node dissection (Clark, 1895; Reis, 1895). Ernst Wertheim in Vienna started his series of *radical abdominal hysterectomies* for cervical cancer in 1893 and greatly popularized the procedure that now bears his name. He reported a series of 500 operations (Wertheim, 1911, 1912).

CONTEMPORARY HYSTERECTOMY

These historical highlights in the development of vaginal and abdominal hysterectomy show that removal of the uterus, although extremely threatening to life, was continually refined and championed as a cure for desperate ills of womankind through the 19th and early 20th centuries. We may not often reflect on the tremendous debt we owe to our enthusiastic surgical predecessors and their patients for their trial-and-error development of proven surgical techniques employed with facility today. As we practice our craft at the end of the 20th century, we truly "stand on their shoulders" (Morley, 1977). We combine this legacy of surgical knowledge with other medical advances only dreamed of or unimagined in the early 19th century (anesthesia, blood transfusion, antibiotics, and the host of support techniques and services available for the critically ill patient). Now there is almost no woman too frail for surgical removal of the uterus. The increased safety of the operation, combined with an increasing availability of medical care and more liberal surgical indications, has resulted in increasing hysterectomy rates around the world. It is estimated that 37% of women in the United States will have a hysterectomy by age 60 (Pokras and Hufnagel, 1988). This chapter reviews current hysterectomy indications and types and presents some alternatives to hysterectomy as medicine moves rapidly into the 21st century.

Age-Specific Hysterectomy Rates and Annual Totals

In the United States during the 9-year period from 1970 to 1978, the hysterectomy rate averaged 8.5 per 1000 women ages 15 to 44 years. Each year hysterectomy rates were highest for the oldest age group (35 to 44 years). The age-specific rates for the 35- to 44-year age group were fairly stable over the study period, averaging 18.4 per 1000 women (Dicker et al,

1982b). This observation was confirmed over the 20-year period 1965 to 1984 by the National Center for Health Statistics (NCHS) as part of the ongoing National Hospital Discharge Survey. The highest hysterectomy rates occurred in the 40- to 44-year age group, with an average age at hysterectomy of 42.7 years (Pokras and Hufnagel, 1987). In 1988 Pokras and Hufnagel observed that the annual number of hysterectomies in the United States could reach about 810,000 in 1995 and 854,000 in 2005 if the age-specific hysterectomy rates remained stable as the "baby boom" population ages (Pokras and Hufnagel, 1988).

Annual hysterectomy rates have actually declined in the United States. Factors accounting for this decline may include second opinions for surgery, quality assurance programs, and increased use of medical and conservative surgical procedures instead of hysterectomy (Wilcox et al, 1994). In 1988 the NCHS reported 578,000 hysterectomies with 133,000 vaginal hysterectomies and 445,000 abdominal operations (Graves, 1989). The total number of hysterectomies increased to 590,000 in 1990 (Graves, 1992). In 1995, the most recent year with complete statistical analysis from the NCHS, 544,000 hysterectomies were performed; 190,000 were vaginal operations and 354,000 were abdominal operations (Graves, 1995). Hysterectomy is the second most common major operation performed on women. Caesarean section ranks first, with 966,000 procedures performed in 1988 (Graves, 1992).

Morbidity and Mortality

Hysterectomy still incurs a notable complication rate, with one fourth to one half of women experiencing one or more complications (Dicker et al, 1982a). Pelvic surgery risks are easily understood, considering the anatomy and technical details. Opening the vaginal cuff contaminates the peritoneal cavity to some degree with the upper vaginal bacterial flora. The bowel, bladder, and ureters are close to the lines of incision, clamping, and suturing (Figs. 45–1 and 45–2). Pelvic surgery predisposes patients to thromboembolism. The magnitude of risk is influenced by many variables, including the patient's age and general health, the indications for hysterectomy, the urgency of the surgical procedure (emergency versus planned), the experience and training of the surgeon, the use of suction drainage, the use of prophylactic antibiotics, and the surgical approach (vaginal versus abdominal).

Risks: Vaginal Versus Abdominal Surgery

Comparative risks of vaginal and abdominal hysterectomy were assessed by the Collaborative Review of Sterilization (CREST) study conducted by the Centers for Disease Control between 1978 and 1981

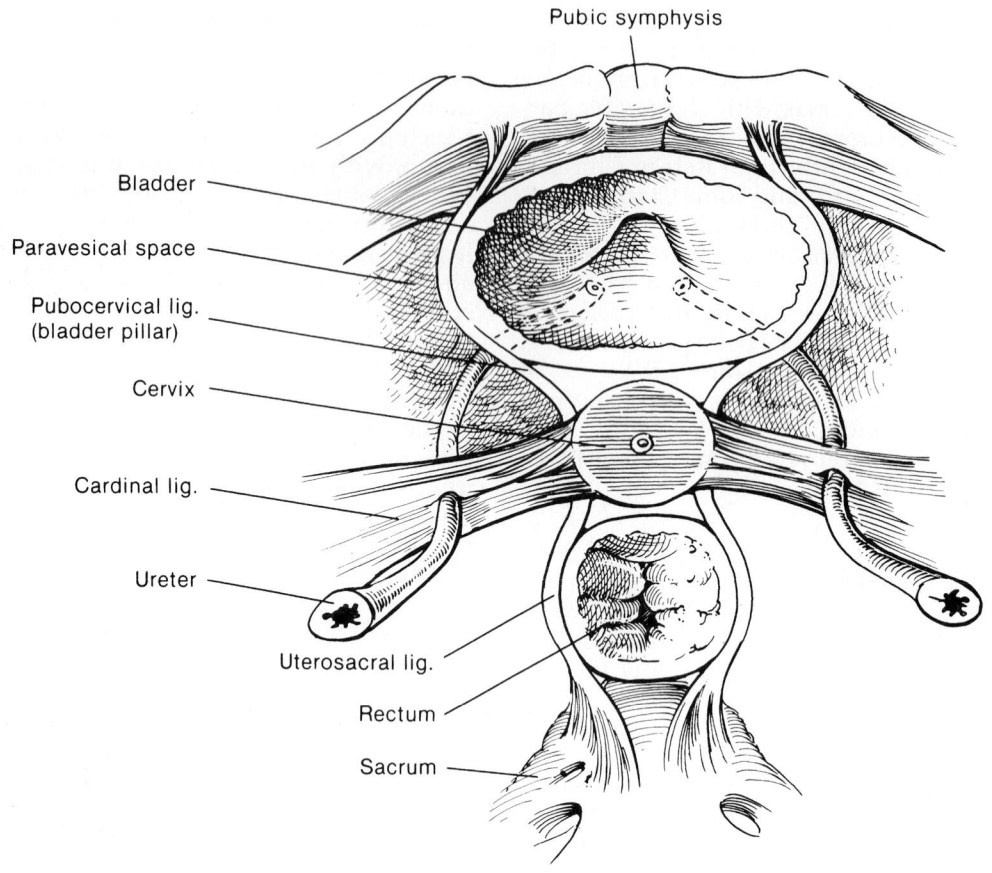

Figure 45–1

Schematic view of pelvic floor showing close anatomic relationships of bladder, ureters, cervix, cardinal and uterosacral ligaments, and rectum.

(Dicker et al, 1982a). The study included women ages 15 to 44 years who had nonemergency, nonradical hysterectomies at nine institutions for all indications excluding pregnancy and gynecologic cancer. A total of 1851 patients were analyzed for 568 vaginal and 1283 abdominal procedures. Surgical complications were grouped into six categories for all patients and compared according to surgical method (Table 45–1).

The overall complication rate was 24.5 per 100 women who had vaginal hysterectomy and 42.8 per 100 women who underwent abdominal hysterectomy. The overall risk for having one or more complications in the abdominal hysterectomy group was 1.7 times the risk for the vaginal hysterectomy group (a 70% higher risk for the abdominal hysterectomy group). Each group had one mortality, resulting in a mortality rate of 2 per 1000 for vaginal hysterectomy and 1 per 1000 for abdominal hysterectomy.

Hysterectomy and Depression

Depression of varied degree is not uncommon after hysterectomy (Melody, 1962; Polivy, 1974; Sloan, 1978). A *posthysterectomy syndrome* has been de-

scribed (Richards, 1974). Clinical studies of this phenomenon show that depression after hysterectomy is more likely in (1) women with a previous history of psychological problems and (2) women who had no organic disease in the extirpated uterus (Barker, 1968; Richards, 1973). However, even excluding women with these features from analysis, depression was still twice as common among women after hysterectomy compared with age-matched women after cholecystectomy or appendectomy (Richards, 1974). At the University of Tennessee colposcopy clinic, we evaluated patient concerns in women undergoing colposcopy, cervical biopsy, and outpatient CO_2 laser surgery for cervical intraepithelial neoplasia (CIN) and found significant patient fears for loss of sexual function, low self-esteem, and high anxiety (McDonald et al, 1989). This demonstrates that outpatient colposcopy and generative tract surgery that is much less extensive than hysterectomy may also cause significant psychological repercussions.

Posthysterectomy depression may stem from a concept that femininity and an intact functioning uterus are one. Perhaps women and men to some degree link the self-image of women with reproductive ability. Menses reminds a woman of her uniqueness, whereas menopause or surgical removal of the

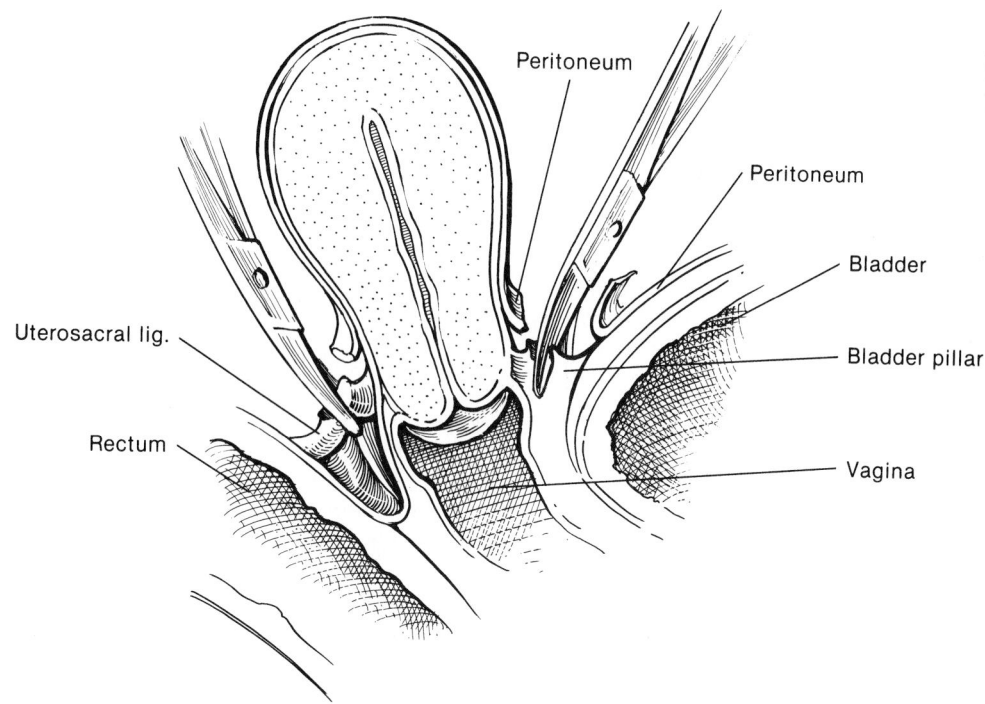

Figure 45–2
Sagittal view of bladder, vagina, uterus, and rectum showing sharp dissection into the vesicocervicovaginal space anteriorly and into the rectovaginal septal space posteriorly during abdominal hysterectomy.

uterus takes away this cue. The essentiality of the uterus and an intact reproductive system may be suppressed in the conscious mind for some individuals who have chosen not to reproduce. However, these same individuals may unconsciously be reassured of their femininity knowing they still have the option to reproduce.

Subconscious and conscious self-image perceptions vary from culture to culture and from person to person within a specific culture. Lost reproductive potential is more likely to cause significant psychological disturbance in a society that regards motherhood and family care as the paramount functions of women. In developed countries the trend toward

equality between men and women with increasing career opportunities open to women may lessen the impact of uterine loss for many (Bunker, 1976). Male attitudes toward women as sexual partners are also linked to the expectations inherent in the society in which they live (Neutens, 1981).

Concomitant factors may potentiate post-hysterectomy depression. Hysterectomy often occurs at a time in the woman's life when other situations are eroding her sense of well-being and femininity. Her children may be having adolescent problems of their own or may have recently left home. Her spouse may be having midlife crisis, may be estranged, or may be insensitive to her needs. She may be coping

Table 45–1. COMPLICATION RATES (PER 100 WOMEN) AMONG WOMEN AGES 15 TO 44 YEARS UNDERGOING VAGINAL AND ABDOMINAL HYSTERECTOMY*

	VAGINAL HYSTERECTOMY	ABDOMINAL HYSTERECTOMY	RISK RATIO
Febrile morbidity	15.3	32.3	2.1
Hemorrhage requiring transfusion	8.3	15.4	1.9
Unintended major surgical procedure	5.1	1.7	0.3
Life-threatening event	0	0.4	—
Rehospitalization	1.8	2.8	1.6
Death	0.2	0.1	0.4
One or more complications	24.5	42.8	1.7

*Vaginal complication $n = 568$; abdominal complication $n = 1283$.
Modified from Dicker RC, Greenspan JR, Strauss LT, et al: Complications of abdominal and vaginal hysterectomy among women of reproductive age in the United States. Am J Obstet Gynecol 1982;144:841, with permission.

with some stigmata of aging (obesity, muscle aches, arthritis, presbyopia) that combine to undermine her youthful self-image.

Before performing a hysterectomy, physicians must strive to recognize all situations that may contribute to posthysterectomy depression. Adverse psychological sequelae are more likely to occur in women with prior depression and/or female identity problems. These issues are explored with the patient and her family before surgery so that she has time to reflect and prepare for complete psychological as well as physical recovery. Time spent carefully discussing these conscious and unconscious concepts may prevent or ameliorate posthysterectomy depression.

Vaginal or Abdominal Hysterectomy?

Vaginal and abdominal hysterectomy each has its advantages and disadvantages, and each method has strong advocates among surgeons today as in the past. The appropriate surgical approach must (1) allow complete evaluation of the particular surgical indication or group of indications and (2) facilitate surgical treatment of the situation. Simply and logically, *these two methods should not be viewed in the light of competition.* Once the decision is made that removal of the uterus will (or is expected to) benefit the patient, the surgical indications usually suggest that one of the two approaches will best fulfill the patient's needs.

Indications for Vaginal Hysterectomy

The surgeon's past experience inevitably colors the decision to proceed vaginally or abdominally. The subjectivity of this decision is highlighted by Joel-Cohen's (1978) observation that, although previous abdominal surgery with adhesive disease constitutes a contraindication to vaginal surgery for many surgeons, he considers previous abdominal surgery associated with peritonitis or intestinal obstruction as an *indication* to try the vaginal approach.

Vaginal hysterectomy should be considered for all patients because of its lower mortality and morbidity compared with abdominal surgery (Dicker et al, 1982a). Heaney (1942) stressed patient benefits from vaginal surgery and advised all gynecologists to ask themselves when considering hysterectomy why the operation could not be performed vaginally.

The vaginal approach is usually selected when hysterectomy is performed for

1. Correction of uterovaginal prolapse
2. Intractable secondary dysmenorrhea
3. Dysfunctional uterine bleeding (DUB) refractory to medical management
4. Symptomatic fibroids appropriate size for safe vaginal removal
5. The very obese patient requiring hysterectomy

Conditions and diagnoses that contraindicate vaginal surgery are

1. A narrow pubic arch
2. Orthopedic problems that make the lithotomy position impossible
3. Severe pelvic adhesive disease
4. Grossly enlarged uterus and/or adnexa
5. Gynecologic cancer

Keep in mind that the above indications and contraindications are not absolute and that certain individual patients and surgeons will be exceptions to these general guidelines. When the ovaries and tubes must be removed with the uterus, this is not always safe or possible by the vaginal approach (Capen et al, 1983). This is more likely with very obese patients when it is very difficult to reach the ovaries and in some elderly postmenopausal patients with ovaries high on the pelvic side wall because of retracted infundibulopelvic ligaments (Porges, 1980). In these situations, the surgeon may have to open the abdomen to remove the ovaries, or it may be possible to save the patient an abdominal incision by removing the ovaries with laparoscopic techniques (Semm, 1986).

Indications for Abdominal Hysterectomy

The abdominal approach is selected for

1. Indications that call for a thorough peritoneal cavity inspection, such as diagnosed gynecologic malignancies and undiagnosed pelvic masses
2. Emergency obstetric situations
3. Removal of uteri and adnexal masses considered too large or too immobile for safe vaginal removal
4. Patients who require other intra-abdominal surgery or evaluation at the time of hysterectomy, such as ventral hernia repair, complex genitointestinal and genitourinary fistulas, extensive adhesiolysis, cholecystectomy, retropubic urethropexy, or sacrocolpopexy

Abdominal hysterectomy may be performed using an *intrafascial technique* when difficult dissection is encountered around the lower uterine segment and cervix. This technique, described in detail by Aldridge and Meredith (1950), hinges on identifying the fascial plane that surrounds the lower uterine segment and cervix.

Richardson (1929) was the first to call attention to the anterior aspect of this tissue, which he called *pubocervical fascia,* in his beautifully illustrated hysterectomy technique publication. He suggested an inverted T-shaped incision in the pubocervical fascia to facilitate distal dissection of the cervix without injury to the bladder and to avoid venous bleeding.

The concept of intrafascial hysterectomy described by Aldridge and Meredith involves a circumferential identification and incision of this fascial plane or "fascial cuff." Surgical dissection is kept medial to or inside of the fascia cuff to avoid injury to the bladder, ureters, and rectum as the cervix is removed. Although a circumferential fascial cuff may not be clearly identified in surgery, the concept of making a circular incision as close as possible to the cervix provides protection against injury to contiguous structures. This fascia, no more than 1 mm thick, contains paracervical vessels and lymphatic vessels that must be removed with the specimen with performing surgery for cervical and uterine cancer. The operation is then properly described as an *extrafascial hysterectomy*. The surgeon should be cognizant of these concepts and should be able to perform both intrafascial and extrafascial dissection as circumstances require.

We expect that the surgeon will not be technically limited to a vaginal or abdominal approach by his or her training. Supervised resident education experience should be sufficient in breadth and quality to produce a physician who can perform both vaginal and abdominal hysterectomy comfortably. The final recommendation for one method over the other should be guided solely by considerations to make the operation the best possible solution for the individual patient's surgical indications.

Pelviscopy/Laparoscopy-Assisted Vaginal Hysterectomy

The term *pelviscopy* was coined by Semm in Kiel, Germany, to describe the laparoscopic surgical procedures that would otherwise require laparotomy to perform. Clinical application has shown that, when proper instrumentation and physician expertise are available, removal of the ovaries and tubes via the laparoscope is a safe alternative to laparotomy (Reich, 1987; Perry and Upchurch, 1990). Removal of the uterus by pelviscopy using a vaginal colpotomy incision was first reported by Reich and colleagues in 1989 and has rapidly become a major technical method of removing the uterus, the *laparoscopy-assisted vaginal hysterectomy* (LAVH). This advanced gynecologic endoscopic procedure offers some patients an alternative to abdominal hysterectomy when it is possible to accomplish vaginal hysterectomy with the assistance of laparoscopy and avoid the morbidity and risks of an abdominal incision.

The initial enthusiasm for LAVH was supported by reports projecting cost savings, decreased hospitalization time, earlier return to work, new developments by the medical technology industry in laparoscopic instrumentation (especially disposable), articles in the popular press and on the Internet supporting this new laparoscopic approach, and of course by the possibility of performing a vaginal procedure in patients who would otherwise be managed by abdominal surgery (Liu, 1992; Padial et al, 1992). However, there was no difference in convalescent time, hospital stay, and operative and postoperative complications between patients prospectively randomized to traditional vaginal hysterectomy and LAVH by Summit and co-investigators (Summitt et al, 1992). Hospital charges were increased for LAVH

related to increased operating room and anesthesia time and use of disposable instrumentation.

More critical reviews of LAVH now question whether the procedure is being overutilized (Weber and Lee, 1996). Twenty-four consecutive patients with an average uterine weight of 270 g were treated with vaginal hysterectomy without complication, with only one patient having laparoscopic assistance (Henry, 1997). Ten patients among this group had uterine leiomyomas with an average uterine weight of 478 g. This series noted that, in the one instance in which laparoscopy was utilized, it was not needed to accomplish vaginal hysterectomy. A group reporting from England suggests that in many instances the laparoscopic portion of the LAVH is a "waste of time" because the operation could have been performed as a routine vaginal hysterectomy (Richardson et al, 1995). Physicians in France reported 126 LAVH procedures with a mean operating time of 72 minutes and emphasized that operating time is reduced by switching to the vaginal stage of the surgery as soon as possible, and that surgeons should always choose vaginal hysterectomy over LAVH unless LAVH is essential to avoid a laparotomy (Aubard et al, 1996).

The decision to perform vaginal hysterectomy versus abdominal hysterectomy may be made more often as the experience and operative skill of the surgeon increases (Kovac, 1995). It is suggested that an individual surgeon may see fewer contraindications to performing vaginal hysterectomy as his or her experience, confidence, and operative skill increase over time. Following his line of thought, perhaps surgeons with less vaginal surgery experience who desire to extend the benefits of a vaginal operation to as many of their patients as possible will choose LAVH, whereas more experienced vaginal surgeons would choose straightforward vaginal surgery for many of these same patients. Among 617 patients operated at one institution between 1989 and 1992, the preoperative decision for route of surgery was compared to the surgical results (Kovac, 1995). Six patients were selected for abdominal hysterectomy, 63 for LAVH procedures, and 548 for vaginal hysterectomy prior to surgery. Thus 98.5% of patients were actually managed by vaginal hysterectomy and 10.2% (63 of 617) were selected for LAVH procedures. One of 548 patients selected for vaginal hysterectomy was converted to abdominal hysterectomy. Only 19% (12 of 63) of patients selected for LAVH procedures actually required laparoscopic techniques to permit vaginal hysterectomy. This series demonstrates that the majority of hysterectomies performed for benign indications may be done vaginally by some operators with about 10% use of LAVH.

Other reports have looked closely at operative time and cost of instrumentation with LAVH. The costs and charges of LAVH compared to total abdominal hysterectomy and vaginal hysterectomy at a large community teaching hospital in Maryland were highest for LAVH (Dorsey et al, 1996). Operative time for LAVH is always increased compared to vaginal hysterectomy and is sometimes increased compared to abdominal hysterectomy. All reviews stress that the increased cost of LAVH compared to vaginal and abdominal hysterectomy is linked to the amount of disposable instrumentation used. Using nondisposable instruments and electrocoagulation rather than disposable stapling devices will aid cost containment (Dorsey et al, 1996; Stovall and Summitt, 1996). The application of LAVH will continue to evolve as this approach finds its proper niche in the repertoire of practitioners. Simply stated, LAVH should be used whenever the surgeon decides the laparoscope is required to remove the uterus vaginally.

Supracervical Hysterectomy

Supracervical hysterectomy is being selected more frequently for patients because this technique is believed by some to offer all the advantages of hysterectomy with less morbidity. Like total hysterectomy, supracervical hysterectomy may be performed via traditional laparotomy or by laparoscopic technique (Semm, 1991). Theoretical advantages of subtotal hysterectomy are less disturbance to bladder and sexual function after hysterectomy because the sympathetic and parasympathetic innervation via the cardinal ligaments and Frankenhauser's plexus are not disturbed during supracervical hysterectomy (Mundy, 1982; Prior et al, 1992). It is also anticipated that there would be decreased operative morbidity from suprecervical hysterectomy versus total hysterectomy or vaginal hysterectomy because most of the surgical injuries to bladder, ureters, and bowel occur during the dissection necessary to remove the cervix and lower uterine segment. Comparison studies between supracervical hysterectomy and total hysterectomy with regard to postoperative urinary tract symptoms and sexual function have to date failed to demonstrate the expected benefits of the supracervical technique (Munro, 1997). Continued investigation using well-designed prospective studies is needed for firm conclusions (Sills et al, 1998). The principal benefit recognized for removing the cervix in the past was the prevention of invasive cervical cancer. Proponents of supracervical hysterectomy point out that current routine screening and office management of preinvasive intraepithelial neoplasia by cryotherapy, laser, or electrical loop excision make removal of the cervix for cancer prophylaxis unnecessary. Some surgeons advise excision or electrodesiccation of the endocervical epithelium during supracervical hysterectomy as additional prophylaxis against the development of cervical cancer (Mettler and Semm, 1995). Developed countries have the resources to detect and treat preinvasive cervical disease which lends support to selection of the technically more simple and safe supracervical hyster-

ectomy rather than total hysterectomy for morbidly obese patients, patients with severe adhesive disease, or patients with no cervical pathology (Jones et al, 1999). However, recognizing the global prevalence of human papillomavirus (HPV) (Bosch et al, 1995) and the fact that invasive cervical cancer is the third most common cancer in women worldwide with about 371,000 new cases reported in 1990 (Parkin et al, 1999), total hysterectomy with removal of the cervix is the best surgical treatment for women who do not benefit from regular screening examinations either because of nonavailability or voluntary nonparticipation.

INAPPROPRIATE INDICATIONS FOR HYSTERECTOMY

Sterilization

Although many hysterectomies in the recent past were performed solely to achieve sterilization, *contraception is now considered an inappropriate indication for hysterectomy* because outpatient treatment (tubal ligation) is safer and more cost-effective (Table 45–2) (Deane and Ulene, 1977). This was demonstrated by Laros and Work (1975), who reported their results with 111 patients who underwent vaginal hysterectomy for sterilization over 5+ years at the University of Michigan Medical Center, contrasted to sterilization by laparoscopic tubal ligation, vaginal tubal ligation, abdominal tubal ligation, and abdominal hysterectomy. Vaginal hysterectomy was associated with significantly greater morbidity, prolonged hospitalization, longer operating time, and greater blood loss than all other sterilization techniques except abdominal hysterectomy. Laros and Work concluded that vaginal hysterectomy is an inappropriate operation for sterilization unless there are other clear gynecologic indications to remove the uterus.

Abdominal hysterectomy, associated with even greater morbidity, is also inappropriate for sterilization. In 1977, Deane and Ulene performed a detailed statistical cost-effectiveness analysis of sterilization accomplished by the Pomeroy procedure versus vaginal or abdominal hysterectomy. They demonstrated the dollar savings accrued by hysterectomy patients as a result of the avoidance of future gynecologic disease and treatments did not offset the higher

Table 45–2. INAPPROPRIATE INDICATIONS FOR HYSTERECTOMY

Sterilization
Cancer prophylaxis*
Cervical intraepithelial neoplasia
Primary dysmenorrhea
Additive indications

*Exception: familial ovarian cancer.

initial cost and risk of death associated with sterilization hysterectomy compared with the Pomeroy procedure. Deane and Ulene concluded that tubal sterilization should always be the procedure of choice compared with hysterectomy sterilization when the patient accepts either method and when there is no other medical reason to recommend hysterectomy.

Cancer Prophylaxis

Cole and Berlin (1977) reported from a public health perspective the projected monetary costs and savings from performing 1 million elective hysterectomies per year in healthy 35-year-old women for indications such as preventing future malignancies of the cervix and endometrium, preventing conception, and preventing menstrual bleeding difficulties. They also considered hysterectomy performed in women at age 45 with bilateral oophorectomy, which would result in additional monetary savings by preventing a certain number of ovarian cancer deaths.

Performing 1 million hysterectomies would cost $2.9 billion. The projected dollar savings over the lifetime of 1 million women was $1.4 billion, resulting in a net cost of $1.5 billion for prophylactic hysterectomies. An estimated 1.3% of 1 million 35-year-old women undergoing hysterectomy would avoid death from cervical and endometrial cancer and would gain 14.3 years of life at a cost of $12,800 per year. If bilateral oophorectomy and hysterectomy were performed on 1 million 45-year-old women, 2.3% would benefit with a gain of 13.9 years of life as a result of eliminating ovarian cancer. The estimated cost per year of life gained was $9800 for the 45-year-old group.

Cole and Berlin (1977) pointed out that they could not assess *possible subjective benefits* from elective hysterectomy, such as elimination of unpredictable bleeding and the fear of pregnancy and a reduction in cancer fears. They expressed concern that oophorectomy in a 45-year-old patient might result in an increased incidence of osteoporosis and atherosclerotic heart disease despite estrogen replacement therapy (Weiss, 1972). Even a 1% or 2% increase in deaths from vascular diseases would offset all gains from uterine and ovarian cancer prevention. Considering all of these variables, Cole and Berlin concluded that *cancer prophylaxis does not justify elective hysterectomy for all women.*

Familial Ovarian Cancer

Familial ovarian neoplasia comprises about 5% to 10% of all ovarian cancers and is recognized as a specific situation that warrants elective prophylactic hysterectomy (Lynch et al, 1993). In 1982 Franceschi and colleagues reported several families in which women of the same or succeeding generations were afflicted with ovarian cancer. The Registry for Fa-

milial Ovarian Cancer established at Roswell Park to study this phenomenon now includes more than 650 families (Piver et al, 1982, 1993). Analysis of this data base shows that families with two first-degree relatives with ovarian cancer are "high-risk" families with regard to epithelial ovarian cancer. All female first-degree relatives in these families have a risk factor of up to 50% for the development of ovarian cancer. The tumor-suppressor gene *BRCA1* was localized to chromosome 17q by genetic linkage studies and cloned in 1994 (Miki et al, 1994). Testing individuals whose pedigree suggests familial breast-ovarian cancer for *BRCA1* identifies carriers who are estimated to have over 90% chance of developing breast or ovarian cancer (Easton et al, 1995). *These women are advised to have prophylactic hysterectomy and oophorectomy as soon as childbearing is completed.* Abdominal hysterectomy has been recommended to allow for cytologic washings and complete inspection of all peritoneal surfaces. The uterus, tubes, and ovaries are completely removed so that no ovarian remnant is left. Another approach is vaginal hysterectomy with complete removal of the tubes and ovaries and laparoscopic evaluation of the peritoneal cavity.

Although this operation does not protect against the occasional ovarian malignancy that seems to arise from am multifocal malignant transformation of the pelvic and abdominal peritoneum, as suggested by Parmley and Woodruff (1974), it is believed to offer significant protection against the more common pattern of ovarian neoplasia for these family members (Tobacman et al, 1982).

Cervical Intraepithelial Neoplasia

Prior to the 1960s, the diagnosis of *carcinoma in situ* (CIS) usually mandated hysterectomy, whereas the diagnosis of cervical dysplasia was poorly understood and often went untreated (Gusberg and Marshall, 1962). Current therapy is based on our understanding that the various grades of dysplasia progress to CIS and then to invasive cancer over a period of time (Richart and Barron, 1969). The term *cervical intraepithelial neoplasia* and the concept that dysplasia and CIS are part of an intraepithelial disease spectrum were introduced in 1966 (Richart, 1967) (see Chapter 55 for a complete discussion of CIN). The disease process is 100% curable while in the intraepithelial state. The depth of cervical tissue that must be excised or destroyed is known from meticulous analysis of conization specimens, as in the study by Anderson and Hartley (1980). They studied 343 cone specimens and observed dysplasia involving endocervical glands at a maximum depth of 5.22 mm, whereas 99.7% of cervical dysplasia and CIS were located within 3.80 mm from the epithelial surface.

Outpatient management of CIN is now well accepted. Colposcopy establishes the diagnosis with rigorous attention to colposcopic protocols designed to avoid missing invasive malignancy (Sevin et al, 1979; Townsend and Richart, 1981). Once the diagnosis is confirmed, treatment involves excisional conization or local cervical destructive therapy. *Hysterectomy is not appropriate therapy for the CIN patient unless there are other indications that call for removal of the uterus* (Burghardt and Holzer, 1980; Goodman et al, 1986; Wilbanks, 1988; Reid, 1989). As emphasized by Boyes and collaborators (1970), all patients need careful lifelong follow-up with attention to the vaginal vault, vulva, and periurethral and perianal regions whether they have been treated by hysterectomy or by conization. An essential part of outpatient management is helping CIN patients understand how essential lifelong follow-up is to prevention of death from invasive cancer. The fact that virtually all patients with CIN have the sexually transmitted HPV integrated into their DNA as an oncogene (Cullen et al, 1991) should be conveyed in understandable terms to give meaning to the recommendation for repetitive, lifelong follow-up visits.

Primary Dysmenorrhea

Primary dysmenorrhea generally presents soon after menarche and is not associated with organic disease. The disorder affects more than 50% of menstruating women and is often sufficiently severe to interfere with daily activities (Sobczyk, 1980). An estimated 10% of adult women are incapacitated for 1 to 3 days per month from dysmenorrhea, which results in an estimated 600 million work-hours lost annually in the United States (Dawood, 1986). The mechanism of cyclic pain is produced by intense uterine contractions and uterine muscle ischemia caused by increased endometrial prostaglandin $F_{2\alpha}$, which occurs in the luteal phase (Halbert et al, 1976; Willman et al, 1976). Because primary dysmenorrhea requires ovulatory cycles, patients who also desire contraception are treated with combination estrogen-progestin birth control, which relieves symptoms in about 90% of patients. Most patients with contraindications to or who fail to respond to oral contraceptive therapy are relieved by specific prostaglandin inhibitors such as indomethacin, ibuprofen, mefenamic acid, and naproxen. These nonsteroidal anti-inflammatory drugs have direct analgesic properties and also suppress menstrual fluid levels of prostaglandin (Halbert et al, 1975; Chan et al, 1981).

Transcutaneous electrical nerve stimulation (TENS) employing high-frequency electrical stimuli significantly relieves primary dysmenorrhea and reduces the amount of pain medications required (Lundeberg et al, 1985; Neighbours et al, 1987; Dawood and Ramos, 1990). Because TENS therapy involves no medication, it may be evaluated for patients in whom medications have been limited by side effects or have brought only partial pain relief.

Hysterectomy has no role in the treatment of primary dysmenorrhea.

Additive Indications

Periodically we see patients who have clusters of desires, complaints, and problems that may seem to indicate hysterectomy as the solution. An example is a 35-year-old woman who requests sterilization, has a fear of ovarian cancer but no familial history, has CIN, has chronic cervicitis with leukorrhea, has premenstrual tension, has mild stress incontinence, and has asymptomatic small fibroids. We readily recognize that each of these conditions is insufficient in itself to warrant hysterectomy, but may they be gathered together to form a valid indication for hysterectomy? The answer is no. Thompson and Birch (1981) addressed this issue and advised that adding patients' insubstantial symptoms, signs, and complaints together does not produce a valid indication for hysterectomy. In these situations we must explain to the patient that hysterectomy is not a panacea and must help her find appropriate remedies for each individual problem.

CONTEMPORARY INDICATIONS FOR HYSTERECTOMY

Contemporary indications for hysterectomy range from crises such as life-threatening obstetric catastrophes to more subtle, subjective, quality-of-life indications, such as pelvic pressure, secondary dysmenorrhea, and dyspareunia. Indications may be categorized for discussion as *anatomic, functional, infectious, emergency* (obstetric and traumatic), and *neoplastic* (both benign and malignant) (Table 45–3). Patients may have surgical indications that overlap several groups in this schema: for example, uterine fibroids (benign neoplastic indication) that cause pelvic pain and DUB (functional indications).

Anatomic Indications

Most anatomic indications for hysterectomy are derangements in pelvic anatomy resulting from pelvic relaxation. Pelvic support loss often stems from tissue or fascial injury during childbirth. The condition is further aggravated by anything that increases intra-abdominal pressure, such as obesity, ascites, chronic pulmonary disease with continual coughing, and uterine enlargement from benign and malignant tumors. Resulting anatomic problems are uterine descensus, cystourethrocele, enterocele, rectocele, and rectal prolapse. Patients may present with one or (often) with combinations of these situations (e.g., cystourethrocele, uterine descensus, and enterocele). *Unless fertility is being preserved, the best surgical correction of these problems involves removal of the uterus*

Table 45-3. CONTEMPORARY INDICATIONS FOR HYSTERECTOMY

Anatomic
Pelvic relaxation
  Uterine descensus
  Cystourethrocele
  Rectocele
  Enterocele
  Rectal prolapse
Abnormal anatomy
  Developmental anomalies
  Uterointestinal fistula
  Pelvic arteriovenous fistula or malformation

Functional
Urinary incontinence
Dysfunctional uterine bleeding
Dyspareunia
Secondary dysmenorrhea
Chronic pelvic pain

Infectious
Chronic pelvic inflammatory disease
Pyometra
Tuberculosis

Emergency
Obstetric
Uterine atony
Uterine rupture
Abdominal pregnancy
Extension of uterine incision
Uterine inversion
Placenta previa
Placenta accreta, increta, percreta
Chorioamnionitis
Septic abortion
Trauma (rare)
Motor vehicle accident
Lower abdominal penetrating injury
Hemorrhage from perforated intrauterine contraceptive
  device

Neoplastic (Benign)
Fibroids
Endometriosis
Adenomyosis
Ovarian tumors

Neoplastic (Malignant)
Endometrial cancer
Ovarian cancer (including familial)
Cervical cancer
Vaginal cancer
Uterine sarcoma
Fallopian tube cancer
Gestational trophoblastic disease
Nongynecologic pelvic cancers
Metastatic cancer to uterus, tubes, and ovaries
Colon/rectal cancer
Bladder cancer

and restoration of pelvic floor support. In most patients, this is accomplished by a vaginal hysterectomy with cystocele, rectocele, and enterocele repair as indicated.

Functional Indications

Hysterectomy is often considered to relieve specific complaints that aggravate and inconvenience pa-

tients. These subjective symptoms and complaints may constitute valid or invalid surgical indications contingent on whether or not the patient's need and desire to correct these conditions warrants surgery. Urinary incontinence, menstrual disturbances (DUB, perimenopausal bleeding), dysmenorrhea, dyspareunia, and chronic pelvic pain (CPP) all fall into this category. Medical management of these subjectively distressing symptoms and complaints must be thoroughly tested using every reasonable alternative before a discussion of hysterectomy. Keeping in mind Finney's (1970) admonition that all surgical procedures should be performed "to save life, to relieve suffering, and to correct deformity," these non–life-threatening conditions call for surgery only if we can hope to relieve suffering or correct function or deformity. However, the variability of both pain perception and its adverse impact on the quality of life from patient to patient makes it very difficult to quantify the need for and possible benefits from hysterectomy for some of these patients.

Dysfunctional Uterine Bleeding

DUB may cause significant patient apprehension and inconvenience and may be associated with pain and anemia (see also Chapter 24). *DUB is a valid indication for removal of the uterus only when it cannot be corrected by medical management.* As discussed by Field (1988) in his excellent review, abnormal uterine bleeding may be categorized into two major etiologic groups: anatomic and functional. Anatomic bleeding (Table 45–4) is caused by a specific lesion in the genital tract. DUB also occurs in patients without genital tract pathology and is associated with ovarian dysfunction and/or anovulation. Approximately 10% of DUB is ovulatory and is most frequently encountered during the adult reproductive years. The remaining 90% of DUB is anovulatory in nature and seen most often at the beginning and end of adult reproductive life, in adolescence and in perimeno-

Table 45-4. ANATOMIC CAUSES OF ABNORMAL UTERINE BLEEDING

Vulvovaginal	**Uterine**
Cancer	Polyps
Trauma	Myomas
Infection	Adenomyosis
Atrophy	Cancer
	Endometritis
Cervical	Intrauterine contraceptive
Polyps	device
Carcinoma	Tuberculosis
Condylomata	
Cervicitis	**Tubal**
	Salpingitis
Gestational	Cancer
Ectopic	
Abortion/retained	**Ovarian**
products	Neoplasia: benign, malignant,
Trophoblastic disease	or steroid producing

Modified from Field CS: Dysfunctional uterine bleeding. Prim Care 1988;15:561, with permission.

Table 45–5. BLEEDING PATTERNS ASSOCIATED WITH OVULATORY AND ANOVULATORY DYSFUNCTIONAL UTERINE BLEEDING

OVULATORY
Mixed etiologic factors
  Short proliferative and/or secretory phases
  Midcycle spotting
  Polymenorrhea (regular intervals of uterine bleeding fewer than 18 days apart)
Corpus uterine insufficiency
  Luteal phase defect
  Premenstrual spotting
  Menorrhagia or hypermenorrhea (excessive uterine bleeding in both amount and duration occurring at regular intervals)
Prolonged corpus luteum activity
  Persistent corpus luteum (Halban's disease)
  Irregular shedding
  Menorrhagia or hypermenorrhea
  Oligomenorrhea (irregular bleeding episodes more than 45 days apart)

ANOVULATORY
Bleeding patterns
  Oligomenorrhea
  Hypermenorrhea
  Menometrorrhagia (excessive uterine bleeding at irregular intervals)

Modified from Kempers RD: Dysfunctional uterine bleeding. Gynecol Obstet 1990;14:1, with permission.

pausal age groups. An outline of ovulatory and anovulatory DUB and the associated bleeding patterns is helpful to the clinician dealing with this important and common gynecologic complaint (Table 45–5) (Kempers, 1990).

A complete history, physical examination, and blood work, including an endocrine profile, may point to diagnoses such as drug-induced hypothalamic dysfunction, anorexia nervosa, pregnancy, ovarian tumor, fibroids, blood dyscrasia, liver disease, estrogen-progesterone imbalance, hyperprolactinemia, adrenal hyperplasia, hypothyroidism, or hyperthyroidism. An endometrial biopsy, hysteroscopy, and/or dilatation and curettage (D&C) may diagnose anovulatory bleeding, endometritis, endometrial polyps, submucous fibroids, endometrial hyperplasia, or endometrial malignancy. *Bleeding from endocrine disturbance, blood dyscrasia, and infection should be medically managed, reserving hysteroscopic endometrial cavity ablation or hysterectomy for patients who fail to respond to medical control* (Goldrath et al, 1981) (see also "Alternatives to Hysterectomy" below).

Secondary Dysmenorrhea

Secondary dysmenorrhea refers to pain associated with menses occurring with pathologic conditions known to cause painful menstruation, such as uterine leiomyomas, endometriosis, endometrial polyps, cervical stenosis, pelvic inflammatory disease (PID), and adenomyosis (see also Chapter 23). Patients with secondary dysmenorrhea are treated symptomatically with prostaglandin inhibitors and antibiotics if appropriate. There should be an attempt to correct the underlying pathologic factors with lesser procedures than hysterectomy, such as D&C, laparoscopic lysis of adhesions, and/or CO_2 laser ablation of endometriosis. *Hysterectomy should be promptly offered if*

these measures fail and if fertility is not desired or possible.

Dyspareunia and Chronic Pelvic Pain

Dyspareunia and CPP are complex diagnostic and therapeutic dilemmas because of the highly subjective emotional and sensory nature of these symptoms and the wide spectrum of organic, somatic, and psychogenic causes from which they may arise. CPP is frequently seen in clinical practice. Up to 20% of all diagnostic laparoscopies are performed for CPP (Levitan et al, 1985; Reiter and Gambone, 1990). In the CREST study, CPP accounted for 12.2% of all indications for hysterectomy, ranking third behind uterine fibroids and bleeding disturbances (Dicker et al, 1982a). Underlying causes of CPP may be organic pathologic factors, such as endometriosis; nongynecologic somatic pathologic factors, such as irritable bowel syndrome (Young et al, 1976); or a psychogenic pain disorder, such as history of sexual abuse (Walker et al, 1988). Alternatively, psychogenic and organic causes may coexist (Reiter, 1990). In fact, all chronic painful physical conditions may cause psychological problems that in turn produce physical manifestations. Testing CPP patients reveals a typical psychological profile in patients both with and without demonstrable tissue pathologic factors (Renaer et al, 1979; Slocumb, 1984). These patients display excessive depression, anxiety, and preoccupation with health.

Laparoscopy is often necessary to exclude intraabdominal causes such as endometriosis, pelvic adhesive disease, chronic PID, or adnexal torsion. In general, on the basis of laparoscopic findings, three groups of patients emerge: (1) those with a normal pelvis (negative laparoscopy), (2) those with endometriosis, and (3) those with pelvic adhesive disease.

The reported percentage of CPP patients with normal pelvic laparoscopic findings varies from 14% to 86% and may be expected to average about 30% (Liston et al, 1972; Goldstein et al, 1980; Lundberg et al, 1984; Cunanan et al, 1983; Kresch et al, 1984; Bahary and Gorodeski, 1987; Kinch, 1987). Approximately 45% of CPP patients with normal laparoscopic examinations have nongynecologic somatic disorders, such as myofascial syndrome, irritable bowel syndrome, or urethral syndrome, and 50% have significant psychopathology. Coexistent somatic and psychological pathologic factors are found in about 20% of patients with normal laparoscopic results (Reiter, 1990).

Management of dyspareunia and CPP often requires the consultation of a clinical psychologist, psychiatrist, anesthesiologist, gastroenterologist, neurologist, and urologist to arrive at a diagnosis and deliver optimal treatment. Multidisciplinary pain clinics have been established to coordinate this comprehensive approach (Rapkin and Kames, 1987; Gambone and Reiter, 1990). *Hysterectomy is appropriate for the CPP patient who has been diagnosed with organic pathologic factors that cannot be controlled by medical therapy.* Clearly, patients with myofascial pain, irritable bowel syndrome, urethral syndrome, and psychogenic causes of pain will not benefit from hysterectomy.

Infectious Indications

Total abdominal hysterectomy with bilateral salpingo-oophorectomy constitutes definitive therapy for severe genital tract infections such as chronic recurrent PID, pyometra, and genital tuberculosis. Extensive extirpative surgery is generally not performed in the acute phase of pelvic infection. Antibiotic therapy is initiated and surgery is reserved for unresponsive infections or drainage of abscess collections. Pelvic abscesses may be successfully drained by percutaneous catheter placement guided by ultrasonography (Gerzof et al, 1981) or laparoscopy (Reich and McGlynn, 1987). The infected uterus (pyometra) is treated with appropriate antibiotics and is drained by placing a small catheter in the endometrial cavity before performing hysterectomy. Genital tuberculosis accounts for 1% to 2% of all pelvic infections. Surgery is not performed on a patient known to have genital tuberculosis without 3 to 4 months of preoperative antibiotics. Genital tuberculosis almost always results in sterility. Total abdominal hysterectomy and bilateral salpingo-oophorectomy combined with extensive preoperative and postoperative drug therapy give the best chance for cure (Schaefer, 1981).

Emergency Indications

Most hysterectomies performed for life-threatening situations involve obstetric indications. In fact, the first successful cesarean hysterectomy was performed for a primigravida dwarf with no possibility of vaginal delivery in 1876 by Eduardo Porro in Milan. A healthy female infant weighing 3300 g was born at term by cesarean section. To control hemorrhage, Porro performed a supracervical hysterectomy by passing a wire snare around the lower uterine segment. The patient was fully recovered in 40 days (Durfee, 1969).

Emergency cesarean hysterectomy is occasionally performed for pregnancies complicated by trauma, such as a motor vehicle accident or gunshot wound. However, most of these desperate obstetric situations stem from uncontrolled intrapartum or postpartum hemorrhage caused by uterine atony, uterine rupture, abdominal pregnancy, extension of the myometrial incision into uterine vessels, uterine inversion, placenta previa, and placenta accreta, increta, and percreta. As the cesarean section rate increased in the 1980s, there was a parallel increase in uterine rupture, placenta previa, and placenta accreta (Haynes and Martin, 1979; Ashton et al, 1985). Chorioamnionitis from prolonged labors and septic abortion are uncommon indications for cesarean hysterectomy in developed nations today.

Cesarean Hysterectomy—Morbidity and Mortality

Generally, the combined-procedure cesarean hysterectomy results in significantly more patient complications than either abdominal hysterectomy or cesarean section performed independently. Analysis of deaths resulting from hysterectomy during 1979 and 1980 in the United States established the mortality rate for abdominal hysterectomy at 0.086% (8.6 per 10,000 procedures) when the indications for surgery excluded obstetrics and cancer (Wingo et al, 1985). In the same study, vaginal hysterectomy performed for indications excluding obstetrics and cancer exhibited a much lower mortality rate of 0.027% (2.7 per 10,000 procedures). The operative mortality rate for cesarean section performed alone is 0.10% (10 per 10,000 procedures) (Barden, 1981). Park and Duff (1980) carefully reviewed 3913 patients who underwent cesarean hysterectomy, finding 28 maternal deaths for an operative mortality rate of 0.71% (71 per 10,000 procedures (Table 45–6). They summarized three other major adverse outcomes from ce-

Table 45–6. PATIENT MORTALITY WITH VAGINAL, ABDOMINAL, AND CESAREAN HYSTERECTOMY

HYSTERECTOMY TYPE	MORTALITY
Vaginal	0.027% (2.7/10,000)*
Abdominal	0.086% (8.6/10,000)*
Cesarean abdominal	0.710% (71/10,000)†

*Data from Wingo PA et al (1985).
†Data from Park and Duff (1980).

sarean hysterectomy: (1) perioperative hemorrhage, (2) infection-related complications, and (3) urinary tract injury.

In addition to true emergency situations, cesarean hysterectomy is performed for elective indications such as endometriosis, dysmenorrhea, fibroids, dysfunctional bleeding, and sterilization. Patients undergoing elective cesarean hysterectomy are usually in much better condition at the time of surgery than emergent patients and therefore have better outcomes. Pletsch and Sandberg (1963) suggested a cesarean hysterectomy classification scheme so that morbidity and mortality could be evaluated in terms of these distinctly different surgical indications. They suggested that cases involving life-threatening hemorrhage, infection, or cancer that require removal of the uterus at the time of delivery be classified as *indicated cesarean hysterectomies*. They called all other cases *elective cesarean hysterectomies*. This classification has generally been used by subsequent investigators and facilitates reporting and comparison of cesarean hysterectomy results.

The increased risk for complications inherent in cesarean hysterectomy needs to be evaluated when the operation is considered. Although indicated cesarean hysterectomies often severely limit the time for choices and deliberations by the patient and physician, the elective cases should be discussed carefully with the patient. Clearly, the decision for elective cesarean hysterectomy exposes the patient to increased risk and must be supported by a valid obstetric indication for cesarean section and a concurrent valid gynecologic indication for hysterectomy (Park and Duff, 1980; Plauche, 1986).

An *interval hysterectomy* may often be the best clinical decision for patients considering the likelihood of mandatory blood transfusion with cesarean hysterectomy. Homologous blood transfusion carries a risk for transmission of hepatitis and the human immunodeficiency virus (HIV) even with modern surveillance. Blood screened negative for HIV may still contain the virus because the test remains negative until the HIV-infected blood donor has been infected about 3 months or longer (Visscher, 1994). Patient counseling and preparations for any elective surgery likely to require transfusion should include alternatives to homologous blood transfusion, such as the use of autologous banked blood, acute normovo-lemic hemodilution, and intraoperative blood salvage (National Institutes of Health, 1990; Toy, 1990).

Benign Neoplastic Indications

Leiomyoma

Most hysterectomies are performed for benign indications. Over a 10-year period Amirikia and Evans (1979) reported that fibroids, adenomyosis, and endometriosis were the surgical indications for 77% of hysterectomies performed at Hutzel Hospital, Detroit, whereas 9% were performed for malignant disease. Leiomyomas were the most common indication for abdominal hysterectomy in the CREST study, accounting for 40.2% of 1283 operations (Dicker et al, 1982a). Approximately 175,000 hysterectomies are performed for leiomyomas in the United States each year (Pokras and Hufnagel, 1987). In Athens, Greece, uterine leiomyomas were the most common indication for hysterectomy for all age groups, especially middle-aged patients (41 to 55 years); 67% of operations over a 16-year period were for myomas (Chryssikopoulos and Loghis, 1986).

Uterine fibroids are the most frequently occurring benign tumors in women and in themselves do not constitute a reason for hysterectomy unless they (1) are large enough to cause pelvic pain, pelvic pressure, bladder urgency, rectal pressure, or ureteral obstruction; (2) cause menorrhagia and anemia uncorrectable by curettage and progestins; (3) are observed to increase in size rapidly (in which case uterine sarcoma is rarely the cause of enlargement); or (4) obscure clinical pelvic examination (Table 45–7). Even with modern imaging techniques we occasionally have the same difficulty as our predecessors 100 years ago distinguishing between an adnexal mass and a large fibroid (Fig. 45–3). Asymptomatic fibroids are usually diagnosed during routine pelvic examination (Romney and Ober, 1981). When the examiner is certain that the enlargement is uterine rather than ovarian, he or she should re-examine the patient in about 3 months to ensure there is no rapid change in size unless previous examinations have documented a stable process. Sarcomatous degeneration of leiomyomas is a rare event, estimated to occur in approximately 0.5% of cases (Novak and Woodruff,

---

☐ **Table 45–7.** LEIOMYOMAS—WHEN TO CONSIDER HYSTERECTOMY

To relieve:	Pelvic pain
	Pelvic pressure
	Bladder symptoms
	Rectal pressure
	Ureteral obstruction
To correct:	Dysfunctional uterine bleeding and anemia unresponsive to curettage and progestins
To diagnose:	Rapid increased size of fibroids
To permit:	Adequate pelvic examination

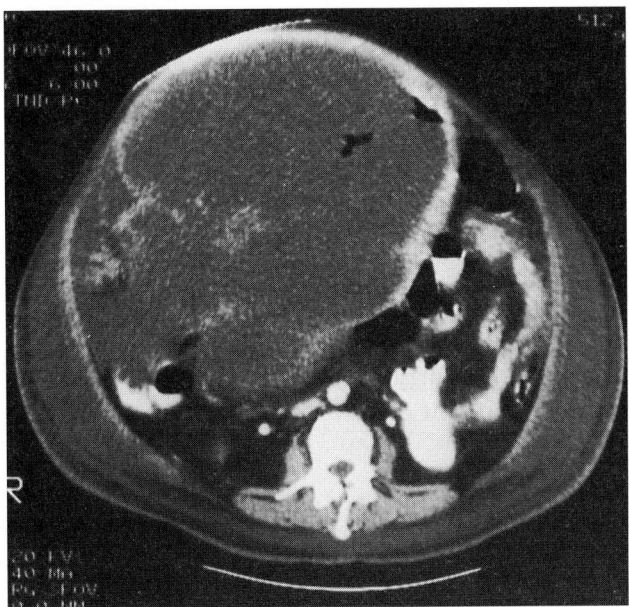

Figure 45–3
This huge abdominopelvic mass appeared to be an ovarian carcinoma that contained gas, suggesting bowel invasion on CT scan. Clinical examination could not discern between an ovarian or uterine mass. Exploratory laparotomy established the diagnosis to be a uterine sarcoma with all bowel intact. An area of intrauterine tumor necrosis with gas formation simulated bowel fistualization. (Courtesy of Dr. T. Morgan, Department of Obstetrics and Gynecology, Gynecologic Oncology Section; and Drs. J. LePage and H. Gould, Department of Radiology, University of Tennessee Medical Center, Knoxville.)

1967). Pelvic ultrasonography enables the clinician to document and observe asymptomatic uterine enlargement.

At some point the uterus becomes so enlarged that both clinical and radiologic examination are unable to distinguish between fibroids and adnexal pathology. Managed care planners strive to pinpoint exactly how large the uterus needs to be to "qualify" for this common clinical diagnostic dilemma; however, the uterus can be no larger than about 14 weeks-size to present this problem in an obese patient. In thinner patients the uterine size is usually somewhat larger. The clinical recommendation is *when uterine fibroid enlargement makes it difficult to rule out other pelvic pathology, then laparoscopic surgery is warranted to establish the diagnosis, and hysterectomy is certainly appropriate in these otherwise healthy asymptomatic patients if the uterine enlargement cannot be followed accurately by noninvasive means* (Thompson and Birch, 1981).

Treatment options now available for women who wish to retain their fertility or their uterus vary according to the patient's age, severity of symptoms, myoma size, and patient preferences. Alternatives to hysterectomy (radical therapy) include (1) observation (expectant therapy), (2) myomectomy (conservative therapy), and (3) medical management with progestins and gonadotropin-releasing hormone analogs (GnRHa). Perimenopausal patients may be observed with the expectation that leiomyomas will regress after menopause. Presurgical treatment with GnRHa agonists (leuprolide acetate [Lupron]) facilitates myomectomy by reduction of myoma size and vascularity (Marut, 1989). Lupron therapy thus reduces surgical risk related to tumor size and may totally eliminate the need for hysterectomy if repetitive treatments are given to shrink leiomyomas until ovarian failure occurs (Friedman, 1989). Myomectomy is considered for patients with symptomatic fibroids who desire children or for women with infertility secondary to leiomyomas (Hilgers, 1986). Approximately 18,000 myomectomies are performed annually in the United States (Pokras and Hufnagel, 1987).

Endometriosis

Endometriosis is the abnormal growth and location of endometrial tissue outside the uterine cavity (see also Chapter 30). Since endometriosis was first described at autopsy by Von Rokitansky (1860), many students of the disease have attempted to explain its pathogenesis. Although a benign process, endometriosis displays some features of malignancy in its ability to proliferate, to locally invade adjacent tissues (Panganiban and Cornog, 1972), and metastasize to lymph nodes (Koss, 1963) and other visceral (Felson et al, 1960) and cutaneous (Steck and Helwig, 1965) sites distant from the pelvis. Endometriosis is a major cause of primary infertility (Surrey and Halme, 1989). It rarely undergoes malignant transformation (Mesko et al, 1988). Pelvic pain, dyspareunia, and dysmenorrhea are the most common complaints associated with endometriosis. When fertility is no longer desired or possible, hysterectomy is performed for symptomatic endometriosis with preservation of normal ovaries. *Hysterectomy is appropriate first-line treatment for severe endometriosis for women who have completed childbearing* (Wheeler and Malinak, 1989).

Adenomyosis

Adenomyosis is a benign invasion of the endometrial basalis layer downward into the myometrium, which undergoes hyperplasia and hypertrophy (Novak and Woodruff, 1979). The diagnosis of adenomyosis rests on the finding of ectopic endometrial glands and stroma within the myometrium. The fact that many women with adenomyosis are asymptomatic, combined with the nonspecific nature of symptoms and varied physical findings, has made correct preoperative diagnosis unlikely. This is confirmed by the CREST study (Lee et al, 1984), which matched preoperative diagnoses with the pathologic findings from hysterectomy. Potentially confirmable preoperative diagnoses were (1) CIN, (2) PID, (3) leiomyomas, (4) adenomyosis, (5) endometriosis, and (6) endometrial hyperplasia. Among these, the least-confirmed preoperative diagnoses were adenomyosis (48%) and endometriosis (47%). Twelve per cent of patients thought to have adenomyosis preoperatively had normal uteri, and 40% had other pathology.

In 1989, Gambone et al reviewed the validity of the preoperative indication for hysterectomy with the diagnoses established after surgery. Adenomyosis was the least-confirmed preoperative diagnosis. They concluded that adenomyosis was not a reliable preoperative indication for hysterectomy because of its low verification rate, and patients with pelvic discomfort and recurrent bleeding suspected to have adenomyosis should undergo appropriate preoperative evaluations (consultation in pelvic pain clinic, attempted medical management, possible laparoscopy, D&C, hormonal treatment) before hysterectomy.

Now adenomyosis has been successfully diagnosed by magnetic resonance imaging (MRI) and transvaginal ultrasound (TVS) prior to surgery. Reinhold et al. (1996) compared the accuracy of TVS and MRI for diagnosis of adenomyosis in 119 consecutive patients prior to hysterectomy and found that the positive predictive value was 71% for TVS and 65% for MRI. They concluded that TVS is as accurate as MRI for the diagnosis of uterine adenomyosis. MRI has been reported to achieve 90% accuracy in distinguishing adenomyosis from leiomyomas (Mark and Hricak, 1987). Because adenomyosis is usually treated by hysterectomy, whereas leiomyomas may be treated by myomectomy, this information can be crucial in preoperative planning.

Symptomatic adenomyosis in patients who wish to preserve fertility may be temporarily treated with danazol and antiprostaglandins. Because there is no satisfactory long-term medical management for adenomyosis, *hysterectomy is definitive treatment and may establish the diagnosis* (Azziz, 1989).

Benign Ovarian Tumors

Benign ovarian tumors frequently lead to laparotomy, which may be accompanied by hysterectomy.

When an ovarian tumor is found, the uncertainty of its histology adds greatly to preoperative anxiety. The absolute determination of benignity versus malignancy is almost always made by frozen section at laparotomy. Exceptional features that strongly suggest malignancy are pleural effusion, ascites, omental cake visible on computerized tomographic (CT) scan, or elevated serum CA-125. The clinician may somewhat alleviate concerns and add direction to patient decisions by reviewing statistical probabilities for various ovarian tumor types occurring at different ages. The patient who is 40 years of age and older is not as likely to be concerned with fertility preservation and is also known to have greater chance for a malignant ovarian tumor than the younger patient.

At one institution, 861 ovarian tumors were reviewed over a 10-year period. There was an increased likelihood for malignant ovarian tumors with increasing age, peaking at ages 60 to 69 years; at this time of life, 49% of ovarian tumors were malignant. Premenopausal women had a 10% chance for malignant ovarian tumors compared with a 45% chance for malignancy among postmenopausal women (Table 45–8). The most frequent benign ovarian tumor in this group was mature cystic teratoma (dermoid), and the most frequent malignant tumor was serous epithelial ovarian cancer (Koonings et al, 1989).

Finding a normal opposite ovary when removing a benign ovarian tumor may present a dilemma. Should it be left in place or prophylactically removed? Some ovarian cancer patients have had prior surgical removal of one ovary for benign reasons. Terz et al (1967) reported that 8.8% of their ovarian cancer patients had undergone previous pelvic surgery and that 3.8% were age 40 or older at the time of their surgery. Similarly, Grundsell and associates (1981) reported that 21 (6%) of 352 ovarian cancer patients had had previous pelvic surgery and that 16 (4.6%) were age 40 or older at the time. Subsequent removal of the retained ovary for benign problems such as pain, or a second benign neoplasm may occur. This was reported in 3.6% of McKenzie's patients (1968), and Christ and Lotze (1975) reported a

Table 45–8. PATIENT AGE AND PROBABILITY FOR MALIGNANT OVARIAN NEOPLASMS

AGE (Years)	% MALIGNANT OVARIAN NEOPLASMS	TOTAL NO. MALIGNANT OVARIAN NEOPLASMS	TOTAL NO. OVARIAN NEOPLASMS
≤19	8.2	5	61
20–29	4.1	12	294
30–39	14.0	24	171
40–49	35.2	45	128
50–59	46.2	48	104
60–69	49.4	39	79
≥70	29.2	7	24
All ages	20.9	180	861

Modified from Koonings PP, Campbell K, Mishell DR, et al: Relative frequency of primary ovarian neoplasms: a 10-year review. Obstet Gynecol 1989;74:921, with permission from the American College of Obstetricians and Gynecologists.

3.3% rate of subsequent oophorectomy in their patients. Functional ovarian tumors and polycystic ovaries are associated with an increased risk for endometrial cancer (McDonald et al, 1977b).

The histology of the ovarian tumor being removed has some relation to the likelihood of bilateral occurrence. Mucinous epithelial cystadenomas are rarely bilateral, whereas serous epithelial tumors are bilateral in up to 10% of patients (DiSaia and Creasman, 1984). About 10% of ovarian fibromas are bilateral, and mature cystic teratomas are bilateral in 15% to 20% of patients (Doss et al, 1977; Gallup and Talledo, 1987).

Once the decision is made to perform bilateral oophorectomy, *the uterus is usually removed because there is no known benefit from its retention and there remains a potential for bleeding disturbances and even malignant change in subsequent years with hormone replacement therapy* (McDonald et al, 1977a). An unusual exception to this approach is the patient who desires intrauterine pregnancy by embryo transfer techniques after removal of her ovaries (Feichtinger and Kemeter, 1985). Some patients insist on retaining the opposite ovary at any age despite all possibilities for future benign and malignant tumors. All options should be discussed in preoperative patient counseling.

Malignant Neoplastic Indications

Endometrial Cancer

Carcinoma of the endometrium is the most frequently diagnosed gynecologic cancer in the United States, with approximately 37,400 new cases and 6400 mortalities expected in 1999 (Landis et al, 1999) (see also Chapter 58). *Surgical removal of the uterus is the principal treatment for endometrial cancer.* In 1989 the International Federation of Gynaecology and Obstetrics (FIGO) replaced the clinical staging of endometrial cancer with a surgical staging system. The uterus is generally removed even in patients with distant metastases if they are medically fit because it increases pelvic disease control. Patients with FIGO stage IA G1 lesions with minimal likelihood for spread beyond the uterus are typically treated by extrafascial abdominal hysterectomy and bilateral salpino-oophorectomy (FIGO Cancer Committee, 1989). Vaginal hysterectomy should be considered for very obese endometrial cancer patients who are medically high risk for abdominal surgery (Malkasian et al, 1980; Peters et al, 1983). Advanced stages require the addition of radiation therapy, which may be given with equal effectiveness preoperatively or postoperatively, to decrease vaginal and pelvic recurrence rates and increase overall cure (Lanciano et al, 1990).

The modern therapeutic approach is initial surgical removal of the uterus in medically fit patients, with thorough inspection of the entire peritoneal cavity, washings for cytology, and sampling of the para-aortic and pelvic lymph nodes. The lymphadenectomy allows some patients without nodal metastases to forego pelvic radiation therapy and may increase survival in patients with pelvic node metastases (Kilgore et al, 1995). Postoperative radiation therapy is given tailored to the surgical findings (Creasman et al, 1987; Hacker, 1989; Peters, 1995). Patients with uterine papillary serous carcinoma of the endometrium, an uncommon histologic type, are all treated with initial complete surgical staging and are found to have over 50% likelihood of extrauterine disease that requires further treatment with radiation therapy and chemotherapy (Goff et al, 1994).

Ovarian Cancer

Ovarian cancer continues to be a major problem among gynecologic malignancies because of late detection (see also Chapter 60). Approximately 75% of all newly diagnosed patients have advanced disease (FIGO stages III and IV) when initially seen (McGarrity et al, 1982). Some 25,200 newly diagnosed patients and 14,500 patient mortalities are estimated for 1999 in the United States by the American Cancer Society (Landis et al, 1999). The cancer usually advances silently in the peritoneal cavity, giving rise to vague abdominal symptoms or no symptoms before it becomes evident with ascites and a large abdominal mass. In the United States, this most lethal gynecologic cancer is estimated to take the life of one woman every 50 minutes. Ovarian cancer develops in 1 of every 70 females (1.4%) during her lifetime (Barber, 1989). Between 5% and 10% of newly diagnosed ovarian cancers in the United States each year are familial and are found to be linked to the *BRCA1* locus of chromosome 17 by genetic analysis (Lynch et al, 1993).

Although early diagnosis is elusive, it is possible to categorize women who have increased risk for ovarian carcinoma (Table 45–9). These women are in the 40- to 60-year age group, may have a history of relative or absolute infertility, and have vague symptoms of gastrointestinal unrest. Women with a family

Table 45–9. WOMEN AT INCREASED RISK FOR OVARIAN CANCER

Age group 40–60 years
Relative or absolute infertility
Vague gastrointestinal complaints
Familial ovarian cancer pedigree
Documented *BRCA1* germline mutation
Peutz-Jeghers syndrome
Gonadal dysgenesis
Thyroid adenomas
Previous therapeutic pelvic radiation
Familial cancers at other sites:
  Breast cancer
  Endometrial cancer
  Colorectal cancer
  Prostate cancer
Postmenopausal pelvic mass syndrome

history of ovarian carcinoma constitute a unique subset of high-risk patients (Piver et al, 1982), as do women with other conditions linked to ovarian tumors, such as Peutz-Jeghers syndrome (papillary cystadenomas and sex cord tumors) (Scully, 1970b); women with gonadal dysgenesis (gonadoblastomas) (Scully, 1970a; Talerman, 1971); women with thyroid adenomas (arrhenoblastomas) (Jensen et al, 1974); and women with previous therapeutic pelvic radiation (Annegers et al, 1979; Boice et al, 1985; Tucker and Fraumeni, 1987). Women whose first-degree relatives have cancers at other sites also have increased risk for epithelial ovarian cancer. A family history of breast cancer increases the risk for epithelial ovarian cancer (Lynch et al, 1978), especially for the endometrioid ovarian cancer histologic type (Schildkraut and Thompson, 1988). There is also increased risk for endometrioid ovarian cancer associated with a family history of endometrial carcinoma (Schildkraut and Thompson, 1988). Ovarian cancer patients have an increased frequency of relatives with colorectal and prostate cancers (Cramer et al, 1983). These observed familial cancer clusters strongly suggested that genetic factors were present in these kindreds.

In 1994, the *BRCA1* gene was identified by the collaborative work of geneticists at the University of Utah and the National Institute of Environmental Health Sciences in North Carolina (Miki et al, 1994). This gene probably functions normally as a tumor-suppressor gene (Merajver et al, 1995). It is located on the long arm of chromosome 17, and mutations of *BRCA1* are seen in over 90% of hereditary ovarian cancer patients (Narod et al, 1995). There is also an increased risk for colon (fourfold) and prostate (threefold) cancer in patients with *BRCA1* mutations (Ford et al, 1994). Testing for *BRCA1* mutation is now available commercially and at academic medical centers. Because published data suggest that 90% to 100% of women with the *BRCA1* mutation have a lifetime risk of developing ovarian or breast cancer, protocols are being developed to manage these patients (Easton et al, 1995).

The clinical outcome of 53 patients with documented *BRCA1* mutations was recently shown to be significantly better than a matched patient control group with sporadic ovarian cancer (Rubin et al, 1996). *BRCA1* patients were younger at diagnosis (average age 48) than the mean diagnosis age of 61 years reported for a large population of ovarian cancer patients by the National Cancer Institute (Miller et al, 1993). The *BRCA1* patients in this report had an actuarial median survival of 77 months compared to 29 months for the control patients matched by age, stage, histologic type, and tumor grade. The value of screening these *BRCA1* carriers with pelvic examination, TVS, and CA-125 determinations needs to be established. Prophylactic oophorectomy should be offered to *BRCA1* carriers if fertility is not an issue or as soon as childbearing is complete (Averette and Nguyen, 1994). It is essential that patient screening take into account all the complex issues of medical testing, psychological consequences of testing, medical insurance coverage after positive testing, confidentiality of testing results, and strategies for management and possible treatment after the results of testing. The physician should be trained in genetic counseling or have access to a multidisciplinary team to offer optimal care for these patients and their families (Berchuck et al, 1996).

Ovarian cancer must be considered in postmenopausal women with a palpable adnexal mass (postmenopausal palpable ovary syndrome) (Barber and Graber, 1971). Women identified to be at high risk require intensive cancer surveillance with mammography, colonoscopy, annual pelvic examination, pelvic ultrasonography, and CA-125 determinations (Bast et al, 1985). *Prophylactic total abdominal hysterectomy with bilateral salpingo-oophorectomy should be performed in high-risk kindreds as soon as their families are complete.*

The surgical approach to ovarian carcinoma is based on the survival advantage afforded by thorough surgical staging and maximal tumor debulking. The ovaries contain bilateral disease in 30% to 60% of cases (Morrow, 1979), and the uterus often harbors gross or microscopic serosal involvement. Patients without obvious intraperitoneal metastases have up to 20% retroperitoneal lymph node involvement (Chen and Lee, 1983). Gross or microscopic involvement of the appendix occurs in roughly 80% of cases (Sonnendecker, 1982; Sonnendecker et al, 1989). *Total abdominal hysterectomy, bilateral salpingo-oophorectomy, omentectomy, and appendectomy are usually performed at initial surgery.* Occasionally, it is necessary to resect portions of the intestine or bladder to achieve optimal debulking, yet the improved survival offered by a maximal surgical effort followed by systemic chemotherapy makes this beneficial for the medically fit patient who gives informed consent (Castaldo et al, 1981; Berek et al, 1982; Hacker et al, 1983).

Cervical Cancer

Invasive cervical cancer ranks third among gynecologic cancers (behind uterine and ovarian cancers) in the United States and is the most common gynecologic malignancy in women younger than 50 years (Boring et al, 1992) (see also Chapter 56). Cervical cancer will develop in 1 of 63 women (1.6%) in her lifetime (Barber, 1989). Prior to cytologic screening in the United States, cervical cancer was the leading cause of cancer deaths among women. In 1995 cervical cancer was the reported second major site contributing to annual cancer deaths in women ages 20 to 39 years, with 12,800 new invasive cervical cancers projected in 1999 for women in all age brackets with approximately 4800 deaths (Landis et al, 1999). The mean age for invasive cervical cancel is 52.2 years, with two peaks at 35 to 39 years and 60 to 64 years (Boring et al, 1991).

In theory, death from invasive cervical cancer is totally preventable by screening and appropriate treatment of all females are risk. Since Rigoni-Stern's observation in 1842 that cervical cancer incidence was significantly higher in women who had married and borne children than in unmarried and celibate women, cervical cancer has repeatedly been linked to sexual activity by epidemiologic studies. In the 1970s, zur Hausen suggested that HPV was the sexually transmitted agent linked to genital tract neoplasms (zur Hausen et al, 1977). Currently DNA hybridization techniques have identified over 70 specific HPV types with more than 30 that infect the anogenital tract of women and men, causing condylomas, intraepithelial neoplasia, and invasive cancer (zur Hausen and Devilliers, 1994; Pfister, 1996). The strong association between HPV infections and cervical (Reid et al, 1982), vaginal (Daling and Sherman, 1992), vulvar (Ikenberg et al, 1983), penile (Gross et al, 1985; Rosemberg et al, 1991), and rectal (Frazer et al, 1986) cancers suggests that HPV infection is a major sexually transmitted carcinogen active with these malignancies (zur Hausen et al, 1977; Lorincz et al, 1987; Nelson et al, 1989).

The role of the immune response in preventing HPV infection is not well understood, but the incidence of HPV-related CIN and cervical cancer is known to be increased in immunodeficient individuals (Nakagawa et al, 1996). Maiman and colleagues (1997) reported 28 cases of invasive cervical cancer among women with acquired immunodeficiency syndrome (AIDS) from New York City over an 8-year period and found that cervical cancer was the most common AIDS-related malignancy. HIV-infected women have been shown to have higher grade cervical lesions with more involvement of the vulva, vagina, and perineum than HIV-negative women. HIV-infected women also had high-grade lesions at an earlier age than HIV-negative women, supporting the hypothesis that HIV infection may enhance tumor progression (Fruchter et al, 1994). These immunosuppressed patients are at increased risk for the development of cervical cancer and require more intensive screening.

FIGO STAGING OF CERVICAL CANCER

Successful treatment of cervical cancer depends on accurately defining the limits of the lesion, which requires coordinating the patient examination with pathologic analysis of the biopsy and/or conization specimen. The latest revision of the FIGO staging for carcinoma of the cervix defines microinvasion (stage IA) for the first time, subdividing it into stages IA1 and IA2. However, the point of division between stages IA1 and IA2 is undefined other than the statement that stage IA1 is "minimal microscopically evident stromal invasion" (FIGO Cancer Committee, 1986). A stage IA2 lesion may invade as deeply as 5 mm beneath the basement membrane and have horizontal spread up to 7 mm. Larger tumors are

designated as stage IB. The current FIGO definition allows more extensive lesions to be classified "microinvasive" than the previous 1974 definition suggested by the Society of Gynecologic Oncologists, which defined a microinvasive lesion as "one in which neoplastic epithelium invades the stroma to a depth of ≤3 mm beneath the basement membrane and in which lymphatic and blood vascular involvement is not demonstrated" (Committee on Nomenclature, 1974).

Cervical conization with uninvolved cervical margins is both diagnostic and therapeutic for microinvasive stage IAI lesions in which there is virtually no incidence of lymph node metastasis (Larsson, 1983; Hatch, 1989). This was demonstrated in a series of 162 patients who were treated with radical hysterectomy and pelvic lymphadenectomy for cervical cancer limited to 1-mm stromal invasion without lymph or vascular space involvement. No lymph node metastases were found (Averette et al, 1976). Tumor invasion between 1 and 3 mm without capillary-lymphatic (CL) space involvement has *less than 1% incidence of pelvic lymph node involvement and may be treated by conization with uninvolved margins if there is a strong desire to preserve fertility.* When fertility is not an important issue, a class I extrafascial hysterectomy or class II "modified radical hysterectomy" without lymphadenectomy would be performed (Table 45–10). For completeness, still another surgical option for an early invasive tumor with no CL space involvement is radical vaginal hysterectomy. This operation, introduced by Schauta (1908) and further refined by Amreich (1924), is still performed in Europe and the Orient for patients at minimal risk for lymph node metastases who are at high medical risk for radical abdominal hysterectomy (Carenza and Villani, 1982; Kudo et al, 1984). The Schauta radical vaginal operation permits wide resection of the parametria without the morbidity of an abdominal operation.

Radical vaginal trachelectomy combined with laparoscopic pelvic lymphadenectomy has been performed as an alternative to standard radical abdominal hysterectomy for about 90 patients reported in the literature with 3 recurrences. A 40% conception rate was reported in a series of 29 patients within 12 months of radical vaginal trachelectomy (Covens and Shaw, 1999). Further evaluation of this procedure with longer follow-up is needed to determine whether radical trachelectomy and laparoscopic lymphadenectomy may be safely offered to select patients desiring to maintain fertility.

Tumors that invade the cervical stroma more than 3 mm or have CL space involvement have been shown to have a significant risk for nodal metastases. These patients are not appropriately managed by conization or simple vaginal or abdominal hysterectomy. This conclusion is supported by the work of Van Nagell and colleagues at the University of Kentucky (1983), who reported 177 cervical cancer patients with invasion up to 5 mm treated with radical hysterectomy and bilateral pelvic lymphadenectomy. There were no nodal metas-

Table 45-10. TREATMENT OF CERVICAL CANCER, INCLUDING FIVE CLASSES OF RADICAL HYSTERECTOMY

LESION	SURGICAL PROCEDURE
Carcinoma in situ	Conization: surgical margins free of disease
Stage IA with up to 1 mm invasion and no CLS invasion	Conization with surgical margins free of disease if further fertility is desired or extrafascial hysterectomy (class I) with lateral retraction of ureters, which allows total removal of the cervix
Stage IA2 with 1–3 mm invasion and no CLS invasion	Conization with free margins if desire further fertility or class I extrafascial hysterectomy or radical vaginal hysterectomy (Schauta)
Stage IA2 with 1–3 mm invasion and with CLS invasion	Class II modified radial hysterectomy with removal of one half of uterosacral and cardinal ligaments, ligation of uterine vessels medial to ureter, and removal of upper one third of vagina; may include pelvic lymph node dissection
Stage IA2 with 3–5 mm invasion and <1 cm diameter tumor	Class II modified radical hysterectomy with pelvic lymphadenectomy
Stage IA2 with 3–5 mm invasion and >1 cm diameter tumor	Class III radical hysterectomy with removal of all cardinal and uterosacral ligaments, ligation of uterine artery at origin from internal iliac artery, removal of one half of vagina, and pelvic
Stages IB and IIA	Class III radical hysterectomy
Postradiation central recurrence not involving bladder or rectum	Class IV radical hysterectomy with removal of all periureteral tissue, removal of superior vesicle artery, and removal of three fourths of vagina
Postradiation central recurrence involving portion of bladder or ureter	Class V extended radical hysterectomy with removal of involved portion of bladder and/or distal ureter with ureteroneocystostomy

Modified from Piver MS, Rutledge F, Smith JP: Five classes of extended hysterectomy for women with cervical cancer. Obstet Gynecol 1974;44:265, with permission from the American College of Obstetricians and Gynecologists.

tases among 57 patients with 3-mm or less stromal invasion and no CL space involvement. However, three (9.41%) of 32 patients with invasion between 3 and 5 mm had lymph node metastases and two died of metastatic disease. A similar 4.8% incidence of pelvic nodal metastases was reported by Simon and co-investigators (1986) with lesions invading between 3 and 5 mm. These patients had nodal metastases only with tumor diameters greater than 1 cm, demonstrating a poorer prognosis as tumor volume increases.

In 1996, the University of Kentucky group reported results with 94 stage IA2 cervical cancer patients treated with primary radical hysterectomy and pelvic lymphadenectomy (Buckley et al, 1996). Seven of 94 patients (7.4%) had lymph node metastases and five patients had recurrent disease despite postoperative radiation therapy. Tumor involvement in lymph vascular spaces was again noted to be associated with an increased risk for tumor recurrence. These studies indicate that stage IA2 patients require radical hysterectomy with pelvic lymphadenectomy or radiation therapy for treatment.

All stages of cervical cancer may be treated with radiation therapy, whereas radical surgery is appropriate only for stage I and IIA tumors. Both modalities yield an approximate 90% 5-year survival, as shown by the 30-year prospective series comparing radiation therapy and radical surgery at the University of Michigan (Morley and Seski, 1976). Surgical treatment is commonly suggested for younger patients to preserve ovarian function and avoid possible radiation-induced dysfunction of the bladder, vagina, and bowel. Postmenopausal patients who are in good health may also be treated surgically, reserving radiation therapy for patients with medical contrain-

dications to surgery or with a preference for radiation treatment.

Recognizing that the extent of surgical therapy used for specific lesions required precise definition to accurately evaluate results and complications and to appropriately modify treatment, Piver et al (1974) described five classes of radical hysterectomy for invasive cervical cancer. As shown in Table 45–10, the class III radical hysterectomy and pelvic lymphadenectomy is used for tumors known to have some risk for nodal metastases (i.e., tumors with 3 mm or more invasion and diameters of 1 cm or more).

Vaginal Cancer

Primary vaginal cancer constitutes only 1% to 2% of gynecologic cancers (Barber, 1989) (see also Chapter 54). Vaginal metastatic lesions from the cervix, endometrium, ovary, vulva, and bowel are more frequent than primary lesions. To be classified a primary vaginal lesion by the rules of FIGO staging, a tumor must be totally confined to the vagina. Tumors contiguous with either the cervix or vulva are considered primary at those sites and metastatic to the vagina.

Colposcopy is used to assess the mucosal extent of vaginal lesions and to direct biopsies. Dysplastic and in situ lesions may be treated with CO_2 laser ablation (Stafl et al, 1977), topical 5-fluorouracil (Ballon et al, 1979), or partial-to-total vaginectomy with split-thickness skin graft vaginoplasty. Radiation therapy is also very effective treatment for in situ lesions but is usually reserved for invasive cancers that cannot be surgically treated because of their location and size or because the general physical condition will not allow surgical treatment (Hernandez-Linares et al, 1980).

Effective treatment of any invasive vaginal cancer is complicated by the proximity of the bladder, ureters, and rectum. Retrospective review of 100 patients treated with surgery, radiation, and combined surgery and radiation showed excellent results in selected patients medically fit for surgical treatment with disease limited to one third of the vaginal canal (Stock et al, 1995). *Surgical treatment is used for stage I vaginal tumors and for recurrences after radiation therapy.* In both of these situations, a radical hysterectomy, pelvic lymphadenectomy, and radical vaginectomy may be performed. The vagina is usually restored by a split-thickness skin graft vaginoplasty. Recurrences after radiation may be too extensive for this approach and require anterior, posterior, or total exenteration to obtain tumor-free margins.

Uterine Sarcomas

Uterine sarcomas make up approximately 3% of uterine cancers and 1% of gynecologic malignancies (Zaloudek and Norris, 1981) (see also Chapter 59). These rare tumors arise from malignant changes in the myometrium as well as in endometrial glands and stroma. As a group, uterine sarcomas are more prone to lymphatic and hematogenous metastases than is endometrial cancer. Therefore, preoperative assessment includes close attention to any sign of metastases beyond the uterus by complete physical examination and CT scan of the liver, abdomen, and pelvis. A CT scan of the lungs may detect metastatic deposits missed by routine chest radiograph.

Extrafascial total abdominal hysterectomy with bilateral salpingo-oophorectomy is performed, along with sampling of pelvic and para-aortic lymph nodes, peritoneal cytology, omental biopsy, and careful inspection of all intra-abdominal peritoneal surfaces for tumor staging. Close to half of all sarcomas are confined to the uterus at the time of diagnosis (Kempson and Bari, 1970; Salazar et al, 1978). These bulky tumors are often accompanied by pelvic pain and bleeding that is relieved or improved by removal of the uterus.

Fallopian Tube Carcinoma

Primary fallopian tube carcinoma is the least common gynecologic cancer, accounting for 0.3% of all female genital tract cancer (Berek et al, 1983) (see also Chapter 62). The fallopian tubes are much more likely to receive metastases from other sites, such as the ovary, endometrium, or gastrointestinal tract, than to be the primary site. Preoperative diagnosis of tubal carcinoma almost never occurs. Diagnosis is usually made during surgery in a woman who is undergoing exploration for suspected uterine fibroids or an adnexal mass. Patients usually present with postmenopausal vaginal bleeding or discharge. They may have lower abdominal cramping pain or

a pressure sensation from tubal distention. The classical sign, *hydrops tubae profluens*, which describes abdominal pain relieved by passage of a watery vaginal discharge, is actually encountered in only 15% to 20% of patients (Sedlis, 1961). Adenocarcinoma cells are occasionally found in cervicovaginal cytology that are not explained by vaginal, endocervical, or endometrial pathologic factors. The tubes and ovaries need to be investigated in this situation (Takashina et al, 1988).

Although there is no official FIGO staging for tubal cancer, in practice the staging and the general management plan are similar to the conventions applied to epithelial ovarian cancer (Podratz et al, 1986; Harrison et al, 1989). *Total abdominal hysterectomy with bilateral salpingo-oophorectomy is performed*, along with complete exploration of the peritoneal cavity, peritoneal washings for cytology, omentectomy, selective para-aortic and pelvic lymph node sampling, and resection of all possible metastatic lesions to achieve optimal debulking (Hershey et al, 1981). After surgery, these patients are usually treated with systemic chemotherapy protocols similar to those used for ovarian cancer (Deppe et al, 1980).

Gestational Trophoblastic Disease

In 1956, Li et al reported the first example of chemotherapeutic cure of a widely metastatic solid tumor using methotrexate. Chemotherapy remains the basis of treatment for gestational trophoblastic disease (GTD), with good expectations for cure dependent on accurate disease staging and appropriate sequencing of chemotherapy, radiotherapy, and surgery for the various GTD stages and risk categories (McDonald and Ruffolo, 1983) (see also Chapter 63).

In certain situations, surgical treatment of GTD is essential. *Initial hysterectomy performed during the first cycle of chemotherapy reduces the number of chemotherapy treatments required to cure GTD patients with uterine disease* (Hammond et al, 1980; Soper, 1994). Torsion of a theca-lutein cyst or intraperitoneal hemorrhage from tumor eroding through the uterine wall may require immediate hysterectomy. Tumor necrosis in response to chemotherapy may result in hemorrhage, necessitating hysterectomy (Lewis et al, 1966; Jones and Lewis, 1974; Berkowitz and Goldstein, 1996). *Hysterectomy is also very appropriate therapy for the patient with hydatidiform mole who does not desire preservation of fertility.* The risk of persistent GTD is less when hysterectomy (Tow, 1966) versus suction curettage is performed. Human chorionic gonadotropin levels are monitored after hysterectomy to detect patients with persistent disease. Suction curettage is the preferred management method for hydatidiform mole when fertility preservation is important (Goldstein and Berkowitz, 1994).

The presence of theca-lutein cysts is associated with greater likelihood for persistent GTD in hydatidiform mole patients (Curry et al, 1975). These large theca-lutein cysts occasionally present with hydatidiform mole (Fig. 45–4) and will spontaneously regress several months after removal of the mole as levels of human chorionic gonadotropin fall. They do not need to be removed unless indicated by pain, torsion, or the patient's age.

Nongynecologic Pelvic Malignancies

The female genital tract often receives metastases from nongynecologic sites that give rise to pelvic symptomatology that warrants *total abdominal hysterectomy with bilateral salpingo-oophorectomy*. This procedure should be performed as part of initial surgical management for most pelvic sigmoid and rectal cancers for several reasons:

1. Patients with colorectal malignancy are at higher risk than the general population for synchronous and metachronous cancers of the ovary and uterus (Enblad et al, 1990).
2. Occult ovarian metastases may be present with colorectal carcinomas (Stearns, 1978).
3. If pelvic radiation therapy has been used, there is increased risk for subsequent malignancy in the retained generative tract (Boice et al, 1985; Tucker and Fraumeni, 1987).
4. After an abdominoperineal resection and possible radiation therapy, it is usually difficult to investigate abnormal uterine bleeding and/or abnormal cervical cytology.
5. Removal of the uterus for any subsequent benign or malignant indication requires a greater surgical effort than removal at the time of the original surgery.

ALTERNATIVES TO HYSTERECTOMY

Office counseling, medical management of symptoms, and surgical procedures short of removing the uterus are alternatives to hysterectomy that may be employed to manage all of the hysterectomy indications listed in Table 45–3 except the emergency and malignant indications, which almost always mandate hysterectomy because they are life threatening. The other indications are all disabling and detrimental to patients' quality of life in various degrees, but the decision to perform hysterectomy for these indications remains elective and nonemergent. The noncancerous, nonemergent patient population accounts for over 90% of hysterectomies performed in the Unites States (Pokras and Hufnagel, 1987). The inner-regional variability of hysterectomy rates in the United States (highest rates in the south and midwest), in addition to the fact that hysterectomy rates in some western European and Scandinavian countries are half the U.S. rate, has resulted in critical review of higher hysterectomy rates in the United States (Walker and Jick, 1979; Van Keep et al, 1983; Kramer and Reiter, 1997).

Hysteroscopic ablation of the endometrial cavity using the neodymium:yittrium-aluminum-garnet (Nd:YAG) laser was introduced by Goldrath and associates in 1981. This new medical approach has evolved as an alternative to hysterectomy to eradicate bleeding resulting from hormonal imbalance, polyps, submucous fibroids, and coagulopathies (Neuwirth, 1983). Hysteroscopic ablation of the endometrium may be performed with laser or electrocautery roller ball technique and has effectively abolished initial bleeding problems in 70% to 90% of patients (Garry, 1990; Gannon et al, 1991). Patients

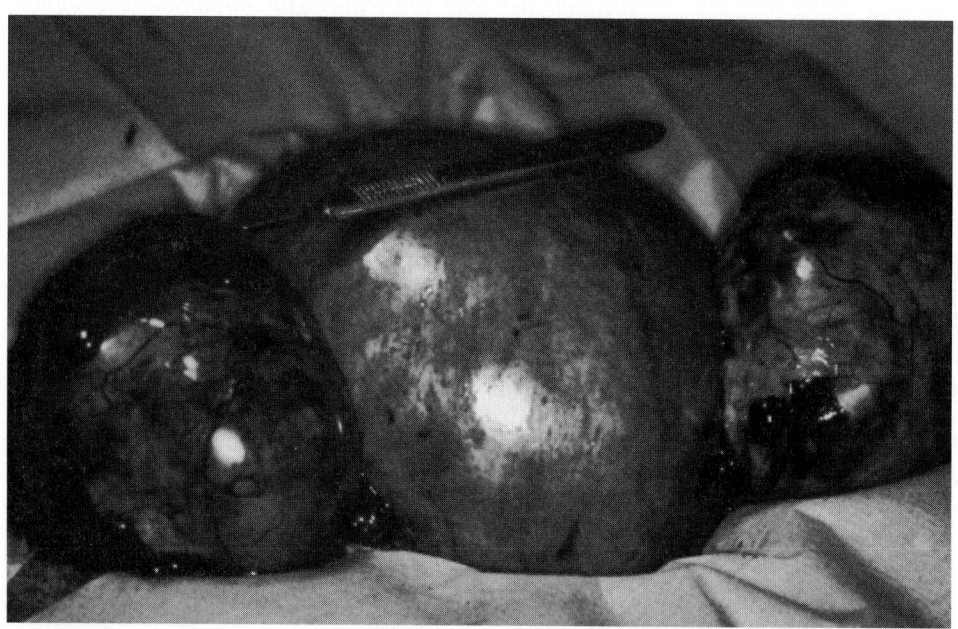

Figure 45–4
A 36-year-old woman, gravida III, para III, with hydatidiform mole and large theca-lutein cysts did not want any more pregnancies. She was therefore treated with abdominal hysterectomy and ovarian preservation. The ovaries and the level of β subunit of human chorionic gonadotropin returned to normal in about 3 months.

may be pretreated with GnRHa therapy for about 1 month prior to endometrial cavity ablation or hysteroscopic myomectomy to facilitate surgery (Philipsen and Naesbol, 1993; Donnez et al, 1995). Recurrent symptomatic bleeding has been reported in 15% to 25% of patients (Pyper and Haeri, 1991). Hysteroscopic ablation is contraindicated for patients with atypical hyperplasias and carcinoma (Loffer, 1988). The presence of endometrial hyperplasia or cancer should be investigated by hysteroscopy and directed biopsy before performing ablation. Baggish and Baltoyannis (1988) reported technical improvements for laser ablation using a dual-channel operating hysteroscope and a high-resolution video camera, which precludes the use of safety lenses by the surgeon. Their patients all had intractable bleeding uncontrolled by hormonal therapy and curettage. Medical problems (coagulopathies, massive obesity, and systemic diseases) increased their risk for traditional hysterectomy. Baggish and Baltoyannis recommended endometrial cavity ablation as an alternative to hysterectomy only for patients medically unfit for hysterectomy and cautioned that major deficiencies of the procedure are the current lack of long-term (>10 years) follow-up and the lack of a surgical specimen for pathologic analysis.

Bleeding from endometrial polyps and submucous fibroids can be managed by hysteroscopy (DeCherney and Polan, 1983) or D&C. Hysteroscopic surgery may be performed in two sessions to remove larger leiomyomas (Donnez et al, 1995). *Benign hyperplasias can usually be reversed with progestins, whereas atypical hyperplasias, large and multiple leiomyomas, and adenocarcinomas should be treated with hysterectomy.*

WHO DECIDES IF HYSTERECTOMY IS APPROPRIATE?

The recommendation for costly medical and surgical therapies is no longer a private issue between the treating physician and the patient and family. In the recent past, these medical recommendations were generally accepted or rejected without outside review and influence. Now there is an ever-increasing involvement by "third-party payers" in the decision-making process regarding costly medical procedures such as hysterectomy. The government, private insurance companies, industry, and hospitals are all concerned with cost containment. Third-party payers naturally tend to look at the financial bottom line because they subsidize the cost of health care.

The entire spectrum of decisions, choices, and options that face the patient and physician dealing with benign pelvic and uterine problems today rapidly increases as our medical practice patterns and techniques continually evolve in response to cost containment issues, critical evaluation of outcomes, and advances in medical and surgical treatments. Consider a typical patient with uterine fibroids followed

for several years and bothered with pain that is attributed to uterine enlargement. The physician assumes with reasonable confidence that the pain is correctly diagnosed at this point in time and proceeds to continue offering nonsurgical medical support of the patient's symptoms or discusses myomectomy via endoscopic or abdominal routes. Months and years may pass as nonhysterectomy treatment options are pursued. Hysterectomy will eventually be elected for some patients, and the decision matrix widens as the route of surgery is selected. Options include total abdominal hysterectomy, vaginal hysterectomy, laparoscopic assisted vaginal hysterectomy, and supracervical hysterectomy either by abdominal or laparoscopic route. All of these techniques have variations employed by individual surgeons, and of course the ovaries may be removed or left in place with all surgical approaches. The information available may seem overwhelming and gives the physician the responsibility and challenge to guide the patient, without paternalism, through this maze to her best available decision. The time devoted to patient-physician discussion of choices and decisions varies and continually challenges the physician to provide adequate time for each patient's needs.

Once the family and physician decide that hysterectomy is the recommended treatment, the patient's third-party payer evaluates the plan by its surgery precertification process. This review determines if the hysterectomy decision fits with the indications acceptable to the particular third-party payer. This review is supposed to protect patients from inappropriate hysterectomies and in this way curtail costs of health care. The good that derives from this extensive oversight is that very few, if any, hysterectomies will be approved for inappropriate indications. This safeguard to patients is worth the cost, trouble, and time required to implement the precertification process.

Although the intent and logic behind this scrutiny of medical decisions are clear, it is a very difficult task to accomplish well, Richardson (1972) estimated that it would require 28 reviewers to make a judgment within 95% confidence limits about the quality of care provided for one gynecology patient! There are many potential conflicts between an individual patient's needs and what the third-party payer algorithm judges to be appropriate and necessary treatment for its entire covered patient population. The third-party payer has to assume a financial perspective on the overall process of hysterectomy approval/disapproval, while the individual patient views the recommended operation as a "benefit" to which she is entitled by the terms of her particular coverage. If the third-party payer disapproves surgery, the physician and family may appeal. Much time, energy and money may be expended by both sides before a final decision is made.

As physicians, we are challenged by the bureaucratic nature of the precertification review process to make sure that it does not become unmanageable and actually increase costs and promote inappropriate care. The varied lists of eligibility criteria and shifting guidelines for hysterectomy imposed by third-party payers may be a significant burden to both patient and physician. This occurs when guidelines become excessively stringent and specific. For example, the third-party payer algorithm may state that hysterectomy is inappropriate treatment unless (1) leiomyomas are larger than a certain size, perhaps 16 weeks' gestational size; (2) patients with dysfunctional bleeding have undergone *multiple* D&Cs; (3) endometriosis patients *have* had a conservative operation prior to hysterectomy; or (4) patients with PID have had two attempts at conservative surgery prior to hysterectomy. These changing guidelines require constant monitoring by practicing physicians to keep them workable. Otherwise the system becomes *meddlesome* and subjects patients to prolonged medical management and multiple pelvic operations by preventing or delaying hysterectomy when it is clearly the appropriate therapy.

The physician's responsibility is always to give his or her best considered medical opinion and then assist the family to obtain approval for the recommended surgery via the guidelines set down by the particular third-party payer. If the guidelines are inappropriate, they must be challenged vigorously on behalf of the patient. Anyone involved in this process knows that it is very time consuming and has become, in fact, a full-time occupation for many in the health care industry.

Second and Third Opinions

The decision to perform hysterectomy has a long tradition of close scrutiny by physicians as well as patients. In his 1946 address to the American Gynecologic Society on its 50th anniversary, entitled "Hysterectomy: Therapeutic Necessity or Surgical Racket?", Norman Miller emphasized the need for standards of care and defined indications for hysterectomy. Today second surgical opinions are mandated by some insurance carriers (Medicaid) and suggested by others. Keeping in mind the significant complications and morbidity that may result from hysterectomy, *a second surgical opinion from another qualified specialist should be obtained whenever there is any question in the patient's or the primary physician's mind about the decision for hysterectomy* (Thompson and Birch, 1981).

The likelihood for disagreement between the first-opinion and second-opinion consultants is readily acknowledged by insurance company forms that reserve a blank space for the "third opinion." This underscores the subjectivity of some decisions for hysterectomy that are based on "quality of life" indications such as dysmenorrhea, dyspareunia, pelvic pressure, and mild yet symptomatic prolapse. These indications are difficult to quantitate, and they vary in significance from woman to woman. The informed patient herself will ultimately make the final judgment for or against hysterectomy in these situations (Pratt, 1980). The gynecologist who has observed the patient for the longest time usually is in the best position to make an accurate medical judgment about hysterectomy and to help the patient in her deliberations.

ACKNOWLEDGMENTS

Thanks to Susan K. Rishworth, History Librarian, The American College of Obstetricians and Gynecologists, for invaluable help with historical citations, and to Charlotte, Tom, Mark, and Paul for inspiration.

REFERENCES

Aldridge AH, Meredith RS: Complete abdominal hysterectomy: a simplified technique and end results in 500 cases. Am J Obstet Gynecol 1950;59:748.

Amirikia H, Evans TN: Ten-year review of hysterectomies: trends, indications, and risks. Am J Obstet Gynecol 1979;134:431.

Amreich I: Zur Anatomic und Technik der erweiterten vaginalen Karzinomoperation. Arch Gynakol 1924;122.

Anderson MC, Hartley RB: Cervical crypt involvement by intraepithelial neoplasia. Obstet Gynecol 1980;55:546.

Annegers FJ, Strome H, Decker DG, et al: Ovarian cancer: incidence and case-control study. Cancer 1979;43:723.

Ashton P, Beischer N, Cullen J, et al: Return to theatre-experience at the Mercy Maternity Hospital, Melbourne 1971–1982. Aust N Z J Obstet Gynaecol 1985;25:159.

Aubard Y, Piver P, Grandjean MH, et al: Laparoscopically assisted vaginal hysterectomy for non-malignant disease of the uterus: report on a personal series of 126 cases. Eur J Obstet Gynecol Reprod Biol 1996;68(1-2):147.

Averette HE, Nelson JH Jr, Ng AB, et al: Diagnosis and management of microinvasive (stage Ia) carcinoma of the uterine cervix. Cancer 1976;38:414.

Averette HE, Nguyen HN: The role of prophylactic oophorectomy in cancer prevention. Gynecol Oncol 1994;55:S38.

Azziz R: Adenomyosis: current perspectives. Obstet Gynecol Clin North Am 1989;16:221.

Baggish MS, Baltoyannis P: New techniques for laser ablation of the endometrium in high-risk patients. Am J Obstet Gynecol 1988;159:287.

Bahary CM, Gorodeski IG: The diagnostic value of laparoscopy in women with chronic pelvic pain. Am Surg 1987;53:672.

Ballon SC, Roberts JA, Lagasse LD: Topical 5-fluorouracil in the treatment of intraepithelial neoplasia of the vagina. Obstet Gynecol 1979;54:163.

Barber HRK: Manual of Gynecologic Oncology. 2nd ed. Philadelphia: JB Lippincott Company, 1989.

Barber HRK, Graber EA: The PMPO syndrome (postmenopausal palpable ovary syndrome). Obstet Gynecol 1971;38:921.

Barden TP: Perinatal care in gynecology and obstetrics: the health care of women. New York: McGraw-Hill, 1981;595.

Barker MG: Psychiatric illness after hysterectomy. Br Med J 1968;2:91.

Bast RC Jr, Siegal FP, Runowicz C, et al: Elevation of serum CA-125 prior to diagnosis of an epithelial ovarian carcinoma. Gynecol Oncol 1985;22:115.

Benrubi G: History of hysterectomy. J Fla Med Assoc 1988;75:533.

Berchuck A, Cirisano F, Lancaster JM, et al: Role of BRCA1 mutation screening in the management of familial ovarian cancer. Am J Obstet Gynecol 1996;175:738.

Berek JS, Hacker NF, Lagasse LD: Ovarian and fallopian tube cancer. In Haskell CM (ed): Cancer Treatment. 2nd ed. Philadelphia: WB Saunders Company, 1983;409.

Berek JS, Hacker NF, Lagasse LD, et al: Lower urinary tract resection as part of cytoreductive surgery for ovarian cancer. Gynecol Oncol 1982;13:87.

Berkowitz RS, Goldstein DP: Chorionic tumors. N Engl J Med 1996;335:1740.

Boice JD, Day NE, Andersen A, et al: Second cancers following radiation treatment for cervical cancer: an international collaboration among cancer registries. J Natl Cancer Inst 1985;74:955.

Boring CC, Squires TS, Tong T: Cancer statistics 1992. CA Cancer J Clin 1992;42:19.

Bosch FX, Manos MM, Munoz N, et al: Prevalence of human papillomavirus in cervical cancer: a worldwide perspective. J Natl Cancer Inst 1995;87:796.

Boyes DA, Worth AJ, Fidler HK: The results of treatment of 4389 cases of pre-clinical cervical squamous carcinoma. J Obstet Gynaecol Br Commonw 1970;77:769.

Buckley SL, Tritz DM, Van Le L, et al: Lymph node metastases and prognosis in patients with stage IA2 cervical cancer. Gynecol Oncol 1996;63:4.

Bunker JP: Elective hysterectomy: pro and con. N Engl J Med 1976;295:264.

Burghardt E, Holzer E: Treatment of carcinoma in situ: evaluation of 1609 cases. Obstet Gynecol 1980;55:539.

Burnham W: Extirpation of the uterus and ovaries for sarcomatous disease. Lancet 1854;8:147.

Capen CV, Irwin H, Magrina J, et al: Vaginal removal of the ovaries in association with vaginal hysterectomy. J Reprod Med 1983;28:589.

Carenza L, Villani C: Schauta radical vaginal hysterectomy. Clin Obstet Gynecol 1982;25:913.

Castaldo TW, Petrilli ES, Ballon SC, et al: Intestinal operations in patients with ovarian carcinoma. Am J Obstet Gynecol 1981;139:80.

Chan WY, Dawood MY, Fuchs F: Prostaglandins in primary dysmenorrhea: comparison of prophylactic and nonprophylactic treatment with ibuprofen and use of oral contraceptive. Am J Med 1981;70:535.

Chen SS, Lee L: Incidence of paraaortic and pelvic lymph node metastasis in epithelial ovarian cancer. Gynecol Oncol 1983;16:95.

Christ JE, Lotze EC: The residual ovary syndrome. Obstet Gynecol 1976;46:551.

Chryssikopoulos A, Loghis C: Indications and results of total hysterectomy. Int Surg 1986;71:188.

Cianfrani T: A Short History of Obstetrics and Gynecology. Springfield, IL: Charles C Thomas, 1960:341.

Clark JG: A more radical method of performing hysterectomy for cancer of the uterus. Johns Hopkins Hosp Bull 52, 53, 1895;52/53:120.

Cole P, Berlin J: Elective hysterectomy. Am J Obstet Gynecol 1977;129:117.

Committee on Nomenclature: Chicago: Society of Gynecologic Oncologists, 1974.

Covens AL, Shaw P: Is radical trachelectomy a safe alternative to radical hysterectomy for early stage IB carcinoma of the cervix? Presented at 30th annual meeting Society of Gynecologic Oncologists, San Francisco, March 22, 1999.

Cramer DW, Hutchison GB, Welch WR, et al: Determinants of ovarian cancer risk: I. Reproductive experiences and family history. J Natl Cancer Inst 1983;71:711.

Creasman WT, Morrow CP, Bundy BN, et al: Surgical pathologic spread patterns of endometrial cancer: a gynecologic oncology group study. Cancer 1987;60:2035.

Cullen AP, Reid R, Champion M, et al: Analysis of the physical state of different human papillomavirus DNAs in intraepithelial and invasive cervical neoplasm. J Virol 1991;65:606.

Cunanan RG Jr, Courey NG, Lippes J: Laparoscopic findings in patients with pelvic pain. Am J Obstet Gynecol 1983;146:589.

Curry SL, Hammond CB, Tyrey L, et al: Hydatidiform mole: diagnosis, management and long-term follow-up of 347 patients. Obstet Gynecol 1975;45:1.

Daling JR, Sherman KJ: Relationship between human papillomavirus infection and tumours of anogenital sites other than the cervix. In Munoz N, Bosch FX, Shah KV, et al (eds): The Epidemiology of Human Papillomavirus and Cervical Cancer. Oxford: Oxford University Press, 1992:223.

Dawood MY: Current concepts in the etiology and treatment of primary dysmenorrhea. Acta Obstet Gynecol Scand Suppl 1986;138:7.

Dawood MY, Ramos J: Transcutaneous electrical nerve stimulation (TENS) for treatment of primary dysmenorrhea: a randomized crossover comparison with placebo TENS and ibuprofen. Obstet Gynecol 1990;75:656.

Deane RT, Ulene A: Hysterectomy or tubal ligation for sterilization: a cost-effectiveness analysis. Inquiry 1977;14:73.

DeCherney A, Polan ML: Hysteroscopic management of intrauterine lesions and intractable uterine bleeding. Obstet Gynecol 1983;61:392.

Deppe G, Bruckner HW, Cohen CJ: Combination chemotherapy for advanced carcinoma of the fallopian tube. Obstet Gynecol 1980;56:530.

Dicker RC, Greenspan JR, Strauss LT, et al: Complications of abdominal and vaginal hysterectomy among women of reproductive age in the United States. Am J Obstet Gynecol 1982a;144:841.

Dicker RC, Scally MJ, Greenspan JR, et al: Hysterectomy among women of reproductive age. JAMA 1982b;248:323.

DiSaia PJ, Creasman WT: The adnexal mass and early ovarian cancer. In: Clinical Gynecologic Oncology. St. Louis: CV Mosby, 1984:254.

Donnez J, Polet R, Anaf V, et al: Treatment of dysfunctional bleeding and fibroids by advanced endoscopic techniques with the Nd:YAG laser: from the present to the future. Baillieres Clin Obstet Gynaecol 1995;9:329.

Dorsey JH, Holtz PM, Griffiths RI, et al: Costs and charges associated with three alternative techniques of hysterectomy. N Engl J Med 1996;335:476.

Doss N, Forney JP, Vellios F, et al: Covert bilaterality of mature ovarian teratomas. Obstet Gynecol 1977;50:651.

Durfee RB: Evolution of cesarean hysterectomy. Clin Obstet Gynecol 1969;12:575.

Easton DF, Ford D, Bishop DT: Breast and ovarian cancer incidence in BRCA1-mutation carriers: Breast Cancer Linkage Consortium. Am J Hum Genet 1995;56:265.

Emge LA, Durfee RB: Pelvic organ prolapse: four thousand years of treatment. Clin Obstet Gynecol 1966;9:997.

Enblad P, Adami HO, Glimelius B, et al: The risk of subsequent primary malignant diseases after cancers of the colon and rectum: a nationwide cohort study. Cancer 1990;65:2091.

Feichtinger W, Kemeter P: Pregnancy after total ovariectomy achieved by ovum donation. Lancet 1985;2:722.

Felson H, McGuire J, Wasserman P: Stromal endometriosis involving the heart. Am J Med 1960;29:1072.

Field CS: Dysfunctional uterine bleeding. Prim Care 1988;15:561.

FIGO Cancer Committee: Staging announcement: West Berlin, September 1985. Gynecol Oncol 1986;25:383.

FIGO Cancer Committee: FIGO stages—1988 revision (announcement). Gynecol Oncol 1989;35:125.

Finney JMT: Preoperative care and complications. In Telinde RW, Mattingly RF (eds): Operative Gynecology. Philadelphia: JB Lippincott Company, 1970:15.

Ford D, Easton DF, Bishop DT, et al: Risks of cancer in BRCA1-mutation carriers: Breast Cancer Linkage Consortium. Lancet 1994;343:692.

Franceschi S, LaVecchia C, Mangioni C: Familial ovarian cancer: eight more families. Gynecol Oncol 1982;13:31.

Frazer IH, Medley G, Crapper RM, et al: Association between anorectal dysplasia, human papillomavirus and human immunodeficiency virus infection in homosexual men. Lancet 1986;2:657.

Freund WA: Eine neue Methode der Exstirpation des ganzen Uterus: Sammlung Klinischer Vortrage No. 133. Gynakologie 1878;41:911.

Freund WA: Z Geburtshilfe Gynakol 1881;6.

Friedman AJ: Clinical experience in the treatment of fibroids with leuprolide and other GnRH agonists. Obstet Gynecol Surv 1989;44:311.

Fruchter RG, Maiman M, Sillman FH, et al: Characteristics of cervical intraepithelial neoplasia in women infected with the human immunodeficiency virus. Am J Obstet Gynecol 1994; 171:531.

Gallup DG, Talledo OE: Benign and malignant tumors. Clin Obstet Gynecol 1987;30:662.

Garry R: Hysteroscopic alternatives to hysterectomy. Br J Obstet Gynaecol 1990;97:199.

Gambone JC, Lench JB, Slesinski MJ, et al: Validation of hysterectomy indications and the quality assurance process. Obstet Gynecol 1989;73:1045.

Gambone JC, Reiter RC: Nonsurgical management of chronic pelvic pain: a multidisciplinary approach. Clin Obstet Gynecol 1990;33:205.

Gannon MJ, Holt EM, Fairbank J, et al: A randomised trial comparing endometrial resection and abdominal hysterectomy for the treatment of menorrhagia. BMJ 1991;303:1362.

Gerzof SG, Robbins AG, Johnson WC, et al: Percutaneous catheter drainage of abdominal abscesses: a five year experience. N Engl J Med 1981;305:653.

Goff BA, Goodman A, Muntz HG, et al: Surgical stage IV endometrial carcinoma: a study of 47 cases. Gynecol Oncol 1994;52:237.

Goldrath MH, Fuller TA, Segal S: Laser photovaporization of endometrium for the treatment of menorrhagia. Am J Obstet Gynecol 1981;140:14.

Goldstein DP, Berkowitz RS: Current management of complete and partial molar pregnancy. J Reprod Med 1994;39:139.

Goldstein DP, deCholnoky C, Emans SJ, et al: Laparoscopy in the diagnosis and management of pelvic pain in adolescents. J Reprod Med 1980;24:251.

Goodman HM, Bowling MC, Nelson JH: Cervical malignancies in gynecologic oncology. In Knapp RC, Berkowitz RS (eds): Gynecologic Oncology. New York: Macmillan, 1986:225.

Graves EJ: National Hospital Discharge Survey, annual summary 1987 (National Center for Health Statistics). Vital Health Stat 13 1989;99.

Graves EJ: National Hospital Discharge Survey: annual summary 1990. Vital Health Stat 13 1992;112.

Graves EJ, Gillum BS: Detailed diagnosis and procedures, National Hospital Discharge Survey, 1995, Vital Health Stat 13 1995;130:1.

Gross G, Ikenberg H, Gissmann L, et al: Papillomavirus infection of the anogenital region: correlation between histology, clinical picture and virus type: proposal of a new nomenclature. J Invest Dermatol 1985;85:147.

Grundsell H, Ekman G, Gulberg B, et al: Some aspects of prophylactic oophorectomy and ovarian carcinoma. Ann Chir Gynaecol 1981;70:36.

Gusberg SB, Marshall D: Intraepithelial carcinoma of the cervix: a clinical reappraisal. Obstet Gynecol 1962;19:713.

Hacker NF: Uterine cancer. In Berek JS, Hacker NF (eds): Practical Gynecologic Oncology. Baltimore: Williams & Wilkins, 1989:285.

Hacker NF, Berek JS, Lagasse LD, et al: Primary cytoreductive surgery for epithelial ovarian cancer. Obstet Gynecol 1983;61:413.

Halbert DR, Demers LM, Fontanta J, et al: Prostaglandin levels in endometrial jet wash specimens in patients with dysmenorrhea before and after indomethacin therapy. Prostaglandins 1975;10:1047.

Halbert DR, Demers LM, Jones DED: Dysmenorrhea and prostaglandins. Obstet Gynecol Surv 1976;31:77.

Hammond CB, Weed JC Jr, Currie JL: The role of operation in the current therapy gestational trophoblastic disease. Am J Obstet Gynecol 1980;136:844.

Harrison CR, Averette HE, Jarrell MA, et al: Carcinoma of the fallopian tube: clinical management. Gynecol Oncol 1989;32:357.

Hatch KD: Cervical cancer. In Berck JS, Hacker NF (eds): Practical Gynecologic Oncology. Baltimore: Williams & Wilkins, 1989:241.

Haynes DM, Martin BJ: Cesarean hysterectomy: a twenty-five year review. Am J Obstet Gynecol 1979,134:393.

Heaney NS: Techniques of vaginal hysterectomy. Surg Clin North Am 1942;22:73.

Heath AM: Case of excision of the uterus by the abdominal section. London Med Gazette 1843;1(NS):309.

Henrotin F: Vaginal hysterectomy. In Kelly H, Noble CP (eds): Gynecology and Abdominal Surgery. Philadelphia: WB Saunders Company, 1907:759.

Henry BL: Expanding indications for vaginal hysterectomy. Paper presented at the 44th Clinical Surgeons' Symposium, Sacramento, CA, 1997.

Hernandez-Linares W, Puthawala A, Nolan JF, et al: Carcinoma in situ of the vagina: past and present management. Obstet Gynecol 1980;56:356.

Hershey DW, Fennell RH, Major FJ: Primary carcinoma of the fallopian tube. Obstet Gynecol 1981;57:367.

Hilgers RD: Myomectomy. In Sciarra JJ (ed): Gynecology and Obstetrics. Philadelphia: Harper & Row, 1986:1.

Ikenberg H, Gissmann L, Gross G, et al: Human papillomavirus type 16 related DNA in genital Bowen's disease and in bowenoid papulosis. Int J Cancer 1983;32:563.

Jensen RD, Norris HJ, Fraumeni JS: Familial arrhenoblastoma and thyroid adenoma. Cancer 1974;33:218.

Joel-Cohen SJ: The place of abdominal hysterectomy. Clin Obstet Gynecol 1978;5:525.

Jones DED, Shackelford DP, Brame RG: Supracervical hysterectomy: back to the future? Am J Obstet Gynecol 1999;180:513.

Jones WB, Lewis JL Jr: Treatment of gestational trophoblastic disease. Am J Obstet Gynecol 1974;120:14.

Kempers RD: Dysfunctional uterine bleeding. In Speroff L, Simpson JL, Sciarra JJ (eds): Gynecology and Obstetrics. Philadelphia: Harper & Row, 1990:1.

Kempson RL, Bari W: Uterine sarcomas: classification, diagnosis, and prognosis. Hum Pathol 1970;1:331.

Kennedy JW: The history of hysterectomy. In Kennedy JA, Campbell AD (eds): Vaginal Hysterectomy. Philadelphia: Davis, 1944:3.

Kilgore LC, Partridge EE, Alvarez RD, et al: Adenocarcinoma of the endometrium: survival comparisons of patients with and without pelvic node sampling. Gynecol Oncol 1995;56:29.

Kimball G: Successful case of extirpation of the uterus. Boston Med Surg J 1855;52(13):249.

Kinch RAH: Enigmatic pelvic pain. Comtemp OB/GYN 1987;30:51.

Koch R: Ueber desinfection. Mitteilungen aus dem Kaiserlichen Gesundheitsamte 1881;1:234.

Koonings PP, Campbell K, Mishell DR, et al: Relative frequency of primary ovarian neoplasms: a 10-year review. Obstet Gynecol 1989;74:921.

Koss LG: Miniature adenoacanthoma arising in an endometriotic cyst in an obturator lymph node. Cancer 1963;16:1369.

Kovac SR: Guidelines to determine the route of hysterectomy. Obstet Gynecol 1995;85:18.

Kramer MG, Reiter RC: Hysterectomy: indications, alternatives and predictors. Am Fam Physician 1997;55:827.

Kresch AJ, Seifer DB, Sachs LB, et al: Laparoscopy in 100 women with chronic pelvic pain. Obstet Gynecol 1984;64:672.

Kudo R, Kusanagi Tk, Hashimoto M: Vaginal semiradical hysterectomy: a new operative procedure of microinvasive carcinoma of the cervix. Obstet Gynecol 1984;64:810.

Lanciano RM, Curran WJ, Greven KM, et al: Influence of grade, histologic subtype, and timing of radiotherapy on outcome among patients with stage II carcinoma of the endometrium. Gynecol Oncol 1990;39:368.

Landis SH, Murray T, Bolden S, Wingo PA: Cancer statistics, 1999. CA Cancer J Clin 1999;49:8.

Langenbeck MA: De totius uteri extirpatione. Gorringen, ex. off. Dieterichiana, 1842.

Laros RK, Work BA: Female sterilization. III. Vaginal hysterectomy. Am J Obstet Gynecol 1975;122:693.

Larsson G: Conization for preinvasive and early invasive carcinoma of the uterine cervix. Acta Obstet Gynecol Scand Suppl 1983;114:1.

Lee NC, Dicker RD, Rubin GL, et al: Confirmation of the preoperative diagnoses for hysterectomy. Am J Obstet Gynecol 1984;150:283.

Levitan Z, Eibschitz I, DeVries K, et al: The value of laparoscopy in women with chronic pelvic pain and a normal pelvis. Int J Gynaecol Obstet 1985;23:71.

Lewis JL Jr, Ketcham AS, Hertz R: Surgical intervention during chemotherapy of gestational trophoblastic neoplasms. Cancer 1966;19:1517.

Li MC, Hertz R, Spencer DB: Effect of methotrexate therapy upon choriocarcinoma and chorioadenoma. Proc Soc Exp Biol Med 1956;93:361.

Lister JB: The antiseptic principle in the practice of surgery. Br Med J 1867;11:246.

Liston WA, Bradford WP, Downie J, et al: Laparoscopy in a general gynecologic unit. Am J Obstet Gynecol 1972;113:672.

Liu CY: Laparoscopic hysterectomy: a review of 72 cases. J Reprod Med 1992;37:351.

Loffer FD: Laser ablation of the endometrium. Obstet Gynecol Clin North Am 1988;15:77.

Lorincz AT, Temple GF, Kurman RJ, et al: Oncogenic association of specific human papillomavirus types with cervical neoplasia. J Natl Cancer Inst 1987;79:671.

Lundberg WI, Wall JE, Mathers JE: Laparoscopy in evaluation of pelvic pain. Obstet Gynecol 1984;42:872.

Lundeberg T, Bondesson L, Lundstrom V: Relief of primary dysmenorrhea by transcutaneous electrical nerve stimulation. Acta Obstet Gynecol Scand 1985;64:491.

Lynch HT, Harris RE, Guirgis HA, et al: Familial association of breast/ovarian carcinoma. Cancer 1978;41:1543.

Lynch HT, Lynch JF, Conway TA: Hereditary ovarian cancer. In Rubin SC, Sutton GP (eds): Ovarian Cancer. New York: McGraw-Hill, 1993:189.

Maiman M, Fruchter RG, Clark M, et al: Cervical cancer as an AIDS-defining illness. Obstet Gynecol 1997;89:76.

Malkasian GD, Annegers JF, Fountain KS: Carcinoma of the endometrium: stage I. Am J Obstet Gynecol 1980;136:872.

Mark AS, Hricak H: Adenomyosis and leiomyoma: differential diagnosis by means of magnetic resonance imaging. Radiology 1987;163:527.

Marut EL: Etiology and pathophysiology of fibroid tumor disease: diagnosis and current medical and surgical treatment alternatives. Obstet Gynecol Surv 1989;44:308.

Mathieu A: The history of hysterectomy. West J Surg Obstet Gynecol 1934;42:1.

McDonald TW, Annegers JF, O'Fallon WM, et al: Exogenous estrogen and endometrial carcinoma: case-control and incidence study. Am J Obstet Gynecol 1977a;127:572.

McDonald TW, Malkasian GD, Gaffey TA: Endometrial cancer associated with feminizing ovarian tumor and polycystic ovarian disease. Obstet Gynecol 1977b;49:654.

McDonald TW, Neutens JJ, Fischer LM, et al: Impact of cervical intraepithelial neoplasia diagnosis and treatment on self-esteem and body image. Gynecol Oncol 1989;34:345.

McDonald TW, Ruffolo EH: Modern management of gestational trophoblastic disease. Obstet Gynecol Surv 1983;38:67.

McDowell E: Three cases of extirpation of diseases ovaria. Eclectic Repertory and Analytical Review, Medical and Philosophical 187;7:242. (Reprinted in Medical Classics 1938;2:651).

McGarrity KA, Pettersson F, Ulfelder H (eds): Annual Report on the Results of Treatment of Gynecologic Cancer. Vol 18. Stockholm: Radiumhemmet, 1982.

McKenzie LL: Discussion of Randall CL, Paloucek FP: The frequency of oophorectomy at the time of hysterectomy: trends in surgical practice, 1928–1953. Am J Obstet Gynecol 1968;100:716.

Melody GF: Depressive reactions following hysterectomy. Am J Obstet Gynecol 1962;83:410.

Merajver SD, Frank TS, Xu J, et al: Germline BRCA1 mutations and loss of the wild-type allele in tumors from families with early onset breast and ovarian cancer. Clin Cancer Res 1995;1:539.

Mesko J, Gates H, McDonald TW, et al: Clear cell ("mesonephroid") adenocarcinoma of the vulva arising in endometriosis: a case report. Gynecol Oncol 1988;29:385.

Mettler L, Semm K: Vaginal supracervical vs. laparoscopic supracervical hysterectomy, with resection of transcervical and transuterine mucosa. Zentralbl Gynakol 1995;117(12):633.

Miki Y, Swensen J, Shattuck-Eidens D, et al: A strong candidate for the breast ovarian cancer susceptibility gene BRCA1. Science 1994;266:66.

Miller BA, Ries LAG, Hankey BF, et al (eds): SEER Cancer Statistics Review, 1973–1990 (NIH publication no 93-2789). Bethesda, MD: National Cancer Institute, 1993.

Miller NF: Hysterectomy: therapeutic necessity or surgical racket? Am J Obstet Gynecol 1946;51:804.

Morley GW: On their shoulders we stand! Gynecol Oncol 1977;5:325.

Morley GW: History of Hysterectomy [videotape]. Washington, DC: American College of Obstetrics and Gynecology, 1988.

Morley GW, Seski JC: Radical pelvic surgery versus radiation therapy for stage I carcinoma of the cervix (exclusive of microinvasion). Am J Obstet Gynecol 1976;126:785.

Morrow CP: Classification and characteristics of ovarian cancer. Clin Obstet Gynecol 1979;22:925.

Mundy AR: An anatomical explanation for bladder dysfunction following rectal and uterine surgery. Br J Urol 1982;54:501.

Munro MG: Supracervical hysterectomy: a time for reappraisal. Obstet Gynecol 1997;89:133.

Nakagawa S, Yoshikawa H, Onda T, et al: Type of human papillomavirus is related to clinical features of cervical carcinoma. Cancer 1996;78:1935.

Narod S, Ford D, Devilee P, et al: Genetic heterogeneity of breast-ovarian cancer revisited. Am J Hum Genet 1995;57:957.

National Institutes of Health: NIH Consensus Statement on Perioperative Red Cell Transfusion. Bethesda, MD: National Institutes of Health, 1990.

Neighbours LE, Clelland J, Jackson JR, et al: Transcutaneous electrical nerve stimulation for pain relief in primary dysmenorrhea. Clin J Pain 1987;3:17.

Nelson JH Jr, Averette HE, Richart RM: Cervical intraepithelial neoplasia (dysplasia and carcinoma in situ) and early invasive cervical carcinoma. CA Cancer J Clin 1989;39:157.

Neutens JJ: Intimacy is not for amateurs. In Pocs O (ed): Annual Editions: Human Sexuality. Guilford, CT: Dushkin Publishing Group, 1981.

Neuwirth RS: Hysteroscopic management of symptomatic submucous fibroids. Obstet Gynecol 1983;62:509.

Novak ER, Woodruff JD: Gynecologic and Obstetric Pathology. Philadelphia: WB Saunders Company, 1967;211.

Novak ER, Woodruff JD: Adenomyosis (adnexomyoma) uteri. In Novak's Gynecologic and Obstetric Pathology. 8th ed. Philadelphia: WB Saunders Company, 1979;280.

Osiander FB: Goettingische Gelehrte Anzeigen. Dietrich, 1816:130.

Padial JG, Sotolongo J, Casey MJ, et al: Laparoscopy-assisted vaginal hysterectomy: report of seventy-five consecutive cases. J Gynecol Surg 1992;8:81.

Palleta G: Storia d'una Matrice Amputata. Milano: Ann Univ di Medicina, 1822.

Panganiban W, Cornog JL: Endometriosis of the intestines and vermiform appendix. Dis Colon Rectum 1972;15:253.

Park RC, Duff WP: Role of cesarean hysterectomy in modern obstetric practice. Clin Obstet Gynecol 1980;23:601.

Parkin DM, Pisani P, Ferlay J: Estimates of the worldwide medicine of 25 major cancers in 1990. Int J Cancer 1999;80:827.

Parmley TH, Woodruff JD: The ovarian mesothelioma. Am J Obstet Gynecol 1974;120:234.

Pean J: De l'hysterectomie vaginale totale appliquee au traitement des tumeurs fibreures multiples de l'uterus; morcellement des tumeurs: pincement definitif des ligaments larges; absence de fermeture du vagin. Gaz des Hopitaux 1886;59:950.

Perry CP, Upchurch JC: Pelviscopic adnexectomy. Am J Obstet Gynecol 1990;162:79.

Peters WA: Management of early endometrial carcinoma. Prim Care Update Obstet Gynecol 1995;2:162.

Peters WA III, Andersen WA, Thornton N Jr, Morley GW: The selective use of vaginal hysterectomy in the management of adenocarcinoma of the endometrium. Am J Obstet Gynecol 1983;146:285.

Pfister H: The role of human papillomavirus in anogenital cancer. Obstet Gynecol Clin North Am 1996;23:579.

Philipsen T, Naesbol C: Electrocoagulation of the endometrium: a new method for the treatment of hemorrhagic disorders in women. Ugeskr Laeger 1993;155(7):484.

Piver MS, Baker TR, Jishi MF, et al: Familial ovarian cancer: a report of 658 families from the Gilda Radner Familial Ovarian Cancer Registry 1981–1991. Cancer 1993;71(Suppl):582.

Piver MS, Barlow JJ, Sawyer DM: Familial ovarian cancer: increasing in frequency? Obstet Gynecol 1982;60;397.

Piver MS, Rutledge F, Smith JP: Five classes of extended hysterectomy for women with cervical cancer. Obstet Gynecol 1974; 44:265.

Plauche WC: Caesarean hysterectomy. In Sciarra JJ (ed): Gynecology and Obstetrics. New York: Harper & Row, 1986:1.

Pletsch TD, Sandberg EC: Caesarean hysterectomy for sterilization. Am J Obstet Gynecol 1963;85:254.

Podratz KC, Podczaski ES, Gaffet TA, et al: Primary carcinoma of the fallopian tube. Am J Obstet Gynecol 1986;154:1319.

Pokras R, Hufnagel VG: Hysterectomy in the United States, 1965–84. Vital Health Stat 13 1987;92.

Pokras R, Hufnagel VG: Hysterectomy in the United States, 1965–84. Am J Public Health 1988;78:852.

Polivy J: Psychological reactions to hysterectomy: A critical review. Am J Obstet Gynecol 1974;118:417.

Porges RF: Changing indications for vaginal hysterectomy. Am J Obstet Gynecol 1980;136:153.

Pratt JH: The unnecessary hysterectomy. South Med J 1980;73: 1360.

Prior A, Stanley K, Smith ARB, et al: Effect of hysterectomy on anorectal and urethrovescial physiology. Gut 1992;33:264.

Pyper RJD, Haeri AD: A review of 80 endometrial resections for menorrhagia. Br J Obstet Gynaecol 1991;98:1049.

Rapkin AJ, Kames LD: The pain management approach to chronic pelvic pain. J Reprod Med 1987;33:323.

Reich H: Laparoscopic oophorectomy and salpingo-oophorectomy in the treatment of benign tubo-ovarian disease. Int J Fertil 1987;32:233.

Reich H, DeCaprio J, McGlynn F: Laparoscopic hysterectomy. J Gynecol Surg 1989;5:213.

Reich H, McGlynn F: Laparoscopic treatment of tuboovarian and pelvic abscess. J Reprod Med 1987;32:747.

Reid R: Preinvasive disease. In Berek JS, Hacker NF (eds): Practical Gynecologic Oncology. Baltimore: Williams & Wilkins, 1989:195.

Reid R, Stanhope CR, Herschman BR, et al: Genital warts and cervical cancer: I. Evidence of an association between subclinical papillomavirus infection and cervical malignancy. Cancer 1982;50:377.

Reinhold C, McCarthy S, Bret PM, et al: Diffuse adenomyosis: comparison of endovaginal US and MR imaging with histopathologic correlation. Radiology 1996;199:151.

Reis E: Eine neue Operationsmethode des Uteruskarzinomes. Z Geburtschilfe Gynakol 1895;32:266.

Reiter RC: Chronic pelvic pain. Clin Obstet Gynecol 1990;33:117.

Reiter RC: Occult somatic pathology in women with chronic pelvic pain. Clin Obstet Gynecol 1990;33:154.

Reiter RC, Gambone JC: Demographic and historical variable in women with idiopathic chronic pelvic pain. Obstet Gynecol 1990;75:428.

Renaer M, Vertommen H, Nijs P, et al: Psychological aspects of chronic pelvic pain in women. Am J Obstet Gynecol 1979;134: 75.

Richards DH: Depression after hysterectomy. Lancet 1973;2:430.

Richards DH: A post-hysterectomy syndrome. Lancet 1974;2:983.

Richardson EH: A simplified technique for abdominal panhysterectomy. Surg Gynecol Obstet 1929;48:248.

Richardson FM: Peer review of medical care. Med Care 1972;10: 29.

Richardson RE, Bournas N, Magos AL: Is laparoscopic hysterectomy a waste of time? Lancet 1995;345:36.

Richart RM: Natural history of cervical intraepithelial neoplasia. Clin Obstet Gynecol 1967;10:748.

Richart RM, Barron BA: A follow-up study of patients with cervical dysplasia. Am J Obstet Gynecol 1969;105:386.

Rigoni-Stern D: Fatti statistici relativi alle malattre cnacerose. Gior Servire Prog Pathol Ther 1842;2:507.

Romney SL, Ober WB: The uterus. In Romney SL (ed): Gynecology and Obstetrics: The Health Care of Women. 2nd ed. New York: McGraw-Hill, 1981:1053.

Rosemberg SK, Herman G, Elfont E: Sexually transmitted papillomaviral infection in the male. 7. Is cancer of penis sexually transmitted? Urology 1991;37:437.

Rubin SC, Benjamin I, Behbakht K, et al: Clinical and pathological features of ovarian cancer in women with germ-line mutations of BRCA1. N Engl J Med 1996;335:1413.

Salazar OM, Bonfiglio TA, Patten SF, et al: Uterine sarcomas: natural history, treatment and prognosis. Cancer 1978;42:1152.

Schaefer G. Tuberculosis of the female genital tract. In Droegemueller W, Sciarra JJ (eds): Gynecology and Obstetrics. Philadelphia: Harper & Row, 1981:1.

Schauta F: Die erweiterten vaginale Totalexstirpation der Uterus beim Kollumcarzinom. Wein Leipzig: J Safar, 1908.

Schildkraut JM, Thompson WD: Relationship of epithelial ovarian cancer to other malignancies within families. Genet Epidemiol 1988;5:355.

Scully RD: Gonadoblastoma: a review of 74 cases. Cancer 1970a; 25:1340.

Scully RD: Sex cord tumor with annular tubules: a distinctive ovarian tumor of the Peutz-Jeghers syndrome. Cancer 1970b; 25:1107.

Sedlis A: Primary carcinomas of the fallopian tube. Obstet Gynecol Surv 1961;16:209.

Semm K: Operative pelviscopy. Br Med Bull 1986;42:284.

Semm K: Hysterectomy via laparotomy or pelviscopy: a new CASH method without colpotomy. Geburtshilfe Frauenheilkd 1991;51:996.

Sevin BU, Ford JH, Girtanner MD, et al: Invasive cancer of the cervix after cryosurgery: pitfalls of conservative management. Obstet Gynecol 1979;53:465.

Sills ES, Saini J, Steiner CA, et al: Abdominal hysterectomy practice patterns in the United States. Int J Gynaecol Obstet 1998; 63:277.

Simon NL, Gore H, Shingleton HM, et al: Study of superficially invasive carcinoma of the cervix. Obstet Gynecol 1986;68:19.

Sloan D: The emotional and psychosexual aspects of hysterectomy. Am J Obstet Gynecol 1978;131:598.

Slocumb JC: Neurological factors in chronic pelvic pain: trigger points and the abdominal pelvic pain syndrome. Am J Obstet Gynecol 1984;149:536.

Sobczyk R: Dysmenorrhea: the neglected syndrome. J Reprod Med 1980;25:198.

Sonnendecker EWW: Is appendectomy mandatory in patients with ovarian carcinoma? S Afr Med J 1982;62:978.

Sonnendecker EWW, Margolius KA, Sonnendecker HEM: Involvement of the appendix in ovarian epithelial cancer–an update. S Afr Med J 1989;76:667.

Soper JT: Surgical therapy for gestational trophoblastic disease. J Reprod Med 1994;39:168.

Stafl A, Wilkinson E, Mattingly RF: Laser treatment of cervical and vaginal neoplasia. Am J Obstet Gynecol 1977;128:128.

Stearns MW: Benign and malignant neoplasms of colon and rectum: diagnosis and management. Surg Clin North Am 1978;58: 605.

Steck WD, Helwig EB: Cutaneous endometriosis. JAMA 1965;191: 167.

Stock RG, Chen ASJ, Seski J: A 30-year experience in the management of primary carcinoma of the vagina: analysis of prognostic factors and treatment modalities. Gynecol Oncol 1995; 56:45.

Stovall TG, Summitt RL: Laparoscopic hysterectomy—is there a benefit? N Engl J Med 1996;335:512.

Summitt RL Jr, Stovall TG, Lipscomb GH, Ling FW: Randomized comparison of laparoscopy-assisted vaginal hysterectory with standard hysterectomy in an outpatient setting. Obstet Gynecol 1992;80:895.

Surrey ES, Halme J: Endometriosis as a cause of infertility. Obstet Gynecol Clin North Am 1989;16:79.

Takashina T, Ono M, Kanda Y: Cervicovaginal and endometrial cytology in ovarian cancer. Acta Cytol 1988;32:159.

Talerman A: Gonadoblastoma and dysgerminoma in two siblings with dysgenetic gonads. Obstet Gynecol 1971;38:218.

Temkin OS: Gynecology. Baltimore: Johns Hopkins Press, 1956.

Terz JJ, Barber HRK, Brunschwig A: Incidence of carcinoma in the retained ovary. Am J Surg 1967;113:511.

Thompson JD, Birch HW: Indications for hysterectomy. Clin Obstet Gynecol 1981;24:1245.

Tilt EJ: Handbook of Uterine Therapeutics. 4th ed. New York: William and Wood Co, 1881:20.

Tobacman JK, Greene MH, Tucker MA, et al: Intra-abdominal carcinomatosis after prophylactic oophorectomy in ovarian cancer-prone families. Lancet 1982;2:795.

Tow WHS: The influence of the primary treatment of hydatidiform mole on its subsequent course. J Obstet Gynaecol Br Commonw 1966;73:544.

Townsend DE, Richart RM: Diagnostic errors in colposcopy. Gynecol Oncol 1981;12:S259.

Toy PRCY, Dzik WH, Gould SA, et al: The use of autologous blood. JAMA 1990;263:414.

Trendelenburg F: Ueber Blasencheidenfisteloperationen und ueber Beckenhochlagerung bei Operationen in der Bauchhohle. In: Sammlung Klinischer Vortrage (Volkmanns). Leipzig: JA Barth, 1890;3373.

Tucker MA, Fraumeni JF: Treatment-related cancers after gynecologic malignancy. Cancer 1987;60:S2117.

Van Keep PA, Wildemeersch D, Lehert P: Hysterectomy in six European countries. Maturitas 1983;5:69.

Van Nagell JR, Greenwell N, Powell BF, et al: Microinvasive carcinoma of the cervix. Am J Obstet Gynecol 1983;145:891.

Visscher HC (ed): Precis V: An Update in Obstetrics and Gynecology. Washington, DC: American College of Obstetricians and Gynecologists, 1994:268.

Von Rokitansky C: Ueber Uterusdrusenneubildung in Uterus and Ovarialsarcomen. Zkk Gesellsch d Aerzte zu Wien 1860;16:577.

Walker AM, Jick H: Temporal and regional variation in hysterectomy rates in the U.S. 1970–1975. Am J Epidemiol 1979;110:41.

Walker E, Katon W, Harrop-Griffiths J, et al: Relationship of chronic pelvic pain to psychiatric diagnosis and childhood sexual abuse. Am J Psychiatry 1988;145:75.

Weber AM, Lee J-C: Use of alternative techniques of hysterectomy in Ohio, 1988–1994. N Engl J Med 1996;335:483.

Weiss NS: Relationship of menopause to serum cholesterol and arterial blood pressure: the United States' Health Examination survey of adults. Am J Epidemiol 1972;96:237.

Wertheim E: Die erweiterte abdominale Operation bei carcinoma colli uteri: auf Grund von 500 Fallen. Berlin: Urban & Schwarzenberg, 1911.

Wertheim E: The extended abdominal operation for carcinoma uterus (based on 500 operative cases). Am J Obstet Dis Women Child 1912;66(2):169.

Wheeler JM, Malinak LR: The surgical management of endometriosis. Obstet Gynecol Clin North Am 1989;16:147.

Wilbanks GD: Cervical intraepithelial carcinoma: History, detection, and treatment. In Buchsbaum HJ, Sciarra JJ (eds): Gynecology and Obstetrics. Philadelphia: Harper & Row, 1988:1.

Wilcox LS, Koonin LM, Pokras R, et al: Hysterectomy in the United States, 1988–1990. Obstet Gynecol 1994;83:549.

Willman EA, Collins WP, Clayton SG: Studies in the involvement of prostaglandins in uterine symptomatology and pathology. Br J Obstet Gynaecol 1976;83:337.

Wingo PA, Huezo CM, Rubin GL, et al: The mortality risk associated with hysterectomy. Am J Obstet Gynecol 1985;152:803.

Young SJ, Alpers DH, Norland CC, et al: Psychiatric illness and the irritable bowel syndrome. Gastroenterology 1976;70:162.

Zaloudek CJ, Norris HJ: Mesenchymal tumors of the uterus. In Fenoglio C, Wolff M (eds): Progress in Surgical Pathology. New York: Masson Publishing, 1981:1.

zur Hausen H, Devilliers EM: Human papillomaviruses. Annu Rev Microbiol 1994;48:427.

zur Hausen H, Meinhof W, Scheiber W, et al: Attempts to detect virus-specific DNA in human tumors: I. Nucleic acid hybridizations with complementary RNA of human wart virus. Int J Cancer 1977;13:650.

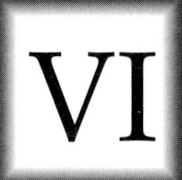

VI

Urogynecological and Pelvic Floor Support Problems

46 | Urinary Incontinence

J. Thomas Benson

HISTORY AND OVERVIEW

Dieffenbach's description of urinary incontinence in 1836 captures the tragic totality of personal calamity suffered by afflicted women:

> A sadder situation can hardly exist than that of a woman afflicted with a vesicovaginal fistula. A source of disgust even to herself, the woman beloved by her husband becomes, in this condition, the object of bodily revulsion to him; and filled with repugnance, everyone else likewise turns his back, repulsed by the intolerable, foul, uriniferous odor. . . . This horrendous evil tears asunder every family bond. The tender mother is rejected from the circle of her children. Indifference overtakes some of these unfortunates; others give themselves over to quiet resignation and pious devotion. Otherwise they would fall victim to despair and would attempt suicide.

Urinary incontinence was not a problem exclusive to the 19th century. Today it constitutes the second most frequent precipitating factor in nursing home placement. At the National Institutes of Health (NIH) Consensus Development Conference on Urinary Incontinence in 1988, it was estimated that at least 10 million adult Americans suffer from incontinence, at an annual overall cost of $10.3 billion (NIH, 1989). That number has now been increased to $16.4 billion according to the 1994 Agency for Health Care Policy and Research update (Agency for Health Care Policy and Research, 1994). This represents an increase of greater than 60% from the previous estimate, rising more rapidly than other medical costs. Greater than 50% of nursing home residents have incontinence and 53% of homebound elderly suffer from incontinence. The Surgeon General's office once estimated the cost of diapering the incontinent women in institutions at $8 billion (Brazda, 1983). This number is certainly higher now and will continue to increase. In a Maryland study, 100,000 nursing home residents nationwide were using chronic urethral catheterization to manage urinary problems, and thus nearly 3 million annual new episodes of bacteriuria with complications of stones, cystitis, pyelonephritis, bacteremia, and death occurred (Warren et al, 1989).

Government studies project that the current figure of 3 million persons age 85 or older may nearly double in another decade (Special Committee on Aging,

1986). Responding to the problem's magnitude, the Residency Review Committee declared in 1990 that obstetrics-gynecology resident education must include diagnosis and management of female urinary incontinence. In addition, the American Board of Obstetrics and Gynecology has begun accrediting fellowships in the field of urogynecology and reconstructive pelvic surgery, which further confirms the pressing need for specialty training in this area.

Historically, gynecologists have been involved with this problem. James Marion Simms is considered by many to be the father of American gynecology despite his ethically debatable experiments on slaves, which did finally cure their vesicovaginal fistulas after 40 failed attempts (Speert, 1958). In the late 19th century, Howard Kelly, the first professor of gynecology at Johns Hopkins University, developed what has been probably the most used operation for stress incontinence in the world: the Kelly plication.

Urinary incontinence in the female should be considered a component of female pelvic floor disorder, often associated with other symptoms of anal incontinence and prolapse. Such pelvic floor disorders are a common cause of disability and distress, their pathogenesis having been poorly understood in the past. We now recognize these disorders to be associated with clinical, electrophysiologic, and histologic features of chronic partial denervation in the muscles of the pelvic floor (Parks et al, 1977; Neill and Swash 1980; Snooks et al, 1984; Gilpin et al, 1989). Damage to this innervation is often initiated by childbirth and progresses until functional disorders become apparent in midlife. The incontinence process in women is, however, multifactorial in origin because even young, nulliparous, physically fit women frequently have stress incontinence symptoms (Nygaard et al, 1994).

ANATOMY

The pelvic floor musculature has long been poorly understood despite decades of debate regarding the significance of "ligaments" and "fascia." A century ago, R. L. Dickinson (1889) stated that "there is no considerable muscle in the body the form and function of which are more difficult to understand that those of the levator ani, and about which such nebulous impressions prevail."

The concept that the pelvic viscera are supported by inert ligamentous structures acting as "guy wires" is erroneous. The support is by tissue that is dynamic and composed largely of muscle, both smooth and skeletal. Smooth muscle fibers are in a constant state of activity, helping to maintain tone but at the same time allowing cellular elongation without increasing tone up to the limits of elasticity. Striated muscle tissue consists of varying compositions of type 1 and type 2 fibers. Type 1 are "slow-twitch," darker, high-oxidative fibers especially useful in maintaining "tone". Type 2 are "fast-twitch" fibers useful for rapid-action responses to stress. The pelvic diaphragm, or levator ani, is mainly skeletal muscle, with portions originating from a membranous insertion on the inner surface of the obturator internus muscle (tendinous arch of the levator ani), higher in amounts of type 1 fibers and functioning mainly for tone. Portions of the levator ani arising from bone, such as the puborectalis and pubococcygeus, have higher concentrations of type 2 fibers and can react reflexly to exert influence on the pelvic viscera in stress situations. All portions of the levator ani join together in a midline raphe just above the anococcygeal junction to form a shelf-like area of the pelvic floor behind the anus and in front of the coccyx. The pelvic viscera rest upon this "shelf," which is called the *levator plate*.

Unlike skeletal muscles elsewhere in the body, which are normally electrically silent at rest, all skeletal muscle acting in pelvic floor support has constant electrical activity. Tissues subjected to stress have a preponderance of elastic fibers that stretch but tend to return to their original state, much like a rubber band. These fibers decrease with aging. Collagen fibers, which contribute little to pelvic floor support, do not stretch but swell and become hyalinized, and are most often found at areas such as the arcus tendineus. Thus the predominant supportive tissue is striated muscle and smooth muscle, the innervation of which is spinal reflex arcs for the former and involuntary through the autonomic nervous system for the latter. The pelvic plexus and the pudendal nerve both carry innervation of a somatic (to skeletal muscle) and an autonomic (to smooth muscle) nature, so that damage in these areas has significance for pelvic visceral support.

Below the levator ani muscle is the urogenital diaphragm, which is now realized to be composed of a perineal membrane associated with the compressor urethra and urethrovaginal sphincter muscles that are part of the striated urogenital sphincter. This perineal membrane has a large opening for the vagina and is attached to the vagina and perineal body. Thus two sheets of tissue extend from the ischial pubic ramus to the perineal body on either side of the vagina: the tonically contracted levator ani muscles and the urogenital diaphragm perineal musculature.

All of the pelvic floor's support depends on its connection to the pelvic bone, which changes, especially as creatures evolve to the upright position. The symphysis was largely responsible for the pelvic visceral support in the pronograde animal, but, in assuming the upright position, the caudal muscles are called on to support the pelvic viscera as the symphysis becomes part of the abdominal wall. The pubococcygeus and coccygeus muscles become attached to the anococcygeal raphe, and the coccygeus muscle becomes more tendinous. The ileococcygeus has lost its origin from the pelvic brim and has moved to the side wall of the pelvis to take origin along the tendinous arch.

Before an infant is able to assume an upright stance, the pelvic organs are located abdominally. Once the newborn becomes upright, the immature pelvis yields to gravitational forces to form a posterior bulging, the sacral concavity (Paramore, 1910), and the pelvic organs descend.

The urethra has both smooth muscle and skeletal muscle compartments. The inner longitudinal smooth muscle is continuous with that of the bladder; the outer circular urethral musculature is both smooth, with fibers throughout the urethra, and striated, with decussating fibers of the surrounding muscles. More bundles of smooth muscle are present anteriorly than laterally or inferiorly. The striated fibers cross laterally and superiorly and encompass both the urethra and the vagina in the lower third of the urethra, but surround the urethra only in the middle third, where they are more prominent on the superior (anterior) surface.

DeLancey's work (1986) ushered in a more modern era of more complete understanding of the periurethral anatomy (Fig. 46–1). The urethra is now divided into fifths instead of thirds, and each part has significant relationships to periurethral structures. The first part (0 to 20th percentile) is intramural, and the 15th to 20th percentile is the area of urethral support afforded by the superior attachment of the vagina to the levator ani musculature, allowing voluntary control of upward and downward motion of the urethra superior to the urogenital diaphragm. The next two fifths (20th to 60th percentile) form both muscular and fascial connections of the urethra to the levator musculature. Fibers in the area of the urogenital diaphragm (60th to 80th percentile) encircle both the vagina and the urethra (urethrovaginal sphincter), while other fibers pass laterally to insert into the pubic rami (the compressor urethrae). The distal fifth, surrounded by nonconnecting bulbocavernosus muscles, lacks skeletal and smooth muscle and is a low-pressure, fibrous conduit.

The vesical neck connects to the pelvic wall by a group of smooth muscle fibers deriving from the detrusor and inserting into the pubic bones (pubovesical muscle); their contraction pulls the anterior bladder neck and proximal urethral anteriorly. Thus the proximal urethra is in a sling, composed of fibromuscular tissue from the anterior vaginal wall, attaching to the levator ani musculature (pelvic diaphragm) and extending caudally to the urogenital

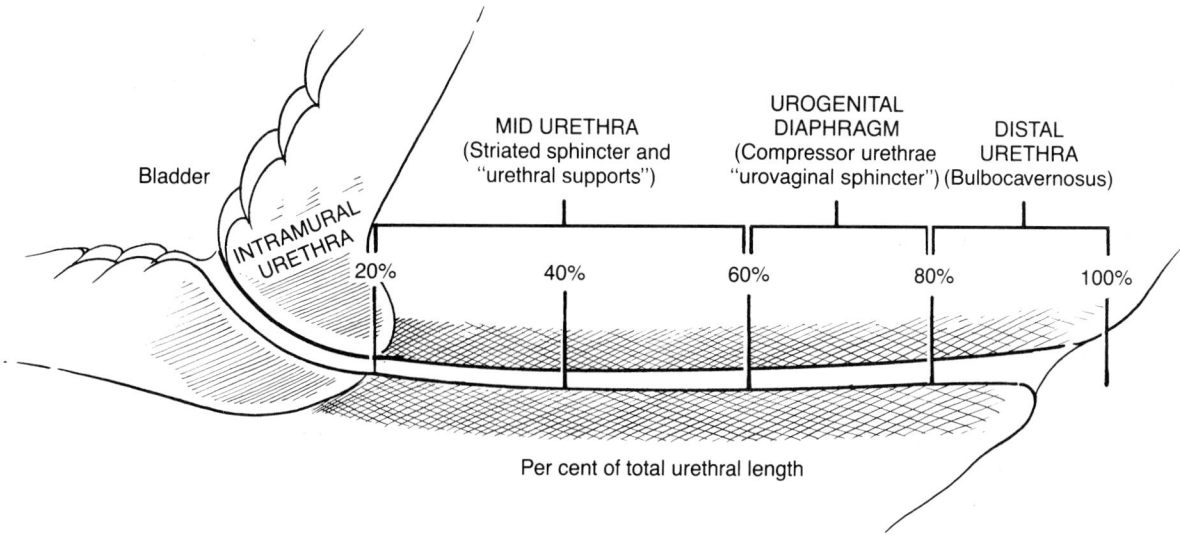

Figure 46 – 1
DeLancey's conceptualized scheme of urethral supports.

diaphragm. This constitutes the previously described "pubourethral ligament," which is not derived from either the urethra or attached pubic bones and should perhaps be called "urethral support."

In the 60th to 80th percentile (urogenital diaphragm area) is the greatest voluntary increase in intraurethral pressure, where (56th percentile) urine flow stops as a woman contracts the pelvic floor (Westby et al, 1982). The urethra enters the urogenital diaphragm at just this point and becomes relatively "fixed," losing the mobility present proximally. This is also the area of greatest pressure "transmission." Sudden increases in intra-abdominal (thus intravesical) pressures are transmitted in continent women to the urethra. In fact, the pressures here in the urethra rise more, and precede the intra-abdominal rise by 0.25 second, suggesting reflex muscle contraction rather than simple "transmission" (Constantinou, 1982).

PHYSIOLOGY

Storage and elimination of urine are accomplished by the coordinated efforts of the bladder and urethra, which compose the lower urinary tract. During storage, the urethra acts as a sphincter while the bladder is the reservoir. With micturition, the bladder contracts and expels its contents through the active conduit represented by the urethra.

STORAGE

Bladder

Urine is delivered to the bladder via the ureters on a continuous basis, the volume varying with the state of hydration. Urine enters the bladder at a rate

of approximately 2 ml/second (Torrens and Morrison, 1987). The bladder wall muscle, called the detrusor, has elastic properties, allowing it to expand during filling without increasing the pressure within its lumen, until it reaches capacity (*accommodation*). The bladder response to filling can be evaluated in terms of sensation, compliance, capacity, and stability. Bladder sensation is generally described in terms of the volume of urine at which the individual first notices sensation to void and the maximum volume tolerated. *Compliance* is defined as a change in bladder pressure for a given change in bladder volume, representing the bladder's ability to "accommodate." Normally, the bladder can fill to 500 to 700 ml with pressure changes less than 15 cm H_2O. Bladder compliance is decreased when the bladder wall is inflamed or has scar formation. Prolonged drainage and motor (efferent) neurologic disorders also can lead to decreased compliance.

During filling, the bladder is termed *stable* if it does not involuntarily contract despite provocation. An unstable bladder is one shown objectively to contract spontaneously or on provocation during the filling phase while the individual is resisting micturition. These contractions can occur without any associated symptoms or can be related to strong sensations of urinary urgency with or without concomitant urinary incontinence (Fantl et al, 1977). The storage phase of bladder function is urodynamically evaluated by cystometrogram.

Urethra

During filling, the entire female urethra acts as the "bladder sphincter," and continence is maintained as long as the intravesical pressure does not exceed the intraurethral resistance. The three main sources of urethral resistance are the periurethral striated muscles, urethral smooth musculature, and elastic connective tissue with submucosal vascular bed. Each contributes approximately one third of the total urethral resistance (Awad and Downie, 1976).

Resting urethral resistance is augmented by the transmission of pressure from the abdomen to the urethra (pressure transmission). Acute increments of intra-abdominal pressure are transmitted to the proximal urethra, maintaining the pressure gradient between the urethra and bladder.

Emptying Phase

Normally, voluntary relaxation of the levator ani and urethral sphincter with subsequent sustained contraction of the bladder leads to complete emptying of the bladder. The bladder neck descends and assumes a funnel shape immediately before the detrusor contraction (Tanagho and Miller, 1970); during this descent of approximately 3 seconds, a progressive drop in intraurethral pressure occurs. Generally, the detrusor contraction does not exceed 50 cm of H_2O, important because greater intravesical pressures may lead to retrograde reflux into ureters. The initiation of urination is voluntary, and the maintenance is autonomic, being mediated by local reflexes. Lower urinary tract dysfunction can occur in either the storage or voiding phases as a result of disorders of the bladder, the urethra, or their neurocontrol.

NEUROANATOMY AND FUNCTION (NEUROPHYSIOLOGY)

The lower urinary tract must accomplish storage in the presence of a closed outlet without increased pressure so that the upper tract is not damaged. In emptying, a complex reflex mechanism under autonomic, central, and peripheral nervous system control must be mediated.

The bladder, if separated from its neuronal relationship with the central nervous system (CNS) and autonomic nervous system, would lose coordination of urethral relaxation and contract weakly. If the bladder is connected to the sacral CNS, more effective detrusor contractions can occur but, again, without coordination. Coordination and detrusor contraction of sufficient temporal duration for emptying the bladder depend on connections to "Barrington's center" in the anterior pontine region of the brain stem.

Bladder contractions are thought to be mediated by sacral parasympathetics originating in S2 through S4 and running in the pelvic nervous plexus, using cholinergic neurotransmitters acting on nicotinic and muscarinic receptors in the ganglia and bladder wall (Fig. 46–2). In storage (Fig. 46–3), lumbar sympathetics originating in the lumbodorsal portion of the cord and traveling in the presacral nervous plexus utilize norepinephrine neurotransmitters to stimulate α-adrenergic and β-adrenergic receptors for

smooth muscle contraction and relaxation, respectively. β-Receptors predominate in the bladder fundus; α-receptors predominate in the base of the bladder. The sympathetic system acts at parasympathetic ganglia to stop transmission. Thus, during storage, there is effective ganglionic cessation of parasympathetic cholinergic activity through α-adrenergic stimulation. Urethral resistance is further augmented by skeletal muscle components innervated through the pudendal nerve and other nerve branches through the pelvic plexus. Thus the autonomic and somatic nervous systems act in harmony (Fig. 46–4). Multiple pelvic floor reflexes to the spinal cord interplay during voiding to allow continuous outlet relaxation and detrusor contraction, with some reflexes going to the sacral cord and others going to Barrington's center in the pons.

Nervous System Relationships to Bladder Function

A summation of the effects of nervous system lesions on lower urinary tract function is given in Figure 46–5.

Brain Lesions

CNS control is effected by voluntary inhibition of the Barrington reflex center from an area in the superior frontal gyrus–septal region. Lesions in this area interfere with voluntary inhibition and result in detrusor hyperreflexia with contractions that are coordinated with urethral relaxation because the pons center is still effective. Such cortical lesions prevent voluntary postponement of voiding, resulting in urge incontinence when sensation is intact. If sensation is not intact, involuntary voiding (enuresis) or "uninhibited neurogenic bladder" occurs. With larger lesions, one's social concern about incontinence is lost.

Located in the paracentral lobule cortical areas is a separate control for upper motor neuron pudendal nerve control. Lesions in this area produce the inability to quiet pelvic floor electrical activity and are characterized by difficulty in initiating micturition.

Spinal Cord Lesions

The nature of disturbance that occurs with spinal cord disease depends on the site and extent of the injury.

SUPRASACRAL CORD AREAS

Lower urinary tract neurons originating in the bladder wall have long, ascending axons reaching Barrington's center in the pons to mediate chiefly facilitative effects for detrusor contraction. Lesions affecting these "sensory" components can lead to detrusor areflexia and increased compliance; corre-

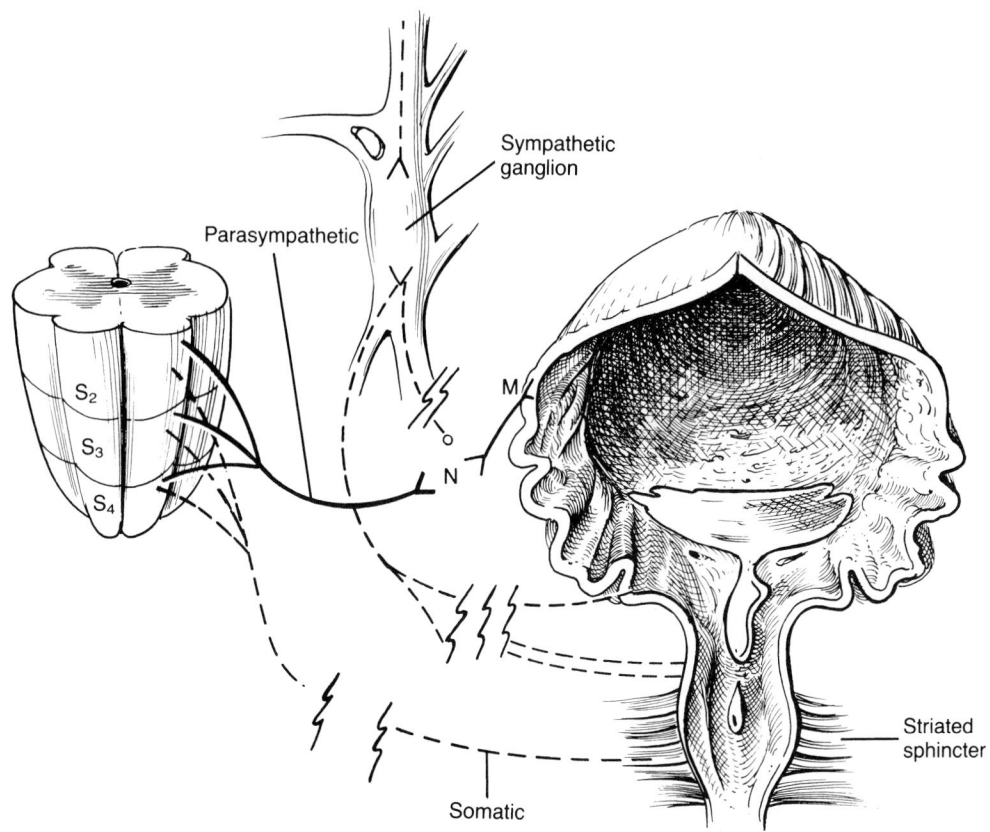

Figure 46–2
Bladder in process of emptying. S2, S3, and S4 make up the sacral cord. Cholinergic neurotransmitters in parasympathetic nerves act at ganglia on nicotinic receptors (N) and at bladder wall on muscarinic receptors (M).

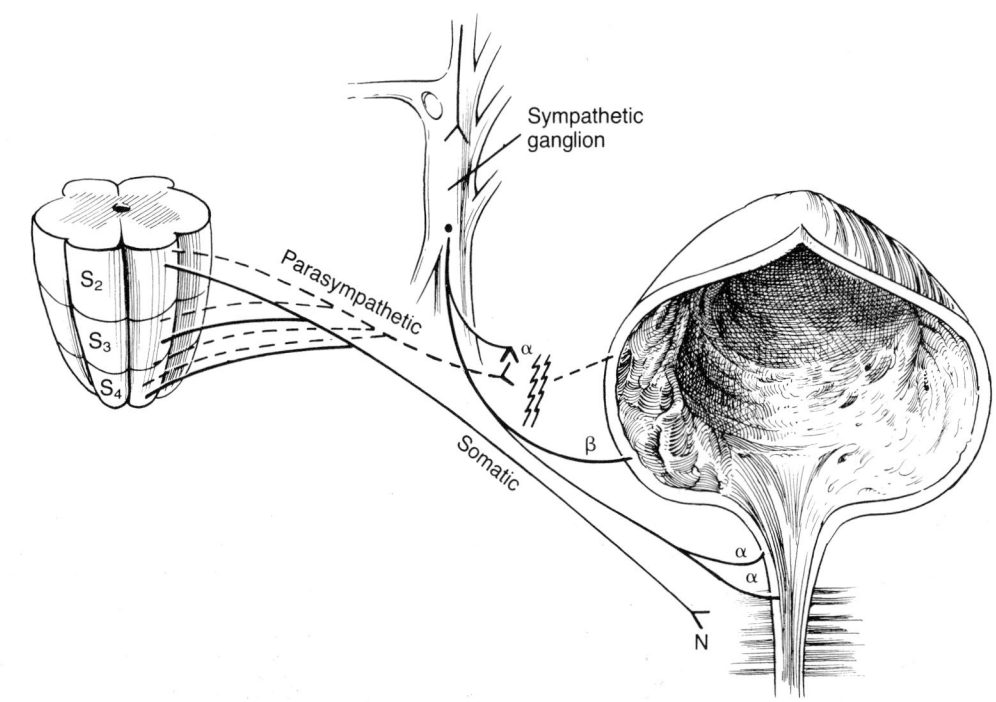

Figure 46–3
Bladder in storage. Norepinephrine neurotransmitter stimulates α- and β-adrenergic receptors at parasympathetic ganglia and at bladder fundus and base. Somatic nerve (pudendal) conveys acetylcholine to activate nicotinic receptors (N) for periurethral skeletal muscle contraction.

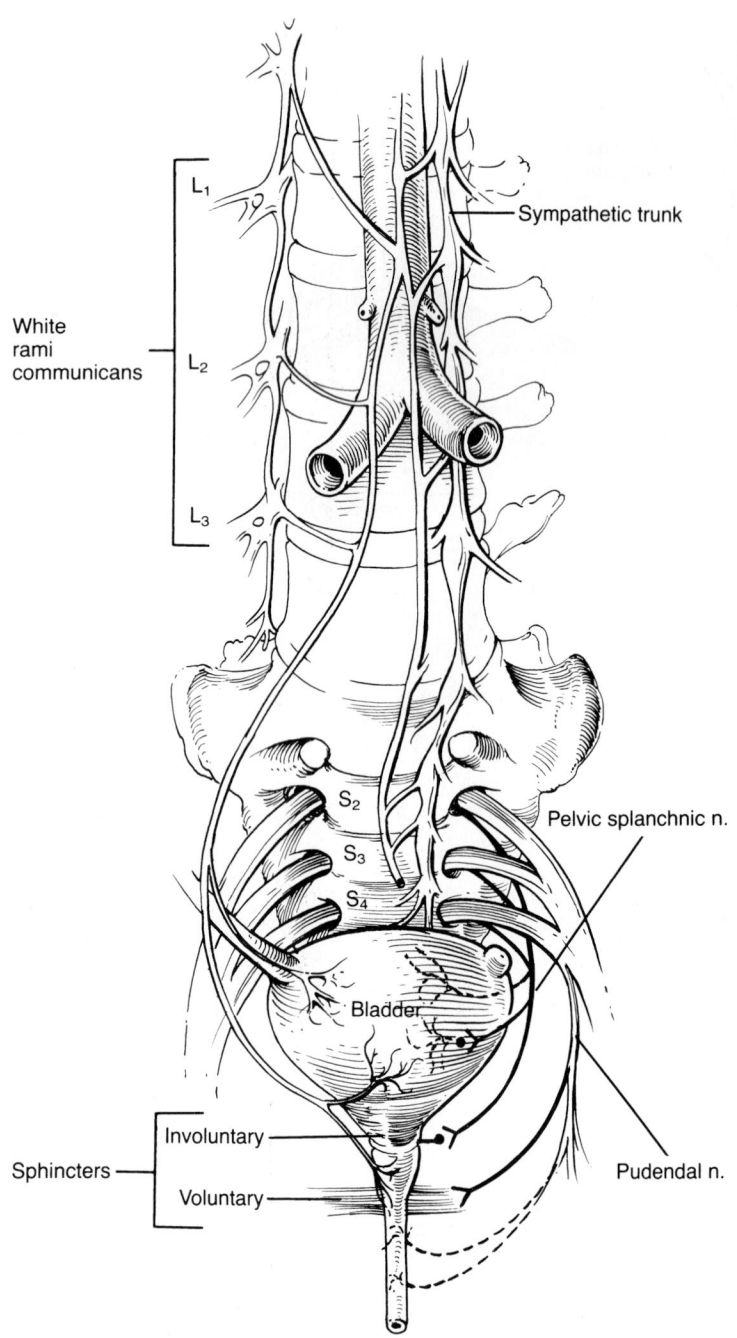

White rami communicans

L₁

L₂

L₃

Sympathetic trunk

S₂

S₃

S₄

Pelvic splanchnic n.

Bladder

Sphincters

Involuntary

Voluntary

Pudendal n.

Figure 46–4
Schematic representation of interaction of autonomic and somatic nervous systems as they affect lower urinary tract. Lumbar sympathetic, pelvic parasympathetics, and pudendal somatic neurons act under corticospinal coordination.

spondingly, intentional sectioning (sacrodorsal rhizotomy) can prevent bladder contractions and increase capacity.

Effector pathways from the pons to the lower cord are chiefly inhibitory, and lesions affecting these areas lead to small, "nonamplified," poorly coordinated detrusor contractions of short duration with resultant increased postvoid residual urine. These contractions occur reflexly in response to bladder filling, a situation called *reflex neurogenic bladder*. Lesions below the pons, then, with resultant loss of bladder and sphincter activity coordination, generally lead to involuntary activity of both the bladder and the outlet, called *detrusor-sphincter dyssynergia*.

This condition further complicates the residual urine problem resulting from the unsustained detrusor contractions.

SACRAL CORD AREAS

Damage in the sacral cord area leads to lower motor neuron disorders with possible absence of both detrusor and urethral sphincteric activity except for feeble intrinsic activity (*autonomic neurogenic bladder*). This type of bladder decentralization may result in loss of subjective sensation of bladder filling. Poor compliance and increased intravesical pressure are common. If the sensory components are affected more than the motor components, increased capacity with elevated residual urine may be seen. When the bladder pressure exceeds urethral closing pressure, incontinence is present.

Cauda Equina Lesions

The cauda equina conveys both afferents and efferents from the sacral cord, and the majority of these patients have autonomic parasympathetic interruption with decreased urinary streams, elevated residual urine, and occasional urinary retention. Loss of urethral competency secondary to lower motor neuron disease of the striated external urethral sphincter may occur. Sensory losses may be detected in the S2 through S4 dermatome area (*saddle anesthesia*). Neuropathy in the cauda equina may be produced by such conditions as disk disease, which frequently is more pronounced on one side, or may be produced by peripheral neuropathies, such as diabetes, with generally more symmetric abnormalities.

Pelvic Plexus Injury

Injury to the pelvic plexus (as with radical surgery or radiation) may show involvement of the sympathetic autonomic system as well as the parasympathetic system and may damage the segmental somatic nervous supply. Sensory disturbances in the bladder with detrusor areflexia may be seen, and the loss of β-adrenergic effect can lead to markedly decreased compliance. α-Adrenergic denervation can lead to incompetency at the bladder neck, so that clinical incontinence may be associated with difficulty in initiating urination.

Pudendal Neuropathy

Distal pudendal neuropathy, now recognized as being produced obstetrically, profoundly affects both the periurethral and perineal musculature and is strongly related to both urinary and fecal incontinence as well as pelvic floor prolapse. Thus, a neurologic understanding of the strong association of childbirth with pelvic floor dysfunction (Snooks et al, 1984) is imperative.

TYPES OF URINARY INCONTINENCE

Functional Incontinence

Many patients with essentially normal lower urinary tract anatomy and function may present with urinary incontinence. It is necessary, especially with elderly patients, to look for possible reversible conditions that cause functional incontinence. Resnick (1989) has helped by creating the mnemonic DIAPPERS:

Delirium – Confusion or psychiatric disease can impair one's awareness that incontinence is undesir-

able or inappropriate. Medicated elderly people are especially vulnerable to this situation.

Infection – This must always be considered in cases of urinary incontinence.

Atrophy – Estrogen plays a vital role in maintenance of lower urinary tract physiology.

Psychology – Many patients complaining of urinary urgency and frequency with no demonstrable abnormality benefit from psychological counseling (Macaulay et al, 1987).

Pharmaceuticals – Many medicines have cholinergic, α-adrenergic, β-adrenergic, or other effects that indirectly affect lower urinary tract function. Such medications include antidepressants, antipsychotics, sedative-hypnotics, and narcotic analgesics.

Endocrine – Endocrine-related causes of incontinence relate primarily to diabetes.

Restricted mobility – Incontinence may actually be a problem with space or with clothing that diminishes the patient's ability to prepare for using the bathroom.

Stool Impaction – Especially in institutionalized elderly patients, impaction commonly causes both urinary and fecal incontinence.

The gynecologist or urogynecologist is more likely to see chronic problems that fall into one or more broad classifications of urge, stress, overflow, or total incontinence.

Urge Incontinence

Urge incontinence occurs when the patient senses urgency during a detrusor contraction and cannot tighten the urinary sphincter enough to stop the flow of urine. Urgency occurring without demonstrable detrusor contractions is referred to as "sensory urgency."

Stress Urinary Incontinence

Stress urinary incontinence (SUI) is a symptom, a sign, and a diagnosis. It is a symptom when a patient loses urine with increased intra-abdominal pressure, as with cough or sneeze; a sign when such urinary loss is observed by the examiner; and a diagnosis when urodynamics demonstrate that, with the increased intra-abdominal pressure, the pressure in the bladder exceeds the pressure in the urethra in the absence of detrusor contraction.

Overflow Incontinence

When the bladder is filled to or beyond capacity, the bladder pressure will rise and, with continued filling, can exceed the resting urethral pressure. Urine then leaks from the urethra in the form of overflow incontinence.

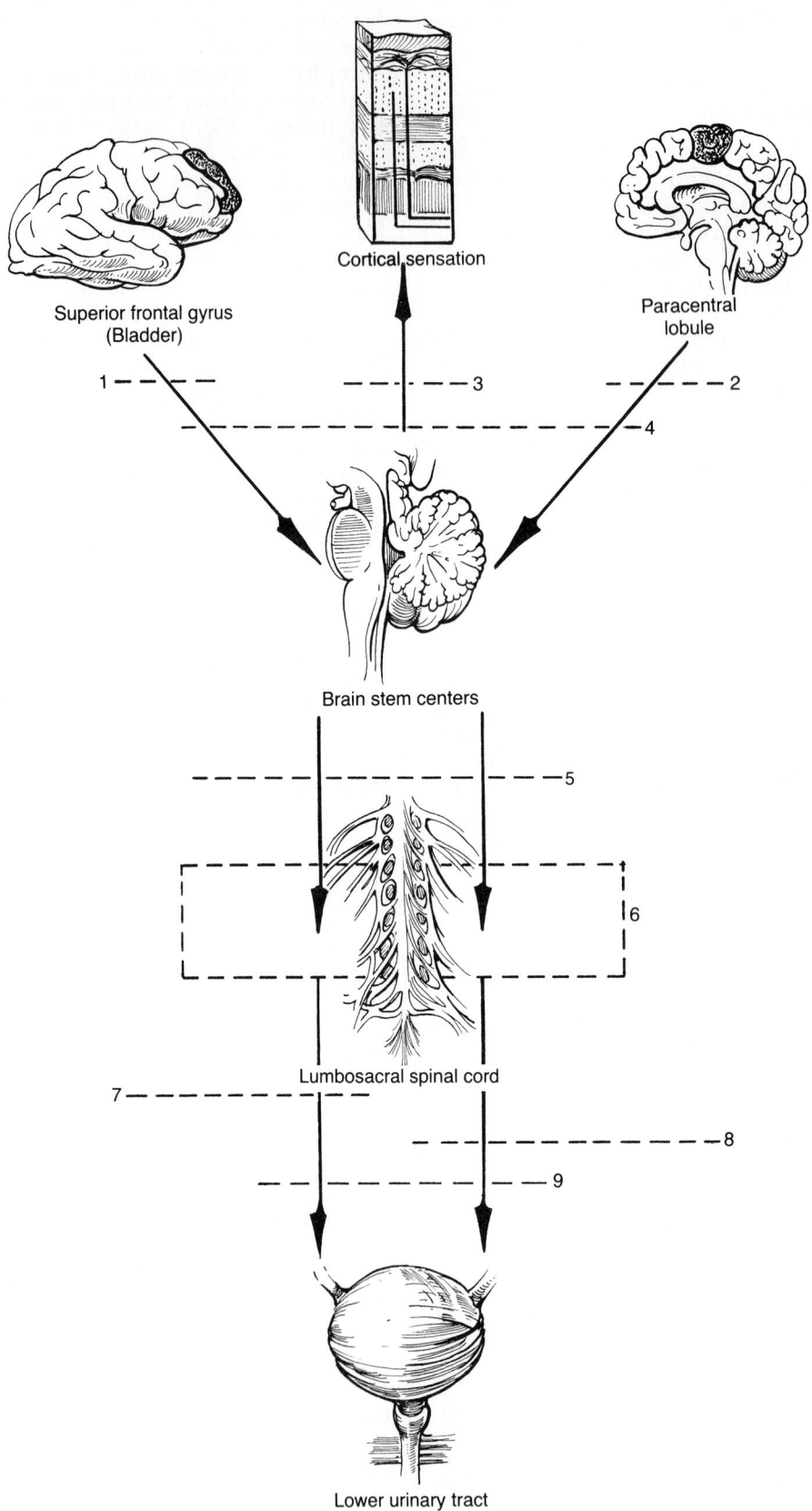

Cortical sensation

Superior frontal gyrus
(Bladder)

Paracentral
lobule

1 — — — — — — — — 3 — — — — — — 2

— — — — — — — — — — — — — — — 4

Brain stem centers

— — — — — — — — — — — — 5

6

Lumbosacral spinal cord

7 — — — — — — —

— — — — — — — — — — 8

— — — — — — — 9

Lower urinary tract

Total Urinary Incontinence

If the resting urethral pressure is so low that there is no resistance to passage of urine, the bladder is not able to store urine and incontinence is continuous. Also, with conditions such as vesicovaginal fistula, urethrovaginal fistula, or congenital ectopic ureter, no mechanism for urine storage exists and total urinary incontinence results.

PATHOPHYSIOLOGY OF INCONTINENCE

For simplicity, the discussion of the pathophysiology involved in the various types of urinary incontinence is divided into *detrusor* and *urethral* dysfunction.

Detrusor Dysfunction

Detrusor Instability

In a newborn infant, the normal bladder fills until a voiding contraction produces urination. The child's ability to voluntarily delay urination occurs when cerebral cortical pathways become myelinated, capable of sending inhibitory messages to the brain stem micturition center and the sacral reflex voiding center to inhibit efferent stimulation of nerves that would result in voiding. Any loss of this CNS control may result in detrusor instability.

Outlet obstruction constitutes another cause of detrusor instability. Obstructive elements are generally more common in men.

Urethral or vesical inflammation, which may lower stretch receptor thresholds, can cause detrusor hyperreflexia and increased sensation of urgency, which may be neurologic by effects upon the parasympathetic ganglia located within the wall of the bladder. Noninfectious inflammatory situations include carcinoma in situ of the bladder and radiation and chemical cystitis. Carcinoma in situ is a malignant change in the urothelium causing irritative voiding and occasionally incontinence. Microhematuria is frequently present. Urine cytologic results may be positive but lack a high degree of sensitivity. If the neoplastic changes within the bladder are widespread, bladder compliance can be reduced. Radiation cystitis can reduce bladder capacity and accommodation and can cause irritative voiding symptoms, including frequency, urgency, and incontinence. Chemical cystitis may occur with toxic drugs, such as cyclophosphamide (Cytoxan).

Particular conditioned reflexes, such as placing a key in the door, or the sight, sound or feel of running water, can lead to conditioned reflex detrusor contractions. Unperceived detrusor contractions, such as with spinal or cortical injury, can also lead to "reflex" urinary incontinence.

Another factor in detrusor hyperreflexia may be the presence of abnormal vesical neck patency ("funneling"), particularly in patients experiencing ur-

---

Figure 46–5

Simplified scheme of interaction of various levels of the nervous system in micturition. The locations of certain possible nervous lesions are denoted by numbers and explained as follows.

1, Lesions isolating the superior frontal gyrus prevent voluntary postponement of voiding. If sensation is intact, this produces urge incontinence. If the lesion is larger, there is additional loss of social concern about incontinence.

2, Lesions isolating the paracentral lobule, sometimes associated with a hemiparesis, cause spasticity of the urethral sphincter and retention. This will be painless if sensation is abolished. Minor degrees of this syndrome may cause difficulty in the initiation of micturition.

3, Pathways of sensation are not known accurately. In theory, an isolated lesion of sensation above the brain stem would lead to unconscious incontinence. Defective central conduction of sensory information would explain nocturnal enuresis.

4, Lesions above the brain stem centers lead to involuntary voiding that is coordinated with sphincter relaxation.

5, Lesions below brain stem centers but above the lumbosacral spinal cord, after a period of bladder paralysis associated with spinal shock, lead to involuntary reflex voiding that is not coordinated with sphincter relaxation (detrusor-sphincter dyssynergia).

6, Lesions destroying the lumbosacral cord of the complete nervous connections between the central and peripheral nervous system result in a paralyzed bladder that contracts only weakly in an autonomous fashion because of its remaining ganglionic innervation. However, if the lumbar sympathetic outflow is preserved in the presence of conus and/or cauda equina destruction, there may be some residual sympathetic tone in the bladder neck and urethra that may be sufficient to be obstructive.

7, A lesion of the efferent fibers alone leads to a bladder of decreased capacity and decreased compliance associated experimentally with an increased number of adrenergic nerves.

8, A lesion confined to the afferent fibers produces a bladder that is areflexic with increased compliance and capacity.

9, Because there are ganglion cells in the bladder wall, it is technically impossible to decentralize the bladder completely, but congenital absence of bladder ganglia may exist producing megacystis.

(From Torrens M, Morrison J: The Physiology of the Lower Urinary Tract. New York: Springer-Verlag, 1987:343, with permission.)

gency with sitting or standing only. The detrusor contractions are triggered by reflex mechanisms when urine enters the proximal urethra.

Finally, a group of patients remains in which no abnormalities can be discerned. Such individuals are said to have idiopathic detrusor hyperreflexia, or simply, "unstable bladders".

Most cases of detrusor instability are presently considered idiopathic, but as ability to diagnose, especially neurophysiologically, increases, "idiopathic" diagnoses should decline.

Low Bladder Compliance

Any condition causing inflammation and/or increased collagenosis (such as scarring from radiation or chronic catheter drainage) can lead to the bladder's loss of ability to accommodate and store urine at low pressure. If bladder pressure is actually higher than the resting closing pressure of the urethra, stress, urge, overflow, or a combination incontinence may occur.

Interstitial cystitis is a condition frequently termed *painful bladder syndrome*. Undulating bladder pain, urinary frequency, urgency, and often dysuria and dyspareunia are symptoms. Urinalysis is normal and specimens for urine culture are negative as a rule. The bladder becomes small and noncompliant, with fine submucosal hemorrhages seen on distention. Pathologic features are nonspecific (Holm-Bentzen and Lose, 1987). Stress and urge incontinence symptomatology is frequently associated. Treatment is difficult and is directed at symptomatic relief. Intravesical instillations of various medications and bladder distention are the most common therapies (Parivar and Bradbrook, 1986).

Motor neurologic disorders can affect bladder compliance as well. The bladder is referred to as "decentralized" when it separates from connection with the CNS. This may occur with lesions in the sacral cord, cauda equina (e.g., lumbosacral disk disease) or pelvic plexus (radical surgery). If the separation, which is rarely complete, primarily affects motor parasympathetic fibers to the bladder, it is termed *motor paralytic bladder. Sensory paralytic bladder*, in which sensory nerves are mainly damaged, frequently occurs in diabetes. If the bladder separates from the sacral micturition center, it functions with very-low-grade, relatively ineffective contractions. This is called *autonomous neurogenic bladder*.

Overflow Incontinence

Sensory nerve pathway interruption common to diabetic neuropathy may lead to overflow incontinence, by both neurogenic (lack of facilitation of pons center) and mechanical effects.

Chronic infrequent voiding can stretch the bladder, causing detrusor musculature to lose its ability to contract effectively. These patients strain to void and carry high residuals. Overflow incontinence can

result from this condition without diagnosable neuropathy.

In the elderly, many situations can cause uninhibited, frequent bladder contractions, but, when they do occur, contractions are inept at emptying the bladder. This is termed *detrusor hyperreflexia with incomplete contractility* (Resnick and Yalla, 1987).

The urethra and supporting structures may be entirely normal in conditions of detrusor dysfunction, and corrective efforts to alter or restore pelvic floor anatomy may well be futile, even harmful.

Urethral Dysfunction

Primary (Genuine) Stress Urinary Incontinence

Weaknesses in urethral supportive structures, now known to be related to neuropathy involving the muscular urethral supports, may result in incontinence. When a patient is subjected to sudden pressure increases, as with coughing or straining, pressure within the bladder lumen becomes temporarily greater than pressure within the urethra and incontinence is demonstrable.

Past theory of genuine stress urinary incontinence (GSUI) held that loss of support led to augmentation of the posterior urethrovesical angle. Stress incontinence was classified as type 1 or type 2, based on the degree of urethral inclination (either more vertical or more horizontal), because it was thought each type could benefit from a different surgical treatment. This theory has largely given way to one involving pressure transmission. That is, pressures generated intra-abdominally and then directly transferred to the bladder must be preferentially and simultaneously transferred to the urethra in order to maintain a higher urethral-bladder pressure gradient and maintain continence (Enhorning, 1961). When the urethrovesical junction (UVJ) has lost its normal retropubic location because of failure of supporting mechanisms, this transference can be decreased. Indeed, the only significant urodynamic parameter consistently improved by urethropexy for GSUI is the pressure transmission ratio.

However, the transference of pressure theory is not without flaw, because many women in whom the UVJs are markedly below the urogenital diaphragm are totally continent. Furthermore, while voiding, a normal woman can increase her flow with an increased Valsalva maneuver, which is inconsistent with simple mechanical pressure transmission, whereby flow would either decrease or not change. Reflex neurologic mechanisms must be involved, wherein "toned" pelvic floor supports provide closure during stress. Conversely, the pelvic floor relaxes and assists with urethral opening during voiding, thus increasing urine flow with a Valsalva maneuver.

Nevertheless, the important clinical finding is that restoring the UVJ to a position behind the pubis is successful in the treatment of classical GSUI. GSUI thus can be thought of as surgically correctable, in that the urethra is essentially normal but is in an abnormal location that can be modified by urethropexy. Careful evaluation is necessary, however, to make certain that there are no intrinsic bladder or urethral abnormalities that would not respond well to surgical relocation.

Incompetent Urethra

The symptom of stress incontinence can occur when the bladder and urethra are in normal anatomic position with normal support but the urethra is not competent. Urethral competence may be thought of as being based on three underlying mechanisms: smooth muscle, skeletal muscle, and mucosal "seal." In animal studies, each factor accounts for roughly one third of the total urethral closing pressure, that is, the urethral pressure above the simultaneously attained pressure in the bladder at rest.

SMOOTH MUSCLE

The smooth muscle component—the internal sphincter—is primarily under sympathetic nervous system innervation, with a preponderance of α-adrenergic receptors to the chief neurotransmitter, norepinephrine. Denervation of the pelvic plexus may affect this; affected patients tend to show open bladder necks on cystourethrogram. Frequently, patients with sacral cord lesions are similarly affected, and unless the more distal sphincter system, primarily dependent on skeletal muscle, is working well, these patients experience stress incontinence. Surgery to relocate the UVJ does not help these patients because the UVJ already has a normal anatomic position.

SKELETAL MUSCLE

Urethral skeletal musculature is supplied through both the pelvic plexus and the pudendal nerve. Neuropathies in these areas may lead to deficiencies in the skeletal muscle. Defects can involve the sacral cord, the cauda equina, the pelvic plexus, or, most commonly, the more peripheral pudendal nerve areas (Smith et al, 1989; Snooks et al, 1990).

Urethral instability, described urodynamically as urethral pressure variations that may allow urine to enter the urethra and precipitate urinary urgency and incontinence (Bereecken and Das, 1985), is thought to be due to a nervous factor. Its actual role in urinary incontinence is still unknown.

Muscular deficiencies become even greater in patients having repeated surgery involving the urethra, including urethral dilatations. Such a urethra might look like an open pipe. The UVJ is in a normal location but the urethra is open at rest, even at its more distal portions. These patients are prone to experience treatment failure if urethropexy is performed.

Such incompetent urethras are now commonly referred to as *intrinsic sphincter deficiency* (Haab et al, 1996).

MUCOSAL SEAL

In addition to smooth muscle and skeletal muscle function and proper urethral positioning, the mucosal seal is also necessary for continence. This rich, vascular network helps coaptation by affording a sponge-like, water-tight seal. This seal may be affected by estrogen because the female urethral mucosa and its richly vascular submucosa have high concentrations of estrogen receptors (Iosif et al, 1981).

In situations of intrinsic urethral weakness, the overall closure pressure is, of course, lowered, and studies suggest that the standard urethropexy is associated with a poor outcome (McGuire, 1981; Sand et al, 1987; Bowen et al, 1989). Because low urethral pressure is associated with increasing age, patient age should be considered and may guide therapy. Whether patients with low urethral closing pressure should undergo a procedure other than urethropexy for urinary incontinence is debatable, especially when low urethral closing pressure is diagnosed without visual evidence of incompetent urethra, such as a "drainpipe" or an open urethra at rest. Certainly, the latter, designated type 3 urethrosphincter incontinence, is known to respond better to procedures such as a sling or periurethral injections, which, unlike urethropexy, elevate closing pressure.

URINARY FISTULAS

Fistulas can occur between the ureter, bladder, or urethra and the vagina. Vesicouterine fistulas can also occur and result in incontinence. Typically, incontinence is continuous and should be suspected in any patient who has had previous pelvic surgery. These fistulas are occasionally difficult to diagnose and must constantly be looked for during the female urinary incontinence work-up.

ECTOPIC URETER

A ureter opening into the vesical neck, urethra, or structures other than the bladder is termed *ectopic*. The ectopic ureter, with an incidence of 1 in approximately 1900 (Campbell, 1970), can cause incontinence if it empties distal to the urethral continence sphincter mechanism. About one third open into the mid and distal urethra, 25% empty into the vagina, and 5% empty into the cervix or uterus (Snider, 1987). The resulting incontinence can be continuous or infrequent, depending on the ureteral orifice location. If the ectopic ureter serves a poorly functioning kidney segment, excretory intravenous pyelogram may not be diagnostic.

PATIENT EVALUATION

History

As with all clinical medicine, the history is first and foremost in evaluating women with urinary incontinence. Patient interviews remain paramount in obtaining the appropriate information and facilitating the essential physician-patient relationship. Computerized forms and questionnaires are very helpful with patient assessment. Four broad categories need to be addressed: (1) symptomatic pelvic relaxation, (2) urinary incontinence, (3) bladder irritability, and (4) anal/rectal disorders.

Complaints not readily offered may be uncovered with such systematic questioning. Pelvic relaxation often causes distressing feelings of "something falling," vaginal heaviness, pressure, or irritation. Symptoms may be more pronounced on standing and may be relieved by resting. A history of recurrent urinary tract infections (UTIs) or a patient's need for digital maneuvers to assist in voiding may be found. Defecation disorders with excessive bearing down and fecal tenesmus are commonly seen, and more than one third of patients, when carefully asked, reveal both urinary and anal incontinence.

Past surgical history is vital because surgery may be associated with scarring, fibrosis, or denervation, resulting in leakage.

History of recurrent UTIs should be explored. If these infections occurred during childhood, congenital abnormalities may be suspected. Association with sexual intercourse may be elicited. Certain barrier methods of contraception (e.g., diaphragm) may be linked to an increased incidence of UTIs (Fihn et al, 1985).

Questions regarding voiding disturbances—urine stream force, the presence or absence of tenesmus, or any associated diseases that may lead to bladder neuropathy (e.g, lumbar disk disease, diabetes)—need to be asked.

Hematuria is an important symptom as well, especially if not resolved after antibiotics, in which case bladder neoplasm and stone formation must be ruled out.

The symptoms of SUI should correspond in amount and timing of the leakage to the stressful event; small amounts directly relating to the event are more suggestive of GSUI. This symptom is very sensitive, with 85% to 100% of GSUI patients complaining of it; however, it is nonspecific because more than half the patients with other urinary disorders complain of this symptom (Walters, 1989). Frequency, urgency, and urge incontinence characteristically suggest unstable bladder, as do symptoms of leakage induced by sound, sight, or feel of running water; rising from a sitting or supine position; or nocturia. Enuresis has a relationship to unstable bladder (Whiteside and Arnold, 1975). Urgency and urge incontinence are very sensitive in the diagnosis of detrusor instability (70% to 95%); again,

however, symptoms are nonspecific because many patients with GSUI complain of urgency. There is a high negative predictive value (82%); that is, patients not complaining of urgency have less than a 20% chance of detrusor instability (Quigley and Harper, 1985).

A urinary diary is very helpful in assessing complaints relative to the lower urinary tract. The diary spans two 24-hour periods in which patients record times and amounts voided, number of pads used, and urinary accidents. The necessity for and amount of absorbent protection are important indicators of the degree of incontinence. The largest voided amount recorded in the diary indicates the patient's maximal bladder capacity, and the total 24-hour urine output may indicate abnormal outflow states. Frequency is defined as more than seven voids in a 24-hour period; nocturia is considered abnormal when two or more episodes occur per night.

Following gynecologic and urologic information gathering, a thorough medical, surgical, and obstetric history is obtained along with a complete list of the patient's medications, which can often greatly influence bladder and bowel symptoms.

Physical Examination

Standing Stress Test

An extremely important test for evaluation of patients is the standing stress test, performed while the patient is upright with a comfortably full bladder. As the patient coughs and performs a Valsalva maneuver, urinary leakage from the urethral meatus is looked for. Direct observation of spurting leakage synchronous with cough is quite suggestive of urethral sphincteric incompetence. Delayed or prolonged loss of urine suggests detrusor instability. A positive stress test has the highest positive and negative predictive value of all office tests (both 89%) for diagnosing GSUI (Fischer-Rasmussen et al, 1986).

Patients having severe uterovaginal prolapse with anterior wall relaxation protruding beyond the vaginal introitus may have a paradoxical continence. When this tissue is surgically replaced to its normal anatomic position, incontinence may result. Thus the stress test should be performed with the prolapsed tissue elevated prior to operation. If results are positive, prolapse correction should include anti-incontinence surgery.

Gross Neurologic Examination

Neurologic examination of the S2 through S4 dermatomes is done by testing sensation over the inner thigh, vulva, and perirectal areas (Bradley, 1985). Deep tendon, Babinski, and bulbocavernosus reflexes (contraction of perianal muscles in response to clitoral touch) are evaluated.

Urethral Axis

The "Q-tip test," introduced in 1972 by Crystle et al, measures UVJ mobility. With the patient in the lithotomy position, a lubricated sterile cotton-tipped swab is inserted through the urethra into the bladder and then withdrawn to the level of the UVJ. By means of a goniometer with an attached level to indicate the true horizontal position, the UVJ axis is measured at rest and at strain. A change in straining angle greater than 30 degrees from resting is considered indicative of urethral hypermobility (Montz and Stanton, 1986). This test alone is not useful in diagnosing SUI; however, it is extremely indicative of incontinence types that can be cured by repositioning the UVJ. The examiner should beware doing urethropexies to reposition a patient with a negative Q-tip test! The negative predictive value of the Q-tip test is very high, especially in patients who have had previous surgery. For them, a negative Q-tip test makes GSUI very likely.

Cystometrography

Simple "eyeball cystometrics" can be accomplished in the office without mechanical equipment. A Foley catheter placed into the bladder can collect postvoiding residual urine, which, after being recorded, undergoes urinalysis. A 50-ml syringe without its plunger is attached to the end of the Foley catheter and held approximately 15 cm above the symphysis pubis. Sterile water is slowly poured into the syringe while the patient verbally indicates sensation to filling, ranging from first sensation to marked fullness and maximal capacity. If, at any point during the examination, the meniscus (which normally descends) rises, the examiner should feel the patient's abdomen to detect a Valsalva maneuver. The absence of palpable abdominal muscle contraction implies detrusor contraction.

Pelvic Examination

Women with urinary incontinence frequently have associated significant gynecologic disorders (Benson, 1985). Furthermore, associated pelvic floor defects in the posterior compartment are also very common, making it necessary to carefully appraise the entire pelvic floor. Performing urethropexy will exacerbate posterior compartment defects because of the anterior relocation of pelvic floor supports. Indeed, 25% of patients having urethropexy return for a subsequent pelvic floor surgery for defects, primarily in the posterior compartment (Wiskind et al, 1991).

Vaginal Examination

The patient's upright position is mandatory in the examination for pelvic relaxation. One can best examine the anterior segment using half a speculum to hold the posterior portion while inspecting the anterior vaginal wall. The "traction" cystocele may occur following loss of lateral attachment to the arcus tendineus. In this condition, the rugae are usually maintained and having the patient "draw in" fails to elevate the lateral walls. "Pulsion" cystoceles, secondary to stretched midline defects, are identified by thinning of the mucosa and loss of rugae. The majority of cystoceles are traction in type, secondary to obstetric injury, and many are combined traction and pulsion type. The type of surgical approach depends on whether the defect is lateral (traction) or central (pulsion).

The posterior vaginal wall is examined next with the half-speculum supporting the anterior wall. Rectocele and enterocele diagnoses can be made with the patient upright, and combined rectovaginal examination is performed. Evacuation proctograms have proved invaluable in radiologically demonstrating significant nonemptying elements of rectocele, whereas clinical examination performed on an empty rectum frequently does not result in appreciation of the degree of deformity.

The superior vaginal segment should be thoroughly examined bimanually, with particular attention to the vaginal axis, which is normally horizontal in the upright patient. Palpating the levator plate by downward traction of the examiner's fingers allows appreciation of the amount of hiatus in the levator plate. This is extremely important because large defects in this area lead to deficiencies in all pelvic visceral support (Fig. 46–6).

To help identify the various pelvic floor defects, a system of defect recognition has now been standardized and should be used to enhance clinical and academic communication (Bump et al, 1996). This system is referred to as pelvic organ prolapse quantification (POP-Q).

Perineal Descent

Concerns that continued perineal descent may cause increasing stretch nerve injury to the pudendal nerve, thereby accentuating the problems with urinary and anal incontinence, are quite real (Jones et al, 1987). Clinically, one can determine perineal descent by observing the perineum "ballooning" below the bony outlet of the pelvis during straining. The anal verge can be measured in relationship to the plane of the ischial tuberosities with a perineometer (Henry et al, 1982).

Necessary Evaluation Before Operation for SUI

Good surgical results can be anticipated for patients having significant SUI with stable, adequate urethral competence and displaced UVJ. These patients should objectively demonstrate a positive standing stress test, a positive cotton-tipped swab (Q-tip) urethral mobility test, a negative simple cystometric evaluation, good bladder emptying without in-

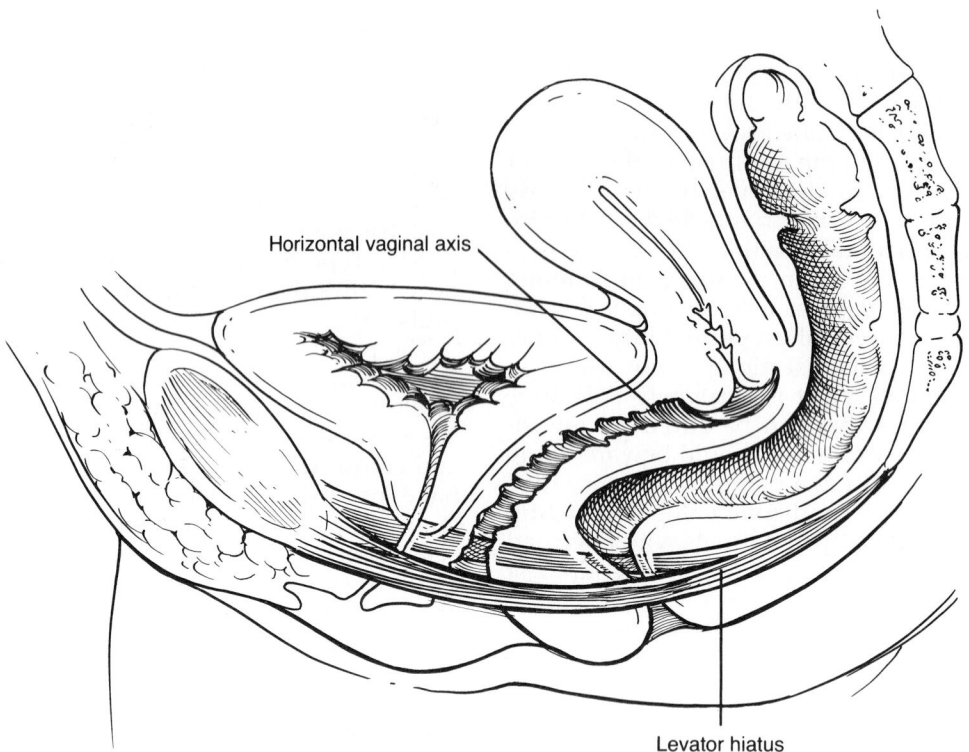

Horizontal vaginal axis

Levator hiatus

Figure 46–6
The levator plate and hiatus. Pelvic visceral descent may accompany "widening" of the hiatus. Perineal descent is associated with levator plate (posterior to hiatus) becoming more vertical.

creased residual urine, and no evidence of markedly incompetent urethra, such as profound urine loss in the supine position or with slightly increased intra-abdominal pressure. Urodynamic evaluation should precede consideration of any surgical therapy if patients have other symptomatology (e.g., significant urge incontinence in addition to stress incontinence, failed previous surgery, history of radiation or radical surgery, history of neurologic disease, diabetes, voiding dysfunctions with increased residual urine volumes, decreased bladder capacity, negative urethral mobility tests, or equivocal or delayed standing stress tests).

Urodynamics

The purpose of urodynamic testing is to identify and quantify the etiologic factors contributing to lower urinary tract dysfunction. It is critical to reproduce symptomatology during the study for objective analysis. This is possible only if the physician personally performs the testing. Thus it is unsatisfactory for testing to be done by technicians while the physician reads and attempts to interpret results.

The cost of urodynamic testing must be considered. Practical urodynamic testing at the office level is probably confined to flow rates and simple cystometry. A retrospective study by Miller et al (1982) suggests that running a complete urodynamic unit is cost-effective provided that more than 200 patients are studied per year.

Cystometry

Bladder storage function is investigated principally by cystometry, which measures the simultaneous pressure and volume relationship during bladder filling. Detrusor activity, sensation, capacity, and compliance are evaluated. Because changes in the intra-abdominal pressure (measured intravaginally or intrarectally) can directly affect bladder pressure, simultaneous recording of these pressures is frequently combined with computer subtraction. Intravaginal and intrarectal techniques for measuring intra-abdominal pressure do vary; therefore, the technique used must be clearly stated and standardized (Weber et al, 1995). Subtracting the abdominal from bladder pressure gives the "detrusor pressure." Simultaneous urethral pressures are recorded, and frequently electromyographic (EMG) activity is measured, generally around the external anal sphincter with surface electrodes. Debate continues over patient position, antegrade versus retrograde bladder filling, the optimal distention medium, temperature of the medium, rate of filling, and indications for electronically subtracted cystometry. Commonly used filling media are carbon dioxide and water. The former offers speed, convenience, and simplicity,

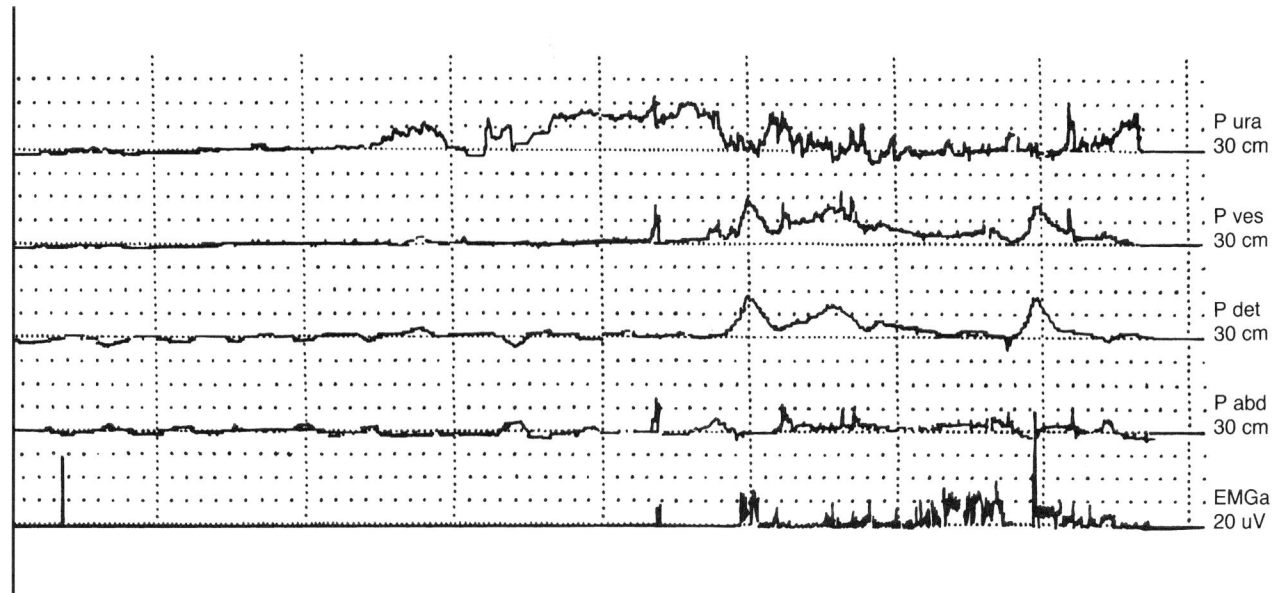

Figure 46–7
Cystometrogram—"unstable bladder." During filling, detrusor contractions associated with urethral relaxation occur. P ura, pressure in the urethra; P ves, pressure in the bladder; P det, true detrusor pressure (bladder pressure minus abdominal pressure); P abd, abdominal pressure; EMGa, perianal surface electromyography.

whereas the latter is more physiologic, providing visible urethral leakage and allowing voiding studies to be performed following cystometric evaluation (Fig. 46–7).

The upright position is the most sensitive for testing (Arnold, 1974). Provocative activating factors such as coughing, straining, heel bouncing, and the sight and sound of running water are used to enhance sensitivity.

Catheters for the study vary from balloon to microtip transducer. The latter is extremely sensitive but expensive and may have rotation artifacts.

Urodynamic diagnosis of GSUI is visual loss of urine simultaneous with coughing or straining in the absence of a detrusor contraction, with no detrusor or urethral instability demonstrated during the test. Patients with urinary loss resulting from nonsuppressible detrusor contraction in the absence of stress incontinence are diagnosed as having pure detrusor instability. About 30% of patients have urodynamic criteria for both conditions, leading to the diagnosis of mixed incontinence (Karram and Bhatia, 1989a). Observed urine loss with cough during multichannel urodynamics is the best examination for diagnosing GSUI (Swift and Ostergard, 1995).

Bladder sensation may be decreased or increased. Hypersensitive bladders not associated with a rise in detrusor pressure are frequently not explained by any inflammatory process (sensory urgency). Multichannel cystourethrometry is not a perfect test. Ambulatory monitoring studies have shown that such monitoring improves the pickup rate of unstable or hyperreflexic bladder diagnosis (Bhatia et al, 1982).

Urinary Flow Rate

Females can void by any combination of detrusor contraction, abdominal straining, and/or urethral relaxation. Because urinary flow rate is dependent on detrusor contraction and urethral relaxation, flow rate dysfunction may reflect abnormality of either component. Flow rate is defined as the volume of fluid expelled per unit of time (expressed in milliliters per second). Extreme regard for the patient's privacy in conducting a uroflow exam diminishes the psychological inhibition that is extremely common in laboratory settings. Flow rate, maximum flow rate, total flow time, total volume voided, average flow rate, and postvoid residual urine levels are determined. Normally a maximum flow rate of about 24 ml/second, appearing as a single, smooth curve over 15 to 20 seconds, with the length of time to maximum flow rate being less than one third the total voiding time, should be demonstrated. Because this test is very volume dependent, studies with less than 200 ml are not interpretable. Empirically stated, flow rates of less than 15 ml/second for voided volumes greater than 200 ml are indicative of abnormally reduced flow. If there is a voiding disorder, instrumented flow studies must be performed to determine the amount of detrusor contraction, compared with flow rate, which is then used to determine if the abnormally reduced flow rate is obstructive in nature or due to insufficient detrusor function.

Urethral Pressure Studies

The urethral pressure profile is a graphic recording of the pressure within the urethra at each point along its length. This study can be performed with balloon catheters or with microtip transducers. Commonly, the catheter has microtransducers at the tip and at 6 cm proximal to the tip. The catheter is inserted into the bladder and is machine-pulled at a constant rate so that the proximal transducer traverses the urethra while the transducer at the tip remains within the bladder, thus providing simultaneous recording of bladder and urethral pressures. On a separate channel, abdominal pressures are obtained for computation of the true detrusor pressure by subtracting the abdominal pressure from the bladder pressure lead. If one pulls the catheter at a constant rate, the portion of the urethra that has pressure above that simultaneously measured in the bladder defines the urethral functional length. The greatest pressure in the urethra during the pull is recorded as the maximum urethral closing pressure.

The test can be done passively and then actively. With active tests, the patient continually coughs during the withdrawal and computer subtraction of the urethral pressure from the bladder pressure can be used to determine transfer of intra-abdominal forces to the urethra. An area where bladder pressure exceeds urethral pressure is said to "negativate" and is associated with clinical loss of urine, which establishes a diagnosis of GSUI in the absence of detrusor contractions (Fig. 46–8).

Considerable debate over the value of urethral pressure profilometry exists and centers on several factors. The primary argument is that one is not actually measuring pressure but instead directed "force." There are no profilometry values that are universally associated with incontinence.

Mean urethral closure pressure appears to show a downward trend with age. The only preoperative clinical index predicting the presence of a markedly incompetent urethra in women with stress incontinence is age over 50 years (Horbach and Ostergard, 1994).

Urethral pressure studies are being replaced by many investigators with "Valsalva leak points." In this test, the pressure at which a Valsalva maneuver produces urethral urinary loss is measured.

Videourodynamics

Anatomic study of the lower urinary tract was once the commonly accepted means of investigation, and lateral chain cystograms were once predominantly used. The urodynamic evaluation has largely replaced anatomic studies in many centers, but the combined benefits of hydrostatic measurements plus anatomic observation are provided by videourody-

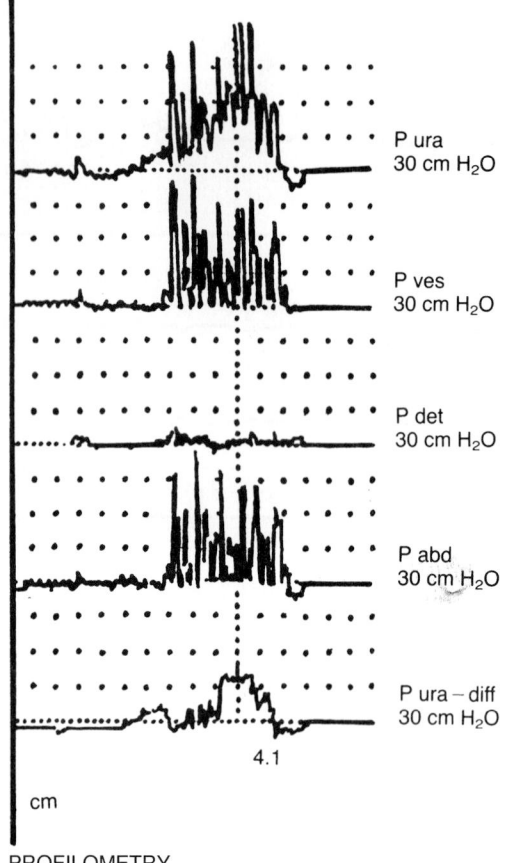

PROFILOMETRY

Figure 46–8
Dynamic cough profile revealing "genuine" stress urinary incontinence. Each vertical "spike" represents a patient cough. P det demonstrates no detrusor contractions, and P ura diff "negativates" (touches baseline or below) when bladder pressure exceeds urethral pressure. P ura, urethral pressure; P ves, bladder pressure; P det, true detrusor pressure (bladder pressure minus abdominal pressure); P abd, abdominal pressure; P ura -diff, urethral pressure minus bladder pressure.

namics. In this technique, radiographic contrast material displays a fluoroscopic image of the bladder and urethra while recording bladder, urethral, and abdominal pressures and, frequently, EMG activity. Major disadvantages of this procedure include radiation exposure (approximately 800 mrad), cost, and support necessary for its use.

The advent of ultrasonography is most exciting, with its technological capability in lower urinary tract examination being almost equal to that of fluoroscopy, but with lengthy ultrasound studies carrying no danger of radiation. The cost is significantly less than that of fluoroscopy and allied personnel are not necessary. Videotaping procedures allow restudy of each parameter. In one setting, then, all hydrostatic and anatomic principles of urodynamics combine with visualization of the lower urinary tract for the safest and most precise evaluation currently available.

Cystourethroscopy

Endoscopy is commonly performed in evaluating female lower urinary tract dysfunction. Although it is not of significant value in patients with primary stress incontinence, endoscopy has import for patients with recurrent incontinence, severe urgency, painful bladder syndromes, and voiding dysfunction.

THERAPY

Most women with urinary incontinence do not need surgical therapy to correct their disorders. As previously discussed, functional reversible types of incontinence should always be looked for and treated appropriately. As for chronic types of urinary incontinence, therapies may be classified as behavioral management, pharmaceutical, functional electrical stimulation, simpler invasive procedures (such as periurethral injection), and, finally, surgical intervention.

Behavioral Management

Biofeedback is a training technique used to alter, in this case, physiologic responses of detrusor and pelvic floor muscles to reverse urinary incontinence. Biofeedback is based soundly on the principles of human behavior and learning and is supported by considerable evidence derived from years of experimental investigation. Through this modality, patients can learn new skills for maintaining continence or can relearn previously acquired control of urination. Biofeedback means simply that learning occurs as a result of feedback, or knowledge of the consequences of one's behavior. In biofeedback a physiologic response is identified and measured. This measured response is amplified, processed, and representationally fed back to the patient by means of visual display, auditory signal, or other sensory modality. The patient is able to equate these tangible signals and symbols to her now conscious physical responses. It is not necessary to make a major distinction between voluntary and involuntary responses.

Biofeedback, then, requires the patient's motivation to be actively involved. The patient must receive a perceptible cue that indicates when the control should be performed; there must be a readily detectable, measurable response and the ability to vary that response with a detectable change.

It is recognized that urinary incontinence occurs when there is inadequate control of the striated muscles of the pelvic floor, which obstructs bladder emptying, or when there is failure to inhibit bladder contractions. Thus the goals of biofeedback training are somewhat different, depending on whether the primary problem is stress or urge incontinence. The primary goal for stress incontinence is to enable the patient to contract the periurethral muscles selectively while inhibiting contraction of the abdominal muscles. For urge incontinence, encouraging the patient to inhibit detrusor contractions by contracting the periurethral muscles selectively until reflex detrusor inhibition is achieved can be effective. Patients acquire these self-control skills in outpatient training sessions. Through repeated practice and implementation, patients can improve muscle strength and control over the reflexes.

Biofeedback is one component of a behavioral training program. Data clearly show that training with biofeedback is an effective and practical method of reducing incontinence in most noninstitutionalized persons who comply with the procedures (Kegel, 1948; Burgio et al, 1985; Burns et al, 1990). Among its advantages are very low risks and absence of documented side effects. Regardless of whether patients are candidates for surgery or for certain medications, behavioral treatment offers a safe alternative that is particularly relevant to the elderly population.

Pharmacologic Therapy

In patients not responding to behavioral modification, pharmacologic therapy may be appropriate. Many evaluated pharmacologic agents have been used in management of urinary incontinence, but the efficacy of most has been somewhat disappointing. Also, because the autonomic nervous system is by necessity affected, the side effects are quite problematic. The mechanisms of actions are multiple and frequently overlap, but for the sake of simplicity, in this text the more commonly used drugs are categorized on the basis of their predominant activity. These categories include medications that tend to (1) promote and relax detrusor contractility and (2) increase and decrease outlet resistance. Many of these drugs are prescribed for indications other than those of the urinary tract, and their actions on the bladder and outlet may produce significant side effects.

Drugs for detrusor stimulation have produced generally disappointing results clinically. Side effects, including malaise, diarrhea, flushing, and bronchial constriction, are bothersome and are contraindicated in patients with asthma, hyperthyroidism, bradycardia, epilepsy, or Parkinson's disease. The muscarinic drugs, such as bethanechol, unfortunately have coincidental α-adrenergic stimulation effect on the urethra. In general, patients whose primary disorder is deficient detrusor contraction with difficult emptying must be treated with mechanical means, such as self-catheterization.

Drugs to relax the detrusor are more widely used. Anticholinergic side effects of dry mouth, blurred vision, drowsiness, constipation, and tachycardia are dosage related. These drugs must be avoided in patients with narrow-angle glaucoma, myasthenia gravis, and urinary tract obstruction.

Increasing outlet resistance by the use of an α-adrenergic agonist has side effects, including anxiety, tachycardia, dry mouth, constipation, and increases in intraocular pressure. In patients with hypertension, hyperthyroidism, or cardiovascular disease, these agents must be used with caution.

Drugs decreasing outlet resistance by α-adrenergic blocking activity have associated effects of orthostatic hypotension, reflex tachycardia, nasal congestion, and diarrhea. Patients should probably have standing and lying blood pressure readings and electrocardiograms obtained before receiving these medications.

Estrogen therapy for urinary incontinence in postmenopausal women has been shown to produce subjective improvement (Fantl et al, 1994).

For patients with mixed incontinence, which includes 20% of all incontinent patients, the consensus is to attempt medical management prior to choosing surgery (Karram and Bhatia, 1989a). The future role of pharmacotherapy for incontinence will probably be expanded as a result of increased selectivity and efficacy of new agents and a growing belief in encouraging first-line pharmacologic management for treatment of incontinence.

Functional Electrical Stimulation

Clinical results with functional electrical stimulation over the past two decades have been encouraging in regard to various types of urinary incontinence (Caldwell et al, 1968; Edwards and Malvern, 1972; Godec et al, 1976; Fall, 1984). Of the many electrodes and types of stimuli, smaller electrodes with short, intermittent stimulation are preferable (Mortimer et al, 1986; Ohlsson et al, 1986). Long-term electrical stimulation (60 to 90 days) almost completely transforms fast, rapidly fatiguing myosin subunits to slow, more fatigue-resistant units (Eriksen, 1989). Recent multicenter trials have shows the effectiveness of this technique as therapy for bladder instability when compared to sham controls (Brubaker et al, 1997).

Pelvic nerve stimulation probably reorganizes the continence system, controlling detrusor activity either centrally or peripherally. Other possible roles of central endorphine conduction and peripheral vasoactive intestinal polypeptide production within the detrusor after maximal stimulation are presently unknown. It is reasonable to suspect that the endogenous opiate system's involvement in the neuromuscular response after electrical stimulation of the pelvic floor is similar to mechanisms observed after transcutaneous electrostimulation for pain relief (Clement-Jones et al, 1980).

Clinical results with female incontinence are successful in 52% to 90% of patients (Conic et al, 1983). A recurrence rate of 25% may be expected.

Contraindications include on-demand heart pacemakers, pregnancy, extraurethral and overflow incontinence, complete peripheral denervation of the pelvic floor, UTIs, and significant prolapse, which may inhibit vaginal application.

Direct electronic stimulation to the sacral nerve roots has also affected both sphincter and detrusor factors. Muscle fibers so stimulated have shown a higher overall oxidative activity and increased glycolytic activity, which may be a factor in increasing fatigue resistance. Inhibitory responses on detrusor activity are also seen (Tanagho, 1990). Continuous frequencies over 35 Hz induce early fatigue, but interrupted stimulation with an "on-off" ratio of 1:2 can be tolerated for long periods of time. Short pulse width (around 200 microseconds) shows better sphincteric response (Bazeed et al, 1982). Therefore, delivering low-frequency, wide pulse width, and intermittent pulsing brings about more resistance to fatigue through an adaptation change in the histochemical composition of the muscle fibers. Fast-twitch glycolytic fibers are converted into fast-twitch oxidative glycolytic fibers without any change in the number of slow-twitch fibers. Detrusor instability is improved (Tanagho and Schmidt, 1988). In these studies a needle is placed at the S3 foramen and an external receiver unit is stimulated and adjusted by the patient. If a good response is obtained, the patient becomes a good candidate for permanent implant.

Invasive Procedures for the Incompetent Urethra

Artificial sphincters and injectables have been used in females with intrinsic sphincter deficiency. Characteristically, these patients have total urinary incontinence in any position. The success of any treatment designed to increase the outflow resistance can be judged by the active leak point pressure: the pressure in the full bladder at which the patient, doing a Valsalva maneuver, leaks. Generally, urethral failure is evidenced by a leak point pressure below 20 cm of H_2O, which, practically speaking, corresponds to the maximal urethral closure pressure. If the urethral mechanism is grossly impaired, repositioning will not restore its competence. Treatment must be designed to increase outflow resistance.

Artificial Sphincters

Artificial urinary sphincters have been placed using a balloon placed around the urethra that is periodically deflated to allow urination. This is contraindicated when there is excessive scarring, often resulting from multiple past surgeries, and in patients with uncontrolled detrusor hyperreflexia and high-grade vesicoureteral reflux. The patients must have manual dexterity, mental capacity, and motivation to work the pump device, placed both transabdominally and transvaginally, which actually enables more than 90% patient continence, although some problems require surgical revision (Donavan et al, 1985; Light and Scott, 1985; Appell, 1988). Only a small number of women have actually received the artificial urinary sphincter, largely because of operating surgeons' concerns over technical difficulties.

Periurethral Injections

Over the past two decades, pressurized transvaginal injections of sclerosing and bulk-enhancing agents (e.g., polytetrafluoroethylene) have been associated with positive reports (Schulman et al, 1983). This is an expensive outpatient procedure, and questionable allergic response and a risk of particle migration have been reported (Malizia et al, 1984). A highly purified, bovine dermocollagen cross-linked with glutaraldehyde and dispersed in phosphate-buffered physiologic saline has been used with great success in clinical trials. The material is easier to deliver than the polytetrafluoroethylene through the 20-gauge spinal needle used under endoscopic guidance. The average volume required to attain continence is 14 ml, and more than 80% of patients are continent within two treatments, averaging an increase of over 25 cm H_2O to reach their leak points.

Surgical Therapy

The goal of the standard surgical approach to the correction of stress incontinence is elevation and support of the UVJ. More than 100 different procedures have been described in the medical literature (Stanton, 1985). In patients with hypermobility of the UVJ, three basic surgical options exist: (1) needle suspension (Pereyra et al, 1982), (2) retropubic urethropexy (Tanagho, 1985), and (3) suburethral sling (Horbach et al, 1988).

The standard anterior colporrhaphy utilizing the Kelly-Kennedy plication has repeatedly shown an increased failure rate (Stanton and Cardoso, 1979), and anterior vaginal repairs are no longer advocated for the surgical treatment of stress incontinence except by those modifying it to do more extensive UVJ elevation. Bergman and colleagues' well-conducted, objectively analyzed, prospectively randomized study (1990), supported by the work of others (Karram and Bhatia, 1989b), suggests that long-term results of the needle suspension are inferior to retropubic urethropexy.

During these surgical procedures, the surgeon should use means such as endoscopy, Q-tip measurement, pressure determination, or manual "touch" to determine the appropriate anatomic elevation of the vesical neck to relieve the incontinence without producing undue obstruction. Also, one must determine that no damage has occurred to either the bladder or ureters. With retropubic urethropexies there is at least a 1% incidence of unrecognized ureteral obstruction. The use of intraoperative cystoscopy transurethrally or transvesically following the instillation of indigo carmine allows intraoperative evaluation of ureteral function.

Postoperatively, a suprapubic catheter permits evaluation of postvoid residual urine. Residuals should be consistently low (<100 ml) for a period of at least 24 hours before the catheter is removed. This system prevents the yo-yo effect so common with repeated removal and reinsertion of Foley catheters.

Surgery to correct urinary incontinence changes force vectors to the remaining pelvic floor. Defects in other areas of the pelvic floor should be appreciated prior to the surgery and corrected simultaneously in an effort to avoid the high number of recurrent anti-incontinence surgeries.

Mechanisms of Successful Surgery

The patient most likely to be cured by urethropexy is one in whom the bladder neck distance to the pubic symphysis is horizontally increased at rest and moves toward the symphysis with strain. The first operative attempt stands the best chance of success; success is highly correlated with a postoperative decrease in bladder neck mobility, especially in the horizontal plane excursion. Abdominal urethropexies tend to stabilize the bladder neck in patients who are cured by the procedure. Patients with vaginal urethropexy, however, may still demonstrate increased mobility, even with cure. The mechanism for continence with the vaginal procedure may be other than simple stabilization. Proper surgical correction elevates the bladder neck more than the bladder's most dependent portion so that the most dependent portion becomes posterior to the UVJ, enabling forces to act posterior to, rather than on, the UVJ.

Bladder instability is affected both positively and negatively by urethropexy. Some have suggested that bladder instability in patients whose detrusor contractions are preceded by urethral relaxation might likely be improved with surgical management that stabilizes the urethra (Bergman et al, 1989). However, emphasis should be on medical treatment of bladder instability in patients with mixed stress incontinence.

Causes of Surgical Failure

Failure rates are higher in patients with preoperatively low urethral pressure (resting maximal urethral pressure of less than 20 cm H_2O on urethral pressure profile performed in the supine position at maximum cystometric capacity). Improper suture location can also cause surgical failure. If the sutures are placed above the UVJ, suspension of the anterior portion of the bladder to the symphysis pubis may occur and symptomatology may actually increase. Sutures placed too far distally are likely to cause troublesome obstructive phenomena. Sutures placed into the muscularis of the urethra may migrate through the epithelium. The best type of suture to be used is debated, but most physicians doing extensive work in this area use permanent sutures.

Transient retention lasting up to a week is common following these procedures and is more marked with vaginal than abdominal urethropexies. The abdominal retropubic urethropexies avoid damage to the urethra, which ought to be an essentially normal structure, and mobility is preserved by the absence of scarring near the urethra. For these reasons, Tanagho's modification of the Burch colposuspension is preferred by many surgeons.

Vaginal urethropexies (needle procedures) are also widely used because they are easy to perform in association with other vaginal procedures. Ureteral obstruction and accidental suture placement through the bladder should be discovered during the surgery by endoscopic visualization. In reviews of Pereyra's original procedure and subsequent modifications, it is noteworthy that procedures involving very little tissue dissection had unacceptably high long-term failure rates. This must be remembered when we read of recent modifications, such as the "incisionless" needle urethropexies, or history may well repeat itself.

Sling Procedures

Abdominal rectus fascia, fascia lata, dura, and synthetic materials all have their advantages and disadvantages in sling procedures. The vertical direction of the fibers of the abdominal rectus fascia make this tissue less preferable than the fascia lata of the leg. Wound herniation can occur after retrieving abdominal fascia, and knee and leg instability can occur after removing segments of fascia lata. Use of dura has been successful in most cases. Synthetic materials can be very advantageous. When there is infection, however, recurrent sinus tract formation occurs and the subsequent course for the patient is quite distressing. All patients undergoing sling procedures risk urinary retention of long duration and the possible necessity of self-catheterization. Manual dexterity and functional vision are important preoperative considerations. Modifications of sling procedures include using a portion of the vaginal wall for the sling or using a piece of material such as rectus fascia suspended by sutures to the overlying rectus musculature.

Summary

Cure rates for anti-incontinence procedures present an overly optimistic picture of efficacy because they focus on the symptoms of stress incontinence and frequently are subjective in nature. Long-term objective follow-up studies show that only about 50% of the women operated on are completely dry with normal voiding at 5 years. Decreased bladder capacity and flow rates as well as increased urethral resistance and flow times, fairly significant urodynamic parameters, are changed by surgery (Eriksen et al,

1990). Furthermore, most lower urinary tract abnormalities leading to incontinence have a demonstrable neurogenic component that is not corrected by surgery.

The surgeon should be familiar with various surgical routes so that the patient is not "tailored" to the surgeon's favorite procedure. Finally, other coexistent defects of the pelvic floor should be recognized and repaired simultaneously.

REFERENCES

Agency for Health Care Policy and Research: U.S. Department of Health and Human Services, Public Health Service Agency for Health Care Policy and Disorder Managing Acute and Chronic Urinary Incontinence, 1994.
Appell RA: Techniques and results in the implantation of the artificial urinary sphincter in women with type 2 stress urinary incontinence by a vaginal approach. Neurourol Urodynam 1988;7:613.
Arnold EP: Cystometry postural effects in incontinence: effects in incontinent women. Urol Int 1974;29:185.
Awad SA, Downie JW: Relative contributions of smooth and striated muscles to the canine urethral pressure profile. Br J Urol 1976;48:347.
Bazeed MA, Thuroff JW, Schmidt RA, et al: Effect of chronic electrostimulation of the sacral roots in the striated urethral sphincter. J Urol 1982;128:1357.
Benson JT: Gynecologic and urodynamic evaluation of women with urinary incontinence. Obstet Gynecol 1985;66:691.
Bereecken RL, Das J: Urethral instability: related to stress and/or urge incontinence? J Urol 1985;134:698.
Bergman A, Ballard CA, Koonings PP: Comparison of three different surgical procedures for genuine stress incontinence: a prospective randomized study. Obstet Gynecol 1990;160:1102.
Bergman A, Koonings PP, Ballard CA: Detrusor instability: is the bladder the cause or the effect? J Reprod Med 1989;34:834.
Bhatia NN, Bradley WE, Haldeman S: Urodynamics: continuous monitoring. J Urol 1982;128:963.
Bø K, Stien R, Kulsent-Hanssen S, Kristofferson M: Clinical and urodynamic assessment of nulliparous young women with and without stress incontinence symptoms: a case controlled study. Obstet Gynecol 1994;84:1028.
Bowen LW, Sand PK, Ostergard DR, Franti CE: Unsuccessful Burch retropubic urethropexy: a case controlled urodynamic study. Am J Obstet Gynecol 1989;160:452.
Bradley WE: Urologic oriented neurologic examination. In Ostergard DR (ed): Gynecologic Urology and Urodynamics. 2nd ed. Baltimore: Williams & Wilkins, 1985:63.
Brazda JF: Washington Report. "Urinary incontinence" transvaginal electrical stimulation for female urinary incontinence. Nation's Health 1983;13:3.
Brubaker LT, Bent A, Clark A, Benson JT: Am J Obstet Gynecol 1997;177:536.
Bump RC, et al: The standardization of terminology of female pelvic organ prolapse and pelvic floor dysfunction. Am J Obstet Gynecol 1996;175:10.
Burgio KL, Whitehead WE, Engel VT: Urinary incontinence in the elderly: bladder sphincter biofeedback and toileting skills training. Ann Intern Med 1985;103:507.
Burns PA, Prankoff K, Nochajski T, et al: Treatment of stress incontinence with pelvic floor muscle exercises and biofeedback. J Am Geriatr Soc 1990;38:341.
Caldwell KPS, Cook PJ, Flack FC: Stress incontinence in females: report on 31 cases treated by electrical implant. J Obstet Gynaecol Br Commonw 1968;75:777.
Campbell MF: Anomalies of the ureter. In Campbell MF, Harrison JH (eds): Campbell's Urology. 3rd ed. Philadelphia: WB Saunders Company, 1970:1487.
Clement-Jones B, McLoughlin L, Tomlin S, et al: Increased beta endorphine but not met-enkephalin levels in human cerebral

spinal fluid after acupuncture for recurrent pain. Lancet 1980;
2:946.

Conic S, Park YC, Yachiku S, Kurita T: Electrical control of urgency and urge incontinence. In: Proceedings of the International Continence Society, 1983:125.

Constantinou CE: Spatial distribution and timing of transmitted and reflexly generated pressure in healthy women. J Urol 1982; 127:964.

Crystle D, Charme L, Copeland W: Q-tip test in stress urinary incontinence. Obstet Gynecol 1972;38:313.

DeLancey JOL: Correlative study of periurethral anatomy. Obstet Gynecol 1986;68:91.

Dickinson RL: Studies of the levator ani muscle. Am J Obstet Dis Women 1889;22:897.

Dieffenbach JF: Ueber die Heilung der Blasen-scheiden-fistein und Zerreissungen der Blase und Scheide. Med Seitung 1836; 5:117, 173, 177.

Donavan MG, Barrett DM, Furlow WL: Use of the artificial urinary sphincter in the management of severe incontinence in females. Surg Gynecol Obstet 1985;161:17.

Edwards L, Malvern J: Electronic control of incontinence: a critical review of the present situation. Br J Urol 1972;44:467.

Enhorning G: Simultaneous recording of the intravesical and intraurethral pressures. Acta Chir Scand 1961;276:1.

Eriksen BC: Electrostimulation of the Pelvic Floor in Female Urinary Incontinence. Trondheim, Norway: University of Trondheim, 1989:20.

Eriksen BC, Hagen B, Eik-Nes SH, et al: Long term effectiveness of the Burch colposuspension in female urinary stress incontinence. Acta Obstet Gynecol Scand 1990;69:451.

Fall M: Does electrostimulation cure urinary incontinence? J Urol 1984;131:664.

Fantl JA, Cordoso L, McClish DK: Estrogen therapy in the management of urinary incontinence in postmenopausal women: a meta-analysis. First report of the Hormones and Urogenital Therapy Committee. Obstet Gynecol 1994;83:8.

Fantl JA, Hurt WG, Dunn LJ: Dysfunctional detrusor control. Am J Obstet 1977;129:299.

Fihn SD, Latham RH, Roberts P: Association between diaphragm use and urinary tract infection. JAMA 1985;254:240.

Fischer-Rasmussen W, Hansen RI, Stage P: Predictive values of diagnostic tests in the evaluation of female urinary stress incontinence. Acta Obstet Gynecol Scand 1986;65:291.

Gilpin SA, Gosling JA, Smith ARB, Warrell DW: The pathogenesis of genitourinary prolapse and stress incontinence of urine: a histological and histochemical study. Br J Obstet Gynaecol 1989;96:15.

Godec C, Cass AS, Ayala GF: Electrical stimulation for incontinence: technique, selection and results. Urology 1976;7:388.

Haab F, Zimmern PE, Leach GE: Female stress urinary incontinence due to intrinsic sphincteric deficiency: recognition and management [review]. J Urol 1996;156:3.

Henry MM, Parks AG, Swash M: The pelvic floor musculature in the descending perineum syndrome. Br J Surg 1982;69:470.

Holm-Bentzen M, Lose G: Pathology and pathogenesis of interstitial cystitis. Urology 1987;29:8.

Horbach NS, Blanco JS, Ostergard DR, et al: A suburethral sling procedure with polytetrafluoroethylene for the treatment of stress incontinence in patients with low urethral closure pressure. Obstet Gynecol 1988;81:648.

Horbach NS, Ostergard DR: Predicting intrinisic urethral sphincter dysfunction in women with stress urinary incontinence. Obstet Gynecol 1994;84:188.

Iosif C, Batra S, Ek A, Astedt B: Estrogen receptors in the human female lower urinary tract. Am J Obstet Gynecol 1981;141:817.

Jones PN, Lubowski DZ, Swash M, Henry MM: Relation between perineal descent and pudendal nerve damage in idiopathic faecal incontinence. Int J Colorectal Dis 1987;2:93.

Karram MM, Bhatia NN: Management of coexistent stress and urge urinary incontinence. Obstet Gynecol 1989a;73:4.

Karram MM, Bhatia NN: Transvaginal needle bladder neck suspension procedures for stress urinary incontinence: a comprehensive review. Onset Gynecol 1989b;73:906.

Kegel AH: Progressive resistance exercise in the functional restoration of the perineal muscles. Am J Obstet Gynecol 1948;56: 238.

Light JK, Scott FB: Management of urinary incontinence in women with the artificial urinary sphincter. J Urol 1985;134: 476.

Macaulay A, Stern R, Holmes D, Stanton S: Micturition and the mind: psychological factors in the aetiology and treatment of urinary symptoms in women. Br Med J 1987;294:540.

Malizia AA Jr, Reimen JM, Meyers RP, et al: Migration and granulomatous reaction after periurethral injection of Polytef. JAMA 1984;251:3277.

McGuire EJ: Urodynamic findings in patients after failure of stress incontinence operations. Prog Clin Biol Res 1981;78:351.

Miller RA, Barod RK, Chapman J, Fergus JN: The clinical value and cost of a district hospital urodynamic unit. Br J Urol 1982; 54:635.

Montz FJ, Stanton SL: Q-tip test in female urinary incontinence. Obstet Gynecol 1986;67:258.

Mortimer J, Benson T, Daroux ML: Electrode and nerve membrane prosthesis during stimulation. In: Proceedings of the 2nd Vienna International Workshop on Functional Electrical Stimulation, Vienna, 1986:13.

National Institutes of Health (NIH): Consensus conference on urinary incontinence in adults. JAMA 1989;261:2685.

Neill ME, Swash M: Increased motor unit fiber density in the external anal sphincter muscle in anorectal incontinence: a single fiber EMG study. J Neurol Neurosurg Psychiatry 1980;43: 343.

Nygaard IE, Thompson FL, Svengalis SL, Albright JP: Urinary incontinence in elite nulliparous athletes. Obstet Gynecol 1994; 84:183.

Ohlsson B, Lindstrom S, Erlandson BE, Fall M: Effects of some different pulse parameters on bladder inhibition and urethral closure during intravaginal electrical stimulation: an experimental study in the cat. Med Biol Eng Comput 1986;24:27.

Paramore RH: The evolution of the pelvic floor in non-mammalian vertebrates and pronograde mammals. Lancet 1910;1:1393.

Parivar F, Bradbrook RA: Interstitial cystitis. Br J Urol 1986;58: 239.

Parks AG, Swash M, Urich H: Sphincter denervation and anorectal incontinence and rectal prolapse. Gut 1977;18:656.

Pereyra AJ, Lebherz TB, Growdon WA, Powers JA: Pubourethral supports and perspective: modified Pereyra procedure for urinary incontinence. Obstet Gynecol 1982;59:643.

Quigley GJ, Harper AC: The epidemiology of urethral-vesical dysfunction in the female patient. Am J Obstet Gynecol 1985; 151:220.

Resnick N: Diagnosis and treatment of incontinence in the institutionalized elderly. Semin Urol 1989;7:117.

Resnick N, Yalla SV: Detrusor hyperactivity with impaired contractility. JAMA 1987;257:3076.

Sand PK, Bowen LW, Panganiban R, Ostergard DR: The low pressure urethra as a factor in failed retropubic urethropexy. Obstet Gynecol 1987;69:399.

Schulman CC, Simon J, Wespas E, Germeau F: Endoscopic injection of Teflon for female urinary incontinence. Eur Urol 1983; 9:246.

Smith ARB, Hosker GL, Worrell DW: The role of partial denervation of the pelvic floor in the aetiology of genitourinary prolapse and stress incontinence of urine: a neurophysiological study. Br J Obstet Gynaecol 1989;96:24.

Snider HM: Anomalies of the ureter. In Gillenwater JY, Grayhack J, Benson T, et al (eds): Adult and Pediatric Urology. Chicago: Year Book Medical Publishers, 1987:1642.

Snooks SJ, Setchell M, Swash M, Henry MM: Injury to innervation of the pelvic floor sphincter musculature in childbirth. Lancet 1984;2:546.

Snooks SJ, Swash M, Mathers SE, Henry MM: Effect of vaginal delivery on the pelvic floor: a five year followup. Br J Surg 1990;77:1358.

Special Committee on Aging: Aging America and Projections (Publication no 1986-498-116-814/42395). Washington, DC: U.S. Senate, 1986.

Speert H: Obstetric and Gynecologic Milestones. New York: Macmillan, 1958:442.

Stanton SL: Stress incontinence: why and how operations work. Urol Clin North Am 1985;12:279.

Stanton SL, Cardoso L: A comparison of vaginal and suprapubic surgery in the correction of incontinence due to urethral sphincter incompetence. Br J Urol 1979;51:497.

Swift SE, Ostergard DR: Evaluation of current urodynamic testing methods in the diagnosis of genuine stress incontinence. Obstet Gynecol 1995;86:85.

Tanagho EA: Retropubic procedures: a physiologic approach to repair of genuine stress incontinence. In Ostergard DR (ed): Gynecologic Urology and Urodynamics. 2nd ed. Baltimore: Williams & Wilkins, 1985;503.

Tanagho EA: Principles and indications of electrical stimulation of the bladder. Urologe A 1990;29:185.

Tanagho EA, Miller ER: Initiation of voiding. Br J Urol 1970;42: 175.

Tanagho EA, Schmidt RA: Electrical stimulation and the clinical management of the neurogenic bladder. J Urol 1988;140:1331.

Torrens M, Morrison J: The Physiology of the Lower Urinary Tract. New York, Springer-Verlag, 1987:343.

Walters MD: The history and physical examination in women with urinary incontinence. Am Urogynecol Soc Q Rep 1989;7: 1.

Warren JW, Steinberg L, Hebel RJ, Tenney JH: The prevalence of urethral catheterization in Maryland nursing homes. Arch Intern Med 1989;149:1535.

Weber AM, Walters MD, Schover LR, Mitchinson A: Sexual function in women with uterovaginal prolapse and urinary incontinence. Obstet Gynecol 1995;85:483.

Westby M, Asmussen M, Ulmsten U: Location of maximal intraurethral pressure in the female subject as studied by simultaneous urethrocystometry and voiding urethrocystography. Am J Obstet Gynecol 1982;144:408.

Whiteside CG, Arnold EP: Persistent primary enuresis: a urodynamic assessment. Br Med J 1975;1:364.

Wiskind AK, Creighton SM, Stanton SL: The incidence of genital prolapse following a Burch colposuspension operation. Neurourol Urodyn 1991;10:453.

47

Linda Brubaker

Abnormalities of Pelvic Support

NORMAL SUPPORT

Each time a physician examines a nulliparous women, there is an important opportunity to study normal anatomy. The majority of pelvic examinations in North America are conducted in the dorsolithotomy position. During this examination, the observant clinician will consciously note the topography of the vaginal supports and the position of the uterus, if present. The site-specific, quantified examination (described later) can record these topographic observations.

The supportive structures themselves cannot be visualized during a pelvic examination, but these tissues have been studied in cadaveric preparations. Older anatomic literature should be interpreted cautiously because older cadaver fixation techniques induced a great deal of artifact on pelvic floor structures as a result of fixation in the supine position. Current techniques suspend the pelvis to more closely mimic the position of the pelvic organs during life (DeLancey, 1996). Artifact remains problematic, because the primary supportive structure, the levator ani muscles, loses contractility after death. These difficulties notwithstanding, significant advances have been made in the anatomic concepts of normal pelvic support.

Apical Support

Normal apical support depends on several anatomic features. The normal vagina is approximately 10 to 11 cm in length. This length allows the upper portion of the vagina to rest on the levator plate in a horizontal fashion, favoring upper vaginal closure during increases in intra-abdominal pressure. Paracolpium fibers originate from the lateral sacrum, the pelvic bones in the region of the sacroiliac articulation, and the region of the greater sciatic foramen over the piriformis muscle. Additionally, support is provided by bilaterally intact uterosacral ligaments. These "ligaments" are not solely made of connective tissue, but are rich in smooth muscle with an autonomic nerve supply. In a woman with normal sup-

port, the top of the vagina (with or without the uterus) should rest at or above the ischial spine (Fig. 47–1).

Midvaginal Support

The supports of the midvagina are provided laterally by the endopelvic fascia, which essentially envelopes the vagina tube, connecting it to the pelvic sidewall. The pubovesical fascia (anteriorly) and the rectovaginal fascia (posteriorly) are continuous at the lateral edges of the vagina (Figs. 47–2 and 47–3).

Distal Vaginal Support

The normal distal 2 to 3 cm of the vagina is near-vertical in orientation. Its supportive structures are in continuity with the supportive structures of the midvagina. The distal vagina is fused with the adjacent anatomic structures. Thus muscle deficits (atrophy of the levator ani) results in clinically apparent enlargement of the vaginal opening (Fig. 47–4). Urethral support is provided by both muscular and connective tissue supports (Fig. 47–5).

INCIDENCE AND PREVALENCE OF SUPPORT ABNORMALITIES

Aside from the rare case of congenital uterovaginal prolapse, the incidence of pelvic organ prolapse is negligible until the reproductive years. It is logical to assume that these abnormalities increase with aging; however, the incidence and prevalence per decade have not yet been studied. Experienced obstetrician-gynecologists are well aware that many asymptomatic women have support abnormalities, particularly anterior and posterior wall defects.

Approximately one of every nine American women will undergo at least one operation for treatment of pelvic organ prolapse and/or urinary incontinence. At least 30% of these patients will have more than one procedure (Olson et al, 1997). These numbers

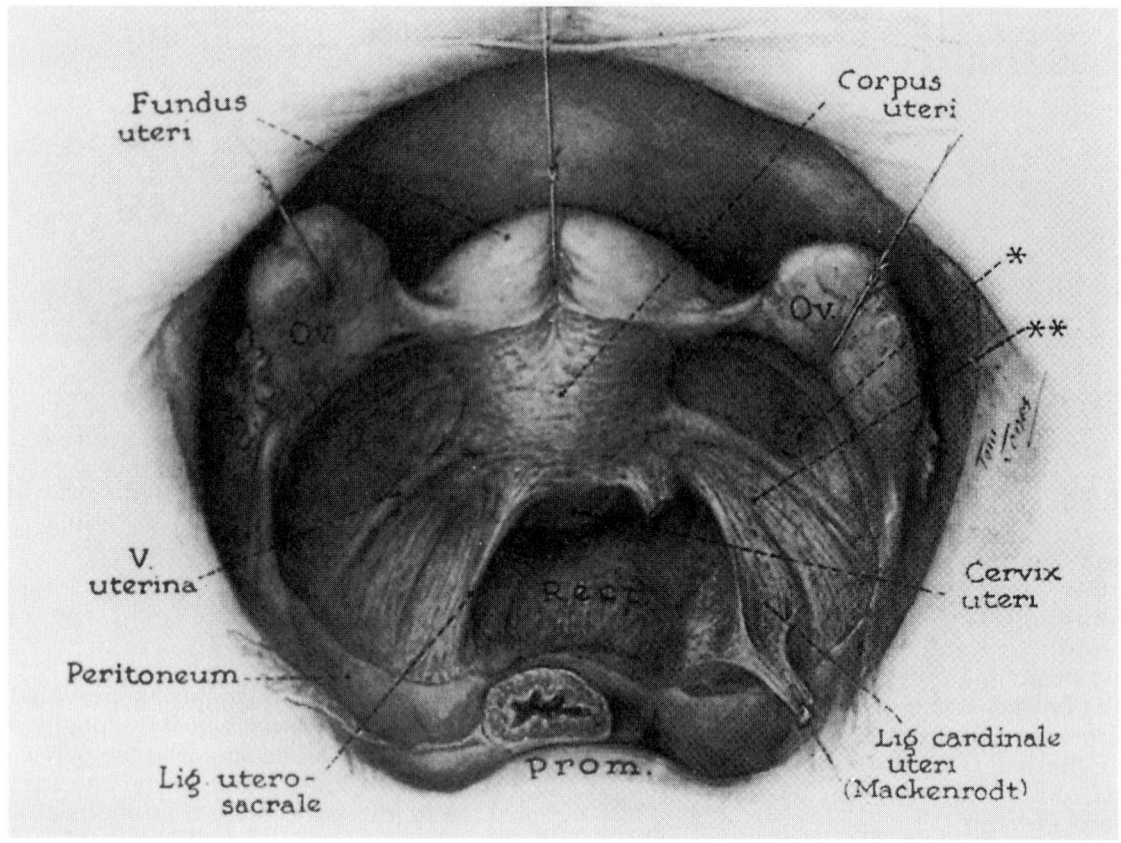

Figure 47–1
The supportive ligaments of the vaginal apex and uterus. In a woman with normal support, the top of the vagina should rest at or above the ischial spine.

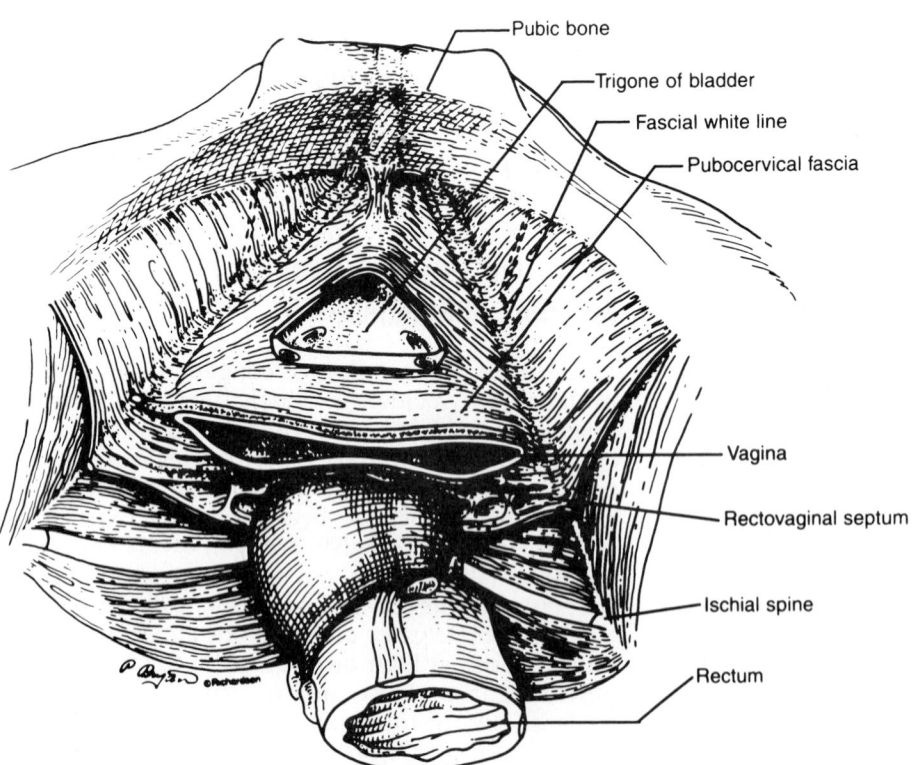

Figure 47–2
The pubovesical fascia is part of the mesh-like connective tissue of the pelvis. It supports the lower urinary tract. The pubovesical and rectovaginal portions of this connective tissue are continuous at the lateral edge of the vagina.

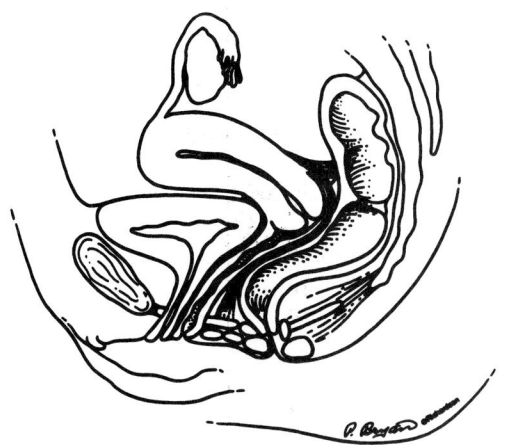

Figure 47–3
Portions of the endopelvic fascia are seen in a midline, sagittal view. Note the superior and inferior attachments of the rectovaginal septum.

probably underestimate the prevalence of pelvic support abnormalities because only those patients presenting for surgical therapy are counted. There are additional women, whose support abnormalities are symptomatic, who decline treatment or who use pessary support.

ETIOLOGY OF SUPPORT ABNORMALITIES

Obstetric

In large part, pelvic organ prolapse is a disorder of vaginally parous women. This well-recognized association has led leading obstetricians to attempt to reduce the level of maternal pelvic floor trauma at the time of delivery. Such efforts have included the use of routine episiotomy with instrumented deliveries. In 1942, a very observant obstetrician, Harold Gainey, reported that significant damage to material support structures is caused by vaginal delivery.

Expert opinion suggests that two important modes of delivery-provoked injury lead to pelvic organ prolapse. There can be damage to multiple connective tissue structures, particularly lateral vaginal and bladder supports. Clinically, this can be recognized as a loss of the vaginal sulcus, unilaterally or bilaterally. Additionally, there can be loss of apical supportive structures, notably the uterosacral ligaments. Clinically, this can be recognized as apical descent, unilaterally or bilaterally.

There can also be neuromuscular injury. As previously discussed, the muscles of the pelvic floor are the primary support mechanism. These muscles can be damaged directly. Alternatively, the innervation

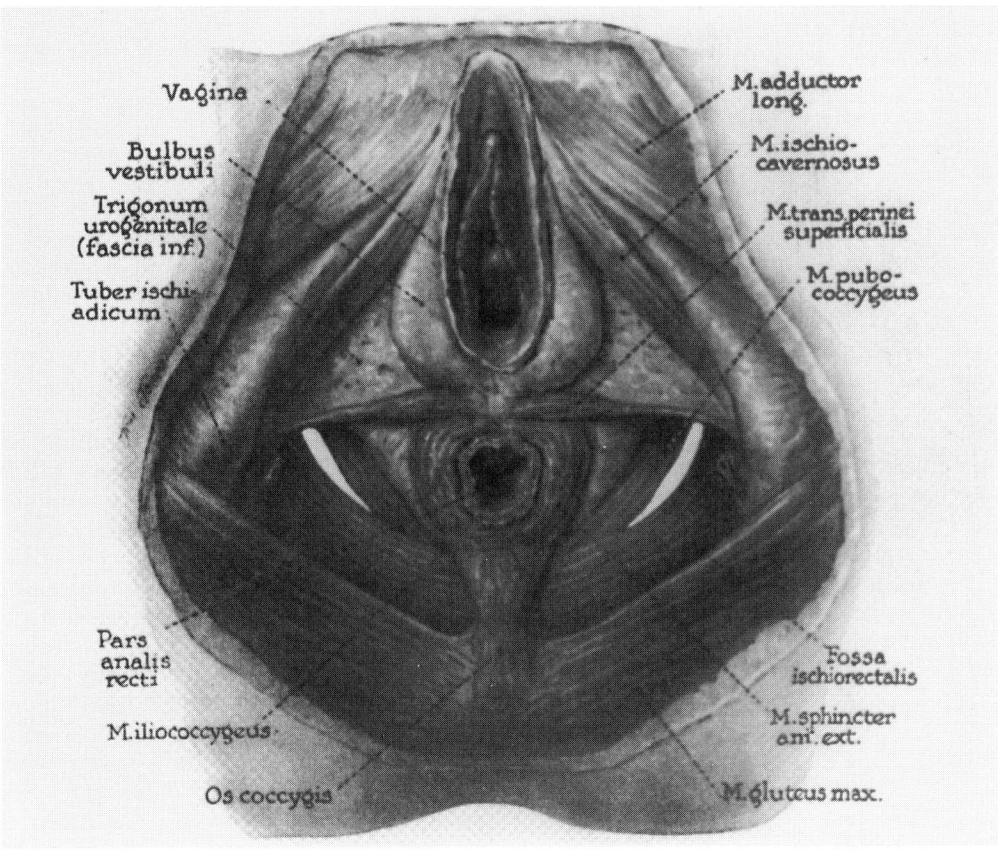

Figure 47–4
The levator ani muscle is the primary support structure for the pelvic organs. This large muscle complex is viewed from below.

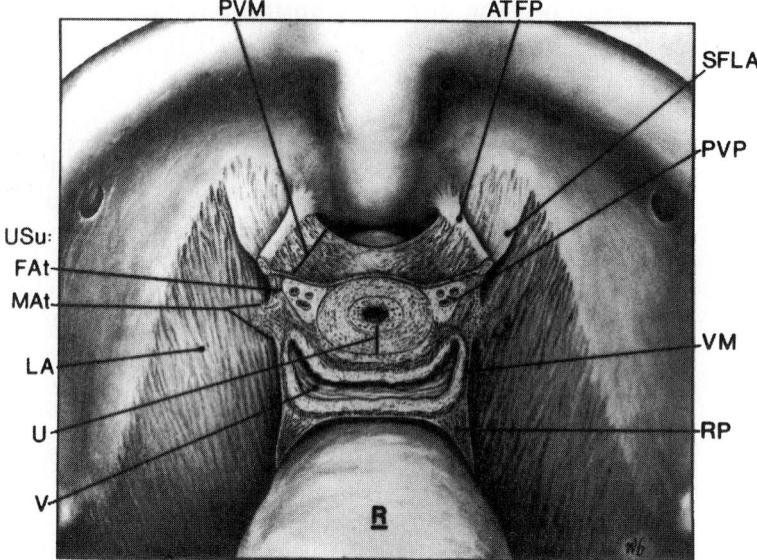

Figure 47–5
Urethral support is provided by both muscular and connective tissue supports, as seen in this cross section to the urethra (U), vagina (V), arcus tendineus fasciae pelvis (ATFP), and superior fascia of levator ani (SFLA) just below the vesical neck (drawn from cadaver dissection). Pubovesical muscles (PVM) lie anterior to the urethra and anterior and superior to the paraurethral vascular plexus (PVP). The urethral supports (Usu) (the pubourethral ligaments) attach the vagina and vaginal surface of the urethra to the levator ani muscles (MAt, muscular attachment) and to the superior fascia of the levator ani (FAt, fascial attachment). R, Rectum; RP, rectal pillar; VM, vaginal wall muscularis.

to the muscle can be damaged. Although human physiology is quite adept at repairing muscle and mild neural injury, more extensive neuromuscular injuries may be incompletely repaired. Studies of peripheral human nerve have documented the many possible mechanisms of nerve injury, including nerve crush (ischemic injury), nerve stretch, and nerve transection. Both crush and stretch occur in the process of normal vaginal deliveries. The pressures in the maternal pelvis can reach 240 mm Hg (Rempen and Kraus, 1991; Brubaker and Benson, 1996). Sustained pressure increases of only 140 mm Hg can lead to irreversible neural injury after 2 hours. It is interesting that this 2 hours mimics the "normal" length of the primigravida second stage. Using electrodiagnostic testing, clinical trials have demonstrated that neural injury is common, affecting approximately 80% of vaginally parous women (Allen et al, 1990). Preliminary studies associate increased infant size, length of second stage, and use of forceps with more severe birth-provoked neuropathy (Allen et al, 1990; Snooks et al, 1996).

The natural history of these connective tissue and neuromuscular injuries has not been studied. Clinically, physicians have observed that many women have initial improvement in symptoms, plateauing at approximately 6 months postpartum. Currently, there are no recommendations for treatment of symptomatic women during this recovery phase. However, in keeping with neuromuscular concepts throughout the body, it is prudent to encourage properly performed pelvic floor contraction exercises.

Other

There is an important subset of nulliparous women who present with pelvic organ prolapse. Such women may mimic the pelvic forces of vaginal delivery by occupational activities that cause repeated heavy lifting (waitresses, parcel/freight workers, etc.) or medical diseases, such as chronic lung disease or refractory constipation. An additional group of women have neural abnormalities that interfere with the innervation of the levator ani. Spinal cord disorders, including congenital abnormalities and tumors, may increase the likelihood of pelvic organ prolapse.

DIAGNOSIS

Physical Examination

In addition to the standard gynecologic speculum and bimanual examination, a detailed evaluation should document the maximum extent of pelvic organ prolapse. This examination can be accomplished in a variety of ways, although it is essential that the patient confirm that the examiner is evaluating the maximum protrusion. Occasionally, the entire vagina is completely everted in the supine position. More commonly, the physician obtains the best information about maximum protrusion when the patient is standing and straining maximally (Fig. 47–6).

The physical examination is the gold standard for assessing the position of the vaginal walls. Although many years of clinical habit are difficult to change, the terms for describing support abnormalities during physical examination should be precise. The terms *urethrocele, cystocele, rectocele,* and *enterocele* should be used only when the examiner is certain that the visceral abnormality accompanies the vaginal wall support abnormality. The findings of the physical examination can be more precisely described using the terminology listed in Table 47–1.

The description of the position of the vagina can be augmented by palpation of some of the supportive structures, particularly rectovaginal fascia. It is

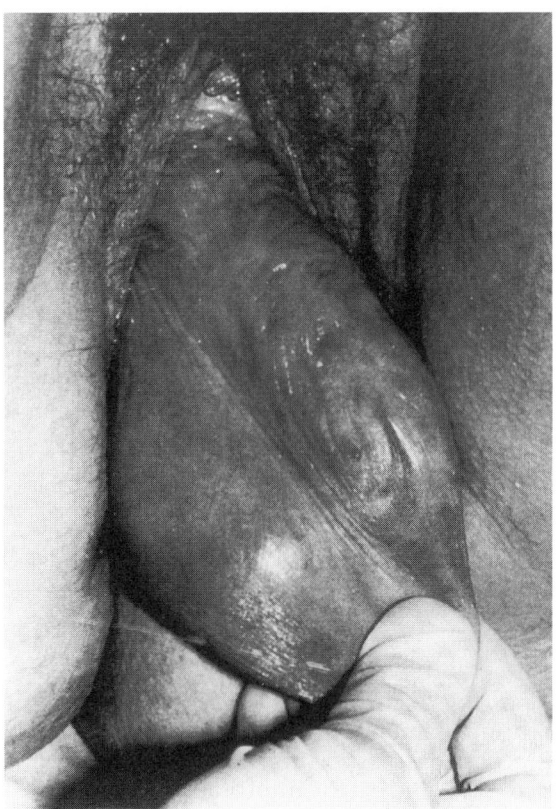

Figure 47–6
The maximum extent of the pelvic organ prolapse is best assessed when the patient stands and strains. This photograph demonstrates the typical findings of a patient with complete loss of vaginal support.

Table 47–1. PHYSICAL EXAMINATION TERMS FOR DESCRIPTION OF SUPPORT ABNORMALITIES

Anterior wall support abnormality (can be further specified as lateral, midline, upper/transverse)
Apical support abnormalities (with or without uterus present)
Posterior wall support abnormality (can be further specified as distal, proximal)

floor fluoroscopy combines aspects of the traditional cystogram and defecating proctogram, which have been used by other specialties for many years. During evaluation of pelvic organ prolapse, in addition to opacification of bladder and rectum, the small bowel and vagina are opacified. Each study consists of static and dynamic images during strain, squeeze, and defecation/urination. When these images are considered with the clinician's knowledge of vaginal topography and visceral function, the planned operation may be more specifically individualized. The advantages of this imaging technique include the ability to ensure maximum strain effort, quantitate visceral descent, assess rectocele function, and discover unusual forms of prolapse, such as sigmoidocele. The disadvantages include the need for a knowledgeable radiologist, use of radiation, and patient inconvenience.

Magnetic resonance imaging of the pelvis provides remarkable anatomic information, particularly when the images can be obtained in the upright position. Both static and dynamic images can be obtained, although the dynamic images are limited by the patient's ability to remain motionless. Although prohibitively expensive for clinical use, this emerging technology may provide additional research information about pelvic support in normal and abnormal circumstances.

common clinical practice to use palpation to diagnose visceral abnormalities, particularly rectocele and enterocele. However, studies document that this practice is unreliable for assessment of posterior wall support abnormalities, even in experienced hands (Kelvin et al, 1994).

NOMENCLATURE OF PELVIC ORGAN PROLAPSE

The evaluation and treatment of pelvic organ prolapse has suffered from a historic lack of standardized nomenclature that has limited surgeons' ability to communicate the pre- and postoperative findings of their patients (Brubaker and Norton, 1996). Previously described systems have been poorly defined, inconsistently used, and randomly modified. A selection of prolapse grading systems are listed in Table 47–2 (Baden and Walker, 1992).

Imaging

The use of imaging is an adjunct to physical examination. At the clinician's discretion, documentation of visceral abnormalities can be easily obtained using a variety of imaging techniques. Ultrasound imaging has been used to document hypermobility of the urethrovesical junction as well as the presence of small bowel in the prolapsed vaginal vault. The transducer may be placed on the perineum, suprapubic area, intravaginally, and intrarectally. Technical considerations include artifact introduced by the pressure of the transducer and the inability to assess the functional abnormalities of rectoceles when present. The advantages of this technique include accessibility of equipment, lack of radiation, and relative inexpense.

Fluoroscopic imaging allows precise localization of the pelvic organs during maximal strain. Pelvic

Table 47–2. SYSTEMS OF PELVIC ORGAN PROLAPSE

Grade 0/1–3/4
Mild/Moderate/Severe
Baden Halfway System (Baden and Walker, 1992)
Pelvic Organ Prolapse–Quantified (Bump et al, 1996)

A newly created, validated system replaces these other systems for quantified descriptions of pelvic organ prolapse. The pelvic organ prolapse–quantified (POP-Q) system measures nine specific aspects of vaginal topography (Bump et al, 1996). If desired, these measurements can be further categorized into clinical stages 1 through 4. This system is shown in Figures 47–7 to 47–9. Several studies have documented the inter- and intrarater reliability of this system (Athanasiou et al, 1995; Kobak et al, 1995; Montella and Cater, 1995; Schussler and Peschers, 1995; Swift and Harring, 1995; Brubaker and Kenton, 1996; Hall et al, 1996). In addition, the system allows the clinician to individualize the examination technique and the use of ancillary studies.

There are important limitations to the POP-Q system. It is not designed to comment upon clinically relevant issues such as the presence of midline versus lateral anterior wall support defects, or volume of vaginal distention. In addition, this system does not predict visceral position. Thus, a specific amount of anterior (or posterior) wall support cannot be equated with the presence of cystocele (or rectocele), particularly in those patients with prior unsuccessful prolapse surgery. Figure 47–10 demonstrates the absence of rectocele formation in a patient with stage 4 pelvic organ prolapse (massive eversion).

Visceral Position

The terms *cystocele*, *rectocele*, and *enterocele* are poorly defined, but generally indicate protrusion of the organ beyond its normal anatomic confines. It is important to recognize that these "cele" entities are not "all or none" phenomena. More appropriately, clinicians should consider the continuum of support abnormalities, ranging from normal support to complete eversion. The combined use of the POP-Q system and imaging techniques is likely to allow appropriate definitions within the next decade.

Assessment of Pelvic Organ Prolapse

Comprehensive symptom assessment is important in the evaluation of patients presenting with pelvic organ prolapse. When the prolapse is stage 1 or 2 (protrusion within 1 cm of the hymen), the patient may be asymptomatic. With increasing protrusion, the rate of symptoms increases. Protrusion-related symptoms include the sensation of "sitting on something," vaginal pressure, and occasionally prolapse-related low back pain/pressure that is relieved by the supine position. The patient may also report the need to replace the prolapse in order to void and/or defecate. A systematic assessment of pelvic floor symptoms increases the opportunity to detect and treat disorders of support, sensation, and visceral function. Table 47–3 lists the "USA" review of systems for pelvic floor disorders.

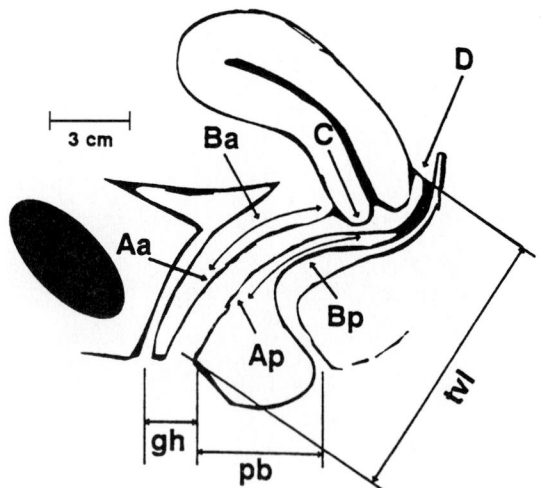

Figure 47–7
Six sites (points Aa, Ba, C, D, Bp, and Ap), genital hiatus (gh), perineal body (pb), and total vaginal length (tvl) used for pelvic organ support quantitation.

Coexisting disorders of visceral function occur frequently in women with pelvic organ prolapse. One well-recognized association is stress urinary incontinence. It is extremely important to detect this abnormality when the patient has selected a surgical correction. Although patients with stage 3-4 pelvic organ prolapse may not report the clinical symptoms of stress incontinence, it is clinically important to test each patient following replacement of her protrusion. Transurethral leakage at the acme of intra-abdominal pressure increase is very sound clinical evidence of genuine stress incontinence, as discussed in Chapter 46. However, when incontinence is not initially demonstrated, the clinician should make additional efforts to detect leakage. The patient should be tested in the upright position with maximum bladder filling and repetitive coughing while the prolapse is replaced. If incontinence is detected, additional testing may be warranted in order to deter-

anterior wall	anterior wall	cervix or cuff
Aa	**Ba**	**C**
genital hiatus	perineal body	total vaginal length
gh	**pb**	**tvl**
posterior wall	posterior wall	posterior fornix
Ap	**Bp**	**D**

Figure 47–8
Three-by-three grid for recording quantitative description of pelvic organ support.

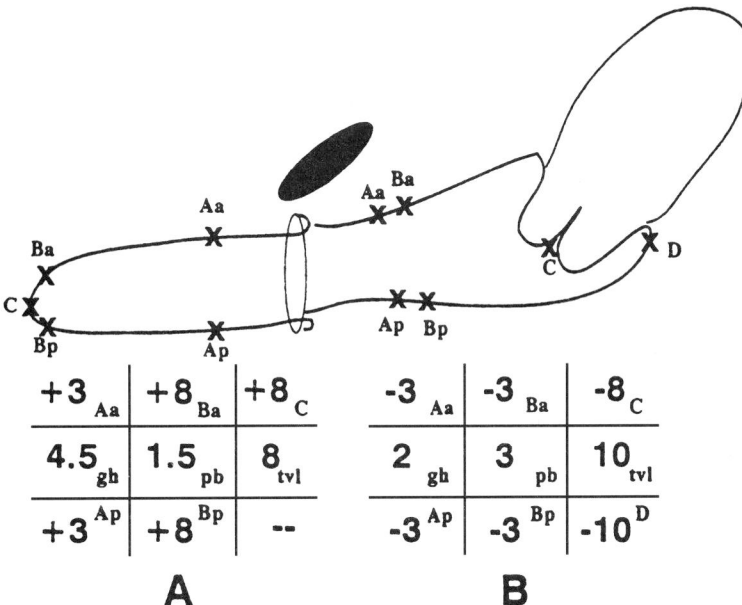

Figure 47–9
A, Grid and line diagram of complete eversion of vagina. Most distal point of anterior wall (point Ba), vaginal cuff scar (point C), and most distal point of the posterior wall (point Bp) are all at same position (+8) and points Aa and Ap are maximally distal (both at +3). Because total vaginal length equals maximum protrusion, this is stage IV prolapse. *B,* Normal support. Points Aa and Ba and points Ap and Bp are all −3 because there is no anterior or posterior wall descent. Lowest point of the cervix is 8 cm above hymen (−8) and posterior fornix is 2 cm above this (−10). Vaginal length is 10 cm and genital hiatus and perineal body measure 2 and 3 cm, respectively. This represents stage 0 support.

mine the appropriate anti-incontinence procedure for that individual patient. The empiric use of anti-incontinence procedures overtreats those patients with adequate continence mechanisms, unnecessarily subjecting them to the morbidity and side effects of these operations.

Approximately one of every five women with urinary incontinence also has some degree of anal incontinence. When the comprehensive symptom assessment detects anorectal disorders, appropriate evaluation should precede surgical decision making. Many women with anorectal disorders who undergo pelvic reconstructive procedures benefit from biofeedback, dietary alterations, and other nonsurgical therapies. An additional subset of women may require anorectal procedures, such as sphincteroplasty or hemorrhoidectomy. The symptom of "constipation" requires preoperative clarification because the etiology of constipation is multifactorial. Colonic motility disorders will not improve following pelvic floor procedures, whereas stool trapping associated with rectocele formation may significantly improve postoperatively.

TREATMENT COUNSELING

Early in the evaluation, the clinician should begin to understand the individual woman's goals for therapy. All patients should initially be given a description of the disorder, as well as an explanation of its progressive nature. Pessary management and surgical options should be discussed. Increasingly, women wish to initially avoid surgical correction. This desire can be accommodated in the vast majority of women, because pelvic organ prolapse is rarely an emergent or painful disorder. However, it is not wise to simply observe patients whose prolapse causes elevated postvoid residuals or hydroureter. Likewise, those women with ulcerated prolapse are at increased risk of evisceration and require treatment.

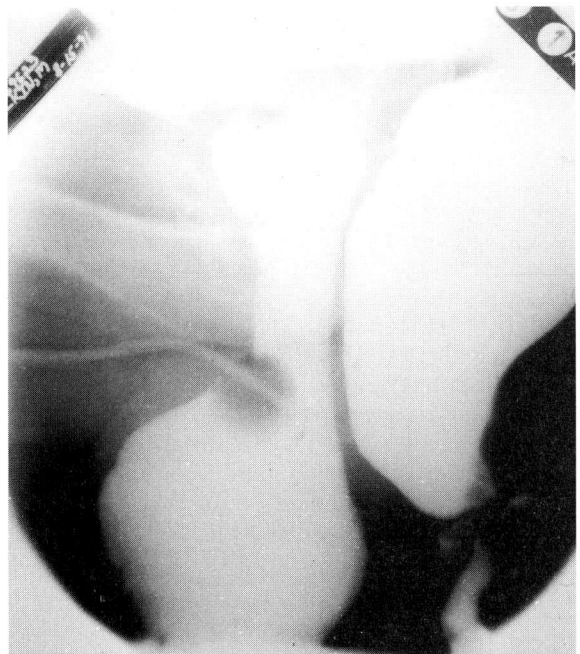

Figure 47–10
Pelvic fluoroscopy demonstrates the visceral position of a woman with stage 4 prolapse (massive eversion). There is no rectocele, despite complete detachment of her posterior vaginal wall.

Observation

Women without symptoms or whose symptoms are minimally bothersome may wish to defer any form

☐ **Table 47-3.** "USA" REVIEW OF SYSTEMS FOR PELVIC FLOOR DISORDERS

Urinary	
Storage phase	Urgency, frequency, nocturia, incontinence (urge, stress, other)
Emptying phase	Voiding dysfunction, postural voiding, urinary retention
Sensation	Increased sensation (pain, constant urge to urinate)
	Decreased sensation
Sexual	
Sexual activity	If yes, ask other questions
	If no, why not
Sexual response	Normal, abnormal
General sensation of protrusion	Increased (pain disorders)
	Decreased
Anorectal	
Storage phase	Urgency, frequency, incontinence (gas, liquid, solid)
Emptying phase	Defecation dysfunction (including manually assisted defecation), postdefecation fullness, "constipation"
Sensation	Increased sensation (pain, constant urge to defecate)
	Decreased sensation (inability to distinguish gas vs. stool)

of therapy. It is reasonable to quantitatively assess these patients on a regular basis, initially 6-month intervals. Annual assessments will suffice when minimal progression has been documented and the patient's symptoms are stable. The use of the POP-Q is extremely helpful for repetitive assessments of the same patient, even when more than one examiner records the measurements, as commonly occurs in busy clinical practices.

Nonsurgical Treatment

Women may select pessary use to avoid surgery altogether or to gain comfort while awaiting a surgical correction. There are several groups of women who may not be optimal candidates for pessary use. Women with unexplained vaginal bleeding or ulcerations should be evaluated for these problems prior to pessary fitting. Likewise, the clinician must consider the degree of hypoestrogenic atrophy against the risk of erosion from the vaginal foreign body. Women with extreme hypoestrogenism who are unable or unwilling to remove the pessary nightly are at increased risk for complications from pessary erosion. Finally, women who cannot comply with frequent follow-up are not well served by pessary placement.

Certain anatomic features may make pessary placement difficult. A woman with a large introital opening and a small/nonexistent perineum often has difficulty retaining the appropriate-size pessary. Protrusion that is predominantly posterior may also be challenging to treat with the pessary.

Women with bothersome urinary incontinence often experience worsening of incontinence when the anterior wall is replaced. This possibility should be discussed with these patients prior to pessary placement.

Pessary fitting is straightforward. The goal is to provide satisfactory reduction of the protrusion, without causing discomfort or adversely affecting bowel or bladder function. Although there are a large number of pessaries available in North America, expert opinion suggests that two pessaries are used commonly. The ring pessary, with or without supportive floor, is similar to a diaphragm and is easy to place and remove (Fig. 47–11). The Gelhorn pessary is also used commonly, although this pessary is somewhat more difficult to remove and replace.

Initial pessary fitting should include choice a device that fits comfortably within the vagina, reducing the prolapse and remaining intravaginal despite increases in intra-abdominal pressure. A follow-up visit should occur within approximately 1 week to ensure that the pessary is satisfactory for prolapse reduction. Additionally, bowel and bladder function should be assessed. Changes in size or type of pessary may be required. Once a satisfactory pessary is obtained, a long-term maintenance plan must be selected. Ideally, a women should be instructed to remove, clean, and replace her own pessary on a nightly or weekly basis in order to reduce the chance for vaginal erosion. Physician follow-up occurs at regular, but infrequent intervals once a successful regimen is established. Some women are unable or unwilling to perform pessary care. In that case, the clinician or ancillary health care worker will need to see the patient at regular intervals for care.

Use of the pessary may be discontinued because the patient wishes surgical treatment or has recurrent vaginal erosions that make continued pessary use unwise. The physician should discuss surgical options and the patient should undergo appropriate presurgical testing.

Surgical Treatment

Prior to a discussion of surgical options, the physician should have a clear understanding of pelvic floor symptoms, vaginal topography, and the functional and support abnormalities of the viscera. It is

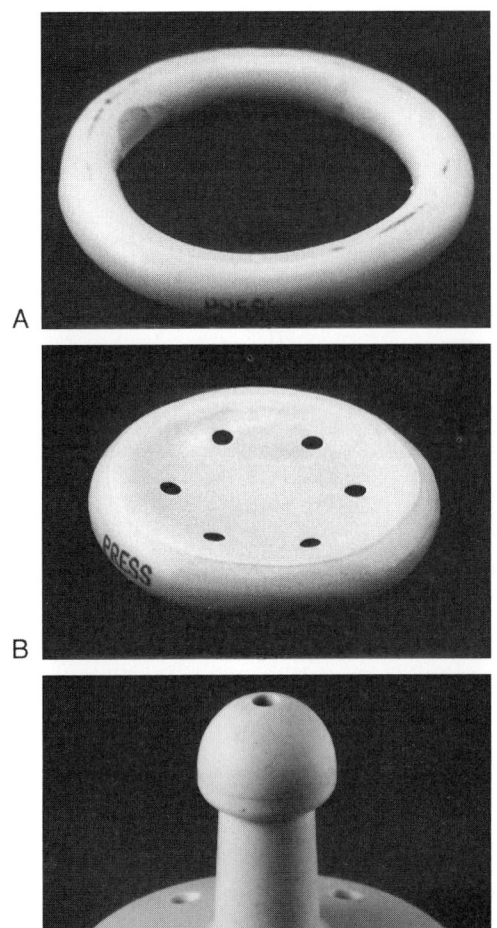

Figure 47-11
The ring (*A*), ring with supportive floor (*B*), and Gelhorn (*C*) pessaries are commonly used devices for nonsurgical management of pelvic organ prolapse.

helpful to list the "problems" to be treated and ensure that the planned surgical procedure addresses as many of the problems as possible. Problems that are not addressed by surgery, such as urge incontinence, should be clearly discussed in the preoperative period. In addition to the standard aspects of the surgical informed consent process, the patient should be told of the success and failure rates for each portion of the planned procedure.

The vast majority of patients should undergo reconstructive procedures. These may be accomplished transvaginally, transabdominally, or by a combined procedure. The route of procedure should be based on the optimal cure for the functional and anatomic disorders to be treated. It is not in patients' best interest to *always* operate vaginally or *always* operate

abdominally. The procedures for treatment of urinary incontinence are addressed in Chapter 46. These procedures are frequently performed concomitantly with the procedures used to correct pelvic organ prolapse.

Transvaginal Repairs

Transvaginal repairs offer the well-recognized advantage of decreased short-term surgical morbidity. Most anatomic aspects can be treated using this route, provided there is sufficient vaginal length and caliber.

ANTERIOR WALL SUPPORT

There are several procedures for treatment of anterior wall support defects. Expert opinion suggests that the anterior wall provides the biggest challenge for long-term success. For almost a century, the anterior colporrhaphy has been performed. This procedure plicates the endopelvic fascia in the midline and provides preferential support to the urethra (Fig. 47-12). The high recurrence rate has led gynecologic surgeons to modify this procedure. Although there are multiple surgical reports that document anterior wall recurrences, there are no clinical trials comparing individual modifications of anterior colporrhaphy. Expert opinion suggests that women whose anterior wall support defect is defective in the midline, traditional plication using delayed absorbable suture material is reasonable. Women with recurrent anterior wall support defects are likely to require alternative materials (permanent sutures) or alternative techniques (paravaginal repair).

Modifications of the traditional anterior colporrhaphy include "pants over vest" technique (Nichols, 1991b), placement of mesh (Pillai-Allen and Benson, 1996), and four-point suspension. None of these specific recommendations has been studied in clinical trials, thus limiting their usefulness for daily clinical practice.

The transvaginal paravaginal repair has been extensively described and studied by Shull et al (1996). This technically challenging procedure replaces the anterolateral vaginal wall to its anatomic position in the white line (arcus tendineus fascia pelvis) (Fig. 47-13). Shull et al reported on 62 women treated with transvaginal repair as a component of their pelvic reconstruction. Fifty-six of these women had a mean follow-up of 1.6 years with a 7% recurrence rate.

APICAL SUPPORT

Transvaginal apical support can be accomplished by several effective procedures. A time-honored treatment is the McCall's culdeplasty, which shortens the uterosacral ligaments and reattaches them to the vaginal apex (Fig. 47-14). Symmonds et al (1981) have reported their success with this procedure.

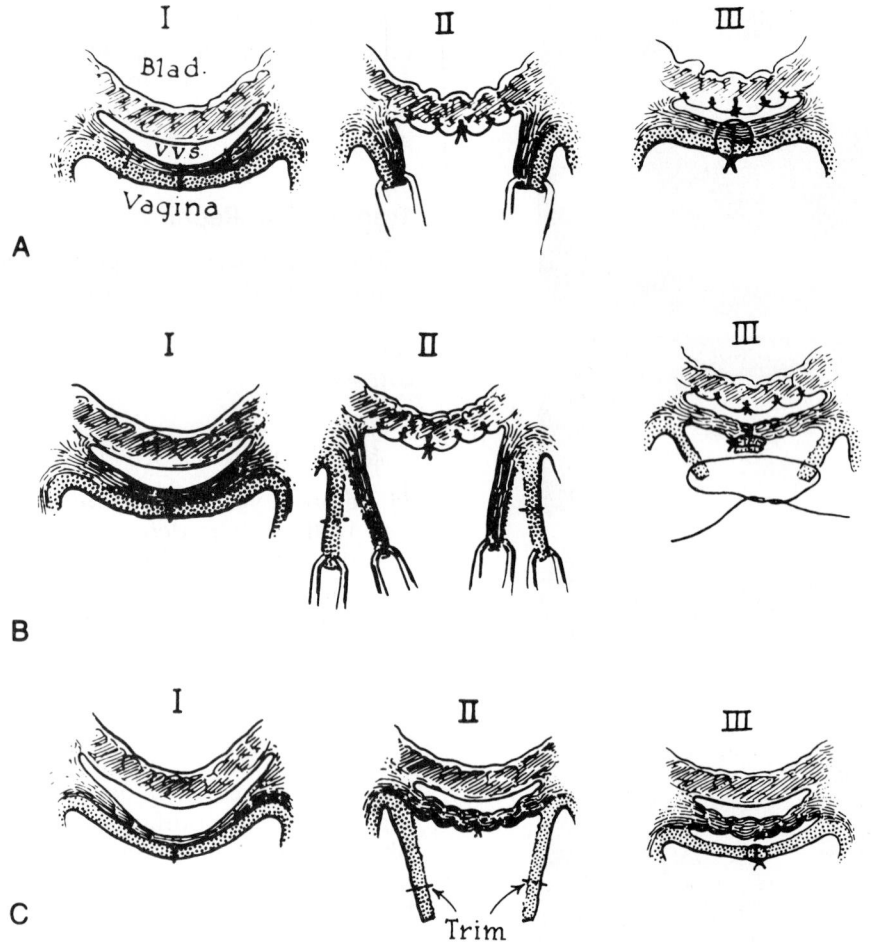

Figure 47–12
Three methods of anterior colporrhaphy. *A, I*: The attenuated anterior vaginal wall to be removed is shown between the *dotted lines*. *II*: The full thickness of this weakened segment has been excised and the fibromuscular bladder capsule has been plicated with some fine absorbable suture, reducing the width of the vesicovaginal space. *III*: The full thickness of the stronger portion of the anterior vaginal walls has been approximated by interrupted subcuticular sutures. *B, I*: A midline incision has been made through the full thickness of the anterior wall into the vesicovaginal space. *II*: The capsule of the bladder has been plicated, reducing the width of the vesicovaginal space, and the fibromuscular layer of the vagina has been gently dissected from the undersurface of the vaginal skin. *III*: Using a synthetic absorbable or nonabsorbable suture, all of this fibromuscular layer is plicated in the midline without resection. The superficial vaginal membrane is trimmed in the appropriated amount, as noted in II, and approximated from side to side with through-and-through or subcuticular sutures. *C*, Drawings depicting a frequent but rather ineffective colporrhaphy in which the vesicovaginal space is never entered. *I*: A superficial midline incision of the vaginal membrane is made. *II*: This is dissected from the underlying fibromuscular layer of the anterior vaginal wall, which is then plicated. *III*: Excess superficial vaginal membrane is trimmed as indicated and the sides approximated with interrupted through-and-through sutures.

Clinically it may be difficult to detect the presence of the uterosacral ligaments, particularly with long-standing stage 3 or 4 vaginal vault prolapse. Many gynecologic surgeons prefer the sacrospinous ligament suspension, popularized in North America by Nichols (1982; Morley and DeLancey, 1988) (Fig. 47–15). This procedure may be performed unilaterally or bilaterally, and modifications include number and type of sutures as well as the specific instrument used for suture placement. A similar technique affixes the vaginal apex to the ileococcygeus fascia in an attempt to more closely approximate the normal vaginal axis (Meeks et al, 1994). Expert consensus suggests that these operations provide good apical support but are troubled by support abnormalities in other portions of the vagina.

POSTERIOR WALL SUPPORT

Posterior wall support defects have been traditionally addressed by posterior colporrhaphy (Fig. 47–16). This procedure mimics the anterior colporrha-

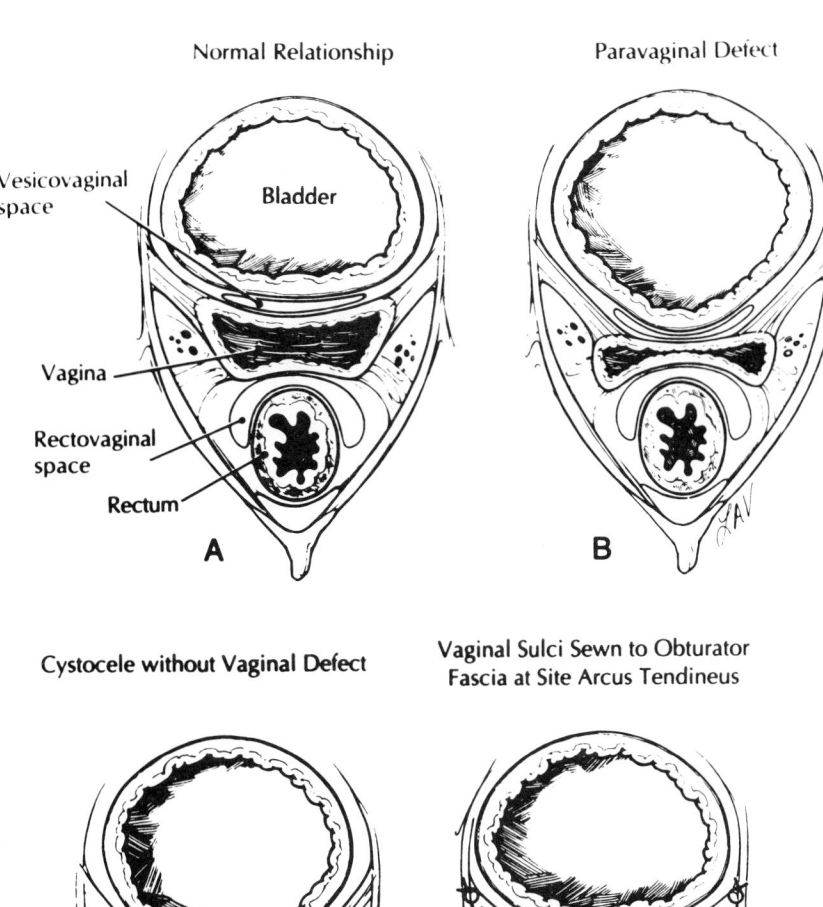

Normal Relationship

Paravaginal Defect

Cystocele without Vaginal Defect

Vaginal Sulci Sewn to Obturator
Fascia at Site Arcus Tendineus

Figure 47–13
Coronal drawings of the pelvis. *A*, A normal relationship between bladder and vagina. Note the connective tissue condensation connecting the anterior vaginal sulci to the arcus tendineus along the pelvic sidewall. *B*, A bilateral paravaginal defect. Note the elongation (or avulsion) of the support of the sulci. *C*, Midline cystocele is noted by the sagging of the anterior vaginal wall. Notice that the connective tissue condensations supporting the sulci are undamaged. *D*, When the vaginal sulci have been sewn directly to the sites of the arcus tendinei, the width of the anterior thin vaginal wall is increased, reducing its sagging and demonstrating how paravaginal repair, even without paravaginal defect, will secondarily elevate the bladder to reduce the cystocele.

phy with a midline plication of endopelvic fascia. Technical variations include plications of levator muscle, reattachment of rectovaginal fascia to perineal body, and use of permanent materials. There are few reports of the anatomic failure rate of this procedure; however, there are multiple reports suggesting that dyspareunia occurs in as many as 30% of these procedures, particularly when levator plication is performed (Arnold et al, 1990; Janssen and van Dijke, 1994; Mellgren et al, 1995).

The usefulness of the rectovaginal fascia is emphasized in an increasingly popular posterior wall reconstructive technique (Brubaker, 1996) (Fig. 47–17). Although initial clinical observations suggest that the dyspareunia rate is decreased, the efficacy of this technique remains to be determined.

Transrectal repair of rectocele formation is described in the colorectal surgery literature and may have some usefulness in a selected group of women with fluoroscopic evidence of an excessively large rectal diameter (Block, 1986; Sarles et al, 1989).

Perineorrhaphy is required when there is a reduced anovaginal distance, generally less than 3 cm. This procedure may also be used when there is insufficient strength to the perineal body and the surgeon wishes to provide additional posterior support. Perineorrhaphy can easily cause dyspareunia. The surgeon must avoid an overzealous vaginal narrowing.

Transabdominal Techniques

Transabdominal procedures are indicated when the added morbidity of this route of surgery is balanced by an increase in cure rate for either a functional or anatomic problem. Certainly, the transabdominal route is indicated whenever the transvaginal route is contraindicated. Additionally, abdominal techniques

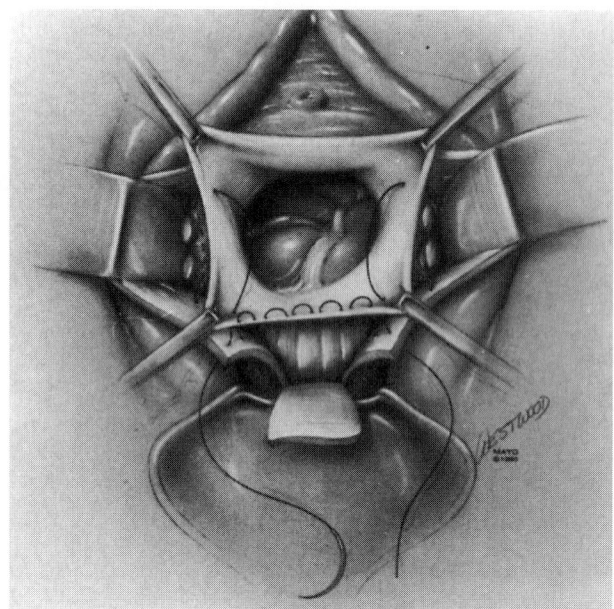

Figure 47–14
McCall's sutures are placed incorporating the pararectal fascia cephalad to the uterosacral ligament but inferior and medial to the ureter. The reperitonealizing suture is brought through the cut edges of the posterior vaginal wall.

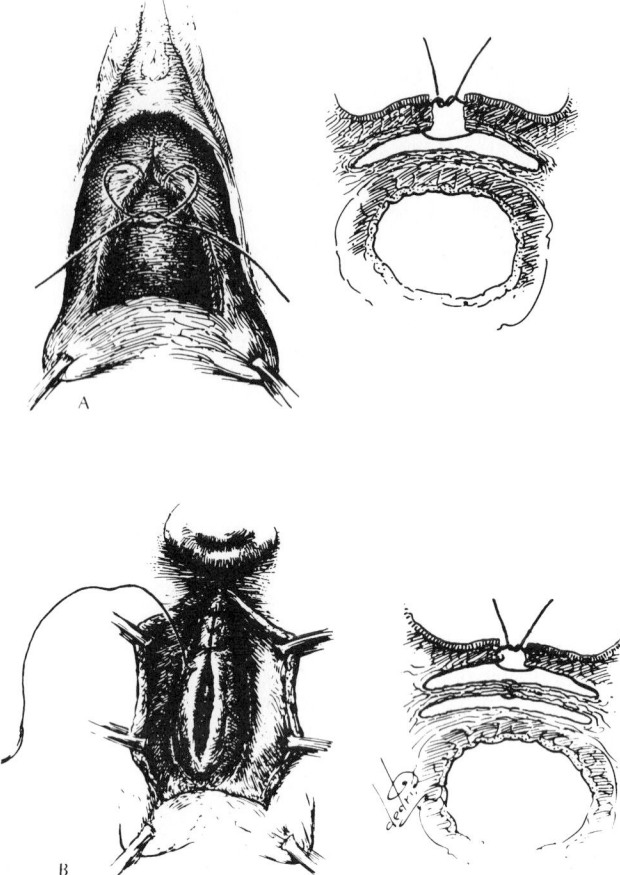

Figure 47–16
Methods of closing the vagina with posterior colporrhaphy. *A,* In the Goff method, an appropriate full-thickness wedge of posterior vaginal wall has been excised, and the tissues, including the fused rectovaginal septum, are closed from side to side. A subcuticular suture is preferred. *B,* In the Bullard modification, the rectovaginal septum has been dissected from the posterior vaginal wall and closed as a separate layer between rectum and vaginal membrane. When this has been accomplished, excess vaginal membrane is trimmed, and the sides are brought together by interrupted suture. A running subcuticular suture may be used.

can be used when there is a concomitant indication for an abdominal approach, such as a pelvic mass. The surgeon must use experience and judgment when determining the best route for treatment of a woman whose prior vaginal repair was unsuccessful. Factors that may have affected the unsuccessful outcome include intrinsic factors, such as patient tis-

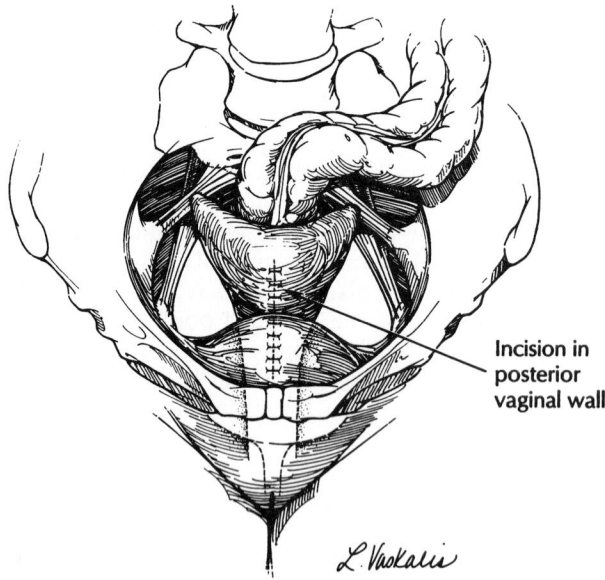

Figure 47–15
Although the sacrospinous ligament suspension is usually performed unilaterally, the bilateral attachment is possible when there is sufficient vaginal width.

sue deficiencies in muscle or connective tissue, co-existing medical disease (chronic lung disease), or extrinsic factors, such as technical factors associated with preoperative diagnosis and/or performance of the procedure.

ANTERIOR WALL SUPPORT

Anterior wall support is best provided with a para-vaginal repair, as described by White (1909) and popularized by Richardson et al (1976). This procedure supports the anterior wall from pubis to ischial spines bilaterally. Midline tissue deficiencies, traditionally treated with anterior colporrhaphy, are sub-optimally treated with this technique. Brubaker (1995) reported the high efficacy of the abdominal route in 65 women. This report also indicated a con-

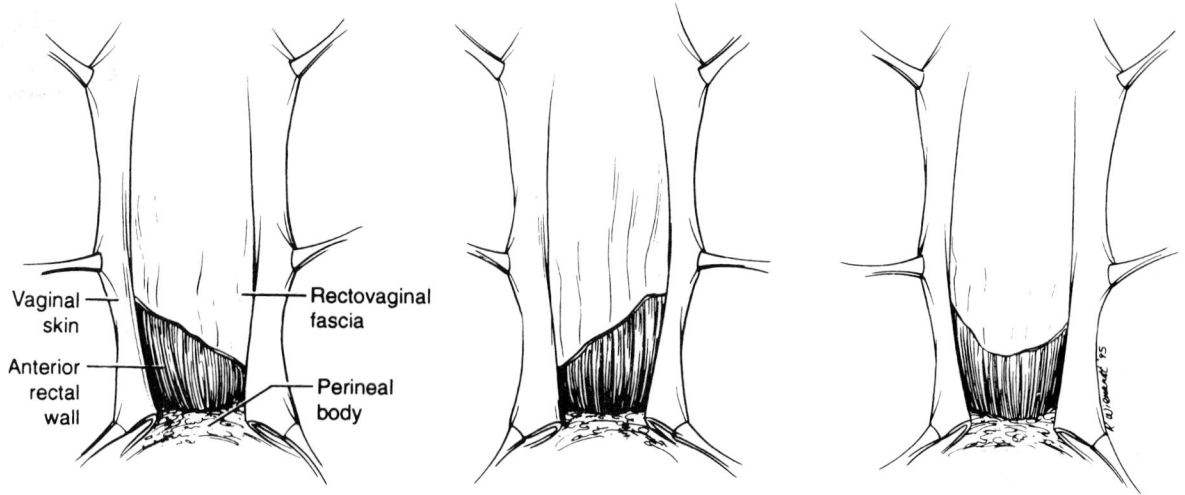

Figure 47–17
Reattachment of rectovaginal fascial defects is an alternative technique that avoids dyspareunia often associated with levator ani plication.

cern of new-onset midline defects, which occurred in 11% of women following the paravaginal repair as a component of extensive reconstruction for stage 3 or 4 prolapse.

Women with voluminous anterior support defects frequently require narrowing of the upper vagina. This is appropriate when the replaced tissue markedly exceeds the distance between the ischial spines. Although no clinical trials have reported efficacy of these techniques, expert opinion suggests that wedging of the anterior wall is essential to a successful reconstructive procedure (Nichols, 1993).

APICAL SUPPORT

Apical support can be accomplished using a variety of techniques. Modified culdeplasties are useful, especially in women with less than stage 4 prolapse. There are distinct advantages of this technique. Technical expertise is required to detect uterosacral remnants and safeguard the ureters. In procedures where uterosacral identification is difficult, it is useful to use the tissue that lies greater than 1 cm medial to the ureter and the lateral boundary of the rectum. Ureteral kinking can occur and should be assessed following these procedures.

When a culdeplasty technique has been unsuccessful, or when available tissue is inadequate, the sacrocolpopexy technique may be considered. This technique suspends the vaginal tube to the sacrum by firmly attaching a graft of tissue or synthetic mesh to the vaginal fascia. Many modifications of this technique have been described (Timmons and Addison, 1996). Regardless of the modification chosen, several essentials are critical to proper resolution of the support defect. The fascial covering of the vaginal tube must be reestablished and reattached to a stable pelvic structure. Frequently, in posthysterectomy vaginal vault prolapse, there is insufficient fas-

cia directly at the apex. It is necessary to attach the graft to the intact fascia, which is typically several centimeters caudal to the apex. Once a graft is secured to the vaginal tube, the superior portion of the graft can be attached to the anterior longitudinal ligament of the sacrum (Fig. 47–18). Multiple studies indicate the efficacy of this procedure for apical support (Timmons et al, 1992). Complications include foreign body risks (infection and rejection) and lower urinary tract injury.

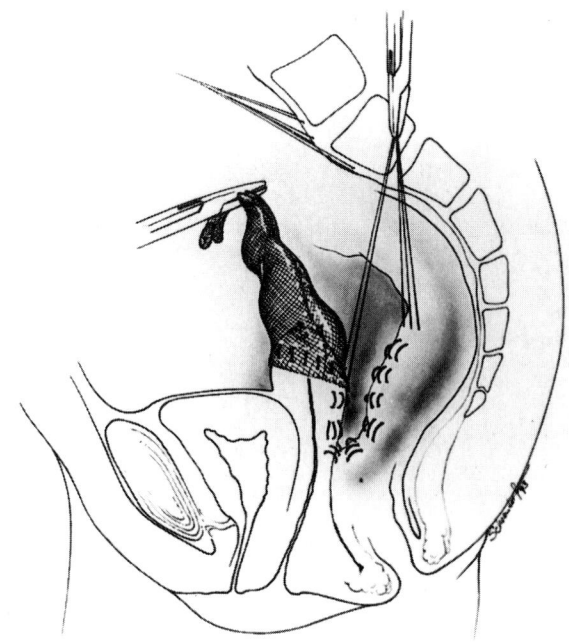

Figure 47–18
Abdominal sacrocolpopexy technique. Attachment of suspensory mesh around the entire vaginal vault and placement of Halban's culdeplasty sutures.

Abdominal techniques for culdeplasty are commonly used to treat and/or prevent enterocele formation. The abdominal McCall or Halban technique (Fig. 47–19) frequently accompanies abdominal colpopexy.

Obliterative Surgery

A minority of women are candidates for obliterative, rather than reconstructive, surgery. These include women who are not currently coitally active and do not anticipate future coital activity, and who find vaginal closure an acceptable surgical option. Vaginal closure (colpocleisis) can be performed regardless of the presence of the uterus. The prudent surgeon must balance the risk of endometrial pathology with the decreased morbidity achieved by avoiding hysterectomy. In many women, this may be accomplished by endometrial curettage with frozen section at the time of operation. The Le-Fort Neugebauer colpocleisis accomplishes vaginal closure, yet preserves small lateral channels for uterine drainage (Ubachs et al, 1973). Alternatively, in women whose prolapse follows hysterectomy, complete colpectomy and vaginal closure can be performed (Hanson and Keettel, 1969).

In this elderly population, lower urinary tract dysfunction is common and may be worsened following vaginal closure. It is preferable to have some understanding of the patient's lower urinary tract function prior to the surgery, in order to minimize subsequent incontinence and/or voiding dysfunction. Routine use of an anti-incontinence procedure, such as suburethral plication, causes voiding dysfunction in a significant minority of these patients.

The Role of Hysterectomy

It is currently common practice to delay pelvic organ prolapse repair until the woman has completed her childbearing. Thus hysterectomy has typically been performed at the time of the repair. There are no clinical trials that report the necessity of hysterectomy in restoring normal support. The more current understanding of support defects suggests that the uterus is simply an innocent passenger in these processes. Several small clinical series have reported reconstructive procedures with uterine preservation (Nichols, 1991a; Kovac and Cruickshank, 1993). The role of hysterectomy in pelvic reconstruction awaits a randomized clinical trial.

The isolated suspension of the uterus is rarely, if ever, indicated. These operations are largely of historical interest because it is widely recognized that abnormalities in support rarely exist at a single anatomic site.

PREVENTION OF PROLAPSE

There is an important opportunity to prevent subsequent pelvic organ prolapse during the performance of hysterectomy for nonprolapse indications. The uterosacral ligaments, which are so critical for apical support, should be firmly reattached to the posterior vaginal cuff following removal of the uterus.

The vaginal technique of the McCall culdeplasty and its modifications take specific, individual steps to optimize pelvic support following the extirpative portions of the procedure. Transabdominally, whether using a laparoscopic or open technique, there is an additional opportunity to identify and tag these lig-

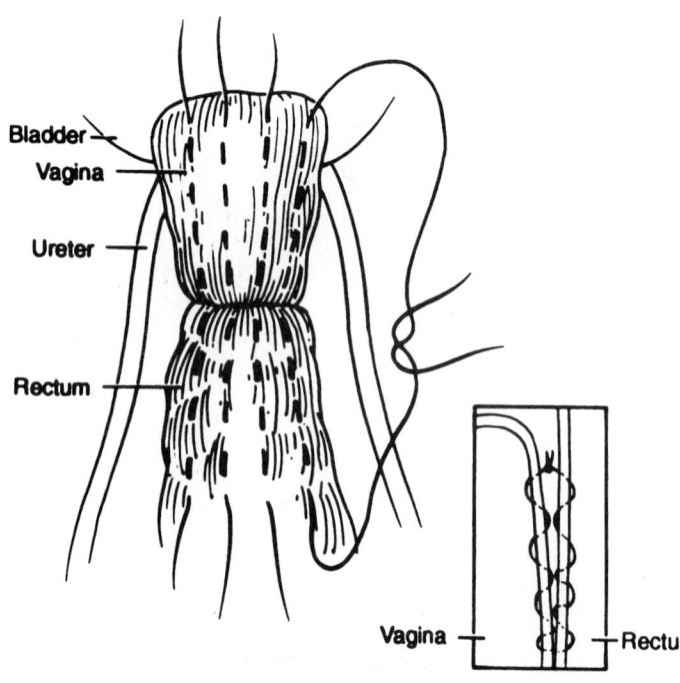

Figure 47–19
Vertical closure of the cul-de-sac using Halban's technique.

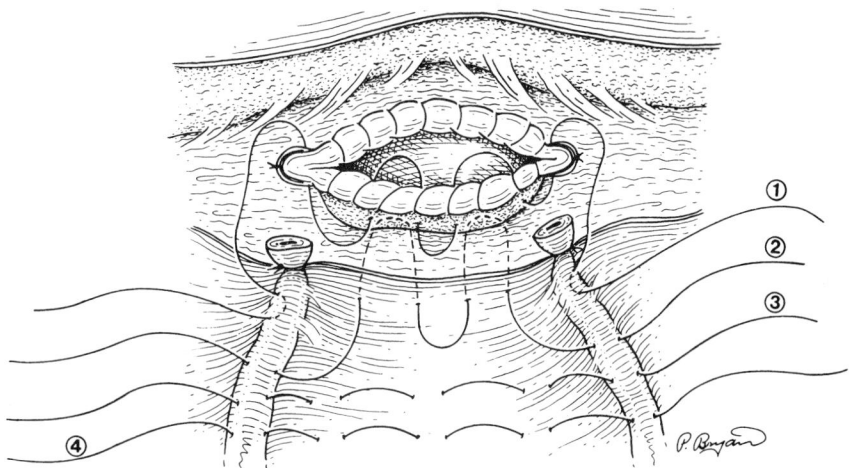

Figure 47−20
A meticulous culdeplasty at the time of hysterectomy is likely to decrease the risk of subsequent vaginal vault prolapse.

aments for lateral attachment. Wall (1994) described an abdominal version of this technique that is likely to add support when the hysterectomy is performed abdominally, either through an open or laparoscopic approach (Fig. 47−20).

ASSESSING SURGICAL OUTCOMES

There is growing interest in less invasive surgical techniques for treatment of pelvic organ prolapse. Efficacy assessment of these interventions should precede the widespread usage. Detailed pre- and postoperative assessment should include quantified anatomic changes as well as comprehensive pelvic symptom history (Table 47−3). Functional assessment of lower urinary tract or anorectal function may also be illuminating. In order to be considered a worthwhile surgical intervention, a procedure should be free of excessive morbidity, likely to cure the problem, and unlikely to cause significant side effects (new symptoms).

Persistent and Recurrent Prolapse

Despite thoughtful preoperative assessment and careful technical performance of reconstructive procedures, pelvic organ prolapse may recur. The overall risk for recurrence is likely to be at least 10% within 5 years. Certain procedures have much higher recurrence rates. When faced with recurrent disorders, the surgeon should determine the level of bothersome symptoms prior to planning further intervention. Not infrequently, an anatomic failure in a single vaginal segment may be minimally symptomatic, not warranting further surgery. However, if there are significant symptomatic or anatomic problems and the patient wishes further intervention, comprehensive assessment should be performed.

Beyond understanding the specific anatomic and functional disorders, the surgeon should give thought to the reasons for initial surgical failure. Are

there modifiable technical factors, such as use of alternative materials or techniques, that may enhance success? Are there modifiable patient factors, such as control of chronic cough, constipation, or occupational lifting, that may improve results? Expert opinion strongly suggests that it is distinctly unusual that performing the same procedure a second time produces successful results. When faced with difficulty in selecting or performing reconstructive techniques, consultation may be helpful.

CONCLUSION

Pelvic organ prolapse is an extremely common disorder, etiologically related to vaginal delivery. The natural history of the disorder remains poorly understood, except for the universal understanding that support defects worsen with time. Treatment options include pessary management and surgical intervention. Effective surgical treatments include transvaginal and transabdominal reconstruction. Symptomatic relief may also be obtained by vaginal closure.

Thoughtful gynecologic surgeons will consider the anatomic defects along with the functional disorders that commonly coexist, including urinary incontinence, voiding dysfunction, and anorectal abnormalities. Optimal treatment is best achieved following an appropriate preoperative assessment designed to allow the surgeon to tailor the operative plan to the individual women.

REFERENCES

Allen RE, Hosker GL, Smith ARB, et al: Pelvic floor damage in childbirth: a neurophysiologic study. Br J Obstet Gynaecol 1990;91:770.

Arnold MW, Stewart WRC, Aguilar PS: Rectocele repair: four years' experience. Dis Colon Rectum 1990;33:684.

Athanasiou S, Hill S, Gleeson C, et al: Validation of the ICS proposed pelvic organ prolapse descriptive system. Neurourol Urodynam 1995;14:414.

Baden WF, Walker T: Surgical Repair of Vaginal Defects. Philadelphia: JB Lippincott Company, 1992.

Block IR: Transrectal repair of rectocele using obliterative suture. Dis Colon Rectum 1986;29:707.

Brubaker L: Sacrocolpopexy and the anterior compartment. Am J Obstet Gynecol 1995;173:1690.

Brubaker L: Posterior colporrhaphy. Oper Tech Gynecol Surg 1996;1:65.

Brubaker L, Benson JT: Clinically relevant neuroanatomy. In Brubaker L, Saclarides TJ (eds): The Female Pelvic Floor: Disorders of Function and Support. Philadelphia: FA Davis, 1996:33.

Brubaker L, Kenton K: Fluoroscopy is necessary to confirm visceral position in women with pelvic organ prolapse. In: Proceedings of the International Continence Society annual clinical meeting, Athens, 1996.

Brubaker L, Norton P: Current clinical nomenclature for description of prolapse. J Pelvic Surg 1996;2:257.

Bump RC, Mattiasson A, Bø K, et al: The standardization of terminology of female pelvic organ prolapse and pelvic floor dysfunction. Am J Obstet Gynecol 1996;175:10.

DeLancey JOL: Standing anatomy of the pelvic floor. J Pelvic Surg 1996;2:1.

Gainey HL: Post-partum observation of pelvic tissue damage. Am J Obstet Gynecol 1942;37:457.

Hall AF, Theofrastous JP, Cundiff GC, et al: Inter- and intraobserver reliability of the proposed International Continence Society, Society of Gynecologic Surgeons and American Urogynecologic Society pelvic organ prolapse classification system. Am J Obstet Gynecol 1996;175:1467.

Hanson GE, Keettel WC: The Neugebauer-LeFort operation: a review of 288 colpocleises. Obstet Gynecol 1969;34:352.

Janssen LWM, van Dijke CF: Selection criteria for anterior rectal wall repair in symptomatic rectocele and anterior rectal wall prolapse. Dis Colon Rectum 1994;37:1100.

Kelvin FM, Maglinte DDT, Benson JT: Evacuation proctography (defecography): an aid to the investigation of pelvic floor disorders. Obstet Gynecol 1994;83:307.

Kobak WH, Rosenberg K, Walters MD: Interobserver variation in the assessment of pelvic organ prolapse using the draft International Continence Society and Baden grading systems. In: Proceedings of the American Urogynecologic Society annual clinical meeting, Seattle, 1995.

Kovac SR, Cruickshank SH: Successful pregnancies and vaginal deliveries after sacrospinous uterosacral fixation in five of 19 patients. Am J Obstet Gynecol 1993;168:1778.

Meeks GR, Washburne JF, McGhee RP, et al: Repair of vaginal vault prolapse by suspension of the vagina to iliococcygeus (prespinous) fascia. Am J Obstet Gynecol 1994;171:1444.

Mellgren A, Anzen B, Nilsson C-Y, et al: Results of rectocele repair: a prospective study. Dis Colon Rectum 1995;38:7.

Montella JM, Cater JR: Comparison of measurements obtained in supine and sitting position in the evaluation of pelvic organ prolapse. In: Proceedings of the American Urogynecologic Society annual clinical meeting, Seattle, 1995.

Morley GW, DeLancey JOL: Sacrospinous ligament fixation for eversion of the vagina. Am J Obstet Gynecol 1988;158:872.

Nichols DH: Sacrospinous fixation for massive eversion of the vagina. Am J Obstet Gynecol 1982;142:901.

Nichols DH: Fertility retention in the patient with genital prolapse. Am J Obstet Gynecol 1991a;164:1155.

Nichols DH: Surgery for pelvic floor disorders. Surg Clin North Am 1991b;71:927.

Nichols DH: Massive eversion of the vagina. In Nichols DH (ed): Gynecologic and Obstetric Surgery. St. Louis: Mosby–Year Book, 1993:431.

Olson AL, Smith VJ, Bergstrom JU, et al: Incidence and clinical characteristics of surgically managed pelvic organ prolapse and urinary incontinence. Obstet Gynecol 1997;89:501.

Pillai-Allen A, Benson JT: Cystocele. In Brubaker L, Saclarides TJ (eds): The Female Pelvic Floor: Disorders of Function and Support. Philadelphia: FA Davis, 1996:269.

Rempen A, Kraus M: Measurement of head compression during labor: preliminary results. J Perinatal Med 1991;19:115.

Richardson AC, Lyon JB, William NL: A new look at pelvic relaxation. Am J Obstet Gynecol 1976;126:568.

Sarles JC, Arnaud A, Selezneff I, et al: Endo-rectal repair of rectocele. Int J Colorect Dis 1989;4:167.

Schussler B, Peschers U: Standardisation of terminology of female genital prolapse according to the new ICS criteria: interexaminer reproducibility. Neurourol Urodynam 1995;14:437.

Shull BL, Benn SJ, Kuehl JJ: Surgical management of prolapse of the anterior vaginal segment: an analysis of support defects, operative morbidity and anatomic outcome. Am J Obstet Gynecol 1996;161:1429.

Snooks SJ, Swash M, Matthews SE, et al: Effect of vaginal delivery on the pelvic floor: a 5-year follow-up. Br J Surg 1996; 77:1358.

Swift SE, Harring MH: Evaluation of the degree of pelvic organ prolapse in the supine versus the standing position employing the International Continence Society's prolapse classification system. In: Proceedings of the American Urogynecologic Society annual clinical meeting, Seattle, 1995.

Symmonds RE, Williams TJ, Lee RA, Webb MJ: Posthysterectomy enterocele and vaginal vault prolapse. Am J Obstet Gynecol 1981;140:852.

Timmons MC, Addison WA: Vaginal vault prolapse. In Brubaker L, Saclarides TJ (eds): The Female Pelvic Floor: Disorders of Function and Support. Philadelphia: FA Davis, 1996:262.

Timmons MC, Addison WA, Addison S, et al: Abdominal sacral colpopexy in 163 women with posthysterectomy vaginal vault prolapse and enterocele: evaluation of operative techniques. J Reprod Med 1992;37:323.

Ubachs JMH, Van Sante TJ, Schellekensla LA: Partial colpocleisis by a modification of LeFort's operation. Obstet Gynecol 1973; 42:415.

Wall LL: A technique for modified McCall culdeplasty at the time of abdominal hysterectomy. J Am Coll Surg 1994;178:507.

White GR: Cystocele: a radical cure by suturing lateral sulci of vagina to white line of pelvic fascia. JAMA 1909;53:1707.

48

Urinary Tract Injury and Fistula

Larry J. Copeland
Kenneth D. Hatch
Jeffrey M. Fowler

Each year an estimated 8000 women will suffer an injury to the urinary tract. Injuries to the bladder or ureter occur in approximately 1% of gynecologic surgeries and cesarean deliveries. More than 75% of these injuries will occur during hysterectomy, and half will result from simple total abdominal or vaginal hysterectomy (Symmonds, 1976). One might expect that the injuries are more likely to occur during difficult dissection of such conditions as endometriosis or pelvic inflammatory disease (PID); however, the majority occur when the surgeon has not anticipated a problem (Lee et al, 1988). Most bladder or ureteral injuries or fistulas are not associated with faulty surgical technique or violations of standard of care. Every gynecologic surgeon should be aware of problems that might arise and should take steps to prevent injury, learn how to recognize injury, and know the principles of repair. A satisfactorily repaired urinary injury rarely leads to subsequent complications.

PREVENTION OF INJURY

Adequate exposure of the operative field and a thorough knowledge of the surrounding anatomy are keys to preventing injury. Exposure begins with an abdominal incision large enough to expose pathologic tissue and includes identifying the ureters from the ovarian pedicle to the uterine arteries. Simple "snapping" of the ureter is not sufficient for identification, especially in conditions that cause limited exposure or anatomic distortion (see Table 48–1). Exposure of the ureter is easily accomplished (Manetta, 1989). The round ligament or peritoneum lateral to the infundibulopelvic ligament is divided and the retroperitoneal pelvic space is opened. Traction is placed on the uterus medially. The ureter is identified lying over the bifurcation of the common iliac artery. Here the dissection is directed medially, lifting the peritoneum off the vessels and carrying the ureter with it. The ureter remains on the peritoneum and under the ovarian vessels. Occasionally, the loose areolar tissue needs to be gently separated with scissors to facilitate mobilization. The ureter can then be followed through the pelvis to the uterine artery, which passes over the ureter.

The bladder is dissected from the cervix and upper vagina by sharp dissection with traction on the bladder ventrally and on the uterus cephalad, allowing the dissection planes to be seen easily. The bladder is advanced 1 cm beyond anticipated vaginal incision. Bleeding at the bladder base should be controlled by (1) pressure and (2) precise cautery of the bleeding vessel, avoiding indiscriminate cautery of a large surface area. The thermal injury induced by cautery is three times as extensive as the visible injury, which may lead to subsequent fistula formation. A simple suture of 3-0 absorbable material is used when light cautery does not suffice.

During procedures requiring full anatomic exposure of the pelvic ureter or with other ureterolysis procedures, it is common to encounter areas of bleeding from the adventitia of the ureter. These bleeders can be controlled by light cautery, suture ligatures, or placement of metallic surgical clips. Because the ureteral blood supply is dependent on the adventitial vascular network, these patients are at risk for delayed complications, including ureteral narrowing from ischemia and necrosis leading to urinoma and fistula formation.

Most obstetric injuries to the bladder and urethra are the result of obstructed labor in developing countries. Obstetric injuries to the urinary tract are the result of operative deliveries (Elkins, 1994).

RECOGNITION AND MANAGEMENT OF INTRAOPERATIVE INJURY

Bladder

Injury to the bladder occurs most often during opening of the abdomen or during dissection of the cervix and upper vagina. Injuries to the dome of the bladder on opening the abdomen rarely lead to significant problems; such injuries are recognized by slight egress of urine and sudden appearance of the Foley bulb in the bladder.

Table 48-1. CONDITIONS THAT CAUSE LIMITED EXPOSURE OR ANATOMICAL DISTORTION AND ARE ASSOCIATED WITH A HIGHER RISK OF URINARY TRACT INJURY

Compromised Surgical Technique
Limited incision
Inadequate retraction
Poor lighting
Visibility limited by hemorrhage
Digression from standard surgical techniques (e.g., laparoscopic procedures)

Anatomic and Physiologic Alterations
Congenital abnormalities (e.g., double ureters, pelvic kidney)
Pregnancy
Morbid obesity
Pelvic floor support abnormalities

Prior Treatments
Prior pelvic surgery
Radiation therapy

Inflammatory Conditions Associated with Pelvic Adhesions
Endometriosis
Pelvic inflammatory disease
Diverticulitis

Masses
Large pelvic masses of any origin
Cervical and broad ligament myomas
Retroperitoneal tumors
Malignant disease

If injury is suspected but not documented, a sterile milk or methylene blue solution can be instilled through the Foley catheter to observe for urinary leaks. Full-thickness injury of the bladder dome is repaired with 2-0 or 3-0 absorbable sutures in two layers. The first layer may be running or interrupted and is placed through the muscularis and mucosal layers. Permanent sutures should never be placed where they will be in contact with urine because they act as a nidus for stone formation. The second layer is a lateral, inverting, interrupted suture, placed in the muscularis and serosa. Foley catheter drainage is instituted for up to 5 days for larger repairs and overnight for smaller repairs.

Injuries at the base of the bladder are repaired by first mobilizing the rest of the bladder base and identifying the ureteral orifices. The ureteral orifices are usually visible and urine efflux is usually noted. If there is significant bladder distortion, intravenous indigo carmine assists in identifying the orifices. If necessary, ureteral catheters can be placed. A two-layer closure is then performed using a 3-0 absorbable suture. The first suture is interrupted or running and contains all layers; the second one is a lateral, imbricating, interrupted suture. If omentum is available, it can be placed between the bladder injury and the vaginal cuff. Sterile milk can be inserted through the Foley catheter to ensure that a watertight repair has been achieved. Suprapubic catheter drainage is preferred to urethral Foley drainage because the bulb of the latter may apply pressure to the repaired area, decreasing the blood supply to the tissue. The suprapubic catheter is left in place for 7 days.

Ureter

Ureteral injuries have been reported in 0.5% to 2.5% of patients undergoing gynecologic surgery (American College of Obstetricians and Gynecologists, 1985). Because some injuries are never recognized, this incidence might actually be underreported. The most common predisposing condition is previous pelvic surgery (Daly and Higgins, 1988; Selzman and Spirnak, 1996). Other factors are pelvic tumors, cervical leiomyomata, endometriosis, PID, and uterine prolapse. Injury occurs primarily at three places: (1) the pelvic brim, where the ovarian vessels are in close proximity to the ureter; (2) at the level of the uterine artery; and (3) the distal ureter just lateral to the vagina. Identification of the ureter during its full course through the pelvis is the most important preventive measure. Preoperative excretory urograms (EXUs) may detect congenital abnormalities and obstruction but often do not reveal information that is not apparent at the time of surgery (Daly and Higgins, 1988; Symmonds, 1976). Placement of ureteral catheters preoperatively has not been an effective preventive tool (Higgins, 1976; Fry et al, 1983). The catheter may actually predispose the ureter to further injury because it makes the ureter more rigid and less able to move away from the dissecting instrument.

Injury to the ureter may consist of transection, laceration, crushing, kinking, ligation, or devascularization. Unfortunately, many of these injuries are not recognized intraoperatively. Simple observation of the ureter to see whether it continues to undergo peristalsis is not proof that it has escaped any of the above injuries. Complete ligation or kinking of the ureter leads to dilatation, which is often evident at the end of the surgery. Complete or partial transection may result in obvious urinary leakage if the ureter has not also been kinked or ligated. Crushing and kinking injuries are the most difficult to recognize and evaluate for need of repair. When a crush injury is suspected intraoperatively, the surgeon should remove the clamp immediately and dissect the ureter free from the surrounding tissue so that it can be inspected. The extent of damage may not be apparent from simple observation. Instillation of 5 ml of indigo carmine dye will disclose extravasation within 10 to 15 minutes. This indicates an extensive injury, which necessitates resection followed by ureteroneocystostomy or ureteroureterostomy, depending on the level of injury. If dye does not extravasate, stenting of the ureter by a double J stent through a cystotomy should be accomplished. An extraperitoneal suction drain should be placed.

Kinking most often involves a suture placed near the ureter. Simple removal of the suture is all that is necessary when this injury is discovered intraoperatively. Complete ligation of the ureter and absence of transection or other injury can be handled intraoperatively by simple deligation and inspection of the involved segment. Indigo carmine dye can be used to determine extent of damage. Once again, consideration should be made for stenting.

A clean partial transection of the ureter that does not interfere with vascularity of the plexus can be repaired with 4-0 absorbable suture and a stent placed for 2 weeks (Symmonds, 1976; Labaski and Leach, 1990). An extraperitoneal drain is placed for 5 to 10 days. Larger or devascularized lacerations are managed by complete transection and either anastomosis or reimplantation into the bladder. The decision to reimplant or to perform anastomosis is based on site of injury. Injuries within 5 cm of the uterine artery are best implanted into the bladder, whereas injuries at the pelvic brim should be managed by anastomosis (Figs. 48–1 and 48–2). Those injuries lying in between can be managed by mobilization of the bladder and reimplantation using a psoas hitch if needed. A segment of small bowel (ureteroileoneocystotomy) can be used to replace a lengthy injury or accidental resection of a large ureteral segment. A transureteroureterostomy can also be considered. However, disruption of the contralateral collecting system is an important disincentive for this technique.

The expanded roles for minimally invasive surgical procedures (laparoscopic procedures or laparoscopy-assisted vaginal surgery) have been accompanied by an apparent increase in urinary tract injuries. Reduction of the occurrence of these injuries requires proper training in the more complex laparoscopic techniques; appropriate mentoring or proctoring; careful adherence to principles of proper visualization and anatomic exposure; and appropriate case selection. A surgical procedure performed by laparoscopic techniques should be done using dissection and exposure similar to what would be done at laparotomy (Grainger et al, 1990; Woodland, 1992; Assimos et al, 1994; Kadar and Lemmerling, 1994).

POSTOPERATIVE URETERAL OBSTRUCTION

Ureteral obstruction from unrecognized ureteral ligation is most often discovered when the patient has persistent postoperative fever with flank pain. Occasionally, there are no symptoms whatsoever and the kidney will die silently. Unilateral ureteral entrapment may be associated with an increase of serum creatinine (mean 0.8 mg/dl) (Stanhope et al, 1991). An EXU will disclose obstruction and probable extravasation of urine in the perinephric fat (Fig. 48–3). The site of obstruction will be apparent by a delayed EXU film. Cystoscopy should be performed and retrograde ureteral stents placed if possible. If

this is unsuccessful, a percutaneous nephrostomy and antegrade passage of the ureteral stent should be attempted (Fig. 48–4). If a stent can be passed, it should be left in place for 4 to 6 weeks. This will avoid an operative repair in most instances. If a stent cannot be passed, a percutaneous nephrostomy should be maintained until operative repair can be attempted. Timing of the repair is dictated by the patient's medical condition, presence of infection or hematoma, and type of repair planned. If the repair needed is simple deligation at the pelvic brim, early reoperation may be indicated. If reimplantation or ureteroureterostomy is planned, a later operation (4 to 6 weeks) may be more advantageous, particularly if there is evidence of pelvic infection.

URINARY FISTULAS

Urinary fistulas usually occur within 2 weeks of the causative injury. The most common indication of fistula is continuous urinary incontinence or leakage of urine from the vagina. One can confirm that the vaginal drainage is urine by collecting it from the posterior vaginal fornix and determining its creatinine content. Lymph fluid, the primary differential, especially after pelvic lymphadenectomy, has the same creatinine level as serum, but urinary drainage is characterized by a high creatinine content. The fistula is localized by a simple speculum examination to see whether an opening can be visualized. Next, a urethral catheter is placed and normal saline, sterile milk, or methylene blue is instilled while the surgeon observes the vagina through the speculum. This may disclose an obvious leak. If this is not successful, a vaginal sponge can be placed in the vagina and methylene blue dye placed in the bladder. After the patient has been ambulating for approximately 30 minutes, she is re-examined to see whether the sponge has been discolored. Occasionally, urethral leakage and retrograde flow into the vagina will give a false-positive result. A second sponge may be placed at the vaginal opening to preclude that possibility.

If the urinary leakage is not from the bladder, its source may be a ureterovaginal fistula. Injection of 5 ml of indigo carmine intravenously discolors the urine blue within 10 to 15 minutes.

Ureterovaginal Fistula

Ureterovaginal (UV) fistulas typically appear within 5 to 14 days of surgery and may be associated with pelvic urinoma, hematoma, or abscess. Ureteral injury with leakage and urinoma formation often presents with a delayed ileus with nausea, vomiting, and abdominal distention. Spontaneous drainage of the urine through the vagina is the next step in the creation of a UV fistula. These fistulas most often result from unrecognized ureteral injury at the time of ab-

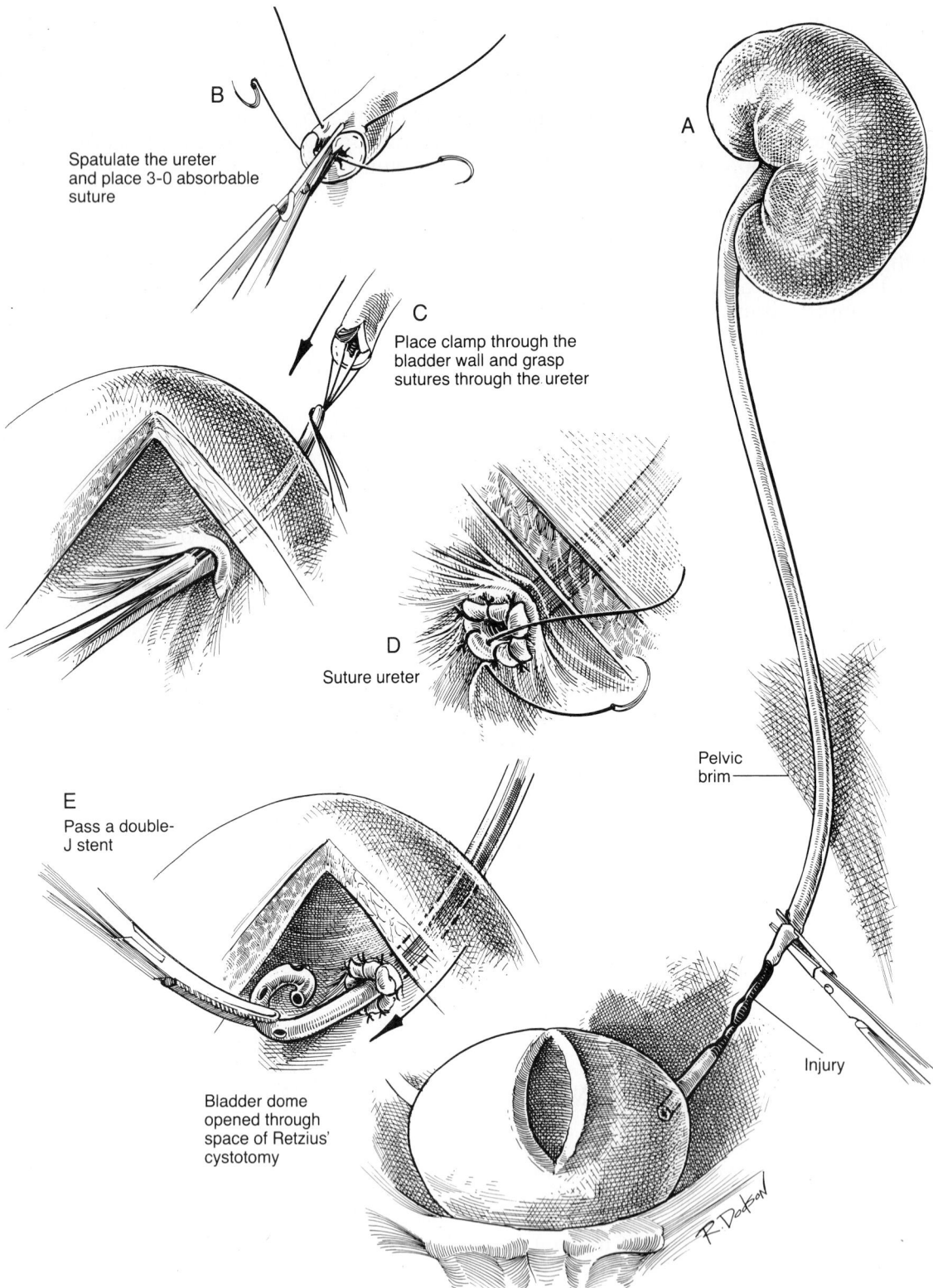

B
Spatulate the ureter
and place 3-0 absorbable
suture

C
Place clamp through the
bladder wall and grasp
sutures through the ureter

D
Suture ureter

E
Pass a double-
J stent

Bladder dome
opened through
space of Retzius'
cystotomy

Pelvic
brim

Injury

R. Dodson

Figure 48–1
Ureteroneocystotomy for injury below the pelvic brim. *Illustration continued on opposite page*

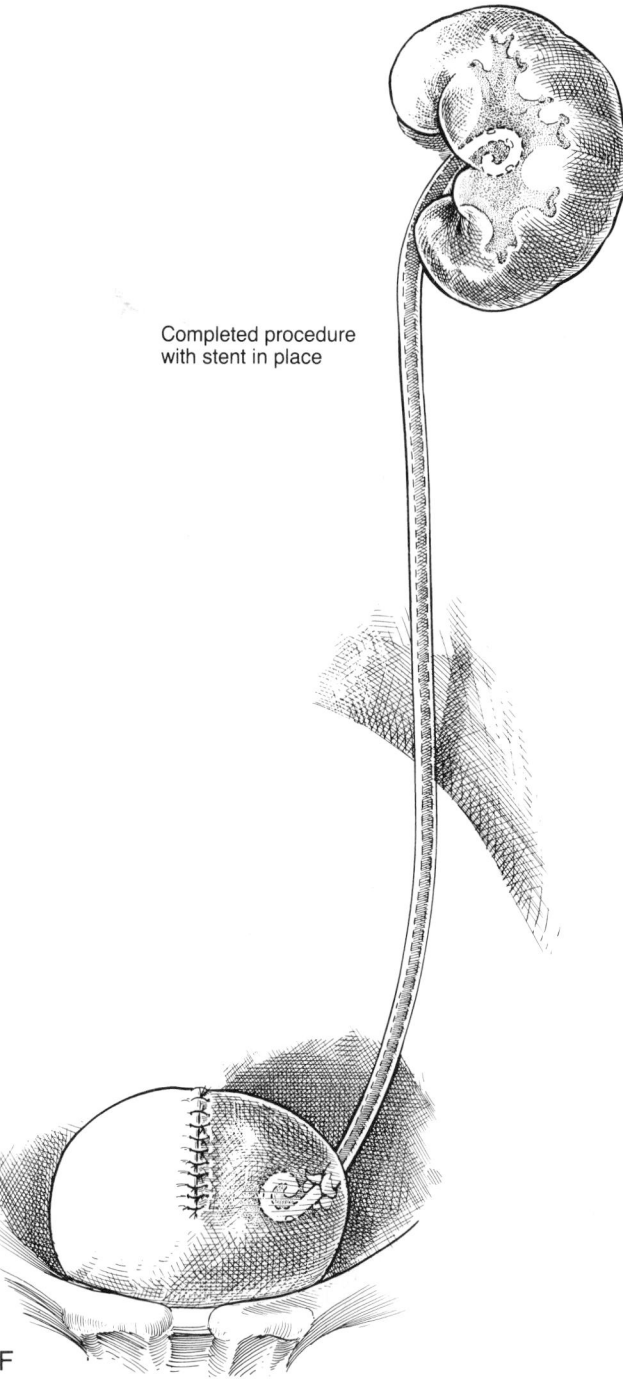

Completed procedure
with stent in place

F

Figure 48-1
Continued

most of the urinary flow of a UV fistula. Most fistulas involve the pelvic ureter (Lee et al, 1988), and reimplantation to the bladder is the correct procedure. The repair can take place as soon as the medical condition allows, without waiting until all of the surrounding inflammatory induration has resolved (Witters et al, 1986; Badenuch et al, 1987; Lee et al, 1988). UV fistulas originating near the pelvic brim should be handled by ureteroureteral anastomosis, by transureteroureteral anastomosis, by a ureteroneocystotomy, or, rarely, by nephrectomy.

Vesicovaginal Fistula

Vesicovaginal fistula appears within 10 days of surgery in two thirds of patients, and 70% occur after abdominal hysterectomy (Lee et al, 1988). After the diagnosis is confirmed by the steps outlined above, cystoscopy is used to evaluate the fistula and to determine its position relative to the ureteral orifices. Next, an EXU is obtained because about 10% of vesicovaginal fistulas are associated with ureterovaginal fistula or obstruction (Goodwin and Scardino, 1980; Symmonds, 1984; Labasky and Leach, 1990). The majority of posthysterectomy fistulas are above the trigone and can be repaired without interfering with ureteral function (Gerber and Schoenberg, 1993). Obstetric fistulas or fistulas that occur after anterior colporrhaphy surgery may be more distal and involve the trigone, ureters, and vesicourethral junction.

Catheter drainage leads to spontaneous closure in many of the small posthysterectomy fistulas (Gorrea et al, 1985). A difference of opinion exists concerning the timing of repair. Some advocate early closure within 2 to 4 weeks of discovery and report primary success rates of 72% to 90% (Collins et al, 1971; Persky et al, 1979; Cruikshank, 1988; Blaivas et al, 1995). However, most advise a waiting period ranging from 6 weeks to 4 months and report primary success rates of up to 98%. The advantage of delay is to allow resolution of edema and infection and return of good blood supply to the damaged tissue. The disadvantage of delay is the discomfort to the patient caused by constant wetness. Attempts to decrease this drainage are usually futile. Foley catheter drainage is usually not left in place longer than the initial 2 to 3 weeks if spontaneous closure does not occur. Catheter drainage can induce inflammation and further delay closure. Urinary collection devices in the vagina have not been successful either and may produce the same problem. Antibiotics should be used, and urinary odor can be reduced by vitamin C tablets, 500 mg three times daily.

Uncomplicated vesicovaginal fistulas following hysterectomy are most amenable to repair by the *Latzko procedure* (Latzko, 1942; Tancer, 1980). Because this procedure is a partial colpocleisis, it is not as successful for larger fistulas or for those that involve the trigone or vesicourethral junction (Elkins et al, 1988). The vaginal epithelium is removed for 1 cm

dominal hysterectomy (Lee et al, 1988). When a ureteral injury is suspected, an EXU should be obtained to evaluate for obstruction, extravasation, urinoma, or fistulization. Cystoscopy and retrograde pyelogram will confirm the site of the fistula. A retrograde or antegrade ureteral stent should be placed if possible. If successful, the stent can be left in place for 4 to 6 weeks and operative repair may be avoided. If unsuccessful, a surgical repair should be planned. A percutaneous nephrostomy may divert

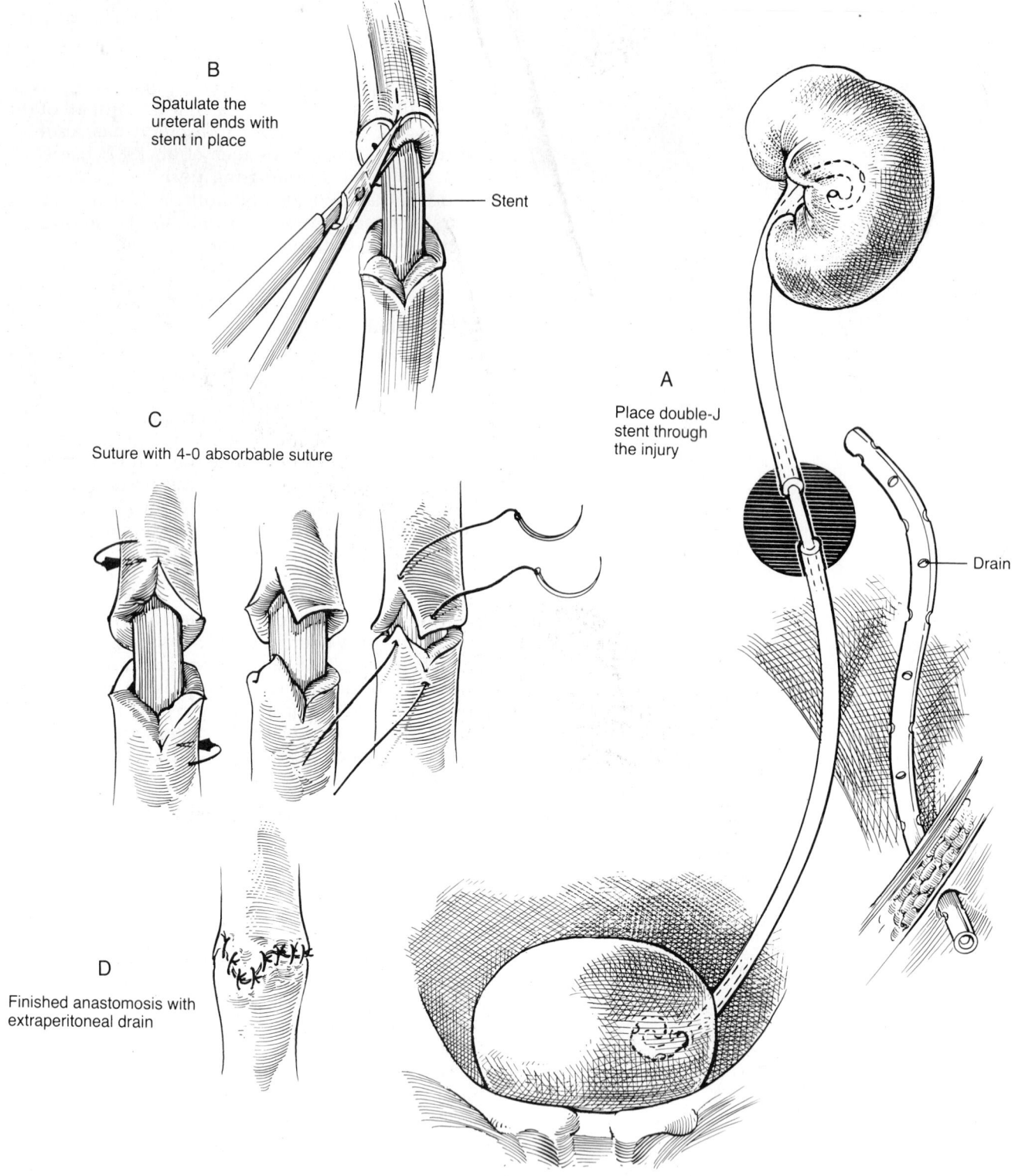

B Spatulate the ureteral ends with stent in place

Stent

A Place double-J stent through the injury

Drain

C Suture with 4-0 absorbable suture

D Finished anastomosis with extraperitoneal drain

Figure 48–2
Ureteroureterotomy for injury at or above the pelvic brim.

around the fistula site, and all vaginal epithelium must be removed from the bladder edge. The bladder edges themselves are not approximated. Instead, the paravaginal tissue is approximated in two layers of 3-0 absorbable suture and the vaginal epithelium

is enclosed. A Foley catheter is left in place for 4 to 5 days (Fig. 48–5).

For larger vesicovaginal fistulas or those occurring more distally in the vagina, the Latzko procedure may result in significant loss of vaginal length. A

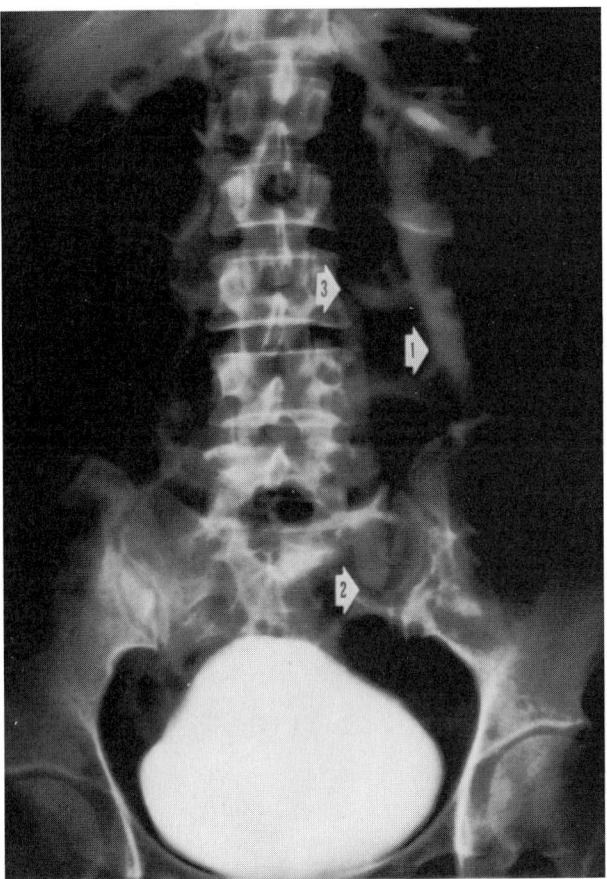

Figure 48–3
Excretory urogram disclosing obstruction of the ureter and extravasation of urine in perinephric fat. *Arrow 1*, Extravasated contrast outlines the psoas muscle. Arrow 2, Site of ligation of the ureter. *Arrow 3*, Tortuous ureter above the ligation.

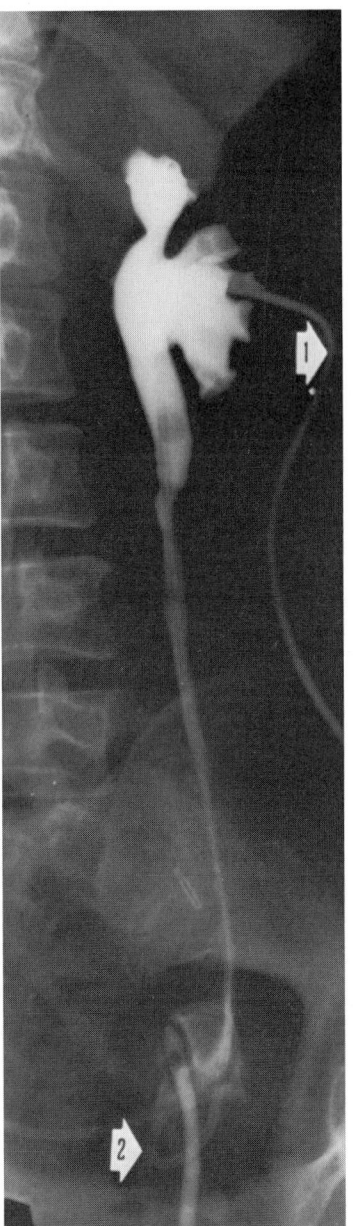

Figure 48–4
Arrow 1, Percutaneous nephrostomy has decompressed the kidney and provided route for antegrade placement of ureteral stent. *Arrow 2*, Double J ureteral catheter in the bladder.

conventional repair (Symmonds, 1984) or a vaginal flap technique (Zimmern et al, 1986) is recommended.

The *conventional repair* includes wide mobilization of the vaginal mucosa from the bladder wall, excision of the scar tissue, and closure of the bladder, paravaginal tissue, and vaginal mucosa without tension (Fig. 48–6). The surgeon makes the incision vertically, encircling the fistula lateral to all scar tissue. After wide mobilization, which might include entry of the peritoneal cavity, the fistula tract is excised. The bladder mucosa is inverted with 3-0 absorbable, interrupted suture. A second layer inverts the first layer, extending laterally beyond the first layer. A watertight closure is necessary, and sterile milk can be inserted through the Foley catheter to test the closure. The vaginal mucosa is then closed. A Foley catheter is placed for 5 days. If the fistula is near the ureterovesical angle, a suprapubic tube is placed instead of a urethral Foley catheter.

The *vaginal flap technique* differs from the conventional closure in that a flap of vagina is raised to overlap the suture lines in the bladder. This repair is

especially indicated for large fistulas (4 cm) (Elkins et al, 1988). A J-shaped incision is used. For apical fistulas, the base is directed toward the vaginal opening; for lower fistulas, it is directed toward the apex (Fig. 48–7). The incision encircles the fistula opening and excises the vaginal mucosa from the fistula tract. The vaginal flaps are elevated, and a layer of 3-0 absorbable sutures is placed to close and invert the bladder edge. A second row of sutures is placed. A portion of the vagina is removed from the smaller of the vaginal flaps, and the larger flap is advanced over the suture layers underneath, producing a non-

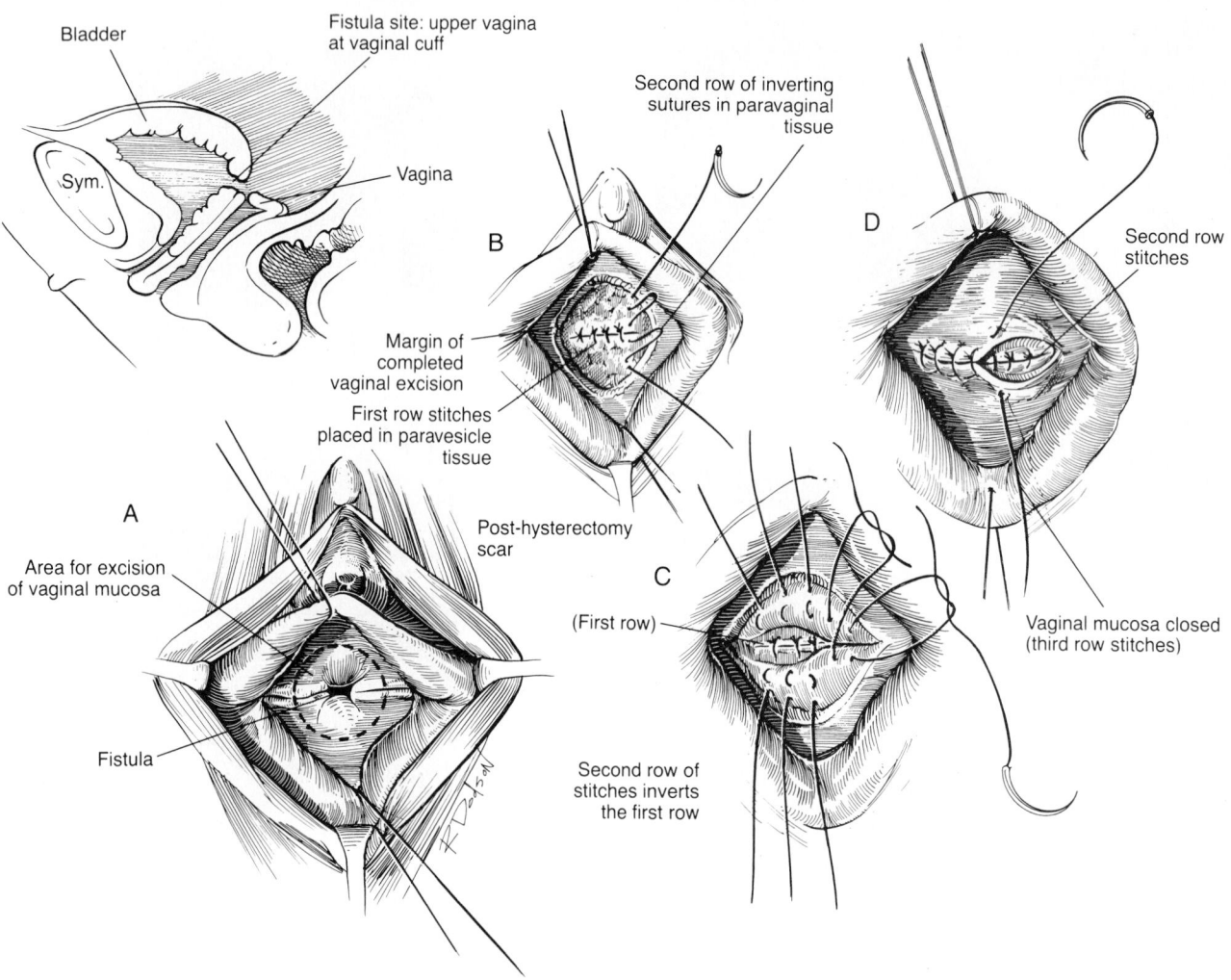

Figure 48–5
Latzko repair of small apical vesicovaginal fistula.

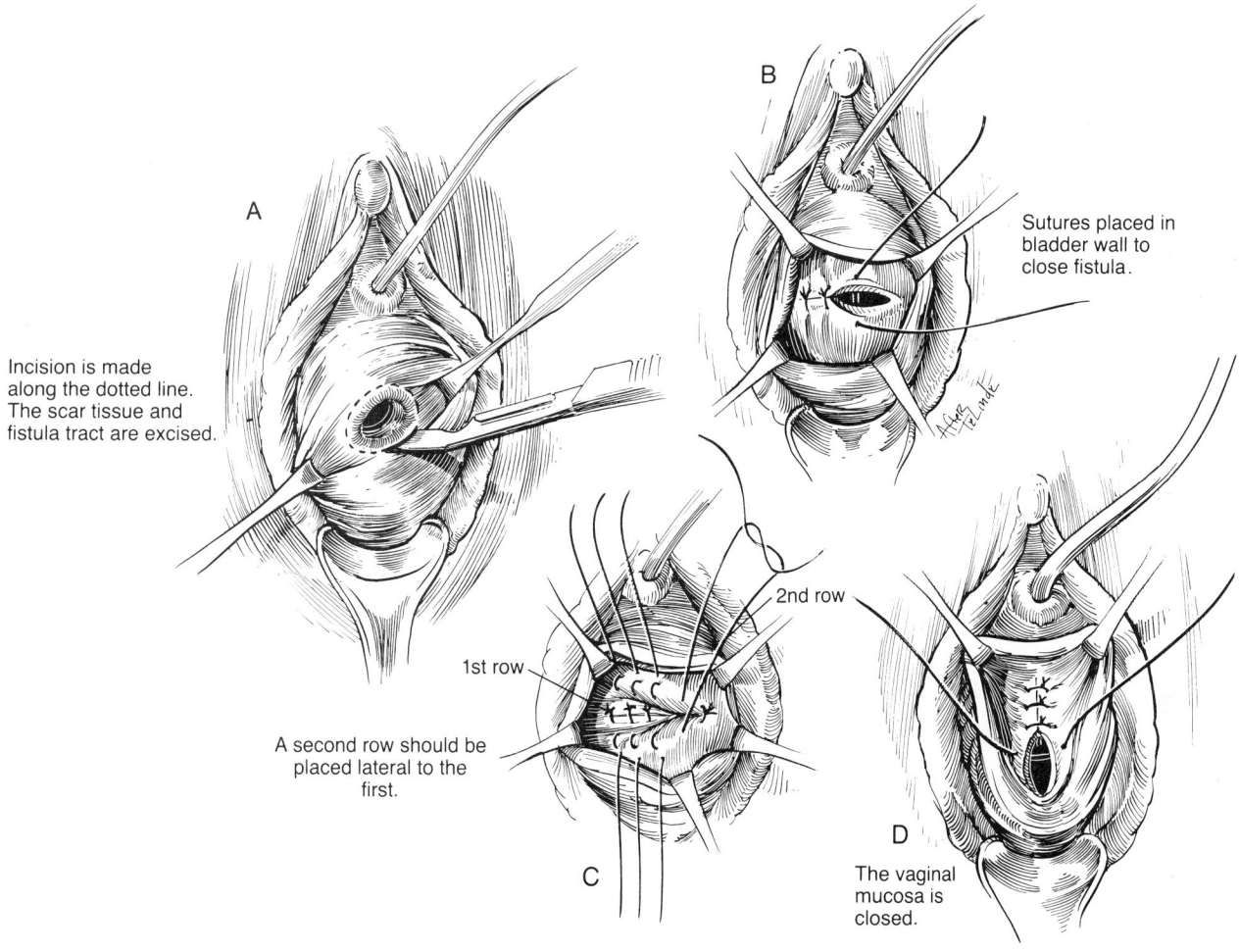

A

Incision is made
along the dotted line.
The scar tissue and
fistula tract are excised.

B

Sutures placed in
bladder wall to
close fistula.

1st row

2nd row

A second row should be
placed lateral to the
first.

C

D

The vaginal
mucosa is
closed.

Figure 48-6
Conventional layered closure of vesicovaginal fistula.

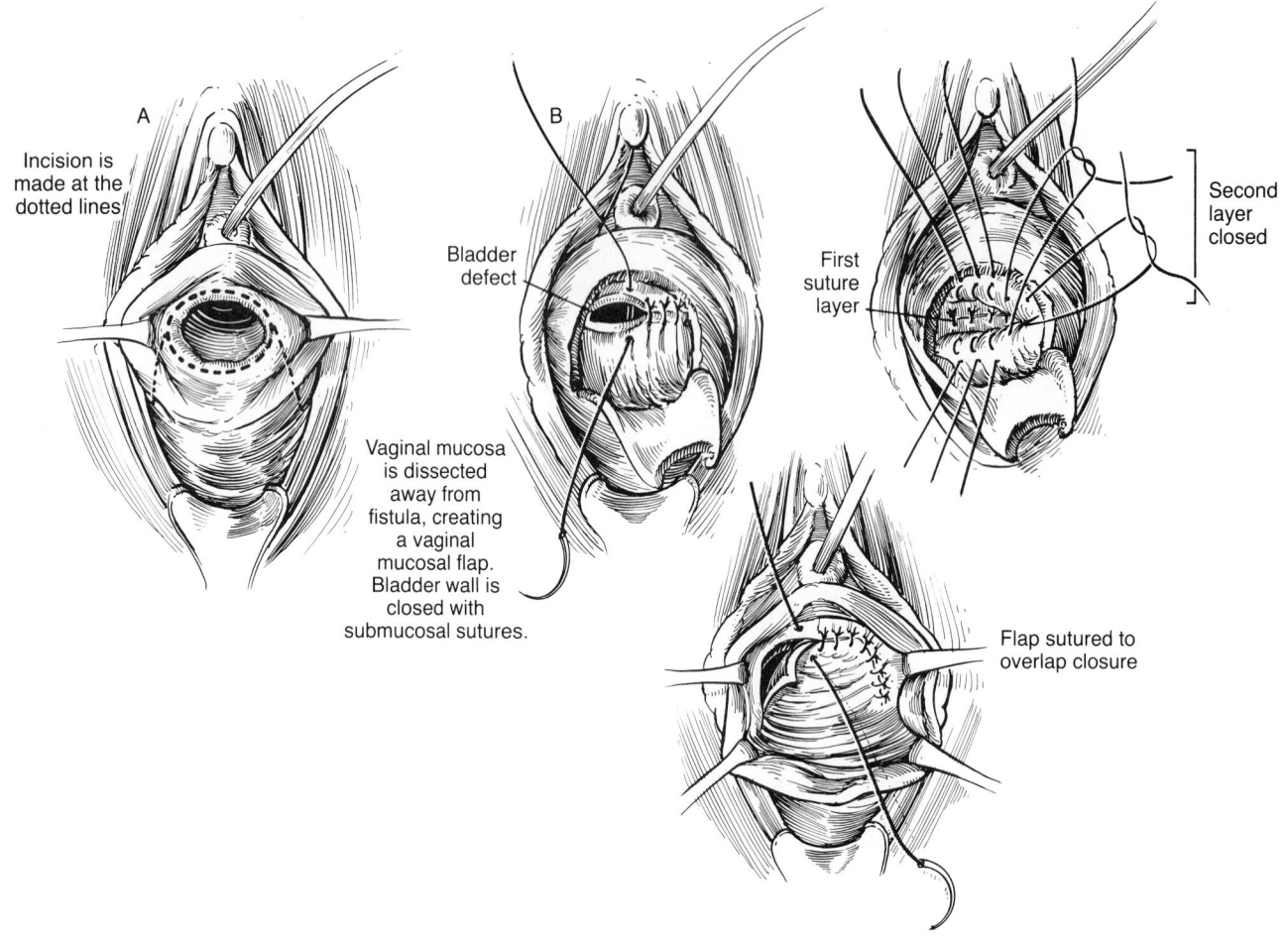

Figure 48–7
Vaginal flap technique for closure of large fistulas or those low in the vagina.

overlapping closure. Bladder drainage is accomplished by suprapubic tube.

Abdominal repair of vesicovaginal fistulas is used when a complex fistula involves the bowel or ureters or when the fistula is affixed high in the vagina and exposure from the vagina is compromised. Principles of repair remain the same. When this technique is used, a pedicle of omentum can be placed between the bladder and the vagina.

Urethrovaginal Fistula

Urethrovaginal and urethrovaginovesical fistulas are uncommon in the United States and usually occur after anterior colporrhaphy or diverticulum repair (Lee et al, 1988). Obstetric trauma continues to be the most common cause in undeveloped countries (Elkins et al, 1988). The technique of repair follows the same principles of wide mobilization, excision of scar tissue, and enclosure without tension (Symmonds, 1984). Occasionally, a Martius graft from the bulbocavernosus muscle is needed (Symmonds, 1984).

REFERENCES

American College of Obstetricians and Gynecologists: Genitourinary Fistula (ACOG Technical Bulletin No. 83). Washington, DC: American College of Obstetricians and Gynecologists, 1985:1.

American College of Obstetricians and Gynecologists: Lower Urinary Tract Operative Injuries (ACOG Educational Bulletin No. 238). Washington, DC: American College of Obstetricians and Gynecologists, 1997:1.

Assimos DG, Patterson C, Taylor CL: Changing incidence and etiology of iatrogenic ureteral injuries. J Urol 1994;152:2240.

Badenoch DF, Tiptaft RC, Thakar DR, et al: Early repair of accidental injury to the ureter or bladder following gynaecological surgery. Br J Urol 1987;59:516.

Blaivas JG, Heritz DM, Romanzi LJ: Early versus late repair of vesicovaginal fistulas: vaginal and abdominal approaches. J Urol 1995;153:1110.

Collins CG, Collins JH, Harrison BR, et al: Early repair of vesicovaginal fistula. Am J Obstet Gynecol 1971;3:524.

Cruikshank SH: Early closure of posthysterectomy vesicovaginal fistulas. South Med J 1988;81:1525.

Cruikshank SH, Kovac SR: Anatomic changes of ureter during vaginal hysterectomy. Contemp Ob/Gyn 1993;38.

Daly JW, Higgins KA: Injury to the ureter during gynecologic surgical procedures. Surg Gynecol Obstet 1988;167:19.

Elkins TE: Surgery for the obstetric vesicovaginal fistula: a review of 100 operations in 82 patients. Am J Obstet Gynecol 1994;170:1108.

Elkins TE, Drescher C, Martey JO, Ford D: Vesicovaginal fistula revisited. Obstet Gynecol 1988;72:307.

Fry DE, Milholen L, Harbrecht PJ: Iatrogenic ureteral injury. Arch Surg 1983;118:454.

Gallup DG, Nolan TE: Prevention, diagnosis, and management of ureteral injuries. The Female Patient 1994;19:73.

Gerber GS, Schoenberg HW: Female urinary tract fistulas. J Urol 1993;149:229.

Goodwin WE, Scardino PT: Vesicovaginal and ureterovaginal fistulas: a summary of 25 years of experience. J Urol 1980;123:370.

Gorrea MA, Zuazu JF, Mompo Sanchis JA, Jimenez-Cruz JF: Spontaneous healing of uretero-vesico-vaginal fistulas. Eur Urol 1985;2:341.

Grainger DA, Soderstrom RM, Schiff SF, et al: Ureteral injuries at laparoscopy: insights into diagnosis, management, and prevention. Obstet Gynecol 1990;75:839.

Higgins CC: Ureteral injuries during surgery: a review of 87 cases. JAMA 1976;199:118.

Kadar N, Lemmerling L: Urinary tract injuries during laparoscopically assisted hysterectomy: causes and prevention. Am J Obstet Gynecol 1994;170:47.

Labasky RF, Leach GE: Prevention and management of urovaginal fistulas. Clin Obstet Gynecol 1990;33:382.

Latzko W: Postoperative vesicovaginal fistulas—genesis and therapy. Am J Surg 1942;58:211.

Lee RA, Symmonds RE, Williams TJ: Current status of genitourinary fistula. Part 1. Obstet Gynecol 1988;72:313.

Manetta A: Surgical maneuver for the prevention of ureteral injuries. J Gynecol Surg 1989;5:291.

Persky L, Herman G, Guerrier K: Nondelay in vesicovaginal fistula repair. Urology 1979;13:273.

Selzman AA, Spirnak JP: Iatrogenic ureteral injuries: a 10-year experience in treating 165 injuries. J Urol 1996;155:878.

Stanhope CR, Wilson TO, Utz WJ, et al: Suture entrapment and secondary ureteral obstruction. Am J Obstet Gynecol 1991;164:1513.

Symmonds RE: Ureteral injuries associated with gynecologic surgery: prevention and management. Clin Obstet Gynecol 1976;19:623.

Symmonds RE: Incontinence: vesical and urethral fistulas. Clin Obstet Gynecol 1984;27:499.

Tancer ML: The post-total hysterectomy (vault) vesicovaginal fistula. J Urol 1980;123:839.

Witters S, Cornelissen M, Vereecken R: Iatrogenic ureteral injury: aggressive or conservative treatment. Am J Obstet Gynecol 1986;155:582.

Woodland MB: Ureter injury during laparoscopy-assisted vaginal hysterectomy with the endoscopic linear stapler. Am J Obstet Gynecol 1992;167:756.

Zimmern P, Schmidbauer CP, Leach GE, et al: Vesicovaginal and urethrovaginal fistulae. Semin Urol 1986;4:24.

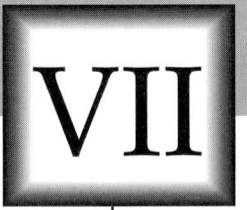

Breast Disease

VII

Breast Disease

49

Benign Breast Disease and Screening for Malignant Tumors

Carolyn D. Runowicz

In order for the obstetrician-gynecologist to provide primary health care for women, knowledge of the entire spectrum of the reproductive tract, including the breast, is essential. The obstetrician-gynecologist is in a position of central importance to educate, screen, and counsel women about benign and malignant conditions of the breast. The physician must have a thorough knowledge of breast embryology, physiology, anatomy, and pathology to properly advise and guide the patient in choosing appropriate therapy and further evaluation. Studies have shown that the obstetrician-gynecologist can confidently and competently provide for the evaluation and treatment of breast disease (Hall et al, 1990).

This chapter provides clinicians with a fund of knowledge in embryology, breast development, physiology, anatomy, and benign breast disease and information on screening for malignant tumors of the breast. Breast cancer is discussed in Chapter 50.

BREAST ANATOMY

On average, the breast is 10 to 12 cm in diameter, with a thickness of 5 to 7 cm (DiSaia and Creasman, 1993). The breast is covered by skin, with a pigmented central area, the nipple and areola. Montgomery glands, the small duct openings of sebaceous glands, are located on the periphery of the areola. The breast is composed of glandular, fatty, and connective tissues. The glandular portion is arranged in a circular manner into 15 to 20 lobes. Each lobe branches into lobules and finally acini. Contractile myoepithelial fibers surround each alveolus or acinus. The lobes, lobules, and acini are connected to the nipple by a complex network of ducts. These ducts enlarge as they enter the nipple into lactiferous sinuses (Fig. 49–1). The majority of glandular tissue is located in the central, upper, and outer quadrants of the breast. A small tongue of glandular tissue penetrates the axilla, the axillary tail of Spence.

The breast, along with the nerves, blood supply, and supporting structures, is enclosed by a superficial and deep fascia. Fibrous bands of connective tissue, Cooper's ligaments (retinacula cutis), surround the lobes, helping to hold the breast in position. Two muscles lie beneath the breast: the pectoralis major and the pectoralis minor (Fig. 49–2). The principal blood supply to the breast is derived from the internal mammary and lateral thoracic arteries. The breast is drained by a chain of axillary and internal mammary lymph nodes. These nodes are of particular importance in malignancies of the breast. A more detailed description of the nodal drainage is provided in Chapter 50.

EMBRYOLOGY

Breast tissue develops from an embryonic ridge of ectoderm known as the milk line. Mammary glands are highly specialized skin derivatives that have evolved from sweat glands. The first visible sign of mammary formation in a human embryo is seen as a thickening of cells within the malpighian layer of the epithelium along the ventrolateral surface at approximately 35 days of development. Mammary buds, specific areas of prominence that develop in the characteristic location, are evident by day 50. By 84 days of development, epithelial outgrowths of the mammary buds can be seen invading the surrounding mesenchyma. As these sprouts continue to develop and invade the mesenchyma, increased pressure under the surface epithelium gives rise to a protuberance of the surface that will further differentiate into a discrete nipple. Branching of the primary sprouts gives rise to the secondary sprouts at approximately 100 days. The secondary sprouts branch to form tertiary sprouts, resulting in the formation of primary and secondary milk ducts. The myoepithelial cells are formed from undifferentiated epithelial cells by 140 days of embryonic development (Brumsted and Riddick, 1990b).

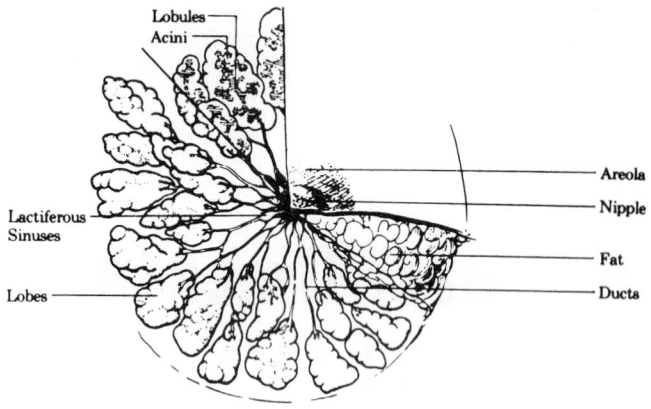

Figure 49-1
Frontal view of breast. (Courtesy of National Cancer Institute.)

Primitive breast tissue is under fetal gonadal control. The mammary prominence and the nipple secretions are the result of the in utero action of fetal prolactin and maternal/placental estrogen. Mammary development is essentially identical in the male and female embryo. The developing mammary bud in the male is affected by androgen, which blocks development at puberty by desensitizing the mammary bud to pubertal estrogen. Nonhormonal influences can also alter breast development. Adipose tis-

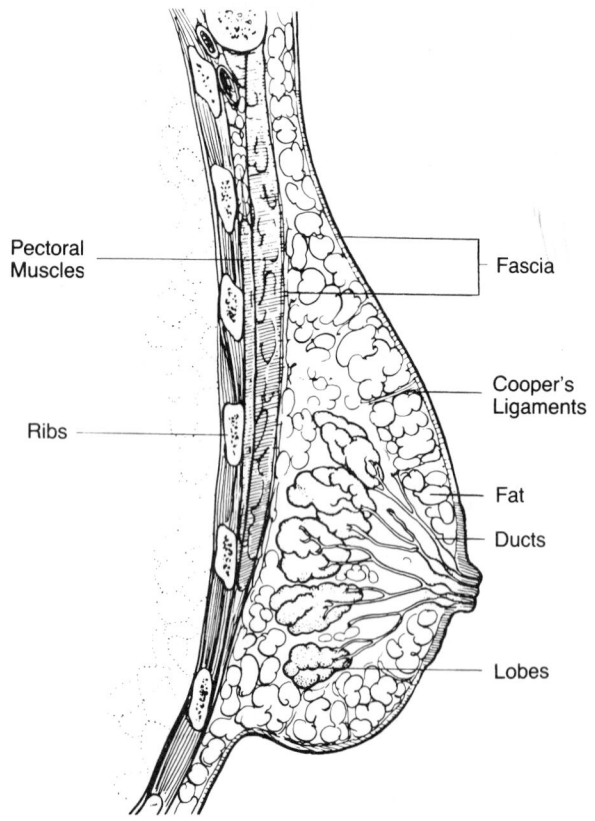

Figure 49-2
Lateral view of breast with supporting structures. (Courtesy of National Cancer Institute.)

sue appears to be critical for normal embryologic differentiation of the breast.

Clinical Correlates

Because breast tissue develops from an embryonic mammary ridge of ectoderm known as the milk line, ectopic breast development can occur in the axilla, abdomen, labia, or, less commonly, the buttocks or back. Accessory nipples (polythelia) or mammary glands (polymastia) are due to differentiation of the mammary bud in an uncharacteristic location or from migration along this line. Polythelia occurs in approximately 1% of the population (Brumsted and Riddick, 1990b). Treatment is not required.

Failure of nipple development (athelia) or failure of development of the entire mammary gland (amastia) may rarely occur. Clinically, this may present as a complete lack of development, unilateral failure, or extreme asymmetry. Although this does not require medical intervention, the patient may elect reconstructive surgery with implants or myocutaneous grafts to correct the congenital anomaly.

Hyperplasia, either symmetric or asymmetric, occurs in about 1% to 4% of all females. The patient may require a reduction mammoplasty for cosmetic or medical reasons.

In the complete form of the testicular feminization syndrome, the biologic action of testosterone is blocked, thus allowing for full mammary development in a genetic male at puberty. The androgens cannot block the development of the mammary bud.

PHYSIOLOGY

Puberty

The breast is a complex endocrine organ whose primary function is milk production. Following birth, breast tissue remains dormant until adolescence. Between the ages of 9 and 14 years, elongation, arborization, and proliferation of the mammary ducts occur, leading to the development of breast lobules. This process requires the synergistic action of estrogen, progesterone, insulin, cortisol, thyroxine, growth hormone, parathyroid hormone, and prolactin. This complex interaction of hormones results in an increase in the fibrous supporting structure, fat deposition, size and pigmentation of the nipple, and the milk duct system. As ovulatory cycles develop, the breast develops its unique alveolar-lobular-ductal growth and there is elastic and lipid deposition, vascular changes, and nipple-areolar pigmentation. Mammary maturation occurs over approximately a 4-year period. About $1\frac{1}{2}$ years after the onset of menstruation, glandular development is complete.

The first sign of breast development is an increase in size of the breast bud (thelarche), which heralds the onset of increased estrogen production. At menarche, the ducts and lobules subdivide, forming the acini. Estrogen stimulates extensive arborization and differentiation of the ductal epithelium. Progesterone, acting in concert with estrogen, produces rapid growth of the alveolar system. Completion of the alveolar-lobular-ductal configuration, with budding of the terminal ductals and differentiation of the alveolar epithelium, requires a synergistic action of estrogen and progesterone on the glandular anlage (Porter, 1974).

The deposition of adequate adipose tissue, under the influence of ovarian estrogen, is necessary to form a loose matrix in which epithelium and ductal proliferation occurs. There is a local steroidogenic hormonal milieu provided by the adipose tissue (Brumsted and Riddick, 1990b).

Menstrual Cycle

During the menstrual cycle, the blood vessels in the breast swell, the cells lining the ducts proliferate, and the ducts expand. Toward the end of the menstrual cycle, as estrogen and progesterone levels begin to fall, prolactin-induced secretory changes become apparent in the alveolar epithelium, with secretory products appearing in the alveolar lumen during the first few days of the menses. There is a peak mitotic activity at about the 25th day of the cycle, evidence that progesterone has a stimulatory effect on the breast (Ferguson and Anderson, 1981; Potten et al, 1988). Increased intracellular and intercellular water, maximum glandular and ductal development, and the accumulation of secretory materials within the alveolar structures cause the breasts to reach their maximum volume, resulting in premenstrual engorgement. With every ovulatory cycle, there is a luteal phase increase in the number of lobules, especially in parous women (Dogliotti et al, 1989). After menstruation, cellular growth regresses.

The breast lobules and acini begin to decrease in all women in their early 20s. The changes continue with age and accelerate with menopause.

Mammogenesis

Mammogenesis, or lactogenesis, is the process of growth and development of the mammary gland in preparation for milk production. Prior to pregnancy, the breast is predominantly adipose tissue, without extensive glandular or ductal development. By the end of pregnancy, the breast has become an almost entirely glandular structure. There is marked enhancement of the vascular supply. The nipples increase in size and pigmentation, and the mammary glands produce secretions important for nipple conditioning and lubrication (Brumsted and Riddick, 1990a). The breast content also increases in water, electrolyte, and fat content.

During the first few weeks of pregnancy, estrogen,

progesterone, and prolactin provide the initial stimuli for mammogenesis. Estrogen stimulates the synthesis and release of prolactin from the pituitary gland. Rising prolactin levels appear to be necessary for estrogen to exert its biologic effects on the mammary gland. Ductal proliferation is predominantly controlled by estrogen, whereas the acinar differentiation reflects the synergistic action of progesterone with estrogen. Prolactin induces the enzymes necessary for the acinar secretory activity. The high plasma concentration of progesterone inhibits the secretory effects of prolactin on the mammary alveolar epithelium until delivery. By the fourth or fifth postpartum day, the concentration of estrogen and progesterone in the plasma is less than in the normal follicular phase of the menstrual cycle. This fall in hormone level facilitates the transition in the acinar epithelium from a presecretory to a secretory state. A woman can nurse following an oophorectomy (Brumsted and Riddick, 1990a). Ovaries are not necessary for this process to occur.

In addition to estrogen, progesterone, and prolactin, lactogenesis requires the synergistic action of growth hormone, insulin, thyroxine, and cortisol. The initiation of milk production requires 2 to 5 days in humans. Prolactin is the principal hormone involved in milk biosynthesis. Suckling facilitates the release of prolactin by inhibiting prolactin inhibiting factor (PIF) and facilitates the release of oxytocin. Oxytocin causes the myoepithelial cells to contract. Eventually, the release of oxytocin becomes a conditioned response. The breast involutes following cessation of lactation. The alveolar-lobular-ductal unit regresses maximally by 3 months. The breasts are slightly larger than their prepregnancy size because they retain some of the fat and connective tissue acquired during breast-feeding (Brumsted and Riddick, 1990a). Adopting mothers occasionally request assistance in initiating lactation (Auerbach and Avery, 1981). Although milk production will not appear for several weeks, successful breast-feeding can be achieved by approximately half of the women by ingestion of 25 mg chlorpromazine tid together with vigorous nipple stimulation every 1 to 3 hours.

If a woman does not wish to breast-feed, there are effective medications to suppress lactation. Bromocriptine (Parlodel), a dopamine agonist, effectively suppresses pituitary prolactin synthesis and release, which inhibits lactation. Its side effects include nausea, vomiting, and a resumption of ovulatory cycles. When used following pregnancy, myocardial infarction, hypertension, seizures, pituitary hemorrhage, and stroke have been reported, especially in women with pregnancy-induced hypertension (Watson et al, 1989; Gittelman, 1991; Eickman, 1992). Bromocriptine is orally administered in a dose of 2.5 mg every 8 hours. Supportive measures for women electing not to breast-feed include fluid restriction, breast binders, ice packs, analgesics, and avoidance of nipple stimulation, tea, coffee, phenothiazines, and tranquilizers.

Menopause

With age the ducts atrophy and the breasts decrease in size. The breasts are increasingly replaced by fatty tissue. This involution of the breast reflects the diminishing levels of estrogen and progesterone.

BREAST SYMPTOMS

Mastodynia or Mastopathy (Breast Pain)

Breast pain is a common symptom affecting most women during their reproductive years. Breast pain can be associated with pregnancy, breast-feeding, trauma, mastitis, and thrombophlebitis. Treatment is directed to the underlying cause. Having excluded these conditions, breast pain is then classified as cyclic, noncyclic, or musculoskeletal. Breast cancer is not characteristically associated with pain. However, 7% to 10% of subclinical breast cancers produce pain as the only presenting symptom (Preece et al, 1982).

Musculoskeletal

Chest wall pain is usually due to injury to the musculoskeletal system. It is unilateral, nonphysiologic, and noncyclic. Tietze's syndrome is an unusual type of chest wall pain. It consists of swelling, pain, tenderness, and erythema in the upper costochondral cartilages (costochondritis). This syndrome may be acute in onset but usually gradually evolves. It is treated with oral anti-inflammatory medications or local steroidal injections. More commonly, anterior chest wall pain is related to trauma or exercise-induced injury and is treated with local therapy or systemic nonsteroidal anti-inflammatory drugs.

Cyclic Mastopathy (Fig. 49–3)

When breast pain is cyclic and bilateral, it is usually physiologic, representing endocrine end-organ sensitivity. The pain has been attributed to nerve irritation by edematous connective tissue and secretory retention in the ducts (Vorheer, 1986; Goodwin et al, 1988). Cyclic mastodynia may be associated with fibrocystic changes of the breast.

Cyclic mastopathy is so common that it may firmly lie within the spectrum of normality. Because of probable underreporting it is alleged that approximately 60% of all premenopausal women experience cyclic mastopathy (BeLieu, 1994). However, most women, if carefully questioned, report some degree of breast tenderness prior to their menses but may not seek medical treatment. Breast pain and nodularity often coexist. Breast swelling, tenderness, and engorgement typically begin during the luteal phase of the cycle and increase in intensity as the menses approach. With the onset of menstruation, the pain and engorgement usually diminish. Approximately 15% of women require treatment (Goodwin et al, 1988). Dietary changes and vitamin and drug therapy have all been used in an attempt to relieve cyclic mastodynia (Fig. 49–3).

NONPRESCRIPTION THERAPY

Some patients report a significant improvement in breast symptoms when dietary fat is reduced from 40% of the caloric intake to 15% to 20%. A randomized study of women with a history of at least 5 years of cyclic mastopathy revealed that the group instructed to reduce the fat content of their daily caloric intake to 15% while increasing the intake of complex carbohydrates demonstrated a significant reduction in breast swelling and tenderness after 6 months of dietary change. The mechanism of action is unclear (Boyd et al, 1988). Such a marked strict

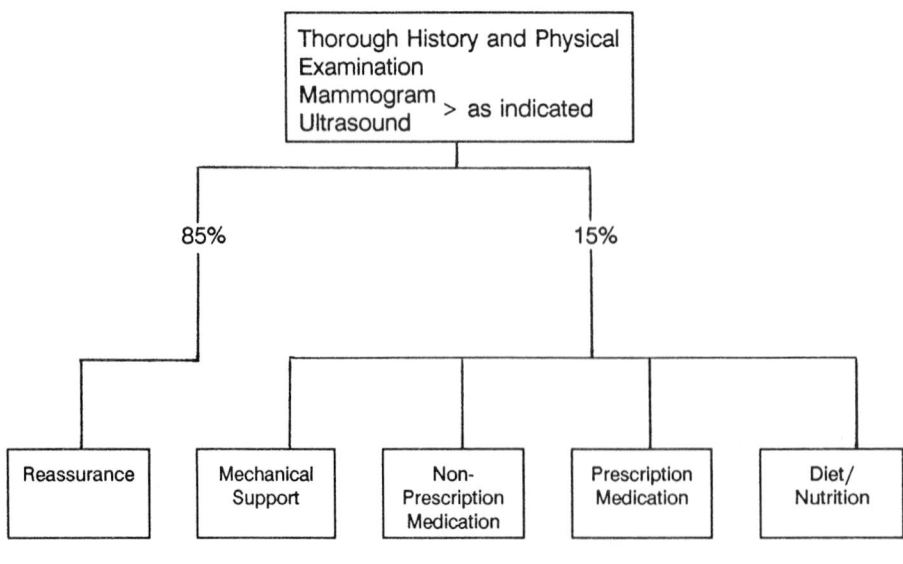

Figure 49–3

Evaluation and treatment of cyclic mastopathy.

restriction of fat intake requires a very motivated patient and is not suitable for most patients.

Vitamins as treatment for breast pain are of no proven benefit. The results of studies reported to date are conflicting and inconclusive. Several uncontrolled small studies have reported reductions in symptoms with vitamin E (α-tocopherol). However, two randomized, double-blind studies failed to demonstrate an improvement in the reported mastodynia (Ernster et al, 1985; London et al, 1985). Vitamin E regulates the synthesis of specific proteins and enzymes. Through this mechanism, it may alter serum gonadotropins. Vitamin E supplementation has been reported to raise high-density lipoprotein (HDL) and lower low-density lipoprotein (LDL) levels (Levy, 1983). Vitamin E supplementation may therefore be most useful in women with lipid abnormalities. Larger controlled studies are necessary to identify whether this subset of women can benefit from vitamin E therapy.

Vitamin A has been reported to be helpful in the management of cyclic mastodynia at an oral dose of 150,000 IU (Ellerhorst-Ryan et al, 1988). The side effects were generally mild and reversible when the drug was discontinued. This study, however, involved only 12 patients treated for 3 months.

Evening primrose oil is a natural product that is an essential fatty acid supplement. The rationale for its use is based on a deficiency of certain fatty acids in some patients with cyclic mastopathy. It has been reported to be effective in about 40% of treated patients (Maddox and Mansel, 1989). The postulated mechanism of action may be through the prostaglandin pathway. It can be obtained over the counter in health food stores. The average recommended dose is 1000 mg tid for a minimum of 3 to 4 months. Side effects include bloating and nausea.

PRESCRIPTION MEDICATIONS

Danazol has also been effective in several studies (Goodwin et al, 1988) and is the only Food and Drug Administration–approved pharmaceutical treatment for mastalgia. It improves breast nodularity as well as symptoms. Danazol is effective in doses ranging from 100 to 400 mg/day, but side effects occur in approximately 25% of patients at these conventional doses. A daily dose is recommended for a period of 6 months. It is also a known teratogen; therefore, effective contraception must be practiced.

Bromocriptine, a dopaminergic agonist, has been shown to be effective in the treatment of cyclic mastopathy when given in the luteal phase of the menstrual cycle (Goodwin et al, 1988). It decreases both breast pain and nodularity. However, it is accompanied by significant side effects, which include nausea, orthostatic hypotension, and dizziness, in approximately 15% of patients. When used following pregnancy to suppress lactation, myocardial infarction, hypertension, seizures, pituitary hemorrhage and stroke have been reported, especially in women with pregnancy-induced hypertension (Watson et al, 1989; Gittelman, 1991; Eickman, 1992). Side effects can be diminished by starting with a lower dose of medication. An incremental dosing protocol begins with 1.25 mg at bedtime, increasing by 1.25 mg every 3 to 4 days until 2.5 mg twice daily is reached (Gateley et al, 1992). The recommended dose is 2.5 to 5 mg/day. A trial of 6 months is recommended to adequately assess efficacy.

Several studies have shown tamoxifen to be effective in the treatment of cyclic mastopathy (Fentiman et al, 1986; Goodwin et al, 1988). It is not currently approved for this indication, and no long-term studies have been reported. Thus it seems premature to recommend tamoxifen until such studies become available. In its use in breast cancer patients, serious side effects, including an increased incidence of endometrial cancer, have been reported (Fisher et al, 1994).

Gestrinone, a 19-nortestosterone derivative, has androgenic, antiestrogenic, and antiprogestagenic properties. Gestrinone acts directly on the pituitary gland, on the ovary, and at the estrogen receptor of the mammary gland (Snyder et al, 1989). A small clinical trial revealed a response rate of approximately 75%. The action and side effects were similar to those of danazol (Peters, 1992). Further trials need to be performed to establish the efficacy and tolerability of this drug.

Gonadotropin-releasing hormone agonists induce a chemical menopause in premenopausal women, which improves cyclic mastalgia (Fentiman and Hamed, 1989; Richardson and Njemanz, 1990; Klijn et al, 1991). Side effects related to inducing a menopausal status may limit the clinical usefulness, especially for long-term treatment. Luteinizing hormone–releasing hormone (LHRH) analogs should be reserved for severe refractory cases of mastalgia and should not be used routinely or for longer than 3 months.

Diuretics have failed to significantly improve breast pain in symptomatic women. Additionally, they can cause electrolytic imbalance, dehydration, and hypotension. The use of diuretics in cyclic mastopathy should be abandoned.

Noncyclic Mastopathy

Noncyclic breast pain is much less common than cyclic breast pain, affecting about one of four women with mastalgia (Wisbey et al, 1983). It tends to occur about a decade later than cyclic mastalgia. On physical examination, approximately half of the patients have diffuse nodularity. The cause of this type of mastopathy is more likely to be anatomic than hormonal. Spontaneous resolution occurs in about 50% of patients (Gateley et al, 1992). The same pharmacologic and nonpharmacologic therapies as used in cyclic mastopathy have been used, although with less efficacy (BeLieu, 1994).

Nipple Discharge

A spontaneous, persistent, nonphysiologic, nonlactational nipple discharge is more commonly associated with an underlying benign breast lesion than with a malignancy. Nipple discharge may also be associated with medications that include oral contraceptive (OC) pills, phenothiazines, rauwolfia alkaloids, amphetamines, opiates, diazepams, butyrophenones, α-methyldopa, and tricyclic antidepressants. Thoracotomy scars, cervical spine lesions, and herpes zoster can also cause nipple discharge. A "pseudonipple" discharge can be associated with inverted nipples, eczematoid lesions of the breast or nipples, traumatic erosion, herpes, a Montgomery gland abscess, or a mammary duct fistula.

Once it is established that a spontaneous, persistent, nonlactational discharge is present, the nature of the discharge should be characterized (Fig. 49–4). It is important to differentiate spontaneous from induced and unilateral from bilateral discharge. Nonspontaneous discharge from multiple ducts of both breasts is generally due to pharmacologic or endocrinologic causes. A unilateral nipple discharge arising from a single duct in a woman more than 50 years of age and serous, serosanguineous, or watery in nature is likely to be malignant.

Seven types of nipple discharge have been described: (1) milky, (2) multicolored and sticky, (3) purulent, (4) clear or watery, (5) yellow or serous, (6) pink or serosanguineous, and (7) bloody or sanguineous (Leis, 1989). After the discharge has been grossly characterized, a slide of the nipple secretion can be made and stained with Wright's stain to evaluate for the presence of pus or blood. The presence of occult blood can also be established with a reagent stick (Hemostix) or by placing the discharge on a white gauze sponge. If blood is present, a red color will appear on the periphery (Leis, 1989).

Galactorrhea

A milky discharge (galactorrhea) is usually bilateral, spontaneous or induced, and from multiple ducts. The final common pathway leading to galactorrhea is an inappropriate augmentation of prolactin release. Dopamine levels are depleted or the dopamine receptor is blocked, resulting in a decrease in PIF. A more comprehensive discussion of prolactin disorders can be found in Chapter 29.

Galactorrhea can be associated with pregnancy, hypothyroidism, or anovulatory syndromes (Chiari-Frommel, Forbes-Albright, Ahumada–del Castillo syndromes). A pituitary adenoma must be ruled out as a cause of galactorrhea. Galactorrhea may be associated with medications such as phenothiazines, tricyclic antidepressants, opiates, methyldopa, OCs, and other medications.

Galactorrhea resulting from a pituitary adenoma can be managed medically, surgically, or with careful surveillance. Management depends on the prolactin level, radiographic findings, and the size and growth of the tumor. Bromocriptine (Parlodel), a dopamine receptor agonist that inhibits prolactin production, can be used for patients with elevated prolactin levels who desire pregnancy. Bromocriptine is useful for the treatment of galactorrhea, even with normal prolactin concentrations and normal radiographic findings. The usual recommended dose is 5.0 to 7.5 mg daily in divided doses.

Purulent Nipple Discharge

A purulent nipple discharge is produced by infection. The patient usually complains of breast pain, and tenderness is elicited on breast examination. The discharge is usually associated with a puerperal mastitis, chronic lactation mastitis, or central duct mastitis. A penicillinase-resistant antibiotic is required because the implicated agent is usually a staphylococcal organism. If an abscess occurs, incision and drainage are required to definitively treat this condition.

Intraductal Papilloma

Intraductal papillomas are the principal cause of nipple discharge in nonpregnant or nonlactating women. They occur most frequently in 45- to 50-year-old women. In 20% to 50% of patients, the lesion is characterized by a bloody or serosanguineous nipple discharge. In the absence of a mass, the most common cause of bloody nipple discharge is an intraductal papilloma. However, a palpable mass can be detected in up to 90% of patients.

Grossly, the lesion appears as a small, fragile, wart-like or finger-line growth in the lining of the mammary duct near the nipple. It usually involves a single duct, and 95% are unilateral. Ductography (galactography) can identify intraductal lesions that cause spontaneous unilateral single-duct discharge. This procedure is usually only available in institu-

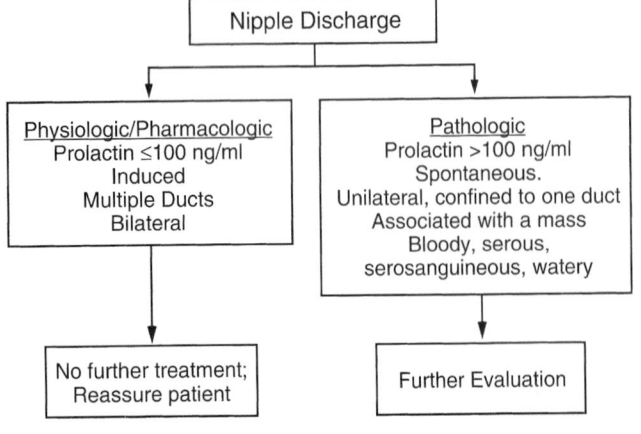

Figure 49–4
Management of nipple discharge.

tions where there is an interest in this technique. Galactography is better than mammography in localizing small intraductal papillomas (Rongione et al, 1996). Treatment is surgical excision of the involved duct.

Pathologically, there is a single cell type that arises from the lining of a terminal duct, arranged in a papillary pattern. An intraductal papilloma usually arises within 1 cm of the areola in more than 90% of patients; however, it can extend 4.5 cm along the duct.

There can be multiple intraductal papillomas, and they can be bilateral in 10% to 15% of patients. Multiple papillomas have been linked with malignant transformation. They usually affect younger women and present as a mass (Haagensen et al, 1981).

Mammary Duct Ectasia

Mammary duct ectasia is the second most common cause of nipple discharge. This entity is discussed in the following section under benign breast disease.

Malignancy

A breast biopsy to rule out an underlying carcinoma is mandatory when there is a clear or watery, yellow or serous, pink, serosanguineous, or bloody discharge (Table 49–1). An associated carcinoma may be found in up to 47% of patients with a nipple discharge (Holleb and Farrow, 1966; Pilnik and Leis, 1978; Haagensen 1986). A mass is usually present when there is cancer, but up to 13% of cancers do not have a palpable mass (Leis, 1989). A slide preparation should be obtained to evaluate the cytologic features of the discharge. However, one should not rely solely on cytology. If there is an underlying carcinoma, 80% of patients will show positive cytologic results (20% false-negative). There is approximately a 2.6% false-positive rate associated with the cytologic interpretation of a nipple discharge. Mammography, in this circumstance, is associated with a false-negative rate of about 10% and a false-positive rate of 1.6% (Zuckerman, 1989).

BENIGN BREAST DISEASE: RISK FACTORS

The OC pill may reduce the risk of benign breast disease, especially in women who have used the pill for more than 2 years. Specifically, it may reduce the risk of fibroadenoma and fibrocystic change (Wang and Fentiman, 1985). The mechanism may be related to the amount of gestagen in the birth control pill. Although the reported studies and reviews cite a lower risk of benign breast disease in patients taking OCs over a long term, this may reflect a physician bias in patient selection. Physicians may be reluctant to prescribe OCs to patients with breast symptoms (Wang and Fentiman, 1985).

A breast biopsy does not increase the risk of benign breast disease. There have been some reports that women who have a breast biopsy performed are at an increased risk for breast cancer. However, when these studies are carefully analyzed, it appears that the risk is related to the underlying histopathology rather than to the surgical procedure (Dupont and Paige, 1985; Wang and Fentiman, 1985; Consensus Statement, 1986). It is important to remember that the vast majority of women with breast cancer have not had a previous breast biopsy performed for benign disease (Ernster, 1981).

Consistent endocrine abnormalities or clearly defined risk factors for benign breast disease have not been elucidated. Risk factors may include nulliparity and methylxanthine intake (caffeine, cola, coffee, tea, chocolate). However, the evidence for methylxanthines in the etiopathogenesis of benign breast disease is quite conflicting, controversial, and inconclusive.

BENIGN BREAST CONDITIONS

Congenital Abnormalities

Amastia and rudimentary breast development are rare and usually unilateral congenital abnormalities. They may be associated with musculoskeletal defects as well as deficiencies in ovarian function. There is a failure of normal breast development. Plastic surgery with augmentation can be offered to the patient once the normal breast has completed its maturation, usually 4 years following menarche.

Accessory breast tissue can occur as supernumerary nipples, areolae, breasts, or any combination. Approximately 1% to 2% of the population has accessory breast tissue. It is frequently reported in females of Asian descent.

Developmental Abnormalities

Precocious breast development is defined as breast development prior to the age of 8 years in the absence of other secondary sexual characteristics. The vast majority of precocious breast development spontaneously resolves by the age of 2. If it develops after the age of 2, a work-up is necessary to rule out an ovarian tumor, adrenal tumor, brain tumor, ingestion of estrogen, or constitutional precocity (Pasquino et al, 1985).

Table 49–1. NIPPLE DISCHARGE: GRAVE SIGNS

Serous, serosanguinous, or watery discharge
Associated with a mass
Unilateral
Single duct
Positive cytology
Positive mammography
Age >50 years

Juvenile (virginal) hypertrophy of the breast is defined as massive unilateral or bilateral enlargement of the breasts in adolescence out of proportion to total body growth. There is excessive growth of fat and connective tissue. The treatment is reduction mammoplasty once the breasts have completed maturation.

Inflammatory Conditions

In *acute mastitis*, the patient presents with breast pain, erythema, and fever. An inflammatory condition is usually associated with breast-feeding, although it can occur in the nonlactating breast. A staphylococcal organism is usually associated with this condition. An antibiotic with activity against this organism is administered. However, if the disease progresses to an unresolved mass, surgical drainage is required. If the patient is nursing, she should stop nursing with the affected breast and use a breast pump until the mastitis resolves.

A *subareolar abscess* requires incision and drainage, which can be temporarily effective. However, the abscess recurs unless the affected duct is excised. The symptoms are due to obstructed dilated ducts. The ducts develop squamous metaplasia in response to the inflammation. The keratin from the desquamated epithelium within the terminal duct obstructs the ducts. Secondary abscess formation occurs at the base of the nipple (Drukker and de Mendonca, 1988).

Mondor's disease, a superficial thrombophlebitis of the thoracoepigastric vein, is an uncommon condition. The patient presents with acute pain localized to the upper lateral portion of the breast. There is a linear, cord-like tender structure, with accompanying erythema. Mondor's disease is usually associated with pregnancy, operative procedures such as augmentation or reduction mammoplasty, and breast trauma. Associated carcinoma has been reported in up to 12.7% of cases (Catania et al, 1992). Histopathologically, there is stromal fibrosis and an inflammatory response in the vein. The treatment is systemic analgesics and local heat. The tenderness usually resolves in 2 to 3 weeks. The cord may last up to 7 months. A mammogram should be performed to rule out an underlying malignancy.

Fat Necrosis

Fat necrosis is an uncommon entity that usually appears as a firm, tender, irregular superficial mass (Fig. 49–5). The majority of patients may recall some breast trauma. Surgical trauma secondary to biopsy and reduction mammoplasty can also lead to fat necrosis (Barber and Libshitz, 1977). Conservative treatment of breast carcinoma with lumpectomy and radiation therapy may also result in fat necrosis (Rostom and El-Sayed, 1987). Patients with transverse rectus abdominis muscle (TRAM) flap recon-

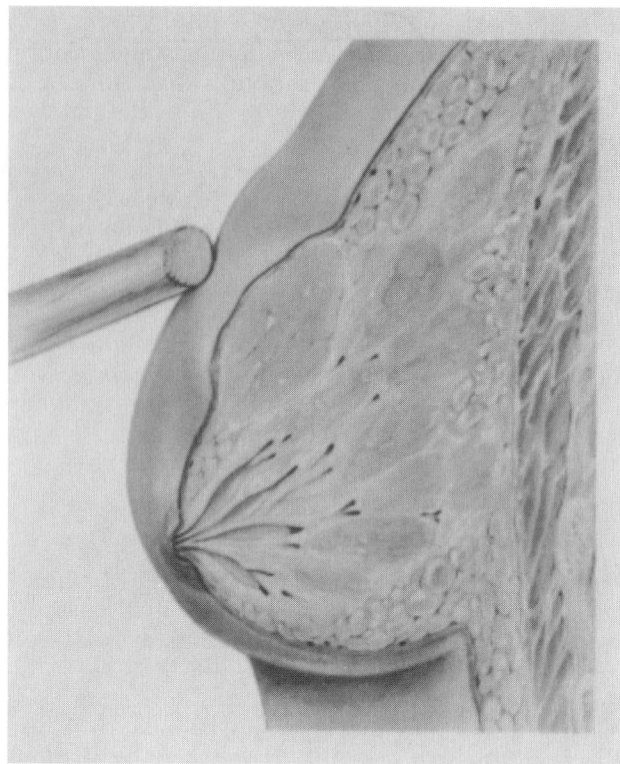

Figure 49–5
Fat necrosis: a mass usually produced by trauma or injury. (Courtesy of Parke-Davis, a Division of Warner-Lambert Company.)

struction following modified radical mastectomy may develop fat necrosis (Hartrampf and Bennett, 1987). Diseases that cause fat necrosis (e.g., Weber-Christian disease) will demonstrate these masses in the breast as well as other parts of the body. A characteristic mammogram reveals a mass (lipid cyst) with a lucent center surrounded by a rim of calcium forming a pseudocapsule (Fig. 49–6).

Patients who present soon after trauma with physical sequelae such as ecchymosis and painful masses in the breast can be safely observed. If patients present with painless masses and histories of trauma that cannot be verified, the diagnosis of fat necrosis must be established by biopsy. Fine-needle aspiration, stereotactic core biopsy, or needle localization and excisional biopsy are mandatory to rule out carcinoma (Magnant, 1996).

An oil cyst, part of the spectrum of fat necrosis, is sonographically characterized by a mass with smooth margins, good through transmission, and a homogeneous echo pattern (Schepps et al, 1994).

Galactocele

A galactocele is a benign tender breast cyst that contains thick, inspissated, milky fluid and desquamated epithelial cells. This is an uncommon condition that usually follows lactation. The patients

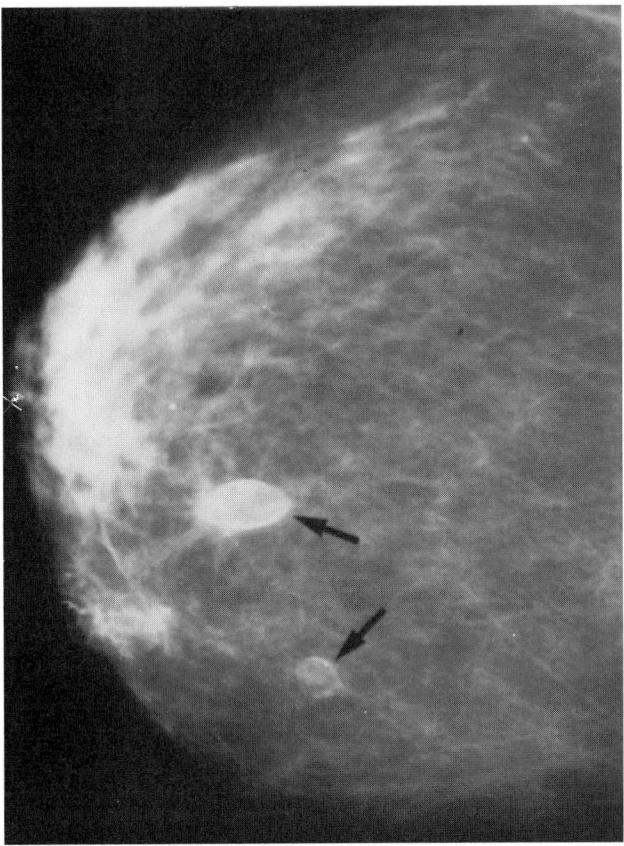

Figure 49-6
Mammogram showing lipid cysts (*arrows*).

present with a tender nodular area or a discrete mass. Diagnostic aspiration is often curative. Surgical resection is required if there is an abscess. If the galactocele has been present for an extended period of time, the clear, milky white collection may become thick and greenish, related to the chronicity of the condition.

Papillomatosis

Papillomatosis is a microscopic entity with no palpable mass present. It is an incidental finding at the time of a breast biopsy. There is ductal hyperplasia of the upper epithelial cells of the duct, which then partially fill the small or medium mammary ducts. Papillomatosis may be caused by estrogen hyperstimulation. This entity is observed in one third of patients with fibrocystic changes of the breast (Vorheer, 1986). Its chief interest lies in the fact that it may be mistaken for an infiltrating glandular carcinoma when accompanied by central sclerosis (Haagensen et al, 1981).

Adenoma

Adenomas account for 1% to 2% of all benign breast disease. The peak incidence is at 20 to 30 years of age. They present as well-circumscribed tumors composed of benign epithelial elements (ductal and alveolar structures) with sparse stroma, thus differentiating them from fibroadenomas. The entity is categorized into two distinct groups: a tubular mobile type, which occurs in young women, and a second type that occurs during pregnancy or in the immediate postpartum period.

Collagenous Spherulosis

This is a rare, benign proliferative duct lesion composed of mixed myoepithelial and epithelial cells with intraluminal spherules (Grignon et al, 1989). It is usually an incidental finding in a breast biopsy or mastectomy specimen; however, it may present as a clinically palpable mass. This lesion is important to recognize because it must be distinguished from adenoid cystic carcinoma and intraductal signet-ring cell carcinoma (Clement et al, 1987).

Diabetic Fibrous Breast Disease (Diabetic Mastopathy)

Diabetic fibrous breast disease, first recognized in 1984, is characterized by a rock-hard, painless, freely mobile mass of dense glandular tissue. It is associated with type I insulin-dependent diabetes. The average duration from the onset of diabetes to the appearance of a breast mass is 23 years. The number and size of lesions increases with age. The condition is bilateral in approximately half the patients. With a mean follow-up of 6 years, breast cancer did not develop in any of the patients in a small study of 36 insulin-dependent diabetic women (Logan and Hoffman, 1989). Recognition of the entity may spare diabetic women a breast biopsy.

For women younger than 25 years, a baseline mammogram, sonographic follow-up, and fine-needle aspiration have been suggested. On ultrasound, there is marked acoustic shadowing of sound waves. On fine-needle aspiration, there is tissue resistance. For women 30 years of age and older, a baseline mammogram followed by yearly mammograms, yearly physical examinations, and sonography are recommended, in addition to a fine-needle aspiration. A mammogram may be difficult to interpret because it can show dense fibrous tissue with microcalcifications (Logan and Hoffman, 1989; Gump and McDermott, 1990). It may not be necessary to obtain biopsy specimens if the lesions are symmetric and if the entity is clinically apparent. If biopsy is performed, a characteristic constellation of histologic features is observed that include dense, keloid-like fibrosis; lymphocytic infiltrates around ducts and lobules; lymphocytic vasculitis; and epithelioid fibroblasts (Tomaszewski et al, 1992; Seidman et al, 1994).

Mammary Duct Ectasia/Periductal Mastitis

Mammary duct ectasia and periductal mastitis accounts for 3% to 12% of benign breast masses (Dixon, 1989). In this condition, dilated ducts are filled with plugs of keratin and stagnant secretions. An inflammatory process, periductal mastitis, surrounds the ducts, with primarily a plasma cell infiltrate. The peak incidence occurs in women between 40 and 49 years of age. It has been observed on microscopic examination in 30% to 40% of women older than 50 years. In approximately 25% of premenopausal patients in whom this entity develops, fibrocystic change is an associated factor.

Mammary duct ectasia may be subclinical or it may present as breast pain, a breast mass, a nipple discharge, nipple retraction, a nonpuerperal breast abscess, or a mammary fistula (Devitt, 1989; Dixon, 1989). The patients can present with fever, chills, and breast hyperemia. The nipple discharge ranges in color from cream to green and it may contain blood.

The cause of mammary duct ectasia is unknown. It remains to be resolved whether the process starts as a retention of secretory material in the ductal system with duct dilation that leads to a periductal mastitis or whether periductal mastitis leads to duct wall damage and subsequent duct dilation.

The treatment of patients with mammary duct ectasia or periductal mastitis varies with clinical presentation. In patients with only nipple discharge, treatment is primarily medical. When inflammatory changes occur without the formation of a mass, bed rest, icepacks, and anti-inflammatory agents may be tried (Issacs, 1994). Broad-spectrum antibiotics are effective in treating the periareolar inflammation associated with this condition (Bundred et al, 1985). A high percentage of patients with duct ectasia have bacteria in their nipple discharge (Dixon et al, 1988). However, this bacterial flora is similar to the endogenous bacterial flora found throughout normal human breast tissue (Issacs, 1994).

Surgical therapy is required in certain circumstances. Patients who present with a mass must undergo biopsy to exclude a diagnosis of carcinoma. Abscesses require drainage. Excision of the involved ducts may be required when associated with inflammatory changes.

If this disease becomes chronic, it may be associated with reactive fibrosis, duct stenosis, obliteration, and/or scar formation, resulting in skin or nipple retraction. Clinically, this may resemble a breast carcinoma (Osuch, 1987).

Mammary Fibromatosis (Desmoid Tumor)

This is an uncommon stromal tumor occurring in patients ranging in age from 14 to 80 years, with a median age of 25 (Rosen and Ernsberger, 1989). It presents as a unilateral, firm to hard, usually discrete, painless mass. Clinically, it may mimic a breast carcinoma on physical examination. A spectrum of microscopic patterns has been observed. The usual spindle-cell pattern is associated with fibroblastic proliferation and infrequent mitoses. The collagenous component can predominate, creating a keloid-like pattern. A few reported cases have been associated with Gardner's syndrome and familial multicentric fibromatosis (Schnitt and Connolly, 1996).

Mammography may reveal a stellate tumor, indistinguishable from carcinoma. Needle aspiration is often inconclusive because of the scanty material obtained. The treatment is wide local excision. Although histologically benign, mammary fibromatosis may recur, particularly if the surgical margins are not clear of the lesion (Rosen and Ernsberger, 1989).

Lipoma

A lipoma is a soft, mobile, fatty tumor most frequently found in postmenopausal women. It is the most common nonepithelial neoplasm of the breast. A thin capsule surrounding a lucent fatty density is the classical mammographic finding. Calcifications are rare (Paulus, 1983). The treatment is surgical excision.

Intramammary Lymph Node

An intramammary lymph node is mammographically characterized by a noncalcified mass usually less than 1.5 cm with a central hilus (Fig. 49–7, small arrow). It may occur in the axilla or in the actual breast tissue. Treatment is not indicated if the characteristic mammographic appearance of the intramammary lymph node is recognized (Homer et al, 1985).

Fibroadenomas

Fibroadenomas account for approximately 15% to 20% of all breast disease and are the most common benign solid tumors of the female breast. They can occur at any age, including in perimenopausal and postmenopausal women, but are most frequently detected in the 20- to 40-year age group. The peak incidence occurs in women in their early 20s. Clinically, these lesions present as discrete, solid masses that are painless, mobile, and rubbery in consistency (Fig. 49–8). They usually present as solitary masses, although up to 20% of patients have multiple fibroadenomas in the involved breast. They may regress, persist, or enlarge.

Fibroadenomas have been noted on routine screening mammograms in up to 25% of patients. Mammographically they are characterized by dense macrocalcifications throughout with sharply marginated borders (Fig. 49–9). The sonographic appear-

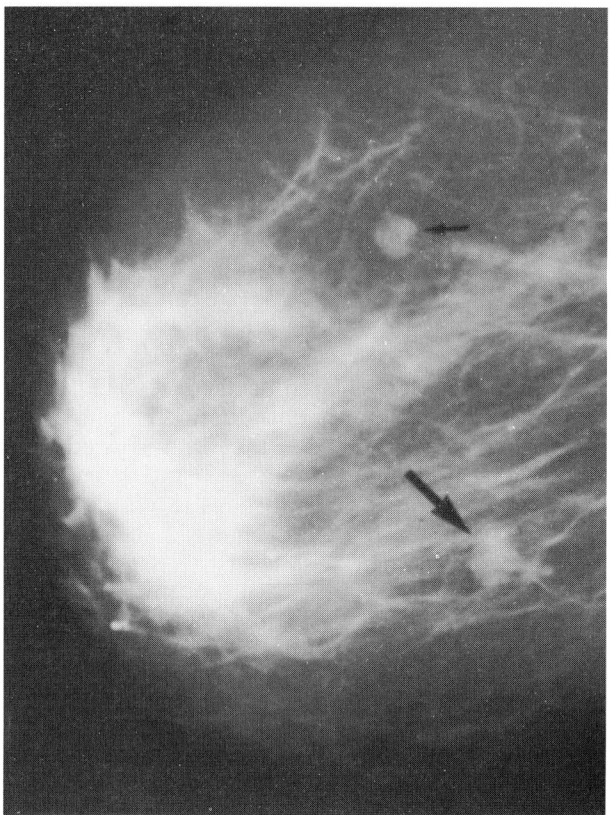

Figure 49-7
Mammogram demonstrating a lymph node (*small arrow*) and a carcinoma (*large arrow*).

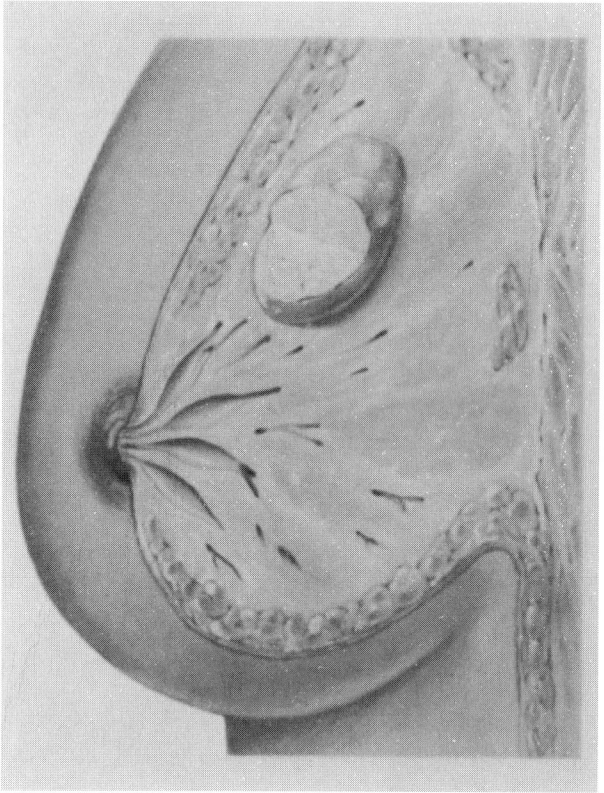

Figure 49-8
Fibroadenoma: a solid benign tumor, usually in young women. (Courtesy of Parke-Davis, a Division of Warner-Lambert Company.)

ance of a fibroadenoma is a solid, homogeneous, smooth-surfaced mass with well-defined borders (Fig. 49-10).

Fibroadenomas are considered to be an abnormality of normal development and involution rather than a true neoplasm, representing a hyperplastic process that involves a terminal ductal-lobular unit and its surrounding connective tissue. Histopathologically, they represent an exuberant overgrowth of stromal and epithelial elements (Hughes et al, 1987). Fibroadenomas have estrogen and progesterone receptors (Kutten et al, 1981). Because fibroadenomas contain the same elements as normal breast tissue, their response to hormonal changes is similar. These lesions tend to enlarge during pregnancy and involute following menopause.

Infrequently, carcinoma may occur in association with a fibroadenoma. The most commonly reported carcinoma is a lobular carcinoma in situ, but infiltrating lobular, intraductal, and infiltrating ductal carcinomas have also been observed. Certain pathologic characteristics of fibroadenomas may serve as markers for increased risk of breast cancer. In a case-control study, patients with complex fibroadenomas (cysts > 3 mm, sclerosing adenosis, epithelial calcifications, or papillary changes) had an increased relative risk of 3.1.

Excisional biopsy remains the procedure of choice. Alternative tissue sampling, such as aspiration cytology or core needle biopsy, may be considered in women under 35 years of age or in patients with multiple fibroadenomas (Wilkinson et al, 1989). Nonpalpable tumors detected by mammography may be watched (Issacs 1994).

There are special variants of fibroadenoma. A giant fibroadenoma is defined as a lesion larger than 5 cm. It is a rapidly enlarging breast mass that can reach 10 to 19 cm. Juvenile fibroadenomas occur in adolescent girls between the ages of 12 and 16 years. They appear to be more common in women of African-American descent. These lesions cause marked breast asymmetry. They can be unilateral or bilateral.

Treatment for both variants is surgical excision. Augmentation mammoplasty may be required to provide satisfactory cosmetic results.

Phyllodes Tumors

Phyllodes tumors are uncommon, usually slowly growing, smooth, rounded, and multinodular tumors (Fig. 49-11). The peak age of incidence is 30 to 55 years; however, they have been reported in all age groups. These tumors produce a spectrum of disease

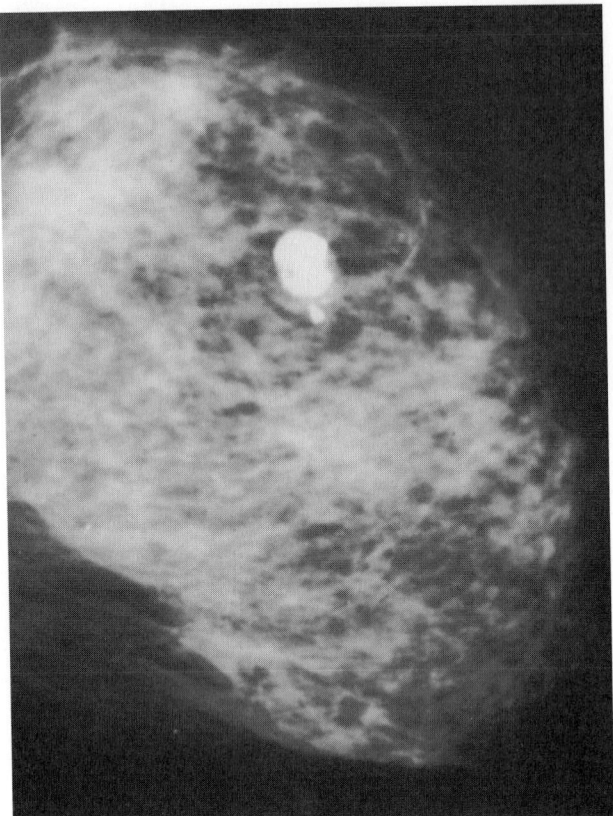

Figure 49–9
Mammogram demonstrating calcified fibroadenoma.

from benign to malignant. Histologically, these tumors are composed of epithelial and stromal elements. Characteristics of the stroma determine whether a phyllodes tumor is benign or malignant. The percentage of all phyllodes tumors classified as malignant ranges from 23% to 50%. Metastases occur in 6% to 22% (Petrek, 1996). If metastatic disease

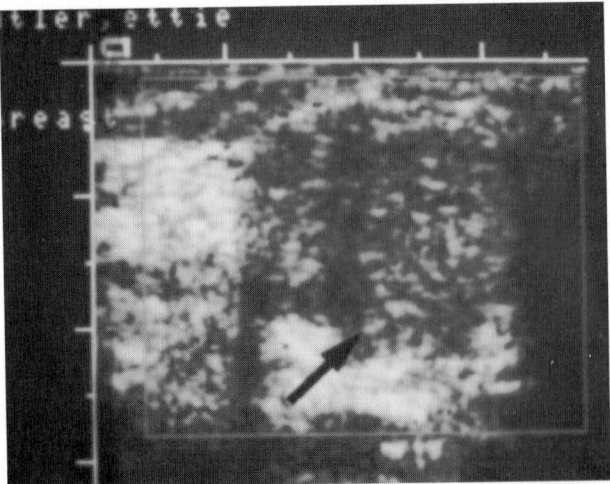

Figure 49–10
Ultrasonography demonstrating fibroadenoma (*arrow*) a solid tumor with smooth borders.

does occur, it is most frequently to the lung. Cure is rare with metastatic tumors (Kinne and DeCosse, 1981).

Phyllodes tumors are often enucleated or excised with close margins. A local recurrence rate of 20% can be expected (Petrek, 1996). In tumors with malignant features, a wide local excision is possible (Reinfuss et al, 1993).

Fibrocystic Change

Fibrocystic disease has been used to describe a spectrum of physiologic and pathologic changes in the breast. In 1985, a consensus meeting advised deleting the term "fibrocystic disease" and substituting "fibrocystic change" or "fibrocystic condition" to more accurately reflect the changes in the breast (Consensus Statement, 1986). At this same meeting, the risk factors for malignancy associated with fibrocystic change were clearly delineated (Table 49–2). The most important pathologic risk factors are the degree and nature (typical or atypical) of the epithelial proliferation (Table 49–2).

Depending on whether one looks at clinical symptoms or histologic/autopsy specimens, the frequency of fibrocystic change can be quite variable. It appears that it is more common in nulliparous women as compared with multiparous women. Women with early menarche, late menopause, and irregular or anovulatory cycles appear to have fibrocystic changes at higher than expected frequencies.

Fibrocystic change is commonly bilateral, with a propensity for the upper outer quadrant, which has the greatest concentration of glandular tissue. The size of the breast and symptoms increase during the premenstrual phase of the menstrual cycle. Patients complain of a dull, heavy pain and a sense of breast fullness. Marked tenderness is elicited on examination. Examination reveals well-delineated, slightly mobile cystic nodules or thickened areas. Needle aspiration of the cysts reveals turbid, nonhemorrhagic fluid.

Histologic Spectrum

Histologically, the spectrum of fibrocystic disease includes microcysts, macrocysts, adenosis, apocrine change, fibrosis, and ductal hyperplasia. Some authorities include the entity of fibroadenoma under this category as well. The histologic changes represent epithelial proliferation within the ductal system and stromal fibrosis. Stromal fibrosis contributes to cyst formation by causing ductal obstruction and retention of alveolar secretions. The most common cystic changes are microcysts, which are smaller than 2 mm (Fig. 49–12). Macrocysts are larger than 3 mm but can occasionally be larger than 3 cm. Cystic changes represent dilated subareolar, lobular, or lobar ducts. Cystic changes occur in 20% to 40% of women with fibrocystic change.

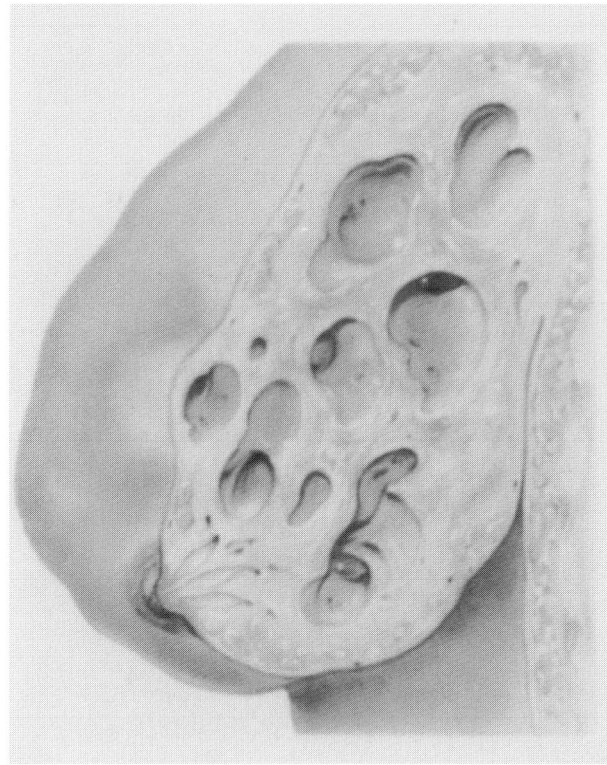

Figure 49–11
Cystosarcoma phyllodes or giant myxoma. (Courtesy of Parke-Davis, a Division of Warner-Lambert Company.)

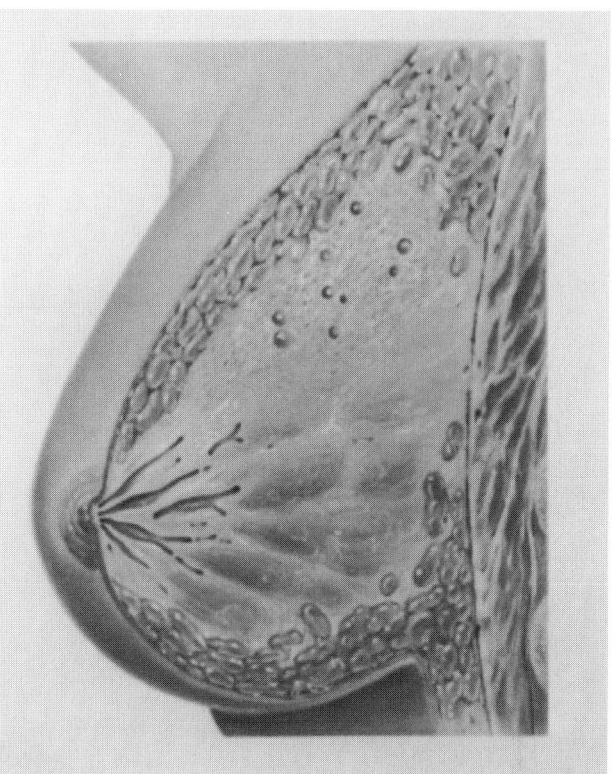

Figure 49–12
Microcysts. On examination, the breasts have a finely nodular character. (Courtesy of Parke-Davis, a Division of Warner-Lambert Company.)

The cystic changes have been described as occurring in three stages (Drukker and deMendonca, 1988). The *early stage* occurs in patients in their 20s to early 30s. The breast tissue become "lumpy," with an increase in premenstrual density and tenderness.

Table 49–2. HISTOPATHOLOGIC RISK FACTORS FOR BREAST CANCER

No Increased Risk
Adenosis, sclerosing or florid
Apocrine metaplasia
Duct ectasia
Fibroadenoma
Fibrosis
Macrocysts or microcysts
Mastitis
Mild hyperplasia (>2 but ≤4 epithelial cells)

1.5–2× Increased Risk
Moderate or florid, solid or papillary hyperplasia
Papilloma with fibrovascular core

5× Increased Risk
Atypical hyperplasia (borderline lesion)
   Ductal
   Lobular

8–10× Increased Risk
Carcinoma in situ

Modified from Consensus statement: is "fibrocystic disease" of the breast precancerous? (Consensus meeting 10/13–10/15, 1985). Arch Pathol Lab Med 1986;110:171, with permission.

It usually affects the upper outer quadrant of the breast and regresses significantly following the menses.

The *second stage* occurs in patients in their fourth decade of life. The pain and tenderness are accentuated 2 to 3 weeks prior to menstrual flow. The cystic areas enlarge in diameter and increase in firmness, which is related to an increase in fibrosis. There is some resolution of symptoms following menses.

The *third stage* occurs in the fifth decade, with multiple, persistent cystic masses. These cystic masses can form "blue dome cysts" (Fig. 49–13) (Vorheer, 1986).

Adenosis represents a proliferation in the acini of the distal mammary lobules. This is prominent in women in their late 30s and 40s. It is usually microscopic without clinical significance. However, if the condition progresses, the ducts become surrounded by dense fibrotic tissue forming a firm mass, producing sclerosing adenosis (Fig. 49–14). These are firm, irregular lesions. Rarely, there may be extensive fibrous change forming a 2- to 3-cm mass. This represents end-stage disease. On gross examination they are irregular, gray to white, and indurated, often simulating a scirrhous carcinoma. They are clinically important because they can simulate a malignancy on physical examination, mammography, and microscopic evaluation. They are treated by local excision (Drukker and de Mendonca, 1988).

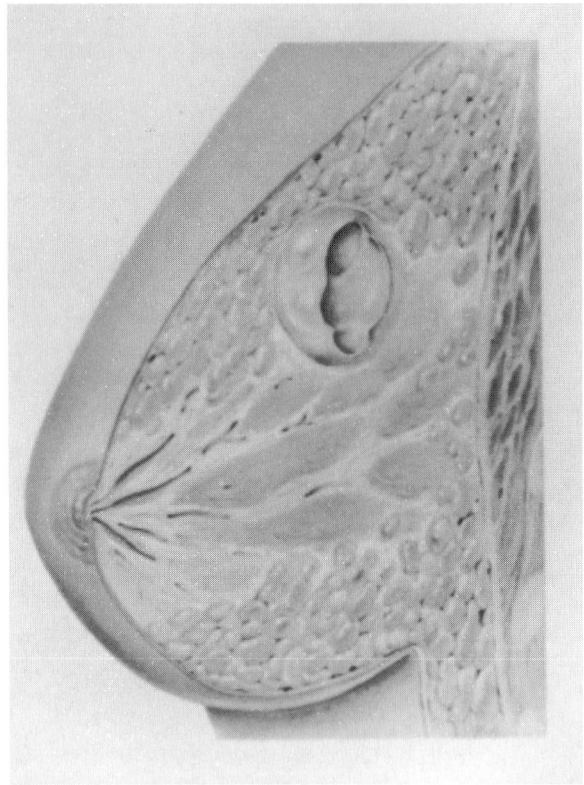

Figure 49–13
A solitary large cyst ("blue dome"). (Courtesy of Parke-Davis, a Division of Warner-Lambert Company.)

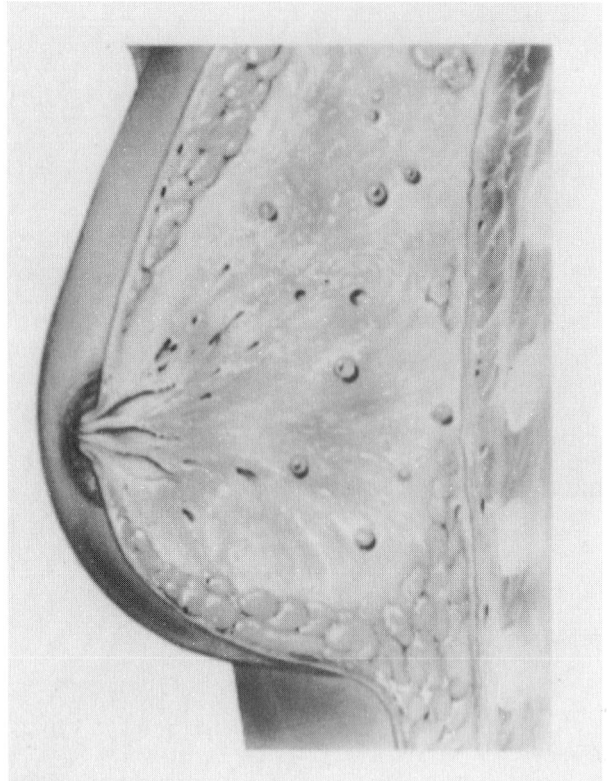

Figure 49–14
Adenosis: a proliferation of the acini in the distal lobules. If the condition progresses, the ducts become surrounded by dense fibrotic tissue, as illustrated in this photo. (Courtesy of Parke-Davis, a Division of Warner-Lambert Company.)

In 20% of patients with fibrocystic change, *mazoplasia* occurs with a peak incidence at 35 to 50 years of age. The pathology reveals focal ductal-alveolar hyperplasia, stromal edema, and epithelial desquamation, with secretory retention and induration or nodularity of the terminal ductal segments, surrounded by a lymphocytic infiltration and fibrosis (Vorheer, 1986).

Etiopathogenesis of Fibrocystic Change

The exact cause of fibrocystic change is unknown. It has been postulated that a relative estrogen excess is involved, perhaps an abnormal production of estrogen or an exaggerated tissue response to a normal level. Conversely, a relative progesterone deficiency may be responsible. Up to 70% of patients with fibrocystic change have a corpus luteum deficiency, ovulatory irregularity, or anovulation (Sitruk-Ware et al, 1979). This relative estrogen excess or progesterone deficiency results in a hyperproliferation of connective and epithelial tissues. There appear to be simultaneous progressive and regressive changes (Vorheer, 1986). The fibrosis ultimately predominates.

The evidence for the role of methylxanthines in the etiopathogenesis of fibrocystic change is controversial and inconclusive (Minton et al, 1979; Ernster et al, 1982). Methylxanthines act as competitive inhib-

itors of the enzyme that breaks down cyclic AMP (cAMP). The amount of cAMP has been correlated with the degree of epithelial proliferation in the breast (Hindi-Alexander et al, 1985).

Treatment

The early diagnosis and treatment of fibrocystic change may arrest and reverse the associated changes. The rationale for treatment is to stop progression and to relieve symptoms. The physician should advise the patients to wear well-fitting brassieres and light, loose clothing. Nonhormonal and hormonal therapies have been used with varying degrees of success in treating symptomatic women. Since methylxanthines (caffeine, theophylline) and nicotine have been implicated in the etiopathogenesis of fibrocystic change, it seems reasonable and harmless to advise symptomatic patients to reduce their methylxanthine intake (coffee, chocolate, tea) and to refrain from smoking. This has been reported to be effective in up to 65% of patients (Minton et al, 1979). However, other authors, although documenting lowered levels of cAMP, report little clinical consequence or benefit associated with these measures (Ernster et al, 1982).

VITAMIN E

In small studies, vitamin E has shown some efficacy in treating fibrocystic change. However, the data are controversial and have not been substantiated in double-blind, randomized, controlled studies (London et al, 1985).

Vitamin E functions as an antioxidant. It also regulates the synthesis of specific proteins and enzymes. Through this mechanism, it may alter serum gonadotropins and adrenal gonadotropins. It has been reported to reduce the risk of atherosclerosis and coronary vascular disease by increasing HDL and decreasing LDL (Levy, 1983). Some patients report significant improvement in breast symptoms when dietary fat is reduced from 40% of the caloric intake to 15% to 20% (Boyd et al, 1988). At least in theory, vitamin E may be most useful in women with fibrocystic breast disease and low plasma levels of HDL and high levels of LDL (Gonzalez, 1980; Vorheer, 1986).

VITAMIN A

Vitamin A has been helpful in more than half of the patients treated for fibrocystic change (Ellerhorst-Ryan et al, 1988). With daily doses of 150,000 IU, side effects were generally mild; however, 25% of the patients required dose adjustment or complete discontinuation of vitamin A because of toxicity. This study involved too few patients, and the results need to be corroborated.

HORMONAL THERAPY

Oral Contraceptives. If the cause of fibrocystic change is a relative estrogen excess or a relative progesterone deficiency, OCs may prove helpful. The pill has been reported to be effective in up to 90% of women within 3 to 6 months of initiation of treatment. Additional advantages of the pill include protection from the development of fibroadenomas (London et al, 1982). Following discontinuation of OCs, 30% to 40% of the patients experience recurrent symptoms.

Progestins. Progestins may be helpful in patients with a luteal-phase deficiency. An oral dose of 5 to 10 mg of medroxyprogesterone acetate administered on the 15th to 25th day of the menstrual cycle has been reported to be effective in up to 85% of treated patients (London et al, 1982). In patients with more pronounced fibrocystic changes, progesterone can be given from the 4th day of the cycle to the 25th day. However, patients may experience metrorrhagia. An alternative approach is to give 10 mg/day of medroxyprogesterone acetate from the 10th day to the 25th day, which will decrease the irregular bleeding. This treatment is maintained for 9 to 12 months. Approximately 40% of the patients experience recurrence following discontinuation of the medication (Vorheer, 1986).

Danazol. This is an antigonadotropin androgen derivative that prevents the midcycle luteinizing hormone surge. It may reduce hormonal stimulation of the breast through suppression of gonadotropins, through enzymatic inhibition of sex steroid synthesis, and by competitively binding sex steroid receptors. It is usually given in doses of 50 to 400 mg/day for 2 to 6 months. Doses up to 600 mg/day have been administered. Side effects are dose related and include menstrual irregularities, weight gain, facial hair, acne, clitoromegaly, and deepening of the voice (Brookshaw, 1979). Other side effects include hot flushes, atrophic vaginitis, hypertension, and liver dysfunction (cholestatic jaundice). Danazol is very expensive. It has been reported effective in 70% to 90% of patients; however, the symptoms may return following discontinuation of the drug, although they may not be as severe.

Bromocriptine. Bromocriptine is a prolactin inhibitor. Plasma prolactin has been found slightly increased in approximately 30% of women with fibrocystic change of the breast. Because most patients have normal levels, its role in the etiopathogenesis of fibrocystic disease is unclear. An alternative mechanism of action may be related to the secondary changes in serum progesterone. In women with borderline hyperprolactinemia, elevated prolactin levels may indirectly increase progesterone secretion. This may be important in women with luteal-phase deficiency.

The recommended dose is 5.0 to 7.5 mg/day. About 60% to 80% of patients will experience subjective and objective improvement. Side effects include nausea, headache, and dizziness. The impact of long-term administration is unknown.

Tamoxifen. This is a triphenylethylene compound that prevents the uptake of radioactive estradiol by estrogen receptors, especially in mammary and uterine tissues. It is absorbed orally, with peak serum concentration obtained after 3 hours. It is currently approved for use in the treatment of breast cancer. A reported, although unapproved, use of tamoxifen is in the treatment or management of cyclic mastalgia. Its efficacy has been documented in both controlled and uncontrolled studies (Eggert-Kruse et al, 1984; Fentiman et al, 1986).

Tamoxifen appears to be as effective as danazol, with perhaps fewer side effects. Side effects are dose related. Relapse rates do not appear to be dose related. With doses of 10 to 20 mg/day, a relapse rate of 50% has been reported for both groups when treated for 3 months. Increasing the duration of treatment has not altered the relapse rate (Fentiman and Caleffi, 1988). The side effects include menstrual irregularity, vaginal discharge, hot flushes, occasional nausea, and bloating. Because administration of this drug has been associated with endometrial cancer, it is not recommended for the treatment of fibrocystic change (Fisher et al, 1994). Tamoxifen can stimulate ovulation; therefore, protected intercourse is necessary to prevent pregnancies.

The side effects of long-term administration are unknown in premenopausal women. It is not approved for use in cyclic mastalgia. Until more studies are available, it seems premature to use tamoxifen in the treatment of fibrocystic disease (Fentiman, 1988).

LHRH Analog. In a small study, LHRH was evaluated for the treatment of chronic fibrocystic changes in women at high risk for breast carcinoma. All patients received intramuscular injections of LHRH agonist for 3 to 6 months. A complete response was observed in half of the treated patients (Monsonego et al, 1991), although some of the patients received other treatments as well. Because LHRH induces a menopausal status, prolonged therapy is not recommended. Larger clinical trials are needed.

SURGICAL THERAPY

A needle aspiration should be performed for patients with macrocysts and whenever clinical examination, ultrasound, or mammography suggests a carcinoma. Surgical excision may be necessary when fluid cannot be aspirated from a cyst or for a residual mass or recurrent cyst following needle aspiration.

BREAST SCREENING

The ability to accurately predict the development of breast cancer is far from optimal. A major prospective study revealed that only 29% of patients with breast cancer in the 55- to 84-year age group had a known risk factor (Seidman et al, 1982). Although it is important to recognize the risk factors associated with this disease, it is clear that most patients do not have detectable or recognizable risk factors. Thus all women need to be carefully screened.

It is estimated that there will have been 180,200 new cases of breast cancer in the United States in 1997 (American Cancer Society [ACS], 1997). Breast cancer develops in approximately one in nine women over a lifetime based on a life expectancy of 85 years. Early detection and improved treatment have kept mortality rates fairly stable. Stage is an important determinant of survival. The 5-year survival rate for localized breast cancer has risen from 78% in the 1940s to 90% in the 1990s. When breast cancer is detected in an in situ stage, the survival rate approaches 100%. To find a cancer in an asymptomatic woman requires periodic screening. Thus it is important that the physician become adept at breast examination, teaching breast self-examination (BSE), and ordering periodic mammograms for eligible patients.

Physical Examination

Women who have had annual medical examinations have significantly smaller tumors and fewer lymph node metastases at the time of detection of breast cancer than those who have not had annual breast examinations (Senie et al, 1981). A breast examination should be performed annually in women older than age 40. Prior to age 40, a breast examination should be performed by the patient's physician or health care provider every 3 years. In a survey of physicians' attitudes and practices conducted by the ACS in 1984, only 11% of primary care physicians followed the accepted guidelines for annual breast examination and mammography in women older than age 40. An updated survey revealed that 37% of primary care physicians followed the accepted guidelines for annual breast examination and mammography (ACS, 1990). A survey completed in 1992 by the Jacobs Institute of Women's Health showed that 56% of women in their 40s and 47% of women in their 50s were in compliance with screening guidelines as recommended by the ACS (Horton et al, 1992). In 1995, these same investigators found 47.4% of women in the United States complying with mammography screening guidelines as recommended by the ACS (Horton et al, 1996). Seventy per cent of the women reported that their health care provider recommended that they have their most recent mammogram. Obstetricians and gynecologists far exceed general internists and family practitioners in following published guidelines for breast cancer screening. In a survey of more than 1000 primary care physicians conducted by the ACS, 81% said they were more inclined to order a screening mammogram in an asymptomatic patient as compared with in 1984 (ACS, 1990).

A careful and well-performed breast examination should include not only the breast but also the axilla and supraclavicular nodal areas. Examination should begin with the patient in the sitting position. The patient's arms are raised above her head and then flexed on her hips. The physician should look for signs of retraction or erythema and marked degrees of asymmetry. The patient should be examined in the sitting and lying positions. The physician must apply firm but gentle pressure using the fingertips to palpate all quadrants of the entire breast, including the area under the nipple. The physical findings should be described as completely and as thoroughly as possible.

In general, a breast lesion must be 1 cm in diameter to be easily palpable. When discovered by professionals, the average size of a palpable lesion is 2.5 cm. With a malignant lesion, the likelihood of lymph node metastasis in a 2.5-cm lesion is approximately 50%. Physician and patient reluctance must be overcome to continue to detect breast cancers in an early stage.

Breast Self-Examination

In theory, a well-trained patient who practices BSE can improve her survival by detecting breast masses when they are very small and presumably at an early stage. However, the magnitude of reduction in mortality attributable to BSE is uncertain. Some reports find that BSE is associated with favorable tumor characteristics and earlier stages of disease, whereas others report no significant advantage (Foster et al, 1978; Baker, 1982). Some physicians have expressed concern that BSE may lead to unwarranted patient anxiety, false reassurance, or unnecessary medical investigations, particularly in patients younger than 35 years (Frank and May, 1985).

The success of BSE is directly related to the instruction given to the patient as well as to the patient's age, education, and income level. The more educated the patient, the more likely she is to perform BSE. Women younger than 35 years seem more receptive to BSE (Mant et al, 1987).

BSE should be performed monthly with systematic examination of the breast and axilla both visually and by palpation. The breasts are easiest to examine immediately following the menses. The California Division of the ACS (1988) has published the seven Ps of BSE: physician, perimeters, palpation, pressure, patterns of search, practice with feedback, and plan of action. The patient should be instructed by the physician or a trained substitute to lie with a pillow under her back. The perimeter should include the boundaries of the breast from the clavicle to the axilla to the sternum and to the bottom of the breast. The patient should palpate carefully with the finger pads, applying the appropriate pressure. The technique of BSE should be observed by a trained health professional. Once the patient detects any abnormality, she should consult a health professional. At least in theory, BSE, together with a physician's examination, should detect cancers that are smaller in size and subsequently result in a better prognosis.

Ultrasonography

Sonography is helpful as an adjunct to clinical examination and mammography. Ultrasonography will reduce the number of biopsies by separating cysts from solid and undeterminate lesions, which require further evaluations. Simple cysts do not require aspiration or biopsy (Jackson, 1995). Sonography was initially used only to differentiate cystic and solid lesions. With the development of 7.5- to 10-MHz linear array transducers, sonography may also be used to characterize both palpable and nonpalpable masses and provide needle guidance for localization, aspiration, and biopsy (Evans, 1995). Indications for breast ultrasound are listed in Table 49–3. Ultrasonic tissue characterization, pulsed Doppler, and color Doppler have all been investigated as methods to differentiate between benign and malignant solid masses. Careful research with large sample sizes is necessary to determine whether these modalities and features are any more reliable than the "classical"

Table 49–3. INDICATIONS FOR BREAST ULTRASOUND

Differentiation of cysts from solid masses
Evaluation of a palpable mass that is not visible in a radiographically dense breast
Assessment of a mass that cannot be completely evaluated with mammography because of location
Evaluation of a young patient with a palpable mass
Evaluation for an abscess

Courtesy of Parke-Davis, a Division of Warner-Lambert Company. Adapted from Jackson VP: The current role of ultrasonography in breast imaging. Radiol Clin North Am 1995;33:1161, with permission.

sonographic findings described in the early 1980s (Jackson, 1995).

Mammography

Mammography is a radiographic procedure used to visualize breast tissue. Available published data demonstrate that widespread use of mammography and clinical examination can reduce the mortality associated with breast cancer in women older than 40 years. In the 1960s, the Health Insurance Plan of New York demonstrated, in a randomized study, that mammography was capable of reducing the mortality associated with breast cancer in women older than 50 years (Shapiro, 1977). A survey in 1995 revealed that only 47.4% of women in the United States were following ACS screening guidelines (Horton et al, 1996). The proportion who reported that they were following guidelines declined with age from a high of 51.8% for women 40 to 49 years of age to as low as 40.4% of women 65 years of age and older.

A joint statement on mammography guidelines was issued in July 1989 from 12 of the nation's largest health care and medical research organizations that recommended that the screening process begin by age 40 and consist of annual clinical examinations and screening mammography at 1- to 2-year intervals; at age 50, women should have both clinical examination and mammography annually (Vanchieri, 1989). However, in December 1993, the National Cancer Institute (NCI) announced that it would no longer recommend routine mammography screening for all women in their 40s and replaced its screening guidelines with a statement of evidence regarding mammography. The statement of evidence specifies the benefits of mammography screening for women of different ages and, rather than providing a specific screening guideline for women in their 40s, advises women under age 50 to speak with their health care providers about their risk for breast cancer and make their own informed decisions about mammography. The NCI based this recommendation on the results of the International Workshop on Screening for Breast Cancer. These results indicated that mammography screening reduced mortality in women ages

50 to 70 by up to 30% but found no significant reduction in mortality for women ages 40 to 49, at 5 to 8 years after screening (Fletcher et al, 1993). In 1997, the NIH Consensus Development Statement on Breast Cancer Screening for Women Ages 40–49 concluded that the available data do not warrant a single recommendation for mammography for all women in their 40s. They recommend that each woman decide for herself. Her decision should be based not only on an objective analysis of the scientific evidence and consideration of her individual medical history, but also on how she perceives and weighs each potential risk and benefit, the values the woman places on each, and how she deals with uncertainty.

However, because breast cancer is the single leading cause of death for women ages 40 to 49 in the United States, not all leading organizations and experts agree with the NIH Consensus Statement. The majority of population-based randomized clinical trials that included women ages 40 to 49 years have shown mortality reductions associated with screening ranging from 22% to 49% for this age group with longer term follow-up (>7 years) (Smart et al, 1995). Critics of these data suggest that this reduction in mortality may be due to other factors such as trial design and the use of mammography after age 49 in the screening group (NIH Consensus Development Conference, 1997).

Although women in their 40s have dense breasts, several studies suggest that faster cancer growth rates are more important reasons for the higher interval rates and consequently lower efficacy of screening in this age group (Tabar et al, 1987; Moskowitz, 1994; Kerlikowske et al, 1996). A higher proportion of invasive cancers among women ages 40 to 49 may be detected by annual screening. Potential adverse consequences of more frequent screening include the consequences of false-positive tests, radiation risk, and cost. However, even for annual screening for women ages 40 to 49 years, radiation risk is negligible compared with expected benefits (Feig, 1995).

Machines dedicated to mammography have been constructed to be more efficient and place less strain on the equipment, patient, and technician. The actual absorbed radiation dose to the breast depends on a number of factors, including the type of recording medium, the target material in the tube, the kilovoltage applied, the radiation filtration, the thickness of the breast, compression techniques, density of the film, and film-processing techniques. With film-screen techniques, the average dose at accredited mammography facilities in the United States was reported to be 1.38 mGy per view (Mettler et al, 1996). Radiation-related breast cancers occur at least 10 years after exposure. Radiation from yearly mammograms during ages 40 to 49 has been estimated to cause one additional breast cancer per 10,000 women (NIH Consensus Development Conference, 1997). For a woman who begins annual screening at age 35

and continues until age 75, the benefit of reduced mortality is projected to exceed the radiation risk by a factor of more than 25 (Mettler et al, 1996).

Two views of each breast are routinely ordered: craniocaudal and mediolateral oblique. If there is a mammographic abnormality, cone-down compression and magnification views are obtained to clarify lesions and improve image quality. On standard views, success in mammography depends on the type of breast being examined as well as the technique. Fatty breasts are more accurately visualized than are dense, fibroglandular breasts. A mammogram may not show a palpable mass, especially in a younger woman with dense breasts, in a woman on hormone replacement therapy, or in the presence of other factors that cause radiographically dense breasts. The literature documents a 10% to 15% false-negative rate in mammography. Thus it is important to obtain biopsy specimens or to perform a needle aspiration on all palpable breast lesions.

The value of breast cancer screening programs is evidenced by an analysis of the Breast Cancer Detection Demonstration Project. These data show an 87% 5-year survival rate and an 81% 8-year survival rate for screened patients with invasive breast cancers compared with an unscreened group with 74% and 65% 5-year and 8-year survival rates, respectively. As expected, the highest survival rate occurred in cases of occult breast cancer detected by mammography alone, with a 94% 8-year survival rate (Seidman et al, 1987).

The vast majority of mammographically detected masses are benign. A positive predictive value for mammography in detecting carcinoma has been reported to be 30% (Ciatto et al, 1987). This means that, for every 100 women undergoing biopsy, 30 have a malignant lesion and 70 have a benign process. To prevent overinterpretation of benign or nonexisting abnormalities, the mammogram must be carefully reviewed. If necessary, another radiologist should review the films. The margin analysis of a mass can be improved with spot compression mammography. Spot compression with magnification can aid in assessment of masses with associated calcifications (Schepps et al, 1994).

An infiltrative mass with a spiculated appearance, numerous (>five) grouped sand-like microcalcifications, and localized areas of trabecular distortion are mammographic signs of malignancy (Figs. 49–7 and 49–15). The microcalcifications represent necrotic intraductal material. They are present in about 30% of breast cancers. Malignancy (excluding lobular carcinoma in situ) was found in 24% of biopsies performed for microcalcifications in one series (Hall et al, 1988). Microcalcifications are not pathognomonic of malignancy because they can occur in benign lesions, such as sclerosing adenosis. Benign microcalcifications are more likely to be round, similar in size and shape, and regional or diffuse/scattered. They often are bilateral even if asymmetric (Monsees, 1995).

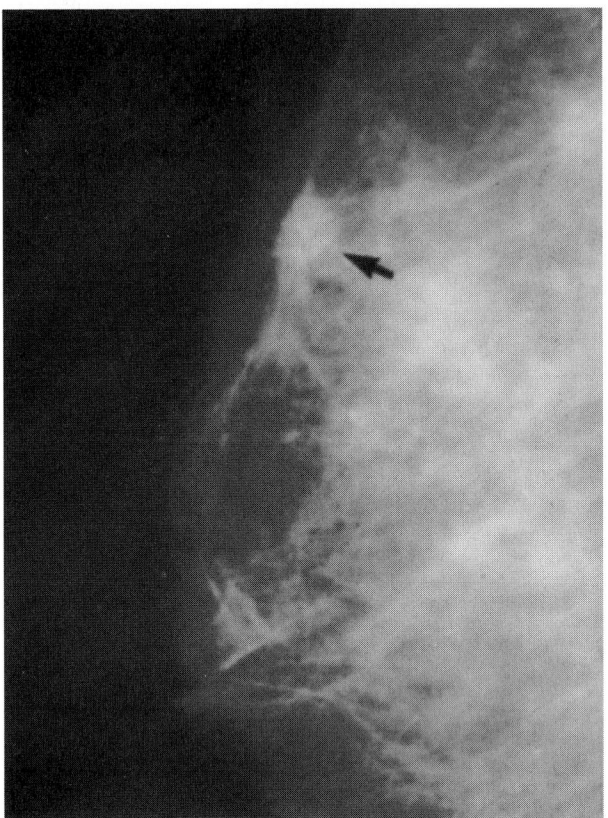

Figure 49–15
Mammogram with characteristic findings of a malignancy. The *arrow* identifies a spiculated mass.

The mammographic appearance of a benign mass is a well-circumscribed, round or oval lesion. These masses displace normal breast tissue. They are homogeneous in density, with occasional large, regular, scattered macrocalcifications. An intraductal papilloma is characteristically seen in the line of the ducts in the subareolar region. A fibroadenoma may calcify in older women and appear as a well-circumscribed, homogeneous mass (see Fig. 49–9). Phyllodes, a variant of fibroadenoma, appears as a well-demarcated, large density. On clinical examination, a lipoma forms a discrete firm mass that has a characteristic mammographic appearance. Fibrocystic changes may appear as symmetric or increased areas of density on mammography.

Film-screen mammography has been used in the imaging evaluation of breast implants. Three views (craniocaudal, mediolateral, axillary) of each breast with spot compression views may be helpful in some patients. A manual rather than phototimer technique may be necessary (Mitnick et al, 1989). Pushing the implant posteriorly to demonstrate the anterior breast parenchyma may improve accuracy but may be difficult in patients with fibrosis. Mammography has two major limitations when evaluating breast implants: (1) the entire implant cannot be consistently displayed and (2) the diagnosis of intracapsular rupture is limited. High-resolution sonography

and magnetic resonance imaging (MRI) are excellent tools for the evaluation of the integrity of breast implants (Jackson, 1990; Reynolds, 1995).

Mammography cannot replace a physician's examination or BSE but should be used in conjunction to most effectively screen for breast cancer in asymptomatic women. With dedicated modern equipment, radiation exposure is minimal.

MRI of the Breast

Breast MRI is undergoing clinical investigation to determine its role in evaluating the breast for benign and malignant changes. Because of the high cost of breast MRI, cost effectiveness is a major hurdle to its widespread use. The dense parenchyma that lowers the sensitivity of film-screen mammography is not a deterrent for lesion detection in contrast-enhanced MRI. The tomographic capability permits visualization of tissues close to implants of the chest wall. MRI cannot detect microcalcifications. Many benign and normal tissues enhance, resulting in a low specificity (Stelling, 1995).

Positron Emission Tomography

Positron emission tomography scanning has been used to evaluate breast masses. Small studies have reported high sensitivity and specificity (over 90%) (Adler et al, 1993). The lack of availability and cost may limit the use of this modality.

MANAGEMENT OF A BREAST MASS

Palpable Breast Mass

Once a breast mass has been detected by the patient or the physician, management is tailored according to the patient's age, physical findings, and risk factors. Under age 30, the most likely cause of a palpable mass is nodular breast tissue, fibrosis, fibroadenoma, or cyst (Palmer and Tsangaris, 1993). In a young menstruating woman, a second physical examination following the menses is recommended before a complete work-up is begun. The initial evaluation should be with sonography or an attempt at aspiration rather than mammography. The management depends on the results of the sonogram. Simple cysts may be followed or aspirated. For suspicious masses, a mammogram is performed prior to aspiration or biopsy. If no mass is identified, the patient may be followed unless the clinical examination is suspicious or suggestive of malignancy. A mammogram followed by a biopsy is necessary in these cases. For solid masses, excisional biopsy is recommended. However, if a needle aspirate is consistent with a fibroadenoma, conservative follow-up is an option.

In patients 30 years of age or older, a mammogram is performed to assess the remainder of the involved breast and the contralateral breast (Fig. 49–16). Supplemental views may improve visualization. Ultrasound may be useful in distinguishing cystic from solid masses. Because of hematoma formation, a mammogram precedes a fine-needle aspiration or follows the cytologic procedure by an interval of at least 2 weeks.

Fine-needle aspiration is an important first step in the evaluation of a palpable breast lesion. It can be performed in the office and may avoid the need for a biopsy. Fine-needle aspiration requires the availability of a trained and skilled cytopathologist. False-positive cytologic findings from needle aspirations may result from atypical epithelial proliferations, fibroadenomas, or inflammatory lesions. False-negative results may occur as a result of technical errors or the underdiagnosis of a low-grade neoplasm. If the cyst fluid is clear, it can be discarded. Malignancies will not be missed if the fluid is clear, if there is no residual mass following aspiration, and if the cyst does not recur. The patient should be re-evaluated in 1 month and again in 2 months (Hamed et al, 1989).

If a specific benign or malignant cytologic diagnosis is not obtained by fine-needle aspiration, a fine-needle biopsy should be performed. With the combination of physical examination, fine-needle aspiration or biopsy, and mammography, open biopsies are rarely needed (Layfield et al, 1989). Although some surgeons perform a mastectomy or segmental resection (lumpectomy) on the basis of a fine-needle aspirate, most surgeons require a tissue diagnosis with either a needle biopsy, open biopsy, or confirmation at surgery with a frozen section analysis (Winchester, 1984).

Fine-needle aspiration is performed with a 22-gauge needle and a 10-ml syringe (Fig. 49–17). The skin is prepared. The needle is inserted into the center of the mass and is moved back and forth. The

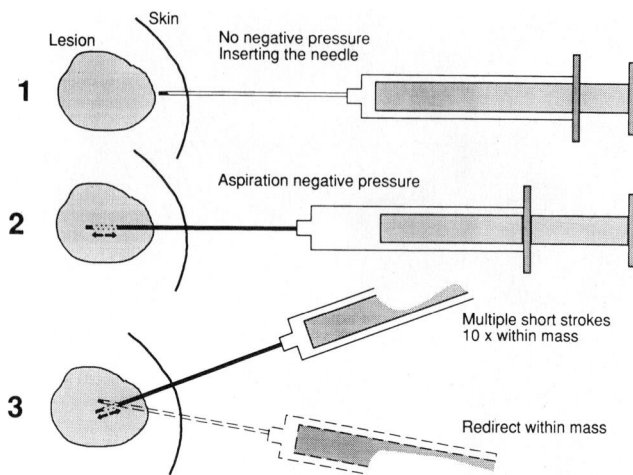

Figure 49–17
Photoillustration demonstrating the technique of needle aspiration of a palpable breast mass.

negative pressure is released prior to withdrawal of the needle. The fluid is put on a slide and fixed as one would fix a Papanicolaou smear. Fine-needle aspiration can be performed with cystic and solid breast lesions; however, some physicians restrict needle aspiration to cystic lesions only. A review of 31,340 fine-needle aspiration biopsies indicates that the sensitivity and specificity vary widely between reporting groups. The reported sensitivity ranged from 65% to 98% and the specificity from 34% to 100% (Hermans, 1992).

A fine-needle biopsy secures a core of tissue for a pathologic diagnosis. An open biopsy requires careful planning of the skin incision. The incision should be periareolar or in Langer's lines to maximize effective healing. Local anesthesia can be used in an outpatient procedure.

Nonpalpable Breast Mass (Fig. 49–18)

A nonpalpable mammographic mass found to be oval, round, or slightly lobulated with relatively well-circumscribed margins may be further evaluated by sonography. Simple cysts need only aspiration and/or routine follow-up. Solid lesions may be evaluated with spot compression films. If significant irregularities are detected, biopsy is recommended (Evans, 1995).

Management of a solid nonpalpable, noncalcified, well-circumscribed mass is controversial. A survey of the Fellows of the Society of Breast Imaging found that periodic mammographic follow-up was appropriate for lesions less than 2.0 cm (Hall, 1993). In a study of more than 3000 women with nonpalpable, probably benign breast lesions followed by serial mammography over a 3- to 3.5-year follow-up, 17 cases of malignancy were detected. Fifteen of the 17 cancers were identified by means of an interval

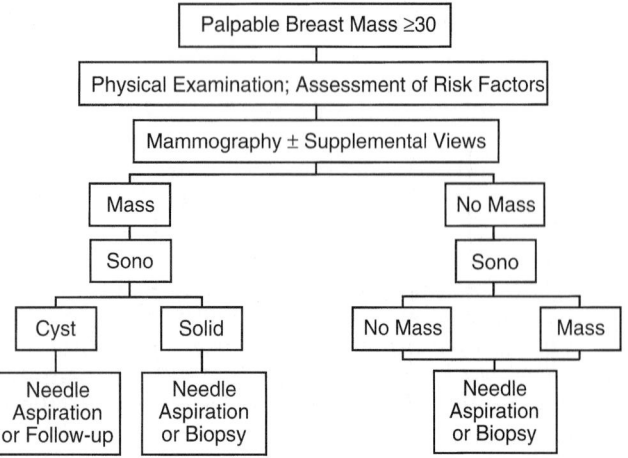

Figure 49–16
Management of palpable breast mass. Sono, ultrasonography.

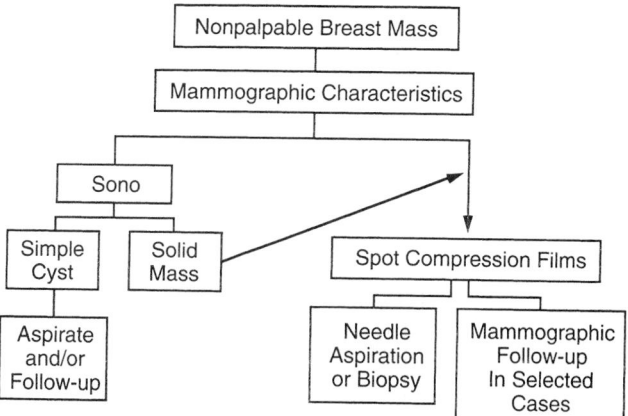

Figure 49–18
Management of nonpalpable breast mass. Sono, ultrasonography.

mammographic change. All 17 cases were Stage 0/I (Sickles, 1991).

Once it has been determined that a biopsy is needed, ultrasound or radiologic guidance is necessary to biopsy a nonpalpable mass. Radiographic localization with a guide wire or a dye injection may

be performed. After the biopsy specimen has been taken, there is a need to confirm radiographically that the lesion, which is not grossly apparent, is present in the tissue specimen. An x-ray film of the removed tissue is required (see Figs. 49–19 and 49–20). Computerized stereotaxic core biopsy of the breast has proved to be a reliable method for evaluation of nonpalpable mammographic lesions. It provides an alternative to open biopsy (Elvecrog et al, 1993). Ultrasonographically guided fine-needle aspiration biopsy is another method that is comparable to mammographic and stereotactic methods (Saarela et al, 1996).

SUMMARY

The obstetrician-gynecologist is in a unique position to provide total health care for the female patient. Studies have documented the competency of the obstetrician-gynecologist in managing breast lesions and screening for breast cancer. This responsibility implies knowledge of breast anatomy, physiology, and pathology. The residency programs in obstetrics and gynecology in the United States are now emphasizing the management of breast disease as part of the training program. However, for clinicians in

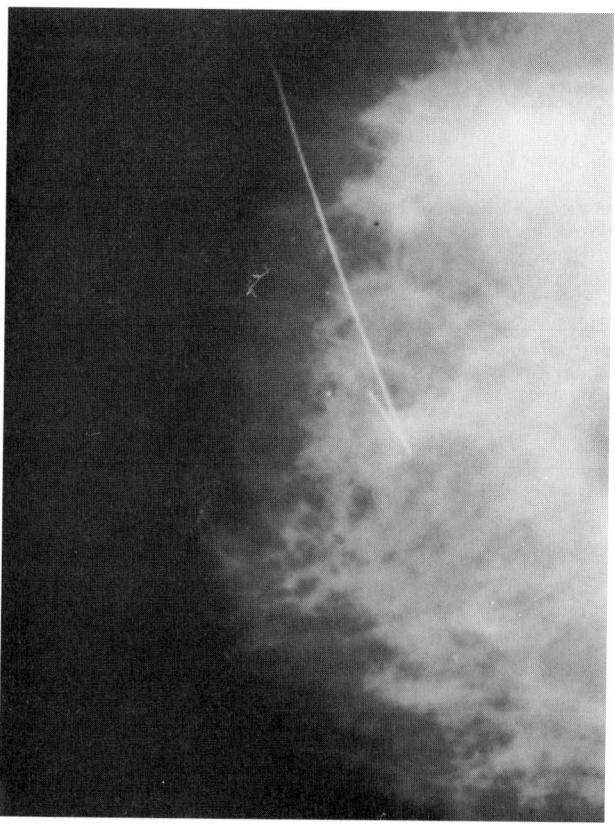

Figure 49–19
A nonpalpable finding on mammography of a cluster of microcalcifications. A needle is placed radiographically, and an open biopsy of the surrounding tissue is performed (needle-directed biopsy). The calcifications are difficult to see in this photograph.

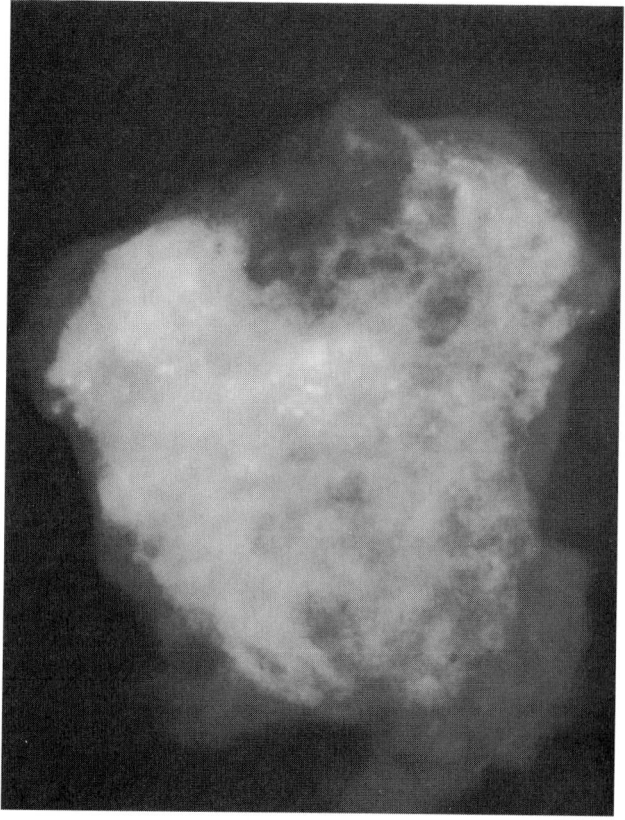

Figure 49–20
A radiograph of the biopsy specimen from Figure 49–19, confirming that the microcalcifications are in the resected specimen.

practice, self-education through journals, textbooks, postgraduate courses, and apprenticeships will be required to maintain current knowledge so that patients can be properly counseled and treated and an impact on the early detection of breast disease can be achieved.

REFERENCES

Adler L, Crowe J, Al-Kaisi N, et al: Evaluation of breast masses and axillary nodes with [F-18] 2-deoxy-2-fluoro-D-glucose PET. Radiology 1993;187:743.

American Cancer Society: Cancer Facts and Figures. Atlanta, GA: American Cancer Society, 1997.

American Cancer Society. (Publication no. 634.42). Oakland: California Division, American Cancer Society, 1988.

American Cancer Society: 1989 survey of physician's attitudes and practices in early cancer detection. CA Cancer J Clin 1990; 40:77.

Auerbach KG, Avery JL: Induced lactation. Am J Dis Child 1981; 135:340.

Baker LH: Breast cancer detection demonstration project: 5-year summary. Cancer 1982;32:194.

Barber C, Libshitz H: Bilateral fat necrosis of the breast following reduction mammoplasty. Am J Roentgenol 1977;128:508.

BeLieu RM: Mastodynia. Obstet Gynecol Clin North Am 1994;21: 461.

Boyd NF, McGuire V, Shannon P, et al: Effect of a low fat, high carbohydrate diet on symptoms of mastopathy. Lancet 1988;2: 128.

Brookshaw JD: Danazol treatment of benign breast disease: a survey of USA multicenter studies. Postgrad Med J Suppl 1979;5: 58.

Brumsted JR, Riddick DH: The breast during pregnancy and lactation. In Sciarra JJ (ed): Gynecology and Obstetrics, Vol 5: Reproductive Endocrinology, Infertility and Genetics (Speroff L, Simpson JL, eds). Philadelphia: JB Lippincott Company, 1990a: 1.

Brumsted JR, Riddick DH: The nonlactating human breast. In Sciarra JJ (ed): Gynecology and Obstetrics, Vol 5: Speroff L, Reproductive Endocrinology, Infertility and Genetics (Speroff L, Simpson JL, eds). Philadelphia: JB Lippincott Company, 1990b:1.

Bundred NJ, Dixon JMJ, Lumsden AB, et al: Are the lesions of duct ectasia sterile? Br J Surg 1985;72:844.

Catania S, Zurrida S, Veronesi P, et al: Mondor's disease in breast cancer. Cancer 1992;69:2267.

Ciatto S, Cataliotti L, Distante V: Nonpalpable breast lesions: accuracy of pre-biopsy. Radiology 1987;165:99.

Clement PB, Young RH, Azzopardi JG: Collagenous spherulosis of the breast. Am J Surg Pathol 1987;11:411.

Consensus statement: is "fibrocystic disease" of the breast precancerous? (Consensus meeting 10/13–10/15, 1985). Arch Pathol Lab Med 1986;110:171.

Devitt JE: Benign breast disease in the postmenopausal woman. World J Surg 1989;13:731.

DiSaia PJ, Creasman WT: Clinical Gynecologic Oncology. 3rd ed. St. Louis; CV Mosby Company, 1993:467.

Dixon JM: Periductal mastitis/duct ectasia. World J Surg 1989;13: 715.

Dixon JM, Anderson TJ, Lumsden AB, et al: Mammary duct ectasia. Br J Surg 1983;70:601.

Dixon JM, Lee ECG, Greenhall MJ: Treatment of periareolar inflammation associated with periductal mastitis using metronidazole and flucloxacillin: a preliminary report. Br J Clin Pract 1988;42:78.

Dogliotti L, Orlandi F, Angeli A: The endocrine basis of benign breast disorders. World J Surg 1989;13:674.

Drukker BH, de Mendonca WC: Benign diseases of the breast. In Sciarra JJ (ed): Gynecology and Obstetrics, Vol 1: Clinical Gynecology. (Droegemueller W, ed). Philadelphia: JB Lippincott Company, 1988:1.

Dupont WD, Page DL: Risk factors for breast cancer in women with proliferative breast disease. N Engl J Med 1985;312:146.

Eggert-Kruse W, VonSurnier D, Legler V, Junkerman H: Comparison of danazol with tamoxifen, gestagen, acupuncture, local treatment and placebo. In Baum M, George WD, Hughes LE (eds): Benign Breast Disease. London: Royal Society of Medicine, 1984.

Eickman FM: Recurrent myocardial infarction in a postpartum patient receiving bromocriptine. Clin Cardiol 1992;15:781.

Ellerhorst-Ryan JM, Turba EP, Stahl DL: Evaluating benign breast disease. Nurse Pract 1988;13:13.

Elvecrog EL, Lechner MC, Nelson MT: Nonpalpable breast lesions: correlation of stereotaxic large-core needle biopsy and surgical biopsy results. Radiology 1993;188:453.

Ernster VL: The epidemiology of benign breast disease. Epidemiol Rev 1981;3:184.

Ernster VL, Goodson WH III, Hunt TK, et al: Vitamin E and benign breast "disease": a double-blind, randomized clinical trial. Surgery 1985;97:490.

Ernster VL, Mason L, Goodson WH III, et al: Effects of caffeine-free diet on benign breast disease: a randomized trial. Surgery 1982;91:263.

Evans WP: Breast masses: appropriate evaluation. Radiol Clin North Am 1995;6:1085.

Feig SA: Mammographic screening of women age 40-49 years: benefit, risk and cost considerations. Cancer 1995;76:2097.

Fentiman IS: Tamoxifen: use in benign conditions. Br J Clin Pract 1988;42:384.

Fentiman IS, Caleffi M: Dosage, duration and effect on bone mineral content of tamoxifen treatment for mastalgia. Br J Clin Pract Suppl 1988;56:18.

Fentiman IS, Caleffi M, Brame K, et al: Double-blind controlled trial of tamoxifen therapy for mastalgia. Lancet 1986;1:287.

Fentiman IS, Hamed H: Clinical assessment of patients with mastalgia. Br J Clin Pract 1989;68:21.

Ferguson D, Anderson T: Morphological evaluation of cell turnover in relation to the menstrual cycle in the "resting" human breast. Br J Cancer 1981;44:177.

Fisher B, Constantino JP, Redmond CK, et al: Endometrial cancer in tamoxifen-treated breast cancer patients: findings from the National Surgical Adjuvant Breast and Bowel Project (NSABP) B-14. J Natl Cancer Inst 1994;86:527.

Fletcher SW, Black W, Harris R, et al: Report of the International Workshop on Screening for Breast Cancer. J Natl Cancer Inst 1993;85:1644.

Foster RS, Lang SP, Constanza MC, et al: Breast self-examination practices and breast cancer stage. N Engl J Med 1978;299:265.

Frank JW, May V: Breast self examination in young women: more harm than good? Lancet 1985;2:654.

Gateley CA, Miers M, Mansel RE, et al: Drug treatments for mastalgia: 17 years experience in the Cardiff mastalgia clinic. J R Soc Med 1992;85:12.

Gittelman DK: Bromocriptine associated with postpartum hypertension, seizures and pituitary hemorrhage. Gen Hosp Psychiatry 1991;73:278.

Gonzalez ER: Vitamin E relieves most cystic breast disease; may alter lipid hormones. JAMA 1980;244:1077.

Goodwin PJ, Neelam M, Boyd NF: Cyclical mastopathy: a critical review of therapy. Br J Surg 1988;75:837.

Grignon DJ, Ro JY, MacKay Bn, et al: Collagenosis spherulous of the breast: immunohistochemical and ultrastructural studies. Am J Clin Pathol 1989;91:386.

Gump FE, McDermott J: Fibrous disease of the breast in juvenile diabetics. N Y State J Med 1990;90:356.

Haagensen CD: Diseases of the Breast. 3rd ed. Philadelphia: WB Saunders Company, 1986.

Haagensen CD, Bodian C, Haagensen DE: Breast Carcinoma: Risk and Detection. Philadelphia: WB Saunders Company, 1981.

Hall F: Statistics, opinions and controversies among expert mammographers. Breast Dis 1993;6:173.

Hall FM, Storella JM, Silverstone DZ, et al: Nonpalpable breast lesions: recommendations for biopsy based on suspicion of carcinoma at mammography. Radiology 1988;167:353.

Hall JA, Hall BR, Murphy DC, Hale KA: Surgical management of breast disease in an obstetrics and gynecology group. Am J Obstet Gynecol 1990;162:1526.

Hamed H, Coady A, Chaudary MA, Fentiman IS: Follow-up of patients with aspirated breast cysts is necessary. Arch Surg 1989;124:253.

Hartrampf CR Jr, Bennett GK: Autogenous tissue reconstruction in the mastectomy patient: a critical review of 300 patients. Ann Surg 1987;205:508.

Hermans J: The value of aspiration cytologic examination of the breast: a statistical review of the medical literature. Cancer 1992;69:2104.

Hindi-Alexander MC, Zielezny MA, Montes N, et al: Theophylline and fibrocystic disease. J Allergy Clin Immunol 1985;75:709.

Holleb AI, Farrow JH: The significance of nipple discharge. CA Cancer J Clin 1966;16:182.

Homer MJ, Pile-Spellman ER, Marchant DJ, Smith TJ: The normal intra-mammary lymph node: mammographic appearance and management. Appl Radiol 1985;14:115.

Horton JA, Cruess DF, Romans MC: Compliance with mammographic screening guidelines: 1995 mammography attitudes and usage study report. Women's Health Issues 1996;6:239.

Horton JA, Romans MC, Cruess DF: Mammography attitudes and usage study, 1992. Women's Health Issues 1992;2:180.

Hughes LE, Mansel RE, Webster DJT: Abnormalities of normal development and involution (ANDI): a new perspective on pathogenesis and nomenclature of benign breast disease. Lancet 1987;2:1316.

Issacs JH: Benign tumors of the breast. Obstet Gynecol Clin North Am 1994;21:487.

Jackson VP: The role of ultrasound in breast imaging. Radiology 1990;177:305.

Jackson VP: The current role of ultrasonography in breast imaging. Radiology Clin North Am 1995;33:1161.

Kerlikowske K, Grady D, Barclay J, et al: Effect of age, breast density and family history on the sensitivity of first screening mammography. JAMA 1996;276:33.

Kinne DW, DeCosse JJ: New developments in the management of breast disease. Surg Annu 1981;13:163.

Klijn JG, Van Geel B, deJong FH, et al: The relation between pharmacokinetics and endocrine effects of buserelin implants in patients with mastalgia. Clin Endocrinol (Oxf) 1991;34:253.

Kutten F, Fournier S, Durand JC, et al: Estradiol and progesterone receptors in human breast fibroadenomas. J Clin Endocrinol Metab 1981;52:1225.

Layfield LJ, Glasgow BJ, Cramer H: Fine-needle aspiration in the management of breast masses. Pathol Annu 1989;24(Pt 2):23.

Leis HP: Management of nipple discharge. World J Surg 1989;13:736.

Levy RI: Current status of the cholesterol controversy. Am J Med 1983;74 (Suppl 5A):1.

Logan WW, Hoffman NY: Diabetic fibrous breast disease. Radiology 1989;172:667.

London RS, Sundaram GS, Goldstein PJ: Medical management of mammary dysplasia. Obstet Gynecol 1982;59:519.

London RS, Sundaram GS, Murphy L, et al: The effect of vitamin E on mammary dysplasia: a double-blind study. Obstet Gynecol 1985;65:104.

Maddox PR, Mansel RE: Management of breast pain and nodularity. World J Surg 1989;13:699.

Magnant CM: Fat necrosis, hematoma and trauma. In Harris JR, Lippman ME, Morrow M, Hellman S (eds): Diseases of the Breast. Philadelphia: Lippincott-Raven, 1996:61.

Mant D, Vessey MP, Neil A, et al: Breast self-examination and breast cancer stage of diagnosis. Br J Cancer 1987;55:207.

Minton JP, Foecking MK, Webster DJ, Matthews RH: Caffeine, cyclic nucleotides and breast disease. Surgery 1979;86:105.

Mitnick JS, Harris MN, Roses DF: Mammographic detection of carcinoma of the breast in patients with augmentation prosthesis. Surg Gynecol Obstet 1989;168:30.

Monsees BS: Evaluation of breast microcalcifications. Radiol Clin North Am 1995;33:1109.

Monsonego J, DeStable MD, Saint Florent G, et al: Fibrocystic disease of the breast in premenopausal women: histohormonal correlation and response to luteinizing hormone releasing hormone analogue treatment. Am J Obstet Gynecol 1991;164:1181.

Moskowitz M: Breast cancer: age-specific growth rates and screening strategies. Radiology 1994;161:37.

National Institutes of Health: Consensus Development Statement: Breast Cancer Screening for Women Ages 40–49. Bethesda, MD: National Institutes of Health, 1997.

Osuch JR: Benign lesions of the breast other than fibrocystic change. Obstet Gynecol Clin North Am 1987;14:702.

Palmer M, Tsangaris T: Breast biopsy in women 30 years old or less. Am J Surg 1993;165:708.

Pasquino AM, Tebaldi L, Cioschi L, et al: Premature thelarche: a follow-up of 40 girls. Natural history and endocrine findings. Arch Dis Child 1985;60:1180.

Paulus DD: Benign diseases of the breast. Radiol Clin North Am 1983;21:36.

Peters F: Multicenter study of gestrinone in cyclical breast pain. Lancet 1992;339:205.

Petrek JA: Phyllodes tumor. In Harris JR, Lippman ME, Morrow M, Hellman S (eds): Diseases of the Breast. Philadelphia: Lippincott-Raven, 1996:863.

Pilnik S, Leis HP Jr: Nipple discharge. In Gallagher HS, Leis HP, Snyderman RK, Urban JA (eds): The Breast. St. Louis: CV Mosby Company, 1978:524.

Potten C, Watson R, Williams G, et al: The effect of age and menstrual cycle upon proliferative activity of the normal human breast. Br J Cancer 1988;58:163.

Porter JC: Hormonal regulation of breast development and activity. J Invest Dermatol 1974;63:85.

Preece PE, Baum M, Mansel RE, et al: Importance of mastalgia in operable breast cancer. Br Med J 1982;284:1299.

Reinfuss M, Mitus J, Smolak K, et al: Malignant phyllodes tumours of the breast: a clinical and pathological analysis of 55 cases. Eur J Cancer 1993;29A:1252.

Reynolds HE: Evaluation of the augmented breast. Radiol Clin North Am 1995;33:1131.

Richardson MR, Njemanze J: Management of severe fibrocystic disease of the breast with leuprolide acetate. Fertil Steril 1990;54:942.

Rongione AJ, Evans BD, Kling KM, McFadden DW: Ductography is a useful technique in evaluation of abnormal nipple discharge. Am Surg 1996;62:785.

Rosen PP, Ernsberger D: Mammary fibromatosis: a benign spindle-cell tumor with significant risk for local recurrence. Cancer 1989;63:1363.

Rostom A, El-Sayed M: Fat necrosis of the breast: an unusual complication of lumpectomy and radiotherapy in breast cancer. Clin Radiol 1987;38:31.

Saarela AO, Kiviniemi HO, Rissanen TJ, Paloneva TK: Nonpalpable breast lesions: pathologic correlation of ultrasonographically guided fine-needle aspiration biopsy. J Ultrasound Med 1996;15:549.

Schepps B, Scola FH, Frates RE: Benign circumscribed breast masses. Obstet Gynecol Clin North Am 1994;21:519.

Schnitt SJ, Connolly JL: Pathology of benign breast disorders. In Harris JR, Lippman ME, Morrow M, Hellman S (eds): Diseases of the Breast. Philadelphia: Lippincott-Raven, 1996:27.

Seidman H, Geld SK, Silverberg E, et al: Survival experience in the Breast Cancer Detection Demonstration Project. CA Cancer J Clin 1987;37:258.

Seidman H, Stillman SD, Moshinski MH: A different perspective on breast cancer risk factors: some implications of the nonattributable risk. CA Cancer J Clin 1982;32:3.

Seidman JD, Schnapper LA, Phillips LE: Mastopathy in insulin-requiring diabetes mellitus. Hum Pathol 1994;25:819.

Senie RT, Rosen PP, Lesser MM, Kinne DW: Breast self-examination and medical examination related to breast cancer state. Am J Public Health 1981;71:583.

Shapiro S: Evidence of screening for breast cancer from a randomized trial. CA Cancer J Clin 1977;29:2772.

Sickles EA: Periodic mammographic follow-up of probably benign lesions: results in 3,184 consecutive cases. Radiology 1991;179:463.

Sitruk-Ware R, Sterkers N, MauVais-Jarvis P: Benign breast disease. I: Hormonal investigation. Obstet Gynecol 1979;53:457.

Smart CR, Hendrick RE, Rutledge JH, Smith RA: Benefit of mammography screening in women ages 40–49: current evidence from randomized controlled trials. Cancer 1995;75:1619.

Snyder BW, Beecham GD, Winnekar RC: Studies on the mechanism of action of danazol and gestrinone. Fertil Steril 1989;51: 705.

Stadel BV, Rubin GL, Webster LA, et al: Oral contraceptives and breast cancer in young women. Lancet 1989;1:973.

Stelling CB: MIR imaging of the breast for cancer evaluation. Current status and future directions. Radiol Clin North Am 1995; 33:1187.

Tabar L, Fagerberg G, Day NE, Holmberg L: What is the optimum interval between mammographic screening examinations? An analysis based on the latest results of the Swedish Two-County Breast Screening Trial. Br J Cancer 1987;55:547.

Tomaszewski JE, Brooks JSJ, Hicks D, et al: Diabetic mastopathy: a distinctive clinicopathologic entity. Hum Pathol 1992;23:780.

Vanchieri C: Medical groups message to women: if 40 or older get regular mammograms. J Natl Cancer Inst 1989;81:1126.

Vorheer H: Fibrocystic breast disease: pathophysiology, pathomorphology, clinical picture and management. Am J Obstet Gynecol 1986;154:161.

Wang DY, Fentiman IS: Epidemiology and endocrinology of benign breast disease. Breast Cancer Res Treat 1985;6:5.

Watson DL, Bhatia RK, Norman GS: Bromocriptine mesylate for lactation suppression: a risk for postpartum hemorrhage. Obstet Gynecol 1989;74:573.

Wilkinson S, Anderson JJ, Rifkind E, et al: Fibroadenoma of the breast: a follow-up of conservative management. Br J Surg 1989;76:390.

Winchester DP: The diagnosis and management of breast disease. In Sciarra JJ (ed): Gynecology and Obstetrics, Vol 1: Clinical Gynecology. (Droegemueller W, ed). Philadelphia: JB Lippincott Company, 1984:1.

Wisbey JR, Kumar S, Mansel RE, et al: Natural history of breast pain. Lancet 1983;2:672.

Zuckerman HC: The role of mammography in the diagnosis of breast disease. In Ariel IM, Cleary JB (eds): Breast Cancer: Diagnosis and Treatment. New York: McGraw-Hill, 1989:152.

50

Douglas J. Marchant
Stephen S. Falkenberry

Breast Cancer

THE PROBLEM

The diagnosis and treatment of breast cancer has changed dramatically during the past two decades, a fact perhaps not fully appreciated by many primary physicians despite numerous scientific publications on the subject and unprecedented media attention. Twenty-five years ago screening programs were not available. The preferred treatment was radical mastectomy, and adjuvant therapy did not exist. This is in marked contrast to the current situation, in which there are well-organized screening programs, effective adjuvant therapy, and alternative treatments.

The most recent figures from the National Cancer Institute (NCI) (1993) reveal that, after a sharp rise in the percentage of women diagnosed with breast cancer from 1980 to 1987, there has been a decline in incidence, especially among women 50 years of age and older. The American Cancer Society (ACS) has indicated that the lifetime risk for developing breast cancer is 1 in 8. This reflects an increase in life expectancy of women, and the fact that breast cancer is a disease of older women. In addition, the increase is the result of the decision to include in the calculations women older than 85 years of age.

The ACS (1999) predicted that, for 1999, there would be 175,000 new cases of breast cancer with 43,300 deaths in the United States. Breast cancer is the leading cause of death for women ages 35 to 54 years and the second leading cause of death for all women. It represents 30% of cancer incidence in women and 17% of cancer deaths (ACS, 1999). The mortality rate for breast cancer has been unchanged since 1930, increasing an average of 0.2% per year from 1973 to 1990, but decreasing in women younger than 65 years of age by an average of 0.3% per year. New data, however, indicate that the breast cancer mortality rate has decreased in whites by almost 5% from 1989 to 1992, probably as a result of the increased diagnosis of localized cancer and the increased use of adjuvant therapy and screening mammography (Landis et al, 1999).

Early detection is associated with increased survival and more cosmetic treatment. Patients at high risk must be identified and appropriately screened for breast cancer. It is essential that the primary care physician provide appropriate risk assessment and timely surveillance.

A number of new health initiatives address women's health, and breast cancer in particular. The Women's Health Initiative has been established by the National Institutes of Health (NIH). The study is based at 16 major research sites selected as Vanguard Clinical Centers. The Women's Health Initiative has been designed to answer several critical questions, including the effects of dietary modifications, hormone therapy, and calcium and vitamin D intake. It is anticipated that about 160,000 women will take part in this study and that data analysis will be completed by the year 2005.

The National Institute of Child Health and Human Development has launched a major study to determine if lifestyle factors are associated with development of breast cancer. This study was launched during Breast Cancer Awareness Month in October 1993 and will include 10,000 women 35 to 64 years of age, with and without breast cancer. The study examines alcohol consumption, smoking, use of medicinal drugs, reproductive factors, and family history.

In 1992 the NCI approved a major clinical trial to test the safety of tamoxifen and its ability to prevent breast cancer. This was a randomized, double-blind, placebo-controlled trial involving 16,000 healthy women at high risk for developing breast cancer. In April of 1998, the study was halted—14 months early having enrolled 13,388 women at this time. It was noted that the incidence of breast cancer was 45% lower in women who received tamoxifen versus the placebo arm (Fisher et al, 1998).

The availability of appropriate therapeutic options is an important consideration for breast cancer patients. A number of organizations have recommended breast conservation therapy as the preferred treatment for early-stage breast cancer. However, there are marked geographic variations in recommended treatment options. Suggestions have included education for physicians and women to increase their familiarity with NIH selection criteria for breast conservation therapy (BCT), encouragement of objective discussions of treatment options during the patient-physician encounter, and patient counseling to help women cope with the diagnosis of breast cancer and to reach a decision about treatment options. Ideally, each patient should be discussed at a prospective, multidisciplinary Tumor Board that includes surgeons, radiation and medical oncologists, radiologists, plastic surgeons, and pathologists.

RISK FACTORS

It is essential for the primary care physician to have a concrete measure of the breast cancer problem, including definitive statements concerning the chances of developing breast cancer and the current information concerning the impact of these facts on the general public.

It is important to define the terms used in discussing cancer risk. The *lifetime risk* is an estimate of an individual's probability of developing cancer from birth until death. Risks are calculated for 5-year intervals and totaled as far as age 85 to approximate a lifetime measure. The *incidence* of a disease, in this case breast cancer, is the number or rate of new cases that are diagnosed during a specific time. *Prevalence* is the number or rate of persons with the disease in the population at any one time. The *cancer rate* is the proportion of cases (or deaths) that occur in a defined population during a specific period. The *relative risk* is the rate of disease, in this case breast cancer, in an exposed group divided by the rate of disease in a nonexposed group. A relative risk of 1 indicates no effect. If the risk is greater than 1, the exposure confers risk. If the relative risk is less than 1, the exposure is considered protective.

Breast cancer incidence, survival, and mortality patterns differ between whites and blacks. The incidence rate in white females is 20% higher than in black females. However, the 5-year relative survival rate for black women is 16% lower than that for white women. The mortality rate in 1990 for white women was 27.4 per 100,000 and the rate for black women 31.7 per 100,000. Data from the NIH note that, in the United States, the death rate from breast cancer dropped by almost 5% from 1989 to 1992 (SEER, 1990). This is the largest short-term decline in the United States for this disease since 1950. It should be noted, however, that among black women the death rate increased to 2.6%. The main reason for this decline appears to be the documented improvement in outcome as a result of adjuvant therapy, especially in young women. A second reason is the increase in the rate of women having routine screening mammography.

Patients are often confused by figures designating the lifetime risk of breast cancer being 1 in 8. This applies, however, to women 90 years or older. A more realistic explanation is that, in the absence of any major risk factors such as breast cancer in first-degree relatives, the chances of getting breast cancer between the ages of 30 and 40 are 1 in 1000, between 40 and 50 2 in 1000, and between 50 and 60 years of age 3 in 1000.

Breast Cancer Risk in Different Populations

Breast cancer incidence has historically been four to seven times higher in the United States than in China or Japan. When Chinese, Japanese or Philippine women migrate to the United States, the breast cancer risk rises across several generations and approaches that among whites in the United States. Given the fact that the risk of breast cancer appears to change with migration, additional studies are needed to clarify the impact of different age categories at migration and for length of residence. Findings from such a study could have implications for targeting and implementing lifestyle modifications. Apparently a region's breast cancer rate is tied to reproductive factors and lifestyle. For example, the Northeast has a higher breast cancer death rate than does the rest of the United States because more women in this area wait until after 20 years of age before having children (Ziegler et al, 1993).

Family History and Genetic Factors

An important component of the risk evaluation is the influence of family history. The physician must attempt to determine the contribution of a hereditable predisposition to an individual patient's risk. One must attempt to distinguish women carrying mutations in breast cancer susceptibility genes, in whom the risk of disease is extremely high, from women in these same families who have not inherited a susceptibility gene. Genetics studies suggest that a significant portion of familial breast cancer may be due to one or more dominantly inherited predisposing genes (Webber and Garber, 1993). The probability that carriers will develop breast or ovarian cancer or both is nearly 60% by 50 years of age, and by 70 years of age may be as high as 85%. This is much higher than the twofold increase in breast cancer risk cited by studies for women with an affected sister or mother. However, even in these families each individual has a 50% probability of *not* carrying the susceptibility allele, and these noncarriers have a lifetime breast cancer risk similar to that of women in the general population, or approximately 70% by 70 years of age.

In terms of breast cancer, there has been a rapid pace of discovery with regard to cancer susceptibility genes, and attention is being given to the unaffected carrier of a mutated gene. These carriers may be at 85% to 90% lifetime risk for cancer of the breast, and, for *BRCA1* heterozygous patients already affected by breast cancer, the risk for subsequent breast or ovarian cancer may be as high as 40% to 60%.

A large number of mutations, perhaps more than 100, have been identified in the *BRCA1* gene. In families with a high incidence rate of breast and ovarian cancer and carrying the *BRCA1* mutation, an estimated lifelong risk of approximately 85% for breast cancer and 50% for ovarian cancer has been noted.

It has been suggested, however, that these penetrance figures may have been overestimated because of bias with respect to families with multiple affected members (Collins, 1996).

How should the primary care physician evaluate this information? Should physicians begin by offering tests for *BRCA1* mutations to women with a family history of breast cancer? Should a test for germline *BRCA1* mutations be offered to all women with newly diagnosed breast or ovarian cancer to identify those with mutations, and as a result to identify relatives who are at risk? False-positive results will complicate this effort, and there will also be false negatives because not every possible mutation will be detected.

A woman with no *BRCA1* mutation still faces the same 12% lifetime risk of breast cancer that any other woman faces, and she could be at high additional risk because of an inherited mutation in *BRCA2*. Thus the value of normal test results is minimal unless an affected relative is known to carry a particular *BRCA1* mutation that can be shown to be absent in the person at risk. Even the most informed in this area are uncertain about the management of women with a mutation. Which breast is involved? Despite the efficacy of mammography for the early detection of breast cancer, physicians have no data suggesting that regular mammography at a young age, together with breast self-examination and clinical evaluation, reduces the risk of metastatic breast cancer among the extremely high-risk women with *BRCA1* mutations (Nelson, 1995).

What is the role of prophylactic mastectomy in those patients with breast cancer and *BRCA1* mutations? What is the preferred method of treatment? Should it be different from the standard recommendations for treatment of early breast cancer (i.e., wide local excision, axillary dissection, and radiation therapy)?

Even if physicians can assume that these issues will be resolved—that is, that the testing can be done with increased sensitivity and specificity, and that eventually appropriate management strategies will be available—discrimination in health insurance based on genetic testing may render women with *BRCA1* mutations uninsurable. The responsibility to provide appropriate genetic counseling is inherent in the recommendation for genetic testing. For the woman with a family history of an identifiable *BRCA1* mutation who is subsequently found not to carry the alteration, this information is beneficial, but the woman who has abnormal test results faces a lifetime of concern. Few, if any, primary care physicians have been educated to provide this type of genetic counseling, and there is urgent need to develop available and well-funded genetic counseling services.

The NCI has advised caution in genetic testing for hereditary cancer genes (Nelson, 1995). Genetic testing until recently has been conducted primarily in university research centers, but, with the availability of genetic testing through commercial laboratories, primary care physicians are confronted with a number of complex medical, ethical, legal, and social issues. Finally, before any widespread *BRCA1* screening is undertaken, provision must be made for education of the medical community and the at-risk public. A complete counseling service must be available, including expertise both in breast and ovarian cancer.

From a practical standpoint, it is important for the physician to obtain an accurate family history. Early age at disease onset and bilateral disease increase patient risk. The occurrence of breast cancer in a premenopausal patient is an indication to conduct a careful family history, including a nuclear pedigree with the reservations previously noted. Families with two or more affected women provide evidence of possible familial clustering. Careful attention must also be directed toward the possibility of paternal transmission in affected families.

Reproductive Factors

For many years certain reproductive characteristics have been associated with the risk of breast cancer. These include nulliparity, early age at onset of menarche, older age at menopause, and older age at first full-term pregnancy. Oophorectomy at an early age, in contrast, has been considered protective, reducing the risk of breast cancer in this age group by almost 70%.

Early menarche is associated with high socioeconomic status and late age at first birth. In underdeveloped countries, whether because of diet deprivation, climate, or other environmental factors, late onset of menarche is the rule, and there is frequently a decreased interval between puberty and the first pregnancy followed by several pregnancies and early menopause. Late age at menopause increases the risk of breast cancer. The incidence is doubled in women with natural menopause after 55 years of age compared with women in whom it occurs before 45 years of age.

Nulliparity and late age at first birth increase the lifetime incidence of breast cancer. Early age at birth of a second child also decreases the risk. The relationship among nulliparity, early age at first birth, and number of pregnancies is complex. Pregnancy before 30 years of age, although it reduces the lifetime risk, may be associated with a transiently increased risk relative to the nulliparous women. This increase may last for one or two decades, followed by a risk that is lower than that of the nulliparous woman later in life (Ewertz et al, 1990).

Does abortion increase breast cancer risk? There is some evidence that there is an increase in breast cancer risk as a result of abortion, but only for women in a specific age group. A number of studies apparently show no demonstrated link between abortion and breast cancer risk (Bradlow et al, 1993). It is acknowledged that there are a number of complexities associated with the abortion–breast cancer issue and that these issues prohibit a consensus at this time. It appears, therefore, that additional studies are required to completely quantify the risk, if any.

As the result of an international case-control study, it had been widely believed that lactation had no effect on the incidence of breast cancer (MacMahon et al, 1973). A more recent study has found that there is a reduction in the risk of breast cancer among premenopausal women who had lactated, but there is no reduction in the risk among postmenopausal women with a history of lactation (Newcomb et al, 1994). The role of lactation, specifically the biologic effect of lactation on breast cells, is unclear. The stronger effect of lactation as a protective factor at an early age suggests that decreased exposure to ovarian hormones at a younger age may be important. This is in keeping with the previous discussion concerning the early age of menarche and the effect of ovarian hormones on the development of breast parenchyma. Of significance is the fact that lactation is a behavior that can be altered, and, whereas the apparent protective effect of lactation is not great, any reduction in breast cancer incidence can be important, especially in younger women.

Estrogen Replacement Therapy

The benefits and risks of estrogen replacement therapy have been debated for many years. It is essential that the physician understand the rationale for estrogen replacement therapy, especially in terms of the prevention of cardiovascular disease and osteoporosis, and at the same time be aware of the lack of solid data to support the unequivocal recommendation for estrogen replacement therapy, particularly in patients treated for breast cancer.

We live in an aging society. Two hundred years ago fewer than 30% of women lived long enough to reach menopause. Now 90% of women reach the climacteric. There are approximately 56 million women older than 35 years of age in the United States, and more than 30 million women have an average postmenopausal life expectancy of 28 years. Furthermore, advances in the treatment of breast cancer have resulted in long-term survival, and premenopausal patients treated for breast cancer often receive adjuvant therapy that in many cases results in premature menopause.

There are two aspects to estrogen replacement therapy: *prevention* (osteoporosis, coronary heart disease) and *treatment* (atrophic changes and vasomotor phenomena). There is no question that in the United States more women die of myocardial infarction than of breast cancer. It is clear that the incidence of cardiovascular disease in women rises after menopause. There have been a number of studies suggesting that estrogen replacement therapy reduces cardiovascular mortality by about 50%. Estrogen lowers low-density lipoprotein cholesterol and raises high-density lipoprotein cholesterol. However, this explains only 35% to 50% of the cardioprotective effect, and there is evidence that preservation of normal endothelial function also plays an important role (Sullivan and Fowlkes, 1996; Wild, 1996). Many investigators are concerned about the validity of these data. The highly touted meta-analyses may have sample sizes too small to show an effect. That is, a priori power calculations should always be done in quantitative clinical research. The physician must weigh these data against the as-yet-unknown information that may be available from the PEPI trial (Healy, 1995) and the large Women's Health Initiative Study (National Institutes of Health, 1994).

In the meantime, there is increasing pressure to prescribe estrogen replacement therapy, but what are the risks? There are a number of interesting observations that suggest a relationship between estrogen and breast cancer. It has been known for many years that oophorectomy in women younger than 35 years of age reduces the risk of breast cancer by 70%. Patients with metastatic cancer treated with aminoglutethimi (an aromatase inhibitor) have a marked reduction in estradiol from 15 to 20 pg/ml to about 5 pg/ml because of the failure of conversion of hormones into estrogen. The level of estradiol is increased to 30 to 35 pg/ml with estrogen replacement therapy. One paper reported that patients on estrogen replacement therapy who developed metastatic breast disease had regression on withdrawal of estrogen therapy (Dhodapker et al, 1995). These data and a number of other studies clearly indicate that there is as-yet-unknown relationship between estrogens and breast cancer.

The literature regarding the primary prevention of coronary heart disease, the risk factors for osteoporosis, the use of estrogens and progestins, and the risk of breast cancer is voluminous and often contradictory. Breast cancer is related to reproductive events. Increasing attention to the contemporary preventive approach to breast cancer focuses on the physiologic effects of the sex steroid hormones and their possible interaction with family history. One researcher has suggested vigorous exercise to delay puberty, followed by hormone treatment to induce artificial menopause (Pike, 1996). Adding to the potential risk of estrogen replacement therapy is the fact that current use of estrogen replacement therapy may be associated with lower specificity and lower sensitivity of screening mammography (Laya et al, 1996). Clearly a risk-benefit analysis must be discussed with the patient, both in terms of prevention, including the uncertainty of the observational data and the lack of information from controlled, randomized trials, and the risk of breast cancer, coupled with the potential decreased accuracy of screening. Given the large numbers of women receiving estrogen replacement therapy, even a small risk could result in a public health problem.

An interesting study discusses the effects of alcohol ingestion on estrogens in postmenopausal women (Ginsberg et al, 1996). There are studies that indicate moderate ingestion of alcohol increases the risk of breast cancer. Apparently acute alcohol ingestion may lead to significant and sustained elevations in circulating estradiol levels to 300% higher than those targeted in the clinical use of estrogen replacement therapy. Thus, although moderate alcohol consumption also appears to decrease the incidence of coronary artery disease, it may increase the incidence of breast cancer, and the combination of estrogen replacement therapy and alcohol ingestion may be additive and increase the risk of breast cancer more than either alone (Ginsberg et al, 1996).

The issue of estrogen replacement therapy in patients treated for breast cancer presents a challenge because of the lack of data. Whereas successful treatment of breast cancer depends on local control, there is always the potential for distant metastases. If the patient is cured, the question is moot.

Unfortunately, not all patients with breast cancer are cured, even with the most effective treatment. The 10-year survival rate for the best patients, those with small tumors and negative nodes, is approximately 70%, indicating that 30% of these patients had metastatic disease that was unknown either at the time of the initial treatment or during the follow-up period. It is the effect of estrogen replacement therapy on occult metastatic disease that is the basis for the caution regarding the use of this therapy in patients treated for breast cancer. Receptor data and other prognostic factors appear to be of little value, at the present time at least, in deciding for or against estrogen replacement therapy in these patients. Finally, if overt metastatic disease is discovered, treatment, however aggressive, is ineffective. That is, none of these patients survive.

In considering estrogen replacement therapy, therefore, the physician must discuss the benefits and risks, including the uncertainty of the available data. Patients must accept an unknown medical risk, and clinicians must accept an unknown medical/legal risk. It is essential that, before estrogen replacement therapy is administered, the oncology team be consulted for an opinion, which in some cases may be surprisingly liberal, particularly if quality-of-life issues are involved (vaginal atrophy and associated dyspareunia). It should be noted that the vaginal administration of estrogen is not without risk. Estrogen is absorbed readily from the atrophic vaginal mucosa. However, there is decreased absorption with increasing vaginal cornification, but perhaps sufficient absorption to stimulate occult micrometastases.

Other Risk Factors

Oral Contraceptives

Soon after the approval of oral contraceptive drugs, a number of epidemiologic studies reported on the risk of breast cancer associated with this therapy (Calache et al, 1983). Review of the recent data concerning oral contraceptive drugs and breast cancer reveals that, despite numerous studies, the question remains unresolved. Data from the NCI presented at the 9th International Breast Society Meeting in May of 1996 suggest that there appears to be increased risk for developing breast cancer for women who begin oral contraceptives within 5 years of their menarche and that this risk is not explained by bias factors (i.e., age at first birth, family history, diet, and body size) (Briton, 1996). If these as-yet-unpublished data are confirmed, this will provide important guidelines for recommending oral contraceptives, particularly in women younger than 20 years of age. Most authorities now believe that the safety and benefits of low-dose oral contraceptive drugs outweigh any potential risk, and as a result no changes have been recommended in the prescribing practice for oral contraceptive drugs.

Benign Breast Disease

There is a large amount of literature dealing with fibrocystic changes, including the risk factors for benign breast disease and the relationship of these changes to the later development of breast cancer (Bodian et al, 1993a, 1993b). It is now believed that the term *benign breast disease* has historically represented a heterogeneous group of histopathologic entities, and there is an increasing attempt to more specifically define these entities. Women with a history of any proliferative epithelial changes appear to have twice the risk of breast cancer, and women with atypical hyperplasia appear to have about four times the risk (Dupont et al, 1989). Lesions without proliferative changes are associated with little or no excess risk. From a practical standpoint, only 4% to 10% of benign breast biopsy specimens show atypical hyperplasia (Hutter, 1985).

Diet and the Risk of Breast Cancer

For many years dietary fat has been suggested as a risk factor for breast cancer. Marked international differences in the rates of breast cancer and the striking increase among populations migrating from low- to high-incidence areas have suggested that environmental factors, possibly dietary, influence the occurrence of breast cancer. A number of studies addressing this issue have produced conflicting results and recommendations (Willett et al, 1987). Obviously clinical trials are needed, and the Women's Intervention Nutrition Study is testing whether a diet with 15% of calories from fat will prevent breast cancer occurrence (Wynder, 1997). Although limiting fat intake may not prevent breast cancer, it may have important implications for survival.

Another possible modifiable environmental determinant is that of vitamins. Most of the studies have found no evidence of a protective influence of vitamins C or E on the incidence of breast cancer (Hunter et al, 1993). In contrast, it was observed that there was a significant inverse association of vitamin A in the risk of this disease. It was noted, however, that vitamin A supplements would be unlikely to influence the risk of breast cancer among women whose dietary intake of his vitamin was already adequate. Because of the potential adverse effects of high-dose supplements of preformed vitamin A, particularly among women who may become pregnant, it has not been recommended that vitamin A supplements be used to prevent breast cancer.

Finally, the relationship between caffeine and related methylxanthenes to the development of fibrocystic changes in the breast requires some comment. Studies do not support any relationship between caffeine and fibrocystic changes (Phelps and Phelps, 1988), and, in the study by Minton and colleagues (1979), no relationship between methylxanthenes and breast cancer was postulated.

Comments

Breast cancer risk factors for which modification would be comfortably acceptable have not yet been established. Nearly all women in the United States are at substantial risk. The majority of women in whom breast cancer will be diagnosed live out their lives without recurrence of the disease. Newer strategies include the development of effective chemopreventive programs. Phase III clinical trials are underway to assess the values of retinoids and tamoxifen. Phase I and II studies have been designed to assess the potential of more specific strategies to inhibit growth factors important in maintaining the malignant phenotype. Obviously more studies are needed to address this major public health problem.

MAKING THE DIAGNOSIS

The diagnostic evaluation begins with a careful history and examination of the breast. During the last decade there have been dramatic changes in the technique of physical examination of the breast: the search for subtle changes that may indicate nonpalpable lesions. The patient must be examined in several positions. The obvious lesion is discovered regardless of the position of the patient, but there are some lesions that can be detected only by employing several maneuvers, including examining the patient in the standing and sitting positions combined with compressing the pectoral muscles and elevating the arms.

Once a dominant mass has been confirmed, it must be resolved. This mass may be cystic, solid, benign, or malignant. An attempt should be made to aspirate the mass with a fine-gauge needle. Local anesthesia is not required. The mass is immobilized, the needle is inserted, and fluid is withdrawn. If no residual mass is palpated immediately following aspiration, follow-up examination is all that is required. If the mass remains or if there is a residual

mass on the first follow-up visit, open biopsy is recommended. For most cases it is not necessary to send the fluid for cytologic evaluation.

The use of *fine-needle aspiration* (FNA) is accurate when applied correctly (Adye et al, 1988). This requires an understanding of the techniques involved and a cytopathologist capable of interpreting the smear. A standard disposable syringe can be used with a 23- to 25-gauge needle, depending on the preference of the cytopathologist. Local anesthesia is helpful because several "passes" may be required to obtain an adequate tissue sample. This technique in essence provides evaluation of "tissue juice." It is therefore important that sufficient material be withdrawn and placed on the slide for appropriate evaluation. The material should not enter the syringe and must be placed directly on the slide. The technique is most useful for the obvious dominant mass with signs suggesting carcinoma. A positive FNA permits immediate treatment planning and discussion of alternative treatments with the therapeutic team. Except in rare instances, this finding must be confirmed by open biopsy at the time of definitive treatment. It must be emphasized that FNA is useful only if positive. A negative finding may be unreliable, particularly if not performed on a regular basis and with the aid of an experienced cytopathologist. To assume that a negative mammogram, ultrasound, and FNA rule out carcinoma is misleading and dangerous. Obviously, in a specialized breast clinic in which thousands of FNAs are performed, and the therapeutic team is dedicated to the diagnosis and treatment of breast disease, the diagnostic evaluation is more reliable.

It is essential to discuss FNA with the radiologist. Some prefer the mammogram be done prior to FNA because of possible distortion of the anatomy and hematoma formation.

In addition to the regular practice of breast self-examination, screening mammography and a complete breast examination, it is now generally accepted that the diagnosis and treatment of breast cancer require a multidisciplinary evaluation. Diagnostic studies, therefore, should represent the optimal approach to establishing the histologic condition without compromising later definitive treatment.

Open biopsy often becomes part of the definitive treatment for breast cancer. In the past the choice of the incision was unimportant because, if cancer was diagnosed, a radical mastectomy or modified radical mastectomy was performed. With the advent of BCT, the placement of the incision is crucial and the appearance of the wound may influence the timing and even the appropriateness of conservative treatment.

With rare exception almost all breast biopsies are performed on a day surgery basis under local anesthesia. It is essential that the patient be told what is going to happen during the procedure. In most cases no sedation is required, and frequently conversation between the nurse and the patient is effective in diverting the patient's attention from the procedure.

The operation is performed using sharp dissection with a minimal number of instruments and appropriate exposure. Bleeding can be controlled with cautery or fine ligatures. The use of cautery for dissection is discouraged because this coagulates the tissue and the determination of free margins may be impossible. An essential component of the procedure is the large pressure dressing applied to the wound following the surgery. This prevents discomfort and avoids hematoma formation.

During the past decade, there has been a significant increase in the number of women availing themselves of *screening mammography* (Martin et al, 1997). The physician recommending the screening mammography must be concerned with at least three issues: safety, cost effectiveness, and quality control. Radiation hazards of mammography have been debated for more than 30 years; however, at present it can be safely stated that modern technology has reduced the radiation exposure to a negligible risk (Harris et al, 1992). Cost effectiveness is more difficult to evaluate. The major issue is periodic screening in younger women, in particular those between the ages of 40 and 49 years. A consensus meeting held at the National Institutes of Health failed to recommend specific guidelines for women in this age group. Women in this age group should decide whether or not to be screened based on their known risk factors and in consultation with their physicians (NIH, 1997). There is little controversy concerning annual screening after the age of 50, although the exact age at which to discontinue annual screening has not been determined. Quality control has been addressed by means of a certification process involving both the American College of Radiology and in many cases local and state government agencies.

A major problem associated with the increase in screening mammography is the discovery of the occult lesion, which presents a challenge both to the radiologist and the surgeon. These lesions include microcalcifications and the asymmetric density. The decision to perform the biopsy is the responsibility of the radiologist. These patients have no symptoms and the physical examination is entirely normal. The management of the occult lesion is one of the most difficult aspects of the diagnosis and treatment of breast disease. If mammography has been performed and the report indicates additional diagnostic studies (spot compression views or magnification views), they should be ordered. It is essential that the primary care physician work with the radiologist to complete the diagnostic evaluation. Once the decision has been made to perform a biopsy, the radiologist usually recommends either an open or a stereotactic procedure. This decision is based on a number of factors, including the experience of the radiology team, the location of the lesion, and the wishes of the patient. For the patient with an abnormal mammogram there are three possibilities: additional studies may be required to clarify the situation, follow-up films in 4 to 6 months may be

requested to assess stability, or localization and biopsy may be required.

For the localization and biopsy procedure, the patient is referred initially to the radiologist, who is responsible for placing the needle in proximity to the occult lesions. The films are reviewed by the radiologist and the operating surgeon and, if they are satisfactory, the patient is taken to the day surgery area where the procedure, as in the open biopsy, is performed with the patient under local anesthesia. The procedure should be performed in a setting in which there is communication between an experienced radiologist and a skillful surgeon. In some cases localization and biopsy may constitute wide local excision resulting in the definitive local treatment of the cancer. Obviously this depends on the site and the size of the lesion and the experience of the operating surgeon. In most cases re-excision is required, and often this is performed with the patient under general anesthesia at the time of the axillary dissection.

An alternative to a needle-guided biopsy is the *stereotactic core biopsy* (Parker et al, 1990). This utilizes sophisticated radiographic equipment employing an automated biopsy "gun" containing a large-bore (12- to 14-gauge) needle (Parker et al, 1991). Several cores may be taken from the area without the need for a surgical incision. Stereotactic biopsy is less costly and the only incision is a small stab wound in the appropriate location in the breast. There is also less scarring in the breast that might interfere with subsequent interpretation of the mammogram.

Several studies are underway to determine the accuracy of the stereotactic core biopsy compared to the traditional needle-guided surgical biopsy (Parker et al, 1993). A significant number of patients is required to obtain the skill necessary to perform the procedure and interpret the core biopsy. There remains considerable debate about the efficacy of the core biopsy in patients with a localized area of microcalcifications. In this situation multiple core biopsies must be taken, both from the area containing the microcalcification and from the adjacent tissue, because occasional carcinomas are found adjacent to the microcalcifications associated with benign fibrocystic changes.

The core biopsy should not be a substitute for careful mammographic follow-up of nonpalpable or occult lesions. The cost of a unilateral follow-up mammogram is about 10% that of a core biopsy.

Improvements in ultrasound equipment have permitted the identification of smaller and smaller masses, and the use of ultrasonography to localize and biopsy nonpalpable lesions is now becoming very popular. *Ultrasound-guided core biopsy* or FNA is very well tolerated and usually takes less time to complete than the traditional stereotactic procedure. It is also less costly (Parker et al, 1993).

Once the diagnosis has been established, patients require pretreatment evaluation—medical clearance, liver function tests, chest radiographs, and, in selected cases, bone scan. The lesion is staged according to the tumor-node-metastasis (TNM) system (Table 50–1).

TREATMENT PLANNING AND ALTERNATIVES IN BREAST CANCER TREATMENT

A number of factors influence the definitive surgical treatment for breast cancer. Important considerations include the size and histologic features of the lesion, the skill and experience of the multidisciplinary team, and the wishes of the patient. The treatment discussed in this chapter includes modified radical mastectomy and BCT—wide local excision with or without axillary dissection.

The conservative approach appeals to most patients; however, statistics clearly indicate that not all patients are treated according to the published guidelines established by the American College of Radiology, the American College of Surgeons, the College of American Pathologists, and the Society of Surgical Oncology (Winchester and Cox, 1992). In 1995, the standards for treating primary breast cancer were updated and the recommendations were published in the *Journal of the National Cancer Institute* (Goldhirsch et al, 1995). In addition, the NIH and the NCI regularly publish PDQ—State-of-the-Art statements. These can be obtained directly from the NIH and NCI (NCI, 1996).

In most cases the patient will have been seen by her primary care physician because of breast symptoms, possibly a mass in the breast or nipple discharge. If the abnormal findings are confirmed, the patient should be referred to a multidisciplinary team dealing with breast cancer. In many areas of the country dedicated breast centers are available for consultation.

Modified Radical Mastectomy (Simple Mastectomy with Axillary Dissection)

This operation, as the name implies, is in essence a total (simple) mastectomy and axillary node dissection with preservation of the pectoral muscles. No attempt is made to clear the axilla of all nodes (i.e., levels 1, 2, and 3). The retrieval of 10 to 15 level 1 and 2 nodes is considered satisfactory for staging purposes. In some cases, when the nodes are clinically involved, extensive axillary dissection may be required.

Modified radical mastectomy is the procedure of choice for large operable lesions, multifocal or multicentric lesions, patients with large lesions and relatively small breasts, and patients who refuse conservative treatment. It is also the procedure of choice for large lesions as demonstrated by mammography and proved by open biopsy.

In our cost-containment-oriented society, the staging work-up is usually obtained on an outpatient ba-

sis. In some centers the operation is performed on a day surgery basis and the patient is discharged home on the same day. Although this is technically feasible, it may not be appropriate for a number of reasons, including the age of the patient, the home environment, and the patient's general medical condition. For most patients, a 48-hour hospital stay is appropriate.

In performing the operation, an attempt is made to use a transverse incision to permit a more cosmetic reconstructive procedure if this is desired by the patient. Following removal of the breast, the axillary dissection is performed dissecting level 1 and 2 nodes. The specimen is carefully marked by the surgeon to facilitate examination by the pathologist. Because of the extensive elevation of skin flaps, suction drainage is required. Most patients can be mobilized soon after the surgical procedure, and usually there is minimal discomfort that can be controlled with analgesics. The patient should be seen by the physiotherapist and instructed in arm and chest wall exercises that should be continued during the postoperative period.

Breast Preservation Procedures (BCT)

As previously noted, a number of consensus development conferences have dealt with the treatment of primary breast cancer in an effort to determine treatment recommendations that provide the best chance for disease-free survival. The use of breast conservation procedures involves the following four important criteria: patient selection, surgery of the primary tumor, surgery of the axilla, and radiotherapy of the retained breast.

The principal advantage of conservation treatment is cosmetic. There are no data to indicate the conservative approach provides improved survival compared with the radical procedure. Poor candidates include patients with widely separated tumors in the same breast, patients whose mammograms reveal diffuse disease in many quadrants, and patients with large tumors in relatively small breasts.

The axillary dissection is performed first. Following this procedure the wound is closed with or without a drain. Wide local excision is then performed. Adequate surgical resection applies grossly clear margins. The pathologist inks the margins and the tissue is submitted for estrogen and progesterone receptor analysis and DNA analysis as well. The majority of patients can be discharged within 24 to 48 hours, at which time the pressure dressing applied at the time of surgery may be removed. Before discharge the patient is instructed in arm and chest exercises in an effort to avoid the fibrosis that may be associated with several weeks of radiation therapy required to complete the local treatment.

For most patients radiation therapy can begin 2 to 3 weeks following surgery and in some cases earlier, depending upon the condition of the wounds. Typ-

Table 50-1. DEFINITION OF TNM* STAGING SYSTEM

STAGE	DEFINITION	STAGE	DEFINITION
Primary Tumor		pN1a	Only micrometastasis (none larger than 0.2 cm)
TX	Primary tumor cannot be assessed	pN1b	Metastasis to lymph node(s), any larger than 0.2 cm
T0	No evidence of primary tumor	pN1bi	Metastasis in 1 to 3 lymph nodes, any more than 0.2 cm and all less than 2 cm in greatest dimension
Tis†	Carcinoma in situ: intraductal carcinoma, lobular carcinoma in situ, or Paget disease of the nipple with no tumor	pN1bii	Metastasis to 4 or more lymph nodes, any more than 0.2 cm and all less than 2 cm in greatest dimension
T1	Tumor 2 cm or less in greatest dimension	pN1biii	Extension of tumor beyond the capsule of a lymph node metastasis less than 2 cm in greatest dimension
T1a	0.5 cm or less in greatest dimension		
T1b	More than 0.5 cm but not more than 1 cm in greatest dimension	pN1biv	Metastasis to a lymph node 2 cm or more in greatest dimension
T1c	More than 1 cm but not more than 2 cm in greatest dimension		
T2	Tumor more than 2 cm but not more than 5 cm in greatest dimension	pN2	Metastasis to ipsilateral axillary lymph nodes that are fixed to one another or to other structures
T3	Tumor more than 5 cm in greatest dimension	pN3	Metastasis to ipsilateral internal mammary lymph node(s)
T4‡	Tumor of any size with direct extension to chest wall or skin		
T4a	Extension to chest wall	**Distant Metastasis (M)**	
T4b	Edema (including peau d'orange) or ulceration of the skin of the breast or satellite skin nodules confined to the same breast	MX	Presence of distant metastasis cannot be assessed
		M0	No distant metastasis
T4c	Both T4a and T4b		
T4d	Inflammatory carcinoma	M1	Distant metastasis (includes metastasis to ipsilateral supraclavicular lymph node(s))
Regional Lymph Nodes (N)			
NX	Regional lymph nodes cannot be assessed (e.g., previously removed)	**Stage Grouping**	
		Stage 0	Tis, N0, M0
N0	No regional lymph node metastasis	Stage I	T1, N0, M0
N1	Metastasis to movable ipsilateral axillary lymph node(s)	Stage IIA	T0, N1, M0 / T1, N1,§ M0 / T2, N0, M0
N2	Metastasis to ipsilateral axillary lymph node(s) fixed to one another or to other structures	Stage IIB	T2, N1, M0 / T3, N0, M0
N3	Metastasis to ipsilateral internal mammary lymph node(s)	Stage IIIA	T0, N2, M0 / T1, N2, M0 / T2, N2, M0 / T3, N1, N2, M0
Pathologic Classification (pN)			
pNX	Regional lymph nodes cannot be assessed (e.g., previously removed or not removed for pathologic study)	Stage IIIB	T4, any N, M0 / Any T, N3, M0
pN0	No regional lymph node metastasis	Stage IV	Any T, any N, M1
pN1	Metastasis to movable ipsilateral axillary lymph nodes(s)		

*Definitions for classifying the primary tumor (T) are the same for clinical and for pathologic classification. The telescoping method of classification can be applied. If the measurement is made by physical examination, the examiner will use the major headings (T1, T2, or T3). If other measurements, such as mammographic or pathologic, are used, the telescoped subsets of T1 can be used.
†Paget disease associated with a tumor is classified according to the size of the tumor.
‡Chest wall includes ribs, intercostal muscles, and serratus anterior muscle but not pectoral muscle.
§The prognosis of patients with pN1a is similar to that of patients with pN0.
From American Joint Committee on Cancer: Manual for Staging of Cancer. 3rd ed. Philadelphia: JB Lippincott Company, 1988.

ically the entire breast and occasionally the draining axillary, internal mammary, and supraclavicular lymphatics are included in the treatment field. Particular attention is paid to technique to minimize the amount of lung and heart that is included in the treatment field.

Treatment is usually administered with 4 to 10 mV x-rays from a linear accelerator. Such megavoltage radiation is "skin sparing" in that some depth of tissue, often several millimeters, is required to achieve the maximal dose, resulting in a somewhat reduced dose to the skin surface. Treatments are given daily, 5 days per week, for a total duration of 5 to 7 weeks to a dose of 45 to 50 Gy. Often this is followed by a boost dose to the tumor bed for an additional 10 to 20 Gy. The side effects typically encountered during the treatment include mild to moderate skin irritation within the treatment field. This occasionally progresses to skin blistering, typically in the inframammary fold or at the site of the high-dose boost. Topical cleansing and antibiotic ointment usually result in complete healing or full-thickness desquamation within 10 to 14 days after completion of radiation. Mild to moderate fatigue may also accompany radiation treatment.

Complications of breast irradiation combined with breast and axillary surgery can develop months to years after treatment and include persistent discoloration of the skin, breast retraction or edema, chronic discomfort in the breast or chest wall, rib fracture, pneumonitis, cardiac injury, brachial plexopathy, arm edema, and secondary tumor formation. These complications are infrequent (<10% to 20% incidence); significant cosmetic deformities and arm edema are rare (<2% to 5% incidence) and pneumonitis and cardiac injury are very rare (<1%).

Tumor control rates with BCT 8 to 10 years after treatment are in the range of 85% to 95% (Haffty et al, 1989; Kurtz et al, 1989; Fowble et al, 1991). The greatest risk for recurrence occurs within the first 5 to 6 years after treatment (Gage et al, 1995).

A number of questions have been raised by both patients and thoughtful physicians concerning local treatment for early invasive cancer. These include

- Why is there marked variation in the United States in the use of breast-conserving surgery for localized breast disease?
- Is menstrual cycle timing of breast cancer resection an important consideration?
- Is the distribution of the cancer in the breast an important consideration for optimizing BCT?
- What is the effect of reexcision on the success of breast-conserving surgery?
- Is axillary lymph node dissection necessary in all cases?
- Is local recurrence a concern in breast-conserving surgery?
- Should age be an important clinical concern in deciding for and against BCT?
- What is the cost of BCT versus modified radical mastectomy?

All are under intensive investigation, and definitive answers are not yet available. As an example, there is intensive investigation regarding the need for axillary dissection, and studies have indicated that lymphatic mapping is technically possible and that the histologic characteristics of the so-called sentinel node probably reflect the histologic characteristics of the axillary nodes (Albertini et al, 1996). These investigations may lead to staging information performed as an outpatient procedure. This would decrease overall morbidity without compromising patient care. As these results are confirmed by other investigators, lymphatic mapping and selective lymphadenectomy could lead to more conservative surgical treatment of women with breast cancer (Krag et al, 1998).

Breast Reconstruction

An increasing number of patients elect reconstructive procedures, either immediately or at a later date following the initial treatment. There are few, if any, contraindications to breast reconstruction. In most cases, for patients requiring a modified radical mastectomy, pretreatment consultation with a plastic surgeon is advisable. Generally accepted contraindications to immediate reconstruction include severe diabetes, vascular disease, smoking, and collagen disease. Adjuvant chemotherapy is not a contraindication to reconstruction.

Currently, approximately one third of women who have undergone reconstruction do so immediately, and this trend is increasing. Immediate reconstruction offers financial, psychological, and physical advantages. It decreases the number of operative procedures required both for the mastectomy and the reconstruction, and it does not extend hospitalization unless a myocutaneous flap is used.

In the past the most popular technique for reconstruction included the placement of an implant if adequate skin is present, and, if not, a soft tissue expander followed by an implant. Obviously, with the controversy concerning the silicone implants, this procedure is reserved for those patients who are part of an ongoing clinical trial directed toward obtaining information concerning the risks and benefits of breast implants. The advantage of the myocutaneous flaps is the use of body tissues to construct the breast mound; however, the operating time is increased severalfold and, as expected, more complications follow this extensive surgical procedure.

Adjuvant Therapy

The decision to employ adjuvant therapy in the treatment of breast cancer must be based on the estimated risk of locoregional and/or systemic relapse that is established by considering numerous prognostic risk factors. The absolute benefit of adjuvant therapy to an individual is determined by the untreated risk of relapse and the effectiveness of the adjuvant therapy in reducing that risk. Adjuvant therapy may be in the form of locoregional therapy (radiation after primary surgery) or systemic therapy (cytotoxic chemotherapy or endocrine therapy). In general, the term *adjuvant therapy* should be restricted to therapy employed to minimize risk of locoregional or systemic recurrence rather than the treatment of known persistent or metastatic disease.

Prognostic Risk Factors

Several factors must be considered in the decision to offer adjuvant therapy.

Lymph Node Status. Of the known prognostic risk factors for systemic relapse, the number of axillary lymph nodes involved with metastatic disease is the most predictive. The risk of axillary lymph node metastases increases with tumor size (Carter et al, 1989; Guiliano et al, 1996), and the risk of systemic relapse increases with the number of axillary lymph nodes involved (Fisher et al, 1983; Nemoto et al, 1983). SEER data from the NCI reveal that 20.6% of women with tumors less than 0.5 cm had axillary lymph node involvement versus 70.1% with tumors greater than 5 cm (Carter et al, 1989). Giuliano et al (1996) found axillary nodal metastases in 10% of T1a and 13% of T1b tumors. Five-year recurrence rates increase from 19% for lymph node–negative patients to 63% for women with 6 to 10 axillary lymph nodes involved (Nemoto et al, 1983).

Tumor Size. Although lymph node status is the most important predictor of systemic relapse, it is known that tumor size is an independent risk factor when nodal status is controlled. For women with tumors less than 1 cm and without axillary lymph node involvement, the estimated risk of systemic relapse is approximately 10%, increasing to approximately 50% for lesions greater than 3 cm in diameter (Mansour et al, 1989; Rosen et al, 1989). For that reason, adjuvant therapy is generally offered to women with tumors greater than 1 cm in diameter either in the form of chemotherapy for premenopausal or estrogen receptor (ER)-negative postmenopausal women, or endocrine therapy (tamoxifen) for ER-positive postmenopausal women.

Hormone Receptor Status. It has been shown that recurrence rates correlate with receptor status, being greater in women with estrogen and progesterone receptor–negative tumors (Clark and McGuire, 1989; McGuire and Clark, 1989). Estrogen and progesterone receptor status correlates directly with menopausal status and inversely with tumor grade. At most centers estrogen and progesterone receptor status are determined by immunohistochemical techniques that can be performed either on fresh tissue or from paraffin-embedded specimens. In addition to prognostic information, estrogen and progesterone

receptor status are used in treatment planning in both the primary and recurrent settings.

Biologic and Genetic Factors. In addition to tumor size, lymph node, and hormone receptor status, many other factors have been demonstrated to correlate with clinical behavior. Among these are DNA ploidy (Clark et al, 1989; Hedley et al, 1993; Wenger et al, 1993), S-phase fraction (Clark et al, 1992; Wenger et al, 1993), and tumor grade (Elston et al, 1991; Schumacher et al, 1993). Overexpression of oncogenes such as *Her-2/neu* (Gusterson et al, 1992; Wright et al, 1992), mutation of tumor suppressor genes such as p-53 (Silverstrini et al, 1993; Mark et al, 1994), and microvessel density (Heimann et al, 1996) have been shown to correlate inversely with prognosis. Her-2 protein, an EGF receptor-related protein, is overexpressed in 25% to 30% of breast cancer and has been shown to negatively influence prognosis. Recent reports have demonstrated the potential to exploit Her-2 overexpression therapeutically by the administration of a Her-2 oncogene receptor antibody (herceptin), in addition to paclitaxel chemotherapy (Slamon et al, 1998).

Types of Adjuvant Therapies

Adjuvant therapy may be in the form of locoregional therapy or systemic therapy.

LOCOREGIONAL THERAPY

Adjuvant radiation therapy is appropriate following breast-conserving surgery after achieving adequate surgical resection margins, and in patients with large tumors involving the skin or chest wall after mastectomy, or, in some cases, in patients with extracapsular or multiple (>3) lymph node involvement. Typically, locoregional radiation therapy is administered in daily 200-cGy fractions to a total dose of 5000 cGy, followed in cases of close surgical margins by tumor bed boost of 1000 cGy. High dose rate (HDR) brachytherapy, treating the tumor excision bed over a short (usually 5 day) period, is currently under investigation as an alternative to 5 to 6 weeks of whole-breast radiotherapy for small lesions.

SYSTEMIC THERAPY

The decision to offer systemic adjuvant therapy is based on the estimated risk of systemic relapse calculated from the prognostic factors previously discussed. In each case a risk-benefit analysis must be performed and the estimated benefit considered relative to the anticipated toxicity of the treatment. As previously stated, the absolute benefit to an individual is determined by the untreated risk of relapse and the effectiveness of the adjuvant therapy in reducing that risk. In general, adjuvant systemic therapy reduces the risk of systemic relapse by approximately 25% (Fisher et al, 1989; Early Breast Cancer Trialists Collaborative Group, 1992, 1998); therefore, a woman with an untreated risk of relapse of 10% (T1a/T1b N0) would have a relatively small (2.5% absolute risk reduction) benefit. This would mean that, for every 100 women treated, 10 would potentially benefit and, in actuality, 2.5 women would derive long-term benefits from the adjuvant therapy. Based on these figures, women with such early-stage cancers are usually not offered adjuvant therapy, while essentially all node-positive and high-risk node-negative women are offered chemotherapy and/or endocrine therapy in the adjuvant setting.

Cytotoxic Chemotherapy. The most commonly employed cytotoxic chemotherapeutic agents in the adjuvant setting are cyclophosphamide, methotrexate, 5-fluorouracil (5-FU), and doxorubicin. Currently, investigational trials are underway evaluating doxorubicin and cyclophosphamide with or without paclitaxel. In women deemed at extremely high risk for systemic relapse ($\geq$10 lymph nodes), dose-intensive chemotherapy with autologous bone marrow transplantation or peripheral stem call rescue is being evaluated.

Endocrine Therapy. Tamoxifen is the standard agent employed in the adjuvant setting for postmenopausal ER-positive breast cancers, and in most cases of premenopausal ER-positive breast cancers following chemotherapy. Tamoxifen competes with estrogen for cellular receptor sites, thereby acting as an antiestrogen in breast tumors. The NSABP-B14 trial demonstrated the efficacy of tamoxifen in the adjuvant setting in women with ER-positive, node-negative breast tumors (Fisher et al, 1989). Subsequent studies, including a meta-analysis, have shown that the benefit of tamoxifen is similar for node-positive patients (Early Breast Cancer Trialists Collaborative Group, 1992). The standard dose of tamoxifen is 20 mg/day. The ideal duration of treatment has not been established. A trial from the Swedish Breast Cancer Cooperative Group (1996) demonstrated that 5 years of tamoxifen is superior to 2 years with regard to disease-free survival. There was an approximately 18% reduction in recurrence and mortality with the longer treatment. An update of the NSABP-B14 data revealed that 5 years of tamoxifen was superior to no tamoxifen; however, no additional advantage was demonstrated by continuing tamoxifen therapy beyond 5 years (Fisher et al, 1996). The major toxicity of tamoxifen is related to its estrogen agonistic activity on the endometrium. There is an approximately 3-fold increased risk of endometrial polyps and a 10-fold increased risk of hyperplasia in women taking tamoxifen (Assikis and Jordan, 1995). The exact risk of endometrial carcinoma in women taking tamoxifen is unknown because of the design of most studies that have addressed this issue. Relative risks have ranged from 0.47 to 15.2 (Morgan, 1997). Although it has been reported that endometrial cancer associated with tamoxifen use has a higher histologic grade and is associated with a poorer prognosis, studies show that

these cancers are similar in grade, stage, and survival to non-tamoxifen-related cancers (Barakat et al, 1994). The value of routine endometrial biopsy and/or ultrasound measurement of endometrial thickness are unproven in asymptomatic women and therefore not recommended in the American Society of Clinical Oncology guidelines.

All women with abnormal bleeding on tamoxifen should undergo endometrial histologic evaluation.

FOLLOW-UP

A standardized follow-up program is essential. The 10-year survival rates for "curative" breast cancer (T1 N0 and T2 N0) are 85% and 75%, respectively. These figures drop sharply to 40% if there is nodal involvement. Most recurrences occur within the first 2 years following treatment. Patients continue to die of breast cancer for periods exceeding 15 to 20 years following adequate treatment and, therefore, they must be observed indefinitely.

TREATMENT OF RECURRENCE

Locoregional recurrences are usually managed with a combination of surgery, radiotherapy, and in many cases systemic therapy. Commonly used agents for treatment of systemic relapse are doxorubicin, cyclophosphamide, paclitaxel, vinorelbine, 5-FU, vincristine, and endocrine therapy.

Patients with metastatic disease are not curable; however, they may be managed with a variety of palliative therapies and, in some cases, for many years with excellent quality of life. A number of diagnostic studies are currently used to detect metastatic disease, including, on an annual basis, liver function tests, carcinoembryonic antigen and CA 15-3 determinations, and a mammogram and chest film. The extent of the follow-up examination has been challenged by a number of investigators. Although more extensive testing leads to earlier diagnosis of recurrence, it does not appear that earlier diagnosis results in improved outcome. Biopsy should be performed to document the recurrence and, if possible, to determine the receptor status. Treatment strategy depends on the extent and location of the disease, the menstrual status of the patient, and the disease-free interval.

Palliation may be achieved with hormonal therapy; however, this should not be used in patients who need a rapid response (i.e., patients with visceral disease). The receptor status can be used to predict the response. About 60% of women with estrogen receptor protein respond to hormonal manipulation, and those with progesterone receptor protein have an 80% or more chance of response to hormones. Tamoxifen produces a response in about one third of the patients with metastatic disease and in two thirds of those with estrogen receptor protein activity. Oophorectomy may be used in an endocrine procedure for premenopausal women. The expected response rate is in the range of 30% to 40%.

Commonly used drugs for palliation include doxorubicin (Adriamycin), cyclophosphamide (Cytoxan), prednisone, methotrexate, 5-FU, and vincristine. Combinations of these cytotoxic agents result in a response rate of 60% to 70%, but all of these patients eventually die of their disease.

Patients with pathologic fractures may be managed with appropriate orthopedic procedures and pamidronate (an osteoclast inhibitor), while radiotherapy may be employed for palliation of pain caused by metastases. Brain metastases are usually managed with palliative radiation therapy. More recent data suggest a role for aromatase inhibitors in the management of ER-positive recurrent or metastatic cancers (Buzdan et al, 1996). Currently, dose-intensive chemotherapy with peripheral stem cell or autologous bone marrow rescue are being employed in the treatment of recurrent metastatic breast cancer. The value of this approach compared to standard combination salvage chemotherapy is unknown at this time.

Metastatic breast cancer, because of the biology of this disease, must be considered a chronic illness. Therefore, the quality of life is important. Continuity of the health care team and a positive attitude are essential to provide the support needed for these patients.

BREAST CANCER WITH SPECIAL FEATURES

Pregnancy

Breast cancer diagnosed during pregnancy is a complex condition requiring a multidisciplinary approach to the management of mother and fetus. Breast cancer occurs in approximately 1 in 3000 pregnancies (Saunders and Baum, 1993). In women under the age of 40 years, 15% of breast cancers occur during or within 1 year of pregnancy (Wallack et al, 1993). As more women delay childbirth into the fourth and fifth decades, greater numbers of gestational breast cancers can be anticipated.

Delay in diagnosis is a major problem in breast cancers associated with pregnancy. It has been demonstrated that pregnant women have larger primary tumors and a higher percentage have axillary lymph node metastases than age-matched nonpregnant women (Petrek et al, 1991; Anderson et al, 1996). It is not clear whether this delay is due to physiologic changes that occur during pregnancy that limit the sensitivity of the breast exam, physician delay in diagnostic evaluation, or the fact that pregnant women do not undergo mammography, thereby eliminating clinically occult lesions from this group.

Breast examination should be part of every new prenatal examination, and any palpable abnormality should be evaluated promptly. A palpable mass in pregnancy is best evaluated initially by ultrasound to distinguish cystic from solid lesions. Cysts may be aspirated and solid lesions evaluated by FNA biopsy as in the nonpregnant woman. Excisional biopsy can be performed under local anesthesia without harm to the fetus.

The treatment of breast cancer in pregnancy depends on the gestational age at diagnosis and the patient's desire to continue the pregnancy. The literature does not support the concept that pregnancy termination improves outcome. The decision to terminate should be based on concerns related to treatment toxicity to the fetus. The recommended local therapy of breast cancer during pregnancy is modified radical mastectomy. Unless the patient intends to terminate an early pregnancy or the gestation is near term, breast conservation is not appropriate. Even with abdominal shielding, radiation therapy is contraindicated in pregnancy because of internal scatter resulting in significant fetal exposure. If the gestation is near term, radiation therapy may be delayed until the postpartum period.

When indicated, adjuvant chemotherapy may be used during the second and third trimesters. With the exception of prematurity and intrauterine growth retardation, there appears to be no increase in adverse fetal outcomes in women treated with systemic chemotherapy during this time (Petrek, 1994). Chemotherapy given during the first trimester results in a fetal malformation rate of 12.7% (Schapira and Chudley, 1984).

Breast cancer has been reported to metastasize to the placenta (Smythe et al, 1973; Davegan, 1983), although no cases of actual fetal metastases have been documented.

The prognosis of breast cancer in pregnancy is related to the usual prognostic factors. When corrected for factors such as lymph node status and tumor size, pregnancy per se does not appear to influence survival or recurrence rate (Smythe et al, 1973; Petrek et al, 1991; Anderson et al, 1996). A subsequent pregnancy does not appear to influence survival in breast cancer patients who have received appropriate treatment, although the possibility of selection bias exists in some of the current studies (Clark and Reid, 1978; Ribiero and Jones, 1986). Continued evaluation of these patients is required to determine the precise influence of a subsequent pregnancy on survival.

In Situ Carcinoma

In situ must be distinguished from infiltrating carcinoma. By definition, in situ carcinoma is confined to the duct and/or lobular epithelium from which it originates without invasion of the surrounding breast stroma. The recognition of this entity as distinct from infiltrating carcinoma is important for treatment planning and prognosis. Generally, two types of in situ carcinoma are recognized: lobular carcinoma in situ (LCIS) or lobular neoplasia, and ductal carcinoma in situ (DCIS).

LCIS, or lobular neoplasia, is usually diagnosed as an incidental finding following biopsy for a dominant mass or an adjacent mammographic lesion. The most important features of the lesion when planning treatment include:

1. Its propensity for bilaterality
2. Multicentricity
3. The relatively low rate of development of subsequent infiltrating lobular carcinoma

The entity is best viewed as a marker for the subsequent development of both ipsilateral and contralateral carcinoma. The annual incidence rate of invasive carcinoma following a diagnosis of LCIS is approximately 1% per year (Haagensen et al, 1981; Salvadon et al, 1991; Zurrida et al, 1996). Subsequent invasive cancers are equally likely to affect the contralateral breast, and the majority of cases are infiltrating ductal carcinomas rather than lobular lesions (Rosen et al, 1978; Hoagenien et al, 1981; Salvadon et al, 1991; Zurrida et al, 1996). Treatment options include surgery or a period of watchful waiting with appropriate follow-up diagnostic studies. A reasonable treatment plan includes reinforcement of breast self-examination, annual physical examination, and annual mammography. It must be said at the outset that these lesions often are not visible by mammography and are usually clinically occult. Because of this possibility, some patients may consider prophylactic mastectomy. Because of the combined risk of ipsilateral and contralateral carcinoma, the recommended procedure, prophylactic mastectomy, is bilateral simple mastectomy. When LCIS is an incidental finding, attempts to obtain clear surgical margins are not necessary.

DCIS is an entirely different lesion and of considerably more significance. If left untreated, infiltrating carcinoma develops in the ipsilateral breast in approximately 50% of the cases (Rosen et al, 1980). Many of the lesions are detected coincidentally associated with an invasive lesion or an occult lesion with microcalcifications. In the past, standard therapy has been total mastectomy with or without conventional axillary dissection. This results in cure in nearly 100% of cases. With the advent of conservative treatment for small invasive cancers, there has been considerable interest in applying a similar surgical approach to the treatment of these in situ lesions. Data suggest that DCIS treated with wide local excision alone results in a local recurrence rate of 8% to 43%, with 20% to 56% of these lesions being invasive cancers (Carpenter et al, 1989; Lagios et al, 1989; Fisher et al, 1991; Silverstein et al, 1992). When wide local excision is followed by radiation therapy, recurrence rates at 5 years have been shown to be 10%, with approximately 2.9% being invasive (Fisher et al, 1993).

Local recurrence rates after mastectomy are generally reported to be less than 1%. Currently women with unifocal DCIS in whom adequate surgical margins can be obtained with acceptable cosmetic results are offered breast-conserving surgery followed by radiation therapy as an alterative to mastectomy. Most series report less than 1% incidence of lymph node metastases in cases of DCIS, and these probably represent unrecognized foci of invasive carcinoma. Currently, axillary lymph node dissection is not recommended in the management of DCIS.

Paget's Disease of the Nipple

Patients with Paget's disease often present with a chronic history of an eczematoid change in the nipple, occasionally with crusting, and "nipple discharge." A mass may be present. Long delays in diagnosis are common because most patients are treated for some time with local medication, including topical antibiotics, various creams, and steroids.

The diagnosis is confirmed by skin biopsy, which can be performed on a day surgery basis with local anesthesia. The diagnosis is confirmed with the identification of the typical Paget cell. This is a large ovoid cell possessive of an abundant clear opaque pale staining cytoplasm with a large round or ovoid nucleus. These changes may be associated either with intraductal or invasive breast carcinoma focal or diffuse. The recommended treatment is modified radical for extensive invasive lesions and wide excision of the nipple-areolar complex for focal lesions, involving the subareolar area (Lagios et al, 1984; Morimoto et al, 1985).

Locally Advanced and Inflammatory Carcinoma

Locally advanced breast carcinoma is usually defined as a lesion greater than 5 cm (T3) and involving the chest wall and/or skin. In mammographically screened populations, locally advanced breast carcinomas generally represent approximately 5% of cases versus 30% to 50% of the cases in nonscreened populations (Seidman et al, 1987). Inflammatory carcinoma is a distinct form of locally advanced breast carcinoma defined *clinically* by diffuse erythema, warmth, edema, and induration of the breast. It is often misdiagnosed as "mastitis" and treated with antibiotics, resulting in a delay in diagnosis. The *pathologic* diagnosis of inflammatory carcinoma is based on the presence of extensive lymphatic infiltration of the dermis and breast stroma. Inflammatory carcinoma represents approximately 2% of breast cancers. In general, modern management of locally advanced breast cancers and inflammatory carcinomas consists of neoadjuvant systemic chemotherapy followed by a combination of radiation and/or surgery. The purpose of neoadjuvant chemotherapy is to (1) treat occult systemic metastases and (2) decrease the extent of local disease, rendering it more amenable to locoregional therapy (surgery and/or radiation therapy). Historically, 5-year survival of women with inflammatory breast carcinoma has been reported to be 0–5% (Jaiyesimi et al, 1992; Singleton et al, 1994). With modern multimodality therapy, 5-year survival rates of over 50% have been reported (Jacquillat et al, 1986; Maloisel et al, 1990).

CASE STUDY

One patient was referred to the Breast Health Center because of a diagnosis of "mastitis" early in her pregnancy (12 weeks). On examination, the right breast was erythematous and edematous and no masses were palpable. Immediate consultation was obtained with the radiologist. An appropriately shielded mammogram revealed skin thickening only and no mass; however, an ultrasound revealed a condensation of "breast tissue" in the upper outer quadrant. FNA was performed in this area, revealing "invasive ductal cancer."

Because of the erythema and edema and the possibility of inflammatory carcinoma, an open biopsy was performed with removal of a portion of dermis. This revealed carcinoma with involvement of intradermal lymphatic vessels, thus confirming the diagnosis of inflammatory carcinoma. ∎

The physician must rule out inflammatory carcinoma in all patients who present with unexplained erythema and edema of the breast. The mammogram usually is noncontributory except for skin thickening, and occasionally ultrasound examination will describe a parenchymal abnormality, as noted in the patient described above. Diagnosis must be confirmed by open biopsy with removal of a portion of skin or punch biopsy. Treatment, as previously discussed, must be multimodal: neoadjuvant chemotherapy, radiation, and surgery.

REFERENCES

Adye B, Jolly PC, Bauermeister DE: The role of fine needle aspiration in the management of solid breast masses. Arch Surg 1988;123:37.

Albertini JJ, Lyman GH, Cox C, et al: Lymphatic mapping and sentinel node biopsy in the patient with breast cancer. JAMA 1996;276:1818.

Anderson BO, Petrek JA, Byrd DR, et al: Pregnancy influences breast cancer stage at diagnosis in women 30 years of age and younger. Ann Surg Oncol 1996;3:204.

Assikis VJ, Jordan VC: Gynecologic effects of tamoxifen and the association with endometrial carcinoma. Int J Gynecol Obstet 1995;49:241.

Barakat RR, Wong G, Curtin JP, et al: Tamoxifen use in breast cancer patients who subsequently develop corpus cancer is not associated with a higher incidence of adverse histologic features. Gynecol Oncol 1994;55:164.

Bodian CA, Perzin KH, Lattes R, et al: Prognostic significance of benign proliferative breast disease. Cancer 1993a;71:3896.

Bodian CA, Perzin KH, Lattes R, et al: Reproducibility and validity of pathologic classifications of benign breast disease and implications for clinical applications. Cancer 1993b;71:3908.

Bradlow L, Briton L, Pike M, et al: Does abortion increase breast cancer risk? J Natl Cancer Inst 1993;85:1987.

Briton L: In: Abstracts of the 9th International Breast Society Meeting, Houston, 1996.

Buzdan A, Jonat W, Howell A, et al: Anastrozole, a potent and selective aromatase inhibitor, versus magistral acetate in postmenopausal women with advanced breast cancer: results of overview analysis of two Phase III trials. J Clin Oncol 1996;14:2000.

Calache A, McPherson K, Barltrop K, et al: Oral contraceptives and breast cancer. Br J Hosp Med 1983;30:278.

Carpenter R, Boulter PA, Cooke T, et al: Management of screen detected ductal carcinoma in situ of the female breast. Br J Surg 1989;76:564.

Carter CL, Allen C, Henson DE: Relation of tumor size, lymph node status, and survival in 24,740 breast cancer cases. Cancer 1989;63:181.

Clark CM, Mathien MC, Owens MA, et al: Prognostic significance of S-phase fraction in good-risk, node-negative breast cancer patients. J Clin Oncol 1992;10:428.

Clark G, McGuire W: Standard receptor and other prognostic factors in primary breast cancer. Semin Oncol 1989;15:20.

Clark GM, Dressler LG, Owens MA, et al: Prediction of relapse as patients in patterns with node-negative breast cancer by DNA flow cytometry. N Engl J Med 1989;320:627.

Clark RM, Reid J: Carcinoma of the breast in pregnancy and lactation. Int J Radiat Oncol Biol Phys 1978;4:693.

Collins FS: BRCA1-1: lots of mutations, lots of dilemmas. N Engl J Med 1996;334:186.

Davegan WL: Cancer and pregnancy. CA Cancer J Clin 1983;33:5.

Dhodapker MV, Ingle JN, Ahmann DL: Estrogen replacement therapy withdrawal and regression of metastatic breast cancer. Cancer 1995;75:43.

Dupont WD, Page DL, Rogers LW, et al: Influence of exogenous estrogens, proliferative breast disease, and other variables on breast cancer risk. Cancer 1989;63:948.

Early Breast Cancer Trialists Collaborative Group: Systemic treatment of early breast cancer by hormonal, cytotoxic, or immune therapy. Cancer 1992;339:71.

Early Breast Cancer Trialists Collaborative Group: Polychemotherapy for early breast cancer: an overview of randomized trials. Lancet 1998;352:930.

Elston CW, Ellis IO: Pathological prognostic factors in breast cancer. I. The value of histologic grade in breast cancer: experience from a large study with long-term follow-up. Histopathology 1991;19:403.

Ewertz M, Duffy SW, Adami HO, et al: Age at first birth, parity and risk of breast cancer: a metaanalysis of eight studies from Nordic countries. Int J Cancer 1990;46:597.

Fisher B, Bauer M, Wickerham DL, et al: Relation of number of positive axillary nodes to the prognosis of patients with primary breast cancer: an NSABP update. Cancer 1983;52:1551.

Fisher B, Costantino J, Redmond C, et al: A randomized clinical trial of tamoxifen in the treatment of patients with node-negative breast cancer who have estrogen receptor-positive tumors. N Engl J Med 1989;320:479.

Fisher B, Costantino J, Redmond C, et al: Lumpectomy compared with lumpectomy and radiation therapy for the treatment of intraductal breast cancer. N Engl J Med 1993;328:1581.

Fisher B, Constantino JP, Wickerham DL, et al: Tamoxifen for prevention of breast cancer: report of National Surgical Breast and Bowel Project P-1 study. J Natl Cancer Inst 1998;90:1371.

Fisher B, Dignan J, Bryant J, et al: Five versus more than five years of tamoxifen therapy for breast cancer patients with negative lymph nodes and estrogen receptor-positive tumors. J Natl Cancer Inst 1996;88:1529.

Fisher B, Leeming R, Anderson S, et al: Conservative management of intraductal carcinoma (DCIS) of the breast. J Surg Oncol 1991;47:139.

Fowble BL, Solin LJ, Schultz, et al: Ten year results of conservative treatment, conservative surgery and irradiation for stage I and II breast cancer. Int J Radiat Oncol Biol Phys 1991;21:269.

Gage I, Recht A, Gelman R, et al: Long term outcome following breast conserving surgery and radiation therapy. Int J Radiat Oncol Biol Phys 1995;33:245.

Ginsburg ES, Mello NK, Mendelson JH, et al: Effects of alcohol ingestion on estrogens in postmenopausal women. JAMA 1996;276:1747.

Giuliano A, Barth A, Spirack B, et al: Incidence and predictors of axillary metastasis for T1 carcinoma of the breast. J Am Coll Surg 1996;183:185.

Goldhirsch A, Wood WC, Senn H-J, et al: Meeting highlights: International Consensus Panel on Treatment of Primary Breast Cancer. J Natl Cancer Inst 1995;87:1441.

Gusterson BA, Gelber RD, Goldbrisch A, et al: Prognostic importance of c-erb B-2 expression in breast cancer: International Ludwig J Breast Cancer Study Group. J Clin Oncol 1992;10:1049.

Haagensen CD, Bodian C, Haagensen DE: Lobular neoplasia (lobular carcinoma in situ) breast carcinoma: risk and detection. Philadelphia: WB Saunders Company, 1981:238.

Haffty BG, Goldberg NB, Fischer D, et al: Conservative surgery and radiation therapy in breast cancer: local recurrence and prognostic implications. Int J Radiat Oncol Biol Phys 1989;17:727.

Harris JR, Lippman ME, Veronesi U, et al: Breast cancer: medical progress. N Engl J Med 1992;327:319.

Healy B, for PEPI: In perspective: good answers spawn pressing questions. JAMA 1995;273:240.

Hedley DW, Clark GM, Comelive CJ, et al: Consensus review of the clinical utility of DNA cytometry in carcinoma of the breast. Cytometry 1993;14:482.

Heimann R, Fergerson D, Pavers C, et al: Angiogenesis as a predictor of long-term survival for patients with node-negative breast cancer. J Natl Cancer Inst 1996;88:1764.

Hunter DJ, Manson JE, Colditz GA, et al: A prospective study of the intake of vitamin C, E, and A and the risk of breast cancer. N Engl J Med 1993;329:234.

Hutter RVP: Goodbye to "fibrocystic disease." N Engl J Med 1985;312:179.

Jacquillat C, Weil M, Auclerc G, et al: Neoadjuvant chemotherapy in the conservative management of breast cancers: study on 205 patients. In Jacquillat C, Weil M, Khayat D (eds): Neoadjuvant Chemotherapy. London: John Libbey, 1986:197.

Jaiyesimi IA, Buzdar AU, Hortobagyi G: Inflammatory breast cancer: a review. J Clin Oncol 1992;10:1014.

Krag D, Weaver D, Ashikaga T, et al: The sentinel node in breast cancer: a multicenter validation study. N Engl J Med 1998;339:941.

Kurtz JM, Amalric R, Brandone H, et al: Local recurrence after breast conserving surgery and radiotherapy: frequency, time, course and prognosis. Cancer 1989;63:1912.

Lagios MD, Margolin FR, Westdahl PR, et al: Mammographically detected duct carcinoma in situ: frequency of local recurrence following tylectomy and prognostic effect of nuclear grade on local recurrence. Cancer 1989;63:618.

Lagios MD, Westdahl PR, Rose MR, et al: Paget's disease of the nipple. Cancer 1984;54:545.

Landis SH, Murray T, Bolden S, Wingo PA: Cancer statistics 1999. CA Cancer J Clin 1999;49:8.

Laya MB, Larson EB, Taplin SH, et al: Effect of estrogen replacement therapy on the specificity and sensitivity of screening mammography. J Natl Cancer Inst 1996;88:643.

MacMahon B, Cole P, Brown J: Etiology of human breast cancer: a review. J Natl Cancer Inst 1973;50:21.

Maloisel F, Dufour P, Bergerat JP, et al: Results of initial doxorubicin, 5-fluorouracil and cyclophosphamide combination chemotherapy for inflammatory carcinoma of the breast. Cancer 1990;65:851.

Mansour E, Gray R, Shatila A, et al: Efficacy of adjuvant chemotherapy in high-risk node-negative breast cancer: an intergroup study. N Engl J Med 1989;320:485.

Mark JR, Humphrey PA, Wu K, et al: Overexpression of p53 and Her-2neu proteins as prognostic markers in early stage breast cancer. Ann Surg 1994;219:332.

Martin LM, Calle E, Wingo PA, et al: Self-reported use of mammography among women aged ≥40 years—United States 1989 and 1995. JAMA 1997;278:1395.

McGuire W, Clark G: Prognostic factors for recurrence and survival in axillary node-negative breast cancer. J Steroid Biochem 1989;34:145.

Minton JP, Foecking MK, Webster DJT: Response of fibrocystic disease to caffeine withdrawal and correlation of cyclic nucleotides with breast cancer. Am J Obstet Gynecol 1979;135:157.

Morgan RW: Risk of endometrial cancer after tamoxifen treatment. Oncology 1997;11(Suppl 1):35.

Morimoto T, Komaki K, Inui K, et al: Involvement of nipple and areola in early breast cancer. Cancer 1985;55:2459.

National Cancer Institute: SEER Cancer Statistics Review 1973–1990. (NIH publication no 93-2789). Bethesda, MD: National Cancer Institute, 1993.

National Cancer Institute: Breast Cancer: PDQ State of the Art Statement. Bethesda, MD: National Cancer Institute, 1996.

National Institutes of Health: Women's Health Initiative. Bethesda, MD: National Institutes of Health, 1994.

National Institutes of Health: Consensus Development Statement: Breast Cancer Screening for Women Ages 40–49. Bethesda, MD: National Institutes of Health, 1997.

Nelson SJ: Caution guides genetic testing for hereditary cancer genes. J Natl Cancer Inst 1995;88:70.

Nemoto T, Natarajian N, Bedwani R, et al: Breast cancer in the medical half: results of the 1978 survey of the American College of Surgeons. Cancer 1983;51:1333.

Newcomb PA, Storer BE, Longnecker MP, et al: Lactation and a reduced risk of premenopausal breast cancer. N Engl J Med 1994;330:81.

Office of Research Reporting: Research Report: Bethesda, MD: The women's health initiative. National Institute of Child Health and Human Development, 1993.

Parker SH, Job WE, Dennis MA, et al: Ultrasound guided automated large core breast biopsy. Radiology 1993;187:507.

Parker SH, Lovin JD, Job WE, et al: Stereotactic breast biopsy with a biopsy gun. Radiology 1990;176:741.

Parker SH, Lovin JD, Job WE, et al: Non-palpable breast lesions, stereotactic automated large core biopsies. Radiology 1991;180:403.

Petrek JA: Breast cancer in pregnancy. Monogr Nat Cancer Inst 1994;16:113.

Petrek JA, Dukoff R, Rogatko A: Prognosis of pregnancy-associated breast cancer. Cancer 1991;67:869.

Phelps HM, Phelps CE: Caffeine ingestion and breast cancer: a negative correlation. Cancer 1988;61:1051.

Pike M: In: Abstracts of the Cancer and Genetics Symposium, 1996.

Ribiero GG, Jones M: Carcinoma of the breast associated with pregnancy. Br J Surg 1986;73:607.

Rosen PP, Braun D, Kinne D: The clinical significance of preinvasive breast carcinoma. Cancer 1980;46:919.

Rosen PP, Groshen S, Saijo P, et al: A long-term follow-up study of survival in stage I ($T_1N_0M_0$) and Stage II ($T_1N_1M_0$) breast carcinomas. J Clin Oncol 1989;7:355.

Rosen PP, Licherman PH, Braun DW Jr, et al: Lobular carcinoma in situ of the breast. Am J Surg Pathol 1978;2:225.

Salvadon B, Bartolic, Zurrida S, et al: Risk of invasive cancer in women with lobular carcinoma in situ of the breast. Eur J Cancer 1991;27:35.

Saunders CM, Baum M: Breast cancer and pregnancy: a review. J R Soc Med 1993;86:162.

Schapira DV, Chudley AE: Successful pregnancy following continuous treatment with combination chemotherapy before conception and throughout pregnancy. Cancer 1984;54:800.

Schumacher M, Schmour C, Squerbret W, et al: The prognostic effect of histologic tumor grade in node-negative breast cancer patients. Breast Cancer Res Treat 1993;25:235.

SEER: Cancer Statistics Review 1973–1990. United States Department of Health and Human Services, Public Health Service, NIH, NCI NIH Publication 1990;93.

Seidman H, Gelb SK, Silverberg E, et al: Survival experience in the Breast Cancer Detection Demonstration Project. CA Cancer J Clin 1987;37:258.

Silverstein MJ, Cohlan BR, Gierson ED, et al: Duct carcinoma in situ: 227 cases without microinvasion. Eur J Cancer 1992;28:630.

Silverstrini R, Benini E, Daidone MG, et al: P53 as an independent prognostic marker in lymph node-negative breast cancer patients. J Natl Cancer Inst 1993;85:965.

Singleton SE, Ames FC, Buzdar AU: Management of inflammatory breast cancer. World J Surg 1994;18:87.

Slamon D, Leyland-Jones B, Shak S, et al: Additional herceptin (humanized anti Her-2 antibody) to first line chemotherapy for

Her-2 overexpression metastatic breast cancer markedly increases anticancer activity. A randomized multinational controlled phase III trial (abstract). Proc Am Soc Clin Oncol 1998; 17:98.

Smythe AR, Underwood PB, Dreutner A: Metastatic placental tumors: report of three cancers. Am J Obstet Gynecol 1973;125:1149.

Sullivan JM, Fowlkes LP: The clinical aspects of estrogen and the cardiovascular system. Obstet Gynecol 1996;87:36.

Swedish Breast Cancer Cooperative Group: Randomized trial of two versus five years of adjuvant tamoxifen for postmenopausal early stage breast cancer. J Natl Cancer Inst 1996;88:1543.

Wallack MK, Wolf JA, Bedwihek J, et al: Gestational carcinoma of the female breast. Curr Probl Cancer 1993;7:1.

Webber BL, Garber JE: Family history and breast cancer: probabilities and possibilities. JAMA 1993;270:1602.

Wenger CR, Beardshee S, Owens MA, et al: DNA ploidy, S-phase and steroid receptors in more than 127,000 breast cancer products. Breast Cancer Res Treat 1993;28:9.

Wild RA: Estrogen: effects on the cardiovascular tree. Obstet Gynecol 1996;87:227.

Willett WC, Stampfer NJ, Colditz GA, et al: Dietary fat and the risk of breast cancer. N Engl J Med 1987;316:22.

Winchester DP, Cox JD: Standards for breast conservation treatment. CA Cancer J Clin 1992;42:134.

Wright C, Nicholson S, Angus B, et al: Relationship between c-erb B-2 protein product expression and response to endocrine therapy in advanced breast cancer. Br J Cancer 1992;65:118.

Wynder EH: Commentary: breast cancer precaution strategies. Oncology 1997;11;1997.

Ziegler RG, Hoover RN, Pike MC, et al: Migration patterns and breast cancer risk in Asian-American Women. J Natl Cancer Inst 1993;85:1819.

Zurrida S, Bartoli C, Galimberti V, et al: Interpretation of the risk associated with the unexpected finding of lobular carcinoma in situ. Ann Surg Oncol 1996;3:57.

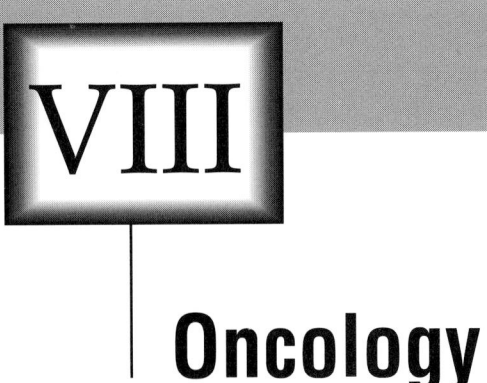

VIII

Oncology

51

Molecular Biology and Applications to Gynecology

Vicki V. Baker

The ability of cells to maintain their structural integrity and function is contingent upon the expression and replication of genetic information. The female reproductive tract provides several models for the identification and characterization of the ways in which these goals are achieved. As examples, the cyclic renewal of the endometrium, the controlled proliferation of the cervical transformation zone, and the indefinite arrest of the primary oocyte in meiosis I with its subsequent development following fertilization all serve as models for the study of the molecular biology of cell growth, differentiation, and function.

METHODOLOGY

The major advances in our understanding of the specific genes and their protein products that regulate cell growth, differentiation, and cell death are a consequence of methodologic advances in basic science. Some of the investigational techniques commonly used in molecular biologic studies are described in Table 51–1. Detailed information concerning these techniques and others may be found in a number of standard texts and manuals.

CELL GROWTH, DIFFERENTIATION, AND DEATH

Cell proliferation and cell death are fundamental events in the life cycle of a cell that are essential to our understanding of normal and abnormal function. Cell proliferation is simplistically defined as an increase in cell number. Cell proliferation is required to balance the loss of senescent cells and to respond to stimuli requiring regulated growth, such as the replacement of cells lost as a consequence of trauma, the clonal expansion of immunologic cells, and placental growth. Cell proliferation is balanced by cell death to maintain a steady state with respect to tissue mass. The physiologic loss of cells occurs as a consequence of programmed cell death or apoptosis, which encompasses a series of genetically regulated events that are energy-dependent processes.

Apoptosis plays a central role in organ development and maintenance of tissue mass. In mammals, examples of apoptosis are found during embryogenesis, endocrine-dependent cellular atrophy, and normal tissue turnover. Apoptosis is the mechanism that accounts for deletion of the interdigital webs (Hammar and Mottet, 1971) and fusion of the palate (Farbman, 1968). The reduction in the number of endometrial cells in response to alterations in steroid hormone levels during the menstrual cycle is in part a consequence of programmed cell death (Pollard et al, 1987). Granulosa cells undergo programmed cell death (e.g., follicular atresia) in response to androgens (Billig et al, 1993).

Apoptosis is a process distinct from necrosis and can be differentiated by a number of histologic and biochemical characteristics (Table 51–2). Although the molecular mechanism of programmed cell death has not been fully defined, characteristic morphologic changes occur in which the cell and its nucleus shrink, condense, and fragment. In contrast, cells that die as a result of acute injury usually swell and burst during the process of necrosis. Apoptosis is a physiologic event that balances cell proliferation to maintain tissue and organ homeostasis. When apoptosis exceeds cell proliferation, the result is atrophy. When cell proliferation exceeds apoptosis, the result is hyperplasia. Neoplastic tissues are often characterized by an increase in cell proliferation and a decrease in apoptosis.

Cell proliferation and programmed cell death are regulated by the coordinate expression of a number of genes in response to internal and external cellular signals (Fig. 51–1). Among the groups of genes that regulate these processes, proto-oncogenes and tumor suppressor genes are particularly important.

1151

Table 51–1. EXPERIMENTAL METHODS COMMONLY USED IN MOLECULAR BIOLOGIC STUDIES

Southern	Analysis of *DNA* for mutations and amplification using restriction endonuclease digestion to detect fragments of varying molecular weight by agarose gel electrophoresis
Northern	Analysis of *RNA* for transcript size and level of gene expression
Western	Detection of specific *proteins* or peptides using antibodies
Single-strand conformational polymorphism analysis	Detection of variations in single-strand *DNA* sequence based upon differences in migration through a nondenaturing gel
Polymerase chain reaction (PCR)	Amplification of 300– to 500–base pair segments of *DNA*
Reverse transcriptase–PCR	Amplification of *mRNA* by converting it to DNA using the enzyme reverse transcriptase
Protein truncation assay	Detection of DNA mutations that encode stop codons based upon an abnormally short *protein* compared to the normal protein product
In situ hybridization	Detection of *genes, mRNA, or protein* in single cells or thin tissue sections using sequence specific probes
Restriction fragment length polymorphism analysis	Detection of normal *DNA* sequences of varying length that encode normal protein products and may be linked with specific diseases or indicate DNA recombination
Methylation analysis	Detection of methylated guanosine-cytosine *DNA* sequences using restriction endonuclease enzymes (increased gene methylation is often associated with decreased gene expression)
Mobility shift DNA-binding assay	Evaluation of *DNA-protein* interactions based upon differences in gel electrophoresis migration

Table 51–2. DIFFERENTIATION OF APOPTOSIS AND NECROSIS

	APOPTOSIS	NECROSIS
Histology	Nuclear fragmentation	Cellular swelling and necrosis
Biochemistry	Energy-dependent, genetically directed event	Energy-independent event
	DNA cleaved into histone-associated fragments	
	ICE-like proteases are activated	

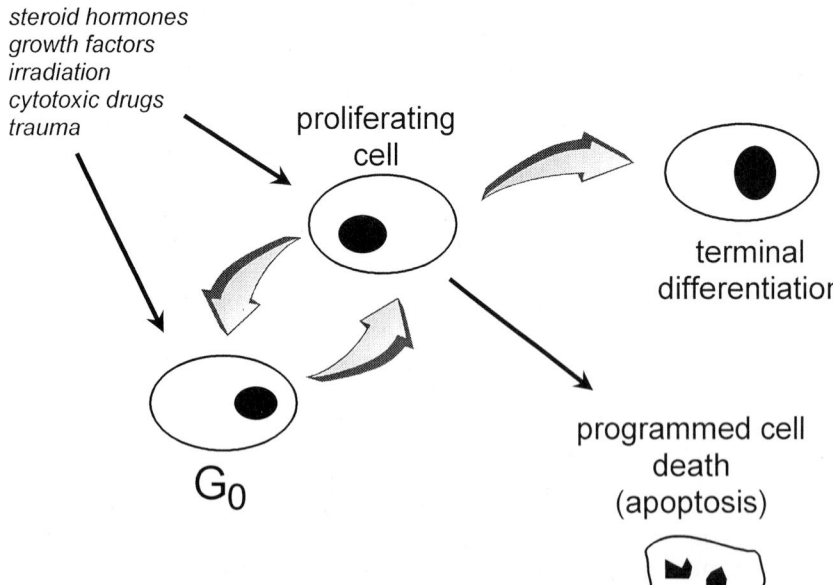

steroid hormones
growth factors
irradiation
cytotoxic drugs
trauma

proliferating cell

terminal differentiation

G_0

programmed cell death (apoptosis)

Figure 51–1
In response to diverse stimuli, cells are induced to proliferate, enter the resting phase (G_0) of the cell cycle, or undergo terminal differentiation or programmed cell death.

Proto-Oncogenes

Proto-oncogenes encode growth factors, membrane and cytoplasmic receptors, and nuclear DNA-binding proteins. As a group, proto-oncogenes typically exert positive effects upon cellular proliferation. More than 50 proto-oncogenes have been identified, all of which play some role in cell growth or cell death (Table 51–3). When a proto-oncogene is mutated, it is referred to as a cellular oncogene (e.g., c-*onc*). Mutations of proto-oncogenes are considered key events in the development of cancer. This is a dominant event in that only one of the two alleles must be mutated to result in abnormal gene activity.

Tumor Suppressor Genes

Tumor suppressor genes exert inhibitory regulatory effects upon cellular proliferation (Table 51–4). As a group, these genes encode DNA-binding proteins. Loss of tumor suppressor gene activity, as opposed to the acquisition of cellular oncogene activity, contributes to neoplastic transformation. Mutations of tumor suppressor genes are often associated with familial cancer syndromes. Unlike the circumstance with proto-oncogenes, mutations of tumor suppressor genes are recessive events and both alleles must be mutated to affect gene activity.

Cell Cycle Regulation

Cells reproduce by duplicating their cytoplasmic and nuclear material and then dividing into two daughter cells through a series of discrete, successive steps. Progression through the proliferative phase of the cell cycle occurs in four distinct phases: G_1, S, G_2, and M (Fig. 51–2). Each phase is highly regulated and must be successfully completed in order to progress to the succeeding phase. The duration of the cell cycle (e.g., the generation time) may be quite variable, although most human cells complete the cell cycle in approximately 24 hours. Variations in cell cycle time generally reflect variations in the duration of the G_1 phase.

The regulation and coordination of the cell cycle requires the interplay of many genes. Of particular importance in the regulation of the cell cycle are the cyclin-dependent kinase (CDK) genes, which are positive regulators (Lee et al, 1988; Murray and Kirschner, 1988). The CDK gene product is thought to associate successively with different cyclins at specific points in the cell cycle to allow or prevent continued progression through the cell cycle. As an example, the accumulation and degradation of cyclins regulate the checkpoint at the G_1/S boundary (Hamel and Hanley-Hyde, 1997). It has been hypothesized that these proteins bind to specific chromosomal sites. When these sites are fully occupied, a critical threshold is exceeded, the free intracellular concentration of cyclin increases, and the cell enters the S phase of the cell cycle. In the presence of DNA damage, cyclins inhibit progression through the cell cycle, causing a G_1 phase arrest. Following the repair of DNA damage, the cell enters the S phase of the cell cycle. In some cell types, the presence of DNA damage triggers cell death rather than delay of the cell cycle to allow time for repair of the damage. The teleologic advantage of a mechanism to prevent the replication of damaged DNA that might contribute to neoplastic transformation is obvious.

The G_0 phase of the cell cycle refers to a temporally arrested state in which the cell is removed from the cell cycle. Cells are released from the G_0 phase to enter the G_1 phase in response to specific external stimuli such as hormones or growth factors.

The G_1 *phase* of the cell cycle is characterized by diverse biosynthetic activities. The synthesis of enzymes and regulatory proteins necessary for DNA synthesis in the S phase occurs during this phase of the cell cycle.

The DNA content of the cell is replicated during the *S phase* of the cell cycle. Once the cell commits to the S phase, the DNA content of the nucleus, which approximates 3 billion base pairs, is replicated in the span of several hours. DNA replication is linked to a proofreading activity to correct copy errors. There are also DNA repair processes to remove mismatched DNA bases. Loss of DNA mismatch repair activity is a predisposing factor in the development of hereditary as well as many sporadic cancers (Fishel and Kolodner, 1995). This defect results in microsatellite instability, which is reflected as altered patterns of short tandem DNA repeat sequences in dividing cells. Among gynecologic cancers, this abnormality is most common in endometrial carcinoma diagnosed in patients with the sporadic nonpolyposis colorectal carcinoma syndrome, although it also occurs in 10% to 25% of cases of sporadic endometrial cancer (Caduff et al, 1996; Kobayashi et al, 1996; Helland et al, 1997). Microsatellite instability has also been found in approximately 10% of sporadic ovarian cancer cases and in ovarian cancers occurring as part of the hereditary nonpolyposis colon cancer syndrome (Arzimanoglou et al, 1996). Of additional interest, defects in DNA mismatch repair have also been associated with in vitro resistance to cisplatin and carboplatin (Aebi et al, 1996; Fink et al, 1996).

RNA and protein synthesis occur during the G_2 *phase* of the cell cycle. This burst of biosynthetic activity provides the metabolic substrates and enzymes required by the two daughter cells. Another important event that occurs during the G_2 phase of the cell cycle is the repair of errors of DNA replication that may have occurred during the S phase. Failure to detect and correct these genetic errors can result in a broad spectrum of adverse consequences for the organism as well as the individual cell (Taylor et al, 1994).

Nuclear division, or mitosis, occurs during the *M phase* of the cell cycle. During this phase, an equal

Table 51–3. REPRESENTATIVE LIST OF PROTO-ONCOGENES

GENERAL FUNCTION	PROTO-ONCOGENE	SPECIFIC FUNCTION*
Growth factors	*sis*	Truncated PDGF
	fgf-5	FGF growth factor
	hst, int-2	
Growth factor receptors	*erb*-B1	EGF receptor
	erb-B2, *kit, ros*	Receptor tyrosine kinase; EGF related
	trk	Nerve growth factor receptor
	kit	Stem cell receptor
	fms	M-CSF receptor
	bek, fig, mas	
Signal transducers	*raf, ral*	GTP-binding protein
	fgr, src, able, yes, fes	Protein tyrosine kinase
	mos, raf, cot	Protein serine-threonine kinase
	Ha-*ras*, Ki-*ras*, N-*ras*	GTP-binding protein
	pim-1	Protein serine kinase
	lck, pks	
Nuclear transcription factors	*fos, myc, ets*-2, *jun, myb, ets*-1, *ski*	Transcription factor
	erb-A	Thyroid hormone receptor

Abbreviations: EGF, epidermal growth factor; FGF, fibroblast growth factor; GTP, guanosine triphosphate; M-CSF, macrophage colony-stimulating factor; PDGF, platelet-derived growth factor.

distribution of nuclear DNA to each of the daughter cells is accomplished. Mitosis provides a diploid (2*n*) DNA complement to each somatic daughter cell. Following *mitosis*, human *somatic* cells normally contain a *diploid* (2*n*) DNA content, reflecting a karyotype that includes 44 somatic chromosomes and an XX or XY sex chromosome complement. Following *meiosis*, human *germ* cells contain a *haploid* (1*n*) genetic complement. Following fertilization, a 46,XX or 46,XY diploid DNA complement is restored. Nuclear division and the equal allocation of replicated DNA to the daughter cells is closely followed by cytoplasmic division (e.g., cytokinesis).

Following completion of the cell cycle, the daughter cells continue in G_1, enter the G_0 phase, undergo terminal differentiation, or undergo programmed cell death. The option that is pursued by the daughter cell has important implications for tissue integrity and organ function.

Cellular Signal Transduction

In order to survive and contribute to the global function of an organ, a cell must be capable of an orchestrated response to the changing extracellular and intracellular milieu. Epigenetic factors, defined as those factors that regulate the expression of gene activity without altering gene structure, include growth factors and steroid hormones. The capability

Table 51–4. REPRESENTATIVE LIST OF TUMOR SUPPRESSOR GENES

GENE	PROPOSED FUNCTION OR DISEASE ASSOCIATION
Tp53	Mutated in as many as 50% of solid tumors; associated with Li-Fraumeni syndrome
RB	Deletions and mutations predispose to the development of retinoblastoma; frequently deleted in sarcomas and osteosarcomas
WT1	Mutations associated with Wilms' tumor
NF1	Neurofibromatosis gene
NF2	Associated with schwannoma
APC	Associated with colon cancer development in patients with familial adenomatous polyposis
DCC	Deleted in colon cancer gene; associated with adenocarcinoma of the colon
BRCA1	Mutations associated with increased risk of breast, breast-ovarian, and hereditary ovarian cancer
BRCA2	Mutations associated with increased risk of prostate cancer, familial breast cancer
MSH1, MLH1, PMS1, PMS2	Associated with hereditary nonpolyposis colorectal cancer
AT	Ataxia-telangiectasia gene
VHL	Associated with von Hippel–Lindau syndrome, renal cell cancer, central nervous system, and retinal hemangioblastomas
MLM	Associated with familial melanoma
NM23	Associated with breast and colorectal cancer

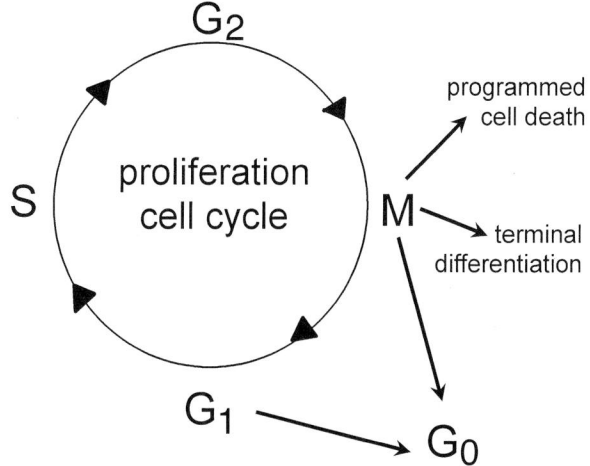

Figure 51–2
The cell cycle is divided into four distinct phases (G_1, S, G_2, and M) that have been characterized morphologically and functionally.

to respond to these factors requires a cell surface recognition system, an intracellular signal transduction system, and a means to elicit the expression of specific genes in coordinate fashion to affect changes in cell function (Fig. 51–3).

Membrane receptors bind extracellular molecules, such as growth factors, to initiate a cascade of events that culminate in altered gene expression and cause specific changes in cellular function. Growth factors are polypeptides that are produced by a variety of cell types and exhibit a wide range of overlapping physiologic and biochemical actions (Pustzal et al, 1993). Growth factors bind to high-affinity cell membrane receptors and trigger complex positive and negative signaling pathways that regulate cell pro-

liferation, differentiation, and apoptosis (Aaronson et al, 1990). Because of their short half-life in the extracellular space, growth factors generally act over limited distances through autocrine or paracrine mechanisms. The autocrine mechanism of growth control involves the elaboration of a growth factor that acts upon the cell that produced it. The paracrine mechanism of growth control involves the elaboration of a growth factor that in turn acts upon another cell in close proximity.

The biologic response of a particular cell to a specific growth factor depends not only upon the type of cell but on the other stimuli that may be concomitantly acting upon the cell. Two growth factors acting in concert may produce a very different effect from either factor acting independently. In addition, the same growth factor may stimulate epithelial cells from one organ to proliferate and inhibit growth in epithelial cells from a different organ.

Following the interaction of a ligand such as platelet-derived growth factor, fibroblast growth factor, epidermal growth factor (EGF), colony-stimulating factor, or insulin-like growth factor with its membrane receptor, the extracellular signal is converted to an intracellular signal. Activation of cell membrane receptors results in the phosphorylation of specific substrates in the cytoplasm that trigger the intracellular transduction system. The intracellular transduction system is responsible for conducting the extracellular signal through the cytoplasm to the nucleus. The intracellular signal transduction system relies upon serine/threonine kinases, *scr*-related kinases, and G proteins, all of which are encoded by proto-oncogenes.

Alternatively, the ligand may translocate across the extracellular membrane and through the cytoplasm into the nucleus, bypassing the membrane re-

Figure 51–3
Cellular transduction allows extracellular stimuli to effect discrete changes in gene expression and cellular function. Following the interaction of a ligand with its membrane receptor (*1*), the signal is transmitted through the cytoplasm to the nucleus (*2*). In the nucleus, specific genes are activated in response to the extracellular signal (*3*), which triggers protein synthesis to effect changes in cell function.

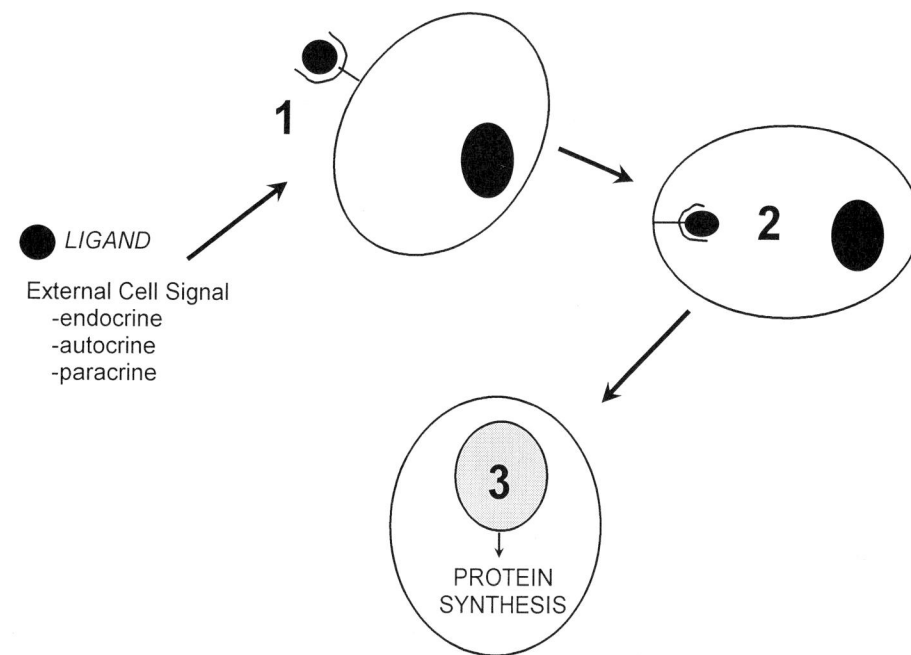

ceptor. As an example, estrogen exerts its effect by diffusing through the cell membrane and cytoplasm to bind to nuclear estrogen receptors. The receptor-steroid complex then binds to DNA at specific sequences designated estrogen-response elements. These steroid-responsive elements are located near the promoter regions of genes that are estrogen sensitive (Landers and Spelsberg, 1992). As is the case for all hormone receptors, specificity of action is conferred by the ligand-binding domain and the DNA-binding domain of the receptor. Mutations of steroid hormone receptors have been identified and correlated with clinical diagnoses. As an example, absence of the estrogen receptor in a male human has been reported (Smith et al, 1994). The clinical sequelae attributed to this mutation include incomplete epiphyseal closure, increased bone turnover, tall stature, and impaired glucose tolerance. Mutations of the androgen receptor result in the androgen insensitivity syndrome (DeBellis et al, 1994). Mutations of the receptors for growth hormone and thyroid-stimulating hormone have also been associated with a spectrum of phenotypic alterations.

Transcription and Translation

The human genome has been estimated to span 3 × 10^9 nucleotide base pairs, organized as 24 chromosomes comprising approximately 100,000 genes. If all of the DNA molecules in a single cell were placed end to end, they would stretch to a total length of 1 meter! The human genome fits into the nuclear package because it is tightly organized into discrete bundles, known as chromosomes. In an individual, all of the somatic cells contain the same genetic material

yet there is considerable tissue and cell specificity with respect to gene expression. It remains one of the marvels of molecular biology that the expression of an individual gene is so accurately regulated in view of the overall complexity of the human genome.

Nuclear proto-oncogenes such as c-*myc*, c-*fos*, *jun*, and *myb* encode DNA-binding proteins that regulate gene transcription and translation in response to signals transmitted via the intracellular signal transduction system to the nucleus. Tumor suppressor genes encode proteins that also regulate gene transcription.

During transcription, DNA is used as a template for the synthesis of mRNA. The information in mRNA is converted into protein during translation (Fig. 51–4). Synthesis of mRNA is initiated from the transcriptional promoter, which is a noncoding, regulatory region of the gene at the 5' end of the gene. Enhancers are auxiliary sequences that may be located some distance from the gene but they coordinate with the promoters to control the overall level and tissue specificity of gene expression. The primary mRNA transcript is composed of coding and noncoding regions, referred to as exons and introns, respectively. Introns are removed or "spliced" from the mRNA before it is transported to the cytoplasm and translated into protein.

The female reproductive tract provides several models of tissue specific gene expression. As an example, germ cell maturation is paralleled by specific changes in proto-oncogene expression. The c-*abl*, c-*mos*, *int*-1, and N-*ras* proto-oncogenes appear to play a role in spermatid maturation based upon discrete levels of gene expression with respect to various stages of germ cell development. The c-*mos* gene

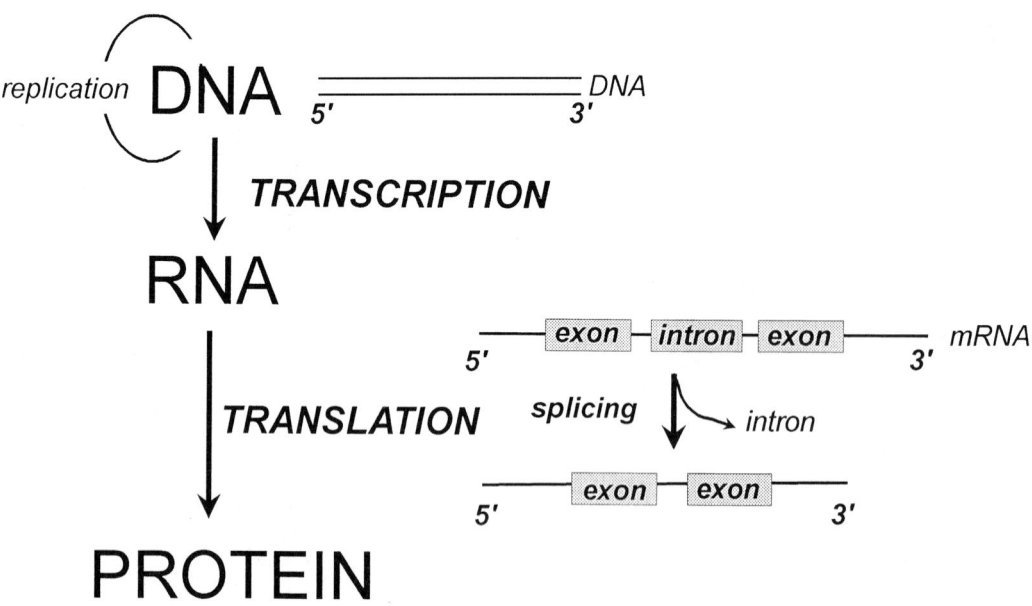

Figure 51–4
Transcription and translation are fundamental events required for cellular replication as well as the cell's response to its environment.

plays a particularly important role in oocyte maturation in that development is accompanied by a rapid increase in the amount of c-*mos* RNA, followed by a prompt decrease during meiosis. The importance of this gene product to normal oocyte development has been demonstrated by experiments in which the injection of antisense oligonucleotides to c-*mos* causes inhibition of meiosis II.

The temporal and cell-specific changes in placental gene expression provide additional examples of highly regulated gene expression. The "pseudomalignant" cytotrophoblast, which is the predominant cell type found in first trimester placental tissue, is characterized by rapid proliferation and the ability to invade the myometrium. The syncytiotrophoblast, which is derived from the cytotrophoblast cell, is a complex functional syncytium that exhibits a myriad of complex metabolic and hormonal functions. The morphologic and functional transition of a cytotrophoblast to syncytiotrophoblast-dominated placental cell population is paralleled by discrete changes in proto-oncogene expression. Normal endometrium also provides an example of changes in gene expression that parallel alterations in cell morphology and function in response to steroid hormones and local growth factors (Baker, 1995).

SEQUELAE OF GENETIC MUTATIONS

In view of the crucial role that genes, particularly proto-oncogenes and tumor suppressor genes, play in normal cell growth, differentiation, and programmed cell death, it is a logical corollary that the abnormal function of these genes as a multistep phenomenon is causally related to the neoplastic phenotype.

Abnormal gene function may be the consequence of gene amplification, structural rearrangements, point mutations, and insertional mutagenesis (Fig. 51–5). A variety of mutations involving proto-oncogenes, tumor suppressor genes, and DNA repair genes have been described in gynecologic cancers.

Gene amplification results in an increase in the copy number of the gene and may be detected cytogenetically as double minutes or as homogeneously staining regions. Amplification results in an increase in the amount of template DNA available for transcription and is often associated with overexpression of the gene. As a group, gynecologic neoplasms often exhibit sporadic amplification of at least one oncogene.

Structural rearrangements of a gene, such as deletions and rearrangements, can result in the synthesis of a markedly altered protein product. The potential consequences of structural rearrangements upon the protein product range from loss of function to potentiation of function. As an example, deletions of the EGF receptor alter tyrosine kinase activity. The mutated receptor is constitutively activated in the absence of bound ligand and transmits a signal to the cytoplasm for cellular proliferation.

Point mutations are single base changes that may result in significant alterations in gene product function when they occur at crucial sites. Point mutations of the *ras* gene occur in approximately 15% of solid tumors. The replacement of a single amino acid in the *ras* gene product as a result of a base mutation at codon 12, 13, or 61 results in the synthesis of a p21 Ras protein with increased transforming ability.

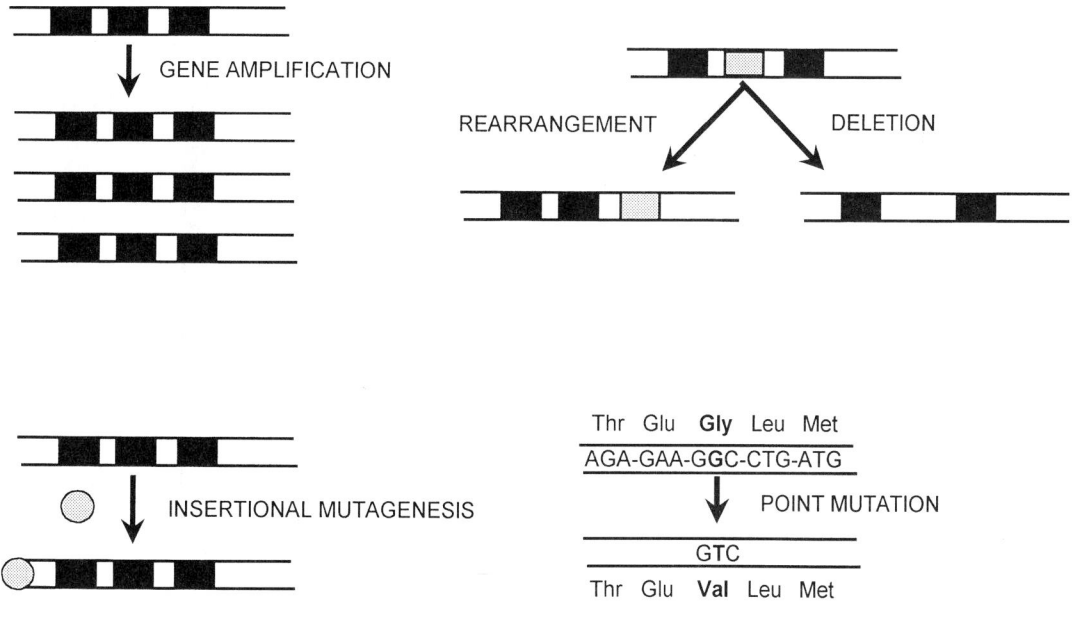

Figure 51–5
The more common mechanisms of proto-oncogene mutation to create an oncogene include amplification, insertional mutagenesis, rearrangements and deletions, and point mutations.

The mutated p21 Ras protein exhibits decreased GTPase activity, and the bound GTP is hydrolyzed to guanosine diphosphate more slowly. As a consequence, the mutant protein is constitutively activated and a continuous signal to proliferate is transduced to the nucleus. Point mutations of the p53 gene are among the most common genetic mutations found in solid human neoplasms. These mutations occur at preferential "hot spots" that coincide with the most highly conserved regions of the gene. Loss of normal p53 gene activity removes one of the endogenous "brakes" on cellular proliferation. In addition, point mutations of the p53 gene impair the ability of the cell to repair DNA damage before entry into the S phase of the cell cycle, thereby increasing the likelihood that DNA damage may be successfully transmitted to daughter cells. Point mutations may also result in loss of function if the nucleotide change signals termination of transcription, producing a shortened or "truncated" protein product.

Combinations of genetic mishaps can eliminate or damage both copies of a gene. For example, the first copy may be lost by chromosomal deletion or inactivated by a point mutation; the second copy may be lost by mitotic recombination. The net result is that the second copy of the gene is either deleted or replaced by a copy of the corresponding region of the first defective chromosome; in other words, the usual heterozygous combination of maternal and paternal alleles of genes in that chromosomal region is lost (e.g., loss of heterozygosity) (Fig. 51–6). This is a common mechanism by which a tumor suppressor gene is activated.

It now appears that genetic abnormalities are progressive in successive generations and increase with loss of differentiation and tumor progression. One genetic error tends to permit additional genetic errors in subsequent generations. One result of these cumulative genetic mutations is defective control of the cell cycle. In a cancer cell, proliferation is not necessarily increased, but the normal constraints upon cell growth are no longer operative and pro-

grammed cell death may fail to occur. A *single* genetic mutation that causes cancer has not been identified. In fact, specific genetic mutations per se may not be as important as the accumulation of a critical number of mutations within a single cell. The discovery of oncogenes and tumor suppressor genes and the functional consequences of their mutations has significantly advanced our understanding of tumorigenesis and tumor progression. In addition, this information has provided opportunities for the development of novel treatment strategies and improved risk assessment. The translation of basic science observations made as a result of advances in molecular genetics is now being realized in the clinical arena.

MOLECULAR ALTERATIONS AND PROGNOSIS

Ovarian Cancer

The prognostic significance of specific genetic alterations in epithelial ovarian cancer is an area of active investigation. Several studies of proto-oncogene and tumor suppressor gene mutations interpreted in the context of prognosis have been published, often with conflicting results.

Foekens et al (1990) have reported that the expression of the EGF receptor, which is encoded by the c-*erb*-B1 gene, predicts disease progression. Scambia et al (1992) reported that EGF receptor expression identified a subset of patients at high risk of progressive disease in both univariate and multivariate analysis. Similar results have been reported by Berchuck et al (1991a).

The expression of the p21 protein, detected by immunohistochemical methods, does not appear to be a prognostic indicator. Yaginuma et al (1992) found no statistically significant difference in survival between stage I and III cases of ovarian cancer that

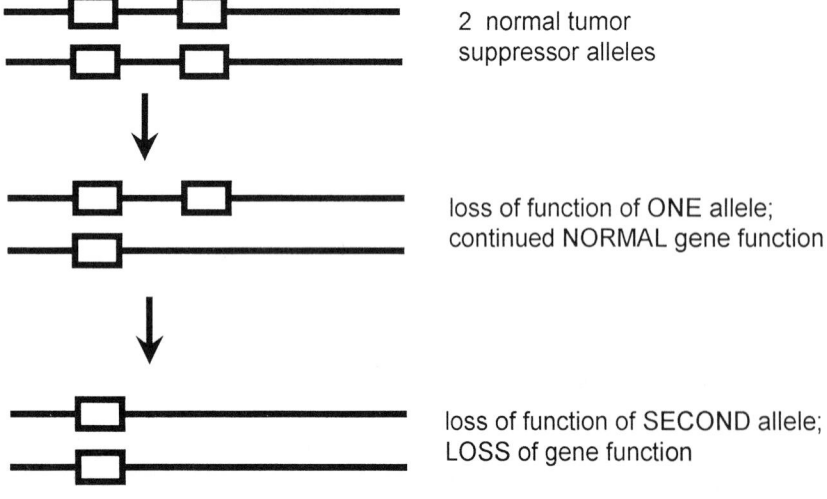

2 normal tumor suppressor alleles

loss of function of ONE allele; continued NORMAL gene function

loss of function of SECOND allele; LOSS of gene function

Figure 51–6
Loss of heterozygosity is a common mechanism by which tumor suppressor gene function becomes vulnerable to the effects of gene mutation.

were Ras p21 positive and those that were negative. Similar results have been reported by Rodenburg et al (1988). However, Scambia et al (1993) reported that p21 expression was a negative prognostic indicator of survival in univariate analysis based on their study of 42 primary ovarian neoplasms and 15 metastatic lesions. In this report, patients with p21-negative neoplasms survived a median of 58 months, and patients with p21-positive lesions survived a median of 17 months (p <0.04). Patients with p21-negative lesions also exhibited a longer progression-free interval when compared with those with p21-positive neoplasms, although the difference was not statistically significant.

The p53 tumor suppressor gene is commonly mutated and overexpressed in advanced-stage ovarian cancer. Marks et al (1991) studied p53 expression in 107 ovarian neoplasms and found no significant relationship with overall survival. Other investigators (Bosari et al, 1993; Henricksen et al, 1994; Levesque et al, 1995) have found that p53 overexpression is associated with poorly differentiated tumors, advanced stage disease, and poor survival. Geisler et al (1997) studied 83 consecutive ovarian neoplasms for p53 expression detected by immunohistochemical staining and quantitated by digital image analysis. In this study, p53 overexpression was also reported to be an independent prognostic indicator of survival. Mutations of the p53 gene have also been associated with resistance to chemotherapy (Buttitta et al, 1997).

The association between abnormalities of HER-2/neu structure and function and prognosis is debated. Slamon et al (1989) first suggested that amplification of HER-2/neu identified a subset of patients with ovarian cancer who had a markedly worse prognosis. Patients with neoplasms that exhibited amplification greater than fivefold the normal gene copy number demonstrated a marked reduction in median survival (243 days) compared with the median survival of patients with abnormal gene copy number (1879 days). A subsequent report by Berchuck et al (1990) indicated that high HER-2/neu expression was associated with a shorter median survival and an incomplete response to primary chemotherapy when compared with moderate or absent HER-2/neu expression. Other investigators, however, have been unable to demonstrate a significant association between HER-2/neu overexpression and prognosis. Haldane et al (1990) studied 104 archival specimens and found no association between HER-2/neu expression and prognosis. Wilkinson et al (1991) found no adverse prognostic significance for HER-2/neu overexpression based on a study of archival specimens. Huettner et al (1992) assessed HER-2/neu expression by enzyme-linked immunosorbent assay, Northern hybridization, and immunohistochemistry. There was no correlation between stage or grade of disease in 57 primary and metastatic ovarian neoplasms. Kacinski et al (1992) subsequently reported an analysis of 66 stage I to IV epithelial ovarian ne-

oplasms. These investigators found no statistically significant association between the intensity of HER-2/neu staining and disease-free or overall survival. Rubin et al (1993) studied frozen sections from 105 epithelial ovarian neoplasms and were unable to demonstrate any prognostic relationship between the immunohistochemical detection of HER-2/neu expression and prognosis. Using the S1 nuclease protection assay, Tanner et al (1996) studied 95 epithelial ovarian cancer specimens for c-erb-B2 (e.g., HER-2/neu) mRNA expression. Based upon follow-up ranging from 3 to 9 years and an analysis of histopathologic and clinical factors, the expression of HER-2/neu mRNA was not a statistically significant prognostic parameter.

The explanation for these disparate observations is not apparent. It has been suggested that the assessment of HER-2/neu expression by immmunohistochemical methods should be done using frozen section material rather than formalin-fixed, paraffin-embedded archival sections. However, more recent studies demonstrate that routine methods of fixation do not significantly diminish the immunohistochemical detection of HER-2/neu expression.

Endometrial Cancer

Numerous oncogene and tumor suppressor gene mutations and/or abnormalities of expression have been described in endometrial carcinoma. Kacinski et al (1988) have reported that high levels of expression of c-fms mRNA is correlated with high International Federation of Gynecology and Obstetrics (FIGO) grade, advanced clinical stage of disease, and deep myometrial invasion, and predicts aggressive clinical behavior and poor outcome. However, Baiocchi et al (1991) were unable to demonstrate a correlation among c-fms expression and these specific clinicopathologic parameters, although overexpression of c-fms did reflect clinically aggressive disease.

Berchuck et al (1991b) reported that overexpression of the HER-2/neu oncoprotein, detected by immunohistochemistry, was associated with an increased incidence of death from persistent or recurrent cancer. Interestingly, overexpression of the HER-2/neu oncoprotein was associated with estrogen receptor–negative tumors. Similar observations concerning the poor prognosis of HER-2/neu–positive, estrogen receptor–negative neoplasms have been reported for patients with breast cancer (McCann et al, 1991). Larger studies must be performed before the clinical significance of this observation can be ascertained.

Mizuuchi et al (1992) analyzed 49 cases of endometrial adenocarcinoma and found mutations of codons 12 or 13 of the Ki-ras gene in 6 cases. Three of the six patients died during follow-up. Using multivariate analysis, the presence of Ki-ras mutations emerged as an independent risk factor for poor prognosis when compared with clinical stage of disease, depth of myometrial invasion, and patient age.

In a series of 221 cases of endometrial adenocarcinoma occurring in Japanese women, mutations of codon 12 of the K-*ras* gene were associated with lymph node metastases and poor overall survival (Ito et al, 1996). Interestingly, K-*ras* mutations in this study were more common in women over the age of 60.

Increased immunostaining of the p53 gene product, reflecting p53 point mutations, occurs in approximately one third of endometrial adenocarcinomas. The prognostic significance of this observation is uncertain. Bur et al (1992) have reported that the intensity of staining determined by image analysis exhibited no correlation with grade or stage of disease. However, a strong diffuse staining pattern was correlated with grade and stage. A subsequent study by Pisani et al (1995) evaluated p53 expression by immunohistochemistry in 104 archival specimens. Overexpression was found in 15% of the tumors, and this was associated with a 5-year survival of 12%. In the subgroup that was p53 negative, the 5-year survival was 90%. Similar results were reported by Kohlberger et al (1996) in a study of 92 patients with stage I endometrial cancer. Significantly poorer survival was observed in those women with tumors that overexpressed the p53 protein.

Geisler et al (1996) studied p53 expression detected by immunohistochemical staining and quantitated by digital image analysis in 46 adenocarcinoma specimens. Increasing histologic grade was associated with overexpression of p53. Using recurrence as an endpoint, FIGO stage and p53 expression emerged as the independent prognostic indicators. Using similar experimental methods for protein detection and quantitation, Hamel et al (1996) also reported that p53 expression was prognostically significant.

Cervical Cancer

Most of the attention has been focused upon c-*myc* as an indicator of prognosis in neoplasms of the cervix. Hendy-Ibbs et al (1987) quantitated c-*myc* expression in formalin-fixed, paraffin-embedded cervical biopsies using flow cytometry and were unable to detect prognostically significant differences in gene expression. However, it is now recognized that the Myc oncoprotein, which has a half-life measured in minutes, is also extremely susceptible to degradation, and tissue specimens must be properly fixed prior to analysis. When using snap-frozen tissue, Hughes et al (1989) reported that 3 of 4 normal cervical biopsies expressed the Myc oncoprotein, 4 of 14 dysplastic lesions were positive, and 0 of 7 invasive cervical carcinoma specimens expressed the c-*myc* antigen.

Studying much larger numbers of invasive cervical cancer specimens, investigators from the Institute Gustave Roussy in France have evaluated c-*myc* expression as a prognostic indicator in cervical cancer (Riou et al, 1987, 1988, 1990a, 1990b; Bourhis et al, 1990). Using Northern hybridization and slot blot analysis, c-*myc* overexpression was found in 33% of 93 cervical carcinoma specimens. There was no apparent relationship among c-*myc* expression and histology, tumor differentiation, status of the surgical margins, or the presence of lymph–vascular space involvement. However, when analyzed with respect to tumor size and nodal status, the overexpression of c-*myc* in node-negative patients was predictive of subsequent relapse. Three-year survival for patients with normal *myc* expression and negative nodes was 93%, compared to only 51% for those with overexpression of *myc* and negative nodes. Patients with nodal metastases who had tumors with normal *myc* expression demonstrated a 3-year survival of 44%, compared to only 15% for those with tumors exhibiting overexpression of c-*myc*.

Sagae et al (1990) have investigated the expression of the Ras protein in dysplastic and invasive lesions of the cervix. Using immunohistochemical techniques upon formalin-fixed, paraffin-embedded biopsy material, these investigators were unable to detect the Ras protein in normal cervical epithelium. Squamous metaplasia was associated with the presence of p21 in 10% of cases, mild dysplasia in 18%, moderate dysplasia in 29%, severe dysplasia in 53%, and invasive carcinoma in 50%. Interestingly, dysplastic lesions that did not express p21 were more likely to spontaneously regress as compared to p21-positive lesions. Hayashi et al (1991) evaluated the prognostic significance of Ras p21 expression in invasive cervical carcinoma. The presence of p21, detected using immunohistochemical techniques, was associated with a greater likelihood of pelvic nodal metastases.

In general, the antibodies used to detect the *ras* gene product cannot differentiate between K-*ras*, N-*ras*, and H-*ras*. Using polymerase chain reaction (PCR) and allele-specific oligonucleotide hybridization, Lee et al (1996) found mutations of codon 12 of the H-*ras* gene in 6 of 27 cases of cervical carcinoma. Examples of positive and negative immunohistochemical staining were found in the group with mutations of the *ras* gene, underscoring the lack of correlation between the two tests. Grendys et al (1997) tested 33 cervical cancer specimens by PCR and dot-blot hybridization and found mutations of the H-, K-, and N-*ras* genes in 24.2% of cases, all at codon 61. Data published by Wong et al (1995) are noteworthy in that all their specimens of invasive cervical cancer exhibited a *ras* gene mutation. In this study, DNA was extracted from 80 archival samples of cervical cancer and analyzed using PCR followed by restriction endonuclease digestion. The H-*ras* gene was mutated at codon 12 in 28 cases, the K-*ras* gene was mutated at codon 12 in 49 cases, and the K-*ras* gene was mutated at codon 13 in 5 cases. Collectively, these data suggest that mutations of the *ras* gene family may play a role in development of cervical cancer.

The role(s) of the human papillomavirus (HPV) E6 and E7 proteins in the pathogenesis of cervical cancer continues to be a subject of active investigation. The E6 and E7 proteins of HPV16 and HPV18 are considered oncoproteins with transforming activity. These proteins interact with nonmutated host genes to disrupt normal cell growth and differentiation. As an example, the E6 oncoprotein binds to the p53 gene product, resulting in accelerated degradation by a ubiquitin-dependent proteolysis pathway (Scheffner et al, 1990). Apart from its accelerated degradation, the p53 protein cannot inhibit cell cycle progression to permit repair of damaged DNA when it is complexed to the E6 protein. Although the p53 gene is the most commonly mutated gene in solid neoplasms, it is uncommonly mutated in cervical cancer. When mutations of the p53 gene are detected in cervical neoplasms, they usually occur in HPV-negative lesions. This suggests that inactivation of the p53 gene may occur by mechanisms other than E6 functional inactivation or point mutations.

TREATMENT STRATEGIES

There are several molecular-based treatment strategies that may be applicable to gynecologic cancer. As a general concept, the goal of genetic therapy is directed toward the restoration of absent gene activity or the abrogation of abnormal gene activity.

As previously noted, expression of a mutated p53 gene product is one of the most common abnormalities diagnosed in solid tumors, including those of the female reproductive tract. Selective inhibition of p53 gene expression can be achieved through the use of antisense oligodeoxynucleotides (Bishop et al, 1996). The p53 gene product can also be used as a potential therapeutic agent. In animal models of head and neck cancer, the introduction of wild-type p53 using an adenoviral vector has been associated with reduction in the size of the tumors and an increase in apoptosis (Liu et al, 1995; Clayman et al, 1996). Clinical trials evaluating the safety and efficacy of p53-based antitumor therapy in human subjects are currently underway (Roth and Cristiano, 1997).

Cervical cancers that are HPV positive exhibit loss of normal p53 activity as a consequence of accelerated degradation resulting from the complex of the HPV E6 protein with wild-type p53 protein. The introduction of excess p53 protein into the cell alters the intracellular ratio and restores p53 activity. Hamada et al (1996b) have shown that the in vitro infection of HeLa cells (which are HPV positive) using an adenoviral vector that carries the p53 gene results in significant growth suppression of the HeLa cells. It is also possible to suppress proliferation of HPV16-positive cells by blocking the synthesis of the E6 gene product. Madrigal et al (1997) achieved growth

inhibition using oligonucleotides specific for the E6 gene. Hamada et al (1996a) reported similar results using an adenoviral vector that released antisense RNA transcripts of the E6 and E7 genes. When studied in the nude mouse model, the tumorigenicity of SiHa cells infected with the antisense RNA adenoviral vector was completely inhibited.

The transfer of adenoviral vectors expressing wild-type p53 to ovarian cancer cells in vitro has been associated with enhanced sensitivity to radiation. When SK-OV-3 cells were implanted into the flanks of immunocompromised mice and injected with adenoviral p53 vector, enhanced radiation responsiveness and improved long-term tumor control was reported (Gallardo et al, 1996).

Abnormal proteins encoded by c-oncogenes can also become the targets of monoclonal antibodies. Deshane et al (1997) have developed a novel treatment strategy using an adenoviral-mediated delivery of an anti–erb-B2 single-chain antibody against tumor cells that overexpress the erb-B2 protein. The Gynecologic Oncology Group is currently investigating this treatment strategy as a Phase II study.

ASSESSMENT OF DISEASE RISK

The insights gained from basic molecular biology are not only providing novel strategies for treatment but diagnostic tests for the identification of individuals who may be at increased risk of cancer development. One of the more promising developments in the past few years that also exemplifies the application of molecular genetics to clinical gynecology relates to mutations of the BRCA1 gene as a predictor of risk for the development of breast cancer and ovarian cancer.

The BRCA1 gene is located on the long arm of chromosome 17(q12-q21). This tumor suppressor gene encodes a protein that appears to play a role in cell growth and differentiation. Over 200 different mutations have been reported. The mutation carrier rate is estimated to be 0.0006% in the general population but is increased to 2% in Ashkenazi Jews (Struewing et al, 1997). Mutations of this gene are also found with increased frequency in women with familial breast cancer and hereditary breast-ovarian cancer (HBOC). The probability of detecting a BRCA1 mutation in an individual was first correlated with the details of the family history by Shattuck-Eidens et al (1995). These data were based upon genetic linkage analyses of large breast and ovarian cancer kindreds. A subsequent study based upon cohorts *without* such extensive family histories of breast and ovarian cancer suggests that the original risk estimates may have been overestimated. Revised estimates suggest that only 7% of women from families with a history of breast cancer carry a BRCA1 mutation. This estimate is increased when the family history is positive for both breast and ovarian cancer (Couch et al, 1997). The probability of developing breast or ovarian cancer increases with age in the presence of a *BRCA1* mutation (Table 51–5).

With the widespread availability of genetic testing, increasing attention has been focused upon the HBOC syndrome and the familial ovarian cancer syndrome. The HBOC syndrome is characterized by an inherited susceptibility to carcinomas of the breast and ovary, with breast tumors generally being much more common. A family history suggestive of HBOC syndrome includes three or more breast cancer cases and one or more cases of ovarian cancer diagnosed before the age of 50, or a family with three or more breast cancer cases diagnosed before the age of 50, or a family with breast cancer diagnosed before the age of 30. The HBOC syndrome is estimated to confer a cumulative lifetime risk of breast or ovarian cancer upon the individual of 59% by age 50 and 82% by age 70.

Familial ovarian cancer syndrome is a variant of the HBOC syndrome. A woman with one first-degree relative diagnosed with ovarian cancer may have a cumulative lifetime risk as great as 1 in 20 of developing this cancer. With two affected first-degree relatives, the cumulative lifetime risk may be increased to 1 in 14. However, it is important to recognize that only approximately 3% of all women with two affected first-degree relatives with ovarian cancer are truly at increased risk of familial ovarian cancer. The distinction between familial and sporadic cancer is often difficult and requires a detailed pedigree analysis that should include at least three generations with confirmation of the cancer diagnoses.

Genetic testing offers an opportunity to refine the risk analysis beyond that based upon family history alone. The technology to test for mutations of the *BRCA1* gene is commercially available to the practicing physician. However, genetic mutation analysis of the *BRCA1* gene is technically challenging because of the genetic and allelic heterogeneity of this large gene. The 5592–base pair coding sequence of the *BRCA1* gene is spread over 100,000 base pairs in 22 exons. Unlike the p53 gene, mutations of the *BRCA1* gene do not preferentially occur at "hot spots." Although approximately 65% of the reported *BRCA1*

mutations do result in the synthesis of truncated proteins that can be detected by mobility shifts on gel electrophoresis, the remainder can only be detected by more labor-intensive techniques.

The implications of *BRCA1* gene testing are still being determined. The routine, indiscriminate application of genetic screening at this time is strongly discouraged because of technical, legal, and clinical practice limitations. Although the influence of a *BRCA1* mutation upon the lifetime risk of cancer based upon population studies has been defined, the implication for the individual patient remains unclear. It is recognized that every patient with a mutation does not develop cancer and, conversely, the absence of a mutation does not predict the absence of cancer development at some time in the future. For women who insist upon genetic testing to detect *BRCA1* mutations, it is important to emphasize several points—precise estimates of cancer risk are not clearly defined for the individual, the specific factors that influence the penetrance and expressivity of these mutations have not been identified, and the recommendations for ovarian cancer screening of "high-risk" individuals remain empirical and are of questionable efficacy.

REFERENCES

Aaronson SA, Rubin JS, Finch PW, et al: Growth-factor-regulated pathways in epithelial cell proliferation. Amer Rev Resp Dis 1990;142:57.

Aebi S, Kurdi-Haidar B, Gordone R, et al: Loss of DNA mismatch repair in acquired resistance to cisplatin. Cancer Res 1996;56:3087.

Arzimanoglou II, Lallas T, Osborne T, et al: Microsatellite instability difference between familial and sporadic ovarian cancers. Carcinogenesis 1996;17:1799.

Baiocchi G, Kavanagh JJ, Talpaz M, et al: Expression of the macrophage colony stimulating factor and its receptor in gynecologic malignancies. Cancer 1991;67:990.

Baker V: Potential criteria for cohort selection in chemoprevention trials of uterine adenocarcinoma. J Cell Biochem 1995;23(Suppl):184.

Berchuck A, Kamel A, Whitaker R, et al: Overexpression of HER-2/neu is associated with poor survival in advanced epithelial ovarian cancer. Cancer Res 1990;50:4087.

Berchuck A, Rodriguez GC, Kamel A, et al: Epidermal growth factor receptor in normal ovarian epithelium and ovarian cancer. I. Correlation of receptor expression with prognostic factors in patients with ovarian cancer. Am J Obstet Gynecol 1991a;164:669.

Berchuck A, Rodiguez G, Kinney RB, et al: Overexpression of HER-2/neu is associated with advanced stage disease. Am J Obstet Gynecol 1991b;164:15.

Billig H, Furutal I, Hsueh AJW: Estrogens inhibit and androgens enhance ovarian granulosa cell apoptosis. Endocrinology 1993;133:2204.

Bishop MR, Iversen PL, Bayever E, et al: Phase I trial of an antisense oligonucleotide OL(1)p53 in hematologic malignancies. J Clin Oncol 1996;14:1320.

Bosari S, Viale G, Radaelli U, et al: p53 Accumulation in ovarian carcinomas and its prognostic implications. Hum Pathol 1993;24:1175.

Bourhis J, Le MG, Barrois M, et al: Prognostic value of c-myc proto-oncogene overexpression in early invasive carcinoma of the cervix. J Clin Oncol 1990;8:1789.

Bur ME, Perlman C, Edelman L, et al: p53 Gene expression in neoplasms of the uterine corpus. Am J Clin Pathol 1992;98:81.

Table 51–5. RISK OF BREAST OR OVARIAN CANCER WITH A FAMILIAL *BRCA1* GENE MUTATION*

AGE	BREAST CANCER	OVARIAN CANCER	EITHER CANCER
30	0.032	0.0017	0.034
40	0.191	0.0061	0.195
50	0.508	0.227	0.619
60	0.542	0.298	0.678
70	0.85	0.633	0.945

*Independent of the location or type of genetic mutation.
From Easton DF, Ford D, Bishop DJ: Breast and ovarian cancer incidence in BRCA1-mutation carriers. Breast Cancer Linkage Consortium. Am J Human Genet 1995;56:265, with permission.

Buttitta F, Marchetti A, Gadducci A, et al: p53 Alterations are predictive of chemoresistance and aggressiveness in ovarian carcinomas: a molecular and immunohistochemical study. Br J Cancer 1997;75:230.

Caduff RF, Johnston DM, Svoboda-Newman SM, et al: Clinical and pathological significance of microsatellite instability in sporadic endometrial carcinoma. Am J Pathol 1996;148:1671.

Clayman GL, Liu TJ, Overholt SM, et al: Gene therapy for head and neck cancer: Comparing the tumor suppressor gene p53 and a cell cycle regulator WAF1/CIP1 (p21). Arch Otolaryngol Head Neck Surg 1996;122:489.

Couch F, DeShano ML, Blackwood MA, et al: BRCA1 mutations in women attending clinics that evaluate the risk of breast cancer. N Engl J Med 1997;336:1409.

DeBellis A, Quigley CA, Marschke KB, et al: Characterization of mutant androgen receptors causing partial androgen insensitivity syndrome. J Clin Endocrinol Metab 1994;78:513.

Deshane J, Seigal GP, Wang M, et al: Transductional efficacy and safety of an intraperitoneally delivered adenovirus encoding an anti-erbB-2 intracellular single-chain antibody for ovarian cancer gene therapy. Gynecol Oncol 1997;64:378.

Farbman AI: Electron microscopic study of palate fusion in mouse embryos. Dev Biol 1968;18:93.

Fink D, Nebel S, Aebi S, et al: The role of DNA mismatch repair in platinum drug resistance. Cancer Res 1996;56:4881.

Fishel R, Kolodner RD: Identification of mismatch repair genes and their role in the development of cancer. Curr Opin Genet Dev 1995;5:382.

Foekens BM, van Putten LJ, Portengen H, et al: Prognostic value of pS2 protein and receptors for epidermal growth factor (EGF-R), insulin-like growth factor-1 (IGF-1-R), and somatostatin (SS-R) in patients with breast ad ovarian cancer. J Steroid Biochem Molec Biol 1990;37:815.

Gallardo D, Drazan KE, McBride WH: Adenovirus-based transfer of wild-type p53 gene increases ovarian tumor radiosensitivity. Cancer Res 1996;56:4891.

Geisler JP, Geisler HE, Wiemmann MC, et al: Quantification of p53 in epithelial ovarian cancer. Gynecol Oncol 1997;66:435.

Geisler JP, Wiemann MC, Zhou Z, et al: p53 As a prognostic indicator in endometrial cancer. Gynecol Oncol 1996;61:245.

Grendys EC, Barnes WA, Weitzel J, et al: Identification of H, K, and N-ras point mutations in stage Ib cervical carcinoma. Gynecol Oncol 1997;65:343.

Haldane JS, Hird V, Hughes CM, et al: c-erbB-2 oncogene expression in ovarian cancer. J Pathol 1990;162:231.

Hamada K, Sakaue M, Alemany R, et al: Adenovirus-mediated transfer of HPV 16 E6/E7 antisense RNA to human cervical cancer cells. Gynecol Oncol 1996a;63:219.

Hamada K, Zhang W-W, Alemany R, et al: Growth inhibition of human cervical cancer cells with the recombinant adenovirus p53 in vitro. Gynecol Oncol 1996b;60:373.

Hamel NW, Sebo TJ, Wilson TO, et al: Prognostic value of p53 and proliferating cell nuclear antigen expression in endometrial carcinoma. Gynecol Oncol 1996;62:192.

Hamel PA, Hanely-Hyde J: G1 cyclins and control of the cell division cycle in normal and transformed cells. Cancer Invest 1997;15:143.

Hammar SP, Mottet NK: Tetrazolium salt and electron microscopic studies of cellular degeneration and necrosis in the interdigital areas of the developing chick limb. J Cell Sci 1971; 8:229.

Hayashi Y, Hachisuga T, Iwasaka T, et al: Expression of the ras oncogene product and EGF receptor in cervical squamous cell carcinoma and its relationship to lymph node involvement. Gynecol Oncol 1991;40:147.

Helland A, Borresen-Dale A-L, Peltomaki P, et al: Microsatellite instability in cervical and endometrial carcinomas. Int J Cancer 1997;70:499.

Hendy-Ibbs P, Cox H, Evan GI, et al: Flow cytometric quantitation of DNA and c-myc oncoprotein in archival biopsies of uterine cervix neoplasia. Br J Cancer 1987;55:275.

Henricksen R, Strang PJ, Wilander E, et al: p53 Expression in epithelial ovarian neoplasms: relationship to clinical and pathological parameters, Ki-67 expression and flow cytometry. Gynecol Oncol 1994;53:301.

Huettner PC, Carney WP, Naber SP, et al: Neu oncogene expression in ovarian tumors: a quantitative study. Mod Pathol 1992; 5:250.

Hughes RG, Neill WA, Norval M: Papillomavirus and c-myc antigen expression in normal and neoplastic cervical epithelium. J Clin Pathol 1989;42:46.

Ito K, Watanabe K, Nasim S, et al: K-ras point mutations in endometrial carcinoma: effect on outcome is dependent on age of patient. Gynecol Oncol 1996;63:238.

Kacinski BM, Carter D, Mittal K, et al: High level of expression of fms proto-oncogene mRNA is observed in clinically aggressive human endometrial adenocarcinomas. Int J Radiat Oncol Biol Phys 1988;5:823.

Kacinski BM, Mayer AG, King BL, et al: NEU protein overexpression in benign, borderline, and malignant ovarian neoplasms. Gynecol Oncol 1992;44:245.

Kobayashi K, Matsushima M, Koi S, et al: Mutational analysis of mismatch repair genes, hMLH1 and hMSH2, in sporadic endometrial carcinomas with microsatellite instability. Jpn J Cancer Res 1996;87:141.

Kohlberger P, Girsch G, Loesche A, et al: p53 Protein overexpression in early stage endometrial cancer. Gynecol Oncol 1996; 62:213.

Landers JP, Spelsberg TC: New concepts in steroid hormone action: transcription factors, proto-oncogenes and the cascade model for steroid regulation of gene expression. Crit Rev Eukaryot Gene Expr 1992;2:19.

Lee J-H, Lee S-K, Yang M-H, et al: Expression and mutation of H-ras in uterine cervical cancer. Gynecol Oncol 1996;62:49.

Lee MG, Norbury CJ, Spurr NK, Nurse P: Regulated expression and phosphorylation of a possible mammalian cell-cycle control protein. Nature 1988;333:257.

Levesque MA, Katsaros D, Hu M, et al: Mutant p53 protein overexpression is associated with poor outcome in patients with well or moderately differentiated ovarian carcinoma. Cancer 1995;75:1327.

Liu TJ, el Naggar AK, McDonnell TJ, et al: Apoptosis induction mediated by wild-type p53 adenoviral gene transfer in squamous cell carcinoma of the head and neck. Cancer Res 1995; 55:3117.

Madrigal M, Janicek MF, Sevin B-U, et al: In vitro antigen therapy targeting HPV 16 E6 and E7 in cervical carcinoma. Gynecol Oncol 1997;64:18.

Marks JR, Davidoff AM, Kerns BJ, et al: Overexpression and mutation of p53 in epithelial ovarian cancer. Cancer Res 1991;51: 2979.

McCann AH, Dervan PA, O'Regan M, et al: Prognostic significance of e-erbB2 and estrogen receptor status in human breast cancer. Cancer Res 1991;51:3296.

Mizuuchi H, Nasim S, Kudo R, et al: Clinical implications of K-ras mutations in malignant epithelial tumors of the endometrium. Cancer Res 1992;52:2777.

Murray AW, Kirschner MW: Dominoes and clocks: the union of two views of the cell cycle. Science 1988;246:614.

Pisani AL, Barbuto DA, Chen D, et al: HER-2/neu, p53 and DNA analysis as prognosticators for survival in endometrial carcinoma. Obstet Gynecol 1995;85:729.

Pollard JW, Pacey J, Cheng SUY, Jordan EG: Estrogens and cell death in murine uterine epithelium. Cell Tissue Res 1987;249: 533.

Pustzal L, Lewis CE, Lorenzen J, McGee JOD: Growth factors: regulation of normal and neoplastic growth. J Pathol 1993;169: 191.

Riou G: Proto-oncogenes and prognosis in early carcinoma of the uterine cervix. Cancer Surv 1988;7:441.

Riou G, Barrois M, Le MG, et al: cMYC proto-oncogene expression and prognosis in early carcinoma of the uterine cervix. Lancet 1987;1:761.

Riou G, Bourhis J, Le MG: The c-myc proto-oncogene in invasive carcinomas of the uterine cervix: clinical relevance of overexpression in early stages of the cancer. Anticancer Res 1990a;10: 1225.

Riou G, Sherg ZM, Zhou D, et al: C-myc and c-Ha-ras protooncogenes in cervical cancer: prognostic value. Bull Cancer 1990b;77:341.

Rodenburg CJ, Koelma IA, Nap M, et al: Immunohistochemical detection of the ras oncogene product p21 in advanced ovarian cancer. Arch Pathol Lab Med 1988;112:151.

Roth JA, Cristiano RJ: Gene therapy for cancer: what have we done and where are we going? J Natl Cancer Inst 1997;89:21.

Rubin SC, Finstad CL, Wong GY, et al: Prognostic significance of HER-2/neu expression in advanced epithelial ovarian cancer: a multivariate analysis. Am J Obstet Gynecol 1993;168:162.

Sagae S, Kudo R, Kuzumaki N, et al: Ras oncogene expression and progression in intraepithelial neoplasia of the uterine cervix. Cancer 1990;66:295.

Scambia G, Cattozzi L, Panici PB, et al: Expression of the ras oncogene p21 protein in normal and neoplastic ovarian tissues: correlation with histopathologic features and receptors for estrogen, progesterone, and epidermal growth factor receptor. Am J Obstet Gynecol 1993;168:71.

Scambia G, Panici PB, Battaglia F, et al: Significance of epidermal growth factor receptor in advanced ovarian cancer. J Clin Oncol 1992;10:529.

Scheffner M, Werness BA, Huibreatse JM, et al: The E6 oncoprotein encoded by human papillomavirus types 16 and 18 promotes the degradation of p53. Cell 1990;63:1129.

Shattuck-Eidens D, McClure M, Simard J, et al: A collaborative survey of 80 mutations in the BRCA1 breast and ovarian cancer susceptibility gene: implications for presymptomatic testing and screening. JAMA 1995;273:535.

Slamon DJ, Godolphin W, Jones LA, et al: Studies of the HER-2/neu proto-oncogene in human breast and ovarian cancer. Science 1989;244:707.

Smith EP, Boyd J, Frank GR, et al: Estrogen resistance caused by a mutation of the estrogen receptor in a man. N Engl J Med 1994;331:1056.

Struewing JP, Hartge P, Wacholder S, et al: The risk of cancer associated with specific mutations of BRCA1 and BRCA2 among Ashkenazi Jews. N Engl J Med 1997;336:1401.

Tanner B, Kreutz E, Weikel W, et al: Prognostic significance of c-erbB-2 mRNA in ovarian carcinoma. Gynecol Oncol 1996;62:268.

Taylor AM, McConville DM, Byrd PJ: Cancer and DNA processing disorders. Br Med Bull 1994;50:708.

Wilkinson N, Todd N, Buckley CH, et al: An immunohistochemical study of the incidence and significance of c-erbB2 oncoprotein overexpression in ovarian neoplasia. Int J Gynecol Cancer 1991;1:285.

Wong YF, Chung TK, Cehung TH, et al: Frequent ras gene mutations in squamous cell cervical cancer. Cancer Lett 1995;95:29.

Yaginuma Y, Yamashita K, Kuzumaki N, et al: ras Oncogene product p21 expression and prognosis of human ovarian tumors. Gynecol Oncol 1992;46:45.

52

Benign and Preinvasive Lesions of the Vulva and Vagina

I. Keith Stone
Edward J. Wilkinson

When Marion Simms published his *Clinical Notes on Uterine Surgery* in 1866, he emphasized "that we should never in our examinations allow any exposure of person not even in hospital practice. When the speculum is used we should see only the neck of the womb and the canal of the vagina" (p. 192). In the 1910 edition of *The Principles of Gynaecology* by William Bell, vulvar disease was addressed, with emphasis on traumatic lesions, cystic abnormalities, and malignant neoplasms. Dermatologic diseases affecting the vulva included herpes, eczema, and leukoplakia. Contrary to the practice in the mid-1800s, when the vulva was rarely examined, and the early 1900s, when it was inadequately studied, today interest in vulvar disease has resulted in improved diagnoses and therapy.

The vulva may not only be involved in generalized dermatologic conditions but may also manifest its own unique pathologic features. In the course of pelvic examination, careful inspection of the vulva and vagina is always in order. Premalignant and malignant lesions are not always symptomatic, nor are they always readily apparent to the unaided eye. In certain conditions such as vulvar intraepithelial neoplasia (VIN), examination limited to the vulva, vagina, and cervix may overlook anal involvement by this process. When observing vulvar pathology, it is important to note location, color, configuration, and consistency. The location of certain conditions is pathognomonic. Hidradenoma tends to occur in the intralabial sulcus, between the labia minora and labia majora. Knife-like ulcerations associated with Crohn's disease occur lateral to the labia majora. Color elicits concern, especially when one is dealing with pigmented lesions on the vulva. The possibility of melanoma, VIN, or atypical nevus must be considered. The smooth, rounded contour and regular consistency of a Bartholin's cyst, hidradenoma, epidermal inclusion cyst, or lipoma suggest an expanding lesion of a benign nature.

To assist the clinician in determining the nature of vulvar disease, it is helpful to examine the patient's skin and mucous membranes. Lichen sclerosus commonly involves the vulva and may involve other skin sites, but typically does not involve the vagina. Lichen planus not only may involve the vulvar skin but also may affect the vagina, oral buccal surfaces, skin, and scalp. A careful history may reveal gastrointestinal symptoms in the patient with vulvar ulcerations, and Crohn's disease should be considered in the differential diagnosis.

Assessment of certain conditions of the vulva is augmented with magnified examination of the vulvar epithelium, which may be performed with a colposcope. The thickened white epithelium associated with intraepithelial neoplasia may be enhanced with the application of 3% acetic acid to the vulva for several minutes before the evaluation. The solution is applied to the vulva and perianal area. Careful examination of vulvar and perianal areas with the colposcope may demonstrate small lesions not apparent to the unaided eye. Historically, topical 1% toluidine blue followed by 1% acetic acid wash has been used to evaluate neoplastic processes. This nuclear stain is readily incorporated into rapidly dividing cells. However, inflamed, eroded, and ulcerated lesions resulting from scratching, and irritated lesions, may also incorporate the stain, diminishing its usefulness, and is currently rarely used in clinical practice.

Although diagnoses may occasionally be made on the basis of the visual findings just mentioned, histopathologic confirmation is often necessary. The thickened white epithelium clinically observed in patients with vulvar candidiasis is also seen in patients with vulvar Paget's disease. The clinical changes associated with squamous cell hyperplasia, including lichen simplex chronicus, may also be seen in patients with VIN. A hyperpigmented lesion is seen in both lentigo simplex and atypical nevus. Biopsies of the vulvar skin can be acceptably performed in the clinic under local anesthesia. Before biopsy, careful assessment must be made to define the area most likely to provide findings upon which to establish the correct diagnosis. Lichen planus lesions should not be subject to biopsy in eroded, erythematous plaques; rather, specimens should be taken from the periphery of the visible lesion where the reticulate pattern is present. Lesions clinically consistent with VIN should undergo biopsy where examination demonstrates the most atypical changes. Multiple diagnostic biopsies are needed if multifocal lesions are present. For small focal abnormalities, excisional biopsy may be diagnostic and therapeutic. Isolated epidermal inclusion cysts may be effectively removed in the clinic. Small, hyperpigmented lesions may also be excised with adequate margins.

Care should be taken to avoid trauma to contiguous structures during vulvar biopsies. A biopsy in the vestibular region may be necessary in the evaluation of vulvar vestibulitis; however, the biopsy should avoid obstructing the duct of the major vestibular gland (Bartholin's gland). To choose the appropriate instrument for biopsy, one must consider the size of the lesion. The 4- or 5-mm Keyes biopsy punch is frequently used to perform diagnostic evaluations; however, a scalpel with a No. 15 blade is more appropriate for larger excisional biopsies (Fig. 52–1). The Keyes biopsy is especially useful in the evaluation of inflammatory dermatoses, where the dermal-epidermal changes need to be seen. A small elevated pigmented lesion is best approached with an excisional biopsy whereas an elevated papular lesion may be best approached using a shave biopsy. Care should be taken when using the Keyes biopsy punch to avoid trauma to deep vessels, which may result in hematoma formation. Not all biopsy sites require suture closure. Small punch biopsies may be coagulated with silver nitrate. Larger incisions or incisions that tend to bleed require suture placement. A 3-0 chromic gut suture on a cutting needle is preferred over the use of polyglactin or polyglycolic acid sutures. The latter suture materials tend to have delayed absorption and require removal of persistent knotted material several weeks after the original biopsy. Larger skin lesions, deep lesions, and lesions in the extremely young patient frequently warrant a more complete evaluation and intervention in the operating suite. One must take care when fixing histologic specimens to ensure proper orientation. The pathologist should be informed of the clinical findings, presumed diagnosis, and the specific site of the biopsy.

Terminology for vulvar and vaginal lesions has undergone change in the classification of non-neoplastic epithelial disorders and in intraepithelial neoplasia. In 1987, the International Society for the Study of Vulvovaginal Disease (ISSVD) and the International Society of Gynecologic Pathologists (ISGP) agreed on the terminology used to classify vulvar non-neoplastic epithelial disorders. The term *lichen sclerosus* had been previously used by the ISSVD to replace the term *lichen sclerosus et atrophicus* (Ridley et al, 1989). *Squamous cell hyperplasia* replaced

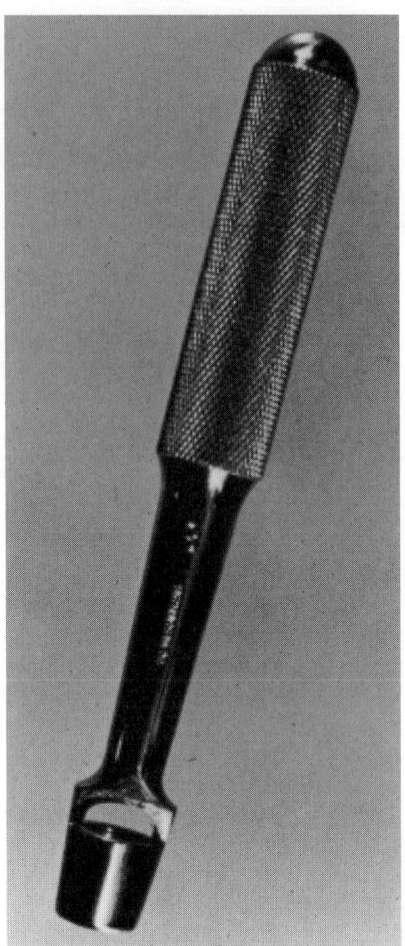

Figure 52–1
Keyes biopsy punch.

the term *hyperplastic dystrophy*. In 1986, the ISSVD and the ISGP committee on non-neoplastic epithelial disorders recommended the term *vulvar intraepithelial neoplasia* (Wilkinson et al, 1986). The recommendation further stated that the terms *Bowen's disease*, *bowenoid papulosis*, *erythroplasia of Queyrat*, *carcinoma in situ*, and *bowenoid dysplasia* should not be used. Although the ISSVD included both Paget's disease and melanoma in situ within the intraepithelial classification, the ISGP group and the World Health Organization classified these abnormalities under their respective invasive tumor categories, specifically Paget's disease under adenocarcinoma and melanoma in situ under malignant melanoma.

VULVA

Non-neoplastic Lesions

Epithelial Disorders

LICHEN SCLEROSUS

First described in 1887 by the French dermatologist Hallopeau, lichen sclerosus has been known by a variety of terms, including *atrophic leukoplakia, kraurosis vulvae, senile atrophy, atrophic vulvitis,* and *lichen sclerosus et atrophicus* (Friedrich, 1983). The ISSVD has recommended the term *lichen sclerosus.*

The disease process may affect males and females. In the male, the glans penis, including the periurethral epithelium, is affected and the condition is termed *balantis xerotica obliterans.* The disease may occur at any age and may persist throughout a person's life; however, it appears to affect women at the two extremes of life: the very young, premenarchal woman and the older, perimenopausal or postmenopausal woman. It has been reported in a 6-month-old female infant (Ridley, 1987). In children it may cause anal stenosis if perianal involvement occurs. This may cause symptoms of painful defecation and blood in the stool. Frequently, apparent remission of symptoms occurs at puberty; however, the physical findings may persist. In the older patient, the disease is chronic and progressive unless there is therapeutic intervention.

Although lichen sclerosus may present on the neck, trunk, and extremities, the most common presentation is on the genital and perianal regions. The cause remains obscure. Reports have demonstrated similarities in major human histocompatibility antigens in patients who are affected with lichen sclerosus. The frequency of human lymphocyte antigen (HLA) types HLA-Aw31 and HLA-B21 has been shown to be increased in patients with lichen sclerosus (Holt and Darke, 1983; Sideri et al, 1988). Patients with lichen sclerosus show an increased frequency of autoantibodies, with as many as 74% of these patients demonstrating one positive autoantibody and 20% of patients demonstrating autoimmune disease, of which thyroiditis is the most common presentation (Meyrick-Thomas et al, 1982). Lichen sclerosus, therefore, may be an autoimmune disease with an HLA linkage.

Currently, topical high-potency corticosteroids (0.5% clobetasol or equivalent) are recommended for initial treatment and can be used for long-term therapy with less frequent application. Topical 2% testosterone proprionate in a petrolatum base is generally not used except occasionally in adults where severe atrophic changes do not adequately respond to the high potency topical corticosteroid (Dalziel and Wojnarowska, 1993).

Supporting the concept of lichen sclerosus as a manifestation of a systemic disease, perhaps autoimmune in nature, is the observation that patients with lichen sclerosus who have been treated with excision of the involved skin have noted the subsequent appearance of lichen sclerosus in the grafted skin (Whimster, 1973; Klein et al, 1984).

The patient typically has symptoms of severe vulvar and/or perianal pruritus. This commonly prompts intense scratching, resulting in ecchymoses and ulceration. Dyspareunia is a common symptom. In advanced cases agglutination of the labia and labial shrinkage may result in stenosis of the vaginal

introitus. Perianal involvement may cause perianal stenosis. In general, the more longstanding the disease, the more advanced the clinical findings. The patient often has a history of topical antifungal therapy with no relief of symptoms.

Upon examination, the involved areas, which may include the perineum, perianal region, and labia minora, appear pale to white and somewhat atrophic (Fig. 52–2). As the disease progresses, the vulvar architecture is altered, with loss and agglutination of the labia minora, prepuce, and frenulum. Continued progression results in diminution of the size of the introitus.

It is important to carefully observe the areas involved by lichen sclerosus for premalignant or malignant conditions. Although lichen sclerosus is not considered to be a premalignant condition, carcinoma of the vulva has been noted in approximately 4% of these patients. Lichen sclerosus has been found as an associated lesion in up to 53% of patients with vulvar invasive carcinoma (Punnonen et al, 1985). It is thought that appropriate topical therapy can reduce the frequency of subsequent carcinoma; however, no controlled prospective studies on this have been published.

Colposcopy of the vulva affected by lichen sclerosus is frequently helpful in evaluating for changes of VIN. Macular or papular areas may be found that may have accentuated surface skin markings, aceto-

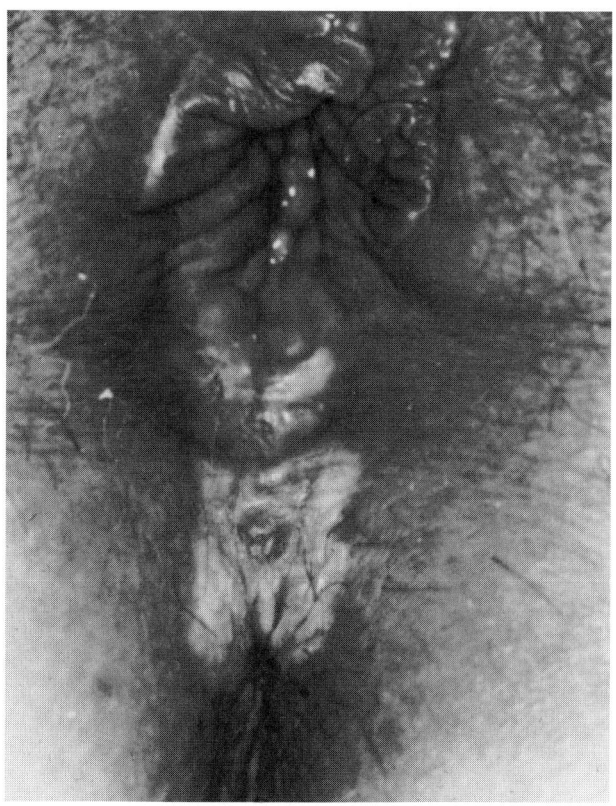

Figure 52–2
Perineal lichen sclerosus.

whitening, and coloration differing from the adjacent epithelium. Palpation of the vulvar skin may disclose regions of thickened, hyperplastic-appearing tissue within fields of lichen sclerosus.

Histopathologic findings include loss of rete ridges with marked thinning of the epithelium. Hyperkeratosis may or may not be present. Within the dermis, there is a loss of vascularity with fibrin deposition and edema. Chronic inflammation is present within the deeper dermis below the zone of prominent edema. Subcutaneous blood, reflecting areas of ecchymosis and superficial ulceration with prominent inflammation, may also be seen. In some cases, adjacent epithelial thickening may be present without atypia. In such cases, a diagnosis of lichen sclerosus with squamous cell hyperplasia should be made. This finding is also referred to as *lichen sclerosus with lichen simplex chronicus*, the latter term being preferred by most dermatopathologists (Carlson et al, 1998).

Lichen sclerosus, with its characteristic architecture, is infrequently confused with other dermatologic conditions of the vulva. Lichen planus may be clinically confused with lichen sclerosus; however, lichen planus involves the introitus and vagina, usually presents as an erythematous process, and in its later stages may result in agglutination of the vaginal wall and loss of the vaginal vault. This does not appear in lichen sclerosus. Vitiligo as well as postinflammatory hypopigmentation may be clinically confused with lichen sclerosus; however, neither one alters the architecture of the vulva (Fig. 52–3). Vitiligo is not associated with symptoms of pruritus.

Treatment is aimed predominantly at alleviation of symptoms. The mainstay in clinical management is the use of topical steroids to decrease the inflammatory response and to control pruritus. A fluorinated high-potency corticosteroid, such as clobetasol ointment applied twice daily to the vulva for approximately 2 to 3 weeks, can control symptoms. The patient may then use the topical steroid periodically as needed and frequently experiences extended periods during which no application is necessary. When more frequent long-term application is required to control symptoms, a less potent steroid should be used (0.1% betamethasone). The ointment preparation is preferred over the cream.

SQUAMOUS CELL HYPERPLASIA

Squamous cell hyperplasia (formerly *hyperplastic dystrophy*) is also characterized by white epithelium, which usually appears thickened with an irregular surface. The change may be unilateral and plaque-like or more diffuse; symmetry, as seen in lichen sclerosus, is rare. Shrinkage and agglutination of the labia are not seen, nor are the focal areas of ecchymosis found that may occur in lichen sclerosus.

The histopathologic diagnosis is one of exclusion. The pathologic changes seen in squamous cell hyperplasia include prominent acanthosis, with elon-

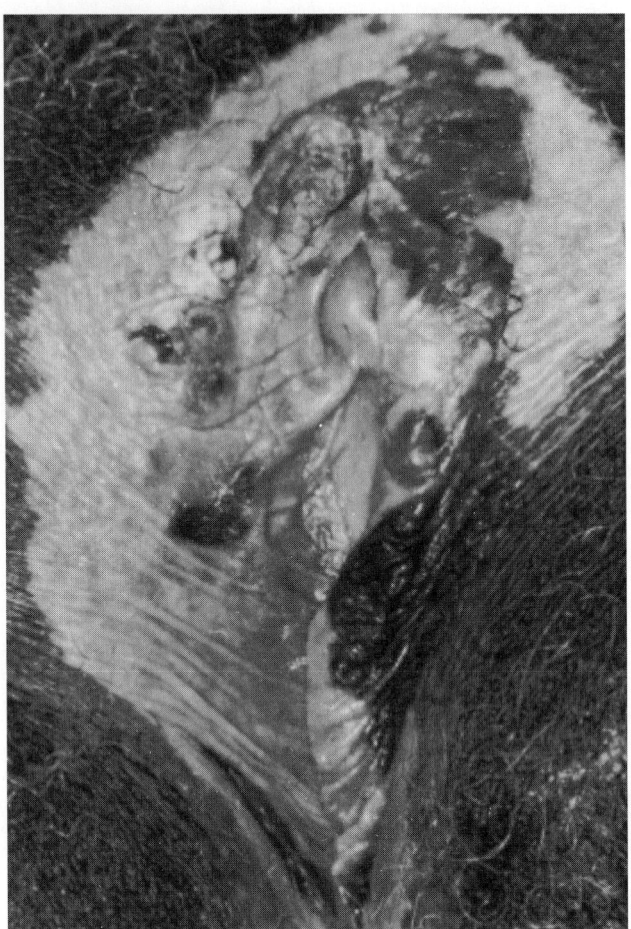

Figure 52–3
Periclitoral hyperplastic lichen sclerosus in a diffuse field of vitiligo.

gation, widening, and deepening of the rete ridges and thickening of the epidermis. There is no epithelial atypia. Hyperkeratosis may be present. A mild, chronic inflammatory infiltrate may be present within the dermis. The term *lichen simplex chronicus* is generally preferred by dermatopathologists (Ambros et al, 1996). This diagnosis is essentially descriptive of the histopathologic epithelial changes present. The term *squamous cell hyperplasia* encompasses changes previously specified as hyperplastic dystrophy but should not be used if a specific dermatosis can be identified (e.g., psoriasis, lichen planus, condyloma acuminatum, lichen simplex chronicus). Chronic monilial or dermatophyte infection may produce similar epithelial changes, and these conditions must be excluded. Those cases demonstrating atypia with changes of vulvar intraepithelial neoplasia are to be classified as VIN. The term *hyperplastic dystrophy with atypia* is not recommended; these cases should be placed in the VIN category. The term *mixed dystrophy* is no longer recommended because it is now appreciated that such cases reflect the spectrum of lichen sclerosus, which may present with adjacent or associated hyperplastic and hyperkeratotic areas (see discussion of lichen sclerosus).

Treatment is directed primarily at control of symptoms. Because pruritus is the usual complaint, steroids are the mainstay of therapy. Topical fluorinated compounds, such as betamethasone 0.1% ointment, almost always control the pruritus. Regression of symptoms is usually evident within 4 to 6 weeks, and long-term cortisteroid therapy is not necessary and may be detrimental in that it can result in atrophic changes. To prevent recurrence, it is important to exclude inciting agents such as residual laundry products in clothing or underwear fabrics that may be occlusive or irritating.

LICHEN PLANUS

Described by Erasmus Wilson in 1869, lichen planus is a disease that is more frequently seen in dermatology or otolaryngology clinics; however, it occasionally involves the vulva or vulva and vagina. The cause of the disease process is poorly understood, although there is a suggestion of an autoimmune basis.

The patient with vulvar or vaginal lichen planus typically presents with burning symptoms, occasionally associated with pruritus. There may be postcoital bleeding. Dyspareunia is a common complaint. On examination of the vulvar region, the initial impression may be that of lichen sclerosus because of the atrophic appearance; however, closer evaluation demonstrates a narrow rim of white reticulation at the periphery of the lesion (Fig. 52–4). Vulvar adhesions may result in obliteration of the labia minora, with absence of the prepuce and clitoris. Vaginal examination may be difficult or impossible because of the occurrence of numerous adhesive bands in the erythematous vagina. In a milder form, erosive erythematous vaginal mucosa may be observed, which bleeds easily when touched. Upon notation of these findings, careful examination of the patient's gingiva may demonstrate changes consistent with the vulvovaginal-gingival syndrome (Pelisse, 1989). The labial aspect of the maxillary gingival surface most frequently demonstrates eroded areas bordered by a thin, white, reticulated pattern. Occasionally, a patient may also demonstrate well-defined areas of alopecia.

Histopathologic examination is necessary for a confirmed diagnosis. Although the tendency is to obtain biopsy specimens of the eroded vaginal or vulvar epithelium, these areas demonstrate inflammation only. It is necessary to obtain the biopsy specimen from the periphery of the desquamated area in the region of the reticulated pattern. This biopsy specimen will show a pattern of acanthosis, basal cell degeneration with formation of necrotic keratinocytes, and heavy, band-like lymphoid infiltrate (Soper et al, 1988).

Treatment is primarily anti-inflammatory with topical steroids. A fluorinated corticosteroid, such as

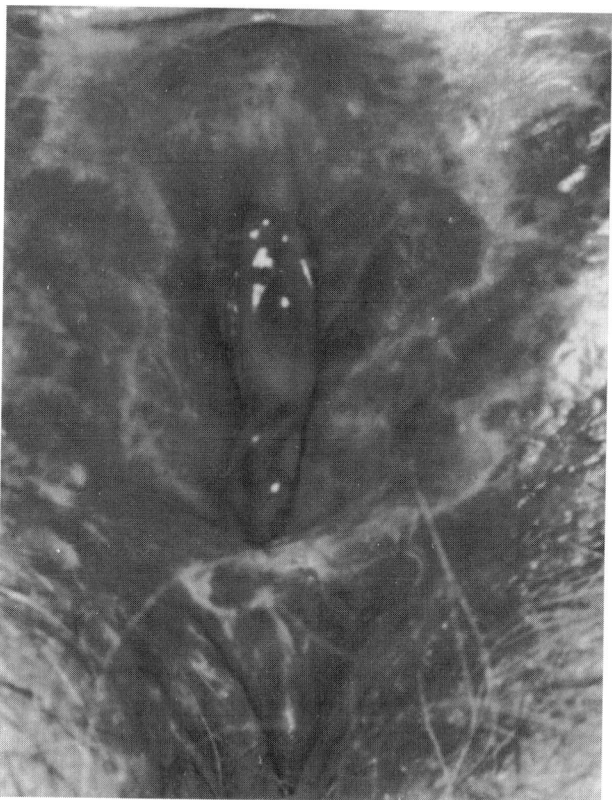

Figure 52–4
Reticulate pattern of lichen planus.

betamethasone 0.1%, is indicated for vulvar involvement. Vaginal involvement may be treated with intravaginal 25-mg hydrocortisone acetate rectal suppositories, inserted daily as needed. Intravaginal hydrocortisone acetate foaming agents (e.g., Colifoam) have recently been observed to provide a therapeutic response in some patients, with reduction of leukorrhea, and prevention of vaginal synechiae (Pelisse, 1999). To decrease the risk of adhesion formation in the vagina, dilators covered with 1% hydrocortisone cream may be necessary. Other therapeutic approaches include the use of oral and topical retinoids, oral griseofulvin, and cytotoxic agents, such as cyclophosphamide.

Lichen planus is difficult to treat effectively, and therapeutic results are often disappointing. Patients require long-term support and management (Edwards, 1989).

Inflammatory Disorders

VESTIBULITIS

Vulvar vestibulitis is a poorly understood, disabling condition that usually results in sexual dysfunction. The vestibule is that region of the vulva that has nonkeratinized squamous mucosa. It begins just caudal (external) to the hymenal ring. It extends from the frenulum of the clitoris posteriorly and laterally to the urethral meatus and circumferentially around the introitus. It is bounded laterally by Hart's line (Hart's line is the junction of the nonkeratinized and keratinized epithelium) on the medial aspects of the labia minora and posteriorly by the perianal body. Within this area, small glands, known as the minor vestibular glands, reside. These are simple tubular glands with mucus-secreting columnar epithelium. The cause of the inflammation in vestibulitis is obscure. The inflammatory process involves the periglandular and subepithelial stroma of the vestibule (Pyka et al, 1988). Human papillomavirus (HPV) infection does not appear to play an etiologic role in this process and has been identified by polymerase chain reaction (PCR) in only 3 of 31 cases studied (Wilkinson et al, 1993). One study has suggested a more frequent association (Turner and Marinoff, 1988).

The typical patient with vestibulitis is in her reproductive years, usually between the ages of 17 and 41 years. The condition may present postmenopausally and has been noted in patients in their 80s. Patients typically are sexually active and will have been engaged in intercourse for a number of years before onset of symptoms. Some patients have noted development of symptoms within the first year of experiencing sexual intercourse and a few virginal patients have been observed with primary vulvar vestibulitis. There is often a history of recurrent vaginal infections, specifically fungal infections. The most common complaint is burning in the region of the vestibule, resulting in painful intercourse. A portion of patients may complain of inability to insert tampons. Pruritus and swelling may also be complaints. Patients who have been referred for evaluation may often have experienced a multitude of unsuccessful therapeutic trials. Spontaneous remission of symptoms may occur; however, long-term prospective studies on the natural history of vulvar vestibulitis are not available currently.

Clinical evaluation includes careful inspection of the vestibule, with pressure applied to numerous sites on the vestibule using the cotton-tipped end of a swab (Q-tip) to determine the degree and locations of tenderness. The vestibule is then examined with the colposcope after application of 3% acetic acid. Regions of distinctly white epithelium, suggesting HPV infection, warrant biopsy after local anesthesia. The vestibule is normally slightly aceto-white, and this finding should not be confused with HPV-associated change (Fig. 52–5). During the biopsy, care should be taken to avoid traumatizing the Bartholin's gland duct. Obstruction of this duct by excisional biopsy may result in the formation of a Bartholin's cyst. Complete examination of the vagina to rule out bacterial vaginosis, candidiasis, or *Trichomonas* should be performed. The observation of atrophic vaginitis in the older patient population may be of therapeutic significance.

Histopathologic features include a superficial chronic inflammatory infiltrate within the subepithelial stroma of the vestibule. The inflammatory cell

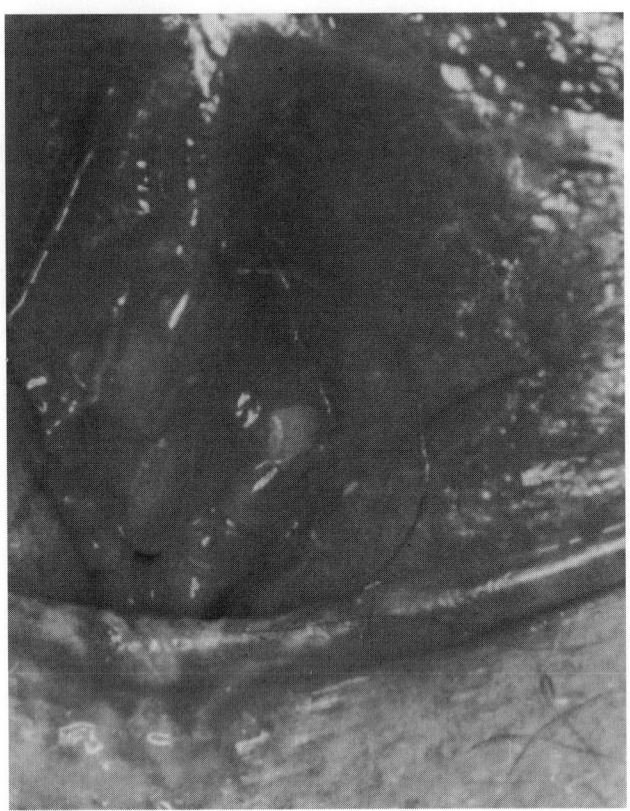

Figure 52–5
White epithelium in the vestibule consistent with human papillomavirus.

population may involve the epithelium and consists predominantly of lymphocytes, although granulocytes, plasma cells, and mast cells may be seen. Minor vestibular glands are not always found in biopsy or vestibulectomy specimens. When present, the inflammation seen is usually periglandular, not intraglandular, and may involve the glandular epithelium (Pyka et al, 1988). The epithelium of the vulvar vestibule, like that of the vagina, is not keratinized, and in women of reproductive age it is glycogenated (Wilkinson and Hardt, 1995). Vulvar vestibular epithelium may have epithelial spongiosis as well as intracellular glycogen, both of which can be misinterpreted as koilocytosis of HPV infection. The epithelium often appears thin, and erosion and ulceration may be noted. Molecular biologic methods, such as DNA in situ hybridization, or PCR studies with HPV probes for the detection of HPV, should be used when the diagnosis of HPV is uncertain.

A multitude of therapies have been attempted to resolve the symptoms associated with vestibulitis. Varying degrees of success have been reported. A reasonable approach to the therapy of vestibulitis should be based on the observations at the initial examination as the patient may be a candidate for interferon injections. Reasonable success rates have been noted with 4-week courses of interferon injections (Horowitz, 1989). The interferon is injected into the vestibule on Mondays, Wednesdays, and Fridays for 4 weeks. On each day, 1 million units of interferon will be injected at a separate site in the vestibule corresponding to the markings on the face of a superimposed clock. Most patients complain of flu-like symptoms during the course of therapy. Observations should be continued for approximately 3 months after completion of injections to determine response. Although the initial use of interferon in vestibulitis was based on the probable cause as HPV, this treatment has given some response in controlled studies where HPV was not a variable.

Progressive vaginal dialation by the patient, employing vaginal dialators and biofeedback techniques, has helped some patients. Topical estrogen has proven to be of some value for women who have associated atrophy or atrophy-like changes. Anesthetics, dapsone, nonsteroidal anti-inflammatory drugs, capsaicin (Zostrix), acyclovir (Zovirax), and trichloroacetic acid applications are rarely successful. Pulsed-dye laser therapy of the vestibule has been inadequately studied. Laser vaporization and topical 5% 5-fluorouracil have not proven effective and may be associated with significant ulceration and post-therapy complications. Before any therapeutic approach is outlined, evidence of vaginitis should be addressed. A history of recurrent vaginitis may suggest an etiologic factor contributing to the patient's discomfort. A thorough fungal and bacteriologic evaluation is appropriate, including cultures for *Candida* species such as *C. glabrata* and *C. tropicalis.*

Patients with vestibulitis often manifest anxiety and/or depression. It is difficult to determine whether these symptoms are a cause or a result of the pain and sexual dysfunction associated with the symptoms of vestibulitis. It is currently thought that depression leads to decreased levels of endorphins and reduces tolerance to pain (Steege, 1989). It is important to determine the degree of depression and anxiety in patients with vestibulitis and to consider psychological support, including antidepressant therapy, in an effort to relieve the chronic pain. The disease process often waxes and wanes and may be related to stress. Verbal and psychological support through these periods of stress and pain assist the patient in dealing with this disabling disease.

In patients who have failed to respond to conservative medical measures, surgical therapy may be considered. Operative procedures include partial vestibulectomy with vaginal advancement, partial vestibulectomy, and total vestibulectomy (Marinoff et al, 1993). The operation and expected success, as well as morbidity and risks, should be carefully discussed with the patient. Although success rates have been reported in the range of 88% to 89%, long-term follow-up is often lacking, and the success rate may be closer to 50% (Ostergard, 1990). Occasionally, patients may require a second vestibulectomy. It is imperative that the region of tenderness be carefully mapped before surgery to ensure removal of all painful areas involved. The surgical procedure necessitates mobilization of the vaginal epithelium to allow approximation of the vagina to the perineal and labial skin. If this is not accomplished, wound breakdown will occur, and healing with then occur by secondary intention. The postoperative discomfort associated with this operation is significant.

HIDRADENITIS SUPPURATIVA

In 1955 Shelley and Cahn produced hidradenitis suppurativa in human volunteers after intentionally obstructing apocrine glands. Obstruction results in autoinoculation of retained apocrine material by skin flora, severe inflammation, rupture of the duct, and spread of the infection to adjacent apocrine glands. Pathologic changes consist of dilated apocrine ducts containing keratin material and deep inflammation.

Although the pathogenesis of the disease is understood, the cause is still speculative. There is some suggestion that Mendelian inheritance may play a role (Fitzsimmons et al, 1985). Patients with moderate or severe clinical disease have been noted to have marked reduction in T lymphocytes and increased frequency of HLA antigens A1 and B8 (O'Loughlin et al, 1988). It has been suggested that the T lymphocytes play a role in the pathogenesis of hidradenitis suppurativa and that HLA-A1 and HLA-B8 may predispose patients to more severe disease. Hormonal studies have demonstrated higher concentrations of total testosterone and free-androgen index than in normal controls (Mortimer et al, 1986b).

Bacteriologic studies in patients with hidradenitis suppurativa have demonstrated multiple organisms, including *Staphylococcus aureus*, anaerobic streptococci, and *Bacteroides* species. It has been suggested that *Streptococcus milleri* may be significantly associated with disease activity (Highet et al, 1988).

The disease affects both males and females, with multiple sites observed in more than 50% of patients. Sites of involvement include the axilla, groin, perineum, perirectal area, and breasts. Patients have chronic recurrent abscesses, draining fistulas, and scarring (Fig. 52–6). The diagnosis should be suspected in patients with suggestive lesions in these sites. Although cultures of these lesions are usually obtained, they have not been demonstrated to be of clinical usefulness. Biopsy typically demonstrates acute and chronic inflammatory changes with keratin plugging of apocrine glands.

Initial therapy for mild disease may consist of avoidance of antiperspirant deodorants and careful attention to local hygiene. Various therapeutic modalities for more advanced disease have been attempted with variable success. Topical clindamycin has been used in an effort to alter the microbiology of the inflammatory process (Clemmensen, 1983). Patients treated with topical clindamycin have reported a significant decrease in the number of abscesses and inflammatory nodules when compared with placebo therapy.

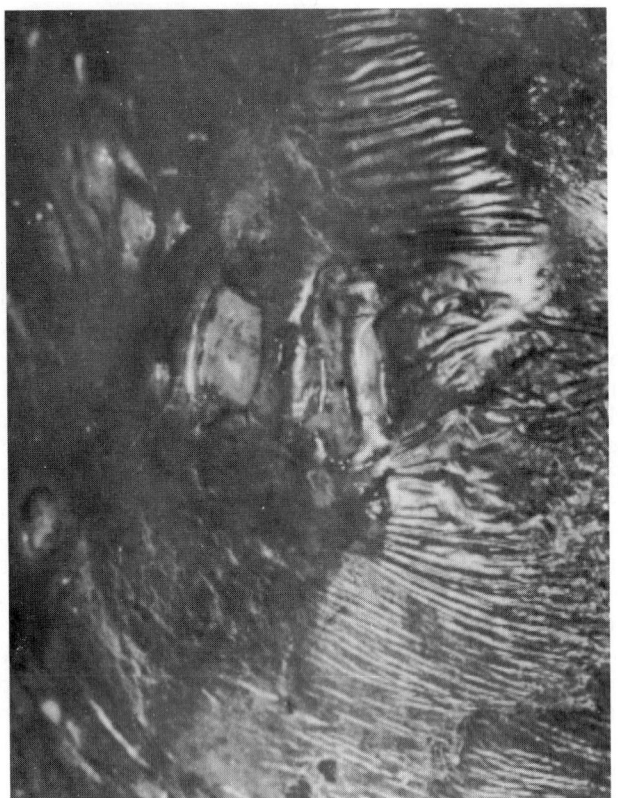

Figure 52–6
Hidradenitis suppurativa.

Isotretinoin, a drug commonly used to treat severe nodulocystic acne, has demonstrated efficacy in the therapy of hidradenitis suppurativa (Dicken et al, 1984). The medication may be prescribed for 4 months at a daily dose of 1 mg/kg, with appropriate instructions concerning the absolute necessity for contraception. Recommended laboratory follow-up with patients treated with isotretinoin should include baseline pregnancy test, complete blood count, and liver function studies. These should be repeated every 4 to 6 weeks (Brown et al, 1988).

The use of oral cyclosporine in the treatment of hidradenitis suppurativa has met with moderate success in a small study (Gupta et al, 1990). Other investigators have noted antiandrogen therapy consisting of cyproterone acetate to be beneficial in the treatment of hidradenitis suppurativa (Mortimer et al, 1986a).

Ultimately, the most consistent response has been noted in patients who have undergone surgical therapy of hidradenitis suppurativa (Bhatiu et al, 1984). Surgery consists of local excision of mild disease. Wide excision is applicable for more extensive disease. Various wound closures, including rhomboid flaps, split-thickness skin grafts, and simple approximation of skin edges, have demonstrated excellent results when appropriately used. Healing by secondary intention usually requires 2 to 5 months and is well tolerated by most patients (Silverber et al, 1987).

CROHN'S DISEASE

Since the original description of Crohn's disease (Crohn et al, 1932), there have been several reports of genital Crohn's disease in the English literature (Baker and Walton, 1988). Genital involvement by Crohn's disease is seen in women of reproductive age, although it has been reported in an 8-year-old girl (Lally et al, 1988). Genital involvement may predate gastrointestinal Crohn's disease by months or years.

Four types of cutaneous Crohn's disease have been described (Schulman et al, 1987). There may be *direct extension* from involved bowel, resulting in perineal ulcerations, abscesses, and fistulas. There may be *extraintestinal involvement*, in which the genital granuloma are separate from the involved gastrointestinal tract. There may be *vascular reactions*, including pyoderma gangrenosum and localized vulvar erythema nodosum. *Skin lesions* secondary to malabsorption may occur. It is important to differentiate the manifestations of extraintestinal Crohn's disease from lymphogranuloma venereum, hidradenitis suppurativa, vulvar tuberculosis, sarcoidosis, and leprosy. Cutaneous Crohn's disease most commonly involves the perineum and is most frequently a manifestation of continuity with anal lesions.

Patients with cutaneous Crohn's disease should undergo appropriate gastrointestinal evaluation. Patients typically are seen with localized vulvar erythema and edema, which result in ulcer formation. The classical finding of vulvar Crohn's disease is the knife-like, sharply demarcated ulceration lateral to the labia majora (Fig. 52–7). These characteristic lesions are not present in all patients with vulvar Crohn's disease. The vulva may be nontender, red, firm, and edematous.

Histopathologic findings include noncaseating granuloma deep within the dermis, often with as-

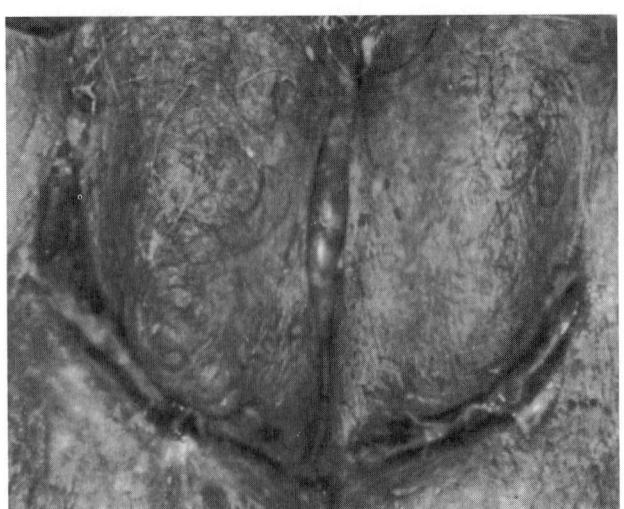

Figure 52–7
Crohn's disease.

sociated abscess formation. Ulceration of the skin may be contiguous with the deep granulomatous reaction. Prominent granulation tissue formation is usually present adjacent to the ulceration. Acid-fast organisms or fungi are not detectable.

Crohn's disease of the vulva can be effectively treated with oral prednisone and oral metronidazole (250 mg three to four times daily). Exacerbations of Crohn's disease of the vulva may occasionally warrant hospitalization for intravenous steroid therapy in association with whirlpool management. Steroid dosages should be tapered gradually after amelioration of symptoms and findings. Remissions may occur, which permit discontinuation of oral steroid therapy altogether.

Hypopigmentary Disorders (Vitiligo; Postinflammatory Hypopigmentation)

An inherited disorder resulting from a dominant gene with variable penetrance, vitiligo is an autoimmune process associated with the progressive loss of melanocytes in the epidermis (Friedrich, 1983). This process is asymptomatic and rarely prompts medical evaluation, provided that it is confined to the genital area. Within the involved hypopigmented area, normal hair, skin surface markings, and texture are maintained. The borders of the involved skin will appear serpiginous. A careful history may reveal that relatives have noted similar areas of hypopigmentation. Autoimmune-related medical conditions that have been associated with vitiligo include thyroid dysfunction, Addison's disease, diabetes mellitus, and pernicious anemia.

The classical appearance of vitiligo generally suffices for a clinical diagnosis, and biopsies are usually not necessary. Although lichen sclerosus is associated with pale skin, it may be differentiated from vitiligo by its association with extreme pruritus, progressive loss of the vulvar architecture, and histopathologic features. Postinflammatory hypopigmentation may occur following severe chronic inflammation, following burns, or after deep laser ablation. When associated with lichen simplex chronicus or squamous hyperplasia, the skin appears hyperkeratotic and pruritus is a chief complaint.

Epithelial Tumors

VESTIBULAR PAPILLOMATOSIS

Vestibular papillomatosis is a poorly understood condition characterized by small papillary-like projections measuring 0.1 to 0.3 cm in length, which may be single or occur in large numbers on the medial aspects of the labia minora (Fig. 52–8). Most commonly, the condition involves both labia minora. The patient may be asymptomatic or complain of pruritus in this region. Micropapillae may be seen in asymptomatic women, and these may reflect a variant of normal vestibular anatomy. On colposcopic examination, these micropapillae are covered with

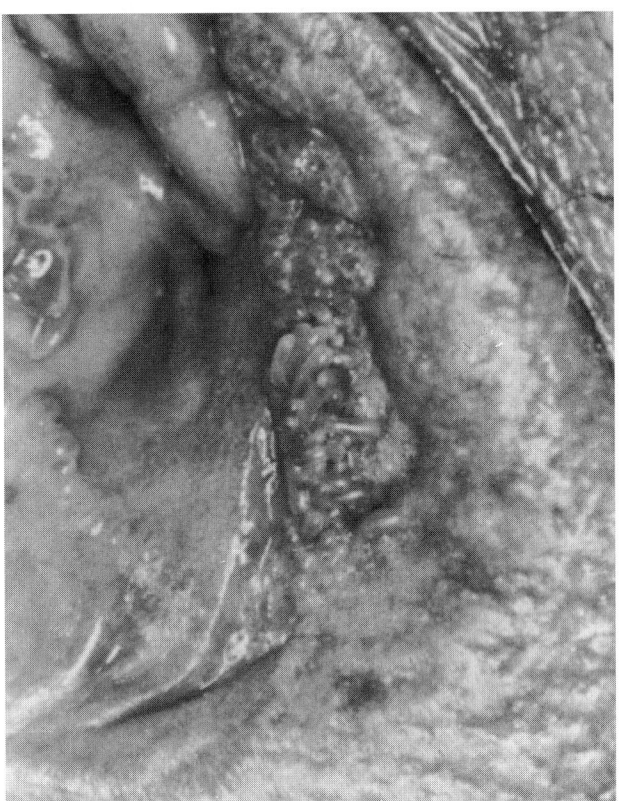

Figure 52–8
Vestibular papillomatosis.

thin epithelium that may be aceto-white. They do not have the typical appearance of condyloma, which usually present with a thick, white epithelium and cauliflower-like appearance.

Histopathologic examination reveals small papillae with a squamous epithelium, which is usually not keratinized. The fibrovascular stalk contains fibromyxomatous connective tissue. Probes for HPV in these micropapillae rarely identify HPV DNA, the reported frequency varying from 0% to 6.9%. However, when clinical findings of associated HPV infection are present, HPV DNA can be found in over half of the cases (Campion et al, 1989). Certainly, the observation of HPV in some of these patients does not establish HPV as the causative agent. Because the cause is unknown in most patients, biopsy of a representative lesion and of any areas suggestive of HPV infection is suggested. HPV probes are of value if the clinical findings suggest HPV; however, if only micropapillae are seen, without HPV changes or symptoms, no therapy or biopsy is needed.

In the symptomatic patient, the application of a caustic agent, such as topical concentrated trichloroacetic acid, results in resolution of the papillomas. However, the patient should be forewarned that the topical application will be painful, and resolution of the papillomas may not necessarily be associated with resolution of her presenting symptoms.

FIBROEPITHELIOMA (ACROCHORDON)

Fibroepithelial polyp or fibroepithelioma is a benign tumor with a stratified squamous epithelial surface and a cellular, myxoid, collagen-rich soft tissue core that is highly vascular (Mucitelli et al, 1990). These polyps may be on the labia minora, on the labia majora, or within the vagina. They present as a polypoid, pedunculated nodular mass that is soft and pliable on palpation. They are typically the color of the adjacent skin or mucosa and may be single or multiple (Fig. 52–9). They may be small or quite large, extending several centimeters from the skin surface. Although this benign tumor is usually asymptomatic when small, the presenting symptoms of a larger tumor relate to the palpable vulvar mass.

Examination demonstrates the typical pedunculated character. A small fibroepithelial polyp may be confused with a compound nevus or a neurofibroma. These benign tumors are treated by local excision.

HIDRADENOMA

Hidradenoma papilliferum is a benign tumor that arises from specialized anogenital glands (Van der Putte and van-Gorp, 1995). The typical vulvar location is noted in the intralabial sulcus, between the labia minora and labia majora. The tumor is usually solitary and asymptomatic. The patient may state that she has palpated a growth on her vulva for several years. On examination, the hidradenoma is mobile, smooth, and nontender. These tumors may erode, resulting in a papillary, ulcerated, exophytic mass that can mimic carcinoma. Occasionally, the hidradenoma may be confused with an epidermal inclusion cyst. Excision is diagnostic and therapeutic. These lesions may be removed in the clinic under local anesthesia.

Histopathologic findings reveal a complex papillary tumor with a two-cell epithelial surface, which includes a superficial secretory epithelial cell layer and a deep myoepithelial cell layer. On microscopic examination, the complex growth pattern may be confused with adenocarcinoma; however, there is no evidence of infiltration of the tumor. Adequate deep excision is of great value to ensure proper diagnosis (Wilkinson, 1994a).

Nonepithelial Tumors

LIPOMAS

Lipomas are slow-growing tumors arising from the fatty tissue in the labia majora or more lateral and inferior regions of the ischiorectal fossa. They may be noted on routine pelvic examination in a patient who states that the tumor has been present for a number of years. With a predominance of fatty tissue, the lipoma is typically soft; however, with increasing amounts of fibrous tissue, the tumor may be firm. These tumors may be broad based and may extend deep into the vulvar tissues.

Most small lipomas can be removed in the clinic. For deeper lesions, excision in the operating room is necessary with adequate anesthesia and hemostasis. Sarcomatous change is rare (Wilkinson, 1994b).

HEMANGIOMAS

Hemangiomas may present as pyogenic granulomas, cherry angiomas, or angiokeratomas.

Pyogenic Granulomas. These may be seen frequently in extragenital regions in children. In adults, this lesion may occasionally be seen in the vulvar region. The typical chief complaint is bleeding associated with contact. The bleeding may be profuse but will typically respond to pressure tamponade. Lesions are well circumscribed and solitary (Wilkinson, 1994b). They may appear red and resemble granulation tissue and may have a crusty surface. Pyogenic granulomas are most expediently treated by local excision, which in adults is also diagnostic and assists in excluding basal cell carcinoma, which may have a similar appearance.

Cherry Angiomas. Cherry angiomas and other asymptomatic superficial vulvar hemangiomas may be managed in a conservative manner. Biopsy is usually unnecessary if the clinical appearance is distinctive. Hemangiomas in children usually regress over time. In adolescents or adults, pulse-dye laser therapy or cryotherapy is effective for larger lesions.

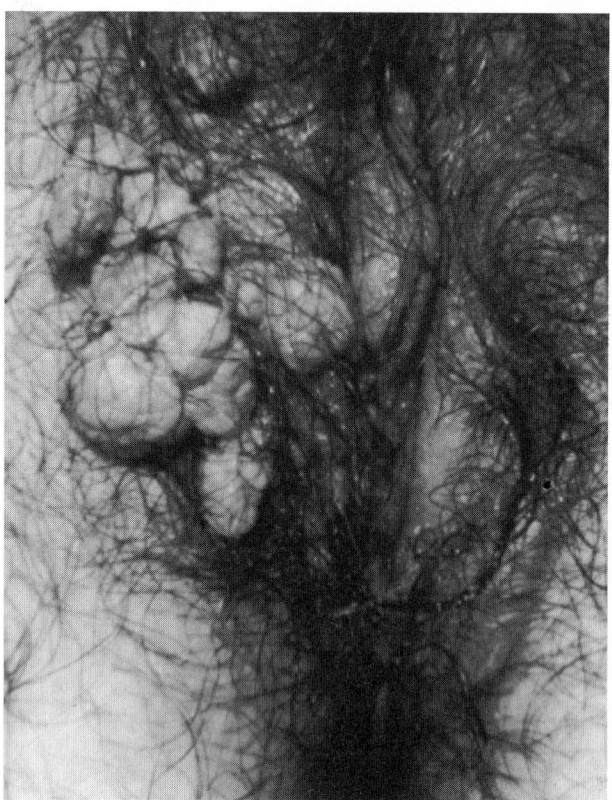

Figure 52–9
Fibroepitheliomas.

Angiokeratomas. Angiokeratomas may present as solitary or multiple lesions. They are usually asymptomatic. Multiple angiokeratomas should raise the suspicion of Fabry's disease. This disease appears in its heterozygous form in the female. Lesions are raised and well circumscribed and have a purple hue. Excisional biopsy is diagnostic and therapeutic for the solitary lesion. Multiple lesions may be treated readily with laser ablation. If Fabry's disease is considered, the diagnosis may be confirmed by an assay for α-glucosidase activity.

Nevomelanocytic Lesions

NEVI

Originating from the neural crest, nevomelanocytic cells migrate to the skin, where they may give rise to nevi. The characteristic development of a nevus begins as nests of cells at the dermal-epidermal junction (e.g., junctional nevus). With maturation, the nevus cells collect in the dermis as well as the epidermis (e.g., compound nevus). With complete progression, all of the nevus cells are found in the dermis (e.g., intradermal nevus). The junctional nevus is typically macular, whereas intradermal (Fig. 52–10) and compound (Fig. 52–11) nevi are elevated and may appear papillomatous (Patterson and Blaylock, 1987). Slightly elevated macular nevi are most frequently compound nevi, whereas polypoid lesions tend to be intradermal nevi. Well-demarcated regular borders and uniform coloration differentiate them from malignant melanoma, which characteristically has irregular borders and irregular coloration.

Histopathologic findings demonstrate nests and cords of rounded nevus cells at the dermal-epidermal junction and in the dermis, depending on the nevus type. These typical nevi must be distinguished from atypical nevomelanocytic nevi, which have nuclear atypia and pleomorphism in the junctional area but retain symmetry and deeper nevus cell maturation. Atypical vulvar nevi can be misinterpreted as superficial spreading malignant melanoma, and adequate biopsy is essential for optimum evaluation. Although most malignant melanomas appear to arise spontaneously, the presence of nevus cells in some melanomas indicates that melanomas can arise in pre-existing nevi. Clinically dysplastic nevi tend to have irregular borders and a mixture of colors. There is a tendency for these nevi to occur in a familial distribution. In the intraepidermal region, there is a proliferation of atypical melanocytes with varying degrees of inflammation and papillary dermal fibrosis.

Because it is often clinically difficult to differentiate nevi from melanomas or other pigmented lesions such as VIN, seborrheic keratoses, and lentigo simplex, excisional biopsy is in order. Histopathologic confirmation of the diagnosis is essential to alleviate concern in the patient and the physician.

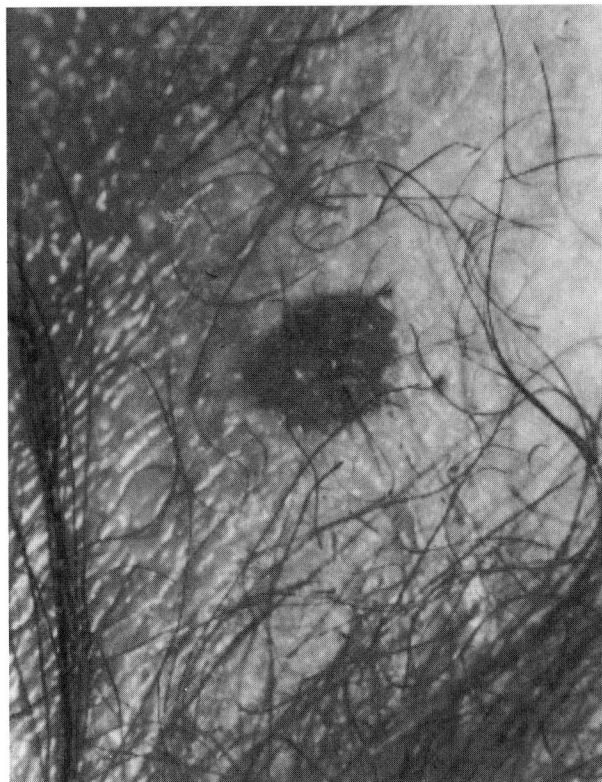

Figure 52–10
Intradermal nevus.

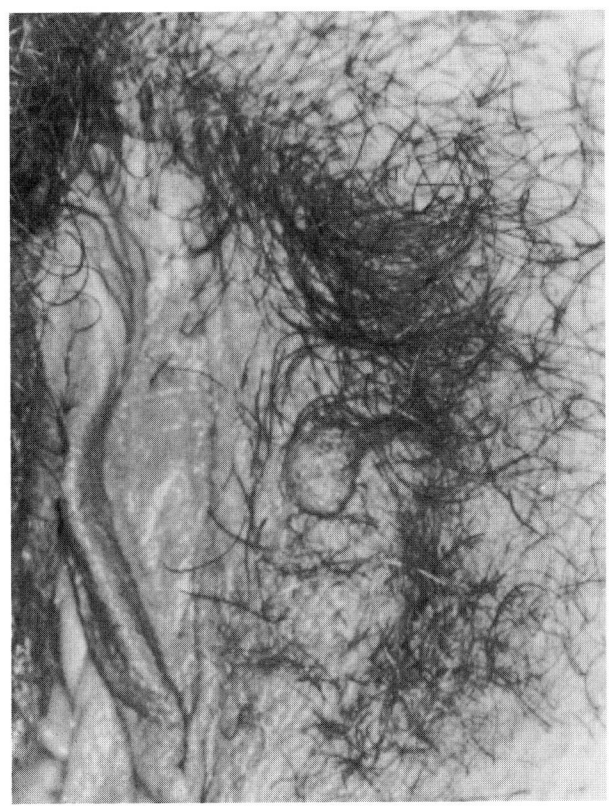

Figure 52–11
Compound nevus.

LENTIGO SIMPLEX

The common pigmented lesion lentigo simplex is frequently discovered during vulvar examination. Macular, irregular, and of variable size, it is found in the vestibule, labia minora, and labia majora. No symptoms are associated with its occurrence. Primary concern rests in differentiating lentigo simplex from an atypical nevus or melanoma. Excisional biopsy of vulvar pigmented lesions is recommended if the pigmented area is larger than 4 mm in diameter, elevated, has an irregular surface contour, or is changing in appearance or symptomatic. Lentigo simplex seldom fill these criteria and rarely need biopsy; however, biopsy is diagnostic and demonstrates increased melanin and downward extension of rete ridges within the lentigo (Wilkinson, 1994a; Wilkinson and Mullins, 1997).

Cysts

EPIDERMAL CYSTS

Epidermal cysts, commonly called *epidermal inclusion cysts*, are the most frequent small cystic tumors of the vulva. Lined by a smooth layer of keratinizing squamous epithelium, they contain keratinized material with a characteristic cheesy appearance, often resulting in their being misinterpreted as *sebaceous cysts*. Their origin is incompletely understood. It is commonly believed that there is entrapment of surface epithelium, resulting in cyst formation.

The patient typically has multiple cysts, usually on the labia majora (Fig. 52–12). These cysts are asymptomatic but may be bothersome to the patient from a cosmetic standpoint. Occasionally, they may erode and become infected. Small, isolated epidermal cysts may be confused with hidradenomas.

Histopathologic findings reveal a stratified squamous epithelial lining within the cyst, with keratinized debris filling the cyst cavity. Sebaceous glands are commonly found adjacent to these cysts (Wilkinson, 1994a; Wilkinson and Mullins, 1997).

Therapy is not indicated in the asymptomatic patient. For the patient with multiple symptomatic lesions, management may be accomplished in the office. To remove multiple lesions, local infiltration with an anesthetic agent is desirable. The surface epithelium may be incised sharply with a scalpel and the cyst excised without entering into the cyst cavity. Should the cyst cavity be entered, an effort should be made to remove the lining epithelium of the cyst to prevent recurrence. These excisional sites may be left to heal by secondary intention; however, if bleeding is a problem, suture closure may be easily accomplished. Smaller cysts need not be removed unless they become symptomatic.

MUCINOUS CYSTS

Mucinous cysts of the vestibule are relatively rare. They arise from obstruction of the minor vestibular

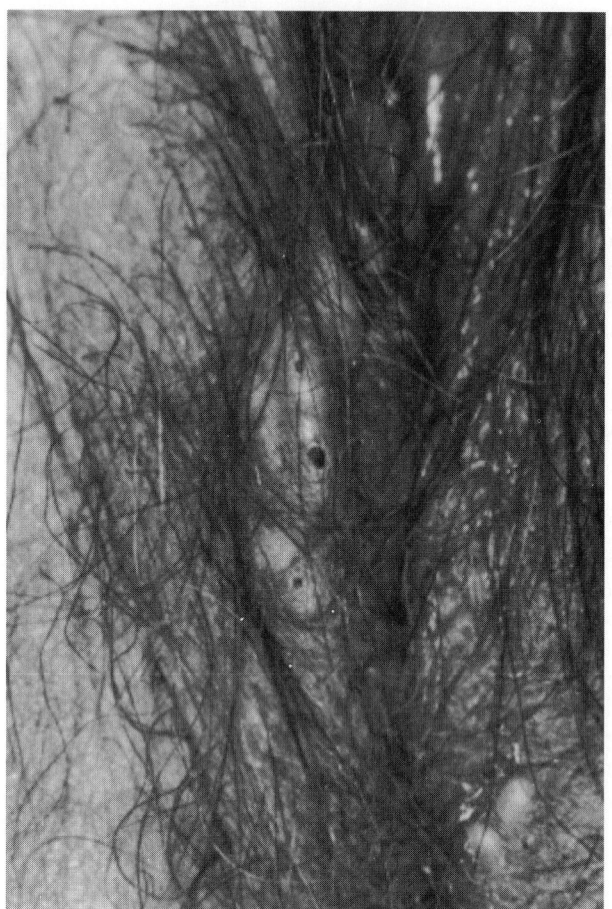

Figure 52–12
Epidermal inclusion cyst.

glands of the vestibule (Fig. 52–13). The inciting event may be infectious or traumatic. Ductal atresia may lead to formation of a vestibular mucous cyst in the newborn. These cysts are typically asymptomatic. They may be encountered on routine examination of a newborn infant or an adult. Symptoms usually result from pressure, especially if the cyst is located just lateral to the urethral meatus. Excision is rarely necessary.

Histopathologic features include a columnar or cuboidal mucus-secreting epithelial lining. Squamous metaplasia may be found within the lining epithelium. The cysts are superficial and, unlike endometriosis, which may be included in the clinical differential diagnosis, lack adjacent endometrial stroma cells or ciliated epithelial lining cells.

Mucous-like cysts and tubal endometrial–like cysts or vaginal or vulvar vestibular epithelium replaced by mucus-secreting columnar epithelium may occasionally be seen in women who have had extensive laser ablation or 5 flurouracil therapy (Sedlacek et al, 1989; Dungar and Wilkinson, 1995). Discontinuation of therapy and topical estrogen therapy will result in healing of the surface epithelium, although the cysts may persist. Columnar metaplasia of the vaginal or vulvar vestibular epithelium is a

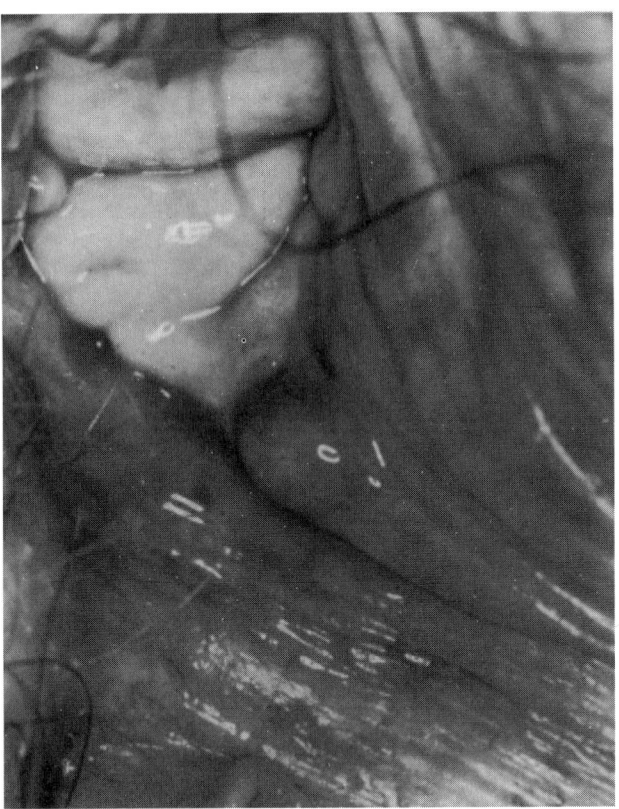

Figure 52–13
Vestibular mucous cyst.

poorly understood process that requires further investigation.

BARTHOLIN'S CYSTS

Bartholin's glands are bilateral and located in the posterior lateral aspect of the vestibule. The acini are lined with mucus-secreting epithelial cells and drain into the Bartholin's duct, which measures approximately 2.5 cm in length. Although the gland contributes to lubrication during intercourse, it is not the primary source of lubrication, nor is it necessary for adequate lubrication. The duct of the gland may become obstructed as a result of trauma, infection, or inspissated material. In the absence of infection, the duct may distend and become cystic, palpable as a nontender, uniform mass protruding into the vestibule. Occasionally, the subsequent cyst may grow to a large size and create pressure symptoms. Concern about these cysts increases in patients older than 40 years. Carcinoma has been noted arising in Bartholin's gland in older women and should be suspected when there is Bartholin's gland enlargement or nodularity in an older patient.

No therapy is required for the asymptomatic Bartholin's cyst. If symptoms warrant therapy, the cyst can be drained in the clinic setting by incising the surface of the cyst in the region of the posterior lateral vestibule just caudal (external) to the hymenal ring. Using local anesthesia, this incision can be ac-

complished with a No. 11 scalpel. A Word catheter may then be inserted into the cyst lumen through this small stab wound and inflated. Sufficient time should be allowed for epithelialization of the surgically created tract, this usually requiring several weeks, after which the Word catheter may be removed. Marsupialization of the Bartholin's cyst may also be accomplished in the clinic setting, provided that the cyst is very superficial. Deep cysts are difficult to isolate and therefore should be managed in the operating room. The cyst is entered in the same region as previously mentioned for insertion of the Word catheter; however, the entry site is expanded and the epithelial lining of the Bartholin's cyst is sutured to the vestibular epithelium, creating a surgically epithelialized tract.

Excellent results have been reported using the laser in an office setting to vaporize a 1.5-cm defect into the Bartholin's cyst, beginning at the vestibular site where incisional drainage is usually performed. This procedure creates a communicating tract (Davis, 1985). In patients who do not respond to conservative attempts to create a draining tract, excision of the Bartholin's gland and duct cyst under appropriate general or regional anesthesia should be considered.

After prior infections of the gland, or prior conservative surgical attempts, there may be significant scarring in the region of Bartholin's gland that will make dissection difficult. It is important to obtain adequate hemostasis to prevent the subsequent development of a hematoma. Surgical excision of the gland is also indicated in older patients in whom changes in a previously existing Bartholin's cyst develop or who note the development of an expanding mass in the region of Bartholin's gland. This specimen should be submitted for pathologic examination to exclude the possibility of a malignant process.

Intraepithelial Squamous Neoplasia

Vulvar Intraepithelial Neoplasia

The prevalence of VIN is increasing (Sturgeon et al, 1992). In women with cytologic evidence of HPV on cervical smears, colposcopic examination has demonstrated 44% to have colposcopic and histologic features of HPV infection on the vulva (Planner and Hobbs, 1988). Over 20 of the over 70 known HPV types infect the genital tract. Analysis of vulvar biopsy specimens containing intraepithelial neoplasia has revealed HPV in 84% of patients with VIN 3. HPV type 16 was identified in 81% of specimens containing VIN 3. HPV types 6 and 11, although recovered in 77% of condyloma acuminatum specimens, have not been demonstrated in VIN 3 (Buscema et al, 1988). Immunocompromised patients are at particular risk for the development of VIN. These patients have an HPV infection rate 17 times greater than a matched immunocompetent population. Their rates of lower genital tract neoplasia have been demonstrated to be as high as 16 times greater than that of the general population (Halpert et al, 1986).

Most patients with HPV-associated VIN have vulvar pruritus and dyspareunia (Planner and Hobbs, 1988). Given the known multicentricity of lower genital tract neoplasia, the observation of VIN should prompt thorough examination of the remainder of the lower genital tract. Although cytology does not lend itself well to the evaluation of vulvar skin, colposcopic examination of the vulva is extremely productive. Prior preparation of the vulva with 3% to 5% acetic acid for several minutes before colposcopic examination will highlight areas of neoplasia. Raised macular, papular, red, white, or hyperpigmented lesions on the vulva will raise suspicion of VIN (Fig. 52–14). Ninety per cent of patients with more advanced intraepithelial neoplasia will have raised lesions, and 80% of flat lesions are hyperpigmented. It is important to evaluate the anal canal as well as the vulva because 22% to 57% of patients with VIN will have perianal or anal involvement. Representative biopsy specimens should be obtained from colposcopically abnormal areas (Sillman et al, 1985).

Histopathologic examination demonstrates lack of epithelial cell maturation with nuclear hyperchromasia and pleomorphism. Multinucleated cells, abnormalities of the nuclear-cytoplasmic ratio, dyskeratosis, abnormal mitoses, mitotic figures above the basal layer, and increased density of cells are all characteristic findings. A *VIN 1* (mild dysplasia) lesion has abnormal cells within the lower one third of the epithelium; a *VIN 2* (moderate dysplasia) lesion has abnormal cells within the lower half of the epithelium; and a *VIN 3* (severe dysplasia, carcinoma in situ) lesion has abnormal cells involving more than the half of the epithelium. Skin appendage involvement, to a depth of approximately 2.5 cm, may occur in hair-bearing skin and should not be interpreted as invasion (Shatz et al, 1989). Although the terms *Bowen's disease, erythroplasia of Queyrat, carcinoma simplex*, and *bowenoid papulosis* have been used clinically to describe intraepithelial neoplasia of the vulva, they are not recognized as histopathologic terms by the ISSVD or the ISGP, nor are they recommended as terms for vulvar pathology by the World Health Organization.

The natural history of VIN is inadequately documented. It is generally believed that progression to invasive carcinoma is infrequent and that, when it occurs, it is a relatively indolent process. Invasive squamous cell carcinoma was found in 3% to 17% of women with clinical VIN (Chafe et al, 1988). Remission has been noted, especially in patients who have been temporarily immunocompromised. An example is the pregnant patient in whom resolution of VIN may be noted after completion of pregnancy. For patients with longstanding immune suppression or Fanconi's anemia, the progression to carcinoma may be accelerated (Sillman et al, 1984).

Treatment necessitates appropriate colposcopic and histologic evaluation. The pregnant patient, who by necessity is temporarily immunocompromised, may be observed throughout her pregnancy and the postpartum period. Resolution of VIN may occur in the patients, especially in the postpartum period. The nonpregnant patient in whom VIN is limited to a small region of the vulva may be managed with an excisional biopsy of the lesion. More extensive disease, especially when classified as VIN 3, has traditionally been treated with wide local excision or partial vulvectomy. The relative infrequency of invasive carcinoma in large fields of high-grade VIN adequately evaluated by colposcopy has resulted in attempts to treat this disease process with vulva-sparing therapeutic modalities.

Laser therapy and topical chemotherapy have been used successfully. When the laser is used, the power density should be at approximately 600 watts/cm^2 and the laser vaporization should be carried to the third surgical plane (Reid, 1985). It is vital to remember before performing laser therapy that multiple biopsies should be obtained to rule out occult invasive disease, which would be appropriately treated surgically (Chafe et al, 1988). Laser therapy is accomplished with concomitant colposcopic examination of the vulva to define all areas of abnormality. The procedure is performed in the operating room with the patient under general or regional anesthesia. The patient is discharged home and is instructed to use frequent sitz baths and topical creams, such as silver sulfadiazine.

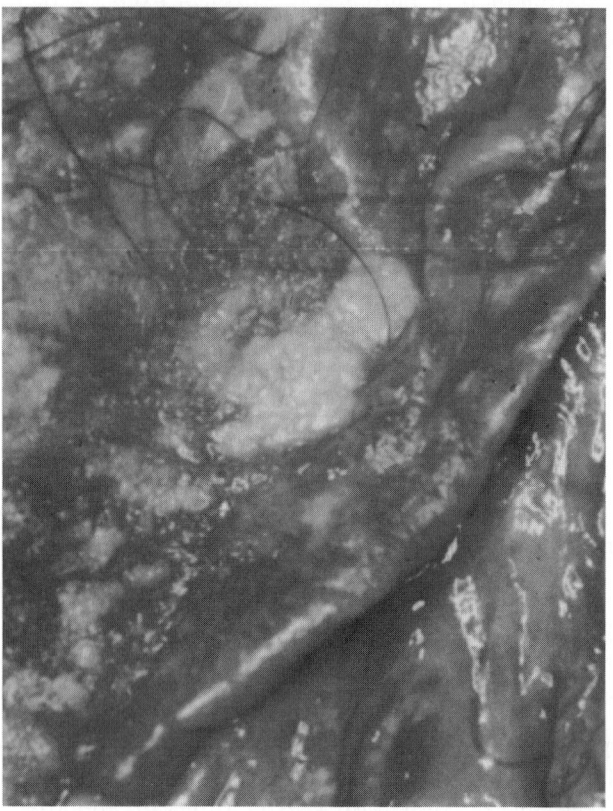

Figure 52–14
Vulvar intraepithelial neoplasia.

For patients with multicentric disease, especially in the immunocompromised patient, frequent recurrences of dysplasia often are the norm. In these patients, repeated returns to the operating room for laser ablation are expensive and pose risks associated with surgery and anesthesia. Alternative therapy in women in whom pregnancy is not a risk may consist of the use of topical 5% 5-fluorouracil. Topical chemotherapy is especially useful for anal lesions and vulvar lesions medial to the pilosebaceous region. It is not approved for this use by the Food and Drug Administration and should not be recommended in women of reproductive age who may become pregnant. Treatment consists of twice-daily applications of 5-fluorouracil for up to 10 days. Typically, these applications produce inflammation, burning, and pain. Approximately 2 days after completion of the topical therapy, the neoplastic epithelium should be loosened from the underlying stroma with fine biopsy forceps, curette, Q-tip, gauze, or a hyfreacator. Postoperative sitz baths and topical silver sulfadiazine may be used. Maintenance therapy is necessary to prevent recurrence. After healing has occurred, 5-fluorouracil is applied to the vulva at least 3 nights per month. Monitoring by colposcopic examination and biopsies as appropriate should occur approximately every 4 months. Recent preliminary studies have demonstrated that the local, typical patient-administered immunostimulant Imiquimod (Aldara) has been effective in small low-grade VIN lesions, as well as in typical genital condyloma acuminatum (Davis et al, 1999). Further studies on this are forthcoming.

Paget's Disease

In 1874 Sir James Paget described the mammary disease associated with his name. Although he suggested a similar disease in extramammary sites, the first pathologic description of extramammary Paget's disease of the vulva was described by Dubreuilh in 1901. In contrast to mammary Paget's disease, which is usually associated with an underlying adenocarcinoma, vulvar Paget's disease is associated with an underlying apocrine gland carcinoma in fewer than 25% of cases (Michael and Roth, 1987). Of note is the observation that vulvar Paget's disease has been associated with carcinoma in extragenital areas, such as the breast and the gastrointestinal tract.

The typical patient with vulvar Paget's disease is in her mid-60s and has delayed for 1 to 2 years seeking medical assistance for a pruritic, inflamed vulva (Friedrich, 1983). A diagnosis of candidiasis or nonspecific dermatitis may be made, and the patient may have a history of being treated with topical corticosteroids or antifungal agents. There is typically no resolution of symptoms with these treatments. Subsequent examination of the vulva reveals no change in the rather diffuse white epithelium with interspersed islands of erythema (Fig. 52–15). Al-

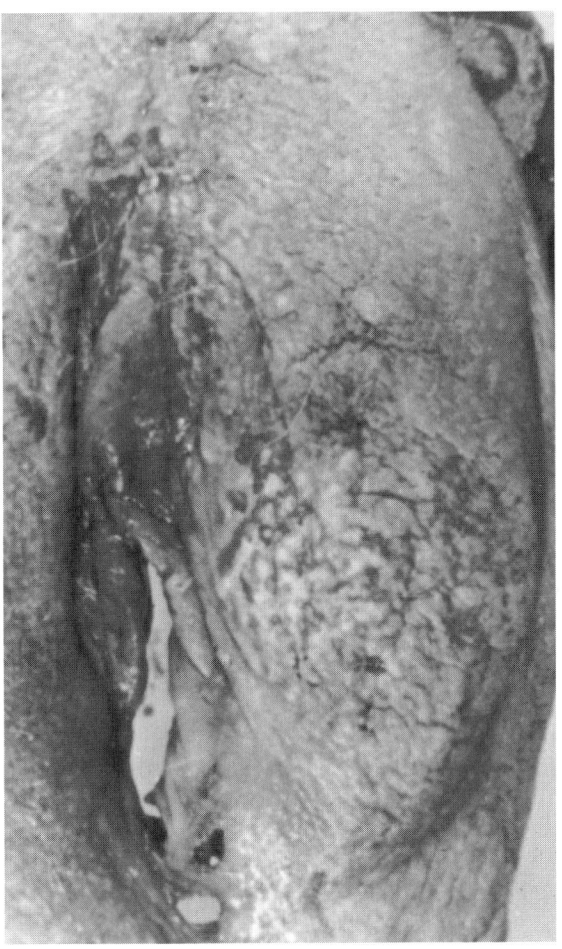

Figure 52–15
Paget's disease.

though candidiasis and Paget's disease have similar clinical appearances, the hyperkeratosis associated with Paget's disease appears much thicker. Candidal infections tend to be more diffuse than Paget's disease. Occasionally, the patient with Paget's disease may be seen with a lesion that resembles eczema with its scaly surface. A biopsy to establish appropriate diagnosis is mandatory.

Histopathologic examination demonstrates the characteristic intraepithelial Paget's cells, which have large, prominent nucleoli and pale, abundant, basophilic and finely granular cytoplasm. These cells tend to form intraepithelial clusters or gland-like nests. Cytoplasmic staining with mucicarmine, aldehyde fuchsin, and periodic acid–Schiff can be seen in most cases. Carcinoembryonic antigen (CEA) immunoreactivity, demonstrable by immunoperoxidase technique, is characteristic. Although Paget cells may be seen at various levels in the epidermis, they are most frequently concentrated in the lower regions. Apocrine gland and hair shaft epithelium infiltrated by Paget's cells should not be interpreted as invasion; underlying adenocarcinoma of the sweat gland or Bartholin's gland or invasion by overlying Paget's disease may be found.

The origin of these cells is controversial. Extramammary Paget's disease is located only in sites containing apocrine glands, such as the anal-genital and axillary regions. Paget's cells bear a greater resemblance to glandular cells than to squamous cells, although cytoplasmic organelles are present, which are consistent with both squamous and secretory skin cells. Paget's cells are frequently arranged in glandular patterns. Histochemical staining of Paget's cells demonstrates enzymes typically found in apocrine gland cells. CEA has been noted in Paget's cells, sweat glands, and underlying adenocarcinoma but not in squamous epithelium, hair follicles, or sebaceous glands (Nadji et al, 1982). Paget's cells represent a population of cells sharing features of glandular epithelium and arise within the epidermis. Their origin may be from undifferentiated epithelial stem cells.

The histologic confirmation of Paget's disease should prompt a complete evaluation of the lower reproductive tract for evidence of disease. The urethra, bladder, ureter, vagina, and cervix have been noted to be involved with this disease process. Although involvement with structures other than the vulva is uncommon, a mammogram and gastrointestinal survey should be obtained to rule out concomitant adenocarcinoma in these areas. The pathologic differential diagnosis of vulvar Paget's disease includes melanoma in situ, pagetoid transitional cell intraepithelial neoplasia (pseudo-Paget's disease), and bowenoid reticulosis (Malik and Wilkinson, 1999).

Melanoma in situ clinically is usually pigmented, and does not resemble Paget's disease; however, morphologically the melanoma in situ resembles Paget's disease. Immunohistochemical studies are needed in that melanoma in situ does not express CEA or keratin, as do Paget cells, but does express S-100 antigens and melanoma specific antigen.

Pagetoid transitional cell intraepithelial neoplasia (PTCIN) may look clinically and pathologically like Paget's disease; however, the cells are neoplastic transitional cells, usually arising from transitional intraepithelial neoplasia and/or carcinoma arising from the bladder or urethra. These cases do not express CEA by immunohistochemistry and do not have associated underlying adenocarcinoma. Such cases do not need total vulvectomy to the fascia because the lesion is entirely intraepithelial, but they do require a careful evaluation of the bladder and urethra and appropriate therapy for the urothelial tumor present there, whether invasive or in situ.

Bowenoid reticulosis is a lymphoproliferative disorder which morphologically can resemble Paget's disease but the cells are immunoreactive for leucocyte common antigen and lack CEA or cytokeratin as seen in Paget's disease.

The therapy of Paget's disease involves a carefully planned surgical approach. Paget's cells may spread horizontally as well as vertically and may be found in normal-appearing skin. The mere excision of abnormal-appearing skin from the vulva of the patient with Paget's disease is therefore suboptimal. Surgical margins may not be as critical as originally suggested (Stacy et al, 1986). The reason excision to the fascia is necessary in Paget's disease is to include the subcutaneous tissues and exclude underlying adenocarcinoma. Paget cells may be found in the epithelium of normal-appearing skin peripheral to the viable lesion. There is no evidence that these cells are at risk to the patient, and radical excision to remove this entirely intraepithelial process is not necessary. Invasive foci do not occur in clinically normal-appearing epithelium, but rather beneath the viable Paget's disease. The frozen section margins have no real significance in improving the identification of underlying adenocarcinoma. Follow-up is imperative, and deep excision of new viable lesions is the treatment of choice to exclude adenocarcinoma. Not only should excisions be wide, but they should also be deep to incorporate all adnexal structures that may contain Paget's cells or underlying adenocarcinoma.

Patients with Paget's disease involving the anus usually have an associated adenocarcinoma of the rectum, requiring an abdominoperineal resection (Stacy et al, 1986). The finding of adenocarcinoma in the biopsy specimen from the patient with Paget's disease warrants a total vulvectomy with bilateral inguinal-femoral groin node dissections. Skinning vulvectomy, laser ablation, cryotherapy, partial excision, and chemotherapy, which are frequently used to treat patients with VIN, are suboptimal in the treatment of primary Paget's disease. These more conservative procedures are of value in the treatment of residual or recurrent disease once underlying adenocarcinoma has been excluded. Destruction of the vulvar skin without proper evaluation for an underlying adenocarcinoma is inappropriate. Likewise, superficial excision without appropriate assessment of the deep adnexal structures will result in either recurrence of disease or the delayed observation that an adenocarcinoma is present.

VAGINA

Non-neoplastic Lesions

Epithelial Disorders (Vaginal Adenosis)

There are two theories concerning the formation of the vagina. One suggests that the upper vagina is formed from the lower ends of the paramesonephric ducts and the lower third originates from the urogenital sinus (Snell, 1975). The alternate theory proposes that the vagina is derived entirely from the urogenital sinus (Moore, 1977). The fused paramesonephric ducts may induce cellular proliferation from the urogenital sinus, which results in formation of a vaginal plate. The cephalic portion of the vaginal vault results in the vagina and the outer portion forms the vestibule. Exposure of the developing vagina to estrogens such as diethylstilbestrol (DES) has resulted in adenosis. Adenosis has also been recorded in adults in association with the Stevens-Johnson syndrome (Marquette et al, 1985) and in association with laser therapy and intravaginal 5-fluorouracil for intraepithelial neoplasia and condyloma acuminatum (Sedlacek et al, 1989; Dungar and Wilkinson, 1993). The neoplastic potential for adenosis as a consequence of intrauterine exposure to estrogen is well known. There is no known neoplastic potential for vaginal adenosis not associated with in utero DES exposure. The observation of glandular areas in the vagina warrants a careful history inquiring about in utero DES exposure, and palpation of the vagina to determine if any subcutaneous nodules are palpable, which may represent clear cell adenocarcinoma. Such nodules, if identified, should be excised, to rule out a neoplastic process.

Inflammatory Disorders of the Vagina of Non-Infectious Type

Desquamative inflammatory vaginitis is a rare condition (Jacobson et al, 1989). Typically, a yellowish mucopurulent discharge is the chief reason the patient consults a physician. On examination, the vagina has large areas of denuded erythematous epithelium. Gram stain usually demonstrates gram-negative bacteria (rather than the usual gram-positive bacteria) (Sobel, 1998). Colposcopic examination may demonstrate atypical vessels. Biopsies reveal epithelial hyperplasia and lymphohistiocytic infiltrates.

Severe erosive vaginitis may be a manifestation of pemphigus vulgaris, erosive lichen planus, or benign mucous membrane pemphigoid. Pemphigus vulgaris may appear initially at mucosal sites including the vulva, but eventually a generalized cutaneous bullous phase ensues. Lichen planus may be differentiated on the basis of histologic evaluation.

Benign mucous membrane pemphigoid is a blistering disease involving mucous membranes and skin that results in permanent scarring. Rarely, it may present initially on the vulva and in the vagina. Histologic examination demonstrates subepithelial bullae formation with a sparse lymphohistiocytic infiltrate. Deposition of linear immunoglobulin G is found with direct immunofluorescence.

Linear immunoglobulin A (IgA) disease is a cutaneous vesiculobullous disease that occurs in young people with a generalized cutaneous eruption, and its histopathology is indistinguishable from dermatitis herpetiformis. Deposition of IgA has been demonstrated rarely in patients with desquamative inflammatory vaginitis.

Therapeutic options for linear IgA disease and pemphigoid include oral dapsone or corticosteroids, applied topically or intralesionally. Topical steroids may ameliorate the symptoms of lichen planus, but results are often disappointing.

Lichenoid vaginitis has been described associated with a nonspecific vaginitis characterized clinically by small focal microscopic hemorrhages and microscopically by atrophic-like erosive changes which are associated with focal lichenoid chronic inflammation consisting predominately of lymphocytes. Submucosal microscopic hemorrhagic areas are also seen (Mullins and Wilkinson et al, 1997). Some of these patients also have similar inflammation and findings in the vulvar vestibule.

Pigmentary Disorders (Melanosis)

Melanosis of the vulva and vagina is a rarely reported condition (Jackson, 1984). Patients are seen for evaluation of dark brown or black lesions of the vulva. On examination, macular hyperpigmented lesions are noted on the inner aspects of the labia majora, labia minora, clitoris, urethra, and vagina. A biopsy demonstrates increased melanin pigmentation in the basal layer and melanophores in the upper portion of the underlying connective tissue. With melanosis the mucosa or skin appear normal other than for the pigmentation. Clinically melanosis and lentigo simplex on the vulva are morphologically identical; however, the pigmented areas of melanosis may be in the vagina alone, involve the vagina and vulva, or involve an area on the vulva of 5 mm or larger, without vaginal involvement. Isolated pigmented areas under 5 mm in diameter on the vulva are classified as lentigo simplex rather than melanosis when the morphology is characteristic of either.

Therapy is not necessary after histologic confirmation of the diagnosis.

Cysts

GARTNER'S DUCT CYST

Gartner's duct cyst is usually asymptomatic and is most commonly discovered on routine pelvic examination. Occasionally, the cyst may be large enough to protrude from the vaginal orifice and cause pressure symptoms. The anterolateral location of the cyst within the vagina differentiates it from a Skene's duct cyst. The majority of Gartner's duct cysts do not require intervention; however, a symptomatic cyst requires excision. The cyst may extend into the vaginal fornix, making excision difficult. Careful attention to hemostasis and to the location of the ureter is warranted. Simple drainage of the cyst is usually ineffective because of recurrence. Rarely, an ectopic ureter may open into a dilated Gartner's duct or Gartner's duct cyst. An ectopic ureter may also open into the vagina or vestibule and have contact with the bladder. This possibility should be considered in a young patient with incontinence, recurrent cystitis, and a vaginal mass.

Although thought by many to be of wolffian origin, some Gartner's duct cysts have ciliated cells within their lining, suggesting a müllerian origin.

Cysts of wolffian origin have a low cuboidal, nonciliated epithelial lining and typically have a demonstrable smooth muscle layer beneath this epithelium.

SKENE'S DUCT CYST

The Skene's glands are located in the vaginal epithelium near the distal urethral meatus. They may become inflamed and obstructed, resulting in cyst or abscess. The cyst may become large enough to create pressure symptoms and may alter the direction of the urinary stream (Fig. 52–16). Small cysts require no therapy; however, larger cysts warrant excision. Urethral diverticulum is included in the differential diagnosis and can be excluded by urethroscopy and a voiding cystourethrogram before an operative approach.

Intraepithelial Squamous Neoplasia: Vaginal Intraepithelial Neoplasia

The true incidence of vaginal intraepithelial neoplasia (VaIN) is unknown; however, it has been estimated that vaginal carcinoma occurs at a rate of 0.2 per 100,000 women (Cramer and Cutler, 1974). The

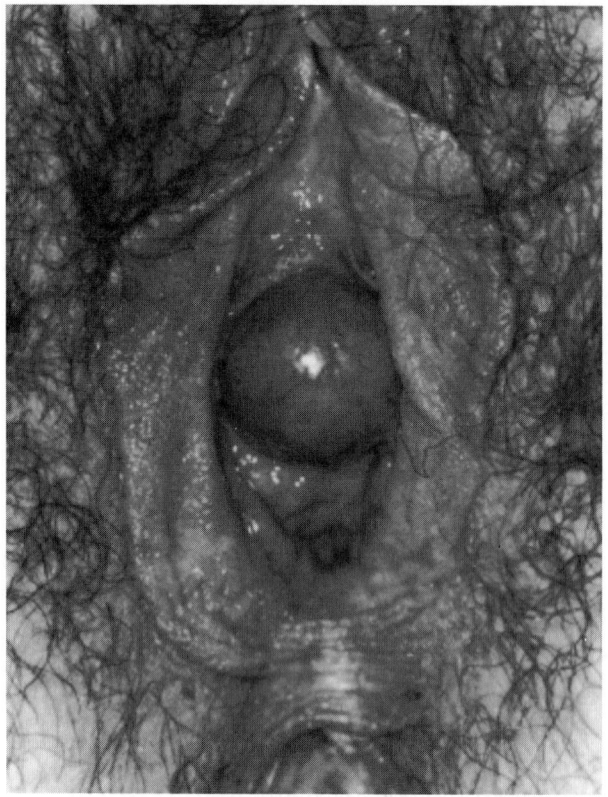

Figure 52–16
Skene's duct cyst.

condition is to be suspected in all patients who have intraepithelial neoplasia of the cervix or vulva. The multicentricity of this process is well recognized. VaIN usually involves the upper one third of the vagina, especially if found after hysterectomy in patients who have been treated for cervical intraepithelial neoplasia (CIN). In such cases the VaIN is often in the apex of the vagina at or near the vaginal cuff margins. It has been demonstrated that 71% of patients with VaIN have associated neoplastic disease elsewhere in the lower genital tract (Lenehan et al, 1986). These findings are commonly associated with HPV type 16.

Evaluation of patients at risk for VaIN or who have abnormal cytologic smears suggesting VaIN consists of colposcopic evaluation after application of 3% acetic acid to the vagina. Hyperkeratotic lesions manifest themselves as white epithelium after acetic acid application. Coarse vascular punctation within aceto-white epithelium is suggestive of a more advanced grade of dysplasia. Representative biopsy specimens should be obtained from these regions. Bleeding from biopsy sites is easily controlled with silver nitrate application.

Thorough evaluation of the vaginal cuff is imperative in patients who have had prior hysterectomy and who are seen with an abnormal vaginal cytologic smear. VaIN may be present within the folds of the vaginal cuff, and meticulous examination is necessary. Occasionally, it may be useful to apply a 50% diluted Lugol's iodine solution to the vagina to define the area of abnormality. Areas demonstrating no iodine staining are productive biopsy sites to identify VaIN.

Small areas of VaIN may be treated with outpatient excisional biopsy. Larger lesions and multicentric lesions require consideration of topical chemotherapy, laser ablation, or extensive resection. Intravaginal treatment with 5% 5-fluorouracil has demonstrated success rates in the range of 80%; however, the therapy is not recommended by the Food and Drug Administration and is not applicable to women who have any risk of pregnancy. Weekly application of 1.5 g of 5% 5-fluorouracil for 10 weeks has been associated with few side effects and an 81% remission rate (Krebs, 1989). Most commonly, patients complain of irritation associated with extravasation of the irritant cream on the sensitive vulvar skin.

Carbon dioxide laser therapy to ablate multifocal VaIN involves ablating all abnormal areas to an approximate depth of 2 to 4 mm. This is usually accomplished in the operating room, unless only a small amount of disease is present. Success rates of 73% to 88% have been reported (Curtin et al, 1985; Krebs, 1989). When considering the option of laser therapy versus intravaginal chemotherapy, cost is a consideration. Excision should be considered in patients who fail to respond to either chemotherapy or laser therapy or in patients with anatomy precluding proper application of the intravaginal 5-fluorouracil or adequate laser vaporization of involved tissue. This may be of particular importance in the patient who is seen with VaIN after a hysterectomy. The infoldings of the vaginal cuff often make the area difficult to assess and treat.

Careful follow-up evaluation is important in all patients with VaIN who have been treated. Recurrence and evolution to a more aggressive lesion are recognized possibilities.

REFERENCES

Baker VV, Walton LA: Crohn's disease of the vulva. South Med J 1988;81:285.

Bell WB: The Principles of Gynaecology. London: Longman's Green and Co, 1910:283, 296, 354, 1323.

Bhatiu NN, Bergman A, Broen EM: Advanced hidradenitis suppurativa of the vulva. J Reprod Med 1984;29:436.

Brown CF, Gallup DG, Brown VM: Hidradenitis suppurative of the anogenital region: response to isotretinoin. Am J Obstet Gynecol 1988;158:12.

Buscema J, Naghashfar Z, Sawada E, et al: The predominance of human papillomavirus type 16 in vulvar neoplasia. Obstet Gynecol 1988;71:601.

Campion MJ, DiPaola FM, Crozier MA, et al: Labial micropapillomatosis: human papillomavirus infection or anatomic variant. In: Proceedings of the 10th International Congress of the International Society of the Study of Vulvar Disease, 1989.

Carlson JA, Lamb P, Malfetano, J, Ambros RA, Mihm MC Jr: Clinicopathologic comparison of vulvar and extragenital lichen sclerosus: histologic variants, evolving lesions and etiology of 141 cases. Mod Pathol 1998;11:844.

Chafe W, Richards A, Morgan LS, Wilkinson EJ: Unrecognized invasive carcinoma in vulvar intraepithelial neoplasia (VIN). Gynecol Oncol 1988;31:154.

Clemmensen OJ: Topical treatment of hidradenitis suppurativa with clindamycin. Int J Dermatol 1983;22:335.

Cramer DW, Cutler SJ: Incidence and histopathology of malignancies of the female genital organs in the United States. Am J Obstet Gynecol 1974;118:443.

Crohn B, Ginzburg L, Oppenheimer GD: Regional ileitis. JAMA 1932;99:1323.

Curtin JP, Twiggs LB, Julian TM: Treatment of vaginal intraepithelial neoplasia with the CO₂ laser. J Reprod Med 1985;30:942.

Dalziel K, Wojnarowska F: Long term control of Lichen sclerosus after treatment with a potent topical steroid cream. J Reprod Med 1993;38:25.

Davis GD: Management of Bartholin duct cysts with the carbon dioxide laser. Obstet Gynecol 1985;65:279.

Davis GD: Vulvar intraepithelial neoplasia, self administered topical treatment. J Reprod Med (in preparation) 1999.

Dicken CH, Powell ST, Spear KL: Evaluation of isotretinoin treatment of hidradenitis suppurativa. J Am Acad Dermatol 1984; 11:500.

Dubreuilh W: Paget's disease of the vulva. Br J Dermatol 1901; 13:407.

Dungar CF, Wilkinson EJ: Vaginal columnar cell metaplasia: an acquired adenosis associated with topical 5-fluorouracil therapy. J Reprod Med 1993;40:361.

Edwards L: Vulvar lichen planus. Arch Dermatol 1989;125:1677.

Fitzsimmons JS, Guilbert PR, Fitzsimmons EM: Evidence of genetic factors in hidradenitis suppurativa. Br J Dermatol 1985; 113:1.

Friedrich EG: Topical testosterone for benign vulvar distrophy. Obstet Gynecol 1971;37:677.

Friedrich EG: Major Problems in Obstetrics and Gynecology: Vulvar Disease. Philadelphia: WB Saunders Company, 1983.

Gupta AK, Ellis CN, Nickoloff BJ, et al: Oral cyclosporine in the treatment of inflammatory and noninflammatory dermatoses. Arch Dermatol 1990;126:339.

Hallopeau M: Leçons cliniques sur les maladies cutanées et syphilitiques. L'Union Med 1887;43:742.

Halpert R, Fruchter RG, Sedlis A, et al: Human papillomavirus and lower genital neoplasia in renal transplant patients. Obstet Gynecol 1986;68:251.

Highet AS, Warren RE, Weeks AJ: Bacteriology and antibiotic treatment of perineal suppurative hidradenitis. Arch Dermatol 1988;124:1047.

Holt PJA, Darke C: HLA antigens and Bf allotypes in lichen sclerosus et atrophicus. Tissue Antigens 1983;22:89.

Horowitz BJ: Interferon therapy for condylomatous vulvitis. Obstet Gynecol 1989;73:446.

Jackson R: Melanosis of the vulva. J Dermatol Surg Oncol 1984; 10:119.

Jacobson M, Krumhola B, Franks A: Desquamative inflammatory vaginitis. J Reprod Med 1989;34:647.

Klein LE, Cohen SR, Weinstein MB: Bullous lichen sclerosus et atrophicus: treatment by tangential excision. J Am Acad Dermatol 1984;10:346.

Krebs HB: Treatment of vaginal intraepithelial neoplasia with laser and topical 5-fluorouracil. Obstet Gynecol 1989;73:657.

Lally MR, Orenstein SR, Cohen BA: Crohn's disease of the vulva in an 8-year-old girl. Pediatr Dermatol 1988;5:103.

Lenehan PM, Meffe F, Lickrish GM: Vaginal intraepithelial neoplasia: biologic aspects and management. Obstet Gynecol 1986; 68:333.

Malik S, Wilkinson EJ: Pseudo-Paget's disease. J Lower Genital Tract 1999;3:201.

Marinoff SC, Turner ML, Hirsch RP, et al: Intralesional alpha interferon: cost effective therapy for vulvar vestibulitis syndrome. J Reprod Med 1993;38:19.

Marquette GP, Su B, Woodruff JD: Introital adenosis associated with Stevens-Johnson syndrome. Obstet Gynecol 1985;66:143.

Meyrick-Thomas RH, Holmes RC, Rowland Payne CME, et al: The incidence of development of autoimmune diseases in women after the diagnosis of lichen sclerosus et atrophicus. Br J Dermatol 1982;107(Suppl 22):29.

Michael H, Roth LM: Congenital and acquired cysts, benign and malignant skin adnexal tumors, and Paget's disease of the vulva. In Wilkinson EJ (ed): Pathology of the Vulva and Vagina. New York: Churchill Livingstone, 1987:25.

Moore KL: The Developing Human: Clinically Oriented Embryology. 2nd ed. Philadelphia: WB Saunders Company, 1977:228.

Mortimer PS, Dawber RPR, Gales MA, et al: A double-blind controlled cross-over trial of cyproterone acetate in females with hidradenitis suppurativa. Br J Dermatol 1986a;115:263.

Mortimer PS, Dawber RPR, Gales MA, et al: Mediation of hidradenitis suppurativa by androgens. Br Med J 1986b;292:245.

Mucitelli DR, Charles EZ, Kraus FT: Vulvovaginal polyps. Int J Gynecol Pathol 1990;9:20.

Mullins D, Wilkinson EJ, Thomasen J: Lichenoid vulvo-vaginitis. J Reprod Med, 1997.

Nadji M, Morales AR, Girtanner RE, et al: Paget's disease of the skin: a unifying concept of histogenesis. Cancer 1982;50:2203.

O'Loughlin S, Woods R, Kirke PN, et al: Hidradenitis suppurativa. Arch Dermatol 1988;124:1043.

Ostergard DR: Vestibulitis: a cause of dyspareunia. Med Aspects Hum Sexuality 1990;24:36.

Patterson JW, Blaylock WK: Tumors and other lesions of the melanocyte system. In A Concise Textbook of Dermatology. New York: Medical Examination Publishing Company, 1987:117.

Pelisse M: The vulvo-vaginal-gingival syndrome. Int J Dermatol 1989;28:381.

Pelisse M: Treatment of erosive vaginal lichen planus with hydrocortisone foam (Colifoam). J Reprod Med (submitted) 1999.

Planner RS, Hobbs JB: Intraepithelial and invasive neoplasia of the vulva in association with human papillomavirus infection. J Reprod Med 1988;33:503.

Punnonen R, Soidinmaki H, Kauppila O, et al: Relationship of vulvar lichen sclerosus et atrophicus to carcinoma. Ann Chir Gynaecol Suppl 1985;197:23.

Pyka R, Wilkinson EJ, Friedrich EG Jr: The histopathology of vulvar vestibulitis syndrome. Int J Obstet Gynecol 1988;7:249.

Reid R: Superficial laser vulvectomy—a new surgical technique for appendage-conserving ablation of refractory condylomas and vulvar intraepithelial neoplasia. Am J Obstet Gynecol 1985; 152:504.

Ridley CM: Lichen sclerosus et atrophicus. Arch Dermatol 1987; 123:457.

Ridley CM, Frankman O, Pincus SH, Wilkinson EJ: New nomenclature in vulvar disease. Am J Obstet Gynecol 1989;160:769.

Schulman D, Beck LS, Roberts IM, et al: Crohn's disease of the vulva. Am J Gastroenterol 1987;82:1328.

Sedlacek TV, Riva JM, Magen A, et al: Vaginal and vulvar adenosis: an unexpected side effect of carbon dioxide laser vaporization. In: Proceedings of the 10th International Congress of the International Society for the Study of Vulvar Disease, City, 1989.

Shatz P, Bergeron C, Wilkinson E, et al: Vulvar intraepithelial neoplasia and skin appendage involvement. Obstet Gynecol 1989; 74:769.

Shelley WB, Cahn MM: Pathogenesis of hidradenitis suppurativa in man: experimental and histologic observations. Arch Dermatol 1955;72:562.

Sideri M, Rognon M, Rizzolo L, et al: Antigens of the HLA system in women with vulvar lichen sclerosus. J Reprod Med 1988;33: 551.

Sillman FH, Sedlis A, Boyce J: A review of lower genital intraepithelial neoplasia and the use of topical 5-fluorouracil. Obstet Gynecol Surv 1985;40:190.

Sillman F, Stanek A, Sedlis A, et al: The relationship between human papillomavirus and lower genital intraepithelial neoplasia in immunosuppressed women. Am J Obstet Gynecol 1984;150:300.

Silverber B, Smoot CE, Landa SJF, et al: Hidradenitis suppurativa: patient satisfaction with wound healing by secondary intention. Plast Reconstr Surg 1987;79:555.

Simms JM: Clinical Notes on Uterine Surgery. London: Robert Hartwicke, 1866:192.

Snell RS: Clinical Embryology for Medical Students. 2nd ed. Boston: Little, Brown, 1975:221.

Sobel J: Vaginitis. New Eng J Med 1997;337:1896.

Soper De, Patterson JW, Hurt WG, et al: Lichen planus of the vulva. Obstet Gynecol 1988;72:74.

Stacy D, Burrell M, Franklin EW: Extramammary Paget's disease of the vulva: use of intraoperative frozen-section margins. Am J Obstet Gynecol 1986;155:519.

Steege JF: Chronic Pelvic Pain (ACOG Technical Bulletin no. 129). Washington, DC: American College of Obstetricians and Gynecologists, 1989.

Sturgeon SR, Brinton LA, Devesa SS, et al: In situ and invasive vulvar cancer incidence trends (1973–1987). Am J Obstet Gynecol 1992;166:1482.

Turner ML, Marinoff SC: Association of human papilloma virus with vulvodynia and the vulvar vestibulitis syndrome. J Reprod Med 1988;33:533.

Van der Putte SCJ, van-Gorp HM: Cysts of mammary-like glands in the vulva. Int J Gynecol Pathol 1995;14:184.

Whimster IW: The natural history of endogenous skin malignancy as a basis for experimental research. Transcripts St. Johns Hosp Dermatol Soc 1973;59:195.

Wilkinson EJ: Benign diseases of the vulva. In: Kurman R (ed): Blaustein's Pathology of the Female Genital Tract. 4th ed. New York: Springer-Verlag, 1994a:31–86.

Wilkinson EJ: Premalignant and malignant tumors of the vulvar. In: Kurman R (ed): Blaustein's Pathology of the Female Genital Tract. 4th ed. New York: Springer-Verlag, 1994b:87–130.

Wilkinson EJ, Hardt NS: Anatomy of the vulva. In: Sternberg S (ed): Histology for Pathologists. Philadelphia: Lippincott-Raven, 1995.

Wilkinson EJ, Mullins D: The vulva and vagina. In: Silverberg S (ed): Principles and Practice of Surgical Pathology and Cytopathology. Vol 3. New York: Churchill Livingstone, 1997:2411–2457.

Wilkinson EJ, Guerrero E, Daniel R, et al: Vulvar vestibulitis is rarely associated with human papillomavirus infection types 6, 11, 16, or 18. Int J Gynecol Pathol 1993;12:344.

Wilkinson EJ, Kneale B, Lynch PJ: Report of the ISSVD Terminology Committee. J Reprod Med 1986;31:973.

Wilson E: Lichen planus. J Cutan Med 1869;3:117.

53

Vulvar Neoplasms

Alan N. Gordon

The vulva is the fourth most common site for cancer to arise within the female genital tract. However, invasive cancer of the vulva accounts for only 3% to 5% of all cancers arising within the female genital tract. The annual age-adjusted incidence rate for invasive cancer of the vulva in the United States has been estimated to be 1.6 per 100,000 women per year (Young et al, 1981).

Invasive squamous carcinoma accounts for approximately 90% of the cancers arising within the vulvar tissue. The bulk of this chapter is therefore dedicated to invasive squamous carcinoma. Other types of cancers can be seen, as listed in Table 53–1. Melanoma is the second most common cancer arising in the vulva and accounts for approximately 5% of all vulvar cancers. Adenocarcinoma can arise within Bartholin's gland, or the apocrine and eccrine glands of the vulva. Primary breast cancer can arise in the vulva as a result of ectopic breast tissue. Of course, virtually any form of sarcoma can be seen to arise in the vulva from the abundant connective tissue present.

SQUAMOUS CELL CARCINOMA

Epidemiology

Squamous carcinoma of the vulva is typically a disease of older postmenopausal patients. The median age at time of presentation is in the 60s, with most series reporting age ranges from 30 to 90 (Green et al, 1958; Franklin and Rutledge, 1972; Mabuchi et al, 1985). Earlier studies had suggested that nulliparity was a risk factor (Green et al, 1958). However, more recent studies have shown parity to be unrelated to risk (Brinton et al, 1990). Although several medical conditions, such as hypertension, diabetes, and obesity, have in the past been related to the occurrence of vulvar carcinoma, more modern epidemiologic techniques have shown that there is no significant association of any of these factors with the development of vulvar cancer (Brinton et al, 1990).

Many authors have long noted an association between carcinoma of the vulva and the development of other cancers. Green et al (1958) reported that 13.4% of their patients had a second primary cancer. Franklin and Rutledge (1972) reported that 20% of their patients developed a second primary cancer and 15% of patients either previously had or developed a cancer of the cervix. More recent attention has therefore focused on the risk factors that may be associated with the development of cervical cancer. In a case-control study, Brinton et al (1990) showed an increased relative risk of 2.5 of developing vulvar cancer in patients with three or more sexual partners. Also reported in that study was the independent risk of development of vulvar cancer with the history of genital warts. Those patients with a history of condylomata had a 15.2 increased relative risk of developing invasive cancer of the vulva. This risk was independent of the number of sexual partners. Of note was that they also found an increased relative risk of 1.8 in patients with a history of an abnormal Pap smear and an increased relative risk of 2.0 in current smokers. Mabuchi et al (1985) did not confirm the increased risk associated with number of sexual partners. However, in that study, coital experience was classified as none versus any and not broken down according to the number of sexual partners. They did, however, confirm the increased risk for current smokers and also noted an increased risk associated with the use of coffee that was associated with a dose-response pattern.

Etiology

On the basis of many retrospective studies, leukoplakia and lichen sclerosis were believed to be precursors of carcinoma of the vulva (Barkley and Bonney, 1909; Taussig, 1940). In fact, Taussig (1940) thought that the incidence of vulvar carcinoma could be cut in half if a complete vulvectomy were performed in all cases of well-developed leukoplakic vulvitis. Green et al (1958) reported 58% of their patients had an associated leukoplakia and thought that this deserved the title of squamous cell carcinoma, grade one-half. Charles (1972), however, reported leukoplakia in association with only 24% of cases and thought that it was probably not as dangerous a precursor as had been reported in the past. Prospective series have not been able to confirm the importance of leukoplakia and lichen sclerosis as precursors to the development of vulvar carcinoma. McAdams and Kistner (1958) found only a 10% in-

Table 53-1. CANCERS OF
THE VULVA

Squamous cell carcinoma	90%
Melanoma	5%
Adenosquamous carcinoma	1%
Bertholin's gland carcinoma	2%
Squamous cell	
Transitional cell	
Adenocarcinoma	
Adenoid cystic	
Sarcoma	2%

cidence (32 of 397 patients) of carcinoma developing in patients with previously existing leukoplakia. Jeffcoate (1966) found that 3% of patients (8 of 269) initially presented with an invasive cancer in association with chronic dystrophy. In that same study, he found that, of 138 patients who were followed, only 4 were found to develop invasive cancer while under follow-up. Kaufman et al (1974) reported a series of 110 patients with dystrophy who were followed. The only patient who developed a vulvar carcinoma had previously been treated for an invasive squamous cell carcinoma. Hart et al (1975) reported a series of 92 patients who were followed for lichen sclerosis. Only one patient developed vulvar carcinoma 12 years later, compared to five patients who developed six other carcinomas. In a review of the literature, they found only 3% of patients (16 of 465) who developed carcinoma while being followed for lichen sclerosis. Most reviewers believe the highest risk for development of carcinoma is in areas of dystrophy associated with atypia (McAdams and Kistner, 1958; Jeffcoate, 1966; Kaufman et al, 1974; Hart et al, 1975). The case-control study by Mabuchi et al (1985) did show a significant association of leukoplakia with invasive cancer of the vulva. However, as the prospective studies have shown, when adequately treated and followed, lichen sclerosis and leukoplakia have a low risk of developing into invasive cancer.

The role of carcinoma in situ as a precursor to invasive cancer of the vulva is also somewhat unclear. In a review of 102 patients with carcinoma in situ, only four examples (4%) were seen of progression to invasive disease (Buscema et al, 1980b). Buscema et al (1980a) also examined the areas adjacent to invasive vulvar carcinomas and found less than 20% of cases demonstrated classic in situ neoplasia in adjacent sections. However, more than 50% showed adjacent histologic alterations consistent with a dystrophy. Therefore, it would appear that patients who have been treated for carcinoma in situ should have a low risk of development of invasive cancer. This risk does appear to be somewhat greater for patients with either immune suppression or advanced age (Buscema et al, 1980b). However, Jones and Rowan (1994) found that seven of eight untreated patients (87.5%) did develop progression to invasive cancer within 8 years.

A viral etiology has been suspected for carcinoma of the vulva because of the similarity of its epidemiologic factors to those of cervical cancer, along with the fact that a large percentage of patients with vulvar cancer have either pre-existing, simultaneous, or subsequent cervical cancer (Franklin and Rutledge, 1972). Kaufman et al (1981) found evidence of herpes simplex virus type 2 antigens in 9 of 10 cases of carcinoma in situ in the absence of infectious viral particles. These findings were confirmed in another study in which herpesvirus antigens were found only in dysplasia, carcinoma in situ, or invasive cancer and not in vulvitis, hyperkeratosis, or condyloma (Cabral et al, 1982).

The failure of herpesvirus to explain all cases has led to an examination of the role of human papillomavirus (HPV) as an etiologic agent just as in cervical cancer. Sutton et al (1987) examined nine carcinomas of the vulva and found 78% contained HPV type 6– or type 11–related DNA, 33% had type 16–related DNA, and 22% had type 18–related DNA. Buscema et al (1988) found HPV DNA in 58% of invasive cancers (7 of 12). Only one case was positive for type 6 or 11 DNA (a verrucous cancer), four cases were positive for type 16 DNA, and two cases for other types. Other reports have also shown that HPV DNA associations in cancer of the vulva are similar to those observed elsewhere in the genital tract (Carson et al, 1988). A significant association between HPV DNA and invasive cancer of the vulva may exist but may not explain all cases. Monk et al (1995) reported that 33 of 55 patients were positive for HPV using polymerase chain reaction techniques. HPV positivity was seen more often in younger patients (<70 years) and in smokers. Warty, verrucous, and basaloid lesions also have a greater proportion of HPV-positive lesions (95% vs. 39%) compared to typical squamous cell cancers (Monk et al, 1995). They also found that both HPV status and node status correlate with recurrence rates and death rates but that HPV was the most important prognostic factor. There may therefore be two types of vulvar cancer: one related to HPV and another that arises via a different pathway.

Clinical Presentation

Currently, the most common presenting complaint of patients with carcinoma of the vulva is pruritis (Table 53–2). This is seen in approximately 70% of patients in more recently reported series (Figge and Gaudenz, 1974; Benedet et al, 1979; Podratz et al, 1983b). The pruritis may be due to either the carcinoma itself or related intraepithelial changes (i.e., dystrophy). Fortunately, because patients are presenting earlier, in more recent years the incidence of patients presenting with either a mass or growth appears to be decreasing. Similarly, fewer patients are being seen on initial presentation with either ulceration or bleeding resulting from the presence of a

Table 53–2. PRESENTING SYMPTOMS

Pruritis	30–70%
Mass/growth	30–70%
Ulcer	15–60%
Bleeding	5–30%
Pain	10–25%
Discharge	15–25%
Urinary symptoms	15–20%

Data from Taussig (1940), Green et al (1958), Collins et al (1971), Franklin and Rutledge (1972), Figge and Gaudenz (1974), Benedet et al (1979), and Podratz et al (1983b).

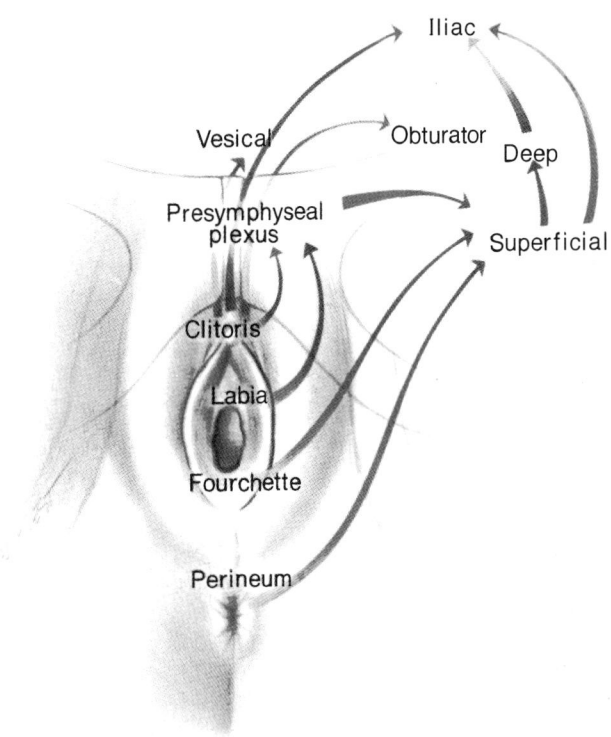

Figure 53–1
Lymphatic drainage of the vulva. (From Plentl AA, Friedman EA: Lymphatic System of the Female Genitalia. Philadelphia: WB Saunders Company, 1971:25, with permission).

significant-sized lesion. Other reported symptoms seen in association with carcinoma of the vulva have been either pain or urinary symptoms (burning, frequency). These last two are usually seen more often in association with a significant-sized growth. Discharge may sometimes be noticed as a result of ulceration or irritation associated with the lesion.

The definitive method of diagnosis is with excisional biopsy. This can almost always be accomplished as an office procedure with just a local anesthetic. After infiltrating the area with 1% lidocaine; a 4- or 6-mm Keyes punch biopsy can be used in a coring motion to delineate an area to be excised. The sample is then grasped with a pickups and cut free from the underlying subcutaneous tissue with scissors. Usually, either silver nitrate sticks or a small amount of Monsel's solution (ferric subsulfate) are all that is necessary to control bleeding. Only in very rare instances will a suture be needed.

Staging and Pattern of Spread

Squamous carcinoma of the vulva tends to spread by continuous growth, with eventual spread to adjacent structures as it continues to enlarge. The primary lesions will tend to stay confined to the vulva, spreading only to adjacent structures after they have tended to achieve significant size. As lesions continue to grow concentrically, they may spread onto the adjacent urethra, vagina, or rectum. With continued growth, spread is even possible beyond the intertriginous folds onto the skin of the thigh in advanced cases.

The secondary spread of carcinoma of the vulva is via embolization to the draining lymphatics. The lymphatic drainage of the vulva has been well described by Parry-Jones (1963) and Plentl and Friedman (1971) (Fig. 53–1). From all areas on the vulva, the lymphatics flow superiorly toward the mons, then course laterally near the pubic tubercle into the femoral triangle. The lymphatics draining the vulva do not extend lateral to the labial-crural fold or cross with the lymphatics in the thigh (Parry-Jones, 1963). There are extensive anastomoses at the midline structures (the clitoris, urethra, and perianal region) that would allow for flow to either side of the vulva.

From the inguinal-femoral nodes, further lymphatic extension can continue along the course of the femoral vein through the inguinal ring to involve the pelvic lymph node groups. Cloquet's node was thought to be the most proximal node in the femoral chain and occupied the "empty space" as the lymphatics coursed through the inguinal space. It was believed that, if Cloquet's node was not involved by tumor, the pelvic nodes would also be free of metastasis. Parry-Jones (1963) also demonstrated a secondary lymphatic pathway directly to the internal iliac group of lymph nodes. It was thought that lesions along the clitoris or perineum could potentially drain to this pelvic node group directly via the dorsal artery of the clitoris and other branches of the internal pudendal vessels.

A staging system for a cancer ideally should be based upon the pattern of spread of the cancer. It attempts to collate cases and then allow separation into groups that have a different prognosis. Taussig (1940) made an initial attempt at staging and analysis of previously untreated cases. The International Federation of Obstetrics and Gynecology (FIGO) recommended a clinical staging system that was adopted in 1971. Although some investigators have questioned the use of a 2-cm limit for stage I disease (Krupp et al, 1975; Donaldson et al, 1981), virtually all other studies have supported the use of this limit. Others have questioned the inclusion of all perianal lesions in stage III (Figge and Gaudenz, 1974). Another problem with the 1971 staging scheme is the assessment of nodal status based on clinical examination. Approximately 40% of clinically positive nodes are found to be negative on histologic assessment, and from 10% to 20% of clinically negative nodes are found to harbor metastatic deposits (Byron et al, 1962; Krupp et al, 1975; Morley, 1976; Sedlis et al, 1987). With these considerations, in 1988 FIGO modified the staging for carcinoma of the vulva into a surgical-pathologic staging system (Table 53–3). Lesion location no longer affects the stage of disease. Histologically documented unilateral groin metastases are now included in stage III, and bilateral groin metastases or metastases to the pelvic lymph nodes are included in stage IV. Several reports reviewing the outcome of previously treated patients have shown that the new staging system places patients into more accurate risk categories and provides for better discrimination of survival between stages (Homesley et al, 1991; Hopkins et al, 1992b; Shanbour et al, 1992).

At the suggestion of the International Society for the Study of Vulvar Disease (ISSVD), stage I was divided into stage IA (lesions with 1 mm or less invasion) and stage IB (lesions with more than 1 mm of invasion). This should not affect prognosis because all cases with positive nodes are included in stage III. The subdivision of stage I may now allow for comparison of different therapies (Creasman, 1995).

Table 53–3. FIGO STAGING OF VULVAR CARCINOMA

T1	Tumor confined to the vulva and/or perineum 2 cm or less in greatest dimension
T2	Tumor confined to the vulva and/or perineum greater than 2 cm in greatest dimension
T3	Tumor of any size with adjacent spread to the lower urethra and/or the vagina and/or the anus
T4	Tumor of any size invading the upper urethra, bladder mucosa, rectal mucosa, or pelvic bone
N0	No lymph node metastasis
N1	Unilateral regional lymph node metastasis
N2	Bilateral regional lymph node metastasis
M0	No clinical metastasis
M1	Distant metastasis (including pelvic lymph node metastasis)

Staging

Stage		
Stage I		T1 N0 M0
	IA	T1 ≤ 1 mm
	IB	T1 > 1 mm
Stage II		T2 N0 M0
Stage III		
	IIIA	T3 N0 M0
	IIIB	T3 N1 M0
		T2 N1 M0
		T1 N1 M0
Stage IV		
	IVA	T4 N0 M0
	IVB	TX N2 M0
		TX NX M1

Table 53–4. FIVE-YEAR SURVIVAL

STAGE	CLINICAL	SURGICAL
I	85–90%	94–98%
II	60–80%	79–85%
III	24–60%	71–74%
IV	20%	31%
A		19%
B		8%

Data from Morley (1976), Benedet et al (1979), Podratz et al (1983b), Figge et al (1985), Homesley et al (1991), and Hopkins et al (1992b).

Prognostic Factors

The stage of disease is still an independent prognostic factor for survival in carcinoma of the vulva (Table 53–4). The 5-year survival rate for clinical stage I disease is essentially in the 85% to 90% range; however, survival is in the range of 94% to 98% for surgically staged patients. This improvement is due to removal of patients with metastatic disease in the inguinal nodes from stage I. Survival tends to decrease with each increase in stage in both systems, and only approximately 20% of stage IV patients survive 5 years.

Even independent of the stage, the presence or absence of metastatic disease in the different lymph node groups is highly prognostic (Table 53–5). Patients with negative nodes exhibit significantly improved survival over those with metastatic disease in the inguinal-femoral lymph nodes (Way, 1960; Morley, 1976; Green, 1978; Benedet et al, 1979; Curry et al, 1980; Donaldson et al, 1981; Hacker et al, 1983a; Podratz et al, 1983b). Additionally, it appears that survival decreases with an increase in the number of involved inguinal-femoral nodes (Morley, 1976; Curry et al, 1980; Hacker et al, 1983a; Podratz et al, 1983b). In fact, Curry et al (1980) reported no survivors with over three positive nodes, and Hacker et al (1983a) reported only 12% survival with three or more positive nodes. A study by the Gynecologic Oncology Group showed that inguinal node status is the most significant prognostic factor for overall survival (Homesley et al, 1991).

The incidence of involvement of the inguinal-femoral nodes by metastatic disease varies by stage (Table 53–6), ranging from 10% to 15% of stage I cases to 80% of stage IV cases (Morley, 1976; Green, 1978; Donaldson et al, 1981; Hacker et al, 1983a; Boyce et al, 1985; Sedlis et al, 1987; Binder et al, 1990). Although the stage appears to be the most im-

Table 53–5. SURVIVAL BY NODAL STATUS (5 YEAR)

Negative nodes	76–96%
Positive inguinal-femoral nodes	33–51%
Positive pelvic nodes	12–20%

Table 53-6. RELATIONSHIP OF STAGE TO POSITIVE INGUINAL-FEMORAL NODES

STAGE	% POSITIVE
I	10–15
II	25–40
III	30–80
IV	60–100

portant predictor of spread to the inguinal-femoral nodes, other factors that correlate with the presence of disease in the lymph nodes include the depth of invasion, the presence of lymph–vascular space involvement, the grade of the lesion, the thickness of the lesion, and the presence of clinically involved nodes (Donaldson et al, 1981; Boyce et al, 1985; Sedlis et al, 1987; Binder et al, 1990).

The ipsilateral inguinal-femoral nodes are highly predictive of involvement of the contralateral lymph nodes by metastatic disease when lesions are located off the midline. Most reports state that there is no involvement of the contralateral node groups unless the ipsilateral nodes contain metastatic disease (Figge and Gaudenz, 1974; Figge et al, 1985; Hoffman et al, 1985). In one series, there were four patients reported to have spread to the contralateral nodes without ipsilateral involvement (Krupp and Bohm, 1978). Although this represents 15% of the patients who had positive nodes in that series, it is only 2% of all patients in that series, indicating that it is an unusual occurrence.

Presence of metastatic disease in the pelvic nodes is an extremely poor prognostic sign: only approximately 15% of patients survive 5 years (Green, 1978; Curry et al, 1980). Fortunately, only 6% of patients will have metastases to the pelvic lymph nodes (Table 53–7). Although there exists the possibility of direct drainage to the pelvic lymph nodes, less than

1% of patients were found to have metastasis to the pelvic lymph nodes bypassing the primary drainage to the groins. It has been pointed out that virtually all patients with involved pelvic nodes have had multiple involved inguinal nodes (Curry et al, 1980; Hacker et al, 1983a; Podratz et al, 1983b). It appears that even midline lesions follow the same pattern of spread as lateral lesions, with primary drainage to the inguinal nodes before they will metastasize to the pelvic nodes (Curry et al, 1980). Therefore, the status of the inguinal-femoral nodes can be used to predict the status of the pelvic nodes in the clinical management of patients.

The presence of metastatic disease in the inguinal-femoral nodes predicts not only the status of the pelvic nodes and contralateral inguinal-femoral nodes but also the pattern of recurrence in cancer of carcinoma of the vulva. Figge et al (1985) found that, when the nodes were negative, 90% of the recurrences were localized to the vulva; however, when the nodes were positive, only 50% of the recurrences involved either the vulva or the groin areas. Hacker et al (1983a) found that, if there were less than three positive inguinal-femoral nodes, there was an approximate 3% incidence of groin or systemic recurrence; however, with three or more positive nodes, there was a 33% incidence of groin recurrence and 66% incidence of systemic recurrence. The higher incidence of groin and systemic recurrence is of significance because recurrences in the vulva can exhibit a 50% 5-year survival, whereas all other occurrences exhibit at best a 10% 5-year survival (Podratz et al, 1982). The high incidence of systemic disease with multiple positive nodes indicates a need for an effective adjuvant therapy for these patients at high risk for occult metastatic disease.

Several investigators have attempted to define an early stage of carcinoma of the vulva that would have a virtually zero incidence of metastasis to the inguinal nodes. Wharton et al (1975) described a group of patients, all of whom had lesions less than

Table 53-7. INCIDENCE OF INGUINAL-FEMORAL (I-F) AND PELVIC NODE METASTASIS

SERIES	NO. OF PATIENTS	POSITIVE I-F NODES*	POSITIVE PELVIC NODES[†]	POSITIVE PELVIC/ NEGATIVE I-F NODES
Podratz et al (1983b)	175	59 (34)	7/114	0
Morley (1976)	222	83 (37)	6/29	0
Green (1978)	142	54 (38)	2/111	0
Hacker et al (1983b)	113	31 (27)	6.18[‡]	0
Curry et al (1989)	191	57 (30)	9/191	0
Figge et al (1985)	123	30 (24)	6/32	0
Way (1960)	143	55 (38)	23/143	5
Krupp and Bohm (1978)	195	40 (21)	9/195	3[§]
Collins et al (1971)	98	31 (32)	11/98	4
Total	1402	440 (31)	79	12

*Number in parenthesis is percentage of patients with positive nodes.
[†]Number with positive nodes/number with pelvic lymphadenectomy.
[‡]Six additional patients developed pelvic recurrence without prior pelvic lymphadenectomy.
[§]Two patients had positive nodes in the contralateral inguinal-femoral nodes.

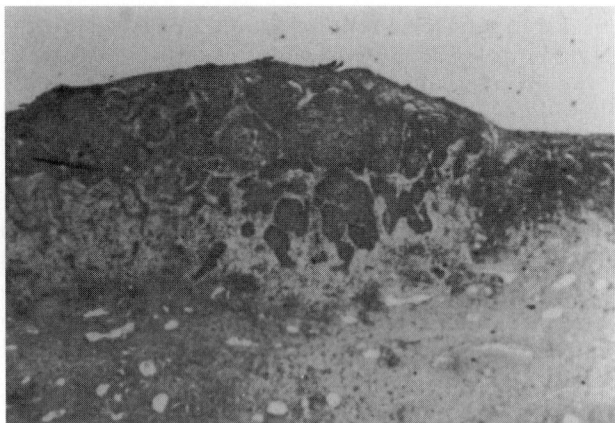

Figure 53-2
An early invasive cancer. The entire lesion is less than 2 mm thick and less than 1 cm in diameter.

2 cm in diameter with less than 5 mm of invasion. In this group categorized as "microinvasive," there were no positive lymph nodes and no recurrences, and no patient died as a result of cancer (Fig. 53-2). However, subsequent reports indicated a significant risk for lymphatic metastasis in similar groups of patients. Parker et al (1975) found 5% of patients had metastases with less than 5 mm of invasion. They suggested that, in addition to the depth of invasion, one needed to consider anaplasia and involvement of lymph-vascular spaces in defining a low-risk group of patients. Buscema et al (1981) reported a 10% incidence of involved inguinal lymph nodes when the depth of invasion was less than 5 mm as measured from the tip of the deepest rete peg. Barnes et al (1980) suggested that only lesions with

a single focus of invasion that is associated with intraepithelial neoplasia be classified as microinvasive.

One of the difficulties in determining at which depth of invasion there is no risk of metastasis to the lymph nodes has been the different points from which invasion was measured. In an effort to provide an improved point from which to measure invasion, Wilkinson et al (1982) suggested measuring from the basement membrane of the adjacent most superficial dermal papilla, which is an easily recognized point (Fig. 53-3). Using this definition, the incidence of nodal involvement was zero in patients with less than 1.5 mm of invasion and 11% with greater than 1.5 mm of invasion. In a subsequent review, Wilkinson (1985) found the depth of invasion to be related to the incidence of nodal involvement. The incidence of involved nodes dropped from 12% in patients with lesions having less than 5 mm of invasion to 4.9% with lesions having less than 3 mm of invasion. Only patients with less than 1 mm of invasion had no nodal involvement. Carcinoma of the vulva does behave differently than carcinoma of the cervix. It has been recommended that the term *microinvasive cancer* not be used when applied to the vulva because of the possibility of nodal metastases even in early cancers (ISSVD Task Force, 1984). The use of the term *early invasive cancer* is probably more appropriate, and now these cases should be included in stage IA.

Tumor Markers

Currently, the role of tumor markers in the management of cancer of the vulva remains investigational. The vast majority of vulvar cancers are squamous

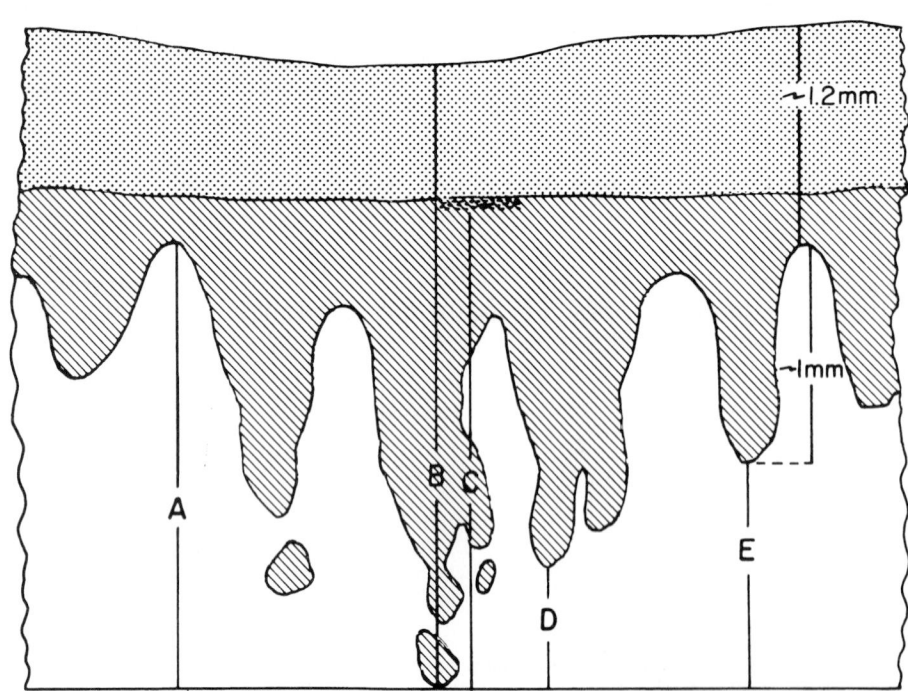

Figure 53-3
The various points from which invasion can be measured. (From Wilkinson EF: Superficial invasive carcinoma of the vulva. Clin Obstet Gynecol 1985;28:188, with permission.)

carcinoma. Therefore, most work has evaluated the role of squamous cell carcinoma antigen (SCCA) as a predictor of nodal metastasis or disease recurrence or progression. There does appear to be a relationship between tumor burden and elevated levels of SCCA. Elevated levels are more often seen in advanced-stage (FIGO III or IV) disease (Kato et al, 1985; van der Sijde et al, 1989). Despite the fact that elevated levels of SCCA are found more often in patients with positive inguinal nodes (37% vs. 16%, van der Sijde et al, 1989), most patients have normal levels, especially in early-stage disease, and preoperative levels do not appear to be sensitive to subclinical metastatic disease in the lymph nodes (Patsner and Mann, 1989). In follow-up of previously treated patients, SCCA elevations have not reliably preceded disease recurrence and were also subject to false-positive elevations as a result of benign skin diseases (van der Sijde et al, 1989).

CA-125 has been used in evaluation and follow-up of adenocarcinoma of the ovary, fallopian tube, and endometrium. However, the vulva is derived from ectodermal tissue, not mesoderm, and it is not known if the capacity to produce CA-125 exists. Metastatic disease to the pelvic peritoneum could result in elevation of CA-125, but this would only be seen in very advanced disease. Therefore, any role for CA-125 in adenocarcinoma of the vulva would be investigational only.

Treatment

For many years, the standard treatment for cancer of the vulva had consisted of a radical vulvectomy with bilateral inguinal-femoral lymphadenectomy and a pelvic lymphadenectomy. This approach was based on the work of Taussig (1940) and Way (1960). Both used a modification of the procedure described by Basset (1912). Way (1960) had noted that the failure to cure patients was due to a totally inadequate attack on the primary lesion along with an inadequate attempt at resecting the draining lymph nodes. The radical approach to therapy was able to produce the excellent cure rates represented in Table 53–4. However, the procedure has significant complication rates: delayed healing and wound breakdown are seen in up to 85% of patients (Podratz et al, 1983b). Most recent series report an increasing proportion of patients being seen with early-stage disease. As many as three fourths of patients currently present with stage I or II disease (Donaldson et al, 1981), and as many as 50% of patients have lesions with less than 5 mm of invasion (Sedlis et al, 1987). Green (1978) has even noted that there seems to be a decreased frequency of involved lymph nodes in more recently treated patients, probably as a result of earlier detection of disease. Podratz et al (1982) has even noted that there has been no improvement in survival noted in the last 30 years. This has prompted many investigators to see if decreasing the radicality

of therapy for earlier stage disease could result in equivalent survival rates while decreasing the morbidity of the therapy.

Lymph Nodes

Most recent studies have shown virtually no role for the pelvic lymphadenectomy in the current management of carcinoma of the vulva. Even though Way (1960) strongly emphasized the need to do a complete lymphadenectomy in the inguinal-femoral area, he recognized that spread to the pelvic nodes did not occur when the inguinal-femoral nodes were negative. The data in Table 53–7 show that less than 1% of patients have been found to have positive pelvic nodes in the absence of spread to the inguinal-femoral nodes. Additionally, patients with spread to the pelvic nodes exhibit no better than a 20% 5-year survival (Green, 1978; Curry et al, 1980). It had been argued by some that the addition of pelvic lymphadenectomy will probably cure an additional 10% to 15% of patients who might have negative nodes on microscopic examination; however, some actually did harbor some microscopic disease in those nodes (Green, 1978). Hacker et al (1983a) believed on reviewing their data, that there was no support for a pelvic lymphadenectomy unless there were three or more positive inguinal nodes. Way (1960) and others (Morley, 1976; Green, 1978; Curry et al, 1980) had thought that the lymphadenectomy should be limited only to those with positive nodes or clinically suspicious nodes. However, the addition of pelvic lymphadenectomy not only adds operative time, it adds to the incidence of lymphedema postoperatively (Figge and Gaudenz, 1974; Parker et al, 1975). The Gynecologic Oncology Group reported the results of a randomized study of radiation therapy versus pelvic lymphadenectomy for patients with positive inguinal-femoral nodes (Homesley et al, 1986). They found that survival was improved in the group that received radical radiation therapy; more importantly, the incidence of complications was less in this same group of patients treated with radiation only. Adjuvant radiation to the pelvis can probably be limited to those patients with two or more positive inguinal-femoral nodes because these seem to be the only patients at high risk for spread to the pelvic nodes (Curry et al, 1980; Hacker et al, 1983a; Hoffman et al, 1985).

Treatment should still include an inguinal-femoral lymphadenectomy. The status of this group of nodes is the most important predictor of survival and the risk of occult distant disease. Lateralized lesions could be treated with unilateral lymphadenectomy only, whereas lesions approaching the midline or involving the clitoris or perineum should have bilateral lymphadenectomies (Figge and Guadenz, 1974; Figge et al, 1985; Iverson et al, 1981; Hoffman et al, 1985). Several different terms have been applied to the group of nodes in this region, including inguinal and inguinal-femoral (Fig. 53–4). The term *superficial*

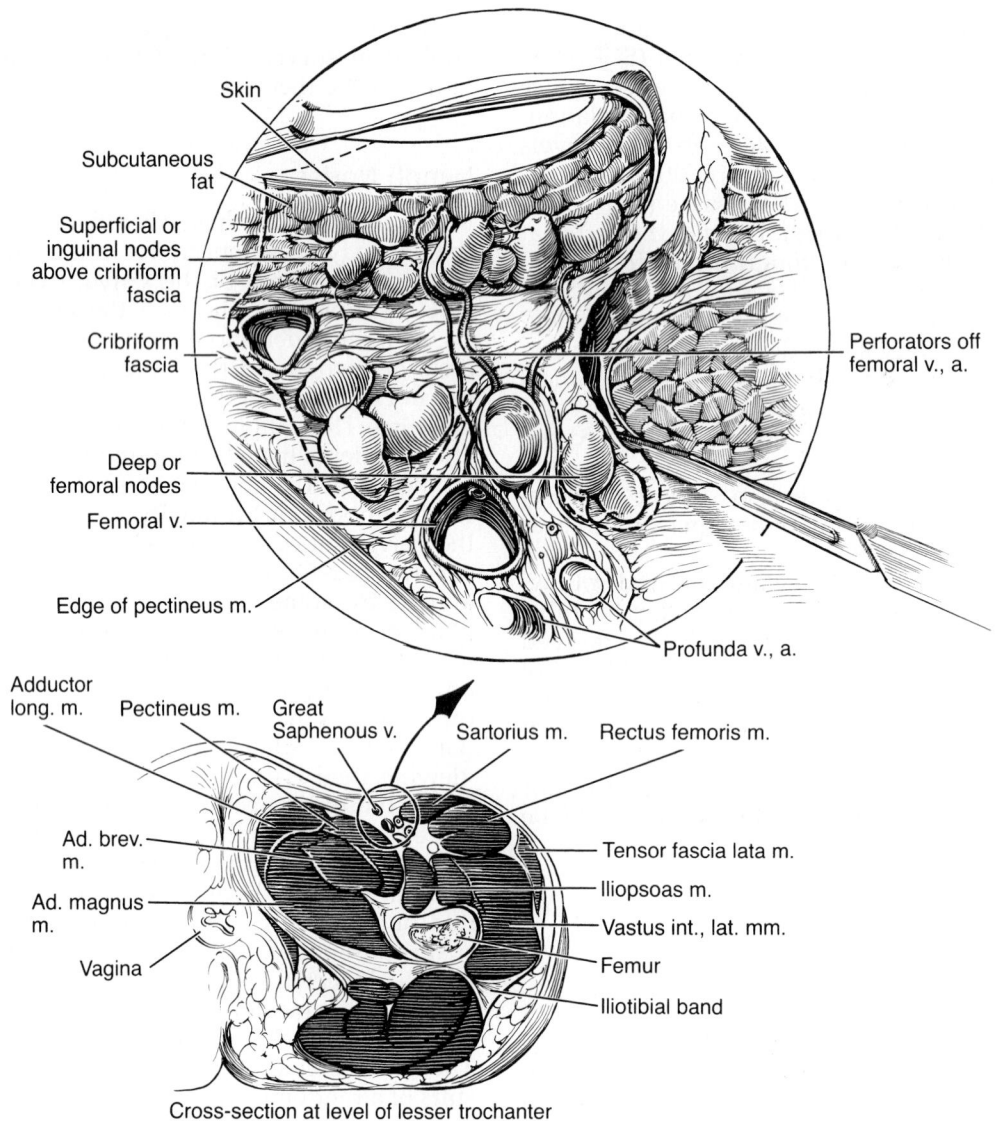

Figure 53–4
Cross-sectional view of the inguinal-femoral nodes demonstrating the superficial and deep nodes. v., vein; m., muscle; a., artery; Ad., adductor; long., longus; int., intermedius; lat., lateralis.

femoral group has been used to refer to those nodes lying deep to the fascia of Camper but superior to the cribriform fascia. The *deep femoral* or femoral nodes are those that lie inferior to the cribriform fascia, surrounding the femoral vessels and then finally entering into the abdomen through the inguinal ring. These nodes are best removed in a "border" approach (Fig. 53–5). After developing the plane beneath Camper's fascia, all the nodes from a point approximately 2 to 3 cm above the inguinal ligament are swept off the fascia of the rectus muscle. The lateral border can then be developed along the medial border of the sartorius muscle by following along its fascial edges. The medial border can then be developed along the lateral edges of the adductor longus by following along its fascial edges. This may require isolating and dividing the saphenous vein. If possible, the saphenous vein should be preserved to

try to decrease or prevent the development of lower extremity edema. The inferior border of the dissection is at the point where the sartorius and adductor muscles meet at Hunter's canal. The cribriform fascia can then be opened along the femoral artery. By staying medial to the lateral edge of the artery, the femoral nerve will be protected in its course under the sartorius muscle. The deep femoral nodes are then excised off the femoral vessels. A cadaver study has suggested that all the femoral nodes are located medial to the femoral vein (Borgno et al, 1990). However, in patients undergoing lymphadenectomy, I have found nodes between the vessels and lateral to the artery. The perforating branches are clamped and ligated as they are encountered. The saphenous vein will again require identification and may require ligation again where it enters the femoral vein at the fossa ovale. The entire lymphatic bundle can

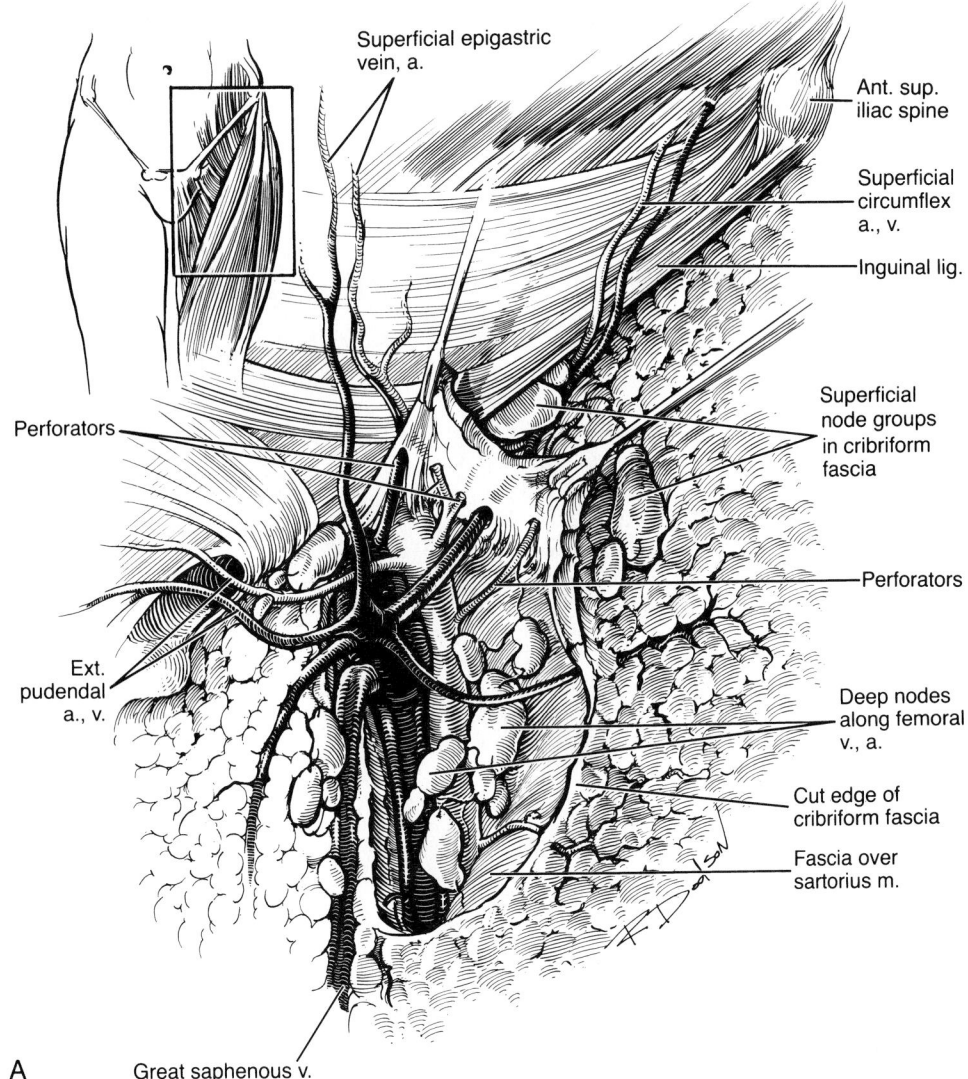

Figure 53–5

Removal of the inguinal-femoral nodes. The borders of the dissection can be seen along with the postoperative results. m., muscle; a., artery; Ant., anterior; sup., superior; v., vein; lig., ligament.
Illustration continued on opposite page

usually be isolated as a pedicle medial to the vein and then ligated where it crosses into the inguinal ring. This is where Cloquet's node will be situated. Transposition of the sartorius muscle over the exposed femoral vessels may be utilized at the completion of the procedure (Byron et al, 1962). If the lymph nodes in a unilateral procedure reveal metastatic disease, consideration must be given to either a delayed lymphadenectomy on the contralateral side (Iverson, 1985) or to radiation treatment to the contralateral nodes (Daly and Million, 1974). A Gynecologic Oncology Group study seemed to indicate that surgery is superior to radiation therapy for a clinically normal groin (Stehman et al, 1992b). However, the dose of radiation used may not have been sufficient at the true location of the nodes or too low for adequate control.

DiSaia et al (1979) have proposed that, for early invasive lesions, the superficial group of nodes can be removed and used as a monitor. They reported that, in patients who had undergone a complete inguinal-femoral lymphadenectomy, no patient was found to have positive deep femoral nodes without involvement of the superficial femoral node group. They did recommend that, if nodal involvement was found on frozen section, a complete inguinal-femoral lymphadenectomy be performed. However, Hacker et al (1983b) reported one patient who was found to have a positive femoral node with negative superficial nodes and an additional patient who had undergone superficial lymphadenectomy and then subsequently developed a groin recurrence. Parker et al (1975) also reported a patient who had positive deep femoral nodes with negative superficial nodes. These

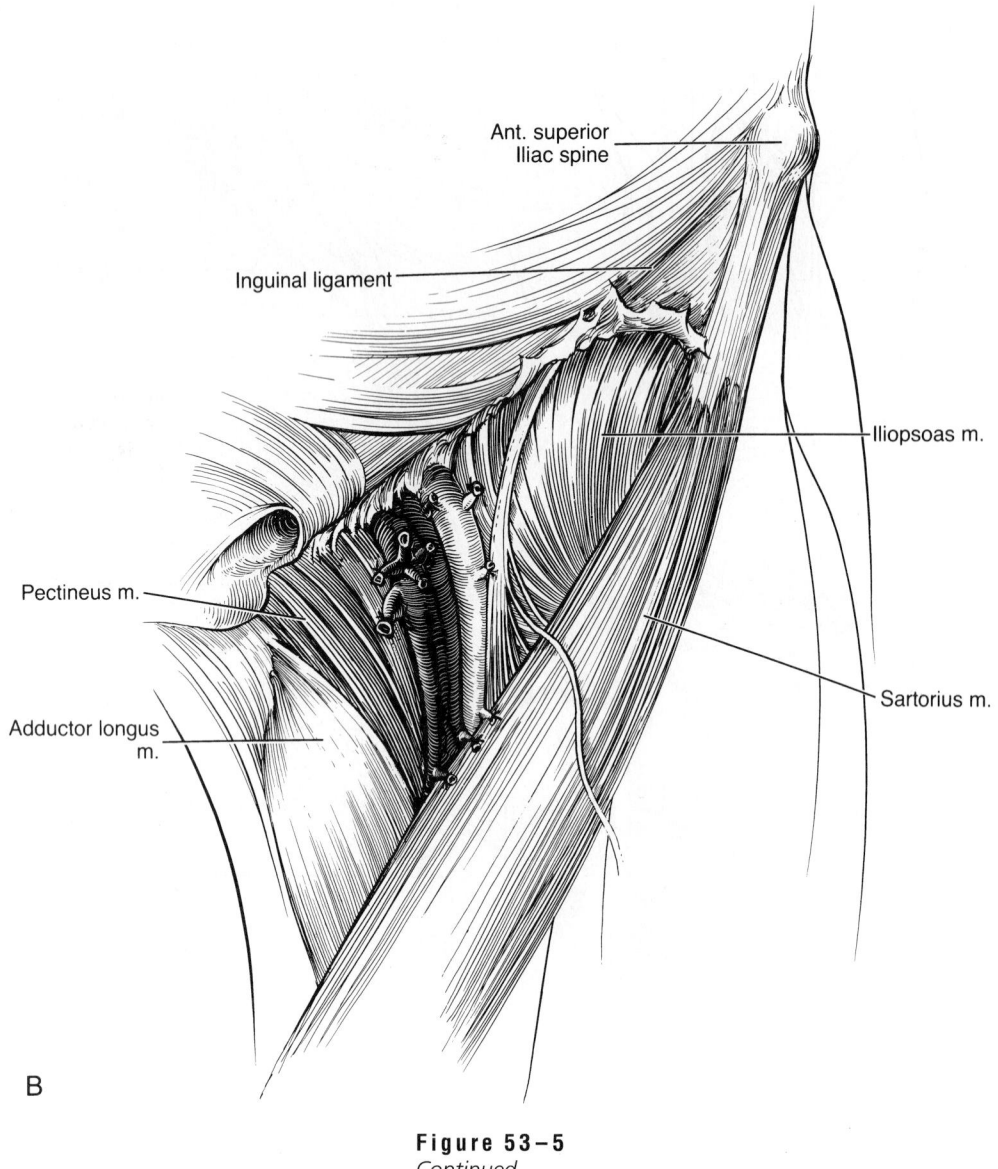

Ant. superior
Iliac spine

Inguinal ligament

Iliopsoas m.

Pectineus m.

Sartorius m.

Adductor longus
m.

B

Figure 53–5
Continued

few cases, however, represent less than 1% of patients overall. It would seem that a superficial lymphadenectomy can be used successfully for most patients with limited invasion (i.e., those with less than 5 mm of invasion and clinically negative nodes) (Berman et al, 1989). Hacker et al (1983b), however, have argued for a complete inguinal-femoral lymphadenectomy based on the small possibility of direct spread to the deeper nodes. The Gynecologic Oncology Group also reported an increased risk of recurrence in the groin with subsequent high mortality following superficial inguinal lymphadenectomy that may be due to failure to remove all the femoral nodes (Stehman et al, 1992a).

It is imperative that, at a minimum, a superficial lymphadenectomy be performed in cases of invasive cancer. There are numerous case reports of "recurrences" in the groin when the lymph nodes were not treated initially (Yazigi et al, 1978; Buscema et al,

1981; Hacker et al, 1984b; Atamdede and Hoogerland, 1989). As Hacker et al (1984b) pointed out, when these patients "recur" in the groin their chance of survival is virtually zero. In an analysis of failure after conservative therapy, the Gynecologic Oncology Group found that groin recurrences tended to occur earlier than local recurrences (7 vs. 36 months) and had significantly shorter survival (9 vs. 52 months) than local recurrences (Stehman et al, 1996).

The identification of a true sentinal node for a patient may allow for modification of the lymphadenectomy to decrease the postoperative morbidity. Local injection of fat-soluble dyes that are then absorbed in the lymphatics has been able to demonstrate lymph channels and nodal uptake in "sentinal" nodes (Levenback et al, 1995). It will remain to be proven that limited resection based on such techniques does not compromise recurrence or survival.

Primary Lesion

The use of radical vulvectomy with en bloc inguinal-femoral lymphadenectomy has produced excellent survival for stage I disease, in the range of 85% to 90% (Morley, 1976; Benedet et al, 1979; Podratz et al, 1983b; Figge et al, 1985). This has, however, produced significant complication rates, the most significant being impaired wound healing. Wound infections or separation may occur in as many as 85% of patients (Podratz et al, 1983b). Postoperative hospitalization can take as long as 21 days (Podratz et al, 1983b). The removal of significant amounts of vulvar tissue along with the resultant postoperative scarring has also resulted in depression, loss of body image, and sexual dysfunction (DiSaia et al, 1979; Anderson and Hacker, 1983). Following radical vulvectomy, prolapse, cystocele, or rectocele can be seen in anywhere from 5% to 16% of patients (Rutledge et al, 1970; Hacker et al, 1981). In most cases, this is probably due to lack of adequate fascial support after radical vulvectomy. Stress urinary incontinence can be seen in 2% to 9% of patients (Benedet et al, 1979; Hacker et al, 1981). Reid et al (1990) reported that radical vulvectomy by itself probably does not cause incontinence. They found that removal of a portion of the urethra often resulted in excision of some of the compressor urethrae muscle and was probably the cause of incontinence in most cases. These complications, combined with the failure to see significant improvement in survival over the last

few decades, has prompted a search for a more conservative treatment, especially for early lesions.

The excision of the skin bridge between the vulva and overlying the lymph nodes was proposed in order to assure complete removal of all the lymphatics. Parry-Jones (1963) proposed that, because there were no lymphatics lateral to the labial-crural fold, excision should not extend any further than that point. Most subsequent investigators began to excise a progressively thinner skin bridge in order to try to decrease the incidence of wound complications (Fig. 53-6). However, carcinoma of the vulva spreads by embolization via the lymphatics and not by permeation through the lymphatics (Parry-Jones, 1963; DiSaia et al, 1979). In one study, multiple random sections of the skin bridge failed to reveal evidence of any undetected disease (DiSaia et al, 1979). With this in mind, several investigators have proposed excising the lymph nodes through separate incisions (Taussig, 1940; Ballon and Lamb, 1975; DiSaia et al, 1979; Hacker et al, 1981; Berman et al, 1989), or through undermining of the skin bridge via the vulvectomy incision (Patsner and Mann, 1988) to avoid removing the skin bridge and decrease postoperative morbidity. There have been isolated reports of skin bridge recurrence (Hacker et al, 1981; Christopherson et al, 1985). However, these seem to be rare events. Limiting the use of separate incisions for inguinal-femoral lymphadenectomy to those patients with clinically negative nodes will probably decrease this low incidence even further (Hacker et

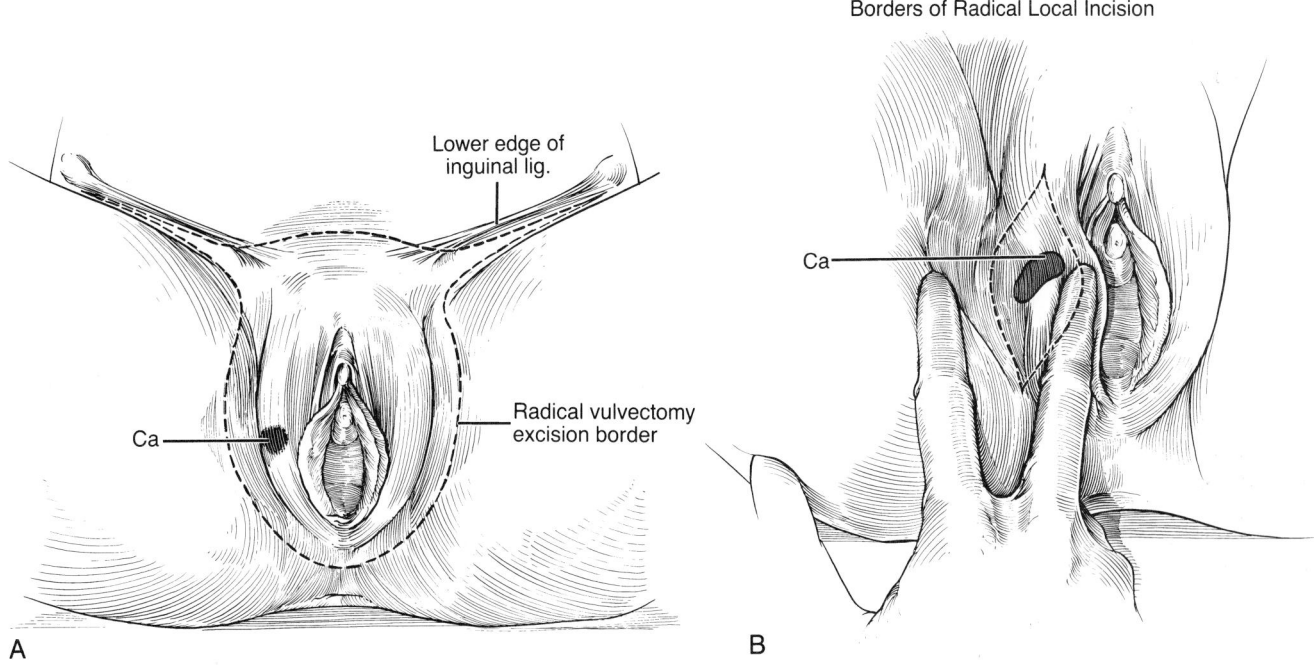

Figure 53-6
Radical vulvectomy compared with radical local excision. *A*, Excision margins for radical vulvectomy. *B*, Excision margins for radical local excision. Significantly less tissue is removed compared with a radical vulvectomy with narrow skin bridges. Ca, cancer; lig., ligament.

al, 1981). In early studies, survival for patients treated with separate incisions has been equivalent to that of patients treated with removal of the skin bridge, attesting to the safety of this approach (Ballon and Lamb, 1975; Hacker et al, 1981). Studies have confirmed that survival following the triple-incision method is not compromised even after stratifying for the stage or size of the lesion (Helm et al, 1992; Hopkins et al, 1993; Siller et al, 1995). Helm et al (1992) and Siller et al (1995) also reported no difference in local or overall recurrence rates. Hopkins et al (1993) did note a slight increase in recurrence rates that was not statistically significant, and stated that the lower complication rate made the triple-incision technique the preferred method.

The use of a radical vulvectomy to remove early lesions, however, still results in the removal of significant amounts of normal tissue. Iverson (1985) has suggested that the optimum treatment is to remove the lesion with free borders. He has proposed the use of a hemivulvectomy in order to spare normal uninvolved tissue (Iverson et al, 1981). However, for most early lesions, removal of the entire lesion with a 2-cm margin of normal tissue along with removing the deep tissue down to the inferior fascia of the urogential diaphragm will probably prove sufficient (DiSaia et al, 1979; Hacker et al, 1984b; Ross and Ehrman, 1987; Berman et al, 1989). The risk of a local recurrence appears to be more related to the adequacy of the excision margins than to the type of procedure performed (Hacker et al, 1984b; Ross and Ehrman, 1987). The use of radical local excisions (Fig. 53–6) has shortened the mean hospital stay to approximately 9 days and significantly reduced complication rates (Berman et al, 1989). Berman et al (1989) reported that the risk of a lymphocyst was only 12% and chronic lymphedema was seen in only 6% of patients who were treated with a radical local excision. Sexual function also appears to be maintained better in patients treated with radical excisions (DiSaia et al, 1979). Therefore, stage I and most stage II patients should be treated with a radical local excision combined with nodal dissections through separate incisions (Fig. 53–7). A more radical excision removing the skin bridge with the nodes should be reserved for those patients with clinically enlarged or suspicious nodes.

For larger or more advanced lesions, the standard of care in the past has been a radical vulvectomy with bilateral inguinal-femoral lymphadenectomy. However, as with smaller lesions, the goal of therapy should be to remove the lesion with free borders, and in many cases a radical procedure can still be performed leaving significant portions of the vulva (Iverson, 1985). In many cases, especially those limited to one side, a hemivulvectomy may prove adequate. Patients with clinically involved nodes appear to be at higher risk for recurrence within the skin bridge (Hacker et al, 1981). Therefore, in patients with clinically involved nodes, the skin bridge should be removed in continuity with the nodes to decrease that risk.

Lesions that have involved the urethra, perineum, rectum, or bone have been more difficult to approach. Portions of the pubic bone can be resected in continuity with the primary lesion in many cases without affecting the stability of the pelvis, and survival of 50% or better can be obtained in cases where the bone is involved (King et al, 1989). Exenterative procedures have been used for patients with extensive involvement of the vulva impinging on either the urethra, vagina, or rectum. The 5-year survival for patients treated with some type of exenteration is in the 50% to 65% range (Morley, 1976; Cavanagh and Shepherd, 1982). A review of patients treated by exenteration revealed that, as with early disease, the presence of lymph node metastasis is strongly correlated with poor survival (Hopkins and Morley, 1992). However, these extensive procedures are usually accompanied by significant postoperative complications and often involve significant psychological adjustment. In some cases, resection can be accomplished removing the perianal skin, but leaving the sphincter intact. However, if there is damage to the sphincter or anal canal during the operation, there is a significant risk of subsequent fecal incontinence (Hoffman et al, 1989). As an alternative to exenteration, preoperative radiation therapy may allow shrinkage of the primary lesion to the extent that its removal can be accomplished by a radical vulvectomy or modified radical vulvectomy with preservation of the rectum, vagina, or bladder. Several investigators have reported satisfactory results when 4000 to 5500 rads are given preoperatively followed by radical vulvectomy (Hacker et al, 1984a; Boronow et al, 1987; Rotmensch et al, 1990). At least 75% of patients will have regression of the tumor during radiation therapy. In order to try to increase response rates, 5-fluorouracil and other agents have been added to radiation therapy both as chemotherapeutic agents and radiation sensitizers. Landoni et al (1996) reported an 80% response rate with a 31% pathologic complete response rate. It is unclear yet whether the added toxicity will also add to survival or disease-free survival. Boronow et al (1987) reported that they were able to preserve 95% of the organs at risk for removal during an exenterative procedure. In that same series, they recorded a 75% 5-year survival by life table analysis for primary therapy of advanced-stage disease. Although some patients may eventually fail or develop radiation complications necessitating exenteration or diversion, it appears the vast majority of patients can be spared an exenterative procedure.

Resections of large portions of the vulva either as part of a radical vulvectomy or as an exenterative procedure may result in a considerable defect on the vulva that is difficult to close. Several techniques have been described to try to allow reconstruction of the vulva and help prevent scarring or other deformities that might result in disfigurement and dyspareunia. The use of full-thickness rhomboid flaps has allowed for closure of large defects, especially in

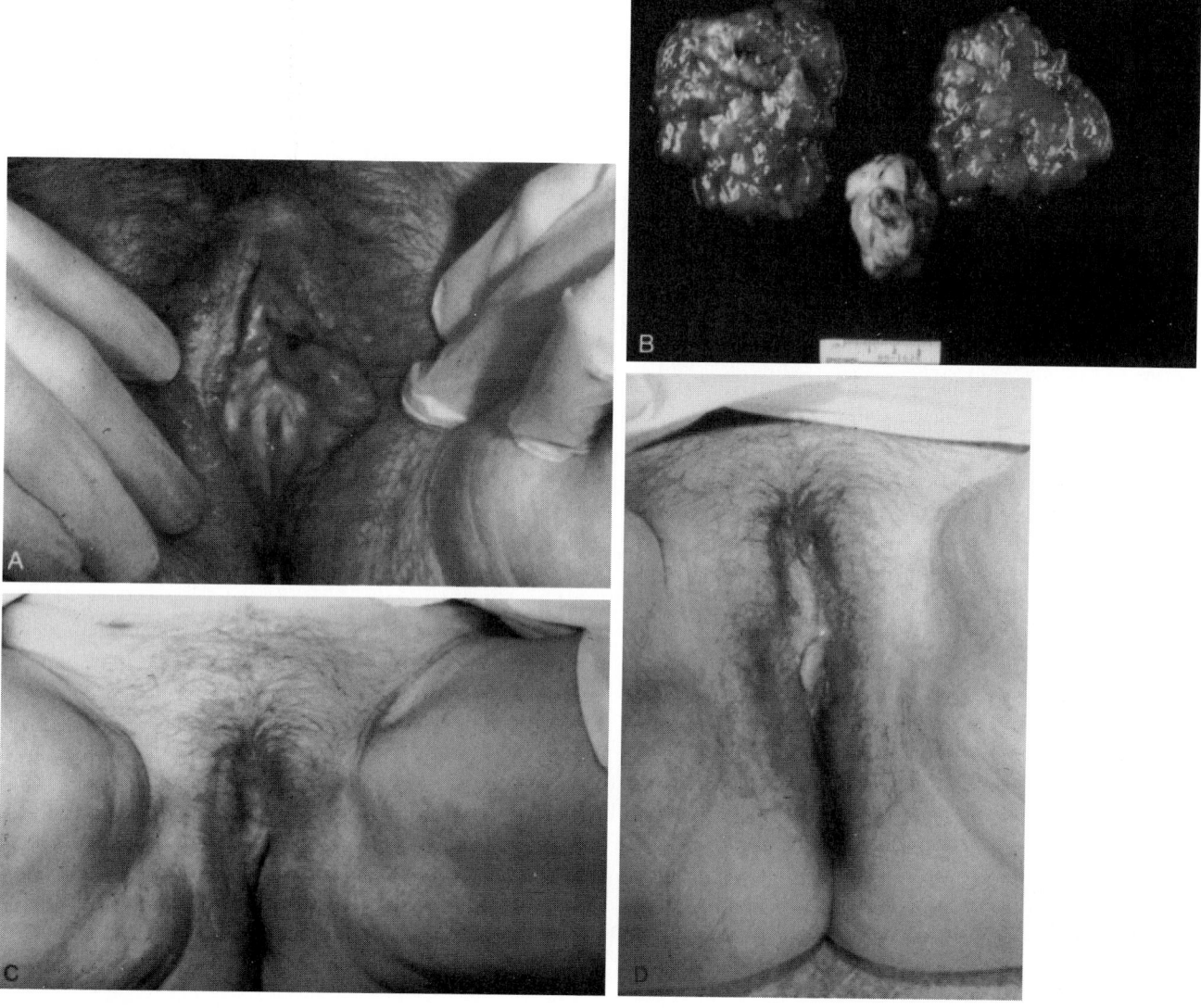

Figure 53–7
Stage I cancer of the vulva. *A*, Preoperative view of the lesion. *B*, The operative specimen. *C*, Postoperative result. *D*, Close-up view of the postoperative result.

the perianeal area (Barnhill et al, 1983; Hoffman et al, 1990b). The use of split-thickness skin grafts to cover extensive vulvar defects has been reported (Caglar et al, 1990). It was thought that the use of a split-thickness skin graft was associated with minimal complications and achieved excellent cosmetic and functional outcomes. If there is a significantly large defect, the use of gracilis myocutaneous flaps may provide not only satisfactory cosmetic results but also a new blood supply to aid healing and allow restoration of a near-normal anatomy (Wheeless et al, 1979; Massey, 1986) (Fig. 53–8). The gracilis flap could also be rotated medially and up into a vaginal defect to aid in vaginal reconstruction after extensive resections or exenteration (Burke et al, 1995). An inferiorly based transverse rectus abdominus flap can

also be used to cover large defects (Patsner and Hetzler, 1994).

Radiation Therapy

In general, radiation therapy has not been used as a primary treatment modality for carcinoma of the vulva because the vulva was thought to tolerate radiation very poorly. The incidence of moist desquamation is very high in treating the vulva with radiation (Fairey et al, 1985; Pao et al, 1988). The development of a moist desquamation will of course require interruption of therapy, and meticulous skin care is necessary during therapy to try to prevent and avoid these interruptions. Radiation may be particularly effective in preventing recurrence in pa-

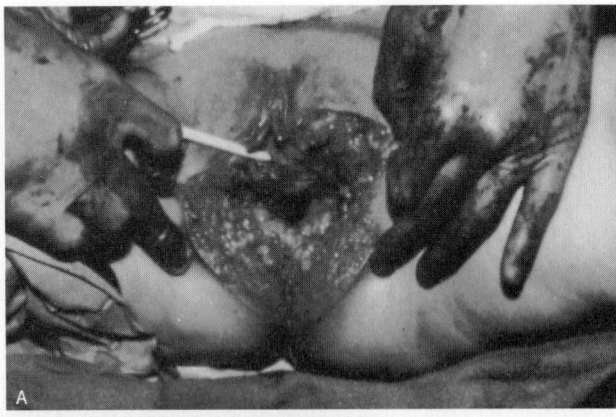
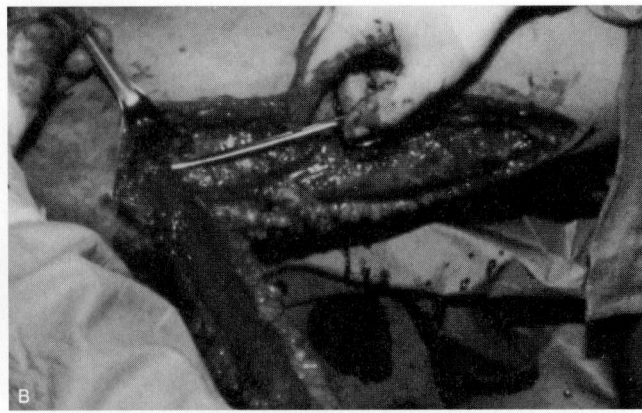
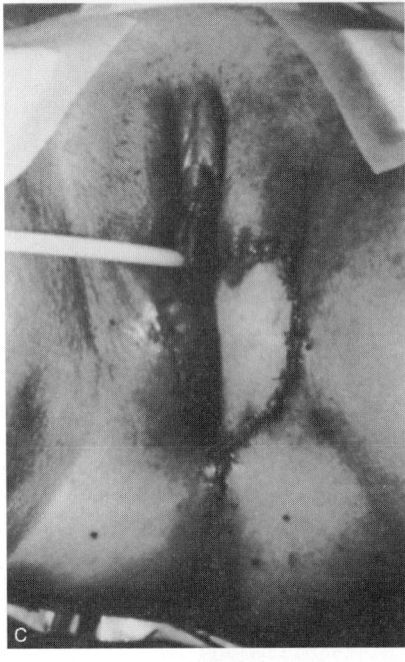

Figure 53–8
Vulvar reconstruction with flaps. *A*, Operative defect. *B*, Gracilis flap being isolated. *C*, Completed reconstruction.

tients who had compromised margins on their initial resection (Fairey et al, 1985; Pao et al, 1988).

Radiation therapy may also be effective as a postoperative adjuvant therapy to treat the groin nodes (Daly and Million, 1974). The report by the Gynecologic Oncology Group appeared to show a poorer result with radiation, but the dose to the inguinal nodes may have been suboptimal (Stehman et al, 1992b). External beam radiation has been shown to be particularly effective in treating the pelvic nodes in patients who have been found to have positive groin nodes (Homesley et al, 1986). Interstitial implants have been used in addition to external radiation in locally advanced cases. Although this has been relatively effective in producing regression of the lesions, the complication rates have been exceedingly high with significant radiation necrosis (Hoffman et al, 1990a).

As discussed earlier, radiation therapy has been effective in reducing the size of the primary lesion to allow performance of a radical vulvectomy in order to clear advanced disease and preserve the rectum, vagina, or bladder (Hacker et al, 1984a; Boronow et al, 1987; Rotmensch et al, 1990).

Chemotherapy

Distant disease may initially be seen on presentation with cancer of the vulva. More often distant disease is seen as a form of recurrent disease, especially in patients who have multiple positive inguinal nodes (Hacker et al, 1983a). The chemotheraputic regimens used in treatment of squamous cell cancer of the vulva have been similar to those used in squamous cell carcinoma of the cervix. *Cis*-platinum has been the most effective single agent used in squamous cell carcinoma of the vulva; unfortunately, multiagent therapies based on *cis*-platinum have not shown any additional efficacy and for the most part have only resulted in increased morbidity.

Chemotherapy has been used as an adjuvant to radiation therapy. Several studies have shown that 5-fluorouracil with or without mitomycin-C could be administered in combination with radiation therapy as a radiation sensitizer to enhance the response (Levin et al, 1986; Thomas et al, 1989). It appears that the addition of chemotherapy to radiation therapy may enhance the radiation effect and allow further reduction in tumor size prior to an operative procedure.

Treatment Planning

The status of the inguinal lymph nodes is the most important prognostic factor for patients with carcinoma of the vulva. Using the clinical status of these nodes as a clinical starting point, an algorithm for the possible management of patients can be developed (Fig. 53–9).

Recurrent Disease

In general, the guidelines for treatment of recurrent carcinoma of the vulva are similar to those for the management of the initial disease. Unfortunately, because of the development of systemic disease in patients with multiple positive inguinal nodes (Hacker et al, 1983a), successful treatment of recurrent carcinoma is usually seen only in patients presenting with a local recurrence, and survival is unusual for patients with either groin or distant recurrences (Podratz et al, 1982; Hacker et al, 1983a; Hopkins et al, 1990). There is an approximately 50% survival for recurrent local disease following surgical resection (Podratz et al, 1982; Hopkins et al, 1990). Hopkins et al (1990) also reported that the status of the lymph nodes at the time of recurrence was highly significant in predicting outcome, with no survivors when lymph nodes were involved compared to an approximately 80% survival in those patients with negative lymph nodes. Radiation therapy alone may occasionally be effective in curing small-volume local disease (Prempree and Amornmarn, 1984). However, radiation therapy has usually been used to reduce lesion size prior to excision (Boronow et al, 1987) or in combination with chemotherapy (as a sensitizing agent) for recurrent disease (Thomas et al, 1989).

MELANOMA

Epidemiology

Malignant melanoma accounts for 5% to 10% of all primary vulvar malignancies (Yackel et al, 1970; Chung et al, 1975). The mean age at presentation is approximately 55, with the majority of patients presenting in the fifth and sixth decades. However, patients have been seen from 17 to 84 (Yackel et al, 1970; Chung et al, 1975).

Unfortunately, many patients often present with a lump, which is the most common presenting symptom and is seen in almost half of patients. Other presenting symptoms include bleeding in about a third of patients and occasionally pruritis (Yackel et, 1970; Chung et al, 1975; Podratz et al, 1983a).

Histology

Histologically, the lesions can consist of any of the cell types typically seen in melanoma: epithelioid, spindle, nevoid, or a mixture (Chung et al, 1975). Amelanotic lesions are occasionally seen. Special stains for either melanin or S-100 protein may help in proving that an amelanotic lesion is actually a melanoma. Various patterns of growth may be seen: superficial spreading melanoma; nodular melanoma (Fig. 53–10); and melanoma of squamous mucosa, which is a variant of the lentigo-maligna melanoma (Chung et al, 1975). Nodular melanoma appears to have a worse 5-year survival rate because of its tendency to invade deeper than superficial spreading melanoma (Podratz et al, 1983a).

Prognostic Factors

In general, the outlook for malignant melanoma is significantly worse than for squamous cell carcinoma, with survival rates ranging from 30% to 55% (Yackel et al, 1970; Chung et al, 1975; Podratz et al, 1983a). As with squamous cell carcinomas, survival is related to involvement of the primary nodes. Yackel et al (1970) found approximately 25% of patients had involved nodes. None of the patients with positive nodes survived 5 years, compared to 44% of patients with negative nodes. Chung et al (1975) found no survivors with clinically positive nodes that were removed, and only 2 of 13 patients with microscopic nodal involvement survived more than 10 years. One of these patients eventually died of disease at 12 years. Jaramillo et al (1985) also found a 25% incidence of involved inguinal-femoral nodes, and all these patients died of disease. Therefore, the presence of metastatic disease in the primary nodes is a very poor prognostic sign.

The most important prognostic indicator for survival with vulvar melanoma appears to be the depth of invasion. This was first reported by Chung et al (1975). They recommended modifying the Clark's levels of invasion that were used in cutaneous melanoma because of differences in the vulvar skin. Chung et al (1975) found that survival was proportional to the described level of invasion. Of the eight patients with level 2 invasion, none died of disease. Sixty percent of those with level 3 or 4 invasion died of disease, and 80% with level 5 invasion died of disease. Other investigators have also found decreasing survival with increasing level of invasion (Podratz et al, 1983a; Jaramillo et al, 1985; Trimble et al, 1992). Podratz et al (1983a) also reported that only patients with level 4 or 5 invasion were found to have positive nodes. Several investigators began to measure the thickness of melanoma as reported by

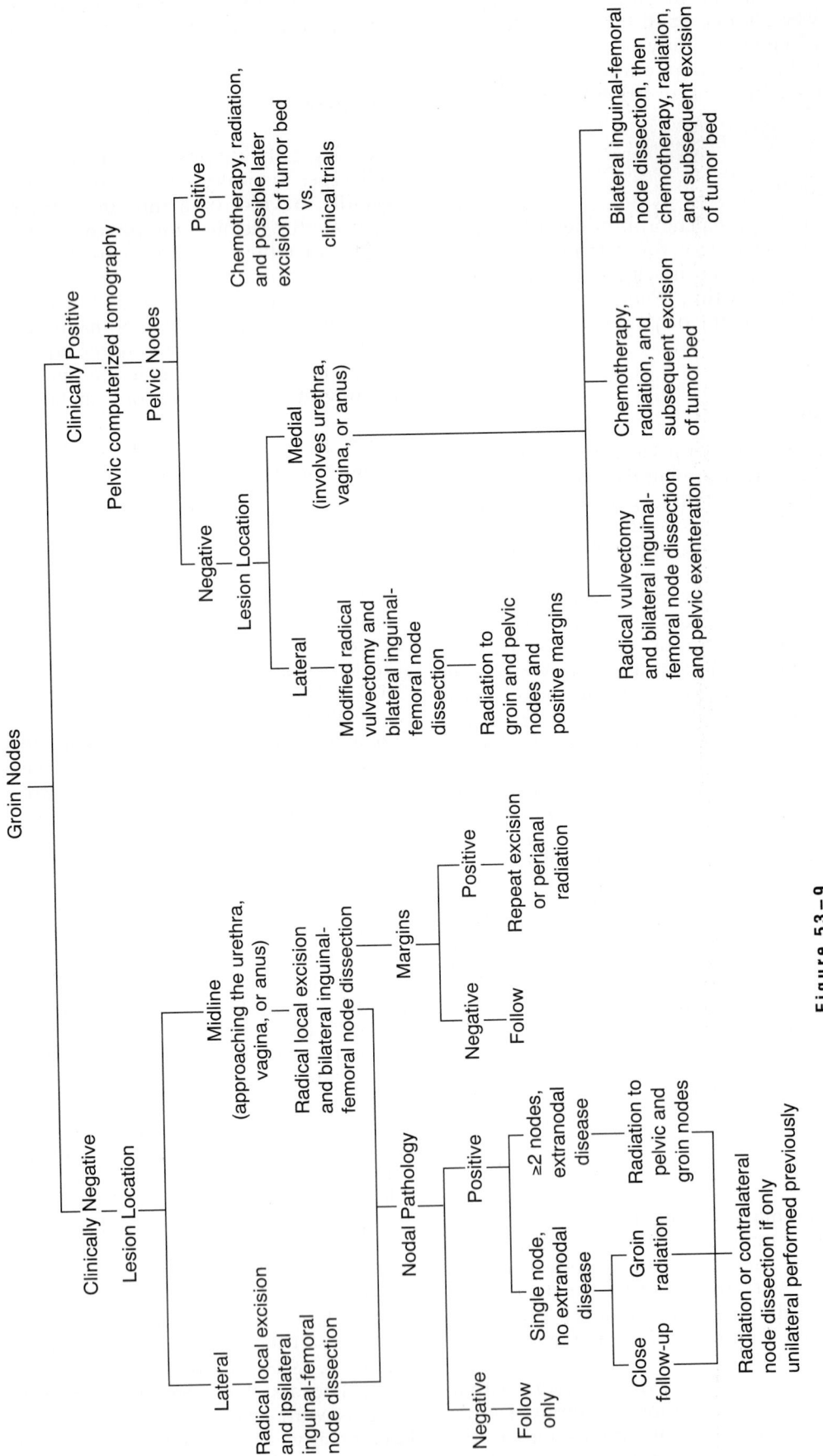

Figure 53-9
Treatment algorithm for management of patients with vulvar cancer.

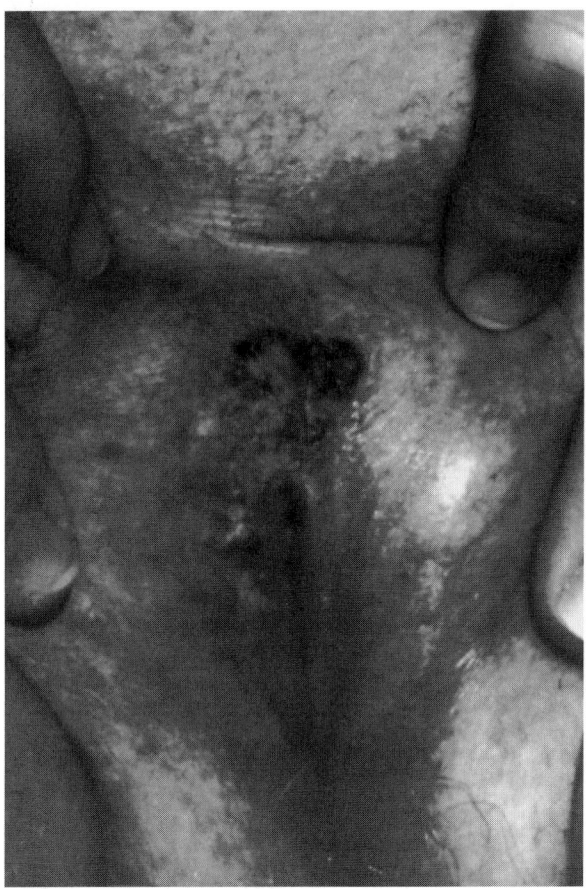

Figure 53-10
Superficial spreading form of melanoma.

Treatment

The standard therapy for malignant melanoma has consisted of radical vulvectomy with bilateral inguinal-femoral lymphadenectomy, along with a pelvic lymphadenectomy in all cases. This recommendation was made because of the poor prognosis of the disease, along with what was believed to be the potential for satellite lesions along the skin and the possibility that melanoma could spread directly to the pelvic nodes (Yackel et al, 1970; Chung et al, 1975; Morley, 1976). It was even thought that, if the lesions impinged upon adjacent structures (i.e., the urethra, vagina, and rectum), exenteration would be indicated rather than compromise the medial margin of resection (Yackel et al, 1970; Podratz et al, 1983a). However, as with squamous carcinoma of the vulva, Jaramillo et al (1985) found no patients had positive pelvic nodes with negative inguinal-femoral nodes. Yackel et al (1970) also found positive pelvic nodes only in patients with involved inguinal-femoral nodes. Therefore, the role of a prophylactic pelvic lymphadenectomy appears to be negligible. The role of the inguinal-femoral lymphadenectomy has also been questioned, especially in early lesions. Podratz et al (1983a) and Jaramillo et al (1985) failed to find any positive nodes in those patients with less than 1.5 mm of invasion. Podratz et al (1983a) also suggested the similarity in behavior of vulvar melanoma to cutaneous melanoma, and studies in cutaneous melanoma have questioned the role of a prophylactic lymphadenectomy in those patients with early disease (Balch et al, 1979). Patients with level 1 disease probably do not require a lymphadenectomy. However, those with level 2 and greater lesions probably should undergo inguinal-femoral lymphadenectomy (Trimble et al, 1992) until there are clear data indicating a lack of efficacy.

The role of the radical vulvectomy has also fallen into question lately. Given the poor prognosis for the disease because of systemic spread, studies have suggested that local excision only may be indicated, as in cutaneous melanoma (Jaramillo et al, 1985). In a retrospective review, Davidson et al (1987) found no difference in local control, disease-free interval, or patient survival according to the extent of the primary resection. Chung et al (1975) recommended radical vulvectomy as primary therapy. However, they reported that three of seven patients treated with wide local excision survived for over 10 years, which is not significantly different from the survival rate of those treated in a more radical manner. Rose et al (1988) reported no difference in survival based on radical versus wide local excisions. There was some suggestion that recurrence was related to the width of the margin because three of six patients with a less than 2-cm margin survived, compared to one of six with a greater than 2-cm margin. However, this result was not statistically significant. Rose et al did, however, believe that this demonstrated that vulvar melanoma is similar to cutaneous melanoma,

Breslow (1970) for cutaneous melanoma (Fig. 53–11). In his report on cutaneous melanoma, he found that thickness was the most significant measure of lesion size. Podratz et al (1983a) found that Breslow's levels were a better predictor than Clark's levels of invasion for vulvar melanoma. They thought that the introduction of Clark's levels or Breslow's thickness as prognostic indicators and staging variables of vulvar melanoma was delayed because these were introduced shortly after the development of the FIGO staging system and therefore initial reports attempted to use the FIGO staging system, which is of little value in melanoma because of the different pattern of spread. Jaramillo et al (1985) and Rose et al (1988) have also reported that survival correlated best with the thickness of invasion. The Gynecologic Oncology Group analyzed 71 patients treated with at least a radical hemivulvectomy and found that the 1992 American Joint Committee on Cancer (AJCC) staging system correlated best with progression-free interval (Phillips et al, 1994). In fact, using regression analysis, the AJCC stage was the only independent prognostic factor. Breslow's levels became the most prognostic factor only in the absence of AJCC stage.

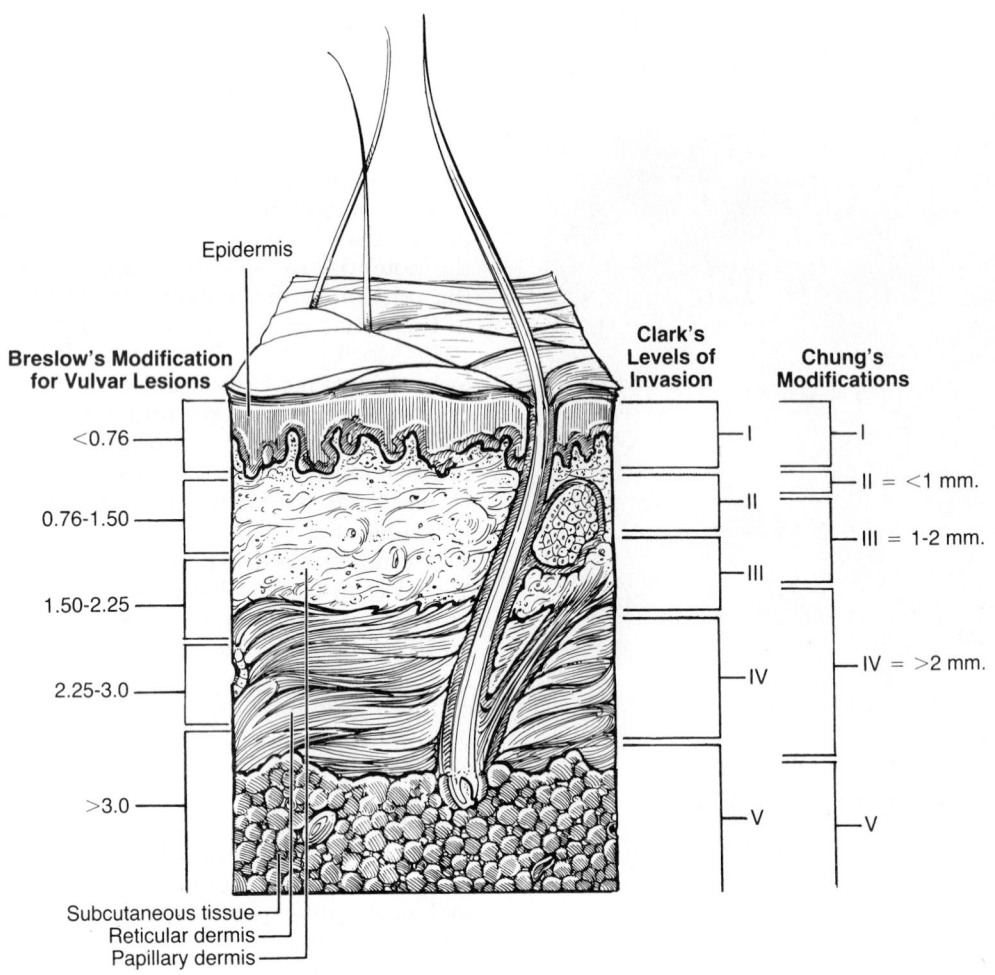

Epidermis

Breslow's Modification
for Vulvar Lesions

Clark's
Levels of
Invasion

Chung's
Modifications

<0.76 — I — I

II = <1 mm.

0.76-1.50 — II

III = 1-2 mm.

1.50-2.25 — III

2.25-3.0 — IV — IV = >2 mm.

>3.0 — V — V

Subcutaneous tissue
Reticular dermis
Papillary dermis

Figure 53–11
Schematic comparison of the different levels of invasion for melanoma.

where margins of over 3 cm have not been shown to improve survival (Aitkin et al, 1983). In cutaneous melanoma, Milton et al (1980) have shown that, in patients treated by wide local excision, the disease-free interval is inversely proportional to the thickness of the lesion; and that patients with thicker lesions are more prone to a local recurrence in the scar, whereas those with thinner lesions who eventually recur are more prone to recurrence in the regional nodes and distant recurrences. A more radical resection will not prevent these distant recurrences. As of yet, no prospective study has confirmed the failure of radical surgery to confer any type of survival advantage. However, because of the significant complications obtained with radical therapy, wide local excisions are being used increasingly in the management of malignant melanoma. Given the similarity in behavior to cutaneous melanoma (Phillips et al, 1994), this similar trend is not surprising.

Radiation therapy may occasionally be employed in the management of symptomatic unresectable metastasis. Usually with systemic or distant disease, management has consisted of chemotherapy. Currently, the chemotherapy for malignant melanoma

has been able to produce responses; however, long-term survival is unusual (Seeger et al, 1986).

BARTHOLIN'S GLAND CARCINOMA

Carcinomas arising within Bartholin's gland have been reported to constitute from 2% to 7% of all cases of vulvar cancer (Wharton and Everett, 1951; Dodson et al, 1970). The criteria used by most authors to diagnose a carcinoma arising in Bartholin's gland are a tumor involving the area of the gland with histologic evidence of transition from normal to neoplastic elements and no evidence of any other primary cancer (Chamblin and Taylor, 1972). This may somewhat underestimate the incidence of cancer arising in this area because in some lesions, especially larger ones where the normal gland has been destroyed, it may be difficult to prove transition (Copeland et al, 1986a).

The mean age at presentation for carcinomas of the vulva is approximately 56, and most patients are seen beyond the age of 50. However, the age range can be from the teens to the 90s (Leuchter et al, 1982).

The presenting symptom generally is a mass in the area of Bartholin's gland, and occasionally pain in the area of the gland is the predominant symptom (Wharton and Everett, 1951; Dodson et al, 1970). In patients with an adenoid cystic carcinoma, pain may be seen somewhat earlier than in other lesions because of extensive perineural involvement in this histologic variant of adenocarcinoma (Copeland et al, 1986b). Patients are misdiagnosed as having a pelvic abscess in as many as 25% of cases (Leuchter et al, 1982). Delay in diagnosis is not uncommon because of misdiagnosis as an abscess, and the average delay in diagnosis may be as long as 11 months (Dodson et al, 1970; Leuchter et al, 1982; Copeland et al, 1986a). The clinician should be suspicious of any persistent vulvar lesion, especially in the older population, and especially of any incision that fails to heal following marsupialization or incision and drainage (Wheelock et al, 1984).

Several histologic variants of carcinoma of Bartholin's gland can be seen. Approximately 45% are adenocarcinomas, which can be either adenocarcinoma, adenosquamous cancer, or adenoid cystic lesions (Wharton and Everett, 1951). Also, squamous carcinoma arising from the duct accounts for approximately 45% of the cancers arising from Bartholin's gland (Wharton and Everett, 1951). Transitional cell carcinoma arising from areas of the duct can account for a small percentage of lesions. Undifferentiated cancers and sarcomas are also occasionally seen.

The status of the inguinal-femoral nodes appears to be highly predictive of survival, as in squamous carcinoma of the vulva. Positive inguinal-femoral nodes are seen in anywhere from 40% to 50% of patients (Leuchter et al, 1982; Wheelock et al, 1984; Copeland et al, 1986a). Leuchter et al (1982) reported 52% 5-year survival with negative inguinal-femoral nodes, compared to 36% survival with positive inguinal-femoral nodes. They also found there was a tendency to decreasing survival with increasing number of nodes involved. Wheelock et al (1984) also confirmed a worse prognosis with positive nodes. There appears to be little risk of spread to the contralateral inguinal-femoral node or to the pelvic nodes unless the ipsilateral inguinal-femoral nodes are already involved by metastatic tumor (Leuchter et al, 1982; Copeland et al, 1986a). Copeland et al (1986a) reported a single patient who was found to have positive contralateral inguinal nodes with negative ipsilateral nodes; in this case, the involved nodes were clinically evident. They also found a single patient to have positive pelvic nodes with negative groin nodes. Leuchter et al (1982) recommended that all lesions be treated with a bilateral inguinal-femoral lymphadenectomy to try to prevent groin recurrence. However, Copeland et al (1986a) have recommended a unilateral inguinal-femoral lymphadenectomy unless there are other clinically apparent nodes, and postoperative radiation to the pelvic and/or groin nodes if metastatic disease is found in the ipsilateral inguinal-femoral node group.

Early treatment recommendations for Bartholin's gland carcinomas were for radical vulvectomy along with inguinal-femoral lymphadenectomy and pelvic lymphadenectomy (Wharton and Everett, 1951). However, as discussed, it appears the ipsilateral inguinal-femoral nodes can be used as a marker with adjuvant radiation therapy given to the groins and/or pelvis as indicated (Copeland et al, 1986a). Wide radical excision, which may necessitate a hemivulvectomy, or excision of portions of the levator muscle may be indicated (Copeland et al, 1986a). If margins are positive or compromised, postoperative adjuvant radiation therapy has been shown to produce excellent local control with recurrence rates that are in the range of 7% (Copeland et al, 1986a). This form of therapy may be effective for all histologic types of Bartholin's gland carcinomas, including the adenoid cystic variant (Copeland et al, 1986b; Rosenberg et al, 1989; Depasquale et al, 1996).

VERRUCOUS CARCINOMA

Verrucous carcinoma is an unusual lesion that can involve the entire genital tract and is occasionally seen arising in the vulva. The average age at time of presentation is in the 50s, and at least 70% of patients are postmenopausal at time of presentation (Japaze et al, 1982; Andersen and Sorensen, 1988). Both grossly and microscopically, these lesions can be confused with condylomata. They differ grossly from condylomata in that verrucous carcinoma is usually unifocal, as opposed to condylomata, which are multifocal (Powell et al, 1978). Grossly they are a warty, fungating, ulcerating, or cauliflower mass (Fig. 53–12) that can involve a significant portion of the vulva (Powell et al, 1978; Japaze et al, 1982). There may be an associated infection of the primary lesion that can cause induration and enlargement of the regional lymph nodes, which may be confused with metastases to the lymph nodes (Powell et al, 1978). Microscopically the lesions will often show fronds of well-differentiated squamous epithelium with an intact basement membrane. There will be pushing, bulbous rete pegs with associated hyperkeratosis and acanthosis, but anaplasia is not present (Powell et al, 1978; Japaze et al, 1982). These may be confused with condylomata; however, verrucous carcinoma will not have a central core of stromal tissue within the papillary fronds (Powell et al, 1978). These lesions may be difficult to diagnose and will require extensive biopsies and communication between the clinician and the pathologist regarding the visible lesion (Japaze et al, 1982). The etiology of these lesions is not clear. However, HPV has been implicated as an etiologic agent (Rando et al, 1986).

These lesions tend to be locally invasive but have generally not been associated with metastatic spread to the lymph nodes (Japaze et al, 1982; Andersen and Sorensen, 1988). In fact, Japaze et al (1982) found no evidence of metastatic disease to the lymph nodes in

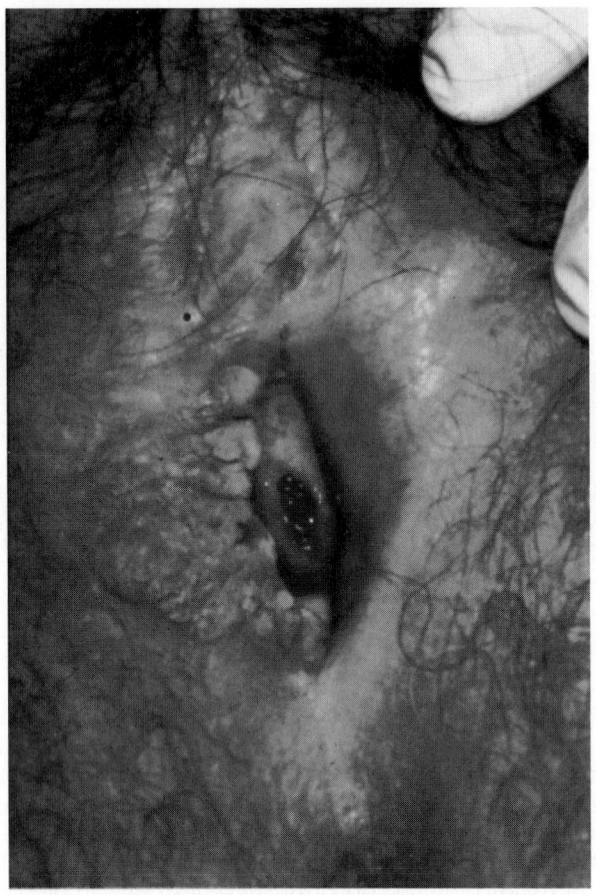

Figure 53-12
Verrucous carcinoma.

17 patients who underwent lymphadenectomy. Recurrent disease may be seen, especially with inadequate margins of excision, and may eventually lead to death (Japaze et al, 1982). However, surgery only may be adequate; Japaze et al (1982) found only one death caused by tumor in 17 patients who were treated with surgery alone. Japaze et al (1982) also failed to find evidence of any beneficial effect with radiation, and several investigators in the past reported that these lesions may become dedifferentiated and behave more aggressively following radiation (Powell et al, 1978). Current therapy for verrucous carcinoma should consist of a wide local excision with adequate resection margins (Japaze et al, 1982; Andersen and Sorensen, 1988). In select cases with hypertrophied lymph nodes, consideration can be given to a lymph node sampling rather than a radical dissection (Japaze et al, 1982).

PAGET'S DISEASE

Extramammary Paget's disease is a well-defined entity, and it appears that most cases of Paget's disease are intraepithelial and may persist as such for long periods of time. These lesions may recur; however, they are usually associated with long-term survival (Parmley et al, 1975). It was previously thought that extramammary Paget's disease was due to intraepidermal spread from an underlying sweat gland carcinoma that could not necessarily be found in all cases (Parmley et al, 1975; Hart and Millman, 1977). In reviewing the literature, Hart and Millman (1977) found that 19% of patients with Paget's disease had an underlying invasive carcinoma. They believed that the actual incidence was probably lower than this figure because of the tendency to overreport unusual cases. Feuer et al (1990) found only one invasive adenocarcinoma in 19 patients seen for Paget's disease over approximately 20 years. Bergen et al (1989) found no cases of invasive adenocarcinoma in 14 patients with Paget's disease seen over a 10-year span. With the small number of reported cases of an apocrine gland carcinoma arising in this area, it is difficult to formulate a treatment recommendation. It is clear that patients who have positive nodes have an exceedingly poor prognosis—all reported patients with metastasis to the inguinal-femoral nodes have died of disease in less than 5 years (Boehm and Morris, 1971; Feuer et al, 1990). It would appear that these patients are probably best managed in a fashion similar to that for squamous cell cancers of the vulva, with a radical local excision along with inguinal-femoral lymphadenectomy on the involved side, or bilateral inguinal-femoral lymphadenectomies for midline lesions.

Although the vast majority of patients with Paget's disease have intraepithelial lesions, occasionally a patient is seen with an invasive form of Paget's disease. Invasive Paget's disease is largely considered a disease of elderly white females (Parmley et al, 1975). The signs and symptoms are similar to those of other vulvar neoplasms in general, with pruritis being the predominant complaint. Usually these patients have a prolonged duration of symptoms that has averaged 6 1/2 years or more. Parmley et al (1975) found that most patients presented with palpable adenopathy. Feuer et al (1990) found that some patients may present with occult invasive disease. Invasion may be difficult to diagnose because histologically it appears very similar to the intraepithelial form of Paget's disease, containing large cells with foamy eosinophilic cytoplasm. These well-differentiated cells tend to arrange themselves in nests and other structures reminiscent of apocrine glands. Stains for mucopolysaccharides and mucicarmine are usually positive. The least differentiated cells are usually small and contain dense hyperchromatic nuclei, and are usually basal in position. Parmley et al (1975) believed that invasion developed from these more undifferentiated areas; a stem cell within the stratum germinativum probably gave rise to the undifferentiated basal cells, which could then differentiate into the more mature and classic Paget's cell. Invasive Paget's disease may be seen on initial presentation or may be found in a subsequent recurrence of what was previously intraepithelial Paget's disease (Hart and Millman, 1977; Feuer et al, 1990).

Parmley et al (1975) thought that the prognosis for these patients was poor and they should all be treated with a radical vulvectomy with nodes. However, of their seven patients, six already had palpable inguinal nodes at the time of presentation and one patient had positive supraclavicular nodes. Only one patient survived over 5 years, and this was the patient with a small ulcer and negative nodes. Feuer et al (1990) also had a patient with invasive Paget's disease who survived over 2 years following a radical vulvectomy with bilateral groin node dissection. They also, however, found two patients who developed what they described as a minimally invasive Paget's lesion; both survived greater than 10 years following a simple vulvectomy in one case and a partial vulvectomy with pelvic radiation in the other. Again, it is difficult to make any treatment recommendations because of the limited number of cases. Because the status of the inguinal-femoral nodes appears to be highly prognostic, it would appear that patients should undergo inguinal-femoral lymphadenectomy for its prognostic information. A radical local excision of the area of the primary lesion probably should be performed with wide margins because of the tendency of Paget's cells to invade laterally along the dermis.

Patients with Paget's disease deserve careful screening for other cancers (especially breast and colon), because several investigators have found anywhere from a 26% to a 29% incidence of other invasive cancers in these patients (Hart and Millman, 1977; Feuer et al, 1990). There also appears to be a somewhat increased propensity for the development of breast cancer in these patients (Boehm and Morris, 1971). Therefore, screening should include mammography along with careful evaluation of the entire genital tract and probably screening for carcinoma of the colon.

ADENOSQUAMOUS CARCINOMA

Adenocarcinomas account for only a small fraction of primary carcinoma of the vulva. Lasser et al (1974) found that 30% of patients with cancer of the vulva had focal adenoid changes. However, in that series, only 4% of patients had a lesion that consisted largely of what they described as adenoid carcinoma. Underwood et al (1978) found that 13% of the patients in their series had an adenosquamous carcinoma. These reviews, which are retrospective in nature, probably overestimate the incidence of adenocarcinoma and adenosquamous carcinoma. Johnson and Helwig (1966) reported an extensive review of 155 patients who had 213 lesions of cutaneous adenocarcinoma; greater than 50% of the lesions were nodular and they often presented with either draining, itching, or tenderness in the area. Johnson and Helwig believed that these lesions probably arose in senile keratosis and usually arose in sun-exposed areas. They believed these lesions

arose from a totipotential cell in the epidermis or from the piliary sheath. Underwood et al (1978), using electron microscopy, confirmed that adenosquamous lesions did indeed produce mucin, and thought they probably arose in the mucin-producing cells of the skin appendages.

The cutaneous lesions in Johnson and Helwig's (1966) series appeared to show a good prognosis, with only 5 of 155 patients dying as a result of the disease. However, lesions arising in the vulva do not appear to have the same excellent outlook. Lasser et al (1974) reported an increased mortality in adenocarcinoma; however, these results were not statistically significant. Underwood et al (1978) found that adenosquamous lesions have an increased proportion of higher stage lesions when compared to squamous carcinomas, and a higher percentage of nodal involvement. Only 1 of the 18 patients in that series survived over 5 years. Based on the poor prognosis, they recommended treating patients with radical vulvectomy with bilateral groin node dissections. However, the poor survival seen would probably be a better argument for treating these lesions similarly to squamous cancers, with radical excision combined with excision of the ipsilateral inguinal-femoral lymph nodes.

SARCOMA

Despite the abundant connective tissue that exists on the vulva, primary sarcomas arising on the vulva are rare. In fact, most of the reports of sarcoma on the vulva are actually case reports. Two series have reported that leiomyosarcoma appears to be the most common form of sarcoma arising on the vulva, followed by malignant fibrous histiocytoma as the second most common form (DiSaia et al, 1971; Davos and Abell, 1976). DiSaia et al (1971) found the mean age at presentation to be 38; however, patients ranged anywhere from 18 to 64 years of age. They also found that the size of the lesion is the most important prognostic factor at time of presentation, similar to sarcomas that arise elsewhere. Although sarcomas have a greater tendency to disseminate hematogeneously, local recurrence appears to be a common problem with vulvar lesions (Davos and Abell, 1976). DiSaia et al (1971) found that only 5 of 12 patients survived without evidence of disease from 18 to 110 months, and all surviving patients had been treated with radical surgery. They therefore recommended surgical excision as the primary treatment of choice, especially for localized disease. Davos and Abell (1976) recommended a wide radical excision or radical vulvectomy, in a manner similar to that for sarcomas that may arise elsewhere. Lymph node resection should be performed at the time of primary therapy.

Copeland et al (1985) reported a series of alveolar rhabdomyosarcomas arising on the vulva. This is a variant of rhabdomyosarcoma, and all patients were in their teens at time of presentation. The only patients to demonstrate long-term survival had localized disease that was completely resected and were then treated with chemotherapy and irradiation. This lesion appears to behave in a very aggressive manner and demonstrates early widespread metastases. It also appears to demonstrate a propensity to metastasize to the breast in these young patients. Early diagnosis along with complete resection and aggressive therapy appears to be indicated in these cases.

Sarcoma botryoides or embryonal rhabdomyosarcoma may also arise in the vulva in the pediatric population. This variant of rhabdomyosarcoma is best treated with a wide excision followed by chemotherapy. The Intergroup Rhabdomyosarcoma Study Group reported that all three patients with this variant survived when treated in this manner (Andrassy et al, 1995).

REFERENCES

Aitkin DR, Clausen K, Klein JP, et al: The extent of primary melanoma excision—how wide is wide? Ann Surg 1983;198:634.

Andersen ES, Sorensen IM: Verrucous carcinoma of the female genital tract: report of a case and review of the literature. Gynecol Oncol 1988;30:427.

Anderson BL, Hacker NF: Psychosexual adjustment after vulvar surgery. Obstet Gynecol 1983;62:457.

Andrassy RJ, Hays DM, Raney RB, et al: Conservative surgical management of vaginal and vulvar pediatric rhabdomyosarcoma: a report from the Intergroup Rhabdomyosarcoma Study III. J Pediatr Surg 1995;30:1034.

Atamdede F, Hoogerland D: Regional lymph node recurrence following local excision for microinvasive vulvar carcinoma. Gynecol Oncol 1989;34:125.

Balch CM, Murad TM, Soong SJ, et al: Tumor thickness as a guide to surgical management of clinical stage I melanoma patients. Cancer 1979;43:883.

Ballon SC, Lamb EJ: Separate inguinal incisions in the treatment of carcinoma of the vulva. Surg Gynecol Obstet 1975;140:81.

Barkley C, Bonney V: Leukoplakia vulvae and its relationship to kraurosis vulvae and carcinoma vulvae. Br Med J 1909;2:1739.

Barnes AE, Crissman JD, Schellhas HG, Azoury RS: Microinvasive carcinoma of the vulva: a clinicopathologic evaluation. Obstet Gynecol 1980;56:234.

Barnhill DR, Hoskins WJ, Metz P: Use of the rhomboid flap after partial vulvectomy. Obstet Gynecol 1983;62:444.

Basset A: Traitement chirurgicale operatoire de l'epithelioma primitif du clitoris: indications-technique-resultats. Rev Chir 1912;46:546.

Benedet JL, Turko M, Fairey RN, Boyes DA: Squamous carcinoma of the vulva: results of treatment, 1938–1976. Am J Obstet Gynecol 1979;134:201.

Bergen S, DiSaia PJ, Liao SY, Berman ML: Conservative management of extramammary Paget's disease of the vulva. Gynecol Oncol 1989;33:151.

Berman ML, Soper JT, Creasman WT, et al: Conservative surgical management of superficially invasive stage I vulvar carcinoma. Gynecol Oncol 1989;35:352.

Binder SW, Huang I, Fu YS, et al: Risk factors for the development of lymph node metastasis in vulvar squamous cell carcinoma. Gynecol Oncol 1990;37:9.

Boehm F, Morris JM: Paget's disease of the vulva. Obstet Gynecol 1971;38:185.

Borgno G, Micheletti L, Barbero M, et al: Topographic distribution of groin lymph nodes: a study of 50 female cadavers. J Reprod Med 1990;35:1127.

Boronow RC, Hickman BT, Reagan MT, et al: Combined therapy as an alternative to exenteration for locally advanced vulvo-vaginal cancer II: results, complications, and dosimetric and surgical considerations. Am J Clin Oncol 1987;10:171.

Boyce J, Fruchter RG, Kasambilides E, et al: Prognostic factors in carcinoma of the vulva. Gynecol Oncol 1985;20:364.

Breslow A: Thickness, cross-sectional areas and depth of invasion in the prognosis of cutaneous melanoma. Ann Surg 1970;172:902.

Brinton LA, Nasca PC, Mallin K, et al: Case-control study of cancer of the vulva. Obstet Gynecol 1990;75,859.

Burke TW, Morris M, Roh MS, et al: Perineal reconstruction using single gracilis myocutaneous flaps. Gynecol Oncol 1995;57:221.

Buscema J, Naghashtar Z, Sawada E, et al: The predominance of human papillomavirus type 16 in vulvar neoplasia. Obstet Gynecol 1988;71:601.

Buscema J, Stern J, Woodruff JD: The significance of the histologic alterations adjacent to invasive vulvar carcinoma. Am J Obstet Gynecol 1980a;137:902.

Buscema J, Stern JL, Woodruff JD: Early invasive carcinoma of the vulva. Am J Obstet Gynecol 1981;140:563.

Buscema J, Woodruff JD, Parmley T, Genadry R: Carcinoma in situ of the vulva. Obstet Gynecol 1980;55:225.

Byron RL, Lamp EJ, Yonemoto RH, Kase S: Radical inguinal node dissection in the treatment of cancer. Surg Gynecol Obstet 1962;114:401.

Cabral GA, Marciano-Cabral F, Fry D, et al: Expression of herpes simplex virus type 2 antigens in premalignant and malignant human vulvar cells. Am J Obstet Gynecol 1982;143:611.

Caglar H, Piver MS, Hreshchyshyn MM: Prevention of infection and wound breakdown with split thickness skin graft reconstruction following radical vulvectomy [abstract]. Gynecol Oncol 1990;36:286.

Carson LF, Twiggs LB, Okagaki T, et al: Human papillomavirus DNA in adenosquamous carcinoma and squamous cell carcinoma of the vulva. Obstet Gynecol 1988;72:63.

Cavanagh D, Shepherd JH: The place of pelvic exenteration in the primary management of advanced carcinoma of the vulva. Gynecol Oncol 1982;13:318.

Chamblin DL, Taylor HB: Primary carcinoma of Bartholin's gland: a report of 24 patients. Obstet Gynecol 1972;39:489.

Charles AH: Carcinoma of the vulva. Br Med J 1972;1:397.

Christopherson W, Buchsbaum HJ, Voet R, Lifschitz S: Radical vulvectomy and bilateral groin lymphadenectomy utilizing separate groin incisions: report of a case with recurrence in the intervening skin bridge. Gynecol Oncol 1985;21:247.

Chung AF, Woodruff JM, Lewis JL Jr: Malignant melanoma of the vulva: a report of 44 cases. Obstet Gynecol 1975;45:638.

Collins CG, Lee FYL, Roman-Lopez JJ: Invasive carcinoma of the vulva with lymph node metastasis. Am J Obstet Gynecol 1971;109:446.

Copeland LJ, Sneige N, Gershenson DM, et al: Bartholin gland carcinoma. Obstet Gynecol 1986a;67:1986.

Copeland LJ, Sneige N, Gershenson DM, et al: Adenoid cystic carcinoma of Bartholin gland. Obstet Gynecol 1986b;67:115.

Copeland LJ, Sneige N, Stringer CA, et al: Alveolar rhabdomyosarcoma of the female genitalia. Cancer 1985;56:849.

Creasman WT: New gynecologic cancer staging. Gynecol Oncol 1995;58:157.

Curry SL, Wharton JT, Rutledge F: Positive lymph nodes in vulvar squamous carcinoma. Gynecol Oncol 1980;9:63.

Daly JW, Million RR: Radical vulvectomy combined with elective node irradiation for TxNo squamous cell carcinoma of the vulva. Cancer 1974;34:161.

Davidson T, Kissin M, Westbury G: Vulvo-vaginal melanoma—should radical surgery be abandoned? Br J Obstet Gynaecol 1987;94:473.

Davos I, Abell MR: Soft tissue sarcomas of the vulva. Gynecol Oncol 1976;4:70.

DePasquale SE, McGuinness TB, Mangan CE, et al: Adenoid cystic carcinoma of Bartholin's gland: a review of the literature and report of a patient. Gynecol Oncol 1996;61:122.

DiSaia PJ, Creasman WT, Rich WM: An alternate approach to early cancer of the vulva. Am J Obstet Gynecol 1979;133:825.

DiSaia PJ, Rutledge F, Smith JP: Sarcomas of the vulva: report of 12 patients. Obstet Gynecol 1971;38:180.

Dodson MG, O'Leary JA, Averette HE: Primary carcinoma of Bartholin's gland. Obstet Gynecol 1970;35:578.

Donaldson ES, Powell DE, Hanson MB, van Nagell JR Jr: Prognostic parameters in invasive vulvar cancer. Gynecol Oncol 1981;11:184.

Fairey RN, MacKay PA, Benedet JL, et al: Radiation treatment of carcinoma of the vulva, 1950–1980. Am J Obstet Gynecol 1985; 151:591.

Feuer GA, Shevchuk M, Calanog A: Vulvar Paget's disease: the need to exclude an invasive lesion. Gynecol Oncol 1990;38:81.

Figge DC, Gaudenz R: Invasive carcinoma of the vulva. Am J Obstet Gynecol 1974;119:382.

Figge DC, Tamimi HK, Greer BE: Lymphatic spread in carcinoma of the vulva. Am J Obstet Gynecol 1985;152:387.

Franklin EW, Rutledge FN: Epidemiology of carcinoma of the vulva. Obstet Gynecol 1972;39:165.

Green TH:. Carcinoma of the vulva: a reassessment. Obstet Gynecol 1978;52:462.

Green TH Jr, Ulfelder H, Meigs JV: Epidermoid carcinoma of the vulva: an analysis of 238 cases. Part 1. Etiology and diagnosis. Am J Obstet Gynecol 1958;73:834.

Hacker NF, Berek JS, Juillard GJF, Lagasse LD. Preoperative radiation therapy for locally advanced vulvar cancer. Cancer 1984a;54:2056.

Hacker NF, Berek JS, Lagasse LD, et al: Management of regional lymph nodes and their prognostic influence in vulvar cancer. Obstet Gynecol 1983;61:408.

Hacker NF, Berek JS, Lagasse LD, et al: Individualization of treatment for stage I squamous cell vulvar carcinoma. Obstet Gynecol 1984b;63:155.

Hacker NF, Leuchter RS, Berek JS, et al: Radical vulvectomy and bilateral inguinal lymphadenectomy through separate groin incisions. Obstet Gynecol 1981;58:574.

Hacker NF, Nieberg RK, Berek JS, et al: Superficially invasive vulvar cancer with nodal metastasis. Gynecol Oncol 1983a; 15:65.

Hart WR, Millman JB: Progress of intraepihtelial Paget's disease of the vulva to invasive carcinoma. Obstet Gynecol 1977;40:2333.

Hart WR, Norris HJ, Helwig EB: Relation of lichen sclerosis et atrophicus of the vulva to development of carcinoma. Obstet Gynecol 1975;45:369.

Helm CW, Hatch K, Austin JM, et al: A matched comparison of single and triple incision techniques for the surgical treatment of carcinoma of the vulva. Gynecol Oncol 1992;46:150.

Hoffman JS, Kumar NB, Morley GW: Prognostic significance of groin lymph node metastases in squamous carcinoma of the vulva. Obstet Gynecol 1985;66:402.

Hoffman M, Greenberg S, Greenberg H, et al: Insterstitial radiotherapy for the treatment of advanced or recurrent vulvar and distal vaginal malignancy. Am J Obstet Gynecol 1990a;162:1278.

Hoffman MS, LaPolla JP, Roberts WS, et al: Use of local flaps for primary anal reconstruction following perianal resection for neoplasia. Gynecol Oncol 1990;36:348.

Hoffman MS, Roberts WS, LaPolla JP, et al: Carcinoma of the vulva involving the perianal or anal skin. Gynecol Oncol 1989; 35:215.

Homesley HD, Bundy BN, Sedlis A, Adcock L: Radiation therapy versus pelvic node resection for carcinoma of the vulva with positive groin nodes. Obstet Gynecol 1986;68:733.

Homesley HD, Bundy BN, Sedlis A, et al: Assessment of current International Federation of Gynecology and Obstetrics staging of vulvar carcinoma relative to prognostic factors for survival (a Gynecologic Oncology Group study). Am J Obstet Gynecol 1991;164:997.

Hopkins MP, Morley GW: Pelvic exenteration for the treatment of vulvar cancer. Cancer 1992a;70:2835.

Hopkins MP, Reid GC, Johnston CM, Morley GW: A comparison of staging systems for squamous cell carcinoma of the vulva. Gynecol Oncol 1992b;47:34.

Hopkins MP, Reid GC, Morley GW: The surgical management of recurrent squamous cell carcinoma of the vulva. Obstet Gynecol 1990;75:1001.

Hopkins MP, Reid GC, Morley GW: Radical vulvectomy: the decision for the incision. Cancer 1993;72:799.

ISSVD Task Force: Microinvasive cancer of the vulva: report of the ISSVD Task Force. J Reprod Med 1984;29:454.

Iverson T: New approaches to treatment of squamous cell carcinoma of the vulva. Clin Obstet Gynecol 1985;28:204.

Iverson T, Abeler V, Aalders J: Individualized treatment of stage I carcinoma of the vulva. Obstet Gynecol 1981;57:85.

Japaze H, Dinh TV, Woodruff JD: Verrucous carcinoma of the vulva: study of 24 cases. Obstet Gynecol 1982;60:462.

Jaramillo BA, Ganjei P, Averette HE, et al: Malignant melanoma of the vulva. Obstet Gynecol 1985;66:398.

Jeffcoate TNA: Chronic vulva dystrophies. Am J Obstet Gynecol 1966;95:61.

Johnson WC, Helwig EB: Adenoid squamous cell carcinoma (adenoacanthoma): a clinicopathologic study of 155 patients. Cancer 1966;19:1639.

Jones RW, Rowan DM: Vulvar intraepithelial neoplasia III: a clinical study of the outcome in 113 cases with relation to the later development of invasive vulvar carcinoma. Obstet Gynecol 1994;84:741.

Kato H, Tamai K, Nagaya T, et al: The use of a tumor antigen TA-4 for the management of squamous cell carcinoma. Cancer Detect Prev 1985;8:155.

Kaufman RH, Driesman GR, Burck J, et al: Herpesvirus-induced antigen in squamous-cell carcinoma of the vulva. N Engl J Med 1981;305,483.

Kaufman RH, Gardner HL, Brown DJ, Beyth Y: Vulvar dystrophies: an evaluation. Am J Obstet Gynecol 1974;120:363.

King LA, Downey GO, Savage JE, et al: Resection of the pubic bone as an adjunct to management of primary, recurrent, and metastatic pelvic malignancies. Obstet Gynecol 1989;73:1022.

Krupp PJ, Bohm JW: Lymph gland metastases in invasive squamous cell cancer of the vulva. Am J Obstet Gynecol 1978;130:943.

Krupp PJ, Lee FYL, Bohm JW, et al: Prognostic parameters and clinical staging criteria in epidermoid carcinoma of the vulva. Obstet Gynecol 1975;46:84.

Landoni F, Maneo A, Zanetta G, et al: Concurrent preoperative chemotherapy with 5-fluorouracil and mitomycin C and radiotherapy (FUMIR) followed by limited surgery in locally advanced and recurrent vulvar carcinoma. Gynecol Oncol 1996; 61:321.

Lasser A, Cornog JL, Morris JM: Adenoid squamous cell carcinoma of the vulva. Cancer 1974;33:224.

Leuchter RS, Hacker NF, Voet RL, et al: Primary carcinoma of the Bartholin gland: a report of 14 cases and review of the literature. Obstet Gynecol 1982;60:361.

Levenback C, Burke TW, Morris M, et al: Potential applications of interoperative lymphatic mapping in vulvar cancer. Gynecol Oncol 1995;59:216.

Levin W, Goldberg G, Altaras M, et al: The use of concomitant chemotherapy and radiotherapy prior to surgery in advanced stage carcinoma of the vulva. Gynecol Oncol 1986;25:20.

Mabuchi K, Bross DS, Kessler II: Epidemiology of cancer of the vulva: a case control study. Cancer 1985;55:1843.

Massey FM: Vulvovaginal reconstruction following radical resections. Clin Obstet Gynecol 1986;29:617.

McAdams AJ, Kistner RW: The relationship of chronic vulvar disease, leukoplakia, and carcinoma in situ to carcinoma of the vulva. Cancer 1958;1:740.

Milton GW, Shaw HM, Farago GA, McCarthy WH: Tumor thickness and the site and time of first recurrence in cutaneous malignant melanoma (stage I). Br J Surg 1980;67:543.

Monk BJ, Burger RA, Lin F, et al: Prognostic significance of human papilloma virus DNA in vulvar carcinoma. Obstet Gynecol 1995;85:709.

Morley GW: Infiltrative carcinoma of the vulva: results of surgical treatment. Am J Obstet Gynecol 1976;124:874.

Pao WM, Perez CA, Kuske RR, et al: Radiation therapy and conservation surgery for primary and recurrent carcinoma of the vulva: report of 40 patients and a review of the literature. Int J Radiat Oncol Biol Phys 1988;14:1123.

Parker RT, Duncan I, Rampone J, Creasman W: Operative management of early invasive epidermoid carcinoma of the vulva. Am J Obstet Gynecol 1975;123:349.

Parmley TH, Woodruff JD, Julian CG: Invasive Paget's disease. Obstet Gynecol 1975;46:341.

Parry-Jones E: The lymphatics of the vulva. J Obstet Gynaecol Br Commonw 1963;70:751.

Patsner B, Hetzler P: Post-radical vulvectomy reconstruction using the inferiorly based transverse rectus abdominis (TRAM) flap: a preliminary experience. Gynecol Oncol 1994;55:78.

Patsner B, Mann WJ: Radical vulvectomy and "sneak" superficial inguinal lymphadenectomy with a single elliptic incision. Am J Obstet Gynecol 1988;158:464.

Patsner B, Mann WJ Jr: Serum squamous cell carcinoma antigen levels in patients with invasive squamous vulvar and vaginal cancer: a preliminary report. Gynecol Oncol 1989;33:323.

Phillips GL, Bundy BN, Okagaki T, et al: Malignant melanoma of the vulva treated by radical hemivulvectomy: a prospective study of the Gynecologic Oncology Group. Cancer 1994;73:2626.

Plentl AA, Friedman EA: Lymphatic System of the Female Genitalia. Philadelphia: WB Saunders Company, 1971.

Podratz KC, Gaffey TA, Symmonds RE, et al: Melanoma of the vulva: an update. Gynecol Oncol 1983a;16:153.

Podratz KC, Symmonds RE, Taylor WF: Carcinoma of the vulva: analysis of treatment failures. Am J Obstet Gynecol 1982;143:340.

Podratz KC, Symmonds RE, Taylor WF, Williams TJ: Carcinoma of the vulva: analysis of treatment and survival. Obstet Gynecol 1983b;61:63.

Powell JL, Franklin EW III, Nickerson JF, Burrell MO: Verrucous carcinoma of the female genital tract. Gynecol Oncol 1978;6:565.

Prempree T, Amornmarn R: Radiation treatment of recurrent carcinoma of the vulva. Cancer 1984;54:1943.

Rando RF, Sedlacek TV, Hunt J, et al: Verrucous carcinoma of the vulva associated with an unusual type 6 human papillomavirus. Obstet Gynecol 1986;67:70S.

Reid GC, DeLancey JO, Hopkins MP, et al: Urinary incontinence following radical vulvectomy. Obstet Gynecol 1990;75:852.

Rose PG, Piver MS, Tsukada Y, Lau T: Conservative therapy for melanoma of the vulva. Am J Obstet Gynecol 1988;159:52.

Rosenberg P, Simonsen E, Risberg B: Adenoid cystic carcinoma of Bartholin gland: a report of five new cases treated with surgery and radiotherapy. Gynecol Oncol 1989;34:145.

Ross MJ, Ehrman RL: Histologic prognosticators in stage I squamous cell carcinoma of the vulva. Obstet Gynecol 1987;70:774.

Rotmensch J, Rubin SJ, Sutton HG, et al: Preoperative radiotherapy followed by radical vulvectomy with inguinal lymphadenectomy for advanced vulvar carcinomas. Gynecol Oncol 1990;6:181.

Rutledge F, Smith JP, Franklin EW: Carcinoma of the vulva. Am J Obstet Gynecol 1970;106:1117.

Sedlis A, Homesly H, Bundy BN, et al: Positive groin lymph nodes in superficial squamous cell vulvar cancer: a Gynecologic Oncology Group study. Am J Obstet Gynecol 1987;156:1159.

Seeger J, Richman SP, Allegra JC: Systemic therapy of malignant melanoma. Med Clin North Am 1986;70:89.

Shanbour KA, Mannel RS, Morris PC, et al: Comparison of clinical versus surgical staging systems in vulvar cancer. Obstet Gynecol 1992;80:927.

Siller BS, Alvarez RD, Conner WD, et al: T2/3 vulva cancer: a case-control study of triple incision versus en bloc radical vulvectomy and inguinal lymphadenectomy. Gynecol Oncol 1995;57:335.

Stehman FB, Bundy BN, Ball H, Clark-Pearson DL: Sites of failure and time to failure in carcinoma of the vulva treated conservatively: a Gynecologic Oncology Group study. Am J Obstet Gynecol 1996;174:1128.

Stehman FB, Bundy BN, Dvoretsky PM, Creasman WT: Early stage I carcinoma of the vulva treated with ipsilateral superficial inguinal lymphadenectomy and modified radical hemivulvectomy: a prospective study of the Gynecologic Oncology Group. Obstet Gynecol 1992a;79:490.

Stehman FB, Bundy BN, Thomas G, et al: Groin dissection versus groin radiation in carcinoma of the vulva: a Gynecologic Oncology Group study. Int J Radiat Biol Phys 1992b;24:389.

Sutton GP, Stehman FB, Ehrlich CE, Roman A: Human papillomavirus deoxyribonucleic acid in lesions of the female genital tract: evidence for type 6/11 in squamous carcinoma of the vulva. Obstet Gynecol 1987;70:564.

Taussig FJ: Cancer of the vulva: an analysis of 155 cases (1911–1940). Am J Obstet Gynecol 1940;40:764.

Thomas G, Dembo A, DePetrillo D, et al: Concurrent radiation and chemotherapy in vulvar carcinoma. Gynecol Oncol 1989;34:263.

Trimble EL, Lewis JL Jr, Williams LL, et al: Management of vulvar melanoma. Gynecol Oncol 1992;45:254.

Underwood JW, Adcock LL, Okagaki T: Adenosquamous carcinoma of skin appendages (adenoid squamous cell carcinoma, pseudoglandular squamous cell carcinoma, adenoacanthoma of sweat gland of Lever) of the vulva. Cancer 1978;42:1851.

van der Sijde R, deBruijn HWA, Krans M, et al: Significance of serum SCC antigen level as a tumor marker in patients with squamous cell carcinoma of the vulva. Gynecol Oncol 1989;35:227.

Way S: Carcinoma of the vulva. Am J Obstet Gynecol 1960;79:692.

Wharton LR Jr, Everett HS: Primary malignant Bartholin gland tumors. Obstet Gynecol Surv 1951;6:1.

Wharton JT, Gallager S, Rutledge FN: Microinvasive carcinoma of the vulva. Am J Obstet Gynecol 1975;118:159.

Wheeless CR Jr, McGibbon B, Dorsey JH, Maxwell GP: Gracilis myocutancous flap in reconstruction of the vulva and female perineum. Obstet Gynecol 1979;54:97.

Wheelock JB, Goplerud DR, Dunn LJ, Oates JF III: Primary carcinoma of the Bartholin gland: a report of ten cases. Obstet Gynecol 1984;63:820.

Wilkinson EJ: Superficial invasive carcinoma of the vulva. Clin Obstet Gynecol 1985;28:188.

Wilkinson EJ, Rico MJ, Pierson KK: Microinvasive carcinoma of the vulva. Int J Gynecol Pathol 1982;1:29.

Yackel DB, Symmonds RE, Kempers RD: Melanoma of the vulva. Obstet Gynecol 1970;35:625.

Yazigi R, Piver MS, Tsukada Y: Microinvasive carcinoma of the vulva. Obstet Gynecol 1978;51:368.

Young JL Jr, Percy CL, Asire AJ (eds): Surveillance, Epidemiology and End Results: Incidence and Mortality Data, 1973–77. (NIH Publication No 81–2330). Bethesda, MD: U.S. Department of Health and Human Services, 1981.

54

Vaginal Neoplasms

Michael P. Hopkins

Vaginal cancer is rare and accounts for only 1% to 2% of all gynecologic malignancies. This malignancy will always be one of the rarest because of the criteria for staging established by the International Federation of Gynecology and Obstetrics (FIGO). These criteria dictate that any malignancy that involves the cervix or the vulva be considered a primary lesion from that site. This malignancy is usually diagnosed in the elderly population, with a mean age in the late 60s and an age range from the 20s to the 90s. Thus vaginal cancer can be seen in any age group. The pathologic cell type is usually of squamous cell origin and accounts for 75% to 85% of these malignancies (Peters et al, 1985b). The remaining 15% to 25% are other cell types, which are discussed later in the chapter. The type that has received the greatest publicity is the clear cell type related to diethylstilbestrol (DES) exposure.

This chapter gives an overview of vaginal malignancies and includes a discussion of epidemiology, symptomatology, diagnosis, embryology, anatomy, staging, survival, pathology, DES-related lesions, and the treatment of vaginal malignancy based on cell type.

EPIDEMIOLOGY

Vaginal malignancy is a disease usually diagnosed in the elderly population. There has been a consistent association with cancer of the cervix and vulva. Women with either an in situ or an invasive cervical or vulvar squamous cell cancer are at increased risk for squamous cell abnormality in the vagina. This is the "field effect" and suggests that the entire genital tract is at risk (Marcus, 1960; Sturgeon et al, 1996). One unifying theory includes the human papillomavirus (HPV) as the etiologic agent. This theory postulates that the virus involves the entire genital tract, leading to vulvovaginal cervical squamous cell abnormalities. Although HPV as a sole carcinogen is an attractive theory, malignant changes do not develop in many women with HPV infection. Thus HPV is probably a co-carcinogen, with other co-carcinogens yet to be identified.

As in cervical cancer, this malignancy is probably associated with sexual activity. The squamous cell lesions are usually located on the upper anterior or the posterior vagina or the apex. Pooling or vaginal secretions and semen in this area may be an etiologic agent. Pessary use has been suggested as a cause of this malignancy, possibly from chronic irritation. However, in combining the reports of Herbst et al (1970), Rutledge (1967), and Way (1948), only 13 of 212 affected patients used pessaries. It is more likely that this elderly age population requires the use of pessaries rather than that the pessaries have caused the malignancy.

Previous radiation therapy has been proposed as a cause. Gallup et al (1987) reported a 14% incidence of patients having previous radiation therapy. Most of these patients received radiation for a cervical cancer. It is likely that the previously described field effect was the reason that vaginal cancer developed, not that it developed as a result of the radiation therapy.

A previous hysterectomy does not appear to be a risk factor for vaginal malignancy. Bell et al (1986) reported 87 patients who had undergone hysterectomy prior to the development of a vaginal malignancy; 31 of these patients had the hysterectomy performed for benign disease. Similarly, Gallup et al (1987) reported that 46% of patients had a hysterectomy performed for previous benign disease. Patients undergoing hysterectomy for malignancy receive close follow-up, and these patients are more likely to be diagnosed with an in situ vaginal lesion compared with those undergoing hysterectomy for benign disease, who are more likely to be diagnosed with an invasive lesion.

There appears to be a continuum from a premalignant state to malignant state. A distinct entity of carcinoma in situ exists, and it is considered a precursor to invasive disease. Peters et al (1985c) reported a microinvasive entity for the vagina. All these microinvasive vaginal squamous cell cancers arose in a field associated with carcinoma in situ. Three of the six patients also had a previous carcinoma in situ or cancer of the cervix. It is logical to assume that the malignancy follows from an in situ to microinvasive to a frankly invasive phase like cervical cancer. Unfortunately, because of the rarity of this lesion, there is little information available on this progression.

The cause for the rare cell types of vaginal cancer is even more obscure. A hormone, DES, has been associated with clear cell adenocarcinoma and is discussed later.

In summary, the only two etiologic factors consistently related to squamous cell cancer of the vagina are advancing age and a previous squamous cell abnormality of the cervix or vulva.

SYMPTOMS AND DIAGNOSIS

Abnormal bleeding is the most common symptom, affecting 65% of patients. This is usually postmenopausal bleeding in the elderly population. Thirty percent of patients will also have a vaginal discharge, prompting them to seek medical attention. Except for the bleeding or discharge, these patients are usually asymptomatic. Symptoms such as pain or vaginal hemorrhage usually represent advanced disease. This disease can be diagnosed at the time of routine cytologic screening (annual Papanicolaou, or Pap, smear). Importantly, if the cervix is present, a routine Pap smear will be taken from the cervix and can be negative when a vaginal lesion is present. Alternatively, a Pap smear may be positive from the pooled secretions or cells present in the vagina. In this situation, an investigation of the cervix with colposcopy will be negative. This will usually lead to a cone biopsy, which also will be nondiagnostic. When this sequence of events is encountered, it is important to consider the vagina as a source of the abnormal cytologic findings. It is especially important, then, to inspect the anterior and posterior walls of the vagina, which are the most common sites. Many speculums, especially metal ones, can obscure a vaginal lesion. Thus it is important to include a four-quadrant visualization of the vagina in a routine examination. Careful palpation of the vagina during bimanual examination is equally important and should be routine.

It is important to continue cytologic screening in patients who have had a hysterectomy, regardless of indications. There is tendency by both patients and physicians to be less concerned and diligent once the uterus is removed. Routine cytologic screening after hysterectomy is not considered to be cost effective by some authors (Piscitelli et al, 1995; Fetters et al, 1996) because of the extremely low yield; others recommend continued screening (Hall et al, 1992). Cytology can be useful in the early diagnosis of vaginal cancer and will identify abnormalities. Bell et al (1984) reported that, in patients who had a previous hysterectomy and in whom vaginal cancer subsequently developed, 65% had positive cytologic findings and another 25% had atypical cytologic results. Therefore, continued screening of patients who have undergone a hysterectomy is necessary. The frequency of the screening after hysterectomy is unclear. Patients who are at low risk should be screened every 2 to 3 years, and those at high risk should be screened more frequently.

The diagnosis of an invasive malignancy is usually

made by visualization of an ulcerative or polypoid lesion. Colposcopy may be necessary to direct the biopsy, but, if an obvious lesion is present, a biopsy specimen can be obtained without colposcopic guidance. Ulcerative lesions are especially prominent when the patient has vaginal prolapse. A component of the ulcerative process is the continued irritation and chronic inflammation of the exposed vagina. Submucosal lesions that do not penetrate into the vagina are more suspicious for metastatic disease. Thus any palpable but nonvisible abnormality should undergo a biopsy for tissue diagnosis. For a patient who is known to have gestational trophoblastic disease, biopsy does not need to be performed. The vagina is a common site of metastases in this disease, and profuse hemorrhage can occur if specimens are taken for biopsy.

In summary, vaginal bleeding is a common symptom. The diagnosis is made either by direct visualization with biopsy or by cytologic evaluation with colposcopy-directed biopsy.

EMBRYOLOGY AND ANATOMY

The vagina is a distensible, tubular, muscular structure lined by an estrogen-sensitive, mucous epithelium. The epithelium is derived from two mesodermal sources. The upper two thirds of the vagina arise from the müllerian tract, whereas the lower one third arises from the urogenital sinus or the cloaca (Fig. 54–1). The müllerian ducts are bilateral and fuse in the midline by the eighth week of intrauterine life (Fig. 54–2). The tip of this fused structure is in close proximity to the urogenital sinus. The müllerian structures are lined by a columnar epithelium. The urogenital sinus differentiates and proliferates into the squamous epithelium, forming the lower part of

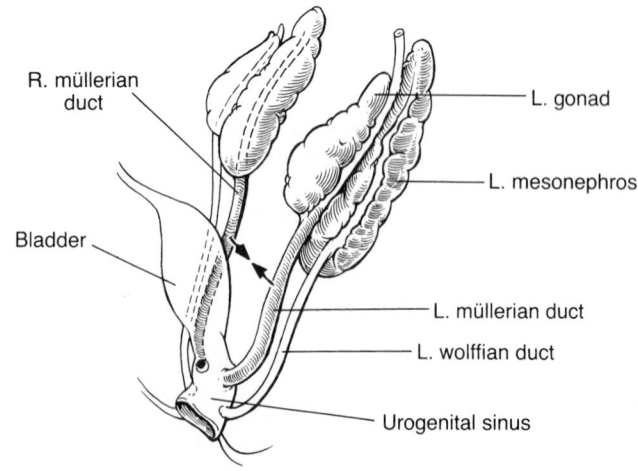

Figure 54–1
Origin of the vagina from the müllerian tract and the urogenital sinus (depicted at around 50 days' gestation, before fusing of right (R.) and left (L.) müllerian ducts).

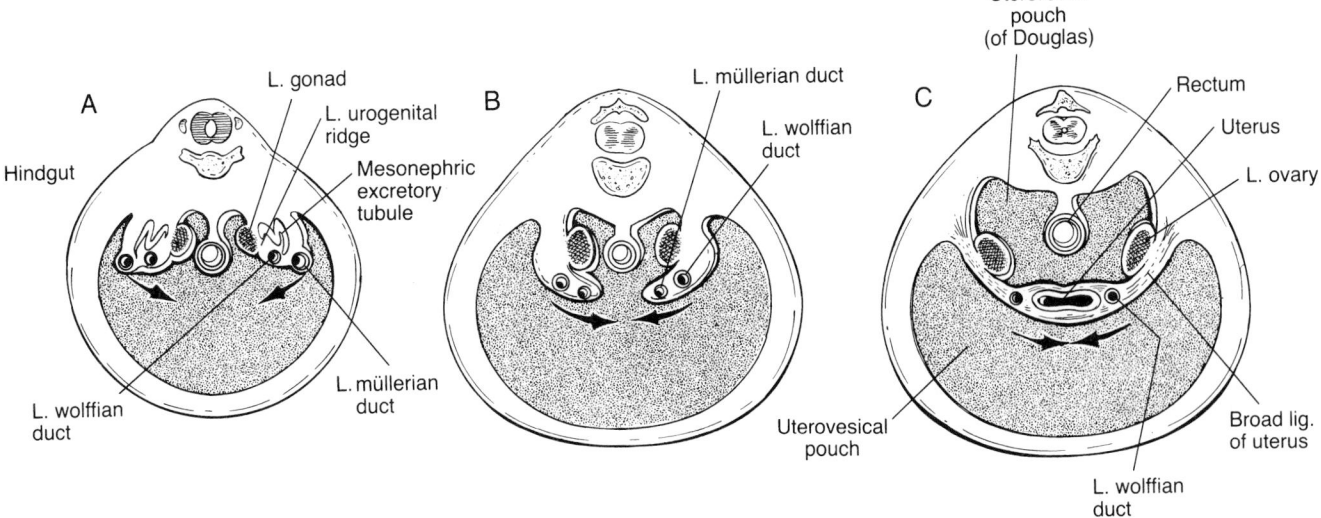

Figure 54-2
Embryologic development of uterus, ovaries, and broad ligament. Fusion in the midline by the bilateral müllerian ducts. *A,* Müllerian ducts migrate toward the midline. *B,* Further migration of müllerian ducts. *C,* Müllerian ducts have fused in the midline and wolffian ducts will degenerate. Fused müllerian ducts from the upper vagina and uterus.

the vagina. During the second trimester of gestation, there is an upgrowth of the urogenital squamous epithelium that covers the columnar glandular müllerian epithelium. This continues onto the vaginal fornices and the cervix. This is usually complete by the 18th week of gestation, thus forming the hollow, epithelialized, cylindrical vagina (Fig. 54-3). In the mature vagina, the cylindrical tube is lined by squamous epithelium and is supported by a smooth muscle layer. There are large numbers of elastic and collagen fibers contributing to the distensibility and elasticity of the vagina (Ulfelder and Robboy, 1976). Thus this development from the müllerian structures and the urogenital sinus, along with its muscular supporting layers, explains the various pathologic origins of vaginal malignancy. The vast majority are squamous cell malignancies arising from the squamous epithelium. Adenocarcinoma is the next most common type, arising from the müllerian columnar epithelium. Other types can arise from the supporting stroma or muscular layers (sarcoma): the rare vaginal melanocyte (melanoma) (Fig. 54-4).

The vascular supply to the vagina is very extensive and arises from a number of sources (Fig. 54-5). The vaginal artery is a branch from the internal iliac artery. The uterine vessels, which also arise from the internal iliac vessels, have a rich anastomosing interchange with the vaginal vessels. The middle rectal artery, which also arises from the internal iliac artery, provides a portion of the blood supply to the mid-vagina. The internal pudendal artery, which arises from the internal iliac vessels, supplies the lower vagina. The lower vagina also receives a blood supply from the external pudendal artery, which arises from the femoral region. The lymphatic drainage of the vagina is complex but, in general, follows

the embryologic development of the vagina (Fig. 54-5). The upper two thirds of the vagina drain to the pelvic lymph nodes, consisting of the internal and external iliac chains. A portion of the upper vagina also can drain directly to the sacral lymph node area. The lower one third of the vagina drains to the inguinal region.

In summary, the vagina is formed from the fused müllerian ducts and the invaginating urogenital sinus. The urogenital squamous epithelium covers the columnar müllerian tissue to the squamocolumnar junction of the cervix. There is a complex anastomosing blood supply to the vagina, and the lymphatic drainage follows the embryologic development of the vagina.

STAGING AND SPREAD PATTERN

Vaginal cancer is staged according to the FIGO guidelines. The staging system is clinical and accounts for local extension of disease as well as the other known methods of spread via the lymphatic or hematogenous routes. The clinical staging is done by pelvic examination. On rectovaginal exam, the paravaginal tissues are evaluated to determine if malignancy has spread to the subvaginal tissue. When disease extends to the pelvic side wall, it is considered to be stage III disease (Fig. 54-6). Similar to cervical cancer, cystoscopy and sigmoidoscopy are performed to ensure there is no invasion into the bladder or rectum.

The distribution of cases by stage of disease is summarized in Table 54-1. Stage II is the most common presentation, with the next most common being stage I. Perez and Camel (1982) proposed a modifi-

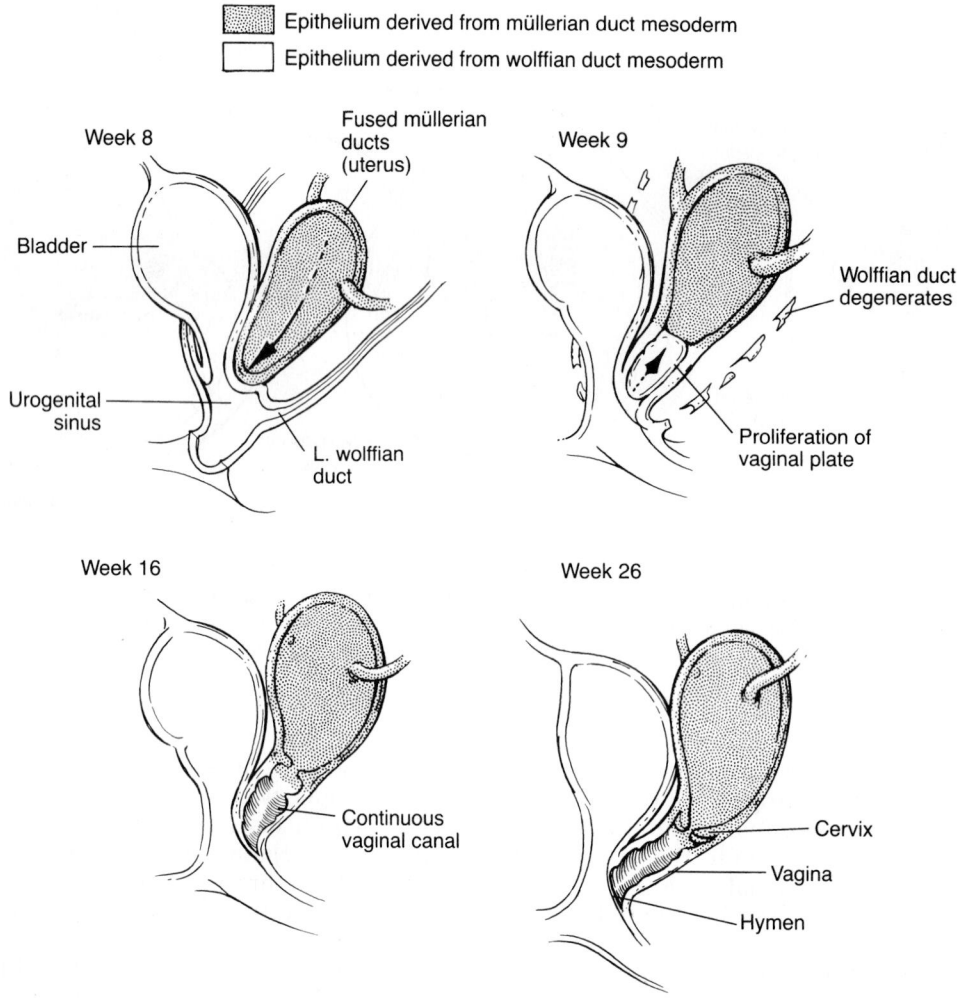

□ Epithelium derived from müllerian duct mesoderm

□ Epithelium derived from wolffian duct mesoderm

Figure 54-3
Embryologic development of cervix and vagina. Upgrowth of the urogenital sinus squamous epithelium to form the epithelialized vagina.

cation of stage II: Stage IIA invades to a minimum depth in the subvaginal area, whereas stage IIB is deeper. In their report, patients with stage IIA disease had a better survival than those with stage IIB. This modification has not gained widespread acceptance, but it is a useful prognostic feature.

Vaginal cancer spreads by both the hematogenous and lymphatic routes. The vagina has a rich blood supply, and a chest radiograph should be performed to rule out metastatic disease. Lymphatic spread depends on the site of the primary lesion. When the lower vagina is involved, the inguinal lymph nodes can be easily palpated to determine if metastatic disease is present. When the upper two thirds of the vagina are involved, the pelvic lymph nodes are at risk for metastatic disease. This area can be evaluated by computerized tomography (CT) scan or lymphangiogram. The incidence of lymph node metastases is not well documented. Pride et al (1979) reported that 16% of patients presented with lymph node metastases, and Rubin et al (1985) reported a 40% incidence of lymph node metastases when lym-

phangiograms were performed. The exact incidence may never be known because these patients are usually treated by radiation. In addition, although surgical staging is ideal to determine the extent of disease, the advanced age of these patients precludes widespread use of surgical staging, which would pose an unacceptable risk.

In summary, vaginal cancer is staged clinically. The primary routes of spread are by direct extension to the subvaginal tissue, by lymphatic spread to inguinal or pelvic lymph nodes, and by the hematogenous route to the lungs.

PROGNOSIS

The survival, stage for stage, in vaginal cancer is thought to be decreased when compared with that for cervical or vulvar cancer. The most important predictor of survival is the stage of disease. Peters et al (1985b) reported that the stage of disease was the most significant predictor of survival, whereas the

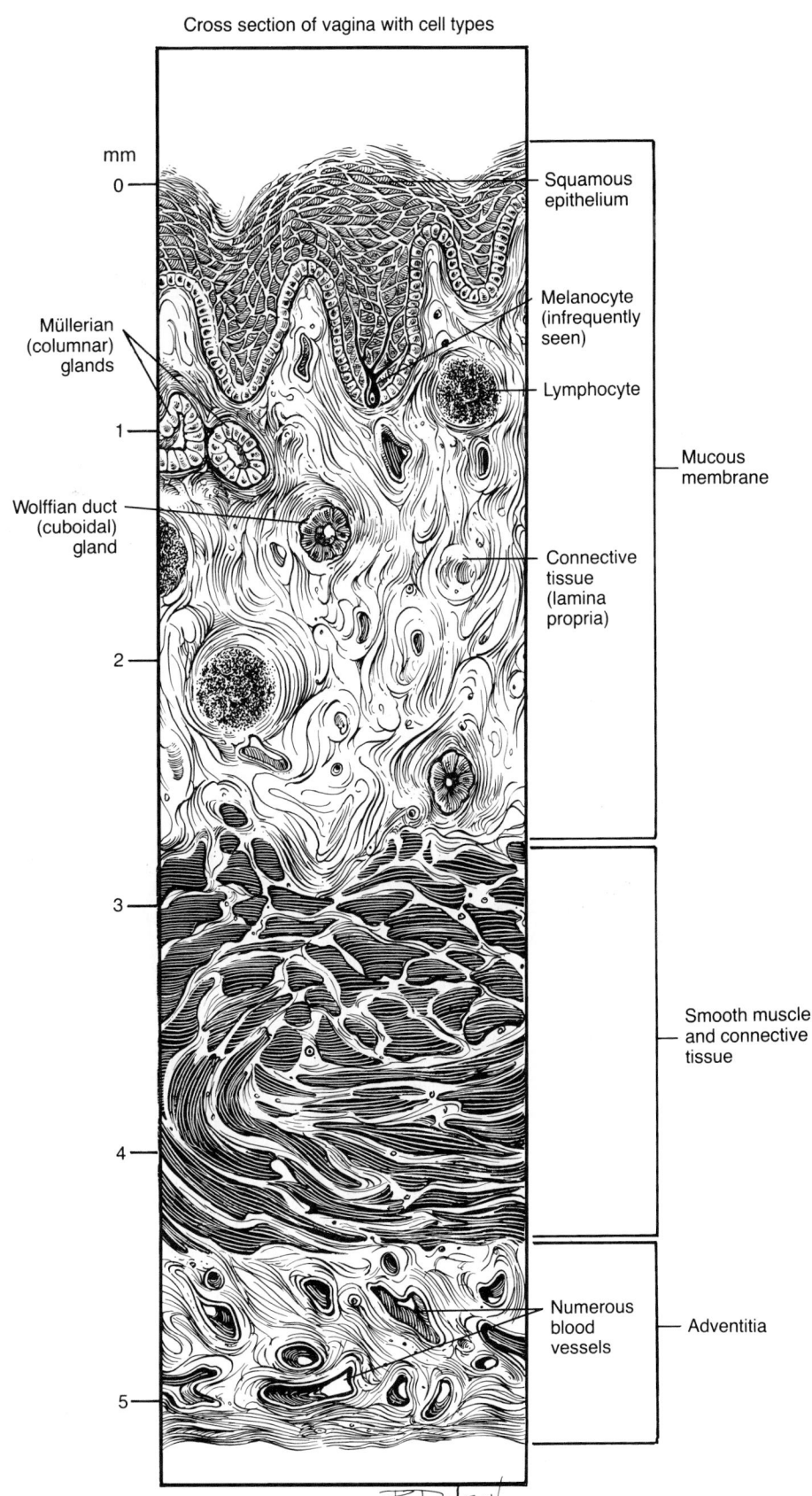

Cross section of vagina with cell types

mm
0 — Squamous epithelium

Müllerian (columnar) glands

Melanocyte (infrequently seen)

Lymphocyte

1 —

Wolffian duct (cuboidal) gland

Connective tissue (lamina propria)

Mucous membrane

2 —

3 —

Smooth muscle and connective tissue

4 —

Numerous blood vessels

Adventitia

5 —

R Dodson

Figure 54–4
Cross section of mature vagina.
Squamous epithelium and various
structures can give rise to malignancy.

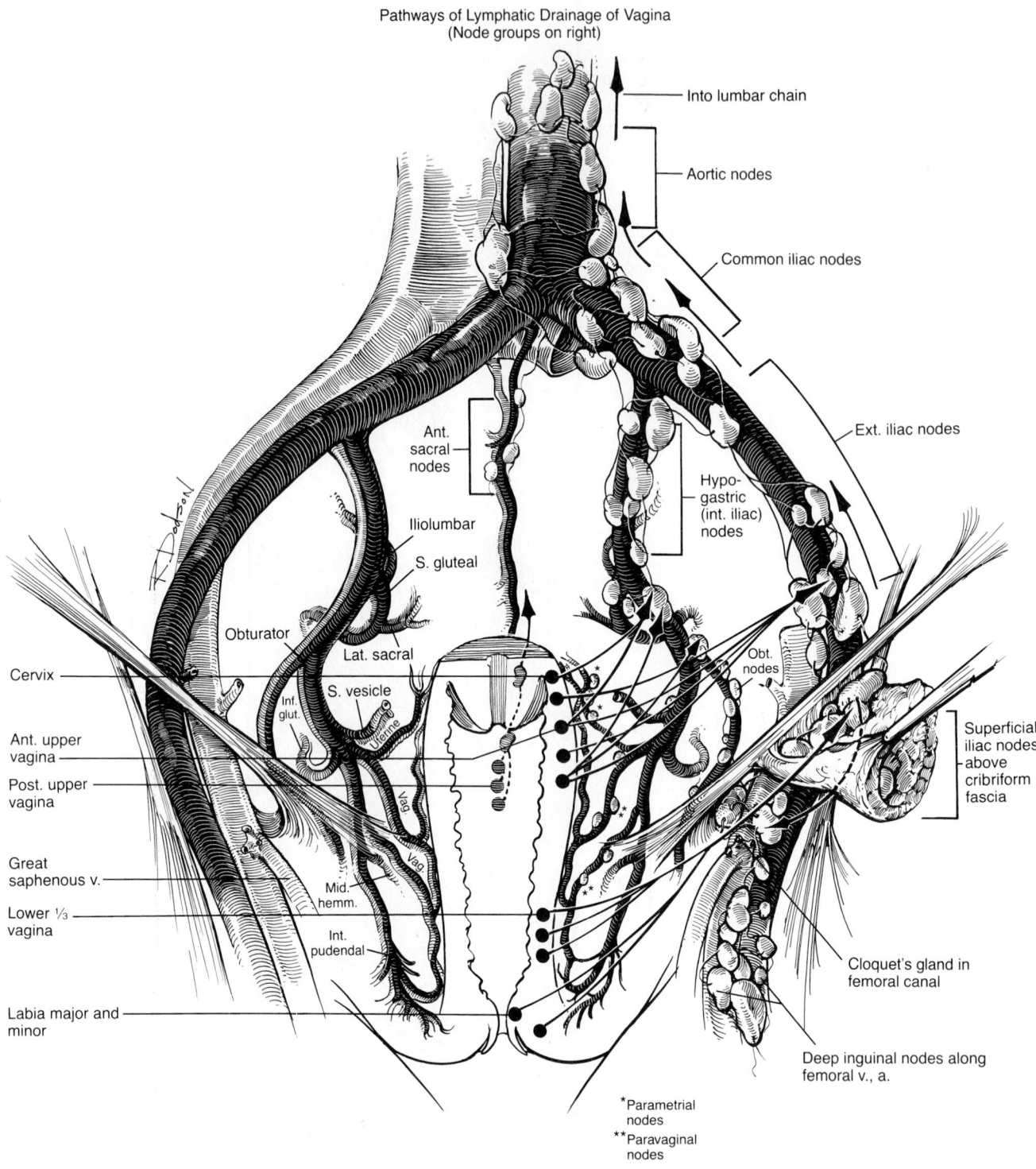

Figure 54–5

Left, Blood supply to vagina is extensive and arises from various sources. *Right,* Lymphatic drainage of the vagina. The upper vagina drains to the pelvis; the lower vagina drains to the inguinal region. Note pneumonic "navel."

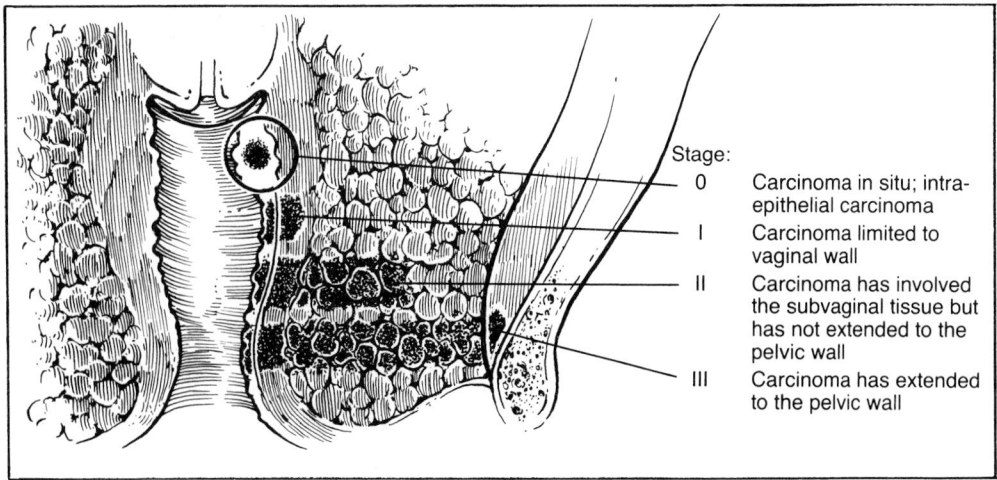

Stage:
0   Carcinoma in situ; intra-epithelial carcinoma

I   Carcinoma limited to vaginal wall

II   Carcinoma has involved the subvaginal tissue but has not extended to the pelvic wall

III   Carcinoma has extended to the pelvic wall

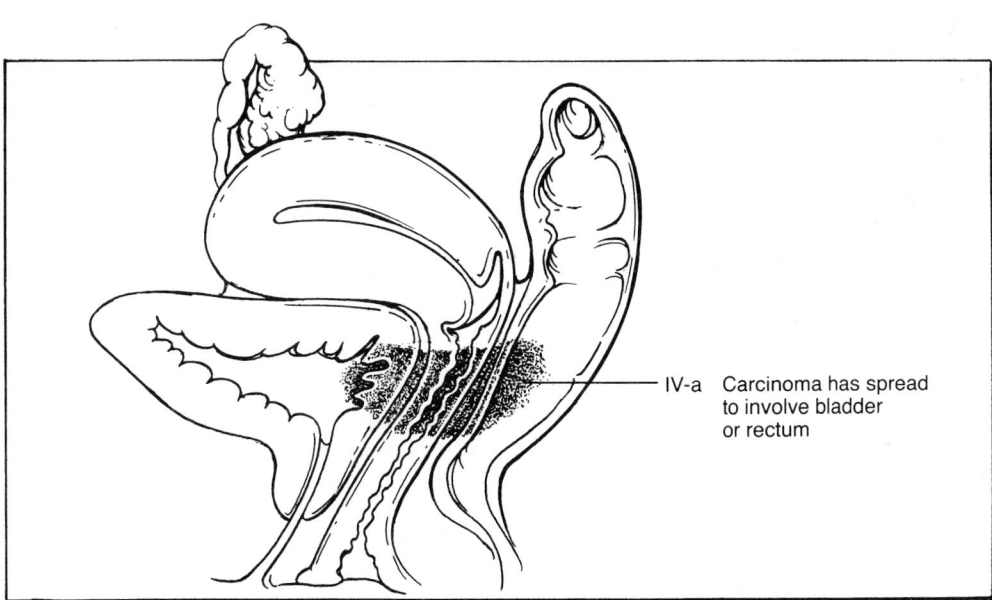

IV-a   Carcinoma has spread to involve bladder or rectum

Figure 54–6
Staging system for vaginal cancer. Metastatic disease beyond the pelvis is stage IVB.

tumor location, cell type, tumor grade, age of the patient, and whether or not a previous hysterectomy had been performed did not influence survival. Ali et al (1996) reported an improved survival for tumors located in the proximal half (80%) when compared to the distal half (40%). The vast majority of patients have squamous cell disease, and thus most of the published series are for patients with this type of cancer. In the compilation of the literature, the overall survival rate is approximately 45% (Table 54–2). This is directly related to the stage of disease: stage I, 69%; stage II, 51%; stage III, 27%; and stage IV, 4.5% (Whelton and Kotmeier, 1962; Herbst et al, 1970; Pride et al, 1979; Pirtoli and Santoni, 1980; Nori et al, 1981; Prempree, 1982; Perez and Camel, 1982;

Benedet et al, 1983; Puthawala et al, 1983; Peters et al, 1985b; Rubin et al, 1985; Gallup et al, 1987; Kirkbride et al 1995). The pathologic cell type is also an important predictor of survival. The prognosis for adenocarcinomas of the vagina is similar to that for squamous cell carcinoma. Melanoma of the vagina is associated with a decreased survival rate when compared with the squamous cell type. Sarcomas of the vagina are rare, but patients also appear to have decreased survival. Small cell carcinoma of the vagina has been reported only in a few patients, all of whom died of the disease. Recurrent vaginal cancer appears to carry a very ominous prognosis. Rubin et al (1985) reported that 30 of 33 patients died when the malignancy recurred.

Table 54-1. DISTRIBUTION FOR VAGINAL CANCERS BY STAGE OF DISEASE

STAGE	PER CENT
I	26
II	40
III	18
IV	16

In summary, the stage of disease is the single most important predictor of survival.

PATHOLOGY

If one considers the embryology and development of the vagina, the various pathologic types of malignancy that involve the vagina can be understood. The pathologic cell types are listed in Table 54–3. The squamous cell type is the most common and accounts for 75% to 85% of vaginal cancers. Squamous cell malignancies have been diagnosed in the in situ or premalignant stage and are called vaginal intraepithelial neoplasia (VAIN). Peters et al (1985c) described six patients with a microinvasive entity, all of whom survived. They considered a microinvasive malignancy to be smaller than 3 mm without angiolymphatic invasion. Eddy et al (1990) reported a further six patients meeting the same criteria, with one case of recurrence. This entity is still not well defined and further reports are necessary. Tumor invasion beyond 3 mm is considered to be frankly invasive.

The next most common cell type is adenocarcinoma, which accounts for 15% to 20% of vaginal malignancies in most series. The clear cell type related to DES exposure is the most common type of adenocarcinoma. The other types of adenocarcinoma include the mesonephric type, which on microscopic examination is very similar to the clear cell type but arises from mesonephric rests in the vagina, and the mucoid type, with an abundant amount of mucus production. Melanomas of the vagina occur rarely and are usually found in the very elderly population. These are very aggressive tumors and, as reported by Reid et al (1989), the survival is related to the

Table 54-2. SURVIVAL RATES FOR CANCER OF THE VAGINA (11 COLLECTED SERIES)

STAGE	PER CENT
I	69.0
II	51.0
III	27.0
IV	4.5
Total	45.0

Table 54-3. PATHOLOGIC CELL TYPES THAT MAY INVOLVE THE VAGINA

Squamous cell
  In situ
  Microinvasive
  Invasive
Adenocarcinoma
  Clear cell
  Mesonephric
  Mucoid
Melanoma
Small cell neuroendocrine
Sarcoma
Neovagina
Metastatic disease
  Endometrial
  Cervix/vulva
  Urothelial/renal
  Colon
  Trophoblastic

depth of invasion. Sarcomas arise from the vagina, but these are very rare. They probably arise from the various tissue elements that form the vagina.

Small cell neuroendocrine carcinoma has been reported in the vagina. Hopkins et al (1989) reported three patients with this entity, all of whom died from the disease. These tumors are similar to the small cell lung cancers, which contain neuroendocrine features and are thought to arise from the APUD (amine precursor uptake and decarboxylation) system.

With the advent of reconstructive pelvic surgery, neovaginas have been recreated most commonly from bowel and skin grafts. Carcinomas arising in the neovagina have been reported. The cell type appears to be related to the type of vagina constructed. When it is constructed of a bowel segment, the malignancy is usually an adenocarcinoma arising from the bowel, and when constructed from a split-thickness skin graft, it is a squamous cell carcinoma. Hopkins and Morley (1987), in reviewing the literature, suggested that exenteration may be the most appropriate treatment because of the high number of recurrences when only radiation therapy was given.

A variety of malignancies can metastasize to the vagina; the three most frequent malignancies are those of the endometrium, cervix, and vulva. An endometrial cancer metastasizes in a submucosal manner, probably through lymphatic channels, whereas malignancies of the cervix or vulva usually metastasize by direct extension. Other tumors that commonly metastasize to the vagina include renal cell carcinoma and gestational trophoblastic disease. With the exception of the direct extension by cervical or vulvar cancer and gestational trophoblastic disease, metastatic lesions to the vagina carry an ominous prognosis.

In summary, squamous cell cancer is the most common pathologic type of malignancy involving the vagina.

DES AND CLEAR CELL CANCER OF THE VAGINA

Clear cell adenocarcinoma of the vagina is a subtype of adenocarcinoma. It deserves special attention because of its association with DES. This was first noted by Herbst et al (1971), who reported on seven young women with clear cell carcinoma. There was a high association in this group with in utero DES exposure. This led to an abundance of literature concerning this malignancy (Ruffolo et al, 1971; Lanier, et al, 1973; Wharton et al, 1975; Noller et al, 1976; Herbst et al, 1997, 1979; Kaminski and Maier, 1983; Jones et al, 1987; Horwitz et al, 1988).

In utero, DES exposure has been associated with a number of abnormalities of the upper vagina and cervix as well as adenosis of the vagina. Diethylstilbestrol appears to cross the placenta and has an effect on the developing müllerian ducts. The effect appears to preserve the normal müllerian cells by preventing the urogenital sinus epithelium upgrowth and squamous metaplasia over the müllerian epithelium. This upgrowth and metaplasia should be completed by the 18th week of gestation, and, thus, the effects of DES are related to the age of gestation when the fetus was exposed. If DES is administered beyond the 22nd week of gestation, it will have little or no effect on the development of the structures because they will be fully formed.

Herbst et al (1977, 1979, 1981, 1986) reported that the number of anomalies were dependent on both the dose of DES administered and the timing of administration. In their reports, the incidence of structural abnormalities was higher when DES was administered prior to 15 weeks of gestation and was dose dependent. When the total dose was 700 mg, the incidence of anomalies was 7%; this increased to 60% when the total dose was 12,000 mg. Thus the effect of DES appears to be related to a large total dose given earlier in pregnancy. When administered after 22 weeks' gestation, the incidence of anomalies is less than 5%. Likewise, when given very early in pregnancy, DES does not seem to have the same effect, and, for equivalent doses, exposure during weeks 13 to 22 is most important.

It is unclear if all the structural changes noted, as well as the increase in clear cell carcinoma, are solely related to DES exposure. Sandberg (1976) reported occult adenosis in autopsy specimens in 41% of young women not exposed to DES. Squamous metaplasia also occurs with puberty and the decrease in pH of the vagina. The incidence of adenosis will thus depend on the age of the patient when she is examined. Vaginal adenosis occurs in 35% to 90% of patients exposed to DES. Forty percent of patients with adenosis have squamous metaplasia and resolution of the problem when followed over time.

Overall, structural abnormalities occur in approximately 20% of women exposed to DES. Cockscombed cervix and vaginal hood are the most common

abnormalities. Transverse cervix and vaginal ridges have also been reported.

The term vaginal epithelial changes has been used to encompass not only adenosis but the structural abnormalities. These structural changes occurred in some women prior to the DES era, but they were rarely clinically detectable. The incidence of these abnormalities depends on whether patients are self-referred and whether all patients exposed to DES are evaluated. There is a higher incidence in the group of women who refer themselves for evaluation (Kaufman et al, 1977; LaBarthe et al, 1978; Robboy et al, 1979; Holt and Herbst, 1982; Noller et al, 1983; Jefferies et al, 1984). There appears to be an increase in the incidence of premalignant squamous cell abnormalities in women exposed to DES. Robboy et al (1978, 1981, 1984) reported that squamous dysplasia and carcinoma in situ are increased almost twofold in women exposed to DES. They reported that the incidence was higher in the DES-exposed women if squamous metaplasia extended to the outer half of the cervix.

The Diethylstilbestrol Adenosis (DESAD) Project has the largest number of patients enrolled and the best available data. The annual incidence of clear cell carcinoma peaked from 1973 to 1975, which also corresponded to the years of peak usage. There appears to be a higher risk in those exposed early in utero, at approximately 9.2 weeks compared with 12 weeks. The mean age of diagnosis is 19.2 years, with a range of 7 to 34 years. The overall 5-year survival rate is 78%, and stage I is associated with a survival rate of 87%. Clear cell carcinoma rarely occurs before the age of 14 years, and the 5-year survival rate is better for those diagnosed after the age of 19. Oral contraceptives have little influence on the development of clear cell carcinoma.

A number of authors have questioned whether or not DES exposure contributes to clear cell malignancy. In the DESAD project, among 4589 women exposed to DES, four clear cell adenocarcinomas of the vagina were diagnosed. The four patients with clear cell cancer were self-referred. Piver et al (1988) reported 500 DES-exposed women without any adenocarcinoma. Kjørstad et al (1989), from Norway, reported 10 cases of clear cell adenocarcinoma of the vagina and none of these patients had been exposed to DES. Kinlen et al (1974) reported 7500 exposed women with no adenocarcinomas of the vagina. Chanen and Pagano (1984) reported no adenocarcinoma in 200 DES-exposed women. Paul et al (1984) reported no adenocarcinoma in 650 DES-exposed women. During a similar time period, Paul et al saw two patients with clear cell adenocarcinoma of the vagina who had not been exposed to DES. Noller et al (1983) reported 20 adenocarcinomas of the vagina between 1930 and 1974, 7 of which were of the clear cell type, and only one of the patients with clear cell carcinoma had been exposed to DES. This malignancy is very rarely diagnosed and, thus, an extremely large number of patients with DES exposure is needed to arrive at incidence figures. The estimated incidence is anywhere from 1 in 1000 to 1 in 10,000.

Women who have been exposed to DES need to be observed carefully, and a variety of regimens have been proposed (Anderson et al, 1979). The most convenient is to perform an initial colposcopy with a cervical and four-quadrant vaginal Pap smear. If the colposcopy is negative and there is no dysplasia present, follow-up should consist of yearly cytology, including a four-quadrant Pap smear of the vagina. The cytology should be labeled by quadrant so that follow-up colposcopy can be performed in the indicated quadrant. Additionally, careful palpation of the vagina should be performed, especially when adenosis is present. A raised, irregular area in the vagina should undergo biopsy.

Treatment of clear cell adenocarcinoma of the vagina is similar to that for other cancers of the vagina, with the exception that, in many of the women, clear cell adenocarcinoma will be diagnosed at a young age. When the cervix and/or vagina are involved in early-stage disease, a radical hysterectomy with vaginectomy can be performed. Pelvic lymphadenectomy is also necessary because of the possibility of regional metastases. With this approach, a split-thickness skin graft can be used to reconstruct the vagina, allowing for adequate sexual function. The radical surgery approach also allows for preservation of the ovaries. Senekjian et al (1987) reported a treatment method using local therapy for 43 patients with very early lesions. When only vaginectomy or local excision was performed, there was a high recurrence rate and this decreased significantly when local irradiation or local excision plus radiation was performed. Thus, when local excision of the vaginal lesion is performed, local radiation therapy should be included. Pelvic lymphadenectomy is necessary when using local therapy to ensure that regional metastases are not present. This is an excellent option for young women who wish to preserve reproductive function. Patients with lesions beyond stage I disease should be treated by radiation therapy, similar to other vaginal cancers.

In summary, the incidence of cervical vaginal abnormalities in DES-exposed women is dose-related and time-related. Adenosis is a benign condition that resolves with expectant management. Clear cell adenocarcinoma in women exposed to DES is extremely rare.

STAGING/PRETHERAPY EVALUATION

The assignment of stage in vaginal cancer consists of clinical examination and radiologic studies. The required studies include chest films, cystoscopy, and sigmoidoscopy. Most patients will undergo CT of the abdomen and pelvis to evaluate the kidneys with their ureteral flow and to rule out metastatic disease to the lymph nodes and to the liver. Lymphangiogram can provide further information on the lymph node status, but this does not influence staging. Cystoscopy and sigmoidoscopy are performed to ensure that disease has not invaded the bladder or the rectum. This extension is more likely to occur with vaginal neoplasms because there is only a thin septa separating the vagina from the bladder and the rectum. Blood work usually consists of a complete blood count and serum chemistry tests. Rarely will this change the planned therapy. If liver enzymes are elevated or a decreased renal function is present, further studies are indicated to evaluate these abnormalities. When anemia is present, the patient should be transfused to maintain her hematocrit in the 30% to 35% range.

THERAPY

Treatment of vaginal cancer is based on the stage of disease. The pathologic type of tumor is also important and modifies treatment. In general, radiation therapy is the primary mode of therapy and surgery is reserved for specific situations. A number of authors have shown that, when radiation therapy is used, the combined approach utilizing external and internal radiation produces better results (Fleming et al, 1980; Perez et al, 1974; Perez and Camel, 1982; Puthawala et al, 1983). Rubin et al (1985) reported that 15 of 29 patients survived when the combined approach was used, compared with 3 of 13 who survived when only external radiation therapy was used. Peters et al (1985b) reported that the combined approach was superior when the total vaginal surface doses exceeded 7500 cG. Kirkbride et al (1995) recommended at least 7000 cG to achieve better survival. Gallup et al (1987) reported that 28% of patients survived with the combined approach, whereas 16% survived when only external radiation was given. None of these are prospective studies. Thus some of the effect is due to patient selection.

The complications with radiation therapy are significant. Pride (Pride and Buchler, 1977; Pride et al, 1979) reported a major complication rate of 18% and a minor complication rate of 23%. Rubin et al (1985) reported an overall complication rate of 25%, with 10% of these being major complications. The complication rates appear higher than those for cervical cancer and may relate to the difficulties involved in irradiating this particular site. The vagina must be treated to the maximum dose tolerable to achieve the desired therapeutic results. There is little distance between the bladder and rectum, giving rise to the higher complication rate. The complications related to the proximity of these other structures include sigmoiditis, cystitis, and enteritis. Additionally, when radiation is given for a vaginal cancer, vaginal stenosis is a significant problem.

Although radiation therapy is the treatment most often used, this must be individualized depend-

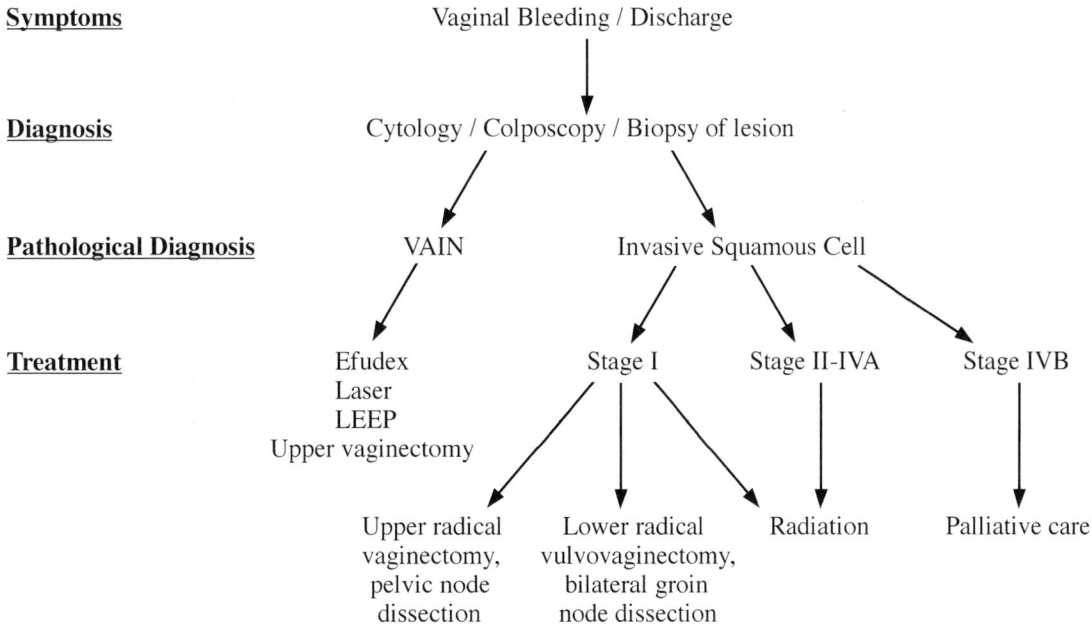

Figure 54–7
Treatment algorithm for management of vaginal cancer. LEEP, loop electrosurgical excision procedure; VAIN, vaginal intraepithelial neoplasia.

ing on the stage of disease and the cell type. The following treatment regimens can be considered (Fig. 54–7).

Squamous Cell Disease

Carcinoma in situ of the vagina can be treated by a number of methods (Benedet and Sanders, 1984; Hernandez-Linares et al, 1990). The easiest and least invasive is application of 5-fluorouracil intravaginal cream (Daly and Ellis, 1980; Sillman et al, 1985; Krebbs, 1989). This produces a sloughing of the squamous epithelium of the vagina and is effective in treating the superficial carcinoma in situ. The effectiveness of this approach obviously depends on the accuracy of the in situ diagnosis. Close follow-up is necessary to ensure that an invasive lesion is not missed and does not develop during the period of follow-up.

Upper vaginectomy, laser ablation of the vagina, or the loop electrosurgical excision procedure is an effective treatment for carcinoma in situ (Townsend et al 1982; Jobson and Homesley, 1983; Hoffman et al, 1992; Patsner, 1993). Often the in situ process occurs after hysterectomy and involves the upper vagina. Thus the bladder and rectum are in close proximity, and care must be taken not to enter these structures. With the surgical approach in early invasive stage I squamous cell cancer of the vagina, a radical hysterectomy with vaginectomy can be effective treatment (Fig. 54–8). This is most appropriate for young patients because sexual function and ovarian function can be retained, and sexual function can be preserved with a split-thickness skin graft. When

malignancy involves the lower posterior vagina, a partial radical vulvovaginectomy can be performed (Fig. 54–9). The lymphatic vessels of the lower vagina drain to the inguinal region, so bilateral groin node dissection should be included. In the elderly patient with stage I disease as well as in patients whose disease extends into the paravaginal tissues, there is little role for surgery prior to radiation. In these patients, radiation should be the primary mode of therapy. When malignancy recurs after radiation therapy, the patient should be evaluated for pelvic

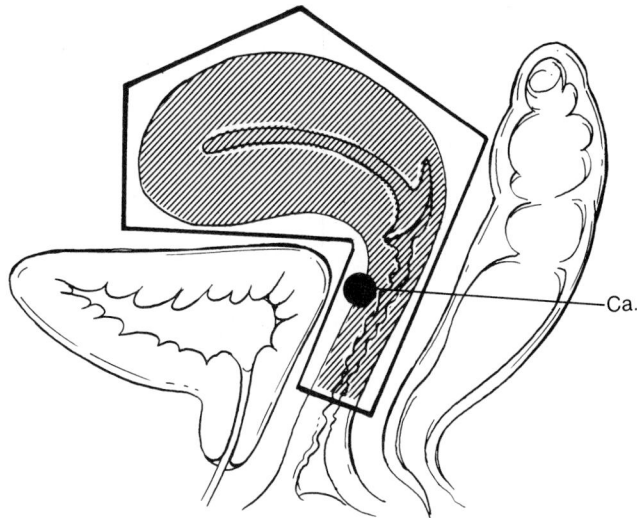

Figure 54–8
Radical hysterectomy, vaginectomy, and pelvic node dissection for treatment of stage I vaginal cancer located in the upper vagina.

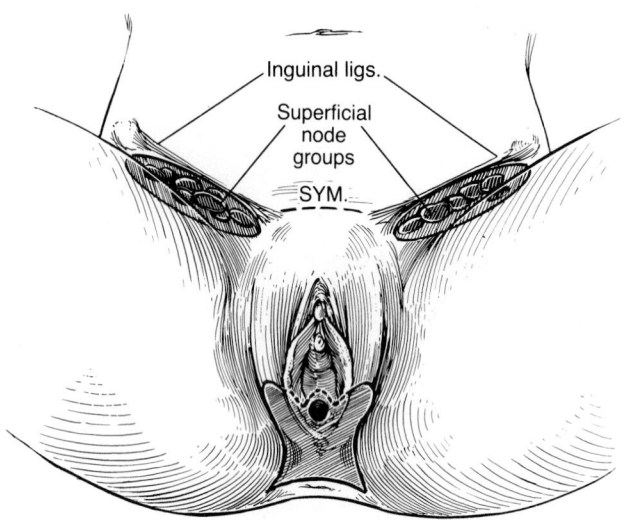

Figure 54–9
Radical vulvovaginectomy with groin node dissection for treatment of stage I vaginal cancer located in the lower vagina.

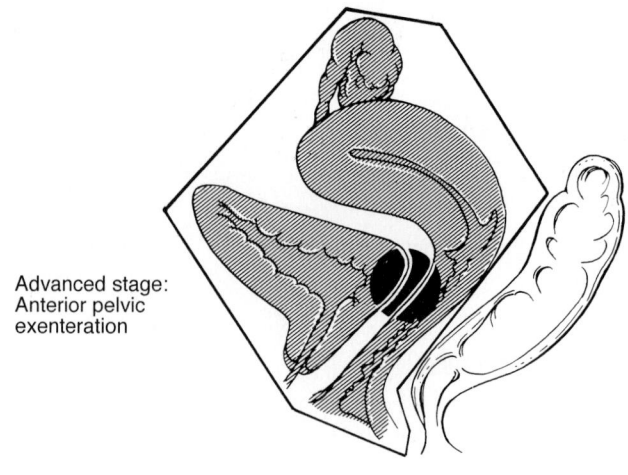

Figure 54–11
Anterior pelvic exenteration with removal of the bladder and vagina. This is most appropriate for recurrent malignancy involving the anterior vaginal wall or the suburethral area.

exenteration (Morley et al, 1989). The type of exenteration required will depend on the location of the malignancy. Usually, a malignancy at the vaginal apex will require a total pelvic exenteration because of the close proximity of the bladder and rectum (Fig. 54–10). An anterior or posterior exenteration can be performed for isolated anterior or posterior lesions (Figs. 54–11 and 54–12). In patients with metastatic disease beyond the pelvic field of radiation, only palliation can be offered. There currently is no active chemotherapeutic agent. The activity of cisplatin reported for squamous cell cancer of the cervix has not been found for squamous cell cancer of the vagina (Thigpen et al, 1986).

Adenocarcinomas

Adenocarcinomas are rare and are usually diagnosed with advanced-stage disease (Strachan, 1932;

Scannel, 1939; Ballon et al, 1979). They are usually approached in a manner similar to that described for squamous cell carcinoma. The exception to this is clear cell adenocarcinoma of the cervix, which often presents in younger women with an earlier stage; thus surgery plays a greater role in their treatment. In these women, adenocarcinomas can be treated with radical hysterectomy, vaginectomy, or local excision with radiation and pelvic lymph node dissection (see "Pathology").

Melanoma

Melanoma of the vagina is very rare and occurs almost exclusively in the elderly population. The gen-

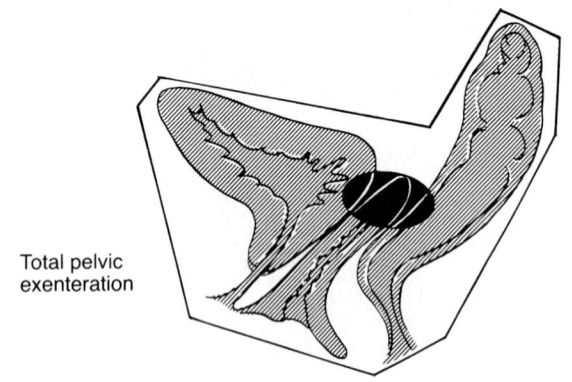

Figure 54–10
Total pelvic exenteration with removal of the bladder, vagina, and rectum. This is most appropriate for recurrent malignancy involving the vaginal apex.

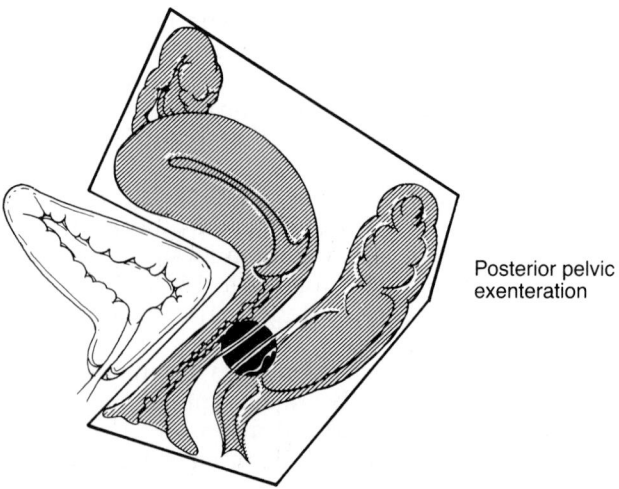

Figure 54–12
Posterior pelvic exenteration with removal of the rectum and vagina. This is most appropriate for recurrent malignancy involving the posterior vaginal wall or the rectal sphincter.

ital tract accounts for 3% of all melanomas in women, and the vagina accounts for only 1%. Thus fewer than 150 patients with vaginal melanoma have been reported in the literature. Melanoblasts, located in the basal layer of the epithelial surface, are present in the vagina in 3% of autopsy specimens. The melanoblasts arise from the neural crest and migrate to all parts of the body (Nigogsyan et al, 1964). They are indistinguishable from mesenchymal cells, and only in the skin do they differentiate and form melanin. Melanomas of the vagina have been treated with radical surgery, often exenteration. Reid et al (1989) reported that 66% of melanomas occurred in the lower one third of the vagina and the 5-year survival rate was 17%. In their report, the size of the lesion significantly influenced survival. The thickness or the depth of the melanoma influenced the disease-free interval but not survival. In Reid et al's review, the age, stage, and location of the melanoma did not influence survival. Importantly, there was no difference in survival on the basis of treatment. Radical exenterative-type surgery did not prove to be superior to radiation therapy or surgery and radiation. The most common sites of recurrence for these patients were the pelvis and the lungs.

Sarcoma

A variety of sarcomas have been reported to arise from the vagina (Table 54–4) (Schram, 1958; Vawter, 1965; Hilgers et al, 1970; Davos and Abell, 1976; Kasai et al, 1980; Harris and Scully, 1984; Andersen et al, 1985; Peters et al, 1985a). Sarcomas represent less than 2% of vaginal malignancies, and they occur in various age groups. In the pediatric population, the sarcoma botryoides or embryonal rhabdomyosarcoma is the most frequent type. Leiomyosarcoma and mixed müllerian and stromal sarcoma can involve the adult vagina (Fig. 54–13). In these patients, radiation therapy with close follow-up for complete resolution is the preferred treatment. When residual disease is present, exenteration can be undertaken. Chemotherapy has little effect on these sarcomas, and radiation followed by radical resection for persistence or recurrence is the only hope of salvage.

Table 54–4. TYPES OF SARCOMA THAT MAY INVOLVE THE ADULT VAGINA

Leiomyosarcoma
Mixed müllerian sarcoma
Endometrial stromal sarcoma
Fibrosarcoma
Alveolar sarcoma
Angiosarcoma
Neurofibrosarcoma
Schwannoma
Synovial cell
Granulocytic sarcoma/lymphoma

Vaginal Malignancy in the Infant

Malignancy can involve the infant vagina and usually presents prior to 3 years of age. The principal types are sarcoma botryoides (polypoid embryonal rhabdomyosarcoma) and endodermal sinus tumor. The embryonal rhabdomyosarcoma has sarcomatous features, whereas the endodermal sinus tumors of the vagina have histologic characteristics similar to endodermal sinus tumor of the ovary. Endodermal sinus tumors of the vagina contain Shiller-Duval bodies, and α-fetoprotein can be demonstrated by immunohistochemical methods. The clinical presentation and therapy are similar for both types of tumors, but a pathologically distinct diagnosis should be established. Additionally, the endodermal sinus tumor will often secrete α-fetoprotein, which can be used to monitor the effectiveness of therapy and detect recurrences. These children usually present with vaginal bleeding and a visible or palpable mass (Aldrich et al, 1984; Kohorn et al, 1985). In the Intergroup Sarcoma Study, Hays et al (1988) reported on 28 patients with rhabdomyosarcoma. Bleeding was the most common symptom, with only 8 of the 28

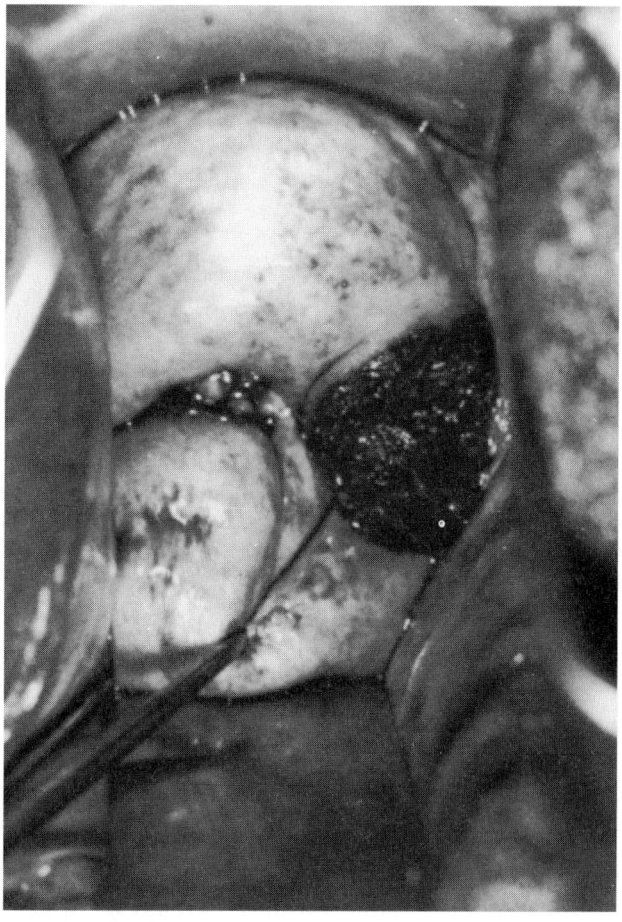

Figure 54–13
Primary polypoid stromal sarcoma involving the upper vaginal apex in a 55-year-old woman. Hysterectomy had been performed many years previously for benign disease.

patients having a visible or protruding mass. The anterior wall was the most common location, and the mass was palpable through the abdomen in seven of these patients. Three patients presented with urethral obstruction, two had lung metastases, and one had bone metastases.

These pediatric malignancies were previously treated with radical exenterative surgery. In the last decade, however, encouraging results with chemotherapy and local resection have been reported (Copeland et al, 1985a, 1985b; Hays et al, 1988; Crist et al, 1990). In these reports, vincristine, actinomycin, and cyclophosphamide (Cytoxan) chemotherapy was followed by surgical resection. Even when the tumor completely resolved preoperatively, there was usually microscopic disease present in the surgical specimen. The modern treatment for these lesions should consist of preoperative chemotherapy, followed by a limited resection preserving the bladder and rectum. Radiation therapy can then be given on the basis of surgical findings. With this approach, approximately 70% to 80% of patients will survive, and only a small percentage will require removal of the bladder or rectum. This is a significant advance when compared with Bell et al's (1986) review of the literature, in which, prior to 1970, less than 15% survived, even with radical exenterative-type surgery.

Small Cell (Neuroendocrine-Type) Malignancy

Only a few patients with small cell (neuroendocrine-type) vaginal malignancy have been reported. Hopkins et al (1989) reported three patients and Chafe (1989) reported one with this malignancy; a total of 10 patients have now been reported (Miliauskas and Leong, 1992; Prasad et al, 1992). These lesions present as a polypoid vaginal lesion. Excellent local control can be achieved with local resection and radiation therapy. Like the small cell neuroendocrine lung cancer or other small cell genital tract cancers, these malignancies rapidly metastasize. Thus adjuvant chemotherapy should be strongly considered. Adjuvant chemotherapy is usually similar to that for small cell lung cancer.

Carcinoma of the Neovagina

Reconstruction of the vagina after treatment for malignancy or for congenital absence is commonly performed. The newly constructed vagina is at risk for malignancy. The usual type of malignancy is related to the type of reconstructed vagina. If a bowel segment has been used, the malignancy will be an adenocarcinoma; if a split-thickness skin graft has been used, the malignancy will be a squamous cell cancer. These are very rare but they can occur. Thus any patient with a neovagina should have periodic pelvic examinations with cytology. Radiation therapy can

be used as primary treatment, but there appears to be a higher failure rate when this modality alone is used. Thus exenteration should be considered for these patients. If disease extends to the side wall, radiation therapy followed by exenteration should be considered (Hopkins and Morley, 1987).

Metastatic Disease

Metastatic disease to the vagina represents an ominous prognosis, with the exception of gestational trophoblastic disease and cervical or vulvar cancer. The treatment of metastatic disease to the vagina depends on the primary site. When cervical or vulvar neoplasm extends onto the vagina, the treatment will be radiation therapy or radical surgery. When endometrial cancer has metastasized to the vagina, it significantly decreases survival and usually signifies that intra-abdominal disease is also present. Surgical exploration and hysterectomy should be performed prior to radiation therapy. Urothelial and renal cell cancer can metastasize to the vagina. If bladder cancer is metastatic to the vagina, radiation or exenteration can be performed. When renal cell cancer is metastatic to the vagina, it usually represents widespread dissemination, and therapy is palliative in nature. The vagina is one of the common sites of metastases for gestational trophoblastic disease. In this situation, metastatic disease to the vagina does not significantly alter the prognosis because chemotherapy is often curative.

Benign Tumors

A variety of benign tumors may involve the vagina (Table 54–5). These usually present as mobile rounded submucosal or polypoid masses. Simple excision will be both diagnostic and therapeutic (Quan and Birnbaum, 1961; Deppisch, 1975; Burt et al, 1976; Gold and Bossen, 1976; Buntine et al, 1979; Naves et al, 1980; Chirayil and Tobon, 1981; Davis and Patton, 1983; Dekel et al, 1988).

SUMMARY

Vaginal cancer is a rare malignancy and represents 1% to 2% of all gynecologic malignancies. Squamous

Table 54–5. BENIGN TUMORS THAT MAY INVOLVE THE VAGINA

Gartner's cyst
Neurofibroma
Capillary hemangioma
Fibroepithelial polyp
Leiomyoma
Benign rhabdomyoma
Müllerian mixed tumor

cell cancer is the most common pathologic type, and adenocarcinoma is the next most common. Other rare malignancies that involve the vagina include melanoma, sarcoma, small cell neuroendocrine-type, and metastatic carcinomas. The usual treatment for vaginal cancer is radiation therapy. A radical surgical approach can be used in selected patients, especially young women and those with early-stage disease. The survival rate for vaginal cancer is decreased when compared with that of the cervix and the vulva, but acceptable survival results can be obtained when therapy is individualized to the stage of disease and the pathologic cell type of cancer.

REFERENCES

Aldrich TE, Glorieux A, Castro S: Florida cluster of five children with endodermal sinus tumors. Oncology 1984;41:233.

Ali MM, Huang DT, Goplerud DR, et al: Radiation alone for carcinoma of the vagina: variation in response related to the location of the primary tumor. Cancer 1996;77:1934.

Andersen WA, Sabio H, Durso N, et al: Endodermal sinus tumor of the vagina. Cancer 1985;56:1025.

Anderson B, Watring WG, Edinger DD, et al: Development of DES-associated clear-cell carcinoma: the importance of regular screening. Obstet Gynecol 1979;53:293.

Ballon SC, Lagasse LE, Chang N, Stehman F: Primary adenocarcinoma of the vagina. Surg Gynecol Obstet 1979;149:233.

Bell J, Averette H, Davis J, Toledano S: Genital rhabdomyosarcoma: current management and review of the literature. Obstet Gynecol Surv 1986;41:257.

Bell J, Sevin BU, Averette H, Nadji M: Vaginal cancer after hysterectomy for benign disease: value of cytologic screening. Obstet Gynecol 1984;64:699.

Benedet JL, Murphy KJ, Fairey RN, Boyes DA: Primary invasive carcinoma of the vagina. Obstet Gynecol 1983;63:715.

Benedet JL, Sanders BH: Carcinoma in situ of the vagina. Am J Obstet Gynecol 1984;148:695.

Buntine DW, Henderson PR, Biggs JSG: Benign müllerian mixed tumor of the vagina. Gynecol Oncol 1979;8:21.

Burt RL, Pritchard RW, Kim BS: Fibroepithelial polyp of the vagina. Obstet Gynecol 1976;47:52S.

Chafe W: Neuroepithelial small cell carcinoma of the vagina. Cancer 1989;64:1948.

Chanen W, Pagano R: Diethylstilboestrol (DES) exposure in utero. Med J Aust 1984;141:491.

Chirayil SJ, Tobon H: Polyps of the vagina: a clinicopathologic study of 18 cases. Cancer 1981;47:2904.

Copeland LJ, Gershenson DM, Saul PB, et al: Sarcoma botryoides of the female genital tract. Obstet Gynecol 1985a;66:262.

Copeland LJ, Sneige N, Ordonez G, et al: Endodermal sinus tumor of the vagina and cervix. Cancer 1985b;55:2558.

Crist WM, Garnesy L, Beltangady MS, et al: Prognosis in children with rhabdomyosarcoma: a report of the Intergroup Rhabdomyosarcoma Studies I and II. J Clin Oncol 1990;8:443.

Daly JW, Ellis GF: Treatment of vaginal dysplasia and carcinoma in situ with topical 5-fluorouracil. Obstet Gynecol 1980;55:350.

Davis GD, Patton WS: Capillary hemangioma of the cervix and vagina: management with carbon dioxide laser. Obstet Gynecol 1983;62:95S.

Davos I, Abell MR: Sarcomas of the vagina. Obstet Gynecol 1976; 47:342.

Dekel A, Avidan D, Barziu J, et al: Neurofibroma of the vagina presenting with urinary retention: review of the literature and report of a case. Obstet Gynecol Surv 1988;43:325.

Deppisch LM: Cysts of the vagina. Obstet Gynecol 1975;45:632.

Eddy GL, Singh KP, Gansler TS: Superficially invasive carcinoma of the vagina following treatment for cervical cancer: a report of six cases. Gynecol Oncol 1990;36:376.

Fetters MD, Fischer G, Reed BD: Effectiveness of vaginal Papanicolaou smear screening after total hysterectomy for benign disease. JAMA 1996;275:94.

Fleming P, Syed N, Neblett D, et al: Description of an afterloading ^{192}Ir interstitial-intracavitary technique in the treatment of carcinoma of the vagina. Obstet Gynecol 1980;40:525.

Gallup DG, Talledo OE, Shah KJ, Hayes C: Invasive squamous cell carcinoma of the vagina: a 14-year study. Obstet Gynecol 1987;69:782.

Gold HJ, Bossen EH: Benign vaginal rhabdomyoma. Cancer 1976; 37:2283.

Hall KL, Dewar MD, Perchalski J: Screening for gynecologic cancer: vulvar, vaginal, endometrial, and ovarian neoplasms. Prim Care 1992;19:607.

Harris NL, Scully RE: Malignant lymphoma and granulocytic sarcoma of the uterus and vagina. Cancer 1984;53:2530.

Hays DM, Shimada H, Raney RB, et al: Clinical staging and treatment results in rhabdomyosarcoma of the female genital tract among children and adolescents. Cancer 1988;61:1893.

Herbst AL, Anderson S, Hubby MM, et al: Risk factors for the development of diethylstilbestrol-associated clear cell adenocarcinoma: a case-control study. Am J Obstet Gynecol 1986;154: 814.

Herbst AL, Cole P, Colton T, et al: Age-incidence and risk of diethylstilbestrol-related clear cell adenocarcinoma of the vagina and cervix. Am J Obstet Gynecol 1977;128:43.

Herbst AL, Cole P, Norusis MJ, et al: Epidemiologic aspects and factors related to survival in 384 registry cases of clear cell adenocarcinoma of the vagina and cervix. Am J Obstet Gynecol 1979;135:876.

Herbst AL, Green TH, Ulfelder H: Primary carcinoma of the vagina. Am J Obstet Gynecol 1970;106:210.

Herbst AL, Hubby M, Azizi F, Makii M: Reproductive and gynecologic surgical experience in diethylstilbestrol-exposed daughters. Am J Obstet Gynecol 1981;141:1019.

Herbst AL, Ulfelder H, Poskanzer DC: Adenocarcinoma of the vagina. N Engl J Med 1971;284:878.

Hernandez-Linares W, Puthawala A, Nolan JF, et al: Carcinoma in situ of the vagina: past and present management. Obstet Gynecol 1990;56:356.

Hilgers RD, Malkasian GD, Soule EH: Embryonal rhabdomyosarcoma (botryoid type) of the vagina. Am J Obstet Gynecol 1970;107:484.

Hoffman MS, De Cesare SL, Roberts WS, et al: Upper vaginectomy for in situ and occult, superficially invasive carcinoma of the vagina. Am J Obstet Gynecol 1992;166(1 Pt 1):30.

Holt LH, Herbst AL: DES-related female genital changes. Semin Oncol 1982;9:341.

Hopkins MP, Kumar NB, Lichter A, et al: Small cell carcinoma of the vagina with neuroendocrine features. J Reprod Med 1989; 34:486.

Hopkins MP, Morley GW: Squamous cell carcinoma of the neovagina. Obstet Gynecol 1987;69:52S.

Horwitz RI, Viscoli CM, Merino M, et al: Clear cell adenocarcinoma of the vagina and cervix: incidence, undetected disease, and diethylstilbestrol. J Clin Epidemiol 1988;41:593.

Jefferies JA, Robboy SJ, O'Brien PC, et al: Structural anomalies of the cervix and vagina in women enrolled in the diethylstilbestrol adenosis (DESAD) project. Am J Obstet Gynecol 1984; 148:59.

Jobson VW, Homesley HD: Treatment of vaginal intraepithelial neoplasia with the carbon dioxide laser. Obstet Gynecol 1983; 62:90.

Jones WB, Koulos JP, Saigo PE, Lewis JL: Clear-cell adenocarcinoma of the lower genital tract: Memorial Hospital 1974–1984. Obstet Gynecol 1987;70:573.

Kaminski PF, Maier RC: Clear cell adenocarcinoma of the cervix unrelated to diethylstilbestrol exposure. Obstet Gynecol 1983; 62:720.

Kasai K, Yoshida Y, Okumura M: Alveolar soft part sarcoma in the vagina: clinical features and morphology. Gynecol Oncol 1980;9:227.

Kaufman RH, Binder GL, Gray PM, Adam E: Upper genital tract changes associated with exposure in utero to diethylstilbestrol. Am J Obstet Gynecol 1977;128:51.

Kinlen LJ, Badaracco MA, Moffett J, Vessey MP: A survey of the use of oestrogens during pregnancy in the United Kingdom and of the genito-urinary cancer mortality and incidence rates in young people in England and Wales. J Obstet Gynaecol Br Emp 1974;81:849.

Kirkbride P, Fyles A, Rawlings GA, et al: Carcinoma of the vagina—experience at the Princess Margaret Hospital (1974–1989). Gynecol Oncol 1995;56:435.

Kjørstad KE, Bergstrøm J, Abeler V: Clear cell adenocarcinoma of the cervix uteri and vagina in young women in Norway. J Norwegian Med Assoc 1989;109:1660.

Kohorn EI, McIntosh S, Lytton B, et al: Endodermal sinus tumor of the infant vagina. Gynecol Oncol 1985;20:196.

Krebbs HB: Treatment of vaginal intraepithelial neoplasia with laser and topical 5-fluorouracil. Obstet Gynecol 1989;73:657.

LaBarthe D, Adam E, Noller KL, et al: Design and preliminary observations of National Cooperative Diethylstilbestrol Adenosis (DESAD) project. Obstet Gynecol 1978;51:453.

Lanier AP, Noller KL, Decker DG, et al: Cancer and stilbestrol: a follow-up of 1,719 persons exposed to estrogens in utero and born 1943–1959. Mayo Clin Proc 1973;48:793.

Marcus S: Multiple squamous cell carcinomas involving the cervix, vagina, and vulva: the theory of multicentric origin. Am J Obstet Gynecol 1960;80:802.

Miliauskas JR, Leong AS: Small cell (neuroendocrine) carcinoma of the vagina. Histopathology 1992;21:371.

Morley GW, Hopkins MP, Lindenauer M, Roberts JA: Pelvic exenteration: University of Michigan 100 patients at 5 years. Obstet Gynecol 1989;74:934.

Naves AE, Monti JA, Chichoni E: Basal cell-like carcinoma in the upper third of the vagina. Am J Obstet Gynecol 1980;90:136.

Nigogsyan G, DeLePava S, Pickren JW: Melanoblasts in vaginal mucosa. Cancer 1964;7:912.

Noller KL, Decker DG, Symmonds RE, et al: Clear-cell adenocarcinoma of the vagina and cervix: survival data. Am J Obstet Gynecol 1976;124:285.

Noller KL, Townsend DE, Kaufman RH, et al: Maturation of vaginal and cervical epithelium in women exposed in utero to diethylstilbestrol (DESAD) project). Am J Obstet Gynecol 1983;146:279.

Nori D, Hilaris BS, Lewis JL: Adenocarcinoma of the vagina: combined surgery and radiation with preservation of genital function. NY State J Med 1981;81:1777.

Patsner B: Treatment of vaginal dysplasia with loop excision: report of five cases. Am J Obstet Gynecol 1993;169:179. (Erratum: Am J Obstet Gynecol 1994;170:701.)

Paul C, Skegg DCG, Seddon RJ: Past use of oestrogens during pregnancy in New Zealand. N Z Med J 1984;97:831.

Perez CA, Arneson AN, Dehner LP, Galakatos A: Radiation therapy in carcinoma of the vagina. Obstet Gynecol 1974;44:862.

Perez CA, Camel HM: Long-term follow-up in radiation therapy of carcinoma of the vagina. Cancer 1982;49:1308.

Peters WA, Kumar NB, Andersen WA, Morley GW: Primary sarcoma of the adult vagina: a clinicopathologic study. Obstet Gynecol 1985a;65:699.

Peters WA, Kumar NB, Morley GW: Carcinoma of the vagina. Cancer 1985b;55:892.

Peters WA, Kumar NB, Morley GW: Microinvasive carcinoma of the vagina: a distinct clinical entity? Am J Obstet Gynecol 1985c;153:505.

Pirtoli L, Santoni R: Radiation therapy of primary vaginal carcinoma. Acta Radiol (Oncol) 1980;19:353.

Piscitelli JT, Bastian LA, Wilkes A, Simel DL: Cytologic screening after hysterectomy for benign disease. Am J Obstet Gynecol 1995;173:424.

Piver MS, Lele SB, Baker TR, Sandecki A: Cervical and vaginal cancer detection at a regional diethylstilbestrol (DES) screening clinic. Cancer Detect Prev 1988;11:197.

Prasad CJ, Ray JA, Kessler S: Primary small cell carcinoma of the vagina arising in a background of atypical adenosis. Cancer 1992;70:2484.

Prempree T: Role of radiation therapy in the management of primary carcinoma of the vagina. Acta Radiol (Oncol) 1982;21:195.

Pride GL, Buchler DA: Carcinoma of vagina 10 or more years following pelvic irradiation therapy. Am J Obstet Gynecol 1977;127:513.

Pride GL, Schultz AE, Chuprevich TW, Buchler DA: Primary invasive squamous carcinoma of the vagina. Obstet Gynecol 1979;53:218.

Puthawala A, Nisar-Syed AM, Nalick R, et al: Integrated external and interstitial radiation therapy for primary carcinoma of the vagina. Obstet Gynecol 1983;62:367.

Quan A, Birnbaum SJ: Vaginal leiomyoma: report of a case and review of the literature. Obstet Gynecol 1961;18:360.

Reid GC, Schmidt RW, Roberts JA, et al: Primary melanoma of the vagina: a clinicopathologic analysis. Obstet Gynecol 1989;74:190.

Robboy SJ, Kaufman RH, Prat J, et al: Pathologic findings in young women enrolled in the National Cooperative Diethylstilbestrol Adenosis (DESAD) project. Obstet Gynecol 1979;53:309.

Robboy SJ, Keh PC, Nickerson RJ, et al: Squamous cell dysplasia and carcinoma in situ of the cervix and vagina after prenatal exposure to diethylstilbestrol. Obstet Gynecol 1978;51:528.

Robboy SJ, Noller KL, O'Brien P, et al: Increased incidence of cervical and vaginal dysplasia in 3,980 diethylstilbestrol-exposed young women. JAMA 1984;252:2979.

Robboy SJ, Szyfelbein WM, Goellner JR, et al: Dysplasia and cytologic findings in 4,589 young women enrolled in diethylstilbestrol-adenosis (DESAD) project. Am J Obstet Gynecol 1981;140:579.

Rubin SC, Young J, Mikuta JJ: Squamous carcinoma of the vagina: treatment, complications, and long-term follow-up. Gynecol Oncol 1985;20:346.

Ruffolo EH, Foxworthy D, Fletcher JC: Vaginal adenocarcinoma arising in vaginal adenosis. Am J Obstet Gynecol 1971;111:167.

Rutledge F: Cancer of the vagina. Am J Obstet Gynecol 1967;97:635.

Sandberg EC: Benign cervical and vaginal changes associated with exposure to stilbestrol in utero. Am J Obstet Gynecol 1976;6:777.

Scannel RC: Primary adenocarcinoma of the vagina. Am J Obstet Gynecol 1939;38:331.

Schram M: Leiomyosarcoma of the vagina. Obstet Gynecol 1958;12:195.

Senekjian EK, Frey KW, Anderson D, Herbst AL: Local therapy in stage I clear cell adenocarcinoma of the vagina. Cancer 1987;609:1319.

Sillman FH, Sedlis A, Boyce JG: A review of lower genital intraepithelial neoplasia and the use of topical 5-fluorouracil. Obstet Gynecol Surv 1985;40:190.

Strachan GI: Adenocarcinoma of the vagina. J Obstet Gynaecol Br Emp 1932;39:566.

Sturgeon SR, Curtis RE, Johnson K, et al: Second primary cancers after vulvar and vaginal cancers. Am J Obstet Gynecol 1996;174:929.

Thigpen JT, Blessing JA, Homesley HD, et al: Phase II trial of cisplatin in advanced or recurrent cancer of the vagina: a Gynecologic Oncology Group study. Gynecol Oncol 1986;23:101.

Townsend DE, Levine RU, Crum CP, Richart RM: Treatment of vaginal carcinoma in situ with the carbon dioxide laser. Am J Obstet Gynecol 1982;143:565.

Ulfelder H, Robboy SJ: The embryologic development of the human vagina. Obstet Gynecol 1976;126:769.

Vawter GF: Carcinoma of the vagina in infancy. Cancer 1965;18:1479.

Way SJ: Primary carcinoma of the vagina. J Obstet Gynecol Br Emp 1948;55:739.

Wharton JT, Rutledge FN, Gallager HS, Fletcher G: Treatment of clear cell adenocarcinoma in young females. Obstet Gynecol 1975;435:365.

Whelton J, Kotmeier HL: Primary carcinoma of the vagina. Acta Obstet Gynecol 1962;41:23.

55

Premalignant Lesions of the Cervix

Hans-B. Krebs

Until 1940, carcinoma of the uterine cervix was the leading cause of death from malignant neoplasms in North American women. Since then, a dramatic reduction in the mortality from cancer of the cervix has occurred, so that cervical carcinoma now ranks sixth in cancer mortality. The decline in incidence and number of women dying from cervical cancer by more than 70% during the last 40 years in the United States is related to the accessibility of the cervix to direct visualization and to cell and tissue study, leading to the recognition of premalignant conditions of the cervix. Consequently, many more preinvasive than invasive cervical lesions are being diagnosed each year. In 1989, for example, there were 44,000 new cases of carcinoma in situ (CIS) in the United States, compared to an estimated 16,000 invasive cervical carcinomas. The incidence of preinvasive changes less severe than CIS is estimated to be several hundred thousand per year. Most of the premalignant lesions of the cervix are eminently treatable by office methods of therapy; extensive surgery and hospitalization are seldom required.

HISTORIC MILESTONES

Recognizing Precursor Lesions

Cullen, in his classic 1900 monograph on cancer of the uterus, first called attention to neoplastic cells confined to the epithelium adjacent to invasive carcinoma. In the ensuing decade, Schauenstein (1908), Pronai (1909), and Rubin (1910) concluded that the superficial neoplastic epithelium represented the earliest stage of squamous carcinoma of the cervix. Schiller (1927) further promoted the concept of preinvasive neoplasia in detailed histologic studies. In addition, in 1928, he reported on the deficient uptake of iodine by abnormal squamous epithelia lacking glycogen. This simple, but useful, clinical test now bears his name.

Defining Precursor Lesions

Broders (1932) is credited for first using the term *carcinoma in situ* for the preinvasive lesions. However, uncertainty remained regarding the precise nature of CIS and the separation from less severe epithelial abnormalities called dysplasia (from the Greek *dys*, abnormal; and *platto*, to form). In 1961, the Committee on Histological Terminology for Lesions of the Uterine Cervix defined CIS at the First International Congress on Exfoliative Cytology as "a lesion of the epithelium in which, throughout its thickness, no differentiation takes place" (Weid, 1961). The same Committee defined dysplasia as "all other disturbances of differentiation of the squamous epithelium of lesser degree than carcinoma in situ" (Weid, 1961). The definition is so broad as to encompass anything apart from a normal epithelium (Ferenczy, 1982).

The grading of dysplastic epithelium into mild, moderate, or severe dysplasia rests upon even more tenuous grounds and, indeed, no criteria have ever been agreed upon for such a grading. As a result, diagnostic uncertainties and disagreements were perpetuated among pathologists concerning the histologic distinction between the various types of intraepithelial abnormalities (Ferenczy, 1982). Concluding that dysplasia and CIS simply represent arbitrarily defined and artificially delineated steps in a single continuous process, Richart in 1967 introduced the term *cervical intraepithelial neoplasia* (CIN). The lesions were numbered from 1 to 3, with CIN 1 corresponding to mild cervical dysplasia, CIN 2 corresponding to moderate cervical dysplasia, and CIN 3 corresponding to severe dysplasia *and* carcinoma in situ (Fig. 55–1).

In the 1980s, the concept of CIN as a continuum became untenable when CIN 1 was found to differ from CIN 2 and 3 in regard to both biologic behavior and associated human papillomavirus (HPV) types. CIN 1 was replaced by the terms *low-grade CIN* or *low-grade squamous intraepithelial lesion* (LGSIL). Correspondingly, CIN 2 and 3 are now jointly being re-

Cervical Intraepithelial Neoplasia

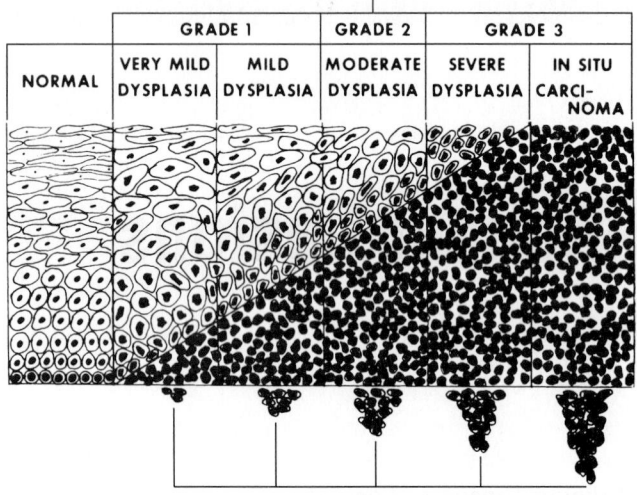

MICRO INVASIVE CARCINOMA

Figure 55-1
Schematic representation of cervical cancer precursors. Cervical intraepithelial neoplasia (CIN) grades 1, 2, and 3 correspond to the traditional terms very mild to mild dysplasia, moderate dysplasia, and severe dysplasia to carcinoma in situ, respectively. They are characterized by a progressive increase in the number of undifferentiated, malignant cells and a decrease in superficial cell differentiation paralleling the increasing severity of CIN. The schema also illustrates that invasion, although more commonly associated with a grade 3 lesion, may also develop directly from any given grade of CIN. The risk of developing invasion from CIN is not necessarily proportional to that illustrated in the schema and should be extremely rare in low-grade lesions. (From Ferenczy A: Cervical intraepithelial neoplasia. In Blaustein A [ed]: Pathology of the Female Genital Tract. 2nd ed. Heidelberg: Springer-Verlag, 1982:158, with permission.)

ferred to as high-grade CIN or *high-grade squamous intraepithelial lesion* (*HGSIL*) (National Cancer Institute, 1989; Richart, 1990).

Detecting the Precursor Lesion

Cytology

The recognition and definition of premalignant lesions of the cervix was paralleled by the development of methods suitable for detection of these early lesions on a mass scale. One method, the identification of abnormal cells exfoliated from the neoplastic cervical epithelium, was championed by George Papanicolaou in New York. Although his early cytologic studies began in 1928, it was not until 1943 that his work on the diagnosis of cervical cancer by vaginal smear was published (Papanicolaou and Traut, 1943). It took 15 to 20 more years until the Papanicolaou (Pap) smear was incorporated into most health care programs in North America.

Colposcopy

Concurrently, in Germany, Hans Hinselmann took a different approach to the detection of cervical cancers. In 1925 he designed the colposcope, an optical device for magnification of lesions too small to be recognized with the naked eye. Although the term *colposcopy* refers to vaginal inspection (from the Greek *colpos*, vagina; and *skopein*, to see), the main object of the examination is the cervix. Application of acetic acid, as proposed by Hinselmann in 1938, extended the diagnostic capability and improved the accuracy of colposcopic methods for detection of intraepithelial changes. Colposcopy was widely used in Europe, South America, and other parts of the world, but did not gain popularity in the United States until the late 1960s. The late acceptance of colposcopy may have been due, in part, to the complicated German terminology and in part to the advent of the Pap test, which provided an efficient alternative to colposcopy in mass screening. A simplified terminology and recent developments in locally ablative therapy of intraepithelial lesions with cryotherapy and electrocautery led to the rebirth of colposcopy as the method of evaluation of women with abnormal Pap smears. Today, colposcopy is no longer regarded as competitive to cytology but as complementary.

EPIDEMIOLOGY

The average age of women with CIS of the cervix is 35 to 40 years, and CIS predates cervical cancer by roughly 10 years. Lower grade cervical dysplasias are usually diagnosed at about 25 to 30 years of age (Sadeghi et al, 1988). In all other aspects, however, the epidemiology of intraepithelial lesions of the cervix is quite similar to that of invasive cervical carcinoma, supporting the concept that the two lesions are different phases of the same disease.

Early Concepts

Presumably, the earliest epidemiologic studies of cervical neoplasia were carried out by Rigoni-Stern. In 1842 he published an analysis of cancer mortality based on deaths in Verona from 1760 to 1839. Observing that cervical cancer was frequent among married or widowed women but quite rare among unmarried women and nuns, he suggested that functional changes of the uterus related to pregnancy or birth may predispose to cancer of the cervix. This theory of carcinogenesis was in support of the work of Broussais, who had previously (1826) speculated on a possible relationship between chronic irritation or trauma and neoplasia. Repeated cervical lacerations, abrasions, and infections associated with poor obstetric care or with multiparity were thought to be causal factors, and would also explain the observation of Weinberg and Gastpar (1904) that women in the lower socioeconomic classes were at higher risk for cervical cancer.

Cervical Neoplasia Among Jews

Jewish women appeared to be an exception to this etiologic concept (Kessler, 1974). Vineberg (1919), a gynecologist in New York City, reviewed records of his patients treated around the turn of the century. He noted that cervical cancer was 20 times more frequent among non-Jewish as compared with Jewish patients, although most of the latter were economically deprived immigrants who lived under poor hygienic conditions and frequently had badly lacerated cervices. The low incidence of cervical cancer among Jewish women was subsequently confirmed by numerous other studies from North America, Europe, and Israel. For many years, the diminished risk was attributed to observance of Mosaic Law on sexual intercourse, to genetic factors, or even to ritual dietary practices (Kessler, 1974).

Role of Circumcision

Circumcision was not seriously considered to be protective of cervical cancer until 1936, when Handley and Walton reported on the low incidence of cervical carcinoma among native women of the Fiji Islands compared to Hindu immigrants from India living on the islands. They speculated that ritual circumcision practiced by the Fijians, but not by the Hindus, may be protective of cervical carcinoma and that Jewish women were afforded protection for the same reason. Moreover, circumcision was also held responsible for the extremely low incidence of penile carcinoma among Jewish men (Handley and Walton, 1936).

Moslems also practice circumcision, although usually at an older age, as well as a less rigid form of menstrual abstinence as compared with Jews. Although population-based incidence data are generally lacking, there is evidence to suggest that cervical cancer is also less frequent in Moslem women (Kessler, 1974). Although the circumcision hypothesis has undergone systematic epidemiologic testing since the 1950s, the results remain inconclusive.

Cervical Neoplasia Among the Amish and Mormons

There are several population groups, including the Amish and Mormons, who do not practice ritual circumcision yet have a low incidence of cervical carcinoma (Cross, 1968; Gardner and Lyon, 1977). Because venereal diseases are also very rare in these groups, it has been suggested that endogamy and strict monogamous sexual behavior may limit the spread of some agent important in the etiology of cervical cancer (Cross, 1968).

Cervical Neoplasia as a Sexually Transmitted Disease

It is now well established that a woman's risk of cervical neoplasia is related to her sexual behavior. Detailed epidemiologic studies have shown that factors associated with an increased risk of this malignancy include marriage, broken marriage, multiple marriages, extramarital sexual activity, premarital sexual activity, early age of first marriage, early age of first intercourse, illegitimacy, multiple sexual partners of the woman and her husband, history of prostitution, history of venereal disease, low socioeconomic status, black race, and urban residence (Beral, 1974). When all of these factors are evaluated by multivariate analysis, early age of first intercourse and multiple sexual partners stand out alone (Harris et al, 1980).

Role of Early Age of First Sexual Intercourse

The association of cervical neoplasia with early age of first intercourse suggests that the cervical epithelium is particularly vulnerable to carcinogens during adolescence. The reason is thought to be the physiologic replacement of cervical glandular epithelium by squamous epithelium (squamous metaplasia), which is particularly active during adolescence (Coppleson and Reid, 1968).

Role of Multiple Sexual Partners

Women with multiple sexual partners are more likely to be exposed to a sexually transmitted carcinogen. Smegma, receiving early consideration as a carcinogen because of the relationship to circumcision, induced cervical carcinoma in mice under experimental conditions, albeit inconsistently (Pratt-Thomas et al, 1956; Heins et al, 1958). The role of smegma and circumcision has recently been deemphasized by studies showing that Jewish women who do develop cervical neoplasia tend to have the same risk factors as non-Jewish women (Pridan and Lilienfeld, 1971). It is more likely that the low risk in Jews is due to a monogamous pattern of sexual behavior (Martin, 1967).

Association with Venereal Diseases

Most known venereal diseases, including syphilis, gonorrhea, trichomoniasis, and chlamydia, were found to be more common in women with cervical neoplasia, but a direct causal relationship has not been established for any of these infections. There is, however, considerable evidence linking herpes simplex virus (HSV) type 2 and HPV infection to cervical neoplasia; this important relationship is discussed below.

Role of Barrier Contraceptives

If cervical neoplasia is caused by an infectious agent transmitted venereally, then one might anticipate a reduced risk among women who use barrier methods of contraception, such as the diaphragm and condoms. Although several studies suggest that such a relationship exists, others remain inconclusive (Kessler, 1974).

Role of the Male Sexual Partner

In a study of cervical dysplasia and carcinoma in women who claim to have had only one partner, the relative risk increased with the number of sexual partners their husbands reported (Buckley et al, 1981). The husbands of affected women were also more likely to have had venereal disease, to have visited prostitutes, and to have had affairs during marriage. It has also been found that, if cervical cancer develops in a man's first wife, his subsequent wife may be at an increased risk (Kessler, 1977). Therefore, the sexual background of each male partner must be of great importance, and would also explain the extremely high incidence of cervical neoplasia in Latin America. Female chastity before marriage and fidelity within marriage are highly valued in many of the Hispanic societies, whereas men tend to have multiple premarital and extramarital encounters, frequently with prostitutes (Skegg et al, 1982). This double standard of sexual morality was characteristic of many European and other societies in the last century, when cervical cancer dominated the female mortality statistics. The "permissive society" that emerged in the 1960s and 1970s in many Western countries is notable for the fact that the incidence of invasive cervical carcinoma has declined and it is now comparatively low, although both men and women in Western societies tend to have several sexual partners during their lives (Skegg et al, 1982). In contrast to Latin American women, most Western women have easy access to cytologic screening and are more likely to have cervical neoplasia detected in the intraepithelial phase. Exceptions are women of the lower socioeconomical strata, in particular black women. It is evident, therefore, that the risk of developing cervical neoplasia is related to sexual practices of a social class, religion, or ethnic group, but it is modified by the availability of health care (see Table 55-1). Immune status, hormonal status (e.g., oral contraceptives), and smoking may be other modifying factors.

ETIOLOGY

Intense research during the past 25 years has produced evidence supporting the role of HSV 2 and, more recently, several HPV types in the development of cervical carcinoma and its precursors.

Herpes Simplex Virus

Serologic Assays and Viral Markers

Studies using serologic assays for detection of antibody to virion envelope glycoproteins have consistently shown a positive correlation between previous HSV infection and development of cervical cancer; however, up to 67% of controls tested also had neutralizing antibodies to HSV 2 (Smith, 1983). Research was therefore directed at detection of an immune response to nonvirion antigens that may have been produced early in the infection and led to transformation of the host cell without completion of the virus cycle. The new assays discriminated more clearly between cancer patients and control groups, with early and nonvirion antigens occurring in over 75% of cancer patients compared to less than 10% of controls (Smith, 1983). One of the HSV 2 nonvirion antigens identified in cervical cancer tissue is ICP 10, also designated AG-4 or VP 143 (Aurelian et al, 1981). ICP 10 expression appears related to tumor growth and may serve as an indicator of successful tumor therapy (Aurelian et al, 1981). In addition, transcripts of viral DNA were detected by in situ hybridization in approximately 60% of preinvasive lesions and in 55% of invasive carcinoma (Jones et al, 1978).

Tumor Induction

The capability of HSV 2 to effect oncogenic transformation has been shown by in vitro and in vivo stud-

---

Table 55-1. INCIDENCE OF CERVICAL CANCER IN FIVE POPULATIONS OR SOCIETIES ACCORDING TO PREVAILING SEXUAL BEHAVIOR AND AVAILABILITY OF HEALTH CARE

POPULATION OR SOCIETY	SEXUAL PARTNERS		INCIDENCE OF CERVICAL CANCER	AVAILABILITY OF HEALTH CARE	EXAMPLES
	Female	Male			
A	0	–	0	Variable	Nuns, virgins
B	+	+	+	Good	Jews, Mormons, Amish
C	+	+++	++++	Poor	Latin Americans, 19th century Europeans
D	+++	+++	++	Good	North Americans, Europeans
E	+++	+++	+++	± Poor	African-Americans, socioeconomically deprived whites

ies. Wentz and colleagues (1983) induced premalignant and malignant cervical lesions in over 75% of mice who were exposed to cotton plugs or tampons saturated with inactivated HSV preparations and inserted into the vagina. Immunization against HSV 2 prevented the oncogenic response of the mouse cervix (Anthony et al, 1989).

In humans, existing data are less compelling for an etiologic relationship between herpes and squamous cell cancer of the cervix. A reproducible assay for transformation of human cells by HSV has yet to be found. In a prospective study of over 10,000 women, patients with HSV 2 infections appeared not to be at higher risk of developing cervical cancer than matched controls (Vonka et al, 1984). HSV has been ascribed the role of a cofactor that may interact with HPV-infected cells by mutating specific host cell genes and destroying the intracellular surveillance of HPV transcription. HSV may also amplify existing HPV genomes and therefore increase the risk for malignant conversion (Zur Hausen, 1989).

Human Papillomavirus

Early Evidence

Isolated cases of conversion of genital warts into squamous cell carcinomas of the vulva and penis were first reported in the previous century. The formation of the neoplasms was not thought to be related to an infectious agent, although the viral origin of warts was postulated in 1907 by Ciuffu. Shope, in 1933, demonstrated the infectious nature of warts by infecting rabbits with papilloma extracts from wild cottontail rabbits. The cottontail rabbit papillomavirus (CRPV) was later named after Shope and was shown to induce rabbit papillomas that developed into malignant squamous cell carcinomas when exposed to chemical mutagens and radiation (Rous and Beard, 1935). Because of the inability to grow human papillomaviruses in tissue culture or to transfer them to suitable animal hosts, progress was minimal until advances were made in molecular biology with hybridization techniques and molecular cloning.

Nonpapillomatous HPV-Associated Genital Lesions

In 1976, Zur Hausen postulated that HPV played a role in anogenital carcinoma. In the same year, Meisels and Fortin (1976), and almost simultaneously Purola and Savia (1977), described epithelial changes on the cervix with cytologic features identical to those of condyloma acuminatum, but without their papillary appearance. These lesions were called "flat condylomas"—a most unfortunate phrase because it constitutes a contradiction in terms (from the Greek condyle, knuckle or protuberance). Flat condylomas were clinically indistinguishable from low-grade cervical dysplasia and were—at least on the cervix—

much more common than papillomatous forms of the infection. The cells in the flat condylomas were called koilocytes. The term (from the Greek koilos, hollow) reflects the hollow or empty appearance of the cell and was originally used by Koss and Durfee in 1956 to describe cells having perinuclear cytoplasmic clearing, or "halos," in cytologic specimens from both cervical cancers and cancer precursors. Because condylomata acuminata were known to be of viral origin, the demonstration of koilocytes in both genital warts and dysplasia suggested that cervical neoplasias also have a viral etiology.

In 1978, Della Torre et al and Laverty et al detected viral particles in flat condylomas using electron microscopy. Direct evidence that the virus was actually HPV was provided by Jenson et al (1980), who developed group-specific antibodies acting against capsid proteins of a wide variety of animal and human papillomaviruses. The immunoperoxidase technique employing these anti-HPV antibodies demonstrated papillomavirus in the superficial layers and in koilocytotic cells of approximately 50% of flat condylomata and mild dysplasias (Shah et al, 1980). Viral assembly is rarely complete in advanced dysplasias and in invasive cancer, so that the viral capsid is not formed. Hence, the immunoperoxidase staining technique is inadequate for HPV detection in these lesions.

Identification of HPV Types

Papillomaviruses are epitheliotropic viruses that infect the surface epithelia and mucous membranes, where they produce warts and epithelial proliferations. They are found in a wide variety of vertebrates and are highly species specific. The classification of papillomaviruses is based on the species of origin and the extent of relatedness between viral genomes. Within a given species there may be a large number of different types of papillomavirus, referred to as genotypes rather than serotypes because they are classified on the basis of DNA composition as opposed to antigenicity. The viruses are assigned numbers according to their order of discovery. It was agreed to designate a new papillomavirus as a different type if its DNA is less than 50% homologous to DNA of other known types of papillomavirus from the same species (Coggin and Zur Hausen, 1979).

The initial isolation and characterization of individual HPV types from genital HPV-associated lesions were achieved by Gissmann and Zur Hausen in 1980. At present more than 90 genotypes of HPV have been characterized; 21 of the HPV types occur predominantly or exclusively in the anogenital tract (Table 55–2). HPV 16 and 18 are most frequently encountered in anogenital cancers and are present in approximately 60% to 95% of tissue samples. Many of the other 21 types have only been sporadically found in individual tumors (Zur Hausen and Schneider, 1987). According to their association with can-

Table 55-2. HPV TYPES AND THEIR ASSOCIATION WITH DISEASES

HPV TYPE	ASSOCIATED DISEASE
1, 2, 4	Plantar and common warts
3, 28, 29	Flat warts
7	Common warts of meat and animal handlers
5, 8, 9, 10, 12, 14, 15, 17, 19, 20, 21, 22, 23, 24, 25, 36, 37, 38, 47, 50	Flat warts, macules and pityriasis, versicolor-like lesions in epidermodysplasia verruciformis (EV) patients, some types occasionally found in keratoacanthoma, solar keratosis, and melanoma
6, 11, 42, 43, 44, 54, 55, 57	Anogenital condylomata acuminata
6, 11	Laryngeal and conjunctival papilloma
6, 11, 16, 18, 30, 31, 33, 34, 35, 39, 40, 42, 43, 44, 45, 51, 52, 56, 57, 58	Cervical intraepithelial neoplasia (CIN), vaginal intraepithelial neoplasia (VAIN), penile intraepithelial neoplasia (PIN), bowenoid papulosis, and genital Bowen's disease
6, 11, 16, 18, 31, 33, 35, 39, 45, 51, 52, 56	Cervical, vulvar, and penile cancer, perianal and anal cancer
13, 32	Oral focal epithelial hyperplasia (Heck's disease)
26, 27, 49	Cutaneous warts from a patient with immune deficiency and from a renal transplant recipient
41, 48	Disseminated warts, squamous cell carcinoma of the skin
46	EV-like lesions in a patient with Hodgkin's disease
53	No specific disease (cloned from cervical scraping)

Modified from Dürst M: The human papillomaviruses: classification and molecular biology. Clin Pract Gynecol 1989;2:29, with permission. Copyright 1989 by Elsevier Science Publishing Co., Inc.

cers, HPV types are often grouped as *low-risk types* (HPV 6, 11, 42, 43, and 44), *medium-risk (or intermediate-risk) types* (HPV 33, 35, 39, 40, 45, 51 through 56, and 58), and *high-risk types* (HPV 16, 18, and 31). Intermediate-risk and high-risk viruses are also referred to as *potentially oncogenic types*.

Methods of HPV Detection (Table 55-3)

FILTER HYBRIDIZATION

Among currently used methods of HPV DNA identification, filter hybridization techniques, including the Southern blot, play a less important role. For these tests, nitrocellulose filters provide the base to which viral and probe DNA are applied (Fig. 55-2). The dot-blot or slot-blot and the filter in situ hybridization (FISH) methods are simplified versions of the Southern blot analysis. Southern blot tests are sensitive and specific and continue to be the gold standard in research studies. HPV testing kits utilizing the FISH technology were the first to be approved by the Food and Drug Administration (FDA) for clinical use and made commercially available. Because of the high cost and low sensitivity and specificity, FISH-based tests have not gained wide popularity.

IN SITU HYBRIDIZATION

In this technique, isotope probes or, more recently, nonradioactive biotin-labeled probes are added directly to cytologic preparations or histologic sections of frozen or fixed materials on a glass slide. The method is therefore suitable for retrospective studies and allows the determination of topographic distribution of viral DNA.

POLYMERASE CHAIN REACTION

The sensitivity of hybridization techniques may be increased by selective enzymatic amplification of minute amounts of specific viral DNA sequences with the polymerase chain reaction (PCR). The amplified DNA increases exponentially with each new cycle and may then be detected by conventional hybridization tests. The early PCR methodology often produced false-positive results by amplifying small amounts of contaminating HPV DNA derived from biopsy forceps or laboratory dust. The extremely high sensitivity makes PCR an outstanding research tool; however, it limits clinical usefulness because it will detect traces of HPV DNA that may be medically meaningless (Reid and Lörincz, 1996). Test kits based on PCR technology have become commercially available for clinical use.

SOLUTION HYBRIDIZATION

Developments in technology have led to a revival of the oldest nucleic acid hybridization methodology, whereby hybridization occurs in solution. The new versions of the solution hybridization are as sensitive and specific as the Southern blot, but much simpler to perform.

Table 55-3. COMPARISON OF DIFFERENT METHODS FOR HUMAN PAPILLOMAVIRUS DETECTION

HYBRIDIZATION METHOD	SENSITIVITY	SPECIFICITY	LABOR AND COST	REMARKS
Southern blot	++	+++	+++	Gold standard
Dot-blot	++	++	++	Suitable for clinical use (first-generation tests)
FISH	+	+	+	Too inaccurate
In situ	+	+	++	For histologic sections
PCR	+++	+++	++	Prone to contamination
Hybrid capture	++	++	+	Suitable for clinical use (second-generation tests)

Abbreviations: FISH, filter in situ hybridization; PCR, polymerase chain reaction.
Key: +, low; ++, moderate; +++, high.
Modified from Schneider A, Grubert T: Diagnosis of HPV infection by recombinant DNA technology. Clin Obstet Gynecol 1989;32:127, with permission.

In the hybrid capture technique, DNA probes are used to bond single-stranded HPV DNA. The hybrids are captured onto the surface of a plastic tube by specific antibodies. The reaction is made visible by the emission of light in direct proportion to the quantity of captured hybrid. A commercial form of the test known as Hybrid Capture (Digene Dragnostics, Silver Spring, MD) has been approved by the FDA. The test detects essentially all HPV types relevant for cervical neoplasia (Reid and Lörincz, 1996).

Clinical Application of HPV Typing

HPV typing may be a useful adjunct to the standard Pap test because it may identify high-risk patients and detect more cervical lesions (Ritter et al, 1988). However, some women would be found to have potentially oncogenic HPV types but no cervical abnormality. The management of these women remains unclear at this time (Crum et al, 1997). In addition, a single negative HPV test may not be reliable because the HPV detection rate varies as a result of laboratory accuracy, essay variability, physiologic changes (e.g., hormonal status), and age (Schiffman, 1990). In a study of adolescent women by Rosenfeld et al (1992), approximately one fourth of women who were HPV negative on the first visit were positive on the second. In older women the rate of HPV positivity is much lower compared to young women, and the predictive value of the test may be higher (Shen et al, 1995).

Another application of HPV DNA testing may be for the evaluation of women with borderline Pap smears. Cox et al (1995) found a high rate of high-grade cervical dysplasias in women with a cytologic diagnosis of atypical squamous cells of undetermined significance (ASCUS), if HPV testing revealed high-risk HPV types. However, some of the concerns about the management of ASCUS may be alleviated more cost-effectively by qualifying the term with statements such as "favor reactive" or "favor intraepithelial neoplasia" rather than performing viral typing (Crum et al, 1997). This is further discussed below.

HPV testing may occasionally also be useful in the management of women with unclear or equivocal histologic diagnosis, low-grade cervical disease, and recurrences after previous treatment, particularly in the presence of immunosuppression. For example, a human immunodeficiency virus–positive women with recurrent dysplasia associated with high-risk HPV types requires more aggressive treatment and follow-up than a woman found to have HPV 6 or 11.

Effects of HPV on Tissue

LATENT INFECTION

Infection with HPV is thought to occur when large numbers of virus particles released from infected superficial cells or keratin fragments gain access to basal cells through epithelial breaks in susceptible individuals. The virus may remain in the basal layer of the epithelium as a separate chromosomal piece of circular DNA termed *episome* (Dürst et al, 1985). Because the infected cells are histologically indistinguishable from uninfected cells, the infection is called latent or occult.

PRODUCTIVE INFECTION

Viral replication may occur after an incubation period ranging from a few weeks to many years. Replication of episomal DNA is highly restricted in the basal layers and occurs only once per cell cycle. As infected epithelial cells mature and migrate toward the surface, constraints to viral replication are released, resulting in production of capsid proteins and assembly of infectious virus. This phase of the viral infection is called *productive infection* and may be associated with a pronounced cytopathic and histopathic effect. The cytopathic effect consists of formation of the characteristic koilocytes exhibiting cytoplasmic vacuolation, chromatin clumping, and hyperchromasia (Fig. 55–3). Histologic changes may occur in permissive epithelia and include proliferation of the basal layer (acanthosis), keratin formation

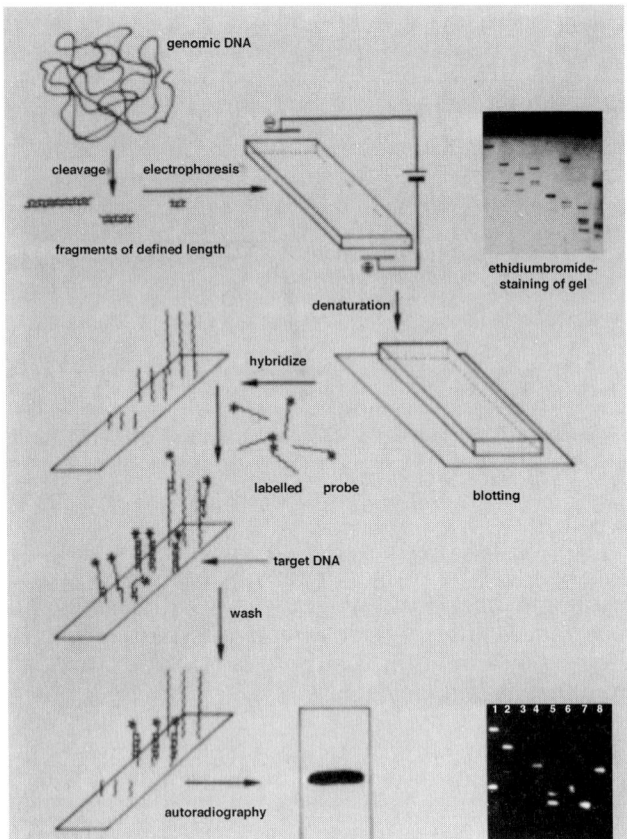

Figure 55–2

Principles of Southern blot hybridization. Cleavage of cellular deoxyribonucleic acid (DNA) by a restriction enzyme produces several DNA fragments of defined length. These fragments are separated by agarose gel electrophoresis according to their length. Long fragments migrate more slowly than shorter ones and remain nearer to the negative electrode. The different bands of DNA in the gel are made visible by staining with ethidium bromide. After denaturation and transfer onto a membrane, the DNA is accessible for the hybridization experiment. Labeled (*asterisks*) single-stranded probes are incubated with the filter, and hybrids are formed. Nonspecifically bound probes are removed by washing under conditions of stringency as defined by the experiment. Thus only the target DNA remains labeled and is made visible by autoradiography, as shown in the example. Photograph in lower right corner documents the hybridization result of the gel electrophoresis illustrated in the upper right corner. (From Schneider A, Grubert T: Diagnosis of HPV infection by recombinant DNA technology. Clin Obstet Gynecol 1989;32: 127, with permission.)

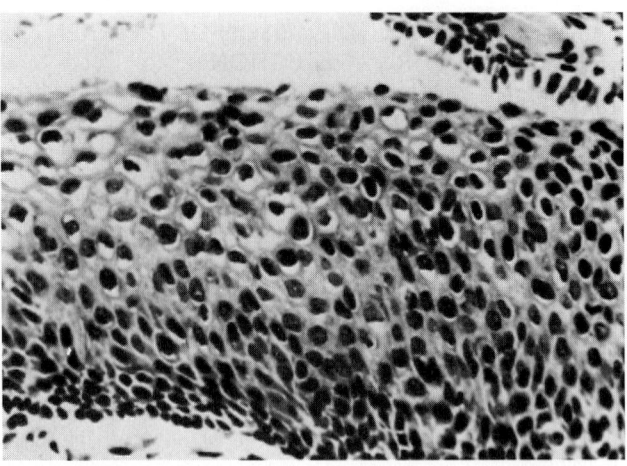

Figure 55–3

Cervical condyloma. Koilocytes exhibiting cytoplasmic vacuolation, chromatin clumping, and hyperchromasia occupy the upper two thirds of the epithelium. (Courtesy of S. M. Kheir, MD, American Medical Laboratories, Inc., Fairfax, VA.)

NONPRODUCTIVE INFECTIONS

In the presence of potentially oncogenic HPV types, the infected cells may fail to differentiate and do not permit completion of the viral life cycle. Such *nonproductive infections* constitute, for the virus, a biologic dead end and occur in high-grade dysplasia and invasive cancer. Koilocytotic changes decrease as the degree of dysplasia increases. Basal cell proliferation, nuclear atypia, pleomorphism, atypical mitotic figures, and progressive loss of base-to-surface maturation are recognized as the hallmarks of HPV-associated neoplasia (Fig. 55–4). Nonproductive infections are, with the exception of invasive cancers, subclinical.

The Role of Cofactors

Only approximately 10% of all genital HPV infections come to clinical attention as condyloma or dysplasia, and cervical cancer will develop in fewer than 1% of women with HPV infection. Therefore, neoplastic cell transformation is not determined by exposure to HPV alone but requires additional factors that modify host cell genes. Several cofactors, such as chemicals, radiation, and genetic traits, have been identified in animal models. Of particular interest is the observation that constituents of cigarette smoke (e.g., nicotine and cotinine) concentrate in the cervical epithelium and may be converted into carcinogenic nitrosamines in the presence of specific bacterial infections (Herrero et al, 1989).

EPIDERMODYSPLASIA VERRUCIFORMIS

Among human models, patients affected with epidermodysplasia verruciformis are best studied. These individuals suffer from a defect in cell-mediated immunity and develop disseminated skin

(parakeratosis, hyperkeratosis), and capillary overgrowth with formation of papillary projections (papillomatosis) that are pathognomonic for the virus. However, on the cervix, nonpapillomatous lesions are more common. These are called *subclinical infections* because they are not recognized by gross inspection, but require exfoliative cytology or magnification for detection. HPV 6 and 11 are detected in 40% to 60% of these lesions, and HPV 16 is isolated from 20% to 35% with considerable geographic variation (Campion et al, 1989).

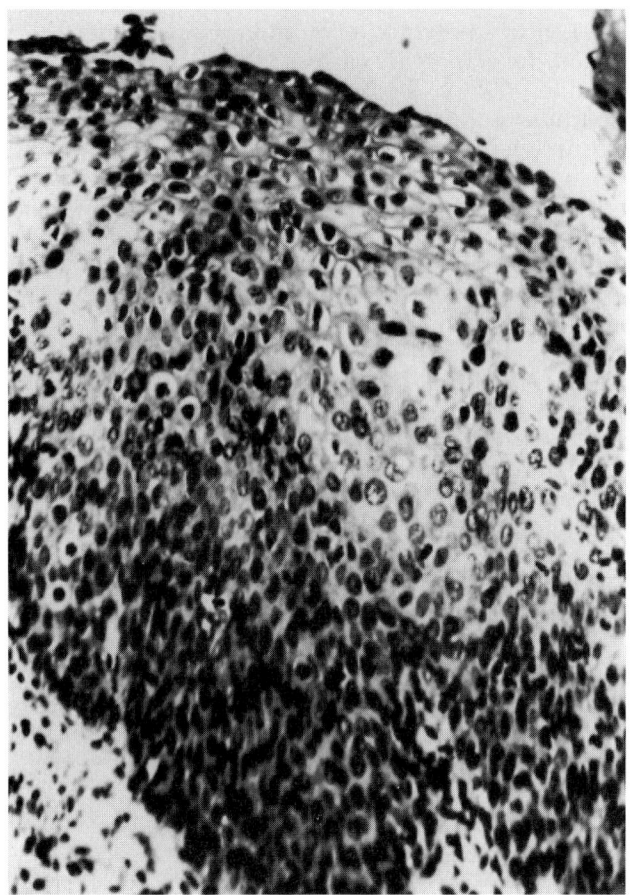

Figure 55–4
Cervical intraepithelial neoplasia, grade 3. The epithelium consists mostly of undifferentiated cells with nuclear atypia, pleomorphism, loss of polarity, and atypical mitotic figures. (Courtesy of S. M. Kheir, MD, American Medical Laboratories, Inc., Fairfax, VA.)

warts. Not infrequently, the warts undergo malignant transformation, particularly in areas exposed to sunlight, indicating a role for ultraviolet irradiation in their development (Orth et al, 1980).

PROGESTERONE

Progesterone has also been considered to promote HPV production and proliferation of infected cells. Indeed, a hormone-responsive element has been found in the noncoding region of genital HPVs. This may explain why long-term contraceptive users appear to have a slightly elevated risk for cancer of the cervix and why women are more likely to test HPV positive during pregnancy compared to their non-pregnant state (Piper, 1985; Schneider et al, 1987).

INVASIVE POTENTIAL

Carcinoma in Situ

In 1952, Galvin et al reported that 10 of 13 women with untreated CIS developed invasive carcinoma 1

to 17 years later. This study convincingly demonstrated that CIS is a precursor of invasive carcinoma. Subsequently, numerous other authors confirmed progression of CIS to invasive cancer in 20% to 100% of patients (Green, 1969). The differences in the reported progression rates reflect not only variable observation periods ranging from 3 to 20 years, but also variations in histologic interpretations and the possibility of altering the normal progression of the lesions by biopsy. Biopsies alone are frequently therapeutic, even if the lesion was not completely removed (Richart and Barron, 1969).

Dysplasia

Most authors describing the fate of dysplasia report a regression to normal in 30% to 50% of cases. The progression rate from dysplasias to CIS is reported to be 10% to 30% in most series, although progression rates of up to 60% have been described (Boronow, 1976). The progression from dysplasia to invasive cancer may be as high as 6% per year (Stern, 1969).

Flat Condyloma

The behavior of flat cervical condyloma not associated with intraepithelial neoplasia appears to be quite similar to that of low-grade cervical dysplasia. Forty per cent to 50% of all flat condylomata resolve spontaneously, 20% to 40% progress to dysplasia or (rarely) carcinoma, and approximately 20% persist over an observation period of 1 year (Evans and Monaghan, 1985; Nash et al, 1987). The findings emphasize that flat condylomata have a definite potential for malignant transformation and should not be ignored. Women with cytologic evidence of HPV in a Pap smear have a relative risk for cervical carcinoma 15.6 times higher than the general population (Mitchell et al, 1986).

CIN Continuum Concept

From carefully executed studies using only cytologic and colpomicroscopic studies for diagnosis and follow-up, Richart and Barron (1969) concluded that dysplasia and CIS are not fundamentally different but represent a spectrum of cervical intraepithelial changes, which they termed CIN. The grade of the lesion would be of relevance only insofar as low-grade CIN generally requires more time to progress to carcinoma than higher grade lesions. However, the transit time from CIN to invasive cancer is unpredictable on an individual basis.

In support of the concept of CIN as a continuum are morphologic and cytogenetic studies that showed that changes occurring in cells of dysplasia and CIS are qualitatively similar and remain constant throughout the disease spectrum. For example, chromosomal aneuploidy representing a specific feature of cancer cells occurs even in some very mild dysplasias (Ferenczy, 1982). It is also known that invasive carcinoma may, on very rare occasions, arise directly from dysplasia (Burghardt and Ostor, 1983). Therefore, CIN may or may not pass through the entire spectrum of intraepithelial changes before invasion occurs (Fig. 55–1).

Low-Grade and High-Grade CIN

A major predictive variable of a lesion's clinical course is its association with potentially oncogenic HPV types. Campion et al (1986) observed progression of CIN 1 to CIN 3 in 26% of cases. In 85% of these cases HPV 16 was present, whereas lesions associated with HPV 6 rarely progressed.

Based on the observation that the biologic course of CIN corresponds to the HPV type, Richart (1990) revised his concept of CIN as a continuum and now distinguishes two categories of lesions. One, designated *low-grade* CIN (CIN 1) or LGSIL, is associated mostly with low-risk HPV types and has malignant potential only in those instances where it is associated with high- and intermediate-risk types. *High-grade* CIN (CIN 2 and 3) or HGSIL contains potentially oncogenic types and would be expected to behave as a precursor lesion.

SITE AND ORIGIN

Transformation Zone

Exact knowledge of the anatomy and physiology of the cervix is fundamental to understanding the pathogenesis of cervical neoplasia, and the principles of screening, colposcopy, and therapy. Of particular importance is the transformation zone (T zone), for it is here that 80% to 85% of precancerous and cancerous squamous lesions of the cervix develop. The remainder of neoplasias develop outside of the transformation zone in original (native) squamous epithelium (Burghardt and Ostor, 1983). The T zone is that area of the cervix where a transformation from columnar to squamous epithelium takes place. This process is called *squamous metaplasia* (from the Greek *metaplatto*, to transform) and is usually initiated when glandular (columnar) epithelium is exposed to the acidity of the vagina. It was believed for many years that columnar epithelium is confined to the endocervix until it is everted to the ectocervix through an estrogen-dependent process active at the time of puberty. Hence, glandular epithelium on the ectocervix was called *eversion* or *ectropion* (from the Greek *ectrepo*, to evert). Although embryologically not entirely correct, the terms *eversion* and *ectropion* are still commonly used.

It is now known that columnar epithelium is present on the ectocervix of most fetuses and newborns (Madile, 1976). Embryologically, the ectocervical glandular epithelium represents the residuum of an incompletely transformed vaginal and cervical müllerian columnar epithelium (Prins et al, 1976). The primary transformation may be inhibited by diethylstilbestrol (DES), by related synthetic estrogens, and by unknown factors so that in some individuals columnar epithelium extends to the periphery of the cervix and even to the vagina (Forsberg, 1973).

Compared to the surrounding multilayered squamous epithelium, the single layer of columnar cells conceals blood vessels within the mucosa poorly, so that the eversion looks distinctly red. For this reason the term *erythroplakia* is sometimes used. Because of the raw, denuded appearance, eversions are often referred to as "erosion" or, in recognition of the actual presence of epithelium, as "pseudo-erosion." It is best to avoid the terms *erythroplakia* and *pseudo-erosion* altogether and to refer to "erosion" in cases where epithelium is actually missing and cervical stroma is exposed. The term *ectopy* suggests that columnar epithelium is out of place when on the ectocervix. The term is misleading and should no longer be a part of modern terminology.

Squamocolumnar Junction

The squamocolumnar junction (SCJ) is the line where squamous epithelium meets columnar epithelium. It is important to differentiate between the original squamocolumnar junction (OSCJ) and the new squamocolumnar junction (NSCJ). The OSCJ, also called the "anatomic SCJ," is the linear junction between the original squamous epithelium of the ectocervix and the columnar epithelium located mostly in the endocervix. When squamous metaplasia occurs, the OSCJ becomes the border between the original and the metaplastic squamous epithelium and is then recognizable only by landmarks such as persistent gland openings or islets of columnar epithelium requiring the help of a magnifying device (e.g., colposcope) (Figs. 55–5 and 55–6). The proximal border of the newly formed (metaplastic) epithelium is the NSCJ, also called the "physiologic SCJ." The area between the OSCJ and NSCJ thus constitutes the transformation zone.

The NSCJ is, strictly speaking, not discernible colposcopically; high magnification, as used in microhysteroscopes or microscopic examinations of histologic sections, is required. The reason is that the most proximal and thus most immature portion of the transformation zone is morphologically insufficiently altered to be differentiated colposcopically from columnar epithelium. *What the colposcopist recognizes as NSCJ is not the upper limit of the transformation zone, but the border between mature and immature squamous metaplastic epithelium.* Therefore, ablation of cervical dysplasia should always be car-

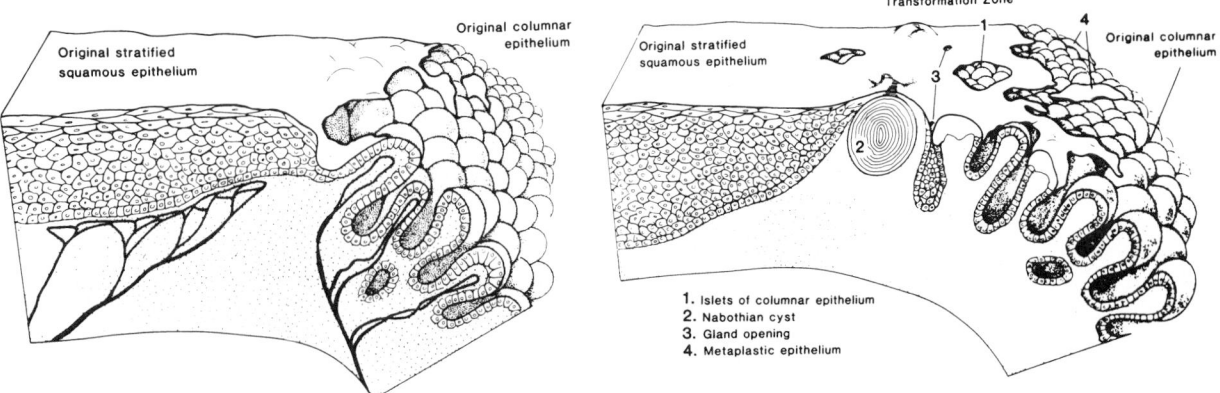

Figure 55–5

Schematic representation of the cervix at the squamocolumnar junction. *Left*, The original squamous epithelium interfaces with the original columnar epithelium at the original squamocolumnar junction. *Right*, Squamous metaplastic epithelium has replaced a portion of the original columnar epithelium, leading to formation of a transformation zone. The new squamocolumnar junction is proximal to the original squamocolumnar junction. Note the presence of nabothian cysts and persistent gland opening. (From Burke L, Antonioli DA, Ducatman BS: Colposcopy Text and Atlas. East Norwalk, CT: Appleton & Lange, 1991:41, and 48, with permission.)

ried a few millimeters into normal-appearing columnar epithelium in order to destroy also potentially oncogen-exposed immature metaplastic epithelium (Coppleson et al, 1978).

Natural History of the Transformation Zone
(Fig. 55–7)

Compared with newborns, the cervix decreases in size during infancy, and the extent of columnar epithelium on the ectocervix diminishes significantly. Nonetheless, small areas of columnar epithelium are found in 40% of prepubertal girls (Linhartova, 1978).

Estrogen stimulation at the time of puberty results in eversion of columnar epithelium from the endocervix to the outside, so that after puberty extensive areas of columnar and metaplastic epithelium are present on the ectocervix of more than 75% of women (Coppleson et al, 1978).

A first pregnancy often leads to a progressive eversion of the endocervical epithelium and rapid squamous metaplasia, especially during the second trimester. Second and subsequent pregnancies exhibit minimal, if any, further metaplastic changes.

During the reproductive years, squamous metaplasia continues to reduce slowly the remaining area of ectocervical columnar epithelium. This process is usually completed in the perimenopausal years. Estrogen deficiency after menopause results in reversion (retraction) of the T zone into the endocervical canal. Therefore, colposcopic examinations are usually unsatisfactory in postmenopausal women.

Histologic Aspects of Squamous Metaplasia

Squamous metaplasia appears to originate from omnipotent müllerian stromal cells, possibly fibroblasts or other cells at the basement membrane. The cells respond to stimuli such as acidity, infections, and unknown factors (Minh et al, 1981). In the most exposed area of the columnar villi, the activated stromal cells gather beneath the columnar epithelium and form *reserve cells*. These cells proliferate to form an immature squamous lining of several layers known as reserve cell hyperplasia (Fig. 55–8). Further maturation results in formation of a multilayered epithelium, which would be indistinguishable from original squamous epithelium by ordinary histologic means were it not for the persistence of columnar epithelial remnants in the stroma beneath the epithelium.

Development of Cervical Dysplasia
(Fig. 55–9)

Squamous metaplasia is a physiologic process resulting in the development of new squamous epithelium and a *typical transformation* zone. Mature metaplastic epithelium appears to be at low risk for development of squamous cancer, whereas immature metaplastic epithelium appears vulnerable to pathogens such as HPV.

Infection with any of the HPV types may begin as a productive infection in which the virus resides in the nucleus in *episomal* form. In the presence of environmental, immunologic, or infectious cofactors, a sequence of events is initiated leading to development of a clone of genetically altered cells in the proximal portion of the T zone. As a result of their unrestricted growth, the abnormal cells replace surrounding metaplastic cells. The cytopathic effect of the virus results in characteristic cytoplasmic and nuclear changes that become apparent as the cells undergo limited maturation and migrate toward the

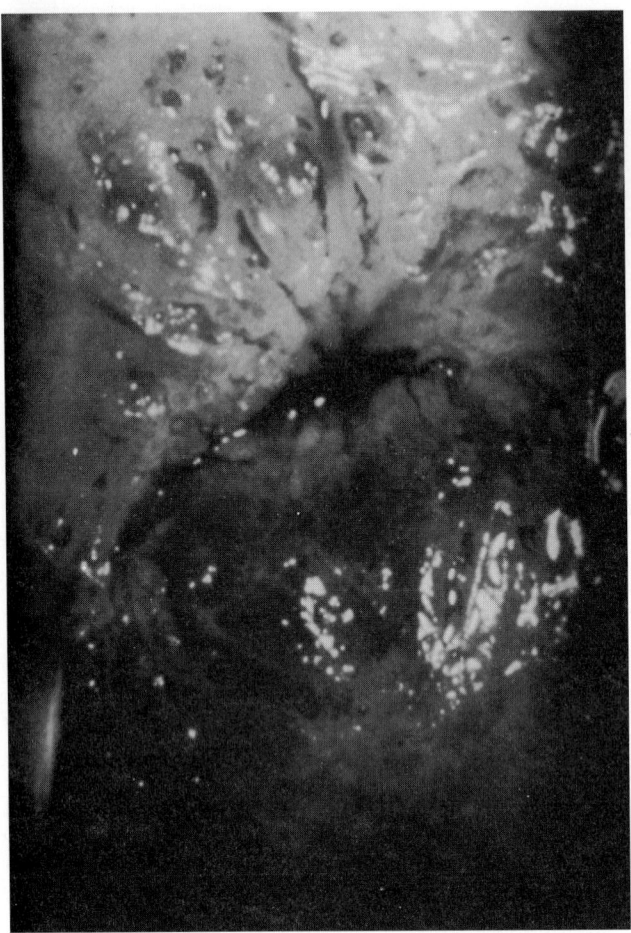

Figure 55–6
Colposcopic view of a cervix in a young woman showing a
normal transformation zone. Villi of columnar epithelium are
visible on the posterior cervical lip near the cervical os.
Squamous metaplastic epithelium in various degrees of
maturity is seen in the periphery of the cervix. Note persistent
gland openings in the proximal portion of the T zone.

surface. Histologically, the early lesion is generally
classified as flat condyloma or mild dysplasia.

If the infectious agent is a potentially oncogenic
virus, then the viral DNA may become *integrated* into
the cellular DNA (Dürst et al, 1985). During integration, the circular viral DNA is disrupted in a specific
region, resulting in loss of viral genes that regulate
transcriptional activity of the viral genome. This may
lead to unrepressed transcription of the intact remaining viral DNA. Some of the gene products appear to mediate proliferative changes in the host cell
and cause abnormalities in host cell DNA replication, resulting in aneuploidy and abnormal chromosomes (Lehn et al, 1988).

Lesions associated with potentially oncogenic
HPV types become progressively less well differentiated as they advance toward the endocervix. The
lesions tend to maintain a grading differentiation
from well differentiated near the original squamocolumnar junction to less well differentiated in the
proximal, or endocervical, portion of their growth

(Richart, 1967). From the diverse genetic pool of
aneuploid cells, a clone may, after a long latency period, be selected to produce invasive carcinoma. It is
assumed that malignant transformation requires further modification of the host cell genome through
mutations in genes that then activate oncogenes and
promote the oncogenic process (Zur Hausen, 1989).

DETECTION AND DIAGNOSIS

Although cytology and instrumentally aided methods of inspection, including colposcopy and cervicography, colpomicroscopy, and microcolpohysteroscopy, are reasonably accurate in experienced
hands in predicting the type and severity of the underlying cervical neoplasia, none of these methods
is sufficient to render a diagnosis. Histologic study
of a tissue specimen obtained by biopsy, cervical
conization, or some other surgical procedure is *always* required for a diagnosis.

Cytology

Since the original description of the Pap smear, several changes in terminology and methods of obtaining the smear have occurred. For example, routine
smears are no longer taken from a pool specimen in
the vaginal fornices, as originally practiced by Papanicolaou, but rather are taken directly from the
cervix. Vaginal smears are limited to documenting
hormonal effects or infections and for screening of
malignancies of noncervical or vaginal origin.

Collection of the Specimen

To obtain an optimal cytologic specimen, physicians
are encouraged to follow the guidelines of the Council of Scientific Affairs of the American Medical Association (AMA) (Table 55–4). The ectocervical sample is best obtained with an Ayre spatula. Numerous
devices are available for collecting the endocervical
specimen, including a pointed Ayre spatula, a moistened cotton swab, endocervical aspiration, or an endocervical brush. Compared to the other methods,
the endocervical brush is particularly effective because it transfers the most cellular material when
spread on the slide (Taylor et al, 1987). Not infrequently, the relatively stiff nylon bristles of the brush
cause bleeding, which may obscure cells in the Pap
smear (AMA, 1989). It is therefore advisable that the
ectocervical specimen be obtained first and that the
examiner proceed very carefully when inserting the
brush and rotating it in the endocervix.

Screening Intervals

In November 1987, the American Cancer Society revised its screening guidelines for cervical cancer and
recommended "that all women who are, or who

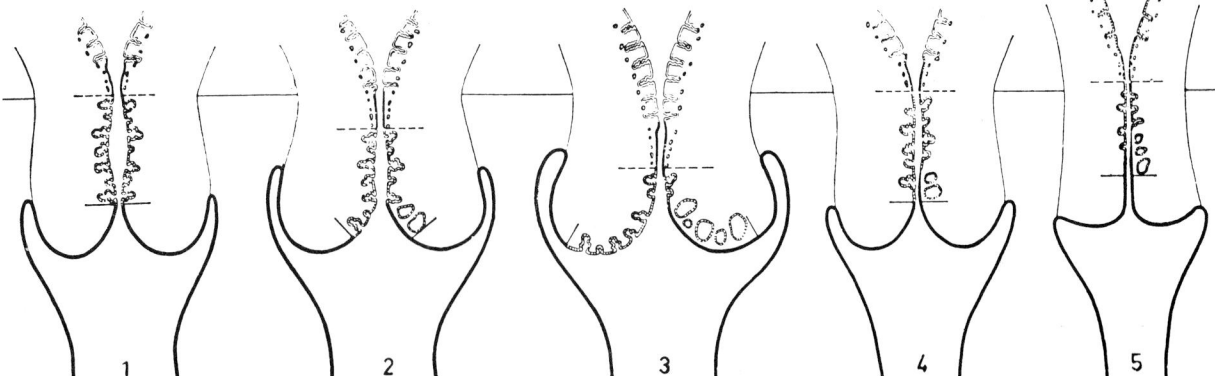

Figure 55-7

Diagram of physiologic cervical changes occurring during the lifetime of women. *1*, Prepubertal cervix. *2*, Postpubertal cervix. *3*, Cervix during pregnancy. *4*, Perimenopausal cervix. *5*, Postmenopausal cervix. Note the change in cervical shape and vaginal vault. The left side of each diagram shows geographic variations of the endocervical glandular area maintaining a constant length throughout all developmental phases. The right side of each diagram depicts changes related to squamous metaplasia. The original squamocolumnar junction is marked by a continuous line. (From Ober KG: Cervix Uteri and Lebensalter. Dtsch Med Wochenschr 1958;83:1661. Courtesy of Georg Thieme Verlag, Stuttgart.)

have been, sexually active, or have reached age 18 years, have an annual Pap test and pelvic examination. After a woman has had three or more consecutive satisfactory normal annual examinations, the Pap test may be performed less frequently at the discretion of her physician" (Fink, 1988).

Lengthening the interval of screening within the guidelines of the American Cancer Society would appear most reasonable in women at low risk for cervical cancer (i.e., those in a lifelong monogamous sexual relationship). However, sensitive information regarding the sexual history of patients is often not obtained accurately. In view of our current understanding of cervical neoplasia as a sexually transmitted disease, it seems necessary that the sexual history of the male partner also be reviewed before the patient can be classified as being at low or high risk for cervical cancer.

Reporting Cytologic Assessments

Several methods of reporting the results of cervical smears are currently in use. Of the systems listed in Table 55-5, the original Papanicolaou classification is the least acceptable because it does not reflect the current understanding of cervical neoplasia and has no equivalent in diagnostic histopathologic terminology (National Cancer Institute, 1989). In an attempt to develop concise, unambiguous, and universal terminology, a group of experts convened in 1988 at the National Institutes of Health in Bethesda, Maryland, and proposed the Bethesda System for reporting cervical or vaginal cytologic diagnoses. The system was simplified in a second workshop held in 1991 and is shown in Table 55-6.

The new system introduced the term *SIL. LGSIL* encompasses mild cervical dysplasia (CIN 1). All higher grade lesions, including moderate and severe

dysplasia and carcinoma in situ (CIN 2 and 3), are designated *HGSIL*. The new terminology corresponds well to current concepts of the biology of cervical cancer precursor lesions and finds its histologic correlation in the new terms *low- and high-grade CIN* (Richart, 1990). HPV-associated changes without features of dysplasia or CIN, the so-called flat condyloma, may be described as "cellular changes associated with HPV," although the Bethesda conference participants recommended that it be included under the designation of "low-grade SIL."

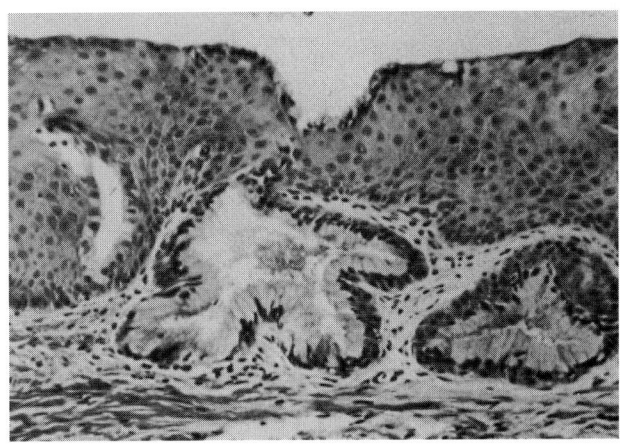

Figure 55-8

Photomicrograph of squamous metaplastic epithelium. The metaplastic epithelium has differentiated into the basal, parabasal, and intermediate cell layers. A duct lined with cuboidal cells still connects the surface with the subepithelial gland. Note the single layer of reserve cells beneath the basement membrane of the central gland. Reserve cell hyperplasia is evident in the periphery of the smaller gland on the right. (×350.)

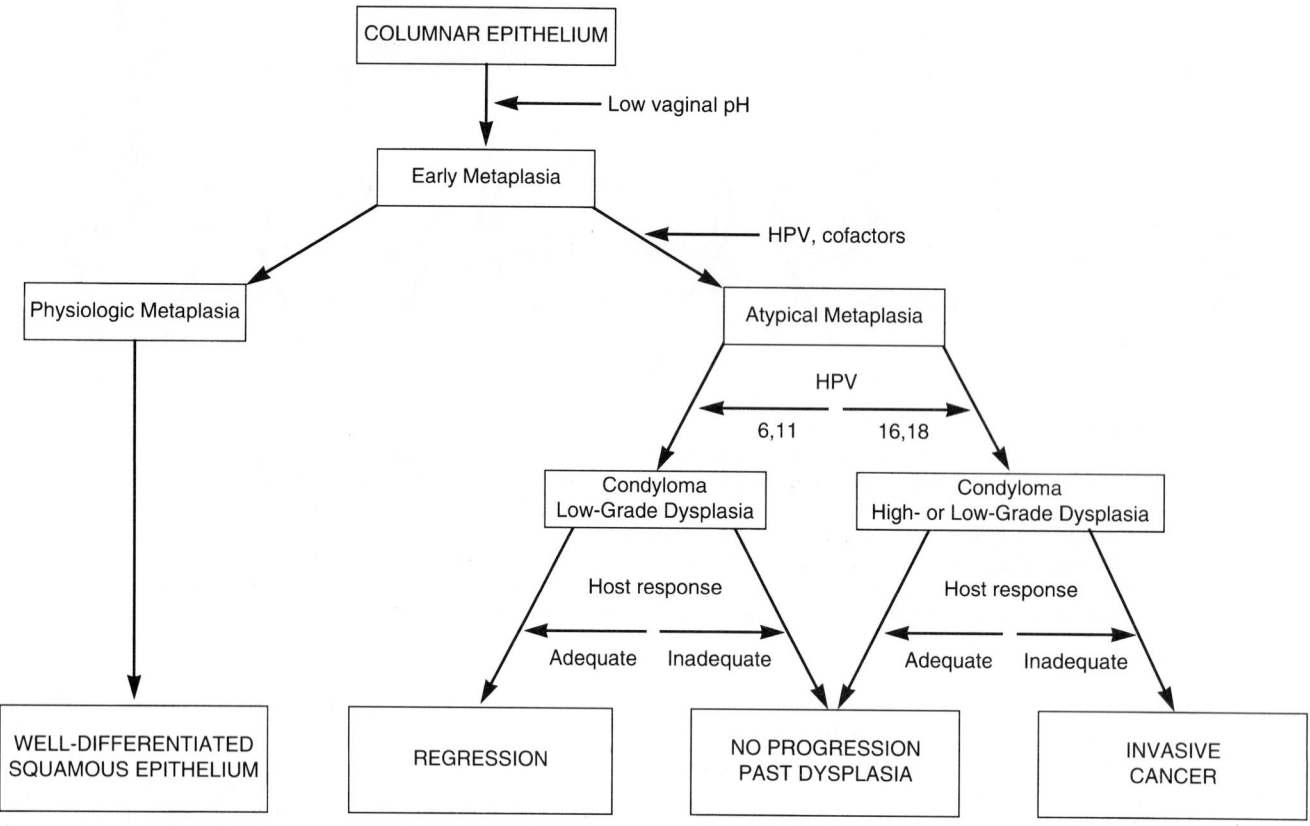

Figure 55–9
Diagrammatic illustration of the theory of development of cervical neoplasia. (Modified from Stafl A, Mattingly RF: Vaginal adenosis: a precancerous lesion? Am J Obstet Gynecol 1974;120:666, with permission.)

Table 55–4. GUIDELINES FOR OBTAINING PAP SMEARS

1. The patient should be instructed not to douche or use any type of vaginal lubricant for 24 hours before having a Pap smear.
2. Cytologic specimens should be obtained with a nonlubricated speculum before the pelvic examination. Moistening the speculum with warm water is usually satisfactory.
3. The cervix must be fully visible when the smear is obtained.
4. The ectocervix and the endocervix should be sampled separately.
5. A wooden or plastic Ayre spatula is rotated with slight pressure over the entire ectocervix.
6. The endocervical sampling device is gently inserted into the endocervix and rotated slowly one to two full turns.
7. The material is rapidly applied to a glass slide with a frosted end and spread evenly. The material on the slide must be spread thinly so that microscopic interpretation is possible. Each sample may be placed on a separate glass slide or, alternatively, placed on a single slide.
8. The slide is fixed immediately to prevent drying either by immersing in a jar of 95% ethyl alcohol and fixing for 15 minutes or spraying with aerosol while holding the spray can at least 10–12 inches from the slide. Slides fixed in 95% ethyl alcohol can be transported to the laboratory in the alcohol bath or allowed to air dry following fixation. Smears fixed with aerosol must be air dried before sending to the laboratory.
9. Once the specimen is collected, it should be properly labeled with complete patient identification and should be accompanied by the appropriate requisition form containing all necessary information and signed by the patient's physician.

Modified from American Medical Association, Council on Scientific Affairs: Quality assurance in cervical cytology: the Papanicolaou smear. JAMA 1989;262:1672, with permission. Copyright 1989, American Medical Association.

Table 55-5. REPORTING SYSTEMS FOR SQUAMOUS CELL NEOPLASIAS OF THE CERVIX

PAPANICOLAOU	WORLD HEALTH ORGANIZATION	CIN SYSTEM	BETHESDA SYSTEM
Class I (normal)	Normal	Normal	Normal
Class II (atypical)	Atypical		Other
			Infection (except HPV)
			Reactive and reparative
Class III (suggestive for cancer)	Dysplasia, mild	CIN 1	Low-grade SIL
Class IV (strongly suggestive for cancer)	Dysplasia, moderate, severe; CIS	CIN 2 CIN 3	High-grade SIL
Class V (conclusive for cancer)	Invasive squamous cell cancer	Invasive squamous cell cancer	Invasive squamous cell cancer

Modified from American Medical Association, Council on Scientific Affairs: Quality assurance in cervical cytology: the Papanicolaou smear. JAMA 1989;262:1672, with permission. Copyright 1989, American Medical Association.

Table 55-6. THE 1991 BETHESDA SYSTEM

Adequacy of the Specimen
Satisfactory for evaluation
Satisfactory for evaluation but limited by (specify reason)
Unsatisfactory for evaluation (specify reason)

General Categorization (optional)
Within normal limits
Benign cellular changes: see descriptive diagnosis
Epithelial cell abnormality: see descriptive diagnosis

Descriptive Diagnosis
Benign cellular changes
  Infection
    Trichomonas vaginalis
    Fungal organisms morphologically consistent with *Candida* species
    Predominance of coccobacilli consistent with shift in vaginal flora
    Bacteria morphologically consistent with *Actinomyces* species
    Cellular changes associated with herpes simplex virus
    Other

  Reactive changes
    Reactive cellular changes associated with:
      Inflammation (includes typical repair)
      Atrophy with inflammation (atrophic vaginitis)
      Radiation
      Intrauterine contraceptive device
      Other
Epithelial cell abnormalities
  Squamous cell
    Atypical squamous cells of undetermined significance (qualify*)
    Low-grade squamous intraepithelial lesion encompassing HPV,[†] mild dysplasia/CIN I
    High-grade squamous intraepithelial lesion encompassing moderate and severe dysplasia, CIS/
      CIN II, and CIN III
    Squamous cell carcinoma
  Glandular cell
    Endometrial cells, cytologically benign, in postmenopausal women
    Atypical glandular cells of undetermined significance (qualify*)
    Endocervical adenocarcinoma
    Endometrial adenocarcinoma
    Extrauterine adenocarcinoma
    Adenocarcinoma, not otherwise specified (NOS)
Other malignant neoplasms (specify)
Hormonal evaluation (applies to vaginal smears only)
  Hormonal pattern compatible with age and history
  Hormonal pattern incompatible with age and history (specify)
  Hormonal evaluation not possible because of (specify)

*Atypical squamous or glandular cells of undetermined significance should be further qualified as to whether a reactive or a premalignant/malignant process is favored.
[†]Cellular changes of HPV—previously termed koilocytosis, koilocytotic atypia, or condylomatous atypia—are included in the category of low-grade squamous intraepithelial lesion.
Modified from Broders S: Report of 1991 Bethesda workshop. JAMA 1992;267:1892, with permission.

Atypical Squamous Cells of Undermined Significance

This category of the Bethesda System does not correspond to the previously used terms *atypia, inflammatory atypia,* or *Class II,* which were replaced by more accurate diagnoses such as "reactive changes" or "infection." The term *ASCUS* is limited to epithelial abnormalities that are of uncertain significance. A 1992 Bethesda workshop concluded that, in most populations, ASCUS may be expected on no more than 5% of Pap test findings. A greater frequency may represent overuse of that diagnosis (Kurman et al, 1994) and result in overtreatment.

It has been found useful to qualify ASCUS by adding the statement "favor reactive" or "favor dysplasia." Less than 5% of women with "ASCUS, favor reactive" will eventually be confirmed histologically to have high-grade lesions. By contrast, women with "ASCUS, favor dysplasia" have biopsy-confirmed high-grade dysplasias in 20% to 30% of cases (Crum et al, 1997).

The 1992 workshop participants developed interim guidelines for the management of women with ASCUS. The guidelines are listed in Table 55–7 and are expected to change as gaps in current knowledge are filled (Kurman et al, 1994).

Atypical Glandular Cells of Undetermined Significance

Atypical glandular cells of undetermined significance (AGUS) may be found in 0.5% to 2.5% of smears and include a variety of lesions ranging from benign reactive changes in endocervical or endometrial cells to advanced adenocarcinoma in situ and invasive adenocarcinoma. Endocervical atypia may be associated with substantial cervical disease in as many as half of the patients (Goff et al, 1992; Nasu et al, 1993). The diagnosis warrants colposcopy, endocervical and endometrial biopsy, and possible hysteroscopy. A persistent finding of AGUS that is not reconciled by these methods usually requires a cone biopsy (Kurman et al, 1994).

Accuracy of the Pap Test

The error rate (false-negative rate) of the Pap test ranges from 15% to 30% in most recent series (AMA, 1989). Laboratory interpretive errors are responsible for approximately one third of errors; the majority are due to sampling errors. Sampling errors may be the result of inadequate sampling techniques and will be higher if endocervical samples are not routinely obtained. In addition, some lesions may not exfoliate abnormal cells as readily as others. Neoplastic cells may also be obscured by inflammatory changes, especially when invasive carcinoma is present. Nearly 50% of women with invasive cancer have negative smears even on subsequent reviews (Van der Graaf et al, 1987). This emphasizes that the Pap smear is a screening device for cervical precursor lesions, and not a diagnostic tool for cervical cancer. Any visible cervical abnormality should be biopsied irrespective of the result of the Pap smear.

Automated Cytology

Efforts to decrease the false-negative rate of Pap smears through automated image analysis systems are over 20 years old, but, until recently, none of the available techniques has gained wide popularity. A major obstacle for automated interpretation of cytology slides was the necessity to prepare monolayer smears. This process may alter the slide-associated tumor diathesis or result in significant cell loss. A promising "semiautomated" system marketed as Papnet (Neuromedical Systems, Inc.) relies on a computer neural network that searches cytology slides for the most abnormal cellular areas and digitally displays them for visual analysis. Preliminary studies suggest that the computerized test may reduce the incidence of false-negative smears (Sherman et al, 1994).

Table 55–7. INTERIM GUIDELINES FOR MANAGEMENT OF ASCUS

1. Follow-up by Pap tests without colposcopy is acceptable for a diagnosis of ASCUS, particularly when the diagnosis is not qualified further or the cytopathologist favors a reactive process. Pap tests should be repeated every 4 to 6 months until there have been three consecutive negative smears. If a second ASCUS report occurs in the 2-year follow-up period, the patient should be considered for colposcopic evaluation.
2. Women with a diagnosis of unqualified ASCUS associated with severe inflammation should be re-evaluated, preferably after 2 to 3 months. If specific infections such as chlamydial or gonorrheal cervicitis or vaginitis caused by *Candida* or *Trichomonas* are identified, re-evaluation should be performed after appropriate treatment.
3. Postmenopausal women with ASCUS should have a repeat Pap smear after a course of topical or systemic estrogen therapy. If the Pap test is still equivocal after estrogen therapy, colposcopy should be considered.
4. If the diagnosis of ASCUS is qualified by a statement indicating that dysplasia is favored, the patient should undergo colposcopy.
5. If the patient with a diagnosis of ASCUS is at high risk (previous positive Pap tests, poor compliance for follow-up), colposcopy should be considered.

Modified from Kurman RJ, Henson DE, Herbst AL, et al for the 1992 National Cancer Institute Workshop: Interim guidelines for management of abnormal cervical cytology. JAMA 1994;271:1866, with permission.

To facilitate the preparation of cytologic samples into thin layers, an automated device called the Thin Prep Processor (Cytec Corporation, Marlborough, MA) has recently been developed. The cytology specimen is collected from the cervix with conventional sampling devices and suspended in a solution for transport and preservation. The cells are mildly dispersed in the cytology laboratory and transferred to a glass slide using filter transfer technology. The cell density on the slide is controlled by the processor. The new method yields clean, uniform samples with better visualization of diagnostic cells (Zahniser and Hurley, 1996). Studies comparing the Thin Prep method with conventional cytology found the preparation of cervical slides from cells in suspension to be more sensitive than the Pap preparation for the detection of cervical lesions. However, the specificity of both methods was equivalent (Sheets et al, 1995). It remains to be seen whether or not the slight gain in diagnostic accuracy with the new tests warrants the increase in cost of approximately $20 per smear.

Colposcopy

Although increasingly used in the assessment of many non-neoplastic conditions of the lower genital tract, the main purpose of colposcopy is to localize the source of the abnormal cells detected by the Pap test, to determine the extent of the lesion for treatment planning, and to select the sites for biopsy in order to establish a histologic diagnosis. Expert colposcopists may also predict the severity of the underlying disease by evaluating several colposcopic parameters.

Colposcopic Examination

The colposcope is a binocular instrument with a working focal length of 300 mm and a powerful coaxial light source allowing stereoscopic inspection of the cervix under magnification (5× to 40×). Most of the examination is carried out under low power (5× to 10×). Higher power settings have little depth of field and are most useful when minute details (e.g., abnormal vessels) are examined. A green filter is helpful to emphasize vascular patterns by giving red vessels a black color against a pale green background.

First, the cervix is fully exposed and cleaned with a large cotton swab moistened with normal saline. If a repeat Pap test is to be obtained, it should be taken before any further manipulation of the cervix takes place. The cervix and surrounding vagina are then carefully examined colposcopically, first without and then with the green filter. Any abnormal vascular pattern or surface changes should be noted.

A 3% to 5% solution of acetic acid is liberally applied to the cervix with cotton swabs. The acid not only precipitates mucus and facilitates its removal but also causes nuclear swelling leading to opacifi-

cation of epithelium containing areas of high nuclear density. Immature squamous metaplastic epithelium and dysplastic epithelium turn white 1 to 2 minutes after application of the acetic acid. The degree of whiteness of the epithelium correlates with the histologic grade of the lesion and the duration of exposure to the acid. Hence, the cervix must be kept moist with acetic acid during the entire colposcopic examination. If abnormal vessels are found, the cervix is re-examined under green light and possibly also under higher magnification. If the T zone or the lesion extends into the endocervix, spreading the endocervical lips with an endocervical speculum may extend the field of vision and help to evaluate concealed portions of the lesion. Occasionally, manipulation of the cervix with a cotton-tipped applicator or an iris hook may be sufficient to inspect the endocervix (Fig. 55–10).

Some colposcopists complete the colposcopic examination by applying iodine solution to the cervix and vagina. The iodine stains normal glycogen-containing epithelium dark brown; other epithelia remain pale. The stain may help to delineate colposcopic findings and is of particular value in the examination of the vagina because of its large surface area. There are many subtleties of the staining that require experience to interpret.

The colposcopist must then decide if the colposcopic examination is "satisfactory" or "adequate." If the T zone and the extent of the lesion cannot be fully visualized, the examination is called "unsatisfactory" or "inadequate."

Colposcopic Findings

The colposcopic terminology adopted by the International Federation of Cervical Pathology and Colposcopy (IFCPC) at its Seventh World Congress in Rome in 1990 is shown in Table 55–8.

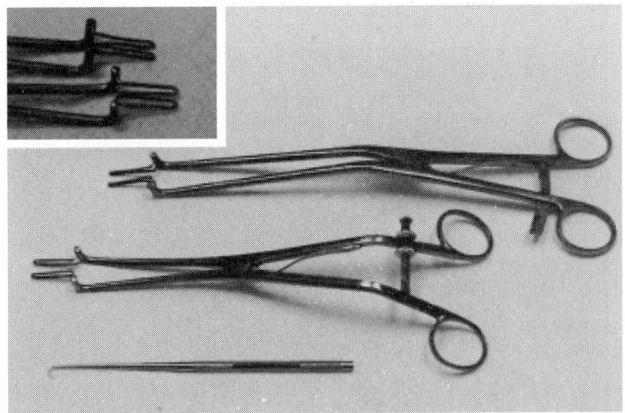

Figure 55–10
Instruments aiding in inspection of the endocervix. *Top,* Narrow and wide endocervical specula. *Bottom,* Emmet hook. *Inset,* Tips of narrow and wide endocervical specula at higher magnification.

Table 55–8. NOMENCLATURE FOR COLPOSCOPY

TERMINOLOGY

I. Normal colposcopic findings
   A. Original squamous epithelium
   B. Columnar epithelium
   C. Normal transformation zone
II. Abnormal colposcopic findings
   A. Within the transformation zone
     1. Aceto-white epithelium*
      a. Flat
      b. Micropapillary or microconvoluted
     2. Punctation*
     3. Mosaic*
     4. Leukoplakia*
     5. Iodine-negative epithelium
     6. Atypical vessels*
   B. Outside the transformation zone (e.g., ectocervix, vagina)
     1. Aceto-white epithelium*
      a. Flat
      b. Micropapillary or microconvoluted
     2. Punctation*
     3. Mosaic*
     4. Leukoplakia*
     5. Iodine-negative epithelium
     6. Atypical vessels*
III. Colposcopically suspect invasive carcinoma
IV. Unsatisfactory colposcopy
   A. Squamocolumnar junction not visible
   B. Severe inflammation or severe atrophy
   C. Cervix not visible
V. Miscellaneous findings
   A. Non–aceto-white micropapillary surface
   B. Exophytic condyloma
   C. Inflammation
   D. Atrophy
   E. Ulcer
   F. Other

DEFINITIONS

I. Normal colposcopic findings
   A. **Original squamous epithelium** is a smooth, pink epithelium originally established on the cervix and vagina.
   B. **Columnar epithelium** is a single-layer, mucus-producing tall epithelium that extends between the endometrium cranially and either the original squamous epithelium or the metaplastic epithelium caudally. The area covered with columnar epithelium has an irregular surface with long stromal papillae and deep clefts. Colposcopically the area has a typical grape-like appearance. Columnar epithelium may be present in the endocervix, on the portio, or even in the vagina (adenosis).
   C. **Normal transformation zone** is the area between original squamous epithelium and columnar epithelium in which metaplastic epithelium in varying degrees of maturity is identified. Components of a normal transformation zone may be islands of columnar epithelium surrounded by metaplastic squamous epithelium, "gland openings," and nabothian cysts.
II. Abnormal colposcopic findings
   A. **Atypical transformation zone:** A transformation zone in which there are colposcopic findings suggestive of cervical neoplasia.
     1. **Aceto-white epithelium** is a focal colposcopic pattern of white epithelium seen after application of acetic acid. The epithelial whitening is a transient phenomenon that is seen in the area of increased nuclear density. The surface of the epithelium may be flat or irregular as a result of micropapillary changes or microconvolutions.
     2. **Punctation** is a focal colposcopic pattern in which capillaries give the epithelium a stippled appearance.
     3. **Mosaic** is a focal colposcopic pattern in which the tissue has a mosaic appearance. The fields of mosaic are separated by reddish borders.
     4. **Leukoplakia** (formerly keratosis) is a focal colposcopic pattern in which hyperkeratosis or parakeratosis is present. It appears as an elevated whitened plaque that is visible before the application of acetic acid. Leukoplakia may be identified outside the transformation zone.
     5. **Iodine-negative epithelium** lacks glycogen and therefore does not take up iodine. It remains pale in contrast to iodine-positive epithelium.
     6. **Atypical vessels** are colposcopically recognizable blood vessels that appear not as punctation, mosaic, or delicately branching vessels, but rather as irregular vessels with abrupt courses appearing as commas, corkscrew capillaries, or spaghetti-like forms.
III. **Colposcopically suspect invasive cancer:** colposcopically obvious invasive cancer that is not evident on clinical examination.
IV. **Unsatisfactory colposcopy:** This term is used in cases where the squamocolumnar junction or the extent of the lesion cannot be visualized, or the findings are obscured by severe inflammation or severe atrophy.

(Table continued on opposite page)

Table 55 – 8. NOMENCLATURE FOR COLPOSCOPY (*Continued*)

V. Miscellaneous findings
   A. **Non–aceto-white micropapillary surface** is often associated with HPV but may represent variants of normal epithelium. The appearance is similar to micropapillary changes but without aceto-whitening.
   B. **Exophytic condyloma** is a papillary growth associated with HPV infection (condyloma acuminatum).
   C. **Inflammation** is a colposcopic pattern of hyperemia in which the blood vessels may appear in a diffused stippled pattern similar to the vascular pattern in punctation, but without aceto-whitening.
   D. **Atrophy** designates estrogen-deprived squamous epithelium in which the vascular pattern is more readily identified because of the relative thinness of the overlying squamous epithelium.
   E. **Ulcer** is an area denuded of epithelium, usually by trauma. In contrast to erosion, there is also a shallow defect of the underlying stroma.
   F. Other

*Indicates minor or major changes. Minor changes: aceto-white epithelium, fine punctation, fine mosaic, thin leukoplakia. Major changes: dense aceto-white epithelium, coarse punctation, coarse mosaic, thick leukoplakia, atypical vessels, erosion.
Modified from Stafl A, Wilbanks GD: An international terminology of colposcopy: report of Nomenclature Committee of the International Federation of Cervical Pathology and Colposcopy. Obstet Gynecol 1991;77:313. Reprinted with permission from the American College of Obstetricians and Gynecologists.

ATYPICAL TRANSFORMATION ZONE

The atypical T zone contains sharply demarcated areas of abnormal epithelium, which the colposcopist identifies as leukoplakia (formerly keratosis) if apparent *before* application of acetic acid. Aceto-white epithelium, punctation, or mosaic pattern becomes apparent after application of acetic acid (Fig. 55–11*A* to *C*). These three patterns are colposcopic hallmarks of dysplasia. However, they may also represent variants of squamous metaplasia, particularly in DES-exposed women with adenosis.

With the beginning of invasion, new vessels form that initially run parallel to and just below the surface. These atypical vessels are called *horizontal capillaries* and often signify microinvasion (Stafl, 1983). With increasing invasion, the vascular pattern becomes more complex as prominent large, irregular vessels form that branch in a random manner. Fully invasive cancer may also be suspected when the surface is highly irregular from exophytic tumor growth, ulceration, or a combination of both.

HPV-ASSOCIATED CERVICAL CHANGES

The discovery of HPV-associated changes of the cervix added a dazzling variety of colposcopic findings to the established patterns of cervical dysplasia. In some patients, islands of aceto-white epithelium (satellite lesions) are found in the periphery of the cervix outside the T zone. The surface may appear micropapillary (spiked), flat, or sometimes microconvoluted to a brain-like epithelial arrangement (Fig. 55–11*D*). Many of the flat lesions have a pure, shiny white color reminiscent of pearls, in contrast to the dull, oyster-white color of high-grade CIN (Fig. 55–11*B*). Some HPV infections produce coarse capillary loops with a horizontal or vertical orientation, giving the appearance of mosaic or punctation. The regular spacing of the vessels helps to differentiate these patterns from invasive carcinomas (Reid and Campion, 1989).

Prominent HPV-associated changes are often over-interpreted, resulting in overly aggressive treatment for these relatively innocuous epithelial changes. Reid and Scalzi (1985) devised a colposcopic grading scheme that is helpful to differentiate low-grade CIN, including flat condylomas, from high-grade CIN (Table 55–9).

Cervicography

As previously discussed, the major deficiency of the Pap smear is the high false-negative rate of up to 30% even when modern sampling methods are used (AMA, 1989). The accuracy of detection of cervical neoplasias can be improved by screening patients by both cytology and colposcopy at the same time. Colposcopy, however, is impractical and not economical for screening purposes. Therefore, Stafl, in 1981, proposed a "snapshot" version of colposcopy that he called "cervicography."

The optical system, called a cervicograph, is a 35-mm camera with a 100-mm fixed focus macrolense and a ring flash. A slide film is used for photographic documentation of the cervix. The photographs (cervicograms) can be made with very little training. After development of the film, the cervicograms are projected on a screen and interpreted by an expert colposcopist (Stafl, 1981).

Several studies have shown that cervicography is more sensitive than cytology in the detection of cervical neoplasias and that the false-negative rate of cytology alone may be significantly reduced. However, approximately 40% of cervicograms are unsatisfactory or unreadable either for technical reasons or because the T zone is not fully displayed (Blythe, 1985). More importantly, 60% to 80% of women with suspicious cervicograms have no demonstrable pathology (Blythe, 1985; Tawa et al, 1988). Because of the unacceptably high false-positive rate, cervicography is unlikely to become a cost-effective adjunct

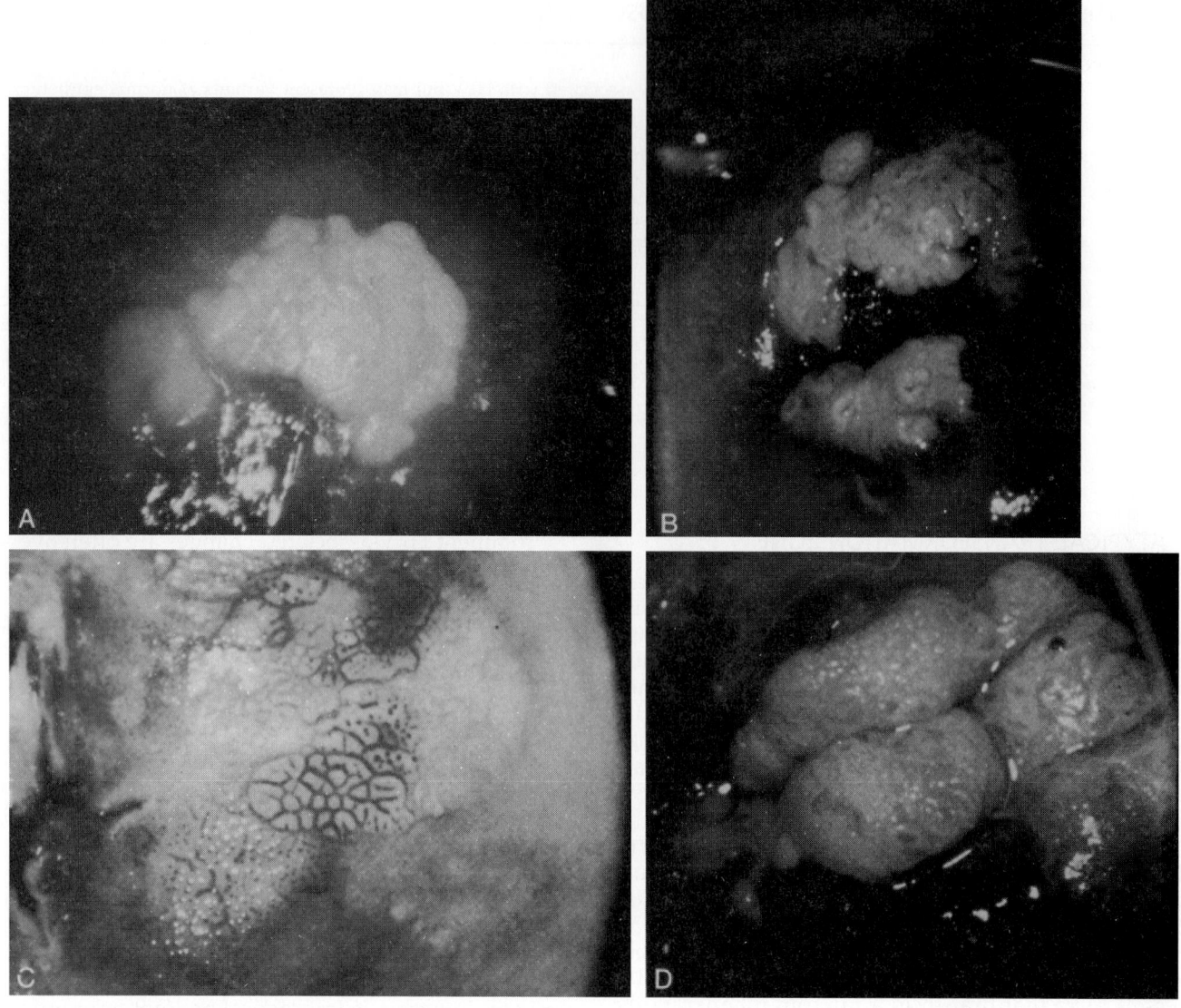

Figure 55–11
Colpophotographs of abnormal transformation zone. *A*, Leukoplakia (keratosis). The prominent, thick white plaque was evident before application of acetic acid. Biopsy showed parakeratosis (dyskeratosis) overlying koilocytotic cellular changes. *B*, Aceto-white epithelium. The lesion surrounds the cervical os. The pearly white, smooth, shiny surface indicates a low-grade lesion. Biopsy showed mild dysplasia associated with condyloma. *C*, Mixed punctate and mosaic pattern consistent with high-grade dysplasia. *D*, Micropapillary pattern. The surface is irregular because of myriad tiny asperites. Biopsy showed condyloma.

to routine cytologic screening (Solomon and Wied, 1989).

Colpomicroscopy

The colpomicroscope was developed by Antoine and Grünberger (1949) in Austria. The instrument is a single-barreled, direct light microscope fitted to a removable obturator that is inserted into the vagina and against the cervix. The exposed area of the cervix may be examined at magnifications of 140× to 280×, depending on the eyepiece used. After vital

staining with 1% toluidine blue or other stains, it is possible to examine the cellular detail of the surface of the cervix in vivo (Wilbanks, 1978).

Colpomicroscopy has limited clinical applications but is a useful tool when cellular details are to be studied in a living patient without disturbing the tissues.

Microcolpohysteroscopy

Microcolpohysteroscopy, like colpomicroscopy, allows in vivo examination of cellular detail at high

Table 55-9. COLPOSCOPIC INDEX*

COLPOSCOPIC SIGN	ZERO POINTS	1 POINT	2 POINTS
Margin	Condylomatous or micropapillary contour Indistinct aceto-whitening Flocculated or feathered margins Angular, jagged lesions Satellite lesions and aceto-whitening that extends beyond transformation zone	Regular lesions with smooth, straight outlines	Rolled, peeling edges Internal demarcations between areas of differing appearance
Color	Shiny, snow white color Indistinct aceto-whitening	Intermediate shade (shiny gray)	Dull, oyster white
Vessels	Fine-caliber vessels, poorly formed patterns Condylomatous or micropapillary lesions	Absent vessels	Definite punctation or mosaicism
Iodine	Positive iodine staining Minor iodine negativity	Partial iodine uptake	Negative staining

*Colposcopic score: 0–2, low-grade CIN; 3–5, indeterminate; 6–8, high-grade CIN.
Modified from Reid R, Scalzi P: Genital warts and cervical cancer. VII. An improved colposcopic index for differentiating benign papillomaviral infections from high-grade cervical intraepithelial neoplasia. Am J Obstet Gynecol 1985;153:611, with permission.

magnification. Unlike the colpomicroscope, however, the microcolpohysteroscope is easily introduced into the endocervix, and may therefore be used to define the extent of the lesion or the T zone within the cervical canal (Fenton et al, 1984). The microcolpohysteroscope is, in fact, an endoscope designed for hysteroscopic examinations, hence the original name "microhysteroscope." The instrument was developed by Hamou in France in 1981. Four magnifications ranging from 1:1 to 150:1 are available and are selected by means of a switch on the ocular. Observations at high magnifications require the application of a supravital stain.

Because microcolpohysteroscopy, like colpomicroscopy, permits only visualization of the superficial cell layers, the diagnosis of invasion cannot be made reliably. Nonetheless, it is possible with this method to predict the underlying pathology in over 80% of the cases. The percentage of correct predictions is even higher when koilocytotic changes are present (Tseng et al, 1987).

Although technically much simpler, quicker, and more convenient than colpomicroscopy, microcolpohysteroscopy is not likely to become a popular diagnostic tool in the work-up of women with abnormal Pap tests because it requires expertise not only in colposcopy but also in cytology and histopathology.

Tissue Diagnosis

Biopsy

The most important prerequisite for office methods of therapy is that a tissue diagnosis be established by biopsy. When performed under colposcopic guidance, tissue specimens can be obtained from the most abnormal appearing area of each separate lesion, resulting in an accurate assessment of the underlying pathology. Biopsies not guided by colposcopy may be entirely sufficient when an obvious lesion is present; they are, however, inadequate when conservative management of the grossly invisible cervical precursor lesions is the issue. Neither multiple random biopsies nor systematic four-quadrant cervical biopsies, even when performed after iodine staining, are precise enough to rule out the presence of invasion.

Because intraepithelial neoplasia is a surface lesion, the objective of the biopsy procedure is to remove a superficial piece of tissue, including the epithelium and some underlying stroma. This is most easily achieved with slightly rounded or square-jawed biopsy forceps (Eppendorfer, Kevorkian) (Fig. 55–12). If the instrument is kept sharp, the cervical biopsy is not painful and sedation or local anesthesia is rarely needed. Provided the patient is not pregnant and has no bleeding diathesis and the biopsy is shallow, bleeding is slight and quickly controlled by pressure or cauterization with silver nitrate or ferrous subsulfate (Monsel's solution). Monsel's solution is most effective, particularly when allowed to air dry, so that it assumes a mustard-like color and consistency. Sexual abstinence for 2 to 3 days following the biopsy is usually sufficient.

The cervical punch biopsy specimens should be placed individually on a small piece of brown paper towel, spread out and oriented so that the epithelium is on the surface. This prevents tangential cutting and loss of surface epithelium during processing. The specimen is then fixed according to the preferences of the examining pathology laboratory.

Endocervical Curettage

It is generally recommended that an endocervical curettage (ECC) be performed in the work-up of an

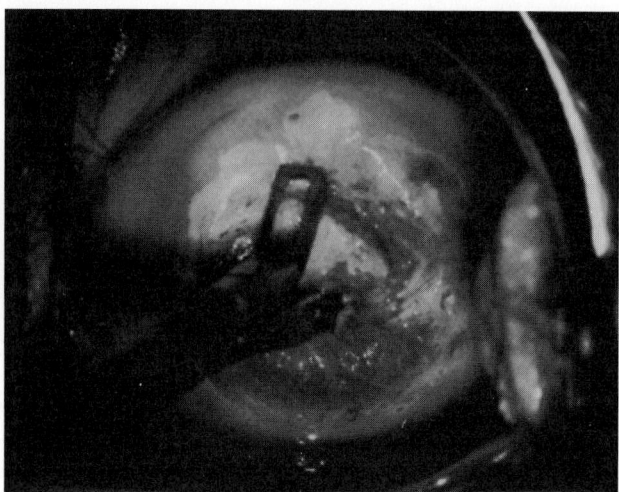

Figure 55–12
Colpophotograph of cervical biopsy under colposcopic guidance. The instrument depicted is a Kevorkian biopsy forceps. Note the aceto-white epithelium on the anterior cervical lip.

abnormal Pap smear to document that the endocervical canal is free of neoplastic epithelium. The need for routine ECC in cases where the lesion and the T zone are confined to the ectocervix has been questioned. However, all but the most experienced colposcopists will be more confident in managing CIN conservatively if they are reassured by a negative ECC.

The endocervical curettage is best carried out by an endocervical curet of the Kevorkian type. The curet has a diameter of 3 mm and may be introduced into the endocervix without dilatation. The tissue fragments obtained are frequently small, devoid of underlying stroma, and impossible to orient. Therefore, the curettings may be unsuitable for histologic grading of the lesion and only a qualitative diagnosis (positive or negative) may be possible. To obtain cohesive strips of epithelium suitable for histologic grading, it is necessary to use a sharp curette and to retrieve it from the endocervix with brisk individual strokes from each quadrant while applying firm pressure against the mucosa. This procedure is perceived as painful and a local anesthetic may be needed.

Diagnostic Conization

Indications

Most women with abnormal Pap smears may be treated in the office. The need for diagnostic conization arises when (1) the colposcopy is unsatisfactory, (2) the ECC is positive, (3) there is a major discrepancy between cytology and histology, and (4) microinvasive cancer is suspected.

UNSATISFACTORY COLPOSCOPY

With increasing age, the T zone regresses into the endocervix so that the SCJ and the extent of the lesion may not be fully visualized. Colposcopic examinations in women over 40 years are unsatisfactory in more than 50% of patients, compared with 10% to 20% in women less than 30 years (Ostergard, 1977). High-grade dysplasias are often larger and extend more commonly into the endocervix than low-grade lesions, resulting in unsatisfactory colposcopy and need for conization in many older women and those with advanced lesions.

POSITIVE ECC

A positive ECC is a common and well-accepted indication for conization. However, when the colposcopic examination is adequate, a positive ECC more often represents a contaminant from a known ectocervical or slightly endocervical lesion than abnormal endocervical epithelium beyond colposcopic visibility. In select patients in whom repeat colposcopy confirms the endocervix to be clear, conservative therapy may be considered.

DISCREPANCY BETWEEN CYTOLOGY AND HISTOLOGY

Sometimes cytology suggests a more advanced lesion than can be verified by colposcopically directed biopsy and ECC. Because the Pap test may have been overread, it is good practice to review the cytology and the biopsy findings with an experienced cytopathologist in light of the available clinical information. If the pathologist maintains that the cellular changes are of concern and not explained by the available evidence, conization is necessary. Otherwise conservative management and close follow-up appear preferable (Krebs and Helmkamp, 1990).

EVALUATION OF MICROINVASION

Diagnostic conization of the cervix is necessary when microinvasive carcinoma is suspected. Microinvasive carcinoma is currently defined both by the depth of invasion (up to 5 mm) and by width at the surface (up to 7 mm). Neither of the two measurements is reliably obtained by simple biopsy.

Contraindications

The presence of an obvious cervical lesion suspicious of invasive carcinoma is an absolute contraindication for cervical conization. The lesion should be biopsied in the office. If invasion is shown, then the visible lesion is most certainly not a microinvasive carcinoma. Conization would do nothing more than add expenses and complications, and delay definitive therapy.

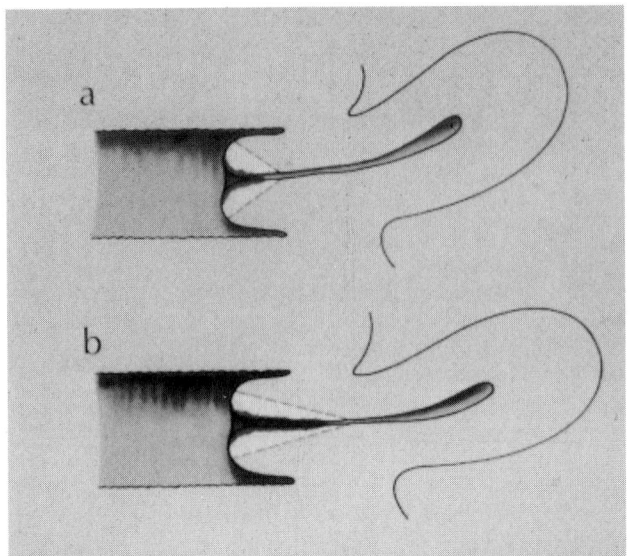

Figure 55-13
Cervical conization. Preoperative assessment determines whether a shallow (a) or deep cone (b) should be excised. (From Helmkamp BF, Krebs HB, Averette HE: Meeting the challenge of cervical cone biopsy. Contemp Obstet Gynecol 1983;December:85, with permission.)

Technical Aspects

Complete excision of the lesion is a prerequisite for exact diagnosis and, at the same time, constitutes definitive therapy if intraepithelial neoplasia is found. To obtain an adequate cone specimen, the surgeon must know the location of the lesion (Fig. 55–13). The external cone margin should be 2 to 3 mm outside the lesion and is easily determined by colposcopic examination or iodine staining. The endocervical extent of the lesion is ascertained by gently exposing the cervical canal with an endocervical speculum. If the expertise is available, the Hamou microcolpohysteroscope may also be used to accurately assess endocervical epithelium and to determine the depth of the cone (Fenton et al, 1984).

Hemostasis is aided by ligating descending branches of the uterine arteries (Fig. 55–14A) and injecting the cervix with a vasoconstricting solution (phenylephrine hydrochloride or vasopressin).

Excision of the cone specimen may be achieved with a scalpel ("cold-knife cone"), electrodiathermy ("hot cone"), or the carbon dioxide (CO_2) laser (Fig. 55–14B). Electrodiathermy may cause extensive tissue necrosis, making the cone margins difficult or impossible to interpret. This problem has recently been largely overcome by improvements in the electrodiathermy equipment and is further discussed below. Laser cone excisions may be associated with the same problem. In skilled hands, however, epithelial burns are acceptable with either electrodiathermy or the CO_2 laser.

After excision of the cone, the remainder of the endocervix should be curetted with an endocervical curette to determine complete clearance of the lesion from the endocervix. A cervical dilation and curettage of the endometrial cavity does not need to be performed routinely but is advisable in peri- and postmenopausal women and in those with irregular uterine bleeding (Helmkamp et al, 1983). Hemostasis is easily obtained by cauterizing the entire cone bed with a suction coagulator, providing electrocoagulation and suction at the same time (Fig. 55–14C). To avoid scarring and distortion of the cervix, sutures are not placed routinely.

When a very large cone is being excised or when troublesome bleeding occurs, the circumferential suture technique (Fig. 55–15) is helpful. It provides excellent hemostasis, reconstructs the cervix, and achieves good anatomic results (Krebs, 1984). The classical Sturmdorf suture of the cervix is more likely to cause cervical stenosis and it is rarely used today unless in modified form.

Complications

Although now routinely performed in outpatient surgery units, cervical conization is not an innocuous procedure. It is, in fact, associated with a higher rate of morbidity and complications than most routine gynecologic operations, including hysterectomy. Up to 30% of women in recent series suffered intraoperative hemorrhage, postoperative hemorrhage, infections, uterine perforation, and cervical stenosis (Krebs, 1984). If large cones are obtained from small cervices, cervical scarring or loss of cervical tissue may be severe and result in infertility. This is particularly of concern in nulliparous women who wish to have children (Claman and Lee, 1974).

Follow-up

Women who have had cervical conization should abstain from sexual intercourse until adequate healing is documented at the 4-week postoperative checkup. At that time, the cervix should be inspected and the endocervical canal probed for patency. Because of persistent inflammation related to the healing process, cytologic examination is best deferred until 3 months after the conization.

Patients with negative cone margins and a negative ECC are, unless invasive carcinoma is found, considered to be adequately treated. However, the chance of persistent or recurrent dysplasia may still be as high as 16% (Husseinzadeh et al, 1989). Therefore, lifelong follow-up examinations with Pap smears are necessary.

Women with positive cone margins pose somewhat of a dilemma. When the external margins are involved, colposcopy should be performed. If an ectocervical lesion is found, it can often be successfully ablated by office methods. Up to 60% of patients with significant dysplasia at the internal cone margins have residual endocervical disease. The ECC may give guidance in regard to further management. If the ECC is negative, the chance of residual endo-

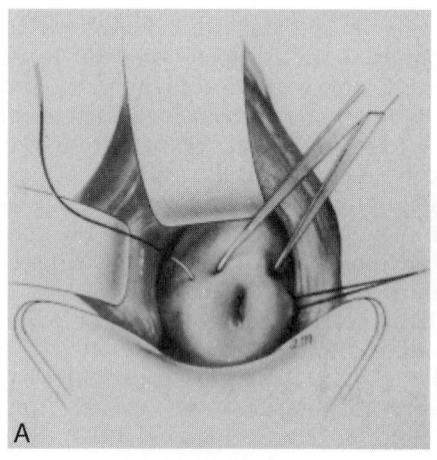 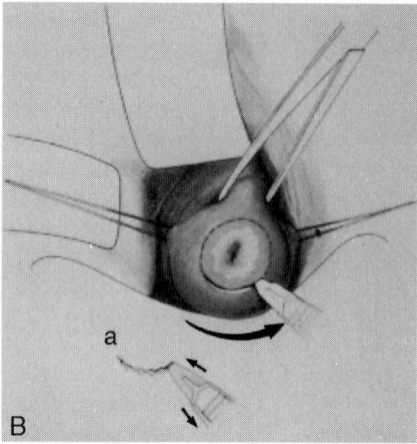 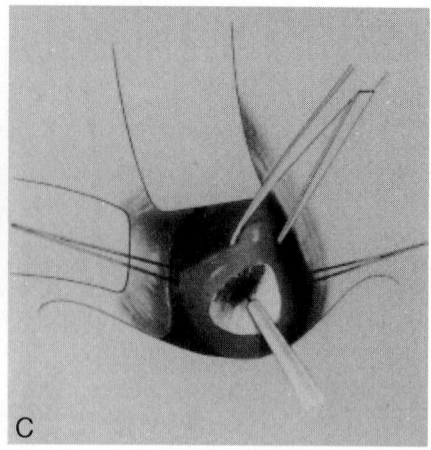

Figure 55-14
Cervical conization. *A,* A suture is placed deeply within the cervical stroma at the level of the internal cervical os to ligate the descending branches of the uterine arteries. *B,* The blade of the knife is "pushed" through the cervical stroma to ensure a smooth cone bed. A "stabbing" or "sawing" motion (*inset "a"*) is more traumatic but may be inevitable in densely fibrotic cervical tissue. *C,* Electrocoagulation of the cone bed at a high-power setting (60 to 80 watts) accomplishes hemostasis. (From Helmkamp BF, Krebs HB, Averette HE: Meeting the challenge of cervical cone biopsy. Contemp Obstet Gynecol 1983;December:85, with permission.)

cervical disease is less than 40% (Husseinzadeh et al, 1989). These women may be managed conservatively if repeat Pap tests and ECCs remain normal during follow-up.

A positive ECC, however, in combination with positive internal margins indicates residual disease

Figure 55-15
Circumferential suturing technique of larger cervical defects after cervical conization. *A,* Placement of the anterior and posterior sutures. *B,* The anterior and posterior sutures are tied together on the right, and the left knot is being tied. *C,* Both sutures are now tied. (From Helmkamp BF, Krebs HB, Averette HE: Meeting the challenge of cervical cone biopsy. Contemp Obstet Gynecol 1983;December:85, with permission.)

in almost 90% of the patients (Husseinzadeh et al, 1989). Further evaluation and therapy are therefore recommended. Although many gynecologists resort directly to hysterectomy, the procedure may not be justified if high-grade dysplasia is found at the cone margins or within the ECC specimen. Invasive carcinoma continues to be a distinct possibility and should again be ruled out (Jones and Buller, 1980). Thus a second, deeper conization is appropriate and most often curative.

Cervical Neoplasia in Pregnancy

The evaluation of a woman with an abnormal Pap smear in pregnancy provides a special challenge for the gynecologist, who is restricted in the use of diagnostic tools and must ascertain the presence or absence of invasive cervical cancer on a hypervascular, congested cervix. This can usually be done with a combination of cytology, colposcopy, and careful use of colposcopically directed biopsy. However, *ECC is contraindicated in pregnancy.*

Colposcopy

The high estrogenic state of pregnancy leads to eversion of the endocervical mucosa and makes the T zone more visible. Therefore, colposcopy is rarely unsatisfactory in early pregnancy. In the second half of pregnancy, hypertrophy and congestion of the cervix, combined with tenacious cervical mucus and redundancy of the vaginal walls, tend to obscure the colposcopic field and prevent adequate visualization of the T zone. A large speculum sheathed with a finger from a latex glove or with a condom from which the tip was cut off is useful to keep the protruding vaginal walls out of the field of vision. Nonetheless, the colposcopic examination is unsatisfactory in 10% to 13% of pregnant women because of inadequate visualization of the T zone (Kohan et al, 1980; LaPolla et al, 1988).

Biopsy

Although some investigators have stated that there is no need to obtain cervical biopsies in the absence of colposcopic features suggesting invasion, even the most experienced examiner will make diagnostic errors on occasion (DePetrillo et al, 1975). Because carefully directed biopsies can be performed with minimal complications, tissue samples should be obtained in all but very minor-appearing cervical lesions.

Conization

Conization of the gravid cervix is associated with complications such as bleeding and pregnancy loss in as many as 32% of patients (Averette et al, 1970). It is therefore recommended that cervical conization be used only when a colposcopically directed biopsy demonstrates microinvasive carcinoma or when abnormal cervical cytologic findings suggestive of invasive carcinoma cannot be explained by colposcopic biopsy (Hannigan et al, 1982). Some patients whose colposcopic evaluation reveals microinvasive carcinoma may be further evaluated and treated by excisional wedge biopsy under colposcopic guidance (DePetrillo et al, 1975).

Most cervical conizations in pregnancy are performed because of deep endocervical location of the lesions, resulting in unsatisfactory colposcopy. To avoid complications, there is a tendency to cut the cones too small and too shallow, resulting in positive cone margins in up to 83% of the cases (Hannigan et al, 1982; LaPolla et al, 1988). Consequently, most of the cones are not adequate to rule out invasive carcinoma, and the need for routine conization of pregnant women with unsatisfactory colposcopy has been questioned. It is strongly recommended that these patients be referred to an expert colposcopist for evaluation.

A possible means of solving the problem of unsatisfactory colposcopy in pregnant women is the use of endocervical endoscopy with the contact hysteroscope or microcolpohysteroscope (Baggish and Dorsey, 1982). The technique can be performed easily on patulous pregnant cervices and allows directed biopsies to be taken from suspicious areas.

Therapy

Unless invasive carcinoma is found, treatment is withheld until after delivery. Biopsy of the lesions during pregnancy, cervical trauma during vaginal delivery, change in the immune status of the patient, and spontaneous regression may all contribute to the fact that a cervical abnormality is no longer demonstrable in 40% or more of patients in the postpartum period. It is therefore necessary that a patient undergo complete re-evaluation with colposcopy, biopsy, and ECC 6 to 8 weeks after delivery to determine whether treatment is still necessary.

Cervical Neoplasia in Postmenopausal Women

The detection and management of cervical neoplasia in postmenopausal women is fraught with great difficulty for three reasons. First, atrophy of the cervical epithelium and inflammatory changes lead to a higher incidence of false-positive cytologic smears. Approximately 30% of postmenopausal women with abnormal smears have no pathologic findings, compared to 10% to 15% of women during their reproductive years. Nonetheless, an abnormal Pap smear is more ominous in older than in younger women: A woman older than 60 years has a 15% chance of having cancer if she has an abnormal Pap smear, whereas a woman younger than 30 has a less than 1% chance (Shingleton et al, 1977).

Second, neoplastic changes are mostly high within the endocervix, so colposcopy is of limited value. Because of a lack of estrogen, the uterine size diminishes after menopause. The cervix loses prominence and eventually becomes flush with the surrounding vaginal epithelium (Fig. 55–7). At the same time, the T zone retracts deeply into the endocervix (Ostergard, 1977). Narrowing of the external cervical os and the cervical canal adds to the difficulties of colposcopic examination. Although colposcopic examination is rarely satisfactory in patients older than 60 years, it should still be attempted, if only to evaluate a possible ectocervical component of the lesion (Krebs et al, 1985). Inflammatory changes related to mucosal atrophy may create confusing colposcopic appearances, and it is often beneficial to repeat the colposcopic examination after 2 to 4 weeks of topical or systemic estrogen therapy. An ECC should also be performed because it provides important information in over 60% of postmenopausal patients (Dinh et al, 1989). Diagnostic conization is necessary in at least one third of postmenopausal women evaluated initially by colposcopy (Shingleton et al, 1977).

Third, cervical cones in postmenopausal women are inadequate in 60% of cases because of the high endocervical location of the lesion and the difficulty in excising a long, narrow cone out of a small, retracted, densely fibrous cervix. It is easier under these circumstances to dissect the vaginal mucosa off the cervix until most of the cervix is exposed. A cervical specimen of sufficient size is then obtained by simply amputating the distal portion of the cervix at the desired level and suturing the vaginal mucosa to the remainder of the cervical stump (Fig. 55–16). With a partial cervicectomy (trachelectomy), as the method is called, it is usually possible to obtain a

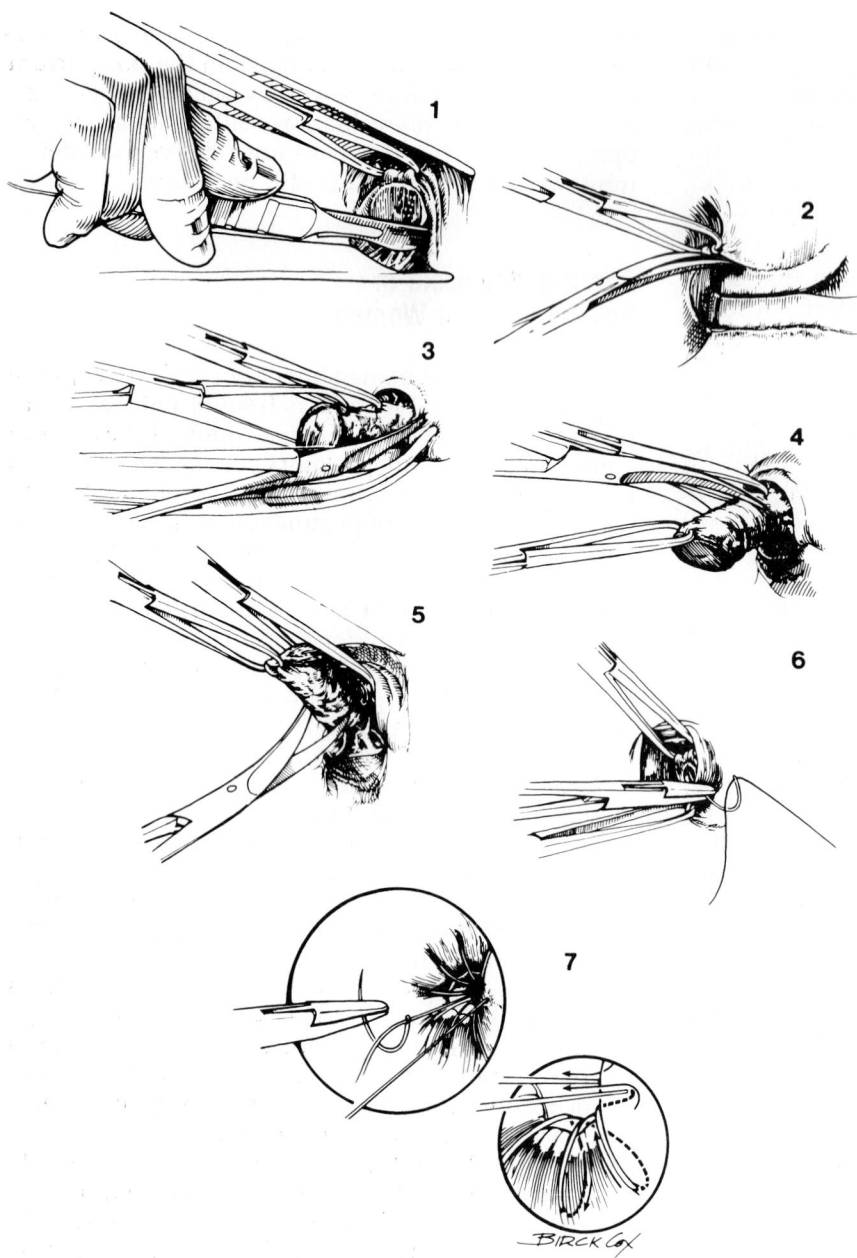

Figure 55-16
Partial cervicectomy (trachelectomy). *1*, The cervix is grasped with a single-toothed tenaculum, and a circumferential incision is made through the vaginal mucosa. *2*, The vaginal mucosa is dissected from the cervix with scissors. *3*, If all of the cervix is removed, the descending cervical branches of the uterine vessels are encountered. The vessels are clamped, cut, and ligated. *4* and *5*, The specimen is removed by cutting across the cervix. A single-toothed tenaculum grasping the remaining portion of the cervix prevents cephalad retraction of the uterus. *6*, Placement of a circumferential suture through vaginal mucosa and the cervical stump. The cervical stump is retracted into the operative field with a single-toothed tenaculum. *7*, Completion of the circumferential suture.

satisfactory tissue sample and to decrease the rate of positive internal margins to 18% (Krebs and Helmkamp, 1990).

Glandular Lesions

Endocervical Glandular Dysplasia

Glandular dysplasia is histologically and cytologically not well defined. It exhibits some of the features of adenocarcinoma in situ (AIS), such as nuclear crowding, stratification, enlargement, irregularity, and slight intraluminal tufting, but intraglandular cribriform patterns, marked papillarity, and multiple mitoses are not observed (Crum et al, 1997).

The clinical significance of glandular dysplasia in the absence of AIS is unknown. Some investigators have found evidence of HPV in such lesions (Higgins et al, 1992; Lee et al, 1993), whereas others have not (Tase et al, 1989). At least the higher grade glandular dysplasias may be precursor to AIS or invasive adenocarcinoma and should be evaluated and treated like AIS (Crum et al, 1997). Low-grade glandular dysplasia may be followed conservatively by repeat Pap smears and endocervical curettage.

Adenocarcinoma in Situ

The evidence of AIS appears to have increased over the past 30 years, but AIS continues to represent less than 5% of all high-grade cervical dysplasias (Andersen and Arffmann, 1984). By contrast, adenocarcinomas constitute up to 25% of invasive cervical carcinomas (Miller et al, 1993). One to four cases of AIS per 100,000 smears are found, but many more cases go undetected because some smears are misinterpreted as CIN or as benign (Ayer et al, 1987). Also, a proportionately higher number of cancers following *documented* normal smears in 3 years were adenocarcinomas compared to squamous cell carcinomas (Janerich et al, 1995). This implies that AIS either may be less readily detected by screening or develops more rapidly than squamous cell carcinomas. The underdiagnosis of AIS has been attributed to the absence of distinct cytologic features and location high in the cervical canal (Benoit et al, 1984). The more rapid transition from precancer to invasive adenocarcinoma may be due to a higher association with HPV 18 compared to squamous lesions, which contain mostly HPV 16 (Hørding et al, 1992). HPV 18 appears to predispose atypical lesions to a more aggressive course with early invasion and rapid spread (Crum et al, 1997).

Notwithstanding the differences, there are sufficient similarities between squamous and glandular cervical lesions to suggest a common origin:

1. The average age of patients with AIS and high-grade CIN is similar (35 to 40 years).
2. Both glandular and squamous lesions are commonly associated with oncogenic HPV types (up to 92% of AIS; Stoler et al, 1992).
3. AIS and HGSIL originate within the T zone contiguous to the SCJ (Andersen and Arffmann, 1989).
4. Squamous dysplasias are seen in association with AIS in up to 70% of cases (Andersen and Arffmann, 1989).

AIS typically involves the surface columnar and underlying glandular epithelium. Deep gland involvement in the absence of superficial gland involvement is rare (Jaworski et al, 1988). It is multifocal in up to 15% of cases and may extend up to 3 cm into the canal (Andersen and Arffmann, 1989; Colgan and Lickrish, 1990).

Women with a cytologic diagnosis of AIS should undergo a colposcopic examination and possibly biopsy and ECC because this may help to detect and delineate an associated squamous lesion. AIS itself looks like normal endocervical epithelium, thereby evading colposcopic diagnosis. A conization is usually necessary.

THERAPY

General Guidelines

The pretreatment evaluation of women with abnormal Pap smears by colposcopy, colposcopically directed biopsies, and ECC has been highly effective in skilled hands in distinguishing among patients who have cancer, CIN, or an indeterminate lesion. Patients with indeterminate lesions because of unsatisfactory colposcopy or other factors outlined previously require a diagnostic conization. Women with invasive carcinoma are treated according to the principles outlined in Chapter 56.

The treatment of CIN depends on the histologic classification of the lesion and the location. Lesions diagnosed by the pathologist as high-grade CIN are associated with potentially oncogenic HPV types and represent the true cancer precursors. These lesions should be removed in the easiest, least costly, and most convenient way possible.

Low-grade CIN, by contrast, is usually associated with low-risk HPV types. It has low potential to progress and frequently regresses. Therefore, patients with low-risk lesions may be followed without therapy. However, the patient may still select to have the lesion treated for two reasons. First, the lesion may be infectious, and there is an as-yet undefined risk of creating new infections if sexual intercourse with new partners takes place. Second, the lesion may be associated with a high-risk virus and it may acquire malignant potential at a later time. Viral typing may provide guidelines in special situations.

There is also a question whether the expense, effort, and complication of treating a patient is greater to, equal to, or less than that of following her periodically for extended periods of time (Richart, 1987). If all factors are weighed, it would appear that the scale tips in favor of therapy if inexpensive, uncomplicated office methods of treatment can be applied. Alternatively, a patient may be followed with repeat Pap smears, colposcopy, biopsy, and ECC every 6 to 12 months until the neoplastic process has resolved or progression is documented.

Prerequisites for Ablative Therapy

Ablative methods of therapy for CIN include cryotherapy, laser vaporization, electrocautery, electrocoagulation diathermy, and cold coagulation. Although effective, inexpensive, and well tolerated, locally destructive treatment methods can be dangerous unless great care is taken in the pretreatment evaluation. The literature is replete with reports of patients who had invasive carcinoma after electrocautery, cryotherapy, or laser ablation (Townsend et al, 1981).

To achieve optimal results with ablative treatment methods, three prerequisites must be met. First, *invasive carcinoma must be ruled out*. Invasive carcinoma is effectively ruled out when neither cytology nor colposcopy suggests invasion, colposcopy is satisfactory, directed biopsy shows CIN, and the ECC is negative.

Secondly, *the lesion must be within reach of the ablating instrument*. The location of the lesion determines whether or not it can be adequately destroyed by the ablating instrument. In cryotherapy, the metal probe must be in contact with the entire lesion. This may not be possible when the lesion extends far into the periphery of the cervix unless multiple applications of the probe are used. If the lesion extends slightly into the cervical canal but the limits are clearly defined, this may not represent a firm contraindication to cryotherapy. In some instances, it may be acceptable to treat these patients with cryotherapy and provide documentation of successful ablation of the lesion by performing an ECC in addition to the Pap test during follow-up. Most women with high-grade dysplasia involving the periphery of the cervix or the endocervix are better treated by loop electrosurgical excision procedure (LEEP) or laser vaporization because these methods are less limited by topographic considerations.

High-grade CINs are usually larger than low-grade CINs and more frequently extend into the endocervix. Therefore, advanced dysplasias are less often amenable to cryotherapy and are more difficult to eradicate than low-grade lesions. Ostergard (1980a) observed a treatment failure rate of 20% for CIN 3 and concluded that cryotherapy is inadequate for treatment of severe dysplasia and CIS. Townsend (1979), by contrast, found that size of the lesion, not histologic grade, was important in predicting the response to cryotherapy. Since then, numerous studies have attested to the adequacy of cryotherapy to eradicate high-grade dysplasia in properly selected patients (Table 55–10).

Third, *the tissue destruction must be sufficiently deep.* Andersen and Hartley (1980) demonstrated in conization specimens that CIN never involved glands deeper than 5.22 mm. More than 99% of lesions would be eliminated if the destructive process penetrated 4 mm from the surface of the epithelium. Although this level of tissue destruction is theoretically obtained by all properly executed locally ablative methods, Savage et al (1982) found that women with cervical gland involvement had a 27% failure rate with cryotherapy as compared with 9% for those women in whom the CIN did not involve glands.

Inadequate patient selection may have been responsible for a high treatment failure rate in that series. Gland involvement is of minimal concern if LEEP or laser vaporization is used because the depth of tissue destruction is directly measurable.

Treatment Methods

Cryotherapy

PRINCIPLES

Cryotherapy, also called cryocautery and cryosurgery, involves the use of a metal probe cooled through isotropic expansion of a compressed gas released from a tank through a small orifice under pressure ranging from 750 to 900 psi (Joule-Thompson effect). The gases most commonly used for cryosurgery (nitrous oxide and CO_2) have a boiling point in the cryogenic range well below the $-20°$ to $-30°C$ necessary for tissue destruction. Nitrous oxide produces a lower temperature ($-89°C$) than CO_2 ($-65°C$) and may therefore be preferable. The destructive effect in the tissue is dependent upon rapid lowering of the temperature resulting in crystallization of cell water and disruption of cell membranes and organelles.

TECHNIQUE

A probe that best fits the anatomy of the cervix and the lesion is coated with a water-soluble jelly to provide good contact and is firmly applied to the cervix. An iceball should form rapidly and extend 4 to 5 mm beyond the end of the probe onto normal tissue. This takes usually 2 to 3 minutes. However, the duration of the exposure appears to be less important than the rapidity of the iceball formation, which depends mostly on adequate fit of the probe, tank pressure, and the refrigerant used. Creasman et al (1973) held a freeze-thaw-freeze approach to be more effective;

Table 55–10. TREATMENT FAILURES ASSOCIATED WITH CRYOTHERAPY (SINGLE TREATMENT)

STUDY	TOTAL PATIENTS TREATED	TREATMENT FAILURES (%)			
		CIN 1	CIN 2	CIN 3	Total
Ostergard (1980a)	344	6.3	7.5	19.6	8.4
Benedet et al (1981a)	516	2.0	4.5	9.8	7.0
Charles et al (1981)	130	18.2	17.0	18.2	17.7
Javaheri et al (1981)	315	4.1	6.7	15.0	7.3
Peckham et al (1982)	385	4.4	8.5	9.8	7.5
Stuart et al (1982)	166	5.6	7.5	17.2	10.8
Van Lent et al (1983)	102	—	—	6.9	—
Creasman et al (1984)	770	5.4	7.2	17.7	10.1
Arof et al (1984)	265	8.3	18.4	28.1	16.1
Bryson et al (1985)	453	—	—	7.1	—
Benedet et al (1987)	1594	4.9	4.3	6.5	5.7
Andersen et al (1988)	135	—	5.1	17.5	—
Einerth (1988)	117	—	5.3	13.5	7.3

however, other authors produced comparable results with a single freeze (Benedet et al, 1981a). It would appear reasonable to limit the double-freeze technique to more complex, high-grade lesions and to treat small, uncomplicated low-grade lesions by the quicker single-freeze technique.

RESULTS AND FOLLOW-UP

Cryotherapy successfully ablates 82% to 92% of all CINs (Table 55–10). The first checkup is usually deferred until 3 months following the treatment to allow inflammatory and reparative changes associated with the healing process to subside. The cervix is then evaluated for stenosis and a Pap smear is taken. Colposcopy and ECC may be indicated in the follow-up of women treated for extensive, high-grade lesions (Lopes et al, 1990).

At least 80% of treatment failures are recognized within the first 12 months after cryotherapy, so further follow-up Pap smears every 3 to 6 months, depending upon the severity of the lesion, are recommended. After a woman treated for CIN has had two or three negative Pap smears, her risk for future intraepithelial neoplasia appears to be no greater than for other high-risk women (Richart et al, 1980). Therefore, routine yearly Pap smears should be sufficient after 1 year of intense follow-up.

Women with an abnormal Pap smear following cryotherapy should again undergo a complete work-up, including colposcopy, directed biopsy, and ECC. Cryotherapy tends to advance the SCJ into the endocervix. Hence, colposcopy is often unsatisfactory and repeat cryotherapy not suitable for most patients with treatment failures.

SIDE EFFECTS AND COMPLICATIONS

Cryotherapy is generally well tolerated but may cause intense uterine cramping during and shortly after treatment. Women with a history of dysmenorrhea are particularly affected and may benefit from taking nonsteroidal anti-inflammatory drugs 15 to 30 minutes before treatment is begun. A paracervical block with a local anesthetic may also be helpful. Vasomotor reactions, including lightheadedness, hot flashes, and pulsating headaches, occur in 20% of patients. Almost all women experience a profuse watery discharge lasting 2 to 4 weeks. Patients should be counseled not to use tampons and to avoid sexual intercourse for 2 weeks or until the vaginal discharge has cleared. Delayed hemorrhage, ascending infection, and cervical stenosis are potentially serious complications but, fortunately, are rare (fewer than 1% of all cases).

Laser (Fig. 55–17)

LASER CONE VAPORIZATION

In the early 1980s, the CO_2 laser emerged as an effective tool for the destruction of dysplastic cervical epithelium. Detailed descriptions of the method may be found in excellent monographs. Proponents of laser therapy advocate the high degree of control over the depth and extent of tissue destruction because the abnormal epithelium is vaporized under colposcopic guidance. Ferenczy (1985) showed that the CO_2 laser produced comparatively better results than cryotherapy in patients with large lesions measuring more than 3 cm in diameter and those extending up to 5 mm into the endocervical canal. For other cervical dysplasias, however, the precision of laser ab-

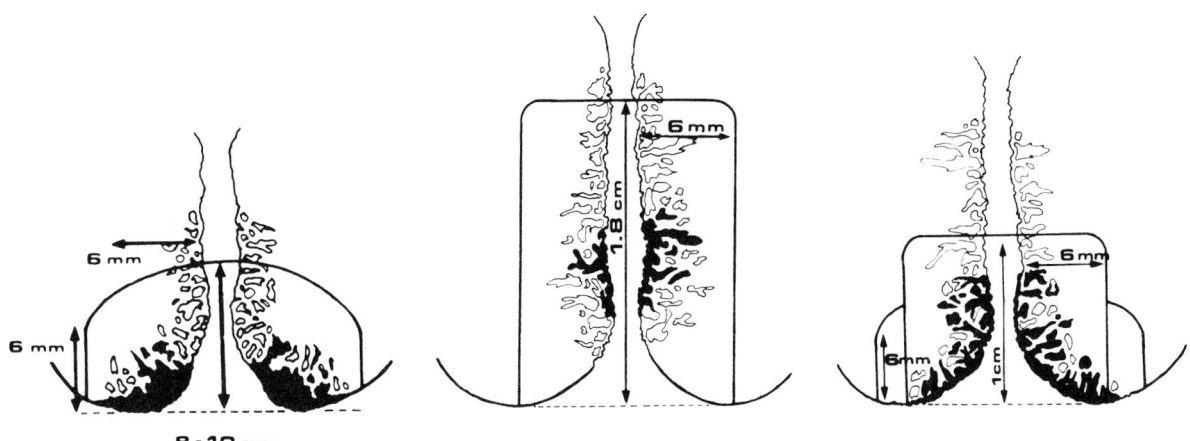

Figure 55–17
Schematic representation of laser treatment methods according to the location of cervical intraepithelial neoplasia on the cervix. *Left,* Ectocervical lesion treated by laser vaporization. *Middle,* Endocervical lesion treated by laser cone (cylinder) excision. *Right,* Ectocervical lesion with endocervical component treated by a laser combination procedure. The central portion of the lesion is excised by laser, providing a specimen for histologic examination. The periphery of the lesion is vaporized. (From Wright VC, Davies E, Riopelle MA: Laser surgery for cervical intraepithelial neoplasia: principles and results. Am J Obstet Gynecol 1983; 145:181, with permission.)

Table 55-11. TREATMENT FAILURES ASSOCIATED WITH LASER VAPORIZATION (SINGLE TREATMENT)

STUDY	TOTAL PATIENTS TREATED	TREATMENT FAILURES (%)			
		CIN 1	CIN 2	CIN 3	Total
Bellina et al (1981)	256	1.1	8.0	13.8	7.0
Benedet et al (1981b)	192	0	13.2	22.0	18.4
Anderson (1982)	337	11.5	19.7	25.6	23.6
Burke (1982)	131	16.3	14.3	22.5	17.6
Bellina et al (1983)	292	6.3	5.4	30.8	7.2
Popkin (1983)	138	11.0	8.5	10.0	9.4
Townsend and Richart (1983)	100	10.0	8.1	13.2	11.0
Caglar et al (1985)	156	10.7	14.3	13.5	12.2
Ferenczy (1985)	147	3.0	4.1	6.5	4.1
Baggish et al (1989)	3070	8.9	6.7	4.1	6.2

lation has not translated into an improved success rate in the treatment of CIN compared with technically simpler and less expensive methods such as cryotherapy or LEEP (Table 55–11).

LASER CONE EXCISION

In experienced hands, a cone or cylindrical piece of tissue may be excised rather than vaporized from the cervix without adding significantly to the time or complications of the operation (Baggish, 1986). This provides a tissue specimen for histologic diagnosis and confirms the absence of invasion and the completeness of excision of the lesion. Laser cone excisions are therefore useful for the treatment of those lesions in which invasion remains a concern in spite of biopsy results, particularly when the lesion extends into the endocervix (Baggish, 1986).

LASER COMBINATION PROCEDURES

A combination of laser cone excision and peripheral laser vaporization may be useful in patients with very large lesions involving the ectocervix and the endocervix. Under these circumstances, the combination procedure is tissue sparing compared with standard conization. The endocervical component of the lesion is excised first and subjected to histologic examination. Subsequently, the ectocervical portion of the lesion is vaporized, resulting in a defect resembling a "cowboy" hat (Wright and Riopelle, 1982).

CURRENT STATUS OF LASER

The cost of laser equipment far exceeds that of other treatment modalities, so the use of a CO_2 laser is rarely cost effective for individual practices. Consequently, CO_2 laser treatments are usually carried out in outpatient surgery centers or hospitals and not infrequently involve general anesthesia, adding considerably to the cost of the treatment. By contrast, LEEP technology is relatively inexpensive and suitable for office use. It has largely replaced laser for the treatment of cervical dysplasia, with the possible exception of those lesions that extend to the vagina or involve the cervix and vagina simultaneously.

Electrocautery and Electrocoagulation Diathermy

Electrocautery ("hot cautery") is the oldest method used in the management of CIN (Younge et al, 1949). The cautery device frequently consists of a resistance-type heating instrument similar to a soldering iron heated to a dull red. The early cautery technique involved radial strokes from the cervical canal out to the periphery of the cervix. The treatment was not very effective because viable islands of dysplasia frequently remained between the radial lines.

Electrocoagulation diathermy (electrodiathermy) devices deliver electrical current from generators of the type routinely used in operating rooms. The cure rate achieved by fulguration of the abnormal epithelium with ball electrodes is comparable to the treatment success obtained with cryotherapy or laser (Table 55–12). Chanen and Rome (1983) in Australia achieved a very high cure rate of 97% by deep coagulation of the cervical stroma with needle electrodes followed by destruction of the remaining surface epithelium with a ball electrode. The procedure, however, is very painful and requires general anesthesia.

Loop Electrosurgical Excision Procedure
(Table 55–13)

Because of the pain and complications such as bleeding and cervical stenosis in 3% of patients, electrocautery and electrocoagulation diathermy became unpopular in the United States when cryotherapy was introduced. However, Cartier (1984) in France rekindled the interest in electrosurgical treatment of CIN when he used small steel wire loop electrodes to strip or cut the affected tissue away. The procedure, also known as "diathermy loop excision" and "large loop excision of the transformation zone" (LLETZ), is more efficient if carried out with much

Table 55–12. TREATMENT FAILURES ASSOCIATED WITH ELECTROCOAGULATION DIATHERMY (SINGLE TREATMENT)

STUDY	TOTAL PATIENTS TREATED	TREATMENT FAILURES (%)			
		CIN 1	CIN 2	CIN 3	Total
Richart and Sciarra (1968)	170	12.3	5.9	40.0	11.1
Ortiz et al (1973)	148	0	0	13.6	8.1
Chanen and Rome (1983)	1864	—	—	—	2.7
Schuurmans et al (1984)	426	10.3	17.7	12.8	14.1
Deigan et al (1986)	772	11.8	9.3	9.0	10.0

larger loop electrodes that allow excision of the entire transformation zone and many CIN lesions in a single pass (Prendville and Cullimore, 1989). The procedure is done under local anesthesia and removes, rather than destroys, the affected tissue. This allows for diagnosis and treatment of many cervical lesions during a single visit to the office or colposcopy clinic and avoids missing an invasive carcinoma—a risk inherent to all ablative methods of therapy (Bigrigg et al, 1990).

When LEEP is used for the evaluation and treatment of *all* women with abnormal Pap smears, as many as one third of specimens will show no evidence of dysplasia and many more have just low-grade dysplasia (Alvarez et al, 1994). In addition, Leep is associated with significant morbidity such as bleeding, pelvic infection, and cervical stenosis in up to 8% of the cases (Hallam et al, 1993). Even injuries to the bladder and rectum have been reported (Krebs et al, 1993). Furthermore, unsuspected invasive carcinoma occurs almost exclusively in women with a Pap smear consistent with a high-grade intraepithelial lesion. The colposcopic finding in case of "missed" invasion is almost always a complex epithelial change, and/or there is extension of the lesion into the endocervix. It follows that ablative therapy is appropriate at least in those circumstances in which the cytology does not suggest the presence of a high-grade intraepithelial lesion, colposcopy reveals a simple lesion not extending into the endocervix, cervical biopsy shows no invasion, and the ECC is negative for dysplasia. These conservative guidelines allow for a selective approach to CIN and avoid overtreatment of women with low-grade lesions. Conization by LEEP or other methods may be avoided in about 75% of patients (Krebs et al, 1993).

Cold Coagulation

The cold coagulator, introduced by Semm in 1966, is still another option for office treatment of CIN. The apparatus generates a probe temperature of 100 to 120°C, which is cold in comparison to electrocautery or electrocoagulation diathermy, hence the name "cold coagulator." The heat is conveyed to the tissues via thermosounds that are held against the lesion in several overlapping applications, each lasting 20 to 30 seconds. Cold coagulation is well tolerated, relatively inexpensive, quick, and convenient and appears to be as effective as other office methods of therapy (Duncan, 1983). The method has not gained wide acceptance in the United States.

Cervical Conization

The effective treatment methods discussed above have largely replaced cold knife conization of the cervix for treatment of CIN. Most conizations are carried out for diagnostic purposes and are considered to be therapeutic if the entire lesion was removed.

Hysterectomy

Hysterectomy is never absolutely indicated for the treatment of cervical dysplasias because the other

Table 55–13. TREATMENT FAILURES ASSOCIATED WITH LEEP

STUDY	TOTAL PATIENTS TREATED	TREATMENT FAILURES (%)			
		CIN 1	CIN 2	CIN 3	Total
Gunasekera et al (1990)	98	—	8.2	7.5	7.8
Whiteley and Olán (1990)	52	—	—	—	5.8
Keijser et al (1992)	424	—	—	—	9.0
Wright et al (1992)	141	4.0	12.5	9.7	6.4
Hallam et al (1993)	967	—	—	—	9.0
Spitzer et al (1993)	237	—	—	—	8.7
Alvarez et al (1994)	195	—	—	—	6.7
Nauman et al (1994)	120	—	—	—	13.3

methods discussed above are suitable for treatment of *any* intraepithel lesion, primary or recurrent. However, of all treatment methods for CIN, hysterectomy has the highest success rate: fewer than 1% of women develop recurrences, mostly as vaginal neoplastic lesions. Hysterectomy is therefore sometimes advocated for women with high-grade CIN who have completed childbearing and are not conscientious about regular follow-up. Hysterectomy may be preferred in patients with severe dysmenorrhea, endometriosis, or other conditions that may require surgery in the future. A simple hysterectomy is also adequate therapy for most microinvasive carcinomas of the cervix. It is, however, inadequate for more deeply invasive lesions (stage IB and greater); thus *invasion must always be ruled out before hysterectomy is performed.*

PROPHYLAXIS

Ablation of the Transformation Zone

If it is true that 80% to 85% of cervical cancers originate in the T zone, then destruction of the T zone should have a prophylactic effect. In a large study of over 400,000 women in Finland, those women subjected to prophylactic electrocoagulation of the cervix had a sixfold lower risk of invasive cancer and a fourfold lower risk of high-grade dysplasia than uncauterized women (Kauraniemi et al, 1978). Because the selection of women participating in the study was not randomized, it is possible that women at low risk for cancer were also more likely treated by electrocoagulation. La Vecchia et al (1985) showed in a small case-control study that the risk estimates of cervical neoplasia among women treated with electrocautery increased when adjustments were made for confounding risk factors. Thus, in the absence of data from randomized trials, routine electrocoagulation for the purpose of cervical cancer prevention cannot be recommended.

Vaccination

In the future, cervical neoplasia may be prevented by polyvalent vaccines directed against various HPV types. Although the classical live, attenuated, and killed virus vaccines cannot be developed until an in vitro culture system for the propagation of HPV is found, the already existing recombinant DNA technology makes it possible to produce proteins derived from any of the viral genes in prokaryotic and eukaryotic vectors. HPV proteins are immunogenic in animals and could be used to induce humoral and cell-mediated immunity in humans.

REFERENCES

Alvarez RD, Helm CW, Edwards RP, et al: Prospective randomized trial of LLETZ versus laser ablation in patients with cervical intraepithelial neoplasia. Gynecol Oncol 1994;52:175.

American Medical Association, Council on Scientific Affairs: Quality assurance in cervical cytology: the Papanicolaou smear. JAMA 1989;262:1672.

Andersen ES, Arffmann E: Adenocarcinoma in situ of the uterine cervix: a clinico-pathologic study of 37 cases. Gynecol Oncol 1984;35:1.

Andersen ES, Thorup K, Larsen G: The results of cryosurgery for cervical intraepithelial neoplasia. Gynecol Oncol 1988;30:21.

Andersen MC, Hartley RB: Cervical crypt involvement by intraepithelial neoplasia. Obstet Gynecol 1980;55:546.

Anderson MS: Treatment of cervical intraepithelial neoplasia with the carbon dioxide laser: report of 543 patients. Obstet Gynecol 1982;59:710.

Anthony DD, Wentz WB, Reagan JW, et al: Induction of cervical neoplasia in the mouse by herpes simplex virus type 2 DNA. Proc Natl Acad Sci U S A 1989;86:4250.

Antoine T, Grünberger V: The incident-light microscopy in gynecology. Klin Med 1949;4:575.

Arof HM, Gerbie MV, Smeltzer J: Cryosurgical treatment of cervical intraepithelial neoplasia: four year experience. Am J Obstet Gynecol 1984;150:865.

Aurelian L, Kessler II, Rosenshein NB, et al: Viruses and gynecologic cancer: herpes virus protein (ICP 10/AG), a cervical tumor antigen that fulfills the criteria for a marker of carcinogenicity. Cancer 1981;48:455.

Averette HE, Nasser N, Yankow SL, et al: Cervical conization in pregnancy. Am J Obstet Gynecol 1970;106:543.

Ayer B, Pacey F, Greenberg M, Bousfield L: The cytologic diagnosis of adenocarcinoma in situ of the cervix uteri and related lesions. I. Adenocarcinoma in situ. Acta Cytol 1987;31:397.

Baggish MS: A comparison between laser excisional conization and laser vaporization for the treatment of cervical intraepithelial neoplasia. Am J Obstet Gynecol 1986;155:39.

Baggish M, Dorsey J: Contact hysteroscopic evaluation of the endocervix as an adjunct to colposcopy. Obstet Gynecol 1982;60:107.

Baggish M, Dorsey JH, Adelson M: A ten year experience treating cervical intraepithelial neoplasia with the CO_2 laser. Am J Obstet Gynecol 1989;161:60.

Bellina JH, Fischer Ross L, Voros J: Colposcopy and the CO_2 laser for treatment of cervical intraepithelial neoplasia: an analysis of seven years' experience. J Reprod Med 1983;28:147.

Bellina JH, Wright VC, Voros J, et al: Carbon dioxide laser management of cervical intraepithelial neoplasia. Am J Obstet Gynecol 1981;141:828.

Benedet JL, Miller DM, Nickerson KG, et al: The results of cryosurgical treatment of cervical intraepithelial neoplasia at one, five, and ten years. Am J Obstet Gynecol 1987;157:268.

Benedet JL, Nickerson KG, Anderson GH: Cryotherapy in the treatment of cervical intraepithelial neoplasia. Obstet Gynecol 1981a;58:725.

Benedet JL, Nickerson KG, White KG: Laser therapy for cervical intraepithelial neoplasia. Obstet Gynecol 1981b;58:188.

Benoit AG, Krepant GV, Lotocki RJ: Results of prior cytologic screening in patients with a diagnosis of stage I carcinoma of the cervix. Am J Obstet Gynecol 1984;148:690.

Beral V: Cancer of cervix: a sexually transmitted infection. Lancet 1974;1:1037.

Bigrigg MA, Codling BW, Pearson P, et al: Colposcopic diagnosis and treatment of cervical dysplasia at a single clinic visit. Lancet 1990;336:229.

Blythe JG: Cervicography: a preliminary report. Obstet Gynecol 1985;152:192.

Boronow RC: Current concepts: cervical intraepithelial neoplasia (carcinoma in-situ and dysplasia). In Rutledge F, Wharton JT, Boronow RC (eds): Gynecologic Oncology. New York: John Wiley & Sons, 1976:3.

Broussais FJV: Histoire des Phlegmasies on Inflammations Chroniques, 4th ed. Paris, 1826.

Bryson SCP, Leneham P, Lickrish GM: The treatment of grade 3 cervical intraepithelial neoplasia with cryotherapy: an 11-year experience. Am J Obstet Gynecol 1985;151:201.

Buckley JD, Harris RWC, Dole R, et al: Case-control study of husbands of women with dysplasia or carcinoma of the cervix uteri. Lancet 1981;2:1010.

Burghardt E, Ostor AG: Site and origin of squamous cervical cancer: a histomorphologic study. Obstet Gynecol 1983;62:117.

Burke L: The use of the carbon dioxide laser in the therapy of cervical intraepithelial neoplasia. Am J Obstet Gynecol 1982;144:337.

Caglar H, Ayhan A, Hreshchyshyn MM: CO_2 laser therapy for cervical intraepithelial neoplasia. Gynecol Oncol 1985;22:46.

Campion MJ, Franklin EW, Stacy LD, et al: Human papillomavirus and anogenital neoplasia: a fresh look at the association. South Med J 1989;82:35.

Campion MJ, McCance DJ, Cuzick J, et al: Progressive potential of mild cervical atypia: prospective cytological colposcopic, and virologic study. Lancet 1986;2:168.

Cartier R: Practical Colposcopy, 2nd ed. Paris: Laboratorie Cartier, 1984:139.

Chanen WL, Rome RM: Electrocoagulation diathermy for cervical dysplasia and carcinoma in situ: a 15-year survey. Obstet Gynecol 1983;61:673.

Charles EH, Savage EW, Hacker N, et al: Cryosurgical treatment of cervical intraepithelial neoplasia. Gynecol Oncol 1981;12:83.

Ciuffu G: Innesto positive confitrado di verruca volgare. Gior Ital Mal Vener 1907;48:12.

Claman AD, Lee N: Factors that relate to complications of cone biopsy. Am J Obstet Gynecol 1974;120:124.

Coggin JR, Zur Hausen H: Workshop on the papillomaviruses and cancer. Cancer Res 1979;39:545.

Colgan TJ, Lickrish GM: The topography and invasive potential of cervical adenocarcinoma in situ with and without associated squamous dysplasia. Gynecol Oncol 1990;36:246.

Coppleson M, Pixley E, Reid B: Colposcopy: A Scientific and Practical Approach to the Cervix and Vagina in Health and Disease. Springfield, IL: Charles C Thomas, 1978.

Coppleson M, Reid B: The etiology of squamous carcinoma of the cervix. Obstet Gynecol 1968;32:432.

Cox JT, Lorincz AT, Schiffman MH, et al: Human papillomavirus testing by hybrid capture appears to be useful in triaging women with a cytologic diagnosis of a typical squamous cells of undetermined significance. Am J Obstet Gynecol 1995;172:946.

Creasman WT, Hinshaw WM, Clarke-Pearson DL: Cryosurgery in the management of cervical intraepithelial neoplasia. Obstet Gynecol 1984;63:145.

Creasman WT, Weed JC, Curry SL, et al: Efficacy of cryosurgical treatment of severe cervical intraepithelial neoplasia. Obstet Gynecol 1973;41:501.

Cross HE, Kennel EF, Lilienfeld AM: Cancer of the cervix in an Amish population. Cancer 1968;21:102.

Crum CP, Cibas ES, Lee KR: Viral pathogenesis and natural history of cervical dysplasia. In Crum CP, Cibas ES, Lee KR (eds): Pathology of Early Cervical Neoplasia. New York: Churchill Livingstone, 1997:7.

Cullen TS: Cancer of the Uterus. New York: D. Appleton & Co, 1900.

Deigan EA, Carmichal JA, Ohlke RN, et al: Treatment of cervical intraepithelial neoplasia with electrocautery: a report of 776 cases. Am J Obstet Gynecol 1986;154:255.

Della Torre G, Pilotti S, De Palo G, et al: Viral particles in cervical condylomatous lesions. Tumori 1978;64:459.

DePetrillo AD, Townsend DE, Morrow CP, et al: Colposcopic evaluation of the abnormal Papanicolaou test in pregnancy. Am J Obstet Gynecol 1975;121:441.

Dinh TA, Dinh TV, Hannigan EV, et al: Necessity for endocervical curettage in elderly women undergoing colposcopy. J Reprod Med 1989;34:621.

Duncan ID: The Semm cold coagulator in the management of cervical intraepithelial neoplasia. Clin Obstet Gynecol 1983;26:996.

Einerth Y: Cryosurgical treatment of CIN I-III: a longterm study. Acta Obstet Gynecol Scand 1988;67:627.

Evans AS, Monaghan JM: Spontaneous resolution of warty atypia: the relevance of clinical and nuclear DNA features: a prospective study. Br J Obstet Gynaecol 1985;92:165.

Fenton DW, Soutter WP, Sharp F, et al: Preliminary experience with microcolpohysteroscopically controlled cone biopsies. Colposcopy Gynecol Laser Surg 1984;1:167.

Ferenczy A: Cervical intraepithelial neoplasia. In Blaustein A (ed): Pathology of the Female Genital Tract, 2nd ed. New York: Springer-Verlag, 1982:156.

Ferenczy A: Comparison of cryo and carbon dioxide laser therapy for cervical intraepithelial neoplasia. Obstet Gynecol 1985;66:793.

Fink D: Change in American Cancer Society checkup guidelines for detection of cervical cancer. CA Cancer J Clin 1988;36:127.

Forsberg JG: Cervicovaginal epithelium: its origin and development. Am J Obstet Gynecol 1973;115:1025.

Galvin GA, Jones HW Jr, TeLinde RW: Clinical relationship of carcinoma in situ and invasive carcinoma of the cervix. JAMA 1952;149:744.

Gardner JW, Lyon JL: Low incidence of cervical cancer in Utah. Gynecol Oncol 1977;5:68.

Gissmann L, Zur Hausen H: Partial characterization of viral DNA from human genital warts (condylomata acuminata). Int J Cancer 1980;25:605.

Goff BA, Atanasoff PT, Brown E, et al: Endocervical glandular atypia in Papanicolaou smears. Obstet Gynecol 1992;79:101.

Green GH: Invasive potential of cervical carcinoma in situ. Int J Gynecol Obstet 1969;7:157.

Gunasekera PC, Phipps JH, Lewis BV: Large loop excision of the transformation zone (LLETZ) compared to carbon dioxide laser in the treatment of CIN: a superior mode of treatment. Br J Obstet Gynecol 1990;97:995.

Hallam NF, West J, Harper C, et al: Large loop excision of the transformation zone (LLETZ) as an alternative to both local ablative and cone biopsy treatment: a survey of 1000 patients. J Gynecol Surg 1993;9:77.

Hamou J: Hysteroscopy and microhysteroscopy with a new instrument: the microhysteroscope. Acta Eur Fertil 1981;12:2.

Handley JE, Walton L: The prevention of cancer. Lancet 1936;1:987.

Hannigan EV, Whitehouse MH III, Atkinson WD: Cone biopsy during pregnancy. Obstet Gynecol 1982;60:450.

Harris RWC, Brinton LA, Cowdell RH, et al: Characteristics of women with dysplasia or carcinoma in situ of the cervix uteri. Br J Cancer 1980;42:359.

Heins HC Jr, Dennis EJ, Pratt-Thomas HR: The possible role of smegma in carcinoma of the cervix. Am J Obstet Gynecol 1958;76:726.

Herrero R, Brinton LA, Reeves WC, et al: Invasive cervical cancer and smoking in Latin America. J Natl Cancer Inst 1989;81:205.

Higgins GD, Phillips GE, Smith LA, et al: High prevalence of human papillomavirus transcripts in all grades of cervical intraepithelial glandular neoplasia. Cancer 1992;70:136.

Hinselmann H: Verbesserung der Inspektionsmöglichkeit von Vulva, Vagina und Portio. Münch Med Wochenschr 1925:1733.

Hinselmann H: Die Essigsäureprobe, ein Bestandteil der erweiterten Kolposkopie. Dtsch Med Wochenschr 1938:1071.

Hørding U, Teglbjaerg CS, Visfeldt J, et al: Human papillomavirus types 16 and 18 in adenocarcinoma of the uterine cervix. Gynecol Oncol 1992;46:313.

Husseinzadeh N, Shbaro L, Wesseler T: Predictive value of cone margins and post-cone endocervical curettage with residual disease on subsequent hysterectomy. Gynecol Oncol 1989;33:198.

Janerich DT, Hadjimichael O, Schwartz PE: The screening history of women with invasive cervical cancer, Connecticut. Am J Public Health 1995;85:79.

Javaheri G, Balin M, Meltzer RM: Role of cryotherapy in the treatment of intraepithelial neoplasia of the uterine cervix. Obstet Gynecol 1981;58:83.

Jaworski RC, Pacy NF, Greeberg ML, Osborn RA: The histologic diagnosis of adenocarcinoma in situ and related lesions of the cervix uteri. Cancer 1988;61:1171.

Jenson AB, Rosenthal JD, Olson C, et al: Immunological relatedness of papillomavirus from different species. J Natl Cancer Inst 1980;64:495.

Jones HW, Buller RE: The treatment of cervical intraepithelial neoplasia by cone biopsy. Am J Obstet Gynecol 1980;137:882.

Jones KW, Genoglio CM, Sherchuk-Chaban M, et al: Detection of herpes simplex virus type 2 in RNA in human cervical biopsies by in situ cytological hybridization. In De The G, Henle W,

Rapp F (eds): Oncogenesis and Herpes Viruses III, Third International Symposium: Part I. Lyon: International Agency for Research on Cancer, 1978:917.

Kauraniemi T, Räsänen-Virtanen U, Hakama M: Risk of cervical cancer among an electrocoagulated population. Am J Obstet Gynecol 1978;131:533.

Keijser KGG, Kenemans P, van der Zanden PHThH, et al: Diathermy loop excision in the management of cervical intraepithelial neoplasia: diagnosis and treatment in one procedure. Am J Obstet Gynecol 1992;166:1281.

Kessler II: Cervical cancer epidemiology in historical perspective. J Reprod Med 1974;12:173.

Kessler II: Venereal factors in human cervical cancer. Cancer 1977;39:1912.

Kohan S, Beckman EM, Bigelow B: The role of colposcopy in the management of cervical intraepithelial neoplasia during pregnancy and postpartum. J Reprod Med 1980;25:279.

Koss LG, Durfee GR: Unusual patterns of squamous epithelium of the uterine cervix: cytologic and pathologic study of koilocytotic atypia. Ann N Y Acad Sci 1956;63:1245.

Krebs HB: Outpatient cervical conization. Obstet Gynecol 1984;63:430.

Krebs HB, Helmkamp BF: Examining the aging cervix. Contemp Obstet Gynecol 1990;November:27.

Krebs HB, Pastore L, Helmkamp B: Loop electrosurgical excision procedures for cervical dysplasia: experience in a community hospital. Am J Obstet Gynecol 1993;160:289.

Krebs HB, Wilstrup MA, Wheelock JB: Partial trachelectomy in the elderly patient with abnormal cytology. Obstet Gynecol 1985;65:579.

Kurman RJ, Henson DE, Herbst AL, et al for the 1992 National Cancer Institute Workshop. Interim guidelines for management of abnormal cervical cytology. JAMA 1994;271:1866.

La Vecchia C, Franceschi S, Decarli A: Electrocoagulation and the risk of cervical neoplasia. Obstet Gynecol 1985;66:703.

LaPolla JP, O'Neill C, Wetrich D: Colposcopic management of abnormal cervical cytology in pregnancy. J Reprod Med 1988;32:301.

Laverty CR, Booth N, Hills E, et al: Noncondylomatous wart virus infection of the postmenopausal cervix. Pathology 1978;10:373.

Lee KR, Howard P, Heintz NH, Collins CC: Low prevalence of human papillomavirus types 16 and 18 in cervical adenocarcinoma in situ, invasive adenocarcinoma and glandular dysplasia by polymerase chain reaction. Mod Pathol 1993;6:433.

Lehn H, Villa LL, Marziona F, et al: Physical state and biological activity of human papillomavirus genomes in precancerous lesions of the female genital tract. J Gen Virol 1988;69:187.

Linhartova A: Extent of columnar epithelium on the ectocervix between the ages of 1 and 13 years. Obstet Gynecol 1978;52:451.

Lopes A, Mor-Yosef S, Pearson S: Is routine colposcopic assessment necessary following laser ablation of cervical intraepithelial neoplasia? Br J Obstet Gynecol 1990;97:175.

Madile BM: The cervical epithelium from fetal age to adolescence. Obstet Gynecol 1976;47:536.

Martin CE: Marital and coital factors in cervical cancer. Am J Public Health 1967;57:803.

Meisels A, Fortin R: Condylomatous lesions of cervix and vagina. I. Cytologic patterns. Acta Cytol 1976;20:505.

Miller BE, Flax SD, Arheart K, Photopulos G: The presentation of adenocarcinoma of the uterus cervix. Cancer 1993;73:128.

Minh H-N, Lecompte D, Smadja A, et al: A hypothesis on the origin of subcylindrical reserve cells of the endocervix. Pathol Res Pract 1981;172:88.

Mitchell H, Drake M, Medley G: Prospective evaluation of risk of cervical cancer after cytological evidence of human papillomavirus infection. Lancet 1986;2:573.

Nash JD, Burke TW, Hoskins WI: Biologic course of cervical human papillomavirus infection. Obstet Gynecol 1987;69:160.

Nasu I, Meurer W, Fu YS: Endocervical glandular atypia and adenocarcinoma: a correlation of cytology and histology. Int J Gynecol Pathol 1993;12:208.

National Cancer Institute: The 1988 Bethesda System for reporting cervical/vaginal cytological diagnoses. JAMA 1989;262:931.

Orth G, Jablonska S, Favre M, et al: Epidermodysplasia verruciformis: a model for viral oncogenesis in man. Cold Spring Harbor Conf Cell Prolif 1980;7:259.

Ortiz R, Newton M, Tsai A: Electrocautery treatment of cervical intraepithelial neoplasia. Obstet Gynecol 1973;41:113.

Ostergard DR: The effect of age, gravidity, and parity on the location of the squamo-columnar junction as determined by colposcopy. Am J Obstet Gynecol 1977;129:59.

Ostergard DR: Cryosurgical treatment of cervical intraepithelial neoplasia. Obstet Gynecol 1980a;56:231.

Ostergard DR: Prediction of clearance of cervical intraepithelial neoplasia by conization. Obstet Gynecol 1980b;56:77.

Papanicolaou GN, Traut HF: Diagnosis of Uterine Cancer by the Vaginal Smear. New York: Commonwealth Fund, 1943.

Peckham BM, Soner MG, Carr WF: Outpatient therapy: success and failure with dysplasia and carcinoma in situ. Am J Obstet Gynecol 1982;142:323.

Piper J: Oral contraceptives and cervical cancer. Gynecol Oncol 1985;22:1.

Popkin DR: Treatment of cervical intraepithelial neoplasia with the carbon dioxide laser. Am J Obstet Gynecol 1983;145:177.

Pratt-Thomas HR, Heins HC, Latham E, et al: The carcinogenic effect of human smegma: an experimental study. I. Preliminary report. Cancer 1956;9:671.

Prendville W, Cullimore NS: Large loop excision of the transformation zone (LLETZ): a new method of management for women with cervical intraepithelial neoplasia. Br J Obstet Gynecol 1989;96:1054.

Pridan H, Lilienfeld AM: Carcinoma of the cervix in Jewish women in Israel, 1960–67. Israel J Med Sci 1971;7:1465.

Prins RP, Morrow CP, Townsend DE, et al: Vaginal embryogenesis, estrogens and adenosis. Obstet Gynecol 1976;48:247.

Pronai K: Zur Lehre von der Histogenese und dem Wachstum des Uteruscarcinoms. Arch Gynäk 1909;89:596.

Purola E, Savia E: Cytology of gynecologic condyloma acuminatum. Acta Cytol 1977;21:26.

Reid R, Campion MJ: HPV-associated lesions of the cervix: biology and colposcopic features. Clin Obstet Gynecol 1989;32:157.

Reid R, Scalzi P: Genital warts and cervical cancer. VII. An improved colposcopic index for differentiating benign papillomaviral infections from high-grade cervical intraepithelial neoplasia. Am J Obstet Gynecol 1985;153:611.

Reid RI, Lörincz AT: New generation of human papillomavirus tests. In Rubin SC, Hoskins WY (eds): Cervical Cancer and Preinvasive Neoplasia. Philadelphia: Lippincott-Raven, 1996:27.

Richart RM: Natural history of cervical intraepithelial neoplasia. Clin Obstet Gynecol 1967;10:748.

Richart RM: Causes and management of cervical intraepithelial neoplasia. Cancer 1987;60:1951.

Richart RM: A modified terminology for cervical intraepithelial neoplasia. Obstet Gynecol 1990;75:131.

Richart RM, Barron BA: A follow-up study of patients with cervical dysplasia. Am J Obstet Gynecol 1969;105:386.

Richart RM, Sciarra JJ: Treatment of cervical dysplasia by outpatient electrocauterization. Am J Obstet Gynecol 1968;101:200.

Richart RM, Townsend DE, Crisp W, et al: An analysis of "long-term" follow-up results in patients with cervical intraepithelial neoplasia treated by cryotherapy. Am J Obstet Gynecol 1980;137:823.

Rigoni-Stern D: Fatti statistici relativi alle malattie cancerose. Gior Servire Progr Path Terap 1842;2:507.

Ritter D, Kadish AS, Vermund SH, et al: Detection of human papillomavirus deoxyribonucleic acid in exfoliated cervicovaginal cells as a predictor of cervical neoplasia in a high-risk population. Am J Obstet Gynecol 1988;159:1517.

Rosenfeld WD, Rose E, Vermund SH, et al: Follow-up evaluation of cervicovaginal human papillomavirus infection in adolescents. J Pediatr 1992;121:307.

Rous P, Beard JW: The progression to carcinoma of virus-induced rabbit papillomas (Shope). J Exp Med 1935;62:523.

Rubin IC: The pathological diagnosis of incipient carcinoma of the uterus. Am J Obstet 1910;62:668.

Sadeghi SB, Sadeghi A, Robboy SJ: Prevalence of dysplasia and cancer of the cervix in a nationwide, Planned Parenthood population. Cancer 1988;61:2359.

Savage EW, Matlock DL, Salem FA, et al: The effect of endocervical gland involvement on the cure rates of patients with cervical intraepithelial neoplasia undergoing cryosurgery. Gynecol Oncol 1982;14:194.

Schauenstein W: Histologische Untersuchung über atypisches Plattenepithel an der Portio und an der Innenfläche der Cervix Uteri. Arch Gynäk 1908;85:576.

Schiffman M: Arguments against routine clinical use of HPV assays. Contemp Obstet Gynecol 1990;April:34.

Schiller W: Untersuchungen zur Entstehung der Geschwülste. I. Collumcarcinom des Uterus. Arch Pathol Anat 1927;263:279.

Schiller W: Zur klinischen Fruhdiagnose der Portiokarzinoms. Zentralbl Gynäk 1928;52:1886.

Schneider A, Holz M, Gissmann L: Prevalence of genital HPV infections in pregnant women. Int J Cancer 1987;40:198.

Schuurmans SN, Ohlke ID, Carmichael JA: Treatment of cervical intraepithelial neoplasia with electrocautery: report of 426 cases. Am J Obstet Gynecol 1984;148:544.

Semm K: New apparatus for the "cold coagulation" of benign cervical lesions. Am J Obstet Gynecol 1966;95:963.

Shah KV, Lewis MG, Jenson AB, et al: Papillomavirus and cervical dysplasia. Lancet 1980;2:1190.

Sheets EE, Constantine NM, Dinisio S, et al: Colposcopically directed biopsies provide a basis for comparing the accuracy of Thin Prep and Papanicolaou smears. J Gynecol Tech 1995;1:27.

Shen L, Rushing L, McLachlin CM, et al: Prevalence and significance of cervical HPV DNA from women at low and high risk for cervical neoplasia. Obstet Gynecol 1995;86:499.

Sherman ME, Mango LJ, Kelly D, et al: PAPNET analysis of reportedly negative smears preceding the diagnosis of a high-grade squamous intraepithelial lesion or carcinoma. Mod Pathol 1994;7:578.

Shingleton HM, Partridge EE, Austin JM: The significance of age in the colposcopic evaluation of women with atypical Papanicolaou smears. Obstet Gynecol 1977;49:61.

Shope RE: Infectious papillomatosis of rabbits. J Exp Med 1933;58:607.

Skegg DCG, Corwin PA, Paul C: Importance of the male factor in cancer of the cervix. Lancet 1982;2:581.

Smith JW: Herpes simplex virus: an expanding relationship to human cancer. J Reprod Med 1983;28:115.

Solomon D, Wied G: Cervicography: an assessment. J Reprod Med 1989;34:321.

Spitzer M, Chernys AE, Seltzer VL: The use of large-loop excision of the transformation zone in an inner-city population. Obstet Gynecol 1993;82:731.

Stafl A: Cervicography—a new approach to cervical cancer detection. Gynecol Oncol 1981;125:5292.

Stafl A: Understanding colposcopic patterns and their clinical significance. Contemp Obstet Gynecol 1983;November:85.

Stern E: Epidemiology of dysplasia. Obstet Gynecol Surv 1969;24:711.

Stoler MH, Rhodes CR, Whitbeck A, et al: Human papillomavirus types 16 and 18 gene expression in cervical enoplasia. Hum Pathol 1992;23:117.

Stuart GCE, Anderson RJ, Corlett BMA, et al: Assessment of failure of cryosurgical treatment in cervical intraepithelial neoplasia. Am J Obstet Gynecol 1982;142:658.

Tase T, Okagaki T, Clark BA, et al: Human papillomavirus DNA in glandular dysplasia and microglandular hyperplasia: presumed precursors of adenocarcinoma of the uterine cervix. Obstet Gynecol 1989;73:1005.

Tawa K, Forsythe A, Cove JK, et al: A comparison of the Papanicolaou smear and the cervicogram: sensitivity, specificity, and cost analysis. Obstet Gynecol 1988;71:229.

Taylor PT, Anderson WA, Barber SR, et al: The screening Papanicolaou smear: contribution of the endocervical brush. Obstet Gynecol 1987;70:734.

Townsend DE: Cryosurgery for CIN. Obstet Gynecol Surv 1979;34:828.

Townsend DE, Richart RM: Cryotherapy and carbon dioxide laser management of cervical intraepithelial neoplasia: a controlled comparison. Obstet Gynecol 1983;61:75.

Townsend DE, Richart RM, Marks E, et al: Invasive cancer following outpatient evaluation and therapy for cervical disease. Obstet Gynecol 1981;57:145.

Tseng P, Hunter V, Reed TP III, et al: Microcolpohysteroscopy compared with colposcopy in the evaluation of abnormal cervical cytology. Obstet Gynecol 1987;69:675.

Van der Graaf Y, Vooijs GP, Gaillaard HLJ, et al: Screening errors in cervical cytology screening. Acta Cytol 1987;31:434.

Van Lent M, Trimbos JB, Heintz APM: Cryosurgical treatment of cervical intraepithelial neoplasia (CIN III) in 102 patients. Gynecol Oncol 1983;16:240.

Vineberg HN: The relative infrequency of cancer of the uterus in women of the Hebrew race. In: Contributions to Medical and Biological Research. Dedicated to Sir William Osler, M.D., in Honor of His Seventieth Birthday, July 12, 1919, by His Pupils and Co-workers, Vol. 2. New York: Paul B. Hoeber, 1919:1223.

Vonka V, Kanka It, Jelinik J, et al: Prospective study on the relationship between cervical neoplasia and herpes simplex type 2 virus: epidemiological characteristics. Int J Cancer 1984;33:49.

Weid GL: Proceedings of the First International Congress on Exfoliative Cytology. Philadelphia: Lippincott, 1961:283.

Weinberg W, Gastpar H: Die bösartigen Neubildungen in Stuttgart 1873–1902. Z Krebsf 1904;2:195.

Wentz WB, Heggie AD, Anthony DD, et al: Effect of prior immunization on induction of cervical cancer in mice by herpes simplex virus type 2. Science 1983;222:1128.

Whiteley PF, Olán KS: Treatment of cervical intraepithelial neoplasia: experience with low-voltage drathermy loop. J Obstet Gynecol 1990;162:1272.

Wilbanks GD: Colpomicroscopy, past, present, and future. Colposcopist 1978;10:1.

Wright TC, Gagnon S, Richart RM, and Ferenczy A: Treatment of cervical intraepithelial neoplasia using the loop electrosurgical excision procedure. Obstet Gynecol 1992;79:173.

Wright VC, Riopelle MA: Gynecologic Laser Surgery: A Practical Handbook. Houston: Biomedical Communications, 1982.

Younge PA, Hertig AT, Armstrong D: A study of 135 cases of carcinoma in situ of the cervix and the Free Hospital for Women. Am J Obstet Gynecol 1949;58:867.

Zahniser DJ, Hurley AA: Automated slide preparation system for the clinical laboratory. Cytometry (Communications Clin Cytometry) 1996;26:60.

Zur Hausen H: Condylomata acuminata and human genital cancer. Cancer Res 1976;36:530.

Zur Hausen H: Papillomaviruses as carcinomaviruses. Adv Viral Oncol 1989;8:1.

Zur Hausen H, Schneider A: The role of papillomaviruses in human anogenital cancer. In Salzman NP, Howley PM (eds): The Papovaviridae. New York: Plenum Press, 1987:245.

56

Mitchell Morris
Diane C. Bodurka-Bevers

Cervical Cancer

Despite the use of large-scale cervical cancer screening programs in industrialized nations, invasive cervical cancer continues to be a worldwide problem. In the United States, the mortality rate from cervical cancer has steadily declined over the last four decades. This trend is largely due to Papanicolaou (Pap) smear screening programs, but improvement in the therapy of invasive disease is also a factor. Even with these advances, the American Cancer Society estimates that there will be approximately 14,500 new cases of invasive cervical carcinoma annually (Parker et al, 1997). Of those women afflicted with the disease, approximately 4800 will die.

Cervical carcinoma ranks among the first malignant diseases that were successfully treated. The exciting discovery of radium by the Curies near the turn of the century led to the observation that ionizing radiation was useful in the treatment of malignancy. The accessibility of the cervix to radioactive implants was soon appreciated, and cures were reported (Abbe, 1913). At this time, Wertheim (1900, 1907) was perfecting his radical operation for removal of the uterus as a treatment for cervical carcinoma. Both radiation and radical surgery developed in a parallel fashion until the latter half of this century, when both therapies have assumed their appropriate role in the treatment of invasive cervical cancer.

EPIDEMIOLOGY AND ETIOLOGY

The association between cervical cancer and sexually transmitted diseases has been noted for many years. Earlier epidemiologists focused on the sexually transmitted diseases of their day, such as syphilis and gonorrhea. Other potential etiologic factors, such as chronic cervical infection or exposure to smegma, have also been suggested as causative agents. As epidemiologic techniques improved, however, it became evident that these were merely associated factors and not causative agents in and of themselves. In the 1960s and 1970s, attention turned to the herpes simplex virus (HSV) with the discovery that many patients with preinvasive lesions of the cervix had concomitant infections with HSV 2 (Naib et al, 1966; Aurelian, 1972). Subsequent studies discovered the presence of HSV 2 RNA in as many as

40% of women with invasive cervical cancer (Maitland et al, 1981; Cabral et al, 1983). However, evidence was lacking to show the presence of DNA in the majority of women with cervical cancer.

In the late 1970s, Meisels and co-workers (1977) noted an association between the human papillomavirus (HPV) infection causing condyloma and cervical dysplasia. Several other lines of evidence connecting HPV with cervical neoplasia were then demonstrated (Durst et al, 1983; Crum et al, 1984; Schwarz et al, 1985). Cervical cancer is unique in that it is the first major solid tumor to have been shown to be virally induced in almost every case. HPV DNA is found in virtually all cases (93%) of cervical cancer and its precursor lesions worldwide (Bosch et al, 1995). HPV infection has been shown to be the major risk factor for squamous intraepithelial lesions and invasive cervical cancer in multiple epidemiologic studies (Koutsky et al, 1992; Schiffman et al, 1993). Research has also demonstrated that the HPV genes E6 and E7 become integrated into the host genome, and that the transforming proteins encoded by these genes are tumorigenic (Dyson et al, 1989; Phelps et al, 1991; Chen et al, 1993). Epidemiologic studies are now concentrating on host factors and cofactors that may help explain the natural history of HPV infections and associated lesions. It is thought that cofactors are essential for the development of disease (Lorincz et al, 1992). Examples include intercourse at an early age, multiple sexual partners, young age at first pregnancy, multiparity, low socioeconomic status, a male sexual partner in a high-risk group, and cigarette smoking (Barron and Richart, 1971; Clarke et al, 1985; Guijon et al, 1985; Peters et al, 1986). A more detailed discussion of HPV and preinvasive disease of the cervix may be found in Chapter 55.

PATHOLOGY

The classification of malignant lesions of the cervix is summarized in Table 56–1 (Scully et al, 1994).

Squamous Cell Carcinoma

Squamous (epidermoid) carcinoma constitutes approximately 85% to 90% of cervical cancers. It is be-

Table 56-1. MODIFIED WORLD HEALTH ORGANIZATION HISTOLOGICAL CLASSIFICATION OF EPITHELIAL TUMORS OF THE UTERINE CERVIX

Squamous cell carninoma
  Microinvasive squamous cell carcinoma
  Invasive squamous cell carcinoma
  Verrucous carcinoma
  Warty (condylomatous) carcinoma
  Papillary squamous cell (transitional) carcinoma
  Lymphoepithelioma-like carcinoma
Adenocarcinoma
  Mucinous adenocarcinoma
    Endocervical type
    Intestinal type
    Signet-ring type
  Endometrioid adenocarcinoma
    Endometrioid adenocarcinoma with squamous
      metaplasia
  Clear cell adenocarcinoma
  Minimal deviation adenocarcinoma
    Endocervical type (adenoma malignum)
    Endometrioid type
  Serous adenocarcinoma
  Mesonephric carcinoma
  Well-differentiated villoglandular adenocarcinoma
Other epithelial tumors
  Adenosquamous carcinoma
  Glassy cell carcinoma
  Mucoepidermoid carcinoma
  Adenoid cystic carcinoma
  Adenoid basal carcinoma
  Carcinoid-like tumor
  Small cell carcinoma
  Undifferentiated carcinoma

From Wright TC, Ferenczy A, Kurman RJ (eds): Carcinoma and other tumors of the cervix. Blaustein's Pathology of the Female Genital Tract. 4th ed. New York: Springer-Verlag, 1994:280, with permission.

lieved that most of these lesions begin as dysplastic lesions that progress to in situ carcinoma and then invasive disease (Fig. 56-1).

When an in situ lesion progresses beyond the basement membrane of the epithelium, it is considered to be invasive, with potential for further growth and the formation of metastatic deposits. The earliest phase of cervical invasion has been termed *microinvasive carcinoma*, a concept first advanced by Mestwerdt in 1947. Since then, numerous investigators have attempted to define an early cervical cancer that has little or no risk of dissemination beyond the cervix and may therefore be treated by more conservative means than a frankly invasive cancer. Definitions of microinvasive carcinoma are usually based on the depth of invasion from the basement membrane, with the maximum depth ranging from 1 to 5 mm. Differences in therapeutic approaches and methods of tumor measurement make it difficult to compare the results of the many clinical reports in the literature. There is information to suggest, however, that when the lesion invades less than 3 mm below the basement membrane, the risk of lymph node metastasis is below 1%. When the lesion invades to a depth of between 3 and 5 mm, however, the risk of spread has been estimated to be between

1% and 13% (Hasumi et al, 1980; van Nagell et al, 1983; Simon et al, 1986).

Insofar as it pertains to staging, microinvasive or microscopic carcinoma of the cervix has been officially defined by the International Federation of Gynecology and Obstetrics (FIGO) and modified by Creasman in 1995. Invasive carcinoma that is less than or equal to 5 mm in depth from the basement membrane and has less than 7 mm in lateral spread may be classified as preclinical or microinvasive carcinoma (stage IA). These lesions are further divided into stage IA1, which refers to invasive lesions up to 3 mm deep and 7 mm wide, and stage IA2, which refers to lesions that have invaded between 3 and 5 mm deep and 7 mm wide. It should be noted that these lesions are not yet clinically apparent; a grossly visible lesion is by definition not microscopic and is at least stage IB.

Because lesions with a depth of invasion between 3 and 5 mm have some risk of lymph node metastasis, the Society of Gynecologic Oncologists (SGO) has developed a functional definition of microinvasion, which uses 3 mm of invasion as the dividing line between those lesions that may be managed conservatively and those that require more radical therapy because of the risk of lymph node metastasis. This definition of microinvasive carcinoma of the cervix also excludes those lesions with lymphatic or vascular space involvement.

The American Joint Committee on Cancer has suggested a pathologic, tumor-node-metastasis (TNM) staging system to be utilized to classify surgically treated patients (Beahrs et al, 1988). This system has not been used to classify patients in any large radiotherapy studies, probably because it cannot be employed in a consistent manner without full surgical assessment of both primary and regional disease.

Histologically, invasive squamous carcinoma is characterized by sheets of flat squamoid cells, occasionally with keratin pearl formation (Fig. 56-2). The presence of keratinization has been associated with a more favorable prognosis (Gauthier et al, 1985). Nuclear atypia and mitotic figures may be prominent. The grading of squamous carcinoma is based on the degree of differentiation. At times, poorly differentiated carcinomas of the cervix of squamous origin may be difficult to distinguish from adenocarcinomas or other poorly differentiated variants.

Verrucous carcinoma is an unusual variant of squamous neoplasia that often has an indolent clinical course. These lesions are exophytic in appearance and may resemble condyloma. Histologically, verrucous carcinoma may be characterized by exuberant proliferation of squamous cells with areas of apparent koilocytosis. It may be difficult to distinguish these lesions from condyloma based on histologic appearance. The interface between the lesion and the normal stroma must be examined for evidence of invasive behavior. Metastasis from verrucous lesions is uncommon. Surgical therapy is preferred because there have been anecdotal reports that these tumors are radioresistant.

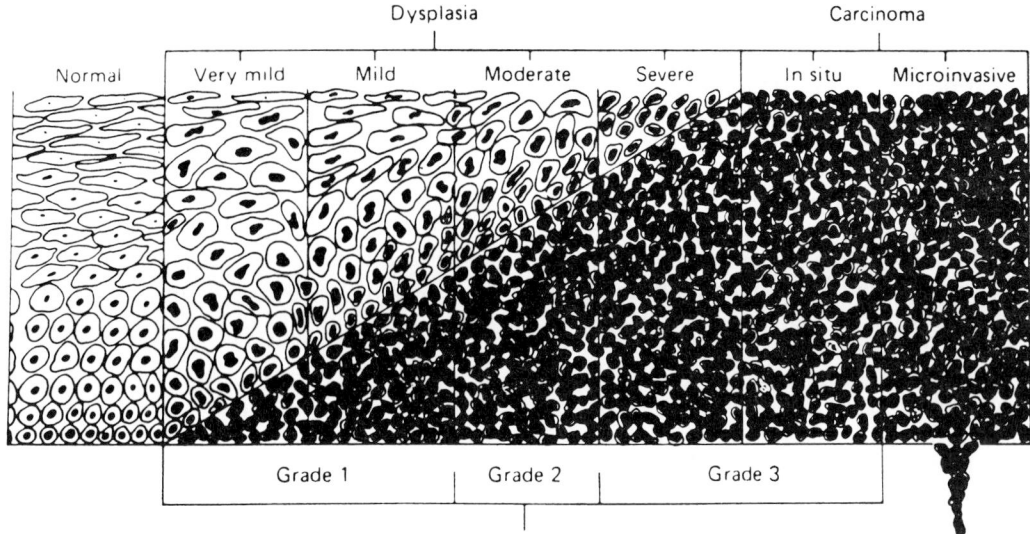

Figure 56–1
Illustration of the continuous spectrum of disease in early neoplasia of the cervix. (From Ferenczy A, Winkler B [eds]: Cervical intraepithelial neoplasia and condyloma. Blaustein's Pathology of the Female Genital Tract. 3rd ed. Heidelberg: Springer-Verlag, 1987:193, with permission.)

Adenocarcinoma

Adenocarcinoma of the cervix accounts for a significant minority of invasive lesions. Previous literature documented a 5% incidence; however, the incidence is more accurately estimated at between 10% and 15% (Shingleton et al, 1981; Eifel et al, 1990). Whether this represents a true increase in the incidence of cervical adenocarcinoma or changing pathologic diagnostic criteria remains unclear.

Grossly, adenocarcinoma of the cervix is, for the most part, indistinguishable from a squamous lesion. The adenocarcinoma may have an increased tendency to be endophytic rather than exophytic. Histologically, lesions range from well to poorly differentiated. Well-differentiated lesions resemble the glandular architecture of the cervix (Fig. 56–3). It is thought that adenocarcinoma of the cervix may have a worse prognosis than squamous lesions, with a tendency to early metastasis. When the lesions are greater than or equal to 4 cm, the rate of recurrence after either radiation therapy or radical hysterectomy significantly increases, primarily reflecting a higher rate of distant metastases in patients with adenocarcinoma versus squamous carcinoma (Eifel et al, 1995).

The term *microinvasion* is usually not applied to adenocarcinoma of the cervix. Depth of invasion is difficult to assess and, because these lesions are less common, the true risk of lymph node metastasis from early lesions has not been well established. One area of particular concern is the management of adenocarcinoma in situ. In a retrospective analysis of 61 patients, Wolf et al (1996) concluded that women

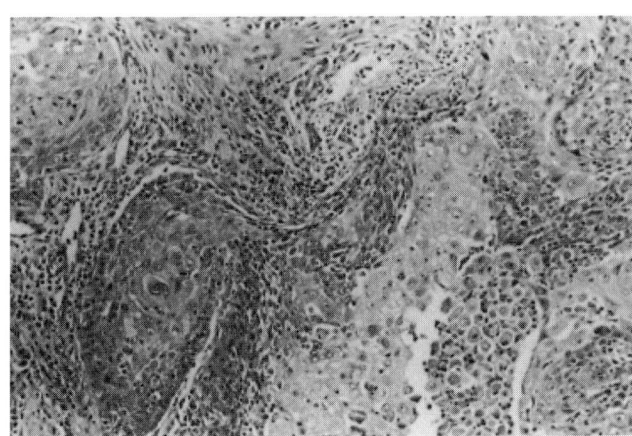

Figure 56–2
Squamous cell carcinoma of the cervix. (Courtesy of Elvio G. Silva, M.D.)

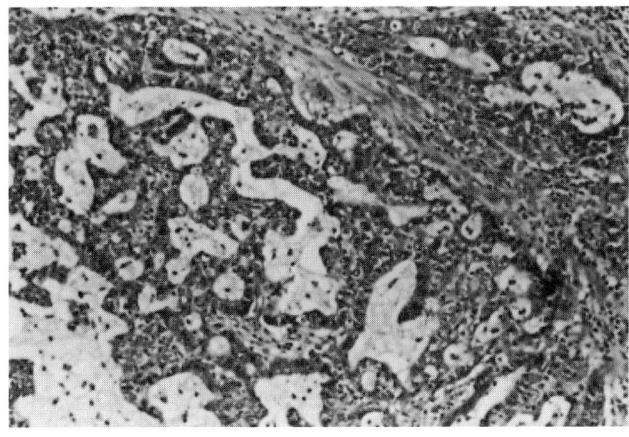

Figure 56–3
Adenocarcinoma of the cervix. (Courtesy of Elvio G. Silva, M.D.)

with adenocarcinoma in situ of the cervix often have residual disease in the uterus, regardless of whether the margins on cone biopsy are positive or negative.

Histologic differentiation between adenocarcinoma in situ and the so-called minimal deviation adenocarcinoma (adenoma malignum) may be difficult. The diagnosis is often based merely on the depth of invasion of abnormal glands. Adenoma malignum may behave malignantly, and some believe it has a worse prognosis than typical adenocarcinoma. This is probably because these lesions are often undertreated and thus more likely to recur.

Adenocarcinoma involving both the endometrial cavity and endocervix can present a clinical dilemma, because differentiating between endometrial and endocervical origin can be difficult. Although the typical endometrioid histologic pattern is more suggestive of an endometrial origin, these lesions can also arise in the cervix. Likewise, adenocarcinoma resembling endocervical glands or mucinous epithelium can arise within the endometrial canal. Careful separate curettage of the endometrial cavity and cervical canal may be helpful. Hysteroscopy and magnetic resonance imaging (MRI) may give additional information regarding the site of origin. Another suggested method for differentiating these lesions is to send a tissue sample for HPV analysis. Those lesions with HPV DNA are more likely to be of cervical than of endometrial origin.

Clear cell carcinoma is a specific variant of cervical cancer that has been associated with intrauterine exposure to diethylstilbestrol (Edelman, 1989) but is not limited to women with such exposure. Histologically, the carcinoma appears as sheets of clear or classical hobnail cells. Routine treatment is indicated.

Adenoid cystic carcinoma is a rare variant that is characterized by a slow growth rate and a tendency to metastasize to the lung.

Mixed Epithelial Carcinoma

Adenosquamous carcinoma of the cervix contains a mixture of malignant squamous and glandular components (Fig. 56–4). The extent of each cell type within a lesion will vary. It has been reported that patients with adenosquamous carcinoma tend to have a worse prognosis than those with pure squamous carcinoma (Wheeless et al, 1970; Gallup et al, 1985). The term *glassy cell carcinoma* refers to a poorly differentiated variant of adenosquamous carcinoma, which tends to have an aggressive course (Tamimi et al, 1988).

Neuroendocrine Carcinoma

Both small cell carcinoma and carcinoid may occur in the uterine cervix. Small cell carcinoma is characterized by small cells with uniform nuclei (Fig. 56–5). These lesions tend to grow rapidly and are

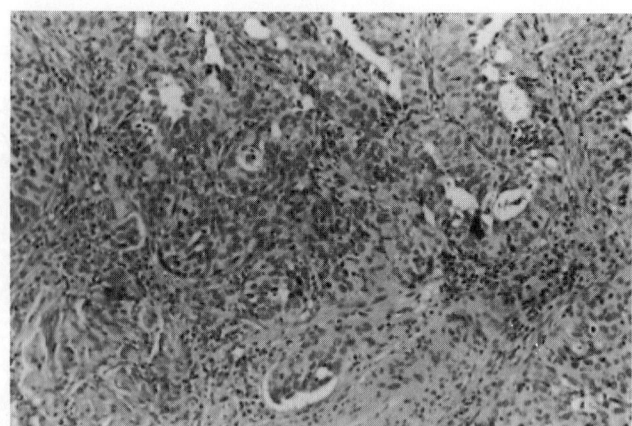

Figure 56–4
Adenosquamous cancer of the cervix. (Courtesy of Elvio G. Silva, M.D.)

prone to distant metastasis through lymphatic and hematogenous dissemination. In a review of 14 patients with early-stage surgically resectable small cell carcinoma of the cervix, Sheets and co-workers (1988) found that 57% had lymph node metastasis. Multimodality therapy has been successfully used in this patient group (Morris et al, 1992). Carcinoid is an unusual primary in the cervix, with histologic features similar to a carcinoid lesion in other areas, such as the appendix. These tumors tend to remain localized for some time, and regional therapy is appropriate. To date, none of these tumors has been associated with the carcinoid syndrome.

Rare Tumors

Other rare tumors of the cervix include melanoma (Jones et al, 1971), choriocarcinoma (Tsukamoto et al, 1980), and a variety of metastatic lesions from other sites, such as uterine corpus, colon, rectum, and

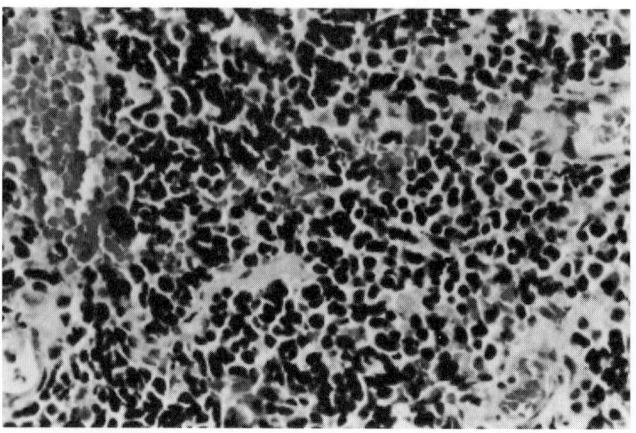

Figure 56–5
Small cell cancer of the cervix. (Courtesy of Elvio G. Silva, M.D.)

bladder. Experience with these lesions has been limited, and therapy should be tailored to the individual situation.

CLINICAL PRESENTATION AND PATTERNS OF SPREAD

In its early stages, cervical carcinoma tends to be asymptomatic. Therein lies the importance of cytologic screening to detect a cancer as early as possible. Early symptoms include vaginal discharge, odor, and abnormal vaginal bleeding. The latter may take on any pattern of menometrorrhagia or postmenopausal bleeding, but the classical complaint of postcoital bleeding is uncommon.

Early-stage lesions are often diagnosed during a routine pelvic examination. When a gross cervical lesion is visible, a biopsy is indicated. The clinician must not be reassured by a normal Pap smear in this situation. Because of the associated inflammation and necrosis, a cytologic smear of an invasive cancer is occasionally reported as inflammatory atypia. A biopsy specimen of every visible cervical lesion should be obtained in order to establish a definitive histologic diagnosis.

Cervical cancers may be characterized by gross appearance as exophytic or endophytic. Exophytic lesions protrude from the cervical surface and can be easily visualized and measured. In contrast, endophytic lesions are more difficult to detect. They may not be visible on speculum examination and may considerably expand the endocervix prior to detection. The only finding on physical examination may be an abnormally firm, expanded cervix. Because adenocarcinomas more often display an endophytic growth pattern, later detection may contribute to their poor prognosis.

Cervical carcinoma has two predominant spread patterns: direct extension and lymphatic dissemination. Cervical cancer will spread from the cervix to adjacent tissues, especially to the upper vagina and the parametrial tissues (cardinal and uterosacral ligaments). These areas are best assessed through a careful pelvic examination. Following speculum examination, vaginal and rectovaginal palpation should be performed to evaluate vaginal or parametrial extension. Extension into the uterine cavity is difficult to detect clinically and has little impact on prognosis or treatment.

The tumor may also involve the pelvic sidewall. It can be difficult to determine whether sidewall disease is a result of direct lateral extension of the cervical tumor or medial growth of metastatic lymph node deposits. Parametrial extension and, more often, sidewall disease can result in pelvic pain, sometimes with an associated radiculopathy in the lower extremity. Lymphatic and venous outflow obstruction can result in unilateral leg edema. An asymptomatic hydroureter is not uncommon with larger cervical cancers and may be diagnosed by intravenous pyelography (IVP) or computerized tomography (CT) imaging. Occasionally, uremia may be the presenting sign in a patient with bilateral ureteral obstruction and an undiagnosed cervical cancer.

The bladder or rectum may also be involved by direct extension of the cervical cancer. This may result in hematuria, rectal bleeding, or obstruction.

The lymphatic spread pattern of cervical cancer is fairly predictable and proceeds in a stepwise fashion (Fig. 56-6). Malignant cells spread via paracervical lymphatic channels into the pelvic node chains associated with the obturator, internal iliac, and external iliac vessels. The cells then spread cephalad to the common iliac chain and the para-aortic lymph nodes. Further extension to the mediastinal and supraclavicular nodes may also be seen.

Metastatic disease resulting from hematogenous dissemination is most often seen in women who have been previously treated for cervical cancer. It is occasionally seen at primary presentation, especially in more aggressive histologic subtypes such as small cell carcinoma. Metastatic disease may involve the lungs, liver, bone, or peritoneal cavity.

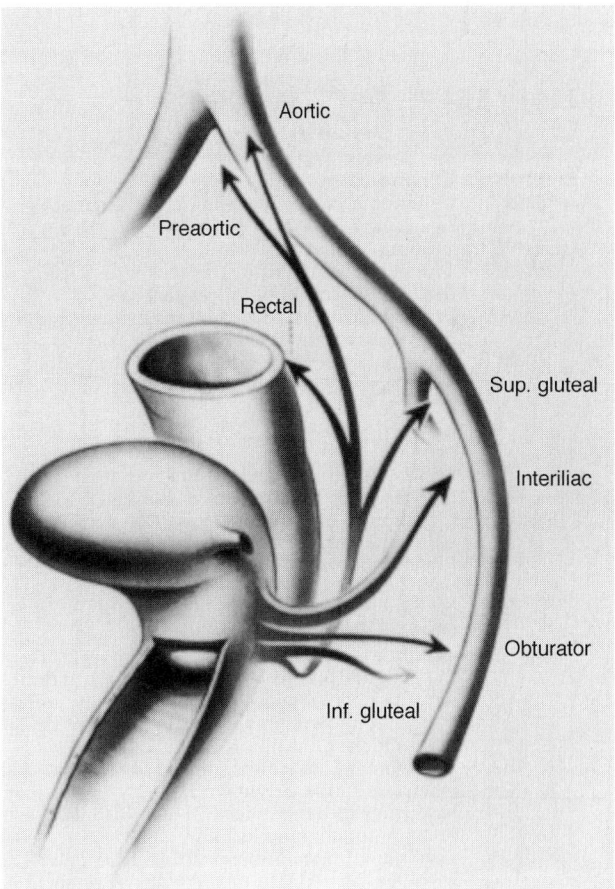

Figure 56-6
Progression of cervical cancer through regional lymph nodes. (From Plentl AA, Friedman EA: Lymphatic System of the Female Genitalia. Philadelphia: WB Saunders Company, 1971: 83, with permission.)

STAGING AND PRETREATMENT EVALUATION

Cervical cancer is staged by clinical evaluation, which allows for comparison of treatment results between centers that use only radiation therapy and those that use surgery. Most patients with cervical cancer are treated with radiation therapy. This is in contrast with the staging methodology for endometrial and ovarian cancer, which is based on surgical criteria because nearly all of these patients undergo surgery. The revised rules for staging cervical cancer have been established by the FIGO and were reported by Creasman in 1995. The staging system used today is presented in Table 56–2. It should be noted that the FIGO system does not incorporate several important prognostic variables such as tumor volume (except in stage I) or surgical or radiographic evidence of lymph node metastasis.

Pretreatment evaluation of a patient with cervical cancer depends upon the extent of disease at the time of initial presentation (Table 56–3). All patients should undergo a thorough history and physical examination; peripheral lymph node chains, such as the supraclavicular, axillary, and inguinal nodes, should be particularly assessed. Pelvic examination, particularly rectovaginal examination, is important

Table 56–2. FIGO STAGING OF CERVICAL CARCINOMA

Preinvasive Carcinoma
Stage 0: Carcinoma in situ; intraepithelial carcinoma

Invasive Carcinoma
Stage I: Carcinoma confined to the cervix (extension to the corpus should be disregarded)
IA: Preclinical invasive carcinoma, diagnosed by microscopy only
IA1: Invasion up to 3 mm deep and 7 mm wide
IA2: Invasion between 3 and 5 mm deep and 7 mm wide
IB: Clinically apparent lesions confined to the cervix
IB1: Lesions no greater than 4 cm in diameter
IB2: Lesions greater than 4 cm in diameter
Stage II: Carcinoma extends beyond the cervix onto either the vagina or parametrium but not to the lower third of the vagina and not to the pelvic wall
IIA: No obvious parametrial involvement
IIB: Obvious parametrial involvement
Stage III: Carcinoma extends to either the lower third of the vagina or to the pelvic wall. Hydronephrosis or a nonfunctioning kidney, unless they are known to be due to another cause, necessitates allocation to stage IIIB
IIIA: Involvement of lower third of vagina. No extension to the pelvic wall
IIIB: Extension to the pelvic wall or hydronephrosis or a nonfunctioning kidney
Stage IV: Carcinoma extends beyond the true pelvis or involves the mucosa of the bladder or rectum. Bullous edema does not permit assignment to stage IV
IVA: Spread to bladder or rectum
IVB: Spread to distant organs

From Creasman WT: New gynecologic cancer staging. Gynecol Oncol 1995;58:157, with permission.

Table 56–3. PRETREATMENT EVALUATION OF CERVICAL CANCER

Studies permitted for staging
 Physical examination
 Routine blood examination
 Chest radiograph
 Intravenous pyelogram
 Barium enema
 Cystoscopy
 Sigmoidoscopy
Optional studies that may not be used for staging
 Computerized tomography
 Magnetic resonance imaging
 Lymphangiogram
 Surgical staging

in determining the size of the lesion and the presence of vaginal or parametrial spread. A history of prior abdominal surgery or pelvic inflammatory disease may influence treatment planning, because this increases the risk for complications of radiation therapy. Other medical conditions, such as hypertension, heart disease, and diabetes, will also affect treatment planning.

All patients should undergo chest radiography. An IVP is a useful study for most patients. Even when the tumor is clinically confined to the cervix, it is not unusual to find a unilateral or bilateral hydroureter that changes the stage and prognosis. Even for those patients who have early lesions, an IVP can serve as a useful baseline examination prior to either radical surgery or radiation therapy, both of which may cause alterations in the urinary tract. An IVP will also confirm the position of the kidneys prior to pelvic radiation.

FIGO staging allows the use of cystoscopy and sigmoidoscopy for evaluation of the bladder and rectum. Because of the proximity of these organs to the cervix, invasion must be ruled out prior to the initiation of therapy. Any change in staging based on involvement of these organs must be based on a biopsy specimen and not on visual impression alone. All patients except those with the earliest and smallest lesions should undergo these procedures.

Barium enema or colonoscopy are useful procedures for patients who are older or who have glandular lesions. The presence of asymptomatic polyps or diverticular disease may influence treatment. Younger patients with smaller squamous lesions probably do not require a barium enema. Plain radiographs are permitted in the staging evaluation but have a low yield and are seldom performed.

Other radiologic tests may be used to aid in the development of a management plan but do not alter the stage. Lymphangiography is extremely useful in determining the presence of pelvic or para-aortic node metastasis (Piver et al, 1971; Wallace et al, 1979; Heller et al, 1990). However, the information gathered from this test does not affect stage. A CT scan may also be used to evaluate nodal status but is not nearly as accurate as lymphangiography. In a prospective trial carried out by the Gynecologic Oncology Group (GDG), 320 patients underwent ultrasound, CT, and lymphangiography prior to surgical staging. Of those patients who had positive para-aortic nodes documented by surgical exploration, 78% were detected by lumphangiography, whereas only 37% were detected by CT and 18% by ultrasound (Heller et al, 1990). Based on these multi-institutional data, lymphangiography is clearly superior in evaluating nodal status. Whenever an abnormal lymph node is detected by any method, confirmation of a metastatic deposit should be obtained by fine-needle aspiration or surgical exploration.

The use of MRI has been reported as helpful in determining the extent of cervical cancer (Powell et al, 1986; Hofmann et al, 1988; Rubens et al, 1988; Burghardt et al, 1989). Preliminary studies comparing MRI with CT scan and/or examination under anesthesia suggest that MRI may be superior to CT scan in assessment of lymph nodes, and more accurate than both modalities in the assessment of parametrial extension (Ho et al, 1992; Kim et al, 1993).

Surgical staging of cervical cancer, although not permitted by FIGO under its staging criteria, is widely performed in the United States. The purpose of surgical staging is to gain additional prognostic information regarding the extent of disease and to tailor therapy appropriately. Initially, surgical staging of cervical cancer patients was performed through a transperitoneal approach to the pelvic and para-aortic lymph nodes. This led to a significant increase in complications from radiation therapy, predominantly radiation bowel injury (Wharton et al, 1977). Surgeons believe that this complication results from the intestine becoming fixed in the pelvis at the sites of transperitoneal entry to the lymph nodes. Because they are adherent, these intestinal segments receive an unacceptably high radiation dose. Accordingly, the preferred approach to the pelvic and para-aortic lymph nodes is via the retroperitoneal space. With a retroperitoneal dissection, lymph node sampling may be accomplished with little increase in morbidity (Potish et al, 1984; Weiser et al, 1989). Although the impact of removal of gross lymph node metastases on survival has yet to be determined, the combination of a preoperative lymphgiogram and intraoperative abdominal radiographs is useful in ensuring that complete resection of abnormal nodes has been accomplished (Coleman et al, 1993).

Surgical staging remains a controversial concept in the treatment of cervical cancer. It does eliminate some of the errors inherent in clinical staging according to FIGO criteria and identifies patients who are likely to benefit from radiation fields extended to the para-aortic area. Some researchers also believe that debulking grossly involved lymph nodes may improve local control in response to radiation. The operation has morbidity of its own, however, and causes a 2- to 4-week delay in the initiation of radi-

ation therapy. Furthermore, there is no evidence that pretreatment surgical staging results in improved survival rates. Proponents of surgical staging indicate that knowledge of pelvic or para-aortic disease leads to use of extended-field radiation therapy for patients with poor prognosis and that some of these women may be salvaged with such an alteration in therapy. However, the additional number of poor-prognosis patients discovered by surgical staging compared with lymphangiography is relatively small and, therefore, many patients must undergo surgery with no apparent benefit in ultimate outcome. Until the therapeutic effect of surgical staging is clarified, it should be considered an investigational technique.

Squamous carcinoma of the cervix may also be evaluated through the use of tumor markers. Squamous cell carcinoma antigen is elevated in 40% to 60% of patients with invasive cervical cancer (Senekjian et al, 1987; Schmidt et al, 1988; Benedetti et al, 1989; Tomas et al, 1991). Other tumor markers such as CA-125, CA-15-3, and CA-19-9 may also predict disease status. Unfortunately, tumor markers for cervical cancer are not as reliable or as predictive as CA-125 is for ovarian cancer. Their use should also be considered investigational.

Although many staging techniques do not alter the FIGO stage, they provide additional prognostic information that will affect the therapy given to the patient. Poor prognostic factors are listed in Table 56–4 (Wentz and Regan, 1959; Boyce et al, 1981; Burke et al, 1987; Buckley et al, 1988; Haas and Friedl, 1988).

TREATMENT OF PRIMARY CERVICAL CANCER

Careful choice of a primary therapy for cervical carcinoma is critical because recurrent disease is seldom curable. The primary approaches are surgery, radiation therapy, and multimodality therapy. Each of these treatment options is subsequently reviewed.

Primary Treatment of Microinvasive Cervical Carcinoma

One can expect excellent results when treating microinvasive carcinoma of the cervix. In this discus-

---

Table 56–4. POOR PROGNOSTIC FACTORS IN CERVICAL CANCER

Advanced FIGO stage
Large tumor volume
Positive pelvic nodes
High-risk histology
Grade
Positive vascular/lymphatic space involvement

Based on Wentz and Reagan (1959), Boyce et al (1981), Burke et al (1987), Buckley et al (1988), and Haas and Friedl (1988).

sion, microinvasive carcinoma of the uterine cervix is limited to squamous lesions. The definition of adenocarcinoma in situ versus microinvasive adenocarcinoma is vague, at best. Many believe that any invasive adenocarcinoma of the cervix should be treated by either radical surgery or radiation therapy.

Microinvasive lesions of the cervix should be documented with either a conization or hysterectomy specimen. A simple punch biopsy is not sufficient to document the presence of microinvasion versus stage IB disease because a single biopsy may miss an adjacent occult invasive cancer.

Most clinicians in the United States utilize the functional definition of microinvasion as described by the SGO; this definition limits the depth of invasion to 3 mm and excludes patients with lymphatic or vascular space involvement. For patients with lesions between 3 and 5 mm, other options, such as radiation therapy or radical surgery with either a type II (modified radical) or type III radical hysterectomy, should be considered. Note that the FIGO definition of stage IA1 carcinoma, as modified by Creasman in 1995, closely resembles the SGO definition of microinvasion.

For those patients who can sacrifice fertility or have questionable margins on the cone biopsy or lymphatic space involvement, hysterectomy by either the vaginal or abdominal route is appropriate. With this approach, the cure rate approaches 100% (Hasumi et al, 1980; Holzer, 1982; Kolstad, 1989). Some women with microinvasive cervical cancer may be of childbearing age and have a strong desire to maintain fertility. In selected cases, some authorities elect to treat with conization alone (Kolstad, 1989; Morris et al, 1993). This is only acceptable when the margins of the conization specimen are

negative for invasive or preinvasive disease, no lymphatic invasion is present, and the patient reliably attends follow-up visits. Continued surveillance with colposcopy, cervical cytology, and endocervical curettage is indicated.

Radical Hysterectomy

For stage IB1 and IIA lesions, radical hysterectomy has long been the standard therapy. Simple hysterectomy had been attempted in women with cervical cancer with poor results. Knowledge of the spread pattern of cervical carcinoma led to the recognition that the uterine ligaments and pelvic lymphatics were at risk. Described in 1900 by Wertheim, the radical hysterectomy was successfully used as a treatment for invasive cervical cancer. In his original series of 500 patients, Wertheim (1907) removed the pelvic lymph nodes only if they were clinically suspicious. Mortality from the operation approached 20%. Enthusiasm for the procedure was limited by the success of radiation therapy as a treatment for cervical cancer. Meigs (1951) modified the radical hysterectomy procedure in the late 1940s, taking a wider margin on the parametrial tissues and routinely dissecting the pelvic lymph nodes. With this approach and the use of blood transfusions and antibiotics, results from the surgical treatment of early cervical cancer equaled those achieved with radiation therapy.

At M. D. Anderson Cancer Center, hysterectomy for cervical cancer is divided into five classes (Table 56–5) (Piver et al, 1974). The procedure of choice for stage IB1 or IIA cervical carcinoma is a type III radical hysterectomy, which involves removal of the uterus, the cardinal and uterosacral ligaments, the

---

Table 56–5. RUTLEDGE CLASSIFICATION OF HYSTERECTOMY

Type I—Treatment for Intraepithelial Lesions or Stage IA1
This extrafascial hysterectomy separates the cervix and upper vagina in a plane outside the pubocervical fascia. The technique assures complete removal of the cervix and 1 to 2 cm of vaginal cuff. The inclusion of some paracervical tissue reduces the risk of dissecting into the cervix, where the cardinal ligaments are attached.

Type II—Treatment for Stage IA2 Lesions
This moderately radical operation preserves the blood supply to the lower ureter and vagina while removing medially two thirds of the parametrium and the upper third of the vagina. The ureters are mobilized, but the uterine artery supply is conserved by ligating the uterine vessels medial to the ureter. The ureteral arteries from the superior vesicle artery remain intact.

Type III—Treatment for Stage IB1 and IIA
This radical hysterectomy may be used as primary treatment for stages I and II cancer of the cervix. The resection follows the pelvic wall to remove the parametrium, the uterosacral ligament, and also about one third of the vaginal length. The extensive resection of the pubocervical ligament sacrifices vasculature to the lower ureter and bladder not lost by the less extended procedures noted above; thus there is a greater risk of fistulas in the Type III operation. The incidence of bladder atony is greater because there is complete resection of the uterosacral ligaments and the rectal pillars.

Types IV and V—Rarely Used for Recurrent Disease in Lieu of Exenteration
These procedures are more extensive than usually implied by radical hysterectomy. When the internal iliac system must be resected, the superior vesicle supply is completely sacrificed. Therefore, this greater resection along with greater reconstruction of a portion of the involved urinary tract are designated as Type IV and V procedures.

pubocervical ligaments, and the upper one third of the vagina (Fig. 56–7). Also performed as part of this procedure is complete pelvic lymphadenectomy, removing the lymph nodes from the obturator, internal iliac, external iliac, and lower common chains. Most surgeons will also remove the upper common iliac and lower para-aortic lymph nodes.

The procedure begins with an abdominal exploration, carefully inspecting the peritoneal surfaces, liver, bowel, ovaries, and other pelvic organs. The pelvic and para-aortic lymph nodes should be carefully palpated for clinically evident metastatic disease. When extrauterine disease is present, most surgeons will discontinue the surgery and treat the patient with radiation or multimodality therapy. If only one or two pelvic lymph nodes are positive, some surgeons will excise them and continue with the radical hysterectomy. The pelvic spaces are then opened, with careful palpation of the cardinal and uterosacral ligaments. If parametrial disease is detected, the procedure is abandoned.

The ideal candidate for radical hysterectomy is a younger patient who is in good health and preferably not obese. The cancer should be confined to the cervix, although some patients with upper vaginal involvement may be adequately treated with radical hysterectomy. Perhaps the most important criteria is that the cervical lesions should not, in most cases, exceed 4 cm in size. Larger lesions are probably best treated by radiation therapy. Because ovarian metastases from early cervical cancer are exceedingly rare, the ovaries may remain in situ when further ovarian function is desired.

Following surgery, further prognostic information can be obtained through analysis of the specimen. When lymph node metastases, close or positive surgical margins, or parametrial spread are detected, most patients are treated with postoperative pelvic radiation therapy. The results of postoperative radiation therapy following radical hysterectomy have been mixed (Morrow, 1980; Hogan et al, 1982; Inoue

and Okamura, 1984; Larson et al, 1987; Kim et al, 1988; Thomas and Dembo, 1991). Pelvic radiation following a radical dissection certainly adds morbidity, but most authorities believe that the potential benefits outweigh the risks in certain high-risk groups of patients. Several prospective randomized trials evaluating the role of postoperative radiation therapy are currently underway.

The results for patients treated with radical hysterectomy are excellent, with 5-year survival rates ranging from 77% to 93% (Park et al, 1973; Underwood et al, 1979; Webb and Symmonds, 1979; Lee et al, 1989). A variety of authors have reported their experiences with laparoscopic lymphadenectomy, laparoscopic modified radical hysterectomy, and laparoscopy-assisted radical vaginal hysterectomy (Nezhat et al, 1992; Melendez and Childers, 1995; Roy et al, 1996). To date, no large prospective randomized trials have compared abdominal radical hysterectomy with laparoscopic radical hysterectomy.

Complications of Radical Hysterectomy

Many of the technical aspects of radical hysterectomy and pelvic lymphadenectomy have been refined in the last few decades, which has led to a reduction in the incidence of serious complications. Great care is now taken in the handling of the ureters and their removal from the cardinal ligament. Some surgeons are able to spare portions of the uterosacral ligament, which may yield less of an effect on the parasympathetic nervous innervation of the bladder and rectum. The use of prophylactic antibiotics has further decreased complications. Nevertheless, a number of problems can occur both in the immediate postoperative period and long term in this group of patients, and the clinician should be familiar with their diagnosis and management.

Acute surgical complications such as hemorrhage or infection are not uncommon. Prior to surgery, we

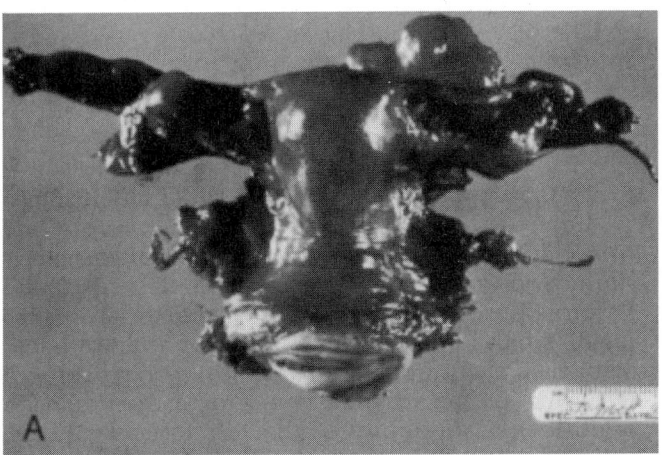 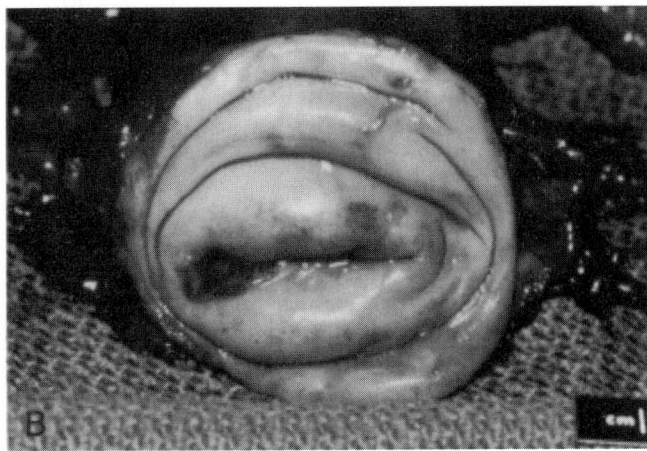

Figure 56–7
Two views of a surgical specimen from a radical hysterectomy.

routinely recommend that a type and screen be obtained. We do not type and cross-match blood unless an extremely unusual antibody is present, requiring that blood be set aside in advance. Prophylactic antibiotics are routinely given by most surgeons to prevent postoperative infectious morbidity. Data from large-scale trials supporting the use of this therapy are lacking.

The patient undergoing radical hysterectomy and pelvic lymphadenectomy is at risk for the usual acute postoperative complications from abdominal surgery, such as prolonged ileus and postoperative bowel obstruction. Particular to this procedure, however, is an increase in the incidence of constipation after surgery. This may be due to transection of the parasympathetic fibers in the uterosacral ligaments. Constipation, when present, may last for many years. The best management approach is to counsel the patient to begin a high-fiber diet, using laxatives only in resistant cases (Griffenberg et al, 1997).

During radical hysterectomy, both the bladder and ureters are at risk for intraoperative injury (Seski and Kiokno, 1977; Kadar et al, 1983; Scotti et al, 1986). As the ureter is separated from its peritoneal attachments and moved lateral to the cardinal ligament, much of the fine anastomotic network of blood vessels that supplies the ureter is divided or traumatized. Division of the superior vesicle artery may exacerbate any injury. With the use of modern antibiotics in a prophylactic setting, the incidence of ureteral fistulas has dropped dramatically. Nevertheless, great care should be taken when handling the ureter to avoid this problem. When a ureteral fistula does occur, management can be expectant and a significant proportion of fistulas will heal spontaneously. Those that do not spontaneously heal may require surgical correction. It is best to wait a minimum of 2 to 3 months after the initial surgery before attempting surgical repair; this will allow any residual inflammation to subside.

The most common alteration in the urinary tract following radical hysterectomy involves the bladder. Women undergoing this procedure often report an altered sensation of bladder fullness, with or without the urge to void. Urinary retention is a common problem during the postoperative period. Some surgeons routinely manage patients with continuous Foley or suprapubic catheter drainage for 6 weeks postoperatively. This regimen has been modified at M. D. Anderson to include 4 days of Foley catheter drainage. The patient then receives instruction in the technique of self-catheterization. The patient is sent home with instructions to spontaneously void every 4 hours followed by self-catheterization and to record the volume of urine remaining. When the postvoid residual has dropped to 25 ml or less for at least 1 week, the patient is told to discontinue self-catheterization. The addition of parasympathomimetics, such as bethanechol (Urecholine), has not been of proven efficacy in the management of these patients. A small percentage of women (1% to 3%)

will have to perform self-catheterization on a chronic basis because of urinary retention.

During radical hysterectomy, up to one half of the vaginal tube may be excised. In most patients, adequate surgical margins can be achieved by removing one third to one quarter of the length of the vagina. In some cases, however, sexual dysfunction may result following radical hysterectomy because of vaginal shortening.

As a result of the interruption of lymphatic channels in the pelvis, some patients develop a collection of lymphatic fluid, which is termed a lymphocyst. Although closed-suction drainage has previously been used in the pelvic dissection beds, we no longer use drains after radical hysterectomy at M. D. Anderson Cancer Center. Support for this policy comes from Patsner (1995), who noted no increase in postoperative pelvic infection, fistula, or lymphocyst formation when he compared 60 patients who had drains after radical hysterectomy versus 60 who did not. Patients with a lymphocyst may present postoperatively with pain, a pelvic mass, or ureteral obstruction. Physical examination may suggest a cystic structure, although at times it is difficult to exclude an ovarian cyst or recurrent cancer. A clinician who believes that a lymphocyst is present can observe the patient for a period of time, because some lymphocysts resolve spontaneously. If patients are symptomatic or have signs of ureteral or intestinal obstruction because of mass effect, lymphocysts can be drained percutaneously. The introduction of a foreign body, however, increases the risk of infection of the lymphocyst. Surgical exploration and excision is a procedure that often gives unsatisfactory results.

Ovarian Transposition

As noted above, radical hysterectomy allows maintenance of ovarian function. A significant minority of women will undergo postoperative pelvic radiation therapy because of the discovery of one or more poor prognostic factors. Because pelvic radiation will result in the loss of ovarian function, many surgeons routinely transpose the ovaries out of the pelvic field of radiation (Fig. 56–8). The procedure can be carried out as part of surgical staging for women who are to undergo primary radiation therapy for cervical cancer. Patients for whom ovarian transposition is not an option are now routinely given hormone replacement therapy following surgery or radiation.

During ovarian transposition, the ovary is divided from the ovarian ligament and mobilized along the infundibulopelvic ligament. Depending on the type and field of radiation therapy planned, the ovary may be mobilized above the level of the renal vessels. Most commonly, the ovary is placed at the anterior level of the anterosuperior iliac spine, well out of the range of pelvic irradiation. The benefit of preserving ovarian function for the additional 20 to 30 years of its expected functional existence justifies this procedure.

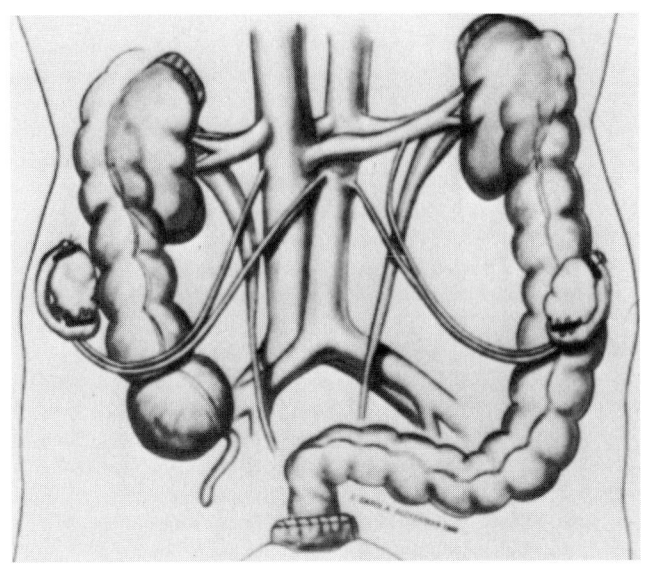

Figure 56–8
Ovarian transposition. (From Di Saia PJ: Surgical aspects of cervical carcinoma. Cancer 1981;48:548, with permission.)

Radiation Therapy

Ionizing radiation is the expected therapy for the majority of women who present with cervical carcinoma. Treatment of cervical carcinoma involves delivery of radiation therapy in two separate phases. Initially, external-beam radiation therapy (EBRT) is given to the pelvic area. The standard treatment area measures 15 × 15 cm, and treatment is divided between two separate fields (anterior and posterior) or by a four-field technique (Fig. 56–9). The lower border of the field is generally placed at the mid-pubis or 4 cm below the lowest level of vaginal disease. The upper border is placed at L4-L5 or L5-S1 unless the para-aortic nodes are believed to be at risk. The lateral borders are placed at least 1 cm lateral to the pelvic margins. The borders of the radiation field are tailored to the distribution of the tumor and the patient's anatomy.

Extended-field EBRT is employed for patients who have known or suspected disease in the para-aortic area. When used for patients with surgically documented *microscopic* disease, extended-field EBRT has the potential to cure nearly 50% of patients. However, the results for patients with *gross* para-aortic metastases are very poor. The results of therapy for patients with biopsy-proven para-aortic metastases are shown in Table 56–6 (Ballon et al, 1981; Piver et al, 1981; Komaki et al, 1983; Berman et al, 1984; Brookland et al, 1984; Nori et al, 1985; Podczaski et al, 1990).

Extended-field therapy may also be useful for patients at risk for occult para-aortic metastases, as shown in a randomized trial for patients with bulky cervical cancer and negative para-aortic nodes (Rotman et al, 1990). When compared with patients who received standard pelvic radiation therapy, women who were treated with extended-field therapy had a significant survival advantage. Because extended-field radiation exposes a greater volume of normal tissue to ionizing radiation, the risk of complications is significantly increased. More patients experience myelosuppression with extended-field therapy. Complications involving the small intestine are also more common.

The purpose of EBRT is twofold. External radiation sterilizes microscopic disease that may exist in pelvic lymph nodes. It also shrinks the central tumor in the cervix and paracervical tissues to provide superior geometry for appropriate placement of the radiation implant. External therapy is given in a series of small fractions, most commonly 1.8 to 2.0 Gy daily, lasting for 4 to 5 weeks for a total of 40 to 50 Gy. Delivery of EBRT in multiple small fractions allows for maximal tumor cell kill with preservation of normal tissues.

Following external radiation, patients usually receive two radiation implants. Intracavitary treatments, also referred to as brachytherapy, may utilize a variety of applicator devices designed to give an intense dose of radiation to the central pelvis while sparing surrounding tissues. Perhaps the most widely used applicator is the Fletcher-Suit-Delclos afterloading tandem and ovoid, which was developed at M. D. Anderson Cancer Center (Fig. 56–10). This system is inserted approximately 1 week after the conclusion of EBRT. Its primary components consist of a curved tandem that is placed within the uterine cavity and two ovoids that lie in the upper vaginal fornices. Together these produce a distribution of high-intensity radiation (Fig. 56–11) that treats the upper vagina, cervix, and uterine cavity. A number of advances have been made to limit the dosage of radiation delivered to the bladder and rectum, most particularly through the shielding present in the ovoids. The placement of the device by an experienced radiation therapist is of vital importance to ensure dose distribution that will improve local control of the cancer without increasing serious complications. The applicators are known as "afterloading" devices because they are hollow and allow the radioactive source to be inserted in the patient's room following verification of proper placement by pelvic radiograph and transfer from the recovery room to a private area. This minimizes the dose of radiation to hospital staff and is a major improvement over the older "hot" systems.

Once inserted, the tandem and ovoids are loaded with either radium or, more commonly, cesium, and are left in place for approximately 48 hours. After a 1- to 2-week rest, a second implant is usually placed for a similar time period. Because the energy from the radiation source decreases over distance by the inverse square law, the major portion of the dose delivered by the implant is to the immediately surrounding tissues.

Treatment results with radiation therapy for stage IB disease are excellent and comparable to those achieved with radical surgery. Cure rates for other stages are listed in Table 56–7 (Horiot et al, 1988).

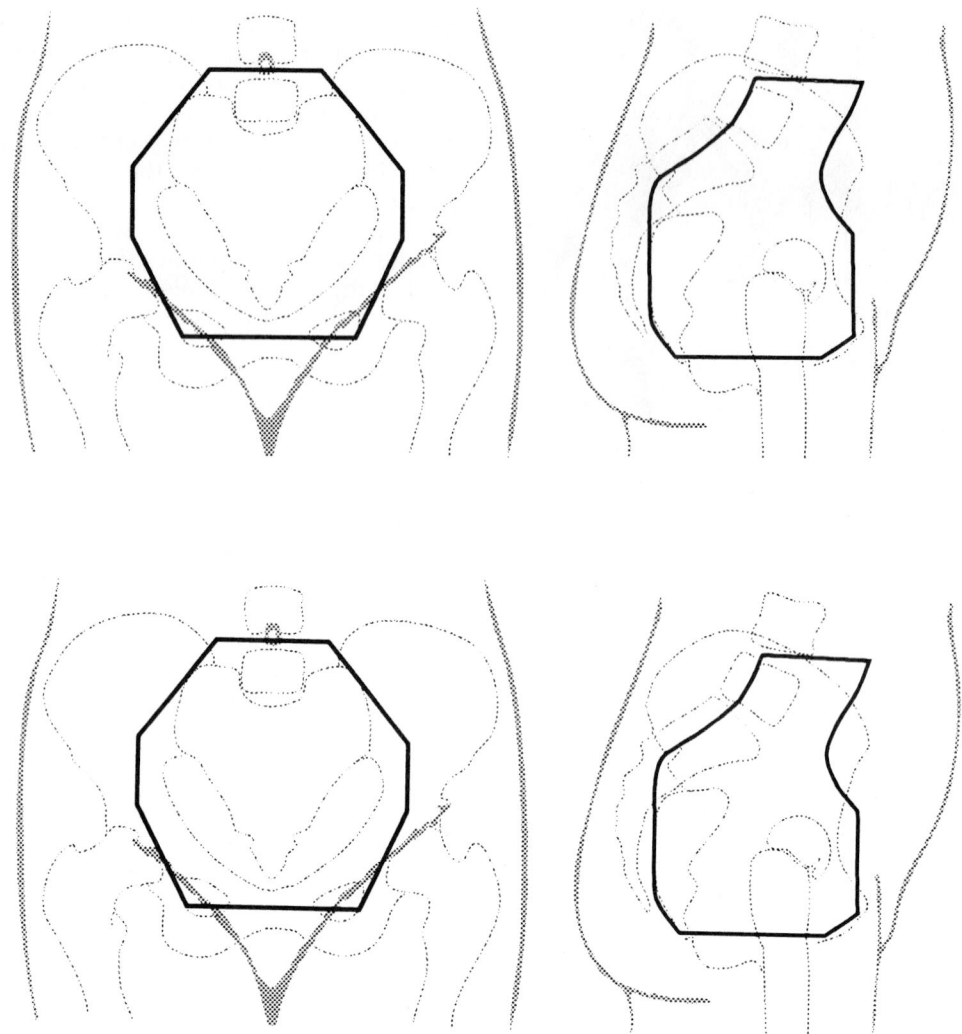

Figure 56–9
Diagram indicating radiation fields by the four-field technique. *Top left*, Anterior-posterior field. *Top right*, Right lateral field. *Bottom left*, Posterior-anterior field. *Bottom right*, Left lateral field.

Intracavitary brachytherapy has traditionally been delivered at a low dose rate (LDR) of 0.4 to 0.8 Gy/hour. There has recently been a dramatic increase in interest, however, in high-dose-rate (HDR) brachytherapy. Although HDR is defined as a dose rate greater than 0.2 Gy/minute, 2 to 3 Gy/minute is usually administered (International Commission on Radiological Units and Measurements, 1985), a rate similar to external beam irradiation. Potential advantages of HDR include the outpatient nature of the procedure (each application lasts only 10 to 15 minutes), decreased costs, decreased anesthetic requirement, and minimization of applicator movement (Dusenbery et al, 1991; Houdek et al, 1991).

Despite these potential benefits, the utility of this technique remains controversial. Because four to seven applications are required, the geometry is not likely to be identical from one session to the next. Furthermore, patients may have difficulty tolerating multiple applications. Finally, convincing evidence

regarding the equivalence of LDR and HDR in terms of tumor control and normal tissue complications has not yet been provided (Eifel, 1992).

SPECIAL SITUATIONS IN RADIATION THERAPY

Treatment of the Pregnant Patient. Cervical carcinoma is the most common malignancy that occurs during pregnancy, and it presents a particular problem for the obstetrician-gynecologist (Prem et al, 1966; Bokhman and Urmancheyeva, 1989; Hannigan, 1990). Therapy must be based on several factors, including the stage and size of the lesion, gestational age of the fetus, and the desire to complete the pregnancy (Hacker et al, 1982).

Staging during pregnancy should be performed as in nonpregnant patients. For patients with advanced lesions who are in the first or second trimester of pregnancy, little regard is usually given to the results

Table 56-6. SURVIVAL OF PATIENTS WITH BIOPSY-PROVEN PARA-AORTIC NODE INVOLVEMENT FOLLOWING EXTENDED-FIELD RADIATION THERAPY

STUDY	NO. OF PATIENTS	SURVIVAL 3-Year	5-Year
Piver et al (1981)	31		10%
Ballon et al (1981)	18		23%
Komaki et al (1983)	15		40%
Berman et al (1984)	98	25%	
Brookland et al (1984)	15	40%	
Nori et al (1985)	27		29%
Podczaski et al (1990	33		31%

of diagnostic radiation on the fetus because the pregnancy will probably be terminated. In earlier cases of cervical cancer, such as stage IA and IB1, numerous staging procedures are not indicated. In women who present with advanced lesions during the third trimester, delivery should be carried out by cesarean section. It may be helpful to conclude staging procedures prior to delivery, however, and this may be accomplished with a minimal dose of radiation to the fetus. Careful physical examination and chest radiography may be performed. An alternative to lymphangiography or CT scan would be MRI. A limited IVP may be carried out with adequate assessment of the collecting system.

Timing of definitive treatment must be individualized for each case. Patients with carcinoma in situ who have satisfactory colposcopy results may be

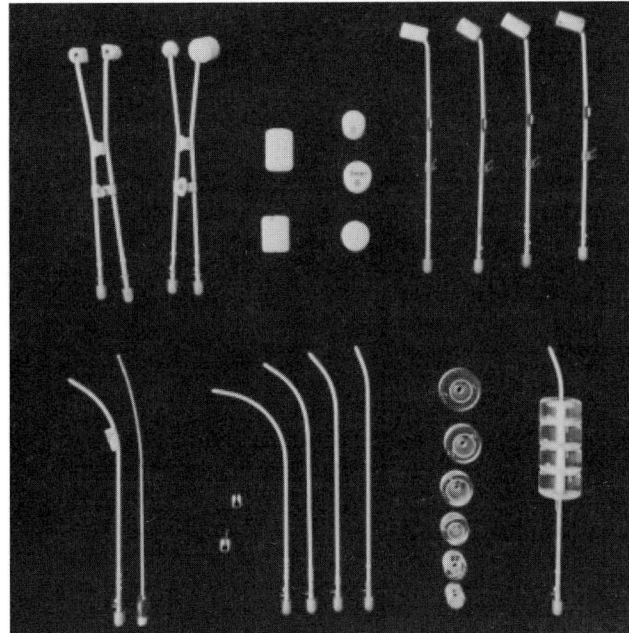

Figure 56-10
Fletcher-Suit-Delclos colpostats and Delclos vaginal cylinder. (Courtesy of Dr. Patricia Eifel.)

managed expectantly without definitive therapy until the pregnancy has been concluded. Patients with a stage IA1 (preclinical) carcinoma should have a conization for definitive diagnosis. If the conization specimen has negative margins and the lesion is less than 3 mm in depth, the patient may complete her pregnancy, if desired, with vaginal delivery. For a stage IB1 lesion or greater, maintenance of a pregnancy that is in the first or second trimester may be hazardous because a delay in definitive therapy could result in an incurable condition. It is therefore suggested that women at this point have an interruption of pregnancy and begin therapy based on the size and distribution of the lesion. Patients who have early lesions may be managed with radical hysterectomy. It is not necessary to terminate the pregnancy prior to this procedure. For lesions best treated with radiation, therapy may begin with EBRT followed by tandem and ovoids. During the first and second trimesters, EBRT will result in spontaneous abortion after 1 to 2 weeks of therapy in the great majority of cases. Occasionally, when a large cervical lesion prevents passage of the fetus, a second-trimester pregnancy may require hysterotomy for evacuation.

Management of invasive cervical carcinoma in the late second or third trimester becomes more complex. Patients who are candidates for radical hysterectomy (see above) may be managed expectantly until fetal lung maturity can be demonstrated. Delivery can then be effected through a radical cesarean hysterectomy. Those patients whose lesions are best treated by radiation therapy should undergo cesarean section through a classical incision as soon as fetal lung maturity is attained. Maneuvers to hasten fetal lung maturity should be undertaken, and, at the first sign of documented maturity, the infant should be delivered.

On the basis of anecdotal experience, it has long been stated that vaginal delivery in women with cervical cancer may hasten the spread of the cancer. Certainly, a large cervical lesion will not adequately dilate during a normal labor process, although certain patients with small stage IA or IB1 lesions may be able to have vaginal delivery without adverse effect. In this day and age, the safety of cesarean section makes experimentation along these lines difficult to justify. Whenever cesarean section is performed, the surgeon should avoid a transverse lower uterine incision because the cancer may have spread to the lower uterine segment. A classical uterine incision is preferred.

Barrel-shaped Lesions of the Cervix. Patients with stage IB lesions that have a barrel shape present a therapeutic dilemma. As tumor size increases, local control with radiation becomes more difficult (Piver and Chung, 1985). It is clear that a 1-cm exophytic lesion on the cervix is more curable than a 6-cm barrel-shaped lesion (Fig. 56-12). With large central lesions, potential for central failure is increased. In 1969, Durrance and colleagues defined a "barrel-

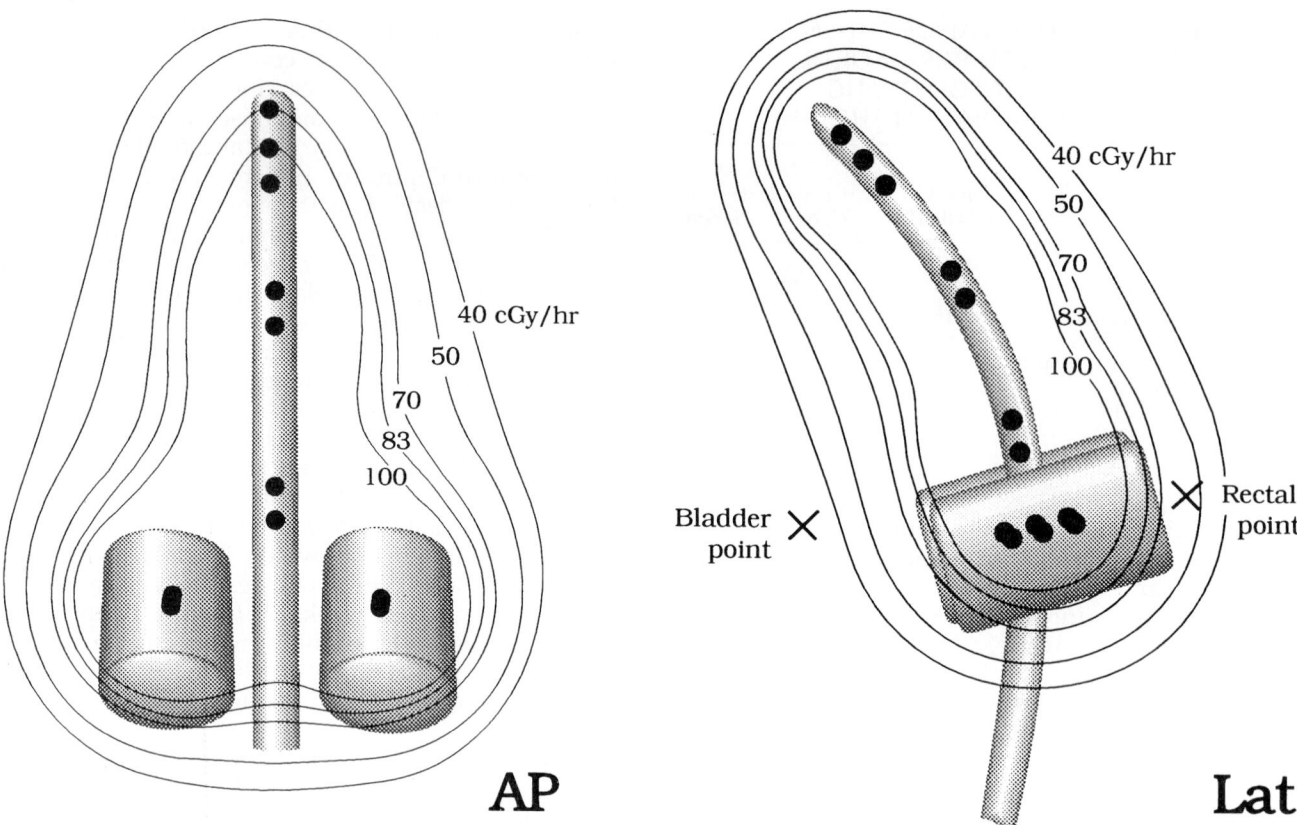

Figure 56–11
Pear-shaped dose distribution obtained with intracavitary therapy.

shaped" lesion as an endocervical cancer 6 cm or greater in size and noted that these cancers had a relatively high central relapse rate after radiation therapy alone. They advocated an extrafascial hysterectomy following pelvic irradiation to decrease the incidence of central failure. Based on this report from M. D. Anderson Cancer Center, many centers adopted a treatment plan for patients with barrel-

shaped lesions that used 40 to 45 Gy whole-pelvic irradiation followed by a 72-hour radium system. After a 6-week rest interval, the patient then underwent an extrafascial hysterectomy. The results of this approach have been difficult to interpret because most studies have been retrospective and have used a variety of definitions of barrel-shaped cancers (O'Quinn et al, 1980; Perez and Kao, 1985; Rotman et al, 1990). There is little question that some additional toxicity results when the surgical procedure is added. Despite the lack of evidence showing superiority to radiation alone, pelvic radiation followed by hysterectomy has been adopted by many practitioners. The GOG performed a randomized Phase III clinical trial to evaluate the role of adjuvant hysterectomy after standard external and intracavitary radiation therapy for patients with barrel-shaped stage IB cervical cancers. Although there was no statistical difference in survival between the two groups, the addition of hysterectomy to standard radiation therapy may have caused some reduction in recurrence (Keys et al, 1997).

Treatment After Inadvertent Simple Hysterectomy.
When simple hysterectomy is performed in the presence of invasive cervical cancer, a condition commonly referred to as a "cut-through" hysterectomy, further treatment with radiation or radical reoperation is advised. Cut-through hysterectomy continues

Table 56–7. PELVIC DISEASE CONTROL RATES AND SURVIVAL RATES OF 1383 PATIENTS WITH CARCINOMA OF THE INTACT UTERINE CERVIX TREATED WITH RADIOTHERAPY ALONE

FIGO STAGE	NUMBER OF PATIENTS	PELVIC DISEASE CONTROL RATE	SURVIVAL RATE
I	229	93%	89%
IIa	315	88%	85%
IIb	314	80%	76%
IIIa	266	63%	62%
IIIb	216	57%	50%
IV	43	18%	20%

Data from Horiot J, Pigneux J, Pourquier H, et al: Radiotherapy alone in carcinoma of the intact uterine cervix according to G. H. Fletcher guidelines: a French cooperative study of 1383 cases. Int J Radiat Oncol Biol Phys 1988;14:605.

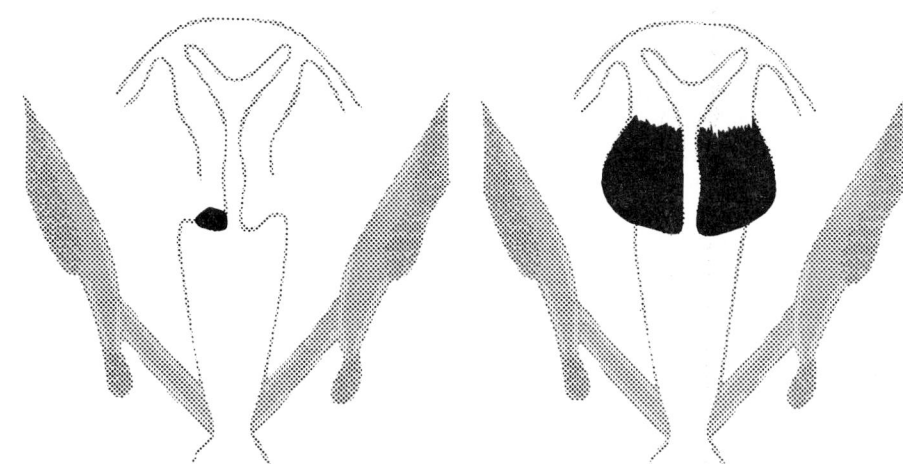

Figure 56-12
Stage IB cervical cancer, showing the comparison of an early exophytic lesion and a more advanced, barrel-shaped lesion. (Courtesy of Dr. Patricia Eifel.)

to be a significant clinical problem despite the widespread use of cervical screening and education of gynecologists in the technique of colposcopy. In one review, Roman and associates (1992) noted that the most common reasons for inappropriate hysterectomy were a false-negative Papanicolaou smear, failure to properly evaluate an abnormal Papanicolaou smear, and failure to perform an indicated conization of the cervix. Patients may be categorized into five classes based on the extent of residual disease present following surgery (Table 56–8).

Although some oncologists have advocated a radical excision of the parametrial tissues and pelvic lymph nodes (Orr et al, 1986), most patients are treated with pelvic radiation. The therapeutic goal is to treat the pelvic lymph nodes, the parametrial tissues, and the vaginal cuff—all of which are at risk for residual disease.

Pretreatment evaluation of patients following cut-through hysterectomy should proceed as described above, including evaluation of the lymph nodes. Because the cervix has been removed, the ability to deliver a high central dose with brachytherapy is somewhat compromised. One must also be concerned that postoperative adhesions may increase the risk of radiation bowel injury. Most patients are treated with 50-Gy EBRT to the whole pelvis followed by a vaginal dome cylinder implant that delivers an additional dose to the vaginal apex. If known residual disease is present, either in the pelvic nodes or at the margin of resection, that area may receive an additional 10-Gy boost.

In a review of patients treated at M. D. Anderson Cancer Center, Roman and co-workers (1992) found

that the outcome for patients who had no residual disease following hysterectomy was excellent, with overall 5-year survival approaching 71% for patients in groups II and III. However, when gross disease remained, the prognosis was poor, with only 41% of group IV patients surviving 5 years or more.

Interstitial Implants. In some cases, it is not possible to insert a tandem and ovoid following EBRT. This is most often due to obliteration of the cervical os from very large tumors. In cases such as this, some radiotherapists utilize interstitial needle implants with a device such as the Syed template (Syed and Fedei, 1977). These needle implants may also allow higher dose treatment to larger lesions that are beyond the effective range of a standard tandem and ovoid.

Cancer of the Cervical Stump. Supracervical hysterectomy is a procedure that is rarely performed. However, cervical cancer occasionally develops in the cervical stump. This presents a special treatment problem because it is difficult to deliver optimal brachytherapy to a cervical stump. Postoperative adhesions may also increase the risk of radiologic complications (Miller et al, 1984). For smaller lesions, radical trachelectomy and bilateral pelvic node dissection may provide the best results.

ALTERNATIVE THERAPIES FOR LARGE LESIONS

The effectiveness of EBRT is directly related to the size and oxygenation of the tumor. Hypoxic tumors tend to be radioresistant, whereas those with a rich blood supply are more radiosensitive. It follows, therefore, that larger tumors that have necrotic centers tend to be more radioresistant. Several strategies have been used to improve the radiosensitivity of such lesions, including hyperbaric oxygen therapy (Fletcher et al, 1977; Brady et al, 1981) and therapy with particles such as neutrons (Maor et al, 1988) as well as radiosensitizers (Hreshchyshyn et al, 1979, Piver et al, 1987, 1989; Stehman et al, 1988; Runowicz

Table 56-8. CUT-THROUGH HYSTERECTOMY PATIENTS BY GROUP

I	Microinvasive cancer
II	Disease confined to cervix, surgical margins negative
III	Surgical margins positive, no gross residual tumor
IV	Gross residual disease present
V	Referred for therapy over 6 months from diagnosis

et al, 1989). None of these therapies has shown a significant advantage, and many increase cost, length of treatment time, and morbidity. Some of these strategies remain areas of active investigation, as described below.

Radiosensitizers potentiate the effect of radiation on tumors. The mechanism of this action is not completely understood. The most commonly used radiosensitizer for cervical cancer has been hydroxyurea. Two other potent radiation sensitizers are fluorouracil and cisplatin. The Radiation Therapy Oncology Group conducted a randomized trial that compared pelvic and paraortic radiation to pelvic radiation administered with concomitant fluorouracil and cisplatin (Morris et al, 1999). The patients on the chemoradiation arm had a 50% improvement in overall survival with no significant increase in morbidity when compared to the radiation treatment group. Another randomized study from the Gynecologic Oncology Group found that radiation with cisplatin or cisplatin with fluorouracil improved survival when compared to women who received hydroxyurea as a sensitizer (Rose et al, 1999). In a third randomized study, women who were at high risk for recurrence after surgery received chemoradiation with cisplatin had an improved survival rate compared to those who received radiation alone (Keys et al, 1999). There is now a strong body of evidence to suggest that women with advanced cervical cancers (bulky Stage Ib and Stage II and over) should be treated with a combination of chemotherapy and radiation.

An alternative to the use of radiosensitizing agents is neoadjuvant chemotherapy. In this setting, chemotherapy is used primarily for its cytotoxic action. It is believed that, when given prior to radiation therapy, chemotherapy will shrink the central tumor and sterilize microscopic metastases outside of the radiation field. Patients are treated prior to radiation with two to four cycles of chemotherapy. Initial studies indicated a good response to chemotherapy, as measured by tumor shrinkage (Goldhirsch et al, 1986; Muss et al, 1987; Lara et al, 1990; Tobias et al, 1990). Randomized studies have failed to demonstrate a significant survival advantage, however (Souhami et al, 1991).

Intra-arterial chemotherapy has also been used prior to radiation with the purpose of shrinking the tumor. In the 1960s, researchers at M. D. Anderson Cancer Center found that intra-arterial chemotherapy prior to or during radiation therapy might improve response (Smith et al, 1972). Because of the morbidity, expense, and complexity of the procedure, however, little further work was done in this regard until the early 1980s. Kavanagh and coworkers (1987) reported that patients receiving intra-arterial cisplatin, mitomycin-C, bleomycin, and floxuridine had good results. Advances in catheter and pump technology have allowed innovative constant intra-arterial infusions during the course of radiation therapy, as reported by Morris and associates (1995).

These procedures are expensive and labor intensive. The role of intra-arterial therapy in the treatment of cervical cancer remains under investigation.

COMPLICATIONS OF RADIATION THERAPY FOR CERVICAL CANCER

Gastrointestinal. Portions of the gastrointestinal tract will inevitably receive a significant radiation dose during the delivery of pelvic radiotherapy.

Sigmoid Colon. The sigmoid colon is within the radiation field, and portions of the small intestine often enter the pelvis as well. With the intimate anatomic relationship of the sigmoid to the cervix, it is not difficult to understand how a tandem and ovoid system with a relatively posterior placement could result in a high dose of radiation to the sigmoid. The acute effects of radiation on the sigmoid are described as proctosigmoiditis. They include diarrhea, at times with passage of blood and mucus, and rarely tenesmus. These effects may occur after 1 to 2 weeks of EBRT and usually subside shortly after EBRT is concluded. A small proportion of patients, however, will have chronic diarrhea, occasionally with enough bleeding to produce profound microcytic anemia. The diagnosis of chronic proctosigmoiditis may be confirmed by flexible sigmoidoscopy. Patients will have a smooth, pale mucosa with prominent friable blood vessels. There is no satisfactory treatment for chronic proctosigmoiditis. Patients who have this problem within the first few months after radiation therapy may be assured that, in many cases, the disorder is self-limited. For some, however, proctosigmoiditis is a progressive illness. It has been suggested that treatment with hydrocortisone enemas may be of some value, although there is little objective evidence that significant improvement results. Chronic proctosigmoiditis can lead to a more serious condition of stricture or obstruction (Fig. 56–13).

Patients with narrowing of the rectosigmoid usually present with diarrhea alternating with constipation. Bloating, gaseousness, and crampy abdominal pain are not uncommon. As a result, patients will often have anorexia and weight loss. One must be careful to distinguish patients with this complication of radiation therapy from those who have recurrent disease. The diagnosis can be confirmed by flexible sigmoidoscopy or barium contrast studies. The involved sigmoid can be narrowed for several centimeters, and the sigmoidoscopist may note that this portion of the colon is relatively fixed. When the stricture is mild, patients may be treated with laxatives. Dilation of the narrowed segment using balloons and other such devices may be hazardous, and perforation may result in tissue with significant ischemia and fibrosis.

Patients with a high-grade obstruction require surgical intervention. In selected cases, it may be possible to resect the narrowed area of colon and perform a reanastomosis. In such resection, it is

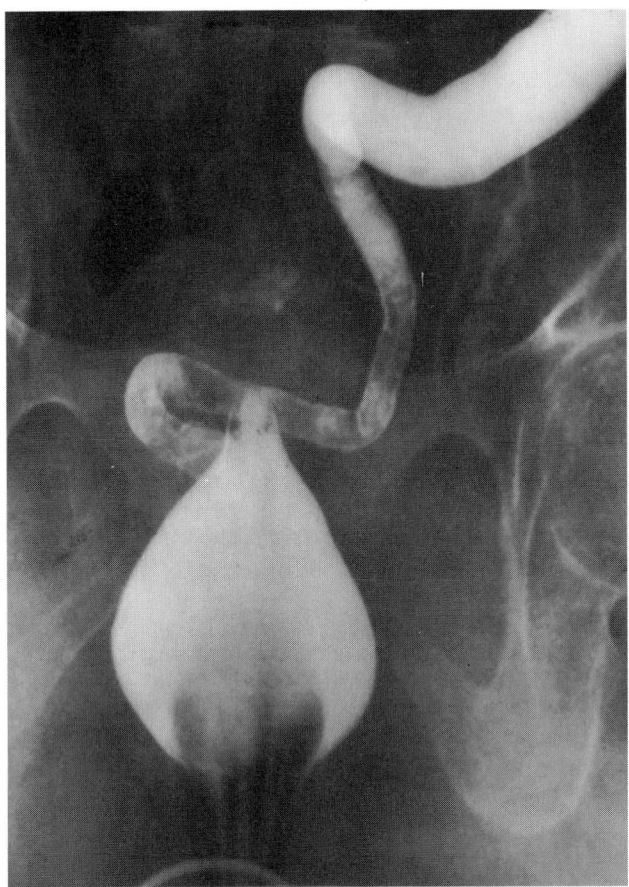

Figure 56–13
Markedly narrowed sigmoid colon with radiation-induced injury seen on barium enema.

important to perform a protective loop colostomy because any anastomosis in a field of irradiated bowel must be considered at high risk for impaired healing, leakage, or stricture. Unfortunately, in most cases of this severity, the remaining sigmoid colon will be found to have severe radiation changes with ischemia, edema, and tethering of the mesentery. These patients are frequently left with a transverse or end descending colostomy with a Hartmann's pouch. The use of an irradiated portion of the colon to form the colostomy stoma can also be hazardous, with stoma stenosis or retraction frequently occurring.

Chronic radiation injury to the sigmoid may also result in progressive ischemia leading to necrosis. Depending upon the site of the greatest injury, necrosis of the intestinal wall can have several effects. Injuries that occur above the peritoneal reflection can result in perforation. This diagnosis can be easily made in the patient who presents with fulminant peritonitis and free air under the diaphragm on chest radiograph. In retrospect, these patients often give a progressive history of chronic crampy abdominal pain and bowel irregularity. Occasionally, the perforation will present in a subacute fashion, having been walled off with subsequent abscess formation.

These patients may present with fevers, a pelvic mass, and pelvic pain. At times, it can be difficult to differentiate this disorder from recurrent cancer or pelvic inflammatory disease. When intestinal necrosis is a consideration, prompt surgical intervention is indicated because the patient with sigmoid perforation will soon develop sepsis.

When necrosis of the sigmoid colon occurs below the peritoneal reflection, patients may develop a rectovaginal fistula. Patients will present with flatus or stool per vagina. Whether the necrosis began primarily in the vagina or rectum is of academic interest only. Fistulas occur because of recurrent tumor as often as they result from radiation injury. Patients should undergo careful examination with indicated biopsies to exclude the possibility of recurrent disease. When caused by radiation, these injuries rarely heal primarily and are difficult to repair. Initial management should include fecal diversion and observation. If there is no evidence of recurrent disease and the area of necrosis does not spread, selected patients may undergo a resection of the involved area with a low reanastomosis of the sigmoid to the anus. Because of the anastomosis in the radiated field, these patients need to maintain their diverting colostomy after surgery. Should the repair be successful, subsequent reversal of the colostomy can be performed. Even in the best of hands, the failure rate is high, and many patients also suffer from fecal incontinence.

Surgical management of sigmoid perforation can be especially difficult in the irradiated patient. It is usually not possible to re-establish intestinal continuity. The necrotic segment should be resected and fecal diversion carried out. Simply performing a loop colostomy and placing a drain will often result in repeated abscess formation. As a result of the intense local fibrosis and ischemia to the surrounding tissues that accompanies these injuries, reanastomosis at a later date is usually not possible. Whereas mortality from sigmoid perforation has been estimated to be as high as 50%, most patients now survive this serious injury with the help of aggressive broad-spectrum antibiotics and intensive care units.

Small Bowel. The acute reaction of the small intestine to radiation therapy is often manifested as diarrhea and abdominal cramping, sometimes associated with nausea and vomiting. These symptoms may arise within 1 to 2 weeks after the initiation of EBRT, and are especially common when the patient is treated with extended-field radiation. Fortunately, this is often a short-lived side effect that promptly disappears with the cessation of irradiation. As with rectosigmoid injury, however, chronic injury can take years to develop. The section of small bowel most prone to injury is the terminal ileum, although other small bowel segments can be involved, especially in patients with prior abdominal surgery. Patients who receive extended-field EBRT are at particular risk for small bowel complications.

Patients with chronic small bowel injury secondary to radiation have a progressive symptom complex that often begins with intermittent distention, nausea, weight loss, and diarrhea. The diarrhea is due to rapid transit and malabsorption. Crampy abdominal pain is often a prominent feature. It is not uncommon for the severity of these symptoms to wax and wane over a period of months to years. Rarely, patients with more severe injuries can progress to focal stricture, obstruction, and, in severe cases, perforation.

The diagnosis of small bowel injury can be confirmed by radiologic studies. The small bowel series has a characteristic appearance, including tethering and narrowing of the bowel lumen (Fig. 56–14). Patients who present with acute exacerbations will often have multiple air-fluid levels or dilated intestinal loops on plain abdominal films. Initial management of these patients should include bowel rest with nasogastric tube decompression, gentle hydration, and close observation. The decision to operatively intervene is often difficult. The surgeon who is experienced with the management of irradiated small bowel recognizes the fact that the surgery is technically difficult and often results in other complications such as inadvertent enterotomy, shortening of an already compromised intestine, and prolonged

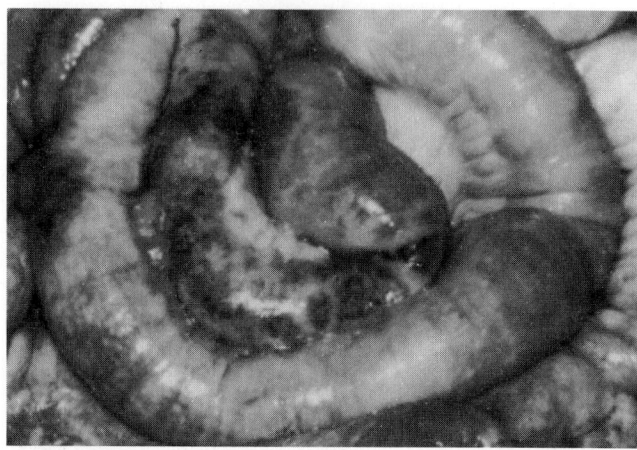

Figure 56–15
Intraoperative photograph of small intestine with diffuse radiation injury manifested by thickening of the intestinal wall, ischemia, and necrosis.

hospitalization, often with serious morbidity. Alternatively, the consequences of prolonged injury in a patient with a complete obstruction are perforation and death.

Patients who have mild to moderate symptoms can often be managed expectantly with a low-residue diet and careful observation. Patients with more severe symptoms, especially repeated episodes of partial obstruction, deserve surgical intervention (Smith et al, 1985). During the procedure, the surgeon may identify areas of injury to the small bowel, with extreme fibrosis and ischemia readily apparent (Fig. 56–15). Care should be taken to identify the narrowed or damaged segment, and resection should be performed. Every attempt should be made to preserve as much length of intestine as possible. Bypass procedures, the operative procedure of choice in the past, should be performed only when resection is not technically feasible. When an anastomosis is performed, it has been the routine at M. D. Anderson Cancer Center to withhold enteral feeding for a minimum of 2 weeks after surgery, allowing the anastomosis and irradiated field adequate time to heal. During this interval, patients are supported with total parenteral nutrition (TPN). Patients who present with preoperative evidence of nutritional depletion may benefit from 1 to 2 weeks of TPN prior to surgery if they are stable and the surgery is elective. Following surgery, patients often require a prolonged recovery period. Nutritional support is important, with patients being slowly weaned from TPN and placed on a low-residue diet. It is not uncommon for tube feedings to be necessary in these individuals, who will often have absorptive impairment of the remaining bowel.

Genitourinary. During EBRT to the pelvis, patients will sometimes note urinary frequency. In most, this is a short-lived side effect of treatment and rapidly resolves upon completion of therapy. A small percentage of patients, however, may develop chronic

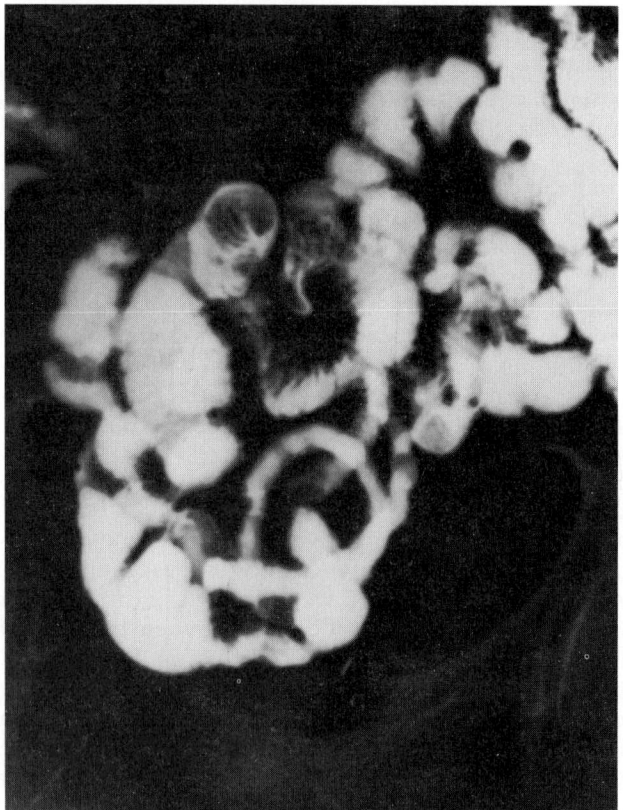

Figure 56–14
Small-bowel roentgenographic series view indicative of severe injury to the small intestine evidenced by numerous areas of narrowing and tethering.

problems: a contracted fibrotic bladder leading to frequent urination and, in some cases, incontinence. Hemorrhagic cystitis may also be present in some women. This may be an incidental microscopic finding, although occasional severe exacerbations with gross hematuria may occur. When the bleeding is significant enough to cause clot formation in the bladder, emergency intervention is indicated (McGuire et al, 1974; van Nagell et al, 1974).

Treatment of hemorrhagic cystitis from radiation therapy is challenging. Cystoscopy with clot evacuation should be carried out. If the bladder can be appropriately visualized, recurrent disease or other lesions should be searched for, with appropriate biopsies taken. Commonly, the surgeon will see an edematous bladder with prominent, friable bleeding vessels. Following clot evacuation, patients may benefit from continuous inpatient irrigation of the bladder using a three-way Foley catheter. A variety of solutions have been proposed for the irrigant; those most commonly used include one-quarter strength acetic acid and potassium permanganate (1:10,000), both of which act as mild oxidizing agents to stop bleeding. Some physicians suggest that simple saline irrigation may be just as effective. Extreme care should be taken to prevent blood clots from obstructing the outflow tract of the catheter during irrigation; continued influx of fluid in this circumstance may lead to bladder perforation. When the urine has cleared, the irrigation may be discontinued.

Those patients with hemorrhagic cystitis who do not respond to irrigation may be treated by a variety of techniques, all of which have varied success. Occasionally, electrocoagulation of bleeding vessels under cystoscopic visualization can be helpful. Tamponade of the bladder using the Helmstein balloon technique is also effective in experienced hands (Schiff and McGuire, 1980). As a last resort, formalin instillation of the bladder can be performed (Behnam et al, 1980). Although formalin instillation often stops the bleeding, the resultant scarred and contracted bladder is frequently nonfunctional. Patients who have persistent bleeding may require cystectomy with urinary diversion.

More severe cases of bladder injury caused by radiation can result in focal necrosis. Depending upon the site of necrosis, this may result in perforation of the bladder and subsequent peritonitis. Most often, necrosis occurs at the interface between the bladder and the vaginal vault, resulting in the formation of a vesicovaginal fistula. As with rectovaginal fistulas, these defects may be very difficult to repair. Initial treatment should include Foley catheter drainage and local care to the perineum to prevent skin breakdown. Indicated biopsies should be performed to eliminate the possibility of recurrent disease. Unfortunately, most cases of radiation-induced vesicovaginal fistulas do not heal spontaneously. Surgical repair can be performed by placing a flap of healthy tissue into the area. In many patients, especially those with larger fistulas, repair cannot be effected,

and urinary diversion by operative means is required.

Ureteral obstruction most often suggests recurrent cervical cancer. In some cases, however, the obstruction is due to radiation fibrosis. The latter is a diagnosis of exclusion; the patient should be evaluated with appropriate diagnostic studies and biopsies to dismiss the possibility of recurrent tumor. Initial management of ureteral obstruction from radiation fibrosis depends upon the function remaining in the occluded renal unit. In women with a longstanding obstruction, salvage of significant function is not likely. Relief of a recent occlusion of 3 months or less may allow the affected kidney to have nearly complete recovery. A nuclear renal scan may be helpful in determining the relative function of the obstructed side.

Initial management of ureteral obstruction involves insertion of a ureteral catheter via cystoscopy. Not surprisingly, this is often unsuccessful, and percutaneous nephrostomy must then be performed. Occasionally, antegrade insertion of a ureteral catheter may be successful. Although such catheters may be left in place for months at a time, problems such as repeated infection and obstruction make definitive repair desirable. At best difficult and often impossible, ureteral repair in the irradiated patient should be attempted only by surgeons who have experience with this challenging situation.

Local Complications. It is expected that patients who undergo a combination of EBRT and brachytherapy will have very high-dose radiation delivery to the superficial vaginal and cervical tissues. It is not uncommon to see some necrosis of these tissues in the weeks following completion of treatment. It may be difficult to differentiate necrosis from recurrent tumor, and numerous biopsies are often performed. Treatment of cervicovaginal necrosis should be conservative. The surgeon who performs aggressive débridements is often left with gaping, uncorrectable defects. The regimen at M. D. Anderson Cancer Center involves cleansing with a solution of 50% peroxide and 50% water two to three times daily. When the defect is in the lower vagina or vulva, this can be accomplished by means of a gentle hand-held spray. When the necrosis is in the upper portion of the vaginal vault or on the cervix, these solutions can be used as a douche. A vigorous examination should be avoided in these patients because it is not uncommon for necrotic areas to develop into either rectovaginal, vesicovaginal, or complex fistulas. Some believe that the addition of estrogen replacement therapy can assist the healing process.

The long-term sequelae of these local changes can have a dramatic impact on the condition of the vagina and surrounding tissues. Patients who are treated with high doses of radiation will frequently have vaginal stenosis, dryness, and shortening of the vaginal vault. These defects can be treated with both systemic and local application of estrogen and the regular use of a vaginal dilator to maintain patency of the canal. The pelvic tissue may develop progressive fibrosis and "woody" induration, particularly in women treated with high doses of EBRT for large lesions, making the interpretation of findings on pelvic examination challenging.

Post-Treatment Surveillance

Seventy-five per cent of cervical cancer recurrences occur within 2 years of therapy. By the end of 5 years, 95% of patients with recurrent disease will have relapsed (Jampolis et al, 1975; van Nagell et al, 1979). In a retrospective study of 1096 women who were treated for stage IB cervical cancer, Bodurka et al (in press) found that early detection of asymptomatic recurrences significantly increased both overall survival and survival from time of initial detection of recurrence. A surveillance program based upon time of asymptomatic recurrence was developed. The surveillance schedule is as follows: pelvic and physical examinations three times a year for the first 2 years post-treatment, then every 6 months for the remaining 3 years; chest radiographs taken twice yearly in year 2 through 4; yearly Pap smears to detect preinvasive disease.

Management of Recurrent Cervical Cancer

The great majority of patients with recurrent disease are incurable. Recurrent cervical cancer may occur in one of three sites. Most commonly, it occurs in the pelvis on the sidewall, presumably in lymph node–bearing areas. Recurrence may also be seen in distant sites, such as para-aortic or other distal lymph node metastasis, lung metastasis, or bony metastasis, most commonly to the vertebral bodies. A few patients will have a central pelvic recurrence. One of the important reasons for careful follow-up after treatment is to identify this last subgroup of patients, because they are candidates for curative therapy through radical surgery.

Treatment of recurrent disease is based on the type of primary therapy delivered. For patients with pelvic recurrence after radical hysterectomy, radiation therapy should be the initial intervention. For central recurrence, radiation may be delivered through a whole-pelvic field and an implant, either needles or a vaginal dome cylinder, if possible. Implants may be delivered through the vaginal route, although exploratory surgery with radioactive gold grain implants or intraoperative radiation are further possibilities. For the patient who has already received pelvic radiation, additional radiation therapy is usually not possible. In some cases, however, when a long interval has passed since primary therapy, re-irradiation of the pelvis can be performed. For disease outside of the pelvis, radiation plays a palliative role in controlling the size and spread of metastatic deposits.

If a patient has a very small cervical recurrence after primary therapy with radiation, radical hysterectomy has been used as a less radical alternative to pelvic exenteration (Rubin et al, 1987). Patients must be carefully selected for this approach because the potential for complications is high. Because the normal pelvic tissues have been irradiated, healing after surgery is impaired. Dissection through tissue planes, especially when mobilizing the ureters, is often difficult and occasionally impossible. Most patients with a central recurrence of cervical cancer following radiation therapy should be considered for pelvic exenteration.

Pelvic Exenteration

Pelvic exenteration is a very radical procedure that involves removal of the pelvic reproductive organs, including the uterus, tubes, ovaries, and vagina; the bladder and distal ureters; the rectum and anus; and the pelvic floor, including the pelvic peritoneum and levator muscles and usually the pelvic lymph nodes as well. Occasionally, a more limited procedure may be performed. In some cases, an anterior exenteration can be used to preserve the rectum and anus or a posterior exenteration can be used to preserve the bladder and ureters. Developed in 1940 by Dr. Alexander Brunschwig at the Memorial Hospital of New York, this surgical procedure was initially envisioned as a palliative measure for women with large ulcerating necrotic lesions. The initial experience with pelvic exenteration had a very high mortality rate, and its palliative effects were questionable. More recently, a number of other investigators made several technical advances and refined patient selection until today, when pelvic exenteration has its current role as a curative operation for women with recurrent pelvic carcinomas (Bricker, 1950, Brunschwig, 1970; Symmonds et al, 1975; Rutledge et al, 1977).

INDICATIONS

There are four specific indications for pelvic exenteration: treatment of primary disease, treatment of recurrent disease, palliation, and management of complications. Each is considered separately.

Certain patients with primary cervical carcinoma may be best treated with pelvic exenteration: for example, a patient with a stage IVA lesion with a large rectovaginal or vesicovaginal fistula that would be unlikely to heal after radiation. In most cases, these patients should also receive primary radiation therapy, usually before pelvic exenteration. Management of complications is another indication for pelvic exenteration in the patient who has received high doses of pelvic radiation. In some cases, extensive pelvic necrosis may result, with vesicovaginal or rectovaginal fistula formation that is not amenable to conservative therapy. Pelvic exenteration may allow these individuals to regain a normal lifestyle. Palliative management would be an unusual indication for pelvic exenteration (Stanhope and Symmonds, 1985). Occasionally, a patient with severe symptoms from a slow-growing, large necrotic lesion may benefit from palliative exenteration. However, the significant morbidity and lengthy recuperative period following such surgery make it difficult to justify in a patient with a relatively short time to live.

The most common and well-accepted indication for pelvic exenteration is a central pelvic recurrence. If no metastatic disease is present, patients with recurrence are potentially curable with radical surgery. Advances in patient selection have led to greater patient acceptance of the procedure and improved cure rates, with lower morbidity and mortality.

Several tumor-associated factors must be satisfied before deciding on pelvic exenteration. The tumor must be localized to the center of the pelvis and not extend to the pelvic sidewall. No distant metastasis should be present. Because unfavorable histologic subtypes such as clear cell carcinoma or small cell carcinoma are unlikely to be cured by exenterative procedures, much thought should be given before performing the procedure in these cases. The presence of lymph node metastasis is a relative contraindication to the procedure. Some surgeons will still perform exenteration when one or two pelvic lymph nodes contain metastatic deposits (Rutledge and McGuffee, 1987); however, when three or more positive pelvic nodes are encountered or para-aortic nodes are positive for metastatic spread, pelvic exenteration should not be performed.

Patient-associated limitations to pelvic exenteration include severe medical illnesses such as end-stage renal, cardiac, or pulmonary disease. Patients who cannot be medically stabilized prior to surgery should not undergo this radical procedure. Age had been thought to be a contraindication, although several investigators have shown that patients with advanced-stage disease can tolerate exenteration very well (Matthews et al, 1992).

PROCEDURE

The operative procedure itself can be broken down into three phases: the operative evaluation, surgical extirpation, and reconstruction.

During the operative evaluation, a vertical midline incision is made with a thorough exploration of the abdominopelvic cavity. Washings are taken to rule out the presence of peritoneal metastases. The liver, spleen, and other abdominal organs are carefully palpated and inspected. Any suspicious areas should be biopsied. Should gross peritoneal disease be discovered or found on positive washings, the procedure should be abandoned. The para-aortic lymph nodes are selectively sampled and pelvic lymph nodes, if not previously removed, should be excised. The paravesicle and pararectal spaces should be opened, and the surgeon should ensure that there is adequate clearance of the tumor from the pelvic si-

dewall. Should any of these operative criteria not be fulfilled, the exenteration should be stopped. It is estimated that approximately 20% to 30% of exploratory laparotomies performed in expectation of exenteration are abandoned because of adverse factors not detected preoperatively.

Surgical extirpation is then carried out with en block removal of the organs described above. Careful anesthesia and blood bank support should be available because significant blood loss often occurs at this point. Surgery is most commonly performed with two teams, one working through the abdominal incision and the other working to excise the surgical specimen through the perineum.

By far the most challenging and interesting portion of the procedure is the reconstructive phase. It is in this area that some of the greatest advances have been made.

In 1950, Bricker first described the urinary conduit (Fig. 56–16). Prior to that, urinary diversion was obtained by implanting the ureters into an active segment of colon or by wet ureterostomy to the skin. Both of these techniques proved unsatisfactory. Use of the ileal conduit or Bricker pouch was a great improvement for many years (Orr et al, 1982; Hancock et al, 1986). Later nonileum intestinal segments were used to avoid an intestinal anastomosis (Fig. 56–17), including sigmoid colon (Mogg, 1967; Gonzales et al, 1977) and transverse colon (Schmidt et al, 1975; Orr et al, 1982; Beddoe et al, 1987).

Some of the greatest advances in urinary diversion have occurred with the advent of both the Kock and Indiana pouches (Kock, 1969; Koch et al, 1978; Rowland et al, 1987). These allow the patient to maintain

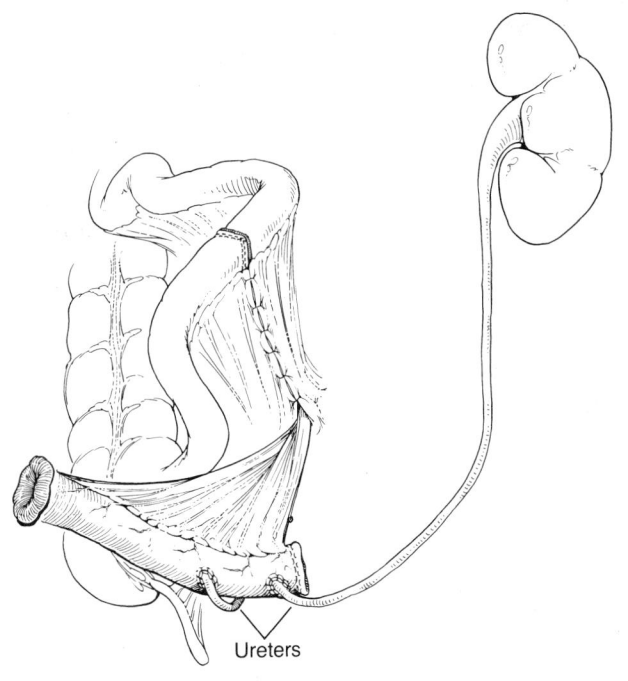

Figure 56–16
Ileal conduit.

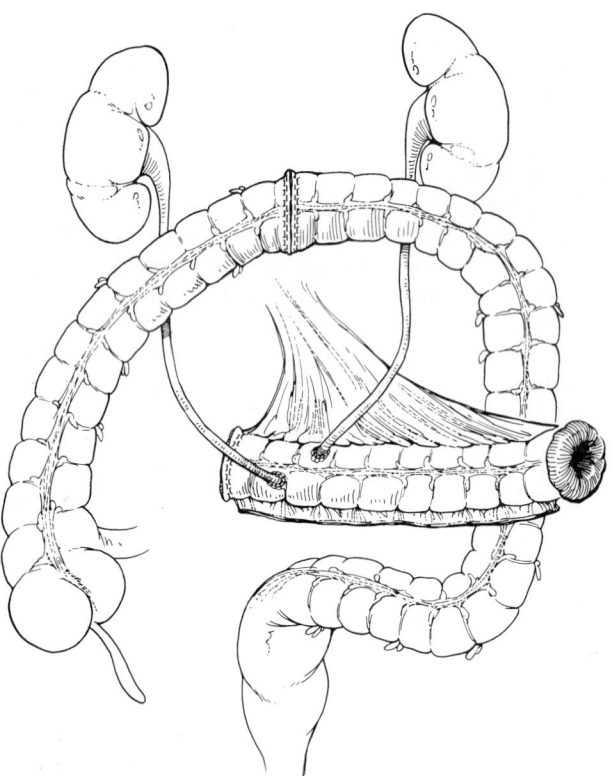

Figure 56–17
Transverse colon conduit.

continence without wearing an appliance, having to use only a catheter to catheterize a small nipple at a time that is socially convenient. The Indiana pouch has been successfully used in patients with gynecologic cancer who have had previous radiation therapy (Penalver et al, 1989).

Another great advance in the reconstructive phase has been the use of stapling instruments and the low rectal anastomosis (Hatch et al, 1990). These have allowed removal of the sigmoid colon with preservation of the anus and anastomosis of the descending colon or even the terminal ileum to a rectal stump. Unfortunately, some patients are incontinent after this procedure and require a diverting colostomy or ileostomy.

Management of the pelvic cavity and vaginal reconstruction presented a major problem to surgeons. Initially, the large raw pelvic cavity left at the conclusion of the procedure was packed with a gauze roll with the end protruding through a perineal defect (Brunschwig, 1940). This was then removed several days postoperatively. The use of the gauze pack proved to be unsatisfactory, with a high incidence of fistula formation and infection. To exclude the small bowel from this raw pelvic cavity, a number of other approaches were then used, including mesenteric slings or artificial substances such as Marlex mesh. These also proved unsatisfactory in most cases. Rutledge and Burns (1965) used the omental flap or carpet to suspend the small bowel out of the pelvis. This procedure was carried out by mobilizing the

omentum from its attachment to the transverse colon and from its short omental branches from the greater curvature of the stomach and right gastroepiploic artery. With the blood supply coming exclusively from the left gastroepiploic artery, the omentum then has sufficient length to be placed along the left gutter to the pelvis to fill the dead space and serve as a sling.

Another important method of pelvic cavity management is the use of myocutaneous flap for vaginal reconstruction (McCraw et al, 1976; Copeland et al, 1989). This serves two purposes. In addition to pelvic cavity management, it also provides the opportunity for preservation of sexual function. Using a graft from the gracilis muscle on the anteromedial portion of each thigh, a vaginal canal lined by skin and supported by subcutaneous fat and muscle can be created. This allows sexual function postoperatively because, in most patients who undergo pelvic exenteration, the labia and clitoris are preserved.

Initial experience with pelvic exenteration reported a high incidence of morbidity and mortality, with a postoperative death rate in the range of 13% (Brunschwig, 1950; Symmonds et al, 1975; Rutledge et al, 1977; Averette et al, 1984). Several advances have lowered this figure, until more recently the death rate reported at M. D. Anderson Cancer Center is 4% or less (Rutledge, 1987). This improvement may be attributed to several factors, including the liberal use of TPN in the postoperative setting, modern antibiotics used prophylactically as well as for treatment of the frequent infectious complications that may occur, and intensive care unit monitoring in the majority of patients in the postoperative setting.

RESULTS

Results of pelvic exenteration can be very satisfactory. Acute complications are those associated with radical surgery, including cardiac decompensation, pulmonary embolism, deep vein thrombosis, and hemorrhage. The average blood loss is between 1 and 2 liters; most patients require blood transfusion. Infectious morbidity, including necrosis of the myocutaneous graft with secondary infection, pyelonephritis, or sepsis, is not uncommon. Complications involving the urinary conduit include obstruction at the ureteral conduit junction, fistula formation, and anastomotic leak. Long-term complications often involve the urinary diversion, with recurring bouts of pyelonephritis noted to be a common feature.

Psychosocial adjustments must also be considered after this surgery. Extensive preoperative and postoperative counseling by both the physician and the support staff can help. The enterostomal therapist plays an important role in preoperative counseling and postoperative teaching, as well as in helping the patient adjust to any appliance that she may require. With the appropriate assistance, most women can resume an essentially normal lifestyle following pelvic exenteration.

The bottom line is survival. Following pelvic exenteration for a recurrent carcinoma of the cervix, 5-year survival, including death from all causes, is 44% (Rutledge, 1987).

Chemotherapy for Recurrent Cervical Cancer

Chemotherapy for recurrent cervical carcinoma should be regarded as a palliative treatment. The opportunity for cure is very small, and the best regimens do not have complete response rates in excess of 10%.

The most active agent in the treatment of recurrent cervical cancer appears to be cisplatin (Thigpen et al, 1981; Bonomi et al, 1985). Used as a single agent, expected response rate is approximately 30%. Other active agents are shown in Table 56–9.

Combination chemotherapy may provide additional chance for response when compared to cisplatin used alone. The use of cisplatin in combination with other agents has provided response rates that range from 30% to 50% (Belinson et al, 1984; Carlson et al, 1984; Jobson et al, 1984; Wheelock et al, 1985; Alberts and Mason, 1989; Bonomi et al, 1989). However, responses tend to be short lived, with median survival in the range of 7 to 10 months. Given this short survival time and the serious toxicity from many forms of chemotherapy, one might legitimately question the benefits of chemotherapy in most patients with recurrent cervical cancer. Response rates to chemotherapy in women who have untreated cervical cancer are significantly higher (Belinson et al, 1984). Once a patient has been pretreated with radiation therapy, however, the results are poor. This may be due to the poor blood supply to the pelvic tumor following radiation, selection of more aggressive tumors that have not been cured with radiation,

and the inherent resistance of squamous carcinoma to radiation therapy.

Palliative Therapy

Perhaps one of the most important roles of a physician for a patient with a recurred cervical cancer is delivering proper palliative treatment. The management of pelvic pain, renal failure, and infection are important aspects of the total care of the patient.

Advanced cervical cancer often results in severe pelvic pain. A lesion on the pelvic sidewall may involve the sacral nerve roots or directly invade the bone. It is not uncommon for patients to have pain that radiates down the leg. Pain may also result from direct invasion of the adjacent pelvic structures, such as the bladder or rectum. Lymphatic and venous outflow obstruction from the leg may also lead to a painful lower extremity.

Pain management should be aggressive, with analgesics given on a regular schedule as opposed to only when pain is severe. We prefer to use a prolonged-release formulation of morphine for this purpose. Narcotic dosage should be escalated as needed. Often the addition of a nonsteroidal anti-inflammatory agent, such as ibuprofen, will provide added benefit. When local pain is resistant to these measures, patients may be helped by the use of epidural analgesia or ambulatory patient-controlled analgesia.

Progressive cervical cancer may result in bilateral ureteral obstruction. The ureters may be blocked in their lower third by pelvic tumor or, less frequently, in the upper third by enlarged para-aortic nodes. In a patient who has not received radiation therapy, urinary diversion by percutaneous nephrostomy or ureteral stenting is indicated (Dudley et al, 1986; de Franca et al, 1987). In the patient with recurrent cancer after radiation, urinary diversion is controversial. With no effective second-line therapy, saving a patient from death by uremia only to have her suffer with progressive pelvic pain may not be helpful. Our approach is to counsel the patient and her family on the severity of the problem and the natural history of cervical carcinoma so that she can make an informed decision regarding urinary diversion.

Table 56–9. RESPONSE RATES TO SINGLE-AGENT CHEMOTHERAPY IN THE TREATMENT OF CERVICAL CARCINOMA

DRUG	RESPONSE RATE
Antimetabolites	
5-Fluorouracil	23%
Methotrexate	20%
Alkylating Agents	
Cyclophosphamide	16%
Melphalan	
	20%
Antibiotics	
Doxorubicin	16%
Mitomycin-C	22%
Bleomycin	10%
Cisplatin	17–38%
Carboplatin	15%

Adapted from DiSaia PJ, Creasman WT: Clinical Gynecologic Oncology. 3rd ed. St. Louis: Mosby, 1989, with permission.

ACKNOWLEDGMENTS

All microscopic pathology figures were provided courtesy of Elvio G. Silva, M.D.

REFERENCES

Abbe R: The use of radium in malignant disease. Lancet 1913;2: 524.
Alberts DS, Mason LN: The role of cisplatin in the management of advanced squamous cell cancer of the cervix. Semin Oncol 1989;18(1, Suppl 3):11.
Aurelian L: Possible role of herpes virus hominis, type 2, in human cervical cancer. Fed Proc 1972;31:1651.

Averette HE, Lichtinger M, Sevin R, Girtanner R: Pelvic exenteration: a 15-year exprience in a general metropolitan hospital. Am J Obstet Gynecol 1984;150:179.

Ballon S, Berman M, Lagasse L, et al: Survival after extraperitoneal pelvic and paraaortic lymphadenectomy and radiation therapy in cervical carcinoma. Obstet Gynecol 1981;57:90.

Barron BA, Richart RM: An epidemiologic study of cervical neoplastic disease. Cancer 1971;27:978.

Beahrs OH, Henson DE, Hutter RVP, Myers MH (eds): Manual for Staging of Cancer. 3rd ed. Philadelphia: JB Lippincott Company, 1988:151.

Beddoe AM, Boyce JG, Remy JC, et al: Stented versus nonstented transverse colon conduits: a comparative report. Gynecol Oncol 1987;27:305.

Behnam K, Patil UB, Mariano E: Intravesical instillation of formalin for hemorrhagic cystitis secondary to radiation for gynecologic malignancies. Gynecol Oncol 1980;16:31.

Belinson JL, Stewart JA, Richards AL, McClure M: Bleomycin, vincristine, mitomycin-c, and cisplatin in the management of gynecological squamous cell carcinomas. Gynecol Oncol 1984; 20:387.

Benedetti PP, Scambia G, Baiocchi G, et al: Circulating tumor markers in cervical cancer. Tumour Biol 1989;10:109.

Berman M, Keys H, Creasman W, et al: Survival and patterns of recurrence in cervical cancer metastatic to periaortic lymph nodes: Gynecologic Oncology Group study. Gynecol Oncol 1984;19:8.

Bodurka-Bevers DC, Morris M, Eifel PJ, et al: Post-therapy surveillance of women with cervical cancer: an outcomes analysis (in press).

Bokhman JV, Urmancheyeva AF: Cervix uteri cancer and pregnancy. Eur J Gynaecol Oncol 1989;10:406.

Bonomi P, Blessing J, Ball H, et al: A Phase II evaluation of cisplatin and 5-fluorouracil in patients with advanced squamous cell carcinoma of the cervix: a Gynecologic Oncology Group study. Gynecol Oncol 1989;34:357.

Bonomi P, Blessing JA, Stehman FB, et al: Randomized trial of three cisplatin dose schedules in squamous cell carcinoma of the cervix: a Gynecologic Oncology Group study. J Clin Oncol 1985;3:1079.

Bosch FX, Manos MM, Munoz N, et al: International Biological Study on Cervical Cancer (IBSCC) Study Group: Prevalence of human papillomavirus in cervical cancer: A worldwide perspective. J Natl Cancer Inst 1995;87:796.

Boyce J, Fruchter R, Nicastri A, et al: Prognostic factors in stage I carcinoma of the cervix. Gynecol Oncol 1981;12:154.

Brady L, Plenk H, Hanley J, et al: Hyperbaric oxygen therapy for carcinoma of the cervix stages IIB, IIIA, IIIB, and IVA: results of a randomized study by the Radiation Therapy Oncology Group. Int J Radiat Oncol Biol Phys 1981;7:990.

Bricker EM: Symposium on clinical surgery: bladder substitution after pelvic eviseeration. Surg Clin North Am 1950;30:1511.

Brookland R, Rubin S, Danoff B: Extended field irradiation in the treatment of patients with cervical carcinoma involving biopsy proven para-aortic nodes. Int J Radiat Oncol Biol Phys 1984;10:1875.

Brunschwig A: A complete excision of the pelvic viscera for advanced carcinoma. Cancer 1940;1:177.

Brunschwig A: Some reflections on pelvic exenterations after twenty years experience. Prog Gynecol 1970;5:416.

Buckley CH, Beards CS, Fox H: Pathological prognostic indicators in cervical cancer with particular reference to patients under the age of 40 years. Br J Obstet Gynaecol 1988;95:47.

Burghardt E, Hofmann HM, Ebner F, et al: Magnetic resonance imaging in cervical cancer: a basis for objective classification. Gynecol Oncol 1989;33:61.

Burke T, Hoskins W, Heller P, et al: Prognostic factors associated with radical hysterectomy failure. Gynecol Oncol 1987;26:153.

Cabral GA, Fry D, Marciano-Cabral F, et al: A herpes virus antigen in human premalignant and malignant cervical biopsies explants. Am J Obstet Gynecol 1983;145:79.

Carlson JA, Day TG, Allegra JC, et al: Methyl-CCNU, doxorubicin, and cis-diaminedichloroplatinum II in the management of recurrent and metastatic squamous carcinoma of the cervix. Cancer 1984;54:211.

Chen TMM, Chen CA, Hsieh CY, et al: The state of p53 in primary human cervical carcinomas and its effects in human papilloma virus-immortalized human cervical cells. Oncogene 1993;8:1511.

Clarke EA, Hatcher J, McKeown-Eyssen GE, et al: Cervical dysplasia: association with sexual behavior, smoking and oral contraceptive use? Am J Obstet Gynecol 1985;151:612.

Coleman RL, Burke TW, Morris M, et al: Intraoperative radiographs to confirm the adequacy of lymph node resection in patients with suspicious lymphangiograms. Gynecol Oncol 1993;51:362.

Copeland LJ, Hancock KC, Gershenson EC, et al: Gracilis myocutaneous vaginal reconstruction concurrent with total pelvic exenteration. Am J Obstet Gynecol 1989;160:1095.

Creasman WT: New gynecologic cancer staging. Gynecol Oncol 1995;58:157.

Crum CP, Ikenberg H, Richart RM, et al: Human papillomavirus type 16 and early cervical neoplasia. N Engl J Med 1984;310:880.

de Franca MA, Graubard Z, Ballot DE: Percutaneous nephrostomy for bilateral ureteric obstruction in carcinoma of the cervix: a case report. S Afr Med J 1987;71:661.

Dudley BS, Gershenson DM, Kavanagh JJ, et al: Percutaneous nephrostomy catheter use in gynecologic malignancy: M. D. Anderson Hospital experience. Gynecol Oncol 1986;24:273.

Durrance F, Fletcher G, Rutledge F: Analysis of central recurrent disease in stages I and II squamous cell carcinomas of the cervix on intact uterus. Am J Roentgenol 1969;106:831.

Durst M, Gissmann L, Ikenberg H, et al: A papillomavirus DNA from a cervical carcinoma and its prevalence in cancer biopsy samples from different geographic regions. Proc Natl Acad Sci U S A 1983;80:3812.

Dusenbery KE, Carson LF, Potish RA: Perioperative morbidity and mortality of gynecologic brachytherapy. Cancer 1991;67:2786.

Dyson N, Howley PM, Munger K, et al: The human papilloma virus-16 E7 oncoprotein is able to bind to the retinoblastoma gene product. Science 1989;243:934.

Edelman DA: Diethylstilbestrol exposure and the risk of clear cell cervical and vaginal adenocarcinoma. Int J Fertil 1989;34:251.

Eifel P: High-dose-rate brachytherapy for carcinoma of the cervix: high tech or high risk? Int J Radiat Oncol Biol Phys 1992;24:383.

Eifel PJ, Burke TW, Morris M, Smith, TL: Adenocarcinoma as an independent risk factor for disease recurrence in patients with stage IB cervical carcinoma. Gynecol Oncol 1995;59:38.

Eifel P, Morris M, Oswald M, et al: Adenocarcinoma of the uterine cervix: prognosis and patterns of failure of 367 cases treated at the M.D. Anderson Cancer Center between 1965 and 1985. Cancer 1990;65:2507.

Fletcher G, Lindberg R, Caderao J, Warton J: Hyperbaric oxygen as a radiotherapeutic adjuvant in advanced cancer of the uterine cervix. Cancer 1977;39:617.

Gallup DG, Harper RH, Stock RJ: Poor prognosis in patients with adenosquamous cell carcinoma of the cervix. Obstet Gynecol 1985;65:416.

Gauthier P, Gore I, Shingleton HM, et al: Identification of histopathologic risk groups in stage IB squamous cell carcinoma of the cervix. Obstet Gynecol 1985;66:569.

Goldhirsch A, Greiner R, Bleher E, et al: Combination of chemotherapy with methotrexate, bleomycin, and cis-platinum, and radiation therapy for locally advanced carcinoma of the cervix. Am J Clin Oncol 1986;9:12.

Gonzales ET Jr, Baum NH, Friedman A, Carlton CE: Sigmoid conduit: review and description of technique. Urology 1977;10:579.

Griffenberg L, Morris M, Atkinson EN, Levenback CL: The effect of dietary fiber on bowel function following radical hysterectomy: a randomized trial. Gynecol Oncol 1997;66:417.

Guijon FB, Paraskevas M, Brunham R: The association of sexually transmitted diseases with cervical intraepithelial neoplasia: a case control study. Am J Obstet Gynecol 1985;151:185.

Haas J, Friedl H: Prognostic factors in cervical carcinoma: a multivariate approach, Baillieres Clin Obstet Gynaecol 1988;2:829.

Hacker NF, Berek JS, Lagasse LD, et al: Carcinoma of the cervix associated with pregnancy. Obstet Gynecol 1982;59:735.

Hancock KC, Copeland LJ, Gershenson DM, et al: Urinary conduits in gynecologic oncology. Obstet Gynecol 1986;67:680.

Hannigan EV: Cervical cancer in pregnancy. Clin Obstet Gynecol 1990;33:837.

Hasumi K, Sakamoto A, Sugano H: Microinvasive carcinoma of the cervix. Cancer 1980;45:928.

Hatch KD, Gelder MS, Soong SJ, et al: Pelvic exenteration with low rectal anastomosis: survival, complications, and prognostic factors. Gynecol Oncol 1990;38:462.

Heller P, Malfetano J, Bundy B, et al: Clinical-pathologic study of stage IIB, III, and IVA carcinoma of the cervix: extended diagnostic evaluation for paraaortic node metastasis—A Gynecologic Oncology Group study. Gynecol Oncol 1990;38:425.

Ho CM, Chien TY, Jeng CM, et al: Staging of cervical cancer: comparison between magnetic resonance imaging, computed tomography and pelvic examination under anesthesia. J Formosan Med Assoc 1992;91:982.

Hofmann HM, Ebner F, Haas J, et al: Magnetic resonance imaging in clinical cervical cancer: pretherapeutic tumour volumetry. Baillieres Clin Obstet Gynaecol 1988;2:789.

Hogan W, Littman P, Griner L, et al: Results of radiation therapy given after radical hysterectomy. Cancer 1982;49:1278.

Holzer E: Microinvasive carcinoma of the cervic—clinical aspects, treatment and follow-up. Clin Oncol 1982;1:315.

Horiot J, Pigneux J, Pourquier H, et al: Radiotherapy alone in carcinoma of the intact uterine cervix according to G. H. Fletcher guidelines: a French cooperative study of 1383 cases. Int J Radiat Oncol Biol Phys 1988;14:605.

Houdek PV, Schwade JG, Abitbol AA, et al: Optimization of high dose-rate cervix brachytherapy. I. Dose distribution. Int J Radiat Oncol Biol Phys 1991;21:1621.

Inoue T, Okumura M: Prognostic significance of parametrial extension in patients with cervical carcinoma stages IB, IIA, and IIB: a study of 628 cases treated by radical hysterectomy and lymphadenectomy with or without postoperative irradiation. Cancer 1984;54:1714.

International Commission on Radiological Units and Measurements: (ICRU): Dose and Volume Specification for Reporting Intracavitary Therapy in Gynecology (ICRU Report 38). Bethesda, MD: ICRU, 1985.

Jampolis S, Andras J, Fletcher G: Analysis of sites and causes of failures of irradiation in invasive squamous cell carcinoma of the intact uterine cervix. Radiology 1975;15:681.

Jobson VW, Muss HB, Thigpen JT, et al: Chemotherapy of advanced squamous carcinoma of the cervix: a Phase I–II study of high-dose cisplatin and cyclophosphamide. Am J Clin Oncol 1984;7:341.

Jones WH, Droegemueller W, Makowski E: A primary melanocarcinoma of the cervix. Obstet Gynecol 1971;111:959.

Kadar N, Saliba N, Nelson JH: The frequency, causes, and prevention of severe urinary dysfunction after radical hysterectomy. Br J Obstet Gynaecol 1983;90:858.

Kavanagh JJ, Delclos L, Wallace S: Arterial chemotherapy prior to radiotherapy in advanced gynecologic cancer. In Rutledge FN (ed): Gynecologic Cancer: Diagnosis and Treatment Strategies. Austin: University of Texas Press, 1989:293.

Keys H, Bundy B, Stehman F, et al: Adjuvant hysterectomy after radiation therapy reduces detection of local recurrence in "bulky" stage IB cervical cancer without improving survival: results of a prospective randomized GOG trial. In: Abstracts of the 1997 American Radium Society Annual Meeting, April 30–May 4, 1997.

Keys HM, Bundy BN, Stehman FB, et al: Cisplatin, radiation, and adjuvant hysterectomy compared with radiation and adjuvant hysterectomy for bulky stage IB cervical carcinoma. N Engl J Med 1999;340:1154.

Kim R, Salter M, Shingleton H: Adjuvant postoperative radiation therapy following radical hysterectomy in stage IB cancer of the cervix: analysis of treatment failures. Int J Radiat Oncol Biol Phys 1988;14:445.

Kim SH, Choi BI, Han JK, et al: Preoperative staging of uterine cervical carcinoma: comparison of CT and MRI in 99 patients. J Comput Assist Tomogr 1993;17:633.

Kock N: Intra-abdominal "reservoir" in patients with permanent ileostomy. Arch Surg 1969;99:223.

Kock N, Nilson A, Norlen L, et al: Urinary diversion via a continent ileum reservoir. Scand J Urol Nephrol 1978;49(Suppl):23.

Kolstad P: Follow-up study of 232 patients with stage Ia1 and 411 patients with stage Ia2 squamous cell carcinoma of the cervix (microinvasive carcinoma). Gynecol Oncol 1989;33:265.

Komaki R, Mattingly R, Hoffman R, et al: Irradiation of paraaortic lymph node metastases from carcinoma of the cervix or endometrium: preliminary results. Radiology 1983;147:245.

Koutsky LA, Holmes KK, Critchlow CW, et al: A cohort study of the risk for cervical intraepithelial neoplasia grade 2 or 3 in relation to papillomavirus infection. N Engl J Med 1992;327:1272.

Lara P, Garcia-Puche J, Pedraza V: Cisplatin-ifosfamide as neoadjuvant chemotherapy in stage IIIB cervical-uterine squamous-cell carcinoma. Cancer Chemother Pharmacol 1990;26(Suppl):36.

Larson D, Stringer C, Copeland L, et al: Stage IB cervical carcinoma treated with radical hysterectomy and pelvic lymphadenectomy: role of adjuvant radiotherapy. Obstet Gynecol 1987;69:378.

Lee YN, Wang KL, Lin MH, et al: Radical hysterectomy with pelvic lymph node dissection for treatment of cervical cancer: a clinical review of 954 cases. Gynecol Oncol 1989;32:135.

Lorincz AT, Reid R, Jenson AB, et al: Human papillomavirus infection of the cervix: relative risk associations of 15 common anogenital types. Obstet Gynecol 1992;79:328.

Maitland NJ, Kinross JH, Busutti IA: The detection of DNA tumor virus-specific RNA sequences in abnormal human cervical biopsies by in situ hybridization. J Gen Virol 1981;55:123.

Maor M, Gillespie B, Peters L, et al: Neutron therapy in cervical cancer: results of a Phase III RTOG study. Int J Radiat Oncol Biol Phys 1988;14:885.

Matthews CM, Morris M, Burke TW, et al: Pelvic exenteration in the elderly patient. Obstet Gynecol 1992;79:1.

McCraw JB, Massey FM, Shamklin KD, et al: Vaginal reconstruction with gracilis myocutaneous flaps. Plast Reconstr Surg 1976;58:176.

McGuire EJ, Weiss RM, Schiff M, Lytton B: Hemorrhagic radiation cystitis: treatment. Urology 1974;3:204.

Meigs JV: Radical hysterectomy with bilateral pelvic node dissections: Report of 100 cases operated on 5 years or more. Am J Obstet Gynecol 1951;62:854.

Meisels A, Fortin R, Roy M: Condylomatous lesions of the cervix II: Cytologic, colposcopic, and histopathologic study. Acta Cytol (Baltimore) 1977;21:379.

Melendez TD, Childers JM: Laparoscopic lymphadenectomy. Curr Opin Obstet Gynecol 1995;7:307.

Mestwerdt G: Probeexision und Kolposkopie in des Fruhdiagnose des Portiokarzinoms. Zentralbl Gynakol 1947;4:326.

Miller BE, Copeland LJ, Hamberger AD, et al: Carcinoma of the cervical stump. Gynecol Oncol 1984;18:100.

Mogg R: Urinary diversion using the colonic conduit. Br J Urol 1967;39:687.

Morris M, Eifel PJ, Burke TW, et al: Treatment of locally advanced cervical cancer with concurrent radiation and intra-arterial chemotherapy. Gynecol Oncol 1995;57:72.

Morris M, Eifel PJ, Lu JD, et al: Pelvic radiation with chemotherapy compared with pelvic and para-aortic radiation for high-risk cervical cancer. N Engl J Med 1999;340:1137.

Morris M, Gershenson DM, Eifel P, et al: Treatment of small cell carcinoma of the cervix with cisplatin, doxorubicin, and etoposide. Gynecol Oncol 1992;47:62.

Morris M, Mitchell MF, Silva EG, et al: Cervical conization as definitive therapy for early invasive squamous carcinoma of the cervix. Gynecol Oncol 1993;51:193.

Morrow C: Is pelvic radiation beneficial in the postoperative management of stage Ib squamous cell carcinoma of the cervix with pelvic node metastases treated by radical hysterectomy and pelvic lymphadenectomy? Gynecol Oncol 1980;10:105.

Muss H, Jobson V, Homesley H, et al: Neoadjuvant therapy for advanced squamous cell carcinoma of the cervix: cisplatin followed by radiation therapy—a pilot study of the Gynecologic Oncology Group. Gynecol Oncol 1987;26:35.

Naib ZM, Nahmias AJ, Josey WE: Cytology and histopathology of cervical herpes simplex infection. Cancer 1966;19:1026.

Nezhat CR, Burrell MO, Nezhat FR, et al: Laparoscopic radical hysterectomy with para-aortic and pelvic node dissection. Am J Obstet Gynecol 1992;166:864.

Nori D, Valentine E, Hilaris B: The role of paraaortic node irradiation in the treatment of cancer of the cervix. Int J Radiat Oncol Biol Phys 1985;11:1469.

O'Quinn A, Fletcher G, Wharton J: Guidelines for conservative hysterectomy after irradiation. Gynecol Oncol 1980;9:68.

Orr JW, Shingleton HM, Hatch KD, et al: Urinary diversion in patients undergoing pelvic exenteration. Obstet Gynecol 1982; 142:883.

Orr JW Jr, Ball GC, Soong SJ, et al: Surgical treatment of women found to have invasive cervix cancer at the time of total hysterectomy. Obstet Gynecol 1986;68:353.

Park RC, Patow WE, Rogers RE, Zimmerman EA: Treatment of stage I carcinoma of the cervix. Obstet Gynecol 1973;41:117.

Parker SL, Tong T, Bolder S, Wingo PA: Cancer statistics, 1997. CA Cancer J Clin 1997;47:8.

Patsner B: Closed-suction drainage versus no drainage following radical abdominal hysterectomy with pelvic lymphadenectomy for stage IB cervical cancer. Gynecol Oncol 1995;57:232.

Penalver MA, Bejany DE, Averette HE, et al: Continent urinary diversion in gynecologic oncology. Gynecol Oncol 1989;343:274.

Perez C, Kao M: Radiation therapy alone or combined with surgery in the treatment of barrel-shaped carcinoma of the uterine cervix (stages IB, IIA, IIB). Int J Radiat Oncol Biol Phys 1985; 11:1903.

Peters RK, Thomas D, Hagan DG, et al: Risk factors for invasive cervical cancer among Latinas and non-Latinas in Los Angeles County. J Natl Cancer Inst 1986;77:1063.

Phelps WC, Bagchi S, Barnes JA, et al: Analysis of trans activation by human papillomavirus type 16 E7 and adenovirus 12S E1A suggests a common mechanism. J Virol 1991;65:6922.

Piver M, Barlow J, Krishnamsetty R: Five-year survival (with no evidence of disease) in patients with biopsy-confirmed aortic node metastases from cervical carcinoma. Am J Obstet Gynecol 1981;139:575.

Piver M, Chung W: Prognostic significance of cervical lesion size and pelvic node metastases in cervical carcinoma. Obstet Gynecol 1975;46:507.

Piver M, Khalil M, Emrich LJ: Hydroxyurea plus pelvic irradiation versus placebo plus pelvic irradiation in nonsurgically staged stage IIIB cervical cancer. J Surg Oncol 1989;42:120.

Piver MS, Rutledge FN, Smith JP: Five classes of extended hysterectomy for women with cervical cancer. Obstet Gynecol 1974;4:265.

Podczaski E, Stryker J, Kaminski P, et al: Extended-field radiation therapy for carcinoma of the cervix. Cancer 1990;66:251.

Potish RA, Twiggs LB, Prem KA, et al: The impact of extraperitoneal surgical staging on morbidity and tumor recurrence following radiotherapy for cervical carcinoma. Am J Clin Oncol 1984;7:245.

Powell MC, Worthington BS, Sokal M, et al: Magnetic resonance imaging—its application to cervical carcinoma. Br J Obstet Gynaecol 1986;93:1276.

Prem KA, Makowski EL, McKelvey JL: Carcinoma of the cervix associated with pregnancy. Am J Obstet Gynecol 1966;95:99.

Roman LD, Morris M, Eifel PJ, et al: Reasons for inappropriate simple hysterectomy in the presence of invasive cancer of the cervix. Obstet Gynecol 1992;79:485.

Rose PG, Bundy BN, Watkins EB, et al: Concurrent cisplatin-based radiotherapy and chemotherapy for locally advanced cervical cancer. N Engl J Med 1999;340:1144.

Rotman M, Choi K, Guze C, et al: Prophylactic irradiation of the para-aortic lymph node chain in stage IIb and bulky stage Ib carcinoma of the cervix, initial treatment results of RTOG 7920. Int J Radiat Oncol Biol Phys 1990;19:513.

Rowland R, Mitichell M, Bihrle R, et al: Indiana continent urinary reservoir. J Urol 1987;137:1136.

Roy M, Plante M, Renaud MC, Tetu B: Vaginal radical hysterectomy versus abdominal radical hysterectomy in the treatment of early-stage cervical cancer. Gynecol Oncol 1966;62:336.

Rubens D, Thornbury JR, Angel C, et al: Stage IB cervical carcinoma: comparison of clinical, MR, and pathologic staging. AJR Am J Roentgenol 1988;150:135.

Rubin SC, Hoskins WJ, Lewis JLJ: Radical hysterectomy for recurrent cervical cancer following radiation therapy. Gynecol Oncol 1987;27:316.

Runowicz CD, Wadler S, Rodriguez RL, et al: Concomitant cisplatin and radiotherapy in locally advanced cervical carcinoma. Gynecol Oncol 1989;34:395.

Rutledge FN: Pelvic exenteration: an update of the U.T. M.D. Anderson Hospital experience and review of the literature. In Rutledge FN (ed): Gynecologic Cancer: Diagnosis and Treatment Strategies. Austin: University of Texas Press, 1987:19.

Rutledge FN, Burns BC Jr: Pelvic exenteration. Am J Obstet Gynecol 1965;91:692.

Rutledge FN, McGuffee VB: Pelvic exenteration: prognostic significance of regional lymph node metastases. Gynecol Oncol 1987;26:374.

Rutledge FN, Smith JP, Wharton JT, O'Quinn AG: Pelvic exenteration: analysis of 296 patients. Am J Obstet Gynecol 1977;129:881.

Schiff M, McGuire EJ: Experience with the use of an intravesical hydrostatic pressure balloon. Surg Gynecol Obstet 1980;150:322.

Schiffman MH, Bauer HM, Hoover RN, et al: Epidemiologic evidence showing that human papillomavirus infection causes most cervical intraepithelial neoplasia. J Natl Cancer Inst 1993;85:958.

Schmidt J, Hawtrey C, Buchsbaum H: Transverse colon conduit: a preferred method of urinary diversion for radiation-treated pelvic malignancies. J Urol 1975;113:308.

Schmidt RP, Schulz KD, Sturm G, et al: Squamous cell carcinoma antigen for monitoring cervical cancer. Int J Biol Markers 1988; 3:87.

Schwarz E, Freese UK, Gissman L, et al: Structure and transcription of human papillomavirus sequences in cervical carcinoma cells. Nature 1985;314:111.

Scotti RJ, Bergman A, Bhatia N, Ostergard DR: Urodynamic changes in urethrovesical function after radical hysterectomy. Obstet Gynecol 1986;68:111.

Scully RE, Poulson H, Sobin LH: International Histological Classification and Histologic Typing of Female Genital Tract Tumors. Berlin: Springer-Verlag, 1994.

Senekjian EK, Young JM, Weiser PA, et al: An evaluation of squamous cell carcinoma antigen in patients with cervical squamous carcinoma. Obstet Gynecol 1987;157:433.

Seski JC, Kiokno AC: Bladder dysfunction after radical abdominal hysterectomy. Am J Obstet Gynecol 1977;128:643.

Sheets EE, Berman ML, Hrountas CK, et al: Surgically treated, early-stage neuroendocrine small-cell cervical carcinoma. Obstet Gynecol 1988;71:10.

Shingleton HM, Gore H, Bradley DH, Soong SJ: Adenocarcinoma of the cervix. I. Clinical evaluation and pathologic features. Obstet Gynecol 1981;139:799.

Simon NL, Gore H, Shingleton HM, et al: Study of superficially invasive carcinoma of the cervix. Obstet Gynecol 1986;68:19.

Smith JP, Randall GE, Castro JR, Lindberg RD: Hypogastric artery infusion and radiation therapy for advanced squamous cell carcinoma of the cervix. Am J Roentgenol Radium Ther Nucl Med 1972;114:110.

Smith S, Seski J, Copeland L, et al: Surgical management of irradiation-induced small bowel damage. Obstet Gynecol 1985; 65:563.

Souhami L, Gil R, Allan S, et al: A randomized trial of chemotherapy followed by pelvic radiation therapy in stage IIIB carcinoma of the cervix. Int J Radiat Oncol Biol Phys 1991;9:970.

Stanhope CR, Symmonds RE: Palliative exenteration: what, when and why? Am J Obstet Gynecol 1985;152:12.

Syed AM, Fedei BH: Technique of afterloading interstitial implant. Radiol Clin North Am 1977;46:458.

Symmonds RE, Pratt JH, Webb MJ: Exenterative operations: experience with 198 patients. Am J Obstet Gynecol 1975;121:907.

Tamimi HK, Ek M, Hesla J, et al: Glassy cell carcinoma of the cervix redefined. Obstet Gynecol 1988;71:837.

Thigpen T, Shingleton H, Homesley H, et al: Cis-platinum in treatment of advanced or recurrent squamous cell carcinoma of the cervix. Cancer 1981;48:899.

Thomas G, Dembo A: Is there a role for adjuvant pelvic radiotherapy after radical hysterectomy in early stage cervical cancer? Int J Gynecol Cancer 1991;1:1.

Thomas G, Dembo A, Fyles A, et al: Concurrent chemoradiation in advanced cervical cancer. Gynecol Oncol 1990;38:446.

Tobias J, Buxton E, Blackledge G, et al: Neoadjuvant bleomycin, ifosfamide and cisplatin in cervical cancer. Cancer Chemother Pharmacol 1990;26(Suppl):59.

Tomas C, Risteli J, Risteli L, et al: Use of various epithelial tumor markers and a stromal marker in the assessment of cervical carcinoma. Obstet Gynecol 1991;77:566.

Tsukamoto N, Nakamura M, Kashimura M, Saito K: Primary cervical choriocarcinoma. Gynecol Oncol 1980;9:99.

Underwood PB, Wilson WC, Kreutner A, et al: Radical hysterectomy: a critical review of twenty-two years' experience. Am J Obstet Gynecol 1979;134:889.

van Nagell JR, Greenwell N, Powell DF, et al: Microinvasive carcinoma of the cervix. Am J Obstet Gynecol 1983;145:981.

van Nagell JR, Parker JC, Maruyama Y, et al: Bladder or rectal injury following radiotherapy for cervical cancer. Obstet Gynecol 1974;119:727.

van Nagell JR Jr, Rayburn W, Donaldson ES, et al: Therapeutic implications of patterns of recurrence in cancer of the uterine cervix. Cancer 1979;44:2354.

Wallace S, Jing B, Zornoza J, et al: Is lymphangiography worthwhile? Int J Radiat Oncol Biol Phys 1979;5:1873.

Webb M, Symmonds R: Wertheim hysterectomy: A reappraisal. Obstet Gynecol 1979;54:140.

Weiser E, Bundy B, Hoskins W, et al: Extraperitoneal versus transperitoneal selective paraaortic lymphadenectomy in the pretreatment surgical staging of advanced cervical carcinoma: a Gynecologic Oncology Group study. Gynecol Oncol 1989;33:283.

Wentz W, Reagan J: Survival in cervical cancer with respect to cell type. Cancer 1959;12:384.

Wertheim E: Zur Frag der radikaloperaton beim uteruskrebs. Arch Gynak 1900;61:627.

Wertheim E: The radical abdominal operation in carcinoma of the cervix uteri. Surg Gynecol Obstet 1907;4:1.

Wharton JT, Jones HW III, Day T, et al: Preirradiation celiotomy and extended field irradiation for invasive carcinoma of the cervix. Obstet Gynecol 1977;49:333.

Wheeless CR, Graham R, Graham JB: Prognosis and treatment of adenoepidermoid carcinoma of the cervix. Obstet Gynecol 1970;35:928.

Wheelock JB, Krebs HB, Goplerud DR, Myers M: Cis-platinum, doxorubicin, and methotrexate treatment for recurrent cervical cancer. Obstet Gynecol 1985;66:410.

Wolf JK, Levenback C, Malpica A, et al: Adenocarcinoma in situ of the cervix: significance of cone biopsy margins. Obstet Gynecol 1996;88:82.

57

Endometrial Hyperplasia

Brigitte M. Ronnett
Robert J. Kurman

Endometrial hyperplasia is an abnormal proliferation, predominantly of the glandular component of the endometrium, which may progress to well-differentiated carcinoma in a small percentage of women. Appropriate management of patients with endometrial hyperplasia depends on a number of clinical and pathologic factors (Gusberg et al, 1954; Nimrod and Ryan, 1957; Campbell and Barter, 1961; Gusberg and Kaplan, 1963; Buehl et al, 1964; Musubuchi and Nemoto, 1972; Gusberg, 1974; Vellios, 1974; Ziel and Finkle, 1975; Gray et al, 1977; Greenwald et al, 1977; Welch and Scully, 1977; Longscope et al, 1978; Beckner et al, 1985; Deligdisch and Cohen, 1985; Kraus, 1985; Silverberg, 1988; Kauppila, 1989). There is a general tendency to overtreat patients with endometrial hyperplasia; however, the development of new histologic criteria for differentiating between well-differentiated endometrial carcinoma and endometrial hyperplasia, the formulation of a new classification of endometrial hyperplasia and carcinoma that will be adopted by the World Health Organization, and the emerging view that there are two different types of endometrial carcinoma, only one of which is related to endometrial hyperplasia, should lead to a more rational approach to the management of this disease (Novak and Rutledge, 1948; Hertig and Sommers, 1949; Robboy et al, 1982).

PATHOLOGIC FEATURES

Endometrial Hyperplasia

Endometrial hyperplasia is characterized by an abnormal proliferation of glands and stroma with the glandular component predominating. The gross appearance of hyperplastic endometrium is not distinctive. Typically, an increased amount of tissue is noted in curettings, and a pale, thick endometrium is noted at the time of hysterectomy. Thus, although the presence of endometrial hyperplasia may be suspected on hysteroscopic examination, the diagnosis is established by microscopic analysis. The International Society of Gynecologic Pathologists under the auspices of the World Health Organization has developed a classification (Table 57–1) in which endometrial hyperplasia is divided into two major categories according to whether cytologic atypia is present. The presence of cytologic atypia is the single most important histologic finding, because only atypical hyperplasia has a significant risk of progression to well-differentiated endometrial carcinoma. Cytologic atypia is characterized by loss of cellular polarity, an increase in the nuclear-cytoplasmic ratio, enlarged round, vesicular nuclei, prominent nucleoli, and coarse chromatin clumping (Fig. 57–1). Increased mitotic activity is often found in association with cytologic atypia. In contrast, the cellular features of hyperplastic endometria that do not display atypia are characterized by tall columnar cells with elongated cigar-shaped nuclei and varying degrees of mitotic activity (Fig. 57–2).

Hyperplasias are further subdivided into simple and complex forms based on architectural abnormalities. The simple form of hyperplasia has an increased number of endometrial glands, some of which have dilated lumens and slightly irregular glandular outlines. The glands are widely spaced and surrounded by abundant stroma. In contrast, the complex form of hyperplasia displays marked back-to-back glandular crowding and highly variable and irregular glandular outlines. The terminology of endometrial hyperplasia is therefore based on both cytologic and architectural features and includes simple hyperplasia (Fig. 57–3), complex hyperplasia (Fig. 57–4), simple atypical hyperplasia (Fig. 57–5), and complex atypical hyperplasia (Fig. 57–6).

At times it may be difficult to distinguish atypical hyperplasia from well-differentiated endometrial carcinoma, but studies have demonstrated that lesions with a significant risk of metastasis can be distinguished from those with little if any risk by the detection of endometrial stromal invasion. Three criteria are useful in the identification of stromal invasion. These include the presence of a desmoplastic (reactive) stromal response (Figs. 57–7 and 57–8), a confluent glandular or cribriform pattern (Figs. 57–9 and 57–10), and a papillary pattern (Kurman and Norris, 1982). More recently, it has been demon-

Table 57-1. CLASSIFICATION OF ENDOMETRIAL HYPERPLASIA*

Simple hyperplasia
Complex hyperplasia
Simple atypical hyperplasia
Complex atypical hyperplasia

*According to the International Society of Gynecological Pathologists and World Health Organization.

strated that clinically significant endometrial proliferations (i.e., those that have a high likelihood of myometrial invasion) can be recognized when either sufficient architectural complexity or nuclear atypia, including prominence of nucleoli, is present (Longacre et al, 1995). In addition, the strong association of a desmoplastic stromal response with a myoinvasive lesion was confirmed.

Endometrial Metaplasia

Metaplasia is defined as the replacement of one type of benign epithelium by another type. A number of endometrial metaplasias have been described, including squamous, papillary, ciliated, eosinophilic, mucinous, and clear cell (Hendrickson and Kempson, 1980). Typically they develop in association with hyperplasia.

Endometrial metaplasias most commonly occur in perimenopausal or postmenopausal women, as a result of unopposed estrogenic stimulation caused by anovulatory cycles. *Squamous* metaplasia is one of the most common types of metaplasias. It is characterized by circumscribed nests of benign squamous epithelium, partially or completely filling glan-

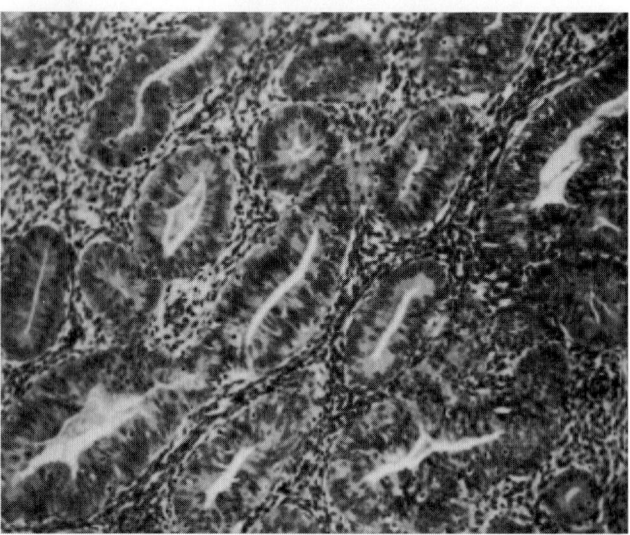

Figure 57-2
Hyperplasia without atypia. The nuclei are cigar-shaped and resemble those in proliferative endometrium.

dular lumens (Figs. 57-11 and 57-12). If it involves a group of glands, it may look ominous, suggesting carcinoma, but unless it is associated with stromal invasion, it should not be interpreted as carcinoma. Another frequent type of metaplasia is the *ciliated* or tubal type, in which endometrial epithelium is replaced by ciliated, tubal-type epithelium. *Papillary* metaplasia most often involves the endometrial surface, and is characterized by papillary structures lined by small, bland cells with pyknotic nuclei and indistinct cytoplasmic borders. *Eosinophilic* metaplasia, characterized by the presence of large, oncocytic cells with deeply eosinophilic cytoplasm and vesicular nuclei, is frequently associated with papillary metaplasia. In and of themselves metaplasias are be-

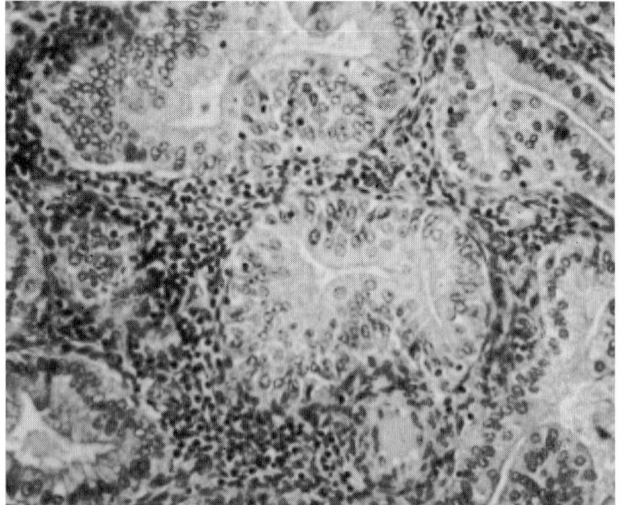

Figure 57-1
Atypical endometrial hyperplasia. Cytologic atypia is characterized by loss of cellular polarity, nuclear enlargement, and rounding with dispersement of the nuclear chromatin resulting in a vesicular appearance.

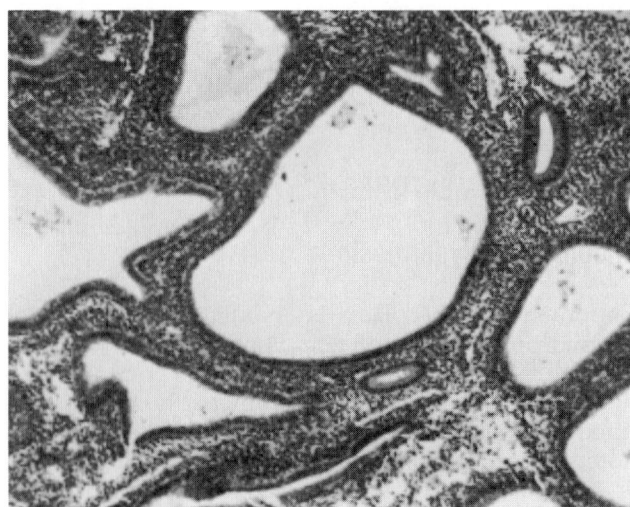

Figure 57-3
Simple hyperplasia is characterized by cystically dilated glands that are separated by abundant stroma. There is no cytologic atypia.

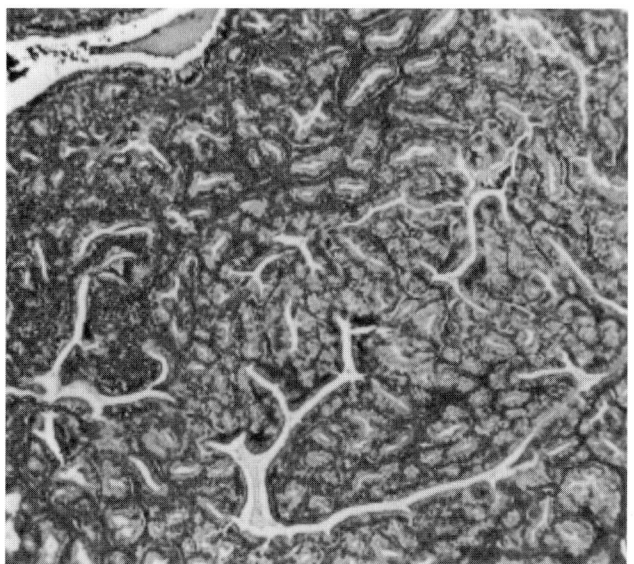

Figure 57-4
Complex hyperplasia is characterized by glands with complex glandular outlines that are markedly crowded. There is no cytologic atypia.

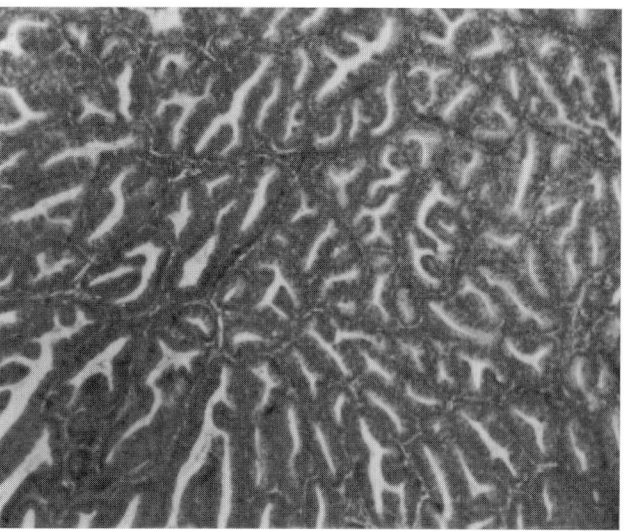

Figure 57-6
Complex atypical hyperplasia is characterized by glands with complex, irregular outlines that are crowded back-to-back. Cytologic atypia is present.

nign processes, but they can occur in association with or on the surface of endometrial adenocarcinomas, particularly the lower grade lesions. Thus further clinical investigation may be indicated in scant specimens from peri- and postmenopausal women (Jacques et al, 1995).

RELATIONSHIP OF ENDOMETRIAL HYPERPLASIA TO CARCINOMA

Endometrial carcinoma can be broadly divided into two types, designated I and II, based on their differ-

ent pathologic features and clinical presentation (Kurman and Norris, 1982; Bokhman, 1983; Deligdisch and Holinka, 1986). Type I is associated with unopposed estrogenic stimulation and endometrial hyperplasia. It occurs most often in perimenopausal white women. Histologically, it is usually a well-differentiated endometrioid adenocarcinoma. Myometrial invasion is usually superficial and confined to the inner half of the uterine wall.

A few subtypes may be found in this group. The most common one is a low-grade endometrioid adenocarcinoma with squamous differentiation (previ-

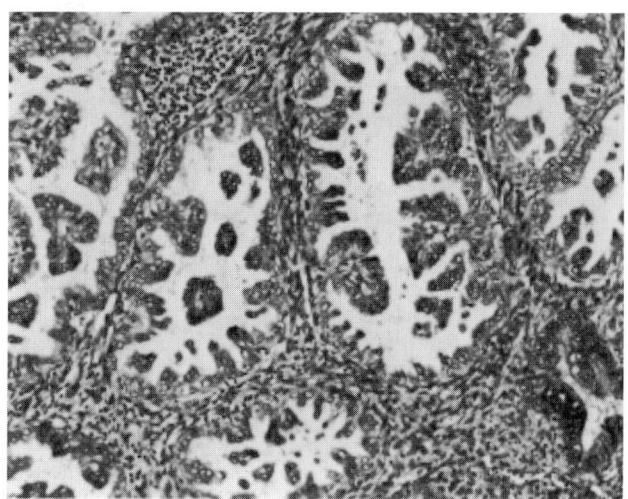

Figure 57-5
Simple atypical hyperplasia is characterized by glands that in this case have intraglandular tufting and are separated by abundant endometrial stroma. Cytologic atypia is present.

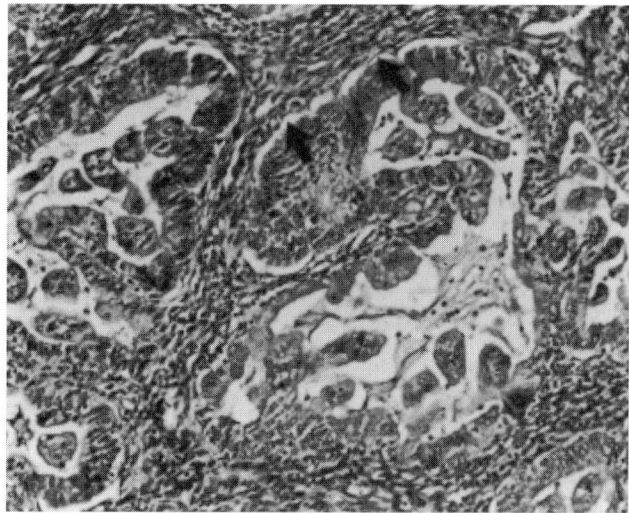

Figure 57-7
Well-differentiated endometrioid adenocarcinoma in which there is a desmoplastic reaction. The endometrial stroma between the glands in the upper part of the field (*arrows*) contains parallel fibroblasts that produce collagen and have an eosinophilic, wavy appearance.

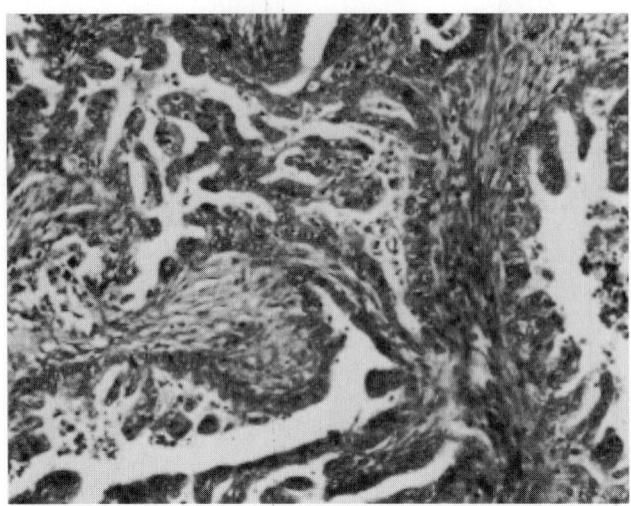

Figure 57-8
Well-differentiated endometrioid adenocarcinoma with an altered desmoplastic stroma, best seen in the stroma separating glands at the right side of the field.

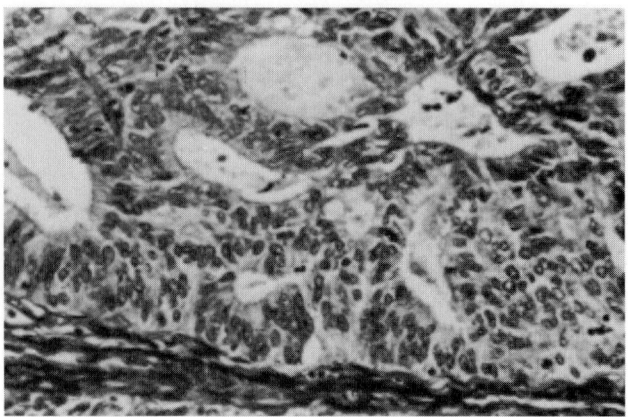

Figure 57-10
Higher magnification of the same case shown in Figure 57-9. The cribriform pattern is distinguished from back-to-back crowding by the absence of endometrial stroma surrounding the lumina.

ously classified as adenoacanthoma), consisting of well-differentiated endometrioid adenocarcinoma with foci of benign-appearing squamous epithelium. Secretory carcinoma is another type characterized by crowded glands showing mild atypia with subnuclear and supranuclear vacuoles, resembling early secretory endometrium. Ciliated carcinoma consists of well-differentiated glands with cilia on the luminal surface. Finally, villoglandular adenocarcinoma is characterized by well-differentiated glandular epithelium lining elongated villous structures. All of these subtypes are slow-growing, low-grade neoplasms with a good prognosis.

Type II endometrial carcinoma is a high-grade neoplasm that occurs in older postmenopausal women. There is usually no history of unopposed estrogenic stimulation, and associated endometrial hyperplasia is extremely unusual. Typically, the adjacent endometrium is atrophic. These tumors are moderately to poorly differentiated endometrioid carcinomas with specific subtypes, including serous, clear cell, and adenosquamous carcinomas. Serous carcinoma is composed of complex, fibrotic, papillary structures or a glandular proliferation lined by highly atypical epithelium with marked nuclear pleomorphism, hyperchromasia, prominent nucleoli, and frequent hobnail-type cells with smudged chromatin. Clear cell carcinoma is composed of clear, hobnail, and eosinophilic cells arranged in solid,

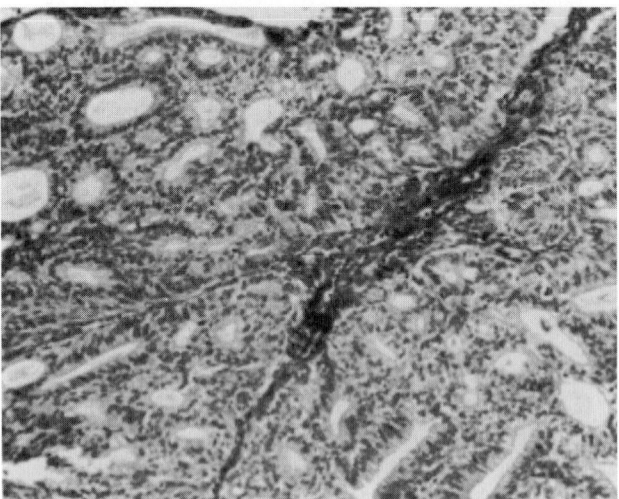

Figure 57-9
Well-differentiated endometrioid adenocarcinoma with a cribriform pattern. The cribriform pattern is characterized by epithelium containing multiple lumina that are not separated by endometrial stroma.

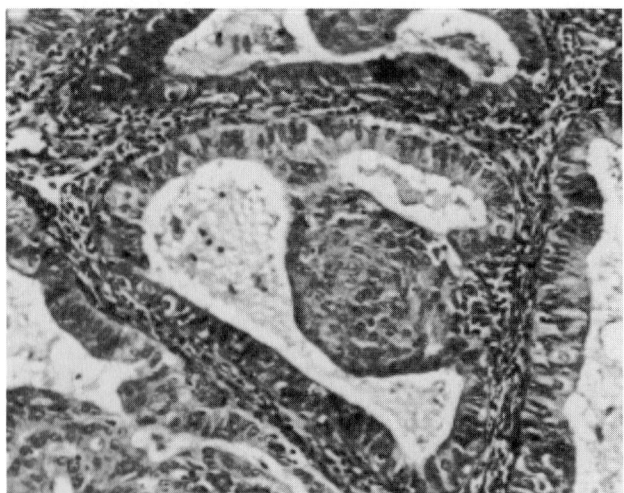

Figure 57-11
Atypical hyperplasia with squamous metaplasia. The squamous epithelium forms what has been termed a "squamous morule" that partially fills the gland lumen. Cytologic atypia is present; however, note that the endometrial stroma is not altered.

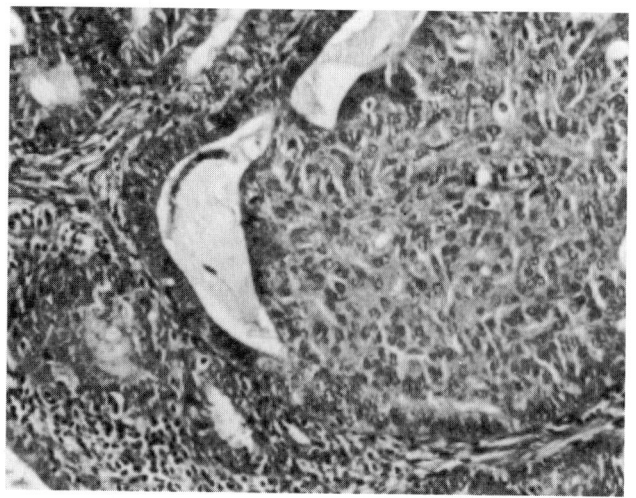

Figure 57-12
Atypical hyperplasia with squamous metaplasia. The squamous morule almost completely fills the gland lumen in this field.

papillary, or tubulocystic patterns. Finally, there are carcinomas with highly atypical glandular and squamous components. In the past these have been termed *adenosquamous carcinomas*, but currently most investigators classify them as poorly differentiated adenocarcinomas with squamous differentiation because the presence of the squamous element per se does not influence the behavior of endometrial carcinomas. Accordingly, endometrial carcinomas with squamous epithelium are classified as adenocarcinomas with squamous differentiation, and are graded based on the appearance of the glandular component.

Type II neoplasms often demonstrate deep myometrial invasion and vascular involvement, and have a poor prognosis. Serous carcinoma is the most common nonendometrioid carcinoma in the type II group of neoplasms. Studies have demonstrated that serous carcinoma is frequently associated with a putative precursor lesion termed *endometrial intraepithelial carcinoma* (EIC), characterized by markedly atypical nuclei lining the surfaces and glands of the atrophic endometrium adjacent to the serous carcinoma (Ambros et al, 1995; Spiegel, 1995). Thus serous carcinoma is clinically and pathologically distinct from the more common endometrioid variety of endometrial carcinoma in that it is an aggressive neoplasm of older women and is associated with EIC rather than endometrial hyperplasia.

ADJUNCTIVE DIAGNOSTIC TECHNIQUES

Electron Microscopy

Electron microscopy findings differ in nonatypical and atypical endometrial hyperplasias (Richart and Ferenczy, 1974; Klemi et al, 1980; Fenoglio et al, 1982). In nonatypical hyperplasias, there is an in-

crease in estrogen-related organelles such as cilia, microvilli, free ribosomes, rough endoplasmic reticulum, Golgi complexes, and mitochondria. These features are present in proliferative endometrium.

In atypical hyperplasias, some cells show diminished numbers of estrogen-related organelles and approach the electron microscopic appearance of cells in well-differentiated adenocarcinoma. They are admixed, however, with cells indistinguishable from those of normal endometrium. Electron microscopy therefore does not assist in the diagnosis of endometrial hyperplasia.

Quantitative Microscopic Methods

Architectural patterns and cytologic atypia can be assessed by histologic sections (Baak et al, 1981; Colgan et al, 1983; Norris et al, 1983; Ausems et al, 1985; Thornton et al, 1989). Cellularity, glandular configurations, and nuclear size and shape can be measured. The value of various morphometric parameters in predicting the outcome of endometrial hyperplasia is controversial. Some studies have shown that the nuclear size is a useful predictor of hyperplasias that will proceed to malignancy (Colgan et al, 1983). Other reports (Skaarland, 1985) have maintained that nuclear size cannot be reliably determined because of overlap. Cell count, in addition to nuclear size, degree of gland formation, and DNA content, have shown to be useful in predicting prognosis (Norris et al, 1989).

Quantitative morphometric analysis is not routinely available in most diagnostic pathology laboratories, and results depend almost entirely on the selection of the appropriate field by the pathologist (Baak et al, 1982; Baak, 1984). Accordingly, this method is currently of little practical value.

DNA Microspectrophotometry and in Vitro Histoaudioradiography

In general, aneuploidy is a feature of malignant cells and diploidy is a feature of benign cells (Richart and Ludwig, 1969; Hustin, 1976). Although some atypical hyperplasias are aneuploid (Katayma and Jones, 1967; Wagner et al, 1967) two thirds of endometrial carcinoma are diploid (Geisinger et al, 1986). Therefore, aneuploidy cannot be reliably used in predicting progression of hyperplasia to carcinoma.

In contrast, it appears that the proliferative activities of endometrial hyperplasias are more useful in predicting their behavior. Proliferative activity is expressed either as the proliferative index or as the percentage of cells in S phase. In vitro DNA labeling shows that atypical hyperplasia has prolonged DNA synthesis (S_1 phase), coupled with a shorter doubling time (Ferenczy, 1982, 1983) and that these features correlate with progression to adenocarcinoma.

Estrogen and Progesterone Receptors

Estrogen and progesterone receptors are concentrated in the nuclei of endometrial cells and have a high affinity for binding to estrogen and progesterone, respectively. When estrogen binds to its receptor and interacts with the DNA of the endometrial cell, there is enhanced synthesis of both estrogen and progesterone receptors and an increase in cellular proliferation. In contrast, binding of progesterone to its receptor and interaction with cellular DNA results in down-regulation of both receptors and decrease in cellular proliferation. The concentration of estrogen and progesterone receptors in the normal endometrium varies during the menstrual cycle, correlating with the change in plasma levels of estradiol and progesterone. The levels of estrogen and progesterone receptors in endometrial hyperplasia are usually increased, but they are decreased in endometrial carcinoma (Bergeron et al, 1988; Contreras Oritz and Sananes, 1988). In one study, estrogen receptors were found in 93% of endometrial hyperplasias and 79% of endometrial carcinomas; progesterone receptors were detected in 73% of endometrial hyperplasias and 56% of endometrial carcinomas (Ehrlich et al, 1981). Immunohistochemical analyses of the subtypes of endometrial carcinoma have demonstrated that well- and moderately differentiated endometrioid carcinomas often express both estrogen and progesterone receptors, whereas poorly differentiated endometrioid tumors usually show only weak expression or are negative. In addition, serous and clear cell carcinomas are almost always hormone receptor negative (Umpierre et al, 1994; Carcangiu et al, 1996; Lax et al, 1998a, 1988b). This explains why well-differentiated endometrioid adenocarcinomas respond better to progestin therapy than poorly differentiated endometrioid, serous, and clear cell carcinomas. Similarly, because progestins decrease the content of female sex steroid hormone receptors in normal tissue, it is likely that they would have a similar effect on endometrial hyperplasia with functioning steroid receptors, resulting in decrease in cellular proliferation (Milgrom et al, 1973; Hsueh et al, 1976; Bayard et al, 1978). Reports of regression of 70% of endometrial hyperplasia treated with progestins (Kjorstad et al, 1978) correlate with elevated progesterone receptor levels in 73% of hyperplastic endometria (Creasman et al, 1980; Ehrlich et al, 1981).

EFFECTS OF TAMOXIFEN THERAPY ON THE ENDOMETRIUM

Tamoxifen is a synthetic, nonsteroidal antiestrogenic drug that is widely used in the adjuvant therapy of breast carcinoma. It acts predominantly as an estrogen antagonist in the breast but has partial agonistic effect in the uterus. Numerous studies have reported that chronic tamoxifen therapy may be associated with the development of endometrial polyps, endometrial hyperplasias, and endometrial malignancies, including carcinomas and mesenchymal and mixed epithelial-mesenchymal tumors (Clement et al, 1996). Polyps have been reported to occur 3 to 11 times more frequently in tamoxifen-treated women than in untreated controls; hyperplasias occur at least 5 times more frequently in treated women (Neven et al, 1989; Lahti et al, 1993; Ismail, 1994, 1996). A statistically significant increase in endometrial cancer among tamoxifen-treated women, with a relative risk of 4.1, has also been documented (Rutqvist et al, 1995) Many, but not all, studies have demonstrated that the relative risk of endometrial carcinoma is related to the cumulative dose and duration of tamoxifen therapy (Fornander et al, 1989, 1993; Magriples et al, 1993; Seoud et al, 1993; Cohen et al, 1994a, 1994b; Fisher et al, 1994; Ingle et al, 1994; van Leeuwen et al, 1994; Cohen et al, 1996). In addition, one study found that women receiving tamoxifen who subsequently developed uterine carcinoma were at risk for high grade cancers that have a poor prognosis (Magriples et al, 1993), whereas another study found no significant differences in the stage, grade, or histologic subtype when comparing breast cancer patients who had received tamoxifen to those who had not (Barakat et al, 1994). Consequently, it is recommended that patients be evaluated for preexisting endometrial lesions before starting tamoxifen therapy. In addition, patients on long-term tamoxifen therapy should be closely followed with endometrial biopsies when they experience symptoms referable to the uterus (Friedl and Jordan, 1994).

MANAGEMENT OF ENDOMETRIAL HYPERPLASIA

The management of patients with endometrial hyperplasia is based on clinical and pathologic factors (Fig. 57–13). The presence or absence of cytologic atypia in endometrial hyperplasia is the single most important histologic feature, but treatment must be individualized, taking into account the patient's age and desire for fertility. Atypical hyperplasia progresses to endometrial carcinoma in 23% of patients, whereas hyperplasia with no atypia progresses to endometrial carcinoma in 2% (Kurman et al, 1985; Kurman and Norris, 1994). The transition time for the progression of hyperplasia to carcinoma in one study was 10 years, compared to 4 years for atypical hyperplasia (Kurman et al, 1985).

Women less than 40 years old with simple and complex hyperplasia and no atypia can be treated conservatively with close follow-up and periodic biopsies. Provera every month or every 2 months may be needed to control bleeding. The vast majority of atypical hyperplasias or well-differentiated adenocarcinomas in women less than 40 years old regress when treated with progestin therapy (Provera or Megace), and therefore conservative treatment should

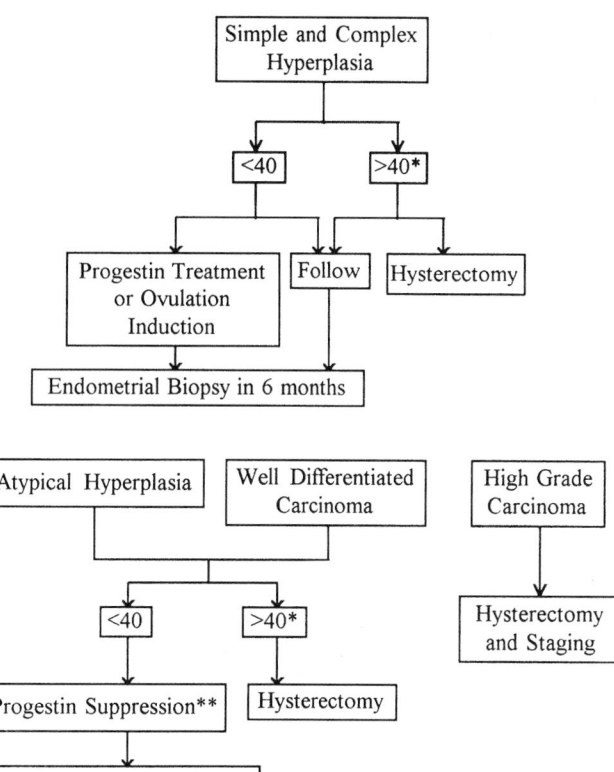

Figure 57–13
Management of endometrial hyperplasia, atypical hyperplasia, and carcinoma. (Modified from Kurman RJ, Norris HJ: Endometrial hyperplasia and related cellular changes. In Kurman RJ [ed]: Blaustein's Pathology of the Female Genital Tract. 4th ed. New York: Springer-Verlag, 1994:411, with permission.)

*Patients age 40-50 may wish to be managed conservatively
**Followed by ovulation induction for women who wish to become pregnant

be strongly considered if preservation of fertility is desired (Randall and Kurman, 1997).

The majority of endometrial hyperplasias in women over 40 years, as in younger women, are associated with anovulatory cycles, and therefore spontaneous regression may occur in up to 80% of hyperplasias with no atypia and 60% of atypical hyperplasia (Hustin, 1976; Lucas and Yen, 1979). In women over 40 years, hyperplasias with no atypia, both simple and complex, can be managed conservatively by observation or suppression with progestins. Repeated episodes of irregular bleeding, unresponsive to hormone treatment, may require hysterectomy.

Treatment of atypical hyperplasias in women in the 40- to 50-year age range may initially consist of observation or suppression with progestins, followed by repeated biopsies until the process has resolved. If the lesion persists, however, hysterectomy may be necessary. Alternatively, hysterectomy is an appropriate initial management in women who prefer a definitive procedure and in women over 50 who have no contraindications for a surgical procedure.

REFERENCES

Ambros RA, Sherman ME, Zahn CM, et al: Endometrial intra-epithelial carcinoma: a distinctive lesion specifically associated with tumors displaying serous differentiation. Hum Pathol 1995;26:1260.

Ausems WEMA, van der Kamp J-K, Baak JAP: Nuclear morphometry in the determination of the prognosis of marked atypical endometrial hyperplasia. Int J Gynecol Pathol 1985;4:180.

Baak JPA: The use and disuse of morphometry in the diagnosis of endometrial hyperplasia and carcinoma. Pathol Res Pract 1984;179:20.

Baak JPA, Kurver PHJ, Boon ME: Computer-aided application of quantitative microscopy in diagnostic pathology. Pathol Annu 1982;17:287.

Baak JPA, Kurver PHJ, Diegenbach PC, et al: Discrimination of hyperplasia and carcinoma of endometrium by quantitative microscopy—a feasibility study. Histopathology 1981;5:61.

Barakat RR, Wong G, Curtin JP, et al: Tamoxifen use in breast cancer patients who subsequently develop corpus cancer is not associated with a higher incidence of adverse histologic features. Gynecol Oncol 1994;55:164.

Bayard F, Damilano S, Robel P: Cytoplasmic and nuclear estradiol and progesterone receptors in human endometrium. J Clin Endocrinol 1978;46:635.

Beckner ME, Mori T, Silverberg SG: Endometrial carcinoma: non-tumor factors in prognosis. Int J Gynecol Pathol 1985;4:131.

Bergeron C, Ferenczy A, Shyamala G: Distribution of estrogen receptors in various cell types of normal hyperplastic, and neoplastic human endometrial tissue. Lab Invest 1988;58:338.

Bokhman JV: Two pathogenic types of endometrial carcinoma. Gynecol Oncol 1983;15:10.

Buehl IA, Vellios F, Carter JE, Hubor CP: Carcinoma in situ of the endometrium. Am J Clin Pathol 1964;42:594.

Campbell PE, Barter RA: The significance of atypical hyperplasia. J Obstet Gynecol Br Commonw 1961;68:668.

Carcangiu ML, Chambers JT, Voynick IM, et al: Immunohistochemical evaluation of estrogen and progesterone receptor content in 183 patients with endometrial carcinoma. Part I. Int J Gynecol Pathol 1996;94:247.

Clement PB, Oliva E, Young RH: Mullerian adenosarcoma of the uterine corpus associated with tamoxifen therapy: a report of six cases and a review of tamoxifen-associated endometrial lesions. Int J Gynecol Pathol 1996;15:222.

Cohen I, Altaras MM, Shapira J, et al: Postmenopausal tamoxifen treatment and endometrial pathology. Obstet Gynecol Survey 1994a;49:823.

Cohen I, Altaras MM, Shapira J, et al: Time-dependent effect of tamoxifen therapy on endometrial pathology in asymptomatic postmenopausal breast cancer patients. Int J Gynecol Pathol 1996;15:152.

Cohen I, Rosen DJD, Shapira J, et al: Endometrial changes with tamoxifen: comparison between tamoxifen-treated and non-treated asymptomatic, postmenopausal breast cancer patients. Gynecol Oncol 1994b;52:185.

Colgan TJ, Norris HJ, Foster W, et al: Predicting the outcome of endometrial hyperplasia by quantitative analysis of nuclear features using a linear discrimination function. Int J Gynecol Pathol 1983;1:347.

Contreras Oritiz O, Sananes CE: Hormonal receptors in endometrial neoplasia. Eur J Gynecol Oncol 1988;9:396.

Creasman WT, McCarty KS, Barton TK, McCarty KS Jr: Clinical correlates of estrogen and progesterone-binding proteins in human endometrial adenocarcinoma. Obstet Gynecol 1980;55:363.

Deligdisch L, Cohen CJ: Histologic correlates and virulence implications of endometrial carcinoma associated with adenomatous hyperplasia. Cancer 1985;56:1452.

Deligdisch L, Holinka CF: Progesterone receptors in two groups of endometrial carcinoma. Cancer 1986;57:1385.

Ehrlich CE, Young PCM, Cleary RE: Cytoplasmic progesterone receptors in normal, hyperplastic, and carcinomatous endometrium: therapeutic implications. Am J Obstet Gynecol 1981; 141:539.

Fenoglio CM, Crum CP, Ferenczy A: Endometrial hyperplasia and carcinoma: are ultrastructural, biochemical and immunohistochemical studies useful in distinguishing between them? Pathol Res Pract 1982;174:257.

Ferenczy A: Cytodynamics of endometrial hyperplasia and neoplasia. Part I. Histology and ultrastructure. Prog Surg Pathol. 1982;4:95.

Ferenczy A: Cytodynamics of endometrial hyperplasia and neoplasia. Part II. In vitro DNA histoautoradiography. Hum Pathol 1983;14:77.

Fisher B, Costantino JP, Redmond CK, et al: Endometrial cancer in tamoxifen-treated breast cancer patients: findings from the National Surgical Adjuvant Breast and Bowel Project (NSABP) B-14. J Natl Cancer Inst 1994;86:527.

Fornander T, Hellstrom A, Moberger B: Descriptive clinicopathologic study of 17 patients with endometrial cancer during or after adjuvant tamoxifen in early breast cancer. J Natl Cancer Inst 1993;85:1850.

Fornander T, Rutqvist LE, Cedermark B, et al: Adjuvant tamoxifen in early breast cancer: occurrence of new primary cancers. Lancet 1989;1:117.

Friedl A, Jordan VC: What do we know and what don't we know about tamoxifen in the human uterus? Breast Cancer Res Treat 1994;31:27.

Geisinger KR, Homesley HD, Morgan TM, et al: Endometrial adenocarcinoma: a multiparameter clinicopathologic analysis including the DNA profile and sex steroid hormone receptors. Cancer 1986;58:1518.

Gray LA, Christopherson WM, Hoover RN: Estrogen and endometrial carcinoma. Obstet Gynecol 1977;49:385.

Greenwald P, Caputo TA, Wolfgang PE: Endometrial cancer after menopausal use of estrogens. Obstet Gynecol 1977;50:239.

Gusberg SB. Precursors of corpus carcinoma: estrogens and adenomatous hyperplasia. Am J Obstet Gynecol 1974;54:905.

Gusberg SB, Kaplan AL: Precursors of corpus cancer. Part IV. Adenomatous hyperplasia as stage 0 carcinoma of the endometrium. Am J Obstet Gynecol 1963;87:661.

Gusberg SB, Moore DB, Martin F: Precursors of corpus cancer. Part II. A clinical and pathological study of adenomatous hyperplasia. Am J Obstet Gynecol 1954;68:1472.

Hendrickson MR, Kempson RL: Endometrial epithelial metaplasias: proliferations frequently misdiagnosed as adenocarcinoma. Am J Surg Pathol 1980;4:525.

Hertig AT, Sommers SC: Genesis of endometrial carcinoma I. Study of prior biopsies. Cancer 1949;2:946.

Hsueh AJW, Peck EJ Jr, Clark JH: Control of uterine estrogen levels by progesterone. Endocrinology 1976;98:438.

Hustin J: Morphology and DNA content of endometrial cancer nuclei under progesterone treatment. Acta Cytol 1976;20:556.

Ingle JN: Tamoxifen and endometrial cancer: new challenges for an "old" drug. Gynecol Oncol 1994;55:161.

Ismail SM: Pathology of endometrium treated with tamoxifen. J Clin Pathol 1994;47:827.

Ismail SM: The effects of tamoxifen on the uterus. Curr Opin Obstet Gynecol 1996;8:27.

Jacques SM, Qureshi F, Lawrence WD: Surface epithelial changes in endometrial adenocarcinoma: diagnostic pitfalls in curettage specimens. Int J Gynecol Pathol 1995;14:191.

Katayma KP, Jones HW: Chromosomes of atypical (adenomatous) hyperplasia and carcinoma of endometrium. Am J Obstet Gynecol 1967;97:978.

Kauppila A: Oestrogen and progestin receptors as prognostic indicators in endometrial cancer. Acta Oncol 1989;28:561.

Kjorstad KE, Welander C, Halvorsen T, et al: Progestagens as primary treatment in pre-malignant changes of endometrium. In Brush MC, King RJB, Taylor RW (eds): Endometrial Cancer. London: Bailliere Tindall, 1978:188.

Klemi PJ, Gronroos M, Rauramo L, Punnonen R: Ultrastructural features of endometrial atypical adenomatous hyperplasia and adenocarcinomas and the plasma levels of estrogens. Gynecol Oncol 1980;9:162.

Kraus FT: High risk and premalignant lesions of endometrium. Am J Surg Pathol 1985;9(Suppl):31.

Kurman RJ, Norris HJ: Evaluation of criteria for distinguishing atypical endometrial hyperplasia from well differentiated carcinoma. Cancer 1982;49:2547.

Kurman RJ, Norris HJ: Endometrial hyperplasia and related cellular changes. In Kurman RJ (ed): Blaustein's Pathology of the Female Genital Tract. 4th ed. New York: Springer-Verlag, 1994: 411.

Kurman RJ, Kaminski PF, Norris HJ: The behavior of endometrial hyperplasia: a long-term study of "untreated" hyperplasia in 170 patients. Cancer 1985;56:403.

Lahti E, Blanco G, Kauppila A, et al: Endometrial changes in postmenopausal breast cancer patients receiving tamoxifen. Obstet Gynecol 1993;81:660.

Lax SF, Pizer E, Ronnett BM, Kurman RJ: P53, Comparison of estrogen and progesterone receptor, Ki-67 and p53 immunoreactivity in uterine endometrioid carcinoma and endometrioid carcinoma with squamous mucinous, secretory, and ciliated cell differentiation. Hum Pathol 1998a;29:924.

Lax SF, Pizer E, Ronnett BM, Kurman RJ: Clear cell carcinoma of the endometrium is characterized by a distinctive profile of p53, Ki-67, estrogen (ER) and progesterone receptor (PR) expression. Hum Pathol 1988b;29:551.

Longacre TA, Chung MH, Jensen DN, Hendrickson MR: Proposed criteria for the diagnosis of well-differentiated endometrial carcinoma. Am J Surg Pathol 1995;19:371.

Longscope S, Pratt JH, Schnedier SH, Fineberg SE: Aromatization of androgens by muscle and adipose tissue in vivo. J Clin Endocrinol Metab 1978;46:146.

Lucas WE, Yen SSC: A study of endocrine and metabolic variables in postmenopausal women with endometrial carcinoma. Am J Obstet Gynecol 1979;134:180.

Magriples U, Naftolin F, Schwartz PE, et al: High grade endometrial carcinoma in tamoxifen-treated breast cancer patients. J Clin Oncol 1993;11:485.

Milgrom E, Thi L, Atger M, et al: Mechanisms regulating the concentration of progesterone receptors in the uterus. J Biol Chem 1973;248:6366.

Musubuchi K, Nemoto H: Epidemiologic studies on uterine cancer at Cancer Institute Hospital, Tokyo, Japan. Cancer 1972;30: 268.

Neven P, De Muylder X, Van Belle Y, et al: Tamoxifen and the uterus and endometrium [letter]. Lancet 1989;1:375.

Nimrod A, Ryan KJ: Aromatization of androgens by human abdominal and breast fat tissue. J Clin Endocrinol Metab 1957;40: 367.

Norris HJ, Becker RL, Mikel UV: A comparative morphometric and cytophotometric study of endometrial hyperplasia, atypical hyperplasia, and endometrial carcinoma. Hum Pathol 1989; 20:219.

Norris HJ, Tavassoli FA, Kurman RJ: Endometrial hyperplasia and carcinoma: diagnostic considerations. Am J Surg Pathol 1983;7:839.

Novak E, Rutledge F: Atypical endometrial hyperplasia stimulating adenocarcinoma. Am J Obstet Gynecol 1948;55:46.

Randall T, Kurman RJ: Progestin treatment of atypical hyperplasia and well differentiated carcinoma of the endometrium in women under age 40. Obstet Gynecol 1997;90:434.

Richart RM, Ferenczy A: Endometrial morphologic response to hormonal environment. Gynecol Oncol 1974;2:180.

Richart RM, Ludwig AS: Alterations in chromosomes and DNA content in gynecologic neoplasms. Am J Obstet Gynecol 1969; 104:463.

Robboy SJ, Miller AW III, Kurman RJ: The pathologic features and behavior of endometrial carcinoma associated with exogenous estrogen administration. Pathol Res Pract 1982;174:237.

Rutqvist LE, Johansson H, Signomklao T, et al: Adjuvant tamoxifen therapy for early stage breast cancer and second primary malignancies. J Natl Cancer Inst 1995;87:645.

Seoud MA-F, Johnson J, Weed JC: Gynecologic tumors in tamoxifen-treated women with breast cancer. Obstet Gynecol 1993; 82:165.

Silverberg SG: Hyperplasia and carcinoma of endometrium. Semin Diagn Pathol 1988;5:135.

Skaarland E: Nuclear size and shape of epithelial cells from the endometrium: lack of value as a criterion for differentiation between normal, hyperplastic, and malignant conditions. J Clin Pathol 1985;38:502.

Spiegel GW: Endometrial carcinoma in situ in postmenopausal women. Am J Surg Pathol 1995;19:417.

Thornton JG, Quirke P, Wells M: Flow cytometry of normal, hyperplastic, and malignant human endometrium. Am J Obstet Gynecol 1989;161:487.

Umpierre SA, Burke TW, Tornos C, et al: Immunocytochemical analysis of uterine papillary serous carcinomas for estrogen and progesterone receptors. Int J Gynecol Pathol 1994;13: 127.

van Leeuwen FE, Benraadt J, Coebergh JWW, et al: Risk of endometrial cancer after tamoxifen treatment of breast cancer. Lancet 1994;343:448.

Vellios F: Endometrial hyperplasia and carcinoma in situ. Gynecol Oncol 1974;2:152.

Wagner D, Richard RM, Terner JY: Deoxyribonucleic acid content of presumed precursors of endometrial carcinoma. Cancer 1967;20:2067.

Welch WR, Scully RE: Precancerous lesions of the endometrium. Hum Pathol 1977;8:503.

Ziel HK, Finkle WD: Increased risk of endometrial carcinoma among users of conjugated estrogens. N Engl J Med 1975;293: 1167.

58

Adenocarcinoma of the Endometrium

Thomas W. Burke
Mitchell Morris

Endometrial carcinomas arise within the glandular epithelium of the uterine lining. With 32,800 cases estimated for 1995, they are the most common gynecologic cancer and the fourth most common malignancy in women (Wingo et al, 1995). Because most patients with endometrial cancer have recognizable symptoms, their disease usually is diagnosed promptly and is localized to the uterine fundus. Surgical therapy is often curative in this setting. Consequently, the projected 1995 death figure of 5900 women is less than deaths expected from either ovarian or cervical cancer, which are considerably less frequent. This has led many physicians to incorrectly view endometrial carcinoma as a "benign" malignancy (Boronow, 1976). Table 58–1 illustrates statistics for stage at diagnosis and survival by clinical stage for patients with endometrial cancer.

Several other categories of malignant neoplastic disease can involve the uterine fundus. Inappropriate stimulation and growth of the endometrium can result in architectural or cytologic atypia within the uterine lining. Some of these endometrial hyperplasias appear to be precursors to adenocarcinoma. Sarcomas arising from endometrial stroma, smooth muscle, or supporting tissue elements (fibroblasts, capillary endothelial cells) occur occasionally. Mixed cancers containing both sarcoma and carcinoma elements are also seen. Metastases or local extension from gastrointestinal, breast, ovarian, and tubal tumors can involve the uterine wall or cavity. Upward extension of cervical cancer is relatively common and sometimes causes a diagnostic dilemma. Endometrial hyperplasias, uterine sarcomas, and cervical carcinomas are described in separate chapters of this text.

EPIDEMIOLOGY

Endometrial cancer is primarily a tumor of postmenopausal women. The peak age-specific incidence is seen in women in their late 50s and early 60s (Wynder et al, 1966; MacMahon, 1974; Davies et al, 1981; Parazzina et al, 1991). Some studies have suggested that patients at the age extremes, less than 40 or

more than 70 years, have a poorer prognosis. However, this age-related concept is not universally accepted; other histopathologic factors may have a greater influence on outcome than age alone.

There is a clear association between prolonged, uninterrupted estrogen exposure and the development of endometrial cancer (Wynder et al, 1966; MacMahon, 1974; Davies et al, 1981; Parazzina et al, 1991; Brinton et al, 1992). Because the glandular epithelial cells of the endometrium normally respond to estrogen stimulation by proliferating, it seems logical that uncontrolled estrogenic stimulation could ultimately result in hyperplastic or malignant growth. The proliferative effects of estrogen are counterbalanced by the maturational and secretory effects of progesterone. Progesterone production by the corpus luteum following ovulation and by the placenta during pregnancy provides natural and cyclic antagonism to estrogen and prevents long-term, unopposed estrogen stimulation. Many of the identified risk factors for endometrial cancer can be tied to this mechanism of chronic unopposed estrogen stimulation. Ovarian hormonal factors that have been associated with a greater risk for endometrial cancer include a history of oligo-ovulation or prolonged anovulation, as is seen in polycystic ovarian disease; presence of an estrogen-secreting neoplasm such as the granulosa cell tumor; early age at menarche and late age at menopause, both of which imply a longer period of ovarian function and estrogen production; and nulliparity, which is significant for the absence of long periods of progestational effect from the placenta. Obesity also appears to increase risk via an estrogen stimulation mechanism. Adipocytes possess the enzymes capable of converting androstenedione (produced in the adrenal gland) to estrone, a weak estrogen. This peripheral conversion results in chronic low-level estrogenic stimulation.

The other major source of estrogen stimulation is endogenous estrogen given to postmenopausal women to maintain bone mineral density, prevent coronary artery disease, and relieve menopausal symptoms. When first popularized in the 1950s and 1960s, estrogen replacement therapy was usually

Table 58–1. STAGE AND SURVIVAL FOR PATIENTS WITH ENDOMETRIAL CANCER*

STAGE	% AT DIAGNOSIS	5-YEAR SURVIVAL
I	75%	90%
II	15%	60%
III	7%	35%
IV	3%	10%

*Pooled data based upon FIGO 1971 clinical staging criteria.

given by continuous daily ingestion of oral estrogens. A sharp rise in the incidence of endometrial adenocarcinoma paralleled widespread use of replacement therapy and subsequently led to the conclusion that chronic estrogen exposure was probably a causative agent (Smith et al, 1975; Ziel and Finkle, 1975; Gray et al, 1977; Antunes et al, 1979). When estrogen replacement is administered in a cyclic fashion or with progestational agents, the risk of endometrial carcinoma is eliminated or even reduced over that seen in women not receiving replacement therapy (Ernster et al, 1988).

Long-term use of oral tamoxifen as an adjuvant breast cancer treatment has also been linked to the occasional development of endometrial polyps, hyperplasia, and cancer (Killackey et al, 1985; Seoud et al, 1993). This agent exhibits both estrogen antagonist and agonist properties. As an agonist, it appears to provide chronic low-level stimulation of the endometrium. An understanding of the role of tamoxifen in endometrial neoplasia is evolving. Current information would suggest that the risk of endometrial carcinoma in tamoxifen users is small—certainly less than the recognized benefit of fewer breast cancer recurrences (Cook et al, 1995; Cuenca et al, 1996). Because the risk of endometrial cancer appears to be related to length of tamoxifen use, current recommendations are to discontinue adjuvant therapy after 5 years (American College of Obstetricians and Gynecologists, 1996). Some reviews have suggested that the endometrial tumors seen in tamoxifen users are often high-risk subtypes (Silva et al, 1994); others have not found this to be true (Fornander et al, 1993; Barakat et al, 1994).

Large epidemiologic studies have suggested several other potential risk factors for the development of endometrial cancer (Wynder et al, 1966; MacMahon, 1974; Davies et al, 1981; Parazzina et al, 1991; Brinton et al, 1992). The incidence seems to be greater in Caucasians of middle or upper socioeconomic class. Societies with high dietary fat intake also demonstrate a higher rate of endometrial tumors. Risk is elevated in women with hypertension and diabetes mellitus. Women with a family history of endometrial cancer are also at increased risk (Lynch et al, 1976). An association between endometrial cancer and malignant tumors of the breast, ovary, and colon has also been described (Lynch et al, 1966). This association between multiple primary cancers has been noted within individuals (i.e., a woman with endometrial cancer is at higher risk for breast cancer) and within families (i.e., a woman whose mother or aunts had endometrial or breast cancer is at increased risk). Epidemiologic factors associated with endometrial carcinoma and their relative risks are summarized in Table 58–2.

PATHOPHYSIOLOGY

The typical adenocarcinoma arises from the glandular epithelium of the endometrium, usually within a background of atypical hyperplastic changes. In fact, it is often difficult to pathologically distinguish early invasive disease from severely atypical hyperplasia. Following development of an early cancer, the tumor's growth involves invasion of the endometrial stroma and exophytic expansion within the uterine cavity. With increasing tumor volume and aggressiveness, there is further extension within the endometrial cavity and invasion of the myometrium. Larger tumors can grow down through the cavity to involve the lower uterine segment and cervix.

Tumors that penetrate the myometrium can invade the myometrial lymphatic channels and metastasize to lymph nodes of the pelvic, para-aortic, or inguinal chains. Some lymphatic channels from the fundal portion of the uterus travel within the upper portion of the broad ligament and tend to drain along routes parallel to the ovarian veins (Burke et

Table 58–2. FACTORS ASSOCIATED WITH INCREASED RISK FOR ENDOMETRIAL CANCER

FACTOR	APPROXIMATE RELATIVE RISK*
Demographic Features	
Increasing age/postmenopause	4–8
Caucasian race	2
High socioeconomic status	1.3
European/North American location	2–3
Medical Conditions	
Diabetes mellitus	2.8
Hypertension	1.5
Gallbladder disease	3.7
Obesity	1.8–4
Pelvic irradiation	8
Family history breast/colon/ endometrial cancer	2
Excess Estrogen Stimulation	
Oligo-ovulation/anovulation	
Estrogen-secreting tumors	
Nulliparity	2–3
Early menarche/late menopause	1.6–4
Unopposed estrogen replacement	2–12

*Compared with normal controls. Compiled from Wynder et al (1966), MacMahon (1974), and Davies et al (1981).

al, 1996). Tumor emboli within these lymphatics reach para-aortic nodes near the level of the renal veins. Lymphatic channels that drain along the course of the uterine veins can deposit metastases in the pelvic nodes. Small lymph channels coursing through the round ligament are thought to transport tumor cells to the inguinal nodes, although this is a rare clinical finding. Because multiple routes of lymphatic drainage from the uterus are available, patients with lymph node metastases can have involvement of any single node group as well as combinations of groups. This situation can be contrasted to that seen in cervical cancer, where lymphatic spread usually follows a stepwise progression from pelvic to para-aortic to scalene node groups.

Advanced regional growth gives rise to direct invasion of adjacent pelvic structures, including the bladder, large bowel, vagina, and broad ligament. Tumors that breach the uterine serosa or shed cells into the fallopian tube can gain access to the peritoneal cavity and produce implanted metastases on peritoneal or serosal surfaces throughout the abdomen. Bulky tumors involving the cervix and upper vagina may invade and obstruct the submucosal lymphatic network of the vagina. In this setting, retrograde lymphatic flow may carry metastatic tumor emboli along the length of the vagina. Suburethral tumor nodules in the distal vagina probably result from this mechanism.

Direct vascular invasion and metastasis is relatively uncommon and is usually associated with highly aggressive or advanced tumors. The more common sites of distant hematogenous spread include the lung, brain, liver, and bone.

CLINICAL PRESENTATION

During the early exophytic growth phase of most endometrial cancers, small segments of the tumor outgrow their available blood supply. The areas of resulting necrosis bleed spontaneously, giving rise to the symptom of postmenopausal bleeding. Most women recognize this bleeding as significant and seek prompt medical evaluation. Similarly, most physicians attach equal importance to this symptom and rapidly obtain diagnostic tissue biopsy. It is estimated that one third to one half of women with postmenopausal bleeding will be found to have an endometrial neoplasm. In the remainder, bleeding will be the result of exogenous hormone use, atrophy, minor trauma, polyps, or other benign causes. However, about 90% of women with endometrial cancer present with postmenopausal bleeding. In some women, disease is diagnosed fortuitously when abnormal endometrial cells are noted on cervical cytology smears obtained as part of a routine screening exam (Fig. 58-1).

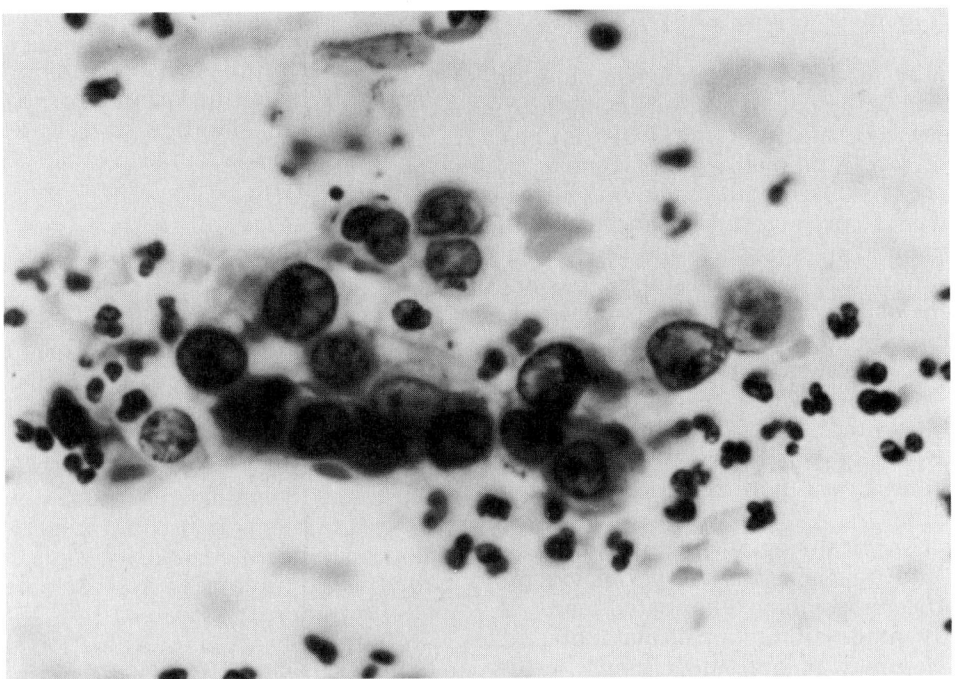

Figure 58-1
Microscopic tumor fragment seen on the Papanicolaou smear of a woman undergoing evaluation for postmenopausal bleeding. Clumps of cells with atypical nuclei, prominent nucleoli, and relatively small amounts of cytoplasm are typical of endometrial adenocarcinomas. Although cervical smears from many endometrial cancer patients contain malignant cells, this method of diagnosis is uncommon in asymptomatic women.

Patients who neglect symptoms or have rapidly progressing tumors demonstrate a wide range of clinical presentations that can be attributed to the extent of regional growth or involvement of other organs by metastases. Lower abdominal pain, pelvic pressure, hematuria, urinary frequency, constipation, rectal bleeding, tenesmus, and hip or back pain may be symptoms of advanced pelvic tumor. Patients with intra-abdominal spread can present with abdominal distention and bloating, early satiety, vague gastrointestinal disturbances, or bowel obstruction. Hematogenous metastases may cause bone pain or fracture, an acute central nervous system event, or hemoptysis.

Most patients with disease limited to the uterine cavity will have minimal or no specific findings on physical examination. Blood or tissue fragments may be seen in the vagina or cervical os and confirm the site of bleeding. If significant exophytic growth has occurred, there may be palpable enlargement of the uterine fundus. Extensive invasion of the cervical stroma will produce an expanded, hard, and irregular cervix that may be difficult to distinguish from a primary cervical cancer. Particular attention should be given to palpation of the superficial inguinal nodes and the vaginal wall. Metastases to these sites, although uncommon, are often missed but easy to feel when a complete detailed examination is performed. Large tumors are simple to detect by examination. The major clinical challenge is to determine the tissue or organ of origin, because a number of advanced pelvic tumors can produce similar examination findings of large mass and obvious erosive tumor.

Diagnosis can be made by histologic sampling of the endometrium by any one of a number of biopsy techniques (Greenwood and Wright 1979; Koss et al, 1982; Grimes, 1986). Traditionally, the diagnosis of endometrial cancer has been made following a fractional dilatation and curettage under anesthesia in the operating room. This approach allowed an accurate pelvic examination under anesthesia, permitted measurement of the length of the endometrial cavity, and obtained separate tissue samples from the endocervix and endometrium. Each of these findings was then incorporated into assigning the patient's disease to a clinical stage category. Additionally, operative curettage was believed to provide a more complete, and hence more accurate, sampling of the uterine lining.

Adoption of a surgical staging system for endometrial cancer and development of specialized instruments for office biopsy have eliminated many of the proposed advantages of fractional dilatation and curettage. The accuracy of outpatient biopsy techniques is virtually identical to that of operative curettage as long as the physician makes a conscientious effort to sample all portions of the uterine cavity. This can be accomplished by making multiple passes with the biopsy instrument and directing the sampling instrument toward each wall of the cavity.

Because most preinvasive and early invasive lesions of the endometrium are proliferative, excess tissue over that normally encountered in the atrophic postmenopausal endometrium should be retrieved by biopsy. Visual inspection of the biopsy specimen to ensure that abundant tissue has been collected is a quick and simple way to assess the adequacy of an outpatient biopsy. Collection of minimal tissue would suggest the absence of a significant endometrial lesion or failure to reach the uterine cavity with the biopsy instrument.

Although office biopsy has become the diagnostic procedure of choice for most patients with endometrial cancer, there are some patients with technical (obese, uncooperative, cervical stenosis) or diagnostic dilemmas who will require a full fractional curettage under anesthesia. In some patients with persistent undiagnosed postmenopausal bleeding, hysteroscopic assessment to target biopsy sites may be advantageous. We do not recommend the use of hysteroscopy for the routine diagnosis of all women with postmenopausal bleeding. However, hysteroscopically directed biopsy may be particularly useful in evaluating the patient whose tumor involves both the endocervix and the endometrium or the patient taking tamoxifen who has an abnormal pelvic examination, ultrasound, or bleeding.

Diagnosis in patients with extensive pelvic tumors can be made with any technique for tissue biopsy. Cervical or vaginal extension can be confirmed by direct or colposcopically directed biopsy. Bladder or rectal invasion can be proven using biopsy through the cystoscope or proctosigmoidoscope. If necessary, metastasis to distant or deep tissue sites can be substantiated by fine-needle aspiration and cytologic evaluation using ultrasound or computerized tomography (CT) (Nordquist et al, 1979; Sevin et al, 1979; Flint et al, 1982; Nash et al, 1987).

PRETHERAPY EVALUATION

Once the diagnosis of endometrial carcinoma has been made, additional pretreatment diagnostic studies should be considered. The focus and complexity of the pretreatment evaluation is tailored to the individual patient presentation. Areas of concern include an attempt to exclude the presence of distant metastases, to evaluate adequate non–tumor-related medical problems that could impact on therapy decision or anticipated toxicity, and, for patients with bulky pelvic tumors, to exclude other pelvic organs as the primary tumor site.

Routine pretreatment evaluation should include a careful history and physical examination, review of biopsy specimens for histologic type and grade, complete blood count, serum electrolytes and glucose, serum renal and hepatic function studies, urinalysis, electrocardiogram, and chest radiograph (Table 58–3). In selected cases, more complex studies may be valuable in confirming the diagnosis or as-

Table 58-3. PRETREATMENT EVALUATION FOR PATIENTS WITH ENDOMETRIAL CANCER

Basic studies
  History and physical examination
  Endometrial biopsy
  Complete blood count
  Serum electrolytes, glucose
  Renal and hepatic serum profiles
  Chest radiograph
  Electrocardiogram
Optional studies
  Cystoscopy
  Proctosigmoidoscopy
  Intravenous pyelogram
  Ultrasonography
  Computerized tomography
  Magnetic resonance imaging
  Lymphangiography
  Fine-needle aspiration

Table 58-4. FIGO CLINICAL STAGING CRITERIA FOR UTERINE CORPUS CANCERS*

Stage IA	Tumor is confined to the uterine corpus. The length of the uterine cavity is 8 cm or less.
Stage IB	Tumor is confined to the corpus. The length of the uterine cavity is greater than 8 cm.
Stage II	The carcinoma has involved the corpus and the cervix, but has not extended outside the uterus.
Stage III	The carcinoma has extended outside the uterus but not outside the true pelvis.
Stage IVA	The carcinoma has spread to the bladder or rectum. Involvement is confirmed by biopsy.
Stage IVB	The carcinoma has spread to distant organs.

*Note: For all stages, the degree of tumor differentiation is evaluated and classified as grade 1 (well differentiated), grade 2 (moderately differentiated), or grade 3 (poorly differentiated).
According to the International Federation of Gynecology and Obstetrics (1971).

sisting in therapy planning. Proctoscopy and cystoscopy should be reserved for patients with large tumors or those with bladder or rectal symptoms. These studies can be used to identify direct invasion of the rectal or bladder mucosa. If suspected, such invasion should be confirmed by biopsy. Intravenous pyelography can identify the presence of ureteral obstruction or urologic anomalies prior to surgical intervention. Barium enema may be helpful in excluding a primary colon tumor or demonstrating extensive diverticular disease. Both CT and lymphangiography can be employed to evaluate pelvic and para-aortic lymph nodes. CT provides a good estimate of nodal size or volume but is inaccurate in identifying small nodal metastases, whereas lymphangiography is a better evaluator of lymph node architecture. Several preliminary studies have suggested that magnetic resonance imaging (MRI) provides a reliable assessment of intrauterine tumor and might be an accurate preoperative predictor of depth of myometrial invasion (Gordon et al, 1989; Yazigi et al, 1989; Harrill et al, 1990). Pelvic ultrasonography appears to be less accurate than MRI for uterine examination (Lehtovirta et al, 1987) and less specific than CT or lymphangiogram for nodal evaluation.

CLINICAL STAGING

The International Federation of Gynecology and Obstetrics (FIGO) adopted its first staging system for endometrial cancer in 1971 (Table 58-4). This clinical staging system uses information obtained from routine pretreatment laboratory and diagnostic studies, careful pelvic examination, uterine sounding, and fractional histologic sampling from the endocervical canal and endometrial cavity. The major prognostic factors incorporated into this system are detectable tumor spread beyond the uterus, tumor extension to

the cervix, and depth of the uterine cavity. Using the clinical staging system, patients are assigned to one of the four FIGO stage groups and receive an additional designation as to the degree of differentiation. Endometrial curettings are examined microscopically and described as well-differentiated (grade 1), moderately differentiated (grade 2), or poorly differentiated (grade 3).

The clinical staging system has the advantage of being based upon relatively simple and straightforward procedures. The required diagnostic evaluation can be adequately performed in a wide variety of clinical settings. This simplicity allows a uniform international approach to staging and permits comparison of treatment results from many different places. However, there are several major problems with the clinical staging of endometrial cancer.

- The criteria for assignment to the major stage groupings are not discriminating. In virtually all large clinical series of patients, 85% to 90% of patients have clinical stage I tumors (Malkasian et al, 1980; Connelly et al, 1982; Hendrickson et al, 1982a; Burke et al, 1990). Within this large collection of patients is a heterogeneous mixture of high-risk subsets not identified by clinical criteria.
- Some components of the clinical staging system have an inherent error rate (Cowles et al, 1985). The depth of the uterine cavity, which was considered to reflect intrauterine tumor volume, is used to distinguish stage IA from IB tumors. Benign uterine pathology such as leiomyomata and adenomyosis may lengthen the cavity but bear no relationship to tumor volume or prognosis. In fact, some have noted no survival differences when comparing clinical stage IA and IB patients (Burke et al, 1990).
- Prehysterectomy sampling techniques generally remove the superficial exophytic fragments of endometrial tumors that project into the cavity. Although these curettings may accurately establish the diagnosis of cancer, they may not accurately

reflect the overall appearance of the tumor. Assignment of histologic grade based upon curettings is often different than that determined by evaluation of tumor from the hysterectomy specimen.

- Similar problems are encountered when trying to assess cervical extension by tumor. Gross invasion of the cervical stroma is usually clinically obvious because the cervix is firm, irregular, and expanded. Surface or microscopic involvement is difficult to detect. Endocervical curettings can easily be contaminated by fragments of tumor that have broken free and are being shed from the endometrial cavity. Extension of the endocervical curet into the lower uterine segment may also result in contamination of the specimen, because the inferior portion of a fundal tumor may be sampled. A precise set of pathologic criteria that is capable of separating contamination from true invasion has been difficult to establish.

SURGICAL STAGING

During the 1970s and early 1980s, an intense effort was made to define additional histopathologic risk factors based upon extended staging procedures done at the time of hysterectomy (Boronow et al, 1984; DiSaia et al, 1985; Morrow et al, 1986). These efforts led to the recognition of a number of prognostic features that were shown to have significant impact on risk of recurrence and survival (Table 58–5). The reliability of these surgically determined factors is thought to be better than that of those used in the clinical staging system.

Detailed analysis of histopathologic variables from the large surgical staging series performed by the Gynecologic Oncology Group demonstrates two key aspects of risk assessment (Morrow et al, 1991). Some factors influence recurrence risk to a greater degree than others: patients with para-aortic lymph node metastases had the poorest outcome. Many patients are found to have multiple high-risk factors; survival is inversely related to the number of risk factors present.

Surgically Determined Prognostic Factors

Histologic Type

Although most endometrial cancers are the typical endometrial adenocarcinomas, a number of rare subtypes are now well described. Each of these variant types have been associated with a treatment failure rate similar to that of the grade 3 adenocarcinomas (Table 58–6). Tumors of variant cell types have a tendency to occur in an older group of postmenopausal women and often demonstrate extrauterine spread at the time of initial diagnosis.

Uterine papillary serous tumors have an exophytic growth pattern with numerous small papillary projections into the endometrial cavity (Fig. 58–2). Psammoma bodies are often present. Histologically, these tumors are identical to papillary serous tumors seen in the ovary or fallopian tube. Despite the well-differentiated histologic appearance of these tumors, they have an aggressive clinical course and commonly present with diffuse intra-abdominal spread or unusual metastases (Fig. 58–3). Five-year survival for clinical stage I patients is only 50% to 60% (Hendrickson et al. 1982b; Jeffrey et al, 1986; Chambers et al, 1987).

Clear cell carcinomas can arise in any female genital tract organ that has a müllerian-derived epithelium. Clear cell tumors comprise a small percentage of cancers of the vagina, cervix, ovary, and uterus. These tumors typically demonstrate clusters of large cells with abundant clear cytoplasm (clear cells), or cystic spaces lined by cells with small amounts of cytoplasm whose nuclei project into the lumen, causing the "hobnail" pattern (Fig. 58–4). Clear cell tumors of the cervix and vagina received great attention during the 1970s, when their association with maternally ingested diethylstilbestrol was recognized. No similar association has been described for endometrial clear cell tumors. Because clear cell tumors can develop in either the endometrium or endocervix, the precise organ of origin can be difficult to establish in more advanced cases. For clinical stage I tumors of known endometrial origin, survival

Table 58–5. SURGICALLY DETERMINED PROGNOSTIC FACTORS

Tumor grade and histology
Depth of myometrial invasion
Extension to cervix or lower uterine segment
Degree of endometrial cavity involvement
Involvement of pelvic and/or para-aortic nodes
Lymph–vascular space invasion
Spread to adnexa
Peritoneal cytology
Intra-abdominal metastasis
Hormone receptor content

Table 58–6. TREATMENT FAILURE FOR VARIOUS HISTOLOGIC TYPES OF ENDOMETRIAL CANCER

HISTOLOGIC TYPE	TREATMENT FAILURE (%)
Endometrial adenocarcinoma	
Grade 1	2.3
Grade 2	5.4
Grade 3	43.6
Papillary adenocarcinoma	32.0
Serous papillary adenocarcinoma	62.5
Clear cell adenocarcinoma	33.3
Adenosquamous carcinoma	16.7

From Burke TW, Heller PB, Woodward JE, et al: Treatment failure in endometrial carcinoma. Obstet Gynecol 1990;75:96, with permission.

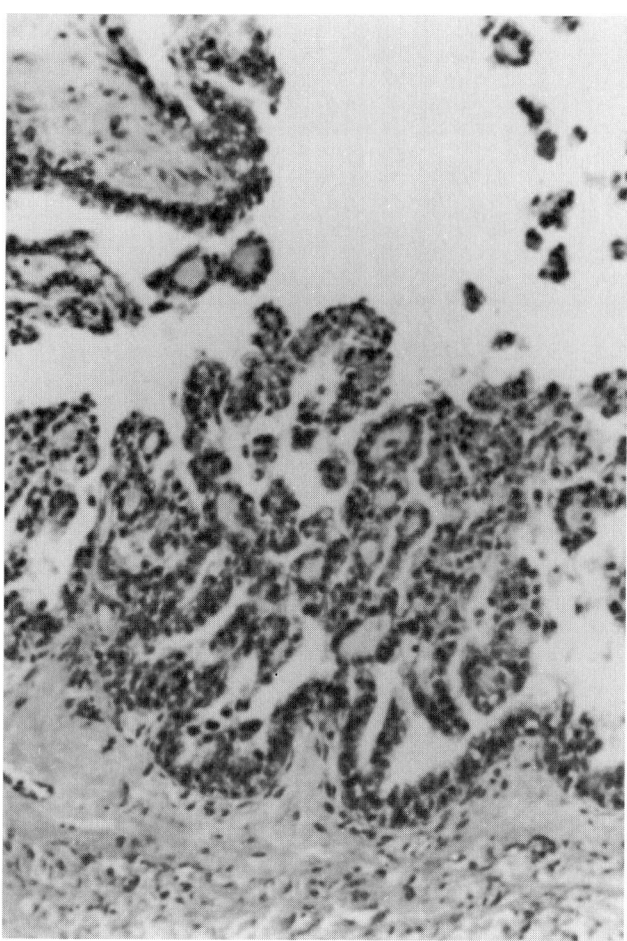

Figure 58–2
Uterine papillary serous carcinoma with an exophytic growth
pattern and small papillary projections similar to those seen in
papillary serous tumors of the ovary. The papillary serous
subtype of endometrial cancer has a propensity for
extrauterine and lymphatic spread.

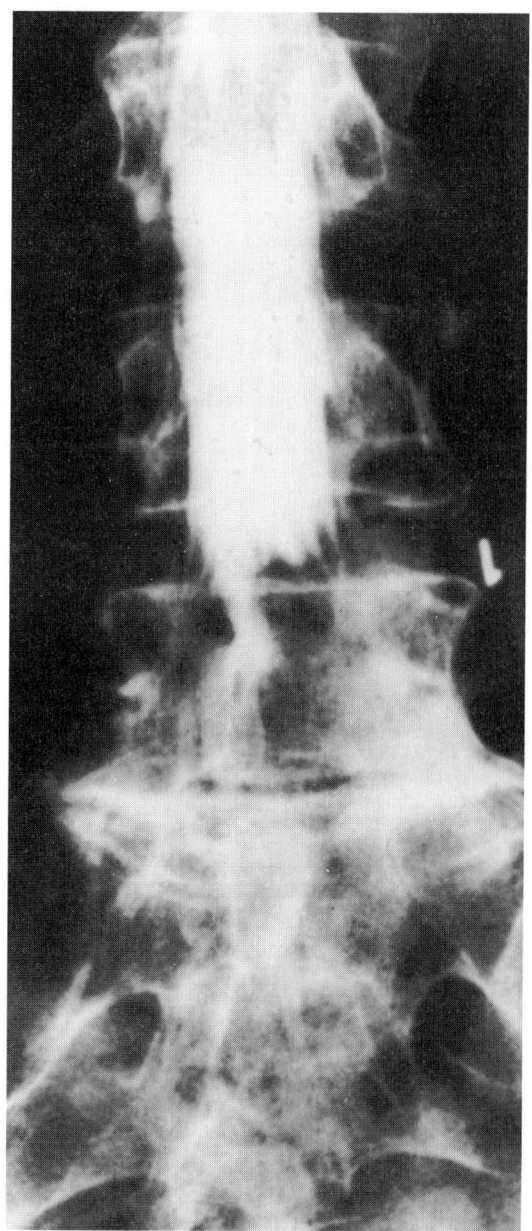

Figure 58–3
Lumbosacral myelogram showing complete occlusion of the
spinal canal at the level of the cauda equina in a patient with
uterine papillary serous carcinoma. Surgical exploration
confirmed the presence of metastatic tumor. These aggressive
endometrial tumors are notorious for their ability to
disseminate widely.

rates of 50% to 70% have been reported (Silverberg
and De Giorgi, 1973; Kurman and Scully, 1976; Christopherson et al, 1982a).

Adenosquamous carcinomas of the endometrium
contain malignant components showing both glandular and squamoid differentiation (Fig. 58–5). It is
currently believed that the squamous elements arise
from metaplastic areas within an adenocarcinoma,
rather than parallel development of two distinct cell
types within one tumor. Prognosis seems to be most
strongly correlated with the histologic grade of the
glandular component. Because most adenosquamous tumors contain poorly differentiated adenocarcinoma, outcomes are comparable to those of
grade 3 typical adenocarcinomas (Ng et al, 1973;
Salazar et al, 1977; Alberhasky et al, 1982).

A more recently described variant is the papillary
endometrioid carcinoma. This tumor has the histologic appearance of typical endometrial adenocarcinoma, but its growth pattern is papillary. It does not
demonstrate the micropapillae or psammoma bodies

seen in the uterine papillar serous tumors. Early
estimates of its clinical behavior suggest an intermediate prognosis between the typical endometrial
adenocarcinoma and the papillary serous variant
(Christopherson et al, 1982b; Sutton et al. 1987).

Histologic Grade

A microscopic evaluation of the degree of tumor differentiation is routinely done for the typical endometrial adenocarcinomas. Two aspects of tumor his-

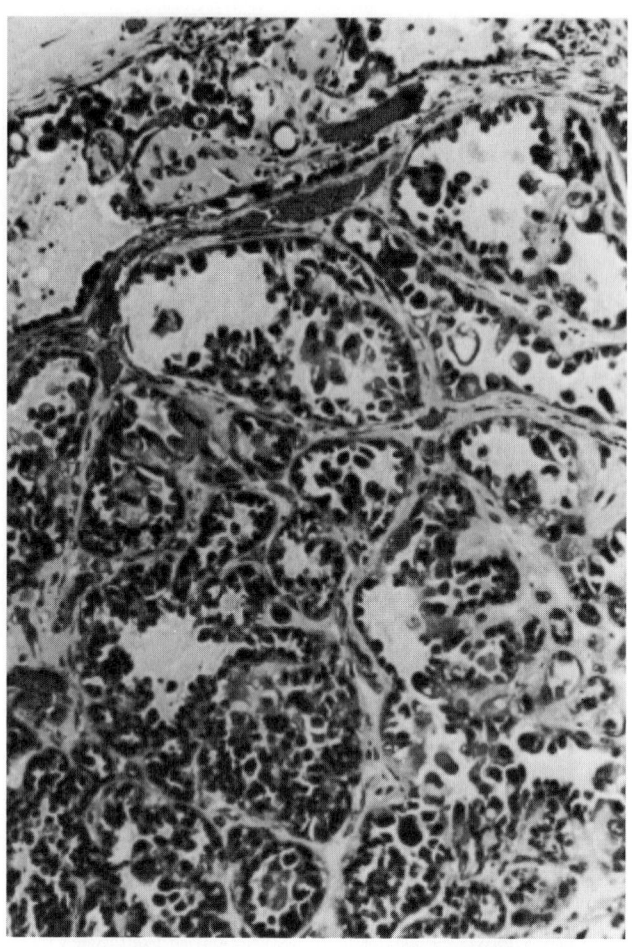

Figure 58–4
Cell nuclei projecting into the lumen of cystic spaces produce the "hobnail" pattern of clear cell carcinoma. Clear cell tumors can arise in any genital tract organ with müllerian epithelium. Endometrial clear cell carcinomas have a high incidence of treatment failure compared to grade 1 adenocarcinomas.

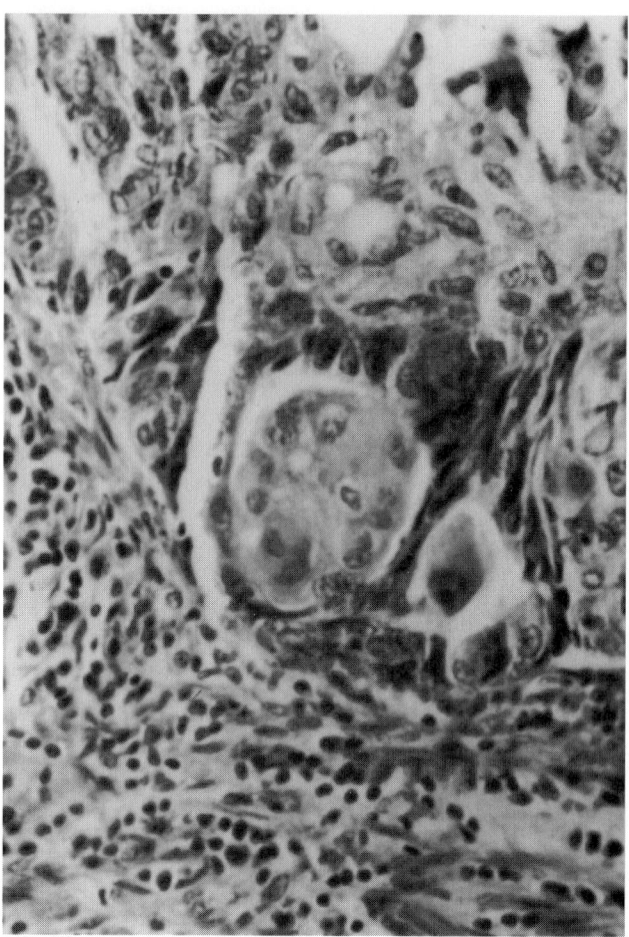

Figure 58–5
Adenosquamous carcinomas contain both malignant glandular (*top*) and squamous (*center*) components. Current thinking is that the squamous elements arise from metaplasia within an adenocarcinoma. Prognosis is probably related to the histologic grade of the glandular component.

tology are normally examined: the portion of the tumor demonstrating a confluent or solid growth pattern and the cytologic atypia of the individual tumor cells (Figs. 58–6 and 58–7). Solid growth component is the major distinguishing characteristic, but surgical staging rules allow for assignment of a higher grade in the presence of significant cytologic atypia. Determination of tumor grade from the hysterectomy specimen allows a more complete examination of the entire tumor and eliminates grading discrepancies based upon uterine curettings. Grade assignment taken from the uterine specimen also permits an averaging of the overall histologic characteristics, because many tumors are heterogeneous and contain both well- and poorly differentiated areas. Staging studies have clearly shown a dramatic and consistent effect of histologic grade upon prognosis, with stage I 5-year survivals of 90% to 95% for grade 1, 80% for grade 2, and 50% for grade 3 (Malkasian, 1978; Malkasian et al, 1980; Connelly et al, 1982; Hendrickson et al, 1982a; Christopherson et al, 1983; Burke et al, 1990). Tumor grading is usually

not possible in patients treated with whole-pelvic external irradiation prior to hysterectomy, because irradiation effects preclude accurate histologic evaluation. Most pathologists do not grade variant cell type tumors, with the exception of assigning a grade to the glandular component of adenosquamous tumors.

Depth of Myometrial Invasion

Risk of lymph node spread, treatment failure, and death from disease are closely related to depth of penetration of the myometrial thickness by tumor (Malkasian et al, 1980; Connelly et al, 1982; Hendrickson et al, 1982a; Christopherson et al, 1983; Burke et al, 1990). Endometrial cancer originates within the endometrial glands, so initial extraglandular growth involves invasion of the endometrial stroma. When further infiltrative growth occurs, the tumor burrows through the muscle of the uterine wall. Most prior studies have categorized endometrial cancers as noninvasive (limited to the endo-

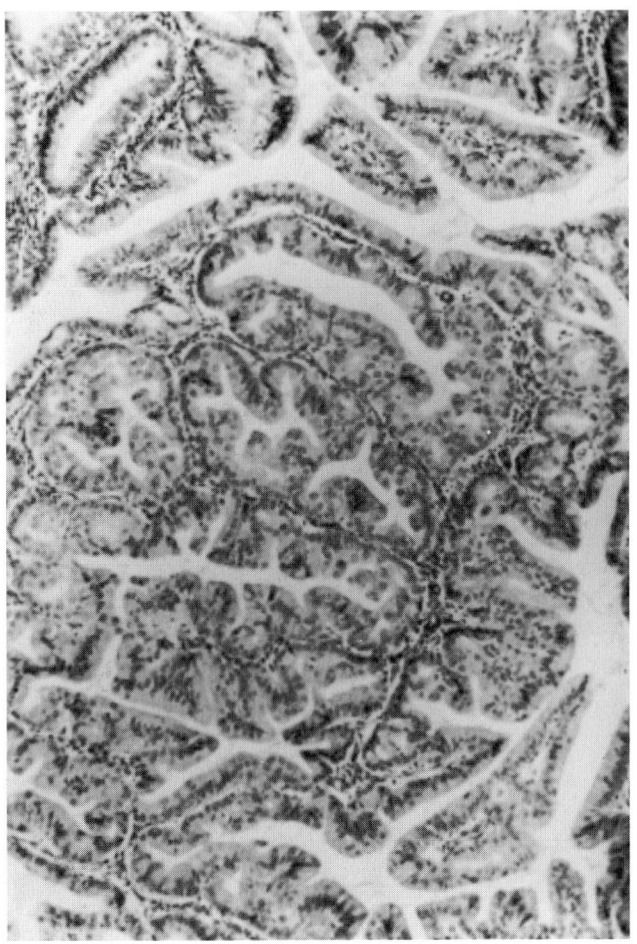

Figure 58–6
Photomicrograph of tumor showing the prominent glandular architecture, intraglandular bridging, and mild atypia that are characteristic of well-differentiated (grade 1) endometrial cancers.

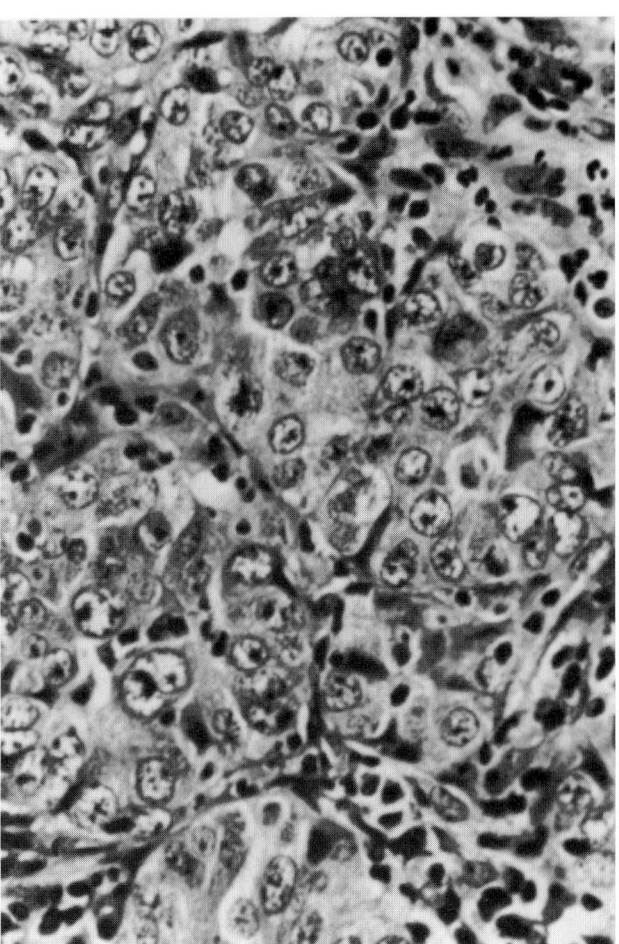

Figure 58–7
Endometrial cancer demonstrating the nuclear atypia and solid growth pattern seen in poorly differentiated tumors. Histologic grade is determined by the percentage of solid growth contained within the tumor.

metrium) or extending to the inner, middle, or outer thirds of the myometrium. This classification is somewhat erroneous in that tumors limited to the endometrium are actually invading stroma and are incorrectly termed *noninvasive*. The new rules for surgical staging separate invasion into endometrium only and inner one half and outer one half of the myometrial thickness. In practice, the most direct approach is to microscopically measure the greatest depth of tumor penetration as well as the total myometrial thickness and report both measurements in the final surgical pathology report.

Depth of invasion can be accurately determined intraoperatively in most cases (Doering et al, 1989). Usually a sharp border between invading tumor and adjacent uterine muscle is visually evident in cut sections from the uterine specimen (Figs. 58–8 and 58–9). Sectioning the uterus in the operating room and grossly measuring an estimated depth of invasion correlates well with final histologic measurement. Frozen section estimates of depth of invasion have also been routinely used intraoperatively or in cases

where the visual estimate is not possible or is difficult to interpret. Intraoperative estimate of depth of invasion can be used to identify patients thought to be low risk on the basis of preoperative assessment but who, in reality, have undetected high-risk features. Detection during surgery allows the surgeon to proceed with a more extensive staging procedure than might be routinely employed in the low-risk case.

Tumor Extension to the Cervix

The clinical staging system relied on endocervical curettage to collect endocervical tumor fragments and predict tumor growth involving the cervix. As discussed earlier, this technique and interpretation of the resulting specimen is highly inaccurate and correlates poorly with results obtained by evaluation of hysterectomy specimens. Surgical staging eliminates these problems and allows precise histologic examination of the cervix using tissue sections. Invasion is classified as involving superficial glands, which

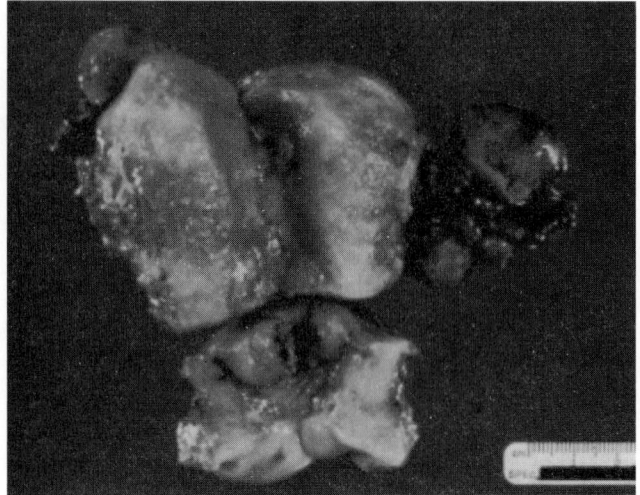

Figure 58-8
Technique for estimating the depth of myometrial invasion intraoperatively. The uterus has been bisected, and a full-thickness segment of myometrium has been excised at the center of the tumor. This tumor arises in the lower uterine segment.

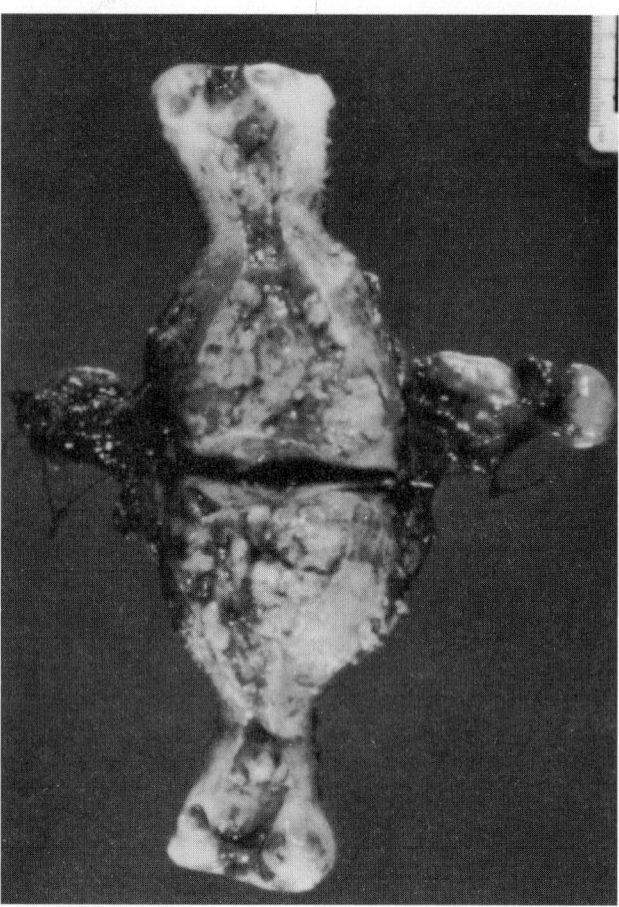

Figure 58-10
The uterus has been bisected to show extensive tumor involvement of the endometrial cavity. Extensive spread within the uterine cavity is a prognostic factor that is easy to assess intraoperatively.

represents surface spreading, or as stromal invasion. Lesions in this latter group are likely to demonstrate clinically detectable evidence of cervical involvement such as barrel-shaped expansion, nodularity, or visible tumor.

Degree of Uterine Cavity Involvement

Several studies have shown that the extent of uterine cavity involvement by tumor can be correlated with outcome (Schink et al, 1987). Complete replacement of the endometrium confers a poorer prognosis (Fig. 58–10). An approximation of percentage of cavity involvement is easy to perform intraoperatively and probably provides an indirect but reliable estimate of tumor volume.

Lymph Node Spread

Uterine fundal lymphatics parallel vessels of the uterine and ovarian systems. Tumors that gain access to the lymphatic system can metastasize to the inguinal, pelvic, and/or para-aortic lymph nodes. The incidence of lymph node spread correlates well with tumor stage, grade, and depth of invasion. Because of the diverse number of possible drainage routes, endometrial tumors can metastasize directly to any node level without involving lower levels. Staging procedures hoping to detect nodal spread must take this into account. Para-aortic node biopsies should be taken near the level of the entry of the ovarian veins into the renal vein and inferior vena cava if this mechanism is suspected. Careful clinical evaluation of inguinal nodes must be done, but, because of the rarity of metastasis to this group, routine bi-

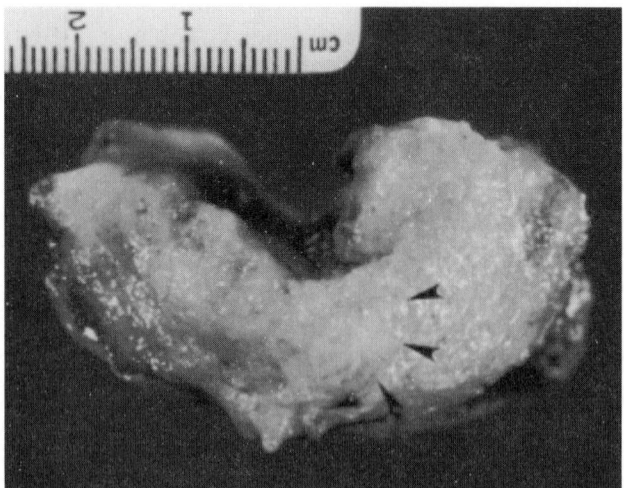

Figure 58-9
The excised segment of uterine wall from Figure 58–8 has an easily identified border between the deeply invasive tumor and adjacent myometrium (*arrows*). Intraoperative estimate of depth of invasion by visual inspection correlates well with final histopathologic results in most cases (Doering et al, 1989).

opsy as part of staging is not recommended. Although any nodal spread is associated with poor prognosis, para-aortic node involvement is associated with a particularly poor prognosis (Morrow et al, 1991). This observation is probably related to the inability to safely deliver effective therapy to this region and the high likelihood of disseminated disease.

Spread to Pelvic Organs

Tumors that have breached the serosal surface of the uterus can directly invade the fallopian tube, ovary, sigmoid colon, or peritoneum (Fig. 58–11). Such extension is usually seen in bulky, locally advanced tumors that can readily be identified at pelvic examination. Extensive regional spread may obstruct regional lymphatic drainage in the vagina. Submucosal vaginal metastases can be seen in this setting and are thought to arise from retrograde lymphatic flow, which carries tumor microemboli away from the uterus and cervix. These vaginal metastases are commonly seen in the vaginal fornices or suburethral areas. Careful palpation of these sites is essential because visible evidence of tumor is often lacking or

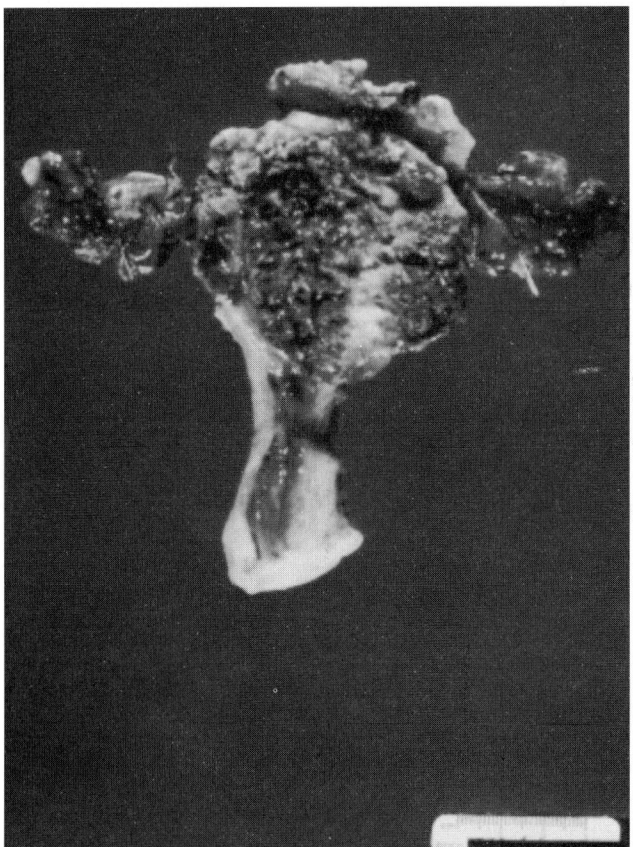

Figure 58–11
This grade 3 adenocarcinoma demonstrates extensive myometrial invasion. The tumor has penetrated the uterine serosa and extends onto the fundus and into the upper left broad ligament.

masked by the position of the speculum. Microscopic involvement of pelvic structures is less common. When seen, microscopic spread is usually associated with multiple other poor prognostic features such as grade 3 histology or deep myometrial invasion.

Intra-abdominal Spread

Tumors extending through the uterine wall can develop implant metastases on any peritoneal or serosal surface in the abdominal cavity. Tumor implants can be detected by careful abdominal exploration and palpation. Attention should be directed to recesses in the pelvic cul-de-sac and lateral pericolic gutters, the omentum, and the diaphragmatic surfaces. This mode of spread is particularly common in papillary serous tumors.

Peritoneal Cytology

Initial reports examining the prognostic influence of malignant cells within abdominal and pelvic washings provided conflicting information (Harouny et al, 1988; Konski et al, 1988; Lurain et al, 1989; Turner et al, 1989). Some series confirmed a negative effect on survival for patients with positive cytology, whereas others documented no effect once other high-risk features were accounted for. Positive peritoneal cytology is seen in about 10% to 15% of clinical stage I cases. The preponderance of available information suggests that this is an independent risk factor for treatment failure.

Exploration for Operative Staging

The inaccuracies of clinical staging, coupled with a greater emphasis on treatment tailored to patient risk assessment, led FIGO to adopt a surgical staging system for endometrial cancer in 1988 (Creasman, 1990) (Table 58–7). This staging system incorporates many of the prognostic factors discussed above, including depth of myometrial invasion, cervical extension, peritoneal cytology, extension to pelvic organs, and lymph node spread (Creasman, 1990). For all stage groups, tumors are graded by the percentage of solid tumor growth pattern: grade 1, 5% or less; grade 2, 6% to 50%; and grade 3, more than 50%. Tumors that demonstrate marked nuclear and cytologic atypia can be upgraded by one grade. Patients who are not candidates for major surgery and those with advanced disease should still be staged using the FIGO clinical criteria from 1971.

Staging Operation

The staging celiotomy for endometrial cancer has two goals: to provide definitive surgical treatment for patients whose tumors are limited to the uterus, and to obtain specimens that provide prognostic information and identify patients with extrauterine

Table 58–7. FIGO SURGICAL STAGING CRITERIA FOR UTERINE CORPUS CANCERS*

Stage I		The tumor is confined to the uterine corpus.
	IA	The tumor is limited to the endometrium.
	IB	The tumor invades to 1/2 or less of the myometrial thickness.
	IC	The tumor invades to more than 1/2 of the myometrial thickness.
Stage II		The tumor extends to the cervix.
	IIA	Endocervical gland involvement only.
	IIB	Cervical stromal invasion.
Stage III		The tumor demonstrates regional spread.
	IIIA	Tumor invades serosa and/or adnexa and/or positive peritoneal cytology.
	IIIB	Vaginal metastases.
	IIIC	Metastases to pelvic and/or para-aortic lymph nodes.
Stage IV		Advanced pelvic or distant disease is present.
	IVA	Tumor invades bladder and/or bowel mucosa.
	IVB	Distant metastases including intraabdominal sites and/or inguinal lymph nodes.

*Note: For all stages, the degree of tumor differentiation is determined by assessing the percentage of solid tumor growth: 5% or less, grade 1; 6% to 50%, grade 2; more than 50%, grade 3. Patients who are not candidates for surgical staging should be clinically staged using 1971 criteria.
According to the International Federation of Gynecology and Obstetrics (1988).

Table 58–8. COMPONENTS OF STAGING CELIOTOMY FOR ENDOMETRIAL CANCER

Peritoneal cytology
Abdominal exploration
Total hysterectomy
Bilateral salpingo-oophorectomy
Pelvic and para-aortic lymph node sampling
Directed biopsies based upon operative findings
  Omentum
  Diaphragm
  Peritoneum
  Bowel surfaces
  Liver

spread who are at risk for recurrence. Our approach is to begin with a midline vertical abdominal incision. Once the abdomen has been entered, saline washings of the peritoneal cavity, particularly the pelvic peritoneum, are taken and forwarded for cytologic examination. Extrafascial hysterectomy with bilateral salpingo-oophorectomy is then performed. The uterine specimen is sent directly to the pathology laboratory, where it is opened. Inspection of the endometrial cavity will give a rapid assessment of the extent of cavity involvement by tumor. Full-thickness sections are then taken, and a gross estimate of depth of invasion is made. Frozen section analysis for depth of myometrial invasion is used for difficult cases or in situations where the myometrial wall is distorted by leiomyomata or suspected adenomyosis. The surgical procedure is terminated at this point for patients with grade 1 tumors that invade superficially. Tumor samples are submitted for measurement of estrogen and progesterone receptor content.

An extended staging procedure is performed if the patient falls into one of the higher risk subsets. These include those with grade 2 or 3 adenocarcinoma, those with one of the more virulent histologic subtypes, those with grade 1 tumors that show significant myometrial invasion, and those in whom abdominal exploration suggests extrauterine spread. The staging scheme published by FIGO does not define a specific set of procedures for surgical staging operations. We have adopted a surgical approach similar to that used in staging ovarian carcinomas that is designed to provide the greatest chance of detecting extrauterine spread. Lymph nodes from the major pelvic node chains are sampled bilaterally.

An attempt is made to obtain the largest identifiable lymph node from each of the external iliac, hypogastric, obturator, and common iliac groups. Additional lymph node biopsies are obtained from the para-aortic group (Chuang et al, 1995). Because some nodal metastases from endometrial cancer parallel the route of the ovarian vessels, we try to obtain some para-aortic nodes at a level well above the bifurcation.

A careful abdominal exploration is then repeated and areas on the peritoneal, diaphragmatic, or serosal surfaces that look or feel abnormal are biopsied. A generous portion of the infracolic omentum is removed as a biopsy and the procedure is completed (Marino et al, 1995). The components of our extended staging operation are summarized in Table 58–8.

Some surgeons perform a laparoscopic staging procedure that includes peritoneal sampling and selective lymphadenectomy in conjunction with assisted vaginal hysterectomy (Childers et al, 1993). The purported advantages of this technique are shorter hospital stay and more rapid recovery. In the hands of appropriately skilled teams, this approach appears to provide staging information equivalent to that obtained at open laparotomy.

Risks of Surgical Staging

The patient risks associated with surgical staging can be grouped into two categories: immediate complications directly attributable to surgery and delayed complications usually associated with additional postoperative external irradiation. Because hysterectomy is usually performed as the "definitive" treatment for endometrial cancer, the operative risks associated with it are not increased in patients undergoing surgical staging. The immediate surgical risks that can be directly connected to extended staging procedures include ureteral and vascular injuries that occur during lymph node sampling. Several studies have shown that major injuries to these structures are uncommon (Moore et al, 1989; Clarke-Pearson et al, 1991; Orr et al, 1991). Surgical infections do not seem to be increased in patients undergoing staging procedures compared with those treated by hysterectomy alone.

An area of greater concern is the risk of radiation injury to the small bowel in patients who have more extensive intraperitoneal procedures and then receive external beam pelvic radiotherapy. This risk has been identified in uterine cancer patients who undergo transperitoneal surgical staging (Weiser et al, 1989; Corn et al, 1994). As more patients undergo surgical staging procedures, a careful evaluation of these complications needs to be made.

Drawbacks to Surgical Staging

The surgical staging system for endometrial cancer has several liabilities. The staging criteria adopted by FIGO do not specify a required set of minimum procedures needed to adequately determine stage. Consequently, the precise details of what constitutes a staging operation are left to the discretion of the surgeon. Our approach is to perform a more limited operation consisting of hysterectomy, abdominal exploration, and peritoneal cytology for low-risk patients with superficially invasive grade 1 tumors. A more extended staging procedure that adds peritoneal biopsies, lymph node sampling, and partial omentectomy is used for patients with grade 2 or 3 and variant cell type tumors. We have chosen to stratify our approach in the belief that the risks of extended staging procedures are greater than the likelihood of identifying extrauterine disease in patients with low-risk tumors.

Surgical staging is most applicable to patients with tumors clinically confined to the uterus. Detection of small-volume subclinical extrauterine disease in this setting is helpful in establishing the need for further treatment as well as selecting an appropriate adjunctive approach. However, patients with clinically obvious extrauterine disease are usually better treated by individualized combined modality therapy. Primary exploration for surgical staging may not be the most appropriate initial approach in these cases.

Although systematic surgical staging and risk assessment provide useful information, a proven survival benefit has not yet been demonstrated. One interesting review has, however, shown a survival advantage for patients undergoing selective lymphadenectomy as part of a staging procedure (Kilgore et al, 1995). Future evaluations of surgically staged patients need to show that additional therapeutic interventions undertaken on the basis of surgical findings result in a survival advantage for the patients that receive such treatment. If survival for high-risk patients is not enhanced, the effort invested in surgical staging is wasted.

ALTERNATE TREATMENT OPTIONS FOR EARLY DISEASE

Some patients with endometrial cancer are poor candidates for an aggressive abdominal staging opera-

tion. Many are elderly and have longstanding and significant medical conditions that increase their surgical and anesthetic risks. Most commonly seen are hypertension, diabetes mellitus, obesity, renal insufficiency, and chronic obstructive pulmonary disease. Some surgeons have advocated vaginal hysterectomy as an alternate surgical approach particularly applicable to the obese patient (Pratt et al, 1964; Peters et al, 1983; Bloss et al, 1991). Presumably the vaginal approach offers a slightly quicker postoperative recovery and eliminates the potential wound complications associated with an abdominal incision. For patients with tumors confined to the uterus, the curative impact of vaginal hysterectomy should be equal to that of abdominal hysterectomy. Of course, intraperitoneal exploration and staging is not possible for patients undergoing vaginal hysterectomy unless simultaneous laparoscopy is performed. It is our impression that vaginal hysterectomy in the obese patient is commonly a difficult operation with exposure problems equal to those encountered by the abdominal approach. Even though lymph node sampling and additional staging biopsies may not be technically possible, we prefer to perform abdominal hysterectomy, which consistently ensures ovarian removal, abdominal exploration, and collection of cytologic specimens. Nevertheless, vaginal hysterectomy is a reasonable option in selected patients, particularly those with grade 1 tumors.

Patients who are thought to be unacceptable candidates for general anesthesia and surgical resection can be treated with radiotherapy alone. Survival rates of 55% to 70% have been reported in patients treated with radiotherapy alone (Landgren et al, 1976; Andersen et al, 1983; Kupelian et al, 1993). Techniques employed usually include multiple brachytherapy applications. Uterine packing techniques, such as Heyman or Simon capsules, appear to provide better results than a linear tandem. Presumably, the dose distribution from the capsule sources provides better coverage and greater delivered dose to the bulk of the tumor present in the uterine fundus (Wollin et al, 1982).

Although radiotherapy alone is often successful in eradicating stage 1 tumors, surgical resection provides superior cure rates and should be the treatment of choice in patients with suspected early disease. Because of this difference in curative potential, we are usually willing to accept a higher rate of surgical morbidity and mortality for the poor-risk patient. Radiotherapy is reserved for the very rare patient whose operative risk is believed to be exorbitantly high.

ADJUVANT THERAPY

A wide variety of adjuvant therapy options have been advocated for patients with early endometrial cancer (Table 58–9). The predominant approach is to identify a high-risk subset of patients on the basis of

Table 58-9. ADJUVANT THERAPY OPTIONS FOR PATIENTS WITH HIGH-RISK TUMORS

Radiotherapy	Brachytherapy
	Whole-pelvis external beam
	Pelvis with extended field
	Whole-abdomen
	Combinations
Hormonal therapy	Progestational agents
	Antiestrogens
	Gonadotropin-releasing hormone analogs
Chemotherapy	Single agent
	Multiple-agent combination
Combined modality	Many possible approaches

one or more clinical, pathologic, or surgical findings. Additional treatment is offered to these patients. The type, timing, and duration of therapy vary considerably depending upon the magnitude of the anticipated risk and the biases of the treating physician. In patients who were clinically staged, decisions regarding adjuvant treatment were usually based upon the perceived risk of recurrence. A possible advantage of surgical staging is that additional treatment can be given to patients with proven extrauterine disease and targeted to specific sites of tumor spread. The suggested adjuvant therapy options can be broadly categorized into three major groups: irradiation, hormonal manipulation, and cytotoxic chemotherapy.

Recognizing that the criteria used to select adjuvant therapy are quite variable, one possible treatment algorithm for women with tumors clinically confined to the uterus is outlined in Figure 58–12.

Radiotherapy

The options for adjuvant radiotherapy include brachytherapy, whole-pelvis external beam therapy with or without extended fields, and whole-abdomen irradiation. These treatments can be delivered preoperatively, postoperatively, or in combination. Because treatment failure in early endometrial cancer is uncommon, prospective randomized comparisons of different radiotherapy approaches do not exist. There is evidence to suggest that preoperative or postoperative brachytherapy can reduce the incidence of vaginal apex recurrence from 5% to 8% to 2% to 4% (Morrow and Townsend, 1987). Radiotherapeutic treatment of the upper vagina by either technique provides excellent results and is associated with few complications (Underwood et al, 1977; Delmore et al, 1987). Some recommend treatment of all patients, whereas others limit treatment to patients with high-grade tumors, deep myometrial invasion, or extension to the lower uterine segment.

Whole-pelvis external beam therapy provides treatment to the pelvic peritoneal surfaces and pelvic

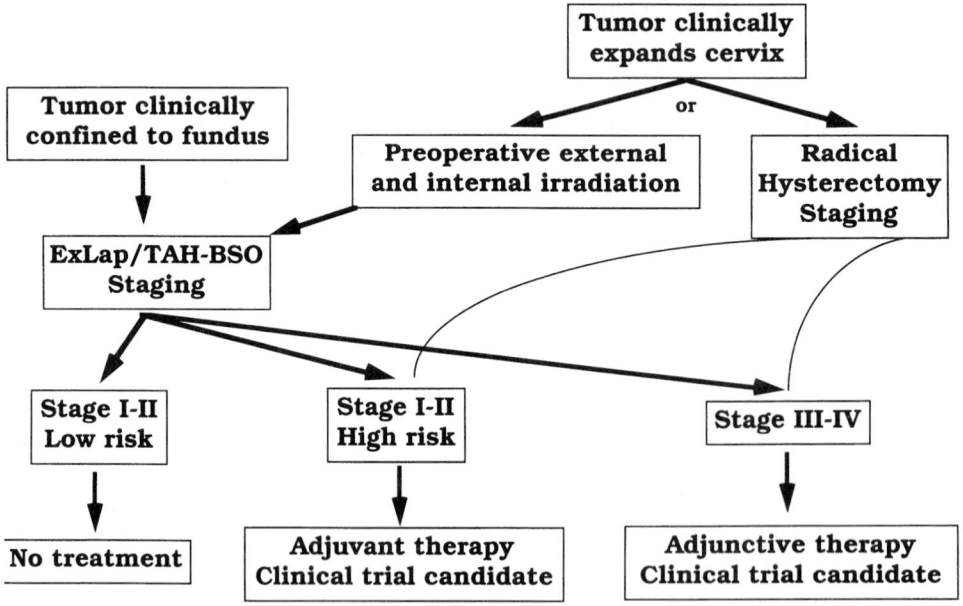

Figure 58-12

Treatment algorithm for women with clinically limited disease (no extrauterine disease detected clinically). Patients with clinically evident endocervical extension receive preoperative irradiation. Following hysterectomy and surgical staging, the FIGO stage assignment is made. Women with low-risk tumors receive no further therapy, whereas those in high-risk categories are candidates for adjuvant therapy trials. Women with advanced surgical stage are considered for adjunctive therapy based upon the location and extent of their disease. ExLap, exploratory laparotomy; TAH-BSO, total abdominal hysterectomy–bilateral salpingo-oophorectomy.

lymph nodes. Advocates of this treatment recommend its use in patients with metastases within the pelvis or positive pelvic nodes (Chung et al, 1981; Ritcher et al, 1981; Chambers et al, 1985; Meerwaldt et al, 1989). A large randomized Norwegian study demonstrated reduced pelvic failures in patients receiving whole-pelvis irradiation, but could not show a significant improvment in survival (Onsrud et al, 1976; Aalders et al 1980). Patients with extrauterine disease often succumb to distant failure even though distant sites of spread are not initially detected. The main impact of whole-pelvis treatment may be improved regional control of tumor.

There are few reports describing patients treated with extended-field (para-aortic) irradiation or whole-abdomen radiotherapy (Komaki et al, 1983; Potish et al, 1985b; Corn et al, 1992; Rose et al, 1992). All report rare patients with proven metastases who achieved long-term survival. The success of large-field irradiation seems to be limited to patients with small tumor volumes (Greer and Hamberger, 1983; Potish et al, 1985a).

Hormonal Manipulation

Some endometrial cancers produce receptor proteins for estrogen and progesterone hormones. In general, low-grade tumors are more likely to be receptor positive (Creasman et al, 1980; Ehrlich et al, 1981; Liao et al, 1986). The normal endometrial gland proliferates in response to estrogen stimulation and matures under progesterone exposure. The therapeutic implications are that estrogenic stimulation has the potential to enhance tumor growth, whereas progestational therapy can arrest or reverse tumor proliferation (Creasman et al, 1985; Ehrlich et al, 1988). Most attempts at therapy have employed an approach that uses chronic high-dose treatment with progestational agents. Progestational therapy is often given empirically to patients following hysterectomy. A large prospective randomized study from the Norwegian Radium Hospital involving over 1100 patients failed to identify a benefit for postoperative adjuvant progesterone therapy (Vergote et al, 1989).

The new gonadotropin-releasing hormone antagonists may offer an additional option for hormonal manipulation by suppressing release of luteinizing and follicle-stimulating hormones. This suppression may modify the hormone receptor content of the tumor and influence growth by an indirect mechanism. These manipulations would be likely to alter the hormonal response of the tumor. At present, the therapeutic value of these newer agents is uncertain.

Chemotherapy

Cytotoxic chemotherapy has been used only rarely as an adjuvant treatment for endometrial cancer. The Gynecologic Oncology Group performed a randomized trial comparing adjuvant whole-pelvis irradiation with or without doxorubicin chemotherapy in patients with high-risk stage I disease (Morrow et al, 1990). They were unable to demonstrate an advantage in the doxorubicin-treated group. A nonrandomized adjuvant study using the combination of cisplatin, doxorubicin, and cyclophosphamide as adjuvant therapy in a similar group of high-risk patients suggested a survival advantage (Stringer et al, 1990). Increased survival was most significant in patients without extrauterine disease. Two additional nonrandomized trials using combination therapy have also reported higher than expected survivals (O'Brien and Killackey, 1994; Jennings et al, 1993). The current role of adjuvant chemotherapy is undefined and requires further study.

TREATMENT OF CLINICALLY ADVANCED DISEASE

The preceding treatment section focused on patients whose tumors were clinically limited to the uterus at the time of presentation. Although some of these patients will be shown to have extrauterine disease at surgical exploration, the volume of such disease is usually small and lends itself to adjuvant or adjunctive therapeutic approaches. Patients with extensive bulky tumors or those with clinically detected metastatic disease at the time of initial presentation offer significant therapeutic challenges. Long-term survival in this group of patients is uncommon. Treatment decision are usually highly individualized. Potential treatment options are outlined in the algorithm shown in Figure 58–13. The primary goals of treatment should focus on control of pelvic tumor and relief of symptoms caused by metastatic disease. A mutlimodality treatment approach is often indicated.

A reasonable attempt at curative therapy can be undertaken in patients with stage II or III tumors confined to the pelvis (Hernandez et al, 1978; Kinsella et al, 1980; Onsrud et al, 1982; Wallin et al, 1984). Despite the adoption of surgical staging criteria, most gynecologic oncologists prefer initial treatment of pelvic disease by external irradiation and brachytherapy. Extrafascial hysterectomy, bilateral salpingo-oophorectomy, and abdominal exploration can be accomplished 4 to 6 weeks after the completion of radiotherapy. The rationale for this approach is that preoperative radiotherapy reduces the volume of the central pelvic disease and simultaneously treats pelvic lymph nodes, adnexal organs, and the pelvic peritoneum. Tumor that has undergone significant regression is more likely to be resectable, and there may be less frequent need to partially or completely resect adjacent pelvic organs, especially the bladder and sigmoid colon. Although the morbidity of combined therapy can be increased, limiting the external therapy dose to 45 Gy and using a

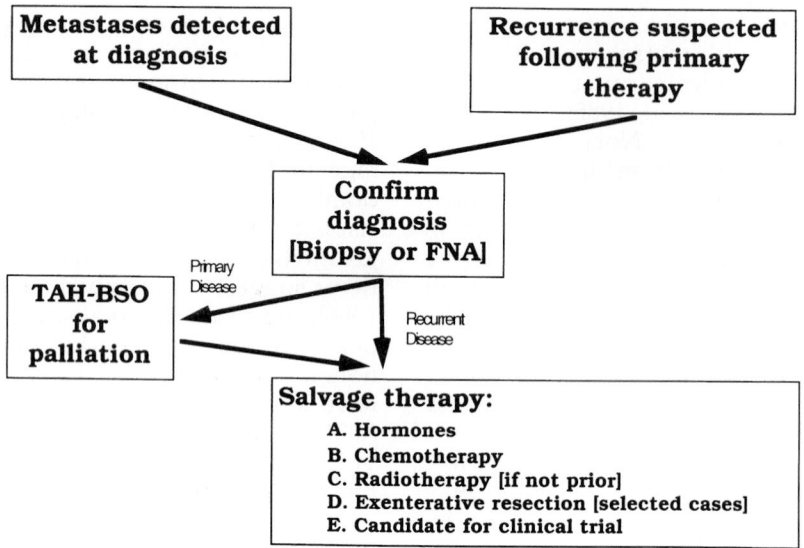

Figure 58-13
Evaluation and treatment algorithm for women with advanced or recurrent endometrial cancer (extrauterine disease detected clinically). Once metastatic disease has been confirmed, salvage therapy can be tailored to the tumor size and location as well as the patient's symptoms. FNA, fine-needle aspiration, TAH-BSO, total abdominal hysterectomy–bilateral salpingo-oophorectomy.

single brachytherapy application result in an acceptable complication rate. Some would argue that patients with disease outside the pelvis will have diagnosis of their extrapelvic disease delayed while they receive pelvic radiotherapy. In truth, the opportunity for long-term cure in patients with substantial extrapelvic disease is neligible with current therapy. Therefore, delay in diagnosis is unlikely to influence outcome. In this setting, control of pelvic disease for palliative benefit is an important consideration and is best achieved with combined treatment.

Some studies describe reasonable survival rates for stage II patients treated by radical hysterectomy alone (Park et al, 1974; Rutledge, 1974). Radical resection has also been attempted in selected stage IVA patients who are candidates for exenterative surgery (Rutledge, 1987). The current trend for advanced disease patients is away from radical surgery and toward combination therapy. Patients who at operation are found to have either extrapelvic or residual pelvic disease can be offered systemic therapy or regional therapy targeted to the operative findings. We generally favor chemotherapy as an initial choice because advanced-stage tumors presenting with bulky disease tend to be poorly differentiated and have a low incidence of steroid hormone receptor positivity.

POST-TREATMENT SURVEILLANCE

If primary therapy for endometrial cancer fails, disease most often recurs within the first 3 years, particularly in patients with advanced stage or high-risk histologic cell types (Burke et al, 1990; Reddoch et al, 1995). Reviews have suggested that routine posttreatment surveillance every 6 to 12 months is appropriate (Shumsky et al, 1994; Berchuck et al, 1995; Reddoch et al, 1995). Physical and pelvic examinations are performed at each visit, as is a Papanicolaou smear taken from the vaginal apex. Serum CA-125 levels are monitored in patients with initial elevations, extrauterine disease, or papillary serous carcinoma and may provide the first hint of recurrence in patients whose tumors produce this antigen (Scambia et al, 1994). Patient education regarding the symptoms of recurrent disease should be provided. Additional diagnostic studies are tailored to patient symptoms, to examination findings, or to sites of perceived recurrence risk based upon initial tumor location.

Patients with endometrial carcinoma have a statistically increased risk for cancers of the breast, ovary, and colon. Part of the follow-up schedule should include careful screening for new tumors at these sites. Each examination should include a diligent physician breast exam, digital rectal exam with stool guaiac test, and bimanual pelvic exam. Breast self-examination should be taught and encouraged. Mammography should be obtained yearly. Colonoscopy should be done about every 5 years.

When an abnormality is detected, additional diagnostic studies and biopsies should confirm the presence of recurrent disease. Pelvic recurrences are usually amenable to direct tissue biopsy of a clinically evident lesion or transvaginal needle biopsy of a low pelvic mass. Deep tissue masses can usually be evaluated with directed fine-needle aspiration biopsy. Cytologic assessment is also helpful in patients presenting with ascites or pleural effusion.

An additional issue related to post-treatment surveillance is the use of estrogen replacement therapy for patients with a history of endometrial cancer. Because estrogenic stimulation has been clearly implicated in the development of these tumors, some have been adamant in recommending that no patient receive estrogen replacement. However, as hormonal replacement therapy has been better evaluated, it seems likely that it provides definite beneficial protection from osteoporosis and heart disease. In patients who have had complete tumor resection by hysterectomy, the neoplastic risk of hormone therapy has been eliminated. In patients with residual disease, there is a theoretical possibility that exogenous estrogen might stimulate growth of residual tumor foci, thus producing symptoms of recurrence and shortening survival time. Exogenous estrogens are not likely to induce new tumor. Two small retrospective studies have examined estrogen replacement therapy in low-risk endometrial cancer patients and shown no apparent increase in recurrence (Creasman et al, 1986; Lee et al, 1990). We believe that patients with low-risk tumors and no extrauterine disease who have been treated by hysterectomy can be safely offered replacement therapy. We routinely use combined estrogen-progestagen or cycled estrogen-progestagen. The addition of a progestational agent may offer protection from breast neoplasms and may reduce the potential to stimulate undetected residual disease. Patients with high-risk tumors or documented extrauterine disease should probably not receive hormonal replacement until risk issues are better clarified.

RECURRENT DISEASE

Recurrent endometrial cancer is a difficult management problem. Rare patients with isolated pelvic recurrences can be salvaged by aggressive therapy. Most patients with extrapelvic recurrence have systemic disease that tends to be refractory to available treatment options. For many patients with recurrence, symptom palliation is the only realistic goal of further therapy. Treatment options and clinical situations for recurrent disease are summarized in Table 58–10.

A small percentage of patients develop single-site recurrences at the vaginal apex or subvaginal tissue beneath the urethra (Brown et al, 1968; Phillips et al, 1982). Presumably these recurrences develop from microemboli in lymphatic channels not included in the primary treatment field or represent implant metastases after hysterectomy. It is important to look for recurrence at these sites, because treatment may still be curative. Depending upon the type and dose of irradiation used in primary treatment, we usually select radiotherapy as the initial option for patients with these recurrences. External beam therapy is given to the region surrounding the recurrence to reduce tumor bulk and sterilize other subclinical metastases. Vaginal cylinders or needle implants can then be placed to deliver a tumoricidal dose of radiation to the residual tumor. Excisional biopsy to reduce initial tumor volume may be valuable in some cases.

Pelvic exenteration can be considered in some patients with central pelvic recurrence, especially when the size or location of the tumor precludes adequate dosing from irradiation (Morris et al, 1996). Older reviews of exenteration for recurrent endometrial cancer suggested that cure rates were substantially lower in patients with recurrent endometrial cancer than those reported for recurrent cervical cancer (Barber and Brunschwig, 1968; Rutledge, 1987). This observation may be related to the different spread patterns of these diseases (i.e., patients with recurrent endometrial cancer are more likely to have disseminated disease), or it may be a function of less-sophisticated preoperative diagnostic studies.

The majority of patients present with distant or disseminated recurrence and are candidates for systemic treatment. Options include hormonal agents or cytotoxic chemotherapy. For most patients these therapies are not curative.

Hormonal Therapy

Hormonal manipulation most often involves the use of progestational agents. Response rates around 30% have consistently been reported for progestins (Reifenstein, 1971; Kohorn, 1976). Response is more likely in patients with grade 1 or receptor-positive tumors; however, responses have been seen in high-

Table 58–10. THERAPY OPTIONS FOR PATIENTS WITH ADVANCED OR RECURRENT ENDOMETRIAL CANCER

THERAPY	INDICATIONS
Radiotherapy	Pelvic failure with no prior irradiation
Radical surgery	Central pelvic failure with prior irradiation, no metastases
Hormonal therapy	Disseminated disease, tumor produces hormone receptors
Chemotherapy	Disseminated disease
Combined modalities	Refractory disseminated disease

grade and receptor-negative tumors. The major advantage of progestational therapy is the ease of administration (oral or parenteral), which allows outpatient management. Side effects are minimal when compared with those from cytotoxic agents. Nevertheless, the risks of deep venous thrombosis and fluid retention should not be ignored, particularly in the elderly patient with cardiovascular disease. Some responses to progestational agents are durable, so therapy should be considered as long as there is no disease progression. Patients who fail one progestational agent are not likely to respond to an alternative drug.

Tamoxifen, an oral antiestrogen used extensively in breast cancer patients, has a 20% to 30% response rate in recurrent endometrial cancer (Swenerton, 1980). Presumably the drug inhibits tumor growth by binding to and tying up the cell's estrogen receptors. Some responses have also been obtained with newer gonadotropin-releasing hormone antagonists. Most responses have been noted in patients with grade 1 tumors that have a long natural history. The mechanism of action for these agents is unclear.

One postulated reason for the lack of response to hormonal therapy is the absence or disappearance of progesterone receptors. Because one of the physiologic functions of estrogen is the stimulation of cell surface progesterone receptors, sequential hormonal therapy employing estrogen or tamoxifen to stimulate receptor production followed by progestational therapy to reverse tumor growth has been proposed. Studies to date have not demonstrated response rates superior to those achievable with progestational therapy alone (Tatman et al, 1989).

Chemotherapy

Evaluation of Chemotherapy

In evaluating the role of systemic chemotherapy in patients with advanced or recurrent endometrial cancers, several basic concepts should be considered, including the observed response rate, type of response, duration of response, and treatment toxicity. Chemotherapeutic response rates are usually expressed as the percentage of patients whose tumors either disappear or shrink significantly during treatment. For recurrent endometrial cancers, response rates above 25% to 30% usually define active drugs or drug combinations. It is important to remember that "response" is not equivalent to "cure."

Duration of response describes the length of time between an observed response to treatment and evidence of further tumor growth. Long response duration is clearly preferable and may provide a significant improvement in survival time for the patient. Short response duration is likely to result in only brief relief of symptoms and minimal increase in survival. Greater emphasis on treatment toxicity and quality-of-life issues has been considered in more recent chemotherapy trials. A toxic drug regimen that produces significant side effects and results in a 4-month partial response may not be particularly valuable to the patient, even though an objective response has occurred.

Success of Chemotherapeutic Agents

A number of chemotherapeutic agents have documented activity against endometrial carcinomas. Single-agent studies from the late 1970s and early 1980s identified cisplatin and doxorubicin as active drugs (Thigpen et al, 1979; Deppe et al, 1980; Seski et al, 1982; Long et al, 1988; Green et al, 1990). Response rates approximated 30% for both drugs, although one study failed to show activity for cisplatin. In subsequent studies that examined the combination of doxorubicin and cyclophosphamide, response rates ranged from 17% to 45% (Muggia et al, 1977; Seski et al, 1981; Horton et al, 1982). More recent studies have concentrated on platinum or platinum combination regimens (Lovecchio et al, 1984; Trope et al, 1984; Pasmantier et al, 1985; Turbow et al, 1985; Edmonson et al, 1987; Burke et al, 1991). Several reports, including our own, have noted excellent response rates for the combination of cisplatin, doxorubicin, and cyclophosphamide. Unfortunately response duration has been short, about 5 to 6 months, and toxicity has been high. In our study the incidence of significant neutropenia was 65%. A recent Gynecologic Oncology Group study using paclitaxel has shown a response rate of 35% in women with untreated recurrent disease (Ball et al, 1996). Further evaluation of paclitaxel combinations is ongoing.

Patients with recurrent endometrial cancer tend to be older and many have pre-existing medical illnesses: they tolerate aggressive chemotherapy poorly. Chemotherapy's benefit to patients with advanced or recurrent disease is unclear. Additional efforts should be directed toward the identification of other active drugs or drug combinations, with particular attention paid to response duration and treatment toxicity issues.

Palliative Treatment

Rare patients with recurrent endometrial cancer will present with local or regional tumor growth that causes severe or life-threatening symptoms. Examples would be a patient with pulmonary metastases compressing a mainstream bronchus or a patient with pelvic wall recurrence eroding or obstructing the sigmoid colon. Judicious use of external irradiation or surgical therapy in these settings may markedly improve quality of life, but it is not curative.

Palliative external irradiation can be delivered to virtually any body site. Typically, doses of 20 to 30 Gy are given over 1 to 2 weeks. The treatment field can be specifically designed to incorporate the tumor site producing the problem. The goal of therapy is to rapidly shrink the tumor and relieve symptoms. This approach is well suited to tumor masses that compress adjacent critical structures; it can often relieve shortness of breath caused by lung or mediastinal metastases and pain from nerve root compression from pelvic or aortic node metastases. Significant symptoms from brain or bone metastases may also be relieved by external beam irradiation.

Palliative radiotherapy may also control bleeding from large pelvic tumors. When bleeding originates from exophytic tumor growth within the vaginal cavity, control can be achieved with transvaginal application of low-energy irradiation. We typically give two 5-Gy doses over 2 days. Bleeding is usually effectively controlled within 5 to 7 days. Bleeding that originates higher in the pelvis may be reduced using a single 10-Gy fraction delivered externally using a high-energy source. The treatment field should be designed to incorporate the major bulk of the tumor. If effective, this technique can be repeated in a month.

Palliative surgical efforts are largely directed toward correction of major gastrointestinal problems. Small bowel obstruction is most often caused by intraperitoneal tumor and usually represents multiple levels of partial obstruction. Surgical intervention in these cases is unrewarding because it is not possible to adequately relieve obstruction, and the patient's life expectancy is limited. However, percutaneous or operative placement of a gastrostomy tube may assist in the management of chronic obstruction and greatly reduce nausea and vomiting as well as the discomfort associated with long-term nasogastric tube drainage.

Large bowel obstruction or fistula formation sometimes occurs when bulky pelvic tumor invades or encircles the rectosigmoid colon. In patients with good functional status and a reasonable life expectancy, usually greater than 2 months, exploration for palliative diversion by colostomy may substantially improve quality of life. If the effluent from a small bowel fistula causes skin erosion and pain, palliative diversion, resection, or bypass can be considered. Patient selection in this situation is critical because small bowel fistulas usually signify extensive abdominal tumor, and surgical correction of these fistulas can be complicated.

In general, palliative surgery should only be considered in the patient with significant symptoms, a reasonable projected survival time, and a problem that is localized. The surgical approach should employ the simplest and most direct method of correcting the immediate problem. Exposing the terminal patient to an extended and potentially morbid operation simply expends her remaining survival time and energy on surgical recover.

REFERENCES

Aalders J, Abeler V, Kolstad P, Onsrud M: Postoperative external irradiation and prognostic parameters in stage I endometrial carcinoma. Obstet Gynecol 1980;56:419.

Alberhasky RC, Connelly PJ, Christopherson WM: Carcinoma of the endometrium. IV. Mixed adenosquamous carcinoma: a clinical-pathological study of 68 cases with long-term follow-up. Am J Clin Pathol 1982;77:655.

American College of Obstetricians and Gynecologists: Tamoxifen and endometrial cancer (ACOG Committee Opinion No. 169). Int J Obstet Gynecol 1996;53:197.

Andersen WA, Peters WA III, Fechner RE, et al: Radiotherapeutic alternatives to standard management of adenocarcinoma of the endometrium. Gynecol Oncol 1983;16:383.

Antunes CMF, Stolley PD, Rosenshein NB, et al: Endometrial cancer and estrogen use: report of a large case-control study. N Engl J Med 1979;300:9.

Ball HG, Blessing JA, Lentz SS, Mutch DG: A Phase II trial of paclitaxel in patients with advanced or recurrent adenocarcinoma of the endometrium: a Gynecologic Oncology Group study. Gynecol Oncol 1996;62:278.

Barakat RR, Wong G, Curtin JP, et al: Tamoxifen use in breast cancer patients who subsequently develop corpus cancer is not associated with a higher incidence of adverse histologic features. Gynecol Oncol 1994;95:164.

Barber HRK, Brunschwig A: Treatment and results of recurrent cancer of corpus uteri in patients receiving anterior and total pelvic exenteration 1947–1963. Cancer 1968;22:949.

Berchuck A, Anspach C, Evans EC, et al: Postsurgical surveillance of patients with FIGO stage I/II endometrial adenocarcinoma. Gynecol Oncol 1995;59:20.

Bloss JD, Berman ML, Bloss LP, Buller RE: Use of vaginal hysterectomy for the management of stage I endometrial cancer in the medically compromised patient. Gynecol Oncol 1991;40:74.

Boronow RC: Endometrial cancer: not a benign disease. Obstet Gynecol 1976;47:630.

Boronow RC, Morrow CP, Creasman WT, et al: Surgical staging in endometrial cancer: clinical-pathologic findings of a prospective study. Obstet Gynecol 1984;63:823.

Brinton LA, Berman ML, Mortel R, et al: Reproductive menstrual, and medical risk factors for endometrial cancer: results from a case control study. Am J Obstet Gynecol 1992;167:1317.

Brown JM, Dockerty MB, Symmonds RE, Banner EA: Vaginal recurrence of endometrial carcinoma. Am J Obstet Gynecol 1968;100:544.

Burke TW, Heller PB, Woodward JE, et al: Treatment failure in endometrial carcinoma. Obstet Gynecol 1990;75:96.

Burke TW, Levenback C, Tornos C, et al: Intraabdominal lymphatic mapping to direct selective pelvic and paraaortic lymphadenectomy in women with high-risk endometrial cancer: results of a pilot study. Gynecol Oncol 1996;62:169.

Burke TW, Stringer CA, Morris M, et al: Prospective treatment of advanced or recurrent endometrial carcinoma with cisplatin, doxorubicin and cyclophosphamide. Gynecol Oncol 1991;40:264.

Chambers JT, Kapp DS, Lawrence R, et al: Immediate versus delayed hysterectomy for endometrial carcinoma: surgical morbidity and hospital stay. Obstet Gynecol 1985;65:245.

Chambers JT, Merino M, Kohorn EI, et al: Uterine serous papillary carcinoma. Obstet Gynecol 1987;69:109.

Childers JN, Brzechffa PR, Hatch KD, Surwitt EA: Laparoscopic assisted surgical staging (LASS) of endometrial carcinoma. Gynecol Oncol 1993;51:33.

Christopherson WM, Alberhasky RC, Conelly PJ: Carcinoma of the endometrium. I. A clinicopathologic study of clear-cell carcinoma and secretory carcinoma. Cancer 1982a;49:1511.

Christopherson WM, Alberhasky RC, Connelly PJ: Carcinoma of the endometrium. II. Papillary adenocarcinoma: a clinical pathological study of 46 cases. Am J Clin Pathol 1982b;77:534.

Christopherson WM, Connelly PJ, Alberhasky RC: Carcinoma of the endometrium. V. An analysis of prognosticators in patients with favorable subtypes and stage I disease. Cancer 1983;51:1705.

Chuang L, Burke TW, Tornos C, et al: Staging laparotomy for endometrial carcinoma: assessment of retroperitoneal lymph nodes. Gynecol Oncol 1995;58:189.

Chung CK, Stryker JA, Nahhas WA, Mortel R: The role of adjunctive radiotherapy for stage I endometrial carcinoma: preoperative vs postoperative irradiation. Int J Radiat Oncol Biol Phys 1981;7:1429.

Clarke-Pearson D, Cliby W, Soper J, et al: Morbidity and mortality of selective lymphadenectomy in early stage endometrial cancer [abstract]. Proc Soc Gynecol Oncol 1991;32:14.

Connelly PJ, Alberhasky RC, Christopherson WM: Carcinoma of the endometrium. III. Analysis of 865 cases of adenocarcinoma and adenoacanthoma. Obstet Gynecol 1982;59:569.

Cook LS, Weiss NS, Schwartz SM, et al: Population-based study of tamoxifen therapy and subsequent ovarian, endometrial, and breast cancers. J Natl Cancer Inst 1995;87:1359.

Corn BW, Lanciano RM, Greven KM, et al: Endometrial cancer with para-aortic adenopathy: patterns of failure and opportunities for cure. Int J Radiat Oncol Biol Phys 1992;24:223.

Corn BW, Lanciano RM, Greven KM, et al: Impact of improved irradiation technique, age, and lymph node sampling on the severe complication rate of surgically staged endometrial cancer patients: a multivariate analysis. J Clin Oncol 1994;12:510.

Cowles TA, Magrina JF, Masterson BJ, Capen CV: Comparison of clinical and surgical staging in patients with endometrial carcinoma. Obstet Gynecol 1985;66:413.

Creasman WT: New gynecologic cancer staging. Obstet Gynecol 1990;75:287.

Creasman WT, Henderson D, Hinshaw W, Clark-Pearson DL: Estrogen replacement therapy in the patient treated for endometrial cancer. Obstet Gynecol 1986;67:326.

Creasman WT, McCarty KS, Barton TK, McCarty KS Jr: Clinical correlates of estrogen and progesterone-binding proteins in human endometrial adenocarcinoma. Obstet Gynecol 1980;55:363.

Creasman WT, Soper JT, McCarty KS Jr, et al: Influence of cytoplasmic steroid receptor content on prognosis of early stage endometrial carcinoma. Am J Obstet Gynecol 1985;51:922.

Cuenca RE, Giachino J, Arredondo MA, et al: Endometrial carcinoma associated with breast carcinoma. Cancer 1996;77:2058.

Davies JL, Rosenshein NB, Antunes CMF, Stolley PD: A review of the risk factors for endometrial carcinoma. Obstet Gynecol Surv 1981;36:107.

Delmore JE, Wharton JT, Hamberger AD, et al: Preoperative radiotherapy for early endometrial carcinoma. Gynecol Oncol 1987;28:34.

Deppe G, Cohen CJ, Bruckner HW: Treatment of advanced endometrial adenocarcinoma with cis-dichlorodiamine platinum (II) after intensive prior therapy. Gynecol Oncol 1980;10:51.

DiSaia PJ, Creasman WT, Boronow RC, Blessing JA: Risk factors and recurrence patterns in stage I endometrial cancer. Am J Obstet Gynecol 1985;151:1009.

Doering DL, Barnhill DR, Weiser EB, et al: Intraoperative evaluation of depth of myometrial invasion in stage I endometrial adenocarcinoma. Obstet Gynecol 1989;74:930.

Edmonson JH, Krook JE, Hilton JF, et al: Randomized Phase II studies of cisplatin and a combination of cyclophosphamide-doxorubicin-cisplatin (CAP) in patients with progestin-refractory advanced endometrial carcinoma. Gynecol Oncol 1987;28:20.

Ehrlich CE, Young PCM, Cleary RE: Cytoplasmic progesterone and estradiol receptors in normal, hyperplastic, and carcinomatous endometria: therapeutic implications. Am J Obstet Gynecol 1981;141:539.

Ehrlich CE, Young PCM, Stehman FB, et al: Steroid receptors and clinical outcome in patients with adenocarcinoma of the endometrium. Am J Obstet Gynecol 1988;158:796.

Ernster VL, Bush TL, Huggins GR, et al: Benefits and risks of menopausal estrogen and/or progestin hormone use. Prev Med 1988;17:201.

Flint A, Terhart K, Murad TM, Taylor PT: Confirmation of metastases by fine needle aspiration biopsy in patients with gynecologic malignancies. Gynecol Oncol 1982;14:382.

Fornander T, Hellstrom A-C, Moberger B: Descriptive clinicopathologic study of 17 patients with endometrial cancer during or after adjuvant tamoxifen in early breast cancer. J Natl Cancer Inst 1993;85:1850.

Gordon AN, Fleischer AC, Dudley BS, et al: Preoperative assessment of myometrial invasion of endometrial adenocarcinoma by sonography (US) and magnetic resonance imaging (MRI). Gynecol Oncol 1989;34:175.

Gray LA, Christopherson WM, Hoover RN: Estrogens and endometrial cancer. Obstet Gynecol 1977;49:385.

Green JB, Green S, Alberts DS, et al: Carboplatin therapy in advanced endometrial cancer. Obstet Gynecol 1990;75:696.

Greenwood SM, Wright DJ: Evaluation of the office endometrial biopsy in the detection of endometrial carcinoma and atypical hyperplasia. Cancer 1979;43:1474.

Greer BE, Hamberger AD: Treatment of intraperitoneal metastatic adenocarcinoma of the endometrium by the whole-abdomen moving-strip technique and pelvic boost irradiation. Gynecol Oncol 1983;16:365.

Grimes DA: Diagnostic office curettage—heresy no longer. Contemp Obstet Gynecol 1986;28:96.

Harouny VR, Sutton GP, Clark SA, et al: The importance of peritoneal cytology in endometrial carcinoma. Obstet Gynecol 1988;72:394.

Harrill CD, Kopecky KK, Weaver SR, Sutton GP: Magnetic resonance imaging in the preoperative assessment of clinical stage I endometrial carcinoma. Comput Med Imaging Graph 1990;14:191.

Hendrickson M, Ross J, Eifel P, et al: Adenocarcinoma of the endometrium: analysis of 256 cases with carcinoma limited to the uterine corpus. Gynecol Oncol 1982a;13:373.

Hendrickson M, Ross J, Eifel P, et al: Uterine papillary serous carcinoma: a highly malignant form of endometrial adenocarcinoma. Am J Surg Pathol 1982b;6:93.

Hernandez W, Nolan JF, Morrow CP, Jernstrom PH: Stage II endometrial carcinoma: two modalities of treatment. Am J Obstet Gynecol 1978;131:171.

Horton J, Elson P, Gordon P, et al: Combination chemothrapy for advanced endometrial cancer. Cancer 1982;49:2441.

International Federation of Gynecology and Obstetrics: Classification and staging of malignant tumors in the female pelvis. Acta Obstet Gynecol Scand 1971;50:1.

Jeffrey JF, Krepart GV, Lotocki RJ: Papillary serous adenocarcinoma of the endometrium. Obstet Gynecol 1986;67:670.

Jennings S, Dottino P, Johnston C, Cohen C: Adjuvant displatin, doxorubicin, and etoposide and pelvic radiotherapy for advanced stage or virulent subtypes of endometrial cancer [abstract]. Proc Am Soc Clin Oncol 1993;12:268.

Kilgore L, Partridge E, Alvarez R, et al: Adenocarcinoma of the endometrium: survival comparisons of patients with and without pelvic node biopsies. Gynecol Oncol 1995;56:29.

Killackey MA, Hakes TB, Pierce VK: Endometrial adenocarcinoma in breast cancer patients receiving antiestrogens. Cancer Treatment Reports 1985;69:237.

Kinsella TJ, Bloomer WD, Lavin PT, Knapp RC: Stage II endometrial carcinoma: 10-year follow-up of combined radiation and surgical treatment. Gynecol Oncol 1980;10:290.

Kohorn EI: Gestagens and endometrial carcinoma. Gynecol Oncol 1976;4:398.

Komaki R, Mattingly RF, Hoffman RG, et al: Irradiation of paraaortic lymph node metastases from carcinoma of the cervix or endometrium. Radiology 1983;147:245.

Konski A, Poulter C, Keys H, et al: Absence of prognostic significance, peritoneal dissemination and treatment advantage in endometrial cancer patients with positive peritoneal cytology. Int J Radiat Biol Phys 1988;14:49.

Koss LG, Schreiber K, Moussouris H, Oberlander SG: Endometrial carcinoma and its precursors: detection and screening. Clin Obstet Gynecol 1982;25:44.

Kupelian PA, Eifel PJ, Tornos C, et al: Treatment of endometrial carcinoma with radiation therapy alone. Int J Radiat Oncol Biol Phy 1993;27:817.

Kurman RJ, Scully RE: Clear cell carcinoma of the endometrium: an analysis of 21 cases. Cancer 1976;37:872.

Landgren RC, Fletcher GH, Delclos L, Wharton JT: Irradiation of endometrial cancer in patients with medical contraindication to surgery or with unresectable lesions. Am J Roentgenol 1976;126:148.

Lee RB, Burke TW, Park RC: Estrogen replacement therapy following treatment for stage I endometrial carcinoma. Gynecol Oncol 1990;36:189.

Lehtovirta P, Cacciatore B, Wahlstrom T, Ylostalo P: Ultrasonic assessment of endometrial cancer invasion. J Clin Ultrasound 1987;15:519.

Liao BS, Twiggs LB, Leung BS, et al: Cytoplasmic estrogen and progesterone receptors as prognostic parameters in primary endometrial carcinoma. Obstet Gynecol 1986;67:463.

Long HJ, Pfeifle DM, Wieand HS, et al: Phase II evaluation of carboplatin in advanced endometrial cancer. J Natl Cancer Inst 1988;80:276.

Lovecchio JL, Averette HE, Lichtinger M, et al: Treatment of advanced or recurrent endometrial adenocarcinoma with cyclophosphamide, doxorubicin, cisplatinum, and megestrol acetate. Obstet Gynecol 1984;63:557.

Lurain JR, Rumsey NK, Schink JC, et al: Prognostic significance of positive peritoneal cytology in clinical stage I adenocarcinoma of the endometrium. Obstet Gynecol 1989;74:175.

Lynch HT, Krush AJ, Larsen AL, Magnuson CW: Endometrial carcinoma: multiple primary malignancies, constitutional factors and heredity. Am J Med Sci 1966;252:381.

Lynch HT, Krush AJ, Thomas RJ, Lynch J: Cancer family syndrome. In Lynch HT (ed): Cancer Genetics. Springfield, IL: Charles C Thomas, 1976:355.

MacMahon B: Risk factors for endometrial cancer. Gynecol Oncol 1974;2:122.

Malkasian GD: Carcinoma of the endometrium: effect of stage and grade on survival. Cancer 1978;41:996.

Malkasian GD, Annegers JF, Fountain KS: Carcinoma of the endometrium: stage I. Am J Obstet Gynecol 1980;136:872.

Marino BD, Burke TW, Tornos C, et al: Staging laparotomy for endometrial carcinoma: assessment of peritoneal spread. Gynecol Oncol 1995;56:34.

Meerwaldt JH, Hoekstra CJM, van Putten WLJ, et al: Endometrial adenocarcinoma, adjuvant radiotherapy tailored to prognostic factors. Int J Radiat Biol Phys 1989;18:299.

Moore DH, Fowler WC Jr, Walton LA, Droegenmueller W: Morbidity of lymph node sampling in cancers of the uterine corpus and cervix. Obstet Gynecol 1989;74:180.

Morris M, Alvarez RD, Kinney WK, Wilson TO: Treatment of recurrent adenocarcinoma of the endometrium with pelvic exenteration. Gynecol Oncol 1996;60:288.

Morrow CP, Bundy BN, Homesley HD, et al: Doxorubicin as an adjuvant following surgery and radiation therapy in patients with high-risk endometrial carcinoma, stage I and occult stage II: a Gynecologic Oncology Group study. Gynecol Oncol 1990; 36:166.

Morrow CP, Bundy BN, Kurman RJ, et al: Relationship between surgical-pathological risk factors and outcome in clinical stage I and II carcinoma of the endometrium: a Gynecologic Oncology Group study. Gynecol Oncol 1991;40:55.

Morrow CP, Creasman WT, Homesley H, et al: Recurrence in endometrial carcinoma as a function of extended surgical staging data. In Morrow CP, Smart G (eds): Gynaecological Oncology: Proceedings of the 2nd International Conference on Gynaecological Cancer. New York: Springer-Verlag, 1986:147.

Morrow CP, Townsend DE: Synopsis of Gynecologic Oncology. New York: Churchill Livingstone, 1987.

Muggia FM, Chia G, Reed LJ, Romney SL: Doxorubicin-cyclophosphamide: effective chemotherapy for advanced endometrial adenocarcinoma. Am J Obstet Gynecol 1977;128:314.

Nash JD, Burke TW, Woodward JE, et al: Diagnosis of recurrent gynecologic malignancy with fine needle aspiration cytology. Obstet Gynecol 1987;71:333.

NG ABP, Reagan JW, Storasli JP, Wentz WB: Mixed adenosquamous carcinoma of the endometrium. Am J Clin Pathol 1973; 59:765.

Nordquist SRB, Sevin BU, Nadji M, et al: Fine-needle aspiration cytology in gynecologic oncology. I. Diagnostic accuracy. Obstet Gynecol 1979;54:719.

O'Brien ME, Killackey M: Adjuvant therapy in "high-risk" endometrial adenocarcinoma [abstract]. Proc Am Soc Clin Oncol 1994;13:249.

Onsrud M, Aalders J, Abeler V, Taylor P: Endometrial carcinoma with cervical involvement (stage II): prognostic factors and value of combined radiological-surgical treatment. Gynecol Oncol 1982;13:76.

Onsrud M, Kolstad P, Normann T: Postoperative external pelvic irradiation in carcinoma of the corpus stage I: a controlled clinical trial. Gynecol Oncol 1976;4:222.

Orr JW, Orr P, Holloway RW: Surgical staging of corpus cancer: perioperative morbidity [abstract]. Proc Soc Gynecol Oncol 1991;32:14.

Parazzina F, La Vecchia C, Bocciolone L, Franceschi S: Review: the epidemiology of endometrial cancer. Gynecol Oncol 1991; 41:1.

Park RC, Patow WE, Petty WM, Zimmerman EA: Treatment of adenocarcinoma of the endometrium. Gynecol Oncol 1974;2:60.

Pasmantier MW, Coleman M, Silver RT, et al: Treatment of advanced endometrial carcinoma with doxorubicin and cisplatin: effects on both untreated and previously treated patients. Cancer Treat Rep 1985;69:539.

Peters WA III, Andersen WA, Thornton WN Jr, Morley GW: The selective use of vaginal hysterectomy in the management of adenocarcinoma of the endometrium. Am J Obstet Gynecol 1983;146:285.

Phillips GL, Prem KA, Adcock LL, Twiggs LB: Vaginal recurrence of adenocarcinoma of the endometrium. Gynecol Oncol 1982; 13:323.

Potish RA, Twiggs LB, Adcock LL, Prem KA: Role of whole abdominal radiation therapy in the management of endometrial cancer: prognostic importance of factors indicating peritoneal metastases. Gynecol Oncol 1985a;21:80.

Potish RA, Twiggs LB, Adcock LL, et al: Paraaortic lymph node radiotherapy in cancer of the uterine corpus. Obstet Gynecol 1985b;65:251.

Pratt JH, Symmonds RE, Welch JS: Vaginal hysterectomy for carcinoma of the fundus. Am J Obstet Gynecol 1964;88:1063.

Reddoch JM, Burke TW, Morris M, et al: Surveillance for recurrent endometrial carcinoma: development of a follow-up scheme. Gynecol Oncol 1995;59:221.

Reifenstein EC: Hydroxyprogesterone caproate therapy in advanced endometrial cancer. Cancer 1971;27:485.

Ritcher N, Lucas WE, Yon JL, Sanford FG: Preoperative whole pelvic external irradiation in stage I endometrial cancer. Cancer 1981;48:58.

Rose PG, Cha SD, Tak WK, et al: Radiation therapy for surgically proven para-aortic node metastasis in endometrial cancer. Int J Radiat Oncol Biol Phys 1992;24:229.

Rutledge F: The role of radical hysterectomy in adenocarcinoma of the endometrium. Gynecol Oncol 1974;2:331.

Rutledge FN: Pelvic exenteration: an update of the U. T. M. D. Anderson Hospital experience and review of the literature. In Rutledge FN, Freedman RS, Gershenson DM (eds): Gynecologic Cancer: Diagnosis and Treatment Strategies. Austin: University of Texas Press, 1987:7.

Salazar OM, DePapp EW, Bonfiglio TW, et al: Adenosquamous carcinoma of the endometrium: an entity with an inherent poor prognosis? Cancer 1977;40:119.

Scambia G, Gadducci A, Panici PB, et al: Combined use of CA 125 and CA 15-3 in patients with endometrial cancer. Gynecol Oncol 1994;54:292.

Schink JC, Lurain JR, Wallemark CB, Chmiel JS: Tumor size in endometrial cancer: a prognostic factor for lymph node metastasis. Obstet Gynecol 1987;70:216.

Seski JC, Edwards CL, Gershenson DM, Copeland LJ: Doxorubicin and cyclophosphamide chemotherapy for disseminated endometrial cancer. Obstet Gynecol 1981;58:88.

Seski JC, Edwards CL, Herson J, Rutledge FN: Cisplatin chemotherapy for disseminated endometrial cancer. Obstet Gynecol 1982;59:225.

Seoud MA-F, Johnson J, Weed JC Jr: Gynecologic tumors in tamoxifen-treated women with breast cancer. Obstet Gynecol 1993;82:165.

Sevin BU, Greening SE, Nadji M, et al: Fine needle aspiration cytology in gynecologic oncology. I. Clinical aspects. Acta Cytol 1979;23:277.

Shumsky AG, Stuart GCE, Brasher PM, et al: An evaluation of routine follow-up of patients treated for endometrial carcinoma. Gynecol Oncol 1994;55:229.

Silva EG, Tornos CS, Mitchell MF: Malignant neoplasms of the uterine corpus in patients treated for breast carcinoma: the effects of tamoxifen. Int J Gynecol Pathol 1994;13:248.

Silverberg SG, De Giorgi LS: Clear cell carcinoma of the endometrium: clinical, pathologic, and ultrasonic findings. Cancer 1973;31:1127.

Smith DC, Prentice R, Thompson DJ, Herrmann WL: Association of exogenous estrogen and endometrial carcinoma. N Engl J Med 1975;293:1164.

Stringer CA, Gershenson DM, Burke TW, et al: Adjuvant chemotherapy with cisplatin, doxorubicin, and cyclophosphamide (PAC) for early stage high risk endometrial cancer: a preliminary analysis. Gynecol Oncol 1990;38:305.

Sutton GP, Brill L, Michael H, et al: Malignant papillary lesions of the endometrium. Gynecol Oncol 1987;27:294.

Swenerton K: Treatment of advanced endometrial cancer with tamoxifen. Cancer Treat Rep 1980;64:805.

Tatman JL, Freedman RS, Scott W, Atkinson EN: Treatment of advanced endometrial adenocarcinoma with cyclic sequential ethinyl estradiol and medroxyprogesterone acetate. Eur J Cancer Clin 1989;25:1619.

Thigpen JT, Buchsbaum HJ, Mangan C, Blessing JA: Phase II trial of Adriamycin in the treatment of advanced or recurrent endometrial carcinoma: a Gynecologic Oncology Group study. Cancer Treat Rep 1979;63:21.

Trope C, Johnson JE, Simonsen E, et al: Treatment of recurrent endometrial adenocarcinoma with a combination of doxorubicin and cisplatin. Am J Obstet Gynecol 1984;149:379.

Turbow MM, Ballon SC, Sikie BI, Koretz MM: Cisplatin, doxorubicin, and cyclophosphamide chemotherapy for advanced endometrial carcinoma. Cancer Treat Rep 1985;69:465.

Turner DA, Gershenson DM, Atkinson N, et al: The prognostic significance of peritoneal cytology for stage I endometrial cancer. Obstet Gynecol 1989;74:775.

Underwood PB, Lutz MH, Kreutner A, et al: Carcinoma of the endometrium: radiation followed immediately by operation. Am J Obstet Gynecol 1977;128:86.

Vergote I, Kjorstad K, Aberler V, Kolstad P: A randomized trial of adjuvant progestogen in early endometrial cancer. Cancer 1989;64:1011.

Wallin TE, Malkasian GD, Gaffey TA, et al: Stage II cancer of the endometrium: a pathologic and clinical study. Gynecol Oncol 1984;18:1.

Weiser EB, Bundy BN, Hoskins WJ, et al: Extraperitoneal versus transperitoneal selective paraaortic lymphadenectomy in the pretreatment surgical staging of advanced cervical carcinoma: a Gynecologic Oncology Group study. Gynecol Oncol 1989;33:283.

Wingo PA, Tong T, Bolden S: Cancer statistics, 1995. CA Cancer J Clin 1995;45:18.

Wollin M, Kagan AR, Kwan DK: Radiation dose calculations in endometrial cancer treated with Heyman capsules or tandem. Gynecol Oncol 1982;13:37.

Wynder EL, Escher GC, Mantel N: An epidemiological investigation of cancer of the endometrium. Cancer 1966;19:489.

Yazigi R, Cohen J, Munoz AK, Sandstad J: Magnetic resonance imaging determination of myometrial invasion in endometrial carcinoma. Gynecol Oncol 1989;34:94.

Ziel HK, Finkle WD: Increased risk of endometrial carcinoma among users of conjugated estrogens. N Engl J Med 1975;293:1167.

59

James L. Nicklin
Larry J. Copeland

Uterine Sarcomas

Sarcomas, by definition, are malignancies that arise from tissues of embryonic mesodermal origin. Uterine sarcomas are uncommon neoplasms that arise from myometrial smooth muscle, the endometrial stroma, or more rarely ubiquitous connective tissue elements. Frequently they arise in conjunction with a malignant epithelial or carcinomatous component. Less often, uterine sarcomas may differentiate along heterologous pathways, highlighting the pleuripotential nature of the uterine primordium (Zaloudek and Norris, 1994). Uterine sarcomas constitute 2% to 6% of all uterine malignancies, or about 1% of all female genital tract malignancies (Lurain and Piver, 1992). Possibly as a result of the low incidence and the poor prognosis of most sarcoma subtypes, these lesions often have been considered and treated as a single entity. This approach depreciates subtle differences in histogenesis, clinical presentation, and response to treatment.

A functional classification of uterine sarcomas that has been widely utilized was published by Ober in 1959 and subsequently modified (Table 59–1). Of note, he defined the admixture of carcinomatous and sarcomatous elements as a *malignant mixed müllerian tumor,* and confined the term *carcinosarcoma* to homologous malignant mixed müllerian tumors. Several authors modified this classification by dividing pure sarcomas and those with carcinomatous elements into homologous and heterologous categories depending on the presence of tissue normally found in the uterus (homologous) or ectopic to the uterus (heterologous) (Clement, 1993). Although this classification and nomenclature persists in the literature, it has been largely superseded by a comprehensive histogenic classification ratified by the World Health Organization and the International Society of Gynecologic Pathologists (Table 59–2). This more semantically correct classification labels all sarcomas mixed with carcinomatous elements as *carcinosarcoma* while annotating the presence or absence of homologous or heterologous elements (Scully et al, 1994). For continuity, the older synonyms of malignant mixed mesodermal tumor and malignant mixed müllerian tumor are recognized. With regard to incidence, and for practical purposes, this comprehensive classification can be condensed to four categories, leiomyosarcoma, carcinosarcoma, endometrial stromal sar-

coma, and "others" (Silverberg and Kurman, 1991). In the largest epidemiologic study to date, carcinosarcomas were found to constitute 48% of all sarcomas, with an incidence of 8.2 per 1 million women per year; leiomyosarcomas 37%, with an incidence of 6.4 per 1 million women per year; endometrial stromal sarcomas 11%, with an incidence of 1.8 per 1 million women per year; and all others combined 4% with an incidence of 0.7 per 1 million women per year (Harlow et al, 1986).

There is no formal separate staging for uterine sarcomas. By convention these lesions have been staged according to the International Federation of Gynecology and Obstetrics (FIGO) system for adenocarcinoma of the endometrium.

LEIOMYOSARCOMA

Pathology

Leiomyosarcomas are malignant smooth muscle tumors that arise from the myometrial smooth muscle or potentially from the smooth muscle in uterine blood vessels. On gross examination they are typically solitary, solid lesions with a median diameter of 10 cm. Approximately 65% are intramural, 20% are submucosal, 10% are subserosal, and 5% arise in the cervix (Clement and Scully, 1992). They are usually less circumscribed than their benign counterpart and cannot be so easily shelled out from the adjacent myometrium. Typically the cut surface is bulging, soft, fleshy, and hemorrhagic, with focal areas of necrosis (Fig. 59–1).

Microscopically, these neoplasms are characterized by interlacing bundles of spindle-shaped cells that may vary in morphology from well-differentiated smooth muscle bundles to bizarre pleomorphic cells associated with necrosis (Hannigan, 1993) (Fig. 59–2). Definitive diagnostic histologic criteria are well established, with mitotic rate the single most important feature in distinguishing malignant from benign lesions. Greater than 10 mitotic figures (MF) per 10 high-power fields (hpf), based on counts of 40 or more consecutive hpf, is considered malignant. When there is marked cellular atypia, tumors with mitotic counts of 5 to 10 MF/10 hpf are also consid-

Table 59-1. MODIFIED OBER CLASSIFICATION OF UTERINE SARCOMAS

I. **Pure sarcomas**
   A. Pure homologous
      1. Endometrial stromal sarcoma
      2. Leiomyosarcoma
      3. Angiosarcoma
   B. Pure heterologous
      1. Liposarcoma
      2. Rhabdosarcoma
      3. Chondrosarcoma
      4. Osteosarcoma
II. **Mixed sarcomas**
   A. Mixed homologous
   B. Mixed with heterologous elements
III. **Malignant mixed müllerian tumors**
   A. Mixed müllerian tumor with homologous elements—carcinosarcoma
   B. Mixed müllerian tumor with heterologous elements
IV. **Unclassified**

Table 59-2. WORLD HEALTH ORGANIZATION AND INTERNATIONAL SOCIETY OF GYNECOLOGIC PATHOLOGISTS CLASSIFICATION OF NONEPITHELIAL TUMORS AND RELATED LESIONS

1. **Nonepithelial Tumors and Related Lesions**
I. Endometrial stromal tumors
   1. Stromal nodule
   2. Low-grade stromal sarcoma
   3. High-grade stromal sarcoma
II. Smooth muscle tumors
   I. Leiomyoma
      Variants
        Cellular
        Epithelioid
        Bizarre (symplastic, pleomorphic)
        Lipomyosarcoma
   2. Smooth muscle tumor of uncertain malignant potential
   3. Leiomyosarcoma
      Variants
        Epithelioid
        Myxoid
   4. Other smooth muscle tumors
      Metastasizing leiomyoma
      Intravenous leiomyomatosis
      Diffuse leiomyomatosis
III. Mixed endometrial stromal and smooth muscle tumors
IV. Adenomatoid tumor
V. Other soft tissue tumors (benign and malignant)
   Homologous
   Heterologous

2. **Mixed Epithelial-Nonepithelial Tumors**
I. Benign
   I. Adenofibroma
   2. Adenomyoma
II. Malignant
   1. Adenosarcoma
      Homologous
      Heterologous
   2. Carcinosarcoma (malignant mixed mesodermal tumor; malignant mixed müllerian tumor)
      Homologous
      Heterologous

3. **Miscellaneous Tumors**
I. Sex cord–like tumors
II. Tumors of germ cell type
III. Neuroectoderm tumors
IV. Lymphomas
V. Others

4. **Secondary Tumors**
5. **Unclassified**

ered malignant (Hendrickson and Kempson, 1995). Finally, tumors with extension beyond the uterus at the time of diagnosis are considered malignant regardless of mitotic count or degree of pleomorphism (Morrow, 1993). A group of tumors with 3 to 5 MF/10 hpf with atypia, or 5 to 9 MF/10 hpf without marked atypia, or (rarely) greater than 15 MF/10 hpf with normal cytology and cellularity have been labeled smooth muscle tumors of uncertain malignant potential, and demonstrate an unpredictable clinical course (Hendrickson and Kempson, 1995; Bell et al, 1994) (Fig. 59–3). Bell and colleagues have further refined the diagnosis of this problematic group by correlating clinical behavior with mitotic index, degree of cytologic atypia, and presence of necrosis (Bell et al, 1994). Of note, the mitotic count in smooth muscle tumors may be spuriously increased in patients who are pregnant or on the oral contraceptive pill; this is believed to be secondary to elevated progestin levels (Tiltman, 1985; Norris et al, 1988).

Clinical Features

The average age at diagnosis is the early 50s (Zaloudek and Norris, 1994). No epidemiologic association has been found with parity, systemic disease, or prior radiation exposure; however, there does appear to be some difference in the race-specific incidence (Fig. 59–4). The relative risk for black women compared with white women is 1.6 (Harlow et al, 1986). There are isolated case reports of leiomyosarcomas arising in patients treated with tamoxifen for breast cancer. There is no evidence that these reports represent an epidemiologically significant association (Silva et al, 1994).

Symptoms include abnormal uterine bleeding, awareness of a mass, pelvic pressure or pain, and rarely vaginal discharge. Cervical cytology is rarely contributory. Diagnosis at dilation and curettage is correctly made in only 15% of cases (Kempson and Bari, 1970; Dihn and Woodruff, 1982), consistent with the observation that leiomyosarcomata arise in the *myometrium* and are therefore largely inaccessible for histologic evaluation with conventional *endometrial* sampling modalities. The majority of cases are diagnosed incidentally on histology following surgery for presumed leiomyomata. In collected series totaling 29,432 patients who underwent laparotomy for presumed fibroids, between 0.21% and 0.7% were found to have a leiomyosarcoma (Corscaden and

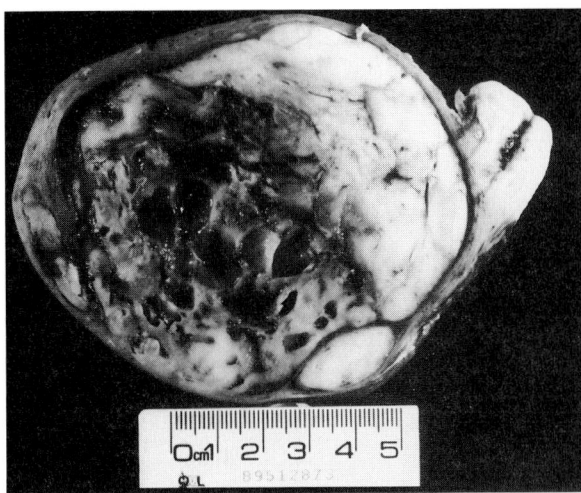

Figure 59–1
Leiomyosarcoma showing areas of necrosis and cystic degeneration. (Courtesy of Dr. R. G. Wright, Queensland Medical Laboratories.)

Singh, 1958; Montague et al, 1965; Leibsohn et al, 1990). Leiomyosarcomas have been estimated to arise in pre-existing leiomyomas in up to 5% to 10% of cases; however, the majority are believed to arise de novo (Hacker, 1994; Morrow, 1993).

Similar to all uterine malignancies, leiomyosarcomas can spread by direct extension, lymphatic embolization, hematogenous embolization, and transperitoneal seeding. Leiomyosarcomas have a propensity for hematogenous and to a lesser extent lymphatic spread (Taylor and Norris, 1966; Fleming et al, 1984). Although there are reports from small series of lymphatic metastases in clinical stage I and II disease ranging from 5% to 75% (Chen, 1989; Morrow, 1993), systematic surgical staging of 59 patients with leiomyosarcomas by members of the Gyneco-

logic Oncology Group (GOG) found only a 3.5% incidence of nodal involvement (Major et al, 1993). In autopsy series, lymph node involvement has been reported in 44% to 50% of patients dying of disease (Taylor and Norris, 1966; Fleming et al, 1984).

The propensity for hematogenous spread is evidenced by the 57% to 72% incidence of distant metastases in patients with recurrent leiomyosarcomas who had clinical stage I disease at the time of initial surgery (Barter et al, 1985; Punnonen et al, 1985; Yu et al, 1989). Fleming and colleagues (1984) found a 97% incidence of extrapelvic disease in patients dying from leiomyosarcoma. Stage is the most important prognostic determinant of outcome (Berchuck et al, 1988; Olah et al, 1992; Gadducci et al, 1996a). Survival for patients with stage I disease approximates 50% (Olah et al, 1992; Morrow, 1993). There are few patients with advanced-stage disease who survive 5 years, and most recurrences occur within 2 years.

Other Prognostic Features

In studies to date, the mitotic index is the only histologic feature found to be independently prognostic of progression-free interval and survival (Major et al, 1993; Gadducci et al, 1996a). However, the following features have been suggested to be associated with improved outcome: pushing margins, hyalinization, absence of necrosis, origin in a fibroid, good histologic differentiation, and size less than 5 cm (Evans, 1988; Morrow, 1993).

Other Histologic Variants

The *epitheloid* leiomyosarcoma is a histologic variant characterized by smooth muscle cells with an epithelial-like appearance. *Myxoid* leiomyosarcomas

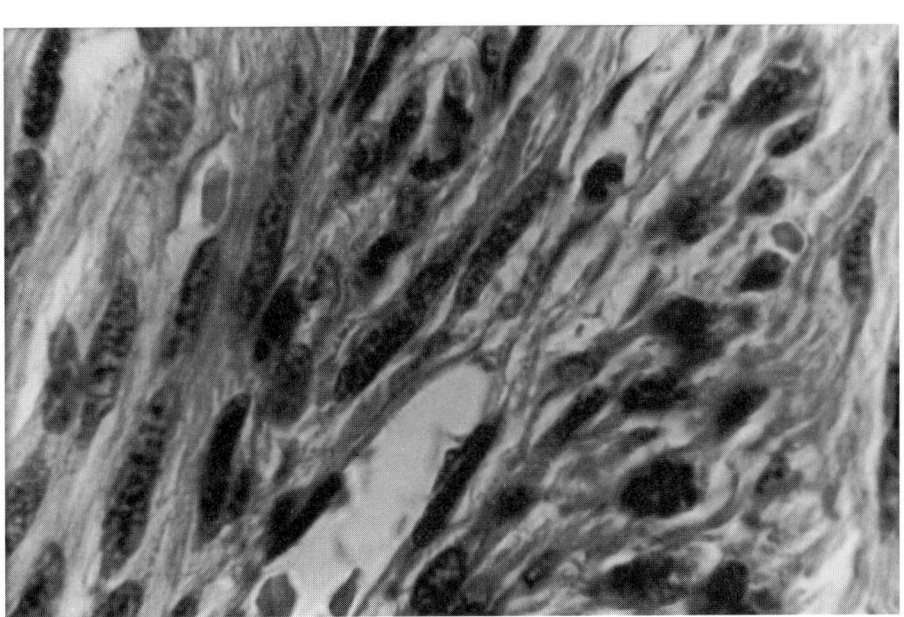

Figure 59–2
High-power photomicrograph of a leiomyosarcoma with a mitotic figure. (Courtesy of Dr. R. G. Wright, Queensland Medical Laboratories.)

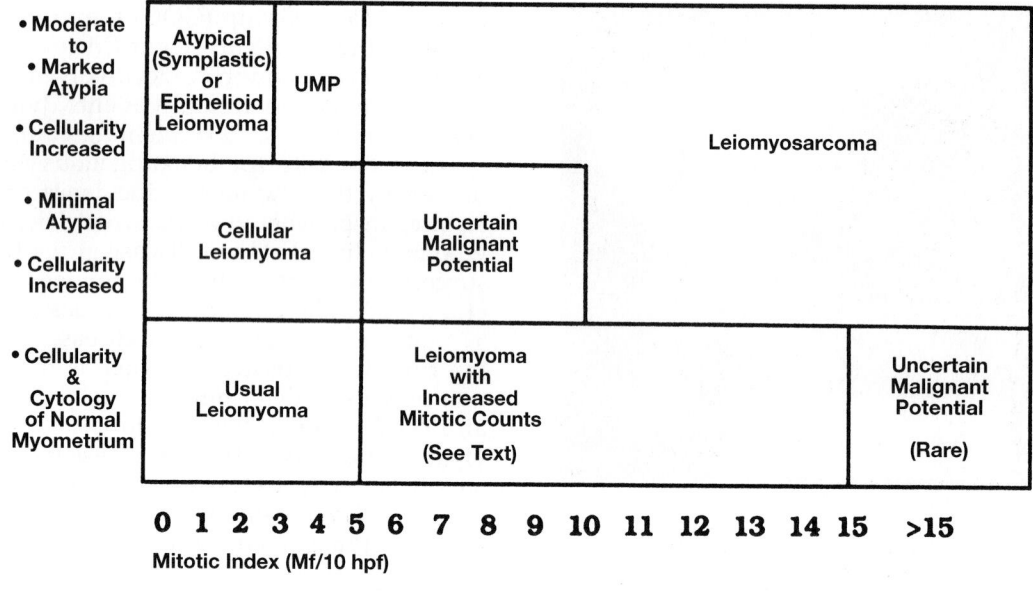

UMP = Uncertain Malignant Potential

Figure 59-3

Diagrammatic representation of the Hendrickson and Kempson classification of uterine smooth muscle neoplasm based on mitotic count, cellularity, and cytologic features.

are grossly gelatinous with a sparsely cellular myxoid appearance on histology. There is a poor correlation between the mitotic index and outcome for these variants, which are usually considered malignant. *Intravenous leimoyomatosis* is a rare and commonly benign tumor characterized by the rubbery cords extending from the primary tumor into the parametrial vessels, sometimes into the inferior vena cava and rarely into the right atrium. *Leiomyomatosis peritonealis disseminata* is another benign condition mimicking malignancy, in which numerous small nodules are found arising from the peritoneal surfaces.

Treatment

The primary modality of treatment for patients with leiomyosarcomas is surgery. Consistent with fundamental oncologic surgical principles, a total abdominal hysterectomy–bilateral salpingo-oophorectomy (TAH-BSO) and surgical staging is recommended (Wain and Hacker, 1993). For clinically evident stage II disease, a radical hysterectomy is recommended to obtain an adequate margin around the primary lesion. Wain and Hacker (1993) advocate staging in the form of peritoneal washings, pelvic and para-aortic lymphadenectomies, biopsy of selected peritoneal sites, and an omental biopsy. This allows eradication of the primary disease and evaluation of possible sites of metastatic spread. Although no randomized prospective trial has been conducted to demonstrate the value of lymphadenectomy, this procedure provides valuable prognostic information, accumulates information about this disease process, allows tai-

lored adjuvant treatment, and causes minimal morbidity. However, when the diagnosis is made on histology some days after the completion of a simple hysterectomy without staging, it is difficult to make a strong case for reoperative staging laparotomy.

The role of radiotherapy is controversial. It has been suggested that adjuvant radiotherapy improves local control of disease without improving overall survival (Salazar et al, 1979; Hacker, 1994; Knocke et al, 1998). Although these observations are often noted in relation to other sarcoma types, most authors have been unable to demonstrate a therapeutic advantage for pure leiomyosarcomas (Belgrad et al, 1975; Gilbert et al, 1975; Hornback et al, 1986; Rose et al, 1987). Furthermore, Berchuck and colleagues (1988) observed no responses to radiation among 10 patients with recurrent leiomyosarcoma.

The role of chemotherapy is also controversial. Many drugs have been evaluated as single agents in the treatment of advanced or recurrent leiomyosarcomas, including ifosfamide, cisplatin, doxorubicin, etoposide, mitoxantrone, piperazinedione, and diaziquone (Slayton et al, 1991; Thigpen, 1992). Only doxorubicin and ifosfamide have demonstrated modest activity. Doxorubicin was found to have a 25% response rate in 28 patients, and ifosfamide a 14% response rate, in a series of 28 patients (Omura et al, 1983; Sutton et al, 1990). There have been two studies comparing single-agent doxorubicin with combination chemotherapy in the treatment of advanced leiomyosarcoma. The first study compared doxorubicin and dimethyltriazinoimidazole carboxamide (DTIC) with doxorubicin (Omura et al, 1983). The second study compared doxorubicin and cyclophosphamide with single-agent doxorubicin therapy

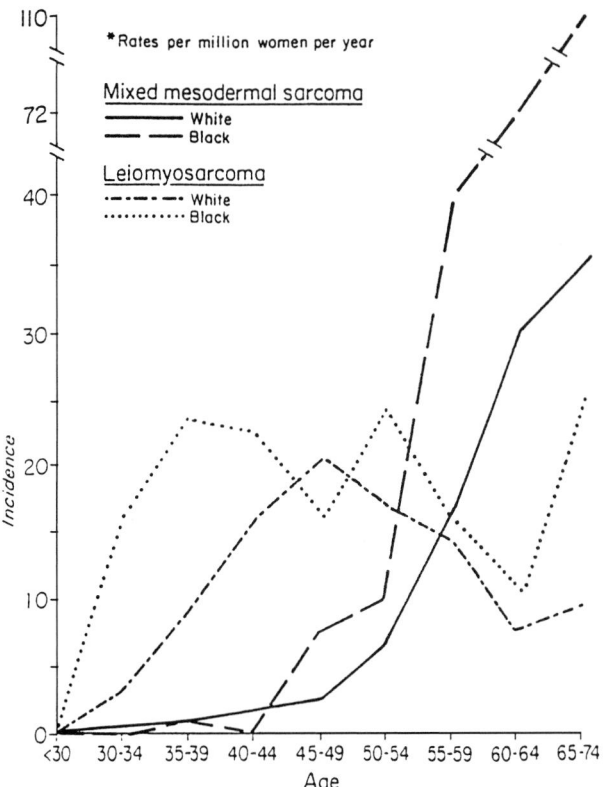

*Rates per million women per year

Mixed mesodermal sarcoma
——— White
– – – Black

Leiomyosarcoma
-·-·-· White
············ Black

Figure 59–4
Incidence of uterine sarcoma among females by age, race, and histology: SEER areas, 1973–81. (From Harlow BL, Weiss NS, Lofton S: The epidemiology of sarcomas of the uterus. J Natl Cancer Inst 1986;76:401, with permission.)

(Muss et al, 1985). Recognizing the statistical limitations of these small studies, there was no significant benefit demonstrated for combination chemotherapy. The GOG has published the results of a Phase II trial of the two most active single agents used in combination, doxorubicin and ifosfamide (Sutton et al, 1996a). They demonstrated a 30% response rate in 33 evaluable patients, with an average response duration of 4 months. This regimen was associated with significant hematologic toxicity, and there were two treatment-related deaths. The GOG published another Phase II study of combination chemotherapy consisting of hydroxyurea, DTIC, and etoposide in the treatment of recurrent and advanced uterine leiomyosarcoma. This demonstrated an 18.4% total response rate in 38 patients with evaluable disease, with markedly less toxicity (Currie et al, 1996b).

The role of adjuvant chemotherapy in completely resected early-stage disease is uncertain. A randomized GOG study comparing eight cycles of doxorubicin, 60 mg/m^2, with no further treatment in patients with completely resected stage I to II leiomyosarcoma showed no statistically significant difference in survival; however, numbers were small and there was a trend toward fewer recurrences (44% compared with 61%) in the treatment arm (Omura et al,

1985). On the basis of this study and data from studies of patients with advanced disease, a case can be made for doxorubicin in the adjuvant setting; however, this treatment must still be considered experimental.

At the present time, there are no studies to support any form of hormonal therapy in the management of leiomyosarcomas. However, there is speculation that the antiprogestin RU 486 (Mifepristone) may demonstrate some therapeutic efficacy (Bonelli, 1992). Molecular biologic investigations are in preliminary stages and clinical applications are pending (Horiuchi et al, 1999).

CARCINOSARCOMA

Pathology

Carcinosarcomas are neoplasms composed of a mixture of both a malignant epithelial (or carcinomatous) component and a malignant mesodermal (or sarcomatous) component. Macroscopically they are often soft, broad-based, fleshy, polypoidal lesions filling the endometrial cavity that frequently will be found protruding through the external os. There may be areas of hemorrhage or necrosis, or occasionally a gritty or hard feel from areas of cartilaginous or osseous differentiation (Fig. 59–5).

Microscopically, either the carcinomatous or the sarcomatous component may predominate. The carinomatous component may differentiate along any of the müllerian epithelial pathways; however, endometrioid-type adenocarcinoma usually predominates and is often poorly differentiated. The sarcomatous component may be homologous or heterologous. It may vary from recognizable, almost mature mesodermal cell lines with atypia (such as rhabdomyosarcoma, chondrosarcoma, and osteosarcoma) to undifferentiated spindle cell forms (Fig. 59–6). Heterologous and homologous sarcomatous components are found with equal frequency and are associated with equivalent survival rates (Silverberg et al, 1990). Mixtures of different types of sarcomatous differentiation are common. Deep myometrial invasion and lymph–vascular space invasion are common. Several investigators note that the majority of lymph node metastases are of the epithelial or the carcinomatous component (Silverberg et al, 1990). This observation is not consistent with earlier studies (Doss et al, 1984; Fleming et al, 1984).

Others have reported stage, age, and the presence of either a serous or clear cell carcinoma component as important prognostic factors (Nordal et al, 1997).

Clinical Features

There is a distinct difference between the age-specific incidence curves for carcinosarcoma and leiomyosarcoma (see Fig. 59–4), highlighting likely differ-

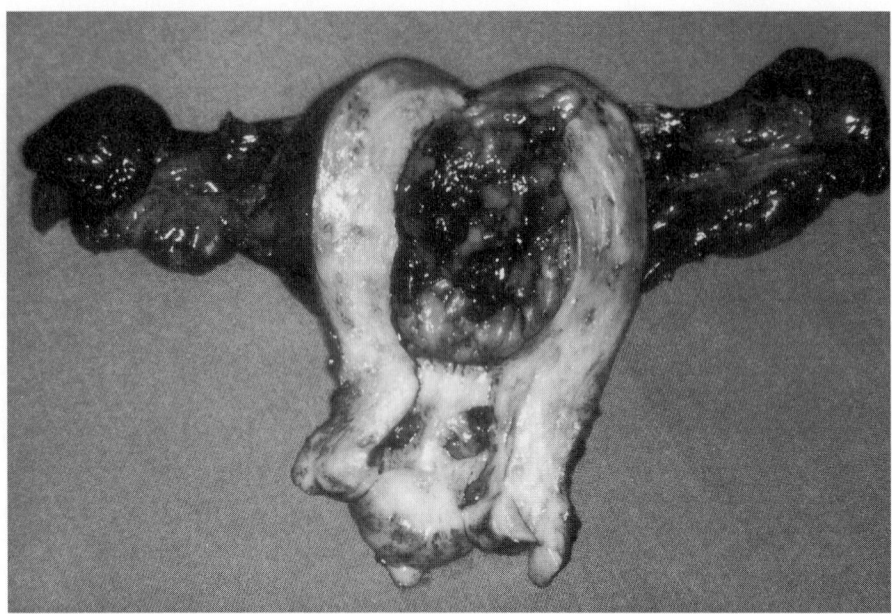

Figure 59–5
Photograph of carcinosarcoma showing typical broad-based, fleshy, polyoidal lesions filling the endometrial cavity.

ences in the histogenesis of these lesions. Carcinosarcoma is uncommon before age 40, after which time the incidence rises steadily. The mean age at diagnosis is the late 60s. There is more marked racial disparity, with black races experiencing a 2.7-fold higher risk (Harlow et al, 1986). There is an association between prior pelvic radiotherapy and the development of carcinosarcomas. Carcinosarcomas have been diagnosed between 2 and 30 years following radiation exposure (Hannigan, 1993), with most occurring between 10 and 20 years later (Perez et al, 1979; Rodriguez and Hart, 1982).

The most common presenting symptoms are vaginal bleeding (85%), abdominal or pelvic pain (25%), abdominal enlargement or mass (10%), and vaginal discharge (Lurain and Piver, 1992; Morrow, 1993;

Olah and Kingston, 1994). Weight loss is sometimes seen in advanced cases. Frequently, polyoidal tumor will be found protruding through the cervical os. Cervical cytology has been reported to be positive in up to 55% of cases (White et al, 1966). Uterine curettings or direct biopsy of visible tumor will usually provide the correct histologic diagnosis. Because the tumor arises from the endometrium, rather than the myometrium as in the case of leiomyosarcoma, adequate histologic sampling is more feasible prior to definitive surgery. Preoperative biopsies can be misleading, however, because biopsies may not be truly representative of the lesion, containing only one of the two tissue types. However, a definitive preoperative diagnosis is available in up to 70% of cases (Boram et al, 1972).

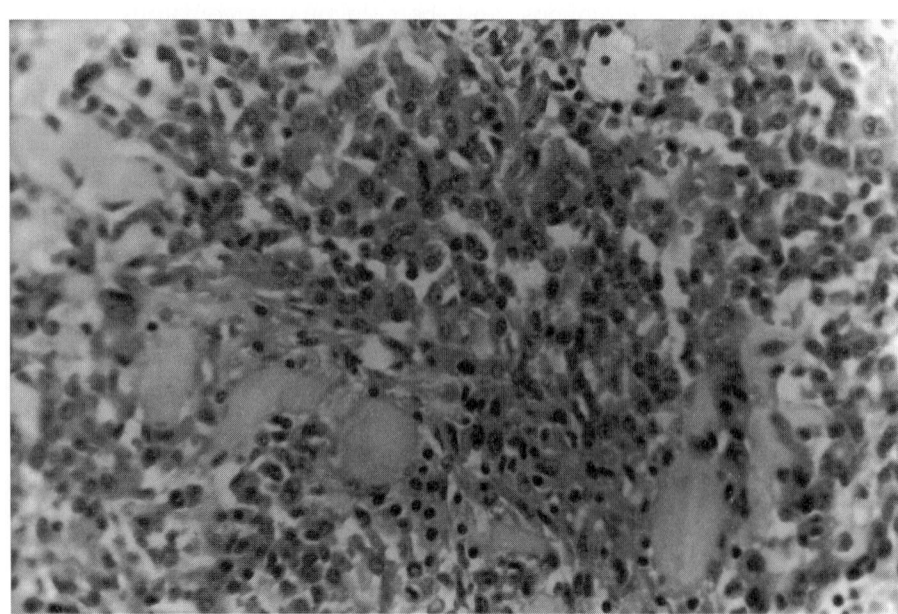

Figure 59–6
Photomicrograph of carcinosarcoma with areas of osteoid present. (Courtesy of Dr. R. G. Wright, Queensland Medical Laboratories.)

Advanced-stage disease is more commonly found in carcinosarcoma than in endometrial adenocarcinoma. Metastatic work-up may reveal pulmonary metastases, retroperitoneal lymphadenopathy, or peripheral lymphadenopathy. Clinical staging of carcinosarcoma is unreliable, with between 16% and 50% of patients with clinical stage I disease upstaged with comprehensive surgicopathologic staging (Doss et al, 1984; Chen, 1989; Dihn et al, 1989; Podczaski et al, 1989; Silverberg et al, 1990). In a series of 203 patients from the GOG, Silverberg and colleagues (1990) found the risk of retroperitoneal lymphadenopathy to be unrelated to features of the sarcomatous component of the lesion, including grade, mitotic index, and presence of heterologous elements. Conversely, high-grade carcinomatous components, deep myometrial invasion, lymph–vascular space invasion, and endocervical involvement were all found to be associated with a higher incidence of lymph node metastases. Others have reported stage, age, and the presence of either a serous or clear cell carcinoma component as important prognostic factors (Nordal et al, 1997). Overall survival is poor. In a combined analysis of several series totaling 399 patients, Morrow (1993) found a 36% survival for stage I disease, 22% for stage II disease, 10% for stage III disease, and 6% for stage IV disease.

Treatment

As with leiomyosarcomas, surgery is the primary modality of treatment. The recommended operative approach is identical to that described for leiomyosarcomas, with TAH-BSO and staging for early-stage disease. Advanced disease should be debulked if possible.

There are no randomized trials evaluating the role of adjuvant radiotherapy in the management of early-stage disease. From analysis of small series using either historical controls or prospective, nonrandomized radiotherapy regimens, there is evidence that adjuvant whole-pelvic radiotherapy improves the rate of local control but has little impact on overall survival (Chuang et al 1970; Perez et al, 1979; Salazar et al, 1979; Lotoki et al, 1982; Spanos et al 1984; Kohorn et al, 1986; Hornback et al, 1986; Chi et al, 1997). Some authors have been able to demonstrate a survival advantage in this setting (Belgrad et al, 1975; Vongtama et al, 1976; Gerszten et al, 1998).

The following drugs have been tested as single agents against recurrent or metastatic carcinosarcoma: ifosfamide, cisplatin, doxorubicin, etoposide, mitoxantrone, piperazinedione, and aminothiadiazole (Thigpen, 1992; Asbury et al, 1996). Ifosfamide has been demonstrated to have a 32% response rate (five complete and four partial responses) in 28 patients (Sutton et al, 1989). cis-Platinum has also been demonstrated to have modest activity. In two series of 28 and 63 patients, response rates of 18% and 19%, respectively, were demonstrated (Thigpen et al, 1986;

Thigpen et al, 1982). In a smaller series of 12 patients, one complete and four partial responses were reported (Gershenson et al, 1987a). Doxorubicin has less apparent activity in the treatment of carcinosarcomas than in leiomyosarcomas. Response rates of 0 to 10% have been reported in series of 9 and 41 patients (Omura et al, 1983; Gershenson et al, 1987b). The remaining drugs have demonstrated negligible activity.

Regarding combination chemotherapy, Peters and colleagues (1989) reported a 62.5% complete response rate among eight patients with advanced carcinosarcoma treated with cis-platinum and doxorubicin. These results have not been duplicated. Doxorubicin has been combined with DTIC, with cyclophosphamide, and with cyclophosphamide-vincristine-DTIC (CYVADIC), producing response rates of 19%, 23%, and 0%, respectively (Muss et al, 1985; Omura et al, 1983; Piver et al, 1982). The combination of vincristine, actinomycin D, and cyclophosphamide has been reported to have a 26% response rate in treating this disease (Hannigan et al, 1983). The combination of hydroxyurea, dacarbazine, and etoposide has been reported to produce a response rate of 15.8% (Currie et al, 1996a). These combinations do not provide significant increases in therapeutic efficacy, but are associated with increased morbidity.

Regarding adjuvant chemotherapy for apparently completely resected disease, the randomized study of the GOG comparing doxorubicin with no further treatment demonstrated a trend toward fewer recurrences in the treatment arm: 17 of 44 treated patients (39%) versus 25 of 49 untreated patients (51%) (Omura et al, 1985). As with the adjuvant treatment of leiomyosarcomas, this difference did not reach statistical significance. Peters and colleagues (1989) reported a 67% survival at a median follow-up of 34 months in 15 patients with no macroscopic residual disease following surgery who were treated with six cycles of adjuvant doxorubicin and cisplatin plus whole-pelvic external beam radiotherapy with or without para-aortic radiotherapy. This included 10 patients with positive washings and/or positive retroperitoneal lymphadenopathy. These figures are the best reported in the literature and should ideally be duplicated in a larger study.

It is apparent that, in the adjuvant setting, a randomized study can be justified comparing either ifosfamide, cisplatin, or doxorubicin (or a combination) with observation. The GOG has completed patient recruitment and is awaiting maturation of data in a Phase II study of adjuvant cisplatin and ifosfamide for patients with completely resected stage I or II carcinosarcoma of the uterus. Based on the currently available literature, the role of adjuvant chemotherapy must still be considered experimental. There is increasingly conclusive evidence that adjuvant radiotherapy improves local control despite showing no consistent significant improvement in long-term survival.

Malignant müllerian mixed tumors of the uterine cervix, compared to the corpus, are more frequently confined to the uterus, may have a better prognosis and the epithelial component is frequently nongrandular (Clement et al, 1998).

Other Mixed Neoplasms

Adenosarcoma

Adenosarcoma is an uncommon variant of the carcinosarcomas demonstrating a benign epithelial component and a malignant stromal component. These neoplasms pursue a more indolent course than carcinosarcomas. The median age of patients is 58 years (range 14 to 89). They usually present with abnormal vaginal bleeding or polyps projecting through the cervix. Other symptoms include abdominopelvic pain, vaginal discharge, and pelvic mass (Clement and Scully, 1990; Kerner and Lichtig, 1993).

Macroscopically these lesions often appear polypoid and fleshy, filling the endometrial cavity. Histologic examination reveals tubular glands or clefts of epithelial cells dispersed throughout a malignant stroma, which typically forms periglandular cuffs of increased cellularity, intraglandular projections, or both (Clement and Scully, 1990). In a GOG study, Kaku and colleagues (1992) reported a 19% incidence of extrauterine disease at presentation. The overall recurrence rate approximates 30%, and late recurrences are well described (Clement and Scully, 1990; Kaku et al, 1992; Olah and Kingston, 1994). In the series reported by Clement and Scully, there was a survival rate of 60.2% with a mean follow-up interval of 5.9 years. Kaku and colleagues noted an 80% survival rate after a mean follow-up of 38 months.

Carcinofibroma

These are extremely rare tumors arising from the uterine corpus or from the cervix, with fewer than 10 cases described in the world literature (Ostor and Fortune, 1980; Thompson and Husemeyer, 1981; Peters et al, 1984; Engdahl and Wolfhagen, 1988; Young et al, 1990). They also appear to behave in a more benign fashion than the carcinosarcomas.

ENDOMETRIAL STROMAL SARCOMAS

Pathology

Endometrial stromal sarcomas represent a spectrum of malignant proliferation of the endometrial stroma that has been broadly classified into three groups. At the benign end of the spectrum is the *benign stromal nodule*. Of intermediate clinical behavior is the *low-grade stromal sarcoma* (LGSS), formerly known as *endolymphatic stromal myosis*. The malignant end of the clinical spectrum is represented by the *high-grade stromal sarcoma* (HGSS).

The benign stromal nodule usually appears as a solitary, well-circumscribed nodule of stromal cells. Tumor margins tend to be "pushing," and central necrosis is rare. Mitotic counts are low, and there is no lymphatic or vascular space invasion.

LGSS most commonly appears as a tan to yellow, poorly demarcated mass merging with the surrounding myometrium, usually with cords of contiguous disease permeating through the myometrium. These infiltrating cords of disease may invade the parametrium and beyond. Macroscopically this can resemble an intravenous leiomyomatosis. Histologically, the lesion appears as a mass of uniform cells resembling stromal cells in proliferative-phase endometrium. They have infiltrating borders, no necrosis, and mitotic activity typically less than 3 MF/10 hpf (Chang et al, 1990). Vascular and lymphatic invasion is common (Olah and Kingston, 1994). They also have a high incidence of both estrogen and progesterone receptors (Dunton et al, 1990).

HGSS macroscopically have a fleshy, polypoid appearance that may bulge into the endometrial cavity, may distort the myometrium, and may invade extrauterine structures (Fig. 59–7). There is usually macroscopically visible hemorrhage and necrosis. Histologically, the cells are larger and more pleomorphic than LGSS, with an infiltrative growth pattern and frequent mitotic figures (Fig. 59–8). There are almost always greater than 10 MF/10 hpf, and frequently greater than 20 MF/10 hpf (Larson et al, 1990). Steroid receptors are rarely found in HGSS. Although endometrial stromal tumors usually can be classified

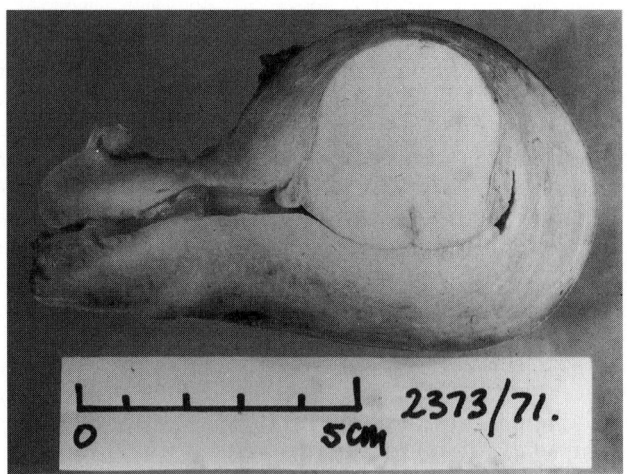

Figure 59–7
High-grade stromal sarcoma. This macroscopic appearance is more consistent with a stromal nodule, because there is an apparent sharp line of demarcation between the tumor and the uterine structures and no evidence of hemorrhage or necrosis. The diagnosis was made on microscopy. This highlights the point that there may be some overlap of histologic features in the spectrum of malignant stromal proliferation; however, stromal sarcomas can usually be classified as either stromal nodule or low-grade or high-grade stromal sarcoma. (Courtesy of Dr. R. G. Wright, Queensland Medical Laboratories.)

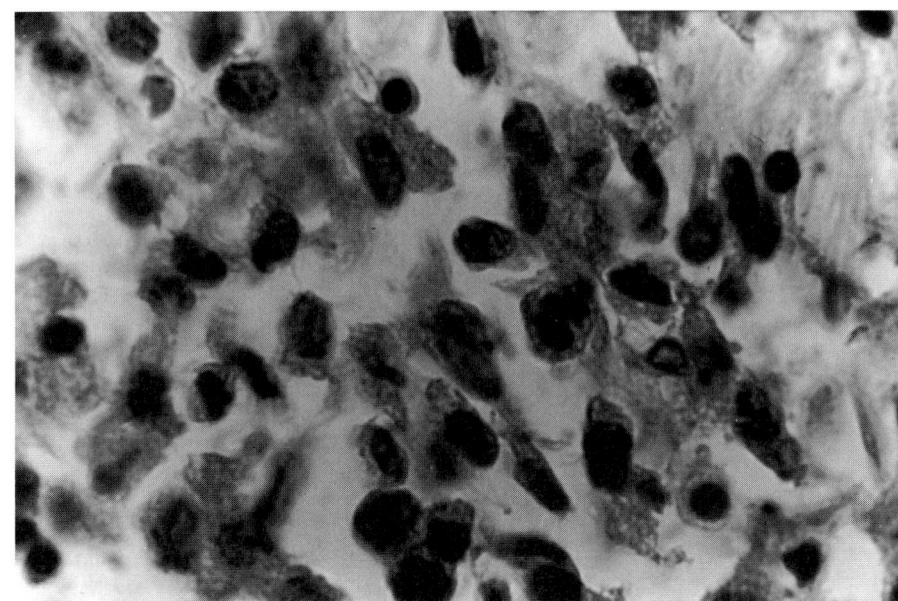

Figure 59–8
High-power photomicrograph of high-grade stromal sarcoma. (Courtesy of Dr. R. G. Wright, Queensland Medical Laboratories.)

as one of the three lesions described, there is a spectrum of disease with some overlap of histologic features.

Clinical Features and Treatment

The mean age of women with endometrial stroma sarcoma is the early 50s (De Fusco et al, 1989; Berchuck et al, 1990; Chang et al, 1990; Larson et al, 1990). There are no epidemiologically proven risk factors for endometrial stromal sarcomas. The most common symptoms of disease are worsening abnormal vaginal bleeding, uterine enlargement, a mass protruding through the cervix, and pelvic pain (De Fusco et al, 1989). Rarely, symptoms from extrauterine metastatic disease can precipitate medical attention.

As distinct from leiomyosarcomas, and in common with carcinosarcomas, endometrial sampling will frequently lead to a correct diagnosis of HGSS. The features of LGSS and benign stromal nodules can be recognized in uterine curettings. However, hysterectomy is usually required to distinguish these two lesions because, by definition, diagnosis is based on the margins and mitotic count (Zaloudek and Norris, 1981). Simple hysterectomy is appropriate treatment for the benign stromal nodule; however, successful treatment of a 12-cm nodule with local resection and uterine conservation is reported (Chang et al, 1990).

In a review of six papers reporting a total of 250 patients with LGSS, Lurain and Piver (1992) noted extrauterine extension in 40% of patients at diagnosis, mostly confined to the pelvis. The mainstay of treatment is TAH-BSO with resection of all macroscopic disease. Conservative surgery, such as subtotal hysterectomy, local resection, and adnexal conservation, has been associated with recurrence in the preserved structures. Recurrence is common. In the review by Lurain and Piver (1992), 44% of patients experienced disease relapse an average of 5 years following primary treatment. Late recurrence is not uncommon, with recurrences up to 25 years later reported. Despite this recurrence rate, only 16% died of disease-related causes. Recurrent disease is frequently amenable to surgical resection. There is a proven role for both progestagen therapy (Piver et al, 1984) and radiotherapy (Norris and Taylor, 1966). Chemotherapy is apparently ineffective in treating LGSS (Berchuck et al, 1990).

HGSS is a more lethal neoplasm (Gadducci et al, 1996b). In the review by Lurain and Piver (1992), a total of 44 patients from five series were found to have a 25% tumor-free 5-year survival. Surgical removal of all macroscopic disease, including TAH-BSO, is the most important component of treatment (Nordal et al, 1996). The role of staging has been questioned (Goff et al, 1993). With small numbers reported, the role of adjuvant therapies is yet to be finally determined (De Fusco et al, 1989). Adjuvant radiotherapy has been reported as beneficial in some series (Larson et al, 1990), but not in others (De Fusco et al, 1989). The prognosis for advanced metastatic or recurrent disease is poor; however, both ifosfamide and doxorubicin have been shown to have modest activity against this neoplasm (Berchuck et al, 1990; Sutton et al, 1996b). Peters and co-workers (1989) reported complete responses in all three patients treated with combination cisplatin-doxorubicin therapy. There are also documented responses to radiotherapy (Berchuck et al, 1990).

OTHER SARCOMAS

This small group of sarcomas mainly comprise the group formerly classified according to the modified

Ober schema as *heterologous pure sarcomas*. They include such neoplasms as rhabdomyosarcomas, osteosarcomas, chondrosarcomas, liposarcomas, and angiosarcomas (formerly classified as *homologous pure sarcoma*). The sparse literature regarding these rare lesions comprises isolated case reports and collated data of isolated cases accumulated over long periods of time. They most commonly present with vaginal bleeding, pelvic mass, or abdominopelvic pain (Clement, 1978; Hart and Craig, 1978; Piscioli et al, 1985; Emoto et al, 1994). Care must be taken in the histologic evaluation to exclude the coexistence of a malignant epithelial component that would change the diagnosis to carcinosarcoma. There is a high incidence of advanced stage at presentation. Long-term survival is unusual despite surgical extirpation and adjuvant therapies.

Alveolar soft part sarcoma of the uterine corpus has been reported in approximately 30 patients (Radig et al, 1998). Patients with these uterine tumors have a better survival than those with the extrauterine counterpart.

CONCLUSION

The uterine sarcomas are an uncommon and heterogeneous group of neoplasms that arise from mesenchymal elements in the uterus. All subtypes have a propensity for distant metastasis, high recurrence rates, and a comparatively poor prognosis. The surgical principles of management are similar for all subtypes. For advanced disease, all macroscopic disease should be resected where possible. For apparent early-stage disease, TAH-BSO plus staging is important to document the true extent of disease, to tailor adjuvant therapy, an to allow valid comparative analysis of treatment regimens based on the most important prognostic feature, stage.

Although the clinical behavior of the uterine sarcomas would suggest an important role for systemic treatment in the form of chemotherapy, trials to date have been somewhat disappointing. On the whole, studies evaluating the role of salvage therapy have reported only modest response rates of limited duration. The place of adjuvant chemotherapy is less defined. In the only randomized trial to date, the authors did not stratify for histologic subtype, and had sufficient numbers to detect only large differences in disease-free interval or survival.

Improvements in survival from uterine sarcoma are unlikely to be achieved by any significant change in surgical management. The greatest likelihood for improved survival is in the area of adjuvant therapy for early-stage disease. As more widespread appreciation develops of the differences in clinical behavior and response to therapy of differing sarcoma subtypes, careful attention can be directed to the design and evaluation of more specific chemotherapy and radiotherapy regimens. The rarity of these neoplasms is such that, of necessity, trials of adjuvant therapies can only be conducted under the auspices of a well-resourced multicenter gynecologic oncology organization.

REFERENCES

Asbury R, Blessing JA, Moore D: A Phase II trial of aminothiadiazole in patients with mixed mesodermal tumors of the uterine corpus: a Gynecologic Oncology Group study. Am J Clin Oncol 1996;19:400.

Barter JF, Smith EB, Szpak CA, et al: Leiomyosarcoma of the uterus: a clinicopathologic study of 21 cases. Gynecol Oncol 1985;21:220.

Belgrad R, Elbadawi N, Rubin P: Uterine sarcomas. Radiology 1975;114:181.

Bell SW, Kempson RL, Hendrickson MR: Problematic uterine smooth muscle neoplasms. Am J Surg Pathol 1994;18:535.

Berchuck A, Rubin SC, Hoskins WJ, et al: Treatment of uterine leiomyosarcoma. Obstet Gynecol 1988;71:845.

Berchuck A, Rubin SC, Hoskins WJ, et al: Treatment of endometrial stromal tumors. Gynecol Oncol 1990;36:60.

Bonelli RM: Mifepristone (RU 486). Wien Med Wochenschr 1992; 142:38.

Boram LH, Erlandson RA, Hajdu SI: Mixed mesodermal tumor of the uterus: a cytologic, histologic, and electron microscopic correlation. Cancer 1972;30:1295.

Chang KL, Crabtree GS, Lim-Tan SK, et al: Primary uterine endometrial stromal neoplasms: a clinicopathological study of 117 cases. Am J Surg Pathol 1990;14:415.

Chen SC: Propensity of retroperitoneal lymph node metastasis in patients with stage I sarcoma of the uterus. Gynecol Oncol 1989;32:215.

Chi DS, Mychalczak B, Saigo PE, Rescigno J, Brown CL: The role of whole-pelvic irradiation in the treatment of early-stage uterine carcinosarcoma. Gynecol Oncol 1997;65:493.

Chuang JT, Van Velden DJJ, Graham JB: Carcinosarcoma and mixed mesodermal tumors of the uterine corpus. Obstet Gynecol 1970;35:769.

Clement PB: Chondrosarcoma of the uterus: report of a case and review of the literature. Hum Pathol 1978;9:726.

Clement PB: Pure mesenchymal tumors. In Clement PB, Young RH (eds): Tumors and Tumorlike Lesions of the Uterine Corpus and Cervix. New York: Churchill Livingstone, 1993:265.

Clement PB, Scully RE: Müllerian adenosarcoma of the uterus: a clinicopathological analysis of 100 cases with a review of the literature. Hum Pathol 1990;21:363.

Clement PB, Scully RE: In Coppleson M (ed): Gynaecologic Oncology, 2nd ed. Edinburgh: Churchill Livingstone, 1992:803.

Clement PB, Zubovits JT, Young RH, Scully RE: Malignant mullerian mixed tumors of the uterine cervix: a report of nine cases of a neoplasm with morphology often different from its counterpart in the corpus. Int J Gynecol Pathol 1998;17:211.

Corscaden JA, Singh BP: Leiomyosarcoma of the uterus. Am J Obstet Gynecol 1958;75:149.

Currie JL, Blessing JA, McGehee R, et al: Phase II trial of hydroxyurea, dacarbazine (DTIC), and etoposide (VP-16) in mixed mesodermal tumors of the uterus: a Gynecologic Oncology Group study. Gynecol Oncol 1996a;61:94.

Currie JL, Blessing JA, Muss HB, et al: Combination chemotherapy with hydroxyurea, dacarbazine (DTIC), and etoposide in the treatment of uterine leiomyosarcoma: a Gynecologic Oncology Group study. Gynecol Oncol 1996b;61:27.

De Fusco PA, Gaffey TA, Malkasian GD Jr, et al: Endometrial stromal sarcoma: review of Mayo Clinic experience, 1945–1980. Gynecol Oncol 1989;35:8.

Dihn TV, Slavin RE, Bhafavan BS, et al: Mixed müllerian tumors of the uterus: clinicopathologic study. Obstet Gynecol 1989;74:388.

Dihn TV, Woodruff JD: Leiomyosarcoma of the uterus. Am J Obstet Gynecol 1982;144:817.

Doss LL, Llorens AS, Hernandez EM: Carcinosarcoma of the uterus: a 40-year experience from the state of Missouri. Gynecol Oncol 1984;18:43.

Dunton CJ, Kelston ML, Brooks SE, et al: Low-grade stromal sarcoma: DNA flow cytometric analysis and estrogen progesterone receptor data. Gynecol Oncol 1990;37:268.

Emoto M, Iwasaki H, Kawarabayashi T, et al: Primary osteosarcoma of the uterus: report of a case with immunohistochemical analysis. Gynecol Oncol 1994;54:385.

Engdahl E, Wolfhagen U: Carcinofibroma—a rare variant of mixed müllerian tumor. Acta Obstet Gynecol Scand 1988;67:85.

Evans HL: Smooth muscle neoplasms of the uterus other than ordinary leiomyoma: a study of 46 cases with emphasis on diagnostic criteria and prognostic factors. Cancer 1988;62:2239.

Fleming WP, Peters WA III, Kumar NB, Morley GW: Autopsy findings in patients with uterine sarcoma. Gynecol Oncol 1984; 16:168.

Gadducci A, Landoni F, Sartori E, et al: Uterine leiomyosarcoma, analysis of treatment failures and survival. Gynecol Oncol 1996a;62:25.

Gadducci A, Sartori E, Landoni F, et al: Endometrial stromal sarcoma: analysis of treatment failures and survival. Gynecol Oncol 1996b;63:247.

Gershenson DM, Kavanagh JJ, Copeland LJ, et al: Cisplatin therapy for disseminated mixed mesodermal sarcoma of the uterus. J Clin Oncol 1987a;5:618.

Gershenson DM, Kavanagh JJ, Copeland LJ, et al: High-dose doxorubicin infusion therapy for disseminated mixed mesodermal sarcoma of the uterus. Cancer 1987b;59:1264.

Gerszten K, Faul C, Kounelis S, et al: The impact of adjuvant radiotherapy on carcinosarcoma of the uterus. Gynecol Oncol 1998;68:8.

Gilbert HA, Kagan AR, Lagasse L, et al: The value of radiation therapy in uterine sarcoma. Obstet Gynecol 1975;45:84.

Goff BA, Rice LW, Fleischhacker D, et al: Uterine leiomyosarcoma and endometrial stromal sarcoma: lymph node metastases and sites of recurrence. Gynecol Oncol 1993;50:105.

Hacker NF: Uterine cancer. In Berek JS, Hacker NF (eds): Practical Gynecologic Oncology. 2nd ed. Baltimore: Williams & Wilkins, 1994:285.

Hannigan EV: Uterine sarcomas. In Copeland LJ (ed): Textbook of Gynecology. Philadelphia: WB Saunders Company, 1993: 1034.

Hannigan EV, Freedman RS, Elder KW, Rutledge FN: Treatment of advanced uterine sarcoma with vincristine, actinomycin-D and cyclophosphamide. Gynecol Oncol 1983;15:224.

Harlow BL, Weiss NS, Lofton S: The epidemiology of sarcomas of the uterus. J Natl Cancer Inst 1986;76:399.

Hart WR, Craig JR: Rhabdomyosarcomas of the uterus. Am J Clin Pathol 1978;70:217.

Hendrickson MR, Kempson RL: The uterine corpus. In Sternberg SS (ed): Diagnostic Surgical Pathology. New York: Raven Press, 1995:1638.

Horiuchi A, Nikaido T, Taniguchi S, Fujii S: Possible role of calponin h1 as a tumor suppressor in human uterine leiomyosarcoma. J Natl Cancer Inst 1999;91:790.

Hornback NB, Omura G, Major FJ, et al: Observations on the use of adjuvant radiation therapy in patients with stage I and II uterine sarcoma. Int J Radiat Oncol Biol Phys 1986;12:2127.

Kaku T, Silverberg SG, Major FJ, et al: Adenosarcoma of the uterus: a Gynecologic Oncology Group study of 31 cases. Int J Gynecol Pathol 1992;11:75.

Kempson RL, Bari W: Uterine sarcomas: classification, diagnosis, and prognosis. Hum Pathol 1970;1:133.

Kerner H, Lichtig C: Müllerian adenosarcoma presenting as cervical polyps: a report of seven cases and review of the literature. Obstet Gynecol 1993;81:655.

Knocke TH, Kucera H, Dorfler D, Pokrajac B, Potter R: Results of postoperative radiotherapy in the treatment of sarcoma of the corpus uteri. Cancer 1998;83:1972.

Kohorn EI, Schwartz PE, Chambers JT, et al: Adjuvant therapy in mixed müllerian tumors of the uterus. Gynecol Oncol 1986;33: 212.

Larson B, Silfversward C, Nisson B, Pettersson F: Endometrial stromal sarcoma of the uterus: a clinical and histolopathological study. The Radiumhemmet series 1936–1981. Eur J Obstet Gynecol Reprod Biol 1990;35:305.

Leibsohn S, d'Ablaing G, Mishell DR, Schlearth JB: Leiomyosarcoma in a series of hysterectomies performed for presumed uterine leiomyomas. Am J Obstet Gynecol 1990;162:968.

Lotoki R, Rosenshein NB, Grumbine F, et al: Mixed müllerian tumors of the uterus, clinical and pathological correlation. Int J Gynecol Obstet 1982;20:237.

Lurain JR, Piver MS: Uterine sarcomas: clinical features and management. In Coppleson M (ed): Gynaecologic Oncology. 2nd ed. Edinburgh: Churchill Livingstone, 1992:827.

Major FJ, Blessing JA, Silverberg SG, et al: Prognostic factors in early-stage uterine sarcoma: a Gynecology Oncology Group study. Cancer 1993;71(Suppl):1702.

Montague AC, Schwartz DP, Woodruff JD: Sarcoma arising in leiomyoma of the uterus. Am J Obstet Gynecol 1965;92:421.

Morrow CP: Uterine sarcomas and related tumors. In Morrow CP (ed): Synopsis of Gynecologic Oncology. 4th ed. New York: Churchill Livingstone, 1993:189.

Muss HB, Bundy BN, DiSaia PJ, et al: Treatment of recurrent or advanced uterine sarcoma: a randomized trial of doxorubicin versus doxorubicin and cyclophosphamide (a Phase III trial of the Gynecologic Oncology Group). Cancer 1985;55:1648.

Nordal RR, Kristensen GB, Kaern J, et al: The prognostic significance of surgery, tumor size, malignancy grade, menopausal status, and DNA ploidy in endometrial stromal sarcoma. Gynecol Oncol 1996;62:254.

Nordal RR, Kristensen GB, Stenwig AE, et al: An evaluation of prognostic factors in uterine carcinosarcoma. Gynecol Oncol 1997;67:316.

Norris HJ, Hilliard GD, Irey NS: Hemorrhagic cellular leiomyomas ("apoplectic leiomyoma") of the uterus associated with pregnancy and oral contraceptives. Int J Gynecol Pathol 1988; 7:212.

Norris HJ, Taylor HB: Mesenchymal tumors of the uterus I: a clinical and pathologic study of 53 endometrial stromal tumors. Cancer 1966;19:1459.

Ober WB: Uterine sarcomas: histogenesis and taxonomy. Ann N Y Acad Sci 1959;75:568.

Olah KS, Dunn JA, Gee H: Leiomyosarcomas have a poorer prognosis than mixed mesodermal tumours when adjusting for known prognostic factors: the result of a retrospective study of 423 cases of uterine sarcoma. Br J Obstet Gynaecol 1992;99: 590.

Olah KS, Kingston RE: Uterine sarcoma. Prog Obstet Gynaecol 1994;11:427.

Omura GA, Blessing JA, Major F, et al: A randomized clinical trial of adjuvant Adriamycin in uterine sarcomas: a Gynecologic Oncologic Group study. J Clin Oncol 1985;3:1240.

Omura GA, Major FJ, Blessing JA, et al: A randomized study of Adriamycin with and without dimethyl triazinoimidazole carboxamide in advanced uterine sarcomas. Cancer 1983;52: 626.

Ostor AG, Fortune DW: Benign and low grade variants of mixed müllerian tumour of the uterus. Histopathology 1980;4:369.

Perez CA, Askin F, Baglan RJ, et al: Effects of irradiation on mixed müllerian tumors of the uterus. Cancer 1979;43:1274.

Peters WA III, Rivkin SE, Smith MR, Tesh DE: Cisplatin and Adriamycin combination chemotherapy for uterine stromal sarcomas and mixed mesodermal tumours. Gynecol Oncol 1989; 34:323.

Peters WM, Wells M, Bryce FC: Müllerian clear cell carcinofibroma of the uterine corpus. Histopathology 1984;8:1069.

Piscioli F, Govoni E, Polla E, et al: Primary osteosarcoma of the uterine corpus: report of a case and critical review of the literature. Int J Gynaecol Obstet 1985;23:377.

Piver MS, De Eulis TG, Lele SB, Barlow JJ: Cyclophosphamide, vincristine, Adriamycin, and dimethyl-triazeno imidazole carboxamide (CYVADIC) for sarcomas of the female genital tract. Gynecol Oncol 1982;14:;319.

Piver MS, Rutledge FN, Copeland L, et al: Uterine endolymphatic stromal myosis: a collaborative study. Obstet Gynecol 1984;64: 173.

Podczaski ES, Woomert CA, Stevens CW Jr, et al: Management of malignant mixed mesodermal tumors of the uterus. Gynecol Oncol 1989;32:240.

Punnonen K, Pystynen P, Kauppila O: Uterine sarcomas. Ann Chir Gynaecol Suppl 1985;197:11.

Radig K, Buhtz P, Roessner A: Alveolar soft part sarcoma of the uterine corpus. Report of two cases and review of the literature. Pathol Res Pract 1998;194:59.

Rodriguez J, Hart WR: Endometrial cancers occurring 10 or more years after pelvic irradiation for carcinoma. Int J Gynecol Pathol 1982;1:125.

Rose PG, Boutselis JG, Sachs L: Adjuvant therapy for stage I uterine sarcoma. Am J Obstet Gynecol 1987;156:660.

Salazar OM, Bonfiglio TA, Pattern SF, et al: Utrine sarcomas: natural history treatment and prognosis. Cancer 1979;42:1152.

Scully RE, Bonfiglio TA, Kurman RJ, et al: Histological Typing of Female Genital Tract Tumours. Berlin: Springer-Verlag, 1994: 1, 18.

Silva EG, Tornos CS, Follen-Mitchell M: Malignant neoplasms of the uterine corpus in patients treated for breast carcinoma: the effects of tamoxifen. Int J Gynecol Pathol 1994;13:248.

Silverberg SG, Kurman RJ: Tumors of the Uterine Corpus and Gestational Trophoblastic Disease. Washington, DC: Armed Forces Institute of Pathology, 1991.

Silverberg SG, Major FJ, Blessing JA, et al: Carcinosarcoma (malignant mixed mesodermal tumor) of the uterus: a Gynecologic Oncology Group pathologic study of 203 cases. Int J Gynecol Pathol 1990;9:1.

Slayton RE, Blessing JA, Look K, Anderson B: A Phase II clinical trial of diaziquone (AZQ) in the treatment of patients with recurrent leiomyosarcoma of the uterus: a Gynecologic Oncology Group study. Invest New Drugs 1991;9:207.

Spanos WJ, Wharton JT, Gomez L, et al: Malignant mixed müllerian tumors of the uterus. Cancer 1984;53:311.

Sutton G, Blessing JA, Malfetano JH: Ifosfamide and doxorubicin in the treatment of advanced leiomyosarcomas of the uterus: a Gynecologic Oncology Group study. Gynecol Oncol 1996a;62: 226.

Sutton G, Blessing J, McGuire W, et al: Phase II trial of ifosfamide and mesna in leiomyosarcomas of the uterus. Gynecol Oncol 1990;36:295.

Sutton G, Blessing J, Park R, et al: Ifosfamide treatment of endometrial stromal sarcomas previously unexposed to chemotherapy: a study of the Gynecologic Oncology Group. Obstet Gynecol 1996b;87:747.

Sutton G, Blessing J, Rosenheim N, et al: Phase II trial of ifosfamide and mesna in mixed mesodermal tumors of the uterus: a Gynecologic Oncology Group study. Am J Obstet Gynecol 1989;161:309.

Taylor HB, Norris HJ: Mesenchymal tumors of the uterus. IV. Diagnosis and prognosis of leiomyosarcomas. Arch Pathol 1966;82:40.

Thigpen JT: Chemotherapy of cancers of the female genital tract. In Perry MC (ed): The Chemotherapy Source Book. Baltimore: Williams & Wilkins, 1992:1039.

Thigpen JT, Blessing JA, Beecham J, et al: Phase II trial of cisplatin as first-line chemotherapy in patients with advanced or recurrent uterine sarcomas: a Gynecologic Oncology Group study. J Clin Oncol 1992;10:1365.

Thigpen JT, Blessing JA, Orr JW Jr, DiSaia PJ: Phase II trial of cisplatin in the treatment of patients with advanced or recurrent mixed mesodermal sarcomas of the uterus: a Gynecologic Oncology Group study. Cancer Treat Rep 1986;70:271.

Thigpen JT, Shingleton H, Homesley H, Blessing J: Phase II trial of cis-diaminedichloroplatinum (DDP) in treatment of mixed mesodermal sarcoma of the uterus. Proc Amer Soc Clin Oncol 1982;1:110.

Thompson M, Husemeyer R: Carcinofibroma—a variant of the mixed müllerian tumour: case report. Br J Obstet Gynaecol 1981;88:1151.

Tiltman AJ: The effect of progestins on the mitotic activity of uterine fibromyomas. Int J Gynecol Pathol 1985;4:89.

Vongtama V, Karten JR, Piver SM, et al: Treatment, results and prognostic factors in stage I and II sarcomas of the corpus uteri. Am J Roentgenol 1976;126:139.

Wain GV, Hacker NF: Genital sarcomas: clinical features and treatment. In Burghardt E (ed): Surgical Gynecologic Oncology. New York: Georg Thieme Verlag, 1993:408.

White TH, Glover JS, Pette CH Jr, Parker RT: A 34-year clinical study of uterine sarcomas, including experience with chemotherapy. Obstet Gynecol 1966;25:657.

Young MPA, Benjamin E, Krausz T: Carcinofibroma—a rare variant of mixed müllerian tumour hitherto unreported at this site. J Pathol 1990;161:353.

Yu KJ, Ho DM, Ng HT, et al: Leiomyosarcoma of the uterus. a review of 14 cases. Chin Med J (Teipei) 1989;44:109.

Zaloudek C, Norris HJ: Mesenchymal tumors of the uterus. Prog Surg Pathol 1981;3:1.

Zaloudek C, Norris HJ: Mesenchymal tumors of the uterus. In Kurman RJ (ed): Blaustein's Pathology of the Female Genital Tract. 4th ed. New York: Springer-Verlag, 1994:487.

60

Epithelial Ovarian Cancer

David M. Gershenson

EPIDEMIOLOGY

Ovarian cancer is the second most common malignancy of the female genital tract in the United States. According to the American Cancer Society, there will be an estimated 25,400 new cases of ovarian cancer in the United States in 1998 (Landis et al, 1998). It is estimated that approximately 1.4%, or 1 of every 70, newborn girls will develop ovarian cancer during her lifetime. It accounts for 4% of all cancers among women. Only cancers of the lung, breast, and colon and rectum result in a higher mortality rate in this country. There will be an estimated 14,500 deaths from ovarian cancer in 1998.

According to data from the Surveillance, Epidemiology, and End Results (SEER) Program (Yancik et al, 1986), the age-specific incidence rate increases from 2 in 100,000 for women in their 20s to 15.7 in 100,000 in the 40- to 44-year age group to a peak rate of 54 in 100,000 in the 75- to 79-year age group. The median age in this data set is 61 years across stages, younger than that of most other studies. The histologic type of tumor varies with age; the majority of tumors in patients younger than 20 are of germ cell origin, whereas most tumors in postmenopausal patients are of epithelial origin.

The etiology of epithelial ovarian cancer remains unknown. Research efforts have focused on the genetic, hormonal, and environmental influences in the carcinogenesis of this group of neoplasms.

Increasing evidence suggests that a woman's lifetime reproductive/hormonal milieu has an effect on her risk of developing ovarian cancer. Increasing parity is associated with a decreasing relative risk of ovarian cancer (Joly et al, 1974; Casagrande et al, 1979; McGowan et al, 1979; Wu et al, 1988; Kvale et al, 1989). For women who are ever pregnant, the risk of ovarian cancer diminishes by 30% to 60% compared with nulliparas. Early age at first pregnancy also seems to be protective (McGowan et al, 1979).

Several studies have also demonstrated a protective effect of oral contraceptives on the development of ovarian cancer (Weiss et al, 1981; Cramer et al, 1982a; Rosenberg et al, 1982; Centers for Disease Control Cancer and Steroid Hormone Study, 1983).

The reduction of risk has been in the range of 30% to 60%, depending on the duration of usage.

The evidence regarding the protective effects of parity and oral contraceptives supports the incessant ovulation hypothesis of Fathalla (1971), which was later expanded by others (Casagrande et al, 1979; Henderson et al, 1982). This hypothesis states that the process involved in repair of traumatized surface epithelium of the ovary from ovulation somehow becomes aberrant, leading to neoplasia. Therefore, the greater the total number of ovulatory cycles in the lifetime of a woman, the greater the risk of developing epithelial ovarian cancer.

Schildkraut et al (1997) found that women whose cancers overexpressed p53 protein had a greater mean number of lifetime ovulatory cycles than women whose cancers did not overexpress p53 protein. More recently, Webb et al (1998) confirmed the association between increased number of ovulatory cycles and risk of ovarian cancer, but their study did not support the hypothesis that this association is due to an increased risk of p53 mutation with a greater number of ovulatory cycles.

In 1981, the Familial Ovarian Cancer Registry was established at Roswell Park Cancer Institute. During most of the 1980s, the Registry collected and collated data on several kindred. Early reports emphasized the laws of mendelian inheritance and described the typical presentation: papillary serous histologic type, poorly differentiated and of advanced stage, usually bilateral, and principally occurring in sister-sister or mother-daughter pedigrees (Piver et al, 1984). In 1989, however, with the death of Gilda Radner, the media catapulted the topic of familial ovarian cancer into the spotlight and escalated the public's awareness of this entity. The implications of this condition have been far-reaching, with a sharper focus on the genetics of ovarian cancer, ovarian cancer screening (see below), and methods of avoiding this disease (i.e., prophylactic oophorectomy).

In fact, familial ovarian cancer probably accounts for no more than 10% of all epithelial ovarian cancers, with the sporadic form comprising the vast majority of cases. Lynch and co-workers have described three separate types of hereditary ovarian cancer: (1)

site-specific familial ovarian cancer; (2) association of familial ovarian and breast cancers; and (3) the Lynch type II cancer family syndrome, in which there is genetic transmission of ovarian cancer, endometrial cancer, and nonpolyposis colorectal cancer (Lynch et al, 1985a, 1985b, 1986, 1990). The inheritance pattern associated with all of these syndromes is one of autosomal dominance with variable penetrance.

For women with two affected first-degree relatives, the risk of developing ovarian cancer may be as high as 50%. For women with only one first-degree relative affected, the precise risk is unknown but probably approximates 2% to 3%. Most experts agree that the risk is not as high as the 25% often mentioned in the literature.

Within the past few years, an epidemiologic characterization of epithelial ovarian cancer has begun to be replaced by a genetic one. Based on current knowledge, it appears that approximately 10% of all ovarian cancers are genetic. *BRCA1* and *BRCA2*, two highly penetrant autosomal dominant susceptibility genes, are responsible. The other 90% of ovarian cancers are sporadic. In 1994, the *BRCA1* gene was isolated by Skolnick and colleagues at the University of Utah, Myriad Pharmaceuticals, and the National Institute of Environmental Health Sciences (Miki et al, 1994). *BRCA1* is a large gene mapped to the long arm of chromosome 17 (17q21). The gene is encoded by 5592 nucleotides spread over 100,000 bases; the 22 coding exons of the gene encode an 1863–amino acid protein. Original estimates were that a *BRCA1* mutation conferred a 60% to 80% lifetime risk of ovarian cancer, but current estimates place the risk at somewhere between 30% and 60%. The *BRCA2* gene has been mapped to chromosome 13q12-13 (Wooster et al, 1994). The lifetime risk of ovarian cancer associated with a *BRCA2* mutation is lower than that of a *BRCA1* mutation and is estimated to be between 10% and 30%.

The incidence of carriers of the *BRCA1* gene in the general population is estimated to be approximately 1 in 800 women. However, specific ethnic groups may have a much greater frequency. In particular, a *BRCA1* mutation called 185delAG is believed to occur in 1 in 100 people of Ashkenzai Jewish descent (Struewing et al, 1995).

Ovarian cancer occurs most frequently in high industrialized Western countries such as England, the Scandinavian countries, and the United States. Although there are some interesting clues regarding the influence of various environmental factors on the development of ovarian cancer, no clear etiologic agent has been found. Talc (Parmley and Woodruff, 1974; Henderson et al, 1979; Longo and Young, 1979; Newhouse, 1979; Cramer et al, 1982b) and asbestos (Graham and Graham, 1967; Newhouse, 1979) have both been implicated as etiologic agents, but existing studies are inconclusive. More recently, Whittemore and associates (1988) found no association between talc and ovarian cancer.

The effect of diet on the development of ovarian cancer has also been studied. Cramer and associates (1984) found a positive correlation between increasing consumption of fat and risk of ovarian cancer. Byers et al (1983), however, reported no such correlation. Several other studies (Stocks, 1970; Trichopoulos et al, 1981; LaVecchia et al, 1984) have suggested a relationship between fat consumption and ovarian cancer. No link has been discovered between the consumption of coffee, tobacco, or alcohol and ovarian cancer (Cramer et al, 1984). Piver and Mettlin (1990) reported a relative risk of 3.1 of developing ovarian cancer for those drinking more than one glass of whole milk per day as compared with those who did not drink whole milk. This increased risk was not apparent for those drinking skim milk or 2% milk, suggesting that the fat content of whole milk may be responsible for the increase in risk.

Viruses have also been incriminated as etiologic agents for ovarian cancer. Cramer and associates (1983) found an association between a history of childhood mumps and the subsequent development of ovarian cancer, although others (West, 1966; McGowan et al, 1979) have noted a protective effect of childhood mumps on the development of ovarian cancer.

TUMOR MARKERS

In the 1980s and 1990s, an increasing amount of research has been conducted in the area of tumor markers for epithelial ovarian cancer. Although considerable progress has been made in this field, the ideal tumor marker for this disease is not yet a reality. There are a number of potential benefits to be derived from such a marker, including the ability to distinguish benign from malignant tumors preoperatively, the ability to distinguish ovarian from other cancers with similar manifestations, the ability to monitor patients for response during therapy and for sustained remission post-therapy, and the potential for replacing second-look laparotomy as part of the standard management of this disease. The ideal marker should possess optimal sensitivity and specificity and be produced by all types of epithelial ovarian tumors. Tumor heterogeneity has been one of the major roadblocks to the development of the ideal marker.

Carcinoembryonic Antigen

One of the best studied oncofetal antigens in epithelial ovarian cancer has been carcinoembryonic antigen (CEA). Several studies (DiSaia et al, 1975; Samaan et al, 1976; Van Nagell et al, 1978; Bast et al, 1984) have documented CEA elevations in 25% to 70% of patients with epithelial ovarian cancer. Unfortunately, the reliability of the test is strongly associated with histologic type and tumor differentiation; patients with mucinous tumors or undifferentiated tumors are more likely to have positive values. Consequently, CEA monitoring has not been used extensively in recent years to monitor patients with ovarian cancer, although it may be helpful in some patients, especially those with mucinous tumors.

CA-125

OC-125 is a murine monoclonal antibody that was raised against an epithelial ovarian cancer cell line and that binds to the determinant CA-125 (Bast et al, 1981). The antigen is present in coelomic epithelium during embryonic development and can be detected in adult tissue-derived coelomic epithelium; it is not detected in normal adult ovarian tissue. An immunoradiometric assay has been developed to monitor CA-125 in serum and body fluids.

Unfortunately, CA-125 is not specific for epithelial ovarian cancer. Elevations have been observed in a variety of benign diseases, including liver disease, acute pancreatitis, peritonitis, renal failure, endometriosis, pelvic inflammatory disease, and early pregnancy (Ruibal et al, 1984; Niloff et al, 1985c; Suzuki et al, 1985). Furthermore, elevated levels have been noted in other gynecologic cancers (adenocarcinomas of the endometrium, endocervix, and fallopian tube [Niloff et al, 1984b]) as well as in nongynecologic cancers (the majority of patients with pancreatic cancer and a minority of patients with colon, breast, and lung cancers [Bast et al, 1983]).

One of the most important potential uses for a serum tumor marker in epithelial ovarian cancer would be in its early detection, because at least two thirds of patients have advanced disease at the time of diagnosis. Niloff et al (1985c) reported a CA-125 level greater than 65 U/ml in 1% of 988 nonpregnant patients with benign gynecologic disorders. Einhorn et al (1986) measured serum CA-125 levels preoperatively in 100 women with palpable adnexal masses and found the level to be greater than 35 U/ml in all 11 patients with frankly malignant nonmucinous ovarian cancers. Although these early reports are promising, it is probable that the ultimate test to detect early ovarian cancer will consist of a panel of two or more monoclonal antibodies (MoAbs) rather than a single one. Furthermore, sensitivity and specificity may be improved by a combination of diagnostic modalities (e.g., sonography and serum tumor markers). With a reliable diagnosis of ovarian cancer preoperatively, patients may be more appropriately referred to gynecologic oncologists trained in aggressive cytoreductive surgery.

Bast et al (1983) initially reported elevated CA-125 levels in 82% of 101 patients with surgically demonstrable ovarian cancer. Studies (Crombach et al, 1983; Dembo et al, 1985; Einhorn et al, 1986; Kivinen et al, 1986; Krebs et al, 1986; Schwartz et al, 1987; Vergote et al, 1987) from many different countries have subsequently confirmed this finding. The majority of these studies have also shown a good correlation between the course of disease—regression, stability, or progression—and CA-125 levels (80% to 95%). Lavin et al (1987) found that the CA-125 level was a critical indicator of response to therapy only 3 months after the initiation of therapy. Mogensen (1992) found that patients with high CA-125 levels (>100 U/ml) 1 month after the third course of chemotherapy had a median survival of only 7 months. Disease recurrence has also been reliably detected with CA-125 monitoring in approximately 80% of patients (Knapp et al, 1985).

Another major potential use of a reliable serum tumor marker is as an alternative to second-look laparotomy in order to avoid the potential morbidity of such a procedure. Although persistently elevated CA-125 levels at completion of therapy have been strongly predictive of the finding of residual tumor at second-look laparotomy (Niloff et al, 1985a; Berek et al, 1986), negative CA-125 levels do not reliably predict negative pathologic findings (Niloff et al, 1984a; Atack et al, 1986; Berek et al, 1986; Patsner and Day, 1987; Schilthuis et al, 1987).

Other tumor markers such as tumor-associated antigens, immune complexes, enzymatic markers, and oncogene products have been studied, but the most promise at present seems to lie in the area of monoclonal technology. Although the CA-125 marker represents a major breakthrough in the diagnosis and management of epithelial ovarian cancer, greater specificity will most likely come from the next generation of markers; these markers will probably consist of a panel of MoAbs aimed at different determinants resulting from tumor heterogeneity (Kamiya et al, 1990; Suzuki et al, 1990; Bast et al, 1991).

OVARIAN CANCER SCREENING

There is currently no reliable screening method for ovarian cancer. An effective screening tool should be safe, inexpensive, and highly sensitive and specific. Whether epithelial ovarian cancer is an ideal disease for screening remains a matter of some debate. Although it is associated with a rather high mortality rate and the prognosis of early-stage disease is clearly superior to that of late-stage disease, it is not among the most common cancers in females and does not have a clearly definable preclinical phase.

Although there is essentially no information on controlled trials in the literature, pelvic exam does not appear to be an adequate screening tool. The use of abdominal sonography has been reported in a British study in which over 5000 women were screened (Campbell et al, 1989). The false-positive rate was 2.3%, and five primary ovarian cancers, all of which were stage Ia, were identified. In a Swedish screening trial (Andolf et al, 1990), 801 women between ages 40 and 70 underwent abdominal sonography. All had high-risk characteristics. Among 163 patients with abnormal scans, 30 patients underwent surgery. There was one borderline ovarian tumor, two endometrial cancers, and 27 benign lesions. The authors concluded that ultrasound probably does not have a role in screening for ovarian cancer.

At the University of Kentucky, transvaginal sonography (TVS) has been used. In one study, 1000 asymptomatic women age 40 or older were screened with this method annually (van Nagell et al, 1990). Thirty-one patients (3.1%) had abnormal sonograms and 24 underwent surgery. On histologic analysis, these 24 tumors included the following: one adenocarcinoma, eight serous cystadenomas, six endometriomas, and two cystic teratomas. In a follow-up report from the same group (van Nagell et al, 1991), 1300 asymptomatic postmenopausal women were screened with TVS. Ovarian abnormalities were noted in 33 (2.5%), and 27 underwent surgery. Ovarian tumors diagnosed at surgery included two primary carcinomas, one metastatic cancer, and 14 serous cystadenomas. Both patients with primary cancers had stage Ia tumors and normal preoperative pelvic exams and CA-125 levels.

Several groups are currently studying the use of color flow Doppler imaging in conjunction with TVS. This technology allows the detection of low-resistance intratumoral blood vessels associated with malignant tumors. In a study of transvaginal color flow imaging of 53 ovarian tumors prior to surgery, Weiner et al (1992) noted a pulsatility index less than 1 in 16 of 17 patients with malignant ovarian tumors and a pulsatility index greater than 1 in 35 of 36 benign tumors. Of the 36 patients with benign tumors, 11 had suspicious sonographic findings and 14 had elevated CA-125 levels.

CA-125 has also been studied as a screening tool. Although CA-125 is elevated in approximately 80% of women with epithelial ovarian cancer, it is also elevated in other gynecologic and nongynecologic malignancies, in approximately 6% of women with benign disease, and in approximately 1% of healthy women. In a Swedish study (Einhorn et al, 1992), serum CA-125 was measured annually in 5500 women over age 40. Among 175 women with elevated CA-125 levels, six ovarian cancers were detected by sonographic or clinical methods. These six ovarian cancers included two stage Ia, two stage IIb, and two stage III patients. In a British study (Jacobs et al, 1988), 1010 postmenopausal women were tested with CA-125, and one case of ovarian cancer was detected. With approximately 2 years' follow-up at the time of the report, no other cases of ovarian cancer had been diagnosed. In this study, the false-positive rate was 3%. Several studies (Finkler et al, 1988; Malkasian et al, 1988; Patsner and Mann, 1988) have analyzed the value of CA-125 in predicting malignancy in women with adnexal masses. All revealed significant false-positive and false-negative rates. Therefore, CA-125 may lack the sensitivity and specificity required of a good screening instrument.

One of the current strategies being investigated to overcome the insensitivity of CA-125 for ovarian cancer screening is the use of a panel of serum markers. Woolas et al (1993) found that CA-125 was abnormal in only 67% of 45 women with stage I ovarian cancer. When two other serum markers—OVX1 and M-CSF—were added, 98% of the women had elevated levels of at least one of the markers. Preliminary studies indicate that lysophosphatidic acid may be a potential biomarker for ovarian and other gynecologic cancers (Xu et al, 1998).

In summary, we currently have not identified the optimal screening technique, the cost-effectiveness remains a question, and we do not yet know, even if screening seems beneficial, who should be screened. There are a few major prospective screening trials ongoing or about to be launched. Some of these trials are targeting high-risk women—those with a family history of ovarian cancer, a personal or family history of breast cancer, or postmenopausal women. It most probably will be a few more years before we have clues about the wisdom of screening for ovarian cancer with the current technology. Women in ovarian cancer families are the focus of the recently established screening programs and methods of preventing ovarian cancer. Screening programs are currently concentrating on pelvic examination, serum CA-125 test, and TVS. It will be a few years, however, before we will have information on the sensitivity and specificity of such screening techniques. Prophylactic oophorectomy has been recommended by some to prevent the development of ovarian cancer in women over age 35 who have completed childbearing. Tobacman et al (1982), however, reported that prophylactic oophorectomy is not fail-safe protection against the subsequent development of primary peritoneal cancer, although this condition appears to be rare. In this study, 3 of 28 women (11%) from 16 families with a high risk of ovarian cancer subsequently developed peritoneal cancer after prophylactic oophorectomy. In another study, reporting the experience of the Gilda Radner Familial Ovarian Cancer Registry, Piver et al (1993) reported that 6 of 324 women (1.9%) in these families developed primary peritoneal cancer after prophylactic oophorectomy. Such a phenomenon probably represents a field effect, with the coelomic epithelium having the same vulnerability as the surface epithelium of the ovary to the etiologic agent.

PATHOLOGY

Common epithelial tumors account for approximately 90% of all ovarian cancers. They arise from the surface epithelium of the ovary, which is closely related to the coelomic epithelium lining of the peritoneal cavity. Table 60–1 shows the current, modified classification system for epithelial ovarian tumors originally outlined by the World Health Organization (WHO) (Serov et al, 1973). These tumors are not uncommonly mixed, with two or more cell types coexisting in the same neoplasm. In addition to being

Table 60-1. MODIFIED WHO CLASSIFICATION OF COMMON EPITHELIAL OVARIAN TUMORS

Serous	
Mucinous	Benign
Endometrioid	Borderline
Clear cell	Malignant
Transitional cell	
Mixed epithelial	
Undifferentiated	
Unclassified	

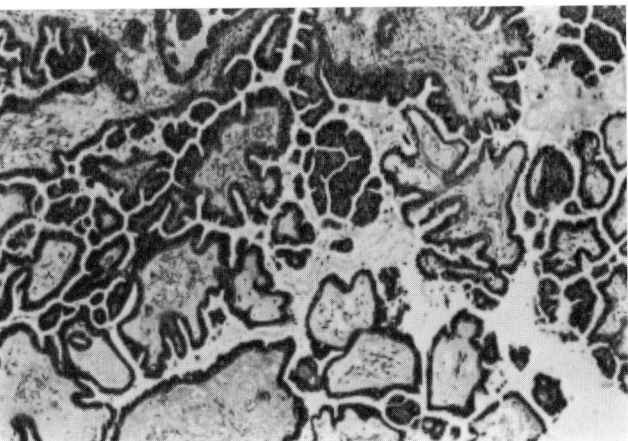

Figure 60-1
Borderline serous tumor. Papillae with stratified serous epithelium without stromal invasion.

classified according to cell type, these tumors are also categorized based on histologic and cytologic features and clinical behavior as benign, borderline, or malignant. Only the latter two categories are discussed in this chapter.

Serous Carcinomas

Serous carcinomas are the most common histologic type of ovarian malignancy, accounting for approximately 50% of all epithelial ovarian cancers. These tumors are usually endophytic, although they may be exophytic. Most tumors are partially cystic and partially solid. The external surface is smooth or may have papillary projections. Surface papillations are very common in borderline tumors. Approximately 33% to 60% of serous borderline tumors are limited to one ovary (Russell, 1979a), whereas frankly malignant tumors are bilateral in about 50% of cases (Janovski and Paramanandhan, 1973). Metastatic disease at diagnosis is noted in 16% to 18% of borderline serous tumors but in over 60% of frankly malignant tumors (Aure et al, 1971).

Grossly, borderline serous tumors typically have surface papillations. Conversely, the surface of malignant serous tumors is quite variable; it may be smooth and multilobulated or covered with exophytic papillations. Malignant tumors are usually mainly solid with occasional cystic areas. Hemorrhage and necrosis are common.

Microscopically, borderline serous tumors are characterized by stratification of the epithelial lining of the papillae, formation of papillary projections or tufts, nuclear atypia, mitotic activity, and the lack of stromal invasion (Fig. 60-1). Frankly malignant serous tumors are graded as well, moderately, and poorly differentiated. They contain disorderly invasive areas and range from glandular or papillary to solid (Fig. 60-2). Psammoma bodies are common in both types of serous carcinoma. Metastatic deposits of borderline serous tumors may represent benign müllerian rests (endosalpingiosis), borderline implants, or invasive implants.

Mucinous Carcinoma

Mucinous tumors represent the second most common type of epithelial ovarian malignancy, accounting for approximately 35% of borderline tumors and 10% to 15% of frankly malignant tumors. Approximately 80% to 90% of borderline tumors are confined to the ovary at diagnosis (stage I) (Russell, 1979a), whereas only about 50% of frankly malignant tumors are stage I. Bilateral ovarian involvement occurs in approximately 5% to 10% of both borderline and frankly malignant tumors (Hart and Norris, 1973).

Grossly, these tumors are large, cystic, and multiloculated with smooth external surfaces. Solid areas and papillary projections are more common in the frankly malignant variant. The criteria outline by Hart and Norris (1973) seem to represent the gold standard by which borderline mucinous tumors are distinguished from invasive mucinous tumors.

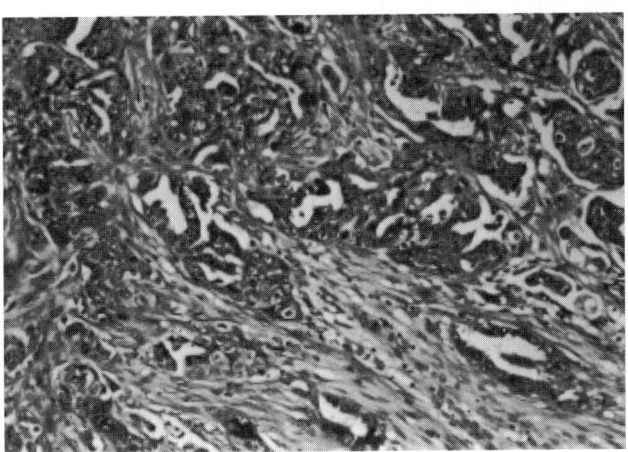

Figure 60-2
Grade 3 serous carcinoma showing highly atypical nuclei and numerous mitoses.

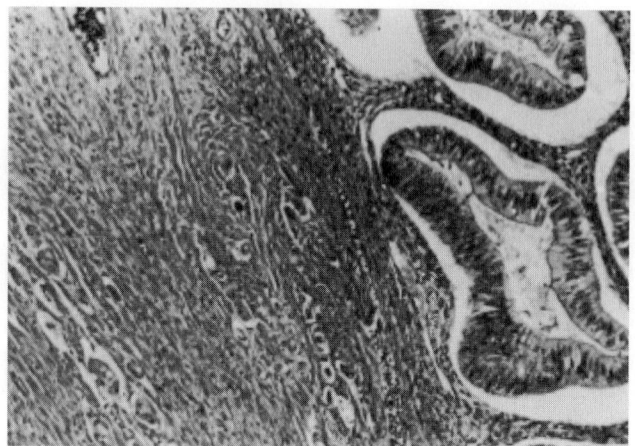

Figure 60-3
Mucinous carcinoma. Single-cell infiltration of stroma close to well-differentiated glands.

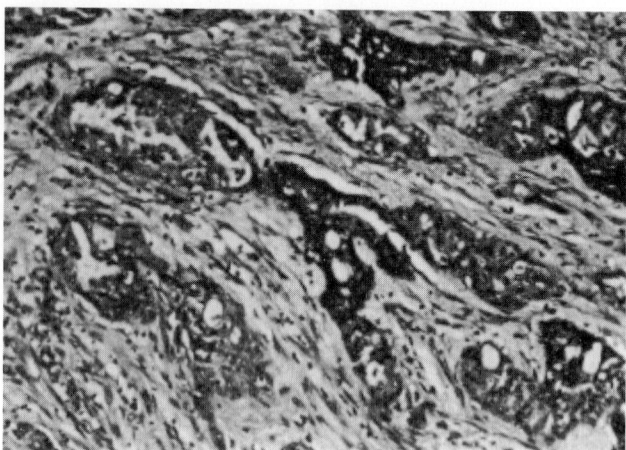

Figure 60-4
Endometrioid carcinoma. Endometrioid-type glands infiltrating stroma with focal squamous metaplasia.

These criteria include (1) the presence or absence of invasion; (2) the degree of stratification of the epithelium; and (3) the degree of atypia. The study by Chaitin et al (1985) essentially agrees with these findings. Figure 60-3 shows a typical invasive mucinous tumor.

Pseudomyxoma peritonei is a rather rare condition associated with mucinous ovarian tumors in which there exists gelatinous mucinous material within the peritoneal cavity, partly free and partly attached to surfaces. Neoplastic cells are intermingled with cysts and pockets surrounded by dense connective tissue. This condition may also be associated with a mucocele of the appendix or an appendiceal carcinoma. The mucinous ascites cannot usually be drained by a paracentesis. Repeat laparotomies may be indicated for severe abdominal distention, pain, or intestinal obstruction. Other than evacuation of the mucinous material at the time of laparotomy, no effective treatment exists.

Endometrioid Carcinoma

Borderline endometrioid tumors are rather rare atypical proliferations that are confined within areas of endometriosis or endometrioid adenofibromas in which the epithelium has low-grade malignant nuclear features without evidence of invasion (Bell and Scully, 1985a).

Endometrioid carcinoma of the ovary was first described in 1925 by Sampson. It accounts for approximately 10% to 25% of all epithelial ovarian cancers (Long and Taylor, 1964; Czernobilsky et al, 1970b). Up to 30% of these tumors coexist with endometrial adenocarcinoma (Eifel et al, 1982). They are found in association with endometriosis in approximately 10% of cases. Grossly, most endometrioid carcinomas are cystic, frequently with papillary structures filling the lumen. Occasionally they are solid. Bilateral involvement occurs in approximately 30% to 50% of

cases, with about 50% of patients having stage I disease (Long and Taylor, 1964; Czernobilsky et al, 1970b; Aure et al, 1971). Microscopically, these tumors closely resemble endometrial adenocarcinoma. Associated squamous metaplasia is very common. Figure 67-4 shows an endometrioid carcinoma.

Clear Cell Carcinomas

Borderline clear cell tumors are adenofibromas with moderate to marked atypia and mitosis but without stromal invasion (Roth et al, 1984; Bell and Scully, 1985b). They account for only 2% of borderline tumors (Russell, 1979b). They are almost always stage I, and the vast majority are unilateral.

Clear cell carcinomas account for approximately 5% of epithelial ovarian malignancies (Kurman and Craig, 1972). As with endometrioid tumors, clear cell carcinoma may be associated with endometriosis or endometrial cancer. Most tumors are partially cystic. Bilaterally occurs in 40% (Czernobilsky et al, 1970a). Almost 50% of cases are stage I (Aure et al, 1971). Microscopically, these tumors contain tubules lined by hobnail cells, glands, papillae, and cysts within varying amounts of stroma (Fig. 60-5).

Brenner Tumor

Proliferating Brenner tumors were first described by Roth and Sternberg in 1971. Other investigators (Hallgrimson and Scully, 1972; Miles and Norris, 1972) confirmed these findings. Most of these tumors are large and cystic, with polypoid masses projecting into the lumen. Microscopic examination reveals intracystic papillary growth that closely resembles low-grade transitional cell carcinoma of the urinary bladder.

Malignant Brenner tumors are usually large and multicystic, with polypoid masses projecting into the

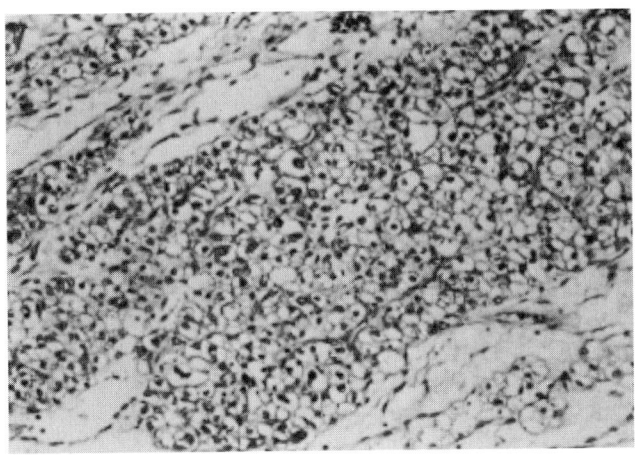

Figure 60–5
Clear cell carcinoma. Solid pattern with cells containing clear cytoplasm.

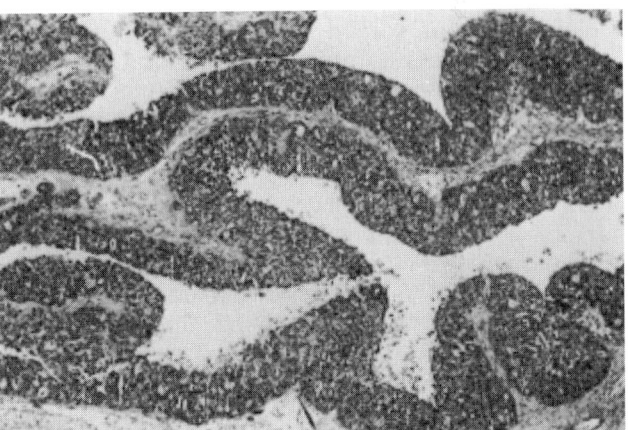

Figure 60–6
Transitional cell carcinoma. Papillary configuration with smooth border projecting into empty cystic spaces.

lumen. Most are unilateral and stage I (Roth and Czernobilsky, 1985). Microscopically, there is malignant squamous or transitional epithelium in dense fibrous stroma.

Transitional Cell Carcinoma

In 1987, Austin and Norris reported their experience with a newly described entity, transitional cell carcinoma of the ovary. Histologically, this tumor differs from malignant Brenner tumor only by the absence of a benign Brenner component. In addition, the transitional cell carcinomas were more likely to spread beyond the ovary (69% vs. 19%), were more likely to result in death even if confined to the ovary (57% vs. 12%), and lacked the prominent stromal calcifications present in most malignant Brenner tumors. Subsequent reports developed from our independent study of these tumors at the M. D. Anderson Cancer Center (MDACC) suggested that transitional cell carcinoma is more chemosensitive and associated with more favorable survival than serous carcinoma (Robey et al, 1989; Silva et al, 1990). The actuarial 5-year survival rate for 88 patients with stages II through IV transitional cell carcinoma treated with surgery and chemotherapy was 37% (Silva et al, 1990). A subsequent matched control study of advanced-stage patients treated with platinum-based chemotherapy found that transitional cell carcinoma of the ovary is significantly more chemosensitive and is associated with a better prognosis than the more common serous carcinoma (Gershenson et al, 1993).

Grossly, transitional cell carcinoma is indistinguishable from other types of epithelial ovarian cancer, with solid areas admixed with cystic areas. Microscopically, it resembles typical transitional cell carcinoma of the bladder, with thick papillary proliferations having a smooth luminal border and projecting into empty cystic spaces. The epithelial cells

forming the papillae are polygonal. Focally, spindle cells and glandular lumina are present. Figure 60–6 shows the typical histologic features of a typical transitional cell carcinoma.

SPREAD PATTERN

The primary mode of dissemination of epithelial ovarian cancer is by implantation on peritoneal surfaces. After invading the ovarian capsule, tumor cells may implant in the pelvis or follow circulatory pathways up the right paracolic gutter to the right hemidiaphragm, with its network of lymphatic capillaries. From there they may traverse the diaphragm and implant on pleural surfaces, resulting in a pleural effusion. Involvement of the omentum is extremely common, occurring in over 80% of autopsied patients. Implantation on the serosa of the small intestine is also common. Ascites not infrequently accompanies peritoneal metastases. The precise mechanism of the formation of ascites remains unclear, although it may be related to either increased production or decreased clearance of peritoneal fluid by obstructed lymphatics.

Direct local extension of ovarian cancer may also occur. Enlargement of the ovarian mass with capsular penetration may result in tumor involvement of surrounding tissues, including cul-de-sac and bladder peritoneum, fallopian tubes, uterus, and rectosigmoid colon. In a small percentage of cases, tumor will infiltrate rather deeply into the wall of the colon. Occasionally, colonic mucosal involvement may be seen. Colonic obstruction may occur as a result of extrinsic compression by the ovarian mass or, less commonly, by tumor penetration and constriction that at times are indistinguishable from an obstructing colon cancer on barium enema. Direct tumor extension may also occasionally involve omentum or small intestine lying in the pelvis in proximity to the ovarian tumor, or cecum or appendix.

Hematogenous spread is rarely noted at the time of diagnosis but is not uncommon as a late manifestation. Liver and lung are most often involved, with bone, spleen, kidneys, skin, and brain being involved less frequently (Bergman, 1966; Julian et al, 1974).

The precise incidence of lymphatic metastases is not known because of inadequate staging information historically, but it is probably considerably higher than previously appreciated. Knapp and Friedman (1974) found positive para-aortic lymph nodes in 18% of 22 women with supposed stage I epithelial ovarian cancer. Musumeci et al (1977), using lymphangiography, found lymph node involvement (either pelvic or para-aortic) in 8% of patients with stage I disease and in 29% of stage III patients. Burghardt et al (1986) noted pelvic nodal involvement in 75% of patients with stages III and IV epithelial ovarian cancer but para-aortic nodal involvement only half as frequently. Factors that seem to be related to the risk of lymphatic dissemination include International Federation of Gynecology and Obstetrics (FIGO) stage, histologic grade, and vascular space involvement.

CLINICAL FEATURES

Signs and Symptoms

As the ovarian tumor enlarges, it causes compression of surrounding pelvic structures, resulting in such symptoms as constipation, urinary frequency, or pelvic pressure. If undetected, pelvic and abdominal pain and distention will eventually occur. Patients may have a variety of vague gastrointestinal complaints as well. Of course, malignant tumors may undergo changes similar to benign tumors, including torsion, hemorrhage, or rupture, which may result in acute abdominal pain and constitute a surgical emergency.

As ascites develops or the tumor metastasizes, abdominal distention becomes more pronounced. Although weight loss associated with chronic anorexia and/or intestinal obstruction is occasionally seen, weight gain associated with progressive ascites is much more common. Menstrual irregularity is also occasionally associated with ovarian malignancies.

Physical Findings

A pelvic or pelvic-abdominal mass is palpable in most patients with ovarian cancer. There are no pathognomonic findings on physical examination that distinguish a malignant from a benign tumor. Benign ovarian tumors tend to be cystic, smooth, unilateral, and mobile, whereas malignant tumors tend to be solid, nodular, and immobile or fixed. A huge mass filling the pelvis and abdomen more often represents a benign tumor or low-grade malignancy. The finding of ascites also favors malignant tumor but may

also be found in Meigs' syndrome. Although ascites may be distinguishable from a pelvic-abdominal mass by percussion, with central tympany in ascites and central dullness and lateral tympany associated with a mass, this distinction is not always possible. Ascites without the presence of a pelvic mass should lead one to consider liver disease or other primary malignancies (e.g., colon, pancreas, stomach, or breast).

Examination of the upper abdomen in patients with advanced disease may reveal hepatomegaly (related to parenchymal involvement), a central abdominal mass signifying massive omental involvement, or a Sister Mary Joseph nodule in the umbilicus. It is also important to examine the peripheral lymph node–bearing areas because these sites may occasionally be involved. Careful chest auscultation and percussion may aid in the diagnosis of pleural effusions. Of course, as with many other disease processes, advances in radiographic techniques have made some of the fine points in physical diagnosis obsolete.

Diagnosis and Preoperative Evaluation

The differential diagnosis of a pelvic mass includes benign ovarian tumors, functional cysts, endometriosis, and pelvic inflammatory disease. Common nongynecologic etiologies include diverticular disease, tumors of the colon or appendix, retroperitoneal tumors, metastatic cancer, and a pelvic kidney. If a functional ovarian cyst is strongly suspected, as evidenced by a unilateral cystic mass less than 8 to 10 cm in diameter (as confirmed by ultrasound) in a young patient, then a period of observation for approximately 6 weeks is indicated. If the mass regresses, no surgical intervention is indicated. If endometriosis is suspected, as evidenced by the symptom complex and physical findings, laparoscopy with biopsy may be indicated to differentiate it from ovarian cancer.

Certain radiographic studies are helpful in the differential diagnosis or preoperative evaluation of patients with a pelvic mass. Plain radiographs of the abdomen may help distinguish a benign cystic teratoma with its associated calcifications and hyperlucency. Psammomatous calcifications of serous carcinoma or related entities or calcification of a myomatous uterus may also be evident. Plain films may also give some indication of associated ascites or dilated loops of small intestine associated with an obstruction.

Chest radiography is useful for detecting the presence of pleural effusions or, rarely, pulmonary metastases. Excretory urography has been routinely performed in patients with a pelvic mass to detect abnormalities such as ureteral displacement or obstruction or a pelvic kidney. However, most of this information can be obtained with the less invasive sonogram. If computerized tomography (CT) is performed, excretory urography is redundant. Therefore, sonography and/or CT have essentially eliminated the necessity for excretory urography.

Barium enema is a valuable study in a patient with a pelvic mass. This test, sometimes in conjunction with proctosigmoidoscopy, will help eliminate such conditions as diverticular disease, cancer of the colon, inflammatory bowel disease, or involvement of the rectosigmoid by ovarian cancer. If the last is suspected, the patient should undergo a mechanical bowel preparation prior to surgery because a colon resection may be necessary. Upper abdominal symptoms, especially in the face of ascites without a definite pelvic mass, may require an upper gastrointestinal series to rule out gastric cancer.

Sonography may be used to differentiate benign from malignant ovarian tumors. Malignant tumors are generally multiloculated, more solid or echogenic, and larger (more than 5 cm), with thick septae and solid nodules. Ascites, if present, is easily detected by sonography; mesenteric or peritoneal involvement may also be noted, but with a high false-negative rate.

The main advantage of CT is its superior ability to detect disease in the liver, retroperitoneum, and omentum. Although it may detect disease in the pelvis, it is not as reliable as sonography. Although CT will demonstrate enlarged retroperitoneal lymph nodes, if present, it will not delineate the architecture of normal-size lymph nodes. Neither sonography nor CT is particularly reliable in detecting intraperitoneal disease smaller than 1 to 2 cm in diameter. However, CT is even superior to surgical exploration in the detection of hepatic metastases and intrauterine disease (Johnson et al, 1983; Kerr-Wilson et al, 1984). When indicated, fine-needle aspiration under CT guidance may be performed.

Magnetic resonance imaging (MRI) is a technique that involves the use of radiofrequency waves in varying magnetic fields. Whether it will prove superior to CT or sonography in the diagnosis and delineation of ovarian cancer is yet to be determined. One clear advantage, however, is its lack of radiation exposure. Comparative studies with CT and sonography will no doubt be forthcoming in the next few years.

Bipedal lymphangiography may be used to delineate lymph node involvement, but it has not been used routinely. Well-designed studies in centers with reliable findings would be of interest. Because of the low incidence of bone metastases, radionuclide bone scans are not indicated in patients suspected of having ovarian cancer. Radionuclide scans of the liver have essentially been replaced by the more reliable CT. Because mucosal involvement of the urinary bladder is exceedingly rare in the absence of symptoms such as hematuria, cystoscopy is not routinely indicated.

In summary, the clinician must consider several factors when planning a preoperative evaluation of a pelvic mass, including potential information gained with possible avoidance of more invasive procedures, possible risks of complications of these procedures, and the associated cost-effectiveness.

PROGNOSTIC FACTORS

Stage

Stage of disease is determined by the extent of tumor at the initial diagnosis. The staging classification for ovarian cancer is a surgicopathologic system, last modified by FIGO in 1985 (Cancer Committee of the International Federation of Gynecology and Obstetrics, 1986) (Table 60–2).

Stage of disease has been shown to have a significant impact on survival in a number of studies. The largest compiled series are those of Tobias and Griffiths (1976) and McGarrity et al (1982). Table 60–3 presents these survival data. Unfortunately, approximately two thirds of patients will present with either stage III or IV disease.

Although early reports suggested that the 5-year survival rate for stage I epithelial ovarian cancer was approximately 60%, more recent data indicate a 90% 5-year survival rate for several subsets of stage I patients (Young et al, 1990). The implication of the subdivisions of stage I is that tumor rupture, surface excrescences, and the presence of ascites are each unfavorable factors. Theoretically, it seems logical to believe that penetration of the ovarian capsule will invariably lead to dissemination of tumor cells throughout the peritoneal cavity. Studies from the Mayo Clinic (Malkasian et al, 1984) have indicated that these factors are associated with a worse prognosis than stage IA disease. However, a number of studies have failed to show an adverse effect of tumor rupture or ascites on survival in stage I disease (Hart and Norris, 1973; Smith and Day, 1979; Sigurdsson et al, 1983; Sevelda et al, 1989; Monga et al, 1991). Some of these studies are undoubtedly confounded by inadequate staging procedures and the effect of histologic grade.

Early studies suggested a 5-year survival of 40% to 60% for patients with stage II disease, although it may be as high as 80% for certain subsets of stage II patients. Of course, over one third of patients reported to have stage II tumors will be upstaged to stage III with repeat laparotomy performed at a referral institution (Young et al, 1983).

The 1985 FIGO revised staging schema also subdivided stage III based on volume of initial tumor. Data that confirm the influence of initial tumor volume on prognosis are beginning to emerge (Partridge et al, 1992); these data confirm the clinical impression that the greater the initial volume of tumor, the worse the prognosis, independent of the effect of debulking. For stage III patients as a whole, the 5-year survival is no better than 15% to 20%; for stage IV patients, the 5-year survival is 5% or less.

1342 / Textbook of Gynecology

Table 60-2. FIGO STAGING FOR PRIMARY CARCINOMA OF THE OVARY

STAGE	DESCRIPTION
I	Growth limited to the ovaries.
	IA — Growth limited to one ovary; no ascites. No tumor on the external surface; capsule intact.
	IB — Growth limited to both ovaries; no ascites. No tumor on the external surfaces; capsule intact.
	IC — Tumor either stage IA or IB but with tumor on surface of one or both ovaries; or with capsule ruptured; or with ascites present containing malignant cells or with positive peritoneal washings.
II	Growth involving one or both ovaries with pelvic extension.
	IIA — Extension and/or metastases to the uterus and/or tubes.
	IIB — Extension to other pelvic tissues.
	IIC — Tumor either stage IIA or IIB, but with tumor on surface of one or both ovaries; or with capsule(s) ruptured; or with ascites present containing malignant cells or with positive peritoneal washings.
III	Tumor involving one or both ovaries with peritoneal implants outside the pelvis and/or positive retroperitoneal or inguinal nodes. Superficial liver metastasis equals stage III. Tumor is limited to the true pelvis but with histologically proven malignant extension to small bowel or omentum.
	IIIA — Tumor grossly limited to the true pelvis with negative nodes but with histologically confirmed microscopic seeding of abdominal peritoneal surfaces.
	IIIB — Tumor of one or both ovaries with histologically confirmed implants of abdominal peritoneal surfaces none exceeding 2 cm in diameter. Nodes are negative.
	IIIC — Abdominal implants greater than 2 cm in diameter and/or positive retroperitoneal or inguinal nodes.
IV	Growth involving one or both ovaries, with distant metastases. If pleural effusion is present, there must be positive cytology to allot a case to stage IV. Parenchymal liver metastasis equals stage IV.

According to Cancer Committee of the International Federation of Gynecology and Obstetrics (1986).

Histologic Grade

Histologic grade is also an extremely important prognostic factor. Many studies (Day et al, 1975; Ozols et al, 1980; Sigurdsson et al, 1983; Malkasian et al, 1984; Wharton et al, 1984; Einhorn et al, 1985; Swenerton et al, 1985) have clearly shown that patients with poorly differentiated tumors have a worse prognosis than those with well-differentiated tumors. Patients with borderline tumors or tumors of low malignant potential (LMP) have a very favorable prognosis; this subject is discussed below.

One of the major problems in interpreting the literature regarding histologic grade has been the lack of uniformity in grading systems. At the MDACC, the pattern-grading system has been used (Day et al, 1975), whereas the Mayo Clinic has employed the Broders' grading system (Broders, 1926; Malkasian et al, 1984). Although there is a need for standardization of histologic grading of epithelial ovarian cancer, this goal may not be attainable because of the unique nature of each histopathologic cell type and interobserver variability (Silva and Gershenson, 1998; Shimizu et al, 1998).

Although the prognostic significance of histologic grade in serous tumors is well defined, the importance in less common histologic types—mucinous, endometrioid, clear cell—is less clear. Our pathologists at MDACC currently grade serous carcinoma as borderline, low grade, or high grade based on mitoses and atypia. All undifferentiated and transitional cell carcinomas are high grade. Clear cell carcinomas are also all high grade. We do not see any value in grading mucinous carcinomas. We grade en-

Table 60-3. FIVE-YEAR SURVIVAL RATES BY STAGE

STAGE	McGARRITY ET AL (1982)		TOBIAS AND GRIFFITHS (1976)	
	No. of Patients	5-Year Survival (%)	No. of Patients	5-Year Survival (%)
IA	940	69.7	528	65
IB	227	63.9	130	52
IC	157	50.3	80	52
IIA	251	51.8	40	60
IIB	672	42.4	205	38
III	2074	13.3	539	5
IV	933	4.1	101	3

dometrioid carcinomas in a fashion similar to endometrial cancers. Carcinomas characterized by mixed patterns are almost always high-grade lesions; in such cases, we specify which one of the components is predominant. Furthermore, histologic grade seems to be a much stronger prognostic variable in early-stage disease than in advanced disease (Day et al, 1975; Wharton et al, 1984; Swenerton et al, 1985).

Residual Tumor

Residual tumor size also appears to exert a strong influence on prognosis in advanced disease. Studies by Griffiths (1975; Griffiths et al, 1979) and Wharton (Wharton and Herson, 1981; Wharton et al, 1984) have established that patients with minimal residual disease have a better prognosis than those with bulky residual disease. Patients who begin chemotherapy with minimal residual disease have a much greater probability of achieving a complete remission than patients who begin chemotherapy with bulky disease (Young et al, 1978; Ehrlich et al, 1979; Greco et al, 1981; Edwards et al, 1983). The aforementioned evidence has been used to support the concept of cytoreductive surgery.

Decline of Serum CA-125 Level

Although preoperative serum CA-125 level has not been shown to be an independent prognostic factor, further study appears to be warranted. However, there are a number of studies that suggest that the rate of decline of serum CA-125 during chemotherapy may be prognostic (Rustin et al, 1989; Mogensen, 1992; Fayers et al, 1993). Based on current information, it may be reasonable to segregate patients into different treatment arms of a study based on the rate of decline of serum CA-125.

Other Factors

There are a number of reports (Friedlander et al, 1983; Blumenfeld et al, 1987; Rosenburg et al, 1987) demonstrating the effect of *DNA content* on prognosis in patients with ovarian cancer; those patients with aneuploid tumors have a significantly worse prognosis than patients with diploid tumors. Proliferative activity as measured in the S-phase fraction has been shown to correlate with prognosis in some studies (Kallioniemi et al, 1988; Kuhn et al, 1989) but not in others (Conte et al, 1989).

Age at diagnosis has inconsistently been reported to be a prognostic factor. Some studies (Sigurdsson et al, 1983; Einhorn et al, 1985) show that patients younger than 40 to 50 years of age survive longer, although other studies (Greco et al, 1981; Swenerton et al, 1985) have not demonstrated this effect. Yancik and associates (1986) reported that, for patients with

stage III and IV disease, 5-year survival rates for women 65 years or older were almost one half of the rate observed for women younger than 65. The influence of age is clearly confounded by the fact that younger patients have a higher proportion of low-grade tumors and less advanced disease.

Existing evidence suggests that *histologic type* has minimal influence on prognosis. Several studies (Wharton et al, 1980; Deligdisch et al, 1982) have documented that, whenever analyzed within specific stage and grade categories, patients with common epithelial tumors have similar prognoses. Conversely, studies of the Gynecologic Oncology Group (GOG) have shown a worse prognosis for advanced-stage patients with mucinous or clear cell tumors compared with other cell types (Omura et al, 1991), whereas other studies have suggested an improved survival rate for patients with advanced-stage endometrioid (Malkasian et al, 1984; Sorbe et al, 1982) and transitional cell (Robey et al, 1989; Silva et al, 1990; Gershenson et al, 1993) carcinomas.

Oncogene amplification has also been studied for its prognostic significance. Slamon and associates (1989) found a significant correlation between *HER-2/neu* oncogene amplification and survival, with patients having one copy of the gene having a mean survival of 1879 days compared with 243 days for patients with more than five copies of the gene. Berchuck and colleagues (1990) reported similar findings. However, Rubin et al (1993a) found no correlation between *HER-2/neu* amplification and survival in a multivariate analysis of patients with advanced ovarian cancer. Nevertheless, the preponderance of evidence suggests that *HER-2/neu* oncogene overexpression is prognostic in advanced ovarian cancer.

The *tumor suppressor gene* p53, which is located on chromosome 17q, has also been studied extensively as a prognostic biomarker in epithelial ovarian cancer (Marks et al, 1991; Kohler et al, 1993; Hartmann et al, 1994; Klemi et al, 1995; Eltabbakh et al, 1997). Although still somewhat controversial, it appears that *p53* overexpression by immunohistochemistry or mutation by genetic analysis is not an independent prognostic factor in ovarian cancer. *p53* Overexpression and mutation do appear to be more common in the advanced stages of epithelial ovarian cancer.

Angiogenesis factors may have prognostic significance in ovarian cancer. Paley et al (1997), in a study of tumor specimens from 68 patients with stage I and II ovarian cancer, found that increased expression of vascular endothelial growth factor was associated with a poorer prognosis.

BRCA1 has also been studied as a prognostic marker in epithelial ovarian cancer. One study suggested that ovarian cancers with a *BRCA1* mutation were associated with a better prognosis than sporadic ovarian cancers (Rubin et al, 1996). However, this study has been criticized on the basis of selection bias, and more recent studies have found no such association (Johannsson et al, 1998).

The above discussion presents a brief summary of the more prominent molecular biomarkers that have been studied in epithelial ovarian cancer. As we approach the new millennium, there has been a true revolution in the study of the molecular pathogenesis of ovarian cancer. A myriad of other biomarkers is currently under investigation.

PRIMARY SURGERY

For a patient suspected of having ovarian cancer, primary surgery accomplishes the following goals:

1. Confirmation of the diagnosis of ovarian cancer
2. Precise determination of extent of disease (i.e., surgical staging)
3. Maximum cytoreductive surgery in patients with advanced disease

Preoperative Assessment and Preparation

Careful patient selection and preoperative evaluation are an important part of the surgical management of ovarian cancer. Current minimal studies for assessment of a patient with a possible or definite mass palpable on pelvic examination include a pelvic sonogram (by either the abdominal or transvaginal approach) and a battery of serum tumor marker determinations. For patients younger than 45 years, recommended serum tumor marker screening includes CA-125, CEA, α-fetoprotein, and human chorionic gonadotropin. For older patients, only the CA-125 and CEA are indicated. If results of these studies suggest a functional ovarian cyst, then conservative management may be indicated. Such clinical management may vary from observation to percutaneous cyst aspiration to diagnostic laparoscopy, depending on several factors, including duration of the condition and characteristics of the cyst—size, consistency, presence and thickness of septae, and so forth. Conversely, if findings suggest the possibility of a malignancy (e.g., elevated levels of tumor markers, sonographic characteristics compatible with malignancy) (Fig. 60–7), then operative intervention is generally indicated. If, after careful evaluation, the physician recommends laparoscopy as an initial procedure, it is critical to ensure that expert frozen section analysis is available and that the surgeon and patient are prepared to proceed immediately to laparotomy if indicated. The report of Maiman et al (1991) has emphasized the potential problems associated with the laparoscopic management of an ovarian mass subsequently found to be malignant.

For a patient for whom surgery is indicated, the preoperative work-up should also include a chest radiograph. Chest radiography is useful for detecting the presence of pleural effusions or, rarely, pulmonary metastases. A barium enema study is valuable in some patients with a pelvic mass. This test, sometimes in conjunction with proctosigmoidoscopy, will

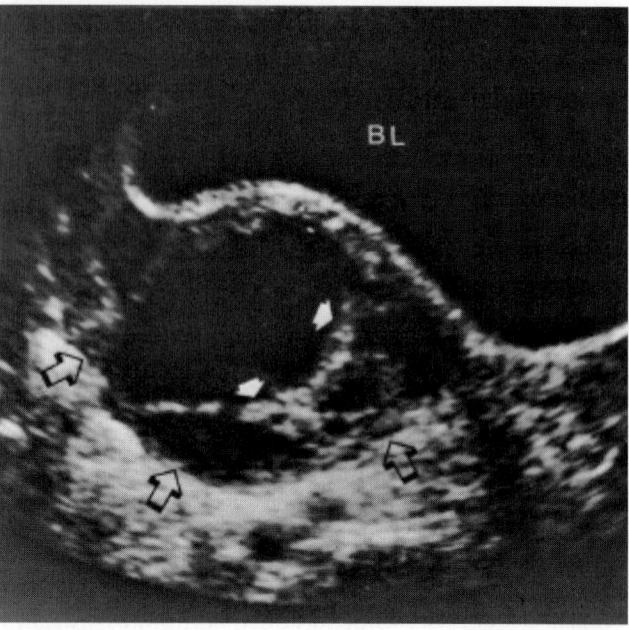

Figure 60–7
Longitudinal sonogram showing a 12-cm predominately cystic mass (*open arrows*) containing thick septations (*closed arrows*) representing a serous carcinoma of the ovary in a 57-year-old woman with ascites and pleural effusion.

help eliminate the possibility of such conditions as diverticular disease, cancer of the colon, inflammatory bowel disease, or involvement of the rectosigmoid colon by ovarian cancer (Fig. 60–8). It may be unnecessary for young patients or those with smaller, freely mobile masses.

Optional preoperative studies include intravenous pyelography, CT or MRI of the abdomen and pelvis, upper gastrointestinal tract series, and bipedal lymphangiography. If CT is performed, intravenous pyelography is redundant. Neither CT nor MRI is reliable in detecting intraperitoneal disease smaller than 1 to 2 cm in diameter. However, both are superior to surgical exploration in the detection of parenchymal hepatic metastases (a rare initial finding).

Although CT or MRI will demonstrate enlarged retroperitoneal lymph nodes, if present, these modalities will not delineate the architecture of normal-size nodes. Bipedal lymphangiography may be used to identify lymph node involvement, but it has not been used routinely.

Only if there is a strong suspicion of a nongynecologic primary cancer or hepatic metastases from ovarian cancer do we routinely obtain a preoperative CT or MRI study. Also, only if the patient has upper gastrointestinal tract symptomatology or a primary gastric cancer is suspected will we recommend endoscopy and upper gastrointestinal tract series.

Once the decision to proceed with surgery is made, the patient and her family are carefully counseled about the procedure, the indications, the possible complications, and the postoperative expectations.

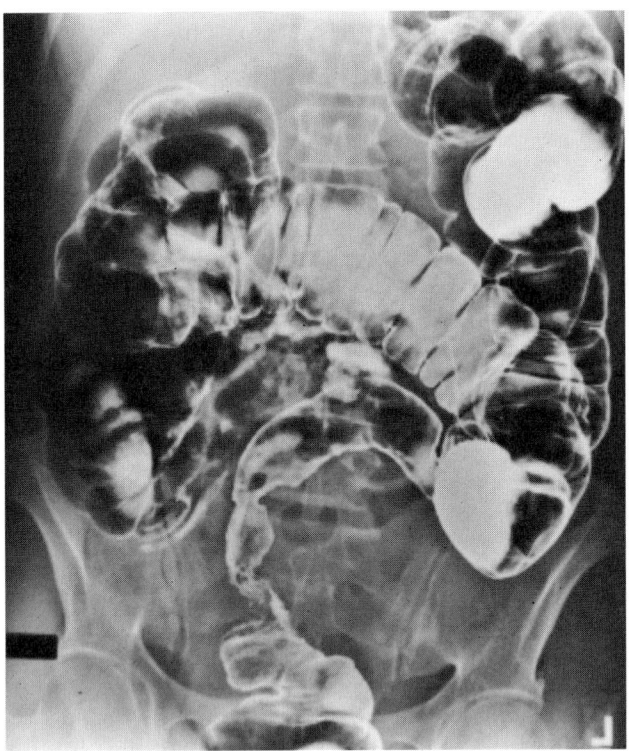

Figure 60-8
Preoperative air-contrast barium enema showing constriction of the rectosigmoid colon related to tumor involvement from ovarian cancer.

In most but not all patients, a mechanical bowel preparation is indicated preoperatively because of the potential for intestinal surgery. Patients for whom intestinal resection is more likely include those with obvious advanced disease, those with a fixed pelvic mass, or those with obvious colonic involvement or compromise found by barium enema study. Our standard bowel preparation at MDACC consists of a 1-day regimen of 3 to 4 liters of Go-LYTELY (polyethylene glycol 3350 and electrolytes). Prophylactic antibiotics are also administered perioperatively. Some type of prophylaxis against thromboembolic phenomena—either subcutaneous heparin or a pneumatic compression device—is also recommended.

A central venous line is inserted preoperatively via either the subclavian or antecubital route; this catheter can be used for hemodynamic monitoring in the perioperative period, for delivery of total parenteral nutrition postoperatively, or for subsequent chemotherapy administration.

Of course, an important component of preoperative preparation includes assessment of the patient's general medical condition. Past history, medications, allergies, and previous medical problems should be carefully reviewed. Cardiopulmonary status is evaluated, especially in elderly patients or those with a pertinent medical history. If massive pleural effusions exist, preoperative thoracentesis may be indicated to allow for better pulmonary expansion. Oc-

casionally, even insertion of a thoracostomy tube is prudent. Likewise, for patients with massive ascites causing excessive pain or pulmonary compromise, preoperative paracentesis may be indicated. In general, routine preoperative paracentesis is not recommended because of the risk of tumor implantation in the site and the small risk of intestinal contamination or bleeding.

Although initial surgery is the obvious choice for patients suspected of having an ovarian malignancy, there are exceptions. Patients who are poor surgical candidates because of massive reaccumulating effusions or severe medical problems may be best served by treatment with initial chemotherapy for two to three cycles prior to surgical intervention, performed after effusions have resolved or the medical condition has improved. In such cases, a presumptive diagnosis of ovarian cancer should be supported by a cytologic diagnosis of the effusion or a sample obtained by fine-needle aspiration. A decision to depart from standard management is often difficult and should be carefully made on an individual basis. The surgeon's previous experience is an important factor. Of course, the options and risks need to be thoroughly discussed with the patient and her family.

Surgical Staging

Stage of disease is determined by the extent of tumor at the time of initial diagnosis. The staging classification for ovarian cancer is a surgicopathologic system, last modified by FIGO in 1985 (Cancer Committee, 1986) (Table 60-2). Several studies have demonstrated a significant impact of FIGO stage on survival. Among the largest are the compiled series of Tobias and Griffiths (1976) and McGarrity et al (1982) (Table 60-3).

The gynecologic literature is replete with inadequate staging information. Several reports (Creasman and Rutledge, 1971; Keettel et al, 1974; Knapp and Friedman, 1974; Rosenoff et al, 1975; Musumeci et al, 1977; Piver et al, 1978; Chen and Lee, 1983; Young et al, 1983) (Table 60-4) have documented occult metastases in patients with apparent stage I or II disease. The problem of inadequate staging in ovarian cancer is illustrated by the collaborative study of Young et al (1983), in which 100 patients with apparent early disease (stages IA through IIB) underwent a variety of restaging procedures upon referral to one of the member institutions. Thirty-one patients were found to have more advanced disease than originally thought, and 23 of the 31 patients (74%) actually had stage III disease. In 61% of patients found to have a more advanced disease stage, procedures other than a second laparotomy (i.e., laparoscopy or lymphangiography) confirmed this evidence.

McGowan et al (1985) reported that only 54% of 291 patients with ovarian cancer received proper staging procedures. The most common examinations

Table 60-4. SITES OF METASTASES IN PATIENTS WITH APPARENT STAGE I OR II EPITHELIAL OVARIAN CANCER

STUDY	NO. PATIENTS WITH METASTASIS AT SITE/TOTAL NO. PATIENTS WITH SITE SAMPLED				
	Peritoneal Cytology	Omentum	Diaphragm	Pelvic Nodes	Para-aortic Nodes
Knapp and Friedman (1974)		1/21		0/9	5/26
Musumeci et al (1977)				2/61	2/61
Creasman and Rutledge (1971)	1/10				
Keettel et al (1974)	16/44				
Rosenoff et al (1975)			7/16		
Piver et al (1978)	8/31	0/5	1/31		0/5
Chen and Lee (1983)				2/21	4/21
Young et al (1983)		6/57	2/58	1/11	6/52
TOTAL	15/85 (29.4%)	7/83 (8.4%)	10/105 (9.5%)	5/102 (4.9%)	17/165 (10.3%)

or procedures missed in incompletely evaluated cases included visualization and palpation of the undersurfaces of the diaphragm, biopsy of the pelvic peritoneum, observation and/or cytologic sampling of peritoneal fluid, and omental biopsy. Moreover, the completeness of the staging procedures varied depending on the type of specialist performing the procedure: gynecologic oncologists, 97%; obstetrician-gynecologists, 53%, and general surgeons, 35%.

In a multicenter trial from the Netherlands, Trimbos and colleagues (1990) reported that surgical staging after one or two laparotomies was complete in only 53% of 86 patients. The most frequently omitted staging steps were biopsy of the paracolic gutter, biopsy of the pelvic peritoneum, and sampling of the retroperitoneal lymph nodes. The authors attributed the incompleteness of the staging procedures either to increased risk or difficulty of the procedure or to lack of knowledge of the sites at risk for metastases. In a survey of 785 ovarian cancer cases diagnosed in 1991, which were selected from the SEER program, Muñoz et al (1997) found that only approximately 10% of women with presumptive stage I and II ovarian cancer received recommended staging and treatment. The absence of lymphadenectomy and assignment of histologic grade were the primary reasons.

A major dilemma facing gynecologic oncologists is the referral of a patient with apparent stage I epithelial carcinoma of the ovary who has had an incomplete staging procedure. We are in the midst of an evolution in which we are attempting to strictly define a subset of patients with early epithelial ovarian cancer who require no adjuvant therapy; inadequate staging information obviously escalates the difficulty in making a decision about the need for postoperative therapy in such patients. In addition to the study by Young et al (1983), other reports (Greer et al, 1980; Helewa et al, 1986) have addressed the rationale for a second laparotomy for patients referred after an initial incomplete surgical staging.

The recent emphasis on surgical staging has heightened our awareness of retroperitoneal nodal involvement associated with epithelial ovarian cancer. In 1974, Knapp and Friedman reported finding aortic nodal involvement with tumor in 19% of 26 patients with apparent stage I ovarian cancer. Since then, other studies (Chen and Lee, 1983; Burghardt et al, 1986; Wu et al, 1986) have shown nodal involvement in over 50% of patients with epithelial ovarian cancer.

Proper staging procedures should consist of the following:

1. Although a transverse abdominal incision is cosmetically superior, a vertical midline incision is preferable to provide adequate exposure for appropriate staging biopsies or resection of metastatic disease in the upper abdomen.
2. Ascites, if present, should be evacuated and submitted for cytologic analysis. If no peritoneal fluid is noted, cytologic washings of the pelvis, bilateral paracolic gutters, and subdiaphragmatic areas should be performed prior to manipulation of the intraperitoneal contents. Cytologic washings are obtained by instilling approximately 50 to 100 ml of normal saline into each area.
3. The entire peritoneal cavity and its structures should be carefully inspected and palpated in a systematic manner. We generally prefer to begin with the subphrenic spaces and move caudad, toward the pelvis. In particular, the subdiaphragmatic areas, hepatic capsule, omentum, colon, all peritoneal surfaces, the entire retroperitoneum, and small intestinal serosa and mesentery should be checked. If any suspicious areas are noted, they should be excised or sampled. During this process, one should be vigilant for nongynecologic primary cancers.
4. The primary ovarian tumor and pelvis should be examined. Both ovaries should be carefully as-

sessed for size, presence of obvious tumor involvement, capsular rupture, external excrescences, and adherence to surrounding structures. If the surgical findings are strongly suggestive of a benign ovarian mass in a young patient desirous of future childbearing, then ovarian cystectomy may be indicated. Otherwise, a unilateral salpingo-oophorectomy should be performed and the specimen submitted for frozen section examination. If bilateral ovarian masses are present, the more suspicious side should be dealt with initially. If frozen section analysis reveals a malignant epithelial tumor, standard surgical therapy consists of hysterectomy and bilateral salpingo-oophorectomy. Exceptions to this rule (i.e., conservative surgery) are discussed below.

5. If disease seems to be limited (i.e., confined to the ovary or localized to the pelvis), then random staging biopsies of structures at risk should be performed. These sites include the omentum (either omentectomy or generous biopsies from multiple areas) and the peritoneal surfaces of the following sites: bilateral paracolic gutters, cul-de-sac, lateral pelvic walls, vesicouterine reflection, and subdiaphragmatic areas. Any adhesions should be generously sampled. Some surgeons, including the authors, prefer cytologic analysis by saline lavage rather than scraping or biopsy of clinically normal subdiaphragmatic surfaces. Others prefer scraping the subdiaphragmatic surfaces with a wooden spatula or tongue depressor and making a cytologic smear. Still others perform biopsies using laparoscopic equipment. The advantage of one technique over another, however, remains unclear and will require further study. In addition, no definitive studies demonstrate that total omentectomy or even infracolic omentectomy is more beneficial in terms of diagnostic accuracy or survival than generous sampling of the omentum in a patient without gross omental tumor.

6. If gross metastatic disease is present, it should be excised if feasible or at least sampled to document disease extent. The concept of cytoreductive surgery and supporting evidence is discussed below.

7. As noted above, the retroperitoneum has historically been the area of greatest neglect. The para-aortic and bilateral pelvic lymph node–bearing areas should be carefully palpated. Any suspicious nodes should be excised or sampled. If no suspicious nodes are detected, we generously sample these areas. There is no evidence at present that a complete para-aortic and/or pelvic lymphadenectomy is advantageous.

TREATMENT OF BORDERLINE TUMORS

Approximately 10% to 15% of all ovarian neoplasms are of the borderline or LMP classification. In 1929, Taylor first described a group of patients with "semi-malignant" or hyperplastic ovarian tumors without

histologic evidence of stromal invasion but with peritoneal implants. He noted that these patients had a better prognosis than those with frankly malignant tumors. However, not until FIGO recognized the distinct clinical entity of "carcinoma of low malignant potential" (International Federation of Gynecology and Obstetrics, 1971) and the WHO adopted the term *borderline malignancies* (Serov et al, 1973) did this group of tumors become fully appreciated. Only in the last decade have we begun to understand their biologic behavior and optimal treatment.

Histologic types include serous (the most common), mucinous, endometrioid, clear cell, and the Brenner tumors. These entities are defined by very strict histologic criteria, the most striking of which is the lack of stromal invasion. Although these tumors are not uncommon in older patients, they are frequently diagnosed in women in the reproductive age group, with a median age some 10 years younger than that for frankly invasive cancer.

The majority of borderline tumors are confined to one or both ovaries. Approximately 33% to 60% of serous tumors of LMP are limited to one ovary (Russell, 1979a). Extraovarian spread is noted in 16% to 18% (Aure et al, 1971). Of mucinous tumors of LMP, at least 80% to 90% are confined to one ovary (Russell, 1979a). Both endometrioid and clear cell LMP tumors are almost always stage I, and the vast majority are unilateral.

For patients with borderline tumors seemingly confined to one ovary, appropriate surgical management includes unilateral salpingo-oophorectomy with surgical staging. For older patients for whom fertility is not an issue, hysterectomy and bilateral salpingo-oophorectomy are acceptable therapy. For young patients with unilateral ovarian involvement, the use of ovarian cystectomy has been reported (Tazelaar et al, 1985; Lim-Tan et al, 1988). Some patients treated in this manner, however, will require repeat surgery for recurrent tumor involvement of the ovary. If bilateral borderline tumors are present, then bilateral salpingo-oophorectomy is appropriate therapy for older patients. For young patients, portions of one or both ovaries may be preserved with ovarian cystectomies, if feasible. In young patients for whom bilateral adnexectomy cannot be avoided, uterine preservation should be considered. Whatever the surgical approach, the 5-year survival of patients with stage I borderline tumors is 95% or better (Aure et al, 1971; Hart and Norris, 1973; Katzenstein et al, 1978; Russell and Merkur, 1979; Genadry et al, 1981; Barnhill et al, 1985, 1995; Chaitin et al; 1985; Bostwick et al, 1986).

For patients with peritoneal implants or supposed metastatic borderline ovarian tumors, the optimal management is less clear. Surgery is also the mainstay of treatment of advanced disease; after frozen section confirmation of borderline tumor, an effort should be made to resect all gross disease. In addition, staging biopsies of peritoneal surfaces and lymph nodes and cytologic washings are indicated.

Even in the face of peritoneal implants, a normal contralateral ovary may be preserved in young patients. In such cases, however, some recommend ovarian biopsy to eliminate the possibility of occult disease. In patients with advanced-stage serous disease, the incidence of bilateral tumors is approximately 75% (Gershenson and Silva, 1990).

The necessity or efficacy of postoperative therapy for patients with advanced-stage disease remains controversial. Some experts recommend only observation, whereas others advocate chemotherapy. A commonly held theory is that these well-differentiated tumors are too slow-growing to respond to chemotherapy. Several reports, however, have surgically documented objective responses, both complete and partial, of borderline tumors to chemotherapy (Barnhill et al, 1985; Kliman et al, 1986; Gershenson and Silva, 1990).

Some investigators have attempted to relate the type of peritoneal implants—benign (endosalpingiosis), noninvasive, or invasive—to survival in advanced-disease patients, but the available literature is confusing and contradictory. Patients with peritoneal implants containing only endosalpingiosis have only stage I disease and can clearly be treated with surgery alone. Some studies (McCaughey et al, 1984; Russell, 1984; Bell et al, 1988) have shown poor survival rates of patients with invasive implants, whereas others (Kliman et al, 1986; Michael and Roth, 1986; Gershenson and Silva, 1990) have not. The varying findings of these studies are potentially confounded by the fact that many patients received postoperative therapy but some did not. In addition, the types of postoperative therapy varied considerably. Other explanations for the disparate conclusions of these studies include differences in definitions of noninvasive and invasive implants and inadequate follow-up times. Until further information becomes available, I currently favor postoperative platinum-based chemotherapy for patients with serous borderline tumors and invasive peritoneal implants, despite the fact that definitive proof of benefit is lacking. In our most recent update of the experience with women with serous borderline tumors with invasive implants, 31% of 39 patients developed progressive or recurrent tumor, and 15% were dead of disease (Gershenson et al, 1998c). In addition, in all but one case, the recurrence was a low-grade invasive serous carcinoma.

For patients with noninvasive peritoneal implants, optimal management remains even less clear. A small, yet significant percentage of these patients (10% to 15%) appear to develop recurrent disease, sometimes despite postoperative treatment. A definitive answer to these very important clinical dilemmas will only come from multicenter randomized clinical trials comparing no postoperative treatment with a consistent postoperative treatment or from reports of excellent disease-free survival in such patients treated with surgery alone. In the most recent update of our experience with these tumors, 30% of patients developed progressive or recurrent tumor, and 8% were dead of disease (Gershenson et al, 1998a). In 70% of the recurrent tumors, the histology was low-grade serous carcinoma, and in 30% it was serous borderline tumor. It is, of course, possible that these apparent recurrences really represent new primary lesions, because the average time from diagnosis to "recurrence" is typically several years. Molecular biomarkers may be helpful in the future in selecting a subset of patients with borderline tumors and peritoneal implants for postoperative therapy.

EARLY-STAGE OVARIAN CANCER

Older studies of ovarian cancer have shown a 5-year survival rate of approximately 60% in patients with stage I disease (Tobias and Griffiths, 1976; Richardson et al, 1985). Unfortunately, many of these early studies were plagued by inaccurate staging and rather imprecise classification of histologic type and grade. Consequently, appropriate treatment of patients with stage I disease remains elusive even to experts in gynecologic oncology, although results of recent studies are helping to clarify this issue.

For older women who have completed childbearing, standard surgical management of apparent early-stage ovarian cancer includes bilateral salpingo-oophorectomy, hysterectomy, and surgical staging. A significant subset of patients with early-stage epithelial malignancies, however, is young and can be managed conservatively. Conservative management is used here to denote surgery that preserves reproductive potential without compromising curability.

When contemplating surgery on a young patient with a suspected ovarian malignancy, it is important to discuss with her all possible operative findings and procedures and long-term implications of the various options. If the patient is a minor, the parents need to clearly understand this information. Comprehensive preoperative counseling can be thwarted by any of a number of circumstances: the chaos that sometimes surrounds an emergency operation for acute abdominal pain; the surgeon's denial of the possibility of malignancy; or the surgeon's lack of understanding of the biology of the variants of ovarian cancer that may afflict young patients.

In most instances, young patients have their initial surgery done outside major university hospitals or cancer centers. Common errors in surgical management include inadequate staging and unnecessary bilateral adnexectomy. In addition, some patients are mismanaged because of an error in the pathologic diagnosis.

The ideal candidate for conservative surgical management is a young patient who has stage Ia disease. If, on initial inspection, the suspected cancer is confined to one ovary, then unilateral salpingo-oophorectomy is appropriate. If the mass is thought to be benign, then ovarian cystectomy may be preferable. The specimen should be sent for frozen section examination. If malignancy is diagnosed, appropriate staging biopsies and cytologic washings should be performed, as discussed above. If the contralateral ovary appears normal, it should be left undisturbed to avoid potential infertility caused by peritoneal adhesions or ovarian failure.

One should not rely too heavily on frozen section examination in making the decision to perform a hysterectomy and bilateral salpingo-oophorectomy. If the histologic diagnosis is in question, it is always preferable to wait for permanent section results for a young patient, even if this requires a repeat laparotomy.

Although strict criteria usually exclude from conservative management patients whose tumors are bilateral, adherent, nonencapsulated, or ruptured and patients with ascites or positive cytologic washings, even with such findings one may consider combining conservative surgery with postoperative adjuvant chemotherapy in selected young patients.

The advent of in vitro fertilization technology should also have an impact on intraoperative management. Convention has dictated that, if a bilateral salpingo-oophorectomy is necessary, a hysterectomy should also be performed. However, current technology for donor oocyte transfer and hormonal support allows a woman without ovaries to sustain a normal intrauterine pregnancy. Similarly, if the uterus and one ovary are resected because of tumor involvement, current techniques allow retrieval of oocytes from the patient's remaining ovary, in vitro fertilization with sperm from her male partner, and implantation of the embryo into a surrogate's uterus. Therefore, traditional guidelines concerning surgical management of ovarian cancer may no longer be applicable in selected young patients.

The major factors in addition to stage that influence the selection process are histologic grade and bilaterality. Serous tumors are bilateral in about 50% of cases. The incidence of bilaterality for mucinous tumors varies widely in reported series from as low as 5% to as high as 50%, but probably is no greater than 10% to 20%. Approximately 30% to 50% of endometrioid and clear cell cancers are bilateral.

For most patients with apparent stage I ovarian cancer, however, childbearing has been completed, and standard surgical management consists of abdominal hysterectomy, bilateral salpingo-oophorectomy, and comprehensive surgical staging. Within the stage I category, histologic grade is the most powerful predictor of outcome (Dembo et al, 1990). Patients with well-differentiated or grade 1 tumors have an excellent prognosis, with a 5-year survival rate of over 90%. In contrast, the 5-year survival rates for patients with grade 2 or 3 tumors are approximately 75% to 80% and 50% to 60%, respectively. Other factors that have been found to have prognostic significance include large-volume ascites (Dembo et al, 1990), dense adherence (Dembo et al, 1990), and clear cell histology (Young et al, 1990;

Monga et al, 1991). Capsular rupture per se has not been found to be a significant independent prognostic factor (Sevelda et al, 1989; Dembo et al, 1990; Monga et al, 1991).

Therefore, for patients with stage I, grade 1 tumors, surgery alone is adequate treatment, and the 5-year survival should be at least 95% (Dembo et al, 1990; Young et al, 1990; Trimbos et al, 1991). In a study conducted by the Ovarian Cancer Study Group and the Gynecologic Oncology Group (Young et al, 1990), 81 patients with stage Iai and Ibi, grade 1 and 2 epithelial ovarian cancer were randomized to either observation or melphalan chemotherapy. There was no significant difference in disease-free survival (91 vs. 98%, respectively). Trimbos and associates (1991) noted tumor recurrence in only 4 of 67 patients (6%) treated with surgery alone for stages Ia through IIa, grade 1 cancer.

For patients with grade 3 tumors, clear cell histology, stage Ic or II, postoperative therapy is probably indicated because of the higher risk of recurrence. Patients with grade 2 tumors are problematic, and opinions vary about the necessity for adjuvant treatment. This controversy is compounded by the lack of uniformity of grading systems. Of course, the key to the appropriate selection of patients for adjuvant therapy is adequate surgical staging information and reliable pathologic analysis.

Once a high-risk subset is defined, the next logical question is the optimal treatment. Treatments studied include single-agent melphalan, intraperitoneal chromic phosphate, and cisplatin-based combination chemotherapy. In prospective randomized trials conducted in the United States, the bias is that all high-risk early-stage ovarian cancer patients ethically require adjuvant treatment because their prognosis is relatively unfavorable. The European philosophy is that there is no proven benefit of postoperative treatment in this group; thus, European randomized trials typically include a study treatment versus observation. Ahmed et al (1996) reported a study in which 194 patients with stage I epithelial ovarian cancer were followed after surgery alone. Five-year survival rates were as follows: stage Ia, 93.7%; stage Ib, 92%; and stage Ic, 84%. Multivariate analysis revealed that histologic grade, presence of ascites, and surface tumor were independent prognostic factors. Intraoperative capsular rupture was not prognostically significant.

In a second randomized trial of the GOG (Young et al, 1990), 141 patients with stages Iaii, Ibii, IIa, IIb, IIc, or stages Ia or Ib with grade 3 histology were randomized to receive either melphalan or intraperitoneal chromic phosphate. The disease-free survival rates for the two groups were identical—80%. Severe toxicities included four patients (6%) who underwent laparotomy for intestinal obstruction in the radioisotope group and two patients who died of leukemia in the melphalan group. Soper et al (1992) reported only a 65% disease-free survival for 23 patients with stage I epithelial ovarian cancer treated with surgery plus intraperitoneal chromic phosphate. They concluded that this adjuvant therapy was ineffective.

The most popular current adjuvant therapy for stage I high-risk patients is cisplatin-based chemotherapy. Piver et al (1989) and Dottino et al (1991) have reported excellent survival rates (>90%) in small series of patients treated with cisplatin-based chemotherapy. Rubin et al (1993b) retrospectively reviewed 62 patients with stage I epithelial ovarian cancer, all of whom underwent comprehensive surgical staging followed by platinum-based chemotherapy. Fifteen patients (24%) relapsed. No patient was rendered disease-free after relapse. Patients with grade 3 tumors and clear cell histology had a higher risk of relapse. Bolis et al (1995) reported the results of two multicenter trials conducted by the Gruppo Italiano Collaborativo in Oncologia Ginecologica. A total of 271 patients were included in these two trials. Trial 1 compared single-agent cisplatin to observation in patients with stage Ia and Ib, grade 2 and 3 cancer. Trial 2 compared single-agent cisplatin to intraperitoneal chromic phosphate in patients with stages Iaii, Ibii, and Ic cancer. In both trials, although the cisplatin groups had a better disease-free survival, overall survival was not significantly different compared with the observation arms. One might conclude from available information that the influence of platinum-based chemotherapy on survival of early-stage ovarian cancer patients remains unclear.

Recently completed and ongoing studies of early ovarian cancer reflect current views. The GOG has recently completed a trial for patients with stage I ovarian cancer in which patients are randomized between intraperitoneal chromic phosphate and three cycles of cisplatin/cyclophosphamide chemotherapy. The results of this trial are not yet mature. The current GOG trial for high-risk early-stage patients is a randomization between three cycles of paclitaxel/carboplatin and six cycles of paclitaxel/carboplatin. Several ongoing randomized trials from the United Kingdom and Europe include randomization between various types of platinum-based chemotherapy and observation.

In summary, although we are much closer to selection of a high-risk subset of patients with stage I disease who may benefit from adjuvant therapy, the optimal treatment remains unclear.

ADVANCED-STAGE OVARIAN CANCER

Primary Cytoreductive Surgery

Cytoreductive or debulking surgery refers to a surgical procedure in which the goal is to reduce the amount of tumor as much as possible in a patient with metastatic ovarian cancer. Early studies (Munnell et al, 1957; Delclos and Quinlan, 1969; Aure et al, 1971) suggested a relationship between the completeness of the surgery or the amount of residual tumor and survival. Griffiths (1975), in a landmark paper, demonstrated an inverse relationship between residual tumor diameter and survival; patients having residual disease less than 1.5 cm in diameter had a significantly improved survival compared with patients with bulky residual disease. More recent reports (Griffiths et al, 1979; Wharton and Herson, 1981; Hacker et al, 1983) subsequently confirmed these findings (Table 60–5). As our philosophy about cytoreductive surgery has evolved over the last two decades, "optimal debulking" has come to denote minimal residual disease no greater than 1.5 to 2.0 cm in diameter; "suboptimal debulking" denotes bulky residual disease greater than 2.0 cm in diameter.

Cytoreductive surgery, of course, must be considered not in a vacuum but rather in the context of responsiveness of residual tumor to postoperative therapies. Both radiotherapy (Delclos and Quinlan, 1969) and chemotherapy (Young et al, 1978; Ehrlich et al, 1979; Greco et al, 1981) trials have shown a higher response rate in patients with minimal residual disease. These observations are supported by basic studies that suggest that larger tumor masses have poorly perfused anoxic areas that are not accessible to cytotoxic agents. Furthermore, larger tumors may have a greater proportion of cells in the resting phase. These nonproliferating cells may be less sensitive to cytotoxic agents. Skipper (1978, 1983) espoused the "fractional cell kill hypothesis," stating that the ability of chemotherapeutic agents to

Table 60–5. SURVIVAL BY RESIDUAL DISEASE FOLLOWING CYTOREDUCTION

| STUDY | NO. OF PATIENTS | OPTIMAL CYTOREDUCTION ACHIEVED | MEDIAN SURVIVAL (MONTHS) | |
			Optimal Cytoreduction	Suboptimal Cytoreduction
Griffiths (1975)	102	72	28.6	11
Wharton and Herson (1981)*	104	43	27.6	15.3
Hacker et al (1983)	47	66	22	6

*Not all patients operated on at authors' institution.
Modified from Hacker et al: Contemp OB GYN, 1983; November:70, with permission.

eradicate cancer cells depends on both the dose of drug and the number of cells present. A given dose of drug kills a constant fraction of cells with each exposure. However, certain factors such as cell repair mechanisms, tumor heterogeneity, the fraction of cells in G_0 phase, and the development of drug resistance serve to counteract this process. Goldie and Coldman (1979) have shown that tumor cells have an intrinsic spontaneous mutation rate; larger tumors that go untreated for an extended period theoretically have a greater probability of containing cell populations resistant to anticancer agents. Therefore, even though patients with advanced ovarian cancer may undergo optimal debulking, the small residual tumor masses may still contain drug-resistant cells that preclude ultimate cure.

Several reports (Griffiths et al, 1979; Wharton and Herson, 1981; Hacker et al, 1983; Chen and Bochner, 1985; Piver and Baker, 1986) have described the accomplishment of optimal cytoreductive surgery in a high percentage of patients, approximately 75% in several series. The morbidity and mortality associated with cytoreductive surgery have also been analyzed (Blyth and Wahl, 1982; Hacker et al, 1983; Chen and Bochner, 1985; Heintz et al, 1986; Piver and Baker, 1986). These studies generally reflect an operative mortality rate of less than 2%, a mean operating time of 3 to 5 hours, and a mean blood loss of approximately 500 to 1500 ml. There is a wide range of postoperative complications, the most common of which are infection, hemorrhage (at times requiring re-exploration), prolonged ileus, and cardiopulmonary problems. The primary question concerning the efficacy of primary cytoreductive surgery is whether improved survival is related more to the biology of the tumor or to the skill and aggressiveness of the surgeon. In other words, are those tumors that can be debulked optimally also tumors that are less invasive, less infiltrative, and more indolent? Available studies (Griffiths et al, 1979; Wharton and Herson, 1981; Hacker et al, 1983) do not suggest that this is the case. All demonstrated that patients who required extensive surgery to achieve minimal residual disease and those who had minimal disease at the outset had similar survival rates. More recent studies (Hoskins et al, 1992b; Partridge et al, 1992), however, suggest that patients with de novo minimal disease have a superior prognosis to those who are debulked to minimal disease, supporting the prognostic influence of substage categories within the stage III classification. Unfortunately, there are no randomized studies to resolve important issues in this area. Moreover, prospects for such studies are not good because of several factors, including deeply established biases, the multiplicity of associated prognostic factors, and the highly individualized nature of each procedure. In the meantime, the efficacy of cytoreductive surgery remains controversial. Better information will ultimately be required to define its role.

Studies indicate that, even for patients with stage IV ovarian cancer, optimal cytoreductive surgery may confer a survival advantage. Three large retrospective reports noted that patients with stage IV disease who were optimally cytoreduced had a statistically superior survival to patients who were suboptimally cytoreduced (Curtin et al, 1997; Liu et al, 1997; Munkarah et al, 1997).

The standard cytoreductive procedure for patients with disseminated epithelial ovarian cancer consists of abdominal hysterectomy (if the uterus is intact), bilateral salpingo-oophorectomy, and omentectomy (Fig. 60–9). In the course of attempting to resect as much tumor as possible, other procedures may be necessary, such as resection of the rectosigmoid colon (Berek et al, 1984a; Soper et al, 1991), small intestinal resection (Hacker et al, 1983; Chen and Bochner, 1985; Piver and Baker, 1986), resection of a portion of the urinary tract (Berek et al, 1982), splenectomy (Deppe et al, 1983; Malfetano, 1986; Sonnendecker et al, 1989; Morris et al, 1991), resection of diaphragmatic metastases (Deppe et al, 1986; Fiorica et al, 1989; Montz et al, 1989; Kapnick et al, 1990), and resection of retroperitoneal lymph nodes (Burghardt et al, 1986; Wu et al, 1986).

Several reports have described innovative techniques of debulking. These include the argon beam coagulator (Brand and Pearlman, 1990), the Cavitron

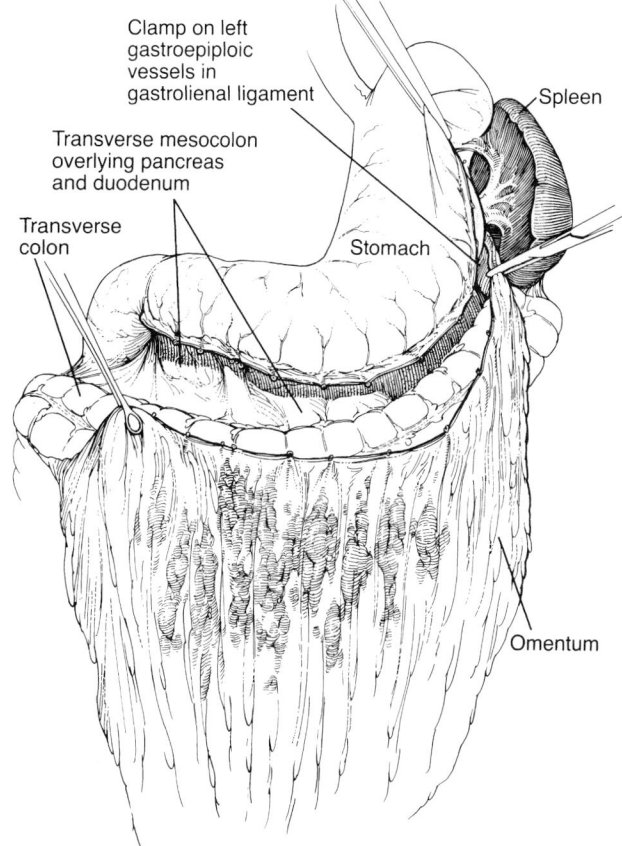

Figure 60–9
Omentectomy. Dissection of omentum with tumor from stomach, with ligation of gastric branches.

ultrasonic surgical aspirator (CUSA) (Adelson et al, 1988; Deppe et al, 1988, 1989, 1990; Adelson, 1991), and various types of laser therapy (Brand et al, 1988). The benefit of any of these new techniques for cytoreductive surgery remains unproved. Further studies will be necessary to elucidate their proper role.

Over the past two decades, the concept of neoadjuvant chemotherapy followed by interval debulking (as a primary cytoreductive procedure after a few cycles of chemotherapy) emerged. Such a primary attempt at cytoreduction should be distinguished from a "secondary" interval debulking, as discussed below. For the most part, neoadjuvant chemotherapy followed by primary surgery, rather than the standard approach of surgery followed by chemotherapy, began to be reported in the late 1970s for certain subsets of patients: (1) patients who were referred to an oncologist after a surgical or nonsurgical biopsy, or (2) patients who initially were poor surgical candidates because of a debilitated state related to massive effusions or comorbid conditions (Griffiths, 1975; Chambers et al, 1990; Jacob et al, 1991). However, this approach has been proposed as a potential alternative for all patients with advanced epithelial ovarian cancer or for certain subsets, such as those predicted to be suboptimally resected (Nelson et al, 1993; Schwartz et al, 1994; Surwitt et al, 1996). European cooperative groups are currently studying this approach in randomized clinical trials.

Chemotherapy

Single-Agent Activity

From the 1950s until the mid-1970s, single-alkylating-agent chemotherapy was standard postoperative treatment for patients with advanced epithelial ovarian cancer. Early reports of alkylating agent activity generally were based on poorly controlled studies and retrospective descriptions without definitions of patient populations, previous therapy, or response criteria. Response rates ranged from 35% to 65% when these agents were employed as first-line therapy (Tobias and Griffiths, 1976). Median survivals of patients receiving alkylating agent therapy, however, were only 8 to 19 months (Gershenson, 1987).

The two most widely used alkylating agents have been melphalan and cyclophosphamide. Melphalan was used as standard postoperative therapy to treat hundreds of patients at MDACC. Cyclophosphamide was mainly popularized by the Mayo Clinic. Other commonly used alkylating agents included chlorambucil and thiotepa. Most of the agents are not associated with many of the untoward side effects—severe nausea and vomiting, alopecia, nephrotoxicity, and neurotoxicity—noted with combination chemotherapy. Myelosuppression has been the principal side effect. The alkylating agents are also well known for their leukemogenic potential (Reimer et al, 1977; Greene et al, 1982, 1986; Kaldor

et al, 1990). With the use of alkylating agent therapy, approximately 10% to 15% of patients achieved long-term survival.

Beginning in the mid-1960s to early 1970s, new nonalkylating agents were introduced into clinical studies involving advanced ovarian cancer. These studies have documented antitumor activity of doxorubicin (O'Bryan et al, 1973; De Palo et al, 1975; Stanhope et al, 1977; Bolis et al, 1978; Wharton et al, 1982), hexamethylmelamine (Johnson et al, 1978; Bolis et al, 1979; Wharton et al, 1979), 5-fluorouracil (Malkasian et al, 1968; Jacobs et al, 1971), and methotrexate (Katz et al, 1981), mostly in patients who had failed alkylating agent therapy. In the early 1970s, cisplatin was introduced into Phase II trials in ovarian cancer patients. The majority of these studies were performed in patients in whom therapy had failed with alkylating agents. Results of the few first-line studies in the literature (Bruckner et al, 1981; Gershenson et al, 1981; Hall et al, 1981; Barlow et al, 1982) reveal response rates of 31% to 83% and median survivals of approximately 21 months. In earlier second-line trials (Bruckner et al, 1978; Wiltshaw et al, 1979; Pesando et al, 1980), cisplatin unquestionably demonstrated significant activity in previously treated patients and has since assumed a very important role in combination studies.

Combination Chemotherapy

Beginning in the mid-1970s, based on the foundation of proven single-agent activity, a large number of combination chemotherapy trials were undertaken. With the advent of combination chemotherapy, the issue of its superiority over single-agent therapy became important. Several clinical trials were therefore designed to explore this important issue. Randomized trials comparing single-agent chemotherapy with both non–platinum-based combinations (Young et al, 1978; Omura et al, 1983) and platinum-based combinations (Decker et al, 1982; Williams et al, 1985) generally showed response and/or survival benefit from the combination regimens.

Results of other clinical trials comparing single-agent therapy (either platinum or nonplatinum) with combination chemotherapy (either platinum or nonplatinum), however, have not confirmed the superiority of the latter (Advanced Ovarian Cancer Trialists Group, 1991). Nevertheless, with the introduction of cisplatin into clinical trials, several randomized and nonrandomized studies of cisplatin-based combination chemotherapy were performed during the 1980s in search of the optimal regimen (Greco et al, 1981; Vogl et al, 1982; Decker et al, 1982; Bruckner et al, 1983; Stehman et al, 1983; Belinson et al, 1984; Neijt et al, 1984; Edmonson et al, 1985; Williams et al, 1985; Gershenson et al, 1989b).

From the mid-1980s until the early-1990s, the most popular chemotherapy regimen in the United States for advanced ovarian cancer was the combination of cisplatin and cyclophosphamide (CP). Others, however, favored the three-drug combination of cisplatin, doxorubicin, and cyclophosphamide (CAP or PAC). In fact, a meta-analysis of four randomized clinical trials (Ovarian Cancer Meta-Analysis Project, 1991) noted a 7% survival advantage of CAP over CP at 6 years. It remains unclear whether this relatively small difference is related to dose intensity or to the doxorubicin itself. Many remain skeptical about this finding and, in addition, hold the opinion that any small survival advantage is overshadowed by the additional toxicity of doxorubicin. Reports have also failed to demonstrate superiority of cisplatin combination therapy over single-agent cisplatin (Advanced Ovarian Cancer Trialists Group, 1991; Gruppo Interegionale Cooperativo Oncologico Ginecologia, 1992).

In the mid-1980s, carboplatin, an analog of cisplatin, was introduced into clinical trials. Early studies demonstrated that carboplatin was less emetogenic, nephrotoxic, ototoxic, and neurotoxic than cisplatin. The dose-limiting toxicity of carboplatin is myelosuppression, particularly thrombocytopenia. A meta-analysis of 11 trials comparing carboplatin with cisplatin either as single agents or in combination revealed no significant differences in survival (Advanced Ovarian Cancer Trialists Group, 1991). Two trials have confirmed findings of similar efficacy for cisplatin and carboplatin combination regimens (Alberts et al, 1992; Swenerton et al, 1992). There was more neuropathy and nephrotoxicity in the cisplatin arm of both studies, although the excessive toxicity associated with cisplatin in one of these trials (Alberts et al, 1992) was most probably a result of the relatively high dose (100 mg/m^2) used.

Based on encouraging results of Phase II studies of paclitaxel in patients with refractory ovarian cancer (see below), the GOG initiated a randomized trial comparing the standard regimen of CP with the combination of paclitaxel and cisplatin in patients with suboptimal advanced epithelial ovarian cancer (McGuire et al, 1996). Although the negative second-look rate was not statistically different—20% versus 26%, respectively—both the progression-free survival and overall survival were superior for patients in the paclitaxel-cisplatin arm. Therefore, when preliminary results of this trial became available in the mid-1990s, paclitaxel-cisplatin rapidly became the standard regimen in the United States. Subsequently, a Phase I study of the combination of 3-hour paclitaxel and carboplatin established this regimen as the most popular postoperative treatment for patients with epithelial ovarian cancer (Ozols et al, 1993). Although equivalent efficacy of this regimen to the paclitaxel-cisplatin combination has not yet been definitively shown, a lower toxicity profile and ease of treatment in the outpatient setting has accelerated this regimen's popularity.

In a subsequent GOG trial in suboptimal advanced ovarian cancer, the paclitaxel-cisplatin regimen was randomized against single-agent paclitaxel and single-agent cisplatin. Surprisingly, preliminary results of this trial reveal no difference in survival between the three arms (Muggia et al, 1997a). The preliminary results of a European trial in which the paclitaxel-cisplatin regimen is being randomized against the combination of paclitaxel and carboplatin indicates that there is no significant difference in efficacy, and the latter regimen appears to be more convenient (Neijt et al, 1998). After completing two trials in patients with optimal advanced epithelial ovarian cancer using intraperitoneal chemotherapy (see below), the GOG is currently conducting a similar trial in this subset comparing paclitaxel-cisplatin with paclitaxel-carboplatin.

The optimal duration of chemotherapy treatment has not been established. Two randomized studies (Hakes et al, 1992; Bertelsen et al, 1993) suggest that more prolonged combination chemotherapy (10 to 12 cycles) provides no survival benefit over chemotherapy of shorter duration (5 to 6 cycles). Furthermore, these and other studies have demonstrated that very few patients who are pathologic partial responders after six or fewer chemotherapy cycles can be converted to complete responders by the use of further systemic chemotherapy. However, Gershenson et al (1992) found that, in patients with optimal advanced ovarian cancer treated with cisplatin-based chemotherapy, those with a planned treatment course of 12 cycles had a significantly longer progression-free survival time than those with a planned course of 6 cycles. Further randomized studies will be necessary to resolve this issue.

Intraperitoneal Chemotherapy

Intraperitoneal chemotherapy has been used in the treatment of ovarian cancer since the 1950s (Green, 1959; Kottmeier, 1968), mainly for the palliation of malignant effusions. It gradually lost popularity as newer, more effective systemic chemotherapeutic agents were discovered, until the late 1970s, when a resurgence of interest occurred. Intraperitoneal chemotherapy has several hypothetical advantages, including the following:

1. Ovarian cancer is primarily a disease confined to the peritoneal cavity.
2. There are several active agents against ovarian cancer, most of which can be safely instilled into the peritoneal cavity.
3. Intracavitary therapy results in a much higher concentration of drug in the peritoneal cavity, with drug levels in the systemic circulation equivalent to or lower than those achieved with systemic administration, thereby allowing for free surface diffusion of the drug as well as for capillary flow.
4. Toxicity might be reduced if the drug were metabolized into a nontoxic form prior to entry into the systemic circulation or if a neutralizing agent

could be administered systemically. Indeed, there is now ample evidence that very high concentrations of drugs can be achieved in the peritoneal cavity with acceptable toxicity.

This rebirth of intraperitoneal chemotherapy has been accompanied by two major advances in drug delivery. First, older studies employed rather low fluid volumes. Investigators discovered that, as with studies involving radioisotopes, large volumes of fluid (approximately 1500 to 2000 ml) are necessary to achieve uniform distribution of drug within the peritoneal cavity (Dunnick et al, 1979; Howell et al, 1982). Second, safe and effective drug delivery systems have been devised. In 1968, Tenckhoff and Scheckter described the use of an implantable silicone catheter for continuous ambulatory dialysis. Since then, the Tenckhoff catheter has been used extensively for the administration of intraperitoneal chemotherapy (Jenkins et al, 1982; Myers, 1984; Lucas et al, 1985). In 1984, Pfeifle et al introduced a subcutaneously implanted portal system: the Port-a-Cath. This system has the theoretical advantages of having a lower incidence of associated infection and greater patient acceptance and seems to be rapidly replacing the Tenckhoff catheter.

The technical and pharmacologic advantages of intraperitoneal chemotherapy do not necessarily translate into therapeutic advantages. Results of Phase I studies (Speyer et al, 1980; Ozols et al, 1982; Howell et al, 1984) have confirmed the pharmacologic advantage with intraperitoneal chemotherapy. Several Phase II studies (Markman et al, 1984; Ozols et al, 1984; ten Bokkel Huinink et al, 1985; Hacker et al, 1987; Howell et al, 1987) have documented responses to a variety of intraperitoneal agents in previously treated patients. The results of these reports suggest that cisplatin is the most active intraperitoneal agent currently available. Also, as with other treatment modalities, intraperitoneal chemotherapy seems to be more effective against minimal residual disease than bulky disease (Markman et al, 1984; Ozols et al, 1984). Hacker et al (1987) treated 18 patients with minimal residual disease (<10 mm) at second-look laparotomy with intraperitoneal cisplatin. Of 15 patients available for pathologic evaluation, 4 (26%) had a complete response, and 2 (13.3%) had a partial response. Howell et al (1987) reported a median survival of more than 49 months in 25 patients with refractory minimal residual disease ovarian cancer treated with intraperitoneal chemotherapy.

Complications associated with intraperitoneal chemotherapy include hemorrhage; bowel perforation; infection; peritonitis; and catheter leakage, dislodgment, or obstruction (Jenkins et al, 1982; Lucas et al, 1985; Piccart et al, 1985; Braly et al, 1986). In the study of Lucas et al (1985), approximately half of the catheters did not allow sufficient drainage because of adhesion formation. Piccart et al (1985), reporting the technical experience with 288 patients at five institutions, noted insufficient drainage in 45%

of patients. For patients with a Tenckhoff catheter, catheter-related peritonitis occurred in 5%, skin infection in 6.6%, and bowel perforation in 3.5%. For patients with Port-A-Cath devices, similar complications occurred in 8%, 0%, and 1.3%, respectively.

Of course, the major issue is the proper role for intraperitoneal chemotherapy. Does it have an advantage over systemic chemotherapy in any clinical setting? It is already clear that, if it does, it is restricted to patients with very minimal tumor burden—probably less than 1 cm.

By the early 1990s, many investigators were rapidly becoming disenchanted with the prospects for improvement in outcome using intraperitoneal chemotherapy. However, this negativism was changed by the report of the Intergroup Study (Alberts et al, 1996). In that study, 654 patients with optimal (≤2 cm) ovarian cancer were randomized to intravenous CP versus intraperitoneal cisplatin plus intravenous cyclophosphamide. The median survival was significantly longer in the group receiving intraperitoneal cisplatin (49 months) than in the group receiving intravenous cisplatin (41 months). In addition, moderate to severe tinnitus, clinical hearing loss, and neurotoxicity were more frequent in the intravenous group. The promising findings of this study have translated into continued pursuit of this approach in patients with optimal ovarian cancer.

A predominant strategy in the continued quest for better treatment for patients with epithelial ovarian cancer is to build on the foundation of the paclitaxel-platinum regimens. This includes the addition of other active agents (see below). Examples of this approach include the GOG Phase I study in which topotecan was added to the combination of paclitaxel and cisplatin and the GOG Phase I study of the combination of oral etoposide, paclitaxel, and carboplatin.

Dose Intensity

Until rather recently, the efficacy of dose intensity, within conventional dose ranges, remained an unresolved issue. Evidence from several studies accumulated over the past few years, however, suggests that doubling the dose of platinum-based chemotherapy does not result in an improved outcome. Levin and Hryniuk (1987) were among the first to address this issue when they analyzed data from 33 first-line chemotherapy studies for advanced ovarian cancer. They found a significant impact of dose intensity of cisplatin on survival. Five randomized trials have shown no advantage of cisplatin or carboplatin dose intensity (Colombo et al, 1993; McGuire et al, 1995; Conte et al, 1996; Dittrich et al, 1996; Gore et al, 1996). A trial from Hong Kong indicated a possible advantage to cisplatin dose intensity, but the population was not well characterized and the study was small (Ngan et al, 1989). A Scottish trial also observed a survival advantage associated with cisplatin dose intensity, but this advantage appeared to diminish over time (Kaye et al, 1996). In summary, it appears that the continued study of platinum dose intensity within the conventional dose ranges is no longer warranted.

Long-term Survival After Platinum-Based Chemotherapy

With the advent of platinum-based combination chemotherapy in the mid-1970s, there was hope that response rates and survival rates for patients with advanced ovarian cancer would dramatically increase. Although results of early randomized trials were encouraging, we now appreciate the fact that long-term survival for patients with advanced epithelial ovarian cancer has not significantly changed over the past three decades. Five-year survival rates have not risen above 15% to 20%. Despite objective response rates of up to 90%, most patients develop progressive tumor and die of their disease; median survival rates range from 18 to 36 months (Greco et al, 1981; Conte et al, 1986; Louie et al, 1986; Bertelsen et al, 1987; Neijt et al, 1987; Sutton et al, 1989b; Gershenson et al, 1992; Gruppo Interegionale Cooperativo Oncologico Ginecologia, 1992; Hoskins et al, 1992a). As noted from large-scale meta-analyses (Advanced Ovarian Cancer Trialists Group, 1991), cisplatin-based combination chemotherapy does not appear to be superior to other forms of chemotherapy in terms of survival time. Although early survival data from paclitaxel-containing clinical trials is encouraging, data are not yet mature enough to define the impact of paclitaxel on long-term survival.

Salvage Chemotherapy

Historically, salvage chemotherapy for patients with epithelial ovarian cancer who have failed initial therapy has been disappointing. Stanhope et al (1977) found that only 6.1% of 347 patients responded to second-line therapy for progressive ovarian cancer. The majority of these patients had received single-agent chemotherapy. Since we have moved into the platinum-based combination chemotherapy era, the results are only slightly better, with a few drugs producing response rates in the 15% to 35% range. Nevertheless, very few patients are cured after failure of initial treatment.

It is generally accepted that there are at least two distinct categories of patients with refractory ovarian cancer receiving salvage chemotherapy—platinum resistant and platinum sensitive. During most of the past two decades, salvage chemotherapy studies included both groups and did not distinguish between them. Platinum-resistant patients include those who develop progressive disease on initial therapy, demonstrate less than a partial response to initial therapy, or relapse 6 months or less from completion of initial treatment. Response to salvage chemotherapy in this group has generally been rather poor. Platinum-sensitive patients include those who responded to a platinum-based regimen initially and who then had a disease-free interval of at least 6 months from completion of chemotherapy. Platinum-sensitive patients generally have at least a 50% response rate to re-treatment with platinum-based chemotherapy (Seltzer et al, 1985; Gershenson et al, 1989a; Gore et al, 1990; Markman et al, 1991).

One of the most promising new drugs to be introduced into Phase I and II trials has been paclitaxel, a diterpene plant product derivative of the western yew tree *Taxus brevifolia*. In three Phase II trials of paclitaxel in refractory ovarian cancer, response rates ranged from 20% to 37% (McGuire et al, 1989; Einzig et al, 1992; Thigpen et al, 1994). Many, but not all of these patients had platinum-resistant tumors. Because of its relatively extraordinary activity, paclitaxel was rapidly introduced into first-line combination regimens in the early 1990s. Further Phase II trials are also being conducted to establish the optimal dose and schedule of paclitaxel in both platinum-resistant and platinum-sensitive patients.

Currently, for platinum-resistant patients there are several drugs available, all of which have a response rate of approximately 15% to 25%. Drug selection for an individual patient is basically empirical. There are no in vitro assays that have yet been shown to be accurate in predicting response to chemotherapy. Therefore, the choice is based on several factors, including drug toxicity, drug schedule, and physician and patient biases. As an overriding principle, patients should generally receive two to three cycles before response can be assessed. The number of cycles and treatment time is dependent on responsiveness and tolerance to the drug. Except in the study setting, most physicians employ single-agent therapy rather than combination regimens because there is no proven benefit to the latter.

At the end of 1998, the menu of drugs for patients with platinum-resistant refractory ovarian cancer included hexamethylmelamine (Bolis et al, 1979; Stehman et al, 1984; Rosen et al, 1987; Manetta et al, 1990; Vergote et al, 1992; Moore et al, 1993), topotecan (Creemers et al, 1996; Kudelka et al, 1996; ten Bokkel Huinink et al, 1997; Hoskins et al, 1998), vinorelbine (George et al, 1989; Bajetta et al, 1996; Gershenson et al, 1998b; Burger et al, 1999), oral etoposide (Rose et al, 1996), doxil (Muggia et al, 1997b), docetaxel (Piccart et al, 1993; Aapro et al, 1994; Kavanagh et al, 1994; Pujade-Lauraine et al, 1994b), and gemcitabine (Kaufmann et al, 1995). Of course, a priority for patients with refractory ovarian cancer is enrollment in innovative clinical trials.

High-Dose Chemotherapy

There are several settings in which high-dose chemotherapy with either bone marrow rescue or peripheral stem cell support has been studied: (1) in refractory platinum-resistant patients; (2) in refractory platinum-sensitive patients; (3) in patients with responding but persistent disease after primary chemotherapy (this group is also theoretically platinum-sensitive); (4) in patients who are pathologically negative after primary chemotherapy (negative second-look); and (5) as first-line treatment in untreated patients.

The introduction of hematopoietic growth factors—erythropoietin, granulocyte or granulocyte-macrophage colony-stimulating factor and thrombopoietin—into clinical trials has enabled clinicians to ameliorate some of the myelosuppressive effects of chemotherapy. These cytokines increase the proliferation of stem cells and in turn shorten the duration or reduce the degree of anemia, neutropenia, or thrombocytopenia. Most commonly, these agents are used with conventional doses of chemotherapy for maintenance of dose intensity. In addition, there are currently several trials combining high-dose chemotherapy with these growth factors in an effort to safely enhance dose intensity. Their precise role in our armamentarium, however, has not yet been defined.

Early trials with high-dose chemotherapy documented promising activity (Maraninchi et al, 1984; Dauplat et al, 1989; Mulder et al, 1989; Shpall et al, 1990). Legros et al (1997) reported 53 patients treated with high-dose chemotherapy after primary surgery and chemotherapy. The 5-year survival was 60%, and the 5-year disease-free survival was 24%. The best outcome was achieved in 19 patients with pathologic complete response at second-look surgery—74% at 5 years. In another study, Stiff et al (1997) reported 100 patients with persistent or recurrent epithelial ovarian cancer treated with high-dose chemotherapy and autologous bone marrow transplantation. The median progression-free survival was 7 months, and the median survival was 13 months. Tumor bulk and chemosensitivity were the best predictors of progression-free survival. Age, tumor bulk, and chemosensitivity provided the best prediction of overall survival. Currently, several groups are continuing to study high-dose chemotherapy in ovarian cancer patients. The GOG is presently conducting a randomized study comparing high-dose chemotherapy with conventional chemotherapy in patients with persistent ovarian cancer.

MOLECULAR AND GENE THERAPIES

With the identification of several molecular biomarkers associated with epithelial ovarian cancer, some of which appear to be prognostic, there is the opportunity for targeting these molecular elements for treatment. Based on preclinical studies, Phase I and II clinical trials are already underway with such agents as intraperitoneal adenovirus vector p53, intraperitoneal E1A (an adenovirus gene product that inhibits HER-2/neu–overexpressing ovarian cancer cells in vitro and in vivo), and Herceptin (a MoAb against HER-2/neu) in ovarian cancer patients. Such studies consist of single-agent trials as well as trials in which these agents are combined with cytotoxic chemotherapeutic agents.

HORMONAL THERAPY

Although hormonal therapy, especially progestational therapy, has been used in the treatment of epithelial ovarian cancer for the past several years, it gained relatively little attention until the initial reports of the presence of estrogen and progesterone receptors in ovarian neoplasms (Holt et al, 1979; Schwartz et al, 1982b; Kauppila et al, 1983). In these studies, approximately 50% to 81% of ovarian cancers were positive for estrogen receptors, and 20% to 76% were positive for progesterone receptors. In a subsequent study, Schwartz et al (1985) reported that the estrogen receptor content of ovarian carcinomas is independent of all histologic parameters with the exception of poorly differentiated tumors, and the progesterone receptor content is independent of all histologic parameters with the exception of lymphocytic infiltration. As with breast and endometrial cancers, this new information has led to a resurgence in hormonal therapy for ovarian cancer.

Progestin therapy has been used in the treatment of ovarian cancer for the past 30 years. Early reports (Jolles, 1962; Varga and Henriksen, 1964; Ward, 1972) described a few objective responses in patients treated with 17α-hydroxyprogesterone caproate (Delalutin). Medroxyprogesterone acetate (Provera) has been extensively investigated in this disease. Studies with oral medroxyprogesterone acetate (Kaufman, 1966; Malkasian et al, 1977; Mangioni et al, 1981; Aabo et al, 1982) demonstrated response rates less than 10%. Reports of intramuscular medroxyprogesterone studies (Mangioni et al, 1981; Slayton et al, 1981; Tropé et al, 1982; Hamerlynck et al, 1985) showed no better results. However, Bergqvist et al (1981) noted objective responses in three of four patients treated with intramuscular medroxyprogesterone acetate. All three responders had mucinous tumors. Rendina et al (1982), using the same medication at high doses, found a 55% response rate in 41 patients with endometrioid ovarian cancers. Furthermore, response to therapy correlated with the presence of positive estrogen or progesterone receptors. Geisler (1985) described six complete responses and four partial responses in 32 patients with ovarian cancer treated with high-dose megestrol acetate (Megace). Other investigators (Ahlgren et al, 1985; Belinson et al, 1987) have reported response rates less than 5% in patients treated with megestrol acetate.

A combination of estrogen and progesterone therapy has also been studied in the treatment of epithelial ovarian cancer. Freedman et al (1986) treated 65 patients with refractory ovarian cancer with a sequential combination of ethinyl estradiol and medroxyprogesterone acetate. Objective responses were noted in 14% of patients (2% complete response, 12%

partial response), and another 20% had stable disease. Vascular complications occurred in three patients. A subsequent report of 23 patients with positive estrogen receptors treated with the same regimen yielded only four (17%) partial responders (Fromm et al, 1991).

Probably the most widely studied hormonal medication for ovarian cancer has been the antiestrogen tamoxifen. Schwartz et al (1982a) treated 13 patients with refractory ovarian cancer with tamoxifen therapy. One patient had a partial response, and four patients had prolonged stabilization of disease. Shirey et al (1985) noted no objective responses in 23 patients with refractory ovarian cancer treated with tamoxifen. Like the study of Schwartz et al (1982a), however, they also observed stabilization of disease; 19 patients had stable disease for a median duration of 17 weeks. Weiner et al (1987) treated 31 evaluable patients with tamoxifen for refractory ovarian cancer. They demonstrated complete responses in one patient (3.2%), partial responses in two patients (6.4%), and stable disease in six patients (19.3%). In a study of the GOG, Hatch et al (1991) treated 105 evaluable patients with tamoxifen for refractory epithelial ovarian cancer. They noted 10 complete responders and 8 partial responders as well as 40 patients who had stable disease. There was no significant difference in response based on estrogen receptor status.

The gonadotropin-releasing hormone analogs leuprolide acetate and goserelin have also been studied in refractory ovarian cancer. In one study (Kavanagh et al, 1989), 4 of 23 patients (17%) with refractory ovarian cancer had a partial response to leuprolide. Three of the four responders had grade 1 tumors and the other had a grade 2 tumor. Subsequent reports have shown only modest activity of these agents in refractory ovarian cancer (Palmer et al, 1988; Bruckner et al, 1989; Jager et al, 1989; Lind et al, 1992; Sevelda et al, 1992; Miller et al, 1992).

BIOLOGIC THERAPY

Because of the rather poor survival rates of patients with advanced ovarian cancer who are treated with conventional modalities, there is considerable interest in a variety of investigational therapies. Foremost among these experimental approaches is biologic therapy. Ovarian cancer is considered a particularly ideal disease for the intraperitoneal administration of biologic response modifiers because the disease is usually confined to the peritoneal cavity, the agents may possess the enhanced ability for tumor penetration, and a variety of agents are capable of evoking a local inflammatory response in the peritoneal cavity.

Nonspecific Immunotherapy

Alberts et al (1979) conducted a prospective randomized study in ovarian cancer patients consisting of doxorubicin and cyclophosphamide with or without bacille bilié de Calmette-Guérin (BCG). The group receiving BCG had a significantly increased progression-free survival and overall survival. In subsequent studies including cisplatin (Alberts et al, 1989a, 1989b), the addition of BCG had no significant effect on pathologic response rates or survival. Gall et al (1986), in a prospective randomized GOG study, found no advantage of melphalan plus *Corynebacterium parvum* over melphalan alone in advanced ovarian cancer patients. Berek et al (1985b) administered *C. parvum* intraperitoneally to 21 patients with epithelial ovarian cancer. Six of 19 patients (31.6%) with surgically measurable disease had a response to therapy (two complete responses and four partial responses). All six responders had 5-mm or smaller maximum diameter tumors.

Interferons

Abdulhay et al (1985) treated 36 patients with refractory ovarian cancer with intramuscular human lymphoblastoid interferon. Of 28 evaluable patients, 2 (7.1%) had complete remissions, 3 (10.8%) had partial remissions, and 14 (50%) had stable disease. In a cooperative Italian study, Rambaldi et al (1985) administered intraperitoneal interferon-β to eight patients with refractory ovarian cancer and noted no objective solid tumor responses; however, ascites completely disappeared in four of seven patients. Berek et al (1985a) reported the treatment of 14 patients with persistent epithelial ovarian cancer documented at second-look laparotomy after combination chemotherapy with intraperitoneal α-recombinant interferon. Of 11 patients undergoing surgical reevaluation, there were 4 (36%) complete responders, 1 (9%) partial responder, and 6 (55%) progressors. All responders had residual disease less than 5 mm prior to interferon therapy.

Adoptive Cellular Immunotherapy

Since publication of the widely read study of Rosenberg et al (1987) outlining the treatment of patients with metastatic cancer with lymphokine-activated killer (LAK) cells and recombinant interleukin-2 (IL-2), there has been considerable interest in adoptive cellular immunotherapy for the treatment of ovarian cancer patients. Stewart et al (1990a) noted one minor response in 10 patients with refractory ovarian cancer who were treated with intraperitoneal LAK plus IL-2. Steis et al (1990) observed two partial responses, as evidence by decreased serum CA-125 and findings at restaging laparotomy, in 10 patients with refractory ovarian cancer. There is currently interest in autologous tumor-infiltrating lymphocytes in the treatment of a variety of tumors, including ovarian cancer. Several studies are in progress.

Monoclonal Antibodies

A number of MoAbs have now been generated to a variety of ovarian cancer cell lines. Current research in this area includes serologic diagnosis, imaging, immunopathology, and therapy of cancer. There has been considerable effort to find a specific and sensitive MoAb serum marker for the diagnosis of asymptomatic women with ovarian cancer and for the monitoring of response to ovarian cancer therapy. Successful imaging of ovarian cancer utilizing radionuclide-labeled MoAbs has already been reported (Davies et al, 1985; Epenetos et al, 1985; Critchley et al, 1986). Preliminary evidence suggests that MoAbs alone are not very potent antineoplastic agents. Consequently, attention has focused on the linkage of MoAbs to drugs, toxins, or radionuclides. Epenetos et al (1987) administered intraperitoneal ^{131}I-conjugated HMFG1, HMFG2, AVA1, and/or HI7E2 to 36 patients with ovarian cancer. They noted antitumor responses in 3 of 6 patients with microscopic tumor, 2 of 15 with less than 2-cm disease, and none of 8 with greater than 2-cm disease. Stewart and co-workers (1990b), using escalating doses of intraperitoneal yttrium-90–labeled HMFG1 in 25 patients with ovarian cancer, noted one partial response in 14 patients with surgically assessable tumor and palliation of ascites in a second patient.

RADIOTHERAPY

Primary Postoperative External Therapy

Despite several decades of treatment of ovarian cancer patients with radiotherapy, its proper role in the management of this disease is not yet established. External beam radiotherapy techniques have varied greatly over the years. Most studies describe either whole-pelvis irradiation or whole-abdominal irradiation. The latter type may be delivered by the open-field technique, treating the entire abdomen with each fraction of therapy using parallel opposed fields, or by the moving strip technique popularized at MDACC (Delclos and Dembo, 1980). Dembo et al (1983) reported the results of a prospective randomized trial comparing the two techniques. They were found to be equally effective, but the open-field technique was simpler, took less time, and was associated with significantly less late toxicity.

Radiotherapy studies in the literature suffer from the same sorts of problems that plague many early studies of ovarian cancer: poor study design, inadequate surgical staging, lack of uniform histologic analysis, and suboptimal statistical methods. These shortcomings make it extremely difficult to interpret treatment results.

A number of studies have investigated the efficacy of pelvic radiotherapy in stage I epithelial ovarian cancer and have demonstrated no survival advantage for this modality (Dembo et al, 1979a; Hreschy-

shyn et al, 1980; Dembo, 1984). For patients with metastatic ovarian cancer, the results are less clear. Delclos and Quinlan (1969) were among the first to observe that tumor control rates with radiotherapy were inversely proportional to the amount of residual disease. It is currently generally accepted that, if radiotherapy has a role, it is in patients with minimal residual disease, mainly because of limitations of normal tissue tolerance.

Smith et al (1975) reported the results of a prospective trial at MDACC in which 149 patients with stages I through III ovarian epithelial cancer were randomized to receive either whole-abdominal radiotherapy with the moving strip technique or 12 cycles of melphalan chemotherapy. All patients had residual disease less than 2 cm. Overall 5-year survival rates were similar (71% for radiotherapy vs. 72% for chemotherapy). Based on a 10% incidence of small intestinal injury in the radiotherapy arm, however, the authors concluded that chemotherapy was just as effective as radiotherapy and also less toxic and more cost effective. In a later study from the Princess Margaret Hospital (Dembo et al, 1979b), abdominopelvic radiotherapy showed a survival benefit over either pelvic radiotherapy or pelvic radiotherapy plus chlorambucil. This survival advantage was true only of those patients who underwent a hysterectomy and bilateral salpingo-oophorectomy. Other randomized studies (Klaassen et al, 1988; Sell et al, 1990) have found no survival differences between abdominopelvic radiotherapy and single-alkylating-agent chemotherapy.

There currently is no randomized study attempting to answer the most germane question—the comparison of abdominopelvic radiotherapy with cisplatin-based combination chemotherapy. Although such studies have been attempted by cooperative groups, they have not been completed because of poor patient accrual related to bias against radiotherapy among several participants. Unless promising information emerges from pilot studies, it is unlikely that such a study will be completed.

Radiotherapy in Multimodality Therapy

Beginning in the early 1980s, there was a revitalization of interest in multimodality therapy, including sequential surgery, cisplatin-based chemotherapy, and radiotherapy. Although results of some studies (Hacker et al, 1985; Cain et al, 1986; Goldhirsch et al, 1988; Kersh et al, 1988; Morgan et al, 1988; Schray et al, 1988; Ledermann et al, 1991) suggested an advantage of this combined approach over chemotherapy alone, other studies (Hainsworth et al, 1983; Hoskins et al, 1985; Coltart et al, 1986; Fuks et al, 1988; Eifel et al, 1991; Rothenberg et al, 1992) found no additional benefit from this approach. The findings of these latter series suggest that abdominopelvic radiotherapy following primary surgery, combination chemotherapy, and second-look laparotomy is difficult to tolerate with regard to myelosuppression, results in a rather low salvage rate, and is associated with small intestinal injury in a relatively high percentage of cases. The failure of this strategy to demonstrate superior results to surgery/chemotherapy is probably related to the fact that there is cross-resistance between cisplatin-based chemotherapy and radiotherapy. Because of this possibility, some investigators are attempting to introduce radiotherapy concomitantly with chemotherapy (King et al, 1991) or after only a few cycles of chemotherapy.

SECONDARY SURGERY

Second-Look Laparotomy

Second-look laparotomy for evaluation of disease status following treatment for cancer of the colon was initially proposed by Wangensteen and associates in 1948 (Wangensteen et al, 1951). Since 1960, second-look laparotomy has been employed extensively in the management of ovarian cancer at MDACC. The procedure has gained popularity over the last two decades as more ovarian cancer patients have been treated with chemotherapy and fewer have received radiotherapy. Within the last 5 years or so, however, there has been increasing skepticism about the benefits of this procedure.

Definition

Interpretation of reports of experience with second-look laparotomy has been complicated by the fact that no standard definition of the procedure exists. Most experts agree that the term *second-look laparotomy* should be restricted to a laparotomy performed on a patient with no clinical evidence of persistent tumor for the purpose of determining disease status after a planned interval of treatment with chemotherapy. The term should not be applied to a surgical procedure performed in patients with clinical evidence of persistent or progressive disease for the primary purpose of debulking or treatment of complications. With current treatment regimens, at least 50% to 60% of patients with advanced ovarian cancer are candidates for second-look laparotomy.

Preoperative Assessment and Technique

Standard preoperative assessment of ovarian cancer patients at completion of the planned interval of chemotherapy includes physical examination, determination of serum tumor marker levels, and CT of the abdomen and pelvis. If these studies clearly document persistent ovarian cancer, then, with rare exceptions, second-look laparotomy is not performed. The operative technique of second-look laparotomy has been well described. It is essentially identical to a staging laparotomy, as discussed above. An adequate vertical midline abdominal incision is made.

Upon entering the abdomen, cytologic washings from the pelvis, bilateral paracolic gutters, and sub-diaphragmatic areas are obtained, and the entire contents of the peritoneal cavity are inspected and palpated. If obvious macroscopic tumor is present, then the procedure is usually limited. However, the extent of disease should be carefully determined, and a few biopsies should be taken for documentation of persistent disease (frozen section as well as permanent section). If no obvious macroscopic disease is noted, then random biopsy specimens are routinely taken from the peritoneal surfaces, including the cul-de-sac, vesicouterine reflection, bilateral pelvic walls, bilateral paracolic gutters, and surfaces of the diaphragm. Omental biopsies and biopsies of the retroperitoneal lymph nodes are also performed. In the process of performing these biopsies, lysis of adhesions is not uncommon. Sites of previously documented tumor and adhesions should be carefully evaluated and generously sampled. An adequate procedure consists of a minimum of 20 to 30 biopsy specimens (Fig. 60–10).

Complications

Second-look laparotomy is a major operative procedure, although it is a very safe one. The average duration of the operation is 2 hours, and the usual hospital stay is 7 days. Operative mortality is a rarity. Operative morbidity is low, and most complications are minor. The most common complications include wound infection and prolonged ileus. Other reported complications include urinary tract infection, small intestinal obstruction, pneumothorax, intestinal injury, hemorrhage, pneumonia, and thromboembolic phenomena (Schwartz and Smith, 1980; Roberts et al, 1982; Webb et al, 1982; Luesley et al, 1984; Smirz et al, 1985; Podczaski et al, 1987).

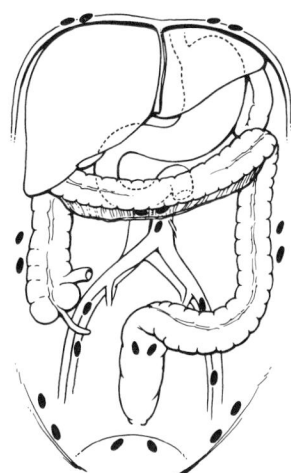

Figure 60–10
Random biopsy sites of peritoneum, residual omentum, and retroperitoneal nodes in standard second-look procedure.

Results

Findings at second-look laparotomy are classified as negative (grossly and pathologically negative), microscopically positive (grossly negative, pathologically positive), and macroscopically positive (grossly and pathologically positive). The clinical variables most consistently associated with findings at second-look laparotomy and survival afterward are histologic grade, amount of residual disease, and FIGO stage (Roberts et al, 1982; Webb et al, 1982; Barnhill et al, 1984; Luesley et al, 1984; Podratz et al, 1985; Miller et al, 1986; Chambers et al, 1988). Patients with low-grade tumors, minimal residual disease, and early-stage disease have a greater probability of having negative findings at second-look laparotomy than do those with high-grade tumors, bulky residual disease, or advanced-stage disease. Other variables found to correlate with second-look findings and subsequent survival in some of these studies are histologic type, type of chemotherapy, amount of disease found at the initial surgery, age, performance status, and peritoneal cytology status.

Findings in approximately 50% of patients with advanced ovarian cancer (and a smaller percentage of those with early-stage disease) will be macroscopically positive at second-look laparotomy. Such patients, with the exception of those with low-grade tumors, have a very poor prognosis; more than 80% will eventually develop progressive disease and die. With rare exceptions, they are candidates for experimental therapies. The issue of cytoreductive surgery in this setting is discussed below.

Approximately 20% of patients with advanced ovarian cancer who undergo second-look laparotomy will have microscopically positive findings. In 1985, Copeland et al reported the experience at MDACC with 50 patients with advanced ovarian cancer who had microscopically positive findings. The 2-year and 5-year actuarial survival rates of these patients were 81% and 70%, respectively—not statistically different from those rates achieved by patients with negative second-look findings (Gershenson et al, 1985). However, most of the patients with microscopic disease received chemotherapy after second-look surgery, whereas those with negative findings did not. Moreover, the microscopic disease group contained a higher percentage of patients with low-grade tumors. After these studies were reported, a detailed pathologic analysis of the microscopic disease group revealed that, in several cases, benign müllerian rests were misinterpreted as representing persistent tumor (Copeland et al, 1988). Another updated analysis of these patients (Copeland and Gershenson, 1986) revealed that, when grade 1 and borderline tumors were excluded, 58% of microscopic disease patients had recurrences. Treatment approaches currently under study for microscopically positive disease include abdominopelvic radiotherapy, intraperitoneal chemotherapy, and radioisotope therapy.

Negative second-look laparotomy findings are noted in approximately 30% of patients with advanced ovarian cancer undergoing this procedure. At MDACC, we initially found a recurrence rate of 24% in 85 patients with advanced ovarian cancer who had negative second-look results (Gershenson et al, 1985). An updated analysis revealed a recurrence rate of 44% in patients with grade 2 and 3 disease. Studies from other large centers (Berek et al, 1984b; Podratz et al, 1985, 1988; Smirz et al, 1985; Rubin et al, 1988, 1991; Luesley et al, 1989) have noted similar recurrence rates. The recurrence rates of 30% to 50% in patients with negative second-look findings after treatment for advanced ovarian cancer have prompted initiation of clinical trials evaluating a variety of therapies to follow negative second-look laparotomy. These treatments include external radiotherapy, intraperitoneal chemotherapy, and radioisotope therapy. It will probably be another 5 years, however, before results of prospective trials become available.

Alternatives

A number of alternatives to second-look laparotomy have been investigated. Laparoscopy has been evaluated as a substitute. With the availability of improved equipment, we may witness a revitalization of interest in this procedure for cancer patients. Approximately 30% to 50% of patients with ovarian cancer undergoing laparoscopy after chemotherapy will have positive findings (Smith et al, 1977; Berek et al, 1981; Ozols et al, 1981; Lele and Piver, 1986), thus avoiding the need for laparotomy. However, second-look laparoscopy is associated with several potential problems:

1. Several areas, including the bowel mesentery, the retroperitoneum, and areas obscured by adhesions, are not accessible with this procedure.
2. If both laparoscopy and laparotomy are performed, total operating time may be significantly longer.
3. Ten to 20% of patients develop complications, including hematomas and intestinal perforation.

The complication rate with the "open" laparoscopy technique is probably lower. With this technique, the surgeon makes a small incision through the abdominal wall layers into the peritoneal cavity and then inserts the scope. A purse-string suture is placed around the incision to avoid rapid escape of carbon dioxide, resulting in the loss of the pneumoperitoneum. Such a maneuver is generally associated with a lower incidence of intestinal perforation. If second-look laparoscopy is employed, it should be recognized that the false-negative rate is approximately 35%. Therefore, a negative laparoscopy should be followed by laparotomy.

CT has also been evaluated as a substitute for second-look laparotomy, but available information confirms the fact that tumor implants smaller than 2 cm in diameter are not reliably imaged (Stern et al, 1981; Goldhirsch et al, 1983; Brenner et al, 1985; Clarke-Pearson et al, 1986; Stehman et al, 1988; Reuter et al, 1989; Lund et al, 1990). Therefore, a negative CT scan does not obviate the need for second-look laparotomy. However, a positive study may avoid second-look laparotomy in approximately 20% of patients. Positive CT studies should always be confirmed with fine-needle aspiration. Whether MRI will prove superior to CT in defining persistent ovarian cancer remains unknown, although preliminary experience suggests that it will not.

The obvious substitute for second-look laparotomy is a reliable serum tumor marker. A negative CA-125 level at completion of chemotherapy, however, does not reliably predict lack of persistent disease. Second-look laparotomy has been negative in only 40% to 50% of patients with normal CA-125 levels (Niloff et al, 1985a; Berek et al, 1986; Patsner et al, 1990). Therefore, a negative CA-125 level is not a substitute for second-look laparotomy. Patsner and associates (1990) reported that size of residual disease at second-look laparotomy did not correlate well with the serum level of CA-125. A positive CA-125 level, however, reliably predicts disease persistence and avoids a surgical procedure. Eventually, a battery of serum tumor markers or a more reliable single marker will most probably replace second-look laparotomy.

Therefore, despite its shortcomings, second-look laparotomy remains the most reliable method for detection of persistent cancer. Theoretically, negative findings allow the clinician to stop potentially toxic therapy, and positive findings prevent premature cessation of therapy. However, for one of several reasons (most commonly patient refusal or physician preference), many patients do not undergo the procedure. Currently, the most widespread alternative to second-look laparotomy is simply discontinuation of chemotherapy after a fixed interval (usually six to nine cycles) for a patient with no clinical evidence of disease.

Perspective

The benefits of second-look laparotomy have been seriously questioned in several articles and editorials (Young, 1987; Sonnendecker, 1988; Friedman and Weiss, 1990; Ho et al, 1987). Few argue that the findings at second-look laparotomy are of prognostic value; patients with macroscopic tumor have a worse survival rate than do those with either microscopic tumor or negative findings. Critics state, however, that although second-look laparotomy is superior to other methods of detecting residual ovarian cancer, the procedure still does not accurately predict the presence or absence of disease. The high recurrence rate after negative second-look laparotomy has essentially eliminated our ability to identify a subgroup of patients for whom therapy can be safely discontinued.

A second major criticism of second-look laparotomy is the lack of evidence that the procedure or the therapeutic decisions made based on the findings enhance survival. No prospective randomized clinical trials have compared patients who undergo second-look laparotomy with those who do not. The greatest impediment to improvement in survival for patients undergoing the procedure is the lack of success of salvage therapies. Few patients with persistent disease found at second-look laparotomy are cured of their disease with second-line therapy. Although there has been a flurry of enthusiasm for such modalities as external radiotherapy and intraperitoneal chemotherapy for patients with minimal persistent tumor, results with the former have been generally quite disappointing, and the benefits of the latter are being questioned increasingly despite reports of responses and prolonged survival.

Proponents of second-look laparotomy claim that resection of residual tumor in this setting improves survival. The issue of debulking at second-look laparotomy is very controversial; it is discussed below. Until randomized clinical trials demonstrate a survival benefit of salvage therapies for patients with negative, microscopic, or macroscopic findings at second-look laparotomy, a cloud will remain over this procedure. Such trials are currently being conducted for patients with negative or microscopically positive findings. To our knowledge, no randomized trials are assigning patients with no clinical evidence of disease after completion of chemotherapy to undergo surgery or not. Such a study might be quite difficult to execute in the present environment. In the meantime, it seems very reasonable to recommend that second-look laparotomy be performed only in a research setting until further information becomes available. For patients with stage I epithelial ovarian cancer, it is very difficult to justify second-look laparotomy because of the high probability of truly negative findings.

Secondary Cytoreductive Surgery

The term *secondary cytoreductive surgery* has no universal definition. It may denote cytoreductive surgery performed in one of several different settings:

1. In patients who are partial responders or nonresponders to primary chemotherapy
2. In patients who have developed recurrent disease after receiving primary therapy and experience a prolonged disease-free interval off therapy (>6 months)
3. In patients who undergo a suboptimal debulking initially followed by three cycles of chemotherapy —so-called interval debulking
4. In patients who have persistent macroscopic tumor at second-look laparotomy

Tumors in these subgroups of ovarian cancer patients may have very different natural histories, principally defined by whether they are "platinum resistant" or "platinum sensitive." For example, patients whose tumor progresses during first-line chemotherapy, whether progression is noted clinically or at second-look laparotomy, are by definition "platinum resistant," whereas patients who have not yet received chemotherapy or are partial responders to chemotherapy, with the response noted clinically or at second-look surgery, or who have developed recurrent disease after a prolonged interval off therapy may well be "platinum sensitive." These subgroups may thus have very different survival rates based on their responsiveness to second-line chemotherapy after secondary cytoreductive surgery. Therefore, it is extremely important for studies designed to assess the impact of these various secondary procedures on survival rates to carefully define their study populations. Because of the lack of prospective randomized studies in this area, it is difficult if not impossible to draw any firm conclusions about the influence of secondary debulking in these settings.

Very little information is available about the possible benefits of secondary surgery for patients who have no or partial response to primary chemotherapy. Morris and associates (1989a) reported the experience at MDACC with 33 ovarian cancer patients who had progressive or stable disease and who subsequently underwent an attempt at secondary cytoreductive surgery. The tumors of 55% of the patients were cytoreduced to a residual diameter of 2 cm or less. Operative morbidity occurred in 24% of patients, mostly in those who underwent bowel resection. The overall median survival after secondary surgery was 9.4 months. The authors concluded that there is no definite evidence that secondary cytoreductive surgery is of significant benefit in most patients with ovarian cancer that is progressive or stable during chemotherapy. This issue can only be resolved by a prospective randomized study, the outcome of which would be significantly influenced by the effectiveness of postoperative second-line therapy. It is quite unlikely, however, that such a randomized study will ever be conducted.

Equally scant information is available about the impact of secondary cytoreductive surgery for recurrent disease. Morris et al (1989b) reported our experience at MDACC with 30 patients who underwent secondary debulking for recurrent ovarian cancer. All had been initially treated with primary cytoreductive surgery and chemotherapy and had a period of clinical remission of at least 6 months thereafter. In 17 patients (57%), residual tumor was smaller than 2 cm. There were no postoperative deaths, but 40% of patients suffered postoperative morbidity, mostly prolonged ileus. The overall median survival after secondary surgery was 16.3 months. In general, the longer the interval from completion of primary chemotherapy to recurrence, the more favorable the survival. Subsequently, three retrospective studies did show an improved survival for patients secondarily cytoreduced to small residual disease compared with patients who were not optimally cytoreduced (Janicke et al, 1992; Segna et al, 1993; Vacarello et al, 1995). Eisenkop et al (1995) reported a prospective study of 36 patients with recurrent ovarian cancer who underwent secondary cytoreductive surgery. Thirty patients (83%) had complete resection of macroscopic tumor; their survival was significantly better than that for patients with macroscopic residual disease (43 vs. 5 months; $p = 0.03$). Clearly, the true value of secondary cytoreductive surgery for recurrent ovarian cancer can be assessed only by a prospective randomized study.

The term *interval cytoreduction* has been used to describe two distinct entities: (1) cytoreduction after a biopsy (performed at surgery or by fine-needle aspiration) and a "few" (typically three) cycles of chemotherapy; or (2) a true secondary cytoreduction performed after primary cytoreduction that is suboptimal (with bulky residual disease remaining) and three cycles of chemotherapy. The former is really neoadjuvant chemotherapy, which is described above. The latter is truly a "secondary" attempt at cytoreduction. These two distinct entities have been confused and used interchangeably in the literature.

Several reports described secondary cytoreductive surgery as interval debulking after a suboptimal primary surgery and a few cycles of chemotherapy (Neijt et al, 1987; Lawton et al, 1990). Van der Burg et al (1995) reported the findings of a large prospective, randomized trial in which 278 patients with greater than 1-cm residual tumor after primary cytoreductive surgery were enrolled. After three cycles of CP chemotherapy, patients were randomized to receive either secondary cytoreduction followed by three more cycles of chemotherapy or three more cycles of chemotherapy alone. Of the 140 patients randomized to the interval cytoreduction arm, 65% still had bulky tumor at the time of this secondary surgery; about 45% of them were able to be cytoreduced optimally. Both progression-free survival and overall survival were modestly improved in the interval cytoreduction group. The GOG is currently conducting a study with an identical study design in an effort to replicate the results of this European trial; the combination of paclitaxel and cisplatin is being used rather than CP.

The issue of cytoreductive surgery at second-look laparotomy is very controversial and its value unproved. No prospective randomized trials exist to resolve this controversy. Whereas some (Raju et al, 1982; Luesley et al, 1984; Wiltshaw et al, 1985) have questioned the value of secondary cytoreduction at second-look laparotomy, several authors (Schwartz and Smith, 1980; Stuart et al, 1982; Berek et al, 1983; Dauplat et al, 1986; Podratz et al, 1988; Hoskins et al, 1989) have suggested a survival benefit associated with tumor resection at second-look laparotomy. In the study of Hoskins et al (1989), the 5-year survival rate of patients found to have microscopic disease at second-look laparotomy was 62%, similar to that of patients whose disease was rendered microscopic by tumor resection—51% ($p = 0.55$). Especially in these retrospective studies, it is extremely difficult to evaluate the influence of all prognostic factors. As with all studies on the subject of cytoreductive surgery, it is virtually impossible to distinguish the effects of secondary tumor resection from the influence of the inherent tumor characteristics. Noninfiltrating tumors may be easier to resect but may also be inherently more indolent. In addition, survival after secondary debulking at second-look laparotomy is intimately linked to the effectiveness of postoperative therapy.

MANAGEMENT OF INTESTINAL OBSTRUCTION

Approximately 25% of ovarian cancer patients will develop intestinal obstruction in the terminal phase of their illness. Signs and symptoms of intestinal obstruction resulting from ovarian cancer include nausea and vomiting, abdominal cramping, abdominal distention, and progressive constipation. In patients who have only partial obstruction, these complaints and findings may be episodic and more subtle. Plain films of the abdomen may support the diagnosis. Dilatation of the small intestine and air-fluid levels suggest involvement of the small bowel. Dilatation of the colon may characterize large bowel obstruction. In patients with early partial obstruction, the radiographic findings may be nonspecific.

Although intestinal obstruction in patients with ovarian cancer may be caused by adhesions, progressive tumor is usually the inciting factor. Of course, if the patient has received abdominopelvic radiotherapy, this cause should also be considered; however, most cases of intestinal obstruction in ovarian cancer patients who have received prior radiotherapy are related primarily to tumor progression.

The site(s) of the obstruction may be solitary or multiple. In 5% to 10% of patients, there is simultaneous obstruction of the small and large bowel. Colon obstruction in the area of the sigmoid portion usually occurs from growth of pelvic tumor and resultant extrinsic compression, although occasionally there may be obstruction of more proximal segments. Small bowel obstruction is usually the result of adherence of loops of bowel by mesenteric or serosal tumor implants.

Once the appropriate evaluation is completed and the diagnosis of intestinal obstruction is made, the gynecologist must outline a plan of management. Many factors influence this decision, including age, nutritional status, and general condition of the patient; the amount of tumor present; the presence or absence of ascites; the options for postoperative salvage therapy; the attitude of the physician; and the wishes of the patient and her family. The decision of whether to operate or manage the patient nonoperatively is also colored by the fact that surgery for patients with refractory ovarian cancer is associated

with significant morbidity and mortality, the obstruction cannot be relieved in almost 20% of those undergoing surgery, and the postoperative survival is disappointingly brief (Castaldo et al, 1981; Krebs and Goplerud, 1983; Clarke-Pearson et al, 1987, 1988; Larson et al, 1989; Rubin et al, 1989). In reported series, the serious complication rate has ranged from 28% to 49% (Castaldo et al, 1981; Clarke-Pearson et al, 1987), and the operative mortality rate is in the range of 12% to 16% (Krebs and Goplerud, 1983; Clarke-Pearson et al, 1987; Larson et al, 1989). The median survival rate for patients who have undergone surgery is in the range of 3 to 5 months (Krebs and Goplerud, 1983; Clarke-Pearson et al, 1987; Larson et al, 1989).

For initial management of a patient with small bowel obstruction, we prefer the insertion of a nasogastric tube rather than a long tube (Cantor, Miller-Abbott, or Dennis) for intestinal decompression. After extensive experience with both, we have found no advantage from the latter. Furthermore, long tubes are associated with considerably greater discomfort. Long intestinal tubes seem to have the greatest success rate in patients with postoperative adhesions but are fairly ineffective in relieving obstruction resulting from cancer. In the study of Krebs and Goplerud (1983), only 10% of patients had their obstruction relieved by tube decompression.

In patients for whom no surgery is planned, we have extensively utilized the technique of percutaneous gastrostomy since 1984 (Malone et al, 1986) (Fig. 60–11). This procedure has resulted in excellent palliation for terminal-stage ovarian cancer patients, avoiding the discomfort of the nasogastric tube and allowing the patient to be easily cared for at home in most cases. With such a device, the patient may even continue to eat some, although, of course, the nutritional benefit is essentially nil. This approach, combined with hospice care, is most appropriate for those patients for whom all effective treatment has been exhausted. There are, however, no universal criteria regarding what constitutes inappropriately prolonged treatment (e.g., number of treatment regimens, performance status), and such clinical situations are emotionally charged and influenced by patient preferences and physician biases. Nevertheless, we do appear to be moving closer to consensus about the characteristics of "futile care."

Colonic obstruction is usually treated by performing a colostomy. The selection of the site of colostomy depends on the area of obstruction. Most commonly, a transverse loop colostomy is indicated in the presence of a sigmoid colon obstruction. For small bowel obstruction, a number of options are available depending on the operative findings. Most commonly, there are multiple sites of obstruction in the terminal ileum, in which case an ileo–ascending colon bypass or ileo–transverse colon bypass is preferable. In such situations, it is usually both unwise and inappropriate to attempt resection and reanastomosis. However, if there is an isolated area of ob-

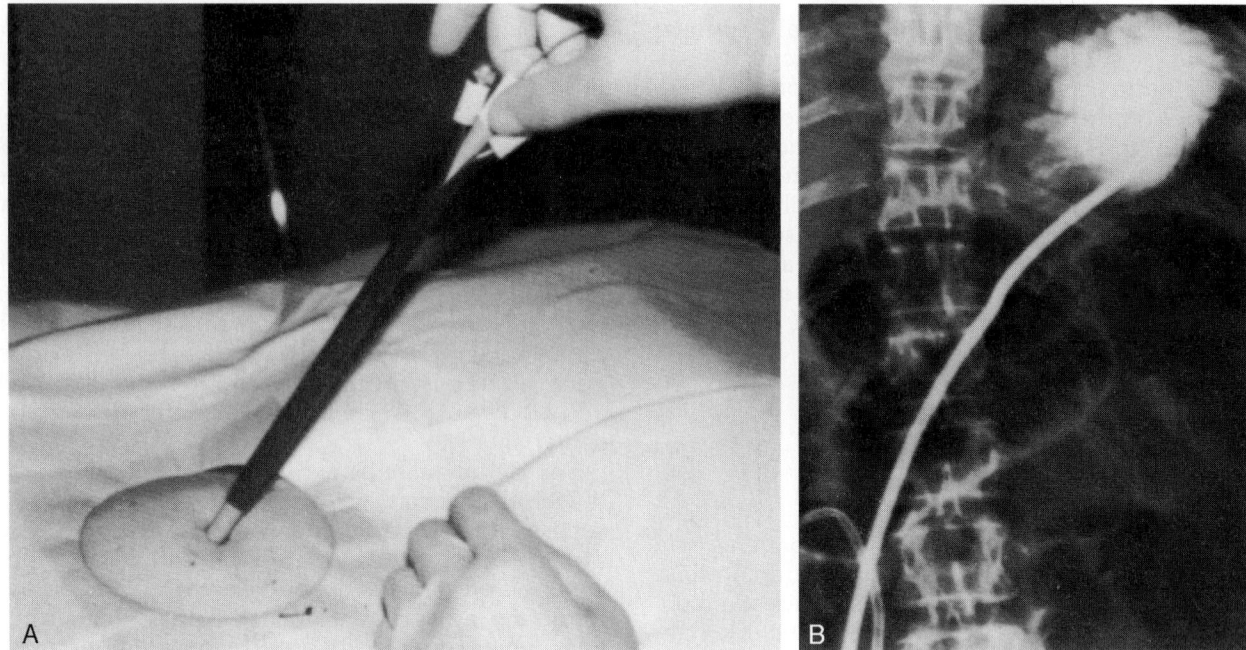

Figure 60-11
A, Percutaneous gastrostomy: 26 French peel-away sheath and dilator inserted over a guidewire prior to passage of Mallecot catheter. *B*, Mallecot catheter in stomach with contrast injected. Dilated loops of small intestine resulting from intestinal obstruction are noted.

struction, a resection and reanastomosis may be indicated. Not infrequently, there may be extensive tumor with multiple areas of obstruction, making both bypass and resection impossible. In such a situation, a tube gastrostomy is indicated, if possible. Procedures such as these are among the most demanding because of the meticulous, often tedious dissection required. Enterotomies are not uncommon and should be repaired as soon as they are identified. Complications of small intestinal procedures include wound infection, intraperitoneal abscess, sepsis, pneumonia, and enterocutaneous fistula.

REFERENCES

Aabo K, Pedersen AG, Hald I, et al: High dose medroxyprogesterone acetate (MPA) in advanced chemotherapy-resistant ovarian carcinoma: a Phase II study. Cancer Treat Rep 1982;66:407.

Aapro M, Pujade-Lauraine E, Lhomme C, et al: EORTC Clinical Screening Group: Phase II study of Taxotere in ovarian cancer. Ann Oncol 1994;5:202.

Abdulhay G, DiSaia PJ, Blessing JA, et al: Human lymphoblastoid interferon in the treatment of advanced epithelial ovarian malignancies: a Gynecologic Oncology Group study. Am J Obstet Gynecol 1985;152:418.

Adelson MD: Cytoreduction of diaphragmatic metastases using the cavitron ultrasonic surgical aspirator. Gynecol Oncol 1991;41:220.

Adelson MD, Baggish MS, Seifer DB, et al: Cytoreduction of ovarian cancer with the cavitron ultrasonic surgical aspirator. Obstet Gynecol 1988;72:140.

Advanced Ovarian Cancer Trialists Group. Chemotherapy in advanced ovarian cancer: an overview of randomised clinical trials. BMJ 1991;303:884.

Ahlgren JD, Thomas D, Ellison N, et al: Phase II evaluation of high dose megestrol acetate in advanced refractory ovarian cancer. Proc Am Soc Clin Oncol 1985;2:124.

Ahmed FY, Wiltshaw E, A'Hern RP, et al: Natural history and prognosis of untreated stage I epithelial ovarian carcinoma. J Clin Oncol 1996;14:2968.

Alberts DS, Green S, Hannigan EV, et al: Improved therapeutic index of carboplatin plus cyclophosphamide versus cisplatin plus cyclophosphamide: final report by the Southwest Oncology Group of a Phase III randomized trial in stages III and IV ovarian cancer. J Clin Oncol 1992;10:706.

Alberts DS, Liu PY, Hannigan EV, et al: Intraperitoneal cisplatin plus intravenous cyclophosphamide versus intravenous cisplatin plus intravenous cyclophosphamide for stage III ovarian cancer. N Engl J Med 1996;335:1950.

Alberts DS, Mason-Liddil N, O'Toole RV, et al: Randomized Phase III trial of chemoimmunotherapy in patients with previously untreated stage III, optimal disease ovarian cancer: a Southwest Oncology Group study. Gynecol Oncol 1989a;32:16.

Alberts DS, Mason-Liddil N, O'Toole RV, et al: Randomized Phase III trial of chemoimmunotherapy in patients with previously untreated stages III and IV suboptimal disease ovarian cancer: a Southwest Oncology Group study. Gynecol Oncol 1989b;32:8.

Alberts DS, Moon T, Stephens RA, et al: Randomized study of chemoimmunotherapy for advanced ovarian carcinoma: a preliminary report of Southwest Oncology Group study. Cancer Treat Rep 1979;63:325.

Andolf E, Jorgensen C, Astedt B: Ultrasound examination for detection of ovarian carcinoma in risk groups. Obstet Gynecol 1990;75:106.

Atack DB, Nisker JA, Allen HH, et al: CA 125 surveillance and second-look laparotomy in ovarian carcinoma. Am J Obstet Gynecol 1986;154:287.

Aure JC, Hoeg K, Kolstad P: Clinical and histological studies of ovarian carcinoma: long term follow-up of 990 cases. Obstet Gynecol 1971;37:1.

Austin RM, Norris HJ: Malignant Brenner tumor and transitional cell carcinoma of the ovary: a comparison. Int J Gynecol Pathol 1987;6:29.

Bajetta E, Di Leo A, Biganzoli L, et al: Phase II study of vinorelbine in patients with pretreated advanced ovarian cancer: activity in platinum-resistant disease. J Clin Oncol 1996;14:2546.

Barlow JJ, Piver MS, Lele SB: Weekly cis-platinum remission "induction" and combination drug consolidation and maintenance in ovarian cancer. Proc Am Soc Clin Oncol 1982;1:119.

Barnhill D, Heller P, Brzozowski P, et al: Epithelial ovarian carcinoma of low malignant potential. Obstet Gynecol 1985;65:53.

Barnhill D, Hoskins W, Heller P, Park R: The second-look surgical reassessment for epithelial ovarian carcinoma. Gynecol Oncol 1984;19:148.

Barnhill DR, Kurman RJ, Brady MF, et al: Preliminary analysis of the behavior of stage I ovarian serous tumors of low malignant potential: a Gynecologic Oncology Group study. J Clin Oncol 1995;13:2752.

Bast RC Jr, Bookman MA, Knapp RC: Concepts of gynecologic tumor immunology. In Knapp RC, Berkowitz R (eds): Gynecologic Oncology. 2nd ed. New York: Macmillan, 1991:97.

Bast RC Jr, Freeney M, Lazarus H, et al: Reactivity of a monoclonal antibody with human ovarian carcinoma. J Clin Invest 1981;68:1331.

Bast RC Jr, Klug TL, Schaetzl E, et al: Monitoring human ovarian carcinoma with a combination of CA 125, CA 19-9, and carcinoembryonic antigen. Am J Obstet Gynecol 1984;149:553.

Bast RC Jr, Klug TL, St John E, et al: A radioimmunoassay using a monoclonal antibody to monitor the course of epithelial ovarian cancer. N Engl J Med 1983;309:883.

Belinson JL, McClure M, Ashikaga T, et al: Treatment of advanced and recurrent ovarian carcinoma with cyclophosphamide, doxorubicin, and cisplatin. Cancer 1984;54:1983.

Belinson JL, McClure M, Badger G: Randomized trial of megestrol acetate vs megestrol acetate/tamoxifen for the management of progressive or recurrent epithelial ovarian carcinoma. Gynecol Oncol 1987;28:151.

Bell DA, Scully RE: Atypical and borderline endometrioid adenofibromas of the ovary: a report of 27 cases. Am J Surg Pathol 1985a;9:205.

Bell DA, Scully RE: Benign and borderline clear cell adenofibroma of the ovary. Cancer 1985b;56:2922.

Bell DA, Weinstock MA, Scully RE: Peritoneal implants of ovarian serous borderline tumors: histologic features and prognosis. Cancer 1988;62:2212.

Berchuck A, Kamel A, Whitaker R, et al: Overexpression of HER-2/neu is associated with poor survival in advanced epithelial ovarian cancer. Cancer Res 1990;50:4087.

Berek JS, Griffiths CT, Leventhal J: Laparoscopy for second-look evaluation in ovarian cancer. Obstet Gynecol 1981;58:192.

Berek JS, Hacker NF, Lagasse LD: Rectosigmoid colectomy and reanastomosis to facilitate resection of primary and recurrent gynecologic cancer. Obstet Gynecol 1984a;64:715.

Berek JS, Hacker NF, Lagasse LD, Leuchter RS: Lower urinary tract resection as part of cytoreductive surgery for ovarian cancer. Gynecol Oncol 1982;13:87.

Berek JS, Hacker N, Lagasse L, et al: Survival of patients following secondary cytoreductive surgery in ovarian cancer. Obstet Gynecol 1983;61:189.

Berek JS, Hacker N, Lagasse L, et al: Second-look laparotomy in stage III epithelial ovarian cancer: clinical variables associated with disease status. Obstet Gynecol 1984b;64:207.

Berek JS, Hacker NF, Lichtenstein A, et al: Intraperitoneal recombinant α-interferon for "salvage" immunotherapy in stage III epithelial ovarian cancer: a Gynecologic Oncology Group study. Cancer Res 1985a;45:4447.

Berek JS, Knapp RC, Hacker NF, et al: Intraperitoneal immunotherapy of epithelial ovarian carcinoma with Corynebacterium parvum. Am J Obstet Gynecol 1985b;152:1003.

Berek JS, Knapp R, Malkasian G, et al: CA-125 serum levels correlated with second-look operations among ovarian cancer patients. Obstet Gynecol 1986;67:685.

Bergman F: Carcinoma of the ovary: a clinicopathological study of 86 autopsied cases with special reference to mode of spread. Acta Obstet Gynecol Scand 1966;45:211.

Bergqvist A, Kullander S, Thorell J: A study of estrogen and progesterone cytosol receptor concentration in benign and malignant ovarian tumors and a review of malignant ovarian tumors treated with medroxyprogesterone acetate. Acta Obstet Gynecol Scand 1981;101:75.

Bertelsen K, Jakobsen A, Andersen J, et al: A randomized study of cyclophosphamide and cisplatinum with or without doxorubicin in advanced ovarian carcinoma. Gynecol Oncol 1987;28:161.

Bertelsen K, Jakobsen A, Kern M, et al: A randomized trial of six cycles versus twelve cycles of cyclophosphamide, Adriamycin, and cis-platinum (CAP) in advanced ovarian cancer. Gynecol Oncol 1993;49:30.

Blumenfeld D, Braly PS, Ben-Ezra J, et al: Tumor DNA content as a prognostic feature in advanced epithelial ovarian carcinoma. Gynecol Oncol 1987;27:389.

Blythe JG, Wahl TP: Debulking surgery: does it increase the quality of survival? Gynecol Oncol 1982;14:396.

Bolis G, Colombo N, Pecorelli S, et al: Adjuvant treatment for early epithelial ovarian cancer: results of two randomised clinical trials comparing cisplatin to no further treatment or chromic phosphate (^{32}P). Ann Oncol 1995;6:887.

Bolis G, D'Incalci M, Grammellini F, et al: Adriamycin in ovarian cancer patients resistant to cyclophosphamide. Eur J Cancer 1978;14:1401.

Bolis G, D'Incalci M, Mangioni C, et al: Hexamethylmelamine in ovarian cancer resistant to cyclophosphamide and Adriamycin. Cancer Treat Rep 1979;63:1375.

Boring CC, Squires TS, Tong T: Cancer statistics [published erratum appears in CA Cancer J Clin 1992;42:127.]. CA Cancer J Clin 1992;42:19.

Bostwick DG, Tazelaar HD, Ballon SC, et al: Ovarian epithelial tumors of borderline malignancy: a clinical and pathologic study of 109 cases. Cancer 1986;58:2052.

Braly P, Doroshow J, Hoff S: Technical aspects of intraperitoneal chemotherapy in abdominal carcinomatosis. Gynecol Oncol 1986;25:319.

Brand E, Pearlman N: Electrosurgical debulking of ovarian cancer: a new technique using the argon beam coagulator. Gynecol Oncol 1990;39:115.

Brand E, Wade ME, Lagasse LD: Resection of fixed pelvic tumors using the Nd:YAG laser. J Surg Oncol 1988;37:246.

Brenner D, Shaff M, Jones H, et al: Abdominopelvic computed tomography: evaluation in patients undergoing second-look laparotomy for ovarian carcinoma. Obstet Gynecol 1985;65:715.

Broders AC: Carcinoma: grading and practical applications. Arch Pathol 1926;2:376.

Bruckner HW, Cohen CJ, Goldberg JD, et al: Improved chemotherapy for ovarian cancer with cis-diamminedi-chloroplatinum and Adriamycin. Cancer 1981;47:2288.

Bruckner HW, Cohen CJ, Goldberg JD, et al: Cisplatin regimens and improved prognosis of patients with poorly differentiated ovarian cancer. Am J Obstet Gynecol 1983;145:653.

Bruckner HW, Cohen CJ, Wallach RC, et al: Treatment of advanced ovarian cancer with cis-dichlorodiammine-platinum (II): poor-risk patients with intensive prior therapy. Cancer Treat Rep 1978;62:555.

Bruckner HW, Motwani BT: Treatment of advanced refractory ovarian carcinoma with gonadotropin-releasing hormone analogue. Am J Obstet Gynecol 1989;161:1216.

Burger RA, DiSaia PJ, Roberts JA, et al: Phase II trial of vinorelbine in advanced epithelial ovarian cancer. Gynecol Oncol 1999;72:148.

Burghardt E, Pickel H, Lahousen M, et al: Pelvic lymphadenectomy in operative treatment of ovarian cancer. Am J Obstet Gynecol 1986;155:315.

Byers T, Marshall J, Graham S, et al: A case-control study of dietary and non-dietary factors in ovarian cancer. J Natl Cancer Inst 1983;7:681.

Cain J, Saigo P, Pierce V, et al: A review of second-look laparotomy for ovarian cancer. Gynecol Oncol 1986;23:14.

Campbell S, Bhan V, Royston P, et al: Transabdominal ultrasound screening for early ovarian cancer. BMJ 1989;299:1363.

Cancer Committee of the International Federation of Gynecology and Obstetrics: Staging announcement: FIGO Cancer Committee. Gynecol Oncol 1986;25:383.

Casagrande JT, Pike MC, Ross RK, et al: "Incessant ovulation" and ovarian cancer. Lancet 1979;2:170.

Castaldo TW, Petrilli ES, Ballon SC, Lagasse LD: Intestinal operations in patients with ovarian carcinoma. Am J Obstet Gynecol 1981;139:80.

Centers for Disease Control Cancer and Steroid Hormone Study: Oral contraceptive use and the risk of ovarian cancer. JAMA 1983;249:1596.

Chaitin BA, Gershsenson DM, Evans HL: Mucinous tumors of the ovary: a clinicopathologic study of 70 cases. Cancer 1985; 55:1958.

Chambers S, Chambers J, Kohorn E, et al: Evaluation of the role of second-look surgery in ovarian cancer. Obstet Gynecol 1988; 72:404.

Chambers JT, Chambers SK, Voynick IM, Schwartz PE: Neoadjuvant chemotherapy in stage X ovarian carcinoma. Gynecol Oncol 1990;37:327.

Chen SS, Bochner R: Assessment of morbidity and mortality in primary cytoreductive surgery for advanced ovarian carcinoma. Gynecol Oncol 1985;20:190.

Chen SS, Lee L: Incidence of para-aortic and pelvic lymph nodes metastases in epithelial carcinoma of the ovary. Gynecol Oncol 1983;16:95.

Clarke-Pearson D, Bandy L, Dudzinski M, et al: Computed tomography in evaluation of patients with ovarian carcinoma in complete clinical remission: correlation with surgical-pathologic findings. JAMA 1986;255:627.

Clarke-Pearson DL, Chin NO, DeLong ER, et al: Surgical management of intestinal obstruction in ovarian cancer. Gynecol Oncol 1987;26:11.

Clarke-Pearson DL, DeLong ER, Chin NE, et al: Surgical management of intestinal obstruction in ovarian cancer. II. Analysis of factors associated with complications and survival. Arch Surg 1988;123:42.

Colombo N, Pittelli MR, Parma G, et al: Cisplatin (P) dose intensity in advanced ovarian cancer (AOC): a randomized study of conventional dose (DC) vs dose-intense (DI) cisplatin monochemotherapy. Proc Am Soc Clin Oncol 1993;12:255.

Coltart RS, Nethersell BW, Brown CH: A pilot study of high-dose abdominopelvic radiotherapy following surgery and chemotherapy for stage III epithelial carcinoma of the ovary. Gynecol Oncol 1986;23:105.

Conte PF, Alama A, Rubagotte A, et al: Cell kinetics in ovarian cancer: relationship to clinicopathologic features, responsiveness to chemotherapy and survival. Cancer 1989;64:1188.

Conte P, Bruzzone M, Carnino F, et al: High-dose versus low-dose cisplatin in combination with cyclophosphamide and epidoxorubicin in suboptimal ovarian cancer: a randomized study of the Gruppo Oncologico Nord-Ovest. J Clin Oncol 1996;14:351.

Conte PF, Bruzzone M, Chiara S, et al: A randomized trial comparing cisplatin plus cyclophosphamide versus cisplatin, doxorubicin and cyclophosphamide in advanced ovarian cancer. J Clin Oncol 1986;4:965.

Copeland L, Gershenson DM: Ovarian cancer recurrences in patients with no macroscopic tumor at second-look laparotomy. Obstet Gynecol 1986;68:873.

Copeland L, Gershenson DM, Wharton JT, et al: Microscopic disease at second-look laparotomy in advanced ovarian cancer. Cancer 1985;55:472.

Copeland L, Silva E, Gershenson DM, et al: The significance of muellerian inclusions found at second-look laparotomy in patients with epithelial ovarian neoplasms. Obstet Gynecol 1988; 71:763.

Cramer DW, Hutchinson GB, Welch WR, et al: Factors affecting the association of oral contraceptives and ovarian cancer. N Engl J Med 1982a;307:1047.

Cramer DW, Welch WR, Cassells S, et al: Mumps, menarche, menopause and ovarian cancer. Am J Obstet Gynecol 1983;147: 1.

Cramer DW, Welch WR, Hutchinson GB, et al: Dietary animal fat in relation to ovarian cancer risk. Obstet Gynecol 1984;63:883.

Cramer DW, Welch WR, Scully RE, et al: Ovarian cancer and talc. Cancer 1982b;50:372.

Creasman WT, Rutledge F: The prognostic value of peritoneal cytology in gynecologic malignant disease. Am J Obstet Gynecol 1971;110:773.

Creemers GJ, Bolis G, Gore M, et al: Topotecan, an active drug in the second-line treatment of epithelial ovarian cancer: results of a large European Phase II study. J Clin Oncol 1996;14:3056.

Critchley M, Brownless S, Paten M, et al: Radionuclide imaging of epithelial ovarian tumors with ^{123}I-labeled monoclonal antibody (H 317) specific for placental-type alkaline phosphatase. Clin Radiol 1986;37:107.

Crombach G, Zippel HH, Wurz H: Clinical significance of cancer antigen 125 (CA125) in ovarian cancer. Cancer Detect Prev 1983;6:623.

Curtin JP, Malik R, Venkatraman ES, et al: Stage IV ovarian cancer: impact of surgical debulking. Gynecol Oncol 1997;64:9.

Czernobilsky B, Silverman BB, Enterline HT: Clear-cell carcinoma of the ovary: a clinicopathologic analysis of pure and mixed forms and comparison with endometrioid carcinoma. Cancer 1970a;25:762.

Czernobilsky B, Silverman BB, Mikuta JJ: Endometrioid carcinoma of the ovary: a clinicopathologic study of 75 cases. Cancer 1970b;26:1141.

Dauplat J, Ferriere JP, Monique G, et al: Second-look laparotomy in managing epithelial ovarian carcinoma. Cancer 1986;57:1627.

Dauplat J, Legros M, Condat P, et al: High-dose melphalan and autologous bone marrow support for treatment of ovarian carcinoma with positive second-look operation. Gynecol Oncol 1989;34:294.

Davies JO, Davies ER, Howe K, et al: Radionuclide imaging of ovarian tumors with ^{123}I-labeled monoclonal antibody (NDOG$_2$) directed against placental alkaline phosphatase. Br J Obstet Gynaecol 1985;92:277.

Day TG, Gallagher HS, Rutledge FN: Epithelial carcinoma of the ovary: prognostic importance of histologic grade. Natl Cancer Inst Monogr 1975;42:15.

Decker DG, Fleming TR, Malkasian GD Jr, et al: Cyclophosphamide plus cis-platinum in combination: treatment program for stage III or IV ovarian carcinoma. Obstet Gynecol 1982;60:481.

Delclos L, Dembo AJ: Ovaries: female pelvis. In Fletcher GH (ed): Textbook of Radiotherapy. 3rd Ed. Philadelphia: Lea & Febiger, 1980:843.

Delclos L, Quinlan EJ: Malignant tumors of the ovary managed with postoperative megavoltage irradiation. Radiology 1969;93: 659.

Deligdisch L, Jacobs AJ, Cohen CJ: Histologic correlates of virulence in ovarian adenocarcinoma. II. Morphologic correlates of host response. Am J Obstet Gynecol 1982;144:885.

Dembo AJ: Radiotherapeutic management of ovarian cancer. Semin Oncol 1984;11:238.

Dembo AJ, Bush RS, Beale FA, et al: The Princess Margaret study of ovarian cancer: stages I, II and asymptomatic III presentations. Cancer Treat Rep 1979a;63:249.

Dembo AJ, Bush RS, Beale FA, et al: Improved survival following abdominopelvic irradiation in patients with a completed pelvic operation. Am J Obstet Gynecol 1979b;134:793.

Dembo AJ, Bush RS, Beale FA, et al: A randomized clinical trial of moving strip versus open field whole abdominal irradiation in patients with invasive epithelial cancer of the ovary. Int J Radiat Oncol Biol Phys 1983;9:97.

Dembo AJ, Chang PL, Urbach GI: Clinical correlations of ovarian cancer antigen NB/70K: a preliminary report. Obstet Gynecol 1985;65:710.

Dembo AJ, Davy D, Stenwig AE, et al: Prognostic factors in patients with stage I epithelial ovarian cancer. Obstet Gynecol 1990;75:263.

De Palo GM, De Lena M, Di Re F, et al: Melphalan versus Adriamycin in the treatment of advanced carcinoma of the ovary. Surg Gynecol Obstet 1975;141:899.

Deppe G, Malviya V, Boike G, Hampson A: Surgical approach to diaphragmatic metastases from ovarian cancer. Gynecol Oncol 1986;24:258.

Deppe G, Malviya V, Boike G, Malone JM: Use of cavitron surgical aspirator for debulking of diaphragmatic metatases in patients with advanced carcinoma of the ovaries. Surg Gynecol Obstet 1989;168:455.

Deppe G, Malviya V, Malone JM: Debulking surgery for ovarian cancer with the cavitron ultrasonic surgical spirator (CUSA)—a preliminary report. Gynecol Oncol 1988;31:223.

Deppe G, Malviya V, Malone JM, Christensen CW: Debulking of pelvic and para-aortic lymph node metastases in ovarian cancer with the cavitron ultrasonic surgical aspirator. Obstet Gynecol 1990;76:1140.

Deppe G, Zbella EA, Skogerson K, Dumitru I: The rare indication for splenectomy as part of cytoreductive surgery in ovarian cancer. Gynecol Oncol 1983;16:282.

DiSaia PJ, Haverback BJ, Dyce BJ, et al: Carcinoembryonic antigen in patients with gynecologic malignancies. Am J Obstet Gynecol 1975;121:159.

Dittrich C, Obermair A, Kurz C, et al: Prospective randomized trial of cisplatin/carboplatin versus conventional cisplatin/cyclophosphamide in epithelial ovarian cancer: first results of the impact of platinum dose intensity on patient outcome. Proc Am Soc Clin Oncol 1996;15:279.

Dottino PR, Plaxe SC, Cohen CJ: A Phase II trial of adjuvant cisplatin and doxorubicin in stage I epithelial ovarian cancer. Gynecol Oncol 1991;43:203.

Dunnick NR, Jones RB, Doppmen JL, et al: Intraperitoneal contrast infusion for assessment of intraperitoneal fluid dynamics. AJR 1979;133:221.

Edmonson JH, McCormack GW, Fleming TR, et al: Comparison of cyclophosphamide plus cisplatin versus hexamethylmelamine, cyclophosphamide, doxorubicin, and cisplatin in combination as initial chemotherapy for stage III and IV ovarian carcinomas. Cancer Treat Rep 1985;69:1243.

Edwards EL, Herson J, Gershenson DM, et al: A prospective randomized clinical trial of melphalan and cisplatinum versus hexamethylmelamine, Adriamycin, and cyclophosphamide in advanced ovarian cancer. Gynecol Oncol 1983;15:261.

Ehrlich CE, Einhorn L, Williams SD, et al: Chemotherapy for stage III-IV epithelial ovarian cancer with cis-dichlorodiammineplatinum II, Adriamycin, and cyclophosphamide: a preliminary report. Cancer Treat Rep 1979;63:281.

Eifel P, Hendrickson M, Ross J, et al: Simultaneous presentation of carcinoma involving the ovary and uterine corpus. Cancer 1982;50:163.

Eifel PJ, Gershenson DM, Delclos L, et al: Twice-daily, split-course abdominopelvic radiation therapy after chemotherapy and positive second-look laparotomy for epithelial ovarian carcinoma. Int J Radiat Oncol Biol Phys 1991;21:1013.

Einhorn N, Bast RC Jr, Knapp RC, et al: Preoperative evaluation of serum CA 125 levels in patients with primary epithelial ovarian cancer. Obstet Gynecol 1986;67:414.

Einhorn N, Nilsson B, Sjovall K: Factors influencing survival in carcinoma of the ovary: study from a well-defined Swedish population. Cancer 1985;55:2019.

Einhorn N, Sjövall K, Knapp RC, et al: Prospective evaluation of serum CA 125 levels for early detection of ovarian cancer. Obstet Gynecol 1992;80:14.

Einzig AI, Wiernik PH, Sasloff J, et al: Phase II study and long-term follow-up of patients treated with taxol for advanced ovarian adenocarcinoma. J Clin Oncol 1992;10:1748.

Eisenkop SM, Friedman RL, Wang, H-J: Secondary cytoreductive surgery for recurrent ovarian cancer. Cancer 1995;76:1606.

Eltabbakh GH, Belinson JL, Kennedy AW, et al: p53 Overexpression is not an independent prognostic factor for patients with primary ovarian epithelial cancer. Cancer 1997;80:892.

Epenetos AA, Hooker G, Durbin H, et al: Indium-III labelled monoclonal antibody to placental alkaline phosphatase in the detection of neoplasms of testis, ovary and cervix. Lancet 1985;2:350.

Epenetos AA, Munro AJ, Stewart S, et al: Antibody-guided irradiation of advanced ovarian cancer with intraperitoneally administered radiolabeled monoclonal antibodies. J Clin Oncol 1987;5:1890.

Fathalla MF: Incessant ovulation—a factor in ovarian neoplasia. Lancet 1971;2:163.

Fayers PM, Rustin G, Wood R, et al: The prognostic value of serum CA125 in patients with advanced ovarian carcinoma: an analysis of 573 patients by the Medical Research Council Working Party on Gynaecological Cancer. 1993;3:285.

Finkler NJ, Benacerraf B, Lavin P, et al: Comparison of serum CA-125, clinical impression, and ultrasound in the preoperative evaluation of ovarian masses. Obstet Gynecol 1988;72:659.

Fiorica JV, Hoffman MS, LaPolla JP, et al: The management of diaphragmatic lesions in ovarian carcinoma. Obstet Gynecol 1989;74:927.

Freedman RS, Saul PB, Edwards CL, et al: Ethinyl estradiol and medroxyprogesterone acetate in patients with epithelial ovarian carcinoma: a Phase II study. Cancer Treat Rep 1986;70:369.

Friedlander ML, Taylor IW, Russel P, et al: Ploidy as a prognostic factor in ovarian cancer. Int J Gynecol Pathol 1983;2:55.

Friedman J, Weiss N: Second thoughts about second-look laparotomy in advanced ovarian cancer. N Engl J Med 1990;322:1079.

Fromm GL, Freedman RS, Fritsche HA, et al: Sequentially administered ethinyl estradiol and medroxyprogesterone acetate in the treatment of refractory epithelial ovarian carcinoma in patients with positive estrogen receptors. Cancer 1991;68:1885.

Fuks Z, Rizel S, Biran S: Chemotherapeutic and surgical induction of pathological complete remission and whole abdominal irradiation for consolidation does not enhance the cure of stage III ovarian carcinoma. J Clin Oncol 1988;6:509.

Gall S, Bundy B, Beecham J, et al: Therapy of stage III optimal epithelial carcinoma of the ovary with melphalan or melphalan and Corynebacterium parvum: a Gynecologic Oncology Group study. Gynecol Oncol 1986;25:26.

Geisler HE: The use of high-dose megestrol acetate in the treatment of ovarian adenocarcinoma. Semin Oncol 1985;12:20.

Genadry R, Poliakoff S, Rotmensch J, et al: Primary, papillary peritoneal neoplasia. Obstet Gynecol 1981;58:730.

George MJ, Heron JF, Kerbrat P, et al: Navelbine in advanced ovarian epithelial cancer: a study of the French Oncology Centers. Semin Oncol 1989;16:30.

Gershenson DM: Chemotherapy for epithelial ovarian cancer. In Rutledge RN, Freedman RS, Gershenson DM (eds): Gynecologic Cancer: Diagnosis and Treatment Strategies. Austin: University of Texas Press, 1987:41.

Gershenson DM, Burke TW, Morris M, Bast RC, Guaspari A, Hohneker J, Wharton JT: A phase I study of a daily × 3 schedule of intravenous vinorelbine for refractory epithelial ovarian cancer. Gynecol Oncol 1998b;70:404.

Gershenson DM, Copeland L, Wharton JT, et al: Prognosis of surgically determined complete responders in advanced ovarian cancer. Cancer 1985;55:1129.

Gershenson DM, Kavanagh JJ, Copeland LJ, et al: Retreatment of patients with recurrent epithelial ovarian cancer with cisplatin-based chemotherapy. Obstet Gynecol 1989a;73:798.

Gershenson DM, Mitchell MF, Atkinson N, et al: The effect of prolonged cisplatin-based chemotherapy on progression-free survival in patients with optimal epithelial ovarian cancer: "maintenance" therapy reconsidered. Gynecol Oncol 1992;47:7.

Gershenson DM, Silva EG: Serous ovarian tumors of low malignant potential with peritoneal implants. Cancer 1990;65:578.

Gershenson DM, Silva EG, Levy L, et al: Ovarian serous borderline tumors with invasive peritoneal implants. Cancer 1998c;82:1096.

Gershenson DM, Silva EG, Mitchell MF, et al: Transitional cell carcinoma of the ovary: a matched control study of advanced stage patients treated with cisplatin-based chemotherapy. Am J Obstet Gynecol 1993;168:1178.

Gershenson DM, Silva EG, Tortolero-Luna G, et al: Ovarian serous borderline tumors with noninvasive peritoneal implants. Cancer 1998a;83:2157.

Gershenson DM, Wharton JT, Copeland LJ, et al: Treatment of advanced epithelial ovarian cancer with cisplatin and cyclophosphamide. Gynecol Oncol 1989b;32:336.

Gershenson DM, Wharton JT, Herson J, et al: Single-agent cisplatinum therapy for advanced ovarian cancer. Obstet Gynecol 1981;58:487.

Goldhirsch A, Greiner R, Dreher E, et al: Treatment of advanced ovarian cancer with surgery, chemotherapy, and consolidation of response by whole abdominal radiotherapy. Cancer 1988;62:40.

Goldhirsch A, Triller J, Greiner R, et al: Computed tomography prior to second-look operation in advanced ovarian cancer. Obstet Gynecol 1983;62:630.

Goldie JH, Coldman AJ: A mathematical model for relating the drug sensitivity of tumors to their spontaneous mutation rate. Cancer Treat Rep 1979;63:1727.

Gore ME, Fryatt I, Wiltshaw E, et al: Treatment of relapsed carcinoma of the ovary with cisplatin or carboplatin following initial treatment with these compounds. Gynecol Oncol 1990; 36:207.

Gore ME, Mainwaring PN, Macfarlane V: A randomized study of high versus standard dose carboplatin in patients (pts) with advanced epithelial ovarian cancer (EOC). Proc Am Soc Clin Oncol 1996;15:284.

Graham J, Graham R: Ovarian cancer and asbestos. Environ Res 1967;1:115.

Greco FA, Julian CG, Richardson RL, et al: Advanced ovarian cancer: brief intensive combination chemotherapy and second-look operation. Obstet Gynecol 1981;58:199.

Green TH: Hemisulfur mustard in the palliation of patients with metastatic ovarian carcinoma. Obstet Gynecol 1959;13:383.

Greene MH, Boice JD Jr, Greer BE, et al: Acute nonlymphocytic leukemia after therapy with alkylating agents for ovarian cancer: a study of five randomized clinical trials. N Engl J Med 1982;307:1416.

Greene MH, Harris EL, Gershenson DM, et al: Melphalan may be a more potent leukemogen than cyclophosphamide. Ann Intern Med 1986;105:360.

Greer BE, Rutledge FN, Gallagher HS: Staging or restaging laparotomy in early-stage epithelial cancer of the ovary. Clin Obstet Gynecol 1980;23:293.

Griffiths CT: Surgical resection of tumor bulk in the primary treatment of ovarian carcinoma: seminar on ovarian cancer. Natl Cancer Inst Monogr 1975;42:101.

Griffiths CT, Parker LM, Fuller AF: Role of cytoreductive surgical treatment in the management of advanced ovarian cancer. Cancer Treat Rep 1979;63:235.

Gruppo Interregionale Cooperativo Oncologico Ginecologia: Long-term results of a randomized trial comparing cisplatin with cisplatin and cyclophosphamide with cisplatin, cyclophosphamide, and Adriamycin in advanced ovarian cancer. Gynecol Oncol 1992;45:115.

Hacker NF, Berek JS, Brunison CM, et al: Whole abdominal radiation as salvage therapy for epithelial ovarian cancer. Obstet Gynecol 1985;65:60.

Hacker NF, Berek JS, Lagasse LD, et al: Primary cytoreductive surgery for epithelial ovarian cancer. Obstet Gynecol 1983;61:413.

Hacker NF, Berek JS, Pretorius RG, et al: Intraperitoneal cisplatinum as salvage therapy for refractory epithelial ovarian cancer. Obstet Gynecol 1987;70:759.

Hainsworth JD, Malcolm A, Johnson DH, et al: Advanced minimal residual ovarian carcinoma: abdominopelvic irradiation following combination chemotherapy. Obstet Gynecol 1983;61:619.

Hakes T, Chalas E, Hoskins W, et al: Randomized prospective trial of 5 versus 10 cycles of cyclophosphamide, doxorubicin, and cisplatin in adanced ovarian carcinoma. Gynecol Oncol 1992;45:284.

Hall DJ, Diasio R, Goplerud DR: cis-Platinum in gynecologic cancer. I. Epithelial ovarian cancer. Am J Obstet Gynecol 1981;141:299.

Hallgrimson J, Scully RE: Borderline and malignant Brenner tumors of the ovary: a report of 15 cases. Acta Pathol Microbiol Scand 1972;A233(Suppl 80):56.

Hamerlynck JV, Maskens AP, Mangioni C, et al: Phase II trial of medroxyprogesterone in advanced ovarian cancer: an EORTC Gynecological Cancer Cooperative Group study. Gynecol Oncol 1985;22:313.

Hart WR, Norris HJ: Borderline and malignant mucinous tumors of the ovary: histologic criteria and clinical behavior. Cancer 1973;31:1031.

Hartmann LC, Podratz KC, Keeney GL, et al: Prognostic significance of p53 immunostaining in epithelial ovarian cancer. J Clin Oncol 1994;12:64.

Hatch KD, Beecham JB, Blessing JA, Creasman WT: Responsiveness of patients with advanced ovarian carcinoma to tamoxifen: a Gynecologic Oncology Group study of second-line therapy in 105 patients. Cancer 1991;68:269.

Heintz APM, Hacker NF, Berek JS, et al: Cytoreductive surgery in ovarian carcinoma: feasibility and morbidity. Obstet Gynecol 1986;67:783.

Helewa ME, Krepart GV, Lotocki R: Staging laparotomy in early epithelial ovarian carcinoma. Am J Obstet Gynecol 1986;154:282.

Henderson BE, Ross RK, Pike MC, et al: Endogenous hormones as a major factor in human cancer. Cancer Res 1982;42:3232.

Henderson WJ, Hamilton TC, Griffiths K: Talc in normal and malignant ovarian tissue. Lancet 1979;1:499.

Ho AG, Beller U, Speyer J, et al: A reassessment of the role of second-look laparotomy for invasive ovarian adenocarcinoma predict size of residual disease? J Clin Oncol 1987;5:1316.

Holt JA, Caputo TA, Kelly KM, et al: Estrogen and progestin binding in cytosols of ovarian adenocarcinomas. Obstet Gynecol 1979;53:50.

Hoskins P, Eisenhauer E, Beare S, et al: Randomized Phase II study of two schedules of topotecan in previously treated patients with ovarian cancer: a National Cancer Institute of Canada clinical trials group study. J Clin Oncol 1998;16:2233.

Hoskins PJ, O'Reilly SE, Swenerton KD, et al: Ten-year outcome of patients with advanced epithelial ovarian carcinoma treated with cisplatin-based multimodality therapy. J Clin Oncol 1992a; 10:1561.

Hoskins W, Bundy B, Thigpen J, Omura G: The influence of initial surgery on progression-free interval (PFI) and survival (S) in optimal (<1 cm) stage III epithelial ovarian cancer (EOC). Society of Gynecologic Oncologists abstract. Gynecol Oncol 1992b;45:76.

Hoskins WJ, Lichter AS, Whittington R, et al: Whole abdominal and pelvic irradiation in patients with minimal disease at second-look surgical reassessment for ovarian cancer. Gynecol Oncol 1985;20:271.

Hoskins WJ, Rubin SC, Dulaney E, et al: Influence of secondary cytoreduction at the time of second-look laparotomy on the survival of patients with epithelial ovarian carcinoma. Gynecol Oncol 1989;34:365.

Howell SB, Pfeifle CE, Wung WE, et al: Intraperitoneal cisplatin with systemic thiosulfate protection. Ann Intern Med 1982;97:845.

Howell SB, Pfeifle CE, Wung WE, et al: Intraperitoneal chemotherapy with melphalan. Ann Intern Med 1984;101:14.

Howell SB, Zimm S, Markman M, et al: Long-term survival of advanced refractory ovarian carcinoma patients with small-volume disease treated with intraperitoneal chemotherapy. J Clin Oncol 1987;5:1607.

Hreshchyshyn MM, Park RC, Blessing JA, et al: The role of adjuvant therapy in stage I ovarian cancer. Am J Obstet Gynecol 1980;138:139.

International Federation of Gynecology and Obstetrics: Classification and staging of malignant tumors in the female pelvis. Acta Obstet Gynecol Scand 1971;50:1.

Jacob JH, Gershenson DM, Morris M, et al: Neoadjuvant chemotherapy and interval debulking for advanced epithelial ovarian cancer. Gynecol Oncol 1991;42:146.

Jacobs EM, Reeves WJ Jr, Wood DA, et al: Treatment of cancer with weekly intravenous 5-fluorouracil: study by the Western Cooperative Cancer Chemotherapy Group (WCCCG). Cancer 1971;27:1302.

Jacobs I, Bridges J, Reynolds C, et al: Multimodal approach to screening for ovarian cancer. Lancet 1988;2:268.

Jager W, Wildt L, Lang N: Some observations on the effect of a GnRH analog in ovarian cancer. Eur J Obstet Gynecol Reprod Biol 1989;32:137.

Janicke F, Holscher M, Kuhn W, et al: Radical surgical procedure improves survival time in patients with recurrent ovarian cancer. Cancer 1992;70:2129.

Janovski NA, Paramanandhan TL: Ovarian Tumors: Tumors and Tumor-like Conditions of the Ovaries, Fallopian Tubes and Ligaments of the Uterus. Stuttgart: Georg Thieme, 1973:32a, 119B.

Jenkins J, Sugarbaker PH, Gianola FJ, et al: Technical considerations in the use of intraperitoneal chemotherapy administered by Tenckhoff catheter. Surg Gynecol Obstet 1982;154:858.

Johannsson OT, Ranstam J, Borg A, et al: Survival of BRCA1 breast and ovarian cancer patients: a population-based study from southern Sweden. J Clin Oncol 1998;16:397.

Johnson BL, Fischer RI, Bender RA, et al: Hexamethylmelamine in alkylating agent-resistant ovarian carcinoma. Cancer 1978; 42:2157.

Johnson RJ, Blackledge G, Eddleston B, et al: Abdominopelvic computed tomography in the management of ovarian carcinoma. Radiology 1983;146:447.

Jolles B: Progesterone in the treatment of advanced malignant tumors of breast, ovary and uterus. Br J Cancer 1962;16:209.

Joly DJ, Lilenfield AM, Diamond EL: An epidemiologic study of the relationship of reproductive experience to cancer of the ovary. Am J Epidemiol 1974;99:190.

Julian CG, Goss J, Blanchard K, et al: Biologic behavior of primary ovarian malignancy. Gynecol Oncol 1974;44:873.

Kaldor JM, Day NE, Pettersson F, et al: Leukemia following chemotherapy for ovarian cancer. N Engl J Med 1990;322:1.

Kallioniemi OP, Punnonen R, Mattila J, et al: Prognostic significance of DNA index multiploidy and S-phase fraction in ovarian cancer. Cancer 1988;61:334.

Kamiya N, Mizuno K, Kawai M, et al: Simultaneous measurement of CA 125, CA 19-9, tissue polypeptide antigen, and immunosuppressive acidic protein to predict recurrence of ovarian cancer. Obstet Gynecol 1990;76:417.

Kapnick SJ, Griffiths CG, Finkler NJ: Occult pleural involvement in stage III ovarian carcinoma: role of diaphragm resection. Gynecol Oncol 1990;39:135.

Katz ME, Schwartz PE, Kapp DS, et al: Epithelial carcinoma of the ovary: current strategies. Ann Intern Med 1981;95:98.

Katzenstein ALA, Mazur MT, Morgan TE, et al: Proliferative serous tumors of the ovary: histologic features and prognosis. Am J Surg Pathol 1978;2:339.

Kaufmann M, Bauknecht T, Jonat W, et al: Gemcitabine (GEM) in cisplatin-resistant ovarian cancer. Proc Am Soc Clin Oncol 1995; 14:272.

Kaufman RJ: Management of advanced ovarian carcinoma. Med Clin North Am 1966;50:845.

Kauppila A, Vierikko P, Kivinen S, et al: Clinical significance of estrogen and progestin receptors in ovarian cancer. Obstet Gynecol 1983;61:320.

Kavanagh J, Kudelka A, Freedman R, et al: Taxotere (docetaxel): activity in platin refractory ovarian cancer and amelioration of toxicity. Proc Am Clin Oncol 1994;13:237.

Kavanagh JJ, Roberts W, Townsend P, Hewitt S: Leuprolide acetate in the treatment of refractory or persistent epithelial ovarian cancer. J Clin Oncol 1989;7:115.

Kaye SB, Paul J, Cassidy J, et al: Mature results of a randomized trial of two doses of cisplatin for the treatment of ovarian cancer. J Clin Oncol 1996;14:2113.

Keettel WX, Pixley EE, Buschbaum HJ: Experience with peritoneal cytology in the management of gynecologic malignancies. Am J Obstet Gynecol 1974;120:174.

Kerr-Wilson RHJ, Shingleton HM, Orr JW Jr, et al: The use of ultrasound and computed tomography scanning in the management of gynecologic cancer patients. Gynecol Oncol 1984; 18:54.

Kersh CR, Randall ME, Constable WC, et al: Whole abdominal radiotherapy following cytoreductive surgery and chemotherapy in ovarian carcinoma. Gynecol Oncol 1988;31:113.

King LA, Downey GO, Potish RA, et al: Concomitant whole-abdominal radiation and intraperitoneal chemotherapy in advanced ovarian carcinoma. Cancer 1991;67:2867.

Kivinen S, Kuoppala T, Leppilampi M, et al: Tumor-associated antigen CA 125 before and during the treatment of ovarian carcinoma. Obstet Gynecol 1986;67:468.

Klaassen D, Shelley W, Starreveld A, et al: Early-stage ovarian cancer: a randomized clinical trial comparing whole abdominal radiotherapy, melphalan, and intraperitoneal chromic phosphate: A National Cancer Institute of Canada Clinical Trials Group report. J Clin Oncol 1988;6:1254.

Klemi PJ, Pylkkanen L, Kiiholma P, et al: p53 protein detected by immunohistochemistry as a prognostic factor in patients with epithelial ovarian carcinoma. Cancer 1995;76:1201.

Kliman L, Rome RM, Fortune DW: Low malignant potential tumors of the ovary: a study of 76 cases. Obstet Gynecol 1986; 68:338.

Knapp RC, Friedman EA: Aortic lymph node metastases in early ovarian cancer. Am J Obstet Gynecol 1974;119:1013.

Knapp RC, Lavin PT, Schaetzel E, et al: Evaluation of CA 125 prior to recurrence of ovarian cancer. Proc Soc Gynecol Oncol 1985;16:30.

Kohler MF, Kerns BJ, Humphrey PA, et al: Mutation and over-expression of p53 in early-stage epithelial ovarian cancer. Obstet Gynecol 1993;81:643.

Kottmeier HL: Treatment of ovarian cancer with thiotepa. Clin Obstet Gynecol 1968;11:447.

Krebs HB, Goplerud DR: Surgical management of bowel obstruction in advanced ovarian carcinoma. Obstet Gynecol 1983;61: 327.

Krebs HB, Goplerud DR, Kolpatrick SJ, et al: Role of CA 125 as tumor marker in ovarian carcinoma. Obstet Gynecol 1986;67: 473.

Kudelka AP, Tresukosol D, Edwards CL, et al: Phase II study of intravenous topotecan as a 5-day infusion for refractory epithelial ovarian carcinoma. J Clin Oncol 1996;14:1552.

Kuhn W, Kaufmann M, Feichter GE, et al: DNA flow cytometry, clinical and morphological parameters as prognostic factors for advanced malignant and borderline tumors. Gynecol Oncol 1989;33:360.

Kurman RJ, Craig JM: Endometrioid and clear cell carcinoma of the ovary. Cancer 1972;29:1653.

Kvale G, Heuch I, Nilssen S, et al: Reproductive factors and risk of ovarian cancer: a prospective study. Int J Cancer 1989;42:246.

Landis SH, Murray T, Bolden SH, et al: Cancer statistics, 1998. CA Cancer J Clin 1998;48:6.

Larson JE, Podczaski ES, Manetta A, et al: Bowel obstruction in patients with ovarian carcinoma: analysis of prognostic factors. Gynecol Oncol 1989;35:61.

LaVecchia C, Franceschi S, Decarli A, et al: Coffee drinking and the risk of epithelial ovarian cancer. Int J Cancer 1984;33:559.

Lavin PT, Knapp RC, Malkasian G: CA 125 for the monitoring of ovarian carcinoma during primary therapy. Obstet Gynecol 1987;69:223.

Lawton FG, Luesley D, Redman C, et al: Feasibility and outcome of complete secondary tumor resection for patients with advanced ovarian cancer. J Surg Oncol 1990;45:14.

Ledermann JA, Dembo AJ, Sturgeon JF, et al: Outcome of patients with unfavorable optimally cytoreduced ovarian cancer treated with chemotherapy and whole abdominal radiation. Gynecol Oncol 1991;41:30.

Legros M, Dauplat J, Fleury J, et al: High-dose chemotherapy with hematopoietic rescue in patients with stage III to IV ovarian cancer: long-term results. J Clin Oncol 1997;15:1302.

Lele S, Piver MS: Interval laparoscopy as predictor of response to chemotherapy in ovarian carcinoma. Obstet Gynecol 1986; 68:345.

Levin L, Hryniuk WM: Dose intensity analysis of chemotherapy regimens in ovarian carcinoma. J Clin Oncol 1987;5:756.

Lim-Tan SK, Cajigas HE, Scully RE: Ovarian cystectomy for serous borderline tumors: a follow-up study of 35 cases. Obstet Gynecol 1988;72:775.

Lind MJ, Cantwell BM, Millward MJ, et al: A Phase II trial of goserelin (Zoladex) in relapsed epithelial ovarian cancer. Br J Cancer 1992;65:621.

Liu PC, Benjamin I, Morgan MA, et al: Effect of surgical debulking on survival in stage IV ovarian cancer. Gynecol Oncol 1997; 64:4.

Long ME, Taylor HC: Endometrioid carcinoma of the ovary. Am J Obstet Gynecol 1964;90:936.

Longo LD, Young RC: Cosmetic talc and ovarian cancer. Lancet 1979;2:349.

Louie KG, Ozols RF, Myers CE, et al: Long-term results of a cisplatin-containing combination chemotherapy regimen for the treatment of advanced ovarian carcinoma. J Clin Oncol 1986;4:1579.

Lucas WE, Markman M, Howell SB: Intraperitoneal chemotherapy for advanced ovarian cancer. Am J Obstet Gynecol 1985; 152:474.

Luesley D, Chan K, Fielding J, et al: Second-look laparotomy in the management of epithelial ovarian carcinoma: an evaluation of fifty cases. Obstet Gynecol 1984;64:421.

Luesley D, Chan K, Lawton F, et al: Survival after negative second-look laparotomy. Eur J Surg Oncol 1989;15:205.

Lund B, Jacobsen K, Rasch L, et al: Correlation of abdominal ultrasound and computed tomography scans with second or third-look laparotomy in patients with ovarian carcinoma. Gynecol Oncol 1990;37:279.

Lynch HT, Bewtra C, Lynch JF: Familial ovarian carcinoma. Am J Med 1986;81:1073.

Lynch HT, Fitzscommons ML, Conway TA, et al: Hereditary carcinoma of the ovary and associated cancers: a study of two families. Gynecol Oncol 1990;36:48.

Lynch HT, Kimberling W, Albano WA, et al: Hereditary nonpolyposis colorectal cancer (Lynch syndrome I and II). I. Clinical description of resource. Cancer 1985a;56:934.

Lynch HT, Schuelke GS, Kimberling WJ, et al: Hereditary neopolyposis colorectal cancer (Lynch syndromes I and II). II. Biomarker studies. Cancer 1985b;56:939.

Maiman M, Seltzer V, Boyce J: Laparoscopic excision of ovarian neoplasms subsequently found to be malignant. Obstet Gynecol 1991;77:563.

Malfetano JH: Splenectomy for optimal cytoreduction in ovarian cancer. Gynecol Oncol 1986;24:392.

Malkasian GD, Decker DG, Jorgensen EO, et al: Medroxyprogesterone acetate for the treatment of metastatic and recurrent ovarian carcinoma. Cancer Treat Rep 1977;61:913.

Malkasian GD, Decker DG, Mussey E, et al: Observations on gynecologic malignancy treated with 5-fluorouracil. Am J Obstet Gynecol 1968;100:1012.

Malkasian GD, Knapp RC, Leving RT, et al: Preoperative evaluation of serum CA 125 in premenopausal and postmenopausal patients with pelvic masses: discrimination of benign from malignant disease. Am J Obstet Gynecol 1988;159:341.

Malkasian GD Jr, Melton LJ III, O'Brien PC, et al: Prognostic significance of histologic classification and grading of epithelial malignancies of the ovary. Am J Obstet Gynecol 1984;149:274.

Malone JM, Koonce T, Larson DM, et al: Palliation of small bowel obstruction by percutaneous gastrostomy in patients with progressive ovarian carcinoma. Obstet Gynecol 1986;68:431.

Manetta A, MacNeill C, Lyter JA, et al: Hexamethylmelamine as a single second-line agent in ovarian cancer. Gynecol Oncol 1990;36:93.

Mangioni C, Franceschi S, LaVecchia C, et al: High-dose medroxyprogesterone acetate (MPA) in advanced epithelial ovarian cancer resistant to first- or second-line chemotherapy. Gynecol Oncol 1981;12:214.

Maraninchi D, Abecassis M, Gastaut G, et al: High-dose melphalan with autologous bone marrow rescue for the treatment of advanced adult solid tumors. Cancer Treat Rep 1984;68:471.

Markman M, Howell SB, Lucas WE, et al: Combination intraperitoneal chemotherapy with cisplatin, cytarabine, and doxorubicin for refractory ovarian carcinoma and other malignancies principally confined to the peritoneal cavity. J Clin Oncol 1984; 2:1321.

Markman M, Rothman R, Hakes T, et al: Second-line platinum therapy in patients with ovarian cancer previously treated with cisplatin. J Clin Oncol 1991;9:389.

Marks JR, Davidoff AM, Kerns BJ, et al: Overexpression and mutation of p53 in epithelial ovarian cancer. Cancer Res 1991;51: 2979.

McCaughey WTE, Kirk ME, Lester W, et al: Peritoneal epithelial lesions associated with proliferative serous tumours of ovary. Histopathology 1984;8:195.

McGarrity KA, Pettersson F, Ulfelder H (eds): Annual Report on the Results of Treatment of Gynecologic Cancer. Vol. 18. State of Results Obtained in 1973 to 1975 Inclusive. Stockholm: Radiumhemmet, 1982.

McGowan L, Lesher LP, Norris HJ, et al: Misstaging of ovarian cancer. Obstet Gynecol 1985;65:568.

McGowan L, Parent L, Lednar W, et al: The woman at risk for developing ovarian cancer. Gynecol Oncol 1979;7:325.

McGuire WP, Hoskins WJ, Brady MF, et al: A Phase III trial of dose intense (DI) versus standard dose (DS) cisplatin (CDDP) and cytoxan (CTX) in advanced ovarian cancer (AOC). J Clin Oncol 1995;13:1589.

McGuire WP, Hoskins WJ, Brady MF, et al: Cyclophosphamide and cisplatin compared with paclitaxel and cisplatin in patients with stage III and stage IV ovarian cancer. N Engl J Med 1996; 334:1.

McGuire WP, Rowinsky EK, Rosenshein NB, et al: Taxol: a unique antineoplastic agent with significant activity in advanced ovarian epithelial neoplasms. Ann Intern Med 1989;111:273.

Michael H, Roth LM: Invasive and noninvasive implants in ovarian serous tumors of low malignant potential. Cancer 1986;57: 1240.

Miki Y, Swensen J, Shattuck-Eidens D, et al: A strong candidate for the breast and ovarian cancer susceptibility gene BRCA1. Science 1994;266:66.

Miles PA, Norris HJ: Proliferative and malignant Brenner tumors of the ovary. Cancer 1972;30:174.

Miller DS, Ballon S, Teng N, et al: A critical reassessment of second-look laparotomy in epithelial ovarian carcinoma. Cancer 1986;57:530.

Miller DS, Brady MK, Barrett RJ: A Phase II trial of leuprolide acetate in patients with advanced epithelial ovarian cancer: a Gynecologic Oncology Group study. Am J Clin Oncol 1992;15: 125.

Mogensen O: Prognostic value of CA 125 in advanced ovarian cancer. Gynecol Oncol 1992;44:207.

Monga M, Carmichael JA, Shelley WE, et al: Surgery without adjuvant chemotherapy for early epithelial ovarian carcinoma after comprehensive surgical staging. Gynecol Oncol 1991;43: 195.

Montz FJ, Schlaerth JB, Berek JS: Resection of diaphragmatic peritoneum and muscle: role in cytoreductive surgery for ovarian cancer. Gynecol Oncol 1989;35:338.

Moore DH, Valea F, Crumpler LS, et al: Hexamethylmelamine/altretamine as second-line therapy for epithelial ovarian carcinoma. Gynecol Oncol 1993;51:109.

Morgan L, Chafe W, Mendenhall W, Marcus R: Hyperfractionation of whole-abdomen radiation therapy: salvage treatment of persistent ovarian carcinoma following chemotherapy. Gynecol Oncol 1988;31:122.

Morris M, Gershenson DM, Burke T, et al: Splenectomy in gynecologic oncology: implications, complications, and technique. Gynecol Oncol 1991;43:118.

Morris M, Gershenson DM, Wharton JT: Secondary cytoreductive surgery in epithelial ovarian cancer: nonresponders to first-line therapy. Gynecol Oncol 1989a;33:1.

Morris M, Gershenson DM, Wharton JT, et al: Secondary cytoreductive surgery for recurrent epithelial ovarian cancer. Gynecol Oncol 1989b;34:334.

Muggia FM, Braly PS, Brady MF, et al: Phase III of cisplatin (P) or paclitaxel (T), versus their combination in suboptimal stage III and IV epithelial ovarian cancer (EOC): Gynecologic Oncology Group (GOG) study #132 [abstract]. Proc Am Soc Clin Oncol 1997a;16:352.

Muggia FM, Hainsworth JD, Jeffers S, et al: Phase II study of liposomal doxorubicin in refractory ovarian cancer: antitumor activity and toxicity modification by liposomal encapsulation. J Clin Oncol 1997b;15:987.

Mulder POM, Willemse PHB, Azalders JG, et al: High-dose chemotherapy with autologous bone marrow transplantation in patients with refractory ovarian cancer. Eur J Clin Oncol 1989; 25:645.

Munkarah AR, Hallum AV, Morris M, et al: Prognostic significance of residual disease in patients with stage IV epithelial ovarian cancer. Gynecol Oncol 1997;64:13.

Munnell EW, Jacob HE, Taylor HC: Treatment and prognosis in cancer of the ovary. Am J Obstet Gynecol 1957;74:1187.

Muñoz KA, Harlan LC, Trimble EL: Patterns of care for women with ovarian cancer in the United States. J Clin Oncol 1997;15: 3408.

Musumeci R, Banfi A, Bolis G: Lymphangiography in patients with ovarian epithelial cancer. Cancer 1977;40:1444.

Myers C: The use of intraperitoneal chemotherapy in the treatment of ovarian cancer. Semin Oncol 1984;11:275.

Neijt JP, Hansen M, Hansen SW, et al: Randomized Phase III study in previously untreated epithelial ovarian cancer FIGO stage IIB, IIC, III, IV, comparing paclitaxel-cisplatin and paclitaxel-carboplatin [abstract]. Proc Am Soc Clin Oncol 1998; 16:352.

Neijt JP, Huinink WW, van der Burg MEL, et al: Randomized trial comparing two combination chemotherapy regimens (CHAP-5 V CP) in advanced ovarian carcinoma. J Clin Oncol 1987;5: 1157.

Neijt JP, Ten Bokkel Huinink W, Van Der Burg ME, et al: Randomized trial comparing two combination chemotherapy regimens (HEXA-CAF vs CHAP-5) in advanced ovarian carcinoma. Lancet 1984;2:594.

Nelson BE, Rosenfeld AT, Schwartz PE: Preoperative abdomino-pelvic computed tomographic prediction of optimal cytoreduction in epithelial ovarian carcinoma. J Clin Oncol 1993;11: 166.

Newhouse ML: Cosmetic talc and ovarian cancer. Lancet 1979;1: 528.

Ngan HYS, Choo YC, Cheung M, et al: A randomized study of high-dose versus low-dose cisplatin combined with cyclophosphamide in the treatment of advanced ovarian cancer. Chemotherapy 1989;35:221.

Niloff JM, Bast RC, Schaetzl EM, et al: Predictive value of CA-125 antigen levels at second-look procedures in ovarian cancer. Am J Obstet Gynecol 1984a;151:981.

Niloff JM, Klug TL, Schaetzl E: Elevation of serum CA 125 in carcinomas of the fallopian tube, endometrium and endocervix. Am J Obstet Gynecol 1984b;148:1057.

Niloff JM, Knapp RC, Schaetzl E, et al: CA 125 antigen levels in obstetric and gynecologic patients. Obstet Gynecol 1985;151: 981.

O'Bryan RM, Luce JK, Talley RW, et al: Phase II evaluation of Adriamycin in human neoplasia. Cancer 1973;32:1.

Omura GA, Brady M, Homesley HD, et al: Long-term follow-up and prognostic factor analysis in advanced ovarian carcinoma: the Gynecologic Oncology Group experience. J Clin Oncol 1991;9:1138.

Omura GA, Morrow CP, Blessing JA, et al: A randomized comparison of melphalan versus melphalan plus hexamethylmelamine versus Adriamycin plus cyclophosphamide in ovarian carcinoma. Cancer 1983;51:783.

Ovarian Cancer Meta-Analysis Project: Cyclophosphamide plus cisplatin versus cyclophosphamide, doxorubicin, and cisplatin chemotherapy of ovarian carcinoma: a meta-analysis. J Clin Oncol 1991;9:1668.

Ozols RF, Fisher R, Anderson T, et al: Peritoneoscopy in the management of ovarian cancer. Am J Obstet Gynecol 1981;140:611.

Ozols RF, Garvin J, Costa J, et al: Correlation of histologic grade with response to therapy and survival. Cancer 1980;45:572.

Ozols RF, Kilparick D, O'Dwyer P, et al: Phase I and pharmacokinetic study of taxol (T) and carboplatin (C) in previously untreated patients (PTS) with adanced epithelial ovarian cancer (OC): a pilot study of the Gynecologic Oncology Group. Proc Am Soc Clin Oncol 1993;12:259.

Ozols RF, Speyer JL, Jenkins J, et al: Phase II trial of 5-FU administered to patients with refractory ovarian cancer. Cancer Treat Rep 1984;68:1229.

Ozols RF, Young RC, Speyer JL, et al: Phase I and pharmacological studies of Adriamycin administered intraperitoneally to patients with ovarian cancer. Cancer Res 1982;42:4265.

Paley PJ, Staskus KA, Gebhard K, et al: Vascular endothelial growth factor expression in early stage ovarian carcinoma. Cancer 1997;80:98.

Palmer H, Rustin G, Lightman SL: Response to D-Trp-6-luteinizing hormone releasing hormone (Decapeptyl) microcapsules in advanced ovarian cancer. Br Med J 1988;296:1229.

Parmley TH, Woodruff JD: The ovarian mesothelioma. Am J Obstet Gynecol 1974;120:234.

Partridge EE, Gunter B, Gelder M, et al: The validity and significance of substages in advanced ovarian carcinoma [abstract]. Gynecol Oncol 1992;45:9.

Patsner B, Day TG Jr: Predictive value of CA-125 levels in advanced ovarian cancer. Am J Obstet Gynecol 1987;156:440.

Patsner B, Mann WJ: The value of preoperative serum CA 125 in patients with a pelvic mass. Am J Obstet Gynecol 1988;159:873.

Patsner B, Orr J, Mann W, et al: Does serum CA-125 level prior to second-look laparotomy for invasive ovarian adenocarcinoma predict size of residual disease? Gynecol Oncol 1990;37: 319.

Pesando JM, Come SE, Stark J, et al: cis-Diamminedichloroplatinum (II) for advanced ovarian cancer. Cancer Treat Rep 1980;64:1147.

Pfeifle CE, Howell SB, Markman M, et al: Totally implantable system for peritoneal access. J Clin Oncol 1984;2:1277.

Piccart MJ, Gore M, Ten Bokkel Huinink W, et al: Taxotere (RP56976, NSC628503): an active new drug for the treatment of advanced ovarian cancer (OVCA). Proc Am Soc Clin Oncol 1993;12:258.

Piccart MJ, Speyer JL, Markman N, et al: Intraperitoneal chemotherapy: technical experience at five institutions. Semin Oncol 1985;12:90.

Piver MS, Baker T: The potential for optimal (≤2 cm) cytoreductive surgery in advanced ovarian carcinoma at a tertiary medical center: a prospective study. Gynecol Oncol 1986;24:1.

Piver MS, Barlow JJ, Lele SB: Incidence of subclinical metastasis in stage I and II ovarian carcinoma. Obstet Gynecol 1978;52: 100.

Piver MS, Jishi MF, Tsukada Y, et al: Primary peritoneal carcinoma after prophylactic oophorectomy in women with a family history of ovarian cancer: a report of the Gilda Radner Familial Ovarian Cancer Registry. Cancer 1993;71:2751.

Piver MS, Malfetano J, Baker TR, et al: Adjuvant cisplatin-based chemotherapy for stage I ovarian adenocarcinoma: a preliminary report. Gynecol Oncol 1989;35:69.

Piver MS, Mettlin CJ: A case-control study of milk drinking and ovary cancer risk. Am J Epidemiol 1990;132:871.

Piver MS, Mettlin CJ, Tsukada Y, et al: Familial ovarian cancer registry. Obstet Gynecol 1984;64:195.

Podczaski E, Stevens C, Manetta A, et al: Use of second-look laparotomy in the management of patients with ovarian epithelial malignancies. Gynecol Oncol 1987;28:205.

Podratz K, Malkasian G, Hilton J, et al: Second-look laparotomy in ovarian cancer: evaluation of pathologic variables. Am J Obstet Gynecol 1985;152:230.

Podratz K, Schwarz MF, Wieand HS, et al: Evaluation of treatment and survival after positive second-look laparotomy. Gynecol Oncol 1988;31:9.

Pujade-Lauraine E, Piccart M, Rustin G, et al: Comparison of CA 125 kinetics and WHO criteria to evaluate chemotherapy response: an EORTC ovarian cancer (O.C.) study with Taxotere (T). Proc Am Soc Clin Oncol 1994;13:269.

Raju KS, McKinna JA, Barker GH, et al: Second-look operations in the planned management of advanced ovarian carcinoma. Am J Obstet Gynecol 1982;144:650.

Rambaldi A, Introna M, Colotta F, et al: Intraperitoneal administration of interferon β in ovarian cancer patients. Cancer 1985; 56:294.

Reimer RR, Hoover R, Fraumeni JF Jr, et al: Acute leukemia after alkylating-agent therapy of ovarian cancer. N Engl J Med 1977; 297:177.

Rendina GM, Donadio C, Giovannini M: Steroid receptors and progestinic therapy in ovarian endometrioid carcinoma. Eur J Gynaecol Oncol 1982;3:241.

Reuter K, Griffith T, Hunter R: Comparison of abdominopelvic computed tomography results and findings at second-look laparotomy in ovarian carcinoma patients. Cancer 1989;63:1123.

Richardson GS, Scully RE, Nikrui N, et al: Common epithelial cancer of the ovary. N Engl J Med 1985;312:415.

Roberts W, Hodel K, Rich W, DiSaia P: Second-look laparotomy in the management of gynecologic malignancy. Gynecol Oncol 1982;13:345.

Robey SS, Silva EG, Gershenson DM, et al: Transitional cell carcinoma in high-grade high-stage ovarian carcinoma. Cancer 1989;63:839.

Rose PG, Blessing JA, Mayer AR, et al: Prolonged oral etoposide as second line therapy for platinum resistant and platinum sensitive ovarian carcinoma: Gynecologic Oncology Group study [abstract]. Proc Am Soc Clin Oncol 1996;15:282.

Rosen GF, Lurain JR, Newton M: Hexamethylmelamine in ovarian cancer after failure of cisplatin-based multiple agent chemotherapy. Gynecol Oncol 1987;27:173.

Rosenberg L, Shapiro S, Slone D, et al: Epithelial ovarian cancer and combination oral contraceptives. JAMA 1982;247:3210.

Rosenberg SA, Lotze MT, Muul LM, et al: A progress report on the treatment of 157 patients with advanced cancer using lymphokine-activated killer cells and interleukin-2 or high-dose interleukin-2 alone. N Engl J Med 1987;316:889.

Rosenburg CJ, Cornelisse CJ, Heintz PA, et al: Tumor ploidy as a major prognostic factor in advanced ovarian cancer. Cancer 1987;59:317.

Rosenoff SH, Young RC, Anderson T, et al: Peritoneoscopy: a valuable staging tool in ovarian carcinoma. Ann Intern Med 1975; 83:37.

Roth LM, Czernobilsky B: Ovarian Brenner tumors. II. Malignant. Cancer 1985;56:592.

Roth LM, Langley FA, Fox H: Ovarian clear cell adenofibromatous tumors: benign, of low malignant potential, and associated with invasive clear cell carcinoma. Cancer 1984;53:1156.

Roth LM, Sternberg WH: Proliferating Brenner tumors. Cancer 1971;27:687.

Rothenberg M, Ozols R, Glatstein E, et al: Dose-intensive induction therapy with cyclophosphamide, cisplatin, and consolidative abdominal radiation in advanced stage epithelial ovarian cancer. J Clin Oncol 1992;10:727.

Rubin SC, Benjamin I, Behbakht K, et al: Clinical and pathological features of ovarian cancer in women with germ-line mutations of BRCA1. N Engl J Med 1996;335:1413.

Rubin SC, Finstad C, Federici M, et al: Prognostic significance of Her-2/neu expression in advanced epithelial ovarian cancer: a multivariate analysis. Am J Obstet Gynecol 1993a;168:162.

Rubin SC, Hoskins WJ, Benjamin I, Lewis JL: Palliative surgery for intestinal obstruction in advanced ovarian cancer. Gynecol Oncol 1989;34:16.

Rubin SC, Hoskins WJ, Hakes T, et al: Recurrence after negative second-look laparotomy for ovarian cancer: analysis of risk factors. Am J Obstet Gynecol 1988;159:1094.

Rubin SC, Hoskins WJ, Saigo P, et al: Prognostic factors for recurrence following negative second-look laparotomy in ovarian cancer patients treated with platinum-based chemotherapy. Gynecol Oncol 1991;42:137.

Rubin SC, Wong GYC, Curtin JP, et al: Platinum-based chemotherapy of high-risk stage I epithelial ovarian cancer following comprehensive surgical staging. Obstet Gynecol 1993b;82:143.

Ruibal A, Encabo G, Capdevila JA, et al: Behavior of serum CA 125 in hepatopathy patients (letter). [Spanish] Medicina Clinica 1984;82:560.

Russell P: The pathological assessment of ovarian neoplasms. I. Introduction to the common "epithelial" tumors and analysis of benign "epithelial" tumors. Pathology 1979a;11:5.

Russell P: The pathological assessment of ovarian neoplasms. II. The proliferating "epithelial" tumors. Pathology 1979b;11:251.

Russell P: Borderline epithelial tumors of the ovary: a conceptual dilemma. Clin Obstet Gynaecol 1984;11:259.

Russell P, Merkur H: Proliferating ovarian "epithelial" tumours: a clinico-pathological analysis of 144 cases. Aust N Z J Obstet Gynaecol 1979;19:45.

Rustin GJ, Gennings JN, Nelstrop AE, et al: Use of CA-125 to predict survival of patients with ovarian carcinoma. North Thames Cooperative Group. J Clin Oncol 1989;7:1667.

Samaan NA, Smith JP, Rutledge FN, et al: The significance of measurement of human placental lactogen, human chorionic gonadotropin, and carcinoembryonic antigen in patients with ovarian carcinoma. Am J Obstet Gynecol 1976;126:186.

Sampson JA: Endometrial carcinoma of the ovary arising in endometrial tissue in that organ. Arch Surg 1925;10:1.

Schildkraut JM, Bastos E, Berchuck A: Relationship between lifetime ovulatory cycles and overexpression of mutant p53 in epithelial ovarian cancer. J Natl Clin Inst 1997;89:932.

Schilthuis MS, Aalders JG, Bouma J, et al: Serum CA 125 levels in epithelial ovarian cancer: relation with findings at second-look operations and their role in the detection of tumour recurrence. Br J Obstet Gynaecol 1987;94:202.

Schray M, Martinez A, Howes A, et al: Advanced epithelial cancer: salvage whole abdominal irradiation for patients with recurrent or persistent disease after combination chemotherapy. J Clin Oncol 1988;6:1433.

Schwartz PE, Chambers SK, Chambers JT, et al: Circulating tumor markers in the monitoring of gynecologic malignancies. Cancer 1987;60:353.

Schwartz PE, Chambers JT, Makuch R: Neoadjuvant chemotherapy for advanced ovarian cancer. Gynecol Oncol 1994;53:33.

Schwartz PE, Keating G, MacLusky N, et al: Tamoxifen therapy for advanced ovarian cancer. Obstet Gynecol 1982a;59:583.

Schwartz PE, Livolsi VA, Hildreth N, et al: Estrogen receptors in ovarian epithelial carcinoma. Obstet Gynecol 1982b;59:229.

Schwartz PE, Merino MJ, Livolsi VA, et al: Histopathologic correlations of estrogen and progestin receptor protein in epithelial ovarian carcinomas. Obstet Gynecol 1985;66:428.

Schwartz PE, Smith J: Second-look operations in ovarian cancer. Am J Obstet Gynecol 1980;138:1124.

Segna RA, Dottino PR, Mandeli JP, et al: Secondary cytoreduction for ovarian cancer following cisplatin therapy. J Clin Oncol 1993;11:434.

Sell A, Bertelsen K, Anderson JE, et al: Randomized study of whole abdomen irradiation versus pelvic irradiation plus cyclophosphamide in treatment of early ovarian cancer. Gynecol Oncol 1990;37:367.

Seltzer V, Vogl S, Kaplan B: Recurrent ovarian carcinoma: retreatment utilizing combination chemotherapy including cisdiamminedichloroplatinum in patients previously responding to this agent. Gynecol Oncol 1985;21:167.

Serov SF, Scully RE, Solvin LH: International Histological Classification of Tumors. No. 9: Histological Typing of Ovarian Tumors. Geneva: World Health Organization, 1973.

Sevelda P, Dittrich C, Salzer H: Prognostic value of the rupture of the capsule in stage I epithelial ovarian cancer. Gynecol Oncol 1989;35:321.

Sevelda P, Vavra N, Fitz R, et al: Goserelin a GnRH-analogue as third-line therapy of refractory epithelial ovarian cancer. Int J Gynecol Cancer 1992;2:160.

Shimizu Y, Kamoi S, Amada S, et al: Toward the development of a universal grading system for ovarian epithelial carcinoma. Gynecol Oncol 1998;70:2.

Shirey DR, Kavanagh JJ Jr, Gershenson DM, et al: Tamoxifen therapy of epithelial ovarian cancer. Obstet Gynecol 1985;66:575.

Shpall EJ, Clarke-Pearson D, Soper JT, et al: High-dose alkylating agent chemotherapy with autologous bone marrow support in patients with stage III/IV epithelial ovarian cancer. Gynecol Oncol 1990;38:386.

Sigurdsson K, Alm P, Gullberg B: Prognostic factors in malignant ovarian tumors. Gynecol Oncol 1983;15:370.

Silva EG, Gershenson DM: Standardized histologic grading of epithelial ovarian cancer: elusive after all these years [editorial]. Gynecol Oncol 1998;70:1.

Silva EG, Robey-Cafferty S, Smith TL, Gershenson DM: Ovarian carcinomas with transitional cell carcinoma pattern. Am J Clin Pathol 1990;93:457.

Skipper HE: Adjuvant chemotherapy. Cancer 1978;41:936.

Skipper HE: Stepwise progress in the treatment of disseminated cancer. Cancer 1983;5:1773.

Slamon DJ, Godolphin W, Jones LA, et al: Studies of the HER-2/neu proto-oncogene in human breast and ovarian cancer. Science 1989;244:707.

Slayton RE, Pagano M, Creech RH: Progestin therapy for advanced ovarian cancer: a Phase II Eastern Cooperative Oncology Group trial. Cancer Treat Rep 1981;65:895.

Smirz L, Stehman F, Ulbright T, et al: Second-look laparotomy after chemotherapy in the management of ovarian malignancy. Am J Obstet Gynecol 1985;152:661.

Smith JP, Day TG: Review of ovarian cancer at the University of Texas System Cancer Center, M. D. Anderson Hospital and Tumor Institute. Am J Obstet Gynecol 1979;135:984.

Smith JP, Rutledge F, Delclos L: Post-operative treatment of early cancer of the ovary: a random trial between post-operative irradiation and chemotherapy. NCI Monogr 1975;42:149.

Smith W, Day T, Smith J: The use of laparoscopy to determine the results of chemotherapy for ovarian cancer. J Reprod Med 1977;18:257.

Sonnendecker EW: Is routine second-look laparotomy for ovarian cancer justified? Gynecol Oncol 1988;31:249.

Sonnendecker EW, Guidozzi F, Margolius KA: Splenectomy during primary maximal cytoreductive surgery for epithelial ovarian cancer. Gynecol Oncol 1989;35:301.

Soper JT, Berchuck A, Dodge R, Clarke-Pearson DL: Adjuvant therapy with intraperitoneal chromic phosphate (^{32}P) in women with early ovarian carcinoma after comprehensive surgical staging. Obstet Gynecol 1992;79:993.

Soper JT, Couchman G, Berchuck A, et al: The role of partial sigmoid colectomy for debulking epithelial ovarian carcinoma. Gynecol Oncol 1991;41:239.

Sorbe B, Frankendal B, Veress B: Importance of histologic grading in the prognosis of epithelial ovarian carcinoma. Obstet Gynecol 1982;59:576.

Speyer JL, Collins JM, Dedrick RL, et al: Phase I and pharmacological studies of 5-fluorouracil administered intraperitoneally. Cancer Res 1980;40:567.

Stanhope CR, Smith JP, Rutledge FN: Second trial drugs in ovarian cancer. Gynecol Oncol 1977;5:52.

Stehman FB, Calkins A, Wass J, et al: A comparison of findings at second-look laparotomy with preoperative computed tomography in patients with ovarian cancer. Gynecol Oncol 1988; 29:37.

Stehman FB, Ehrlich CE, Callangan MF: Failure of hexamethylmelamine as salvage therapy in ovarian epithelial adenocarcinoma resistant to combination chemotherapy. Gynecol Oncol 1984;17:189.

Stehman FB, Erhlich CE, Einhorn LH, et al: Long-term follow-up and survival in stage II-IV epithelial ovarian cancer treated with cis-dichlorodiammineplatinum, Adriamycin, and cyclophosphamide (PAC). Proc Am Soc Clin Oncol 1983;3:147.

Steis RG, Urba WJ, VanderMolen LA, et al: Intrapeirtoneal lymphokine-activated killer cell and interleukin-2 therapy for malignancies limited to the peritoneal cavity. J Clin Oncol 1990; 8:1618.

Stern J, Buscema J, Rosenshein N, Siegelman S: Can computed tomography substitute for second-look operation in ovarian carcinoma? Gynecol Oncol 1981;11:82.

Stewart JA, Belinson JL, Moore AL, et al: Phase I trial of intraperitoneal recombinant interleukin-2/lymphokine-activated killer cells in patients with ovarian cancer. Cancer Res 1990a; 50:6302.

Stewart JSW, Hird V, Snook D, et al: Intraperitoneal yttrium-90-labeled monoclonal antibody in ovarian cancer. J Clin Oncol 1990b;8:1941.

Stiff PJ, Bayer R, Kerger C, et al: High-dose chemotherapy with autologous transplantation for persistent/relapsed ovarian cancer: a multivariate analysis of survival for 100 consecutively treated patients. J Clin Oncol 1997;15:1309.

Stocks P: Cancer mortality in relation to national consumption of cigarettes, solid fuel, tea, and coffee. Br J Cancer 1970;24:215.

Struewing JP, Abeliovich D, Peretz T, et al: The carrier frequency of the BRCA1 185delAG mutation is approximately 1 percent in Ashkenazi Jewish individuals. Nat Genet 1995;11:198.

Stuart GC, Jeffries M, Stuart JL, Anderson RJ: The changing role of "second-look" laparotomy in the management of epithelial carcinoma of the ovary. Am J Obstet Gynecol 1982;142:612.

Surwit E, Childers J, Atlas I, et al: Neoadjuvant chemotherapy for advanced ovarian cancer. Int J Gynecol Cancer 1996;6:356.

Sutton GP, Stehman FB, Einhorn LH, et al: Ten-year follow-up of patients receiving cisplatin, doxorubicin, and cyclophosphamide chemotherapy for advanced epithelial ovarian carcinoma. J Clin Oncol 1989b;7:223.

Suzuki M, Sekiguchi I, Ohwada M, et al: Clinical evaluation of a cancer antigen CA 125 associated with ovarian cancer. IV. Serum CA 125 levels through normal menstrual cycle and in benign disease. Rinsho Biyori–Japanese J Clin Pathol 1985;33:285.

Suzuki M, Sekiguchi I, Tamada T: Clinical evaluation of tumor-associated mucin-type glycoprotein CA 54/61 in ovarian cancers: comparison with CA 125. Obstet Gynecol 1990;76:422.

Swenerton KD, Hislop TG, Spinelli J, et al: Ovarian carcinoma: a multivariate analysis of prognostic factors. Obstet Gynecol 1985;65:264.

Swenerton KD, Jeffrey J, Stuart G, et al: Cisplatin-cyclophosphamide versus carboplatin-cyclophosphamide in advanced ovarian cancer: a randomized Phase III study of the National Cancer Institute of Canada Clinical Trials Group. J Clin Oncol 1992;10:718.

Taylor HC Jr: Malignant and semimalignant tumors of the ovary. Surg Gynecol Obstet 1929;48:204.

Tazelaar HD, Bostwick DG, Ballon SC, et al: Conservative treatment of borderline ovarian tumors. Obstet Gynecol 1985;66: 417.

ten Bokkel Huinink WW, Dubbelman R, Aartsen E, et al: Experimental and clinical results with intraperitoneal cisplatin. Semin Oncol 1985;12:43.

ten Bokkel Huinink WW, Gore M, Carmichael J, et al: Topotecan versus paclitaxel for the treatment of recurrent epithelial ovarian cancer. J Clin Oncol 1997;15:2183.

Tenckhoff H, Scheckter H: A bacteriologically safe peritoneal access device. Am Soc Artif Organs 1968;12:181.

Thigpen T, Blessing J, Ball H, et al: Phase II trial of paclitaxel in patients with progressive ovarian carcinoma after platinum-based chemotherapy: a Gynecologic Oncology Group study. J Clin Oncol 1994;12:1748.

Tobacman JK, Tucker MA, Kase R, et al: Intra-abdominal carcinomatosis after prophylactic oophorectomy in ovarian-cancer-prone families. Lancet 1982;2:795.

Tobias JS, Griffiths CT: Management of ovarian carcinoma: current concepts and future prospects. N Engl J Med 1976;15:818.

Trichopoulos D, Papapostolou M, Polychromopoulou A: Coffee and ovarian cancer. Int J Cancer 1981;28:691.

Trimbos JB, Schueler JA, van der Burg M, et al: Watch and wait after careful surgical treatment in well-differentiated early ovarian cancer. Cancer 1991;67:597.

Trimbos JB, Schueler JA, vanLent M, et al: Reasons for incomplete surgical staging in early ovarian carcinoma. Gynecol Oncol 1990;37:374.

Tropé C, Johnson JE, Sigurdsson K, et al: High-dose medroxyprogesterone acetate for the treatment of advanced ovarian carcinoma. Cancer Treat Rep 1982;66:1441.

Vacarello L, Rubin SC, Vlamis V, et al: Cytoreductive surgery in ovarian carcinoma patients with a documented previously complete surgical response. Gynecol Oncol 1995;57:61.

van der Burg MEL, van Lent M, Buyse M, et al: The effect of debulking surgery after induction chemotherapy on the prognosis in advanced epithelial ovarian cancer. N Engl J Med 1995; 332:629.

Van Nagell JR Jr, DePriest PD, Puls LE, et al: Ovarian cancer screening in asymptomatic postmenopausal women by transvaginal sonography. Cancer 1991;68:458.

Van Nagell JR Jr, Donaldson ES, Gay EC, et al: Carcinoembryonic antigen in ovarian epithelial cystadenocarcinomas: the prognostic value of tumor and serial plasma determinations. Cancer 1978;41:2335.

Van Nagell JR Jr, Higgins RV, Donaldson ES, et al: Transvaginal sonography as a screening method for ovarian cancer: a report of the first 1000 cases screened. Cancer 1990;65:573.

Varga A, Henriksen E: Effect of 17-alpha-hydroxyprogesterone 17-n-caproate on various pelvic malignancies. Obstet Gynecol 1964;23:51.

Vergote I, Himmelmann A, Frankendal B, et al: Hexamethylmelamine as second-line therapy in platin-resistant ovarian cancer. Gynecol Oncol 1992;47:282.

Vergote IB, Bormer OP, Abeler VM: Evaluation of serum CA 125 levels in the monitoring of ovarian cancer. Am J Obstet Gynecol 1987;157:88.

Vogl S, Kaplan B, Pagano M: Diamminedichloroplatinum-based combination chemotherapy is superior to melphalan for advanced ovarian cancer when age >50 and tumor diameter >2 cm. Proc Am Soc Clin Oncol 1982;1:119.

Wangensteen OH, Lewis FJ, Tongen LA: The "second-look" in cancer surgery. Lancet 1951;71:303.

Ward HW: Progesterone therapy for ovarian carcinoma. J Obstet Gynaecol Br Commonw 1972;79:55.

Webb M, Synder J, Williams T, Decker D: Second-look laparotomy in ovarian cancer. Gynecol Oncol 1982;14:285.

Webb PM, Green A, Cummings MC, et al: Relationship between number of ovulatory cycles and accumulation of mutant p53 in epithelial ovarian cancer. J Natl Cancer Inst 1998;90:1729.

Weiner SA, Alberts DS, Surwit EA, et al: Tamoxifen therapy of epithelial ovarian cancer. Obstet Gynecol 1987;66:575.

Weiner Z, Thaler I, Beck D, et al: Differentiating malignant from benign ovarian tumors with transvaginal color flow imaging. Obstet Gynecol 1992;79:159.

Weiss NS, Lyon JKL, Liff JM, et al: Incidence of ovarian cancer in relation to the use of oral contraceptives. Int J Cancer 1981;28:669.

West RO: Epidemiologic study of malignancies of the ovaries. Cancer 1966;19:1001.

Wharton JT, Edwards CL, Rutledge FN: Long-term survival after chemotherapy for advanced epithelial ovarian carcinoma. Am J Obstet Gynecol 1984;148:997.

Wharton JT, Herson J: Surgery for common epithelial tumors of the ovary. Cancer 1981;48:582.

Wharton JT, Herson J, Edwards CL, et al: Long-term survival following chemotherapy for advanced epithelial ovarian carcinoma. In van Oosterom AT, Muggia FM, Cleton FJ (eds): Therapeutic Process in Ovarian Cancer, Testicular Cancer and the Sarcomas. The Hague: Martinus Nijhoff, 1980:96.

Wharton JT, Herson J, Edwards CL, et al: Single-agent Adriamycin followed by combination hexamethylmelamine-cyclophosphamide for advanced ovarian carcinoma. Gynecol Oncol 1982;14:262.

Wharton JT, Rutledge FN, Smith JP, et al: Hexamethylmelamine: an evaluation of its role in the treatment of ovarian cancer. Am J Obstet Gynecol 1979;133:833.

Whittemore AS, Wu ML, Paffenbarger RS, et al: Personal and environmental characteristics related to epithelial ovarian cancer II. Exposure to talcum powder, tobacco, alcohol and coffee. Am J Epidemiol 1988;128:1228.

Williams CJ, Mead GM, Macbeth FR, et al: Cisplatin combination chemotherapy versus chlorambucil in advanced ovarian carcinoma: mature results of a randomized trial. J Clin Oncol 1985;3:1455.

Wiltshaw E, Raju KS, Dawson I: The role of cytoreductive surgery in advanced carcinoma of the ovary: an analysis of primary and second surgery. Br J Obstet Gynecol 1985;92:522.

Wiltshaw E, Subramarian S, Alexopoulos C, et al: Cancer of the ovary: a summary of experience with cis-dichlorodiammineplatinum (II) at the Royal Marsden Hospital. Cancer Treat Rep 1979;63:1545.

Woolas RP, Xu FJ, Jacobs IJ, et al: Elevation of multiple serum markers in patients with stage I ovarian cancer. J Natl Cancer Inst 1993;85:1748.

Wooster R, Neuhausen SL, Mangion, et al: Localization of a breast cancer susceptibility gene, BRCA2, to chromosome 13q12-13. Science 1994;265:2088.

Wu ML, Whittemore AS, Paffenbarger RS, et al: Personal and environmental characteristics related to epithelial ovarian cancer. Am J Epidemiol 1988;128:1216.

Wu P-C, Qu J-Y, Lang J-H, et al: Lymph node metastasis of ovarian cancer: a preliminary survey of 74 cases of lymphadenectomy. Am J Obstet Gynecol 1986;155:1103.

Xu Y, Zhongzhou S, Wiper DW, et al: Lysophosphatidic acid as a potential biomarker for ovarian and other gynecologic cancers. JAMA 1998;280:719.

Yancik R, Ries LG, Yates JW: Ovarian cancer in the elderly: an analysis of surveillance, epidemiology and end results program data. Am J Obstet Gynecol 1986;154:639.

Young RC: A second look at second-look laparotomy [editorial]. J Clin Oncol 1987;5:1311.

Young RC, Chabner BA, Hubbard SP, et al: Advanced ovarian adenocarcinoma: a prospective clinical trial of melphalan (l-Pam) versus combination chemotherapy. N Engl J Med 1978;299:1261.

Young RC, Decker DG, Wharton JT, et al: Staging laparotomy in young early ovarian cancer. JAMA 1983;250:3072.

Young RC, Walton LA, Ellenberg SS, et al: Adjuvant therapy in stage I and II epithelial ovarian cancer: results of two prospective randomized trials. N Engl J Med 1990;322:1021.

61

Papillary Serous Carcinoma of the Peritoneum

Alberto E. Selman
Theodore H. Niemann
Larry J. Copeland

Primary peritoneal adenocarcinoma (PPA) is rare (Gitsch et al, 1992). The incidence varies from 7% to 21% among cases of epithelial ovarian carcinoma (EOC) or papillary serous ovarian carcinoma (PSOC) assessed retrospectively (Kannerstein et al, 1977a; Lele et al, 1988; Mills et al, 1988; Feuer et al, 1989; Wick et al, 1989; Fromm et al, 1990; Altaras et al, 1991; Fowler et al, 1994). Basically, PPA is an adenocarcinoma that develops in the peritoneum and spreads widely throughout the peritoneal cavity with minimal or no ovarian involvement (Fig. 61–1). There is no identifiable primary tumor. Most of PPA cases reported have been of serous histology, and in many cases, the malignancy developed following bilateral oophorectomy for reasons other than cancer (Kannerstein et al, 1977a; Kemp et al, 1992; Yamakazi et al, 1995). Histopathologic, immunohistochemical, and clinical similarities have been observed between PPA and EOC—specifically the serous variety (Resta et al, 1988; Raju et al, 1989; Truong et al, 1990)—but PPA involves the ovarian surface only minimally (microscopic disease) or spares the ovaries entirely (Ulbright et al, 1983). Molecular and epidemiologic studies (Kowalski et al, 1997; Eltabbakh et al, 1998a) have reported some differences between the two diseases.

Disagreement and controversy continue to exist in the literature among authorities who consider PPA a different clinical entity from EOC (Strand et al, 1989; Fromm et al, 1990; Fox, 1993) and others who cannot find any justification for this distinction (Gooneratne et al, 1982). Most investigators consider these entities to be similar in clinical presentation and course, except that all PPA patients by disease definition present at an advanced stage.

HISTORY

Numerous terms have been used to describe this entity, including serous surface carcinoma of the peritoneum, papillary tumor of the peritoneum, serous surface papillary carcinoma, serous papillary surface carcinoma of the ovary, serous borderline tumor of the peritoneum, extraovarian pelvic serous tumor, multifocal extraovarian serous carcinoma, extraovarian papillary serous carcinoma, mesothelioma, and papillary serous carcinoma of the peritoneum (PSCP).

In a 1959 case report, Swerdlow first described "malignant mesothelioma" with diffuse involvement of the peritoneum, no obvious primary site, and grossly normal ovaries in a 27-year-old woman. Since then, many authors have reported similar cases (Kannerstein et al, 1977a; Foyle et al, 1981; Chen and Flam, 1986; Resta et al, 1988; Fromm et al, 1990; Bloss et al, 1993). Kannerstein et al (1977a) pointed out the importance of distinguishing PPA from malignant mesothelioma. Since its first description by Swerdlow, PPA has been recognized in females (Swerdlow, 1959); its histologic similarities to malignant mesothelioma and PSOC have caused difficulties in classifying it as an independent clinicopathologic entity (Kannerstein et al, 1977a; Bollinger et al, 1989; Gitsch et al, 1992). It is recognized as a distinct clinicopathologic tumor that arises from mesothelial cells under müllerian influences (Lauchlan, 1972; Parmley, 1987). Some authors (Hertig, 1952; Rosenbloom and Foster, 1961) have regarded the term *mesothelioma* and PSCP as synonymous. Parmley and Woodruff (1974) also proposed that all tumors arising from the pleural and peritoneal cavities be classified as mesotheliomas. In 1981, Foyle et al described 25 peritoneal tumors in women and divided them histologically into five groups: mesothelial hyperplasia, well-differentiated diffuse papillary mesothelioma, diffuse papillary mesothelioma, atypical diffuse mesothelioma, and papillary carcinoma. Only three tumors closely resembled papillary or tubopapillary diffuse malignant mesothelioma, the type associated with asbestos, which occurs in the pleural cavities in both sexes. There were eight well-differentiated mesotheliomas, and these were associated to indolent behavior. However, in 10 cases,

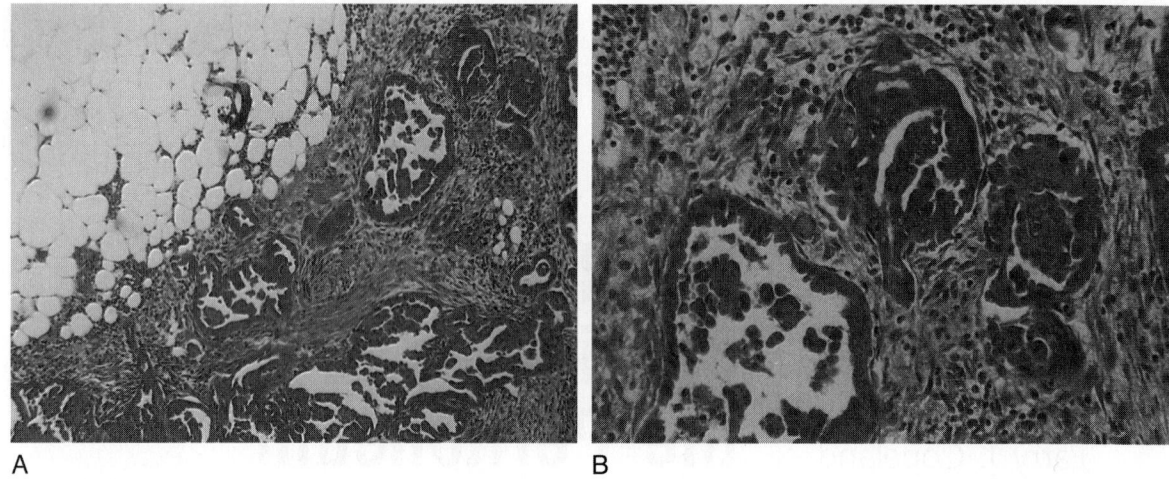

Figure 61-1
Primary peritoneal serous carcinoma resembles its ovarian counterpart and is characterized by glands, papillary clusters, and solid nests (*A*) lined by cells with varying degrees of cytologic atypia (*B*). By definition, there is destructive stromal invasion.

tumor resembled PSOC; these tumors were different and progressed rapidly. Foyle et al (1981) concluded that PSCP should not be merged with the general group of diffuse mesotheliomas. Other authors (Kannerstein et al, 1977a; Fromm et al, 1990) have also opposed the grouping of PSCP and mesothelioma of the peritoneum because of important epidemiologic, histologic, ultrastructural, and biologic differences between the mesothelioma and the PSCP. Researchers have demonstrated the link between peritoneal mesotheliomas and asbestos exposure (Selikoff et al, 1965), which is not present in PSCP. Furthermore, peritoneal mesotheliomas have a male predilection and are rarely seen in women (Kannerstein and Churg, 1977).

HISTOGENESIS

The histogenesis of this tumor is not known with certainty, but its origin may be a metaplastic process in the secondary müllerian system (Lauchlan, 1972). Lauchlan included the female peritoneum in the definition of the secondary müllerian system. Since then, PPA is better understood as a neoplasm that arises from mesothelial cells under müllerian influence. In 1974, Parmley and Woodruff demonstrated that pelvic peritoneum had the potential to differentiate into a müllerian type of epithelium. Ovarian surface epithelium and the peritoneum share a common embryonic origin, and tumors with various histologic types resembling EOC can develop primarily in the peritoneum (Gompel and Silverberg, 1994). Embryologically, the coelomic epithelium invaginates to form the müllerian ducts and also gives rise to the layer of mesothelial cells that line the peritoneal cavity and cover the cortical surfaces of the ovaries (Clement, 1987; Parmley, 1987). PPA may thus arise from the multipotential mesothelial cells lining the peritoneal cavity. During fetal development, before the secretion of müllerian inhibiting factor by the fetal testes, the müllerian ducts develop in male fetuses (Parmley, 1987). Müllerian inhibiting factor subsequently inhibits their development and they degenerate and completely disappear by 9 to 12 weeks. This müllerian influence, however brief, may account for the rare occurrence of lesions resembling PPA in the male peritoneum (Shah et al, 1998), including lesions involving the tunica vaginalis testis and epididymis (Remmle et al, 1992; Jones et al, 1995).

PATHOLOGY

Histopathologic similarities have been drawn between PPA and PSOC (Resta et al, 1988; Raju et al, 1989). For study purposes the Gynecologic Oncology Group (GOG) developed a set of criteria for PPA diagnosis (Bloss et al, 1993):

1. The ovaries are either absent or normal in size (<4.0 cm largest diameter).
2. The involvement in the extraovarian sites is greater than that of the surface of either ovary.
3. Microscopically, the ovaries are either not involved with tumor or exhibit only serosal or cortical implants less than 5 mm in depth (Fig. 61-2).
4. The histopathologic and cytologic characteristics of the tumor are predominantly of the serous type.

Other types of PPA have been described (Table 61-1), including endometrioid (Clark et al, 1979), mucinous (Banerjee and Gough, 1988), clear cell (Lee et al, 1991; Altaras et al, 1991), Brenner (Hampton et al, 1992), and malignant mixed müllerian (Mirc et al, 1995). Eltabbakh et al (1998b) reported that the me-

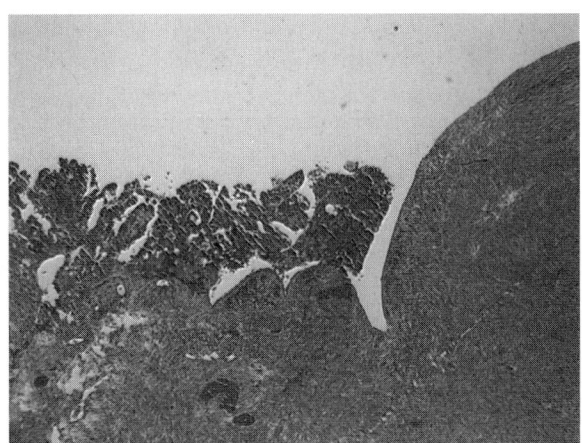

Figure 61–2
One of the defining features of primary peritoneal serous carcinoma is absent or limited involvement of the ovaries. This photomicrograph demonstrates an ovary with a small (<0.5-cm) implant confined to the surface of the ovary. There was no involvement of the contralateral ovary or the endometrium; consequently this was regarded as a primary peritoneal serous carcinoma.

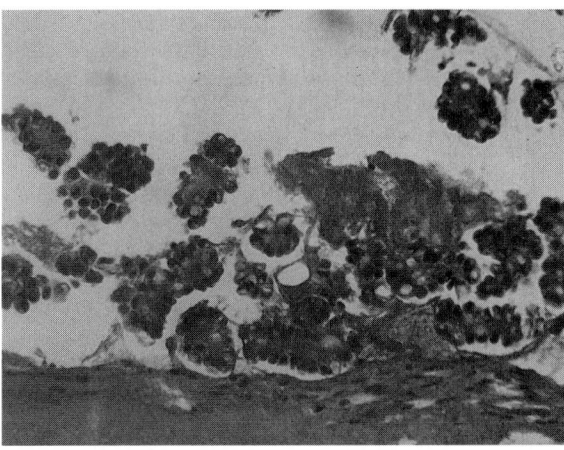

Figure 61–3
Serous borderline tumor of the peritoneum is characterized by papillary clusters lined by cells with mild to moderate cytologic atypia. By definition, there is no evidence of destructive stromal invasion.

dian survival of patients who had nonserous histology was not significantly different from that of patients with serous histology. In 1991, Altaras et al reported one patient with papillary clear cell PPA alive without evidence of disease 76 months following diagnosis.

Two PPA variations appear less virulent (Bell et al, 1988; Bell and Scully, 1990; Killackey and Davis, 1993). The *peritoneal serous borderline tumors* (PSBT) behave similarly to their ovarian counterparts. These PSBT have an excellent prognosis, although in rare cases transformation to carcinoma has been observed on follow-up examination (Bell and Scully, 1990; Weir et al, 1998). Forty-one to 99% of PSBT are accompanied by endosalpingiosis, suggesting an origin therein (Bell and Scully, 1990; Biscotti and Hart, 1992; Weir et al, 1998). Histologically, PSBT are identical to peritoneal implants found in association with ovarian serous borderline tumors (Fig. 61–3). Although patients with PSBT are typically under 35 years old, and often infertile (Bell and Scully, 1990), malignant tumors are rare in young women (Dalrymple et al, 1989; Truong et al, 1990). Second are the *serous psammocarcinomas of the peritoneum*. This latter group has a proportionately larger number of psammoma bodies and less-aggressive cytologic ap-

pearance, with absent or moderate nuclear atypicality and rare mitotic figures (Fig. 61–4). Conservative management, both surgical—possible fertility preserving and withholding adjuvant chemotherapy, should be considered in the management of this disease (Whitcomb et al, 1999; Munkarah et al, 1999).

The presently accepted criteria for making the distinction between EOC and PPA are based on minimal scientific evidence. Therefore, it is likely that some tumors designated as PPA according to current criteria are actually small ovarian cancers that find the peritoneum a more hospitable site for growth than the ovary. Possible reasons why the peritoneum may provide a more favorable environment for carcinoma is the greater density of the ovarian tissue,

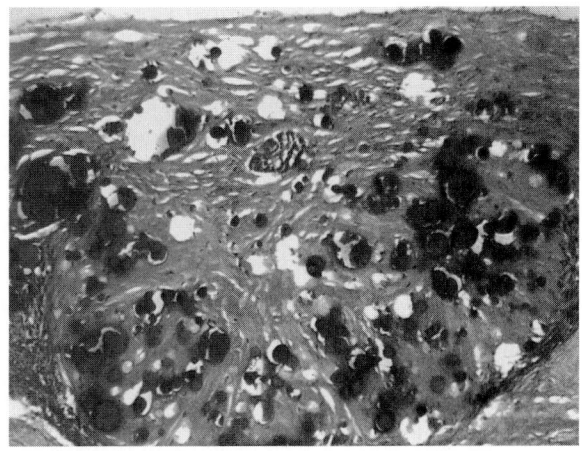

Figure 61–4
Serous psammocarcinoma is a low-grade carcinoma that can arise from the ovary or peritoneum. By definition the tumor forms numerous psammoma bodies, contains nests of tumor cells no more than 15 cells across, shows no more than moderate cytologic atypia, and shows areas of stromal or lymphovascular space invasion.

Table 61–1. HISTOPATHOLOGIC TYPES OF PPA

Serous (predominantly)
Endometrioid
Mucinous
Clear cell
Brenner
Mixed müllerian

Table 61-2. DIFFERENTIAL DIAGNOSIS OF PPA

Variations of PPA
   Peritoneal serous borderline tumors
   Psammocarcinomas of the peritoneum
Endosalpingosis
Florid mesothelial hyperplasia
Malignant mesotheliomas
Metastatic adenocarcinoma

which may inhibit invasion of tumor cells originating within its superficial layers; and the production of a tumor-inhibitory substance by the ovarian stroma (Scully, 1998), which has been demonstrated in vitro (Karlan et al, 1995).

Besides separating PPA and EOC, there are different entities that need to be distinguished (Table 61–2). Histologically, PPA should be included in the differential diagnosis of all papillary serous lesions of the peritoneum, including endosalpingosis, mesothelial hyperplasia, malignant mesothelioma, and metastatic adenocarcinoma (Bell and Scully, 1990; Biscotti and Hart, 1992; Kemp et al, 1992).

1. *Endosalpingiosis*: Refers to the presence of histologically benign glands lined by tubal-type epithelium outside the confines of the fallopian tube (Fig. 61–5). This disorder is often associated with chronic salpingitis and ovarian serous borderline tumors. The association with chronic salpingitis suggests that shedding of tubal epithelial cells onto the peritoneum is a route of development of endosalpingosis. Endosalpingosis is also a legitimate candidate for a precursor to PPA. In one series, 2 of 14 carcinomas of this type were associated with this disorder (Weir et al, 1998).
2. *Florid mesothelial hyperplasia*: Hyperplasia of mesothelial cells is a common response to inflamma-

tion and chronic effusions. Psammoma bodies may be present but rarely are as numerous as in PPA (Clement, 1987).
3. *Malignant mesotheliomas*: Under light microscopy, differentiation between the two types of tumor may be difficult (Fig. 61–6). Kannerstein et al (1977a) and Kannerstein and Churg (1977) described some morphologic and histochemical differences between the mesothelioma and PSCP. Although not of absolute differential diagnostic value, the presence of psammoma bodies, epithelial mucin, and columnar cells and the absence of hyaluronic acid favors the diagnosis of PSCP over mesothelioma. In 1982, Warhol et al compared the ultrastructural features of malignant mesothelioma and EOC, which are clinically similar to PSCP. They found that the mesotheliomas were characterized ultrastructurally by a greater content of tonofilaments, lack of mucin, fewer cilia, and dense core granules of the neurosecretory type. Mesotheliomas may exactly mimic PPA, and definitive distinction requires immunohistochemistry and/or electron microscopy (Eyden et al, 1996). Although the signs and symptoms of peritoneal mesothelioma and PSCP are similar, the response to treatment and survival are generally poorer in patients with peritoneal mesothelioma. Malignant mesotheliomas of the pleura are approximately 10 times as frequent as those of the peritoneum (Kannerstein et al, 1977b; Stauffer and Carbone, 1986; Ascoli et al, 1996), and malignant mesothelioma of the peritoneum is extremely rare in the absence of pleural malignant mesothelioma and a history of asbestos exposure. Epidemiologically, malignant mesothelioma is more common in older men, especially men with a history of asbestos exposure. PPA is likely to be overlooked in men unless it is considered in the differential diagnosis. In males, another malignant

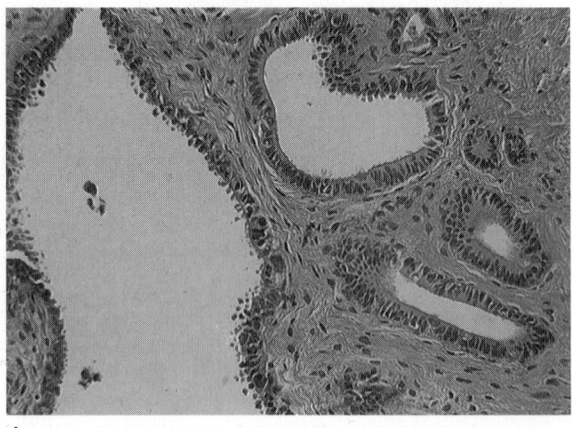
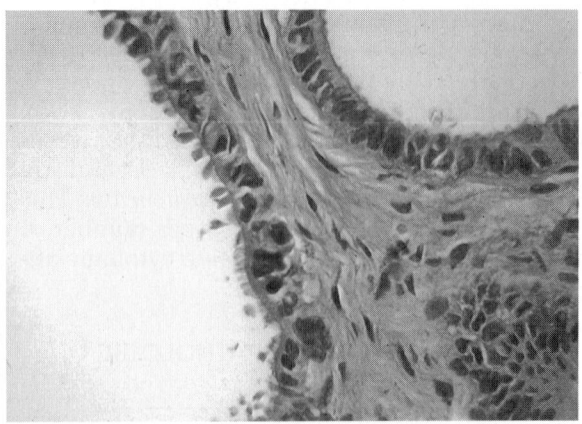

A   B

Figure 61-5
Endosalpingosis is characterized by small groups of subserosal glands (*A*) lined by a single layer of bland, ciliated (tubal) epithelium (*B*). The glands are surrounded by fibrous stroma. This process is distinguished from endometriosis by the absence of investing endometrial stroma.

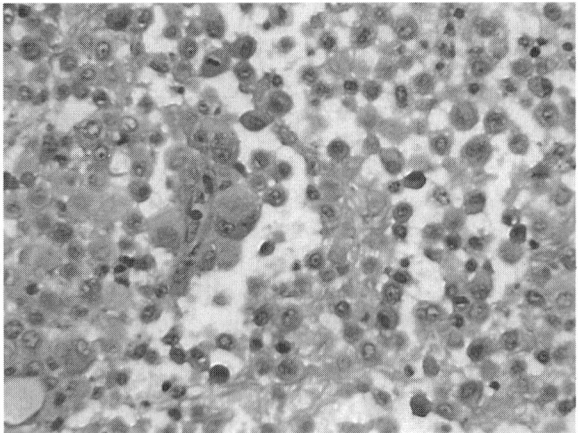

Figure 61–6
Peritoneal mesothelioma, like its pleural component, may assume an epithelioid, spindled sarcomatoid, or mixed pattern. This photomicrograph shows loose clusters of epithelioid cells characteristic of an epithelioid mesothelioma. Generally, special studies are required to separate epithelioid mesothelioma from carcinoma.

tumor that can mimic PPA is malignant mesothelioma of the tunica vaginalis testis (Jones et al, 1995; Ascoli et al, 1996).
4. *Metastatic adenocarcinoma*: This is ruled out by the absence of a primary tumor elsewhere.

Moll et al (1997) demonstrated *p53* overexpression in 83% of 29 PPA patients. The authors did not discuss the significance of *p53* overexpression on survival. Kowalski et al (1997) described *p53* overexpression in 48% of 44 PPA patients, similar to the 59% incidence in patients with EOC. The authors did not find that *p53* overexpression was predictive of prognosis within the PPA or the EOC groups. Ben-Baruch et al (1996), using immunohistochemistry of archival material, demonstrated *p53* overexpression in 42.4% of 75 PPA patients. PPA patients whose tumors demonstrated *p53* overexpression had a shorter median survival than those whose tumors did not (11.0 vs. 23.5 months, respectively). However, the difference did not achieve statistical significance.

CLINICAL PRESENTATION

Although several studies (Kannerstein and Churg, 1977; Kannerstein et al, 1977a; Gooneratne et al, 1982; Chen and Flam, 1986; Lele et al, 1988; Mills et al, 1988; Resta et al, 1988; Feuer et al, 1989; Raju et al, 1989; Bollinger et al, 1989; Dalrymple et al, 1989; Fromm et al, 1990; Ransom et al, 1990; Altaras et al, 1991; Bloss et al, 1993; Killackey and Davis 1993; Eltabbakh et al, 1998b) have described the clinicopathologic features of this tumor entity, the clinical behavior of PPA remains obscure. It is still not clear whether PPA patients differ from PSOC patients with regard to epidemiologic characteristics. It has been suggested that these tumors biologically be-

Table 61–3. CLINICAL PRESENTATION OF PPA

- Mean age 60 years (range 57–67)
- Abdominal pain
- Abdominal distention
- Ascites
- Pelvic abdominal mass
- Peripheral edema
- Constipation
- Nausea
- Vomiting
- Loss of weight
- Loss of appetite
- Malaise
- Dispareunia
- Urinary symptoms

have similarly to EOC of similar stage (Khoury et al, 1990). The natural history is similar to the ovarian counterpart (Table 61–3), with the disease occurring mostly in women between 57 and 67 years old and with a clinical presentation that does not differ from that of advanced stages of EOC (Altaras et al, 1991). Ben-Baruch et al (1996) did not find significant differences in patient characteristics between PPA and EOC with regard to mean age at diagnosis, parity, and menopausal status. The mean age at diagnosis of PPA was 61.1 years, similar to that reported by Ransom et al (1990), Fromm et al (1990), Altaras et al (1991), and Fowler et al (1994), who found a mean age of 60, 57.4, 61.2, and 61.4 years, respectively. Ben-Baruch et al did not demonstrate significant differences between EOC and PPA in the operative findings. The risk of ascites fluid volume exceeding 1000 ml and the proportion of patients with stage IV disease was the same between these two entities. The rate of stage IV disease was found to be 28%, which is similar to the rates of 29% and 32% reported by Altaras et al (1991) and Killackey and Davis (1993), respectively. To our knowledge, there have been two reports of this tumor occurring in children. In 1983, Ulbright et al described an 11-year-old girl with an extraovarian serous carcinoma of the retroperitoneum, and Wall et al (1995) reported an adolescent girl with PSCP whose tumor responded to paclitaxel after showing limited response to two other chemotherapeutic regimens, one of which included carboplatin.

The most common presenting symptoms are abdominal pain and distention (Moertel, 1972; Foyle et al, 1981; Gooneratne et al, 1982; Chen and Flam, 1986; Lele et al, 1988; Mills et al, 1988; Dalrymple et al, 1989; Raju et al, 1989; Fromm et al, 1990; Ransom et al, 1990; Truong et al, 1990; Altaras et al, 1991; Bloss et al, 1993; Killackey and Davis 1993; Eltabbakh et al, 1998b). Other PPA patients also presented with constipation, nausea, vomiting, loss of weight, loss of appetite, malaise, dispareunia and urinary symptoms (Kannerstein and Churg, 1977; Fromm et al, 1990). Common signs include ascites (Moertel, 1972), pelvic-abdominal mass (Kannerstein and Churg,

1977; Fromm et al, 1990), and peripheral edema (Kannerstein and Churg, 1977). The presence of psammoma bodies in the cervicovaginal smear of a PPA patient has also been documented (Shapiro and Nunez, 1983). The common sites of disease at the time of laparotomy are the omentum, abdominal and pelvic peritoneum, ovaries, and serosa of the bowel (Fromm et al, 1990; Rose and Reale, 1991; Eltabbakh et al, 1998b). Eltabbakh et al (1997) suggested that the incidence of central nervous system metastases in PPA patients (1.4%) is similar to that of EOC patients. A case of syndrome of inappropriate antidiuretic hormone secretion in a patient with suboptimally cytoreduced stage III PSCP has also been described (Resnik and Bender, 1996).

Altaras et al (1991) and Rose and Reale (1991) reported the usefulness of CA-125 in diagnosis and follow-up of PSCP patients. In patients whose preoperative CA-125 values are known, this tumor marker was elevated in 94.4% of cases (Eltabbakh et al, 1998b). Mills et al (1988) reported elevated CA-125 values in eight PPA patients. Altaras et al (1991) described elevated CA-125 values in three patients and found that CA-125 measurements correlated with the clinically determined status of disease. Similar to the situation in EOC patients, CA-125 values may be useful in the diagnosis of PPA patients and follow-up of their response to therapy.

The prognostic significance of estrogen and progesterone receptor analysis in patients with PPA is controversial (Bizzi et al, 1988, Sevelda et al, 1990; Kommos et al, 1992; Geisler et al, 1996). A confounding problem when comparing studies on estrogen and progesterone receptors from different institutes is the different ways in which different laboratories determine estrogen and progesterone receptor status. Eltabbakh et al (1998b) employed immunohistochemistry, a technique that reduces the number of falsely elevated results (Kommos et al, 1992). In their study of PPA patients, estrogen and progesterone receptors were positive in 50.0% and 6.3% of the cases, respectively. Estrogen and progesterone receptor positivity did not correlate significantly with survival. However, the median survival of PPA patients whose tumors were progesterone receptor positive was almost twice that of patients whose tumors were progesterone receptor negative (40.0 vs. 21.2 months).

In practice, the difficulty is to identify PPA patients without subjecting patients with other less treatable malignancies to invasive procedures. In this group of patients, exhaustive investigations are usually carried out, including computerized tomography of the abdomen and pelvis, barium studies, and endoscopy of the gastrointestinal tract. In patients who present with ascites as the sole clinical feature (absence of a pelvic or abdominal mass), a diagnostic paracentesis is performed, and malignant cells may be seen on cytology. Some authors (Della-Fiorentina et al, 1996) have suggested that the detection of signet-ring cells in ascites can be taken to exclude primary ovarian or peritoneal carcinoma. In the absence of these findings, all women with ascites containing adenocarcinoma cells should undergo laparoscopy and/or laparotomy as a diagnostic and potentially therapeutic debulking procedure. If during surgery no primary site is found but there are peritoneal tumor deposits, then we have to manage the patient as for PPA with a total hysterectomy, bilateral salpingo-oophorectomy, omentectomy, and cytoreductive surgery, followed by adjuvant chemotherapy (Fig. 61–7). In short, the surgical management is as for ovarian cancer.

STAGING

There is no separate staging system for PPA. Most investigators have used the International Federation of Gynecology and Obstetrics (FIGO) staging system for ovarian cancer (Cancer Committee of the International Federation of Gynecology and Obstetrics, 1986). Most cases reported in the literature have been stage III or IV.

TREATMENT

Raju et al (1989) suggested that PPA should be treated as are ovarian tumors of similar grade and stage. Their clinical behavior, including response to treatment, is equivalent to that of EOC with a comparable extent of disease (Raju et al 1989; Fromm et al, 1990; Altaras et al, 1991). Accordingly, the standard regimen used in the treatment of EOC is generally administered to PPA patients (Fromm et al, 1990; Ransom et al, 1990). The goal of surgical treatment is cytoreduction to no gross residual disease (Ransom et al, 1990). Chemotherapy is commonly administered after cytoreductive surgery. It is generally agreed that these patients should be managed following the aggressive chemotherapeutic regimens established for patients with advanced ovarian carcinoma. However, because of the rarity of this tumor, reported experience with chemotherapeutic agents is limited (Table 61–4). Since 1979, cisplatin-based multiagent chemotherapy has been the standard treatment for EOC patients and, consequently, for PPA patients. Several authors (Chen and Flam, 1986; Lele et al, 1988; Dalrymple et al, 1989; Strand et al, 1989; Fromm et al, 1990; Ransom et al, 1990; Altaras et al, 1991; Bloss et al, 1993; Mulhollan et al, 1994) have reported that the response of patients with PPA to platinum-based chemotherapy is similar to that of patients with PSOC and have subsequently recommended treating patients with PPA in a fashion similar to that used in patients with EOC. Other investigators (Gooneratne et al, 1982; Mills et al, 1988), however, have failed to confirm these findings. Long-term survival has been reported predominantly in patients with optimal cytoreduction and platinum-based chemotherapy (Chen and Flam,

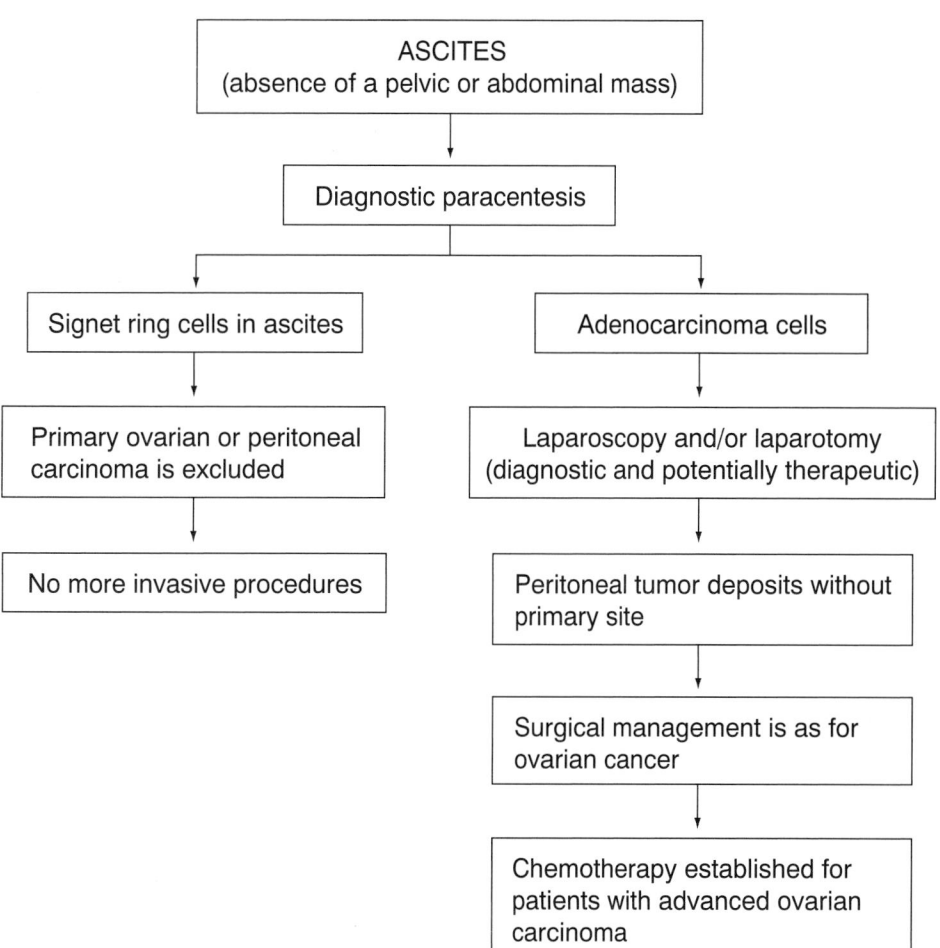

Figure 61–7
Treatment algorithm for PPA.

1986; Ransom et al, 1990). Numerous regimens have been utilized with varying degrees of success. The majority of clinical responses have occurred with cisplatin-based regimens, usually in conjunction with alkylating agents.

The response to platinum-based therapy has been evaluated in four retrospective studies. In one report

(Altaras et al, 1991), seven cases of PSCP were analyzed. All patients received cisplatin-based combination chemotherapy, with four of seven exhibiting complete responses. The median survival of the group was 34.5 months (range, 6 to 67). The authors concluded that these tumors may be treated and followed up just like EOC. Another study (Mulhollan

Table 61–4. RESPONSE OF PPA TO FIRST-LINE CHEMOTHERAPY

STUDY	NO. OF PATIENTS	REGIMEN*	OVERALL RESPONSE (%)
August et al (1985)	8	PAC (n = 3), PC (n = 1), melphalan (n = 4)	37.5
Chen and Flam (1986)	3	PAC (n = 2), DC (n = 1)	100
Lele et al (1988)	23	Platinum-based (n = 20), MeCy (n = 2), MFP (n = 1)	65
Mills et al (1988)	10	PAC (n = 3), PC (n = 4), P (n = 1) alkylators (n = 2)	80
Dalrymple et al (1989)	31	Platinum-based (n = 26), chlorambucil (n = 5)	32.3
Fromm et al (1990)	44	PC, P, M (n = 44)	63.6
Altaras et al (1991)	7	PAC (n = 5), PC (n = 2)	100
Bloss et al (1993)	33	PAC (n = 29), PC (n = 4)	63.6
Menzin et al (1996)	4	TP (n = 4)	100
Piver et al (1997)	46	PAC (n = 25),	62.5
		TP (n = 21)	70
Bloss et al (1998)	33	Platinum-based	65
Kennedy et al (1998)	38	Paclitaxel/Ca (n = 26), TP (n = 12)	87

*Ca, carboplatin; DC, doxorubicin-cisplatin; melphalan; MeCY, methotrexate-cyclophosphamide with leucovorin rescue; MFP, melphalan-fluorouracil-provera; P, cisplatin; PAC, cisplatin-doxorubicin-cyclophosphamide; PC, cisplatin-cyclophosphamide; TP, paclitaxel-cisplatin.

et al, 1994) evaluated 33 cases of PSCP and compared them with 54 cases of EOC. With at least a 4-year follow-up period, no differences in the median survival time (17 vs. 18 months) were noted. Another report consisted of a retrospective, case-controlled study comparing the response and survival to cytoreductive surgery followed by cisplatin-based chemotherapy of 33 women with PSCP versus 33 women with EOC (Bloss et al, 1993). The authors concluded that there was no significant difference in median survival between the cases (20.8 months) and controls (27.8 months).

Chen and Flam (1986) described three patients treated with cisplatin and doxorubicin, with or without cyclophosphamide and reported long-term survivals of at least 5 years. They concluded that perhaps the long-term prognosis of this disease could be modified by chemotherapeutic regimens with cisplatin and doxorubicin. Ransom et al (1990) reported an 18.8% surgical response rate and a median survival of 17 months in 33 patients with PPA treated with cisplatin-based chemotherapy. Fromm et al (1990) described 74 patients treated with surgery and postoperative chemotherapy, of whom 29.2% received single-agent therapy while 70.8% were given a multiagent regimen. Half of all patients received cisplatin, either singly or in combination with other cytotoxic drugs. An overall response rate to first-line chemotherapy (multiple regimens) of 63.6% was achieved, with a median survival of 24 months. They achieved a complete response in 22.7% and a partial response in 40.9% of patients. In 31.8% of cases, the disease progressed despite chemotherapy. They demonstrated that patients who received cisplatin-based regimens had a median survival of 31.5 months, whereas those who did not had a median survival of 19.5 months. This difference was not statistically significant. Survival rate was not influenced by residual tumor at primary surgery. Strand et al (1989) reported 18 patients with peritoneal carcinomatosis and unknown primary treated with laparotomy, maximal cytoreductive surgery, and postoperative cisplatin-based chemotherapy. They reported a median survival of 23 months, with three long-term survivors with 41, 59, and 77 months. Patients with minimal disease after cytoreductive surgery experienced longer median survival (31 months as opposed to 11 months), suggesting that successful debulking surgery may provide survival advantage. Similar results have been reported in other series (Chen and Flam, 1986; Lele et al, 1988; Dalrymple et al, 1989; Altaras et al, 1991). Lele et al (1988) reported a 65% response rate in 20 patients using cisplatin-based first-line chemotherapy. Killackey and Davis (1993) reported a median disease-free survival of 3.4 months and a median survival of 19 months. Altaras et al (1991) reported a 100% response rate and a median survival of 34.5 months in five patients who received cisplatin-doxorubicin-cyclophosphamide (PAC) following cytoreductive surgery. Eltabbakh et al (1998b) described a retrospective analysis of 75 women diagnosed with PPA. Following cytoreductive surgery, 43 patients received platin-based chemotherapy that did not include paclitaxel: 26 patients received combination PAC, 7 patients combination cisplatin-cyclophosphamide (PC), 6 patients combination cisplatin-doxorubicin-ifosfamide, and 4 patients single-agent cisplatin. Twenty-four patients received cisplatin-paclitaxel and three received carboplatin-paclitaxel. One patient received single-agent alkeran. In their study, the median survival of patients who received platin-based multiagent chemotherapy without paclitaxel (mostly PC or PAC) was almost identical to that of patients who received cisplatin-paclitaxel as first-line therapy (23.1 vs. 24.0 months).

In 1996, a randomized GOG trial demonstrated a significant survival advantage in patients with advanced EOC whose residual disease was greater than 1.0 cm treated with cisplatin-paclitaxel compared to similar patients who were treated with PC (McGuire et al, 1996). As a result of this study, paclitaxel was advanced to first-line chemotherapy for patients with EOC. The impact on response and survival of this combination, and the relative contribution of adding a taxane to the first-line therapy in PPA patients, have not been thoroughly evaluated. To date four PPA patients treated with paclitaxel (135 mg/m^2) and cisplatin (50 to 75 mg/m^2) for six cycles have been reported (Menzin et al, 1996). Reassessment surgery demonstrated complete surgical response in one and partial surgical response in three patients. Kennedy et al (1998) treated 38 PPA patients (36 stage IIIC and 2 stage IV). All patients received paclitaxel (135 or 175 mg/m^2), and 12 received cisplatin and 26 carboplatin. Median progression-free survival was 15 months and median overall survival 40 months. Survival for optimally debulked patients was significantly better than for suboptimally debulked patients (median 32.8 months). Bloss et al (1998) demonstrated a similar response to treatment of PSCP compared to PSOC in a Phase II GOG study of PC.

Piver et al (1997) described 46 PPA patients treated with PAC (n = 25) or cisplatin-paclitaxel (n = 21) following cytoreductive surgery in two sequential trials. In trial 1, patients received weekly cisplatin induction (1 mg/kg) for 4 cycles followed by monthly cisplatin (50 mg/m^2), cyclophosphamide (750 mg/m^2), and doxorubicin (50 mg/m^2) for 10 cycles. In trial 2, patients received weekly cisplatin induction (1 mg/kg) for four cycles followed by monthly cisplatin and paclitaxel (135 mg/m^2) over 24 hours for six cycles. Surgical assessment of response was performed in 15 (60%) and 13 (61.9%) patients in PAC and cisplatin-paclitaxel trials, respectively. The median overall survival for all patients was 23.1 months. There was no statistically significant difference in overall survival or progression/recurrence time between patients in the PAC and cisplatin-paclitaxel groups.

Because in preclinical (Nicoletti et al, 1993) and clinical (Einzig et al, 1992) trials paclitaxel has been effective in advanced and platinum-refractory EOC, it should be considered in the treatment of patients with platinum-resistant PPA (Wilailak et al, 1995). El-tabbakh et al (1998b) reported that patients who received paclitaxel alone or in combination as second-line chemotherapy had significantly longer survival than patients who received chemotherapy without paclitaxel (median survival 23.0 vs. 8.2 months, $P = 0.026$). A high dose of paclitaxel (250 mg/m^2) was reported to have a 48% response rate in platinum-resistant ovarian cancer (Sevelda et al, 1990; Wall et al, 1995). In one report (Wilailak et al, 1995), a paclitaxel dose of 250 mg/m^2 given as a 24-hour continuous intravenous infusion resulted in a rapid partial response with good palliation of symptoms. Another study (Wall et al, 1995) reported a complete response after therapy with a paclitaxel dose of 420 mg/m^2 also given over 24 hours as a continuous intravenous infusion in a Phase I trial. The fact that paclitaxel may exhibit a dose-response relationship in the treatment of EOC (Eisenhauer et al, 1994; Holmes et al, 1995) can explain the presence of a complete response in the case that used 420 mg/m^2 and only a partial response when a 210 to 250-mg/m^2 dose was used. Further studies are required to determine the best dose of paclitaxel.

Carboplatin may be active in paclitaxel-resistant PPA. This clinical phenomenon has been reported in patients with EOC previously treated with paclitaxel and whose most recent platinum-based therapy was 12 months prior to carboplatin re-induction (Kavanagh et al, 1995). It has also been reported in patients with ovarian carcinoma whose primary treatment was single-agent paclitaxel (Thigpen et al, 1996). Carboplatin therapy should be considered in patients with paclitaxel-refractory PPA without platinum chemotherapy for 12 months (Herrada et al, 1997).

Other forms of treatment have also been described, including radiotherapy and hormonal treatments with estrogen and progesterone preparations (Fromm et al, 1990). However, their roles in treatment are as yet undefined.

PROGNOSIS

The prognosis for patients with PSCP is generally poor (Table 61–5). Although most investigators (Lele et al, 1988; Resta et al, 1988; Dalrymple et al, 1989; Strand et al, 1989; Ransom et al, 1990; Fromm et al, 1990; Bloss et al, 1993) have described similar behavior for PPA and PSOC, this finding has not been uniformly accepted. Some investigators reported worse (Foyle et al, 1981; Gooneratne et al, 1982; Mills et al, 1988; Killackey and Davis, 1993; Rothacker et al, 1995) or better (Chen and Flam, 1986; Mulhollan et al, 1994) prognosis (Table 61–6).

Although the prognostic factors in patients with EOC are well defined, those of patients with PPA are still obscure. Multivariate analysis of 21,240 cases with primary EOC showed that stage, histology, grade, age, presence of ascites, lymph node status, and race were predictors of survival (Kosary, 1994). Eltabbakh et al (1998b) demonstrated that age, surgical stage, performance status, and degree of cytoreductive surgery are significant prognostic factors in PPA patients; performance status and primary debulking surgery are independent factors. Mulhollan et al (1994) investigated the significance of ovarian involvement in the survival of PPA patients. These authors demonstrated that size of the ovarian tumor and amount of ovarian stromal invasion had no significant effect on survival.

The amount of residual disease may be an important prognostic determining factor for both PPA and EOC patients (Strand et al, 1989; Petru et al, 1992; Ben-Baruch et al, 1996). However, controversy exits concerning the ability to perform optimal surgical debulking, and its clinical significance in PPA. Optimal cytoreductive surgery, defined as less than 2.0 cm of residual tumor, has been accomplished in 33% to 69% of patients with PPA (Mills et al, 1988; Fromm et al, 1990; Ransom et al, 1990). Strand et al (1989) found that successful surgical cytoreduction resulted in better response to chemotherapy and prolonged survival. Fromm et al (1990) were able to accomplish optimal debulking surgery only in 41.2% of 74 pa-

Table 61–5. REPORTED SURVIVAL OF PPA PATIENTS

STUDY	NO. OF PATIENTS	MEDIAN SURVIVAL (months)	5-YEAR SURVIVAL RATE* (%)
Foyle et al (1981)	7	7	0
White et al (1985)	11	16.4	N/A
Dalrymple et al (1989)	31	11.3	20
Truong et al (1990)	22	16	20
Fromm et al (1990)	74	24	22
Ransom et al (1990)	33	17	20
Altaras et al (1991)	7	24.1	14.3
Killackey and Davis (1993)	29	19	10
Bloss et al (1993)	33	20	15
Fowler et al (1994)	34	17.8	12
Ben-Baruch et al (1996)	25	21	N/A
Kowalski et al (1997)	44	27.8	15
Eltabbakh et al (1998b)	75	23.5	26.5

*N/A, not available.

Table 61-6. COMPARISON OF SURVIVAL OF PATIENTS WITH PPA AND EOC

STUDY	NO. OF PATIENTS WITH PPA	SURVIVAL VS. PATIENTS WITH EOC
Foyle et al (1981)	25	Worse
Gooneratne et al (1982)	16	Worse
Chen and Flam (1986)	3	Better
Lele et al (1988)	23	Similar
Mills et al (1988)	10	Worse
Dalrymple et al (1989)	31	Similar
Fromm et al (1990)	74	Similar
Ransom et al (1990)	33	Similar
Bloss et al (1993)	33	Similar
Killackey and Davis (1993)	29	Worse
Mulhollan et al (1994)	33	Better
Rothacker et al (1995)	57	Worse
Ben-Baruch et al (1996)	25	Similar

tients with PPA. They demonstrated that patients receiving multiagent chemotherapy (i.e., PC) had a statistically greater median survival rate compared to those receiving a single-agent regimen (melphalan). The median survival of PPA patients treated with combination chemotherapy was very similar to that of EOC patients who received the same treatment. Fromm et al observed, that, neither age nor the presence of residual disease 2 cm or greater after cytoreductive surgery was predictive of survival. Among the pathologic factors that these authors examined, only the absence of mitosis was significantly predictive in survival. The presence of vascular invasion and the proportion of papillary areas in the tumor failed to predict survival.

Mills et al (1988) as well as Fromm et al (1990) did not find a significant prognostic value in optimal cytoreductive surgery in PPA patients. White et al (1985) reported removal of grossly identifiable disease in 9 of 11 patients with PPA. In the study by Ransom et al (1990), only three patients who had long-term survival had optimal tumor cytoreduction. Fowler et al (1994) found that patients who underwent optimal cytoreduction had an increased survival rate, although the difference did not reach statistical significance. These results are similar to those of Ben-Baruch et al (1996). In their study comparing 25 PPA patients with stages III and IV PSOC, the survival was significantly better in patients with optimal debulking only in the EOC group. The survival curve for patients with residual disease 2 cm or greater was almost identical for PPA and EOC patients. Ben-Baruch et al's rate of successful debulking, and the result of postoperative aggressive treatment with platinum-based combination chemotherapy, were the same in both groups. This is in contrast to a previous report of a lower rate of optimal cytoreduction and decreased response to platinum-based chemotherapy in the PPA group (Killackey and Davis, 1993). Eltabbakh et al (1998b) demonstrated that optimal cytoreductive surgery, defined as cytoreductive surgery resulting in less than 1.0 cm of residual tumor, was achieved in 65.3%

of their study population. Optimal cytoreductive surgery was a favorable prognostic factor in both univariate and multivariate analyses. The difference in the results of these investigators could be explained by difference in number of patients and the definition of optimal cytoreductive surgery. Eltabbakh et al also suggested a possible value of secondary cytoreductive surgery in PPA patients that was not discussed in previous reports. They found that patients who underwent cytoreductive surgery following recurrence or progression of disease had a longer survival rate than patients who did not undergo secondary cytoreductive surgery (median survival 12.2 vs. 3.1 months, respectively).

The overall 5-year survival of PPA patients is about 20%, which is similar to the survival rate of patients with advanced ovarian cancer (Dalrymple et al, 1989; Ransom et al, 1990; Truong et al, 1990). These results were achieved with surgery without lymphadenectomy (Winter, 1993). The question remains whether retroperitoneal lymphadenectomy improves the survival rate of PPA patients. In addition, the inclusion of paclitaxel into adjuvant treatment protocols and/or the use of high-dose chemotherapy may improve the survival in PPA patients and has to be proven in clinical trials. Median survivals of 19 (Dalrymple et al, 1989), 23 (Strand et al, 1989), 17 (Ransom et al, 1990), 24 (Fromm et al, 1990), 17.8 (Fowler et al, 1994), 21 (Ben-Baruch et al, 1996), and 23.5 (Eltabbakh et al, 1998b) months of PPA patients has been documented. However, long-term survival after chemotherapy of more than 5 years has been documented in the literature (Chen and Flam, 1986). In 1992, Petru et al reported a median survival of only 10 months for 14 PPA patients. However, because 7 of these patients did not undergo surgical debulking, Petru et al concluded that the amount of residual disease may represent an important prognostic factor (Ransom et al, 1990). Foyle et al (1981) reported that, of nine patients with documented follow-up, eight were dead 1.5 years after the diagnosis was made. White et al, in a 1985 publication of 11 cases, found that 8 patients were dead within 3 years of diagnosis despite chemotherapy. They reported a median survival of 15 and 16 months for single- (*n* = 3) and multiple- (*n* = 8) agent chemotherapy regimens given as first-line treatment.

One of the important issues regarding ovarian cancer is familial occurrence. Mutations of the tumor-suppressor gene *BRCA1* have been implicated in the development of familial ovarian and breast cancer (Miki et al, 1994; Shattuck-Eidens et al, 1995). The role of *BRCA1* gene mutations in the development of PPA is uncertain (Eltabbakh and Piver, 1998). Bandera et al (1997) found *BRCA1* germline mutations in 3 (17.6%) of 17 PPA patients. Karlan et al (1998) reported that three PPA patients who underwent genetic testing carried *BRCA1* mutations. They developed the disease at the ages of 38, 39, and 55. In one case, the ovaries were without any histologic evidence of malignancy, whereas in the other two cases the two ovaries and each of the metastatic sites studied differed in patterns of oncogene overexpression. Bandera et al (1998) identified in 2 of 17 PPA patients the 185delAG germline *BRCA1* mutation described in the Ashkenazi Jewish population. The family history of one patient was notable: a mother and five aunts had breast or ovarian cancer. The other patient had a personal history of breast cancer. Both patients exhibited allelic loss of the normal *BRCA1* allele in their tumor. A third patient was found to have a previously undescribed exon 11 single basepair substitution at nucleotide 1239 (CAG → CAC) resulting in a missense mutation (Gln → His). The patient had no family or personal history of breast or ovarian cancer, and her tumor did not exhibit loss of heterozygosity.

Karlan et al (1998) suggested that PPA may be a phenotypic variant of hereditary ovarian cancer. The risk of developing intraperitoneal carcinomatosis after prophylactic oophorectomy has raised questions about the value of prophylactic surgery in women at high risk of developing ovarian cancer. To date, at least 12 cases of PPA have been reported after prophylactic oophorectomies in women with family histories of ovarian cancer (Tobacman et al, 1982; Lynch et al, 1986, 1991; Kemp et al, 1992; Piver et al, 1993). Tobacman et al (1982), from the National Cancer Institute, reported that 3 of 28 women with a family history of ovarian cancer developed intra-abdominal malignancies 1, 5, and 11 years after undergoing prophylactic oophorectomies. Piver et al (1993) performed prophylactic oophorectomies in 324 women with family histories of ovarian cancer; 6 (1.8%) developed PPA 1, 2, 5, 13, 15, and 27 years after prophylactic oophorectomies. Although data about the efficacy of prophylactic oophorectomy are limited, two statistical studies using the Markov model suggested that prophylactic oophorectomy may provide long-term benefits to patients with high risk of cancer (Grann et al, 1997; Schrag et al, 1997). Currently, the National Institutes of Health and the Society of Gynecologic Oncology recommend prophylactic oophorectomies for women from high-risk families after childbearing or at the age of 35 to 40 at the latest.

SUMMARY

PPA is similar in clinical presentation, histologic appearance, and response to EOC. However, molecular and epidemiologic studies suggest that PPA may be a separate entity. We may never be able to distinguish on scientific grounds between primary ovarian and primary peritoneal serous carcinomas in every case. PPA patients should be reported separately from those with ovarian carcinoma but should be treated in a similar fashion.

REFERENCES

Altaras MM, Aviram R, Cohen I, et al: Primary peritoneal papillary serous adenocarcinoma: clinical and management aspects. Gynecol Oncol 1991;40:230.

Ascoli V, Taccogna S, Bosman C, et al: Malignant mesothelioma of the tunica vaginalis testis in a young adult. J Urol Pathol 1996;5:75.

August CZ, Murad TM, Newton M: Multiple focal extraovarian serous carcinoma. Int J Gynecol Pathol 1985;4:11.

Bandera CA, Muto MG, Schorge JO, et al: BRCA1 gene mutations in women with papillary serous carcinoma of the peritoneum. Obstet Gynecol 1998;92:596.

Bandera CA, Muta MG, Berkowitz RS, et al: Germline BRCA1 mutations in women with papillary serous carcinoma of the peritoneum (PSCP). Proc Am Assoc Cancer Res 1997;38:82.

Banerjee R, Gough F: Cystic mucinous tumors of the mesentery and retroperitoneum: report of three cases. Histopathology 1988;12:527.

Bell DA, Scully RE: Serous borderline tumors of the peritoneum. Am J Surg Pathol 1990;14:230.

Bell DA, Weinstock MA, Scully RE: Peritoneal implants of ovarian serous borderline tumors: histopathological features and prognosis. Cancer 1988;62:2212.

Ben-Baruch G, Sivan E, Moran O, et al: Primary peritoneal serous papillary carcinoma: a study of 25 cases and comparison with stage III-IV ovarian papillary serous carcinoma. Gynecol Oncol 1996;60:393.

Biscotti CV, Hart WR: Peritoneal serous papillomatosis of low malignant potential (serous borderline tumors of the peritoneum): a clinicopathologic study of 17 cases. Am J Surg Pathol 1992;16:467.

Bizzi A, Codegoni AM, Landoni F, et al: Steroid receptors in epithelial ovarian carcinoma: relation to clinical parameters and survival. Cancer Res 1988;48:622.

Bloss JD, Brady M, Rocereto T, et al: A Phase II trial of cisplatin and cyclophosphamide in the treatment of extraovarian peritoneal serous papillary carcinoma with comparison to papillary serous ovarian carcinoma: a Gynecologic Oncology Group study. Gynecol Oncol 1998;68:109.

Bloss JD, Liao SY, Buller RE, et al: Extraovarian peritoneal serous papillary carcinoma: a case-control retrospective comparison to papillary adenocarcinoma of the ovary. Gynecol Oncol 1993;50:347.

Bollinger DJ, Wick MR, Dehner LP, et al: Peritoneal malignant mesothelioma versus serous papillary adenocarcinoma: a histochemical and immunohistochemical comparison. Am J Surg Pathol 1989;13:659.

Cancer Committee of the International Federation of Gynecology and Obstetrics: Staging announcement: FIGO Cancer Committee. Gynecol Oncol 1986;25:383.

Chen KT, Flam MS: Peritoneal papillary serous carcinoma with long-term survival. Cancer 1986;58:1371.

Clark JE, Wood H, Jaffurs WJ, Fabro S: Endometrioid-type cystadenocarcinoma arising in the mesosalpinx. Obstet Gynecol 1979;54:656.

Clement PB: Endometriosis, lesions of the secondary müllerian system, and pelvic mesothelial proliferation. In Kurman RJ (ed): Blaustein's Pathology of the Female Genital Tract. 3rd ed. New York: Springer-Verlag, 1987:516.

Dalrymple JC, Bannatyne P, Russell P, et al: Extraovarian peritoneal serous papillary carcinoma: a clinicopathologic study of 31 cases. Cancer 1989;64:110.

Della-Fiorentina SA, Jaworski RC, Crandon AJ, Harnett PR: Primary peritoneal carcinoma: a treatable subset of patients with adenocarcinoma of unknown primary. Aust N Z J Surg 1996;66:124.

Einzig AI, Wiernik P, Sasloff J, et al: Phase II study and long-term follow-up of patients treated with Taxol for advanced ovarian adenocarcinoma. J Clin Oncol 1992;10:1748.

Eisenhauer EA, Ten Bokkel-Huinink WW, Swenerton KD, et al: European-Canadian randomized trial of paclitaxel in relapsed ovarian cancer: high-dose verus low-dose and long versus short infusion. J Clin Oncol 1994;12:2654.

Eltabbakh GH, Piver MS: Extraovarian primary peritoneal carcinoma. Oncology 1998;12:813.

Eltabbakh GH, Piver MS, Natarajan N, Metlin CJ: Epidemiologic differences between women with extra-ovarian primary peritoneal carcinoma and women with epithelial ovarian cancer. Obstet Gynecol 1998a;91:254.

Eltabbakh GH, Piver MS, Werness BA: Primary peritoneal adenocarcinoma metastatic to the brain. Gynecol Oncol 1997;66:160.

Eltabbakh GH, Werness BA, Piver MS, Blumenson LE: Prognostic factors in extra-ovarian primary peritoneal carcinoma [abstract]. Gynecol Oncol 1998b;68:112.

Eyden BP, Banik S, Harris M: Malignant epithelial mesothelioma of the peritoneum: observation on a problem case. Ultrastruct Pathol 1996;20:337.

Feuer GA, Shevchuk M, Calanog A: Normal-sized ovary carcinoma syndrome. Obstet Gynecol 1989;73:786.

Fowler JM, Nieberg RK, Schooler TA, Berek JS: Peritoneal adenocarcinoma (serous) of müllerian type: a subgroup of women presenting with peritoneal carcinomatosis. Int J Gynecol Cancer 1994;4:43.

Fox H: Primary neoplasia of the female peritoneum. Histopathology 1993;23:103.

Foyle A, Al-Jabi M, Mc Caughey WTE: Papillary peritoneal tumors in woman. Am J Surg Pathol 1981;5:241.

Fromm GL, Gershenson DM, Silva EG: Papillary serous carcinoma of the peritoneum. Obstet Gynecol 1990;75:89.

Geisler JP, Wiemann MC, Miller GA, Geisler HE: Estrogen and progesterone receptor status as prognostic indicators in patients with optimally cytoreduced stage IIIC serous cystoadenocarcinoma of the ovary. Gynecol Oncol 1996;60:424.

Gitsch G, Tabery U, Feigl W, Breitarecker G: The differential diagnosis of primary peritoneal papillary tumors. Arch Gynecol Obstet 1992;251:139.

Gompel C, Silverberg SG: The female peritoneum. In Gompel C, Silverberg SG (eds): Pathology in Gynecology and Obstetrics. Philadelphia: JB Lippincott, 1994:414.

Gooneratne S, Sassone M, Blaustein A, Taleman A: Serous papillary carcinoma of the ovary: a clinicopathologic study of 16 cases. Int J Gynecol Pathol 1982;1:258.

Grann VR, Panageas K, Whang W: A decision analysis of prophylactic treatments in BRCA1 gene positive patients [abstract]. Proc Am Soc Clin Oncol 1997;16:532.

Hampton HL, Hufman HT, Meeks GR: Extraovarian Brenner tumor. Obstet Gynecol 1992;79:844.

Herrada J, Kudelka AP, Tornos C, et al: Remission with carboplatin of paclitaxel resistant primary peritoneal papillary serous carcinoma: case report. Eur J Gynaecol Oncol 1997;18:39.

Hertig AT: Proceedings of the 18th Seminar of the American Society of Clinical Pathology. Chicago: American Society of Clinical Pathology, 1952:49.

Holmes FA, Kudelka AP, Kavanagh JJ, et al: Current status of clinical trials with paclitaxel and docetaxel. In George GI, Chen TC, Ojima I, Vyas DM (eds): ACS Symposium: Taxane Anticancer Agent: Basic Science and Current Status. Washington, DC: American Cancer Society, 1995:3.

Jones MA, Yooung RH, Scully RE: Malignant mesothelioma of the tunica vaginalis: a clinicopathologic analysis of 11 cases with review of the literature. Am J Surg Pathol 1995;19:815.

Kannerstein M, Churg J: Peritoneal mesothelioma. Hum Pathol 1977;8:83.

Kannerstein M, Churg J, McCaughey WTE, Hill DP: Papillary tumors of the peritoneum in women: mesothelioma or papillary carcinoma? Am J Obstet Gynecol 1977a;127:306.

Kannerstein M, McCaughey WTE, Churg J, SelikoffI J: A critique of the criteria for the diagnosis of diffuse malignant mesothelioma. Mt Sinai J Med 1977b;44:485.

Karlan BY, Baldwin RL, Cirisano ED, et al: Secreted ovarian stromal substance inhibits ovarian epithelial cell proliferation. Gynecol Oncol 1995;59:67.

Karlan BY, Baldwin RL, Lopez-Luevanos E, et al: Peritoneal serous papillary carcinoma, a phenotypic variant of familial ovarian cancer: implications for ovarian cancer screening. Am J Obstet Gynecol 1999;180:917.

Kavanagh JJ, Tresukosol D, Edwards C, et al: Carboplatin reinduction after Taxane in patients with platinum-refractory epithelial ovarian cancer. J Clin Oncol 1995;13:1584.

Kemp GM, Hsiu JG, Andrews MC: Papillary peritoneal carcinomatosis after prophylactic oophorectomy: case report. Gynecol Oncol 1992;47:395.

Kennedy AW, Markman M, Webster K, et al: Experience with platinum-paclitaxel chemotherapy in the initial management of papillary serous carcinoma of the peritoneum. Gynecol Oncol 1998;71:288.

Khoury N, Raju U, Crissman JD, et al: A comparative immunohistochemical study of peritoneal and ovarian serous tumors, and mesotheliomas. Hum Pathol 1990;21:811.

Killackey MA, Davis AR: Papillary serous carcinoma of the peritoneal surface: matched-case comparison with papillary serous ovarian carcinoma. Gynecol Oncol 1993;51:171.

Kommos F, Pfisterer J, Thome M, et al: Steroid receptors in ovarian carcinoma: immunohistochemical determination may lead to new aspects. Gynecol Oncol 1992;47:317.

Kosary CL: FIGO stage, histologic grade, age, and race as prognostic factors in determining survival for cancers of the female gynecological system: an analysis of 1973–87 SEER cases of cancers of the endometrium, cervix, ovary, vulva, and vagina. Semin Surg Oncol 1994;10:31.

Kowalski LD, Kanbur AI, Price FV, et al: A matched-case comparison of extraovarian versus primary ovarian adenocarcinoma. Cancer 1997;79:1587.

Lauchlan SC: The secondary müllerian system. Am J Obstet Gynecol 1972;27:133.

Lee KR, Verma U, Belinson JL: Primary clear cell carcinoma of the peritoneum. Gynecol Oncol 1991;41:259.

Lele SB, Piver MS, Matharu J, Tsukada Y: Peritoneal papillary carcinoma. Gynecol Oncol 1988;31:315.

Lynch HT, Bewtra C, Lynch JF: Familial ovarian cancer: clinical nuances. Am J Med 1986;81:1073.

Lynch HT, Watson P, Bewtra C, et al. Hereditary ovarian cancer. Cancer 1991;67:1460.

McGuire WP, Hoskins WJ, Brady MF, et al: Cyclophosphamide and cisplatin compared with paclitaxel plus cisplatin in patients with stage III and IV ovarian cancer. N Engl J Med 1996;334:1.

Menzin AW, Aikins JK, Wheeler JE, Rubin SC: Surgically documented responses to paclitaxel and cisplatin in patients with primary peritoneal carcinoma. Gynecol Oncol 1996;62:55.

Miki Y, Swensen J, Shattuck-Eidens D, et al: A strong candidate for the breast and ovarian susceptibility gene BRCA1. Science 1994;266:66.

Mills SE, Andersen WA, Fechner RE, Austin MB: Serous surface papillary carcinoma: a clinicopathologic study of 10 cases and comparison with stage III-IV ovarian serous carcinoma. Am J Surg Pathol 1988;12:827.

Mirc JL, Fenoglio-Preiser CM, Husseinzadeh N: Malignant mixed müllerian tumor of extraovarian secondary müllerian system: report of two cases and review of the literature. Arch Pathol Lab Med 1995;119:1044.

Moertel CG: Peritoneal mesothelioma. Gastroenterology 1972;63:346.

Moll UM, Valea F, Chumas J: Role of p53 alteration in primary peritoneal carcinoma. Int J Gynecol Pathol 1997;16:156.

Mulhollan TJ, Silva EG, Tornos C, et al: Ovarian involvement by serous surface papillary carcinoma. Int J Gynecol Pathol 1994;13:120.

Munkarah AR, Jacques SM, Qureshi F, Deppe G: Conservative surgery in a young patient with peritoneal psammocarcinoma. Gynecol Oncol 1999;73:312.

Nicoletti MI, Lucchini V, Massazza G, et al: Antitumor activity of taxol (NSC-125973) in human ovarian carcinomas growing in the peritoneal cavity of nude mice. Ann Oncol 1993;4:151.

Parmley T: Embryology of the female genital tract. In Kurman RJ (ed): Blaustein's Pathology of the Female Genital Tract. 3rd ed. New York: Springer-Verlag, 1987:1.

Parmley TH, Woodruff JD: The ovarian mesothelioma. Am J Obstet Gynecol 1974;120:234.

Petru E, Heydarfadai M, Pickel H, et al: Primary papillary serous carcinoma of the peritoneum: a report of experiences. Geburt Frauen 1992;5:533.

Piver MS, Eltabbakh GH, Hempling RE, et al: Two sequential studies for primary peritoneal carcinoma: induction with weekly cisplatin followed by either cisplatin-doxorubicin-cyclophosphamide or paclitaxel-cisplatin. Gynecol Oncol 1997;67:141.

Piver MS, Jishi MF, Tsukada Y, Nava G: Primary peritoneal carcinoma after prophylactic oophorectomy in women with a family history of ovarian cancer. Cancer 1993;7:2751.

Raju U, Fine G, Greenwald KA, Ohrodnik JM: Primary papillary serous neoplasia of the peritoneum: a clinico-pathological and ultrastructural study of eight cases. Hum Pathol 1989;20:426.

Ransom DT, Patel SR, Keeney GL, et al: Papillary serous adenocarcinoma of the peritoneum: a review of 33 cases treated with platin-based chemotherapy. Cancer 1990;66:1091.

Remmle W, Kaiserling E, Zerban U, et al: Serous papillary cystic tumor of borderline malignancy with focal carcinoma arising in testis: a case report with immunohistochemical and ultrastructural observations. Hum Pathol 1992;23:75.

Resnik E, Bender D: Syndrome of inappropriate antidiuretic hormone secretion in papillary serous surface carcinoma of the peritoneum. J Surg Oncol 1996;61:63.

Resta L, Maiorano E, Zito FA, et al: Multifocal extraovarian serous carcinoma: a histochemical and immunohistochemical study. Eur J Gynecol Oncol 1988;IX:474.

Rose PG, Reale FR: Papillary serous carcinoma of the peritoneum following endometrial cancer. Obstet Gynecol 1991;78:980.

Rosenbloom MA, Foster RB: Probable pelvic mesothelioma. report of a case and review of literature. Obstet Gynecol 1961;18:213.

Rothacker D, Mobius G: Varieties of serous surface papillary carcinoma of the peritoneum in Northern Germany: a thirty-year autopsy study. Int J Gynecol Pathol 1995;14:310.

Schrag D, Kuntz KM, Garber JE, Weeks JC: Decision analysis-effects of prophylactic mastectomy and oophorectomy expectancy among women with BRCA1 or BRCA2 mutations. N Engl J Med 1997;336:1465.

Scully RE: The Eltabbakh/Piver article reviewed. Oncology 1998;12:820.

Selikoff IJ, Churg J, Hammond EC: Relation between exposure to asbestos and mesothelioma. N Engl J Med 1965;272:560.

Sevelda P, Denison U, Schemper M, et al: Estrogen and progesterone receptor content as a prognostic factor in advanced epithelial ovarian carcinoma. Br J Obstet Gynecol 1990;97:706.

Shah IA, Jayram L, Gani O, et al: Papillary serous carcinoma of the peritoneum in a man. Cancer 1998;82:860.

Shapiro SP, Nunez C: Psammoma bodies in the cervicovaginal smear in association with papillary tumor of the peritoneum. Obstet Gynecol 1983;61:130.

Shattuck-Eidens D, McClure M, Simrad J, et al: A collaborative survey of 80 mutations in the BRCA1 breast and ovarian cancer susceptiblity gene. JAMA 1995;273:535.

Stauffer JL, Carbone JE: Pulmonary diseases. Curr Med Diagn Treat 1986;7:151.

Strand CM, Grosh WW, Baxter J, et al: Peritoneal carcinomatosis of unknown primary site in women. a distinct subset of adenocarcinoma. Ann Intern Med 1989;111:213.

Swerdlow M: Mesothelioma of the pelvic peritoneum resembling papillary cystadenocarcinoma of the ovary: case report. Am J Obstet Gynecol 1959;77:197.

Thigpen T, Blessing J, Homesley H, et al: Cisplatin as salvage therapy in ovarian carcinoma treated initially with single agent paclitaxel: a Gynecologic Oncology Group study. Proc Am Soc Clin Oncol 1996;15:778.

Tobacman JK, Tucker MA, Kose R, et al: Intra-abdominal carcinomatosis after prophylactic oophorectomy in ovarian-cancer prone families. Lancet 1982;2:795.

Truong LD, Maccato ML, Awalt H, et al: Serous surface carcinoma of the peritoneum: a clinicopathologic study of 22 cases. Hum Pathol 1990;21:99.

Ulbright TM, Morley DJ, Roth LM, Berkow RL: Papillary serous carcinoma of the retroperitoneum. Am J Clin Pathol 1983;79:633.

Wall JE, Mandrell BN, Jenkins JJ III, et al: Effectiveness of paclitaxel in treating papillary serous carcinoma of the peritoneum in an adolescent. Am J Obstet Gynecol 1995;172:1049.

Warhol MJ, Hunter NJ, Corson JM: An ultrastructural comparison of mesotheliomas and adenocarcinomas of the ovary and endometrium. Int J Gynecol Pathol 1982;1:125.

Weir MM, Bell DA, Young RH: Grade 1 peritoneal serous carcinoma: a report of 14 cases and comparison with 7 peritoneal serous psammocarcinomas and 19 peritoneal serous borderline tumors. Am J Surg Pathol 1998;22:849.

Whitcomb BP, Kost ER, Hines JF, Zahn CM, Hall KL: Primary peritoneal psammocarcinoma: A case presenting with an upper abdominal mass and elevated CA-125. Gynecol Oncol 1999;73:331.

White PF, Merino MJ, Barwick KW: Serous surface papillary carcinoma of the ovary: a clinical, pathological, ultrastructural, and immunohistochemical study of 11 cases. Pathol Annu 1985;20:403.

Wick M, Mills S, Dehner L, et al: Serous papillary carcinomas arising from the peritoneum and ovaries: a clinicopathologic and immunochemical comparison. Int J Gynecol Pathol 1989;8:179.

Wilailak S, Kudelka AP, Donner LR, et al: Peritoneal papillary serous carcinoma: response to taxol in a platinum resistant disease. Eur J Gynaecol Oncol 1995;16:187.

Winter R: Lymphadenectomy. In Burghardt E, Webb M, Monaghan J, Kindermann G (eds): Surgical Gynecologic Oncology. Stuttgart: Thieme, 1993:281.

Yamakazi T, Hatano H, Suzuki A, et al: Normal-sized ovarian carcinoma syndrome: histopathological analysis of 14 cases. Acta Obstet Gynecol Jpn 1995;42:27.

62

Germ Cell, Stromal, and Miscellaneous Ovarian Neoplasms

Larry J. Copeland

In addition to the epithelial ovarian tumors, two other major categories are the ovarian *germ cell tumors*, arising from the primitive germ cells of the embryonic gonad, and the *sex cord–stromal tumors*, arising from the specialized gonadal stroma. The other ovarian neoplasms discussed in this chapter include *metastatic tumors to the ovary* and the less common *nonspecific mesenchymal ovarian tumors*. The germ cell tumors, especially the malignant variants, tend to occur in women under age 40, and the sex cord–stromal tumors, although found in women of all ages, are most common in the over-50 age group.

GERM CELL TUMORS

Germ cell neoplasms are second only to the epithelial ovarian tumors in frequency, constituting approximately 15% to 20% of all primary ovarian neoplasms. Table 62–1 outlines a simplified version of the World Health Organization (WHO) classification of germ cell tumors (Serov et al, 1973; Talerman, 1987a). Approximately 75% of malignant germ cell tumors are diagnosed with early stage (I or II) disease, in contrast to epithelial ovarian cancer where 75% of patients have advanced disease (stage III or IV). The germ cell tumors can be classified into general categories as benign and malignant. Both the benign germ cell tumors—the mature teratoma and the gonadoblastoma—have the potential to degenerate into malignant variants. Most of the malignant germ cell tumors (dysgerminoma and nondysgerminomatous variants) occur in young women between the ages of 13 and 30 years although exceptions exist (Doss et al, 1999). Serum tumor marker analysis (Table 62–2) may be useful for confirming diagnosis, for following treatment efficacy, and for surveillance for recurrence in the patient free of disease by clinical and imaging evaluations.

While most commonly arising from the gonads, various types of germ cell tumors also develop in other midline structures from the pineal gland to the sacrum, vagina, or vulva (Park et al, 1999). Each type of germ cell tumor is discussed with regard to its clinical and pathologic features, and comments regarding treatment and prognosis follow.

Types of Germ Cell Tumors

Dysgerminoma

Dysgerminoma, homologous to the male seminoma, is the most common malignant ovarian germ cell tumor, constituting a little less than half of all the malignant germ cell tumors (Kurman and Norris, 1977). Most patients with a dysgerminoma have a normal karyotype. However, because the most common malignant germ cell tumor to arise from a dysgenetic gonad or a gonadoblastoma is the dysgerminoma, karyotype analysis is appropriate, especially in young or amenorrheic patients. Patients with a dysgenetic gonad and a Y chromosome are at high risk for a malignant germ cell tumor. Although this risk has been quoted from 25% to 50%, it may actually be higher with advancing age.

The two clinical features unique to the dysgerminoma, in comparison to the nondysgerminomatous germ cell tumors, are the incidence of bilaterality and radiosensitivity. About 10% to 15% of dysgerminomas and 1% or less of the pure nondysgerminomas are associated with synchronous bilateral disease. The dysgerminomas tend to be exquisitely radiosensitive, whereas the responsiveness of the nondysgerminomas to radiation is notably less. Dysgerminoma tumors not uncommonly reach a significant size before a diagnosis is made, and 15% to 20% are diagnosed in association with pregnancy (Krepart et al, 1978). Symptomatic presentation is usually related to tumor size and pressure on adjacent organs. These tumors tend to be solid, and tumor rupture, producing an acute presentation, is uncommon. Characteristically, the pure dysgerminoma has no reliable serum tumor marker. The two fast fractions of serum lactate dehydrogenase (LDH) may

Table 62–1. MODIFIED WHO CLASSIFICATION OF GERM CELL TUMORS OF THE OVARY

I. Germ cell tumors
  A. Dysgerminoma
  B. Endodermal sinus tumor
  C. Embryonal cell carcinoma
  D. Polyembryoma
  E. Choriocarcinoma
  F. Teratoma
    1. Immature
    2. Mature (dermoid cyst)
    3. Monodermal (struma ovarii, carcinoid)
  G. Mixed forms (any combination of types A–F)
II. Tumors composed of germ cells and sex cord stromal derivatives
  A. Gonadoblastoma
  B. Mixed germ cell–sex cord stromal tumor

be elevated in patients with dysgerminoma and may be a useful tumor marker (Sheiko and Hart, 1982; Awais, 1983; Pressley et al, 1992). Macrophase colony-stimulating factor has been reported as a highly sensitive and specific tumor marker for dysgerminoma (Suzuki et al, 1998). Serum inhibin may also provide useful marker information (Santala et al, 1998). Approximately 8% of dysgerminoma tumors have human chorionic gonadotropin (hCG) production from focal multinucleated syncytial giant cells (Fig. 62–1). These tumors are not considered to be mixed tumors with a choriocarcinoma component because cytotrophoblastic cells are absent. Neither hCG nor LDH can be considered a clinically reliable tumor marker for dysgerminomas. Metastatic spread to liver or lung is rare. Lymph node involvement, usually aortic, is much more common than intraperitoneal surface metastases (Gordon et al, 1981).

Pathologically, these tumors are characterized grossly as large, solid, and lobulated (Fig. 62–2). The external surface is usually smooth, and the cut surface reveals a solid white or cream-colored appearance. Areas of hemorrhage and necrosis may be present, but they are usually small and focal. It is important, however, for these focal areas of hemorrhage to undergo careful pathologic examination because they represent areas most likely to contain nondysgerminomatous tumor. Microscopically, these tumors are composed of aggregates of large round or polygonal cells with a prominent cell membrane and abundant glycogen. Characteristically, the germ cells are divided by thin, fibrous septa with adjacent lymphocytes (Fig. 62–3). Syncytial giant cells may be present (Fig. 62–1).

Endodermal Sinus Tumor

The second most common malignant germ cell tumor of the ovary is the endodermal sinus tumor (EST). First described as a tumor of mesonephric origin (Schiller, 1939), the endodermal sinus tumor was later correctly identified as a germ cell tumor (Teilum, 1946, 1959). Teilum (1965) also noted that the endodermal sinus tumor resembled the endodermal sinus of Duval in the rodent placenta. This tumor has occasionally been referred to as the "yolk sac tumor of the ovary," terminology that is outdated.

The EST is characterized by very rapid growth. Although bilateral synchronous ovarian tumor development is extremely rare, metastatic spread to the contralateral ovary is more common. These tumors tend to be solid and cystic, and the presence of hemorrhagic ascitic fluid is not uncommon. Approximately one third of these tumors rupture prior to or during surgery. Intraperitoneal metastatic spread is more frequent than lymph node involvement; however, both spread modalities occur. Recurrent tumor is often characterized by retroperitoneal lymph node and liver metastases (Gershenson et al, 1983).

α-Fetoprotein (AFP) appears to be a relatively reliable tumor marker for the EST. Serum AFP levels obtained preoperatively may provide a clue to the nature of the tumor. However, the greatest value of the AFP marker is in monitoring efficacy of chemotherapy and in monitoring for evidence of occult recurrence. Recurrent EST and normal AFP values have been reported (Curtin et al, 1989), but these case reports have been questioned with regard to their clinical significance (Gershenson, 1989).

The gross appearance of these tumors may resemble a simple epithelial cystic tumor with a smooth and glistening cystic capsule. As previously noted, capsule tears and rupture are common. The cut surface usually reveals solid and cystic components with areas of hemorrhage and necrosis. Microscopi-

Table 62–2. OVARIAN GERM CELL TUMOR MARKERS

TUMOR	hCG	AFP	OTHERS
Dysgerminoma	+(8%)/−	−	LDH, M-CSF, Inhibin
Endodermal sinus tumor	−	+	−
Immature teratoma	−	−/+ (rarely)	−
Mixed germ cell tumor	+/−	+/−	hPL/LDH
Embryonal carcinoma	+	+ (70%)/−	+/−
Choriocarcinoma	+	−	+/−
Polyembryoma	+	+/−	hPL

Abbreviations: AFP, α-fetoprotein; hCG, human chorionic gonadotropin; hPL, human placental lactogen; LDH, lactate dehydrogenase; M-CSF, macrophage colony stimulating factor.

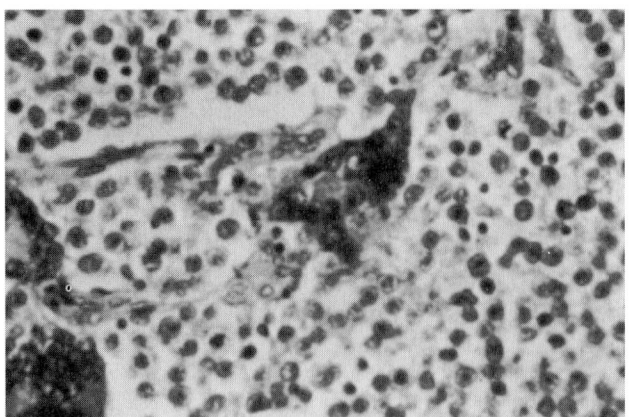

Figure 62–1
Dysgerminoma with multinucleated syncytial giant cells. Immunoperoxidase staining for β-human chorionic gonadotropin (β-hCG) may be positive. Without cytotrophoblastic cells, this focus is not considered a focus of choriocarcinoma.

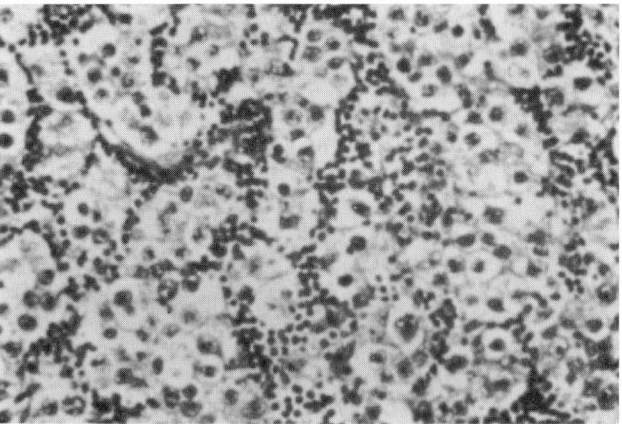

Figure 62–3
Dysgerminoma: large round or polygonal cells with lymphocytic infiltrate.

cally, at least 10 histologic patterns may be observed (Talerman, 1987a); however, the most common patterns are the reticular and festoon patterns (Schiller-Duval bodies). Schiller-Duval bodies are characterized by a simple papillary tuff protruding into a sinus-like space. A central capillary is usually present within the protruding papilla (Fig. 62–4). Hyaline bodies, intracellular or extracellular, are present in most patterns, and immunoperoxidase staining of these bodies is positive for AFP. The pure polyvesicular vitelline pattern tends to be AFP-negative and may carry a better prognosis (Nogales et al, 1978).

Immature Teratoma

Pure immature teratomas constitute approximately 20% of the malignant germ cell tumors. The imma-

ture teratoma is characterized by variable amounts of immature tissues derived from one of the three germ cell layers: ectoderm, mesoderm, or endoderm. Immature neural tissue, neuroepithelium, or glia is usually the most common type of immature tissue found. Mature (adult) tissue may predominate. The immature teratoma is the only germ cell tumor for which histologic grading carries prognostic significance. The immature components of an immature teratoma are capable of spontaneous maturation to grade 0 tissue (mature). Although this maturation process may occur spontaneously, it occurs more predictably under the influence of chemotherapy. Prior areas of immature glia, under the influence of chemotherapy, are frequently found at second-look laparotomy as mature glia. The presence of multiple nodules of mature glia throughout the peritoneal cavity is termed *gliomatosis peritoni* (Robboy and Scully, 1970). Likewise, benign heterogeneous im-

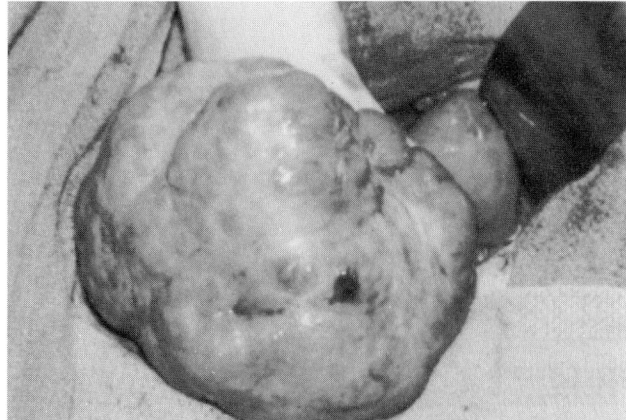

Figure 62–2
Dysgerminoma approximately 12 cm in greatest dimension. This tumor developed in the left ovary of a 22-year-old woman, 6 years after a right oophorectomy and "tailored" conservative pelvic and aortic irradiation for a right-sided dysgerminoma. She had a normal 46,XX karyotype.

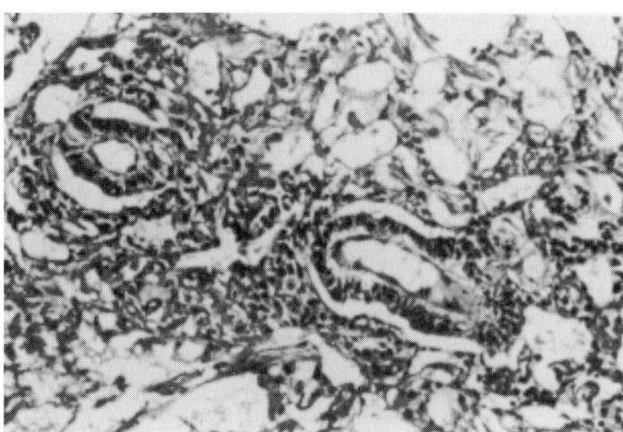

Figure 62–4
Endodermal sinus tumor demonstrating two Schiller-Duval bodies. (From Copeland LJ: Malignant gynecologic tumors. In Sutow WW, Fernbach DJ, Vietti TJ [eds]: Clinical Pediatric Oncology. 3rd ed. St. Louis: CV Mosby Company, 1984:749, with permission.)

plants may develop into dermoid cyst–like structures a number of years after initial therapy for immature teratoma. This process, although it may simulate a malignant progression, is responsive to simple excisional surgery.

Bilateral ovarian involvement with immature teratomas is uncommon; however, the contralateral ovary in 10% to 15% of patients may contain a mature teratoma (dermoid cyst). In a small percentage of cases, AFP levels (Ihara et al, 1984; Taylor et al, 1985; Kawai et al, 1991) and serum LDH levels (Liu et al, 1984) may be elevated.

The gross appearance of these tumors is principally solid with variable cystic areas. Mature tissues, such as bone or cartilage, may be grossly apparent. Microscopically, a range of maturity and cell types may be present. Immature neuroepithelium or mesenchyme may predominate. The grading system for this tumor is outlined in Table 62–3. The major determinant for metastatic spread is the grade of the primary tumor. When spread has occurred, the predominant prognostic factor is the grade of the metastatic disease (Norris et al, 1976).

Embryonal Carcinoma

Previously, the embryonal carcinoma tumor was miscategorized to be included with either the EST or immature teratoma; however, it should be regarded as a separate pathologic entity. Only a few cases of pure embryonal carcinoma have been reported. Embryonal carcinoma is more commonly found as a component of a mixed germ cell tumor. This tumor usually produces hCG, and approximately 70% of patients have detectable levels of AFP. Embryonal cell carcinoma tends to occur at a slightly younger age than most of the other germ cell tumors, with the median age being 15 years (Kurman and Norris, 1976a).

Pathologically, these tumors are characterized as relatively solid with small areas of cysts and areas of hemorrhage and necrosis. Histologically, the tumor consists of solid sheets of primitive anaplastic cells with areas of cleft-like spaces. Hyaline bodies and clusters of syncytial giant cells are not uncommon.

Choriocarcinoma

Ovarian choriocarcinoma is very rare in the pure form. Choriocarcinoma is more commonly a component of a mixed germ cell tumor. As a result of the possibility of an ovarian ectopic pregnancy giving rise to choriocarcinoma, one could make the argument that a pure nongestational choriocarcinoma can be diagnosed with confidence only in a prepubertal female. Only about 50 cases of choriocarcinoma of the ovary have been reported in the world literature (Gerbie et al, 1975; Jacobs et al, 1982; Axe et al, 1985). When choriocarcinoma develops in a prepubertal female, pseudoprecocious puberty may ensue.

Table 62–3. GRADING FOR IMMATURE TERATOMA

GRADE	DEFINITION
0	All tissues mature; mitoses rare or absent
1	Mature tissue predominates; some immature tissue but neuroepithelium absent or limited to 1 lpf (×40) per slide
2	More immature neuroepithelium, not exceeding 3 lpf per slide
3	Prominence of immature tissue with immature neuroepithelium in 4 lpf per slide

Abbreviations: lpf, low-power field.
Adapted from Norris HJ, Zirkin HJ, Benson WL: Immature (malignant) teratoma of the ovary. Cancer 1976;37:2359, with permission.

Grossly, these tumors are unilateral and solid, with areas of hemorrhage and necrosis on the cut surface. Microscopically, cytotrophoblastic and syncytiotrophoblastic cells should be identified.

Polyembryoma

The rarest of germ cell tumors, the polyembryoma is composed of embryoid bodies of various differentiation and size (Fig. 62–5). As with the other germ cell tumors, this tumor is more commonly found as a component of a mixed tumor rather than as a pure germ cell tumor. Three tumor markers—AFP, hCG, and placental lactogen—have been reported (Takeda et al, 1982). While limited successful management without adjuvant therapy has been reported (Chapman et al, 1994), the general management of non-dysgerminomatas would dictate that limited adjuvant therapy should be considered.

Mixed Germ Cell Tumors

Mixed germ cell tumors contain two or more malignant germ cell components and occur with a frequency similar to that of the immature teratoma

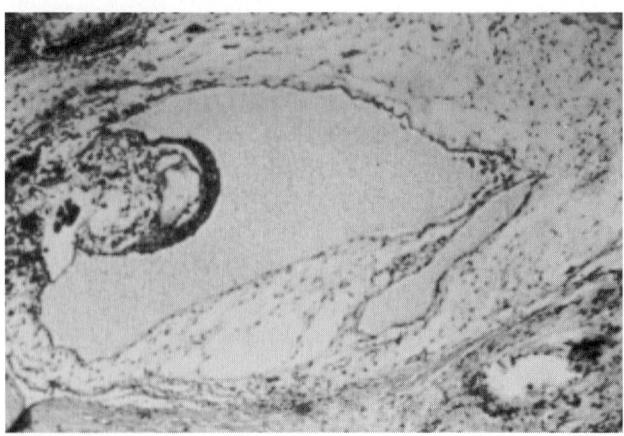

Figure 62–5
Polyembryoma, one of the rarest of the pure germ cell tumors, characterized by embryoid bodies.

(10% to 15% of all germ cell malignancies). To not miss or overlook a mixed component, it is necessary to sample germ cell tumors carefully. Sampling guidelines suggest that at least one tissue block be cut for every centimeter in greatest tumor diameter. Likewise, it is important to sample the various areas that exhibit different gross appearances. These tumors may be bilateral, and it is unclear as to whether the presence of a dysgerminoma component is influential in the likelihood of bilateral ovarian involvement (Kurman and Norris, 1976b; Jimerson and Woodruff, 1977). On the basis of the various elements present, serum AFP and hCG levels may be elevated (Gershenson et al, 1984; Wax and Segna, 1997).

Benign Germ Cell Tumors

GONADOBLASTOMA

Both germ cell and sex cord stromal elements are present in a gonadoblastoma. The gonadoblastoma, however, is usually categorized with the germ cell tumors because the germ cell element has the propensity to undergo malignant degeneration. These tumors are usually small, and bilateral ovarian involvement occurs in about 30% of cases. The rare patient with a gonadoblastoma may have an apparently normal karyotype (Bergher de Bacalao and Dominguez, 1969), but most patients are sex chromatin–negative, with 46,XY, 45,XO, or 46,XX/46,XY karyotypes. Fine calcifications are frequently present, and these may be evident on pelvic roentgenogram.

The aspect of greatest clinical significance in management of patients with the gonadoblastoma is the propensity for malignant germ cell tumors to develop (Scully, 1953). Although gonadoblastomas most commonly give rise to dysgerminomas, other types of germ cell tumors have been reported (Talerman, 1974; Luzzato et al, 1979). Because of the risk of malignant degeneration, both gonads should be excised, with the exception of the rare patient who may have a contralateral normal ovary (Hart and Burkons, 1979). One must be careful not to consider a streaked ovary, enlarged to the size of a normal ovary by gonadoblastoma, to be a normal ovary. Retention of the uterus for possible in vitro fertilization should be considered (Jarrell, 1990).

MATURE TERATOMA

Whereas chromosomal studies suggest that teratomas arise from a single germ cell (Linder et al, 1975), they are composed of elements from one or more of all three germ cell layers. The terminology for teratomas has been very confusing. Mature teratomas have been described as "cystic," "adult," and "benign." In contrast, immature teratomas have been described as "malignant," "fetal," and "solid." Unfortunately, these descriptive terms can be misleading because mature teratomas can occur in the fetus or the very young, they can transform into a malig-

nant tumor, and the monodermal variants are frequently solid. Likewise, the immature teratomas can be cystic in nature, commonly occur in adults, and may undergo maturation (either with time or under the influence of chemotherapy) to benign tissues. For this reason, it is best to limit the terminology used to describe teratomas to either "mature" or "immature."

Mature teratomas account for approximately 25% of all ovarian neoplasms and approximately 95% of all ovarian teratomas. Although the mature teratoma is the most common ovarian neoplasm of childhood, more than 50% occur during the reproductive years and 10% to 20% occur in postmenopausal women.

Mature teratomas with prominent ectodermal components are commonly referred to as *dermoid cysts* or *dermoid tumors*. Nodular thickening on the cyst walls is commonly referred to as a *dermoid process*, or Rokitansky's protuberance. These areas should be thoroughly sampled to rule out the presence of immature or malignant tissues. Dermoids are bilateral in 10% to 15% of patients, but it is uncommon for a normal-appearing contralateral ovary to contain an occult focus of teratoma (Doss et al, 1977). Therefore, routine bivalving or wedging of a normal-appearing contralateral ovary is not recommended. If a cystic area of the contralateral ovary is at all suspicious, it can be aspirated. If the aspirate is clear or serous, no further intervention is recommended. However, if the aspirate is mucoid, excision of the cystic area is advised.

Dermoid tumors are usually asymptomatic and are often detected on routine pelvic examination, but it is possible for them to present with acute symptoms secondary to torsion or spontaneous rupture, leading to various degrees of peritonitis (Waxman and Boyce, 1976; Stern et al, 1981; Stuart and Smith, 1983). The mature teratoma may be associated with autoimmune hemolytic anemia not responsive to steroids or splenectomy. Removal of the tumor may lead to resolution of this syndrome (Payne et al, 1981).

Monodermal and Specialized Teratomas. Thyroid tissue may be present in about 10% of mature teratomas; when thyroid tissue constitutes more than 50% of the tumor, it is usually called a *struma ovarii*. Struma ovarii tumors may be associated with hyperthyroidism (Kempers et al, 1970), and a small percentage can develop metastatic thyroid carcinoma, usually of a follicular type (Yannopoulos et al, 1976; Scully, 1979; Devaney et al, 1993). While most of these tumors are relatively small and solid, there is a cystic subset that are frequently undiagnosed. They may be unilocular or multilocular and immunohistochemical staining for thyroglobulin may assist in establishing the diagnosis (Szyfelbein et al, 1994).

Carcinoid. Primary carcinoid tumors of the ovary may occur, and, because ovarian venous drainage is not portal, the carcinoid syndrome may present without metastatic disease. Ovarian carcinoids are usually unilateral, although a contralateral dermoid or mucinous cystadenoma may be present. In a small percentage of these patients (5%), recurrent disease develops that characteristically progresses very slowly (Robboy et al, 1975, 1977). Gastrointestinal carcinoid metastatic to the ovary must be considered in the differential diagnosis of these patients. In such situations, the prognosis is more guarded. Bilateral ovarian disease is more common, and no other germ cell neoplasm is usually present in either ovary (Robboy et al, 1974).

When thyroid tissue is present with a carcinoid tumor, the entity is usually referred to as a *strumal carcinoid*. More than 95% of these can be expected to act in a benign fashion (Robboy and Scully, 1980) and serum tumor markers (CA-125; CA19-9; CEA) have been reported and if elevated may be useful to follow (Takomori et al, 1995).

Benign Teratomas Undergoing Malignant Transformation. Seen in 1% to 2% of patients with mature teratoma, this complication occurs most frequently in postmenopausal women (Gordon et al, 1980). Features suspicious of malignancy include rupture, necrosis, adhesions to adjacent structures, and solid areas within cyst walls. The most common tumor is a squamous carcinoma (Pins et al, 1996). The overall cure rate for these tumors is approximately 75%, but this is attributable to the fact that approximately half of these patients have apparent stage IA disease and the carcinoma is an incidental pathologic finding. Patients with more advanced disease tend to do very poorly, with most dying within 1 year. Other types of malignancies can develop from the various constituents of a mature teratoma.

Treatment

Surgery

The surgical management of ovarian germ cell tumors should focus on preservation of normal ovarian tissue, accurate staging (see Chapter 60 for surgical staging of ovarian tumors), and effective tumor reduction. The frequency of bilateral and ovarian involvement varies with the histologic type. Ten per cent to 15% of dysgerminoma tumors are bilateral at the time of initial surgery. Because conservative management and contralateral ovarian preservation in patients with dysgerminoma tumors are relatively recent developments, the percentage of patients in whom a dysgerminoma tumor subsequently develops in the contralateral ovary is not precisely known; however, estimates are 15% to 20% (Casey et al, 1996). Although the malignant nondysgerminomatous tumors rarely show synchronous bilateral tumor development, 5% to 10% of these patients have a coexisting mature teratoma involving the ipsilateral or contralateral ovary. If possible, a contralateral mature teratoma should be managed with an ovarian cystectomy rather than oophorectomy. When the contralateral ovary is involved with tumor of a

nondysgerminomatous type, it is most frequently secondary to spread from the original ovarian primary. Because the germ cell tumors are very sensitive to chemotherapy and cure rates are high, even in the presence of metastatic disease to other pelvic and abdominal structures, every effort should be made to preserve normal ovarian tissue and the uterus. Even in rare circumstances in which both ovaries must be excised secondary to tumor involvement, the uterus should be left in place for the possibility of in vitro fertilization if the patient has childbearing expectations.

Because the volume of residual disease may adversely affect outcome (Williams et al, 1989; Ablin et al, 1991), tumor-reductive surgery is recommended for patients with metastatic disease. However, there are no prospective trials that address the impact of aggressive tumor-reductive surgery for metastatic germ cell tumors. Salvage surgery for chemorefractory ovarian germ cell tumors should be considered in select circumstances (Munkarah et al, 1994).

Adjuvant Therapy

Although most germ cell malignancies are stage I at the time of initial surgery, all patients with malignant germ cell tumors require postoperative adjuvant therapy except those with stage IA, grade I immature teratomas or stage IA dysgerminomas comprehensively staged.

RADIOTHERAPY

Historically, radiotherapy was the cornerstone of adjuvant therapy for metastatic dysgerminoma. Adjuvant chemotherapy has replaced the role of radiotherapy for dysgerminoma (Williams et al, 1991), but there may still exist situations in which radiotherapy should be considered. Although radiotherapy with tailored ports has provided adequate treatment for metastatic disease with preservation of fertility, the most desirable treatment to retain fertility in a patient with a preserved contralateral ovary and uterus is chemotherapy (Thomas et al, 1987). Radiotherapy remains satisfactory for a patient who has metastatic dysgerminoma and has undergone extirpation of both fallopian tubes and the ovaries and uterus, presumably for appropriate indications. For disease limited to the ovary and retroperitoneal lymph nodes, standard treatment fields would be to the pelvis and an aortic port. Tumor rupture or the presence of peritoneal metastases is an indication for treatment to the whole abdomen. In select clinical situations, radiotherapy treatment to the mediastinum and supraclavicular areas may be indicated. Because dysgerminoma is very radiosensitive, the dose of radiation therapy is usually modest and radiation therapy complications should be avoided. Other than loss of reproductive capabilities and an increase in frequence of bowel movements, morbidity from treating dysgerminoma patients with irradiation is not usually serious (Mitchell et al, 1991).

Radiotherapy for patients with nondysgerminomatous germ cell tumors is usually not indicated. These patients are effectively treated with chemotherapy. There may be rare situations in which small radiation therapy fields might play a palliative role in patients who have demonstrated resistance to chemotherapy.

CHEMOTHERAPY

Combination chemotherapy is the postoperative treatment of choice for patients with malignant germ cell tumors. Treatments with surgery alone or adjuvant treatment with radioisotopes, radiation, or alkylating agents have yielded dismal results (Kurman and Norris, 1976a, 1976b; Norris et al, 1976; Gershenson et al, 1983). One of the first active combinations for the management of metastatic malignant germ cell tumors was vincristine, actinomycin D, and cyclophosphamide (VAC). Numerous studies have demonstrated good efficacy of VAC for malignant germ cell tumors, especially for patients with stage I disease (Malkasian et al, 1974; Smith and Rutledge, 1975; Curry et al, 1978; Gallion et al, 1979, 1983; Schwartz, 1984; Gershenson et al, 1985; Micha et al, 1985; Slayton et al, 1985). However, for those with more advanced disease (stages II through IV), VAC therapy is inferior to the platinum-containing combinations (Gershenson et al, 1985, 1986b; Schwartz et al, 1992).

The combination of vinblastine, bleomycin, and cisplatin (VBP), first recorded as successful in the management of testicular tumors (Einhorn and Donohue, 1977), was subsequently adopted for management of malignant ovarian germ cell tumors (Julian et al, 1980; Carlson et al, 1983; Gershenson et al, 1986b). Patients with stage I disease usually receive three to four cycles and patients with advanced disease usually receive four to six cycles. Treatment with VBP or etoposide combinations has demonstrated the potential for salvage of about 50% of the patients who fail to respond to VAC treatment (Jacobs et al, 1982; Carlson et al, 1983; Smith et al, 1984; Gershenson et al, 1986a). The replacement of vinblastine in VBP with etoposide (BEP) has produced a regimen with equal efficacy and less toxicity (Williams et al, 1980). Numerous other reports support the efficacy of this combination (Pinkerton et al, 1986; Smales and Peckham, 1987; Gershenson et al, 1990). Etoposide-containing therapy carries a risk of the induction of acute leukemia (see Chapter 64, p 1424).

Additional treatment combinations include vinblastine, cisplatin, and ifosfamide or etoposide, cisplatin, and ifosfamide (Loehrer et al, 1988; Harstrick et al, 1991). Cisplatin or bleomycin appear to be key ingredients in most active regimens (Loehrer et al, 1995; Culine et al, 1997). Also, carboplatin appears to be an inferior substitute for cisplatin in the management of germ cell tumors (Bajorin et al, 1993). High-dose chemotherapy with autologous bone marrow rescue should be considered for refractory tumors.

Second-Look Laparotomy

When one considers the development of effective chemotherapy, the frequent availability of excellent tumor markers, and the better understanding of the overall nature of these tumors, the role of second-look laparotomy in the management of patients with malignant germ cell tumors is questioned (Creasman and Soper, 1985; Gershenson et al, 1986a). It remains controversial as to whether a second-look laparotomy should play a role in patients who have no reliable tumor markers and in patients with EST, because there are isolated reports of marker-negative recurrences (Maeyama et al, 1984; Pippit et al, 1988; Curtin et al, 1989; Marina et al, 1991; Gershenson, 1989).

Prognosis

Modern-day therapy for the malignant germ cell tumors offers excellent survival rates. Patients who have a stage I malignant germ cell tumor who receive appropriate adjuvant therapy have a 5-year cure rate of 95% to 100%. Analysis of reports using VBP or BEP for primary therapy suggest a cure rate of up to 80% for patients with stage II, III, or IV malignant germ cell tumors (Williams, 1994). Most recurrences present within two years after attaining clinical complete response and almost always within five years, with rare exceptions (Bekail-Saab et al, 1999).

Menstrual and Reproductive Potential After Chemotherapy

The majority of women with malignant germ cell tumors cured with the use of chemotherapy resume normal menses (80%) and reproductive function (75%) (Gershenson, 1988). Factors adversely related to future gonadal function include older age at initiation of therapy, greater cumulative drug dose, and longer duration of treatment.

Chemotherapy Treatment During Pregnancy

Because malignant germ cell tumors can demonstrate very rapid growth, it is occasionally necessary to administer postoperative chemotherapy when these tumors are diagnosed during pregnancy. Cisplatin combination chemotherapy has been reported effective and safe in isolated reports (Copeland and Landon, 1996).

SEX CORD–STROMAL TUMORS

Ovarian stromal tumors constitute 5% or fewer of all ovarian neoplasms. Although they can occur in women of all ages, they tend to have a peak inci-

Table 62–4. CLASSIFICATION OF SEX CORD STROMAL NEOPLASMS

I. Granulosa-stromal cell tumors
  A. Granulosa cell tumor
    1. Adult type
    2. Juvenile type
  B. Theca-fibroma
    1. Thecoma
    2. Fibroma
    3. Fibrosarcoma
    4. Sclerosing stromal tumor
II. Sertoli-stromal cell tumors (androblastomas)
  A. Sertoli cell tumor
  B. Leydig cell tumor
  C. Sertoli-Leydig tumor
    (well differentiated; intermediate differentiation; poorly differentiated; retiform; with heterologous elements; mixed)
III. Gynandroblastoma
IV. Sex cord tumor with annular tubules
V. Unclassified

dence in those over age 50. These tumors have frequently been referred to as the "functioning tumors" because a small percentage (15% to 30%) produce estrogen, progesterone, testosterone, or other androgens. However, most of these tumors are hormonally inert, and hormonal production cannot be relied on either to classify these tumors or to utilize hormonal levels as tumor markers. The production of hormones by ovarian neoplasms is not exclusive to stromal tumors. Other ovarian neoplasms, either primary or metastatic, have been reported to stimulate adjacent non-neoplastic ovarian stroma, with the resultant production of gonadal sex steroids (Aiman et al, 1977, 1986a, 1986b).

The primitive gonadal stroma possesses sexual bipotential, and consequently tumors developing from gonadal stroma may be of a male-directed cell type (Sertoli or Leydig cell) or a female-directed cell type (granulosa or theca cells). The homologous pairings are Sertoli-granulosa and Leydig-theca (Teilum, 1977). Table 62–4 contains a modification of the WHO classification for the ovarian sex cord–stromal tumors.

Types of Sex Cord–Stromal Tumors

Granulosa Cell Tumors

Both the granulosa and theca cell tumors represent approximately 2% of all ovarian neoplasms, and approximately 50% of the cases of granulosa cell occur in postmenopausal women. Only about 5% of granulosa cell tumors occur in prepubertal females, and approximately 85% of these patients have the juvenile granulosa cell variant.

Because the granulosa cell tumor has a propensity to rupture, patients often present with sudden onset of abdominal pain, simulating a ruptured ectopic pregnancy, abruptio placentae, ruptured appendix, ovarian torsion, or other acute pelvic conditions. In a prepubertal female, presenting symptoms may be related to hormonal production, causing isosexual pseudoprecocious puberty. Patients may also present during the reproductive years with menorrhagia or irregular bleeding, or in the postmenopausal years with bleeding secondary to endogenous estrogen production.

Breast enlargement or breast tenderness may be a presenting feature. There is an increased incidence of breast cancer (Ohel et al, 1983). Likewise, there is a significant association with endometrial carcinoma (5% to 15%) or endometrial hyperplasia (50%) (Norris and Taylor, 1968; Fox et al, 1975; Evans et al, 1980). The presence of endometrial hyperplasia in a nonobese postmenopausal woman who is not receiving exogenous estrogens should raise suspicion for the possibility of an estrogen-producing stromal tumor. If no palpable adnexal mass is found, additional investigations, such as transvaginal ultrasound or serum estradiol level (greater than 30 pg/ml), may be indicated. Progesterone or androgen production during the reproductive years can manifest with defeminizing signs such as amenorrhea. The majority of patients (85% to 90%) are diagnosed with stage I disease, and fewer than 5% of cases are bilateral (Björkholm and Silfverswärd, 1981). Although recurrences 10 to 20 years after initial diagnosis are not uncharacteristic, most patients who experience recurrent disease do so within 2 to 3 years. Follicular regulatory protein (inhibin), normally produced by granulosa cells, may be a clinically useful tumor marker for granulosa cell tumors, possibly predictive of recurrences months to years before they are clinically evident (Lappohn et al, 1989; Boggess et al, 1997).

Pathologically, granulosa tumors on gross appearance are usually solid and cystic with areas of hemorrhage. Occasionally, they may be simple or complex, thin-walled cysts. One characteristic microscopic feature is the Call-Exner body (Fig. 62–6). A number of microscopic patterns, including the microfollicular, macrofollicular, trabecular, insular, and

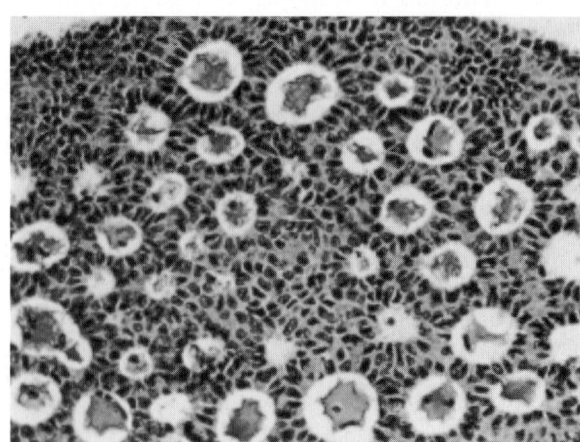

Figure 62–6
Granulosa cell tumor: Call-Exner body characterized by a rosette arrangement of cells around an eosinophilic fluid space. (From Scully RE, Morris JMcL: Functioning ovarian tumors. In Meigs J, Sturgis SH [eds]: Progress in Gynecology III. New York: Grune & Stratton, 1957, with permission.)

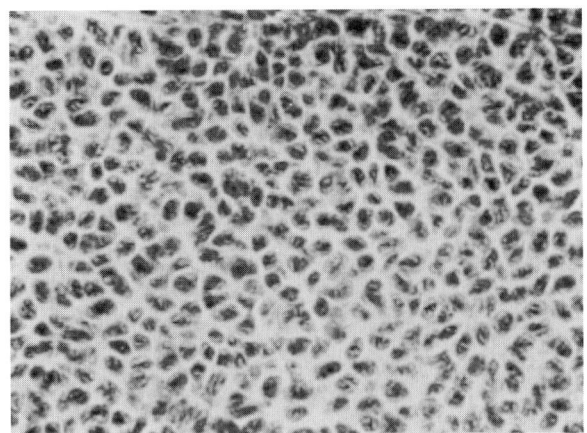

Figure 62–7

Granulosa cell tumor. Note the pale nuclei and prominent grooves ("coffee bean" nuclei). (From Young RH, Scully RE: Ovarian sex cord stromal and steroid cell tumors. In Roth LM, Czernobilsky B [eds]: Tumors and Tumor-like Conditions of the Ovary. New York: Churchill Livingstone, 1985, with permission.)

diffuse (formerly called sarcomatoid), may be seen. The various pathologic patterns do not correlate well with prognosis. Tumor cell nuclei are of variable configuration but are always pale and usually grooved, "coffee bean" nuclei (Fig. 62–7). A variety of other ovarian tumors, especially poorly differentiated adenocarcinoma, are frequently misdiagnosed as granulosa cell tumors.

JUVENILE GRANULOSA CELL TUMOR

This distinct histologic variant accounts for 75% to 85% of granulosa cell tumors in women under age 20 (Scully, 1977; Young et al, 1984). In the prepubertal female, the juvenile granulosa cell tumor may present with signs and symptoms of pseudoprecocious puberty. This tumor appears to have an association with Ollier's disease (multiple endochondromatosis).

Grossly, these tumors are similar to the adult types of granulosa cell tumors; however, their microscopic features are somewhat unique (Fig. 62–8), characterized by cuboidal cells forming nodules and cords. Cytoplasm is abundant, and, in contrast to the adult type, the nuclei are darker and lack grooves. These tumors may be confused with endodermal sinus tumor or embryonal cell carcinoma. Most lesions (98%) are stage IA, and, despite their aggressive histologic appearance, treatment is usually surgery alone.

Thecoma-Fibroma Tumor

The thecoma and fibroma tumors are histologically similar and are often combined for descriptive purposes. The fibroma is hormonally inert and may be associated with Meigs' syndrome (pelvic mass, ascites, pleural effusion—usually right-sided) (Meigs et al, 1943; Dockerty and Masson, 1944; Samanth and Black, 1970), or Gorlin's syndrome (basal cell nevus syndrome/basal cell nevi, carcinomas, dental and bone cysts, soft tissue calcification). Fibromas with a mitotic count greater than 3 mitoses per 10 high-power fields (hpf) are considered to be fibrosarcomas (Prat and Scully, 1981).

Because thecomas may be hormonally active, patients may present with hormonally related symptoms similar to those in patients with granulosa cell tumors. Accordingly, there is an increased frequency of breast and endometrial pathology (Norris and Taylor, 1968). However, thecomas are usually solid and are not associated with rupture or the acute symptoms common with granulosa cell tumors.

Pathologically, the thecoma and the fibroma are very similar. They are both solid, lobulated tumors that are usually 6 cm or smaller in greatest dimensions. The larger fibromas are more likely to be associated with Meigs' syndrome. The cut surface of the ovarian fibroma is usually white to gray; the cut surface of the thecoma is usually white, yellow, or orange. The presence of a yellow color suggests that the tumor may be hormonally active. Fat stains may be necessary to help clarify the nature of the tumor. The microscopic appearance consists of a predominant spindle cell pattern. Nests of plump luteinized theca cells may be identified.

SCLEROSING STROMAL TUMOR

See Chapter 31.

Sertoli-Leydig Cell Tumors (Androblastoma, Arrhenoblastoma)

Sertoli-Leydig cell tumors most commonly occur in women in their late teens, 20s, or early 30s. They constitute fewer than 1% of all ovarian tumors (Young and Scully, 1985). The arrhenoblastoma is the classical virilizing ovarian neoplasm, but only about 30% are androgen-producing. Early signs and symptoms in the young female include defeminizing symptoms, including oligomenorrhea progressing to amenorrhea, breast atrophy, and loss of body contour. Defeminization is followed by masculinization, including acne, deepening of the voice, hirsutism, temporal balding, altered libido, and clitoromegaly.

Grossly, Sertoli-Leydig cell tumors are solid or cystic. On cut surface, they vary in color from gray to yellow with focal areas of hemorrhage. Bilaterality is uncommon (Young and Scully, 1985). Microscopically, Sertoli-Leydig cell tumors contain hollow or solid tubules with intervening bands of fibrous tissue. Poorly differentiated tumors or tumors with heterologous elements, such as skeletal muscle or cartilage, are associated with a higher rate of recurrence.

SERTOLI CELL TUMOR

The pure Sertoli cell tumor (Sertoli cell–only tumor; Pick's adenoma; folliculoma lipidique) is rare and more likely to be feminizing than virilizing (Tavassoli and Norris, 1980; Young and Scully, 1984).

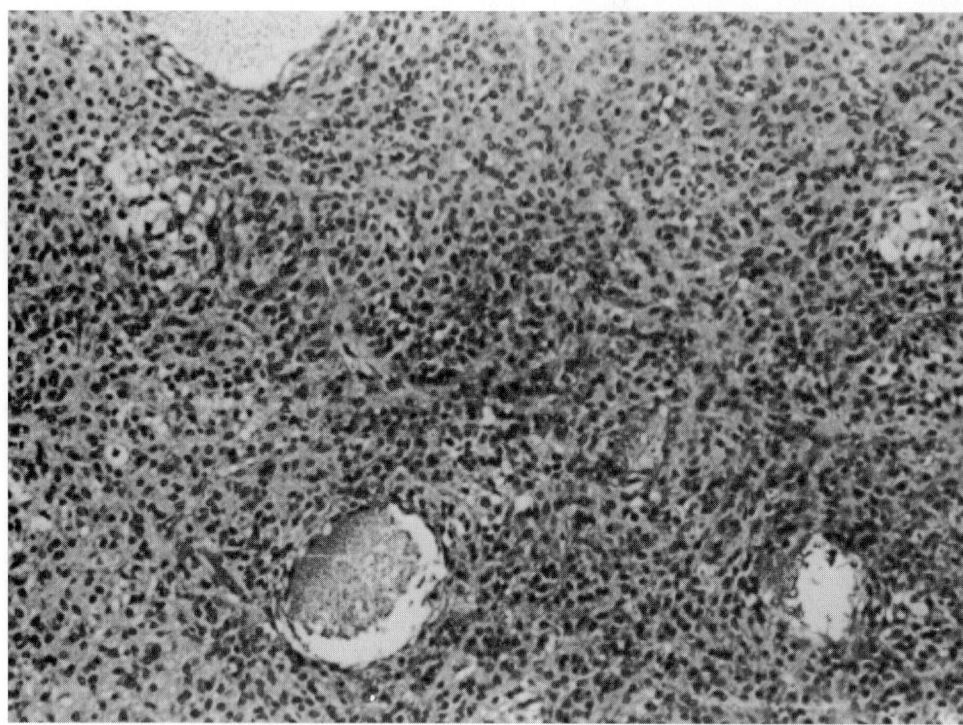

Figure 62–8
Juvenile granulosa cell tumor. Follicles of various shapes separated by cellular areas. In contrast to the adult granulosa cell tumor, note the dark pyknotic nuclei. (Courtesy of Elvio G. Silva, MD.)

Leydig Cell and Lipid Cell Tumors

The Leydig cell tumors (hilus cell tumors) (Fig. 62–9) are usually unilateral, benign, and testosterone-producing. These tumors are usually small and solid. On cut surface, they have a yellow-orange appearance. Microscopically, Reinke crystals may be present; if so, this assures a benign behavior.

These tumors usually occur in postmenopausal women and need to be differentiated from the lipid (lipoid; adrenal rest) cell tumor that behaves in a malignant fashion in about 20% of cases. Lipid (lipoid) cell tumors may be very difficult to differentiate from the Leydig cell tumor. They tend to occur at a younger age. Virilization tends to be more rapid and severe. Cellular atypia mitosis and a large size are suggestive features of malignant behavior. Reinke crystals are absent.

Gynandroblastoma

This combined granulosa cell and Leydig cell tumor is very rare and may be associated with either androgen or estrogen production (Chalvardjian and Derzko, 1982).

Sex Cord Tumor with Annular Tubules

Sex cord tumor with annular tubules is associated with Peutz-Jeghers syndrome (oral and cutaneous pigmentation and gastrointestinal polyps) in about one third of cases. When associated with this syndrome, the tumor is usually bilateral but benign. Adenoma malignum of the cervix occurs in about 15% of these patients. When these tumors occur independently of Peutz-Jeghers syndrome, approximately 20% act in a malignant fashion (Scully, 1970; Young and Scully, 1982; Young et al, 1982).

Unclassified

Seidman reported 32 tumors that could not be classified more specifically and the stage and prognosis were similar to the well differentiated sex cord stromal tumors (Seidman, 1996).

Treatment

Ovarian stromal tumors occurring in the perimenopausal or postmenopausal patient should be surgi-

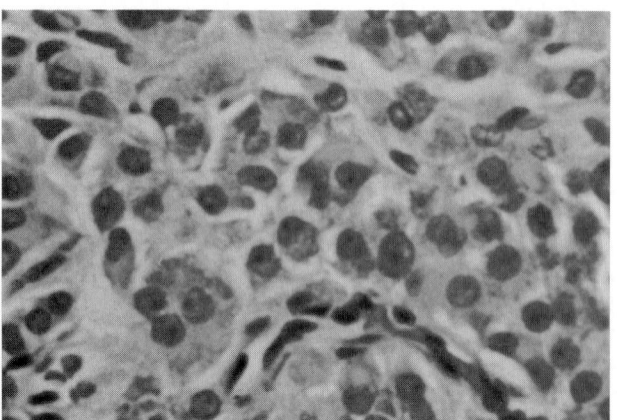

Figure 62–9
Hilus cell tumor. Patient presented with hirsutism and temporal balding.

cally managed with hysterectomy and bilateral salpingo-oophorectomy. Most patients with recurrent granulosa cell tumor experience the recurrence in preserved genital tract tissue (Evans et al, 1980). Stromal tumors may be difficult to interpret histologically on frozen section. Therefore, in the young patient, excision of the tumor and a comprehensive staging procedure are recommended. Cytoreductive surgery should be performed for metastatic disease. The possibility of a concurrent endometrial cancer or endometrial hyperplasia should be evaluated by a uterine curettage if the uterus is retained in patients with a known estrogen-producing tumor.

Although the efficacy of adjuvant therapy in patients with stage I disease has never been assessed, adjuvant therapy should be considered for patients with stromal tumors with tumor rupture, mitoses greater than 2 per 10 hpf, extraovarian spread, or tumors greater than 10 cm in diameter. Adjuvant therapy is also recommended for Sertoli-Leydig tumors with poor differentiation or heterologous elements. Lipid cell tumors with pleomorphism, with increased mitoses, or greater than 8 cm in size should undergo adjuvant treatment. Metastatic or recurrent disease is usually treated with combination chemotherapy regimes such as VAC (Schwartz and Smith, 1976; Slayton, 1984), VBP (Colombo et al, 1986; Gershensen et al, 1996) or platinum, doxorubicin, and cyclophosphamide (Camlibel and Caputo, 1983; Kaye and Davies, 1986; Gershenson et al, 1987). It also should be noted that granulosa cell tumors appear to have good sensitivity to radiation therapy (Schwartz and Smith, 1976).

Prognosis

Granulosa cell tumors carry an overall good prognosis, with a 75% to 90% survival for all stages. Only 5% to 10% of patients with stage I disease experience a recurrence, and many of these tumors recur more than 5 years after diagnosis. Juvenile granulosa cell tumors are also associated with a good prognosis, with only 1% to 2% of patients with stage IA disease and only 10% to 15% of patients with stage IC disease experiencing recurrence. Tumor size (Fox et al, 1975; Stenwig et al, 1979) and tumor rupture (Björkholm and Silfverswärd, 1981) adversely affect survival.

For patients with Sertoli-Leydig tumors, the prognosis is decreased with the less differentiated tumor types and advanced-stage disease, including tumor rupture. In patients with stage I disease but intermediate or poor tumor differentiation, the expected recurrence rate is 3% to 7% (Roth et al, 1981; Zaloudek and Norris, 1984; Young and Scully, 1985).

METASTATIC TUMORS TO THE OVARY

Primary tumors most commonly metastasizing to the ovary include other gynecologic (fallopian tube, endometrium), breast, and gastrointestinal tract tumors (stomach, colon, gallbladder, pancreas). Metastatic spread to the ovaries usually involves both ovaries. Krukenberg, although his name is affixed to ovarian neoplasms demonstrating classic signet-ring cells (Fig. 62–10), actually thought he was describing a primary ovarian mucin-producing sarcoma. In 1902, 6 years after Krukenberg's report, Schlaggenhoffer identified the correct origins of these metastatic tumors.

In most patients with Krukenberg's tumors, the prognosis is poor, with the median survival being less than a year (Hale, 1968). In rare instances, no primary site can be identified and the Krukenberg's tumor may be a primary tumor (Joshi, 1968). However, microscopic primary tumors of the breast or stomach may remain clinically occult for years (Ulbright and Roth, 1985). Tumors metastatic from many primary sites have been reported (Young and Scully, 1987) and must be considered when atypical ovarian histology is encountered.

NONSPECIFIC MESENCHYMAL OVARIAN TUMORS

The nonspecific benign mesenchymal ovarian tumors are reviewed in Chapter 31.

Fibroma

The fibroma, although a nonspecific mesenchymal ovarian tumor, has been included with thecomas in this chapter because of its similarity to the thecoma.

Lymphoma

Ovarian lymphomas are rare and may be primary or from disseminated lymphoma. On occasion the ovarian tumors can be the presenting manifestation of disseminated disease (Osborne and Robboy, 1983).

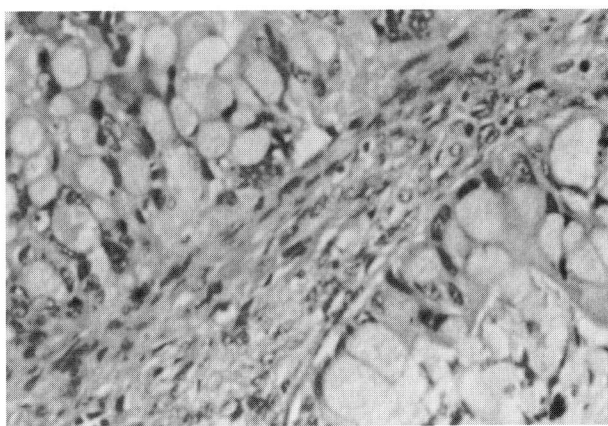

Figure 62–10
Krukenberg's tumor: a colon carcinoma metastatic to ovaries. High-power view of signet-ring cells.

After the jaws, the second most common site for Burkitt's lymphoma is the ovary. All patients with ovarian lymphoma require accurate staging and adequate therapy, usually consisting of regional irradiation and chemotherapy.

A variety of other ovarian tumors can be confused with the ovarian lymphoma, including the dysgerminoma, granulosa cell tumor, leukemia, neuroblastoma, embryonal rhabdomyosarcoma, and metastatic carcinoma from breast or lung (small cell) (Talerman, 1987b).

SMALL CELL CARCINOMA

This rare aggressive ovarian tumor tends to develop in young patients, age 9 to 43 (average 24) years of age (Young et al, 1994). In approximately two-thirds of cases, there is an associated hypercalcemia secondary to a parathyroid hormone-related protein. There may be some association between p53 gene mutations and the evolution of this tumor (Seidman, 1995). Similar to the malignant nondysgerminomatous germ cell tumors, patients with stage IA disease without adjuvant chemotherapy have an estimated survival of about 30% (Young et al, 1994). Since a few patients with more advanced disease have been salvaged with aggressive adjuvant treatment (Young et al, 1994; Reed, 1995; Powell et al, 1998), it seems reasonable that adjuvant chemotherapy should be standard management in all patients with this disease.

REFERENCES

Ablin AR, Krailo NKC, Ramsay MH, et al: Results of treatment of malignant germ cell tumors in 93 children: a report from the Children's Cancer Study Group. J Clin Oncol 1991;9:1782.

Aiman J, Forney JP, Parker CR Jr: Androgen and estrogen secretion by normal and neoplastic ovaries in premenopausal women. Obstet Gynecol 1986a;68:327.

Aiman J, Forney JP, Parker CR Jr: Secretion of androgens and estrogens by normal and neoplastic ovaries in postmenopausal women. Obstet Gynecol 1986b;68:1.

Aiman J, Nalick RH, Jacobs A, et al: The origin of androgen and estrogen in a virilized postmenopausal woman with bilateral benign cystic teratomas. Obstet Gynecol 1977;49:695.

Awais GM: Dysgerminoma and serum lactic dehydrogenase levels. Obstet Gynecol 1983;61:99.

Axe SR, Klein VR, Woodruff JD: Choriocarcinoma of the ovary. Obstet Gynecol 1985;66:111.

Bajorin DF, Sarosdy MF, Pfister DG, et al: Randomized trial of etoposide and cisplatin versus etoposide and carboplatin in patients with good-risk germ cell tumors: a multi-institutional study. J Clin Oncol 1993;11:598.

Bekaii-Saab T, Einhorn LH, Williams SD: Late relapse of ovarian dysgerminoma: case report and literature review. Gynecol Oncol 1999;72:111.

Bergher de Bacalao E, Dominguez I: Unilateral gonadoblastoma in a pregnant woman. Am J Obstet Gynecol 1969;105:1279.

Björkholm E, Silverswärd C: Prognostic factors in granulosa cell tumors. Gynecol Oncol 1981;11:261.

Boggess JF, Soules MR, Goff BA, Greer BE, Cain JM: Serum inhibin and disease status in women with ovarian granulosa cell tumors. Gynecol Oncol 1997;64:64.

Camlibel FT, Caputo TA: Chemotherapy of granulosa cell tumors. Am J Obstet Gynecol 1983;145:763.

Carlson RW, Sikie BI, Turbow MM, Ballon SC: Combination cis-platin, vinblastine, and bleomycin chemotherapy (PVB) for malignant germ cell tumors of the ovary. J Clin Oncol 1983;1:645.

Casey AC, Bhodauria S, Shapter A, et al: Dysgerminoma: the role of conservative surgery. Gynecol Oncol 1996;63:352.

Chalvardjian A, Derzko C: Gynandroblastoma: its ultrastructure. Cancer 1982;50:710.

Chapman DC, Grover R, Schwartz PE: Conservative management of an ovarian polyembryoma. Obstet Gynecol 1994;83:879.

Colombo N, Sessa C, Landoni F, et al: Cisplatin, vinblastine, and bleomycin combination chemotherapy in metastatic granulosa cell tumor of the ovary. Obstet Gynecol 1986;67:265.

Copeland LJ, Landon MB: Malignant diseases and pregnancy. In Gabbe SG, Niebyl JR, Simpson JL (eds). Obstetrics: Normal and Problem Pregnancies, 3rd ed. New York: Churchill Livingstone 1996:1157.

Creasman WT, Soper JT: Assessment of contemporary management of germ cell malignances of the ovary. Am J Obstet Gynecol 1985;153:828.

Culine S, Lhomme C, Kattan J, et al: Cisplatin-based chemotherapy in the management of germ cell tumors of the ovary: The Institut Gustave Roussy experience. Gynecol Oncol 1997;64:160.

Curry SL, Smith JP, Gallagher HS: Malignant teratoma of the ovary: prognostic factors and treatment. Am J Obstet Gynecol 1978;131:845.

Curtin JP, Rubin SC, Hoskins WJ, et al: Second-look laparotomy in endodermal sinus tumor: a report of two patients with normal levels of alpha-fetoprotein and residual tumor at reexploration. Obstet Gynecol 1989;73:893.

Devaney K, Snyder R, Norris HS, Tavassoli FA: Proliferative and histologically malignant struma ovarii: a clinicopathologic study of 54 cases. Int J Gynecol Pathol 1993;12:333.

Dockerty MB, Masson JC: Ovarian fibromas: a clinical and pathologic study of two hundred and eighty-three cases. Am J Obstet Gynecol 1944;47:741.

Doss N Jr, Forney JP, Vellios F: Covert bilaterality of mature ovarian teratomas. Obstet Gynecol 1977;50:651.

Doss BJ, Jacques SM, Qureshi F, et al: Immature teratomas of the genital tract in older women. Gynecol Oncol 1999;73:433.

Einhorn LH, Donohue JP: Cisdiammine dichloroplatinum, vinblastine, and bleomycin combination chemotherapy in disseminated testicular cancer. Ann Intern Med 1977;87:293.

Evans AT, Gaffey TA, Malkasian GD Jr, Annegers JF: Clinicopathologic review of 118 granulosa and 82 theca cell tumors. Obstet Gynecol 1980;55:231.

Fox H, Agrawal K, Langley FA: A clinicopathologic study of 92 cases of granulosa cell tumor of the ovary with special reference to the factors influencing prognosis. Cancer 1975;35:231.

Gallion H, van Nagell JR Jr, Donaldson ES, et al: Immature teratoma of the ovary. Am J Obstet Gynecol 1983;146:361.

Gallion H, van Nagell JR Jr, Powell DF, et al: Therapy of endodermal sinus tumor of the ovary. Am J Obstet Gynecol 1979;135:447.

Gerbie MV, Brewer JI, Tamimi H: Primary choriocarcinoma of the ovary. Obstet Gynecol 1975;46:720.

Gershenson DM: Menstrual and reproductive function after treatment with combination chemotherapy for malignant ovarian germ cell tumors. J Clin Oncol 1988;6:270.

Gershenson DM: Second-look laparotomy in endodermal sinus tumor: a report of two patients with normal levels of alpha-fetoprotein and residual tumor at reexploration [letter]. Obstet Gynecol 1989;74:683.

Gershenson DM, Copeland LJ, Del Junco G, et al: Second-look laparotomy in the management of malignant germ cell tumors of the ovary. Obstet Gynecol 1986a;67:789.

Gershenson DM, Copeland LJ, Kavanagh JJ, et al: Treatment of malignant nondysgerminomatous germ cell tumors of the ovary with vincristine, dactinomycin, and cyclophosphamide. Cancer 1985;56:2756.

Gershenson DM, Copeland LJ, Kavanagh JJ, et al: Treatment of metastatic stromal tumors of the ovary with cisplatin, doxorubicin, and cyclophosphamide. Obstet Gynecol 1987;70:765.

Gershenson DM, Del Junco G, Copeland LJ, Rutledge FN: Mixed germ cell tumors of the ovary. Obstet Gynecol 1984;64:200.

Gershenson DM, Del Junco G, Herson J, Rutledge FN: Endodermal sinus tumor of the ovary: the M. D. Anderson experience. Obstet Gynecol 1983;61:194.

Gershenson DM, Kavanagh JJ, Copeland LJ, et al: Treatment of malignant nondysgerminomatous germ cell tumors of the ovary with vinblastine, bleomycin, and cisplatin. Cancer 1986b; 57:1731.

Gershenson DM, Morris M, Burke TW, et al: Treatment of poor prognosis sex cord stromal tumors of the ovary with the combination of bleomycin, etoposide, and cisplatin. Obstet Gynecol 1996;87:527.

Gershenson DM, Morris M, Cangir A, et al: Treatment of malignant germ cell tumors of the ovary with bleomycin, etoposide and cisplatin. J Clin Oncol 1990;8:715.

Gordon A, Lipton D, Woodruff JD: Dysgerminoma: a review of 158 cases from the Emil Novak Ovarian Tumor Registry. Obstet Gynecol 1981;58:497.

Gordon A, Rosenshein N, Parmley T, Bhagavan D: Benign cystic teratomas in postmenopausal women. Am J Obstet Gynecol 1980;138:1120.

Hale RW: Krukenberg tumor of the ovaries: a review of 81 records. Obstet Gynecol 1968;32:221.

Harstrick A, Schmoll HJ, Wilke H, et al: Cisplatin, etoposide and ifosfamide salvage therapy for refractory or relapsing germ cell carcinoma. J Clin Oncol 1991;9:1549.

Hart WR, Burkons DM: Germ cell neoplasms arising in gonadoblastomas. Cancer 1979;43:668.

Ihara T, Ohama K, Satoh H, et al: Histologic grade and karyotype of immature teratoma of the ovary. Cancer 1984;54:2988.

Jacobs AJ, Newland JR, Green RK: Pure choriocarcinoma of the ovary. Obstet Gynecol Surv 1982;37:603.

Jarrell JF: Reproductive conservation. Can J Surg 1990;33:337.

Jimerson GK, Woodruff JD: Ovarian extraembryonal teratoma: 2. Endodermal sinus tumor mixed with other germ cell tumors. Am J Obstet Gynecol 1977;127:302.

Joshi VV: Primary Krukenberg tumor of ovary: review of literature and case report. Cancer 1968;22:1199.

Julian CG, Barrett JM, Richardson RL, Greco FA: Bleomycin, vinblastine and cisplatinum in the treatment of advanced endodermal sinus tumor. Obstet Gynecol 1980;56:396.

Kawai M, Kano T, Furuhashi Y, et al: Immature teratoma of the ovary. Gynecol Oncol 1991;40:133.

Kaye SB, Davies E: Cyclophosphamide, Adriamycin, and cisplatinum for the treatment of advanced granulosa cell tumor, using serum estradiol as a tumor marker. Gynecol Oncol 1986; 24:261.

Kempers RD, Dockerty MD, Hoffman DI: Struma ovarii-ascitic, hyperthyroid, and asymptomatic syndromes. Ann Intern Med 1970;72:883.

Krepart G, Smith JP, Rutledge F, Declos L: The treatment of dysgerminoma of the ovary. Cancer 1978;42:986.

Kurman RJ, Norris HJ: Embryonal carcinoma of the ovary. Cancer 1976a;38:2420.

Kurman RJ, Norris HJ: Malignant mixed germ cell tumors of the ovary: a clinical and pathologic analysis of 30 cases. Obstet Gynecol 1976b;48:579.

Kurman RJ, Norris HJ: Malignant germ cell tumors of the ovary. Hum Pathol 1977;8:551.

Lappohn RE, Burger HG, Bouma J, et al: Inhibin as a marker for granulosa-cell tumors. N Engl J Med 1989;321:790.

Linder D, McCaw BK, Hecht F: Parthenogenic origin of benign ovarian teratoma. N Engl J Med 1975;292:63.

Liu TL, Linn IJ, Deppe G: Serum lactic dehydrogenase (SLDH) in germ cell malignancies of the ovary. Gynecol Oncol 1984;19: 355.

Loehrer PJ, Johnson D, Elson P, Einhorn LH, Trump D: Importance of bleomycin in favorable-prognosis disseminated germ cell tumors: an Eastern Cooperative Oncology Group trial. J Clin Oncol 1995;13:470.

Loehrer PJ, Lauer R, Roth BJ, et al: Salvage therapy with VP-16 or vinblastine plus ifosfamide plus cisplatin in recurrent germ cell cancer. Ann Intern Med 1988;109:540.

Luzzato R, Murray JM, Gallagher HS: Gonadoblastomas associated with malignant teratoma. South Med J 1979;72:624.

Maeyama M, Tayama C, Inoue S, et al: Serial serum determination on α-fetoprotein as a marker of the effect of postoperative chemotherapy in ovarian endodermal sinus tumor. Gynecol Oncol 1984;17:104.

Malkasian GD, Webb MJ, Jorgensen EO: Observations on chemotherapy of granulosa cell carcinomas and malignant ovarian teratomas. Obstet Gynecol 1974;44:885.

Marina NM, Rao B, Etcubanas E, et al: The role of second-look surgery in the management of advanced germ cell malignancies. Cancer 1991;68:309.

Meigs JV, Armstrong SH, Hamilton HH: A further contribution to the syndrome of fibroma of the ovary with fluid in the abdomen and chest: Meigs' syndrome. Am J Obstet Gynecol 1943; 46:19.

Micha JP, Kucera PR, Berman ML, et al: Malignant ovarian germ cell tumors: a review of thirty-six cases. Am J Obstet Gynecol 1985;152:842.

Mitchell MF, Gershenson DM, Soeters R-P, et al: The long-term effects of radiation therapy on patients with ovarian dysgerminoma. Cancer 1991;67:1084.

Munkarah A, Gershenson DM, Levenback C, et al: Salvage surgery for chemorefractory ovarian germ cell tumors. Gynecol Oncol 1994;54:217.

Nogales FF Jr, Matilla A, Nogales-Ortiz F, Galera-Davidson HL: Yolk sac tumors with pure and mixed polyvesicular vitelline patterns. Human Pathol 1978;9:553.

Norris HJ, Taylor HB: Prognosis of granulosa-theca tumors of the ovary. Cancer 1968;21:255.

Norris HJ, Zirkin HJ, Benson WL: Immature (malignant) teratoma of the ovary. Cancer 1976;37:2359.

Ohel G, Kaneti H, Schenker JG: Granulosa cell tumors in Israel: a study of 172 cases. Gynecol Oncol 1983;15:278.

Osborne BM, Robboy SJ: Lymphomas or leukemia presenting as ovarian tumors: an analysis of 42 cases. Cancer 1983;52:1933.

Park NH, Ryu SY, Park IA, Kang SB, Lee HP: Primary endodermal sinus tumor of the omentum. Gynecol Oncol 1999;72:427.

Payne D, Muss HB, Homesley HD, et al: Autoimmune hemolytic anemia and ovarian dermoid cysts: case report and review of the literature. Cancer 1981;48:721.

Pinkerton CR, Pritchard J, Spitz L: High complete response rate in children with advanced germ cell tumors using cisplatin-containing combination chemotherapy. J Clin Oncol 1986;4:194.

Pins MR, Young RH, Daly WJ, Scully RE: Primary squamous cell carcinoma of the ovary. Report of 37 cases. Am J Surg Pathol 1996;20:823.

Pippitt CH, Cain JM, Hakest B, et al: Primary chemotherapy and the role of second-look laparotomy in nondysgerminomatous germ cell malignancies of the ovary. Gynecol Oncol 1988;31: 268.

Powell JL, McAfee RD, McCoy RC, Shiro BS: Uterine and ovarian conservation in advanced small cell carcinoma of the ovary. Obstet Gynecol 1998;91:846.

Prat J, Scully RE: Cellular fibromas and fibrosarcomas of the ovary: a comparative clinicopathologic analysis of seventeen cases. Cancer 1981;47:2663.

Pressley RH, Muntz HG, Falkenberry S, Rice LW: Case Report: serum lactic dehydrogenase as a tumor marker in dysgerminoma. Gynecol Oncol 1992;44:281.

Reed WC: Small cell carcinoma of the ovary with hypercalcemia: report of a case of survival without recurrence 5 years after surgery and chemotherapy. Gynecol Oncol 1995;56:452.

Robboy SJ, Norris HJ, Scully RE: Insular carcinoid primary in the ovary—a clinicopathologic analysis of 48 cases. Cancer 1975; 36:404.

Robboy SJ, Scully RE: Ovarian teratoma with glial implants on the peritoneum. Hum Pathol 1970;1:643.

Robboy SJ, Scully RE: Strumal carcinoid of the ovary: an analysis of 50 cases of distinctive tumor composed of thyroid tissue and carcinoid. Cancer 1980;46:2019.

Robboy SJ, Scully RE, Norris HJ: Carcinoid metastatic to the ovary: a clinicopathologic analysis of 35 cases. Cancer 1974;33: 798.

Robboy SJ, Scully RE, Norris HJ: Primary trabecular carcinoid of the ovary. Obstet Gynecol 1977;49:202.

Roth LM, Anderson MC, Govan ADT, et al: Sertoli-Leydig cell tumors: a clinicopathologic study of 34 cases. Cancer 1981;48: 187.

Samanth KK, Black WC: Benign ovarian stromal tumors associated with free peritoneal fluid. Am J Obstet Gynecol 1970;107: 538.

Santala M, Burger H, Ruokonen A, Stenback F, Kauppila A: Elevated serum inhibin and tumor-associated trypsin inhibitor concentrations in a young woman with dysgerminoma of the ovary. Gynecol Oncol 1998;71:465.

Schiller W: Mesonephroma ovarri. Am J Cancer 1939;35:1.

Schwartz PE: Combination chemotherapy in the management of ovarian germ cell malignancies. Obstet Gynecol 1984;64:564.

Schwartz PE, Chambers SK, Chambers JT, et al: Ovarian germ cell malignancies: the Yale University experience. Gynecol Oncol 1992;45:26.

Schwartz PE, Smith JP: Treatment of ovarian stromal tumors. Am J Obstet Gynecol 1976;125:402.

Scully RE: Gonadoblastoma: a gonadal tumor related to the dysgerminoma (seminoma) and capable of sex hormone production. Cancer 1953;6:455.

Scully RE: Sex cord tumor with annular tubules, a distinctive ovarian tumor of the Peutz-Jeghers syndrome. Cancer 1970;25: 1107.

Scully RE: Ovarian tumors: a review. Am J Pathol 1977;87: 686.

Scully RE: Tumors of the ovary and maldeveloped gonads. In Atlas of Tumor Pathology. 2nd series, Fasc 16. Washington, DC: Armed Forces Institute of Pathology, 1979.

Seidman JD: Small cell carcinoma of the ovary with hypercalcemic type: p53 protein accumulation and clinicopathologic features. Gynecol Oncol 1995;59:283.

Seidman JD: Unclassified ovarian gonadal stromal tumors: a clinicopathologic study of 32 cases. Am J Surg Pathol 1996;20:699.

Serov SF, Scully RE, Sobin LH: International Histologic Classification of Tumors, No. 9: Histologic Typing of Ovarian Tumors. Geneva: World Health Organization, 1973.

Sheiko MC, Hart WR: Ovarian germinoma (dysgerminoma) with elevated serum lactic dehydrogenase: case report and review of literature. Cancer 1982;49:994.

Slayton RE: Management of germ cell and stromal cell tumors of the ovary. Semin Oncol 1984;11:299.

Slayton RE, Park RC, Silverberg SG, et al: Vincristine, dactinomycin, and cyclophosphamide in the treatment of malignant germ cell tumors of the ovary—a Gynecologic Oncology Group study. Cancer 1985;56:1341.

Smales E, Peckham MJ: Chemotherapy of germ cell ovarian tumors: first-line treatment with etoposide, bleomycin and cisplatin or carboplatin. Eur J Cancer Clin Oncol 1987;23:469.

Smith EB, Clarke-Pearson DL, Creasman WT: A VP16-231- and cisplatin-containing regimen for treatment of refractory ovarian germ cell malignancies. Am J Obstet Gynecol 1984;150:927.

Smith JP, Rutledge F: Advances in chemotherapy for gynecologic cancer. Cancer 1975;36:669.

Stenwig JT, Hazekamp JT, Beecham JB: Granulosa cell tumors of the ovary: a clinicopathological study of 118 cases with long-term follow-up. Gynecol Oncol 1979;7:136.

Stern JL, Buscema J, Rosenshein NB, Woodruff JD: Spontaneous rupture of benign cystic teratomas. Obstet Gynecol 1981;57: 363.

Stuart GC, Smith JP: Rupture of benign cystic teratomas mimicking gynecologic malignancy. Gynecol Oncol 1983;16:139.

Suzuki M, Kobayashi H, Ohwada M, Terao T, Sato I: Macrophage colony-stimulating factor as a marker for malignant germ cell tumors of the ovary. Gynecol Oncol 1998;68:35.

Szyfelbein WM, Young RH, Scully RE: Cystic struma ovarii: a frequently unrecognized tumor. A report of 20 cases. Am J Surg Pathol 1994;18:785.

Takeda A, Ishizuka T, Goto T, et al: Polyembryoma of ovary producing alpha-fetoprotein and hCG: immunoperoxidase and electron microscopic study. Cancer 1982;49:1878.

Takemori M, Nishimura R, Sugimura K, Obayashi C, Yasuda D: Ovarian strumal carcinoid with markedly high serum levels of tumor markers. Gynecol Oncol 1995;58:266.

Talerman A: Gonadoblastoma associated with embryonal carcinoma. Obstet Gynecol 1974;43:138.

Talerman A: Germ cell tumors of the ovary. In Kurman RJ (ed): Blaustein's Pathology of the Female Genital Tract. 3rd ed. New York: Springer-Verlag, 1987a:659.

Talerman A: Nonspecific tumors of the ovary. In Kurman RJ (ed): Blaustein's Pathology of the Female Genital Tract. 3rd ed. New York: Springer-Verlag, 1987b:735.

Tavassoli FA, Norris HJ: Sertoli tumors of the ovary: a clinicopathologic study of 28 cases with ultrastructural observations. Cancer 1980;46:2281.

Taylor MH, DePetrillo AD, Turner AR: Vinblastine, bleomycin, and cisplatin in malignant germ cell tumors of the ovary. Cancer 1985;56:1341.

Teilum G: Gonocytoma: homologous ovarian and testicular tumors. 1. With discussion of "mesonephroma ovarii" (Schiller: Am J Cancer 1939). Acta Pathol Microbiol Scand 1946;23:242.

Teilum G: Endodermal sinus tumors of the ovary and testis: comparative morphogenesis of the so-called mesonephroma ovarii (Schiller) and extra-embryonic (yolk sac allantoic) structures of the rat placenta. Cancer 1959;12:1092.

Teilum G: Classification of endodermal sinus tumor (mesoblastoma vitellinum) and so-called "embryonal carcinoma" of the ovary. Acta Pathol Microbiol Scand 1965;64:407.

Teilum G: Special Tumors of Ovary and Testis and Related Extragonadal Lesions. Comparative Pathology and Histological Identification. 2nd ed. Philadelphia: JB Lippincott Company, 1977.

Thomas GM, Dembo AJ, Hacker NF, DePetrillo AD: Current therapy for dysgerminoma of the ovary. Obstet Gynecol 1987;70: 268.

Ulbright TM, Roth LM: Secondary tumors of the ovary. In Roth LM, Czernobilsky B (eds): Tumors and Tumor-like Conditions of the Ovary (Contemporary Issues in Surgical Pathology. No. 6). New York: Churchill Livingstone, 1985:129.

Wax JR, Segna RA: Recurrent mixed germ cell tumor of the ovary manifest as an unexplained elevated maternal serum alpha-fetoprotein. J Matern Fetal Med 1997;6:338.

Waxman M, Boyce JG: Intraperitoneal rupture of benign cystic ovarian teratoma. Obstet Gynecol 1976;49:9s.

Williams SD: Current management of ovarian germ cell tumors. Oncology 1994;8:53.

Williams SD, Blessing JA, Hatch KD, Homesley HD: Chemotherapy of advanced dysgerminoma: trials of the Gynecologic Oncology Group. J Clin Oncol 1991;9:1950.

Williams SD, Blessing JA, Moore DH, et al: Cisplatin, vinblastine, and bleomycin in advanced and recurrent ovarian germ cell tumors. Ann Intern Med 1989;111:22.

Williams SD, Einhorn LH, Greco FA, et al: VP-16-213 salvage therapy for refractory germinal neoplasms. Cancer 1980;46: 2154.

Yannopoulous D, Yannopoulous K, Ossowski R: Malignant struma ovarii. Pathol Ann 1976;11:403.

Young RH, Scully RE: Ovarian sex cord-stromal tumors: recent progress. Int J Gynecol Pathol 1982;1:101.

Young RH, Scully RE: Ovarian Sertoli cell tumors: a report of 10 cases. Int J Gynecol Pathol 1984;2:349.

Young RH, Scully RE: Ovarian Sertoli-Leydig cell tumors: a clinicopathological analysis of 207 cases. Am J Surg Pathol 1985;9: 543.

Young RH, Scully RE: Metastatic tumors of the ovary. In Kurman RJ (ed). Blaustein's Pathology of the Female Genital Tract. 3rd ed. New York: Springer-Verlag, 1987:742.

Young RH, Dickersin GR, Scully RE: Juvenile granulosa cell tumor of the ovary. Am J Surg Pathol 1984;8:575.

Young RH, Oliva E, Scully RE: Small cell carcinoma of the ovary, hypercalcemic type. A clinicopathological analysis of 150 cases. Am J Surg Pathol 1994;18:1102.

Young RH, Welch WR, Dickersin GR, Scully RE: Ovarian sex cord tumor with annular tubules. Cancer 1982;50:1384.

Zaloudek C, Norris HJ: Sertoli-Leydig tumors of the ovary: a clinicopathologic study of 64 intermediate and poorly differentiated neoplasms. Am J Surg Pathol 1984;8:405.

63 | Fallopian Tube Neoplasms

L. Stewart Massad
David G. Mutch

HISTORY

Carcinoma of the fallopian tube was first described by Renaud in 1847 (Doran, 1896). Orthmann (1888) published the first case report, but standard diagnostic criteria were not developed until the series of 478 cases described by Hu et al in 1950. Dodson and colleagues (1970) proposed the staging system that became accepted. To date, reports of more than 1500 cases of fallopian tube cancer have been published.

EPIDEMIOLOGY

Fallopian tube cancer is one of the rarest cancers of the female genital tract, comprising only 0.1% to 1.0% of female genital malignancies in series reported from referral centers. Because this cancer is so rare, there are no epidemiologic studies describing this disease. The average patient presents in her sixth decade, but there have been reports of this disease developing in teenagers and octogenarians. In some series, tubal cancer appeared to be associated with low parity, but many patients who develop this disease are multiparous. More than 1500 cases of this disease have been reported in the literature, but this comprises most case reports and small case series; this makes comparative analysis between series difficult (Gurney et al, 1990).

Nonetheless, in a review of the literature in 1994, Nordin calculated that the mean age at presentation was 56.7 years, which is similar to reports by other authors (Sedlis, 1978; Schink and Lurain, 1991) who quoted 52 and 53 years, respectively. The age-specific incidence of fallopian tube carcinoma is similar to that of ovarian cancer, suggesting a common etiologic factor. Both ovarian and fallopian tube carcinoma appear to associated with nulliparity (Rosenblatt et al, 1989; Nordin, 1994.) The nulliparity rate is about 27%, compared to 34% calculated from U.S. tumor registries, with mean parity of 1.7 (Nordin, 1994).

In some early reports, an association with tubal inflammation or tuberculous pelvic infection was described, but this appears to be either coincidental or secondary to the tumor itself. Therefore no etiologic role related to prior infection can be assumed.

PATHOLOGY

The majority of fallopian tube carcinomas are papillary serous adenocarcinomas, but adenocarcinomas of other histologic types, such as squamous carcinomas, transitional cell carcinomas, and sarcomas, have been reported. A group of 26 endometrioid adenocarcinomas of the fallopian tube were described by Navani et al (1996). This histologic type was believed to carry a slightly better prognosis than the papillary serous histology. The distal tube is most commonly involved, but disease can involve the isthmic and intramural portions of the tube as well. Obstruction of the fimbria and the uterotubal junction by tumor or by prior inflammation can cause massive distention with resulting hydrosalpinx. Bilateral disease occurs in about 25% of cases (Sedlis, 1961).

Primary cancers of the fallopian tube are rare and must be distinguished from metastases, especially those arising from an ovarian cancer. Criteria for distinguishing ovarian cancer from fallopian tube carcinoma were established by Hu et al (1950). First, in fallopian tube carcinoma, the bulk of the cancer must be in the fallopian tube. Second, mucosal involvement should predominate microscopically, with a papillary pattern. Third, if the tubal wall is extensively involved, there should be an observed transition between benign and malignant epithelium in the tubal wall. Finally, if ovarian or endometrial metastases are present, they must contain less tumor than the tube or have only superficial implants.

Hu et al (1950) also defined three grades of fallopian tube cancer. Papillary, alveolar, and medullary growth patterns were considered to be progressively more advanced grades of disease, showing increasing amounts of solid growth, atypia, and mitotic figures. These authors attempted to correlate grade with prognosis. At the time of their report, none of five patients with grade 3 disease and six of seven patients with grades 1 and 2 disease had survived. However, later retrospective series with larger numbers have shown that tumor grade has no prognostic value. To date there have been no prospective trials that evaluate this characteristic.

Pfeiffer et al (1989) found that 83% of patients without lymphvascular space invasion survived 5 years after diagnosis, whereas only 29% of patients whose tumors invaded lymphvascular spaces survived 5 years. The incidence of second primary malignancies also appears to be increased for patients with cancer of the fallopian tube. Peters et al (1988), in their review of 115 women with tubal cancer, found a 15% incidence of second cancers, with breast and endometrial cancers being the most common. One report distinguished "multifocal upper genital tract malignancy" from true fallopian tube cancer as defined by the above criteria (Rose and Piver, 1990).

Pathologic examination of fallopian tubes removed for reasons other than suspicion of carcinoma sometimes reveals areas of cellular proliferation and atypia that are histologically similar to in situ carcinomas found in other organs. The significance of these lesions is controversial. Moore and Enterline (1975) exhaustively sectioned fallopian tubes from all 124 salpingectomy specimens submitted to their laboratory during a 6-month period. They found that almost 20% of patients had proliferative lesions and suggested, based on these findings and the known low incidence of fallopian tube carcinoma, that these could not be malignant precursors. Stern and colleagues (1981) found no recurrences in the follow-up of five patients diagnosed with carcinoma in situ after partial unilateral salpingo-oophorectomy. However, Schiller and Silverberg (1971) reported two patients who died with "intra-abdominal carcinomatosis" after salpingectomy showed "intramucosal carcinoma." At present, close follow-up but no further therapy appears indicated in patients with atypical epithelial lesions of the fallopian tube. Tubes that show atypical proliferation should be evaluated with multiple histologic sections to exclude an adjacent microscopic focus of invasive cancer.

DIAGNOSIS

Late-stage fallopian tube carcinoma often presents like ovarian cancer. Because of its rarity, early-stage fallopian tube cancer is usually considered in the differential diagnosis of a pelvic mass. Therefore fallopian tube carcinoma is not often diagnosed preoperatively. The correct preoperative diagnosis was made in only 2 of 71 patients in the series published by Eddy et al (1984b). The two classical diagnostic triads for fallopian tube cancer are vaginal discharge, irregular vaginal bleeding and a pelvic mass, or pelvic pain, a pelvic mass, and serosanguinous vaginal discharge (Latzko's triad). However, most patients with fallopian tube carcinoma have nonspecific symptoms, and therefore patients are usually diagnosed with the disease after laparotomy. Typical symptoms include discharge and bleeding as well as pelvic pain from tubal distention, weight loss, fatigue, and vague gastrointestinal or urinary tract symptoms. Many patients with early fallopian tube cancer are diagnosed incidentally at the time of laparotomy for other diseases.

Hydrops tubae profluens, the discharge of serous or serosanguinous fluid from the vagina associated with resolution of a painful pelvic mass, has been considered pathognomonic for tubal cancer. It occurs when fluid accumulates in a tube obstructed by tumor, causing pain that is relieved by release of fluid through the lower genital tract. This sign has proved to be quite rare because it requires complete distal and partial proximal tubal obstruction. It was reported in only 11 of 122 cases where this symptom was evaluated (Henderson et al, 1977; Raju and Wiltshaw, 1981; Semrad et al, 1986; Muntz et al, 1989; Nordin, 1994). Furthermore, it has been specifically reported as not occurring in several series (Tamimi and Figge, 1981; Roberts and Lifschitz, 1982; Pfeiffer et al, 1989).

Most patients with cancer of the fallopian tube have a pelvic mass and present with bleeding or abdominal pain (Nordin, 1994). Ascites, sometimes massive, is seen with advanced disease. Pleural effusions suggest transdiaphragmatic spread of malignant cells. Inguinal and supraclavicular adenopathy usually occurs only in combination with widespread intraperitoneal cancer. None of these findings are specific for fallopian tube cancer.

Laboratory tests are similarly nonspecific. Abnormal vaginal cytology has been touted as useful in the diagnosis of fallopian tube cancer, but large series have found it to be neither sensitive nor specific. CA-125 antigen levels may be elevated preoperatively (Tokunaga et al, 1990), but this occurs more commonly in association with ovarian cancer. When elevated in a patient with fallopian tube cancer, CA-125 may be used as a reliable tumor marker because it reflects volume of disease.

Imaging studies, including computerized tomography and ultrasonography, lack the ability to distinguish tubal from ovarian masses reliably and cannot differentiate tubal cancers from inflammatory diseases or endometriomas of the tube. However, a fusiform or sausage-shaped cystic mass with solid luminal projections distinct from the ovary is highly suggestive of primary tubal cancer (Meyer et al, 1987). Hysterosalpingography has been reported to identify tubal carcinoma accurately by demonstrating an intraluminal mass causing distal dilation (Hinton et al, 1988), but the test is useless when the tumor causes proximal obstruction. Most authors advise against this test to avoid lavage of malignant cells from the tubal lumen into the peritoneal cavity (Sedlis, 1978).

STAGING

Fallopian tube carcinoma is similar to ovarian carcinoma in its propensity to metastasize by exfoliation of cells into the abdominal cavity. Unlike ovarian cancer, however, fallopian tube cancer begins in a hollow viscus, and early lesions may be less likely to be associated with extensive intraperitoneal carcinoma. This is particularly so if distal tubal occlusion occurs, blocking the passage of shed malignant cells into the peritoneal cavity. As a result of this, extraperitoneal recurrence is not uncommon, as described by Semrad et al (1986) and confirmed by others. Tubal cancer also has a propensity for metastasis to lymph nodes, especially those in the para-aortic chain (Tamimi and Figge, 1981).

No system of staging has been defined by the International Federation of Gynecology and Obstetrics (FIGO), but categories have been defined by convention that are analogous to the FIGO staging of ovarian cancer (Table 63–1). This staging system has been shown to have prognostic importance. Momtazee and Kempson (1968) combined 8 patients from their institution with 31 others previously reported and found 3-year survival rates of 60% among patients with stage I disease, 40% among patients with stage II disease, and 9% among patients with stage III/IV disease. Denham and MacLennan's (1984) review of seven combined series showed 5-year survival rates of 71.6% in stage I disease, 37.6% in stage II, 17.7% in stage III, and 0 in stage IV. The M. D. Anderson series of 51 patients reported by Eddy et al (1984b) showed median survival to be 51 months in stage I disease, 21 months in stage II, 15 months in stage III, and 29 months in stage IV. Peters et al (1988), in a report of the long-term follow-up of 115 patients with fallopian tube carcinoma, found that the majority of women died from their cancers.

Other factors that suggest a favorable prognosis are invasion of less than 50% of the muscularis of the fallopian tube in stage I disease, the use of adjuvant chemotherapy regimens containing cisplatin and minimal residual disease after initial surgery.

MANAGEMENT

Appropriate management of patients with cancer of the fallopian tube begins with adequate surgical staging. Exploration must include examination of all peritoneal surfaces for evidence of metastasis and, therefore, generally requires a vertical incision. Peritoneal cytology should be obtained because it has been shown that 5-year survival drops from 67% among patients with negative washings to 20% among those with positive washings (Podratz et al, 1986). Hysterectomy with bilateral salpingo-oophorectomy, standard therapy for many years, is no longer sufficient. Omentectomy, pelvic and para-aortic lymph node sampling, and biopsy of the peritoneum of the diaphragm, colic gutters, and cul-de-sac must be undertaken to precisely stage the patient and guide postoperative management. All adhesions and areas suspicious for involvement by tumor must be biopsied. Pleural effusions must be evaluated cytologically as well. Intrahepatic and other distant metastases can often be evaluated by fine-needle aspiration.

Therapy for tubal cancer requires maximal efforts to remove visible tumor. Eddy et al (1984b) found that 5-year survival among patients with advanced disease fell from 29% among patients with no gross residual disease to 15% among those with less than 2 cm residual disease and to 7% among those with more than 2 cm residual disease. Podratz and colleagues (1986), in reviewing the Mayo Clinic experience with tubal cancers, found that patients with residual tumor less than 1 cm in diameter had a median survival of more than 5 years, whereas those with larger residual disease had a median survival of less than 2 years. Peters et al (1988) found stage and volume of residual disease to be the only factors determining prognosis in their series.

Chemotherapy appears to have improved survival of patients with fallopian tube carcinoma, although controlled trials have not been conducted. Regimens containing cisplatin seem to provide the most benefit. Therapy with paclitaxel in this disease has not been evaluated but may also provide survival benefit when used with cisplatin in this setting. Peters et al (1989) observed that only 9% of patients with fallopian tube cancer responded to single-agent chemotherapy, whereas 29% of those receiving multiagent chemotherapy without cisplatin and 81% of those receiving cisplatin-containing regimens showed an initial response. In their series, patients with stage III/

Table 63–1. STAGING SYSTEM FOR FALLOPIAN TUBE CARCINOMA

Stage I Growth limited to the tubes
  Ia Growth limited to one tube; no ascites; intact serosa
  Ib Growth limited to both tubes; no ascites; intact serosa
  Ic Growth limited to one or both tubes; malignant ascites or pelvic washings; serosa involvement
Stage II Growth involving one or both tubes with pelvic extension
  IIa Extension and/or metastasis to the uterus or ovary
  IIb Extension to other pelvic tissues
  IIc Tumor limited to pelvis with malignant ascites or pelvic washings
Stage III Growth involving one or both tubes with intra-abdominal metastasis
  IIIa Microscopic intraperitoneal metastasis only; negative lymph nodes
  IIIb Intraperitoneal metastasis smaller than 2 cm; negative lymph nodes
  IIIc Intraperitoneal metastasis larger than 2 cm or metastasis to retroperitoneal lymph nodes
Stage IV Growth involving one or both tubes with intrahepatic or extraperitoneal metastasis

IV disease who received cisplatin-based combination therapy showed an improved survival. Maxson and colleagues (1987) found a 92% response rate (nine complete, two partial) among 12 patients who received cisplatin and cyclophosphamide therapy. Response in these series did not always correlate with improved long-term survival. Jacobs et al (1986) reported on three patients treated with cisplatin, doxorubicin, and cyclophosphamide who had surgically documented complete responses and sustained clinical remissions for up to 56 months.

The growth of endometrial carcinomas can be arrested by progestin therapy, and some tubal carcinomas appear to have histologic similarities. Furthermore, normal endosalpinx contains progestin receptors. Despite these theoretical considerations, however, no data exist to support the use of progestational or antiestrogen therapy in the management of fallopian tube cancer. Peters et al (1989) found no clinical responses among five patients treated with progestational agents. These hormones may have a role in palliation of disease in patients who have failed platinum-based chemotherapy.

After chemotherapy has been administered, second-look laparotomy can be performed on patients with no evidence of persistent disease to assess the need for second-line therapy and to assign prognosis. As with ovarian cancer, this procedure is controversial, and CA-125 levels, which reflect disease status, may allow one to avoid this therapeutic option. Eddy et al (1984a) reported on findings and outcome in eight patients who underwent second-look surgery. Two of five patients experienced recurrent disease after negative second-look operations, one at 41 months and one at 69 months after surgery. Both later died with disease despite treatment with alkylating agents or cisplatin. One patient had microscopic disease at laparotomy. She was alive without recurrence more than 4 years later. Both patients with macroscopic persistent tumor died within 3 years of second surgery. As with ovarian cancer, the clinical benefit of this procedure is unclear, and second-look laparotomy should be used in protocol settings or in unusual situations where the findings might help guide clinical treatment.

The value of adjuvant radiation therapy in fallopian tube cancer is controversial. No randomized controlled trials have been performed to assess the value of radiotherapy, and most recommendations come from the authors of institutional case series that used a variety of treatment schemes. Pfeiffer et al (1989) observed no statistically significant difference in survival among 17 patients who received postoperative pelvic radiotherapy and 18 patients who received no treatment. The 6-year survival in both groups was less than 50%, suggesting that most patients with disease grossly limited to the pelvis have occult abdominal metastasis. For this reason, most authors agree that treatment of the entire abdominal cavity is required for benefit. Schray et al (1987) found that 7 of 11 patients treated with pelvic

or pelvic and para-aortic irradiation died of recurrent disease, whereas 8 of 10 patients who received whole-abdominal radiation (including two who received intraperitoneal radioactive chromic phosphate) survived. Some have argued for the intraperitoneal administration of radioactive chromic phosphate as an adjuvant in early-stage patients without macroscopic residual disease, malignant ascites, or positive pelvic washings, but such therapy does not treat retroperitoneal lymph nodes and should not be administered to patients with nodal involvement by tumor or with nodes that have not been sampled (DiSaia and Creasman, 1989). Roberts and Lifshitz (1982) found no benefit to patients with early disease when intraperitoneal radioisotopes were administered. No study has compared whole-abdominal radiation with chemotherapy.

RECURRENCE

Recurrent fallopian tube cancer has been reported more than 10 years after initial treatment. When elevated preoperatively, CA-125 levels appear to rise with recurrence and decline with remission (Tokunaga et al, 1990). As in ovarian cancer, frequent examination and imaging studies directed at sites suggested by symptomatology appear to be the most effective means for diagnosing recurrent tubal cancer.

Intraperitoneal recurrence appears to be most common, especially in patients initially diagnosed at later stages. McMurray et al (1986) found, in their series of 30 patients treated at Washington University, that all patients with recurrent stage III cancer presented with intraperitoneal disease, whereas half of patients with stage I/II disease had extraperitoneal recurrence. Sites of extraperitoneal recurrence in their series included the liver (four patients), vagina (two), lung (two), pleura (two), kidney (one), brain (one), and axilla (one). Henderson et al (1977) reported extraperitoneal metastases in the lung (three patients), breast (one), brain (one), and spine (one). In their series, Semrad et al (1986) found metastases in extraperitoneal sites in 10 of 14 patients in whom recurrence developed. Half of their recurrences were to lymph nodes, including those in the inguinal and supraclavicular regions. Both chemotherapy and radiotherapy may increase the frequency with which extraperitoneal recurrence is observed.

Therapy for recurrent cancer of the fallopian tube is undefined. However, long-term survival has been reported after whole-abdominal irradiation or chemotherapy regimens containing cisplatin.

Henderson et al (1977) reported the cause of death in patients with fallopian tube carcinoma. Bronchopneumonia and intestinal obstruction were common diagnoses. Congestive heart failure, leukemia, and sepsis resulting from myelosuppression have resulted from chemotherapy for fallopian tube carcinoma, and fatal bowel perforation resulting from radiation bowel injury has been reported, indicating that adjuvant treatment for fallopian tube cancer is not without hazard.

SUMMARY

Although similar to ovarian cancer in many aspects of its behavior, its response to surgical debulking, and its sensitivity to platinum-based chemotherapy, carcinoma of the fallopian tube remains a unique entity. The rarity of tubal cancer has so far precluded detailed research into the etiology, natural history, and optimal treatment of this disease. Current understanding depends entirely on retrospective, often poorly controlled case series, leaving many areas of controversy unresolved. Considerable latitude remains to those managing and investigating this troublesome cancer.

REFERENCES

Denham J, MacLennan KA: The management of primary carcinoma of the fallopian tube: experience of 40 cases. Cancer 1984; 53:166.

DiSaia PJ, Creasman WT: Clinical Gynecologic Oncology. St. Louis: CV Mosby Company, 1989.

Dodson MG, Ford JH, Averette HE: Clinical aspects of fallopian tube carcinoma. Am J Obstet Gynecol 1970;36:935.

Doran A: Primary cancer of the fallopian tubes. Trans Obstet Soc London 1896;38:322.

Eddy GL, Copeland LJ, Gershenson DM: Second look laparotomy in fallopian tube carcinoma. Gynecol Oncol 1984a;19:182.

Eddy GL, Copeland LJ, Gershenson DM, et al: Fallopian tube carcinoma. Obstet Gynecol 1984b;64:546.

Gurney H, Murphey D, Crowther D: The management of primary fallopian tube carcinoma. Br J Obstet Gynaecol 1990;97: 822.

Henderson SR, Harper RC, Salazaar OM, Rudolph JH: Primary carcinoma of the fallopian tube: difficulties of diagnosis and treatment. Gynecol Oncol 1977;5:168.

Hinton A, Bea C, Winfield AC, Entman SS: Carcinoma of the fallopian tube. Urol Radiol 1988;10:113.

Hu CT, Taylor ML, Hertig AT: Primary carcinoma of the fallopian tube. Am J Obstet Gynecol 1950;59:58.

Jacobs AJ, McMurray EH, Parham P, et al: Treatment of carcinoma of the fallopian tube using cisplatin, doxorubicin, and cyclophosphamide. Am J Clin Oncol 1986;9:436.

Maxson WZ, Stehman FB, Ulbright TM, et al: Primary carcinoma of the fallopian tube: evidence for activity of cisplatin based chemotherapy. Gynecol Oncol 1987;26:305.

McMurray EH, Jacobs AJ, Perez CA, et al: Carcinoma of the fallopian tube: management and sites of recurrence. Cancer 1986; 58:2070.

Meyer JS, Kim CS, Price HM, Cooke JK: Ultrasound presentation of primary carcinoma of the fallopian tube. J Clin Ultrasound 1987;15:132.

Momtazee S, Kempson RL: Primary adenocarcinoma of the fallopian tube. Obstet Gynecol 1968;32:649.

Moore SW, Enterline HT: Significance of proliferative epithelial lesions of the uterine tube. Obstet Gynecol 1975;45:385.

Muntz HG, Tarraza HM, Granai CO: Primary adenocarcinoma of the fallopian tube. Eur J Gynaecol Oncol 1989;10:239.

Navani SS, Alvarado-Cabero I, Young RH, Scully RE: Endometrioid carcinoma of the fallopian tube: a clinicopathologic analysis of 26 cases. Gynecol Oncol 1996;63:371.

Nordin AJ: Primary carcinoma of the fallopian tube: a 20-year literature review. Obstet Gynecol Surv 1994;23:349.

Orthmann EC: Ueber carcinoma tubal. Gerbutsch Gynakol 1888; 15:212.

Peters WA, Andersen WA, Hopkins MP: Results of chemotherapy in advanced carcinoma of the fallopian tube. Cancer 1989;63: 836.

Peters WA, Andersen WA, Hopkins MP, et al: Prognostic features of carcinoma of the fallopian tube. Obstet Gynecol 1988;71:757.

Pfeiffer P, Mogensen H, Amtrup F, Honore E: Primary carcinoma of the fallopian tube: a retrospective study of patients reported to the Danish Cancer Registry in a five year period. Acta Oncol 1989;28:7.

Podratz KC, Pocczaski ES, Gaffey TA, et al: Primary carcinoma of the fallopian tube. Am J Obstet Gynecol 1986;154:1319.

Raju KS, Wiltshaw E: Primary carcinoma of the fallopian tube: a report of 22 cases. Br J Obstet Gynaecol 1981;88:1124.

Roberts JA, Lifschitz S: Primary adenocarcinoma of the fallopian tube. Gynecol Oncol 1982;13:301.

Rose PG, Piver MS: Fallopian tube cancer: the Roswell Park experience. Cancer 1990;66:2661.

Rosenblatt KA, Weiss NS, Schwartz SM: Incidence of malignant fallopian tube tumors. Gynecol Oncol 1989;35:236.

Schiller HM, Silverberg SG: Staging and prognosis in primary carcinoma of the fallopian tube. Cancer 1971;28:389.

Schink JC, Lurain JR: Rare gynecologic malignancies. Curr Opin Obstet Gynecol 1991;3:78.

Schray MF, Podratz KC, Malkasian GD: Fallopian tube cancer: the role of radiation therapy. Radiother Oncol 1987;10:267.

Sedlis A: Primary carcinoma of the fallopian tube. Obstet Gynecol Surv 1961;16:208.

Sedlis A: Primary carcinoma of the fallopian tube. Surg Clin North Am 1978;58:121.

Semrad N, Watring W, Fu Y-S, et al: Fallopian tube adenocarcinoma: common extraperitoneal recurrence. Gynecol Oncol 1986;24:230.

Stern J, Buscema J, Parmley T, et al: Atypical epithelial proliferations of the fallopian tube. Am J Obstet Gynecol 1981;140:309.

Tamimi HK, Figge DC: Adenocarcinoma of the uterine tube: potential for lymph node metastases. Am J Obstet Gynecol 1981; 141:132.

Tokunaga T, Miyazaki K, Matsumaya S, Okamura H: Serial measurement of CA 125 in patients with primary carcinoma of the fallopian tube. Gynecol Oncol 1990;36:335.

64

Gestational Trophoblastic Neoplasia

Larry J. Copeland

The clinical diseases encompassed within the spectrum of gestational trophoblastic neoplasia (GTN) present a range of neoplastic potential that confronts the clinician with numerous diagnostic and treatment challenges. Although the histologic features permit allocation to one of the pathologic entities—hydatidiform mole (partial or complete), invasive mole (chorioadenomatous destruens), placental site trophoblastic tumor (PSTT), or choriocarcinoma (chorioepithelioma)—diagnosis and management may be based solely on history, β-human chorionic gonadotropin (β-hCG) assay, and metastatic work-up. This clinical situation of treating a metastatic tumor with potentially lethal cytotoxic drugs is a unique deviation from the usual requirement of documenting tumor by histology prior to treatment. The treatment of GTN is more dependent on the clinical classification of a given tumor than on the pathologic classification (Fig. 64–1).

HYDATIDIFORM MOLE (COMPLETE)

The precise incidence of hydatidiform moles is difficult to define. Although it is generally accepted that the frequency of molar pregnancy is increased in the Far East, this may be the result of the bias of reporting hospital-based studies rather than population-based studies. Population-based studies should be corrected for the segment of population not at risk for pregnancy. The best denominator would be pregnancies at risk. Reports from Southeast Asia and Latin America are usually hospital-based studies, and, because many "normal" deliveries occur at home, this type of study results in a bias overestimation of the true incidence of hydatidiform mole. These factors may explain why the incidence of hydatidiform moles appears to have great geographic variability, reported in Indonesia to be as frequent as 1 in 85 pregnancies and reported in the United States to be approximately 1 in 1000 to 1 in 1500 pregnancies (Buckley, 1984).

A number of clinical factors (Table 64–1) appear to correlate with molar pregnancy occurrence (Yen and MacMahon, 1968; Bandy et al, 1984; Grimes,

1984; Matsuura et al, 1984; Sand et al, 1984; Berkowitz et al, 1985; Messerli et al, 1985; Parazzini et al, 1985, 1986; Atash et al, 1986; Palmer, 1994; Palmer et al, 1999). In addition to these risk factors, there are reported cases of familial molar pregnancies (Ambani et al, 1980; Parazzini et al, 1984). Paternal age over 45 years may also increase the relative risk for complete mole to 3 to 5 (Parazzini et al, 1986). A significant percentage of pregnancies in women over age 50 will result in hydatidiform mole; there is a 300- to 400-fold increased risk compared to women between the ages of 25 and 29 (Parazzini et al, 1986; Mazzanti et al, 1986). Unconfirmed risk factors include Rh-positive blood type, artificial insemination, nulliparity, consanguinity, and professional occupation. Clinical risk factors that appear to reduce the risk are a prior term pregnancy with no prior spontaneous abortion and adequate dietary vitamin A. Multiple gestations complicated by complete moles are rare, and ovulation induction has been reported in about one quarter of cases (Stellar et al, 1994).

Etiology (Cytogenetics)

In cases of complete hydatidiform moles, all chromosomes are paternal in origin (Kajii and Ohama, 1977). Approximately 95% of complete molar gestations have a 46,XX pattern homologous chromosomal pattern (diandric diploidy). One explanation for this pattern is *androgenesis*, the development of an ovum under the influence of a sperm nucleus when the nucleus of the egg is absent or inactive (the "empty egg" theory). It has been proposed that the rare hydatidiform mole with a 46,XY karyotype arises from dispermic fertilization (Ohama et al, 1981; Surti et al, 1982). The risk of persistent GTN appears to be similar for both chromosomal types.

Pathology

Invariably, with complete moles there is no gross or microscopic evidence of embryo, membranes, or cord. The absence of fetal tissue is essential for the

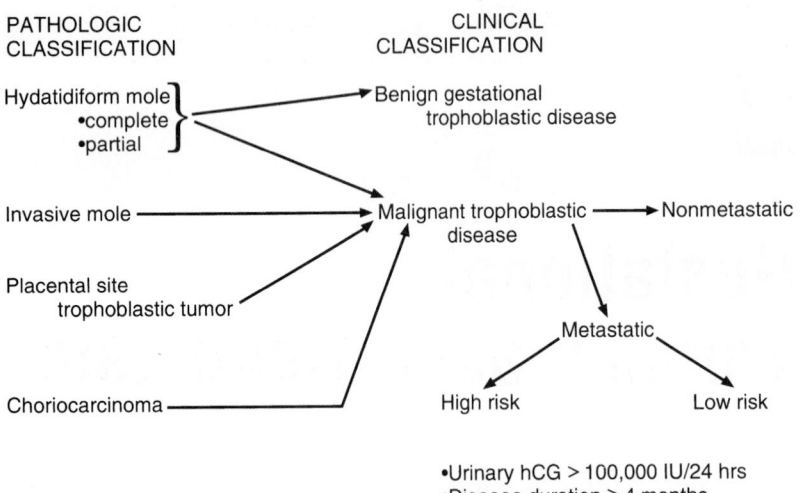

PATHOLOGIC
CLASSIFICATION

CLINICAL
CLASSIFICATION

Hydatidiform mole
•complete
•partial
→ Benign gestational
trophoblastic disease

Invasive mole ——→ Malignant trophoblastic ——→ Nonmetastatic
disease

Placental site
trophoblastic tumor

Choriocarcinoma ——

Metastatic

High risk   Low risk

•Urinary hCG > 100,000 IU/24 hrs
•Disease duration > 4 months
•Liver metastasis
•Brain metastasis
•Serum hCG > 40,000 mIU/ml
•Term pregnancy
•Failed prior chemotherapy
•WHO score ≥ 8

Figure 64–1
Pathologic and clinical classifications for gestational trophoblastic disease (see "Staging and Prognostic Factors" for additional discussion). (Data from Hertz et al [1961] and Ross GT et al [1965].)

diagnosis of hydatidiform mole, but the possibility always exists for a twin pregnancy with one gestation representing a complete mole and the other gestation representing normal or abnormal fetal development.

Gross inspection of a hydatidiform mole reveals vesicles (hydropic villi) of various size (Fig. 64–2). Areas of hemorrhage and necrosis may be grossly evident among the hydropic villi. The microscopic appearance of a hydatidiform mole reveals hydropic swelling of all villi. No normal-appearing villi are present. The mesenchyme of the villi is usually immature and undifferentiated. Although vessels are usually absent within the villi, they can be found occasionally. If vessels are found, however, their lumina should be absent of erythrocytes. Sheets of cytotrophoblastic and syncytiotrophoblastic cells will show evidence of hyperplasia and anaplasia. Hertig (1968) attempted to classify postevacuation curettings into a grading system that would predict the subsequent risk of malignancy. Subsequent studies

failed to demonstrate a correlation between the Hertig grade and clinical behavior (Elston, 1977).

The typical vesicular appearance of the complete mole may be less apparent in patients diagnosed by ultrasound at an early stage. In these cases, the presence of polypoid villi and the abnormal pattern of trophoblastic proliferation become key diagnostic factors (Paradinas, 1994).

Clinical Features

Although it has been stated that only 50% of hydatidiform moles are diagnosed prior to expulsion of the typical grape-like vesicles, it is probable that 80% to 90% are currently diagnosed either prior to the appearance of symptoms or before vesicles are

Table 64–1. CLINICAL RISK FACTORS FOR MOLAR PREGNANCY

Age (extremes of reproductive years)
    <15
    >40
Reproductive history
    Prior hydatidiform mole
    Prior spontaneous abortion
Diet
    Vitamin A deficiency
Birthplace
    Outside North America
Long duration of oral contraceptive use

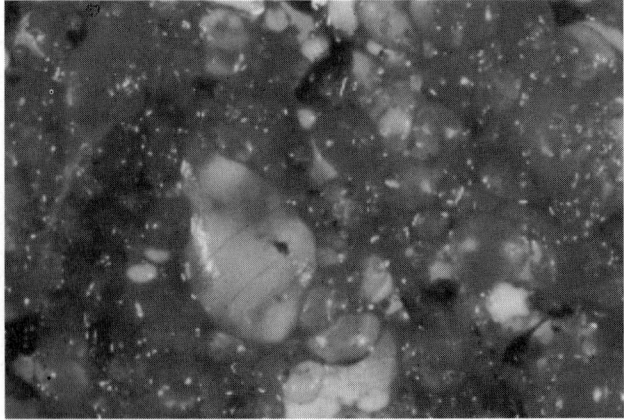

Figure 64–2
Complete mole characterized grossly by hydropic villi of various sizes.

passed. In developed countries, the widespread use of sonography to assess early pregnancy and bleeding in early pregnancy has contributed to a more timely diagnosis of molar pregnancy. As a result, many molar pregnancies are now diagnosed in very early gestation, prior to presentation with the usual signs and symptoms. The most common clinical presentation is that of a threatened abortion with painless vaginal bleeding. This can be followed with painful contractions and passage of molar tissue. Other clinical features that may increase suspicion that a molar pregnancy is present include a uterus large for dates (about 50% of patients) and hyperemesis (15% to 25% of patients) (Curry et al, 1975; Berkowitz et al, 1987b). The hyperemesis appears related to the high levels of β-hCG. Symptoms of toxemia are present in 5% to 10% of patients with complete moles, and, in patients presenting with toxemia prior to 24 weeks' gestation, the diagnosis of hydatidiform mole should be excluded. Fetal heart tones will be absent in a patient with a complete mole, with the exception, of course, of the rare situation of a coexisting twin pregnancy. Clinical hyperthyroidism is seen in 2% to 7% of molar pregnancies (Curry et al, 1975; Berkowitz et al, 1987b). Although previously believed to be the result of high hCG levels, the total thyroxine (T_4) or free T_4 index values are elevated above normal pregnancy levels in 25% and 50% of cases. This elevation does not appear to be the result of a high hCG level (Amir et al, 1984).

Patients with a molar pregnancy may present with a variety of other medical complications, including anemia, high-output cardiac failure, sepsis, and acute pulmonary insufficiency. The pulmonary insufficiency can be secondary to high-output cardiac failure or pulmonary edema, related to excessive fluid administration (Twiggs et al, 1979; Cotton et al, 1980; Twiggs, 1984). The sudden onset of dyspnea should also raise the possibility of trophoblastic tissue embolization. Deportation of trophoblastic tissue to the pulmonary vasculature occurs most commonly when the uterus is markedly enlarged, contracting, and undergoing mechanical manipulation. Although rare, trophoblastic embolization has been reported to cause death, documented by autopsy findings (Llewellyn-Jones, 1967).

Diagnosis and Evaluation

The diagnostic method of choice for confirming the diagnosis of hydatidiform mole in a patient presenting with clinical features is ultrasonography. Figure 64–3 illustrates the sonographic findings of a molar pregnancy. The characteristic "snowstorm" pattern is usually easy to identify in a uterus greater than 14 weeks in size. In a uterus smaller than 14 weeks in size, ultrasound findings may be similar to a missed or incomplete abortion (Woodward et al, 1980). Other clinical entities that may present diagnostic confusion include uterine fibroids, hydramnios, and hyperplacentosis (especially from multiple gestation). In clinical situations in which sonographic findings are not convincing, serial hCG determinations may support the diagnosis of molar pregnancy. Should ultrasound and serial β-hCG assays be inconclusive, one can consider amniography. An amniocentesis is performed, and, if amniotic fluid is withdrawn, a normal pregnancy is presumed. Submission of cells for karyotype analysis should be

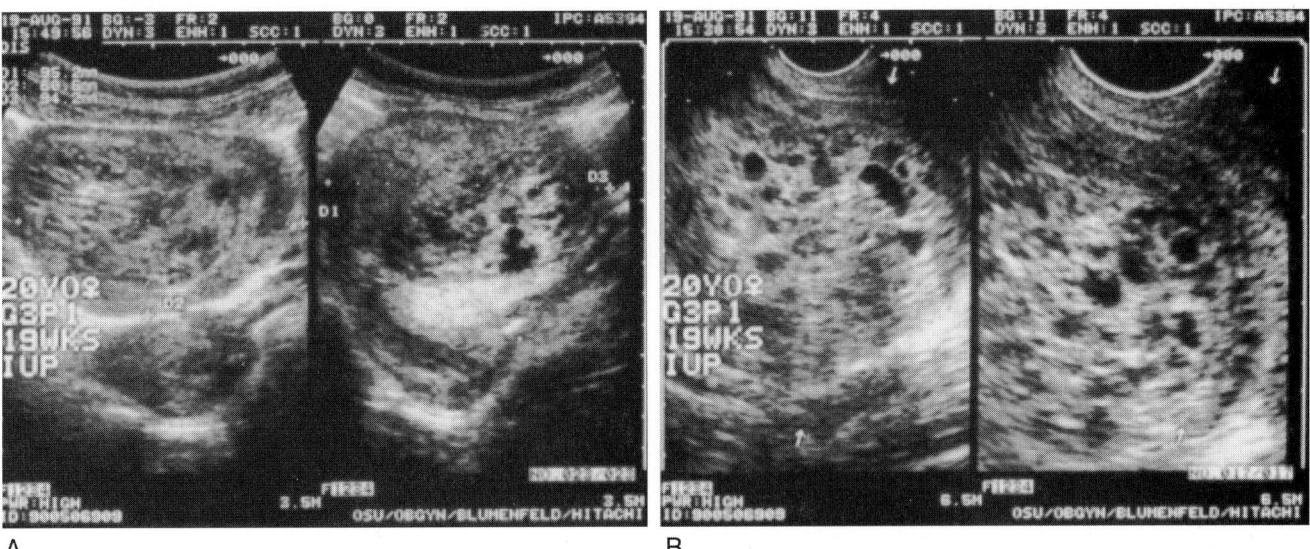

A   B

Figure 64–3
A, Sonographic findings of a molar pregnancy. The characteristic "snowstorm" pattern is evident. Transverse view (*left*) and sagittal view (*right*) demonstrate cervix posterior to fundus. The uterus is anteverted with molar gestation at 19 weeks. B, Magnification of molar gestation with transvaginal view demonstrating hydropic villi. (Courtesy of Michael Blumenfeld, MD.)

considered if a partial mole is in the differential diagnosis. If no amniotic fluid is obtained, contrast material may be injected into the uterine cavity. The outline of the multiple vesicles produces a honeycomb appearance on a flat plate of the abdomen. For the most part, amniography has been abandoned because of the accuracy of current ultrasonography.

Prior to treatment, a number of baseline studies should be considered. A chest film may reveal evidence of metastatic disease, pulmonary edema, or trophoblastic emboli. If a patient has an abnormality on chest radiography or any respiratory distress, baseline blood gas determinations should be obtained. Cardiac abnormalities, secondary to either hyperthyroidism or severe pregnancy-induced hypertension, may exist. Patients with supraventricular tachycardia may benefit from treatment with a β-blocking agent prior to surgical evacuation. Prior to evacuation, screening for coagulation problems should also be performed. Blood replacement therapy may be indicated on the basis of clinical findings and the presence of anemia.

Theca-lutein cysts occur in approximately 25% of patients with hydatidiform mole, and rupture and hemorrhage may necessitate surgical management (Fig. 64–4). These theca-lutein cysts are the result of high levels of hCG producing an exaggerated physiologic response in the ovary. These cysts may regress slowly following serum hCG regression, and neither removal nor decompression at the time of hysterectomy is necessary (Montz et al, 1988).

Treatment

The urgency of uterine evacuation is dependent on the clinical setting. In patients who present with bleeding and evidence of uterine contraction, evacuation should be performed promptly, assuming that the patient is stable. In patients who are asympto-

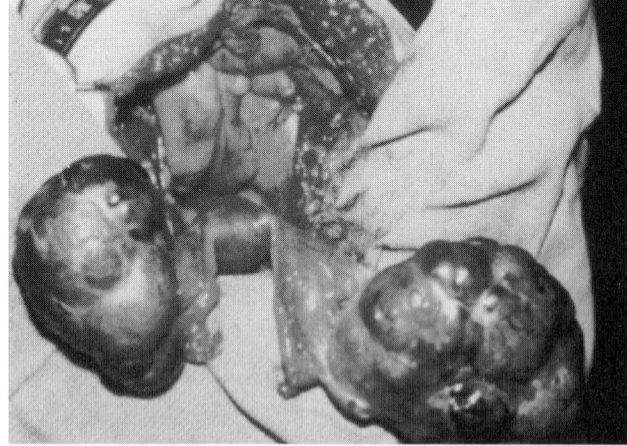

Figure 64–4
Large bilateral theca-lutein cysts resembling ovarian germ cell tumors. With resolution of the human chorionic gonadotropin (hCG) stimulation, they return to normal-appearing ovaries.

matic, with the diagnosis made by routine antenatal sonography, evacuation should be done within 24 to 48 hours.

The evacuation method of choice is suction curettage. If uterine bleeding is absent or mild, intravenous oxytocin is not started until the suction curettage procedure has been initiated. In the patient with heavy vaginal bleeding, it may be necessary to start oxytocin before the surgical evacuation. Although the oxytocin may assist in decreasing the bleeding, it may also increase the risk of trophoblastic embolization, especially in a patient with a large uterus.

The suction curettage technique should be specific for hydatidiform mole. After dilation of the cervix to permit insertion of a 10- to 12-mm suction curette just past the internal os, the suction is initiated and the uterine contents are evacuated by gently rotating the curette without inserting it further. This technique limits the risk of uterine perforation. There is a significant risk of uterine perforation in patients with hydatidiform mole, especially if there is a focus of invasive molar disease. An oxytocin infusion should be started concurrently with the suction procedure. After completion of the suction evacuation, a large curette can be used to gently remove any remaining molar tissue. Evacuation of a hydatidiform mole without the availability of a suction curette is potentially problematic. Evacuation of a very large molar pregnancy with traditional curettage instruments may place a very young patient at risk for serious uterine injury and hysterectomy. This risk exists because of the possibility of the molar disease being extensively invasive into the myometrium, potentially full-thickness. On the basis of this risk, in the absence of a suction apparatus, hysterotomy is recommended for evacuation of a large uterus (>14 weeks in size). If uterine perforation occurs, suction should immediately be discontinued and the suction canula removed. Laparoscopy or laparotomy should be performed to assess the site of perforation and to rule out injury to other viscera. Curettage is then completed under direct visualization of the pelvis. Bleeding from a perforation site of deep myometrial invasion, depending on the site and extent, may require segmental resection or hysterectomy.

For patients who are good surgical candidates and who desire no further children, termination of a molar pregnancy by primary hysterectomy should be considered. Although the patients remain at risk for persistent GTN, the risk is significantly less than that for the patient undergoing evacuation. Also, if chemotherapy is subsequently indicated, fewer cycles are required for successful treatment (Hammond et al, 1980).

Prophylactic chemotherapy (administration of single-agent chemotherapy immediately prior to or immediately after evacuation of a hydatidiform mole) has been suggested. This approach reduces the risk of neoplastic sequelae (from 15% to 20% to 1% to 2%). These patients still require serial β-hCG determinations. In other words, prophylactic chemotherapy is not a substitute for appropriate post-evacuation surveillance follow-up. However, prophylactic chemotherapy should be considered in patients who are considered at risk for poor compliance, especially if high-risk factors for recurrence are present (Kim et al, 1986). Concern has been expressed about the toxicity and mortality from chemotherapy at the time of evacuation. Additionally, there is concern regarding the possible induction of chemotherapy resistance in patients who develop choriocarcinoma (Ratnam et al, 1971). Because 100% of patients are treated with chemotherapy, in contrast to only 20% who do not receive prophylaxis, the use of prophylactic chemotherapy has not gained widespread acceptance.

With regard to coexisting twin fetus/mole situations, a comprehensive obstetric ultrasound study may be valuable to assess for fetal malformations and to characterize the placenta. Overmanagement of coexisting twin pregnancies with complete mole should be avoided until the situation is fully evaluated because the differential diagnosis with partial molar disease may be difficult. A significant percentage of multiple gestations with fetus/mole can result in a viable fetus and, although malignant postmolar disease is more common, the response to chemotherapy reported to date has been excellent (Stellar et al, 1994).

Post-Treatment Surveillance

Following evacuation of the molar tissue, patients require weekly β-hCG determinations until the hCG titer is within normal limits for 3 weeks. The titers are then observed at monthly intervals for 6 to 12 months. An algorithm for postmolar follow-up is illustrated in Figure 64–5. Figure 64–6 illustrates a normal regression curve for patients with spontaneous remission after evacuation of a hydatidiform mole. Such curves may provide early recognition of patients who will eventually require chemotherapy for malignant sequelae of hydatidiform mole (Morrow et al, 1985; Shigematsu et al, 1998). Within the first 8 weeks of follow-up, 65% to 70% of patients should have entered into spontaneous regression. Of the remaining patients, 10% to 15% will continue to show a decline in titers, whereas 15% to 20% will show a plateau or rise (Brewer et al, 1968). This latter group requires chemotherapy, as discussed later in this chapter.

After evacuation, patients require effective contraception. In the absence of a contraindication for the use of oral contraceptives, this method is preferred. In early retrospective studies, oral contraceptives were incriminated as causing a higher likelihood of persistent GTN (Stone et al, 1976; Brewer et al, 1979; Ho Yuen and Burch, 1983). Subsequent retrospective reports in the early 1980s failed to support the relationship between oral contraceptives and persistent molar disease (Berkowitz et al, 1981; Ho Yuen and Burch, 1983; Morrow et al, 1985). A prospective randomized study conducted by the Gynecologic Oncology Group (GOG) revealed no association between the use of oral contraceptives and an increased risk of requiring chemotherapy (Curry et al, 1989b). A more recent report suggests that there may be an outcome advantage in patients using oral contraceptives after evacuation (Deicas et al, 1991).

Several clinical features of molar pregnancy appear to be related to a higher likelihood of persistent molar disease. These are outlined in Table 64–2 (Curry et al, 1975; Morrow et al, 1977; Morrow and Townsend, 1987; Montz et al, 1988; Newman and Eddy, 1989; Stellar et al, 1994; Goldstein and Berkowitz, 1994). Multiple gestation complicated by mole is also more likely to develop metastatic disease than singleton moles (Stellar et al, 1994; Fishman et al, 1998).

Assays for free alpha or beta subunits may provide new prognostic information on the risk for persistent disease. Some reports (Nishimura et al, 1979; Quigley et al, 1980) suggest an association between abnormal free alpha subunit clearance and persistent disease; however, other reports fail to support these findings (Kohorn et al, 1981). Free beta subunits have also been correlated with a higher likelihood of persistent disease (Khazaeli et al, 1986, 1989). Again, other studies have failed to support this association (Berkowitz et al, 1989). A prospective GOG study is currently evaluating the prognostic value of free β-hCG ratios. Aneuploidy identified by flow cytometry has not reliably provided prognostic information (Martin et al, 1989; Cheung et al, 1993).

PARTIAL HYDATIDIFORM MOLE

The frequency with which partial hydatidiform mole occurs is generally regarded to be significantly less than that of the complete hydatidiform mole. However, the incidence varies, depending on diagnostic criteria. For example, if the only pathologic characteristic considered necessary to make a diagnosis of partial hydatidiform mole is presence of vessel-like structures within the villi, the incidence of partial hydatidiform mole may be quite high. However, if more appropriately rigid criteria (presence of blood components within the vessel structures, coexistence of normal adjacent villi, or coexistence of other products of conception) are used, the frequency of partial hydatidiform mole probably represents 10% to 20% of that of complete hydatidiform mole.

The etiology of partial hydatidiform mole is not clearly understood. Chromosomal abnormalities are common, with most partial hydatidiform moles having a triploid karyotype, incorporating an extra haploid paternal chromosomal complement (diandric triploidy) (Szulman, 1988). The next most common karyotype is that of trisomy, most commonly trisomy 16. A minority of partial moles exhibit a normal diploidy. When normal karyotype analysis is present, the possibility exists of a twin gestation—one nor-

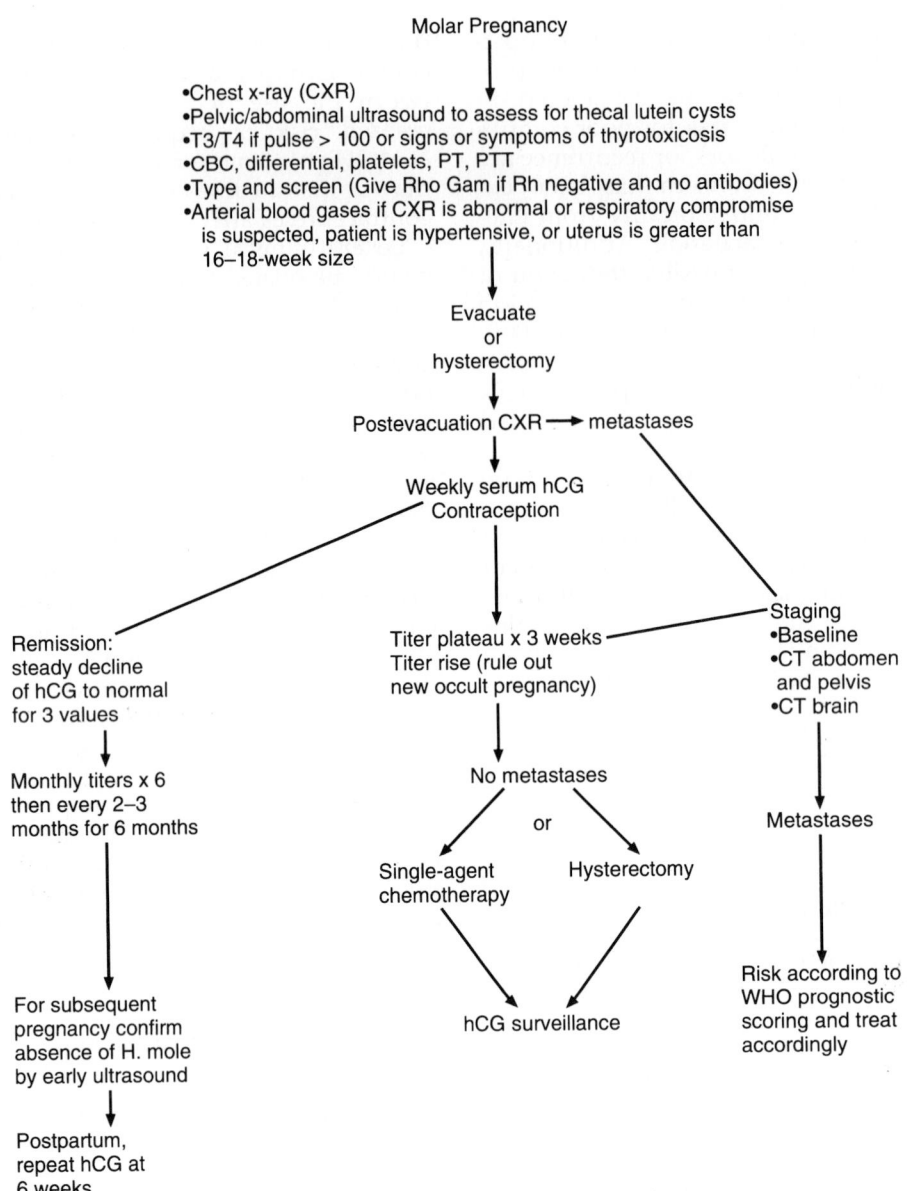

Figure 64–5
Algorithm for molar pregnancy management.

mally developing fetus and one molar pregnancy (Miller et al, 1993). Also, the overdiagnosis of degenerative changes (hydropic villi) and aborted tissue, sometimes referred to as a "transitional mole," may lead to the diagnosis of partial hydatidiform mole with a diploid conceptus (Vejerslev et al, 1986).

There appears to be no maternal or paternal age-associated risk for partial hydatidiform mole (Parazzini et al, 1986).

Pathology

The comparative pathologic features of complete mole and partial mole are listed in Table 64–3 (Vassilakos et al, 1977; Szulman and Surti, 1978).

Clinical Features

Most patients with partial hydatidiform moles present with signs and symptoms suggestive of a threatened or spontaneous abortion. Most patients with complete moles usually present during the first trimester or very early second trimester, but patients with partial moles tend to present a little later, any time from late first trimester throughout the second trimester. Although patients with complete hydatidiform moles tend to present with a uterus that is large for dates, this occurs in only approximately 11% of patients with the partial molar syndrome. Approximately two thirds present with a small-for-gestational-age uterus. Like the complete mole, the

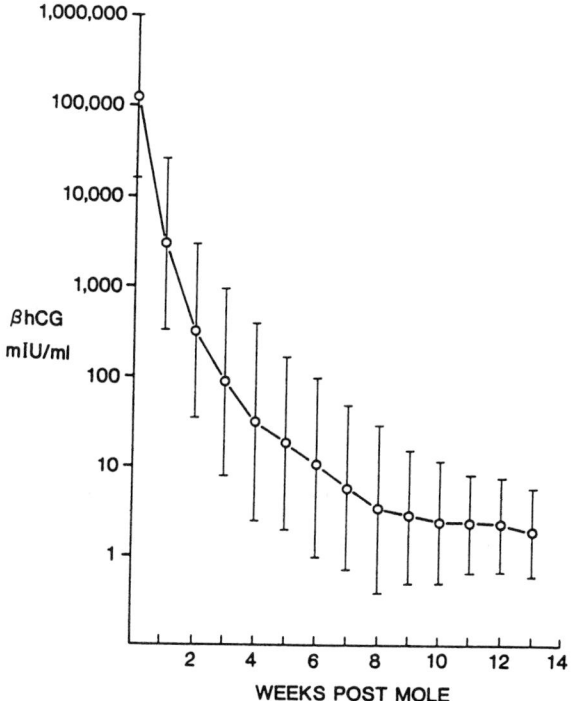

Figure 64–6
Postmolar human chorionic gonadotropin regression curve with 95% confidence limits. (From Morrow CP, Kletzky OA, DiSaia PJ, et al: Clinical and laboratory correlates of molar pregnancy and trophoblastic disease. Am J Obstet Gynecol 1977;128:424, with permission.)

partial mole may present with other associated clinical signs, including pre-eclampsia and hyperemesis.

Diagnosis

Like the complete hydatidiform mole, the partial mole diagnosis is based primarily on an ultrasound assessment. Whereas most patients with partial mo-

Table 64–2. CLINICAL FEATURES OF MOLAR PREGNANCY AND ESTIMATED RISK OF PERSISTENT TROPHOBLASTIC DISEASE (PER CENT)*

CLINICAL FEATURE	PER CENT
Eclampsia	90
Delayed hemorrhage	75
Acute pulmonary insufficiency	60
Theca-lutein cysts >5 cm	55
Uterus >20 weeks size	55
Coexistent twin fetus	55
Uterus large for dates	45
Serum human chorionic gonadotropin >100,000 mIU/ml	45
Uterus >16 weeks size	35
Maternal age >40 years	25

*Overall, approximately 20% of all patients with molar pregnancies develop persistent gestational disease and require chemotherapy.

lar syndrome present with a dead fetus in the late first trimester (Fig. 64–7), the presentation may be that of a live fetus with adjacent molar tissue. The presence on sonographic study of a living fetus demonstrating an abnormality consistent with a partial hydatidiform mole presents a challenging clinical situation, especially if the diagnosis is made in the late mid-trimester. Consideration should be given to performing a karyotype analysis on the apparent viable fetus. The presence of a grossly abnormal karyotype may facilitate clinical decision making. However, because other abnormalities, including benign abnormalities of the uterus or placenta, must be considered in the differential diagnosis, the presence of a normal diploid karyotype supports a more expectant management. Mesenchymal dysplasia associated with placentomegaly with hydropic villous transformation (Beckwith-Wiedemann syndrome) is an example of this situation (Jauniaux et al, 1997). Baseline and serial β-hCG titers should be obtained.

Treatment

A partial hydatidiform mole presents a more complex problem regarding uterine evacuation than does the complete mole. If the fetal parts appear very small or degenerated, consideration can be given to using suction curettage in a technique similar to that described for complete mole. If the fetus is intact and 15 to 16 weeks in size or greater, the surgical evacuation method of choice is hysterotomy. Pharmaceutically induced contractions put the patient at risk for trophoblastic embolization.

Follow-Up

Like the patient with a complete mole, an effective form of contraception, preferably an oral contraceptive, is recommended during the postevacuation surveillance. Although the risk for persistent GTN is much lower in the case of the partial hydatidiform mole compared with the complete mole (5% to 7% vs. 15% to 20%) (Rice et al, 1990), the postevacuation surveillance program should be similar. The chemotherapy for these patients is discussed later.

INVASIVE MOLE (CHORIOADENOMA DESTRUENS)

It is estimated that between 5% (Delfs, 1959) and 10% (Brewer et al, 1968) of all molar pregnancies contain myometrial invasion by molar villi. Because this process is clinically occult and the diagnosis is usually made on the basis of hysterectomy, it is difficult to assess accurately the frequency of this clinical entity.

Table 64-3. COMPARATIVE PATHOLOGIC FEATURES OF COMPLETE AND PARTIAL HYDATIDIFORM MOLES

FEATURE	COMPLETE MOLE	PARTIAL MOLE
Karyotype	Usually 46,XX (paternal homologous)	Usually triploidy, 69,XXY most common Occasional trisomy (e.g., trisomy 16); rarely diploidy; paternal and maternal
Villi	All villi hydropic; no normal adjacent villi	Normal adjacent villi may be present
Villous vessels	Usually absent; when present they contain no fetal blood cells	Usually present; may contain fetal blood cells
Fetal tissue	None present	Usually present
Trophoblast	Hyperplasia usually present to variable degrees	Hyperplasia mild and focal

Data from Vassilakos et al (1977) and Szulman and Surti (1978).

Pathology

Pathologically, the invasive mole is similar to choriocarcinoma, with one exception: there are persistent hydropic villi within the invading tumor (Fig. 64–8).

Clinical Features

The clinical hallmark is hemorrhage. Like normal trophoblastic tissue, the invasive mole has the propensity to seek out and rupture maternal arterioles. This may result in sudden onset of severe vaginal or intraperitoneal hemorrhage. Metastatic invasive molar disease most frequently involves the lung or vagina. Patients with metastatic invasive moles may undergo spontaneous remission without therapy (Wilson et al, 1961); patients with metastatic trophoblastic disease are usually treated with chemotherapy regardless of histologic findings.

Diagnosis and Evaluation

Because invasive mole is usually clinically occult, the diagnosis is most often an incidental finding follow-

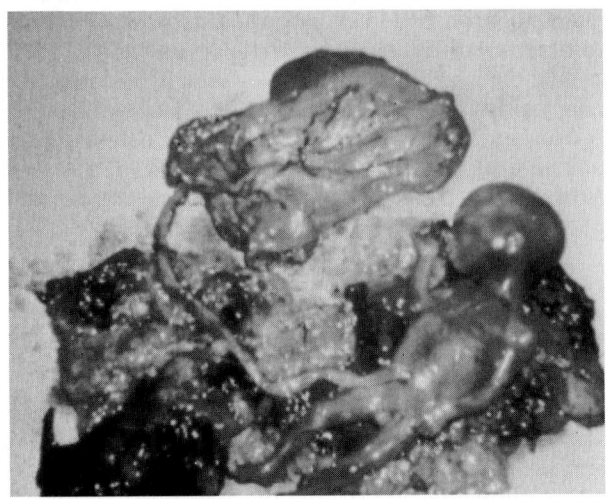

Figure 64-7
Partial mole with dead fetus of abnormal karyotype.

ing hysterectomy for hemorrhagic complications. In the absence of metastatic disease, patients require postsurgical surveillance and treatment similar to the management of patients with complete or partial moles.

Treatment

Treatment indications, not only hysterectomy, are based on hemorrhagic complications. Additional treatment in the form of chemotherapy is based on whether metastases are present or on β-hCG surveillance. Chemotherapy is discussed later in this chapter.

PLACENTAL SITE TROPHOBLASTIC TUMOR

PSTT probably represents an incidence of no more than 1% of all patients with GTN. If the incidence is higher, the disease is clinically occult and undergoes spontaneous resolution. This disease was first described in 1976 as a trophoblastic *pseudotumor* and was thought to be a non-neoplastic syncytial endometritis (Kurman et al, 1976). Subsequent reports (Scully and Young, 1981; Young and Scully, 1984, 1994) identified the malignant potential of this tumor, noting that 10% to 20% of patients develop metastases and most of these patients succumb to their disease.

Pathology

Initially, this tumor grows locally with infiltration of the myometrium or with polypoid growth into the uterine cavity. In contrast to choriocarcinoma, hemorrhage and necrosis are focal or absent. Microscopically (Fig. 64–9), these tumors are composed of solid sheets of a monomorphic cell population of intermediate trophoblastic cells (Kurman et al, 1984). Immunocytochemical staining demonstrates large amounts of human placental lactogen (hPL) and only focal areas positive for hCG.

Because mitotic counts vary substantially between

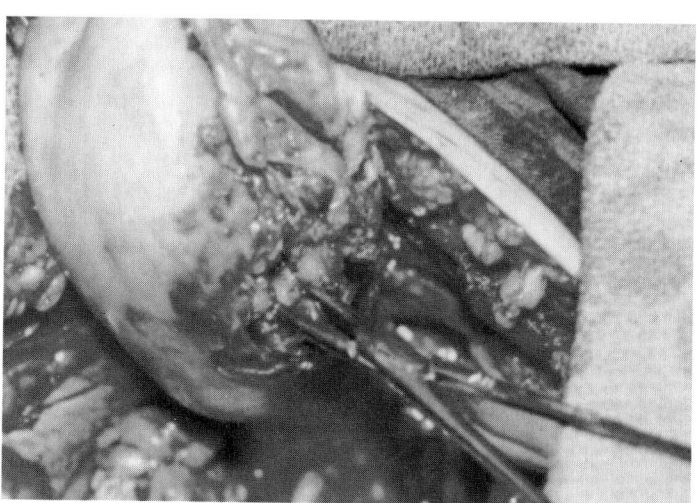

Figure 64–8
Invasive mole eroding through uterus. The surgical instrument points to hydropic villi.

endometrial curettings and hysterectomy specimens, conservative therapeutic decisions based on a low mitotic count on an endometrial sampling present a risk of treatment failure (Young and Scully, 1994).

Clinical Features

Patients with PSTT usually present with abnormal vaginal bleeding. Most patients with this disease present following a term pregnancy, but PSTT can also be a sequel to a molar pregnancy or abortion. During the postpartum period, the patient presents with a slightly enlarged uterus, persistent postpartum bleeding or sometimes amenorrhea, and a slightly elevated β-hCG level. The hCG value may not be a reliable marker reflecting disease progression. Serial serum hPL measurements may be a use-

ful marker; hLP is more useful as a histologic staining target for confirming the diagnosis. Nephrotic syndrome and virilization have also been reported to be associated with some cases of PSTT (Eckstein et al, 1982; Nagelberg and Rosen, 1985; Young et al, 1985). In the general course of this disease, metastases usually occur late. Because PSTTs are "well-differentiated" tumors, tend to metastasize late, and are usually resistant to chemotherapy, they are conceptually considered the "low-malignant-potential" portion of the spectrum of GTN.

Diagnosis

A high index of suspicion for PSTT can be based on the characteristic clinical presentation. The histologic diagnosis may be obtained by uterine dilatation and

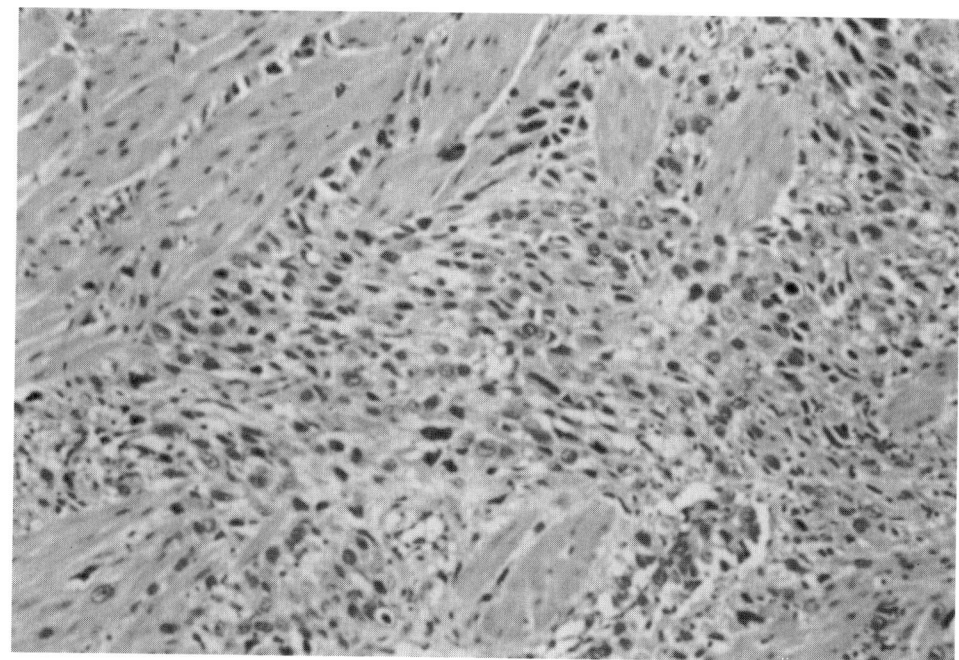

Figure 64–9
Placental site trophoblastic disease with solid sheets of intermediate cells. Note the clean interface between tumor and myometrium with no hemorrhage or necrosis.

curettage. Hysteroscopic assistance in directing tissue sampling may be of some value. Because of the clinically occult nature of the disease and the problem with persistent bleeding, many patients are assigned this diagnosis on the basis of a hysterectomy specimen. When the diagnosis is suspected, a metastatic work-up should be performed and hCG and hPL assays should be obtained at regular intervals.

Vaginal ultrasonography may reveal additional nonspecific features of PSTT: a decrease of resistance to flow, an increase in overall uterine vascularity, an irregular endomyometrial interface, and occasionally intramural cystic structures (Heintz et al, 1985; Jaffe, 1993; Abulafia et al, 1994). Although ultrasonographic features may increase the index of suspicion for PSTT, the absence of these features is not reassuring that the disease is not present.

Treatment

Uterine curettage or selective hysteroscopic endomyometrial resection may be curative in patients with focal trophoblastic proliferations of the placental site.

Because this disease tends to metastasize late and tends to be somewhat resistant to chemotherapy, surgical excision (hysterectomy) is recommended (Finkler et al, 1988). Management in a patient desirous of future childbearing is more difficult. Treatment considerations could include systemic chemotherapy, regional infusion chemotherapy, and uterine curettage, which has been reported with some success. In patients with metastatic disease, hysterectomy may offer little or nothing to improving long-term survival.

Follow-Up

Because there has been a report of a metastatic recurrence after 5 years, it is advisable to observe these patients for an extended period of time (Heintz et al, 1985).

CHORIOCARCINOMA

Choriocarcinoma develops in one of 20,000 to 40,000 term pregnancies (Brinton et al, 1986); in contrast, it develops in approximately 3% to 5% of patients with a molar pregnancy disease. In approximately 50% of patients with choriocarcinoma, disease develops following a hydatidiform mole; in approximately 15%, following a term pregnancy; and in 25%, following an abortion (spontaneous, therapeutic, or ectopic). Trophoblastic disease following a normal pregnancy is either choriocarcinoma or PSTT and not a benign or invasive mole.

Pathology

The gross appearance of choriocarcinoma often resembles that of a friable segment of placenta. The tissue is often dark red or purple. Microscopically, choriocarcinoma is characterized by hemorrhage and necrosis, by large sheets of poorly differentiated syncytiotrophoblastic and cytotrophoblastic cells, and by the absence of hydropic villi. Immunoperoxidase staining demonstrates β-hCG within the syncytiotrophoblastic giant cells. Attempts to histologically document the presence of choriocarcinoma may be difficult. It is not uncommon to obtain only evidence of hemorrhage and necrosis on tissue sampling from uterus or metastatic sites. As mentioned previously, the usual requirement for histologic documentation of the neoplasia is not necessary for the management of metastatic GTN.

Clinical Features

Choriocarcinoma is well known for its tendency to masquerade as other disease processes; as a result, delays in diagnosis are common. The natural history for choriocarcinoma is rapid progression and spread, with death occurring within a few weeks to a few months of clinical presentation. The immediate cause of death is usually hemorrhage-related. Because of a propensity for hematogenous spread, all the blood-rich organs are at significant risk for metastatic disease (Table 64–4). The strong propensity of trophoblastic cells to disrupt normal vascular integrity, leading to focal hemorrhage, usually leads to the first symptoms of this disease. The imitation of other disease processes is predominantly secondary to hemorrhagic metastasis present in a variety of organ systems (hematuria, hemophysis, hematemesis, hematochezia, stroke, and vaginal bleeding). The diagnosis of metastatic GTN must be considered in any woman of reproductive age who presents with metastatic disease from an unknown or poorly documented primary tumor.

Diagnosis

The diagnosis of choriocarcinoma is usually based on history, imaging studies, and serum hCG de-

Table 64–4. COMMON SITES FOR METASTATIC CHORIOCARCINOMA*

SITE	PER CENT
Lung	60–95
Vagina	40–50
Vulva/cervix	10–15
Brain	5–15
Liver	5–15
Kidney	0–5
Spleen	0–5
Gastrointestinal	0–5

*Frequency varies depending on whether data are based on autopsy studies or are obtained from pretreatment imaging.

terminations. Although histologic confirmation is sometimes available, it is neither essential for the diagnosis nor a prerequisite to treatment of metastatic GTN. In addition to the unnecessary general surgical morbidity, surgical intervention such as craniotomy or thoracotomy is seldom justifiable as a diagnostic procedure. Two hazards are associated with attempts to obtain histologic confirmation: One is the risk that the biopsy site may bleed profusely, and this hemorrhage may be difficult to control (Fig. 64–10); the other risk is that the biopsy or fine-needle aspirate obtained may fail to provide satisfactory tissue to illustrate the neoplastic process. Hemorrhage and necrosis are so prominent that a clear demonstration of the trophoblastic tumor may be difficult. Unnecessary and dangerous delays in therapy have resulted from such false-negative biopsy specimens. It is important to exclude the presence of a new pregnancy as the source of an elevated serum β-hCG level prior to extensive diagnostic imaging or therapeutic intervention.

An investigational diagnostic technique for identifying occult metastatic disease is radioimmunoscintigraphy with ^{131}I-labeled anti-hCG antibodies (Quinones et al, 1971; Begent et al, 1980; Hatch et al, 1980).

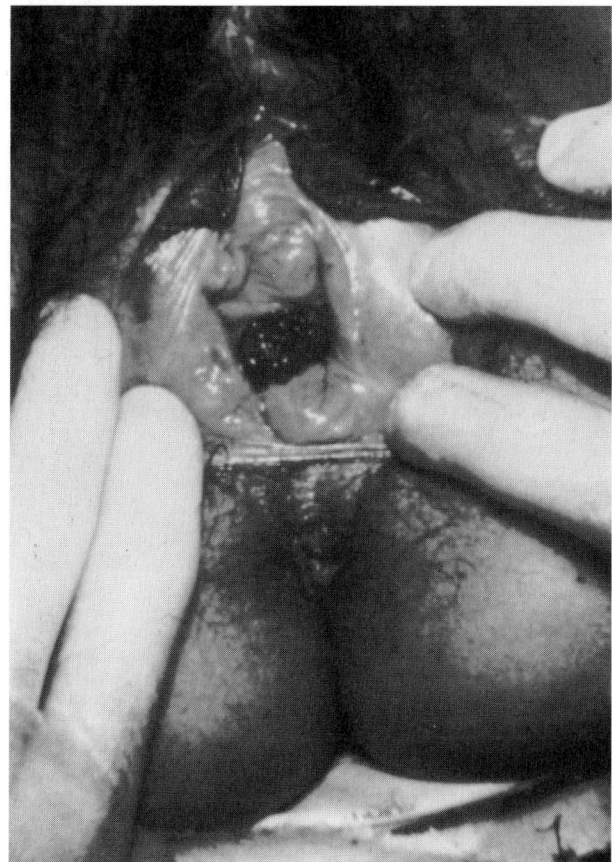

Figure 64–10
Choriocarcinoma metastatic to the vagina. Shortly after this photograph, a biopsy specimen was obtained and excessive vaginal bleeding resulted.

Treatment

Although chemotherapy is the cornerstone of the treatment of metastatic GTN, optimal treatment results may depend on the addition of surgery and irradiation in select circumstances. Women with high-risk or complicated trophoblastic disease should be treated by physicians with special interest and experience in the complexities of this multifaceted disease. The old adage—"the first shot is the best shot"—is true for the management of many malignancies, but it is particularly true for trophoblastic disease.

Central nervous system (CNS), hepatic, and extensive pulmonary disease and transplacental metastases deserve special diagnostic and treatment considerations.

Surgery

Hysterectomy may play a primary role in the management of nonmetastatic or low-risk metastatic GTN. Primary hysterectomy followed by chemotherapy has been reported to reduce the average number of chemotherapy cycles (from 5.9 to 3.8) (Hammond et al, 1980). However, because historically surgery alone cured only about 40% of patients with nonmetastatic disease (Brewer et al, 1961), it is important that all of these patients also receive chemotherapy.

Hysterectomy may also be indicated to treat focal disease resistant to chemotherapy. Prior to hysterectomy, it is important to demonstrate persistent uterine disease by either curettage or angiography. Also, the absence of significant metastatic disease should be confirmed.

Other foci of chemoresistant disease, including pulmonary, brain, hepatic, or unilateral renal metastases, should be considered for resection in isolated circumstances (Shirley et al, 1972; Liftshitz et al, 1977; Sink et al, 1978; Tomoda et al, 1980; Weed et al, 1982; Xu et al, 1985; Barnard et al, 1986; Soper et al, 1988). One should keep in mind that persistent pulmonary nodules do not necessarily represent persistent active tumor, because radiographic regression may lag behind the actual biologic (hCG) response (Wong and Ma, 1983).

Surgical intervention may be indicated for supportive care (e.g., indwelling central venous catheters) or for management of hemorrhagic or other complications. Arteriography with embolization may be useful for the control of focal excessive bleeding (Fig. 64–11A and B).

Radiation Therapy

Radiation therapy plays a limited role in the management of choriocarcinoma. Historically, irradiation has been incorporated into the management of brain or liver metastasis. In most treatment centers, brain metastasis continues to be treated with irradiation,

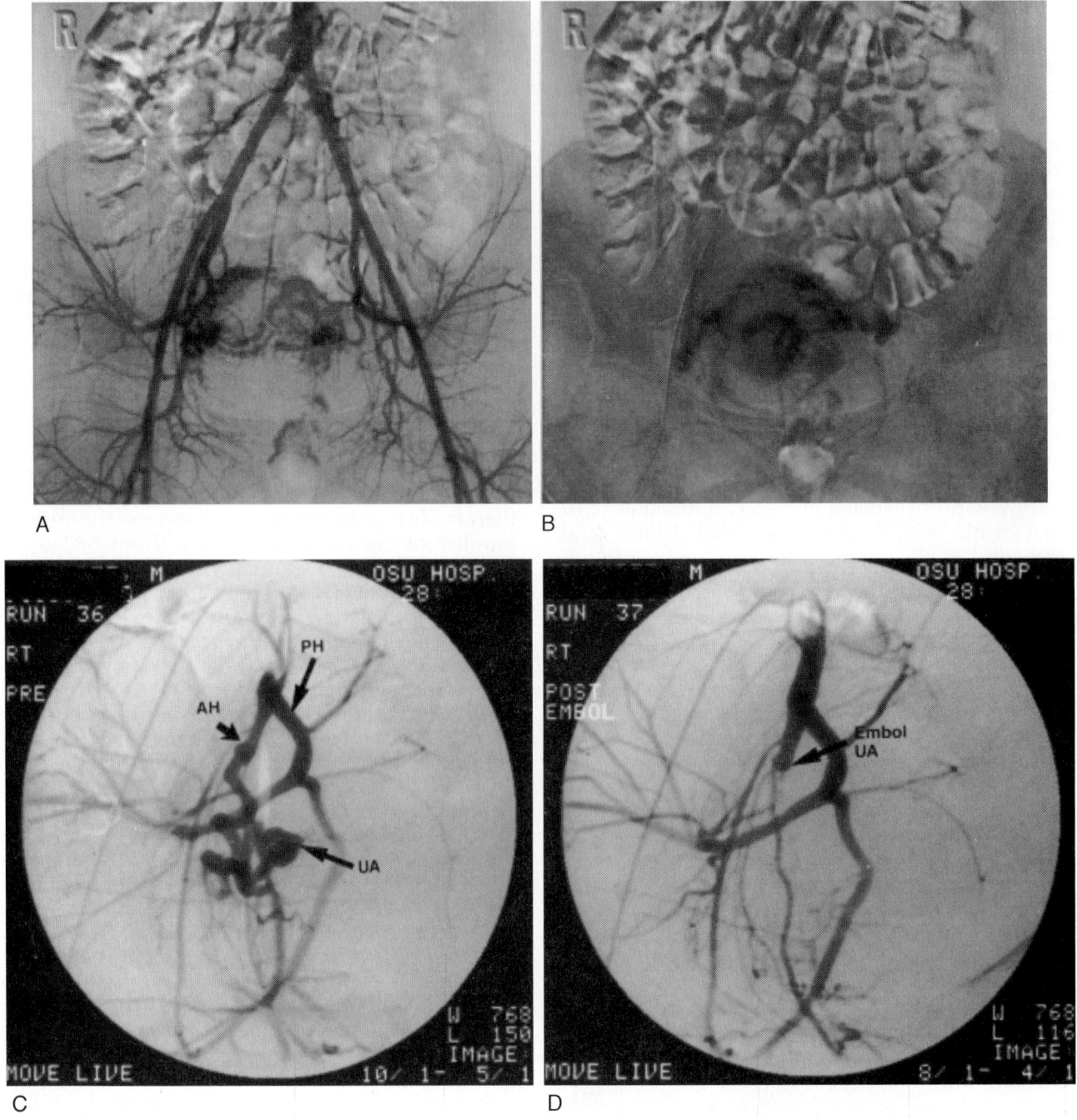

Figure 64–11

A 23-year-old patient was referred with acute vaginal hemorrhage following primary chemotherapy for choriocarcinoma. She requested uterine preservation if possible. Angiographic studies were performed. The arterial phase (A) revealed a hypervascular uterus with extensive neovascularization. There was moderate arteriovenous shunting, and delayed films demonstrated pooling of contrast and tumor blush (B). Selective bilateral uterine artery embolization was performed. Digital subtraction films of the right pelvic vessels prior to embolization are shown (C). Postembolization digital subtraction arteriograms demonstrated total occlusion of the uterine arteries (D). The vaginal bleeding abated, and additional nonsurgical treatment was initiated. AH, anterior hypogastric artery; PH, posterior hypogastric artery; UA, uterine artery (right); Embol UA, embolized uterine artery (right). (Courtesy of Dr. Alfred Stockum, Ohio State University.)

usually 3000 cGy over 3 weeks, but the use of irradiation for hepatic metastasis has declined in popularity.

Metastatic Disease

CENTRAL NERVOUS SYSTEM METASTASES

About 1 of 10 patients with metastatic choriocarcinoma have CNS metastasis. Brain involvement (Fig. 64–12) is more common than spinal metastasis, but either can be responsible for the presenting symptoms. Lung metastases precede or coexist with CNS involvement in most, but not all, cases (Athanassiou et al, 1983). Corticosteroid therapy should be initiated concurrently with the diagnosis and continued through treatment.

The presence of CNS involvement may be evaluated by either computerized tomography scanning or magnetic resonance imaging. Prior to the availability of these techniques, reliance was placed on radioisotope brain scans and cerebrospinal fluid (CSF) hCG levels. A serum-to-CSF ratio of less than 60 is suggestive of CNS metastases (Bagshawe and Harland, 1976).

Following the diagnosis of CNS metastases, radiation therapy is generally initiated promptly to decrease the risk of hemorrhage. In addition to hemorrhagic prophylaxis, the irradiation has tumoricidal effects (Brace, 1968). Whether the irradiation also renders the blood-brain barrier more permeable to chemotherapeutic agents is speculative. Complications of radiation therapy appear limited (Sheline et al, 1980); however, a secondary glioblastoma has been reported (Barnes et al, 1982).

Brain irradiation combined with multiagent chemotherapy is reported to cure 70% to 90% of patients with brain metastases when primary therapy is initiated (Schink et al, 1992). However, salvage treatment for brain metastasis is much less successful, with reported success rates ranging from 0% to 30% (Ross et al, 1965; Brace, 1968; Yordan et al, 1987; Bakri et al, 1994; Evans et al, 1995). Similar success rates have been reported with primary systemic and intrathecal chemotherapy (Athanassiou et al, 1983; Rustin et al, 1989). Anatomically accessible brain metastasis can also be considered for resection in conjunction with primary chemotherapy or in the management of refractory disease. Surgical intervention may also be indicated for the management of elevated intracranial pressure from hemorrhage or edema.

HEPATIC METASTASES

Liver metastases contribute to the high-risk profile of patients with metastatic choriocarcinoma. Hemorrhagic sequelae can be catastrophic; this is not surprising, considering the vasculature of the liver and the propensity for trophoblastic cells to disrupt local blood vessels. Hemorrhagic prophylaxis with whole-liver irradiation has previously been advocated (Hammond and Soper, 1984). However, this may not prevent bleeding (Lacey et al, 1983), and control by interventional radiology may be an acceptable alternative (Grumbine et al, 1980; Heaton et al, 1986). Also, postirradiation hepatitis, although uncommon, can be life-threatening (Barnard et al, 1986).

Approximately 27% to 63% of patients with significant liver metastases have been reported cured (Soper et al, 1986; Bakri et al, 1993; Crawford et al, 1997). One report, in which two thirds of the patients had lesions no larger than 1 cm, claimed an 80% (12/15) survival (Wong et al, 1986a). Correct interpretation of this report must include the possibilities that

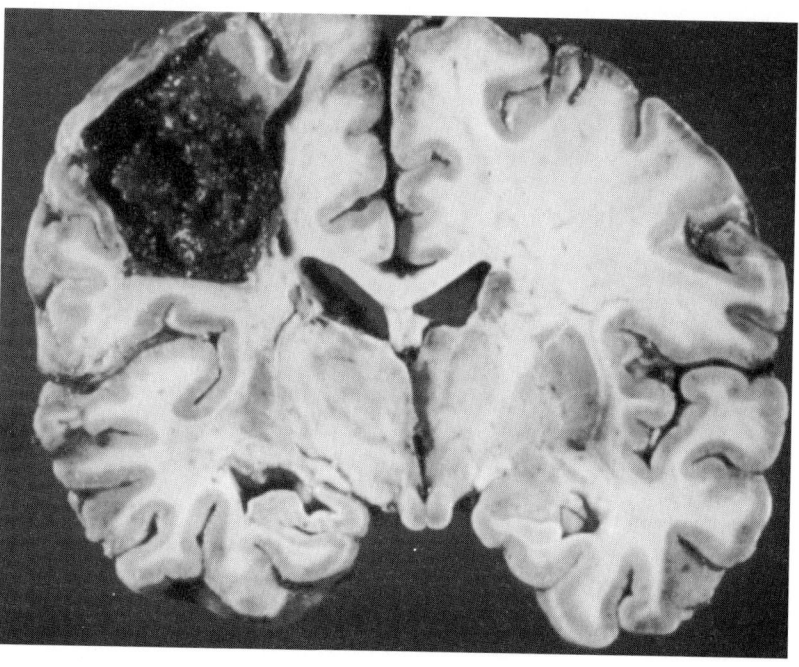

Figure 64–12
Large right parietal metastasis with hemorrhage was the cause of a sudden left-sided hemiparesis manifestation.

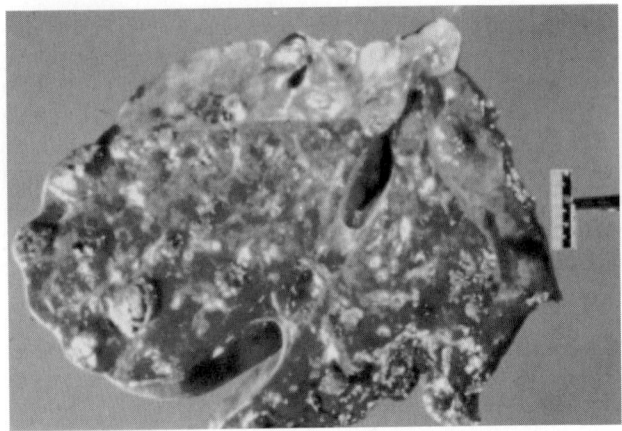

Figure 64–13
Extensive pulmonary metastasis.

smaller liver lesions are more treatable or that patients with multiple small liver hemangiomas were misdiagnosed as having metastasis.

EXTENSIVE PULMONARY METASTASES

Patients who present with extensive pulmonary disease (Fig. 64–13), characterized by more than 50% lung opacification, anemia, or angina, are at risk for an early respiratory death after the initiation of chemotherapy (Kelly et al, 1990). Progressive hypoxia may be related to interstitial bleeding or edema. Correction of the anemia and extracorporeal perfusion have been identified as important aspects of management. Unfortunately, extracorporeal perfusion requires complete therapeutic anticoagulation, a situation of great peril for the patient with metastatic choriocarcinoma (Figs. 64–14 and 64–15). The roles

of reduced-dose chemotherapy and ventilation remain uncertain.

TRANSPLACENTAL METASTASES

Considering the facility with which choriocarcinoma invades the vascular system, it is surprising that fetal metastases are not seen more frequently. This event is rare, but, when it occurs, the prognosis is poor. Consideration should be given to hCG testing of the infant when the maternal diagnosis is made (Witzleben and Bruninga, 1968).

STAGING AND PROGNOSTIC FACTORS

Following the early success in treating choriocarcinoma with methotrexate and actinomycin D, National Institutes of Health (NIH) investigators recognized that a subset of patients with particular features experienced a remission rate under 50%. In contrast, patients without these features showed a remission rate above 90% (Hertz et al, 1961; Ross et al, 1965). These features became known as the "high-risk metastatic disease" group, and patients with these features were subject to more aggressive treatment. In addition to urinary hCG excretion greater than 100,000 IU in 24 hours, duration of disease longer than 4 months, brain or liver metastases, and previously failed or inadequate therapy, additional criteria have been added by various investigators over recent decades. These additional poor-prognostic criteria include antecedent term pregnancy (Miller et al, 1979) and a serum hCG level greater than 40,000 mIU/ml (Surwit and Hammond, 1980), a figure similar to that of a patient who excretes 100,000 IU per liter in a 24-hour urine collec-

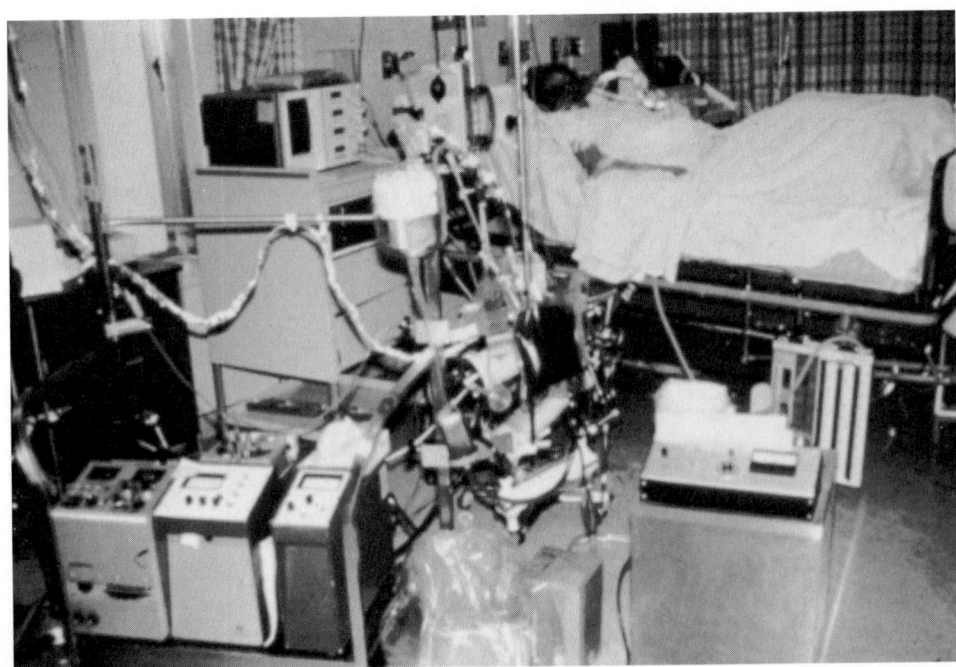

Figure 64–14
Extracorporeal membrane oxygenization in a patient with extensive pulmonary metastases. Although the human chorionic gonadotropin titers reflected an excellent response to chemotherapy, the clinical course was one of progressive respiratory failure.

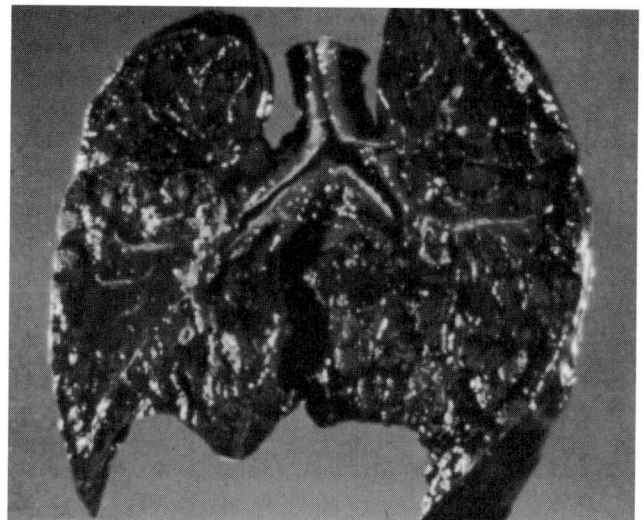

Figure 64-15
Autopsy photograph of lungs of the patient in Figure 64-14. The lungs are heavily saturated with blood and fluid, related to the disease process, the chemotherapy, the anticoagulation, or a combination of these.

tion. These high-risk criteria are listed in Figure 64–1. Patients with only a high pretherapy hCG level of long duration of disease may be at lesser risk than patients with liver or brain metastasis or prior treatment failure (Lewis, 1979; Jones et al, 1997).

On the basis of the Charing Cross Hospital experience (Bagshawe, 1976), the World Health Organization (WHO) in 1983 adopted a scoring system based on numerous prognostic factors (Table 64–5). The WHO scoring system appears to add additional stratification to patients considered "high risk" by the traditional NIH criteria. The WHO system can predict which patients with a high-risk profile are most likely to fail to respond to conventional combination therapy (DuBeshter et al, 1988; Gordon et al, 1989).

An anatomic staging system (Table 64–6) developed by the International Federation of Gynecology and Obstetrics (FIGO) was modified in 1992 to incorporate prognostic factors related to hCG level and duration of disease. However, the FIGO system is not routinely utilized to identify patients who need multiagent chemotherapy (Dubuc-Lissoir et al, 1992).

A comparison of survival for the various staging or risk classification systems for untreated patients is listed in Table 64–7.

CHEMOTHERAPY

Since the 1956 report by Li and colleagues, the cornerstone of treatment for persistent molar disease or metastatic trophoblastic tumors is chemotherapy. The aggressiveness of the chemotherapy treatment is influenced by determining whether the disease is metastatic and by the associated prognostic scoring factors (Hertz et al, 1961; Ross et al, 1965; Hammond et al, 1973). Patients with good prognostic features generally receive single-agent therapy; combination therapy is given to patients with more aggressive disease. In general, following each cycle of chemotherapy, a 1-log drop in LCG is anticipated. A drop of less than 25% may represent relative resistance and a change in the regimen should be considered (Soper et al, 1994).

Single-Agent Therapy

Patients with nonmetastatic and low-risk metastatic disease are treated with single-agent chemotherapy. Remission rates of 75% to 100% are expected; for those patients who fail to respond to primary therapy, almost all (98% to 100%) are cured with subsequent therapy. Table 64–8 outlines the most commonly used single-agent regimens for persistent molar disease or low-risk metastatic GTN. Methotrexate is the most commonly used single agent. The decreased toxicity associated with the alternate-day folinic acid treatments may be attributed as much to the scheduling interval of methotrexate as to the res-

▢ Table 64-5. WHO PROGNOSTIC SCORING SYSTEM

	SCORE*			
PROGNOSTIC FACTOR	0	1	2	4
Age (years)	≤39	>39	—	—
Antecedent pregnancy	Hydatidiform mole	Abortion, ectopic	Term pregnancy	—
Interval (months) of treatment	<4	4–6	7–12	>12
Initial hCG (mIU/ml)	$<10^3$	10^3–10^4	10^4–10^5	$>10^5$
Blood groups	—	OxA	B or AB	—
Largest tumor (cm)	<3	3–5	>5	—
Sites of metastasis	Lung	Spleen, kidney	GI tract, liver	Brain
No. of metastases	—	1–4	4–8	8
Previous (treatment)	—	—	Single drug	2 or more

*Low risk = 4 or lower; medium risk = 5–7; high risk = 8 or higher.
Abbreviations: GI, gastrointestinal; hCG, human chorionic gonadotropin.
Modified from World Health Organization Scientific Group on Gestational Trophoblastic Disease (Technical Report Series No. 692). Geneva: World Health Organization, 1983, with permission.

Table 64-6. FIGO STAGING SYSTEM FOR GESTATIONAL TROPHOBLASTIC TUMORS

STAGE	DESCRIPTION
I	Limited to the uterine corpus
II	Extends to the adnexae, outside the uterus, but limited to the genital structures
III	Extends to the lungs with or without genital tract involvement
IV	All other metastatic sites

Substages assigned for each stage as follows:
  A. No risk factors present
  B. One risk factor
  C. Both risk factors

Risk factors used to assign substages:
  1. Pretherapy serum hCG > 100,000 mIU/ml
  2. Duration of disease > 6 mo

FIGO Oncology Committee Report, 1992, with permission.

cue effect of the folinic acid (Rotmensch et al, 1984). Alternating the 5-day methotrexate and 5-day actinomycin D regimens will yield similar response rates, and cumulative toxicity is reduced.

Patients with nonmetastatic and low-risk metastatic disease are treated with single-agent therapy at 12- to 21-day intervals, waiting for the major toxicities (usually granulocytopenia and stomatitis) to clear. Chemotherapy is continued until the β-hCG titers are down to normal. Usually, at least one additional treatment cycle is then given before discontinuing treatment and the patient is observed with close surveillance of β-hCG values.

Combination Therapy

For patients with poor-prognostic metastatic GTN, therapy should be directed by physicians who are

Table 64-7. SURVIVAL BY STAGING AND RISK CLASSIFICATION

STAGING OR RISK CLASSIFICATION	ESTIMATED SURVIVAL (%)
FIGO Staging System	
I	100
II	100
III	75–80
IV	50–75
Clinical Traditional Criteria	
No metastatic	100
Metastatic, low risk	100
Metastatic, high risk	80
WHO Prognostic Scoring	
Low risk, ≤4	100
Medium risk, 5–7	95
High risk, 8–12	70
Very high risk, >12	65

Modified from Soper JT, Evans AC, Conoway MR, et al: Evaluation of prognostic factors and staging of gestational trophoblastic tumors. Obstet Gynecol 1994;84:969, with permission.

both very knowledgeable and experienced in the management of this disease. Although multidrug chemotherapy will play an integral treatment role, opportunities for the incorporation of surgery and irradiation therapy may be critical to achieve a curative outcome.

For patients with poor-prognostic disease, on the basis of either traditional criteria or more contemporary scoring methods, initial treatment is with multiagent chemotherapy (Hammond et al, 1973). Despite the recent introduction of a number of etoposide- or cisplatin-containing chemotherapy combinations, methotrexate, actinomycin D, and cyclophosphamide (MAC) (Table 64-9) remains the standard regimen in most centers throughout North America. Sustained remission rates with MAC therapy for high-risk metastatic disease range from 60% to 80% (Hammond et al, 1973; Lewis, 1979; Surwit and Hammond, 1980; Lurain and Brewer, 1985; DuBeshter et al, 1987; Curry et al, 1989a; Gordon et al, 1989).

The Bagshawe or CHAMOMA regimen (cyclophosphamide, hydroxyurea, actinomycin D, methotrexate, vincristine [Oncovin], melphalan, and doxorubicin [Adriamycin]) is reported to yield a 75% remission rate. Subsequently, the GOG performed a prospective trial comparing MAC and CHAMOMA (Curry et al, 1987). The MAC regimen had a more favorable therapeutic index. Primary remissions for MAC and CHAMOMA were similar, but the survival after salvage therapy favored the patients treated with MAC (96% vs. 70%). In addition, the CHAMOMA regimen with significantly more toxic and the study was closed early for this reason.

The combination proposed by the Charing Cross Hospital in London (Newlands et al, 1986, 1998), EMA-CO (Table 64-10), has shown promise with a primary sustained remission rate of about 77% to 90% in previously untreated patients and a 68% to 86% survival rate in patients subjected to prior treatment (Newlands et al, 1986; Schink et al, 1992; Soper et al, 1994; Kim et al, 1996). The toxicity is similar to that reported by the GOG for MAC (Bolis et al, 1988; Curry et al, 1989a). The risk of the development of a secondary leukemia related to etoposide is estimated to be at least 0.6%, and possibly higher (95% upper confidence bound of 5.9%) when used in combination with alkylating agents or dactinomycin (Smith et al, 1999). This risk should also be considered in treatment planning.

The reported experience with variations of EMA-CO, including the substitution of CO with etoposide and cisplatin, is limited (Surwit and Childers, 1991). Newer combinations of cisplatin, dactinomycin, and etoposide have demonstrated good efficacy in the management of high-risk GTN (Theodore et al, 1989; Bakri et al, 1993; Bakri et al, 1994). In general, treatment delays secondary to leukopenia should be minimized with the use of granulocyte colony-stimulating factor.

Effective second-line regimens yield significant responses and contribute to our high expectations for

Table 64-8. SINGLE-AGENT CHEMOTHERAPY

AGENT	DOSE AND ROUTE*	TOXICITIES Common	TOXICITIES Less Common	COMMENTS	REFERENCES
Methotrexate	0.3–0.4 mg/kg IM or IV daily × 5, repeat q 12–14 days	Myelosuppression Gastrointestinal Muscositis Nausea Alopecia Skin rashes	Hepatotoxicity Nephrotoxicity Pleuritis Pulmonary fibrosis	Contraindicated with parenchymal liver disease or renal function impairment	Hertz et al (1961) Ross et al (1965)
	0.4 mg/kg PO (max 25 mg) daily × 5, repeat q14d	Toxicities as above but less severe		Compliance and erratic absorption potential problems	Barter et al (1987)
	30 mg/m^2 IM weekly with dose escalation to 50 mg/m^2	Toxicities as above but reported minimal		Effective for postmolar GTN; efficacy for low-risk metastatic GTN not established	Homesley et al (1988)
Methotrexate (MTX) and folinic acid (FA)	MTX 1 mg/kg IM days 1, 3, 5, 7 FA 0.1 mg/kg IM days 2, 4, 6, 8 (24-hr delay)	Myelotoxicity—less than 5 days Gastrointestinal—less than 5 days Hepatotoxicity		Single cycle	Berkowitz et al (1986)
	Same as above but repeated q14d (Wong et al, 1985); MTX 0.5 mg/kg and FA 0.15 mg/kg and 30-hour FA delay	Hepatotoxicity similar to 5-day regimen (Wong et al, 1985)		Repetitive cycles; efficacy 70–75% Wong et al (1985): higher doses increased hepatic toxicity	Smith et al (1982) Wong et al (1985) Bagshawe et al (1989)
	MTX 500–600 mg/m^2 (1000-mg fixed dose) 6–15 hr infusion FA 30 mg IV 24-hr delay, 15 mg q6h × 7	Minimal hematologic or gastrointestinal toxicity		82% remission rate	Elit et al (1994)
Actinomycin D	10–12 μg/kg (IV/day × 5 (average-sized patient usually receives 0.5 mg/day × 5 days)	Myelosuppression Gastrointestinal Nausea/vomiting Stomatitis Alopecia	Severe vesicant	Less systemic toxicity than methotrexate	Goldstein et al (1972)
	40 μg/kg (1.25 mg/m^2) IV q2wk	Similar		GOG study—94% remission after average of 4.4 cycles	Pertrilli and Morrow (1980), Twiggs (1983), Schlaerth et al (1984), Petrilli et al (1987) (GOG)
5-Fluorouracil	28–30 mg/kg continuous IV infusion over 10 days q 24–31 days	Gastrointestinal Nausea/vomiting Stomatitis Diarrhea Pseudomembranous colitis Hepatotoxicity	Cerebellar ataxia	Widely used in Southeast Asia	Sung et al (1984)
Etoposide (VP-16)	200 mg/m^2 PO daily for 5 days q 12–14 days	Myelosuppression Gastrointestinal Nausea and vomiting Alopecia	Acute leukemia (0.6%; chromosomal damage: 11q23)		Wong et al (1986), Smith et al (1999)

*Chemotherapy for GTN should be prescribed and administered under the supervision of someone experienced with chemotherapy and the nuances of GTN, usually by a gynecologic oncologist. Dosages and intervals of treatment will vary according to many factors, including patient's weight, blood counts, liver and hepatic functions, prior toxicities, and other considerations.

Table 64-9. MAC THERAPY FOR METASTATIC GTN

Methotrexate	0.3 mg/kg	IV or IM daily × 5 days	(15 mg/day maximum)
Actinomycin D	8–10 μg/kg	IV daily × 5 days	(0.5 mg/day maximum)
Cyclophosphamide	3–5 mg/kg	IV daily × 5 days	(250 mg/day maximum)
Chlorambucil (as a substitute for cyclophosphamide)	0.2 mg/kg	PO daily × 5 days	(12 mg/day maximum)

Repeat every 14 to 21 days as toxicity permits.

curative therapy. By substituting etoposide and cisplatin for cyclophosphamide and vincristine (EMA-EP) (Newlands et al, 1991), over 75% of patients with disease refractory to EMA-CO have been reported to be cured. Cisplatin-etoposide combinations have been employed for the management of disease refractory to methotrexate and actinomycin (Theodore et al, 1989), and most recently ifosfamide has been added, commonly referred to as the VIP protocol (Sutton et al, 1992; Garris et al, 1992). When the cisplatin is replaced with carboplatin, the ICE protocol is useful in patients with renal or neurologic toxicities (Table 64–11). High-dose chemotherapy and the use of paclitaxel are the future areas of exploration for the management of refractory choriocarcinoma (Lotz et al, 1995; Jones et al, 1996).

Patients with high-risk trophoblastic disease usually receive at least two and often three cycles of additional chemotherapy after normalization of the hCG value. This is recommended to reduce the risk of recurrence.

REPRODUCTIVE POTENTIAL

Concerns about future reproductive potential are usually expressed by young patients after evaluation of a hydatidiform mole or after receiving chemotherapy for persistent or metastatic disease. Having seen their last pregnancy go from what they thought would be a joyous event culminating in a new addition to the family to a potentially life-threatening rare disease of which they had never heard, it is understandable that they will be apprehensive about subsequent fertility and their ability to have a normal pregnancy. Appropriate counseling allays most patients' fears.

The risk for development of a second molar pregnancy is between 1% and 4% (Matalon and Modan, 1972; Lurain et al, 1982; Berkowitz et al, 1987a, 1998; Woolas et al, 1998; Kim et al, 1998a). However, after two hydatidiform moles, the risk of a third is approximately 6% to 25% (Sand et al, 1984; Berkowitz et al, 1998; Woolas et al, 1998). Although the genetic abnormality has not been identified, there are rare cases of familial molar disease manifesting in sisters with repetitive molar pregnancies.

Infertility or ovarian failure rate does not seem to be increased, even in patients receiving chemotherapy (Berkowitz et al, 1987a; Amr, 1999). Retention of ovarian function is probably attributable in part to the usual short durations of chemotherapy and to the fact that most of these patients are in their early reproductive years. There is one report that expresses concern that treatment with etoposide (VP-16) may be associated with a higher risk of ovarian failure (Choo et al, 1985). The Charing Cross experience with 1313 pregnancies and 1000 subsequent live births reports no difference in pregnancy rate or outcome among women of the various risk groups, nor did the treatment regimen impact subsequent reproductive outcome (Woolas et al, 1998). Both the role of a 1-year pregnancy delay from treatment to permit "clearance" of damaged ova and the protective role of oral contraceptives during chemotherapy are speculative.

Subsequent pregnancies should be confirmed to be normal with a first-trimester ultrasound examination. Numerous reports claim no apparent increase

Table 64-10. EMA-CO CHEMOTHERAPY FOR POOR PROGNOSTIC DISEASE

Etoposide (VP-16)	100 mg/m²	IV daily × 2 days (over 30–45 min)
Methotrexate	100 mg/m²	IV loading dose, then 200 mg/m² over 12 hr day 1
Actinomycin D	0.5 mg	IV daily × 2 days
Folinic acid		15 mg IM or PO q12h × 4 starting 24 hr after starting methotrexate
Cyclophosphamide	600 mg/m²	IV on day 8
Oncovin (vincristine)	1 mg/m²	IV on day 8

Repeat every 15 days as toxicity permits.

Table 64-11. VIP AND ICE CHEMOTHERAPY FOR REFRACTORY DISEASE

VIP		
Etoposide (VP-16)	75 mg/m²	IV daily × 4
Ifosfamide (Mesna)	1.2 g/m²	IV daily × 4
	120 mg/m² IV bolus and 1.2 g/m²	IV daily over 12 hr after ifosfamide
Cisplatin	20 mg/m²	IV daily × 4
ICE		
Ifosfamide (Mesna)	Same as VIP but for only 3 days	
Carboplatin	300 mg/m² IV (or AUC of 4)	IV day 1
Etoposide (VP-16)	Same as VIP but for only 3 days	

Repeat every 21 days as toxicity permits.

in the risks of spontaneous abortion, prematurity, stillbirth, or congenital anomalies (Walden and Bagashawe, 1976; Goldstein et al, 1984; Berkowitz et al, 1987a; Song et al, 1988; Kim et al, 1998a). The Charing Cross experience reports a rate of stillbirth significantly higher than that for the general population (Woolas et al, 1998). Pregnancies occurring before completion of hGG follow-up tend to do well but they are at risk for delayed diagnosis of a relapse (Tuncer et al, 1999). An hCG test 6 to 8 weeks after completion of any future pregnancy is generally recommended. The risk of placenta accreta has been reported to be increased in patients who have received chemotherapy (Van Thiel et al, 1972).

One recent report suggests chemotherapy for GTN hastens menopause by an average of 3 years (Bower et al, 1999).

RECURRENCES

The risk of recurrent disease—elevation of titers after three consecutive normal titers—correlates with the severity of the initial disease (Mutch et al, 1990). Patients with nonmetastatic GTN face a 2.5% risk of recurrence; with "good-prognosis" metastatic disease, 3.7%; and with "poor-prognosis" disease, 12%. The risk of recurrence after 12 months of normal hCG levels is less than 1%. Although most patients are receiving hormonal contraception during the treatment and surveillance period, it is important to rule out the existence of a new pregnancy when a recurrent elevation of hCG occurs. The reinstitution of potentially teratogenic treatment necessitates exclusion of a normal intrauterine pregnancy or cautious counseling with regard to the inherent risks of therapy.

Salvage therapy for recurrent disease has improved significantly since the late 1970s. Mutch and colleagues (1990) have reported a 40% salvage rate prior to 1978 and a salvage rate of 83% since 1978. Improved cure rates for recurrent disease can be attributed to new and effective chemotherapeutic agents and to the combination of aggressive treatment modalities (Theodore et al, 1989; Mutch et al, 1990).

REFERENCES

Ambulafia O, Sherer D, Fultz P, et al: Unusual endovaginal ultrasonography and magnetic resonance imaging of placental site trophoblastic tumor. Am J Obstet Gynecol 1994;170:750.

Ambani LM, Vaidya RA, Rao CS, et al: Familial occurrence of trophoblastic disease: report of recurrent molar pregnancies in sisters in three families. Clin Genet 1980;18:27.

Amir SM, Osathanoudh R, Berkowitz RS, Goldstein DP: Human chorionic gonadotropin and thyroid function in patients with hydatidiform mole. Am J Obstet Gynecol 1984;150:723.

Amr MF: Return to fertility after successful chemotherapy treatment of gestational trophoblastic tumors. Int J Fertil Womens Med 1999;44:146.

Athanassiou A, Begent RHJ, Newlands ES, et al: Central nervous system metastases of choriocarcinoma: 23 years experience at Charing Cross Hospital. Cancer 1983;52:1728.

Atrash HK, Hogue CJR, Grimes DA: Epidemiology of hydatidiform mole during early gestation. Am J Obstet Gynecol 1986;154:906.

Bagshawe KD: Risk and prognostic factors in trophoblastic neoplasia. Cancer 1976;38:1373.

Bagshawe KD, Dent J, Newlands ES, Begent RHJ: The role of low-dose methotrexate and folinic acid in gestational trophoblastic tumors. Br J Obstet Gynecol 1989;96:795.

Bagshawe KD, Harland S: Immunodiagnosis and monitoring of gonadotropin producing metastases in the central nervous system. Cancer 1976;38:112.

Bakri YN, Berkowitz RS, Goldstein DP, et al: Brain metastases of gestational trophoblastic tumor. J Reprod Med 1994;39:179.

Bakri YN, Subhi J, Amer M, et al: Liver metastases of gestational trophoblastic tumor. Gynecol Oncol 1993;48:110.

Bandy LC, Clarke-Pearson DL, Hammond CB: Malignant potential of gestational trophoblastic disease at the extreme ages of reproductive life. Obstet Gynecol 1984;64:395.

Barnard DE, Woodward KT, Yancy SG et al: Hepatic metastases of choriocarcinoma: a report of 15 patients. Gynecol Oncol 1986;25:73.

Barnes AE, Liwnicz BH, Schellhas HF, et al: Case Report: successful treatment of placental choriocarcinoma metastatic to brain followed by primary brain glioblastoma. Gynecol Oncol 1982;13:108.

Barter JF, Soong SJ, Hatch KD, et al: Treatment of nonmetastatic gestational trophoblastic disease with oral methotrexate. Am J Obstet Gynecol 1987;157:1166.

Begent RHJ, Searle F, Stanway G, et al: Radioimmunolocalization of tumors by external scintigraphy after administration of ^{131}I antibody to human chorionic gonadotropin: preliminary communication. J R Soc Med. 1980;73:624.

Berkowitz RS, Im S, Bernstein MR, Goldstein DP: Gestational trophoblastic disease: subsequent pregnancy outcome, including repeat molar pregnancy. J Reprod Med 1998;43:81.

Berkowitz R, Ozturk M, Goldstein DP, et al: Human chorionic gonadotropin and free subunits serum levels in patients with partial and complete hydatidiform moles. Obstet Gynecol 1989;74:212.

Berkowitz RS, Cramer DW, Bernstein MR, et al: Risk factors for complete molar pregnancy from a case-control study. Am J Obstet Gynecol 1985;152:1016.

Berkowitz RS, Goldstein DP, Bernstein MR: Ten years' experience with methotrexate and folinic acid as primary therapy for gestational trophoblastic disease. Gynecol Oncol 1986;23:111.

Berkowitz RS, Goldstein DP, Bernstein MR, Sablinska B: Subsequent pregnancy outcomes in patients with molar pregnancies and gestational trophoblastic tumors. J Reprod Med 1987a;32:680.

Berkowitz RS, Goldstein DP, DuBeshter BE, Bernstein R: Management of complete molar pregnancy. J Reprod Med 1987b;32:634.

Berkowitz RS, Goldstein DP, Marean AR, Bernstein M: Oral contraceptives and postmolar trophoblastic disease. Obstet Gynecol 1981;58:474.

Bolis G, Bonazzi C, Landoni F, et al: EMA/CO regimen in high risk gestational trophoblastic tumor (GTT). Gynecol Oncol 1988;31:439.

Bower M, Rustin GL, Newlands ES, et al: Chemotherapy for gestational trophoblastic tumours hastens menopause by 3 years. Eur J Cancer 1998;34:1204.

Brace KD: The role of irradiation in the treatment of metastatic trophoblastic disease. Radiology 1968;91:540.

Brewer JI, Halpern B, Torok EE: Gestational trophoblastic disease: selected clinical aspects and chorionic gonadotropin test methods. Curr Prob Cancer 1979;3:1.

Brewer JI, Rinehart JJ, Dunbar RW: Choriocarcinoma report of the 5 or more years survival from the Albert Mathieu Chorionepithelium Registry. Am J Obstet Gynecol 1961;21:574.

Brewer JI, Torok EE, Webster A, Dolkart RE: Hydatidiform mole: a follow-up regimen for identification of invasive mole and choriocarcinoma and for selection of patients for treatment. Am J Obstet Gynecol 1968;101:557.

Brinton LA, Braken MB, Connelly RR: Choriocarcinoma incidence in the United States. Am J Epidemiol 1986;123:1094.

Buckley JD: The epidemiology of molar pregnancy and chorio-carcinoma. Clin Obstet Gynecol 1984;27:153.

Cheung AN, Ngan HY, Chen WZ, et al: The significance of pro-liferating cell nuclear antigen in human trophoblastic disease: an immunohistochemical study. Histopathology 1993;22:265.

Choo YC, Chan SYW, Wong LJC, Ho K: Ovarian dysfunction in patients with gestational trophoblastic neoplasia treated with short intensive courses of etoposide (VP 16–213). Cancer 1985; 55:2348.

Cotton DB, Bernstein SG, Reed JA, et al: Hemodynamic obser-vations in evacuation of molar pregnancy. Am J Obstet Gynecol 1980;138:6.

Crawford RA, Newlands E, Rustin GJ, et al: Gestational tropho-blastic disease with liver metastases: the charing Cross expe-rience. Br J Obstet Gynaecol 1997;104:105.

Curry SL, Blessing J, DiSaia P, et al. A prospective randomized comparison of methotrexate, actinomycin D, and chlorambucil (MAC) versus modified Bagshawe regimen in "poor progno-sis" gestational trophoblastic disease [SGO abstract]. Gynecol Oncol 1987;26:407.

Curry SL, Blessing JA, DiSaia PJ, et al: A prospective, randomized comparison of methotrexate, dactinomycin, and chlorambucil versus methotrexate, dactinomycin, cyclophosphamide, doxo-rubicin, melphalan, hydroxyurea, and vincristine in "poor prognosis" metastatic gestational trophoblastic disease: a Gy-necologic Oncology Group study. Obstet Gynecol 1989a;73:357.

Curry SL, Hammond CB, Tyrey L, et al: Hydatidiform mole: di-agnosis, management, and long-term follow-up of 347 patients. Obstet Gynecol 1975;45:1.

Curry SL, Schlaerth JB, Kohorn EI, et al: Hormonal contraception and trophoblastic sequelae after hydatidiform mole: a Gyne-cologic Oncology Group study. Am J Obstet Gynecol 1989b;160: 805.

Deicas RE, Miller DS, Rademaker AW, Lurain JR: The role of con-traception in the development of postmolar gestational tropho-blastic tumor. Obstet Gynecol 1991;78:221.

Delfs E: Chorionic gonadotropin determinations in patients with hydatidiform mole and choriocarcinoma. Ann N Y Acad Sci 1959;80:125.

DuBeshter BE, Berkowitz RS, Goldstein DP, Bernstein MR: Anal-ysis of treatment failure in high risk metastatic gestational tro-phoblastic disease. Gynecol Oncol 1988;29:199.

DuBeshter BE, Berkowitz RS, Goldstein DP, et al: Metastatic ges-tational trophoblastic disease at the New England Trophoblas-tic Disease Center, 1965 to 1985. Obstet Gynecol 1987;689:390.

Dubuc-Lissoir J, Swelzig S, Schlaerth JB, Morrow CP: Metastatic gestational trophoblastic disease: a comparison of prognostic classification systems. Gynecol Oncol 1992;45:40.

Eckstein RP, Paradinas FJ, Bagshawe KD: Placental site tropho-blastic tumour (trophoblastic pseudotumour): a study of four cases requiring hysterectomy, including one fatal case. Histo-pathology 1982;6:211.

Elit L, Covens A, Osborne R, et al: High-dose methotrexate for gestational trophoblastic disease. Gynecol Oncol 1994;54:282.

Elston CW: The histopathology of trophoblastic tumours. J Clin Pathol 1977;29(Suppl):111.

Evans AC Jr, Soper JT, Clarke-Pearson DL, et al: Gestational tro-phoblastic disease metastatic to the central nervous system. Gynecol Oncol 1995;59:226.

Finkler NS, Berkowitz RS, Driscoll SG, et al: Clinical experience with placental site trophoblastic tumors at the New England Trophoblastic Disease Center. Obstet Gynecol 1988;71:854.

Fishman DA, Padilla LA, Keh P, et al: Management of twin preg-nancies consisting of a complete hydatidiform mole and nor-mal fetus. Obstet Gynecol 1998;91:546.

Garris PD, Gallup DG, Melton K: Long-term remission of previ-ously resistant choriocarcinoma with a combination of etopo-side, ifosfamide, and cisplatin. Gynecol Oncol 1995;57:254.

Giacalone PL, Benos P, Donnadio D, Laffargue F: High-dose che-motherapy with autologous bone marrow transplantation for refractory gestational trophoblastic disease. Gynecol Oncol 1995;58:383.

Goldstein DP, Berkowitz RS: Current management of complete and partial molar pregnancy. J Reprod Med 1994;39:139.

Goldstein DP, Berkowitz RS, Bernstein MR: Reproductive perfor-mance after molar pregnancy and gestational trophoblastic tu-mors. Clin Obstet Gynecol 1984;27:221.

Goldstein DP, Winig P, Shirley RL: Actinomycin D as initial ther-apy of gestational trophoblastic disease: a re-evaluation. Obstet Gynecol 1972;39:341.

Gordon AN, Gershenson DM, Copeland LJ, et al: High-risk met-astatic gestational trophoblastic disease: further stratification into two clinical entities. Gynecol Oncol 1989;34:54.

Grimes DA: Epidemiology of gestational trophoblastic disease. Am J Obstet Gynecol 1984;150:309.

Grumbine FC, Rosenschein NB, Brewerton MD, Kaufman SL: Management of liver metastasis from gestational trophoblastic neoplasia. Am J Obstet Gynecol 1980;137:959.

Hammond CB, Borchert LG, Tyrey L, et al: Treatment of meta-static trophoblastic disease: good and poor prognosis. Am J Obstet Gynecol 1973;115:451.

Hammond CB, Soper JT: Poor prognosis metastatic gestational trophoblastic neoplasia. Clin Obstet Gynecol 1984;27:228.

Hammond CB, Weed JC Jr, Currie JL: The role of operation in the current therapy of gestational trophoblastic disease. Am J Ob-stet Gynecol 1980;136:844.

Hatch KD, Mann WJ Jr, Boots LR, et al: Localization of chorio-carcinoma by ^{131}I-hCG antibody. Gynecol Oncol 1980;10:253.

Heaton GE, Matthews TH, Christopherson WH: Malignant tro-phoblastic tumors with massive hemorrhage presenting as liver primary: a report of two cases. Am J Surg Pathol 1986;10:342.

Heintz APM, Schaberg A, Englesman E, van Hall EV: Placental-site trophoblastic tumor: diagnosis, treatment and biological behavior. Int J Gynecol Pathol 1985;4:75.

Hertig AT: Human Trophoblast. Springfield, IL: Charles C Tho-mas, 1968.

Hertz R, Lewis J Jr, Lipsett MB: Five years' experience with the chemotherapy of metastatic choriocarcinoma and related tro-phoblastic tumors in women. Am J Obstet Gynecol 1961;82:631.

Ho Yuen B, Burch P: Relationship of oral contraceptives and the intrauterine contraceptive devices to the regression of concen-trations of the beta subunit of human chorionic gonadotropin and invasive complications after molar pregnancy. Am J Obstet Gynecol 1983;145:214.

Homesley HD, Blessing JA, Rettenmaier M, et al: Weekly intra-muscular methotrexate for nonmetastatic gestational tropho-blastic disease. Obstet Gynecol 1988;72:413.

Jaffe R: Investigation of abnormal first-trimester gestation by color Doppler imaging. J Clin Ultrasound 1993;21:521.

Jauniaux E, Nicolaides KH, Hustin J: Perinatal features associated with placental mesenchymal dysplasia. Placenta 1997;18:701.

Jones WB, Cardinale C, Lewis JL Jr: Management of high-risk gestational trophoblastic disease: the Memorial Hospital ex-perience. Int J Gynecol Cancer 1997;7:27.

Jones WB, Schneider J, Shapiro F, et al: Treatment of resistant gestational choriocarcinoma with Taxol: a report of two cases. Gynecol Oncol 1996;61:126.

Kajii T, Ohama K: Androgenetic origin of hydatidiform mole. Na-ture 1977;268:633.

Kelly MP, Rustin GJS, Ivory C: Respiratory failure due to chorio-carcinoma: a study of 103 dyspneic patients. Gynecol Oncol 1990;38:149.

Khazaeli MB, Buchina ES, Patillo RA, et al: Radioimmunoassay of free beta-subunit of human chorionic gonadotropin in di-agnosis of high risk and low risk gestational trophoblastic dis-ease. Am J Obstet Gynecol 1989;160:444.

Khazaeli MB, Hedyaat MM, Hatch KD, et al: Radioimmunoassay of free β-subunit of human chorionic gonadotropin as a prog-nostic test for persistent trophoblastic disease in molar preg-nancy. Am J Obstet Gynecol 1986;155:520.

Kim DS, Moon H, Kim KT, Moon YJ, Hwang YY: Effects of pro-phylactic chemotherapy for persistent trophoblastic disease in patients with complete hydatidiform mole. Obstet Gynecol 1986;67:690.

Kim JH, Park DC, Bae SN, et al: Subsequent reproductive expe-rience after treatment for gestational trophoblastic disease. Gy-necol Oncol 1998a;71:108.

Kim SJ, Bae SN, Kim JH, Kim CJ, Jung JK: Risk factors for the prediction of treatment failure in gestational trophoblastic tumors treated with EMA/CO regimen. Gynecol Oncol 1998b;71: 247.

Kohorn EI, Caldwell BV, Cortes JM: Alpha-subunit in gestational trophoblastic disease. Placenta 1981;3:231.

Kurman RJ, Scully RE, Norris HJ: Trophoblastic pseudotumor of the uterus: an exaggerated form of "syncytial endometritis" simulating a malignant tumor. Cancer 1976;38:1214.

Kurman RJ, Young RH, Norris HJ, et al: Immunocytochemical localization of placental lactogen and chorionic gonadotropin in the normal placenta and trophoblastic tumors, with emphasis on intermediate trophoblast and the placental site trophoblastic tumor. Int J Gynecol Pathol 1984;3:101.

Lacey CG, Barnard D, Degefu S, Witty JB, Eisenman E: Irradiation of liver metastases due to gestational choriocarcinoma. Obstet Gynecol 1983;61:71S.

Lewis JL Jr: Treatment of metastatic trophoblastic neoplasms. Am J Obstet Gynecol 1979;136:163.

Li MD, Hertz R, Spencer DB: Effect of methotrexate therapy upon choriocarcinoma and chorioadenoma. Proc Soc Exp Biol Med 1956;93:361.

Liftshitz H, Barber CE, Hammond CB: The pulmonary metastases of choriocarcinoma. Obstet Gynecol 1977;49:412.

Llewellyn-Jones D: Management of benign trophoblastic tumors. Am J Obstet Gynecol 1967;99:589.

Lotz J-P, Andre T, Donsimoni R, et al: High dose chemotherapy with ifosfamide, carboplatin, and etoposide combined with autologous bone marrow transplantation for the treatment of poor-prognosis germ cell tumors and metastastic trophoblastic disease in adults. Cancer 1995;75:874.

Lurain JR, Brewer JL: Treatment of high-risk gestational trophoblastic disease with methotrexate, actinomycin D, and cyclophosphamide chemotherapy. Obstet Gynecol 1985;65:830.

Lurain JR, Brewer JL, Turok EE, Halpern B: Gestational trophoblastic disease: treatment results at the Brewer Trophoblastic Disease Center. Obstet Gynecol 1982;60:354.

Martin DA, Sutton GP, Ulbright TM, et al: DNA content as a prognostic index in gestational trophoblastic neoplasia. Gynecol Oncol 1989;34:385.

Matalon M, Modan B: Epidemiologic aspects of hydatidiform mole in Israel. Am J Obstet Gynecol 1972;112:107.

Matsuura J, Chiu D, Jacobs PA, Szulman AE: Complete hydatidiform mole in Hawaii: an epidemiological study. Genet Epidemiol 1984;1:271.

Mazzanti P, LaVecchia C, Parazzini F, et al: Frequency of hydatidiform mole in Lombardy, Italy. Gynecol Oncol 1986;24:337.

Messerli M, Rosenshein N, Lilienfield A: Risk factors for gestational trophoblastic neoplasia. Gynecol Oncol 1985;20:261.

Miller D, Jackson R, Ehein T, McMuurtrie E: Complete hydatidiform mole coexistent with a twin live fetus: clinical course of four cases with complete cytogenetic analysis. Gynecol Oncol 1993;50:119.

Miller JM, Surwit EA, Hammond CB: Choriocarcinoma following term pregnancy. Obstet Gynecol 1979;53:207.

Montz FJ, Schlaerth JB, Morrow CP: The natural history of theca lutein cysts. Obstet Gynecol 1988;72:247.

Morrow CP, Kletzky OA, DiSaia PJ, et al: Clinical and laboratory correlates of molar pregnancy and trophoblastic disease. Am J Obstet Gynecol 1977;128:424.

Morrow CP, Nakamura R, Schlaerth J, et al: The influence of oral contraceptives on the postmolar human chorionic gonadotropin regression curve. Am J Obstet Gynecol 1985;151:906.

Morrow CP, Townsend DE: Synopsis of Gynecologic Oncology. 3rd ed. New York: John Wiley & Sons, 1987:367.

Mutch DG, Soper JT, Babcock CS, et al: Recurrent gestational trophoblastic disease: experience of the Southeastern Regional Trophoblastic Disease Center. Cancer 1990;66:978.

Nagelberg SB, Rosen SW: Clinical and laboratory investigation of a virilized woman with placental site trophoblastic tumor. Obstet Gynecol 1985;65:527.

Newlands ES, Bagshawe KD, Begent RHJ, et al: Developments in chemotherapy for medium- and high-risk patients with gestational trophoblastic tumours (1979–1984). Br J Obstet Gynaecol 1986;93:63.

Newlands ES, Bagshawe KD, Begent RHJ, et al: Results with EMA/CO (etoposide, methotrexate, actinomycin D, cyclophosphamide, vincristine) regimen in high risk gestational trophoblastic tumors, 1979–1989. Br J Obstet Gynaecol 1991;98:550.

Newlands ES, Bower M, Holden L, et al: The management of high-risk gestational trophoblastic tumours. Int J Gynaecol Obstet 1998;60:S65.

Newman RB, Eddy GL: Eclampsia as a possible risk factor for persistent trophoblastic disease. Gynecol Oncol 1989;34:212.

Nishimura R, Ashitaka Y, Tojo S: The clinical evaluation of the simultaneous measurements of human chorionic gonadotropin (hCG) and its alpha subunit in sera of patients with trophoblastic diseases. Endocrinol Jpn 1979;26:575.

Ohama K, Kajii T, Okamoto E, et al: Dispermic origin of XY hydatidiform moles. Nature 1981;292:551.

Palmer JR: Advances in the epidemiology of gestational trophoblastic disease. J Reprod Med 1994;39:155.

Palmer JR, Driscoll SG, Rosenberg L, et al: Oral contraceptive use and risk of gestational trophoblastic tumors. J Natl Cancer Inst 1999;97:635.

Paradinas FJ: The histological diagnosis of hydatidiform moles. Curr Diag Pathol 1994;1:24.

Parazzini F, LaVecchia C, Franceschi S, Mangili G: Familial trophoblastic disease: case report. Am J Obstet Gynecol 1984;149: 382.

Parazzini F, LaVecchia C, Pampallona S: Parental age and risk of complete and partial hydatidiform mole. Br J Obstet Gynaecol 1986;93:582.

Parazzini F, LaVecchia C, Pampallona S, Fraceschi S: Reproductive patterns and the risk of gestational trophoblastic disease. Am J Obstet Gynecol 1985;152:866.

Petrilli ES, Morrow CP: Actinomycin D toxicity in the treatment of trophoblastic disease: a comparison and the five-day course to single-dose administration. Gynecol Oncol 1980;9:18.

Petrilli ES, Twiggs LB, Blessing JA, et al: Single-dose actinomycin D treatment for nonmetastatic gestational trophoblastic disease: a prospective phase II trial of the Gynecologic Oncology Group. Cancer 1987;60:2173.

Quigley MM, Tyrey L, Hammond CB: Utility of assay of alpha subunit of human chorionic gonadotropin in management of gestational trophoblastic malignancies. Am J Obstet Gynecol 1980;138:545.

Quinones J, Mizejewski G, Beirwaltes WH: Choriocarcinoma scanning using radiolabelled antibody to chorionic gonadotropin. J Nucl Med 1971;12:69.

Ratnam SS, Teoh ES, Dawood MY: Methotrexate for prophylaxis of choriocarcinoma. Am J Obstet Gynecol 1971;111:1021.

Rice LW, Berkowitz RS, Lage JM, et al: Persistent gestational trophoblastic tumor after partial hydatidiform mole. Gynecol Oncol 1990;36:358.

Ross GT, Goldstein DP, Hertz R, et al: Sequential use of methotrexate and actinomycin D in the treatment of metastatic choriocarcinomas and related trophoblastic tumors in women. Am J Obstet Gynecol 1965;93:223.

Rotmensch J, Rosenshein N, Donehower R, et al: Plasma methotrexate levels in patients with gestational trophoblastic neoplasia treated by two methotrexate regimens. Am J Obstet Gynecol 1984;148:730.

Rustin GJ, Newlands ES, Begent RH, et al: Weekly alternating etoposide, methotrexate and actinomycin/vincristine and cyclophosphamide chemotherapy for the treatment of CNS metastases of choriocarcinoma. J Clin Oncol 1989;7:900.

Sand PK, Lurain JR, Brewer JI: Repeat gestational trophoblastic disease. Obstet Gynecol 1984;63:140.

Schink JC, Singh DK, Rademaker AW, et al: Etoposide, methotrexate, actinomycin D, cyclophosphamide, and vincristine for the treatment of metastatic high-risk gestational trophoblastic disease. Obstet Gynecol 1992;80:817.

Schlaerth JB, Morrow CP, Nalick RH, Gaddis O Jr: Single-dose actinomycin D in the treatment of postmolar trophoblastic disease. Gynecol Oncol 1984;19:53.

Scully RE, Young RH: Trophoblastic pseudotumor: reappraisal. Am J Surg Pathol 1981;5:75.

Sheline GE, Wara WM, Smith V: Therapeutic irradiation and brain injury. Int J Radiat Oncol Biol Phys 1980;6:1215.

Shigematsu T, Kamura T, Saito T, et al: Identification of persistent trophoblastic diseases based on a human chorionic gonadotropin regression curve by means of a stepwise piecewise linear regression analysis after the evacuation of uneventful moles. Gynecol Oncol 1998;71:376.

Shirley RL, Goldstein DP, Collins JJ Jr: The role of thoracotomy in management of patients with chest metastases from gestational trophoblastic disease. J Thorac Cardiovasc Surg 1972;63:545.

Sink JD, Hammond CB, Young WG: Pulmonary resection in the management of metastases from choriocarcinoma. J Thorac Cardiovasc Surg 1978;81:830.

Smith EB, Weed JC Jr, Tyrey L, Hammond CB: Treatment of nonmetastatic gestational trophoblastic disease: results of methotrexate alone versus methotrexate-folinic acid. Am J Obstet Gynecol 1982;44:88.

Smith MA, Rubinstein L, Anderson JR, et al: Secondary leukemia or myelodysplastic syndrome after treatment with epipodophyllotoxins. J Clin Oncol 1999;17:569.

Song H, Wu P, Wong Y, et al: Pregnancy outcomes after successful chemotherapy for choriocarcinoma and invasive mole: long-term follow-up. Am J Obstet Gynecol 1988;158:538.

Soper JT, Evans AC, Clarke-Pearson DL, et al: Alternating weekly chemotherapy with etoposide-methotrexate-dactinomycin/cyclophosphamide-vincristine for high-risk gestational trophoblastic disease. Obstet Gynecol 1994;84:113.

Soper JT, Mutch DG, Chin N, et al: Renal metastases of gestational trophoblastic disease: a report of eight cases. Obstet Gynecol 1988;72:796.

Stellar MA, Genest DR, Bernstein MR, et al: Natural history of twin pregnancy with complete hydatidiform mole and coexistent fetus. Obstet Gynecol 1994;83:35.

Stone M, Dent J, Kardena A, Bagshawe KD. Relationship of oral contraception to development of trophoblastic tumor after evacuation of a hydatidiform mole. Br J Obstet Gynaecol 1976;83:913.

Sung H, Wu P, Yan H: Re-evaluation of 5-fluorouracil as a single therapeutic agent for gestational trophoblastic neoplasms. Am J Obstet Gynecol 1984;150:69.

Surti U, Szulman AE, O'Brien S: Dispermic origin and clinical outcome of three complete hydatidiform moles with 46 XY karyo-type. Am J Obstet Gynecol 1982;144:84.

Surwit EA, Childers JM: High-risk metastatic gestational trophoblastic disease: a new dose-intensive, multiagent chemotherapeutic regimen. J Reprod Med 1991;36:45.

Surwit EA, Hammond CB: Treatment of metastatic trophoblastic disease with poor prognosis. Obstet Gynecol 1980;55:565.

Sutton GP, Soper JT, Blessing JA, Hatch KD, Barnhill DR: Ifosfamide alone and in combination in the treatment of refractory malignant gestational trophoblastic disease. Am J Obstet Gynecol 1992;167:489.

Szulman AE: Trophoblastic disease: clinical pathology of hydatidiform moles. Obstet Gynecol Clin North Am 1988;15:433.

Szulman AE, Surti U: The syndromes of hydatidiform mole. I. Cytogenetics and morphologic correlations. Am J Obstet Gynecol 1978;131:665.

Theodore C, Azab M, Droz JP, et al: Treatment of high-risk gestational trophoblastic disease with chemotherapy combinations containing cisplatin and etoposide. Cancer 1989;64:1824.

Tomoda Y, Arii Y, Kaseki S, et al: Surgical indications for resection in pulmonary metastasis of choriocarcinoma. Cancer 1980;46:2723.

Tuncer ZS, Bernstein MR, Goldstein DP, Berkowitz RS: Outcome of pregnancies occurring before completion of human chorionic gonadotropin follow-up in patients with persistent gestational trophoblastic tumor. Gynecol Oncol 1999;73:345.

Twiggs LB: Pulse actinomycin D scheduling in nonmetastatic gestational trophoblastic disease: cost-effective chemotherapy. Gynecol Oncol 1983;16:190.

Twiggs LB: Non-neoplastic complications of molar pregnancy. Clin Obstet Gynecol 1984;27:199.

Twiggs LB, Morrow DP, Schlaerth JB: Acute pulmonary complications of molar pregnancy. Am J Obstet Gynecol 1979;135:189.

Van Thiel DH, Grodin JM, Ross GT, Lipsett MB: Partial placenta accreta in pregnancies following chemotherapy for gestational trophoblastic neoplasms. Am J Obstet Gynecol 1972;112:54.

Vassilakos P, Riotton G, Kajii T: Hydatidiform mole: two entities. A morphologic and cytogenetic study with some clinical considerations. Am J Obstet Gynecol 1977;127:167.

Vejerslev LO, Dueholm M, Nielsen FH: Hydatidiform mole: cytogenetic marker analysis in twin gestation. Am J Obstet Gynecol 1986;155:614.

Walden PAM, Bagshawe KD: Reproductive performance of women successfully treated for gestational trophoblastic tumors. Am J Obstet Gynecol 1976;125:1108.

Weed JC, Woodward KT, Hammond CB: Choriocarcinoma metastatic to the brain: therapy and prognosis. Semin Oncol 1982;9:208.

Wilson RB, Hunter JS, Dockerty MB: Chorioadenoma destruens. Am J Obstet Gynecol 1961;81:546.

Witzleben CL, Bruninga G: Infantile choriocarcinoma: a characteristic syndrome. J Pediatr 1968;73:374.

Wong LC, Choo YC, Ma HK: Hepatic metastases in gestational trophoblastic disease. Obstet Gynecol 1986a;67:107.

Wong LC, Ma HK: Persistent chest opacity in trophoblastic disease: is thoracotomy justified? Aust N Z J Obstet Gynaecol 1983;23:237.

Wong MA, Choo YC, Ma HK: Methotrexate with citrovorum factor rescue in gestational trophoblastic disease. Am J Obstet Gynecol 1985;152:59.

Wong MA, Choo YC, Ma HK: Primary oral etoposide therapy in gestational trophoblastic disease: an update. Cancer 1986b;58:14.

Woodward RM, Filly RA, Callen PW: First trimester molar pregnancy: nonspecific ultrasonographic appearance. Obstet Gynecol 1980;55:1S.

Woolas RP, Bower M, Newlands ES, et al: Influence of chemotherapy for gestational trophoblastic disease on subsequent pregnancy outcome. Br J Obstet Gynaecol 1998;105:1032.

Xu LT, Suu CF, Wang YE, Song HZ: Resection of pulmonary metastatic choriocarcinoma in 43 drug-resistant patients. Ann Thorac Surg 1985;39:25.

Yen S, MacMahon B: Epidemiologic features of trophoblastic disease. Am J Obstet Gynecol 1968;101:126.

Yordan EL Jr, Schlaerth J, Gaddis O, Morrow CP: Radiation therapy in the management of gestational choriocarcinoma metastatic to the central nervous system. Obstet Gynecol 1987;69:627.

Young RH, Scully RE: Placental-site trophoblastic tumors: current status. Clin Obstet Gynecol 1984;27:248.

Young RH, Scully RE, McCluskey RT: A distinctive glomerular lesion complicating placental site trophoblastic tumor: report of two cases. Hum Pathol 1986;161:35.

65

Psychological Adjustment for the Gynecologic Cancer Patient*

Barbara L. Andersen

Although the diagnosis of cancer is a devastating experience, the majority of women and men cope successfully. In fact, many individuals report renewed vigor in their approach to life and also describe other positive outcomes such as stronger interpersonal relationships and a "survivor" mentality (e.g., Taylor, 1983). These outcomes do not, however, describe the *process* of the experience, which includes the emotional turmoil at diagnosis, the emotions of fear and sadness, and the adjustment to permanent changes in one's life. For decades the understanding of the psychological processes and outcomes was largely clinical, consisting of case studies of patients and clinical descriptions of the phenomena (e.g., Sutherland et al, 1952). The message from these reports was that the psychological trajectory was, at best, guarded.

However, controlled psychological and behavioral research has specified the difficulties that cancer patients face, offered hypotheses of the mechanisms leading to "better" adjustment or more favorable disease outcomes, and tested interventions for improving the psychological adjustment and, possibly, the disease outcomes. In much of this research, breast cancer patients have been studied (for reviews, see Andersen, 1989; *Cancer* 1992 (supplement, whole issue), and these findings can be applied, in part, to the experiences of other female cancer patients.

To overview the psychological processes of adjustment to cancer in general and gynecologic cancer in particular, a disease time line approach organizes the content. Within this framework, descriptive as well as experimental data are included on central areas of adjustment: psychological, social, marital, and sexual. When interventions are discussed, a model for predicting which women will be at risk for difficulty following treatment is highlighted.

PSYCHOLOGICAL AND BEHAVIORAL COURSE

Diagnosis

Responses to Cancer Symptoms

Much of cancer incidence and premature death can be prevented through changes in behavior. Shortening delay in seeking a diagnosis once symptom/sign awareness has occurred directly impacts morbidity and may also affect mortality. For endometrial, ovarian, and vulvar diseases, this is the only type of prevention that is currently available and/or feasible. To the extent that spread of major or microscopic disease is limited, morbidity and mortality may be reduced.

Research has examined the psychological and behavioral aspects of delay in seeking a medical diagnosis of gynecologic cancer (Andersen et al, 1995). It appears there is a series of decision steps or stages that an individual experiences, from his or her first awareness of symptoms to the point when he or she finally appears before a physician. The stages include the following:

- *Appraisal delay*: days from the detection of a symptom to the individual's decision that he or she is ill
- *Illness delay*: days from the above illness inference and a decision to seek medical attention
- *Behavioral delay*: days from the decision to seek medical attention to the person acting on this decision by making an appointment

*This work was supported by the U.S. Army Medical Research Acquisition Activity (Grant DAMD 17-96-1-6294) and the National Institute of Mental Health (Grant 1 RO1 MH14887).

- *Scheduling delay*: days elapsed between the person making an appointment and first receiving medical attention

These stages are differentially important. Our analysis has also focused on the delay processes of symptom interpretation—that is, appraisal delay—because this interval accounts for the majority (e.g., 75%) of the delay in seeking a gynecologic cancer diagnosis (Andersen et al, 1995). We have examined the possible role in symptom appraisal and delay of specific decisions and inferences women draw when relating their symptoms to their prior expectations and knowledge about the physiologic aspects of cancer (e.g., Does vaginal bleeding mean that one has cancer? Does a vulva sore mean one may have cancer?). We tested the model of patient delay with a sample of gynecology patients.

We studied 50 women with initial or recurrent gynecologic cancer at diagnosis (Andersen et al, 1995). The period of symptom appraisal accounted for 80% of the total delay from the day of the first symptom/sign appearance to the day of arrival before a physician. For example, a common scenario was a 45-year-old woman who took about 3 months to decide that her irregular vaginal bleeding may indicate something more serious (possibly cancer?) rather than her first hypothesis of a normal condition, such as menopause. Women's appraisal delay was also related to their drive to explain their unexpected symptoms, which in turn was predicted by the specificity (e.g., Was the symptom only bleeding as opposed to bleeding and pain with intercourse), salience (e.g., How heavy was the bleeding? How many days did it last?), and perceived consequences of the symptoms (e.g., Did she lose interest in or avoid intercourse because of the pain or bleeding?). These data directly counter popular notions that individuals deny cancer symptomatology and/or delay because of fears of the disease or treatment. Instead, the data suggest that individuals "delay" because they are trying to interpret and generate hypotheses about their symptoms—that is, they are trying to "figure out" what is wrong or what the symptoms indicate, and, in turn, they are delaying while engaged in this effort.

Other data suggested that the appearance of some gynecologic cancer signs and symptoms produce sexual disruption (Andersen et al, 1986). When sexual functioning adversely changes, this may provide additional evidence to a woman of the "non-normality" of a symptom picture and further prompt her regarding the need for medical evaluation. We studied 41 women with early-stage cervical or endometrial cancer and a matched group (i.e., age, menopausal and sexually active status) of healthy women in no gynecologic distress. They provided data on the range and frequency of sexual behavior, level of sexual responsiveness, and presence of sexual dysfunction. Analyses indicated that, prior to the onset of cancer signs and symptoms, the gynecologic cancer patients reported similar patterns of sexual activity and responsiveness as the healthy sample. With the appearance of disease signs/symptoms (i.e., fatigue, postcoital bleeding, vaginal discharge, pain), the women who would subsequently receive a gynecologic cancer diagnosis reported significant sexual dysfunctions. There was a four- to fivefold increase in the frequency of sexual dysfunctions such as lowered desire and orgasmic dysfunction from pre- to postappearance of cancer signs/symptoms. Moreover, 75% of the women with cancer experienced these changes. This suggests that such obvious and disruptive sexual problems may have been additional warning signs that influenced the women to seek medical consultation.

Responses to the Diagnosis

The diagnosis of cancer, whether initial or recurrent, is the maximally stressful time for the cancer patient. This crisis period is defined by the emotions of sadness (depression), fear (anxiety), confusion, and, on some occasions, anger. Each emotion is important for understanding the process patients undergo when learning their diagnosis, completing the tumor evaluation, and beginning treatment.

Surveys cite *depression* as the most prevalent affective problem for patients, with estimates of unipolar diagnoses in the order of 5% to 6% (Derogatis et al, 1983; Lansky et al, 1985). When major depression and adjustment disorder with depressed mood are considered, prevalence rates are higher (16% in the study by Derogatis et al [1983]). In a study of gynecologic cancer patients, Evans et al (1986) reported that 23% of the women had major depression. In general, higher rates of depression are found for those patients in active treatment rather than on follow-up, in those receiving palliative rather than curative treatment, in those with pain or other disturbing symptoms rather than not, and in those with a history of affective disorder. The latter attributes represent risk factors. Among women not having these characteristics, the base rate of major depression is likely to be in the range of 6%, comparable to that of the general population.

Not surprisingly, it can be difficult to make a diagnosis of depression in cancer patients, as it is for patients with other serious illnesses; however, some indications may be noted. First, a determination should be made about the vegetative symptoms: poor appetite, which may lead to weight loss; insomnia or hypersomnia; loss of energy or fatigue; and loss of sexual desire or interest. The diagnostician must determine if such symptomatology is representative of depression, disease-related events, or some combination of factors. For example, if the disease is disseminated or accompanied with pain, the case would be stronger for disease-initiated symptoms rather than a psychological source. Conversely, if a woman presents with localized disease and nonpainful symptoms/signs, the likelihood of a psychological etiology might be higher.

Another difficult issue is distinguishing between the symptoms of depression (e.g., dysphoric mood, loss of interest or pleasure, guilt, hopelessness) and the normal reactions to a life-threatening illness. This is particularly difficult because depression for cancer patients is reactive; that is, it occurs soon after the diagnosis, and the content of the depressive ruminations reflect the diagnostic event (Noyes and Kathol, 1986). When depressive symptoms are present, they tend to be intermittent and rarely persist for more than a few weeks once treatment has begun or is concluded. Our controlled longitudinal studies indicate that emotional "rebound" for gynecologic patients is rapid—usually occurring by 3 to 4 months following treatment—when recovery proceeds smoothly (Andersen et al, 1989b). However, because cancer is a realistic health stressor, patients and physicians alike regard some type of depressive reaction to the diagnosis as "normal." Therefore, patients may not feel comfortable (or able) to complain about their feelings, even when they are extreme. Similarly, physicians or nurses may not recognize severe depressive reactions because of their infrequency and the commonality of less severe, transitory reactions. In combination, these circumstances conspire to the underrecognition and undertreatment (Derogatis et al, 1979) of major depression among cancer patients.

When depression does occur, some symptoms may be more or less characteristic. In addition to dysphoric mood, other common symptoms may include loss of interest or pleasure, loss of energy or fatigue, and difficulty thinking or concentrating (e.g., feeling confused or bewildered). Other common feelings include intermittent anxiety, helplessness, and concern about the future (Lansky et al, 1985). Endicott (1984) has suggested that other possibilities, including fearful or depressed appearance, social withdrawal or decreased talkativeness, brooding or pessimism, and mood that is not reactive (i.e., the patient cannot be cheered up, does not smile, and/or does not react to good news), should be considered as symptoms/signs of major depression in medical patients. In contrast, common psychological characteristics of depressed psychiatric patients that are uncommon for cancer patients include feelings of low self-esteem and guilt. Finally, it is rare for cancer patients to be psychotic or suicidal (Plumb and Holland, 1977; Bukberg et al, 1984).

Anxiety disorder is the affective problem second in frequency among cancer patients. In an early study of 44 breast cancer patients interviewed at the time of diagnosis, Hughes (1981) estimated that 25% of the sample had severe anxiety reactions. Anxiety-related problems are typically manifested by the symptoms of generalized anxiety. That is, there are the classical responses such as fear, worry, and rumination, but other symptoms include motor tension (e.g., feeling shaky, muscle tension, restless, and easy fatigability), autonomic hyperactivity (e.g., abdominal distress, frequent urination), and/or indications of vigilance and scanning (e.g., difficulty concentrating, trouble falling or staying asleep, feeling on edge). Much of the content of the anxiety-provoking thoughts is focused on medical examinations and cancer treatments (e.g., fear of pain or disfigurement) and the short- and long-term disruption they may produce (see discussion below). Other targets include the life disruption and change that may occur because the individual has cancer. The most common spheres of worry include family, money, work, and illness—for example, Who will care for the children when I am in the hospital? What if our insurance does not cover the bills? Will I be able to go back to work? What if I never get well?).

Finally, *anger* has been hypothesized as relevant to the etiology and progression of cancer (e.g., Schmale and Iker, 1971). However, in our longitudinal studies of emotions at diagnosis (see below), we have not found any evidence of elevated anger at initial diagnosis, but there may be higher levels reported at the time of cancer recurrence. Clinical reports of the foci for the anger include anger and frustration with the treatment failure.

To examine the emotional responses at diagnosis, we assessed the moods of 65 cancer patients within 5 to 10 days of learning their diagnosis, which was during their tumor work-up prior to treatment (Andersen et al, 1989b). All had clinical stage I or II gynecologic cancer. Their responses on a self-report questionnaire (Profile of Mood States; McNair et al, 1971) were compared to those of women from two age-matched comparison groups, a group of women with recently diagnosed benign gynecologic disease and gynecologically healthy women receiving routine examinations. Also, the cancer patients were followed for approximately 4 years, and during that time a subset of the women with cancer recurred and moods were reassessed at this second diagnosis.

For depression, there was a significant elevation for the cancer patients only at the time of the initial diagnosis, and a further, significant increment in distress at recurrence. In combination, these data indicate the unique and significant role of depressed affect for the cancer patient at diagnosis. In contrast, anxiety is a common affective experience for those with a medical diagnosis and anticipating medical treatment, whether or not the disease is malignant. This pattern would suggest that the anxiety may be prompted in part by treatment-related fears. Anger was present to a significant degree for the cancer patients only at the time of recurrence. These data indicate that the initial diagnosis is characterized by depressed affect, whereas recurrence may be characterized by even greater depression and the addition of anger.

Treatment

A certain component of the emotional distress occurring at diagnosis is the anticipation of undergoing difficult treatment(s). Surgery with or without radiotherapy is the treatment mainstay for the majority, whereas women with ovarian cancer usually receive surgery and lengthy, combination chemotherapy. All treatments are preceded and followed with physical examinations, tumor surveys, and/or laboratory studies. Thus cancer treatments are significant stressors, and supporting data consistently portray more distress (particularly fear and anxiety), slower rates of emotional recovery, and, perhaps, additional behavioral difficulties (e.g., conditioned anxiety reactions) than is found with relatively healthy women also undergoing medical treatment (e.g., hysterectomy, cholecystectomy).

Surgery

There have been few investigations of cancer surgery, and no studies of women facing gynecologic cancer surgery. However, there are numerous descriptive and intervention studies of the reactions of healthy women undergoing surgery for benign conditions (e.g., uterine fibroid; see Anderson and Masur, 1983, for an early review). The latter studies are consistent in their portrayal of high levels of self-reported preoperative anxiety predictive of lowered postoperative anxiety and postoperative anxiety predictive of recovery (e.g., time out of bed, pain reports). What may distinguish cancer surgery patients are higher overall levels of distress and slower emotional rebound (Gottesman and Lewis, 1982). Considering these data, the interactions of patients with their medical caregivers may be especially important. However, Blanchard et al (1987) found attending physicians on a cancer unit to be less likely to engage in supportive behaviors and address patients needs than physicians treating general medical patients. The heavier volume and more seriously ill patients common to cancer units may be sources for this unfortunate relationship. Related findings indicate that oncology nurses may find their job significantly more stressful than other assignments (e.g., cardiac, intensive care, or operating room nursing) (Stewart et al, 1982). Taken together, these findings suggest that the interactions between oncologists, oncology nurses, and gynecologic patients may be even more important than is commonly acknowledged in terms of influencing patient's recovery and adjustment during difficult treatment periods.

Radiotherapy

Although radiation therapy can be used for all gynecologic sites of disease, the majority of patients receiving radiotherapy have either cervix or endometrial disease. Clinical descriptions of women's concerns and fears are available (Karlsson and Andersen, 1986). We have studied both intracavitary (vaginal) radiotherapy and external beam treatment for gynecologic patients, and the former treatment is particularly difficult and painful (Andersen et al,

1984). High levels of anxiety in anticipation of beginning radiotherapy are found, and, if interventions to reduce distress are not conducted (Rainey, 1985), post-treatment anxiety is also evident (Andersen and Tewfik, 1985) and may be maintained for as long as 3 months post-therapy, particularly when treatment symptoms (e.g., diarrhea, fatigue) linger (King et al, 1985). When acute side effects resolve (usually by 12 months post-treatment), there appears to be no higher incidence of emotional difficulties for radiotherapy patients than for surgery patients (Hughson et al, 1987).

Chemotherapy

Early behavioral research in cancer focused on the psychological reactions to chemotherapy, particularly the side effects of nausea and vomiting. A classical conditioned conceptualization has been offered to explain anticipatory reactions. That is, the administration of chemotherapy (an unconditioned stimulus) produces post-treatment nausea and/or vomiting (the unconditioned response). Each chemotherapy infusion, however, is paired with environmental stimuli—conditioned stimuli such as visual (the sight of the nurse), olfactory (the smell of rubbing alcohol), or gustatory (the lingering taste of recently eaten foods or drinks). With sufficient pairings of the stimuli and severe post-treatment nausea and vomiting, the conditioned stimuli, such as the sight of the chemotherapy nurse, may alone come to elicit the same or a related response (i.e., nausea/vomiting—the conditioned response). Thus, even after only one difficult cycle of chemotherapy, patients may report nausea and/or vomiting *prior* to chemotherapy administration (usually on the first day) of the second or subsequent cycles.

Research progressed from this theoretical understanding of the etiology of such reactions to investigations focused on eliminating or reducing disruptive side effects through hypnosis, progressive muscle relaxation with guided imagery, systematic desensitization, attention diversion or redirection, and biofeedback (see Carey and Burish, 1988, for a review). Research also uncovered important individual differences in patients that may put them at higher risk for the development of such reactions. For example, women reporting very high initial anxiety about beginning chemotherapy, or women who have severe vomiting in the early cycles are at risk for conditioned nausea and vomiting. With this psychological research and the improvement in antiemetic drugs and efforts to reduce drug toxicity, many anticipatory reactions have been reduced or eliminated. There are, however, other problematic psychological and behavioral side effects of chemotherapy that remain. Appetite and weight loss are significant clinical problems for gynecologic cancer patients, particularly women with ovarian disease receiving chemotherapy, women treated with extended-field abdominal radiotherapy, and/or individuals susceptible to tumor-induced aversions. Learned food aversions, particularly from chemotherapy, appear to be robust, with rapid acquisition (usually after a single trial) and maintenance after long delays between presentations of the conditioned stimulus (the taste of food) and the onset of the unconditioned stimulus (aversive internal sensations) (Bernstein, 1986). This important research has pointed the way, for example, to interventions employing novel tastes to "block" conditioning to familiar diet items, reducing food intake prior to drug administration, and ingesting carbohydrate rather than protein source meals.

Recovery

For the long-term survivor, there may be two types of continuing stressors (Cella and Tross, 1986). The first comprises residual sequelae, including lingering emotional distress from the trauma of diagnosis, treatment, and, more generally, life threat. This could include such common reactions as dreading follow-up physical examinations or ruminating about recurrence upon learning of cancer diagnoses or deaths among other family or friends. The second class of stressors comprises continuing sequelae, including confrontation with the changes to one's premorbid life (e.g., sterility; inorgasmia following radical hysterectomy) and adjustment requiring new behaviors/emotions (e.g., consideration of adoption) and/or coping with losses (e.g., a sexual relationship that does not include intercourse following pelvic exenteration).

Writings from the 1950s to the 1980s suggested that the psychological trajectory for women was, at best, difficult, with somatic problems, psychological distress (Bard and Sutherland, 1952), impaired relationships (Dyk and Sutherland, 1956; Wortman and Dunkle-Schetter, 1979), preoccupation with death (e.g., Gullow et al, 1974), and/or general life disruption, such as reduced employment or career opportunities (Schonfield, 1972). Many of these pioneering reports (of primarily breast cancer patients) were clinical in focus and, in general, uncontrolled on disease variables now recognized as moderators of adjustment. By the end of this same period, cancer had become more public, and more survivable for some (cervical cancer patients in particular), and clinical trials were able to examine treatment toxicity following the establishment of effectiveness. These important changes may account, in part, for the positive findings emerging in the study of long-term adjustment.

Emotional Adjustment

If the disease is controlled and recovery from treatment proceeds unimpaired, longitudinal data indicate that, by 1 year post-treatment, the severe distress of diagnosis has dissipated and emotions have stabilized. Our controlled, prospective longitudinal study indicated no differences between the levels of emotional distress of women with cancer and either those with benign disease or healthy comparison subjects (Andersen et al, 1989b). Longitudinal study of breast cancer patients with benign comparison subjects reveals the same pattern (Bloom, 1987). The consistency of findings for the studies conducted during the 1980s are important because they represent replications across site and, to some degree, treatment toxicity, for women with cancer.

Interpersonal Relationships

The majority of close relationships remain intact, satisfactory, and, on occasion, stronger (Meyerowitz et al, 1983; Baider and Sarell, 1984; Lichtman and Taylor, 1986). Our longitudinal data with stage I and II women indicated, on average, no significant disruption in social or marital disruption. When problems do occur, they include estrangement and distress that was originally hypothesized for the majority of patients (Wortman and Dunkel-Schetter, 1979). For example, a woman may want to discuss her feelings in an attempt to cope with the cancer stressor, but her husband may be more inclined to advise her to "put the experience behind you" (Lichtman and Taylor, 1986). For other couples, the distress of kin (e.g., spouse) may approach that of the patient's (Cassileth et al, 1985). Also, for women with young children, the family is at heightened risk for emotional distress (Vess et al, 1985).

Sexual Outcomes

A variety of data have documented sexual outcomes, because this is the life area at greatest risk for difficulty for women with gynecologic cancer. Andersen and colleagues (1989a, 1989b) compared low- to moderate-risk women with clinical stage I or II gynecologic cancer ($N = 47$) with two matched comparison groups, women diagnosed and treated for benign gynecologic disease ($N = 18$) and gynecologically healthy women ($N = 57$). All women were assessed after their diagnosis but prior to treatment and then reassessed at 4, 8, and 12 months post-treatment. Global sexual behavior disruption did not occur, but the frequency of intercourse declined for women treated for disease, whether malignant or benign. Considering the sexual response cycle, diminution of sexual excitement was pronounced for women with disease; however, this difficulty was more severe and distressing for the women with cancer, possibly due to significant coital and postcoital pain, premature menopause, and/or treatment side effects. Changes in desire, orgasm, and resolution phases of the sexual response cycle occurred, but they were of lesser magnitude and/or duration. Approximately 30% of the women treated for cancer were diagnosed with a sexual dysfunction. The nature, early timing, and maintenance of sexual functioning morbidity suggested the instrumental role that cancer and cancer treatments play in these deficits (particularly arousal problems).

Additional data assessed other quality-of-life outcomes, including mood, marital and social adjustment, and employment and occupational status, and provide a complete context for interpreting the sexual outcome data. The data indicated that the emotional response to the life-threatening diagnosis and anticipation of treatment was characterized by depressed, anxious, and confused moods, whereas the response for women with benign disease was anxious only. In both cases, the responses were transitory and resolved post-treatment. There was no evidence for a higher incidence of relationship dissolution or poorer marital adjustment; however, 30% of the women treated for disease reported that their sexual partners may have had some difficulty in reaching orgasm (i.e., delayed ejaculation) during the recovery year. There was no evidence for impaired social adjustment. Finally, women treated for gynecologic cancer retained their employment and occupations; however their involvement (e.g., hours worked per week) was significantly reduced during recovery. In combination, the sexual and psychological data documented that significant sexual disruption, ranging from mild to moderate severity and of a transitory to continuing frequency, occurs, and sexual functioning is the life area at greatest risk for disruption for women with early-stage disease.

Even though women with early-stage disease have significant sexual problems, they pale in severity to those of women receiving radical pelvic and/or genital surgery. For the latter women, the majority (80% to 90% of those surveyed) report significant morbidity. With the exception of one Canadian report, all of the reports come from the United States, and they replicate a discouraging scenario for sexual outcomes (e.g., Andersen and van der Dos, 1994). For the majority of women and couples, the prospect of ending their sexual life (most couples cease all sexual activity when intercourse becomes impossible) is distressing and may be a source of continuing marital discord and may even lead to divorce.

Vaginal reconstruction (e.g., with a loop of bowel or portions of inner thigh muscle) is a possibility for some and enables a woman to maintain sexual activity that includes intercourse; however, many sexual difficulties often remain. Some women have difficulties with the physical characteristics of the new vagina (e.g., the cavity is too large or too narrow); others have general problems with arousal, orgasm, or dyspareunia or bleeding with intercourse (Andersen and Hacker, 1983a). Regardless of whether or not women with pelvic exenteration undergo vaginal reconstruction, these women face the greatest disruption to their sexual body and functioning of any female cancer group. It is remarkable that so little systematic descriptive or intervention work has been done with these women in view of the curative intent of this surgery.

A related picture comes from women treated for vulvar cancer. Individualized (and, consequently, more conservative) approaches for treatment of the vulva have been advocated (Hacker, 1994). Andersen and colleagues (1988) have provided data on the sexual outcomes for women treated with wide local excision and related treatments for in situ disease. In situ patients as a group are more likely to be sexually inactive at follow-up, whether or not they have available sexual partners, than age-matched healthy counterparts. However, if the women have a sexual relationship, the rates of sexual dysfunction appear only slightly higher than those for healthy women. Additional analyses contrasting treatment methods (e.g., surgery vs. laser vs. combined treatment) found no significant differences.

The outcomes for women with in situ disease contrast markedly with those for women with invasive disease. Although all of these reports are limited by their small sample sizes (ranging from 9 to 25) and retrospective evaluations, the general trend of the data is consistent: at least 30% to 50% of patients become sexually inactive and, of the women remaining active, 60% to 70% have multiple sexual dysfunctions (Andersen and van der Dos, 1994). For the women who become sexually inactive, many factors may be contributory. For some this is due to negative feelings (by the woman or her partner) about the physical changes to the body, and for others it may be due to severe dyspareunia, such as may occur with a narrowed introitus. When queried, the majority of women would have preferred to remain sexually active rather than have all intimacy end (e.g., Andersen and Hacker, 1983a).

Predicting Risk for Sexual Morbidity

Thus data have documented the significant sexual morbidity that occurs for women; more important for the future is to predict which women will be at risk for sexual difficulties and provide preventive or rehabilitative care (Andersen, 1994b). In addition to disease and treatment variables (Andersen, 1994a), one psychological variable, sexual self-schema, appears important as well (Andersen and Cyranowski, 1994). Specifically, a sexual self-schema (or sexual self-concept) is a cognitive view about sexual aspects of oneself; it is derived from past experience, manifests in current experience, and guides the processing of domain-relevant social information. When well articulated, it functions not only as a quick referent of one's sexual history, but also as a point of origin for information—judgments, decisions, inferences, predictions, and behaviors—about the current and future sexual self. In addition to regulating intrapersonal processes, the sexual self-schema also appears to mediate interpersonal processes, the most obvious being sexuality within relationships.

We measured this psychological variable with a 24-item trait adjective measure (Andersen and Cyranowski, 1994). Following a series of psychometric studies providing extensive reliability and validity information, our research indicates that women who differ in the valence of their sexual self views—that is, women with a positive versus a negative sexual self-schema—have very different sexual lives. Women with a positive sexual self-schema enter sexual relationships more willingly, have a more extensive behavioral repertoire, evidence more positive emotions when in sexual relationships, and anticipate having positive sexual relationships in the future. Also, the affects and behaviors indicative of loving, intimate attachments are central to women with a positive sexual self-schema. In contrast, women with a negative sexual self-schema tend to describe themselves as emotionally cold or unromantic; also, they are behaviorally inhibited in their sexual and romantic relationships. They may describe themselves as self-conscious, embarrassed, or inexperienced in sexual matters. Importantly, our longitudinal data indicate that these are stable self-views, impervious, for example, to the passage of time or the waxing and waning of specific sexual or romantic relationships.

We tested the importance of this variable in predicting which women would be at risk for sexual difficulties following gynecologic cancer treatment (Andersen et al, 1997). As noted above, approximately 50% of women treated for gynecologic cancer have sexual dysfunctions as they recover and become cancer survivors. This outcome occurs in the context of satisfactory quality of life in other domains. We compared gynecologic cancer survivors ($N = 61$) and gynecologically healthy women ($N = 74$), and found that the groups did not differ in important quality-of-life areas (i.e., general, depressive symptoms, social contacts and stress), whereas significantly poorer sexual functioning was found for the survivors.

Of added importance were the analyses focused on variables that may predict risk for sexual morbidity. Specifically, we tested sexual self-schema as a potentially important, sexually relevant individual difference. We predicted two different sexual outcomes—sexual responsiveness (e.g., desire, excitement, orgasm, and resolution) and sexual behavior. We also included three important controls: a marker of pretreatment sexuality (frequency of intercourse), extent of disease/treatment, and menopausal symptomatology were selected in view of their general relevance to sexuality and their specific relevance to data on the sexual outcomes following cancer. In multiple regression analyses, sexual self-schema accounted for a significant and large portion of the variance (28%) in the prediction of current sexual responsiveness. In the prediction of sexual behavior, other components of the model were singly and in combination also powerful contributors, accounting for 42% of the variance. Still, sexual self-schema contributed an additional, significant 6% for a final total of 48% of the variance.

The findings are supportive for the consideration of sexual self-schema construct in understanding sexual outcomes following gynecologic cancer. Consistent with the schema definition, we anticipated that women with a more negative sexual self-concept, in contrast to women with a more positive view, would have greater sexual morbidity. Women with a more negative sexual self-schema were expected to have more difficulties because they are, in general, less romantic/passionate in their emotions, less open to sexual experiences, and more likely to have negative feelings about their sexuality. Thus, in the context of cancer, with disease or treatment factors causing direct changes to the sexual body and/or sexual responses and symptoms of premature menopause, we anticipated that women with negative sexual self-schemas would evidence lower rates of activity and less responsiveness. We suggested that women with negative self-views of their sexuality might find, for example, that their sexual arousability may have lessened further, that they are less apt to try new sexual activities as a way to cope with their sexual difficulties, or they may be prone to negative cognitions or feelings, such as embarrassment, about any body changes. Further research will need to confirm these hypotheses about additional cognitive and behavioral processes of sexual dysfunction. In earlier efforts (e.g., Andersen and Elliot, 1993), we have detailed a process model of the occurrence and maintenance of "dysfunctional" and "nondysfunctional" sexual response patterns in women with cancer. Based on our empirical findings, the "dysfunctional" pattern is characterized by low arousal, behavioral inhibition, and negativity—a constellation of responses relevant to sexual self-schema.

Finally, these data would suggest that preventive or rehabilitative interventions would be particularly important for the woman with a less positive (more negative) view of her sexuality, and, moreover, the schema construct could give theoretical guidance to such efforts. A schema-guided intervention could, for example, challenge the woman's typical self-view. Techniques could be designed to enhance sexual self-concept, such as ones providing a woman with strategies for enhancing arousal, increasing the sexual behavioral repertoire, and specifically lowering negative affects, such as embarrassment. Such possibilities, along with traditional behavioral strategies (Wincze and Carey, 1991) might provide the needed, important assistance to the woman who survives gynecologic cancer but must cope with the resulting sexual difficulties.

Recurrence and Death

Cancer recurrence is devastating. As noted above, the magnitude of distress is even greater than that found with the initial diagnosis, and studies contrasting cancer patients with no evidence of disease with those receiving palliative treatment (e.g., Cassileth et al, 1985) report the greatest distress for those with disseminated disease (Bloom, 1987). Difficult decisions (e.g., beginning a regimen that offers little chance for cure and has side effects vs. no treatment) are made in a context of extreme emotional distress and physical debilitation. A frequent complication of disseminated disease is pain, because it is common and less controllable for those with metastatic disease (Ahles et al, 1984). When palliative therapy is of little use and/or brings further debilitation, psychological interventions may provide pain control and, secondarily, prevent or treat pain sequelae, such as sleep disturbances, reduced appetite, irritability, and other behavioral difficulties.

PSYCHOLOGICAL INTERVENTIONS TO PREVENT OR REDUCE MORBIDITY

To organize the review of the psychological intervention literature, a model of risk for psychological/behavioral morbidity is offered (Andersen, 1994a). In this conceptualization, three characteristics and correlates of disease are considered: extent, magnitude of treatment, and prognosis. In formulating this risk categorization, facts about cancer (e.g., staging of disease) as well as descriptive data documenting adjustment patterns without psychological intervention (such as that reviewed above) were considered. Such conceptual frameworks are important for research and clinical efforts with gynecology cancer patients. Women at *low risk* may have disease/treatment scenarios of localized disease at diagnosis, treatment consisting of one modality (e.g., surgery), and/or disease for which the prognosis is good (e.g., 5-year survival estimates of 70% to 95%). Women at *moderate risk* may be characterized as having regional disease, oftentimes combination therapy (e.g., surgery and follow-up radiotherapy; surgery and chemotherapy), and/or a 50-50 chance of survival, usually ranging from 40% to 60% for 5-year estimates. Because the ability to predict survival and other disease end points is reduced, psychosocial adjustment appears to be more variable. Women at *high risk* may be characterized by advanced disease at diagnosis (e.g., stage III ovarian cancer), recurrent disease, or disease that rapidly progresses to death. Patients must suddenly confront a lifetime line of months, because survival for the next year is a possible but unlikely event (e.g., 3-year observed survival rates for metastatic cervical, endometrial, and ovarian cancer are 21%, 18%, and 33%, respectively [Menck et al, 1991]). The following discussion is limited to methodologically stronger studies with quasi-experimental (i.e., the nonequivalent control group) or experimental designs. Detailed coverage of studies, including gynecology patients, is provided here and other sources are available for more comprehensive coverage (e.g., Andersen, 1992).

Low Morbidity Risk

Two nonequivalent control group designs have provided brief interventions to gynecologic cancer pa-

tients. Capone and colleagues (1980) provided a crisis-oriented intervention that assisted women to express feelings related to their diagnosis or upcoming treatments, provided information about treatment sequelae, and attempted to enhance self-esteem, femininity, and interpersonal relationships. For sexually active women, a sexual therapy component included sexual information and methods to cope and reduce anxiety when resuming intercourse. The format was at least four individual sessions during the surgical hospitalization; the length of each session or total therapy time was not specified. Fifty-six newly diagnosed women were included; 51% were stage I, 22% stage II, 15% stage III, and 12% stage IV or unstaged. A nonequivalent control group was obtained by recruiting previously treated women as they returned for post-treatment follow-up. Standardized outcome measures assessed emotional distress and self-concept and were supplemented with self-reports of return to employment and frequency of intercourse. Analyses indicated no differences between groups or within the intervention group on the measures of emotional distress. A trend in the percentages of women returning to work favored the intervention participants (e.g., 50% vs. 25% at 3 months). In contrast to these weak findings, substantial differences were found between the groups in the return to and frequency of intercourse across all post-treatment assessments (e.g., 16% of the intervention vs. 57% of the control women reported less or no sexual activity at 12 months post-treatment).

The second quasi-experimental investigation was reported by Houts et al (1986), who examined the efficacy of a peer counseling model. The structured intervention included encouragement to maintain interpersonal relationships; to make positive plans for the future; to query the medical staff regarding treatments, side effects, and sexual outcomes; and to maintain normal routines. These interventions were delivered in three telephone contacts (one pretreatment and at 5 and 10 weeks post-treatment) and with provision of a booklet and audiotape description of the coping strategies at the pretreatment hospital visit. Two former cancer patients also trained as social workers were the peer counselors. Thirty-two newly diagnosed (stage not specified) women, 14 intervention and 18 control, participated. No intervention comparison subjects were recruited on alternate weeks. A standardized outcome measure assessed emotional distress and an experimenter-derived measure assessed coping strategies at pretreatment and 6 and 12 weeks post-treatment. Analyses indicated no differences between groups at any point in time.

These and other intervention studies for low-risk patients (Andersen, 1994a) suggest that broad-based interventions produced limited, if any, gains in psychological or behavioral outcomes, but, in contrast, significant improvement was found in sexual functioning (Capone et al, 1980; Davis, 1986; Houts et al,

1986). The descriptive data of Andersen et al (1989b) and findings of Capone et al and Houts et al confirm the hypothesized profile of lowered psychosocial morbidity but heightened sexual morbidity. The emotional rebound that occurs following cancer treatment may contribute to the findings of no differential outcome or only modest improvement (Christensen, 1983; Fawzy et al, 1990a) in emotional distress. Longer term follow-up data suggest some consolidation of intervention effects across time (upward of 6 months post-treatment), with lowered emotional distress and/or enhanced coping (Fawzy, Cousins et al, 1990) coupled with confirming biologic outcomes (Davis, 1986; Fawzy, Kemeny et al, 1990). If the long-term outcomes are replicable across investigators, they are made more impressive by their achievement with very brief therapy (e.g., 10 therapy hours).

Moderate Morbidity Risk

The only intervention study with moderate-risk gynecologic cancer patients is that of Cain and colleagues (1986) comparing individual and group therapy formats. The intervention had eight components, including discussion of the causes of cancer at diagnosis, impact of the treatment(s) on body image and sexuality, relaxation training, emphasis on good dietary and exercise patterns, communication difficulties with medical staff and friends/family, and setting goals for the future to cope with uncertainty and fears of recurrence. The eight-session program was conducted during individual sessions in the hospital or the woman's home or in weekly groups of four to six patients at the hospital. Seventy-two women (21 individual intervention, 22 group intervention, and 29 no-treatment control) with gynecologic cancer (disease stage not specified) completed the study. Outcome measures were standardized and included the Hamilton depression and anxiety rating scales and the Psychosocial Adjustment to Illness Scale administered pre- and post-treatment and at a 6-month follow-up. Post-treatment analyses indicated all groups improved with time; however, interview-rated anxiety was significantly lower for the individual therapy subjects only. Gains for the intervention subjects were more impressive with the 6-month follow-up data. At that time there were no differences between the intervention formats, but both groups reported less depression and anxiety and better psychosocial adjustment (including health perspectives, sexual functioning, and use of leisure time) than the no-treatment control group. In sum, the brief intervention, delivered either in individual or groups format, appeared to be immediately effective, with gains enhanced during the early recovery months.

With moderate-risk patients, there is continuing distress with their lengthy treatments. Unlike the weak effects at post-treatment for low-risk intervention subjects, more impressive gains could be found and effects appeared stronger with continued follow-up (e.g., Maguire et al, 1983; Forester et al, 1985; Cain et al, 1986). Interventions with an informational component could also improve patients knowledge about their disease and/or treatment(s). Outcomes in other areas, such as activities of daily living, are more difficult to detect. Some interventions appear to lower symptom levels either directly (e.g., Maguire et al, 1983) or indirectly (e.g., Forester et al, 1985).

High Morbidity Risk

No published studies have included high-risk gynecology patients, but two studies included all or at least a majority of women. Ferlic and colleagues (1979) provided an interdisciplinary crisis intervention program that included patient education (introduction to the hospital, cancer as a disease, cancer treatments, etc.); presentations by medical team members (physician, nurse, social worker, chaplain, dietician); and supportive group therapy (including topics of emotional distress, coping, sexuality, and strain on family/social relationships). The format was group meetings for six sessions. Sixty adults (50% female) with "advanced cancer at varying stages of their treatment" with a mean of 7 weeks since diagnosis participated. Analyses indicated the intervention group improved in adjustment across all areas, whereas the controls improved in the areas of relationship strength, cancer information, and death perceptions only. Also, the self-concept score for the intervention group significantly increased, whereas that for the control group significantly decreased.

Several papers have described the outcomes of the group support intervention for women with breast cancer developed by Spiegel, Bloom, and colleagues (Spiegel et al, 1981; Spiegel and Bloom, 1983). Women were randomized to no treatment or a group treatment intervention that included discussion of death and dying, family problems, communication problems with physicians, and living fully in the context of a terminal illness. The intervention subjects were also randomized a second time to two conditions; no additional treatment or self-hypnosis for pain problems (Spiegel and Bloom, 1983), which was incorporated into the support group format. All intervention groups met for weekly meetings for 1 year, for a total of 75 therapy hours. Eighty-six women, 50 intervention and 36 no-treatment control, with metastatic breast cancer and referred to the intervention from their oncologists, participated. Following random assignment, there was subject loss (e.g., refusal, too weak, death), with the study beginning with 34 intervention and 24 control participants; however, the survival data are reported for the original sample of 86.

Analyses indicated that the intervention group reported significantly fewer phobic responses and lower anxiety, fatigue, and confusion and higher vigor than the controls. There was also a significant decrease in the use of maladaptive coping responses by the intervention group. There were no significant differences on the remaining measures. Regarding the findings from the hypnosis substudy, women receiving hypnosis within the group support intervention reported no change in their pain sensations during the year, whereas pain sensations significantly increased for the other women in group support who did not receive hypnosis. It is important to note that pain sensation scores for both groups were, however, significantly lower than those for the no-intervention controls, suggesting that the hypnosis component provided an additive analgesic effect to other group treatment components. The most startling data from this project were reported in a survival analysis (Spiegel et al, 1989), which indicated a difference of 18.9 months for the control subjects and 36.6 months for the intervention subjects from study entry until death.

Despite the challenges of studying these patients, well-controlled investigations have been conducted, albeit none with women with gynecologic cancer. The positive outcomes for high-risk cancer patients are notable considering their patients' worsening pain and/or increasing debilitation. Measures of emotional distress were sensitive to initial post-treatment gains as well as changes with continued follow-up. In addition, change in other areas—self-esteem/concept, death perceptions, life satisfaction, and/or locus of control—were found (e.g., Ferlic et al, 1979; Linn et al, 1982); these effects were not detected in studies with low-risk patients. Important for quality of life, psychological interventions could also lower or stabilize pain reports (Spiegel and Bloom, 1983).

Summary

Although there appear to be unique intervention components for different phases in cancer, there are some commonalities. Studies with newly diagnosed cancer patients focus on the trauma of learning one has a potentially life-threatening illness. Both descriptive and intervention data suggest a crisis intervention or brief therapy model as the "best fit" for this period. These models are similar in terms of their rapid early assessment, present-day focus, limited goals, therapist direction, and prompt interventions. When applied in the context of cancer, therapy components have included an *emotionally supportive context* to address fears and anxieties about the disease, information about the disease and treatment, *behavioral coping strategies* (e.g., role playing difficult discussions with family or the medical staff), *cognitive coping strategies*, and *relaxation training* to lower "arousal" and/or enhance one's sense of control. The components noted above appear more important to improved outcome than procedural varia-

tions. For example, therapy format, such as individual or group, appears to have little impact. Involvement of significant others such as a spouse may have some positive effects, but his or her participation appears to be unnecessary to achieve psychological gains for patients. Furthermore, direct benefit for a spouse may be minimal unless the focus of treatment is on a mutually important issue, such as sexual problems (Christensen, 1983). Finally, there were null findings for (group) interventions that included no structured content, suggesting that reliance on group support is insufficient to produce any measurable benefit.

The descriptive data also highlight the need for *focused interventions* for sexual functioning for women treated for gynecologic cancer, and the intervention data attest to the effectiveness of this specific component. We have previously described sexual therapy interventions (Andersen and Elliot, 1993). Briefly, at least three components appear essential for a preventive intervention. First, sexuality information (e.g., male and female sexual anatomy, the sexual response cycle, sexual dysfunctions and potential sources of difficulty) is needed. Furthermore, explication of the specific sexual changes following cancer treatment may prevent problems resulting from ignorance or misconceptions or decrease the severity of problems that arise from other factors. Second, medical interventions are central (see Berek and Andersen, 1997, for a discussion) and, as the model indicates, they may directly reduce morbidity risk. Several examples can be cited, but common ones include hormonal therapy, the use of dilators to reduce adhesions following radiotherapy, or reconstructive surgery.

Third, the delivery of *specific sex therapy suggestions* is often necessary. Interventions for specific sexual behaviors or phases of the response cycle may be needed. For example, interventions for desire problems can include (1) determining what circumstances for sexual activity are more or less appealing, with encouragement that sexual activity occur under the most desirable circumstances; (2) increasing the frequency of a range of intimate activities (not only sexual behaviors) that the woman might find pleasurable; and (3) increasing the frequency and variety of the woman's sexual fantasies during sexual activity. Interventions of this ilk are designed to increase the frequency of positive sexual cognitions, intimate occasions with the partner, and optimal times and circumstances for sexual activity for the woman. Alternatively, women may not have sexual dysfunctions, per se, but may have other difficulties that impact on sexual functioning, such as reacting negatively to their body after cancer treatment. Such reactions have been described following radical surgeries—vulvectomy or pelvic exenteration—and have included anxiety or disgust when looking at the site or fear of being seen by one's spouse, among others. Although these responses are difficult, they are not unique and may be expressed by healthy women with sexual difficulties, for example. For such women, anxiety reduction techniques, systematic desensitization, or individual sensate focus exercises have proven effective. Such activities may not change a woman's negative body feelings to positive, but these feelings may achieve neutrality or no longer be disruptive of the woman's sexual activity or mood.

CONCLUSIONS AND FUTURE DIRECTIONS

Major advances in understanding psychological and behavioral aspects of gynecologic cancer have been made. First, descriptive clinical reports, and in some cases, controlled prospective longitudinal investigations, have traced the development of psychological and behavioral sexual problems among treated female cancer patients (see Andersen and van der Dos, 1994, for an international review). While providing estimates of the magnitude of quality of life problems, these data can be used for models which predict which women might be at greatest risk for adjustment difficulties. The latter is an important step toward designing interventions tailored to the difficulties and circumstances of women with gynecologic cancer. Second, reliability and validity data have been published on measures of sexual functioning such that any behavioral scientist in collaboration with a gynecologic oncologist could implement assessment of sexual responses and difficulties of women.

An extensive literature on the use of psychological interventions to improve the quality of life for cancer patients exists (see Andersen, 1992, for a review). The effectiveness of these interventions is robust, because they have reduced distress and enhanced the quality of life of many cancer patients differing on disease stage as well as disease site. These gains have also been achieved through remarkably short therapies, such as 6 to 15 hours. Unfortunately, the area of greatest morbidity for the woman with gynecologic cancer, sexual functioning, has received lesser intervention study. However, it would be expected that brief interventions for sexuality could also result in significantly improved outcomes.

REFERENCES

Ahles TA, Ruckdeschel JC, Blanchard EG: Cancer related pain—I. Prevalence in an outpatient setting as a function of stage of disease and type of cancer. J Psychosom Res 1984;28:115.

Andersen BL: Health psychology's contribution to addressing the cancer problem: update on accomplishments. Health Psychol 1989;8:683.

Andersen BL: Psychological interventions for cancer patients to enhance the quality of life. J Consult Clin Psychol 1992;60:552.

Andersen BL: Surviving cancer. Cancer 1994a;74:1484.

Andersen BL: Yes, there are sexual problems. Now, what can we do about them? Gynecol Oncol 1994b;52:10.

Andersen BL, Anderson B, deProsse C: Controlled prospective longitudinal study of women with cancer: I. Sexual functioning outcomes. J Consult Clin Psychol 1989a;57:683.

Andersen BL, Anderson B, deProsse C: Controlled prospective longitudinal study of women with cancer: II. Psychological outcomes. J Consult Clin Psychol 1989b;57:692.

Andersen BL, Cacioppo JT, Roberts DC: Delay in seeking a cancer diagnosis: delay stages and psychophysiologic comparison processes. Br J Soc Psychol 1995;34:33.

Andersen BL, Cyranowski JC: Women's sexual self schema. J Pers Soc Psychol 1994;67:1079.

Andersen BL, Elliot M: Sexuality for women with cancer: assessment, theory and treatment. J Sexuality Disabil 1993;11:7.

Andersen BL, Hacker NF: Psychosexual adjustment after vulvar surgery. Obstet Gynecol 1983a;62:457.

Andersen BL, Hacker NF: Psychosexual adjustment following pelvic exenteration. Obstet Gynecol 1983b;61:331.

Andersen BL, Karlsson JA, Anderson B, Tewfik HH: Anxiety and cancer treatment: response to stressful radiotherapy. Health Psychol 1984;3:535.

Andersen BL, Lachenbrach PA, Anderson B, deProsse C: Sexual dysfunction and signs of gynecologic cancer. Cancer 1986;57:1880.

Andersen GL, Tewfik HH: Psychological reactions to radiation therapy: reconsideration of the adaptive aspects of anxiety. J Pers Soc Psychol 1985;48:1024.

Andersen BL, Turnquist D, LaPolla JP, et al: Sexual functioning after treatment of in situ vulvar cancer: preliminary report. Obstet Gynecol 1988;71:15.

Andersen BL, van der Dos J: Sexual morbidity following gynecologic cancer: an international problem. Int J Gynecol Cancer 1994;4:225.

Andersen BL, Woods XA, Copeland LJ: Sexual self schema and sexual morbidity among gynecologic cancer survivors. J Consult Clin Psychol 1997;65:221.

Anderson KO, Masur FT: Psychological preparation for invasive medical and dental procedures. J Behav Med 1983;6:1.

Baider L, Sarell M: Couples in crisis: patient-spouse differences in perception of interaction patterns and the illness situation. Fam Ther 1984;11:115.

Bard M, Sutherland AM: Adaptation to radical mastectomy. Cancer 1952;8:656.

Berek J, Andersen BL: Sexual rehabilitation: surgical and psychological approaches. In Hoskins WJ, Perez CA, Young RC (eds): Principles and Practice of Gynecologic Oncology. 2nd ed. Philadelphia: JB Lippincott Company, 1997:551.

Bernstein LL: Etiology of anorexia in cancer. Cancer 1986;58:1881.

Blanchard CG, Ruckdeschel JC, Labrecque MS, et al: The impact of a designated cancer unit on house staff behaviors toward patients. Cancer 1987;60:2348.

Bloom JR: Psychological Aspects of Breast Cancer Study Group: psychological response to mastectomy. Cancer 1987;59:189.

Bukberg J, Penman D, Holland JC: Depression in hospitalized cancer patients. Psychosom Med 1984;46:199.

Cain EN, Kohorn EI, Quinlan DM, et al: Psychosocial benefits of a cancer support group. Cancer 1986;57:183.

Capone MA, Good RS, Westie KS, Jacobson AF: Psychosocial rehabilitation of gynecologic oncology patients. Arch Phys Med Rehabil 1980;61:128.

Carey MP, Burish TG: Etiology and treatment of the psychological side effects associated with cancer chemotherapy. Psychol Bull 1988;104:307.

Cassileth BR, Lusk EJ, Strouse TB, et al: A psychological analysis of cancer patients and their next-of-kin. Cancer 1985;55:72.

Cella DF, Tross S: Psychological adjustment to survival from Hodgkin's disease. J Consult Clin Psychol 1986;54:616.

Christenen DN: Postmastectomy couple counseling: an outcome study of a structured treatment protocol. J Sex Marital Ther 1983;9:266.

Davis H: Effects of biofeedback and cognitive therapy on stress in patients with breast cancer. Psychol Rep 1986;59:967.

Derogatis LR, Feldstein M, Morrow G, et al: A survey of psychotropic drug prescriptions in an oncology population. Cancer 1979;44:1919.

Derogatis LR, Morrow GR, Fetting J, et al: The prevalence of psychiatric disorders among cancer patients. JAMA 1983;249:751.

Dyk RB, Sutherland AM: Adaptation of the spouse and other family members to the colostomy patient. Cancer 1956;9:123.

Endicott J: Measurement of depression in patients with cancer. Cancer 1984;53:2243.

Evans DW, McCartney CF, Nemeroff CB, et al: Depression in women treated for gynecologic cancer: clinical and neuroendocrine assessment. Am J Psychiatry 1986;143:447.

Fawzy FI, Cousins N, Fawzy N, et al: A structured psychiatric intervention for cancer patients: I. Changes over time in methods of coping and affective disturbance. Arch Gen Psychiatry 1990;47:720.

Fawzy FI, Kemeny ME, Fawzy N, et al: A structured psychiatric intervention for cancer patients: I. Changes over time in immunological measures. Arch Gen Psychiatry 1990;47:729.

Ferlic M, Goldman A, Kennedy BJ: Group counseling in adult patients with advanced cancer. Cancer 1979;43:760.

Forester B, Kornfeld DS, Fleiss JL: Psychotherapy during radiotherapy: effects on emotional and physical distress. Am J Psychiatry 1985;142:22.

Gottesman D, Lewis M: Differences in crisis reactions among cancer and surgery patients. J Consult Clin Psychol 1982;50:381.

Gullo V, Cherico J, Shadick R: Suggested stages and response styles in life threatening illness: a focus on the cancer patient. In Schoenberg L, Carr E, Kutscher C, et al (eds): Anticipatory Grief. New York: Columbia University Press, 1974:153.

Hacker NF: Vulvar cancer. In Berek JS, Hacker NF (eds): Practical Gynecological Oncology. Baltimore: Williams & Wilkins, 1994:403.

Houts PS, Whitney CW, Mortel R, Bartholomew MJ: Former cancer patients as counselors of newly diagnosed cancer patients. J Natl Cancer Inst 1986;76:793.

Hughes J: Emotional reactions to the diagnosis and treatment of early breast cancer. J Psychosom Res 1981;26:277.

Hughson AVM, Cooper AF, McArdle CS, Smith DC: Psychosocial effects of radiotherapy after mastectomy. Br Med J 1987;294:1515.

Karlsson JA, Andersen BL: Radiation therapy and psychological distress in gynecologic oncology patients: outcomes and recommendations for enhancing adjustment. J Psychosom Obstet Gynecol 1986;5:283.

King KB, Nail LM, Kreamer K, et al: Patients' descriptions of the experience of receiving radiation therapy. Oncol Nurs Forum 1985;12:55.

Lansky SB, List MA, Herrmann CA, et al: Absence of major depressive disorders in female cancer patients. J Clin Oncol 1985;3:1553.

Lichtman RR, Taylor SE: Close relationships and the female cancer patient. In BL Andersen (ed), Women with Cancer: Psychological Perspectives. New York: Springer-Verlag, 1986:233.

Linn MW, Linn BS, Harris R: Effects of counseling for late stage cancer patients. Cancer 1982;49:1048.

Maguire P, Brooke M, Tait A, et al: The effect of counselling on physical disability and social recovery after mastectomy. Clin Oncol 1983;9:319.

McNair DM, Lorr M, Droppleman LF: Profile of Mood States. San Diego: Educational Testing Service, 1971.

Menck HR, Garfinkel L, Dodd GD: CA Cancer J Clin 1991;41:7.

Meyerowitz BE, Watkins IK, Sparks FC: Psychosocial implications of adjuvant chemotherapy: a two year follow up. Cancer 1983;52:1541.

Noyes R, Kathol RG: Depression and cancer. Psychiatr Dev 1986;2:77.

Plumb MM, Holland J: Comparative studies of psychological functioning in patients with advanced cancer. I. Self-reported depressive symptoms. Psychosom Med 1977;39:264.

Proceedings of the Second Workshop on Methodology in Behavioral and Psychosocial Cancer Research. Cancer 1991;67(3) (whole issue).

Rainey LC: Effects of preparatory patient education for radiation oncology patients. Cancer 1985;56:1056.

Schmale AH, Iker H: Hopelessness as a predictor of cervical cancer. Soc Sci Med 1971;5:95.

Schonfield J: Psychological factors related to delayed return to an earlier life-style in successfully treated cancer patients. J Psychosom Res 1972;16:41.

Spiegel D, Bloom JR: Group therapy and hypnosis reduce metastatic breast carcinoma pain. Psychosom Med 1983;45:333.

Spiegel D, Bloom JR, Kraemer HC, Gottheil E: Effect of psychosocial treatment on survival of patients with metastatic breast cancer. Lancet, 1989;2:888.

Spiegel D, Bloom JR, Yalom I: Group support for patients with metastatic cancer: a randomized outcome study. Arch Gen Psychiatry 1981;38:527.

Stewart BE, Meyerowitz BE, Jackson LE, et al: Psychological stress associated with outpatient oncology nursing. Cancer Nurs 1982;October:383.

Sutherland AM, Orbach CF, Dyk RB, Bard M: The psychological impact of cancer and cancer surgery. I. Adaptation to the dry colostomy. Cancer 1952;5:857.

Taylor SE: Adjustment to threatening events: a theory of cognitive adaptation. Am Psychol 1983;38:1161.

Vess JD, Moreland JR, Schwebel AI: A follow up study of role functioning and the psychosocial environment of families of cancer patients. J Psychosoc Oncol 1985;3:1.

Wincze JP, Carey MP: Sexual Dysfunction: A Guide for Assessment and Treatment. New York: Guilford Press, 1991.

Wortman CB, Dunkel-Schetter C: Interpersonal relationships and cancer: a theoretical analysis. J Soc Issues 1979;35:120.

66

Basic Principles of Radiation Therapy

Vernon J. King
Henry Wagner, Jr.
Henry M. Keys

Radiation therapy is one of the three principal treatment modalities in current cancer management and, as such, plays a critical role in the treatment of a high percentage of patients with gynecologic malignancies. Either used alone or integrated with surgery and cytotoxic chemotherapy (the other two modalities), it contributes to the control and/or cure of many cancers.

Radiation therapy represents the application of a physical mode of treatment to achieve a cytotoxic end. Like cytotoxic chemotherapy, it acts by interfering with cellular structures and metabolic processes necessary for cell division and survival. Like other cytotoxic agents, its efficacy depends on such factors as total dose and schedule of administration. Like other physical treatments such as surgery, radiation therapy can be delivered to a localized volume, which allows the potential of treatment of the tumor-containing volume while preserving adjacent normal tissues. Also like surgery, it is ineffective against disease that has already spread beyond its volume of treatment.

The effective treatment of any disease requires not only an understanding of the normal biology and pathophysiology of the involved organ system, but also a knowledge of the various means available for its treatment. Nowhere is this more the case than in the treatment of malignant disease. Here the differences between normal and pathologic biology are subtle, particularly at the molecular level, and the achievement of a therapeutic advantage may require the careful exploitation of such small differences.

SCOPE OF RADIATION ONCOLOGY IN THE TREATMENT OF GYNECOLOGIC MALIGNANCIES

The development of clinical radiation oncology has been linked with the treatment of a number of malignancies whose clinical characteristics have made them particularly well suited to this modality of treatment. Gynecologic neoplasms, particularly squamous cell carcinoma of the cervix, as well as squamous cell carcinomas of the head and neck re-

gion have been important in this development because of their accessibility, amenability to early detection efforts, and the use of radiation therapy as an approach to treatment with curative intent. Radiation is used in the treatment of many gynecologic malignancies, including carcinomas of the cervix, uterus, ovaries, vagina, fallopian tubes, and vulva.

NUMBER OF PATIENTS TREATED

About 50% of all patients with cancer (of all sites of origin) are given radiation therapy at some point during their treatment course. Of these, about half are treated with curative intent, using radiation therapy either alone or as a component of multimodality treatment (Kramer, 1982; Hall, 1984). Half of these patients are, in fact, cured, and about one half who are not cured still achieve control of local tumor. The early success in cancer of the cervix was particularly important in the continued development of radiation oncology and in forging a continuing close relationship between the gynecologic surgeon and the radiation oncologist.

TREATMENT INTENT

The rational development of a treatment plan for an individual patient requires the clear understanding of the desired and expected outcomes of treatment. In some cases this is simple. Patients with early-stage disease who are in good general health with no medical contraindications to aggressive treatment should be treated in this manner, with the intent and reasonable expectation of cure. Conversely, patients with disseminated solid tumors, with rare exceptions such as ovarian and testicular germ cell tumors and malignant lymphomas, are not curable with any current therapies and should be treated with the intent of either palliating present symptoms or preventing the development of symptoms that would likely result from the unchecked progression of disease and that, once established, are more difficult to palliate than they are to prevent. In selected cases, patients

1443

wishing to receive aggressive treatment may be offered experimental therapies such as high-dose chemotherapy with bone marrow transplantation. The more difficult, but not uncommon, situation arises with patients who have a disease of intermediate prognosis, with a cure rate of perhaps 10% to 15%, and substantial morbidity (physical, emotional, logistic, financial) associated with radical treatment. In such situations, it is essential that decisions about the treatment approach be made by the patient in the context of a full and compassionate presentation of all available information by the physicians involved in her care (Holland et al, 1987).

Even considering only those patients being treated with curative intent, the outcome of patients receiving radiation therapy varies considerably with the histologic type of tumor and stage of the disease. Small tumors of epithelial origin, such as squamous cell carcinomas of the upper aerodigestive tract or of the cervix, fare well with radiation therapy as the sole treatment modality. Local control of nonbulky disease is readily achieved with tolerable doses of radiation and the risk of occult metastases is low, so cure rates are high. The high-grade malignant lymphomas represent a somewhat different situation, because although the probability of local control with radiation therapy is good, these tumors will often have disseminated systemically even when they appear localized. Achieving local control is not necessarily equivalent to cure, and a systemic component of therapy is needed. Finally, there are a small number of cell types, perhaps best represented by the high-grade malignant gliomas, that are rarely, if ever, controlled locally by even high doses of radiation. The reasons for this radiation resistance presumably lie in intrinsic cellular processes that are as yet poorly understood.

GENERAL PRINCIPLES OF CLINICAL RADIATION ONCOLOGY

In developing the rationale for the therapeutic use of ionizing radiation, we first review some basic physics of the production of these radiations and their absorption by matter, then turn to the biology of their interactions with living cells, and finally discuss the application of this process to the clinic. We conclude with a brief look at several areas of current research interest.

Electromagnetic Spectrum

The electromagnetic spectrum encompasses radiations ranging from radio waves to microwaves, visible light, x-rays, and gamma rays. These differ in their wavelength and frequency and, consequently, in their energy according to Planck's relationship, in which the photon's energy, E, is related to its wavelength, λ, by the following equation:

$$E = hc/\lambda$$

where c is the speed of light and h is Planck's constant. X-rays and gamma rays are physically indistinguishable and differ only in that x-rays are generated by changes in electron energy levels, whereas gamma rays are produced by changes in nuclear energy levels. Only x-rays and gamma rays have sufficient quantal energy to produce ionization of target molecules, and they are the forms of electromagnetic radiation of concern in radiation therapy. Although the absolute amount of energy transferred to a cell by ionization events is small, it is transferred in large enough packets to produce the disruption of important molecules. A similar amount of energy transferred by infrared radiation serves only to warm the cell slightly.

The x-rays and gamma rays used in radiation therapy are forms of electromagnetic radiation with energies commonly ranging from 50,000 volts (50 kV) up to 50 million volts (50 MV). Particulate radiations—both charged particles, such as electrons, protons, and negative pi-mesons, and uncharged particles, such as neutrons—have also been used in radiation therapy. Aside from electrons, which are widely used, their availability is limited and their use still investigational. Neutron radiation has been explored more thoroughly than some of the other particulate radiation entities and is discussed later.

Production of X-ray Beams

A fundamental method of producing a beam of x-rays is to accelerate a particle to energy high enough so that, when it collides with an appropriate target, part of the kinetic energy will be converted to electromagnetic radiation in the x-ray range. For clinical purposes, the accelerated particles are commonly electrons. Electrons are produced by heating a metal filament and then accelerated to speeds approaching the velocity of light. When the electrons impact on a metal—usually tungsten—target, they collide inelastically with atoms of this target, giving rise to lower energy electrons and x-rays that carry off the energy difference. This "braking radiation," or *bremsstrahlung*, accounts for essentially all of the x-ray production from an x-ray tube (Khan, 1994). Different types of x-ray–generating equipment vary in the means used to accelerate the electron beam to high energy before striking the target, but share this common method of x-ray generation.

In low-energy diagnostic or superficial therapy units, which produce x-rays with energies of 50 to 150 kV, the target is simply the anode in an evacuated glass tube. X-ray generation from the impact of the electrons with the target is very inefficient, and most of the kinetic energy of the electron beam is converted to heat. These low-energy x-rays have very little penetration of tissue and are useful therapeutically only for treating the most superficial skin lesions.

Orthovoltage x-rays in the energy range of 150 to 500 kV were commonly used in the treatment of many malignancies during the 1930s to 1950s. They were more penetrating than superficial x-rays and could be used to treat deep-seated tumors. However, they gave the highest dose at the skin entry surface, and the reaction of the skin was often a limiting factor in tolerance to treatment. Orthovoltage x-rays are still frequently used for the treatment of skin cancer.

The betatron, developed in 1941, and the linear accelerator, developed initially in 1928, extensively modified during World War II with advances in microwave technology, and developed for medical applications in the early 1950s, both approached the generation of highly energetic electron beams without the use of high-voltage gradients. In the betatron, the electrons are accelerated in a circular orbit by an alternating magnetic field. In the linear accelerator, electrons are accelerated to low energy and then introduced into a series of resonant chambers where they are accelerated to relativistic energies by radiofrequency microwaves. The high-energy electron beam produced in either of these devices may then be directed against a tungsten target to produce a beam of x-rays or used directly for electron-beam therapy. Although betatrons and linear accelerators can produce x-ray beams of identical energies and tissue penetration characteristics, the dose rates, stability, and mechanical flexibility of linear accelerators surpass those of betatrons and have led to the wide adoption of linear accelerators for both clinical and research use.

Radioisotopes and Radioactive Decay

Each element in the periodic table of elements is characterized by a specific number of protons in its nucleus, which defines its atomic number. A variable number of neutrons are associated with these protons and held to them by short-range attractive forces. Atoms with the same number of protons but a different number of neutrons are called *isotopes* of each other.

Many elements occur naturally in several isotopic forms. Others may be produced by the bombardment of materials with beams of neutrons, protons, or other particles. Isotopes may be stable, such as carbon-12 (^{12}C) or hydrogen-1 (^{1}H), or unstable and subject to radioactive decay as their nucleus rearranges to a structure of lower energy. During this process of nuclear rearrangement, energy may be released in several decay pathways. In the first of these, *alpha decay*, an alpha particle or helium nucleus consisting of two protons and two neutrons is ejected. Alpha particles have only a short range in matter of normal tissue density and produce dense ionization during this short distance. Because of their short tissue penetration, alpha particles are unsuitable for use in external beam radiation therapy but are being considered for use for therapy in which

antibodies directed against determinants preferentially present on tumor cells are radioactively labeled and used to target radioactivity to these tumor cells. In this situation, the short range and dense ionization of alpha particles may present therapeutic advantages.

In *beta decay*, an electron is emitted from the nucleus, which gains in atomic number as a result. One may think of this as the conversion of a neutron to a proton and an electron. The range of these electrons in tissue is dependent on their energy, and, for typical beta-decay electrons, such as those released in the decay of ^{32}P to ^{32}S, in which electrons with energies up to 1.7 million electron volts (MeV) are released, the electron range in tissue is about 0.6 cm. This depth of penetration makes such radiation useful for the treatment of superficial tumors for example, by instillation of the radioactive substance into the peritoneal or pleural space to treat malignant ascites or pleural effusions.

In many nuclear decay processes, the initial alpha or beta decay leaves the daughter nucleus in an energetic or excited state. In returning to the ground state, this excess energy is released as one or more *gamma rays*. Unlike the rays produced by the impact of a beam of accelerated electrons impacting a tungsten target, which give a continuous spectrum of energies up to a maximum value defined by the incident electron energy, gamma rays are produced at specific energies corresponding to the differences in the binding energies of the nuclei. For radioisotopes of clinical use, these energies range from several hundred kilovolts to several million volts.

In addition to its predominant mode of decay, each isotope is characterized by its *half-life*, the time that it will take for half of the nuclei in a sample population to undergo radioactive decay. For nuclei that may undergo radioactive decay by more than one pathway, the half-life reflects the combined contribution of these different processes to the decay of the parent radionuclide.

Radioisotopes of Clinical Significance

Radium-226 (^{226}RA) is an alpha-emitting isotope that historically has had a large place in the development of radiation oncology. It occurs naturally and its isolation by the Curies in 1898 provided the first opportunity for the use of radioactive isotopes in cancer treatment. It is produced by the decay of ^{230}Th.

Radium 226 itself then decays according to the following scheme:

$$^{226}\text{Ra} \rightarrow {}^{222}\text{Rn} + {}^4\text{He}$$

Its half-life is 1622 years, and it decays by release of a 4.79-MeV gamma ray (98.8% of disintegrations) or by release of a gamma ray of 4.61 MeV followed by a 0.18-MeV ray. Radon, the initial decay product, is a chemically inert gas that is unstable and undergoes alpha decay, which proceeds through isotopes of polonium, lead, and bismuth before reaching the stable isotope of ^{206}Pb. In this process, a large number of gamma rays of various energies as well as alpha and beta particles of several energies are emitted.

Several factors make radium less than ideal for clinical use. Its initial decay product, radon, is a gas that is itself radioactive. This requires that radium sources be sealed in impermeable containers, usually made of platinum, to prevent release of the radon to the surroundings. Such encapsulation of the source also serves to absorb most of the beta particles released in the decay, so that most of the clinically useful radiation emitted in the decay of radium is from the gamma-ray component. Radium sources must be carefully checked to ensure that the encapsulation is not leaking, which would result in both a lower source strength and environmental contamination. The higher energy gamma rays emitted by radium also require more shielding to limit personnel exposure than is needed with other isotopes.

Particularly for use in standard gynecologic application, cesium-137 (^{137}Cs) has almost completely replaced radium. It decays through two mechanisms. One is by pure beta decay, releasing a beta particle of 1.17 MeV. In 92% of disintegrations, decay is through the release of a beta particle of 0.51 MeV, leaving the resultant barium nucleus in an excited state, which returns to its ground state by the emission of a photon of energy 0.662 MeV. The half-life of ^{137}Cs is 30 years.

Phosphorus-32 (^{32}P) undergoes beta decay, with a half-life of 14.3 days. Electrons are released with energies up to a maximum of 1.70 MeV. The major therapeutic use of ^{32}P is in the treatment of patients with malignant pleural, pericardial, and peritoneal effusions. It has also been used intravenously in the treatment of patients with polycythemia vera and some other hematoproliferative diseases.

Gold-198 (^{198}Au) has a relatively short half-life of 2.7 days. This allows almost all of its activity to have decayed within a period of a few days and makes it suitable for permanent intraoperative implants. It decays by two pathways, both involving beta emission to excited states of ^{198}Hg and the subsequent emission of gamma rays of 0.667 and 0.4122 MeV.

Iridium 192 (^{192}Ir) has become very widely used for interstitial implants in a variety of anatomic locations. It is physically available as thin wires or seeds and, as a reactor product, may be custom-ordered in the desired specific activity. Its decay scheme is complicated, with both beta and gamma emissions. The average gamma energy is 0.340 MeV, and the half-life, 74.3 days.

Interactions of Radiation with Matter

Both diagnostic and therapeutic uses of ionizing radiation depend on the interaction of this radiation with the tissues of the patient undergoing imaging or treatment. In diagnostic applications, it is desir-

able to obtain maximum differences in radiation absorption by different tissues to produce an image with a high degree of contrast. For therapy, however, such differential absorption is undesirable.

Photons interact with matter by several processes. At the energies used in radiation therapy, the major modes of interaction are the photoelectric effect, the Compton effect, and pair production. As shown in Table 66–1, which one of these will predominate depends on the x-ray energy and the composition of the target material (Krasin and Wagner, 1988).

The *photoelectric effect* is the main mode of interaction at low photon energies, below 50 kV, and remains important at energies up to about 90 kV. It involves the bound electrons of the inner orbitals of target atoms, and its probability is maximal with photon energies just energetic enough to knock these electrons from their orbitals. The probability of interaction varies approximately as E^{-3}, where E is the photon energy, and as Z^3, where Z is the atomic number of the target material. The photoelectric effect is very important in the production of diagnostic images, and is less so in radiation therapy.

The *Compton effect* is the predominant interaction at energies between 100 kV and 10 MV. It occurs between the incident photon and the outer orbital "free" electrons of target atoms. Its probability is independent of atomic number of the target material and decreases with the energy of the photon. Radiation is both absorbed and scattered, and the scattered radiation is sufficiently energetic to interact further within the target material.

Pair production entails the conversion of some of the energy of an incident photon to formation of an electron and positron. A minimum photon energy equal to twice the rest mass of the electron, or 1.022 MeV, is required. Photons more energetic than this divide their additional energy as kinetic energy between the newly produced electron and positron. The positron created in pair production combines with an electron in the target to produce two photons. This usually occurs when the positron is almost at rest, and the energy of the photons produced is 511 kV.

The common result of these absorptive processes is the transfer of sufficient energy from the incident photon to atoms of the target to allow orbital elec-

Table 66–1. TYPES OF PHOTON INTERACTIONS

INTERACTION	DEPENDENCE ON TARGET Z	DEPENDENCE ON PHOTON ENERGY
Photoelectric	Z^3	Greatest at electron's binding energy
Compton effect	Independent	Inverse
Pair production	Independent	Threshold at 1.022 MeV, then rapid increase

trons to be freed from their nuclei. The resulting ionized electron may have sufficient energy to produce secondary ionizations in neighboring molecules.

The positively charged ions that result from the electron loss of ionization are not stable and undergo a variety of chemical reactions. Many of these involve an initial loss of a hydrogen ion, and with it the positive charge, resulting in a reactive free radical.

The effects of ionizing radiation on biologic systems are produced both by the direct damage to biologically critical molecules such as DNA and by the secondary reaction of ions and free radicals produced by the ionization of other intracellular and extracellular molecules with these critical targets. Because the predominant cellular molecule is water, accounting for 70% to 80% of cellular weight, the radiolysis products of water account for the majority of initially formed species after ionizing radiation. These include highly reactive molecular species such as hydroxyl ions, which mediate much of the damage to cellular macromolecules.

There is considerable evidence that DNA represents a critical cellular target for radiation damage and that the risk of such damage may be influenced by the association of DNA with protein and/or the cell membrane. Four major categories of DNA damage are produced by ionizing radiation: (1) crosslinks between the DNA strands or between DNA and protein, (2) damage to DNA bases without altering of the sugar-phosphate chain backbone, (3) single-strand breaks, and (4) double-strand breaks.

DNA Repair

The number of DNA strand breaks produced by direct and indirect ionization far exceeds the number of cells that are killed. This implies either that more than one break—in fact, a rather large number of breaks—is required for cell death or that processes exist that can repair radiation-induced DNA damage. There is clear evidence that most cells possess rather extensive mechanisms for the detection and repair of DNA damage, whether caused by ionizing radiation, ultraviolet radiation, or chemical damage through compounds such as alkylating agents. These mechanisms have been reviewed, and their biochemical mechanisms are not detailed here (Friedberg, 1985; Goffman et al, 1990). For practical purposes, it is sufficient to remember that these repair processes are highly efficient and usually accurate, so that about 1000 single-strand breaks and 100 double-strand breaks are produced for each lethal event. Agents that can inhibit these DNA repair processes can increase cell killing and, if even relatively selective for tumor cells, may have a role in clinical treatment.

Operationally, two types of repair after ionizing radiation damage have been described in mammalian cells. The first, *sublethal damage repair* (SLDR), is

inferred from the increase in surviving fraction that occurs when a dose of radiation is split into two smaller doses. The half-time for such repair is approximately 1 hour.

A second manifestation of cellular repair processes is seen when cells are irradiated with a single radiation fraction and either plated immediately in growth medium or held for some time in a nutritionally depleted condition that inhibits progression of cells through the growth cycle before plating. Net survival is increased by this delay in active cell growth following irradiation. This phenomenon is termed *potentially lethal repair damage* (PLDR).

These processes of repair are of considerable potential significance in clinical radiation therapy. Typical courses of treatment are given with multiple radiation doses over several days, allowing repair processes to occur. In many tumors, regions of cells that are far from their vasculature are nutritionally depleted as well as hypoxic, factors that will modify their radiation sensitivity. Attempts are being made for the rational clinical exploitation of these conditions (Peters and Ang, 1986; Goffman et al, 1990; Peters et al, 1990).

Although operationally PLDR and SLDR are defined as separate processes, the molecular mechanisms of both remain incompletely understood. They may well represent not two distinct processes but, rather, two ways of looking at a single underlying set of molecular events or overlapping and possibly competing processes.

Radiation Dosimetry and Radiation Therapy Planning

As a result of the processes of absorption and scattering that have just been discussed, the intensity of a beam of x-rays decreases as it penetrates into an absorbing material. The resulting dose profile depends on the x-ray beam energy and the density of the absorbing material. Figure 66–1 shows the dose profiles for photon beams of various energies. As the energy increases, there is a reduced dose to the entry skin surface, a shift to a greater depth for the point of maximum dose, and a decreased rate of dose decrease with depth. These features, particularly the greater skin sparing and higher dose to deeply seated tissues, have led to the adoption of high-energy beams (4 to 20 MV) in the vast majority of clinical uses.

The depth-dose profiles of electron beams differ greatly from those of photons. There is relatively little skin sparing, but this decreases with increasing electron energy rather than increases, as it does with photons. Instead of a relatively constant decrease in beam intensity with depth, the dose from the electron beam has a region over which the dose changes relatively slowly, followed by a region in which it declines very rapidly, as shown in Figure 66–2. The depth at which this rapid decrease in dose occurs

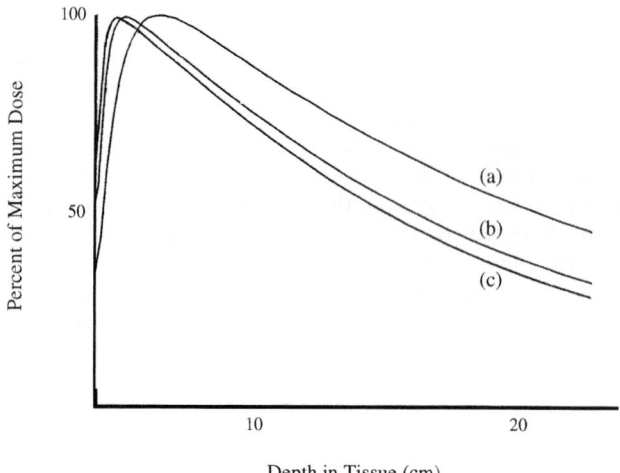

Figure 66-1
Representative depth-dose curves for 18-MV photons (*a*), 6-MV photons (*b*), and 4-MV photons (*c*).

depends on the energy of the electron beam, increasing with increasing energy. These characteristics of relatively uniform dose over a region of several centimeters followed by a rapid decline in dose make the electron beam very useful for the treatment of relatively superficial lesions that overlie vital structures. This has been valuable in the treatment of tumors on the chest wall and tumors in the posterior cervical triangle that overlie the spinal cord.

Dose Units

The basic dose units used in radiation therapy have dimensions of amount of energy transferred per gram of matter. The presently defined Système International (SI) unit is the gray (Gy), which repre-

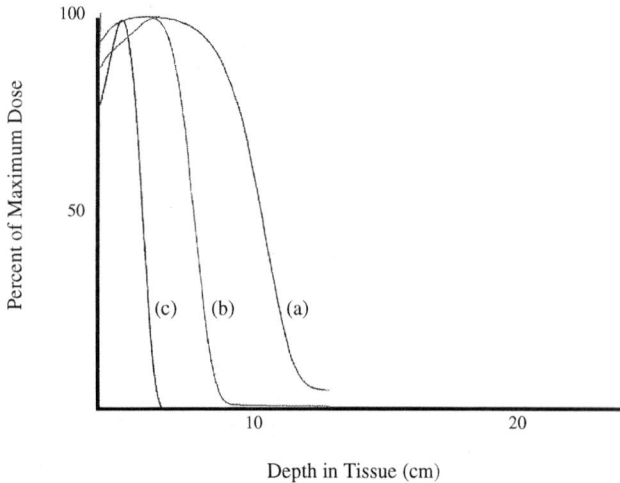

Figure 66-2
Representative depth-dose curves for 20-MeV electrons (*a*), 12-MeV electrons (*b*), and 6-MeV electrons (*c*).

sents 1 joule per kilogram. For many years, the rad was the commonly used unit of dose; this represents 100 erg per gram or 1/100 Gy. One now often hears doses expressed in centigray (cGy), a hybrid unit that bows to the SI standard while retaining numeric equivalence with the familiar dose in rad.

The gradual and sometimes overlapping change in units has occasioned some satirical verse:

> *The Rad will soon have had its day And then for dose we'll use the GRAY But Grays are bigger as we've said So talk of centi-grays instead That brings us right back to the start You can't tell these and rads apart*

Newing, cited in Hall (1984)

Relative Biologic Effectiveness and Microdosimetry

Although the absorbed dose is a sufficient unit for physical dosimetry, it does not adequately describe the biologic effectiveness of the radiation. As is described later, the place of cells in the mitotic cycle, their nutritional and oxygenation state, and the fractionation of the total radiation dose play important roles in determining the biologic effect of a radiation dose. However, even with these factors held constant, 1 Gy of neutron radiation and 1 Gy of gamma radiation will have quite different biologic effects. Under oxic conditions and with cells randomly distributed in their growth cycle, the neutron radiation produces about three times as much cell killing per rad as the photon treatment. The ratio of the biologic effect produced for a physical unit of absorbed dose is referred to as the relative biologic effectiveness (RBE) of the radiation, with 250 kV photons as the reference energy. The RBE of a typical photon beam for a 6-MV linear accelerator is about 0.85; that is, the same dose in gray produces less cell kill with this beam than with the reference 250-kV beam.

The discrepancy occurs because, although the physical dose describes the net amount of energy transfer, it does not include any consideration of the distribution of ionizations over a local region of interest. In fact, the density of ionizations varies considerably for different types of radiations. For example, with x-rays and gamma rays of 250 kV, the density of ionizations following the track of a single photon is rather sparse; the rate of energy transfer per unit distance, or linear energy transfer (LET), is small (about 3 keV/μm); and the range of the photon is great. For alpha particles, whose range is short, the density of ionization is much higher and the rate of energy transfer is approximately 95 keV/μm. Such dense ionization is more likely to produce double-strand DNA breaks or multiple single breaks in close proximity, lesions that are thought to be more likely to lead to cell death than widely spaced single-strand breaks. LET values have been measured for a variety of types of radiation. Up to a LET value of about 100 keV/μm, the RBE increases; beyond this it begins to decline. The likely explanation for this decline is that the additional ionizations produced are not leading to any greater cell death (i.e., the ratio of ionizations produced to lethal events decreases). Cells cannot be killed twice no matter how dense the ionization.

Radiation Dose Delivery

Once the decision to include radiation therapy as a part of the care of a patient has been reached, the patient must undergo a series of procedures designed to plan the manner in which the radiation dose is to be delivered and to establish the location of the radiation fields on the skin surface. The planning of a course of radiation therapy is a complex process that often involves the combined work of the radiation oncologist, simulator therapist, and radiation physicist or dosimetrist. The radiation oncologist determines which tissues are to be treated, to what dose, and the limits of dose that any nearby normal tissues may receive. The dosimetrist determines, from these requirements and constraints and from information about the patient's anatomy, a suitable arrangement of external beams, or combination of external beam plus radioisotope implantation into the tumor, to meet these conditions. Finally, the simulator therapist converts this plan to a set of marks on the patient indicating the size, position, and angulation of each of these treatment beams.

Immobilization Devices

In designing a treatment plan, what is being designed is not merely a geometric exercise but the treatment of a patient who will, at the least, breathe during the course of each day's treatment. Sometimes, patients not only breathe but also fidget, move from the position in which they were placed on the treatment table, lose weight, blur their skin marks when they sweat, and in other ways make it clear that millimeter precision in routine treatment planning is not a realistic goal. Immobilization devices, such as custom-made plastic or rubber molds to place around the patient, can help to make treatment setups more rapid, comfortable, and accurate, but allowances are made for the inevitable day-to-day variations in treatment setup and delivery.

Treatment Planning

The goal of radiation treatment planning is to deliver a specified dose of radiation uniformly to a desired target volume while keeping the dose to surrounding tissues as low as possible. Although this may seem to be a simple and obvious goal, its implementation can be, at times, most difficult. Broadly speaking, there are two component approaches used in treatment planning: approaches to maximize dose uniformity in a moderate to large treatment volume and approaches to deliver a high dose to a small volume with rapid decrease in dose outside this volume. The first approach is exemplified by external beam treatment planning, the second by intracavitary or interstitial implants.

External Beam Plans

A single photon beam rarely produces a dose distribution useful for giving definitive high-dose treatment. As seen in the depth-dose curves in Figure 66–1, the dose within any reasonable volume of tissue will be quite nonuniform. Such a degree of dose heterogeneity may be acceptable for a limited course of palliative treatment; vertebral metastases are, for example, often treated quite effectively with a single beam. This is successful because the total doses required are low and adjacent normal tissues will tolerate a dose 10% to 15% higher than the tumor dose.

An arrangement of two colinear beams pointing in opposite directions, termed a *parallel opposed pair*, is a commonly used beam arrangement in a large number of clinical settings. This simple arrangement may suffice for many treatment situations. When the separation between the two patient surfaces is relatively small, on the order of 20 cm, the dose distribution is reasonably uniform throughout the treatment volume. As separation increases, the dose at midplane becomes significantly less than that at shallower depths, which would lead to overtreatment of normal tissues. As patient size increases, more complex field arrangements become necessary.

For pelvic malignancies, such as carcinomas of the cervix and endometrium, the use of four treatment beams—anterior, posterior, and right and left laterals—is the most common field arrangement. Such a four-field "box" arrangement allows delivery of a uniform dose to a large volume, which in these cases will typically cover the primary tumor, known and possible parametrial extensions, and lymph node chains along the pelvic side walls, while delivering a significantly lower dose to most of the bladder and rectum, which are the dose-limiting normal organs in the region. The contribution of the lateral beams to this field arrangement must be limited to avoid overdose to the femoral heads, but this is generally not a major concern.

Dose distributions can be further shaped to conform to the target volume and spare normal tissue by shielding portions of the basic rectangular beams into more intricate shapes and by differentially absorbing one part of the x-ray beam with wedge-shaped devices or compensators. Such devices are particularly useful in treating sloping portions of the patient's anatomy of uneven thickness, such as the breast.

A logical extension to the use of multiple stationary beams is a continuous rotation of the radiation source around a fixed point or isocenter located within the tumor volume (although not necessarily at its center). Treatment may be delivered throughout the entire 360-degree rotation or may be omitted for certain arcs to protect normal tissues. Such arc therapy is sometimes used to irradiate the prostate while sparing the more anteriorly located bladder and posteriorly located rectum. Such a dose distribution is rarely used alone but, rather, for a portion of an overall treatment plan, which might also include a four-field box to irradiate the pelvic nodes. A similar technique can be used as part of the treatment of carcinoma of the cervix and its lateral extensions into the parametria.

Intracavitary and Interstitial Therapy

The placement of radioactive sources in or against a tumor volume is an effective way to give a very high dose to the tumor-containing tissue and a much lower dose to adjacent normal tissues. In addition to the possible geometric superiority of such dose distributions, these distributions are less sensitive to patient motion, which is an important consideration in real patients as opposed to geometric phantoms used to plan hypothetic dose distributions.

Treatment of cervical cancer has long relied on the use of *intracavitary therapy* to deliver a high radiation dose to the cervix, lower uterine segment, and vaginal fornices with sparing of the bladder and rectum. Several appliances have been devised to allow the accurate and stable positioning of radioisotope sources adjacent to the cervix. One of these, the applicator designed by Fletcher and Suit, consists of a hollow tube, the *tandem*, which passes through the cervical os and into the endometrial cavity. The rounded *ovoids* are placed in the lateral vaginal fornices. After confirmation of the proper positioning of these holders, radioactive sources are placed in them after the patient has returned to her hospital room. Figure 66–3 shows anteroposterior and lateral views of such an intracavitary application with the radiation dose distribution superimposed. The lines connect points of equal dose rate and are thus termed *isodose lines*. There is a rapid decrease in dose rate as one moves several centimeters from the center of the implant.

Another approach to brachytherapy, used when the organ to be treated does not have a natural cavity to hold the radioactive sources, is *interstitial therapy*. In this method, narrow sources are inserted directly into the tumor-bearing organ. In past years, these were often radium needles enclosed in pointed platinum shells. The platinum shells served both to absorb the low-energy electrons produced in the decay of the radium and to enclose the radon produced. Radium needles for interstitial implants have been almost completely replaced by ^{192}Ir in afterloading catheters. The surgical portion of the procedure involves placement of hollow catheters through the tumor or tumor bed. This may be done as an open surgical procedure or through percutaneous trocars

through which the catheters are threaded. The proper placement of the catheters is confirmed radiographically using nonradioactive dummy sources. Only then are the radioactive sources, usually ^{192}Ir, threaded into the catheters. This two-step approach allows as much time as needed to be spent in ensuring a properly positioned implant without concern for radiation exposure of the physician and other operating room and dosimetry staff during this phase of the procedure.

With typical brachytherapy loadings, for intracavitary or interstitial treatment, radiation dose rates to the target volume are on the order of 50 to 70 cGy/hour. To deliver a dose of 25 Gy to the designated volume, the implant must be in place for about 2 days. During this time, the patient must be hospitalized in a private room with limited care by nursing personnel to decrease their cumulative radiation exposure. Because of the gradual rate of tumor treatment secondary to the activity of the radioactive source, these treatments are sometimes called low dose rate (LDR).

High-Dose-Rate Brachytherapy

Over the 1990s, high-dose-rate (HDR) brachytherapy has been increasingly reported in the literature and used in the clinic. This technique allows the remote placement of the radioactive source into the implant through catheters and then its removal into a shielded lead container following treatment, all by computerized remote control, thus reducing occupational radiation exposure to the patient's caregivers. The high-activity source can deliver a target dose rate of 100 cGy/minute. Depending on tumor location, either interstitial or intracavitary treatments can be delivered. In addition to cervix cancer, HDR brachytherapy is being used to treat endobronchial carcinoma, endometrial carcinoma, esophageal cancers, primary brain tumors, breast tumors, prostate cancers, soft tissue sarcomas, and others (Speiser, 1993).

An enhancement of this remote afterloading technique is to vary the position of the sources within the patient during the time of the implant, in effect producing a customized dose distribution that depends on the intensity of the sources and the length of time they remain at any given point. Radiation dose distributions produced by this method can be tailored to follow irregular tumor and/or normal tissue contours in a more individualized manner than those produced with standard applicators. Such techniques have the potential to improve the therapeutic ratio of brachytherapy treatments by increasing tumor dose while reducing normal tissue dose.

Because of the high specific activity of the radioactive source, the dose can be delivered over a period of several minutes as opposed to the several days required for LDR brachytherapy. Such treatment avoids the need for hospitalization. Some of the initial impetus for the development of this tech-

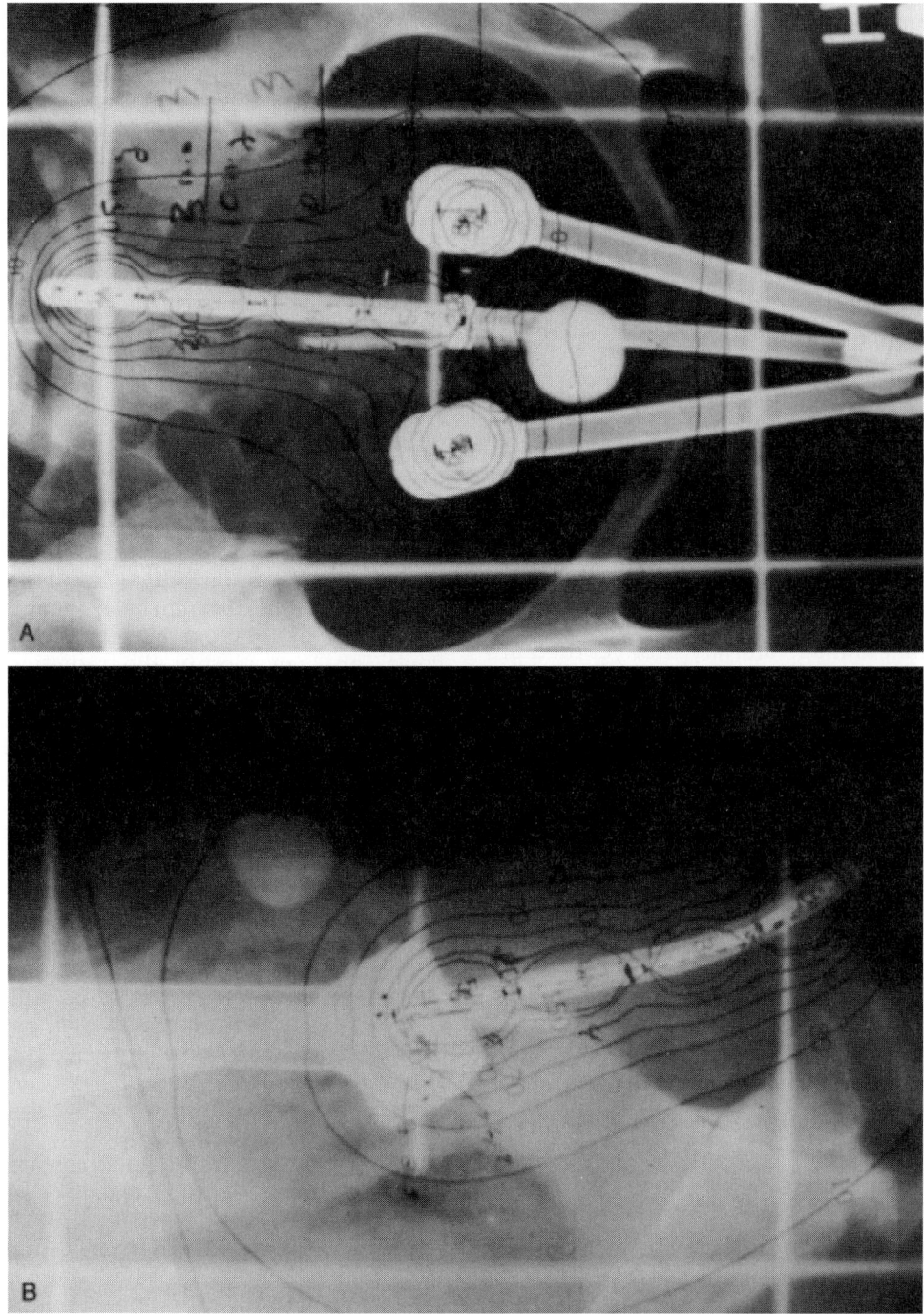

Figure 66–3
Anteroposterior (*A*) and lateral (*B*) views of a tandem and ovoid application for carcinoma of the cervix with superimposed isodose curves. Dose rates are in centigray per hour.

nique came from the need to treat large populations of women with cervical carcinoma in parts of the world with limited medical resources in which hospital-based treatment was economically and logistically impossible. With the dose rate of HDR so much higher than LDR, the acute and especially the long-term toxicity of this relatively new modality are debated by radiobiologists and others, with some ar-

guing that HDR has less side effects than LDR, and some insisting that the opposite is true. To the extent that sparing of normal tissue is partly due to that tissue's ability to repair sublethal and potentially lethal damage, HDR treatment will abrogate this. It is hoped that high dose rates, at least in gynecologic malignancies, may allow better positioning of the source for a 10-minute treatment than is possible (or tolerable by a nonsedated patient) for a 48-hour treatment, and thus compensate for any radiobiologic disadvantage. Undoubtedly, as the use of HDR continues, additional data and time will allow its role, effectiveness, and potential long-term side effects to be further elucidated.

RADIATION BIOLOGY AS A BASIS OF CLINICAL PRACTICE

Radiation Sensitivity

The effect of radiation that is of greatest therapeutic use is its ability to damage cells in such a way as to destroy their reproductive capability. The loss of this potential for clonogenicity will lead to cessation of growth of the tumor and eventually to its destruction. Whereas lethally damaged cells may remain alive for some time and in some cases even go through one or more rounds of mitosis, their daughter cells eventually all die out. Cells that have sustained such lethal damage but have not yet died are referred to as "doomed" cells. They have no distinctive morphologic characteristics that allow them to be distinguished reliably from viable cells. The appearance of tumor cells in biopsy specimens obtained shortly (e.g., a few weeks) after a course of radiation treatment thus cannot be taken as a sure indication of the presence of residual viable tumor that would lead to a recurrence unless excised.

The sensitivity of clonogenic tumor cells to ionizing radiation has been studied for a variety of tumor systems in vitro. When single-cell suspensions are irradiated with graded doses of radiation and their clonogenic survival determined, curves that relate cell survival to radiation dose may be plotted. If one plots the logarithm of the surviving cell fraction against the radiation dose, the resulting curves usually show an initial region of very shallow slope, which then becomes steeper and remains linear at least to doses of several thousand centigray. These data can be fit reasonably well to a simple second-order equation of the form

$$\text{effect} = \alpha D + \beta D^2$$

where α and β are experimentally determined constants.

Small but reproducible differences in these parameters can be measured for cell lines derived from different tumor types and for different individual tumors of the same cell type (Peters and Ang, 1986; Weichselbaum et al, 1986; Peters, 1990). Another parameter that has been used to characterize cellular radiation sensitivity is the fraction of cells surviving a dose of 200 cGy, the S_{200}. This has been correlated with the clinical likelihood of obtaining tumor control and shows some promise as an indicator of prognosis following radiation therapy. Differences in these parameters (α, β, S_{200}) are small, and there is considerable overlap between tumors of different types and between values obtained for tumor and normal tissue cells. In addition to these small differences in intrinsic radiation sensitivity, the location of tumor cells in a particular microenvironment with characteristic pH and oxygen tension will also influence radiation sensitivity. One generally valid observation is that the survival curves for late-responding tissues, typically normal tissues of organs that are not usually undergoing frequent cell division, are more strongly curved than those of rapidly proliferating tissues, either tumors or rapidly regenerating normal tissues such as intestinal mucosa. Mathematically, this is expressed as a greater α/β ratio. This has implications for the choice of fraction size in clinical treatment, indicating that a greater differential protection of important late-responding tissues can be obtained by treating with a larger number of small fractions and that treatment with regimens of a small number of large fractions (3 Gy or more), even if the total dose is adjusted to give acceptable acute toxicity, may produce severe late effects.

In addition to differences in the intrinsic radiation sensitivity of their stem cells, local environmental conditions can modify the radiation sensitivity of cells in vitro and in vivo. Several factors have been identified that modify radiation sensitivity in ways that may be clinically significant (Table 66–2).

If a synchronized cell population is irradiated at different times from the previous mitosis, the surviving fraction of cells will depend on their position in the cell cycle. Cells are most sensitive to radiation during mitosis and least sensitive during S phase. With radiation doses of 2 to 3 Gy, the difference in surviving fraction for cells in M phase and S phase is approximately 10-fold. This differential radiation sensitivity means that a dose of radiation will produce partial synchronization of the surviving cells, which will be enriched in those cells that were in the more radioresistant portions of the cell cycle. As these cells progress through the cell cycle, they will become more radiosensitive.

In addition to their metabolic state, the degree of oxygenation of a population of cells at the time at which they are irradiated is an important determinant of radiation sensitivity. The magnitude of this oxygen effect varies a bit with the dose of radiation given and with the radiation dose rate, but with typical fraction sizes of 2 to 3 Gy is on the order of 3.

Molecular oxygen can react with free radicals produced by the radiolysis of water or in biologically

Table 66–2. MODIFIERS OF CELLULAR RADIATION SENSITIVITY

FACTOR	MAGNITUDE OF EFFECT
Oxygen	3-fold
Position in cell cycle	10-fold
Repair	3-fold

important target molecules. The reaction of oxygen with aqueous free radicals can lead to the production of highly reactive chemical species such as hydroperoxide radicals and hydrogen peroxide. Reaction of oxygen with free radicals in biologic organic compounds occurs more rapidly than the reconstitution of these molecules by hydrogen abstraction from cysteine or glutathione and represents a pathway for fixation of this biologic damage. Oxygen-dependent radiosensitization requires that oxygen be present at the time of radiation; subsequent oxygenation is ineffective. Similarly, transient hypoxia is radioprotective.

Processes Occurring Between Fractions

Since the seminal observation by Coutard in the 1920s—that, although it was not possible to use a single dose of radiation to sterilize a ram without massive damage to the overlying skin, this could be achieved by dividing the dose into several fractions—the role of fractionation of the total radiation dose has attracted much clinical interest. It has become evident that fractionated treatment is superior to treatment using a large single dose in most clinical situations. In addition to clinical experience that such fractionated treatment produces superior outcomes to those obtained from a single dose, there is a developing understanding of the radiobiologic processes behind this observation. Several processes occur during a fractionated course of treatment that modify the net effect of the radiation on both the tumor and normal tissues (Hall, 1994).

Repair

When cells in tissue culture are irradiated with two doses of radiation, the resultant cell survival depends on the interval between fractions. As the interval between fractions is increased from a few minutes to several hours, the overall survival fraction increases. The half-time for this increase is on the order of 1 hour for most cell types. This increase in survival with increasing separation of doses is attributed to the repair of sublethal radiation damage, mostly single-strand DNA breaks, which could combine with subsequently incurred damage to produce a lethal lesion. Incubation of cells in conditions that inhibit such repair increases cell lethality (Friedberg, 1985).

Repopulation

In the interval between fractions, cells that have not been lethally damaged are inhibited in their progression through the cell cycle. If fractions are sufficiently closely spaced, treatment may successfully reduce the number of clonogens. However, if the rate of cell proliferation is sufficiently rapid, the tumor may increase in number during the course of radiation treatment despite the killing of a large number of cells. This phenomenon of increased proliferation is of particular concern because there is evidence, in several human tumors, that the rate of proliferation of surviving stem cells may accelerate after several weeks of a course of fractionated treatment. Because this is also the period when the acute toxicity of treatment is making side effects more difficult for patients to tolerate and patients are often eager to interrupt treatment, it is important to avoid such interruptions.

Data have emerged that prolongation of treatment time for cervical carcinoma is associated with decreased local control and survival (Petereit et al, 1995). Conversely, shorter treatment times have been associated with increased local control. It is believed that the cause of local failure after a protracted course of radiation therapy is proliferation of surviving tumor clonogens during the prolonged period over which treatment is delivered.

Redistribution of Cells in the Cell Cycle

The sensitivity of cells to radiation varies with their position in the cell cycle. Cells are most sensitive during mitosis and least sensitive during S phase or in the long G_1 phase of cells that are not actively proliferating. In tumor tissues, such slowly proliferating cells are also often in regions of relative hypoxia, which will further protect them from radiation lethality.

Reoxygenation

If oxic and nutritionally repleted cells are preferentially killed by clinically significant doses of radiation, the remaining cells may become better oxygenated during a course of fractionated treatment and thus become more susceptible to killing by subsequent fractions. There is experimental and clinical evidence that this occurs in some tumors, although its overall significance in most clinical treatments is uncertain. The rate at which such reoxygenation can occur depends on the number and radiation sensitivity of the tumor cells as well as the rate at which doomed cells die and cease to consume oxygen.

RADIORESPONSIVENESS

In distinction from radiation sensitivity, which is an expression of survival of clonogenic cells, radioresponsiveness refers to the effect of radiation on a measurable tumor mass, for example, a palpable tumor mass or a lesion visualized by imaging techniques such as chest x-ray films, computerized tomography (CT), or magnetic resonance imaging (MRI). In the clinic, we have no direct way of measuring radiation sensitivity and are, in fact, making frequent inferences about radiation sensitivity based on radioresponsiveness.

DISTINCTION BETWEEN RATE AND EXTENT OF RESPONSE

In the early development of radiation oncology, it was noted that different tumors regressed at different rates when treated in a similar manner. This led to two practices that subsequent radiobiologic consideration has shown to be ill-founded. One of these was the titration of total dose of radiation according to the rate of tumor regression. The other was to assume that those tumors that regressed slowly were inherently radioresistant and unlikely to be controlled by even high doses of radiation. Both of these practices were based on a confusion of the rate of tumor regression with the extent of kill of stem cells. This latter parameter is what is important in determining whether or not the tumor will recur following radiation therapy. The rate of regression, while dependent in part on the extent of stem cell kill, is also determined by the rate at which cells that have received lethal damage from radiation die, and, having died, are cleared from the body by processes of necrosis and/or apoptosis. As a first approximation, tumors that were growing rapidly prior to the institution of radiation therapy will regress rapidly with successful treatment, but this rapid regression does not ensure local control and should not be used as an indication to reduce the total planned treatment dose. Conversely, tumors that often have relatively slow growth rates, such as many adenocarcinomas of the gastrointestinal and genitourinary tracts, regress slowly following radiation and yet seem to be as likely to be controlled as other epithelial tumors (e.g., squamous cell carcinomas) of similar bulk.

RADIOCONTROLLABILITY

The availability of a test predicting the ability of radiation to control a local tumor, analogous to antibiotic sensitivity testing, would be a major aid in choosing appropriate therapy for patients with cancer, particularly those in whom there is a reasonable choice between surgery and radiation therapy. Extensive research to develop such a test has been performed for the past 50 years, unfortunately without yet producing a clinically useful test. Research has indicated several promising avenues for further exploration (Peters, 1990).

Tumor cells differ subtly in their sensitivity to ionizing radiation, not by the several logarithms of cell kill that drug-sensitive and drug-resistant cell lines may differ in their resistance to chemotherapy, but by perhaps 10% to 20% in the surviving fraction after a radiation dose in the clinically relevant range of 1.8 to 3.0 Gy. Although this difference is small, when it is accumulated over a course of 30 to 35 treatments, it can lead to a substantial difference in the final probability of cell survival and local control. Such relatively radioresistant cells exist in many tumor types, and such variations in radiation sensitivity appear to be at least as great within tumor types (e.g., squamous cell carcinoma of the cervix) as between tumor types. Several laboratories have now reported that they have been able to identify such radioresistant cells in the pretreatment biopsies of some patients with head and neck cancers and that the identification of such cells predicts a low probability of local control.

The number of stem cells present per gram of tumor tissue has also been shown to vary between tumors. Because higher doses of radiation are expected to be required to control a tumor with a greater number of stem cells, for a given radiation dose, the greater the number of stem cells, the lower the probability of achieving local control. Assays to measure the density of such stem cells in human tumors prior to treatment have been developed and are being tested.

At present, the prediction of tumor radiocontrollability is not yet a clinical reality, and it is questionable whether there will be a single test that will ever have high predictive value. However, the integration of such information with other clinical factors may help to refine our ability to choose the most appropriate treatment for individual patients.

ANALYSIS OF PATTERNS OF FAILURE

Improvement of the results of present methods of cancer treatment requires an understanding of their deficiencies. It is not enough to know simply whether or not a patient with cancer remains alive 5 years after treatment. If the patient has died, the cause of death should be known. If death is due to tumor, is this from local tumor progression or the development of systemic metastatic disease? If there has been local tumor recurrence, where is this in relation to the areas treated by surgery and/or radiation therapy? In patients treated with radiation therapy, a recurrence at the center of the treatment volume suggests that the dose was insufficient, whereas a recurrence at the margin of the treatment volume suggests that the volume was too small. Failure in distant sites with control of local disease indicates that radiation therapy had successfully met the local need but that the natural history of the disease in question was such as to require systemic therapy as well.

RADIOCURABILITY

The best outcome that can be achieved with the use of a local treatment such as radiation therapy or surgery is the control of local disease, the primary tumor and its regional nodal metastases. Whether or not this will result in the cure of the disease will depend on other factors, including the natural history of the disease in question and the expected survival of the patients. Some tumors are quite readily controlled in their local extent by radiation therapy but are virtually never cured by local means because of near-universal systemic dissemination. The corollary is that the use of survival rates as the sole assessment of the effectiveness of radiation therapy is inappropriate.

It is essential also to determine whether or not local tumor control has been achieved. If so, radiation therapy has achieved all that could reasonably be expected from a local treatment modality, and the problem lies in the capacity of the tumor for subclinical dissemination. Conversely, if there is failure to achieve local control, this implies a need to consider a change in radiation therapy dose or technique or the use of another local treatment modality. The ability to achieve local control of tumor does not guarantee a good clinical outcome but is generally a prerequisite. Although in a few selected malignancies there is a meaningful possibility of curative salvage therapy by other modalities if patients relapse locally following radiation therapy, this is usually not the case.

DOSE-RESPONSE RELATIONS

Increasing doses of radiation produce increasing effects in tumor and normal tissue (Table 66–3). The relation between dose and effect is not a simple linear one, but rather a complex function of the total radiation dose, the size and number of fractions in which it is delivered, and the overall time during which treatment is given. The precise nature of this relation appears to differ for rapidly and slowly proliferating tissues, which is partly the basis for fractionating the radiation dose to spare the relatively slowly proliferating normal tissues while effectively killing more rapidly proliferating tumor cells. Some of the earliest attempts to codify this were in carcinoma of the skin as described by Strandquist in the 1930s. He showed that tumor control depended on at least three treatment factors: the total dose, the number of fractions in which it was divided, and the overall time (in days) elapsed between the start and completion of treatment. Similar relations have been established for a number of other relatively common tumor types, including head and neck and cervical carcinomas, particularly in which the effects of radiation dose on local control are not obscured by the emergence of metastatic disease. Several attempts have been made to create isoeffect formulas relating total dose, number of fractions, and time of treatment, but it is hazardous to generalize these across different tissue types.

CLINICAL FRACTIONATION SCHEDULES

It is desirable but not yet possible to customize the total dose, fractionation, and duration of a treatment course based on characteristics (size, histology,

Table 66–3. CARCINOMA OF THE TONSILLAR REGION (T3): LOCAL CONTROL AND COMPLICATIONS BY DOSE

TOTAL DOSE (Gy)	LOCAL CONTROL	COMPLICATIONS	
		Grade 2	Grade 3
55–59	0/2	0	0
60–69	2/5 (40%)	2	0
70–79	6/10 (60%)	1	1
80+	7/8 (88%)	3	0

From Million RR, Cassisi NJ, Mancuso AA: The unknown primary. In Million RR, Cassisi NJ (eds): Management of Head and Neck Cancer: A Multidisciplinary Approach. Philadelphia: JB Lippincott Company, 1984:311, with permission.

growth rate, oxygenation, and so on) of an individual tumor that would predict its individual radiation sensitivity and radiocontrollability. From decades of clinical experience, several guidelines for radiation dose and fractionation have been learned:

1. Palliation of symptoms, in which tumor control and cure are not treatment goals and the expected survival of the patient is relatively short, can often be achieved with modest total doses of radiation given over a relatively brief time period (e.g., 30 Gy in 10 fractions over 2 to $2^{1}/_{2}$ weeks).
2. When long-term disease control and possible cure are the treatment goals, radiation doses must be higher and must depend on the volume of disease present. To achieve control, large tumors require higher radiation doses than do small tumors of the same histology. To achieve high total doses and minimize long-term damage to normal tissues, the radiation must be given in a relatively large number of small fractions (e.g., 1.8 to 2.0 Gy per day; see Table 66–4).
3. With the exception of a few tumor types, such as lymphomas or germ cell tumors, which are controlled by relatively low total radiation doses, and malignant gliomas, which are rarely controlled by even very high doses, there is not a great or a clinically predictable variation in the radiation doses required to control different tumors of similar bulk, and radiation doses should not vary

Table 66–4. RADIATION DOSE REQUIRED FOR CONTROL VERSUS TUMOR BULK*

TUMOR SIZE (cm)	DOSE (Gy)
Microscopic	45–50
<2	60
2–4	70
4–6	70–75
>6	75–80

*Dose required for 90% probability of local control; daily fraction size: 1.8 to 2.0 Gy.
Modified from Fletcher GH: Clinical dose-response curves of human malignant epithelial tumors. Br J Radiol 1973;46:1, with permission.

much with histology. Different histologic tumor types may have other features that influence the radiation therapy technique or the combination of radiation with other treatment modalities (e.g., the frequency of bulky endocervical involvement by adenocarcinoma of the cervix is greater than that for squamous cell carcinoma and requires either care that this area is irradiated to a high dose or the addition of a simple extrafascial hysterectomy to radiation therapy. This is a statistical difference, however, and an equally bulky squamous cell tumor showing a similar pattern of spread should also be managed in this way).

DISSOCIATION BETWEEN EARLY AND LATE EFFECTS

The acute toxicities of radiation exposure are seen in tissues that are normally rapidly proliferating, such as skin, mucosa of the respiratory or gastrointestinal tract, and bone marrow. The tissues that limit long-term tolerance, however, are more often slowly proliferating ones such as the spinal cord, muscular wall of the esophagus or other viscera, or vascular endothelium. Extensive clinical experience indicates that the extent of the acute reaction does not predict the late effects of treatment and that the dependence of early and late effects on the radiation dose per fraction are different. With daily small fractions, the acute toxicity may be quite brisk in tissues such as oral mucosa and there may be little in the way of late effects. Attempts to shorten the overall treatment time by increasing the daily radiation dose and reducing the total dose may give no greater acute toxicity but a high incidence of late damage.

Other toxicities, such as the incidence of leukemias or solid tumors in irradiated tissues, are clearly not well correlated with the extent of the early reaction.

COMBINATIONS OF RADIOTHERAPY WITH OTHER TREATMENT MODALITIES

Surgery

The limitations of both radiation and surgery in curing patients with locally advanced carcinomas led to the thought of combining these modalities in the hopes of improving local control and thus survival. Initial attempts to combine radical surgery and radical (in radiation dose and treatment volume) radiation therapy often resulted in severe complications, although they were successful in demonstrating the improvements in local control. Fletcher (1976, 1985) advocated and popularized the concept of associating less-than-radical surgery with less-than-radical radiation therapy, so long as each component of disease was treated with adequate intensity. Surgery was used to remove macroscopic disease without removing wide margins of normal tissue. Radiation

therapy was used to treat the volume of normal tissue surrounding the main tumor mass at risk for harboring microscopic disease, limiting the radiation dose to a level, usually 45 to 55 Gy, capable of controlling such small tumor burdens. This approach has produced good results in the treatment of a number of malignancies in which it has allowed good local control with less morbidity than seen with either modality given alone. The treatment of localized breast cancer with a planned combination of excision of all known macroscopic tumor (local excision, lumpectomy, tylectomy) results in excellent local control and far better cosmesis than that achieved either by mastectomy (with or without subsequent reconstructive surgery) or by radiation alone without resection of the gross disease, in which much higher radiation doses have to be used.

Chemotherapy

As a locoregional modality, radiation therapy does not ordinarily treat the issue of systemic disease, occult or overt. In special circumstances, wide-field irradiation, including total-body irradiation, has been used in conjunction with programs of autologous or allogeneic bone marrow transplantation in the treatment of patients with leukemias, lymphomas, and some solid tumors. With relatively few exceptions, radiation therapy is a local modality. Its combination with chemotherapy has been explored in the hope that effective cell kill with chemotherapy might both enhance the probability of local control and delay or prevent the emergence of systemic disease. At a minimum, the success of such efforts requires that both modalities have independent toxicity against the tumor in question. In many cases, it is believed or hoped that the combined effects of radiation and chemotherapy on local control will be greater than additive, possibly through the sensitization by one modality to the effects of the other or the interference by certain chemotherapeutic agents with cellular repair processes. This area is currently one of rather intense clinical application and clinical and laboratory investigation. Although good clinical results can be obtained, the mechanisms behind these and the real existence of synergistic toxicity remain somewhat conjectural (Bellamy, 1990).

The combination of radiation therapy with chemotherapy allows several possible sequences. Chemotherapy may be given first in hopes of reducing the size of the tumor, possibly enhancing oxygenation prior to irradiation, as well as addressing, from the beginning of treatment, possible dissemination of the tumor outside the radiation portal. Radiation may be given first, particularly for tumors in which the results of treatment with radiation alone are rather good, the tumor proliferation rate is low, and the advantages of adding the chemotherapy are uncertain. One argument against this sequence is that it delays the treatment of distant disease, and the delivery of drug to the site of the primary tumor may be impaired by postirradiation edema and/or fibrosis.

Simply from the standpoint of tumor cell killing, the concurrent application of radiation therapy and chemotherapy should be most effective because there is no delay in the start of either modality. If there are subpopulations of cells that have developed resistance to either modality, they are not given the opportunity to proliferate. If there are sensitizing effects of chemotherapy on radiation therapy or vice versa, these will be maximized. Unfortunately, all of these factors may also work to enhance the toxicity of the combined treatment to normal tissue, so a net clinical advantage cannot be assumed. However, the concept of organ preservation by combined modality treatment is increasing, with results that are sometimes equal to or better than traditional approaches (e.g., surgery). Example tumor sites include the anus (Nigro et al, 1989), the larynx (Wolf et al, 1991), and the bladder (Tester et al, 1996).

To avoid some of the toxicity of concurrent treatment approaches to chemoradiotherapy, several groups have devised schedules in which short courses of radiation therapy and chemotherapy are rapidly alternated. In this manner, the overall time required to complete both modalities is about the same as if they were given concurrently but patients do not receive both modalities on any given day. There are animal model systems in which such a rapid alternation of modalities gives results that are clearly superior to either sequential or concurrent treatment. Human studies in small cell carcinoma of the lung, high-grade lymphomas, and squamous cell carcinoma of the head and neck have established the feasibility of this approach, but randomized studies are required to determine any advantage over other treatment schedules.

EFFECTS OF RADIATION ON NORMAL TISSUES

All normal tissues studied can be shown to be affected by clinically relevant doses of radiation. The extent and significance of this reaction depend on several factors: tissue irradiated, volume of tissue (or percentage of the total organ volume) irradiated, radiation dose and fractionation, time since radiation, and whether or not other treatment modalities, such as surgery and/or chemotherapy, have also damaged tissue integrity.

Ionizing radiation possesses no inherent selectivity in its toxicity to tumor or normal tissue. Whatever difference in the effects to these tissues that is achieved in treatment occurs through targeting of the radiation to deliver a higher dose to the tumor than to surrounding tissues and through exploiting any differences in the proliferation kinetics of these tissues. It is impossible, however, to avoid all damage to normal tissue, and the sequelae of radiation

therapy have become well characterized in the decades of its clinical use.

Because radiation damage is expressed at the time of cell division, and cells in mitosis are inherently more radiosensitive than nondividing cells, radiation toxicity is seen first in rapidly dividing tissues such as bone marrow and gastrointestinal mucosa. These effects are typically seen during a course of radiation therapy. The rapid renewal of such systems, however, allows them to recover rapidly after completion of the course of treatment so long as the total radiation dose has not been excessive. More slowly proliferating normal tissues can express radiation damage, and severe damage to these tissues may not produce any symptoms during the course of treatment. This late normal tissue damage is produced both by direct cytotoxicity against the normal organ stem cells and by secondary changes resulting from radiation damage to vascular endothelial cells, leading to intimal hyperplasia and endarteritis. Fibrosis developing months after radiation is common after administration of doses of 45 Gy or more.

The delay in clinical expression of much normal tissue damage means that short-term toxicity cannot be used as a guide to a safe total radiation dose. Lack of toxicity during a course of treatment does not imply that the total dose may be safely increased. Conversely, brisk acute toxicity does not necessarily indicate a higher risk of severe late effects.

NEW DEVELOPMENTS AND RESEARCH DIRECTIONS

Clinical radiation treatment is currently a modality with real but limited success. It is most effective in treating patients with small tumors that have relatively few clonogenic cells in the primary tumor mass and are unlikely to have metastasized to remote sites outside the treatment volume. Although there are a small number of diseases that, by virtue of unusual intrinsic radiation sensitivity or low tumor burden at the time of diagnosis are curable in the majority of patients, many common malignancies are as yet poorly controlled with radiation therapy or progress in distant sites despite local tumor control. Research activities in radiation oncology are aimed at finding ways to enhance local control and to combine radiation therapy with systemic treatment methods to treat micrometastases before they become clinically evident.

Radiolabeled Immunoglobulins

We have so far discussed delivery of radiation therapy to a relatively large (by cellular dimensions) volume through radiation sources that are located far from the tumor cells. A very different approach is to deliver a radiation source in close proximity to the target cells, preferably in a manner that is selective for these as compared with normal tissues. One move in this direction has been the development of heterogeneous and/or monoclonal antibodies directed at determinants preferentially expressed on tumor cells. If a suitable radionuclide is stably attached to such an immunoglobulin or immunoglobulin fragment, this conjugate can be used to deliver a high dose of radiation to the tumor with considerable sparing of normal tissues. The relative sparing depends on the chemical stability of the conjugate, the clearance of the conjugate from various organs, the degree to which the antigen to which the antibody has been produced is preferentially expressed on tumor cells, and the avidity of the antibody. Many of these difficulties are being overcome, and this approach is now being evaluated in clinical trials for patients with several tumor types, including lung cancer and malignant lymphomas (Magerstadt, 1991).

Dose-Modifying Agents: Radiosensitizers and Radioprotectors

The observation that molecular oxygen was a potent cellular radiosensitizer and that tumors, even those of relatively small size, contain regions that are poorly vascularized and at low partial pressure of oxygen, have led to the hypothesis that a drug that mimicked oxygen's electron affinity and radiosensitization, but that could reach these poorly vascularized regions of the tumor in good concentration, could be a clinically useful radiation sensitizer. Over the past several decades, there has been extensive laboratory and clinical research in trying to identify such compounds, demonstrate their clinical efficacy, and optimally integrate their combination with radiation therapy. To date, the results of such efforts have not yielded as great success as had been hoped for a variety of reasons.

Most of the compounds that have been in extensive clinical trial to date have been electron-affinic nitroimidazoles, such as metronidazole, misonidazole, and etanidazole. They have had potencies as radiosensitizers (measured with a single radiation fraction) of a factor of 1.4 to 1.8 at maximally achievable concentrations, somewhat less than oxygen. They have also had significant toxicity, particularly peripheral neuropathy with the less polar of these, such as metronidazole, which has prevented their use with each fraction. Even with the newer sensitizers, such as etanidazole, which have been designed to be more hydrophilic and less neurotoxic, it has not been possible to give sensitizer with each daily treatment of a 30- to 35-fraction treatment course, so only about one third of the fractions are given with sensitizer.

The converse approach to selective radiation sensitization of tumor cells is selective protection of normal tissues. It has been known since the 1940s that certain compounds with free thiol groups, such as cystamine, were radioprotective of cells in vitro and

of whole organisms given total-body radiation. The most likely mechanism of this protection is scavenging of radiation-produced free radicals, preventing them from reacting with vital target molecules. Many simple thiol compounds will accomplish this but without any selectivity for normal tissues over tumor cells. Such nonselective radioprotection is of no more clinical use than nonselective radiation sensitization. A number of compounds have been developed, however, that appear to be preferentially accumulated in normal cells compared with tumor cells, possibly because of differences in cellular membrane transport. One of these compounds, WR2721, has been entered in clinical trials and has been shown to protect some but not all normal tissues. It is not an ideal drug for a number of reasons, primarily its cardiovascular toxicity, and more tolerable analogous compounds are being tested. It is also being investigated as a chemoprotective agent with high doses of cis-platinum and has shown some interesting results in this system.

Hyperthermia

There is a long history of interest in the use of elevated temperatures in the treatment of malignancy. Coley, in the early 1900s, reported treatment of patients with disseminated malignancies with a bacterial toxin preparation that induced high fevers. This has been claimed as a historic precedent for both hyperthermia and the use of biologic response modifiers. In subsequent years, there has been both a greater development of hyperthermic treatment and a clearer understanding of its mechanisms of action (Dewey, 1984). Most cells grow well within a rather narrow range of temperatures. Lower temperatures are reasonably well tolerated with slowing but with no irreversible interferences with processes of cellular maintenance and growth. Elevated temperatures are more damaging. For mammalian cells accustomed to grow at a temperature of 37°C, temperatures of even a few degrees higher will induce cell death in a time-dependent manner. If one plots the reciprocal of the time required for a given level of cell killing against the reciprocal of the temperature (an Arrhenius plot, used to determine the energy of activation, n, of a biochemical process), the resultant plot changes slope at approximately 42°C, suggesting that different mechanisms of action are operative above and below this temperature.

In addition to its direct cytotoxicity, elevated temperature can interfere with the ability of cells to repair radiation damage. Because, under normal conditions, the vast majority of cellular DNA damage is repaired, with lethality resulting from the few remaining unrepaired or misrepaired breaks, a small impairment of repair can result in a large difference in cell survival.

There does not appear to be a great difference in the intrinsic sensitivity to heat, either for direct cell killing or radiation sensitization, between most normal tissue and tumor cells. For a useful therapeutic gain to be achieved by combining radiation and hyperthermia, differences in the local environment of the cells appear to be important. To the extent that some regions of tumors are poorly perfused compared with normal tissues, they may be less able to dissipate heat applied by external heating by ultrasound or microwaves. Poorly vascularized hypoxic areas of the tumor may also have a lower pH, which will render them more sensitive to hyperthermic killing.

Altered Fractionation: Accelerated and Hyperfractionated Treatment

Skeptics have suggested that the clinical basis of radiation fractionation rests equally on the sciences of radiation biology and astronomy and that fractionation schedules are based more on the period of the earth's rotation on its axis than on anything having to do with cell kinetics. There may be some truth to this allegation. Although there is clear clinical evidence that fractionation is of great benefit, there is little evidence to suggest that giving five fractions per week at 24-hour intervals between the weekday fractions is a schedule designed to optimize more than patient, physician, and therapist convenience.

There has been considerable interest in exploring fractionation schedules that allow either a higher total tumor dose to be delivered or the administration of a relatively conventional total tumor dose in a shorter elapsed time (Peters and Ang, 1986). In the former approach, termed *hyperfractionation*, the size of each treatment fraction is reduced and two fractions are given each treatment day. With an interval of 6 hours between fractions, the majority of sublethal damage can be repaired. Because of the greater dose sparing of late tissues with reduction in fraction size, a higher total tumor dose is expected to be tolerated for a similar incidence of acute effects and tumor control. If one then increases the total dose to the maximum tolerated late complication level, the maximum local control should be achieved.

A different approach to fractionation has been explored for those tumors expected to have a high proliferation rate, in which it is advantageous to shorten the overall treatment time. In this *accelerated fractionation*, the fraction size is reduced only slightly from the usual 1.8 to 2.0 Gy range, typically to 1.5 to 1.6 Gy, two fractions given per day. The aim is to deliver a "standard" dose over a shortened period of time, reducing the amount of repopulation that can occur.

Three-Dimensional Treatment Planning/ Conformal Therapy

Although both tumors and their surrounding normal organs are three-dimensional structures, until recently treatment planning in three dimensions has not been possible. Plans were generally developed for a plane through the central axis of the treatment beams, which were coplanar. At best, several points of interest, typically dose-limiting structures such as the spinal cord, would have off-axis dose calculations performed.

With recent developments in three-dimensional imaging and computational speed, it is now feasible to perform true three-dimensional planning and to examine radiation dose distributions throughout a volume of tissue. This has also spurred interest in computer control of treatment machines so that the field angle, size, isocenter, and dose rate may be varied during the course of each daily treatment.

Three-dimensional treatment planning can now be done on essentially all tumor sites. Information from CT scans or MRI is directly input to the three-dimensional treatment software where target volumes and normal tissue volumes can be fully outlined in their position in three-dimensional space. Treatment plans are then designed through comparison of different combinations of multiple beams. With this "conformal" type of treatment, dose plans can be optimized in a way to maximize the dose to the tumor volume and minimize dose to normal structures. In order to reach the full potential of this technique, patient immobilization is critical. Once achieved, the therapeutic dose of radiation delivered can be increased (dose escalation) and the theoretical ability to sterilize an increased number of tumor cells and gain local control may be realized. Conformal therapy is increasingly being used in the clinic, and major academic centers are proceeding with large protocols involving dose escalation and evaluating for effectiveness and side effects of treatment. One particular area of widespread present interest is conformal therapy for prostate cancer. Another application of this technology is delivery of pinpoint radiation treatments to lesions in the brain. Patients are immobilized using a stereotactic head frame. Treatments are delivered either with a linear accelerator rotating through multiple arcs around the patients's head (stereotactic radiosurgery) or by carefully positioning the patient within a helmet that contains 201 small cobalt sources focused on a single isocenter (the Gamma Knife). Amazingly, these highly complex treatments are frequently done on an outpatient basis.

Intraoperative Radiation Therapy

With all the good work done in devising elegant and complicated—and, some claim, impractical—treatment plans for the external beam treatment of deep-seated tumors, the fact remains that adjacent organs will usually receive a dose not greatly dissimilar from that received by the target volume. If there were a way of physically separating, even for a time, the tumor volume and dose-limiting normal tissues, higher doses could safely be given to the target volume with a correspondingly increased probability of local tumor control. One direct approach to this problem has been with the use of intraoperative radiation therapy. At the time of surgical exploration, as much of the tumor as possible is resected. The remaining tumor, or tumor bed with presumed residual microscopic disease, is then irradiated with a direct radiation beam while adjacent local organs are held out of the radiation fields with retractors. To limit the depth of penetration of the radiation beam, orthovoltage x-rays or electrons are usually used for intraoperative treatment (Tepper et al, 1985).

The advantage of physical separation of the target volume and dose-limiting normal tissues is partially offset by the loss of the advantages of fractionation in intraoperative treatment. For this reason, most efforts in the United States have been directed to using intraoperative treatment for only a portion of the entire treatment course, as an additional dose (boost) to the gross tumor volume or tumor bed, while treating a larger volume with conventional fractionated external beam. Attempts are also being made to combine unfractionated intraoperative treatment with hypoxic cell sensitizers and/or chemotherapeutic agents to increase the therapeutic ratio.

Neutron and Other Particle Radiation

An interest in using forms of radiation other than x-rays and electrons has existed since the availability of generators of these particles in the 1930s. Hope-Stone conducted the first such trials, which indicated that even rather severely advanced tumors might respond well to neutron irradiation. He also observed severe late radiation effects in patients who were long-term survivors, a finding that, together with the rather primitive equipment available at the time, dampened enthusiasm for further research. In the 1950s and 1960s, developments in cell culture allowed a much better understanding of the radiation biology of neutron irradiation and suggested several ways in which it might show clinical superiority to photon treatment. These included a decreased dependence on oxygen for cell killing, decreased repair of sublethal and potentially lethal radiation damage, and less variation in cell killing with the position in the cell cycle (possibly as a reflection of less repair).

Dose distributions achievable with available neutron beams have been, at best, comparable to what can be achieved with low-energy photons. Any advantage of neutron treatment is thus due to radiobiologic rather than dosimetric superiority. Despite these limitations, there are indications that, for a few tumor types, particularly slowly proliferating salivary gland tumors, there may be clinical superiority for neutron treatment (Griffin, 1989).

There has been relatively little work on the use of external beam neutron therapy for patients with gynecologic malignancies. The relatively poor beam characteristics and resulting dose distributions for external beam treatment of the pelvis have been a discouragement to such efforts. Maruyama et al (1991) have explored the use of californium-251 (^{251}Cf) for intracavitary treatment of carcinoma of the cervix. The limited availability of this isotope and the problems associated with achieving adequate shielding from neutrons have delayed further trials of this modality.

Interestingly, there is now a greater interest developing with proton beam therapy, with recent increased clinical application and additional research advancing at centers that have this capability. The advantage of proton irradiation is the ability to accurately and precisely direct the beam onto the tumor. This improved dose localization, combined with a sharp dose fall-off and limited scatter, make this type of particle an interesting one for further exploration.

CONCLUSIONS

With properly defined treatment goals and expectations, radiation therapy is a valuable component in the treatment of patients with most malignancies. Radiation is highly effective in curing disease in patients who present with early-stage epithelial malignancies in most anatomic sites, as well as those with Hodgkin's disease and malignant lymphomas. In conjunction with surgery and chemotherapy, radiation therapy provides an intensification of local treatment for patients who are at high risk of local tumor recurrence following treatment with a single modality. For patients with metastatic disease, relatively brief courses of radiation therapy are highly effective in palliating such distressing symptoms as bleeding, pain of bone metastases, and neurologic deficits from central nervous system metastases.

Current progress in radiation oncology is directed along two main fronts. A better integration of newer imaging modalities such as CT and MRI, computer-controlled linear accelerators, and precise patient immobilization will allow better dose distributions and possible escalation of radiation dose delivered to the tumor without an increase in dose to normal tissues or complications. Similar improvements may be achieved by the use of moving sources in brachytherapy applications. A second approach is through a better understanding of the intrinsic radiation biology of tumor and normal tissues and the exploitation of small differences in their radiation sensitivity or through the modification of radiation sensitivity through tissue-selective radiation sensitizers or protectors. A combination of these approaches, along with improvements in the planned combination of local irradiation and systemic therapy, will, it is hoped, lead to further improvements in treatment effectiveness.

REFERENCES

Bellamy AS: Fundamental concepts associated with combining cytotoxic drugs and x-irradiation. In Hill BT, Bellamy AS (eds): Anti-tumor Drug-Radiation Interactions. Boca Raton, FL: CRC Press, 1990:1.

Dewey WC: Interaction of heat with radiation and chemotherapy. Cancer Res 1984;44:4714.

Fletcher GH: Indications for combination of irradiation and surgery. J Radiol Electrol 1976;57:379.

Fletcher GH: The association of irradiation with less-than-radical surgery in various types of cancer. Texas Med 1985;81:27.

Friedberg EC: DNA Repair. New York: WH Freeman, 1985:459.

Goffman TE, Raubitschek A, Mitchell JB, Glatstein E: The emerging biology of modern radiation oncology. Cancer Res 1990;50:7735.

Griffin TW: Status of clinical trials with neutron irradiation. Important Adv Oncol 1989:221.

Hall EJ: Radiation and Life. 2nd ed. New York: Pergamon Press, 1984:12.

Hall EJ: Radiobiology for the Radiologist. 4th ed. Philadelphia: JB Lippincott Company, 1994:91.

Holland JC, Marchini A, Tross S: An international survey of physician attitudes and practice in regard to revealing the diagnosis of cancer. Cancer Invest 1987;5:151.

Khan FM: The Physics of Radiation Therapy. 2nd ed. Baltimore: Williams & Wilkins, 1994:39.

Kramer S: Assessment of the patterns and quality of care in radiation therapy in the United States of America. In Karcher KH, Kogelnik HD, Reinartz G, et al (eds): Progress in Radio-oncology II. New York: Raven Press, 1982:3.

Krasin F, Wagner H Jr: Biological effects of ionizing radiation. In Webster JG (ed): Encyclopedia of Medical Devices. New York: John Wiley & Sons, 1988:260.

Magerstadt M: Antibody Conjugates and Malignant Disease. Boca Raton, FL: CRC Press, 1991.

Maruyama Y, Donaldson E, van Nagell JR, et al: Specimen findings and survival after preoperative ^{252}Cf neutron brachytherapy for stage II cervical carcinoma. Gynecol Oncol 1991;43:252.

Nigro ND, Vaitkevicus VK, Herskovic AM: Preservation of function in the treatment of cancer of the anus. Important Adv Oncol 1989:161.

Petereit D, Sarkaria J, Chappell R, et al: The adverse effect of treatment prolongation in cervical carcinoma. Int J Radiat Oncol Biol Phys 1995;32:1301.

Peters LJ: Inherent radiosensitivity of tumor and normal tissue cells as a predictor of human tumor response. Radiother Oncol 1990;17:177.

Peters LJ, Ang KA: Unconventional fractionation schemes in radiotherapy. Important Adv Cancer Ther 1986:269.

Peters LJ, Brock WA, Travis EL: Radiation biology at clinically relevant fractions. Important Adv Cancer Ther 1990:65.

Speiser BL: High dose rate brachytherapy. In: American Society for Therapeutic Radiology and Oncology Refresher Course No. 409, 1993:1.

Tester W, Caplan R, Heaney J, et al: Neoadjuvant combined modality program with selective organ preservation for invasive bladder cancer: results of Radiation Therapy Oncology Group Phase II Trial 8802. J Clin Oncol 1996;14:119.

Tepper JE, Wood WDC, Cohen AM, et al: Intraoperative radiation therapy. Important Adv Cancer Ther 1985:226.

Weichselbaum RR, Dahlberg W, Beckett M, et al: Radioresistant and repair-proficient human tumor cells may be associated with radiotherapy failure in head and neck cancer patients. Proc Natl Acad Sci U S A 1986;83:2684.

Wolf GT, Hong WK, Fisher SG, et al: Induction chemotherapy plus radiation compared with surgery plus radiation in patients with advanced laryngeal cancer. N Engl J Med 1991;324:1685.

Maurie Markman | # Chemotherapy

A t the turn of the century, Paul Ehrlick coined the term *chemotherapy* to refer to toxic substances he was examining as a treatment for syphilis. Thus began the search for drugs, or "magic bullets," that could cure illnesses as diverse as bacterial infection and malignancy.

The modern cancer chemotherapeutic area developed in the late 1940s, following the observation that certain agents being examined for their potential use in chemical warfare during World War II were effective in killing malignant cells in in vitro testing. Several of the earliest drugs examined ultimately were found to be useful agents in treating human malignancies. These included nitrogen mustard, a drug used today in the treatment of Hodgkin's disease, and aminopterin, and analog of the important cytotoxic agent methotrexate.

PRINCIPLES OF ANTINEOPLASTIC DRUG DEVELOPMENT (Schilsky et al, 1996)

As a group, cytotoxic chemotherapeutic agents are potent drugs with the potential to produce profound side effects. In general, the *therapeutic ratio* (i.e., relative anticipated benefit of a therapeutic strategy compared to its potential toxicity) is quite narrow. Therefore, it is important that any new agent undergo rigorous preclinical and clinical testing before it can be accepted as a standard treatment option in the management of human cancers.

The testing of new drugs or combination chemotherapy regimens follows a well-defined drug development pathway. If a pharmaceutical agent is demonstrated in preclinical testing to possess "promising" activity against human cancers, either in vitro or in vivo in animal tumors, Phase I clinical trials of the agent will be initiated.

It is the purpose of *Phase I trials* to examine the safety of the drug and learn about its pharmacokinetics (i.e., where the agent goes in the patient, how it is metabolized and/or eliminated from the body). Based on toxicity considerations, the initial patients entered on a Phase I trial of a new antineoplastic agent are treated at very low dose levels (as determined from data obtained during preclinical testing). If an acceptable degree of toxicity is observed, subsequent patients will receive higher doses of the

drug. This process is continued until "dose-limiting toxicity" (i.e., an unacceptable level of side effects) is encountered.

If the results of Phase I testing suggest both a favorable toxicity profile and at least limited evidence of an antineoplastic effect, further testing will likely be pursued. In *Phase II clinical trials*, patients with a single tumor type are generally treated at the "maximally tolerated dose" (determined in Phase I testing) to evaluate the efficacy of the new agent. Efficacy is usually defined in cancer chemotherapy trials as objective evidence of tumor shrinkage of a predetermined magnitude (e.g., 50% reduction in the size of a measurable tumor). In Phase II trials additional information regarding toxicity in a larger patient population is obtained.

If the results of Phase II testing indicate a major degree of antitumor activity, a randomized *Phase III trial* comparing the new agent to a previously defined standard drug or regimen might be indicated. It is only through the conduct of a randomized trial that the true therapeutic superiority of a new drug can be evaluated. In general, in the absence of such trials, it is not possible to know if even the most promising results in Phase II testing reflect an improvement in treatment or simply the selection of patients whose ultimate survival would have been favorable independent of the specific treatment program selected (e.g., younger age, superior medical condition prior to treatment, slower growing tumor). Evidence of clinical benefit for drugs obtained through the conduct of Phase III randomized trials is generally more favorably regarded than such evidence obtained in even multiple smaller Phase II (noncomparative) studies.

GENERAL PRINCIPLES OF CYTOTOXIC CHEMOTHERAPY (Haskell, 1995; DeVita et al, 1997)

The major defining characteristic of cancer is the failure of malignant cells to undergo normal regulation of growth. Although cancers may replicate rapidly, this is not a requirement for the presence of a malignancy, because many neoplasms actually exhibit rather slow growth, although this growth is uncontrolled by normal cellular regulatory mechanisms. The goal of administering cancer chemotherapeutic agents is to preferentially interfere with the replication and growth of malignant cells, compared to the effects of these agents on normal cell populations.

Both normal and malignant cells undergo five individual phases of development, during which specific metabolic activities occur. When a cell that is in the resting phase (G_0) starts to divide, it will enter the G_1 phase. Resting (G_0) cells are capable of performing all biochemical functions except cell reproduction. In G_1, RNA and other proteins necessary for cellular division are produced. During the next phase (S), DNA is synthesized. This phase is often the most sensitive to interruption by cytotoxic agents. With the completion of DNA synthesis, the cell enters G_2, during which RNA and other necessary proteins are synthesized for mitosis. Finally, in the mitotic phase (M), two daughter cells are created with identical genetic material.

The cell will then enter G_0 for a highly variable period of time, based on the tissue type (for normal cells) and the rate of tumor growth (for malignant cells). For example, normal white blood cells have a short survival in the circulation, measured in hours. Thus granulocyte precursor cells will have a relatively short doubling time. Normal tissues with little cellular turnover (e.g., liver) in the absence of injury to the organ will have a much lower cellular growth rate. (Because most chemotherapeutic agents are more effective against actively dividing cells, it should not be surprising that one of the major toxicities of cancer chemotherapy is *bone marrow suppression*, including the development of granulocytopenia, thrombocytopenia, and anemia.)

Similarly, well-differentiated tumors (i.e., maintenance of many of the morphologic appearances of the normal tissue of origin) generally have a slower growth rate, whereas poorly differentiated cancers, which maintain few, if any, normal regulatory pathways, exhibit more rapid growth and spread of cancer. In general, cancer chemotherapeutic agents are most effective in producing major tumor cell kill against cancers that have at least a moderately high growth fraction. Conversely, tumors with very slow growth rates are rarely favorably influenced by cytotoxic antineoplastic agents.

Cytotoxic drugs that are effective exclusively in cells actively undergoing the process of division are called *cell cycle specific* (e.g., inhibitors of mitosis), whereas drugs that can influence cellular functions independent of cell division are called *cell cycle nonspecific* (e.g., alkylating agents).

It is important to note that experimental and clinical observations indicate that the cell kill produced by cytotoxic chemotherapy follows *first-order kinetics*. This principle implies that a constant *fraction* rather than a constant number of cancer cells is killed per unit of time. Highly effective chemotherapeutic agents against a particular tumor type kill a higher percentage of cancer cells with each treatment. How-

ever, in general, multiple treatments will be required to eliminate all viable tumor.

Because the individual antineoplastic agents currently available for the treatment of malignant disease possess only limited potential to preferentially kill cancer cells, combination chemotherapy has become accepted as the standard therapeutic strategy for the treatment of most cancers for which cytotoxic agents are employed. It is hypothesized that the use of two (or more) drugs that produce their cytotoxic effects and develop resistance by different mechanisms will be more successful in erradicating the cancer, or at least prolonging disease-free and overall survival, compared to treatment with a single agent.

Resistance develops to cytotoxic agents by a variety of mechanisms. It is highly likely that cancer cells that are either inherently resistant to the currently available chemotherapeutic agents, or develop resistance following an initial response to therapy, have established several mechanisms to overcome the cytotoxic effects of the drugs.

Table 67–1 lists a number of resistance mechanisms that may be operative in gynecologic cancer patients with resistant tumors. One of the major research questions confronting basic cancer investigators is how to pharmacologically overcome resistance to chemotherapy without increasing the toxicity of treatment.

COMMON SIDE EFFECTS OF CHEMOTHERAPY

As previously noted, cytotoxic chemotherapeutic agents have the potential to be associated with the development of distressing and life-threatening toxicities. Physicians administering these drugs must be thoroughly familiar with both the expected and the rarer but more serious side effects of the treatment programs.

Bone Marrow Suppression

Bone marrow suppression is a common and potentially severe toxicity of cytotoxic chemotherapy. All marrow elements can be affected, although neutropenia is generally of greatest concern. Patients experiencing moderate degrees of bone marrow suppression (e.g., granulocyte nadir counts >1200/mm^3, platelet nadir counts >50,000/mm^3) are generally at low risk for serious complications of treatment. However, with granulocyte nadirs of less than 500/mm^3 and platelet nadirs of less than 20,000/mm^3, there is a major risk for infection and bleeding, respectively.

The development of any fever (>38°C) in a patient with a low granulocyte nadir count following chemotherapy (e.g., neutrophils <1000/mm^3) is a genuine medical emergency, and a broad-spectrum antibiotic(s) must be initiated as rapidly as possible to

Table 67-1. POTENTIAL MECHANISMS OF DRUG RESISTANCE AND AGENTS IN WHICH THESE PROCESSES HAVE BEEN OBSERVED

MECHANISM	AGENTS
Decreased drug transport into tumor cells	Methotrexate, melphalan
Increased drug transport out of cells	Vincristine, doxorubicin, etoposide
Reduced activation of drug	Methotrexate, 5-fluorouracil
Increased inactivation of drug	Cyclophosphamide, melphalan, ifosfamide
Increased DNA repair	Etoposide, cisplatin, cyclophosphamide, ifosfamide, doxorubicin
Use of alternative pathways as source of metabolites	Methotrexate, 5-fluorouracil
Gene amplification of enzyme target for action of drug	Methotrexate, 5-fluorouracil
Alteration of target to reduce drug binding	Vincristine, methotrexate, doxorubicin, etoposide

prevent the development of sepsis and subsequent endotoxic shock (Pizzo, 1993). In general, because fever is an excellent warning sign for the presence of infection, in the absence of fever, patients with severe granulocytopenia do not need to have antibiotics initiated.

In patients experiencing severe reductions in granulocyte counts (with or without the development of fever), subsequent treatment courses should either be administered at lower dose levels or with the use of a granulocyte stimulating factor (e.g., granulocyte colony-stimulating factor, granulocyte-macrophage colony-stimulating factor) to reduce the severity of bone marrow suppression. In general, unless there are data available to demonstrate that reductions in dose for a particular tumor type will be associated with an unfavorable influence on quality of life or ultimate survival, doses of chemotherapy should be reduced in subsequent courses in patients experiencing unacceptable degrees of bone marrow suppression.

Emesis

The nausea and vomiting induced by the delivery of cytotoxic chemotherapeutic agents are the side effects of cancer treatment most often associated by the public with the "horrors" of chemotherapy (Grunberg and Hesketh, 1993). Although many of the commonly employed cytotoxic agents produce minimal emesis, it is important to note that, even with agents capable of producing severe emesis, the currently available antiemetic drugs are highly effective in reducing both the incidence and severity of this side effect of treatment. This statement is true even for cisplatin, one of the most commonly utilized cytotoxic agents in the treatment of gynecologic malignancies, and one of the most emetogenic anticancer drugs.

At the present time the most frequently utilized and effective antiemetic agents belong to the class of drugs known as *serotonin receptor antagonists*. Two commercially available serotonin receptor antagonists are ondansetron (Zofran) and granisetron (Ky-

tril). These agents are generally administered with a corticosteroid (frequently dexamethasone), which has been shown in randomized trials to potentiate the antiemetic effects of the serotonin receptor antagonists.

Alopecia

Hair loss is a common complication of a number of cytotoxic chemotherapeutic agents, and is a particularly distressing side effect of treatment for females. Although certainly not a life-threatening toxicity of therapy, the emotional impact of hair loss can be extremely negative, particularly for individuals who have recently been informed they have a potentially fatal disease and must receive treatment with all the potential toxicities of cytotoxic chemotherapy.

However, it is extremely important to point out that, in essentially all circumstances, hair loss from chemotherapy is only temporary and excellent wigs are available. In addition, many insurance companies now pay for the costs associated with such wigs if indicated for hair loss caused by cancer chemotherapy. Unfortunately, although various methods have been advocated to prevent hair loss following chemotherapy, none has been shown to be effective and some can be quite uncomfortable (e.g., cooling the scalp during chemotherapy delivery). In addition, there is legitimate concern that any method that has the potential to prevent hair loss may actually interfere with the ability of the cytotoxic agent(s) to reach the hair follicles and, at least in theory, negatively influence the ability of the antineoplastic agents to kill circulating tumor cells.

Mucositis, Stomatitis, and Diarrhea

Several cytotoxic agents active in the treatment of gynecologic malignancies can kill rapidly dividing cells in the gastrointestinal tract. Although these symptoms are generally mild in severity, and completely reversible, they can be quite debilitating.

Dose reductions with subsequent treatments will usually result in fewer symptoms.

The development of mucositis, stomatitis, or diarrhea in the presence of nadir fever is a cause of concern because the loss of barrier function of the gastrointestinal mucosa can lead to the introduction of bacteria into the bloodstream and the development of sepsis. Patients in this clinical state must be carefully monitored and appropriate broad-spectrum antibiotics rapidly initiated at the first indication of fever.

Fatigue

Fatigue is one of the most common, although nonspecific, side effects of cytotoxic chemotherapy. It results from a number of factors, including recovery from surgery (commonly employed modality in the treatment of gynecologic cancers), anemia (from blood loss, cancer-associated anemia of chronic disease, and chemotherapy-associated bone marrow suppression), nutritional factors (partial or complete bowel obstruction, poor appetite secondary to disease or chemotherapy), muscle wasting, emotional distress, and disease progression. To the extent that fatigue is related to chemotherapy in an individual demonstrating a response to the therapeutic pro-

gram, the patient can be provided reasonable assurance the fatigue will substantially improve within several months of discontinuing chemotherapy.

CYTOTOXIC AGENTS EMPLOYED IN THE TREATMENT OF GYNECOLOGIC MALIGNANCIES

(Haskell, 1995; Krakoff, 1996; DeVita et al, 1997) (Table 67–2)

Alkylating Agents

Alkylating agents possess one or more reactive alkyl groups that are capable of forming ionized, highly reactive, positively charged intermediates that can covalently bond to a negatively charged (nucleophilic) group on a protein or nucleic acid. The drugs cross-link the strands of DNA, preventing DNA replication and the transcription of RNA. The major site of action is on the 7-N position of the nucleic acid guanine. The alkylating agents are not phase specific, although they exert their maximum cytotoxic potential in cells actively synthesizing DNA.

The most commonly used drugs in this class in the gynecologic malignancies include *cyclophosphamide* (used in the treatment of ovarian cancer and ges-

Table 67–2. POSSIBLE CHEMOTHERAPY PROGRAMS IN THE TREATMENT OF GYNECOLOGIC CANCERS

CANCER TYPE	CHEMOTHERAPY REGIMEN
Ovarian cancer (Cannistra, 1993; McGuire et al, 1996)	
Initial therapy	Cisplatin plus paclitaxel
	Carboplatin plus paclitaxel
Second-line therapy	Topotecan (single agent)
	Oral etoposide (single agent)
	Liposomal doxorubicin (single agent)
	Altretamine (single agent)
	Ifosfamide (single agent)
	Gemcitabine (single agent)
Endometrial cancer (Rose, 1996)	Cisplatin plus doxorubicin
	Cisplatin plus paclitaxel
	Carboplatin plus paclitaxel
	Doxorubicin plus paclitaxel
	Paclitaxel (single agent)
	Doxorubicin (single agent)
Cervical cancer (Vermorken, 1993) (squamous cell)	Cisplatin plus ifosfamide
	Cisplatin plus ifosfamide plus bleomycin
	Cisplatin (single agent)
	Carboplatin (single agent)
	Paclitaxel (single agent)
Germ cell tumors (Williams et al, 1994)	Cisplatin plus etoposide plus bleomycin
Gestational trophoblastic tumors (Berkowitz and Goldstein, 1996)	
"Low risk"	Methotrexate
	Actinomycin D
"High risk"	EMA-CO (etoposide, methotrexate, actinomycin D, cyclophosphamide, vincristine)

tational trophoblastic disease), *melphalan* (ovarian cancer), *chlorambucil* (ovarian cancer), and *ifosfamide* (sarcomas, germ cell tumors, cervix and endometrial cancers). Chlorambucil is administered orally, while both cyclophosphamide and melphalan can be delivered both orally and intravenously. Ifosfamide is only administered by the intravenous route.

Until relatively recently, several of the alkylating agents were commonly employed as first-line treatment of ovarian cancer, either as single agents (melphalan, chlorambucil) or in a combination chemotherapy regimen (e.g., cyclophosphamide plus cisplatin; cyclophosphamide plus carboplatin).

Ifosfamide is one of the two most active agents in the treatment of gynecologic sarcomas (the other being doxorubicin), is commonly employed in the BIP (bleomycin, ifosfamide, and cisplatin) regimen for cervix cancer, and is an active drug in the salvage therapy (second-line setting) in women with refractory germ cell tumors. Ifosfamide also has modest activity (10% to 15% response rate) in women with ovarian cancer who have failed initial platinum-based chemotherapy.

The major toxicity of all the alkylating agents is bone marrow suppression. This can involve all marrow elements, but most commonly influences the granulocyte series. Other common toxicities of the alkylating agents include emesis and alopecia.

Both cyclophosphamide and, more commonly, ifosfamide are associated with the development of a hemorrhagic cystitis. Mesna (2-mercapto-ethane sulfonate) is administered along with standard-dose levels of ifosfamide and high-dose cyclophosphamide regimens to inactivate the cytotoxic agents in the urinary tract and prevent this complication of therapy.

Ifosfamide can also be associated with the development of neurotoxicity, characterized by confusion, lethargy, and somnolence, which rarely can be fatal. This toxicity of treatment is more often observed in individuals with pre-existing renal insufficiency, poor performance status, a low serum albumin, or taking narcotic analgesia or sedatives at the time of delivery of this cytotoxic agent. Ifosfamide should be administered with great caution in individuals with any of these clinical characteristics.

Although not a classical alkylating agent, *altretamine* (hexamethylmelamine) is often considered with this class of cytotoxic drugs. Altretamine is administered orally and possesses modest activity in the treatment of platinum-refractory ovarian cancer. Its side effects include the development of emesis and a peripheral neuropathy.

Platinum Compounds

The platinum compounds have a mechanism of action similar to that of the alkylating agents in that they intercalate between DNA base pairs and sub-

sequently cause cross-linking of DNA nucleic acid strands.

Cisplatin, introduced into the clinic in the late 1970s, has proven itself to be one of the most active antineoplastic agents against gynecologic cancers. It has been the major drug in combination chemotherapy regimens in the treatment of ovarian cancer (Cannistra, 1993), and is the single most active cytotoxic agent in the treatment of advanced cervical cancer (Vermorken, 1993).

Cisplatin is also an important component of the curative chemotherapy program in ovarian germ cell tumors (along with etoposide and bleomycin) (Williams et al, 1994), and has been shown, in a randomized controlled Phase III trial, to add to the favorable effects of doxorubicin in the treatment of metastatic endometrial cancer.

In addition, in women with very-small-volume residual advanced ovarian cancer following initial surgical tumor cytoreduction, the use of cisplatin delivered by the intraperitoneal route has been shown in a randomized trial to improve both disease-free and overall survival, compared to intravenous delivery of the agent (Alberts et al, 1996). Because this study demonstrating the clinical utility of intraperitoneal cisplatin was conducted in women also receiving intravenous cyclophosphamide, it remains uncertain at present if this added benefit for regional drug delivery will also be observed in patients receiving paclitaxel (see later information regarding this drug) instead of the alkylating agent.

Unfortunately, despite its major clinical utility, cisplatin is one of the most toxic antineoplastic agents. Side effects include emesis (which can be severe), nephrotoxicity (elevated serum creatinine, renal magnesium, calcium and potassium wasting), neurotoxicity (peripheral neuropathy, hearing loss, tinnitus, visual disturbances), and hypersensitivity reactions (uncommon).

Vigorous hydration prior to, during, and following cisplatin administration has been shown to reduce substantially the potential for developing renal dysfunction, although magnesium wasting and hypomagnesemia remain common problems following therapy with this agent. It should also be noted that the risk of experiencing cisplatin-induced peripheral neuropathy increases with the total cumulative dose, significantly influencing the duration of treatment with this valuable antineoplastic drug.

Carboplatin was initially developed as a second platinum agent that would hopefully demonstrate activity in cisplatin-resistant cancers. Although clinical trials have demonstrated essentially complete cross-resistance between the two platinum drugs, carboplatin has been shown to be as active as the older drug in several clinical settings with a more favorable toxicity profile.

The major side effect of carboplatin is bone marrow suppression, with a much lower incidence of nephrotoxicity and neurotoxicity compared to cisplatin. Significant thrombocytopenia can be observed with carboplatin administration, especially following multiple treatment cycles.

Although emesis is common following carboplatin administration, its severity is generally less than that experienced with cisplatin. In particular, the development of severe delayed emesis (occurring more than 24 hours after cytotoxic drug delivery), a particularly troublesome side effect of cisplatin, is far less common with carboplatin.

Several randomized trials have revealed that carboplatin- and cisplatin-based combination chemotherapy regimens result in similar activity in advanced ovarian cancer (Alberts et al, 1992). Although definitive comparative trials have not been conducted in other gynecologic cancers, carboplatin has been employed in endometrial and cervix cancer in patients whose medical status precludes the use of the more toxic platinum agent.

In one gynecologic cancer the use of carboplatin should be avoided. Cisplatin is a major component of highly curative treatment of both female and male germ cell tumors. Data from randomized clinical trials have revealed that the substitution of carboplatin for cisplatin in *male* germ cell cancers results in an inferior clinical outcome. Although comparative trials have not been conducted in the less common female germ cell tumors, it is reasonable to conclude that carboplatin should not be substituted for cisplatin in this clinical situation unless use of the older platinum drug is contraindicated (e.g., presence of pre-existing renal insufficiency).

Mitotic Inhibitors

Cytotoxic agents in this class produce their effect by binding to microtubular proteins within cells, interfering with mitosis. There are several components of this complex process that have been successfully influenced to produce tumor cell kill. *Vincristine* and *vinblastine* cause metaphase arrest and disaggregation of the mitotic spindles. In contract, *paclitaxel* results in stabilization of the spindles with subsequent cell death. *Etoposide* inhibits topoisomerase II, a critically important enzyme in cell division.

Vincristine and vinblastine, the initial mitotic inhibitors in clinical practice, have limited current indications in the treatment of gynecologic malignancies. Vincristine is an important component of the EMA-CO regimen (etoposide, methotrexate, actinomycin D, cyclophosphamide, and vincristine), standard therapy for gestational trophoblastic tumors (Berkowitz and Goldstein, 1996). Vinblastine had previously been a component of the CVB (cisplatin, vinblastine, and bleomycin) program for the treatment of germ cell tumors, but *vinblastine* has been replaced with etoposide because of an improved toxicity profile. The major side effects of vincristine are the development of a peripheral neuropathy and constipation, while vinblastine's major toxicity is bone marrow suppression.

Etoposide is employed in the EMA-CO regimen (Berkowitz and Goldstein, 1996), as a major component of the BEP (bleomycin, etoposide, and cisplatin) program for germ cell tumors (Williams et al, 1994), and as a single agent in second-line treatment of refractory ovarian cancer. The major toxicity of etoposide treatment is bone marrow suppression and the development of hypersensitivity reactions.

It has been recognized that patients treated with high cumulative dose levels of etoposide experience a significant risk of developing secondary acute leukemia (Rustin et al, 1996). These data have led investigators to suggest that the total dose of etoposide delivered to patients with gynecologic and other cancers should be kept within an acceptable level to minimize the risk for developing this serious, and usually fatal, complication of therapy.

Clinical experience has revealed paclitaxel to be one of the most important antineoplastic agents in the management of malignant disease in general and gynecologic cancers in particular (Rowinsky and Donehower, 1995). The two-drug regimen of paclitaxel and cisplatin (or carboplatin) is considered the current standard treatment program for advanced ovarian cancer (McGuire et al, 1996).

Paclitaxel is also one of the most active agents in the treatment of endometrial cancer (Rose, 1996), and has activity in cervical cancer and germ cell tumors. Clinical trials are in progress to define the role of paclitaxel in the standard management of these gynecologic cancers, either as a single agent or in a combination chemotherapy program.

The major toxicity of paclitaxel is bone marrow suppression, the severity of which is related to both the dose and schedule of administration of the drug. Paclitaxel is also associated with a high incidence of hypersensitivity reactions. A three-drug regimen to prevent these reactions (including steroids plus histamine$_1$ and histamine$_2$ blocking agents) is administered prophylactally prior to all infusions of paclitaxel.

Additional side effects include alopecia (which can involve all body hair), arthralgias (which commonly develop 24 to 48 hours after treatment and last 3 to 5 days), peripheral neuropathy (which is dose related), and cardiac toxicity (uncommon).

Docetaxel, a cytotoxic agent closely related to paclitaxel, has been demonstrated to be an active agent in several human malignancies, including platinum-resistant ovarian cancer. This drug has a toxicity profile similar, although not identical, to that of paclitaxel.

Antimetabolites

Antimetabolites are structural analogs of normal metabolites essential for cell replication and growth. By incorporating into DNA or RNA, these drugs can block the production of enzymes necessary for synthesis of essential compounds. Antimetabolites are principally active in the synthetic phase of the cell cycle.

Methotrexate is the major antimetabolite used in the treatment of gynecologic malignancies. It is employed as a single agent in the treatment of "low-risk" gestational trophoblastic disease, and as an important component of the combination regimen EMA-CO for women with this malignancy at "high risk" (Berkowitz and Goldstein, 1996). *Leucovorin* (folinic acid) is frequently administered with higher dose regimens of methotrexate, beginning 24 hours after administration of the cytotoxic drug, to reduce the potential toxicity of this agent.

Side effects of methotrexate include bone marrow suppression, stomatitis, mucositis, hepatic fibrosis, and renal tubular necrosis.

5-Fluorouracil, one of the oldest cytotoxic agents, is rarely used in the treatment of gynecologic malignancies, although it has definite activity in cancers of the cervix and ovary. The combination of cisplatin and 5-fluorouracil may be used in the treatment of cervical cancer, particularly in association with radiation, because both agents have been suggested to potentiate the effects of this modality of treatment.

The potential side effects of 5-fluorouracil include diarrhea, stomatitis, bone marrow suppression, a characteristic skin rash, photosensitivity, and cerebellar ataxia (high-dose regimens).

Gemcitabine is a new chemotherapeutic agent in this therapeutic class, which has been shown in several series to be an active drug in platinum-refractory ovarian cancer.

Antibiotics

This class of cytotoxic agents was derived from microorganisms. Antibiotics affect the function or synthesis of nucleic acids.

Doxorubicin is one of the two most active single agents in the treatment of endometrial cancer (the other being paclitaxel) (Rose, 1996). Based on the results of a recently completed randomized trial, the "standard chemotherapy regimen" for this malignancy employs a combination of doxorubicin and cisplatin. Current trials are attempting to combine doxorubicin and paclitaxel in the treatment of advanced endometrial cancer.

Doxorubicin and ifosfamide are the major active agents in the treatment of gynecologic sarcomas. There is currently no evidence that combination therapy is superior to single-agent doxorubicin in the treatment of any gynecologic sarcoma.

Although doxorubicin is an active drug in ovarian cancer, it is not currently commonly employed as treatment of this malignancy. However, a meta-analysis of long-term follow-up of randomized trials comparing patients treated with or without doxorubicin has suggested a small survival benefit associated with the use of this agent (A'Hern and Gone, 1995). These data have stimulated renewed interest in a potential role for doxorubicin, or closely related drugs, in the treatment of cancer of the ovary.

The major side effects of doxorubicin include bone marrow suppression, alopecia, stomatitis and the development of a cumulative dose-related cardiomyopathy. Patient age, prior history of radiation to the chest or cardiac dysfunction, and concomitant use of cyclophosphamide appear to increase the risk for the development of serious doxorubicin-induced cardiac damage (Shan et al, 1996). The drug is also a vesicant and can cause severe tissue injury if accidentally infused subcutaneously.

A commercially available doxorubicin preparation contained within liposomes (Doxil) has been shown to be active in a small Phase II clinical trial in platinum-refractory ovarian cancer. This novel method of drug delivery has stimulated interest in examining this preparation as a component of initial therapy of ovarian cancer.

Mitoxantrone, a cytotoxic agent closely related to doxorubicin, had demonstrated only modest activity against ovarian cancer when delivered at conventional dose levels. However, the drug demonstrates the steepest dose-response curve against ovarian cancer cells in in vitro testing, and is one of the agents contained in a combination chemotherapy regimen being examined in a multi-institutional randomized trial conducted to determine the role of very-high-dose chemotherapy in the management of ovarian cancer.

Bleomycin is commonly employed along with cisplatin and ifosfamide in the treatment of metastatic cervix cancer (Murad et al, 1994), and is an integral component of the curative regimen for germ cell tumors, which also includes cisplatin and etoposide. In addition, the agent can be administered intrapleurally to control malignant pleural fluid reaccumulation.

Side effects of bleomycin include fever and chills, which can be quite severe; stomatitis; skin hyperpigmentation; and pulmonary fibrosis, which rarely can be fatal. All patients receiving bleomycin undergo pulmonary function testing. With evidence of a significant decrease in oxygen diffusion capacity, the agent is discontinued.

Actinomycin D may be used as an alternative single agent to methotrexate in the treatment of "low-risk" gestational trophoblastic tumors. Toxicities include the development of emesis and alopecia. Actinomycin D is also a vesicant and should be administered with great caution.

Camptothecin Derivatives

Camptothecin derivatives are a new class of pharmaceutical agents that establish covalent bonds with the critical enzyme topoisomerase I. This process, which occurs during single-strand DNA cleavage, causes an interruption of replication and eventual cell death.

Topotecan has been demonstrated to possess a level of activity similar to paclitaxel in the treatment of platinum-refractory ovary cancer. Clinical trials are in progress examining the use of this agent as a component of initial therapy in this malignancy. Bone marrow suppression is the major toxicity of topotecan.

There is less experience in the treatment of gynecologic malignancies with a second camptothecin derivative, *irinotecan*, but the drug appears to be active in cancers of both the cervix and ovary. The major side effect of irinotecan is diarrhea, which can be severe.

REFERENCES

A'Hern RP, Gone ME: Impact of doxorubicin on survival in advanced ovarian cancer. J Clin Oncol 1995;13:726.

Alberts DS, Green S, Hannigan EV, et al: Improved therapeutic index of carboplatin plus cyclophosphamide versus cisplatin plus cyclophosphamide: final report by the Southwest Oncology Group of a Phase III randomized trial in stages III and IV ovarian cancer. J Clin Oncol 1992;10:706.

Alberts DS, Liu JY, Hannigan EV, et al: Intraperitoneal cisplatin plus intravenous cyclophosphamide versus intravenous cisplatin plus intravenous cyclophosphamide for stage III ovarian cancer. N Engl J Med 1996;335:1950.

Berkowitz RS, Goldstein DP: Chorionic tumors. N Engl J Med 1996;335:1740.

Cannistra SA: Cancer of the ovary. N Engl J Med 1993;329:1550.

DeVita VT Jr, Hellman S, Rosenberg SA: Cancer: Principles and Practice of Oncology. 5th ed. Philadelphia: Lippincott-Raven, 1997.

Grunberg SM, Hesketh PJ: Control of chemotherapy-induced emesis. N Engl J Med 1993;329:1790.

Haskell CM: Cancer Treatment. 4th ed. Philadelphia: WB Saunders Company, 1995.

Krakoff IH: Systemic treatment of cancer. CA Cancer J Clin 1996; 46:134.

McGuire WP, Hoskins WJ, Brady MF: Cyclophosphamide compared with paclitaxel and cisplatin in patients with stage III and stage IV ovarian cancer. N Engl J Med 1996;334:1.

Murad AM, Triginelli SA, Ribalta JCL: Phase II trial of bleomycin, ifosfamide, and carboplatin in metastatic cervical cancer. J Clin Oncol 1994;12:55.

Pizzo PA: Management of fever in patients with cancer and treatment-induced neutropenia. N Engl J Med 1993;328:1323.

Rose PG: Endometrial carcinoma. N Engl J Med 1996;335:640.

Rowinsky EK, Donehower RC: Paclitaxel (Taxol). N Engl J Med 1995;332:1004.

Rustin GJS, Newlands ES, Lutz J-M, et al: Combination but not single-agent methotrexate chemotherapy for gestational trophoblastic tumors increases the incidence of second tumors. J Clin Oncol 1996;14:2769.

Schilsky RL, Milano GA, Ratain MJ (eds): Principles of Antineoplastic Drug Development and Pharmacology. New York: Marcel Dekker, 1996.

Shan K, Lincoff AM, Young JB: Anthracyclin-induced cardiotoxicity. Ann Intern Med 1996;125:47.

Vermorken JB: The role of chemotherapy in squamous cell carcinoma of the uterine cervix: a review. Int J Gynecol Cancer 1993;3:129.

Williams S, Blessing JA, Liao S-Y, et al: Adjuvant therapy of ovarian germ cell tumors with cisplatin, etoposide and bleomycin: a trial of the Gynecologic Oncology Group. J Clin Oncol 1994; 12:701.

68

Immunology and Immunotherapy in Gynecologic Oncology

Oliver Dorigo
Otoniel Martínez-Maza
Jonathan S. Berek

This chapter reviews the organization and regulation of the human immune system. A discussion of the immunologic mechanisms involved in the control of tumor growth and immunotherapy in gynecologic oncology follows.

ORGANIZATION AND REGULATION OF THE IMMUNE SYSTEM

The immune system plays an important role in maintaining organismal integrity in a hostile and complex environment that contains many infectious agents. Another function of the immune system is to respond to neoplastic growth. Several types of cells with different phenotypes and functional properties, whose activities and interactions are coordinated to respond to the host's environment and to regulate aberrant cell growth, are involved in immune responses.

It is clear that the immune system is essential in the defense of the host against invading pathogens. Individuals with primary or acquired forms of immune deficiency are rapidly overwhelmed by viral or microbial infection, including infections by opportunistic infectious agents that do not normally cause clinical disease in healthy individuals. The immune system also can respond to host cells that have undergone transformation to become neoplastic cells. However, the role of immune responses in controlling neoplastic growth is not totally clear. There is no doubt that many effective antitumor immune mechanisms exist, and these have been described in various study systems. However, the relative importance of immune responses in protecting the host from cancer, as described in the concept of immune surveillance, is still not clear (Benjamini et al, 1984). Although immune-deficient patients undoubtedly have a higher frequency of clinically apparent tumors, the tumors that develop in these patients tend to be lymphoproliferative, such as lymphoma, or unusual forms of cancer, such as Kaposi's sarcoma in the acquired immunodeficiency syndrome (AIDS) (Ziegler and Levy, 1985). In any case, it is clear that the immune system can respond to tumors in various ways and that these responses, whether natural or induced, can in some cases lead to tumor regression. Also, immunodiagnostic procedures, using antitumor marker antibodies, show great promise as diagnostic and/or prognostic tools.

Components of the Immune System

The cells of the human immune system can respond to antigens or molecules that are foreign to the organism. Some of these immune responses occur in an innate, or non–antigen-specific, manner, whereas other immune responses are adaptive, or antigen specific. Adaptive responses not only are specific for a given antigen but also result in the establishment of memory, allowing a more rapid and vigorous response to that same antigen in future encounters (Roitt, 1988; Roitt et al, 1989).

Adaptive, or specific, immune responses can be classified as *humoral* or *cellular* responses. Humoral responses refer to the production of antibodies. Antibodies are antigen-reactive, soluble molecules. Antibody molecules are bifunctional molecules that are composed of specific antigen-binding sites that react with foreign antigens, combined with a constant portion that directs the biologic activities of the antibody, such as the binding of antibody molecules to cells (e.g., phagocytes) or the activation of complement. Cellular immune responses are antigen-specific immune responses mediated directly by activated immune cells rather than by the production of antibodies. The distinction between humoral and cellular responses originates from the observation in experimental animal model systems that humoral immune function can be transferred by serum, whereas cellular immune function requires the transfer of cells. In nature, responses to antigens usually involve both humoral and cellular responses.

Several types of cells, including those from both the myeloid and lymphoid lineages, make up the immune system. Specific humoral and/or cellular immune responses to foreign antigens involve the coordinated action of populations of lymphocytes operating in concert with each other and with phagocytic cells (macrophages). These cellular interactions include both direct cognate interactions, involving cell-cell contact, and cellular interactions involving the secretion of, and response to, cytokines and lymphokines. Lymphoid cells are found in lymphoid tissues, such as lymph nodes or spleen, or in the peripheral circulation. The cells that make up the immune system originate from stem cells in the bone marrow.

B Lymphocytes and Antibodies

The cells that synthesize and secrete antibodies are B lymphocytes. Mature, antigen-responsive B cells develop from pre-B cells (committed B-cell progenitors) and differentiate to become plasma cells, which are cells that produce large quantities of antibodies. Pre-B cells originate from bone marrow—stem cells in adults. After these cells become committed to the B-cell lineage, an event that is associated with the rearrangement of immunoglobulin genes from their germ cell configuration to that seen in B cells, they become pre-B cells. Pre-B cells contain intracellular immunoglobulin heavy-chain molecules but do not express cell-surface immunoglobulin. Mature B cells express cell-surface immunoglobulin molecules, which these cells use as their receptors for antigen. Mature B cells can respond to antigen to become antibody-producing cells in the presence of antigenic stimulus and the appropriate cell-cell interactions.

Antibody molecules are composed of two types of polypeptide chains: heavy chains and light chains (Nisonoff, 1982; Roitt, 1988; Roitt et al, 1989). Each B cell produces antibodies specific for a given antigen, made up of two identical heavy chains and two identical light chains. Immunoglobulin genes, which are rearranged during B-cell maturation, yield a functional immunoglobulin heavy-chain or light-chain gene. Immunoglobulins are found in solution in serum and body fluids and secretions and on the surface of mature B cells, where they function as the receptor for antigen.

There are five classes of immunoglobulins (Igs): IgG, IgA, IgM, IgD, and IgE. Immunoglobulin class is determined by the characteristics of the constant portions of the heavy-chain molecule. These classes correspond to gamma, alpha, mu, delta, and epsilon heavy-chain types, respectively. There are two classes of light chain—kappa and lambda—and either of these types of light chain can associate with any of five types of heavy chains to form a complete immunoglobulin molecule. A given immunoglobulin molecule, however, contains only one type of heavy chain and one type of light chain. Different antibodies of a given class share similar biologic properties

(e.g., binding to cell surface Fc receptors, or complement activation), albeit with different antigen-binding properties.

IgG, which is the major class of immunoglobulin found in human serum, makes up approximately 70% of total serum immunoglobulin. IgG is the predominant form of antibody produced in secondary immune responses, and it is the only class of immunoglobulin that crosses the placenta, and therefore is important in the transfer of passive immunity to the newborn.

IgA makes up about 20% of total serum immunoglobulin. IgA is the predominant form of immunoglobulin found in seromucous secretions, including saliva, milk colostrum, and genitourinary secretions. Secretory IgA exists primarily in dimeric form (two complete antibody molecules plus a joining [J] chain and one secretory component), whereas most serum IgA is monomeric.

IgM represents about 10% of total serum immunoglobulin. It has a pentameric structure, composed of five complete antibody molecules and one J chain. Because of its very large size, IgM is restricted to the intravascular pool. IgM is the predominant antibody type produced early in humoral immune responses and is the most efficient class of immunoglobulin in activating complement.

IgD accounts for less than 1% of total serum immunoglobulin but is found in relatively larger quantities on the surface of B cells. The precise biologic role of IgD is not defined. However, it may play a role in the process by which antigen triggers the activation of B lymphocytes. *IgE* is found in extremely low levels in serum. This antibody class is associated with immediate hypersensitivity and infection with parasites.

T Lymphocytes and Cellular Immunity

T lymphocytes are one of the cells types that mediate cellular immunity. T cells also play a central role in the generation of immune responses by acting as helper cells in both humoral and cellular immune responses (Figs. 68–1 through 68–3). T-cell precursors originate in bone marrow and home to the thymus, where they mature into functional T cells. During this thymic maturation, T cells learn to recognize antigen in the context of the major histocompatibility type of the individual. Also, it appears that T cells with the capability of responding to self can be removed during thymic development.

T cells can be distinguished from other types of lymphocytes by their cell surface phenotype (the pattern of expression of various molecules on the cell surface) as well as by differences in their biologic functions. All mature T cells express certain cell surface molecules. These include the CD3 molecular complex (Kan et al, 1983) and the T-cell antigen receptor (Ti) (Hedrick et al, 1984; Williams, 1984; Yanagi et al, 1984; Hood et al, 1985; Marx, 1985), which is found in close association with the CD3 complex

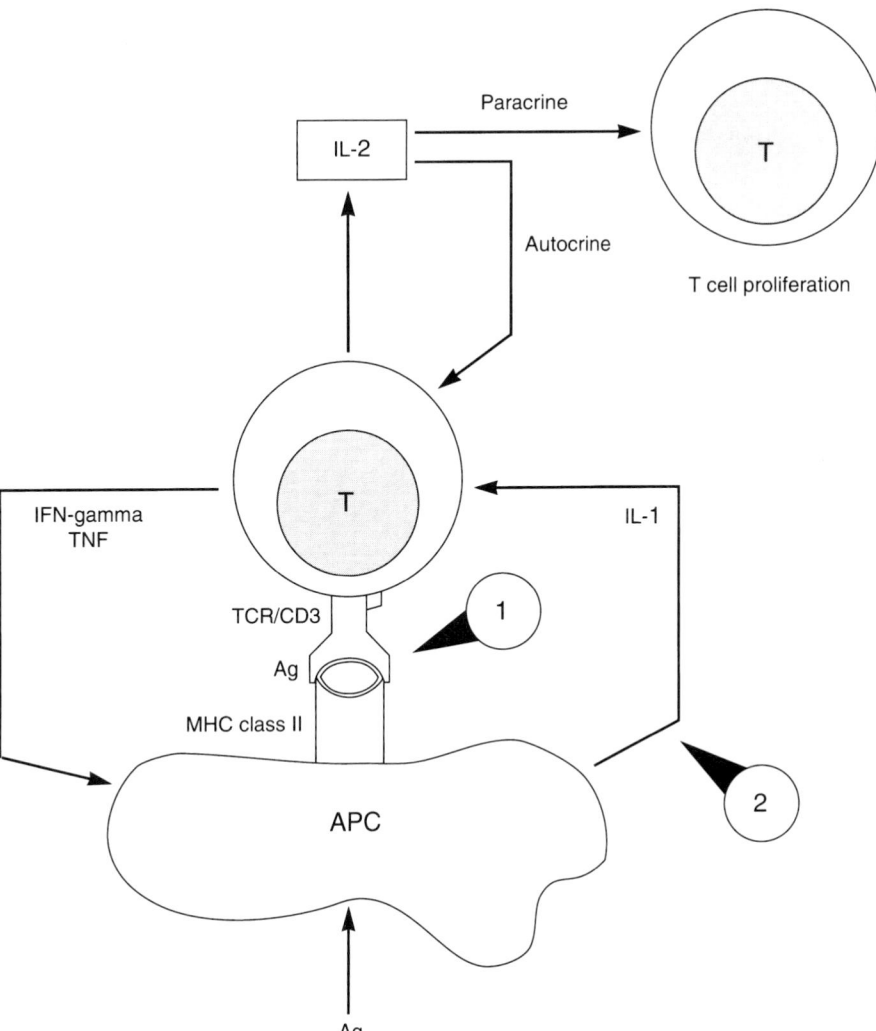

Figure 68–1
Antigen (Ag) presentation and T cell activation. T-cell activation requires two signals: (1) presentation of processed antigen by an antigen-presenting cell (APC), in the context of self major histocompatibility complex (MHC) class II molecules, and (2) a co-stimulatory signal (in this case provided by interleukin-1 [IL-1] secreted by the APC). Following this, the activated T cell secretes interleukin-2 (IL-2), which can act as an autocrine and/or paracrine growth factor, inducing T-cell proliferation. IFN-gamma, interferon-γ; TCR, T-cell receptor; TNF, tumor necrosis factor.

(Figs. 68–1 through 68–3). The expression of these cell surface molecules can be quantified using monoclonal antibodies specific for these molecules. The availability of monoclonal antibody reagents specific for such markers has led to great progress in understanding the organization of the immune system in recent years. Certainly, such monoclonal antibodies are of great value in understanding the clinical immunology of immune-deficiency disorders and in following the effects of experimental treatment, with biologic response modifiers or cytokines, on the human immune system.

T cells recognize antigen via the cell surface T-cell antigen receptor (Williams, 1984; Hood et al, 1985; Marx, 1985). In terms of its structure and molecular organization, this molecule is similar to antibody molecules, which are the B-cell receptor for antigen. The T-cell receptor gene undergoes gene arrangements during T-cell development similar to those seen in B cells (Hood et al, 1985; Marx, 1985; Roitt, 1988; Roitt et al, 1989). However, there are important differences between the antigen receptors on B cells and T cells. For instance, the T-cell receptor is not secreted, and its structure is different from that of

antibody molecules in some ways. Also, the way in which the B-cell and T-cell receptors interact with antigens is quite different.

There are two major subsets of mature T cells, which are phenotypically and functionally distinct: T helper/inducer cells, which express the CD4 cell-surface marker, and T suppressor/cytotoxic cells, which express the CD8 marker (Kotzin et al, 1981). The expression of these markers is acquired during the passage of T cells through the thymus. CD4 T cells can provide help to B cells, resulting in the production of antibodies by B cells. Also, CD4 T cells can act as helper cells for other T cells. CD8 T cells include cells that are cytotoxic (cells that can kill target cells bearing appropriate antigens). The CD8 T-cell subset also contains suppressor T cells. Suppressor T cells are cells that can inhibit the biologic functions of B cells or other T cells.

Natural Killer Cells

A third major population of lymphocytes includes natural killer (NK) cells. NK cells do not consistently bear cell surface markers characteristic of T or B

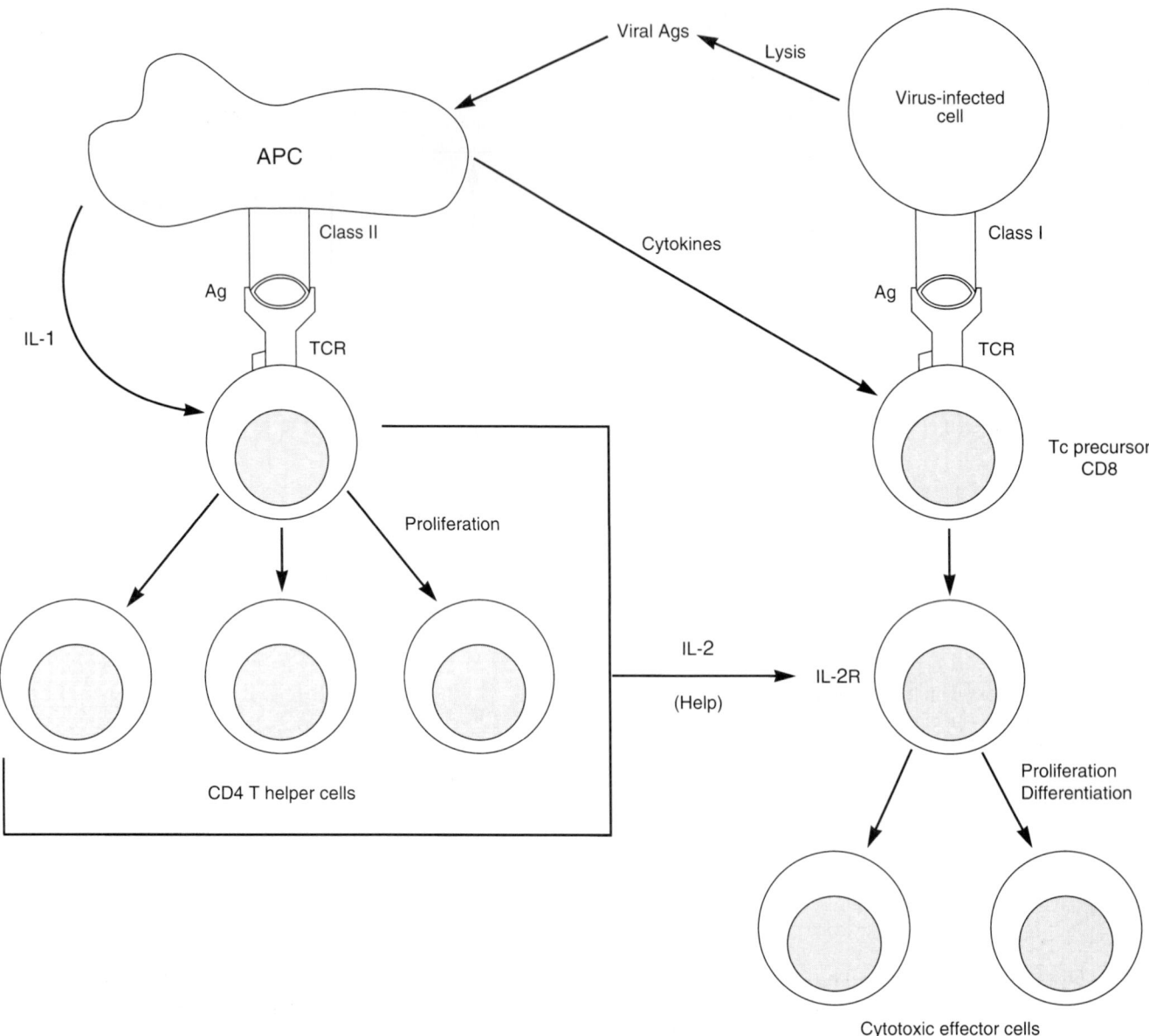

Figure 68–2

Cytotoxic T-cell responses. Cytotoxic T cells (CD8+) most often "see" antigen (Ag) in association with major histocompatibility complex class I molecules, expressed on the surface of the target cell. Helper T cells (CD4+), activated by antigen presented by antigen-presenting cells (APCs), enhance cytotoxic T-cell responses by secreting interleukin-2 (IL-2). This results in the proliferation and expansion of cytotoxic effector cells. IL-1, interleukin-1; IL-2R, interleukin-2 receptor. TCR, T-cell receptor.

cells, although they can share certain cell surface molecules with other types of lymphocytes. NK-type cells have in the past been called null cells, or third-population cells. NK cells characteristically have a large granular lymphocyte morphology (Ortaldo and Herberman, 1984). The NK cells are effector cells in an innate type of immune response: the nonspecific killing of tumor cells and/or virus-infected cells. Also, some reports indicate that NK cells may have a role in the regulation of some immune responses. Although NK cells can express certain cell surface receptors, particularly a receptor for the Fc portion

of antibodies, and other NK-associated markers, it appears that cells with NK function are phenotypically heterogeneous, at least when compared with T or B cells. The cells that can carry out antibody-dependent cellular cytotoxicity (ADCC), or antibody-targeted cytotoxicity, appear to be NK-like cells.

Monocytes and Macrophages

Monocytes and macrophages, which are myeloid cells, play important roles in both innate and adaptive immune responses. In fact, macrophages can

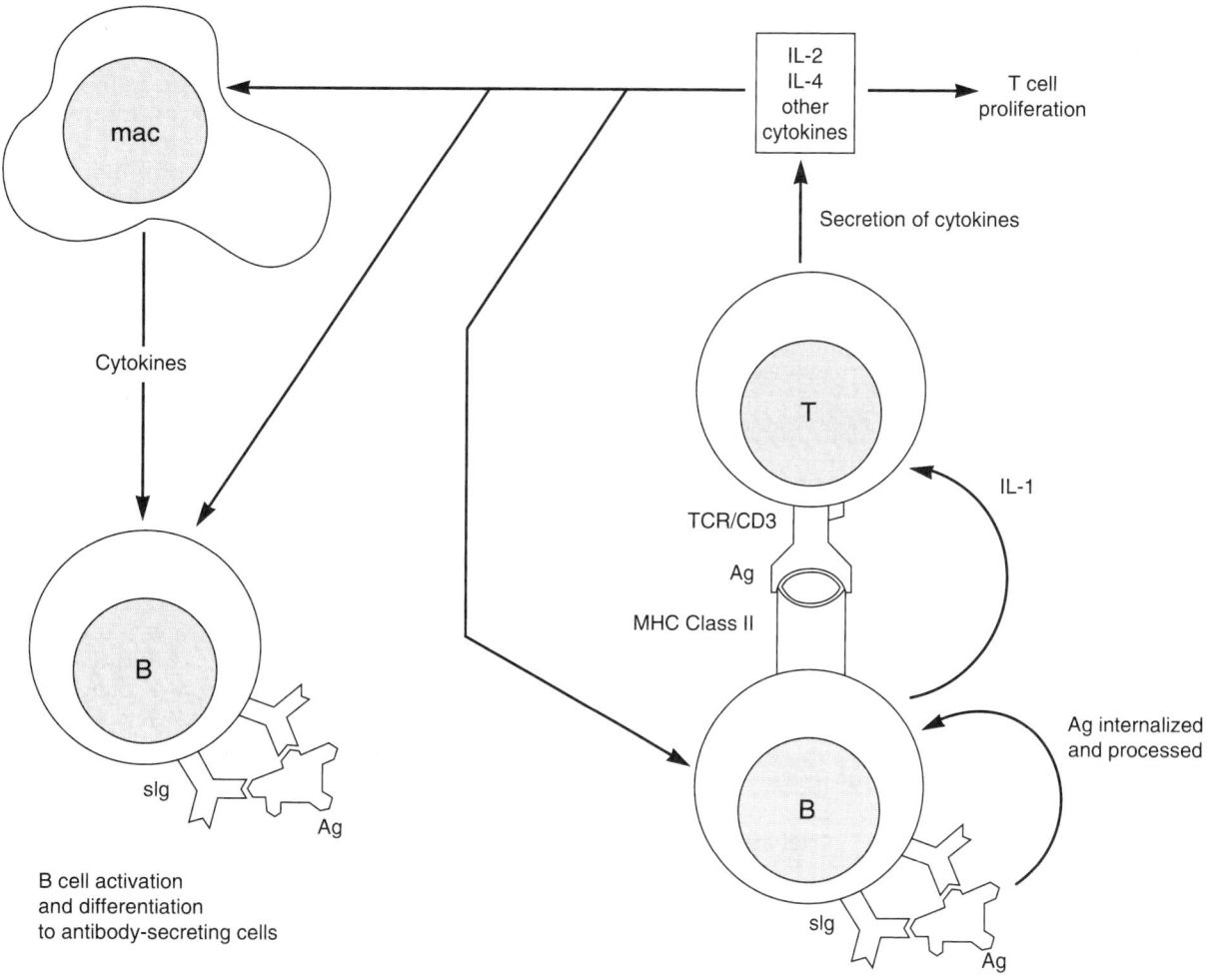

Figure 68–3

Cytokines and B-cell activation and differentiation. B cells can act as antigen-presenting cells (APCs). B cells use immunoglobulin as their cell-surface antigen receptor and can present antigen to T cells in association with major histocompatibility complex (MHC) class II molecules. On interaction with antigen (Ag) and in the presence of various cytokines, B cells are activated, proliferate, and differentiate to immunoglobulin-secreting cells. T-helper cells, which have recognized processed antigen on the surface of APCs, provide help to B cells by secreting cytokines. This can result both in enhanced antigen-presenting ability and in immunoglobulin production. Monocytes and macrophages (mac) also produce cytokines that enhance B-cell differentiation. IL-1, interleukin-1; IL-2, interleukin-2; IL-4, interleukin-4; sig, signal; TCR, T-cell receptor.

play a key role in the generation of immune receptors. T cells do not respond to foreign antigens unless these antigens are processed and presented by antigen-presenting cells. Macrophages (and B cells) can serve as antigen-presenting cells (Lanzavecchia, 1985; Chestnut and Grey, 1986; Unanue and Allen, 1987). After being processed, antigen is presented to T cells in an appropriate form on the surface of macrophages. Helper/inducer (CD4) T cells, bearing a T-cell receptor of appropriate antigen and self specificity, are activated by this antigen-presenting cell to provide help (various factors—lymphokines—that induce the activation of other lymphocytes). In addition to their role as antigen-presenting cells, macrophages can play an important role in innate responses by ingesting and killing microorganisms or

by becoming activated to become cytotoxic for tumor cells.

Dendritic Cells

Dendritic cells (DCs) were first identified in 1973 as a cell population in murine spleens (Steinman and Cohn, 1973). These cells were found to be morphologically and functionally different from monocytes and macrophages. They lacked most of the lineage-associated surface antigens of monocytes/macrophages or lymphocytes but expressed major histocompatibility complex (MHC) class I and class II molecules at high density. Human interstitial DCs were first described by Hart and Fabre in 1981. They are found in a variety of tissues, such as skin (Langerhans' cells), thymus, blood, lymph nodes, and parenchymatous organs such as the liver, kidney, and pancreas, with the exception of brain and central cornea (Daar et al, 1983; Hart et al, 1989). DCs show abundant expression of human leukocyte antigen (HLA) locus products. They express the leukocyte common (CD45) antigen and are therefore most likely hematopoietic cells derived from the bone marrow.

The most important identifying feature of DCs is their powerful ability to stimulate naive or primary T-lymphocyte proliferation (Young et al, 1990). DCs have been shown to exhibit between 10 and 100 times more potent allostimulatory activity than other cell populations and were found to induce significant T-cell proliferation at stimulator-responder ratios as low as 1:100. DCs can elicit both CD4+ and CD8+ T-cell responses (Young et al, 1990). In order to function as efficient antigen-presenting cells, DCs acquire antigen, process it into antigenic fragments by proteolysis in lysosomes; present this processed fragment, in conjunction with MHC class I and MHC class II molecules, to T lymphocytes; and provide co-stimulatory signals to the T cells.

DCs have been used to present specific tumor-associated antigen and induce efficient antitumor responses in vivo (Flamand et al, 1994). This approach is most effective when tumor-specific antigens are used. In ovarian cancer, a variety of tumor-associated antigens are potential candidates for this immune stimulatory approach, including CA125, HER/2-neu (p185), EGFR (p170), and MDR1 (gp170) (Kuiper et al, 1995).

Major Histocompatibility Complex

MHC molecules are a family of genetically polymorphic molecules, originally described as antigens involved in graft rejection after tissue transplantation (hence the term *histocompatibility antigens*). MHC molecules now are known to play a central role in immunoregulation (Auffray and Strominger, 1986).

The MHC gene complex, which in humans is found on chromosome 6, contains several individual genes. There are three general classes of MHC products, based on structural and functional similarities. Class I MHC proteins are composed of two polypeptides, only one of which is encoded by a gene within the MHC. The other molecule that associates with the MHC-encoded product to form a class I molecule is β_2-microglobulin. In humans, MHC class I molecules are termed *human leukocyte antigen-A* (HLA-A) and HLA-B region products. Class II MHC molecules are made up of two different peptides, an alpha chain and a beta chain, both of which are encoded by genes within the MHC gene locus. In humans, MHC class II molecules are called *HLA-D molecules*. Class III molecules include *complement* components encoded by genes within the MHC.

MHC class I molecules are expressed nearly ubiquitously; most nucleated cells express MHC class I antigens. MHC class II antigens have a much more restricted tissue distribution, and MHC class III molecules are expressed primarily on cells of the immune system: B cells, macrophages, monocytes, and activated T cells. Interestingly, certain HLA types are associated with increased susceptibility to various diseases.

Cytokines, Lymphokines, and Immune Mediators

Many events in the generation of immune responses that involve cellular proliferation and/or differentiation appear to require, or to be enhanced by, a variety of soluble mediators, or cytokines (Roitt, 1988; Roitt et al, 1989). These cytokines tend to have multiple biologic functions, depending on the target cell type or the maturational status of the target cell. *Lymphokines* are cytokines produced by lymphocytes. *Interleukins* are cytokines that exert their actions among leukocytes. *Interferons* are cytokines that have antiviral effects. *Monokines* are cytokines produced by monocytes and macrophages. These agents, which are produced by a wide variety of cell types, seem to play important roles in many biologic responses. Also, they may be involved in the pathophysiology of a wide range of diseases and are potentially exploitable as therapeutic agents.

Cytokines are a heterogeneous group of proteins, and they share few specific characteristics. However, although heterogeneous, cytokines do share some characteristics. For instance, most cytokines are low-molecular-weight to intermediate-molecular-weight (10 to 60 kDa) glycosylated secreted proteins. Also, cytokines are involved in immunity and inflammation, are produced transiently and locally (they do not act in an endocrine manner), are extremely potent, and interact with high-affinity cellular receptors. The cell-surface binding of cytokines by specific receptors ultimately leads to a change in the cellular proliferation and/or in the pattern of RNA and protein synthesis, resulting in altered cell behavior.

Various cytokines are involved in the regulation of immune responses. Many lymphokines and cytokines active on, or produced by, the cells of the immune system have been described and cloned, including several interleukins (ILs), interferons (IFNs), colony-stimulating factors, and lymphotoxin and tumor necrosis factor (TNF).

INTERLEUKINS

IL-1 constitutes several polypeptides with a wide range of biologic activities, including direct effects on several cells involved in immune responses (Di Giovine and Duff, 1990). IL-1 plays important roles as a mediator of host innate and adaptive immune responses. Also, IL-1 is involved in fever and inflammatory responses and may be involved in the pathogenesis of several diseases, such as rheumatoid arthritis and immune complex glomerulonephritis (Smith, 1984; Strober and James, 1988).

There are two defined forms of IL-1: IL-1-α and IL-1-β. Although these molecules have similar biologic functions, IL-1-α and IL-1-β show only distant (about 25%) amino acid homology. However, certain overall structural features are shared. Both forms of IL-1 are synthesized as a 31-kDa propeptide and cleaved to produce a 17-kDa mature form of IL-1, which is a stable globular protein. The overall structure of the IL-1-α and IL-1-β genes also is strikingly similar, with seven exons (six exons containing coding regions), suggesting their evolution from a common ancestral gene. Both forms of IL-1 bind to the same cellular receptor with similar binding affinities. Also, the bioactive portions of both forms of IL-1 map to the C-terminal half of their precursor propeptides. IL-1 can be released as a soluble form or can be found as a cell-associated molecule on the cell surface of macrophages. All cell-associated IL-1 remains in the propeptide form. Most IL-1-α remains cell associated, whereas most IL-1-β is released.

The primary sources of IL-1 production are macrophages, the phagocytic cells of the liver and spleen, some B cells, epithelial cells, certain brain cells, and the cells lining the synovial spaces. IL-1 has a broad range of target cells and biologic activities, as do most lymphokines. In addition to its effects as a lymphocyte-activating factor, IL-1 can induce fever, is highly inflammatory (IL-1 increases the concentrations of arachidonic acid pathway metabolites), can induce the production of acute-phase reactants by hepatocytes (probably indirectly by stimulating IL-6 production), can induce proliferative responses in a variety of tissues, and can cause the resorption of cartilage and bone.

IL-2 is a lymphokine that was originally called T-cell growth factor, which indicates one of the major biologic activities of this molecule (Grimm et al, 1983). Failure of T cells to produce IL-2 (and helper T cells do most of this production) results in the absence of a T-cell immune response and a diminution of the antibody response. Natural human IL-2 is a glycoprotein with a molecular weight of about 15 kDa and is encoded by a single gene consisting of four exons. IL-2 is produced primarily by activated T cells.

In order for IL-2 to exert its proliferation-inducing effects, it has to interact with a specific receptor on the surface of the target cell; this molecule is termed the IL-2 receptor and consists of two polypeptides: the alpha (75-kDa) and beta (55-kDa) chains (de Totero et al, 1995). The beta chain alone is a low-affinity receptor for IL-2, which is not effective at driving T-cell growth in the presence of IL-2. The alpha chain alone is an IL-2 receptor with intermediate affinity, which can result in cellular activation in the presence of very high concentrations of IL-2 (Greene et al, 1986). Resting T cells have relatively small numbers of alpha chains and no beta chains on their surface. Following activation, activated T cells express greatly increased numbers of beta chains and increased numbers of alpha chains. The heterodimer of alpha and beta chains is a high-affinity receptor for IL-2, the expression of which is required for driving T-cell growth.

IL-3 is a factor involved in the early differentiation of hematopoietic cells (Shrader, 1986). Various cytokines are involved in the process of B-cell activation and development from resting B cells to immunoglobulin-secreting plasma cells, including IL-1 and IL-2. However, several cytokines were originally described as unique B-cell–stimulating factors, distinct from IL-1 or IL-2. These include the lymphokines that are now called IL-4, IL-5, and IL-6. After further study, it became clear that these cytokines are not exclusively involved in the process of B-cell activation and differentiation and that they have a wider range of biologic activities, with biologic effects extending outside of the immune system. The most intensively studied of these factors have been IL-4 and IL-6.

IL-4 is a 15- to 20-kDa factor that acts as a proliferation-inducing factor for B cells (Snapper et al, 1988). Because IL-4 can play a role in inducing cytotoxic T cells; can act as a growth factor for T cells, thymocytes, and mast cells; and can activate macrophages and hematopoietic progenitor cells, its biologic effects are clearly not restricted to B cells. IL-4 is produced primarily by T cells.

IL-5 is a 45- to 60-kDa factor that can act as a proliferation-inducing and differentiation-inducing factor for B cells. Also, IL-5 can induce the differentiation of eosinophils (Sanderson, 1988). IL-5 is produced by T cells and is able to enhance IL-2–mediated lymphokine-activated killer (LAK) activity (Aoki et al, 1989).

IL-6 is a 20- to 25-kDa factor that can induce B-cell differentiation to immunoglobulin-secreting cells. However, IL-6 is a pleiotropic factor, with a wide range of biologic activities (Wong et al, 1988a). These include the induction of thymocyte proliferation and the induction of the production of acute-phase reactants by hepatocytes. Also, IL-6 has activity as a colony-stimulating factor for hematopoietic progenitor cells (Wong et al, 1988b). IL-6 is produced primarily by activated monocytes and macrophages, although T and B cells can produce this lymphokine. Interestingly, several types of tumor cells produce IL-6, and IL-6 has been proposed to act as an autocrine growth factor for different types of neoplasms.

IL-7 can stimulate the proliferation of progenitor B cells, thymocytes, T-cell progenitors, and mature CD4+ and CD8+ T cells. IL-7 can induce the formation of LAK cells as well as the development of cytotoxic T lymphocytes. It can up-regulate the production of proinflammatory cytokines and stimulate the tumoricidal activity of monocytes and macrophages. IL-7 is expressed by adherent stromal cells from various tissues. IL-7 bioactivities are mediated by the binding of IL-7 to functional high-affinity receptor complexes. Furthermore, the gamma chain of the IL-2 receptor complex has been shown to be an essential component for IL-7 signal transduction. Both IL-7 receptor (IL-7 R) and IL-2 R gamma are members of the hematopoietin receptor superfamily. Cells known to express IL-7 receptors include pre-B cells, T cells, and bone marrow cells.

IL-8 is a T-cell activating factor and has chemotactic effects on neutrophils, monocytes, and granulocytes. A variety of hematopoietic and mesenchymal cells as well as various tumor cell lines can produce IL-8 in response to a wide variety of proinflammatory stimuli such as exposure to IL-1, TNF, lipopolysaccharide, and viruses. Additional effects of IL-8 include degranulation of neutrophil granules, induction of expression of the cell adhesion molecules, and promotion of adherence of neutrophils to endothelial cells.

IL-9 is produced by human T-lymphotrophic virus type I– or type II–transformed T-cell lines, activated human peripheral blood lymphocytes, and Hodgkin and Reed-Sternberg cells, suggesting a possible role for IL-9 in the development of the pathophysiology of Hodgkin's disease (Renauld, 1995). IL-9 is capable of enhancing in vitro survival of human T-cell lines and supports erythroid colony formation. The specific high-affinity functional IL-9 receptor complex has been found to contain the IL-2 R gamma chains as well as an IL-9 receptor (IL-9 R) that is a member of the hematopoietin receptor superfamily (Houssiau et al, 1995). Cells known to express IL-9 R include T cells, neutrophils, mast cells, and macrophages.

IL-10 was originally identified as a product of murine T helper 2 (Th2) clones that inhibited the cytokine production by Th1 clones (Fiorentino et al, 1989). IL-10 is produced by CD4+ T-cell clones as well as by some CD8+ T-cell clones. In addition, human B cells, Epstein-Barr virus–transformed lymphoblastoid cell lines, and monocytes can also produce IL-10 upon activation. IL-10 is a potent immunosuppressant of the cytotoxic function of macrophages, for example, by inhibiting the monocyte-macrophage–dependent, antigen-stimulated cytokine synthesis (Bogdan et al, 1991). It inhibits the antigen-presenting capacity of monocytes by down-regulating class II MHC expression. As an immunostimulatory cytokine, IL-10 can act on B cells to enhance their viability, cell proliferation, immunoglobulin secretion, and class II MHC expression (Defrance et al, 1992). IL-10 is also a growth co-stimulator for thymocytes and mast cells, as well as an enhancer of cytotoxic T-cell development. IL-10 binds specifically and with high affinity to cell surface receptors. The IL-10 receptors are structurally related to the IFN-γ receptor. Recombinant IL-10 soluble receptor, consisting of the extracellular domain of IL-10 R, binds IL-10 with high affinity in solution and is a potent IL-10 antagonist.

The human *IL-11* cDNA encodes a 199-amino-acid residue precursor polypeptide with a 21-amino-acid residue hydrophobic signal that is processed proteolytically to generate the 178-amino-acid residue mature protein (Quesniaux et al, 1993). The biologic effects of IL-11 are similar to those for IL-6. In vitro, IL-11 can synergize with other cytokines to shorten the G_0 period of early hematopoietic progenitors. IL-11 can enhance megakaryocyte colony formation, stimulate the T-cell–dependent development of specific immunoglobulin-secreting B cells, and stimulate erythropoiesis. IL-11 exerts its biologic activities through binding to a specific high-affinity receptor that, similarly to IL-6, utilizes the signal transducer gp130 for signal transduction.

IL-12 is produced by macrophages and B lymphocytes and is a mediator of the cell-mediated immune responses (Lotze, 1996). It induces the production of IFN-γ and TNF by T and NK cells, enhances their cytotoxic activity, and stimulates the generation of LAK cells. In its role as the initiator of cell-mediated immunity, it has been suggested, that IL-12 has therapeutic potential as a stimulator of cell-mediated immune responses to microbial pathogens, metastatic cancers, and viral infections such as AIDS (Tahara et al, 1996). IL-12 consists of a p40 and p35 subunit. The p40 subunit of IL-12 has been shown to have extensive amino acid sequence homology to the extracellular domain of the human IL-6 receptor, while the p35 subunit shows distant but significant sequence similarity to IL-6 and granulocyte colony-stimulating factor (G-CSF).

Human *IL-13* cDNA encodes a 132-amino-acid protein containing a proposed 20-amino-acid signal peptide. IL-13 also shares approximately 30% amino acid sequence homology to human IL-4, and the two cytokines exhibit overlapping biologic activities (Zurawski and de Vries, 1994). It is produced by activated CD4+ and CD8+ T cells. The gene for human IL-13 has been mapped to chromosome 5, closely linked to the genes for IL-3, IL-4, IL-5, and granulocyte-macrophage colony-stimulating factor (GM-CSF). Similar to IL-4, IL-13 has multiple effects on the differentiation and functions of monocytes and macrophages (DeFife et al, 1997). It can suppress the cytotoxic functions of monocytes and macrophages, and inhibit the production of proinflammatory cytokines.

IL-15 is a novel cytokine that shares many biologic properties with, but lacks amino acid sequence homology to, IL-2 (Giri et al, 1995). High-affinity cell surface receptors for IL-15 have been detected on a variety of T cells and B cells, as well as nonlymphoid cells (Nishimura et al, 1996; Lucy et al, 1997). It has been demonstrated that the beta and gamma common chain subunits of the IL-2 high-affinity receptor complex are also required for IL-15 signal transduction and efficient internalization. IL-15 mRNAs have been detected in a number of human tissues and cell types, including heart, lung, liver, placenta, skeletal muscle, adherent peripheral blood mononuclear cells (PBMCs), and epithelial and fibroblast cell lines. However, IL-15 mRNA is not detectable in activated peripheral blood T cells that contain high levels of IL-2 mRNA. Similar to IL-2, IL-15 can stimulate the growth of NK cells, activated peripheral blood T lymphocytes, tumor-infiltrating lymphocytes (TILs), and B cells (Munger et al, 1995).

IL-17 is a novel cytokine produced by T cells (Yao et al, 1995). An IL-17–specific mouse cell surface receptor (IL-17 R) has been cloned. Whereas the expression of IL-17 mRNA is restricted to activated T cells, the expression of mIL-17 R mRNA has been detected in virtually all cells and tissues tested. IL-17 exhibits multiple biologic activities on a variety of cells, including the induction of IL-6 and IL-8 production in fibroblasts, the enhancement of surface expression of intercellular adhesion molecule-1 in fibroblasts, activation of nuclear factor-κB and co-stimulation of T cell proliferation (Fossiez et al, 1996).

COLONY-STIMULATING FACTORS

GM-CSF was initially characterized as a growth factor that can stimulate the growth of granulocyte-macrophage progenitors (Gasson et al, 1984). GM-CSF is also a growth factor for erythroid, megakaryocyte, and eosinophil progenitors (Souza et al, 1986). It is produced by a number of different cell types, including activated T cells, B cells, macrophages, mast cells, endothelial cells, and fibroblasts, in response to cytokine or immune and inflammatory stimuli. GM-CSF can also induce human endothelial cells to migrate and proliferate as well as stimulating the proliferation of a number of tumor cell lines, including adenocarcinoma cell lines. GM-CSF exerts its biologic effects through binding to specific cell surface receptors. The high-affinity receptors required for human GM-CSF signal transduction have been shown to be heterodimers consisting of a GM-CSF–specific alpha chain and a common beta chain that is shared by the high-affinity receptors for IL-3 and IL-5.

Human macrophage colony-stimulating factor (M-CSF), was originally described as a factor that can stimulate the formation of macrophage colonies from bone marrow hematopoietic progenitor cells (Metcalf et al, 1985). M-CSF can be produced by, for example, fibroblasts, activated macrophages, or secretory epithelial cells of the endometrium. M-CSF effects include stimulating of macrophage proliferation and cytotoxic activity and regulation of release of cytokines and other inflammatory modulators from macrophages. Elevated levels of mouse uterine M-CSF levels observed during pregnancy suggest a possible role for M-CSF in the formation and differentiation of the placenta. M-CSF is synthesized as a membrane-bound propeptide that is subsequently proteolytically cleaved. Both the soluble form and the membrane-anchored form are biologically active. Natural M-CSFs are glycosylated, disulfide-linked, homodimeric proteins with molecular weights ranging from 40 to 70 kDa. The C-terminal end of the soluble form of M-CSF is highly variable.

INSULIN-LIKE GROWTH FACTOR

Insulin-like growth factor I and II (IGF-I and IGF-II) belong to the family of growth factors that are structurally homologous to proinsulin (Zapf and Froesch, 1986). Mature IGF-I and IGF-II share approximately 70% sequence identity. IGF-I is a potent mitogenic growth factor that among other functions mediates the growth-promoting activities of growth hormone postnatally. A role for IGF-I during embryonic growth and differentiation has been described. Two cell surface receptors for IGF-I and IGF-II have been identified. The type I IGF, a disulfide-linked hetero-tetrameric transmembrane glycoprotein with an intracellular tyrosine kinase domain receptor, participates in IGF signaling and is structurally related to the insulin receptor. Type I IGF receptor binds IGF-I with higher affinity than IGF-II, whereas the type II IGF receptor binds IGF-II with much higher affinity than IGF-I. Circulating IGFs exist in complexes bound to a variety of IGF-binding proteins (Baxter, 1986).

EPIDERMAL GROWTH FACTOR

Epidermal growth factor (EGF) was originally discovered in crude preparations of nerve growth factor from mouse submaxillary glands as an activity that induced early eyelid opening, incisor eruption, hair growth inhibition, and stunting of growth when injected into newborn mice. Human EGF was isolated from urine based on its inhibitory effect on gastric secretion, and named urogastrone accordingly (Gregory, 1975). EGF belongs to a family of growth factors that are characterized by the presence of at least one EGF structural unit in their extracellular domain, defined by the presence of a conserved 6-cysteine motif that forms three disulfide bonds. EGF is initially synthesized as a 130-kDa precursor transmembrane protein containing nine EGF units (Scott et al, 1983). The membrane EGF precursor is capable of binding to the EGF receptor and was reported to be biologically active. In vitro, EGF predominantly stimulates proliferation and differentiation of mesenchymal and epithelial cells. In vivo, EGF induces epithelial development, promotes angiogenesis, and inhibits gastric acid secretion.

Transforming growth factor-α (TGF-α) is a member of the EGF family of cytokines. The soluble forms of these cytokines are released from the transmembrane protein by proteolytic cleavage. Membrane-bound pro–TGF-α is biologically active and plays a role in mediation of cell-cell adhesion and in paracrine stimulation of adjacent cells. Expression of TGF-α is found in a variety of tumor cell lines, but also in normal tissues during embryogenesis and in adult tissues, including pituitary, brain, keratinocytes, and macrophages. TGF-α binds to the EGF receptor and activates the receptor tyrosine kinase. It shows a potency similar to EGF as a mitogen for fibroblasts and as an inducer of epithelial development in vivo. TGF-α has potent angiogenic effects in vivo.

Transforming growth factor-β (TGF-β) is a multifunctional polypeptide growth factor (Lawrence, 1996). Specific TGF-β receptors have been found on almost all mammalian cell types. Although the effects of TGF-β vary according to the cell line and in vitro conditions, it is generally stimulatory for cells of mesenchymal origin and inhibitory for cells of epithelial or neuroectodermal origin (Kehrl, 1991). A number of more closely related proteins exist that are designated TGF-β 1, TGF-β 1.2, TGF-β 2, TGF-β 3, TGF-β 4, and TGF-β 5. TGF-β 1 and TGF-β 2 have been found in the highest concentration in human platelets and mammalian bone, but are produced by many cell types in smaller amounts. The heterodimer, TGF-β 1.2, has been found in small amounts in porcine platelets. TGF-β 3 has been detected in human, porcine, and avian sources, mainly in cells of mesenchymal origin, suggesting a different role for this protein than for TGF-β 1 or TGF-β 2. TGF-β 4 has been detected so far only in chick embryo chondrocytes, and its distribution in other types of cells has not yet been characterized. TGF-β 5 has been detected only in *Xenopus* embryos. TGF-β 1, TGF-β 2, and TGF-β 1.2 have similar biologic activities, although differences in binding to certain types of receptors and differential responses to TGF-β 1 and TGF-β 2 have been reported.

TUMOR NECROSIS FACTOR

TNF-α and TNF-β are two related proteins that bind to the same cell surface receptors (TNF RI and TNF RII) and produce a variety of similar effects (Hill and Lunec, 1996). An important effect is the ability to kill certain tumor cells directly (Rink and Kirchner, 1996). TNF is expressed in activated T and B lymphocytes. In addition to its cytotoxic action on tumor cells, TNF has been shown to be a mediator of inflammation and autoimmune function (Kunkel et al, 1989).

INTERFERON

IFN-α, IFN-β, and IFN-γ interfere with viral production. These factors have a variety of effects on the immune system and direct antitumor effects (Golub, 1984). For example, IFN-γ is a T-cell–produced lymphokine with direct effects on immune function: IFN-γ is a potent inducer of the expression of MHC class II molecules on monocytes and macrophages (Nathan et al, 1983; Schreiber et al, 1983; Schultz and Kleinschmidt, 1983). Because of this activity, it has been implicated as an important factor in enhancing the activity of antigen-presenting cells. Therefore, IFN-γ might act as a positive feedback signal for T-cell activation. IFN-γ also has effects on B-cell activation and differentiation.

COMMENTS

As research on the biologic activities of cytokines has progressed, it has become clear that most of these factors are pleiotropic and have a wide variety of biologic activities (Kishimoto and Hirano, 1988; Strober and James, 1988). Some of these factors have potent antitumor and/or immune-enhancing effects, and several of these factors have been used in experimental treatment of cancer and immune deficiency.

Initiation and Regulation of Immune Responses

The initiation and regulation of immune responses involve the coordinated activities of various types of cells and include cell-cell communication mediated by signals transmitted by direct cell-cell contact and/or by soluble mediators (lymphokines) (Figs. 68–1 through 68–3).

Role of MHC in the Genesis of Immune Responses

The MHC molecules play a central role in the genesis of immune responses. Specifically, MHC class II molecules on macrophages or B cells are intimately involved in antigen presentation, a process that is required for the generation of immune responses (see Fig. 68–1) (Lanzavecchia, 1985; Chestnut and Grey, 1986; Unanue and Allen, 1987).

Processed antigen, which had been taken up by macrophages by phagocytosis or by B cells by specific binding of antigen to surface antibody, is presented in an appropriate form on the surface of the antigen-presenting cell (see Fig. 68–1). This involves the association of a short stretch of peptide from the antigen with an MHC class II molecule. This processed bit of antigen appears to bind to a cleft in the surface of the MHC class II molecule. T cells (of the helper/inducer T subset) bearing a T-cell receptor of appropriate binding specificity for antigen, in combination with self MHC class II molecules, are activated by this interaction with the antigen-presenting cell. This process of helper T-cell activation appears to involve a signal delivered on binding of the antigen plus MHC class II complex via the T-cell receptor plus CD3 complex. Also, other interactions and signals appear to be important (see Fig. 68–1). The delivery of a second signal to the T cell, either by the production of a lymphokine (IL-1) by the antigen-presenting cell and/or by the delivery of accessory signals by the interactions of cell surface molecules other than MHC class II and the T-cell receptor, such as adhesion molecules or the interaction of CD4 on the T cell with MHC class II on the antigen-presenting cell, appears to be important for efficient T-cell activation (see Fig. 68–1). In any case, the interaction of the antigen-presenting cell and the helper T cell results in the activation of the T cell and thus in the production of a variety of factors (lymphokines) that induce the activation of other B and T lymphocytes (Figs. 68–1 through 68–3).

The MHC class I molecules also play an important role in the generation of immune responses. However, they are involved in responses of a different sort, namely cytotoxic immune responses (see Fig. 68–2). Virus-infected cells usually express viral antigens on their surface. Some viral antigens are expressed on the surface of infected cells in association with MHC class I molecules (see Fig. 68–2). The MHC class I–associated antigens are recognized by CD8 cytotoxic T cells (Zinkernagel and Doherty, 1979). Cytotoxic T cells are the immune cells responsible for the elimination of virus-infected cells and recognize foreign viral antigens on autologous cells in combination with MHC class I determinants. Although many details of the molecular interaction of viral antigen with MHC class I and the CD8 cytotoxic cell receptors are not yet clarified, this interaction appears to involve binding of the T-cell antigen receptor plus CD3 complex on T cells with the viral antigen plus MHC class I complex on the virus-infected target cell.

Role of Cytokines in Initiation and Expansion of Immune Responses

As mentioned, IL-1 is involved in initiating early events in immune responses. IL-1 functions by inducing antigen-responsive T cells to transcribe and translate the gene for IL-2; these T cells will then express the IL-2 receptor and will respond to IL-2 with increased proliferation. Therefore, stimulation of resting T cells with antigen presented in the context of self (i.e., antigen associated with an MHC molecule on the surface of an antigen-presenting cell) and with IL-1 induces the synthesis and secretion of IL-2. During this activation process, responding T cells undergo a change or alteration in their cell surface receptors, including the expression of cell surface receptors for IL-2. Continuing exposure to IL-2 then leads to the proliferation of T cells bearing the IL-2 receptor, thereby acting as an activation and response-amplification stage in the generation of immune responses. Activated T cells not only respond to IL-2 but also produce IL-2. Therefore, IL-2 can act in an autocrine manner (i.e., the cells producing the lymphokine then respond to it) or in a paracrine manner (i.e., the IL-2 produced by a T cell is taken up and responded to by neighboring cells).

IL-1 has other direct effects on cells of the immune system. For instance, IL-1 can act as a B-cell activation-inducing factor. Also, IL-1 can induce the production of other lymphokines that are involved in immune responses, such as IL-6. Since its original description as a T-cell growth hormone, IL-2 has been shown to have a variety of other immune activities, including the promotion of B-cell activation and maturation and monocyte and NK cell activation. Also, IL-2 can lead directly or indirectly to the stimulation of the production of IFN and other cytokines.

T-helper cells, as well as macrophages, also can help induce and expand B-cell responses by producing B-cell activating factors, which include IL-4, IL-5, and IL-6, as well as IL-1 and IL-2 (see Fig. 68–3). On exposure to antigen, mature B cells become receptive to these B-cell–stimulating factors and in their presence proliferate and differentiate to become antibody-secreting cells (see Fig. 68–3).

IMMUNOLOGIC MECHANISMS INVOLVED IN THE CONTROL OF TUMOR GROWTH

Various innate and adaptive immune mechanisms are involved in responses to tumors, including cytotoxicity directed to tumor cells, mediated by cytotoxic T cells, NK cells, macrophages, or LAK cells, and antibody-dependent cytotoxicity mediated by complement activation, or ADCC (Benjamini et al, 1984; Boyer et al, 1989a).

The immune status of patients with gynecologic cancers has been determined in many studies. This has taken the form of the quantification of mitogen-induced in vitro proliferation of mononuclear cells, the use of skin tests to assess in vivo responses to microbial antigens or contact allergens, the enumeration of lymphocyte subsets, and the measurement of immunoglobulin levels (Zighelboim et al, 1988; Boyer et al, 1989a). However, because of the complex and relatively insensitive nature of the tests used and the lack of appropriate controls, the results of these studies have been difficult to assess. It is hoped that the future study of immune function and immune mechanisms in gynecologic cancers will benefit from new technologies and by a more stringent experimental design and analysis.

Cytotoxic T Cells

Cytotoxic immune T cells can be involved in anti-tumor responses. These cells can recognize and kill tumor cells. The ability of cytotoxic T cells to kill tumor cells in vitro is most commonly measured by the release of ^{51}Cr from isotope-labeled target cells. Presumably, cytotoxic T cells first recognize antigens on tumor cells via their antigen-specific T-cell receptor; then a series of events occur that ultimately result in the lysis of the target cell.

NK Cells, ADCC and Macrophage Cytotoxicity

NK cells can recognize and lyse tumor cells in vitro. NK activity is an innate form of immunity that does not require an adaptive memory response for optimal biologic function. However, NK antitumor activity can be augmented by exposure to several agents, especially cytokines. It has been shown that ADCC by NK-like cells results in the lysis of tumor cell targets in vitro. The mechanisms of tumor cell killing in ADCC are not clearly understood, although close cellular contact between the ADCC effector cell and the target cell appears to be required. Activated macrophages, in addition to their many other functional capabilities, can also effect cytotoxicity of tumor cell targets.

Adoptive Immunotherapy: LAK Cells and TILs

Exposure of PBMCs to IL-2, or other cytokines, in vitro leads to the generation of cytotoxic effect cells called LAK cells (Grimm et al, 1982). These cells are effective cytotoxic cells for a variety of tumor cells, including tumor cells resistant to NK cell– or T-cell–mediated lysis.

The treatment of patients with such ex vivo–activated autologous cells forms the basis of adoptive immunotherapy. Experimental treatment of human subjects with ex vivo–generated autologous LAK cells and IL-2 has yielded tumor regression in some cases (Rosenberg, 1984a, 1984b; Lotze et al, 1986). Expansion of TILs, isolated from tumors and activated and expanded in vitro by exposure to IL-2, to obtain tumor-specific cytotoxic cells has been explored (Strober and James, 1988). Adoptive immunotherapy is a very active area of study and may lead to effective forms of antitumor therapy based on modified forms of antitumor immune responses.

Antitumor Effects of Cytokines

Various cytokines appear to have antitumor effects in vitro and in vivo. However, in many instances it has been difficult to discern whether these effects are the direct result of a cytokine-mediated antitumor effect or an indirect effect induced in some manner by cytokine exposure, such as activation of immune effector cells or the induction of the secretion of other cytokines. Clearly, some cytokines, such as TNF, can have potent direct antitumor cytotoxic effects. Other cytokines, including some IFNs, may inhibit tumor growth by cytostatic and cytotoxic effects.

IMMUNOTHERAPY IN GYNECOLOGIC CANCER

Most immunotherapeutic agents used in the treatment of cancer have been nonspecific agents that, when introduced into the human system, elicit a generalized inflammatory reaction and immune response. Because of the diverse and broad biologic effects of such agents, they are often referred to as immunomodulators or biologic response modifiers (BRMs). The response of a given patient to such

treatment depends on the ability of such an individual to react to the immunomodulator or BRM with a generalized immune response. In fact, some elements of the immune response elicited by immunotherapeutic agents or BRMs may be counterproductive, possibly causing immune suppression or some other unfavorable or inappropriate immune response.

Biologic Response Modifiers

BRMs are agents that can modulate, induce, modify, or alter inflammatory and immune responses. Nonspecific immunotherapies with BRMs have been used in most previous trials for the treatment of gynecologic cancer. Such trials have involved the inoculation of the patient with BRMs, including inactivated bacteria, such as *Corynebacterium parvum*, which is a heat-killed, gram-negative anaerobic bacillus; bacille Calmette-Guérin (BCG), which is a live, attenuated strain of *Mycobacterium bovis*; or Freund's complete adjuvant. Modifications can be made in these agents by extracting fractions of these organisms using biochemical techniques. Fractionation, typically by acid or phenol extraction, can lead to the isolation of active components (glycolipids or carbohydrates) that might more selectively elicit desirable immunologic responses while sparing less desirable immune reactions or side effects (Muruhata et al, 1980). For example, methanol-extracted residue of BCG retains significant immunomodulatory activity while potentially avoiding some of the problems associated with viable BCG.

Exposure to *C. parvum* results in a variety of immune responses (Halpern, 1975), including an acute inflammatory response, predominantly the induction and infiltration of neutrophils, and macrophage attraction, activation, and cytotoxicity. NK cytotoxicity is enhanced, and T-lymphocyte activation also results from exposure to *C. parvum* (Herberman, 1980). *Corynebacterium parvum* has been shown to be active in many animal systems (Scott, 1984), with tumor rejection being temporally associated with a cellular response. Studies of a murine teratocarcinoma model examining biochemically fractionated *C. parvum* showed that tumor rejection in animals treated with intraperitoneal (IP) injection of the residue of pyridine-extracted *C. parvum*, a fraction that contains the bacterial cell walls (Berek et al, 1984b), is comparable to the rejection observed after IP administration of whole, unmodified *C. parvum*. The sequential administration of these *C. parvum* fractions in combination with bacterial endotoxins resulted in an even greater antitumor effect (Berek et al, 1985c).

BCG has been widely used in many tumor systems and has been administered systemically, by intralesional injection, or by escarification (Bast et al, 1974). Occasionally BCG has been mixed with whole irradiated tumor cells and injected into the patient as a vaccine. In a large series (Borstein et al, 1973), melanoma lesions intracutaneously injected with BCG demonstrated some active tumor rejection in patients with cutaneous recurrence. However, visceral or parenchymal metastatic disease has been resistant to this therapy. Although there have been some preliminary observations obtained examining the use of BCG as an adjuvant in children with acute lymphocytic leukemia and with stage II melanoma, randomized studies have not revealed significant responses. In ovarian cancer, BCG has been used in combination with cytotoxic agents in a randomized prospective study (Alberts et al, 1978), and an apparent increase in survival was detected. However, this observation has not yet been substantiated. It is important to note that, in most experimental animal systems in which immunotherapy and chemotherapy are combined, tumor rejection is augmented most often when the administration of the immunostimulant precedes the administration of cytotoxic agents by a sufficient interval to permit some positive immunomodulation (Hanna and Key, 1982).

Another immunomodulator is AS101 (ammonium trichloro[dioxoethylene-O,O']tellurate), which was found to stimulate mouse and human cells to proliferate and secrete a variety of cytokines. A clinical trial evaluated the ability of AS101 to modulate cytokine responses in patients with advanced cancer, including ovarian cancer (Sredni et al, 1996). Treatment of patients with AS101 resulted in a clear predominance of TH1 responses, with a concomitant decrease in the TH2-type response. This was reflected by a significant enhancement in IL-2 and IFN-γ levels paralleled by a substantial decrease in IL-4 and IL-10. Moreover, the concentration of IL-12 was significantly increased in AS101-treated patients, who also showed enhanced levels of NK and LAK cell-mediated cytotoxicity.

Cytokines and Adoptive Immunotherapy

IFNs have received much attention because of their ability to act as immunomodulators. These small glycoproteins are natural cellular products that have been shown to be elicited by a variety of stimuli, particularly viral infections. Interferons are potent inducers of NK cell function in vitro and in vivo, and this has been associated with antitumor activity in animal models (Stewart, 1979). The precise role of IFNs in relation to other components of immune responses has not been completely elucidated. The mechanisms by which these molecules exert antitumor effects could include both direct antitumor activities and induction of antitumor immune responses. Clinical trials of IFNs have been undertaken in gynecologic malignancies.

The effectiveness of IFN-α in patients with lung and metastatic breast and ovarian cancer was evaluated in 25 patients with malignant pleural or peritoneal effusions (Stathopoulos et al, 1996). After drainage of pleural or peritoneal fluid, patients received 10 million units of IFN-α by intrapleural or IP injection at weekly intervals. A group of patients showed an increase in amount of ascites-infiltrating mononuclear cells. In this group of patients the administration of IFN-α was associated with 25% complete response and 75% partial response rates. NK cell activity and MHC class I antigen expression on effusion-associated tumor cells were also enhanced during treatment.

ILs, have been studied extensively and have been documented to produce tumor regression in a variety of animal and human tumors. IL-1α has been used in patients with recurrent ovarian carcinoma treated with carboplatin. In a Phase I study (Verschraegen et al, 1996), IL-1α treatment showed minor but objective antitumor effects in 2 of 18 patients. IL-2 has shown antitumor effects in melanoma and renal cell carcinoma, in conjunction with the adoptive transfer of autologous LAK cells (Rosenberg, 1984a, 1984b). In patients with advanced ovarian cancer, IL-2 has been administered IP in escalating doses via a Tenckhoff catheter. Considerable stimulation of IP immune cells was observed without severe toxic side effect (Schroder et al, 1995).

The tolerability and efficacy of human IL-3 and recombinant human G-CSF were studied during paclitaxel and ifosfamide plus cisplatin chemotherapy in patients with ovarian cancer (Veldhuis et al, 1997). Patients treated with IL-3 showed a tendency to a faster platelet recovery, allowing a greater cisplatin dose intensity. Six of the nine evaluable patients had a tumor response. Another study used the GM-CSF/IL-3 fusion protein PIXY321 in patients with a variety of malignancies (Gheilmini et al, 1996). A biphasic modest increase of white blood cell count and platelets was seen, accompanied by an increased bone marrow cellularity and an increase in circulating progenitors. In a Phase I/II study, PIXY321 was subcutaneously administered after the second cycle of chemotherapy in ovarian cancer patients (Runowicz et al, 1996). The study showed that PIXY321 could be safely administered. However, aggressive dosing of cyclophosphamide and carboplatin could not be maintained for six cycles in the majority of patients. The use of recombinant human IL-6 was studied in a randomized Phase Ib study in patients with ovarian carcinoma (D'Hondt et al, 1995). IL-6 was administered during an initial 7-day cycle before chemotherapy and at day 4 through day 17 at escalating dose levels from 0.5 to 10 μg/kg/day. During the prechemotherapy cycle of IL-6, a dose-dependent increase in platelet count was observed from day 12 to day 15 and was maximal on day 15. A significant decrease in hemoglobin level occurred rapidly after initiation of IL-6 therapy and was maximal on day 8 ($p < 0.001$). When given after chemotherapy, IL-6 accelerated platelet recovery after chemotherapy cycles two through six. Toxicity of IL-6 appeared mild, with systemic symptoms such as fever, headache, and myalgia.

Adoptive immunotherapy involves the administration of ex vivo IL-2–generated LAK cells, along with the concomitant administration of IL-2. This sort of treatment has resulted in some complete responses (Rosenberg et al, 1985), with a combined response rate of 27% in 146 cancer patients treated in two separate studies (Rosenberg et al, 1987; West et al, 1987). However, the overall response rate to LAK treatment is low, and this type of adoptive immunotherapy results in high morbidity (Rosenberg et al, 1985; West et al, 1987; Berek, 1990). Also, the cost of LAK treatment is high, and this type of treatment is impractical in most medical settings. Much current experimental work aims at developing more efficient and practical applications of adoptive immunotherapy. One approach involves the ex vivo generation of immune effector cells from TILs, which are then administered concurrently with IL-2 (Topalian et al, 1988). However, this approach is hampered by the need to expand a limited number of TILs in vitro to generate enough effector cells for treatment. Another promising approach that has been explored in animal studies involves the targeting of activated T lymphocytes with a bifunctional monoclonal antibody that binds to both the CD3/T-cell receptor complex (on the activated effector T cell) and a tumor-associated antigen (on the target tumor cell) (Garrido et al, 1990). This approach has the potential advantage of allowing a large fraction of the activated lymphocytes to target their effects directly on tumor cells, thereby reducing the need to amplify a large number of effector cells from TILs. Also, this approach has the potential to reduce some of the side effects associated with LAK treatment, which is a more nonspecific form of adoptive immunotherapy. There is in vitro evidence to suggest that LAK cells and IL-2 are effective in the induction of cytotoxicity against ovarian cancer cells (Boyer et al, 1989b; Nio et al, 1990). TILs may represent an active immune response of the host directed against the tumor cells, because these T-cell lines may either exhibit tumor-specific cytotoxicity against autologous tumor cells, or produce immunostimulatory cytokines (Freedman and Platsoucas, 1996).

Intraperitoneal application of TILs possibly combined with low-dose IL-2 in patients with advanced ovarian carcinoma may present an effective therapeutic alternative, in particular in patients with disease refractory to platinum-based chemotherapy. In an effort to redirect T lymphocytes against specific tumor cell targets, chimeric antibody/T-cell receptor genes were designed that are composed of the variable domains from monoclonal antibodies joined to the T-cell receptor-signaling chains. T cells transduced with these genes can recognize antibody-defined antigens on tumor cells and are subsequently activated to lyse the tumor cells and release cytokines (Hwu et al, 1995).

The monoclonal antibody OC/TR, which is directed to the CD3 molecule on T lymphocytes and to the folate receptor on ovarian carcinoma cells, was used in a Phase II trial in ovarian cancer patients (Canevari et al, 1995). Patients received two cycles of five daily IP infusions of autologous in vitro–activated peripheral blood T lymphocytes retargeted with OC/TR plus recombinant IL-2. Of 19 patients, who could be evaluated by surgery and histology, three showed complete response, one showed complete IP response with progressive disease in retroperitoneal lymph nodes, three showed partial response, seven had stable disease, and five had progressive disease. The overall IP response rate was 27%.

Monoclonal Antibodies

Kohler and Milstein (1978) developed monoclonal antibody technology more than 20 years ago. More recently, there has been considerable interest in the use of monoclonal antibodies for tumor detection and monitoring and for therapy. Monoclonal antibodies reactive with tumor-associated antigens may provide new therapeutic agents for ovarian cancer. However, many obstacles limit the clinical utility of monoclonal antibodies: tumor cell antigenic heterogeneity, modulation of tumor-associated antigens, and cross-reactivity of normal host and tumor-associated antigens. In fact, no unique tumor-specific antigens have been identified. All tumor antigens identified to date are tumor related, because these antigens have been seen to be expressed to some extent on nonmalignant tissues. However, normal tissues may display a lower level of antigen expression than tumor tissues, which can express high levels of these cell-surface tumor antigens. Also, because most monoclonal antibodies are murine, the host's immune system can recognize and respond to these foreign mouse proteins. The use of genetically engineered monoclonal antibodies composed of human constant regions with specific antigen-reactive murine variable regions should result in reduced antigenicity to the host and might help eliminate many of the problems associated with the administration of murine monoclonal antibodies.

OC-125, a monoclonal antibody reactive with a molecule produced by human epithelial ovarian carcinoma cells (OC-125), is widely used to monitor the blood CA-125 antigen level in women with ovarian cancer (Bast et al, 1981, 1983b). Monoclonal antibodies have also been used in gynecologic oncology patients for radioimmunodetection. Monoclonal antibodies that recognize tumor-associated antigens on epithelial ovarian cancer cells labeled with radioactive tracers have been used to detect primary and recurrent lesions (Davies et al, 1985; Epenetos et al, 1985, 1986a, 1986b; Symonds et al, 1985; Granowska et al, 1986).

Monoclonal antibodies can kill tumor cells by complement activation and tumor cell lysis; by direct antiproliferative effects, enhancing the activity of nonspecific phagocytic cells that recognize the murine immunoglobulin on the surface of the tumor cell; or by ADCC. However, most monoclonal antibodies are not cytotoxic and fail to activate human immune effector systems. Radionuclide-conjugated monoclonal antibodies, given by IP injection, have been used as experimental treatment in patients with advanced ovarian cancer (Epenetos et al, 1985). This approach has the potential to reduce exposure of the monoclonal antibody to normal body tissue that might express antigens reactive with the monoclonal antibody. Another approach has been to link monoclonal antibodies to toxins, such as ricin A or *Pseudomonas* exotoxin (Fitzgerald et al, 1986), or detoxified *Salmonella* endotoxin, in combination with another agent (Berek et al, 1985c). The efficacy of the clinical use of monoclonal antibodies and immunotoxins in humans requires further evaluation.

Studies evaluating the efficacy of monoclonal antibody–directed radiotherapy in gynecologic malignancies are limited. Epenetos et al used two different murine antibodies labeled with ^{131}I (Hammersmith Oncology Group and Imperial Cancer Research Fund, 1984; Epenetos et al, 1986a). Prospective studies using new monoclonal antibody and different energy sources (particularly rhenium) are ongoing. The most successful studies using toxin-conjugated monoclonal antibodies in ovarian cancer have used an antitransferrin receptor (a cell-surface molecule expressed mainly by rapidly growing cells) antibody linked to *Pseudomonas* exotoxin (anti-TFR-PE) (Pirker et al, 1985).

Bispecific Antibodies and Idiotypic Network

MDX-210 is a bispecific antibody that recognizes Fc gamma R1 on monocytes and macrophages and the cell surface product of the *HER-2/neu* oncogene. It has been used in a number of clinical trials and found to be well tolerated and immunologically and clinically active (Valone et al, 1995). Optimization of the dose and schedule of MDX-210 and development of combination treatments with cytokines that modulate immune effector cells is currently underway and may enhance the efficacy of this novel therapeutic approach in, for example, *HER-2/neu*-overexpressing ovarian cancers.

Another concept of immunotherapy comprises the attempt to trigger the immune system of the host into a response against tumor cells via the anti-idiotypic network. Anti-idiotypic antibodies present the internal image of an antigen expressed on the surface of the tumor and can generate humoral and cellular antitumor immune responses. Activation of the idiotypic network has been attempted in a number of clinical trials in ovarian cancer. A radiolabeled antibody (131J-F(Ab)2 OC 125 Mab) against the tumor antigen CA-125 was used for diagnostic purposes in 62 patients with ovarian carcinoma (Schmolling et al, 1995). A significant anti-idiotypic antibody (Ab2) level was found in 28 patients that increased with repetitive applications. Interestingly, 20 patients with Ab2 concentrations greater than

10,000 U/ml had a significantly higher survival rate than the patients who had lower levels of Ab2. In another study, 26 of 50 ovarian cancer patients receiving anti–CA-125 murine monoclonal antibody B43.13 were found to have elevated anti-idiotypic antibodies (Madiyalakan et al, 1995).

Human anti-mouse antibodies (HAMA) are observed frequently after immunoscintigraphy with monoclonal antibodies directed against CA-125. In an analysis of 32 patients, a HAMA frequency of 34% was found (Baum et al, 1994). Although all these patients had advanced disease, seven patients with anti-idiotypic HAMA responses after OC-125 immunoscintigraphy remained free of tumor over 2 to 32 months. Similar observations were made in 58 patients with advanced ovarian carcinomas who had received monoclonal antibody (OC-125) against the cancer-associated antigen CA-125 for diagnostic purposes (Wagner et al, 1994). This study showed that the induction of anti-idiotypic antibodies leads to a prolongation of the survival rate and induction of antitumoral immunity. It is possible that anti-idiotypic immune responses may trigger an antitumor effect either by suppressing the growth of CA-125–expressing cancer cells directly, or by activating the patient's immune response via induction of Ab3.

Immunotherapy of Ovarian Cancer

There has been great interest in examining the potential role of immunotherapy in ovarian cancer. Because long-term survival in patients with ovarian epithelial malignancies is poor and most patients present with metastatic disease, there is a great need to develop useful biologic therapies. Furthermore, patients with advanced disease are significantly immunocompromised (Khoo and MacKay, 1974), suggesting a role for immune-enhancing therapies.

Only anecdotal evidence exists for responses using vaccines in ovarian cancer. Graham and Graham (1962) treated 232 patients with gynecologic malignancies, 48 of whom had ovarian cancer, with Freund's complete adjuvant. Freund's complete adjuvant was mixed either with DNA-protein extract of the tumor or viable tumor cells. Systemic reactions to these agents were low in most patients who had tumor progression. However, this vaccine did not control tumor growth. Ten patients with stage III or IV ovarian cancer received BCG combined with an allogenic tumor cell vaccine. Administration of alkylating agents along with the BCG and vaccine of 107 irradiated allogenic tumor cells resulted in prolonged survival compared retrospectively with historic controls (Hudson et al, 1976). Although these reports suggested some improvement in survival, they were all uncontrolled and retrospective and involved a very small number of patients. Also, patients have been treated (Julliard et al, 1978) with irradiated tumor cells injected intralymphatically, a technique referred to as active specific intra-lymphatic immunotherapy (ASILI). A complete response, with the patient free of clinical evidence of disease at 13 months, was reported in seven patients with epithelial ovarian carcinoma treated with ASILI. Unfortunately, most patients with ovarian cancer have bulky, persistent tumors located in the peritoneal cavity and do not respond to this type of therapy.

Most studies in metastatic ovarian cancer have used nonspecific immunotherapies. *Corynebacterium parvum* and BCG have been used in the largest single retrospective series to date. Phase I studies of *C. parvum* have demonstrated that toxicity generally includes systemic chills, fever, malaise, nausea, and vomiting in most patients (Rao et al, 1977; Alberts et al, 1978; Gall et al, 1978; Webb et al, 1978; Montovani et al, 1981; Bast et al, 1983a). Serious toxicity, including hypotension, prolonged elevated temperatures, and chest pain, is not common. In early studies in patients with ovarian cancer, subcutaneously administered *C. parvum* was combined in escalating doses with cyclophosphamide, doxorubicin, and 5-fluorouracil (CAF) administered monthly (Rao et al, 1977). Pretreatment immune parameters were normal in patients who responded to therapy, compared with decreased immune parameters in those who did not. However, immune function was not augmented by therapy. In a randomized trial of CAF chemoimmunotherapy, with or without intravenously administered *C. parvum*, there was no difference in response rates, disease progression-free intervals, or survival (Wanebo and Ochoa, 1977).

Creasman et al (1979) reported a series of patients retrospectively treated with either melphalan or melphalan plus *C. parvum*. The study evaluated 108 patients with untreated stage III ovarian epithelial malignancies. The melphalan plus *C. parvum* combination group had a 53% total response rate, compared with 29% in the group treated with melphalan alone. However, a prospective, randomized study attempting to confirm these findings showed no significant differences between melphalan, 7 mg/m^2/day for 5 days orally every 4 weeks, and the same regimen plus *C. parvum* given IV on day 7 after chemotherapy.

In a randomized, prospective study by Alberts et al (1978), 66 patients with stages III and IV epithelial ovarian carcinomas were treated with either a combination of cyclophosphamide and doxorubicin or these two agents plus concomitant intravenous BCG. Doxorubicin was given at 40 mg/m^2 on day 1, cyclophosphamide at 200 mg/m^2 on days 3 through 6, and BCG on day 8 and day 15. This cycle was repeated every 4 weeks. Of the 32 patients who were treated with a combination of chemotherapy and immunotherapy, the total response rate was 56%, with 2 of 32 evaluable patients having a complete response. The median duration of response was 45 weeks; the median survival, 93 weeks. This is compared with the 34 patients treated with doxorubicin and cyclophosphamide alone; only 11 patients (32%) had a partial response. The median duration of response in this group was 26 weeks, and the median survival was 59 weeks. Thus the immunotherapy combined with chemotherapy did not improve the survival of patients with ovarian carcinoma. The unpublished results of a prospective, randomized Gynecologic Oncology Group (GOG) study that compared doxorubicin, cyclophosphamide, and cisplatin with or without BCG administered by escarification in patients with suboptimal stage III disease confirm these data.

Systemically administered cytokine therapy has been applied in Phase I-II trials of patients with ovarian cancer. Purified or recombinant IFN-α or IFN-β was administered systemically to patients with advanced ovarian cancer, most of whom had persistent or recurrent metastatic epithelial cancers, in five studies (Einhorn et al, 1982; Ezaki et al, 1983; Freedman et al, 1983; Abdulhay et al, 1985; Niloff et al, 1985). The combined response rate of these clinical trials was only 10%.

Intraperitoneal Immunotherapy

Because the most successful immunomodulators in many animal models are those that can be brought into direct contact with regional tumors, the IP administration of immunotherapeutic agents in ovarian cancer is appealing. Patients with ovarian cancer have been treated with IP immunotherapy. In patients with minimal residual epithelial ovarian carcinoma after treatment with combination cytotoxic chemotherapy, Bast et al (1983a) and Berek et al (1985b) reported a total of 21 patients treated with IP immunotherapy. Of the 19 evaluable patients, there were six responders, including two complete responses. All of the responding patients had macroscopic disease of less than 5 mm maximum tumor diameter at the initiation of therapy. ADCC is significantly augmented during the course of therapy (Bast et al, 1983a), as is NK cytotoxicity (Berek et al, 1984a; Lichtenstein et al, 1984). The increase of cytotoxic effectors in the peritoneal cavity correlates well with the response to the agent *C. parvum* administered every 2 weeks in escalating doses starting at 0.25 mg/m^2 and rising to 4 mg/m.^{2}

The IP administration of *C. parvum* has been noted by Mantovani et al (1981) to be useful for the palliation of ascites in women with advanced ovarian cancer. In eight patients, IP administration of 7 to 14 mg of *C. parvum* on days 0, 7, and 28 resulted in complete disappearance of ascites in three patients and a marked reduction of the effusion in two others. The palliative effect was noted to be sustained for 6 to 13 months.

Hernandez et al (1980) reported the treatment of nine patients with advanced ovarian epithelial malignancies with IP administration of sterile, pyrogen-free rabbit-derived human ovarian antitumor serum (HOATS). Although the study had short follow-up, the clinical response rate was 80%, with a 1-year survival of 87%. A trial of passive serotherapy using the rabbit heteroantiserum is being studied prospectively (Order et al, 1981). Patients are being treated with IP ^{32}P, total abdominal irradiation, and melphalan, with or without 150 to 200 ml of serum. After a 2-year follow-up in 13 patients, there is no difference in survival between the two groups.

There has been considerable interest in the IP administration of cytokines. Most studies have used the IFNs, especially recombinant IFN-α. In a favorable group of patients, most of whom had minimal residual disease (less than 5 mm maximum tumor dimension), the IP administration of recombinant IFN-α augmented peritoneal NK cytotoxicity and resulted in a surgically documented complete response in 4 of 11 (36%) patients (Berek et al, 1985a). This observation was replicated by Willemse and colleagues (1990) in a series of 19 patients in whom five (26%) complete responses were documented by a third-look laparotomy. No responses have been observed after the IP administration of recombinant IFN-β or IFN-γ treatment in patients with larger tumor burdens (Rambaldi et al, 1985; D'Acquisto et al, 1988). The combined response rate of about 25% for IP recombinant IFN therapy is similar to that observed with IP C. parvum therapy. A Phase I trial of IP IL-2 also has been conducted in patients with residual peritoneal cancer, and the agent is well tolerated (Chapman et al, 1988). The results of these several trials suggest that, if regionally administered cytokines are to be useful in ovarian cancer, they can be used only in patients with minimal residual disease or in an adjuvant or consolidation protocol. Pharmacokinetic analyses of the IP administration of both IFN-α and IL-2 showed that there was a significant advantage for this route of administration and that the high peritoneal levels persisted for more than 24 hours.

There is evidence that the IFNs can produce a greater cytotoxicity effect in vitro when combined with several chemotherapeutic agents (Aapro et al, 1983). The combined use of IP cisplatin and IFN-α has been reported in two trials (Nardi et al, 1990; Berek et al, 1991). In one study (Berek et al, 1991), the cisplatin and IFN were given within 12 hours of one another every other week for up to 12 cycles, and, of the eight patients who underwent a third-look laparotomy, there were two (25%) complete responses documented. The maximum tolerated doses in this trial was cisplatin, 60 mg/m^2, and IFN, 25 million units given every other week. In a second trial (Nardi et al, 1990), the cisplatin and IFN were administered IP on alternating weeks, and, of the 14 patients who underwent a third-look laparotomy, there were 7 (50%) who had a complete response to the therapy. In all of the responding patients in these four studies, the maximum residual tumor size was less than 5 mm, and most patients initiated therapy with microscopic disease only.

A group of researchers from Tokyo (Ohkawa and Ohkawa, 1981) studied the use of IP administration of semisynthesized acid polysaccharides, BCG, and OK432 (Picibanil, which is a streptococcal preparation). These agents were administered IP for 4 days in a row, with weekly IP injections of doxorubicin, 5-fluorouracil, Endoxan, bleomycin, and mitomycin C. Although this is an uncontrolled study, the 60 evaluable patients treated between 1970 and 1977 had a 5-year survival of 40%. These results further suggest that locoregional immunotherapy combined with chemotherapy may play a role in the control of ovarian cancer confined to the peritoneal cavity.

Adoptive Immunotherapy

Studies using adoptive immunotherapy with LAK cells, with the concomitant administration of IL-2, in gynecologic malignancies are in progress (Boyer et al, 1989b; Berek, 1990). One study (Urba et al, 1989) reported the IP administration of IL-2 and autologous LAK cells in 12 patients with persistent ovarian or colon cancer confined to the peritoneal cavity. Two of six evaluable ovarian cancer patients had partial responses documented, and three of eight evaluable colon cancer patients had a partial response. In a more recent report updating this experience (Steiss et al, 1990), in which 22 patients with tumors confined to the peritoneal cavity were treated IP with IL-2 and LAK cell therapy, six responses were seen. However, a major problem encountered with this approach has been excessive regional toxicity, especially peritoneal fibrosis. Also, hypotension and sepsis developed in several patients. This LAK plus IL-2–induced peritoneal fibrosis might result from the release of various growth factors and cytokines capable of inducing collagen synthesis by fibroblasts. Such side effects might be reduced either by modification of LAK plus IL-2 regimens or by the development of more targeted and less nonspecific forms of adoptive immunotherapy (Berek, 1990).

Gene Therapy

In the last few years, advances in molecular biology and technologies that allow the modification of genetic material have generated a more profound understanding of the structure, regulation, and function of many genes. The ability to transfer genes into cells either to replace a missing or malfunctioning gene or to provide a new function to a cell has opened a new spectrum of therapeutic possibilities (Sobol et al, 1995). Various novel molecular strategies have been developed to inhibit tumor growth directly or stimulate a systemic immune response against the cancer.

Several methods are currently used to transfer genes into mammalian cells (Vile and Russell, 1995). These methods differ in accuracy, efficiency, and stability of gene expression. The expression level of the transgene inside the host cell is dependent on the transferred DNA construct and may vary depending on the cell system.

Physical methods like electroporation or the use of a gene gun and chemical methods like calcium-phosphate or DEAE-Dextran transfection have been used in a variety of cell systems (Kriegler, 1990). The DNA transferred by these techniques is usually in form of plasmid DNA. In general, physical methods yield low gene transfer efficiencies.

Liposomes consist of positively charged lipid molecules that possess the ability to bind negatively charged DNA (Puyal et al, 1995). This lipid-DNA complex subsequently fuses with the membrane of the host cell to release the DNA into the cytoplasm or is taken up by the cell via endocytosis. Some of the DNA molecules relocate into the nucleus and use the host cell's transcription machinery to express the foreign gene. This technique is easy to use and can be applied to a variety of cell lines (Hofland and Huang, 1995).

Infective particles such as retroviruses (Miller, 1993), recombinant adenoviruses, adeno-associated viruses (Kremer et al, 1995), herpesviruses (Anderson et al, 1992), and adenovirus-polylysine-DNA (Curiel et al, 1994) complexes are able to effectively transfer genes (Jolly, 1994). The viral gene transfer systems most widely used in vitro and in vivo are retroviruses and adenoviruses. Retroviral transfer vectors are generated by deleting the structural genes, namely *pol*, *env*, and *gag*, from the retroviral genome and replacing these sequences with the transgene of interest (Danos and Mulligan, 1988). A helper cell line provides the necessary structural proteins to yield an intact but replication-incompetent retroviral vector (Markowitz et al, 1988). These retroviral vectors bind to most human cells via a receptor. Fusion between the viral envelope and the target cell membrane releases the viral core particle into the cytoplasm. The viral RNA is reverse transcribed into proviral DNA that subsequently translocates into the cell nucleus. Integration of proviral DNA into the cell's genome is only possible if the host cell undergoes a cell division shortly after the infection. Such integration yields stable transfectants that can be selected in vitro via drug resistance genes and maintain transgene expression over an extended period of time. The efficiency of retroviral gene transfer and subsequent transgene expression in vivo is low, mainly because of inactivation by complement (Welsh et al, 1975).

Adenoviruses have been used either in recombinant form with the transgene inserted into the viral genome or complexed to polylysine-transferrin-DNA complexes (Kremer et al, 1995; Berns and Giraud, 1995). Current adenoviral vectors are deleted in the E1 and/or E3 regions of the 36-kbp DNA genome and can accept up to 7 kbp of foreign sequence. In the absence of the E1a coding sequence, the other adenovirus genes are not expressed. A helper cell line provides the necessary structural proteins for the production of a recombinant adenoviral particle (Graham and Prevec, 1995). Adenoviruses attach to the cells via a fiber-like structure whose structure is still under investigation. Most cells, including non-dividing cells, are readily and efficiently infected with adenoviruses. Expression of the transgene is usually transient, but prolonged expression has been reported in liver, skeletal muscle, bronchial epithelial, and brain cells. In contrast to retroviruses, adenoviruses are not subject to complement inactivation and have been used in vivo with better transfection efficiency than other vector systems (Addison et al, 1995). However, immune responses against viral proteins can interfere with the effectiveness of subsequent injections of adenoviruses in vivo.

Immuno-Gene Therapy

Stimulation of effective immune response against cancer cells involves the presentation of tumor-associated antigens and production of cytokines necessary to stimulate immune effector cells capable of tumor cell killing. In clinical trials, the administration of cytokines to cancer patients has resulted in objective antitumor responses (Steiss et al, 1990). However, severe toxicities limit the dose and efficacy of systemic cytokine administration.

In order to circumvent the problem of severe toxicity associated with high doses of cytokines, several investigators have used the transfer of cytokine genes into tumor cells to co-present tumor-associated antigen and the immunostimulatory cytokine (Miller et al, 1994). The injection of cytokine gene-modified tumor cells has resulted in significant antitumor immune responses in several animal tumor models. In these studies, the transfer of cytokine genes into tumor cells has reduced or abrogated the tumorigenicity of the cells after implantation into syngeneic hosts. Furthermore, treated animals developed systemic antitumor immunity and were protected against subsequent tumor challenges with the unmodified parental tumor (Dorigo and Berek, 1997; Shawler et al, 1995).

The stimulation of antitumor immune responses by cytokine gene modified tumor cell vaccines involves presentation of tumor-associated antigen and an immunostimulatory cytokine at the injection site (Fig. 68–4). Tumor cells can be genetically modified to express, for example, IL-2. Injection of IL-2–secreting tumor cells (e.g., subcutaneously) is thought to stimulate circulating CD8+ T-killer cells at the injection site. The CD4+ T-helper cell function is being bypassed, because IL-2, one of the main immunostimulatory cytokines generated by CD4+ cells, is produced directly by the genetically modified tumor cell vaccine (Fearon et al, 1990). The stimulated killer cells subsequently circulate, recognize tumor cells at distant sites, and elicit tumor cell killing. An alternative concept describes the stimulation of antigen-presenting cells at the tumor cell vaccine site. Tumor-associated antigens are ingested by, for

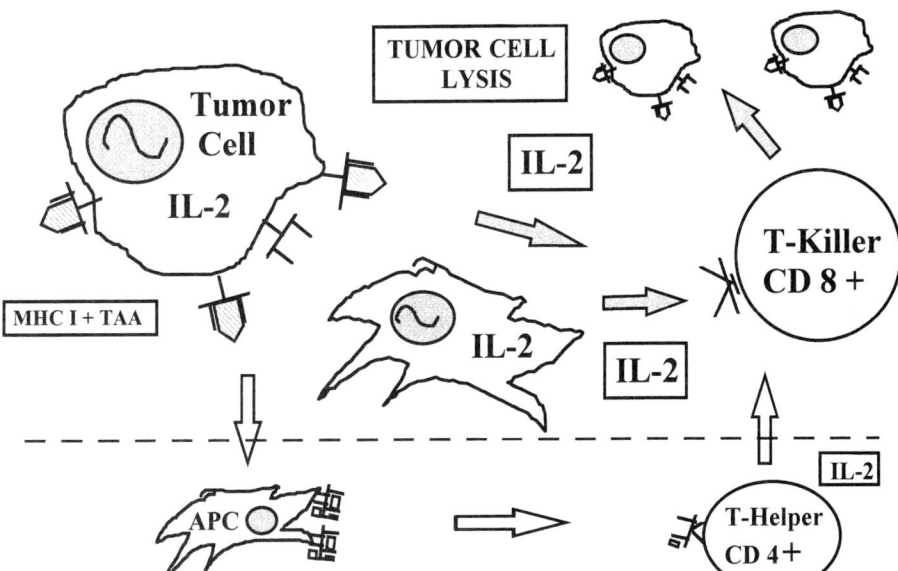

Figure 68-4
The stimulation of antitumor immune reponses by IL-2 gene-modified tumor cell vaccines. Tumor-associated antigen (TAA) in conjunction with MHC class I and IL-2 as secreted by either genetically modified tumor cells or genetically modified fibroblasts stimulates CD8+ helper cells directly. The CD4+ T-helper cell function is being bypassed, because IL-2, one of the main immunostimulatory cytokines generated by CD4+ cells, is produced directly by the genetically modified tumor cell vaccine.

example, macrophages at the tumor cell vaccine site and processed into antigenic fragments. Subsequently, these stimulated macrophages migrate to the local lymph nodes and present antigen to naive T cells. Stimulated, tumor antigen-specific T cells leave the lymph node to systemically circulate and kill distant tumor cells.

Clinical responses using TILs in, for example, ovarian cancer have only shown limited efficacy, mainly because of lack of specificity and/or activity of injected TILs. Attempts are currently being made to increase specificity by redirecting TILs against ovarian cancer cells through specific ligands (Hwu et al, 1993, 1995). A chimeric single-chain antibody–T-cell receptor construct that combines antigen specificity via the variable portion of an antibody recognition site with the signaling components of a T-cell receptor has been used to redirect TILs against ovarian cancer cells. TILs expressing the chimeric protein on the cell surface are subsequently able to recognize tumor-associated antigen on ovarian cancer cells. Upon linking to the appropriate ligand, the TILs are activated via the signaling pathways of the attached T-cell receptor component.

Stimulation of antitumor immune responses against gynecologic malignancies with, for example, genetically modified tumor cell vaccines is a promising gene therapy approach (Dorigo et al, 1997). The stimulation of systemic antitumor immunity has the potential to eradicate metastases at distant sites. Preliminary data from ongoing clinical immuno-gene therapy trials in a variety of cancers indicate that the injection of genetically modified tumor cell vaccines in patients is tolerated without significant toxicity. However, the most effective approaches have yet to be identified.

Treatment of Cervical Cancer

The treatment of stages IIB, IIIB, and IVA cervical carcinoma confined to the pelvis and/or para-aortic lymph nodes was evaluated in a study undertaken by the GOG (Gynecologic Oncology Group, 1983). Radiotherapy to the pelvis was compared with the same therapy plus intravenous C. parvum. The most common and limiting toxicity was moderate to severe chills and fever in the patients receiving C. parvum, along with occasional elevations of the total white blood cell count. In a study of 132 patients taking C. parvum, only 9 patients had no significant adverse effects and dose modification was required in 47 patients. Preliminary analysis of these data suggests that C. parvum does not add any therapeutic effect as an adjuvant to radiotherapy in these patients (Gynecologic Oncology Group, 1983). A Phase I-II trial of intracervical injection of C. parvum in patients with stages IB and IIA carcinoma of the cervix has been reported (Minot et al, 1981). This prospective, randomized trial indicated a relapse rate of only 5% of patients (1 of 22) who received both an intralesional injection of 2 mg of C. parvum 10 days before a radical hysterectomy, compared with 29% of patients (6 of 21 patients) who had a radical hysterectomy only ($p < 0.05$). These data have not been subsequently confirmed, and the incidence of lymph node involvement and lesion size in each group have not been controlled. Although there are theoretical reasons to suggest that it might be an appropriate means of therapy, primarily because of the direct intralesional injection of the agent into a locally grown tumor, other BRMs have not been tested as adjuvants in stage I disease.

Several agents have been used for the treatment of

intraepithelial neoplasia, which can be easily eradicated by the intracervical injection of human leukocyte or fibroblast interferon (Ikic et al, 1981; Moller et al, 1983; Hsu et al, 1984; Choo et al, 1985) and *cis*-retinoic acid (Surwit and Meyskens, 1982). There is some interest as to whether or not these agents might be prophylactic against the development of dysplasia in the cervix.

In addition, 15 patients with invasive squamous cell carcinoma of the cervix (stages IA, IB, and IIA) have been treated with topical human leukocyte IFN 3 weeks before surgery, and 9 these patients also received IFN intramuscularly (Ikic et al, 1981). The authors reported significant tumor shrinkage in six patients and complete disappearance of tumor in three, although accurate tumor dimensions were not reported.

Human Papillomavirus and Cervical Cancer

Human papillomavirus (HPV) infection has been found to be associated with cervical cancer. Approximately 90% of cervical cancer contain HPV DNA, particularly the HPV serotypes 16 and 18 (Munoz et al, 1996). In one study, 137 newly diagnosed cervical cancer patients were evaluated for evidence of HPV infection (Fisher et al, 1996). Elevated antibody titers to HPV 16 E6 and E7 were detected in 16.8% and 32.8% of the women, respectively. Although no difference across disease stage was detected for E6, increasing proportions of positivity to E7 with stage of disease were detected.

Two of the main HPV proteins, E6 and E7, are consistently expressed in tumor cells. The association of carcinoma of the uterine cervix with human papillomavirus suggests that vaccine strategies that target the virus could be useful in the control of disease progression. The immune response might be directed to prevention of infection, to virus-infected cells, and to virally transformed cells (Tindle, 1996).

A live recombinant vaccinia virus expressing the E6 and E7 proteins of HPV 16 and 18 was used in a Phase I/II trial in eight patients with late-stage cervical cancer (Borysiewicz et al, 1996). Vaccination resulted in no significant clinical side effects. All patients mounted an anti-vaccinia antibody response, and three of the eight patients developed an HPV-specific antibody response as a result of the vaccination. HPV-specific cytotoxic T lymphocytes were detected in one of three evaluable patients. Although HPV vaccines might be useful in preventing or even treating cervical cancer, further studies are needed to optimize this strategy and investigate the clinical effectiveness.

Treatment of Vaginal and Vulvar Cancer

Vaginal intraepithelial neoplasia has been shown to regress after local exposure to topical agents. Six

women without evidence of invasive cancer were treated with dinitrochlorobenzene (DNCB) (Guthrie and Way, 1975), and all patients had normal cytology with 2 to 35 months' follow-up. One study (Spirtos et al, 1990) reported a 50% complete response rate in patients with vulvar carcinoma in situ treated with topically applied IFN gel. This experience suggested that the topical IFN was well tolerated and may be less toxic than topical 5-fluorouracil.

Another report (Freedman and Bowen, 1980) studied the use of a virus-modified homologous tumor cell extract in eight patients with invasive vulvar carcinoma and two or more positive groin lymph nodes. The patients were initially vaccinated three times a week and then twice a week for up to 2 years. All patients studied were free of disease 2 to 24 months later, whereas historic controls treated with surgery alone had a median time to recurrence of 14.8 months. Delayed hypersensitivity and antiviral antibody titers were elevated in most patients. These findings have not been confirmed in a controlled study.

Treatment of Gestational Trophoblastic Neoplasia

Although extensive research using immunotherapy has not been performed in patients with gestational trophoblastic neoplasia (GTN), principally because most tumors respond to cytotoxic chemotherapies, the immunobiology of trophoblastic tissue has been the subject of considerable interest. Paternal histocompatibility antigens have been noted to be present in metastatic GTN, and this has prompted the notion that immunotherapy may play a role in the treatment of patients whose tumors are refractory to chemotherapy or as an adjunct in chemotherapy "high-risk" metastatic GTN. One study used systemic immunotherapy with paternal leukocytes in a patient with choriocarcinoma and pulmonary metastases, and a complete response was seen (Cinander et al, 1961). Also, spontaneous regression of metastasis of choriocarcinoma has been reported to occur after surgical resection of the primary tumor, suggesting that cytoreduction may enhance the ability of the host mechanisms to reject metastatic lesions (Goldstein and Berkowitz, 1982).

CONCLUSION

Various immune mechanisms can be involved in effective antitumor responses, including direct cytotoxicity directed against tumor cells, as well as other mechanisms, such as the production of cytotoxic or immune-enhancing lymphokines. Immunotherapy for gynecologic malignancies has been limited in scope and responses. Preliminary studies indicate that immune enhancement leading to tumor rejection can most likely occur when the various biologic response modifiers are brought into direct contact with tumors, when the tumor burden is minimal, such as in an adjuvant setting, and/or when combined with cytotoxic chemotherapy.

Advances in recombinant technology have provided large amounts of relatively pure biologics that can be used for clinical trials. Thus newly described cytokines and monoclonal antibodies can be made available in sufficient quantities to permit appropriate clinical trials of these agents. We are now entering a period of extensive development and testing of these agents both alone and in combination with adoptive immunotherapy.

REFERENCES

Aapro MS, Alberts DS, Salmon SE: Interaction of human leukocyte interferon with vinca alkaloids and other chemotherapeutic agents against human tumors in clonogenic assay. Cancer Chemother Pharmacol 1983;10:161.

Abdulhay G, DiSaia PJ, Blessing JA, Creasman WT: Human lymphoblastoid interferon in the treatment of advanced epithelial ovarian malignancies: a gynecologic oncology group study. Am J Obstet Gynecol 1985;152:418.

Addison CL, Braciak T, Ralston R, et al: Intratumoral injection of an adenovirus expressing interleukin 2 induces regression and immunity in a murine breast cancer model. Proc Natl Acad Sci U S A 1995;92:8522.

Alberts DS, Salmon SE, Moon TE: Chemoimmunotherapy for advanced ovarian carcinoma with adriamycin-cyclophosphamide +/− BCG: early report of a Southwest Oncology Group study. Recent Results Cancer Res 1978;68:160.

Anderson JK, Garber DA, Meaney CA, Breakefield XO: Gene transfer into mammalian central nervous system using herpes virus simplex vectors: extended expression of bacterial lacZ in neurons using the neuron-specific enolase promoter. Hum Gene Ther 1992;3:487.

Aoki T, Kikuchi H, Miyatake S, et al: Interleukin 5 enhances interleukin 2-mediated lymphokine-activated killer activity. J Exp Med 1989;170:583.

Auffray C, Strominger JL: Molecular genetics of the human major histocompatibility complex. Adv Hum Genet 1986;15:197.

Bast RC, Berek JS, Obrist R, et al: Intraperitoneal immunotherapy of human ovarian carcinoma with Corynebacterium parvum. Cancer Res 1983a;43:1395.

Bast RC, Feeney M, Lazarus H, et al: Reactivity of a monoclonal antibody with human ovarian carcinoma. J Clin Invest 1981;68:1331.

Bast RC, Klug T, St. John E, et al: Monitoring growth of human ovarian carcinoma with a radioimmunoassay for antigen(s) defined by a murine monoclonal antibody (OC125). N Engl J Med 1983b;309:883.

Bast RC, Zbar B, Borsos T, Rapp RJ: BCG and cancer. N Engl J Med 1974;290:1413, 1458.

Baum RP, Niesen A, Hertel A, et al: Activating anti-idiotypic human anti-mouse antibodies for immunotherapy of ovarian carcinoma. Cancer 1994;73(3 Suppl):1121.

Baxter RC: The somatomedins: insulin-like growth factors. Adv Clin Chem 1986;25:49.

Benjamini E, Rennick DM, Sell S: Tumor immunology. In Stites DP, Stobo JD, Fudenberg HH, et al (eds): Basic and Clinical Immunology. Los Altos, CA: Lange, 1984:223.

Berek JS: Intraperitoneal adoptive immunotherapy for peritoneal cancer. J Clin Oncol 1990;8:1610.

Berek JS, Bast RC, Hacker NF, et al: Lymphocyte cytotoxicity in the peritoneal cavity and blood of patients with ovarian cancer. Obstet Gynecol 1984a;64:708.

Berek JS, Cantrell JL, Lichtenstein AK, et al: Immunotherapy with biochemically dissociated fractions of Proprionebacterium acnes in a murine ovarian cancer model. Cancer Res 1984b;44:1871.

Berek JS, Hacker NF, Lichtenstein AK, et al: Intraperitoneal recombinant alpha-interferon for salvage immunotherapy in

stage III epthelial ovarian cancer: a Gynecologic Oncology Group study. Cancer Res 1985a;45:4447.

Berek JS, Knapp RC, Hacker NF, et al: Intraperitoneal immunotherapy of epithelial ovarian carcinoma with Corynebacterium parvum. Am J Obstet Gynecol 1985b;152:1003.

Berek JS, Lichtenstein AK, Knox RM, et al: Synergistic effects of combination sequential immunotherapies in a murine ovarian cancer model. Cancer Res 1985c;45:4215.

Berek JS, Welander CE, Schink JC, et al: A Phase I-II trial of intraperitoneal cisplatin and alpha-interferon in patients with persistent epithelial ovarian cancer. Gynecol Oncol 1991;40:237.

Berns KI, Giraud C: Adenovirus and adeno-associated virus as vectors for gene therapy. Ann N Y Acad Sci 1995;772:95.

Bogdan C, Vodovotz Y, Nathan C: Macrophage deactivation by interleukin 10. J Exp Med 1991;174:1549.

Borstein RS, Mastrangelo MJ, Sulit H: Immunotherapy of melanoma with intralesional BCG. Natl Cancer Inst Monogr 1973;39:213.

Borysiewicz LK, Fiander A, Nimako M, et al: A recombinant vaccinia virus encoding human papillomavirus types 16 and 18, E6 and E7 proteins as immunotherapy for cervical cancer [see comments]. Lancet 1996;347:1523.

Boyer CM, Knapp RC, Bast RC: Immunology and immunotherapy. In Berek JS, Hacker NF (eds): Practical Gynecologic Oncology. Baltimore: Williams & Wilkins, 1989a:73.

Boyer P, Berek JS, Zigelboim J: Lymphocyte activation by recombinant interleukin-2 in ovarian cancer patients. Obstet Gynecol 1989b;73:793.

Canevari S, Stoter G, Arienti F, et al: Regression of advanced ovarian carcinoma by intraperitoneal treatment with autologous T lymphocytes retargeted by a bispecific monoclonal antibody. J Natl Cancer Inst 1995;87:1463.

Chapman PB, Kolitz JE, Hakes T, et al: A Phase I trial of intraperitoneal recombinant interleukin-2 in patients with ovarian cancer. Invest New Drugs 1988;6:179.

Chestnut RW, Grey HM: Antigen presentation by B cells and its significance in T-B interactions. Adv Immunol 1986;39:51.

Choo YC, Hsu C, Seto WH, et al: Intravaginal application of leukocyte interferon gel in the treatment of cervical intraperitoneal neoplasia. Arch Gynecol 1985;237:51.

Cinander B, Hayler MA, Rider WD, Warwick OH: Immunotherapy of a patient with choriocarcinoma. Can Med Assoc J 1961;84:306.

Creasman WT, Gall SA, Blessing JA, et al: Chemoimmunotherapy in the management of primary stage III ovarian cancer: a Gynecologic Oncology Group study. Cancer Treat Rep 1979;68:319.

Curiel DT: High-efficiency gene transfer mediated by adenovirus-polylysine-DNA complexes. Ann N Y Acad Sci 1994;716:36; discussion 56.

D'Acquisto R, Markman M, Hakes T, et al: A Phase I trial of intraperitoneal recombinant gamma-interferon in advanced ovarian carcinoma. J Clin Oncol 1988;6:689.

Daar SA, Fuggle SV, Hart DNJ, Dalchau R: Demonstration and phenotypic characterization of HLA-DR-positive interstitial dendritic cells widely distributed in human connective tissues. Transplant Proc 1983;1:311.

Danos O, Mulligan RC: Safe and efficient generation of recombinant retroviruses with aphotropic and ecotroic host range. Proc Natl Acad Sci U S A 1988;85:6460.

Davies JO, Davies ER, Howe K, et al: Radionuclide imaging of ovarian tumors with 123I-labeled monoclonal antibody (NDOG2) directed against placental alkaline phosphatase. Obstet Gynecol 1985;93:277.

de Totero D, Francia di Celle P, Cignetti A, Foa R: The IL-2 receptor complex: expression and function on normal and leukemic B cells. Leukemia 1995;9:1425.

DeFife KM, Jenney CR, McNally AK, et al: Interleukin-13 induces human monocyte/macrophage fusion and macrophage mannose receptor expression. J Immunol 1997;158:3385.

Defrance T, Vanbervliet B, Briere F, et al: Interleukin 10 and transforming growth factor beta cooperate to induce anti-CD40-activated naive human B cells to secrete immunoglobulin A. J Exp Med 1992;175:671.

D'Hondt V, Humblet Y, Guillaume T, et al: Thrombopoietic effects and toxicity of interleukin-6 in patients with ovarian cancer before and after chemotherapy: a multicentric placebo-controlled, randomized Phase Ib study. Blood 1995;85:2347.

Di Giovine FS, Duff GW: Interleukin 1: the first interleukin. Immunol Today 1990;11:13.

Dorigo O, Berek JS: Gene therapy for ovarian cancer—development of novel treatment strategies. Int J Gynecol Cancer 1997;7:1.

Dorigo O, Fakhrai H, Shawler DL, et al: Development of a genetically modified tumor cell vaccine for ovarian cancer using IL-2 gene transfer combined with TGF-β antisense modification. Soc Gynecol Oncol 1997;7:40.

Einhorn N, Cantrell K, Einhorn S, Strander H: Human leukocyte interferon for advanced ovarian carcinoma. Am J Clin Oncol 1982;5:167.

Epenetos AA: Antibody guided lymphangiography in the staging of cervical cancer. Br J Cancer 1985;51:805.

Epenetos AA, Carr D, Johnson PM, et al: Antibody-guided radiolocalization of tumors in patients with testicular or ovarian cancer using two radioiodinated monoclonal antibodies to placental alkaline phosphatine. Br J Radiol 1986a;59:117.

Epenetos AA, Hooker L, Krausz T, et al: Antibody-guided irradiational malignant ascites in ovarian cancer: a new therapeutic method possessing specificity against cancer cells. Obstet Gynecol 1986b;68:715.

Epenetos AA, Shepherd J, Britton K, et al: 123I radioiodinated antibody imaging of occult ovarian cancer. Cancer 1985;55:984.

Ezaki K, Okabe K, Domyo M, et al: Effect of human fibroblast interferon on the cytotoxic activity of natural killer cells and lymphocytes against autochthonous and allogenic tumor cells. Jpn J Cancer Res 1983;74:723.

Fearon ER, Pardoll DM, Itaya T, et al: Interleukin-2 production by tumor cells bypasses T helper function in the generation of an antitumor response. Cell 1990;60:397.

Fiorentino DF, Bond MW, Mosmann TR: Two types of mouse T helper cell. IV. Th2 clones secrete a factor that inhibits cytokine production by Th1 clones. J Exp Med 1989;170:2081.

Fisher SG, Benitez-Bribiesca L, Nindl I, et al: The association of human Papillomavirus type 16 E6 and E7 antibodies with stage of cervical cancer. Gynecol Oncol 1996;61:73.

Fitzgerald DJ, Willingham MC, Pastan I, et al: Antitumor effects of an immunotoxin made with Pseudomonas exotoxin in a nude mouse model of human ovarian cancer. Proc Natl Acad Sci U S A 1986;83:6627.

Flamand V, Sornasse T, Thielemans K, et al: Murine dendritic cells pulsed in vitro with tumor antigen induce tumor resistance in vivo. Eur J Immunol 1994;24:605.

Fossiez F, Djossou O, Chomarat P, et al: T cell interleukin-17 induces stromal cells to produce proinflammatory and hematopoietic cytokines [see comments]. J Exp Med 1996;183:2593.

Freedman RS, Bowen JM: Virus-modified homologous tumor cell extract in the treatment of vulvar cancer. Cancer Immunol Immunother 1980;8:33.

Freedman RS, Gutterman JV, Wharton JT, Rutledge FN: Leukocyte interferon (IFN-a) in patients with epithelial ovarian carcinoma. J Biol Response Mod 1983;2:133.

Freedman RS, Platsoucas CD: Immunotherapy for peritoneal ovarian carcinoma metastasis using ex vivo expanded tumor infiltrating lymphocytes. Cancer Treat Res 1996;82:115.

Gall SA, DiSaia PJ, Schmidt H, et al: Toxicity manifestation following intravenous Corynebacterium parvum administration to patients with ovarian and cervical carcinoma. Am J Obstet Gynecol 1978;132:555.

Garrido MA, Valdayo MJ, Winkler DR, et al: Targeting human T-lymphocytes with bispecific antibodies to react against human ovarian carcinoma cells growing in nu/nu mice. Cancer Res 1990;50:4227.

Gasson JC, Weisbart RH, Kaufman SE, et al: Purified human granulocyte-macrophage colony-stimulating factor: direct action on neutrophils. Science 1984;226:1339.

Gheilmini M, Pettengell R, Coutinho LH, et al: The effect of the GM-CSF/IL-3 fusion protein PIXY321 on bone marrow and circulating haemopoietic cells of previously untreated patients with cancer. Br J Haematol 1996;93:6.

Giri JG, Anderson DM, Kumaki S, et al: IL-15, a novel T cell growth factor that shares activities and receptor components with IL-2. J Leukoc Biol 1995;57:763.

Goldstein DD, Berkowitz RS: Gestational Trophoblastic Neoplasm: Clinical Principles of Diagnosis and Management. Philadelphia: WB Saunders Company, 1982.

Golub SH: Immunological and therapeutic effects of interferon treatment of cancer patients. Clin Immunol Allergy 1984;4:377.

Graham FL, Prevec L: Methods for construction of adenovirus vectors. Mol Biotechnol 1995;3:207.

Graham JB, Graham RM: The effect of vaccine on cancer patients. Surg Gynecol Obstet 1962;114:1.

Granowska M, Britton KE, Shepherd JH, et al: A prospective study of 123I-labelled monoclonal antibody imaging in ovarian cancer. J Clin Oncol 1986;4:730.

Greene WC, Depper JM, Kronke M, Leonard WJ: The human interleukin-2 receptor: analysis of structure and function. Immunol Rev 1986;92:29.

Gregory H: Isolation and structure of urogastrone and its relationship to epidermal growth factor. Nature 1975;257:325.

Grimm EA, Mazumder A, Zhang HZ, Rosenberg SA: The lymphokine activated killer cell phenomenon: lysis of NK resistant fresh solid tumor cells by IL-2 activated autologous human peripheral blood lymphocytes. J Exp Med 1982;155:1823.

Grimm EA, Robb RJ, Roth JA, et al: Lymphokine-activated killer cell phenomenon. III. Evidence that IL-2 is sufficient for direct activation of peripheral blood lymphocytes into lymphokine-activated killer cells. J Exp Med 1983;158:1356.

Guthrie D, Way S: Immunotherapy of non-clinical vaginal cancer. Lancet 1975;2:1242.

Gynecology Oncology Group (GOG): Statistical Report, 1983.

Halpern B: Corynebacterium parvum: Applications in Experimental and Clinical Oncology. New York: Plenum Press, 1975.

Hammersmith Oncology Group and Imperial Cancer Research Fund: Antibody-guided irradiation of malignant lesions: three cases illustrating a new method of treatment. Lancet 1984;1:1441.

Hanna MG, Key ME: Immunotherapy of metastases enhances subsequent chemotherapy. Science 1982;217:367.

Hart DNJ, Fabre JW: Demonstration and characterization of Ia-positive dendritic cells in the interstitial connective tissues of rat heart and other tissues, but not brain. J Exp Med 1981;153:347.

Hart, DNJ, Prickett RCR, McKenzie JL, et al: Characterization of interstitial dendritic ells in human tissues. Transplant Proc 1989;21:401.

Hedrick SM, Cohen DI, Nielsen EA, Davis MM: Isolation of cDNA clones encoding T cell-specific membrane-associated proteins. Nature 1984;308:149.

Herberman RB: Natural Cell-Mediated Immunity Against Tumors. New York: Academic Press, 1980:973.

Hernandez E, Rosenshein NB, Pino y Torres J, et al: IP immunotherapy and chemotherapy in advanced epithelial ovarian cancer. Cancer Treat Rep 1980;66:1981.

Hill CM, Lunec J: The TNF-ligand and receptor superfamilies: controllers of immunity and the Trojan horses of autoimmune disease? Mol Aspects Med 1996;17:455.

Hofland H, Huang L: Inhibition of human ovarian carcinoma cell proliferation by liposome-plasmid DNA complex. Biochem Biophys Res Commun 1995;207:492.

Hood L, Kronenberg M, Hunkapiller T: T cell antigen receptors and the immunoglobulin supergene family. Cell 1985;40:225.

Houssiau FA, Schandene L, Stevens M, et al: A cascade of cytokines is responsible for IL-9 expression in human T cells. involvement of IL-2, IL-4, and IL-10. J Immunol 1995;154:2624.

Hsu C, Choo YC, Seto WH, et al: Exfoliative cytology in the evaluation of interferon treatment of cervical intraepithelial neoplasia. Acta Cytol 1984;28:111.

Hudson CN, Levin L, McHaudy JE, et al: Active specific immunotherapy for ovarian cancer. Lancet 1976;2:877.

Hwu P, Shafer GE, Treisman J, et al: Lysis of ovarian cancer cells by human lymphocytes redirected with a chimeric gene composed of an antibody variable region and the Fc receptor g chain. J Exp Med 1993;178:361.

Hwu P, Yang JC, Cowherd R, et al: In vivo antitumor activity of T cells redirected with chimeric antibody/T-cell receptor genes. Cancer Res 1995;55:3369.

Ikic D, Krusic J, Kirhmajer V, et al: Application of human leukocyte interferon in patients with carcinoma of the uterine cervix. Lancet 1981;9:1027.

Jolly D: Viral vectors systems for gene therapy. Cancer Gene Ther 1994;1:51.

Julliard GJF, Boyer PJ, Yamashiro CH: A Phase I study of active specific intralymphatic immunotherapy (ASILI). Cancer 1978; 41:2215.

Kan EAR, Wang CY, Wang LC, Evans RL: Non-covalently bonded subunits of 22 and 28 Kd are rapidly internalized by T cells reacted with anti-Leu-4 antibody. J Immunol 1983;131:536.

Kehrl JH: Transforming growth factor-beta: an important mediator of immunoregulation. Int J Cell Cloning, 1991;9:438.

Khoo SK, MacKay EV: Immunologic reactivity of female patients with genital cancer: status in preinvasive, locally invasive and disseminated disease. Am J Obstet Gynecol 1974;119:1018.

Kishimoto T, Hirano T: Molecular regulation of B lymphocyte response. Annu Rev Immunol 1988;6:485.

Kohler G, Milstein C: Continuous cultures of fused cells secreting antibody of predefined specificity. Nature 1978;256:495.

Kotzin BL, Benike CJ, Engleman EG: Induction of immunoglobulin secreting cells in the allogenic mixed leukocyte reaction: regulation by helper and suppressor lymphocyte subsets in man. J Immunol 1981;127:931.

Kremer EJ, Perricaudet M: Adenovirus and adeno-associated virus mediated gene transfer. Br Med Bull 1995;51:31.

Kriegler M: Gene Transfer and Expression: A Laboratory Manual. New York: Stockton Press, 1990.

Kuiper M, Peakman M, Farzanek F: Ovarian tumour antigens as potential targets for immune gene therapy. Gene Ther 1995;2:7.

Kunkel SL, Remick DG, Strieter RM, Larrick JW: Mechanisms that regulate the production and effects of tumor necrosis factor-alpha. Crit Rev Immunol 1989;9:93.

Lanzavecchia A: Antigen-specific interaction between T and B cells. Nature 1985;314:537.

Lawrence DA: Transforming growth factor-beta: a general review. Eur Cytokine Network 1996;7:363.

Lichtenstein A, Berek JS, Bast RC, et al: Activation of peritoneal lymphocyte cytotoxicity in patients with ovarian cancer by intraperitoneal treatment with Corynebacterium parvum. J Biol Response Mod 1984;3:1.

Lotze MT: Interleukin 12: cellular and molecular immunology of an important regulatory cytokine: introduction. Ann N Y Acad Sci 1996;795:xiii.

Lotze MT, Chang AE, Seipp CA, et al: High-dose recombinant IL-2 in the treatment of patients with disseminated cancer: responses, treatment related morbidity, and histologic findings. JAMA 1986;256:3117.

Lucey DR, Pinto LA, Bethke FR, et al: In vitro immunologic and virologic effects of interleukin 15 on peripheral blood mononuclear cells from normal donors and human immunodeficiency virus type 1-infected patients. Clin Diagn Lab Immunol 1997;4:43.

Madiyalakan R, Sykes TR, Dharampaul S, et al: Antiidiotype induction therapy: evidence for the induction of immune response through the idiotype network in patients with ovarian cancer after administration of anti-CA125 murine monoclonal antibody B43.13. Hybridoma 1995;14:199.

Mantovani A, Sessa C, Peri G, et al: Intraperitoneal administration of Corynebacterium parvum by chemical fractionation. Int J Immunopharmacol 1981;2:437.

Markowitz D, Goff S, Bank A: Construction and use of a safe and efficient amphotropic packaging cell line. Virology 1988;167: 400.

Marx JL. The T-cell receptor—the genes and beyond. Science 1985;227:733.

Metcalf D: Multi-CSF-dependent colony formation by cells of a murine hemopoietic cell line: specificity and action of multi-CSF. Blood 1985;65:357.

Miller AD: Retroviral vectors. Curr Top Microbiol Immunol 1993; 3:102.

Miller AR, McBride WH, Hunt K, Economou JS: Cytokine-mediated gene therapy for cancer. Ann Surg Oncol 1994;1:436.

Minot MH, Len JW, Drexhage HA, et al: Lower relapse rate after neighborhood injection of Corynebacterium parvum in operable cervix carcinoma. Br J Cancer 1981;44:856.

Moller BR, Johannesen P, Osther K, et al: Treatment of dysplasia of the cervical epithelium with an interferon gel. Obstet Gynecol 1983;62:625.

Munger W, DeJoy SQ, Jeyaseelan R Sr, et al: Studies evaluating the antitumor activity and toxicity of interleukin-15, a new T cell growth factor: comparison with interleukin-2. Cell Immunol 1995;165:289.

Munoz N, Bosch FX: The causal link between HPV and cervical cancer and its implications for prevention of cervical cancer. Bull Pan Am Health Organ 1996;30:362.

Muruhata RI, Cantrell J, Lichtenstein A, Zighelboim J: Disassociation of biological activities of Corynebacterium parvum by chemical fractionation. Int J Immunopharmacol 1980;2:47.

Nardi M, Cognetti F, Pollera CF, et al: Intraperitoneal recombinant alpha-2-interferon alternating with cisplatin as salvage therapy for minimal residual disease ovarian cancer: a Phase II study. J Clin Oncol 1990;8:1036.

Nathan CF, Murray HW, Wiebe ME, Rubin BY: Identification of g-interferon as the lymphokine that activates human macrophage oxidative metabolism and antimicrobial activity. J Exp Med 1983;158:670.

Niloff TM, Knapp RC, Jones G, et al: Recombinant leukocyte alpha interferon in advanced ovarian carcinoma. Cancer Treat Rep 1985;69:895.

Nio Y, Zigelboim J, Berek JS, et al: Augmentation of cytotoxicity of lymphokine-activated killer cells on ovarian tumor cells by various biologic response modifiers. Anticancer Res 1990;10: 441.

Nishimura H, Hiromatsu K, Kobayashi N, et al: IL-15 is a novel growth factor for murine gamma delta T cells induced by Salmonella infection. J Immunol 1996;156:663.

Nisonoff A: Introduction to Molecular Immunology. Oxford, England: Blackwell Scientific, 1982.

Ohkawa K, Ohkawa R: Locoregional immunotherapy and chemotherapy in advanced ovarian cancer cytotoxicity. Asian Oceania Fed Obstet Gynecol 1981;Oct:352.

Order SE, Rosenshein N, Klein JL, et al: The integration of new therapies and radiation in management of ovarian cancer. Cancer 1981;48(2 Suppl):590.

Ortaldo JR, Herberman RB: Heterogeneity of natural killer cells. Annu Rev Immunol 1984;2:359.

Pirker R, Fitzgerald DJP, Hamilton TC, et al: Anti-transferrin receptor antibody linked to Pseudomonas exotoxins as a model immunotoxin in human ovarian carcinoma cell lines. Cancer Res 1985;45:751.

Puyal C, Milhaud P, Bienvenue A, Philippot JR: A new cationic liposome encapsulating genetic material: a potential delivery system for polynucleotides. Eur J Biochem 1995;228:697.

Quesniaux VF, Mayer P, Liehl E, et al: Review of a novel hematopoietic cytokine, interleukin-11. Int Rev Exp Pathol 1993; 34(Pt A):205.

Rambaldi A, Introna M, Colotta F, et al: Intraperitoneal administration of interferon in ovarian cancer patients. Cancer 1985; 56:294.

Rao B, Wanebo HJ, Ochoa M, et al: Intravenous C. parvum: an adujvant to chemotherapy for resistant advanced ovarian carcinoma. Cancer 1977;39:514.

Renauld JC: Interleukin-9: structural characteristics and biologic properties. Cancer Treat Res 1995;80:287.

Renauld JC, Houssiau F, Louahed J, et al: Interleukin-9. Adv Immunol 1993;54:79.

Rink L, Kirchner H: Recent progress in the tumor necrosis factor-alpha field. Int Arch Allergy Immunol 1996;111:199.

Roitt I: Essential Immunology. 6th ed. Oxford, England: Blackwell Scientific, 1988.

Roitt I, Brostoff J, Male D: Immunology. 2nd ed. St. Louis: CV Mosby, 1989.

Rosenberg SA: Adoptive immunotherapy of cancer, accomplishments and prospects. Cancer Treat Rep 1984a;68:233.

Rosenberg SA: Immunotherapy of cancer by systemic administration of lymphoid cells plus interleukin-2. J Biol Response Mod 1984b;3:501.

Rosenberg SA, Lotze MT, Muul LM, et al: Observations on the systemic administration of autologous lymphokine-activated killer cells and recombinant interleukin-2 to patients with metastatic cancer. N Engl J Med 1985;313:1485.

Rosenberg SA, Lotze MT, Muul LM, et al: A progress report on the treatment of 157 patients with advanced cancer using lymphokine-activated killer cells and interleukin-2 or high-dose interleukin-2 alone. N Engl J Med 1987;316:889.

Runowicz CD, Mandeli J, Speyer JL, et al: Phase I/II study of PIXY321 in combination with cyclophosphamide and carboplatin in the treatment of ovarian cancer. Am J Obstet Gynecol 1996;174:1151; discussion 1159.

Sanderson CJ: Interleukin-5: an eosinophil growth and activation factor. Dev Biol Stand 1988;69:23.

Schmolling J, Wagner U, Reinsberg J, et al: [Immune reactions and survival of patients with ovarian carcinomas after administration of 131I-F(Ab)2 fragments of the OC 125 monoclonal antibody]. Geburtshilfe Frauenheilk 1995;55:200.

Schreiber RD, Pace JL, Russell SW, et al: Macrophage-activating factor produced by a T cell hybridoma: physiochemical and biosynthetic resemblance to g-interferon. J Immunol 1983;131:826.

Schroder W, Schwulera U, Lissner R, Bender HG: [Animal experiment, pharmacokinetic and clinical studies of intraperitoneal therapy with interleukin-2 (n Il-2) in patients with ovarian carcinoma]. Gynakologisch-Geburtshilfliche Rundschau, 1995;35(Suppl 1):46.

Schultz RM, Kleinschmidt WJ: Functional identity between murine interferon and macrophage activating factor. Nature 1983;305:239.

Scott J, Urdea M, Quiroga M, et al: Structure of a mouse submaxillary messenger RNA encoding epidermal growth factor and seven related proteins. Science 1983;221:236.

Scott MT: Corynebacterium parvum as an immunotherapeutic anti-cancer agent. Semin Oncol 1984;1:367.

Shawler DL, Dorigo O, Gjerset RA, et al: Comparison of gene therapy with interleukin-2 (IL-2) gene modified fibroblasts and tumor cells in the murine CT-26 model of colorectal carcinoma. J Immunother 1995;17:201.

Shrader JW: The panspecific hemopoietin of activated T lymphocytes (interleukin-3). Annu Rev Immunol 1986;4:205.

Smith KA: Lymphokine regulation of T cell and B cell function. In Paul WE (ed): Fundamental Immunology. New York: Raven Press, 1984:559.

Snapper CM, Finkelman FD, Paul WE: Regulation of IgG1 and IgE production by interleukin 4. Immunol Rev 1988;102:51.

Sobol RE, Shawler DL, Dorigo O, et al: Immunogene therapy of cancer. In Sobol RE, Scanlon KJ (eds): The Internet Book of Gene Therapy. Norwalk, CT: Appleton and Lange, 1995;175.

Souza LM, Boone TC, Gabrilove J, et al: Recombinant human granulocyte colony-stimulating factor: effects on normal and leukemic myeloid cells. Science 1986;232:61.

Spirtos NM, Smith LH, Teng NH: Prospective randomized trial of topical alpha interferon (alpha interferon gels) for the treatment of vulvar intraepithelial neoplasia. Gynecol Oncol 1990;37:34.

Sredni B, Tichler T, Shani A, et al: Predominance of TH1 response in tumor-bearing mice and cancer patients treated with AS101. J Natl Cancer Inst 1996;88:1276.

Stathopoulos GP, Baxevanis CN, Papadopoulos NG, et al: Local immunotherapy with interferon-alpha in metastatic pleural and peritoneal effusions: correlation with immunologic parameters. Anticancer Res 1996;16(6B):3855.

Steinman RM, Cohn ZA: Identification of a novel cell type in peripheral lymphoid organs of mice. I. Morphology, quantitation, tissue distribution. J Exp Med 1973;137:1142.

Steiss RG, Urba WJ, Vander Molen LA, et al: Intraperitoneal lymphokine-activated killer cell and interleukin-2 therapy for malignancies limited to the peritoneal cavity. J Clin Oncol 1990;8:1618.

Stewart WE: The Interferon System. New York: Springer-Verlag, 1979.

Strober W, James SP: The interleukins. Pediatric Res 1988;24:549.

Surwit EA, Meyskens FL: Chemoprevention of intraepithelial neoplasia of the cervix with locally applied beta-trans-retinoic acid: a Phase I/II trial. Proc West Assoc Gynecol Oncol 1982;10:10.

Symonds EM, Perkins AC, Pim MV, et al: Clinical implications for immunoscintigraphy in patients with ovarian malignancy: a preliminary study using monoclonal antibody 791T/36. Br J Obstet Gynaecol 1985;92:270.

Tahara H, Zitvogel L, Storkus WJ, et al: Murine models of cancer cytokine gene therapy using interleukin-12. Ann N Y Acad Sci 1996;795:275.

Tindle RW: Human papillomavirus vaccines for cervical cancer. Curr Opin Immunol 1996;8:643.

Topalian SL, Solomon D, Avis FP, et al: Immunotherapy of patients with advanced cancer using tumor infiltrating lymphocytes and recombinant interleukin 2: a pilot study. J Clin Oncol 1988;6:839.

Unanue ER, Allen PM: The basis for the immunoregulatory role of macrophages and other accessory cells. Science 1987;236:551.

Urba W, Clark JW, Steis RG, et al: Intraperitoneal lymphokine-activated killer cell/interleukin-2 therapy in patients with intra-abdominal cancer: immunologic considerations. J Natl Cancer Inst 1989;81:602.

Valone FH, Kaufman PA, Guyre PM, et al: Clinical trials of bispecific antibody MDX-210 in women with advanced breast or ovarian cancer that overexpresses HER-2/neu. J Hematother 1995;4:471.

Veldhuis GJ, Willemse PH, Beijnen JH, et al: Paclitaxel, ifosfamide and cisplatin with granulocyte colony-stimulating factor or recombinant human interleukin 3 and granulocyte colony-stimulating factor in ovarian cancer: a feasibility study. Br J Cancer 1997;75:703.

Verschraegen CF, Kudelka AP, Termrungruanglert W, et al: Effects of interleukin-1 alpha on ovarian carcinoma in patients with recurrent disease. Eur J Cancer 1996;32A:1609.

Vile R, Russell SJ: Gene transfer technologies for the gene therapy of cancer. Gene Ther 1995;1:88.

Wagner U, Reinsberg J, Schmidt S, et al: Monoclonal antibodies and idiotypic network activation for ovarian carcinoma. Cell Biophys 1994;24–25:237.

Wanebo HJ, Ochoa M: Randomized chemoimmunotherapy trial of CAF and intravenous C. parvum for resistant ovarian cancer—preliminary results. Proc Am Assoc Cancer Res 1977;18:225.

Webb HE, Oaten SW, Pike CP: Treatment of malignant ascitic and pleural effusions with Corynebacterium parvum. Br Med J 1978;1:338.

Welsh RM, Cooper NR, Jensen FC, Oldstone MBA: Human serum lyses RNA tumour viruses. Nature 1975;257:612.

West WH, Tauer KW, Yannelli JR, et al: Constant-infusion recombinant interleukin-2 in adoptive immunotherapy of advanced cancer. N Engl J Med 1987;316:898.

Willemse PHB, DeVries EGE, Aalders JG, et al: Intraperitoneal human recombinant interferon alpha-2b in minimal residual ovarian cancer. Eur J Cancer 1990;26:353.

Williams AF: The T-lymphocyte receptor—elusive no more. Nature 1984;308:108.

Wong GG, Clark SC: Multiple actions of interleukin 6 within a cytokine network. Immunol Today 1988a;9:137.

Wong GG, Witek-Giannotti J, Hewick RM, et al: Interleukin 6: identification as a hematopoietic colony-stimulating factor. Behring Inst Mitteilung 1988b;Aug(83):40.

Yanagi Y, Yoshikai Y, Legget K, et al: A human T cell–specific cDNA clone encodes a protein having extensive homology to immunoglobulin chains. Nature 1984;308:145.

Yao Z, Painter SL, Fanslow WC, et al: Human IL-17: a novel cytokine derived from T cells. J Immunol 1995;155:5483.

Young JW, Steinman RM: Dendritic cells stimulate primary human cytolytic lymphocyte responses in the absence of CD4+ helper cells. J Exp Med 1990;171:1315.

Zapf J, Froesch ER: Insulin-like growth factors/somatomedins: structure, secretion, biological actions and physiological role. Horm Res 1986;24:121.

Ziegler JL, Levy JA: Acquired immunodeficiency syndrome and cancer. Adv Viral Oncol 1985;5:239.

Zighelboim J, Nio Y, Berek JS, Bonavida B: Immunologic control of ovarian cancer. Nat Immun Cell Growth Regul 1988;7:216.

Zinkernagel RM, Doherty PC: MHC-restricted cytotoxic T cells: studies on the biological role of polymorphic major transplantation antigens determining T cell restriction specificity, function, and responsiveness. Adv Immunol 1979;27:51.

Zurawski G, de Vries JE: Interleukin 13 elicits a subset of the activities of its close relative interleukin 4. Stem Cells 1994; 12:169.

69

Palliative Care and End-of-Life Care in Gynecology

Joanna M. Cain

The term *palliative care* conjures up a number of images and definitions. Cicely Saunders (1993) gives a description that embodies the scope of this chapter: "All the work of the professional team—the increasingly skilled symptom control, the supportive nursing, the social work, the home care, and the mobilization of community resources—are to enable the dying person to live until s(he) dies, at (her) own maximum potential, performing to the limit of (her) physical activity and mental capacity with control and independence wherever possible . . . to what has deepest meaning to (her) and end (her) life with a sense of completion."

As physicians and caregivers to women with gynecologic malignancies and fatal diseases, the goals of medicine we aspire to include not only cure of disease, but equally the amelioration of suffering and the quest to bring functional quality of life to the terminal phase of our patients' existence. To do so, we must face the fact that there is a point where further therapy to achieve a "cure" or even a longer term remission is futile. The likelihood of its success are so remote as to be medically implausible. In short, the goal of our treatment is "not merely to cause an effect on some portion of the patient's anatomy, physiology, or chemistry, but to benefit the patient as a whole" (Schneiderman et al, 1990). The focus of care turns to the medical goals of alleviating suffering and symptoms of disease. This is an active affirmation of our role in making the process of dying become a time of purpose for patient and families, of knitting up unraveled edges of life and leaving this life with the sense of completion that Dr. Saunders speaks of. This goal of medicine demands a great deal professionally of physicians—it is often the most technically and personally difficult task we will have as health professionals. It is also the most potentially rewarding.

Some of these women die in an intensive care setting, some on floor care units, some in extended care facilities, some in hospice, and some at home. For each site and with each addition of other disciplines involved in care, the amount of involvement that individual practitioners have in the palliative terminal care of a patient changes. We often find circumstances where initial acute care is given by one physician or team, but palliative terminal care is given by another physician or team. The consequences of this discontinuity of care are difficult to assess for the patient and for the surrounding family unit. As physicians we have variable skills in dealing with the shift of care from acute settings to palliative settings, and variable skills in dealing with the psychosocial context of that change. This chapter is intended to first examine what ethical obligations might be relevant to making choices about terminal, palliative care and, second, to explore what issues are relevant as information and skills for terminal, palliative care for gynecologic-related terminal disease processes.

THE ETHICAL FOUNDATION OF PALLIATIVE, TERMINAL CARE

The choice to focus medical interventions toward palliation rather than cure has a broad basis in medical ethics. Patients have the ethical and legal right to set the goals and specifics of their own medical care (unless it would cause harm to others). Even if they do not have terminal illness, they have the right to refuse treatment or resuscitation as long as they are capable of making such decisions. In order to make decisions and enter into a conversation about the goals of therapy for individual patients, health caregivers must give the patient an accurate understanding of the status and probable progression of her disease. This is one of the most delicate obligations that the profession of medicine carries—to give accurate information at a pace and timing that allows informed decision making by patients. Merely to baldly state that a patient has a fatal illness or that resuscitation efforts will fail and should not be initiated does not discharge this duty. In fact, for some

1497

patients such an approach may be a breach of the obligation to do no harm (nonmaleficence) by leading to reactions that harm the patient (Gillon, 1989; Schade and Muslin, 1989). This discussion is best initiated by eliciting an individual's understanding of her disease process and clarifying with her what the actual status is, over time and with care. It is a discussion held by sitting (not standing) with the patient, with adequate time allotted to complete whatever portion of the discussion meets the needs of the patient at that time. Some patients may not wish to have explicit discussions or may defer their decisions to family members—both are entirely within their rights as patients. The majority, however, want and need accurate information to participate in decision making for terminal care. Because this conversation is emotionally and intellectually taxing, it can be easier to obscure the underlying discussion by offering additional attempts at "cure" without clarifying the likelihood of success. It is often easier to cave in to demands for treatment or resuscitation that are clearly futile by assuaging our discomfort with the offer by identifying a remote possibility that it "might" in some rare event work. As Schneiderman et al (1990) pointed out, "Reports of one or two 'miraculous' successes do not counter the notion of futility, if these successes were achieved against a background of hundreds or thousands of failures." When these exceptionally rare events are pointed to in our rationale for continuing aggressive, "curative" treatment—or even life-extending treatment—it is often the potential for such rare events rather than the fact of such rare events that we identify, leaving us on even more morally perilous grounds.

Respect for autonomy—the right of patients to determine the course of their medical care—demands that we assure that our patients' desires regarding health care are represented beyond their ability to make such choices. That the public also shares this concern is evident in the Patient Self-Determination Act that outlines a hospital admissions-based procedure to assure that advance directives (such as living wills and durable powers of attorney) are identified and placed in the admitted patient's chart or information is offered if no such documents exist (LaPuma et al, 1991). Advance directives are usually encoded in state law and allow individuals to state their preferences for such interventions as cardiopulmonary resuscitation, nutrition, and hydration at the end of life should they not be able to speak for themselves. Durable powers of attorney allow individuals to identify who should make such choices for patients when they are unable to do so for themselves. This is particularly important for elderly patients who may not wish to have their elderly spouse face the burden of making such decisions or whose ability to make such decisions is impaired in some way (Lambert et al, 1990). If such a document exists, the state hierarchy for surrogate decision makers does not apply. Regardless of these documents, however, if a surrogate decision maker must be used for

decision making by the medical team, it must be clear that those decisions must be made in the framework that the patient herself would have made them and for her best interests. Only if there is a serious concern that the surrogate is not representing the best interests of the patient or her framework of decision making should consideration of a court-appointed guardian be entertained, and even then only with extensive efforts to promote such decision-making function in the surrogate.

Finally, a tandem obligation of terminal care is assuring that interventions of no benefit and potential harm, such as cardiopulmonary resuscitation, are not carried out on the patient's behalf. There is no ethical obligation for physicians to offer interventions of no benefit. The hospital setting has become the site of frequent "codes" where the sequenced intervention to restore cardiopulmonary function is applied to individual patients. To present this intervention, do-not-attempt-resuscitation (DNAR) policies have been promulgated; each individual hospital has differing policies, including whether or not a DNAR policy exists in the operating theater. The initiation of such DNAR orders when the predictable outcome of resuscitation is immediate failure or success with return to a painful (now even more so) and fatal condition adds to the burden of suffering for the patient and her family (Cohen and Cohen, 1996; Snider, 1991).

MANAGING PAIN

The most feared aspect of dying is rarely death itself, but always the pain that might be experienced. The assurance and demonstration that an individual patient's health caregiver will aggressively pursue the best of pain control on her behalf in itself alleviates suffering by decreasing fear. Pain control, however, is not to be undertaken lightly, nor is it something to be left to rare appointments for management. It is often more demanding than any other aspect of care. Unfortunately, the major cause of pain at the end of life is undermedication or underutilization of pain control resources by physicians.

The tenets of pain control are relatively simple. The physician can start with a careful elucidation of the type or types of pain and the amount the individual is experiencing and then follow the World Health Organization pain control ladder in addressing it. Were it this simple, however, pain control would be absolute for all patients at all times. It is often the side effects of the various drugs and treatments used balanced against the particular goals of a patient and the quality of her life that becomes the pivotal elements for success, so a clear understanding of the goals and values of the patient are critical to success. Is it acceptable to be less ambulatory if clarity is preserved? Is attendance at a wedding so critical a goal that any therapy that lessens the patient's ambulatory status is unacceptable? Can it be

Table 69–1. CLINICAL APPROACH TO PAIN MANAGEMENT

A	*Ask about pain regularly.* *Assess pain systematically.*
B	*Believe the patient and family in their reports of pain and what relieves it.*
C	*Choose pain control options appropriate for the patient, family, and setting.*
D	*Deliver interventions in a timely, logical, and coordinated fashion.*
E	*Empower patients and their families.* *Enable them to control their course to the greatest extent possible.*

From Jacox A, Carr DB, Payne R, et al: Management of Cancer Pain (Clinical Practice Guideline No. 9; AHCPR Publication No. 94-1592). Rockville, MD: Agency for Health Care Policy and Research, 1994.

managed at home by the caregivers she has access to? These are all important elements in the choice of pain control.

To identify and treat pain successfully, the routine clinical approach summarized by the mnemonic "ABCDE" is best (Table 69–1) (Jacox et al, 1994). Pain may be a product of local tumor progression or local tissue damage (nociceptive pain), it may be the product of nerve injury (neuropathic), or it may be simply a case of lack of use—such as muscle atrophy with chronic limitation of mobility. The elucidation of the type of pain can be helpful in the choice of therapy. The initial pain assessment is critical to this approach and must be repeated when new pain symptoms appear—it cannot be assumed they arise from the same source as the previous pain. An appreciation of the type of pain described is also critical for therapy (Table 69–2).

The choice of therapy for individual patients *must* be individualized based on this careful review of the pain experienced and its likely cause. It is always best to start with an oral medication, the simplest dosage schedule, and the least invasive and lowest side effect modality first. Maximal management of pain may require rapid ascent up the World Health Organization ladder (Ventafridda et al, 1990; Grond et al, 1991), steady increases in narcotic medications to levels far above those used for standard postoperative pain, and consideration of multiple alternatives and combinations to treat an individual pattern of pain initially and as it changes through the course of disease. There is *no* place in the management of pain for the terminal patient for inadequate pain relief based on concerns about "addiction," or for trials of placebos.

All pain treatment strategies should utilize an around-the-clock and by-the-clock pattern with additional "as needed" doses for breakthrough pain. For mild to moderate pain, nonsteroidal anti-inflammatory drugs (NSAIDs), acetaminophen, or aspirin may be adequate. If not, the next step up the ladder adds opioids such as codeine or hydrocodone to these drugs. These combinations are limited by the side effects and dose limitations of the nonopioids—so the next step would focus on increasing opioid potency and/or dosages. If oral pain medication can be tolerated, sustained-release morphine on an every-12-hour basis with additional rapid release for breakthrough pain may be the best solution. Analysis of the patient's requirements for breakthrough pain control will allow for adjustment of the base regimen, including the consideration of increase in dose or decrease in interval to every 8 hours if breakthroughs consistently occur near the end of the dose. The last steps include invasive procedures such as periodic or permanent nerve root destruction (Table 69–3).

Table 69–2. PAIN DESCRIPTIONS AND ASSOCIATED THERAPIES

DESCRIPTION	TYPE OF PAIN	TREATMENT APPROACH
Constant burning pain, often dysesthesia	Peripheral nerve damage	Anticonvulsant or antidepression class
Painful paresthesias, hyporeflexia	Chemotherapy (taxol, cisplatin, vinca alkaloids) nerve damage	Same
Shock-like paroxysmal pain, burning, constant aching, paresthesia and dysesthesia	Acute and chronic postherpetic neuropathy	Same for chronic syndrome Antiviral therapy for acute WHO pain scale for analgesia
Sharp, deep, persistent postoperative pain	Tissue damage	R/O other acute treatable sources of pain (e.g., obstruction, infection) WHO pain scale for analgesia Consider epidural or nerve block if needed
Pelvic and groin pain, aching, occasionally burning, occasionally sharp	Tissue and nerve damage (usually related to progressive malignancy; can also be post–high-dose radiation)	Same as above, but more likely to require continuous epidural or nerve block for progressive disease and pain syndromes
Localized pinpoint pain, intercostal or abdominal	Single nerve or group with peripheral damage (possibly postoperative)	Local nerve (area) infiltration Nerve block if unresolved

Abbreviations: R/O, rule out; WHO, World Health Organization.

Table 69-3. STEPS TO PAIN CONTROL AND PROBLEMS OF METHODS

CATEGORY/STEP/COST	LEVEL OF PAIN	PROBLEMS
Oral analgesics (NSAIDs, aspirin, acetaminophen): step I ($ to $$$$)	Mild to moderate	Side effects of different members limit use (bleeding, gastritis, renal toxicity)
Oral opioids (codeine, hydrocodone): step II ($$)	Moderate: use round the clock, may need second for rescue	Constipation, sedative effects (can be benefit)
Transdermal opioids (fentanyl): step II–III ($$$$)	Moderate to severe: adjunct or replace oral if needed	Long duration, slow onset—must use other backup over first 3 days at least
Rectal opioids: step II ($$)	Same	Local trauma (could be considered through stoma)
Subcutaneous/IV infusions: step II–III ($$$$)	Severe pain: rapid relief and titration; for problems with oral route therapy	Infection, difficulty in using method in home setting, usual opioid side effects
Invasive techniques ($$$$$$)	Intractable pain: include epidural, intrathecal, regional, and ablative techniques	Infection, urinary retention, irreversible, special expertise required, may increase need for specialized caregivers

Neuropathic pain is particularly resistant to opioid medications, although an initial trial is warranted (Asbury and Fields, 1984; Portenoy, 1991). Trials of antidepressants or anticonvulsants, which may significantly improve the pain, need to be undertaken with caution because of the potential for increased side effects with liver dysfunction, renal dysfunction, and mental disorientation of the patient. Transcutaneous electrical nerve stimulation units may provide additional short-term relief. However, if the neuropathic pain is resistant to all these approaches, long-term relief may require invasive methods.

Two particularly difficult areas of pain problems are pelvic pain and abdominal pain associated with ascites with or without bowel obstruction. Pelvic pain can be neuropathic, originating with involvement of the sacral plexus and from local pressure (nociceptive) and spasm of bowel or bladder in the area. Opioids may help, but addition of calcium channel blockers as antispasmodic agents could also be considered (Castell, 1985). Neuropathic perineal pain that is unresponsive to these measures might be well treated by a saddle block. For both sites, visceral pain, which can stimulate autonomic reflexes that add to already existent nausea and terminal weakness, can be the most difficult to treat. Relief of bowel obstruction or ascites, if technically possible, may decrease this pain somewhat. Because this type of pain is generally widespread, the best approach is opioid use coupled with antinausea regimens.

Adjuvant approaches to pain control with imagery, biofeedback, relaxation techniques, hypnosis, and even music or art therapy may all improve the overall pain control achieved by pharmacologic means and should be encouraged. However, although the relaxation or distraction provided by these methods may be of some value, the additive effect of these approaches in treating pain itself may not be significant (Syrjala et al, 1995).

GASTROINTESTINAL-BASED PALLIATIVE CARE NEEDS

Nausea and Vomiting

The majority of needs for control of nausea and vomiting are related to obstruction or peritoneal irritation related to the gynecologic process. Anorexia is a usual companion to nausea and vomiting, but may additionally require palliation for some patients. There are relatively few studies that document the prevalence and prevention of these symptoms in a palliative care setting, although one study suggests up to 60% of patients will have such symptoms (Dunlop, 1989).

There are two potential mechanisms for emesis and nausea, the leading theory being an emetic center (Andrews and Hawthorne, 1988); however, a description of the sequence of events may provide a better illustration of the mechanisms and pathway. The majority of nausea in terminal gynecologic patients is from peripheral stimuli. It is rare that nausea and vomiting as terminal problems are related to central disease, such as brain metastasis, in gynecology. However, the central triggering of the emetic center can be from fear and anxiety, metabolic problems, afferent stimulation from bowel obstruction, or drugs (such as for pain relief) themselves. These stimulate the limbic system, cortex, and chemoreceptor trigger zone and begin the sequence. Gastric stasis and radiation stimulate both central and peripheral structures. The peripheral triggers can be anywhere from the taste buds through the gastrointestinal mucosa, smooth muscle, and nerve endings in the peritoneal cavity. The neurophysiology of emesis is multisequential, and occasionally a part of the sequence is missed.

Therapy depends on the etiology of the problem,

so the hallmark of good palliative care—the careful history and physical—is just as necessary here. This should include the entire alimentary tract as well as consideration of central lesions, although rare. Poor oral hygiene with thrush or herpes simplex infection should receive direct treatment for the infection. Alteration of taste, common with cytotoxic chemotherapy agents (such as cisplatin) may require careful nutritional counseling and trial and error to overcome. Ruling out gastric irritation from other medications (e.g., NSAIDs) is also important in evaluation. Bowel obstruction and site of obstruction (high or low) will have an impact on the methods used for relief of emesis, and clarity about site and type of obstruction is an important element of the history and physical examination.

Bowel obstruction, if complete, may be amenable to surgical relief if the patient is an appropriate candidate both temporally (she will survive long enough to benefit from the surgery) and medically (Chan and Woodruff, 1992; Markman, 1995). Additionally, distal obstructions may be amenable to endoscopic therapy (Rupp et al, 1995; Tan et al, 1995). Bowel obstruction in the terminal phase can be particularly difficult to treat, if not surgically correctable. Not only must nausea and vomiting related to sympathetic afferent stimulation be dealt with, but the modalities for therapy (tolerance of oral medication) are limited as well. In some studies butyrophenones (haloperidol) and phenothiazines (prochlorperazine, chlorpromazine) were effective antiemetics without concurrent nasogastric suction (Baines et al, 1985). Additionally, octreotide has been reported to be of benefit as a single agent in bowel obstruction in terminal ovarian cancer (Mangili et al, 1996). Smooth muscle relaxants such as hyoscine hydrobromide may help relieve the crampy discomfort that triggers the emesis reflex. Antihistamines (promethazine) also may be effective. Although metoclopramide and ondansetron are staples of chemotherapy-induced nausea therapy, it is worthwhile remembering that they have a gastrokinetic effect that may compound the symptoms rather than relieve symptoms from bowel obstruction. If at all possible, avoidance of the placement of a nasogastric tube will allow the patient more mobility and less local irritation. For many patients, occasional emesis is more acceptable than a nasogastric or gastrostomy tube, and the option should be considered with the patient's input. If the obstruction is high, however, the only feasible option may be some form of venting procedure (Baines, 1994).

For nausea related to metabolic causes—most often uremia or electrolyte imbalances in this population—a central sedative to diminish neurologic irritability may be appropriate. Correction of electrolyte imbalances or uremia directly to decrease nausea must be balanced against the temporal benefits and alterations in quality of life for such things as nephrosotomies or intravenous lines when not otherwise required. Trials of IV hydration or reple-

tion may be appropriate to assess the proportion of the nausea referable to electrolyte imbalance. If no benefit can be assessed, then further IV therapy has little value. The idea that nutrition and hydration may be unnecessary forms of therapy for terminal care in and of themselves has both ethical and clinical research support ("American College of Physicians," 1992; Burge, 1993; McCann et al, 1994). Of particular interest is the study by McCann et al, who documented the loss of normal appetite in dying patients and the concurrent lack of hunger in this group. Thirst and dry mouth were adequately relieved by mouth care and sips of liquids, and no quality-of-life benefit could be derived from more aggressive attempts to rehydrate or to increase food intake beyond the amount desired by the individual.

Constipation

Constipation alone can be a source of discomfort and emesis. Considering the multitude of constipating medications used for pain symptom relief, particularly opioids, it is a common problem in palliative care (Sykes, 1994). The best approach is prevention with a laxative protocol begun concurrently with pain control. This must be understood to be as important as any other palliative care regimen, and the therapy escalated as needed. Regularity of diet and activity or changes in both need to be considered in developing such a regimen. For example, if a patient is taking decreasing amounts of fluids, a bulk stool softener is more likely to harm than help because of the lack of water.

Gastrointestinal Bleeding and Tumor-Related Hemorrhage: Interventional Radiology Versus Transfusions

The primary means of addressing gastrointestinal bleeding is through interventional radiology or transfusion. The choice to intervene must again be made by clarifying the goals of intervention. If there is gastrointestinal bleeding from radiation injury or direct tumor progression, and there is an expectation that resolution would return the patient to a stable and adequate quality of life, then consideration for interventional embolization would be appropriate (Broadley et al, 1995; Jones, 1995). Transfusion itself can have palliative benefits by addressing weakness, respiratory problems, and an overall sense of well-being in similar settings. Furthermore, transfusion, rather than interventional embolization, may be the best option with chronic low-grade bleeding problems (Gleeson and Spencer, 1995). Transfusion merely for decreased red blood cell mass, however, without concurrently addressing symptoms referable to the anemia, is questionable in the palliative care setting. Similar arguments apply to the use of platelet transfusions.

RESPIRATORY SYMPTOMS

Problems of air hunger and difficulty breathing can be the most distressing symptomatology faced by patients and families. The common problems in gynecology include airflow obstruction with local compression from direct tumor infiltration or nodal disease as well as diminished volumes for oxygen exchange produced by conditions such as pleural effusions, pulmonary edema, or pulmonary embolism. These conditions are often superimposed on pulmonary problems of long standing, such as emphysema or asthma, not only compounding the respiratory status problems but altering the pain management needs by causing pleural pain as well. Evaluation of the patient should include chest radiography if pleural effusion or edema secondary to heart failure is suspected. Additional studies such as ventilation-perfusion scans, oxygen saturation measurements, or pulmonary function tests are dependent upon the present status of the patient and the potential for symptomatic relief and benefit from treating the condition being pursued. For example, if a pulmonary embolus is suspected but there is no intention to treat with anticoagulation, there is no value in a ventilation-perfusion scan.

Both pleural and pericardial effusions (leading to cardiac failure and secondary pulmonary compromise) have the potential for treatment. Pleural effusion can be managed by simple aspiration on an intermittent basis if survival time is limited. If a more durable solution is required, pleurodesis is the appropriate procedure, with a good response rate (McAlpine et al, 1990). For pericardial effusions, although rare with gynecologic malignancies, sclerosis and the surgical creation of a window may be appropriate in some patients.

Therapy is generally directed toward the underlying causes of dyspnea. For airway sensitivity, bronchodilators or corticosteroids may be helpful. For heart failure, diuretics, digoxin, or other interventions may be helpful. When all the underlying causes are maximally treated, however, the only alternative left for the suffering of awareness of air hunger is some form of respiratory sedative. Unfortunately, many of the drugs that maximally impact the awareness of air hunger also depress respiratory drive themselves. The balance must be carefully individualized. Opioids are the most widely used in the control of dyspnea. Not all opioids are effective, however. Dihydrocodeine is, but codeine itself is not. Morphine is particularly effective; however, results of studies focused on individuals with chronic obstructive pulmonary disease may not directly translate for oncology patients (Light et al, 1989). Morphine is also helpful with oxygen and benzodiazepines for episodes of respiratory panic. Additional research in the area of management of terminal dyspnea and respiratory distress is needed and would benefit patients and their families significantly (Davis, 1994).

At the very end of life, the "death rattle" of hypoventilation and lack of ability to clear respiratory mucus and fluids is distressing to family and staff. It is rare that this has an impact on the patient, who is usually semiconscious. Hyoscine or atropine and gentle suction may be adequate to eliminate this.

HYPERCALCEMIA/BONE PAIN

Although rare, hypercalcemia and bone pain can occur with gynecologic malignancies, including choriocarcinoma, melanoma, cervical cancers (all grades and types), endometrial cancers, and rarely ovarian cancers. In addition, local extension to the bone (e.g., vulvar cancer) may be the major source of pain. For bony disease, options include local radiation (Maher et al, 1992), which is quite effective when adequate local doses can be delivered, as well as the use of isotopes such as strontium-89 (Nightengale et al, 1995). Strontium-89, a calcium analog, can be injected intravenously and is rapidly cleared from the bloodstream to deposit primarily in metastatic sites in the bone—thereby delivering very local radiation and sparing normal bone. Given the previous exposure to chemotherapeutic agents and radiation in many of these patients, the potential for bystander impact on stem cells requires monitoring complete blood counts.

Hypercalcemia from bone destruction and decreased renal clearance is a rare complication of gynecologic malignancies. Furthermore, the comments regarding the benefits of normalizing electrolytes pertain here—correction of hypercalcemia is of value if the patient has time to enjoy an increased quality of life, but not if the remaining life is a short time of increased pain. The standard initial approach is intravenous hydration with the use of bisphosphonates to provide a stable fall in calcium over a few days. Failures with this regimen may warrant further intervention with calcitonin. The use of mithramycin has been virtually replaced by the bisphosphonates because of the associated cumulative nephrotoxicity, thrombocytopenia, and nausea as well as the potential for hepatotoxicity with mithramycin. This intervention should be reserved for circumstances where other efforts fail.

LOCAL CARE ISSUES: SKIN AND ORAL HEALTH

Although the issues outlined heretofore are ones commanding greater physician intervention, the issues of oral and skin care are often the most vexing and difficult for caregivers. Problems with cutaneous metastases, poorly fitted ostomy appliances, pressure sores, lymphedema, or simply the odor of necrotic tissue are the elements of daily living that prevent families and patients from achieving the best life that can be had in the terminal phase of the disease process.

Fungating metastatic skin lesions may be treated with local electron beam therapy, excision, or local care. Local care should be as simple as possible—such as normal saline wash and nontraumatic dressing. The alginate dressings manufactured from seaweed react with tissue fluids to provide a gel-like coating that allows for easy removal, yet still absorbs a significant amount of exudate.

Fistulas, particularly enterocutaneous fistulas, can result in skin damage with ulceration and chronic infection in addition to the loss of electrolytes and fluid with high fistulas. The first approach is to work with a stoma therapist to facilitate the best application of an appliance that can be found. The usual stoma care patterns apply, with careful skin cleaning, drying, and application of local antifungal therapy as necessary before applying the appliance. Odor control during changing and around dressings is a major palliative care concern because the odors not only are unpleasant but can themselves stimulate the emetic center. Use of stomal deodorants, charcoal tablets, or aromatherapy oils may all help alleviate this problem (Miller et al, 1993).

A special problem of pelvic malignancy progression is perineal drainage from vesicovaginal or rectovaginal extensions of tumor. Surgical diversion to a colostomy for rectal fistula is generally well tolerated. Urinary diversions generally are more physically demanding surgery for the patient and have had a smaller role in management of urinary tract fistulas. Proximal diversion with nephrostomies may occasionally be warranted. Local care of the skin, with copious and frequent irrigation with normal saline, and efforts to allow diverting drainage with Foley or suprapubic catheters or continuous suction may all be required to bring some measure of comfort for this difficult problem.

Lymphadema is a difficult problem with many roots in gynecologic palliative care. Radiation or surgery to groin and pelvic lymph node chains can impact lymphatic flow. Local pelvic compression from progressive malignancy can decrease return flow. Finally, low serum proteins with chronic wasting can impact tissue swelling and cause aggravation of existing lymphadema. Fluid restriction and diuretics generally give minimal assistance. Local therapy such as gentle massage and compression bandages and hosiery specifically designed for graduated compression are the most helpful. Passive movement in bed, if ambulation is not possible, can also aid in management.

THE LAST DAYS OF LIFE

The last days of life are usually marked by intensification in comfort care. Pain needs to be continually assessed and local measures for pain from specific sites (bedsores, bladder discomfort) needs to be ag-

gressively pursued. About half of patients will experience new pain, different from previously treated pain, in the last day of life, and increase in pain medication is likely (Lichter and Hunt, 1990). Terminal restlessness is disturbing to the patient and those attending her. Alternatives include methotrimeprazine IM as well as benzodiazepines (subcutaneous midazolam may be particularly helpful, and is the drug of choice if delirium is absent) and anticonvulsants for muscle twitching and jerking (Enck, 1992). Acute exacerbation of respiratory symptoms may also occur, with panic that could be alleviated with a rapid-acting anxiolytic and encouragement to breathe slowly and deeply. If the last few hours of life are to occur at home, adequate planning for anticipated changes and crises must happen beforehand. At no time should families be left to their own devices with no ability to address changes in pain or other symptoms and no access to help. Furthermore, if it is clear to all concerned that the best symptom control could be achieved by hospital admission, this should be available for the patient and her family. At the end of life, the only goal of medicine to be achieved may be the relief of suffering for the patient and family, supplemented by the knowledge that the physician and the health caregivers will not desert them—even if no active intervention other than support is medically required.

PSYCHOSOCIAL ASPECTS OF PALLIATIVE CARE

Approach to the Patient

It is common in terminal care that hope and despair alternate during the terminal phase (Doyle, 1993). There is often a significant element of depression, which can be treated pharmacologically but also warrants attention to clarifying any issues of confusion about the future course of disease and identifying what goals a patient might reasonably meet. It is a time to be clear about expected symptoms or problems, what the response to those problems might be, and what cannot be treated. Furthermore, it is important to address where terminal care should be given and what resources—financial and caregiver—can be mobilized in each site. The majority of patients would prefer to be cared for at home (Townsend et al, 1990), but disease progression and symptomatology may progress too rapidly for adequate support to be established—further supporting the need for careful planning prospectively. Additional issues such as insurance coverage for respite care, hospice care, stabilization of pain control, and adequate provision of at-home health caregivers continue to vex the most careful planning process. The greater the time for planning before the most labor- and emotion-intensive period of terminal care, the more likely the barriers to adequate at-home care at the end of life will be overcome (Rhymes, 1991).

Obligations to Families, Intimate Others, and Health Care Providers

With dying patients, the goals of medicine are clearly focused on the relief of pain and suffering. The experience of suffering is far more than simply the experience of a constellation of symptoms. It is the individual interpretation of those symptoms and the environment and social network that impact on that interpretation that produce suffering. The interplay between the individual and her support environment is critical to alleviating suffering at the end of life and the individual's ability to achieve her terminal goals. Furthermore, there is an increasing recognition that, although respect for an individual's right to make choices regarding her own medical care (the principle of autonomy) has held a dominant position in medical ethics, those choices can have harmful influences on the surrounding family. The converse is also true, that families can have adverse effects on the individual's ability to choose.

The recognition that the context of decision making and daily living rarely consists of the individual alone has increasingly raised the issue of what role families and social networks can and should have in the decision-making process and what obligations these ties imply for health caregivers to families and intimate others themselves. It is not uncommon that, with a semiconscious patient, the goal of medicine to be achieved might be a sense of completion and closure for the family members of the patient as well as for the individual herself. How families grieve and how they participate in care decisions are surprisingly poorly researched (Kissane et al, 1996a, 1996b). Yet, "Grief, an experience confronting all of us as individuals and, of necessity, our families, is a process of adjustment in which the growth of everyone involved can be facilitated. On the other hand, failure to grieve in an adaptive manner potentially paves the way for substantial morbidity" (Kissane et al, 1996a). This is also true of health caregivers, including physicians. As Mount (1996) points out "The weight of . . . repeated losses may lead to a burden that is increasingly intolerable and frequently difficult to define," with real consequences in the lives of health caregivers for their own marriages, drug addictions, or creation of cynicism and personal devaluation. For all these reasons, health caregivers may find themselves in the position of treating terminal conditions that do not directly impact the individual dying but impact those staying, such as quieting "death rattles" or prolonging mechanical ventilation to allow a child to say a final good bye to a parent.

The duty we owe to the patient extends to a degree to those who care about and care for that individual. It is a societal duty to assure that, in managing the terminal phase of one individual's illness, we also practice disease prevention for those who stay after that individual is gone. There are, of course, cost limits on this approach arising from the same obligation to the greater good (societal well-being). However, limited interventions to this end will undoubtedly have long-term health benefits for society and should be considered within the scope of obligations of physicians caring for the dying patient.

REFERENCES

American College of Physicians Ethics Manual, Third Edition. Ann Intern Med 1992;117:947.
Andrews PL, Hawthorne J: The neurophysiology of vomiting. Baillieres Clin Gastroenterol 1988;2:141.
Asbury AK, Fields HL: Pain due to peripheral nerve damage: an hypothesis. Neurology 1984;34:1587.
Baines MJ: Intestinal obstruction. Cancer Surv 1994;21:147.
Baines M, Oliver DJ, Carter RL: Medical management of intestinal obstruction in patients with advanced malignant disease. Lancet 1985;339:990.
Broadley KE, Kurowska A, Dick R, et al: The role of embolization in palliative care. Palliat Med 1995;9:331.
Burge FI: Dehydration symptoms of palliative care cancer patients. J Pain Symptom Manage 1993;8:454.
Castell DO: Calcium channel blocking agents for gastrointestinal disorders. Am J Cardiol 1985;55:210B.
Chan A, Woodruff R: Intestinal obstruction in patients with widespread intraabdominal malignancy. J Pain Symptom Manage 1992;7:339.
Cohen CB, Cohen PJ: Do-not-resuscitate orders in the operating room. Anesthesiology 1996;85:1190.
Davis CL: The therapeutics of dyspnoea. Cancer Surv 1994;21:85.
Doyle D: The stages of dying—a new conceptual framework. In Doyle D, Hanks G, MacDonald N (eds): Oxford Textbook of Palliative Medicine. Oxford, England: Oxford University Press, 1993:51.
Dunlop GM: A study of the relative frequency and importance of gastrointestinal symptoms and weakness in patients with far advanced cancer. Palliat Med 1989;4:37.
Enck RE: The last few days. Am J Hosp Palliat Care 1992;July/August:11.
Gillon R: Deciding not to resuscitate. J Med Ethics 1989;15:171.
Gleeson C, Spencer D: Blood transfusion and its benefits in palliative care. Palliat Med 1995;9:307.
Grond S, Zech D, Schug SA, et al: Validation of World Health Organization guidelines for cancer pain relief during the last days and hours of life. J Pain Symptom Manage 1991;6:411.
Jacox A, Carr DB, Payne R, et al: Management of Cancer Pain (Clinical Practice Guideline No. 9; AHCPR Publication No. 94-1592). Rockville, MD: Agency for Health Care Policy and Research, 1994.
Jones SN: Interventional radiology in a palliative care setting. Palliat Med 1995;9:319.
Kissane DW, Bloch S, Dowe DL, et al: The Melbourne Family Grief Study, I: perceptions of family functioning in bereavement. Am J Psychiatry 1996a;53:650.
Kissane DW, Bloch S, Onghena P, et al: The Melbourne Family Grief Study II: psychosocial morbidity and grief in bereaved families. Am J Psychiatry 1996b;153:659.
Lambert P, Gibson JM, Nathanson P: The values history: an innovation in surrogate medical decision-making. Law Med Health Care 1990;18:202.
LaPuma J, Orentlicher D, Moss RJ: Advance directives on admission: clinical implication and analysis of the Patient Self-determination Act of 1990. JAMA 1991;266:402.
Lichter I, Hunt E: The last 48 hours of life. J Palliat Care 1990;6:7.
Light RW, Muro JR, Sato RI, et al: Effects of oral morphine on breathlessness and exercise tolerance in patients with chronic obstructive pulmonary disease. Am J Respir Dis 1989;139:126.
Maher EJ, Coia L, Duncan G, Lawton PA: Treatment strategies in advanced and metastatic cancer: differences in attitude between the USA, Canada and Europe. Int J Radiat Oncol Biol Phys 1992;23:239.

Mangili G, Franchi M, Mariani A, et al: Octreotide in the management of bowel obstruction in terminal ovarian cancer. Gynecol Oncol 1996;61:345.

Markman M: Surgery for support and palliation in patients with malignant disease. Semin Oncol 1995;22:91.

McAlpine LG, Hulks G, Thomson NC: Management of recurrent malignant pleural effusion in the United Kingdom: survey of clinical practice. Thorax 1990;45:699.

McCann RM, Hall WH, Groth-Juncker A: Comfort care for terminally ill patients: the appropriate use of nutrition and hydration. JAMA 1994;272:1263.

Miller CM, O'Neill A, Mortimer PS: Skin problems in palliative care: nursing aspects. In Doyle D, Hanks G, MacDonald (eds): Oxford Textbook of Palliative Medicine. Oxford, England: Oxford University Press, 1993:395.

Mount BM: Dealing with our losses. J Clin Oncol 1986;4:1127.

Nightengale B, Brune M, Blizzard SP, et al: Strontium chloride Sr 89 for treating pain from metastatic bone disease. Am J Health Syst Pharm 1995;52:2890.

Portenoy RK: Issues in the management of neuropathic pain. In Basbaum A, Besson JM (eds): Towards a New Pharmachotherapy of Pain. New York: John Wiley & Sons, 1991:393.

Rhymes JA: Home hospice care. Clin Geriatr Med 1991;7:803.

Rupp KD, Dohmoto M, Meffert R, et al: Cancer of the rectum—palliative endoscopic treatment. Eur J Surg Oncol 1995;32:644.

Saunders C: Foreword. In Doyle D, Hanks G, MacDonald N (eds): Oxford Textbook of Palliative Medicine. Oxford, England: Oxford University Press, 1993:8.

Schade S, Muslin H: Do not resuscitate decisions: discussion with patients. J Med Ethics 1989;15:186.

Schneiderman LJ, Jecker NS, Jonsen AR: Medical futility: its meaning and ethical implications. Ann Intern Med 1990;112: 949.

Snider GL: The do-not-resuscitate order: ethical and legal imperative or medical decision? Am Rev Respir Dis 1991;143:665.

Sykes NP: Current approaches to the management of constipation. Cancer Surv 1994;32:137.

Syrjala KL, Donaldson GW, Davis MW, et al: Relaxation and imagery and cognitive-behavioral training reduce pain during cancer treatment: a controlled clinical trial. Pain 1995; 63:189.

Tan CC, Iftikhar SY, Allan A, Freeman JG: Local effects of colorectal cancer are well palliated by endoscopic laser therapy. Eur J Surg Oncol 1995;21:648.

Townsend J, Frank AO, Fermont D, et al: Terminal cancer care and patients' preference for place of death: a prospective study. BMJ 1990;301:415.

Ventafridda V, Caraceni A, Gamba A: Field-testing of the WHO Guidelines for Cancer Pain Relief: summary report of demonstration projects. Adv Pain Res Ther 1990;16:451.

Index

Note: Page numbers in *italics* indicate figures; page numbers followed by t indicate tables.

Urethrovaginal fistula, 1102
Urinary bladder. See *Bladder.*
Urinary diversion. See *Pelvic exenteration.*
Urinary fistula, 1065
  diagnosis of, 1095
  ureterovaginal, 1095, 1097
  urethrovaginal, 1102
  vesicovaginal, catheter drainage of, 1097
    conventional repair of, 1099, *1101*
    Latzko repair of, 1097–1098, *1100*
    vaginal flap technique in, 1099, *1102*
Urinary flow rate, 1069–1070
Urinary incontinence, 1061, 1063
  etiology of, 1061
    cauda equina lesions in, 1061
    detrusor dysfunction in, 1063–1064
    detrusor hyperreflexia with incomplete contractility in, 1064
    DIAPPERS mnemonic in, 1061
    ectopic ureter in, 1065
    low bladder compliance in, 1064
    overflow, 1061, 1064
    painful bladder syndrome in, 1064
    pelvic plexus injury in, 1061
    pudendal neuropathy in, 1061
    spinal cord lesions and, 1058, 1060–1061
    urethral dysfunction in, 1065
    urinary fistulas and, 1065
  evaluation of, cystometrography in, 1067
    cystometry in, 1068–1069, *1069*
    cystourethroscopy in, 1071
    gross neurologic examination in, 1066
    medical history in, 1066
    pelvic examination in, 1067
    perineal descent in, 1067
    Q-tip test in, 1067
    standing stress test in, 1066
    urethral axis in, 1067
    urethral pressure studies in, 1070, *1070*
    urinary flow rate in, 1069–1070
    urodynamics testing in, 1068
    vaginal examination in, 1067, *1068*
    videourodynamics in, 1070
  functional, 1061
  funneling in, 1063–1064
  history and overview of, 1055
  pathophysiology of, 1063–1065
  pelvic floor anatomy and, 1055–1057, *1057*
  stress, 1061, 1064–1065
    Kegel's exercises for, 23
    paravaginal suspension for, 42
    treatment of, pelvic spaces in, 46
    urogenital diaphragm trauma and, 23
  treatment of, artificial sphincters in, 1072–1073
    biofeedback in, 1071
    functional electrical stimulation in, 1072
    pelvic spaces in, 46
    periurethral injections in, 1073
    pharmacologic, 1071–1072
    sling procedures in, 1074
    surgical, 1067–1068, 1073–1074
    vaginal urethropexies in, 1074
  urge, 1061
Urinary system, anatomy of, *1026–1027*, 1055–1057, *1057*
  bladder in, 1057
  brain lesions and, 1058
  emptying phase in, 1058

Urinary system (*Continued*)
  neurophysiology of, 1058, *1059–1060*, 1060–1061, *1062–1063*
  physiology of, 1057
  radiation complications in, 1278–1279
  urethra in, 1057–1058
Urinary tract infections, causes of, 905, 906t
  diagnosis of, 905–906
  in pregnancy, 906t, 907–908
  treatment of, 906t, 906–907
Urinary tract injury, in gynecologic surgery, 1002–1003
  incidence of, 1093
  intraoperative, 1094t
    to bladder, 1093–1094
    to ureter, 1094–1095, *1096–1099*
  prevention of, 1093
Urogenital diaphragm, anatomy of, *21, 23*
  clinical correlates of, 23–24
Urogenital sinus, anomalous, 201, *201*
  repair of, *202*
Urogenital structure, embryonic, adult derivatives and vestigial remains of, 14t
Urogenital system, after menopause, 612–613
Urogenital triangle. See also *Perineum, muscles of; Urogenital diaphragm; Vulva.*
  anatomy of, 17–24, *18–21*
Urologic disorders, sexual functioning and, 482t
Uterine adenosarcoma, 1327–1328
Uterine artery, path of, 48
Uterine bleeding, dysfunctional, anovulatory, 534–535
  causes of, 533–534, 534t, 1033t
    endocrinologic, 536t, 536–537
    organic, 535–536, 536t
    systemic disease as, 536t, 537
  definition of, 533
  diagnosis of, 533, 537–538, 538t
    imaging in, 113–114, *119–124*
  in adenomyosis, 713
  in adolescent, anovulatory, 595, 595t
    causes of, 595t, 595–596
    coagulation disorders and, 595, 595t
    defining normal and abnormal in, 594, 595t
    diagnosis of, 594–596
    laboratory tests in, 596
    physical examination in, 596
    prognosis of, 598
    treatment of, 596–598, 597t
  in endometriosis, 692
  in ovulatory cycles, 539
  initial evaluation of, 535
  leiomyomas and, 728
  ovulatory, 535
  pathophysiology of, 534–535
  patterns of, 535t, 1034t
  profuse, 538–539
    after induced abortion, 350–351
    oral contraceptives and, 317
  pseudo-dysfunctional uterine bleeding, 534t
  recurrent, 539
  treatment of, hysterectomy in, 539, 596–598, 597t, 1033–1034
    pharmacologic, 538–539
Uterine cancer. See also *Gynecologic cancer-related infection.*
  adenomyosis with, 715–716

Uterine carcinofibroma, 1328
Uterine carcinosarcoma, clinical features of, 1325–1327
  pathology of, 1325, *1326*
  treatment of, 1327
Uterine endometrium. See *Endometrium.*
Uterine leiomyosarcomas, clinical features of, 1322–1323, *1325*
  histologic variants of, 1323–1324
  pathology of, 1321–1322, *1323–1324*
  prognosis of, 1323
  treatment of, 1324–1325
Uterine ligament, 44, *44, 49*
  as surgical landmark, 46
  pain in, 46
Uterine sarcomas. See also specific type, e.g., *Uterine leiomyosarcoma.*
  adenosarcoma as, 1327–1328
  carcinofibroma as, 1328
  carcinosarcoma as, 1325–1327, *1326*
  classification of, 1321, 1322t
  endometrial stromal sarcomas as, 1328–1329, *1328–1329*
  heterologous pure, 1329–1330
  hysterectomy for, 1043
  incidence of, 1321
  metastasis of, 1330
  prognosis of, 1330
Uterine suspension operation, 46
Uterine tubes, development of, 8–9, *11*
Uterovaginal agenesis. See also *Mayer-Rokitansky-Kuster-Hauser syndrome.*
  amenorrhea and, 560
Uterus. See also *Endometrial* entries; *Endometrium.*
  adenomatoid mesothelioma of, 729
  adenomyomas in, 726
  adhesions in, cervicoisthmic, 248
    classification of, 248
    corporal, 248
    diagnosis of, 248, *248*
    dysmenorrhea and, 514t
    etiology of, 247
    lysis of, 248–249
    post-treatment verification of normal cavity in, 249
    prevention of, 249
  anatomy of, 47–48, *48–50*
  anomalies of, 210–211, *211*
    abdominal metroplasty for, 240, *241–242, 242*
    arcuate, 239
    arteriovenous malformation as, 729
    bicornuate, 129, *138, 145*, 240, *241*
    bivalved, endometrial cancer with, 178, *178*
    cervical incompetence with, 238
    classification of, 236, *237*
    diagnosis of, 235–236, 238
    didelphys, 239
    diethylstilbestrol-related, 239–240. See also *Diethylstilbestrol exposure in pregnancy.*
    dysmenorrhea and, 514t
    etiology of, 236
    habitual abortion and, 235t, 235–236
    hysterosalpingography of, 129, *138–139*
    hysteroscopic metroplasty for, reproductive outcome after, 243, 243t
    infertility and, 363–366, *364–365*, 365t
    MRI of, 144–145, *145*
    reproductive outcome associated with, 239t
    septate, 240, *242*, 242–243

ISBN 0-7216-5552-1